Laboratory Test	Conventional Units	Conversion Factor	Système International Units
	2.26–2.56 mEq/L	0.50	1.13–1.28 mmol/L
Carbamazepine, therapeutic	4–12 mg/L	4.23	17–51 μmol/L
Carboxyhemoglobin (nonsmoker)	< 2%	0.01	< 0.02
Carcinoembryonic antigen (CEA)			
Nonsmokers	< 2.5 ng/mL	1	[illegible]
Smokers	< 5 ng/mL	1	[illegible]
CD4 lymphocyte count	31%–61% of total lymphocytes	0.01	[illegible]
CD8 lymphocyte count	18%–39% of total lymphocytes	0.01	[illegible]
Cerebrospinal fluid (CSF)			
Pressure	75–175 mm H_2O	0.0098	[illegible]
Glucose	40–70 mg/dL	0.0555	[illegible]
Protein	15–45 mg/dL	0.01	[illegible]
White blood cell (WBC) count	< 10/mm³	1	[illegible]
Ceruloplasmin	18–45 mg/dL	10	[illegible]
Chloride	97–110 mEq/L	1	97–110 mmol/L
Cholesterol			
Desirable	< 200 mg/dL	0.0259	< 5.18 mmol/L
Borderline high	200–239 mg/dL	0.0259	5.18–6.19 mmol/L
High	≥ 240 mg/dL	0.0259	≥6.2 mmol/L
Chorionic gonadotropin (β-hCG)	< 5 mIU/mL	1	< 5 IU/L
Clozapine, minimum trough	300–350 ng/mL or mcg/L	3.06	918–1,071 nmol/L
		0.00306	0.92–1.07 μmol/L
CO_2 content	22–30 mEq/L	1	22–30 mmol/L
Complement component 3 (C3)	70–160 mg/dL	0.01	0.70–1.60 g/L
Complement component 4 (C4)	20–40 mg/dL	0.01	0.20–0.40 g/L
Copper	70–150 mcg/dL	0.157	11–24 μmol/L
Cortisol (fasting, morning)	5–25 mcg/dL	27.6	138–690 nmol/L
Creatine kinase			
Male	30–200 IU/L	0.01667	0.50–3.33 μkat/L
Female	20–170 IU/L	0.01667	0.33–2.83 μkat/L
MB fraction	0–7 IU/L	0.01667	0.0–0.12 μkat/L
Creatinine clearance (CrCl)	85–135 mL/min/1.73 m²	0.00963	0.82 1.30 mL/s/m²
		0.01667	85–135 mL/s/1.73 m²
Creatinine			
Male 4–20 years	0.2–1.0 mg/dL	88.4	18–88 μmol/L
Female 4–20 years	0.2–1.0 mg/dL	88.4	18–88 μmol/L
Male (adults)	0.7–1.3 mg/dL	88.4	62–115 μmol/L
Female (adults)	0.6–1.1 mg/dL	88.4	53–97 μmol/L
Cyclosporine			
Renal, cardiac, liver, or pancreatic transplant	100–400 ng/mL or mcg/L	0.832	83–333 nmol/L
Cryptococcal antigen	Negative		
D-dimers	< 250 ng/mL	1	< 250 mcg/L
Desipramine	75–300 ng/mL or mcg/L	3.75	281–1125 nmol/L
Dexamethasone suppression test (DST) (overnight), 8:00 am cortisol	< 5 mcg/dL	27.6	< 138 nmol/L
DHEAS (dehydroepiandrosterone sulfate)			
Male	170–670 mcg/dL	0.0272	4.6–18.2 μmol/L
Female			
Premenopausal	50–540 mcg/dL	0.0272	1.4–14.7 μmol/L
Postmenopausal	30–260 mcg/dL	0.0272	0.8–7.1 μmol/L
Digoxin, therapeutic (heart failure)	0.5–0.8 ng/mL or mcg/L	1.28	0.6–1.0 nmol/L
Therapeutic (atrial fibrillation)	0.8–2.0 ng/mL or mcg/L	1.28	1.0–2.6 nmol/L
Erythrocyte count (blood)			
See under red blood cell (RBC) count			
Erythrocyte sedimentation rate (ESR)			
Westergren			
Male	0–20 mm/h		
Female	0–30 mm/h		
Wintrobe			
Male	0–9 mm/h		
Female	0–15 mm/h		
Erythropoietin	2–25 mIU/mL	1	2–25 IU/L
Estradiol			
Male	10–36 pg/mL	3.67	37–132 pmol/L
Female	34–170 pg/mL	3.67	125–624 pmol/L
Ethanol, legal intoxication (depends on location)	≥ 50–100 mg/dL	0.217	≥10.9–21.7 mmol/L
	≥ 0.05–0.1%	217	≥10.9–21.7 mmol/L
Ethosuximide, therapeutic	40–100 mg/L or mcg/mL	7.08	283–708 μmol/L
Factor VIII or factor IX			
Severe hemophilia	< 1 IU/dL	0.01	< 0.01 IU/mL
Moderate hemophilia	1–5 IU/dL	0.01	0.01–0.05 IU/mL
Mild hemophilia	> 5 IU/dL	0.01	> 0.05 IU/mL
Usual adult levels	60 to 140 IU/dL	0.01	0.60–1.40 IU/mL
Ferritin			
Male	20–250 ng/mL	1	20–250 mcg/L
		2.25	45-562 pmol/L
Female	10–150 ng/mL	1	10–150 mcg/L
		2.25	22-337 pmol/L
Fibrin degradation products (FDP)	2–10 mg/L		
Fibrinogen	200–400 mg/dL	0.01	2.0–4.0 g/L
Folate (plasma)	3.1–12.4 ng/mL	2.266	7.0–28.1 nmol/L
Folate (RBC)	125–600 ng/mL	2.266	283–1,360 nmol/L
Follicle-stimulating hormone (FSH)			
Male	1–7 mIU/mL	1	1–7 IU/L
Female			
Follicular phase	1–9 mIU/mL	1	1–9 IU/L
Midcycle	6–26 mIU/mL	1	6–26 IU/L
Luteal phase	1–9 mIU/mL	1	1–9 IU/L
Postmenopausal	30–118 mIU/mL	1	30–118 IU/L
Free thyroxine index (FT_4I)	6.5–12.5		
Gamma glutamyltransferase (GGT)	0–30 U/L	0.01667	0–0.50 μkat/L
Gastrin (fasting)	0–130 pg/mL	1	0–130 ng/L
Gentamicin, therapeutic (traditional dosing)			
Peak	4–10 mg/L	2.09	8.4–21 μmol/L
Trough	≤ 2 mg/L	2.09	≤ 4.2 μmol/L
Globulin	2.3–3.5 g/dL	10	23–35 g/L
Glucose (fasting, plasma)	65–109 mg/dL	0.0555	3.6–6.0 mmol/L
Glucose, 2-hour postprandial blood (PPBG)	< 140 mg/dL	0.0555	< 7.8 mmol/L
Granulocyte count	1.8–6.6 × 10³/mm³	10⁶	1.8–6.6 × 10⁹/L

(Continued on back inside cover)

Pharmacotherapy
Principles & Practice

NOTICE

Medicine is an ever-changing science. As new research and clinical experience broaden our knowledge, changes in treatment and drug therapy are required. The authors and the publisher of this work have checked with sources believed to be reliable in their efforts to provide information that is complete and generally in accord with the standards accepted at the time of publication. However, in view of the possibility of human error or changes in medical sciences, neither the authors nor the publisher nor any other party who has been involved in the preparation or publication of this work warrants that the information contained herein is in every respect accurate or complete, and they disclaim all responsibility for any errors or omissions or for the results obtained from use of the information contained in this work. Readers are encouraged to confirm the information contained herein with other sources. For example and in particular, readers are advised to check the product information sheet included in the package of each drug they plan to administer to be certain that the information contained in this work is accurate and that changes have not been made in the recommended dose or in the contraindications for administration. This recommendation is of particular importance in connection with new or infrequently used drugs.

Pharmacotherapy Principles & Practice

FOURTH EDITION

Editors

Marie A. Chisholm-Burns, PharmD, MPH, MBA, FCCP, FASHP
Dean and Professor
College of Pharmacy
University of Tennessee
Memphis, Knoxville, and Nashville, Tennessee

Terry L. Schwinghammer, PharmD, FCCP, FASHP, FAPhA, BCPS
Professor and Chair
Department of Clinical Pharmacy
School of Pharmacy
West Virginia University
Morgantown, West Virginia

Barbara G. Wells, PharmD, FASHP, FCCP
Dean Emeritus and Professor Emeritus
School of Pharmacy
The University of Mississippi
University, Mississippi

Patrick M. Malone, PharmD, FASHP
Professor and Associate Dean, Internal Affairs
College of Pharmacy
The University of Findlay
Findlay, Ohio

Jill M. Kolesar, PharmD, BCPS, FCCP
Professor
School of Pharmacy
University of Wisconsin
Director, 3P Analytical Instrumentation Laboratory
University of Wisconsin Comprehensive Cancer Center
Madison, Wisconsin

Joseph T. DiPiro, PharmD, FCCP
Dean, Professor, and Archie. O. McCalley Chair
School of Pharmacy
Virginia Commonwealth University
Richmond, Virginia

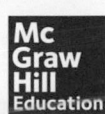

Mc Graw Hill Education

New York Chicago San Francisco Athens London Madrid Mexico City
Milan New Delhi Singapore Sydney Toronto

Pharmacotherapy Principles & Practice, Fourth Edition

1 2 3 4 5 6 7 8 9 0 DSS/DSS 20 19 18 17 16

ISBN 978-0-07-183502-2
MHID 0-07-183502-4

This book was set in Minion by Cenveo® Publisher Services India, LLC.
The editors were Michael Weitz and Peter J. Boyle.
The production supervisor was Catherine H. Saggese.
Art management was by Armen Ovsepyan.
Project management was provided by Shruti Awasthi, Cenveo Publisher Services India, LLC.
The designer was Alan Barnett.
RR Donnelley/China was printer and binder.

This book was printed on acid-free paper.

Library of Congress Cataloging-in-Publication Data

Names: Chisholm-Burns, Marie A., editor.
Title: Pharmacotherapy principles & practice / editors, Marie A. Chisholm-Burns, Terry L. Schwinghammer, Barbara G. Wells, Patrick M. Malone, Jill M. Kolesar, Joseph T. DiPiro.
Other titles: Pharmacotherapy principles and practice
Description: Fourth edition. | New York : McGraw-Hill Education, [2016] | Includes bibliographical references and index.
Identifiers: LCCN 2015041158| ISBN 9780071835022 (hardcover : alk. paper)| ISBN 0071835024 (hardcover : alk. paper)
Subjects: | MESH: Drug Therapy.
Classification: LCC RM262 | NLM WB 330 | DDC 615.5/8—dc23 LC record available at http://lccn.loc.gov/2015041158

CONTENTS

SI unit conversions were produced by Ed Randell, PhD, DCC, FCACB, Division Chief and Professor of Laboratory Medicine, Department of Laboratory Medicine, Eastern Health Authority and Faculty of Medicine, Memorial University of Newfoundland, St. John's, Newfoundland, Canada

ABOUT THE EDITORS

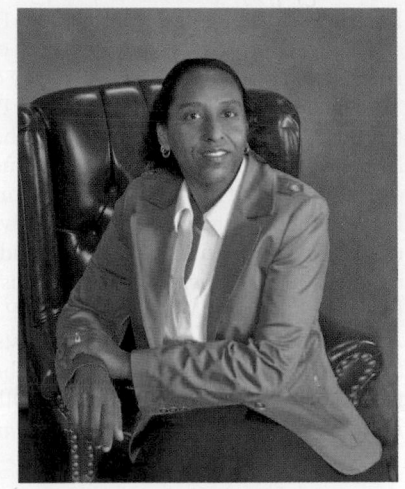

Marie A. Chisholm-Burns, BS Pharm, PharmD, MPH, MBA, FCCP, FASHP, is Dean and Professor at the University of Tennessee College of Pharmacy. She received her BS and PharmD degrees from the University of Georgia, and completed a residency at Mercer University Southern School of Pharmacy and at Piedmont Hospital in Atlanta, Georgia. She has served in elected positions in numerous professional organizations. Dr. Chisholm-Burns has greater than 280 publications and approximately $10 million in external funding as principal investigator. In 2008 and 2011, textbooks co-edited by Dr. Chisholm-Burns, *Pharmacotherapy Principles and Practice* and *Pharmacy Management, Leadership, Marketing, and Finance,* respectively, received the Medical Book Award from the American Medical Writers Association. She has also received numerous awards and honors, including the Robert K. Chalmers Distinguished Pharmacy Educator Award from the American Association of Colleges of Pharmacy (AACP), Clinical Pharmacy Education Award from the American College of Clinical Pharmacy, Daniel B. Smith Practice Excellence Award from the American Pharmacists Association (APhA), Nicholas Andrew Cummings Award from the National Academies of Practice, Award of Excellence from the American Society of Health-System Pharmacists (ASHP), Pharmacy Practice Research Award (2011 and 2014) and Award for Sustained Contributions to the Literature from the ASHP Foundation, Research Achievement Award from the APhA, Clinician of Distinction Award from the American Society of Transplantation, Paul R. Dawson Biotechnology Award from AACP, Chauncey I. Cooper Pharmacist Leadership Award from the National Pharmaceutical Association and Rufus A. Lyman Award for most outstanding publication in the *American Journal of Pharmaceutical Education* (in 1996 and 2007). Dr. Chisholm-Burns lives in Memphis, is married, and has one child, John Fitzgerald Burns Jr. She enjoys writing, cycling, and playing chess.

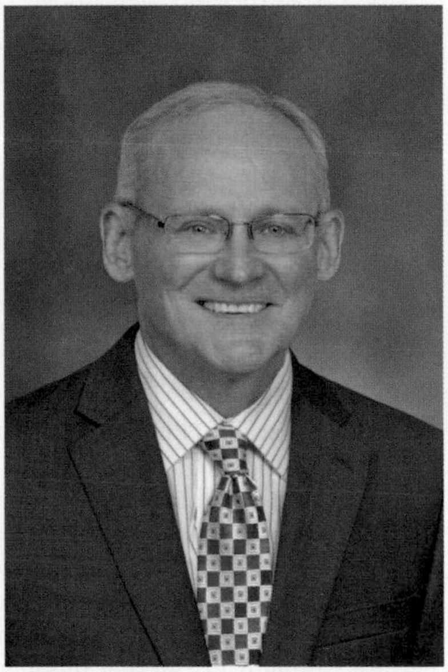

Terry L. Schwinghammer, BS Pharm, PharmD, BCPS, FCCP, FASHP, FAPhA, is Professor and Chair of the Department of Clinical Pharmacy and holds the Arthur I. Jacknowitz Distinguished Chair in Clinical Pharmacy at the West Virginia University School of Pharmacy. He received his BS and PharmD degrees from Purdue University and completed a pharmacy residency at Indiana University Hospitals. He is a Board Certified Pharmacotherapy Specialist and has practiced in adult inpatient and ambulatory care settings. Dr. Schwinghammer is a recipient of the American Pharmacists Association-APPM Distinguished Achievement Award in Clinical/Pharmacotherapeutic Practice and is a Distinguished Practitioner in the National Academies of Practice. His teaching focuses on development of clinical skills, case-based learning, and pharmacotherapy of rheumatic diseases. He is a member of the Academy of Excellence in Teaching and Learning of the WVU Health Sciences Center. In addition to authoring over 75 research papers and journal articles, he is a co-editor of the *Pharmacotherapy Casebook* and *Pharmacotherapy Handbook* and is Editor-in-Chief of McGraw-Hill's AccessPharmacy (www.AccessPharmacy.com). Dr. Schwinghammer has served the American Association of Colleges of Pharmacy as Chair of the Pharmacy Practice Section, Chair of the Council of Faculties, and member of the Board of Directors. He is a past president of the Pennsylvania Society of Health-System Pharmacists and received both the Pharmacist of the Year and Sister M. Gonzales Lecture Awards from the organization. He has served as Chair of the Board of Pharmacy Specialties and elected member of the Board of Regents of the American College of Clinical Pharmacy. He is a Fellow of ACCP, ASHP, and APhA and has been elected to membership in the Rho Chi Pharmaceutical Honor Society and the Phi Lambda Sigma Pharmacy Leadership Society. He was named a Distinguished Alumnus of Purdue University in 2004. His hobby is collecting apothecary antiques, and he enjoys spending time with his wife Donna and their two children and three grandchildren.

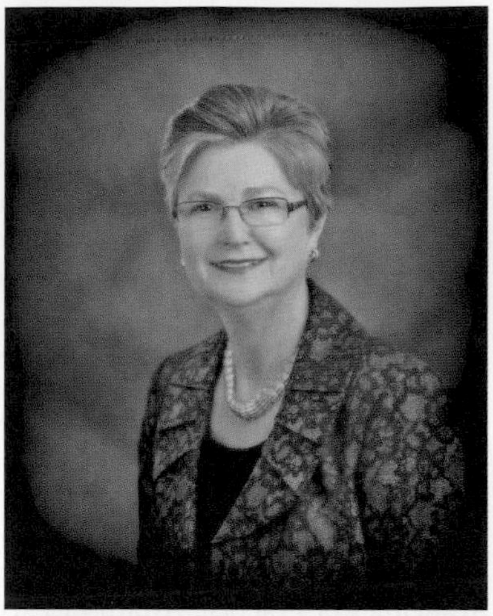

Barbara G. Wells, BS Pharm, PharmD, FCCP, FASHP, is Dean Emeritus and Professor Emeritus at the University of Mississippi School of Pharmacy and Executive Director Emeritus of the Research Institute of Pharmaceutical Sciences. She earned her BS Pharm and PharmD degrees at the University of Tennessee and completed a residency in psychiatric pharmacy practice at the University of Tennessee and Memphis Mental Health Institute. She is past president of the College of Psychiatric and Neurologic Pharmacists Foundation (CPNPF). She is a past president and chair of the Board of the American Association of Colleges of Pharmacy (AACP) and the American College of Clinical Pharmacy (ACCP). She is a past member of the NIH Advisory Committee on Research on Women's Health and of the FDA Psychopharmacologic Drugs Advisory Committee. Her primary instructional interests are in psychiatric therapeutics, and she has received seven teaching awards. She is the recipient of the Robert K. Chalmers Distinguished Pharmacy Educator Award from AACP, the Paul F. Parker Medal from ACCP, the Gloria Niemeyer Francke Leadership Mentor Award from the American Pharmacists Association, and the Career Achievement Award from the CPNPF. She is a member of the National Academy of Practice of Pharmacy within the National Academies of Practice. Other books that she co-edits are *Pharmacotherapy: A Pathophysiologic Approach* and the *Pharmacotherapy Handbook.*

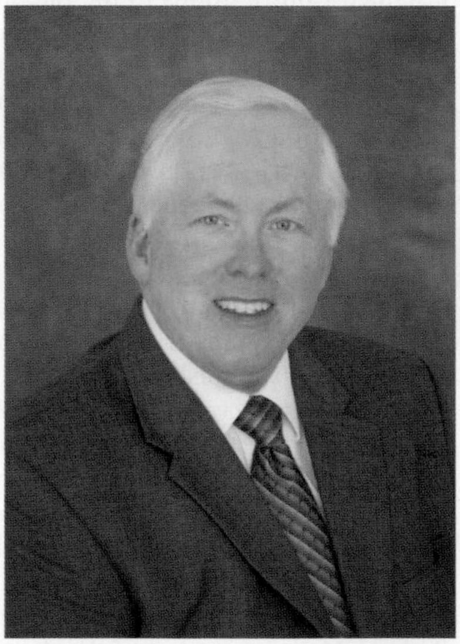

Patrick M. Malone, BS Pharm, PharmD, FASHP, is Professor and Associate Dean of Internal Affairs at the University of Findlay College of Pharmacy. Dr. Malone received his BS in Pharmacy from Albany College of Pharmacy and PharmD from the University of Michigan. He completed a clinical pharmacy residency at the Buffalo General Hospital, Drug Information Fellowship at the University of Nebraska Medical Center, and U.S. West Fellowship in Academic Development and Technology at Creighton University. His practice and teaching have centered on drug information, and he is the first author for all five editions of *Drug Information—A Guide for Pharmacists.* Dr. Malone was also the drug information pharmacist at the XIII Winter Olympics. He has approximately 100 publications and numerous presentations and has held various offices in national organizations. He was the Director of the Web-Based Pharmacy Pathway at Creighton University Medical Center, from its initial establishment until after graduation of the first class. His hobby is building and flying radio-controlled aircraft.

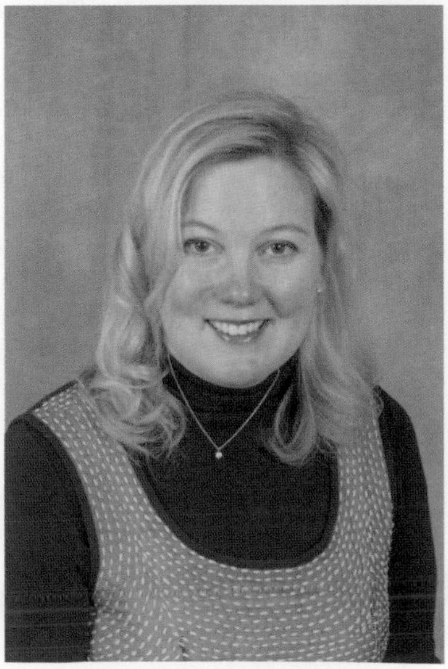

Jill M. Kolesar, BS Pharm, PharmD, BCPS, FCCP, is a Professor at the University of Wisconsin and the Director of the 3P Laboratory, Co-Leader Cancer Therapy Discovery and Development, Co-Chair, and Molecular Tumor Board at the University of Wisconsin Carbone Comprehensive Cancer Center. She received a BS in pharmacy from the University of Wisconsin and a PharmD from the University of Texas. Dr. Kolesar also completed an oncology residency and fellowship at the University of Texas Health Science Center in San Antonio. Dr. Kolesar is the author of more than 125 peer reviewed publications and has received more than $1.2 million in external funding as a co and principal investigator. She holds two US and international patents for novel technologies invented in her laboratory and founded Helix Diagnostics based on this technology. She is a member of National Cancer Institute Cancer Prevention and Control Central IRB, and is currently a member of the Pharmacology Taskforce, an advisory group to the Investigational Drug Steering Committee of the NCI. She also co-chairs the Lung Biology Subcommittee for the Thoracic Committee of the Eastern Cooperative Oncology Group. Dr. Kolesar received the Innovations in Teaching Award from AACP, and has served in multiple elected offices of national and international pharmacy organizations. Other books she co-edits are *Top 300 Pharmacy Flash Cards, Top 100 Nonprescription Flash Cards,* and *The Pharmacogenomics Handbook.* Dr. Kolesar loves to read, run, ski, and travel with her husband and five children. She has completed 2 marathons and 16 half-marathons.

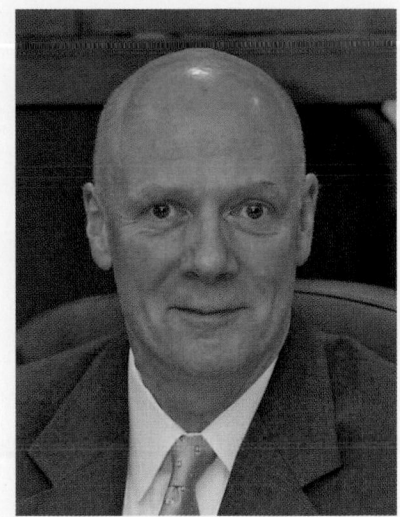

Joseph T. DiPiro, BS Pharm, PharmD, FCCP, is Dean, Professor, and Archie O. McCalley Chair at the Virginia Commonwealth University School of Pharmacy. From 2005 to 2014, he was Executive Dean of the South Carolina College of Pharmacy. He received his BS in pharmacy (Honors College) from the University of Connecticut and Doctor of Pharmacy from the University of Kentucky. He served a residency at the University of Kentucky Medical Center and a fellowship in Clinical Immunology at Johns Hopkins University. From 1981 to 2005, Dr. DiPiro was a faculty member at the University of Georgia College of Pharmacy and the Medical College of Georgia.

He is Past Chair of the American Association of Colleges of Pharmacy Council of Deans and served as President of the American College of Clinical Pharmacy. He is a Fellow of the College and has served on the Research Institute Board of Trustees. He has been a member of the American Society of Health-System Pharmacists, having served on the Commission on Therapeutics and the Task Force on Science. In 2002, the American Association of Colleges of Pharmacy selected Dr. DiPiro for the Robert K. Chalmers Distinguished Educator Award. He has also received the Russell R. Miller Literature Award and the Education Award from the American College of Clinical Pharmacy, the Award for Sustained Contributions to the Literature from the American Society of Health-System Pharmacists, and was named in 2013 as the national Rho Chi Distinguished Lecturer. Dr. DiPiro was elected a Fellow in the American Association for the Advancement of Science.

Dr. DiPiro served as editor of *The American Journal of Pharmaceutical Education* for 12 years. He is an editor for *Pharmacotherapy: A Pathophysiologic Approach,* now in its ninth edition. He is also the author of *Concepts in Clinical Pharmacokinetics* and editor of the *Encyclopedia of Clinical Pharmacy.* He has published over 200 journal papers, books, book chapters, and editorials in academic and professional journals, mainly related to antibiotics, drug use in surgery, and pharmacy education. His papers have appeared in *Antimicrobial Agents and Chemotherapy, Pharmacotherapy, Critical Care Medicine, JAMA, Annals of Surgery, Archives of Surgery, American Journal of Surgery, Journal of Pharmacology and Experimental Therapeutics,* and *Surgical Infections.*

CONTRIBUTORS

Shirley Abraham, MD
Assistant Professor, Department of Pediatrics, University of New Mexico, Albuquerque, New Mexico
Chapter 95

Val Adams, PharmD, FCCP, BCOP
Associate Professor, Pharmacy Practice, College of Pharmacy, University of Kentucky, Lexington, Kentucky
Chapter 90

Daniel S. Aistrope, PharmD, BCACP
Director of Clinical Practice Advancement, American College of Clinical Pharmacy, Lenexa, Kansas
Chapter 102

Ronda L. Akins, PharmD
Infectious Diseases Clinical Pharmacy Specialist, Methodist Charlton Medical Center, Dallas, Texas; Adjunct Associate Professor, Department of Biological Sciences, University of Texas at Dallas, Richardson, Texas
Chapter 74

Samson Amos, RPh, PhD
Associate Professor of Pharmaceutical Science, Cedarville University School of Pharmacy, Cedarville, Ohio
Chapter 64

J. V. Anandan, PharmD
Pharmacy Specialist, Department of Pharmacy Services, Henry Ford Hospital, Detroit Michigan
Chapter 78

Emily Anastasia
Clinical Pharmacy Specialist, Cardiology, Durham Veterans Affairs Medical Center, Durham, North Carolina
Chapter 5

Miriam Ansong, PharmD, E. MBA
Director, Drug Information, Associate Professor of Pharmacy Practice, Cedarville University School of Pharmacy, Cedarville, Ohio
Chapter 64

David A. Apgar, PharmD
Assistant Professor, Department of Pharmacy Practice and Science, College of Pharmacy, University of Arizona, Tucson, Arizona
Chapter 63

Justin M. Balko, PharmD, PhD
Assistant Professor, Department of Medicine, Ingram Cancer Center, Vanderbilt University, Nashville, Tennessee
Chapter 90

Katie E. Barber, PharmD
Assistant Professor of Pharmacy Practice, School of Pharmacy, University of Mississippi, Mississippi
Chapter 74

Marianne Billeter, PharmD, BCPS
Clinical Pharmacy Coordinator, McLeod Health, Florence, South Carolina
Chapter 86

Christopher M. Bland, PharmD, BCPS
Clinical Assistant Professor, College of Pharmacy, University of Georgia, Athens, Georgia
Chapter 82

P. Brandon Bookstaver, PharmD
Associate Professor, Vice Chair, Department of Clinical Pharmacy and Outcomes Sciences, South Carolina College of Pharmacy, Columbia, South Carolina
Chapter 70

Jill S. Borchert, PharmD, BCACP, BCPS, FCCP
Vice-Chair and Professor of Pharmacy Practice, Chicago College of Pharmacy, Midwestern University, Chicago, Illinois
Chapter 60

Emily B. Borders, PharmD, BCOP
Assistant Professor, Clinical and Administrative Sciences, College of Pharmacy, University of Oklahoma, Oklahoma City, Oklahoma
Chapter 91

Sheila R. Botts, PharmD, FCCP, BCCP
Chief, Clinical Pharmacy Research and Academic Affairs, Kaiser Permanente Colorado, Aurora, Colorado
Chapter 40

Bradley A. Boucher, PharmD, FCCP, FCCM
Professor, Department of Clinical Pharmacy, Associate Dean of Strategic Initiatives and Operations, College of Pharmacy, University of Tennessee, Memphis, Tennessee
Chapter 13

Catherine A. Bourg, PharmD, BCPS, BCACP
Clinical Assistant Professor, Clinical and Administrative Pharmacy, College of Pharmacy, University of Georgia, Athens, Georgia
Chapter 18

Trisha N. Branan, PharmD, BCPS
Clinical Assistant Professor, Clinical and Administrative Pharmacy, College of Pharmacy, University of Georgia, Athens, Georgia
Chapter 82

Evans Branch III, PharmD, CPh
Professor, College of Pharmacy and Pharmaceutical Sciences, Florida A&M University, Miami, Florida
Chapter 80

Gretchen M. Brophy, PharmD, BCPS, FCCP, FCCM, FNCS
Professor of Pharmacotherapy and Outcomes Science and Neurosurgery, Virginia Commonwealth University, Medical College of Virginia, Richmond, Virginia
Chapter 32

Susan P. Bruce, PharmD, BCPS
Associate Dean for Pharmacy Education and Interprofessional Studies, Chair and Professor of Pharmacy Practice, College of Pharmacy, Northeast Ohio Medical University, Rootstown, Ohio
Chapter 57

Karim Anton Calis, PharmD, MPH, FASHP, FCCP
Adjunct Senior Clinical Investigator, *Eunice Kennedy Shriver* National Institute of Child Health and Human Development, National Institutes of Health, Bethesda, Maryland; Clinical Professor, University of Maryland School of Pharmacy, Baltimore, Maryland; Clinical Professor, Virginia Commonwealth University School of Pharmacy, Richmond, Virgina
Chapters 45 and 46

Diane M. Cappelletty, PharmD
Associate Professor of Clinical Pharmacy, Chair, Department of Pharmacy Practice, Co-Director, The Infectious Disease Research Laboratory, College of Pharmacy and Pharmaceutical Sciences, University of Toledo, Toledo, Ohio
Chapter 71

Christina Carracedo, PharmD, BCOP
BMT/Hematology Clinical Pharmacist, University of Kentucky HealthCare; Assistant Adjunct Professor, Pharmacy Practice and Science, College of Pharmacy, University of Kentucky, Lexington, Kentucky
Chapter 98

Nicholas W. Carris, PharmD, BCPS
Assistant Professor, Department of Pharmacotherapeutics & Clinical Research, College of Pharmacy; Department of Family Medicine, Morsani College of Medicine, University of South Florida, Tampa, Florida
Chapter 58

Marshall E. Cates, PharmD, BCPP, FASHP
Professor of Pharmacy Practice, McWhorter School of Pharmacy, Samford University, Birmingham, Alabama
Chapter 38

Larisa H. Cavallari, PharmD, BCPS, FCCP
Associate Professor and Associate Chair, Department of Pharmacotherapy and Translational Research, Director, Center for Pharmacogenomics, Associate Director, Personalized Medicine Program, University of Florida, Gainesville, Florida
Chapter 7

Kevin W. Chamberlin, PharmD
Associate Clinical Professor, Assistant Head, Department of Pharmacy Practice, School of Pharmacy, University of Connecticut, Farmington, Connecticut
Chapter 29

Juliana Chan, PharmD, FCCP, BCACP
Clinical Associate Professor, Gastroenterology and Hepatology, Clinical Pharmacist, Ambulatory Pharmacy Services, Clinical Associate Professor, Pharmacy Practice, Colleges of Pharmacy and Medicine, University of Illinois, Chicago, Illinois
Chapter 24

Sallie H. Charles, PMHNP-BC, MS, MBA
Advanced Practice Nurse, Psychiatry, Hidden Lake Medical Offices, Kaiser Permanente Colorado, Westminster, Colorado
Chapter 40

Judy T. Chen, PharmD, BCPS, CDE, FNAP
Clinical Associate Professor, Pharmacy Practice, Purdue University College of Pharmacy, Indianapolis, Indiana
Chapters 45 and 46

Marie A. Chisholm-Burns, PharmD, MPH, MBA, FCCP, FASHP
Dean and Professor, College of Pharmacy, University of Tennessee, Memphis, Knoxville, and Nashville, Tennessee
Chapter 17

Kevin W. Cleveland, PharmD
Associate Professor and Assistant Dean for Experiential Education, Department of Pharmacy Practice and Administrative Sciences, College of Pharmacy, Idaho State University, Pocatello, Idaho
Chapter 42

Amanda H. Corbett, PharmD, BCPS, FCCP, AAHIVE
Clinical Associate Professor, Eshelman School of Pharmacy, University of North Carolina at Chapel Hill, Chapel Hill, North Carolina
Chapter 87

Brian L. Crabtree, PharmD, BCPP
Professor and Chair, Department of Pharmacy Practice, Eugene Applebaum College of Pharmacy and Health Sciences, Wayne State University, Detroit, Michigan
Chapter 39

Nicole S. Culhane, PharmD, FCCP, BCPS
Director, Experiential Education, Associate Professor, Clinical and Administrative Sciences, School of Pharmacy, Notre Dame of Maryland University, Baltimore, Maryland
Chapter 50

Clarence E. Curry Jr., PharmD
Associate Professor Emeritus of Pharmacy Practice, College of Pharmacy, Howard University, Washington, DC
Chapter 21

Devra K. Dang, PharmD, BCPS, CDE
Associate Clinical Professor, Pharmacy Practice, University of Connecticut School of Pharmacy, Storrs, Connecticut
Chapters 45 and 46

Simon de Denus, BPharm, MSc(Pharm), PhD
Beaulieu-Saucier Chair in Pharmacogenomics, Pharmacist, Montreal Heart Institute; Associate Professor, Faculty of Pharmacy, Université de Montréal, Montreal, Canada
Chapter 8

Robert J. DiDomenico, PharmD
Clinical Professor, Department of Pharmacy Practice, College of Pharmacy, University of Illinois at Chicago, Chicago, Illinois
Chapter 7

Joseph T. DiPiro, PharmD, FCCP
Professor and Dean, Archie O. McCalley Chair, School of Pharmacy, Virginia Commonwealth University, Richmond, Virginia
Chapter 77

John M. Dopp, PharmD
Associate Professor, School of Pharmacy, University of Wisconsin-Madison, Madison, Wisconsin
Chapter 41

Megan J. Ehret, PharmD, MS, BCPP
Behavioral Health Clinical Pharmacist, Department of Defense, Fort Belvoir Community Hospital, Fort Belvoir, Virginia
Chapter 29

Lori J. Ernsthausen, PharmD, BCPS
Associate Professor and Chair, Department of Pharmacy Practice, University of Findlay College of Pharmacy, Findlay, Ohio
Chapter 65

John Erramouspe, PharmD, MS
Professor, Pharmacy Practice and Administrative Sciences, College of Pharmacy, Idaho State University, Pocatello, Idaho
Chapter 42

Edward Faught, MD
Professor, Department of Neurology, School of Medicine, Emory University, Atlanta, Georgia
Chapter 31

Ema Ferreira, BPharm, MSc, PharmD, FCHSP
Pharmacist, Clinical Professor, Associate Dean, Academics, CHU Ste-Justine, Université de Montréal, Montreal, Quebec, Canada
Chapter 47

Jack E. Fincham, PhD, RPh
Professor, Pharmaceutical and Administrative Sciences, School of Pharmacy, Presbyterian College, Clinton, South Carolina
Chapter 1

Shannon W. Finks, PharmD, FCCP, BCPS
Associate Professor, Department of Clinical Pharmacy, College of Pharmacy, University of Tennessee, and Clinical Pharmacy Specialist, Cardiology, VA Medical Center, Memphis, Tennessee
Chapter 8

Joshua W. Fleming, PharmD, BCACP
Clinical Assistant Professor, Department of Pharmacy Practice, University of Mississippi School of Pharmacy, Jackson, Mississippi
Chapter 35

Steven Gabardi, PharmD, FAST, FCCP, BCPS
Abdominal Organ Transplant Clinical Specialist, Brigham and Women's Hospital; Assistant Professor of Medicine, Harvard Medical School, Boston, Massachusetts
Chapter 55

Heather L. Girand, PharmD
Professor, Pharmacy Practice, College of Pharmacy, Ferris State University, Big Rapids, Michigan
Chapter 72

Maqual R. Graham, PharmD
Professor and Associate Dean for Academic Affairs, University of Missouri School of Pharmacy, Kansas City, Missouri
Chapter 102

John G. Gums, PharmD, FCCP
Professor of Pharmacy and Medicine, Associate Dean for Clinical Affairs, Department of Pharmacotherapy and Translational Research, College of Pharmacy, University of Florida, Gainesville, Florida
Chapter 58

Tracy M. Hagemann, PharmD, FCCP, FPPAG
Associate Dean and Professor, College of Pharmacy, University of Tennessee, Nashville, Tennessee
Chapter 68

Stuart T. Haines, PharmD, BCPS, BC-ADM
Professor and Vice Chair for Clinical Services, Department of Pharmacy Practice and Science, University of Maryland School of Pharmacy, Baltimore, Maryland
Chapter 10

Kim Hawkins, PhD, APRN-NP
Assistant Professor, Creighton University College of Nursing, Omaha, Nebraska
Appendix D

Kathleen B. Haynes, PharmD, BCPS, CDE
Clinical Coordinator, Bridges to Health, Community Health Network, Indianapolis, Indiana
Chapter 48

Keith A. Hecht, PharmD, BCOP
Associate Professor, Department of Pharmacy Practice, School of Pharmacy, Southern Illinois University, Edwardsville, Illinois
Chapter 97

Nancy Heideman, PharmD, BCPS
Clinical Specialist-Pediatrics, University of New Mexico Hospital, Albuquerque, New Mexico
Chapter 95

Emily L. Heil, PharmD
Clinical Assistant Professor, School of Pharmacy, University of Maryland Medical Center, Baltimore, Maryland
Chapter 87

Brian A. Hemstreet, PharmD, FCCP, BCPS
Associate Professor and Assistant Dean for Student Affairs, Regis University School of Pharmacy, Denver, Colorado
Chapter 19

Gerald Higa, PharmD
Professor, Schools of Pharmacy and Medicine, West Virginia University, Morgantown, West Virginia
Chapter 89

Michelle L. Hilaire, PharmD, CDE, BCPS
Clinical Associate Professor of Pharmacy Practice, University of Wyoming School of Pharmacy, Laramie, Wyoming
Chapter 62

Marlon S. Honeywell, PharmD
Professor, College of Pharmacy and Pharmaceutical Sciences, Florida A&M University, Tallahassee, Florida
Chapter 80

Jaime R. Hornecker, PharmD, BCPS
Clinical Associate Professor of Pharmacy Practice, School of Pharmacy, University of Wyoming, Laramie, Wyoming
Chapter 73

Melissa L. Hunter, PharmD
Drug Information Director, School of Pharmacy, University of Wyoming, Laramie, Wyoming
Chapter 62

Jill Isaacs, MS, APRN-NP
Charleston Southern University, Charleston, South Carolina
Appendix D

Matthew K. Ito, PharmD, FCCP, FNLA, CLS
Professor, Department of Pharmacy Practice, Oregon State University/Oregon Health and Science University College of Pharmacy, Portland, Oregon
Chapter 12

Cherry W. Jackson, PharmD, BCPP, FASHP, FCCP
Professor, Department of Pharmacy Practice, Auburn University; Clinical Professor, Department of Psychiatric and Behavioral Neurobiology, School of Medicine, University of Alabama, Birmingham, Alabama
Chapter 38

Mikael D. Jones, PharmD, BCPS
Clinical Associate Professor, Pharmacy Practice and Science, College of Pharmacy, University of Kentucky, Lexington, Kentucky
Chapter 61

Michael D. Katz, PharmD
Professor and Director, International Education, Department of Pharmacy Practice and Science, College of Pharmacy, University of Arizona, Tucson, Arizona
Chapter 44

Deanna L. Kelly, PharmD, BCPP
Professor of Psychiatry, Director and Chief, Treatment Research Program, Maryland Psychiatric Research Center, University of Maryland School of Medicine, Baltimore, Maryland
Chapter 37

Jacqueline M. Klootwyk, PharmD, BCPS
Assistant Professor of Pharmacy Practice, Division of Clinical, Social, and Administrative Sciences, Mylan School of Pharmacy, Duquesne University, Pittsburgh, Pennsylvania
Chapter 49

Emily Knezevich, PharmD, BCPS, CDE
Associate Professor of Pharmacy Practice, School of Pharmacy and Health Professions, Creighton University, Omaha, Nebraska
Appendix D

Jon Knezevich, PharmD, BCPS
Pharmaceutical Care Pharmacist, Think Whole Person Healthcare, Omaha, Nebraska
Appendix D

Julia M. Koehler, PharmD, FCCP
Associate Dean for Clinical Education and External Affiliations, Professor of Pharmacy Practice, Butler University College of Pharmacy and Health Sciences, Indianapolis, Indiana
Chapter 48

Jill M. Kolesar, PharmD, BCPS, FCCP
Professor, School of Pharmacy, University of Wisconsin; Director, 3P Analytical Instrumentation Laboratory, University of Wisconsin Comprehensive Cancer Center Madison, Wisconsin
Chapter 93

Michael D. Kraft, PharmD, BCNSP
Clinical Associate Professor, University of Michigan College of Pharmacy; Assistant Director—Education and Research, University of Michigan Health System, Ann Arbor, Michigan
Chapter 100

Kelly R. Kroustos, PharmD
Associate Professor of Pharmacy Practice, Raabe College of Pharmacy, Ohio Northern University, Ada, Ohio
Chapter 4

Sum Lam, PharmD
Associate Clinical Professor, Department of Clinical Pharmacy Practice, College of Pharmacy and Allied Health Professions, St. John's University, Queens, New York; Clinical Specialist in Geriatric Pharmacy, Divisions of Geriatric Medicine and Pharmacy, Winthrop University Hospital, Mineola, New York
Chapter 53

Michael Lauzardo, MD
Chief, Division of Infectious Diseases and Global Medicine, College of Medicine, University of Florida, Gainesville, Florida
Chapter 75

Amber P. Lawson, PharmD, BCOP
Clinical Pharmacy Specialist, Hematology/Oncology, University of Kentucky Healthcare, Lexington, Kentucky
Chapter 98

Ellyn M. Lee, MD, FACP
Director, Palliative Care Services Swedish Medical Center, Seattle, Washington
Chapter 2

Jeannie K. Lee, PharmD, BCPS
Assistant Head, Department of Pharmacy Practice and Science, Associate Professor, Colleges of Pharmacy and Medicine, University of Arizona, Tucson, Arizona
Chapter 2

Mary Lee, PharmD, BCPS, FCCP
Professor of Pharmacy Practice, Chicago College of Pharmacy, Vice President and Chief Academic Officer, Midwestern University, Chicago, Illinois
Chapter 52

Russell E. Lewis, PharmD, FCCP, BCPS
Associate Professor, Department of Medical and Surgical Sciences, University of Bologna, Bologna, Italy
Chapter 84

Teresa V. Lewis, PharmD, BCPS
Assistant Professor, Department of Pharmacy, Clinical and Administrative Sciences, College of Pharmacy, University of Oklahoma Health Sciences Center, Oklahoma City, Oklahoma
Chapter 68

Cara Liday, PharmD, BCPS, CDE
Associate Professor, Department of Pharmacy Practice, College of Pharmacy, Idaho State University; Clinical Pharmacist, InterMountain Medical Clinic, Pocatello, Idaho
Chapter 51

Susanne E. Liewer, PharmD, BCOP
Pharmacy Coordinator, Blood and Marrow Transplant; Clinical Assistant Professor, College of Pharmacy, University of Nebraska Medical Center, Omaha, Nebraska
Chapter 97

Kenneth H. Lin, MAT
Student Pharmacist, School of Pharmacy, University of Wisconsin, Madison, Wisconsin
Chapter 93

Melissa Lipari, PharmD, BCACP
Clinical Assistant Professor, Wayne State University Eugene Applebaum College of Pharmacy and Health Sciences; Clinical Pharmacy Specialist, Ambulatory Care, St. John Hospital and Medical Center, Detroit, Michigan
Chapter 20

Mark A. Malesker, PharmD, FCCP, FCCP, FASHP, BCPS
Professor of Pharmacy Practice and Medicine, Creighton University, Omaha, Nebraska
Chapters 27 and 28

Michelle T. Martin, PharmD, BCPS, BCACP
Clinical Pharmacist, University of Illinois Hospital and Health Sciences System; Clinical Assistant Professor, University of Illinois at Chicago College of Pharmacy, Chicago, Illinois
Chapter 14

Spencer T. Martin, PharmD, BCPS
Solid Organ Transplant Specialist, Department of Pharmacy Services, Hartford Hospital, Hartford, Connecticut
Chapter 55

Dianne May, PharmD, BCPS
Campus Director for Pharmacy Practice Experiences, Division of Experience Programs; Clinical Professor, Department of Clinical and Administrative Pharmacy, University of Georgia College of Pharmacy, Augusta, Georgia
Chapters 17 and 18

J. Russell May, PharmD, FASHP
Clinical Professor, Department of Clinical and Administrative Pharmacy, University of Georgia College of Pharmacy, Augusta, Georgia
Chapter 54

Joseph E. Mazur, PharmD, BCPS, BCNSP
Critical Care Clinical Specialist, Medical Intensive Care Unit; Clinical Associate Professor, South Carolina College of Pharmacy, Charleston, South Carolina
Chapter 77

Trevor McKibbin, PharmD, MS, BCOP
Clinical Pharmacy Specialist, Medical Oncology, Winship Cancer Institute, Emory University, Atlanta, Georgia
Chapter 92

Patrick J. Medina, PharmD, BCOP
Professor, College of Pharmacy, University of Oklahoma, Oklahoma City, Oklahoma
Chapter 91

Damian M. Mendoza, PharmD, CGP
Clinical Instructor in Pharmacy Practice and Science, University of Arizona College of Pharmacy; Clinical Pharmacy Specialist, Geriatrics, Southern Arizona VA Health Care System, Tucson, Arizona
Chapter 2

Sarah J. Miller, PharmD, BCNSP
Professor, Department of Pharmacy Practice, University of Montana Skaggs School of Pharmacy; Pharmacy Clinical Coordinator, Saint Patrick Hospital, Missoula, Montana
Chapter 101

Beverly C. Mims, PharmD
Associate Professor of Pharmacy Practice, Howard University, College of Pharmacy, Clinical Pharmacist, Howard University Hospital, Washington, DC
Chapter 21

M. Jane Mohler, RN, MPH, PhD
Associate Professor, Section of Geriatrics, General and Palliative Medicine, University of Arizona, Tucson, Arizona
Chapter 2

Caroline Morin, BPharm, MSc
Pharmacist in Obstetrics and Gynecology, Associated Clinician, CHU Ste-Justine, Université de Montreal Pharmacist, Montreal, Quebec, Canada
Chapter 47

Lee E. Morrow, MD, MSc
Professor, Division of Pulmonary, Critical Care, and Sleep Medicine, Creighton University School of Medicine, Omaha, Nebraska
Chapters 27 and 28

Milap C. Nahata, PharmD, MS
Professor Emeritus of Pharmacy, Pediatrics and Internal Medicine; Director, of the Institute of Therapeutic Innovations and Outcomes, College of Pharmacy, Ohio State University; Columbus, Ohio
Chapter 3

Rocsanna Namdar, PharmD
Lecturer, School of Pharmacy, University of Colorado, Denver, Colorado
Chapter 75

Melinda M. Neuhauser, PharmD, MPH
National PBM Clinical Pharmacy Program Manager, Infectious Diseases, Department of Veterans Affairs Pharmacy Benefits Management Services, Hines, Illinois
Chapter 81

Douglas A. Newton, MD, MPH
Child and Adolescent Psychiatrist, Colordao Permanente Medical Group, Denver, Colorado
Chapter 40

Tien M.H. Ng, PharmD, FCCP, BCPS AQ-C
Associate Professor, Clinical Pharmacy, School of Pharmacy, University of Southern California, Los Angeles, California
Chapter 6

Kimberly J. Novak, PharmD, BCPS
Clinical Pharmacy Specialist, Pediatric Pulmonary Medicine, Nationwide Children's Hospital; Clinical Assistant Professor, Ohio State University College of Pharmacy, Columbus, Ohio
Chapter 16

Edith A. Nutescu, PharmD, MS, FCCP
Associate Professor, Department of Pharmacy Systems, Outcomes and Policy, and Director, Center for Pharmacoepidemiology and Pharmacoeconomic Research, College of Pharmacy, University of Illinois, Chicago, Illinois
Chapter 10

Catherine M. Oliphant, PharmD
Associate Professor and Assistant Chair, Department of Pharmacy Practice and Administrative Sciences, College of Pharmacy, Idaho State University, Meridian, Idaho
Chapter 69

Ali J. Olyaei, PharmD
Professor, Department of Medicine and Pharmacy Practice, Oregon State University and Oregon Health and Sciences University, Portland, Oregon
Chapter 55

Christine Karabin O'Neil, BS, PharmD, BCPS, CGP, FCCP
Professor of Pharmacy Practice, Division of Clinical, Social, and Administrative Sciences, Duquesne University, School of Pharmacy, Pittsburgh, Pennsylvania
Chapter 34

Dennis Ownby, MD
Professor of Pediatrics and Chief, Section of Allergy and Immunology, Georgia Regents Medical Center, Georgia Regents University, Augusta, Georgia
Chapter 54

Victor Padron, PhD
Associate Professor, Department of Pharmacy Sciences, Creighton University School of Pharmacy and Health Professions, Omaha, Nebraska
Chapter 64

Vinita B. Pai, PharmD, MS
Associate Professor of Clinical Pharmacy, Ohio State University, College of Pharmacy; Clinical Pharmacy Specialist, Pediatric Blood and Marrow Transplant Program, Nationwide Children's Hospital, Columbus, Ohio
Chapter 3

David Parra, PharmD, FCCP, BCPS
Clinical Pharmacy Program Manager in Cardiology, Veterans Integrated Service Network 8, Pharmacy Benefits Management, Bay Pines, Florida; Clinical Associate Professor, Department of Experimental and Clinical Pharmacology, College of Pharmacy, University of Minnesota, Minneapolis, Minnesota
Chapter 5

Princy A. Pathickal, PharmD, BCPS
Clinical Pharmacy Specialist, Good Samaritan Regional Medical Center, Suffern, New York
Chapter 56

Charles Peloquin, PharmD, FCCP
Professor, Department of Pharmacotherapy and Translational Research, School of Pharmacy, University of Florida, Gainesville, Florida
Chapter 75

Susan L. Pendland, MS, PharmD
Adjunct Associate Professor, University of Illinois at Chicago, Chicago, Illinois
Chapter 81

Laura A. Perry, PharmD, BCPS
Associate Professor, Department of Pharmacy Practice, University of Findlay College of Pharmacy, Findlay, Ohio
Chapter 65

Hanna Phan, PharmD, BCPS
Assistant Professor, Department of Pharmacy Practice and Science, Assistant Professor, Department of Pediatrics, Colleges of Pharmacy and Medicine, University of Arizona; Clinical Pharmacy Specialist, Pediatric Pulmonary Medicine, Arizona Respiratory Center, University of Arizona Medical Center, Tucson, Arizona
Chapter 3

Beth Bryles Phillips, PharmD, FCCP, BCPS
Rite Aid Professor, University of Georgia College of Pharmacy; Director VAMC/UGA Ambulatory Care Residency Program, Athens, Georgia
Chapter 56

Bradley G. Phillips, PharmD, FCCP, BCPS
Millikan-Revee Professor and Head, Department of Clinical and Administrative Pharmacy, University of Georgia College of Pharmacy, Athens, Georgia
Chapter 41

Amy M. Pick, PharmD, BCOP
Associate Professor of Pharmacy Practice, Creighton University School of Pharmacy and Health Professions, Omaha, Nebraska
Chapter 96

Melissa R. Pleva, PharmD, BCPS, BCNSP
Clinical Pharmacist and Adjunct Clinical Assistant Professor, University of Michigan Health System and College of Pharmacy, Ann Arbor, Michigan
Chapter 100

Frank Pucino, Jr., PharmD, MPH
New Market, Maryland
Chapters 45 and 46

April Miller Quidley, PharmD, BCPS
Critical Care Pharmacist and Critical Care Residency Program Director, Vidant Medical Center, Greenville, North Carolina
Chapter 70

Kelly R. Ragucci, PharmD, FCCP, BCPS, CDE
Professor and Chair, Clinical Pharmacy and Outcome Sciences, South Carolina College of Pharmacy, Medical University of South Carolina Campus, Charleston, South Carolina
Chapter 50

Évelyne Rey, MD
Internist, Department of Obstetrics and Gynecology, CHU Sainte-Justine, Montreal, Quebec, Canada
Chapter 47

Anastasia Rivkin, PharmD, BCPS
Assistant Dean for Faculty and Professor of Pharmacy Practice, School of Pharmacy, Fairleigh Dickinson University, Florham Park, New Jersey
Chapter 67

Kelly C. Rogers, PharmD, FCCP
Professor, Department of Clinical Pharmacy, College of Pharmacy, University of Tennessee, Memphis, Tennessee
Chapter 8

P. David Rogers, PharmD, PhD, FCCP
First Tennessee Endowed Chair of Excellence in Clinical Pharmacy, Vice Chair for Research, Director, Clinical and Experimental Therapeutics, and Professor of Clinical Pharmacy and Pediatrics, College of Pharmacy, University of Tennessee Memphis, Tennessee
Chapter 84

Youssef M. Roman, PharmD
Pharmacist and Clinical Toxicologist, Safetycall International; Research Assistant, University of Minnesota, Minneapolis, Minnesota
Chapter 5

Warren E. Rose, PharmD
Associate Professor, Pharmacy Practice Division, School of Pharmacy, University of Wisconsin, Madison, Wisconsin
Chapter 79

Brendan S. Ross, MD
Staff Physician, G.V. (Sonny) Montgomery Veterans Affairs Medical Center; Clinical Associate Professor, Department of Pharmacy Practice, University of Mississippi School of Pharmacy, Jackson, Mississippi
Chapter 35

Leigh Ann Ross, PharmD, BCPS, FCCP, FASHP
Associate Dean for Clinical Affairs, Professor and Chair, Department of Pharmacy Practice, University of Mississippi School of Pharmacy, Jackson, Mississippi
Chapter 35

John C. Rotschafer, PharmD, FCCP
Professor, College of Pharmacy, University of Minnesota, Minneapolis, Minnesota
Chapter 85

Laurajo Ryan, PharmD, MSc, BCPS, CDE
Clinical Associate Professor, University of Texas at Austin College of Pharmacy, University of Texas Health Science Center, Department of Medicine, Pharmacotherapy Education Research Center, Austin, Texas
Chapter 22

Melody Ryan, PharmD, MPH
Professor, Department of Pharmacy Practice and Science, College of Pharmacy, and Associate Professor, Department of Neurology, College of Medicine, University of Kentucky, Lexington, Kentucky
Chapter 30

Sarah L. Scarpace, PharmD, MPH, BCOP
Associate Professor, Pharmacy Practice, Albany College of Pharmacy and Health Sciences, St. Peter's Health Partners Cancer Care Center, Albany, New York
Chapter 99

Lauren S. Schlesselman, MEd, PharmD
Associate Clinical Professor of Pharmacy Practice, Assistant Dean of Academic and Strategic Initiatives, and Director of Assessment and Accreditation, University of Connecticut School of Pharmacy, Storrs, Connecticut
Chapter 83

Kristine S. Schonder, PharmD
Assistant Professor, Department of Pharmacy and Therapeutics, University of Pittsburgh School of Pharmacy, Pittsburgh, Pennsylvania
Chapter 26

Julie Sease, PharmD, FCCP, BCPS, CDE, BCACP
Professor of Pharmacy Practice and Associate Dean for Academic Affairs, School of Pharmacy, Presbyterian College, Clinton, South Carolina
Chapter 43

Roohollah Sharifi, MD
Section Head of Urology, Jesse Brown Veterans Administration Hospital, and Department of Medicine, University of Illinois at Chicago College of Medicine, Chicago, Illinois
Chapter 52

Kayce Shealy, PharmD, BCPS
Assistant Professor of Pharmacy Practice, Director, Center for Entrepreneurial Development, School of Pharmacy, Presbyterian College, Clinton, South Carolina
Chapter 43

Devon A. Sherwood, PharmD, BCPP
Assistant Professor, Psychopharmacology, Department of Pharmacy Practice, College of Pharmacy, University of New England, Portland, Maine
Chapter 36

Bradley W. Shinn, PharmD
Professor of Pharmacy Practice, University of Findlay College of Pharmacy, Findlay, Ohio
Chapter 76

Judith A. Smith, PharmD, BCOP, CPHQ, FCCP, FISOPP
Associate Professor, Department of Obstetrics, Gynecology and Reproductive Sciences, University of Texas Medical School at Houston, Houston, Texas
Chapter 94

Steven M. Smith, PharmD, MPH, BCPS
Assistant Professor, Departments of Pharmacotherapy and Translational Research and Community Health & Family Medicine, Colleges of Pharmacy and Medicine, University of Florida, Gainesville, Florida
Chapter 58

Thomas R. Smith, PharmD
Assistant Professor of Pharmacy Practice, College of Pharmacy, Natural, and Health Sciences, Manchester University, Fort Wayne, Indiana
Chapter 33

Mary K. Stamatakis, PharmD
Associate Dean for Academic Affairs and Educational Innovation and Professor, West Virginia University School of Pharmacy, Morgantown, West Virginia
Chapter 25

Robert J. Straka, PharmD, FCCP
Professor and Head, Experimental and Clinical Pharmacology Department, University of Minnesota College of Pharmacy, Minneapolis, Minnesota
Chapter 5

S. Scott Sutton, PharmD, BCPS
Professor, South Carolina College of Pharmacy, University of South Carolina, Columbia, South Carolina
Chapter 82

Marc A. Sweeney, PharmD, MDiv
Professor and Dean, School of Pharmacy, Cedarville University, Cedarville, Ohio
Chapter 4

Robert K. Sylvester, PharmD
Professor Emeritus, Department of Pharmacy Practice, College of Health Professions North Dakota State University; Fargo, North Dakota
Chapter 66

Sharon Ternullo, PharmD
Assistant Professor of Pharmacy Practice, University of Findlay College of Pharmacy, Findlay, Ohio
Chapter 76

Eljim P. Tesoro, PharmD, BCPS
Clinical Associate Professor, College of Pharmacy, Clinical Pharmacist, Neurosciences, Director, PGY2 Critical Care Residency, University of Illinois Hospital and Health Sciences System, Chicago, Illinois
Chapter 32

Christian J. Teter, PharmD, BCPP
Associate Professor, Psychopharmacology, Department of Pharmacy Practice, College of Pharmacy, University of New England, Portland, Maine
Chapter 36

Heather M. Teufel, PharmD, BCPS
Clinical Pharmacy Specialist, Emergency Medicine, University of Pennsylvania Health System, Chester County Hospital, West Chester, Pennsylvania

Janine E. Then, PharmD, BCPS
Lead Pharmacist–Clinical Services, University of Pittsburgh Medical Center, Presbyterian-Shadyside Hospital, Pittsburgh, Pennsylvania
Chapter 23

Katherine Theriault, MD
Fellow in Maternal Fetal Medecine, Department of Obstetrics-Gynecology, CHU Ste-Justine, Université de Montréal, Montreal, Canada
Chapter 47

Maria Miller Thurston, PharmD, BCPS
Clinical Assistant Professor, Department of Pharmacy Practice, Mercer University College of Pharmacy, Atlanta, Georgia
Chapter 59

James E. Tisdale, PharmD, BCPS, FCP, FAPhA, FAHA
Professor, College of Pharmacy, Purdue University; Adjunct Professor, School of Medicine, Indiana University, Indianapolis, Indiana
Chapter 9

Christine Trezza, PharmD
Division of Pharmacotherapy and Experimental Therapeutics, Eshelman School of Pharmacy, University of North Carolina, Chapel Hill, North Carolina
Chapter 87

Mary A. Ullman, PharmD
Pharmacist, Regions Hospital, St. Paul, Minnesota
Chapter 85

Elena M. Umland, PharmD
Associate Dean for Academic Affairs, Associate Professor of Pharmacy, Thomas Jefferson School of Pharmacy, Thomas Jefferson University, Philadelphia, Pennsylvania
Chapter 49

Sandeep Vansal, PharmD
Associate Professor and Director, Pharmaceutical Sciences, School of Pharmacy, Fairleigh Dickinson University, Florham Park, New Jersey
Chapter 67

Orly Vardeny, PharmD, MS, FCCP, BCACP
Associate Professor, School of Pharmacy, University of Wisconsin, Madison, Wisconsin
Chapter 6

Mary L. Wagner, PharmD, MS
Associate Professor, Department of Pharmacy Practice and Administration, Ernest Mario School of Pharmacy, Rutgers University, Piscataway, New Jersey
Chapter 33

Heidi J. Wehring, PharmD, BCPP
Assistant Professor, Department of Psychiatry, Maryland Psychiatric Research Center, University of Maryland School of Medicine, Washington, DC
Chapter 37

Elaine Weiner, MD
Assistant Professor, Department of Psychiatry, University of Maryland Medical School, Catonsville, Maryland
Chapter 37

Lydia E. Weisser, DO
Director, Inpatient Mental Health Services, William Jennings Bryan Dorn Veterans Affairs Medical Center, Columbia, South Carolina
Chapter 39

Timothy E. Welty, PharmD, MA, FCCP, BCPS
Professor and Chair, Department of Clinical Sciences, College of Pharmacy and Health Sciences, Drake University, Des Moines, Iowa
Chapter 31

Tara R. Whetsel, PharmD, BCACP, BC-ADM
Clinical Associate Professor, West Virginia University School of Pharmacy, Morgantown, West Virginia
Chapter 15

Jon P. Wietholter, PharmD, BCPS
Clinical Associate Professor, West Virginia University School of Pharmacy; Internal Medicine Clinical Pharmacist, WVU Medicine Ruby Memorial Hospital, Morgantown, West Virginia
Chapter 15

Sheila Wilhelm, PharmD, FCCP, BCPS
Clinical Associate Professor, Department of Pharmacy Practice, Eugene Applebaum College of Pharmacy and Health Sciences, Wayne State University; Clinical Pharmacy Specialist, Internal Medicine, Harper University Hospital, Detroit, Michigan
Chapter 20

Lori Wilken, PharmD, BCACP, AE-C
Clinical Pharmacist, University of Illinois Hospital and Health Sciences System, Clinical Assistant Professor, Pharmacy Practice, University of Illinois at Chicago College of Pharmacy, Chicago, Illinois
Chapter 14

Amy Robbins Williams, PharmD, BCOP
Adjunct Professor of Pharmacy Practice, Union University School of Pharmacy, Jackson, Tennessee
Chapter 88

Susan R. Winkler, PharmD, FCCP, BCPS
Professor and Chair, Department of Pharmacy Practice, Midwestern University Chicago College of Pharmacy, Downers Grove, Illinois
Chapter 11

Ann K. Wittkowsky, PharmD, CACP, FASHP, FCCP
Director, Anticoagulation Services, Department of Pharmacy, UWMedicine; Clinical Professor, School of Pharmacy, University of Washington, Seattle, Washington
Chapter 10

G. Christopher Wood, PharmD, FCCP
Associate Professor, Department of Clinical Pharmacy, College of Pharmacy, University of Tennessee, Memphis, Tennessee
Chapter 13

REVIEWERS

Julie Akens, PharmD, BCPS
Clinical Pharmacy Specialist, Spinal Cord Injury, Louis Stokes Cleveland VA Medical Center, Cleveland, Ohio

Rita R. Alloway, PharmD, FCCP
Research Professor of Medicine; Director, Transplant Clinical Research; Director, Transplant Pharmacy Residency and Fellowship, University of Cincinnati, Cincinnati, Ohio

Jennifer H. Austin, PharmD, BCPS
Clinical Pharmacy Specialist—Internal Medicine, University of Chicago School of Medicine, Chicago, Illinois

Carmela Avena-Woods, BS Pharm, PharmD, CGP
Associate Clinical Professor, Department of Clinical Health Professions, College of Pharmacy and Health Sciences, St. John's University, Queens, New York

Deborah Berlekamp, PharmD, BCPS
Assistant Professor of Pharmacy Practice, University of Findlay, Findlay, Ohio

Martha Blackford, PharmD, BCPS
Pediatric Clinical Pharmacologist and Toxicologist, Akron Children's Hospital, Akron, Ohio

Mary Brennan, DNP, ACNP-BC, ANP, CNS, RN
Clinical Associate Professor, College of Nursing, New York University, New York, New York

Denise Buonocore, MSN, ACNPC, CCNS, CCRN, CHFN
Acute Care Nurse Practitioner for HF Services, St. Vincent's Multispecialty Group, Bridgeport, Connecticut

Katie E. Cardone, PharmD, BCACP, FNKF
Associate Professor, Department of Pharmacy Practice, Albany College of Pharmacy and Health Sciences, Albany, New York

Kimberly Joy L. Carney, DNP, APRN, FNP-BC, CDE
Doctor of Nursing Practice Graduate Faculty, Eleanor Mann School of Nursing, University of Arkansas, Fayetteville, Arkansas

Amber N. Chiplinski, PharmD, BCPS
Clinical Pharmacy Coordinator, Meritus Medical Center, Hagerstown, Maryland

Jennifer Confer, PharmD, BCPS
Clinical Associate Professor, West Virginia University School of Pharmacy; Critical Care Clinical Pharmacy Specialist, Cabell Huntington Hospital, Huntington, West Virginia

Kelli Coover, PharmD, CGP, FASCP
Associate Professor and Vice-Chair of Pharmacy Practice, Creighton University School of Pharmacy and Health Professions, Omaha, Nebraska

Sandra Cuellar, PharmD, BCOP
Clinical Assistant Professor, Department of Pharmacy Practice, University of Illinois at Chicago College of Pharmacy, Chicago, Illinois

Bonnie A. Dadig, EdD, PA-C
Professor and Chair, Physician Assistant Department, College of Allied Health Sciences, Augusta University, Physician Assistant, Department of Family Medicine, Medical College of Georgia, Augusta, Georgia

Lawrence W. Davidow, PhD, RPh
Director, Pharmacy Skills Laboratory, University of Kansas School of Pharmacy, Lawrence, Kansas

Thomas Dowling, PharmD, PhD
Assistant Dean and Department Head-Pharmacy Practice, College of Pharmacy, Ferris State University

David P. Elliott, PharmD, CGP, FASCP, FCCP, AGSF
Professor and Associate Chair of Clinical Pharmacy, School of Pharmacy, West Virginia University, Charleston, West Virginia

Jingyang Fan, PharmD, BCPS
Clinical Associate Professor, Southern Illinois University Edwardsville, School of Pharmacy; Cardiovascular Clinical Pharmacist, Mercy Hospital, St. Louis, Missouri

Karen M. Fancher, PharmD, BCOP
Assistant Professor of Pharmacy Practice, Duquesne University Mylan School of Pharmacy, Clinical Pharmacy Specialist, University of Pittsburgh Medical Center at Passavant Hospital, Pittsburgh, Pennsylvania

Shannon W. Finks, PharmD, FCCP, BCPS
Associate Professor, Department of Clinical Pharmacy, College of Pharmacy, University of Tennessee, and Clinical Pharmacy Specialist, Cardiology, VA Medical Center, Memphis, Tennessee

Thomas S. Franko II, PharmD, BCACP
Assistant Professor of Pharmacy Practice, Wilkes University Nesbitt School of Pharmacy; Ambulatory Care/Pain Management Clinical Pharmacist, The Wright Center for Graduate Medical Education, Clarks Summit, Pennsylvania

Maisha Freeman, PharmD, MS, BCPS, FASCP
Professor of Pharmacy Practice, Samford University McWhorter School of Pharmacy, Birmingham, Alabama

Lisa R. Garavaglia, PharmD, BCPS
Pediatric Clinical Pharmacist, WVU Medicine; Adjunct Assistant Professor, West Virginia University School of Pharmacy, Morgantown, West Virginia

Justine S. Gortney, PharmD, BCPS
Assistant Professor of Pharmacy Practice, Wayne State University, Eugene Applebaum College of Pharmacy and Health Sciences, Detroit, Michigan

Leslie Hamilton, PharmD, BCPS
Associate Professor, Department of Clinical Pharmacy, College of Pharmacy, University of Tennessee, Knoxville, Tennessee

Jin Han, PharmD, PhD, BCPS
Clinical Pharmacist and Clinical Assistant Professor, Department of Pharmacy Practice, University of Illinois at Chicago College of Pharmacy, Chicago, Illinois

Cara A. Harshberger, PharmD, BCOP
Clinical Assistant Professor of Pharmacy Practice, School of Pharmacy, University of Wyoming, Laramie, Wyoming

Deborah A. Hass, PharmD, BCOP, BCPS
Oncology Pharmacist, Mt. Auburn Hospital Cambridge, Massachusetts

Lisa M. Holle, PharmD, BCOP
Assistant Clinical Professor, Department of Pharmacy Practice, University of Connecticut School of Pharmacy, Storrs, Connecticut; Assistant Professor, Department of Medicine, University of Connecticut School of Medicine, Farmington, Connecticut

Irma O. Jordan, DNP, APRN, FNP/PMHNP-BC
Assistant Professor, Retired, University of Tennessee, College of Nursing, Hayden, Kentucky

Michelle D. Lesé, PharmD, BCPS
Assistant Professor of Pharmacy Practice, Lloyd L. Gregory School of Pharmacy, Palm Beach Atlantic University, West Palm Beach, Florida

Jennifer M. Malinowski, PharmD
Associate Professor, Pharmacy Practice, Nesbitt School of Pharmacy, Wilkes University, Wilkes-Barre, Pennsylvania; Director, Clinical Pharmacy Services Integration, The Wright Center for Primary Care, Jermyn, Pennsylvania

Michael A. Mancano, PharmD
Chair, Department of Pharmacy Practice; Clinical Professor of Pharmacy Practice, Temple University School of Pharmacy, Philadelphia, Pennsylvania

Rupal Mansukhani, PharmD
Clinical Assistant Professor, Rutgers University, Piscataway, New Jersey; Clinical Pharmacist, Morristown Medical Center, Morristown, New Jersey

Mary Mihalyo, PharmD, BCPS, CGP, CDE
Assistant Professor Pharmacy Practice, Division of Clinical, Social and Administrative Science, Duquesne University School of Pharmacy, Pittsburgh, Pennsylvania

Rima A. Mohammad, PharmD, BCPS
Clinical Assistant Professor, Department of Clinical, Social, and Administrative Services, College of Pharmacy and Health System, University of Michigan, Ann Arbor, Michigan

Anne Moore, DNP, APN, FAANP
Nurse Practitioner, Women's Health and Adult Certification, Division of Family Health and Wellness, Tennessee Department of Health, Nashville, Tennessee

Candis M. Morello, PharmD, CDE
Professor of Clinical Pharmacy, Skaggs School of Pharmacy, University of California, San Diego, La Jolla, California

Jadwiga Najib, BS, PharmD
Professor of Pharmacy Practice, Long Island University, Arnold and Marie Schwartz College of Pharmacy and Health Sciences, Brooklyn, New York, Clinical Pharmacist, Mount Sinai Roosevelt Hospital Center, New York

Stephen Orr, MD
Ophthalmologist, Spectrum Eye Care, Inc., Findlay, Ohio

Victor Padron, RPh, PhD
Associate Professor of Pharmacy Practice, Creighton University, Omaha, Nebraska

Robert B. Parker, PharmD
Professor, Department of Clinical Pharmacy, University of Tennessee College of Pharmacy, Memphis, Tennessee

Maribel A. Pereiras, PharmD, BCPS, BCOP
Clinical Assistant Professor, Pharmacy Practice and Administration, Ernest Mario School of Pharmacy, Rutgers University, Piscataway, New Jersey; Clinical Pharmacist, John Theurer Cancer Center, Hackensack University Medical Center, Hackensack, New Jersey

Stephanie A. Plummer, DNP, APRN, PMHNP-BC, FNP
Assistant Professor, College of Nursing, University of Tennessee Health Science Center, Memphis, Tennessee; Veterans Healthcare System of the Ozarks, Fayetteville, Arkansas

Jeremy J. Prunty, PharmD, BCPS
Clinical Assistant Professor, West Virginia University School of Pharmacy; Internal Medicine Clinical Pharmacy Specialist, Cabell Huntington Hospital, Huntington, West Virginia

Shaunta' M. Ray, PharmD
Associate Professor, Department of Clinical Pharmacy, College of Pharmacy, University of Tennessee, Knoxville, Tennessee

Michael Reed, PharmD, FCCP, FCP
Director, Rainbow Clinical Research Center, Rainbow Babies and Children's Hospital, Cleveland, Ohio

Kelly C. Rogers, PharmD, FCCP
Professor, Department of Clinical Pharmacy, College of Pharmacy, University of Tennessee, Memphis, Tennessee

Carol Rollins, MS, RD, PharmD, BCNSP, FASPEN, FASHP
Clinical Professor, University of Arizona, College of Pharmacy, Tucson, Arizona

Tricia M. Russell, PharmD, BCPS, CDE
Medicare Formulary Clinical Pharmacist, OptumRx, Mountain Top, Pennsylvania; Adjunct Instructor, Department of Pharmacy, Nesbitt School of Pharmacy, Wilkes University, Wilkes-Barre, Pennsylvania

Aline Saad, PharmD
Clinical Assistant Professor, Department of Pharmacy Practice, School of Pharmacy, Lebanese American University, Byblos, Lebanon

Maha Saad, PharmD, CGP, BCPS
Associate Clinical Professor, St. John's University College of Pharmacy and Health Sciences, Queens, New York

JoAnne M. Saxe, DNP, ANP-BC, MS, FAAN
Health Sciences Clinical Professor, Department of Community Health Systems, School of Nursing, University of California San Francisco, San Francisco, California

Denise Schentrup, DNP, ARNP-BC
Associate Dean for Clinical Affairs, College of Nursing, University of Florida, Gainesville, Florida

Catherine N. Shull, PA-C, MPAS
Assistant Professor, Department of Physician Assistant Studies, Department of Family and Community Medicine, Wake Forest School of Medicine, Winston-Salem, North Carolina

J. Andrew Skirvin, PharmD, BCOP
Associate Clinical Professor, Department of Pharmacy and Health System Sciences, School of Pharmacy, Northeastern University, Boston, Massachusetts

April Smith, PharmD, BCPS
Assistant Professor of Pharmacy Practice, Creighton University, Omaha, Nebraska

Michael A. Smith, PharmD, BCPS
Assistant Professor of Clinical Pharmacy, Philadelphia College of Pharmacy, University of the Sciences, Philadelphia, Pennsylvania

Jacqueline Jordan Spiegel, MS, PA-C
Associate Professor, College of Health Sciences, Director, Clinical Skills and Simulation, Midwestern University, Glendale, Arizona

Sneha Baxi Srivastava, PharmD, BCACP
Clinical Associate Professor, Pharmacy Practice, Chicago State University College of Pharmacy, Chicago, Illinois

Javad Tafreshi, PharmD, BCPS-AQ Cardiology, FAHA
Professor and Chair, Department of Pharmacy Practice, Director, PGY2 Cardiology Pharmacy Practice Residency Program, Loma Linda University School of Pharmacy, Loma Linda, California

Justin B. Usery, PharmD, BCPS
Internal Medicine/Infectious Disease Pharmacy Specialist, Methodist University Hospital; Associate Professor, College of Pharmacy, University of Tennessee, Memphis, Tennessee

Kurt Wargo, PharmD, BCPS(AQ-ID)
Associate Clinical Professor, Auburn University Harrison School of Pharmacy, Huntsville, Alabama

Kimberly M. Welch, PharmD, BCPS
Inpatient Clinical Pharmacist, James H. Quillen Veterans Affairs Medical Center, Mountain Home, Tennessee

Christine M. Werner, PhD, PA-C, RD
Professor, Department of Physician Assistant Education, Doisy College of Health Sciences, Saint Louis University, St. Louis, Missouri

Thomas White, JD, PA-C
Associate Professor, Physician Assistant Program, Westbrook College of Health Professions, University of New England, Portland, Maine

Jon P. Wietholter, PharmD, BCPS
Clinical Associate Professor, West Virginia University School of Pharmacy; Internal Medicine Clinical Pharmacist, WVU Medicine Ruby Memorial Hospital, Morgantown, West Virginia

Monty Yoder, PharmD, BCPS
Clinical Specialist, Department of Pharmacy, Wake Forest Baptist Health; Assistant Clinical Professor, Wake Forest School of Medicine, Winston-Salem, North Carolina

PREFACE

Use of effective and safe pharmacotherapy is a cornerstone of appropriate patient care for both acute and chronic medical conditions. Although the biomedical research enterprise continues to provide medications that have enormous potential to improve individual patient and population health outcomes, these agents are too often applied inappropriately and ineffectively. Consequently, many patients do not achieve the best possible outcomes or incur harm from their drug therapy.

Appropriate implementation and management of high-quality, cost-effective pharmacotherapy by health care providers requires an integration of scientific knowledge and clinical practice skills combined with a fiduciary responsibility to put the patient's needs first. The development of mature, independent pharmacotherapists occurs through structured learning processes that include formal coursework, independent study, mentorship, and direct involvement in the care of actual patients in interprofessional settings.

The fourth edition of *Pharmacotherapy Principles & Practice* is designed to provide student learners and health care practitioners with essential knowledge of the pathophysiology and pharmacotherapeutics of disease states likely to be encountered in routine practice. Chapters are written by content experts and peer reviewed by clinical pharmacists, nurse practitioners, physician assistants, and physicians who are authorities in their fields.

Pharmacotherapy Principles & Practice, fourth edition, opens with an introductory chapter followed by chapters on pediatrics, geriatrics, and palliative care. The remainder of the book consists of 98 disease-based chapters that review disease etiology, epidemiology, pathophysiology, and clinical presentation, followed by clear therapeutic recommendations for drug selection, dosing, and patient monitoring. The following features were designed in collaboration with educational design specialists to enhance learning and retention:

- *Structured learning objectives* at the beginning of each chapter, with information in the text that corresponds to each learning objective identified by a vertical rule in the margin, allowing the reader to quickly find content related to each objective.
- *Key concepts related to patient assessment and treatment* highlighted with an easily identifiable icon throughout the chapter.
- *Patient encounters* that facilitate development of critical thinking skills and lend clinical relevance to the scientific foundation provided.
- A new section on the *patient care process* that provides specific recommendations about the process of care for an individual patient, from the initial patient assessment through therapy evaluation, care plan development, and follow-up monitoring.
- *Up-to-date literature citations* for each chapter to support treatment recommendations.
- *Tables, figures, and algorithms* that enhance understanding of pathophysiology, clinical presentation, medication selection, pharmacokinetics, and patient monitoring.
- *Medical abbreviations and their meanings* at the end of each chapter to facilitate learning the accepted shorthand used in real-world health care settings.
- *Self-assessment questions and answers for each chapter* in the Online Learning Center to facilitate self-evaluation of learning.
- *Laboratory values* expressed as both conventional units and Système International (SI) units.
- *Appendices* that contain: (1) conversion factors and anthropometrics; (2) common medical abbreviations; (3) glossary of medical terms (the first use of each term in a chapter appears in bold, colored font); and (4) prescription writing principles.
- *A table of common laboratory tests and reference ranges* appears on the inside covers of the book.

A companion textbook, *Pharmacotherapy Principles and Practice Study Guide: A Case-Based Care Plan Approach,* is available to further enhance learning by guiding students through the process of applying knowledge of pharmacotherapy to specific patient cases. This study guide contains approximately 100 patient cases that correspond to chapters published in the textbook.

The Online Learning Center at www.ChisholmPharmacotherapy.com provides self-assessment questions, grading and immediate feedback on the questions, and reporting capabilities. The complete textbook and study guide are now available to subscribers of the publisher's AccessPharmacy site (www.accesspharmacy.com), an online educational resource for faculty and students of the health professions.

We acknowledge the commitment and dedication of more than 185 contributing authors and more than 65 peer reviewers of the chapters in this new edition. We are also grateful to many educators and institutions that have adopted this text in their courses. Finally, we extend our sincere thanks to the McGraw-Hill Professional editorial team, especially Michael Weitz, Peter Boyle, and Laura Libretti, for their dedication in bringing this new edition to you.

The Editors
February 2016

Part I

Basic Concepts of Pharmacotherapy Principles and Practices

1 Introduction

Jack E. Fincham

INTRODUCTION

Health professionals are given significant responsibilities in our health care system. These roles may be taken for granted by patients until a pharmacist, nurse practitioner, physician assistant, physician, or others perform assigned tasks that make major impacts upon patients and patients' families lives in countless ways. The exemplary manner in which health professionals provide necessary care to patients is a hallmark of health professional practice and delivery of US health care. Patients are thus well served, and fellow health professionals share knowledge and expertise specific to their profession. However, there are significant problems remaining in the US health care system from a structural standpoint. The United States spends 17% to 18% of the gross domestic product (GDP) on health care, yet the United States ranks 37th in the world considering outcomes of care. Comparing the United States to similar industrialized countries, we rank 11th out of 11 comparator contries.[1]

The uninsured remain a major concern. There were close to 45.2 million uninsured individuals in the United States in 2012, representing 16.9% of the population.[2] This significant number exists despite the institution of health care reform in the United States beginning in 2010. Even with health care reform, the number of uninsured younger than 65 years has decreased only 1.3%. Simply stated, this uninsured segment of the US population is simply staggering in scope and implications for the future collective health of the US population.

Countless other Americans in our midst are underinsured. They may have partial coverage after a fashion, but for these Americans the high price of deductibles, co-pays, and monthly payments for insurance create an economic dilemma for individuals each time they seek care or pay premiums. Recent expenditure data indicate that in 2013, $3.8 trillion was spent on health care in the United States during 2013[3] and $329.2 billion was spent for prescriptions.[4]

There are tremendous opportunities for health professionals due to the implementation the Patient Protection and Affordable Care Act (PPACA). For the first time in the structure of the US health care system, there is a tangible, significant effort to enhance the quality and outcomes of health care delivered. Now payment mechanisms are in place to demand the evidence of quality of health care delivered, regardless of point of delivery of services. If the quality is not there, reimbursement will be decreased, increased, or stay static in monetary values provided to providers.[5] The intent of these measures is to reduce and/or eliminate unnecessary expenditures and duplicative health care service in the United States.

The use of medications in the health care system provides enormous help to many; lives are saved or enhanced, and life spans are lengthened. Many other uses of medications lead to significant side effects, worsening states of health, and premature deaths. So, how to separate these disparate pictures of drug use outcomes? You, within your practices and within your networks in the health care workplace, can help to promote the former and diminish the latter. The authors of the chapters in this book have written informative, current, and superb chapters that can empower you to positively influence medication use.

DRUG USE IN THE HEALTH CARE SYSTEM

Spending on drugs, as a percentage of what was spent on health care in total, increased 3.2% in 2013 compared to the previous year.[6] Drivers for this significant increase include increasing numbers of therapy innovative products and price increases for agents not facing patent expirations.

Prescription medications are used daily; 48.5% of the population uses one prescription drug daily, 21.7% use three or more drugs daily, and 10.6% use five or more prescription drugs daily.[2] Problems occurring with the use of drugs can include:

- Medication errors
- Suboptimal drug, dose, regimen, dosage form, and duration of use
- Unnecessary drug therapy
- Therapeutic duplication
- Drug–drug, drug–disease, drug–food, or drug–nutrient interactions
- Drug allergies
- Adverse drug effects, some of which are preventable

Clinicians are often called upon to resolve problems that occur due to undertreatment, overtreatment, or inappropriate treatment. Individuals can purchase medications through numerous outlets. Over-the-counter (OTC) medications can be purchased virtually anywhere. OTCs are widely used by all age groups. Prescription medications can be purchased through traditional channels (community chain and independent pharmacies), from mail-order pharmacies, through the Internet, from physicians, from health care institutions, and elsewhere. Herbal remedies are marketed and sold in numerous outlets. The monitoring of positive and negative outcomes of the use of these drugs, both prescription and OTC, can be disjointed and incomplete. Clinicians and health professionals need to take ownership of these problems and improve patient outcomes resulting from drug use.

Although clinicians are the gatekeepers for patients to obtain prescription drugs, patients obtain prescription medications from numerous sources. Patients may also borrow from friends, relatives, or even casual acquaintances. In addition, patients obtain OTC medications from physicians through prescriptions, on advice from pharmacists and other health professionals, through self-selection, or through the recommendations of friends or acquaintances. Through all of this, it must be recognized that there are both formal (structural) and informal (word-of-mouth) components at play. Health professionals may or may not be consulted regarding the use of medications, and in some cases are unaware of the drugs patients are taking.

External variables may greatly influence patients and their drug-taking behaviors. Coverage for prescribed drugs allows those with coverage to obtain medications with varying cost-sharing requirements. However, many do not have insurance coverage for drugs or other health-related needs.

Self-Medication

Self-medication can be broadly defined as a decision made by a patient to consume a drug with or without the approval or direction of a health professional. The self-medication activities of patients have increased dramatically in the late 20th and early 21st centuries. Many factors affecting patients have continued to fuel this increase in self-medication. There have been many prescription items switched to OTC classification in the last 50 years, which is dramatically and significantly fueling the rapid expansion of OTC drug usage. In addition, patients are increasingly comfortable with self-diagnosing and self-selection of OTC remedies.

Through the rational use of drugs, patients may avoid more costly therapies or expenditures for other professional services. Self-limiting conditions, and even some chronic health conditions (eg, allergies and dermatologic conditions), if appropriately treated through patient self-medication, allow the patient to have a degree of autonomy in health care decisions.

Compliance Issues

Noncompliance with prescription regimens is one of the most understated problems in the health care system. Approximately 10% of initial prescriptions written by physicians are never filled.[6] Reasons can include trying too soon to obtain a new prescription, prior approval requirements, the prescribed drug may not be covered under the patient's insurance, etc. The effects of noncompliance have enormous ramifications for patients, caregivers, and health professionals. Noncompliance is a multifaceted problem with a need for interprofessional, multidisciplinary solutions. Interventions that are organizational (how clinics are structured), educational (patient counseling, supportive approach), and behavioral (impacting health beliefs and expectations) are necessary. Compliant behavior can be enhanced through your actions with the patients for whom you provide care. Sometimes what is necessary is referral to specific clinicians for individualized treatment and monitoring to enhance compliance. The case histories provided in this textbook will allow you to follow what others have done in similar situations to optimally help patients succeed in improving compliance rates and subsequent positive health outcomes.

Drug Use by the Elderly

The major source of payment for prescription drugs for those aged 65 years and older in the United States is the Medicare Part D Drug Benefit. Seniors have benefitted tremendously from this component. Estimates place the expenditure for Medicare Part D to be $58 billion in 2014; this is 11% of Medicare expenditures.[7] Since the inception of Medicare Part D, recipients have had to pay costs after initial minimum threshold amounts are reached, then enter the so-called "donut hole" requiring payment out of pocket until a certain amount would be paid, and then coverage for payment would ensue. This so called donut hole closes in 2020, which will provide more benefits for more enrollees. At that point, estimates place Medicare Part D payments to account for 16% of Medicare expenditures.[7] Enhanced use of pharmacoeconomic tenets to select appropriate therapy, while considering cost and therapeutic benefits for seniors and others, will become even more crucial for clinicians in the future.

Unnecessary drug therapy and overmedication are problems with drug use in the elderly. Cost estimates are projected to be $1.3 billion per year for elderly patient polypharmacy alone.[4] A joint effort by health professionals working together is the best approach to aiding seniors in achieving optimal drug therapy. Evaluation of all medications taken by seniors at each patient visit can help prevent polypharmacy from occurring.[8]

IMPACTING THE PROBLEMS OF DRUG USE

Medication Errors

There is a tremendous opportunity in medication use and monitoring for working to reduce medication errors. Untold morbidity and mortality occur due to the many errors occurring in medication use. Studies have shown that reconciling the medications that patients take, with coordination by various caregivers providing care, can help reduce medication errors in patient populations.[11] Current changes in how drugs are prescribed, such as electronic prescribing, bar code identification of patients, and electronic medication records, can and have helped to reduce medication errors.[9,10]

The incorporation of three key interventions (computerized physician order entry [CPOE], additional staffing, and bar coding) have been shown in an institutional setting to help reduce medication errors.[10] Being able to track drug ordering, dispensing, and administration electronically has been shown to be cost-effective in the long run.[11] Nurses and office staff have been proven as a valuable resource for reporting prescribing errors, especially with ongoing reminders to scrutinize orders.[12]

HEALTH CARE REFORM

The potential for health care reform to enhance patient outcomes and the quality of care provided to Americans is very significant. The inclusion of health professionals in segments of the innovative medical homes and accountable care organizations will help all health care providers reach more patients needing care.[13]

DiPiro and Davis[14] noted that now and in the future, there will be an important and expectant need for pharmacists to focus on health outcomes and documentation of quality to fully participate in the new health care models that are a focus of health care reform. These authors point to accountable care organizations and patient centered medical homes as innovative models for health professionals to more fully participate.

There are also covered preventive aspects enabled by the PPACA that include immunizations, screenings, and other offering. The provision of these preventive activities by health professionals will serve patients over the long term and work to prevent costly care later on.

SUMMARY

Health professionals are at a crucial juncture facing an uncertain, yet promising future. Technological advances, including electronic prescribing, may stem the tide of medication errors and inappropriate prescribing. These technological enhancements for physician order entry (via personal data assistants or through web access to pharmacies) have been implemented to reduce drug errors. The skills and knowledge that enable effective practice have never been more daunting among the numerous health professions. Technology can further empower health professionals to play an effective role in helping patients and fellow health professionals to practice safe and effective medicine. Health care reform has the potential to dramatically impact your practices in the health care system for the length of your careers. There is also current, and no doubt future, enhanced use of health care apps available to consumers. Consumer computer apps have pervaded many aspects of society, including health care.[15] Consumer apps, although many in number, have not gained widespread use at present; it may be that there are simply too many in number and their utility has not yet been widely adopted.

The use of this text, which incorporates materials written by the finest minds in pharmacy practice and education, can enable the reader to play a crucial role in improving the drug use process for patients, providers, payers, and society. The thorough analysis of common disease states, discussion of therapies to treat these conditions, and specific advice for patients will help you in your practices. The purpose of this book is to help you make a real improvement in the therapies you provide to your patients. Current and future clinicians can rely on the information laid out here to enhance your knowledge and allow you to assist your patients with the sound advice that they expect you to provide. Use the text, case histories, and numerous examples here to expand your therapeutic skills, and to help positively impact your patients in the years to come.

You can help to reverse medication-related problems, improve outcomes of care both clinically and economically, and enable drug use to meet stated goals and objectives. This text provides a thorough analysis and summary of treatment options for commonly occurring diseases and the medications or alternative therapies used to successfully treat these conditions.

Abbreviations Introduced in This Chapter

CPOE	computerized physician order entry
GDP	gross domestic product
OTC	over-the-counter
PPACA	Patient Protection and Affordable Care Act

REFERENCES

1. Davis K, Stremikis K, Schoen C, Squires D. Mirror, mirror on the wall, 2014 update: how the U.S. health care system compares internationally. New York: The Commonwealth Fund, June 2014.
2. National Center for Health Statistics. Health, United States, 2013: with special feature on prescription drugs. Hyattsville, MD: National Center for Health Statistics; 2014.
3. Munro D. Annual U.S. health care spending hits $3.8 trillion. Forbes PHARMA and Health Care [Internet]. Jersey City(NJ): Forbes; 2014 Feb 2 [cited 2015 Jul 7]. Available from: http://www.forbes.com/sites/danmunro/2014/02/02/annual-u-s-healthcare-spending-hits-3-8-trillion/.
4. Aitken H, Valkova S. Exhibit 1: avoidable U.S. healthcare costs add up to $213 billion. Avoidable costs in U.S. Healthcare: the $200 billion opportunity from using medicines more responsibly. Report by the IMS Institute for Healthcare Informatics. Parsippany (NJ): IMS Institute for Healthcare Informatics; June 2013: p. 3.
5. Emanuel EJ. Reinventing American health care: how the Affordable Care Act will improve our terribly complex, blatantly unjust, outrageously expensive, grossly inefficient, error prone system. New York, NY: PublicAffairs, 2014.
6. Aitken M, Kleinrock, M, Lyle J, Caskey L. Introduction. Medicine use and shifting costs of healthcare. Report by the IMS Institute for Healthcare Informatics. Parsippany (NJ): IMS Institute for Healthcare Informatics; April 2014: p. 2.
7. The Medicare Part D Prescription Drug Benefit [Internet]. Menlo Park (CA): The Henry J. Kaiser Family Foundation; 2013 Nov [cited 2015 Jul 7]. Available from: http://kaiserfamilyfoundation.files.wordpress.com/2013/11/7044-14-medicare-part-d-fact-sheet.pdf.
8. Hajjar ER, Cafiero AC, Hanlon JT. Polypharmacy in elderly patients. Am J Geriatr Pharmacother. 2007;5:345–351.
9. Fincham JE. e-prescribing: The Electronic Transformation of Medicine. Sudbury, MA: Jones and Bartlett Publishers, 2009.
10. Franklin BD, O'Grady K, Donyai P, Jacklin A, Barber N. The impact of a closed-loop electronic prescribing and administration system on prescribing errors, administration errors and staff time: a before-and-after study. Qual Saf Health Care. 2007;16:279–284.
11. Karnon J, McIntosh A, Dean J, et al. Modelling the expected net benefits of interventions to reduce the burden of medication errors. J Health Serv Res Policy. 2008;13:85–91.
12. Kennedy AG, Littenberg B, Senders JW. Using nurses and office staff to report prescribing errors in primary care. Int J Qual Health Care. 2008;20:238–245.
13. Smith M, Bates DW, Bodenheimer T, Cleary PD. Why pharmacists belong in the medical home. Health Aff. 2010;29(5):906–913.
14. DiPiro JT, Davis RE. New questions for pharmacists in the health care system. Am J Pharm Educ. 2014;78(2):26.
15. Aitken M, Gauntlett C. Profiling widely available consumer health-care apps. Patient Apps for Improved Healthcare: From Novelty to Main-stream. Report by the IMS Institute for Healthcare Informatics. Parsippany, NJ: IMS Institute for Healthcare Informatics; October 2013, Chap. 1: p. 6.

2 Geriatrics

Jeannie K. Lee, Damian M. Mendoza, M. Jane Mohler, and Ellyn M. Lee

LEARNING OBJECTIVES

Upon completion of the chapter, the reader will be able to:

1. Explain changing aging population demographics.
2. Discuss age-related pharmacokinetic and pharmacodynamic changes.
3. Identify drug-related problems and associated morbidities commonly experienced by older adults.
4. Describe major components of geriatric assessment.
5. Recognize interprofessional patient care functions in various geriatric practice settings.

INTRODUCTION

The growth of the aging population and increasing lifespan require that health care professionals gain knowledge necessary to meeting the needs of this patient group. Despite the availability and benefit of numerous pharmacotherapies to treat their diseases, older patients commonly experience drug-related problems resulting in additional morbidities. Therefore, it is essential for clinicians serving older adults across all health care settings to understand the epidemiology of aging, age-related physiological changes, drug-related problems prevalent in the elderly, comprehensive geriatric assessment, and interprofessional approaches to geriatric care.

EPIDEMIOLOGY AND ETIOLOGY

As humans age, they are at increasing risk of disease, disability, and death for three reasons: (a) genetic predisposition; (b) reduced immunological surveillance; and (c) the accumulated effects of physical, social, environmental, and behavioral exposures over the life course. All elders experience increasing vulnerability (**homeostenosis**) as they age, resulting in considerable heterogeneity in health states and care requirements. While resilient elders can maintain high levels of physical and cognitive functioning, others suffer functional decline, **frailty**, disability, or premature death. There is an urgent need for all clinicians to better understand the epidemiology of aging to comprehensively provide high-value services to optimize functioning and health-related quality of life of older adults.[1]

Sociodemographics

▶ Population

KEY CONCEPT *Our population is rapidly growing older.* In 2010, 40.3 million US residents were 65 years and older (13% of the total population), nearly 5.5 million people were 85 years or older (the "oldest-old"), and over 53,000 were centenarians.[2] The baby boomers (those born between 1946 and 1964) began turning 65 years in 2011; their numbers will double to 83.7 million in the year 2050, representing over 20% of the total US population.[3] In 2010, there were a total of 22.9 million women and 17.4 million men (an average ratio of 100 women to 77.3 men) 65 years and older; this ratio widens as elders age. The oldest-old are projected to increase from 5.3 million in 2006 to nearly 21 million in 2050.[3] In addition, minority elders are projected to increase to 12.9 million in 2020.[3] Surviving baby boomers will be disproportionally female, more ethnically/racially diverse, better educated, and have more financial resources than were elders in previous generations.

▶ Economics

More elders are enjoying higher economic prosperity than ever before, although major inequalities persist, with older blacks and those without high school diplomas reporting fewer financial resources.[4] Considerable disparities exist, and may prevent less advantaged elders from being able to purchase all prescribed medications.

▶ Education and Health Literacy

By 2007, more than 75% of US elders had graduated from high school, and nearly 20% had a bachelor's degree or higher. Still, substantial educational differences exist among racial and ethnic minorities. While more than 80% of non-Hispanic white elders had high school degrees in 2007, 72% of Asians, 58% of blacks, and 42% of Hispanic elders were graduates. Nearly 40% of people 75 years or older have low **health literacy**, more than any other age group.[4] Despite these limitations, the Pew Trust reports that more than 8 million Americans (22%) 65 years or older increasingly use the Internet,[5] and large health care systems are increasingly offering online health information to older health consumers. These advances are important because communication between health care providers and elders is vital in providing quality care, supporting self-care, and in negotiating transitions of care.

Health Status

► *Life Expectancy*

Although Americans are living longer than ever before, an estimated average of 78.14 years overall in 2008, US life expectancy lags behind that of many other industrialized nations.[6] There is nearly a 6-year gap between 2008 estimated life expectancy in men (75.29 years) and women (81.13 years).[6] Disparities in mortality persist, with estimated 2008 life expectancy in the white population nearly 5 years higher than that of the black population.[6] Nearly 35% of US deaths in 2000 were attributed to three risk behaviors: smoking, poor diet, and physical inactivity. Currently, only 9% of Americans older than 65 years smoke; however, nearly 54% of men and 21% of women are former smokers.[7] Overweight elders 65 to 74 years of age increased from 57% to 73% in 2004 largely due to inactivity and a diet high in refined foods, saturated fats, and sugared beverages.[4] Despite the proven health benefits of regular physical activity, more than half of the older population is sedentary; 47% of those 65 to 74 years and 61% older than 75 years report no physical activity.[8]

The 2007 National Health Interview Survey indicated that 39% of non-Hispanic white elders reported "very good" or "excellent" health, compared with 29% of Hispanics and 24% of blacks.[9] Approximately 80% of older adults have at least one chronic condition, and 50% have at least two. The prevalence of certain chronic conditions differs by sex, with women reporting higher levels of arthritis (54% vs 43%), and men reporting higher levels of heart disease (37% vs 26%) and cancer (24% vs 19%).[5] Among the 15 leading causes of death, age-adjusted death rates decreased significantly from 2004 to 2005 for the top three leading causes: heart disease (33%), cancer (22%), and stroke (8%); while rates of chronic lower respiratory diseases, unintentional injuries, Alzheimer disease, influenza and pneumonia, hypertension, and Parkinson disease increased.[6] Figure 2–1 specifies the most common chronic conditions of older adults by sex. Frailty is a common biological syndrome in the elderly. Once frail, elders may rapidly progress toward failure to thrive and death. Only 3% to 7% of elders between the ages of 65 and 75 years are frail, increasing to more than 32% in those older than 90 years.[10]

Patient Encounter, Part 1

CC is an 80-year-old woman who lived in Mexico until just after her 67th birthday when she moved to the United States to take care of her grandchildren. Her daughter was promoted at work and required more travel, so asked CC for help with the children. CC finished eighth grade in Mexico, speaks almost no English, therefore has low health literacy. She was referred to the Interprofessional Geriatrics Clinic for a comprehensive care of multiple chronic conditions, including hypertension, diabetes, stroke, seizure disorder, arthritis, depression, insomnia, and glaucoma. CC uses 14 medications for the described conditions and supplements from Mexico for "general health." She is overweight and reports eating high amount of refined foods because she cooks for her grandchildren only. She watches TV most of the day while the kids are at school.

What information is consistent with epidemiology of aging?

Which of CC's medical conditions are commonly found in older adults?

What additional information do you need before conducting a comprehensive medication review?

► *Health Care Utilization and Cost*

KEY CONCEPT *Older Americans use more health care services than younger Americans do.* Although hospital stays for those 65 years and older decreased by half from 1970 to 2010 (12.6 vs 5.5 days), they accounted for more than 65% of hospitalizations overall, with longer lengths of stay corresponding to increasing age.[11] In 2010 there were 1.3 million (3.6%) US nursing home residents aged 65 and older, and as the aged live longer, more will require assistance, which will be increasingly performed in the home. Health care costs among older Americans are three to five times greater than the cost for someone younger than 65 years.

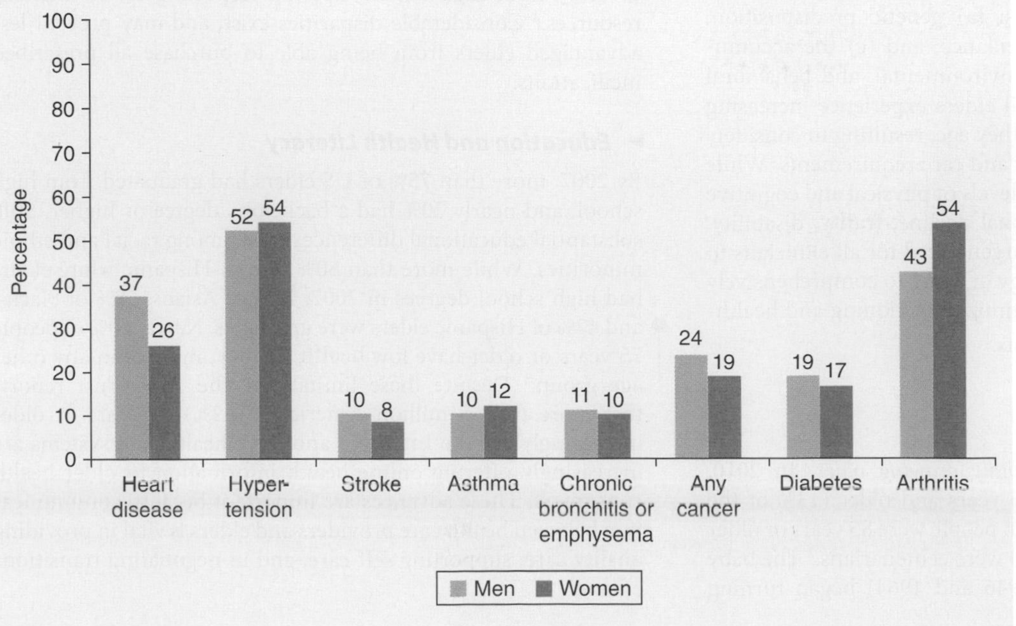

FIGURE 2–1. Percentage of people 65 years and older who reported having selected chronic conditions, by sex, 2005 to 2006. Note: Data are based on a 2-year average from 2005 to 2006. Reference population: These data refer to the noninstitutionalized population. (From Centers for Disease Control and Prevention, National Center for Health Statistics, National Health Interview Survey.)

Medicare plays a major role in health care costs, accounting for 20% of total US health spending in 2012, 27% of spending on hospital care, and 23% of spending on physician services.[12]

By applying the epidemiology of aging, clinicians can better intervene with pharmacotherapy to postpone disease, disability, and mortality, and promote health, functioning, and health-related quality of life.

AGE-RELATED CHANGES

In basic terms, pharmacokinetics is what the body does to the drug, and pharmacodynamics is what the drug does to the body. KEY CONCEPT *All four components of pharmacokinetics—absorption, distribution, metabolism, and excretion—are affected by aging; the most clinically important and consistent is the reduction of renal elimination of drugs.*[13] As people age, they can become more frail and are more likely to experience altered and variable drug pharmacokinetics and pharmacodynamics. Even though this alteration is influenced more by a patient's clinical state than their chronological age, the older patient is more likely to be malnourished and suffering from diseases that affect pharmacokinetics and pharmacodynamics.[14] Clinicians have the responsibility to use pharmacokinetic and pharmacodynamic principles to improve the care of older patients and avoid adverse effects of pharmacotherapy.

Pharmacokinetic Changes

▶ *Absorption*

Multiple changes occur throughout the gastrointestinal (GI) tract with aging, but little evidence indicates that drug absorption is significantly altered. The changes include decreases in overall surface of the intestinal epithelium, gastric acid secretion, and splanchnic blood flow.[13] Peristalsis is weaker and gastric emptying delayed. These changes slow absorption in the stomach, especially for enteric-coated and delayed-release preparations. Delays in absorption may lead to a longer time required to achieve peak drug effects, but it does not significantly alter the amount of drug absorbed, and drug movement from the GI tract into circulation is not meaningfully changed.[13,14] However, relative **achlorhydria** can decrease the absorption of nutrients such as vitamin B_{12}, calcium, and iron.[14]

Aging facilitates atrophy of the epidermis and dermis along with a reduction in barrier function of the skin. Tissue blood perfusion is reduced, leading to decreased or variable rates of transdermal, subcutaneous, and intramuscular drug absorption. Therefore, intramuscular injections should generally be avoided in the elderly due to unpredictable drug absorption.[13] Additionally, because saliva production decreases with age, medications that need to be absorbed rapidly by the buccal mucosa are absorbed at a slower rate.[14] Yet, for most drugs, absorption is not significantly affected in older patients and the changes described are clinically inconsequential.[15]

▶ *Distribution*

Main physiological changes that affect distribution of drugs in older adults are changes in body fat and water, and in protein binding. Lean body mass can decrease by 12% to 19% through loss of skeletal muscle in the elderly. Thus, blood levels of drugs primarily distributed in muscle increase (eg, digoxin), presenting a risk for overdose.[14] While lean muscle mass decreases, adipose tissue can increase with aging by 18% to 36% in men and 33% to 45% in women. Therefore, fat-soluble drugs (eg, diazepam, amiodarone, and verapamil) have increased volume of distribution (V_d), leading to higher tissue concentrations and prolonged duration of action. Greater V_d leads to increased half-life and time required to reach steady-state serum concentration.[13,14]

Total body water decreases by 10% to 15% by age 80. This lowers V_d of hydrophilic drugs (eg, aspirin, lithium, and ethanol) leading to higher plasma drug concentrations than in younger adults when equal doses are used.[13,14] Toxic drug effects may be enhanced when dehydration occurs and when the extracellular space is reduced by diuretic use.

Likewise, plasma albumin concentration decreases by 10% to 20%, although disease and malnutrition contribute more to this decrease than age alone.[13] In patients with an acute illness, rapid decreases in serum albumin can increase drug effects. Examples of highly protein-bound drugs include warfarin, phenytoin, and diazepam.[14] For most chronic medications, these changes are not clinically important because although the changes affect peak level of a single dose, mean serum concentrations at steady state are not altered unless clearance is affected.[14] For highly protein-bound drugs with narrow therapeutic indices (eg, phenytoin), however, it is important to appropriately interpret serum drug levels in light of the older patient's albumin status. In a malnourished patient with hypoalbuminemia, a higher percentage of the total drug level consists of free drug than in a patient with normal serum albumin. Thus, if a hypoalbuminemic patient has a low total phenytoin level and the phenytoin dose is increased, the free phenytoin concentration may rise to a toxic level.[15]

▶ *Metabolism*

Drug metabolism is affected by age, acute and chronic diseases, and drug–drug interactions. The liver is the primary site of drug metabolism, which undergoes changes with age; though the decline is not consistent, older patients have decreased metabolism of many drugs.[13,15] Liver mass is reduced by 20% to 30% with advancing age, and hepatic blood flow is decreased by as much as 40%. These changes can drastically reduce the amount of drug delivered to the liver per unit of time, reduce its metabolism, and increase the half-life.[14] Metabolic clearance of some drugs is decreased by 20% to 40% (eg, amiodarone, amitriptyline, warfarin, and verapamil), but it is unchanged for drugs with a low hepatic extraction.[14] Drugs that have high **extraction ratios** have significant first-pass metabolism, resulting in higher bioavailability for older adults. For example, the effect of morphine is increased due to a decrease in clearance by around 33%. Similar increases in bioavailability can be seen with propranolol, levodopa, and statins. Thus, older patients may experience a similar clinical response to that of younger patients using lower doses of these medications.[14]

The effect of aging on liver enzymes (cytochrome P-450 system [CYP450]) may lead to a decreased elimination rate of drugs that undergo oxidative phase I metabolism, but this is controversial.[13] Originally, it was thought that the CYP450 system was impaired in the elderly, leading to decreased drug clearance and increased serum half-life, but studies have not consistently confirmed this. Thus, variations in the CYP450 activity may not be due to aging but to lifestyle (eg, smoking), illness, or drug interactions.[14,15] A patient's nutritional status plays a role in drug metabolism as well. Frail elderly have a more diminished drug metabolism than those with healthy body weight.[13] Aging does not affect drugs that undergo phase II hepatic metabolism, known as conjugation or glucuronidation, but conjugation is reduced with frailty. Temazepam and lorazepam are examples of drugs that undergo phase II metabolism.[14]

► Elimination

The clinically most important pharmacokinetic change in the elderly is the decrease in renal drug elimination.[13] As people age, renal blood flow, renal mass, glomerular filtration rate, filtration fraction, and tubular secretion decrease. After age 40, there is a decrease in the number of functional glomeruli, and renal blood flow declines by approximately 1% yearly. From age 25 to 85 years, average renal clearance declines by as much as 50% and is independent of the effects of disease.[13–15] Still, the impact of age on renal function is variable and not always linear.[15] Longitudinal studies have suggested that a percentage (up to 33%) of older adults do not experience this age-related decline in renal function. Clinically significant effects of decreased renal clearance include prolonged drug half-life, increased serum drug level, and increased potential for **adverse drug reactions** (ADRs).[13] Special attention should be given to renally eliminated drugs with a narrow therapeutic index (eg, digoxin, aminoglycosides). Monitoring serum concentration and making appropriate dose adjustment for these agents can prevent serious ADR resulting from drug accumulation.[14] It is important to note that despite a dramatic decrease in renal function (creatinine clearance) with aging, serum creatinine may remain fairly unchanged and remain within normal limits. This is because elderly patients, especially the frail elderly, have decreased muscle mass resulting in less creatinine production for input into circulation.[13,14] Because chronic kidney disease can be overlooked if a clinician focuses only on the serum creatinine value, overdose and ADR can occur.

Thus, creatinine clearance should be calculated when starting or adjusting pharmacotherapy in older adults. Clearance measure using 24-hour urine collection is impractical, costly, and often done inaccurately. The Cockcroft–Gault equation is the most widely used formula for estimating renal function and adjusting drug doses. See Chapter 25 (Table 25–2) for more details.

$$\text{Creatinine clearance} = \frac{(140-\text{Age})\times \text{Weight (kg)}}{\text{Serum creatinine}\times 72}\times(0.85 \text{ if female})$$

when serum creatinine is expressed in mg/dL,

$$\text{CrCl(mL/min)} = \frac{(140-\text{Age})\times 1.23\times(\text{BW})}{(\text{SCr})}(\times 0.85 \text{ if women})$$

When serum creatinine is expressed in μmol/L, and converted to units of mL/s by multiplying by 0.167.

This equation is also used by drug manufacturers to determine renal dosing guidelines. The Cockcroft–Gault equation provided the best balance between predictive ability and bias in a study that compared it with the Modification of diet in renal disease (MDRD) and Jelliffe "bedside" clearance equations.[14] Understand that the predictive formulas can significantly overestimate actual renal function in chronically ill, debilitated older patients.

Pharmacodynamic Changes

Pharmacodynamics refers to the actions of a drug at its target site and the body's response to that drug. KEY CONCEPT *In general, the pharmacodynamic changes that occur in the elderly tend to increase their sensitivity to drug effects.* Most pharmacodynamic changes in the elderly are associated with a progressive reduction in homeostatic mechanisms and changes in receptor properties. Although the end result of these changes is an increased sensitivity to the effects of many drugs, a decrease in response can also occur.[16] The changes in the receptor site include alterations in binding affinity of the drug, number or density of active receptors at the target organ, structural features, and postreceptor effects (biochemical processes/signal transmission). These include receptors in the adrenergic, cholinergic, and dopaminergic systems, as well as γ-*aminobutyric acid* (GABA) and opioid receptors.[13,14]

► Cardiovascular System

Decreased homeostatic mechanisms in older adults increase their susceptibility to orthostatic hypotension when taking drugs that affect the cardiovascular system and lower the arterial blood pressure. This is explained by a decrease in arterial compliance and baroreceptor reflex response, which limits their ability to compensate quickly for postural changes in blood pressure. It has been estimated that 5% to 33% of the elderly experience drug-induced orthostasis. Examples other than typical antihypertensives that have a higher likelihood of causing orthostatic hypotension in geriatric patients are tricyclic antidepressants, antipsychotics, loop diuretics, direct vasodilators, and opioids.[13,14,16] Older patients have a decreased β-adrenergic receptor function, and they are less sensitive to β-agonists and β-adrenergic antagonists effects in the cardiovascular system and possibly in the lungs, but their response to α-agonists and antagonists is unchanged.[14,16] Increased hypotensive and heart rate response (to a lesser degree) to calcium channel blockers (eg, verapamil) are reported. Increased risk of developing drug-induced QT prolongation and **torsade de pointes** is also present.[16] Therefore, clinicians must start medications at low doses and titrate slowly, closely monitoring the patient for any adverse effects.

► Central Nervous System

Overall, geriatric patients exhibit a greater sensitivity to the effects of drugs that gain access to the CNS. In most cases, lower doses result in adequate response, and higher incidence of adverse effects may be seen with standard and high doses. For example, lower doses of opioids provide sufficient pain relief for older patients, whereas conventional doses can cause oversedation and respiratory depression.[13,14,16] The blood-brain barrier becomes more permeable as people age; thus, more medications can cross the barrier and cause CNS adverse effects. Examples of problematic medications include benzodiazepines, antidepressants, neuroleptics, and antihistamines. There is a decrease in the number of cholinergic neurons as well as nicotinic and muscarinic receptors, decreased choline uptake from the periphery, and increased acetylcholinesterase.[14,16] The elderly have a decreased ability to compensate for these imbalances of the neurotransmitters, which can lead to movement and memory disorders. Older adults have an increased number of dopamine type 2 receptors, making them more susceptible to delirium from anticholinergic and dopaminergic medications. At the same time, they have a reduced number of dopamine and dopaminergic neurons in the substantia nigra of the brain, resulting in higher incidence of extrapyramidal symptoms from antidopaminergic medications (eg, antipsychotics).[13,16]

► Fluids and Electrolytes

Fluid and electrolyte homeostatic mechanism is decreased in the geriatric population. The elderly experience more severe dehydration with equal amounts of fluid loss compared with younger adults.

The multitude of factors involved include decreased thirst and cardiovascular reflexes, decreased fluid intake, decreased ability of the kidneys to concentrate urine, increased atrial natriuretic peptide, decreased aldosterone response to hyperkalemia, and decreased response to antidiuretic hormone. The result is an increased incidence of hyponatremia, hyperkalemia, and prerenal azotemia, especially when the older patient is taking a diuretic (eg, hydrochlorothiazide, furosemide). Angiotensin-converting enzyme inhibitors have an increased potential to cause hyperkalemia and acute renal failure in older adults. Thus, these agents need to be started with low doses, titrated slowly, and monitored frequently.[13,16]

▶ *Glucose Metabolism*

An inverse relationship between glucose tolerance and age has been reported. This is likely due to reduced insulin secretion and sensitivity (greater insulin resistance). Consequently, the incidences of hypoglycemia are increased when using sulfonylureas (eg, glyburide, glipizide) from age-related impairment to counter-regulate the hypoglycemic response.[13] Due to an impaired autonomic nervous system, elderly patients may not distinguish symptoms of hypoglycemia such as sweating, palpitations, or tremors. They do experience neurological symptoms of syncope, ataxia, confusion, or seizures.

▶ *Anticoagulants*

Older people are more sensitive to anticoagulant drug effects compared to younger people. When similar plasma concentrations of warfarin are attained, there is greater inhibition of vitamin K–dependent clotting factors in older patients than in younger counterparts. Overall, the risk of bleeding is increased in the elderly, and when overanticoagulated, the likelihood of morbidity and mortality is higher. This is further complicated by the presence of **polypharmacy**, drug–drug interactions, non-adherence, and acute illness. Close monitoring of the **international normalized ratio** (INR) and appropriate use is paramount. In contrast, there is no association between age and response to heparin.[13]

DRUG-RELATED PROBLEMS

KEY CONCEPT *Comorbidities and polypharmacy complicate elderly health status, particularly inappropriate medications that lead to drug-related problems.* It is reported that 28% of hospitalizations in older adults are due to medication-related problems, including nonadherence and ADRs. Studies also indicate that 14% to 40% of the frail elderly are prescribed at least one inappropriate drug, and unnecessary medication use was detected in 44% of older veterans at the time of hospital discharge.[17] A decision-tree model estimated the overall cost of drug-related morbidity and mortality in 2000 as greater than $177.4 billion, with $121.5 billion (almost 70%) for hospital admissions and $32.8 billion (18%) for long-term care admissions.[18] Collaboration among interprofessional providers and older patients can ensure appropriate therapy, minimize adverse drug events, and maximize medication adherence.

Polypharmacy

Polypharmacy is defined as taking multiple medications concurrently (four to nine medications or more have been used as criteria in studies). Polypharmacy is prevalent in older adults who compose 14% of the US population but receive 36.5% of all prescription drugs.[17] An estimated 50% of the community-dwelling elderly take five or more medications, and 12% of them take 10 or more.[19] Also, common use of dietary supplements and herbal products in this population adds to polypharmacy. In nursing home settings, patients receiving nine or more chronic medications increased from 17% in 1997 to 27% in 2000.[17] Among various reasons for polypharmacy, an apparent one is a patient receiving multiple medications from different providers who treat the patient's comorbidities without coordinated care. Thus, medication reconciliation becomes increasingly important as the aging population continues to grow.

A review analyzing studies aimed at reducing polypharmacy in elderly emphasized complete evaluation of all medications by health care providers at each patient visit to prevent inappropriate polypharmacy.[20] Efforts should be made to reduce polypharmacy by discontinuing any medication without indication. However, clinicians should also understand that appropriate polypharmacy is indicated for older adults who have multiple diseases, and support should be provided for optimal adherence. Drug-related problems associated with polypharmacy can be identified by performing a comprehensive medication review (see Patient Care Process).

Patient Encounter, Part 2

CC was recently hospitalized for dehydration and is recovering from "low kidney function." CC's daughter (interpreter) states that one of the providers thought CC may need to double her phenytoin dose. CC's current chronic medications include: (1) losartan 50 mg by mouth twice daily, (2) amlodipine 5 mg by mouth twice daily, (3) hydrochlorothiazide 25 mg by mouth every morning, (4) sertraline 50 mg by mouth at bedtime, (5) glyburide 5 mg by mouth twice daily, (6) phenytoin 100 mg by mouth three times a day, (7) zolpidem 10 mg by mouth at bedtime, (8) calcium-vitamin D 600 mg–500 units by mouth twice daily, (9) oxycodone-acetaminophen 5–325 mg two tablets by mouth every 4 hours for pain, (10) brimonidine 0.1% one drop in each eye twice daily, (11) brinzolamide 1% one drop in each eye twice daily, (12) timolol 0.5% one drop in each eye twice daily, (13) bimatoprost 0.3% one drop in each eye at bedtime, (14) diphenhydramine 25 mg by mouth at bedtime. She is allergic to penicillin (hives) and experienced cough with lisinopril. CC does not smoke or drink alcohol.

VS: BP: 102/52, P: 68 beats/min, RR: 14, T: 38.4°C (101.1°F)

Ht: 5′2″ (157 cm), Wt: 66 kg, Pain: 0/10

Labs: Na 141 mEq/L (141 mmol/L), K 4.2 mEq/L (4.2 mmol/L), Cl 98 mEq/L (98 mmol/L), CO_2 25 mEq/L (25 mmol/L), BUN 55 mg/dL (19.6 mmol/L), creatinine 1.6 mg/dL (141 μmol/L), glucose 98 mg/dL (5.4 mmol/L), albumin 2.7 g/dL (27 g/L), $HgbA_{1c}$ 6.6% (0.066; 49 mmol/mol Hgb), phenytoin 10 mcg/mL (mg/L, 40 μmol/L)

What is CC's estimated creatinine clearance?

What steps should be taken prior to increasing CC's phenytoin dose?

What drug-related problems does CC have per her medication list?

Inappropriate Prescribing

Inappropriate prescribing is defined as prescribing medications that cause a significant risk of an adverse event when there is an effective and safer alternative. The incidence of prescribing potentially inappropriate drugs to elderly patients has been reported to be 12% in those living in the community and 40% in nursing home residents.[21,22] A systematic review in 2012 reported that the median rate of inappropriate medication prescribing among elderly patients in the primary care setting was 19.6%.[23] At times, medications are continued long after the initial indication has resolved. The clinician prescribing for older adults must understand the rate of adverse reactions and drug–drug interactions, the evidence available for using a specific medication, and patient use of over-the-counter (OTC) medications and herbal supplements.[21]

Screening tools have been developed to help the clinician identify potentially inappropriate medications in older adults. The most utilized is the Beers criteria,[24] first developed in 1991. The current Beers criteria include 53 medications or medication classes that are potentially inappropriate in elderly patients, listed in three categories: (a) medications that should be avoided regardless of disease/condition, (b) potentially inappropriate medications when used in older adults with certain diseases/syndromes, and (c) medications to use with caution.[24]

Common medications referred to in the Beers criteria are as follows:[24]

- Tertiary tricyclic antidepressants (TCAs) like amitriptyline (strong anticholinergic and sedative properties)
- Benzodiazepines including diazepam (increased risk of falls, fractures, and cognitive impairment)
- First-generation antihistamines like diphenhydramine (confusion and fall risk with prolonged effect)
- Nonsteroidal anti-inflammatory drugs (NSAIDs) (increased risk of GI bleeding, exacerbate heart failure, and cause kidney injury)

Examples of drug/disease combinations reported as potentially inappropriate:

- Anticholinergic drugs in patients with bladder outlet obstruction or benign prostatic hyperplasia
- Metoclopramide and antipsychotics in patients with Parkinson disease and antipsychotics in patients with dementia
- Benzodiazepines, anticholinergics, antispasmodics, and muscle relaxants with cognitive impairment

Practical strategies for appropriate medication prescribing include establishing a partnership with patients and caregivers to enable them to understand and self-monitor their medication effects. Providers should perform drug–drug and drug–disease interaction screening, use time-limited trials to evaluate the benefits and risks of new regimens, and trial off medications to assess need.[23]

Undertreatment

Much has been written about the consequences of overmedication and polypharmacy in the elderly. However, underutilization of medications is just as harmful, resulting in reduced functioning, and increased morbidity and mortality. There are instances when a drug is truly contraindicated, when a lower dose is indicated, or when prognoses dictate withholding therapy. Outside of these scenarios, many elders do not receive therapeutic interventions that would provide benefit.[25] This occurs for many reasons, including belief that treatment of primary problem is enough intervention, cost, concerns of nonadherence, fear of adverse effects and associated liability, starting low and failing to increase to an appropriate dose, skepticism regarding secondary prevention benefits, or ageism. A study found underprescribing in 64% of older patients, and those on more than eight medications at the highest risk. Interestingly, the lack of proven beneficial therapy did not depend on age, race, sex, comorbidity, cognitive status, and dependence in activities of daily living.[26] Common categories of geriatric undertreatment are listed in Table 2–1.

Table 2–1

Common Categories of Geriatric Undertreatment

Therapy	Concern
Anticoagulation in patients with atrial fibrillation	Overly concerned with risk of bleeding or the risk of falls if anticoagulated
Malignant and nonmalignant pain complaints	Hesitant to prescribe opioids due to possible cognitive and bowel side effects, concerns about addiction; patients may often be hesitant to take opioids
Antihypertensive therapy	Underestimate the benefit on stroke and cardiovascular event prevention, and/or fail to add the second or third medication needed to attain control
β-Blocker treatment in heart failure	Concerned about complications in high-risk patients despite the substantial evidence of mortality benefit
Statin treatment for ASCVD	Underestimate benefit or have concerns about adverse events

ASCVD, atherosclerotic cardiovascular disease.

A clinical assessment to weigh the potential benefit versus harm of the older patient's complete medication regimen is required. Once obvious contraindications have been dismissed, the patient's (a) goals and preferences, (b) prognosis, and (c) time to therapeutic benefit should be taken into consideration to determine whether the pharmacotherapy meets treatment goals. Underprescribing can best be avoided by using clinical assessment strategies, improving adherence support, and liberalizing financial coverage of drugs.

Adverse Drug Reaction

ADR is defined by the World Health Organization as a reaction that is noxious and unintended, which occurs at dosages normally used in humans for prophylaxis, diagnosis, or therapy. (See the glossary for the American Society of Health-System Pharmacists' definition of an ADR.[27]) ADRs increase with polypharmacy use and are the most frequently occurring drug-related problem among elderly nursing home residents. The yearly occurrence in outpatient older adults is 5% to 33%.[28]

Seven predictors of ADRs in older adults have been identified[28]: (a) taking more than four medications; (b) more than 14-day hospital stay; (c) having more than four active medical problems; (d) general medical unit admission versus geriatric ward; (e) alcohol use history; (f) lower Mini Mental State Examination

Table 2–2

Strategies to Prevent Adverse Drug Reactions in Older Adults

- Evaluating comorbidities, frailty, and cognitive function
- Identifying caregivers to take responsibility for medication management
- Evaluating renal function and adjusting doses appropriately
- Monitoring drug effects
- Recognizing that clinical signs or symptoms can be an ADR
- Minimizing number of medications prescribed
- Adapting treatment to patient's life expectancy
- Realizing that self-medication and nonadherence are common and can induce ADRs

ADR, adverse drug reaction.

Adapted, with permission, from Merle L, Laroche ML, Dantoine T, et al. Predicting and preventing adverse drug reactions in the very old. Drugs Aging. 2005;22(5):375–392.

score (confusion, dementia); and (g) two to four new medications added during a hospitalization. Similarly, there are four predictors for severe ADRs experienced by the elderly[29]: (a) use of certain medications, including diuretics, NSAIDs, antiplatelet medications, and digoxin; (b) number of drugs taken; (c) age; and (d) comorbidities. Suggested strategies to preventing ADRs in older adults are described in Table 2–2.[29] Particular caution must be taken when prescribing drugs that alter cognition in the elderly, including antiarrhythmics, antidepressants, antiemetics, antihistamines, anti-Parkinson, antipsychotics, benzodiazepines, digoxin, histamine-2 receptor antagonists, NSAIDs, opioids, and skeletal muscle relaxants.[29]

One of the most damaging ADRs that frequently occur in older adults is medication-related falls. Falls are associated with a poor prognosis ranging from premature institutionalization to early death, and polypharmacy is a risk factor. A systematic review concluded that psychotropic medications, including benzodiazepines, antidepressants, and antipsychotics have a strong association with increased risk of falls, while antiepileptics and antihypertensives have a weak association.[30] Comprehensive fall prevention strategies should include medication simplification and modification to prevent or resolve ADRs.

Nonadherence

America's other drug problem is the term given to medication nonadherence by the National Council on Patient Information and Education.[31] Nonadherence to chronic medications is prevalent and escalates health care costs associated with worsening disease and increased hospitalization.[31] *Medication adherence* describes a patient's medication-taking behavior, generally defined as the extent to which one adheres to an agreed regimen derived from collaboration with their health care provider.[32]

KEY CONCEPT *Older adults are at greater risk for medication nonadherence due to the high prevalence of multimorbidities, cognitive deficit, polypharmacy, and financial barriers.* Numerous barriers to optimal medication adherence exist and include patient's lack of understanding, provider's failure to educate, polypharmacy leading to **complex regimen** and inconvenience, treatment of asymptomatic conditions (such as hypertension and dyslipidemia), and cost of medications.[31] Factors influencing medication nonadherence are listed in Table 2–3.

Table 2–3

Factors Influencing Medication Nonadherence

Three or more chronic medical conditions	Significant cognitive or physical impairments
Five or more chronic medications	Recent hospital discharge
Three times or more per day dosing or 12 or more medication doses per day	Caregiver reliance
Four or more medication changes in past 12 months	Low health literacy
Three or more prescribers	Medication cost
	History of medication nonadherence
	Living alone in the community

Following is a list of six "how" questions to ask when assessing medication adherence[33]:

1. How do you take your medicines?
2. How do you organize your medicines to help you remember to take them?
3. How do you schedule your meal and medicine times?
4. How do you pay for your medicines?
5. How do you think the medicines are working for your conditions?
6. How many times in the last week/month have you missed your medicine?

Although no single intervention has found to improve adherence consistently, patient-centered multicomponent interventions such as combining education, convenience, and regular follow-up have resulted in a positive impact on medication adherence and associated health outcomes.[34] Future research needs include adherence studies evaluating belief-related variables, such as personal and cultural beliefs, in larger and more ethnically diverse samples of older populations.

Patient Encounter, Part 3

CC is now 90 years old and has been living at a long-term care facility for a year. Even though she was overweight most of her life, she has lost 5 kg in the past 6 months and developed a new coccyx ulcer. She is currently on multiple medications, including (1) aspirin 81 mg by mouth daily, (2) hydrochlorothiazide 25 mg by mouth twice daily, (3) metformin 500 mg by mouth twice daily, (4) levothyroxine 25 mcg by mouth daily, (5) ibuprofen 600 mg by mouth daily, (6) docusate sodium 100 mg by mouth twice daily, (7) lorazepam 2 mg by mouth three times daily, (8) diphenhydramine 25 mg by mouth at bedtime, and (9) amitriptyline 10 mg by mouth at bedtime. Today her pain score is 7/10.

What recommendations can be made about CC's medication regimen at this time?

Which quality indicators should be of concern in CC?

GERIATRIC ASSESSMENT

The term *geriatric assessment* is used to describe the interprofessional team evaluation of the frail, complex elderly patient. Such a team may include but is not limited to a geriatrician, nurse, pharmacist, case manager/social worker, physical therapist, occupational therapist, speech therapist, psychologist, dietician, dentist, optometrist, and audiologist. Assessment may be performed in a centralized geriatric clinic or by a series of evaluations performed in separate settings after which the team may conduct an interprofessional case conference to discuss the patient's assessment and plan.

Patient Interview

KEY CONCEPT *The clinical approach to assessing older adults frequently goes beyond a traditional "history and physical" used in general internal medicine practice.*[35] Functional status must be determined, which includes the activities of daily living (ADLs) and instrumental activities of daily living (IADLs), see Table 2–4. Evidence of declining function in specific organ systems is sought. Of particular importance is cognitive assessment, which may require collateral history from family, friends, or other caregivers, and is important in determining the patient's capacity to consent to medical treatment.[36] The mini-cog mental status examination,[37] shown in Figure 2–2, is a quick tool to assess patient's cognitive impairment. Commonly there is decreased visual acuity, hearing loss, dysphagia, and impaired dexterity. Decreased skin integrity, if present, greatly increases risk for pressure ulcers. Sexual function is a sensitive but important area and should be specifically inquired about. Cardiac, renal, hepatic, and digestive insufficiencies can have significant implications for pharmacotherapy. Inadequate nutrition may lead to weight loss and impaired functioning at the cellular or organ level. See Table 2–5 for common problems experienced by older adults.

It is important to recognize "geriatric syndromes" such as frailty, falls, osteoporosis, insomnia, and incontinence that have an impact on quality of life. Common diseases present with atypical symptoms, such as thyroid dysfunction and depression presenting as delirium. It is also important to assess for caregiver

Table 2–4

Activities of Daily Living and Instrumental Activities of Daily Living

ADLs			
Transfers	Dressing	Mobility	Eating
Bathing	Toileting	Grooming	

IADLs	
Using transportation	If still driving, assess driving ability (including cognitive function, medications that can impair driving ability, vision, neuromuscular conditions that may interfere with reaction time, ability to turn head) at the time of license renewal
Using the telephone	Check for emergency phone numbers located near the telephone
Management of finances	Assess the ability to balance checkbook and pay bills on time
Cooking	Check for safe operation of appliances and cooking tools as well as ability to prepare balanced meals
Housekeeping	Check for decline in cleanliness or neatness
Medication administration	Assess organization skills and adherence

ADL, activity of daily living; IADL, instrumental activity of daily living.

Three-item recall
1. Ask the patient if you may test his or her memory.
2. Give the patient three words (eg, apple, table, penny) to repeat and remember.
3. Have the patient repeat the three words from memory later (eg, after the clock drawing test).

Clock drawing test
1. Have the patient draw the face of a clock, including numbers.
2. Instruct the patient to place the hands at a specific time, such as 11:10.

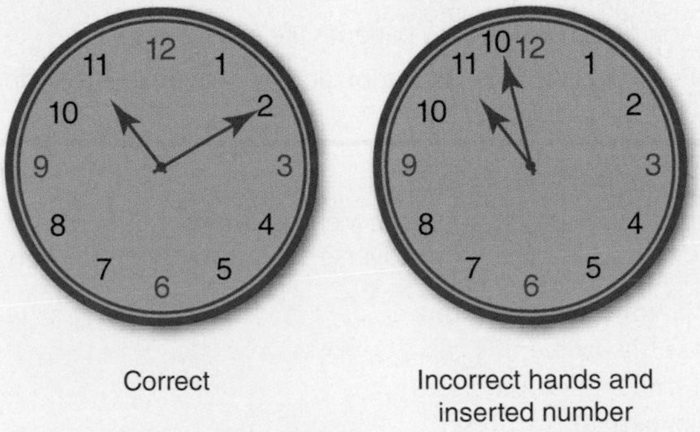

A positive dementia screen
1. Failure to remember all three words.
2. Failure to remember one or two words plus an abnormal clock drawing.

FIGURE 2–2. The mini-cog mental status examination. (Adapted from Borson S, Scanlan J, Brush M, Vitaliano P, Dokmak A. The mini-cog: A cognitive "vital signs" measure for dementia screening in multi-lingual elderly. Int J Geriatr Psychiatry. 2000;15(11):1021–1027.)

Table 2–5

The *I*s of Geriatrics: Common Problems in Older Adults

Immobility	Instability
Isolation	Intellectual impairment
Incontinence	Impotence
Infection	Immunodeficiency
Inanition (malnutrition)	Insomnia
Impaction	Iatrogenesis
Impaired senses	

Reprinted with permission from DiPiro JT, Talbert RL, Yee GC, Matzke GR, Wells BG, Posey L. eds. Pharmacotherapy: A Pathophysiologic Approach, 9th ed. New York, NY: McGraw-Hill; 2014. http://accesspharmacy.mhmedical.com/content.aspx?bookid=689&Sectionid=48811433. Accessed November 03, 2014.

stress and be aware of older patients' support systems. These may include family, friends, religious and social networks, as well as home health aides, homemakers, or sitters. Such networks may facilitate older adults to continue to live independently. Home safety assessment is often necessary for the frail elderly. In addition, look for signs and symptoms of elder abuse, neglect, or exploitation. Health professionals are required to report suspicion of elder mistreatment to Adult Protective Services.[38]

Drug Therapy Monitoring

Geriatric patients often are frail and have multiple medications, medical comorbidities, and prescribers. It is essential that there be a single provider who oversees the patient's pharmacotherapy. The providers need to be aware of the patient's Medicare Part C or D plan, and what type of coverage these plans afford. What is the copayment for generic, preferred, and nonpreferred drugs? Is the patient responsible for all drug costs during the Medicare "donut hole" period? (The first $2250 of medication is partially subsidized, but the patient pays 100% of the next $2850.[39]) Many Medicare patients, especially the socioeconomically challenged, have limited understanding of the complex Medicare drug benefit. This problem is compounded when the prescriber also does not understand the patient's insurance program.[40] Providers can assist patients by prescribing generic medications that are offered through retail pharmacy discount plans ($4 retail pharmacy programs do not bill insurance, thus are not counted toward the $2250 Medicare benefit) and help patients apply for the medication assistance programs offered by drug manufacturers. Particularly challenging in the geriatric population is identifying the cause(s) of nonadherence. Providers assessing older patients' medication regimens should keep the following questions in mind:

- Are medications skipped or reduced due to cost?
- Can the patient benefit from sample drugs? Starting a patient on a free drug sample may increase patient costs in the long term because samples typically are newer, expensive drugs.[40]
- Is there an educational barrier such as low health literacy?
- Does the patient speak English but only read in another language?
- Can the patient see labels and written instructions?
- Does the patient have hearing problems? Patients might not admit they cannot hear instructions.
- Can the patient manipulate pill bottles, syringes, inhalers, eye/ear drops?
- Has the patient's cognitive functioning worsened over time such that they can no longer follow the medication regimen?

Homeostenosis and comorbidities require more frequent monitoring for adverse effects: symptoms, abnormal laboratory results, drug interactions, and drug levels.

Documentation

A clear, current, and accurate medication list must be available to the patient and all individuals involved with their care. It is particularly important for geriatric patients to bring medication containers for reconciliation by a provider. Medications taken may require verification with the pharmacist, caregivers, or family. Transitions in patient care, such as hospital to subacute nursing facility or home, are points of vulnerability for medication errors because medications may have been deleted or added.[41] It is now standard of care to conduct medication reconciliation upon hospital admission and discharge to ensure that the medication list is up to date.

Patient Education

Poor adherence in the geriatric age group could be related to inadequate patient education. "Ask me 3" cues the patient to ask three important questions of their providers to improve health literacy[42]:

1. What is my main problem?
2. What do I need to do?
3. Why is it important for me to do this?

The provider can assess patient grasp of medication instructions by asking the patient to repeat instructions initially and again in 3 minutes (teach-back method).

KEY CONCEPT *Consideration of geriatric patients' vision, hearing, swallowing, cognition, motor impairment, and education and health literacy during counseling and education can lead to enhanced medication adherence.* Specific drug formulations, such as metered-dose inhalers, ophthalmic/otic drops, and subcutaneous injections, will require detailed education and practice. More time needs to be spent on advising the patient and/or caregivers of potential ADRs and when to notify the provider about ADRs also. (See Patient Care Process box for detailed information regarding patient education.)

GERIATRIC PRACTICE SITES

Ambulatory Clinic and Home-Based Primary Care

Ambulatory geriatric clinics are established to provide a multitude of primary care needs specifically tailored to the older population. Home-based primary care brings primary care into the patient's home for homebound patients to facilitate independent living at home as long as possible. Patients are usually referred by their primary care physicians due to the desire for increased access to services (patients-to-physician ratio), complex care needs due to multimorbidity and polypharmacy, and need for geriatric treatment competencies. It is common for the appearance of cognitive impairment to be the catalyst for a referral to such services. Interprofessional team care is the norm in these settings, which benefits patients with varied needs. The interprofessional teams hold regular meetings to discuss care plans of the patients. The geriatrician, who has specialized training in treating the older population encompassing patient's physical, medical, emotional, and social needs assumes the overall care of the patient. The clinical pharmacist focuses on optimizing medication regimen by conducting comprehensive medication review, making evidence-based disease state management recommendations, screening and resolving drug-related problems, and educating patients, caregivers and members of the health care team about pharmacotherapy and monitoring parameters. Clinical pharmacists' effectiveness can be enhanced with the specialty certification in geriatrics. Nurses provide medical triage and day-to-day patient care activities such as obtaining vitals, providing wound care, educating patients, and ensuring adherence. Social workers are involved in various aspects from assessing mood and cognitive status of patients to obtaining placement in higher levels of care. Physical/occupational therapists are often involved in improving the patient's functional status, providing fall prevention interventions, and maintaining a safe home environment. They provide adaptive equipment such as grab bars, raised toilet seat and shower bench for the bathroom, and cane or walker for ambulation. Dieticians evaluate the patient's nutritional status and educate on proper diet and weight management. Using these team collaborations, specialty geriatric clinics have developed including a multidisciplinary geriatric oncology clinic[43] and a community-based memory clinic.[44]

Long-Term Care

Long-term care provides support for people who are dependent to varying degrees in ADLs and IADLs, numbering about 9 million people older than 65 years in 2008.[45] Care is provided in the patient's home, in community settings such as adult care homes or assisted living facilities, and in nursing homes. Long-term care is expensive, typically several thousand dollars per month. Most care is provided at home by unpaid family members or friends. Medicare covers all or part of the cost of skilled nursing care for a limited period posthospitalization.[45,46] Medicare does not cover long-term care. Financing of long-term care comes from patients' and family savings and/or private long-term care insurance. When a patient's assets have been depleted, Medicaid provides basic nursing home care.[46] However, this care is heavily discounted, often resulting in economizing such as lower caregiver-to-patient ratios and higher number of patients per room. Nursing homes are highly regulated by state and federal government through the Center for Medicare and Medicaid Services.[47] Initial and continuing certification of the facility depends on periodic state and federal review of the facility. Auditors' ratings are available to consumers in an online Nursing Home Report Card.[47] **Quality indicators** are used by facility administrators and government overseers to identify problem areas, including[48]:

- Use of nine or more medications in single patient
- Prevalence of indwelling catheters
- Prevalence of antipsychotic, anxiolytic, and hypnotic use
- Use of physical restraints
- Prevalence of depression in patients without antidepressant therapy
- Clinical quality measures such as pressure ulcers
- Moderate daily pain or excruciating pain in residents

Long-term care geriatric practices emphasize the interprofessional team approach. The medical director leads regular meetings with all disciplines delivering care. These may include director of nursing, rehabilitation services (physical, occupation, and speech therapy), pharmacist, social worker, nutritionist, case manager, and psychologist. The pharmacist conducts a monthly drug review of each patient's medication list.[41] The physician is alerted to medication concerns and approves the patient's orders every 60 days. Such a team approach is vital to coordinate care for the typical frail, complex long-term care patient.

Patient Care Process

1. Identify drug-related problems in the older patient by performing a comprehensive medication review.
2. Have the patient bring all medication bottles to the visit, including prescription medications, OTC medications, vitamins, supplements, and herbal products.
3. Identify the indication for all medications used by the patient.
4. Review medication doses to determine any underdose and/or overdose.
5. Screen for drug–drug, drug–disease, drug–vitamin/herbal, drug–food interactions.
6. Ensure that patient is not using any agents to which they have allergies or intolerance.
7. Assess medication adherence by using combination methods (whenever possible): tablet/capsule count, refill history, self-report, and demonstration of use of nonoral agents.
8. Inquire about ADRs experienced.
9. Identify untreated indication or undertreatment, including preventive use of aspirin and calcium plus vitamin D.
10. Assess vital signs, including pain.
11. Evaluate laboratory findings to assess renal function, hepatic function, therapeutic drug monitoring (eg, digoxin, warfarin, phenytoin), and therapeutic goals for chronic diseases (eg, $HgbA_{1c}$).
12. Perform medication regimen tailoring when indicated: discontinue unnecessary medications/supplements/herbals, simplify dosing times to minimize complex regimen, and tailor regimen to individual's daily routine to improve adherence.
13. Solve any physical/functional barriers to medication use such as providing non–child-resistant caps and tablet cutters.
14. Provide education and adherence aid:
    - Verbal and written information about medications and/or disease states in health literacy-sensitive manner
    - Specific product education for nonoral agents (eg, inhalers, insulin, ophthalmic/otic drops)
    - Medication chart/list to include generic and brand names, indication, dose, direction for use, timing of dose, etc.
    - Medication storage, expiration date, and refill status
    - Medication organizer (eg, pillbox, blister packs) when indicated
    - List of future appointments
15. Promote self-monitoring and lifestyle modification by promoting use of blood pressure monitoring device and glucometer, diet and exercise, smoking cessation, immunization.
16. Formulate a patient-centered and interprofessional team-based follow-up plan to track patient response and health outcomes, and to prevent adverse events.

Abbreviations Introduced in This Chapter

ADL	Activities of daily living
ADR	Adverse drug reaction
GABA	γ-aminobutyric acid
$HgbA_{1c}$	Hemoglobin A_{1c}
IADL	Instrumental activities of daily living
INR	International normalized ratio
MDRD	Modification of diet in renal disease
NSAID	Nonsteroidal anti-inflammatory drug
OTC	Over the counter
V_d	Volume of distribution

REFERENCES

1. Institute of Medicine. Retooling for an Aging America: Building the Health Care Workforce. Washington, DC: National Academies Press, 2008.
2. U.S. Census Bureau. The 2010 Census Summary File 1 [Internet]. Washington, DC: U.S. Census Bureau; 2000 [updated 2010; cited 2011 Oct 20]. http://www.census.gov/prod/cen2010/briefs/c2010br-03.pdf.
3. U.S. Census Bureau. The 2012 National Population Projections. Washington, DC. 2012b. www.census.gov/population/projections/data/national/2012.html. Accessed August 13, 2014.
4. Federal Interagency Forum on Aging-Related Statistics. Older Americans 2008: Key Indicators of Well-Being. Federal Interagency Forum on Aging-Related Statistics. Washington, DC: U.S. Government Printing Office, 2008.
5. Centers for Disease Control and Prevention and the Merck Company Foundation. The State of Aging and Health in America. Whitehouse Station, NJ: The Merck Company Foundation, 2007.
6. U.S. National Center for Health Statistics, National Vital Statistics Reports (NVSR), Deaths: Preliminary Data for 2008, Vol. 59, No. 2, December 2010.
7. U.S. Department of Health and Human Services. Health Consequences of Smoking: A Report of the Surgeon General [Internet]. Atlanta, GA: U.S. Department of Health and Human Services, Centers for Disease Control and Prevention, National Center for Chronic Disease Prevention and Health Promotion, Office on Smoking and Health; 2004 [cited 2011 Oct 20]. http://www.surgeongeneral.gov/library/Smokingconsequences/.
8. National Committee for Quality Assurance (NCQA). HEDIS 2008: Healthcare Effectiveness Data & Information Set. Vol. 2, Technical Specifications for Health Plans. Washington, DC: National Committee for Quality Assurance (NCQA), 2007.
9. Pleis JR, Lucas JW. Summary Health Statistics for U.S. Adults: National Health Interview Survey, 2007 [Vital Health Stat 10-240-2009]. Washington, DC: National Center for Health Statistics, 2009.
10. Ahmed N, Mandel R, Fain MJ. Frailty: an emerging geriatric syndrome. Am J Med. 2007;120(9):748–753.
11. DeFrances CJ, Hall MJ. 2005 National Hospital Discharge Survey: Advance Data from Vital and Health Statistics [Report No. 385]. Hyattsville, MD: National Center for Health Statistics, 2007.
12. Centers for Medicare & Medicaid Services, Office of the Actuary, National Health Statistics Group, National Health Expenditures Tables, January 2014.
13. Delafuente JC. Pharmacokinetic and pharmacodynamic alterations in the geriatric patient. Consult Pharm. 2008;23:324–334.
14. Sera LC, McPherson ML. Pharmacokinetics and pharmacodynamic changes associated with aging and implications for drug therapy. Clin Geriatr Med. 2012;28:273–286.
15. Hilmer SN, McLachlan AJ, Le Couteur DG. Clinical pharmacology in the geriatric patient. Fundam Clin Pharmacol. 2007;21(3):217–230.
16. Hutchison LC, O'Brien CE. Changes in pharmacokinetics and pharmacodynamics in the elderly patient. J Pharm Pract. 2007;20(1):4–12.
17. Chutka DS, Takahashi PY, Hoel RW. Inappropriate medications for elderly patients. Mayo Clin Proc. 2004;79:122–139.
18. Ernst FR, Grizzle AJ. Drug-related morbidity and mortality: updating the cost-of-illness model. J Am Pharm Assoc. 2001;41(2):192–199.
19. Cannon KT, Choi MM, Zuniga MA. Potentially inappropriate medication use in elderly patients receiving home health care: a retrospective data analysis. Am J Geriatr Pharmacother. 2006;4(2):134–143.
20. Hajjar ER, Cafiero AC, Hanlon JT. Polypharmacy in elderly patients. Am J Geriatr Pharmacother. 2007;5:345–351.
21. Gallagher P, Barry P, O'Mahony D. Inappropriate prescribing in the elderly. J Clin Pharm Ther. 2007;32:113–121.
22. Hajjar ER, Gray SL, Slattum PW, et al. eChapter 8. Geriatrics. In: DiPiro JT, Talbert RL, Yee GC, Matzke GR, Wells BG, Posey L, eds. Pharmacotherapy: A Pathophysiologic Approach, 9th ed. New York, NY: McGraw-Hill, 2014. http://accesspharmacy.mhmedical.com/content.aspx?bookid=689&Sectionid=48811433. Accessed November 03, 2014.
23. Opondo D, Eslami S, Visscher S, et al. Inappropriateness of medication prescriptions to elderly patients in the primary care setting: a systematic review. PLoS ONE. 2012;7(8):e43617.
24. The American Geriatrics Society 2012 Beers Criteria Update Expert Panel. American Geriatrics Society updated Beers Criteria for potentially inappropriate medication use in older adults. J Am Geriatr Soc. 2012;60:616–631.
25. Barry PJ, Gallagher P, Ryan C, et al. START (screening tool to alert doctors to the right treatment): an evidence based screening tool to detect prescribing omissions in elderly patients. Age Aging. 2007;36:632–638.
26. Singer DE, Chang Y, Fang MC, et al. The net clinical benefit of warfarin anticoagulation in atrial fibrillation. Ann Intern Med. 2009;151:297–305.
27. American Society of Health-System Pharmacists. ASHP guidelines on adverse drug reaction monitoring and reporting. Am J Health Syst Pharm. 1995;52:417–419.
28. Gurwitz JH, Field TS, Harrold LR, et al. Incidence and preventability of adverse drug events among older persons in the ambulatory setting. JAMA. 2003;289:1107–1116.
29. Merle L, Laroche ML, Dantoine T, et al. Predicting and preventing adverse drug reactions in the very old. Drugs Aging. 2005;22(5):375–392.
30. Hartikainen S, Lonnroos E, Louhivuori K. Medication as a risk factor for falls: critical systematic review. J Gerontol Med Sci. 2007;62A(10):1172–1181.
31. Sokol MC, McGuigan KA, Verbrugge RR, Epstein RS. Impact of medication adherence on hospitalization risk and healthcare cost. Med Care. 2005;43:521–530.
32. Osterberg L, Blaschke T. Adherence to medication. N Engl J Med. 2005;353:487–497.
33. MacLaughlin EJ, Raehl CL, Treadway AK, et al. Assessing medication adherence in the elderly: which tools to use in clinical practice? Drugs Aging. 2005;22(3):231–255.
34. Lee JK, Grace KA, Taylor AJ. Effect of a pharmacy care program on medication adherence and persistence, blood pressure, and low-density lipoprotein cholesterol: a randomized controlled trial. JAMA. 2006;296:2563–2571.
35. Miller KE, Zylstra RG, Standridge JB. The geriatric patient: a systematic approach to maintaining health. Am Fam Physician. 2000;61:1089–1104.

36. Appelbaum PS. Clinical practice. Assessment of patients' competence to consent to treatment. N Engl J Med. 2007;357(18): 1834–1840.
37. Borson S, Scanlan J, Brush M, Vitaliano P, Dokmak A. The mini-cog: A cognitive "vital signs" measure for dementia screening in multi-lingual elderly. Int J Geriatr Psychiatry. 2000;15(11):1021–1027.
38. Armstrong J, Mitchell E. Comprehensive nursing assessment in the care of older people. Nurs Older People. 2008;20(1):36–40.
39. Center for Medicare & Medicaid Service. Prescription Drug Coverage: Basic Information [Internet]. Washington, DC: Centers for Medicare & Medicaid Services 2008 [cited 2011 Oct 20]. http://www.medicare.gov/pdp-basic-information.asp/. Accessed July 29, 2014.
40. Piette JD, Heisler M. The relationship between older adults' knowledge of their drug coverage and medication cost problems. J Am Geriatr Soc. 2006;54:91–96.
41. Levenson SA, Saffel DA. The consultant pharmacist and the physician in the nursing home: roles, relationships, and a recipe for success. J Am Med Dir Assoc. 2007;8:55–64.
42. National Patient Safety Foundation. Ask Me 3 [Internet]. Boston, MA: National Patient Safety Foundation; 2007 [updated 2014; cited 2014 August]. http://www.npsf.org/for-healthcare-professionals/programs/ask-me-3/. Accessed July 29, 2014.
43. Lynch MP, Marcone D, Kagan SH. Developing a multidisciplinary geriatric oncology program in a community cancer center. Clin J Oncol Nurs. 2004;11:929–933.
44. Grizzell M, Fairhurst A, Lyle S, Jolley D, Willmott S, Bawn S. Creating a community-based memory clinic for older people. Nurs Times. 2006;102:32–34.
45. Centers for Medicare & Medicaid Services. Long Term Care [Internet]. Washington, DC: Centers for Medicare & Medicaid Services; 2007 [updated 2008; cited 2011 Oct]. http://www.medicare.gov/LongTermCare/Static/Home.asp/.
46. Gozalo PL, Miller SC, Intrator O, et al. Hospice effect on government expenditures among nursing home residents. Health Serv Res. 2008;43(1):134–153.
47. Centers for Medicare & Medicaid Services. Nursing Home Compare [Internet]. Washington, DC: Centers for Medicare & Medicaid Services; 2008 [cited 2011 Oct]. http://www.medicare.gov/NHCompare/. Accessed July 29, 2014.
48. Hawes C, Mor V, Phillips CD, et al. The OBRA-87 nursing home regulations and implementation of the resident assessment instrument: Effects on process quality. J Am Geriatr Soc. 1997;45: 977–985.

3 Pediatrics

Hanna Phan, Vinita B. Pai,
and Milap C. Nahata

LEARNING OBJECTIVES

Upon completion of the chapter, the reader will be able to:

1. Define different age groups within the pediatric population.
2. Explain general pharmacokinetic and pharmacodynamic differences in pediatric versus adult patients.
3. Identify factors that affect selection of safe and effective drug therapy in pediatric patients.
4. Identify strategies for appropriate medication administration to infants and young children.
5. Apply pediatric pharmacotherapy concepts to make drug therapy recommendations, assess outcomes, and effectively communicate with patients and caregivers.

INTRODUCTION

Pediatric clinical practice involves care of infants, children, and adolescents with the goal of optimizing health, growth, and development toward adulthood. Clinicians serve as advocates for this unique and vulnerable patient population to optimize their well-being. Care for pediatric patients is relevant in both inpatient and outpatient settings and requires additional considerations with regards to selection and monitoring of drug therapy.

KEY CONCEPT *Despite the common misconception of pediatric patients as "smaller adults" where doses are scaled only for their smaller size, there are multiple factors to consider when selecting and providing drug therapy for patients in this specific population.* Pediatric patients significantly differ within their age groups and from adults regarding drug administration, psychosocial development, and organ function development, which affect the efficacy and safety of pharmacotherapy.

FUNDAMENTALS OF PEDIATRIC PATIENTS

Classification of Pediatric Patients

Pediatric patients are those younger than 18 years, although some pediatric clinicians may care for patients up to age 21. Unlike an adult patient, whose age is commonly measured in years, a pediatric patient's age can be expressed in days, weeks, months, and years. Patients are classified based on age and may be further described based on other factors, including birth weight and prematurity status (Table 3–1).[1]

Growth and Development

Children are monitored for physical, motor, cognitive, and psychosocial development through clinical recognition of timely milestones during routine well-child visits. As a newborn continues to progress to infant, child, and adolescent stages, different variables are monitored to assess growth compared with the general population of similar age and size. Growth charts are used to plot head circumference, weight, length or stature, weight for length, and body mass index for a graphical representation of a child's growth compared with the general pediatric population. These markers of growth and development are both age and gender dependent; thus, the use of the correct tool for measurement is important. For children younger than 2 years, one should use the World Health Organization (WHO) growth standards (Figure 3–1).[2] For children 2 years and older, the Centers for Disease Control and Prevention (CDC) growth charts (Figure 3–2) are used.[3] These tools assess whether a child is meeting the appropriate physical growth milestones, thereby allowing identification of nutritional issues such as poor weight and height gain (eg, failure to thrive).

Differences in Vital Signs

Normal values for heart rate and respiratory rate vary based on age. Normal values for blood pressure vary based on gender and age for all pediatric patients, and also height percentile for patients older than 1 year. Respiratory rates are also higher in neonates and infants (30–60 breaths/min), decreasing with age to adult rates around 15 years of age (12–16 breaths/min).

Normal values for blood pressure in pediatric patients can be found in various national guidelines and other pediatric diagnostic references.[4–7] In general, blood pressure increases with age, with average blood pressures of 70/50 in neonates, increasing throughout childhood to 110/65 in adolescents.[6] Heart rates are highest in neonates and infants, ranging from 85 to 205 beats/min and decrease with age, reaching adult rates (60–100 beats/min) around 10 years of age.

Another vital sign commonly monitored in children by their caregivers is body temperature, especially when they seem "warm to the touch." The American Academy of Pediatrics (AAP) supports the use of rectal measurement of body temperature as it is most accurate when appropriate technique is used; however, for other routes, the AAP offers an age-specific guideline on routes of measurement.[8] For patients aged less than 3 months, axillary temperature is safest for initial measurement, followed by rectal

Table 3–1

Pediatric Age Groups, Age Terminology, and Weight Classification

Age Group	Age
Neonate	≤ 28 days (4 weeks) of life
Infant	29 days to ≤ 12 months
Child	1–12 years
Adolescent	13–17 years (most common definition)
Age Terminology	**Definition**
GA	Age from date of mother's first day of last menstrual period to date of birth
Full term	Describes infants born at 37-week gestation or greater
Premature	Describes infants born before 37-week gestation
Small for GA	Neonates with birth weight below the 10th percentile among neonates of the same GA
Large for GA	Neonates with birth weight above the 90th percentile among neonates of the same GA
Chronological or postnatal age	Age from birth to present, measured in days, weeks, months, or years
Corrected or adjusted age	May be used to describe the age of a premature child up to 3 years of age: Corrected age = Chronological age in months – [(40 – GA at birth in weeks) × 1 month ÷ 4 weeks]. For example, if a former 29-week GA child is now 10 months old chronologically, his corrected age is approximately 7 months: 10 months – [(40 – 29 weeks) × 1 month ÷ 4 weeks] = 7.25 months
Weight Classification	**Definition**
LBW infant	Premature infant with birth weight between 1500 and 2500 g
VLBW infant	Premature infant with birth weight 1000 g to < 1500 g
ELBW infant	Premature infant with birth weight < 1000 g

ELBW, extremely low birth weight; GA, gestational age; LBW, low birth weight; VLBW, very low birth weight.

Based on defined terms in American Academy of Pediatrics, Committee on Fetus and Newborn. Age terminology during the perinatal period. Pediatrics. 2004;114:1362–1364.

measurement if axillary result is above 99°F (37.2°C), for more accurate measurement and determining need for additional medical assessment in case of defined fever. For patients age 3 months to 5 years, oral measurement is reliable with an option to use otic or temporal artery measurement alternatively, after 6 months of age. Axillary measurement is not considered first line in this age group, as proper technique in this age group is important for accurate measurement and other accurate options are available. Generally, fever is defined as temperature 100.4°F (38°C) and greater measured via rectal, otic, or temporal artery technique. For oral and axillary measurement, fever is defined as temperature 100°F (37.8°C) and 99°F (37.2°C) and greater, respectively.[8] Low-grade fevers range from 37.8°C to 39°C (100–102°F), with antipyretic treatment (eg, acetaminophen) considered by most pediatricians in cases of temperature greater than 38.3°C (101°F, any measurement route) accompanied by patient discomfort. Formal definition of fever, like other vital signs, is also age dependent, with a lower temperature threshold for neonates (38°C or 100.4°F) and infants (38.2°C or 100.7°F).[8,9]

Also sometimes considered as the fifth vital sign, pain assessment is more challenging to assess in neonate, infants, and young children due to their inability to communicate symptoms. Indicators of possible pain include physiological changes, such as increased heart rate, respiratory rate, and blood pressure, decreased oxygen saturation, as well as behavior changes such as prolonged, high-pitch crying, and facial expressions.[10] Such indicators are used in validated assessment scales, such as the FACES scale and FLACC (Face, Legs, Activity, Cry, Consolability) scale behavioral tools.[11,12]

Fluid Requirements

Fluid requirement and balance are important to monitor in pediatric patients, especially in premature neonates and infants. Maintenance fluid requirement can be calculated based on body surface area for patients weighing more than 10 kg, with a range of 1500 to 2000 mL/m²/day. However, a weight-based method of determining normal maintenance fluid requirement for children is often used (Table 3–2).[13]

EFFECTS OF PHARMACOKINETIC AND PHARMACODYNAMIC DIFFERENCES ON DRUG THERAPY

Drug selection strategy may be similar or different depending on age and disease state, as a result of differences in pathophysiology of certain diseases and pharmacokinetic and pharmacodynamic parameters among pediatric and adult patients. It is noteworthy that pediatric patients may require the use of different medications from those used in adults affected by certain diseases. For example, phenobarbital is commonly used for treatment of neonatal seizures but seldom used for seizure treatment in adults, due to differences in seizure etiology and availability of extensive data regarding its use in neonates compared with newer antiepileptic medications. There also exist commonalities between pediatric and adult patients, such as therapeutic serum drug concentrations required to treat certain diseases. For example, gentamicin peak and trough serum concentrations needed for bacteremia treatment are the same in children and adults. Appropriate selection and dosing of drug therapy for a pediatric patient depends on a number of specific factors, such as age, weight, height, disease, comorbidities, developmental pharmacokinetics, and available drug dosage forms. Pediatric drug doses are often calculated based on body weight (eg, mg/kg/dose) compared with uniform dosing (eg, mg/day or mg/dose) for adult patients. Thus, accurate weight should be available while prescribing or dispensing medications

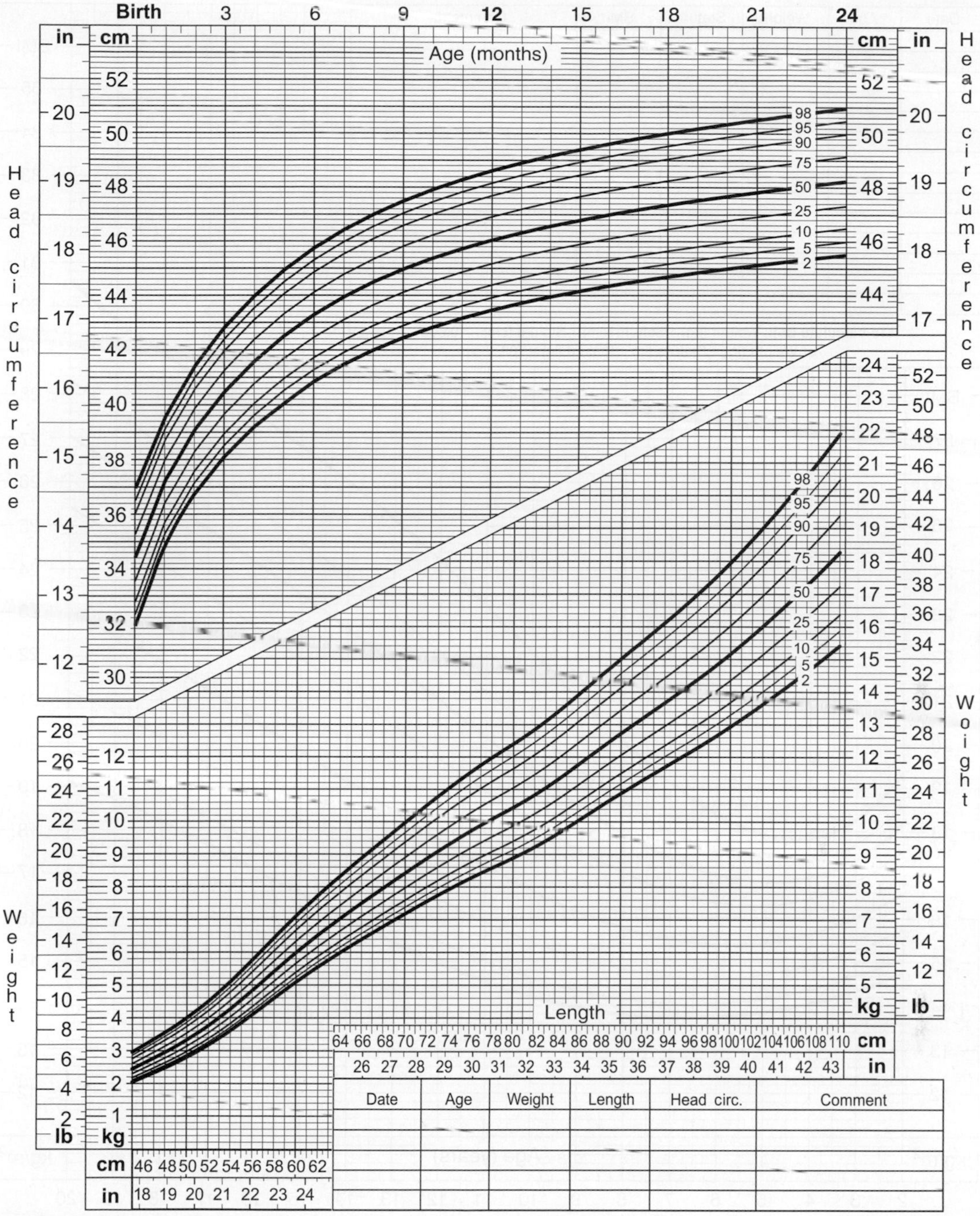

FIGURE 3–1. Example of WHO growth chart of girls, birth to 24 months: Head circumference-for-age and weight-for-length percentile, 2000. (From Centers for Disease Control and Prevention from the WHO Growth Standards. World Health Organization [WHO] Growth Standards, 2009 [updated September 9, 2010], http://www.cdc.gov/growthcharts/who_charts.htm.)

for this patient population. Pediatric doses may exceed adult doses by body weight for certain medications due to differences in pharmacokinetics and pharmacodynamics; hence, the use of pediatric drug dosing guides is recommended.

KEY CONCEPT *Due to multiple differences, including age-dependent development of organ function in pediatric patients, the pharmacokinetics, efficacy, and safety of drugs often differ between pediatric and adult patients; thus, pediatric dosing should not be calculated based on a single factor of difference.* Equations proposed to estimate pediatric doses based on adjusted age or weight, such as the Clark's, Fried's, or Young's rule should not be routinely used to calculate pediatric doses because they account for only one factor of difference (eg, age or weight), and they lack integration of the effect of growth and development on drug pharmacokinetics and pharmacodynamics in this population. For off-label medication dosing, when no alternative treatment is available and limited dosage guidelines have been published, clinicians may estimate a pediatric dose based on body surface area ratio.

$$\textbf{Approximate pediatric dose} = \textbf{Adult dose} \times [\textbf{BSA (in m}^2) \div \textbf{1.73 m}^2]$$

Limitations for this dose-estimating approach include the need for the patient to be of normal height and weight for age,

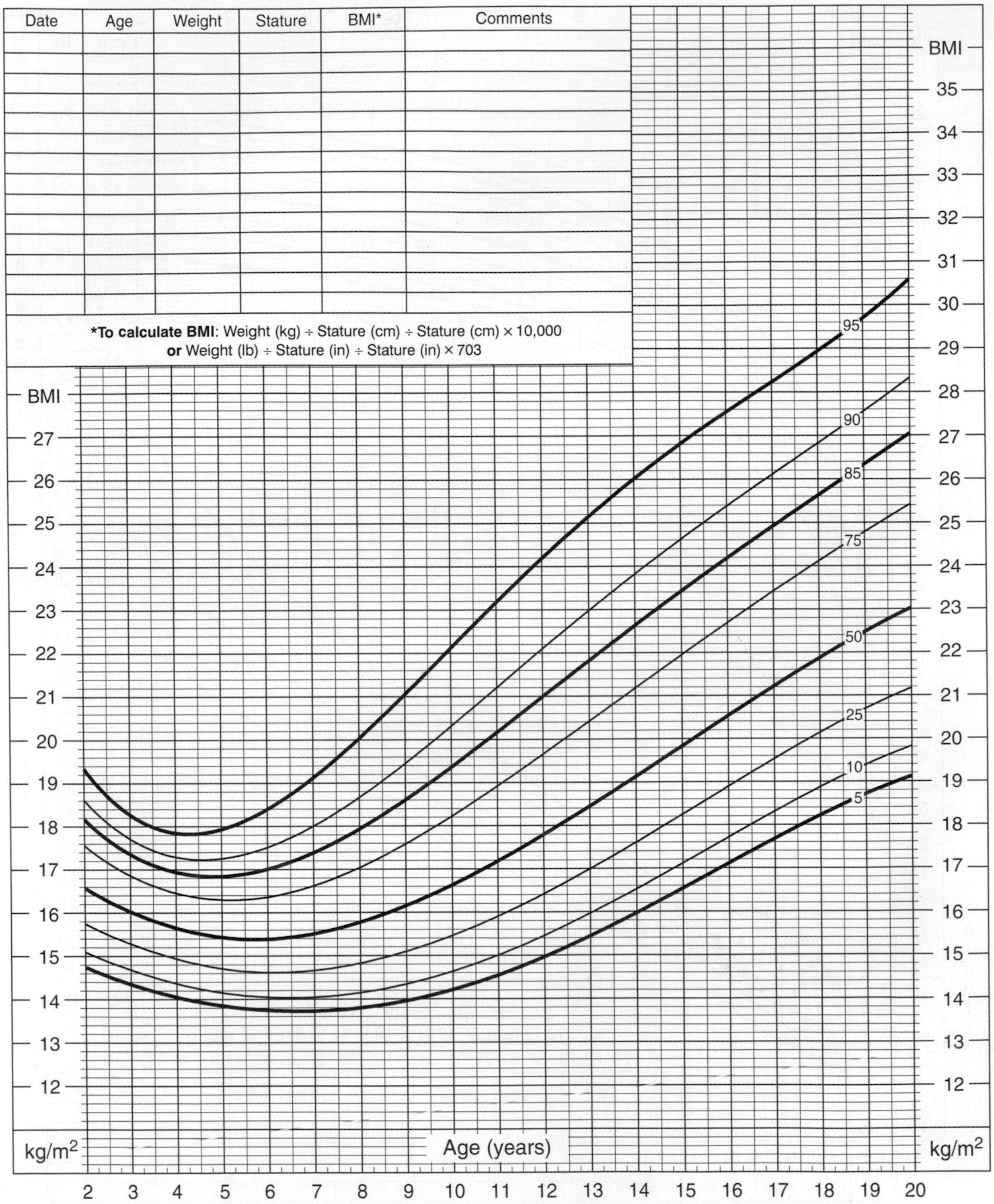

FIGURE 3–2. Example of CDC growth chart of boys, 2 to 20 years: Body mass index for age percentile, 2000. (From National Center for Health Statistics and National Center for Chronic Disease Prevention and Health Promotion. Center for Disease Control Growth Charts, 2000 [updated September 9, 2010], http://www.cdc.gov/growthcharts.)

and lack of incorporation of exact pharmacokinetic differences regarding each medication.[14]

Absorption

Oral absorption may be different in premature infants and neonates due to differences in gastric acid secretion and pancreatic and biliary function. Neonates and infants have increased gastric pH (eg, pH 6–8) due to lower gastric acid output by body weight, reaching adult values by approximately 2 years of age.[15] Low gastric acid secretion can result in increased serum concentrations of weak bases and acid-labile medications, such as penicillin, and decreased serum concentrations of weak acid medications, such as phenobarbital, due to increased ionization. Additionally, gastric emptying time and intestinal transit time are delayed in premature infants, increasing drug contact time with the gastrointestinal mucosa and drug absorption.[15,16] Diseases, such as gastroesophageal reflux, respiratory distress syndrome, and congenital heart disease may further delay gastric emptying time. Pancreatic exocrine and biliary function are also reduced in newborns, with about 50% less secretion of amylase and lipase than adults, reaching adult values as early as the end of the first year and as late as 5 years of age. Deficiency in pancreatic secretions and bile salts in newborns can decrease bioavailability of prodrug esters, such as erythromycin, which requires solubilization or

Table 3–2

Maintenance Fluid Calculations by Body Weight

Patient Body Weight	Maintenance Fluid Requirement
< 10 kg	100 mL/kg/day
11–20 kg	1000 mL + 50 mL/kg over 10 kg
> 20 kg	1500 mL + 20 mL/kg over 20 kg

intraluminal hydrolysis.[15] Due to limited data on oral bioavailability of medications in infants and children for newer agents, some drug dosing recommendations may be extrapolated from adult safety and efficacy studies and case reports.

Topical or percutaneous absorption in neonates and infants is increased due to a thinner stratum corneum, increased cutaneous perfusion, and greater body surface-to-weight ratio. Hence, application of topical medications, such as corticosteroids, should be limited to the smallest amount possible. Limiting exposure can help minimize serum concentrations of active drug as well as inactive, yet potentially harmful additives such as propylene glycol.

Intramuscular absorption in premature and full-term infants can be erratic due to variable perfusion, poor muscle contraction, and decreased muscle mass compared with older patients.[19] Intramuscular administration may be appropriate for some medications; however, use of this route of administration can be painful and is usually reserved when other routes are not accessible, for example, initial IV doses of ampicillin and gentamicin for neonatal sepsis.

Intrapulmonary absorption and disposition is largely due to anatomical size of the lungs and drug delivery. The smaller airways of neonates and lower inspiratory volume can result in greater drug concentrations in the upper and central airways. Particle size, breathing pattern, and route (eg, oral vs nasal) can impact the amount of drug absorbed and should be considered when utilizing pulmonary drug delivery devices such as nebulizers or inhalers.[17]

Rectal absorption can also be erratic due to uncontrollable pulsatile contraction and risk of expulsion in younger patients (ie, infants and young children).[18] Thus, it is not commonly recommended if other routes are available. This route is useful in cases of severe nausea and vomiting or seizure activity. For medications that undergo extensive first-pass metabolism, bioavailability increases as the blood supply bypasses the liver from the lower rectum directly to the inferior vena cava. Availability of rectal dosage forms varies and use of oral medications or other dosage forms rectally is based on limited studies and case reports.

Patient Encounter, Part 1

TS is a 32-week GA premature baby boy weighing 2 kg, length 42 cm, born to a 21-year-old woman this morning.

What is TS's weight classification as a neonate?

Calculate TS's corrected age for TS 8 months from today.

How much maintenance fluid would you recommend for TS at birth?

Volume of Distribution

In pediatric patients, apparent volume of distribution (V_d) is normalized based on body weight and expressed as L/kg. Extracellular fluid and total body water per kilogram of body weight are increased in neonates and infants, resulting in higher V_d for water-soluble drugs, such as aminoglycosides, and decreases with age. Therefore, neonates and infants often require higher doses by weight (mg/kg) than older children and adolescents to achieve the same therapeutic serum concentrations.[15,18] The use of extracorporeal membrane oxygenation (ECMO) can further effect V_d of medications in patients due to the added volume from the circuit and potential fluid changes (eg, edema) while on the circuit. Thus, the use of additional, close clinical and, when available, therapeutic drug monitoring is recommended for those patients requiring ECMO.[19] Neonates and infants have a lower normal range for serum albumin (2–4 g/dL, 20–40 g/L), reaching adult levels after 1 year of age. Highly protein bound drugs, such as sulfamethoxazole-trimethoprim, are not typically used in neonates due to theoretical concern for bilirubin displacement. This displacement may result in a complication known as kernicterus, from bilirubin encephalopathy.[20]

Although neonates have lower body adipose composition compared with older children and adults, their overall V_d for many lipid-soluble drugs (eg, lorazepam) is similar to infants and adults. Some medications (eg, vancomycin, phenobarbital) may also reach higher concentrations in the central nervous system of neonates due to an immature blood-brain barrier.[18]

Metabolism

Hepatic drug metabolism is slower at birth in full-term infants compared with adolescents and adults, with further delay in premature neonates. Phase 1 reactions and enzymes, such as oxidation and alcohol dehydrogenase, are impaired in premature neonates and infants and do not fully develop until later childhood or adolescence. Accordingly, the use of products containing ethanol or propylene glycol can result in increased toxicities, including respiratory depression, hyperosmolarity, metabolic acidosis, and seizures, thus should be avoided in neonates and infants. Age at which cytochrome P450 isoenzymes (eg, CYP3A4, CYP2C19) activity reaches adult values varies, depending on the isoenzyme, with delayed development in premature infants. Increased dose requirements by body weight (eg, mg/kg) for some hepatically metabolized medications (eg, phenytoin, valproic acid) in young children (ie, ages 2–4 years) is theorized due to an increased liver mass to body mass ratio.[21] This increase in metabolism slows to adult levels as the child goes through puberty into adulthood.[15,21]

Among phase 2 reactions, sulfate conjugation by sulfotransferases is well developed at birth in term infants. Glucuronidation by the uridine diphosphate glucuronosyltransferases, in contrast, is immature in neonates and infants, reaching adult values at 2 to 4 years of age.[15,21] In neonates, this deficiency results in adverse effects including cyanosis, ash gray color of the skin, limp body tone, and hypotension, also known as "gray baby syndrome" with use of chloramphenicol.[22] Products containing benzyl alcohol or benzoic acid should be avoided in neonates due to immature glycine conjugation, resulting in accumulation of benzoic acid. This accumulation can lead to "gasping syndrome," which includes respiratory depression, metabolic acidosis, hypotension, seizures or convulsions, and gasping respirations.[23] Acetylation via *N*-acetyltransferase reaches adult maturation at around 1 year of life; however, overall activity is dependent on genotypic variability.[15]

Elimination

Nephrogenesis completes at approximately 36-week gestation; thus, premature neonates and infants have compromised glomerular and tubular function that may correlate with a glomerular filtration rate (GFR). This reduction in GFR affects renal drug clearance; thereby necessitating longer dosing intervals for renally cleared medications, such as vancomycin, to prevent accumulation. GFR increases with age and exceeds adult values in early childhood, after which there is a gradual decline to approximate adult value during adolescence. For example, vancomycin is often given every 18 to 24 hours in a low birth weight (LBW) premature neonate, every 6 hours in children with normal renal function, and every 8 to 12 hours in adult patients with normal renal function. Children with cystic fibrosis also present with greater renal clearance of drugs such as aminoglycosides, compared with children without the disease, requiring higher doses by weight and more frequent dosing intervals.[24]

Pediatric GFR, also referred to as "creatinine clearance," informally by clinicians, is normalized due to variable body size (mL/min/1.73 m²). The Cockroft–Gault, Jelliffe, or modification of diet in renal disease (MDRD) equations for estimating GFR in adults should not be used for evaluating patients younger than 18 years.[25,26] The Schwartz equation is a common method of estimating pediatric GFR from infancy up to 21 years of age (**Figure 3–3**). This equation uses patient length (cm), serum creatinine (mg/dL) (or μmol/L × 0.0113), and a constant, *k*, which depends on age (including LBW status for infants) for all patients and also gender for those older than 12 years.[27] There is also a simplified version of this equation, validated for ages 1 to 16 years old, commonly referred to as the "bedside" Schwartz equation.[28]

$$\textbf{Estimated GFR} = [0.413 \times \text{height (in cm)}] \div \text{serum creatinine (in mg/dL)}$$

Or

$$\textbf{Estimated GFR} = [36.5 \times \text{height (in cm)}] \div \text{serum creatinine (in μmol/L)}$$

$$\text{GFR} = \frac{kL}{SCr}$$

Age	k
Low birth weight < 1 year	0.33
Full term < 1 year	0.45
1–12 year	0.55
13–21 year (female)	0.55
13–21 year (male)	0.70

k = Proportionality constant
L = Length in cm
SCr = Serum creatinine in mg/dL
GFR = estimated glomerular filtration rate (i.e., creatinine clearance) in mL/min/1.73 m²

FIGURE 3–3. Schwartz equation for estimation of glomerular filtration rate (GFR) in pediatric patients up to 21 years of age. (Schwartz GJ, Brion LP, Spitzer A. The use of plasma creatinine concentration for estimating glomerular filtration rate in infants, children, and adolescents. Pediatr Clin North Am. 1987;34(3):571–590.)

Patient Encounter, Part 2

TS is now 8 weeks old (weight: 3.5 kg) and presents to the community pharmacy with a 3-day history of lethargy, poor oral intake, and low-grade fever. The pharmacist refers the child to seek medical attention at the emergency department. TS is admitted to the general pediatric ward for further assessment including a neonatal sepsis and meningitis rule-out. Blood samples, cerebral spinal fluid, and urine were collected for Gram stain and culture, still pending results. He was empirically started on ampicillin 175 mg (50 mg/kg/dose) IV q 6 h, cefuroxime 175 mg IV q 6 h (50 mg/kg/dose). Given his poor oral intake on admission, the team requests addition of maintenance IV fluids and a nutrition consultation.

BB's Laboratory Values	Normal Ranges
WBC 18 × 10³/mm³ (18 × 10⁹/L)	6–17 × 10³/mm³ (6–17 × 10⁹/L)
Bands 7% (0.07)	4%–12% (0.04–0.12)
Segs 36% (0.36)	13%–33% (0.13–0.33)
Lymphs 51% (0.51)	41%–71% (0.41–0.71)
Monocytes 6% (0.06)	4%–7% (0.04–0.07)

Serum creatinine 0.5 mg/dL (44 μmol/L) ≤ 0.6 mg/dL (53 μmol/L)

How much maintenance fluid would you recommend for TS now?

The team decides to change cefotaxime to gentamicin (ie, meningitis ruled out). Because gentamicin can affect renal function, TS's GFR should be assessed. Using the most appropriate method, calculate an estimated GFR for TS.

Because serum creatinine is a crude marker of GFR, the Schwartz equation, as with other estimation calculations, carries limitations including the potential for overestimating GFR in patients with moderate to severe renal insufficiency.[29,30] Urine output is also a parameter used to assess renal function in pediatric patients, with a urine output more than 1 to 2 mL/kg/hour considered normal.

SPECIFIC CONSIDERATIONS IN DRUG THERAPY

In addition to differences in pharmacokinetics and pharmacodynamic parameters, other factors, including dosage formulations, medication administration techniques, and parent/caregiver education, should be considered when selecting drug therapy.

Off-Label Medication Use

Currently, there is a lack of pediatric dosing, safety, and efficacy information for more than 75% of drugs approved in adults.[31] Off-label use of medications occur in both outpatient and inpatient settings. Off-label use of medication is the use of a drug outside of its approved labeled indication. This includes the use of a medication in the treatment of illnesses not listed on the manufacturer's package insert, use outside the licensed age range, dosing outside those recommended, or use of a different route of administration.[32,33] KEY CONCEPT *It is appropriate to use a drug off-label when no alternatives are available; however, clinicians should refer to published studies and case reports for available safety, efficacy, and dosing information.* FDA regulatory changes, such as extended patent exclusivity, provide incentives for a pharmaceutical manufacturer to market new drugs for pediatric patients. However, such incentives are not available for generic drugs.

Routes of Administration and Drug Formulations

Depending on age, disease, and disease severity, different routes of administration may be considered. The rectal route of administration is reserved for cases where oral administration is not possible and IV route is not necessary. Topical administration is often used for treatment of dermatologic ailments. Transdermal routes are often not recommended, unless it is an approved indication such as the methylphenidate transdermal patch for treatment of attention deficit hyperactivity disorder. The injectable route of administration is used in patients with severe illnesses or when other routes of administration are not possible. As done with adult patients, IV compatibility and access should be evaluated when giving parenteral medications. Dilution of parenteral medications may be necessary to measure smaller doses for neonates. However, a higher concentration of parenteral medications may be necessary for patients with fluid restrictions, such as premature infants and patients with cardiac anomalies and/or renal disease. Appropriate stability and diluent selection data should be obtained from the literature.

When oral drug therapy is needed, one must also consider the dosage form availability and child's ability to swallow a solid dosage form. Children younger than 6 years are often not able to swallow oral tablets or capsules and may require oral liquid formulations. Not all oral medications, especially those unapproved for use in infants and children, have a commercially available liquid dosage form. Use of a liquid formulation compounded from a solid oral dosage form is an option when data are available. Factors such as drug stability, suspendability, dose uniformity, and palatability should be considered when compounding a liquid formulation.[34] Commonly used **suspending agents** include methylcellulose and carboxymethylcellulose (eg, Ora-Plus). Palatability of a liquid formulation can be enhanced by using simple syrup or Ora-Sweet. If no dietary contraindications or interactions exist, doses can be mixed with food items such as pudding, fruit-flavored gelatin, chocolate syrup, applesauce, or other fruit puree immediately before administration of individual doses. Honey, although capable of masking unpleasant taste of medication, may contain spores of *Clostridium botulinum* and should not be given to infants younger than 1 year due to increased risk for developing botulism. Most hospitals caring for pediatric patients compound formulations in their inpatient pharmacy. Limited accessibility to compounded oral liquids in community pharmacies poses a greater challenge. A list of community pharmacies with compounding capabilities should be maintained and provided to the parents and caregivers before discharge from the hospital.

Common Errors in Pediatric Drug Therapy

Prevention of errors in pediatric drug therapy begins with identification of possible sources. The error rate for medications is as high as 1 in 6.4 orders among hospitalized pediatric patients.[35] Off-label use of medications increases risk of medication error and has been attributed to difference in frequency of errors compared with adults. One of the most common reasons for medication errors in this specialized population is incorrect dosing such as calculation error.[36,37] KEY CONCEPT *Medication errors among pediatric patients are possible due to differences in dose calculation and preparation; it is important to identify potential errors through careful review of orders, calculations, dispensing, and administration of drug therapy to infants and children.* It is crucial to verify accurate weight, height, and age for dosing calculations and dispensing of prescriptions because pediatric patients are a vulnerable population for medication error. Consistent units of measurements in reporting patient variables, such as weight (kg) and height (cm), should be used. Dosing units such as mg/kg, mcg/kg, mEq/kg, mmol/kg, or units/kg should also be used accurately. Given the age-related differences in metabolism of additives, such as propylene glycol and benzyl alcohol, careful consideration should be given to the active and inactive ingredients when selecting a formulation.

Decimal errors, including trailing zeroes (eg, 1.0 mg misread as 10 mg) and missing leading zeroes (eg, .5 mg misread as 5 mg) in drug dosing or body weight documentation are possible, resulting in several-fold overdosing. Strength or concentration of drug should also be clearly communicated by the clinician in prescription orders. Similarly, labels that look alike may lead to drug therapy errors (eg, mistaking a vial of heparin for insulin). Dosing errors of combination drug products can be prevented by using the right component for dose calculation (eg, dose of sulfamethoxazole/trimethoprim is calculated based on the trimethoprim component).

Use of standardized concentrations and programmable infusion pumps, such as smart pumps with built-in libraries, is encouraged to minimize errors with parenteral medications, especially those for continuous infusions such as inotropes. Computer physician order entry (CPOE) systems and bar coding technology, with ability for dose range checks by weight for pediatric medication orders and accurate matching of correct ordered medication to patient, respectively, have decreased medication errors.[37]

Prevention of medication errors is a joint effort between health care professionals, patients, and parents/caregivers. Obtaining a complete medication history, including over-the-counter (OTC) and complementary and alternative medicines (CAMs), simplification of medication regimen, clinician awareness for potential errors, and appropriate patient/parent/caregiver education on measurement and administration of medications, are essential in preventing medication errors.

Complementary and Over-the-Counter Medication Use

Between 30% and 70% of children with a chronic illnesses (eg, asthma, attention deficit hyperactivity disorder, autism, cancer) or disability use CAMs.[38] CAMs can include mind-body therapy (eg, imagery, hypnosis), energy field therapies (eg, acupuncture, acupressure), massage, antioxidants (eg, vitamins C and E), herbs (eg, St. John's wort, kava, ginger, valerian), prayer, immune modulators (eg, echinacea), or other folk/home remedies. It is important to encourage communication about CAM use, including interdisciplinary discussion between CAM providers and pediatric health care providers.[38] It is critical to appreciate that there are limited data establishing efficacy of various CAM therapies in children. For example, colic is a condition of unclear etiology in which an infant cries inconsolably for over a few hours in a 24-hour period, usually during the same time of day. Symptoms of excessive crying usually improve by the third month of life and often resolve by 9 months of age. No medication has been approved by the FDA for this condition. Some parents are advised by family and friends to use alternative treatments, such as gripe water, to treat colic. Gripe water is an oral solution containing a combination of ingredients, such as chamomile and sodium bicarbonate, not regulated by the FDA. In addition, some gripe water products may contain alcohol, which is not recommended for infants due to their limited metabolism ability (ie, alcohol dehydrogenase). Further, some CAM products (eg, St. John's wort) can interact with prescription drugs and produce undesired outcomes. It is important to assess OTC product use in pediatric patients. For example, treatment of the common cold in children is similar to adults, including symptom control with adequate fluid intake, rest, use of saline nasal spray, and acetaminophen (10–15 mg/kg/dose every 6–8 hours) or ibuprofen (4–10 mg/kg/dose every 8 hours) for relief of discomfort and fever. Other products, such as a topical vapor rub or oral honey, have demonstrated some potential for alleviation of symptoms, such as cough, based on survey studies of parents for children of 2 years and older.[39,40] Unlike adults, symptomatic relief through the use of pharmacologic agents, such as OTC combination cold remedies, is not recommended for pediatric patients younger than 4 years. Currently, the FDA does not recommend the use of OTC cough and cold medications (eg, diphenhydramine and dextromethorphan) in children younger than 2 years; however, the Consumer Healthcare Products Association, with the support of the FDA, has voluntarily changed product labeling of OTC cough and cold medications to state "do not use in children under 4 years of age." This is due to increased risk for adverse effects (eg, excessive sedation, respiratory depression) and no documented benefit in relieving symptoms. It has also been noted that these medications may be less effective in children younger than 6 years compared with older children and adults.[41,42] Also noteworthy is the potential for medication error with use of OTC products in older children, such as cold medications containing diphenhydramine and acetaminophen. A parent/caregiver may inadvertently overdose a child on one active ingredient, such as acetaminophen, by administering acetaminophen suspension for fever and an acetaminophen-containing combination product for cold symptoms. The use of aspirin in patients younger than 18 years with viral infections is not recommended due to the risk of Reye syndrome. While making an appropriate recommendation for an OTC product for a pediatric patient, the parent/caregiver should always be referred to their pediatrician for further advice and evaluation when severity of illness is a concern.

Clinicians should respect parents'/caregivers' beliefs in the use of CAM and OTC products and encourage open discussion with the intention of providing information regarding their risks and benefits to achieve desired health outcomes as well as optimize medication safety.

Medication Administration to Pediatric Patients and Caregiver Education

Considering the challenges in cooperation from infants and younger children, medication administration can become a difficult task for any parent or caregiver. One should also consider factors that may affect adherence to prescribed therapy including caregiver and/or patient's personal beliefs, socioeconomic limitation(s), and fear of adverse drug effects. One common factor to consider is ease of measurement and administration when selecting and dosing pediatric drug therapy. Clinicians should check concentrations of available products and round doses to a measurable amount. For example, if a patient were to receive an oral formulation, such as amoxicillin 400 mg/5 mL suspension, and the dose was calculated to be 4.9 mL, the dose should be rounded to 5 mL for ease of administration. Rounding the dose by 10% to the closest easily measurable amount is commonly practiced for most medications (eg, antibiotics); however, drugs with narrow therapeutic indices (eg, anticoagulants) are exceptions to this guideline.

The means or devices for measuring and administering medications should also be closely considered. Special measuring devices as well as clear and complete education about their use are essential. Oral syringes are accurate and offered at most community pharmacies for the measurement of oral liquid medications. Oral droppers included specifically with a medication may be appropriate for use in infants and young children. Medicine cups are not recommended for measuring doses for infants and young children due to the possible inaccuracy of measuring smaller doses. Household dining or measuring spoons are not accurate or consistent and should not be used for the administration of oral liquids.

KEY CONCEPT *Comprehensive and clear parent/caregiver education improves medication adherence, safety, and therapeutic outcomes and is essential in care of infants and young children.* Information about the drug, including appropriate and safe storage away from children, possible drug interactions, duration of therapy, importance of adherence, possible adverse effects, and expected therapeutic outcomes should be provided. Parent/caregiver education is important in both inpatient and outpatient care settings and should be reviewed at each point of care.

Because parents/caregivers are often sole providers of home care for ill children, it is important to demonstrate appropriate dose preparation and administration techniques to the caregivers before medication dispensing. First, a child should be calm for successful dose administration. Yet, calming a child is often a challenge during many methods of administration (eg, otic, ophthalmic, rectal). Parents/caregivers should explain the process in a simple and understandable form to the child because this may decrease the child's potential anxiety. In addition, it is also recommended to distract younger children using a favorite item such as toy or to reward cooperative or "good" behavior during medication administration. Helpful tips regarding administration of selected dosage forms in pediatric patients are listed in Table 3–3.[43]

Accidental Ingestion in Pediatric Patients

Pediatric accidental ingestions most often occur in the home.[44] Various factors account for incidence of accidental ingestions in young children, including hand-to-mouth behaviors as well as new and increased mobility resulting in easier access areas where

Patient Encounter, Part 3

TS is now 18 months old, and his mother calls the clinic and tells you that her son is "just miserable" with a runny nose, cough, and a fever (axillary temperature) of 37.8°C (100°F). She wanted to know if she could use baby aspirin instead of the acetaminophen that does not seem to help. She also wanted to know which cough and cold preparation would be most appropriate for TS.

What additional information would you need to help TS and his mom?

What is your recommendation regarding use of aspirin for TS's fever?

What would you recommend for TS's cold symptoms?

Table 3–3

Helpful Tips for Medication Administration for Selected Dosage Forms[43]

Dosage Form	Recommendations
Ophthalmic drops or ointment	• Wash hands thoroughly prior to administration • Position child laying down in supine position • Avoid contact of applicator tip to surfaces, including the eye • Drops should be placed in the pocket of the lower eyelid • Ointment strip should be placed along the pocket of the lower eyelid

Otic drops	• Wash hands thoroughly prior to administration
	• Position child laying down in prone position
	• Tilt head to expose treated ear, gently pull outer ear outward, then due to age-dependent change in angle of Eustachian tube:
	  • If child < 3 years of age, gently pull downward and back; apply drops
	  • If child > 3 years of age, gently pull upward and back; apply drops

Nasal drops	• Wash hands thoroughly prior to administration • Position child laying down in supine position • Slightly tilt head back; place drops in nostril(s) • Remain in position for appropriate distribution of medication
Rectal suppository	• Similar to adult administration; challenging route for administration • For younger patients (ie, < 3 years), a smaller finger (eg, pinky finger) should be used to insert suppository
Metered-dose inhalers (MDI)	• Use a spacer • For younger children, use one with a mask, be sure the mask is secured/placed closely up against the child's face, avoiding gaps between face and mask and creating a seal to ensure medication delivery • Child should take slow breaths in with each dose • Wait at least 1 minute between doses

Patient Encounter, Part 4

TS is now 4 years old, brought by his father to the pediatrician. He has a 4-day history of left ear pain, excessive crying, decreased appetite, and difficulty sleeping over the past 2 days. The child's temperature last night was 39°C (102.2°F) by electronic axial thermometer. The father gave the child several doses of ibuprofen, but the pain or temperature did not improve and none was given this morning. He has considerable recurrences of acute otitis media each year often treated with amoxicillin. He has had three episodes in the last 8 months, with the last episode treated 2 months ago using oral amoxicillin 90 mg/kg/day divided every 12 hours but developed a rash. He is also presenting with wheeze and cough. Dad states that he was recently diagnosed with allergic rhinitis, but lost the prescription for his son's allergy medication (cetirizine) and so never started it.

Home medications: Ibuprofen suspension (100 mg/5 mL) as needed for pain and fever.

PE:

General: crying, tugging on his left ear, coughing with wheeze

VS: T 39°C (102.2°F), BP 93/50 mm Hg, HR 115 beats/min, RR 30 beats/min, Wt 24.2 lb (11.0 kg), Ht 32.3 in (82 cm)

HEENT: Tympanic membranes erythematosus (L > R); left ear is bulging and nonmobile. Throat erythematous; nares patent

Pulmonary: Wheeze bilaterally, no congestion noted

Diagnosis: (1) Acute otitis media, left ear and (2) newly diagnosed allergic rhinitis, untreated

You and the pediatrician decide to start TS on oral cefdinir suspension (250 mg/5 mL) at 7 mg/kg/dose q 12 h for a total of 10 days and continue ibuprofen (100 mg/5 mL) at 10 mg/kg/dose every 6 to 8 hours as needed for fever or pain. In addition to treatment for acute otitis media, he needs treatment of allergic rhinitis with cetirizine 2.5 mg by mouth daily. TS's dad also asks about the use of an herbal supplement (from his traditional Eastern medicine herbalist) advertised for allergies because his brother-in-law uses it in addition to his prescribed allergy therapy.

Based on the information available, create a care plan for TS. The plan should include:

(a) Statement of the drug-related needs and/or problems,

(b) Patient-specific detailed therapeutic plan with specific dosing,

(c) Parent/caregiver education points, and

(d) Approach to Dad's inquiry about herbal supplement use for TS's allergic rhinitis.

Patient Care Process

Patient Assessment:

- For patients up to 2 years of age, review the patient's birth history, including gestational age, birth weight, medical complications, postnatal age, and corrected age.
- Review the patient's past medical history, comorbidities.
- Assess this patient's (or patient's caregiver) history of medication adherence and health care beliefs.

Therapy Evaluation:

- Review all current medication therapy, including CAM and OTC. Is the patient on appropriate drug therapy for current diagnoses? Are the doses of current medications appropriate (ie, for age, weight, etc)? Any medications without indication?
- Assess current therapy for safety and efficacy. Is the medication effective for this patient? Is the patient experiencing any adverse effects?

Care Plan Development:

- Consider the patient's medication allergies and/or intolerances.
- Consider the available data regarding safe and effective dosing of selected drug.
- Consider the available routes of administration. What is the most appropriate route? If IV medication is needed, what types of IV accesses are available? For example, does the patient have a central or peripheral line? Determine if IV medication needs to be further diluted or concentrated based on patient's comorbidities and fluid status.
- Evaluate the patient's organ function (renal and hepatic), including use of appropriate equations (eg, Schwartz).
- Consider ease of administration for the patient and/or caregiver. Is the dose easily measurable? Is the dosing frequency reasonable for their family schedule?
- Verify accuracy of dose calculations. Verify current weight and dosing units (eg, mg/kg/day, mg/kg/dose). Is the dosing interval appropriate?
- Determine what drug–drug/drug–food interactions are possible with this new therapy. How can they be managed?
- Educate parent/caregiver/patient regarding selected drug therapy including purpose, dose, administration, duration therapy, possible side effects, etc.

Follow-up Evaluation:

- Monitor signs and symptoms of clinical outcomes (improvement and decline). Measure drug serum concentrations when appropriate. Monitor for possible adverse drug events.
- Reinforce patient/caregiver education.

harmful substances are stored (eg, medication cabinets). Indeed, caregivers are encouraged to use "child-safe" devices to lock closets and cabinets to reduce risk of accidental ingestions; however, this is not a substitute for appropriate caregiver supervision.

Ingested substances can vary from household cleaning solutions to prescription and nonprescription medications. The most common exposures in children age younger than 5 years were cosmetics/personal care products, analgesics, household cleaning substances, foreign bodies (eg, small toys), and topical preparations.[44] Management of accidental ingestions varies depending on the ingested substance, the amount, and the age and size of the child. Inducing emesis is not recommended for any type of ingestion. The American Academy of Clinical Toxicology and the AAP do not recommend the use of ipecac syrup for treatment of accidental ingestion.[45] Clinicians receiving calls regarding management of accidental ingestions, depending on severity of case, should direct them to the emergency department for evaluation and/or the local or regional poison control center for specific recommendations, which can reached via a universal contact number (1-800-222-1222), with additional information located through the American Association of Poison Control Centers (*www.aapcc.org*).[46]

Abbreviations Introduced in This Chapter

AAP	American Academy of Pediatrics
CAM	Complementary and alternative medicine
CDC	Centers for Disease Control and Prevention
CFR	Creatinine clearance
CPOE	Computer physician order entry
ELBW	Extremely low birth weight
GA	Gestational age
GFR	Glomerular filtration rate
LBW	Low birth weight
MDRD	Modification of diet in renal disease
MDI	Metered-dose inhaler
OTC	Over-the-counter
V_d	Volume of distribution (apparent)
VLBW	Very low birth weight

REFERENCES

1. American Academy of Pediatrics, Committee on Fetus and Newborn. Age terminology during the perinatal period. Pediatrics. 2004;114:1362–1364.
2. Centers for Disease Control and Prevention from the WHO Growth Standards. World Health Organization (WHO) Growth Standards, 2009 [updated 2010 Sept 9; cited 2011 Sept 23]. http://www.cdc.gov/growthcharts/who_charts.htm.
3. National Center for Health Statistics and National Center for Chronic Disease Prevention and Health Promotion. Center for Disease Control Growth Charts, 2000 [updated 2010 Sept 9; cited 2011 Sept 23]. http://www.cdc.gov/growthcharts.
4. National High Blood Pressure Education Program Working Group on High Blood Pressure in Children and Adolescents. The fourth report on the diagnosis, evaluation, and treatment of high blood pressure in children and adolescents. NIH Publication No. 05-5268. Bethesda, MD: National Heart, Lung, and Blood Institute. Pediatrics. 2004;114(2 Suppl 4th Report):555–576.

5. American Heart Association. Pediatric advanced life support provider manual. Dallas, TX: American Heart Association; 2006:273.
6. Kaelber DC, Pickett F. Simple table to identify children and adolescents needing further evaluation of blood pressure. Pediatrics. 2009;123(6):e972–e974.
7. Task Force on Blood Pressure Control in Children. Report of the Second Task Force on Blood Pressure Control in Children—1987. National Heart, Lung, and Blood Institute, Bethesda, Maryland. Pediatrics. 1987;79(1):1–25.
8. Schmidt BD. American Academy of Pediatrics. Fever-How to take the temperature. [updated 2011 May 24; cited 2014 Nov 18]. http://www.healthychildren.org/English/tips-tools/Symptom-Checker/Pages/Fever-How-to-Take-the-Temperature.aspx.
9. Section on Clinical Pharmacology and Therapeutics; Committee on Drugs, Sullivan JE, Farrar HC. Fever and antipyretic use in children. Pediatrics. 2011;127(3):580–587.
10. Lawrence J, Alcock D, McGrath P, Kay J, MacMurray SB, Dulberg C. The development of a tool to assess neonatal pain. Neonatal Netw. 1993;12(6):59–66.
11. Wong DL, Baker CM. Pain in children: comparison of assessment scales. Pediatr Nurs. 1988;14(1):9–17.
12. Merkel SI, Voepel-Lewis T, Shayevitz JR, Malviya S. The FLACC: a behavioral scale for scoring postoperative pain in young children. Pediatr Nurs. 1997;23(3):293–297.
13. Holliday MA, Segar WE. The maintenance need for water in parenteral fluid therapy. Pediatrics. 1957;19(5):823–832.
14. Shirkey HC. Drug dosage for infants and children. JAMA. 1965; 193:443–446.
15. Anderson GD, Lynn AM. Optimizing pediatric dosing: a developmental pharmacologic approach. Pharmacotherapy. 2009; 29(6):680–690.
16. Ramirez A, Wong WW, Shulman RJ. Factors regulating gastric emptying in preterm infants. J Pediatr. 2006;149(4):475–479.
17. Everard ML. Inhalation therapy for infants. Adv Drug Deliv Rev. 2003;55:869–878.
18. Sage DP, Kulczar C, Roth W, Liu W, Knipp GT. Persistent pharmacokinetic challenges to pediatric drug development. Front Genet. 2014;5:281. Published online 2014 August 27. doi: 10.3389/fgene.2014.00281. Accessed October 30, 2014.
19. Buck ML. Pharmacokinetic changes during extracorporeal membrane oxygenation: implications for drug therapy of neonates. Clin Pharmacokinet. 2003;42(5):403–417.
20. Thyagarajan B, Deshpande SS. Cotrimoxazole and neonatal kernicterus: a review. Drug Chem Toxicol. Apr 2014;37(2):121–129. doi: 10.3109/01480545.2013.834349. Epub 2013 Oct 7.
21. de Wildt SN, Tibboel D, Leeder JS. Drug metabolism for the paediatrician. Arch Dis Child. 2014;99(12):1137–1142. doi: 10.1136/archdischild-2013-305212. Epub 2014 Sep 3.
22. Mulhall A, de Louvois J, Hurley R. Chloramphenicol toxicity in neonates: Its incidence and prevention. Br Med J. (Clin Res Ed) 1983;287(6403):1424–1427.
23. Menon PA, Thach BT, Smith CH, et al. Benzyl alcohol toxicity in a neonatal intensive care unit. Incidence, symptomatology, and mortality. Am J Perinatol. 1984;1(4):288–292.
24. Prestidge C, Chilvers MA, Davidson AG, Cho E, McMahon V, White CT. Renal function in pediatric cystic fibrosis patients in the first decade of life. Pediatr Nephrol. Apr 2011;26(4):605–612.
25. Cockroft DW, Gault MH. Prediction of creatinine clearance from serum creatinine. Nephron. 1976;16:31–41.
26. Jelliffe RW. Creatinine clearance: Bedside estimate. Ann Intern Med. 1973;79(4):604–605.
27. Schwartz GJ, Brion LP, Spitzer A. The use of plasma creatinine concentration for estimating glomerular filtration rate in infants, children, and adolescents. Pediatr Clin North Am. 1987;34(3): 571–590.
28. Staples A, LeBlong R, Watkins CW, Brandt J. Validation of the revised Schwartz estimating equation in a predominantly non-CKD population. Pediatr Nephrol. 2010;25:2321–2326.
29. Seikaly MG, Browne R, Bajaj G, Arant BS Jr. Limitations to body length/serum creatinine ratio as an estimate of glomerular filtration in children. Pediatr Nephrol. 1996;10(6):709–711.
30. Filler G, Lepage N. Should the Schwartz formula for estimation of GFR be replaced by cystatin C formula? Pediatr Nephrol. 2003;18(10):981–985.
31. Shah SS, Hall M, Goodman DM, et al. Off-label drug use in hospitalized children. Arch Pediatr Adolesc Med. 2007;161(3): 282–290.
32. American Academy of Pediatrics, Committee on Drugs. Uses of drugs not described in the package insert (off-label uses). Pediatrics. 2002;110:181–183.
33. Conroy S. Unlicensed and off-label drug use: Issues and recommendations. Pediatr Drugs. 2002;4:363–369.
34. Nahata MC, Pai VB. Pediatric Drug Formulations. 6th ed. Cincinnati, OH: Harvey Whitney Books; 2011:385.
35. Marino BL, Reinhardt K, Eichelberger WJ, Steingard R. Prevalence of errors in a pediatric hospital medication system: implications for error proofing. Outcomes Manag Nurs Pract. 2000;4:129–135.
36. Stucky ER, American Academy of Pediatrics, Committee on Drugs and Committee on Hospital Care. Prevention of medication errors in the pediatric inpatient setting. Policy Statement. Pediatrics. 2003;112(2):431–436.
37. Conroy S, Sweis D, Planner C, et al. Interventions to reduce dosing errors in children: A systematic review of the literature. Drug Saf. 2007;30(12):1111–1125.
38. Kemper KJ, Vohra S, Walls R. Task Force on Complementary and Alternative Medicine. Provisional Section on Complementary, Holistic, and Integrative Medicine, American Academy of Pediatrics. The use of complementary and alternative medicine in pediatrics. Pediatrics. 2008;122(6):1374–1386.
39. Paul IM, Beiler J, McMonagle A, Shaffer ML, Duda L, Berlin CM Jr. Effect of honey, dextromethorphan, and no treatment on nocturnal cough and sleep quality for coughing children and their parents. Arch Pediatr Adolesc Med. 2007;161(12):1140–1146.
40. Paul IM, Beiler JS, King TS, Clapp ER, Vallati J, Berlin CM Jr. Vapor rub, petrolatum, and no treatment for children with nocturnal cough and cold symptoms. Pediatrics. 2010;126(6):1092–1099.
41. US Food and Drug Administration. Public Health Advisory: FDA recommends that over-the-counter (OTC) cough and cold products not be used for infants and children under 2 years of age [updated 2011 Dec 8; cited 2011 Sept]. http://www.fda.gov/ForConsumers/ConsumerUpdates/ucm051137.htm.
42. US Food and Drug Administration. FDA Statement Following CHPA's Announcement on Nonprescription Over-the-Counter Cough and Cold Medicines in Children [updated 2009 June 18; cited 2011 Sept 23]. http://www.fda.gov/NewsEvents/Newsroom/PressAnnouncements/2008/ucm116964.htm.
43. Buck ML, Hendrick AE. Pediatric Medication Education Text. 5th ed. American College of Clinical Pharmacy, 2009; Sec1: xvii–xxvii.
44. Mowry JB, Spyker DA, Cantilena LR Jr, Bailey JE, Ford M. 2012 Annual Report of the American Association of Poison Control Centers' National Poison Data System (NPDS): 30th Annual Report. Clin Toxicol (Phila). 2013;51(10):949–1229.
45. Höjer J, Troutman WG, Hoppu K, et al. American Academy of Clinical Toxicology. European Association of Poison Centres and Clinical Toxicologists. Position paper update: ipecac syrup for gastrointestinal decontamination. Clin Toxicol (Phila). 2013; 51(3):134–139.
46. American Association of Poison Control Centers. [cited 2014 Nov 18]. www.aapcc.org.

4 Palliative Care

Kelly R. Kroustos and Marc A. Sweeney

LEARNING OBJECTIVES

Upon completion of the chapter, the reader will be able to:

1. Describe the philosophy of palliative care including hospice care and its impact on medication therapy management.
2. Discuss the therapeutic management of palliative care patients and how it differs from and is similar to traditional patient care at the end of life.
3. List the most common symptoms experienced by the terminally ill patient.
4. Explain the pathophysiology of the common symptoms experienced in the terminally ill patient.
5. Assess the etiology of symptoms in the patient with a life-limiting illness.
6. Describe the pharmacologic rationale of medication therapy used for symptom management in the terminally ill patient.
7. Recommend nonpharmacologic and pharmacologic management of symptoms in a terminally ill patient.
8. Develop a patient-specific palliative care management plan.
9. Educate patients and caregivers regarding palliative care management plan, including rationale of treatment, importance of medication adherence, and assessment and monitoring of desired outcomes.

INTRODUCTION

KEY CONCEPT *According to the World Health Organization (WHO), "Palliative care is an approach that improves the quality of life of patients and their families facing the problem associated with life-threatening illness, through the prevention and relief of suffering by means of early identification and impeccable assessment and treatment of pain and other problems, physical, psychosocial and spiritual."* The goal of **palliative care** is to achieve the best **quality of life** for patients and their families.[1] "Palliate" literally means "to cloak." The WHO goal of achieving high quality of life depends on a team approach to manage disease-related symptoms while honoring the patient's goals for care.[2] Palliative care focuses on patients and their families and the challenges they face associated with life-threatening illness.[3] The goal is to prevent and relieve suffering by means of early identification, assessment, and treatment of pain and other physical symptoms including associated psychosocial, emotional, and spiritual concerns.[1] Palliative medicine is rapidly becoming a well-recognized medical specialty[4] and is much needed due to the increased number of patients with chronic, slowly debilitating diseases.[2]

The term *palliative care* is frequently used synonymously with **hospice**, and although hospice programs provide palliative care, palliative care has a much broader application. In the United States, hospice is defined by Medicare and other third-party payers as a benefit available to individuals who have less than or equal to 6 months life expectancy if the disease runs its typical course.[5] Hospice care guidelines and regulations are primarily defined by federal regulations. Palliative care outside of the umbrella of hospice care, in contrast, is neither currently regulated nor have the same reimbursement structure. Palliative care services may be provided at any point during the disease process and are not limited to the last 6 months of life; therefore, patients and families may receive benefits from palliative care services beginning at the time of diagnosis of life-limiting illness. Palliative care, may be delivered to patients in all care settings.[6] The foundation for providing quality palliative care centers around active participation of an interdisciplinary team of professionals working closely together to meet the goals of the patient and family.[7] Palliative care team members include representatives from medicine, nursing, social work, pastoral or related counseling, pharmacy, nutrition, rehabilitation, and other professional disciplines providing a holistic approach to the patient's care. KEY CONCEPT *The goals of palliative care include enhancing quality of life while maintaining or improving functionality.*[7,8] Palliative care should most logically be delivered to patients from the onset of any chronic, life-altering disease. Before many of our modern medical and therapeutic advancements were developed, curative treatments were not normally available.[9] Provision of comfort was considered the mainstay for patient care. Advances in medical care, nutrition, public health, and trauma care resulted in fewer patient deaths and medical management shifted focus from comfort to a death-denying approach with prolonging life as the primary goal. With this shift, palliative care became less emphasized until 1967 when the first modern hospice was established in London, England.

Today the palliative care philosophy attempts to combine enhanced quality of life, compassionate care, and patient and family support with modern medical advances.

EPIDEMIOLOGY AND ETIOLOGY

The first hospice in the United States was founded in 1974. Since then, hospice acceptance and utilization has increased in the United States. The number of Medicare beneficiaries enrolled in hospice increased by 100% between 2000 and 2005.[10] Medicare spending for hospice care tripled during that same time period, reflecting a greater number of patients receiving this type of care. Currently, approximately 5000 hospice agencies care for patients across the United States.[11] In 2013, approximately 66% of hospice patients were cared for in the home, and 84% of hospice patients were older than 65 years.[12]

According to a study published in 2007, hospice patients live 29 days longer than nonhospice patients, with the largest difference noted in chronic heart failure (CHF) patients.[13] Lung cancer patients receiving early palliative care survived 23% longer than those with delayed palliative care, according to a 2010 study.[14] Early referrals to hospice appear to improve the overall care of the patient and offer prolonged survival in some patients. The integration of palliative care prior to the patient's eligibility for hospice care may prove to even further benefit the survival and quality of life and care of patients.

Because health care providers have an increasing recognition of the benefit of palliative care for patients with all life-limiting illness, increased integration of this model of care has extended to other disease states beyond cancer.

PATHOPHYSIOLOGY

Understanding the pathophysiology of multiple end-stage disease states is daunting, yet in palliative care, the emphasis is not so much on the disease state management as it is on the assessment and appropriate treatment of associated physical, psychological, social, and spiritual symptoms. Palliative care focuses on symptom management for patients with progressive life-limiting illnesses from diagnosis through death where the pathophysiological impact of disease on a patient's symptoms may vary greatly depending on the stage of a patient's illness. KEY CONCEPT *Palliative care is appropriate for all life-limiting diseases including cancer; chronic obstructive pulmonary disease (COPD); dementia, including Alzheimer disease; Parkinson disease; chronic cardiac disease; stroke; renal failure; hepatic failure; multiorgan failure; diabetes mellitus; etc.*

For the purpose of this chapter, pathophysiology is not a primary focus. Rather, the philosophy of managing physical, psychological, social, and spiritual symptoms to maintain quality of life and prevent suffering is discussed within the context of progressively incurable illnesses. Although palliative may coexist with aggressive disease state management to extend life, as the patient approaches the end of life, philosophy and management generally moves away from those principles related to the disease state management of patients where prolonging life is the goal.

CLINICAL PRESENTATION AND DIAGNOSIS

Cancer

Palliative care is most commonly associated with cancer patients. Regardless of whether or not the cancer is curable, most patients have various degrees of physical, psychological, social, and spiritual symptoms that arise once a diagnosis is confirmed. Once a cancer patient has failed curative and life-prolonging therapy, prognosis and disease trajectory is easier to determine than in patients with other life-limiting diseases. The change in focus from cure to symptom control becomes apparent and therefore more acceptable. Symptoms associated with cancer depend on both the primary tumor site and the location of metastatic spread. Symptoms may also result from the effects of cancer treatments such as chemotherapy and radiation. (See Chapters 88–99 for specific cancers and their treatments.)

End-Stage Heart Failure

Many forms of heart disease result in sudden death; however, the disease progression of heart failure is protracted yet unpredictable. Advanced heart failure (class III–IV or stage C or D) is characterized by persistent symptoms that limit activities of daily living despite optimal drug therapy. Common symptoms include fatigue, breathlessness, anxiety, fluid retention, and pain. In heart failure, standard medication management is intended to reduce the progression of cardiac remodeling and is considered disease modifying. However, as patients approach the final months of life, with the exception of cholesterol-lowering agents, these same cardiac medications are also palliative and should not be discontinued prematurely without cause (Figure 4–1). Exacerbations of heart failure symptoms should be aggressively treated as long as the patient is responsive to therapy and wishes to receive treatment. In hospice, this can often be accomplished through medication manipulation in the patient's home without the need for hospitalization (see Chapter 6).

Chronic Obstructive Pulmonary Disease

Chronic obstructive pulmonary disease (COPD) has a prolonged and variable course. Patients with COPD have a high number of physician visits and hospital admissions. Palliative care treatment is directed at reducing symptoms, reducing the rate of decline in lung function, preventing and treating exacerbations, and maintaining quality of life. In end-stage COPD, bronchodilators and anti-inflammatory agents become less effective. As patients decline, their ability to use inhalers appropriately becomes more difficult. Utilizing a nebulizer to administer bronchodilators allows for more reliable drug delivery to the site of action. Symptoms of late-stage disease include wheezing, chronic sputum production, cough, frequent respiratory infections, **dyspnea** with exertion progressing to dyspnea at rest, fatigue, pain, hypoxia, and weight loss. Pulmonary hypertension may also occur and can lead to cor pulmonale or right-sided heart failure (see Chapter 15).

End-Stage Kidney Disease

Chronic kidney disease is progressive and leads to renal failure. In end-stage kidney disease, the only life-sustaining treatments are dialysis or renal transplant. Without treatment, kidney failure causes uremia, oliguria, hyperkalemia and other electrolyte disorders, fluid overload and hypertension unresponsive to treatment, anemia, hepatorenal syndrome, and uremic pericarditis. Symptoms associated with chronic kidney disease (stage 5) include fatigue, pruritus, nausea, vomiting, constipation, dysgeusia, muscle pain, agitation, and bleeding abnormalities. Palliative care in these patients includes the minimization of these symptoms; however, because many options for drug therapy will be cleared through the kidneys, agents should be chosen cautiously to avoid other complications (see Chapter 26).

End-Stage Liver Disease

Like kidney disease, the only treatment to prolong life in advanced liver disease is transplant. Patients with end-stage liver disease typically present with ascites, jaundice, pruritus, or

	Mortality Benefit	Functional Benefit	Renal Dosing Adjustments	Risk vs. Benefit Considerations
Diuretics *(furosemide, torsemide, bumetanide)*	–	✓	✓	Continue for symptom management (edema, dyspnea) Caution: dehydration, hypokalemia
ACEI *(lisinopril, enalapril)*	✓	✓	✓	Caution: Dehydration, sepsis, concurrent NSAID use and renal artery stenosis can increase renal toxicity
Aldosterone antagonists *(spironolactone)*	✓	–/✓	✓	Primary benefit for reducing mortality Caution: Hyperkalemia risk with renal insufficiency
β-blockers *(carvedilol, metoprolol)*	✓	✓	–	Taper doses prior to discontinuation Caution: May cause hypotension and bradycardia
Inotrope PO *(digoxin)*	–	✓	✓	Caution: Digoxin toxicity (N/V, anorexia, confusion, arrhythmia)

FIGURE 4–1. Drugs, their use in class III to IV heart failure, and their effects on mortality, hospital admissions, and functional status. Checkmark indicates a positive impact on specified parameter, and—indicates no significant impact on specified parameter. (Data from Strickland JS. Palliative Pharmacy Care. Bethesda, MD: American Society of Health-Systems Pharmacists, 2009. and Grauer PA, Shuster J, Protus BM. Palliative Care Consultant, 3rd ed. Dubuque, IA: Kendall-Hunt, 2008.)

encephalopathy, and frequently all four symptoms. Additionally, bleeding disorders are common, and associated esophageal or gastric varices bleeds are the cause of death in about one-third of those who die from liver disease. Palliative care in these patients focuses on the symptom management of end-stage liver disease complications.

Human Immunodeficiency Virus/Acquired Immune Deficiency Syndrome (HIV/AIDS)

Pharmacologic advances have changed prognosis and progression of HIV/AIDS. Palliative care is predominantly directed toward patients without access to drug therapy in the early stages of disease. Patients with progressed HIV/AIDS are susceptible to acquire opportunistic infections and cancer that may hasten their death. Common symptoms observed in individuals with HIV/AIDS at the end of their life include fatigue, profound weight loss, breathlessness, nausea, gastrointestinal (GI) disturbances, and pain. The goal of palliative care in these patients is to minimize common AIDS-related symptoms (see Chapter 87).

Stroke/Cerebral Vascular Accident

Stroke result from hemorrhage or ischemia. The prognosis of cerebral vascular accident (CVA) patients is unpredictable and may be extended, resulting in caregiver fatigue. Approximately one-third of patients who have a stroke will die within 2 years. Patients with stroke deal with loss of physical and cognitive function, poststroke pain, and frequent depression. Incontinence, aphasia, **dysphagia**, and seizures are also common. Patients who have dysphagia have a high incidence of aspiration pneumonia, which often is the cause of death (see Chapter 11).

Parkinson Disease

Parkinson disease is a degenerative neurologic disease with a long chronic, progressive course evidenced by akinesia, rigidity, and tremor. The goal of therapy is to reduce symptoms and maintain or improve quality of life. Palliative care provides support to both the patient and caregiving system as patients become more disabled and as neuropsychiatric problems arise. Frequent symptoms are skin infections and breakdown, constipation, pain, depression, hallucinations, and confusion. Individuals with Parkinson disease often die from bronchial pneumonia due to dysphagia or complication from falls (see Chapter 33).

Amyotrophic Lateral Sclerosis (Lou Gehrig Disease)

Amyotrophic lateral sclerosis (ALS) is a chronic neurodegenerative disorder characterized by progressive loss of motor neurons. The median survival is approximately 3 years from the symptom onset with less than 15% of patients surviving 10 years. Initially symptoms of ALS present as limb weakness, with other symptoms developing in no particular order including cramps, spasticity, pain, dysarthria, sialorrhea, fatigue, insomnia, depression, fear and anxiety, involuntary emotional expression disorder, constipation, aspiration, and laryngospasm. Many patients do not have cognitive impairment; however, one-fourth to one-half of patients with ALS may have associated frontal lobe dementia. Disease progression eventually involves all systems except sphincter control and eye movement. Unless the individual has long-term mechanical ventilation, the cause of death is typically respiratory failure.

Alzheimer Disease and Other Dementia

Dementia is a progressive, nonreversible deterioration in cognitive function with associated behavioral dysfunction. Alzheimer disease accounts for the majority of dementia cases; vascular, Parkinson disease, dementia with Lewy body, and frontotemporal dementias are less prevalent. Drug therapy is targeted at slowing the progression of the cognitive symptoms and preserving the patient's function. As patients progress toward end-stage dementia, in addition to memory loss and personality and behavioral changes, they require assistance in basic activities of daily living such as feeding, dressing, and toileting. At this point, they may not respond to their surroundings, may not communicate, or have impaired movements and dysphagia. Depression, agitation, delusions, compulsions, confusion, hallucinations, incontinence, and disruption of sleep/wake cycles are all common symptoms in end-stage dementias. Assessment of symptoms is challenging due to the cognitive impairment and frequent aphasia. Palliative care is not only directed toward the patient, but also emotional support for those close to them (see Chapter 29).

TREATMENT

KEY CONCEPT *Following a complete assessment of the patient, developing a comprehensive therapeutic plan that utilizes the fewest number of medications to achieve the highest quality of life is essential.* Many times, one drug may relieve multiple symptoms, resulting in better patient care, lower costs, and decreased medications. Cost-effective drug recommendations are essential to control costs. Avoiding polypharmacy will reduce adverse drug events related to drug interactions, excessive side effects, and duplications of therapy. The following list of symptoms includes common symptoms observed in palliative and end-of-life care; however, it is not comprehensive. KEY CONCEPT *Palliative care is more than just pain management. It includes the treatment of symptoms resulting in the discomfort for the patient, which may include nausea and vomiting, agitation, anxiety, depression, delirium, dyspnea, anorexia and cachexia, constipation, diarrhea, pressure ulcers and edema.*

Note that many drugs used to treat symptoms in palliative and end-of-life care are often prescribed for unapproved uses, administered by unapproved routes or in dosages higher than that recommended by the package insert. This "off-label" use of medication is not unique to palliative care.

Anxiety

A comprehensive review of anxiety disorders may be found in Chapter 40.

▶ *Palliative Care Considerations*

- Anxiety is "a state of fearfulness, apprehension, worry, emotional discomfort, or uneasiness resulting from an unknown internal stimulus, is excessive, or is otherwise inappropriate to a given situation."[15]
- Anxiety is closely related to fear, but fear has an identified cause or source of worry (eg, fear of death). Fear may be more responsive to counseling than anxiety that the patient cannot attribute to a particular fearful stimulus. Anxiety disorders are the most prevalent class of mental disorders, so it is not surprising that anxiety is a common cause of distress at life's end.

In addition to anxiety disorders, a variety of conditions can cause, mimic, or exacerbate anxiety.[16,17] Delirium, particularly in its early stages, can easily be confused with anxiety. Physical complications of illness, especially dyspnea and undertreated pain, are common precipitants. Significant anxiety is present in most patients with advanced lung disease and is closely related to periods of oxygen desaturation. Medication side effects, especially akathisia from older antipsychotics and antiemetics (including metoclopramide), can present as anxiety. Interpersonal, spiritual, or existential concerns can mimic and exacerbate anxiety. Patients with an anxious or dependent coping style are at high risk of anxiety as a complication of advanced illness. Short of making a diagnosis of a formal anxiety disorder, differentiating normal worry and apprehension from pathologic anxiety requires clinical judgment.

Behaviors indicative of pathological anxiety include intense worry or dread, physical distress (eg, tension, jitteriness, or restlessness), maladaptive behaviors, and diminished coping and inability to relax.

Pathological anxiety may be complicated by insomnia, depression, fatigue, GI upset, dyspnea, or dysphagia. Anxiety can also worsen these conditions if they are already present. Untreated anxiety may lead to numerous complications, including withdrawal from social support, poor coping, limited participation in palliative care treatment goals, and family distress. Reassess the patient for anxiety with any change in behavior or any change in the underlying medical condition. Assessment for formal anxiety disorders or other contributing factors is key to management. A comprehensive review of insomnia may be found in Chapter 41.

▶ *Nonpharmacologic Treatment*

Regardless of treatment approach chosen, the following principles apply. Ask questions and listen to patients' concerns and fears. Offer emotional support and reassurance when appropriate. Err on the side of treatment—be willing to palliate anxiety. Assess treatment response and side effects frequently. Aim to provide maximum resolution of anxiety and educate patients and families about anxiety and its treatments.

Psychotherapies can help manage anxiety, although availability of trained therapists willing to make home visits, and limited stamina and attention span of seriously ill patients, typically make such therapies impractical in the hospice setting. Cognitive and behavioral therapies can be beneficial, including simple relaxation exercises or distraction strategies (ie, focusing on something pleasurable or at least emotionally neutral). Encourage pastoral care visits, especially if spiritual and existential concerns predominate.

When an underlying cause of anxiety can be identified, treatment is initially aimed at the precipitating problem, with monitoring to see if anxiety improves or resolves as the underlying cause is addressed.

▶ *Pharmacotherapy*

In most cases, management of pathological anxiety in the hospice setting involves pharmacologic therapies. Benzodiazepines are the standard for treatment; however, selective serotonin reuptake inhibitors (SSRIs), typical and atypical antipsychotics, may be appropriate based on the patient's life expectancy.[18] The primary goal of therapy for anxiety in hospice is patient comfort. Aim to prevent anxiety, not just treat it with as needed medications. Think of pain management as an analogy. As with all medications that act in the central nervous system (CNS), anxiolytics such as benzodiazepines should be dosed at the lower end of the dose range to prevent unnecessary sedation, particularly in the frail and elderly. However, recognize that standard or higher doses may be required. Avoid use of bupropion and psychostimulants for anxiety. Although effective for depression, they are ineffective for anxiety and may make anxiety worse. Many patients have difficulty swallowing as they approach the end of life. Lorazepam, alprazolam, and diazepam tablets are commonly crushed and placed under the tongue with a few drops of water if the liquid formulations are not readily available. Low-dose haloperidol is also used to treat anxiety in palliative care, particularly if delirium is present. Chapter 40 provides more detailed information on appropriate use of anxiolytic agents.

Delirium

▶ Palliative Care Considerations

Delirium is very common in hospice, occurring in more than 80% of terminally ill patients, most often in the last few days of life.[14] Potential causes of delirium in the hospice setting include, but are not limited to, medical illness, dehydration, hypoxia, sleep deprivation, metabolic disturbances, sepsis, side effects of drugs (particularly anticholinergic agents, benzodiazepines, opioids, corticosteroids, tricyclic antidepressants), urinary retention, urinary tract infection, constipation or impaction, uncontrolled pain, or alcohol or drug withdrawal.[19,20]

A classic symptom of delirium is clouding of consciousness. This can be manifested by an inability to either maintain or shift attention. Patients also have impaired cognitive functioning, which may or may not include memory disturbances. "Sundowning" is very common phenomenon at the end of life, especially in the presence of delirium. It presents as daytime sleepiness and nighttime agitation and restlessness. Another common characteristic is fluctuation in severity of delirium symptoms during the course of the day. This can even occur within the course of a single hour or also from day to day. Patients exhibiting agitation from their delirium are easy to identify, but those who present as withdrawn and with diminished responsiveness ("quiet" delirium) are more difficult to diagnose. It is not uncommon for patients to exhibit both quiet and agitated delirium. Treatment is the same for both types of delirium. Delirium is difficult to distinguish from dementia. Delirium more commonly presents as a sudden onset (eg, hours to days), with an altered level of consciousness and a clouded sensorium. However, dementia more commonly presents gradually and with an unimpaired level of consciousness.

▶ Nonpharmacologic Treatment

Establishing a safe, soothing environment including familiar objects such as photographs and familiar music can be helpful to calm the patient. Minimizing risk of injury is important when the patient is agitated. Providing education to families and caregivers about the causes of delirium, signs and symptoms, and how to best manage it will help reduce their anxiety and distress when it occurs.

▶ Pharmacotherapy

The most important initial step is to determine the goal of care. If possible, reverse the underlying cause of delirium to restore the patient to a meaningful cognitive status.[14,19] If the precipitating factors cannot be reversed, initiate to treat the symptoms. If the patient is irreversibly delirious and agitated, drug therapy is generally indicated.

Antipsychotic (neuroleptic) drugs (conventional or atypical antipsychotics) are the drugs most commonly used to treat confusion and agitation associated with delirium. However, treatment of delirium with these drugs is an "off-label" indication. Atypical antipsychotics including risperidone, olanzapine, quetiapine, ziprasidone, paliperidone, and aripiprazole are also an option for management of delirium.[21]

Haloperidol, when given in doses less than 2 mg/day is well tolerated and nonsedating. Doses greater than 4.5 mg/day are associated with increased incidence of extrapyramidal symptoms.[22] Cumulative doses of 35 mg or single IV doses greater than 20 mg have been associated with QTc prolongation.[23] When sedation is beneficial for terminal aggressive, agitated delirium, chlorpromazine provides more sedation as compared with low-dose haloperidol. When patients are bedbound and in the final stages of life, orthostatic hypotension common with chlorpromazine is not a concern. Haloperidol and chlorpromazine are commonly given sublingually or rectally if swallowing becomes difficult, although these are not approved routes of administration. Haloperidol, but not chlorpromazine, can be given subcutaneously.[24]

Administering benzodiazepines alone in a patient with delirium can actually make the delirium and confusion worse. While addition of benzodiazepines with antipsychotics is not routinely used, delirium induced by withdrawal or untreated anxiety may benefit from addition of a benzodiazepine.[17]

Patient Encounter 1

JP is an 86-year-old man diagnosed with lung cancer (right upper lobe) with metastases to the right shoulder and brain. He is following up today at the outpatient palliative care clinic for uncontrolled symptoms. Past medical history includes hypercholesterolemia, CHF, and depression. No known allergies. JP's reports right shoulder pain rating 6/10 on the visual analog pain scale (0–10) which is constant, dull, aching and exacerbated by movement. JP reports a dull, aching, constant pain in his right upper right chest region rated 4/10 on the visual analog pain scale (0–10) and minor diffuse, and lower abdominal cramping. JP reports uncontrolled nausea and vomiting, headache, constipation and dizziness upon standing. JP's caregiver reports two fall within the past 2 weeks without injury.

VS: BP 98/60, RR 19, P 62, Wt 69 kg (152 lbs), Ht 5′10″ (178 cm)

Medications: carvedilol 12.5 mg by mouth twice daily, lisinopril 20 mg by mouth daily, sertraline 25 mg by mouth daily, simvastatin 20 mg by mouth daily, spironolactone 25 mg by mouth daily, furosemide 40 mg by mouth twice daily, ferrous gluconate 324 mg by mouth twice daily, multivitamin by mouth once daily, oxycodone/acetaminophen 5/325 1 tablet by mouth every 6 hours as needed, docusate 100 mg by mouth twice daily as needed.

What are potential etiologies of the nausea and vomiting JP is experiencing?

What type of the pain is JP experiencing?

What questions would you ask JP during your assessment?

What potential drug–drug interactions may exist, and how would you monitor the patient for them?

What medications should be added, changed, or discontinued?

List nonpharmacologic interventions that the practitioner should make to improve the care of JP.

Dyspnea

▶ Palliative Care Considerations

Dyspnea is described as an uncomfortable awareness of breathing. It is a subjective sensation, and patient self-report is the only reliable indicator. Respiratory rate or po_1 may not correlate with the feeling of breathlessness.[25] Respiratory effort and dyspnea are not the same. Patients may report substantial relief of dyspnea from opioids with no change in respiratory rate. The prevalence of dyspnea varies from 12% to 74%, worsening during the last week of life in terminally ill cancer patients to between 50% and 70%. History and physical examination should be taken and reversible causes of dyspnea should be identified and treated, if present.

▶ *Nonpharmacologic Treatment*

Provide information, anticipate and proactively prepare the patient and family for worsening symptoms. Identify and attempt to minimize triggers that cause episodes of dyspnea. Educate patient and family regarding treatment of dyspnea, including the use of opioids and benzodiazepines for dyspnea-associated anxiety. Prevent isolation and address spiritual issues that can worsen symptoms. Encourage relaxation and minimize the need for exertion.

Reposition to comfort, usually to a more upright position or with the compromised lung down. Avoid strong odors, perfumes, and smoking in the patient's presence or in close proximity. Improve air circulation/quality: provide a draft, use fans, or open windows and adjust temperature/humidity with air conditioner or humidifier.

▶ *Pharmacotherapy*

If no treatable causes can be identified or when treatments do not completely alleviate distressing symptoms, opioids are first-line agents for treating dyspnea.[26] Opioids suppress respiratory awareness, decrease response to hypoxia and hypercapnia, vasodilate, and have sedative properties. Low-dose opioids (eg, starting oral dose of morphine ~5 mg) have been shown to be safe and effective in the treatment of dyspnea. Opioid doses should be titrated judiciously. Once an effective dose of an opioid has been established, converting to an extended-release preparation may simplify dosing. When using opioids, anticipate side effects and prevent constipation by initiating a stimulant laxative/stool softener combination.

Nebulized opioids for treatment of dyspnea are controversial. Study results have been inconsistent.[27,28] Nonrandomized studies, case reports, and chart reviews describe anecdotal improvement in dyspnea using nebulized opioids; however, several controlled studies using nebulized opioids have provided inconclusive or negative results. However, nebulized opioids may be an alternative in patients who are not able or willing to take an oral agent or cannot tolerate adverse effects of systemic administration.

Nebulized furosemide appears effective for dyspnea refractive to other conventional therapies.[29] The hypothesized mechanism of action of nebulized furosemide is its ability to enhance pulmonary stretch receptor activity, inhibition of chloride movement through the membrane of the epithelial cell, and its ability to increase the synthesis of bronchodilating prostaglandins.[29]

Because anxiety can exacerbate dyspnea, benzodiazepines and antidepressants that have anxiolytic properties are frequently beneficial. Not all dyspnea is caused by low oxygen saturation. However, oxygen therapy is useful and beneficial for dyspnea if hypoxia is present.

For known etiologies of dyspnea, consider the following:

Bronchospasm or COPD exacerbation: Albuterol, ipratropium, and/or oral steroids are effective for symptoms management. Nebulized bronchodilators are more effective than handheld inhalers in patients who are weak and have difficulty controlling breathing.

Patient Encounter 2

LP is a 52-year-old man admitted to hospice with a diagnosis of liver failure secondary to alcoholic liver cirrhosis. Comorbidities include type 2 diabetes mellitus, hyperlipidemia, and hypothyroidism. LP consumes 2 to 4 beers per day. No known drug allergies. Liver associated symptoms include moderate-severe ascites with dependent leg edema, jaundice, pruritus and shortness of breath upon exertion. LP has been recently hospitalized for paracentesis (1–2 L drained). His appetite is poor and he is bedbound.

VS: BP 135/50, RR 40, P 80, Wt 76.2 kg (168 lb), Ht 5′5″ (165 cm)

Meds: insulin glargine 80 units subcutaneously daily; regular insulin administered on a sliding scale for fasting blood glucose of 250 mg/dL (13.9 mmol/L); potassium chloride 10 mEq (10 mmol) by mouth daily; furosemide 20 mg by mouth daily; spironolactone 25 mg by mouth once daily, lactulose 10 g/15 ml take 15 ml by mouth daily as needed, nadolol 40 mg by mouth once daily, levothyroxine 125 mcg daily; simvastatin 20 mg by mouth daily.

What potential interventions could the practitioner make to improve LP's care?

What medications could be added, changed, or discontinued?

What potential drug–drug interactions may exist? How would you monitor the patient for them?

Thick secretions: If cough reflex is strong, loosen secretions by increasing fluid intake. Guaifenesin may thin secretions; however, its efficacy in the absence of hydration is controversial. Nebulized saline may also help loosen secretions. If the patient is unable to cough, hyoscyamine, glycopyrrolate, or scopolamine patch can effectively dry secretions.[26]

Anxiety associated with dyspnea: Consider benzodiazepines (eg, lorazepam, diazepam).

Effusions: Thoracentesis may be necessary.

Low hemoglobin: Red blood cell transfusion (controversial) or erythropoietin (rarely used in hospice but might have larger role in palliative care).

Infections: Antibiotic therapy as appropriate.

Pulmonary emboli: Anticoagulants for prevention and treatment or vena cava filter placement (rarely used in hospice but might have a larger role in palliative care).

Rales due to volume overload: Reduction of fluid intake or diuretic therapy as appropriate.

Nausea and Vomiting

A comprehensive review of nausea and vomiting may be found in Chapter 20.

▶ *Palliative Care Considerations*

Up to 71% of palliative care patients will develop nausea and vomiting with approximately 40% experiencing these symptoms

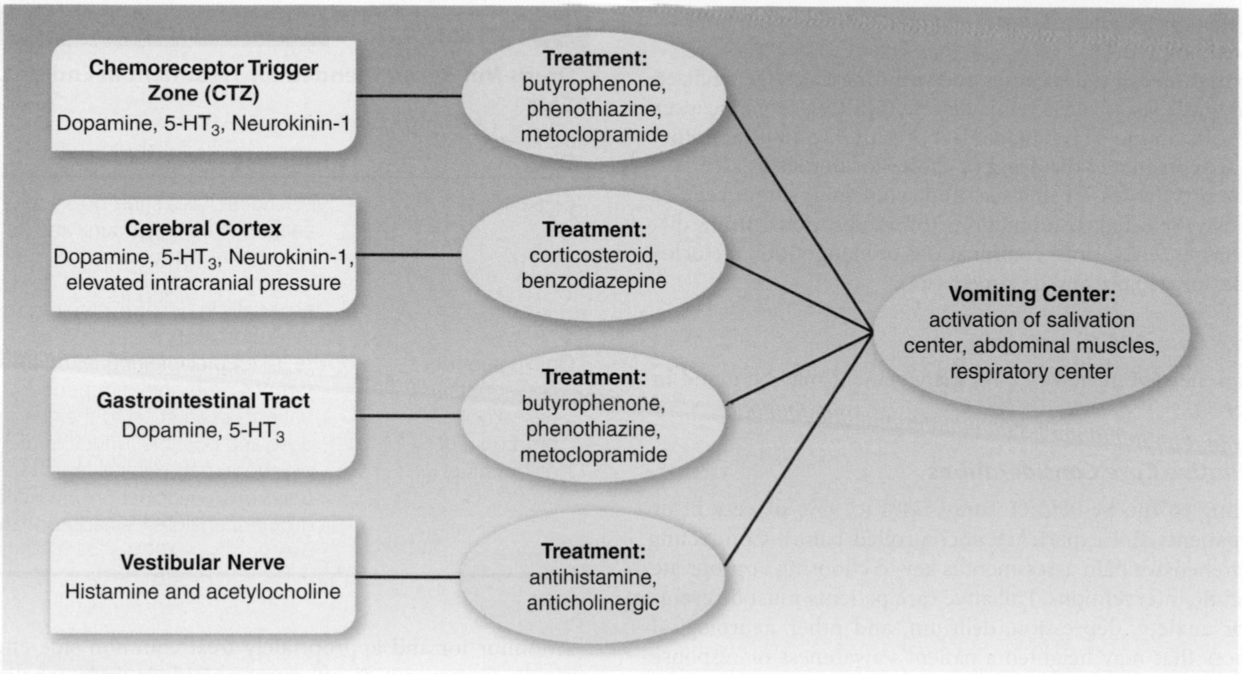

FIGURE 4–2. Mechanisms and associated neurotransmitters involved in nausea and vomiting.

in the last 6 weeks of life. Chronic nausea can be defined as lasting longer than a week and without a well-identified or self-limiting cause such as chemotherapy, radiation, or infection.[30] Four major mechanisms are correlated with the stimulation of the vomiting center (Figure 4–2). Potentially reversible causes of nausea and vomiting should not be overlooked. Causes of chronic nausea in end-of-life patients may include autonomic dysfunction, constipation, antibiotics, nonsteroidal anti-inflammatory drugs (NSAIDs), other drugs, infection, bowel obstruction, metabolic abnormalities (eg, renal or hepatic failure, hypercalcemia), increased intracranial pressure, anxiety, radiation therapy, chemotherapy, or untreated pain.

▸ *Nonpharmacologic Treatment*

Relaxation techniques may prove beneficial. Strong foods or odors should be avoided and eliminate offending medications.

▸ *Pharmacotherapy*

Clinical features of nausea and vomiting should guide the choice of antiemetics used (for a more comprehensive review, see Chapter 20).

Chemoreceptor trigger zone (CTZ)-induced nausea and vomiting are caused by chemotherapeutic agents, bacterial toxins, metabolic products (eg, uremia), and opioids. Dopamine (D_2), serotonin (5-HT), and neurokinin-1 are the primary neurotransmitters involved in this process. Therapy is based on blocking D_2 with D_2-antagonists including butyrophenones (eg, haloperidol), phenothiazines, and metoclopramide.

Due to receptor specificity, serotonin$_3$ (5-HT$_3$) antagonists such as ondansetron, granisetron, dolasetron, and palonosetron have limited usefulness in nausea and vomiting at the end of life.[31] They are typically indicated with emetogenic chemotherapy and up to 10 to 14 days posttreatment. Aprepitant is a neurokinin-1 antagonist indicated for the treatment of nausea due to highly emetogenic chemotherapy in combination with a 5-HT$_3$ antagonist and corticosteroid. Aprepitant should not be used as monotherapy.

Cerebral cortex–induced nausea and vomiting can be caused by anxiety, taste, and smell, and also secondary to increased intracranial pressure. Corticosteroids decrease intracranial pressure due to tumor involvement. Corticosteroids have been found to be effective in nonspecific nausea and vomiting. The mechanism of this action is unknown. Anxiolytics such as benzodiazepines are used to treat anxiety and "anticipatory" gustatory and olfactory stimulation.

Vestibular nausea and vomiting is triggered by motion. Opioids can sensitize the vestibular center resulting in movement-induced nausea. Since histamine and acetylcholine are the predominant neurotransmitters, antihistamines and anticholinergics are the drugs of choice in movement-induced nausea and vomiting.

GI tract stimulation occurs through vagal and sympathetic pathways. These pathways are triggered by stimulation of mechanoreceptors or chemoreceptors located in the gut. Gastric stasis, GI obstruction, drugs, metastatic disease, bacterial toxins, chemotherapeutic agents, and irradiation may cause nausea and vomiting. Glossopharyngeal or vagus nerve stimulation in the pharynx by sputum, mucosal lesions, or infection (eg, *Candida*) can also evoke nausea. The major neurotransmitters in the upper GI tract are D_2, acetylcholine, and 5-HT. Metoclopramide is a 5-HT$_4$ agonist and increases gastric motility above the jejunum, whereas anticholinergics decrease GI spasticity and motility in nausea induced by gut hyperactivity. In high doses, metoclopramide also acts as a 5 HT$_3$ antagonist.[8]

Autonomic failure causes gastroparesis resulting in anorexia, nausea, early satiety, and constipation. Delayed gastric emptying occurs in patients with diabetes mellitus, chronic renal failure, and neurological disorders. Malnutrition, cachexia, lung and pancreatic cancers, HIV, radiotherapy, and drugs such as opioids, anticholinergics, antidepressants, and vasodilators have been associated with autonomic failure and resulting chronic nausea, poor performance, tachycardia, and malnutrition. Evaluate underlying causes, including multiple drugs that may cause gastroparesis.

If drug therapy is indicated, metoclopramide is effective in improving gastric emptying.[8]

GI irritation can cause nausea and vomiting due to generalized gastritis, gastroesophageal reflux disease (GERD), or peptic ulcer disease. Histamine$_2$ (H_2) antagonists or proton pump inhibitors (PPIs) are considered the drugs of choice for ongoing gastritis.

Refractory cases of nausea and vomiting often require judiciously selected combinations of medications from different classes (eg, various combinations of haloperidol, metoclopramide, lorazepam, and dexamethasone).

Pain

A comprehensive review of pain management may be found in Chapter 34.

▸ *Palliative Care Considerations*

According to the SUPPORT study, 74% to 95% of very ill or dying patients still experience uncontrolled pain.[32] Conducting a comprehensive pain assessment is key to choosing appropriate therapeutic interventions. Palliative care patients must be evaluated for anxiety, depression, delirium, and other neurological influences that may heighten a patient's awareness or response to pain.

▸ *Nonpharmacologic Treatment*

Nonpharmacologic treatment is essential. Physical, complementary, and cognitive behavioral interventions reduce the perception of pain and decrease the dose requirements of medications. Examples of such strategies may include providing education, massage, ice, heat, physical therapy, music therapy, imagery, pet therapy, and psychotherapy.

▸ *Pharmacotherapy*

Pain should be assessed thoroughly and frequently, especially at the onset of treatment. The WHO approach to pain management addresses nociceptive pain (see Chapter 34). Although opioid analgesics are not always necessary or appropriate for all types of pain, most patients with cancer-related pain require opioids. For chronic, constant pain, around-the-clock dosing of analgesics (preferably long-acting agents) is usually necessary and preferred.[33] When titrating opioid doses, increase daily maintenance doses by 25% to 50% if patients are routinely requiring three or more breakthrough doses per 24 hours as a result of around-the-clock maintenance dose failure. The around-the-clock maintenance doses should not be increased if breakthrough doses are used only for incident pain such as increased activity or dressing changes.

Fentanyl transdermal patches may be appropriate in some patients; however, many patients at the end-of-life experience fat and muscle wasting and dehydration, resulting in reduced and variable absorption. Fentanyl transdermal patches have a slow onset of action, contributing to difficulty in dose titration.

Only short-acting opioids should be used for breakthrough pain (eg, immediate-release morphine, oxycodone, and hydromorphone are common examples). The dose of short-acting opioids for the treatment of breakthrough pain should be equal to 5% to 20% of the total daily maintenance dose. Frequencies for breakthrough dosing should not exceed the following:

- **Oral:** Every 1 to 2 hours
- **Subcutaneous:** Every 20 to 30 minutes
- **IV:** Every 8 to 20 minutes

Table 4–1

Drugs Not Recommended for Treatment in End-of-Life Care

Drug	Rationale
Meperidine	Meperidine has a short duration of analgesia (eg, 2–3 hours) and its metabolite, normeperidine, may accumulate with repeated dosing, especially in geriatric patients, resulting in neurotoxicity
Opioid agonist-antagonists (eg, pentazocine, butorphanol, nalbuphine)	The risk of precipitating withdrawal symptoms in opioid-dependent patients in addition to their ceiling dose and possible induction of psychomimetic effects (eg, dysphoria, delusions, hallucinations) make this group of analgesics inappropriate for use

Monitor for and appropriately treat common side effects of opioids. Common side effects of opioids include constipation, nausea and vomiting, itching, and transient sedation. Because constipation occurs with all chronic opioid therapy, prevention is imperative. Stimulant laxatives (senna or bisacodyl) with or without a stool softener (docusate) are the drugs of choice for opioid-induced constipation. Myoclonus, delirium, hallucinations, and hyperalgesia are possible signs of opioid-induced neurotoxicity and require rotation to another opioid or dose reduction. Respiratory depression is uncommon with the appropriate opioid dose titration. However, if dangerous opioid-induced respiratory depression does occur, small doses (0.1 mg) of the μ-receptor antagonist naloxone are appropriate and can be repeated as necessary. The goal is to increase respirations to a safe level while preventing the patient from experiencing a loss of pain control.

Drugs that should not be used for treatment of pain during end-of-life care are listed in Table 4–1.

Different types of pain may require specific types of analgesics or adjuvant medications. Examples of pain types commonly seen in patients with advanced illness are as follows:

Visceral pain (nociceptive pain induced by stretching or spasms of visceral organs including the GI tract, liver, and pancreas) should be treated with an adjuvant such as an anticholinergic agents or, if inflammation is associated with the pain, corticosteroids.

Bone pain (metastatic site of cancer) is best treated with NSAIDs or corticosteroids in addition to standard opioid therapy.

Neuropathic pain (pain caused by damage to the afferent nociceptive fibers) can be managed with tricyclic antidepressants, antiepileptic drugs, tramadol, tapentadol or *N*-methyl-D-aspartate antagonists such as ketamine. Methadone is an opioid μ-agonist that has a role in neuropathic pain given its added *N*-methyl-D-aspartate antagonist activity.

Terminal Secretions

▸ *Palliative Care Considerations*

Terminal secretions, or death rattle, is the noise produced by the oscillatory movements of secretions in the upper airways in association with the inspiratory and expiratory phases of respiration.[34,35]

As patients lose their ability to swallow and clear oral secretions, accumulation of mucus results in a rattling or gurgling sound produced by air passing through mucus in the lungs and air passages. The sound does not represent any discomfort for the patient. However, the sound is sometimes so distressing to the family that it should be treated. Terminal secretions are typically seen only in patients who are obtunded or are too weak to expectorate. Drugs that decrease secretions are best initiated at the first sign of death rattle because they do not affect existing respiratory secretions. These agents have limited or no impact when the secretions are secondary to pneumonia, pulmonary congestion or edema.

▶ *Nonpharmacologic Treatment*

Position the patient on their side or in a semiprone position to facilitate drainage of secretions. If necessary, place the patient in the Trendelenburg position (lowering the head of the bed); this allows fluids to move into the oropharynx, facilitating an easy removal. Do not maintain this position for long due to the risk of aspiration. Oropharyngeal suctioning is another option but may be disturbing to the patient and visitors. Fluid intake can also be decreased, as appropriate.

▶ *Pharmacotherapy*

Anticholinergic drugs remain the standard of therapy for prevention and treatment of terminal secretions due to their ability to effectively dry secretions.[34–36] Drugs used for this indication are similar pharmacologically, and one can be selected by anticholinergic potency, onset of action, route of administration, alertness of patient, and cost. The most commonly used anticholinergic agents are atropine, hyoscyamine, scopolamine, and glycopyrrolate.

Anticholinergic side effects include blurred vision, constipation, urinary retention, confusion, delirium, restlessness, hallucinations, dry mouth, and heart palpitations. Unlike the other anticholinergics, glycopyrrolate does not cross the blood-brain barrier and is associated with fewer CNS side effects. Glycopyrrolate is a potent drying agent when compared with others agents and has the potential to cause excessive dryness.[36]

Advanced Heart Failure

▶ *Palliative Care Considerations*

Heart failure symptoms at the end of life may include hypotension, volume overload, edema, and fatigue. Patients should be assessed to confirm symptoms are related to heart failure rather than other disease states to ensure appropriate treatment.[37,38]

Goals for advanced heart failure treatment differ from traditional heart failure management. Drug therapy focuses on symptom management rather than improving mortality. Prevention of cardiovascular disease through cholesterol reduction is no longer necessary at this point.

▶ *Nonpharmacologic Treatment*

Patients should be maintained in a comfortable position with feet elevated to minimize lower leg fluid accumulation. Minimizing high-salt foods and limiting fluid intake can help reduce fluid accumulation. At this stage in heart failure, comfort becomes the primary initiative.

▶ *Pharmacotherapy*

As patients approach the end of life, it is difficult to determine when certain medications for heart failure should be dose reduced or discontinued. The following general principles may help serve as a guide. However, each individual's history, prognosis, and current condition should be evaluated to determine appropriateness.

If a patient becomes symptomatic due to hypotension, angiotensin-converting enzyme (ACE) inhibitor, angiotensin receptor blocker (ARB), and/or β-adrenergic blocker doses should be reduced or discontinued. For β-adrenergic blockers, in particular, this should be done gradually to avoid significant clinical deterioration. If volume overload occurs or persists while taking β-adrenergic blocker therapy, consider tapering off the medication. Likewise, for patients experiencing fatigue while taking a β-adrenergic blocking agent, consider tapering down the dose *only if* their heart rate does not increase with exertion. Consider discontinuing the ACE inhibitor (or the angiotensin receptor blocker) if the patient's renal function deteriorates (eg, cardiorenal syndrome).

In patients with excessive fluid overload where sodium and water intake restrictions are not effective or not possible, consider increasing the dose of diuretic. However, vascular dehydration can occur in some patients with end-stage heart failure if the dose of diuretic is excessive.

Digoxin toxicity is common; therefore, patients should be carefully monitored and therapy adjusted or discontinued as appropriate. The symptoms of digoxin toxicity including complaints of anorexia, nausea and vomiting, visual disturbances, disorientation, confusion, or cardiac arrhythmias.

Hydroxymethylglutaryl coenzyme-A (HMG-CoA) reductase inhibitors (and other cholesterol-lowering medications) are likely to have a long-term effect rather than a palliative effect. If patients are eligible for hospice admission, consider discontinuing lipid lowering therapy.

Figure 4–1 provides a list of agents that improve functional status in advanced heart failure patients.

OUTCOME EVALUATION

KEY CONCEPT *Involving the patient, family, and caregivers in the development of the therapeutic plan demonstrates responsible palliative care.* Before the implementation of drug therapy, the patient, family, and caregiver should be involved with the decision-making process. The practitioner should provide information about all reasonable options for care so that the patient, family, and caregivers can collaborate with the health care team to meet their combined goals. KEY CONCEPT *Positive therapeutic outcomes include resolution of symptoms while minimizing adverse drug events.* When treating symptoms pharmacologically, adverse drug events must be avoided or minimized to prevent negative outcomes.

Patients with life-limiting diseases have emotional and spiritual issues that deserve attention by trained professionals. Addressing these concerns and providing support and coping skills can dramatically reduce the medication requirements for symptom control. Psychosocial and spiritual support is not only directed toward the patient in palliative care but also supports the family during the time of the illness and after the death of their loved one.

KEY CONCEPT *Patient and caregiver education is vital to ensuring positive outcomes.* If the patient and caregiver are unaware of the purpose and goals for interventions used in palliative medicine, adherence to regimens will be hindered and outcomes will be compromised. Education regarding the role and value of the palliative care team will allow the patient and family to understand why palliative care is important to their overall quality of life. Patients will achieve the best possible outcomes when practitioners incorporate the interdisciplinary palliative care approach to care early in the disease progression of patients with life-limiting illnesses.

Patient Encounter 3

ST is a 45-year-old woman recently diagnosed with pancreatic cancer. She received several rounds of palliative chemotherapy with localized radiation over the past few months. The interventions were unsuccessful in limiting tumor growth which has now metastasized to liver, brain, and right hip bone. Patient is jaundice with mild ascites with no reported pruritus. ST's chief complaint today is uncontrolled nausea and vomiting which worsens with meals and has been going on for a week. The oncologist prescribed ondansetron 8 mg by mouth every 8 hours as needed. Patient has prescription filled and at home but has not taken any yet. Comorbidities include hypertension, depression with recent anxiety. Allergy: Codeine (reaction unknown). Medications include: hydrocodone/acetaminophen 5/325 1 to 2 tablets by mouth every 4 to 6 hours as needed for pain, ibuprofen 200 mg 1 to 2 tablets by mouth every 4 to 6 hours as needed for pain and acetaminophen 500 mg 1 to 2 tablets by mouth every 6 hours as needed.

What questions would you ask ST during your assessment of her nausea and vomiting?

What are potential causes of ST's nausea and vomiting?

What potential drug–drug interactions and side effects exist in this patient?

What medications could be added, changed, and/or discontinued?

How does the patient's reported allergy to codeine impact potential treatment options?

Abbreviations Introduced in This Chapter

5-HT	5-Hydroxytriptophan (serotonin)
ACE	Angiotensin-converting enzyme
ALS	Amyotrophic lateral sclerosis
ARB	Angiotensin receptor blocker
CHF	Chronic heart failure
CNS	Central nervous system
COPD	Chronic obstructive pulmonary disease
CTZ	Chemoreceptor trigger zone
CVA	Cerebrovascular accident
ESRD	End-stage renal disease
GERD	Gastroesophageal reflux disease
HMG-CoA	Hydroxymethylglutaryl coenzyme-A
NSAID	Nonsteroidal anti-inflammatory drug
PEG	Percutaneous endoscopic gastrostomy
PICC	Peripherally inserted central catheter
PPI	Proton pump inhibitors
SSRI	Selective serotonin reuptake inhibitor
WHO	World Health Organization

Patient Care Process

Patient Assessment:

- Evaluate the patient's physical exam, review of systems, and assess for uncontrolled symptoms related to, or worsened by their current hospice diagnosis.
- Perform a medication reconciliation (prescription, OTC medications, herbals) to determine medications taken by the patient.
- Determine the patient's goals of care as it relates to their hospice plan of care.

Therapy Evaluation:

- Based on anticipated prognosis of a specific disease state, determine if continuing medication for preventative or long-term management of a disease state is appropriate.
- If the patient's goals of care include discontinuing laboratory monitoring, then medications with a narrow therapeutic index or a lab guided toxicity indicator should be discontinued.
- Ensure that medications are appropriate for the patient's functional status.
- Evaluate adherence strategies and monitor for adverse drug effects.
- Before adding a medication to manage an uncontrolled symptom, evaluate that the specific symptom is not attributable to current drug therapy.
- Verify the patient's prescription coverage or institutional formulary when adding medications.

Care Plan Development:

- Involve the patient, family, and caregivers in the development of a pharmacologic and nonpharmacologic plan of care that is built upon the patient's goals of care.
- Ensure that current medications confer benefit for functional status rather than only increasing survival (Example seen in Figure 4–1) and that this medication management approach is in line with the patient's goals of care.
- Continue to evaluate current therapy as the patient's functional status (ie, ambulation, swallowing, continence) changes, and ensure that all medications are safe and effective while avoiding adverse drug effects.
- Offer patients and family psychosocial support.

Follow-Up Evaluation:

- Encourage the patient, family, and caregivers to contact the hospice or palliative care team with questions or concerns.
- Bimonthly reviews of the patient's medical condition, current medication and goals of care will occur during the hospice interdisciplinary team meeting.

REFERENCES

1. World Health Organization. WHO definition of palliative care. Geneva, Switzerland: World Health Organization [cited 2014 June 12]. http://www.who.int/cancer/palliative/definition/en.
2. Centers for Medicare & Medicaid Services. Medicare Hospice Benefits. Centers for Medicare and Medicaid Services. Washington, DC: Centers for Medicare and Medicaid Services, 2013 [cited 2014 June 12]. http://www.medicare.gov/Publications/Pubs/pdf/02154.pdf.
3. National Consensus Project for Quality Palliative Care. Clinical Practice Guidelines for Quality Palliative Care, 2nd ed. Pittsburgh, PA: National Consensus Project for Quality Palliative Care, 2009 [cited 2014 Aug 7]. http://nationalconsensusproject.org/guideline.pdf.
4. Butterfield S. Growing specialty offers opportunity for hospitalists. ACPHospitalist. February 2009 [cited 2014 Aug 7]. http://www.acphospitalist.org/archives/2009/02/cover.htm.
5. Sepúlveda C, Marlin A, Yoshida T, Ullrich A. Palliative care: The World Health Organization's global perspective. J Pain Symptom Manage. 2002;24:91.
6. Hill RR. Clinical pharmacy services in a home-based palliative care program. Am J Health Syst Pharm. 2007;64:806–810.
7. Teno JM, Connor SR. Referring a patient and family to high-quality palliative care at the close of life: "We met a new personality … with this level of compassion and empathy." JAMA. 2009;301:651.
8. Grauer P, Shuster J, Protus BM. Palliative Care Consultant, 3rd ed. Dubuque, IA: Kendall/Hunt Publishing, 2008.
9. Goldstein NE, Fischberg D. Update in palliative medicine. Ann Intern Med. 2008;148:135–140.
10. Strickland JS. Palliative Pharmacy Care. Bethesda, MD: American Society of Health-Systems Pharmacists, 2009.
11. Hospice care. Health Letter. Cambridge, MA: Harvard Health Publications, July 2008.
12. Facts and Figures on Hospice Care in America: 2014. National Hospice and Palliative Care Organization, 2014.
13. Connor SR, Pyenson B, Fitch K, Spence C, Iwasaki K. Comparing hospice and nonhospice patient survival among patients who die within a three year window. J Pain Symptom Manage. 2007;33(3):238–246.
14. Ternel JS, Greer JA, Muzinkansky A, et al. Early palliative care for patients with metastatic non-small-cell lung cancer. N Engl J Med. 2010;363(8):733–742.
15. Breitbart W, Alici Y. Agitation and delirium at the end of life "We can't manage him." JAMA 2008;300(24):2898–2910.
16. Desplenter F, Bond C, Watson M, et al. Incidence and drug treatment of emotional distress after cancer diagnosis: a matched primary care case-control study. Br J Cancer. 107:1644–1651.
17. Bush SH, Pereira JL, Currow DC, et al. Treating an established episode of delirium in palliative care: expert opinion and review of the current evidence base with recommendations for future development. J Pain Symptom Manage. 2014 Aug;48(2):231–248.
18. Wilson KG, Chochinov, HM, Skirko MG, et al. Depression and anxiety disorders in palliative cancer care. J Pain Symptom Manage. 2007;33:118–129.
19. Grauer PA, Shuster J, Protus BM. Palliative Care Consultant, 3rd ed. Dubuque, IA: Kendall-Hunt, 2008:29–31, 40–47, 78–85.
20. Bush SH, Leonard MM, Spiller JA, et al. End-of-life delirium: issues regarding recognition, optimal management, and the role of sedation in the dying phase. J Pain Symptom Manage. 2014;48(2):215–230.
21. Gareri P, De Fazio P, Manfredi VG, et al. Use and safety of antipsychotics in behavioral disorders in elderly people with dementia. J Clinical Psychopharmacol. 2014;34(1):109–123.
22. Lonergan E, Britton AM, Luxenberg J Antipsychotics for delirium. Cochrane Reviews[Internet]. 2009 Jan 21 [cited 2012 Mar 2]. http://www2.cochrane.org/reviews/en/ab005594.html.
23. Haloperidol Monograph. Lexicomp Online. Hudson (OH): Lexi-Comp Inc. [cited 2014 June 12]. http://www.crlonline.com/crlsql/servlet/crlonline.
24. Breitbart W, Marotta R, Platt MM, et al. A double-blind trial of haloperidol, chlorpromazine, and lorazepam in the treatment of delirium in hospitalized AIDS patients. Am J Psychiatry. 1996;153:231–237.
25. Storey P, Knight CF. UNIPAC Four: Management of Selected Non-Pain Symptoms in the Terminally Ill, 2nd ed. New York, NY: Mary Ann Liebert, 2003:29–35.
26. Brennan CW, Mazanec P. Dyspnea management across the palliative care continuum. J Hosp Palliat Nurs. 2011;13(3):130–139.
27. Kallet RH. The role of inhaled opioids and furosemide for the treatment of dyspnea. Respir Care. 2007;52(7):900–910.
28. Emanuel LL, von Gunten CF, Ferris FD, Hauser JM, eds. The education for physicians on end-of-life Care (EPEC) curriculum. Module 10: Common Physical Symptoms. 2003:5–10.
29. Kamal AH, Maguire JM, Wheeler JL, et al. Dyspnea review for the palliative care professional: treatment goals and therapeutic options. J Palliat Med. 2012;15(1):106–114.
30. Schaefer KG, Chittenden EH, Sullivan AM, et al. Raising the bar for care of seriously ill patients: results of a national survey to define essential palliative care competencies for medical students and residents. Acad Med. 2014;89(7):1024–1031.
31. Vella-Brincat J, Macleod AD. Haloperidol in palliative care. Palliat Med. 2004;18:195–201.
32. American Pain Society. Principles of Analgesic Use in Treatment of Acute Pain and Cancer Pain, 6th ed. Glenview, IL: American Pain Society, 2009.
33. McCaffery M, Pasero C. Pain: Clinical Manual, 2nd ed. St. Louis, MO: Elsevier Mosby, 1999.
34. Lokker ME, van Zuylen L, van der Rijt, C. Prevalence, impact, and treatment of death rattle: a systematic review. J Pain Symptom Manage. 2014;47(1):105–122.
35. Curtis JR. Palliative and end-of-life care for patients with severe COPD. Eur Respir J. 2008;32:796–803.
36. Protus BM, Grauer PA, Kimbrel JM. Evaluation of atropine 1% ophthalmic solution administered sublingually for the management of terminal respiratory secretions. Am J Hosp Palliat Care. 2012;30(4):388–392.
37. Whellan DJ, Goodlin SJ, Dickinson MG, et al. End-of-life care in patients with heart failure. Consensus Statement. J Card Fail. 2014;20(2):121–134.
38. McPherson ML. Palliative Care and Appropriate Medication Use in End-Stage Heart Failure. Medscape Nurses. 2007 [cited 2014 June 12]. http://www.medscape.com/viewarticle/556035.

Part II

Disorders of Organ Systems

5 Hypertension

David Parra, Youssef M. Roman,
Emily Anastasia, and Robert J. Straka

LEARNING OBJECTIVES

Upon completion of the chapter, the reader will be able to:

1. Classify blood pressure (BP) levels and treatment goals.
2. Recognize underlying causes and contributing factors in the development of hypertension.
3. Describe the appropriate measurement of BP.
4. Recommend appropriate lifestyle modifications and pharmacotherapy for patients with hypertension.
5. Identify populations requiring special consideration when designing a treatment plan.
6. Construct an appropriate monitoring plan to assess hypertension treatment.

INTRODUCTION

Despite blood pressure (BP) being a surrogate target for reducing cardiovascular risk, it has been well established that reducing elevated BP in patients at sufficient risk provides a significant cardiovascular benefit. However, in spite of efforts to promote awareness, treatment, and the means available to aggressively manage high BP, global control remains suboptimal. Worldwide, only about one-third of adults have their BP controlled, and in the United States, slightly over one-half of adults experience BP control.[1] Based on clinical evidence, national and international organizations continually refine recommendations on the management of patients with high BP. The purpose of this chapter is to: (a) provide a summary of key issues associated with the management of hypertension; (b) discuss the basic approach to treating hypertension and provide a functional summary of the currently prevailing themes of recent guidelines; and (c) summarize salient pharmacotherapeutic issues essential for clinicians to consider when treating hypertension. In doing so, we hope to provide the practicing clinician with a contemporary view on a defensible approach to managing BP and therefore risk in patients with elevated BP.

Various algorithms recommend nonpharmacologic and pharmacologic management, with the underlying premise that lowering elevated BP reduces end-organ damage leading to reductions in stroke, myocardial infarction (MI), end-stage renal disease, and heart failure (HF). Although other guidelines are mentioned, this chapter focuses primarily on two recent guidelines: the American Society of Hypertension (ASH) and the International Society of Hypertension (ISH) Joint Clinical Practice Guidelines for the Management of Hypertension in the Community,[2] and the 2014 Evidence-Based Guideline for the Management of High BP in Adults by the former panel members appointed to the Eighth Joint National Committee (JNC 8).[3] Guidelines from the American Heart Association and American College of Cardiology are anticipated to be released in 2015.

The ASH/ISH hypertension guidelines classify BP and provide guidance on nonpharmacologic and pharmacologic approaches to managing hypertension. These guidelines state that the lowest risk of adverse cardiovascular or renal outcomes is at a BP of around 115/75 mm Hg, with risk rising as BP increases. They further classify elevations in BP beyond specific thresholds as prehypertension, stage 1 hypertension, and stage 2 hypertension (Table 5–1). These classifications imply different levels of risk and thus the need for varying intensities of intervention with drug therapy.[2] Recommendations for drug therapy typically begin with one or two (in the case of stage 2 hypertension) antihypertensive drugs as an initial step. Compelling indications, such as HF with reduced ejection fraction (HFrEF), post-MI, diabetes, and chronic kidney disease (CKD), are examples of specific conditions for which explicit evidence in the literature exists to document the utility of a particular agent or class of agents. Selection of drug therapy consequently involves an iterative process of adding antihypertensive drugs as needed to achieve target BP, otherwise known as a stepped approach. An example of an approach by the ASH/ISH guidelines is contained within Figure 5–1 and Table 5–2. Others have argued for greater personalization in selecting drug

Table 5–1

Classification of Hypertension[2]

Classification	Systolic Blood Pressure (mm Hg)	Diastolic Blood Pressure (mm Hg)
Prehypertension	120–139	80–89
Stage 1	140–159	90–99
Stage 2	≥ 160	≥ 100

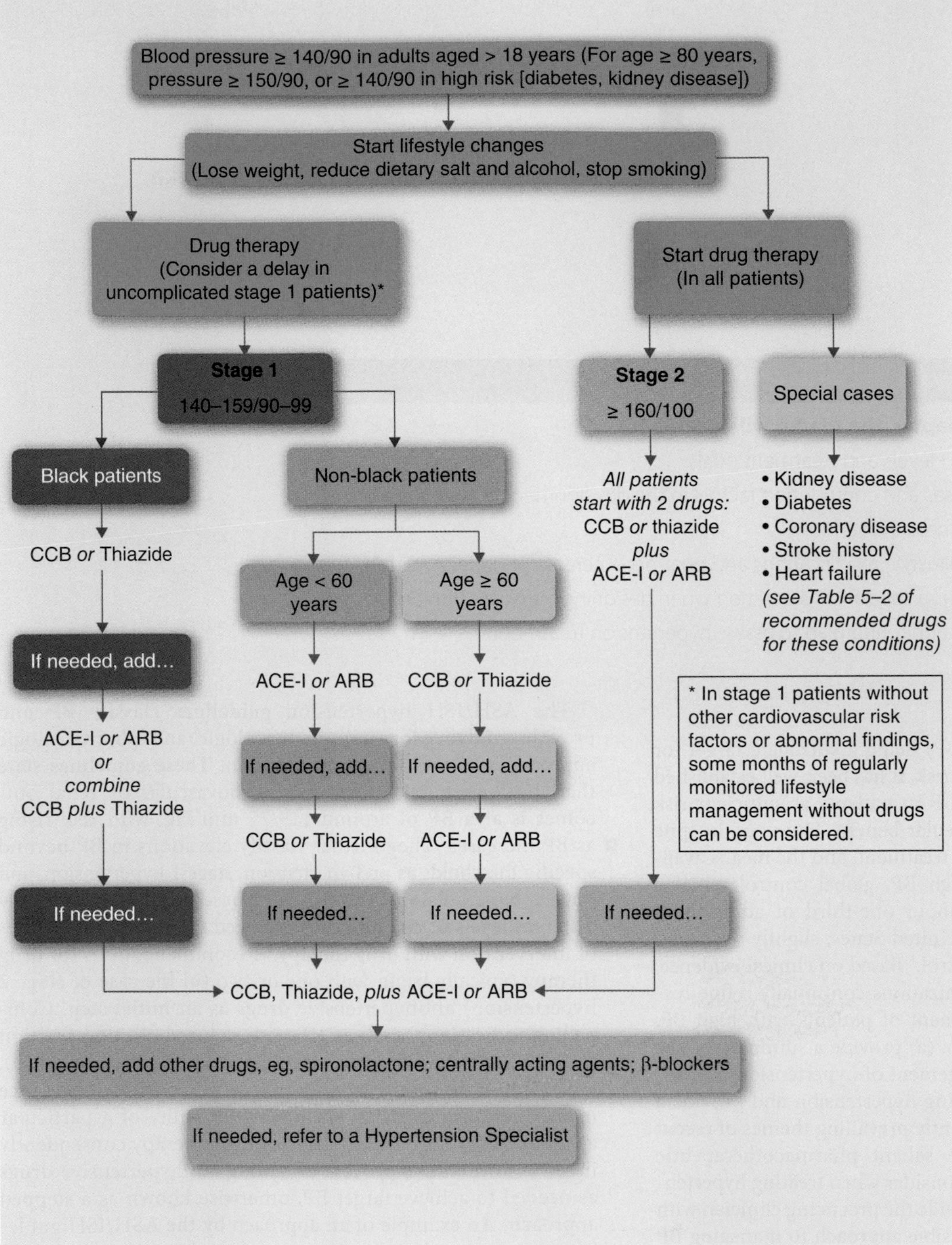

FIGURE 5–1. Algorithm of the main recommendations of the American Society of Hypertension/International Society of Hypertension (ASH/ISH) guidelines. At any stage, it is entirely appropriate to seek help from a hypertension expert if treatment is proving difficult. In patients with stage 1 hypertension in whom there is no history of cardiovascular, stroke, or renal events or evidence of abnormal findings and who do not have diabetes or other major risk factors, drug therapy can be delayed for some months. In all other patients (including those with stage 2 hypertension), it is recommended that drug therapy should be started when the diagnosis of hypertension is made. Blood pressure values are in mm Hg. (ACE-I, angiotensin-converting enzyme inhibitors; ARB, angiotensin receptor blocker; CCB, calcium channel blocker; thiazide, thiazide or thiazide-like diuretics.) (Reprinted with permission from James PA, Oparil S, Carter BL, et al. 2014 evidence-based guideline for the management of high blood pressure in adults: report from the panel members appointed to the Eighth Joint National Committee (JNC 8). JAMA. Feb 5 2014;311(5):507–520.)

therapy.[4] Recently, the roles of 24-hour ambulatory BP monitoring (ABPM), home BP (HBP) monitoring, and ambulatory office-based BP (AOBP) monitoring have been more clearly defined.[2,5] Although current versions of major guidelines differ slightly in terms of their thresholds for initiating drug therapy, target BPs, and recommendations for initial selection of drug therapy, they have each relaxed their BP targets based on existing clinical evidence.[2,3,6]

Table 5 3 summarizes key elements of recent guidelines, including BP goals/targets.[7,8] Regardless of the guideline used, it is imperative that clinicians consider patient-specific characteristics and preferences among other considerations when establishing BP targets and drug selection.

EPIDEMIOLOGY

KEY CONCEPT *Hypertension is widely prevalent and significantly contributes to cardiovascular-related morbidity, mortality, and their associated health care costs.* Worldwide in 2008, nearly 1 billion adults aged 25 and older (40% of the adult population) had hypertension.[9,10] Globally, 51% of all strokes and 45% of ischemic heart disease deaths are attributable to hypertension. Furthermore, hypertension is the leading noncommunicable disease risk factor for death and for ischemic heart disease disability-adjusted life years.[10] The following summary of contemporary statistics relevant to the United States underscores the importance of hypertension to public health.[1] In the United States, the prevalence of hypertension is estimated to include nearly

Table 5–2

Drug Selection in Hypertensive Patients With or Without Other Major Conditions

Patient Type	First Choice Drug	Add Second Drug If Needed to Achieve a BP < 140/90 mm Hg	If Third Drug Is Needed to Achieve a BP < 140/90 mm Hg
A. When hypertension is the only or main condition			
Black patients (African Ancestry): all ages	CCB[a] or thiazide diuretic	ARB[b] or ACE-I (if unavailable can add alternative first choice drugs)	Combination of CCB + ACE-I or ARB + thiazide diuretic
White and other non-black patients: Younger than 60	ARB[b] or ACE-I	CCB[a] or thiazide diuretic	Combination of CCB + ACE-I or ARB + thiazide diuretic
White and other non-black patients: 60 and older	CCB[a] or thiazide diuretic (although ACE-Is or ARBs are also usually effective)	ARB[b] or ACE-I (or CCB or thiazide if ACE-I or ARB used first)	Combination of CCB + ACE-I or ARB + thiazide diuretic
B. When hypertension is associated with other conditions			
Hypertension and diabetes	ARB or ACE-I; Note: in black patients, it is acceptable to start with CCB or thiazide	CCB or thiazide diuretic; Note: in black patients, if starting with a CCB or thiazide, add an ARB or ACE-I	Alternative second drug (thiazide or CCB)
Hypertension and chronic kidney disease	ARB or ACE-I; Note: in black patients, good evidence for renal protective effects of ACE-Is	CCB or thiazide diuretic[c]	Alternative second drug (thiazide or CCB)
Hypertension and clinical coronary artery disease[d]	β-blocker plus ARB or ACE-I	CCB or thiazide diuretic	Alternative second step drug (thiazide or CCB)
Hypertension and stroke history[e]	ACE-I or ARB	Thiazide diuretic or CCB	Alternative second drug (CCB or thiazide)
Hypertension and heart failure	Patients with symptomatic heart failure should usually receive an ARB or ACE-I + β-blocker + diuretic + spironolactone regardless of blood pressure. A dihydropyridine CCB can be added if needed for BP control.		

ACE-I, angiotensin-converting enzyme inhibitor; ARB, angiotensin receptor blocker; BP, blood pressure; CCB, calcium channel blocker.

[a]CCBs are generally preferred, but thiazides may cost less.

[b]ARBs can be considered because ACE-I can cause cough and angioedema, although ACE-Is may cost less.

[c]If estimated glomerular filtration rate (eGFR) < 40 mL/min/1.73 m^2, a loop diuretic (eg, furosemide or torsemide) may be needed.

[d]Note: If history of myocardial infarction, a β-blocker plus ACE-I or ARB are indicated regardless of BP.

[e]Note: If using a diuretic, there is good evidence for indapamide (if available).

Reprinted with permission from Weber MA, Schiffrin EL, White WB, et al. Clinical practice guidelines for the management of hypertension in the community: a statement by the American Society of Hypertension and the International Society of Hypertension. J Clin Hypertens (Greenwich). Jan 2014;16(1):14–26.

78 million individuals (one in three adults 20 years of age or older), with an estimated $46.4 billion spent annually in direct and indirect costs. The prevalence of hypertension differs based on age, sex, and ethnicity. As individuals become older, risk of systolic hypertension increases. Hypertension is slightly more prevalent in men than women before the age of 45 years, similar between the ages of 45 and 64 years, and more prevalent in women than men thereafter. Age-adjusted prevalence of hypertension is highest in non-Hispanic blacks (42.6%–47%) when compared with non-Hispanic whites (30.7%–33.4%) and Hispanic Americans (28.8%–30.1%).[1]

ETIOLOGY

KEY CONCEPT *In most patients (more than 90%), the cause of hypertension is unknown and referred to as primary hypertension. However, in some patients there is an identifiable cause of hypertension, referred to as secondary hypertension. Common causes of secondary hypertension include:*[11]

- CKD
- Coarctation of the aorta
- Cushing syndrome and other glucocorticoid excess states
- Drug induced/related (Table 5–4)
- Pheochromocytoma
- Primary aldosteronism and other mineralocorticoid excess states
- Renovascular hypertension
- Sleep apnea
- Thyroid or parathyroid disease

Identification of a secondary cause of hypertension is often not initially pursued unless suggested by routine clinical and laboratory evaluation of the patient or a failure to achieve BP control.[6,11]

In addition to primary and secondary hypertension, the clinician may encounter what is referred to as resistant hypertension. KEY CONCEPT *Patients failing to achieve goal BP despite adherence to optimal doses of three antihypertensive agents of different classes (ideally, one being a diuretic) have resistant hypertension and should be evaluated for secondary causes of hypertension.*[12] Several causes

Table 5–3

Summary of Key Aspects of Recent Hypertension Guidelines

	ESH/ESC 2013[6]	James et al. JAMA 2013[3]	ASH/ISH 2013[2]
When to initiate BP lowering medications in general population[a]	General population: ≥ 160/100 mm Hg or ≥140/90 mm Hg if high cardiovascular risk (ie, organ damage, CVD, DM or CKD, or if low to moderate risk after implementation of lifestyle changes for several months) Elderly (≥ 80 years old): SBP ≥ 160 mm Hg	General population: ≥ 60 years: ≥ 150/90 mm Hg < 60 years, > 18 years with CKD or DM: ≥ 140/90 mm Hg	General population: ≥ 160/100 mm Hg (or ≥ 140/90 mm Hg if lifestyle interventions not effective) Elderly (≥ 80 years): ≥ 150/90 mm Hg
BP targets	General population: < 140/90 mm Hg Patients with DM: < 140/85 mm Hg Elderly (≥ 80 years old): 140–150/90 mm Hg	General population: ≥ 60 years: < 150/90 mm Hg[a] < 60 years, ≥ 18 years: < 140/90 mm Hg ≥ 18 years with DM or CKD: < 140/90 mm Hg	General population: < 140/90 mm Hg Elderly (≥ 80 years old): < 150/90 mm Hg, but can consider < 140/90 if DM or CKD
Initial BP-lowering agent suggested[b]	Diuretic (ie, chlorthalidone, indapamide), β-blocker, CCB, ACE-I, ARB	Non-black population including those with DM: Thiazide-type diuretic, CCB, ACE-I, ARB Black population including those with DM: Thiazide-type diuretic, CCB CKD population: ACE-I, ARB	BP 140-159/90-99 mm Hg: 1 drug Black patients: CCB, Thiazide Non-Black patients: Age < 60 years: ACE-I or ARB Age ≥ 60 years: CCB or thiazide BP ≥ 160/100 mm Hg: 2 Drugs (CCB or thiazide and ACE-I or ARB)

ACE-I, angiotensin-converting enzyme inhibitor; ARB, angiotensin receptor blocker; ASH, American Society of Hypertension; BP, blood pressure; CCB, calcium channel blocker; CKD, chronic kidney disease; CVD, cardiovascular disease; DM, diabetes mellitus; ESC, European Society of Cardiology; ESH, European Society of Hypertension; ISH, International Society of Hypertension; JAMA, Journal of the American Medical Association; SBP, systolic blood pressure.

[a]The authors of these guidelines did not agree upon the age threshold of 60 for a relaxed BP goal and several of the authors published a dissenting opinion supporting an age threshold of 80 instead.[8]

[b]Compelling indications may change initial recommendations; specific guideline should be consulted in these circumstances.

Adapted from Parra D, Hough A. Current therapeutic approaches to cardio-protection in hypertension. Curr Hypertens Rep. Aug 2014;16(8):457.

of resistant hypertension are listed in Table 5–4 and should be carefully considered in such patients.[13]

PATHOPHYSIOLOGY

KEY CONCEPT *The pathophysiology of primary hypertension is heterogeneous but ultimately exerts its effects through the two primary determinants of BP: cardiac output (CO) and peripheral resistance (PR).* The processes influencing these two determinants are numerous and complex, and although the underlying cause of primary hypertension remains unknown, it is most likely multifactorial. As a review of these mechanisms is beyond the scope of this text, readers are referred to other sources.[11]

The development of primary hypertension involves interplay between genetic and environmental factors interacting with multiple physiological systems including neural, renal, hormonal, and vascular. Further complicating this is that an individual's phenotype of primary hypertension (eg, diastolic hypertension in middle-aged individuals, isolated systolic hypertension in the elderly, and obesity-related hypertension) may have different contributing mechanisms.[11] Because of these complexities, no final common pathway has been identified and a single target for the treatment of primary hypertension remains elusive. Therefore, guidelines for the selection of specific therapeutic agents allow the clinician some flexibility in choices.

Genetic Factors

Although multiple genetic polymorphisms have been associated with relatively small effects on systolic BP (SBP), diastolic BP (DBP), and response to antihypertensive medications, replications of these findings in large populations are elusive. Consequently, the information available to date is far from sufficient to provide any practical guidance for clinicians.[11] Nevertheless, genetic basis of variability in response to drug therapy continues to be pursued.

Environmental Factors

In contrast with genetic factors, environmental factors contributing to hypertension are well characterized. Cigarette smoking

Patient Encounter 1

A 64-year-old white male comes into your clinic with concerns about his BP. He arrived after his morning BP measurements at home were 149/90 mm Hg and when repeated 160/100 mm Hg. Upon examination in your clinic, seated BP in the left arm is 153/96 mm Hg and 157/89 mm Hg in the right arm. You request that the patient return to your clinic in 1 week for a follow-up BP. His seated BPs in the left arm 1 week later were 156/92 mm Hg and 150/87 mm Hg. The patient's physical examination was unremarkable, but his past medical history was significant for dyslipidemia and depression. His previous cholesterol panel revealed a high-density lipoprotein level of 52 mg/dL (1.34 mmol/L), triglyceride level of 180 mg/dL (2.03 mmol/L), and total cholesterol of 198 mg/dL (5.12 mmol/L). Calculated low-density lipoprotein level is 110 mg/dL (2.84 mmol/L). All other laboratory values were within normal limits. Current medications include aspirin and citalopram.

Based on the information above, what stage of hypertension does this patient have according to the ASH/ISH Hypertension Guidelines?

What is the patient's BP target according to ASH/ISH guidelines and by the evidence-based guidelines from the former JNC 8 panel?

What steps are involved in assuring that the patient's BP measurements are accurate?

(cigars and smokeless tobacco) and caffeine cause transient increases in BP via norepinephrine release and, in the case of caffeine, by its antagonism of vasodilatory adenosine receptors. Acute alcohol ingestion may have a variable effect (increased due to sympathetic nerve activity or lowering due to vasodilation) which is transient, whereas chronic heavy consumption of alcohol and binge drinking raises the risk of hypertension.[11,14] Many other environmental factors have been shown or been proposed to influence BP and, in some cases, contribute to the development of hypertension. These include obesity, physical inactivity, fetal environment (eg, maternal malnutrition, increased fetal exposure to maternal glucocorticoids), postnatal weight gain, premature birth and low birth weight, potassium and magnesium depletion, vitamin D deficiency, and environmental toxins (eg, lead).[11]

Neural Mechanisms

Overactivity of the sympathetic nervous system (SNS) in the early stages of primary hypertension manifests as increased heart rate, CO, and peripheral vasoconstriction. Despite this, recent outcome trials of agents targeting the SNS (α- and β-adrenergic blockers) have not performed as well as other classes of drugs. Nevertheless, strategies aimed at targeting the SNS continue to be pursued with specific interest in invasive strategies aimed at resistant hypertension.[11]

Renal Mechanisms

The contribution of sodium to the development of primary hypertension is related to excess sodium intake and/or abnormal sodium excretion by the kidneys.[11] However, it is generally accepted that dietary salt is associated with increases in BP that can be lowered with reduction of sodium intake,[15] particularly in individuals deemed salt sensitive.[16] For example, 29% of participants in the Dietary Approaches to Stop Hypertension (DASH)-Sodium trial were deemed to be salt sensitive and responded to reductions in salt intake.[16,17] Current guidelines suggest there is a threshold effect of sodium intake on BP in the range of 50 to 100 mmol/day (1.2–2.4 g). However, these recommendations may require modification based on contemporary investigations.[18] Although population-wide based reduction in dietary sodium intake via global policies has been widely advocated as an approach to reduce hypertension and cardiovascular disease (CVD), the need for further scientific investigation of salt restriction persists.

Table 5–4

Causes of Resistant Hypertension[13]

Apparent Resistance
Improper blood pressure measurement
Failure to receive or take antihypertensive medication appropriately (nonadherence)
Inadequate doses (subtherapeutic)
Improper antihypertensive selection or combination
White coat hypertension
True Resistance
Secondary hypertension
Drug effects and interactions
Adrenal steroid hormones
Amphotericin B
Cocaine, amphetamines, and other illicit drugs
Cyclosporine and tacrolimus
Erythropoietin
Fluid retention from kidney disease or potent vasodilators (eg, minoxidil)
Herbal products (ma huang, guarana, bitter orange, blue cohosh)
Highly active antiretroviral therapy (HAART)
Inadequate diuretic therapy
Natural licorice (including some chewing tobacco)
Neurologic and psychiatric agents (eg, venlafaxine, modafinil)
Nonsteroidal anti-inflammatory medications
Oral contraceptive hormones
Recent caffeine or nicotine intake
Sympathomimetics (decongestants, anorectics, and stimulants)
Vascular endothelial growth factor inhibitors (bevacizumab, sorafenib, sunitinib)
Volume overload
Excess sodium intake
Comorbidities
Obesity
Excess alcohol intake
Chronic pain syndromes
Intense vasoconstriction (arteritis)
Anxiety-induced hyperventilation/panic attacks
Genetic variation
Genetic differences in drug efficacy or metabolism

Hormonal Mechanisms

Renin is produced and stored in the juxtaglomerular cells of the kidney, and its release is stimulated by impaired renal perfusion, salt depletion, and β_1-adrenergic stimulation. The release of renin is the rate-limiting step in the eventual formation of angiotensin II, which is a potent vasoconstrictor (Figure 5–2).[11] The role of the renin-angiotensin-aldosterone system (RAAS) in primary hypertension is supported by the presence of high levels of renin, suggesting the system is inappropriately activated. Proposed mechanisms include increased sympathetic drive, defective regulation of the RAAS (nonmodulation), and the existence of a subpopulation of ischemic nephrons that release excess renin.[11] However, there are also patients with primary hypertension and low levels of renin which suggests alternative mechanisms, unrelated to renin levels or activity, may be in play. Thus, although uncommon in general practice, plasma renin activity (PRA) measurements may be utilized to guide antihypertensive therapy selection. In fact, it has been demonstrated that patients with low PRA (less than 0.65 ng/mL/hour [0.18 ng/L/s]) respond preferentially to diuretics, aldosterone antagonists, and calcium channel blockers (CCBs), whereas those with higher PRA levels respond preferentially to renin-mediated therapies such as β-blockers, angiotensin-converting enzyme inhibitors (ACE-Is), angiotensin receptor blockers (ARBs), and direct renin inhibitors.[4] However, use of PRA measurements to guide therapy is not without controversy and the reader is referred to other sources for more information on the subject.[7]

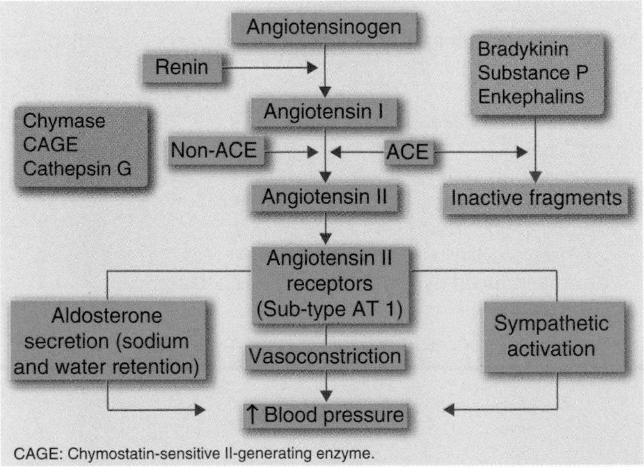

FIGURE 5–2. Diagram of the renin-angiotensin-aldosterone system (RAAS), a key system involved in the modulation of blood pressure. The diagram depicts the pathways involved in the action of various antihypertensive agents including angiotensin-converting enzyme (ACE) inhibitors, ARBs, diuretics, and aldosterone antagonists. By inhibiting the action of ACE, ACE inhibitors reduce both the formation of the vasoconstrictors angiotensin II and the degradation of vasodilation substances including bradykinin. ARBs primarily act through inhibition of the action of angiotensin II on the angiotensin-I receptors that modulate vasoconstriction. Aldosterone antagonists directly inhibit the action of aldosterone; diuretics affect sodium and water retention at a renal level. (ARB, angiotensin receptor blockers; AT1, angiotensin-1.) (From Victor RG, Kaplan NM. Kaplan's Clinical Hypertension, 10th ed. Philadelphia, PA: Wolters Kluwer Lippincott Williams & Wilkins Health, 2010.)

Vascular Mechanisms

Elevated peripheral arterial resistance is the hemodynamic hallmark of primary hypertension. The increase in PR typically observed may be due to a reduction in arterial lumen size as a result of vascular remodeling. This remodeling, or change in vascular tone, may be modulated by various endothelium-derived vasoactive substances, growth factors, and cytokines. This increase in arterial stiffness or reduced compliance results in the observed increase in systolic BP.[11]

Contributing Comorbidities

Several comorbidities have a high concurrence with the presence of hypertension leading to a higher risk of target organ damage, cardiovascular morbidity and mortality, and overall health care costs. Specifically, these include the presence of diabetes mellitus (DM), dyslipidemia, obesity, and CKD. As such, the assessment of global cardiovascular risk in all patients with hypertension should be part of the management plan while also pursuing target BPs through nonpharmacologic and pharmacologic means.[6]

MEASUREMENT OF BLOOD PRESSURE

KEY CONCEPT *Appropriate technique in measuring BP is a vital component to the diagnosis and management of hypertension.* Accurate measurement of a patient's BP requires the control of factors that may influence variability in the measure. Failure to consider these factors, including body position, cuff size, device selection, auscultatory technique and dietary intake prior to the visit, may lead to misclassification and thus inaccurate assessments of risk. Clinicians should instruct patients to avoid exercise, alcohol, caffeine, or nicotine consumption 30 minutes before BP measurement. Patients should be sitting comfortably with their back supported and arm free of constrictive clothing with legs uncrossed and feet flat on the floor for a minimum of 5 minutes before the first reading. Systolic and diastolic BP tend to increase when the cuff size is too small. Ideally, the cuff bladder should encircle at least 80% of the arm's circumference to ensure a more accurate measurement of BP.[19]

To reduce deviations in BP measurement in the clinic, the patient and clinician should not talk during BP readings. The measurement arm is supported and positioned at heart level. If a mercury or aneroid device is used, then the palpatory method must be used first to estimate the SBP.[20] If an automated device is used, this is not necessary. After the patient's cuff is inflated above the systolic pressure, the pressure indicator should drop at a rate of 2 to 3 mm Hg/s. A stethoscope placed over the brachial artery in the antecubital fossa identifies the first and last audible Korotkoff sounds, which should be taken as systolic and diastolic pressure, respectively. A minimum of two readings at least 1 minute apart are then averaged. If measurements vary by more than 5 mm Hg between the two readings, then one or two additional BP measurements are collected and the multiple readings averaged. BP classification is based on the average of two or more properly measured BP readings on each of two or more office visits. Details and further recommendations for accurate measurement of BP in special populations can be found elsewhere.[6,19] Finally, the measurement of clinic or office BPs is often poorly correlated with assessments of BP in other settings. Consequently, under select circumstances, clinicians are increasingly using 24-hour ABPM, AOBP monitoring and HBP monitoring. These tools are useful in identifying patients with *white coat hypertension* or in the case of 24-hour ABPM, elevations of BP during the night. They may also aid in the management of refractory hypertension with minor target organ damage, those with suspected autonomic neuropathy, those with hypotensive symptoms, and patients with large differences between home and clinic BP measurements. Benefits derived from these additional modes of BP monitoring may be of greater prognostic significance than traditional office-based measurements.[5,20]

TREATMENT

Desired Outcomes

The goal of BP management is to reduce the risk of CVD and target organ damage such as MI, HF, stroke, and kidney disease associated morbidity and mortality. Targeting a specific BP is actually a surrogate goal that has been associated with reductions in CVD and target organ damage.

General Approach to Treatment

KEY CONCEPT *Drug selection for the management of patients with hypertension should be considered as adjunctive to nonpharmacologic approaches for BP lowering. Ultimately, the attainment of target BP in many cases may be more important than the antihypertensive agent used.* Previous clinical research has established the value of using individual antihypertensive drugs versus placebo to achieve reduction in morbidity and mortality by lowering BP. However, as newer antihypertensive agents are developed, contemporary large outcome-based multicenter trials have had to be designed to compare one specific agent-based therapy (along with options to add others) versus another agent-based therapy (along with options to add others of a different class). These attempts at "head-to-head" comparisons and meta-analyses of multidrug regimen trials have, in general, provided evidence

Clinical Presentation and Diagnosis of Primary Hypertension

General

Age: Prevalence of hypertension is likely to be highest with middle-aged or older patients

Gender: In the United States, hypertension is slightly more prevalent in men than women before the age of 45 years, similar between the ages of 45 and 64 years, and higher in women than men thereafter

Symptoms

The patient with primary hypertension may be asymptomatic yet still have major CVD risk factors

Signs

Adult patients have an average of two or more BP readings (SBP and DBP) on two separate occasions indicating:

	SBP (mm Hg)	*DBP (mm Hg)*
Normal	less than 120	less than 80
Prehypertension	120–139	or 80–89
Stage 1 hypertension	140–159	or 90–99
Stage 2 hypertension	greater than or equal to 160	greater than or equal to 100

Laboratory Tests (not necessarily indicative of hypertension but should be measured in patients with hypertension)

Fasting lipid panel:

- Low-density lipoprotein cholesterol greater than 160 mg/dL (4.14 mmol/L)
- Total cholesterol greater than 240 mg/dL (6.21 mmol/L)
- High-density lipoprotein cholesterol less than 40 mg/dL (1.03 mmol/L)
- Triglycerides greater than 200 mg/dL (2.26 mmol/L)

Fasting plasma glucose or hemoglobin A1c (does not need to be fasting):

- Impaired fasting glucose 100–125 mg/dL (5.6–6.9 mmol/L)
- Diagnosis of diabetes with fasting glucose greater than or equal to 126 mg/dL (7.0 mmol/L) or hemoglobin A1c greater than or equal to 6.5% (0.065; 48 mmol/mol Hb) on two separate occasions, or random plasma glucose reading of greater than or equal to 200 mg/L (11.1 mmol/L) with symptoms of diabetes

The following abnormal tests may indicate hypertension-related damage:

- Serum creatinine elevated (greater than 1.2 mg/dL [106 μmol/L])
- Microalbuminuria, which is diagnosed either from a 24-hour urine collection (20–200 mcg/min) or from elevated concentrations (30–300 mg/L) on at least two occasions. Use of the albumin-to-creatinine ratio (ACR) in a spot urine sample is becoming more common, and microalbuminuria is defined by this measure as 30 to 300 mg/g creatinine (3.4–34 mg/mmol creatinine)

Common Comorbidities and Factors Contributing to Cardiovascular Risk

DM

Metabolic syndrome

Insulin resistance

Dyslipidemia

Microalbuminuria/CKD

Family history

Central obesity

Physical inactivity

Tobacco use

Target Organ Damage

Heart (left ventricular hypertrophy, angina, prior acute coronary syndrome [ACS], prior coronary revascularization, HF)

Brain (stroke or transient ischemic attack, dementia)

CKD

Peripheral arterial disease

Retinopathy

supporting the position that the main benefits of pharmacologic therapy are related to the achievement of BP lowering and are generally largely independent of the selection of an individual drug regimen. Inherent in this position is the realization that nonpharmacologic approaches alone are rarely successful in attaining target BPs, and multidrug therapy (sometimes as many as three or more agents) is necessary for most patients with hypertension.[2,21] Conversely, chronotherapy, or adjusting administration timing of certain pharmacotherapy for therapeutic benefit, has been shown to confer significant cardiovascular event reduction. Specifically, the Ambulatory Blood Pressure Monitoring for Prediction of Cardiovascular Events (MAPEC) study and subsequent subgroup analyses in CKD and diabetes demonstrated that moving the administration time of one antihypertensive agent to bedtime dosing significantly reduced composite cardiovascular events compared to administering all antihypertensive agents at one time in the morning.[22]

Although there are several approaches currently used to manage patients with hypertension, this chapter focuses on using the ASH/ISH hypertension guidelines[2] as well as the evidence-based guidelines by the JNC 8 panel,[3] while acknowledging important recommendations found in other guidelines and documents.

Nonpharmacologic Treatment: Lifestyle Modifications

Therapeutic lifestyle modifications consisting of nonpharmacologic approaches to BP reduction should be part of all treatment plans for patients with hypertension. The most widely studied interventions demonstrating effectiveness include:

- Dietary sodium restriction
- Low-fat diet, high in vegetables and fruits
- Weight reduction in overweight or obese individuals
- Regular physical activity
- Moderation of alcohol consumption

KEY CONCEPT *Implementation of these lifestyle modifications successfully lowers BP (Table 5–5), often with results similar to those of therapy with a single antihypertensive agent.*[2,6] Combining multiple lifestyle modifications can have even greater BP lowering effects. Sodium restriction to 2.4 g (100 mmol) of elemental sodium (6 g of sodium chloride or one teaspoon of table salt) per day lowers BP and has been recommended for the general population, especially individuals with hypertension. Although controversy surrounds the optimal level of sodium intake and its cardiovascular benefits and risks,[15,18,23,24] adoption of an optimal dietary pattern that includes consuming less processed foods is expected to afford overall cardiovascular benefits.

Compared to the general population, BP lowering through sodium restriction is more pronounced in salt-sensitive individuals (low PRA), persons with diabetes, metabolic syndrome, or CKD, as well as older individuals and black people.[4,6] Simple dietary advice and instructions on reading nutrition labels should be introduced to patients initially and assessed and reinforced at subsequent visits. The DASH trial demonstrated that a diet high in fruits, vegetables, and low-fat dairy products, along with a reduced intake of total and saturated fat, significantly reduced BP in as little as 8 weeks.[25] Weight reduction by only 4.5 kg (10 lb) may lower BP in overweight patients. Similarly, small changes in physical activity can have a significant effect on BP. It is generally accepted that 30 minutes of moderately intense aerobic activity (eg, brisk walking) most days of the week will lower BP.[26] The acute effects of alcohol on BP are variable as previously described. Reduction in alcohol intake in heavy drinkers reduces BP.[11] Furthermore, alcohol attenuates the effects of antihypertensive therapy, which is mostly reversible within 1 to 2 weeks with moderation of intake.

Lifestyle modifications also have a favorable effect on other risk factors for cardiovascular events including dyslipidemia and insulin resistance, which are commonly encountered in the hypertensive population. Smoking cessation should also be encouraged for overall cardiovascular health despite its lack of chronic effects on BP.[6] Although BP-lowering lifestyle modifications have never been documented to reduce cardiovascular morbidity and mortality in patients with hypertension, they do effectively lower BP in most hypertensive patients. This may obviate the need for drug therapy in those with mild elevations in BP or minimize the doses or number of antihypertensive agents required in those with greater elevations in BP.[6]

Table 5–5

Lifestyle Modifications to Manage Hypertension[a,19]

Modification	Recommendation	Approximate Systolic BP Reduction (Range)
Weight reduction	Maintain normal body weight (body mass index: 18.5–24.9 kg/m^2)	5–20 mm Hg/10 kg
Adopt DASH eating plan	Consume a diet rich in fruits, vegetables, and low-fat dairy products with a reduced content of saturated and total fat	8–14 mm Hg
Dietary sodium restriction	Reduce dietary sodium intake to no more than 100 mmol/day (2.4 g sodium or 6 g sodium chloride)	2–8 mm Hg
Physical activity	Engage in regular aerobic physical activity such as brisk walking (at least 30 min/day, most days of the week)	4–9 mm Hg
Moderation of alcohol consumption	Limit consumption to no more than two standard drinks per day in most men and to no more than one standard drink per day in women and lighter weight persons[b]	2–4 mm Hg

BP, blood pressure; DASH, Dietary Approaches to Stop Hypertension.

[a]For overall cardiovascular risk reduction, stop smoking. The effects of implementing these modifications are dose and time dependent and could be greater for some individuals.

[b]One standard drink is defined as 12 oz (355 mL) beer, 5 oz (148 mL) wine, or 1.5 oz (45 mL) 80-proof whiskey.

Pharmacologic Treatment

KEY CONCEPT *An approach to selection of drugs for the treatment of patients with hypertension should be evidence based with considerations regarding the individual's comorbidities, coprescribed medications, and practical patient-specific issues including cost.* The evidence-based guideline by the former JNC 8 panel members[3] and statements from other global organizations recommend drug therapy that is largely grounded in the best available evidence for superiority in outcomes—specifically morbidity and mortality.[2,6] The approach is often tempered with practical considerations related to competing options for specific comorbidities and issues regarding a patient's experience or tolerance for side effects and, in some cases, the cost of medications.

Landmark trials such as the Antihypertensive and Lipid-Lowering Treatment to Prevent Heart Attack Trial (ALLHAT) have provided some objective basis for comparisons between initiating antihypertensive drug therapy with one class of antihypertensives versus another; however, there is room for criticism of these studies.[21,27,28] Consequently, practical interpretations of their conclusions must always leave room for individualization based on clinical judgment. Overall, current clinical guidelines provide a reasonable basis for guiding the selection of drug classes for individuals based on their stage of hypertension, comorbidities, and special circumstances. The following section summarizes key features of specific drug classes and guideline recommendations for patients with hypertension. Finally, an overview of the specific oral antihypertensive drug classes in common use is summarized in Table 5–6.[19,26]

Diuretics

Guidelines advocating for the use of diuretics as initial therapy for uncomplicated patients with hypertension do so based on their practical attributes including cost, availability as combination agents and overall years of experience, as well as favorable outcomes in well-controlled landmark clinical trials for select populations. For example, patients randomized to chlorthalidone, a thiazide-type diuretic, as initial antihypertensive had similar outcomes to those randomized to receive initial therapy with either amlodipine or lisinopril.[21] However, in some cases, differences in outcomes for select secondary end points or special populations demonstrated superiority of chlorthalidone-based therapy over either ACE-I or CCB-based regimens. Criticism of the differential BPs achieved in the various treatment groups, the artificial construct guiding the use of add-on drugs to base therapy, and the overrepresentation of African Americans exhibiting select end points have weakened the interpretability of this trial. Furthermore, other studies have challenged the status of diuretics as an ideal baseline choice for initial antihypertensive drug therapy for all patients[27,28] and even the choice of diuretic used,[29] supporting the debate over whether the means by which BP is lowered (specific drug selected) is more or less important than the extent and/or time taken to lower BP. Nonetheless, diuretics remain supported by many as acceptable baseline initial therapy for hypertensive patients without compelling indications to the contrary.

Key differences in the features of various subtypes of diuretics may also play a role in selection. The four subtypes include thiazides, loop diuretics, potassium-sparing agents, and aldosterone antagonists. The latter will be specifically discussed as a separate entity. Each diuretic subtype has clinically based properties that distinguish their roles in select patient populations. Thiazide diuretics are by far the most commonly prescribed subtype with the greatest number of outcome-based studies supporting their use. In the United States, hydrochlorothiazide and chlorthalidone represent the most commonly prescribed thiazide-type diuretics and have been the subject of most large outcome-based studies. Although subtle differences in pharmacokinetics between these agents exist, practical differences are limited to their relative diuretic potency, with chlorthalidone being considered approximately 1.5 to 2 times more potent than hydrochlorothiazide for BP reduction.[29] Several recent analyses have demonstrated the superiority of chlorthalidone over hydrochlorothiazide,[29] leading some national guidelines to prefer chlorthalidone.[30]

Because the relationship between antihypertensive efficacy and metabolic/electrolyte-related side effects of thiazide diuretics is dose related, attention to the differential in potency may be important. Specifically, select metabolic effects (hyperlipidemic and hyperglycemic) and electrolyte-related effects (hypokalemic, hypomagnesemic, hyperuricemic, and hypercalcemic) increase with higher doses. These metabolic effects may complicate the management of higher risk patients with common comorbidities such as dyslipidemia or diabetes, or even those likely to be sensitive to complications from hyperuricemia and the potassium- or magnesium-wasting effects of diuretics (patients with dysrhythmias or those taking digoxin). Whether presumed thiazide diuretic-induced development of new-onset diabetes is of clinical significance is in question since the ALLHAT and Systolic Hypertension in the Elderly Program (SHEP) showed no significant adverse cardiovascular events from new diuretic-associated diabetes, whereas a smaller trial contradicts this finding.[31] Nonetheless, clinicians should generally not exceed 25 to 50 mg/day of hydrochlorothiazide or 25 mg/day of chlorthalidone.[3] In addition, regardless of the dose used, careful assessment of the potential for metabolic- or electrolyte-based effects is essential. In this way, optimization of BP-lowering potential may be achieved while minimizing potential adverse outcomes.

Additionally, it is important to recognize that when estimated creatinine clearance approaches or is less than 30 mL/min (0.50 mL/s), thiazide diuretics have limited efficacy and loop diuretics may be preferred. Clinicians are advised to reevaluate the use of thiazide diuretics prescribed to individuals whose renal function has been declining with age and whose risk for the consequences of metabolic effects, such as increased uric acid and insulin resistance, may be more significant.[32] Loop diuretics, such as furosemide, bumetanide, torsemide, and ethacrynic acid, have a common site of action in the thick ascending limb of the loop of Henle. As this region reabsorbs over 35% to 45% of filtered sodium, their diuretic efficacy is superior to that of thiazides, potassium-sparing diuretics, and aldosterone antagonists. With the exception of torsemide, which has a longer half-life, the loop diuretics should be administered twice daily versus once when utilized primarily for their antihypertensive (vs diuretic) effect. The most significant adverse effect of loop diuretic use is excessive diuresis leading to hyponatremia or hypotension. Additionally, hypokalemia, hypomagnesemia, and hypocalcemia may develop over time and contribute to the potential for cardiac arrhythmias. Overall, relevance of drug–drug interactions and potential for aggravating select conditions (hyperglycemia, dyslipidemias, and hyperuricemia) should be routinely monitored.[11]

Potassium-sparing diuretics that do not act through mineralocorticoid receptors include triamterene and amiloride. These agents are often prescribed with potassium-wasting diuretics to mitigate potassium losses. When administered as a single entity or as a combination product, these agents result in modest diuresis since they act on the late distal tubule and collecting ducts

Table 5–6

Commonly Used Oral Antihypertensive Drugs by Pharmacologic Class[19,26]

Class	Drug Name and Usual Oral Dosage Range (mg/day)	Select Adverse Events	Comments[a]
Thiazides	Chlorthalidone (Hygroton) 12.5–25 Indapamide (Lozol) 1.25–5 Hydrochlorothiazide 12.5–50 Metolazone (Zaroxolyn) 2.5–5	Hypokalemia and other electrolyte imbalances Negative effect on glucose and lipids	Thiazide diuretics are generally more effective antihypertensive agents than loop diuretics Not first-line agents in pregnancy, but may be used with close monitoring for hypokalemia Monitor electrolytes (ie, decreased serum potassium) and metabolic abnormalities (ie, dyslipidemia, hyperglycemia) Use caution in patients with gout and severe renal impairment Contraindications include hypersensitivity and anuria
Loops	Bumetanide (Bumex) 0.5–2 Furosemide (Lasix) 20–80 Torsemide (Demadex) 2.5–10 Ethacrynic acid (Edecrin) 25–100	Hypokalemia and other electrolyte imbalances	Monitor electrolytes (ie, decreased potassium) and metabolic abnormalities (ie, dyslipidemia, hyperglycemia) Use with caution in patients with gout Contraindications include hypersensitivity, anuria, acute renal insufficiency
Potassium-sparing aldosterone antagonists	Amiloride (Midamor) 5–10 Triamterene (Dyrenium) 50–100 Spironolactone (Aldactone) 25–100 Eplerenone (Inspra) 50–100	Hyperkalemia Gynecomastia (spironolactone) Potassium-sparing diuretics may enhance hyperkalemic effects of drug therapies (eg, ACE inhibitor, aldosterone antagonist)	Monitor electrolytes (ie, potassium) Contraindications include hypersensitivity, acute renal insufficiency, hyperkalemia Eplerenone contraindicated as an antihypertensive in patients with estimated creatinine clearance less than 50 mL/min (0.83 mL/s) or serum creatinine greater than 1.8 mg/dL (159 μmol/L) for women or 2 mg/dL (177 μmol/L) in men as well as type 2 diabetes mellitus with microalbuminuria. Also contraindicated in patients concomitantly receiving strong CYP3A4 inhibitors or a serum potassium greater than 5.0 mEq/L (5.0 mmol/L) at initiation
β-Blocker			
Cardioselective	Atenolol (Tenormin) 25–100 Bisoprolol (Zebeta) 2.5–10 Metoprolol tartrate (Lopressor) 50–100 Metoprolol succinate (Toprol XL) 25–100	Bradycardia Heart block Heart failure Dyspnea, bronchospasm Fatigue, dizziness, lethargy, depression	Caution with heart rate less than 60 and respiratory disease Selectivity of β_1 agents is diminished at higher doses Abrupt discontinuation may cause rebound hypertension May mask signs/symptoms of hypoglycaemia in diabetic patients
Nonselective	Nadolol (Corgard) 20–120 Nebivolol (Bystolic) 5–40 Propranolol (Inderal) 40–160 Propranolol long-acting (Inderal LA, InnoPran XL) 60–180 Timolol (Blocadren) 20–60	Hyper/hypoglycemia, hyperkalemia, hyperlipidemia	Contraindicated in hypersensitivity, sinus node dysfunction or severe sinus bradycardia (in the absence of a pacemaker), heart block (greater than first-degree), cardiogenic shock, acute decompensated heart failure
Mixed α- and β-blocker	Carvedilol (Coreg) 12.5–50 Carvedilol CR (Coreg CR) 20–80 Labetalol (Trandate) 200–800		
CCB			
Nondihydropyridines	Diltiazem long-acting (Cardizem SR, Cardizem CD, others) 180–420 Verapamil sustained-release (Calan SR, Isoptin SR, Verelan) 120–360	Bradycardia, heart block (nondihydropyridines) Constipation (nondihydropyridines) Peripheral edema, headache, flushing	Caution with heart rate < 60 (verapamil, diltiazem) Use caution in concomitant use with β-blocker; may potentiate heart block Extended-release formulations are preferred for once- or twice-daily medication administration
Dihydropyridines	Amlodipine (Norvasc) 2.5–10 Felodipine (Plendil) 2.5–10 Isradipine SR (DynaCirc SR) 1.25–10 Nicardipine SR (Cardene SR) 60–120 Nifedipine long-acting (Adalat CC, Procardia XL) 30–60 Nisoldipine (Sular) 10–40	Gingival hyperplasia (dihydropyridines) Reflex tachycardia (dihydropyridines)	Contraindicated in hypersensitivity, sinus node dysfunction, or severe sinus bradycardia (in the absence of a pacemaker) (nondihydropyridines), heart block (greater than first degree) in the absence of a pacemaker [nondihydropyridines], atrial fibrillation/flutter associated with accessory bypass tract (nondihydropyridines), reduced ejection fraction (most CCBs except amlodipine)

(Continued)

Table 5–6

Commonly Used Oral Antihypertensive Drugs by Pharmacologic Class[19,26] (*Continued*)

Class	Drug Name and Usual Oral Dosage Range (mg/day)	Select Adverse Events	Comments[a]
ACE inhibitors	Benazepril (Lotensin) 10–40 Captopril (Capoten) 25–100 Enalapril (Vasotec) 2.5–40 Fosinopril (Monopril) 10–40 Lisinopril (Prinivil, Zestril) 5–40 Moexipril (Univasc) 7.5–30 Perindopril (Aceon) 4–8 Quinapril (Accupril) 10–80 Ramipril (Altace) 2.5–20 Trandolapril (Mavik) 1–4	Cough Hyperkalemia Renal insufficiency Angioedema	Monitor electrolytes (ie, serum potassium) Monitor renal function Initial dose may be reduced in renal impairment, the elderly, patients who are volume depleted or maintained on diuretic therapy Use with caution in patients with baseline hyperkalemia Contraindicated in pregnancy and hypersensitivity, bilateral renal artery stenosis or unilateral renal artery stenosis in a solitary functional kidney
ARBs	Azilsartan (Edarbi) 40–80 Candesartan (Atacand) 8–32 Eprosartan (Teveten) 400–800 Irbesartan (Avapro) 150–300 Losartan (Cozaar) 25–100 Olmesartan (Benicar) 20–40 Telmisartan (Micardis) 20–80 Valsartan (Diovan) 80–320	Hyperkalemia Renal function deterioration Angioedema Hypotension/syncope	Above comments to ACE inhibitors also apply to ARBs
Direct renin inhibitors	Aliskiren (Tekturna) 150–300	Hyperkalemia Hypotension	Use caution in patients with severe renal impairment and in patients with deteriorating renal function or renal artery stenosis, both bi- and unilateral Contraindicated in combination with ACE-Is or ARBs in patients with diabetes
Central α-2 agonists	Methyldopa 250–1000 Clonidine (Catapres) 0.1–0.8 Clonidine patch (Catapres TTS) 0.1–0.3 Guanabenz 4–32 Guanfacine 1–2	Transient sedation initially Hepatotoxicity, hemolytic anemia, peripheral edema (methyldopa) Orthostatic hypotension (methyldopa, clonidine) Dry mouth, muscle weakness (clonidine)	First-line agent in pregnancy (methyldopa) Tolerance may occur 2–3 months after initiation of methyldopa; increase dose or add diuretic Contraindications include hypersensitivity, concurrent use of MAO inhibitor (methyldopa), hepatic disease [methyldopa], pheochromocytoma (methyldopa)
α-1 Blockers	Doxazosin (Cardura) 1–16 Prazosin (Minipress) 2–20 Terazosin (Hytrin) 1–20	Syncope, dizziness, palpitations, orthostatic hypotension	Contraindicated in hypersensitivity
Direct vasodilator	Isosorbide dinitrate 20 mg and hydralazine 37.5 (BiDil) 1–2 tablets three times a day Hydralazine (Apresoline) 25–100 Minoxidil (Loniten) 2.5–80	Edema, hypertrichosis (minoxidil) Tachycardia Lupus-like syndrome (hydralazine)	Give minoxidil with diuretic and β-blocker to mitigate side effects Contraindicated in hypersensitivity, pheochromocytoma (minoxidil), increased intracranial pressure [isosorbide dinitrate + hydralazine]
Peripheral sympathetic inhibitors	Reserpine 0.05–0.25	Mental depression Orthostatic hypotension Nasal congestion, fluid retention, peripheral edema Diarrhea, increased gastric secretion	Contraindications include hypersensitivity, peptic ulcer disease or ulcerative colitis, history of mental depression or electroconvulsive therapy

ACE, angiotensin-converting enzyme; ARB, angiotensin receptor blocker; MAO, monoamine oxidase

[a]Comments listed are not intended to be inclusive of all adverse effects, monitoring parameters, cautions, or contraindications, and may vary by source.

Data from Lexi-Comp OnlineTM, American Hospital Formulary Service Drug Information OnlineTM, Hudson, Ohio: Lexi-Comp, Inc.; August 29, 2014.

where there exists a limited ability to affect sodium reabsorption. Their most significant risk is the potential to contribute to hyperkalemia. This is especially relevant in the context of those patients with moderate to severe renal impairment or those receiving other agents with potassium-sparing properties, such as ACE-Is, ARBs, and potassium supplements, as well as nonsteroidal anti-inflammatory drugs (NSAIDs).[11]

Aldosterone Antagonists

Aldosterone antagonists such as spironolactone and eplerenone modulate vascular tone through a variety of mechanisms besides diuresis (Figure 5–2). Their potassium-sparing effects mediated through aldosterone antagonism counteract the potassium-wasting effects of other diuretics such as thiazide or loop diuretics. Patients with resistant hypertension (with or without primary aldosteronism) experience significant BP reductions with the addition of low-dose spironolactone (12.5–50 mg/day) to diuretics, ACE-Is, and ARBs.[33] Although a positive attribute, it is important to recognize the risk for hyperkalemia in patients with impaired or fluctuating renal function, or those who are receiving ACE-Is, ARBs, direct renin inhibitors, potassium supplements, potassium-containing salt substitutes, or NSAIDs. In addition, spironolactone is associated with gynecomastia, whereas eplerenone rarely causes this complication, presumably because of its greater specificity than spironolactone to block aldosterone while minimally affecting androgens and progesterone and milder hyperkalemia compared with spironolactone.[2,11]

β-Blockers

Most contemporary guidelines refrain from supporting the use of β-blockers as first-line antihypertensive agents.[2,3,6] The basis of this position varies but often cites studies indicating inferior outcomes[34] and a lack of positive outcomes in elderly patients when compared to other classes of agents. These analyses were conducted with a limited number of β-blockers (usually atenolol), and thus their findings may or may not apply to newer formulations of existing agents (eg, metoprolol succinate) or agents with unique properties such as carvedilol or nebivolol.[34] However, the role of β-blockers in patients with specific select comorbidities is well established (Table 5–7).[19] Specific outcome-based studies conducted in patients with comorbidities such as HF or recent MI have clearly demonstrated a benefit from β-blocker use.[35] Their hemodynamic effects and antiarrhythmic properties make them desirable agents for hypertensive patients who suffer from ischemic conditions including acute coronary syndromes (ACS). The mechanisms through which β-blockers affect BP are complex but most certainly include their modulation of renin, which appears to result in a reduction in CO and/or reduction in PR along with their negative inotropic/chronotropic actions (Figure 5–2).

The specific pharmacologic properties of β-blockers are varied and diverse. An understanding of these properties may assist in the selection of one agent over others given a patient's specific condition(s) or comorbidities. One of these properties is cardioselectivity: the property of some β-blockers that preferentially block β_1-receptor versus β_2-receptor. Some β-blockers exhibit membrane stabilization activity, which relates to the β-blocker's capacity to exhibit certain antiarrhythmic properties. Some β-blockers, as shown in Figure 5–3, possess properties referred to as intrinsic sympathomimetic activity (ISA). β-Blockers possessing this property effectively block the β-receptor at higher circulating catecholamine levels, such as during exercise, while having modest β-blocking activity at times of lower catecholamine levels, such as at rest.[36]

Cardioselectivity represents the most clinically relevant property of β-blockers, but β-blockers with ISA are not recommended for use in the post-ACS patient.[36] With regard to cardioselectivity, consider a patient with asthma, chronic obstructive pulmonary disease, or peripheral vascular disease (intermittent claudication). A β-blocker with relative cardioselectivity to block β_1-receptors may be more desirable in such a patient, whereas a nonselective β-blocker may be potentially disadvantageous. In such a patient, low doses of cardioselective β-blockers may achieve adequate blockade of β_1-receptors in the heart and kidneys while minimizing the undesirable effects of β_2-receptor blockade on the smooth muscle lining the bronchioles. In doing so, hypertension may be managed while avoiding complications of the coexisting reactive airway disease, which is mediated by β_2-receptor stimulation. Similarly, either because of a reduction in the β_2-mediated vascular blood flow or by enhanced unopposed α-agonist–mediated vasoconstriction, a patient with intermittent claudication may experience a worsening of symptoms with use of a nonselective β-blocker (Figure 5–3). It is important to remember that cardioselectivity depends on dose, with diminished selectivity exhibited with higher doses.

A limited number of β-blockers also possess vasodilatory properties that are either mediated through α_1-receptor blockade (carvedilol, labetalol) or via L-arginine/nitric oxide-induced release from endothelial cells, with subsequent increased nitric oxide bioavailability in the endothelium (nebivolol). Although theoretically of benefit, there has been no proven evidence of superior outcomes from use of β-blockers with these vasodilatory properties.

Table 5–7

Compelling Indications for Individual Drug Classes[19]

	Recommended Drug Class						
Compelling Indication	**Diuretic**	**Ald Ant**	**BB**	**CCB**	**ACE-I**	**ARB**	**Dir Vaso**
Heart Failure with Reduced Ejection Fraction	X	X	X		X	X	X
Post-MI		X	X		X		
High Coronary Disease Risk	X		X	X	X		
Diabetes	X		X	X	X	X	
Chronic Kidney Disease					X	X	
Recurrent Stroke Prevention	X				X		
Peripheral Vascular Disease				X			
Isolated Systolic Hypertension	X			X			
Atrial Fibrillation			X	X[a]			

ACE-I, angiotensin-converting enzyme inhibitor; Ald Ant, aldosterone antagonist; ARB, angiotensin receptor blocker; BB, β-blocker; CCB, calcium channel blocking agent; Dir Vaso, direct vasodilator; MI, myocardial Infarction.

[a]nondihydropridine CCBs.

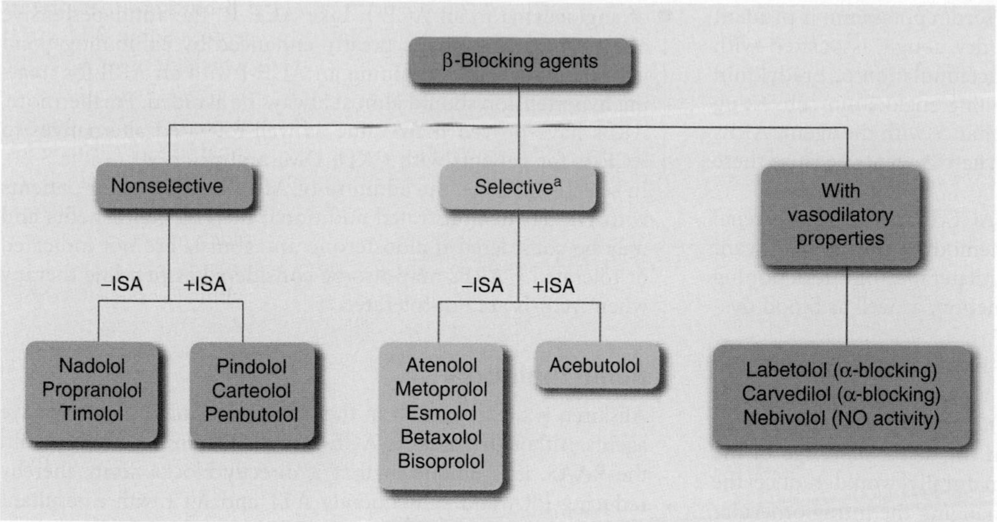

FIGURE 5–3. Flowchart listing various β-blocking agents separated by β-receptor activity and intrinsic sympathomimetic activity. [a]β-1 Cardioselective. (ISA, intrinsic sympathomimetic activity; NO, nitrous oxide.)

The adverse effects of β-blockers logically follow their pharmacology. Their potential to precipitate bradycardia, various degrees of heart block, or signs and symptoms of HF may be of concern to those with a subclinical diagnosis, the elderly or those with reduced left ventricular ejection fraction. Conversely, abrupt discontinuation of β-blockers has been cited as a precipitating factor in the development of ischemic syndromes, especially for those patients in whom β-blockers were used for extended periods of time, at higher doses, or who had underlying ischemic heart disease. In such cases, tapering the dose over a period of several days to perhaps 1 or even 2 weeks is recommended. β-Blocker use in diabetics is usually a complex decision requiring consideration of their consequential effects on insulin, glucose availability, and effects on blocking the signs and symptoms of hypoglycemia against their potential for morbidity/mortality benefits for select candidates with comorbidities such as HFrEF. Lastly, β-blockers, particularly first-generation agents (ie, those other than carvedilol, nebivolol) have a greater effect on glucose metabolism as well as other metabolic effects, and they should be used cautiously if at all with diuretics unless compelling indications exist for both.

Calcium Channel Blockers

Exhibiting considerable interclass diversity, CCBs are recognized as effective antihypertensives, particularly in the elderly.[2] Although the Valsartan Antihypertensive Long-term Use Evaluation (VALUE) trial,[28] which compared valsartan-based with amlodipine-based therapy, failed to achieve its primary end point of cardiac morbidity and mortality, the more pronounced early BP-lowering effect of amlodipine may have conferred a benefit in regards to some secondary end points (stroke and MI). In addition, in the Anglo-Scandinavian Cardiac Outcomes Trial-Blood Pressure Lowering Arm (ASCOT-BPLA),[27] which compared amlodipine-based versus atenolol-based therapy, achievement of greater BP-lowering with amlodipine-based therapy appeared to confer protection against stroke and MI in hypertensive patients. These two trials provide evidence that regardless of the agents used, event reduction may be more strongly associated with achieved BP than the specific agents or combinations of agents used to achieve it.

The diversity of pharmacologic properties among the subclasses of CCBs is significant and categorizes their expected effects on the cardiovascular system and potential risk of toxicities. Dihydropyridine CCBs such as nifedipine and amlodipine are commonly associated with edema, especially when used at higher doses. Nondihydropyridine CCBs such as verapamil and diltiazem are recognized for their electrophysiological effects, negative chronotropic effects, and negative inotropic effects. These pharmacologic properties may be exploited for their specific clinical utility. Given that verapamil and diltiazem effectively block cardiac conduction through the atrioventricular node, their value in the management of patients with atrial fibrillation in addition to hypertension is obvious, whereas secondary to their negative inotropic effects, they should be avoided in patients with reduced ejection fraction. In contrast, the dihydropyridine subclass of agents has no utility in managing atrial dysrhythmias but may be used safely (exception being nifedipine) in patients with reduced ejection fraction. Similarly, all CCBs possess some coronary vasodilating properties and, therefore, may be used in select patients for the management of patients with angina, in addition to their antihypertensive benefits.[11]

ACE Inhibitors

ACE-Is have been extensively studied for the treatment of hypertension, and outcome-based trials generally support their use for a wide array of patients, especially with select comorbidities. These compelling indications include their qualified role in managing patients with hypertension who have type 1 or 2 DM, HF, prior-MI, CKD, or recurrent stroke prevention.[6] Comparative trials between ACE-Is and diuretics as initial drug therapy have demonstrated diuretics may be superior to ACE-Is in regard to combined incidence of new onset CVD and HF (ALLHAT),[21] but diuretics and ACE-Is may be similar in overall outcomes.[37] As such, it is reasonable to conclude that both diuretics and ACE-Is represent appropriate choices as either first- or second-line hypertensive therapies that effectively achieve a target BP goal for most patients with or without comorbidities.

Although generally well tolerated, ACE-Is are associated with two hallmark side effects: hyperkalemia and a persistent dry cough. Modest elevations in serum potassium should be anticipated when starting or increasing the dose of an ACE-I, particularly in patients with compromised renal function, those receiving concurrent NSAIDs, those taking potassium supplementation, or those using a potassium-containing salt substitute. Hyperkalemia is rarely a reason for discontinuation of therapy.

Nonetheless, periodic monitoring of serum potassium is prudent for patients receiving ACE-Is. The dry cough associated with ACE-Is is thought to be caused by accumulation of bradykinin resulting from a direct effect of inhibiting angiotensin-converting enzyme. If a cough jeopardizes compliance with the agent, ARBs should be considered as possible alternative agents because there is less incidence of cough.

Less common adverse effects of ACE-Is include acute renal failure, particularly in patients with hemodynamically significant bilateral renal artery stenosis (or unilateral if one functioning kidney) or preexisting kidney dysfunction, as well as blood dyscrasias and angioedema.

In general, the effects of ACE-Is on renal function and potassium can be predicted given an understanding of their pharmacologic actions (Figure 5–2). Inhibition of angiotensin II synthesis through ACE inhibition (or direct blockage of the angiotensin II receptor by ARBs) naturally would reduce the efferent renal artery tone, thereby changing the intraglomerular pressure. Although changes in the afferent renal artery tone also occur, the overall effects usually produce a reduction in glomerular filtration rate (GFR), with resulting elevations of up to 30% in serum creatinine values.[11] Such elevations in serum creatinine are not usually indications to discontinue use of the ACE-I; however, continued monitoring for further increases in serum creatinine and consideration of dose reduction remains prudent. Alternatively, should elevations in serum creatinine exceed 30%, dose reduction or discontinuation is warranted until further evaluation can be made.

Angiotensin Receptor Blockers

ARBs are inhibitors of the angiotensin-1 (AT1) receptors (Figure 5–2). AT1 receptor stimulation evokes a pressor response via a host of accompanying effects on catecholamines, aldosterone, and thirst.[11] Consequently, inhibition of AT1 receptors directly prevents this pressor response and results in upregulation of the RAAS. Upregulation of the RAAS results in elevated levels of angiotensin II, which have the added effect of stimulating the angiotensin-2 (AT2) receptors. AT2-receptor stimulation is generally associated with antihypertensive activity; however, long-term effects of AT2-receptor stimulation that involve cellular growth and repair are relatively unknown. While the pharmacologic differences between ARBs and ACE-Is are clear, the therapeutic relevance resulting from these differences remains ambiguous. Previously, the clinical benefits of ARBs were considered less robust as compared to ACE-Is, but the Ongoing Telmisartan Alone and in Combination with Ramipril Global End-point Trial (ONTARGET) has demonstrated that in high-risk patients, telmisartan is noninferior to ramipril for the reduction of death from cardiovascular causes, MI, stroke, or hospitalization for HF.[38] This study also demonstrated that an ACE-I in combination with an ARB reduces proteinuria to a greater extent than either agent as monotherapy but increases the composite of dialysis, doubling of serum creatinine, and death.[39] Although better tolerated than ACE-Is, ARBs have not been shown to demonstrate superiority of outcomes relative to ACE-Is.

At this point, ARBs have emerged as an effective class of antihypertensives whose low incidence of side effects and demonstrated clinical role in patients with specific comorbidities have afforded them an attractive position in the antihypertensive armamentarium. However, as with ACE-Is, patients may develop angioedema and, although estimates of cross-reactivity are reportedly low,[40] one should always exercise caution when considering the use of an ARB in a patient with a known history of angioedema to an ACE-I. Like ACE-Is, the antihypertensive effectiveness of ARBs is greatly enhanced by combining them with diuretics, but combining an ACE-I with an ARB for treating hypertension should almost always be avoided. Furthermore, ARBs have proven their value as well-tolerated alternatives to ACE-Is for patients with CKD, DM, and prior MI (Table 5–7). In select situations, the addition of ARBs to ACE-Is for patients with HF has demonstrated additional incremental benefits and may be considered if aldosterone antagonists are not indicated or tolerated.[40] ARBs may also be considered as first line therapy when ACE-Is are not tolerated.[40]

Renin Inhibitors

Aliskiren is the first agent in the newest class of antihypertensive agents. Although similar to ACE-Is and ARBs in that it acts within the RAAS, it is unique in that it directly blocks renin, thereby reducing PRA and subsequently AT1 and AT2 with a resultant reduction in BP. This disruption of the negative feedback loop results in a compensatory increase in pro-renin and renin levels, the significance of which is not well established. Aliskiren has been shown to be well tolerated and effective in reducing BP when used as monotherapy and in combination with other antihypertensive agents, including thiazide diuretics, ARBs, and CCBs.[6] However, long-term clinical trials evaluating efficacy and safety have not been completed, and thus the effects of aliskiren on morbidity and mortality are as yet unknown. Additionally, the Aliskiren Trial In Type 2 Diabetes Using Cardio-renal End points (ALTITUDE), which compared ACE-I or ARB monotherapy to that in combination with alkiskiren, was stopped prematurely as the combination therapy did not reduce cardiovascular end points.[41] With this

Patient Encounter 2

A 48-year-old Hispanic male returns to your clinic for a follow-up visit. His seated BP measurements are 156/92 mm Hg and 150/88 mm Hg. His heart rate is 52 beats/min. He is currently on metoprolol tartrate 100 mg twice daily, chlorthalidone 12.5 mg once daily, and amlodipine 10 mg daily. He states that he has been adherent with all medication. He smokes one pack per day of cigarettes and consumes 3 to 4 beers several times a week. He is overweight, does not exercise, and consumes mostly processed and/or fast foods. Past medical history is significant for prior MI, hypertension and osteoarthritis. Physical examination was unremarkable. Laboratory values were significant for serum creatinine of 0.8 mg/dL (71 μmol/L), a potassium level of 3.4 mEq/L (3.4 mmol/L), fasting glucose of 120 mg/dL (6.7 mmol/L) total cholesterol of 170 mg/dL (4.40 mmol/L), HDL cholesterol of 40 mg/dL (1.03 mmol/L), triglyceride level of 125 mg/dL (1.41 mmol/L), and calculated LDL cholesterol of 105 mg/dL (2.72 mmol/L).

Based on the information provided, does the patient have resistant hypertension?

Based on the information presented, create a care plan for this patient's hypertension. This should include (a) goals of therapy, (b) a patient-specific therapeutic plan, and (c) a plan for appropriate monitoring to achieve goals and avoid adverse effects.

evidence, and the results of the ONTARGET trial, combining two or more RAAS blocking agents (ACE-Is, ARBs, and renin inhibitor) for the treatment of hypertension is not recommended.[39,41] Because of aliskiren's role in the RAAS, recommendations and precautions for monitoring serum potassium and kidney function should be similar to those of ACE-Is and ARBs.

α-Blockers

Generally, α_1-blockers are considered inferior agents and should not be used as monotherapy. The ALLHAT trial discontinued the α_1-blocker arm prematurely because doxazosin was associated with an increase in cardiovascular events.[21] However, α_1-blockers may be considered as add-on therapy to other agents (eg, fourth or fifth line) when hypertension is not adequately controlled. In addition, they may have a specific role in the antihypertensive regimen for elderly men with prostatism; however, their use is often curtailed by complaints of syncope, dizziness, or palpitations following the first dose and orthostatic hypotension with chronic use. The roles of doxazosin, terazosin, and prazosin in management of patients with hypertension are limited due to the paucity of outcome data and absence of a unique role for special populations or compelling indications.[6]

Central α_2-Agonists

Limited by their tendency to cause orthostasis, sedation, dry mouth, and vision disturbances, clonidine, methyldopa, guanfacine, and guanabenz represent rare choices in contemporary treatment of patients with hypertension. Their central α_2-adrenergic stimulation is thought to reduce sympathetic outflow and enhance parasympathetic activity, thereby reducing heart rate, CO, and total PR. Occasionally used for cases of resistant hypertension, these agents may have a role when other more conventional therapies appear ineffective. The availability of a transdermal clonidine patch applied once weekly may offer an alternative to hypertensive patients with adherence problems. Of particular importance is the issue of severe rebound hypertension when clonidine is abruptly discontinued. The dose of this agent should be gradually reduced when being discontinued. In patients concurrently taking a β-blocker, the β-blocker should be tapered to discontinuation first, ideally several days before initiating the clonidine taper. Because clonidine withdrawal results in an increase in SNS activity, patients withdrawing from clonidine while on a β-blocker could experience unbalanced α-mediated vasoconstriction.[11]

Other Agents

Direct vasodilators such as hydralazine and minoxidil represent alternative agents used for patients with resistant hypertension. They primarily act to relax smooth muscles in arterioles and activate baroreceptors. Because of the reflex tachycardia and fluid retention they cause, their use in the absence of concurrently administered β-blockers and diuretics is uncommon. Rare adverse effects include hydralazine-induced lupus-like syndrome and hypertrichosis from minoxidil. References describing the appropriate use and monitoring of these infrequently used agents should be consulted before use.[11] Finally, reserpine, although slow to act, reduces sympathetic tone and thus PR by depleting norepinephrine from sympathetic nerve endings. Although included in the SHEP and ALLHAT trials,[21,42] reserpine's numerous side effects, including gastric ulceration, depression, and sexual side effects, have limited its utility. Two additional agents, guanethidine and guanadrel, act as postganglionic sympathetic inhibitors inhibiting the release of norepinephrine as well as depleting norepinephrine from these nerve terminals. However, these agents have little role in the management of hypertension because of significant adverse effects.[11]

SPECIAL PATIENT POPULATIONS

Compelling Indications and Special Considerations

KEY CONCEPT *Specific antihypertensive therapy is warranted for certain patients with comorbid conditions that may elevate their level of risk for CVD.* Clinical conditions and patient factors for which there is compelling evidence supporting one or more classes of drug therapy include:

- Ischemic heart disease
- HFrEF
- Diabetes
- CKD
- Cerebrovascular disease
- Age 60 years or older
- Race

Compelling indications for specific drug therapies are summarized in Table 5–7.[2] The basis for their recommendations for select patient populations may follow their pharmacology and, in some cases, evidence of specific value in select patient populations. For example, in patients with hypertension and angina, β-blockers and long-acting CCBs are indicated due to their antihypertensive and antianginal effects. β-Blockers and ACE-Is are indicated for post-MI patients due to their proven reduction of cardiovascular morbidity/mortality in this population. Aldosterone antagonists are also indicated for the post-MI patient with reduced ejection fraction and either diabetes or symptoms of HF.[40]

Patients with reduced ejection fraction and hypertension should be treated with β-blockers, ACE-Is, ARBs, or aldosterone antagonists as each have evidence supporting their morbidity/mortality benefits for such patients. In contrast, diuretics are

Patient Encounter 3

A 65-year-old black male patient with history of hypertension, gout, and CKD presents to clinic for his annual exam. Upon reviewing his medication history you see the patient has been taking hydrochlorothiazide 25 mg daily and allopurinol 100 mg daily. Physical exam is unremarkable. Laboratory values are remarkable for potassium 3.4 mEq/L (3.4 mmol/L), serum creatinine 1.2 mg/dL (106 μmol/L), serum uric acid 7.5 mg/dL (446 μmol/L), and proteinuria 600 mg/24hrs (0.6 g/day). Patient's average seated BP was 148/94 mm Hg with HR of 78 beats/min.

Based on the Evidence-Based Guidelines by the former JNC 8 Panel, is this patient achieving his blood pressure goal?

What therapeutic options would you explore given the patient's BP, laboratory values, and medical history?

How would you assess the effectiveness of your therapeutic recommendation for this patient?

Table 5–8

Parenteral Antihypertensive Agents for Hypertensive Emergency[a]

Drug	Dose Range	Onset of Action	Duration of Action	Adverse Effects[b]	Special Indications
Vasodilators					
Sodium nitroprusside	0.25–10 mcg/kg/min as IV infusion[c]	Immediate	1–2 minutes	Nausea, vomiting, muscle twitching, sweating, thiocyanate and cyanide intoxication	Most hypertensive emergencies; use with caution with high intracranial pressure or azotemia
Nicardipine hydrochloride	5–15 mg/hour IV	5–10 minutes	15–30 minutes, may exceed 4 hours	Tachycardia, headache, flushing, local phlebitis	Most hypertensive emergencies except acute heart failure; use with caution with coronary ischemia
Fenoldopam mesylate	0.1–0.3 mcg/kg/min as IV infusion[c]	< 5 minutes	30 minutes	Tachycardia, headache, nausea, flushing	Most hypertensive emergencies; use with caution with glaucoma
Nitroglycerin	5–100 mcg/kg/min as IV infusion	2–5 minutes	5–10 minutes	Headache, vomiting, methemoglobinemia, tolerance with prolonged use	Coronary ischemia
Enalaprilat	1.25–5 mg every 6 hours IV	15–30 minutes	6–12 hours	Precipitous fall in pressure in high-renin states; variable response	Acute left ventricular failure; avoid in acute MI
Hydralazine hydrochloride	10–20 mg IV 10–40 mg IM	10–20 minutes 20–30 minutes	1–4 hours IV 4–6 hours IM	Tachycardia, flushing, headache, vomiting, aggravation of angina	Eclampsia
Clevidipine	1–21 mg/hour IV	2–4 minutes	5–15 minutes	Atrial fibrillation, fever, insomnia, nausea, headache, vomiting, post-procedural hemorrhage, acute renal failure, respiratory failure	*Caution*: Avoid use if hypersensitivity to soy or egg products, pathologic hyperlipidemia, lipoid nephrosis, or acute pancreatitis if accompanied by hyperlipidemia, severe aortic stenosis exists
Diazoxide	1–3 mg/kg or 50–100 mg every 5–15 minutes	2 minutes	3–12 hours	Hyperglycemia, sodium and water retention	Preeclampsia, eclampsia, impaired renal function
Furosemide	10–40 mg/hour IV, maximum 80–160 mg/hour IV	5 minutes	2 hours	Hypotension, electrolyte abnormalities, hearing impairment	Heart failure, fluid overload, adjunct therapy to vasodilators
Adrenergic inhibitors					
Labetalol hydrochloride	20–80 mg IV bolus every 10 minutes	5–10 minutes	3–6 hours	Vomiting, scalp tingling, dizziness, bronchoconstriction, nausea, heart block, orthostatic hypotension	Most hypertensive emergencies, pregnancy except acute heart failure
Esmolol hydrochloride	250–500 mcg/kg/min IV bolus, then 50–100 mcg/kg/min by infusion; may repeat bolus after 5 minutes or increase infusion to 300 mcg/min	1–2 minutes	10–30 minutes	Hypotension, nausea, asthma, first-degree heart block, heart failure	Aortic dissection, perioperative
Phentolamine	5–15 mg IV bolus	1–2 minutes	10–30 minutes	Tachycardia, flushing, headache	Catecholamine excess

IM, intramuscular; IV, intravenous; MI, myocardial infarction.

[a]These doses may vary from those in the *Physicians' Desk Reference*.

[b]Hypotension may occur with all agents.

[c]Requires special delivery system.

Adapted from Saseen JJ, Maclaughlin EJ. Hypertension. In: DiPiro JT, Talbert RL, Yee GC, et al, eds. Pharmacotherapy: A Pathophysiologic Approach, 8th ed. New York, NY: McGraw-Hill, 2011:131, with permission.

recommended in HF patients with evidence of volume overload for symptom relief. African Americans with HFrEF are ideal candidates for combination therapy with isosorbide dinitrate and hydralazine based on morbidity and mortality benefits and their beneficial effects on lowering BP.[40] The dihydropyridine CCBs amlodipine or felodipine may be used in patients with HFrEF for uncontrolled BP; however, they offer no beneficial effect on morbidity and mortality and may increase the risk of edema.[40] For patients with HF with preserved ejection fraction (HFpEF), use of select CCB is not discouraged.[40] In summary, antihypertensive therapies beneficial for patients with concurrent HFrEF include diuretics, β-blockers, ACE-Is, ARBs, and possibly amlodipine to control BP.

According to evidence-based guidelines by the former JNC 8 panel,[3] patients with diabetes and hypertension without CKD (regardless of age) represent a target population whose initial drug therapy depends on if they are Black or non-Black. Specifically, Black patients with diabetes and no CKD should be treated initially with thiazide-type diuretics or CCBs alone or in combination. Non-Black patients with diabetes and no CKD, are candidates for the same starting therapies but with expanded options to include ACE-Is or ARBs.

In patients with CKD and hypertension (regardless of age or presence of diabetes), ACE-Is and ARBs alone or in combination with other agents are preferred.[3] ACE-Is in combination with a thiazide diuretic are also preferred in patients with a history of prior stroke or transient ischemic attack. This therapy reduces the risk of recurrent stroke, making it particularly attractive in these patients for BP control.

The target for BP in patients 60 years and older remains highly debated with the release of the evidence-based guidelines by the former JNC 8 panel members[3] who recommend a systolic BP target less than 150 mm Hg for this population. This relaxed BP goal triggered a spiral of critics indicating the possibility of increasing the risk for cardiovascular events and accelerating the development of CKD.[43] The post-hoc analysis of the International Verapamil-Trandolapril Study (INVEST) trial has shown that hypertensive patients 60 years of age or older with coronary artery disease (CAD) had higher risk of cardiovascular mortality achieving SBP less than 150 to 140 mm Hg compared to SBP less than 140 mm Hg.[44] However, the implications of the INVEST trial should be judiciously analyzed given the study's primary design and main objective.[45]

There are several situations in the management of hypertension requiring special considerations including, but not limited to:

- Hypertensive crisis
- Elderly populations
- Isolated systolic hypertension
- CAD
- Minority populations
- Pregnancy
- Pediatrics

Hypertensive crisis can be divided into hypertensive emergencies and hypertensive urgencies. A hypertensive emergency occurs when severe elevations in BP are accompanied by acute or life-threatening target organ damage such as ACS, unstable angina, encephalopathy, intracerebral hemorrhage, acute left ventricular failure with pulmonary edema, dissecting aortic aneurysm, rapidly progressive renal failure, accelerated malignant hypertension with papilledema, and eclampsia, among others. BP is generally greater than 180/120 mm Hg, although a hypertensive emergency can occur at lower levels, particularly in individuals without previous hypertension. The goal in a hypertensive emergency is to reduce mean arterial pressure by up to 25% to the range of 160/100 to 110 mm Hg in minutes to hours.[19] Intravenous (IV) therapy is generally required and may consist of the agents listed in Table 5–8. A hypertensive urgency is manifested as a severe elevation in SBP greater than 179 mm Hg and DBP greater than 109 mm Hg without evidence of acute or life-threatening target organ damage.[46] In these individuals, BP can usually be managed with orally administered short-acting medications (ie, captopril, clonidine, or labetalol) and observation in the emergency department over several hours, with subsequent discharge on oral medications and follow-up in the outpatient setting within 24 hours.[19,46]

The treatment of elderly patients (greater than or equal to 65 years of age) with hypertension, as well as those with isolated systolic hypertension, should follow the same approach as with other populations with the exception that lower starting doses may be warranted to avoid adverse effects. Special attention should be paid to postural hypotension. This should include a careful assessment of orthostatic symptoms, measurement of BP in the upright position upon standing for 1 to 3 minutes, and caution to avoid volume depletion and rapid titration of antihypertensive therapy.[19] The general recommended BP goal in uncomplicated hypertension in the very elderly is less than 150/90 mm Hg.[2,3] However, it is unclear whether the target SBP should be the same in those older than 80 years, and an achieved SBP of 140 to 145 mm Hg, if tolerated, can be acceptable, as well as attempts to avoid SBP of less than 130 mm Hg and a DBP of less than 65 mm Hg.[32] The Hypertension in the Very Elderly Trial (HYVET) documented the benefits of antihypertensive therapy in patients older than 80 years because they experienced a significant reduction in all-cause mortality, fatal stroke, and HF when treated with a diuretic (indapamide) with or without an ACE-I (Perindopril) to a target SBP of less than 150 mm Hg.[47] In individuals with isolated systolic hypertension, the optimal level of diastolic pressure is not known, and although treated patients who achieve diastolic pressures less than 60 to 70 mm Hg had poorer outcomes in a landmark trial, their cardiovascular event rate was still lower than those receiving placebo.[32] While the treatment approach of hypertension in minority populations is similar, special consideration should be paid to socioeconomic and lifestyle factors that may be important barriers to BP control. In addition, in patients of African origin, diminished BP responses have been seen with ACE-Is and ARBs compared with diuretics or CCBs.[19]

Hypertension in pregnancy is a major cause of maternal, fetal, and neonatal morbidity and mortality. There are four different categories of hypertension in pregnancy: preexisting chronic hypertension, gestational hypertension, preeclampsia-eclampsia, and preeclampsia superimposed on chronic hypertension, which are treated slightly differently. The therapeutic selection of an oral antihypertensive agent in a pregnant patient with chronic hypertension is summarized in Table 5–9. Also refer to the American College of Obstetricians and Gynecologists task force on hypertension in pregnancy article for detailed therapeutic options for acute severe hypertension in preeclampsia.[48]

In children and adolescents, three or more BP readings are compared with tables listing the 90th, 95th, and 99th percentile for BPs based on age, height, and gender that classify BP as normal, prehypertension, and stage 1 and stage 2 hypertension.[49] The prevalence of hypertension in adolescent populations is increasing and associated with obesity, sedentary lifestyle, or a positive family history, which increases the risk of CVD. The

Table 5–9

Treatment of Chronic Hypertension in Pregnancy[19,48]

Agent	Comments
Methyldopa	Preferred first-line therapy on the basis of long-term follow-up studies supporting safety after exposure in utero. Surveillance data do not support an association between drug and congenital defects when the mother took the drug early in the first trimester
Labetalol	Increasingly preferred to methyldopa because of reduced side effects. The agent does not seem to pose a risk to the fetus, except possibly in the first trimester
β-Blockers	Generally acceptable on the basis of limited data. Reports of intrauterine growth restriction with atenolol in the first and second trimesters
Clonidine	Limited data; no association between drug and congenital defects when the mother took the drug early in the first trimester, but number of exposures is small
Calcium channel antagonists	Limited data; nifedipine in the first trimester was not associated with increased rates of major birth defects, but animal data were associated with fetal hypoxemia and acidosis. This agent should probably be limited to mothers with severe hypertension
Diuretics	Not first-line agents; probably safe; available data suggest that throughout gestation, a diuretic is not associated with an increased risk of major fetal anomalies or adverse fetal-neonatal events
Angiotensin-converting enzyme inhibitors and angiotensin II receptor antagonists	Contraindicated; reported fetal toxicity and death

clinician should be aware that secondary causes are common in adolescents with hypertension and the identification and aggressive modification of risk factors with nonpharmacologic and pharmacologic interventions is paramount for risk reduction of target organ damage. The 2004 National High Blood Pressure Education Program (NHBPEP) Working Group Report on Hypertension in Children and Adolescents provides specific recommendations to modify and treat risk factors in this population of patients. The *Nelson Textbook of Pediatrics* is also recommended for a comprehensive review of treatment of congenital and pediatric hypertension, which is beyond the scope of this chapter.[50]

OUTCOME EVALUATION

- Short-term goals are to achieve reduction in BP safely through the iterative process of using pharmacologic therapy, along with nonpharmacologic therapy or lifestyle changes.

Patient Care Process

Patient Assessment:

- Measure BP. Evaluate both office and home BP readings. Consider the use of 24-hour ABPM or AOBP monitoring as described previously.
- Identify if the patient is experiencing signs or symptoms of elevated BP and comorbidities that may alter approach to treatment. (See Clinical Presentation and Diagnosis of Primary Hypertension.)
- Perform a detailed medication reconciliation including over-the-counter medications and supplements. Inquire about allergies and previous adverse drug reactions.
- Evaluate laboratory values, serum electrolytes, renal function, and target organ damage.

Therapy Evaluation:

- If patient is not currently on an antihypertensive regimen, determine if immediate initiation of antihypertensive pharmacotherapy is warranted. Figure 5–1 presents the recommendations from the ASH/ISH, but guidelines from other organizations may be considered as well.[2,3,6,30]
- If patient is already receiving pharmacotherapy but BP is not at target despite pharmacotherapy, evaluate current antihypertensive regimen regarding efficacy, safety, and patient adherence.
- Evaluate patient's lifestyle factors as well as possible drug causes of elevated BP.
- Determine whether the patient has prescription coverage.

Care Plan Development:

- Select lifestyle modifications (Table 5–5) and antihypertensive therapy (Table 5–6) that are likely to be effective and safe.
- Determine whether drug doses are optimal (Table 5–6). Use combination therapy when appropriate to take advantage of complementary mechanisms of action and to reduce side effects.
- Address any patient concerns about hypertension and its management.
- Discuss the importance of medication adherence and lifestyle modifications to reduce BP.

Follow-up Evaluation:

The frequency of follow-up visits for patients with hypertension varies but is influenced by the severity of hypertension, comorbidities, and choice of agent selected.

- At a minimum, assessment of response to medications should be done at 1-month intervals.[3] In patients with stage 2 hypertension or those with comorbidities (eg, diabetes, vascular disease, HF, or CKD), shorter time frame of less than or equal to 2 weeks is more appropriate.[2]
- Once BP is controlled, annual or semiannual monitoring of serum biochemistries such as serum creatinine or potassium are recommended, unless more frequent follow-up is indicated based on comorbidities.

- Lifestyle changes should address risk factors for CVD including obesity, physical inactivity, insulin resistance, dyslipidemia, smoking cessation, and others.
- Monitoring for efficacy, adverse events, and adherence to therapy is key to achieving the long-term goals of reducing the risk of morbidity and mortality associated with CVD.

Abbreviations Introduced in This Chapter

ABPM	Ambulatory blood pressure monitoring
ACE-I	Angiotensin-converting enzyme inhibitor
ACR	Albumin-to-creatinine ratio
ACS	Acute coronary syndromes
ALLHAT	Antihypertensive and Lipid-Lowering Treatment to Prevent Heart Attack Trial
ALTITUDE	Aliskiren Trial In Type 2 Diabetes Using Cardio-renal End points
AOBP	Ambulatory office-based blood pressure
ARB	Angiotensin receptor blocker
ASCOT-BPLA	Anglo-Scandinavian Cardiac Outcomes Trial-Blood Pressure Lowering Arm
ASH	American Society of Hypertension
AT1	Angiotensin-1
AT2	Angiotensin-2
BP	Blood pressure
CAD	Coronary artery disease
CCB	Calcium channel blocker
CKD	Chronic kidney disease
CO	Cardiac output
CVD	Cardiovascular disease
DASH	Dietary Approaches to Stop Hypertension
DBP	Diastolic blood pressure
DM	Diabetes Mellitus
GFR	Glomerular filtration rate
HAART	Highly active antiretroviral therapy
HBP	Home blood pressure
HF	Heart failure
HFpEF	Heart failure with preserved ejection fraction
HFrEF	Heart failure with reduced ejection fraction
HYVET	Hypertension in the Very Elderly Trial
IM	Intramuscular
INVEST	International Verapamil-Trandolapril Study
ISA	Intrinsic sympathomimetic activity
ISH	International Society of Hypertension
IV	Intravenous
JNC 8	Eighth Joint National Committee
MAPEC	Monitorización ambulatoria para predicción de eventos cardiovasculares; translated to English, Ambulatory blood pressure monitoring for prediction of cardiovascular events
MI	Myocardial infarction
NHBPEP	National High Blood Pressure Education Program
NSAID	Nonsteroidal anti-inflammatory drug
ONTARGET	Ongoing Telmisartan Alone and in combination with Ramipril Global Endpoint Trial
PR	Peripheral resistance
PRA	Plasma renin activity
RAAS	Renin-angiotensin-aldosterone system
SBP	Systolic blood pressure
SHEP	Systolic Hypertension in the Elderly Program
SNS	Sympathetic nervous system
VALUE	Valsartan Antihypertensive Long-term Use Evaluation

REFERENCES

1. Go AS, Mozaffarian D, Roger VL, et al. Heart disease and stroke statistics—2014 update: a report from the American Heart Association. Circulation. Jan 21 2014;129(3):e28–e292.
2. Weber MA, Schiffrin EL, White WB, et al. Clinical practice guidelines for the management of hypertension in the community: a statement by the American Society of Hypertension and the International Society of Hypertension. J Clin Hypertens (Greenwich). Jan 2014;16(1):14–26.
3. James PA, Oparil S, Carter BL, et al. 2014 evidence-based guideline for the management of high blood pressure in adults: report from the panel members appointed to the Eighth Joint National Committee (JNC 8). JAMA. Feb 5 2014;311(5):507–520.
4. Laragh JH, Sealey JE. The plasma renin test reveals the contribution of body sodium-volume content (V) and renin-angiotensin (R) vasoconstriction to long-term blood pressure. Am J Hypertens. Nov 2011;24(11):1164–1180.
5. O'Brien E, Parati G, Stergiou G, et al. European Society of Hypertension position paper on ambulatory blood pressure monitoring. J Hypertens. Sep 2013;31(9):1731–1768.
6. Mancia G, Fagard R, Narkiewicz K, et al. 2013 ESH/ESC Guidelines for the management of arterial hypertension: the Task Force for the management of arterial hypertension of the European Society of Hypertension (ESH) and of the European Society of Cardiology (ESC). J Hypertens. Jul 2013;31(7):1281–1357.
7. Parra D, Hough A. Current therapeutic approaches to cardio-protection in hypertension. Curr Hypertens Rep. Aug 2014;16(8):457.
8. Wright JT, Jr, Fine LJ, Lackland DT, Ogedegbe G, Dennison Himmelfarb CR. Evidence supporting a systolic blood pressure goal of less than 150 mm Hg in patients aged 60 years or older: the minority view. Ann Intern Med. Apr 1 2014;160(7):499–503.
9. Global Status Report on Noncommunicable Diseases 2010, 1st ed. World Health Organization, 2011.
10. Lim SS, Vos T, Flaxman AD, et al. A comparative risk assessment of burden of disease and injury attributable to 67 risk factors and risk factor clusters in 21 regions, 1990-2010: a systematic analysis for the Global Burden of Disease Study 2010. Lancet. Dec 15 2012;380(9859):2224–2260.
11. Victor RG, Kaplan NM. Kaplan's clinical hypertension. 10th ed. Philadelphia, PA: Wollters Kluwer Lippincott Williams & Wilkins Health; 2010.
12. Calhoun DA, Jones D, Textor S, et al. Resistant hypertension: diagnosis, evaluation, and treatment: a scientific statement from the American Heart Association Professional Education Committee of the Council for High Blood Pressure Research. Circulation. Jun 24 2008;117(25):e510–e526.
13. Grossman E, Messerli FH. Drug-induced hypertension: an unappreciated cause of secondary hypertension. Am J Med. Jan 2012;125(1):14–22.
14. Kloner RA, Rezkalla SH. To drink or not to drink? That is the question. Circulation. Sep 11 2007;116(11):1306–1317.
15. Mozaffarian D, Fahimi S, Singh GM, et al. Global sodium consumption and death from cardiovascular causes. N Engl J Med. Aug 14 2014;371(7):624–634.
16. Franco V, Oparil S. Salt sensitivity, a determinant of blood pressure, cardiovascular disease and survival. J Am Coll Nutr. Jun 2006;25(3 Suppl):247S–255S.

17. Obarzanek E, Proschan MA, Vollmer WM, et al. Individual blood pressure responses to changes in salt intake: results from the DASH-Sodium trial. Hypertension. Oct 2003;42(4):459–467.
18. Mente A, O'Donnell MJ, Rangarajan S, et al. Association of urinary sodium and potassium excretion with blood pressure. N Engl J Med. Aug 14 2014;371(7):601–611.
19. Chobanian AV, Bakris GL, Black HR, et al. Seventh report of the Joint National Committee on Prevention, Detection, Evaluation, and Treatment of High Blood Pressure. Hypertension. Dec 2003;42(6):1206–1252.
20. Pickering TG, Hall JE, Appel LJ, et al. Recommendations for blood pressure measurement in humans and experimental animals: part 1: blood pressure measurement in humans: a statement for professionals from the subcommittee of professional and public education of the american heart association council on high blood pressure research. Circulation. Feb 8 2005;111(5): 697–716.
21. Major outcomes in high-risk hypertensive patients randomized to angiotensin-converting enzyme inhibitor or calcium channel blocker vs diuretic: The Antihypertensive and Lipid-Lowering Treatment to Prevent Heart Attack Trial (ALLHAT). JAMA. 2002;288(23):2981–2997.
22. Hermida RC, Ayala DE, Mojon A, Fernandez JR. Influence of circadian time of hypertension treatment on cardiovascular risk: results of the MAPEC study. Chronobiol Int. Sep 2010;27(8):1629–1651.
23. Mitka M. IOM report: evidence fails to support guidelines for dietary salt reduction. JAMA. Jun 26 2013;309(24):2535–2536.
24. O'Donnell M, Mente A, Rangarajan S, et al. Urinary sodium and potassium excretion, mortality, and cardiovascular events. N Engl J Med. Aug 14 2014;371(7):612–623.
25. Sacks FM, Svetkey LP, Vollmer WM, et al. Effects on blood pressure of reduced dietary sodium and the Dietary Approaches to Stop Hypertension (DASH) diet. DASH-Sodium Collaborative Research Group. N Engl J Med. 2001;344(1):3–10.
26. Izzo JL, Jr, Black HR. Hypertension Primer. The Essentials of High Blood Pressure. 3rd ed. Philadelphia, PA: Lippincott Williams & Wilkins; 2003.
27. Dahlof B, Sever PS, Poulter NR, et al. Prevention of cardiovascular events with an antihypertensive regimen of amlodipine adding perindopril as required versus atenolol adding bendroflumethiazide as required, in the Anglo-Scandinavian Cardiac Outcomes Trial-Blood Pressure Lowering Arm (ASCOT-BPLA): a multicentre randomised controlled trial. Lancet. 2005;366(9489):895–906.
28. Julius S, Kjeldsen SE, Weber M, et al. Outcomes in hypertensive patients at high cardiovascular risk treated with regimens based on valsartan or amlodipine: the VALUE randomised trial. Lancet. 2004;363(9426):2022–2031.
29. Ernst ME, Carter BL, Goerdt CJ, et al. Comparative antihypertensive effects of hydrochlorothiazide and chlorthalidone on ambulatory and office blood pressure. Hypertension. 2006;47(3):352–358.
30. NICE. Hypertension: NICE Clinical Guideline 127. 2011; www.nice.org.uk/guidance/CG127. Accessed September 30, 2011.
31. Carter BL, Einhorn PT, Brands M, et al. Thiazide-induced dysglycemia: call for research from a working group from the national heart, lung, and blood institute. Hypertension. Jul 2008;52(1):30–36.
32. Aronow WS, Fleg JL, Pepine CJ, et al. ACCF/AHA 2011 expert consensus document on hypertension in the elderly: a report of the American College of Cardiology Foundation Task Force on Clinical Expert Consensus Documents. Circulation. May 31 2011;123(21):2434–2506.
33. de Souza F, Muxfeldt E, Fiszman R, Salles G. Efficacy of spironolactone therapy in patients with true resistant hypertension. Hypertension. Jan 2010;55(1):147–152.
34. Lindholm LH, Carlberg B, Samuelsson O. Should beta blockers remain first choice in the treatment of primary hypertension? A meta-analysis. Lancet. Oct 29–Nov 4 2005;366(9496):1545–1553.
35. Bangalore S, Messerli FH, Kostis JB, Pepine CJ. Cardiovascular protection using beta-blockers: a critical review of the evidence. J Am Coll Cardiol. Aug 14 2007;50(7):563–572.
36. Weber MA. The role of the new beta-blockers in treating cardiovascular disease. Am J Hypertens. Dec 2005;18(12 Pt 2): 169S–176S.
37. Wing LM, Reid CM, Ryan P, et al. A comparison of outcomes with angiotensin-converting enzyme inhibitors and diuretics for hypertension in the elderly. N Engl J Med. 2003;348(7):583–592.
38. ONTARGET Investigators, Yusuf S, Teo KK, et al. Telmisartan, ramipril, or both in patients at high risk for vascular events. N Engl J Med. Apr 10 2008;358(15):1547–1559.
39. Mann JF, Schmieder RE, McQueen M, et al. Renal outcomes with telmisartan, ramipril, or both, in people at high vascular risk (the ONTARGET study): a multicentre, randomised, double-blind, controlled trial. Lancet. Aug 16 2008;372(9638):547–553.
40. Yancy CW, Jessup M, Bozkurt B, et al. 2013 ACCF/AHA guideline for the management of heart failure: executive summary: a report of the American College of Cardiology Foundation/ American Heart Association Task Force on practice guidelines. Circulation. Oct 15 2013;128(16):1810–1852.
41. Parving HH, Brenner BM, McMurray JJ, et al. Cardiorenal end points in a trial of aliskiren for type 2 diabetes. N Engl J Med. Dec 6 2012;367(23):2204–2213.
42. Prevention of stroke by antihypertensive drug treatment in older persons with isolated systolic hypertension. Final results of the Systolic Hypertension in the Elderly Program (SHEP). SHEP Cooperative Research Group. JAMA. Jun 26 1991;265(24): 3255–3264.
43. Reisin E, Harris RC, Rahman M. Commentary on the 2014 BP Guidelines from the Panel Appointed to the Eighth Joint National Committee (JNC 8). JASN. 2014 Nov;25(4):2419–2424.
44. Bangalore S, Gong Y, Cooper-DeHoff RM, Pepine CJ, Messerli FH. 2014 Eighth Joint National Committee Panel Recommendation for Blood Pressure Targets Revisited: results from the INVEST Study. J Am Coll Cardiol. Aug 26 2014;64(8):784–793.
45. Gradman AH. Optimal blood pressure targets in older adults: how low is low enough? J Am Coll Cardiol. Aug 26 2014;64(8):794–796.
46. Marik PE, Varon J. Hypertensive crises: challenges and management. Chest. Jun 2007;131(6):1949–1962.
47. Beckett NS, Peters R, Fletcher AE, et al. Treatment of hypertension in patients 80 years of age or older. N Engl J Med. May 1 2008;358(18):1887–1898.
48. American College of Obstetricians and Gynecologists, Task Force on Hypertension in Pregnancy. Hypertension in Pregnancy. Report of the American College of Obstetricians and Gynecologists' Task Force on Hypertension in Pregnancy. Obstet Gynecol. Nov 2013;122(5):1122–1131.
49. The fourth report on the diagnosis, evaluation, and treatment of high blood pressure in children and adolescents. Pediatrics. Aug 2004;114(2 Suppl 4th Report):555–576.
50. Kliegman R, Nelson WE. Nelson textbook of pediatrics. 18th ed. Philadelphia, PA: Saunders; 2007.

6 Heart Failure

Orly Vardeny and Tien M. H. Ng

LEARNING OBJECTIVES

Upon completion of the chapter, the reader will be able to:

1. Differentiate between the common underlying etiologies of heart failure (HF), including ischemic, nonischemic, and idiopathic causes.
2. Describe the pathophysiology of HF as it relates to neurohormonal activation of the renin-angiotensin-aldosterone system (RAAS) and the sympathetic nervous system (SNS).
3. Identify signs and symptoms of HF and classify a given patient by New York Heart Association Functional Classification and American College of Cardiology/American Heart Association Heart Failure Staging.
4. Describe the goals of therapy for a patient with acute or chronic HF.
5. Develop a nonpharmacologic treatment plan that includes patient education for managing HF.
6. Develop a specific evidence-based pharmacologic treatment plan for a patient with acute or chronic HF based on disease severity and symptoms.
7. Formulate a monitoring plan for the nonpharmacologic and pharmacologic treatment of a patient with HF.

INTRODUCTION

Heart failure (HF) is defined as the inadequate ability of the heart to pump enough blood to meet the blood flow and metabolic demands of the body.[1] High-output HF is characterized by an inordinate increase in the body's metabolic demands that outpaces an increase in **cardiac output** (CO) of a generally normally functioning heart. More commonly, HF is a result of low CO secondary to impaired cardiac function. The term *heart failure* refers to low-output HF for the purposes of this chapter.

HF is a clinical syndrome characterized by a history of specific signs and symptoms related to congestion and hypoperfusion. Because HF can occur in the presence or absence of fluid overload, the term *heart failure* is preferred over the former term *congestive heart failure*. HF results from any structural or functional cardiac disorder that impairs the ability of the ventricle to fill with or eject blood.[1] Many disorders, such as those of the pericardium, epicardium, endocardium, or great vessels, may lead to HF, but most patients develop symptoms due to impairment in left ventricular (LV) myocardial function.

The term *acute heart failure* (AHF) is used to signify either an acute decompensation of a patient with a history of chronic HF or to refer to a patient presenting with new-onset HF symptoms. Terms commonly associated with HF, such as *cardiomyopathy* and *LV dysfunction,* are not equivalent to HF but describe possible structural or functional reasons for the development of HF.

EPIDEMIOLOGY AND ETIOLOGY

Epidemiology

HF is a major public health concern affecting approximately 5.1 million people in the United States. An additional 825,000 new cases are diagnosed each year. HF manifests most commonly in adults older than 60 years.[2] The growing prevalence of HF corresponds to (a) better treatment of patients with acute myocardial infarctions (MIs) who will survive to develop HF later in life, and (b) the increasing proportion of older adults due to the aging baby boomer population. The relative incidence of HF is lower in women compared with men, but there is a greater prevalence in women overall due to their longer life expectancy. Acute HF accounts for 12 to 15 million office visits per year and 6.5 million hospitalizations annually, and HF is the most common hospital discharge diagnosis for Medicare patients and the most costly diagnosis in this population.[2] According to national registries, patients presenting with AHF are older (mean age: 75 years) and have numerous comorbidities such as coronary artery disease (CAD), renal insufficiency, and diabetes. Total estimated direct and indirect costs for managing both chronic and acute HF in the United States for 2012 was approximately $30.7 billion. Medications account for approximately 10% of that cost.[2]

The prognosis for patients hospitalized for AHF remains poor. Average hospital length of stay is estimated to be between 4 and 6 days, a number that has remained constant over the past decade.[3] In-hospital mortality rate has been estimated at approximately 4%, with ranges from 2% to 20%.[4] Readmissions are also high, with up to 30% to 60% of patients readmitted within 6 months of initial discharge date.[4] The 5-year mortality rate for chronic HF remains greater than 50%. Survival strongly correlates with severity of symptoms and functional capacity. Sudden cardiac death is the most common cause of death, occurring in approximately 40% of patients.[2] Although therapies targeting the upregulated neurohormonal response contributing to the pathophysiology of HF have clearly impacted morbidity and mortality, long-term survival remains low.

Etiology

HF is the eventual outcome of numerous cardiac diseases or disorders (Table 6–1).[5] HF can be classified by the primary underlying etiology as ischemic or nonischemic, with 70% of HF related to ischemia. KEY CONCEPT *The most common causes of HF are CAD, hypertension, and dilated cardiomyopathy.* CAD resulting in acute MI and reduced ventricular function is a common presenting history.

HF can also be classified based on the main component of the cardiac cycle leading to impaired ventricular function. A normal cardiac cycle depends on two components: systole and diastole. Expulsion of blood occurs during systole or contraction of the ventricles; diastole relates to filling of the ventricles. Ejection fraction (EF) is the fraction of the volume present at the end of diastole that is pushed into the aorta during systole. Abnormal ventricular filling (diastolic dysfunction) and/or ventricular contraction (systolic dysfunction) can result in a similar decrease in CO and cause HF symptoms. Most HF is associated with evidence of LV systolic dysfunction (evidenced by a reduced EF and also known as heart failure with reduced ejection fraction, or HFrEF) with or without a component of diastolic dysfunction, which coexists in up to two-thirds of patients. Isolated diastolic dysfunction, occurring in approximately one-third to one-half of HF patients, is diagnosed when a patient exhibits impaired ventricular filling without accompanying HF symptoms but normal systolic function. When isolated diastolic dysfunction occurs with symptoms of HF, this is referred to as heart failure with preserved ejection fraction (HFpEF). Long-standing hypertension is the leading cause of HFpEF. Ventricular dysfunction can also involve either the left or right chamber of the heart or both. This has implications for symptomatology because predominant right-sided failure manifests as systemic congestion, whereas predominant left-sided failure results in pulmonary symptoms.

Table 6–1

Causes of Heart Failure

Systolic Dysfunction (Decreased Contractility)
- Reduction in muscle mass (eg, myocardial infarction)
- Dilated cardiomyopathies
- Ventricular hypertrophy
  - Pressure overload (eg, systemic or pulmonary hypertension, aortic or pulmonic valve stenosis)
  - Volume overload (eg, valvular regurgitation, shunts, high-output states)

Diastolic Dysfunction (Restriction in Ventricular Filling)
- Increased ventricular stiffness
- Ventricular hypertrophy (eg, hypertrophic cardiomyopathy, pressure and/or volume overload)
- Infiltrative myocardial diseases (eg, amyloidosis, sarcoidosis, endomyocardial fibrosis)
- Myocardial ischemia and infarction
- Mitral or tricuspid valve stenosis
- Pericardial disease (eg, pericarditis, pericardial tamponade)

Non-Ischemic Etiologies
- Hypertension
- Viral illness
- Thyroid disease
- Excessive alcohol use
- Illicit drug use
- Pregnancy-related heart disease
- Familial congenital disease
- Valvular disorders such as mitral or tricuspid valve regurgitation or stenosis.

From Parker RB, Nappi JM, Cavallari LH. Systolic heart failure. In: DiPiro JT, Talbert RL, Yee GC, et al., eds. Pharmacotherapy: A pathophysiologic approach, 9th ed. New York, NY: McGraw-Hill, 2014:86, with permission.

PATHOPHYSIOLOGY

A basic grasp of normal cardiac function sets the stage for understanding the pathophysiological processes leading to HF and selecting appropriate therapy for HF. CO is defined as the volume of blood ejected per unit of time (L/min) and is a major determinant of tissue perfusion. CO is the product of heart rate (HR) and stroke volume (SV): CO = HR × SV. The following sections describe how each parameter relates to CO.

HR is controlled by the autonomic nervous system, where sympathetic stimulation of β-adrenergic receptors results in an increase in HR and CO. SV is the volume of blood ejected with each systole. SV is determined by factors regulating preload, afterload, and contractility. Preload is a measure of ventricular filling pressure, or the volume of blood in the left ventricle (also known as LV end-diastolic volume). Preload is determined by venous return as well as atrial contraction. An increase in venous return to the left ventricle results in the stretch of cardiomyocyte sarcomeres (or contractile units) and a subsequent increase in the number of cross-bridges formed between actin and myosin myofilaments. This results in an increase in the force of contraction based on the Frank-Starling mechanism.[6] Afterload is the resistance to ventricular ejection and is regulated by ejection impedance, wall tension, and regional wall geometry. Thus, elevated aortic and systemic pressures result in an increase in afterload and reduced SV. Contractility, also known as the inotropic state of the heart, is an intrinsic property of cardiac muscle incorporating fiber shortening and tension development. Contractility is influenced to a large degree by adrenergic nerve activity and circulating catecholamines such as epinephrine and norepinephrine.

Compensatory Mechanisms

In the setting of a sustained loss of myocardium, a number of mechanisms aid the heart when faced with an increased hemodynamic burden and reduced CO. They include the Frank-Starling mechanism, tachycardia and increased afterload, and cardiac hypertrophy and remodeling (Table 6–2).[5,7]

► *Preload and the Frank-Starling Mechanism*

In the setting of a sudden decrease in CO, the natural response of the body is to decrease blood flow to the periphery to maintain perfusion to vital organs such as the heart and brain. Therefore, renal perfusion is compromised due to both decreased CO as well as shunting of blood away from peripheral tissues. This results in activation of the renin-angiotensin-aldosterone system (RAAS).

Table 6–2

Beneficial and Detrimental Effects of the Compensatory Responses in Heart Failure

Compensatory Response	Beneficial Effects of Compensation	Detrimental Effects of Compensation
Increased preload (through sodium and water retention)	Optimizes stroke volume via Frank-Starling mechanism	Pulmonary and systemic congestion and edema formation Increased MVO_2
Vasoconstriction	Maintains BP and perfusion in the face of reduced cardiac output	Increased MVO_2 Increased afterload decreases stroke volume and further activates the compensatory responses
Tachycardia and increased contractility (due to SNS activation)	Increases cardiac output	Increased MVO_2 Shortened diastolic filling time β_1-Receptor downregulation, decreased receptor sensitivity Precipitation of ventricular arrhythmias Increased risk of myocardial cell death
Ventricular hypertrophy and remodeling	Maintains cardiac output Reduces myocardial wall stress Decreases MVO_2	Diastolic dysfunction Systolic dysfunction Increased risk of myocardial cell death Increased risk of myocardial ischemia Increased arrhythmia risk

BP, blood pressure; MVO_2, myocardial oxygen consumption; SNS, sympathetic nervous system.

The decrease in renal perfusion is sensed by the juxtaglomerular cells of the kidneys leading to the release of renin and initiation of the cascade for production of angiotensin II. Angiotensin II stimulates the synthesis and release of aldosterone. Aldosterone in turn stimulates sodium and water retention in an attempt to increase intravascular volume and hence preload. In a healthy heart, a large increase in CO is usually accomplished with just a small change in preload. However, in a failing heart, alterations in the contractile filaments reduce the ability of cardiomyocytes to adapt to increases in preload. Thus, an increase in preload actually impairs contractile function in the failing heart and results in a further decrease in CO. See Figure 6–1.

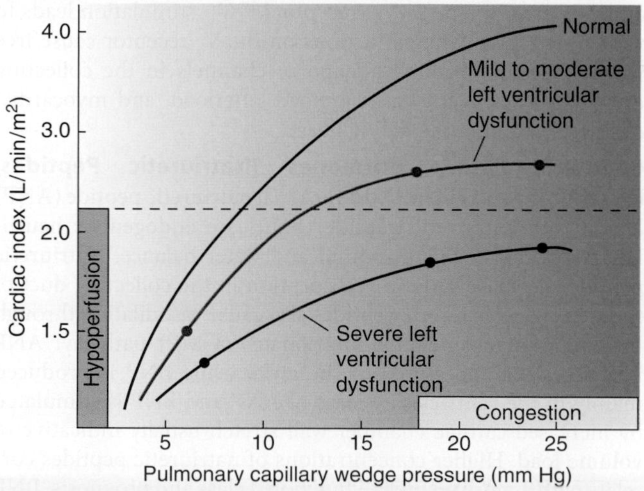

FIGURE 6–1. Relationship between cardiac output (shown as cardiac index) and preload (shown as pulmonary capillary wedge pressure). Cardiac index is expressed in conventional units of L/min/m^2, and can be converted to SI units of L/s/m^2 by multiplying by 0.0167. (Reproduced, with permission, from Rodgers JE, Reed BN. Acute decompensated heart failure. In: DiPiro JT, Talbert RL, Yee GC, et al., eds. *Pharmacotherapy: A Pathophysiologic Approach,* 9th ed. New York, NY: McGraw-Hill, 2014:129.)

▶ *Tachycardia and Increased Afterload*

Another mechanism to maintain CO when contractility is low is to increase HR. This is achieved through sympathetic nervous system (SNS) activation and the agonist effect of norepinephrine on β-adrenergic receptors in the heart. Sympathetic activation also enhances contractility by increasing cytosolic calcium concentrations. SV is relatively fixed in HF; thus HR becomes the major determinant of CO. Although this mechanism increases CO acutely, the chronotropic and inotropic responses to sympathetic activation increase myocardial oxygen demand, worsen underlying ischemia, contribute to proarrhythmia, and further impair both systolic and diastolic function.

Activation of both the RAAS and SNS also contribute to vasoconstriction in an attempt to redistribute blood flow from peripheral organs such as the kidneys to coronary and cerebral circulation.[7] However, arterial vasoconstriction leads to impaired forward ejection of blood from the heart due to an increase in afterload. This results in a decrease in CO and continued stimulation of compensatory responses, creating a vicious cycle of neurohormonal activation.

▶ *Cardiac Hypertrophy and Remodeling*

Ventricular hypertrophy, an adaptive increase in ventricular muscle mass due to the growth of existing myocytes, occurs in response to an increased hemodynamic burden such as volume or pressure overload.[5] Hypertrophy can be concentric or eccentric. Concentric hypertrophy occurs in response to pressure overload such as in long-standing hypertension or pulmonary hypertension, whereas eccentric hypertrophy occurs after an acute MI. Eccentric hypertrophy involves an increase in myocyte size in a segmental fashion, as opposed to the global hypertrophy occurring in concentric hypertrophy. Although hypertrophy helps to reduce cardiac wall stress in the short term, continued hypertrophy accelerates myocyte cell death through an overall increase in myocardial oxygen demand.

Cardiac remodeling occurs as a compensatory adaptation to a change in wall stress and is largely regulated by neurohormonal activation, with angiotensin II and aldosterone being key stimuli.[7] The process entails changes in myocardial and extracellular matrix composition and function that results in both structural and functional alterations to the heart. In HF, the changes in cardiac size, shape, and composition are pathological and detrimental to heart function. In addition to myocyte size and extracellular matrix changes, heart geometry shifts from an elliptical to a less efficient spherical shape. Even after remodeling occurs, the heart can maintain CO for many years. However, heart function continues to deteriorate until progression to clinical HF. The timeline for remodeling varies depending on the cardiac insult. For example, in the setting of an acute MI, remodeling starts within a few days.[6] Chronic remodeling, however, is what progressively worsens HF, and therefore is a major target of drug therapy.

Models of Heart Failure

▶ *Neurohormonal Model*

KEY CONCEPT *Development and progression of HF involves activation of neurohormonal pathways including the SNS and the RAAS.* This model begins with an initial precipitating event or myocardial injury resulting in a decline in CO, followed by the compensatory mechanisms previously discussed. This includes activation of neurohormonal pathways with pathological consequences including the RAAS, SNS, endothelin, and vasopressin, and those with counterregulatory properties such as the natriuretic peptides and nitric oxide. This model currently guides our therapy for chronic HF in terms of preventing disease progression and mortality.

Angiotensin II Angiotensin II is a key neurohormone in the pathophysiology of HF. The vasoconstrictive effects of angiotensin II lead to an increase in systemic vascular resistance (SVR) and blood pressure (BP). The resulting increase in afterload contributes to an increase in myocardial oxygen demand and opposes the desired increase in SV. In the kidneys, angiotensin II enhances renal function acutely by raising intraglomerular pressure through constriction of the efferent arterioles.[6] However, the increase in glomerular filtration pressure may be offset by a reduction in renal perfusion secondary to angiotensin II's influence over the release of other vasoactive neurohormones such as vasopressin and endothelin-1 (ET-1). Angiotensin II also potentiates the release of aldosterone from the adrenal glands and norepinephrine from adrenergic nerve terminals. Additionally, angiotensin II induces vascular hypertrophy and remodeling in both cardiac and renal cells. Clinical studies show that blocking the effects of the RAAS in HF is associated with improved cardiac function and prolonged survival. Thus, angiotensin-converting enzyme (ACE) inhibitors and angiotensin receptor blockers (ARBs) are the cornerstone of HF treatment.

Aldosterone Aldosterone's contribution to HF pathophysiology is multifaceted. Renally, aldosterone causes sodium and water retention in an attempt to enhance intravascular volume and CO. This adaptive mechanism has deleterious consequences because excessive sodium and water retention worsen the already elevated ventricular filling pressures. Aldosterone also contributes to electrolyte abnormalities seen in HF patients. Hypokalemia and hypomagnesemia contribute to the increased risk of arrhythmias. In addition, evidence supports the role of aldosterone as an etiological factor for myocardial fibrosis and cardiac remodeling by causing increased extracellular matrix collagen deposition and cardiac fibrosis.[6] Aldosterone potentially contributes to disease progression via sympathetic potentiation and ventricular remodeling. In addition, the combination of these multiple effects is likely responsible for the increased risk of sudden cardiac death attributed to aldosterone. As elevated aldosterone concentrations have been associated with a poorer prognosis in HF, its blockade has become an important therapeutic target for improvement of long-term prognosis.

Norepinephrine Norepinephrine is a classic marker for SNS activation. It plays an adaptive role in the failing heart by stimulating HR and myocardial contractility to augment CO and by producing vasoconstriction to maintain organ perfusion. However, excess levels are directly cardiotoxic. In addition, sympathetic activation increases the risk for arrhythmias, ischemia, and myocyte cell death through increased myocardial workload and accelerated apoptosis. Ventricular hypertrophy and remodeling are also influenced by norepinephrine.[8]

Plasma norepinephrine concentrations are elevated proportionally to HF severity, with highest levels correlating to the poorest prognosis. Several mechanisms relate to diminished responsiveness to catecholamines (eg, norepinephrine) as cardiac function declines.[6] Adrenergic receptor desensitization and downregulation (decreased receptor number and postreceptor responses and signaling) occurs under sustained sympathetic stimulation. The desensitization contributes to further release of norepinephrine. β-adrenergic blocking agents, although intrinsically negatively inotropic, have become essential therapy for chronic HF.

Endothelin ET-1, one of the most potent physiological vasoconstrictors, is an important contributor to HF pathophysiology.[9] ET-1 binds to two G-protein coupled receptors, endothelin-A (ET-A) and endothelin-B (ET-B). ET-A receptors mediate vasoconstriction and are prevalent in vascular smooth muscle and cardiac cells. ET-B receptors are expressed on the endothelium and in vascular smooth muscle, and receptor stimulation mediates vasodilation and endothelin clearance. Levels of ET-1 correlate with HF functional class and mortality.

Arginine Vasopressin Higher vasopressin concentrations are linked to dilutional hyponatremia and a poor prognosis in HF. Vasopressin exerts its effects through vasopressin type 1a (V_{1a}) and vasopressin type 2 (V_2) receptors.[5,7] V_{1a} stimulation leads to vasoconstriction, whereas actions on the V_2 receptor cause free water retention through aquaporin channels in the collecting duct. Vasopressin increases preload, afterload, and myocardial oxygen demand in the failing heart.

Counterregulatory Hormones (Natriuretic Peptides, Bradykinin, and Nitric Oxide) Atrial natriuretic peptide (ANP) and B-type natriuretic peptide (BNP) are endogenous neurohormones that regulate sodium and water balance. Natriuretic peptides decrease sodium reabsorption in the collecting duct of the kidney.[10] Natriuretic peptides also cause vasodilation through the cyclic guanosine monophosphate (cGMP) pathway. ANP is synthesized and stored in the atria, while BNP is produced mainly in the ventricles. Release of ANP and BNP is stimulated by increased cardiac chamber wall stretch usually indicative of volume load. Higher concentrations of natriuretic peptides correlate with a more severe HF functional class and prognosis. BNP is sensitive to volume status; thus the plasma concentration can be used as a diagnostic marker in HF.[10]

Bradykinin is part of the kallikrein-kinin system, which shares a link to the RAAS through ACE. Bradykinin is a vasodilatory peptide that is released in response to a variety of stimuli, including neurohormonal and inflammatory mediators known to be activated in HF.[9] As a consequence, bradykinin levels are elevated in HF patients and thought to partially antagonize the vasoconstrictive peptides.

Nitric oxide, a vasodilatory hormone released by the endothelium, is found in higher concentrations in HF patients and provides two main benefits in HF: vasodilation and neurohormonal antagonism of endothelin.[9] Nitric oxide's production is affected by the enzyme inducible nitric oxide synthetase (iNOS), which is upregulated in the setting of HF, likely due to increased levels of angiotensin II, norepinephrine, and multiple cytokines. In HF, the physiological response to nitric oxide appears to be blunted, which contributes to the imbalance between vasoconstriction and vasodilation.

▶ *Cardiorenal Model*

There is growing evidence of a link between renal disease and HF.[8] Renal insufficiency is present in one-third of HF patients and is associated with a worse prognosis. In hospitalized HF patients, the presence of renal insufficiency is associated with longer lengths of stay, increased in-hospital morbidity and mortality, and detrimental neurohormonal alterations. Conversely, renal dysfunction is a common complication of HF or results from its treatment. Renal failure is also a common cause for HF decompensation.

▶ *Proinflammatory Cytokines*

Inflammatory cytokines have been implicated in the pathophysiology of HF.[9] Several proinflammatory (eg, tumor necrosis factor [TNF]-α, interleukin-1, interleukin-6, and interferon-γ) and anti-inflammatory cytokines (eg, interleukin-10) are overexpressed in the failing heart. The most is known about TNF-α, a pleiotropic cytokine that acts as a negative inotrope, stimulates cardiac cell apoptosis, uncouples β-adrenergic receptors from adenylyl cyclase, and is related to cardiac cachexia. The exact role of cytokines and inflammation in HF pathophysiology continues to be studied.

Precipitating and Exacerbating Factors in Heart Failure

HF patients exist in one of two clinical states. When a patient's volume status and symptoms are stable, their HF condition is said to be "compensated." In situations of volume overload or other worsening symptoms, the patient is considered "decompensated." Acute decompensation can be precipitated by numerous etiologies (Table 6–3).[5]

Table 6–3

Exacerbating or Precipitating Factors in Heart Failure

Cardiac	Metabolic	Patient-Related
Acute ischemia Arrhythmia Endocarditis Myocarditis Pulmonary embolus Uncontrolled hypertension Valvular disorders	Anemia Hyperthyroidism/thyrotoxicosis Infection Pregnancy Worsening renal function	Dietary/fluid nonadherence HF therapy nonadherence Use of cardiotoxins (cocaine, chronic alcohol, amphetamines, sympathomimetics) Offending medications (NSAIDs, COX-2 inhibitors, steroids, lithium, β-blockers, calcium channel blockers, antiarrhythmics, alcohol, thiazolidinediones)

COX-2, cyclooxygenase-2; HF, heart failure; NSAID, nonsteroidal anti-inflammatory drug.

KEY CONCEPT *The clinician must identify potential reversible causes of HF exacerbations including prescription and nonprescription drug therapies, dietary indiscretions, and medication nonadherence.* Nonadherence with dietary restrictions or chronic HF medications deserves special attention because it is the most common cause of acute decompensation and can be prevented. As such, an accurate history regarding diet, food choices, and the patient's knowledge regarding sodium and fluid intake (including alcohol) is valuable in assessing dietary indiscretion. Nonadherence with medical recommendations such as laboratory and other appointment follow-up can also be indicative of nonadherence with diet or medications.

CLINICAL PRESENTATION AND DIAGNOSIS OF HEART FAILURE

In low-output HF, symptoms are generally related to either congestion behind the failing ventricle(s), or hypoperfusion (decreased tissue blood supply), or both. For example, a failing left ventricle causes fluid to back up in the lungs, and a patient with right ventricular failure (RVF) would exhibit systemic symptoms of congestion. Congestion is the most common symptom in HF, followed by symptoms related to decreased perfusion to peripheral tissues including decreased renal output, mental confusion, and cold extremities. Activation of the compensatory mechanisms occurs in an effort to increase CO and preserve blood flow to vital organs. However, the increase in preload and afterload in the setting of a failing ventricle leads to elevated filling pressures and further impairment of cardiac function, which manifests as systemic and/or pulmonary congestion. It is important to remember that congestion develops behind the failing ventricle, caused by the inability of that ventricle to eject the blood that it receives from the atria and venous return. As such, signs and symptoms may be classified as left sided or right sided. KEY CONCEPT *Symptoms of left-sided HF include dyspnea, orthopnea, and paroxysmal nocturnal dyspnea (PND), whereas symptoms of right-sided HF include fluid retention, gastrointestinal (GI) bloating, and fatigue.* Although most patients initially have left ventricular failure (LVF; pulmonary congestion), the ventricles share a septal wall; because LVF increases the workload of the right ventricle, both ventricles eventually fail and contribute to the HF syndrome. Because of the complex nature of this syndrome, it has become exceedingly more difficult to attribute a specific sign or symptom as caused by either RVF (systemic congestion) or LVF. Therefore, the numerous signs and symptoms associated with this disorder are collectively attributed to HF rather than to dysfunction of a specific ventricle.

General Signs and Symptoms

Refer to the Clinical Presentation and Diagnosis of Chronic Heart Failure textbox for a description of signs and symptoms. It is important to note that in chronic severe HF, unintentional weight loss can occur that leads to a syndrome of cardiac cachexia, defined as a nonedematous weight loss more than 6% of the previous normal weight over a period of at least 6 months. HF prognosis worsens considerably once cardiac cachexia has been diagnosed, regardless of HF severity. This results from several factors including loss of appetite, malabsorption due to GI edema, elevated metabolic rate, and elevated levels of norepinephrine and proinflammatory cytokines. Absorption of fats is especially affected, leading to deficiencies of fat-soluble vitamins.

Patients can experience a variety of symptoms related to buildup of fluid. The most recognized finding of systemic venous congestion related to RVF is peripheral edema. It usually occurs in dependent areas of the body, such as the ankles (pedal edema) for ambulatory patients or the sacral region for bedridden patients. Patients may complain of swelling of their feet and ankles, which can extend up to their calves or thighs. Abdominal congestion may cause a bloated feeling, abdominal pain, early satiety, nausea, anorexia, and constipation. Often patients may have difficulty fitting into their shoes or pants due to edema. Weight gain often precedes signs of overt peripheral edema. Therefore, it is crucial for patients to weigh themselves daily even in the absence of symptoms to assess fluid status.

A clinically validated measure of venous congestion is assessment of the jugular venous pressure (JVP). This is performed by examining the right internal jugular vein for distention or elevation of the pulsation while reclining at a 45-degree angle. A JVP more than 4 cm above the sternal angle is indicative of elevated right atrial pressure. JVP may be normal at rest, but if application of pressure to the abdomen can elicit a sustained elevation of JVP, this is defined as hepatojugular reflux (HJR). A positive finding of HJR indicates hepatic congestion and results from displacement of volume from the abdomen into the jugular vein because the right atrium is unable to accept this additional blood. Hepatic congestion can cause abnormalities in liver function, which can be evident in liver function tests and/or clotting times. Development of hepatomegaly occurs infrequently and is caused by long-term systemic venous congestion. Intestinal or abdominal congestion can also be present, but it usually does not lead to characteristic signs unless overt ascites is evident. In advanced RVF, evidence of pulmonary hypertension may be present (eg, right ventricular heave).

Dyspnea, or shortness of breath, can result from pulmonary congestion or systemic hypoperfusion due to LVF. Exertional dyspnea occurs when patients experience breathlessness

Clinical Presentation and Diagnosis of Chronic Heart Failure

General

Patient presentation may range from asymptomatic to cardiogenic shock.

Symptoms

- Dyspnea, particularly on exertion
- Orthopnea
- Shortness of breath (SOB)
- Paroxysmal nocturnal dyspnea
- Exercise intolerance
- Tachypnea
- Cough
- Fatigue
- Nocturia and/or polyuria
- Hemoptysis
- Abdominal pain
- Anorexia
- Nausea
- Bloating
- Ascites
- Mental status changes (confusion, hallucinations)
- Weakness
- Lethargy
- Insomnia

Signs

- Pulmonary rales
- Pulmonary edema
- S_3 gallop
- Pleural effusion
- Cheyne-Stokes respiration
- Tachycardia
- Cardiomegaly
- Peripheral edema (eg, pedal edema, which is swelling of feet and ankles)
- Jugular venous distension (JVD)
- Hepatojugular reflux (HJR)
- Hepatomegaly
- Cyanosis of the digits
- Pallor or cool extremities

Laboratory Tests

- BNP greater than 100 pg/mL (greater than 100 ng/L or 28.9 pmol/L) or N-terminal proBNP (NT-proBNP) greater than 300 pg/mL (greater than 300 ng/L or greater than 35.4 pmol/L).
- Electrocardiogram (ECG): May be normal or could show numerous abnormalities including acute ST-T–wave changes from myocardial ischemia, atrial fibrillation, bradycardia, and LV hypertrophy.
- Serum creatinine: May be increased owing to hypoperfusion; preexisting renal dysfunction can contribute to volume overload.
- Complete blood count: Useful to determine if HF is due to reduced oxygen-carrying capacity.
- Chest x-ray: Useful for detection of cardiac enlargement, pulmonary edema, and pleural effusions.
- Echocardiogram: Used to assess LV size, valve function, pericardial effusion, wall motion abnormalities, and ejection fraction.

induced by physical activity or a lower level of activity than previously known to cause breathlessness. Patients often state that activities such as stair climbing, carrying groceries, or walking a particular distance cause shortness of breath. Severity of HF is inversely proportional to the amount of activity required to produce dyspnea. In severe HF, dyspnea is present even at rest.

Orthopnea is dyspnea that is positional. Orthopnea is present if a patient is unable to breathe while lying flat on a bed (ie, in the recumbent position). It manifests within minutes of a patient lying down and is relieved immediately when the patient sits upright. Patients can relieve orthopnea by elevating their head and shoulders with pillows. The practitioner should inquire as to the number of pillows needed to prevent dyspnea as a marker of worsening HF. PND occurs when patients awaken suddenly with a feeling of breathlessness and suffocation. PND is caused by increased venous return and mobilization of interstitial fluid from the extremities leading to alveolar edema, and usually occurs within 1 to 4 hours of sleep. In contrast to orthopnea, PND is not relieved immediately by sitting upright and often takes up to 30 minutes for symptoms to subside.

Pulmonary congestion may also cause a nonproductive cough that occurs at night or with exertion. In cases of pulmonary edema, the most severe form of pulmonary congestion, patients may produce pink frothy sputum and experience extreme breathlessness and anxiety due to feelings of suffocation and drowning. If not treated aggressively, patients can become cyanotic and acidotic. Severe pulmonary edema can progress to respiratory failure, necessitating mechanical ventilation. Not all patients with LVF will exhibit signs of pulmonary congestion if lymphatic clearance is intact.

▸ *Patient History*

A thorough history is crucial to identify cardiac and noncardiac disorders or behaviors that may lead to or accelerate the development of HF. Past medical history, family history, and social history are important for identifying comorbid illnesses that are risk factors for the development of HF or underlying etiological factors. A complete medication history (including prescription and nonprescription drugs, herbal therapy, and vitamin supplements) should be obtained each time a patient is seen to evaluate adherence, to assess appropriateness of therapy, to eliminate drugs that may be harmful in HF (Table 6–4), and to determine additional monitoring requirements.[5] For newly diagnosed HF, previous use of radiation or chemotherapeutic agents as well as current or past use of alcohol and illicit drugs should be assessed. In addition, for patients with a known history of HF, questions related to symptomatology and exercise tolerance are essential for assessing any changes in clinical status that may warrant further evaluation or adjustment of the medication regimen.

Heart Failure Classification

There are two common systems for categorizing patients with HF. The New York Heart Association (NYHA) Functional Classification (FC) system is based on the patient's activity level and exercise tolerance. It divides patients into one of four classes, with functional class I patients exhibiting no symptoms or limitations of daily activities, and functional class IV patients who are symptomatic at rest (Table 6–5). The NYHA FC system reflects a subjective assessment by a health care provider and can change frequently over short periods of time. Functional class correlates poorly with EF; however, EF is one of the strongest predictors of prognosis. In general, anticipated survival declines in conjunction with a decline in functional ability.

The American College of Cardiology/American Heart Association (ACC/AHA) have proposed another system based on the development and progression of the disease. Instead of classifications, patients are placed into stages A through D (Table 6–5).[1] Because the staging system is related to development and progression of HF, it also proposes management

Table 6–4

Drugs That May Precipitate or Exacerbate Heart Failure

Agents Causing Negative Inotropic Effect
Antiarrhythmics (eg, disopyramide, flecainide, and others)
β-blockers (eg, propranolol, metoprolol, atenolol, and others)
Nondihydropyridine calcium channel blockers (eg, verapamil)
Itraconazole
Terbinafine

Cardiotoxic Agents
Doxorubicin
Daunomycin
Cyclophosphamide

Agents Causing Sodium and Water Retention
Nonsteroidal anti-inflammatory drugs
COX-2 inhibitors
Glucocorticoids
Androgens
Estrogens
Salicylates (high dose)
Sodium-containing drugs (eg, carbenicillin disodium, ticarcillin disodium)
Thiazolidinediones (eg, pioglitazone)

COX-2, cyclooxygenase-2.

Adapted from Parker RB, Nappi JM, Cavallari LH. Systolic heart failure. In: DiPiro JT, Talbert RL, Yee GC, et al., eds. Pharmacotherapy: A pathophysiologic approach, 9th ed. New York, NY: McGraw-Hill, 2014:92.

Patient Encounter Part 1

A 68-year-old man with a history of known CAD and type 2 diabetes mellitus presents for a belated follow-up clinic visit (his last visit was 2 years ago). His most bothersome complaint is SOB at night when lying down flat; he has to sleep on three pillows to get adequate rest and sometimes even that does not help. Although he used to be able to walk a few blocks and two to three flights of stairs comfortably before getting breathless, he has had increasing symptoms after one flight of stairs. He also notes his ankles are always swollen and his shoes no longer fit; therefore he only wears slippers. Additionally, he has difficulty finishing his meals due to bloating and nausea, and overall his appetite is decreased.

What information is suggestive of a diagnosis of HF?

What additional information do you need to know before creating a treatment plan?

Table 6–5

New York Heart Association (NYHA) Functional Classification and American College of Cardiology/American Heart Association (ACC/AHA) Staging

NYHA Functional Class	ACC/AHA Stage	Description
N/A	A	Patients at high risk for heart failure but without structural heart disease or symptoms of heart failure.
I	B	Patients with cardiac disease but without limitations of physical activity. Ordinary physical activity does not cause undue fatigue, dyspnea, or palpitation.
II	C	Patients with cardiac disease that results in slight limitations of physical activity. Ordinary physical activity results in fatigue, palpitations, dyspnea, or angina.
III	C	Patients with cardiac disease that results in marked limitation of physical activity. Although patients are comfortable at rest, less than ordinary activity will lead to symptoms.
IV	C, D	Patients with cardiac disease that results in an inability to carry on physical activity without discomfort. Symptoms of heart failure are present at rest. With any physical activity, increased discomfort is experienced. Stage D refers to end-stage heart failure patients.

strategies for each stage including risk factor modification. The staging system is meant to complement the NYHA FC system; however, patients can move between NYHA functional classes as symptoms improve with treatment, whereas HF staging does not allow for patients to move to a lower stage (eg, patients cannot be categorized as stage C and move to stage B after treatment). Currently, patients are categorized based on both systems. Functional classification and staging are useful from a clinician's perspective, allowing for a longitudinal assessment of a patient's risk and progress, requirements for nonpharmacologic interventions, response to medications, and overall prognosis.

TREATMENT OF CHRONIC HEART FAILURE

Desired Therapeutic Outcomes

There is no cure for HF. KEY CONCEPT *The general therapeutic management goals for chronic HF include preventing the onset of clinical symptoms or reducing symptoms, preventing or reducing hospitalizations, slowing progression of the disease, improving quality of life, and prolonging survival.* The ACC/AHA staging system described earlier provides a guide for application of these goals based on the clinical progression of HF for a given patient. The goals are additive as one moves from stage A to stage D.[1] For stage A, risk factor management is the primary goal. Stage B includes the addition of pharmacologic therapies known to slow the disease progression in an attempt to prevent the onset of clinical symptoms. Stage C involves the use of additional therapies aimed at controlling symptoms and decreasing morbidity. Finally, in stage D, the goals shift toward palliative care and quality-of-life related issues. Only with aggressive management throughout all the stages will the ultimate goal of improving survival be realized. Attainment of these goals is based on designing a therapeutic approach that encompasses strategies aimed at control and treatment of contributing disorders, nonpharmacologic interventions, and optimal use of pharmacologic therapies.[11]

Control and Treatment of Contributing Disorders

All causes of HF must be investigated to determine the etiology of cardiac dysfunction in a given patient. Because the most common etiology of HF in the United States is ischemic heart disease, coronary angiography is warranted in most patients with a history suggestive of underlying CAD, and may be considered in patients who newly exhibit reduced left ventricular ejection fraction (LVEF). Revascularization of those with significant CAD may help restore some cardiac function in patients with reversible ischemic defects. Aggressive control of hypertension, diabetes, and obesity is also essential because each of these conditions can cause further cardiac damage. Surgical repair of valvular disease or congenital malformations may be warranted if detected. Clinical HF partly depends on metabolic processes, so correction of imbalances such as thyroid disease, anemia, and nutritional deficiencies is required. Other more rare causes such as autoimmune disorders or acquired illnesses may have specific treatments. Identifying and discontinuing medications that can exacerbate HF is also an important intervention.

Nonpharmacologic Interventions

It is imperative that patients recognize the role of self-management in HF. KEY CONCEPT *Nonpharmacologic treatment involves dietary modifications such as sodium and fluid restriction, risk factor reduction including smoking cessation, timely immunizations, and supervised regular physical activity.* Patient education regarding monitoring symptoms, dietary and medication adherence, exercise and physical fitness, risk factor reduction, and immunizations are important for the prevention of AHF exacerbations.

Patients should be encouraged to become involved in their own care which includes self-monitoring. Home monitoring should include daily assessment of weight and exercise tolerance. Daily weights should be done first thing in the morning upon arising and before any food intake to maintain consistency. Patients should record their weight daily in a journal and bring this log to each clinic or office visit. Changes in weight can indicate fluid retention and congestion prior to onset of peripheral or pulmonary symptoms. Individuals who have an increase of 3 pounds (1.4 kg) in a single day or 5 pounds (2.3 kg) over a week should alert their HF care provider. Some patients may be educated about self-adjusting diuretic doses based on daily weights. In addition to weight changes, a marked decline in exercise tolerance should also be reported to the HF care provider.

Nonadherence is an important issue because it relates to acute exacerbations of HF. Ensuring an understanding of the importance of each medication used to treat HF, proper administration, and potential adverse effects may improve adherence. Stressing the rationale for each medication is important,

Patient Encounter Part 2

Medical History, Physical Examination, and Diagnostic Tests

PMH: Dyslipidemia × 20 years, type 2 diabetes mellitus × 15 years, coronary artery disease × 10 years (MIs in 1999 and 2002), history of alcohol abuse × 30 years, history of migraines × 40 years

Allergies: No known drug allergies

Meds: Diltiazem CD 240 mg once daily, nitroglycerin 0.4 mg sublingual as needed (last use yesterday after showering), glipizide 10 mg twice daily for diabetes, metformin 1000 mg twice daily for diabetes, atorvastatin 40 mg once daily for dyslipidemia, naproxen 220 mg twice daily as needed for headaches, vitamin B_{12} once daily, multivitamin daily, aspirin 81 mg once daily

FH: Significant for early heart disease in mother (MI at age 63)

SH: He is disabled from a previous accident; he is married, has three children, and runs his own business; he drinks 10 to 12 beers nightly

PE:

BP 126/84 mm Hg, pulse 60 beats/min and regular, respiratory rate 16/min, Ht 5′8″ (173 cm), Wt 251 lb (114 kg), body mass index (BMI): 38.2 kg/m²

Lungs are clear to auscultation with a prolonged expiratory phase

CV: Regular rate and rhythm with normal S_1 and S_2; there is an S_3 and a soft S_4 present; there is a 2/6 systolic ejection murmur heard best at the left lower sternal border; point of maximal impulse is within normal limits at the midclavicular line

Abd: Soft, nontender, and bowel sounds are present, (+) hepatojugular reflux

Ext: 2+ pitting edema extending to below the knees is observed. JVP 11 cm

Chest x-ray: Bilateral pleural effusions and cardiomegaly

Echocardiogram: EF = 25% (0.25)

Laboratory Values:

Hct: 41.1% (0.411)

WBC: 5.3 × 10³/μL (5.3 × 10⁹/L)

Sodium: 136 mEq/L (136 mmol/L)

Potassium: 3.2 mEq/L (3.2 mmol/L)

Bicarb: 30 mEq/L (30 mmol/L)

Chloride: 90 mEq/L (90 mmol/L)

Magnesium: 1.5 mEq/L (0.75 mmol/L)

Fasting blood glucose: 120 mg/dL (6.7 mmol/L)

Uric acid: 8 mg/dL (476 μmol/L)

BUN: 40 mg/dL (14.3 mmol/L)

SCr: 1.6 mg/dL (141 μmol/L)

Alk Phos: 120 IU/L (2.00 μKat/L)

Aspartate aminotransferase: 100 IU/L (1.67 μKat/L)

What other laboratory or diagnostic tests are required for assessment of the patient's condition?

How would you classify his NYHA FC and ACC/AHA HF stage?

Identify exacerbating or precipitating factors that may worsen his HF.

What are your treatment goals for the patient?

especially for NYHA FC I or ACC/AHA stage B patients who are asymptomatic yet started on drugs that may worsen symptoms initially. A clinician's involvement in emphasizing medication adherence, offering adherence suggestions such as optimal timing of medications or use of weekly pill containers, and providing intensive follow-up care has been shown to reduce AHF hospitalizations.

Dietary modifications in HF consist of initiation of an AHA step II diet as part of cardiac risk factor reduction, sodium restriction, and sometimes fluid restriction. Because sodium and water retention is a compensatory mechanism that contributes to volume overload in HF, salt and fluid restriction is often necessary to help avoid or minimize congestion. The normal American diet includes 3 to 6 g of sodium per day. Most patients with HF should limit salt intake to a maximum of 2 g/day. Patients should be educated to avoid cooking with salt and to limit intake of foods with high salt content, such as fried or processed food (lunch meats, soups, cheeses, salted snack foods, canned food, and some ethnic foods). Salt restriction can be challenging for many patients. The clinician should counsel to restrict salt slowly over time. Drastic dietary changes may lead to nonadherence due to an unpalatable diet. Substituting spices to flavor food is a useful recommendation. Salt substitutes should be used judiciously because many contain significant amounts of potassium that can increase the risk of hyperkalemia. Fluid restriction may not be necessary in many patients. When applicable, fluid intake is generally limited from all sources to less than 2 L/day.

Exercise, although discouraged when the patient is acutely decompensated to ease cardiac workload, is recommended when patients are stable. The heart is a muscle that requires activity to prevent atrophy. In addition, exercise improves peripheral muscle conditioning and efficiency, which may contribute to better exercise tolerance despite the low CO state. Regular low intensity, aerobic exercise that includes walking, swimming, or riding a bike is encouraged; heavy weight training is discouraged. The prescribed exercise regimen needs to be tailored to the individual's functional ability, and thus it is suggested that patients participate in cardiac rehabilitation programs, at least initially. It is important that patients not overexert themselves to fatigue or exertional dyspnea.

Modification of classic risk factors, such as tobacco and alcohol consumption, is important to minimize the potential for further aggravation of heart function. Data from observational studies suggest that patients with HF who smoke have a mortality rate 40% higher than those who do not consume tobacco products.[1] All HF patients who smoke should be counseled on the importance of tobacco cessation and offered a referral to a cessation program. Patients with an alcoholic cardiomyopathy should abstain from alcohol. Whether all patients with other forms of HF should abstain from any alcohol intake remains controversial. Proponents of moderation of alcohol base their rationale on the potential cardioprotective effects. However, opponents to any alcohol intake point out that alcohol is cardiotoxic and should be avoided.

In general, it is suggested that patients remain up-to-date on standard immunizations. Patients should be counseled to receive yearly influenza vaccinations. Additionally, pneumococcal vaccines are recommended.

Pharmacologic Treatment

In addition to determining therapeutic goals, the ACC/AHA staging system delineates specific therapy options based on disease progression.[1] For patients in stage A, every effort is made to minimize the impact of diseases that can injure the heart. Antihypertensive and lipid-lowering therapies should be utilized when appropriate to decrease the risk for stroke, MI, and HF. ACE inhibitors should be considered in high-risk vascular disease patients. For stage B patients, the goal is to prevent or slow disease progression by interfering with neurohormonal pathways that lead to cardiac damage and mediate pathological remodeling. The goal is to prevent the onset of HF symptoms. The backbone of therapy in these patients includes ACE inhibitors or ARBs and β-blockers. In stage C patients with symptomatic LV systolic dysfunction (EF less than 40% [0.40]), the goals focus on alleviating fluid retention, minimizing disability, slowing disease progression, and reducing long-term risk for hospitalizations and death. Treatment entails a strategy that combines diuretics to control intravascular fluid balance with neurohormonal antagonists (including ACE inhibitors or ARBs, β-adrenergic blockers, and aldosterone receptor antagonists) to minimize the effects of the RAAS and SNS. Digoxin may be added to improve symptoms. If a patient continues to exhibit evidence of disease progression, other therapies can be used. In some cases, these include the combination of ACE inhibitors and ARBs, although the evidence for this option is limited. Another option is combination of hydralazine and isosorbide dinitrate in African American patients. Patients with advanced stage D disease are offered more modest goals, such as improvement in quality of life. Enhancing quality of life is often achieved at the expense of expected survival. Treatment options include mechanical support, transplantation, and continuous use of intravenous (IV) vasoactive therapies, in addition to maintaining an optimal regimen of chronic oral medications.

► *Diuretics*

Diuretics have been the mainstay for HF symptom management for many years. KEY CONCEPT *Diuretics are used for relief of acute symptoms of congestion and maintenance of euvolemia.* These agents interfere with sodium retention by increasing urinary sodium and free water excretion. No prospective data exist on the effects of diuretics on patient outcomes. Therefore, the primary rationale for the use of diuretic therapy is to maintain euvolemia in symptomatic or stages C and D HF. Diuretic therapy is recommended for all patients with clinical evidence of fluid overload. In mild HF, diuretics may be used on an as-needed basis. However, once the development of edema is persistent, regularly scheduled doses will be required.

Two types of diuretics are used for volume management in HF: thiazides and loop diuretics. Thiazide diuretics such as hydrochlorothiazide, chlorthalidone, and metolazone block sodium and chloride reabsorption in the distal convoluted tubule. Thiazides are weaker than loop diuretics in terms of effecting an increase in urine output and therefore are not utilized frequently as monotherapy. They are optimally suited for patients with hypertension who have mild congestion. Additionally, the action of thiazides is limited in patients with renal insufficiency (creatinine clearance less than 30 mL/min [0.50 mL/s]) due to reduced secretion into their site of action. An exception is metolazone, which retains its potent action in patients with renal dysfunction. Metolazone is often used in combination with loop diuretics when patients exhibit diuretic resistance, defined as edema unresponsive to loop diuretics alone.

Loop diuretics are the most widely used diuretics in HF. These agents, including furosemide, bumetanide, and torsemide, exert their action at the thick ascending loop of Henle. Loop diuretics are not filtered through the glomerulus, but instead undergo active transport into the tubular lumen via the organic acid pathway. As a result, drugs that compete for this active transport (eg, probenecid and organic by-products of uremia) can lower efficacy of loop diuretics. Loop diuretics increase sodium and water excretion and induce a prostaglandin-mediated increase in renal blood flow that contributes to their natriuretic effect. Unlike thiazides, they retain their diuretic ability in patients with poor renal function. The various loop diuretics are equally effective when used at equipotent doses, although there are intrinsic differences in pharmacokinetics and pharmacodynamics (Table 6–6).[5] The choice of which loop diuretic to use and the route of administration depends on clinical factors such as the presence of intestinal edema and rapidity of the desired effect. Oral diuretic efficacy may vary based on differing bioavailability, which is almost complete for torsemide and bumetanide but averages only 50% for furosemide. Oral torsemide can be considered an alternative to the IV route of administration for patients who do not respond to oral furosemide in the setting of profound edema. Onset of effect is slightly delayed after oral

Table 6–6

Loop Diuretics Used in Heart Failure

	Furosemide	Bumetanide	Torsemide
Usual daily dose (oral)	20–160 mg	0.5–4 mg	10–80 mg
Ceiling dose:			
Normal renal function	80–160 mg	1–2 mg	20–40 mg
CrCL 20–50 mL/min (0.33–0.83 mL/s)	160 mg	2 mg	40 mg
CrCL < 20 mL/min (0.33 mL/s)	400 mg	8–10 mg	100 mg
Bioavailability	10%–100% (average 50%)	80%–90%	80%–100%
Affected by food	Yes	Yes	No
Half-life	0.3–3.4 hours	0.3–1.5 hours	3–4 hours

CrCL, creatinine clearance.

From Parker RB, Cavallari LH. Systolic heart failure. In: DiPiro JT, Talbert RL, Yee GC, et al., eds. Pharmacotherapy: A Pathophysiologic Approach, 8th ed. New York, NY: McGraw-Hill, 2011:152, with permission.

administration but occurs within a few minutes with IV dosing. Consequently, bioequivalent doses of IV furosemide are half the oral dose, whereas bumetanide and torsemide IV doses are generally equivalent to the oral doses.

In patients with evidence of mild to moderate volume overload, diuretics should be initiated at a low dose and titrated to achieve a weight loss of up to 2 pounds (0.9 kg) per day. Patients with severe volume overload should be managed in an inpatient setting. Once diuretic therapy is initiated, dosage adjustments are based on symptomatic improvement and daily body weight. Because body weight changes are a sensitive marker of fluid retention or loss, patients should continue to weigh themselves daily. Once a patient reaches a euvolemic state, diuretics may be cautiously tapered and then withdrawn in appropriate patients. In stable, educated, and adherent patients, another option is self-adjusted diuretic dosing. Based on daily body weight, patients may temporarily increase their diuretic regimen to reduce the incidence of overt edema. This also avoids overuse of diuretics and possible complications of overdiuresis such as hypotension, fatigue, electrolyte imbalances, and renal impairment.

The maximal response to diuretics is reduced in HF, creating a "ceiling dose" above which there is limited added benefit. This diuretic resistance is due to a compensatory increase in sodium reabsorption in the distal tubules, which decreases the effect of blocking sodium reabsorption in the loop of Henle. In addition, there is a simultaneous increase in the reabsorption of sodium from the proximal tubule, allowing less to reach the site of action for loop diuretics. Apart from increasing diuretic doses, strategies to improve diuretic efficacy include increasing the frequency of dosing to two or three times daily, utilizing a continuous infusion of a loop diuretic, and/or combining a loop diuretic with a thiazide diuretic. The latter strategy theoretically prevents sodium and water reabsorption at both the loop of Henle and the compensating distal convoluted tubule. Metolazone is used most often for this purpose because it retains its activity in settings of low creatinine clearance. Metolazone can be dosed daily or as little as once weekly. This combination is usually maintained until the patient reaches his or her baseline weight. The clinician must use metolazone cautiously because its potent activity predisposes a patient to metabolic abnormalities as outlined next.

Diuretics cause numerous adverse effects and metabolic abnormalities, with severity linked to diuretic potency. A particularly worrisome adverse effect is hypokalemia which can predispose patients to arrhythmias and sudden death. Hypomagnesemia often occurs concomitantly with diuretic-induced hypokalemia, and therefore both should be assessed and replaced in patients needing correction of hypokalemia. Magnesium is an essential cofactor for movement of potassium intracellularly to restore body stores. Patients taking diuretics are also at risk for renal insufficiency due to overdiuresis and reflex activation of the renin-angiotensin system. The potential reduction in renal blood flow and glomerular pressure is amplified by concomitant use of ACE inhibitors or ARBs.

▸ *Neurohormonal Blocking Agents*

KEY CONCEPT *Agents with proven benefits in improving symptoms, slowing disease progression, and improving survival in chronic HF target neurohormonal blockade. These include ACE inhibitors, ARBs, β-adrenergic blockers, and aldosterone receptor antagonists.*

Angiotensin-Converting Enzyme Inhibitors ACE inhibitors are the cornerstone of treatment for HF. ACE inhibitors decrease neurohormonal activation by blocking the conversion of angiotensin I (AT_1) to angiotensin II (AT_2), a potent mediator of vasoconstriction and cardiac remodeling. The breakdown of bradykinin is also reduced. Bradykinin enhances the release of vasodilatory prostaglandins and histamines. These effects result in arterial and venous dilatation, and a decrease in myocardial workload through reduction of both preload and afterload. ACE inhibitors demonstrate favorable effects on cardiac hemodynamics, such as long-term increases in **cardiac index** (CI), stroke work index, and SV index, as well as significant reductions in LV filling pressure, SVR, mean arterial pressure, and HR.

There is extensive clinical experience with ACE inhibitors in systolic HF. Numerous clinical studies show ACE inhibitor therapy is associated with improvements in clinical symptoms, exercise tolerance, NYHA FC, LV size and function, and quality of life as compared with placebo.[12–14] ACE inhibitors significantly reduce hospitalization rates and mortality regardless of underlying disease severity or etiology. ACE inhibitors are also effective in preventing HF development in high-risk patients. Studies in acute MI patients show a reduction in new-onset HF and death with ACE inhibitors whether they are initiated early (within 36 hours) or started later. In addition, ACE inhibition decreases the risk of HF hospitalization and death in patients with asymptomatic LV dysfunction. The exact mechanisms for decreased HF progression and mortality are postulated to involve both the hemodynamic improvement and the inhibition of AT_2's growth promoting and remodeling effects. All patients with documented LV systolic dysfunction, regardless of existing HF symptoms, should receive ACE inhibitors unless a contraindication or intolerance is present.

There is no evidence to suggest that one ACE inhibitor is preferred over another. ACE inhibitors should be initiated using low doses and titrated up to target doses over several weeks depending on tolerability (adverse effects and BP). The ACC/AHA 2013 guidelines advocate using doses that were proven to decrease mortality in clinical trials as the target doses (Table 6–7).[1] If the target dose cannot be attained in a given patient, the highest tolerated dose should be used chronically. Although there is incremental benefit with higher doses of ACE inhibitors, it is accepted that lower doses provide substantial if not most of the effect.[15] Because ACE inhibitors are only one component of a mortality-reducing treatment plan in HF, targeting a high ACE inhibitor dose should be used cautiously to avoid a hypotensive effect that precludes starting a β-blocker or aldosterone receptor antagonist.

Despite their clear benefits, ACE inhibitors are still underutilized in HF. One reason is undue concern or confusion regarding absolute versus relative contraindications for their use. Absolute contraindications include a history of angioedema, bilateral renal artery stenosis, and pregnancy. Relative contraindications include unilateral renal artery stenosis, renal insufficiency, hypotension, hyperkalemia, and cough. Relative contraindications provide a warning that close monitoring is required, but they do not necessarily preclude their use.

Clinicians are especially concerned about the use of ACE inhibitors in patients with renal insufficiency. It is important to recognize that ACE inhibitors can potentially contribute to the preservation or decline of renal function depending on the clinical scenario. Through preferential efferent arteriole vasodilation, ACE inhibitors can reduce intraglomerular pressure. Reduced glomerular pressures are renoprotective chronically; however, in situations of reduced or fixed renal blood flow, this leads to a reduction in filtration. In general, ACE inhibitors can be used in patients with serum creatinine less than 2.5 to 3.0 mg/dL (221–265 μmol/L). In HF, their addition can result in improved

Table 6–7

Dosing and Monitoring for Neurohormonal Blocking Agents

Drug	Initial Daily Dose	Target or Maximum Daily Dose	Monitoring
ACE Inhibitors[a]			
Captopril	6.25 mg three times	50 mg three times	BP
Enalapril	2.5 mg twice	10–20 mg twice	Electrolytes (K^+, BUN, SCr) at baseline, 2 weeks, and after dose titration, CBC periodically
Fosinopril	5–10 mg once	40 mg once	
Lisinopril	2.5–5 mg once	20–40 mg once	Adverse effects: cough, angioedema
Perindopril	2 mg once	8–16 mg once	
Quinapril	5 mg once	20 mg twice	
Ramipril	1.25–2.5 mg twice	5 mg twice	
Trandolapril	1 mg once	4 mg once	
Angiotensin Receptor Blockers[a]			
Candesartan	4–8 mg once	32 mg once	BP
Losartan	25–50 mg once	50–100 mg once	Electrolytes (K^+, BUN, SCr) at baseline, 2 weeks, and after dose titration, CBC periodically
Valsartan	20–40 mg once	160 mg twice	Adverse effects: cough, angioedema
Aldosterone Antagonists			
Spironolactone	12.5–25 mg once	25 mg once or twice	BP
Eplerenone	25 mg once	50 mg once	Electrolytes (K^+) at baseline and within 1 week of initiation and dose titration Adverse effects: gynecomastia or breast tenderness, menstrual changes, hirsutism
β-Blockers			
Bisoprolol	1.25 mg once	10 mg once	BP, HR baseline and after each dose titration, ECG
Carvedilol	3.125 mg twice	25 mg twice (50 mg twice for patients > 85 kg or 187 lb)	Adverse effects: worsening HF symptoms (edema, SOB, fatigue), depression, sexual dysfunction
Metoprolol succinate	12.5–25 mg once	200 mg once	

[a]Use lower dose listed in patients with renal failure.

ACE, angiotensin-converting enzyme; BP, blood pressure; BUN, blood urea nitrate; CBC, complete blood cell count; ECG, electrocardiogram; HF, heart failure; HR, heart rate; K^+, potassium; SCr, serum creatinine; SOB, shortness of breath.

renal function through an increase in CO and renal perfusion. Although a small increase in serum creatinine (less than 0.5 mg/dL [44 μmol/L]) is possible with the addition of an ACE inhibitor, it is usually transient or becomes the patient's new serum creatinine baseline level. However, ACE inhibition can also worsen renal function because glomerular filtration is maintained in the setting of reduced CO through AT_2's constriction of the efferent arteriole. Patients most dependent on AT_2 for maintenance of glomerular filtration pressure, and hence most susceptible to ACE inhibitor worsening of renal function, include those with hyponatremia, severely depressed LV function, or dehydration. The most common reason for creatinine elevation in a patient without a history of renal dysfunction is overdiuresis. Therefore, clinicians should consider decreasing or holding diuretic doses if an elevation in serum creatinine occurs concomitantly with a rise in blood urea nitrogen (BUN).

Hypotension occurs commonly at the initiation of therapy or with dosage increases but may happen anytime during therapy. Hypotension can manifest as dizziness, lightheadedness, presyncope, or syncope. The risk of hypotension due to possible volume depletion increases when ACE inhibitors are initiated or used concomitantly in patients on high diuretic doses. Therefore, in euvolemic patients, diuretic doses may often be decreased or withheld during ACE inhibitor dose titration. Initiating at a low dose and titrating slowly can also minimize hypotension. It may be advisable to initiate therapy with a short-acting ACE inhibitor, such as captopril, and subsequently switch to a longer-acting agent, such as lisinopril or enalapril, once the patient is stabilized.

Hyperkalemia results from reduced angiotensin II–stimulated aldosterone release. The risk of hyperkalemia with ACE inhibitors is also increased in HF due to a propensity for impaired renal function and additive effects with aldosterone receptor antagonists. ACE inhibitor dose may need to be decreased or held if serum potassium increases above 5 mEq/L (5 mmol/L). Persistent hyperkalemia in the setting of renal insufficiency may preclude the use of an ACE inhibitor.

Cough is commonly seen with ACE inhibitors (5%–15%) and may be related to accumulation of tissue bradykinins.[5] It can be challenging to distinguish an ACE inhibitor–induced cough from cough caused by pulmonary congestion. A productive or wet cough usually signifies congestion, whereas a dry, hacking cough is more indicative of a drug-related etiology. If a cough is determined to be ACE inhibitor–induced, its severity should be evaluated before deciding on a course of action. If the cough is truly bothersome, a trial with a different ACE inhibitor or switching to an ARB is warranted.

Angiotensin Receptor Blockers ARBs selectively antagonize the effects of AT_2 directly at the AT_1 receptor. AT_1 receptor stimulation is associated with vasoconstriction, release of aldosterone, and cellular growth promoting effects, whereas AT_2 stimulation causes vasodilation. By selectively blocking AT_1 but leaving AT_2 unaffected, ARBs block the detrimental AT_1 effects on cardiac function while allowing AT_2-mediated vasodilation and inhibition of ventricular remodeling. ARBs are considered an equally effective replacement for ACE inhibitors in patients who are intolerant or have a contraindication to an ACE inhibitor.

Prospective randomized trials suggest the clinical efficacy of ARBs is similar to that of ACE inhibitors for reduction of hospitalizations for HF, sudden cardiac death, and all-cause mortality.[16–18] Despite poorer suppression of AT_2, comparable efficacy of ACE inhibitors may be due to the additional effects on the kallikrein-kinin system. Although ARBs produce hemodynamic and neurohormonal effects similar to those of ACE inhibitors, they are considered second-line therapy due to the overwhelming clinical trial experience with ACE inhibitors.

Because the mechanism for long-term benefit appears different for ACE inhibitors and ARBs, the combination has been studied for additive benefits. In one study, candesartan reduced the combined incidence of cardiovascular death and hospitalization for HF; however, the greatest benefit was noted in those not on an ACE inhibitor. Candesartan also significantly decreased mortality compared with placebo. Based on this study, the addition of an ARB to ACE inhibitor therapy can be considered in patients with evidence of disease progression despite optimal ACE inhibitor therapy and when aldosterone receptor antagonists are not tolerated, although this strategy is not widely applied.[1]

ARBs show similar tolerability to ACE inhibitors with regard to hypotension and hyperkalemia, but they are less likely to induce cough because ARBs do not cause an accumulation of bradykinin. ARBs can be considered in patients with ACE inhibitor–induced angioedema, but should be initiated cautiously because cross-reactivity has been reported. Many of the other considerations for use of ARBs are similar to those of ACE inhibitors, including the need for monitoring renal function, BP, and potassium. Contraindications are similar to those of ACE inhibitors. In patients truly intolerant or contraindicated to ACE inhibitors or ARBs, the combination of hydralazine and isosorbide dinitrate should be considered.

Hydralazine and Isosorbide Dinitrate Complementary hemodynamic actions originally led to the combination of nitrates with hydralazine. Nitrates reduce preload by causing primarily venous vasodilation through activating guanylate cyclase and a subsequent increase in cGMP in vascular smooth muscle. Hydralazine reduces afterload through direct arterial smooth muscle relaxation via an unknown mechanism. More recently, nitric oxide has been implicated in modulating numerous pathophysiological processes in the failing heart including inflammation, cardiac remodeling, and oxidative damage. Supplementation of nitric oxide via administration of nitrates has also been proposed as a mechanism for benefit from this combination therapy. The beneficial effect of an external nitric oxide source may be more apparent in the African American population, which appears to be predisposed to having an imbalance in nitric oxide production. In addition, hydralazine may reduce the development of nitrate tolerance when nitrates are given chronically.

The combination of hydralazine and isosorbide dinitrate was the first therapy shown to improve long-term survival in patients with systolic HF, but it has largely been supplanted by AT_2 antagonist therapy (ACE inhibitors and ARBs).[19,20] Therefore, until recently, this combination therapy was reserved for patients intolerant to ACE inhibitors or ARBs secondary to renal impairment, angioedema, or hyperkalemia. New insight into the pathophysiological role of nitric oxide has reinvigorated research into this combination therapy.

The nitrate–hydralazine combination was first shown to improve survival compared with placebo.[19] However, when compared with an ACE inhibitor, enalapril produced a 28% greater decrease in mortality.[20] Therefore, the combination is considered a third-line vasodilatory option for patients truly intolerant of ACE inhibitors and ARBs.

More recently, the value of adding the combination of isosorbide dinitrate 40 mg and hydralazine 75 mg three times daily to therapy including ACE inhibitors, β-blockers, digoxin, and diuretics was shown in a prospective randomized trial in African American patients.[21] KEY CONCEPT *Combination therapy with hydralazine and isosorbide dinitrate is an appropriate substitute for AT_2 antagonism in those unable to tolerate an ACE inhibitor or ARB or as add-on therapy in African Americans.* The ACC/AHA HF guidelines now recommend considering the addition of isosorbide dinitrate and hydralazine in African Americans already on ACE inhibitors or ARBs.[1] Combination therapy with isosorbide dinitrate and hydralazine should be initiated and titrated as are other neurohormonal agents such as ACE inhibitors and β-blockers. Low doses are used to initiate therapy with subsequent titration of the dose toward target doses based on tolerability. Adverse effects such as hypotension and headache cause frequent discontinuations in patients taking this combination, and full doses often cannot be tolerated. Patients should be monitored for headache, hypotension, and tachycardia. Hydralazine is also associated with a dose-dependent risk for lupus.

The frequent dosing of isosorbide dinitrate (eg, three to four times daily) is not conducive to patient adherence; therefore, a once-daily isosorbide mononitrate is commonly substituted for isosorbide dinitrate to simplify the dosing regimen. A nitrate-free interval is still required when using nitrates for HF.

β-Adrenergic Antagonists β-adrenergic antagonists, or β-blockers, competitively block the influence of the SNS at β-adrenergic receptors. As recently as 15 to 20 years ago, β-adrenergic blockers were thought to be detrimental in HF due to their negative inotropic actions, which could potentially worsen symptoms and cause acute decompensations. Since then, the benefits of inhibiting the SNS have been recognized as far outweighing the acute negative inotropic effects. Chronic β-blockade reduces ventricular mass, improves ventricular shape, and reduces LV end-systolic and diastolic volumes.[6,8] β-blockers also exhibit antiarrhythmic effects, slow or reverse catecholamine-induced ventricular remodeling, decrease myocyte death from catecholamine-induced necrosis or apoptosis, and prevent myocardial fetal gene expression. Consequently, β-blockers improve EF, reduce all-cause and HF-related hospitalizations, and decrease all-cause mortality in patients with systolic HF.[22–24]

The ACC/AHA recommends that β-blockers be initiated in all patients with NYHA FC I to IV or ACC/AHA stages B through D HF if clinically stable.[1] To date, only three β-blockers have been shown to reduce mortality in systolic HF including the selective β_1-antagonists bisoprolol and metoprolol succinate, and the nonselective β_1-, β_2-, and α_1-antagonist carvedilol.[22–24] The positive findings of β-blockers are not a class effect because bucindolol did not exhibit a beneficial effect on mortality when studied for HF, and there is limited information with propranolol and atenolol.

Although metoprolol succinate and carvedilol are the most commonly used β-antagonists in HF, it is unknown whether one agent should be considered first line. Carvedilol was shown to lower all-cause mortality significantly more than metoprolol tartrate, but carvedilol has not been directly compared to metoprolol succinate.[25]

The key to utilizing β-blockers in systolic HF is initiation with low doses and slow titration to target doses over weeks to months. It is important that the β-blocker be initiated when a patient is clinically stable and euvolemic. Volume overload at the time of β-blocker initiation increases the risk for worsening symptoms. β-blockade should begin with the lowest possible dose (Table 6–7), after which the dose may be doubled every 2 to 4 weeks depending on patient tolerability. β-blockers may cause an acute decrease in LVEF and short-term worsening of HF symptoms upon initiation and at each dosage titration. After each dose titration, if the patient experiences symptomatic hypotension, bradycardia, orthostasis, or worsening symptoms, further increases in dose should be withheld until the patient stabilizes. After stabilization, attempts to increase the dose should be reinstituted. If mild congestion ensues as a result of the β-blocker, an increase in diuretic dose may be warranted. If moderate or severe symptoms of congestion occur, a reduction in β-blocker dose should be considered along with an increase in diuretic dose. Dose titration should continue until target clinical trial doses are achieved (Table 6–7) or until limited by repeated hemodynamic or symptomatic intolerance. Patient education regarding the possibility of acutely worsening symptoms but improved long-term function and survival is essential to ensure adherence.

Apart from possible clinical differences between the β-blockers approved for HF, selection of a β-blocker may also be affected by pharmacologic differences. Carvedilol exhibits a more pronounced BP lowering effect, and thus causes more frequent dizziness and hypotension as a consequence of its β_1- and α_1-receptor blocking activities. Therefore, in patients predisposed to symptomatic hypotension, such as those with advanced LV dysfunction (LVEF less than 20% [0.20]) who normally exhibit low systolic BP, metoprolol succinate may be the more desirable first-line β-blocker. In patients with uncontrolled hypertension, carvedilol may provide additional antihypertensive efficacy.

β-blockers may be used by those with reactive airway disease or peripheral vascular disease but should be used with considerable caution or avoided if patients display active respiratory symptoms. Care must also be used in interpreting shortness of breath in these patients because the etiology could be either cardiac or pulmonary. A selective β_1-blocker such as metoprolol succinate is a reasonable option for patients with reactive airway disease. The risk versus benefit of using any β-blocker in peripheral vascular disease must be weighed based on the severity of the peripheral disease, and a selective β_1-blocker is preferred.

Both metoprolol and carvedilol are metabolized by the liver through cytochrome P-450 (CYP450) 2D6 and undergo extensive first-pass metabolism. β-blockers should not be used in patients with severe hepatic failure. Bisoprolol is not as commonly used since it is not Food and Drug Administration (FDA) approved for HF.

There is some debate regarding which class of agents should be initiated first in a patient with HF, namely, ACE inhibitors or β-blockers. A recent study evaluated whether the order of initiation affects all-cause mortality or hospitalization and found no difference but that more events occurred during the 6-month single-treatment phase part of the study.[26] These findings reinforce the importance of using both ACE inhibitors and β-blockers in the HF patient. As such, doses of the agent initiated first should not prohibit initiation of the second class of agents.

Mineralocorticoid Receptor Antagonists (MRAs) The MRAs currently available are spironolactone and eplerenone. Both agents are inhibitors of aldosterone that produce weak diuretic effects while sparing potassium concentrations. Eplerenone is selective for the mineralocorticoid receptor and hence does not exhibit the endocrine adverse effect profile commonly seen with spironolactone. The initial rationale for specifically targeting aldosterone for treatment of HF was based on the knowledge that ACE inhibitors do not suppress the chronic production and release of aldosterone. Aldosterone is a key pathological neurohormone that exerts multiple detrimental effects in HF. Similar to norepinephrine and AT_2, aldosterone levels are increased in HF and have been shown to correlate with disease severity and patient outcomes.

MRAs have been shown to improve clinical outcomes, including mortality, across the spectrum of HF in three separate clinical trials. These comprised patients who were post-MI with LVEF less than 40% (0.40), patients with NYHA FC II HF, and patients with NYHA FC III-IV HF.[27–29] It is postulated that MRAs reduce mortality at least in part through prevention of sudden cardiac death. Based on these studies, the ACC/AHA guidelines recommended MRAs in NYHA FC II through IV patients with LVEF less than 35% (0.35), unless contraindicated, in addition to patients post-MI with evidence of LV dysfunction. For individuals with mild symptoms (NYHA FC II), it is recommended they also exhibit a history of hospitalization or elevated BNP levels.[1]

The major risk related to MRAs is hyperkalemia. Therefore, the decision for use of these agents should balance the benefit of decreasing death and hospitalization from HF and the potential risks of life-threatening hyperkalemia. Before and within 1 week of initiating therapy, two parameters must be assessed: serum potassium and creatinine clearance (or serum creatinine). MRAs should not be initiated in patients with potassium concentrations greater than 5.0 mEq/L (5.0 mmol/L). Likewise, these agents should not be given when creatinine clearance is less than 30 mL/min (0.50 mL/s) or serum creatinine is greater than 2.5 mg/dL (221 μmol/L).

In patients without contraindications, spironolactone is initiated at a dose of 12.5 to 25 mg daily, or occasionally on alternate days for patients with baseline renal insufficiency. Eplerenone is used at a dose of 25 mg daily, with the option to titrate up to 50 mg daily. Doses should be halved or switched to alternate-day dosing if creatinine clearance falls below 50 mL/min (0.83 mL/s). Potassium supplementation is often decreased or stopped after MRAs are initiated, and patients should be counseled to avoid high-potassium foods. At any time after initiation of therapy, if potassium concentrations exceed 5.5 mEq/L (5.5 mmol/L), the dose of the MRA should be reduced or discontinued. In addition, worsening renal function dictates consideration for stopping the MRA. Other adverse effects observed mainly with spironolactone include gynecomastia for men and breast tenderness and menstrual irregularities for women. Gynecomastia leads to discontinuation in up to 10% of patients on spironolactone. Eplerenone is a CYP3 A4 substrate and should not be used concomitantly with strong inhibitors of 3A4.

▸ Digoxin

Digoxin has been used for several decades in the treatment of HF. Traditionally, it was considered useful for its positive inotropic effects, but more recently its benefits are thought to be related to neurohormonal modulation. Digoxin exerts positive inotropic effects through binding to sodium- and potassium-activated adenosine triphosphate (ATP) pumps, leading to increased intracellular sodium concentrations and subsequently more available intracellular calcium during systole. The mechanism of digoxin's neurohormonal blocking effect is less well understood but may be related to restoration of baroreceptor sensitivity and reduced central sympathetic outflow.[5]

The exact role of digoxin in therapy remains controversial largely due to disagreement on the risk versus benefit of routinely using this drug in patients with systolic HF. Digoxin was shown to decrease HF-related hospitalizations but did not decrease HF progression or improve survival.[30] Moreover, digoxin was associated with an increased risk for concentration-related toxicity and numerous adverse effects. Post hoc study analyses demonstrated a clear relationship between digoxin plasma concentration and outcomes. Concentrations below 1.2 ng/mL (1.5 nmol/L) were associated with no apparent adverse effect on survival, whereas higher concentrations increased the relative risk of mortality.[31]

Current recommendations are for the addition of digoxin for patients who remain symptomatic despite an optimal HF regimen consisting of an ACE inhibitor or ARB, β-blocker, and diuretic. In patients with concomitant atrial fibrillation, digoxin may occasionally be added to slow ventricular rate, however, β-blockers are more effective at controlling ventricular rate, especially in the setting of exercise. Clinicians may also consider adding digoxin in patients with severe HF who have not responded symptomatically to neurohormonal blockade.

Digoxin is initiated at a dose of 0.125 to 0.25 mg daily depending on age, renal function, weight, and risk for toxicity. The lower dose should be used if the patient satisfies any of the following criteria: older than 65 years, creatinine clearance less than 60 mL/min (1.0 mL/s), or ideal body weight less than 70 kg (154 lb). The 0.125-mg daily dose is adequate in most patients. Doses are halved or switched to alternate-day dosing in patients with moderate to severe renal failure. The desired concentration range for digoxin is 0.5 to 0.9 ng/mL (0.6–1.2 nmol/L), preferably with concentrations at or less than 0.8 ng/mL (1.0 nmol/L). Routine monitoring of serum drug concentrations is not required but recommended in those with changes in renal function, suspected toxicity, or after addition or subtraction of an interacting drug.

Digoxin toxicity may manifest as nonspecific findings such as fatigue or weakness and other central nervous system (CNS) effects such as confusion, delirium, and psychosis. GI manifestations include nausea, vomiting, or anorexia, and visual disturbances may occur such as halos, photophobia, and color perception problems (red-green or yellow-green vision). Cardiac findings include numerous types of arrhythmias related to enhanced automaticity, slowed or accelerated conduction, or delayed after-depolarizations. These include ventricular tachycardia and fibrillation, atrioventricular nodal block, and sinus bradycardia. Risk of digoxin toxicity, in particular, the cardiac manifestations, are increased with electrolyte disturbances such as hypokalemia, hypercalcemia, and hypomagnesemia. To reduce the proarrhythmic risk of digoxin, serum potassium and magnesium should be monitored closely and supplemented when appropriate to ensure adequate concentrations (potassium greater than 4.0 mEq/L [4.0 mmol/L] and magnesium greater than 2.0 mEq/L [1.0 mmol/L]). In patients with life-threatening toxicity due to cardiac or other findings, administration of digoxin-specific Fab antibody fragments usually reverses adverse effects within an hour in most cases.

▶ *Calcium Channel Blockers*

Treatment with nondihydropyridine calcium channel blockers (diltiazem and verapamil) may worsen HF and increase the risk of death in patients with advanced LV systolic dysfunction due to their negative inotropic effects. Conversely, dihydropyridine calcium channel blockers, although negative inotropes in vitro, do not appear to decrease contractility in vivo. Amlodipine and felodipine are the two most extensively studied dihydropyridine calcium channel blockers for systolic HF.[32,33] These two agents have not been shown to affect patient survival, either positively or negatively. As such, they are not routinely recommended as part of a standard HF regimen; however, amlodipine and felodipine can safely be used in HF patients to treat uncontrolled hypertension or angina once all other appropriate drugs are maximized.

▶ *Antiplatelets and Anticoagulation*

Patients with HF are at an increased risk of thromboembolic events secondary to a combination of hypercoagulability, relative stasis of blood, and endothelial dysfunction. However, the role of antiplatelets and anticoagulants remains debatable due to a lack of prospective clinical trials.

Aspirin is generally used in HF patients with an underlying ischemic etiology, a history of ischemic heart disease, or other compelling indications such as history of embolic stroke. Routine use in nonischemic cardiomyopathy patients is currently discouraged because of a lack of data supporting any long-term benefit, as well as the potential negative drug–drug interaction with ACE inhibitors and ARBs. If aspirin is indicated, the preference is to use a low dose (81 mg daily).

Current guidelines support chronic anticoagulation in patients with reduced LV systolic dysfunction and a compelling indication such as atrial fibrillation or prosthetic heart valves. For atrial fibrillation, a stronger level of evidence is given for use of anticoagulation in patients with an additional risk factor for cardioembolic stroke, such as history of hypertension, diabetes mellitus, previous stroke or transient ischemic attack, or age 75 years or older.[1] Patients with HF often have difficulty maintaining a therapeutic international normalized ratio (INR) due to fluctuating volume status and varying drug absorption. The choice of anticoagulant (warfarin vs novel anticoagulants) should be based on risk factors, tolerability, cost, and potential for drug–drug interactions.

▶ *LCZ696*

LCZ696 is a first in class angiotensin receptor neprilysin inhibitor.[34] Neprilysin is a neutral endopeptidase responsible for the breakdown of natriuretic peptides, in addition to substance P, adrenomedullin, bradykinin, and AT_2. Blockade of neprilysin increases circulating natriuretic peptide levels. Because neprilysin inhibition would also result in elevated levels of AT_2, combination of a neprilysin inhibitor with an ARB negates this potentially deleterious effect. LCZ696 is a crystalline complex composed of equal parts of the neprilysin inhibitor sacubitril and the ARB valsartan. Shortly after ingestion, LCZ696 breaks apart into sacubitril, a prodrug which is cleaved to the active form LBQ657, and valsartan. LCZ696 dosed at 200 mg twice daily was found to reduce the combined end point of cardiovascular death and hospitalization for HF by 20% compared to enalapril 10 mg twice daily in patients with symptomatic HF and reduced LVEF.[35] It is anticipated that HF guidelines will incorporate this drug, but whether LCZ696 will replace ACE inhibitors as first-line therapy will be clarified following additional research.

▶ *Complementary and Alternative Medications*

Complementary and alternative medications (CAMs) are treatment strategies not commonly used in Western medicine and are considered nutrition supplements by the FDA. Some patients with HF use CAM for heart problems, weight loss, anxiety, and arthritis. Fish oils, n-3 polyunsaturated fatty acids, or omega-3 fatty acids were recently studied for HF and found to mildly decrease cardiovascular admissions and mortality without significant adverse effects. Fish oils are more commonly used for treatment of hypertriglyceridemia. Their mechanism in HF is incompletely understood but postulated to involve decreased membrane excitability (thus reducing arrhythmias), decreased inflammation and platelet aggregation, and favorable changes in autonomic tone. Hawthorn is another CAM studied in HF and shown to increase exercise capacity and reduce HF symptoms. Its benefits are thought to be due to flavonoids that increase force of contraction and CO. The ACC/AHA guidelines do not currently advocate the use of fish oils and hawthorn for HF. It is important to counsel patients to remain on their other HF medications if they decide to initiate a CAM, and to let their health care providers know when starting a new supplement. As with any therapy, it is important to monitor for adverse events and therapeutic outcomes.

Heart Failure with Preserved Left Ventricular Ejection Fraction

It is now recognized that a significant number of patients exhibiting HF symptoms have normal systolic function or preserved LVEF (40%–60% [0.40–0.60]). It is believed the primary defect in these patients is impaired ventricular relaxation and filling, commonly referred to as HF with preserved EF (HFpEF). HFpEF is more prevalent in older women and closely associated with hypertension or diabetes and, to a lesser extent, CAD and atrial fibrillation. Morbidity in HFpEF is comparable to those with depressed EF because both are characterized by frequent, repeated hospitalizations. However, HFpEF appears to be associated with slightly lower mortality. The diagnosis is based on findings of typical signs and symptoms of HF, in conjunction with echocardiographic evidence of abnormal diastolic function, absence of significant LV chamber dilation, and no valvular disease.

Unlike systolic HF, few prospective trials have evaluated the safety and efficacy of various cardiac medications in patients with HFpEF. The PEP-CHF (Perindopril in Elderly People with Chronic Heart Failure) study did not find differences in mortality and hospitalizations between perindopril and placebo, but premature withdrawal of many patients after 1 year could have contributed to the neutral findings.[36] The Candesartan in Heart Failure Assessment of Reduction in Mortality and Morbidity (CHARM) study demonstrated that angiotensin receptor blockade with candesartan resulted in beneficial effects on HF morbidity in patients with preserved LVEF similar to those seen in depressed LV function.[18] However, the largest clinical trial in HFpEF, the I-PRESERVE (Irbesartan in Patients with Heart Failure and Preserved Ejection Fraction) study did not find a reduction in the primary composite outcome of death or hospitalizations between irbesartan and placebo.[37] In the TOPCAT (Treatment of Preserved Cardiac Function Heart Failure with an Aldosterone Antagonist) trial, spironolactone did not reduce the composite end point of cardiovascular death, aborted cardiac arrest, or HF hospitalizations, but resulted in reduced hospitalizations due to HF.[38] In the absence of more landmark clinical studies, the current treatment approach for HFpEF is: (a) correction or control of underlying etiologies (including optimal treatment of hypertension and CAD and maintenance of normal sinus rhythm); (b) reduction of cardiac filling pressures at rest and during exertion; and (c) increased diastolic filling time. Diuretics are frequently used to control congestion. β-blockers and calcium channel blockers can theoretically improve ventricular relaxation through negative inotropic and chronotropic effects. Unlike in systolic HF, nondihydropyridine calcium channel blockers (diltiazem and verapamil) may be especially useful in improving diastolic function by limiting the availability of calcium that mediates contractility. A recent study did not find favorable effects with digoxin in patients with mild to moderate diastolic HF. Therefore, the role of digoxin for symptom management and HR control in these patients is not well established.

Patient Encounter Part 3

Based on the information presented and your problem-based assessment, create a care plan for the patient's HF. Your plan should include:

- *Nonpharmacologic treatment options.*
- *Acute and chronic treatment plans to address symptoms and prevent disease deterioration.*
- *Monitoring plan for acute and chronic treatments.*

Outcome Evaluation of Chronic Heart Failure

- The evaluation of therapy is influenced by the ability of treatment to successfully reduce symptoms, improve quality of life, decrease frequency of hospitalizations for acute HF, reduce disease progression, and prolong survival (Figure 6–2).
- The major outcome parameters focus on (a) volume status, (b) exercise tolerance, (c) overall symptoms/quality of life, (d) adverse drug reactions, and (e) disease progression and cardiac function. Assess quality of life by evaluating patients' ability to continue their activities of daily living.
- Assess symptoms of HF such as dyspnea on exertion, orthopnea, weight gain, and edema, and abdominal manifestations such as nausea, bloating, and loss of appetite.
- If diuretic therapy is warranted, monitor for therapeutic response by assessing weight loss and improvement of fluid retention, as well as exercise tolerance and presence of fatigue.
- Once therapy for preventing disease progression is initiated, monitoring for symptomatic improvement continues.
- It is important to keep in mind that patients' symptoms can worsen with β-blockers, and it may take weeks or months before patients notice improvement.
- Monitor BP to evaluate for hypotension caused by drug therapy.
- To assess for prevention of disease progression, practitioners may utilize serial echocardiograms every 6 months to assess cardiac function and evaluate the effects of drug therapy.
- Occasional exercise testing is conducted to ascertain disease prognosis or suitability for heart transplant. Even though these tests can demonstrate improvement in heart function and therefore slowed disease progression, patient symptoms may not improve.

ACUTE AND ADVANCED HEART FAILURE

Clinical Presentation and Diagnosis of Acute Heart Failure

Patients with AHF present with symptoms of worsening fluid retention or decreasing exercise tolerance and fatigue (typically worsening of symptoms presented in the chronic HF clinical presentation text box). These symptoms reflect congestion behind

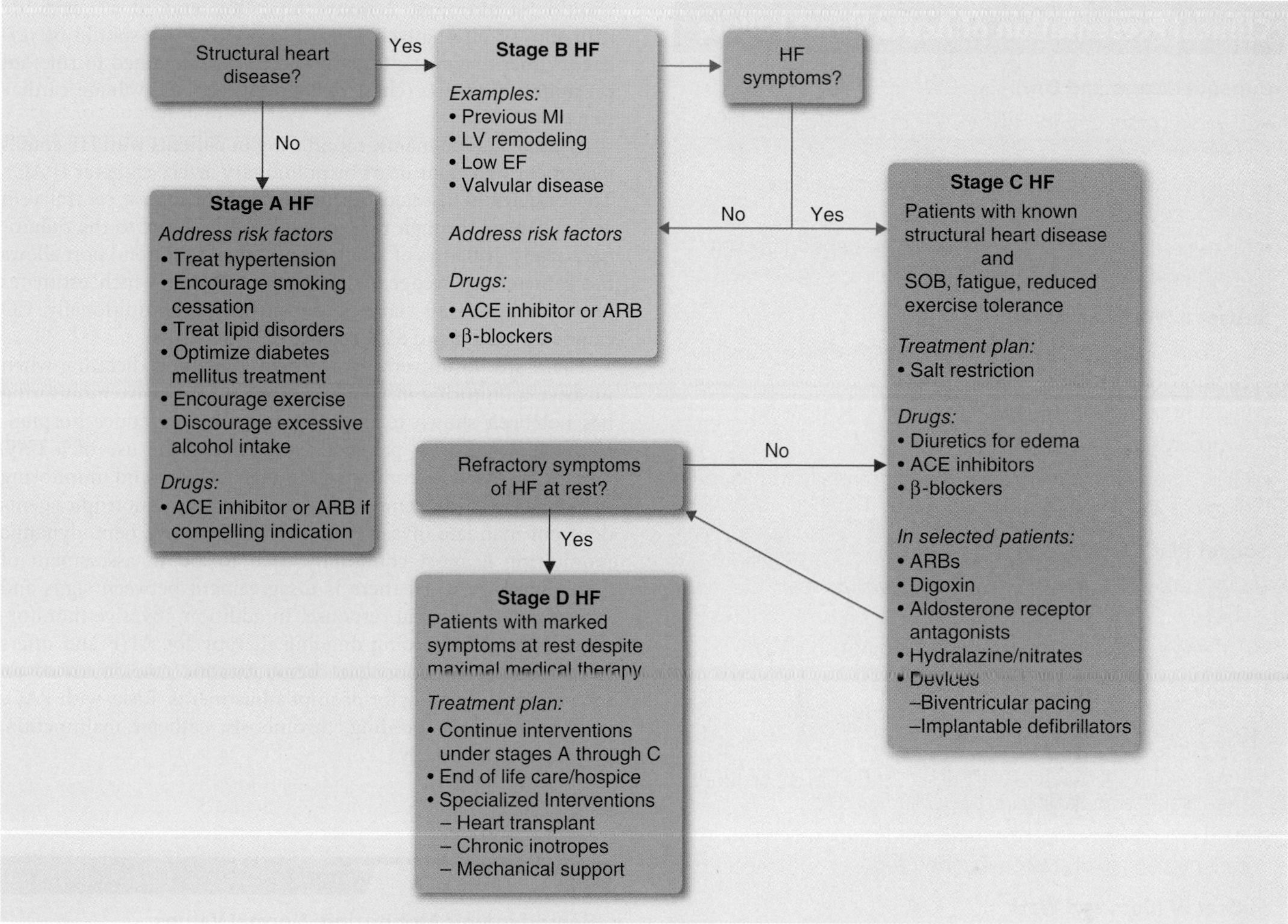

FIGURE 6–2. Treatment algorithm for chronic heart failure. (ACE, angiotensin-converting enzyme; ARB, angiotensin receptor blocker; EF, ejection fraction; HF, heart failure; LV, left ventricular; MI, myocardial infarction; SOB, shortness of breath.) Table 6–5 describes the staging of heart failure.

the failing ventricle and/or hypoperfusion. Patients can be categorized into hemodynamic subsets based on assessment of physical signs and symptoms of congestion and/or hypoperfusion.[39] Patients can be described as "wet" or "dry" depending on volume status, as well as "warm" or "cool" based on adequacy of tissue perfusion. "Wet" refers to patients with volume/fluid overload (eg, edema and jugular venous distension [JVD]), whereas "dry" refers to euvolemic patients. "Warm" refers to patients with adequate CO to perfuse peripheral tissues (and hence the skin will be warm to touch), whereas "cool" refers to patients with evidence of hypoperfusion (skin cool to touch with diminished pulses). Additionally, invasive hemodynamic monitoring can be used to provide objective data for assessing volume status (pulmonary capillary wedge pressure [PCWP]) and perfusion (CO). A CI below 2.2 L/min/m^2 is consistent with hypoperfusion and reduced contractility, and a PCWP above 18 mm Hg (2.4 kPa) correlates with congestion and an elevated preload. The four possible hemodynamic subsets a patient may fall into are "warm and dry," "warm and wet," "cool and dry," or "cool and wet."

▸ *Precipitating Factors*

KEY CONCEPT *It is important for the clinician to identify the cause(s) of AHF to maximize treatment efficacy and reduce future disease exacerbations. Cardiovascular, metabolic, and lifestyle factors can all precipitate AHF.* The most common precipitating factors for acute decompensation and how they contribute pathophysiologically are listed in Table 6–3.

▸ *Laboratory Assessment*

Routine laboratory testing of patients with AHF includes electrolytes and blood glucose, as well as serum creatinine and BUN to assess renal function. Complete blood cell count is measured to determine if anemia or infection is present. Creatine kinase and/or troponin concentrations are used to diagnose ischemia, and hepatic transaminases are measured to assess hepatic congestion. Thyroid function tests are measured to assess hyperthyroidism or hypothyroidism as causes of AHF. A urinalysis is attained in patients with an unknown history of renal disease to rule out nephrotic syndrome. Lastly, a toxicology screen is obtained in patients in whom the use of illicit drugs is suspected.

Assays measuring BNP and its degradation product N-terminal proBNP (NT-proBNP) are being used with greater frequency in clinical practice. BNP is synthesized, stored, and released from the ventricles in response to increased ventricular filling pressures. Hence plasma levels of BNP can be used as a marker for volume overload. The most widely accepted indication for BNP

Clinical Presentation of Acute Heart Failure

Subset I (Warm and Dry)

- CI *greater than* 2.2 L/min/m², PCWP *less than* 18 mm Hg (2.4 kPa)
- Patients considered well compensated and perfused, without evidence of congestion
- No immediate interventions necessary except optimizing oral medications and monitoring

Subset II (Warm and Wet)

- CI *greater than* 2.2 L/min/m², PCWP *greater than* or equal to 18 mm Hg (2.4 kPa)
- Patients adequately perfused and display signs and symptoms of congestion
- Main goal is to reduce preload (PCWP) carefully with loop diuretics and vasodilators

Subset III (Cool and Dry)

- CI *less than* 2.2 L/min/m², PCWP *less than* 18 mm Hg (2.4 kPa)
- Patients are inadequately perfused and not congested
- Hypoperfusion leads to increased mortality, elevating death rates fourfold compared with those who are adequately perfused
- Treatment focuses on increasing CO with positive inotropic agents and/or replacing intravascular fluids
- Fluid replacement must be performed cautiously because patients can rapidly become congested

Subset IV (Cool and Wet)

- CI *less than* 2.2 L/min/m², PCWP *greater than* 18 mm Hg (2.4 kPa)
- Patients are inadequately perfused and congested
- Classified as the most complicated clinical presentation of AHF with the worst prognosis
- Most challenging to treat; therapy targets alleviating signs and symptoms of congestion by increasing CI as well as reducing PCWP while maintaining adequate mean arterial pressure
- Treatment involves a delicate balance between diuretics, vasodilators, and inotropic agents
- Use of vasopressors is sometimes necessary to maintain BP

measurement is as an adjunctive aid for diagnosing a cardiac etiology for dyspnea.[10] The current values for ruling out a cardiac etiology for dyspnea are a BNP less than 100 pg/mL (100 ng/L or 28.9 pmol/L) or an NT-proBNP less than 300 pg/mL (300 ng/L or 35.4 pmol/L). BNP measurements require cautious interpretation because numerous conditions can also elevate BNP concentrations. These include older age, renal dysfunction, pulmonary embolism, and chronic pulmonary disease. Nesiritide, a recombinant BNP drug, has an identical structure to native BNP and will interfere with the commercial BNP assay, resulting in a falsely elevated level. Therefore, blood for BNP determination should be obtained 2 hours after the end of a nesiritide infusion, or alternatively the NT-proBNP assay should be utilized. Other diagnostic tests should also be obtained to rule out precipitating factors (chest radiograph) and to evaluate cardiac function (ECG).

Invasive hemodynamic monitoring in patients with HF entails placement of a right heart or pulmonary artery catheter (PAC). The catheter is inserted percutaneously through a central vein and advanced through the right side of the heart to the pulmonary artery. Inflation of a balloon proximal to the end port allows the catheter to "wedge," yielding the PCWP, which estimates pressures in the left ventricle during diastole. Additionally, CO can be estimated and SVR calculated (Table 6–8).

There are no universally accepted guidelines dictating when invasive monitoring in HF is required, and invasive monitoring has not been shown to improve mortality or reduce hospitalizations in high-risk patients. Nonetheless, the use of a PAC remains an essential component of management and monitoring of patients in cardiogenic shock; however, use of inotropic agents does not mandate invasive monitoring. Invasive hemodynamic monitoring is most commonly used to aid in assessment of hemodynamics when there is disagreement between signs and symptoms and clinical response. In addition, invasive monitoring is helpful in guiding ongoing therapy for AHF and offers the advantage of immediate hemodynamic assessment of an intervention, allowing for prompt adjustments. Risks with PACs include infection, bleeding, thrombosis, catheter malfunction, and ventricular ectopy.

Table 6–8

Hemodynamic Monitoring: Normal Values

Hemodynamic Variable	Normal Value
Central venous (right atrial) pressure, mean	< 5 mm Hg[a] (0.67 kPa)
Right ventricular pressure	25/0 mm Hg[a]
Pulmonary artery pressure	25/10 mm Hg[a]
Pulmonary artery pressure, mean	< 18 mm Hg[a] (2.4 kPa)
Pulmonary artery occlusion pressure, mean	< 12 mm Hg[a] (1.60 kPa)
Systemic arterial pressure	120/80 mm Hg[a]
Mean arterial pressure	90–120 mm Hg[a] (12.0–16.0 kPa)
Cardiac index	2.8–4.2 L/min/m²
Stroke volume index	30–65 mL/beat/m²[a] (0.030–0.065 L·beat⁻¹·m⁻²)
Systemic vascular resistance	900–1400 dyn·s·cm⁻⁵[b] (90–140 MPa·s·m⁻³)
Pulmonary vascular resistance	150–250 dyn·s·cm⁻⁵[b] (15–25 MPa·s·m⁻³)
Arterial oxygen content	20 mL/dL[b] (200 mL/L)
Mixed venous oxygen content	15 mL/dL[b] (150 mL/L)
Arteriovenous oxygen content difference	3–5 mL/dL[b] (30–50 mL/L)

[a]1 mm Hg = 0.133 kPa; 1 mL/beat per square meter = 0.001 L·beat⁻¹·m⁻².

[b]1 dyn·s·cm⁻⁵ = 0.1 MPa·s·m⁻³; 1 mL/dL = 10 mL/L.

From Rodgers JE, Reed BN. Acute decompensated heart failure. In: DiPiro JT, Talbert RL, Yee GC, et al., eds. Pharmacotherapy: A pathophysiologic approach, 9th ed. New York, NY: McGraw-Hill, 2014:127, with permission.

Desired Therapeutic Outcomes

The goals of therapy for AHF are to: (a) correct the underlying precipitating factor(s); (b) relieve the patient's symptoms; (c) improve hemodynamics; (d) optimize a chronic oral medication regimen; and (e) educate the patient, reinforcing adherence to lifestyle modifications and the drug regimen. The ultimate goal for a patient hospitalized for AHF is return to a compensated HF state and discharge to the outpatient setting on oral medications. Only through aggressive management to achieve all of these goals will a patient's prognosis be improved and future hospitalizations for acute decompensations be prevented.

Removal or control of precipitating factors is essential for an optimal response to pharmacologic therapy. Relief of symptoms should occur rapidly to minimize length of hospitalization. Although a rapid discharge from the hospital is desirable, a patient should not be discharged before ensuring that he or she is in a euvolemic, or nearly euvolemic, state with a body weight and functional capacity similar to before the acute decompensation. Oral agents such as β-blockers, ACE inhibitors or ARBs, and aldosterone antagonists should be initiated as soon as possible during the hospitalization. These chronic oral medications not only improve mortality and prevent readmissions, acutely they also contribute to improvement in hemodynamics. Patient education prior to discharge from the hospital is recommended to assist in minimizing adverse effects and nonadherence. Dissemination of written information, in addition to verbal information, is helpful for patient comprehension and retention. This can include therapy goals, lifestyle modifications, drug regimen, dosage information, and relevant adverse effects, as well as symptom and diary cards.

Pharmacologic Approaches to Treatment

KEY CONCEPT *Treatment of AHF targets relief of congestion and optimization of CO utilizing oral or IV diuretics, IV vasodilators, and, when appropriate, inotropes based on presenting hemodynamics. Current treatment strategies in AHF target improving hemodynamics while preserving organ function.* A specific treatment approach is formulated depending on the patient's symptoms (congestion versus hypoperfusion) and hemodynamic indices (CI and PCWP).[40] If the patient primarily exhibits signs and symptoms of congestion, treatment entails use of diuretics as first-line agents to decrease PCWP. Additionally, IV vasodilators are added to provide rapid relief of congestion and additional reductions in PCWP. By reducing congestion in the heart, cardiac contractile function may improve, which results in an increase in SV and CO, and hence perfusion to vital organs. The patient's presenting BP can also help guide the clinician on choice of diuretic, vasodilator, or both. For the patient with a systolic BP of 120 to 160 mm Hg in the setting of progressive worsening of chronic HF with pulmonary and systemic congestion, aggressive diuresis can be beneficial. In the patient with systolic BP greater than 160 mm Hg and abrupt onset of pulmonary congestion, IV vasodilators may be indicated in addition to diuretics. For patients primarily displaying symptoms of hypoperfusion, treatment relies on use of agents that increase cardiac contractility, known as positive inotropes. Some patients display both symptoms of congestion as well as hypoperfusion and thus require use of combination therapies. One of the current challenges to the treatment of AHF is achieving hemodynamic improvement without adversely affecting organ function. In the case of inotropes, the increased contractility occurs at the expense of an increase in cardiac workload and proarrhythmia. In addition, high-dose diuretic therapy is associated with worsened renal function and possibly neurohormonal activation.

► *Diuretics*

Loop diuretics, including furosemide, bumetanide, and torsemide, are the diuretics of choice in the management of AHF. Furosemide is the most commonly used agent. Diuretics decrease preload by functional venodilation within 5 to 15 minutes of administration and subsequently by an increase in sodium and water excretion. This provides rapid improvement in symptoms of pulmonary congestion. Diuretics reduce PCWP but do not increase CI like positive inotropes and arterial vasodilators. Patients who have significant volume overload often have impaired absorption of oral loop diuretics because of intestinal edema or altered transit time. Therefore, doses are usually administered via IV boluses or continuous IV infusions (Table 6–9). Higher doses may be required for patients with renal insufficiency due to decreased drug delivery to the site of action in the loop of Henle.

There is limited clinical trial evidence comparing the benefit of diuretics with other therapies for symptom relief or long-term outcomes. Careful monitoring of diuresis is needed as excessive preload reduction can lead to a decrease in CO resulting in reflex increase in sympathetic activation, renin release, and the expected consequences of vasoconstriction, tachycardia, and increased myocardial oxygen demand. Also, it is important to avoid overdiuresis. Monitoring of serum electrolytes such as potassium, sodium, and magnesium is done frequently to identify and correct imbalances. Monitor serum creatinine and BUN daily at a minimum to assess volume depletion and renal function.

Occasionally, patients with HF do not respond to a diuretic, defined as failure to achieve a weight reduction of at least 0.5 kg (or negative net fluid balance of at least 500 mL) after several increasing bolus doses. Several strategies are used to overcome diuretic resistance. These include using larger oral

Table 6–9

Intravenous Diuretics Used to Treat Heart Failure–Related Fluid Retention

	Onset of Action (minutes)	Duration of Action (hours)	Relative Potency	Intermittent Bolus Dosing (mg)	Continuous Infusion Dosing (bolus/infusion)
Furosemide	2–5	6	40	20–200+	20–40/2.5–10
Torsemide	< 10	6–12	20	10–100	20/2–5
Bumetanide	2–3	4–6	0.5	1–10	1–4/0.5–1
Ethacrynic acid	5–15	2–7		0.5–1 mg/kg per dose up to 100 mg/dose	

doses, converting to IV dosing, or increasing the frequency of administration. A small study using low-dose continuous infusions of furosemide and torsemide have shown an increase in urine output compared with intermittent bolus dosing, but newer evidence suggests there may be little difference between intermittent bolus dosing and continuous infusion strategies on symptom relief at 72 hours.[41] Nonetheless, many regimens include a bolus dose followed by a maintenance infusion (Table 6–9). Another useful strategy is to combine two diuretics with different sites of action within the nephron. The most common combination is the use of a loop diuretic with a thiazide diuretic such as metolazone. Combining diuretics should be used with caution due to an increased risk for cardiovascular collapse due to rapid intravascular volume depletion. Strict monitoring of electrolytes, vital signs, and fluid balance is warranted. Also, poor CO may contribute to diuretic resistance. In these patients, it may become necessary to add vasodilators or inotropes to enhance perfusion to the kidneys. Care must be taken because vasodilators can decrease renal blood flow despite increasing CO through dilation of central and peripheral vascular beds.

▸ *Vasodilators*

IV vasodilators cause a rapid decrease in arterial tone, resulting in a decrease in SVR and a subsequent increase in SV and CO. Additionally, vasodilators reduce ventricular filling pressures (PCWP) within 24 to 48 hours, reduce myocardial oxygen consumption, and decrease ventricular workload. Vasodilators are commonly used in patients presenting with AHF accompanied by moderate to severe congestion. This class includes nitroglycerin, nitroprusside, and nesiritide. Hemodynamic effects and dosages for these agents are included in Tables 6–10 and 6–11, respectively. Although vasodilators are generally safe and effective, identification of the proper patient for use is important to minimize the risk of significant hypotension. In addition, vasodilators are contraindicated in patients whose cardiac filling (and hence CO) depends on venous return or intravascular volume, as well as patients who present with shock.

Nitroglycerin Nitroglycerin acts as a source of nitric oxide, which induces smooth muscle relaxation in venous and arterial vascular beds. Nitroglycerin is primarily a venous vasodilator at lower doses, but it exerts potent arterial vasodilatory effects at higher doses. Thus, at lower doses, nitroglycerin causes decreases in preload (or filling pressures) and improved coronary blood flow. At higher doses (greater than 100 mcg/min), additional reduction in preload is achieved, along with a decrease in afterload and subsequent increase in SV and CO. IV nitroglycerin is primarily used as a preload reducer for patients exhibiting pulmonary congestion or in combination with inotropes for congested patients with severely reduced CO.

Continuous infusions of nitroglycerin should be initiated at a dose of 5 to 10 mcg/min and increased every 5 to 10 minutes until symptomatic or hemodynamic improvement. Effective doses range from 35 to 200 mcg/min. The most common adverse events reported are headache, dose-related hypotension, and tachycardia. A limitation to nitroglycerin's use is the development of tachyphylaxis, or tolerance to its effects, which can be evident within 12 hours after initiation of continuous infusion and necessitate additional titrations to higher doses.

Nitroprusside Nitroprusside, like nitroglycerin, causes the formation of nitric oxide and vascular smooth muscle relaxation. In contrast to nitroglycerin, nitroprusside is both a venous and arterial vasodilator regardless of dosage. Nitroprusside causes a pronounced decrease in PCWP, SVR, and BP, with a modest increase in CO. Nitroprusside has been studied to a limited extent in AHF, and no studies have evaluated its effects on mortality. Nitroprusside is initiated at 0.1 to 0.25 mcg/kg/min, followed by dose adjustments in 0.1 to 0.2 mcg/kg/min increments if necessary to achieve desired effect. Because of its rapid onset of action and metabolism, nitroprusside is administered as a continuous infusion that is easy to titrate and provides predictable hemodynamic effects. Nitroprusside requires strict monitoring of BP and HR. Nitroprusside's use is limited in AHF due to recommended hemodynamic monitoring with an arterial line and mandatory

Table 6–11

Usual Doses and Monitoring of Commonly Used Hemodynamic Medications

Drug	Dose	Monitoring Variables[a]
Dopamine	0.5–10 mcg/kg/min	BP, HR, urinary output and kidney function, ECG, extremity perfusion (higher doses only)
Dobutamine	2.5–20 mcg/kg/min	BP, HR, urinary output and function, ECG
Milrinone	0.375–0.75 mcg/kg/min	BP, HR, urinary output and function, ECG, changes in ischemic symptoms (eg, chest pain), electrolytes
Nitroprusside	0.25–3 mcg/kg/min	BP, HR, liver and kidney function, blood cyanide and/or thiocyanate concentrations if toxicity suspected (nausea, vomiting, altered mental function)
Nitroglycerin	5–200+ mcg/min	BP, HR, ECG, changes in ischemic symptoms
Nesiritide	Bolus: 2 mcg/kg; Infusion: 0.01 mcg/kg/min	BP, HR, urinary output and kidney function, blood BNP concentrations

[a]In addition to pulmonary capillary wedge pressure and cardiac output.

BNP, B-type natriuretic peptide; BP, blood pressure; ECG, electrocardiogram; HR, heart rate.

Table 6–10

Usual Hemodynamic Effects of Commonly Used Intravenous Agents for Treatment of Acute or Severe Heart Failure

Drug	CO	PCWP	SVR	BP	HR
Diuretics	↑/↓/0	↓		↓	0
Nitroglycerin	↑	↓↓	↓	↓↓	↑/0
Nitroprusside	↑	↓↓↓	↓↓↓	↓↓↓	↑
Nesiritide	↑	↓↓	↓↓	↓↓	0
Dobutamine	↑↑	↓/0	↓/0	↓/0	↑↑
Milrinone	↑↑	↓↓	↓	↓	↑

BP, blood pressure; CO, cardiac output; HR, heart rate; PCWP, pulmonary capillary wedge pressure; SVR, systemic vascular resistance; ↑, increase; ↓, decrease; 0, no or little change.

intensive care unit admission at many institutions. Abrupt withdrawal of therapy should be avoided because rebound neurohormonal activation may occur. Therefore, the dose should be tapered slowly. Nitroprusside has the potential to cause cyanide and thiocyanate toxicity, especially in patients with hepatic and renal insufficiency, respectively. Toxicity is most common with use longer than 3 days and with higher doses. Nitroprusside should be avoided in patients with active ischemia because its powerful afterload-reducing effects within the myocardium can "steal" coronary blood flow from myocardial segments that are supplied by epicardial vessels with high-grade lesions.

Nesiritide BNP peptide is an endogenous neurohormone that is synthesized and released from the ventricles in response to chamber wall stretch or increased filling pressures. Recombinant BNP, or nesiritide, is the newest compound developed for AHF. Nesiritide binds to guanylate cyclase receptors in vascular smooth muscle and endothelial cells, causing an increase in cGMP concentrations leading to vasodilation (venous and arterial) and natriuresis. Nesiritide also antagonizes the effects of the RAAS and endothelin. Nesiritide reduces PCWP, right atrial pressure, and SVR. Consequently, it also increases SV and CO without affecting HR. Continuous infusions result in sustained effects for 24 hours without tachyphylaxis, although experience with its use beyond 72 hours is limited.

Nesiritide has been shown to improve symptoms of dyspnea and fatigue. In a randomized clinical trial, nesiritide was found to significantly decrease PCWP more than nitroglycerin and placebo over 3 hours.[42] Nesiritide improved patients' self-reported dyspnea scores compared with placebo at 3 hours, but there was no difference compared with nitroglycerin. In another study, nesiritide did not decrease death or rehospitalization for HF within 30 days, worsen renal function, or increase the risk for mortality, despite previous concerns regarding its association with elevations in serum creatinine.[43]

Currently, nesiritide is indicated for patients with AHF exhibiting dyspnea at rest or with minimal activity. The recommended dose regimen is a bolus of 2 mcg/kg, followed by a continuous infusion for up to 24 hours of 0.01 mcg/kg/min. Because nesiritide's effects are predictable and sustained at the recommended dosage, titration of the infusion rate (maximum of 0.03 mcg/kg/min) is not commonly required nor is invasive hemodynamic monitoring. Nesiritide should be avoided in patients with systolic BP less than 90 mm Hg. Although nesiritide's place in AHF therapy is not firmly defined, it can be used in combination with diuretics for patients presenting in moderate to severe decompensation, and it offers a unique mechanism of action. One potential disadvantage compared with other vasodilators is its longer half-life. If hypotension occurs, the effect can be prolonged (2 hours).

▸ *Inotropic Agents*

Currently available positive inotropic agents act via increasing intracellular cyclic adenosine monophosphate (cAMP) concentrations through different mechanisms. β-agonists activate adenylate cyclase through stimulation of β-adrenergic receptors, which subsequently catalyzes the conversion of ATP to cAMP. In contrast, phosphodiesterase inhibitors reduce degradation of cAMP. The resulting elevation in cAMP levels leads to enhanced phospholipase activity, which then increases the rate and extent of calcium influx during systole, thereby enhancing contractility. Additionally, during diastole, cAMP promotes uptake of calcium by the sarcoplasmic reticulum, which improves cardiac relaxation.

Dobutamine Dobutamine has historically been the inotrope of choice for AHF. As a synthetic catecholamine, it acts as an agonist mainly on β_1- and β_2-receptors and minimally on α_1-receptors. The resulting hemodynamic effects are due to both receptor- and reflex-mediated activities. These effects include increased contractility and HR through β_1- (and β_2-) receptors and vasodilation through a relatively greater effect on β_2- than α_1-receptors. Dobutamine can increase, decrease, or cause little change in mean arterial pressure depending on whether the resulting increase in CO is enough to offset the modest vasodilation. Although dobutamine has a half-life of approximately 2 minutes, its positive hemodynamic effects can be observed for several days to months after administration. The use of dobutamine is supported by several small studies documenting improved hemodynamics, but large-scale clinical trials in AHF are lacking.

Dobutamine is initiated at a dose of 2.5 to 5 mcg/kg/min, which can be gradually titrated to 20 mcg/kg/min based on clinical response. There are several practical considerations to dobutamine therapy. First, owing to its vasodilatory potential, monotherapy with dobutamine is reserved for patients with systolic BP greater than 90 mm Hg. However, it is commonly used in combination with vasopressors in patients with lower systolic BP. Second, due to downregulation of β_1-receptors or uncoupling of β_2-receptors from adenylate cyclase with prolonged exposure to dobutamine, attenuation of hemodynamic effects has been reported to occur as early as 48 hours after initiation of a continuous infusion, although tachyphylaxis is more evident with use spanning longer than 72 hours. Full sensitivity to dobutamine's effects can be restored 7 to 10 days after the drug is withdrawn. Third, many patients with AHF will be taking β-blockers chronically. Because of β-blockers' high affinity for β-receptors, the effectiveness of β-agonists such as dobutamine will be reduced. In patients on β-blocker therapy, it is recommended that consideration be given to the use of phosphodiesterase inhibitors such as milrinone, which do not depend on β-receptors for effect.[44,45] Although commonly practiced, use of high doses of dobutamine to overcome the β-blockade should be discouraged because this negates any of the protective benefits of the β-blocker and may increase risk for arrhythmias.

Dopamine Dopamine is most commonly reserved for patients with low systolic BP and those approaching cardiogenic shock. Dopamine exerts its effects through direct stimulation of adrenergic receptors, as well as release of norepinephrine from adrenergic nerve terminals. Dopamine produces hemodynamic effects that differ based on dosing. At lower doses, dopamine stimulates dopamine type 1 (D1) receptors and thus increases renal perfusion. Positive inotropic effects are more pronounced at doses of 3 to 10 mcg/kg/min. CI is increased due to increased SV and HR. At doses higher than 10 mcg/kg/min, chronotropic and α_1-mediated vasoconstriction effects are evident. This causes an increase in mean arterial pressure due to higher CI and SVR. The ultimate effect on cardiac hemodynamics will depend largely on the dosage prescribed and must be individually tailored to the patient's clinical status. Dopamine is generally associated with an increase in CO and BP, with a concomitant increase in PCWP. Dopamine increases myocardial oxygen demand and may decrease coronary blood flow through vasoconstriction and increased wall tension. As with other inotropes, dopamine is associated with a risk for arrhythmias.

Phosphodiesterase Inhibitors Milrinone and inamrinone work by inhibiting phosphodiesterase III, the enzyme responsible for the breakdown of cAMP. The increase in cAMP levels leads to increased intracellular calcium concentrations and enhanced contractile force generation. Milrinone has replaced inamrinone as the phosphodiesterase inhibitor of choice due to the higher frequency of thrombocytopenia seen with inamrinone.

Milrinone has both positive inotropic and vasodilating properties and as such is referred to as an "inodilator." Its vasodilating activities are especially prominent on venous capacitance vessels and pulmonary vascular beds, although a reduction in arterial tone is also noted. IV administration results in an increase in SV and CO, and usually only minor changes in HR. Milrinone also lowers PCWP through venodilation. Routine use of milrinone during acute decompensations in NYHA FC II to IV HF is not recommended, and milrinone use remains limited to patients who require inotropic support.[46]

Dosing recommendations for milrinone include a loading dose of 50 mcg/kg, followed by an infusion beginning at 0.5 mcg/kg/min (range: 0.23 mcg/kg/min for patients with renal failure up to 0.75 mcg/kg/min). A loading dose is not necessary if immediate hemodynamic effects are not required or if patients have low systolic BP (less than 90 mm Hg). Decreases in BP during an infusion may necessitate dose reductions as well. Lower doses are also used in patients with renal insufficiency.

Milrinone is a good option for patients requiring an inotrope who are also chronically receiving β-blockers because the inotropic effects are achieved independent of β-adrenergic receptors. However, milrinone exhibits a long distribution and elimination half-life compared with β-agonists, thus requiring a loading dose when an immediate response is desired. Potential adverse effects include hypotension, arrhythmias, and, less commonly, thrombocytopenia. Additionally, milrinone has been associated with increased risk for death in some studies. Milrinone should not be used in patients in whom vasodilation is contraindicated.

Mechanical, Surgical, and Device Therapies

▸ *Intraaortic Balloon Counterpulsation*

Intraaortic balloon counterpulsation (IABC) or intraaortic balloon pumps (IABPs) are widely used mechanical circulatory assistance devices for patients with cardiac failure who do not respond to standard therapies. An IABP is placed percutaneously into the femoral artery and advanced to the high descending thoracic aorta. Once in position, the balloon is programmed to inflate during diastole and deflate during systole. Two main beneficial mechanisms are: (a) inflation during diastole increases aortic pressure and perfusion of the coronary arteries; and (b) deflation just prior to the aortic valve opening reduces arterial impedance (afterload). As such, IABC increases myocardial oxygen supply and decreases oxygen demand. This device has many indications, including cardiogenic shock, high-risk unstable angina in conjunction with percutaneous interventions, preoperative stabilization of high-risk patients prior to surgery, and in patients who cannot be weaned from cardiopulmonary bypass. Possible complications include infection, bleeding, thrombosis, limb ischemia, and device malfunction. The device is typically useful for short-term therapy due to its invasiveness, need for limb immobilization, and requirement for anticoagulation.

▸ *Ventricular Assist Device*

The ventricular assist device (VAD) is a surgically implanted pump that reduces or replaces the work of the right, left, or both ventricles. VADs are indicated for short-term support in patients refractory to pharmacologic therapies, as long-term bridge therapy (a temporary transition treatment) in patients awaiting cardiac transplant, or in some instances as destination therapy (for patients who are not appropriate candidates for

Patient Encounter Part 4

After 6 months, the patient returns to the clinic complaining of extreme SOB with any activity, as well as at rest. He sleeps sitting up due to severe orthopnea, can only eat a few bites of a meal and then feels full and nauseous, and states he has gained 22 lb (10 kg) from his baseline weight. He is also profoundly dizzy when standing up from a chair and bending over. He states that he does not feel his furosemide therapy is working. He is admitted to the cardiology unit.

SH: Admits to resuming previous alcohol intake; additionally, he has been eating out in restaurants more often in the past 2 weeks

Meds: Atorvastatin 40 mg once daily, lisinopril 10 mg once daily, furosemide 80 mg twice daily, glipizide 10 mg twice daily for diabetes, metformin 1000 mg twice daily for diabetes, nitroglycerin 0.4 mg sublingual as needed, multivitamin daily, aspirin 325 mg daily

VS: BP 96/54 mm Hg, pulse 102 beats/min and regular, respiratory rate 22/minute, temperature 37°C (98.6°F), Wt 273 lb (124 kg), BMI 41.5 kg/m²

Lungs: There are rales present bilaterally

CV: Regular rate and rhythm with normal S_1 and S_2; there is an S_3 and an S_4; a 4/6 systolic ejection murmur is present and heard best at the left lower sternal border; point of maximal impulse is displaced laterally; jugular veins are distended, JVP is 11 cm above sternal angle

Abd: Hard, tender, and bowel sounds are present; 3+ pitting edema of extremities is observed

CXR: Bilateral pleural effusions and cardiomegaly

Echo: EF = 20% (0.20)

Pertinent labs: BNP 740 pg/mL (740 ng/L; 214 pmol/L), K: 4.2 mEq/L (4.2 mmol/L), BUN 64 mg/dL (22.8 mmol/L), SCr 2.4 mg/dL (212 μmol/L), Mg 1.8 mEq/L (0.9 mmol/L); A pulmonary catheter is placed, revealing the following: PCWP 37 mm Hg (4.9 kPa); CI 2.3 L/min/m²

What NYHA functional class, ACC/AHA stage, and hemodynamic subset is the patient currently in?

What are your initial treatment goals?

What pharmacologic agents are appropriate to use at this time?

Identify a monitoring plan to assess for efficacy and toxicity of the recommended drug therapy.

Once symptoms are improved, how would you optimize oral medication therapy for this patient's HF?

transplantation).[1] The most common complications are infection and thromboembolism. Other adverse effects include bleeding, air embolism, device failure, and multiorgan failure.

▶ *Surgical Therapy*

Heart transplantation represents the final option for refractory end-stage HF patients who have exhausted medical and device therapies. Heart transplantation should be considered a trade between a life-threatening syndrome and the risks associated with the operation and long-term immunosuppression. Assessment of appropriate candidates includes comorbid illnesses, psychosocial behavior, available financial and social support, and patient willingness to adhere to lifelong therapy and close medical follow-up.[1] Overall, the transplant recipient's quality of life may be improved, but not all patients receive this benefit. Posttransplant survival continues to improve due to advances in immunosuppression, treatment and prevention of infection, and optimal management of patient comorbidities.

Outcome Evaluation of Acute Heart Failure

- Focus on (a) acute improvement of symptoms and hemodynamics due to IV therapies, (b) criteria for a safe discharge from the hospital, and (c) optimization of oral therapy.
- Initially, monitor patients for rapid relief of symptoms related to the chief complaint on admission. This includes improvement of dyspnea, oxygenation, fatigue, JVD, and other markers of congestion or distress.
- Monitor for adequate perfusion of vital organs through assessment of mental status, creatinine clearance, liver function tests, and a stable HR between 50 and 100 beats/min. Additionally, adequate skin and muscle blood perfusion and normal pH is desirable.
- Monitor changes in hemodynamic variables if available. CI should increase, with a goal to maintain it above 2.2 L/min/m^2. PCWP should decrease in volume-overloaded patients to a goal of less than 18 mm Hg (2.4 kPa).
- Closely monitor BP and renal function while decreasing preload with diuretics and vasodilators.
- Ensure patients are euvolemic or nearly euvolemic prior to discharge.
- Because oral therapies can both improve symptoms and prolong survival, optimizing outpatient HF management is a priority when preparing a patient for hospital discharge. Ensure the patient's regimen includes a vasodilator, β-blocker, a diuretic at an adequate dose to maintain euvolemia, and digoxin or aldosterone antagonist if indicated.

Patient Care Process

Patient Assessment:

- Assess the severity and duration of the patient's symptoms of HF and hypoperfusion, including limitations in activity. Rule out potential exacerbating factors. See Clinical Presentation and Diagnosis of Chronic Heart Failure textbox and Tables 6–1 and 6–3.
- Obtain a thorough history of prescription, nonprescription, and herbal medication use.
- Review available diagnostic information from the chest radiograph, ECG, and echocardiogram. Investigate the patient's underlying etiology of HF.
- Review the patient's lifestyle habits including salt and alcohol intake, tobacco product use, exercise routine, weight gain, swelling in extremities, etc.

Therapy Evaluation:

- Based on evaluation of the patient's current prescription, nonprescription, and herbal medication use, is the patient taking any medications that can exacerbate HF (Table 6–4)?
- If patient is already receiving pharmacotherapy for HF and symptom relief, assess efficacy, safety, and adherence. Are there significant drug interactions?
- Determine whether additional adjustment or new therapy is needed to address patient's acute and chronic conditions.

Care Plan Development:

- Develop a treatment plan to alleviate symptoms and maintain euvolemia with diuretics (Tables 6–6 and 6–7). Daily weights to assess fluid retention are recommended.
- Develop a medication regimen to slow the progression of HF with the use of neurohormonal blockers such as vasodilators (ACE inhibitors, ARBs, or hydralazine/ isosorbide dinitrate), β-blockers, and aldosterone receptor antagonists (Table 6-7). Utilize digoxin if the patient remains symptomatic despite optimization of the therapies just described.
  - Is the patient at goal or maximally tolerated doses of vasodilator and β-blocker therapy (Table 6–7)?
  - Are aldosterone receptor antagonists utilized in appropriate patients with proper electrolyte and renal function monitoring (Table 6–7)?
- Educate the patient on lifestyle modifications such as salt restriction (maximum 2 g/day), fluid restriction if appropriate, limitation of alcohol, tobacco cessation, participation in a cardiac rehabilitation and exercise program, and proper immunizations such as the pneumococcal vaccine and yearly influenza vaccine.
- Stress the importance of adherence to the therapeutic regimen and lifestyle changes for maintenance of a compensated state and slowing of disease progression.

Follow-Up Evaluation:

- Monitor patient, including appropriate hemodynamic monitoring for AHF (Table 6–8), for desired outcomes.
- Evaluate the patient for presence of adverse drug reactions, drug allergies, and drug interactions.
- Provide patient education with regard to disease state and drug therapy, and reinforce medication adherence and self-monitoring for symptoms of HF (eg, daily weights). Emphasize follow-up with health care practitioners.
- Assess changes in echocardiographic parameters from a follow up echocardiography, ideally performed 2 months after medication optimization. Has the LVEF risen to above 40% (0.40)?

Abbreviations Introduced in This Chapter

ACC/AHA	American College of Cardiology/American Heart Association
ACE	Angiotensin-converting enzyme
AHF	Acute heart failure
ANP	Atrial natriuretic peptide
ARB	Angiotensin receptor blocker
AT_1	Angiotensin type I
AT_2	Angiotensin type II
ATP	Adenosine triphosphate
BMI	Body mass index
BNP	B-type natriuretic peptide
BP	Blood pressure
BUN	Blood urea nitrogen
CAD	Coronary artery disease
CAM	Complementary and alternative medication
cAMP	Cyclic adenosine monophosphate
CBC	Complete blood cell count
cGMP	Cyclic guanosine monophosphate
CHARM	Candesartan in Heart Failure Assessment of Reduction in Mortality and Morbidity
CI	Cardiac index
CNS	Central nervous system
CO	Cardiac output
COX-2	Cyclooxygenase-2
CrCL	Creatinine clearance
CYP450	Cytochrome P-450 isoenzyme
D1	Dopamine receptor type 1
ECG	Electrocardiogram
EF	Ejection fraction
ET-1	Endothelin-1
ET-A	Endothelin-A
ET-B	Endothelin-B
FDA	Food and Drug Administration
GI	Gastrointestinal
HF	Heart failure
HFpEF	Heart failure with preserved ejection fraction
HFrEF	Heart failure with reduced ejection fraction
HJR	Hepatojugular reflux
HR	Heart rate
IABC	Intraaortic balloon counterpulsation
IABP	Intraaortic balloon pump
iNOS	Inducible nitric oxide synthetase
INR	International normalized ratio
I-PRESERVE	Irbesartan in Patients with Heart Failure and Preserved Ejection Fraction
IV	Intravenous
JVD	Jugular venous distention
JVP	Jugular venous pressure
K	Potassium
LV	Left ventricular
LVEF	Left ventricular ejection fraction
LVF	Left ventricular failure
MI	Myocardial infarction
MRA	Mineralocorticoid receptor antagonist
MVO_2	Myocardial oxygen consumption
NSAID	Nonsteroidal anti-inflammatory drug
NT-proBNP	N-terminal proBNP
NYHA FC	New York Heart Association Functional Class
PAC	Pulmonary artery catheter
PCWP	Pulmonary capillary wedge pressure
PEP-CHF	Perindopril in Elderly People with Chronic Heart Failure
PND	Paroxysmal nocturnal dyspnea
RAAS	Renin-angiotensin-aldosterone system
RVF	Right ventricular failure
SCr	Serum creatinine
SNS	Sympathetic nervous system
SOB	Shortness of breath
SV	Stroke volume
SVR	Systemic vascular resistance
TNF-α	Tumor necrosis factor-α
TOPCAT	Treatment of Preserved Cardiac Function Heart Failure with an Aldosterone Antagonist
V_{1a}	Vasopressin type 1a
V_2	Vasopressin type 2
VAD	Ventricular assist device

REFERENCES

1. Yancy CW, Jessup M, Bozkurt B, et al. 2013 ACCF/AHA guideline for the management of heart failure: A report of the American College of Cardiology Foundation/American Heart Association Task Force on practice guidelines. Circulation. Oct 15 2013;128(16):e240–e327. Jun 5 2013.
2. Go AS, Mozaffarian D, Roger VL, et al. Heart disease and stroke statistics—2014 update: A report from the American Heart Association. Circulation. Jan 21 2014;129(3):e28–e292.
3. Nieminen MS, Harjola VP. Definition and epidemiology of acute heart failure syndromes. Am J Cardiol. Sep 19 2005;96(6A): 5G–10G.
4. Bonow RO, Bennett S, Casey DE, Jr, et al. ACC/AHA Clinical Performance Measures for Adults with Chronic Heart Failure: a report of the American College of Cardiology/American Heart Association Task Force on Performance Measures (Writing Committee to Develop Heart Failure Clinical Performance Measures): endorsed by the Heart Failure Society of America. Circulation. Sep 20 2005;112(12):1853–1887.
5. Parker RB, Cavallari LH. Systolic heart failure. Pharmacotherapy: a pathophysiologic approach, 8th ed. New York: McGraw-Hill; 2011:137–172.
6. Jessup M, Brozena S. Heart failure. New Eng J Med. May 15 2003; 348(20):2007–2018.
7. Schrier RW, Abraham WT. Hormones and hemodynamics in heart failure. N Engl J Med. Aug 19 1999;341(8):577–585.
8. Mann DL. Mechanisms and models in heart failure: A combinatorial approach. Circulation. Aug 31 1999;100(9):999–1008.
9. Mann DL. Inflammatory mediators and the failing heart: past, present, and the foreseeable future. Circulation research. Nov 29 2002;91(11):988–998.
10. Silver MA, Maisel A, Yancy CW, et al. BNP Consensus Panel 2004: A clinical approach for the diagnostic, prognostic, screening, treatment monitoring, and therapeutic roles of natriuretic peptides in cardiovascular diseases. Congest Heart Fail. Sep–Oct 2004;10(5 Suppl 3):1–30.
11. Lindenfeld J, Albert NM, Boehmer JP, et al. HFSA 2010 Comprehensive Heart Failure Practice Guideline. J Card Fail. Jun 2010;16(6):e1–e194.
12. Effects of enalapril on mortality in severe congestive heart failure. Results of the Cooperative North Scandinavian Enalapril Survival Study (CONSENSUS). The CONSENSUS Trial Study Group. New Eng J Med. Jun 4 1987;316(23):1429–1435.
13. Effect of enalapril on survival in patients with reduced left ventricular ejection fractions and congestive heart failure. The SOLVD Investigators. New Eng J Med. Aug 1 1991;325(5):293–302.
14. Effect of enalapril on mortality and the development of heart failure in asymptomatic patients with reduced left ventricular ejection fractions. The SOLVD Investigators. New Eng J Med. Sep 3 1992;327(10):685–691.
15. Packer M, Poole-Wilson PA, Armstrong PW, et al. Comparative effects of low and high doses of the angiotensin-converting enzyme inhibitor, lisinopril, on morbidity and mortality in chronic heart

failure. ATLAS Study Group. Circulation. Dec 7 1999;100(23): 2312–2318.
16. Pitt B, Poole-Wilson PA, Segal R, et al. Effect of losartan compared with captopril on mortality in patients with symptomatic heart failure: randomised trial—the Losartan Heart Failure Survival Study ELITE II. Lancet. May 6 2000;355(9215):1582–1587.
17. Cohn JN, Tognoni G. A randomized trial of the angiotensin-receptor blocker valsartan in chronic heart failure. New Eng J Med. Dec 6 2001;345(23):1667–1675.
18. Pfeffer MA, Swedberg K, Granger CB, et al. Effects of candesartan on mortality and morbidity in patients with chronic heart failure: the CHARM-Overall programme. Lancet. Sep 6 2003;362(9386):759–766.
19. Cohn JN, Archibald DG, Ziesche S, et al. Effect of vasodilator therapy on mortality in chronic congestive heart failure. Results of a Veterans Administration Cooperative Study. New Eng J Med. Jun 12 1986;314(24):1547–1552.
20. Cohn JN, Johnson G, Ziesche S, et al. A comparison of enalapril with hydralazine-isosorbide dinitrate in the treatment of chronic congestive heart failure. New Eng J Med. Aug 1 1991;325(5): 303–310.
21. Taylor AL, Ziesche S, Yancy C, et al. Combination of isosorbide dinitrate and hydralazine in blacks with heart failure. New Eng J Med. Nov 11 2004;351(20):2049–2057.
22. Packer M, Bristow MR, Cohn JN, et al. The effect of carvedilol on morbidity and mortality in patients with chronic heart failure. U.S. Carvedilol Heart Failure Study Group. New Eng J Med. May 23 1996;334(21):1349–1355.
23. The Cardiac Insufficiency Bisoprolol Study II (CIBIS-II): A randomised trial. Lancet. Jan 2 1999;353(9146):9–13.
24. Effect of metoprolol CR/XL in chronic heart failure: Metoprolol CR/XL Randomised Intervention Trial in Congestive Heart Failure (MERIT-HF). Lancet. Jun 12 1999;353(9169): 2001–2007.
25. Poole-Wilson PA, Swedberg K, Cleland JG, et al. Comparison of carvedilol and metoprolol on clinical outcomes in patients with chronic heart failure in the Carvedilol Or Metoprolol European Trial (COMET): Randomised controlled trial. Lancet. Jul 5 2003; 362(9377):7–13.
26. Funck-Brentano C, van Veldhuisen DJ, van de Ven LL, Follath F, Goulder M, Willenheimer R. Influence of order and type of drug (bisoprolol vs. enalapril) on outcome and adverse events in patients with chronic heart failure: a post hoc analysis of the CIBIS-III trial. Eur J Heart Fail. Jul 2011;13(7):765–772.
27. Pitt B, Zannad F, Remme WJ, et al. The effect of spironolactone on morbidity and mortality in patients with severe heart failure. Randomized Aldactone Evaluation Study Investigators. New Eng J Med. Sep 2 1999;341(10):709–717.
28. Pitt B, Remme W, Zannad F, et al. Eplerenone, a selective aldosterone blocker, in patients with left ventricular dysfunction after myocardial infarction. New Eng J Med. Apr 3 2003;348(14):1309–1321.
29. Zannad F, McMurray JJ, Krum H, et al. Eplerenone in patients with systolic heart failure and mild symptoms. New Eng J Med. Jan 6 2011;364(1):11–21.
30. The effect of digoxin on mortality and morbidity in patients with heart failure. The Digoxin Investigation Group. New Eng J Med. Feb 20 1997;336(8):525–533.
31. Rathore SS, Curtis JP, Wang Y, Bristow MR, Krumholz HM. Association of serum digoxin concentration and outcomes in patients with heart failure. JAMA. Feb 19 2003;289(7):871–878.
32. Packer M, O'Connor CM, Ghali JK, et al. Effect of amlodipine on morbidity and mortality in severe chronic heart failure. Prospective Randomized Amlodipine Survival Evaluation Study Group. New Eng J Med. Oct 10 1996;335(15):1107–1114.
33. Packer M, Carson P, Elkayam U, et al. Effect of amlodipine on the survival of patients with severe chronic heart failure due to a nonischemic cardiomyopathy: results of the PRAISE-2 study (prospective randomized amlodipine survival evaluation 2). JACC Heart Fail. Aug 2013;1(4):308–314.
34. Vardeny O, Miller R, Solomon SD. Combined neprilysin and renin-angiotensin system inhibition for the treatment of heart failure. JACC Heart Fail. Sep 27 2014.
35. McMurray JJ, Packer M, Desai AS, et al. Angiotensin-neprilysin inhibition versus enalapril in heart failure. New Eng J Med. Aug 30 2014.
36. Cleland JG, Tendera M, Adamus J, Freemantle N, Polonski L, Taylor J. The perindopril in elderly people with chronic heart failure (PEP-CHF) study. Eur Heart J. Oct 2006;27(19):2338–2345.
37. Massie BM, Carson PE, McMurray JJ, et al. Irbesartan in patients with heart failure and preserved ejection fraction. New Eng J Med. Dec 4 2008;359(23):2456–2467.
38. Pfeffer MA, Pitt B, McKinlay SM. Spironolactone for heart failure with preserved ejection fraction. New Eng J Med. Jul 10 2014;371(2):181–182.
39. Stevenson LW. Tailored therapy to hemodynamic goals for advanced heart failure. Eur J Heart Fail. Aug 1999;1(3):251–257.
40. Nohria A, Lewis E, Stevenson LW. Medical management of advanced heart failure. JAMA. Feb 6 2002;287(5):628–640.
41. Felker GM, Lee KL, Bull DA, et al. Diuretic strategies in patients with acute decompensated heart failure. New Eng J Med. Mar 3 2011;364(9):797–805.
42. Intravenous nesiritide vs nitroglycerin for treatment of decompensated congestive heart failure: A randomized controlled trial. Publication Committee for the VMAC Investigators. JAMA. Mar 27 2002;287(12):1531–1540.
43. O'Connor CM, Starling RC, Hernandez AF, et al. Effect of nesiritide in patients with acute decompensated heart failure. New Eng J Med. Jul 7 2011;365(1):32–43.
44. Stevenson LW. Clinical use of inotropic therapy for heart failure: looking backward or forward? Part I: Inotropic infusions during hospitalization. Circulation. Jul 22 2003;108(3):367–372.
45. Stevenson LW. Clinical use of inotropic therapy for heart failure: looking backward or forward? Part II: Chronic inotropic therapy. Circulation. Jul 29 2003;108(4):492–497.
46. Cuffe MS, Califf RM, Adams KF, Jr, et al. Short-term intravenous milrinone for acute exacerbation of chronic heart failure: A randomized controlled trial. JAMA. Mar 27 2002;287(12): 1541–1547.

7 Ischemic Heart Disease

Robert J. DiDomenico and Larisa H. Cavallari

LEARNING OBJECTIVES

Upon completion of the chapter, the reader will be able to:

1. Identify risk factors for the development of ischemic heart disease (IHD).
2. Differentiate between the pathophysiology of chronic stable angina and acute coronary syndromes.
3. Recognize symptoms and diagnostic criteria of IHD in a specific patient.
4. Compare and contrast the diagnostic criteria of IHD and acute coronary syndrome.
5. Identify treatment goals of IHD.
6. Identify appropriate lifestyle modifications and pharmacologic therapy to address each treatment goal.
7. Design an appropriate therapeutic regimen for the management of IHD based on patient-specific information.
8. Formulate a monitoring plan to assess effectiveness and adverse effects of an IHD drug regimen.

INTRODUCTION

Ischemic heart disease (IHD) is also called coronary heart disease (CHD) or coronary artery disease (CAD). The term *ischemic* refers to a decreased supply of oxygenated blood to the heart muscle. IHD is caused by stenosis, or narrowing, in one or more of the major coronary arteries that supply blood to the heart, most commonly by atherosclerotic plaques. Atherosclerotic plaques may impede coronary blood flow to the extent that cardiac tissue distal to the coronary artery narrowing is deprived of sufficient oxygen to meet oxygen demand. KEY CONCEPT *Ischemic heart disease results from an imbalance between myocardial oxygen supply and oxygen demand (Figure 7–1). Common clinical manifestations of IHD include chronic stable angina and the acute coronary syndromes (ACS) of unstable angina, non–ST-segment elevation myocardial infarction (MI), and ST-segment elevation MI.*

Angina pectoris, or simply angina, is the most common symptom of IHD. Angina is discomfort in the chest that occurs when the blood supply to the myocardium is compromised. Chronic stable angina is a chronic occurrence of chest discomfort due to transient myocardial ischemia with physical exertion or other conditions that increase oxygen demand. The primary focus of this chapter is the management of chronic stable angina. However, some information is also provided related to ACS, given the overlap between the two disease states. The American College of Cardiology (ACC), the American Heart Association (AHA), and several other organizations have jointly published practice guidelines for the management of chronic stable angina. Refer to these guidelines for further information.[1]

EPIDEMIOLOGY AND ETIOLOGY

IHD affects over 15 million Americans and is the leading cause of death for both men and women in the United States.[2] The incidence of IHD is higher in middle-aged men compared with women. However, the rate of IHD increases twofold to threefold in women after menopause. Chronic stable angina is the initial manifestation of IHD in about 50% of patients, whereas ACS is the first sign of IHD in other patients. Chronic stable angina is associated with considerable morbidity and frequently requires hospitalization for ACS. In addition, chronic stable angina negatively impacts health-related quality of life. Thus, in patients with chronic stable angina, it is important to optimize pharmacotherapy to reduce symptoms, improve quality of life, slow disease progression, and prevent ACS.

Conditions Associated with Angina

Figure 7–2 shows the anatomy of the coronary arteries. The major epicardial coronary arteries are the left main, left anterior descending, left circumflex, and right coronary arteries. Atherosclerosis leading to obstructive lesions in one or more of the major coronary arteries or their principal branches is the major cause of angina. Vasospasm at the site of an atherosclerotic plaque may further constrict blood flow and contribute to angina. Less commonly, vasospasm in coronary arteries with no or minimal atherosclerotic disease can produce angina and even precipitate ACS. This uncommon form of angina is referred to as variant or Prinzmetal angina. Other nonatherosclerotic conditions that can cause angina-like symptoms are listed in Table 7–1.[1] It is important to differentiate the etiology of chest discomfort because treatment varies depending on the underlying disease process.

Risk Factors

Factors that predispose an individual to IHD are listed in Table 7–2. Optimization of modifiable risk factors can significantly reduce the risk of MI.[1] Hypertension, diabetes,

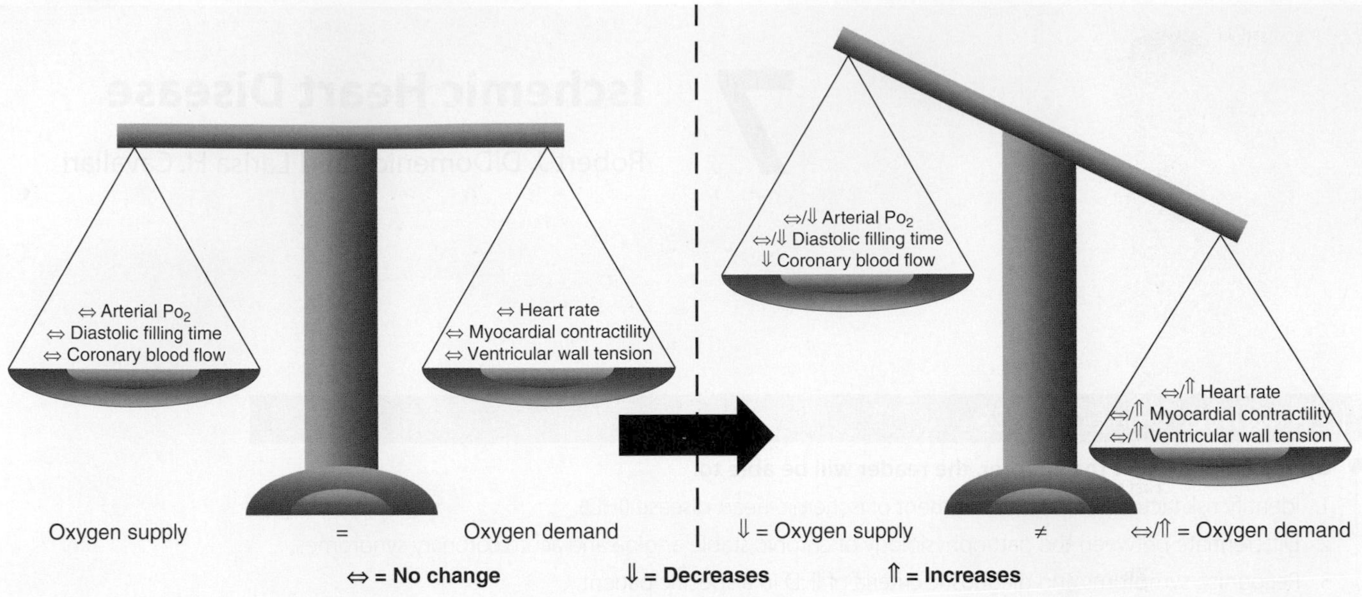

FIGURE 7–1. This illustration depicts the balance between myocardial oxygen supply and demand and various factors that affect each. It should be noted that diastolic filling time is not an independent predictor of myocardial oxygen supply per se, but rather a determinant of coronary blood flow. On the left is myocardial oxygen supply and demand under normal circumstances. On the right is the mismatch between oxygen supply and demand in patients with IHD. In patients without IHD, coronary blood flow increases in response to increases in myocardial oxygen demand. However, in patients with IHD, coronary blood flow cannot sufficiently increase (and may decrease) in response to increased oxygen demand resulting in angina. (IHD, ischemic heart disease; Po_2, partial pressure of oxygen.)

dyslipidemia, and cigarette smoking are associated with endothelial damage and dysfunction and contribute to atherosclerosis of the coronary arteries. Physical inactivity and obesity independently increase the risk for IHD, in addition to predisposing individuals to hypertension, dyslipidemia, and diabetes.

Patients with multiple risk factors, particularly those with diabetes, are at the greatest risk for IHD, experiencing fivefold to sevenfold higher risk compared to individuals without risk factors.[2] Although alternative definitions exist, **metabolic syndrome** is generally considered a constellation of common cardiovascular risk factors including hypertension, abdominal obesity, dyslipidemia, and insulin resistance. Metabolic syndrome increases the risk of developing IHD and related complications by twofold.[3] According to a joint statement from several large organizations, including the AHA, patients must meet at least three of the following criteria for the diagnosis of metabolic syndrome:[3]

- Increased waist circumference (40 inches [102 cm] or greater in men and 35 inches [89 cm] or greater in women).
- Triglycerides of 150 mg/dL (1.70 mmol/L) or greater or active treatment to lower triglycerides.
- Low high-density lipoprotein (HDL) cholesterol (less than 40 mg/dL [1.03 mmol/L] in men and less than 50 mg/dL [1.29 mmol/L] in women) or active treatment to raise HDL cholesterol.
- Systolic blood pressure (BP) of 130 mm Hg or greater, diastolic BP of 85 mm Hg or greater, or active treatment with antihypertensive therapy.
- Fasting blood glucose of 100 mg/dL (5.6 mmol/L) or greater or active treatment for diabetes.

KEY CONCEPT *Early detection and aggressive modification of risk factors are among the primary strategies for delaying IHD progression and preventing IHD-related events including death.*

PATHOPHYSIOLOGY

The determinants of oxygen supply and demand are shown in Figure 7–1. Increases in heart rate, cardiac contractility, and left ventricular wall tension increase the rate of myocardial oxygen consumption (MVO_2). Ventricular wall tension is a function of BP, left ventricular end-diastolic volume, and ventricular wall thickness. Physical exertion increases MVO_2 and commonly precipitates symptoms of angina in patients with significant coronary atherosclerosis.

Reductions in coronary blood flow (secondary to atherosclerotic plaques, vasospasm, or **thrombus** formation) and arterial oxygen content (secondary to hypoxia) decrease myocardial oxygen supply. Because the coronary arteries fill during diastole, decreases in diastolic filling time (eg, tachycardia) can also reduce coronary perfusion and myocardial oxygen supply. Anemia, carbon monoxide poisoning, and cyanotic congenital heart disease are examples of conditions that reduce the oxygen-carrying capacity of the blood, potentially causing ischemia in the face of adequate coronary perfusion.

Coronary Atherosclerosis

The normal arterial wall is illustrated in panel A of **Figure 7–3**. The intima consists of a layer of endothelial cells that line the lumen of the artery and form a selective barrier between the vessel wall and blood contents. Vascular smooth muscle cells are found in the media. The vascular adventitia comprises the artery's outer layer. Atherosclerotic lesions form in the subendothelial space in the intimal layer.

Endothelial damage and dysfunction, commonly caused by hypertension, diabetes, and smoking, allow low-density lipoprotein (LDL) cholesterol and inflammatory cells (eg, monocytes and T lymphocytes) to migrate from the plasma to the subendothelial space, as illustrated in Figure 12–5 in Chapter 12,

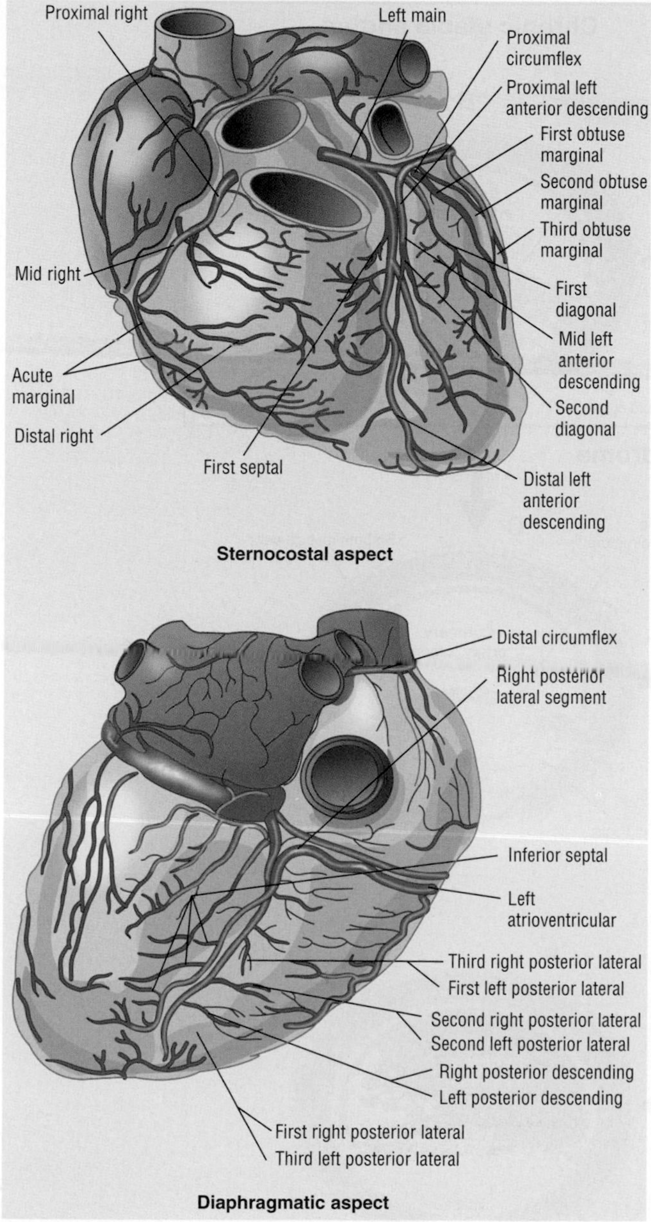

FIGURE 7–2. Coronary artery anatomy with sternocostal and diaphragmatic views. (Reproduced from Talbert RL. Ischemic heart disease. In: DiPiro JT, Talbert RL, Yee GC, et al, eds. Pharmacotherapy: A Pathophysiologic Approach, 6th ed. New York, NY: McGraw-Hill, 2005:263, with permission.)

Table 7–1

Nonatherosclerotic Conditions That Can Cause Angina-Like Symptoms[1]

Organ System	Condition
Cardiac	Aortic dissection, aortic stenosis, coronary artery vasospasm, pericarditis, valvular heart disease, severe uncontrolled hypertension
Noncardiac	Anemia, anxiety disorders, carbon monoxide poisoning, chest wall trauma, cocaine use, esophageal reflux or spasm, generalized anxiety disorder, peptic ulcer, pleuritis, pneumonia, pneumothorax, pulmonary embolus, pulmonary hypertension, thyrotoxicosis

"Dyslipidemias." The process is initiated with monocyte-derived macrophages ingesting lipoproteins to form foam cells. Macrophages also secrete growth factors that promote smooth muscle cell migration from the media to the intima. The development of early atherosclerosis in the form of a fatty streak consisting of lipid-laden macrophages and smooth muscle cells is formed.

The fatty streak enlarges as foam cells, smooth muscle cells, and necrotic debris accumulate in the subendothelial space. A collagen matrix forms a fibrous cap that covers the lipid core of the lesion to establish an atherosclerotic plaque. The atherosclerotic plaque may progress until it protrudes into the artery lumen and impedes blood flow. When the plaque occludes 70% or more of a major coronary artery or 50% or more of the left main coronary artery, the patient may experience angina during activities that increase myocardial oxygen demand.

Compared with men, women with angina are more likely to present with microvascular disease. Microvascular angina, also called cardiac syndrome X, refers to disease of the smaller coronary vessels causing typical angina in the absence of obstructive CAD of the epicardial arteries. Endothelial dysfunction and reduced smooth muscle relaxation, resulting in reduced vasodilation and enhanced vasoconstriction, are proposed to contribute to microvascular disease.[4]

Stable versus Unstable Atherosclerotic Plaques

The hallmark feature in the pathophysiology of chronic stable angina is an established atherosclerotic plaque in one or more of the major coronary arteries that impedes coronary blood flow such that myocardial oxygen supply can no longer meet myocardial oxygen demand. In contrast, the hallmark feature in the pathophysiology of ACS is atherosclerotic plaque rupture with subsequent thrombus formation. Plaque rupture refers to fissuring of the fibrous cap and exposure of the plaque contents to elements in the blood. Plaque composition, rather than the

Table 7–2

Major Risk Factors for Ischemic Heart Disease

Modifiable	Nonmodifiable
Cigarette smoking	Age ≥ 45 years for men, age ≥ 55 years for women
Dyslipidemia • Elevated LDL or total cholesterol • Reduced HDL cholesterol	Gender (men and postmenopausal women)
Diabetes mellitus	Family history of premature cardiovascular disease, defined as cardiovascular disease in a male first-degree relative (ie, father or brother) < 55 years or a female first-degree relative (ie, mother or sister) < 65 years
Hypertension	
Physical inactivity	
Obesity (body mass index ≥ 30 kg/m²)	
Low daily fruit and vegetable consumption	
Alcohol overconsumption	

HDL, high-density lipoprotein; LDL, low-density lipoprotein.

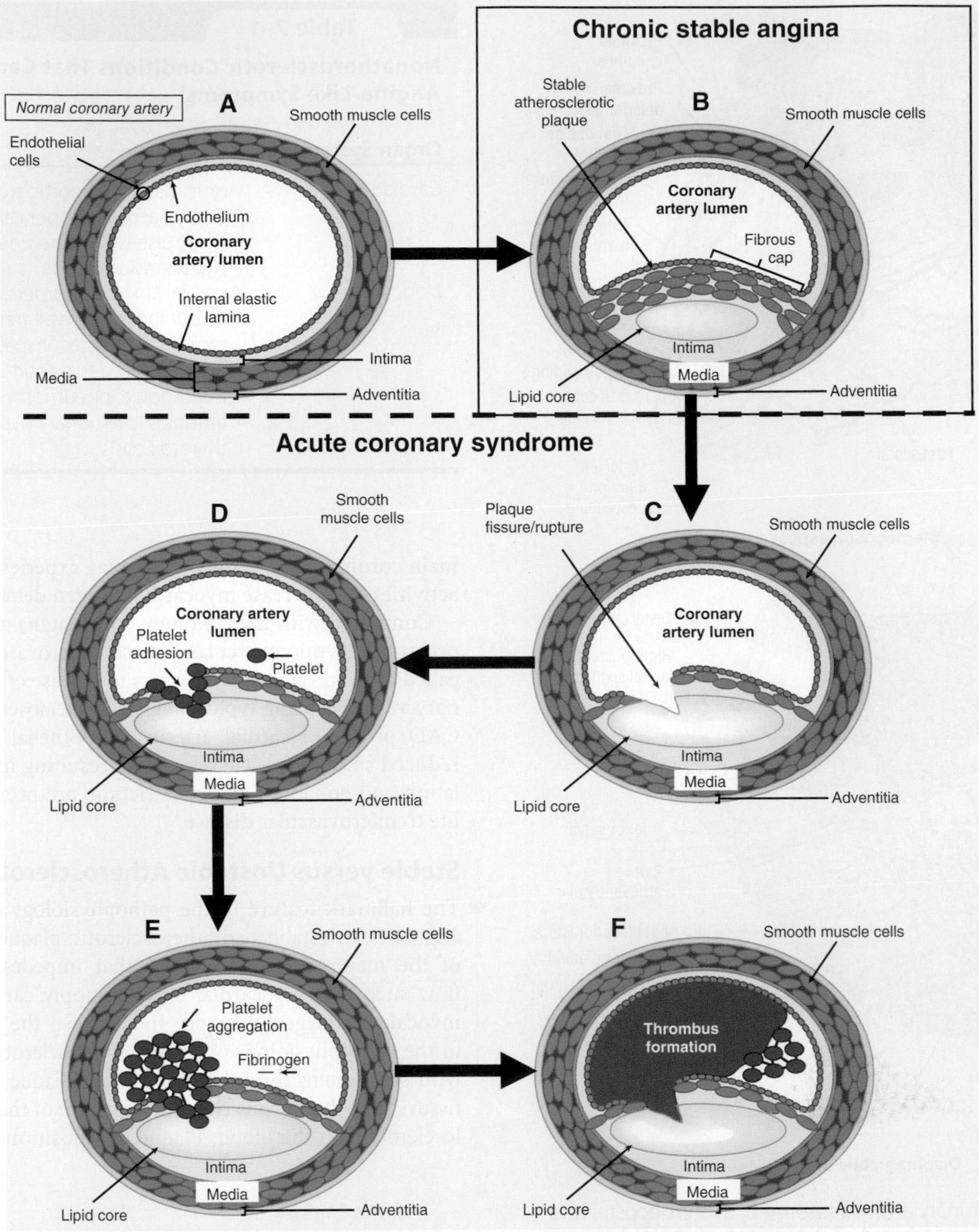

FIGURE 7–3. Pathophysiology of chronic stable angina versus acute coronary syndromes. **Panel A** depicts the cross-section of a normal coronary artery. **Panel B** depicts the cross-section of a coronary artery with a stable atherosclerotic plaque. Note that the lipid core is relatively small in size and the fibrous cap is made up of several layers of smooth muscle cells. **Panel C** depicts an unstable atherosclerotic plaque with a larger lipid core, and a thin fibrous cap composed of a single layer of smooth muscle cells with a fissure or rupture. **Panel D** depicts platelet adhesion in response to the fissured plaque. Platelet activation may ensue, leading to platelet aggregation as fibrinogen binds platelets to one another to form a mesh-like occlusion in the coronary lumen (**Panel E**). At this stage, patients may experience symptoms of acute coronary syndrome. If endogenous anticoagulant proteins fail to halt this process, platelet aggregation continues and fibrinogen is converted to fibrin, resulting in an occlusive thrombus (**Panel F**).

degree of coronary stenosis, determines the stability of the plaque and the likelihood of rupture and ACS. As depicted in Figure 7–3B, a stable lesion characteristic of chronic stable angina consists of a small lipid core surrounded by a thick fibrous cap that protects the lesion from the shear stress of blood flow. In contrast, an unstable plaque consists of a thin, weak cap covering a large lipid-rich core that renders the plaque vulnerable to rupture (Fig. 7–3C). The transformation of a stable plaque into an unstable plaque involves the degradation of the fibrous cap by substances released from macrophages and other inflammatory cells. Following plaque rupture, platelets adhere to the site of rupture, aggregate, and generate thrombin leading to the development of a fibrin clot (Figures 7–3D, 7–3E, and 7–3F). Coronary thrombi extend into the vessel lumen, where they partially or completely occlude blood flow, potentially resulting in unstable angina or MI.

Unstable plaque often produces minimal occlusion of the coronary vessel, and the patient remains asymptomatic until

Clinical Presentation and Diagnosis of Ischemic Heart Disease

General

- Patients with chronic stable angina will generally be in no acute distress. In patients presenting in acute distress, the clinician should be suspicious of ACS.

Symptoms of Angina Pectoris

- The five components commonly used to characterize chest pain are: quality, location, and duration of pain, factors that provoke pain, and factors that relieve pain.
- Patients typically describe pain as a sensation of pressure, heaviness, tightness, or squeezing in the anterior chest area. Sharp pain is not a typical symptom of IHD.
- Pain may radiate to the neck, jaw, shoulder, back, or arm.
- Pain may be accompanied by dyspnea, nausea, vomiting, or diaphoresis.
- Pain typically persists for several minutes.
- Symptoms are often provoked by exertion (eg, walking, climbing stairs, and doing yard or housework) or emotional stress and relieved within minutes by rest or sublingual nitroglycerin. Other precipitating factors include exposure to cold temperatures and heavy meals. Pain that occurs at rest (without provocation) or that is prolonged and unrelieved by sublingual nitroglycerin is indicative of ACS.
- Some patients, most commonly women, the elderly, and patients with diabetes, may present with atypical symptoms including indigestion, gastric fullness, back pain, and shortness of breath. Patients with diabetes and the elderly may experience associated symptoms, such as dyspnea, diaphoresis, nausea, fatigue, and dizziness, without having any of the classic chest pain symptoms.
- In some cases, ischemia may not produce any symptoms and is termed "silent ischemia."

Signs

- Findings on physical examination are often normal with chronic stable angina. However, during episodes of ischemia, patients may present with abnormal heart sounds, such as paradoxical splitting of the second heart sound, a third heart sound, or a loud fourth heart sound.

Laboratory Tests

- Cardiac enzymes (creatine kinase [CK], CK-MB fraction, troponin I, and troponin T) are elevated in MI but normal in chronic stable angina and unstable angina.
- Hemoglobin, fasting glucose, and fasting lipid profile should be determined for assessing cardiovascular risk factors and establishing the differential diagnosis.

Other Diagnostic Tests

- A 12-lead electrocardiogram (ECG) recorded during rest is often normal in patients with chronic stable angina in the absence of active ischemia. Significant Q waves may indicate prior MI. ST-segment changes (ST-segment depression or elevation) or T-wave inversion in two or more contiguous leads during symptoms of angina support the diagnosis of IHD. ST-segment depression or T-wave inversion may be observed in chronic stable angina, unstable angina, and non–ST-segment elevation MI, whereas ST-segment elevation occurs with ST-segment elevation MI and Prinzmetal (variant) angina.
- Treadmill or bicycle exercise ECG, commonly referred to as a "stress test," is considered positive for IHD if the ECG shows at least a 1-mm deviation of the ST-segment (depression or elevation).
- Wall motion abnormalities or left ventricular dilation with stress echocardiography or cardiac magnetic resonance (MR) (exercise or pharmacological) are indicative of IHD.
- Perfusion abnormalities can be detected by stress myocardial perfusion imaging using either radionuclides technetium-99m sestamibi or thallium-201 or cardiac MR (with or without late gadolinium enhancement).
- Coronary angiography detects the location and degree of coronary atherosclerosis and is used to evaluate the potential benefit from revascularization procedures. Stenosis of at least 70% of the diameter of at least one of the major epicardial arteries (≥ 50% for the left main coronary artery) on coronary angiography is indicative of significant IHD.
- Coronary angiography may be normal with microvascular angina.

the plaque ruptures. In fact, many acute coronary syndromes arise from vulnerable plaques that occlude less than 50% of the coronary lumen.[5]

Coronary Artery Vasospasm

Prinzmetal or variant angina results from spasm (or vasoconstriction) of a coronary artery in the absence of significant atherosclerosis. Variant angina usually occurs at rest, especially in the early morning hours. Although vasospasm is generally transient, vasospasm may persist long enough to cause MI. Patients with variant angina are typically younger than those with chronic stable angina and often do not possess the classic risk factors for IHD. The cause of variant angina is unclear but appears to involve vagal withdrawal, endothelial dysfunction, and paradoxical response to agents that normally cause vasodilation. Precipitants of variant angina include cigarette smoking, cocaine or amphetamine use, hyperventilation, and exposure to cold temperatures. The management of variant angina differs from that of classic angina, and thus it is important to distinguish between the two.

CLINICAL PRESENTATION AND DIAGNOSIS

History

The evaluation of a patient with suspected IHD begins with a detailed history of symptoms. KEY CONCEPT *The classic presentation of angina is described in the Clinical Presentation and Diagnosis text box.* Chronic stable angina should be distinguished from unstable angina because the latter is associated with a greater risk for MI and death and requires hospitalization for more aggressive treatment. Because the pathophysiology of chronic stable angina is due primarily to increases in oxygen demand rather

Table 7–3

Presentations of Acute Coronary Syndromes[6]

- Angina at rest that is prolonged in duration, usually lasting over 20 minutes.
- Angina of recent onset (within 2 months) that markedly limits usual activity.
- Angina that increases in severity (ie, by Canadian Cardiovascular Society Classification System Class of one level or greater), frequency, or duration, or that occurs with less provocation over a short time period (ie, within 2 months).

than acute changes in oxygen supply, symptoms are typically reproducible when provoked by exertion, exercise, or stress. The exception may be a patient with coronary artery vasospasm, in whom symptoms may be more variable and unpredictable. In contrast to chronic stable angina, ACS is due to an acute decrease in coronary blood flow leading to inadequate oxygen supply. Consequently, ACS is marked by prolonged symptoms, often occurring at rest, or an escalation in the frequency or severity of angina over a short period of time. The presentation of unstable angina is described in Table 7–3.[6]

Canadian Cardiovascular Society Classification System

The Canadian Cardiovascular Society Classification System (Table 7–4) is commonly used to assess the degree of disability resulting from IHD.[7] Patients are categorized into one of four classes depending on the extent of activity that produces angina. Grouping patients according to this or a similar method is commonly used to assess changes in IHD severity over time and the effectiveness of pharmacologic therapy.

Physical Findings and Laboratory Analysis

A thorough medical history, physical examination, and laboratory analysis are necessary to ascertain cardiovascular risk factors and to exclude nonischemic and noncardiac conditions that could mimic angina-like symptoms. Laboratory analyses should assess for glycemic control (ie, fasting glucose, glycated hemoglobin), fasting lipids, hemoglobin, and organ function (ie, blood urea nitrogen, creatinine, liver function tests, thyroid function tests). For patients with ACS, serial measurements of cardiac enzymes (usually three measurements within 12 hours) are performed to exclude the diagnosis of an acute MI. Cardiac findings on the physical examination are often normal in patients with chronic stable angina. However, findings such as carotid bruits, abdominal and/or renal bruits, or abnormal peripheral pulses would indicate atherosclerosis in other vessel systems and raise the suspicion for IHD.

Table 7–4

Canadian Cardiovascular Society Classification System of Angina[7]

Class	Description
I	Able to perform ordinary physical activity (eg, walking and climbing stairs) without symptoms. Strenuous, rapid, or prolonged exertion causes symptoms.
II	Symptoms slightly limit ordinary physical activity. Walking rapidly or for more than two blocks, climbing stairs rapidly, or climbing more than one flight of stairs causes symptoms.
III	Symptoms markedly limit ordinary physical activity. Walking less than two blocks or climbing one flight of stairs causes symptoms.
IV	Angina may occur at rest. Any physical activity causes symptoms.

Patient Encounter Part 1

A 64-year-old white female with a history of hypertension, diabetes, dyslipidemia, and a cerebral vascular accident presents to your clinic complaining of chest pain that occurred several times over the past few weeks. She describes her chest pain as "a heaviness," and states the discomfort first occurred while carrying her granddaughter to her second floor bedroom. Since then, she experienced the same heavy sensation while walking in the shopping mall and carrying laundry upstairs. The pain was located in the substernal area and was associated with tingling down the left arm and dyspnea. In each instance, the pain resolved after about 5 minutes of rest.

What information is suggestive of angina?

What tests would be beneficial in establishing a diagnosis?

What additional information do you need to create a treatment plan for this patient?

Diagnostic Tests

A resting 12-lead ECG is indicated in all patients with new or worsening symptoms of ischemia. Patients with characteristic chest discomfort, accompanied by ST-segment elevation in two or more contiguous leads, or a new left bundle branch block are at the highest risk of death. Most of these patients are diagnosed with MI (ST-segment elevation MI) which is treated as a medical emergency, often requiring expeditious percutaneous coronary intervention (PCI) or fibrinolytic therapy to restore blood flow in the occluded artery and reperfuse the myocardium. For patients with ACS, cardiac enzymes are measured serially to distinguish between MI (elevated cardiac enzymes) and either unstable angina or noncardiac causes of chest discomfort (normal cardiac enzymes); troponin is the most sensitive and thus preferred biomarker.

"Stress" testing with either exercise or pharmacologic agents increases myocardial oxygen demand and is commonly used to evaluate the patient with suspected IHD. Approximately 50% of patients with IHD who have a normal ECG at rest will develop ECG changes with exercise on a treadmill (most commonly) or bicycle ergometer. Dobutamine is a common pharmacologic agent used in patients who are unable to exercise. Dobutamine increases oxygen demand by stimulating the β_1-receptor, increasing heart rate and contractility. Echocardiography is commonly performed along with exercise or dobutamine (eg, treadmill or dobutamine stress echocardiography) to identify stress-induced wall motion abnormalities of the left ventricle indicative of IHD.

Exercise or pharmacologic agents are also commonly combined with radionuclide myocardial perfusion imaging (nuclear imaging studies) or cardiac magnetic resonance (MR) to detect IHD. An intravenous (IV) radioactive tracer is administered and extracted by the myocardium in proportion to coronary blood flow. Adenosine, dipyridamole, and regadenoson are coronary vasodilators that increase coronary blood flow in healthy arteries but not in atherosclerotic vessels. Radionuclide myocardial perfusion imaging is performed at rest and following exercise or pharmacologic stressor to detect perfusion defects indicative of IHD. Positive emission tomography, which utilizes a radioactive tracer that emits γ rays, is an alternative to conventional myocardial perfusion imaging that may be preferred in obese patients. Similar to other myocardial perfusion imaging, stress cardiac MR can detect wall motion abnormalities as well as perfusion defects, the latter often performed using late gadolinium enhancement, to determine the extent and severity of myocardial scarring that may be present.

Coronary artery calcium scoring via computed tomography (CT), also known as electron beam CT (EBCT) or "ultra-fast CT," may be performed as a noninvasive means to assess for CAD. Calcium deposits within the atherosclerotic coronary arteries are detected on CT, a calcium score is calculated, and the risk for IHD-related events is estimated.

Coronary angiography (also referred to as a cardiac catheterization or "cardiac cath") is indicated when stress testing results are abnormal or symptoms of angina are poorly controlled. Angiography involves catheter insertion into either the femoral or radial artery with advancement of the catheter into the ascending aorta near the coronary ostia. Contrast medium is injected through the catheter into the coronary arteries and fluoroscopy is performed to visualize the coronary anatomy and detect IHD. Contrast medium must be used cautiously in patients with preexisting renal disease (especially in those with diabetes) to avoid contrast-induced nephropathy and often warrants prophylactic hydration periprocedurally.

TREATMENT

Desired Outcomes

Once the diagnosis of IHD is established in a patient, the clinician should provide counseling on lifestyle modifications, institute appropriate pharmacologic therapy, and evaluate the need for revascularization. Optimal medical therapy is essential for managing patients with IHD. KEY CONCEPT *The major goals for the treatment of IHD are to:*

- *Prevent acute coronary syndrome and death*
- *Alleviate acute symptoms of myocardial ischemia*
- *Prevent recurrent symptoms of myocardial ischemia*
- *Prevent progression of the disease*
- *Reduce complications of IHD*
- *Avoid or minimize adverse treatment effects*

The treatment approach to address these goals is illustrated in Figure 7–4.

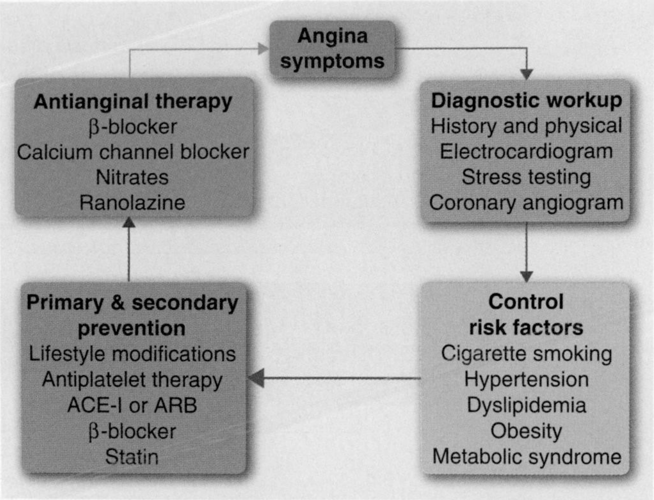

FIGURE 7–4. General treatment strategies for angina follow in clockwise fashion from the top center. (ACE-I, angiotensin-converting enzyme inhibitor; ARB, angiotensin receptor blocker.)

General Approach to Treatment

The primary strategies for preventing ACS and death (eg, primary or secondary prevention) are to:

- Aggressively modify cardiovascular risk factors
- Slow the progression of coronary atherosclerosis
- Stabilize existing atherosclerotic plaques

The treatment algorithm in Figure 7–5 summarizes the appropriate management of IHD. Risk factor modification is accomplished through lifestyle changes and pharmacologic therapy. KEY CONCEPT *Both 3-hydroxy-3-methylglutaryl coenzyme A reductase inhibitors (HMG-CoA reductase inhibitors or statins) and angiotensin-converting enzyme (ACE) inhibitors are believed to provide vasculoprotective effects (eg, anti-inflammatory effects, antiplatelet effects, improvement in endothelial function, and/or improvement in arterial compliance and tone). Together with aspirin, these drugs have been shown to reduce the risk of acute coronary events and death in patients with IHD. In select patients with IHD (following hospitalization for ACS ± PCI and/or following intracoronary stent placement), dual antiplatelet therapy with aspirin and a $P2Y_{12}$ antagonist has also been shown to reduce ischemic events. Angiotensin receptor blockers (ARBs) may be used in patients who cannot tolerate ACE inhibitors because of side effects (eg, chronic cough). β-blockers have been shown to decrease morbidity and improve survival in patients who have suffered an MI.*

Therapies to alleviate and prevent angina are aimed at improving the balance between myocardial oxygen demand and supply. Drug treatment is primarily aimed at reducing oxygen demand whereas revascularization by PCI and coronary artery bypass graft (CABG) surgery effectively restore coronary blood flow, improving myocardial oxygen supply. Coronary revascularization is generally reserved for patients with symptoms despite optimal medical therapy and those hospitalized for ACS.

Adverse treatment effects can be averted by avoiding drug interactions and the use of drugs that may have unfavorable effects on comorbid diseases. Appropriate drug dosing and monitoring reduces the risk for adverse treatment effects. Drugs should be initiated in low doses, with careful up-titration as necessary to control symptoms of angina and cardiovascular risk factors.

Lifestyle Modifications

Lifestyle modifications (smoking cessation, avoidance of secondhand smoke, dietary modifications, increased physical activity, and weight loss) reduce cardiovascular risk factors, slow the progression of IHD, and decrease the risk for IHD-related complications. Cigarette smoking is the single most preventable

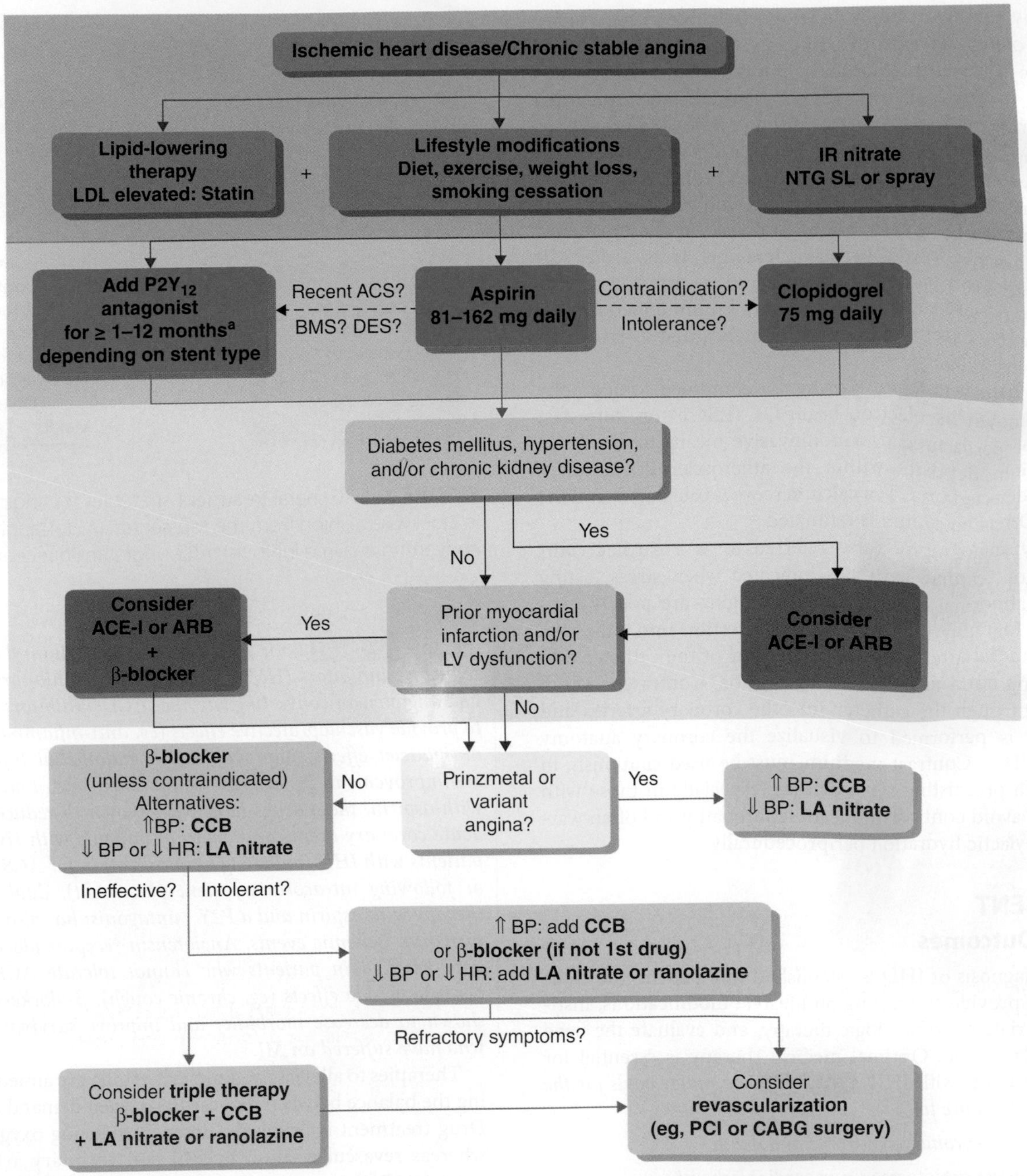

FIGURE 7–5. The treatment algorithm for ischemic heart disease. It begins at the top (blue section), which suggests risk factor modifications as the first treatment modality. Moving down to the green section, appropriate antiplatelet therapy is selected. The purple section identifies patients at high risk for major adverse cardiac events (MACE) and suggests appropriate drug therapy to decrease cardiovascular risk. The orange section at the bottom recommends appropriate antianginal therapy. [a]The minimum duration of clopidogrel therapy following intracoronary stent placement is as follows: at least 1 month for bare metal stents and at least 12 months for drug-eluting stents. (ACE-I, angiotensin-converting enzyme inhibitor; ACS, acute coronary syndrome; ARB, angiotensin receptor blocker; BMS, bare metal stent; BP, blood pressure; CABG, coronary artery bypass graft; CCB, calcium channel blocker; DES, drug-eluting stent; HR, heart rate; IR, immediate release; LA, long acting; LDL, low-density lipoprotein; LV, left ventricular; NTG, nitroglycerin; PCI, percutaneous coronary intervention; SL, sublingual.)

cause of IHD and IHD-related death. Smoking may also attenuate the antianginal effects of drug therapy. Clinicians should counsel patients and/or family members who smoke on the importance of smoking cessation at each encounter and offer referral to special smoking cessation programs. There are several pharmacologic aids for smoking cessation. Transdermal nicotine replacement therapy and bupropion have been studied in patients with IHD and appear safe and effective.[8,9] Varenicline, a partial nicotine receptor agonist, is similarly efficacious but has been associated with worsening of preexisting depression and suicidal ideation.[10] Thus, it should be used cautiously, particularly in patients treated for depression, and the risk:benefit ratio

Patient Encounter Part 2: Medical History, Physical Examination, and Diagnostic Tests

PMH: Hypertension, diagnosed 13 years ago; diabetes, diagnosed 8 years ago; dyslipidemia, diagnosed 8 years ago; cerebral vascular accident, diagnosed 3 years ago

FH: Father with coronary artery disease, died of myocardial infarction at age 50 years; mother alive and well

SH: Active smoker, 48-year pack history; denies alcohol or illicit drug use; no regular exercise program

Meds: Aspirin 81 mg po daily, hydrochlorothiazide 25 mg po once daily, metformin 500 mg po twice daily, pravastatin 20 mg po at bedtime, vitamin E 200 IU po daily, fish oil 1000 mg po twice daily

Allergies/intolerances (reaction): Lisinopril (cough)

PE:

VS: Blood pressure 152/98 mm Hg, HR 54 beats/min, RR 22 breaths/min, T 37°C (98.6°F), height 5'5" (165 cm), weight 212 lb (96.4 kg)

Cardiovascular: Regular rate and rhythm, normal S_1 and S_2, no S_3 or S_4; no murmurs, rubs, gallops

Lungs: Clear to auscultation and percussion

Abd: Nontender, nondistended, + bowel sounds

Ext: no clubbing, cyanosis, or edema

Labs: Fasting lipid profile: total cholesterol 206 mg/dL (5.33 mmol/L), HDL cholesterol 38 mg/dL (0.98 mmol/L), LDL cholesterol 119 mg/dL (3.08 mmol/L), triglycerides 246 mg/dL (2.78 mmol/L); fasting glucose 217 mg/dL (12.0 mmol/L); other labs within normal limits

Dobutamine stress echocardiography: regional wall motion abnormalities during peak exercise suggestive of ischemia

Identify the patient's risk factors for ischemic heart disease.

How might her current drug regimen adversely affect the patient's ischemic heart disease?

What therapeutic alternatives are available to manage her ischemic heart disease?

should be discussed with patients. Weight loss, through caloric restriction and increased physical activity, should be encouraged in patients who have a body mass index greater than 25 kg/m^2. Dietary counseling should be provided to all patients with newly diagnosed angina regardless of weight. The AHA recommends a diet that includes a variety of fruits, vegetables, grains, low-fat or nonfat dairy products, fish, legumes, poultry, and lean meats.[11] The addition of plant stanols/sterols (2 g/day) and/or viscous fiber (over 10 g/day) are effective in lowering LDL cholesterol.[12] Specific dietary recommendations for patients with IHD should include the following:[1,11]

- Limit cholesterol intake to less than 200 mg/day.
- Limit consumption of saturated fat to less than 7% and trans fatty acids to less than 1% of total calories.
- Limit daily sodium intake to 2.4 g (6 g of salt) for BP control.

Exercise facilitates weight loss, BP reduction, and glycemic control. In addition, regular exercise improves functional capacity and symptoms in chronic stable angina.[13] Guidelines recommend moderate intensity aerobic activity, such as brisk walking, ideally for 30 to 60 minutes at least 5 and preferably 7 days weekly.[1] Medically supervised cardiac rehabilitation programs are recommended for high-risk patients.

Interventional Approaches to Revascularization

▶ *Percutaneous Coronary Intervention*

For patients with stable IHD, optimal medical therapy is equivalent to PCI in reducing major adverse cardiac events (MACE) and is the preferred initial strategy.[14] However, when optimal medical therapy fails, symptoms are unstable, or extensive coronary atherosclerosis is present (eg, greater than 70% occlusion of coronary lumen), PCI is often performed to restore coronary blood flow and relieve symptoms. Several catheter-based interventions may be used during PCI, including:

- Percutaneous transluminal coronary angioplasty (PTCA)
- Intracoronary bare metal stent placement
- Intracoronary drug-eluting stent placement
- Rotational atherectomy

During PCI, a catheter is advanced into the diseased coronary artery, as described for cardiac catheterization. If PTCA is performed, a balloon at the end of the catheter is inflated inside the artery at the site of the critical stenosis, compressing the atherosclerotic plaque from the coronary lumen and restoring normal myocardial blood flow. Most PCI procedures involve the placement of a stent, a small metal scaffold-like device similar in size and shape to the spring at the tip of a ballpoint pen, at the site of angioplasty. Coronary stents are contained on special balloon catheters that are inflated at the site of stenosis to deploy the stent in the wall of the coronary artery, forming a sort of bridge to maintain a patent artery and improve coronary blood flow. Either a bare metal stent or a drug-eluting stent may be used. Drug-eluting stents are impregnated with low concentrations of an antiproliferative drug (paclitaxel, everolimus, sirolimus, or zotarolimus), which is released locally over a period of weeks to inhibit **restenosis** of the coronary artery after PCI. Compared to bare metal stents, drug-eluting stents have been associated with a significant reduction in all-cause mortality for patients with IHD.[15] Stents are thrombogenic, especially until they become endothelialized (covered in endothelial cells like a normal coronary artery). Dual antiplatelet therapy (discussed later) is required until the stent becomes endothelialized, generally a period of 12 months to reduce the risk for stent thrombosis, MI, or death. Lastly, rotational atherectomy may be performed wherein a special catheter is used to essentially cut away the atherosclerotic plaque, restoring coronary blood flow.

▶ *Coronary Artery Bypass Graft Surgery*

As an alternative to PCI, CABG surgery, or open-heart surgery, may be performed if the patient is found to have extensive coronary atherosclerosis (generally greater than 70% occlusion of three or more coronary arteries) or is refractory to optimal medical treatment. In the former case, CABG surgery has been shown to reduce the need for revascularization, but not death, compared with PCI.[16] During CABG surgery, veins from the leg (ie, saphenous veins) and/or arteries from the chest wall (ie, internal mammary arteries) or less commonly from the arm (ie, radial artery) or stomach (gastroepiploic artery) are harvested and used as conduits to restore coronary blood flow. A median sternotomy, in which an incision the length of the sternum is made, is commonly required to gain access to the thoracic cavity and expose the heart. As the "new" blood vessels are being engrafted, the patient is typically placed on cardiopulmonary bypass (ie, heart-lung machine) to maintain appropriate myocardial and systemic perfusion. Alternative surgical approaches for advanced IHD may be used in some settings including "off-pump" CABG (cardiopulmonary bypass is not required) and minimally invasive CABG (ie, thorascopic surgery), although these techniques are uncommon. Because of its extremely invasive nature, CABG surgery is generally reserved for patients with extensive coronary disease or as a treatment of last resort in patients with symptoms refractory to medical therapy.

Pharmacologic Therapy

▶ *Pharmacotherapy to Prevent Acute Coronary Syndromes and Death*

Control of Risk Factors A major component of any IHD treatment plan is control of modifiable risk factors, including dyslipidemia, hypertension, and diabetes. Treatment strategies for dyslipidemia and hypertension in the patient with IHD are summarized in the following paragraphs. Visit chapters in this textbook on the management of hypertension (see Chapter 5) and dyslipidemias (see Chapter 12) for further information.

Because lipoprotein metabolism and the pathophysiology of atherosclerosis are closely linked, treatment of dyslipidemias is critical for both primary and secondary prevention of IHD-related cardiac events. In 2013, the ACC/AHA revised guidelines for the management of patients with dyslipidemia.[17] Unlike previous guidelines for dyslipidemia, current guidelines no longer recommend specific targets for LDL and non-HDL cholesterol and de-emphasize the use of non-statin therapies for the treatment of dyslipidemia. Rather, current guidelines focus on the use of statins stratified by presence of or 10-year risk for atherosclerotic cardiovascular disease (ASCVD). Recommendations for initiation of statin therapy for dyslipidemia include[17]:

- High-intensity statin therapy in the presence of clinical ASCVD and for patients without clinical ASCVD in whom LDL cholesterol is 190 mg/dL (4.91 mmol/L) or greater; moderate-intensity therapy for elderly patients (age greater than 75 years) or those for whom safety concerns exist.
- Moderate to high-intensity statin therapy for patients at least 40 years of age with diabetes.
- Moderate to high-intensity statin therapy for patients with LDL cholesterol less than 190 mg/dL (4.91 mmol/L) who are at least 40 years of age and have a 10-year ASCVD risk of 7.5% in the absence of diabetes; consideration may be given to moderate-intensity statin therapy in patients with a 10-year ASCVD risk between 5% and 7.5%.

Hypertension is another major, modifiable risk factor for the development of IHD and related complications. Aggressive identification and control of hypertension is warranted in patients with IHD to minimize the risk of MACE. Recent guidelines recommend a BP goal of less than 140/90 mm Hg in most patients with IHD.[1,18] Because of their cardioprotective benefits, ACE inhibitors (or ARBs in ACE inhibitor–intolerant patients), either alone or in combination with calcium channel blockers (CCBs) or thiazide diuretics, are appropriate for most patients with both hypertension and IHD.[18]

Antiplatelet Agents Platelets play a major role in the pathophysiology of ACS. Thromboxane A2 (TXA2) is a potent platelet activator. Aspirin inhibits cyclooxygenase, an enzyme responsible for the production of TXA2, thereby inhibiting platelet activation and aggregation. In patients with stable or unstable angina, aspirin has been consistently shown to reduce the risk of major adverse cardiac events, particularly MI.[19] KEY CONCEPT *Antiplatelet therapy with aspirin should be considered for all patients without contraindications, particularly in patients with a history of MI. Aspirin doses of 75 to 162 mg daily are recommended in patients with or at risk for IHD.[1,19,20] Doses above 162 mg offer no additional benefit but increase bleeding risk. If aspirin is contraindicated (eg, aspirin allergy) or is not tolerated by the patient, an alternative antiplatelet agent such as clopidogrel should be considered.*[1]

Binding of adenosine diphosphate to the $P2Y_{12}$ receptors on platelets activates glycoprotein IIb/IIIa receptors leading to platelet aggregation and thrombus formation. KEY CONCEPT *Inhibition of the $P2Y_{12}$ receptor with either a thienopyridine (clopidogrel, prasugrel) or ticagrelor prevents platelet aggregation and is indicated in combination with aspirin in select patients with IHD.* Ticlopidine is a $P2Y_{12}$ receptor inhibitor used historically in combination with aspirin, but is rarely used in practice because of hematologic toxicity. Dual antiplatelet therapy with aspirin and a $P2Y_{12}$ inhibitor is recommended following hospitalization for ACS and/or following PCI with stent placement to prevent ischemic events, although indications for specific drugs differ slightly.[21–23] Following stent placement, prolonged treatment with dual antiplatelet therapy (often greater than or equal to 12 months) is often necessary to prevent in-stent thrombosis.

Clopidogrel is a prodrug that must be converted via a two-step process to its active thiol metabolite. The CYP2C19 enzyme is involved in both steps of the biotransformation. Individuals with reduced CYP2C19 activity, either from inherited deficiencies of CYP2C19 or use of CYP2C19 inhibitors (eg, proton pump inhibitors), may produce less of the active thiol metabolite. These individuals are at increased risk for stent thrombosis and MACE during clopidogrel treatment compared with those with "normal" CYP2C19 activity.[24] The clopidogrel labeling now warns of reduced effectiveness in CYP2C19 poor metabolizers, who carry two dysfunctional *CYP2C19* gene alleles. The *CYP2C19*2* and *CYP2C19*3* alleles are the most common alleles leading to reduced CYP2C19 activity.

Prasugrel is a thienopyridine that also requires biotransformation to its active metabolite. However, unlike clopidogrel, CYP2C19 deficiency does not alter its effectiveness. Ticagrelor is a direct-acting $P2Y_{12}$ inhibitor that does not require biotransformation to exert its antiplatelet effects and is unaffected by CYP2C19 activity.[25] Thus, prasugrel or ticagrelor may be suitable alternatives to clopidogrel when reduced CYP2C19 activity is suspected.

Antiproliferative drugs in drug-eluting stents delay endothelialization, and thus a longer period of dual antiplatelet therapy is recommended for drug-eluting stents compared with bare metal stents to prevent thrombosis. Guidelines advocate dual antiplatelet therapy for 12 months after stent placement.[21–23] The duration of dual antiplatelet therapy may be abbreviated in select patients with bare metal stents (ie, high risk for bleeding, history of nonadherence, need for invasive procedures or major surgery), whereas some data support indefinite use of combination antiplatelet therapy following stent placement. Because of the risk for stent thrombosis with premature discontinuation of dual antiplatelet therapy, it is imperative for clinicians to educate patients on this risk and the need for continuation of combination antiplatelet therapy for the recommended duration.

Clopidogrel, prasugrel, and ticagrelor are all indicated in combination with aspirin for at least 1 year in patients with ACS who undergo PCI.[21–23] Both clopidogrel and ticagrelor are also indicated in combination with aspirin in ACS patients who do not undergo PCI.[21,23] In patients with ACS, dual antiplatelet therapy with aspirin and either clopidogrel, prasugrel, or ticagrelor more effectively reduces the risk of death, MI, and stroke compared with aspirin alone even in patients who are managed medically (eg, in the absence of PCI).[26–28] Compared to clopidogrel, prasugrel and ticagrelor provide greater protection against cardiovascular events in ACS but increase risk for bleeding.[26,27] For more information regarding the use of dual antiplatelet therapy in the setting of ACS, see Chapter 8.

Statins Statins are the preferred drugs to lower LDL cholesterol based on their potency and efficacy in preventing cardiac events. Several studies in tens of thousands of patients with or at high-risk for IHD demonstrate that lowering cholesterol with statins reduces the risk of MACE by 21%.[29]

In addition to their LDL cholesterol–lowering effect, statins likely confer additional benefits in patients with IHD.[30] Prompted by evidence that patients with "normal" LDL cholesterol derived benefit from statins, studies suggest statins modulate the following characteristics thought to stabilize atherosclerotic plaques and contribute to the cardiovascular risk reduction seen with these drugs:

- Shift LDL cholesterol particle size from predominantly small, dense, highly atherogenic particles to larger, less atherogenic particles.
- Improve endothelial function leading to more effective vasoactive response of the coronary arteries.
- Prevent or inhibit inflammation by lowering C-reactive protein and other inflammatory mediators thought to be involved in atherosclerosis.
- Possibly improve atherosclerotic plaque stability.

KEY CONCEPT *In summary, to control risk factors and prevent MACE, statin therapy should be considered in all patients with IHD, particularly in those with elevated LDL cholesterol or diabetes.* Statins are potent lipid-lowering agents, possess non–lipid-lowering effects that may provide additional benefit to patients with IHD, and have been shown to reduce morbidity and mortality in patients with and at high risk for IHD. Moreover, because statins improve outcomes in patients with IHD and "normal" LDL cholesterol, statins should be considered in all patients with IHD, regardless of baseline LDL cholesterol.

ACE Inhibitors and Angiotensin Receptor Blockers

Angiotensin II, a neurohormone produced primarily in the kidney, is a potent vasoconstrictor and stimulates the production of aldosterone. Together, angiotensin II and aldosterone increase BP and sodium and water retention (increasing ventricular wall tension), cause endothelial dysfunction, promote thrombus formation, and cause myocardial fibrosis.

ACE inhibitors decrease angiotensin II production and have consistently been shown to decrease morbidity and mortality in patients with heart failure or history of MI.[31,32] In addition, there is evidence that ACE inhibitors reduce the risk of vascular events in patients with chronic stable angina or risk factors for IHD.[33,34] In patients with vascular disease (including IHD) or risk factors for vascular disease, both ramipril and perindopril reduced the risk of MACE by 20% or more in separate studies.[33,34]

KEY CONCEPT *In the absence of contraindications, ACE inhibitors should be considered in all patients with IHD, particularly those individuals who also have hypertension, diabetes mellitus, chronic kidney disease, left ventricular dysfunction, history of MI, or any combination of these.[1] Additionally, ACE inhibitors should also be considered in patients at high risk for developing IHD based on findings from the studies summarized above. ARBs may be used in patients with indications for ACE inhibitors but who cannot tolerate them due to side effects (eg, chronic cough).* ARBs also antagonize the effects of angiotensin II. In one large trial, valsartan was as effective as captopril at reducing morbidity and mortality in post-MI patients.[31] However, there are far more data supporting the use of ACE inhibitors in IHD. Therefore, ACE inhibitors are preferred in patients with a history of MI, diabetes, chronic kidney disease, or left ventricular dysfunction. The ACE inhibitors and ARBs with indications for patients with or at risk for IHD or IHD-related complications are listed in Table 7–5.

Table 7–5

Doses of Angiotensin-Converting Enzyme Inhibitors and Angiotensin Receptor Blockers Indicated in Ischemic Heart Disease (IHD)

Drug	Indications	Usual Dosage in IHD[a]
Angiotensin-Converting Enzyme Inhibitors		
Captopril	HTN, HF, post-MI, diabetic nephropathy	6.25–50 mg three times daily
Enalapril	HTN, HF	2.5–40 mg daily in one to two divided doses
Fosinopril	HTN, HF	10–80 mg daily in one to two divided doses
Lisinopril	HTN, HF, post-MI	2.5–40 mg daily
Perindopril	HTN, IHD	4–8 mg daily
Quinapril	HTN, HF, post-MI	5–20 mg twice daily
Ramipril	HTN, high-risk for IHD, HF, post-MI	2.5–10 mg daily in one to two divided doses
Trandolapril	HTN, HF, post-MI	1–4 mg daily
Angiotensin Receptor Blockers		
Candesartan	HTN, HF	4–32 mg daily
Valsartan	HTN, HF, post-MI	80–320 mg daily in one to two divided doses
Telmisartan	HTN, high-risk for IHD	20–80 mg daily

HF, heart failure; HTN, hypertension; MI, myocardial infarction.

[a]Reduce initial dose and gradually titrate upward as tolerated in renal impairment.

Side effects with ACE inhibitors and ARBs include hyperkalemia, deterioration in renal function, and angioedema. Serum potassium increases are secondary to aldosterone inhibition and are more likely in the presence of preexisting renal impairment, diabetes, or concomitant therapy with nonsteroidal anti-inflammatory drugs (NSAIDs), potassium supplements, or potassium-sparing diuretics. Reductions in glomerular filtration may occur during ACE inhibitor or ARB initiation or up-titration due to inhibition of angiotensin II-mediated vasoconstriction of the efferent arteriole. This type of renal impairment is usually temporary and more common in patients with preexisting renal dysfunction or unilateral renal artery stenosis. Bilateral renal artery stenosis is a contraindication for ACE inhibitors and ARBs because of the risk for overt renal failure. Angioedema is a potentially life-threatening adverse effect that occurs in less than 1% of white patients but up to 8% of African Americans treated with ACE inhibitors. Angioedema may also occur with the administration of ARBs. Patients treated with ACE inhibitors may develop a chronic cough secondary to bradykinin accumulation. For patients who develop a persistent ACE inhibitor-induced cough, substitution of an ARB for an ACE inhibitor is appropriate. Both ACE inhibitors and ARBs can cause fetal injury and death and are contraindicated in pregnancy.

► *Nitroglycerin to Relieve Acute Symptoms*

Short-acting nitrates are first-line treatment to terminate acute episodes of angina. KEY CONCEPT *All patients with a history of angina should have sublingual nitroglycerin tablets or spray to relieve acute ischemic symptoms.* Nitrates undergo biotransformation to nitric oxide. Nitric oxide activates smooth muscle guanylate cyclase, leading to increased intracellular concentrations of cyclic guanosine monophosphate (cGMP), release of calcium from the muscle cell, and ultimately, to smooth muscle relaxation. Nitrates primarily cause venodilation, leading to reductions in preload. The resultant decrease in ventricular volume and wall tension leads to a reduction in myocardial oxygen demand. In higher doses, nitrates cause arterial dilation and reduce afterload and BP. In addition to reducing oxygen demand, nitrates increase myocardial oxygen supply by dilating the epicardial coronary arteries and collateral vessels, as well as relieving vasospasm.

Short-acting nitrates are available in tablet and spray formulations for sublingual administration. Sublingual nitroglycerin tablets are well absorbed across the oral mucosa, produce an antianginal effect within 1 to 3 minutes, and are less expensive than the spray. However, the spray is preferred for patients who have difficulty opening the tablet container or produce insufficient saliva for rapid dissolution of sublingual tablets. At the onset of an angina attack, a 0.3 to 0.4 mg dose of nitroglycerin (tablet or spray) should be administered sublingually, and repeated every 5 minutes up to three times or until symptoms resolve. Standing enhances venous pooling and may contribute to hypotension, dizziness, or lightheadedness. Sublingual nitroglycerin may be used to prevent effort- or exertion-induced angina. In this case, the patient should use sublingual nitroglycerin 2 to 5 minutes prior to an activity known to cause angina, with the effects persisting for approximately 30 minutes. Isosorbide dinitrate, also available in sublingual form, has a longer half-life with antianginal effects lasting up to 2 hours. The use of short-acting nitrates alone, without concomitant long-acting antianginal therapy, may be acceptable for patients who experience angina symptoms once every few days. However, for patients with more frequent attacks, other antianginal therapies are recommended.

The use of nitrates within 24 to 48 hours of a phosphodiesterase type 5 inhibitor (eg, sildenafil, vardenafil, and tadalafil), commonly prescribed for erectile dysfunction, is contraindicated. Phosphodiesterase degrades cGMP, which is responsible for the vasodilatory effects of nitrates. Concomitant use of nitrates and phosphodiesterase type 5 inhibitors enhances cGMP-mediated vasodilation and can result in serious hypotension, decreased coronary perfusion, and even death. All patients with IHD should be prescribed sublingual nitroglycerin and educated regarding its use. Points to emphasize when counseling a patient on sublingual nitroglycerin use include:

- The seated position is generally preferred when using nitroglycerin because the drug may cause dizziness.
- Call 911 if symptoms are unimproved or worsen 5 minutes after the first dose.
- Keep nitroglycerin tablets in the original glass container and close the cap tightly after use.
- Nitroglycerin should not be stored in the same container as other medications because this may reduce nitroglycerin's effectiveness.
- Repeated use of nitroglycerin is not harmful or addictive and does not result in any long-term side effects. Patients should not hesitate to use nitroglycerin whenever needed.
- Nitroglycerin should not be used within 24 hours of taking sildenafil or vardenafil or within 48 hours of taking tadalafil because of the potential for life-threatening hypotension.

► *Pharmacotherapy to Prevent Recurrent Ischemic Symptoms*

The overall goal of antianginal therapy is to allow patients with IHD to resume normal activities without symptoms of angina and to experience minimal to no adverse drug effects. The drugs used to prevent ischemic symptoms are β-blockers, CCBs, nitrates, and ranolazine. These drugs exert their antianginal effects by improving the balance between myocardial oxygen supply and demand, with specific effects listed in Table 7–6. β-Blockers, CCBs, nitrates, and ranolazine decrease the frequency of angina and delay the onset of angina during exercise. However, there is no evidence that any of these agents prevent ACS or improve survival

Table 7–6

Effects of Antianginal Medications on Myocardial Oxygen Demand and Supply

Antianginal Agent	Oxygen Demand: Heart Rate	Oxygen Demand: Wall Tension	Oxygen Demand: Cardiac Contractility	Oxygen Supply
β-blockers	↓	↔ or ↑	↓	↔
Calcium channel blockers				
Verapamil, diltiazem	↓	↓	↓	↑
Dihydropyridines	↔ or ↑	↓	↓	↑
Nitrates	↑	↓	↔	↑
Ranolazine[a]	↔	↓	↔	↔

[a]The exact mechanism of the antiischemic effects of ranolazine is not known.

↓ decreases; ↔, no change; ↑, increases.

in patients with chronic stable angina. Combination therapy with two or three antianginal drugs is often needed.

β-Blockers β-blockers antagonize β_1- and β_2-adrenergic receptors in the heart, reducing heart rate and cardiac contractility, and decreasing myocardial oxygen demand. β-Blockers may also reduce oxygen demand by lowering BP and ventricular wall tension through inhibition of renin release from juxtaglomerular cells. By slowing heart rate, β-blockers prolong diastole, thus increasing coronary blood flow. However, β-blockers do not improve myocardial oxygen supply.

β-blockers with intrinsic sympathomimetic activity (eg, acebutolol, pindolol, and penbutolol) have partial β-agonist effects and cause lesser reductions in heart rate at rest. As a result, β-blockers with intrinsic sympathomimetic activity may produce lesser reductions in myocardial oxygen demand and should be avoided in patients with IHD. Other β-blockers appear equally effective at controlling symptoms of angina. The properties and recommended doses of various β-blockers used to prevent angina are summarized in Table 7–7. The frequency of dosing and drug cost should be taken into consideration when choosing a particular drug. Most β-blockers are available in inexpensive generic versions. β-blockers should be initiated in doses at the lower end of the usual dosing range, with titration according to symptom and hemodynamic response. The β-blocker dose is commonly titrated to achieve the following:

- Resting heart rate between 55 and 60 beats/min.
- Maximum heart rate with exercise of 100 beats/min or less or 20 beats/min above the resting heart rate.

KEY CONCEPT *In the absence of contraindications, β-blockers are the preferred initial therapy to prevent symptoms of angina in patients with IHD because of their potential cardioprotective effects [eg, after MI and/or in patients with heart failure with reduced ejection fraction (HFrEF)].* The long-term effects of β-blockers on morbidity and mortality in patients with chronic stable angina are largely unknown. Yet, β-blockers have been shown to decrease the risk of reinfarction and death by 23% in patients who have suffered an MI.[35] However, controversy exists regarding the role of β-blockers as first-line therapy for all patients with IHD. In a recent observational study, β-blockers did not lower the risk of MACE in patients with IHD or IHD risk factors.[36] Additionally, recommendations for using β-blockers for risk reduction in patients with IHD or other vascular disease, in the absence of MI or heart failure, was recently downgraded (IIb recommendation).[37]

β-blockers are contraindicated in patients with severe bradycardia (heart rate less than 50 beats/min) or atrioventricular (AV) conduction defects in the absence of a pacemaker. β-blockers should be used with particular caution in combination with other agents that depress AV conduction (eg, digoxin, verapamil, and diltiazem) because of the increased risk for bradycardia and heart block. Relative contraindications include asthma, bronchospastic disease, and severe depression. β_1-selective blockers are preferred in patients with asthma or chronic obstructive pulmonary disease. However, selectivity is dose dependent, and β_1-selective agents may induce bronchospasm in higher doses.

There are several precautions to consider with the use of β-blockers in patients with diabetes or heart failure. All β-blockers may mask the tachycardia and tremor (but not sweating) that commonly accompany episodes of hypoglycemia in diabetes. In addition, nonselective β-blockers may alter glucose metabolism and slow recovery from hypoglycemia in insulin-dependent diabetes. β_1-selective agents are preferred because they are less likely to prolong recovery from hypoglycemia. Importantly, β blockers should not be avoided in patients with IHD and diabetes, particularly in patients with a history of MI who are at high risk for recurrent cardiovascular events. β-blockers are indicated in patients with chronic HFrEF who are euvolemic due to their mortality benefit in this population. However, β-blockers are negative inotropes (ie, they decrease cardiac contractility). Therefore, β-blockers may worsen symptoms of heart failure in patients with left ventricular dysfunction (ie, ejection fraction less than 40% [0.40]) and initiation or titration should be delayed in patients with acute heart failure until symptoms have resolved. In particular, when used for the management of IHD in a patient with heart failure, β-blockers should be initiated in very low doses with slow up-titration to avoid worsening heart failure symptoms.

Other potential adverse effects from β-blockers include fatigue, sleep disturbances, malaise, depression, and sexual dysfunction. Abrupt β-blocker withdrawal may increase the frequency and severity of angina, possibly because of

Table 7–7

Properties and Dosing of β-Blockers in Ischemic Heart Disease

Drug	Receptor Affinity	Usual Dose Range	Dose Adjust in Hepatic Impairment	Dose Adjust in Renal Impairment
Atenolol	β_1-selective	25–200 mg once daily	No	Yes
Betaxolol	β_1-selective	5–20 mg once daily	No	Yes
Bisoprolol	β_1-selective	2.5–10 mg once daily	Yes	Yes
Carvedilol	α_1, β_1, and β_2	3.125–25 mg twice daily	Avoid in severe impairment	No
Carvedilol phosphate	α_1, β_1, and β_2	10-80 mg once daily	Avoid in severe impairment	No
Labetalol	α_1, β_1, and β_2	100–400 mg twice daily	Yes	No
Metoprolol	β_1-selective	50–200 mg twice daily (once daily for extended release)	Yes	No
Nadolol	β_1 and β_2	40–120 mg once daily	No	Yes
Propranolol	β_1 and β_2	20–120 mg twice daily (60–240 mg once daily for long-acting formulation)	Yes	No
Timolol	β_1 and β_2	10–20 mg twice daily	Yes	Yes

increased receptor sensitivity to catecholamines after long-term β-blockade. If the decision is made to stop β-blocker therapy, the dose should be tapered over several days to weeks to avoid exacerbating angina.

Calcium Channel Blockers CCBs inhibit calcium entry into vascular smooth muscle and cardiac cells, resulting in the inhibition of the actin-myosin complex and contraction of the cell. Inhibition of calcium entry into the vascular smooth muscle cells leads to systemic vasodilation and reductions in afterload. Inhibition of calcium entry into the cardiac cells leads to reductions in cardiac contractility. Thus, CCBs reduce myocardial oxygen demand by lowering both wall tension (through reductions in afterload) and cardiac contractility. The nondihydropyridine CCBs, verapamil and diltiazem, slow sinoatrial and AV nodal conduction, decrease heart rate, and further decrease myocardial oxygen demand. Because of their negative chronotropic effects, verapamil and diltiazem are generally more effective antianginal agents than the dihydropyridine CCBs. In contrast, dihydropyridine CCBs, nifedipine, in particular, inhibit calcium in the vasculature, and are potent vasodilators that can cause baroreflex-mediated increases in sympathetic tone and heart rate. In addition to decreasing myocardial oxygen demand, all CCBs increase myocardial oxygen supply by dilating coronary arteries, thus increasing coronary blood flow and relieving vasospasm.

CCBs are as effective as β-blockers at preventing ischemic symptoms. KEY CONCEPT *Calcium channel blockers are recommended as alternative treatment in IHD when β-blockers are contraindicated or not tolerated. In addition, CCBs may be used in combination with β-blockers when initial treatment is unsuccessful.* The combination of a β-blocker and a dihydropyridine CCB may improve symptoms better than either drug used alone.[38] However, the combination of a β-blocker with either verapamil or diltiazem should be used with extreme caution because both drugs decrease AV nodal conduction, increasing the risk for severe bradycardia or AV block when used together. If combination therapy is warranted, a long-acting dihydropyridine CCB is preferred. β-Blockers will prevent reflex increases in sympathetic tone and heart rate with the use of CCBs with potent vasodilatory effects. For patients with variable and unpredictable occurrences of angina, indicating possible coronary vasospasm, CCBs may be more effective than β-blockers in preventing angina episodes. The dosing of CCBs in IHD is described in Table 7–8.

Verapamil and diltiazem are contraindicated in patients with bradycardia and preexisting conduction disease in the absence of a pacemaker. As previously noted, verapamil and diltiazem should be used with particular caution in combination with other drugs that depress AV nodal conduction (eg, β-blockers and digoxin). Because of their negative inotropic effects, CCBs may cause or exacerbate heart failure in patients with HFrEF and should be avoided in this population. The exceptions are amlodipine and felodipine that have less negative inotropic effects compared with other CCBs and appear to be safe in patients with left ventricular systolic dysfunction.[39,40] Finally, there is some evidence that short-acting CCBs (particularly short-acting nifedipine and nicardipine) may increase the risk of cardiovascular events.[41] Therefore, short-acting agents should be avoided in the management of IHD.

Long-Acting Nitrates Nitrate products are available in both oral and transdermal formulations for chronic use. Commonly used products are listed in Table 7–9. All long-acting nitrate products produce effects within 30 to 60 minutes and are equally effective at preventing the recurrence of angina when used appropriately.

The major limitation of nitrate therapy is the development of tolerance with continuous use. The loss of antianginal effects may occur within the first 24 hours of continuous nitrate therapy. Although the cause of tolerance is unclear, several mechanisms have been proposed, including the generation of free radicals that

Table 7–8

Dosing of Calcium Channel Blockers in Ischemic Heart Disease

Drug	Usual Dose Range
Nondihydropyridines	
Diltiazem, extended release	120–360 mg once daily; consider dose adjustment in hepatic dysfunction
Verapamil, extended release	180–480 mg once daily; use initial dose of 120 mg in hepatic dysfunction
Dihydropyridines	
Amlodipine	5–10 mg once daily
Felodipine	5–10 mg once daily; use initial dose of 2.5 mg once daily in hepatic dysfunction
Nifedipine, extended release	30–90 mg once daily; dose adjust and monitor closely in hepatic dysfunction
Nicardipine	20–40 mg three times daily; dose twice daily in hepatic dysfunction and up-titrate slowly in both hepatic and renal dysfunction

Table 7–9

Nitrate Formulations and Dosing for Chronic Use

Formulation	Dose
Oral	
Nitroglycerin extended-release capsules	2.5 mg three times daily initially, with up-titration according to symptoms and tolerance; allow a 10- to 12-hour nitrate-free interval
Isosorbide dinitrate tablets	5–20 mg two to three times daily, with a daily nitrate-free interval of at least 14 hours (eg, dose at 7 AM, noon, and 5 PM)
Isosorbide dinitrate slow-release capsules	40 mg one to two times daily, with a daily nitrate-free interval of at least 18 hours (eg, dose at 8 AM and 2 PM)
Isosorbide mononitrate tablets	5–20 mg two times daily initially, with up-titration according to symptoms and tolerance; doses should be taken 7 hours apart (eg, 8 AM and 3 PM)
Isosorbide mononitrate extended-release tablets	30–120 mg once daily
Transdermal	
Nitroglycerin extended-release film	0.2–0.8 mg/hour, on for 12–14 hours, off for 10–12 hours

degrade nitric oxide. The most effective method to avoid tolerance and maintain the antianginal efficacy of nitrates is to allow a daily nitrate-free interval of at least 8 to 12 hours. Nitrates do not provide protection from ischemia during the nitrate-free period. Therefore, the nitrate-free interval should occur when the patient is least likely to experience angina, which is generally during the nighttime hours when the patient is sleeping and myocardial oxygen demand is reduced. Thus, it is common to dose long-acting nitrates so that the nitrate-free interval begins in the evening. For example, isosorbide dinitrate is typically dosed on awakening and again 6 to 7 hours later.

Monotherapy with nitrates for the prevention of ischemia should generally be avoided. Reflex increases in sympathetic activity and heart rate, with resultant increases in myocardial oxygen demand, may occur secondary to nitrate-induced venodilation. In addition, patients are unprotected from ischemia during the nitrate-free interval. β-blockers and CCBs are dosed to provide 24-hour protection from ischemia. KEY CONCEPT *Treatment with long-acting nitrates should be added to baseline therapy with either a β-blocker or CCB or a combination of the two.* β-blockers attenuate the increase in sympathetic tone and heart rate that occurs during nitrate therapy. As a result, the combination of β-blockers and nitrates is particularly effective at preventing angina and provides greater protection from ischemia than therapy with either agent alone. Monotherapy with nitrates may be appropriate in patients who have low BP at baseline or who experience symptomatic hypotension with low doses of β blockers or CCBs.

Common adverse effects of nitrates include postural hypotension, dizziness, flushing, and headache secondary to venodilation. Headache often resolves with continued therapy and may be treated with acetaminophen. Hypotension is generally of no serious consequence. However, in patients with hypertrophic obstructive cardiomyopathy or severe aortic valve stenosis, nitroglycerin may cause serious hypotension and syncope. Therefore, long-acting nitrates are relatively contraindicated in these conditions. Because life-threatening hypotension may occur with concomitant use of nitrates and phosphodiesterase type 5 inhibitors, nitrates should not be used within 24 hours of taking sildenafil or vardenafil or within 48 hours of taking tadalafil. Skin erythema and inflammation may occur with transdermal nitroglycerin administration and may be minimized by rotating the application site.

Ranolazine Ranolazine is an anti-ischemic agent indicated for the management of chronic angina. The mechanism of action is unclear, but it is believed to inhibit the late inward sodium current during the plateau phase of the cardiac action potential. Under ischemic conditions, excess sodium may enter the myocardial cell during systole. The resultant intracellular sodium overload leads to intracellular calcium accumulation (calcium overload) through a sodium/calcium exchange mechanism. Calcium overload results in increases in left ventricular wall tension and myocardial oxygen consumption. By reducing intracellular sodium concentrations in ischemic myocytes, ranolazine decreases intracellular calcium overload, left ventricular wall tension, and myocardial oxygen consumption.

Similar to other antianginal drugs, ranolazine reduces angina and increases exercise capacity but does not reduce incidence of MACE. Ranolazine has minimal effects on heart rate or BP; thus, it may be an option in IHD patients with low baseline BP or heart rate. Ranolazine is indicated as a first-line treatment for chronic stable angina. However, it is often reserved for patients

Table 7–10

Contraindications and Precautions with Ranolazine

Contraindications	Precautions
Liver cirrhosis increases ranolazine plasma concentrations by 30%–80%, resulting in increased risk for QT interval prolongation	Treatment with moderate CYP3A4 inhibitors including diltiazem, verapamil, grapefruit juice, erythromycin, and fluconazole increases ranolazine plasma concentrations (twofold with diltiazem and verapamil)
Treatment with potent CYP3A4 inhibitors (including ketoconazole, clarithromycin, and nelfinavir) increases ranolazine concentrations (3.2-fold with ketoconazole)	Preexisting QT prolongation, history of torsades de pointes, or treatment with other QT-prolonging drugs as QT interval prolongation may occur with ranolazine
Treatment with CYP3A4 inducers (including rifampin, phenobarbital, phenytoin, carbamazepine, and St. John's wart) may significantly decrease the efficacy of ranolazine (by 95% with rifampin)	Treatment with a P-gp inhibitor, such as cyclosporine, may increase ranolazine absorption
	Up to a 50% increase in ranolazine plasma concentration has been observed in renal impairment
	Ranolazine may increase bioavailability of P-gp substrates (increases digoxin plasma concentrations by 1.5-fold)
	Ranolazine may cause reduced metabolism of CYP2D6 substrates
	Ranolazine may increase exposure to drugs transported by OCT2; metformin doses should not exceed 1700 mg/day in patients treated with ranolazine 1000 mg twice daily
	Ranolazine may reduce the metabolism of CYP3A3 substrates; the dose of simvastatin should not exceed 20 mg in patients treated with ranolazine

CYP, cytochrome P450; OCT2, organic cation transporter 2; P-gp, P-glycoprotien.

with angina refractory to other antianginal medications due to its excessive cost. Ranolazine can prolong the QT interval. However, when used at recommended doses, the mean prolongation of QT interval is minimal (2.4 milliseconds [ms]).[42] The risk for QT interval prolongation is elevated in patients with hepatic impairment or taking other medications known to interact with ranolazine or prolong QT interval. Ranolazine should be started at a dose of 500 mg twice daily and increased to 1000 mg twice daily if needed for symptom relief. Higher doses are poorly tolerated and should be avoided. Contraindications to ranolazine are shown in Table 7–10. Common adverse effects with ranolazine include dizziness, constipation, headache, and nausea. Syncope may occur infrequently. Ranolazine is a CYP3A4 substrate, weak CYP2D6 substrate, CYP2D6 inhibitor, OCT2 inhibitor, and both an inhibitor and substrate of P-glycoprotein (P-gp). Concomitant use of ranolazine with potent CYP3A4 inhibitors (eg, ketoconazole, clarithromycin, and nelfinavir) or inducers (eg, rifampin) is contraindicated. The use of ranolazine is contraindicated in patients with significant hepatic disease. The ranolazine dose should be limited to 500 mg twice daily when combined with moderate CYP3A4 inhibitors including diltiazem and verapamil. Ranolazine should be used cautiously with P-gp inhibitors (eg, cyclosporine) and substrates (eg, digoxin). The maximum doses of simvastatin (20 mg daily) and metformin (1700 mg daily) are lower during concomitant treatment with ranolazine.

▶ *Pharmacotherapy with No Benefit or Potentially Harmful Effects*

Hormone Replacement Therapy, Folic Acid, and Antioxidants Current guidelines recommend against the use of hormone replacement therapy (HRT), folic acid, or antioxidants for reducing cardiovascular risk.[1] Early evidence from observational studies with each of these suggested potential benefit in IHD. However, no benefit was observed in randomized controlled clinical trials.[43–47] In the case of HRT, there was evidence of harm, with an increased risk of thromboembolic events and breast cancer with HRT in postmenopausal women.[44,45] Clinicians should consider discontinuing HRT therapy in women who suffer an acute coronary event while receiving such therapy.

Herbal Supplements Herbal products are widely used for their purported cardiovascular benefits; examples of such products include danshen, dong quai, feverfew, garlic, hawthorn, and hellebore. However, strong evidence supporting their benefits in cardiovascular disease is generally lacking. Furthermore, the potential for drug interactions and the lack of standardization limits the products' usefulness in clinical practice. Safety with herbal supplements in patients with IHD is a major concern. Numerous case reports of adverse cardiovascular events led the Food and Drug Administration (FDA) to ban ephedra-containing products (eg, Ma huang) in 2004. However, other herbal supplements with potentially serious adverse cardiovascular effects remain easily accessible. Some herbal supplements, such as feverfew and garlic, may interact with antiplatelet and antithrombotic therapy and increase bleeding risk. Dietary supplements purported to enhance sexual performance may contain phosphodiesterase-like chemicals and increase risk for serious hypotension with nitroglycerin. Other agents may reduce the effectiveness of antianginal medications, such as St. John's wart with ranolazine. Thus, it is important to assess the use of herbal products in patients with IHD and to counsel patients about the potential for drug interactions and adverse events with herbal therapies.

Cyclooxygenase-2 Inhibitors and Nonsteroidal Anti-inflammatory Drugs Data suggest that cyclooxygenase-2 (COX-2) inhibitors and nonselective NSAIDs may increase the risk for MI and stroke.[48] The cardiovascular risk with COX-2 inhibitors and NSAIDs may be greatest in patients with a history of, or with risk factors for, cardiovascular disease. The COX-2 inhibitors rofecoxib and valdecoxib were withdrawn from the market because of safety concerns. Product labeling for other COX-2 and nonselective NSAIDs (prescription and over-the-counter) now includes boxed warning about potential adverse cardiovascular effects. The AHA recommends the use of COX-2 inhibitors be limited to low-dose, short-term therapy in patients for whom there is no appropriate alternative.[48] Patients with cardiovascular disease should consult a clinician before using over-the-counter NSAIDs.

Patient Encounter Part 3: Creating a Care Plan

Based on the information presented, create a specific plan for the management of the patient's ischemic heart disease. Your plan should include (a) the goals of therapy, (b) specific nonpharmacologic and pharmacologic interventions to address these goals, and (c) a plan for follow-up to assess drug tolerance and whether the therapeutic goals have been achieved.

SPECIAL POPULATIONS

Variant Angina

Vasospasm as the sole etiology of angina (Prinzmetal or variant angina) is relatively uncommon. As a result, treatment options are not well studied. Nevertheless, based on the pharmacology of available drugs, several recommendations can be made. First, β-blockers should be avoided in patients with variant angina because of their potential to worsen vasospasm due to unopposed α-adrenergic receptor stimulation. In contrast, both CCBs and nitrates are effective in relieving vasospasm and are preferred in the management of variant angina. Because nitrates require an 8- to 12-hour nitrate-free interval, their role as monotherapy for prophylaxis of anginal attacks due to vasospasm is limited. However, immediate-release nitroglycerin is effective at terminating acute anginal attacks due to vasospasm. Therefore, all patients diagnosed with variant angina should be prescribed immediate-release nitroglycerin. CCBs are effective for monotherapy of variant angina. Because short-acting CCBs have been associated with increased risk of adverse cardiac events, they should be avoided.[41] Long-acting nitrates may be added to CCB therapy if needed.

Microvascular Angina

There are limited data on optimal therapy in patients with microvascular disease. Both ACE inhibitors and statins may produce beneficial effects on endothelial function and improve microvascular angina.[4] Short-acting nitrates remain the treatment of choice for relieving acute symptoms, although they may be less effective in microvascular disease. Similar to obstructive CAD, β-blockers are first line to control symptoms of angina in patients with microvascular disease and may be more effective than CCBs and long-acting nitrates in this setting.[4] Ranolazine may also produce favorable antianginal effects for patients with continued symptoms.

Elderly Patients with IHD

Elderly patients are more likely than younger patients to have other comorbidities that may influence drug selection for the treatment of angina. As a result, polypharmacy is more common in elderly patients, increasing the risk of drug–drug interactions, and perhaps decreasing medication adherence. Additionally, elderly patients are often more susceptible to adverse effects of antianginal therapies, particularly the negative chronotropic and inotropic effects of β-blockers and CCBs. Therefore, drugs should be initiated in low doses with close monitoring of elderly patients with IHD.

Acute Coronary Syndromes

Management of ACS is discussed in further detail in Chapter 8, "Acute Coronary Syndromes." It is important to educate patients with IHD on the signs of ACS and steps to take if signs or symptoms occur. Importantly, patients should be instructed to seek emergent care if symptoms of angina last longer than 20 to 30 minutes, do not improve after 5 minutes of using sublingual nitroglycerin, or worsen after 5 minutes of using sublingual nitroglycerin. In patients with a history of ACS, it is crucial to select appropriate pharmacotherapy to prevent recurrent ACS and death. Appropriate pharmacotherapy for patients with a history of ACS includes aspirin (perhaps in combination with a $P2Y_{12}$ inhibitor), ACE inhibitors or ARBs, β-blockers, statins, and sublingual nitroglycerin. In addition, control of cardiovascular risk factors (eg, dyslipidemia, hypertension, and diabetes) with lifestyle modifications and pharmacotherapy is critical.

OUTCOME EVALUATION

Assessing for Drug Effectiveness and Safety

- KEY CONCEPT *Monitor symptoms of angina at baseline and at each clinic visit for patients with IHD to assess the effectiveness of antianginal therapy. In particular, assess the frequency and intensity of anginal symptoms.* Determining the frequency of sublingual nitroglycerin use is helpful in making this assessment. If angina is occurring with increasing frequency or intensity, adjust antianginal therapy and refer the patient for additional diagnostic testing (eg, coronary angiography) and possibly coronary intervention (eg, PCI or CABG surgery), if indicated.
- Assess the patient for IHD-related complications, such as heart failure. The presence of new comorbidities may indicate worsening IHD requiring additional workup or pharmacologic therapy.
- Routinely monitor hemodynamic parameters to assess drug tolerance. Assess BP at baseline, after drug initiation and after dose titration. BP should be monitored periodically in patients treated with β-blockers, CCBs, nitrates, ACE inhibitors, and/or ARBs.
- BP reduction may be particularly pronounced after initiation and dose titration of β-blockers that also possess α-blocking effects (eg, labetalol and carvedilol).
- Because of the potential for postural hypotension, warn patients that dizziness, presyncope, and even syncope may result from abrupt changes in body position during initiation or up-titration of drugs with α-blocking effects.
- Closely monitor heart rate in patients treated with drugs that have negative chronotropic effects (eg, β-blockers, verapamil, or diltiazem) or drugs that may cause reflex tachycardia (eg, nitrates or dihydropyridine CCBs).
- Treatment with β-blockers, verapamil, or diltiazem can usually be continued in patients with asymptomatic bradycardia. However, reduce or discontinue treatment with these agents in patients who develop symptomatic bradycardia or serious conduction abnormalities.
- Regularly assess control of existing risk factors and the presence of new risk factors for IHD. Routine screening for the presence of metabolic syndrome will help in assessing the control of known major risk factors and identifying new risk factors. If new risk factors are identified and/or the presence of metabolic syndrome is detected, modify the pharmacotherapy regimen, as discussed previously, to control these risk factors and lower the risk of IHD and IHD-related adverse events.

Patient Care Process

Patient Assessment:

- Assess the patient's symptoms. (See Table 7–4.)
    - Determine quality, location, and duration of pain.
    - Determine factors that provoke and relieve pain.
    - Are symptoms characteristic of angina?
- If available, review findings from diagnostic tests performed to evaluate for IHD. (See Figure 7–4.)
    - Have any of the following diagnostic tests been performed: ECG, stress test, coronary angiogram? If so, did the results suggest or confirm IHD? Was PCI performed?
- Identify risk factors for IHD. (See Table 7–2 and Figure 7–4.)
    - Are there any modifiable risk factors?
- Obtain a thorough history of prescription drug, nonprescription drug, and herbal product use.
    - Is the patient taking any medications that may exacerbate angina or interact with antianginal drug therapy?

Therapy Evaluation:

- Is the patient taking appropriate drug therapy to prevent ACS and death (see Figure 7–4)? If not, why?
- Is the patient taking appropriate antianginal therapy? If not, why?

Care Plan Development:

- Refer patients with unstable signs and symptoms of angina (eg, ACS) to the hospital, if appropriate. (See Table 7–3.)
- Develop a therapeutic plan to control modifiable risk factors, and initiate or optimize therapy to prevent ACS and death and prevent and treat symptoms of angina. (See Figure 7–5.)
- Stress the importance of adherence with the therapeutic regimen including lifestyle modifications.
- Provide patient education regarding disease state, lifestyle modifications, and drug therapy. Review the following with the patient:
    - Consequences of untreated IHD
    - Lifestyle modifications
    - Timing of medication administration
    - Potential adverse drug effects
    - Potential drug interactions
    - Importance and mechanisms to monitor heart rate and BP
    - Signs and symptoms of worsening angina
    - When to seek emergent care
- Develop a plan to assess effectiveness of anti-ischemic therapy after 1 to 2 weeks.

Follow-Up Evaluation:

- During each subsequent visit, assess control of modifiable risk factors; control of angina symptoms; and detect adverse drug reactions, drug intolerance, and drug interactions.

  Revise therapeutic plan accordingly in response to each follow-up evaluation.

- In patients treated with ACE inhibitors and/or ARBs, routinely monitor renal function and potassium levels at baseline, after drug initiation, post dose titration, and periodically thereafter. This is particularly important when using these therapies in patients with preexisting renal impairment or diabetes because they may be more susceptible to these adverse events.

Duration of Therapy

- Drugs that modify platelet activity, lipoprotein concentrations, and neurohormonal systems reduce the risk for coronary events and death. However, these therapies do not cure IHD.
- Treatment with antiplatelet (aspirin or clopidogrel), lipid-lowering, and neurohormonal-modifying therapy for IHD is generally lifelong. Similarly, antianginal therapy with a β-blocker, CCB, and/or nitrate is usually long term.
- A patient with severe symptoms managed with combination antianginal drugs who undergoes successful coronary revascularization may be able to reduce antianginal therapy. However, treatment with at least one agent that improves the balance between myocardial oxygen demand and supply is usually warranted.

Abbreviations Introduced in This Chapter

ACC	American College of Cardiology
ACE	Angiotensin-converting enzyme
ACE-I	Angiotensin-converting enzyme inhibitor
ACS	Acute coronary syndromes
AHA	American Heart Association
ARB	Angiotensin receptor blocker
ASCVD	Atherosclerotic cardiovascular disease
AV	Atrioventricular
BMS	Bare metal stent
BP	Blood pressure
CABG	Coronary artery bypass graft
CAD	Coronary artery disease
CCB	Calcium channel blocker
cGMP	Cyclic guanosine monophosphate
CHD	Coronary heart disease
CK	Creatine kinase
CK-MB	Creatine kinase, MB fraction
COX-2	Cyclooxygenase-2
CT	Computed tomography
CYP	Cytochrome P450
DES	Drug-eluting stent
EBCT	Electron beam computed tomography
ECG	Electrocardiogram
FDA	Food and Drug Administration
HDL	High-density lipoprotein
HF	Heart failure
HFrEF	Heart failure with reduced ejection fraction
HMG-CoA	3-hydroxy-3-methylglutaryl coenzyme A
HR	Heart rate
HRT	Hormone replacement therapy
HTN	Hypertension
IHD	Ischemic heart disease
IR	Immediate release
IV	Intravenous
LA	Long acting
LV	Left ventricular
LDL	Low-density lipoprotein
MACE	Major adverse cardiac events
MI	Myocardial infarction
MR	Magnetic resonance
ms	Milliseconds
MVO_2	Myocardial oxygen consumption
NSAID	Nonsteroidal anti-inflammatory drug
NTG	Nitroglycerin
OCT2	Organic cation transporter 2
PCI	Percutaneous coronary intervention
P-gp	P-glycoprotein
Po_2	Partial pressure of oxygen
PTCA	Percutaneous transluminal coronary angioplasty
SL	Sublingual
TXA2	Thromboxane A2

REFERENCES

1. Fihn SD, Gardin JM, Abrams J, et al. 2012 ACCF/AHA/ACP/AATS/PCNA/SCAI/STS Guideline for the diagnosis and management of patients with stable ischemic heart disease: a report of the American College of Cardiology Foundation/American Heart Association Task Force on Practice Guidelines, and the American College of Physicians, American Association for Thoracic Surgery, Preventive Cardiovascular Nurses Association, Society for Cardiovascular Angiography and Interventions, and Society of Thoracic Surgeons. J Am Coll Cardiol. 2012;60(24):e44–e164.
2. Go AS, Mozaffarian D, Roger VL, et al. Heart disease and stroke statistics—2014 update: A report from the American Heart Association. Circulation. 2014;129(3):e28–e292.
3. Alberti KG, Eckel RH, Grundy SM, et al. Harmonizing the metabolic syndrome: a joint interim statement of the International Diabetes Federation Task Force on Epidemiology and Prevention; National Heart, Lung, and Blood Institute; American Heart Association; World Heart Federation; International Atherosclerosis Society; and International Association for the Study of Obesity. Circulation. 2009;120(16):1640–1645.
4. Lanza GA, Crea F. Primary coronary microvascular dysfunction: clinical presentation, pathophysiology, and management. Circulation. 2010;121(21):2317–2325.
5. Stone GW, Maehara A, Lansky AJ, et al. A prospective natural-history study of coronary atherosclerosis. N Engl J Med. 2011;364(3):226–235.
6. Braunwald E, Jones RH, Mark DB, et al. Diagnosing and managing unstable angina. Agency for Health Care Policy and Research. Circulation. 1994;90(1):613–622.
7. Sangareddi V, Chockalingam A, Gnanavelu G, Subramaniam T, Jagannathan V, Elangovan S. Canadian Cardiovascular Society classification of effort angina: An angiographic correlation. Coron Artery Dis. 2004;15(2):111–114.
8. Tonstad S, Farsang C, Klaene G, et al. Bupropion SR for smoking cessation in smokers with cardiovascular disease: A multicentre, randomised study. Eur Heart J. 2003;24(10):946–955.
9. Tzivoni D, Keren A, Meyler S, Khoury Z, Lerer T, Brunel P. Cardiovascular safety of transdermal nicotine patches in patients with coronary artery disease who try to quit smoking. Cardiovasc Drugs Ther. 1998;12(3):239–244.
10. Kuehn BM. Varenicline gets stronger warnings about psychiatric problems, vehicle crashes. JAMA. 2009;302(8):834.
11. Eckel RH, Jakicic JM, Ard JD, et al. 2013 AHA/ACC guideline on lifestyle management to reduce cardiovascular risk: A report of the American College of Cardiology/American Heart Association Task Force on Practice Guidelines. J Am Coll Cardiol. 2014;63(25 Pt B):2960–2984.

12. Chen JT, Wesley R, Shamburek RD, Pucino F, Csako G. Meta-analysis of natural therapies for hyperlipidemia: Plant sterols and stanols versus policosanol. Pharmacotherapy. 2005;25(2):171–183.
13. Gibbons RJ, Abrams J, Chatterjee K, et al. ACC/AHA 2002 guideline update for the management of patients with chronic stable angina—summary article: A report of the American College of Cardiology/American Heart Association Task Force on practice guidelines (Committee on the Management of Patients With Chronic Stable Angina). J Am Coll Cardiol. 2003;41(1):159–168.
14. Boden WE, O'Rourke RA, Teo KK, et al. Optimal medical therapy with or without PCI for stable coronary disease. N Engl J Med. 2007;356(15):1503–1516.
15. Shishehbor MH, Goel SS, Kapadia SR, et al. Long-term impact of drug-eluting stents versus bare-metal stents on all-cause mortality. J Am Coll Cardiol. 2008;52(13):1041–1048.
16. Serruys PW, Morice MC, Kappetein AP, et al. Percutaneous coronary intervention versus coronary-artery bypass grafting for severe coronary artery disease. N Engl J Med. 2009;360(10): 961–972.
17. Stone NJ, Robinson JG, Lichtenstein AH, et al. 2013 ACC/AHA guideline on the treatment of blood cholesterol to reduce atherosclerotic cardiovascular risk in adults: A report of the American College of Cardiology/American Heart Association Task Force on Practice Guidelines. J Am Coll Cardiol. 2014;63(25 Pt B):2889–2934.
18. James PA, Oparil S, Carter BL, et al. 2014 evidence-based guideline for the management of high blood pressure in adults: report from the panel members appointed to the Eighth Joint National Committee (JNC 8). JAMA. 2014;311(5):507–520.
19. Patrono C, Baigent C, Hirsh J, Roth G. Antiplatelet drugs: American College of Chest Physicians Evidence-Based Clinical Practice Guidelines (8th Edition). Chest. 2008;133 (6 Suppl):199S–233S.
20. Vandvik PO, Lincoff AM, Gore JM, et al. Primary and secondary prevention of cardiovascular disease: Antithrombotic Therapy and Prevention of Thrombosis, 9th ed: American College of Chest Physicians Evidence-Based Clinical Practice Guidelines. Chest. 2012;141(2 Suppl):e637S–e668S.
21. Anderson JL, Adams CD, Antman EM, et al. 2012 ACCF/AHA focused update incorporated into the ACCF/AHA 2007 guidelines for the management of patients with unstable angina/non-ST-elevation myocardial infarction: A report of the American College of Cardiology Foundation/American Heart Association Task Force on Practice Guidelines. J Am Coll Cardiol. 2013;61(23):e179–e347.
22. Levine GN, Bates ER, Blankenship JC, et al. 2011 ACCF/AHA/SCAI Guideline for Percutaneous Coronary Intervention. A report of the American College of Cardiology Foundation/American Heart Association Task Force on Practice Guidelines and the Society for Cardiovascular Angiography and Interventions. J Am Coll Cardiol. 2011;58(24):e44–e122.
23. O'Gara PT, Kushner FG, Ascheim DD, et al. 2013 ACCF/AHA guideline for the management of ST-elevation myocardial infarction: A report of the American College of Cardiology Foundation/American Heart Association Task Force on Practice Guidelines. J Am Coll Cardiol. 2013;61(4):e78–e140.
24. Mega JL, Simon T, Collet JP, et al. Reduced-function CYP2C19 genotype and risk of adverse clinical outcomes among patients treated with clopidogrel predominantly for PCI: A meta-analysis. JAMA. 2010;304(16):1821–1830.
25. Wallentin L, James S, Storey RF, et al. Effect of CYP2C19 and ABCB1 single nucleotide polymorphisms on outcomes of treatment with ticagrelor versus clopidogrel for acute coronary syndromes: A genetic substudy of the PLATO trial. Lancet. 2010;376(9749):1320–1328.
26. Wallentin L, Becker RC, Budaj A, et al. Ticagrelor versus clopidogrel in patients with acute coronary syndromes. N Engl J Med. 2009;361(11):1045–1057.
27. Wiviott SD, Braunwald E, McCabe CH, et al. Prasugrel versus clopidogrel in patients with acute coronary syndromes. N Engl J Med. 2007;357(20):2001–2015.
28. Yusuf S, Zhao F, Mehta SR, Chrolavicius S, Tognoni G, Fox KK. Effects of clopidogrel in addition to aspirin in patients with acute coronary syndromes without ST-segment elevation. N Engl J Med. 2001;345(7):494–502.
29. Baigent C, Keech A, Kearney PM, et al. Efficacy and safety of cholesterol-lowering treatment: Prospective meta-analysis of data from 90,056 participants in 14 randomised trials of statins. Lancet. 2005;366(9493):1267–1278.
30. Liao JK. Effects of statins on 3-hydroxy-3-methylglutaryl coenzyme a reductase inhibition beyond low-density lipoprotein cholesterol. Am J Cardiol. 2005;96(5A):24F–33F.
31. Pfeffer MA, McMurray JJ, Velazquez EJ, et al. Valsartan, captopril, or both in myocardial infarction complicated by heart failure, left ventricular dysfunction, or both. N Engl J Med. 2003;349(20):1893–1906.
32. Rodrigues EJ, Eisenberg MJ, Pilote L. Effects of early and late administration of angiotensin-converting enzyme inhibitors on mortality after myocardial infarction. Am J Med. 2003;115(6): 473–479.
33. Fox KM. Efficacy of perindopril in reduction of cardiovascular events among patients with stable coronary artery disease: randomised, double-blind, placebo-controlled, multicentre trial (the EUROPA study). Lancet. 2003;362(9386):782–788.
34. Yusuf S, Sleight P, Pogue J, Bosch J, Davies R, Dagenais G. Effects of an angiotensin-converting-enzyme inhibitor, ramipril, on cardiovascular events in high-risk patients. The Heart Outcomes Prevention Evaluation Study Investigators. N Engl J Med. 2000;342(3):145–153.
35. Freemantle N, Cleland J, Young P, Mason J, Harrison J. beta Blockade after myocardial infarction: systematic review and meta regression analysis. BMJ. 1999;318(7200):1730–1737.
36. Bangalore S, Steg G, Deedwania P, et al. Beta-blocker use and clinical outcomes in stable outpatients with and without coronary artery disease. JAMA. 2012;308(13):1340–1349.
37. Smith SC, Jr., Benjamin EJ, Bonow RO, et al. AHA/ACCF secondary prevention and risk reduction therapy for patients with coronary and other atherosclerotic vascular disease: 2011 update: A guideline from the American Heart Association and American College of Cardiology Foundation endorsed by the World Heart Federation and the Preventive Cardiovascular Nurses Association. J Am Coll Cardiol. 2011;58(23):2432–2446.
38. Klein WW, Jackson G, Tavazzi L. Efficacy of monotherapy compared with combined antianginal drugs in the treatment of chronic stable angina pectoris: A meta-analysis. Coron Artery Dis. 2002;13(8):427–436.
39. Cohn JN, Ziesche S, Smith R, et al. Effect of the calcium antagonist felodipine as supplementary vasodilator therapy in patients with chronic heart failure treated with enalapril: V-HeFT III. Vasodilator-Heart Failure Trial (V-HeFT) Study Group. Circulation. 1997;96(3):856–863.
40. Packer M, O'Connor CM, Ghali JK, et al. Effect of amlodipine on morbidity and mortality in severe chronic heart failure. Prospective Randomized Amlodipine Survival Evaluation Study Group. N Engl J Med. 1996;335(15):1107–1114.
41. Psaty BM, Smith NL, Siscovick DS, et al. Health outcomes associated with antihypertensive therapies used as first-line agents.

A systematic review and meta-analysis. JAMA. 1997;277(9):739–745.
42. Koren MJ, Crager MR, Sweeney M. Long-term safety of a novel antianginal agent in patients with severe chronic stable angina: the Ranolazine Open Label Experience (ROLE). J Am Coll Cardiol. 2007;49(10):1027–1034.
43. Cook NR, Albert CM, Gaziano JM, et al. A randomized factorial trial of vitamins C and E and beta carotene in the secondary prevention of cardiovascular events in women: results from the Women's Antioxidant Cardiovascular Study. Arch Intern Med. 2007;167(15):1610–1618.
44. Heiss G, Wallace R, Anderson GL, et al. Health risks and benefits 3 years after stopping randomized treatment with estrogen and progestin. JAMA. 2008;299(9):1036–1045.
45. Hulley S, Grady D, Bush T, et al. Randomized trial of estrogen plus progestin for secondary prevention of coronary heart disease in postmenopausal women. Heart and Estrogen/progestin Replacement Study (HERS) Research Group. JAMA. 1998;280(7):605–613.
46. Marti-Carvajal AJ, Sola I, Lathyris D, Salanti G. Homocysteine lowering interventions for preventing cardiovascular events. Cochrane Database Syst Rev. 2009(4):CD006612.
47. Vivekananthan DP, Penn MS, Sapp SK, Hsu A, Topol EJ. Use of antioxidant vitamins for the prevention of cardiovascular disease: meta-analysis of randomised trials. Lancet. 2003;361(9374):2017–2023.
48. Bennett JS, Daugherty A, Herrington D, Greenland P, Roberts H, Taubert KA. The use of nonsteroidal anti-inflammatory drugs (NSAIDs): A science advisory from the American Heart Association. Circulation. 2005;111(13):1713–1716.

8 Acute Coronary Syndromes

Kelly C. Rogers, Simon de Denus, and Shannon W. Finks

LEARNING OBJECTIVES

Upon completion of the chapter, the reader will be able to:

1. Define the role of atherosclerotic plaque, platelets, and the coagulation system in an acute coronary syndrome (ACS).
2. List key electrocardiographic and clinical features identifying a patient with non–ST-segment elevation (NSTE), ACS, and ST-segment elevation myocardial infarction (STEMI).
3. Devise a pharmacotherapy treatment and monitoring plan for a patient undergoing percutaneous coronary intervention (PCI) in NSTE-ACS and STEMI given patient-specific data.
4. Devise a pharmacotherapy treatment and monitoring plan for a patient with NSTE-ACS or STEMI not undergoing PCI given patient-specific data.
5. Develop a pharmacotherapy and risk factor modification treatment plan for secondary prevention of coronary heart disease (CHD) events in a patient following NSTE-ACS or STEMI.

INTRODUCTION

Cardiovascular disease (CVD) is the leading cause of death in the United States and one of the major causes of death worldwide. **Acute coronary syndromes** (ACS), including **unstable angina** (UA) and **myocardial infarction** (MI), are a form of coronary heart disease (CHD) that comprises the most common cause of CVD death.[1] KEY CONCEPT *ACS is primarily caused by rupture of an atherosclerotic plaque with subsequent platelet adherence, activation, aggregation, and the activation of the clotting cascade. Ultimately, a thrombus composed of fibrin and platelets may develop, resulting in incomplete or complete occlusion of a coronary artery.*[2] *The American Heart Association (AHA) and the American College of Cardiology Foundation (ACCF) recommend strategies or guidelines for ACS patient care for* **ST-segment elevation MI** (STEMI) and **non–ST-segment elevation** (NSTE)-ACS which includes both UA and non–ST-elevation MI (NSTEMI). In collaboration with the Society for Cardiovascular Angiography and Interventions (SCAI), the ACCF and AHA issue joint guidelines for **percutaneous coronary intervention** (PCI), including PCI in the setting of ACS. These practice guidelines are based on a review of available clinical evidence, have graded recommendations based on evidence and expert opinion, and are updated periodically. These guidelines form the cornerstone for quality care of the ACS patient.[3–5]

EPIDEMIOLOGY

Each year, approximately 620,000 Americans will have a new "coronary attack," a first hospitalized MI or CHD death, while 295,000 will have a recurrent event.[1] The risks of CHD events, such as death, recurrent MI, and stroke, are higher for patients with established CHD and a history of MI than for patients with no known CHD.

The incidence rates of MIs in the United States have been decreasing.[1] In particular, the number of patients presenting with STEMI has significantly decreased (from 133 to 50 cases per 100,000 person-years). Nevertheless, 122,071 Americans died of an MI in 2010.[1] One in six deaths is secondary to CHD, which is the leading cause of hospitalization in the United States, with 1,346,000 hospitalizations listing it as the first cause of hospitalization in 2010. This is nevertheless a marked improvement from the 2,165,000 reported in 2000.[1]

In patients with STEMI, in-hospital death rates are approximately 3% in patients receiving primary PCI, 7% for patients who are treated with fibrinolytics, and 16% for patients who do not receive reperfusion therapy. In patients with NSTEMI, in-hospital mortality is less than 5%. Mortality rates have been declining since the 1990s. Improvements in care that may have contributed to this reduction include greater use of guideline-recommended drugs (eg, aspirin [ASA], β-blockers, angiotensin-converting enzyme [ACE] inhibitors, angiotensin receptor blockers [ARBs], statins, clopidogrel); reductions in the median times for administering fibrinolytics and performing primary PCI; and increased use of early coronary angiography and PCI for high-risk patients with NSTE-ACS.[1] Other than persistent ST-segment changes and troponin, other predictors of in-hospital mortality include older age, elevated serum creatinine (SCr), tachycardia, and heart failure (HF).[6]

The cost of CHD is high, with estimated direct and indirect costs of more than $204 billion.[1] Even more concerning, these costs are expected to double by 2030. The median length of hospital stay is 3.2 days.[7]

ETIOLOGY

Endothelial dysfunction, inflammation, and formation of fatty streaks contribute to the formation of atherosclerotic coronary artery plaques, the underlying cause of coronary artery disease (CAD).[8] KEY CONCEPT *The predominant cause of ACS in more than 90% of patients is atheromatous plaque rupture, fissuring, or erosion of an unstable atherosclerotic plaque.*[2,8] This is called an MI type 1, which generally occurs in coronary arteries where the stenosis occludes less than 50% of the lumen prior to the event, rather than a more stable 70% to 90% stenosis of the coronary artery.[5,9] Stable stenoses are characteristic of stable angina. MI type 2 is related to a reduction in myocardial oxygen supply or an increase in myocardial demand in the absence of a coronary artery process. MI type 3 is defined as MI resulting in death without the possibility of measuring biomarkers, while MI types 4 and 5 occur during revascularization procedures.[9]

PATHOPHYSIOLOGY

Spectrum of ACS

The term ACS encompasses all clinical syndromes compatible with acute myocardial ischemia and/or MI resulting from an imbalance between myocardial oxygen demand and supply. In contrast to stable angina, an ACS results primarily from diminished myocardial blood flow secondary to an occlusive or partially occlusive coronary artery thrombus. ACS are classified according to electrocardiographic (ECG) changes into STEMI or NSTE-ACS (NSTEMI and UA) (Figure 8–1).[4,5] An injury that transects the entire thickness of the myocardial wall results in an STEMI. A NSTEMI is limited to the subendocardial myocardium and is usually smaller and not as extensive as an STEMI. NSTEMI differs from UA in that ischemia is severe enough to produce myocardial necrosis resulting in the release of biomarkers, mainly **troponins** T or I, from the necrotic myocytes into the bloodstream. The clinical significance of serum markers is discussed in greater detail in later sections of this chapter.

Plaque Rupture and Clot Formation

Plaques that rupture are generally characterized by a soft lipid-rich necrotic core, a thin fibrous cap, adventitial and perivascular inflammation, intraplaque hemorrhage, angiogenesis, and expansive vascular remodeling. The latter explains why these plaques only show minimal luminal obstruction, despite being larger than plaques that characterize stable angina which are associated with more severe luminal narrowing.[2,8] Following plaque rupture, a clot (a partially or completely occlusive thrombus) forms on top of the ruptured plaque. The thrombogenic

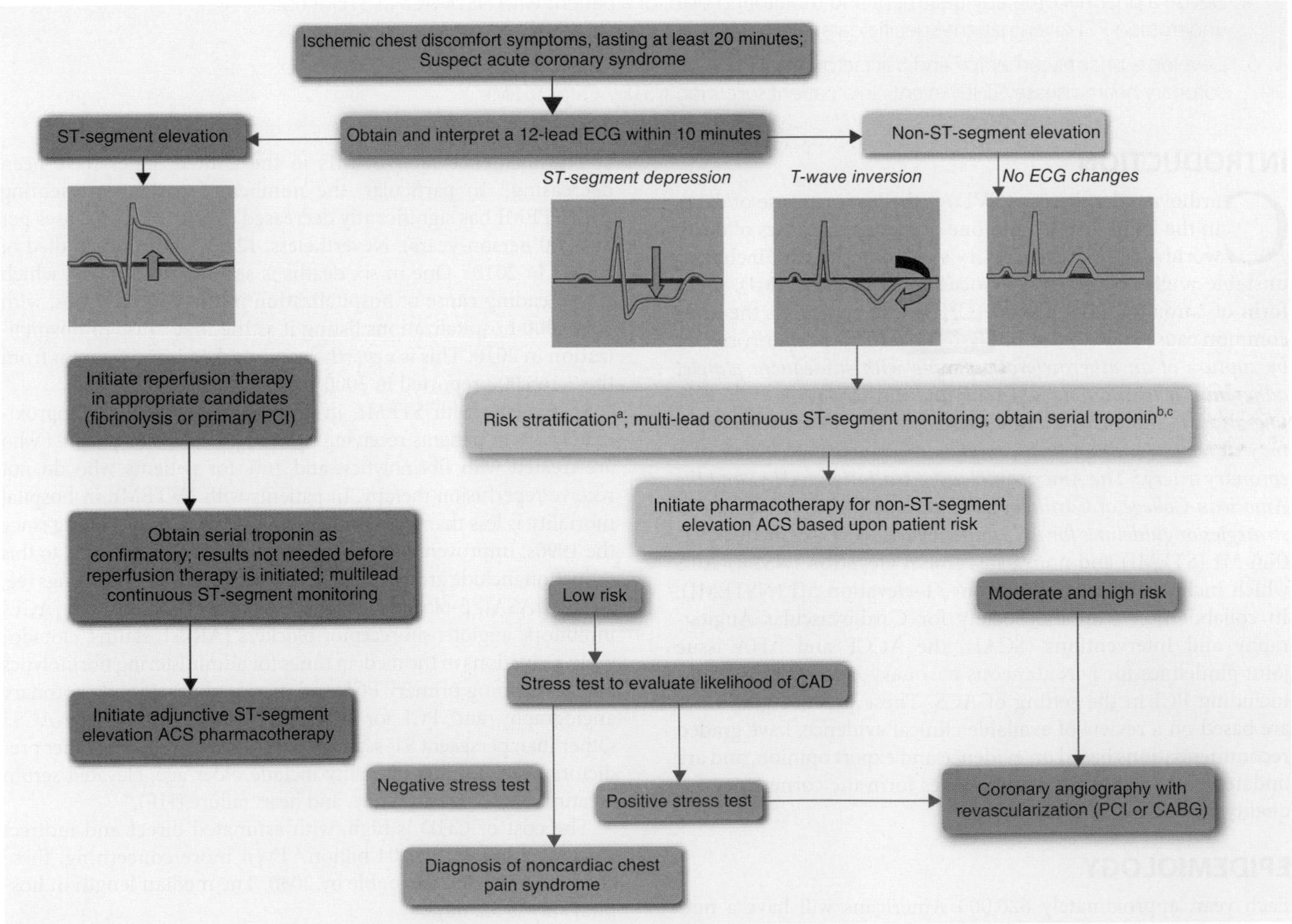

FIGURE 8–1. Evaluation of the acute coronary syndrome patient. [a]As described in Table 8–1. [b]"Positive": Above the myocardial infarction decision limit. [c]"Negative": Below the myocardial infarction decision limit. (ACS, acute coronary syndrome; CABG, coronary artery bypass graft; CAD, coronary artery disease; ECG, electrocardiogram; PCI, percutaneous coronary intervention.) Reproduced with permission from DiPiro JT, Talbert RL, Yee GC, et al. Pharmacotherapy: A Pathophysiologic Approach, 9th ed. New York, NY: McGraw-Hill; 2014:177.

contents of the plaque are exposed to blood elements. Exposure of collagen and tissue factor induce platelet adhesion and activation, which promote the release of platelet-derived vasoactive substances, including adenosine diphosphate (ADP) and thromboxane A_2 (TXA_2).[8] These produce vasoconstriction and potentiate platelet activation. Furthermore, during platelet activation, a change in the conformation in the glycoprotein (GP) IIb/IIIa surface receptors of platelets occurs that cross-links platelets to each other through fibrinogen bridges. This is considered the final common pathway of platelet aggregation. Inclusion of platelets gives the clot a white appearance. Simultaneously, the extrinsic coagulation cascade pathway is activated as a result of exposure of blood components to the thrombogenic lipid core and disrupted endothelium, which are rich in tissue factor. This leads to the production of thrombin (factor IIa), which converts fibrinogen to fibrin through enzymatic activity. Fibrin stabilizes the clot and traps red blood cells, which gives the clot a red appearance. Therefore, the clot is composed of cross-linked platelets and fibrin strands.[2,8]

Ventricular Remodeling Following an Acute MI

Ventricular remodeling is a process that occurs in several cardiovascular (CV) conditions including HF and following an MI. It is characterized by left ventricular dilation and reduced pumping function of the left ventricle, leading to cardiac failure.[10] Because HF represents one of the principal causes of morbidity and mortality following an MI, preventing ventricular remodeling is an important therapeutic goal.

Use of ACE inhibitors, ARBs, β-blockers, and aldosterone antagonists can slow down or reverse ventricular remodeling through inhibition of the renin-angiotensin aldosterone system and/or through improvement in hemodynamics (decreasing preload or afterload).[10] These agents also improve survival.

At some point during hospitalization but prior to discharge, patients with a definite ACS should have their left ventricular function (LVF) evaluated.[4,5] The most common way LVF is measured is using an echocardiogram to calculate the patient's left ventricular ejection fraction (LVEF). LVF is one of the strongest predictors of mortality following MI. Patients with LVEF less than 40% (0.40) are at high risk of death, and LVEF is an important factor to consider when contemplating the use of several drugs, such as ACE inhibitors and aldosterone antagonists. Patients with ventricular fibrillation or sustained ventricular tachycardia occurring more than 2 days following MI (which are not due to transient and reversible ischemia, reinfarction, or metabolic abnormalities), those with LVEF less than 30% (0.30; measured at least 40 days after STEMI) regardless of symptoms, or those with LVEF less than or equal to 35% (0.35) with New York Heart Association functional classes II to III benefit from placement of an implantable cardioverter defibrillator (ICD).[4]

Complications

This chapter focuses on management of the uncomplicated ACS patient. However, it is important for clinicians to recognize complications of an acute MI due to an increased risk of mortality. The most serious early complication of MI is cardiogenic shock, occurring in approximately 7% of hospitalized patients presenting with STEMI.[11,12] Mortality in cardiogenic shock patients with MI is high, approaching 60%.[12] Other complications that may result from MI are HF, valvular dysfunction, bradycardia, heart block, pericarditis, stroke secondary to left ventricular thrombus embolization, venous thromboembolism, left ventricular free wall rupture, and ventricular and atrial tachyarrhythmias.[4] In fact, more than a quarter of MI patients die, presumably from ventricular fibrillation, prior to reaching the hospital.[1]

CLINICAL PRESENTATION AND DIAGNOSIS

Symptoms and Physical Examination Findings

The classic symptom of an ACS is substernal anginal chest discomfort, most often occurring at rest, with severe new onset, or an increasing angina that is at least 20 minutes in duration. The pain may radiate to the shoulder, down the left arm, and to the back or jaw. Associated symptoms include nausea, vomiting, **diaphoresis**, or shortness of breath. Although similar to stable angina, the duration may be longer and the intensity greater.[4,5] All health care professionals should review these warning symptoms with patients at high risk for CHD. On physical examination, no specific features are indicative of ACS. Patients with suspected ACS should be referred immediately to an emergency department (ED).

12-Lead ECG

KEY CONCEPT *There are key features of a 12-lead ECG that identify and risk-stratify a patient with an ACS. Within 10 minutes of presentation to an ED with symptoms of ischemic chest discomfort, a 12-lead ECG should be obtained and interpreted.* If the first ECG is not diagnostic, additional ECGs should be performed every 15 to 30 minutes for the first hour if the patient is still symptomatic and the clinician has a high suspicion of ACS.[5] KEY CONCEPT *When possible, an ECG should be performed by emergency medical system providers to reduce the delay until myocardial reperfusion.* If available, a prior ECG should be reviewed to identify whether or not ischemic changes are new or old, with new findings being more indicative of an ACS. Key findings on review of an ECG that indicate myocardial ischemia or infarction are STE (ST-segment elevation), ST-segment depression, and T-wave inversion (see Figure 8–1).[4,5] ST-segment and/or T-wave changes in certain groupings of ECG leads help to identify the location of the coronary artery that is the cause of the ischemia or infarction. In addition, the appearance of a new left bundle-branch block accompanied by chest discomfort is highly specific for acute STEMI. Approximately one-third of patients diagnosed with MI present with STE on their ECG, with the remainder having ST-segment depression, T-wave inversion, or, in some instances, no ECG changes.[5] According to the latest guidelines, the diagnosis of STE, in the absence of left bundle-branch block or left ventricular hypertrophy, is a new STE in at least two contiguous leads of greater than or equal to 2 mm in men and greater than or equal to 1.5 mm in women in leads V_2-V_3 and/or of greater than or equal to 1 mm in other leads. Some parts of the heart are more "electrically silent" than others, and myocardial ischemia may not be detected on an ECG. Therefore, it is important to review findings from the ECG in conjunction with biochemical markers of myocardial necrosis, such as troponin I or T, clinical symptoms, and other risk factors for CHD to determine the patient's risk for experiencing a new MI or having other complications.

Biochemical Markers/Cardiac Enzymes

Biochemical markers of myocardial cell death are important for confirming the diagnosis of MI. KEY CONCEPT *The diagnosis of MI is confirmed when the following conditions are met in a clinical setting consistent with myocardial ischemia: "Detection of a rise and/or fall of cardiac biomarkers with at least one value above the*

Clinical Presentation and Diagnosis

General

- The patient is typically in acute distress and may develop or present with acute HF, cardiogenic shock, or cardiac arrest.

Symptoms

- The classic symptom of ACS is substernal chest pain or discomfort. Accompanying symptoms may include radiation of pain to arm, back, or jaw, nausea, vomiting, diaphoresis, anxiety, or shortness of breath.
- Elderly, women, and diabetics are less likely to present with classic symptoms.

Physical Signs

- There are no "classic" signs for ACS.
- Patients with ACS may present with signs of acute HF, including edema, jugular venous distention, an S_3 sound on auscultation, or pulmonary edema on a chest X-ray.
- Patients may also present with arrhythmias such as tachycardia, bradycardia, or heart block.

Laboratory Tests

- Troponin I or T are measured at presentation and repeated 2–3 times at 6- to 8-hour intervals to ascertain heart muscle damage; confirmatory for the diagnosis of an infarction. For patients with NSTE-ACS, an elevated troponin is diagnostic for MI, differentiating NSTEMI from UA. Patients presenting with suspected NSTE-ACS who do not have an MI undergo further diagnostic testing to determine whether they have UA or are not experiencing an ACS.
- Blood chemistry tests are performed with particular attention given to potassium and magnesium, which may affect heart rhythm.
- SCr is measured and creatinine clearance (CrCl) is used to identify patients who may need dosing adjustments for medications, as well as those who are at high risk of morbidity and mortality.
- Baseline complete blood count (CBC) and coagulation tests (activated partial thromboplastin time [aPTT] and international normalized ratio [INR]) should be obtained because most patients will receive antithrombotic therapy that increases the risk for bleeding.
- Fasting lipid panel within 24 hours is recommended.

Other Diagnostic Tests

- The 12-lead ECG is the first step in management. Patients are risk stratified into two groups: STEMI or NSTE-ACS.
- High-risk ACS patients, especially those with STEMI and those with recurrent chest discomfort will undergo coronary angiography via a left heart catheterization and injection of contrast dye into the coronary arteries to determine the presence and extent of coronary artery stenosis with possible PCI.
- During hospitalization, a measurement of LVF, such as an echocardiogram, is performed to identify patients with EF less than or equal to 40% (0.40) who are at high risk of death following hospital discharge.
- Selected low-risk patients may undergo early stress testing.

Modified with permission from Spinler SA, de Denus S. Acute coronary syndromes. In: DiPiro JT, Talbert RL, Yee GC, et al, eds. Pharmacotherapy: A Pathophysiologic Approach, 9th ed. New York, NY: McGraw-Hill, 2014:178.

99th percentile of the upper reference limit and with at least one of the following: (a) symptoms of ischemia; (b) ECG changes of new ischemia or development of pathological Q waves; (c) imaging evidence of new loss of viable myocardium; (d) new regional wall motion abnormality; or (e) identification of an intracoronary thrombus by angiography or autopsy."[9] The most recent guidelines indicate that only the use of troponin assays is recommended to assess myocardial necrosis. Typically, troponin levels are obtained at presentation, then 3 to 6 hours later in patients with a high suspicion of MI to identify variations (increase or decrease greater than or equal to 20% if the initial value is increased). In patients with normal troponin levels with an intermediate or high suspicion of ACS, additional levels should be obtained after 6 to 8 hours.[5] A single measurement of troponin is not adequate to exclude a diagnosis of MI, as up to 15% of values that were initially below the level of detection (a "negative" test) rise to the level of detection (a "positive" test) in subsequent hours. Measurement of N-terminal pro B-type natriuretic peptide may help predict long-term risk of mortality in patients with ACS but does not aid with acute diagnosis.[5]

Risk Stratification

KEY CONCEPT *Patient symptoms, past medical history, ECG, and troponins are utilized to stratify patients into low, medium, or high risk of death, MI, or likelihood of failing pharmacotherapy and needing urgent coronary angiography and PCI* (Table 8–1). Initial treatment according to risk stratification is depicted in Figure 8–1.[4,5] Patients with STEMI are at the highest risk of death; therefore, immediate reperfusion strategies should be initiated. The ACCF/AHA/SCAI PCI guidelines define a target time to initiate reperfusion treatment as within 30 minutes of hospital arrival for fibrinolytics (eg, alteplase, reteplase, and tenecteplase) and within 90 minutes from presentation for primary PCI.[3] The sooner the infarct-related coronary artery is opened, the lower the mortality and the greater the amount of myocardium that is preserved.[3] Although all patients should be evaluated for reperfusion therapy, not all patients may be eligible. Indications and contraindications for fibrinolytic therapy are described in the treatment section of this chapter. If patients with STEMI are not eligible for reperfusion therapy, additional pharmacotherapy should be initiated in the ED and the patient transferred to a coronary intensive care unit.

Risk-stratification of the patient with NSTE-ACS is more complex because outcomes vary. Patients with a high likelihood of coronary ischemia have a greater risk of adverse cardiac events.[5] Not all patients presenting with suspected NSTE-ACS have CAD. Some are eventually diagnosed with nonischemic chest discomfort. In general, among NSTE-ACS

Table 8–1

Risk Stratification for Acute Coronary Syndromes[5]

TIMI Risk Score for NSTE-ACS

One point is assigned for each of the seven medical history and clinical presentation findings below. The point total is calculated, and the patient is assigned a risk for experiencing the composite endpoint of death, MI, or urgent need for revascularization.

- Age 65 years or older
- Three or more CHD risk factors: smoking, hypercholesterolemia, HTN, DM, family history of premature CHD death/events
- Known CAD (50% or greater stenosis of at least one major coronary artery on coronary angiogram)
- Aspirin use within the past 7 days
- Two or more episodes of chest discomfort within the past 24 hours
- ST-segment depression 0.5 mm or greater
- Positive biochemical marker for infarction

High-Risk	Medium-Risk	Low-Risk
TIMI Risk Score 5–7 points	TIMI Risk Score 3–4 points	TIMI Risk Score 0–2 points

TIMI Risk Score	Mortality, MI, or Severe Recurrent Ischemia Requiring Urgent Revascularization Through 14 days
0/1	4.7%
2	8.3%
3	13.2%
4	19.9%
5	26.2%
6/7	40.9%

GRACE Risk Factors for Increased Mortality and the Composite of Death or MI in ACS

Signs and symptoms of HF
Low systolic BP
Elevated heart rate
Older age
Elevated SCr
Baseline risk factors on clinical evaluation: cardiac arrest at admission, ST-segment deviation, elevated troponin
A high-risk patient is defined as a GRACE Risk Score more than 140 points

ACS, acute coronary syndromes; BP, blood pressure; CAD, coronary artery disease; CHD, coronary heart disease; DM, diabetes mellitus; GRACE, Global Registry of Acute Coronary Events; HF, heart failure; HTN, hypertension; MI, myocardial infarction; NSTE, non–ST-segment elevation; SCr, serum creatinine; TIMI, thrombolysis in myocardial infarction.

An online calculator for the GRACE Risk Model is available at http://www.outcomes-umassmed.org/GRACE/acs_risk/acs_risk_content.html (Accessed January 6, 2015).

Reproduced with permission from DiPiro JT, Talbert RL, Yee GC, et al. Pharmacotherapy: A pathophysiologic Approach, 9th ed. New York, NY: McGraw-Hill; 2014:179.

patients, those with ST-segment depression (see Figure 8–1) and/or elevated biomarkers are at higher risk of death or recurrent infarction. Various risk scores are available and should be used to assess the prognosis of patients presenting with NSTE-ACS (see Table 8-1).[5]

Based on this risk assessment, a management strategy is chosen and patients are either treated using: (1) an invasive strategy, which involves coronary angiography, or (2) an ischemia-guided strategy in which patients undergo an invasive evaluation only if they fail medical therapy (eg, continued ischemia despite optimal medical treatment), have objective evidence of ischemia on non-invasive stress testing, or are later stratified as being at very high risk of CV events based on clinical characteristics (eg, high TIMI [Thrombolysis in myocardial infarction] score).[5] The ischemia-guided strategy is generally reserved for low-risk individuals. The timing of the diagnostic angiography in moderate- to high-risk patients is generally guided by the short-term risk of the patients, with an earlier angiography generally preferred in high-risk individuals.[5]

TREATMENT

Desired Outcomes

Short-term desired outcomes in a patient with ACS are: (a) early restoration of blood flow to the infarct-related artery to prevent infarct expansion (in the case of MI) or prevent complete occlusion and MI (in UA); (b) prevention of death and other MI complications; (c) prevention of coronary artery reocclusion; (d) relief of ischemic chest discomfort; and (e) resolution of ST-segment and T-wave changes on the ECG.

Long-term desired outcomes are control of CV risk factors, prevention of additional CV events, including reinfarction, stroke, and HF, and improvement in quality of life.

General Approach to Treatment

Selecting evidence-based therapies described in the guidelines for patients without contraindications results in lower mortality.[4,5] General treatment measures for all STEMI and high- and

Patient Encounter 1, Part 1

A 58-year-old, 85-kg (187-lb) African American woman developed lower back pain accompanied by nausea and vomiting while at work. Local paramedics were summoned and ST-segment elevation was found on ECG. She was given three 0.4 mg sublingual nitroglycerin tablets by mouth, 325 mg ASA by mouth, and morphine 2-mg IV push without relief of discomfort upon transport to the emergency department (ED). She was taken to a facility with a cardiac catheterization laboratory with the intent of performing primary PCI.

PMH: Hypertension (HTN) for 5 years; dyslipidemia for 6 years; diabetes mellitus (DM) type 2 for 2 years

FH: Father with stroke at age 65; mother with HTN; no siblings

SH: Smoked one pack per day for 30 years, quit 6 years ago

Allergies: NKDA

Meds: Amlodipine 10 mg by mouth once daily; ASA 81 mg by mouth once daily; simvastatin 20 mg by mouth once daily at bedtime

ROS: general malaise; lower back pain 7/10; shortness of breath

PE:

HEENT: Normocephalic atraumatic

CV: Regular rate and rhythm; S_1, S_2, no S_3, no S_4; no murmurs or rubs

VS: BP 130/75 mm Hg; HR 88 beats/min; T 37°C (98.6°F)

Lungs: Clear to auscultation and percussion

Abd: Nontender, nondistended

GI: Normal bowel sounds

GU: Stool guaiac negative

Exts: No bruits, pulses 2+, femoral pulses present, good range of motion

Neuro: Alert and oriented × 3, cranial nerves intact

Labs: Sodium 138 mEq/L (138 mmol/L), potassium 3.8 mEq/L (3.8 mmol/L), chloride 102 mEq/L (102 mmol/L), bicarbonate 24 mEq/L (24 mmol/L), SCr 1.3 mg/dL (115 μmol/L), glucose 135 mg/dL (7.5 mmol/L), WBC $9.9 \times 10^3/mm^3$ ($9.9 \times 10^9/L$), hemoglobin 15.7 g/dL (157 g/L or 9.74 mmol/L), hematocrit 47% (0.47), platelets $220 \times 10^3/mm^3$ ($220 \times 10^9/L$), troponin I 3.8 ng/mL (3.8 mcg/L; 3800 ng/L), oxygen saturation 96% (0.96) on room air

ECG: Normal sinus rhythm, PR 0.16 seconds, QRS 0.08 seconds, QTc 0.38 seconds, 3-mm ST-segment elevation in anterior leads

CXR: No active disease

Echo: Anterior wall dyskinesis, LVEF 45% (0.45)

What information is suggestive of acute MI?

Are any complications of MI present?

intermediate-risk NSTE-ACS patients include admission to hospital, oxygen administration (if oxygen saturation is low, less than 90% [0.90] or respiratory distress), continuous multilead ST-segment monitoring for arrhythmias and ischemia, frequent measurement of vital signs, bed rest for 12 hours in hemodynamically stable patients, avoidance of the Valsalva maneuver (prescribe stool softeners routinely), and pain relief (Figures 8–2 and 8–3).[4,5]

Because risk varies and resources are limited, it is important to triage and treat patients according to their risk category. Initial approaches to treatment of STEMI and NSTE-ACS patients are outlined in Figures 8–2 and 8–3. Patients with STE are at high risk of death, and efforts to reestablish coronary perfusion as well as adjunctive pharmacotherapy should be initiated immediately (see Figure 8–2). Features identifying low-, moderate-, and high-risk NSTE-ACS patients are described in Table 8–1 and treatment efforts are outlined in Figure 8–3.[5]

Reperfusion Strategies for ACS

▶ Reperfusion Strategies for STEMIs

KEY CONCEPT *Early reperfusion therapy with primary PCI of the infarct artery within 90 minutes from time of hospital presentation is the reperfusion treatment of choice for patients with STEMI who present within 12 hours of symptom onset* (see Figure 8–2).[4] Patients may not often recognize the importance of seeking immediate medical care for a variety of reasons, which include self-treatment and preconception regarding the importance or presentation of a heart attack. Thus, education to patients and their families is paramount to reduce delays in reperfusion.

For primary PCI, the patient is taken from the ED to the cardiac catheterization laboratory and undergoes coronary angiography with either balloon angioplasty or placement of a bare metal or drug-eluting intracoronary stent in the artery associated with the infarct.[3] Results from a meta-analysis of trials comparing fibrinolysis with primary PCI indicate a lower mortality rate with primary PCI.[13] One reason for the superiority of primary PCI compared with fibrinolysis is that more than 90% of occluded infarct-related coronary arteries are opened with primary PCI compared with fewer than 60% with fibrinolytics.[3,4] In addition, intracranial hemorrhage (ICH) and major bleeding risks from primary PCI are lower than the risks of severe bleeding events following fibrinolysis.[14] An invasive strategy of primary PCI is generally preferred in patients presenting to institutions with skilled interventional cardiologists and a catheterization laboratory immediately available, those in cardiogenic shock, those with contraindications to fibrinolytics, and those with continuing symptoms 12 to 24 hours after symptom onset.[4,15] Current guidelines indicate that the time from first medical contact to device should be less than or equal to 90 minutes, with every effort made to ensure the time to reperfusion is as short as possible.[4]

Patients presenting to facilities that do not have interventional cardiology services can be transferred when a protocol that minimizes delays has been established between institutions and if primary PCI can be performed within the first 120 minutes of first medical contact.[4] Immediate transfer to a PCI-capable facility is recommended for patients who develop cardiogenic shock or acute severe HF, irrespective of the timing of presentation. PCI during hospitalization for STEMI, or transfer to a PCI-capable hospital, is also appropriate in those in whom fibrinolysis is not successful and those with persistent rest ischemia or signs of ischemia on stress testing following MI.[3,4]

▶ Fibrinolytic Therapy

Administration of a fibrinolytic agent is indicated in patients with STEMI who present to the hospital within 12 hours of the onset of chest discomfort, who are initially seen at a non-PCI-capable

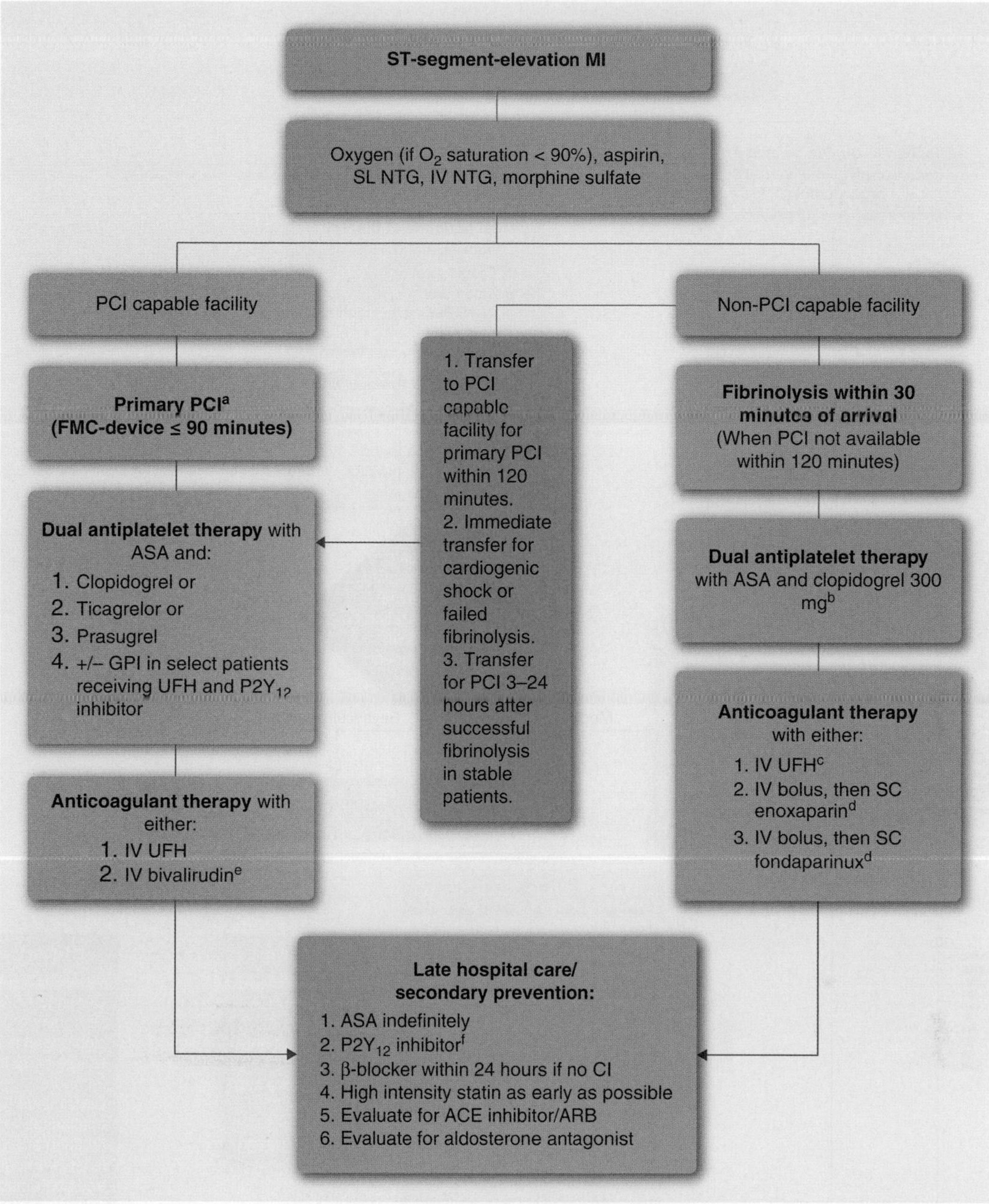
ST-segment-elevation MI
Oxygen (if O2 saturation < 90%), aspirin, SL NTG, IV NTG, morphine sulfate
PCI capable facility
Non-PCI capable facility
Primary PCI[a] (FMC-device ≤ 90 minutes)
1. Transfer to PCI capable facility for primary PCI within 120 minutes. 2. Immediate transfer for cardiogenic shock or failed fibrinolysis. 3. Transfer for PCI 3–24 hours after successful fibrinolysis in stable patients.
Fibrinolysis within 30 minutes of arrival (When PCI not available within 120 minutes)
Dual antiplatelet therapy with ASA and: 1. Clopidogrel or 2. Ticagrelor or 3. Prasugrel 4. +/– GPI in select patients receiving UFH and P2Y12 inhibitor
Dual antiplatelet therapy with ASA and clopidogrel 300 mg[b]
Anticoagulant therapy with either: 1. IV UFH 2. IV bivalirudin[e]
Anticoagulant therapy with either: 1. IV UFH[c] 2. IV bolus, then SC enoxaparin[d] 3. IV bolus, then SC fondaparinux[d]
Late hospital care/ secondary prevention: 1. ASA indefinitely 2. P2Y12 inhibitor[f] 3. β-blocker within 24 hours if no CI 4. High intensity statin as early as possible 5. Evaluate for ACE inhibitor/ARB 6. Evaluate for aldosterone antagonist

FIGURE 8–2. Initial pharmacotherapy for ST-segment elevation myocardial infarction. See Table 8–3 for dosing recommendations and contraindications to specific therapies. [a]Options after coronary angiography also include medical management alone or CABG surgery. [b]Clopidogrel preferred $P2Y_{12}$ when fibrinolytic therapy is utilized. No loading dose recommended if age older than 75 years. [c]Given for up to 48 hours or until revascularization. [d]Given for the duration of hospitalization, up to 8 days or until revascularization. [e]If pretreated with UFH, stop UFH infusion for 30 minutes prior to administration of bivalirudin (bolus plus infusion). [f]In patients with STEMI receiving a fibrinolytic or who do not receive reperfusion therapy, administer clopidogrel for at least 14 days and ideally up to 1 year. (ACE, angiotensin-converting enzyme; ARB, angiotensin receptor blocker; ASA, aspirin; CI, contraindication; FMC, first medical contact; GPI, glycoprotein IIb/IIIa inhibitor; IV, intravenous; MI, myocardial infarction; NTG, nitroglycerin; PCI, percutaneous coronary intervention; SC, subcutaneous; SL, sublingual; UFH, unfractionated heparin.)

hospital and who have an anticipated time from first medical contact-to-device greater than 120 minutes if transferred to a PCI capable hospital (see Figure 8–2).[4] The reduction in mortality with fibrinolysis is greatest with early administration and diminishes after 12 hours. The use of fibrinolytics between 12 and 24 hours after symptom onset should be limited to patients with ongoing ischemia. Fibrinolytic therapy is preferred over primary PCI when there is no cardiac catheterization laboratory in a hospital and the delay from first medical contact-to-device would exceed 120 minutes if the patient was transferred to a PCI-capable hospital.[4] Guidelines recommend that the fibrinolytic agent be administered within 30 minutes of arrival.[4] All hospitals should have protocols addressing fibrinolysis eligibility, dosing, and monitoring. Indications and contraindications for

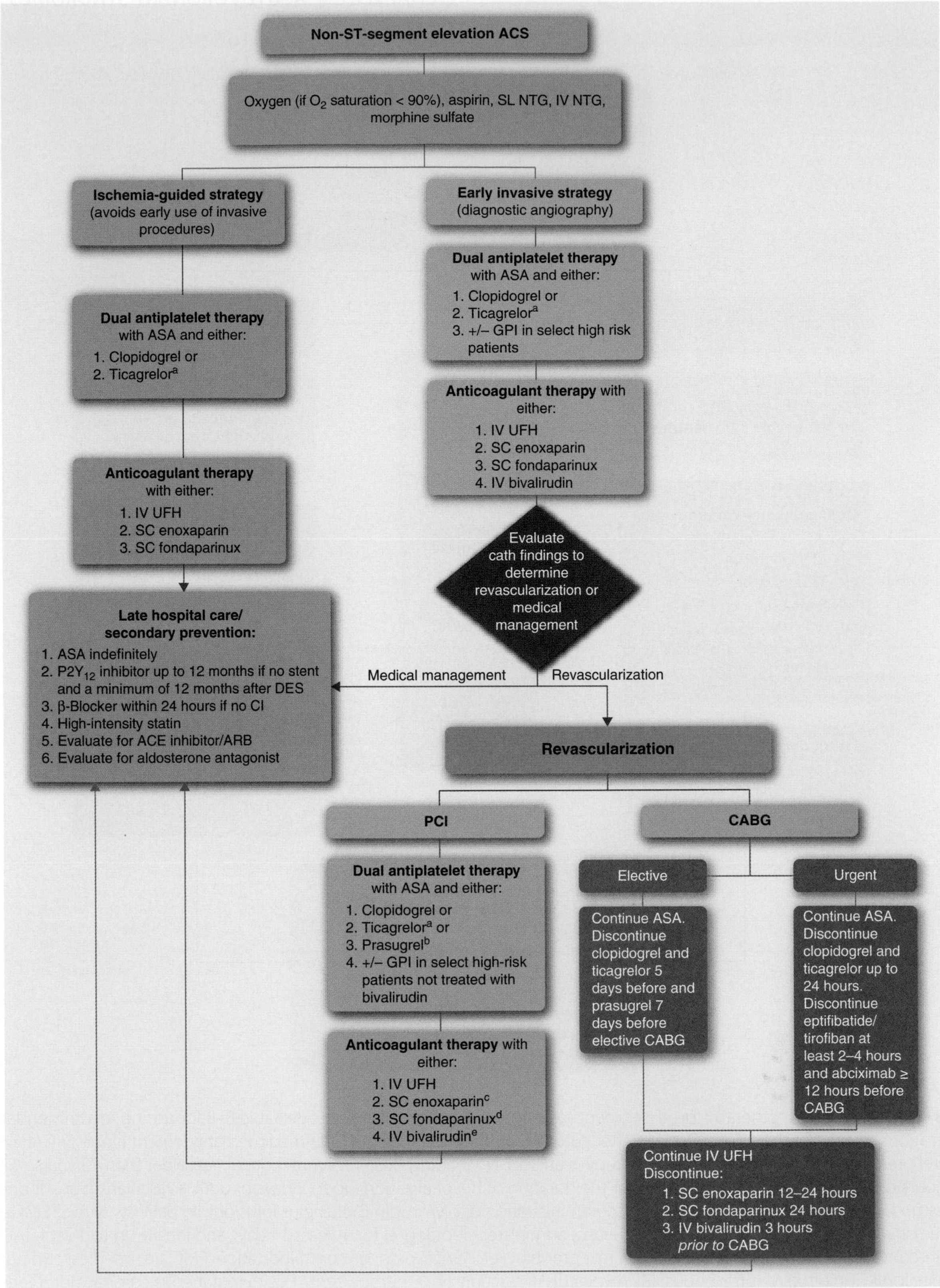

FIGURE 8–3. Initial pharmacotherapy for non–ST-segment elevation (NSTE) ACS. See Table 8–3 for dosing recommendations and contraindications to specific therapies. [a]Reasonable to choose ticagrelor over clopidogrel for maintenance $P2Y_{12}$ for NSTE-ACS patients treated with an early invasive or ischemia-guided strategy. [b]Reasonable to choose prasugrel over clopidogrel for maintenance $P2Y_{12}$ for NSTE-ACS patients undergoing PCI who are not at high risk for bleeding. Do not use if prior history of stroke/transient ischemic attack (TIA), age older than 75 years, or body weight less than or equal to 60 kg (132 lb). [c]May require IV supplemental dose of enoxaparin; see Table 8–2. [d]Not to be used as the sole anticoagulant during PCI. Give additional 85 units/kg IV without GPI and 60 Units/kg IV with GPI. [e]If pretreated with UFH, stop UFH infusion for 30 minutes prior to administration of bivalirudin bolus plus infusion. (ACE, angiotensin-converting enzyme; ACS, acute coronary syndrome; ARB, angiotensin receptor blocker; ASA, aspirin; CABG, coronary artery bypass graft; CI, contraindication; DES, drug-eluting stent; GPI, glycoprotein IIb/IIIa inhibitor; IV, intravenous; NTG, nitroglycerin; PCI, percutaneous coronary intervention; SC, subcutaneous; SL, sublingual; UFH, unfractionated heparin).

Patient Encounter 1, Part 2

Identify your acute treatment goals for this patient with STEMI.

What adjunctive pharmacotherapy should be administered in the emergency department prior to proceeding to the cardiac catheterization laboratory?

What additional pharmacotherapy should be initiated on the first day of this patient's hospitalization following successful PCI/intracoronary stenting?

fibrinolysis are listed in Table 8–2.[4] It is not necessary to obtain the results of biochemical markers before initiating fibrinolytic therapy.

Because administration of fibrinolytics result in clot lysis, patients who are at high risk of major bleeding (including ICH) presenting with an absolute contraindication should not receive fibrinolytic therapy; primary PCI is preferred.

Generally, a more fibrin-specific agent such as alteplase, reteplase, or tenecteplase is preferred over a nonfibrin-specific agent such as streptokinase.[4] Fibrin-specific fibrinolytics open a greater percentage of infarcted arteries. In a large clinical trial, administration of alteplase resulted in a 1% absolute reduction in mortality and cost about $30,000 per year of life saved compared with streptokinase.[16] Other trials compared alteplase with reteplase and alteplase with tenecteplase and found similar mortality between agents.[17,18] Therefore, either alteplase, reteplase, or tenecteplase is acceptable as a first-line agent. ICH and major bleeding are the most serious side effects of fibrinolytic agents. The risk of ICH is higher with fibrin-specific agents than with streptokinase.[19] However, the risk of systemic bleeding other than ICH is higher with streptokinase than with other more fibrin-specific agents and was higher with alteplase versus tenecteplase in one study.[4,17,19]

Fibrinolytic therapy is not indicated and should not be used in patients with NSTE-ACS because increased mortality has been reported with these agents compared with controls in clinical trials.[4]

Table 8–2

Indications and Contraindications to Fibrinolytic Therapy for Management of ST-Segment Elevation Myocardial Infarction[4]

Indications

1. Ischemic chest discomfort at least 20 minutes in duration but 12 hours or less since symptom onset
   and
   ST-segment elevation of at least two contiguous leads of ≥ 2 mm in men and ≥ 1.5 mm in women in leads V_2-V_3 and/or of ≥ 1 mm in other leads, or new or presumed new left bundle-branch block
2. Ongoing ischemic chest discomfort at least 20 minutes in duration 12–24 hours since symptom onset
   and
   ST-segment elevation of at least two contiguous leads of ≥ 2 mm in men and ≥ 1.5 mm in women in leads V_2-V_3 and/or of ≥ 1 mm in other leads

Absolute Contraindications

- Active internal bleeding (not including menses)
- Previous intracranial hemorrhage at any time; ischemic stroke within 3 months (except acute ischemic stroke within 4.5 hours)
- Known intracranial neoplasm
- Known structural cerebral vascular lesion (eg, arteriovenous malformation)
- Suspected aortic dissection
- Significant closed head or facial trauma within 3 months
- Intracranial or intraspinal surgery within 2 months
- Severe uncontrolled hypertension (unresponsive to emergency therapy)
- For streptokinase, prior treatment within the previous 6 months

Modified with permission from: DiPiro JT, Talbert RL, Yee GC, et al. Pharmacotherapy: A Pathophysiologic Approach, 9th ed. New York, NY: McGraw-Hill; 2014:190.

▸ *Early Invasive Therapy for NSTE-ACS*

KEY CONCEPT *Clinical practice guidelines recommend coronary angiography followed by either PCI or coronary artery bypass graft (CABG) surgery revascularization as an early treatment (early invasive strategy) for patients with NSTE-ACS at an elevated risk for death or MI, including those with a high risk score (see Table 8–1) or patients with refractory angina, hemodynamic instability or electrical instability* (see Figure 8–3).[3,5] Several clinical trials support an "invasive" interventional strategy with early angiography and PCI or CABG versus an ischemia-guided approach, whereby coronary angiography with revascularization is reserved for patients with symptoms refractory to pharmacotherapy and patients with signs of ischemia on stress testing.[5,20] An early invasive approach results in a long-term reduction in the rates of CV death or MI, with the largest absolute effect seen in higher-risk patients.[5] Several studies have also shown less angina, fewer hospitalizations, and improved quality of life with an invasive strategy.[5]

All patients undergoing PCI should receive ASA therapy indefinitely. A $P2Y_{12}$ inhibitor antiplatelet (clopidogrel, prasugrel, or ticagrelor) should be administered concomitantly with ASA for at least 12 months following PCI for a patient with ACS (Table 8–3).[4,5] A longer duration of $P2Y_{12}$ inhibitor therapy may be considered for select patients with a low bleeding risk receiving a drug-eluting stent (DES) because the risk of stent thrombosis is greater upon cessation of dual antiplatelet therapy (DAPT).[4,5] This is because although DESs reduce the rate of smooth muscle cell growth causing stent restenosis, they induce a delay in endothelial cell regrowth at the site of the stent that places the patient at higher risk of thrombotic events following PCI. This explains why DAPT may be beneficial for a longer period of time following PCI with a DES. Nevertheless, recent trials have provided uncertain evidence regarding the benefit of continuing DAPT beyond 12 months, while the risk of bleeding persists.[21] Until data from larger trials evaluating the need for an extended duration (greater than 12 months) of $P2Y_{12}$ inhibitor therapy following PCI are available, the preferred duration of $P2Y_{12}$ therapy is at least a year regardless of whether or not a patient with NSTE-ACS receives a stent.[5]

Ischemia-Guided Therapy for NSTE-ACS

For patients with NSTE-ACS, an initial ischemia-guided strategy is recommended for patients with a low risk score, normal ECGs, and negative troponin tests who are without recurrence of chest discomfort (see Figure 8–3).[5] An ischemia-guided strategy

Table 8–3

Evidence-Based Pharmacotherapy for ST-Segment Elevation Myocardial Infarction and Non–ST-Segment Elevation Acute Coronary Syndrome[4,5]

Drug	Clinical Condition and Guideline Recommendations[a]	Contraindications[b]	Dose and Duration of Therapy
Aspirin	STEMI, class I recommendation for all patients. NSTE-ACS, class I recommendation for all patients.	Hypersensitivity, active bleeding, severe bleeding risk	160–325 mg orally once on hospital day 1. 81–325 mg once daily orally starting hospital day 2 and continued indefinitely in all patients. Aspirin dose of 81 mg is preferred. Limit dose to < 100 mg if using ticagrelor.
Clopidogrel	NSTE-ACS, class I recommendation added to aspirin. STEMI, class I recommendation added to aspirin. PCI in STE and NSTE-ACS, class I recommendation. In patients with aspirin allergy, class I recommendation.	Hypersensitivity, active bleeding, severe bleeding risk	300- to 600-mg oral loading dose on hospital day 1 followed by a maintenance dose of 75 mg once daily starting on hospital day 2 in patients with NSTE-ACS. 300-mg oral loading dose followed by 75 mg orally daily in patients receiving a fibrinolytic or who do not receive reperfusion therapy with an STEMI, avoid loading dose in patients ≥ 75 years. 600-mg (class I recommendation) loading dose before or when PCI performed (unless within 24 hours of fibrinolytic therapy, a dose of 300 mg should be given). Discontinue at least 5 days before CABG surgery if bleeding risk outweighs benefit (class I recommendation). Administer indefinitely in patients with aspirin allergy (class I recommendation). Continue for at least 12 months (class I recommendation) and possibly beyond 12 months (class IIb recommendation) in patients with ACS managed with PCI/stent. In patients with NSTE-ACS treated medically, administer for up to 1 year (class I recommendation). In patients receiving a fibrinolytic or who do not receive reperfusion therapy, administer for at least 14 days (class I recommendation) and up to 1 year. Genetic testing might be considered to identify patients at high risk of poor response (class IIb recommendation). In these patients, an alternative $P2Y_{12}$ inhibitor might be considered (class IIb recommendation). The routine use of genetic testing is not recommended (class III recommendation).
Prasugrel	PCI in STE and NSTE-ACS, added to aspirin, class I recommendation.	Active bleeding, prior stroke or TIA	Initiate in patients with known coronary artery anatomy only (so as to avoid use in patients needing CABG surgery; class I recommendation). Give no later than 1 hour after PCI. Patients who have history of prior stroke or TIA or are 75 years of age or more or weigh < 60 kg (132 lb) have higher risk of bleeding and no added benefit compared with clopidogrel. 60-mg oral loading dose followed by 10 mg once daily for patients weighing 60 kg (132 lb) or more. Consider 5 mg once daily in patients weighing < 60 kg (132 lb) (based on limited data). Discontinue at least 7 days prior to CABG surgery if bleeding risk outweighs benefit (class I recommendation). Continue for at least 12 months (class I recommendation) and possibly beyond 12 months (class IIb recommendation) in patients with ACS managed with PCI/stent.
Ticagrelor	PCI in STEMI and NSTE-ACS, added to aspirin, class I recommendation. Class IIa as preference over clopidogrel.	Active bleeding	180-mg (class I recommendation) oral loading dose in patients undergoing PCI or ischemia-guided management, followed by 90 mg twice daily for at least 12 months (class I recommendation) and possibly beyond 12 months (class IIb recommendation) in patients with ACS managed with PCI/stent. Current data are too limited to recommend use in patients with STEMI not undergoing primary PCI. Discontinue at least 5 days prior to CABG surgery if bleeding risk outweighs benefit (class I recommendation).

Cangrelor	PCI-adjunct in patients not treated with oral $P2Y_{12}$ inhibitor or GPI. Newly FDA approved agent without guideline recommendations	Active bleeding	30 mcg/kg IV bolus initiated prior to PCI followed by 4 mcg/kg/min IV infusion for duration of PCI or 2 hours, whichever is longer. To maintain platelet inhibition after infusion, initiate oral $P2Y_{12}$ agent as follows: Ticagrelor 180 mg at any time during or immediately after infusion; prasugrel 60 mg or clopidogrel 600 mg immediately after discontinuation of infusion. Do not administer prasugrel or clopidogrel during infusion of cangrelor.
Unfractionated heparin	STEMI, class I recommendation in patients undergoing PCI and for those patients treated with fibrinolytics. NSTE-ACS, class I recommendation in combination with antiplatelet therapy for ischemia-guided or early invasive approach PCI, class I recommendation (NSTE-ACS and STEMI).	Active bleeding, history of heparin-induced thrombocytopenia, severe bleeding risk, recent stroke	For STEMI with fibrinolytics, administer 60-Units/kg IV bolus (maximum 4000 Units) heparin followed by a constant IV infusion at 12-Units/kg/hour (maximum 1000 Units/hour). For STEMI primary PCI, administer 50- to 70-Units/kg IV bolus if a GP IIb/IIIa inhibitor planned; 70–100 Units/kg IV bolus if no GP IIb/IIIa inhibitor planned and supplement with IV bolus doses to maintain target ACT. For NSTE-ACS, administer 60-Units/kg IV bolus (maximum 4000 Units) followed by a constant IV infusion at 12 Units/kg/hour (maximum 1000 Units/hour). Titrated to maintain an aPTT of 1.5–2.0 times control (approximately 50–70 seconds) for STEMI with fibrinolytics and for NSTE-ACS. Titrated to ACT of 250–350 seconds for primary PCI without a GP IIb/IIIa inhibitor and 200–250 seconds in patients given a concomitant GP IIb/IIIa inhibitor. The first aPTT should be measured at 4–6 hours for NSTE-ACS and STE ACS in patients not treated with fibrinolytics or undergoing primary PCI. The first aPTT should be measured at 3 hours in patients with STE ACS who are treated with fibrinolytics. Continue for 48 hours or until the end of PCI.
Enoxaparin	STEMI class I recommendation in patients receiving fibrinolytics and class IIa for patients not undergoing reperfusion therapy. NSTE-ACS, class I recommendation in combination with aspirin for conservative or invasive approach. For PCI, class IIa recommendation as an alternative to UFH in patients with NSTE-ACS. For primary PCI in STEMI, class IIb recommendation as an alternative to UFH.	Active bleeding, history of heparin-induced thrombocytopenia, severe bleeding risk, recent stroke, avoid enoxaparin if CrCl < 15 mL/min (< 0.25 mL/s), avoid if CABG surgery planned	Enoxaparin 1 mg/kg SC every 12 hours for patients with NSTE-ACS (CrCl ≥ 30 mL/min ≥ 0.50 mL/s]). Enoxaparin 1 mg/kg SC every 24 hours (CrCl 15–29 mL/min [0.25–0.49 mL/s]) for NSTE or STEMI. For all patients undergoing PCI following initiation of SC enoxaparin for NSTE-ACS, a supplemental 0.3-mg/kg IV dose of enoxaparin should be administered at the time of PCI if the last dose of SC enoxaparin was given 8–12 hours prior to PCI or received < 2 therapeutic SC doses. For patients with STEMI receiving fibrinolytics: • Age < 75 years: Administer enoxaparin 30-mg IV bolus followed immediately by 1 mg/kg. • SC every 12 hours (first two doses administer maximum of 100 mg for patients weighing > 100 kg). • Age ≥ 75 years: Administer enoxaparin 0.75-mg/kg SC every 12 hours (first two doses administer maximum of 75 mg for patients weighing > 75 kg). Continue throughout hospitalization or up to 8 days for STEMI. Continue for 24–48 hours for NSTE-ACS or until the end of PCI for NSTEMI. Discontinue at least 12–24 hours after CABG surgery.
Bivalirudin	NSTE-ACS class I recommendation for invasive strategy. PCI in STEMI (Class I recommendation).	Active bleeding, severe bleeding risk	For NSTE-ACS, administer 0.1 mg/kg IV bolus followed by 0.25-mg/kg/hour infusion. For PCI in NSTE-ACS, administer a second bolus of 0.5 mg/kg IV and increase infusion rate to 1.75 mg/kg/hour. For PCI in STEMI, administer 0.75-mg/kg IV bolus followed by 1.75-mg/kg/hour infusion. If prior UFH given, discontinue UFH and wait 30 minutes before initiating bivalirudin. Dosage adjustment for severe renal failure and hemodialysis. Discontinue at end of PCI or continue at 0.25 mg/kg/hour if prolonged anticoagulation necessary. Lower bleeding rates are mitigated when administered with a GP inhibitor. Clopidogrel should be administered at least 6 hours before if a GP inhibitor is not used. Discontinue at least 3 hours prior to CABG surgery.

(Continued)

Table 8–3

Evidence-Based Pharmacotherapy for ST-Segment Elevation Myocardial Infarction and Non–ST-Segment Elevation Acute Coronary Syndrome[4,5] (*Continued*)

Drug	Clinical Condition and Guideline Recommendations[a]	Contraindications[b]	Dose and Duration of Therapy
Fondaparinux	STEMI class I recommendation receiving fibrinolytics and IIa for patients not undergoing reperfusion therapy. NSTE-ACS class I recommendation for invasive or conservative approach. Class III as sole agent in PCI.	Active bleeding, severe bleeding risk, SCr ≥ 3.0 mg/dL (≥ 265 μmol/L) or CrCl < 30 mL/min (< 0.50 mL/s)	For STEMI, 2.5-mg IV bolus followed by 2.5-mg SC once daily starting on hospital day 2. For NSTE-ACS, 2.5-mg SC once daily. Continue until hospital discharge or up to 8 days. For PCI, give additional 85 Units/kg IV without and 60 Units/kg IV with GP IIb/IIIa inhibitor. Discontinue at least 24 hours prior to CABG surgery.
Fibrinolytic therapy	STEMI, class I recommendation for patients presenting within 12 hours following the onset of symptoms, class IIa in patients presenting between 12 and 24 hours following the onset of symptoms with continuing signs of ischemia. NSTE-ACS, class III recommendation.	Any prior ICH, known structural cerebrovascular lesions, such as an arterial venous malformation, known intracranial malignant neoplasm, ischemic stroke within 3 months, active bleeding (excluding menses), significant closed head or facial trauma within 3 months	Streptokinase: 1.5 MU IV over 60 minutes. Alteplase: 15-mg IV bolus followed by 0.75 mg/kg IV over 30 minutes (maximum 50 mg) followed by 0.5 mg/kg (max 35 mg) over 60 minutes (maximum dose 100 mg). Reteplase: 10 Units IV × 2, 30 minutes apart. Tenecteplase: • < 60 kg (< 132 lb), 30-mg IV bolus • 60–69.9 kg (132–153 lb), 35-mg IV bolus • 70–80 kg (154–176 lb), 40-mg IV bolus
Glycoprotein IIb/IIIa receptor inhibitors	NSTE-ACS PCI, class I recommendation for abciximab, high-bolus dose tirofiban or double-bolus eptifibatide at the time of PCI in high-risk patients already receiving aspirin and not adequately pretreated with a $P2Y_{12}$ inhibitor and not receiving bivalirudin as the anticoagulant; class IIa at the time of PCI for high-risk patients already receiving aspirin and pretreated with a $P2Y_{12}$ inhibitor; class IIb for upstream use in high-risk patients already receiving aspirin and pretreated with a $P2Y_{12}$ inhibitor and not receiving bivalirudin as the anticoagulant; class I for upstream use in addition to aspirin without $P2Y_{12}$ inhibitor pretreatment for moderate- to high-risk patients. NSTE-ACS for patients not undergoing PCI (ischemia guided management), class IIb recommendation (eptifibatide or tirofiban). STEMI primary PCI, class IIa recommendation for abciximab, high-bolus dose tirofiban or double-bolus eptifibatide.	Active bleeding, thrombocytopenia, prior stroke, renal dialysis (eptifibatide)	**Drug** / **Dose** / **Dosing Adjustment for CKD** Abciximab / 0.25-mg/kg IV bolus followed by 0.125 mcg/kg/min (maximum 10-mcg/min) for 12 hours / None Eptifibatide / 180-mcg/kg IV bolus × 2, 10 minutes apart with an infusion of 2 mcg/kg/min for 18–24 hours after PCI / Reduce maintenance infusion to 1 mcg/kg/min for CrCl < 50 mL/min (< 0.83 mL/s); contraindicated if patient dependent on dialysis. Patients weighing 121 kg (267 lb) or more should receive a maximum infusion rate of 22.6 mg per bolus and a maximum rate of 15 mg/hour Tirofiban / 25-mcg/kg IV bolus followed by an infusion of 0.15 mcg/kg/min for up to 18 hours / Reduce maintenance infusion to 0.075 mcg/kg/min for patients with CrCl ≤ 60 mL/min

Nitroglycerin	STEMI and NSTE-ACS, class I recommendation in patients with ongoing ischemic discomfort, control of HTN, or management of HF.	Hypotension, sildenafil, or vardenafil within 24 hours or tadalafil within 48 hours	0.4-mg SL, repeated every 5 minutes × 3 doses then assess need for IV infusion. 5- to 10-mcg/min IV infusion titrated up to 75–100 mcg/min until relief of symptoms or limiting side effects (headache) with a systolic BP < 90 mm Hg or more than 30% below starting mean arterial pressure levels if significant HTN is present. Topical patches or oral nitrates are acceptable alternatives for patients without ongoing or refractory symptoms. Discontinue IV infusion after 24–48 hours.
β-blockers[c]	STEMI and NSTE-ACS, class I recommendation for oral β-blockers in all patients without contraindications in the first 24 hours, class IIa for IV β-blockers in STEMI patients with HTN or those with ongoing ischemia. Class III for IV β-blockers in patients with risk factors for shock.	PR ECG interval > 0.24 seconds, second-degree or third-degree atrioventricular heart block, heart rate < 60 beats/min, systolic BP < 90 mm Hg, shock, left ventricular failure with decompensated HF, severe reactive airway disease	Metoprolol 5-mg slow IV push (over 1–2 minutes), repeated every 5 min for a total of 15 mg followed in 1–2 hours by 25–50 mg orally every 6 hours; if a very conservative regimen is desired, initial doses can be reduced to 1–2 mg. Propranolol 0.5- to 1-mg IV dose followed in 1–2 hours by 40–80 mg orally every 6–8 hours. Atenolol 5-mg IV dose followed in 5 minutes by a second 5-mg IV dose for a total of 10 mg followed in 1–2 hours by 50–100 mg orally once daily. Alternatively, initial IV therapy can be omitted and treatment started with oral dosing. For dosing of carvedilol, metoprolol succinate, and bisoprolol in patients with systolic HF, please refer to Chapter 6. Continue oral β-blocker for 3 years and possibly indefinitely.
Calcium channel blockers	NSTE-ACS class I recommendation for patients with ongoing ischemia who are already taking adequate doses of nitrates and β-blockers or in patients with contraindications or intolerance to β-blockers (diltiazem or verapamil preferred during initial presentation if EF > 40% [0.40]). NSTE-ACS, class IIb recommendation for diltiazem for patients with AMI.	Pulmonary edema, evidence of left ventricular dysfunction, systolic BP < 100 mm Hg, PR ECG segment to > 0.24 seconds second- or third-degree atrioventricular heart block for verapamil or diltiazem, pulse rate < 60 beats/min for diltiazem or verapamil	Diltiazem 120–360 mg sustained release orally once daily. Verapamil 180–480 mg sustained release orally once daily. Amlodipine 5–10 mg orally once daily. Continue as indicated to manage angina, HTN, or arrhythmias.
ACE inhibitors	NSTE-ACS and STEMI, class I recommendation for patients with HF, left ventricular dysfunction and EF < 40% (0.40), type 2 DM or CKD in the absence of contraindications. Consider in all patients with CAD (class I recommendation, class IIa in low-risk patients). Indicated indefinitely for all patients with EF < 40% (0.40) (class I recommendation).	Systolic BP < 100 mm Hg, history of intolerance to an ACE inhibitor, bilateral renal artery stenosis, serum potassium > 5.5 mEq/L (> 5.5 mmol/L), acute renal failure, pregnancy	**Drug** / **Initial Dose (mg)** / **Target Dose (mg)** Captopril / 6.25–12.5 / 50 twice daily orally to 50 three times daily Enalapril / 2.5–5.0 / 10 twice daily orally Lisinopril / 2.5–5.0 / 10–20 once daily orally Ramipril / 1.25–2.5 / 5 twice daily or 10 once daily orally Trandolapril / 1.0 / 4 once daily orally
Angiotensin receptor blockers	NSTEMI and STEMI, class I recommendation in patients with HF or left ventricular EF < 40% (0.40) and intolerant of an ACE inhibitor, class IIa recommendation in patients with clinical signs of HF or EF < 40% (0.40) and no documentation of ACE inhibitor intolerance. Class I in other ACE inhibitor–intolerant patients with HTN.	Systolic BP < 100 mm Hg, bilateral renal artery stenosis, serum potassium more than 5.5 mEq/L (> 5.5 mmol/L), acute renal failure, pregnancy	**Drug** / **Initial Dose (mg)** / **Target Dose (mg)** Candesartan / 4–8 / 32 once daily orally Valsartan / 40 / 160 twice daily orally Losartan / 12.5–25 / 150 daily Continue indefinitely.

(Continued)

Table 8–3

Evidence-Based Pharmacotherapy for ST-Segment Elevation Myocardial Infarction and Non–ST-Segment Elevation Acute Coronary Syndrome[4,5] (*Continued*)

Drug	Clinical Condition and Guideline Recommendations[a]	Contraindications[b]	Dose and Duration of Therapy		
			Drug	**Initial Dose (mg)**	**Target Dose (mg)**
Aldosterone antagonists	NSTEMI and STEMI class I recommendation in patients with EF < 40% (0.40) and either DM or HF who are already receiving an ACE inhibitor and β-blocker.	Hypotension, hyperkalemia, serum potassium > 5.0 mEq/L (> 5 mmol/L), SCr > 2.5 mg/dL (221 μmol/L) for men and > 2.0 mg/dL (177 μmol/L) for women and/or CrCl < 30 mL/min (< 0.50 mL/s)	Eplerenone	25	50 once daily orally
			Spironolactone	12.5	25–50 once daily orally
			Continue indefinitely.		
Morphine sulfate	STEMI and NSTE-ACS (class IIb) recommendation for patients whose chest pain persists despite treatment with maximally tolerated anti-anginal drugs.	Hypotension, respiratory depression, confusion, obtundation	1- to 5-mg IV bolus dose. May be repeated every 5–30 minutes as needed to relieve symptoms and maintain patient comfort.		
Statins	NSTE-ACS and STEMI class I recommendation to initiate or continue high-intensity statin therapy during early hospital care.	Caution with use of fibrate and statin-specific drug interactions	Atorvastatin 40–80 mg daily. Rosuvastatin 20–40 mg daily.		

[a]Class I recommendations are conditions for which there is evidence and/or general agreement that a given procedure or treatment is useful and effective.

Class II recommendations are those conditions for which there is conflicting evidence and/or divergence of opinion about the usefulness/efficacy of a procedure or treatment. For Class IIa recommendations, the weight of the evidence/opinion is in favor of usefulness/efficacy. Class IIb recommendations are those for which usefulness/efficacy is less well established by evidence/opinion. Class III recommendations are those where the procedure or treatment is not useful and may be harmful.

[b]Allergy or prior intolerance contraindication for all categories of drugs listed in this chart.

[c]Choice of the specific agent is not as important as ensuring that appropriate candidates receive this therapy. If there are concerns about patient intolerance due to existing pulmonary disease, especially asthma, selection should favor a short-acting agent, such as metoprolol, or the ultra short-acting agent, esmolol. Mild wheezing or a history of chronic obstructive pulmonary disease should prompt a trial of a short-acting agent at a reduced dose (eg, 2.5-mg IV metoprolol, 12.5-mg oral metoprolol, or 25-mcg/kg/min esmolol as initial doses) rather than complete avoidance of β-blocker therapy.

ACE, angiotensin-converting enzyme inhibitor; ACS, acute coronary syndrome; ACT, activated clotting time; AMI, acute myocardial infarction; aPTT, activated partial thromboplastin time; BP, blood pressure; CABG, coronary artery bypass graft; CAD, coronary artery disease; CKD, chronic kidney disease; CrCl, creatinine clearance; DM, diabetes mellitus; ECG, electrocardiogram; EF, ejection fraction; GP, glycoprotein IIb/IIIa; HF, heart failure; HTN, hypertension; ICH, intracranial hemorrhage; IV, intravenous; MI, myocardial infarction; NSTE, non–ST-segment elevation; PCI, percutaneous coronary intervention; SC, subcutaneous; SCr, serum creatinine; SL, sublingual; STE, ST-segment elevation; STEMI, ST-segment elevation myocardial infarction; TIA, transient ischemic attack; UFH, unfractionated heparin.

Modified with permission from DiPiro JT, Talbert RL, Yee GC, et al. Pharmacotherapy: A Pathophysiologic Approach, 9th ed. New York, NY: McGraw-Hill; 2014:183-189.

may also be the preferred approach in patients with extensive comorbidities in which the cumulative risks of comorbidities and revascularization would outweigh the potential benefits of revascularization.

Stress testing (see Figure 8–1) is indicated in patients with NSTE-ACS when an initial ischemia-guided strategy is selected and for patients with STEMI where primary PCI was not performed and who do not have high-risk clinical characteristics for which earlier coronary angiography would be warranted.[4,5] Following the stress test, patients experiencing recurrent ischemia or symptoms despite optimal medical treatment or who are considered high-risk (see Table 8–1) should undergo left heart catheterization with coronary angiography and revascularization as indicated.[4,5] Patients with NSTE-ACS at low risk for recurrent CHD events following stress testing should be given ASA indefinitely and either clopidogrel or ticagrelor for up to 12 months following hospital discharge in addition to other secondary preventative pharmacotherapy described later in this chapter.[5] Patients with STEMI at low risk for recurrent CHD events should receive ASA indefinitely and clopidogrel for at least 14 days and up to 12 months in addition to other secondary preventative pharmacotherapy (see Figure 8–2).[4]

Early Pharmacologic Therapy for ACS

Pharmacotherapy for early treatment of ACS is outlined in Figures 8–2 and 8–3 and Table 8–2.[3–5] KEY CONCEPT *According to the ACCF/AHA STEMI and NSTE ACS practice guidelines, additional pharmacotherapy that all patients should receive within the first day of hospitalization, and preferably in the ED, are intranasal oxygen (if oxygen saturation is low), sublingual (SL) nitroglycerin (NTG), ASA, a P2Y$_{12}$ inhibitor (agent dependent on reperfusion strategy), and anticoagulation (agent dependent on reperfusion strategy). A GP IIb/IIIa inhibitor (GPI) may be administered with unfractionated heparin (UFH) for patients with STEMI undergoing primary PCI. High-risk patients with NSTE-ACS should proceed to early angiography (within 24 hours) and select high-risk patients may receive a GPI. Intravenous (IV) NTG may be given in select patients still experiencing pain despite SL NTG. It is reasonable to administer* morphine to patients with refractory angina as an analgesic and a venodilator that lowers preload. *Oral β-blockers should be initiated within the first day in patients without cardiogenic shock or other contraindications.*[4,5] ACE inhibitors (or ARB in ACE inhibitor-intolerant patients) should be initiated in select patients during hospitalization with ACS.[4] High-intensity statin therapy should be initiated or continued during hospitalization in all patients without contraindications. Dosing and contraindications for SL and IV NTG, ASA, clopidogrel, β-blockers, ACE inhibitors, statins, anticoagulants, and fibrinolytics are listed in Table 8–2.[4,5]

▶ *Nitrates*

Nitrates promote the release of nitric oxide from the endothelium, which results in venous and arterial vasodilation. Venodilation lowers preload and myocardial oxygen demand. Arterial vasodilation may lower blood pressure (BP), thus reducing myocardial oxygen demand. Arterial vasodilation also relieves coronary artery vasospasm, dilating coronary arteries to improve myocardial blood flow and oxygenation. Randomized clinical trials failed to show a mortality benefit for IV nitrate therapy followed by oral nitrate therapy in acute MI.[5]

In patients presenting with ACS, one SL NTG tablet should be administered every 5 minutes for up to three doses to relieve myocardial ischemia, unless contraindicated. IV NTG may be initiated in patients who have persistent ischemia, HF, or uncontrolled high BP in the absence of contraindications.[4,5] IV NTG is typically continued until revascularization is performed or for approximately 24 hours following ischemia relief.

The most significant adverse effects of nitrates are tachycardia, flushing, headache, and hypotension. Nitrate administration is contraindicated in patients who have received

Patient Encounter 2, Part 1

A 66-year-old, 90-kg (198-lb) man presents to the ED by ambulance complaining of 3 hours of continuous chest pressure that started while mowing his lawn. His symptoms were not relieved with rest. Local paramedics were called who gave the patient three 0.4 mg sublingual nitroglycerin tablets by mouth, 325 mg ASA by mouth, and morphine 2-mg IV push without relief of chest discomfort. The patient is transferred to the hospital where an early invasive strategy is chosen.

PMH: HTN for 5 years; type 2 diabetes mellitus (DM) for 5 years; dyslipidemia for 2 years

FH: Father died after myocardial infarction at age 70; mother and brother alive with type 2 DM and HTN

SH: Nonsmoker

Allergies: NKDA

Meds: Metformin 1000 mg by mouth twice daily; ASA 325 mg by mouth once daily; lisinopril 20 mg by mouth once daily; simvastatin 20 mg by mouth once daily at bedtime

ROS: 10/10 chest pressure/squeezing

PE:

HEENT: Normocephalic atraumatic

CV: Regular rate and rhythm; S_1, S_2, no S_3, no S_4; no murmurs or rubs

VS: BP 150/92; HR 88 beats/min; T 37°C (98.6°F)

Lungs: Fine crackles in lower lung bases

Abd: Nontender, nondistended

GI: Normal bowel sounds

GU: Stool guaiac negative

Exts: 2+ pitting edema, no bruits, pulses 2+, femoral pulses present, fair range of motion

Neuro: Alert and oriented × 3, cranial nerves intact

Labs: Sodium 131 mEq/L (131 mmol/L), potassium 3.4 mEq/L (3.4 mmol/L), chloride 105 mEq/L (105 mmol/L), bicarbonate 22 mEq/L (22 mmol/L), SCr 1.0 mg/dL (88 μmol/L), glucose 160 mg/dL (8.9 mmol/L), WBC 6.9 × 10^3/mm^3 (6.9 × 10^9/L), hemoglobin 14.7 g/dL (147 g/L or 9.12 mmol/L), hematocrit 42% (0.42), platelets 226 × 10^3/mm^3 (226 × 10^9/L), troponin I 1.0 ng/mL (1.0 mcg/L; 1000 ng/L), oxygen saturation 99% (0.99) on room air, BNP 8600 pg/mL (2485 pmol/L)

ECG: Normal sinus rhythm, PR 0.16 seconds, QRS 0.08 seconds, QT_c 0.38 seconds, 1-mm ST-segment depression in anterior leads

CXR: Normal

Echo: Anterior wall dyskinesis, LVEF 35% (0.35)

What type of ACS is this?

What information is suggestive of acute MI?

oral phosphodiesterase-5 inhibitors, such as sildenafil and vardenafil, within the past 24 hours, and tadalafil within the past 48 hours (see Table 8–2).[5]

▶ *Aspirin*

Aspirin (ASA) is the preferred antiplatelet agent in the treatment of ACS.[4,5] The antiplatelet effects of ASA are mediated by inhibiting the synthesis of TXA_2 through an irreversible inhibition of platelet cyclooxygenase-1.

In patients receiving fibrinolytics, ASA reduces mortality, and its effects are additive to fibrinolysis alone.[22] In patients undergoing PCI, ASA prevents acute thrombotic occlusion during the procedure. Additionally, in patients undergoing PCI, ASA, in addition to a $P2Y_{12}$ inhibitor, reduces the risk of stent thrombosis. ASA reduces the risk of death or MI by approximately 50% compared with no antiplatelet therapy in patients with NSTE-ACS.[22] Therefore, ASA remains the cornerstone of early treatment for all ACS.

In patients experiencing an ACS, an initial dose equal to or greater than 160 mg nonenteric-coated ASA is recommended to achieve a rapid platelet inhibition.[4,5] Current guidelines for STEMI and NSTE-ACS recommend an initial ASA dose of 162 to 325 mg (see Table 8–3).[4,5] This first dose can be chewed in order to achieve high blood concentrations and platelet inhibition rapidly. Current data suggest that although an initial dose of 162 to 325 mg is required, long-term therapy with doses of 75 to 150 mg daily are as effective as higher doses. Therefore, a daily maintenance dose of 81 to 162 mg is generally preferred in most patients with ACS, including those patients also receiving a $P2Y_{12}$ inhibitor, to inhibit the 10% of the total platelet pool that is regenerated daily.[4,5,22] In patients receiving ticagrelor, the recommended maintenance dose of ASA is 81 mg.[5] ASA should be continued indefinitely following either STEMI or NSTE-ACS.[4,5]

The most frequent side effects of ASA are dyspepsia and nausea. Patients should be counseled about the risk of bleeding, especially gastrointestinal (GI) bleeding, with ASA (see Table 8–2).[22]

Nonsteroidal anti-inflammatory agents other than ASA, as well as cyclooxygenase-2 (COX-2) selective anti-inflammatory agents, are contraindicated and should be discontinued at the time of ACS secondary to increased risk of death, reinfarction, HF, and myocardial rupture.[4,5]

▶ *Platelet $P2Y_{12}$ Inhibitors*

Clopidogrel, prasugrel, and ticagrelor block the $P2Y_{12}$ receptor, a subtype of ADP receptor, on platelets which prevents the binding of ADP to the receptor and subsequent expression of platelet GP IIb/IIIa receptors, and reduces platelet activation and aggregation. Both clopidogrel and prasugrel are thienopyridines and prodrugs that are converted to an active metabolite by a variety of cytochrome P-450 (CYP) isoenzymes, the most critical appearing to be CYP2C19 for clopidogrel (Table 8–4).[22] Both of these agents bind irreversibly to $P2Y_{12}$ receptors. Ticagrelor, which is not a thienopyridine, is a reversible, noncompetitive $P2Y_{12}$ receptor inhibitor. Ticagrelor's parent compound has antiplatelet effects and is also metabolized primarily by CYP3A to an active metabolite producing its antiplatelet effects.

Both prasugrel and ticagrelor are more potent ADP inhibitors than clopidogrel. Prasugrel has the fewest significant drug–drug interactions. Moderate and strong inhibitors of CYP2C19 reduce the production of clopidogrel's active metabolite and consequently its antiplatelet effect, whereas strong inhibitors of CYP3A reduce ticagrelor's concentration. A more detailed discussion of the drug interactions with clopidogrel and proton pump inhibitors (PPI) may be found in Chapter 7, "Ischemic Heart Disease."

Genetic variations in the gene coding for *CYP2C19* significantly modulate the antiplatelet effects of clopidogrel. Specifically, carriers of reduced-function allele (ie, *2 or *3) are not able to convert clopidogrel to its active metabolite to the extent of carriers of the wild-type allele. This results in decreased antiplatelet effects, which could translate into higher rates of CV events, especially stent thrombosis and MI around the time of PCI.[22,23] Prasugrel and ticagrelor efficacy are not associated with *CYP2C19* genotype.[4,5,22] Hence, ticagrelor or prasugrel may theoretically be considered preferred agents in carriers of *CYP2C19* reduced function alleles.[24] Nevertheless, in the absence of a large randomized trial demonstrating the benefit of such genotype-based approach, the most recent clinical practice guidelines of the ACCF/AHA/SCAI have not endorsed routine genotyping to guide the prescription of $P2Y_{12}$ inhibitors.[4,5] Ongoing clinical trials should clarify the benefits of genotype-guided use of $P2Y_{12}$ receptor inhibitors.

Administration of a $P2Y_{12}$ receptor inhibitor, in addition to ASA, is recommended for all patients with ACS.[4,5] For patients with STEMI undergoing primary PCI, clopidogrel, prasugrel, or ticagrelor, in addition to ASA, should be administered to prevent subacute stent thrombosis and long-term CV events (see Table 8–3 and Figure 8–2).[3–5] Although the most recent PCI and STEMI guidelines give no preference for one agent over the other, the NSTE-ACS guidelines indicate that ticagrelor may be preferred over clopidogrel for patients treated with either an ischemia-guided or early invasive approach, and both ticagrelor and prasugrel may be preferred over clopidogrel post PCI if patients are not at high risk of bleeding.[3–5]

A large randomized double-blind study demonstrated that, compared to clopidogrel, the addition of prasugrel to ASA for patients undergoing PCI significantly reduced the risk of CV death or MI by 19% (9.9% vs 12.1%), as well as MI and stent thrombosis, but increased the risk of major bleeding (not ICH) by 32% (2.4% vs 1.8%).[25] Patients with a history of prior stroke or transient ischemic attack (TIA) had an increased risk of ICH and net harm from prasugrel; therefore, prior stroke or TIA are contraindications to prasugrel.[5] Patients 75 years and older as well as those weighing less than 60 kg (132 lb) are at increased risk of bleeding with prasugrel compared with clopidogrel and received no net clinical benefit from prasugrel.[25]

In a large randomized clinical trial, ticagrelor significantly reduced the rate of CV death, MI, stroke, and stent thrombosis compared with clopidogrel.[26] Although no increase in study-defined major bleeding was noted with ticagrelor, the frequency of non-CABG major bleeding was increased compared with clopidogrel. Therefore, both of the more potent $P2Y_{12}$ inhibitors are more efficacious than clopidogrel but are also associated with an increased risk of bleeding. Patients with diabetes mellitus (DM) or those with STEMI appear to have a greater ischemic benefit with prasugrel and ticagrelor without an increase in major bleeding compared to clopidogrel.[27–30] No large randomized trial has directly compared ticagrelor to prasugrel. Figures 8–2 and 8–3 and Table 8–4 outline the role of antiplatelets and anticoagulants in ACS.[4,5]

A clopidogrel loading dose of 600 mg is recommended over administration of 300 mg for patients undergoing PCI. A systematic review and meta-analysis of randomized and nonrandomized trials in more than 25,000 patients demonstrated a reduction in CV ischemic events with a loading dose of 600 mg compared with 300 mg in patients undergoing PCI.[31] Although a modest

Table 8–4

Clinical Considerations When Choosing an Oral $P2Y_{12}$ Receptor Inhibitor[3–5,22]

	Clopidogrel	Prasugrel	Ticagrelor
Pharmacologic class	Thienopyridine	Thienopyridine	Cyclopentyl triazolopyrimidine
ADP receptor binding	Irreversible	Irreversible	Reversible
Pharmacokinetics	Prodrug Converted twice to active metabolite primarily through CYP2C19 Peak platelet inhibition occurs within 2 hours after 600 mg load and 6 hours after 300 mg load Elimination half-life of active metabolite is approximately 30 minutes after a 75-mg dose Excretion is 50% urinary and 46% fecal	Prodrug Converted to active metabolite through CYP 3A4 and 2B6 Peak platelet inhibition reached within 1–1.5 hours after 60-mg load Median elimination half-life of the active metabolite approximately 7.4 hours Excretion is primarily urinary (approximately 70%); fecal excretion < 30%	Active moiety Converted to active metabolite through CYP 3A4/5 Peak platelet inhibition within 1 hour after 180 mg load Median elimination half-life of the parent compound is approximately 7 hours and active metabolite approximately 9 hours Excretion is primarily metabolism (84%); fecal excretion 58%, urinary excretion (26%)
Dosing	300- to 600-mg loading dose; 75 mg daily	60-mg loading dose; 10 mg daily	180-mg loading dose; 90 mg twice daily
Drug and Disease considerations	Genetic polymorphisms may influence efficacy; Enhanced bleeding with NSAIDs; avoid use Enhanced bleeding with warfarin; monitor carefully for bleeding; target INR to 2.0–2.5 for most indications Avoid use with moderate or strong CYP2C19 inhibitors (omeprazole, esomeprazole, chloramphenicol, cimetidine, efavirenz, etravirine felbamate, fluoxetine, fluconazole, fluvoxamine, isoniazid, oxcarbazepine, ketoconazole, voriconazole); select alternative noninteracting $P2Y_{12}$ inhibitor or alternative noninteracting drug	Enhanced bleeding with warfarin and NSAIDs, avoid use	Enhanced bleeding with warfarin and NSAIDs Use aspirin doses < 100 mg daily Avoid use with strong CYP3A inhibitors (atazanavir, clarithromycin, indinavir, itraconazole, nefazodone, nelfinavir, ketoconazole, ritonavir, saquinavir, telithromycin, voriconazole) Avoid use with potent CYP3A inducers (carbamazepine, dexamethasone, phenobarbital, phenytoin, rifampin) Avoid simvastatin and lovastatin doses more than 40 mg daily (ticagrelor inhibits CYP3A4 and increases statin concentration) Monitor digoxin serum concentrations with any change in ticagrelor dose (ticagrelor inhibits P-glycoprotein) Unique side-effects including dyspnea and bradycardia
Contraindications	Any active pathological bleeding	Any active pathological bleeding; any history of TIA/stroke	Any active pathological bleeding; ICH or severe hepatic disease
Surgery hold time	5 days for elective surgery; 24 hours for urgent	7 days	5 days for elective surgery; 24 hours for urgent
NSTE-ACS indication	May be used regardless of treatment strategy; additional non-ACS indications	Reasonable over clopidogrel in patients treated with PCI who are not at high risk for bleeding	Preferable to clopidogrel for NSTE-ACS patients treated with early or invasive or ischemia-guided approach
STEMI indication	Preferred when fibrinolytics used	Superior to clopidogrel in STEMI or in other high risk patients like DM; not studied in patients receiving fibrinolytic therapy	Superior to clopidogrel; not studied in patients receiving fibrinolytic therapy
Risk benefit considerations	Gold standard for reducing CV death and stent thrombosis compared to placebo; consider alternative if documented clopidogrel ineffectiveness (ie, poor metabolism, stent thrombosis during clopidogrel therapy)	Superior to clopidogrel with a significant increase in bleeding risk (driven mainly by reductions in MI and stent thrombosis); no clinical benefit when age ≥ 75 years or weight < 60 kg (132 lb); net harm in patients with history of TIA or stroke	Superior to clopidogrel with modest increase in major non-CABG related bleeding; associated with an all-cause mortality reduction; consider compliance with twice daily dosing

ADP, adenosine diphosphate; CABG, coronary artery bypass graft; CV, cardiovascular; CYP, cytochrome P-450; DM, diabetes mellitus; ICH, intracranial hemorrhage; INR, international normalized ratio; MI, myocardial infarction; NSAIDs, nonsteroidal anti-inflammatory drugs; NSTE-ACS, Non–ST-segment elevation acute coronary syndrome; PCI, percutaneous coronary intervention; STEMI, ST-segment elevation myocardial infarction; TIA, transient ischemic attack.

benefit of using a 7-day course of clopidogrel 150 mg compared to 75 mg daily has been suggested, it is also associated with a higher risk of major bleeding.[32] Thus, routine use of such dosing is not recommended in current clinical guidelines.[4,5]

In STEMI patients receiving fibrinolysis, early therapy with clopidogrel 75 mg once daily administered during hospitalization and up to 28 days (mean: 14 days) reduced mortality and reinfarction without increasing the risk of major bleeding.[22] In adult patients 75 years or younger receiving fibrinolytics, a 300-mg loading dose (omit the load in those greater than 75) of clopidogrel followed by 75 mg daily is recommended.[4] Clopidogrel should be continued for at least 14 days (and up to 1 year in the absence of bleeding) for patients presenting with STEMI who undergo reperfusion therapy with fibrinolysis.[4] Although prasugrel and ticagrelor are recommended in the setting of STEMI and primary PCI, no studies have evaluated their use in conjunction with fibrinolytics.

For patients with NSTE-ACS with an initial ischemia-guided approach, either clopidogrel (a 300- or 600-mg loading dose followed by 75 mg daily) or ticagrelor can be used (ticagrelor preferred). If an invasive management strategy is selected, either clopidogrel or ticagrelor can be used (ticagrelor may be preferred) either prehospital or in the ED. Following PCI, in patients not already treated with a $P2Y_{12}$ inhibitor, either clopidogrel, prasugrel, or ticagrelor can be used (ticagrelor and prasugrel in patients not at high risk of bleeding may be preferred) and should be initiated within 1 hour following PCI. Specific dosing and contraindications of the $P2Y_{12}$ inhibitors are described in Tables 8–3 and 8–4.[4,5,22]

The recommended duration of $P2Y_{12}$ inhibitors for a patient undergoing PCI for ACS, either STEMI or NSTE-ACS, is at least 12 months for patients receiving either a bare metal stent (BMS) or a DES.[4,5,22] The benefit of prolonging treatment beyond 12 months is uncertain.[4,5,22] For patients who are treated using an ischemia-guided approach, $P2Y_{12}$ inhibitors should be given for up to 12 months.

Nonadherence to $P2Y_{12}$ inhibitors is a major risk factor for stent thrombosis; therefore, the likelihood of compliance with DAPT (ASA and a $P2Y_{12}$ inhibitor) should be assessed prior to angiography.[3] The use of a BMS over a DES should be considered in patients who are anticipated to be nonadherent to 12 months of DAPT.[3] Compliance to twice daily ticagrelor should also be a consideration.

To minimize the risk of CV events, elective noncardiac surgery should be delayed 4 to 6 weeks after angioplasty or BMS implantation, or 12 months after DES implantation if the discontinuation of the $P2Y_{12}$ inhibitor is required.[3] If elective CABG surgery is planned, clopidogrel and ticagrelor should be withheld preferably for 5 days, and prasugrel at least 7 days, to reduce the risk of postoperative bleeding, unless the need for revascularization outweighs the bleeding risk.[3] If urgent CABG is necessary, discontinue clopidogrel and ticagrelor up to 24 hours to reduce the risk of major bleeding.[5]

Although a variety of blood tests can assess functional platelet aggregation inhibition to $P2Y_{12}$ inhibitors, especially clopidogrel, there is no one gold standard test. Moreover, their benefit to personalize antiplatelet regimens has not been demonstrated.[3–5] Therefore, the most recent practice guidelines do not recommend routine platelet aggregation testing to determine $P2Y_{12}$ inhibitor strategy.[3–5]

Bleeding should be carefully monitored when using $P2Y_{12}$ inhibitors.[25–27] Rarely, thrombotic thrombocytopenic purpura (TTP) has been reported with clopidogrel.[33] In addition, the use of ticagrelor is associated with dyspnea and, rarely, ventricular pauses and bradyarrhythmias.[5] Small non-clinically significant increases in SCr and serum uric acid have also been reported with ticagrelor.[26]

► *Glycoprotein IIb/IIIa Receptor Inhibitors*

GP IIb/IIIa receptor inhibitors block the final common pathway of platelet aggregation, namely cross-linking of platelets by fibrinogen bridges between the GP IIb and IIIa receptors on the platelet surface. In patients with STEMI undergoing primary PCI who are treated with UFH, abciximab, eptifibatide, or tirofiban may be administered on an individual basis.[34] Investigations of GPIs precede the widespread use of oral DAPT and thus their benefit in modern settings is not as clear. Their use appears most appropriate and beneficial in patients who are not adequately treated with a $P2Y_{12}$ receptor antagonist or in those with a large thrombus burden.[4] Routine use of a GPI is not recommended in patients who have received fibrinolytics or bivalirudin secondary to increased bleeding risk. For patients treated with bivalirudin as the anticoagulant, GPIs should be only used as "bail-out" in select cases.[4] These agents should not be administered for medical management of patients with STEMI who will not be undergoing PCI.

The role of GPIs in NSTE-ACS is diminishing as $P2Y_{12}$ inhibitors are used earlier in therapy, and bivalirudin is selected more commonly as the anticoagulant in patients receiving an early intervention approach. Current evidence indicates no benefit of routine use of GPIs in patients treated with an ischemia-guided approach because the bleeding risk exceeds the benefit.[5] Nevertheless, in select patients treated with an ischemia-guided approach who experience recurrent ischemia (chest discomfort and ECG changes), HF, or arrhythmias after initial medical therapy necessitating a change in strategy to angiography and revascularization, a GPI may be added to ASA prior to the angiogram, particularly if the patient is (1) not adequately treated with clopidogrel or ticagrelor and (2) not treated with bivalirudin.

In patients who undergo an early invasive strategy and are adequately treated with clopidogrel or ticagrelor, routine upstream (prior to coronary angiography) administration of a GPI is not recommended, although eptifibatide or tirofiban may be considered in select high-risk patients (eg, troponin positive). Indeed clinical trials have shown that eptifibatide (added to ASA and clopidogrel) prior to angiography and PCI (ie, "upstream" use) in NSTE-ACS does not reduce ischemic events and increases bleeding risk.[5,35] In patients undergoing PCI, a GPI (abciximab, double-bolus eptifibatide, or high-dose bolus tirofiban) should be used in patients presenting high-risk features who are not adequately pretreated with clopidogrel or ticagrelor (and who are not treated with bivalirudin as the anticoagulant), and may be considered in select individuals adequately pretreated with clopidogrel.[5]

Dosing and contraindications for GPIs are described in Table 8–3.[4,5] Bleeding is the most significant adverse effect associated with administration of GPIs; therefore, they should not be administered to patients with a prior history of hemorrhagic stroke or recent ischemic stroke. The risk of bleeding is increased in patients with chronic kidney disease (CKD). Eptifibatide is contraindicated in patients dependent on dialysis and requires a 50% reduced infusion rate in patients with creatinine clearance (CrCl) less than 50 mL/min (0.83 mL/s).[4] The rate of tirofiban infusion should also be halved in patients with CrCl less than 30 mL/min (0.50 mL/s).[4] No dosage adjustment for renal function is necessary for abciximab. An immune-mediated thrombocytopenia occurs in approximately 5% of patients with abciximab and less than 1% of patients receiving eptifibatide or tirofiban.[36]

► Anticoagulants

All patients should receive an anticoagulant in addition to DAPT regardless of ACS type or initial treatment strategy. Options for anticoagulant therapy are outlined in Figures 8–2 and 8–3.[4,5] For patients with STEMI undergoing primary PCI, either UFH or bivalirudin is preferred.[4] Bivalirudin monotherapy reduces CV and overall mortality while minimizing bleeding compared to UFH plus a GPI. However, direct head-to-head comparisons of monotherapy with UFH and bivalirudin have not shown this bleeding advantage.[37–39] Anticoagulant therapy is generally discontinued after primary PCI unless a compelling reason to continue exists. When fibrinolytic therapy is utilized in STEMI, UFH, enoxaparin, and fondaparinux are options. In this case, anticoagulant therapy should be maintained for a minimum of 48 hours (for UFH) and preferably for the duration of the hospitalization (with enoxaparin and fondaparinux) up to 8 days after fibrinolysis or until reperfusion is performed to support patency and prevent reocclusion of the affected artery.[4] Enoxaparin dosing is adjusted for body weight and renal function, and when administered in combination with fibrinolysis, it has special dosing requirements for older patients and those weighing more than 100 kg (see Table 8–3).

The choice of anticoagulant for a patient with NSTE-ACS is guided by risk stratification and initial treatment strategy, either an early invasive approach with coronary angiography and PCI or an ischemia-guided strategy with angiography in select patients guided by relief of symptoms and stress testing (see Figure 8–3). For patients treated by an early invasive strategy, UFH, enoxaparin, fondaparinux or bivalirudin are options.[5] These same anticoagulants are continued after angiography if the decision is made to revascularize with PCI with one exception. Fondaparinux should not be used as the sole anticoagulant during PCI due to an increased risk of catheter-related thrombosis. Additional heparin must be administered during PCI if fondaparinux was initially chosen for anticoagulation. Clinical trials with bivalirudin have demonstrated similar efficacy in preventing CV ischemic events with a lower bleeding rate compared to UFH or enoxaparin plus a GPI in moderate- and high-risk patients with NSTE-ACS undergoing an early invasive strategy.[22] Use of enoxaparin during PCI is considered reasonable in patients treated with upstream subcutaneous enoxaparin. Dosing considerations for initial treatment and during PCI are outlined in Table 8–3.[5]

In NSTE-ACS patients in whom an initial ischemia-guided strategy is planned, enoxaparin, UFH, or low-dose fondaparinux is recommended.[5] Bivalirudin has not been studied as initial therapy in this setting. When added to ASA, UFH and low-molecular-weight heparins (LMWHs) reduce the frequency of death or MI in patients presenting with NSTE-ACS compared with control/placebo in patients primarily managed with an ischemia-guided strategy.[5,22] Compared with enoxaparin, fondaparinux showed similar ischemic outcomes with a lower bleeding rate in patients with NSTE-ACS primarily managed with an ischemia-guided strategy and may be preferred in patients at high risk for bleeding.[22] However, if fondaparinux is chosen for a patient who subsequently undergoes angiography and PCI, it should be administered in combination with UFH to avoid catheter thrombosis.[5] Guideline-recommended dosing and contraindications are described in Table 8–3.

UFH is preferred following angiography in patients proceeding to CABG during the same hospitalization because it has a short duration of action following discontinuation. Because enoxaparin is eliminated renally and patients with renal insufficiency generally have been excluded from clinical trials, UFH should be considered for patients with CrCl rates of less than 30 mL/min (0.50 mL/s) based on total patient body weight using the Cockroft–Gault equation.[5] Although recommendations for dosing adjustment of enoxaparin in patients with CrCl between 10 and 30 mL/min (0.17 and 0.50 mL/s) are listed in the product manufacturer's label, the safety and efficacy of enoxaparin in this patient population remain vastly understudied. Administration of enoxaparin should be avoided in dialysis patients with ACS. While the duration of bivalirudin infusion is generally short (several hours only), few patients with significant renal impairment have been included in clinical trials. Dose adjustments for bivalirudin in patients with CrCl less than 30 mL/min (0.50 mL/s) or on hemodialysis is recommended. Patients with SCr greater than 3.0 mg/dL (265 μmol/L) were excluded from ACS trials with fondaparinux. Fondaparinux is contraindicated in patients with CrCl less than 30 mL/min (0.50 mL/s).[5]

UFH is monitored and the dose adjusted to a target activated partial thromboplastin time (aPTT), whereas the dose of enoxaparin is based on actual body weight without routine monitoring of antifactor Xa levels. Some experts recommend antifactor Xa monitoring for LMWHs (eg, enoxaparin, fondaparinux) in patients with renal impairment during prolonged courses of administration of more than several days. No monitoring of coagulation is recommended for bivalirudin and fondaparinux.

Besides bleeding, the most serious adverse effect of UFH and enoxaparin is **heparin-induced thrombocytopenia**. ACS registry data indicate the frequency of heparin-induced thrombocytopenia is rare (less than 0.5%).[11] Bivalirudin would be the preferred anticoagulant for patients with a history of heparin-induced thrombocytopenia undergoing PCI.[3]

► β-Blockers

Oral β-blockers should be administered early in the care of patients with an ACS and continued for at least 3 years in patients with normal LVF.[4,5,40] In ACS, the benefit of β-blockers results mainly from the competitive blockade of β_1-adrenergic receptors located on the myocardium. β_1-blockade produces a reduction in heart rate, myocardial contractility, and BP, decreasing myocardial oxygen demand. In addition, the reduction in heart rate increases diastolic time, thus improving ventricular filling and coronary artery perfusion. As a result of these effects, β-blockers reduce the risk for recurrent ischemia, infarct size, risk of reinfarction, and occurrence of ventricular arrhythmias in the hours and days following MI.[4,5]

The role of early β-blocker therapy in reducing MI mortality was established in the 1970s and 1980s before routine use of early reperfusion therapy. Data in the reperfusion era are derived mainly from a large clinical trial that suggests IV initiation followed by oral β-blockers early in the course of MI is associated with a lower risk of reinfarction or ventricular fibrillation. However, there may be an early risk of cardiogenic shock, particularly with IV β-blockers especially in patients presenting with advanced age (greater than 70 years), heart rate greater than 100 beats/min, systolic BP less than 120 mm Hg, or late presentation.[5,41] Therefore, initiation of β-blockers (oral preferred) should be limited to patients who are hemodynamically stable, not at increased risk for cardiogenic shock, and without signs or symptoms of acute HF.[4,5] Careful assessment for any contraindications to β-blockers should be performed following initiation and prior to any dose titration. The most serious side effects of β-blocker administration early in ACS are hypotension, acute HF, bradycardia, and heart block.

Patients already taking β-blockers can continue taking them. Patients with contraindications to their use in the first 24 hours of presentation should be reevaluated and treated with β-blockers at a later time if they become eligible. In patients presenting with acute HF, use of β-blockers should be delayed until they are stabilized. Initiation of β-blockers may be attempted before hospital discharge in most patients following resolution of acute HF. Patients with HF secondary to reduced LVF should receive one of three β-blockers: bisoprolol, sustained-release metoprolol succinate, or carvedilol.[4,5]

▸ *Additional Therapies*

Oral ACE inhibitors have been shown to decrease nonfatal and fatal major CV events.[4,5] The benefit of ACE inhibitors in patients with MI most likely comes from their ability to prevent cardiac remodeling and ultimately development of HF. The largest reduction in mortality is observed in patients with left ventricular dysfunction (low LVEF) or HF symptoms. Early initiation (within 24 hours) of an oral ACE inhibitor is recommended as benefit can be seen as early as 24 hours post MI.[4,5] However, these agents should be used cautiously in the first 24 hours to avoid renal dysfunction or hypotension.[5] The use of IV ACE inhibitors is not recommended because mortality may be increased. Administration of ACE inhibitors should be continued indefinitely. Hypotension should be avoided because coronary artery filling may be compromised.

The administration of high-intensity statins prior to PCI may reduce the risk of periprocedural MI, and hence statins should be initiated as early as possible in ACS.[3] Additionally, statins reduce the risk of CV death, recurrent MI, stroke, and the need for revascularization when initiated early in the treatment of ACS.[4,5] Although the primary effect of statins is to decrease low-density lipoprotein (LDL) cholesterol, statins are believed to produce many non-lipid-lowering or "pleiotropic" effects such as anti-inflammatory and antithrombotic properties. Based on current evidence, the most recent guidelines for the treatment of cholesterol in adults recommend that patients who experience an ACS should receive high-intensity statin therapy (atorvastatin 40–80 mg daily; rosuvastatin 20–40 mg daily) if they are less than or equal to 75 years of age, and moderate-intensity statin therapy (eg, atorvastatin 10–20 mg; pravastatin 40–80 mg; simvastatin 20–40 mg) if they are older than 75 years or not a candidate for high-intensity statins because of contraindications, at risk for statin intolerance, or have a history of statin-associated adverse drug reactions. Select patients older than 75 years may be candidates for high-intensity therapy to lower LDL cholesterol. High- and moderate-intensity statins are respectively defined as daily statin doses required to reduce LDL cholesterol greater than or equal to 50% and 30% to 49%, respectively.[42] Thus, in the absence of contraindications and depending on age, moderate- to high-intensity statin therapy should be initiated early during hospitalization to all patients experiencing ACS.

▸ *Calcium Channel Blockers*

Calcium channel blockers in the setting of ACS are used for relief of continued ischemia despite β-blocker and nitrate therapy, vasospastic angina, additional need for BP lowering (ie, amlodipine), or in patients with contraindications to β-blockers. Data suggest little benefit on clinical outcomes beyond symptom relief for calcium channel blockers in the setting of ACS especially in patients with reduced LVEF.[4,5] Therefore, calcium channel blockers should be avoided in the acute management of ACS unless there is a clear symptomatic need or contraindication to β-blockers. Agent selection is based on presenting heart rate and left ventricular dysfunction (diltiazem and verapamil are contraindicated in patients with bradycardia, heart block, or reduced LVEF). Immediate-release nifedipine should be avoided because it has demonstrated reflex sympathetic activation, tachycardia, and worsened myocardial ischemia.[4,5] Dosing and contraindications are described in Table 8–3.

> **Patient Encounter 2, Part 2**
>
> *Is reperfusion therapy with fibrinolysis indicated at this time for this patient?*
>
> *What adjunctive pharmacotherapy should be administered to this patient in the emergency department?*
>
> *What additional pharmacotherapy should be initiated on the first day of this patient's hospitalization following successful reperfusion with PCI?*

Secondary Prevention Following MI

The long-term goals following ACS are to: (a) control modifiable CHD risk factors; (b) prevent the development of HF; (c) prevent new or recurrent MI and stroke; (d) prevent death, including sudden cardiac death; and (e) prevent stent thrombosis following PCI. Pharmacotherapy, which has been proven to decrease mortality, HF, reinfarction, stroke, and stent thrombosis should be initiated prior to hospital discharge for secondary prevention. KEY CONCEPT *Secondary prevention guidelines suggest that following MI, all patients should receive long-term treatment with ASA, a β-blocker, an ACE inhibitor, and a statin for secondary prevention of death, stroke, or recurrent infarction.*[40] *A P2Y$_{12}$ inhibitor should be continued for at least 12 months for patients undergoing PCI and for patients with NSTE-ACS receiving an ischemia-guided treatment strategy.*[3-5] *Clopidogrel should be continued for at least 14 days and up to 1 year in patients with STEMI receiving thrombolytics. Other P2Y$_{12}$ inhibitors have not been studied in combination with thrombolytics; however, prasugrel may be an alternative to clopidogrel in patients who undergo delayed PCI after thrombolytics.*[4] *An ARB and an aldosterone antagonist should be given to select patients. Dosing and contraindications of medication therapy are described in detail in* Table 8–3. *For all patients with ACS, treatment and control of modifiable risk factors such as hypertension (HTN), dyslipidemia, obesity, smoking, and DM are essential.*[4,5,40] Patients should receive proper counseling and education, both verbal and written, regarding these treatments and recommendations prior to discharge. At follow-up appointments, medication reconciliation and dose optimization improve drug adherence.[43] Use of ICDs for the prevention of sudden cardiac death following MI in patients with reduced LVF and nonsustained ventricular arrhythmias is discussed in more detail in Chapter 9, "Arrhythmias."

▸ *Aspirin*

ASA decreases the risk of death, recurrent infarction, and stroke following MI. All patients should receive daily ASA 81 to 325 mg indefinitely; those patients with a contraindication to ASA should receive clopidogrel.[4,5,40] The risk of major bleeding from chronic ASA therapy is approximately 2% and is dose related.

Higher doses of ASA, 160 to 325 mg, are not more effective than ASA doses of 75 to 81 mg but have higher rates of bleeding.[44] Therefore, the guidelines recommend 81 mg daily as a preferred strategy in ACS patients with or without PCI.[4,5]

▶ $P2Y_{12}$ Inhibitors

For patients with either STEMI or NSTE-ACS, clopidogrel decreases the risk of CV events and stent thrombosis compared with placebo. Compared with clopidogrel, either prasugrel or ticagrelor lowers the risk of CV death, MI, or stroke by an additional 20% to 30% depending on the patient population studied. The frequency of stent thrombosis following PCI is also lower with prasugrel or ticagrelor compared with clopidogrel. However, the rate of bleeding not related to CABG surgery is higher with both prasugrel and ticagrelor compared with clopidogrel.[25,26]

The PCI guidelines recommend continuation of a $P2Y_{12}$ inhibitor for at least 12 months following PCI.[3] For medically managed patients with STEMI, clopidogrel should be continued for at least 14 days and up to 1 year.[4] For medically managed NSTE-ACS patients, clopidogrel or ticagrelor should be continued up to 1 year.[5]

Bleeding is an inherent risk with long-term DAPT. In fact, oral antiplatelet agents are the third leading cause of adverse drug reaction–associated hospital admissions after ED visits among seniors.[45] Therefore, patients should be counseled on the risks and sites of potential bleeding and should be told to seek medical care immediately if significant bleeding is noticed. Some patients who are at increased risk of GI bleeding may benefit from the addition of a proton pump inhibitor (PPI).[46]

▶ β-Blockers, Nitrates, and Calcium Channel Blockers

Current treatment guidelines recommend that following an ACS, patients with normal LVF should receive a β-blocker for at least three years and indefinitely for those with reduced LVF.[4,5,40] Overwhelming data support the use of β-blockers in patients with a previous MI to improve long-term survival. Currently, there are no data to support the superiority of one β-blocker over another in the absence of HF with reduced LVF. Whether the use of β-blockers beyond 3 years after an MI in patients without angina or HF is beneficial is debatable but is unlikely to be tested in a randomized controlled trial.[47]

Although β-blockers should be avoided in patients with decompensated HF from left ventricular systolic dysfunction complicating an MI, clinical trial data suggest it is safe to initiate β-blockers prior to hospital discharge in these patients once HF symptoms have resolved.[4,5] In patients who cannot tolerate or have a contraindication to a β-blocker, a calcium channel blocker can be used to prevent anginal symptoms but nondihydropyridines should not be used in patients with reduced LVF.[4,5]

Chronic long-acting nitrate therapy has not been shown to reduce CHD events following MI and is not indicated in ACS patients who have undergone revascularization, unless the patient has stable ischemic heart disease, refractory angina, coronary vasospasms, or significant coronary stenoses that were not revascularized. All patients should be prescribed short-acting SL NTG tablets or spray to relieve any anginal symptoms when necessary and instructed on its use.[4,5] If ischemic chest discomfort persists for more than 5 minutes after the first dose, the patient should be instructed to contact emergency medical services. Nitrates should not be administered to patients with hypotension or who have recently received a phosphodiesterase inhibitor (see Table 8–3).[4,5,48]

▶ ACE Inhibitors and ARBs

ACE inhibitors reduce mortality, decrease reinfarction, and prevent the development of HF with recent ACS, especially in those with reduced LVF.[4,5,40] Additional trials suggest that most patients with CAD, not just ACS or HF patients, benefit from ACE inhibitors. Therefore, ACE inhibitors should be considered in all patients (eg, those with HTN, DM, or CKD) following an ACS in the absence of a contraindication.

Besides hypotension, the most frequent adverse reaction to an ACE inhibitor is cough, which may occur in up to 30% of patients. Patients who cannot tolerate an ACE inhibitor may be prescribed an ARB. Other, less common but more serious adverse effects of ACE inhibitors and ARBs include acute renal failure, hyperkalemia, and angioedema.[4,5,40]

▶ Aldosterone Antagonists

Aldosterone plays an important role in HF and in MI because it promotes vascular and myocardial fibrosis, endothelial dysfunction, HTN, left ventricular hypertrophy, sodium retention, potassium and magnesium loss, and arrhythmias. Aldosterone antagonists have been shown to attenuate these adverse effects and reduce mortality in patients who are already receiving an ACE inhibitor (or ARB) and β-blocker and have an LVEF less than or equal to 40% (0.40) and either HF symptoms or DM.[4,5]

Eplerenone and spironolactone are aldosterone antagonists that block the mineralocorticoid receptor. In contrast to spironolactone, eplerenone has no effect on the progesterone or androgen receptor, thereby minimizing the risk of gynecomastia, sexual dysfunction, and menstrual irregularities. In a large clinical trial, eplerenone significantly reduced mortality as well as hospitalization for HF in post–MI patients with an LVEF less than 40% (0.40) and symptoms of HF at any time during hospitalization.[49]

The risk of hyperkalemia increases with the use of aldosterone antagonists when added to an ACE inhibitor or ARB. Therefore, patients with serum potassium concentrations greater than 5.0 mmol/L (5.0 mEq/L) should not receive these agents. Specific contraindications for spironolactone include SCr greater than or equal to 2.5 mg/dL (221 μmol/L) for men or 2.0 mg/dL (177 μmol/L) for women, or CrCl less than or equal to 30 mL/min (0.50 mL/s). Contraindications for eplerenone include SCr greater than or equal to 2.0 mg/dL (177 μmol/L) for men or 1.8 mg/dL (159 μmol/L) for women, or CrCl less than or equal to 50 mL/min (0.83 mL/s). Currently, there are no data to support that eplerenone is superior or preferred to spironolactone unless a patient has experienced gynecomastia, breast pain, or impotence while receiving spironolactone.

▶ Lipid-Lowering Agents

Following MI, statins reduce total mortality, CV mortality, and stroke. According to the most recent practice guidelines, all patients post ACS should receive moderate to high-intensity statin therapy as well as dietary counseling.[42] A major change in these new guidelines is that no specific LDL cholesterol goals are recommended. Rather, the guidelines focus on identifying patients most likely to benefit from lipid-lowering agents, mostly statins, and the targeted LDL cholesterol reductions. Patients with atherosclerotic CV disease, including those who experience an ACS, represent one of the groups in which the benefit of statins clearly outweighs their risk. Indeed, results from landmark clinical trials have unequivocally demonstrated the value of statins in secondary prevention following MI. A meta-analysis of randomized controlled clinical trials in almost 18,000 patients with recent ACS found that statin therapy reduces mortality by 19%, with benefits observed after approximately 4 months of treatment.[50] The current evidence indicates that higher-dose statin therapy, such as atorvastatin 40 to 80 mg daily and rosuvastatin 10 to 20 mg daily, produces a greater reduction in CV events such as MI, ischemic stroke, and revascularization than less intensive statin regimens (such as simvastatin 20–40 mg daily).

These most recent guidelines emphasize that no data support the routine use of nonstatin lipid-lowering drugs in patients taking statins or in statin-intolerant patients. Thus, the use of fibrate derivatives, niacin, or fish oil are only considered in select high-risk patients who present a "less-than anticipated therapeutic response" to statins in whom the benefits outweigh the potential risks, and in patients who are completely intolerant to statins.[42]

► *Other Modifiable Risk Factors*

Smoking cessation, managing HTN, weight loss, exercise, and glucose control for patients with DM, in addition to treatment of

Table 8–5

Therapeutic Drug Monitoring of Pharmacotherapy for Acute Coronary Syndromes

Drug	Adverse Effects	Monitoring
Aspirin	Dyspepsia, bleeding, gastritis	Clinical signs of bleeding[a]; GI upset; baseline and every 6 months: Hgb, HCT, platelet count
Clopidogrel and prasugrel	Bleeding, diarrhea, rash, TTP (rare)	Clinical signs of bleeding[a]; baseline and every 6 months: Hgb, HCT, platelet count
Ticagrelor	Bleeding, dyspnea, diarrhea, rash, elevated SCr, elevated serum uric acid	Clinical signs of bleeding[a]; baseline and every 6 months: Hgb, HCT, platelet count
Unfractionated heparin	Bleeding, heparin-induced thrombocytopenia	Clinical signs of bleeding[a]; baseline aPTT, INR, Hgb, HCT, and platelet count; aPTT every 6 hours until target then every 24 hours; daily Hgb, HCT, and platelet count
Enoxaparin	Bleeding, heparin-induced thrombocytopenia	Clinical signs of bleeding[a]; baseline SCr, aPTT, INR, Hgb, HCT, and platelet count; daily SCr, Hgb, HCT, and platelet count
Fondaparinux	Bleeding	Clinical signs of bleeding[a]; baseline SCr, aPTT, INR, Hgb, HCT, and platelet count; daily SCr, Hgb, HCT, and platelet count
Bivalirudin	Bleeding	Clinical signs of bleeding[a]; baseline SCr, aPTT, INR, Hgb, HCT, and platelet count
Fibrinolytics	Bleeding, especially ICH	Clinical signs of bleeding[a]; baseline aPTT, INR, Hgb, HCT, and platelet count; mental status every 2 hours for signs of ICH; daily Hgb, HCT, and platelet count
GPIs	Bleeding, acute profound thrombocytopenia	Clinical signs of bleeding[a]; baseline SCr (for eptifibatide and tirofiban), Hgb, HCT, and platelet count; platelet count at 4 hours after initiation; daily Hgb, HCT, and platelet count (and SCr for eptifibatide and tirofiban)
IV nitrates	Hypotension, flushing, headache, tachycardia	BP and HR every 2 hours
β-blockers	Hypotension, bradycardia, heart block, bronchospasm, acute HF, fatigue, depression, sexual dysfunction	BP, RR, HR, 12-lead ECG, and clinical signs of HF every 5 minutes with bolus IV dosing; BP, RR, HR, and clinical signs of HF every shift with oral therapy, then BP and HR every 6 months following hospital discharge
Diltiazem and verapamil	Hypotension, bradycardia, heart block, HF, gingival hyperplasia	BP and HR every shift with oral therapy, then every 6 months following hospital discharge; dental examination and teeth cleaning every 6 months
Amlodipine	Hypotension, dependent peripheral edema, gingival hyperplasia	BP every shift with oral therapy, then every 6 months following hospital discharge; dental examination and teeth cleaning every 6 months
ACE inhibitors and ARBs	Hypotension, cough (with ACE inhibitors), hyperkalemia, prerenal azotemia, acute renal failure, angioedema (ACE inhibitors more so than ARBs)	BP every 4 hours × 3 for first dose, then every shift with oral therapy, then once every 6 months following hospital discharge; baseline SCr and potassium; daily SCr and potassium while hospitalized, then every 6 months (or 1–2 weeks after each outpatient dose titration); closer monitoring required in patients receiving spironolactone or eplerenone or if renal insufficiency; counsel patient on throat, tongue, and facial swelling
Aldosterone antagonists	Hypotension, hyperkalemia, increased SCr	BP and HR every shift with oral therapy, then once every 6 months; baseline SCr and serum potassium concentration then at 48 hours, at 7 days, monthly for 3 months, then every 3 months thereafter
Morphine	Hypotension, respiratory depression	BP and RR 5 minutes after each bolus dose
Statins	GI upset, myopathy, hepatotoxicity	Liver function tests at baseline. CK if indicated. Only repeat if patients present with sign/symptoms of liver failure or muscle symptoms; counsel patient on myalgia; consider CK at baseline if adding a fibrate or niacin

[a]Clinical signs of bleeding include bloody stools, melena, hematuria, hematemesis, bruising, and oozing from arterial or venous puncture sites.

ACE, angiotensin-converting enzyme; aPTT, activated partial thromboplastin time; ARB, angiotensin receptor blocker; BP, blood pressure; CK, creatine kinase; ECG, electrocardiogram; GI, gastrointestinal; GPI, glycoprotein IIb/IIIa inhibitor; Hgb, hemoglobin; HCT, hematocrit; HF, heart failure; HR, heart rate; ICH, intracranial hemorrhage; INR, international normalized ratio; IV, intravenous; RR, respiratory rate; SCr, serum creatinine; TTP, thrombotic thrombocytopenic purpura.

Modified with permission from DiPiro JT, Talbert RL, Yee GC, et al. Pharmacotherapy: A Pathophysiologic Approach, 9th ed. New York, NY: McGraw-Hill; 2014:199.

Patient Encounter 2, Part 3

The patient undergoes coronary angiography and is found to have a 90% stenosis in his left anterior descending coronary artery. PCI is performed and a drug-eluting stent is placed without complications.

Identify the long-term treatment goals for this patient.

What additional pharmacotherapy should be initiated prior to hospital discharge?

Create a care plan for this patient for hospital discharge that includes pharmacotherapy, desired treatment outcomes, and monitoring for efficacy and adverse effects.

dyslipidemia, are important treatments for secondary prevention of CHD events.[40] Referral to a comprehensive CV risk reduction program for cardiac rehabilitation is recommended.[4,40] HTN should be strictly controlled according to published guidelines.[40] Patients who are overweight, hypertensive, or who require cholesterol lowering should be educated on the importance of regular exercise, healthy eating habits, and reaching and maintaining an ideal weight.[34] Moderate-intensity aerobic exercise for at least 40 minutes, 3 to 4 days per week is recommended. Because patients with DM have up to a fourfold increased mortality risk compared with patients without DM, the importance of blood glucose control, as well as other CHD risk factor modifications, cannot be overstated.[40] Finally, influenza vaccination is recommended in all patients with CV disease. Additionally, vaccination with the 13- and 23-valent pneumococcal polysaccharide vaccines is recommended in those 65 years and older, as well as all high-risk individuals presenting with CV disease.[5,40]

In patients who require treatment for musculoskeletal pain, a stepped-care approach should be taken in the selection of treatment. Acetaminophen, tramadol, and nonacetylated salicylates are preferred. Use of small doses of narcotics for short periods can be added if the aforementioned are not adequate to relieve the patient.[5] If these agents are insufficient, nonselective nonsteroidal anti-inflammatory drugs (NSAIDS) can be considered, and should be used at the lowest effective dose and for the shortest possible time. Existing evidence suggests that naproxen may have the most modest risk to induce CV ischemic events, but the quality of the evidence available limits the definitiveness of assessment of its safety, particularly when it is used for long term. Importantly, all NSAIDs increase the risk of HF. If NSAIDs are used, a PPI should be added to reduce risk of GI bleeding.[46]

OUTCOME EVALUATION

- KEY CONCEPT *To determine the efficacy of nonpharmacologic and pharmacotherapy for both STEMI and NSTE-ACS, monitor patients for: (a) relief of ischemic discomfort; (b) return of ECG changes to baseline; and (c) absence or resolution of HF signs and symptoms.*
- Monitoring parameters for recognition and prevention of adverse effects from ACS pharmacotherapy are described in Table 8–5. KEY CONCEPT *In general, the most common adverse reactions from ACS therapies are hypotension and bleeding.* To treat bleeding and hypotension, discontinue the offending agent(s) until symptoms resolve. Severe bleeding resulting in

Patient Care Process

Patient Assessment:

- A 12-lead ECG should be performed and interpreted within 10 minutes (see Figure 8-1).
- Based on symptoms indicative of chest pain and/or other symptoms and review of ECG and initial troponin measurements, determine if the patient is experiencing an ACS (see Figure 8-1, Clinical Presentation and Diagnosis textbox).
- Obtain serial cardiac troponin levels at presentation and 3 to 6 hours after symptom onset. Serial troponin measurements are not necessary if the patient is experiencing an STEMI (see Figure 8-1).
- Conduct a medication history (including prescriptions, over-the-counter medications, and dietary supplements) to identify possible causes of ACS (eg, HTN, hyperlipidemia).
- Does the patient have any drug allergies? Is the patient experiencing side effects from therapy?

Therapy Evaluation:

- If patient is already receiving pharmacotherapy for ACS, assess efficacy, safety, and patient adherence. Are there any significant drug interactions? Document existing contraindications to medications (eg, aspirin, $P2Y_{12}$ inhibitors, β-blockers, ACE inhibitors, or aldosterone antagonists) in the medical record.
- If patient is diagnosed with ACS, determine what pharmacotherapy is indicated.
- Discuss prescription coverage with the patient to determine any barriers to paying for medications.
- Determine whether recommended agents are included on the institution's formulary.

Care Plan Development:

- Select an appropriate strategy for treatment, either immediate reperfusion for those with STEMI or risk stratification using available risk calculators for those with NSTE-ACS (see Table 8-1).
- Assess for contraindications for fibrinolytic therapy for STEMI patients in non-PCI facilities if patient cannot be transferred and undergo PCI within 120 minutes.
- Use risk stratification to select site of care, antithrombotic therapies, and invasive management for patients with NSTE-ACS (see Figure 8–3).
- Discontinue NSAIDs and select COX-2 inhibitor agents taken prior to ACS.
- Ensure that patients receive anti-ischemic (nitroglycerin [NTG], β-blockers), antiplatelet (aspirin), and analgesic (morphine) medications where appropriate early in care.
- Evaluate for potential contraindications for antiplatelet (active bleeding, history of TIA/stroke, renal function) and anticoagulant therapies (SCr, hemoglobin/hematocrit, platelet function). See Table 8–3.

(*Continued*)

Patient Care Process (*Continued*)

- Choose appropriate antiplatelet and anticoagulant medications based on ACS type (STEMI vs NSTE-ACS) and strategy chosen (early invasive vs ischemia guided) (see Figures 8–2 and 8–3). If a patient has received fondaparinux and is going to the catheterization or cath laboratory, ensure that additional anticoagulation with UFH is given at time of intervention (see Figure 8–3).
- Review renal function and baseline coagulation tests (aPTT, platelets) to make appropriate dosing adjustments in antiplatelet and anticoagulant therapies given during early ACS.
- Appropriately adjust all medications based on renal function (see Table 8–3).
- Monitor for signs and symptoms of bleeding during hospitalization and prior to discharge.
- Ensure all patients without contraindications receive oral β-blockers, preferably within the first 24 hours.
- Patients with initial contraindications to β-blockers in the first 24 hours should be reevaluated for therapy prior to discharge.
- Ensure all patients receive aspirin and statins at discharge and continue indefinitely as long as no contraindication exists.
- Review discharge prescription for DAPT (with aspirin 81 mg plus a $P2Y_{12}$ inhibitor), which should be given for 12 months after ACS regardless of stenting. Also, discuss with the patient the importance of DAPT (especially in the patient receiving a stent).
- Evaluate for indication of ACE inhibitors (or ARBs) and aldosterone antagonists before discharge.
- Evaluate for prescription of PPI therapy for those requiring triple therapy with aspirin, a $P2Y_{12}$ receptor inhibitor, and a vitamin K antagonist.
- Ensure patients receive a prescription for SL NTG at time of discharge with verbal and written instructions for use.
- Continue anti-ischemic medications at discharge in those with recurrent symptoms or in patients who do not undergo revascularization.
- Educate patients about appropriate cholesterol management, blood pressure goals, smoking cessation, and lifestyle management with easily understandable and culturally sensitive verbal and written instruction.
- Evaluate for appropriate vaccinations prior to discharge.
- Address musculoskeletal pain control prior to discharge.
- Refer all patients to a comprehensive CV rehabilitation program.

Follow-Up Evaluation:

- Follow up within 2 weeks to assess angina symptoms and interventional success if applicable.
- Review medical history and physical examination findings, laboratory tests, and results of other diagnostic workup.
- Discuss adherence with medications and discover if the patient is experiencing any adverse events from medications.

hypotension secondary to hypovolemia may require blood transfusion.

- Because poor medication adherence of secondary prevention medications following MI leads to worsened CV outcomes, patients should receive medication counseling (including counseling prior to hospital discharge) and be monitored for medication persistence.[4,5,43] Counseling should include assessment of health literacy level, assessment of barriers to adherence, assessment of access to medications, written and verbal instructions about the purpose of each medication, changes to previous medication regimen, optimal time to take each medication, new allergies or medication intolerances, need for timely prescription fill after discharge, anticipated duration of therapy, consequences of nonadherence, common and/or serious adverse reactions that may develop, drug–drug and drug–food interactions, and an assessment of instruction understanding.

ACKNOWLEDGMENT

The authors and editors wish to acknowledge and thank Dr. Sarah A. Spinler, the primary author of this chapter in the first, second, and third editions of this book.

Abbreviations Introduced in This Chapter

ACCF	American College of Cardiology Foundation
ACE	Angiotensin-converting enzyme
ACS	Acute coronary syndrome
ADP	Adenosine diphosphate
AHA	American Heart Association
aPTT	Activated partial thromboplastin time
ARB	Angiotensin receptor blocker
ASA	Aspirin
BMS	Bare metal stent
BP	Blood pressure
CABG	Coronary artery bypass graft (surgery)
CAD	Coronary artery disease
CBC	Complete blood count
CHD	Coronary heart disease
CKD	Chronic kidney disease
COX-2	Cyclooxygenase-2
CrCl	Creatinine clearance
CV	Cardiovascular
CVD	Cardiovascular disease
CYP	Cytochrome P-450
DAPT	Dual antiplatelet therapy
DES	Drug-eluting stent
DM	Diabetes mellitus
ECG	Electrocardiogram
ED	Emergency department
GI	Gastrointestinal
GP	Glycoprotein
GPI	Glycoprotein IIb/IIIa inhibitor
HF	Heart failure
HTN	Hypertension
ICD	Implantable cardioverter defibrillator
ICH	Intracranial hemorrhage
INR	International normalized ratio
IV	Intravenous
LDL	Low density lipoprotein
LMWH	Low molecular weight heparin
LVEF	Left ventricular ejection fraction
LVF	Left ventricular function

MI	Myocardial infarction
NSAID	Nonsteroidal anti-inflammatory drug
NSTE	Non–ST segment elevation
NSTEMI	Non–ST-elevation MI
NTG	Nitroglycerin
PCI	Percutaneous coronary intervention
PPI	Proton pump inhibitor
SCAI	Society for Cardiovascular Angiography and Interventions
SCr	Serum creatinine
SL	Sublingual
STE	ST-segment elevation
STEMI	ST-segment elevation myocardial infarction
TIA	Transient ischemic attack
TIMI	Thrombolysis in myocardial infarction
TTP	Thrombotic thrombocytopenic purpura
TXA_2	Thromboxane A_2
UA	Unstable angina
UFH	Unfractionated heparin

REFERENCES

1. Go AS, Mozaffarian D, Roger VL, Benjamin EJ, et al. Heart disease and stroke statistics--2014 update: A report from the American Heart Association. Circulation. 2014;129(3):e28–e292.
2. Bentzon JF, Otsuka F, Virmani R, Falk E. Mechanisms of plaque formation and rupture. Circ Res. 2014;114(12):1852–1866.
3. Levine GN, Bates ER, Blankenship JC, et al. 2011 ACCF/AHA/SCAI guideline for percutaneous coronary intervention. A report of the American College of Cardiology Foundation/American Heart Association Task Force on Practice Guidelines and the Society for Cardiovascular Angiography and Interventions. J Am Coll Cardiol. 2011;58(24):e44–e122.
4. O'Gara PT, Kushner FG, Ascheim DD, et al. 2013 ACCF/AHA guideline for the management of ST-elevation myocardial infarction: a report of the American College of Cardiology Foundation/American Heart Association Task Force on Practice Guidelines. J Am Coll Cardiol. 2013;61(4):e78–e140.
5. Amsterdam EA, Wenger NK, Brindis RG, et al. 2014 AHA/ACC Guideline for the management ofpatients with non-ST-elevation acute coronary syndromes: A report of the American College of Cardiology/American Heart Association Task Force on Practice Guidelines. J Am Coll Cardiol. 2014;64(24):e139–e228.
6. Chin CT, Chen AY, Wang TY, et al. Risk adjustment for in-hospital mortality of contemporary patients with acute myocardial infarction: The acute coronary treatment and intervention outcomes network (ACTION) registry-get with the guidelines (GWTG) acute myocardial infarction mortality model and risk score. Am Heart J. 2011;161(1):113–22.e2.
7. Go AS, Mozaffarian D, Roger VL, et al. Heart disease and stroke statistics--2013 update: a report from the American Heart Association. Circulation. 2013;127(1):e6–e245.
8. Borissoff JI, Spronk HM, ten Cate H. The hemostatic system as a modulator of atherosclerosis. N Engl J Med. 2011;364(18):1746–1760.
9. Thygesen K, Alpert JS, Jaffe AS, et al. Third universal definition of myocardial infarction. J Am Coll Cardiol. 2012;60(16):1581–1598.
10. Gajarsa JJ, Kloner RA. Left ventricular remodeling in the post-infarction heart: a review of cellular, molecular mechanisms, and therapeutic modalities. Heart Fail Rev. 2011;16(1):13–21.
11. Goodman SG, Huang W, Yan AT, et al. The expanded Global Registry of Acute Coronary Events: Baseline characteristics, management practices, and hospital outcomes of patients with acute coronary syndromes. Am Heart J. 2009;158(2):193–201.e1–e5.
12. Awad HH, Anderson FA, Jr, Gore JM, Goodman SG, Goldberg RJ. Cardiogenic shock complicating acute coronary syndromes: Insights from the Global Registry of Acute Coronary Events. Am Heart J. 2012;163(6):963–971.
13. Huynh T, Perron S, O'Loughlin J, et al. Comparison of primary percutaneous coronary intervention and fibrinolytic therapy in ST-segment-elevation myocardial infarction: Bayesian hierarchical meta-analyses of randomized controlled trials and observational studies. Circulation. 2009;119(24):3101–3109.
14. Bagai A, Dangas GD, Stone GW, Granger CB. Reperfusion strategies in acute coronary syndromes. Circ Res. 2014;114(12):1918–1928.
15. Krumholz HM, Herrin J, Miller LE, et al. Improvements in door-to-balloon time in the United States, 2005 to 2010. Circulation. 2011;124(9):1038–1045.
16. Mark DB, Hlatky MA, Califf RM, et al. Cost effectiveness of thrombolytic therapy with tissue plasminogen activator as compared with streptokinase for acute myocardial infarction. N Engl J Med. 1995;332(21):1418–1424.
17. Van De Werf F, Adgey J, Ardissino D, et al. Single-bolus tenecteplase compared with front-loaded alteplase in acute myocardial infarction: the ASSENT-2 double-blind randomised trial. Lancet. 1999;354(9180):716–722.
18. A comparison of reteplase with alteplase for acute myocardial infarction. The Global Use of Strategies to Open Occluded Coronary Arteries (GUSTO III) Investigators. N Engl J Med. 1997;337(16):1118–1123.
19. Indications for fibrinolytic therapy in suspected acute myocardial infarction: collaborative overview of early mortality and major morbidity results from all randomised trials of more than 1000 patients. Fibrinolytic Therapy Trialists' (FTT) Collaborative Group. Lancet. 1994;343(8893):311–322.
20. Hoenig MR, Aroney CN, Scott IA. Early invasive versus conservative strategies for unstable angina and non-ST elevation myocardial infarction in the stent era. Cochrane Database Syst Rev. 2010(3):Cd004815.
21. Mauri L, Kereiakes DJ, Yeh RW, et al. Twelve or 30 months of dual antiplatelet therapy after drug-eluting stents. N Engl J Med. 2014;371(23):2155–2166.
22. Bhatt DL, Hulot JS, Moliterno DJ, Harrington RA. Antiplatelet and anticoagulation therapy for acute coronary syndromes. Circ Res. 2014;114(12):1929–1943.
23. Sofi F, Giusti B, Marcucci R, Gori AM, Abbate R, Gensini GF. Cytochrome P450 2C19*2 polymorphism and cardiovascular recurrences in patients taking clopidogrel: A meta-analysis. Pharmacogenomics J. 2011;11(3):199–206.
24. Scott SA, Sangkuhl K, Stein CM, et al. Clinical Pharmacogenetics Implementation Consortium guidelines for CYP2C19 genotype and clopidogrel therapy: 2013 update. Clin Pharmacol Ther. 2013;94(3):317–323.
25. Wiviott SD, Braunwald E, McCabe CH, et al. Prasugrel versus clopidogrel in patients with acute coronary syndromes. N Engl J Med. 2007;357(20):2001–2015.
26. Wallentin L, Becker RC, Budaj A, et al. Ticagrelor versus clopidogrel in patients with acute coronary syndromes. N Engl J Med. 2009;361(11):1045–1057.
27. Montalescot G, Wiviott SD, Braunwald E, et al. Prasugrel compared with clopidogrel in patients undergoing percutaneous coronary intervention for ST-elevation myocardial infarction (TRITON-TIMI 38): Double-blind, randomised controlled trial. Lancet. 2009;373(9665):723–731.
28. Wiviott SD, Braunwald E, Angiolillo DJ, et al. Greater clinical benefit of more intensive oral antiplatelet therapy with prasugrel in patients with diabetes mellitus in the trial to assess improvement in therapeutic outcomes by optimizing platelet inhibition with prasugrel-Thrombolysis in Myocardial Infarction 38. Circulation. 2008;118(16):1626–1636.

29. James S, Angiolillo DJ, Cornel JH, et al. Ticagrelor vs. clopidogrel in patients with acute coronary syndromes and diabetes: A substudy from the PLATelet inhibition and patient Outcomes (PLATO) trial. Eur Heart J. 2010;31(24):3006–3016.
30. Wallentin L, James S, Storey RF, et al. Effect of CYP2C19 and ABCB1 single nucleotide polymorphisms on outcomes of treatment with ticagrelor versus clopidogrel for acute coronary syndromes: A genetic substudy of the PLATO trial. Lancet. 2010;376(9749):1320–1328.
31. Siller-Matula JM, Huber K, Christ G, et al. Impact of clopidogrel loading dose on clinical outcome in patients undergoing percutaneous coronary intervention: A systematic review and meta-analysis. Heart. 2011;97(2):98–105.
32. Mehta SR, Tanguay JF, Eikelboom JW, et al. Double-dose versus standard-dose clopidogrel and high-dose versus low-dose aspirin in individuals undergoing percutaneous coronary intervention for acute coronary syndromes (CURRENT-OASIS 7): A randomised factorial trial. Lancet. 2010;376(9748):1233–1243.
33. Mangalpally KK, Kleiman NS. The safety of clopidogrel. Expert Opin Drug Saf. 2011;10(1):85–95.
34. Eckel RH, Jakicic JM, Ard JD, et al. 2013 AHA/ACC guideline on lifestyle management to reduce cardiovascular risk: A report of the American College of Cardiology/American Heart Association Task Force on Practice Guidelines. Circulation. 2014;129(25 Suppl 2):S76–S99.
35. Giugliano RP, White JA, Bode C, et al. Early versus delayed, provisional eptifibatide in acute coronary syndromes. N Engl J Med. 2009;360(21):2176–2190.
36. Dasgupta H, Blankenship JC, Wood GC, Frey CM, Demko SL, Menapace FJ. Thrombocytopenia complicating treatment with intravenous glycoprotein IIb/IIIa receptor inhibitors: A pooled analysis. Am Heart J. 2000;140(2):206–211.
37. Stone GW, Witzenbichler B, Guagliumi G, et al. Heparin plus a glycoprotein IIb/IIIa inhibitor versus bivalirudin monotherapy and paclitaxel-eluting stents versus bare-metal stents in acute myocardial infarction (HORIZONS-AMI): Final 3-year results from a multicentre, randomised controlled trial. Lancet. 2011;377(9784):2193–2204.
38. Shahzad A, Kemp I, Mars C, et al. Unfractionated heparin versus bivalirudin in primary percutaneous coronary intervention (HEAT-PPCI): An open-label, single centre, randomised controlled trial. Lancet. 2014;384(9957):1849–1858.
39. Cavender MA, Sabatine MS. Bivalirudin versus heparin in patients planned for percutaneous coronary intervention: A meta-analysis of randomised controlled trials. Lancet. 2014;384(9943):599–606.
40. Smith SC, Jr., Benjamin EJ, Bonow RO, et al. AHA/ACCF secondary prevention and risk reduction therapy for patients with coronary and other atherosclerotic vascular disease: 2011 update: A guideline from the American Heart Association and American College of Cardiology Foundation endorsed by the World Heart Federation and the Preventive Cardiovascular Nurses Association. J Am Coll Cardiol. 2011;58(23):2432–2446.
41. Chen ZM, Pan HC, Chen YP, et al. Early intravenous then oral metoprolol in 45,852 patients with acute myocardial infarction: Randomised placebo-controlled trial. Lancet. 2005;366(9497):1622–1632.
42. Stone NJ, Robinson JG, Lichtenstein AH, et al. 2013 ACC/AHA guideline on the treatment of blood cholesterol to reduce atherosclerotic cardiovascular risk in adults: A report of the American College of Cardiology/American Heart Association Task Force on Practice Guidelines. J Am Coll Cardiol. 2014;63(25 Pt B):2889–2934.
43. Ho PM, Lambert-Kerzner A, Carey EP, et al. Multifaceted intervention to improve medication adherence and secondary prevention measures after acute coronary syndrome hospital discharge: A randomized clinical trial. JAMA Intern Med. 2014;174(2):186–193.
44. Serebruany VL, Steinhubl SR, Berger PB, et al. Analysis of risk of bleeding complications after different doses of aspirin in 192,036 patients enrolled in 31 randomized controlled trials. Am J Cardiol. 2005;95(10):1218–1222.
45. Budnitz DS, Lovegrove MC, Shehab N, Richards CL. Emergency hospitalizations for adverse drug events in older Americans. N Engl J Med. 2011;365(21):2002–2012.
46. Abraham NS, Hlatky MA, Antman EM, et al. ACCF/ACG/AHA 2010 Expert Consensus Document on the concomitant use of proton pump inhibitors and thienopyridines: a focused update of the ACCF/ACG/AHA 2008 expert consensus document on reducing the gastrointestinal risks of antiplatelet therapy and NSAID use: A report of the American College of Cardiology Foundation Task Force on Expert Consensus Documents. Circulation. 2010;122(24):2619–2633.
47. Steg PG, De Silva R. Beta-blockers in asymptomatic coronary artery disease: No benefit or no evidence? J Am Coll Cardiol. 2014;64(3):253–255.
48. Fihn SD, Gardin JM, Abrams J, et al. 2012 ACCF/AHA/ACP/AATS/PCNA/SCAI/STS Guideline for the diagnosis and management of patients with stable ischemic heart disease: A report of the American College of Cardiology Foundation/American Heart Association Task Force on Practice Guidelines, and the American College of Physicians, American Association for Thoracic Surgery, Preventive Cardiovascular Nurses Association, Society for Cardiovascular Angiography and Interventions, and Society of Thoracic Surgeons. J Am Coll Cardiol. 2012;60(24):e44–e164.
49. Pitt B, Remme W, Zannad F, et al. Eplerenone, a selective aldosterone blocker, in patients with left ventricular dysfunction after myocardial infarction. N Engl J Med. 2003;348(14):1309–1321.
50. Hulten E, Jackson JL, Douglas K, George S, Villines TC. The effect of early, intensive statin therapy on acute coronary syndrome: A meta-analysis of randomized controlled trials. Arch Intern Med. 2006;166(17):1814–1821.

9 Arrhythmias

James E. Tisdale

LEARNING OBJECTIVES

Upon completion of the chapter, the reader will be able to:

1. Describe the phases of cardiac action potential, compare and contrast cardiac myocyte ion changes corresponding to each phase, and explain the relationship between the cardiac action potential and the electrocardiogram (ECG).
2. Describe the modified Vaughan Williams classification of antiarrhythmic drugs, and compare and contrast the effects of available antiarrhythmic drugs on ventricular conduction velocity, refractory period, automaticity, and inhibition of ion flux through specific myocardial ion channels.
3. Compare and contrast risk factors for and features, mechanisms, etiologies, symptoms, and goals of therapy of (a) sinus bradycardia, (b) atrioventricular (AV) nodal block, (c) atrial fibrillation (AF), (d) paroxysmal supraventricular tachycardia (PSVT), (e) ventricular premature depolarizations (VPDs), (f) ventricular tachycardia (VT, including torsades de pointes [TdP]), and (g) ventricular fibrillation (VF).
4. Compare and contrast appropriate nonpharmacologic and pharmacologic treatment options for sinus bradycardia and AV nodal block.
5. Compare and contrast mechanisms of action of drugs used for ventricular rate control, conversion to sinus rhythm and maintenance of sinus rhythm in patients with AF, and explain the importance of anticoagulation for patients with AF.
6. Discuss nonpharmacologic methods for termination of PSVT, and compare and contrast mechanisms of action of drugs used for acute termination of PSVT.
7. Compare and contrast the role of drug therapy versus nonpharmacologic therapy for long-term prevention of PSVT recurrence.
8. Describe the role of drug therapy for management of asymptomatic and symptomatic VPDs.
9. Compare and contrast mechanisms of action of drugs used for treatment of acute episodes of VT, and describe options and indications for nonpharmacologic treatment of VT and VF.
10. Design individualized drug therapy treatment plans for patients with (a) sinus bradycardia, (b) AV nodal block, (c) AF, (d) PSVT, (e) VPDs, (f) VT (including TdP), and (g) VF.

NORMAL AND ABNORMAL CARDIAC CONDUCTION AND ELECTROPHYSIOLOGY

The heart functions via both mechanical and electrical activity. Mechanical activity of the heart refers to atrial and ventricular contraction, the mechanism by which blood is delivered to tissues. When circulated blood returns to the heart via venous circulation, blood enters the right atrium. Right atrial contraction and changes in right ventricular pressure result in delivery of blood to the right ventricle through the tricuspid valve. Right ventricular contraction pumps blood through the pulmonic valve through the pulmonary arteries to the lungs, where blood becomes oxygenated. The blood then flows through the pulmonary veins into the left atrium. Left atrial contraction and changes in left ventricle (LV) pressure result in delivery of blood through the mitral valve into the LV. Contraction of the LV results in pumping of blood through the aortic valve and to the tissues of the body.

Mechanical activity of the heart (contraction of the atria and ventricles) occurs as a result of the electrical activity of the heart. The heart possesses an intrinsic electrical conduction system (Figure 9–1). Normal myocardial contraction cannot occur without proper and normal function of the heart's electrical conduction system. Depolarization of the atria results in atrial contraction, and ventricular depolarization is followed by ventricular contraction. Malfunction of the heart's electrical conduction system may result in dysfunctional atrial and/or ventricular contraction and may reduce cardiac output.

Cardiac Conduction System

Under normal circumstances, the sinoatrial (SA) node (also known as the sinus node), located in the upper portion of the right atrium, serves as the **pacemaker** of the heart and generates the electrical impulses that subsequently result in atrial and **ventricular depolarization** (see Figure 9–1). The SA node serves

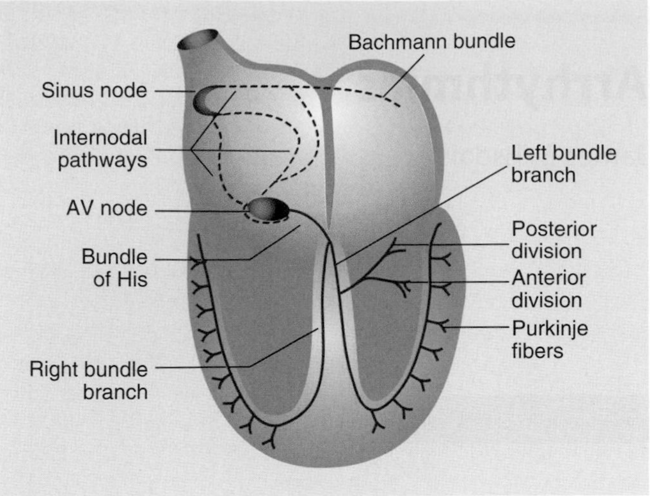

FIGURE 9–1. The cardiac conduction system. (AV, atrioventricular.)

as the heart's dominant pacemaker because it has the greatest degree of **automaticity**, which is defined as the ability of a cardiac fiber or tissue to initiate depolarizations spontaneously. In adults at rest, the normal intrinsic depolarization rate of the SA node is 60 to 100 per minute. Other cardiac fibers also possess the property of automaticity, but normally the intrinsic depolarization rates are slower than that of the SA node. For example, the normal intrinsic depolarization rate of the atrioventricular (AV) node is 40 to 60 per minute; that of the ventricular tissue is 30 to 40 per minute. Therefore, because of greater automaticity, the SA node normally serves as the pacemaker of the heart. However, if the SA node fails to generate depolarizations at a rate faster than that of the AV node, the AV node may take over as the pacemaker. If both the SA node and AV node fail to generate depolarizations at a rate more than 30 to 40 per minute, ventricular tissue may take over.

Following initiation of the electrical impulse from the SA node, the impulse travels through internodal pathways of the specialized atrial conduction system and Bachmann bundle. The atrial conducting fibers do not traverse the entire breadth of the left and right atria; impulse conduction occurs across the internodal pathways, and when the impulse reaches the end of Bachmann bundle, atrial depolarization spreads as a wave, conceptually similar to that which occurs upon throwing a pebble into water. As the impulse is conducted across the atria, each depolarized cell excites and depolarizes the surrounding connected cells, until both atria have been completely depolarized. Atrial contraction follows normal atrial depolarization.

Following atrial depolarization, impulses are conducted through the AV node, located in the lower right atrium (see Figure 9–1). The impulse then enters the bundle of His and is conducted through the ventricular conduction system, consisting of the left and right bundle branches. The left ventricle requires a larger conduction system than the right ventricle due to its larger mass; therefore, the left bundle branch bifurcates into the left anterior and posterior divisions (also known as "fascicles"). The bundle branches further divide into the **Purkinje fibers** through which impulse conduction results in ventricular depolarization, initiating ventricular contraction.

Ventricular Action Potential

Ventricular **action potential** is depicted in Figure 9–2. Ventricular myocyte resting membrane potential is usually –70 to –90 mV, due to the action of the sodium–potassium adenosine triphosphatase (ATPase) pump, which maintains relatively high extracellular sodium concentrations and relatively low extracellular potassium concentrations. During each action potential cycle, the potential of the membrane slowly increases to a threshold potential due to a slow influx of sodium into the cell, raising the threshold to –60 to –80 mV. When the membrane potential reaches this threshold, the fast sodium channels open, allowing sodium ions to enter the cell rapidly. This rapid influx of positive ions creates a vertical upstroke of the action potential, such that

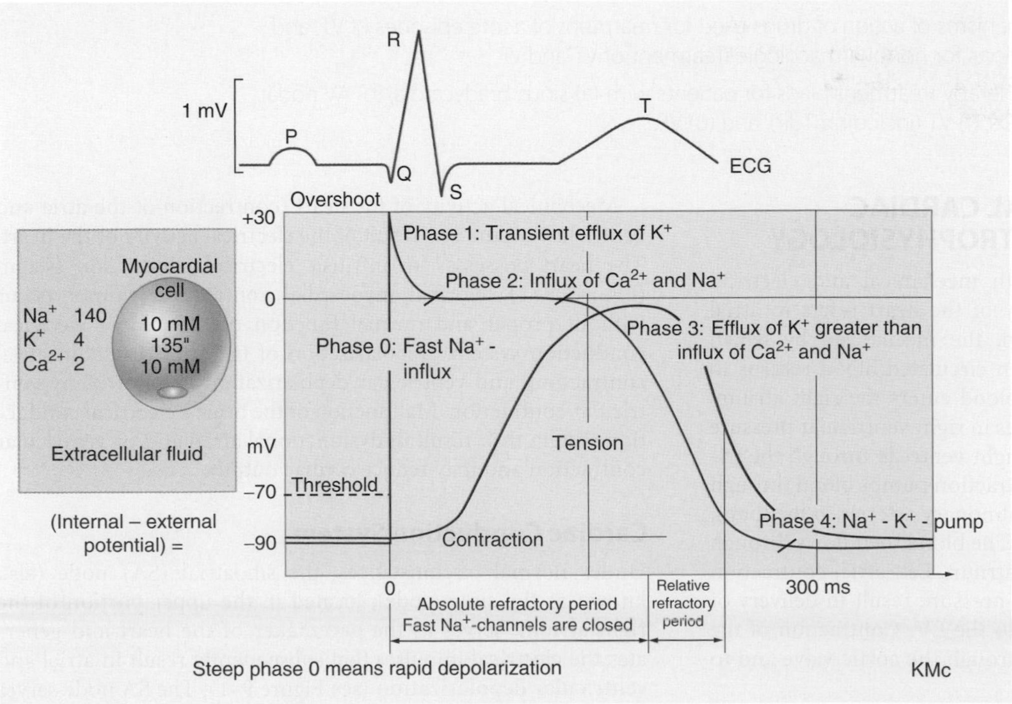

FIGURE 9–2. The ventricular action potential depicting the flow of specific ions responsible for each phase. The phases of the action potential that correspond to the absolute and relative refractory periods are portrayed, and the relationship between phases of the action potential and the electrocardiogram (ECG) are shown. (Ca, calcium; K, potassium; Na, sodium.)

the potential reaches 20 to 30 mV. This is phase 0, which represents ventricular depolarization. At this point, the fast sodium channels become inactivated, and ventricular repolarization begins, consisting of phases 1 through 3 of the action potential. Phase 1 repolarization occurs primarily as a result of an efflux of potassium ions. During phase 2, potassium ions continue to exit the cell, but the membrane potential is balanced by an influx of calcium and sodium ions, transported through slow calcium and slow sodium channels, resulting in a plateau. During phase 3, the efflux of potassium ions greatly exceeds calcium and sodium influx, resulting in the major component of ventricular repolarization. During phase 4, sodium ions gradually enter the cell, increasing the threshold again to −60 to −80 mV and initiating another action potential. An understanding of the ion fluxes that are responsible for each phase of the action potential facilitates understanding of the effects of specific drugs on the action potential. For example, drugs that primarily inhibit ion flux through sodium channels influence phase 0 (ventricular depolarization), whereas drugs that primarily inhibit ion flux through potassium channels influence the repolarization phases, particularly phase 3.

Electrocardiogram

The electrocardiogram (ECG) is a noninvasive means of measuring the electrical activity of the heart. The relationship between the ventricular action potential and the ECG is depicted in Figure 9–2. The P wave on the ECG represents atrial depolarization (atrial depolarization is not depicted in the action potential shown in Figure 9–2, which shows only the ventricular action potential). Phase 0 of the action potential corresponds to the QRS complex; therefore, the QRS complex on the ECG is a noninvasive representation of ventricular depolarization. The T wave on the ECG corresponds to phase 3 ventricular repolarization. The interval from the beginning of the Q wave to the end of the T wave, known as the QT interval, is used as a noninvasive marker of ventricular repolarization time. Atrial repolarization is not visible on the ECG because it occurs during ventricular depolarization and is obscured by the QRS complex.

Several ECG intervals and durations are routinely measured. The PR interval represents the time of conduction of impulses from the atria to the ventricles through the AV node; the normal PR interval in adults is 0.12 to 0.2 seconds. The QRS duration represents the time required for ventricular depolarization, which is normally 0.08 to 0.12 seconds in adults. The QT interval, measuring 0.32 to 0.4 seconds, represents the time required for ventricular repolarization. The QT interval varies with heart rate—the faster the heart rate, the shorter the QT interval, and vice versa. Therefore, the QT interval is corrected for heart rate using Bazett's equation:

$$QT_c = \frac{QT}{\sqrt{RR}}$$

where QT_c is the QT interval corrected for heart rate, and RR is the interval from the onset of one QRS complex to the onset of the next QRS complex, measured in seconds (ie, the heart rate, expressed in different terminology). The normal QT_c interval in adults is 0.36 to 0.47 seconds in men and 0.36 to 0.48 seconds in women.[1]

Refractory Periods

After an electrical impulse is initiated and conducted, there is a period of time during which cells and fibers cannot be depolarized again. This period of time is referred to as the absolute refractory period (see Figure 9–2) and corresponds to phases 1, 2, and approximately one-third of phase 3 repolarization of the action potential. The absolute refractory period also corresponds to the period from the Q wave to approximately the first half of the T wave on the ECG (see Figure 9–2). During this period, if there is a premature stimulus for an electrical impulse, this impulse cannot be conducted because the tissue is absolutely refractory. However, there is a period of time following the absolute refractory period during which a premature electrical stimulus can be conducted and is often conducted abnormally. This period of time is called the relative refractory period, which corresponds roughly to the latter two-thirds of phase 3 repolarization on the action potential and to the latter half of the T wave on the ECG. If a new (premature) electrical stimulus is initiated during the relative refractory period, it can be conducted abnormally, potentially resulting in an arrhythmia.

Mechanisms of Cardiac Arrhythmias

KEY CONCEPT *In general, cardiac arrhythmias are caused by (a) abnormal impulse initiation, (b) abnormal impulse conduction, or (c) both.*

▸ Abnormal Impulse Initiation

Abnormal initiation of electrical impulses occurs as a result of abnormal automaticity. If SA node automaticity decreases, this results in a reduced rate of impulse generation and a slow heart rate (sinus bradycardia). Conversely, if SA node automaticity increases, this results in an increased rate of generation of impulses and a rapid heart rate (sinus tachycardia). If other cardiac fibers become abnormally automatic, such that the rate of spontaneous impulse initiation exceeds that of the SA node, or premature impulses are generated, other tachyarrhythmias may occur. Many cardiac fibers possess the capability for automaticity, including atrial tissue, the AV node, the Purkinje fibers, and the ventricular tissue. In addition, fibers with the capability of initiating and conducting electrical impulses are present in the pulmonary veins. Abnormal atrial automaticity may result in premature atrial contractions or may precipitate atrial tachycardia or atrial fibrillation (AF); abnormal AV nodal automaticity may result in "junctional tachycardia" (the AV node is also sometimes referred to as the AV junction). Abnormal automaticity in the ventricles may result in ventricular premature depolarizations (VPDs) or may precipitate ventricular tachycardia (VT) or ventricular fibrillation (VF). In addition, abnormal automaticity originating from the pulmonary veins is a precipitant of AF.

Automaticity of cardiac fibers is controlled in part by activity of the sympathetic and parasympathetic nervous systems. Enhanced sympathetic nervous system activity may result in increased automaticity of the SA node or other automatic cardiac fibers. Enhanced parasympathetic nervous system activity suppresses automaticity, while inhibition of parasympathetic nervous system activity increases automaticity. Other factors may lead to increases in automaticity of extra-SA nodal tissues, including hypoxia, atrial or ventricular stretch (such as following long-standing hypertension or during and after development of heart failure [HF]), and electrolyte abnormalities such as hypokalemia or hypomagnesemia.

▸ Abnormal Impulse Conduction

The mechanism of abnormal impulse conduction is traditionally referred to as reentry. KEY CONCEPT *Reentry is often initiated as a result of an abnormal premature electrical impulse (abnormal automaticity); therefore, in these situations, the mechanism of the arrhythmia is both abnormal impulse formation (automaticity) and abnormal impulse conduction (reentry)*. For reentry to occur, three conditions must be present. There must be (a) at least two pathways down which an electrical impulse may travel (which is the case in most cardiac fibers); (b) a "unidirectional block" in one of the conduction pathways (this "unidirectional block" reflects prolonged refractoriness in this pathway, or increased "dispersion of refractoriness," defined as substantial variation in refractory periods between cardiac fibers); and (c) slowing of the velocity of impulse conduction down the other conduction pathway.

The process of reentry is depicted in Figure 9–3.[2] Under normal circumstances, when a premature impulse is initiated, it cannot be conducted in either direction down either pathway because the tissue is in its absolute refractory period from the previous impulse. A premature impulse may be conducted down both pathways if it is only slightly premature and arrives after the tissue is no longer refractory. However, when refractoriness is prolonged down one of the pathways, a precisely timed premature beat may be conducted down one pathway but cannot be conducted in either direction in the pathway with prolonged refractoriness because the tissue is still in its absolute refractory period.[2] Refractoriness may be prolonged to a greater degree in one pathway than in the other as a result of increased dispersion of repolarization. When the third condition for reentry is present, that is, when the velocity of impulse conduction in one pathway is slowed, the impulse traveling forward down the other pathway still cannot be conducted. However, because the impulse in one pathway is traveling more slowly than normal, by the time it circles around and travels upward along the other pathway, sufficient time has passed so the pathway is no longer in its absolute refractory period, and now the impulse may travel upward in that pathway. In other words, the electrical impulse "reenters" a previously stimulated pathway in the reverse (retrograde) direction. This results in circular movement of electrical impulses; as the impulse travels in this circular fashion, it excites each cell around it, and if the impulse is traveling at a rate faster than the intrinsic rate of the SA node, a tachycardia occurs in the tissue in question. Reentry may occur in numerous tissues, including the atria, the AV node, and the ventricles.

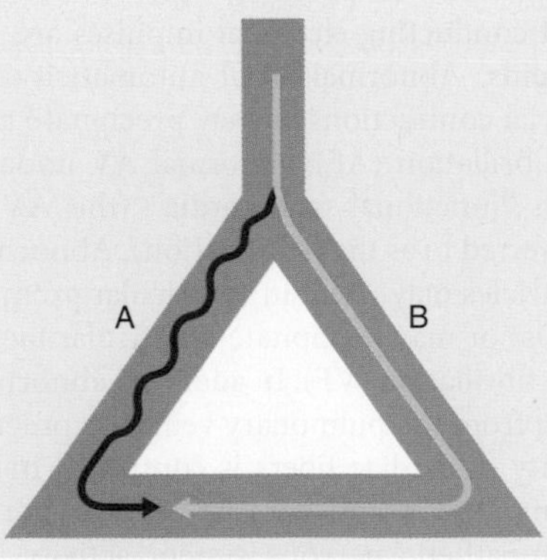

FIGURE 9–3. The process of initiation of reentry. There are two pathways for impulse conduction, slowed impulse conduction down pathway A and a longer refractory period in pathway B. A precisely timed premature impulse initiates reentry; the premature impulse cannot be conducted down pathway B because the tissue is still in the absolute refractory period from the previous, normal impulse. However, because of dispersion of refractoriness (ie, different refractory periods down the two pathways), the impulse can be conducted down pathway A. Because conduction down pathway A is slowed, by the time the impulse reaches pathway B in a retrograde direction, the impulse can be conducted retrogradely up the pathway because the pathway is now beyond its refractory period from the previous impulse. This creates reentry, in which the impulse continuously and repeatedly travels in a circular fashion around the loop.

Prolonged refractoriness and/or slowed impulse conduction velocity may be present in cardiac tissues for a variety of reasons. Myocardial ischemia may alter ventricular refractory periods or impulse conduction velocity, facilitating ventricular reentry. In patients with past myocardial infarction (MI), the infarcted myocardium is dead and cannot conduct impulses. However, there is typically a border zone of tissue that is damaged and in which refractory periods and conduction velocity are often aberrant, facilitating ventricular reentry. In patients with left atrial or LV hypertrophy as a result of long-standing hypertension, refractory periods and conduction velocity are often perturbed. In patients with HF with reduced ejection fraction (HFrEF), ventricular refractoriness and conduction velocity are often altered due to LV hypertrophy, collagen deposition, and other anatomical and structural changes.

Vaughan Williams Classification of Antiarrhythmic Drugs

The Vaughan Williams classification of antiarrhythmic drugs is presented in Table 9–1.[3–5] This classification is based on the effects of specific drugs on ventricular conduction velocity, repolarization/refractoriness, and automaticity. Class I drugs primarily inhibit ventricular automaticity and slow conduction velocity. However, due to differences in the potency of the drugs to slow conduction velocity, the class I drugs are subdivided into classes IA, IB, and IC. The class IC drugs have the greatest potency for slowing ventricular conduction, class IA drugs have intermediate potency, and class IB drugs have the lowest potency, with minimal effects on conduction velocity at normal heart rates. Class II drugs are the adrenergic β-receptor inhibitors (β-blockers), class III drugs are those that inhibit ventricular repolarization and prolong refractoriness, and class IV drugs are the calcium channel blockers (CCBs), diltiazem and verapamil.

The Vaughan Williams classification of antiarrhythmic drugs has been criticized for a number of reasons. The classification is based on the effects of drugs on normal, rather than diseased, myocardium. In addition, many of the drugs may be placed into more than one class. For example, the class IA drugs prolong repolarization/refractoriness, either via the parent drug[6] or an active metabolite,[7] and therefore may also be placed in class III. Sotalol is also a β-blocker and therefore fits into class II. Amiodarone inhibits sodium and potassium conductance, is a noncompetitive inhibitor of β-receptors, and inhibits calcium channels, and therefore, it may be placed into any of the four classes. For this reason, drugs within each class cannot be considered "interchangeable." Nonetheless, despite attempts to develop mechanism-based classifications that better distinguish the actions of antiarrhythmic drugs, the Vaughan Williams classification continues to be widely used because of its simplicity and the fact that it is relatively easy to remember and understand.

CARDIAC ARRHYTHMIAS

Cardiac arrhythmias are classified into two broad categories: supraventricular (those occurring above the ventricles) and ventricular (those occurring in the ventricles). Names of specific arrhythmias are generally composed of two words: the first

Table 9–1

Vaughan Williams Classification of Antiarrhythmic Agents[a]

Class	Drug	Conduction Velocity[b]	Repolarization/Refractoriness[b]	Automaticity[b]
IA	Quinidine Procainamide Disopyramide	↓	↑	↓
IB	Lidocaine Mexiletine	0/↓	↓/0	↓
IC	Flecainide Propafenone	↓↓	0	↓
II	β-blockers[c] Acebutolol Atenolol Betaxolol Bisoprolol Carteolol Carvedilol[d] Esmolol Labetalol[d] Metoprolol Nadolol Nebivolol Penbutolol Pindolol Propranolol Timolol	0	0	0
III	Amiodarone[e] Dofetilide Dronedarone[e] Ibutilide Sotalol	0	↑	0
IV	CCBs[c] Diltiazem Verapamil	0	0	0

CCB, calcium channel blocker; ↑, increase/prolong; ↓, decrease; 0, no effect; 0/↓, does not change or may decrease: ↓/0, decreases or does not change.

[a]Adenosine and digoxin are agents used for the management of arrhythmias that do not fit into the Vaughan Williams classification.

[b]In ventricular tissue only; effects may differ in atria, sinus node, or atrioventricular node.

[c]Slow conduction, prolong refractory period, and reduce automaticity in sinoatrial node and atrioventricular node tissue but generally not in the ventricles.

[d]Combined α- and β-blockers.

[e]Amiodarone and dronedarone also slow conduction velocity and inhibit automaticity.

indicates the location of the electrophysiological abnormality resulting in the arrhythmia (sinus, AV node, atrial, or ventricular), and the second describes the arrhythmia as abnormally slow (bradycardia) or fast (tachycardia), or the type of arrhythmia (block, fibrillation, or flutter).

SUPRAVENTRICULAR ARRHYTHMIAS

Sinus Bradycardia

Sinus bradycardia, originating in the SA node, is defined by a sinus rate less than 60 beats/min.[8]

▶ *Epidemiology and Etiology*

Many individuals, particularly those who engage in regular vigorous exercise, have resting heart rates less than 60 beats/min. For those individuals, sinus bradycardia is normal and healthy, and it does not require evaluation or treatment. However, some individuals may develop symptomatic sinus node dysfunction. In the absence of correctable underlying causes, idiopathic sinus node dysfunction is referred to as sick sinus syndrome and occurs with greater frequency in association with advancing age.[8] The prevalence of sick sinus syndrome is approximately 1 in 600 individuals older than 65 years.[8] Sinus node dysfunction may also manifest as the bradycardia-tachycardia syndrome (also known as tachy-brady syndrome), characterized by alternating periods of supraventricular tachyarrhythmias and bradycardia.[8,9]

Sick sinus syndrome leading to sinus bradycardia may be caused by degenerative changes in the sinus node that occur with advancing age. KEY CONCEPT *However, there are other possible etiologies of sinus bradycardia, including drugs* (Table 9–2).[8–10]

Table 9–2

Etiologies of Sinus Bradycardia[8–10]

Idiopathic ("sick sinus syndrome")
Myocardial ischemia
Carotid sinus hypersensitivity
Neurocardiac syncope
Electrolyte abnormalities: hypokalemia or hyperkalemia
Hypothyroidism
Hypothermia
Amyloidosis
Sarcoidosis
Systemic lupus erythematosus
Scleroderma
Sleep apnea
Drugs:

Adenosine	Fluoxetine
Amiodarone	Halothane
β-blockers	Isradipine
Cisplatin	Ketamine
Citalopram	Neostigmine
Clonidine	Nicardipine
Cocaine	Nitroglycerin
Dexmedetomidine	Paclitaxel
Digoxin	Propafenone
Diltiazem	Propofol
Dipyridamole	Remifentanil
Disopyramide	Sotalol
Donepezil	Succinylcholine
Dronedarone	Thalidomide
Flecainide	Verapamil

Clinical Presentation and Diagnosis of Sinus Bradycardia

Symptoms

- Many patients are asymptomatic, particularly those with normal resting heart rates less than 60 beats/min as a result of physical fitness due to regular vigorous exercise
- Susceptible patients may develop symptoms, depending on the degree of heart rate lowering
- Symptoms include dizziness, fatigue, light-headedness, syncope, chest pain (in patients with underlying coronary artery disease [CAD]), and shortness of breath and other symptoms of HF (in patients with underlying LV dysfunction)

Diagnosis

- Cannot be made on the basis of symptoms alone because the symptoms of all bradyarrhythmias are similar
- History of present illness, presenting symptoms, and 12-lead ECG that reveals sinus bradycardia
- Assess possible correctable etiologies, including myocardial ischemia, serum potassium concentration (for hyperkalemia), thyroid function tests (for hypothyroidism)
- Determine whether patient is taking any drugs known to cause sinus bradycardia. If the patient is currently taking digoxin, determine the serum digoxin concentration and ascertain whether it is supratherapeutic (greater than 2 ng/mL [2.6 nmol/L])

► *Pathophysiology*

Sick sinus syndrome leading to sinus bradycardia occurs as a result of fibrotic tissue in the SA node, which replaces normal SA node tissue.[8]

► *Treatment*

Desired Outcomes Desired outcomes of treatment are to restore normal heart rate and alleviate patient symptoms.

Pharmacologic Therapy Treatment of sinus bradycardia is only necessary in patients who become symptomatic. KEY CONCEPT *If the patient is taking any medication(s) that may cause symptomatic sinus bradycardia, they should be discontinued whenever possible.* If the patient remains in sinus bradycardia after drug discontinuation and after five half-lives of the drug(s) have elapsed, then the drugs(s) can usually be excluded as the etiology of the arrhythmia. In certain circumstances, however, discontinuation may be undesirable, even if the drug may be the cause of symptomatic sinus bradycardia. For example, if the patient has a history of MI or HFrEF, discontinuation of a β-blocker may be necessary in the short term but undesirable long term because β-blockers have been shown to reduce mortality and prolong life in patients with those diseases, and benefits of therapy with β-blockers outweigh the risks associated with sinus bradycardia. In this situation, clinicians and patients may elect to implant a permanent pacemaker to allow continuation of therapy with β-blockers.

Acute treatment of the symptomatic and/or hemodynamically unstable patient with sinus bradycardia includes administration of the anticholinergic drug atropine, which should be given in doses of 0.5 mg intravenous (IV) every 3 to 5 minutes. The maximum recommended total dose of atropine is 3 mg.[11] Atropine is generally used as a method of achieving acute symptom control while awaiting placement of a transcutaneous or transvenous pacemaker. Where necessary, transcutaneous pacing can be initiated during atropine administration. Atropine should be used cautiously in patients with myocardial ischemia or MI because increasing heart rate and myocardial oxygen demand may aggravate ischemia or extend the infarct.

In patients with hemodynamically unstable sinus bradycardia unresponsive to atropine, transcutaneous pacing may be initiated. In patients with hemodynamically unstable or severely symptomatic sinus bradycardia unresponsive to atropine and in whom temporary or transvenous pacing is not available or is ineffective, or while awaiting placement of a pacemaker, dopamine (2–10 mcg/kg/min, titrate to response), epinephrine (2–10 mcg/min, titrate to response), or isoproterenol (2–10 mcg/min, titrate to response) may be administered to increase heart rate.[11]

In patients with sinus bradycardia due to underlying correctable disorders (such as electrolyte abnormalities or hypothyroidism), management consists of correcting those disorders.

Nonpharmacologic Therapy Long-term management of patients with sick sinus syndrome requires implantation of a permanent pacemaker.[8]

► *Outcome Evaluation*

- Monitor the patient's heart rate and alleviation of symptoms.
- Monitor for adverse effects of medications such as atropine (dry mouth, mydriasis, urinary retention, and tachycardia).

AV Nodal Block

AV nodal block occurs when conduction of electrical impulses through the AV node is impaired to varying degrees. AV nodal block is classified into three categories. First-degree (1°) AV block is defined simply as prolongation of the PR interval to greater than 0.2 seconds. During 1° AV block, all impulses initiated by the SA node resulting in atrial depolarization are conducted through the AV node; the abnormality is simply that the impulses are conducted more slowly than normal, resulting in prolongation of the PR interval.[9] Second-degree (2°) AV block is further distinguished into two types: Mobitz type I (also known as Wenckebach) and Mobitz type II. In both types, some of the impulses initiated by the SA node are not conducted through the AV node. This often occurs in a regular pattern; for example, there may be absence of AV nodal conduction of every third or fourth impulse generated by the SA node. During third-degree (3°) AV block, which is also referred to as "complete heart block," none of the impulses generated by the SA node are conducted through the AV node. This results in AV dissociation, during which the atria continue to depolarize normally as a result of normal impulses initiated by the SA node; however, the ventricles initiate their own depolarizations because no SA node–generated impulses are conducted to the ventricles. Therefore, on the ECG, there is no relationship (dissociation) between the P waves and the QRS complexes.

▸ *Epidemiology and Etiology*

Overall incidence of AV nodal block is unknown. AV nodal block may be caused by degenerative changes in the AV node. KEY CONCEPT *In addition, there are many other possible etiologies of AV nodal block including drugs* (Table 9–3).[8–10]

▸ *Pathophysiology*

1° AV nodal block is due to inhibition of conduction within the upper portion of the node.[11] Mobitz type I 2° AV nodal block results from inhibition of conduction further down within the node.[8,9] Mobitz type II 2° AV nodal block is caused by inhibition of conduction within or below the level of the bundle of His.[8,9] 3° AV nodal block may be a result of inhibition of conduction either within the AV node or within the bundle of His or the His-Purkinje system.[8,9] AV nodal block may occur as a result of age-related AV node degeneration.

Clinical Presentation and Diagnosis of AV Nodal Block

Symptoms

- 1° AV nodal block is rarely symptomatic because it rarely results in bradycardia
- 2° AV nodal block may cause bradycardia because not all impulses generated by the SA node are conducted through the AV node to the ventricles
- In 3° AV nodal block, or complete heart block, the heart rate is often 30 to 40 beats/min, resulting in symptoms
- Symptoms consist of dizziness, fatigue, light-headedness, syncope, chest pain (in patients with underlying coronary artery disease [CAD]), and shortness of breath and other symptoms of HF (in patients with underlying HF)

Diagnosis

- Made on the basis of patient presentation, including history of present illness and presenting symptoms, as well as a 12-lead ECG that reveals AV nodal block
- Assess potentially correctable etiologies, including myocardial ischemia, serum potassium concentration (for hyperkalemia), and thyroid function tests (for hypothyroidism)
- Determine whether the patient is taking any drugs known to cause AV nodal block
- If the patient is currently taking digoxin, determine the serum digoxin concentration and ascertain whether it is supratherapeutic (greater than 2 ng/mL [2.6 nmol/L])

Table 9–3

Etiologies of AV Nodal Block[8–10]

Idiopathic degeneration of the AV node	
Myocardial ischemia or infarction	
Neurocardiac syncope	
Carotid sinus hypersensitivity	
Electrolyte abnormalities: hypokalemia or hyperkalemia	
Hypothyroidism	
Hypothermia	
Infectious diseases: Chagas disease or endocarditis	
Amyloidosis	
Sarcoidosis	
Systemic lupus erythematosus	
Scleroderma	
Sleep apnea	
Drugs:	
Adenosine	Hydroxychloroquine
Amiodarone	Paclitaxel
β-blockers	Phenylpropanolamine
Bupivacaine	Propafenone
Carbamazepine	Propofol
Chloroquine	Sotalol
Digoxin	Thioridazine
Diltiazem	Tricyclic antidepressants
Dronedarone	Verapamil
Flecainide	

AV, atrioventricular.

▸ *Treatment*

Desired Outcomes Desired outcomes of treatment are to restore normal sinus rhythm and alleviate patient symptoms.

Pharmacologic Therapy Treatment of 1° AV nodal block is rarely necessary because symptoms rarely occur. However, the ECGs of patients with 1° AV nodal block should be monitored to assess the possibility of progression of 1° AV nodal block to 2° or 3° block. 2° or 3° AV nodal block requires treatment because bradycardia often results in symptoms. If the patient is taking any medication(s) that may cause AV nodal block, the drug(s) should be discontinued whenever possible. If the patient's rhythm still exhibits AV nodal block after discontinuing the medication(s) and after five half-lives of the drug(s) have elapsed, then the drug(s) can usually be excluded as the etiology of the arrhythmia. However, in certain circumstances, discontinuation of a medication that is inducing AV nodal block may be undesirable. For example, if the patient has a history of MI or HFrEF, discontinuation of a β-blocker is undesirable because β-blockers have been shown to reduce mortality and prolong life in patients with those diseases, and the benefits of therapy with β-blockers outweigh the risks associated with AV nodal block.

In these patients, clinicians and patients may elect to implant a permanent pacemaker to allow the patient to continue therapy with β-blockers.

Acute treatment of patients with 2° or 3° AV nodal block consists primarily of administration of atropine, which may be administered in the same doses as recommended for management of sinus bradycardia. In patients with hemodynamically unstable or severely symptomatic AV nodal block that is unresponsive to atropine and in whom temporary or transvenous pacing is not available or is ineffective, epinephrine (2–10 mcg/min, titrate to response) and/or dopamine (2–10 mcg/kg/min) may be administered.[11]

In patients with 2° or 3° AV block due to underlying correctable disorders (such as electrolyte abnormalities or hypothyroidism), management consists of correcting those disorders.

Nonpharmacologic Therapy Long-term treatment of patients with 2° or 3° AV nodal block due to idiopathic AV node degeneration requires implantation of a permanent pacemaker.[8]

▶ *Outcome Evaluation*

- Monitor the patient for termination of AV nodal block and restoration of normal sinus rhythm, heart rate, and alleviation of symptoms.
- If atropine is administered, monitor the patient for adverse effects, including dry mouth, mydriasis, urinary retention, and tachycardia.

Atrial Fibrillation

AF is the most common arrhythmia encountered in clinical practice. It is important for clinicians to understand AF because it is associated with substantial morbidity and mortality, and because many strategies for drug therapy are available. Some drugs used to treat AF have a narrow therapeutic index and a broad adverse effect profile.

▶ *Epidemiology and Etiology*

Approximately 2.2 million Americans have AF, and as many as 4.5 million in the European Union. The prevalence of AF increases with advancing age; roughly 8% of patients between the ages of 80 and 89 years have AF.[12] Similarly, the incidence of AF increases with age, and it occurs more commonly in men than women.[12]

Etiologies of AF are presented in Table 9–4.[12–17] The common feature of the majority of etiologies of AF is the development of left atrial hypertrophy. Hypertension may be the most important risk factor for development of AF. However, AF also occurs commonly in patients with CAD. In addition, HF is increasingly recognized as a cause of AF; approximately 25% to 30% of patients with New York Heart Association (NYHA) class III HF have AF,[13] and the arrhythmia is present in as many as 50% of patients with NYHA class IV HF.[14]

Drug-induced AF is relatively uncommon but has been reported (see Table 9–4).[10,15,16] Acute ingestion of large amounts of alcohol may cause AF; this phenomenon has been referred to as the "holiday heart" syndrome.[15] Recent evidence suggests that chronic moderate alcohol intake also may be associated with an increased risk of AF. In addition, recent reports have associated use of some bisphosphonate drugs with new-onset AF.[16] The potential relationship between bisphosphonate use and new-onset AF requires further study.

Table 9–4

Etiologies of AF[12–17]

Hypertension
Coronary artery disease
Heart failure
Diabetes
Hyperthyroidism
Rheumatic heart disease
Diseases of the heart valves:
Mitral stenosis or regurgitation
Mitral valve prolapse
Acute myocardial infarction
Obesity
Sleep apnea
Pericarditis
Amyloidosis
Myocarditis
Pulmonary embolism
Idiopathic ("lone" AF)
Familial AF
Genetic predisposition
Thoracic surgery:
Coronary artery bypass graft surgery
Pulmonary resection
Thoracoabdominal esophagectomy
Drugs:
Adenosine
Albuterol
Alcohol
Alendronate
Dobutamine
Enoximone
Ipratropium bromide
Methylprednisolone
Milrinone
Mitoxantrone
Paclitaxel
Propafenone
Theophylline
Verapamil
Zoledronic acid

AF, atrial fibrillation.

▶ *Pathophysiology*

KEY CONCEPT *AF may be caused by both abnormal impulse formation and abnormal impulse conduction.* Traditionally, AF was believed to be initiated by premature impulses initiated in the atria. However, it is now understood that in many patients AF is triggered by electrical impulses generated within the pulmonary veins.[18] These impulses initiate the process of reentry within the atria, and AF is believed to be sustained by multiple reentrant wavelets operating simultaneously within the atria. Some believe that, at least in some patients, the increased automaticity in the pulmonary veins may be the sole mechanism of AF and that the multiple reentrant wavelet hypothesis may be incorrect. However, the concept of multiple simultaneous reentrant wavelets remains the predominant hypothesis regarding the mechanism of AF.[19]

AF leads to electrical remodeling of the atria. Episodes of AF that are of longer duration and occur with increasing frequency result in progressive shortening of atrial refractory periods, further potentiating atrial reentry.[20] Therefore, it is often said that "atrial fibrillation begets atrial fibrillation"; that is, AF causes atrial electrophysiologic alterations that further promote AF.[19,20]

Patient Encounter, Part 1

A 67-year-old man presents to the emergency department (ED) complaining that he can feel his heart fluttering and pounding in his chest. He states that this started several hours ago, and he waited to see if it would stop, but it has not. He also complains of feeling light-headed and says that he "nearly passed out." His pulse is irregular, with a rate of 145 beats/min.

What information is suggestive of AF?

What additional information do you need to develop a treatment plan?

AF is associated with chaotic, disorganized atrial electrical activity, resulting in no completed atrial depolarizations and therefore no atrial contraction.

AF occurs when structural and/or electrophysiologic abnormalities occur that promote abnormal atrial automaticity and/or reentry.[17] Structural abnormalities of the atria may include fibrosis, dilation, ischemia, infiltration, and hypertrophy.[17] Other contributing factors may include inflammation, oxidative stress, activation of the renin-angiotensin-aldosterone system, autonomic nervous system activation, and variants in myocardial ion channels and those leading to cardiomyopathy.[17]

A substantial amount of the atrial electrical activity occurring during AF is conducted through the AV node into the ventricles, resulting in ventricular rates ranging from 100 to 200 beats/min.

AF is categorized into specific classifications.[17] Paroxysmal AF is defined as that which terminates spontaneously or with interventions within 7 days of onset.[17] Patients with paroxysmal AF have episodes that begin suddenly and spontaneously, last minutes to hours, or sometimes as long as 7 days, and often terminate suddenly and spontaneously. Episodes may recur with variable frequency. Persistent AF is defined as continued AF that lasts longer than 7 days.[17] Long-standing persistent AF is defined as continuous AF lasting 12 months or longer.[17] The term permanent AF is used when patient and clinician jointly decide to terminate further attempts to restore and/or maintain sinus rhythm.[17] Acceptance of AF represents a therapeutic attitude from the patient and clinician, rather than a pathophysiological feature of the AF, and may change as symptoms, efficacy of treatments, and patient and clinician preferences develop and evolve.[17]

AF is associated with substantial morbidity and mortality. This arrhythmia is associated with a risk of ischemic stroke of approximately 5% per year.[21] The risk of stroke is increased two- to sevenfold in patients with AF compared to patients without this arrhythmia.[21] AF is the cause of roughly one of every six strokes. During AF, atrial contraction is absent. Because atrial contraction is responsible for approximately 30% of LV filling, this blood that is not ejected from the left atrium to the left ventricle pools in the atrium, particularly in the left atrial appendage. Blood pooling facilitates the formation of a thrombus, which subsequently may travel through the mitral valve into the left ventricle and may be ejected during ventricular contraction. The thrombus then may travel through a carotid artery into the brain, resulting in an ischemic stroke. Patients with AF are also at increased risk for systemic thromboembolism.

AF is associated with a threefold increase in the risk of HF as a result of tachycardia-induced cardiomyopathy.[17] AF increases the risk of dementia and mortality approximately twofold compared to patients without AF;[17] causes of death are likely stroke or HF.

Clinical Presentation and Diagnosis of AF

Symptoms

- Approximately 20% to 30% of patients with AF remain asymptomatic
- Symptoms include palpitations, dizziness, light-headedness, shortness of breath, chest pain (if underlying CAD is present), near-syncope, and syncope. Patients commonly complain of palpitations; often the complaint is "I can feel my heart beating fast" or "I can feel my heart fluttering" or "It feels like my heart is going to beat out of my chest"
- Other symptoms depend on the degree to which cardiac output is diminished, which in turn depends on ventricular rate and the degree to which stroke volume is reduced by the rapidly beating heart
- In some patients, the first symptom of AF is stroke

Diagnosis

- Because symptoms of all tachyarrhythmias depend on heart rate and are therefore essentially the same, the diagnosis depends on the presence of AF on the ECG
- AF is characterized on ECG by an absence of P waves, an undulating baseline that represents chaotic atrial electrical activity, and an irregularly irregular rhythm, meaning the intervals between the R waves are irregular and there is no pattern to the irregularity
- AF is sometime first diagnosed in patients presenting with ischemic stroke

▶ *Treatment*

Desired Outcomes KEY CONCEPT *The goals of individualized therapy for AF are: (a) ventricular rate control; (b) termination of AF and restoration of sinus rhythm (commonly referred to as "cardioversion" or "conversion to sinus rhythm"); (c) maintenance of sinus rhythm, or reduction in the frequency of episodes of paroxysmal AF; and/or (d) prevention of stroke and systemic thromboembolism.* These goals of therapy do not necessarily apply to all patients; the specific goal(s) that apply depend on the patient's AF classification (Table 9–5).

Hemodynamically Unstable AF For patients who present with an episode of AF that is hemodynamically unstable, emergent conversion to sinus rhythm is necessary using direct current cardioversion (DCC). Hemodynamic instability may be defined as the presence of any one of the following: (a) acutely altered mental status; (b) hypotension (systolic blood pressure less than 90 mm Hg) or other signs of shock; (c) ischemic chest discomfort; and/or (d) acute HF.[11]

DCC is the process of administering a synchronized electrical shock to the chest. The purpose of DCC is to simultaneously depolarize all of the myocardial cells, resulting in interruption and termination of the multiple reentrant circuits and restoration of normal sinus rhythm. The recommended initial energy level for conversion of AF to sinus rhythm is 120 to 200 joules (J)

Table 9–5

Treatment Goals According to AF Classification

Paroxysmal AF	Persistent AF	Long-Standing Persistent AF	Permanent AF
Ventricular rate control Prevention of thromboembolism Maintenance of sinus rhythm *if ventricular rate control is not sufficient to control symptoms*	Ventricular rate control Prevention of thromboembolism Conversion to sinus rhythm	Ventricular rate control Prevention of thromboembolism Conversion to sinus rhythm	Ventricular rate control Prevention of thromboembolism

AF, atrial fibrillation.

for biphasic shocks or 200 J for monophasic shocks. If the DCC attempt is unsuccessful, DCC energy should be increased in a stepwise fashion.[11] Delivery of the shock is synchronized to the ECG by the cardioverter machine, such that the electrical charge is not delivered during the latter portion of the T wave (ie, the relative refractory period), to avoid delivering an electrical impulse that may be conducted abnormally, which may result in a life-threatening ventricular arrhythmia.

The remainder of this section is devoted to pharmacologic management of hemodynamically stable AF.

Ventricular Rate Control Ventricular rate control can be achieved by inhibiting the proportion of electrical impulses conducted from the atria to the ventricles through the AV node. Therefore, drugs that are effective for ventricular rate control are those that inhibit AV nodal impulse conduction: β-blockers, diltiazem, verapamil, digoxin, and amiodarone (Tables 9–6[17] and 9–7).

In patients who present to the emergency department (ED) with an episode of symptomatic persistent AF or paroxysmal AF for which intervention is desired, ventricular rate control is usually initially achieved using IV drugs. A decision algorithm for selecting a specific drug for ventricular rate control is presented in Figure 9–4.[17] In general, an IV CCB or β-blocker is preferred for ventricular rate control in patients with normal LV function because ventricular rate control can often be achieved within several minutes. In patients with HFrEF, IV diltiazem and verapamil should be avoided, as these drugs confer negative inotropic effects and may exacerbate HFrEF.[17,21] In patients with HFrEF, an IV β-blocker may be administered, but only following stabilization of acute decompensated HF, due to the potential for acute HF exacerbation. IV digoxin is also a therapeutic option for patients with HFrEF.

For patients with paroxysmal or permanent AF requiring long-term rate control with oral medications, the treatment algorithm is the same (see Figure 9–4). In general, although digoxin is effective for ventricular rate control in patients at rest, it is less effective than CCBs or β-blockers for ventricular rate control in patients undergoing physical activity, including activities of daily living. This is likely because activation of the sympathetic nervous system during exercise and activity overwhelms the stimulating effect of digoxin on the parasympathetic nervous system. It should be noted that some recent evidence suggests that digoxin therapy may be independently associated with an increased risk of mortality in patients with AF.[22] These data should be considered hypothesis-generating, and the influence of digoxin on mortality in patients with AF requires study in a prospective, randomized trial. Overall, in patients with normal LV function, CCBs or β-blockers are preferred for long-term ventricular rate control. Diltiazem may be preferable to verapamil in older patients due to a lower incidence of constipation. However, in patients with HFrEF, oral diltiazem and verapamil are contraindicated as a result of their negative inotropic activity and propensity to exacerbate HFrEF. Therefore, the options in this population are β-blockers or digoxin. Most patients with HFrEF should be receiving therapy with an oral β-blocker with the goal of achieving mortality risk reduction. In patients with HFrEF who develop rapid AF while receiving therapy with β-blockers, digoxin can be administered for purposes of ventricular rate control. Fortunately, studies have found the combination of digoxin and β-blockers to be effective for ventricular rate control, likely as a result of β-blocker–induced attenuation of the inhibitory effects of the sympathetic nervous system on the efficacy of digoxin.

Conversion to Sinus Rhythm Termination of AF in hemodynamically stable patients may be performed using antiarrhythmic drug therapy or elective DCC. Drugs that may be used for conversion to sinus rhythm are presented in Table 9–8;[17] these agents slow atrial conduction velocity and/or prolong

Patient Encounter, Part 2: Medical History, Physical Examination, and Diagnostic Tests

PMH: Hypertension × 19 years; Myocardial infarction 4 years ago

Meds: Aspirin 81 mg once daily; lisinopril 20 mg orally once daily; metoprolol tartrate 50 mg orally twice daily

PE:

Ht 5′9″ (175 cm), Wt 88 kg (194 lb), BP 95/58 mm Hg, P 145 beats/min, RR 18 breaths/min; remainder of physical examination noncontributory

Labs: All within normal limits. Serum creatinine 1.1 mg/dL (97 μmol/L)

CXR: No pulmonary edema

ECG: Atrial fibrillation

What is your assessment of the patient's condition?

What are your treatment goals?

What pharmacologic or nonpharmacologic alternatives are available for each treatment goal?

Table 9–6

Drugs for Ventricular Rate Control in AF[17]

Drug	Mechanism of Action	Intravenous Administration	Usual Oral Maintenance Dose	Drug Interactions
Amiodarone	β-blocker CCB	300 mg over 1 hour, then 10–50 mg/hour over 24 hours via continuous infusion	100–200 mg po once daily	Inhibits clearance of digoxin, warfarin, some statins, and other drugs
β-blockers[a]	Inhibit AV nodal conduction by slowing AV nodal conduction and prolonging AV nodal refractoriness	Esmolol 500 mcg/kg over 1 minute, then 50–300 mcg/kg/min continuous infusion Propranolol 1 mg over 1 minute, up to 3 doses at 2 minute intervals Metoprolol tartrate 2.5–5 mg over 2 minutes; up to 3 doses	Atenolol 25–100 mg once daily Bisoprolol 2.5–10 mg once daily Carvedilol 3.125–25 mg twice daily Metoprolol tartrate 25–100 mg twice daily Metoprolol XL (succinate) 50–400 mg once daily Nadolol 10–240 mg once daily Propranolol 10–40 mg three or four times daily	
Diltiazem	Inhibits AV nodal conduction by slowing AV nodal conduction and prolonging AV nodal refractoriness	0.25-mg/kg bolus over 2 minutes, then 5–15 mg/hour continuous infusion	120–360 mg once daily (extended release)	Increases carbamazepine, cyclosporine, midazolam, triazolam, theophylline, atorvastatin, cerivastatin, lovastatin, simvastatin concentrations Cimetidine, ranitidine, diazepam, grapefruit juice may increase serum diltiazem concentrations Dantrolene (combination may lead to ventricular arrhythmias)
Verapamil	Inhibits AV nodal conduction by slowing AV nodal conduction and prolonging AV nodal refractoriness	0.075–0.15-mg/kg bolus over 2 minutes. If no response after 30 min, may give an additional 10 mg, then 0.005 mg/kg/min continuous infusion	180–480 mg daily (extended release)	Increases digoxin, carbamazepine, cyclosporine, theophylline, atorvastatin, cerivastatin, lovastatin, simvastatin concentrations Dantrolene (combination may lead to ventricular arrhythmias)
Digoxin	Inhibits AV nodal conduction by (a) vagal stimulation (b) directly slowing AV nodal conduction, and (c) prolonging AV nodal refractoriness	0.25 mg every 2 hours, up to 1.5 mg over 24 hours	0.125–0.25 mg once daily	Amiodarone, verapamil inhibit digoxin elimination

AF, atrial fibrillation; AV, atrioventricular; CCB, calcium channel blocker.

[a]Although oral β-blockers are important agents for mortality reduction in patients with heart failure, intravenous β-blockers are generally avoided due to the potential for heart failure exacerbation.

refractoriness, facilitating interruption of reentrant circuits and restoration of sinus rhythm. DCC is generally more effective than drug therapy for conversion of AF to sinus rhythm. However, patients who undergo elective DCC must be sedated and/or anesthetized to avoid the discomfort associated with delivery of 120 to greater than or equal to 200 J of electricity to the chest. Therefore, it is important that patients scheduled to undergo elective DCC do not eat within approximately 8 to 12 hours of the procedure to avoid aspiration of stomach contents during the period of sedation/anesthesia. This often factors into the decision as to whether to use elective DCC or drug therapy for conversion of AF to sinus rhythm. If a patient presents with AF

Table 9–7

Adverse Effects of Drugs Used to Treat Arrhythmias

Drug	Adverse Effects
Adenosine	Chest pain, flushing, shortness of breath, sinus bradycardia/AV block
Amiodarone	IV: Hypotension, sinus bradycardia Oral: Blue-gray skin discoloration, photosensitivity, corneal microdeposits, pulmonary fibrosis, hepatotoxicity, sinus bradycardia, hypo- or hyperthyroidism, peripheral neuropathy, weakness, AV block
Atenolol	Hypotension, bradycardia, AV block, heart failure exacerbation[a]
Atropine	Tachycardia, urinary retention, blurred vision, dry mouth, mydriasis
Bisoprolol	Hypotension, bradycardia, AV block, heart failure exacerbation[a]
Carvedilol	Hypotension, bradycardia, AV block, heart failure exacerbation[a]
Digoxin	Nausea, vomiting, anorexia, green-yellow halos around objects, ventricular arrhythmias
Diltiazem	Hypotension, sinus bradycardia, heart failure exacerbation, AV block
Dofetilide	Torsades de pointes
Dronedarone	Diarrhea, asthenia, nausea and vomiting, abdominal pain, bradycardia, GI distress, hepatotoxicity
Esmolol	Hypotension, sinus bradycardia, AV block, heart failure exacerbation
Flecainide	Dizziness, blurred vision, heart failure exacerbation
Ibutilide	Torsades de pointes
Metoprolol	Hypotension, sinus bradycardia, AV block, fatigue, heart failure exacerbation[a]
Mexiletine	Nausea, vomiting, GI distress, tremor, dizziness, fatigue, seizures (if dose too high)
Nadolol	Hypotension, bradycardia, AV block, heart failure exacerbation[a]
Procainamide	Hypotension, torsades de pointes
Propafenone	Dizziness, blurred vision
Propranolol	Hypotension, bradycardia, AV block, heart failure exacerbation[a]
Sotalol	Sinus bradycardia, AV block, fatigue, torsades de pointes
Verapamil	Hypotension, heart failure exacerbation, bradycardia, AV block, constipation (oral)

AV, atrioventricular; GI, gastrointestinal; IV, intravenous.

[a]Associated with intravenous administration (metoprolol, propranolol), inappropriately high oral doses at initiation of therapy, or overly aggressive and rapid dose titration.

requiring nonemergent conversion to sinus rhythm, and the patient has eaten a meal that day, then pharmacologic conversion methods must be used on that day, or DCC must be postponed to the following day to allow for a period of fasting prior to the procedure.

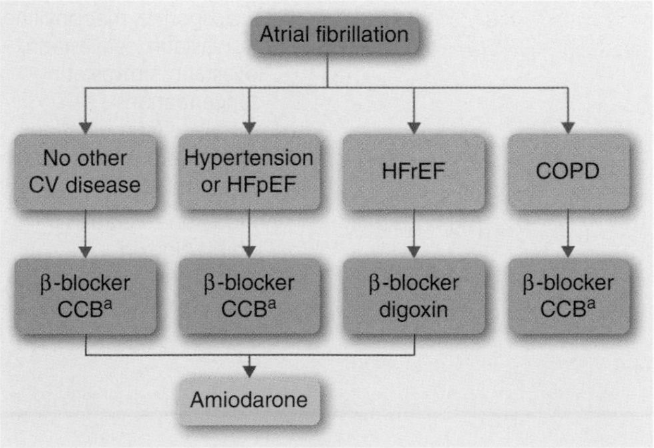

FIGURE 9–4. Decision algorithm for selecting drug therapy for ventricular rate control. (Adapted with permission from January CT, Wann LS, Alpert JS, et al. 2014 AHA/ACC/HRS guideline for the management of patients with atrial fibrillation. J Am Coll Cardiol 2014; dpi: 10.1016/j.jacc.2014.03.022). [a]When administered intravenously, diltiazem is generally preferred over verapamil because of a lower risk of severe hypotension. CCB, calcium channel blocker (diltiazem or verapamil); COPD, chronic obstructive pulmonary disease; CV, cardiovascular; HFpEF, heart failure with preserved ejection fraction; HFrEF, heart failure with reduced ejection fraction.

A decision strategy for conversion of AF to sinus rhythm is presented in Figure 9–5.[17] The cardioversion decision strategy depends greatly on the duration of AF. If the AF episode began within 48 hours, conversion to sinus rhythm is safe and may be attempted with elective DCC or specific drug therapy (see Figure 9–5). However, if the duration of the AF episode is 48 hours or longer, or if there is uncertainty regarding the duration of the episode, two strategies for conversion may be considered. Data indicate that a thrombus may form in the left atrium during AF episodes of 48 hours or longer; if an atrial thrombus is present, the process of conversion to sinus rhythm, whether with DCC or drugs, can dislodge the atrial thrombus, leading to embolization and a stroke. Therefore, in patients experiencing an AF episode of 48 hours or longer, conversion to sinus rhythm should be deferred unless it is known that an atrial thrombus is not present. One option in patients with AF of duration 48 hours or longer is to anticoagulate with warfarin [maintaining an **international normalized ratio** (INR) of 2–3], dabigatran, rivaroxaban, or apixaban for 3 weeks, after which cardioversion may be performed. Patients should subsequently be anticoagulated for a minimum of 4 weeks following the restoration of sinus rhythm. An alternative approach is, rather than send patients with ongoing AF home for 3 weeks of anticoagulation, to perform a **transesophageal echocardiogram** (TEE) to determine whether an atrial thrombus is present; if such a thrombus is not present, DCC or pharmacologic cardioversion may be performed. If this strategy is selected, hospitalized patients should undergo anticoagulation with IV unfractionated heparin, with the dose targeted to a partial thromboplastin time (PTT) of 60 seconds (range: 50–70 seconds), low molecular weight heparin, or oral anticoagulation therapy with warfarin (target INR: 2.5; range: 2–3), dabigatran, rivaroxaban, or apixaban during the hospitalization

Table 9–8

Drugs for Conversion of AF to Normal Sinus Rhythm[17]

Treatment	IV Administration	Oral Administration	Drug Interactions
Amiodarone	150 mg over 10 minutes, then 1 mg/min for 6 hours, then 0.5 mg/min for 18 hours or change to oral dosing	600–800 mg daily in divided doses up to a total load of 10 g, then maintenance dose of 200 mg daily	Inhibits elimination of digoxin, warfarin, some statins, and other drugs
Dofetilide	Not available IV	CrCl (mL/min)[a,b]: > 60 500 mcg twice daily 40–60 250 mcg twice daily 20–40 125 mcg twice daily < 20 Not recommended	Cimetidine, hydrochlorothiazide, ketoconazole, medroxyprogesterone, promethazine, trimethoprim, verapamil (all inhibit dofetilide elimination)
Flecainide	Not available IV in the United States	200–300 mg × one dose[c]	Quinidine, fluoxetine, tricyclic antidepressants increase flecainide concentrations
Ibutilide	1 mg IV over 10 minutes, followed by a second 1 mg IV dose if necessary. If weight < 60 kg (132 lb), dose should be 0.01 mg/kg	Not available orally	—
Propafenone	Not available IV	450–600 mg × one dose[c]	Quinidine, fluoxetine, tricyclic antidepressants increase propafenone concentrations Increases serum digoxin concentrations Inhibits CYP2C9, inhibits warfarin metabolism

AF, atrial fibrillation; CrCl, creatinine clearance; IV, intravenous.

[a]Creatinine clearance of > 60, 40–60, 20–40, and < 20 mL/min corresponds to > 1.0, 0.67–1.0, 0.33–0.67, and < 0.33 mL/s, respectively.

[b]Dofetilide therapy must be initiated in the hospital, due to the risk of QT interval prolongation that may lead to torsades de pointes.

[c]It is recommended that a β-blocker or nondihydropyridine calcium channel blocker be administered ≥ 30 minutes prior to administering flecainide or propafenone.

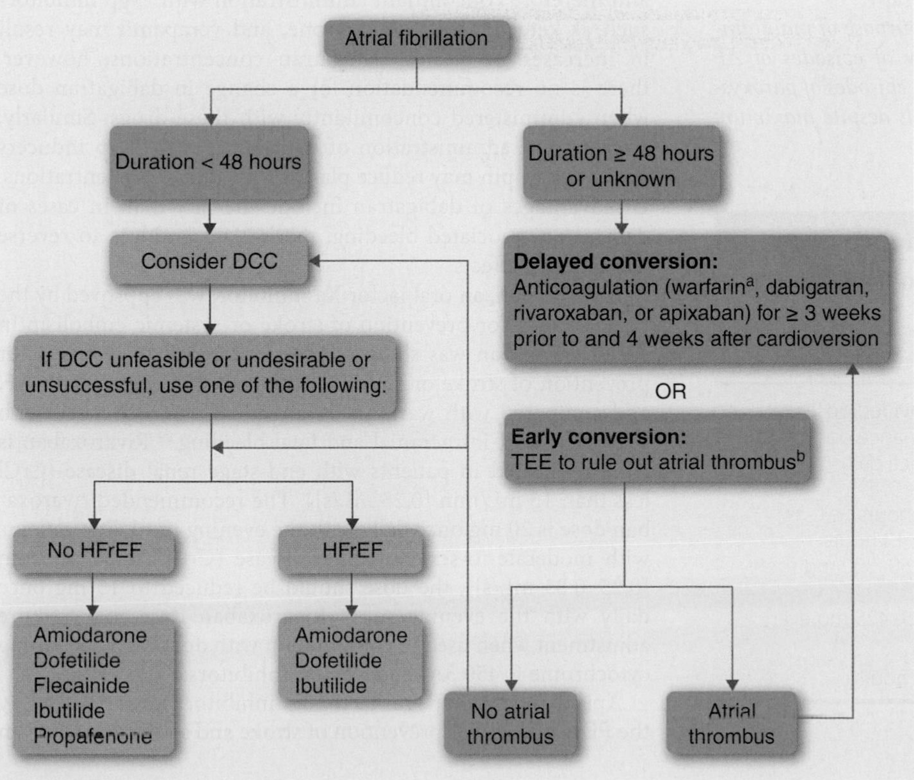

FIGURE 9–5. Decision algorithm for conversion of hemodynamically stable atrial fibrillation to normal sinus rhythm. DCC, direct current cardioversion; HFrEF, heart failure with reduced ejection fraction; TEE, transesophageal echocardiogram [a]International normalized ratio (INR) of 2–3. [b]Anticoagulation must be achieved prior to TEE and maintained for more than or equal to 4 weeks after TEE.

period prior to the TEE and cardioversion procedure. If a thrombus is not present during TEE and cardioversion is successful, patients should maintain oral anticoagulation for at least 4 weeks. If a thrombus is observed during TEE, then cardioversion should be postponed and anticoagulation should be continued indefinitely. Another TEE should be performed prior to a subsequent cardioversion attempt.[17]

Conversion of hemodynamically stable AF to sinus rhythm may be performed in patients with a symptomatic episode of persistent or paroxysmal AF. In patients who have been designated as being in permanent AF, there has been a joint decision by the patient and clinician to terminate further attempts to restore and/or maintain sinus rhythm.[17] Therefore, in patients with permanent AF, conversion to sinus rhythm is not attempted.

Maintenance of Sinus Rhythm/Reduction in the Frequency of Episodes of Paroxysmal AF In many patients, permanent maintenance of sinus rhythm after cardioversion is an unrealistic goal. Many patients experience recurrence of AF after cardioversion. Similarly, in patients with paroxysmal AF, complete maintenance of sinus rhythm without recurrent AF episodes is unrealistic. Therefore, a more realistic goal for many patients is not permanent maintenance of sinus rhythm, but rather reduction in the frequency of episodes of paroxysmal AF. Maintenance of sinus rhythm is more likely to be successful in patients with AF duration of less than 6 months.

In recent years, numerous studies have been performed to determine whether drug therapy for maintenance of sinus rhythm is preferred to drug therapy for ventricular rate control.[23-27] In these studies, patients have been assigned randomly to receive therapy either with drugs for rate control or with drugs for rhythm control (Table 9–9). These studies have found no significant differences in mortality in patients who received rhythm control therapy versus those who received rate control therapy.[23-27] However, patients assigned to the rhythm control strategy were more likely to be hospitalized[23,25-27] and to experience adverse effects associated with drug therapy.[23,24]

KEY CONCEPT *Therefore, drug therapy for the purpose of maintaining sinus rhythm or reducing the frequency of episodes of AF should be initiated only in those patients with episodes of paroxysmal AF who continue to experience symptoms despite maximum tolerated doses of drugs for ventricular rate control.* A decision strategy for maintenance therapy of sinus rhythm is presented in Figure 9–6.[17] Drug therapy for maintenance of sinus rhythm and/or reduction in the frequency of episodes of paroxysmal AF should not be initiated in patients with underlying correctable causes of AF, such as hyperthyroidism; rather, the underlying cause of the arrhythmia should be corrected. Drug therapy for maintenance of sinus rhythm should be discontinued when AF becomes designated as permanent.

Table 9–9

Drugs for Maintenance of Sinus Rhythm/Reduction in the Frequency of Episodes of AF

Drug	Dose
Amiodarone	400–600 mg po in divided doses for 2–4 weeks; maintenance dose 100–200 mg po once daily
Dofetilide	As described in Table 9–8
Dronedarone	400 mg po every 12 hours
Flecainide	50–200 mg po every 12 hours
Propafenone	Immediate release: 150–300 mg every 8 hours Extended release: 225–425 mg every 12 hours
Sotalol	40–160 mg every 12 hours

AF, atrial fibrillation.

Prevention of Stroke and Systemic Thromboembolism Most patients with paroxysmal, persistent, or permanent AF should receive therapy for prevention of thromboembolism unless compelling contraindications exist. A decision strategy for assigning patients to receive anticoagulation for prevention of thromboembolism in AF is presented in Table 9–10.[17] KEY CONCEPT *In general, most patients require oral anticoagulation; however, in patients with nonvalvular AF and a CHA_2DS_2-VASc[28] score of 0, anticoagulation is not recommended.*

The landscape of anticoagulation for stroke prevention in AF has changed with the availability of dabigatran, rivaroxaban, and apixaban. Dabigatran, approved by the Food and Drug Administration (FDA) in October 2010, is a direct thrombin inhibitor for stroke prevention in patients with nonvalvular AF. Dabigatran should not be used in patients with end-stage renal disease (creatinine clearance [CrCl] under 15 mL/min [0.25 mL/s]) or advanced liver disease (impaired baseline clotting function). The recommended dabigatran dose is 150 mg twice daily, except for patients with severe kidney disease (CrCl: 15 to 30 mL/min [0.25–0.50 mL/s]), for whom the recommended dose is 75 mg twice daily. Advantages of dabigatran include the fact that INR monitoring is not required, and the drug's onset of action is rapid, eliminating the need for bridging with unfractionated or low molecular weight heparins. In addition, there is a lower likelihood of drug interactions with dabigatran than with warfarin. Dabigatran is a P-glycoprotein (P-gp) substrate, and therefore concomitant administration with P-gp inhibitors such as ketoconazole, amiodarone, and verapamil may result in increases in plasma dabigatran concentrations; however, there is no recommendation for a change in dabigatran dose when administered concomitantly with these drugs. Similarly, concomitant administration of dabigatran with P-gp inducers such as rifampin may reduce plasma dabigatran concentrations. Disadvantages of dabigatran include the fact that, in cases of dabigatran-associated bleeding, there is no antidote to reverse dabigatran's effects.

Rivaroxaban, an oral factor Xa inhibitor, was approved by the FDA in 2011 for prevention of stroke or systemic embolism in AF. Rivaroxaban was shown to be noninferior to warfarin for prevention of stroke or systemic embolism in patients with AF, and compared with warfarin, rivaroxaban was associated with a lower risk of intracranial and fatal bleeding.[29] Rivaroxaban is contraindicated in patients with end-stage renal disease (CrCl less than 15 mL/min [0.25 mL/s]). The recommended rivaroxaban dose is 20 mg once daily with the evening meal. For patients with moderate-to-severe kidney disease (CrCl 15–50 mL/min [0.25–0.83 mL/s]), the dose should be reduced to 15 mg once daily with the evening meal. Rivaroxaban dose may require adjustment when used in combination with dual P-gp and strong cytochrome P-450 3A4 inducers or inhibitors.

Apixaban, another oral factor Xa inhibitor, was approved by the FDA in 2012 for prevention of stroke and systemic embolism

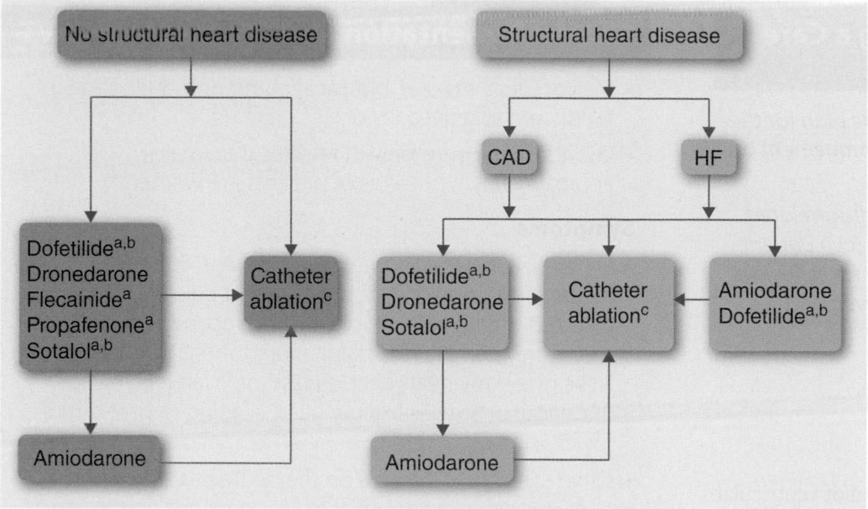

FIGURE 9–6. Decision algorithm for maintenance of sinus rhythm/reduction in the frequency of episodes of atrial fibrillation (AF) for patients with symptomatic paroxysmal or persistent AF despite rate control therapy. (Adapted with permission from January CT, Wann LS, Alpert JS, et al. 2014 AHA/ACC/HRS guideline for the management of patients with atrial fibrillation. J Am Coll Cardiol 2014; dpi: 10.1016/j.jacc.2014.03.022). Drugs are listed alphabetically, not in order of preference. CAD, coronary artery disease; HF, heart failure. [a]Not recommended in patients with severe left ventricular hypertrophy. [b]Should be used cautiously in patients at risk for torsades de pointes. [c]Catheter ablation is only recommended as first-line therapy in patients with paroxysmal AF and is recommended depending on patient preference when performed at experienced centers.

Table 9–10

American Heart Association/American College of Cardiology/Heart Rhythm Society Recommendations for Prevention of Thromboembolism in Patients with Nonvalvular AF[a,17]

CHA_2DS_2-VASc Score	Recommended Stroke Prevention Strategy
0	Antithrombotic therapy is not recommended
1	No antithrombotic therapy or treatment with an oral anticoagulant or aspirin may be considered
≥ 2	Oral anticoagulation recommended. Options include: Warfarin (INR: 2.0–3.0) Dabigatran Rivaroxaban Apixaban

CHA_2DS_2-VASc score calculated as follows:[28]

Congestive heart failure	1 point
Hypertension	1 point
Age ≥ 75 years	2 points
Diabetes mellitus	1 point
History of **s**troke, TIA or thromboembolism	2 points
Vascular disease (prior MI, PAD or aortic plaque)	1 point
Age 65–74 years	1 point
Female **s**ex	1 point
Maximum score	9 points

[a]Patients with AF who have mechanical heart valves should receive warfarin titrated to an INR of 2.0–3.0 or 2.5–3.5 depending on the type and location of the prosthetic heart valve.

AF, atrial fibrillation; INR, international normalized ratio; MI, myocardial infarction; PAD, peripheral arterial disease; TIA, transient ischemic attack.

in patients with AF. Apixaban may be superior to warfarin for prevention of stroke or systemic embolism in patients with AF, with lower bleeding risk.[30] The recommended dose of apixaban is 5 mg orally twice daily. In patients with moderate kidney disease (CrCl 30–50 mL/min [0.50–0.83 mL/s]), the dose should be reduced to 2.5 mg orally twice daily. There are no data or dosage recommendations for patients with CrCl less than 30 mL/min (0.50 mL/s). Apixaban dose should be reduced to 2.5 mg orally twice daily when any two of the following characteristics are present: serum creatinine greater than 1.5 mg/dL (133 μmol/L), 80 years of age or older, body weight less than or equal to 60 kg (132 lb). Apixaban should not be administered to patients with severe liver disease.

For patients for whom warfarin is preferred over other oral anticoagulants (such as in patients with mechanical prosthetic heart valves, those with valvular AF, and patients with end-stage renal disease), specific genetic tests to guide the initiation of therapy have been approved by the FDA. These tests assess single nucleotide polymorphisms of the gene that encodes cytochrome P-450 2C19, the primary hepatic enzyme responsible for warfarin metabolism, and the gene *VKORC1*, which encodes vitamin K epoxide reductase, the enzyme that is inhibited by warfarin as its mechanism of anticoagulation. Some advocate that all patients in whom warfarin therapy is being initiated should undergo genetic testing to guide the initiation of therapy; patients with specific polymorphisms of one or both of these genes may require adjustment of the initial warfarin dose to achieve adequate anticoagulation or avoid over-anticoagulation and toxicity.[31] Genetic testing to guide the initiation of warfarin therapy has not yet become standard practice, and many have questioned the efficacy and cost effectiveness of incorporation of routine genetic testing into warfarin therapy. The role of routine genetic testing in selecting initial warfarin doses is likely to continue to evolve but at the present time appears limited.

Algorithms for estimating the initial dose of warfarin have been developed incorporating clinical and pharmacogenetic information.[32,33] One widely used algorithm, which provides warfarin dose computations with clinical data even if pharmacogenetic information is not obtainable, is available at http://www.warfarindosing.org.

Patient Encounter, Part 3: Creating a Care Plan

Based on the information presented, create a care plan for the patient's acute AF episode and for long-term management of his AF.

Your plan should include (a) a statement of the drug-related needs and/or problems, (b) the goals of therapy, (c) a patient-specific detailed therapeutic plan, and (d) a plan for follow-up to determine whether the goals have been achieved and adverse effects avoided.

► *Outcome Evaluation*

- Monitor the patient to determine whether the goal of ventricular rate control is met: heart rate less than 80 beats/min for most patients, though a target heart rate of less than 110 beats/min may be reasonable as long as patients remain asymptomatic and LV systolic function is preserved.
- Monitor ECG to assess continued presence of AF and to determine whether conversion to sinus rhythm has occurred.
- In patients receiving warfarin, monitor INR approximately monthly to make sure it is therapeutic (target: 2.5; range: 2.0–3.0).
- Monitor patients for adverse effects of specific drug therapy (see Table 9–7). Monitor patients receiving oral anticoagulation for signs and symptoms of bruising or bleeding.

Clinical Presentation and Diagnosis of PSVT

- May occur at any age, but most commonly during the fourth and fifth decades of life[34]
- Occurs more commonly in females than males; approximately two-thirds of patients are women[34]

Symptoms

- Symptoms include palpitations, dizziness, light-headedness, shortness of breath, chest pain (if underlying CAD is present), near-syncope, and syncope. Patients commonly complain of palpitations; often the complaint is "I can feel my heart beating fast" or "I can feel my heart fluttering" or "It feels like my heart is going to beat out of my chest"
- Other symptoms depend on the degree to which cardiac output is diminished, which in turn depends on the heart rate and degree to which stroke volume is reduced by the rapidly beating heart

Diagnosis

- Because the symptoms of all tachyarrhythmias depend on heart rate and are therefore essentially the same, diagnosis depends on the presence of PSVT on the ECG, characterized by narrow QRS complexes (less than 0.12 seconds). P waves may or may not be visible, depending on heart rate
- PSVT is a regular rhythm and occurs at rates ranging from 100 to 250 beats/min

Paroxysmal Supraventricular Tachycardia

Paroxysmal supraventricular tachycardia (PSVT) is a term that refers to a number of arrhythmias that originate above the ventricles and require atrial or AV nodal tissue for initiation and maintenance.[34] The most common of these arrhythmias is known as AV nodal reentrant tachycardia, in which the arrhythmia is caused by a reentrant circuit that involves the AV node or tissue adjacent to the AV node. Other types of PSVT include the relatively uncommon Wolff-Parkinson-White syndrome, which is caused by reentry through an accessory extra-AV nodal pathway. For the purposes of this section, the term *PSVT* refers to AV nodal reentrant tachycardia.

► *Epidemiology and Etiology*

Although PSVT can occur in patients experiencing myocardial ischemia or MI, it often occurs in young individuals with no history of cardiac disease. The overall incidence of PSVT is unknown.

► *Pathophysiology*

KEY CONCEPT *PSVT is caused by reentry that includes the AV node as a part of the reentrant circuit.* Typically, electrical impulses travel forward (antegrade) down the AV node and then travel back up the AV node (retrograde) in a repetitive circuit. In some patients, the retrograde conduction pathway of the reentrant circuit may exist in extra-AV nodal tissue adjacent to the AV node. One of these pathways usually conducts impulses rapidly while the other usually conducts impulses slowly. Most commonly, during PSVT the impulse conducts antegrade through the slow pathway and retrograde through the faster pathway; in approximately 10% of patients, the reentrant circuit is reversed.[35]

► *Treatment*

Desired Outcomes The desired outcomes for treatment are to terminate the arrhythmia, restore sinus rhythm, and prevent recurrence. Drug therapy is used to terminate the arrhythmia and restore sinus rhythm; nonpharmacologic measures are used to prevent recurrence.

Termination of PSVT Hemodynamically unstable PSVT should be treated with immediate synchronized DCC, using an initial energy level of 50 to 100 J; if the initial DCC attempt is unsuccessful, the shock energy should be increased in a stepwise fashion.[11]

The primary method of termination of hemodynamically stable PSVT is inhibition of impulse conduction and/or prolongation of the refractory period within the AV node. Because PSVT is propagated via a reentrant circuit involving the AV node, inhibition of conduction within the AV node interrupts and terminates the reentrant circuit.

Prior to initiation of drug therapy for termination of hemodynamically stable PSVT, some simple nonpharmacologic methods known as vagal maneuvers may be attempted.[11,35] Vagal maneuvers stimulate the activity of the parasympathetic nervous system, which inhibits AV nodal conduction, facilitating termination of the arrhythmia. Vagal maneuvers alone may terminate PSVT in up to 25% of cases.[11] Perhaps the simplest vagal maneuver to perform is cough, which stimulates the vagus nerve. Instructing the patient to cough two or three times may successfully terminate the PSVT. Another vagal maneuver that may be attempted is carotid sinus massage; one of the carotid sinuses, located in the neck in the vicinity of the carotid arteries, may be gently massaged, stimulating vagal activity. Carotid sinus massage should not be performed in patients with a history of stroke or transient ischemic attack, or in those in whom carotid bruits may be heard on auscultation. The **Valsalva maneuver**, during which patients bear down against a closed glottis, may also be attempted.

If vagal maneuvers are unsuccessful, IV drug therapy should be initiated.[11,34,35] Drugs that may be used for termination of hemodynamically stable PSVT are presented in Table 9–11.[11] A decision strategy for pharmacologic termination of hemodynamically stable PSVT is presented in Figure 9–7.[11,35]

KEY CONCEPT *Adenosine is the drug of choice for pharmacologic termination of PSVT and is successful in 90% to 95% of patients.* Adenosine inhibits conduction transiently and is associated with adverse effects (see Table 9–7), including flushing, sinus bradycardia or AV nodal block, and bronchospasm in susceptible patients. In addition, adenosine may cause chest pain that mimics the discomfort of myocardial ischemia but is not actually associated with ischemia. The half-life of adenosine is approximately 10 seconds, due to deamination in the blood; therefore, in the vast majority of patients, adverse effects are of short duration.

If adenosine therapy is unsuccessful for termination of PSVT, subsequent choices of therapy depend on whether the patient has HFrEF.

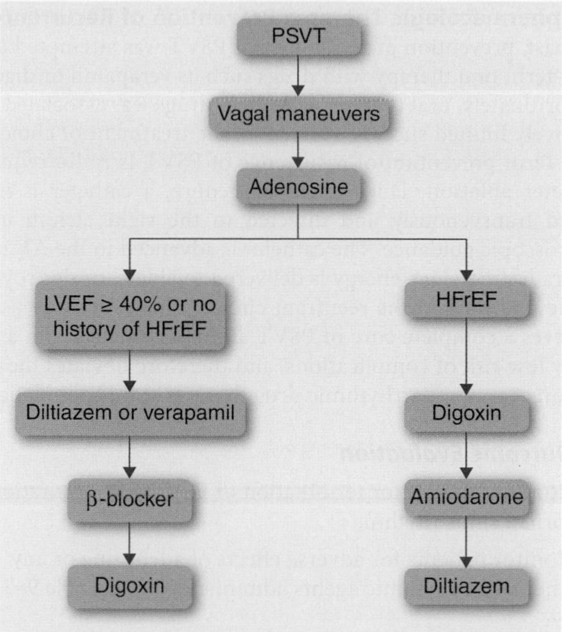

FIGURE 9–7. Decision algorithm for termination of PSVT. (HFrEF, heart failure with reduced ejection fraction; LVEF, left ventricular ejection fraction; PSVT, paroxysmal supraventricular tachycardia; LVEF of 40% can also be expressed as 0.40.)

Table 9–11

Drugs for Termination of PSVT[11]

Drug	Mechanism of Action	Dose	Drug Interactions
Adenosine	Direct AV nodal inhibition	6-mg IV rapid push followed by 20-mL saline flush. If no response in 1–2 minutes, 12-mg IV rapid push followed by 20-mL saline flush	Dipyridamole and carbamazepine accentuate response to adenosine
Diltiazem	Direct AV nodal inhibition	0.25 mg/kg IV over 2 minutes If insufficient response in 15 minutes, give second dose (0.35 mg/kg) IV over 2 minutes Maintenance infusion 5–15 mg/hour	
Verapamil	Direct AV nodal inhibition	(1) 2.5–5.0 mg IV over 2 minutes (2) May repeat as 5–10 mg IV every 15–30 minutes to total dose of 20–30 mg	
Digoxin	(1) Vagal stimulation (2) Direct AV nodal inhibition	8–12 mcg/kg total loading dose, half of which should be administered over 5 minutes, with the remaining portion administered as 25% fractions at 4- to 8-hour intervals	Slow onset of action
β-blockers	Direct AV nodal inhibition	Esmolol 500 mcg/kg IV over 1 minute then 50-mcg/kg/min continuous infusion. If inadequate response, give second loading dose of 500 mcg/kg and increase maintenance infusion to 100 mcg/kg/min. Increment dose increases in this manner as necessary to maximum infusion rate of 200 mcg/kg/min Propranolol 0.5–1.0 mg IV over 1 minute; repeat as necessary to a total dose of 0.1 mg/kg Metoprolol 5 mg IV over 1–2 minutes; repeat as necessary every 5 minutes to a total dose of 15 mg	
Amiodarone	β-blocker CCB	150 mg IV over 10 minutes; repeat if necessary. Follow with continuous infusion of 1 mg/min for 6 hours, followed by 0.5 mg/min. Total dose over 24 hours should not exceed 2.2 g	Inhibits elimination of digoxin, warfarin and some statins

AV, atrioventricular; CCB, Calcium channel blocker; IV, intravenous; PSVT, paroxysmal supraventricular tachycardia.

Nonpharmacologic Therapy: Prevention of Recurrence In the past, prevention of recurrence of PSVT was attempted using long-term oral therapy with drugs such as verapamil or digoxin. Unfortunately, oral therapy with these drugs was associated with relatively limited success. Currently, the treatment of choice for long-term prevention of recurrence of PSVT is radiofrequency catheter ablation. During this procedure, a catheter is introduced transvenously and directed to the right atrium under fluoroscopic guidance. The catheter is advanced to the AV node, and radiofrequency energy is delivered to ablate, or destroy, one of the pathways of the reentrant circuit. This procedure usually achieves a complete cure of PSVT and is associated with a relatively low risk of complications, and therefore obviates the need for long-term antiarrhythmic drug therapy in this population.

▶ *Outcome Evaluation*

- Monitor patients for termination of PSVT and restoration of normal sinus rhythm.
- Monitor patients for adverse effects of adenosine or any other antiarrhythmic agents administered (see Table 9–7).

VENTRICULAR ARRHYTHMIAS

Ventricular Premature Depolarizations

VPDs are ectopic electrical impulses originating in ventricular tissue, resulting in wide, misshapen, abnormal QRS complexes. VPDs are also commonly known by other terms, including premature ventricular contractions (PVCs), ventricular premature beats (VPBs), and ventricular premature contractions (VPCs).

Clinical Presentation and Diagnosis of VPDs

- VPDs are usually categorized as simple or complex: simple VPDs are those that occur as infrequent, isolated single abnormal beats; complex VPDs are those that occur more frequently and/or in specific patterns
- Two consecutive VPDs are referred to as a couplet. The term *bigeminy* refers to a VPD occurring with every other beat; *trigeminy* means a VPD occurring with every third beat; *quadrigeminy* means a VPD occurring every fourth beat

Symptoms

- Most patients who experience simple or complex VPDs are asymptomatic. Occasionally, patients with complex or frequent VPDs may experience symptoms of palpitations, light-headedness, fatigue, near-syncope, or syncope

▶ *Epidemiology, Etiology, and Pathophysiology*

VPDs occur with variable frequency, depending on underlying comorbid conditions. The prevalence of complex or frequent VPDs is approximately 33% and 12% in men with and without CAD, respectively;[36] in women, the prevalence of complex or frequent VPDs is 26% and 12% in those with and without CAD, respectively.[37] VPDs occur more commonly in patients with ischemic heart disease, a history of MI, and HFrEF. They may also occur as a result of hypoxia, anemia, and following cardiac surgery. KEY CONCEPT *VPDs occur as a result of abnormal ventricular automaticity due to enhanced activity of the sympathetic nervous system and altered electrophysiological characteristics of the heart during myocardial ischemia and following MI.*

In patients with underlying CAD or a history of MI, the presence of complex or frequent VPDs is associated with an increased risk of mortality due to sudden cardiac death.[38]

▶ *Treatment*

Desired Outcomes Desired outcomes are to alleviate patient symptoms.

Pharmacologic Therapy KEY CONCEPT *Asymptomatic VPDs should not be treated with antiarrhythmic drug therapy.* Based on the knowledge that complex or frequent VPDs increase the risk of sudden cardiac death in patients with a history of MI, the Cardiac Arrhythmia Suppression Trials (CAST I and II) tested the hypothesis that suppression of asymptomatic VPDs with the drugs flecainide, encainide, or moricizine in patients with a relatively recent history of MI would lead to a reduction in the incidence of sudden cardiac death.[39,40] However, the results of the trial showed that not only did these antiarrhythmic agents not reduce the risk of sudden cardiac death, there was a significant *increase* in risk of death in patients who received therapy with encainide or flecainide compared with those who received placebo.[39] During the continuation of the study with moricizine, a trend was found toward an increase in the incidence of death in patients who received this antiarrhythmic drug as well.[40]

Additional evidence suggests that other Vaughan Williams class I agents, including quinidine, procainamide, and disopyramide, increase the risk of death in patients with complex VPDs following MI.[41] Thus, evidence indicates that patients with complex VPDs following MI do not benefit from therapy with antiarrhythmic agents and that many of these drugs increase risk of death. KEY CONCEPT *Therefore, asymptomatic VPDs should not be treated.*

Patients with symptomatic VPDs should be treated with β-blockers because the majority of patients with symptomatic VPDs have underlying CAD. β-blockers have been shown to reduce mortality in this population and to be effective for VPD suppression.[42]

▶ *Outcome Evaluation*

- Monitor patients for relief of symptoms.
- Monitor for adverse effects of β-blockers: bradycardia, hypotension, fatigue, masking symptoms of hypoglycemia, glucose intolerance (in diabetic patients), wheezing or shortness of breath (in patients with severe asthma or chronic obstructive pulmonary disease [COPD]).

Ventricular Tachycardia

VT is a series of three or more consecutive VPDs at a rate greater than 100 beats/min. VT is defined as nonsustained if it lasts less than 30 seconds and terminates spontaneously; sustained VT lasts greater than 30 seconds and does not terminate spontaneously but rather requires therapeutic intervention for termination.

▶ *Epidemiology, Etiology, and Pathophysiology*

Etiologies of VT are presented in Table 9–12. The incidence of VT is variable, depending on underlying comorbidities. Up to 20% of patients who experience acute MI experience ventricular arrhythmias.[43] Approximately 2% to 4% of patients with MI develop VT during the period of hospitalization.[43] Nonsustained VT occurs in 20% to 80% of patients with HF.[44] Other etiologies

Table 9–12

Etiologies of VT and VF

Coronary artery disease	
Myocardial infarction	
Heart failure	
Electrolyte abnormalities: hypokalemia, hypomagnesemia	
Drugs:	
Adenosine	Procainamide
Amiodarone	Propafenone
Chlorpromazine	Sotalol
Cocaine	Terbutaline
Digoxin	Thioridazine
Disopyramide	Trazodone
Flecainide	Venlafaxine
Ibutilide	

VF, ventricular fibrillation; VT, ventricular tachycardia.

of VT include electrolyte abnormalities such as hypokalemia, hypoxia, and drugs.

KEY CONCEPT *VT is usually initiated by a precisely timed VPD, occurring during the relative refractory period, which provokes reentry within ventricular tissue.*

Sustained VT requires immediate intervention, because if untreated, the rhythm may cause sudden cardiac death via hemodynamic instability and the absence of a pulse (pulseless VT) or via degeneration of VT into VF.

Clinical Presentation and Diagnosis of VT

Symptoms

- Symptoms associated with VT depend primarily on heart rate and include palpitations, dizziness, light-headedness, shortness of breath, chest pain (if underlying CAD is present), near-syncope, and syncope
- Patients with nonsustained VT may be asymptomatic if the duration of the arrhythmia is sufficiently short. However, if the rate is sufficiently rapid, patients with nonsustained VT may experience symptoms
- Patients with sustained VT are usually symptomatic, provided the rate is fast enough to provoke symptoms. Patients with rapid sustained VT may be hemodynamically unstable
- In some patients, sustained VT results in the absence of a pulse or may deteriorate to VF, resulting in the syndrome of sudden cardiac death

Diagnosis

- Diagnosis of VT requires ECG confirmation of the arrhythmia
- VT is characterized by wide, misshapen QRS complexes, with the rate varying from 140 to 250 beats/min
- In most patients with VT, the shape and appearance of the QRS complexes are consistent and similar, referred to as monomorphic VT. However, some patients experience polymorphic VT, in which the shape and appearance of the QRS complexes vary

Table 9–13

Drugs for Termination of VT[11]

Drug	Loading Dose	Maintenance Dose
Procainamide	20- to 50-mg/min continuous IV infusion until arrhythmia suppressed, hypotension occurs, QRS duration increases > 50%, or maximum dose of 17 mg/kg is reached	1- to 4-mg/min continuous IV infusion
Amiodarone	150 mg IV over 10 minutes. Repeat as needed if VT recurs.	1-mg/min continuous infusion for 6 hours, 0.5 mg/min for 18 hours

IV, intravenous; VT, ventricular tachycardia.

▶ *Treatment*

Desired Outcomes Desired outcomes are to terminate the arrhythmia and restore sinus rhythm, and to prevent sudden cardiac death.

Pharmacologic Therapy Hemodynamically unstable VT should be terminated immediately using synchronized DCC beginning with 100 J (for monophasic shocks) and increasing subsequent shocks to 200, 300, and 360 J.[11] In the event that VT is present but the patient does not have a palpable pulse (and therefore no blood pressure), asynchronous defibrillation should be performed, at 360 J for monophasic waveforms and starting at 120 to 200 J for biphasic waveforms.[10]

Drugs used for the termination of hemodynamically stable VT are presented in Table 9–13.[11] IV drug administration is required. A decision algorithm for management of hemodynamically stable VT is presented in Figure 9–8. The initial choice of drug depends on whether the patient has normal LV function or HFrEF. If the patient has normal LV function with no history of HFrEF, the drug of choice is procainamide, followed by amiodarone in refractory cases.[11] However, if the patient has HFrEF, therapy with procainamide should be avoided due to the drug's negative inotropic effects and its propensity to cause hypotension and QT interval prolongation, for which patients

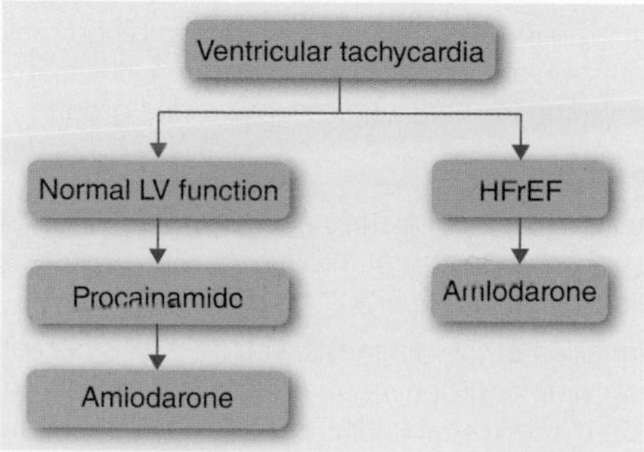

FIGURE 9–8. Decision algorithm for termination of hemodynamically stable ventricular tachycardia. (HFrEF, heart failure with reduced ejection fraction; LV, left ventricular.)

with HF are at increased risk. Therefore, for patients with hemodynamically stable VT and concomitant HFrEF, IV amiodarone is recommended.[11]

Nonpharmacologic Therapy: Prevention of Sudden Cardiac Death KEY CONCEPT *In patients who have experienced VT and are at risk for sudden cardiac death, an implantable cardioverter-defibrillator (ICD) is the treatment of choice.*[45] An ICD is a device that provides internal electrical cardioversion of VT or defibrillation of VF; the ICD does not prevent the patient from developing the arrhythmia, but it reduces the risk that the patient will die of sudden cardiac death as a result of the arrhythmia. Whereas early versions of ICDs required a thoracotomy for implantation, these devices now may be implanted transvenously, similarly to pacemakers, markedly reducing the incidence of complications.

ICDs are significantly more effective than antiarrhythmic drugs such as amiodarone or sotalol for reducing the risk of sudden cardiac death, and therefore are preferred therapy.[45–47] However, many patients with ICDs receive concurrent antiarrhythmic drug therapy to reduce the frequency with which patients experience the discomfort of shocks and to prolong battery life of the devices. Combined pharmacotherapy with amiodarone and a β-blocker is more effective than monotherapy with sotalol or β-blockers for reduction in the frequency of ICD shocks.[48]

► *Outcome Evaluation*

- Monitor patients for termination of VT and restoration of normal sinus rhythm.
- Monitor patients for adverse effects of antiarrhythmic drugs (see Table 9–7).

Ventricular Fibrillation

VF is irregular, disorganized, chaotic electrical activity in the ventricles resulting in absence of ventricular depolarizations, and consequently, lack of pulse, cardiac output, and blood pressure.

► *Epidemiology and Etiology*

Approximately 400,000 people die of sudden cardiac death annually in the United States. Although some of these deaths occur as a result of asystole, the majority occur as a result of primary VF or VT that degenerates into VF. Etiologies of VF are presented in Table 9–12 and are similar to those of VT.

Clinical Presentation and Diagnosis of VF

Symptoms

- VF results in immediate loss of pulse and blood pressure. Patients who are in the standing position at the onset of VF suddenly and immediately collapse to the ground

Diagnosis

- The absence of a pulse does not guarantee VF because pulse may also be absent in patients with asystole, VT, or pulseless electrical activity
- Confirmation of the diagnosis with an ECG is necessary to determine appropriate treatment. ECG reveals no organized, recognizable QRS complexes. If treatment is not initiated within a few minutes, death will occur, or at best, resuscitation of the patient with permanent anoxic brain injury

► *Treatment*

Desired Outcomes Desired outcomes are to: (a) terminate VF, (b) achieve return of spontaneous circulation, and (c) achieve patient survival to hospital admission (in those with out-of-hospital cardiac arrest) and to hospital discharge.

Pharmacologic and Nonpharmacologic Therapy VF is by definition hemodynamically unstable, due to the absence of a pulse and blood pressure. Initial management includes provision of basic life support, including calling for help and initiation of cardiopulmonary resuscitation (CPR).[11] Oxygen should be administered as soon as it is available. Most importantly, defibrillation should be performed as soon as possible. It is critically important to understand that the only means of successfully terminating VF and restoring sinus rhythm is electrical defibrillation. Defibrillation should be attempted using 360 J for monophasic defibrillators, and 120 to 200 J for biphasic shocks, after which CPR should be resumed immediately while the defibrillator charges; if the first shock was unsuccessful, subsequent defibrillation attempts should be performed at equivalent or higher energy doses.[11]

If VF persists following two defibrillation shocks, drug therapy may be administered. KEY CONCEPT *The purpose of drug administration for treatment of VF is to facilitate successful defibrillation. Drug therapy alone will not result in termination of VF.* Drugs used for facilitation of defibrillation in patients with VF are listed in Table 9–14.[11] Drug administration should occur during CPR, before or after delivery of a defibrillation shock. The vasopressor agents epinephrine or vasopressin are administered initially because it has been shown that a critical factor in successful defibrillation is maintenance of coronary perfusion pressure, which is achieved via the vasoconstricting effects of these drugs. A decision algorithm for the treatment of VF is presented in Figure 9–9. Epinephrine and vasopressin are equally effective for facilitation of defibrillation leading to survival to hospital admission in patients with out-of-hospital cardiac arrest due to VF. Amiodarone is effective for facilitation of defibrillation leading to survival to hospital admission in patients with VF.[49] Note that amiodarone doses recommended for administration during a resuscitation attempt for VF (see Table 9–14) are different than those recommended for administration for termination of VT (see Table 9–13).

► *Outcome Evaluation*

- Monitor the patient for return of pulse and blood pressure, and for termination of VF and restoration of normal sinus rhythm.
- After successful resuscitation, monitor the patient for adverse effects of drugs administered (see Table 9–7).

Table 9–14

Drugs for Facilitation of Defibrillation in Patients with VF[11]

Drug	Dose
Epinephrine	1 mg IV every 3–5 minutes
Vasopressin	40 units IV single dose
Amiodarone	300 mg IV diluted in 20–30 mL D_5W. One subsequent dose of 150 mg IV may be administered

D_5W, 5% dextrose in water; IV, intravenous; VF, ventricular fibrillation.

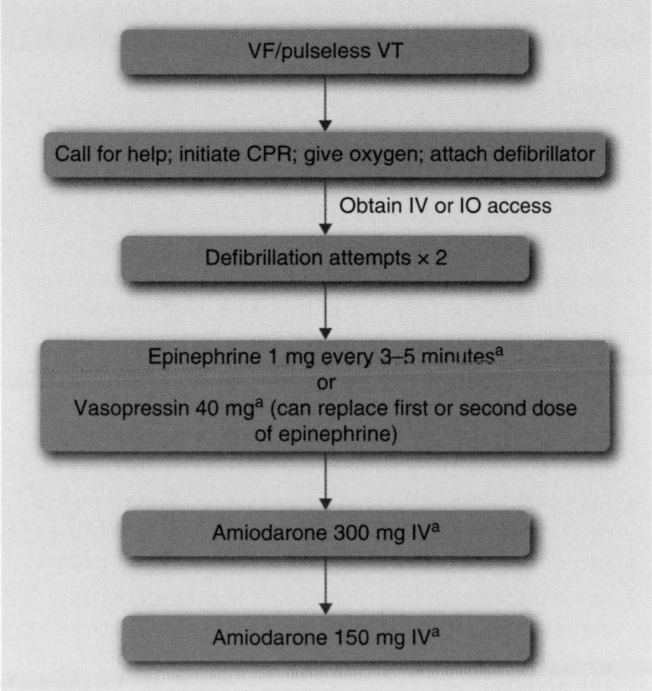

FIGURE 9–9. Decision algorithm for resuscitation of VF or pulseless VT. (CPR, cardiopulmonary resuscitation; IO, intraosseous; IV, intravenous; VF, ventricular fibrillation; VT, ventricular tachycardia.) [a]Defibrillation attempt should be made after every dose of drug.

Torsades de Pointes

Torsades de Pointes (TdP) is a specific polymorphic VT associated with prolongation of the QT interval in the sinus beats that precede the arrhythmia.[1,50]

▸ *Epidemiology and Etiology*

The incidence of TdP in the population at large is unknown. The incidence of TdP associated with specific drugs ranges from less than 1% to as high as 8% to 10%, depending on dose and plasma concentration of the drug and the presence of other risk factors for the arrhythmia.

TdP may be inherited or acquired. Patients with specific genetic mutations may have an inherited long QT syndrome, in which the QT interval is prolonged, and these patients are at risk for TdP. Acquired TdP may be caused by numerous drugs (Table 9–15);[1,50] the list of drugs known to cause TdP continues to expand.

▸ *Pathophysiology*

TdP is caused by circumstances, often drugs, that lead to prolongation in the repolarization phase of the ventricular action potential (see Figure 9–2) manifested on the ECG by prolongation of the QT interval. Prolongation of ventricular repolarization occurs via inhibition of efflux of potassium through potassium channels; therefore, drugs that inhibit conductance through potassium channels may cause QT interval prolongation and TdP. KEY CONCEPT *Prolongation of ventricular repolarization promotes the development of early ventricular afterdepolarizations during the relative refractory period, which may provoke reentry leading to TdP.*

Table 9–15

Some Drugs That Have Been Reported to Cause Torsades de Pointes[1,50]

Amiodarone	Levofloxacin
Amitriptyline	Levomethadyl
Arsenic	Methadone
Chloroquine	Metoclopramide
Chlorpromazine	Moxifloxacin
Ciprofloxacin	Ondansetron
Citalopram	Pentamidine
Clarithromycin	Pimozide
Disopyramide	Procainamide
Dofetilide	Propafenone
Doxepin	Quetiapine
Droperidol	Quinidine
Erythromycin	Risperidone
Famotidine	Sertraline
Flecainide	Sotalol
Fluconazole	Tacrolimus
Fluoxetine	Thioridazine
Haloperidol	Trazodone
Ibutilide	Voriconazole
Indapamide	Ziprasidone
Ketoconazole	

KEY CONCEPT *Drug-induced TdP rarely occurs in patients without specific risk factors for the arrhythmia (Table 9–16).*[1,50] In most cases, administration of a drug known to cause TdP is unlikely to cause the arrhythmia; however, the likelihood of the arrhythmia increases in patients with concomitant risk factors.

The onset of TdP associated with oral drug therapy is somewhat variable and in some cases may be delayed; often, a patient can be taking a drug known to cause TdP for months or longer without problem until another risk factor for the arrhythmia becomes present, which then may trigger the arrhythmia.

In some patients, TdP may be of short duration and may terminate spontaneously. However, TdP may not terminate on its

Table 9–16

Risk Factors for Drug-Induced Torsades de Pointes[1,50]

QT_c interval > 500 ms
Increase in QT_c interval by > 60 ms compared with the pretreatment value
Female sex
Age > 65 years
Heart failure
Electrolyte abnormalities: hypokalemia, hypomagnesemia, hypocalcemia
Bradycardia
Elevated plasma concentrations of QT interval-prolonging drugs due to drug interactions or absence of dose adjustment for organ dysfunction
Rapid IV infusion of torsades-inducing drugs
Concomitant administration of more than one agent known to cause QT interval prolongation/torsades de pointes
Concomitant administration of loop diuretics
Genetic predisposition
Previous history of drug-induced torsades de pointes

IV, intravenous; ms, milliseconds; QT_c, corrected QT interval.

Clinical Presentation and Diagnosis of Torsades de Pointes

Symptoms

- Symptoms associated with TdP depend primarily on heart rate and arrhythmia duration, and include palpitations, dizziness, light-headedness, shortness of breath, chest pain (if underlying CAD is present), near-syncope, and syncope
- TdP may be hemodynamically unstable if the rate is sufficiently rapid
- Like sustained monomorphic VT, TdP may result in the absence of a pulse or may rapidly degenerate into VF, resulting in the syndrome of sudden cardiac death

Diagnosis

- Diagnosis of TdP requires examination of the arrhythmia on ECG
- TdP, or "twisting of the points," appears on ECG as apparent twisting of the wide QRS complexes around the isoelectric baseline
- Associated with heart rates from 140 to 280 beats/min
- Characteristic feature: a "long-short" initiating sequence that occurs as a result of a VPD followed by a compensatory pause followed by the first beat of the TdP
- Episodes of TdP may self-terminate, with frequent recurrence

own, and if left untreated, it may degenerate into VF and result in sudden cardiac death.[1,50] Several drugs, including terfenadine, astemizole, and cisapride, have been withdrawn from the US market as a result of causing deaths due to TdP.

▶ *Treatment*

Desired Outcomes Desired outcomes include (a) prevention of TdP, (b) termination of TdP, (c) prevention of recurrence, and (d) prevention of sudden cardiac death.

Pharmacologic and Nonpharmacologic Therapy KEY CONCEPT *In patients with risk factors for TdP, drugs with the potential to cause QT interval prolongation and TdP should be avoided or used with extreme caution, and diligent QT interval monitoring should be performed.*

Management of drug-induced TdP includes discontinuation of the potentially causative agent. Patients with hemodynamically unstable TdP should undergo immediate synchronized DCC. In patients with hemodynamically stable TdP, electrolyte abnormalities such as hypokalemia, hypomagnesemia, or hypocalcemia should be corrected. Hemodynamically stable TdP is often treated with IV magnesium sulfate, irrespective of whether the patient is hypomagnesemic; magnesium has been shown to terminate TdP in normomagnesemic patients.[11] Magnesium sulfate should be administered IV in doses of 1 to 2 g, diluted in 50 to 100 mL 5% dextrose in water (D_5W), administered over 5 to 10 minutes; doses may be repeated to a total of 12 g.

Alternatively, a continuous magnesium infusion (0.5 to 1 g/hour) may be initiated after the first bolus. Other treatments include transvenous insertion of a temporary pacemaker for overdrive pacing, which shortens the QT interval and may terminate TdP

Patient Care Process

Patient Assessment:

- Perform a thorough medication history to determine whether the patient is receiving prescription or nonprescription drugs that may cause or contribute to the development of an arrhythmia. See Tables 9–2, 9–3, 9–4, 9–12, and 9–15.
- Determine the patient's serum electrolyte concentrations to determine the presence of hypokalemia, hyperkalemia, hypomagnesemia, hypermagnesemia, or hypocalcemia.
- Consider the patient's heart rate, blood pressure, and symptoms to determine whether he or she is hemodynamically stable or unstable, and the degree to which symptoms are limiting function and quality of life.
- Assess the patient's 12-lead ECG or single rhythm strips to determine if an arrhythmia is present and to identify the specific arrhythmia, and evaluate and monitor symptoms.
- Assess information from the chest X-ray, transthoracic or transesophageal echocardiograms, and other physical examination and diagnostic information pertinent to arrhythmias.

Therapy Evaluation:

- Evaluate the patient for the presence of drug-induced diseases, drug allergies, and drug interactions.
- For patients with preexisting arrhythmias, assess the current drug therapy regimen for efficacy, side effects, and adherence.
- In patients currently receiving warfarin for AF, determine the INR and evaluate for appropriateness, adverse effects, and drug–drug and drug–food interactions.
- Assess adherence to current drug therapy regimens.

Care Plan Development:

- Develop drug therapy treatment plans for management of the pertinent arrhythmia: sinus bradycardia, AV nodal block, AF, PSVT, VPDs, VT (including TdP), or VF. See Figures 9–4 through 9–9 and Tables 9–6, 9–8, 9–9, 9–10, 9–11, 9–13, and 9–14.
- Determine whether the patient has prescription coverage and/or whether recommended agents are included on the institution's formulary.

Follow-Up Evaluation:

- Develop specific drug therapy monitoring plans, including assessment of symptoms, ECG, adverse effects of drugs, and potential drug interactions.
- Monitor QT_c interval in patients receiving QT-prolonging drugs.
- Provide information regarding safe and effective oral anticoagulation:
  - Notify clinicians in the event of severe bruising, blood in urine or stool, **melena**, **hemoptysis**, **hematemesis**, or frequent **epistaxis**.
  - Patients taking warfarin should avoid radical changes in diet.

(Continued)

Patient Care Process (*Continued*)

- Avoid alcohol.
- Do not take nonprescription medications or herbal/alternative/complementary medicines without notifying physician, pharmacist, and/or health care team members.
- Stress the importance of adherence to therapy.
- Provide patient education regarding disease state and drug therapy.

and reduce the risk of recurrence; or IV isoproterenol 2 to 10 mcg/min, to increase the heart rate and shorten the QT interval.

▶ *Outcome Evaluation*

- Monitor vital signs (heart rate and blood pressure).
- Monitor the ECG to determine the QT_c interval (maintain less than 470 milliseconds [ms] in males and 480 ms in females)[1] and for the presence of TdP.
- Monitor serum potassium, magnesium, and calcium concentrations.
- Monitor for symptoms of tachycardia.

Abbreviations Introduced in This Chapter

1°	First-degree
2°	Second-degree
3°	Third-degree
AF	Atrial fibrillation
ATPase	Adenosine triphosphatase
AV	Atrioventricular
Ca	Calcium
CAD	Coronary artery disease
CAST	Cardiac Arrhythmia Suppression Trial
CCB	Calcium channel blocker
COPD	Chronic obstructive pulmonary disease
CPR	Cardiopulmonary resuscitation
CrCl	Creatinine clearance
CV	Cardiovascular
DCC	Direct current cardioversion
D_5W	5% Dextrose in water
ECG	Electrocardiogram
ED	Emergency department
FDA	Food and Drug Administration
GI	Gastrointestinal
HF	Heart failure
HFpEF	Heart failure with preserved ejection fraction
HFrEF	Heart failure with reduced ejection fraction
ICD	Implantable cardioverter-defibrillator
INR	International normalized ratio
IO	Intraosseous
IV	Intravenous
J	Joule
K	Potassium
LV	Left ventricle
LVEF	Left ventricular ejection fraction
MI	Myocardial infarction
ms	Milliseconds
Na	Sodium
NYHA	New York Heart Association
P-gp	P-glycoprotein
PAD	Peripheral arterial disease
PSVT	Paroxysmal supraventricular tachycardia
PTT	Partial thromboplastin time
PVC	Premature ventricular contraction
QT_c	Corrected QT interval
SA	Sinoatrial
TdP	Torsades de pointes
TEE	Transesophageal echocardiogram
TIA	Transient ischemic attack
VF	Ventricular fibrillation
VPB	Ventricular premature beat
VPC	Ventricular premature contraction
VPD	Ventricular premature depolarization
VT	Ventricular tachycardia

REFERENCES

1. Drew BJ, Ackerman MJ, Funk M, et al. On behalf of the American Heart Association Acute Cardiac Care Committee of the Council on Clinical Cardiology, the Council on Cardiovascular Nursing, and the American College of Cardiology Foundation. Prevention of torsades de pointes in hospital settings: a scientific statement from the American Heart Association and the American College of Cardiology Foundation. Circulation. 2010;121:1047–1060.
2. Fogoros RN. Electrophysiologic testing, 4th ed. Malden, MA: Blackwell, 2006:17.
3. Vaughan Williams EM. Classification of anti-arrhythmic drugs. In: Sandoe E, Flensted-Jansen E, Olesen KH, eds. Symposium on Cardiac Arrhythmias. Sodertalje, Sweden: AB Astra, 1970: 449–472.
4. Singh BN, Vaughan Williams EM. A third class of anti-arrhythmic action. Effects on atrial and ventricular intracellular potentials, and other pharmacological actions on cardiac muscle, of MJ 1999 and AH 3474. Br J Pharmacol. 1970;39:675–687.
5. Singh BN, Vaughan Williams EM. A fourth class of anti-arrhythmic action? Effect of verapamil on ouabain toxicity, on atrial and ventricular intracellular potentials, and on other features of cardiac function. Cardiovasc Res. 1972;6:109–119.
6. Snyders J, Knoth KM, Roberds SL, Tamkun MM. Time-, voltage-, and state-dependent block by quinidine of a cloned human cardiac potassium channel. Mol Pharmacol. 1992;41:322–330.
7. Komeichi K, Tohse N, Nakaya H, et al. Effects of N-acetylprocainamide and sotalol on ion currents in isolated guinea-pig ventricular myocytes. Eur J Pharmacol. 1990;187: 313–322.
8. Mangrum JM, DiMarco JP. The evaluation and management of bradycardia. N Engl J Med. 2000;342:703–709.
9. Ufberg JW, Clark JS. Bradydysrhythmias and atrioventricular conduction blocks. Emerg Med Clin North Am. 2006;24:1–9.
10. Tisdale JE. Supraventricular arrhythmias. In: Tisdale JE, Miller DA, eds. Drug-Induced Diseases: Prevention, Detection and Management, 2nd ed. Bethesda, MD: American Society of Health-System Pharmacists, 2010:445–484.
11. Neumar RW, Otto CW, Link MS, et al. Part 8: Adult advanced cardiovascular life support: 2010 American Heart Association Guidelines for Cardiopulmonary Resuscitation and Emergency Cardiovascular Care. Circulation. 2010;122(Suppl 3):S729–S767.
12. Kannel WB, Wolf PA, Benjamin EJ, Levy D. Prevalence, incidence, prognosis, and predisposing conditions for atrial fibrillation: Population-based estimates. Am J Cardiol. 1998;82:2N–9N.

13. Torp-Pedersen C, Moller M, Bloch-Thomsen PE, et al. Dofetilide in patients with congestive heart failure and left ventricular dysfunction. Danish Investigations of Arrhythmia and Mortality on Dofetilide Study Group. N Engl J Med. 1999;341:857–865.
14. Maisel WH, Stevenson LW. Atrial fibrillation in heart failure: epidemiology, pathophysiology, and rationale for therapy. Am J Cardiol. 2003;91:2D–8D.
15. Rich EC, Siebold C, Campion B. Alcohol-related acute atrial fibrillation. A case-control study and review of 40 patients. Arch Intern Med. 1985;145:830–833.
16. Sharma A, Einstein AJ, Vallakati A, et al. Risk of atrial fibrillation with use of oral and intravenous bisphosphonates. Am J Cardiol. 2014;113:1815–1821.
17. January CT, Wann LS, Alpert JS, et al. 2014 AHA/ACC/HRS guideline for the management of patients with atrial fibrillation. J Am Coll Cardiol. 2014; doi: 10.1016/j.jacc.2014.03.022.
18. Haissaguerre M, Jais P, Shah DC, et al. Spontaneous initiation of atrial fibrillation by ectopic beats originating in the pulmonary veins. N Engl J Med. 1998;339(10):659–666.
19. Cohen M, Naccarelli GV. Pathophysiology and disease progression of atrial fibrillation: Importance of achieving and maintaining sinus rhythm. J Cardiovasc Electrophysiol. 2008;19: 885–890.
20. Wijffels MC, Kirchhof CJ, Dorland R, Allessie MA. Atrial fibrillation begets atrial fibrillation. A study in awake chronically instrumented goats. Circulation. 1995;92:1954–1968.
21. Wann LS, Curtis AB, January CT, et al., writing on behalf of the 2006 ACC/AHA/ESC Guidelines for the Management of Patients with Atrial Fibrillation Writing Committee. 2011 ACCF/AHA/HRS focused update on the management of patients with atrial fibrillation (updating the 2006 guideline): A report of the American College of Cardiology Foundation/American Heart Association Task Force on Practice Guidelines. Circulation. 2011;123:104–123.
22. Turakhia MP, Santangeli P, Winkelmayer WC, et al. Increased mortality associated with digoxin in contemporary patients with atrial fibrillation: findings from the TREAT-AF study. J Am Coll Cardiol. 2014;64:660–668.
23. The Atrial Fibrillation Follow-up Investigation of Rhythm Management (AFFIRM) Investigators. A comparison of rate control and rhythm control in patients with atrial fibrillation. N Engl J Med. 2002;347:1825–1833.
24. Van Gelder IC, Hagens VE, Bosker HA, et al., for the Rate Control versus Electrical Cardioversion for Persistent Atrial Fibrillation Study Group. A comparison of rate control and rhythm control in patients with recurrent persistent atrial fibrillation. N Engl J Med. 2002;347:1834–1840.
25. Carlsson J, Miketic S, Windeler J, et al. Randomized trial of rate-control versus rhythm-control in persistent atrial fibrillation: the Strategies of Treatment of Atrial Fibrillation (STAF) study. J Am Coll Cardiol. 2003;41:1690–1696.
26. Opolski G, Torbicki A, Kosior D, et al. Rhythm control versus rate control in patients with persistent atrial fibrillation. Results of the HOT CAFE Polish Study. Kardiol Pol. 2003;59:1–16.
27. Roy D, Talajic M, Nattel S, et al. Rhythm control versus rate control for atrial fibrillation and heart failure. N Engl J Med. 2008;358:2667–2677.
28. Lip GY, Nieuwlaat R, Pisters R, et al. Refining clinical risk stratification for predicting stroke and thromboembolism in atrial fibrillation using a novel risk factor-based approach: the euro heart survey on atrial fibrillation. Chest. 2010;137: 263–72.
29. Patel MR, Mahaffey KW, Garg J, et al. Rivaroxaban versus warfarin in nonvalvular atrial fibrillation. N Engl J Med. 2011;365:883–891.
30. Granger CB, Alexander JH, McMurray JJV, et al., for the ARISTOTLE committee and investigators. Apixaban versus warfarin in patients with atrial fibrillation. N Engl J Med. 2011;365;981–992.
31. Johnson JA, Whirl-Carrilo M, Gage BF, et al. Clinical pharmacogenetics implementation consortium guidelines for CYP2C9 and VKORC1 genotypes and warfarin dosing. Clin Pharmacol Ther. 2011;90:625–629.
32. Gage BF, Johnson JA, Deych E, et al. Use of pharmacogenetics and clinical factors to predict the therapeutic dose of warfarin. Clin Pharmacol Ther. 2008;84:326–331.
33. International Warfarin Pharmacogenetics Consortium, Klein TE, Altman RB, Eriksson N, et al. Estimation of warfarin dose with clinical and pharmacogenetics data. N Engl J Med. 2009;360:753–764.
34. Ganz LI, Friedman PL. Supraventricular tachycardia. N Engl J Med. 1995;332:162–173.
35. Blomstrom-Lundqvist C, Scheinman MM, Aliot EM, et al., for the Writing Committee to Develop Guidelines for the Management of Patients with Supraventricular Arrhythmias. ACC/AHA/ESC guidelines for the management of patients with supraventricular arrhythmias—Executive summary: A report of the American College of Cardiology/American Heart Association Task Force on practice guidelines and the European Society of Cardiology Committee for Practice Guidelines (Writing Committee to Develop Guidelines for the Management of Patients with Supraventricular Arrhythmias). J Am Coll Cardiol. 2003;42:1493–1531.
36. Bikkina M, Larson MG, Levy D. Prognostic implications of asymptomatic ventricular arrhythmias: The Framingham Heart Study. Am J Cardiol. 1994;74:232–235.
37. Lown B, Wolf M. Approaches to sudden death from coronary heart disease. Circulation. 1971;44:130–144.
38. Ruberman W, Weinblatt E, Goldberg JD, et al. Ventricular premature beats and mortality after myocardial infarction. N Engl J Med. 1977;297:750–757.
39. Echt DS, Liebson PR, Mitchell LB, et al. Mortality and morbidity in patients receiving encainide, flecainide, or placebo. The Cardiac Arrhythmia Suppression Trial. N Engl J Med. 1991;324:781–788.
40. The Cardiac Arrhythmia Suppression Trial II Investigators. Effect of the antiarrhythmic agent moricizine on survival after myocardial infarction. N Engl J Med. 1992;327:227–233.
41. Teo KK, Yusuf S, Furberg CD. Effects of prophylactic anti-arrhythmic drug therapy in acute myocardial infarction. An overview of results from randomized controlled trials. JAMA. 1993;270:1589–1595.
42. Chandraratna PA. Comparison of acebutolol with propranolol, quinidine, and placebo: Results of three multicenter arrhythmia trials. Am Heart J. 1985;109:1198–1204.
43. Al-Khatib SM, Stebbins AL, Califf RM, et al. Sustained ventricular arrhythmias and mortality among patients with acute myocardial infarction: results from the GUSTO-III trial. Am Heart J. 2003;145:515–521.
44. Saltzman HE. Arrhythmias and heart failure. Cardiol Clin. 2014;32:125–133.
45. Epstein AE, DiMarco JP, Ellenbogen KA, et al. ACC/AHA/HRS 2008 guidelines for device-based therapy of cardiac rhythm abnormalities: A report of the American College of Cardiology/American Heart Association Task Force on Practice Guidelines (Writing Committee to Revise the ACC/AHA/NASPE 2002 Guideline Update for Implantation of Cardiac Pacemakers and Antiarrhythmia Devices). J Am Coll Cardiol. 2008;51: e1–62.
46. The Antiarrhythmics versus Implantable Defibrillators (AVID) Investigators. A comparison of antiarrhythmic-drug therapy with

implantable defibrillators in patients resuscitated from near-fatal ventricular arrhythmias. N Engl J Med. 1997;337:1576–1583.

47. Connolly SJ, Gent M, Roberts RS, et al. Canadian implantable defibrillator study (CIDS): A randomized trial of the implantable cardioverter defibrillator against amiodarone. Circulation. 2000;101:1297–1302.
48. Connolly SJ, Dorian P, Roberts RS, et al. Comparison of β-blockers, amiodarone plus β-blockers, or sotalol for prevention of shocks from implantable cardioverter-defibrillators. The OPTIC study: A randomized trial. JAMA. 2006;295:165–171.
49. Dorian P, Cass D, Schwartz B, et al. Amiodarone as compared with lidocaine for shock-resistant ventricular fibrillation. N Engl J Med. 2002;346:884–890.
50. Tisdale JE. Ventricular arrhythmias. In: Tisdale JE, Miller DA, eds. Drug-Induced Diseases: Prevention, Detection and Management, 2nd ed. Bethesda, MD: American Society of Health-System Pharmacists, 2010:485–515.

10 Venous Thromboembolism

Edith A. Nutescu, Stuart T. Haines, and Ann K. Wittkowsky

LEARNING OBJECTIVES

Upon completion of the chapter, the reader will be able to:

1. Identify risk factors and signs and symptoms of deep vein thrombosis (DVT) and pulmonary embolism (PE).
2. Describe the processes of hemostasis and thrombosis.
3. Determine a patient's relative risk of developing venous thrombosis.
4. Formulate an appropriate prevention strategy for a patient at risk for DVT.
5. Select and interpret laboratory test(s) to monitor antithrombotic drugs.
6. Identify factors that place a patient at high risk of bleeding while receiving antithrombotic drugs.
7. State at least two potential advantages of newer anticoagulants (ie, low molecular weight heparins, fondaparinux, oral direct thrombin inhibitors, and oral direct factor Xa inhibitors) over traditional anticoagulants (ie, unfractionated heparin and warfarin).
8. Manage a patient with an elevated international normalized ratio with or without bleeding.
9. Identify anticoagulant drug–drug and drug–food interactions.
10. Formulate an appropriate treatment plan for a patient who develops a DVT or PE.

INTRODUCTION

Venous thromboembolism (VTE) is one of the most common cardiovascular disorders in the United States. VTE is manifested as **deep vein thrombosis** (DVT) and **pulmonary embolism** (PE) resulting from **thrombus** formation in the venous circulation (**Figure 10–1**).[1,2] It is often provoked by prolonged immobility and vascular injury and most frequently seen in patients hospitalized for a serious medical illness, trauma, or major surgery. VTE can also occur with little or no provocation in patients who have an underlying hypercoagulable disorder.

Although VTE may initially cause few or no symptoms, the first overt manifestation of the disease may be sudden death from PE, which can occur within minutes, before effective treatment can be given.[2,3] A history of VTE is a significant risk factor for recurrent thromboembolic events.[4–7] Postthrombotic syndrome (PTS) is a complication of VTE that occurs due to damage to the vein caused by a blood clot and leads to development of symptomatic venous insufficiency such as chronic lower extremity swelling, pain, tenderness, skin discoloration, and ulceration.

The treatment of VTE is fraught with substantial risks.[8] KEY CONCEPT *Antithrombotic therapies (**thrombolytics** and anticoagulants) require precise dosing and meticulous monitoring, as well as ongoing patient assessment and education.*[4,9–10] *Well-organized anticoagulation management services improve quality of care and reduce overall cost.* A systematic approach to drug therapy management reduces risks, but bleeding remains a common and serious complication.[10,11] Therefore, preventing VTE is paramount to improving outcomes. When VTE is suspected, a rapid and accurate diagnosis is critical to making appropriate treatment decisions. The optimal use of antithrombotic drugs requires not only an in-depth knowledge of their pharmacology and pharmacokinetic properties but also a comprehensive approach to patient management.[3,12]

EPIDEMIOLOGY AND ETIOLOGY

The true incidence of VTE in the general population is unknown because many patients, perhaps more than 50%, have no overt symptoms or go undiagnosed.[1,12,13] An estimated 2 million people in the United States develop VTE each year, of whom 600,000 are hospitalized and 60,000 die. The estimated annual direct medical costs of managing the disease are well over $1 billion. The incidence of VTE nearly doubles in each decade of life older than 50 years of age and is slightly higher in men. As the population ages, the total number of DVT and PE cases continues to rise.[1,2,13,14]

KEY CONCEPT *The risk of VTE is related to several factors including age, history of VTE, major surgery (particularly orthopedic procedures of the lower extremities), trauma, malignancy, pregnancy, estrogen use, and **hypercoagulable states*** (**Table 10–1**).[5–7] VTE risk factors can be categorized in one of the three elements of Virchow triad: stasis in blood flow, vascular endothelial injury, and inherited or acquired changes in blood constituents resulting in hypercoagulation states.[16,17] These risk factors are additive, and some can be easily identified in clinical practice.[1,3] A prior history of venous **thrombosis** is perhaps the strongest risk factor for recurrent VTE, presumably because of damage to venous valves

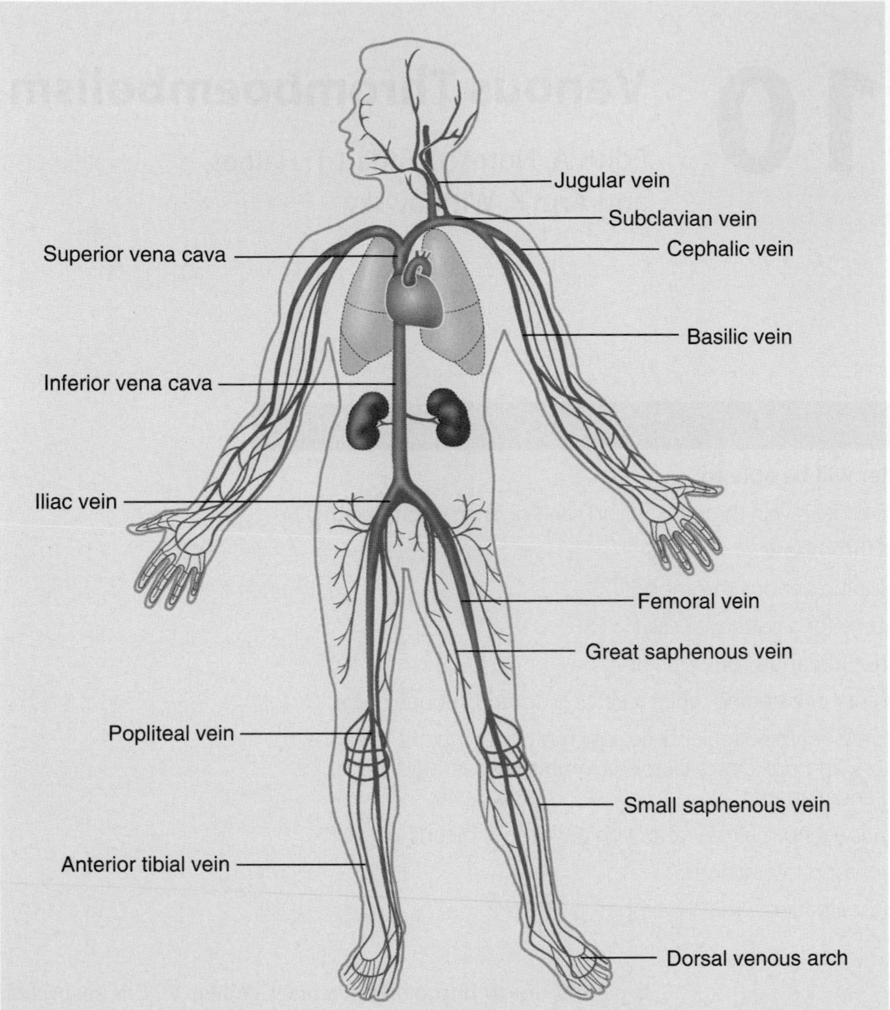

FIGURE 10–1. Venous circulation. (From Witt DM, Clark NP. Venous thromboembolism. In: DiPiro JT, Talbert RL, Yee GC, et al., eds. Pharmacotherapy: A Pathophysiologic Approach, 9th ed. New York, NY: McGraw-Hill, 2014:246.)

and obstruction of blood flow caused by the initial event.[5–7] Rapid blood flow has an inhibitory effect on thrombus formation, but a slow rate of flow reduces the clearance of activated clotting factors in the zone of injury and slows the influx of regulatory substances. Stasis tips the delicate balance of procoagulation and anticoagulation in favor of thrombogenesis. The rate of blood flow in the venous circulation, particularly in the deep veins of the lower extremities, is relatively slow. Valves in the deep veins of the legs, as well as contraction of the calf and thigh muscles, facilitate the flow of blood back to the heart and lungs. Damage to the venous valves and periods of prolonged immobility result in venous stasis. Vessel obstruction, either from a thrombus or external compression, promotes clot propagation. Numerous medical conditions and surgical procedures are associated with reduced venous blood flow and increase the risk of VTE. Greater than normal blood viscosity, seen in myeloproliferative disorders like polycythemia vera, may also contribute to slowed blood flow and thrombus formation.[5–7,16,17]

A growing list of hereditary deficiencies, gene mutations, and acquired diseases have been linked to hypercoagulability (Table 10–1).[18–21] Hereditary deficiencies include activated protein C resistance also known as factor V Leiden, the prothrombin gene 20210A mutation, deficiencies of the natural anticoagulants protein C, protein S, and antithrombin (AT), and high concentrations of factors VIII, IX, and XI. Some patients may have multiple genetic defects. Acquired disorders of hypercoagulability include malignancy, antiphospholipid antibodies, estrogen use, and pregnancy.[22–25] Estrogen-containing contraceptives, estrogen replacement therapy, and many of the selective estrogen receptor modulators (SERMs) increase the risk of venous thrombosis.[23,26] Although the mechanisms are not clearly understood, estrogens increase serum clotting factor concentrations and induce activated protein C resistance. Increased serum estrogen concentrations may explain, in part, the increased risk of VTE during pregnancy and the postpartum period.[23,26]

PATHOPHYSIOLOGY

Hemostasis, the arrest of bleeding following vascular injury, is essential to life.[27] Within the vascular system, blood remains in a fluid state, transporting oxygen, nutrients, plasma proteins, and waste. When a vessel is injured, a dynamic interplay between thrombogenic (activating) and antithrombotic (inhibiting) forces result in the local formation of a hemostatic plug that seals the vessel wall and prevents further blood loss (Figures 10–2 and 10–3). A disruption of this delicate system of checks and balances may lead to inappropriate clot formation within the blood vessel that can obstruct blood flow or embolize to a distant vascular bed.

Table 10–1

Risk Factors for VTE

Risk Factor	Example
Age	Risk doubles with each decade after age 50
History of VTE	Strongest known risk factor for DVT and PE
Venous stasis	Major medical illness (eg, heart failure, acute myocardial infarction, ischemic stroke, acute infection)
	Major surgery (eg, general anesthesia for > 30 minutes)
	Paralysis (eg, due to stroke or spinal cord injury)
	Polycythemia vera
	Obesity
	Varicose veins
	Immobility (eg, bedrest for ≥ 3 days during hospital admission)
Vascular injury	Major orthopedic surgery (eg, knee and hip replacement)
	Trauma (especially fractures of the pelvis, hip, or leg)
	Indwelling venous catheters
Hypercoagulable states	Malignancy, diagnosed or occult
	Activated protein C resistance/factor V Leiden
	Prothrombin (20210A) gene mutation
	Protein C deficiency
	Protein S deficiency
	AT deficiency
	Factor VIII excess (> 90th percentile)
	Factor XI excess (> 90th percentile)
	Antiphospholipid antibodies
	Dysfibrinogenemia
	PAI-I excess
	Pregnancy/postpartum
Drug therapy	Estrogen-containing oral contraceptive pills
	Estrogen replacement therapy
	SERMs
	HIT
	Chemotherapy

AT, antithrombin; DVT, deep vein thrombosis; HIT, heparin-induced thrombocytopenia; PAI-I, plasminogen activator inhibitor; PE, pulmonary embolism; SERMs, selective estrogen receptor modulators; VTE, venous thromboembolism.

Under normal circumstances, the endothelial cells that line the inside of blood vessels maintain blood flow by producing a number of substances that inhibit platelet adherence, prevent the activation of the coagulation cascade, and facilitate **fibrinolysis**.[16,17,27] Vascular injury exposes the subendothelium. Platelets adhere to the subendothelium, using glycoprotein (GP) Ib receptors found on their surfaces and facilitated by von Willebrand factor (vWF). This causes platelets to become activated, releasing a number of procoagulant substances that stimulate circulating platelets to expose GP IIb and IIIa receptors and allow platelets to adhere to one another, resulting in platelet aggregation. The damaged vascular tissue releases tissue factor that activates the extrinsic pathway of the coagulation cascade (Figure 10–3).

The **clotting cascade** is a stepwise series of enzymatic reactions that result in the formation of a fibrin mesh.[12] Clotting factors circulate in the blood in inactive forms. Once a precursor is activated by specific stimuli, it activates the next precursor in the sequence. The final steps in the cascade are the conversion of

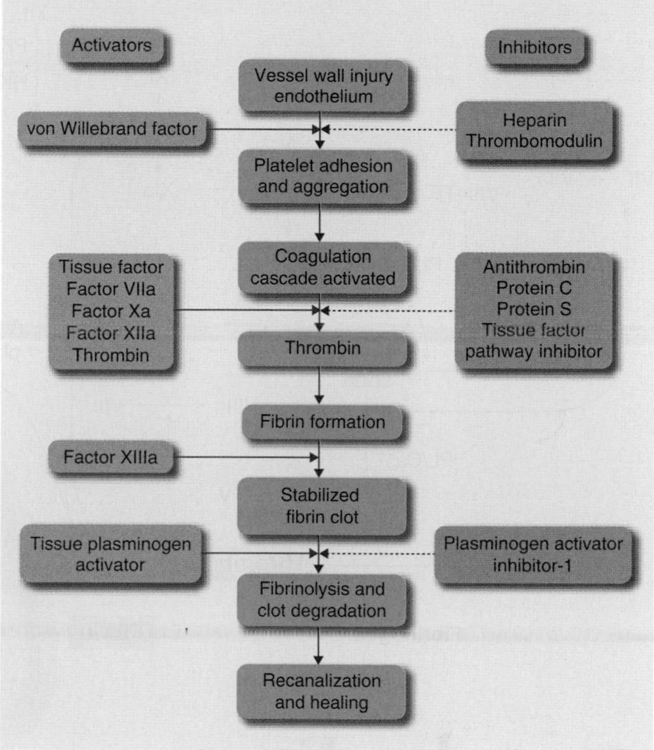

FIGURE 10–2. Hemostasis and thrombosis. (From Witt DM, Clark NP. Venous thromboembolism. In: DiPiro JT, Talbert RL, Yee GC, et al., eds. Pharmacotherapy: A Pathophysiologic Approach, 9th ed. New York, NY: McGraw-Hill, 2014:248.)

prothrombin (factor II) to **thrombin** (factor IIa) and fibrinogen to **fibrin**. Thrombin plays a key role in the coagulation cascade; it is responsible not only for the production of fibrin, but also for the activation of factors V and VIII, creating a positive feedback loop that greatly accelerates the entire cascade. Thrombin also enhances platelet aggregation. Traditionally, the coagulation cascade has been divided into three distinct parts: the intrinsic, the extrinsic, and the common pathways. This artificial division is misleading because there are numerous interactions between the three pathways.[16,17,27] A number of tempering mechanisms control coagulation (Figure 10–2).[27–30] Without effective self-regulation, the coagulation cascade would proceed unabated until all the clotting factors and platelets are consumed.

CLINICAL PRESENTATION AND DIAGNOSIS

Although a thrombus can form in any part of the venous circulation, most begin in the lower extremities. Once formed, a venous thrombus may behave in multiple ways including: (a) remain asymptomatic, (b) spontaneously lyse, (c) obstruct the venous circulation, (d) propagate into more proximal veins, (e) embolize, and/or (f) slowly incorporate into the endothelial layer of the vessel.[1,3,16] Most patients with VTE never develop symptoms.[3,31] However, even those who initially experience no symptoms may suffer long-term consequences, such as PTS and recurrent VTE.

Given that VTE can be debilitating or fatal, it is important to treat it quickly and aggressively.[1,2,12] However, because major bleeding induced by antithrombotic drugs can be equally harmful, it is important to avoid treatment when the diagnosis is not

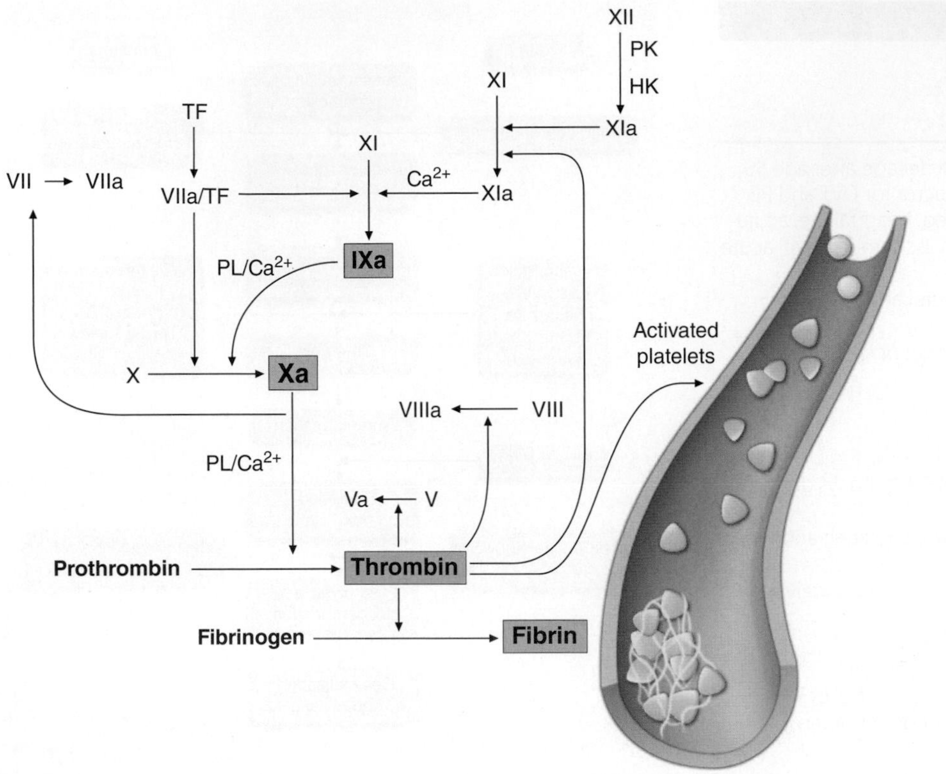

FIGURE 10–3. Summary of coagulation pathways. Specific coagulation factors ("a" indicates activated form) are responsible for the conversion of soluble plasma fibrinogen into insoluble fibrin. This process occurs via a series of linked reactions in which the enzymatically active product subsequently converts the downstream inactive protein into an active serine protease. In addition, the activation of thrombin leads to stimulation of platelets. (HK, high molecular weight kininogen; PK, prekallikrein; TF, tissue factor.) (From Freedman JE, Loscalzo J. Arterial and venous thrombosis. In: Longo DL, Fauci AS, Kasper DL, et al., eds. Harrison's Principles of Internal Medicine, 18th ed. New York, NY: McGraw-Hill, 2012:985.)

reasonably certain. Assessment should focus on patient specific risk factors during the medical history (Table 10–1).[1,2,12] Venous thrombosis is uncommon in the absence of risk factors, and the effects of these risks are additive. If a patient has multiple risk factors, VTE should be strongly suspected even when the symptoms are very subtle.

KEY CONCEPT *The symptoms of DVT or PE are nonspecific, and it is extremely difficult to distinguish VTE from other disorders on clinical signs alone.*[1–3,31] *Therefore, objective tests are required to confirm or exclude the diagnosis.* Patients with DVT frequently present with unilateral leg pain, swelling that can persist after a night's sleep, and cyanosis of the skin in the affected leg (Table 10–2). Similarly, PTS, a long-term complication of DVT caused by damage to the venous valves, produces chronic lower extremity swelling, pain, and tenderness that lead to skin discoloration and ulceration. To distinguish acute DVT from PTS and other possible diagnoses, a clinical prediction rule that incorporates signs, symptoms and risk factors can be used to categorize the patient as at low, intermediate, or high probability of having acute DVT. This model, known as the Wells Criteria, is summarized in Table 10–2.[2,3,12] If the clinical probability of DVT is low, the D-dimer test can be used to confirm the patient does not have DVT. The D-dimer test is a quantitative measure of fibrin breakdown in the serum, and it is a marker of acute thrombotic activity. D-dimer assays are sensitive but not specific markers for VTE, so a negative D-dimer test can be used to rule out the diagnosis of DVT.

If the D-dimer test is positive in a low probability patient, or if the patient has a moderate or high probability of DVT, then an objective test is used to confirm the diagnosis of DVT. Contrast venography allows visualization of the entire venous system in the lower extremities. This radiographic contrast study is the most accurate and reliable method for diagnosis of DVT and considered the gold standard in clinical trials.[3,31–32] However, venography is an expensive, invasive procedure that is technically difficult to perform and evaluate. Severely ill patients may be unable to tolerate the procedure, and many develop hypotension and cardiac arrhythmias. Furthermore, the contrast material

Table 10–2

Clinical Model/Modified Wells Criteria for Evaluating the Pretest Probability of Deep Vein Thrombosis (DVT)[a]

Clinical Characteristic	Score
Active cancer (cancer treatment within previous 6 months or currently on palliative treatment)	+1
Paralysis, paresis, or recent plaster immobilization of the lower extremities	+1
Recently bedridden for 3 days or more, or major surgery within the previous 12 weeks requiring general or regional anesthesia	+1
Localized tenderness along the distribution of the deep venous system	+1
Entire leg swollen	+1
Calf swelling at least 3 cm larger than that on the asymptomatic side (measured 10 cm below tibial tuberosity)	+1
Pitting edema confined to the symptomatic leg	+1
Collateral superficial veins (nonvaricose)	+1
Previously documented DVT	+1
Alternative diagnosis at least as likely as DVT	−2

[a]Assess the patient for the presence of any of the 9 clinical characteristics listed in Table 10-2. Assign a score of "+1" for each characteristic that is present. Tally the total score. If an alternative diagnosis is at least as likely as DVT, then substract 2 points from the total points tallied above. The clinical probability of DVT is low if the score is 0 or less; moderate if the score is 1 or 2; high if the score is 3 or greater. In patients with symptoms in both legs, the more symptomatic leg is used.

Clinical Presentation and Diagnosis of DVT

General

- Most commonly develops in patients with identifiable risk factors (Table 10–1) during or following a hospitalization. Many, perhaps most, patients have asymptomatic disease.

Symptoms

- Patient may complain of leg swelling, pain, warmth, and/or skin discoloration. Symptoms are nonspecific, and objective testing must be performed to establish the diagnosis.

Signs

- Superficial veins may be dilated and a "palpable cord" may be felt in the affected leg.
- May experience unilateral leg edema with measurable difference in leg circumference, erythema, increase in warmth, and tenderness with palpation of calf muscles.
- May experience pain in back of the knee or calf in the affected leg when the examiner dorsiflexes the foot while the knee is slightly bent (Homans sign).
- Note: The physical examination signs can be unreliable. Homans sign (a positive test is pain in the calf or popliteal region with dorsiflexion of the foot) can also be unreliable.

Clinical Probability

- Apply the Wells criteria to determine the probability that the patient's signs, symptoms, and risk factors are the result of DVT (Table 10–2).

Laboratory Tests

- The initial laboratory evaluation should include complete blood count (CBC) with differential, coagulation studies (such as prothrombin time [PT]/international normalized ratio [INR], activated partial thromboplastin time [aPTT]), serum chemistries with renal and liver function, and urinalysis.
- Serum concentrations of D-dimer, a by-product of thrombin generation, will be elevated in an acute event. A negative D-dimer in a patient with low clinical probability of DVT can be used to rule out DVT.
- Patient may have an elevated erythrocyte sedimentation rate (ESR) and white blood cell (WBC) count.

Diagnostic Tests

- Duplex ultrasonography is the most commonly used test to diagnose DVT. It is a noninvasive test that can measure the rate and direction of blood flow and visualize clot formation in proximal veins of the legs. It cannot reliably detect small blood clots in distal veins. Coupled with a careful clinical assessment, it can rule in or out (include or exclude) the diagnosis in most cases. Repeat testing may be necessary if the first test is negative and the patient is still symptomatic.
- Venography (also known as phlebography) is the gold standard for the diagnosis of DVT. However, it is an invasive test that involves injection of radiopaque contrast dye into a foot vein. It is expensive and can cause anaphylaxis and nephrotoxicity.

is irritating to vessel walls and toxic to the kidneys. For these reasons, noninvasive testing using duplex ultrasonography is preferred. See the Clinical Presentation and Diagnosis of DVT textbox for further information.

Like DVT, the nonspecific nature of the signs and symptoms of PE requires further evaluation. Table 10–3 describes a validated prediction model that can be used to stratify patients into high, moderate, and low probability of PE.[3,31–33] In patients with a low clinical probability of PE, diagnosis of PE can be ruled out if D-dimer testing is negative. If D-dimer testing is positive, or if the patient has a moderate or high clinical probability of PE, diagnostic imaging studies should be performed. Pulmonary angiography allows visualization of the pulmonary arteries. Diagnosis of VTE can be made if there is a persistent intraluminal filling defect observed on multiple x-ray films. However, as with DVT, a noninvasive test is preferred, such as computed tomographic pulmonary angiography, magnetic resonance imaging (MRI), and ventilation/perfusion (V/Q) scans. See the Clinical Presentation and Diagnosis of PE textbox for further information.

Table 10–3

Clinical Model/Wells Criteria for Evaluating the Pretest Probability of Pulmonary Embolism (PE)[a]

Clinical Characteristic	Score
Cancer	+1
Hemoptysis	+1
Previous PE or DVT	+1.5
Heart rate greater than 100 beats/min	+1.5
Recent surgery or immobilization	+1.5
Clinical signs of DVT	+3
Alternative diagnosis less likely than PE	+3

DVT, deep vein thrombosis.

[a]Clinical probability of PE: low, 0–1; moderate, 2–6; high, 7 or greater.

PREVENTION

Given that VTE is often clinically silent and potentially fatal, prevention strategies have the greatest potential to improve patient outcomes.[5–7]

The goal of an effective VTE prophylaxis program is to identify all patients at risk, determine each patient's level of risk, and select and implement regimens that provide sufficient protection for the level of risk.[5–7] KEY CONCEPT *At the time of hospital admission, change in level of care, and prior to discharge, all patients should be evaluated for risk of VTE, and appropriate prophylaxis strategies should be routinely used. Prophylaxis should be continued throughout the period of risk.*

There are several risk assessment models available for estimating VTE risk specific to hospitalized medical and surgical patients.[5–7,12] While none of these models have been

Clinical Presentation and Diagnosis of PE

General

- Most commonly develops in patients with risk factors for VTE (Table 10–1) during or following a hospitalization. Although many patients will have symptoms of DVT prior to developing a PE, many do not and some patients can be asymtomatic. Patients may die suddenly before effective treatment can be initiated.

Symptoms

- May complain of cough, pleuritic chest pain, chest tightness, shortness of breath with or without exertion, wheezing, or palpitations.
- May present with **hemoptysis** (spit or cough up blood).
- May complain of dizziness or lightheadedness.
- May be confused for a myocardial infarction (MI) or pneumonia, and objective testing must be performed to establish the diagnosis.

Signs

- May have tachypnea (increased respiratory rate) and tachycardia (increased heart rate).
- May appear diaphoretic (sweaty) and may have fever.
- Neck veins may be distended reflecting increased jugular venous pressure.
- The examiner may hear diminished breath sounds, crackles, wheezes, or pleural friction rub, right ventricular S_3, or parasternal lift during auscultation of the lungs.
- In massive PE, the patient may appear cyanotic and hypotensive and may appear to have signs of right-sided heart failure. In such cases, oxygen saturation by pulse oximetry or arterial blood gas will likely indicate the patient is hypoxic.
- In the worst cases, the patient may go into circulatory shock and die within minutes.

Clinical Probability

- Apply the Wells Criteria to determine the probability that the patient's signs, symptoms, and risk factors are the result of PE (Table 10–3).

Laboratory Tests

- Serum concentrations of D-dimer, a by-product of thrombin generation, will be elevated. A negative D-dimer in a patient with low clinical probability of PE can be used to rule out PE.
- In patients with a low probability for PE, the PE rule-out criteria ("PERC rule") is an alternative to sensitive D-dimer testing. In patients who fulfill the following eight criteria the likelihood of PE is low and no further testing is required: age less than 50 years; heart rate less than 100 beats/min; oxyhemoglobin saturation at or above 95% (0.95); no hemoptysis; no estrogen use; no prior DVT or PE; no unilateral leg swelling; and no surgery/trauma requiring hospitalization within the prior 4 weeks.
- May have an elevated ESR and WBC count.
- May have elevated serum lactate dehydrogenase (LDH) or aspartate aminotransferase (AST; serum glutamic-oxaloacetic transaminase [SGOT]) with normal bilirubin.
- Serum troponin I and troponin T can be elevated in a large PE. These typically resolve within 40 hours if due to PE but persist longer after acute MI.
- Electrocardiogram may show nonspecific ST-segment and T-wave changes and tachycardia.

Diagnostic Imaging Tests

- A computed tomography (CT) scan is the most commonly used test to diagnose PE, but some institutions still use a ventilation/perfusion (V/Q) scan. Spiral CT scans can detect emboli in the pulmonary arteries. A V/Q scan measures the distribution of blood and air flow in the lungs. When there is a large mismatch between blood and air flow in one area of the lung, there is a high probability the patient has a PE.
- Pulmonary angiography is the gold standard for diagnosis of PE. However, it is an invasive test that involves injection of radiopaque contrast dye into the pulmonary artery. The test is expensive and associated with significant risk of mortality.

extensively validated, the Padua Prediction score is recommended for assessment of medical patients **(Table 10–4)** and the Caprini score is recommended for assessment of general surgical patients **(Table 10–5)**. Bleeding risk should also be assessed to help identify patients in whom the risk of bleeding may outweigh benefits of pharmacologic prophylaxis.[5–7] Table 10–6 lists general and procedure-specific risk factors for major bleeding complications. Patients with moderate to high risk of VTE should receive pharmacologic prophylaxis. If pharmacologic prophylaxis is contraindicated, such as in patients actively bleeding or at high risk of bleeding, nonpharmacologic prophylaxis should be used **(Table 10–7)**.

Several pharmacologic and nonpharmacologic methods are effective for preventing VTE, and these can be used alone or in combination (Table 10–7).[5–7,34] Nonpharmacologic methods improve venous blood flow by mechanical means; drug therapy prevents thrombus formation by inhibiting the coagulation cascade.

Nonpharmacologic Therapy

Ambulation as soon as possible following surgery lowers the incidence of VTE in low-risk patients.[5–7,34] Walking increases venous blood flow and promotes the flow of natural antithrombotic factors into the lower extremities. All hospitalized patients should be encouraged to ambulate as early as possible, and as frequently as possible.

Graduated compression stockings (GCS) are specialized hosiery that provide graduated pressure on the lower legs and feet to help prevent thrombosis. Compared with anticoagulant

Table 10–4

Risk Factors for Predicting Venous Thromboembolism (VTE) in Hospitalized Medical Patients (Padua Prediction Score)

Risk Factor	Points
Active cancer[a]	3
Previous VTE (with the exclusion of superficial vein thrombosis)	3
Reduced mobility[b]	3
Already known thrombophilic condition[c]	3
Recent (≤ 1 month) trauma and/or surgery	2
Elderly age (≥ 70 years)	1
Heart and/or respiratory failure	1
Acute myocardial infarction or ischemic stroke	1
Acute infection and/or rheumatologic disorder	1
Obesity (body mass index ≥ 30)	1
Ongoing hormonal treatment	1
Cumulative score of ≥ 4 points indicates high risk of VTE	

[a]Patients with local or distant metastases and/or in whom chemotherapy or radiotherapy had been performed in the previous 6 months.

[b]Anticipated bed rest with bathroom privileges (either because of patient's limitations or on physician's order) for at least 3 days.

[c]Carriage of defects of antithrombin, protein C or S, factor V Leiden, G20210A prothrombin mutation, antiphospholipid syndrome.

Adapted with permission from Kahn SR, Lim W, Dunn AS, et al. Prevention of VTE in nonsurgical patients: Antithrombotic Therapy and Prevention of Thrombosis, 9th ed: American College of Chest Physicians Evidence-Based Clinical Practice Guidelines. Chest. 2012;141(2 suppl):e195S–e226S.

drugs, GCS are relatively inexpensive and safe; however, they are less effective and not recommended in moderate to higher risk patients.[2] They offer an alternate choice in low- to moderate-risk patients when pharmacologic interventions are contraindicated. When combined with pharmacologic interventions, GCS have an additive effect. However, some patients are unable to wear compression stockings because of the size or shape of their legs, and some patients may find them hot, confining, and uncomfortable.

Similar to GCS, intermittent pneumatic compression (IPC) devices increase the velocity of blood flow in the lower extremities.[5–7,34] These devices sequentially inflate a series of cuffs wrapped around the patient's legs from the ankles to the thighs and then deflate in 1- to 2-minute cycles. Although IPC has been shown to reduce the risk of VTE in surgical patients, most studies failed to define the type of device used. IPC was frequently used in combination with other prophylaxis methods, making it difficult to quantify their efficacy. Although IPC is safe to use in patients who have contraindications to pharmacologic therapies, it does have a few drawbacks: it is more expensive than GCS, it is a relatively cumbersome technique, some patients may have difficulty sleeping while using it, and some patients find the devices hot, sticky, and uncomfortable. To be effective, IPC needs to be used throughout the day. In practice, this is difficult to achieve, and special efforts should be made to ensure the devices are worn and operational for most of the day.

Inferior vena cava (IVC) filters, also known as Greenfield filters, provide short-term protection against PE in very high-risk patients by preventing the **embolization** of a thrombus formed in the lower extremities into the pulmonary circulation.[5–7,34] Insertion of a filter into the IVC is a minimally invasive procedure. Despite the widespread use of IVC filters, there are very limited data regarding their effectiveness and long-term safety. The evidence suggests that IVC filters, particularly in the absence of effective antithrombotic therapy, are thrombogenic themselves and increase the long-term risk of recurrent DVT and of filter thrombosis. Although IVC filters can reduce the short-term risk of PE in patients at highest risk, they should be reserved for patients in whom other prophylactic strategies cannot be used. To further reduce the long-term risk of VTE in association with IVC filters, pharmacologic prophylaxis is necessary in patients with IVC filters in place, and warfarin therapy should begin as soon as the patient is able to tolerate it.[2] If used, retrievable filters are preferred, which can be removed once pharmacologic prophylaxis can be safely administered or once the patient is no longer at risk for VTE.

Pharmacologic Therapy

Appropriately selected drug therapies can dramatically reduce the incidence of VTE in medical and surgical patients (Table 10–7). The choice of medication and dose to use for VTE prevention must be based on the patient's level of risk for thrombosis and bleeding risk, as well as the cost and availability of an adequate drug therapy monitoring system.[5–7,34]

The most extensively studied drugs for the prevention of VTE are unfractionated heparin (UFH), the low molecular weight heparins (LMWHs; dalteparin and enoxaparin), fondaparinux, and warfarin.[5–7,34] Generally the LMWHs provide improved protection against VTE when compared with low-dose UFH in most medical and surgical patients and when compared to low-dose UFH and warfarin in major orthopedic surgery patients. Fondaparinux is more effective than LMWH in patients undergoing high-risk orthopedic surgery, but it has a heightened risk of bleeding.

For hospitalized general surgical and medical patients, the available evidence supports the use of UFH (5000 Units every 12 or 8 hours), enoxaparin 40 mg subcutaneously (SC) daily, dalteparin 2500 to 5000 Units SC daily, or fondaparinux 2.5 mg SC daily.

For the prevention of VTE following major orthopedic surgery, current evidence supports the use of UFH, LMWH, fondaparinux, adjusted dose warfarin, aspirin, and the newer direct oral anticoagulants (DOACs) apixaban, dabigatran and rivaroxaban. However, dabigatran is not yet approved by the Food and Drug Administration (FDA) for this indication. Additionally, the role of aspirin for VTE prevention is controversial as it produces a very modest reduction in VTE following orthopedic surgeries of the lower extremities.[5,34]

The effectiveness of UFH, aspirin, and warfarin is lower than LMWH, thus current American College of Chest Physicians (ACCP) guidelines recommend the use of LMWH or fondaparinux preferentially over other pharmacologic options in major orthopedic surgery patients.[5,34] The appropriate prophylactic dose for each LMWH product in orthopedic surgery is indication specific; however, enoxaparin 30 mg SC twice daily, enoxaparin 40 mg SC daily, and dalteparin 5000 Units SC daily are the most commonly used regimens. The dose of fondaparinux is 2.5 mg SC daily.

The dose of warfarin, another commonly used option for prevention of VTE following orthopedic surgery, must be adjusted to maintain an INR between 2 and 3.[5,34] Oral administration and low drug acquisition cost give warfarin some advantages over the LMWHs and fondaparinux. However, warfarin does not achieve its full antithrombotic effect for several days and requires

Table 10–5

Risk Factors for Predicting VTE in General Surgical Patients (Modified Caprini Risk Assessment Model for VTE in General Surgical Patients)

Risk Score			
1 Point	**2 Points**	**3 Points**	**5 Points**
Age 41–60 years Minor surgery BMI > 25 kg/m² Swollen legs Varicose veins Pregnancy or postpartum History of unexplained or recurrent spontaneous abortion Oral contraceptives or hormone replacement Sepsis (< 1 month) Serious lung disease, including pneumonia (< 1 month) Abnormal pulmonary function Acute myocardial infarction Heart failure (< 1 month) History of inflammatory bowel disease Medical patient at bed rest	Age 61–74 years Arthroscopic surgery Major open surgery (> 45 minutes) Laparoscopic surgery (> 45 minutes) Malignancy Confined to bed (> 72 hours) Immobilizing plaster cast Central venous access	Age ≥ 75 years History of VTE Family history of VTE Factor V Leiden Prothrombin 20210A Lupus anticoagulant Anticardiolipin antibodies Elevated serum homocysteine Heparin-induced thrombocytopenia Other congenital or acquired thrombophilia	Stroke (< 1 month) Elective arthroplasty Acute spinal cord injury (< 1 month)

Risk Score Interpretation

Total Risk Score	Risk of VTE
0	Very low (< 0.5%)
1–2	Low (1.5%)
3–4	Moderate (3%)
≥ 5	High (6%)

BMI, body mass index; VTE, venous thromboembolism.

Adapted with permission from Gould MK, Garcia DA, Wren SM, et al. Prevention of VTE in nonorthopedic surgical patients: Antithrombotic Therapy and Prevention of Thrombosis, 9th ed: American College of Chest Physicians Evidence-Based Clinical Practice Guidelines. Chest. 2012;141(2 suppl):e227S–e277S.

Patient Encounter 1

A 75-year-old obese man (BMI 40 kg/m²) with a history of DVT and diverticulosis is admitted to the hospital after a 3-day period of severe abdominal pain, fever, nausea, and constipation. He is diagnosed with peritonitis and started on antibiotic therapy.

PMH: DVT in left lower extremity 12 years ago; diverticulosis × 10 years; depression × 5 years; chronic knee pain × 3 years; hypertension × 2 years

FH: Father died at 55 years due to MI; Mother died at 74 years due to breast cancer

SH: Occasional alcohol use. Employed in county government. Lives at home with spouse and pets

Home Meds: Aspirin 81 mg by mouth once daily; metoprolol 50 mg by mouth twice daily; bupropion XL 300 mg by mouth once daily

Allergies: NKDA

VS: BP 135/70 mm Hg, HR 72 beats/min, RR 16 breaths/min, T 38.7°C (101.6°F), Wt 90 kg (198 lb)

Labs: WBC 22.4 × 10^3/mm³ (22.4 × 10^9/L); estimated glomerular filtration rate (eGFR) 80 mL/min/1.73 m² (0.77 mL/s/m²)

Hospital Treatment: Bowel rest with nothing by mouth; metronidazole 500 mg IV every 8 hours; ceftriaxone 1 gm IV every 24 hours

Which risk factor(s) predispose this patient to VTE?

What is his estimated risk for developing VTE?

Given his presentation and history, create an appropriate VTE prophylaxis plan including the pharmacologic agent, dose, route and frequency of administration, duration of therapy, and monitoring parameters.

Table 10–6

Risk Factors for Major Bleeding Complications

General Risk Factors	Procedure-Specific Risk Factors	Procedures in Which Bleeding Complications May Have Especially Severe Consequences
Active bleeding Previous major bleeding Known, untreated bleeding disorder Severe renal or hepatic failure Thrombocytopenia Acute stroke Uncontrolled systemic hypertension Lumbar puncture, epidural, or spinal anesthesia within previous 4 hours or next 12 hours Concomitant use of anticoagulants, antiplatelet therapy, or thrombolytic drugs	**Abdominal Surgery** Male sex, preoperative hemoglobin level < 13 g/dL (130 g/L; 8.07 mmol/L), malignancy, and complex surgery defined as two or more procedures, difficult dissection, or more than one anastomosis **Pancreaticoduodenectomy** Sepsis, pancreatic leak, sentinel bleed **Hepatic Resection** Number of segments, concomitant extrahepatic organ resection, primary liver malignancy, lower preoperative hemoglobin level, and platelet counts **Cardiac Surgery** Use of aspirin Use of clopidogrel within 3 days before surgery BMI > 25 kg/m^2, nonelective surgery, placement of five or more grafts, older age renal insufficiency, operation other than CABG, longer bypass time **Thoracic Surgery** Pneumonectomy or extended resection	Craniotomy Spinal surgery Spinal trauma Reconstructive procedures involving free flap

BMI, body mass index; CABG, coronary artery bypass graft.

Adapted with permission from Gould MK, Garcia DA, Wren SM, et al. Prevention of VTE in nonorthopedic surgical patients: Antithrombotic Therapy and Prevention of Thrombosis, 9th ed: American College of Chest Physicians Evidence-Based Clinical Practice Guidelines. Chest. 2012;141(2 suppl):e227S–e277S.

frequent monitoring and periodic dosage adjustments, making therapy cumbersome. Warfarin should only be used when a systematic patient monitoring system is available.

The oral factor Xa inhibitors rivaroxaban and apixaban are newer options for VTE prevention following hip and knee replacement surgery and offer a convenient alternative to traditional anticoagulants.[5,34–36] Both agents have shown superior efficacy compared to LMWH with a similar rate of bleeding complications. Rivaroxaban is given at a fixed dose of 10 mg once daily, and apixaban is given at a fixed dose of 2.5 mg twice daily. Both are given without the need for routine laboratory monitoring and dosing adjustments (as with warfarin) and without the inconvenience of administration by injection (as with LMWH and fondaparinux).

The optimal duration for VTE prophylaxis is not well established but should be given throughout the period of risk. For patients who have undergone total knee replacement, total hip replacement, or hip fracture repair, prophylaxis is recommended for a minimum of 10 to 14 days; however, extending it up to 35 days is recommended due to continued VTE risk up to one month postsurgery.[5–7,34]

TREATMENT

Desired Therapeutic Outcomes

The goal of VTE treatment is to prevent short- and long-term complications of the disease. The aim of initial therapy is to prevent propagation or local extension of the clot, embolization, hemodynamic collapse, and death. The goal of long-term and extended therapy is to prevent complications such as PTS, pulmonary hypertension, and recurrent VTE.[2,12]

General Treatment Principles

Anticoagulant drugs are considered the mainstay of therapy for patients with VTE, and the therapeutic strategies for DVT and PE are similar.[2,12] Management decisions are guided by balancing the risks and benefits of various treatment options. The treatment of VTE can be divided into three phases: acute (first 5–10 days), long term (first 3 months), and extended (beyond 3 months).[12] The acute treatment phase of VTE is typically accomplished by administering a fast-acting parenteral or a DOAC (Table 10–8). The long-term and extended phase treatments of VTE are usually accomplished using oral anticoagulant agents such as warfarin, or one of the DOACs (apixaban, dabigatran, and rivaroxaban).[2,12] In certain populations, such as patients with cancer and women who are pregnant, the LMWHs are the preferred agents during long-term and extended treatment phases due to better safety or efficacy.[2] The etiology of VTE will guide the duration of therapy. VTE can be provoked (by transient risk factors), unprovoked (or idiopathic) and cancer associated. Patients with unprovoked or cancer associated VTE have a significantly higher risk of recurrence compared to patients with provoked VTE.[2,12]

KEY CONCEPT *In the absence of contraindications, the treatment of VTE should initially include a rapid-acting injectable anticoagulant (eg, UFH, LMWH, fondaparinux) or a rapidly acting DOAC (eg, apixaban, rivaroxaban). If warfarin is used for oral anticoagulation, it should be initiated on the same day as the parenteral anticoagulant, and the parenteral agent should be overlapped for a minimum of 5 days and until the INR is greater than or equal to 2 for at least 24 hours. Anticoagulation therapy should*

Table 10–7[5–7]

Thrombosis Risk Classification and Recommended VTE Prevention Strategies

Indication and Level of Risk	Prevention Strategies
Hospitalized Medical Patients	
Low thrombosis risk	Early ambulation
High thrombosis risk[a] (Padua Score > 4)	LMWH, LDUH, fondaparinux
Critically Ill Patients	
High thrombosis risk[a]	LMWH, LDUH
General Surgical Patients	
Very low thrombosis risk (Caprini Score 0)	Early Ambulation
Low thrombosis risk (Caprini Score 1–2)	IPC
Moderate thrombosis risk[b] (Caprini Score 3–4)	LMWH, LDUH, IPC
High thrombosis risk[b] (Caprini Score ≥ 5)	LMWH, LDUH, plus GCS or IPC
Cancer Surgery	LMWH
Major Orthopedic Surgery	
Hip fracture surgery[b]	LMWH, fondaparinux, LDUH, adjusted dose warfarin, ASA
Hip and knee arthroplasty[b]	LMWH, fondaparinux, LDUH, warfarin, ASA, apixaban, dabigatran, rivaroxaban

ASA, aspirin; GCS, graduated compression stockings; IPC, intermittent pneumatic compression; LDUH, low-dose unfractionated heparin; LMWH, low molecular weight heparin; VTE, venous thromboembolism.

[a]Mechanical methods of prophylaxis with IPC or GCS should be used in patients actively bleeding or those at high risk of bleeding complications (See Table 10–6 for risk factors for major bleeding).

[b]Mechanical methods of prophylaxis with IPC should be used in patients actively bleeding or those at high risk of bleeding complications (See Table 10–6 for risk factors for major bleeding).

Table 10–8

Pharmacologic Options for the Acute Phase Treatment of VTE

Parenteral Anticoagulants

UFH

IV administration:[a] use weight-based dosing nomogram (Table 10–10)

Or

SC administration: 17,500 units (250 units/kg) given every 12 hours (an initial 5000 unit IV bolus dose is recommended to obtain rapid anticoagulation)

Adjust subsequent doses to attain a goal aPTT based on the institution-specific therapeutic range

Or

SC administration: 333 units/kg followed by 250 units/kg given every 12 hours (fixed-dose unmonitored dosing regimen)

LMWHs

Dalteparin: 200 units/kg SC once daily *or* 100 units/kg SC twice daily

Enoxaparin: 1.5 mg/kg SC once daily *or* 1 mg/kg SC twice daily; if CrCl < 30 mL/min (0.50 mL/s): 1 mg/kg SC once daily

Factor Xa Inhibitor

Fondaparinux[b]:

For body weight < 50 kg (110 lb), use 5 mg SC once daily

For body weight 50–100 kg (110–220 lb), use 7.5 mg SC once daily

For body weight > 100 kg (220 lb), use 10 mg SC once daily

Direct Oral Anticoagulants

Apixaban: 10 mg po twice daily for the initial 7 days, then 5 mg po twice daily[c]

Rivaroxaban: 15 mg po twice daily for the initial 21 days, then 20 mg po daily[d]

aPTT, activated partial thromboplastin time; CrCl, creatinine clearance; IV, intravenous; LMWHs, low molecular weight heparins; SC, subcutaneous; UFH, unfractionated heparin; VTE, venous thromboembolism.

[a]IV administration preferred due to improved dosing precision.

[b]Contraindicated in patients with CrCl < 30mL/min (0.50 mL/s).

[c]After the initial 6 months of therapy, the dose is reduced to 2.5 mg po twice daily.

[d]Avoid in patients with CrCl < 30mL/min (0.50 mL/s).

Patient Encounter 2

A 64-year-old woman with a new diagnosis of squamous cell cancer of the tongue is admitted to the hospital for extensive surgical resection of her tongue, feeding tube placement and Port-a-Cath placement for future chemotherapy.

PMH: Dyslipidemia × 8 years; history of hip fracture 3 years ago with subsequent lower left extremity DVT, treated with LMWH and warfarin for 3 months

FH: Brother 47 years old with type 2 diabetes; maternal grandfather died at 65 years due to pancreatic cancer.

SH: Smoked half a pack per day for 25 years, quit 15 years ago; occasional alcohol use. Lives alone and expects to be discharged to a rehabilitation facility postoperatively before returning home

Home Meds: Simvastatin 40 mg by mouth daily; oxycodone 5 to 10 mg by mouth every 5 hours as needed for pain; docusate 250 mg by mouth twice daily

Allergies: NKDA

VS: BP 110/60 mm Hg, HR 55 beats/min, RR 18 breaths/min, T 37.0°C (98.6°F), Wt 127 kg (280 lb), BMI 40 kg/m^2

Labs: All within normal limits; eGFR 96 mL/min/1.73 m^2 (0.92 mL/s/m^2)

Which risk factor(s) predispose this patient to VTE?

How should postoperative VTE be prevented?

How long should she receive VTE prophylaxis?

What education about VTE prophylaxis should she receive?

be continued for a minimum of 3 months. However, the duration of anticoagulation therapy should be based on the patient's risk of VTE recurrence and major bleeding.[2,12]

Pharmacologic Therapy

▶ *Thrombolytics*

The role of thrombolysis in the treatment of VTE is controversial.[2,12,37] Compared with anticoagulants, thrombolytics restore venous patency more quickly; however, the bleeding risk associated with their use is significantly higher. In patients with DVT, thrombolytics decrease short-term pain and swelling and prevent destruction of the venous valves. While they may decrease the incidence and severity of PTS, clinical trials have failed to show reduction in recurrent DVT, PE or death[37]; therefore, their use in most patients is not recommended.[2,12] In a select group of high-risk patients with massive iliofemoral DVT who are at risk of venous gangrene and limb loss, thrombolysis may be considered. See Table 10–9.

In patients with acute PE, the use of thrombolytics provides short-term benefits such as restoring pulmonary artery patency and hemodynamic stability.[2,12,37] However, systemic thrombolysis does not reduce mortality and is associated with a greater risk of major bleeding.[12] Given the relative lack of data to support their routine use, thrombolytics should be reserved for select high-risk circumstances. Candidates for thrombolytic therapy are patients with acute massive embolism who are hemodynamically unstable (systolic blood pressure [SBP] less than 90 mm Hg) and at low risk for bleeding. Current guidelines recommend a short infusion time (2 hours) over prolonged infusion times (24 hours) and administration through a peripheral vein over a pulmonary artery catheter.[2,12]

▶ *Unfractionated Heparin*

UFH has traditionally been the drug of choice for indications requiring a rapid anticoagulation including the acute treatment of VTE. Unlike thrombolytics, UFH and other anticoagulants will not dissolve a formed clot but prevent its propagation and growth.[2,9] Heparin exerts its anticoagulant effect by augmenting the natural anticoagulant, AT. See Figure 10–4.

UFH can be administered via the intravenous (IV) or subcutaneous (SC) route.[2,9] See Table 10–8. When rapid anticoagulation is required, UFH should be administered IV and an initial bolus dose should be given. For the treatment of VTE, UFH is generally given as a continuous IV infusion. The half-life of UFH is dose dependent and ranges from 30 to 90 minutes but may be significantly longer, up to 150 minutes, with high doses. UFH is eliminated by two mechanisms: (a) enzymatic degradation via a saturable zero-order process, and (b) renally via a first-order process. Lower UFH doses are primarily cleared via enzymatic processes, whereas higher doses are primarily renally eliminated. Clearance of UFH can be impaired in patients with renal and hepatic dysfunction. Patients with active thrombosis may require higher UFH doses due to a more rapid elimination or variations in the plasma concentrations of heparin-binding proteins. AT deficiency and elevated factor VIII levels are common in pregnant patients. AT deficiency has been linked to higher UFH dose requirements. The requirement of these higher UFH doses is termed *heparin resistance*. Factor VIII elevations can result in altered activated partial thromboplastin time (aPTT) response to UFH, and monitoring with antifactor Xa levels is recommended.[2,9,10]

The dose of UFH required to achieve a therapeutic anticoagulant response is correlated to the patient's weight.[2,9] Weight-based dosing regimens should be used to exceed the therapeutic threshold in the first 24 hours after initiating treatment.[9,10] Achieving a therapeutic aPTT in the first 24 hours after initiating UFH is critical because it has been shown to lower the risk of recurrent VTE. For nonobese patients, the actual body weight should be used to calculate the initial UFH dose (Table 10–10). For obese patients, using the actual body weight to calculate the initial dose is also generally recommended; however, data are limited in morbidly obese patients, that is, weight more than 150 kg (330 lb). Some experts recommend using an adjusted body weight (ABW) in these patients instead. The infusion rate is then adjusted based on laboratory monitoring of the patient's response.[9,10]

Table 10–9

Thrombolysis for the Treatment of VTE

- Thrombolytic therapy should be reserved for patients who present with shock, hypotension, or massive DVT with limb gangrene
- Diagnosis must be objectively confirmed before initiating thrombolytic therapy
- Thrombolytic therapy is most effective when administered as soon as possible after PE diagnosis, but benefit may extend up to 14 days after symptom onset

FDA-Approved PE Thrombolytic Regimens

  - Streptokinase 250,000 units IV bolus over 30 minutes followed by 100,000 units/hour for 12–24 hours[a]
  - Urokinase 4400 units/kg IV bolus over 10 minutes followed by 4400 units/kg/hour for 12–24 hours[a]
  - Alteplase (rt-PA) 100 mg IV over 2 hours

Non-FDA Approved Thrombolytic Regimens

  - Reteplase two 10-unit IV boluses given 30 minutes apart
  - Tenecteplase weight-adjusted IV bolus over 5 seconds (30–50 mg with a 5-mg step every 10 kg from < 60 to > 90 kg)

- Factors that increase the risk of bleeding must be evaluated before thrombolytic therapy is initiated (ie, recent surgery, trauma or internal bleeding, uncontrolled hypertension, recent stroke, or ICH)
- Baseline labs should include CBC and blood typing in case transfusion is needed
- UFH should not be used during thrombolytic therapy. Neither the aPTT nor any other anticoagulation parameter should be monitored during the thrombolytic infusion
- aPTT should be measured following the completion of thrombolytic therapy:
  - If aPTT < 2.5 times the control value, UFH infusion should be started and adjusted to maintain aPTT in therapeutic range
  - If aPTT > 2.5 times the control value, remeasure every 2–4 hours and start UFH infusion when aPTT is < 2.5
- Avoid phlebotomy, arterial puncture, and other invasive procedures during thrombolytic therapy to minimize the risk of bleeding

aPTT, activated partial thromboplastin time; CBC, complete blood count; DVT, deep vein thrombosis; FDA, Food and Drug Administration; ICH, intracranial hemorrhage; IV, intravenous; PE, pulmonary embolism; rt-PA, recombinant tissue plasminogen activator; UFH, unfractionated heparin; VTE, venous thromboembolism.

[a]Two-hour infusions of streptokinase and urokinase are as effective and safe as alteplase; 2-hour infusion times are preferred over longer infusion times.

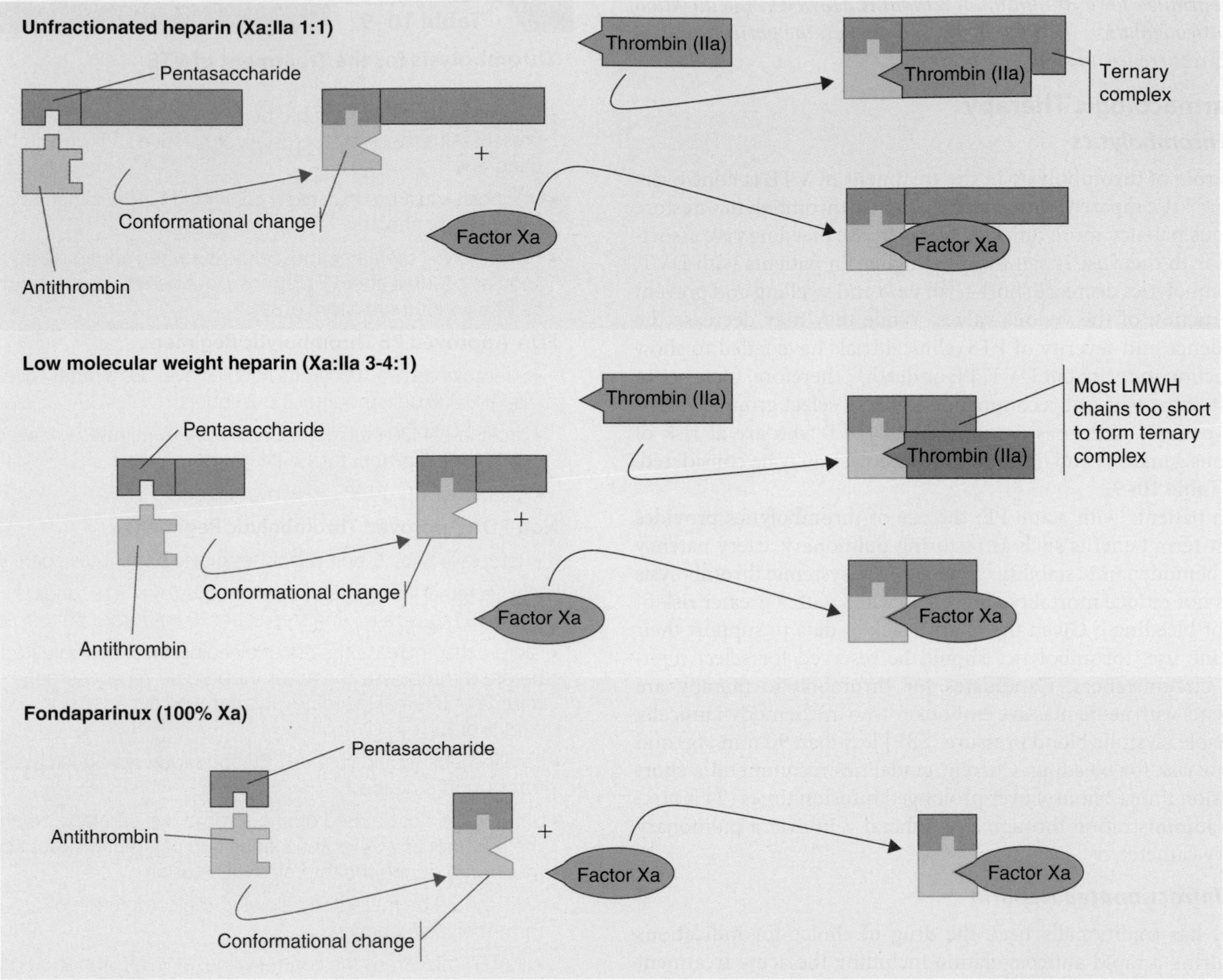

FIGURE 10–4. Mechanism of action of unfractionated heparin, low molecular weight heparin (LMWH), and fondaparinux. (From Witt DM, Clark NP. Venous thromboembolism. In: DiPiro JT, Talbert RL, Yee GC, et al., eds. Pharmacotherapy: A Pathophysiologic Approach, 9th ed. New York, NY: McGraw-Hill, 2014:266.)

KEY CONCEPT *Due to significant variability in interpatient response and changes in patient response over time, UFH requires close monitoring and periodic dose adjustment.* The response to UFH can be monitored using a variety of laboratory tests including the aPTT, the whole blood clotting time, activated clotting time (ACT), antifactor Xa activity, and the plasma heparin concentration.[9,10] Although it has several limitations, the aPTT is the most widely used test in clinical practice to monitor UFH. Traditionally, therapeutic aPTT range is defined as 1.5 to 2.5 times the control aPTT value. However, due to variations in reagents and instruments used to measure the aPTT in different laboratories, each institution should establish a therapeutic range for UFH. The institution-specific therapy range should correlate with a plasma heparin concentration of 0.2 to 0.4 units/mL (0.2–0.4 kU/L) by protamine titration or 0.3 to 0.7 units/mL (0.3–0.7 kU/L) by an amidolytic antifactor Xa assay.[4,33] An aPTT should be obtained at baseline, 6 hours after initiating the heparin infusion, and 6 hours after each dose change because this is the time required to reach steady state. UFH dose is then adjusted based on the aPTT measurement and institutional-specific therapeutic range (Table 10–10). In patients with heparin resistance, antifactor Xa concentrations may be a more accurate method of monitoring the patient's response.[9,10]

Side effects associated with UFH include bleeding, thrombocytopenia, hypersensitivity reactions, and, with prolonged use, alopecia, hyperkalemia, and osteoporosis.[9,10] KEY CONCEPT *Bleeding is the most common adverse effect associated with antithrombotic drugs including UFH therapy.*[8] *A patient's risk of major hemorrhage is related to the intensity and stability of therapy, age, concurrent drug use, history of gastrointestinal bleeding, risk of falls or trauma, and recent surgery.* Several risk factors can increase the risk of UFH-induced bleeding (Table 10–11). The risk of bleeding is related to intensity of anticoagulation. Higher aPTT values are associated with an increased risk of bleeding. The risk of major bleeding is 1% to 5% during the first few days of treatment.[2,9,10] In addition to the aPTT, hemoglobin, hematocrit, and blood pressure should be monitored. Concurrent use of UFH with other antithrombotic agents, such as thrombolytics and antiplatelet agents, also increases bleeding risk. Patients receiving UFH therapy should be closely monitored for signs and symptoms of bleeding, including epistaxis, hemoptysis, hematuria, **hematochezia**, **melena**, severe headache, and joint pain. If major

Table 10–10

Weight-Based[a] Dosing for UFH Administered by Continuous IV Infusion for VTE

Initial Loading Dose	Initial Infusion Rate
80 units/kg (maximum = 10,000 units)	18 units/kg/hour (maximum = 2300 units/hour)
	Maintenance Infusion Rate
aPTT (seconds)	*Dose Adjustment*
< 37 (or < 12 seconds below institution-specific therapeutic range)	80 units/kg bolus then increase infusion by 4 units/kg/hour
37–47 (or 1–12 seconds below institution-specific therapeutic range)	40 units/kg bolus then increase infusion by 2 units/kg/hour
48–71 (within institution-specific therapeutic range)	No change
72–93 (or 1–22 seconds above institution-specific therapeutic range)	Decrease infusion by 2 units/kg/hour
> 93 (or > 22 seconds above institution-specific therapeutic range)	Hold infusion for 1 hour then decrease by 3 units/kg/hour

aPTT, activated partial thromboplastin time; IV, intravenous; UFH, unfractionated heparin; VTE, venous thromboembolism.

[a]Use actual body weight for all calculations. Adjusted body weight (ABW) may be used for morbidly obese patients (> 130% of ideal body weight [IBW]).

ABW = IBW + (Actual body weight − IBW) × 0.7

bleeding occurs, UFH should be stopped immediately and the source of bleeding treated.[9,10] If necessary, use protamine sulfate to reverse the effects of UFH. The usual dose is 1 mg protamine sulfate per 100 units of UFH, up to a maximum of 50 mg, given as a slow IV infusion over 10 minutes. The effects of UFH are neutralized in 5 minutes, and the effects of protamine persist for 2 hours. If bleeding is not controlled or the anticoagulant effect rebounds, repeated doses of protamine may be administered.[9,10]

Heparin-induced thrombocytopenia (HIT) is a very serious adverse effect associated with UFH use. Platelet counts should be monitored every 2 to 3 days during the course of UFH therapy.[9,10] HIT should be suspected if the platelet count drops by more than 50% from baseline or to below 150 × 10^3/mm^3 (150 × 10^9/L). HIT should also be suspected if thrombosis occurs despite UFH use. Immediate discontinuation of all heparin-containing products including the use of LMWHs is in order. Alternative anticoagulation with direct thrombin inhibitors (DTIs) should be initiated. In patients with contraindications to anticoagulation therapy, UFH should not be administered (Table 10–12).

UFH is FDA pregnancy category C and may be used to treat VTE during pregnancy. UFH should be used with caution in the peripartum period due to risk of maternal hemorrhage. UFH is not secreted into breast milk and is safe for use by women who wish to breastfeed.[2,9,10,23] For treatment of VTE in children, the UFH dose is 50 units/kg bolus followed by an infusion of 20,000 units/m^2 per 24 hours. Alternatively, a loading dose of 75 units/kg followed by

Table 10–11

Risk Factors for Major Bleeding While Taking Anticoagulation Therapy

- Anticoagulation intensity (eg, INR > 5, aPTT > 120 seconds)
- Initiation of therapy (first few days and weeks)
- Unstable anticoagulation response
- Age older than 65 years
- Concurrent antiplatelet drug use
- Concurrent nonsteroidal anti-inflammatory drug or aspirin use
- History of gastrointestinal bleeding
- Recent surgery or trauma
- High risk for fall/trauma
- Heavy alcohol use
- Renal failure
- Cerebrovascular disease
- Malignancy

aPTT, activated partial thromboplastin time; INR, international normalized ratio.

Table 10–12

Contraindications to Anticoagulation Therapy

General
- Active bleeding
- Hemophilia or other hemorrhagic tendencies
- Severe liver disease with elevated baseline PT
- Severe thrombocytopenia (platelet count < 20 × 10^3/mm^3 [20 × 10^9/L])
- Malignant hypertension
- Inability to meticulously supervise and monitor treatment

Product-Specific Contraindications
- UFH
  - Hypersensitivity to UFH
  - History of HIT
- LMWHs
  - Hypersensitivity to LMWH, UFH, pork products, methylparaben, or propylparaben
  - History of HIT or suspected HIT
- Fondaparinux
  - Hypersensitivity to fondaparinux
  - Severe renal insufficiency (CrCl < 30 mL/min [0.50 mL/s])
  - Body weight < 50 kg (110 lb)
  - Bacterial endocarditis
  - Thrombocytopenia with a positive in vitro test for antiplatelet antibodies in the presence of fondaparinux
- Lepirudin
  - Hypersensitivity to hirudins
- Argatroban
  - Hypersensitivity to argatroban
- Warfarin
  - Hypersensitivity to warfarin
  - Pregnancy
  - History of warfarin-induced skin necrosis
  - Inability to obtain follow-up PT/INR measurements
  - Inappropriate medication use or lifestyle behaviors
- Dabigatran
  - Mechanical prosthetic heart valves
  - Hypersensitivity to dabigatran
- Apixaban
  - Hypersensitivity to apixaban
- Rivaroxaban
  - Hypersensitivity to rivaroxaban

CrCl, creatinine clearance; HIT, heparin-induced thrombocytopenia; INR, international normalized ratio; LMWHs, low molecular weight heparins; PT, prothrombin time; UFH, unfractionated heparin.

an infusion of 28 units/kg/hour if younger than 12 months old and 20 units/kg/hour if older than 1 year may be considered.[38]

▸ *Low Molecular Weight Heparins*

Compared with UFH, LMWHs have improved pharmacodynamic and pharmacokinetic properties.[9,10,12] They exhibit less binding to plasma and cellular proteins, resulting in a more predictable anticoagulant response. Consequently, routine monitoring of anticoagulation activity and dose adjustments are not required in most patients. LMWHs have longer plasma half-lives, allowing once- or twice-daily administration, improved SC bioavailability, and dose-independent renal clearance. In addition, LMWHs have a more favorable side-effect profile than UFH. They are also associated with a lower incidence of HIT and osteopenia. Two LMWHs are currently available in the United States: dalteparin and enoxaparin.

Like UFH, LMWHs prevent the propagation and growth of formed thrombi.[9] The anticoagulant effect is mediated through a specific pentasaccharide sequence that binds to AT. The primary difference in the pharmacologic activity of UFH and LMWH is their relative inhibition of thrombin (factor IIa) and factor Xa. Smaller heparin fragments cannot bind AT and thrombin simultaneously (Figure 10–4). The SC bioavailability of the LMWHs is greater than 90%. Peak anticoagulant effect of the LMWHs is reached 3 to 5 hours after a SC dose. The elimination half-life is 3 to 6 hours and is agent specific. In patients with renal impairment, the half-life of LMWHs is prolonged.[9,10,12]

The dose of LMWHs for the treatment of VTE is determined based on the patient's weight and is administered SC once or twice daily (Table 10–8). The dose of enoxaparin is expressed in milligrams, whereas the dose of dalteparin is expressed in units of antifactor Xa activity. Due to their predictable anticoagulant effect, routine monitoring is not necessary in most patients.[9] LMWHs have been evaluated in a large number of randomized trials and have been shown to be at least as safe and effective as UFH for the treatment of VTE.[2,12] Indeed, the rate of mortality was lower in patients treated with a LMWH in clinical trials. This mortality benefit was primarily seen in patients with cancer.[39]

Prior to initiating treatment with a LMWH, baseline laboratory tests should include PT/INR, aPTT, complete blood count (CBC), and serum creatinine. Monitor the CBC with platelet count every 3 to 5 days during the first 2 weeks of therapy, and every 2 to 4 weeks with extended use.[9,10] Use LMWHs cautiously in patients with renal impairment due to the potential of drug accumulation and risk of bleeding. Specific dosing recommendations for patients with a creatinine clearance (CrCl) less than 30 mL/min (0.50 mL/s) are currently available for enoxaparin but are lacking for other LMWH agents (Table 10–8). Current guidelines recommend the use of UFH over LMWH in patients with severe renal dysfunction (CrCl less than 30 mL/min [0.50 mL/s]).[2]

KEY CONCEPT *Most patients with an uncomplicated DVT can be managed safely at home.*[2] LMWHs can be easily administered in the outpatient setting, thus enabling the treatment of VTE at home. Several large clinical trials have demonstrated the efficacy and safety of LMWHs for outpatient treatment of DVT.[2,39] Acceptance of this treatment approach has increased substantially over the last several years among clinicians. Patients with DVT with normal vital signs, low bleeding risk, no other comorbid conditions requiring hospitalization, and who are stable may have anticoagulant initiated at home. Although the treatment of patients with PE in the outpatient setting is controversial, patients with submassive PE who are hemodynamically stable can be safely treated in the outpatient setting as well.[12] Patients considered for outpatient therapy must be reliable or have adequate caregiver support and must be able to strictly adhere to the prescribed treatment regimen and recommended follow-up visits. Close patient follow-up is critical to the success of any outpatient DVT treatment program. Home DVT treatment results in cost savings and improved patient satisfaction and quality of life.[2,12,39]

Laboratory methods of measuring a patient's response to LMWH may be warranted in certain situations.[9,40] Although controversial, measurement of antifactor Xa activity has been the most widely used method in clinical practice. Monitoring of antifactor Xa activity may be considered in adult patients who are morbidly obese (weight greater than 150 kg [330 lb] or body mass index [BMI] greater than 50 kg/m^2), weigh less than 50 kg (110 lb), or have significant renal impairment (CrCl less than 30 mL/min [0.50 mL/s]). Laboratory monitoring may also be useful in children and pregnant women.[40]

Similar to UFH, bleeding is the major complication associated with LMWHs. The incidence of major bleeding reported in clinical trials is less than 3%.[8,9] Minor bleeding, especially bruising at the injection site, occurs frequently. Protamine sulfate will partially reverse the anticoagulant effects of the LMWHs and should be administered in the event of major bleeding. Due to its limited binding to LMWH chains, protamine only neutralizes 60% of their antithrombotic activity. If the LMWH was administered within the previous 8 hours, give 1 mg protamine sulfate per 1 mg of enoxaparin or 100 antifactor Xa units of dalteparin. If bleeding is not controlled, give 0.5 mg of protamine sulfate for every antifactor Xa 100 units of LMWH. Give smaller protamine doses if more than 8 hours have lapsed since the last LMWH dose.

The incidence of HIT is lower with LMWHs than with UFH.[9,10] However, LMWHs cross-react with heparin antibodies in vitro and should not be given as an alternative anticoagulant in patients with a diagnosis or history of HIT. Monitor platelet counts every few days during the first 2 weeks and periodically thereafter.

In patients undergoing spinal and epidural anesthesia or spinal puncture, spinal and epidural hematomas have been linked to the use of LMWHs. In patients with in-dwelling epidural catheters, concurrent use of LMWHs and all other agents that impact hemostasis should be avoided. When inserting and removing the in-dwelling epidural catheters, the timing of LMWH administration around catheter manipulation should be carefully coordinated. Catheter manipulation should only occur at minimal or trough anticoagulant levels.[9,10]

LMWHs are an excellent alternative to UFH for the treatment of VTE in pregnant women.[9,23] The LMWHs do not cross the placenta, and they are FDA pregnancy category B. Because the pharmacokinetics of LMWHs may change during pregnancy, monitoring of antifactor Xa activity every 4 to 6 weeks to make dose adjustments is recommended.[40] LMWHs have also been used to treat VTE in pediatric patients. Children younger than 1 year require higher doses (eg, enoxaparin 1.5 mg/kg SC every 12 hours). Monitor antifactor Xa activity to guide dosing in children.[38]

▸ *Factor Xa Inhibitors*

Parenteral Fondaparinux is an indirect inhibitor of factor-Xa and exerts its anticoagulant activity by accelerating AT.[9,41,42] Due to its small size, fondaparinux exerts inhibitory activity specifically against factor-Xa and has no effect on thrombin (Figure 10–4). After SC administration, fondaparinux is completely absorbed, and peak plasma concentrations are reached within 2 to 3 hours.[9,41,42] It has a half-life of 17 to 21 hours, permitting once-daily administration, but the anticoagulant effects of fondaparinux will persist for 2 to 4 days after stopping the drug. In patients with renal impairment, the anticoagulant effect persists even longer. Fondaparinux does not require routine coagulation monitoring or dose adjustments.

Fondaparinux is not metabolized in the liver and therefore has few drug interactions.[9,41,42] However, concurrent use with other antithrombotic agents increases the risk of bleeding. Unlike the heparins, factor Xa inhibitors do not affect platelet function and do not react with the heparin platelet factor (PF)-4 antibodies seen in patients with HIT. Thus, they have a theoretical role in treatment and prevention of HIT. A few small observational studies report fondaparinux use in the management of patients with HIT. Based on these data some centers use fondaparinux in patients with subacute HIT or a history of HIT who require anticoagulation therapy.[9,41,42]

Fondaparinux is as safe and effective as IV UFH for the treatment of PE and SC LMWH for the treatment of DVT.[9,41,42] The recommended dose for fondaparinux in the treatment of VTE is based on the patient's weight (Table 10–8). Fondaparinux is renally eliminated, and accumulation can occur in patients with renal dysfunction. Due to the lack of specific dosing guidelines, fondaparinux is contraindicated in patients with severe renal impairment (CrCl less than 30 mL/min [0.50 mL/s]). Baseline renal function should be measured and monitored closely during the course of therapy. Based on limited data at this time, monitoring antifactor Xa activity to guide fondaparinux dosing is not recommended.[9,41,42]

As with other anticoagulants, the major side effect associated with fondaparinux is bleeding. Fondaparinux should be used with caution in elderly patients because their risk of bleeding is higher. Patients receiving fondaparinux should be carefully monitored for signs and symptoms of bleeding. A CBC should be obtained at baseline and monitored periodically to detect the possibility of occult bleeding. In the event of major bleeding, fresh-frozen plasma and factor concentrates should be given. Fondaparinux is not reversed by protamine.[9,41,42]

Fondaparinux is pregnancy category B, but there are very limited data regarding its use during pregnancy. Use in pediatric patients has not been studied.[41]

Oral Apixaban and rivaroxaban are direct inhibitors of factor-Xa, part of a newer generation of oral anticoagulants also referred to as direct oral anticoagulants (DOACs).[35,36,42,43] Both agents have been evaluated and approved by the FDA for the treatment of VTE (DVT and PE) and reduction in the risk of recurrence of DVT and PE. Rivaroxaban had similar efficacy and safety when compared to traditional therapy with LMWH and a vitamin K antagonist in the treatment of patients with VTE. Apixaban was noninferior in preventing recurrent VTE or VTE-related death but resulted in lower major bleeding events when compared to LMWH and warfarin therapy. Therefore, both agents can be used as monotherapy without parenteral anticoagulation overlap, allowing for a single oral regimen approach in the treatment and prevention of recurrent VTE. See Table 10–13.

The DOACs inhibit a serine protease single target within the common pathway of the coagulation cascade during the final stages of clot formation. See Figure 10–5. This specificity provides a linear dose response and wider therapeutic index that allows for fixed dosing and precludes the need for routine coagulation monitoring.[4,12,35,36,42,43] Apixaban and rivaroxaban are competitive, selective and potent direct inhibitors of factor Xa that bind in a reversible manner to the active site of both free-floating factor Xa and factor Xa within the prothrombinase complex, thereby attenuating thrombin generation. These agents have intrinsic anticoagulant activity, and do not require a cofactor to exert their effect.[4,12,35,36,42,43]

The pharmacokinetic and pharmacodynamic properties of DOACs are significantly different than those of warfarin. See Table 10–14. They have a more rapid onset and offset of action and shorter half-lives compared to warfarin. However, missed doses may be more prone to result in therapy complications than longer half-life therapies such as warfarin. They are all eliminated renally to varying degrees (see Table 10-14), and dose adjustment or avoidance in patients with renal impairment may be needed.[4,12,35,36,42,43] See Table 10–13. All DOACs are substrates of the P-glycoprotein (P-gp) transport system, and the Xa inhibitors are also substrates of the hepatic cytochrome P-450 (CYP) isoenzyme system. Any inhibition or induction of these metabolic systems will alter their absorption.[44] There are currently no readily available standardized laboratory assays to measure the anticoagulant effect of the DOACs, nor are there specific antidotes to reverse their anticoagulant effects. This can cause challenges in situations where rapid reversal of anticoagulation is required such as in cases of major bleeding or need for emergent surgery.[12,35,36,45]

Apixaban undergoes oxidative metabolism primarily via hepatic isoenzymes CYP3A4/5 and to a lesser degree CYP 1A2 and CYP 2J2.[35,42] Apixaban has dual pathways of elimination,

Table 10–13

Dosing of the Direct Oral Anticoagulants in the Treatment of VTE

	Dabigatran	Rivaroxaban	Apixaban
Acute VTE	150 mg BID after 5–10 days of parenteral anticoagulation	15 mg BID × 3 weeks then 20 mg once daily with food	10 mg BID for 7 days, then 5 mg BID
Prevention of VTE recurrence	150 mg BID	20 mg once daily with food	2.5 mg BID
Dosage adjustments and/or thresholds for avoidance	Any P-gp *inducer*: avoid concurrent use Any P-gp *inhibitor* with CrCl < 50 mL/min (0.83 mL/s): avoid concurrent use CrCl < 30 mL/min (0.50 mL/s): avoid use	CrCl 30–50 mL/min (0.50–0.83 mL/s): use with caution CrCl < 30 mL/min (0.50 mL/s): avoid use	Dual strong CYP3A4 and P-gp inhibitors: If dose > 2.5 mg BID, decrease by 50% If already taking 2.5 mg BID and dual strong CYP3A4 and P-gp inhibitor: avoid use No dose adjustment in renal impairment required

CrCl, creatinine clearance; CYP, cytochrome P-450; P-gp, P-glycoprotein; VTE, venous thromboembolism.

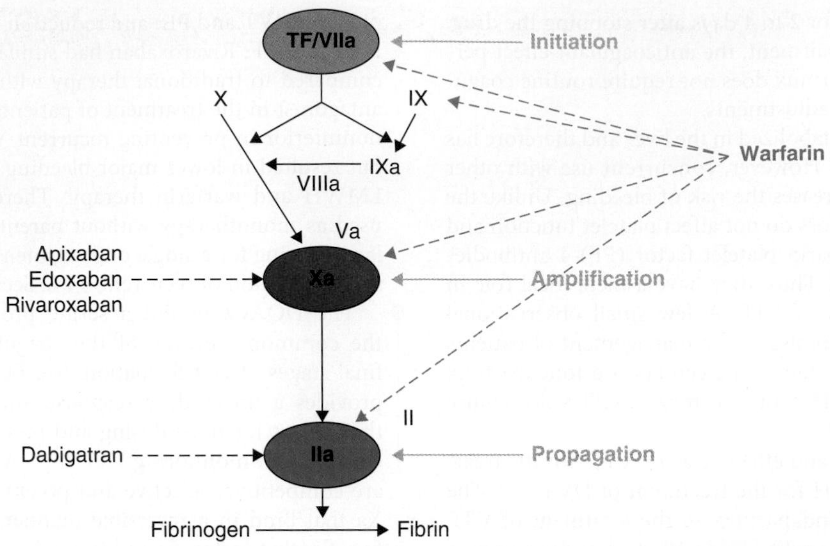

FIGURE 10–5. Mechanism of action of the oral anticoagulants. (From Weitz JI, Bates SM. J Thromb Haemost. 2005;3:1843–53.)

with approximately 27% being cleared renally and the remainder eliminated via the fecal route. Elderly, low weight (less than 50 kg [110 lb]), and patients with renal impairment can have increased exposure to apixaban, while gender and race do not appear to have clinically relevant influence. Apixaban pharmacokinetics are not significantly altered in patients with mild (Child Pugh A) to moderate (Child Pugh B) hepatic impairment. However, apixaban has not been studied in patients with severe hepatic impairment and is not recommended for use in these patients. Apixaban is pregnancy category B, but there are no adequate studies in pregnant women and its use during pregnancy is likely to increase bleeding risk. Use in pediatric patients has not been studied.[35,42,43]

Table 10–14

Pharmacologic and Pharmacokinetic Characteristics of Direct Oral Anticoagulants

Property	Apixaban	Dabigatran	Rivaroxaban
Mechanism of action	Factor Xa inhibitor	Direct thrombin inhibitor	Factor Xa inhibitor
Bioavailability (%)	50%	3%–7%	80%–100% for 10-mg dose 66% for 20-mg dose[a]
T_{max} (hours)	1–3	1–3	2–4
Onset of effect	Within 3 hours	Within 3 hours	Within 4 hours
Half-life (hours)	8–15	12–17	5–13
Renal excretion	27%	80%	35%
CYP mediated metabolism	25% CYP3A4/5, CYP2J2 (minor), CYP1A2 (minor)	No	30% CYP3A4/5, CYP2J2 (equal)
Drug transporter	P-gp, BCRP	P-gp	P-gp, BCRP
Drug–drug interactions	Potent CYP3A4 and P-gp inhibitors; affecting absorption, metabolism, and excretion	Potent P-gp inhibitors; affecting absorption	Potent CYP3A4 and P-gp inhibitors; affecting absorption, metabolism, and excretion
Food effect	No effect reported	Delayed absorption with food but no influence on bioavailability	Delayed absorption with food with increased (+39%) bioavailability Take with largest meal of the day (usually dinner)
Age	Lower clearance as age increases	Lower clearance as age increases	No effect reported
Body weight	Higher exposure with low body weight (< 50 kg)	No effect reported	No effect reported
Sex	Lower clearance in women	Lower clearance in women	No effect reported
Ethnicity	No effect reported	No effect reported	Lower dose in Japanese patients
Gastrointestinal tolerability	No effect reported	Dyspepsia 5%–10%	No effect reported
Coagulation measurement	anti-FXa	ECT > dTT > aPTT	anti-FXa > PT

aPTT, activated partial thromboplastin time; BCRP, breast cancer resistance protein; CYP, cytochrome P-450; dTT, diluted thrombin time; ECT, ecarin clotting time; FXa, factor Xa; P-gp, P-glycoprotein; PT, prothrombin time; T_{max}, time to maximum plasma concentration

[a]Bioavailability is dependent on food intake for doses > 10 mg. Rivaroxaban doses > 10 mg should be administered with food.

Table 10–15

Drug Interactions and Monitoring Recommendations for Direct Oral Anticoagulants

	Apixaban	Rivaroxaban	Dabigatran
Drug interactions	Avoid concomitant use with strong dual inhibitors of CYP3A4 and P-gp (eg, ketoconazole, ritonavir, erythromycin) or reduce apixaban dose Avoid concomitant use with strong dual inducers of CYP3A4 and P-gp (eg, rifampin, phenytoin, carbamazepine) Concomitant use with antiplatelet agents, fibrinolytics, heparin, aspirin, and chronic NSAID increases bleeding risk	Avoid concomitant use with strong dual inhibitors of CYP3A4 and P-gp (eg, ketoconazole, ritonavir, erythromycin) Avoid concomitant use with strong dual inducers of CYP3A4 and P-gp (eg, rifampin, phenytoin, carbamazepine) Avoid concomitant use with other anticoagulants	Avoid concomitant use with P-gp inducers (eg, rifampin) P-gp inhibitors and impaired renal function can lead to increased exposure to dabigatran: Avoid concomitant use with severe renal impairment (CrCl < 30 mL/min [0.50 mL/s]) For moderate renal impairment reduce dose to 75 mg twice daily when used concomitantly with dronedarone or systemic ketoconazole or avoid concomitant use
Monitoring	Baseline laboratory assessment: Hemoglobin/hematocrit, liver function, renal function, PT/INR At every visit: Adherence, signs/symptoms of bleeding or thromboembolism, side effects, concomitant medications (including over-the-counter) Annual laboratory assessment: Hemoglobin/hematocrit, renal function, liver function If CrCl 30–60 mL/min (0.50–1.0 mL/s), > 75 years, or fragile: renal function every 6 months If CrCl 15–30 mL/min (0.25–0.50 mL/s): renal function every 3 months If condition changes that might impact anticoagulation therapy: check renal and/or liver function		

CrCL, creatinine clearance; CYP, cytochrome P-450; INR, International Normalized Ratio; NSAID, nonsteroidal anti-inflammatory drug; P-gp, P-glycoprotein; PT, prothrombin time.

Apixaban is a substrate of both the CYP 3A4/5 and P-gp systems, and it may be subject to a number of drug interactions (Table 10–15).[35,44] See Tables 10–13, 10–14, and 10–15 for pertinent drug interactions, monitoring and dosing recommendations.

As with any anticoagulant, concomitant administration of apixaban and additional antithrombotic agents will increase risk of bleeding and caution or avoidance should be exercised. While routine anticoagulation monitoring is not required, there may be clinical scenarios where knowing the patient's degree of anticoagulation may be necessary.[42,43,45] A drug-specific chromogenic anti-Xa assay may be used to measure apixaban plasma concentrations, however, this assay is not readily available in most laboratories. Other tests such as the PT, aPTT, and INR are not recommended to assess the anticoagulant effects of apixaban.[35] Baseline and periodic patient assessment including adherence, side effects, and renal and liver function should be conducted (Table 10–15).[46]

Rivaroxaban's bioavailability is dose dependent.[36,42] At a dose of 10 mg, bioavailability is 80% to 100% and may be taken without regard for food. At higher doses, bioavailability is approximately 66% in the fasted state, which is increased to greater than 80% by food intake. Thus, rivaroxaban 15 mg and 20 mg tablets should be taken with the largest meal of the day. See Table 10–14. Approximately two-thirds of an administered dose of rivaroxaban undergoes biotransformation to inactive metabolites. It is subject to oxidative degradation via CYP 3A4/5 and to a lesser extent CYP 2J2, as well as non-CYP mediated hydrolysis.[36,42] Like apixaban, rivaroxaban does not induce or inhibit CYP-450 isoenzymes, but may be affected by medications that are substrates for this enzymatic pathway.[26,44] Rivaroxaban has a dual mode of elimination, with approximately 35% excreted unchanged in the urine and the remaining two-thirds (in the form of inactive metabolites) excreted fairly equally between the renal and hepatobiliary route.[36] Rivaroxaban is a P-gp substrate, not only at the level of gut absorption, but also at the level of elimination in the kidney. Medications that are substrates for the P-gp transport system may impact plasma concentrations of rivaroxaban.[44,46]

While patients with renal impairment can have increased exposure to rivaroxaban, gender, race, age and extremes of weight (less than 50 kg [110 lb] or greater than 120 kg [265 lb]) have not been shown to significantly impact its pharmacokinetics or pharmacodynamics. Rivaroxaban should be avoided in patients with CrCl less than 30 mL/min (0.50 mL/s) when used in VTE treatment.[36,42,43] See Table 10–13. Mild hepatic impairment has minimal impact on the pharmacokinetics and pharmacodynamics of rivaroxaban. Patients with moderate hepatic impairment (Child-Pugh B) have significantly increased exposure to rivaroxaban and its use in patients with severe liver disease has not been studied.[36] Rivaroxaban is pregnancy category C. There are no well controlled studies in pregnant women and dosing in these patients has not been established. Its use in pediatric patients has not been studied.[36,42]

Rivaroxaban should not be used concomitantly with medications that are dual P-gp and strong CYP3A4 inhibitors or inducers.[44,46] See Table 10–15. Use with weaker combined P-gp and CYP3A4 substrates should be undertaken with caution and only if benefit of use outweighs risk. Concomitant use of rivaroxaban with antiplatelet and nonsteroidal anti-inflammatory agents should be done with extreme caution due to the additive antithrombotic effects and heightened risk of bleeding. As with apixaban, a drug-specific chromogenic anti-Xa assay may be used to measure rivaroxaban activity, but is not yet widely available or standardized. Rivaroxaban prolongs the aPTT and PT in a dose-dependent manner, but the PT is more sensitive to rivaroxaban than the aPTT.[35,45,46] Because it is widely available and has a low level of complexity, the PT may be used in a qualitative manner to quickly determine the presence of rivaroxaban. A normal result with most PT reagents would exclude clinically significant anticoagulant activity. The prothrombin time (PT) and INR are is not suitable for measurement of rivaroxaban activity.

► Direct Thrombin Inhibitors

Given that thrombin is the central mediator of coagulation and amplifies its own production, it is a natural target for pharmacologic intervention.[9,42] Direct thrombin inhibitors (DTIs) bind thrombin and prevent interactions with their substrates (Figure 10–6).

Parenteral Parenteral DTIs are considered the drugs of choice for the treatment of VTE in patients with a diagnosis or history of HIT.[9,42,47] Several injectable DTIs are approved for use in the US including lepirudin, bivalirudin, argatroban, and desirudin. All have been used to treat thrombosis in patients with HIT, but only lepirudin and argatroban are FDA-approved for this indication. However, as of 2012, lepirudin is no longer commercially available in the United States. Data with some of the DTIs (desirudin, bivalirudin) in the treatment HIT is limited and there are no high-quality studies that directly compare one DTI with another. DTIs differ in terms of their chemical structure, binding to the thrombin molecule and pharmacokinetic profiles. See Table 10–16. Unlike heparins, DTIs do not require AT as a cofactor and do not bind to plasma proteins. Therefore, they produce a more predictable anticoagulant effect. DTIs have a targeted specificity for thrombin, the ability to inactivate clot-bound thrombin, and an absence of platelet interactions that can lead to HIT.[9,42,47]

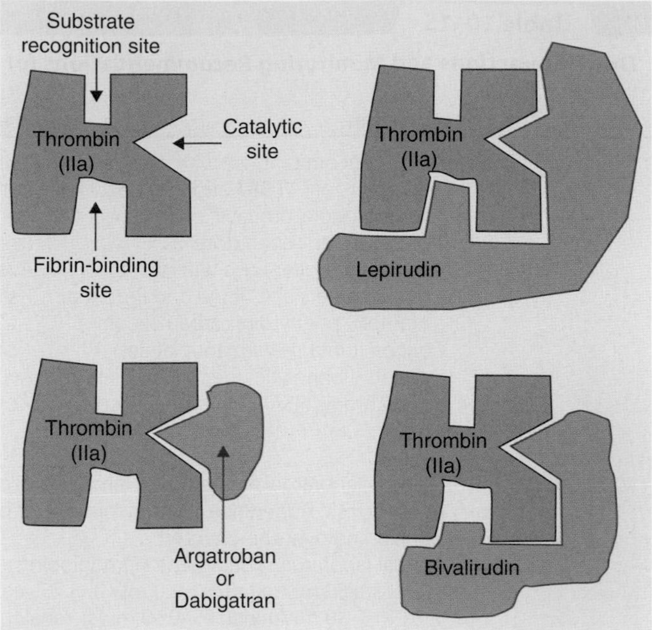

FIGURE 10–6. Mechanism of action of direct thrombin inhibitors. (From Witt DM, Nutescu EA, Haines S. Venous thromboembolism. In: DiPiro JT, Talbert RL, Yee GC, et al., eds. Pharmacotherapy: A Pathophysiologic Approach, 8th ed. New York, NY: McGraw-Hill, 2011:326.)

Table 10–16

Pharmacologic and Clinical Properties of DTIs used in Treatment of Thrombosis in Patients with HIT

	Lepirudin	Desirudin	Bivalirudin	Argatroban
Route of administration	IV	SC	IV	IV
FDA approved indication	Treatment of thrombosis in patients with HIT	VTE prevention after THA	Patients with UA undergoing PTCA; PCI with provisional use of GPI; patients with or at risk of HIT or HITTS undergoing PCI	Prophylaxis or treatment of thrombosis in adult patients with HIT; patients with or at risk of HIT undergoing PCI
Binding to thrombin	Irreversible Catalytic site and exosite-1	Irreversible Catalytic site and exosite-1	Partially reversible Catalytic site and exosite-1	Reversible Catalytic site
Half-life in healthy subjects	80 minutes	2–3 hours	25 minutes	40–50 minutes
Monitoring	aPTT (IV) SCr/CrCl	aPTT SCr/CrCl	aPTT/ACT SCr/CrCl	aPTT/ACT Liver function
Elimination	Renal	Renal	Enzymatic (80%) and renal (20%)	Hepatobiliary
Antibody development	Anti-hirudin antibodies in up to 40%–60% of patients	Not reported	May cross-react with anti-hirudin antibodies	No
Effect on INR	+	+	++	+++

+ minimal effect

++ moderate effect

+++ significant effect

ACT, activated clotting time; aPTT, activated partial thromboplastin time; CrCl, creatinine clearance; DTI, direct thrombin inhibitor; FDA, Food and Drug Administration; GPI, glycoprotein IIb-IIIa inhibitor; HIT, heparin induced thrombocytopenia; HITTS, heparin induced thrombocytopenia and thrombosis syndrome; INR, International Normalized Ratio; IV, intravenous; PCI, percutaneous coronary intervention; PTCA, percutaneous transluminal coronary angioplasty; SC, subcutaneous; SCr, serum creatinine; THA, total hip arthroplasty; UA, unstable angina; VTE, venous thromboembolism.

Oral Small molecule DTIs have been structurally modified for oral administration.[42] One agent, dabigatran, is currently approved in the United States for treatment of VTE.[48] Dabigatran was found to be as effective and safe as warfarin in the treatment and prevention of recurrent VTE.[12,43] Unlike apixaban and rivaroxaban, dabigatran is not used as monotherapy in the acute phase of VTE treatment. Patients should be anticoagulated with UFH or LMWH for the initial 5 to 10 days of therapy and then transitioned to dabigatran.[2,12,43] See Table 10–13. Similar to other DOACs, dabigatran can be given in fixed doses without the need for routine coagulation monitoring and has a fast onset and offset of action, offering more convenient anticoagulation options for patients and providers.[28,42]

Dabigatran is a direct reversible, competitive inhibitor of thrombin and an oral prodrug of dabigatran etexilate.[42,48] Dabigatran is converted to its active form dabigatran etexilate by serum esterases that are independent of CYP-450 pathways. See Table 10–14. Dabigatran has an oral bioavailability of approximately 3% to 7% and requires an acidic environment for absorption. The prodrug is contained in small pellets coated with an acid core. These pellets are enclosed in a capsule shell. This specific capsule formulation improves the dissolution and absorption of the prodrug, independent of gastric pH. Therefore the capsules should not be broken, chewed, or opened before administration. Dabigatran demonstrates 35% protein binding and is a substrate of the efflux transporter P-gp. Although the absence of CYP-450 metabolism decreases potential for many drug interactions, co-administration with P-gp substrates, inhibitors, or inducers may affect the efficacy of dabigatran.[44,46] See Table 10–15.

Approximately 80% of dabigatran is eliminated in the urine, and its use is not recommended in the treatment of VTE in patients with a CrCl less than 30 mL/min (0.50 mL/s) due to increased risk of drug exposure and bleeding.[48] Subjects with severe liver disease were excluded from clinical trials of dabigatran. In those with moderate hepatic impairment (Child-Pugh B), the pharmacokinetic profile of dabigatran is not affected. Gender, age, race or extremes of weight (less than 50 kg [110 lb] or greater than 110 kg [243 lb]) do not significantly impact dabigatran pharmacology.[48]

Dabigatran prolongs the aPTT, PT, thrombin time (TT) and ecarin clotting time (ECT) assays in a dose-dependent manner.[45,46] Peak values greater than 2.5 times control may indicate supratherapeutic levels. A normal aPTT would indicate a lack of clinically relevant anticoagulant activity. The aPTT may be used in a qualitative manner to determine the presence of anticoagulation with dabigatran. It should not be used to quantitate dabigatran plasma concentrations. The PT is relatively insensitive to dabigatran, and the INR is not suitable for measurement of dabigatran due to significant variability. The TT, diluted thrombin time (dTT), and ECT exhibit a linear dose-response with therapeutic dabigatran plasma concentrations. Unfortunately, none of these assays are widely available in practice. It is important to note that quantitative thresholds beyond which a patient would be at increased risk of clotting or bleeding have not been established for any of the DOACs.[42,45,46,48]

Contraindications to the use of DTIs and risk factors for bleeding are similar to those of other antithrombotic agents (Tables 10–11 and 10–12). Bleeding is the most common side effect reported. Concurrent use of DTIs with thrombolytics or antiplatelet agents significantly increases bleeding complications.[47] Currently, there are no commercially available antidotes to reverse the effects of dabigatran or other DTIs. Fresh-frozen plasma, factor concentrates, or recombinant factor VIIa may be given in the event of a major life-threatening bleed; however, their efficacy for this use has not been established. DTIs can increase PT/INR and interfere with the accuracy of monitoring and dosing of warfarin therapy. Data on use of DTIs in pregnancy are very limited. Argatroban, bivalirudin, and lepirudin are pregnancy category B, while desirudin and dabigatran are pregnancy category C. Use of DTIs in pediatric patients has not been established.[47]

▶ *Warfarin*

KEY CONCEPT *Warfarin has been the primary oral anticoagulant used in the US when long-term or extended anticoagulation is required.* Warfarin is FDA approved for prevention and treatment of VTE.[49] Although very effective, warfarin has a narrow therapeutic index, requiring frequent dose adjustments and careful patient monitoring.[4,10,11,49]

Warfarin exerts its anticoagulant effect by inhibiting production of the vitamin K–dependent coagulation factors II (prothrombin), VII, IX, and X, as well as the anticoagulant proteins C and S (Figure 10–7). Warfarin has no effect on circulating coagulation factors that have been previously formed, and its therapeutic antithrombotic activity is delayed for 5 to 7 days, and potentially longer in slower metabolizers. This delay is related to half-lives of the clotting factors: 60 to 100 hours for factor II (prothrombin), 6 to 8 hours for factor VII, 20 to 30 hours for factor IX, and 24 to 40 hours for factor X. Proteins C and S, the natural anticoagulants, are inhibited more rapidly due to their shorter half-lives, 8 to 10 hours and 40 to 60 hours, respectively. Reductions in the concentration of natural anticoagulants before the clotting factors are depleted can lead to a paradoxical hypercoagulable state during the first few days of warfarin therapy. It is for this reason that patients with acute thrombosis should receive a fast-acting anticoagulant (heparin, LMWH, or fondaparinux) while transitioning to warfarin therapy.[4,10,11,49]

Warfarin is metabolized in the liver via several isoenzymes including CYP 1A2, 3A4, 2C9, 2C19, 2C8, and 2C18 (Figure 10–7).[4,10–11,49] Hepatic metabolism of warfarin varies greatly among patients, leading to large interpatient differences in dose requirements and genetic variations in these isoenzymes. Multiple studies have demonstrated that VKORC1 and CYP2C9 genotypes influence the interpatient variability in warfarin dose requirements, together explaining up to 45% of overall dose variance. Several algorithms that incorporate CYP2C9 genotype and VKORC1 haplotype with other patient characteristics to predict warfarin maintenance dosing requirements have been developed and showed efficacy in better predicting warfarin stable doses when compared to clinical algorithms. Based on these data, the FDA recommends incorporating patient's genotype information in guiding warfarin dosing when such information is available.[49] See Table 10–17. However, randomized studies to date showed mixed results of pharmacogenomic-based dosing on clinical and health utilization outcomes. Therefore, pharmacogenomic-based dosing has not yet been widely adopted in clinical practice and some guidelines recommend against routine ordering of genetic testing.[2,4]

Warfarin does not follow linear kinetics. Small-dose adjustments can lead to large changes in anticoagulant response.[4,10,11,49] The dose of warfarin is determined by each patient's individual response to therapy and the desired intensity of anticoagulation. In addition to hepatic metabolism and genotype, warfarin dose requirements are influenced by diet, drug–drug interactions, and health status. Therefore, warfarin dose must be determined by frequent clinical and laboratory monitoring. Although there are

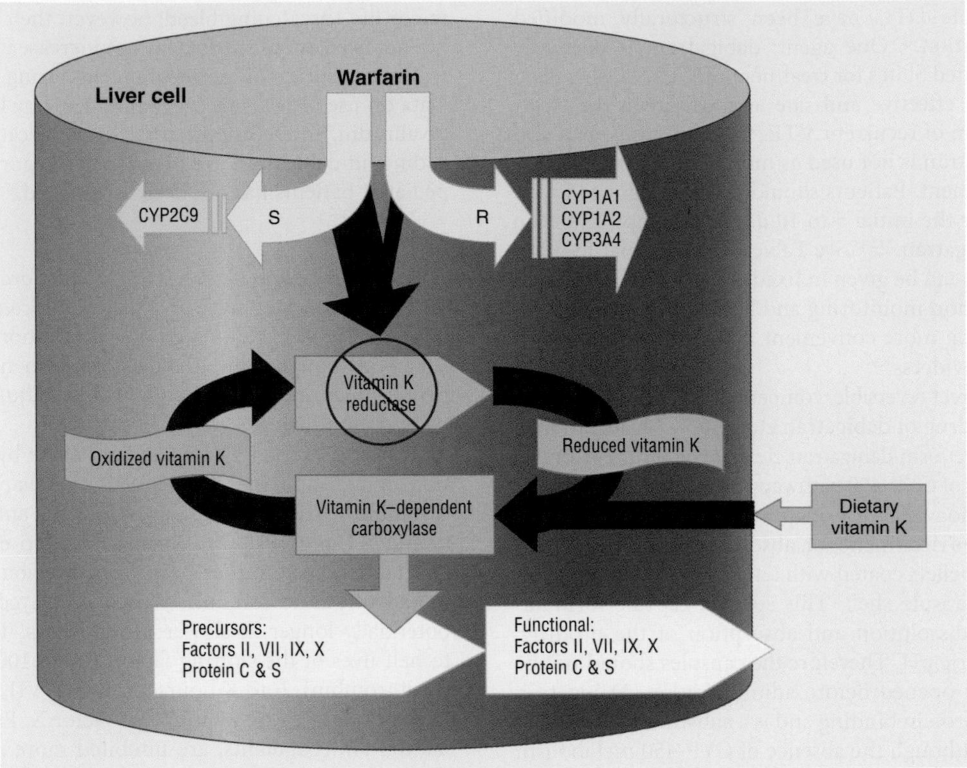

FIGURE 10–7. Pharmacologic activity and metabolism of warfarin. (CYP, cytochrome P-450 isoenzyme.) (From Witt DM, Nutescu EA, Haines S. Venous thromboembolism. In: DiPiro JT, Talbert RL, Yee GC, et al., eds. Pharmacotherapy: A Pathophysiologic Approach, 8th ed. New York, NY: McGraw-Hill, 2011:328.)

conflicting data regarding the optimal warfarin induction regimen, when the patient's genotype is not known, most patients can start with 5 mg daily and subsequent doses are determined based on INR response (Figure 10–8). When initiating therapy, it is difficult to predict the precise warfarin maintenance dose a patient will require. Patients who are younger (less than 55 years) and otherwise healthy can safely use higher warfarin "initiation" doses (eg, 7.5 or 10 mg). A more conservative "initiation" dose (eg, 4 mg or less) should be given to patients older than 75 years, patients with heart failure, liver disease, or poor nutritional status, and patients who are taking interacting medications or are at high risk of bleeding.[5,23] Loading doses of warfarin (eg, 15–20 mg) are not recommended. These large doses can lead to the false impression that a therapeutic INR has been achieved in 2 to 3 days and lead to potential future overdosing.[4,10,11,49] Before initiating therapy, screen the patient for any contraindications to anticoagulation therapy and risk factors for major bleeding (Tables 10–11 and 10–12). Conduct a thorough medication history including the use of prescription and nonprescription drugs, and any herbal supplements to detect interactions that may affect warfarin dosing requirements.

In patients with acute VTE, a rapid-acting anticoagulant (UFH, LMWH, or fondaparinux) should be overlapped with warfarin for a minimum of 5 days and until the INR is greater than 2 and stable. This is important because the full antithrombotic effect will not be reached until 5 to 7 days or even longer after initiating warfarin therapy.[2,4,12] The typical maintenance dose of warfarin for most patients will be between 25 and 55 mg per week, although some patients require higher or lower doses. Adjustments in the maintenance warfarin dose should be determined based on the total weekly dose and by reducing or increasing the weekly dose by increments of 5% to 25%. When adjusting the maintenance dose, wait at least 7 days to ensure a steady

Table 10–17

Food and Drug Administration Recommended Warfarin Initial Doses Based on CYP2C9 and VKORC1 Genotypes

	CYP2C9					
VKORC1	*1/*1	*1/*2	*1/*3	*2/*2	*2/*3	*3/*3
GG	5–7 mg	5–7 mg	3–4 mg	3–4 mg	3–4 mg	0.5–2 mg
AG	5–7 mg	3–4 mg	3–4 mg	3–4 mg	0.5–2 mg	0.5–2 mg
AA	3–4 mg	3–4 mg	0.5–2 mg	0.5–2 mg	0.5–2 mg	0.5–2 mg

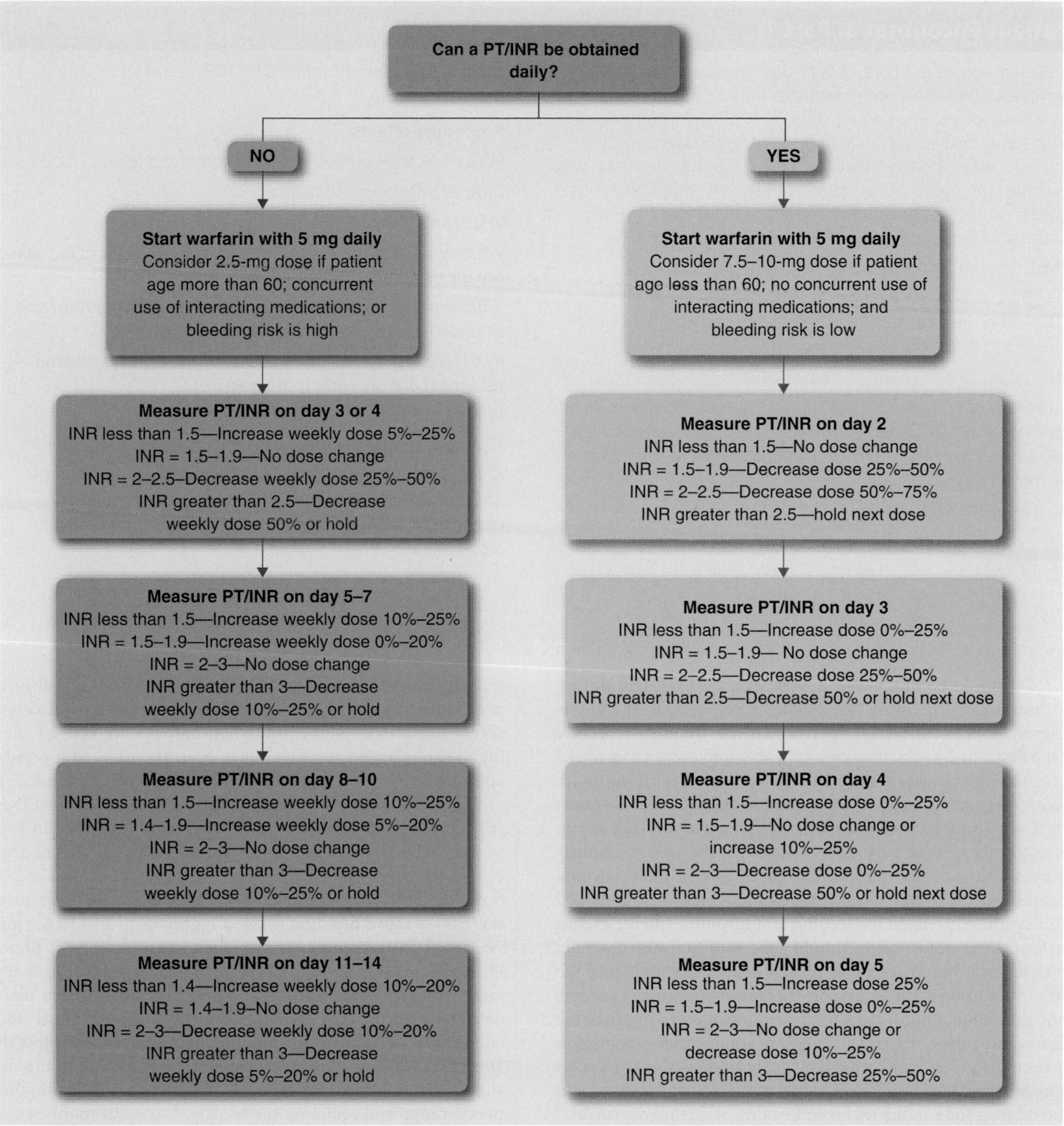

FIGURE 10–8. Initiation of warfarin therapy. (INR, international normalized ratio; PT, prothrombin time.) (From Witt DM, Clark NP. Venous thromboembolism. In: DiPiro JT, Talbert RL, Yee GC, et al., eds. Pharmacotherapy: A Pathophysiologic Approach, 9th ed. New York, NY: McGraw-Hill, 2011:261.)

state has been attained on the new dose before checking the INR again. Checking the INR too soon can lead to inappropriate dose adjustments and unstable anticoagulation status.[4,10,11,49]

KEY CONCEPT *Warfarin requires frequent laboratory monitoring to ensure optimal outcomes and minimize complications.* The PT is the most frequently used test to monitor warfarin's anticoagulant effect. The PT measures biological activity of factors II, VII, and X. Due to wide variation in reagent sensitivity, different **thromboplastins** will result in different PT results, potentially leading to inappropriate dosing decisions.[4,10,11,49] To standardize result reporting, the World Health Organization (WHO) developed a reference thromboplastin and recommended the INR to monitor warfarin therapy. The INR corrects for the differences in thromboplastin reagents. Goal or target INR for each patient is based on the indication for warfarin therapy. For treatment and prevention of VTE, the INR target is 2.5 with an acceptable range of 2 to 3. Before initiating warfarin therapy, a baseline PT/INR and CBC should be obtained. After initiating warfarin therapy,

Patient Encounter 3, Part 1

A 38-year-old woman presents to the emergency department complaining of chest pain, shortness of breath, and lightheadedness. The patient states that her symptoms started with some mild left calf pain approximately 5 days ago. She started feeling short of breath and experiencing chest pain last evening. She could not sleep and her shortness of breath has gotten progressively worse in the last several hours. She was hospitalized because she was suspected to have a PE.

PMH: Obesity × 12 years; chronic obstructive pulmonary disease

FH: Mother died of a stroke; paternal grandmother had clots (deep vein thrombosis) in her legs

SH: The patient is a full-time bus driver

Current Meds: Albuterol (salbutamol) metered-dose inhaler as needed; ortho-Tri-Cyclen Lo by mouth daily; echinacea one to two tablets by mouth daily as needed; multivitamin one tablet by mouth daily

Allergies: Shellfish, NKDA

PE:

VS: BP 104/64 mm Hg, HR 102 beats/min, RR 20 breaths/min, T 38.0°C (100.4°F), Wt 96 kg (211 lb), Ht 65 in (165 cm)

Labs: Within normal limits; eGFR 101 mL/min/1.73 m^2 (0.97 mL/s/m^2)

Procedures/Tests

ECG: Normal sinus rhythm; no ischemic changes

CXR: Slightly enlarged heart

V/Q scan: High probability of PE

What symptoms are consistent with the diagnosis of PE? What are the most likely etiologies for PE in this case?

What are appropriate initial acute phase and long-term and extended treatment options for this patient?

If UFH is chosen as the initial acute phase anticoagulation treatment option, what is the goal aPTT?

What is patient's goal INR for warfarin therapy?

How long should she remain on anticoagulation therapy?

Given the list of medications this patient took prior to hospitalization, should any of these be discontinued or changed? If changed, what alternative therapy would you recommend?

the INR should be monitored at least every 2 to 3 days during the first week of therapy. Once a stable response to therapy is achieved, INR monitoring is performed less frequently, weekly for the first 1 to 2 weeks, then every 2 weeks, and every 4 to 6 weeks thereafter if the warfarin dose and the patient's health status are stable.[5,48] At each encounter, the patient should be carefully questioned regarding any factors that may influence the INR result. These factors include adherence to therapy, the use of interacting medications, consumption of vitamin K–rich foods, alcohol use, and general health status. Patients should also be questioned about symptoms related to bleeding and thromboembolic events. Warfarin dose adjustments should take into account not only the INR result but also patient-related factors that influence the result. Structured anticoagulation therapy management services (anticoagulation clinics) have been demonstrated to improve the efficacy and safety of warfarin therapy. Some patients engage in self-testing and self-management by using a point-of-care PT/INR device approved for home use. Highly motivated and well-trained patients are good candidates for self-testing or self-management.[50]

KEY CONCEPT *Similar to other anticoagulants, warfarin's primary side effect is bleeding.*[8] Warfarin can unmask an existing lesion. Incidence of warfarin-related bleeding appears to be highest during the first few weeks of therapy. The annual incidence of major bleeding ranges from 1% to 10% depending on the quality of warfarin therapy management. Bleeding in the gastrointestinal tract is most common. Intracranial hemorrhage (ICH) is one of the most serious complications because it often causes severe disability and death. The intensity of anticoagulation therapy is related to bleeding risk. Higher INRs result in higher bleeding risk, and risk of ICH increases when the INR exceeds 4.[4,10–11] Instability and wide fluctuations in the INR are also associated with higher bleeding risk. In cases of warfarin overdose or overanticoagulation, vitamin K may be used to reverse warfarin's effect.[5] Vitamin K can be given by IV or oral route; the SC route is not recommended. When given SC, vitamin K is erratically absorbed and frequently ineffective. The IV route is reserved for cases of severe warfarin overdose and when patients are actively bleeding. Anaphylactoid reactions have been reported with rapid IV administration; therefore, slow infusion is recommended. An oral dose of vitamin K will reduce INR within 24 hours. If INR is still elevated after 24 hours, another dose of oral vitamin K can be given. The dose of vitamin K should be based on the degree of INR elevation and whether bleeding is present. A dose of 2.5 to 5 mg orally is recommended when INR is greater than 10 and there is no active bleeding, while a higher dose 5 to 10 mg given via slow IV is recommended in cases when bleeding is present. Higher doses (eg, 10 mg) can lead to prolonged warfarin resistance. In cases of life-threatening bleeding, fresh-frozen plasma or clotting factor concentrates should also be administered, in addition to IV vitamin K. In patients in whom INR is less than 10 and there is no active bleeding or imminent risk of bleeding, simply withholding warfarin until INR decreases to within therapeutic range and reducing the weekly dose with more frequent monitoring is appropriate.[4,10,11,49]

Nonhemorrhagic side effects related to warfarin are rare but can be severe when they occur. Warfarin-induced skin necrosis presents as an eggplant-colored skin lesion or a maculopapular rash that can progress to necrotic gangrene. It usually manifests in fatty areas such as the abdomen, buttocks, and breasts. The incidence is less than 0.1%, and it generally appears during the first week of therapy. Patients with protein C or S deficiency or those who receive large loading doses of warfarin are at greatest risk.[49] The mechanism is thought to be due to imbalances between procoagulant and anticoagulant proteins early in the course of warfarin therapy. Warfarin-induced purple toe syndrome is another rare side effect; patients present with a purplish discoloration of their toes. If these side effects are suspected, warfarin therapy should be discontinued immediately and an

alternative anticoagulant given. There is a theoretical risk that warfarin may cause accelerated bone loss with long-term use, but to date there is no evidence to support this concern. Warfarin is teratogenic and FDA pregnancy category X. It should be avoided during pregnancy, and women of childbearing potential should be instructed to use an effective form of contraception.

KEY CONCEPT *Warfarin is prone to numerous clinically significant drug–drug and drug–food interactions* (Tables 10–18, 10–19, and 10–20).[10,11,49] Patients on warfarin should be questioned at every

Table 10–18

Clinically Significant Warfarin Drug Interactions

Increase Anticoagulation Effect (↑ INR)	Decrease Anticoagulation Effect (↓ INR)	Increase Bleeding Risk
Acetaminophen	Amobarbital	Argatroban
Alcohol binge	Butabarbital	Aspirin
Allopurinol	Carbamazepine	Clopidogrel
Amiodarone	Cholestyramine	Danaparoid
Cephalosporins (with MTT side chain)	Dicloxacillin	Dipyridamole
Chloral hydrate	Griseofulvin	LMWHs
Chloramphenicol	Nafcillin	Nonsteroidal anti-inflammatory drugs
Cimetidine	Phenobarbital	Ticlopidine
Ciprofloxacin	Phenytoin	UFH
Clofibrate	Primidone	
Danazol	Rifampin	
Disulfiram	Secobarbital	
Doxycycline	Sucralfate	
Erythromycin	Vitamin K	
Fenofibrate		
Fluconazole		
Fluorouracil		
Fluoxetine		
Fluvoxamine		
Gemfibrozil		
Influenza vaccine		
Isoniazid		
Itraconazole		
Lovastatin		
Metronidazole		
Miconazole		
Moxalactam		
Neomycin		
Norfloxacin		
Ofloxacin		
Omeprazole		
Phenylbutazone		
Piroxicam		
Propafenone		
Propoyxphene		
Quinidine		
Sertraline		
Sulfamethoxazole		
Sulfinpyrazone		
Tamoxifen		
Testosterone		
Vitamin E		
Zafirlukast		

INR, international normalized ratio; LMWHs, low molecular weight heparins; MTT, methyl-tetrazole-thiomethyl; UFH, unfractionated heparin.

Table 10–19

Potential Warfarin Interactions with Herbal and Nutritional Products

Increase Anticoagulation Effect (Increase Bleeding Risk or ↑ INR)		Decrease Anticoagulation Effect (↓ INR)
Amica flower	Ginkgo	Coenzyme Q_{10}
Angelica root	Horse chestnut	Ginseng
Anise	Licorice root	Green tea
Asafoetida	Lovage root	St. John's wort
Bogbean	Meadowsweet	
Borage seed oil	Onion	
Bromelain	Papain	
Capsicum	Parsley	
Celery	Passionflower herb	
Chamomile	Poplar	
Clove	Quassia	
Danshen	Red clover	
Devil's claw	Rue	
Dong quai	Sweet clover	
Fenugreek	Turmeric	
Feverfew	Vitamin E	
Garlic	Willow bark	
Ginger		

INR, international normalized ratio.

Table 10–20

Vitamin K Content of Select Foods[a]

Very High (> 200 mcg)	High (100–200 mcg)	Medium (50–100 mcg)	Low (< 50 mcg)
Brussels sprouts	Basil	Apple, green	Apple, red
Chickpea	Broccoli	Asparagus	Avocado
Collard greens	Canola oil	Cabbage	Beans
Coriander	Chive	Cauliflower	Breads and grains
Endive	Coleslaw	Mayonnaise	Carrot
Kale	Cucumber (unpeeled)	Pistachios	Celery
Lettuce, red leaf	Green onion/scallion	Squash, summer	Cereal
Parsley	Lettuce, butterhead		Coffee
Spinach	Mustard greens		Corn
Swiss chard	Soybean oil		Cucumber (peeled)
Tea, black			Dairy products
Tea, green			Eggs
Turnip greens			Fruit (varies)
Watercress			Lettuce, iceberg
			Meats, fish, poultry
			Pasta
			Peanuts
			Peas
			Potato
			Rice
			Tomato

[a]Approximate amount of vitamin K per 100 g (3.5 oz) serving.

Patient Encounter 3, Part 2

The patient is discharged home on warfarin therapy. She was referred to a local area antithrombosis center for monitoring of her oral anticoagulation therapy and has been maintained on warfarin 6 mg daily for the last 3 months. The patient presents today for a routine visit for anticoagulation monitoring and her INR is 10.3. She reports that 6 days ago she was started on ciprofloxacin 500 mg by mouth twice daily, which was prescribed by her primary care physician for a urinary tract infection. In addition, the primary care physician told the patient that her thyroid gland was enlarged and ordered some lab tests to determine if she has a thyroid problem. The patient has not heard what the results are. She also reports that her intake of vitamin K-rich foods (spinach, broccoli, and cabbage) has increased significantly over the last month because she is trying to lose weight. She has no other complaints today and denies any signs or symptoms of bleeding.

What is the most likely explanation for elevated INR?

Should she be given vitamin K? If yes, discuss the dose, route of administration, and an appropriate patient monitoring plan.

How will you manage this patient's warfarin therapy? Outline a plan including specific dose changes, timing of monitoring, and patient education.

encounter to assess for any potential interactions with foods, drugs, herbal products, and nutritional supplements. When an interacting drug is initiated or discontinued, more frequent monitoring should be instituted. In addition, the dose of warfarin can be modified (increased or decreased) in anticipation of the expected impact on the INR.[5,49] Warfarin-related drug interactions can generally be divided into two major categories: pharmacokinetic and pharmacodynamic. Pharmacokinetic interactions are most commonly due to changes in hepatic metabolism or binding to plasma proteins. Drugs that affect the CYP2C9, CYP3A4, and CYP1A2 have the greatest impact on warfarin metabolism. Interactions that impact the metabolism of the S-isomer result in greater changes in the INR than interactions affecting the R-isomer. Pharmacodynamic drug interactions enhance or diminish the anticoagulant effect of warfarin, increasing the risk of bleeding or clotting, but may not alter the INR. There are increasing reports regarding dietary supplements, nutraceuticals, and vitamins that can interact with warfarin. Patients on warfarin may experience changes in the INR due to fluctuating intake of dietary vitamin K. Patients should be instructed to maintain a consistent diet and avoid large fluctuations in vitamin K intake rather than strictly avoiding vitamin K–rich foods.[4,10,11,49]

Nonpharmacologic Therapy

▶ *Thrombectomy*

Most cases of VTE can be successfully treated with anticoagulation. In some cases, removal of the occluding thrombus by surgical intervention may be warranted. Surgical or mechanical thrombectomy can be considered in patients with massive iliofemoral DVT when there is a risk of limb gangrene due to venous occlusion.[2,12] The procedure can be complicated by recurrence of thrombus formation. In patients who present with massive PE, pulmonary embolectomy can be performed in patients with contraindications to thrombolytic therapy, when thrombolysis has failed clinically or will not have sufficient time to take effect. Administer heparin by IV infusion to achieve a therapeutic aPTT during the operation and postoperatively. Thereafter, give warfarin for the usual recommended duration.[2,12,39]

▶ *Inferior Vena Cava Filters*

An inferior vena cava (IVC) filter is indicated in patients with newly diagnosed proximal DVT or PE who have a contraindication to anticoagulation therapy.[2,12] IVC interruption is accomplished by inserting a filter through the internal jugular vein or femoral vein and advancing it into the IVC using ultrasound or fluoroscopic guidance. One of the risks associated with these filters is development of thrombosis on the filter itself. Therefore, anticoagulation therapy should be resumed as soon as contraindications resolve. Temporary or removable filters are now increasingly used and filters should be removed once therapy is completed.[15]

▶ *Compression Stockings*

Postthrombotic syndrome (PTS) occurs in 20% to 50% of patients within 8 years after a DVT. Wearing graduated compression stockings (GCS) after a DVT reduces the risk of PTS by as much as 50%. Current guidelines recommend the use of GCS with an ankle pressure of 30 to 40 mm Hg for 2 years after a DVT. To be effective, GCS must fit properly. Traditionally, strict bed rest has been recommended after a DVT, but this approach has now been refuted, and patients should be encouraged to ambulate as tolerated.[2,12]

APPROACH TO TREATING PATIENTS WITH VTE

A treatment algorithm for VTE is presented in Figure 10–9. Note that LMWH or fondaparinux are preferred over UFH for acute VTE treatment; however, in patients with CrCl less than 30 mL/min (0.50 mL/s), UFH is the preferred treatment approach. For the long-term and extended treatment phases, an oral anticoagulant (ie, warfarin, apixaban, dabigatran, rivaroxban) is the preferred approach to prevent recurrent thrombosis. However, in patients with cancer, the LMWHs are recommended for the acute, long-term and extended phases of treatment due to better efficacy in preventing recurrent thromboembolic events.[2,39] When warfarin is used for treatment of VTE, it is important to initiate warfarin on the first day of therapy after the first dose of parenteral rapid-acting anticoagulant is given and overlap the two therapies for a minimum of 5 days. Warfarin should be dosed to achieve a goal INR range of 2 to 3. Once the INR is stable and above 2, the parenteral anticoagulant should be discontinued. Historically, initial acute phase VTE treatment required hospitalization to administer UFH. However, the availability of LMWH and the DOACs have enabled management of VTE in the outpatient setting, resulting in reduced health care costs and improved patient quality of life.[2,12,39]

Anticoagulation therapy is continued for a minimum of 3 months but should be given longer depending on the underlying etiology of the VTE and the patient's risk factors.[2,12] Determining the optimal duration of anticoagulation involves weighing the risk of recurrent VTE against the risk of bleeding associated with anticoagulation therapy and determining patient preference regarding treatment duration. Patient with provoked VTE by transient risk factors (eg, surgery, trauma) require therapy for 3 months. Extended treatment for more than 3 to 6 months

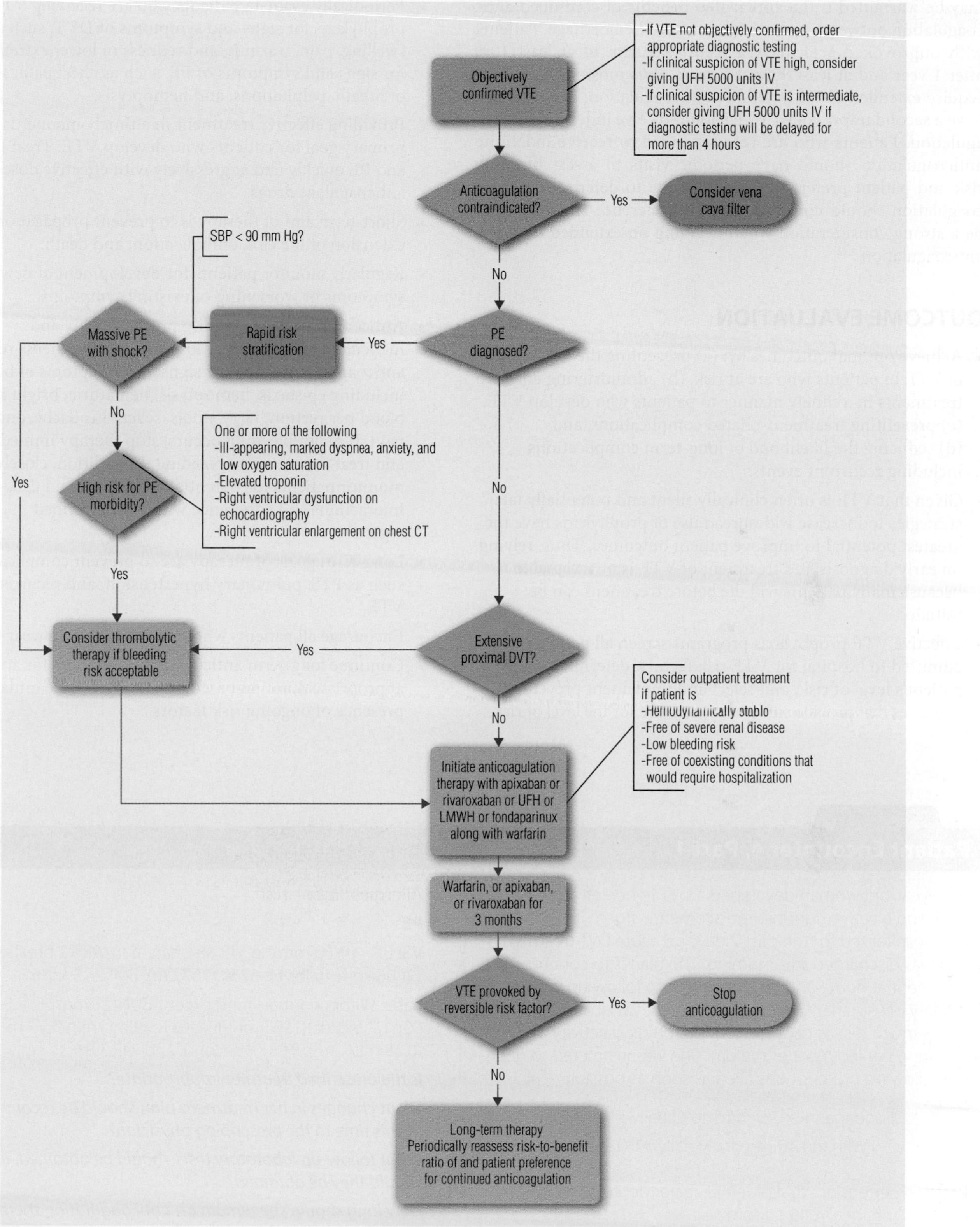

FIGURE 10–9. Treatment of VTE. (CT, computed tomography; DVT, deep vein thrombosis; IV, intravenous; LMWH, low molecular weight heparin; PE, pulmonary embolism; SBP, systolic blood pressure; UFH, unfractionated heparin; VTE, venous thromboembolism.) (From Witt DM, Clark NP. Venous thromboembolism. In: DiPiro JT, Talbert RL, Yee GC, et al., eds. Pharmacotherapy: A Pathophysiologic Approach, 9th ed. New York, NY: McGraw-Hill, 2014:254.)

may be warranted if the anticipated benefits of continued anticoagulation outweigh potential harm from hemorrhage. Patients with unprovoked VTE have a recurrence risk of at least 10% after 1 year and at least 30% at 5 years, thus most such patients require extended if not indefinite anticoagulation. Patients who have a second unprovoked VTE should receive indefinite anticoagulation. Patients who are recommended to receive indefinite anticoagulation should have periodic visits to assess bleeding risk and patient preference/quality of life to determine if anticoagulation should continue. Patient preference should always be a strong consideration when deciding on extended duration anticoagulation.[2,12]

OUTCOME EVALUATION

- Achieve optimal outcomes by: (a) preventing the occurrence of VTE in patients who are at risk, (b) administering effective treatments in a timely manner to patients who develop VTE, (c) preventing treatment-related complications, and (d) reducing the likelihood of long-term complications including recurrent events.
- Given that VTE is often clinically silent and potentially fatal, strategies to increase widespread use of prophylaxis have the greatest potential to improve patient outcomes. Thus, relying on early diagnosis and treatment of VTE is unacceptable because many patients will die before treatment can be initiated.
- Effective VTE prophylaxis programs screen all patients admitted to hospital for VTE risk factors, determine each patient's level of risk, and select and implement prevention strategies that provide sufficient protection for the level of risk.
- Periodically evaluate patients who are receiving VTE prophylaxis for signs and symptoms of DVT, such as swelling, pain, warmth, and redness of lower extremities, and for signs and symptoms of PE, such as chest pain, shortness of breath, palpitations, and hemoptysis.
- Providing effective treatment in a timely manner is the primary goal for patients who develop VTE. Treat DVT and PE quickly and aggressively with effective doses of anticoagulant drugs.
- Short-term aim of therapy is to prevent propagation or local extension of the clot, embolization, and death.
- Regularly monitor patients for development of new symptoms or worsening of existing symptoms.
- Anticoagulant drugs require precise dosing and meticulous monitoring. Closely monitor patients receiving anticoagulant therapy for signs and symptoms of bleeding including epistaxis, hemoptysis, hematuria, bright red blood per rectum, tarry stools, severe headache, and joint pain. If major bleeding occurs, stop therapy immediately and treat the source of bleeding. In addition, closely monitor patients for potential drug–drug and drug–food interactions and adherence with the prescribed regimen.
- Long-term goals of therapy are to prevent complications such as PTS, pulmonary hypertension, and recurrent VTE.
- Encourage all patients who have had DVT to wear GCS.
- Continue long-term anticoagulation therapy for an appropriate duration based on etiology of the initial clot and presence of ongoing risk factors.

Patient Encounter 4, Part 1

A 77-year-old woman developed a DVT in her left leg 5 weeks following elective right hip replacement surgery. The patient was hospitalized for the past 2 days for acute DVT treatment and was discharged this morning. The plan is to continue treatment at home and for the patient to follow up with her primary physician in 2 weeks. The patient was instructed to get as much rest as possible, limiting physical activity and elevating her leg most of the day. She was instructed to get the following prescriptions filled as soon as possible:

Fondaparinux 7.5 mg Sub-Q daily #14 refill 0

Warfarin 10 mg orally daily #30 refill 2

PMH: Hypertension; dyslipidemia; major depressive disorder; gastroesophageal reflux disorder

FH: Father died of "old age"; Mother died of cancer; brother (age 72) has hypertension and had MI (age 66)

SH: Patient is a retired college professor

Current Meds: Lisinopril 20 mg/HCTZ 12.5 mg orally daily; amlodipine 5 mg orally daily; simvastatin 20 mg orally daily; fluoxetine 20 mg orally daily; omeprazole 20 mg orally daily; Aspirin 81 mg orally daily for stroke prevention

Allergies: Sulfa—rash

PE:

VS: BP 144/60 mm Hg, HR 88 beats/min, RR 12 breaths/min, Wt 66 kg (146 lb), Ht 62 in (157 cm), BMI 26.5 kg/m^2

Labs: Within normal limits; except BUN 21 mg/dL (7.5 mmol/L), SCr 1.7 mg/dL (150 μmol/L), eGFR 29 mL/min/1.73 m^2 (0.28 mL/s/m^2), PT 17.8 second, and INR 1.8

Is the prescribed treatment appropriate?

What changes in her treatment plan should be recommended at this time to the prescribing physician?

What follow-up laboratory tests should be obtained, and when should they be obtained?

How long should she remain on anticoagulation therapy?

Given the current list of medications that the patient is taking, should any be discontinued or changed? If changed, what alternative therapy would you recommend?

Develop a patient education plan including appropriate techniques for self-administering injectable anticoagulants.

Patient Encounter 4, Part 2

The patient has been taking warfarin for the past 2 months. Her INR has been in goal range and no changes in warfarin dose have been made. She states that she is currently taking warfarin 5 mg every day except 2.5 mg on Wednesdays and Saturdays. She states she has had two nosebleeds in the past month and notices that she bruises more easily, but has had no major bleeding episodes. Her DVT symptoms essentially resolved within the first month after her diagnosis, but she's noticed some mild pain and swelling in her left leg the past 2 weeks. She states that she has been taking naproxen sodium 220 mg twice daily for her leg pain. Given that the patient has been tolerating the treatment well and is able to obtain the necessary laboratory tests in a timely manner, her primary care physician has recommended that she continue warfarin therapy for another 6 months. She is not very pleased about this recommendation because she finds it difficult to moderate her vitamin K intake ("I love kale!") and the frequent blood tests are annoying.

PE:

VS: BP 136/62 mm Hg, HR 74 beats/min, Wt 64 kg (142 lb), BMI 26.2 kg/m^2

Labs: CBC within normal limits; PT 21.8 seconds, and INR 3.1 (drawn this morning)

How should the patient's recurrent symptoms (ie, pain and swelling in left leg) be evaluated and addressed?

Outline a patient education plan to prevent and manage nosebleeds.

Is the current treatment plan appropriate? Outline a plan including specific medication changes, nonpharmacologic treatment recommendations, and a follow-up plan.

Assume that anticoagulation therapy is appropriate. Is she a good candidate for dabigatran therapy? Justify your answer.

Patient Care Process

Patient Assessment:

- Confirm diagnosis of VTE
  - Clinical assessment: risk factors for VTE; use the Wells criteria to determine probability of VTE (Tables 10–2 and 10–3)
  - If DVT symptoms are present, obtain a venous ultrasound
  - If PE is suspected, obtain a V/Q or CT scan
  - D-dimer: may be a helpful adjunct to rule out VTE
  - In patients with a low probability for PE, the PERC rule is an alternative to D-dimer testing
- Obtain baseline laboratory tests prior to initiating anticoagulation therapy:
  - PT and calculated INR, aPTT or antifactor Xa activity, serum creatinine, serum albumin, and blood urea nitrogen (BUN), liver function tests, CBC with platelets
- Assess risk of bleeding and check for any contraindications to anticoagulation therapy
- Screen dietary and medication profile including over-the-counter medications and herbal therapies used at home for potential drug–drug interactions with anticoagulation therapy
- Assess severity of VTE and whether patient is a candidate for outpatient therapy

Therapy Evaluation:

- If patient is already receiving anticoagulation pharmacotherapy, assess efficacy, safety, and adherence. Are there any drug–drug or drug–food interactions?

Care Plan Development:

- Once diagnosis of VTE has been confirmed with an objective test, promptly start anticoagulation therapy in full therapeutic doses. If there is high clinical suspicion of VTE, anticoagulation therapy may be initiated while waiting for results of diagnostic tests.
- Determine the most appropriate anticoagulant therapy option based on patient clinical characteristics, insurance coverage, plans for outpatient therapy, complexity of anticoagulation management and patient preferences.
- When warfarin is used for treatment of VTE, initiate on the first day of therapy after the first dose of parenteral rapid-acting anticoagulant is given and overlap the two therapies for a minimum of 5 days. Warfarin should be dosed to achieve a goal INR range of 2 to 3. Once INR is stable and above 2, the parenteral anticoagulant should be discontinued.
- Determine optimal duration of anticoagulation therapy by weighing the risk of recurrent VTE against the risk of bleeding and considering patient preferences regarding treatment duration.
- Devise a structured plan for long-term monitoring of anticoagulation therapy; refer the patient to a specialized anticoagulation clinic if available or another designated provider.
- Educate the patient on purpose of therapy and importance of proper monitoring, potential drug–drug and drug–food interactions, dietary consistency with vitamin K-containing foods if treated with warfarin, taking appropriate birth

(Continued)

Patient Care Process (*Continued*)

control measures in females, adherence with anticoagulants and with laboratory monitoring, potential side effects and procedures to follow in case of emergency.

Follow-Up Evaluation:

- Follow a structured plan for periodic long-term monitoring of anticoagulation therapy.
- Reevaluate risks and benefits of continuing anticoagulation therapy beyond the initial 3 months; patients who are recommended to receive indefinite anticoagulation should have periodic visits to assess bleeding risk and patient preference/quality of life to determine if anticoagulation should continue.
- Periodically reassess patient adherence, concurrent medications to screen for drug interactions, and renal and liver functions tests.
- If patient is being treated with warfarin, measure PT/INR at least every 4 weeks based on the stability of INR and patient's health status. Adjust warfarin dose as needed to maintain INR between 2 and 3.
- Interview the patient to determine if there is worsening or new symptoms related to VTE. Ask the patient about overt bruising or bleeding, as well as changes in stool or urine color.

Abbreviations Introduced in This Chapter

ABW	Adjusted body weight
ACCP	American College of Chest Physicians
ACT	Activated clotting time
aPTT	Activated partial thromboplastin time
AST	Aspartate aminotransferase
AT	Antithrombin
BMI	Body mass index
BUN	Blood urea nitrogen
CBC	Complete blood count
CrCl	Creatinine clearance
CT	Computed tomography
CYP	Cytochrome P-450
DOAC	Direct oral anticoagulants
DTI	Direct thrombin inhibitor
dTT	Diluted thrombin time
DVT	Deep vein thrombosis
ECT	Ecarin clotting time
eGFR	Estimated glomerular filtration rate
ESR	Erythrocyte sedimentation rate
FDA	Food and Drug Administration
GCS	Graduated compression stockings
GP	Glycoprotein
HIT	Heparin-induced thrombocytopenia
ICH	Intracranial hemorrhage
INR	International normalized ratio
IPC	Intermittent pneumatic compression (device)
IV	Intravenous
IVC	Inferior vena cava
LDH	Lactate dehydrogenase
LMWH	Low molecular weight heparin
MI	Myocardial Infarction
MRI	Magnetic resonance imaging
PE	Pulmonary embolism
PF	Platelet factor
P-gp	P-glycoprotein
PT	Prothrombin time
PTS	Postthrombotic syndrome
SBP	Systolic blood pressure
SC	Subcutaneous
SGOT	Serum glutamic-oxaloacetic transaminase
SERM	Selective estrogen receptor modulator
TT	Thrombin time
UFH	Unfractionated heparin
V/Q	Ventilation/perfusion (scan)
VTE	Venous thromboembolism
vWF	von Willebrand factor
WBC	White blood cell
WHO	World Health Organization

REFERENCES

1. Goldhaber SZ, Bounameaux H. Pulmonary embolism and deep vein thrombosis. Lancet 2012;379(9828):1835–1846.
2. Kearon C, Akl EA, Comerota AJ, et al. Antithrombotic therapy for VTE disease: Antithrombotic Therapy and Prevention of Thrombosis, 9th ed: American College of Chest Physicians Evidence-Based Clinical Practice Guidelines. Chest. 2012;141(2 suppl):e419S–e494S.
3. Bates SM, Jaeschke R, Stevens SM, et.al. Diagnosis of DVT: Antithrombotic Therapy and Prevention of Thrombosis, 9th ed: American College of Chest Physicians Evidence-Based Clinical Practice Guidelines. Chest. 2012 Feb;141(2 suppl):e351S–e418S.
4. Ageno W, Gallus AS, Wittkowsky A, Crowther M, Hylek EM, Palareti G. Oral anticoagulant therapy: Antithrombotic Therapy and Prevention of Thrombosis, 9th ed: American College of Chest Physicians Evidence-Based Clinical Practice Guidelines. Chest. 2012;141(2 suppl):e44S–e88S.
5. Falck-Ytter Y, Francis CW, Johanson NA, et al. Prevention of VTE in orthopedic surgery patients: Antithrombotic Therapy and Prevention of Thrombosis, 9th ed: American College of Chest Physicians Evidence-Based Clinical Practice Guidelines. Chest. 2012;141(2 suppl):e278S–e325S.
6. Gould MK, Garcia DA, Wren SM, et al. Prevention of VTE in nonorthopedic surgical patients: Antithrombotic Therapy and Prevention of Thrombosis, 9th ed: American College of Chest Physicians Evidence-Based Clinical Practice Guidelines. Chest. 2012;141(2 suppl):e227S–e277S.
7. Kahn SR, Lim W, Dunn AS, et al. Prevention of VTE in nonsurgical patients: Antithrombotic Therapy and Prevention of Thrombosis, 9th ed: American College of Chest Physicians Evidence-Based Clinical Practice Guidelines. Chest. 2012;141(2 suppl):e195S–e226S.
8. Schulman S, Beyth RJ, Kearon C, Levine MN; Hemorrhagic complications of anticoagulant and thrombolytic treatment: American College of Chest Physicians Evidence-Based Clinical Practice Guidelines, 8th ed. Chest. 2008;133:257S–298S.
9. Garcia DA, Baglin TP, Weitz JI, Samama MM. Parenteral anticoagulants: Antithrombotic Therapy and Prevention of Thrombosis, 9th ed: American College of Chest Physicians

Evidence-Based Clinical Practice Guidelines. Chest. 2012;141(2 suppl):e24S–e43S.
10. Holbrook A, Schulman S, Witt DM, et.al. Evidence-based management of anticoagulant therapy: Antithrombotic Therapy and Prevention of Thrombosis, 9th ed: American College of Chest Physicians Evidence-Based Clinical Practice Guidelines. Chest. 2012;141(2 suppl):e152S–e184S.
11. Ansell J, Hirsh J, Hylek E, et al. Pharmacology and management of the vitamin K antagonists: American College of Chest Physicians Evidence-Based Clinical Practice Guidelines, 8th ed. Chest. 2008; 133:160S–198S.
12. Wells PS, Forgie MA, Rodger MA. Treatment of venous thromboembolism. JAMA. 2014;311(7):717–728.
13. Huang W, Goldberg RJ, Anderson FA, Kiefe CI, Spencer FA. Secular trends in occurrence of acute venous thromboembolism: The Worcester VTE study (1985–2009). Am J Med. 2014;127(9): 829–839.
14. Tagalakis V, Patenaude V, Kahn SR, Suissa S. Incidence of and mortality from venous thromboembolism in a real-world population: The Q-VTE Study Cohort. Am J Med. 2013;126(9): e13–e21.
15. Reitsma PH, Versteeg HH, Middeldorp S. Mechanistic view of risk factors for venous thromboembolism. Arterioscler Thromb Vasc Biol. 2012;32(3):563–568.
16. Kearon C. Natural history of venous thromboembolism. Circulation. 2003;107(23 suppl 1):I22–I30.
17. Furie B, Furie BC. Mechanisms of thrombus formation. N Engl J Med. 2008;359(9):938–949.
18. Anderson JA, Weitz JI. Hypercoagulable states. Crit Care Clin. 2011;27(4):933–952, vii.
19. Dalen JE. Should patients with venous thromboembolism be screened for thrombophilia? Am J Med. 2008;121(6):458–463.
20. Rosendaal FR, Reitsma PH. Genetics of venous thrombosis. J Thromb Haemost. 2009;7(suppl 1):301–304.
21. Crowther MA, Kelton JG. Congenital thrombophilic states associated with venous thrombosis: A qualitative overview and proposed classification system. Ann Intern Med. 2003;138(2): 128–134.
22. Giannakopoulos B, Passam F, Rahgozar S, Krilis SA. Current concepts on the pathogenesis of the antiphospholipid syndrome. Blood. 2007;109(2):422–430.
23. Bates SM, Greer IA, Middeldorp S, et.al. VTE, thrombophilia, antithrombotic therapy, and pregnancy: Antithrombotic Therapy and Prevention of Thrombosis, 9th ed: American College of Chest Physicians Evidence-Based Clinical Practice Guidelines. Chest. 2012;141(2 suppl):e691S–e736S.
24. Khorana AA. Cancer and coagulation. Am J Hematol. 2012; 87(suppl 1):S82–S87.
25. Buller HR, van Doormaal FF, van Sluis GL, Kamphuisen PW. Cancer and thrombosis: From molecular mechanisms to clinical presentations. J Thromb Haemost. 2007;5(suppl 1): 246–254.
26. Canonico M, Plu-Bureau G, Lowe GDO, Scarabin P-Y. Hormone replacement therapy and risk of venous thromboembolism in postmenopausal women: Systematic review and meta-analysis. BMJ. 2008;336:1227–1231.
27. Aird WC. Coagulation. Crit Care Med. 2005;33:S485–S487.
28. Crawley JT, Zanardelli S, Chion CK, Lane DA. The central role of thrombin in hemostasis. J Thromb Haemost. 2007;5(suppl 1): 95–101.
29. Monroe DM, Hoffman M. What does it take to make the perfect clot? Arterioscler Thromb Vasc Biol. 2006;26(1): 41–48.
30. Rijken DC, Lijnen HR. New insights into the molecular mechanisms of the fibrinolytic system. J Thromb Haemost. 2009; 7(1):4–13.
31. Wells PS. Integrated strategies for the diagnosis of venous thromboembolism. J Thromb Haemost. 2007;5(suppl 1):41–50.
32. Sinert R, Foley M. Clinical assessment of the patient with a suspected pulmonary embolism. Ann Emerg Med. 2008;52: 76–79.
33. Bauersachs RM. Clinical presentation of deep vein thrombosis and pulmonary embolism. Best Pract Res Clin Haematol. 2012; 25(3):243–251.
34. Jobin S, Kalliainen L, Adebayo L, et.al. Institute for Clinical Systems Improvement. Venous Thromboembolism Prophylaxis. http://bit.ly/VTEProphy1112. November 2012. Last accessed December 1, 2014.
35. Apixaban Prescribing Information. Bristol-Myers Squibb/Pfizer. August 2014. http://packageinserts.bms.com/pi/pi_eliquis.pdf. Last accessed December 1, 2014.
36. Rivaroxaban Prescribing Information. Janssen Pharmaceuticals Inc. March 2014. http://www.xareltohcp.com/sites/default/files/pdf/xarelto_0.pdf. Last accessed December 1, 2014.
37. Watson LI, Armon MP. Thrombolysis for acute deep vein thrombosis. Cochrane Database Syst Rev. 2004:CD002783.
38. Monagle P, Chan AK, Goldenberg NA, et al. Antithrombotic therapy in neonates and children: Antithrombotic Therapy and Prevention of Thrombosis, 9th ed: American College of Chest Physicians Evidence-Based Clinical Practice Guidelines. Chest. 2012;141(2 suppl):e737S–e801S.
39. Segal JB, Streiff MB, Hofmann LV, et al. Management of venous thromboembolism: A systematic review for a practice guideline. Ann Intern Med. 2007;146(3):211–222.
40. Nutescu EA, Spinler SA, Wittkowsky AK, Dager WE. Low Molecular weight heparins in renal impairment and obesity: available evidence and clinical practice recommendations across medical and surgical settings. Ann Pharmacother. 2009; 43(6):1064–1083.
41. Arixtra Prescribing Information. GlaxoSmithKline. September 2013, https://www.gsksource.com/gskprm/htdocs/documents/ARIXTRA-PI-PIL.PDF. Last accessed December 1, 2014.
42. Weitz JI, Eikelboom JW, Samama MM. New antithrombotic drugs: Antithrombotic Therapy and Prevention of Thrombosis, 9th ed: American College of Chest Physicians Evidence-Based Clinical Practice Guidelines. Chest. 2012;141(2 suppl):e120S–e51S.
43. Yeh CH, Gross PL, Weitz JI. Evolving use of new oral anticoagulants for treatment of venous thromboembolism. Blood. 2014 Aug 14;124(7):1020–1028.
44. Nutescu E, Chuatrisorn I, Hellenbart E. Drug and dietary interactions of warfarin and novel oral anticoagulants: An update. J Thromb Thrombolysis. 2011;31(3):326–343.
45. Garcia D, Barrett YC, Ramacciotti E, Weitz JI. Laboratory assessment of the anticoagulant effects of the next generation of oral anticoagulants. J Thromb Haemost. 2013 Feb;11(2):245–252.
46. Heidbuchel H, Verhamme P, Alings M, et.al. European Heart Rhythm Association Practical Guide on the use of new oral anticoagulants in patients with non-valvular atrial fibrillation. Europace. 2013 May;15(5):625–651.
47. Nutescu EA, Shapiro NL, Chevalier A. New anticoagulant agents: Direct thrombin inhibitors. Cardiol Clin. 2008;26(2):169–187.
48. Dabigatran Prescribing Information. Boehringer-Ingelheim. April 2014. http://bidocs.boehringer-ingelheim.com/BIWebAccess/ViewServlet.ser?docBase=renetnt&folderPath=/Prescribing%20Information/PIs/Pradaxa/Pradaxa.pdf. Last accessed December 1, 2014.
49. Warfarin Prescribing Information. Bristol-Myers Squibb. October 2011. http://packageinserts.bms.com/pi/pi_coumadin.pdf. Last accessed December 1, 2014.
50. Garcia DA, Witt DM, Hylek E, et al. Delivery of optimized anticoagulant therapy: Consensus statement from the Anticoagulation Forum. Ann Pharmacother. 2008;42(7):979–988.

11 Stroke

Susan R. Winkler

LEARNING OBJECTIVES

Upon completion of the chapter, the reader will be able to:

1. Differentiate types of cerebrovascular disease including transient ischemic attack, ischemic stroke (cerebral infarction), and hemorrhagic stroke.
2. Identify modifiable and nonmodifiable risk factors associated with ischemic stroke and hemorrhagic stroke.
3. Explain the pathophysiology of ischemic stroke and hemorrhagic stroke.
4. Describe the clinical presentation of transient ischemic attack, ischemic stroke, and hemorrhagic stroke.
5. Evaluate various treatment options for acute ischemic stroke.
6. Determine whether fibrinolytic therapy is indicated in a patient with acute ischemic stroke.
7. Formulate strategies for primary and secondary prevention of acute ischemic stroke.
8. Evaluate treatment options for acute hemorrhagic stroke.

EPIDEMIOLOGY

Cerebrovascular disease, or stroke, is the second most common cause of death worldwide. It is the fourth leading cause of death in the United States, declining from third most common cause of death due to a decrease in both stroke incidence and stroke case fatality rates. This decline is a result of decades of progress in treatment and prevention of stroke, especially improved control of hypertension and other risk factors.[1] Approximately 795,000 strokes occur in the United States each year. New strokes account for 610,000 of this total; recurrent strokes account for the remaining 185,000. Stroke is the leading cause of long-term disability in adults, with 90% of survivors having residual deficits. Moderate to severe disability is seen in 70% of survivors. An estimated 15% to 30% of stroke survivors are permanently disabled, and 20% require institutional care at 3 months after the stroke. The American Heart Association estimates that there are currently over 7 million stroke survivors in the United States. Societal impact and economic burden is great, with total costs of $36.5 billion reported in the United States in 2010. Stroke mortality has declined due to improved recognition and treatment of risk factors; however, risk factor management is still inadequate. Stroke incidence increases with age, especially after age 55 years, resulting in an increased incidence in the elderly population.[2]

ETIOLOGY

Strokes can either be ischemic (87% of all strokes) or hemorrhagic (13% of all strokes). KEY CONCEPT *Ischemic stroke, which may be thrombotic or embolic, is the abrupt development of a focal neurological deficit that occurs due to inadequate blood supply to an area of the brain.* A thrombotic occlusion occurs when a **thrombus** forms inside an artery in the brain. An embolic stroke typically occurs when a piece of thrombus, originating either inside or outside of the cerebral vessels, breaks loose and is carried to the site of occlusion in the cerebral vessels. An extracerebral source of emboli is often the heart, leading to cardioembolic stroke.

KEY CONCEPT *Hemorrhagic stroke is a result of bleeding into the brain and other spaces within the central nervous system (CNS) and includes subarachnoid hemorrhage (SAH), intracerebral hemorrhage (ICH), and subdural* ***hematomas.*** SAH results from sudden bleeding into the space between the inner and middle layers of the **meninges**, most often due to trauma or rupture of a cerebral **aneurysm** or **arteriovenous malformation** (AVM). ICH is bleeding directly into the brain parenchyma, often as a result of chronic uncontrolled hypertension. Subdural hematomas result from bleeding under the dura that covers the brain and most often occur as a result of head trauma.

Risk Factors

Assessment of risk factors for ischemic stroke and hemorrhagic stroke is an important component of stroke prevention, diagnosis, and treatment. A major goal in the long-term management of ischemic stroke involves primary prevention (prevention of first stroke) and prevention of a recurrent stroke through reduction and modification of risk factors. Risk factors for ischemic stroke are divided into modifiable and nonmodifiable (Table 11–1). Every patient should have risk factors assessed and treated, if possible, because management can decrease the occurrence and/or recurrence of stroke.[3,4]

CLASSIFICATION

Cerebral Ischemic Events

There are two main classifications of cerebral ischemic events: **transient ischemic attack** (TIA) and ischemic stroke (cerebral infarction). A TIA is a transient episode of neurological

Table 11–1

Nonmodifiable and Modifiable Risk Factors for Ischemic Stroke

Nonmodifiable Risk Factors
- Age (> 55 years)
- Gender (males more than females)
- Race and ethnicity (American Indian/Alaska Natives, African American, Asian/Pacific Islander, Hispanic)
- Genetic predisposition
- Low birth weight

Well Documented and Modifiable Risk Factors
- Hypertension (most important risk factor)
- Atrial fibrillation (most important and treatable cardiac cause of stroke)
- Cardiac disease
  - Mitral stenosis
  - Mitral annular calcification
  - Left atrial enlargement
  - Structural abnormalities such as atrial-septal aneurysm
  - Acute MI
- Transient ischemic attacks or prior stroke (major independent risk factor)
- Diabetes (independent risk factor)
- Dyslipidemia
- Asymptomatic carotid stenosis
- Oral contraceptive use (with estrogen content greater than 50 mcg)
- Postmenopausal hormone therapy
- Sickle cell disease
- Lifestyle factors
  - Cigarette smoking
  - Excessive alcohol use
  - Physical inactivity
  - Obesity
  - Diet
  - Cocaine and intravenous drug use
  - Low socioeconomic status

Less Well Documented or Potentially Modifiable Risk Factors
- Increased hematocrit
- Metabolic syndrome
- Hyperhomocysteinemia (less well documented)
- Migraine (risk not clear)
- Sleep disordered breathing

MI, myocardial infarction.

dysfunction caused by focal brain, spinal cord, or retinal ischemia without acute infarction. TIAs have a rapid onset and short duration, typically lasting less than 1 hour and often less than 30 minutes. The symptoms vary depending on the area of the brain affected; however, no deficit remains after the attack. The classic definition of TIA was based on symptom duration of less than 24 hours; symptoms lasting 24 hours or greater were categorized as ischemic stroke. Improved neuroimaging techniques have revealed that clinical symptoms lasting more than 1 hour are often ischemic stroke based on evidence of tissue infarction. Using the classic definition of TIA would potentially miscategorize the event in up to one-third of cases. For this reason, the definition of TIA has been changed to eliminate the focus on time and encourage prompt diagnosis and classification of the event.[5]

KEY CONCEPT *TIAs are a risk factor for acute ischemic stroke, preceding acute ischemic stroke in approximately 15% of cases; therefore, preventive measures are the same for both TIA and ischemic stroke.*[6]

Ischemic stroke is similar to TIA; however, tissue injury and infarction are present, and in many patients, residual deficits remain after the event. A standardized tissue-based definition of cerebral infarction has been established defining cerebral infarction as brain, spinal cord, or retinal cell death attributable to ischemia, based on neuropathological, neuroimaging, and/or clinical evidence of permanent injury.[7]

Hemorrhagic Events

For hemorrhagic events associated with stroke, refer to the Clinical Presentation and Diagnosis of Stroke textbox.

PATHOPHYSIOLOGY

Ischemic Stroke

In ischemic stroke, there is an interruption of the blood supply to an area of the brain either due to thrombus formation or an embolism. Loss of cerebral blood flow results in tissue hypoperfusion, tissue hypoxia, and cell death. Thrombus formation usually starts with lipid deposits in the vessel wall that cause turbulent blood flow. This leads to vessel injury and vessel collagen becoming exposed to blood. This vessel injury initiates the platelet aggregation process due to the exposed subendothelium. Platelets release adenosine diphosphate (ADP), which causes platelet aggregation and consolidation of the platelet plug. Thromboxane A_2 is released, contributing to platelet aggregation and vasoconstriction. The vessel injury also activates the coagulation cascade, which leads to thrombin production. Thrombin converts fibrinogen to fibrin, leading to clot formation as fibrin molecules, platelets, and blood cells aggregate. Refer to Figures 7–3, 10–3, and 10–4 for a depiction of these processes.

After the initial event, secondary events occur at the cellular level that contribute to cell death. Regardless of the initiating event, the cellular processes that follow may be similar. Excitatory amino acids such as glutamate accumulate within the cells, causing intracellular calcium accumulation. Inflammation occurs and oxygen free radicals are formed resulting in the common pathway of cell death.

There is often a core of ischemia containing unsalvageable brain cells. Surrounding this core is an area termed the **ischemic penumbra**. In this area, cells are still salvageable; however, this is

Patient Encounter Part 1

A 78-year-old (84.1 kg [185.0 lb], 5′10″ [178 cm]) white man presents to the emergency department with weakness in his left arm and leg and difficulty speaking. His symptoms began approximately 2 hours ago, prompting his wife to call the paramedics. His past medical history is significant for hypertension, dyslipidemia, and a previous stroke 2 years ago. He experienced a transient ischemic attack 1 week ago, but did not seek medical care. Social history is significant for moderate alcohol use and cigarette smoking half pack per day for the past 50 years. Current medications include perindopril 4 mg once daily, simvastatin 40 mg daily, aspirin 81 mg daily, and a multivitamin tablet once daily.

What signs and symptoms does the patient have that are suggestive of stroke?

What nonmodifiable and modifiable risk factors does he have for acute ischemic stroke?

a time-sensitive endeavor. Without restoration of adequate perfusion, cell death continues throughout a larger area of the brain, ultimately leading to neurological deficits.

Hemorrhagic Stroke

The pathophysiology of hemorrhagic stroke is not as well studied as that of ischemic stroke; however, it is more complex than previously thought. Much of the process is related to the presence of blood in the brain tissue and/or surrounding spaces resulting in compression. The hematoma that forms may continue to grow and enlarge after the initial bleed, and early growth is associated with a poor outcome. Brain tissue swelling and injury is a result of inflammation caused by thrombin and other blood products. This can lead to increased intracranial pressure (ICP) and herniation.[8,9]

CLINICAL PRESENTATION AND DIAGNOSIS

Refer to the Clinical Presentation and Diagnosis of Stroke textbox for information on the signs and symptoms of stroke. It is important to note that hypertension is one of the major risk factors for both ischemic and hemorrhagic stroke. For ICH specifically, hypertension has been shown to increase risk by a factor of 3.68.[10] Other risk factors for hemorrhagic stroke include trauma, cigarette smoking, cocaine use, heavy alcohol use, anticoagulant use, and cerebral aneurysm and AVM rupture.[4,8]

DESIRED TREATMENT OUTCOMES

The short-term treatment goals for acute ischemic stroke include reducing secondary brain damage by reestablishing and maintaining adequate perfusion to marginally ischemic areas of the brain and protecting these areas from the effects of ischemia (ie, neuroprotection). KEY CONCEPT *Long-term treatment goals for acute ischemic stroke include prevention of a recurrent stroke through reduction and modification of risk factors and by use of appropriate treatments.*

Short-term treatment goals for hemorrhagic stroke include rapid neurointensive care to maintain adequate oxygenation, breathing, and circulation. Management of increased ICP and blood pressure (BP) are important in the acute setting. Long-term management includes prevention of complications and of a recurrent bleed and delayed cerebral ischemia.

Prevention of long-term disability and death related to stroke are important regardless of stroke type.

GENERAL APPROACH TO TREATMENT

KEY CONCEPT *All patients should have a brain CT or MRI scan to differentiate an ischemic stroke from a hemorrhagic stroke because treatment differs and fibrinolytic therapy must be avoided until hemorrhagic stroke is ruled out.* A CT or MRI scan is the most important diagnostic test in patients with acute stroke. For those with an ischemic stroke, an evaluation should be done to

Clinical Presentation and Diagnosis of Stroke

General

- Patient may not be able to reliably report history owing to cognitive or language deficits. A reliable history may have to come from a family member or another witness.

Symptoms

- The patient may complain of weakness on one side of the body, inability to speak, loss of vision, vertigo, headache, or falling.

Signs

- Patients usually have multiple signs of neurologic dysfunction, and specific deficits are determined by the area of the brain involved.
- Hemiparesis or monoparesis occur commonly, as does a hemisensory deficit.
- Patients with vertigo and double vision are likely to have posterior circulation involvement.
- Aphasia is seen commonly in patients with anterior circulation strokes.
- Patients may also suffer from dysarthria, visual field defects, and altered levels of consciousness.

Signs and Symptoms of Hemorrhagic Stroke

- A sudden severe headache, nausea, vomiting, and photophobia may be the first signs and symptoms. Patients may complain the headache is "the worst headache of my life," especially if the cause is a SAH.
- Neck pain and nuchal rigidity may also be experienced at the time of the hemorrhage.

**It is important to note that a diagnosis of type of stroke cannot be made solely on signs and symptoms because overlap occurs between types of stroke.

Laboratory Tests

- There are no specific laboratory tests for stroke.
- Tests for hypercoagulable states, such as protein C deficiency and antiphospholipid antibody, should be done only when cause of stroke cannot be determined based on presence of well-known risk factors.

Other Diagnostic Tests

- Computed tomography (CT) scan of the head will reveal an area of hyperintensity (white) identifying that a hemorrhage has occurred. The CT scan will either be normal or hypointense (dark) in an area where an infarction has occurred. It may take 24 hours (and rarely longer) to reveal the area of infarction on a CT scan.
- Magnetic resonance imaging (MRI) of the head will reveal areas of ischemia earlier and with better resolution than a CT scan. Diffusion-weighted imaging can reveal an evolving infarct within minutes.
- Carotid Doppler studies will determine whether the patient has a high degree of stenosis in the carotid arteries supplying blood to the brain (extracranial disease).
- Electrocardiogram (ECG) will determine whether the patient has AF, a major risk factor for cardioembolic stroke.
- Transthoracic echocardiogram will identify whether there are heart valve abnormalities or problems with wall motion of the heart resulting in emboli to the brain.

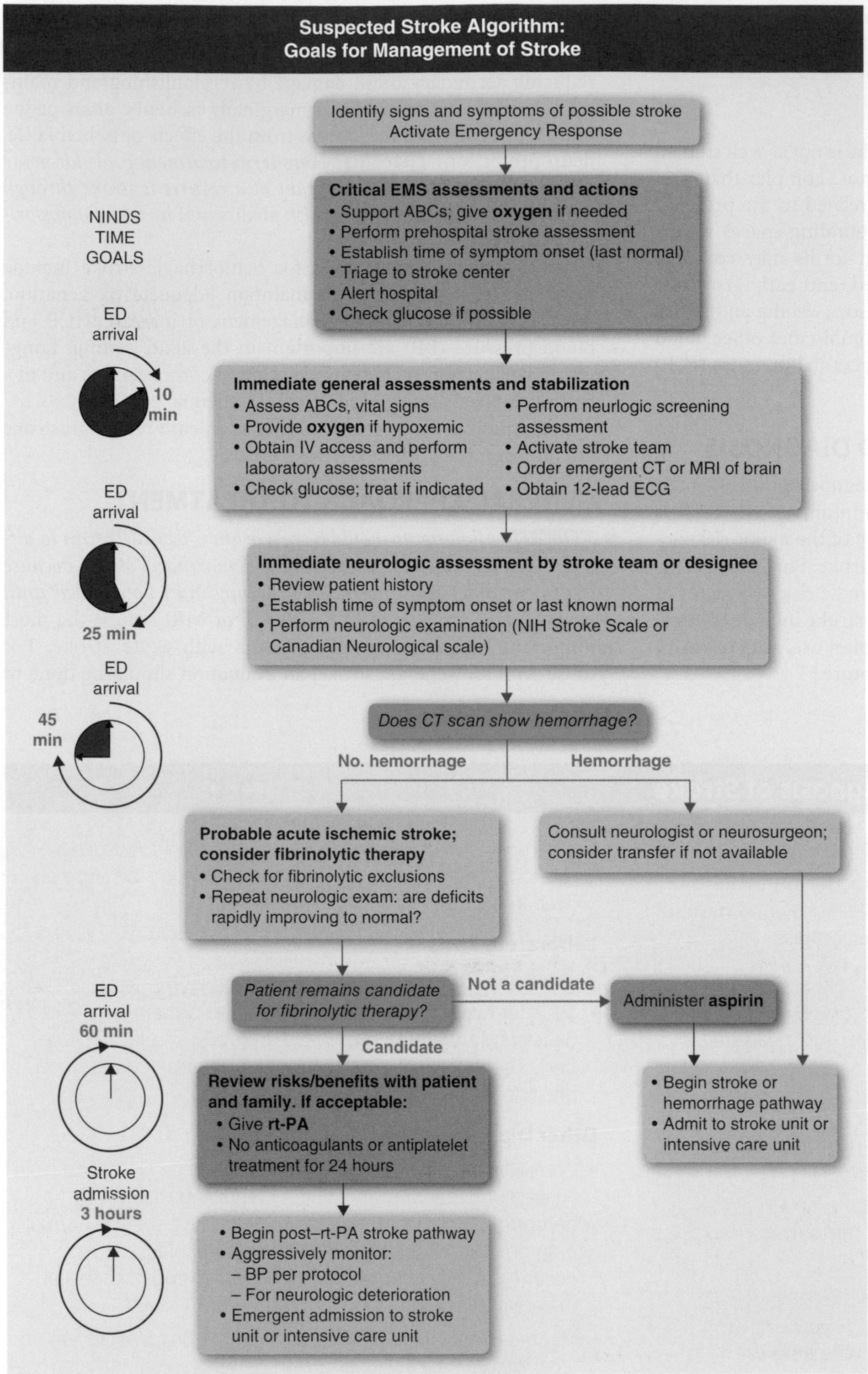
Suspected Stroke Algorithm:
Goals for Management of Stroke
Identify signs and symptoms of possible stroke
Activate Emergency Response
Critical EMS assessments and actions
• Support ABCs; give oxygen if needed
• Perform prehospital stroke assessment
• Establish time of symptom onset (last normal)
• Triage to stroke center
• Alert hospital
• Check glucose if possible
NINDS TIME GOALS
ED arrival
10 min
Immediate general assessments and stabilization
• Assess ABCs, vital signs
• Provide oxygen if hypoxemic
• Obtain IV access and perform laboratory assessments
• Check glucose; treat if indicated
• Perfrom neurlogic screening assessment
• Activate stroke team
• Order emergent CT or MRI of brain
• Obtain 12-lead ECG
ED arrival
25 min
Immediate neurologic assessment by stroke team or designee
• Review patient history
• Establish time of symptom onset or last known normal
• Perform neurologic examination (NIH Stroke Scale or Canadian Neurological scale)
ED arrival
45 min
Does CT scan show hemorrhage?
No. hemorrhage
Hemorrhage
Probable acute ischemic stroke; consider fibrinolytic therapy
• Check for fibrinolytic exclusions
• Repeat neurologic exam: are deficits rapidly improving to normal?
Consult neurologist or neurosurgeon; consider transfer if not available
ED arrival 60 min
Patient remains candidate for fibrinolytic therapy?
Not a candidate
Administer aspirin
Candidate
Review risks/benefits with patient and family. If acceptable:
• Give rt-PA
• No anticoagulants or antiplatelet treatment for 24 hours
• Begin stroke or hemorrhage pathway
• Admit to stroke unit or intensive care unit
Stroke admission 3 hours
• Begin post–rt-PA stroke pathway
• Aggressively monitor:
– BP per protocol
– For neurologic deterioration
• Emergent admission to stroke unit or intensive care unit

FIGURE 11–1. Suspected stroke treatment algorithm. 2011 American Heart Association, with permission. ABC, airway, breathing, and circulation; BP, blood pressure; CT, computed tomography; ECG, electrocardiogram; ED, emergency department; EMS, emergency medical services; IV, intravenous; MRI, magnetic resonance imaging; NIH, National Institutes of Health; NINDS, National Institute of Neurological Disorders and Stroke rt-PA, alteplase.

determine the appropriateness of reperfusion therapy. In hemorrhagic stroke, a surgical evaluation should be completed to assess the need for surgical clipping of an aneurysm or other procedure to control the bleeding and prevent rebleeding and other complications. Figure 11–1 provides an algorithm for initial management of the acute stroke patient.

TREATMENT OF ACUTE ISCHEMIC STROKE

Acute ischemic stroke is a medical emergency. Identification of the time and manner of stroke onset is an important determinant in treatment. The time the patient was last without symptoms is used as the time of stroke onset. Because patients typically do not experience pain, determining the onset time can be difficult. It is also important to document risk factors and previous functional status to assess current disability due to stroke.

Supportive Measures

Acute complications of ischemic stroke include cerebral edema, increased ICP, seizures, and **hemorrhagic conversion**. In the acute setting, supportive interventions and treatments to prevent acute complications should be initiated. Cardiac monitoring, most commonly with a Holter monitor, should be continued for the first 24 hours to screen for atrial fibrillation (AF) and other cardiac diseases.[11] Tissue oxygenation should be maintained acutely. Measure the oxygen saturation using pulse oximetry and supplement the patient with oxygen if necessary. Oxygen saturation should be maintained at 94% (0.94) or greater.[12] Volume status and electrolytes should be corrected. If required, blood glucose should be corrected because both hyperglycemia and hypoglycemia may worsen brain ischemia. When blood glucose less than 60 mg/dL (3.3 mmol/L) is present, bolus with 25 mL of 50% dextrose immediately. Patients with elevated blood glucose poststroke have been documented to have worse outcomes; therefore, lowering the blood glucose to between 140 and 180 mg/dL (7.8–10.0 mmol/L) with subcutaneous insulin is a reasonable approach.[13,14] If the patient is febrile, treat with acetaminophen because fever is associated with brain ischemia and increased morbidity and mortality after stroke. Alternatively, cooling devices can be used.[13,15] Low-dose unfractionated heparin (UFH) or low-dose low molecular weight heparin (LMWH) administered subcutaneously significantly decrease the risk of developing venous thromboembolism (VTE) poststroke. UFH 5000 units subcutaneously every 8 to 12 hours or low-dose LMWH should be given for VTE prophylaxis in patients who are not candidates for intravenous (IV) alteplase. In patients receiving IV alteplase, the administration of subcutaneous UFH or LMWH should be delayed until 24 hours after the administration of alteplase to avoid bleeding complications.

In the setting of acute ischemic stroke, up to 75% of patients have an elevated BP in the first 24 to 48 hours. BP should be optimized; however, hypertension should generally not be treated in the acute period (12–24 hours) because it may cause decreased blood flow in ischemic areas, potentially increasing the infarction size. The cautious use of antihypertensive medications may be necessary in patients who are otherwise candidates for fibrinolytic therapy, including those with severely elevated BP (systolic BP greater than 220 mm Hg or diastolic BP [DBP] greater than 120 mm Hg), and those with other medical disorders requiring immediate lowering of BP. Tables 11–2 and 11–3 provide recommendations on BP management in those eligible and not eligible for alteplase. In those not eligible for alteplase, when BP is lowered, aim for a 15% reduction in systolic BP and diastolic BP in the first 24 hours after stroke onset. BP should be checked three times with each reading taken 5 minutes apart.

Nonpharmacologic Therapy

► *Carotid Endarterectomy and Other Surgical Procedures*

It is not well established whether carotid endarterectomy (CEA) is of value when performed emergently or urgently after stroke, meaning within the first 24 hours after symptom onset.[13] Recent trials have concluded that patients with TIA or mild to moderate stable stroke undergoing CEA within 48 hours may have an acceptable surgical risk. However, patients with unstable neurological status and more severe strokes demonstrated worse outcomes.[13,16] Emergency extracranial-intracranial bypass is not recommended in acute ischemic stroke as it has not been shown to provide a benefit. Due to lack of proven efficacy of these procedures when performed emergently or urgently in acute ischemic stroke, they are not routinely recommended. More research is needed to determine optimal timing of surgery and to delineate the role of CEA in acute treatment.

Table 11–2

Blood Pressure (BP) Recommendations for Ischemic Stroke (Eligible for Alteplase)

Before treatment: If systolic BP > 185 mm Hg or diastolic BP > 110 mm Hg	Labetalol 10–20 mg IV over 1–2 minutes (may repeat after 10 minutes) or nicardipine infusion 5 mg/hour (titrate up by 2.5 mg/hour every 5–15 minutes; maximum dose 15 mg/hour) or may consider other agents (hydralazine, enalaprilat)
During and after treatment to maintain BP ≤ 180/105 mmHg:	
If systolic BP > 180–230 mm Hg or diastolic BP > 105–120 mm Hg	Labetalol 10 mg IV over 1–2 minutes followed by labetalol infusion 2–8 mg/min or nicardipine infusion 5 mg/hour (titrate up by 2.5 mg/hour every 5–15 minutes; maximum dose 15 mg/hour)
If BP not controlled or diastolic BP > 140 mm Hg	Nitroprusside 0.3–0.5 mcg/kg/min titrated by 0.5 mcg/kg/min to response; maximum dose 10 mcg/kg/min

IV, intravenous.

Fibrinolytic Therapy

► *Alteplase*

American Stroke Association guidelines include alteplase (rt-PA; Activase) as the only Food and Drug Administration (FDA)-approved acute treatment for ischemic stroke and strongly encourage early diagnosis and treatment of appropriate patients.[13] Alteplase is an IV fibrinolytic that was approved for acute ischemic stroke treatment in 1996 based on the results of the National Institute of Neurological Disorders and Stroke (NINDS) rt-PA Stroke Trial.[17] Patients treated with alteplase were 30% more likely to have minimal or no disability at 3 months compared with patients given placebo. Alteplase treatment resulted in an 11% to 13% absolute increase in patients with excellent outcomes at 3 months, independent of patient age, stroke subtype, stroke severity, or prior use of aspirin (ASA).[18] ICH within 36 hours after stroke onset occurred in 6.4% of those

Table 11–3

Blood Pressure (BP) Recommendations for Ischemic Stroke (Not Eligible for Alteplase)

Systolic BP < 220 mm Hg and diastolic BP < 120 mm Hg	Observe unless other end-organ involvement
Systolic BP > 220 mm Hg or diastolic BP 121–140 mm Hg	Labetalol 10–20 mg IV over 1–2 minutes (may repeat every 10–20 minutes; maximum dose 300 mg) or nicardipine infusion 5 mg/hour titrated to response
Diastolic BP > 140 mm Hg	Nitroprusside 0.3–0.5 mcg/kg/min titrated by 0.5 mcg/kg/min to response; maximum dose 10 mcg/kg/min

IV, intravenous.

given alteplase versus 0.6% in those given placebo. There was no significant difference in mortality between the two groups at 3 months or 1 year. A dose of 0.9 mg/kg (maximum 90 mg) is recommended; the first 10% is given as an IV bolus, and the remainder is infused over 1 hour.

Subsequent studies that followed the NINDS trial protocol have supported alteplase use in acute ischemic stroke and have shown similar rates for both response and ICH occurrence. When the clinical trials are pooled, study results show that the sooner alteplase is given after the onset of stroke symptoms, the greater the benefit seen in neurological outcome.[18] KEY CONCEPT *Current guidelines recommend alteplase use within 3 hours after stroke onset in appropriate patients and within 3 to 4.5 hours in select patients meeting criteria.* The guidelines further recommend that alteplase be started as soon as possible within this window of time.[13,18,19] A **door-to-needle** time of 60 minutes is recommended for patients eligible to receive alteplase. Further research is needed to evaluate alteplase use in patients with minor or rapidly improving stroke symptoms. Alteplase is commonly withheld in this group of patients; however, as many as one-third may go on to have a poor outcome.[20] Research to evaluate combination treatments and new fibrinolytic agents are underway in an effort to improve outcomes after ischemic stroke.[21] Table 11–4 details the inclusion and exclusion criteria for administration of alteplase in acute ischemic stroke.

Antiplatelet agents, anticoagulants, and invasive procedures such as insertion of a central line, placement of a nasogastric tube, and bladder catheterization should be avoided for 24 hours after infusion of alteplase to prevent bleeding complications. A CT scan should be obtained 24 hours after IV infusion of alteplase before initiating anticoagulants or antiplatelet agents.

Efficacy is measured by elimination of existing neurological deficits and long-term improvement in neurological status and functioning based on neurological examinations and other outcome measures. BP measurements and neurological examinations should be completed every 15 minutes during and after the infusion of alteplase for 2 hours, every 30 minutes for the next 6 hours, and then every hour until 24 hours after alteplase administration. In the NINDS trial, neurological function was assessed 24 hours after administration of alteplase using the National Institutes of Health Stroke Scale (NIHSS). This 42-point scale quantifies neurological deficits in patients who have had a stroke and is easily performed. Use of a standardized stroke scale such as the NIHSS is recommended at baseline and 24 hours after the administration of alteplase.

The major adverse effects of fibrinolytic therapy are bleeding, including ICH and serious systemic bleeding. Mental status changes and a severe headache may indicate ICH. Signs of systemic bleeding include easy bruising; hematemesis; guaiac-positive stools; black, tarry stools; hematoma formation; hematuria; bleeding gums; and nosebleeds. Angioedema is a potential side effect that may cause airway obstruction.

▶ *Other Fibrinolytics*

Fibrinolytics, other than alteplase, are not indicated for use in acute ischemic stroke. Trials evaluating streptokinase were stopped early due to a high incidence of hemorrhage in the streptokinase-treated patients. Other fibrinolytic agents, including tenecteplase, reteplase, desmoteplase, and urokinase, and the defibrinogenating agents, including ancrod, are not recommended for treatment unless associated with a clinical trial. Results with these agents have been mixed and clinical trials are currently ongoing.[13,21]

Table 11–4

Inclusion and Exclusion Criteria for Alteplase (rt-PA) Use in Acute Ischemic Stroke

Inclusion Criteria
- 18 years of age or older (> 80 years old relative exclusion for extended treatment time)
- Clinical diagnosis of ischemic stroke causing a measurable neurological deficit
- Time of symptom onset well established to be less than 4.5 hours before treatment would begin

Exclusion Criteria
- Evidence of multilobar infarction on CT scan of the brain (> 1/3 cerebral hemisphere) prior to treatment
- Clinical presentation suggestive of SAH even with a normal head CT
- Active internal bleeding
- Known bleeding diathesis, including but not limited to: (a) platelet count less than $100 \times 10^3/mm^3$ ($100 \times 10^9/L$); (b) heparin within 48 hours with an elevated aPTT; or (c) current oral anticoagulant use (eg, warfarin) or recent use with an elevated PT (> 15 seconds) or INR (> 1.7)
- Current use of direct thrombin inhibitors or direct factor Xa inhibitors with elevated sensitive laboratory tests (aPTT, INR, platelet count, and ECT; TT; or appropriate factor Xa activity assays)
- Blood glucose concentration < 50 mg/dL (2.8 mmol/L)
- Recent intracranial or intraspinal surgery, significant head trauma, or previous stroke within 3 months
- Recent arterial puncture at a noncompressible site in previous 7 days
- Lumbar puncture within 7 days
- History of previous intracranial hemorrhage
- Intracranial neoplasm, known AVM or aneurysm
- SBP > 185 mm Hg or DBP > 110 mm Hg at time of treatment, or patient requires aggressive treatment to reduce BP to within these limits

Relative Exclusion Criteria
- Consider risk to benefit of IV rt-PA if any relative contraindications are present:
  - Only minor or rapidly improving stroke symptoms
  - Pregnancy
  - Witnessed seizure at onset of stroke symptoms with postictal residual neurological impairments
  - Major surgery or serious trauma within 14 days
  - Recent gastrointestinal or urinary tract hemorrhage (within previous 21 days)
  - Recent acute MI (within previous 3 months)

aPTT, activated partial thromboplastin time; AVM, arteriovenous malformation; CT, computed tomography; DBP, diastolic blood pressure; ECT, ecarin clotting time; INR, international normalized ratio; IV, intravenous; MI, myocardial infarction; PT, prothrombin time; SAH, subarachnoid hemorrhage; SBP, systolic blood pressure; TT, thrombin time.

▶ *Intraarterial Fibrinolytics*

Intraarterial (IA) fibrinolytics may improve outcomes in select patients with acute ischemic stroke due to large-vessel occlusion, if administered within 6 hours of symptom onset. Patients in two clinical trials received pro-urokinase (r-pro UK) plus heparin or heparin alone within 6 hours of symptom onset.[22,23] Results from the first trial were not statistically significant but favored r-pro UK, whereas results of the second trial showed a statistically significant benefit to r-pro UK. No difference in mortality was found, although incidence of ICH was greater in the r-pro UK plus heparin group versus heparin alone. Note that r-pro UK is not FDA approved and not available for clinical use. A recent meta-analysis evaluating IA fibrinolytics found comparable results.[24] The treatment group was found to have a statistically significant benefit for either a good outcome or an excellent outcome. The incidence of ICH was increased; however, no difference in mortality was observed. Additionally, earlier treatment with IA fibrinolysis has been associated with better clinical outcomes.[13] IA fibrinolysis with alteplase may be an option for patients who have contraindications to IV alteplase. It may be considered in patients with middle cerebral artery occlusion within 6 hours of symptom onset who are not candidates for IV alteplase. IA fibrinolysis should be performed by qualified personnel and should not delay treatment with IV alteplase in eligible patients.

Heparin

Full-dose IV UFH has been previously used in acute stroke therapy; however, no adequately designed trials have been conducted to establish its efficacy and safety. Current acute ischemic stroke treatment guidelines do not recommend routine, urgent full-dose anticoagulation with UFH due to lack of a proven benefit in improving neurological function and the risk of intracranial bleeding.[13,18,25] Full-dose UFH may prevent early recurrent stroke in patients with large-vessel atherothrombosis or those thought to be at high risk of recurrent stroke (eg, cardioembolic stroke); however, more study is required.

The major complications of heparin include conversion of ischemic stroke into hemorrhagic stroke, bleeding, and thrombocytopenia. Occurrence of severe headache and mental status changes may indicate ICH. Signs of bleeding mirror those listed for alteplase therapy. Hemoglobin, hematocrit, and platelet count should be obtained at least every 3 days to detect bleeding and thrombocytopenia.

LMWHs and Heparinoids

Full-dose LMWHs and heparinoids are not recommended in the treatment of acute ischemic stroke.[13,18,26] Studies with these agents have generally been negative, with no convincing evidence of improved outcomes after ischemic stroke. Increased risk of bleeding complications and hemorrhagic transformation has been observed.

Thrombin Inhibitors

Several thrombin inhibitors have been approved for stroke prevention in patients with AF and may have a potential benefit in acute stroke treatment. Currently, use of these agents in acute stroke treatment is not well established, and it is recommended that their use be in conjunction with a clinical trial.[13]

Antiplatelet Agents

Aspirin use in acute ischemic stroke has been studied in two large randomized trials. Patients who received ASA within 48 hours of onset of acute ischemic stroke symptoms were less likely to suffer early recurrent stroke, death, and disability. **KEY CONCEPT** *ASA therapy with an initial dose of 160 to 325 mg is recommended in most patients with acute ischemic stroke within 24 to 48 hours after stroke symptom onset.* ASA dose may then be decreased to 75 to 100 mg daily to reduce bleeding complications.[18] Administration of ASA should not replace other acute stroke treatments and should be delayed for 24 hours in patients receiving alteplase. Clopidogrel is not recommended in acute ischemic stroke. Glycoprotein IIb/IIIa receptor inhibitors are not recommended except in the setting of research.[13]

PREVENTION OF ACUTE ISCHEMIC STROKE

Primary Prevention

► Aspirin

Use of ASA in patients with no history of stroke or ischemic heart disease reduced the incidence of nonfatal myocardial infarction (MI) but not stroke. Primary prevention guidelines recommend ASA for general cardiovascular prophylaxis (not specific to stroke) in men and women with a 10-year risk of cardiovascular events of 6% to 10% and in older women who are at high risk for stroke. The benefits must be weighed against the risk of major bleeding. Due to lack of benefit observed in clinical trials, ASA is not recommended for primary prevention in patients with diabetes and asymptomatic peripheral arterial disease, or in those at low risk.[3]

► Diabetes

Diabetes is an independent risk factor for stroke. Intensive glycemic control has not been shown to reduce stroke risk in either type 1 or type 2 diabetes mellitus. Adequate control of BP and management of dyslipidemia are recommended in individuals with diabetes.[3,27] Hypertension guidelines recommend initial therapy that includes a thiazide-type diuretic, calcium channel blocker (CCB), angiotensin-converting enzyme inhibitor (ACE-I) or angiotensin receptor blocker (ARB).[27] Although a weaker recommendation, the guidelines suggest that in black patients with diabetes, initial antihypertensive therapy should include a thiazide-type diuretic or a CCB.[27] The use of a statin to prevent a first stroke is also recommended.[3]

► Dyslipidemia

Recent studies have found a relationship between total cholesterol levels and stroke rate.[3] Statin use may reduce the incidence of a first stroke in high-risk patients (eg, hypertension, coronary heart disease, or diabetes) including patients with normal lipid levels. Patients with a history of MI, coronary artery disease (CAD), elevated lipid levels, diabetes, and other risk factors benefit from treatment with a statin, including patients with normal lipid levels. The benefit of other lipid-lowering therapies on stroke risk has not been established.[3]

Patient Encounter Part 2

The patient arrives in the emergency department 3 hours after the onset of his symptoms. In the emergency department, an IV line is placed, a physical and neurological examination is completed, and he is moved to the stroke unit. A head CT scan is negative for hemorrhagic stroke. His BP on admission to the stroke unit is 198/112 mm Hg. The patient denies other exclusions to IV alteplase. The neurologist is evaluating him for alteplase administration.

Identify your acute treatment goals for the patient.

Is he a candidate for IV alteplase at this time?

What acute management would be appropriate for the patient in the stroke unit?

▶ *Hypertension*

Hypertension is the most important and well-documented risk factor for stroke. Lowering BP in hypertensive patients has been shown to reduce the relative risk of stroke, both ischemic and hemorrhagic, by 35% to 44%.[28] All patients should have BP monitored and controlled appropriately based on current guidelines for BP management. The JNC 8 guidelines do not specifically address stroke patients, but recommend a BP goal of less than 150/90 mm Hg in the general population older than 60 years with high BP, and less than 140/90 mm Hg in patients older than 60 years and adults of any age with renal disease or diabetes.[27] Many patients require two or more drug therapies to achieve BP control. For primary prevention of stroke, reduction in BP is the main goal because one antihypertensive agent has not been clearly shown to be more beneficial than any other.

▶ *Smoking Cessation*

The relationship between smoking and both ischemic and hemorrhagic stroke is clear. Smoking status should be assessed at every patient visit. Patients should be assisted and encouraged in smoking cessation as stroke risk after cessation has been shown to decline over time. Effective treatment options are available including counseling, nicotine replacement products, and oral agents.

▶ *Other Treatments*

A number of other disease states and lifestyle factors should be addressed as primary prevention of stroke. AF is an important and well-documented risk for stroke. See Chapter 9 for information on stroke prevention in AF. Asymptomatic carotid stenosis, cardiac disease, sickle cell disease, obesity, excessive alcohol use, and physical inactivity are other risks that should be assessed and managed appropriately.

Secondary Prevention

▶ *Nonpharmacologic Therapy*

Carotid Endarterectomy The benefit of carotid endarterectomy (CEA) for prevention of recurrent stroke has been studied in major clinical trials including a meta-analysis and systematic review combining clinical trials to evaluate 6092 patients.[29,30] CEA is recommended to prevent ipsilateral stroke in patients with symptomatic carotid artery stenosis of 70% or greater when the surgical risk is less than 6%. In patients with symptomatic stenosis of 50% to 69%, a moderate reduction in risk is seen in clinical trials. CEA is recommended when anesthesia risk is low based on patient factors including age, sex, and comorbidities, and surgical risk is less than 6%. CEA is not beneficial for symptomatic carotid stenosis less than 50% and should not be considered in these patients. Patients with asymptomatic carotid artery stenosis of 70% or more may benefit from CEA if surgical complication rates for stroke, MI, and death are low.[31]

Carotid Angioplasty Carotid angioplasty with stenting has evolved as a less invasive procedure with shorter recovery times for appropriate patients. Several trials have compared carotid angioplasty with stenting to CEA in symptomatic patients. Carotid angioplasty with stenting is an alternative to CEA in high-risk surgical candidates with greater than 50% stenosis by angiography and greater than 70% stenosis by noninvasive imaging when performed by skilled clinicians.[32] Age is an important factor when deciding between carotid angioplasty with stenting and CEA. Patients older than 70 years may have improved outcomes with CEA compared to carotid angioplasty with stenting. In patients younger than 70 years, CEA and carotid angioplasty with stenting have similar risks for stroke, MI, and death and also similar rates for ipsilateral stroke.[32]

▶ *Pharmacologic Therapy*

Aspirin In a meta-analysis including 144,051 patients with previous MI, acute MI, previous TIA or stroke, or acute stroke, as well as others at high risk, ASA was found to decrease the risk of recurrent stroke by approximately 25%.[33] ASA decreases risk of subsequent stroke by approximately 22% in both men and women with previous TIA or stroke.[33] Therefore, ASA is an option for initial therapy for secondary prevention of ischemic stroke. A wide range of doses have been used (50–1500 mg/day); however, the FDA has approved doses of 50 to 325 mg for secondary ischemic stroke prevention. Current guidelines recommend varying ASA doses including 75 to 100 mg daily and 50 to 325 mg daily.[18,32] Lower ASA doses are currently recommended to decrease the risk of bleeding complications. Adverse effects of ASA include gastrointestinal (GI) intolerance, GI bleeding, and hypersensitivity reactions.

Ticlopidine Ticlopidine was found to be slightly more beneficial in secondary stroke prevention than ASA in men and women in one study, while another trial found no benefit over aspirin therapy.[32] Due to the adverse effect profile and costly laboratory monitoring required, ticlopidine is typically avoided clinically.

Clopidogrel Clopidogrel is slightly more effective than ASA and similar in efficacy to the combination of extended-release (ER) dipyridamole plus aspirin.[34,35] The usual dose is 75 mg orally taken once daily. Clopidogrel has a lower incidence of diarrhea and neutropenia than ticlopidine, and laboratory monitoring is not required. There have been 11 case reports of thrombotic thrombocytopenic purpura (TTP) occurring secondary to clopidogrel. Most occurred within the first 2 weeks of therapy; therefore, clinicians need to be aware of the potential for the development of TTP with clopidogrel. Proton pump inhibitors may decrease the effectiveness of clopidogrel. An H_2-blocker may be preferred in patients who require both acid suppression and clopidogrel.[36] Patients with a genetic variant of CYP2C19 classified as poor metabolizers may have a decrease in the active metabolite of clopidogrel.[37] Clopidogrel may be used as monotherapy for secondary stroke prevention. It is an option for initial therapy for secondary prevention of ischemic stroke and is considered first-line therapy in patients who also have peripheral arterial disease or are allergic to aspirin.

Extended-Release Dipyridamole Plus Aspirin Combination therapy with ER dipyridamole plus ASA has been found to be more effective in preventing stroke than either agent alone.[38,39] Headache and diarrhea were common adverse effects of dipyridamole; bleeding was more common in all treatment groups that included ASA. A trial comparing the combination of ER dipyridamole plus ASA to clopidogrel found no difference in outcomes; however, adverse events occurred more frequently in the combination of ER dipyridamole plus ASA group.[35] The currently available formulation is a combination product containing 25 mg ASA and 200 mg ER dipyridamole. This combination is an option for initial therapy for secondary stroke prevention, but is not appropriate for patients who are intolerant to ASA.

Current Clinical Trials Recent trials have been completed to evaluate other combinations of antiplatelet agents and to compare them against one another. Low-dose ASA plus clopidogrel combination therapy did not show a significant benefit in reducing recurrent stroke compared with clopidogrel alone in one large trial.[40] This trial found the addition of ASA to clopidogrel increased the risk of major bleeding. Another large trial compared the combination of clopidogrel plus low-dose ASA to low-dose ASA alone in patients with cardiovascular disease or multiple risk factors.[41] The combination did not show a benefit over monotherapy in prevention of cardiovascular events. An increased bleeding risk was observed in the stroke subgroup. Two trials have evaluated the use of the combination of aspirin and clopidogrel in the months following a TIA or minor stroke.[42,43] One trial demonstrated a trend toward a reduction in ischemic events; however, the trial was stopped early due to low enrollment. The second trial demonstrated a benefit to combination therapy compared to aspirin alone. Based on this trial, the combination of ASA and clopidogrel may be considered within 24 hours of a TIA or minor stroke and continued for 90 days. Continuation beyond 90 days is not recommended due to an increased risk of hemorrhage.

Antiplatelet Therapy Summary KEY CONCEPT *Current stroke treatment guidelines recommend ASA or combination therapy with ER dipyridamole plus ASA as initial antiplatelet therapy for the secondary prevention of stroke. Clopidogrel is another option for initial treatment and is recommended in patients unable to tolerate ASA.*[18,32] KEY CONCEPT *Initial choice of agent should be individualized based on patient factors and cost.* Therapeutic failure in this patient population is challenging because no data are available to guide a treatment decision. When a patient is on therapeutic doses of ASA, yet experiences a recurrent TIA or stroke, switching to either clopidogrel or the combination of ER dipyridamole and ASA is a reasonable option. If failure occurs on either clopidogrel or the combination of ASA and ER dipyridamole, switching to the alternate drug may be appropriate.

Oral Anticoagulants Recent clinical trials have not found oral anticoagulation to be better than antiplatelet therapy in those patients without AF or carotid stenosis. In patients without AF, antiplatelet therapy is recommended over oral anticoagulants. Patients with AF and a previous TIA or stroke have the highest risk of recurrent stroke. Long-term anticoagulation with warfarin or other newer agents is effective and therefore recommended in the primary and secondary prevention of cardioembolic stroke.[18,32] The newer oral anticoagulants have been studied for stroke prevention in nonvalvular AF. The goal international normalized ratio (INR) when monitoring warfarin for this indication is 2 to 3.

▸ ***Blood Pressure Management***

Hypertension is a major risk factor for stroke, and BP control is an important strategy for secondary stroke prevention. A recent meta-analysis evaluating antihypertensive trials documented that BP control reduced the risk of recurrent TIA or stroke.[44] Current stroke guidelines recommend initiation of antihypertensive treatment for untreated patients with TIA or stroke and an established BP of greater than 140/90 mm Hg. Patients previously treated with antihypertensives should be reinitiated on therapy several days after acute ischemic stroke. The optimal regimen to achieve the BP goal has not been established. Diuretics, either alone or in combination with an ACE-I, have been shown to be beneficial.[32]

Patient Encounter Part 3

The patient's BP responds to the antihypertensive agent within 40 minutes and his current BP is 178/100 mm Hg. He is still experiencing weakness in the left arm and leg and difficulty speaking at times. The neurologist decides to administer IV alteplase because it is now almost 4 hours after the onset of symptoms, and the patient is being managed in the stroke unit.

What recommendations would you make regarding the administration of IV alteplase in this patient?

What treatments would you recommend at this time to reduce risk of another stroke?

▸ ***Other Recommendations***

Management of diabetes and lipids based on treatment guidelines, cessation of smoking, increased physical activity, and reducing alcohol use in heavy drinkers are additional recommendations for management of patients with previous stroke or TIA.[32] Statin therapy is recommended in patients with previous stroke or TIA, regardless of history of coronary heart disease.

Table 11–5 provides drug and dosing recommendations for treatment of ischemic stroke.

TREATMENT OF ACUTE HEMORRHAGIC STROKE

Supportive Measures

Acute hemorrhagic stroke is considered to be a medical emergency due to intracerebral hemorrhage (ICH), subarachnoid hemorrhage (SAH), or subdural hematoma. Initially, patients experiencing a hemorrhagic stroke should be transported to a neurointensive care unit. KEY CONCEPT *There is no proven treatment for ICH. Management is based on neurointensive care treatment and prevention of complications.* Treatment should be provided to manage the needs of the critically ill patient including management of increased ICP, seizures, infections, and prevention of rebleeding and delayed cerebral ischemia. In those with severely depressed consciousness, rapid endotracheal intubation and mechanical ventilation may be necessary. BP is often elevated after hemorrhagic stroke; appropriate management is important to prevent rebleeding and expansion of the hematoma. Two trials in ICH patients have been completed evaluating early intensive BP management. Treatment guidelines have been updated to suggest that in patients with a systolic BP between 150 and 220 mm Hg, lowering the systolic BP to 140 mm Hg is a reasonable approach.[45] BP can be controlled with IV boluses of labetalol 10 to 80 mg every 10 minutes up to a maximum of 300 mg or with IV infusions of labetalol (0.5–2 mg/min) or nicardipine (5–15 mg/hour). Deep vein thrombosis prophylaxis with intermittent compression stockings should be implemented early after admission. In those patients with SAH, once the aneurysm has been treated, heparin may be instituted. In ICH patients with lack of mobility after 1 to 4 days, heparin or LMWH may be started.[8,45]

Nonpharmacologic Therapy

Patients with hemorrhagic stroke are evaluated for surgical treatment of SAH and ICH. In SAH, either clipping of the aneurysm or coil embolization is recommended within 72 hours after the initial event to prevent rebleeding. Coil embolization, also called

Table 11–5

Recommendations for Pharmacotherapy of Ischemic Stroke

	Primary Agents	Alternatives
Acute treatment	Alteplase 0.9 mg/kg IV (maximum dose 90 mg); 10% as IV bolus, remainder infused over 1 hour in selected patients within 3 hours of onset	Alteplase 0.9 mg/kg IV (maximum dose 90 mg); 10% as IV bolus, remainder infused over 1 hour in selected patients between 3 and 4.5 hours of onset
	ASA 160–325 mg started within 48 hours of onset; hold for 24 hours if alteplase given (may reduce dose to 50–100 mg daily after 48 hours)	Alteplase (various doses) intraarterially up to 6 hours after onset in selected patients
Secondary prevention	ASA 50–325 mg daily	Ticlopidine 250 mg twice daily
	ASA 25 mg + ER dipyridamole 200 mg twice daily	Clopidogrel 75 mg daily
Cardioembolic	Warfarin (INR 2–3)	Rivaroxaban 20 mg daily with the evening meal; decrease to 15 mg daily with the evening meal if creatinine clearance 15–50 mL/min (0.25–0.83 mL/s)
	Dabigatran 150 mg twice daily; decrease to 75 mg twice daily if creatinine clearance is 15–30 mL/min (0.25–0.50 mL/s)	
	Apixaban 5 mg twice daily; decrease to 2.5 mg twice daily if patient has two of the following: age ≥ 80, weight ≤ 60 kg or serum creatinine ≥ 1.5 mg/dL (133 μmol/L)	
All patients	BP control	
	Statin therapy	

ASA, aspirin; BP, blood pressure; ER, extended-release; INR, international normalized ratio; IV, intravenous.

coiling, is a minimally invasive procedure in which a platinum coil is threaded into the aneurysm. The flexible coil fills up the space to block blood flow into the aneurysm thereby preventing rebleeding. Surgical removal of the hematoma in patients with ICH is controversial because trials have not consistently shown improved outcomes. Minimally invasive clot removal techniques with or without fibrinolytic therapy aspiration have been evaluated; however, these procedures are considered investigational because outcomes are not certain. Current guidelines note that surgical treatment of ICH is uncertain and is not recommended except in specific patient situations.[45]

Pharmacologic Therapy

▶ *Calcium Antagonists*

Oral nimodipine is recommended in SAH to prevent delayed cerebral ischemia. It is recommended to begin oral nimodipine promptly after the initial event, but no later than 96 hours following SAH. Delayed cerebral ischemia occurs 4 to 14 days after the initial aneurysm rupture and is a common cause of neurological deficits and death. A meta-analysis of 12 studies was conducted and concluded that oral nimodipine 60 mg every 4 hours for 21 days following aneurysmal SAH reduced the risk of a poor outcome and delayed cerebral ischemia.[46]

▶ *Hemostatic Therapy*

Recombinant factor VIIa has been shown to have a benefit in the treatment of ICH. In one clinical trial, hematoma growth was decreased at 24 hours, mortality was decreased at 90 days, and overall functioning was increased at 90 days in the treatment group. However, an increased incidence of thromboembolic events was seen in the treatment group.[47] A phase 3 trial showed that recombinant factor VIIa decreased growth of the hematoma, but did not improve survival or functional outcome. Intraventricular hemorrhage was more likely in the higher dose treatment group.[48] Current guidelines do not recommend treatment with recombinant factor VIIa due to an uncertain benefit and increased risk of thromboembolic events. Further trials are warranted to determine specific patients who may benefit from therapy.[45]

OUTCOME EVALUATION

- Stroke outcomes are measured based on neurological status and functioning of the patient after the acute event. The NIHSS is a measure of daily functioning used to assess patient status following a stroke.
- Early rehabilitation can reduce functional impairment after a stroke. Recent stroke rehabilitation guidelines have been endorsed by the American Heart Association and American Stroke Association. These guidelines recommend that patients receive care in a multidisciplinary setting or stroke unit, receive early assessment using the NIHSS, and that rehabilitation is started as soon as possible after the stroke. Other recommendations include screening for **dysphagia** and aggressive secondary stroke prevention treatments.[49]
- Table 11–6 provides monitoring guidelines for the acute stroke patient.

Table 11–6

Monitoring the Stroke Patient

Treatment	Parameter(s)	Monitoring Frequency	Comments
Ischemic Stroke			
Alteplase	CT scan	Before and 24 hours after alteplase infusion	
	BP	Every 15 minutes × 2 hours, every 30 min × 6 hours, every 1 hour × 16 hours; then every shift	
	Neurologic function	Neurological exam every 15 minutes × 2 hours, every 30 min × 6 hours, every 1 hour × 16 hours; NIHSS 24 hours after alteplase infusion and at discharge	
	Bleeding	Clinical signs of bleeding every 2 hours × 24 hours	
ASA	Bleeding Hb/Hct, platelets[a]	Daily	
Clopidogrel	Bleeding Hb/Hct, platelets[a]	Daily	
ASA/ER dipyridamole	Headache, bleeding Hb/Hct, platelets[a]	Daily	
Warfarin	Bleeding, INR, Hb/Hct[a]	INR daily × 3 days; weekly until stable; then monthly	
New Oral Anticoagulants	Bleeding	Each visit	
	Hb/Hct, renal and liver function	Yearly; if decreased renal function every 3–6 months	
Hemorrhagic Stroke			
	BP, neurologic function, ICP	Every 2 hours in ICU	May require treatments to lower BP to < 180 mm Hg systolic
Nimodipine for SAH	BP, neurologic function, fluid status	Every 2 hours in ICU	

ASA, aspirin; BP, blood pressure; CT, computed tomography; ER, extended-release; Hb, hemoglobin; Hct, hematocrit; ICP, intracranial pressure; ICU, intensive care unit; INR, international normalized ratio; NIHSS, National Institutes of Health Stroke Scale; SAH, subarachnoid hemorrhage.

[a]Hb/Hct and platelets should be monitored at baseline and every 6 months for ASA, clopidogrel, ASA/ER dipyridamole, and warfarin treatment.

Patient Care Process for Stroke

Patient Assessment:

- Determine if patient is experiencing an acute ischemic or hemorrhagic stroke.
- Assess signs and symptoms including time of symptom onset and time of arrival in the emergency department.
- Perform a thorough neurological and physical examination evaluating for potential causes of stroke.
- Perform a comprehensive medication history.
- Perform a CT or MRI scan to rule out hemorrhagic stroke prior to administering any fibrinolytic treatment if indicated.

Therapy Evaluation:

- Evaluate inclusion and exclusion criteria for fibrinolytic therapy to determine appropriateness.
- Transfer the patient to a stroke center if available and develop a plan for acute management.
- Determine the patient's risk factors for stroke.

Care Plan Development:

- If fibrinolytic therapy is indicated, initiate treatment protocol for alteplase administration and follow recommended monitoring plan.
- Develop a plan for long-term management of risk factors to prevent a recurrent stroke.

Follow-Up Evaluation:

- Educate the patient on:
  - Appropriate lifestyle modifications that will reduce stroke risk.
  - Medication regimen, stressing the importance of adherence.

Abbreviations Introduced in This Chapter

ACE-I	Angiotensin-converting enzyme inhibitor
ADP	Adenosine diphosphate
AF	Atrial fibrillation
ARB	Angiotensin receptor blocker
ASA	Aspirin
AVM	Arteriovenous malformation
BP	Blood pressure
CAD	Coronary artery disease
CCB	Calcium channel blocker
CEA	Carotid endarterectomy
CNS	Central nervous system
CT	Computed tomography
DBP	Diastolic blood pressure
ECG	Electrocardiogram
ER	Extended release
FDA	Food and Drug Administration
GI	Gastrointestinal
IA	Intraarterial
ICH	Intracerebral hemorrhage
ICP	Intracranial pressure
INR	International normalized ratio
IV	Intravenous
LMWH	Low molecular weight heparin
MI	Myocardial infarction
MRI	Magnetic resonance imaging
NIHSS	National Institutes of Health Stroke Scale
NINDS	National Institute of Neurological Disorders and Stroke
rt-PA	Alteplase
r-pro UK	Pro-urokinase
SAH	Subarachnoid hemorrhage
SBP	Systolic blood pressure
TIA	Transient ischemic attack
TTP	Thrombotic thrombocytopenic purpura
UFH	Unfractionated heparin
VTE	Venous thromboembolism

REFERENCES

1. Lackland DT, Roccella EJ, Deutsch, et al; on behalf of the American Heart Association Stroke Council, Council on Cardiovascular and Stroke Nursing, Council on Quality of Care and Outcomes Research, and Council on Functional Genomics and Translational Biology. Factors influencing the decline in stroke mortality: a statement from the American Heart Association/American Stroke Association. Stroke. 2014;45:315–353.
2. Go AS, Mozaffarian D, Roger VL, et al; on behalf of the American Heart Association Statistics Committee and Stroke Statistics Subcommittee. Heart disease and stroke statistics – 2014 update: a report from the American Heart Association. Circulation. 2014;129:e28–e292.
3. Goldstein LB, Bushnell CD, Adam R, et al; on behalf of the American Heart Association Stroke Council, Council on Cardiovascular Nursing, Council on Epidemiology and Prevention, Council for High Blood Pressure Research, Council on Peripheral Vascular Disease, and Interdisciplinary Council on Quality of Care and Outcomes Research. Guidelines for the primary prevention of stroke: A guideline for healthcare professionals from the American Heart Association/American Stroke Association. Stroke. 2011;42:517–584.
4. Grysiewicz RA, Thomas D, Pandey DK. Epidemiology of ischemic and hemorrhagic stroke: Incidence, prevalence, mortality and risk factors. Neurol Clin. 2008;26:871–895.
5. Easton JD, Saver JL, Albers GW, et al. Definition and evaluation of transient ischemic attack: A scientific statement for healthcare professionals from the American Heart Association/American Stroke Association Stroke Council; Council on Cardiovascular Surgery and Anesthesia; Council on Cardiovascular Radiology and Intervention; Council on Cardiovascular Nursing; and the Interdisciplinary Council on Peripheral Vascular Disease. Stroke. 2009;40:2276–2293.
6. Rothwell PM, Warlow CP. Timing of TIAs preceding stroke: Time window for prevention is very short. Neurology. 2005;64:817–820.
7. Sacco RL, Kasner SE, Broderick JP, et al; on behalf of the American Heart Association Stroke Council, Council on Cardiovascular Surgery and Anesthesia, Council on Cardiovascular Radiology and Intervention, Council on Cardiovascular and Stroke Nursing, Council on Epidemiology and Prevention, Council on Peripheral Vascular Disease, and Council on Nutrition, Physical Activity and Metabolism. An updated definition of stroke for the 21st century: A statement for healthcare professionals from the American Heart Association/American Stroke Association. Stroke. 2013;44:2064–2089.
8. Connelly ES, Rabinstein AA, Carhuapoma JR; on behalf of the American Heart Association Stroke Council, Council on Cardiovascular Radiology and Intervention, Council on Cardiovascular Nursing, Council on Cardiovascular Surgery and Anesthesia, and Council on Clinical Cardiology. Guidelines for the management of aneurysmal subarachnoid hemorrhage: a guideline for healthcare professionals from the American Heart Association/American Stroke Association. Stroke. 2012;43:1711–1737.
9. Testai FD, Aiyagari V. Acute hemorrhagic stroke pathophysiology and medical interventions: blood pressure control, management of anticoagulant-associated brain hemorrhage and general management principles. Neurol Clin. 2008;26:963–985.
10. Ariesen MJ, Claus SP, Rinkel GJE, Algra A. Risk factors for intracerebral hemorrhage in the general population: A systematic review. Stroke. 2003;34:2060–2065.
11. Lazzaro MA, Krishnan K, Prabhakaran S. Detection of atrial fibrillation with concurrent Holter monitoring and continuous cardiac telemetry following ischemic stroke and transient ischemic attack. J Stroke Cerebrovasc Dis. 2012;21:89–93.
12. Jauch EC, Cucchiara B, Adeoye O, et al. Part 11: adult stroke: 2010 American Heart Association guidelines for cardiopulmonary resuscitation and emergency cardiovascular Care [published correction appears in Circulation. 2011;124:e404]. Circulation. 2010;122(suppl 3):S818–S828.
13. Jauch EC, Saver JL, Adams HP, et al; on behalf of the American Heart Association Stroke Council, Council on Cardiovascular Nursing, Council on Peripheral Vascular Disease, and Council on Clinical Cardiology. Guidelines for the early management of adults with ischemic stroke: a guideline from the American Heart Association/American Stroke Association. Stroke. 2013;44:870–914.
14. Baker L, Juneja R, Bruno A. Management of hyperglycemia in acute ischemic stroke. Curr Treat Options Neurol. 2011;13:616–628.
15. Kallmunzer B, Kollmar R. Temperature management in stroke—an unsolved, but important topic. Cerebrovasc Dis. 2011;31:532–543.
16. Barbetta I, Carmo M, Mercandalli G. Outcomes of urgent carotid endarterectomy for stable and unstable acute neurologic deficits. J Vasc Surg. 2014;59(2):440–446.
17. National Institute of Neurological Disorders and Stroke rt-PA Stroke Study Group. Tissue plasminogen activator for acute ischemic stroke. N Engl J Med. 1995;333:1581–1587.
18. Lansberg MG, O'Donnell MJ, Khatri P, et al. Antithrombotic and thrombolytic therapy for ischemic stroke. Antithrombotic therapy and prevention of thrombosis: American College of Chest Physicians evidence-based clinical practice guildelines. 9th ed. Chest. 2012;141(2 supp):e601S–e636S.

19. del Zoppo GJ, Saver JL, Jauch ED, Adams HP, Jr. Expansion of the time window for treatment of acute ischemic stroke with intravenous tissue plasminogen activator: a science advisory from the American Heart Association/American Stroke Association. Stroke. 2009;40:2945–2948.
20. Rajajee V, Kidwell C, Starkman S, et al. Early MRI and outcomes of untreated patients with mild or improving ischemic stroke. Neurology. 2006;67:980–984.
21. Barreto AD. Intravenous thrombolytics for ischemic stroke. Neurotherapeutics. 2011;8:388–399.
22. del Zoppo GJ, Higashida RT, Furlan AJ, et al. PROACT: A phase II randomized trial of recombinant pro-urokinase by direct arterial delivery in acute middle cerebral artery stroke. Stroke. 1998;29:4–11.
23. Furlan A, Higashida R, Wechsler L, et al. Intra-arterial prourokinase for acute ischemic stroke. The PROACT II study: A randomized controlled trial. Prolyse in acute cerebral thromboembolism. JAMA. 1999;282:2003–2011.
24. Lee M, Hong KS, Saver JL. Efficacy of intra-arterial fibrinolysis for acute ischemic stroke: Meta-analysis of randomized controlled trials. Stroke. 2010;41:932–937.
25. Sandercock PA, Counsell C, Kamal AK. Anticoagulants for acute ischaemic stroke. Cochrane Database Syst Rev. 2008;8(4):CD000024.
26. Sandercock PA, Counsell C, Tseng MC. Low-molecular-weight heparins or heparinoids versus standard unfractionated heparin for acute ischaemic stroke. Cochrane Database Syst Rev. 2008;16(3):CD000119.
27. James PA, Oparil S, Carter BL, et al. 2014 evidence-based guideline for the management of high blood pressure in adults: report from the panel members appointed to the eighth Joint National Committee (JNC 8). JAMA. 2014;311(5):507–520.
28. Neal B, MacMahon S, Chapman N; Blood Pressure Lowering Treatment Trialists' Collaboration. Effects of ACE inhibitors, calcium antagonists, and other blood-pressure-lowering drugs: Results of prospectively designed overviews of randomized trials. Blood Pressure Lowering Treatment Trialists' Collaboration. Lancet. 2000;356:1955–1964.
29. Rothwell PM, Eliasziw M, Fox AJ, et al; for the Carotid Endarterectomy Trialists' Collaboration. Analysis of pooled data from the randomised controlled trials of endarterectomy for symptomatic carotid stenosis. Lancet. 2003;361:107–116.
30. Rerkasem K, Rothwell PM. Carotid endarterectomy for symptomatic carotid stenosis. Cochrane Database Syst Rev. 2011;4:CD001081.
31. Brott TG, Halperin JL, Abbara S, et al; American College of Cardiology; American Stroke Association; American Association of Neurological Surgeons; American College of Radiology; American College of Radiology; Society of NeuroInterventional Surgery; Society for Vascular Medicine; Society for Vascular Surgery. 2011 ASA/ACCF/AHA/AANN/AANS/ACR/ASNR/CNS/SAIP/SCAI/SIR/SNIS/SVM/SVS guideline on the management of patients with extracranial carotid and vertebral artery disease: a report of the American College of Cardiology Foundation/American Heart Association Task Force on Practice Guidelines, and the American Stroke Association, American Association of Neuroscience Nurses, American Association of Neurological Surgeons, American College of Radiology, American Society of Neuroradiology, Congress of Neurological Surgeons, Society of Atherosclerosis Imaging and Prevention, Society for Cardiovascular Angiography and Interventions, Society of Interventional Radiology, Society of NeuroInterventional Surgery, Society for Vascular Medicine, and Society for Vascular Surgery. Circulation. 2011;124(4): e54–e130.
32. Kernan WN, Ovbiagele B, Black HR, et al; on behalf of the American Heart Association Stroke Council, Council on Cardiovascular and Stroke Nursing, Council on Clinical Cardiology, and Council on Peripheral Vascular Disease. Guidelines for the prevention of stroke in patients with stroke or transient ischemic attack: a guideline for healthcare professionals from the American Heart Association/American Stroke Association. Stroke. 2014;45:2160–2236.
33. Collaborative meta-analysis of randomised trials of antiplatelet therapy for prevention of death, myocardial infarction, and stroke in high risk patients. BMJ. 2002;324:71–86.
34. CAPRIE Steering Committee. A randomized, blinded, trial of clopidogrel versus aspirin in patients at risk of ischaemic events. Lancet. 1996;348:1329–1339.
35. Sacco RL, Deiner HC, Yusuf S, et al; PRoFESS Study Group. Aspirin and extended-release dipyridamole versus clopidogrel for recurrent stroke. N Engl J Med. 2008;359:1238–1251.
36. Ho PM, Maddox TM, Wang L, et al. Risk of adverse outcomes associated with concomitant use of clopidogrel and proton pump inhibitors following acute coronary syndrome. JAMA. 2009; 301(9):937–944.
37. Mega JL, Close SL, Wiviott SD, et al. Cytochrome P-450 polymorphisms and response to clopidogrel. N Engl J Med. 2009;360:354–362.
38. Diener HC, Cunha L, Forbes C, et al. European Stroke Prevention Study 2. Dipyridamole and acetylsalicylic acid in the secondary prevention of stroke. J Neurol Sci. 1996;143:1–13.
39. The ESPRIT Study Group. Aspirin plus dipyridamole versus aspirin alone after cerebral ischaemia of arterial origin (ESPRIT): randomized controlled trial. Lancet. 2006;367:1665–1673.
40. Deiner HC, Bogousslavsky J, Brass LM, et al; for the MATCH Investigators. Aspirin and clopidogrel compared with clopidogrel alone after recent ischaemic stroke or transient ischaemic attack in high-risk patients (MATCH): randomised, double-blind, placebo-controlled trial. Lancet. 2004;364:331–337.
41. Bhatt DL, Fox KA, Hacke W, et al; CHARISMA Investigators. Clopidogrel and aspirin versus aspirin alone for the prevention of atherothrombotic events. N Engl J Med. 2006;354(16):1706–1717.
42. Kennedy J, Hill MD, Ryckborst KJ, et al; FASTER Investigators. Fast assessment of stroke and transient ischaemic attack to prevent early recurrence (FASTER): a randomized controlled pilot trial. Lancet Neurol. 2007;6(11):961–969.
43. Wang Y, Zhao X, Liu L, et al; CHANCE Investigators. Clopidogrel with aspirin in acute minor stroke or transient ischemic attack. N Engl J Med. 2013;369:11–19.
44. Liu L, Wang Z, Gong L, et al. Blood pressure reduction for the secondary prevention of stroke: a Chinese trial and a systematic review of the literature. Hypertens Res. 2009;32:1032–1040.
45. Morgenstern LB, Hemphill JC 3rd, Anderson C, et al; on behalf of the American Heart Association Stroke Council and Council on Cardiovascular Nursing. Guidelines for the management of spontaneous intracerebral hemorrhage: A guideline for healthcare professionals from the American Heart Association/American Stroke Association. Stroke. 2010;41:1–22.
46. Dorhout Mees SM, Rinkel GJ, Feigin VL, et al. Calcium antagonists for aneurysmal subarachnoid haemorrhage. Cochrane Database Syst Rev. 2007;3:CD000277.
47. Mayer SA, Brun NC, Begtrup K, et al, for the Recombinant Activated Factor VII Intracerebral Hemorrhage Trial Investigators. Recombinant activated factor VII for acute intracerebral hemorrhage. N Engl J Med. 2005;352:777–785.
48. Mayer SA, Brun NC, Begtrup K, et al; FAST Trial Investigators. Efficacy and safety of recombinant activated factor VII for acute intracerebral hemorrhage. N Engl J Med. 2008;358:2127–2137.
49. Miller EL, Murray L, Richards L, et al; on behalf of the American Heart Association Council on Cardiovascular Nursing and Stroke Council. Comprehensive overview of nursing and interdisciplinary rehabilitation care of the stroke patient: A scientific statement from the American Heart Association. Stroke. 2010;41:2402–2448.

12 Dyslipidemias

Matthew K. Ito

LEARNING OBJECTIVES

Upon completion of the chapter, the reader will be able to:

1. Identify the common types of lipid disorders.
2. Identify the statin-benefit groups and intensity of statin therapy according to the American College of Cardiology/American Heart Association.
3. Recommend appropriate therapeutic lifestyle changes (TLC) and pharmacotherapy interventions for dyslipidemia.
4. Determine a patient's atherosclerotic cardiovascular disease risk and corresponding treatment goals according to the National Lipid Association.
5. Identify diagnostic criteria and treatment strategies for metabolic syndrome.
6. Describe components of a monitoring plan to assess effectiveness and adverse effects of pharmacotherapy for dyslipidemias.
7. Educate patients about the disease state, appropriate TLC, and drug therapy required for effective treatment.

INTRODUCTION

Coronary heart disease (CHD) is the leading cause of death in adults in the United States and most industrialized nations. It is also the chief cause of premature, permanent disability in the US workforce. KEY CONCEPT *Hypercholesterolemia and other abnormalities in serum lipids play a major role in atherosclerosis and plaque formation leading to CHD as well as other forms of atherosclerotic cardiovascular disease (ASCVD), such as carotid and peripheral artery disease.*[1]

EPIDEMIOLOGY AND ETIOLOGY

Annually, approximately 515,000 Americans experience a new heart attack and 205,000 will have a recurrent event.[2] Lowering cholesterol reduces atherosclerotic progression and mortality from CHD and stroke. The development of CHD is a lifelong process. Except in rare cases of severely elevated serum cholesterol levels, years of poor dietary habits, sedentary lifestyle, and life-habit risk factors (eg, smoking and obesity) contribute to the development of atherosclerosis.[3]

PATHOPHYSIOLOGY

Cholesterol and Lipoprotein Metabolism

Cholesterol, an essential substance manufactured by most cells in the body, is used to maintain cell wall integrity and for the biosynthesis of **bile acids** and steroid hormones. Cholesterol, triglycerides and phospholipids circulate in the blood as lipoproteins (**Figure 12–1**). The major lipoproteins are chylomicrons, very low-density lipoprotein (VLDL), intermediate-density lipoprotein (IDL), low-density lipoprotein (LDL), and high-density lipoprotein (HDL). A measured total cholesterol is the total cholesterol molecules in all these major lipoproteins. The estimated value of LDL cholesterol is found using the following equation (after fasting for 9 to 12 hours):

LDL cholesterol (mg/dL) = total cholesterol – (HDL cholesterol + triglycerides/5), when lipids are expressed in units of mg/dL;

or

LDL cholesterol (mmol/L)= total cholesterol – (HDL cholesterol + triglycerides/2.2), when lipids are expressed in units of mmol/L

Where triglycerides/5 or triglycerides/2.2 estimate VLDL cholesterol in units of mg/dL or mmol/L, respectively.

This formula becomes inaccurate if serum triglycerides are greater than 400 mg/dL (4.52 mmol/L), if chylomicrons are present, or the patient has type III hyperlipoproteinemia. In each of these cases, LDL cholesterol must be directly measured.[3] Non-HDL cholesterol is carried by all atherogenic apolipoprotein B-containing lipoproteins including VLDL, IDL, and LDL. It is calculated as:

Non-HDL cholesterol = total cholesterol – HDL cholesterol

Non-HDL cholesterol can be determined in a nonfasting state.

Each lipoprotein has various proteins called apolipoproteins (Apos) embedded on the surface (Figure 12–1) that serve four main purposes: (a) required for assembly and secretion of lipoproteins; (b) serve as major structural components of lipoproteins; (c) act as ligands for binding to receptors on cell surfaces; and (d) can be cofactors for inhibition of enzymes involved in the breakdown of triglycerides from chylomicrons and VLDL.[4]

Cholesterol from the diet as well as from bile enters the small intestine and is emulsified by bile salts into **micelles** (**Figure 12–2**). These micelles interact with the **duodenal**

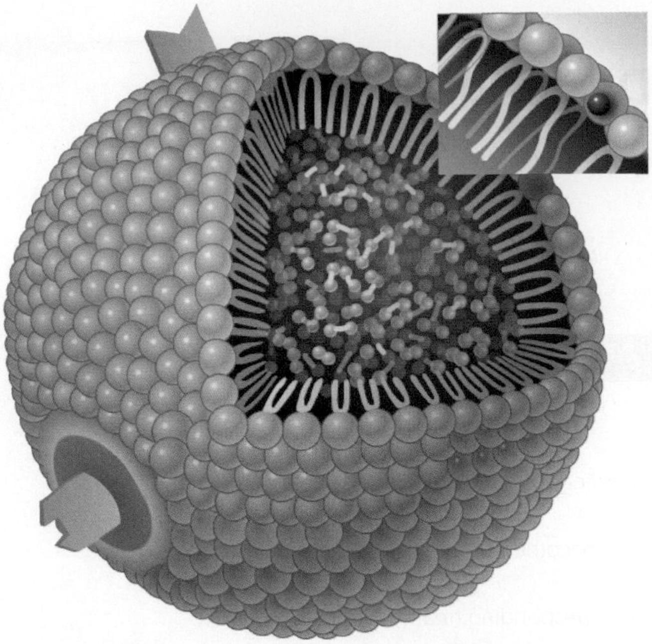

FIGURE 12–1. Lipoprotein structure. Lipoproteins are a diverse group of particles with varying size and density. They contain variable amounts of core cholesterol esters and triglycerides, and have varying numbers and types of surface apolipoproteins. The apolipoproteins function to direct the processing and removal of individual lipoprotein particles.

enterocyte and jejunal enterocyte surfaces, and cholesterol is transported from the micelles into these cells by the Niemann-Pick C1 Like 1 (NPC1L1) transporter. Cholesterol within enterocytes is esterified and packaged into chylomicrons along with triglycerides, phospholipids, and apolipoproteins, which are then released into the lymphatic circulation. In the lymph and blood, chylomicrons are converted to chylomicron remnants. During this process, chylomicrons also interact with HDL particles (Figure 12–3) and exchange triglyceride and cholesterol content (facilitated by cholesterol ester transfer protein, or CETP), and HDL particles acquire Apos A and C. Chylomicron remnant particles are then taken up by LDL-related protein (LRP).

In the liver, cholesterol and triglycerides are incorporated into VLDL along with phospholipids and Apo B-100 (Figure 12–4). VLDL loses its triglyceride content through interaction with lipoprotein lipase (LPL) to form VLDL remnant and IDL. IDL can be cleared from the circulation by hepatic LDL receptors or further converted to LDL (by further depletion of triglycerides) through the action of hepatic lipases (HLs). Approximately 50% of IDL is converted to LDL. LDL particles are cleared from the circulation primarily by hepatic LDL receptors by interaction with Apo B-100. They can also be taken up by extrahepatic tissues or enter the arterial wall, contributing to atherogenesis.

Cholesterol is transported from the arterial wall or other extrahepatic tissues back to the liver by HDL (Figure 12–3). Triglyceride-rich HDL is hydrolyzed by HL, generating fatty acids and nascent HDL particles, or mature HDL can bind to scavenger receptors (SR-BI) on hepatocytes and transfer their cholesterol ester content for excretion in the bile.

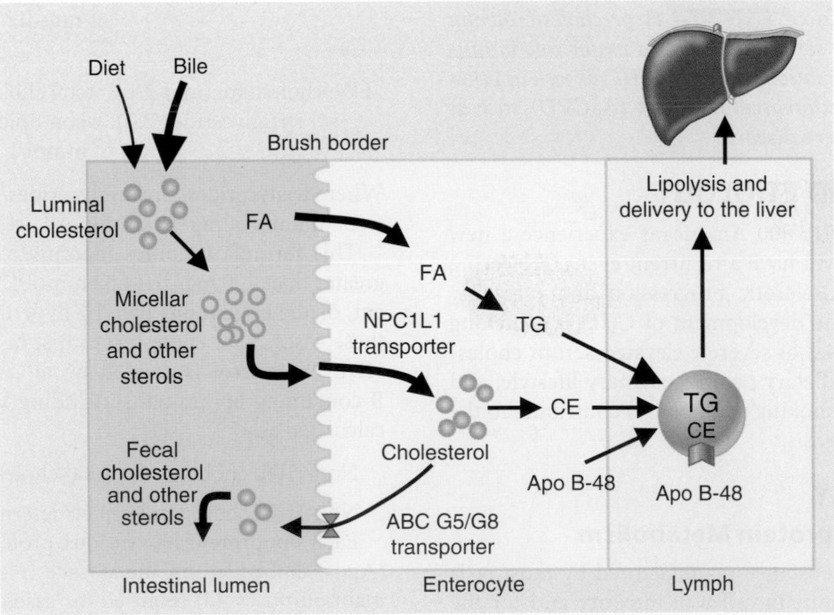

FIGURE 12–2. Intestinal cholesterol absorption and transport. Cholesterol from food and bile enter the gut lumen and are emulsified by bile acids into micelles. Micelles bind to the intestinal enterocytes, and cholesterol and other sterols are transported from the micelles into the enterocytes by a sterol transporter. Triglycerides synthesized by absorbed fatty acids, along with cholesterol and apolipoprotein B-48, are incorporated into chylomicrons. Chylomicrons are released into the lymphatic circulation and converted to chylomicron remnants (through loss of triglyceride), and then taken up by the hepatic LDL receptor-related protein (LRP). (ABC G5/G8, ATP-binding cassette G5/G8; Apo, apolipoprotein; CE, cholesterol ester; FA, fatty acid; LDL, low-density lipoprotein; NPC1L1, Niemann-Pick C1 Like 1; TG, triglyceride.)

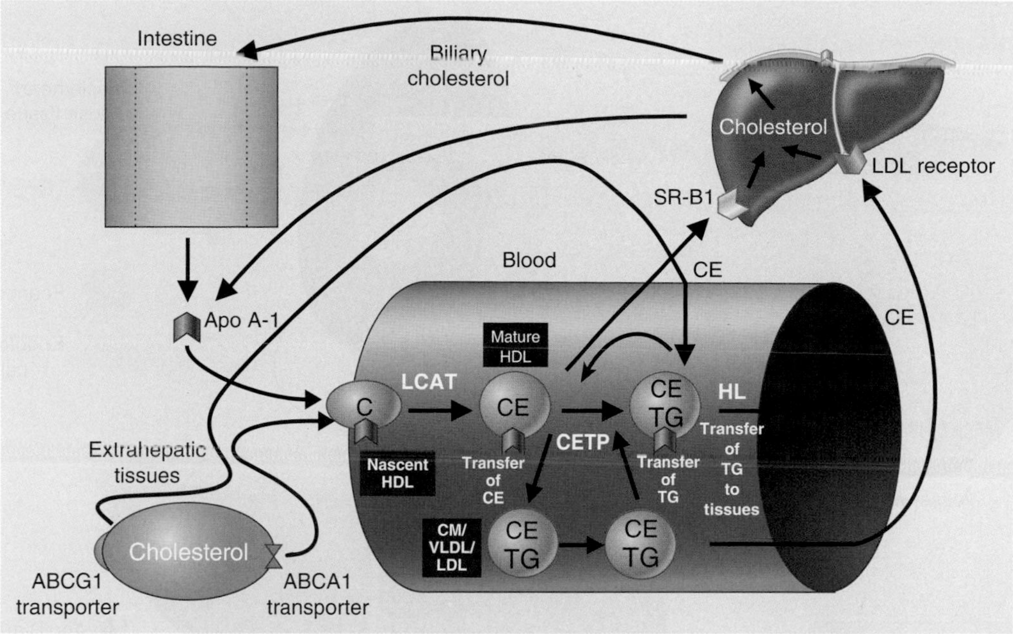

FIGURE 12–3. Reverse cholesterol transport. Cholesterol is transported from the arterial wall or other extrahepatic tissues back to the liver by HDL. Esterified cholesterol from HDL can be transferred to apolipoprotein B–containing particles in exchange for triglycerides. Cholesterol esters transferred from HDL to VLDL and LDL are taken up by hepatic LDL receptors or delivered back to extrahepatic tissue. (ABCA1, ATP-binding cassette A1; ABCG1, ATP-binding cassette G1; Apo, apolipoprotein; C, cholesterol; CE, cholesterol ester; CETP, cholesterol ester transfer protein; CM, chylomicrons; HDL, high-density lipoprotein; HL, hepatic lipase; LCAT, lecithin-cholesterol acyltransferase; LDL, low-density lipoprotein; SR-B1, scavenger receptors; TG, triglyceride; VLDL, very low-density lipoprotein.)

A variety of genetic mutations can occur during lipoprotein synthesis and metabolism that cause lipid disorders. The major genetic disorders and their effect on serum lipids are presented in Table 12–1. Disorders that increase serum cholesterol are generally those that affect the number or affinity of LDL receptors and are known as familial hypercholesterolemia (FH). These patients commonly present with corneal arcus of the eye and xanthomas of extensor tendons of the hand and Achilles tendon, and premature CHD. Elevations in triglycerides are generally associated with overproduction of triglyceride-rich VLDL, mutations in

Clinical Presentation and Diagnosis

Lipid Panel

- Non-HDL cholesterol exceeding 130 mg/dL (3.36 mmol/L) or LDL cholesterol exceeding 100 mg/dL (2.59 mmol/L) should be evaluated for high cholesterol in conjunction with assessment of ASCVD risk.
- Serum triglycerides exceeding 150 mg/dL (1.70 mmol/L) and serum HDL cholesterol less than 40 mg/dL (1.03 mmol/L) in men and less than 50 mg/dL (1.29 mmol/L) in women may suggest metabolic syndrome and should be evaluated.

Physical Findings

- Corneal arcus of the eye and xanthomas may be seen in patients with genetic disorders that cause a marked increase in serum LDL cholesterol (greater than 250 mg/dL [6.47 mmol/L])
- Those with extremely elevated serum triglycerides (greater than 1000 mg/dL [11.3 mmol/L]) can develop pancreatitis and tuberoeruptive xanthomas.

Indications for Lipid Panel

- All adults more than 20 years of age should be screened at least every 5 years using a fasting blood sample to obtain a lipid profile (total cholesterol, non-HDL cholesterol, LDL cholesterol, HDL cholesterol, and triglycerides). A fasting lipid profile is preferred so an accurate assessment of LDL cholesterol can be performed.
- Children between 2 and 20 years old should be screened for high cholesterol if their parents have premature CHD or if one of their parents has a total cholesterol greater than 240 mg/dL (6.21 mmol/L). Early screening will help identify children at highest risk of developing CHD in whom early education and dietary intervention is warranted.

Indications for Other Tests

- Conditions that may produce lipid abnormalities (such as those listed in Table 12–2) should be screened for using appropriate tests. If present, these conditions should be properly addressed.

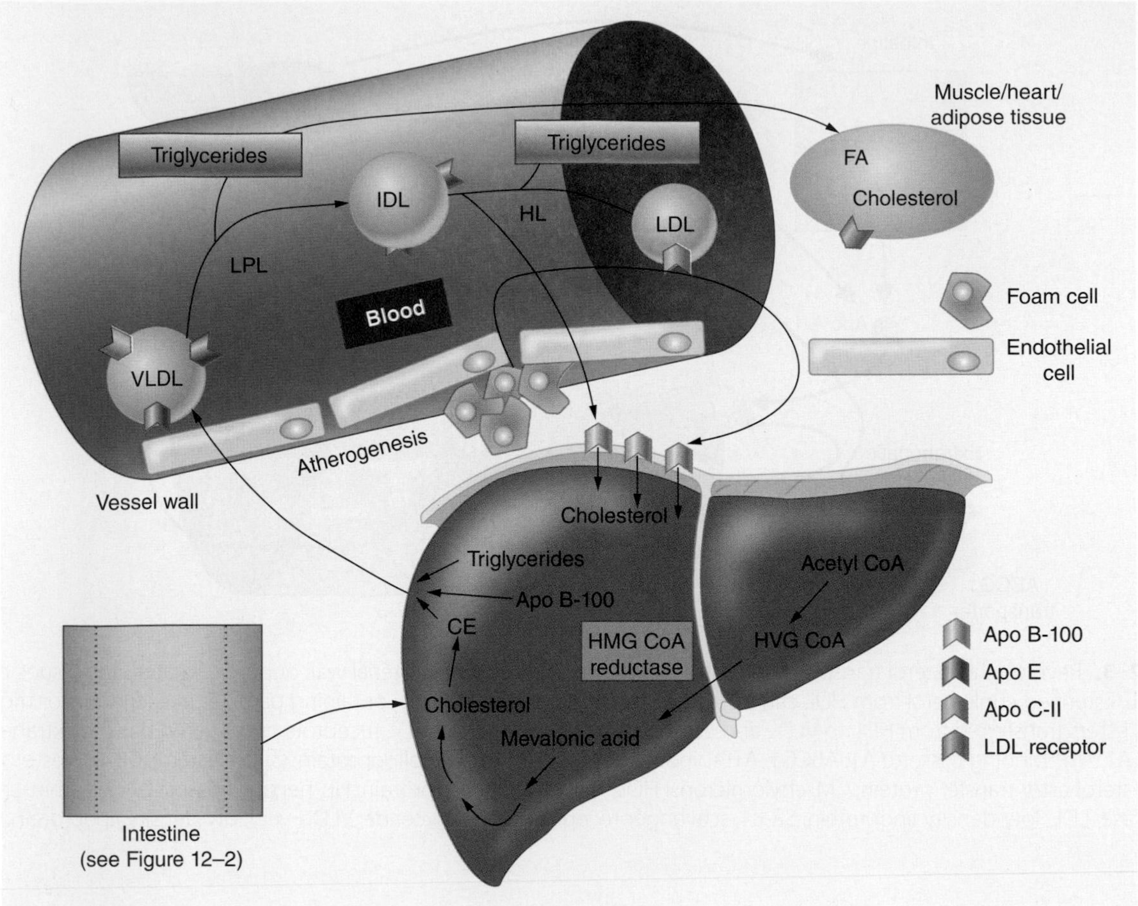

FIGURE 12–4. Endogenous lipoprotein metabolism. In liver cells, cholesterol and triglycerides are packaged into VLDL particles and exported into blood where VLDL is converted to IDL. Intermediate-density lipoprotein can be either cleared by hepatic LDL receptors or further metabolized to LDL. LDL can be cleared by hepatic LDL receptors or can enter the arterial wall, contributing to atherosclerosis. (Acetyl CoA, acetyl coenzyme A; Apo, apolipoprotein; CE, cholesterol ester; FA, fatty acid; HL, hepatic lipase; HMG-CoA, 3-hydroxy-3-methylglutaryl coenzyme A; IDL, intermediate-density lipoprotein; LDL, low-density lipoprotein; LPL, lipoprotein lipase; VLDL, very low-density lipoprotein.)

Table 12–1

Selected Characteristics of Primary Dyslipidemias

Disorder	Estimated Frequency	Metabolic Defect	Main Lipid Parameter
Autosomal Dominant Hypercholesterloemia			
Familial hypercholesterolemia homozygous	1/250,000–1/1 million	LDL-receptor negative	LDL-C > 500 mg/dL (12.93 mmol/L)
Heterozygous	1/300–1/500	Reduction in LDL receptors	LDL-C 250–500 mg/dL (6.47–12.93 mmol/L)
Familial defective Apo B-100	1/1000	Single nucleotide mutation	LDL-C 250–500 mg/dL (6.47–12.93 mmol/L)
PCSK9 gain of function mutations	Rare	Single nucleotide mutations	LDL-C 250–500 mg/dL (6.47–12.93 mmol/L)
Polygenic hypercholesterolemia	Common	Metabolic and environmental	LDL-C 160–250 mg/dL (4.14–6.47 mmol/L)
Familial combined dyslipidemia	1/200–300	Overproduction of VLDL and/or LDL	LDL-C 250–350 mg/dL (6.47–9.05 mmol/L) TG 200–800 mg/dL (2.26–9.04 mmol/L)
Familial hyperapobetalipoproteinemia	5%	Increase Apo B production	Apo B > 125 mg/dL (1.25 g/L)
Familial dysbetalipoproteinemia	0.5%	Apo E2/2 phenotype	LDL-C 300–600 mg/dL (7.76–15.52 mmol/L) TG 400–800 mg/dL (4.52–9.04 mmol/L)
Familial hypertriglyceridemia			
Type I	1/500,000–1/1 million	LPL-Apo CII system	TG > 1000 mg/dL (11.3 mmol/L)
Type IV	1/300	Unknown	TG 200–500 mg/dL (2.26–5.65 mmol/L)
Type V	1/205,000	Metabolic and environmental	TG > 1000 mg/dL (11.3 mmol/L)
Hypoalphalipoproteinemia	3%–5%	Defect in HDL catabolism	HDL-C < 35 mg/dL (0.91 mmol/L)

Apo, apolipoprotein; C, cholesterol; HDL, high-density lipoprotein; LDL, low-density lipoprotein; LPL, lipoprotein lipase; PCSK9, proprotein convertase subtilisin/kexin type 9; TG, triglyceride; VLDL, very low-density lipoprotein.

Table 12–2

Secondary Conditions and Drugs That May Cause Hyperlipidemias

	↑ LDL Cholesterol	↑ Triglycerides	↓ HDL Cholesterol
Other Conditions			
Diabetes		√	√
Hypothyroidism	√	√	
Obstructive liver disease/biliary cirrhosis	√		
Renal disease		√	
Nephrotic syndrome	√	√	
Chronic renal failure		√	
Hemodialysis patients		√	
Obesity		√	√
Drugs			
Estrogen		√	
Progestins	√		√
Protease inhibitors		√	√
Anabolic steroids	√		√
Corticosteroids	√	√	
Isotretinoin		√	√
Cyclosporine	√		
Atypical antipsychotics		√	√
Thiazide diuretics	√	√	
β-blockers		√	√

LDL, low-density lipoprotein; HDL, high-density lipoprotein.

Apo E, or lack of LPL or Apo CII, which causes hyperchylomicronemia. Most individuals have mild to moderate elevations in cholesterol known as polygenic hypercholesterolemia, thought to be caused by various more subtle genetic defects as well as environmental factors such as diet, lack of physical activity, and obesity.[3]

Pathophysiology of Clinical Atherosclerotic Disease

Lipoproteins are the "root cause" of atherosclerosis. The process begins when lipoproteins migrate between the endothelial cells into the arterial wall where they are modified by oxidation (Figure 12–5). Oxidized lipoproteins promote endothelial dysfunction by disturbing the production of nitric oxide that maintains vasomotor tone, as well as increasing expression of cell-adhesion molecules on vascular endothelial cells leading to recruitment of monocytes into the intima. The monocytes differentiate into macrophages and express scavenger receptors, allowing enhanced uptake of these oxidized lipoproteins. The macrophages continue to accumulate lipoproteins and ultimately develop into lipid-laden foam cells. Accumulation of foam cells leads to formation of a lipid-rich core, which marks the transition to a more complicated atherosclerotic plaque. Such plaques may result in ischemic heart disease and acute coronary syndromes, further discussed in Chapters 7 and 8, respectively. Aggressive lipid lowering can restore endothelial function, decrease cardiovascular disease risk, and improve patient outcomes.[3,5]

TREATMENT

The rate-limiting enzyme in cholesterol biosynthesis is 3-hydroxy-3-methylglutaryl coenzyme A (HMG-CoA) reductase. Isolation of a specific inhibitor of this enzyme resulted in the first marketed statin called lovastatin.[6,7] By reducing cholesterol synthesis, statins were shown to up-regulate the LDL receptor. Statins have now become the mainstay therapy for both familial and nonfamilial hypercholesterolemia.

The last version of the National Heart, Lung, and Blood Institute's (NHLBI) National Cholesterol Education Program (NCEP) guidelines was published in 2004 and provided an optional LDL cholesterol goal of less than 70 mg/dL (1.81 mmol/L) in very high risk patients.[8] In November 2013, the American College of Cardiology (ACC) and American Heart Association (AHA) released new guidelines for treating high blood cholesterol to reduce risk of ASCVD in adults.[9] These guidelines represent a paradigm shift in how clinicians have traditionally managed patients. Some of the major changes include removal of cholesterol treatment goals, non-statin therapies are not generally recommended due to lack of data supporting reduced ASCVD, and guidance for other lipid disorders such as hypertriglyceridemia is not provided. The guidelines also depart markedly from those issued by other major medical organizations, as shown in Table 12–3.[8–15] In this chapter, the ACC/AHA guidelines[9] and the National Lipid Association (NLA) recommendations[15] will be reviewed.

The ACC/AHA Guidelines identify four groups of patients targeted for statin treatment (Figure 12–6), including:

- Established clinical ASCVD (secondary prevention)
- Primary elevation of LDL levels 190 mg/dL (4.91 mmol/L) or higher
- Diabetes mellitus (DM), age 40 to 75 years, with LDL levels 70 to 189 mg/dL (1.81–4.89 mmol/L)
- Primary prevention without DM, age 40 to 75 years, with an estimated 10-year risk of 7.5% or greater, and LDL levels 70 to 189 mg/dL (1.81–4.89 mmol/L)

A new pooled cohort risk estimator was developed to assist with decisions regarding initiation of statin therapy for primary prevention (http://my.americanheart.org/professional/StatementsGuidelines/Prevention-Guidelines_UCM_457698_SubHomePage.jsp). It should be emphasized that this risk estimator is part of the patient-clinician discussion regarding potential benefit of statin therapy and not the sole determinant for initiation of therapy. Clinical judgment, which includes risk and benefits, cost, and potential drug–drug interactions, must be exercised. This is especially important since the risk estimator has been shown to overestimate or underestimate risk in some patient populations. If initiation of statin therapy is uncertain based on quantitative risk assessment, additional factors such as LDL cholesterol 160 mg/dL (4.14 mmol/L) or higher, family history of premature ASCVD, high-sensitivity C-reactive protein (hs-CRP) of 2.0 mg/L or higher, coronary artery calcium (CAC) score of 300 Agatston units or higher, ankle-brachial index (ABI) less than 0.9, or elevated lifetime ASCVD risk can be considered.

Once the decision to initiate statin therapy is made, dose intensity is based on which statin benefit group the patient fits (Figure 12–6). High-intensity statin therapy on average lowers

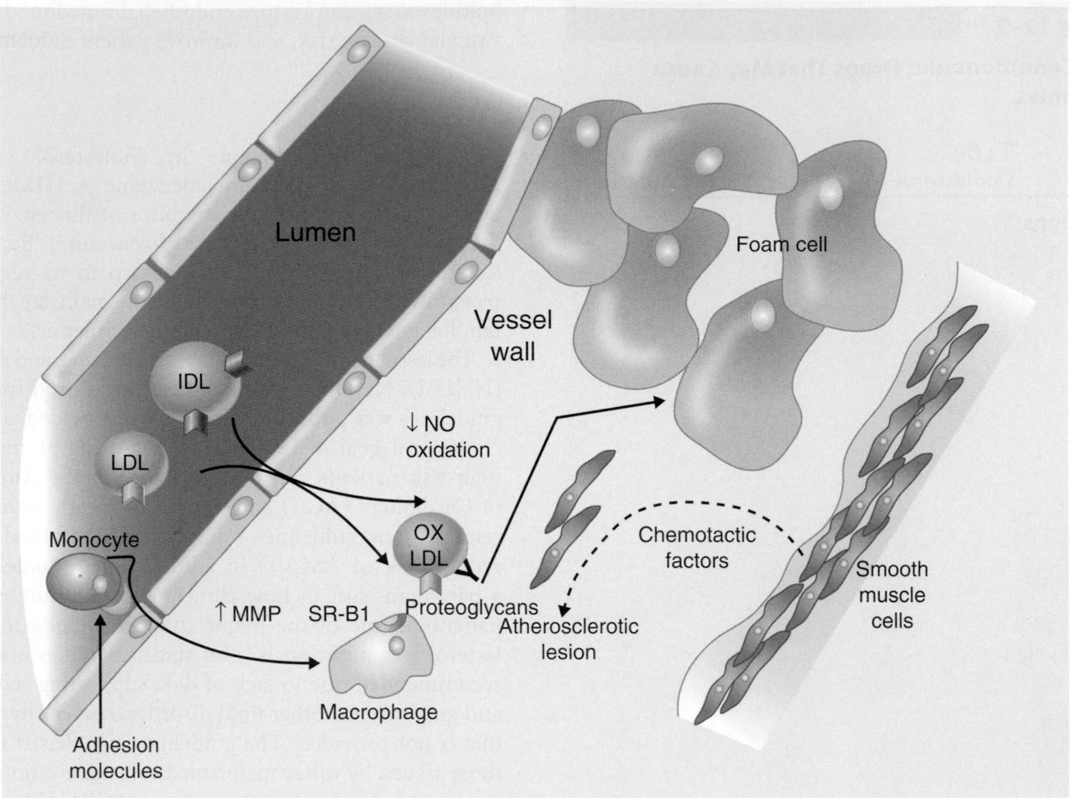

FIGURE 12–5. The process of atherogenesis. Atherosclerosis is initiated by the migration and retention of LDL and remnant lipoprotein particles into the vessel wall. These particles undergo oxidation and are taken up by macrophages in an unregulated fashion. The oxidized particles participate to induce endothelial cell dysfunction, leading to a reduced ability of the endothelium to dilate the artery and cause a prothrombotic state. The unregulated uptake of cholesterol by macrophages leads to foam cell formation and the development of a blood clot–favoring fatty lipid core. The enlarging lipid core eventually causes an encroachment of the vessel lumen. Early in the process, smooth muscle cells are activated and recruited from the media to the intima, helping to produce a collagen matrix that covers the growing clot protecting it from circulating blood. Later, macrophages produce and secrete matrix metalloproteinases that degrade the collagen matrix, leading to unstable plaque that may cause a myocardial infarction. (IDL, intermediate-density lipoprotein; LDL, low-density lipoprotein; MMP, matrix metalloproteinases; NO, nitric oxide; SR-BI, scavenger receptors.)

LDL cholesterol by approximately 50% and moderate-intensity statin therapy lowers LDL cholesterol approximately 30% to 50% (see Table 12–4). The ACC/AHA expert panel concluded they could not find evidence for or against titration of drug therapy to specific LDL cholesterol and/or non-HDL cholesterol goals, thus no recommendations are given.[9] This is one of the most controversial features of the ACC/AHA Guidelines. A follow-up LDL cholesterol is used only to assess response and statin adherence, and not for determining if goals have been achieved.

In 2014, the NLA issued its recommendation for patient-centered management of dyslipidemia and reaffirmed the importance of setting cholesterol goals for prevention of ASCVD.[13] The NLA emphasized that non-HDL cholesterol is a better primary target for modification than LDL cholesterol, and is now considered a cotarget with LDL cholesterol. KEY CONCEPT *The NLA recommendations for "desirable" cholesterol levels are presented in Table 12–5.*

KEY CONCEPT *Both the NLA and ACC/AHA emphasize that lifestyle therapies are an important element of risk reduction efforts in ASCVD prevention, whether or not pharmacotherapy is also used.* Therapeutic lifestyle changes (TLC) should be the first approach tried in all patients (Table 12–6), but pharmacotherapy should be instituted concurrently in higher-risk patients. TLC includes dietary restrictions as well as regular exercise and weight reduction. Additionally, consumption of plant stanols/sterols and dietary fiber should be encouraged as they may reduce LDL cholesterol by 20% to 25%.

Recommendations for Treatment

▸ *Step 1: Screening and Classification of Initial Lipoprotein Lipid Levels*

Determine lipoprotein profile after fasting for 9 to 12 hours. KEY CONCEPT *The NLA recommends that all adults older than 20 years are screened at least every 5 years to obtain a lipid profile (see Clinical Presentation and Diagnosis).* Children between 2 and 20 years old should be screened for high cholesterol if their parents have premature CHD or if one of their parents has total cholesterol greater than 240 mg/dL (6.21 mmol/L).

▸ *Step 2: Rule Out Secondary Causes of Dyslipidemia*

Certain drugs and diseases can cause abnormalities in serum lipids and should be evaluated (Table 12–2). Every effort should be made to correct or control underlying diseases such as hypothyroidism and DM. Concurrent medications known to

Table 12–3

International and US Guidelines for Management of Dyslipidemias

Source	Fasting Lipid Panel Measurement for Risk Assessment	Recommended Lipoprotein Target of Therapy	Treatment Goals
National Cholesterol Education Program Adult Treatment Panel III Update[8] (2004)	Yes	LDL cholesterol Non-HDL cholesterol (secondary target)	LDL cholesterol: < 70 mg/dL (1.81 mmol/L) is an optional goal for very high-risk patients < 100 mg/dL (2.59 mmol/L) for high-risk patients < 130 mg/dL (3.36 mmol/L) for moderate-risk patients < 160 mg/dL (4.14 mmol/L) for lower-risk patients Non-HDL cholesterol: In patients with high serum triglycerides, goal can be set 30 mg/dL (0.78 mmol/L) higher than LDL goal
International Atherosclerosis Society[10] (2014)	Yes	Non-HDL cholesterol LDL cholesterol (alternate target)	"Treatment goals" not specified. Identifies optimal levels of atherogenic cholesterol and makes the general statement that intensity of cholesterol-lowering therapy should be adjusted to long-term risk. Potency of cholesterol-lowering therapy relative to optimal levels must be left to clinical judgment.
European Society of Cardiology/European Atherosclerosis Society[11] (2011)	Yes	LDL cholesterol Non-HDL cholesterol and Apo B (secondary targets)	LDL cholesterol: < 70 mg/dL (1.81 mmol/L) or a ≥ 50% reduction in baseline LDL cholesterol for very high-risk patients < 100 mg/dL (2.59 mmol/L) for high-risk patients < 115 mg/dL (2.97 mmol/L) for moderate-risk patients Non-HDL cholesterol: Can be set 30 mg/dL (0.78 mmol/L) higher than LDL goal Apo B: Targets for subjects at very high or high risk are < 80 mg/dL (0.80 g/L) and < 100 mg/dL (1.00 g/L), respectively
Canadian Cardiovascular Society[12] (2013)	Yes	LDL cholesterol Non-HDL cholesterol and Apo B (secondary targets)	LDL cholesterol: ≤ 77 mg/dL (1.99 mmol/L) or 50% reduction of LDL cholesterol from baseline for high and intermediate-risk patients ≥ 50% reduction in LDL cholesterol from baseline in low-risk patients Non-HDL cholesterol: ≤ 100 mg/dL (2.59 mmol/L) for high and intermediate-risk patients Apo B: ≤ 80 mg/dL (0.80 g/L) for high and intermediate-risk patients
2013 American College of Cardiology/American Heart Association: Blood Cholesterol Guidelines for ASCVD Prevention[9] (2013)	No Used to evaluate for more severe forms and secondary dyslipidemias and to assess anticipated therapeutic response and adherence to statin therapy	No recommendation	No recommendation
National Lipid Association Recommendations for Patient-Centered Management of Dyslipidemia[13] (2014)	Yes	Non-HDL cholesterol and LDL cholesterol Apo B (secondary target)	LDL cholesterol: < 70 mg/dL (1.81 mmol/L) for very high-risk patients < 100 mg/dL (2.59 mmol/L) for high-risk, moderate-risk and low-risk patients Non-HDL cholesterol: < 100 mg/dL (2.59 mmol/L) for very high-risk patients < 130 mg/dL (3.36 mmol/L) for high-risk, moderate-risk and low risk patients Apo B: < 80 mg/dL (0.80 g/L) for very high risk patients < 90 mg/dL (0.90 g/L) for high-risk, moderate-risk, and low-risk patients

Apo, apolipoprotein; ASCVD, atherosclerotic cardiovascular disease; LDL, low-density lipoprotein; non-HDL, non–high-density lipoprotein.

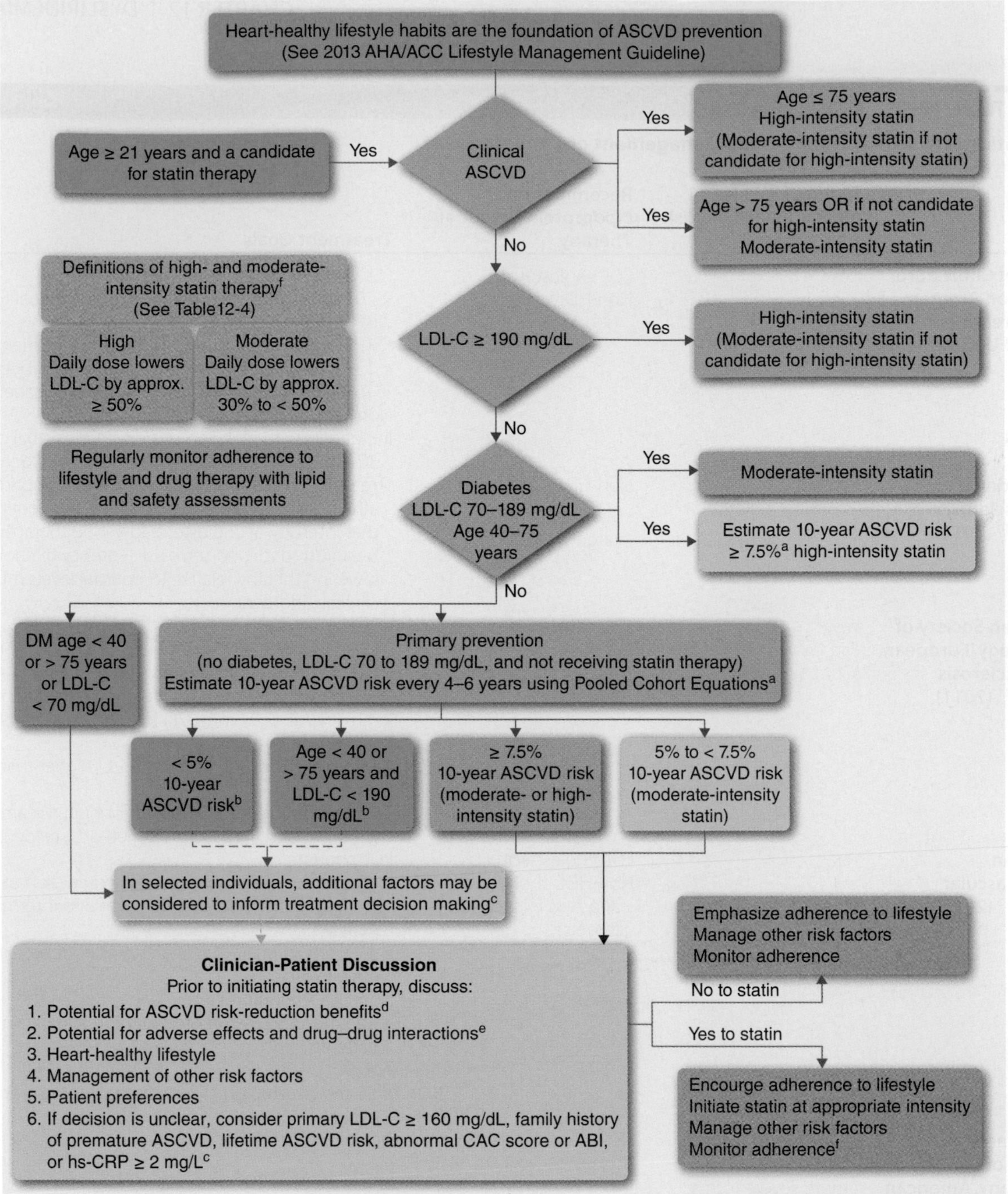

FIGURE 12–6. Summary of statin initiation recommendations for the treatment of blood cholesterol to reduce ASCVD risk in adults. [a]The Pooled Cohort Equation can be used to estimate 10-year ASCVD risk in individuals with and without diabetes. The estimator within this application should be used to inform decision making in primary prevention patients not on a statin. [b]Consider moderate-intensity statins as more appropriate in low-risk individuals. [c]For those in whom a risk assessment is uncertain, consider factors such as primary LDL-C ≥ 160 mg/dL (4.14 mmol/L) or other evidence of genetic hyperlipidemias, family history of premature ASCVD with onset < 55 years of age in a first-degree male relative or < 65 years of age in a first-degree female relative, hs-CRP ≥ 2 mg/L, CAC score ≥ 300 Agatston units, or ≥ 75th percentile for age, sex, and ethnicity, ABI < 0.9, or lifetime risk of ASCVD. [d]Potential ASCVD risk reduction benefits. The absolute reduction in ASCVD events from moderate- or high-intensity statin therapy can be approximated by multiplying the estimated 10-year ASCVD risk by the anticipated relative-risk reduction from the intensity of statin initiated (~30% for moderate-intensity statin or ~45% for high-intensity statin). [e]Potential adverse effects. The excess risk of diabetes is the main consideration in ~0.1 excess cases per 100 individuals treated with a moderate-intensity statin for 1 year and ~0.3 excess cases per 100 individuals treated with a high-intensity statin for 1 year. In randomized controlled trials, both statin-treated and placebo-treated participants experienced the same rate of muscle symptoms. The actual rate of statin-related muscle symptoms in the clinical population is unclear. Muscle symptoms attributed to statin therapy should be evaluated. [f]Percent reduction in LDL-C can be used as an indication of response and adherence to therapy, but is not in itself a treatment goal. ABI, ankle-brachial index; ACC, American College of Cardiology; AHA, American Heart Association; ASCVD, atherosclerotic cardiovascular disease; CAC, coronary artery calcium; DM, diabetes mellitus; hs-CRP, high-sensitivity C-reactive protein; LDL-C, low-density lipoprotein cholesterol. The algorithm LDL-C values expressed in mmol/L are 4.91 mmol/L for 190 mg/dL, 4.89 mmol/L for 189 mg/dL, and 1.81 mmol/L for 70 mg/dL. (From Stone NJ, Robinson JG, Lichtenstein AH, et al. 2013 ACC/AHA guideline on the treatment of blood cholesterol to reduce atherosclerotic cardiovascular risk in adults: a report of the American College of Cardiology/American Heart Association Task Force on Practice Guidelines. J Am Coll Cardiol. 2014 Jul 1;63(25 Pt B):2889–2934, with permission.)

Table 12–4

High, Moderate, and Low-Intensity Statin Therapy as Indicated by the ACC/AHA

High-Intensity Statin Therapy	Moderate-Intensity Statin Therapy	Low-Intensity Statin Therapy
Daily dose lowers LDL cholesterol, on average, by approximately ≥ 50%	Daily dose lowers LDL cholesterol, on average, by approximately 30% to < 50%	Daily dose lowers LDL cholesterol, on average, by < 30%
Atorvastatin (40[a])–80 mg	**Atorvastatin 10 (*20*) mg**	*Simvastatin 10 mg*
Rosuvastatin 20 (*40*) mg	**Rosuvastatin (*5*) 10 mg**	**Pravastatin 10–20 mg**
	Simvastatin 20–40 mg	**Lovastatin 20 mg**
	Pravastatin 40 (*80*) mg	*Fluvastatin 20–40 mg*
	Lovastatin 40 mg	*Pitavastatin 1 mg*
	Fluvastatin XL 80 mg	
	Fluvastatin 40 mg twice daily	
	Pitavastatin 2–4 mg	

ACC, American College of Cardiology; AHA, American Heart Association; LDL, low-density lipoprotein.

Boldface type indicates specific statins and doses that were evaluated in randomized controlled trials (RCTs) by the ACC/AHA guideline committee.

Italic type indicates statins and doses that have been approved by the Food and Drug Administration but were not tested in RCTs reviewed by the ACC/AHA guidelines.

[a]Evidence from 1 RCT only: down-titration if unable to tolerate atorvastatin 80 mg.

Table 12–5

National Lipid Association Classifications of Cholesterol and Triglyceride Levels in mg/dL (mmol/L)

Lipids	
Non-HDL Cholesterol[a]	
< 130 (3.36)	Desirable
130–159 (3.36–4.11)	Above desirable
160–189 (4.14–4.89)	Borderline high
190–219 (4.91–5.66)	High
≥ 220 (5.69)	Very high
LDL Cholesterol	
< 100 (2.59)	Desirable
100–129 (2.59–3.34)	Above desirable
130–159 (3.36–4.11)	Borderline high
160–189 (4.14–4.89)	High
≥ 190 (4.91)	Very high
HDL Cholesterol	
< 40 (1.03)(men)	Low
< 50 (1.29)(women)	Low
Triglycerides	
< 150 (1.70)	Normal
150–199 (1.70–2.25)	Borderline
200–499 (2.26–5.64)	High
≥ 500 (5.65)	Very high[b]

HDL, high-density lipoprotein; LDL, low-density lipoprotein; non-HDL, non–high-density lipoprotein.

[a]Non-HDL-C = total cholesterol minus HDL cholesterol.

[b]Severe hypertriglyceridemia is another term used for very high triglycerides in pharmaceutical product labeling.

induce lipid abnormalities should be evaluated for discontinuation prior to instituting long-term lipid-modifying therapy.[13]

► *Step 3: Identify Patients with Very High-Risk Conditions*

Individuals with established ASCVD (Table 12–7) or DM with greater or equal to two ASCVD risk factors (Table 12–8) or evidence of end-organ damage are considered very high risk. The NLA set non-HDL cholesterol and LDL cholesterol goals for very high-risk patients at less than 100 mg/dL (2.59 mmol/L) and less than 70 mg/dL (1.81 mmol/L), respectively. Pharmacotherapy can be considered when non-HDL cholesterol or LDL cholesterol are equal to or above these goals. For patients with ASCVD or DM, consideration can be given to use of moderate or high-intensity statin therapy, irrespective of baseline cholesterol levels.

► *Step 4: Identify Patients with High-Risk Conditions*

Criteria for being considered high risk are described in Table 12–7. The NLA set non-HDL cholesterol and LDL cholesterol goals for high-risk patients at less than 130 mg/dL (3.36 mmol/L) and less than 100 mg/dL (2.59 mmol/L), respectively. Pharmacotherapy can be considered when non-HDL cholesterol or LDL cholesterol are equal to or above these goals. If it is not possible to attain desirable cholesterol levels in patients with severe hypercholesterolemia phenotype, a reduction of at least 50% is recommended.[13,14] For FH patients with multiple or poorly controlled other major ASCVD risk factors, clinicians may consider attaining even lower levels of atherogenic cholesterol.[13]

► *Step 5: Identify Patients with Two Or Less ASCVD Risk Factors*

For individuals with two major ASCVD risk factors, quantitative risk scoring should be considered and additional risk indicators

Table 12–6

Essential Components of Therapeutic Lifestyle Changes

Component	Recommendation
LDL-raising nutrients	
Dietary cholesterol	< 200 mg/day
Saturated fats	Total fat range should be 25%–35% for most cases
	< 7% of total calories and reduce intake of trans fatty acids
Therapeutic options for LDL-lowering plant stanols/sterols	2 g/day
Increased viscous (soluble) fiber	10–25 g/day
Total calories	Adjust caloric intake to maintain desirable body weight and prevent weight gain
Physical activity	≥ 150 minutes per week of moderate or higher intensity activity

LDL, low-density lipoprotein.

Table 12–7

National Lipid Association Criteria for ASCVD Risk Assessment, Treatment Goals, and Levels at Which to Consider Drug Therapy

Risk Category	Criteria	Cholesterol Treatment Goal	Consider Drug Therapy
Very High Risk	ASCVD • Myocardial infarction or other acute coronary syndrome • Coronary or other revascularization procedure • Transient ischemic attack • Ischemic stroke • Atherosclerotic peripheral arterial disease (Includes ankle/brachial index, 0.90) • Other documented atherosclerotic diseases such as: coronary atherosclerosis, renal atherosclerosis, aortic aneurysm secondary to atherosclerosis, carotid plaque, ≥ 50% stenosis DM (type 1 or 2) • ≥ 2 other major ASCVD risk factors or • Evidence of end-organ damage[a]	Non-HDL = < 100 mg/dL (2.59 mmol/L) LDL = < 70 mg/dL (1.81 mmol/L)	Non-HDL = ≥ 100 mg/dL (2.59 mmol/L) LDL = ≥ 70 mg/dL (1.81 mmol/L)
High Risk	≥ 3 major ASCVD risk factors DM (type 1 or 2)[b] • 0–1 other major ASCVD risk factors and • No evidence of end organ damage CKD stage 3B or 4[c] LDL ≥ 190 mg/dL (4.91 mmol/L) (severe hypercholesterolemia)[d] Quantitative risk score reaching the high-risk threshold[e]	Non-HDL = < 130 mg/dL (3.36 mmol/L) LDL = < 100 mg/dL (2.59 mmol/L)	Non-HDL = ≥ 130 mg/dL (3.36 mmol/L) LDL = ≥ 100 mg/dL (2.59 mmol/L)
Moderate Risk	Two major ASCVD risk factors • Consider quantitative risk scoring • Consider other risk indicators[f]	Non-HDL = < 130 mg/dL (3.36 mmol/L) LDL = < 100 mg/dL (2.59 mmol/L)	Non-HDL = ≥ 160 mg/dL (4.14 mmol/L) LDL = ≥ 130 mg/dL (3.36 mmol/L)
Low Risk	0–1 major ASCVD risk factor • Consider other risk indicators, if known	Non-HDL= < 130 mg/dL (3.36 mmol/L) LDL = < 100 mg/dL (2.59 mmol/L)	Non-HDL = ≥ 190 mg/dL (4.91 mmol/L) LDL = ≥ 160 mg/dL (4.14 mmol/L)

ASCVD, atherosclerotic cardiovascular disease; CKD, chronic kidney disease; DM, diabetes mellitus; LDL, low-density lipoprotein; non-HDL, non–high-density lipoprotein.

For patients with ASCVD or DM, consideration should be given to use of moderate or high-intensity statin therapy, irrespective of baseline atherogenic cholesterol levels.

[a]End-organ damage indicated by increased albumin/creatinine ratio (≥ 30 mg/g [3.4 mg/mmol]), CKD, or retinopathy.

[b]For patients with DM plus 1 major ASCVD risk factor, treating to a non-HDL-C goal of 100 mg/dL or 2.59 mmol/L (LDL, 70 mg/dL [1.81 mmol/L]) is considered a therapeutic option.

[c]For patients with CKD Stage 3B (glomerular filtration rate [GFR] 30–44 mL/min/1.73 m^2 [0.29–0.42 mL/s/m^2]) or Stage 4 (GFR 15–29 mL/min/1.73 m^2 [0.14–0.28 mL/s/m^2]), risk calculators should not be used because they may underestimate risk. Stage 5 CKD (or on hemodialysis) is a very high-risk condition, but results from randomized controlled trials of lipid-altering therapies have not provided convincing evidence of reduced ASCVD events in such patients. Therefore, no treatment goals for lipid therapy have been defined for stage 5 CKD.

[d]If LDL is ≥ 190 mg/dL (4.91 mmol/L), consider severe hypercholesterolemia phenotype, which includes familial hypercholesterolemia (FH). Lifestyle intervention and pharmacotherapy are recommended for adults with the severe hypercholesterolemia phenotype. If it is not possible to attain desirable levels of atherogenic cholesterol, a reduction of at least 50% is recommended. For FH patients with multiple or poorly controlled other major ASCVD risk factors, clinicians may consider attaining even lower levels of atherogenic cholesterol. Risk calculators should not be used in such patients.

[e]High-risk threshold is defined as ≥ 10% using Adult Treatment Panel III Framingham Risk Score for hard coronary heart disease (CHD; myocardial infarction or CHD death), ≥15% using the 2013 Pooled Cohort Equations for hard ASCVD (myocardial infarction, stroke, or death from CHD or stroke), or ≥ 45% using the Framingham long-term (to age 80) cardiovascular disease (CVD; myocardial infarction, CHD death or stroke) risk calculation. Clinicians may prefer to use other risk calculators, but should be aware that quantitative risk calculators vary in clinical outcomes predicted (eg, CHD events, ASCVD events, cardiovascular mortality); the risk factors included in their calculation; and the timeframe for their prediction (eg, 5 years, 10 years, or long term or lifetime). Such calculators may omit certain risk indicators that can be important in individual patients, provide only an approximate risk estimate and require clinical judgment for interpretation.

[f]For those at moderate risk, additional testing may be considered for some patients to assist with decisions about risk stratification.

Table 12–8

Risk Factors for Atherosclerotic Cardiovascular Disease According to the National Lipid Association[a]

Risk Factor	Definition
Age (years)	Male ≥ 45; female ≥ 55
Family history of premature CHD events[b]	Male first-degree relative at < 55 years Female first-degree relative at < 65 years
Hypertension	SBP ≥ 140 mm Hg DBP ≥ 90 mm Hg
Low HDL cholesterol	< 40 mg/dL (1.03 mmol/L) in males < 50 mg/dL (1.29 mmol/L) in females
Cigarette smoking	Current

[a]Levels of non-HDL cholesterol and LDL cholesterol are not listed because these risk factors are used to assess risk category and treatment goals for atherogenic lipoprotein cholesterol levels. Diabetes is not listed because it is considered a high- or very high-risk condition for ASCVD risk assessment purposes.

[b]CHD is defined as myocardial infarction, coronary death, or a coronary revascularization procedure.

CHD, coronary heart disease; DBP, diastolic blood pressure; HDL, high-density lipoprotein; LDL, low-density lipoprotein; SBP, systolic blood pressure.

Table 12–9

Risk Indicators (Other Than Major ASCVD Risk Factors) That Might Be Considered for Refinement[a]

Component
1. A severe disturbance in a major ASCVD risk factor, such as multipack per day smoking or strong family history of premature CHD
2. Indicators of subclinical disease, including coronary artery calcium ≥ 300 Agatston units[b] is considered high risk
3. LDL cholesterol ≥ 160 mg/dL (4.14 mmol/L) and/or non-HDL cholesterol ≥ 190 mg/dL (4.91 mmol/L)
4. High-sensitivity C-reactive protein ≥ 2.0 mg/L[c]
5. Lipoprotein (a) ≥ 50 mg/dL (500 mg/L; 125 nmol/L) using an isoform insensitive assay
6. Urine albumin/creatinine ratio ≥ 30 mg/g (3.4 mg/mmol)

ASCVD, atherosclerotic cardiovascular disease; CHD, coronary heart disease; non-HDL, non–high-density lipoprotein; LDL, low-density lipoprotein.

[a]The presence of 1 or more of the risk indicators listed may be considered, in conjunction with major ASCVD risk factors, to reclassify an individual into a higher risk category. Except in the case of evidence of subclinical disease defining the presence of ASCVD, reclassification to a higher risk category is a matter of clinical judgment. Doing so will alter the threshold for consideration of pharmacotherapy and/or the treatment goals for atherogenic cholesterol.

[b]Or coronary artery calcium 75th percentile for age, sex, and ethnicity.

[c]Because of high intraindividual variability, multiple high sensitivity C-reactive protein (hs-CRP) values should be obtained before concluding that the level is elevated; hs-CRP should not be tested in those who are ill, have an infection, or are injured. If hs-CRP level is 0.10 mg/L, consider other etiologies such as infection, active arthritis, or concurrent illness.

(Table 12–9) may be useful for some patients. If quantitative risk score reaches the high-risk threshold, assign patient to high-risk category. If other risk indicators are present, consider assigning to the high-risk category. If no indication is present to assign to high risk, assign to moderate-risk category, with NLA goals for non-HDL cholesterol and LDL cholesterol of less than 130 mg/dL (3.36 mmol/L) and less than 100 mg/dL (2.59 mmol/L), respectively. Pharmacotherapy can be considered when non-HDL cholesterol or LDL cholesterol are equal to or above 160 mg/dL (4.14 mmol/L) and 130 mg/dL (3.36 mmol/L), respectively. For individuals with one or no major ASCVD risk factors, the NLA set goals for non-HDL cholesterol and LDL cholesterol level at less than 130 mg/dL (3.36 mmol/L) and less than 100 mg/dL (2.59 mmol/L), respectively. Pharmacotherapy can be considered when non-HDL cholesterol or LDL cholesterol are equal to or above 190 mg/dL (4.91 mmol/L) and 160 mg/dL (4.14 mmol/L), respectively. Consider assigning to a higher risk category based on other known risk indicators, when present.

► *Step 6: Identify Patients with Metabolic Syndrome*

Diagnosis of metabolic syndrome is made when three or more of the following risk factors are present[3,14]:

- Waist circumference greater than or equal to 40 inches (102 cm) in men (35 inches [89 cm] in Asian men), or 35 inches (89 cm) in women (31 inches [79 cm] in Asian women)
- Triglycerides greater than or equal to 150 mg/dL (1.70 mmol/L) or on drug treatment for elevated triglycerides
- HDL cholesterol less than 40 mg/dL (1.03 mmol/L) in men or 50 mg/dL (1.29 mmol/L) in women or on drug treatment for reduced HDL cholesterol
- Blood pressure greater than or equal to 130/85 mm Hg or on drug treatment for hypertension
- Fasting blood glucose greater than or equal to 100 mg/dL (5.6 mmol/L) or on drug treatment for elevated glucose

Patients with metabolic syndrome are twice as likely to develop type 2 DM and four times more likely to develop ASCVD.[3,13] These individuals are usually insulin resistant, obese, have hypertension, are in a prothrombotic state, and have atherogenic dyslipidemia characterized by low HDL cholesterol, elevated triglycerides, and an increased proportion of small and dense LDL particles.[3]

KEY CONCEPT *The NLA identified metabolic syndrome as an important target for further reducing ASCVD risk.* Treatment starts with increased physical activity, weight reduction (which also enhances LDL cholesterol lowering and insulin sensitivity), and moderation of ethanol and carbohydrate intake, which effectively reduces many of the associated risk factors. Each of the risk factors should be addressed independently as appropriate, including treatment of hypertension and use of aspirin in CHD patients to reduce the prothrombotic state.

► *Step 7: Treatment of Elevated Triglycerides*

KEY CONCEPT *Patients with serum triglycerides exceeding 500 mg/dL (5.65 mmol/L) are at increased risk of pancreatitis, especially when levels exceed 1000 mg/dL (11.3 mmol/L).[3] Reducing triglycerides in these individuals becomes the primary target for*

Patient Encounter 1, Part 1

A 44-year-old, nonsmoking man presents to your clinic for a physical exam. He states that he is worried since his younger brother was recently diagnosed with CHD. He has never had his cholesterol evaluated. He denies having chest pain or history of myocardial infarction (MI), stroke, or peripheral artery disease. He has tendon xanthomas on both hands. His sister is 52 and healthy; however, his mother had an MI when she was 47 and has elevated cholesterol. He is married with three children. He does not smoke and exercises regularly. He ate breakfast (eggs and bacon) approximately 1 hour ago.

Can the patient be evaluated today for non-HDL cholesterol?

Should an assessment of his risk factors for ASCVD be conducted?

What additional information do you need to evaluate the patient?

intervention. Reduction in fats and carbohydrates and abstaining from ethanol should be considered, and secondary causes (Table 12–2) should be assessed. Increase in exercise should be encouraged. Weight loss should also be encouraged if individual is overweight. When pharmacotherapy is instituted, the goal is to reduce triglycerides to less than 150 mg/dL (1.70 mmol/L). Once triglycerides are less than 500 mg/dL (5.65 mmol/L) and the risk of pancreatitis is reduced, the primary focus of intervention should once again be on non-HDL and LDL cholesterol. Individuals with triglycerides between 200 and 499 mg/dL (2.26 and 5.64 mmol/L) have increased triglyceride-rich remnant lipoproteins and small-dense LDL particles. Niacin, fibrates, and long-chain omega-3 fatty acids are the most effective agents in patients with fasting triglyceride concentrations greater than 1000 mg/dL (11.3 mmol/L).[3] For patients with triglycerides 500 to 999 mg/dL (5.65–11.29 mmol/L), a triglyceride-lowering agent or a statin (if no history of pancreatitis) may be reasonable. For patients with high triglycerides between 200 and 499 mg/dL (2.26 and 5.64 mmol/L), statins will generally be first line since they are most effective in reducing non-HDL and LDL-cholesterol levels.

Pharmacotherapy

► *Statins (HMG-CoA Reductase Inhibitors)*

KEY CONCEPT *Statins are very effective LDL-lowering medications and are proven to reduce the risk of CHD, stroke, and death. Thus, ACC/AHA and NLA consider statins the preferred LDL-lowering medications.* Statins are effective in reducing ASCVD and in some cases, mortality. This effectiveness has been demonstrated in both genders, the elderly, patients with DM and hypertension, those with or without preexisting ASCVD, and following an acute coronary syndrome.[15–26] Statins inhibit conversion of HMG-CoA to L-mevalonic acid and subsequently cholesterol. Statins lower LDL cholesterol levels by approximately 25% to 62% (Table 12–10), are moderately effective at reducing triglycerides, and modestly raise HDL cholesterol. Additionally, statins also inhibit other important by-products in the cholesterol biosynthetic pathway that affect intracellular transport, membrane trafficking, and gene transcription. This may explain some of the cholesterol-independent benefits (so-called pleiotropic effects) of statins such as reducing lipoprotein oxidation, enhancing endothelial synthesis of nitric oxide, and inhibiting thrombosis. These pleiotropic effects are thought to contribute to the early benefits of statins on CHD risk, while the decrease in serum lipids accounts for the later benefits.

KEY CONCEPT *Statins are well tolerated, with less than 4% of patients in clinical trials discontinuing therapy due to adverse side effects* (Table 12–11). Elevations in liver function tests (LFTs) and myopathy, including rhabdomyolysis, are important adverse effects associated with statins. Liver toxicity, defined as LFT elevations greater than three times the upper limit of normal, is reported in less than 2% of patients. Incidence is higher at higher doses, but the progression to liver failure is exceedingly rare. LFTs should be obtained at baseline and as clinically indicated thereafter. Myopathy, defined as muscle symptoms with creatine kinase (CK) 10 times the upper limit of normal, is reported to range from 0% to less than 0.5% for the currently marketed statins at approved doses. Rhabdomyolysis, defined as muscle symptoms with marked elevation in CK at 10 times the upper limit of normal and creatinine elevation usually associated with myoglobinuria and brown urine, is very rare.[27] The risks associated with statin-induced myopathy are[28]

- Small body frame and frailty
- Multisystem disease (eg, chronic renal insufficiency, especially due to DM)
- Perioperative periods
- Multiple medications (see next bullet)
- Specific concomitant medications or consumptions (check specific statin package insert for warnings): fibrates (especially gemfibrozil, but other fibrates too), nicotinic acid (rarely), cyclosporine, azole antifungals, macrolide antibiotics, protease inhibitors, nefazodone, verapamil, amiodarone, large quantities of grapefruit juice (usually more than 1 quart [about 950 mL] per day), and alcohol abuse (independently predisposes to myopathy).

It is reasonable to check a baseline CK in patients at risk for myopathy. Follow-up CK should only be obtained in patients complaining of muscle pain, weakness, tenderness, or brown urine. Patient assessment for symptoms of myopathy should be done 6 to 12 weeks after starting therapy and at each visit.

Some evidence suggests that statins increase the risk for development of DM. The Food and Drug Administration (FDA) warns of increased blood sugar and glycosylated hemoglobin (HbA1c) levels in statin labels. In addition, the FDA has added to statin labels that cognitive impairment, such as memory loss, forgetfulness and confusion, has been reported by some statin users. The FDA continues to believe the cardiovascular benefits of statins outweigh these small increased risks.

With the exception of pravastatin and pitavastatin, the other statins undergo biotransformation by the cytochrome P-450 system. Therefore, drugs known to inhibit statin metabolism should be used cautiously or avoided. Medications such as cyclosporine and gemfibrozil can inhibit drug transporters in the gut and liver that can increase statin concentrations. The time until maximum effect on lipids for statins is generally 4 to 6 weeks.

► *Cholesterol Absorption Inhibitors*

Ezetimibe blocks biliary and dietary cholesterol as well as phytosterol (plant sterol) absorption by interacting with the NPC1L1 transporter (Figure 12–2).[5] Less cholesterol is delivered to the liver which leads to an upregulation of LDL receptors.

Table 12–10

Effects of Lipid-Lowering Drugs on Serum Lipids at FDA-Approved Doses

Lipid-Lowering Drug	LDL Cholesterol	HDL Cholesterol	Triglycerides	Total Cholesterol
Statins				
Atorvastatin	−26% to −60%	+5% to +13%	−17% to −53%	−25% to −45%
Fluvastatin	−22% to −36%	+3% to +11%	−12% to −25%	−16% to −27%
Fluvastatin ER	−33% to −35%	+7% to +11%	−19% to −25%	−25%
Lovastatin	−21% to −42%	+2% to +10%	−6% to −27%	−16% to −34%
Lovastatin ER	−24% to −41%	+9% to +13%	−10% to −25%	−18% to −29%
Pitavastatin	−31% to −45%	+1% to +8%	−13% to −22%	−23% to −31%
Pravastatin	−22% to −34%	+2% to +12%	−15% to −24%	−16% to −25%
Rosuvastatin	−45% to −63%	+8% to +14%	−10% to −35%	−33% to −46%
Simvastatin	−26% to −47%	+8% to +16%	−12% to −34%	−19% to −36%
Bile Acid Sequestrants				
Cholestyramine	−15% to −30%	+3% to +5%	May increase in patients with elevated triglycerides	−10% to −25%
Colesevelam	−15% to −18%	+3% to +5%		−70% to −10%
Colestipol	−15% to −30%	+3% to +5%		−10% to 25%
Cholesterol Absorption Inhibitor				
Ezetimibe	−18%	+1% to +2%	−7% to −9%	−12% to −13%
Nicotinic Acid				
Niacin ER	−5% to −17%	+14% to +26%	−11% to −38%	−3% to −12%
Niacin IR	−5% to −25%	+15% to +39%	−20% to −60%	−3% to −25%
Fibric Acid Derivatives				
Fenofibrate	−31% to +45%	+9% to +23%	−23% to −54%	−9% to −22%
Gemfibrozil	−30% to +30%	+10% to +30%	−20% to −60%	−2% to −16%
Combination Products				
Niacin ER and lovastatin	−30% to −42%	+20% to +30%	−32% to −44%	Not stated
Niacin ER and simvastatin[a]	−12% to −14%	+21% to +29%	−27% to −38%	−9% to −11%
Simvastatin and ezetimibe	−46% to −59%	+8% to +12%	−25% to −26%	−34% to −43%
Omega-3-Fatty Acids				
Lovaza	+45%	+9%	−45%	−10%
Vascepa	−5%	−4%	−27%	−7%
Epanova	+26%	+5%	−31%	−6%
OMTRYG	+20% to +45%	0% to +9%	−25% to -45%	−8% to −10%
Micosomal Transfer Protein Inhibitors				
Lomitapide	−40%	−7%	−45%	−36%
Antisense Oligonucleotide				
Mipomersen	−25%	+15%	−18%	−21%

ER, extended-release; FDA, Food and Drug Administration; HDL, high-density lipoprotein; LDL, low-density lipoprotein.

[a]Percent change relative to simvastatin 20 mg.

This causes a reduction in serum cholesterol and a compensatory increase in cholesterol biosynthesis. Because statins inhibit cholesterol biosynthesis, this compensatory increase by ezetimibe can be blocked when coadministered with a statin.

KEY CONCEPT *Ezetimibe reduces LDL cholesterol by an average of 18%.* However, larger reductions can be seen in some individuals, presumably due to higher absorption of cholesterol. These individuals appear to have a blunted response to statin therapy. Ezetimibe lowers triglycerides by 7% to 9% and modestly increases HDL cholesterol. (See Table 12–10.)

Ezetimibe is contraindicated in patients with active liver disease or unexplained persistent elevations in LFTs. Since statins are the standard of care, a placebo controlled randomized trial of the effects of ezetimibe monotherapy on CHD morbidity and mortality has never been conducted. Ezetimibe combined with simvastatin and simvastatin monotherapy were not associated with a reduction in carotid intima-media thickness in patients with heterozygous FH.[29] However, ezetimibe combined with simvastatin was associated with a reduced incidence of ischemic cardiovascular events in low-risk patients with mild to moderate asymptomatic aortic stenosis compared with placebo,[30] as well as reduced incidence of major atherosclerotic events in a wide range of patients with advanced chronic kidney disease.[71] Most recently, ezetimibe combined with simvastatin was shown to further reduce ASCVD events in patients who have suffered a recent MI compared to simvastatin alone (http://www.cardiosource.org/science-and-quality/clinical-trials/i/improve-it.aspx?w_nav=RI). Ezetimibe is primarily used in combination with a statin when

Table 12–11

Formulation, Dosing, and Common Adverse Effects of Lipid-Lowering Drugs

Lipid-Lowering Drug	Dosage Forms	Usual Adult Maintenance Dose Range	Adverse Effects
Statins			
Atorvastatin	10-, 20-, 40-, 80-mg tablets	10–80 mg once daily (at any time of day). Dose adjustment in patients with renal dysfunction is not necessary	Most frequent side effects are constipation, abdominal pain, diarrhea, dyspepsia, and nausea. Statins should be discontinued promptly if serum transaminase levels (liver function tests) rise to three times upper limit of normal or if patient develops signs or symptoms of myopathy. Approximate equivalent doses of HMG-CoA reductase inhibitors are: atorvastatin 10 mg, fluvastatin 80 mg, lovastatin 40 mg, pitavastatin 2 mg, pravastatin 40 mg, simvastatin 20 mg, and rosuvastatin 5 mg
Fluvastatin	20-, 40-mg capsules; 80-mg extended-release tablets	20–40 mg/day as a single dose (evening) or 40 mg twice daily; 80 mg once daily (evening). Dose adjustments for mild to moderate renal impairment are not necessary	
Lovastatin	10-, 20-, 40-mg tablets	10–80 mg/day as a single dose (with evening meal) or divided twice daily with food. In patients with severe renal insufficiency (creatinine clearance less than 30 mL/min [0.5 mL/s]), dosage increases above 20 mg/day should be carefully considered and, if deemed necessary, implemented cautiously	
Lovastatin ER	20-, 30-, 60-mg tablets	20–60 mg/day as a single dose. In patients with severe renal insufficiency (creatinine clearance < 30 mL/min [0.5 mL/s]), dosage increases above 20 mg/day should be carefully considered and, if deemed necessary, implemented cautiously	
Pravastatin	10-, 20-, 40-, 80-mg tablets	10–80 mg/day as a single dose at bedtime. In patients with a history of significant renal or hepatic dysfunction, a starting dose of 10 mg daily is recommended	
Pitavastatin	1-, 2-, 4-mg tablets	1–4 mg/day as a single dose can be taken with or without food, at any time of day. Moderate renal impairment (glomerular filtration rate 30–60 mL/min/1.73 m^2 [0.29–0.58 mL/s/m^2]) and end-stage renal disease on hemodialysis: Starting dose of 1 mg once daily and maximum dose of 2 mg once daily	
Rosuvastatin	5-, 10-, 20-, 40-mg tablets	5–40 mg/day (at any time of day); 40 mg reserved for those who do not achieve LDL cholesterol goal on 20 mg. In patients with history of significant renal or hepatic dysfunction, starting dose of 10 mg daily is recommended	
Simvastatin	5-, 10-, 20-, 40-mg tablets	5–40 mg/day as a single dose in the evening, or divided. Recommended starting dose for patients at high risk of CHD is 40 mg/day. In patients with mild to moderate renal insufficiency, dosage adjustment is not necessary. However, caution should be exercised in patients with severe renal insufficiency; such patients should be started at 5 mg/day and be closely monitored. Due to increased risk of myopathy, including rhabdomyolysis, use of the 80-mg dose should be restricted to patients who have been taking simvastatin 80 mg chronically (eg, for 12 months or more) without evidence of muscle toxicity. Because of an increased risk for myopathy in Chinese patients taking simvastatin 40 mg coadministered with lipid-modifying doses (≥ 1 g/day niacin) of niacin-containing products, caution should be used when treating Chinese patients with simvastatin doses exceeding 20 mg/day coadministered with lipid-modifying doses of niacin-containing products. Because the risk for myopathy is dose related, Chinese patients should not receive simvastatin 80 mg coadministered with lipid-modifying doses of niacin-containing products	

(Continued)

Table 12–11

Formulation, Dosing, and Common Adverse Effects of Lipid-Lowering Drugs (*Continued*)

Lipid-Lowering Drug	Dosage Forms	Usual Adult Maintenance Dose Range	Adverse Effects
Bile Acid Sequestrants			
Cholestyramine	4-g packets	4–24 g/day in two or more divided doses	Main side effects are nausea, constipation, bloating, and flatulence, although these may be less with colesevelam. Increasing fluid and dietary fiber intake may relieve constipation and bloating. Impair absorption of fat-soluble vitamins
Colesevelam	625-mg tablets	3750–4375 mg/day as a single dose or divided twice daily, with meals	
	3.75-g oral suspension packet	One packet once a day with meals	
Colestipol	5-g packets	5–30 g/day as a single dose or divided	
	1-g tablets	2–16 g/day as a single dose or divided	
Cholesterol Absorption Inhibitors			
Ezetimibe	10 mg tablets	10 mg once daily. No dosage adjustment is necessary in patients with renal or mild hepatic insufficiency	Overall incidence of adverse events reported with ezetimibe alone was similar to that reported with placebo and generally similar between ezetimibe with a statin and statin alone. The frequency of increased transaminases was slightly higher in patients receiving ezetimibe plus a statin compared with those receiving statin monotherapy (1.3% vs 0.4%)
Nicotinic Acid (Prescription Products)			
Niacin ER (Niaspan)	500-, 750-, 1000-mg extended-release tablets	1000–2000 mg once daily at bedtime. Use with caution in patients with renal impairment	Side effects include flushing, itching, gastric distress, headache, hepatotoxicity, hyperglycemia, and hyperuricemia
Niacin IR (Niacor)	500-mg tablets	1–6 g/day in two to three divided doses. Do not exceed 6 g daily	
Fibric Acid Derivatives			
Fenofibrate	54-, 160-mg tablets[a]	54–160 mg/day; the dosage should be minimized in severe renal impairment	Most common side effects are nausea, diarrhea, abdominal pain, and rash. Increased risk of rhabdomyolysis when given with a statin. Fibric acids are associated with gallstones, myositis, and hepatitis
Gemfibrozil	600-mg tablets	1200 mg/day in two doses, 30 minutes before meals; should be avoided in hepatic or severe renal impairment	
Omega-3-Fatty Acids			
Lovaza	1-g capsule containing at least 0.9 g of OM3FA ethyl ester (EPA~0.465 g and DHA~0.375 g)	4 g/day taken as single 4 g dose (four capsules) or two 2 g doses (two capsules twice daily)	All products are obtained from oil of fish. Should be used with caution in patients with known hypersensitivity to fish and/or shellfish. Side effects include: Lovaza/Omtryg • Eructation, 4% • Dyspepsia, 3% • Taste perversion, 4% Vascepa • Arthralgia, 2.3% Epanova • Diarrhea, 15% • Nausea, 6% • Abdominal pain or discomfort, 5%
Vascepa	1-g capsule containing 1 g of icosapent ethyl	4 g/day taken as 2 g doses (two capsules twice daily)	
Epanova	1-g capsule containing at least 0.85 g OM3FFA (EPA~0.550 g and DHA~0.2 g)	2 or 4 g/day taken as single 2 g dose (2 capsules) or single 4 g doses (four capsules)	
Omtryg	1-g capsule containing at least 0.9 g of OM3FA ethyl ester (EPA~0.465 g and DHA~0.375 g)	4 g/day taken as single 4 g dose (four capsules) or two 2 g doses (two capsules twice daily)	

(*Continued*)

Table 12–11

Formulation, Dosing, and Common Adverse Effects of Lipid-Lowering Drugs (*Continued*)

Lipid-Lowering Drug	Dosage Forms	Usual Adult Maintenance Dose Range	Adverse Effects
Micosomal Transfer Protein Inhibitors			
Lomitapide	5-, 10-, and 20-mg capsules	5 mg once daily. Titrate dose based on acceptable safety/tolerability: increase to 10 mg daily after at least 2 weeks; and then, at a minimum of 4-week intervals, to 20 mg, 40 mg, and up to the maximum recommended dose of 60 mg daily	Gastrointestinal side effects and elevation in liver enzymes and hepatic fat are common
Antisense Oligonucleotide			
Mipomersen	200 mg subcutaneous injection	200 mg once weekly as a subcutaneous injection	Injection site reactions, hepatic fat, and liver enzyme elevations are common
Combination Products			
Niacin ER and lovastatin	500 mg/20 mg, 750 mg/20 mg, 1000 mg/20 mg tablets	500 mg/20 mg to 2000 mg/40 mg daily, at bedtime	See previous entries for each drug (niacin ER and lovastatin)
Niacin ER and simvastatin	500 mg/20 mg, 500 mg/40 mg, 750 mg/20 mg, 1000 mg/20 mg, 1000 mg/40 mg	500 mg/20 mg to 2000 mg/40 mg daily, at bedtime	See previous entries for each drug (niacin ER and simvastatin)
Ezetimibe and atorvastatin	10 mg/10 mg, 10 mg/20 mg, 10 mg/40 mg, 10 mg/80 mg	Dosage range is 10/10 mg/day through 10/80 mg/day. Recommended usual starting dose is 10/10 or 10/20 mg/day. Recommended starting dose is 10/40 mg/day for patients requiring a > 55% reduction in LDL cholesterol	See previous entries for each drug (ezetimibe and atorvastatin)
Ezetimibe and simvastatin	10 mg/10 mg, 10 mg/20 mg, 10 mg/40 mg, 10 mg/80 mg	Dosage range is 10/10 mg/day through 10/40 mg/day. Recommended usual starting dose is 10/10 or 10/20 mg/day. Initiation of therapy with 10/10 mg/day may be considered for patients requiring less aggressive LDL cholesterol reductions. Due to increased risk of myopathy, including rhabdomyolysis, use of the 10/80 mg dose of Vytorin should be restricted to patients who have been taking Vytorin 10/80 mg chronically (eg, for 12 months or more) without evidence of muscle toxicity. Because of an increased risk for myopathy in Chinese patients taking simvastatin 40 mg coadministered with lipid-modifying doses (≥ 1 g/day niacin) of niacin-containing products, caution should be used when treating Chinese patients with Vytorin doses exceeding 10/20 mg/day coadministered with lipid-modifying doses (≥ 1 g/day niacin) of niacin-containing products. Because the risk for myopathy is dose-related, Chinese patients should not receive Vytorin 10/80 mg coadministered with lipid-modifying doses of niacin-containing products	See previous entries for each drug (ezetimibe and simvastatin)

CHD, coronary heart disease; DHA, docosahexaenoic acid; ER, extended release; EPA, eicosapentaenoic acid; HMG-CoA, 3-hydroxy-3-methylglutaryl coenzyme A; IR, immediate-release; LDL, low-density lipoprotein; OM3FA, omega-3 fatty acid; OM3FFA, omega-3 free fatty acid.

[a]Dose strengths vary depending on brand.

adequate reductions in atherogenic cholesterol is not achieved or in those patients who are intolerant to statin therapy. The time until maximum effect on lipids for ezetimibe is generally 2 weeks.

► *Bile Acid Sequestrants*

Cholestyramine, colestipol, and colesevelam are the bile acid-binding resins or sequestrants (BAS) currently available in the United States. Resins are highly charged molecules that bind to bile acids in the gut. The resin–bile acid complex is then excreted in the feces. The loss of bile causes a compensatory conversion of hepatic cholesterol to bile, reducing hepatocellular stores of cholesterol and resulting in an upregulation of LDL receptors which then results in a decrease in serum cholesterol. Resins have been shown to reduce CHD events in patients without CHD.[32]

KEY CONCEPT *Resins are moderately effective in lowering LDL cholesterol but do not lower triglycerides. Moreover, in patients with elevated triglycerides, the use of a resin may worsen the condition.* This may be due to a compensatory increase in HMG-CoA reductase activity which results in an increase in secretion of VLDL. The increase in HMG-CoA reductase activity can be blocked

Patient Encounter 1, Part 2: Medical History, Physical Examination, and Diagnostic Tests

PMH: Unremarkable

FH: Father and mother both alive. Mother had MI at age 47. Brother recently diagnosed with CHD

SH: Works as an insurance agent and plays golf regularly. He exercises at a gym three to four times per week; drinks alcohol (glass of wine most nights)

Meds: Multivitamin once daily

ROS: No chest pain, shortness of breath, or dizziness

PE:

VS: BP 130/83 mm Hg, pulse 71 beats/min, RR 16 breaths/min, T 98.6°F (37°C), waist circumference 35 in (89 cm)

CV: RRR, normal S_1, S_2; no murmurs, rubs, or gallops

Abd: Soft, nontender, nondistended; positive for bowel sounds, no hepatosplenomegaly or abdominal aortic aneurysm

Exts: ABI 1.1

Neck: No carotid and basilar bruits

EENT: Corneal arcus in both eyes

Labs: Total cholesterol 376 mg/dL (9.72 mmol/L), triglycerides 290 mg/dL (3.28 mmol/L), HDL cholesterol 42 mg/dL (1.09 mmol/L), non-HDL cholesterol 334 mg/dL (8.64 mmol/L), LDL cholesterol unable to determine since nonfasting, and glucose 98 mg/dL (5.4 mmol/L), all other labs within normal limits

Given this additional information, what is your assessment of the patient's CHD risk?

What type of lipid disorder does he have?

Identify your treatment goals for the patient based on the NLA guidelines.

What nonpharmacologic and pharmacologic alternatives are available for the patient?

Should his children be screened for high cholesterol and why?

Develop a care plan for the patient.

with a statin, resulting in enhanced reductions in serum lipids. Resins reduce LDL cholesterol from 15% to 30%, with a modest increase in HDL cholesterol (3%–5%) (Table 12–10). Resins are most often used as adjuncts to statins in patients who require additional lowering of atherogenic cholesterol. Because these drugs are not absorbed, adverse effects are limited to the gastrointestinal (GI) tract (Table 12–11). About 20% of patients taking cholestyramine or colestipol report constipation and symptoms such as flatulence and bloating. A large number of patients stop therapy because of this. Resins should be started at the lowest dose and escalated slowly over weeks to months as tolerated until the desired response is obtained. Patients should be instructed to prepare the powder formulations in 6 to 8 ounces (~180–240 mL) of noncarbonated fluids, usually juice (enhances palatability) or water. Fluid intake should be increased to minimize constipation. Colesevelam is better tolerated with fewer GI side effects, although it is more expensive.[33] All resins have the potential to prevent absorption of other drugs such as digoxin, warfarin, thyroxine, thiazides, β-blockers, fat-soluble vitamins, and folic acid. Potential drug interactions can be avoided by taking a resin either 1 hour before or 4 hours after these other agents. The time until maximum effect on lipids for resins is generally 2 to 4 weeks.

► *Niacin*

Niacin (vitamin B_3) has broad applications in the treatment of lipid disorders when used at doses higher than those used as a nutritional supplement. Niacin inhibits fatty acid release from adipose tissue and fatty acid and triglyceride production in liver cells. This results in a reduction in the number of VLDL particles secreted (Figure 12–4), which leads to an overall reduction in LDL cholesterol and a decrease in the number of small dense LDL particles. Niacin also reduces the uptake of HDL-Apo A1 particles and increases uptake of cholesterol esters by the liver, thus improving the efficiency of reverse cholesterol transport between HDL particles and vascular tissue (Figure 12–4). Niacin is indicated for patients with elevated triglycerides, low HDL cholesterol, and elevated LDL cholesterol.[3]

Several different niacin formulations are available: niacin immediate-release (IR), niacin sustained-release (SR), and niacin extended-release (ER).[34,35] These formulations differ in terms of dissolution and absorption rates, metabolism, efficacy, and side effects. Limitations of niacin IR and SR are flushing and **hepatotoxicity**, respectively. These differences appear related to the dissolution and absorption rates of niacin formulations and their subsequent metabolism. Niacin IR is available by prescription (Niacor) as well as a dietary supplement, which is not regulated by the FDA.[34] Currently, all SR products are available only as dietary supplements.[36]

Niacin ER (Niaspan) was developed as a once-daily formulation to be taken at bedtime, with the goal of reducing the incidence of flushing without increasing the risk of hepatotoxicity. Niaspan is the only long-acting niacin product approved by the FDA for dyslipidemia.

Niacin use is limited by cutaneous reactions such as flushing and pruritus of the face and body. The use of aspirin or a nonsteroidal anti-inflammatory drug (NSAID) 30 minutes prior to taking niacin can help alleviate these reactions because they are mediated by an increase in prostaglandin D2.[3] In addition, taking niacin with food and avoiding hot liquids or alcohol at the time niacin is taken is helpful in minimizing flushing and pruritus.

In general, niacin reduces LDL cholesterol from 5% to 25%, reduces triglycerides by 20% to 50%, and increases HDL cholesterol by 15% to 35% (Table 12–10). Niacin monotherapy has been shown to reduce CHD events and total mortality,[37] as well as the progression of atherosclerosis when combined with a statin.[38] However, a recent trial that tested the effects of adding niacin ER or placebo in patients with CHD optimally treated (LDL cholesterol ~70 mg/dL [1.81 mmol/L]) on a statin was stopped earlier than planned because no apparent benefits by adding niacin ER were found. Moreover, a small and unexplained increase in ischemic stroke in the niacin ER group was seen.[39] Another trial also found no benefit by the addition of niacin ER plus an antiflush medication (laropiprant).[40] These two trials have resulted in ambiguity in the role of niacin in lipid management. However, niacin is still a useful agent in the management of high triglycerides and patients with FH.

Although niacin can raise uric acid levels and serum glucose levels, it can be used safely and effectively in patients with DM.[41] Due to the high cardiovascular risk of patients with DM, the benefits of improving the lipid profile appear to outweigh the risk.[42]

Niacin should be instituted at the lowest dose and gradually titrated to a maximum dose of 2 g daily for ER and SR products and no more than 6 g daily for IR products. FDA-approved niacin products are preferred because of product consistency. Moreover, niacin products labeled as "no flush" do not contain nicotinic acid and therefore have no therapeutic role in the treatment of lipid disorders.[34] The time until maximum effect on lipids for niacins is generally 3 to 5 weeks.

▶ Fibrates

KEY CONCEPT *The predominant effects of fibrates are a decrease in triglyceride levels by 20% to 50% and an increase in HDL cholesterol levels by 9% to 30% (Table 12–10).* The effect on LDL cholesterol is less predictable. In patients with high triglycerides, however, LDL cholesterol may increase. Fibrates increase the size and reduce the density of LDL particles much like niacin. KEY CONCEPT *Fibrates are the most effective triglyceride-lowering drugs and are used primarily in patients with elevated triglycerides and low HDL cholesterol.*

Fibrates work by activating peroxisome proliferator-activated receptor-alpha (PPAR-α), a nuclear receptor involved in cellular function. This results in a reduction in triglyceride-rich lipoproteins (VLDL and IDL) and an increase in HDL.

Clinical trials of fibrate therapy in patients with elevated cholesterol and no history of CHD demonstrated a reduction in CHD incidence, although less than the reduction attained with statin therapy.[43] In addition, a large study of men with CHD, low HDL cholesterol, low LDL cholesterol, and elevated triglycerides demonstrated a 24% reduction in risk of death from CHD, nonfatal myocardial infarction (MI), and stroke with gemfibrozil.[44] Fibrates may be appropriate in prevention of CHD events for patients with established CHD, low HDL cholesterol, and triglycerides below 200 mg/dL (2.26 mmol/L). However, LDL-lowering therapy with statins should be the primary target if non-HDL and LDL cholesterol are elevated. Evidence of a reduction in CHD risk among patients with established CHD has not been demonstrated with fenofibrate.

The fibric acid derivatives are generally well tolerated. The most common adverse effects include dyspepsia, abdominal pain, diarrhea, flatulence, rash, muscle pain, and fatigue (Table 12–11). Myopathy and rhabdomyolysis can occur, and the risk appears to increase with renal insufficiency or concurrent statin therapy. If a fibrate is used with a statin, fenofibrate is preferred because it appears to inhibit the glucuronidation of the statins less than gemfibrozil.[27,45] A CK level should be checked before therapy is started and if symptoms occur. Liver dysfunction has been reported, and LFTs should be monitored. Fibrates increase cholesterol in the bile and have caused gallbladder and bile duct disorders, such as cholelithiasis and cholecystitis. Unlike niacin, these agents do not increase glucose or uric acid levels. Fibrates are contraindicated in patients with gallbladder disease, liver dysfunction, or severe kidney dysfunction. The risk of bleeding is increased in patients taking both a fibrate and warfarin. The time until maximum effect on lipids is generally 2 weeks for fenofibrate and 3 to 4 weeks for gemfibrozil.

▶ Long-Chain Omega-3 Fatty Acids

Long-chain omega-3 fatty acids (eicosapentaenoic acid and docosahexaenoic acid), the predominant long-chain fatty acids in the oil of cold-water fish, lower triglycerides by as much as 45% (Table 12–10) when taken in large amounts (2–4 g). Long-chain omega-3 fatty acids may be useful for patients with high triglycerides despite diet and weight loss, alcohol restriction, and fibrate therapy. This effect may be modulated through reduction in hepatic synthesis and release of VLDL triglycerides, increased β-oxidation of fatty acids, and enhanced triglyceride clearance from triglyceride-rich lipoproteins. Long-chain omega-3 fatty acids have other cardiac effects such as reduced platelet aggregation and antiarrhythmic properties. The current AHA Scientific Statement on fish consumption, fish oil, omega-3 fatty acids and cardiovascular disease recommends an increased intake of omega-3 fatty acids in the diet.[46]

Prescription-grade long-chain omega-3 fatty acid ethyl esters and free fatty acid formulations are FDA approved at a dose of 2 to 4 g daily for the treatment of elevated triglycerides (greater than or equal to 500 mg/dL [5.65 mmol/L]). Use of high-quality omega-3 fatty acids free of contaminants such as mercury and organic pollutants should be encouraged when using these agents. Common side effects associated with long-chain omega-3 fatty acids are diarrhea and excess bleeding (Table 12–11). Patients taking anticoagulant or antiplatelet agents should be monitored more closely when consuming these products because excessive amounts of long-chain omega-3 fatty acids (eg, greater than 3 g daily) may lead to bleeding and may increase risk of hemorrhagic stroke.

▶ Microsomal Triglyceride Transport Inhibitors

Lomitapide is an oral inhibitor of microsomal triglyceride transfer protein, thereby inhibiting the normal transfer of triglycerides to Apo B in the lumen of the endoplasmic reticulum and preventing the assembly of Apo B–containing lipoproteins in enterocytes and hepatocytes.[13] Lomitapide reduces LDL cholesterol levels on average by 40% (Table 12–10) in homozygous FH patients on maximum tolerated lipid-lowering therapy and LDL apheresis. However, given its mechanism of action, GI side effects and elevation in liver enzymes and hepatic fat are common (Table 12–11). Because of the risk of hepatotoxicity, lomitapide is available only through the Risk Evaluation and Mitigation Strategy program (REMS) and is currently FDA approved for the management of patients with homozygous FH. Gastrointestinal side effects are managed by strict adherence to a low-fat diet (less than 20% of total calories from fat) and gradual dose escalation based on acceptable safety and tolerability. Lomitapide is metabolized extensively by the liver primarily by the cytochrome P-450 system. Lomitapide interacts with numerous agents such as strong and moderate cytochrome P-450 3A4 inhibitors, warfarin, lovastatin and simvastatin. Lomitapide is classified as Pregnancy Category X.

▶ Antisense Oligonucleotide Inhibitor of Apo B-100 Synthesis

Mipomersen is a once-weekly subcutaneous injectable antisense inhibitor of Apo B synthesis. When given in combination with maximum tolerated doses of lipid-lowering therapy, it can reduce LDL cholesterol by an additional 25% in homozygous FH patients (Table 12–10).[13] Injection site reactions, flu-like symptoms, hepatic fat, and liver enzyme elevations are common

(Table 12–11). Because of the risk of hepatotoxicity similar to lomitapide, mipomersen is available only through a REMS program. Mipomersen is not a substrate for cytochrome P-450 metabolism and is metabolized by endonucleases and exonucleases. Therefore, mipomersen has minimal clinically relevant drug–drug interactions. Mipomersen is Pregnancy Category B.

▶ *Investigational Agents*

Numerous investigational drugs are in development for the treatment of lipid disorders and the prevention of atherosclerosis. Many of these will likely be used in combination with currently available lipid-modulating drugs or in patients who are statin-intolerant. The most promising are the proprotein convertase subtilisin/kexin type 9 (PCSK9) inhibitors using monoclonal antibodies.[13] In clinical trials, these agents have produced an additional 50%–60% decrease in LDL levels when used in combination with statin therapy, compared with statin monotherapy. If shown to be safe and efficacious, it may make attainment of cholesterol goal levels practical for a greater fraction of patients with more severe forms of hypercholesterolemia. Alirocumab was recently the first in class to be approved by the FDA for use in adults with heterozygous familial hypercholesterolemia or ASCVD who require additional lowering of LDL cholesterol and are on a maximally tolerated statin. Evolocumab is the next PCSK9 inhibitor expected to be approved.

Combination Pharmacotherapy

A large proportion of the US population will not achieve their NLA-recommended cholesterol targets for a variety of reasons.[47] These include inadequate patient adherence, adverse events, inadequate starting doses, lack of dose escalation, and lower treatment targets.[31,48] Moreover, patients with concomitant elevations in triglycerides may need combination drug therapy to normalize their lipid profile. KEY CONCEPT *Combination drug therapy is an effective means to achieve greater reductions in non-HDL and LDL cholesterol (statin plus ezetimibe or bile acid resin, bile acid resin plus ezetimibe, or three-drug combinations) as well as lowering serum triglycerides (statin plus niacin, long-chain omega-3 fatty acids or fibrate).*

▶ *Combination Therapy for Elevated LDL Cholesterol*

For patients who do not achieve their non-HDL and LDL cholesterol goals with statin monotherapy and lifestyle modifications, including those unable to tolerate high doses due to adverse effects, combination therapy may be appropriate. Resins or ezetimibe combine effectively with statins to augment further cholesterol reduction. When added to a statin, ezetimibe can reduce LDL cholesterol levels by an additional 18% to 21% or up to 65% total reduction with maximum doses of the more potent statins. Ezetimibe and simvastatin or atorvastatin are available as a combination tablet and indicated as adjunctive therapy to diet for the reduction of elevated total cholesterol, LDL cholesterol, Apo B, triglycerides, and non-HDL cholesterol, and to increase HDL cholesterol. Adverse events are similar to those of each product taken separately; however, the percentage of patients with LFT elevations greater than three times normal is slightly higher than with a statin alone. The time until maximum effect on lipids for this combination is generally 2 to 6 weeks.

A statin combined with a resin results in similar reductions in LDL cholesterol as those seen with ezetimibe. However, the magnitude of triglyceride reduction is less with a resin compared with ezetimibe, and this should be considered in patients with higher baseline triglyceride levels. In addition, GI-adverse events and potential drug interactions limit the utility of this combination.

Ezetimibe and a resin can also be combined. A study that assessed the effects of adding ezetimibe to ongoing resin therapy showed an additional 19% reduction in LDL cholesterol and 14% reduction in triglycerides. This combination was well tolerated.[49]

Some patients, in particular those with genetic forms of hypercholesterolemia such as FH (Table 12–1), require three or more drugs to manage their disorder. It is recommended that patients with FH obtain a minimum of greater than or equal to 50% reduction in LDL cholesterol.[13,14]

▶ *Combination Therapy for Elevated Cholesterol and Triglyceridemia With or Without Low HDL Cholesterol*

Fibrates are the most effective triglyceride-lowering agents and also raise HDL cholesterol levels. Combination therapy with a fibrate, particularly gemfibrozil, and a statin has been found to increase the risk for myopathy. Therefore, more frequent monitoring, thorough patient education, and consideration of factors that increase risk as reviewed previously should be considered.

KEY CONCEPT *The evidence of reducing non-HDL and LDL cholesterol while substantially raising HDL cholesterol (statin plus niacin or fibrate) to reduce the risk of CHD related events to a greater degree than statin monotherapy remains in question.* A recent trial found the combination of fenofibrate and simvastatin did not reduce the overall rate of fatal cardiovascular events, nonfatal MI, or nonfatal stroke, as compared with simvastatin alone. However in a prespecified subgroup analysis, incremental benefits of adding a fenofibrate to simvastatin therapy were noted in patients with triglycerides greater than or equal to 204 mg/dL (2.31 mmol/L) and HDL cholesterol less than or equal to 34 mg/dL (0.88 mmol/L).[50] Combining niacin with a statin augments the non-HDL and LDL cholesterol lowering potential of niacin

Patient Encounter 2

A 43-year-old woman with type 2 diabetes and obesity (BMI: 32 kg/m^2) has been referred to you for a follow-up of her cholesterol. She is taking pravastatin 10 mg once daily in the evening for her cholesterol. Her blood glucose is 130 mg/dL (7.2 mmol/L). Her laboratory test results are within normal limits, except her albumin/creatinine ratio is 40 mg/g (4.5 mg/mmol). Her fasting lipid profile: total cholesterol 175 mg/dL (4.53 mmol/L), triglycerides 257 mg/dL (2.90 mmol/L), HDL cholesterol 43 mg/dL (1.11 mmol/L), non-HDL cholesterol 132 mg/dL (3.41 mmol/L), and LDL cholesterol 81 mg/dL (2.09 mmol/L).

What is your assessment of the patient's cholesterol results?

What diagnostic parameters does she have for metabolic syndrome?

What statin-benefit group does she fit according to the ACC/AHA guidelines?

Identify treatment goals for the patient based on the NLA guidelines.

Assess her risk for statin-induced side effects.

Design a treatment plan for the patient.

Patient Care Process

Patient Assessment:

- Obtain fasting cholesterol profile and assess any abnormal lipid levels.
- Assess for the presence of very high-risk or high-risk conditions (Table 12–7).
- Assess major risk factors for ASCVD (Table 12–8). Assign patient to risk category based on assessment and risk scoring as previously described (eg, Tables 12–7 and 12–9).
- Obtain a thorough history of prescription, nonprescription, and natural drug product use.
- Assess if taking any medications that may contribute to abnormal lipid levels (Table 12–2).
- Assess concomitant diseases that may contribute to abnormal lipid levels (Table 12–2).
- Assess risk factors for metabolic syndrome.

Therapy Evaluation:

- Determine what treatments for cholesterol the patient has used in the past (if any). If already receiving pharmacotherapy for dyslipidemia, assess efficacy, safety, and adherence. Are there any significant drug interactions?
- Determine treatment goal for non-HDL cholesterol and LDL cholesterol based on risk category (Table 12–7).

Care Plan Development:

- Discuss importance of family screening if patient has FH.
- Select TLCs and educate patient on importance of TLCs and regular physical activity (Table 12–6).
- Consider starting pharmacotherapy in very high-risk and high-risk patients.
- For patients with ASCVD or DM, consideration should be given to use of moderate or high-intensity statin therapy (Table 12–4), irrespective of baseline atherogenic cholesterol levels.
- Determine patient's prescription coverage.
- Assess potential disease and drug interactions that may affect choice or intensity of pharmacotherapy (Table 12–11).
- Provide patient education and address concerns associated with ASCVD, hyperlipidemia, drug therapy, and therapy adherence.

Follow-up Evaluation:

- Follow up at regular intervals to assess cholesterol levels, side effects, and adherence (Table 12–11).
- If not meeting treatment goals, assess adherence.
- For patients with FH, if it is not possible to attain desirable levels of atherogenic cholesterol levels, a reduction of at least 50% is recommended.
- Intensify TLC for those patients above cholesterol targets.
- Titrate therapy or add additional drug as needed.

while enhancing both the HDL cholesterol–raising effects and triglyceride-lowering effects of the statin. A statin combined with niacin appears to offer greater benefits for reducing atherosclerosis progression compared with a statin alone[33]; however, the incremental benefits on reducing CHD events remains in question.[40] Similar to fenofibrate, a subset of patients in both the highest triglyceride and lowest HDL cholesterol tertiles showed a trend toward benefit with addition of ER niacin. Formulations combining ER niacin and lovastatin (Advicor) and ER niacin and simvastatin (Simcor) are available, and they are indicated for treatment of primary hypercholesterolemia and mixed dyslipidemia. The time until maximum effect on lipids for this combination is generally 3 to 6 weeks.

Niacin can be combined with a fibrate in patients with high elevations in serum triglycerides. The combination may increase risk of myopathy compared with either agent alone.

Compared with monotherapy, combination therapy may reduce patient adherence through increased side effects and increased costs. When used appropriately and with proper precautions, however, combination therapy is effective in normalizing lipid abnormalities, particularly in patients who cannot tolerate adequate doses of statin therapy for more severe forms of dyslipidemia.

OUTCOME EVALUATION

- The successful outcome in cholesterol management is to reduce cholesterol and triglycerides below the NLA goals in an effort to alter the natural course of atherosclerosis and decrease future cardiovascular events and pancreatitis.
- Use an adequate trial of TLC in all patients, but institute pharmacotherapy concurrently in higher-risk patients.
  - For patients in whom lipid-lowering drug therapy is indicated, statin treatment is the primary modality for reducing ASCVD risk because of their ability to substantially reduce non-HDL and LDL cholesterol, ability to reduce morbidity and mortality from atherosclerotic disease, convenient once-daily dosing, availability of inexpensive generics, and low risk of side effects.
- Use an individualized patient monitoring plan in an effort to minimize side effects, maintain treatment adherence, and achieve lipid goals.

Abbreviations Introduced in This Chapter

ABI	Ankle brachial index
ACC	American College of Cardiology
AHA	American Heart Association
Apo	Apolipoprotein
ASCVD	Atherosclerotic cardiovascular disease
BAS	Bile acid sequestrant
CAC	Coronary artery calcium
CETP	Cholesterol ester transfer protein
CHD	Coronary heart disease

CK	Creatine kinase
DM	Diabetes mellitus
ER	Extended-release
FA	Fatty acid
FDA	Food and Drug Administration
FH	Familial hypercholesterolemia
GI	Gastrointestinal
HbA1c	Glycosylated hemoglobin
HDL	High-density lipoprotein
HMG-CoA	3-hydroxy-3-methylglutaryl coenzyme A
HL	Hepatic lipase
hs-CRP	High-sensitivity C-reactive protein
IDL	Intermediate-density lipoprotein
IR	Immediate-release
LDL	Low-density lipoprotein
LFT	Liver function test
LPL	Lipoprotein lipase
LRP	LDL-related protein
MI	Myocardial infarction
NCEP	National Cholesterol Education Program
NHLBI	National Heart, Lung, and Blood Institute
NLA	National Lipid Association
NPC1L1	Niemann-Pick C1 Like 1
NSAID	Nonsteroidal anti-inflammatory drug
PPAR-α	Peroxisome proliferator-activated receptor-alpha
PCSK9	Proprotein convertase subtilisin/kexin 9
REMS	Risk evaluation and mitigation strategy
SR	Sustained-release
SR-BI	Scavenger receptors
TLC	Therapeutic lifestyle changes
VLDL	Very low-density lipoprotein

REFERENCES

1. Kronmal RA, Cain KC, Ye Z, Omenn GS. Total serum cholesterol levels and mortality risk as a function of age. A report based on the Framingham data. Arch Intern Med. 1993;153:1065–1073.
2. Go AS, Mozaffarian D, Roger VL, et al. Heart disease and stroke statistics—2014 update: A report from the American Heart Association. Circulation. 2014 Jan 21;129(3):e28–e292.
3. Third Report of the National Cholesterol Education Program (NCEP) Expert Panel on Detection, Evaluation, and Treatment of High Blood Cholesterol in Adults (Adult Treatment Panel III) Final Report. Circulation. 2002;106(25):3143–3421.
4. Genest J. Lipoprotein disorders and cardiovascular risk. J Inherit Metab Dis. 2003;26:267–287.
5. Brown BG, Zhao XQ, Chait A, et al. Simvastatin and niacin, antioxidant vitamins, or the combination for the prevention of coronary disease. N Engl J Med. 2001;345:1583–1592.
6. Endo A. The discovery and development of HMG-CoA reductase inhibitors. J Lipid Res. 1992;33(11):1569–1582.
7. Brown MS, Faust JR, Goldstein JL, Kaneko I, et al. Induction of 3-hydroxy-3-methylglutaryl coenzyme A reductase activity in human fibroblasts incubated with compactin (ML-236B), a competitive inhibitor of the reductase. J Biol Chem. 1978 Feb 25;253(4):1121–1128.
8. Grundy SM, Cleeman JI, Bairey Merz CN, et al., for the Coordinating Committee of the National Cholesterol Education Program endorsed by the National Heart, Lung, and Blood Institute, American College of Cardiology Foundation, and American Heart Association. Update implications of recent clinical trials for the national cholesterol education program adult treatment panel III guidelines. Circulation. 2004;110:227–239.
9. Stone NJ, Robinson JG, Lichtenstein AH, et al. 2013 ACC/AHA guideline on the treatment of blood cholesterol to reduce atherosclerotic cardiovascular risk in adults: A report of the American College of Cardiology/American Heart Association Task Force on Practice Guidelines. J Am Coll Cardiol. 2014 Jul 1;63(25 Pt B):2889–2934.
10. Grundy SM, Arai H, Barter P, et al. An International Atherosclerosis Society position paper: global recommendations for the management of dyslipidemia: Executive summary. Atherosclerosis. 2014 Feb;232(2):410–413.
11. Catapano AL, Reiner Z, De Backer G, et al. ESC/EAS Guidelines for the management of dyslipidaemias: The Task Force for the management of dyslipidaemias of the European Society of Cardiology (ESC) and the European Atherosclerosis Society (EAS). Atherosclerosis. 2011 Jul;217(1):3–46.
12. Anderson TJ, Grégoire J, Hegele RA, et al. 2012 update of the Canadian Cardiovascular Society guidelines for the diagnosis and treatment of dyslipidemia for the prevention of cardiovascular disease in the adult. Can J Cardiol. 2013 Feb;29(2):151–167.
13. Jacobson TA, Ito MK, Maki KC, et al. National Lipid Association recommendations for patient-centered management of dyslipidemia: Part 1 - executive summary. J Clin Lipidol. 2014 Sep-Oct;8(5):473–488.
14. Goldberg AC, Hopkins PN, Toth PP, et al. Familial hypercholesterolemia: Screening, diagnosis and management of pediatric and adult patients: Clinical guidance from the National Lipid Association Expert Panel on Familial Hypercholesterolemia. J Clin Lipidol. 2011;5(3):133–140.
15. Ridker PM, Danielson E, Fonseca FA, et al. Rosuvastatin to prevent vascular events in men and women with elevated C-reactive protein. N Engl J Med. 2008;359(21):2195–2207.
16. Shepherd J, Cobbe SM, Ford I, et al., for The West of Scotland Coronary Prevention Study Group. Prevention of coronary heart disease with pravastatin in men with hypercholesterolemia. N Engl J Med. 1995;333:1301–1307.
17. Sever PS, Dahlof B, Poulter NR, et al. Prevention of coronary and stroke events with atorvastatin in hypertensive patients who have average or lower-than-average cholesterol concentrations, in the Anglo-Scandinavian Cardiac Outcomes Trial—Lipid-Lowering Arm (ASCOT-LLA): A multicentre randomised controlled trial. Lancet. 2003;361:1149–1158.
18. The ALLHAT Officers and Coordinators for the ALLHAT Collaborative Research Group. Major outcomes in moderately hypercholesterolemia, hypertensive patients randomized to pravastatin vs usual care: The Antihypertensive and Lipid-Lowering Treatment to Prevent Heart Attack Trial (ALLHAT-LLT). JAMA. 2002;288:2998–3007.
19. Calhoun HM, Betteridge DJ, Durrington PN, et al. Primary prevention of cardiovascular disease with atorvastatin in type 2 diabetes in the Collaborative Atorvastatin Diabetes Study (CARDS): Multicentre randomised placebo-controlled trial. Lancet. 2004;364:685–696.
20. Scandinavian Simvastatin Survival Study Group. Randomised trial of cholesterol lowering in 4444 patients with coronary heart disease: The Scandinavian Simvastatin Survival Study (4S). Lancet. 1994; 344:1383–1389.
21. Sacks FM, Pfeffer MA, Moye LA, et al., for the Cholesterol and Recurrent Events Trial Investigators. The effect of pravastatin on coronary events after myocardial infarction in patients with average cholesterol levels. Cholesterol and Recurrent Events Trial investigators. N Engl J Med. 1996;335:1001–1009.
22. Heart Protection Study Collaborative Group. MRC/BHF Heart Protection Study of cholesterol lowering with simvastatin in 20,536 high-risk individuals: A randomized placebo-controlled trial. Lancet. 2002;360(9326):7–22.
23. The Long-Term Intervention with Pravastatin in Ischemic Disease (LIPID) Study Group. Prevention of cardiovascular events and death with pravastatin in patients with coronary heart disease and a broad range of initial cholesterol levels. N Engl J Med. 1998;399(19):1349–1357.

24. Cannon CP, Braunwald E, McCabe CH, et al. Intensive versus moderate lipid-lowering with statins after acute coronary syndromes. N Engl J Med. 2004;350:1495–1504.
25. LaRosa JC, Grundy SM, Waters DD, et al. Treating to New Targets (TNT) Investigators. Intensive lipid lowering with atorvastatin in patients with stable coronary disease. N Engl J Med. 2005;352:1425–1435.
26. Downs JR, Clearfield M, Weis S, et al., for the AFCAPS/TexCAPS Research Group. Primary prevention of acute coronary events with lovastatin in men and women with average cholesterol levels: Results of AFCAPS/TexCAPS. JAMA. 1998;270:1615–1622.
27. Pasternak RC, Smith SC, Jr, Bairey-Merz CN, et al. ACC/AHA/NHLBI clinical advisory on the use and safety of statins. J Am Coll Cardiol. 2002;40:568–573.
28. Staffa JA, Chang J, Green L. Cerivastatin and reports of fatal rhabdomyolysis. New Engl J Med. 2002;346(7):539–540.
29. Kastelein JJ, Akdim F, Stroes ES, et al. Simvastatin with or without ezetimibe in familial hypercholesterolemia. N Engl J Med. 2008;358(14):1431–1443.
30. Rossebø AB, Pedersen TR, Boman K, et al. Intensive lipid lowering with simvastatin and ezetimibe in aortic stenosis. N Engl J Med. 2008;359:1343–1356.
31. Baigent C, Landray MJ, Reith C, et al. The effects of lowering LDL cholesterol with simvastatin plus ezetimibe in patients with chronic kidney disease (Study of Heart and Renal Protection): A randomised placebo-controlled trial. Lancet. 2011;377(9784):2181–2192.
32. The Lipid Research Clinics Coronary Primary Prevention Trial results. II. The relationship of reduction in incidence of coronary heart disease to cholesterol lowering. JAMA. 1984;251:365–374.
33. Sankyo Pharma, Inc. Welchol [prescribing information]. Parsippany, NJ: Author. 2011.
34. Meyers CD, Carr MC, Park S, et al. Varying cost and free nicotinic acid content in over-the-counter niacin preparations for dyslipidemia. Ann Intern Med. 2003;139:996–1002.
35. McKenney JM, Proctor JD, Harris S, et al. A comparison of the efficacy and toxic effects of sustained- vs immediate-release niacin in hypercholesterolemic patients. JAMA. 1994;271:672–677.
36. Dunatchik AP, Ito MK, Dujovne CA. A systematic review on evidence of the effectiveness and safety of a wax-matrix niacin formulation J Clin Lipidol. 2012;6:121–131.
37. Canner PL, Berge GK, Wender NK, et al. Fifteen-year mortality in Coronary Drug Project patients: Long-term benefit with niacin. J Am Coll Cardiol. 1986;18:1245–1255.
38. Taylor AJ, Sullenberger LE, Lee HJ, et al. Arterial biology for the investigation of the treatment effects of reducing cholesterol (ARBITER) 2. A double-blind, placebo-controlled study of extended-release niacin on atherosclerosis progression in secondary prevention patients treated with statins. Circulation. 2004;110:3512–3517.
39. AIM-HIGH Investigators, Boden WE, Probstfield JL, Anderson T, et al. Niacin in patients with low HDL cholesterol levels receiving intensive statin therapy. N Engl J Med. 2011 Dec 15; 365(24):2255–2267.
40. HPS2-THRIVE Collaborative Group, Landray MJ, Haynes R, Hopewell JC, et al. Effects of extended-release niacin with laropiprant in high-risk patients. N Engl J Med. 2014 Jul 17; 371(3):203–212.
41. Bays HE, Dujovne CA, McGovern ME, et al. ADvicor versus Other Cholesterol-Modulating Agents Trial Evaluation. Comparison of once-daily, niacin extended-release/lovastatin with standard doses of atorvastatin and simvastatin (the ADvicor versus Other Cholesterol-Modulating Agents Trial Evaluation [ADVOCATE]). Am J Cardiol. 2003;91(6):667–672.
42. Canner PL, Furberg CD, Terrin ML, et al. Benefits of niacin by glycemic status in patients with healed myocardial infarction (from the Coronary Drug Project). Am J Cardiol. 2005;95: 254–257.
43. Frick MH, Elo O, Haapa K, et al. Helsinki Heart Study: Primary prevention trial with gemfibrozil in middle aged men with dyslipidemia. Safety of treatment, changes in risk factors, and incidence of coronary heart disease. N Engl J Med. 1987;317:1237–1245.
44. Robins SJ, Collins D, Wittes JT, et al., for the VA-HIT Study Group. Veterans Affairs High-Density Lipoprotein Intervention Trial. Relation of gemfibrozil treatment and lipid levels with major coronary events: VA-HIT: A randomized controlled trial. JAMA. 2001;285(12):1585–1591.
45. Prueksaritanont T, Zhao JJ, Ma B, et al. Mechanistic studies on metabolic interactions between gemfibrozil and statins. J Pharmacol Exp Ther. 2002;301(3):1042–1051.
46. Kris-Etherton PM, Harris WS, Appel LJ, for the Nutrition Committee: Fish consumption, fish oil, omega-3 fatty acids, and cardiovascular disease. Circulation. 2002;106:2747–2757.
47. Pearson TA, Laurora I, Chu H, et al. The lipid treatment assessment project (L-TAP): A multicenter survey to evaluate the percentages of dyslipidemic patients receiving lipid-lowering therapy and achieving low-density lipoprotein cholesterol goals. Arch Intern Med. 2000;160:459–467.
48. Ito MK, Lin JC, Morreale AP, et al. Effect of pravastatin-to-simvastatin conversion on reducing low-density lipoprotein cholesterol. Am J Health Syst Pharm. 2001;58:1734–1739.
49. Xydakis AM, Guyton JR, Chiou P, et al. Effectiveness and tolerability of ezetimibe add-on therapy to a bile acid resin-based regimen for hypercholesterolemia. Am J Cardiol. 2004;94(6): 795–797.
50. The ACCORD Study Group. Effects of combination lipid therapy in type 2 diabetes mellitus. N Engl J Med. 2010;362(17): 1563–1574.

13 Hypovolemic Shock

Bradley A. Boucher and G. Christopher Wood

LEARNING OBJECTIVES

Upon completion of the chapter, the reader will be able to:

1. List the most common etiologies of decreased intravascular volume in hypovolemic shock patients.
2. Describe the major hemodynamic and metabolic abnormalities that occur in patients with hypovolemic shock.
3. Describe the clinical presentation including signs, symptoms, and laboratory test measurements for the typical hypovolemic shock patient.
4. Prepare a treatment plan with clearly defined outcome criteria for a hypovolemic shock patient that includes both fluid management and pharmacologic therapy.
5. Compare and contrast relative advantages and disadvantages of crystalloids, colloids, and blood products in the treatment of hypovolemic shock.
6. Formulate a stepwise monitoring strategy for a hypovolemic shock patient

INTRODUCTION

The primary function of the circulatory system is to supply oxygen and vital metabolic compounds to cells throughout the body, as well as removal of metabolic waste products. Circulatory shock is a life-threatening condition whereby this principal function is compromised resulting in inadequate cellular oxygen utilization.[1,2] When circulatory shock is caused by a severe loss of blood volume or body water, it is called hypovolemic shock. KEY CONCEPT *Regardless of etiology, the most distinctive clinical manifestations of hypovolemic shock are arterial hypotension, clinical signs of hypoperfusion, and metabolic acidosis.*[2] *Metabolic acidosis is a consequence of an accumulation of lactic acid resulting from tissue hypoxia and anaerobic metabolism. If the decrease in arterial blood pressure (BP) is severe and protracted, such hypotension will inevitably lead to severe hypoperfusion and organ dysfunction.* Rapid and effective restoration of circulatory homeostasis using fluids, pharmacologic agents, and/or blood products is imperative to prevent complications of untreated shock and ultimately death.

ETIOLOGY AND EPIDEMIOLOGY

Practitioners must have a good understanding of cardiovascular physiology to diagnose, treat, and monitor circulatory problems in critically ill patients. The interrelationships among the major hemodynamic variables are depicted in Figure 13–1.[3] These variables include arterial BP, cardiac output (CO), systemic vascular resistance (SVR), heart rate (HR), stroke volume (SV), left ventricular size, afterload, myocardial contractility, and preload. Although an oversimplification, Figure 13–1 is beneficial in conceptualizing where the major abnormalities occur in patients with circulatory shock as well as predicting the body's compensatory responses.

Hypovolemic shock is caused by a loss of intravascular volume either by hemorrhage or fluid loss (eg, dehydration). In essence, there is a profound deficit in preload, defined as the volume in the left ventricle at the end of diastole. Decreased preload results in subsequent decreases in SV, CO, and eventually, mean arterial pressure (MAP). As such, restoration of preload becomes an overarching goal in the management of hypovolemic shock.

The prognosis of shock patients depends on several variables, including severity, duration, underlying etiology, preexisting organ dysfunction, and reversibility.[4] Data are not readily available on the incidence of hypovolemic shock, although hypovolemia due to hemorrhage is a major factor in 40% to 50% of trauma deaths annually.[5]

PATHOPHYSIOLOGY

The total amount of water in a typical 70-kg (154-lb) adult is approximately 42 L (Figure 13–2). About 28 of the 42 L are inside the cells of the body (intracellular fluid); the remaining 14 L are in the extracellular fluid space (fluid outside of cells, ie, interstitial fluid and plasma). Circulating blood volume for a normal adult is roughly 5 L (70 mL/kg) and is composed of 2 L of red blood cell fluid (intracellular) and 3 L of plasma (extracellular).

KEY CONCEPT *By definition, hypovolemic shock occurs as a consequence of inadequate intravascular volume to meet the oxygen and metabolic needs of the body.* Diminished intravascular volume can result from severe external or internal bleeding, profound fluid losses from gastrointestinal (GI) sources such as diarrhea or vomiting, or urinary losses such as diuretic use, diabetic ketoacidosis, or diabetes insipidus (Table 13–1).[1] Other sources of intravascular fluid loss can occur through damaged skin, as seen with burns, or via capillary leak into the interstitial space or peritoneal

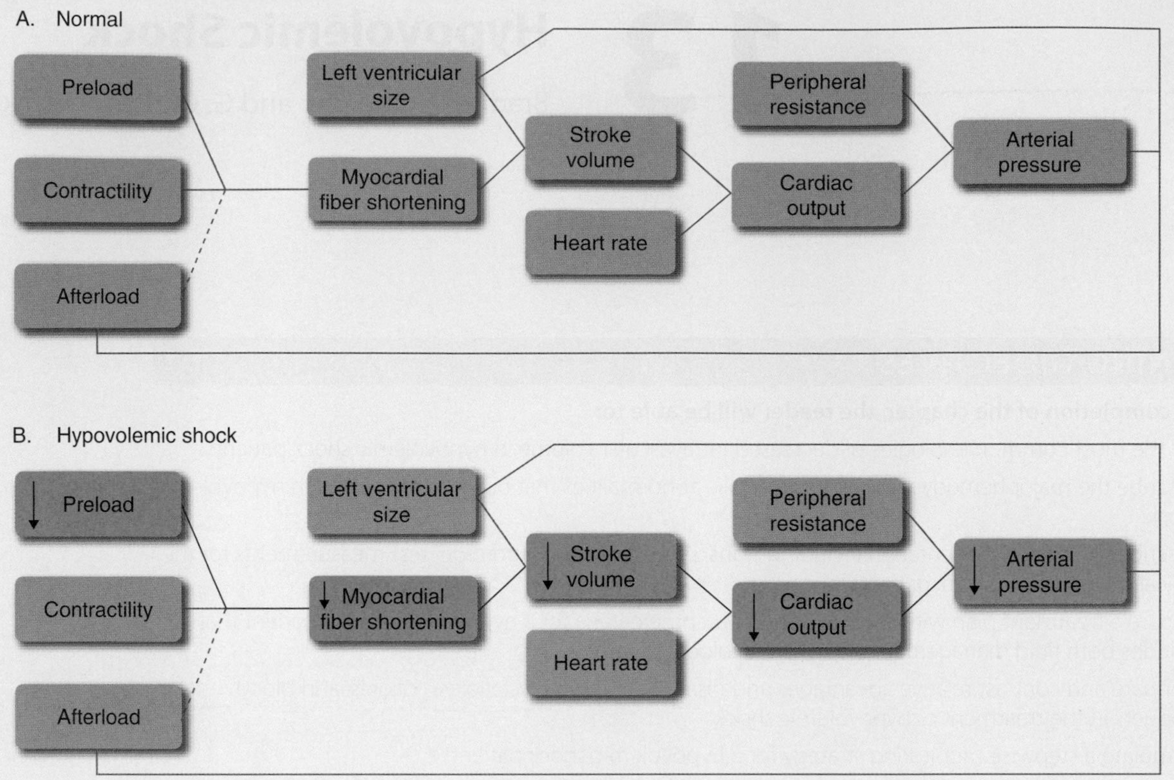

FIGURE 13–1. Hemodynamic relationships among key cardiovascular parameters (A). Solid lines represent a direct relationship; the broken line represents an inverse relationship. In (B), the alterations typically observed in hypovolemic shock are highlighted with arrows depicting the likely direction of the alteration. (Panel A from Braunwald E. Regulation of the circulation. I. N Engl J Med. 1974;290:1124–1129, with permission.)

cavity, as seen with edema or ascites. This latter phenomenon is often referred to as **third spacing** because fluid accumulates in the interstitial space disproportionately to the intracellular and extracellular fluid spaces. Regional ischemia may also develop as blood flow is naturally shunted from organs such as the GI tract or the kidneys to more immediately vital organs such as the heart and brain.

Hypovolemic shock symptoms begin to occur with decreases in intravascular volume in excess of 750 to 1500 mL (about 1.5–3 pints) or 15% to 30% of the circulating blood volume (20–40 mL/kg in pediatric patients).[6] Decreases in preload result in decreases in SV. Initially, CO may be partially maintained by compensatory tachycardia. Similarly, reflex increases in SVR and myocardial contractility may diminish arterial hypotension. Regardless, rapid losses (eg, minutes) undoubtedly have more profound effects than losses over a longer period (eg, hours). This neurohumoral response to hypovolemia is mediated by the sympathetic nervous system in an attempt to preserve perfusion to vital organs such as the heart and brain. Two major end points of this response are to conserve water to maximize intravascular volume and to improve tissue perfusion by increasing BP and CO (oxygen delivery). The body attempts to maximize its fluid status by decreasing water and sodium excretion through release of antidiuretic hormone (ADH), aldosterone, and cortisol. BP is maintained by peripheral vasoconstriction mediated by catecholamine release and the renin-angiotensin system.[1] CO is augmented by catecholamine release and fluid retention.[1,7] Unfortunately, the increased sympathetic drive may become detrimental as tissue ischemia occurs with inconsistent microcirculatory flow.[1] Regardless, when intravascular volume losses exceed 1500 mL (about 3 pints), the compensatory mechanisms are inadequate, typically resulting in a fall in CO and arterial BP; acute losses greater than 2000 mL (about 4 pints) are life threatening (35 mL/kg in pediatric patients).[8] The decrease in CO results in a diminished delivery of oxygen to tissues within the body and activation of an acute inflammatory response.[1,5] Oxygen delivery can be further compromised by inadequate blood hemoglobin levels due to hemorrhage and/or diminished hemoglobin saturation due to impaired ventilation. Decreased delivery of oxygen and other vital nutrients results in diminished production of the energy substrate, adenosine triphosphate (ATP). Lactic acid is then produced as a by-product of anaerobic metabolism within tissues throughout the body.[7] Hyperglycemia produced during the stress response from cortisol release is also a contributing factor in the development of lactic acidosis. Lactic acidosis indicates that inadequate tissue perfusion has occurred.[7]

KEY CONCEPT *Protracted tissue hypoxia sets in motion a downward spiral of events leading to organ dysfunction and eventual failure if untreated.* Table 13–2 describes the effects of shock on the body's major organs. Relative failure of more than one organ is

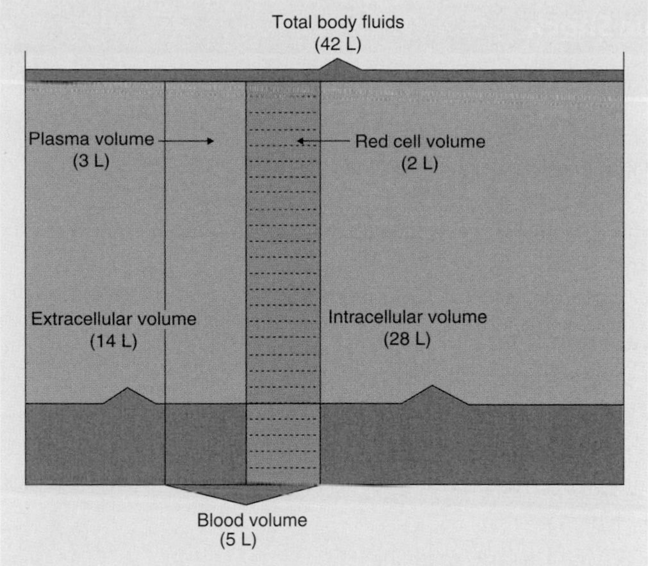

FIGURE 13–2. Distribution of body fluids showing the extracellular fluid volume, intracellular body fluid volume, and total body fluids in a 70-kg (154-lb) adult. Extracellular volume (ECV) comprises 14 L of total body fluid (42 L). Plasma volume makes up approximately 3 L of the 14 L of ECV. Intracellular volume accounts for the remaining 28 L of total body fluids, with roughly 2 L located within the red blood cells. Blood volume (~5 L) is also depicted and made up of primarily red blood cells and plasma. (From Guyton AC, Hall JE. Textbook of Medical Physiology, 8th ed. Philadelphia, PA: Saunders, 1991:275, with permission.)

referred to as the multiple organ dysfunction syndrome (MODS). Involvement of the heart is particularly devastating considering the central role it plays in oxygen delivery and the potential for myocardial dysfunction to perpetuate the shock state. Preexisting organ dysfunction and buildup of inflammatory mediators can also exacerbate the effects of hypovolemic shock to the point of irreversibility.[5] For example, acute or chronic heart failure can lead to pulmonary edema, further aggravating gas exchange in the lungs and ultimately tissue hypoxia. Only about one-third of early-onset MODS is quickly reversible (within 48 hours) with proper fluid resuscitation. Thus it is imperative that hypovolemic shock be treated quickly to avoid MODS.[9]

Table 13–1

Major Hypovolemic Shock Etiologies[1,2]

I. Hemorrhagic
- Trauma
- GI bleeding
- Abdominal aortic aneurysm

II. Nonhemorrhagic (dehydration)
- Vomiting
- Diarrhea
- Third spacing
- Burns
- Fistulae

GI, gastrointestinal.

Table 13–2

Hypovolemic Shock Manifestations on Major Organs

Heart
- Myocardial ischemia
- Dysrhythmias

Brain
- Restlessness, confusion, obtundation
- Global cerebral ischemia

Liver
- Release of liver enzymes
- Biliary stasis

Lungs
- Pulmonary edema
- ARDS

Kidneys
- Oliguria
- Decreased glomerular filtration
- Acute kidney injury

GI tract
- Stress-related mucosal disease
- Bacterial translocation

Hematologic
- Thrombocytopenia
- Coagulopathies

ARDS, acute respiratory distress syndrome; GI, gastrointestinal.

TREATMENT

Desired Outcomes

KEY CONCEPT *The major goals in treating hypovolemic shock are to restore effective circulating blood volume, as well as manage its underlying cause.* In achieving this goal, the downward spiral of events that can perpetuate severe or protracted hypovolemic shock is interrupted. This is accomplished through the delivery of adequate oxygen and metabolic substrates such as glucose and electrolytes to the tissues throughout the body that will optimally bring about a restoration of organ function and return to homeostasis. Evidence of the latter is a return to the patient's baseline vital signs, relative normalization of laboratory test results, and alleviation of other signs and symptoms of hypovolemic shock previously discussed. Concurrent supportive therapies are also warranted to avoid exacerbation of organ dysfunction associated with the hypovolemic shock event.

General Approach to Therapy

Securing an adequate airway and ventilation is imperative in hypovolemic shock patients consistent with the "VIP Rule" of resuscitation: Ventilate (oxygen administration), Infuse (fluid resuscitation, and Pump (administration of vasoactive agent).[2] Any compromise in ventilation only accentuates the tissue hypoxia occurring secondary to inadequate perfusion. Thus, early sedation with tracheal intubation and mechanical ventilation typically occurs at this stage of resuscitation (Figure 13–3). Intravenous (IV) access is also essential for administration of fluids and medications that can be facilitated through the placement of peripheral IV lines or catheterization with central venous lines if rapid or large volumes of resuscitative fluids are indicated. Placement of an arterial catheter is advantageous to allow for accurate and continual monitoring of BP, as well as

Clinical Presentation and Diagnosis of Hypovolemic Shock

General

Patients will be in acute distress, although symptoms and signs will vary depending on the severity of the hypovolemia and whether the etiology is hemorrhagic versus nonhemorrhagic.

Symptoms

- Thirst
- Weakness
- Light-headedness

Signs

- Hypotension, arterial SBP less than 90 mm Hg or fall in SBP greater than 40 mm Hg
- Tachycardia
- Tachypnea
- Hypothermia
- Oliguria
- Dark, yellow-colored urine
- Skin color: pale to ashen; may be cyanotic in severe cases
- Skin temperature: cool to cold
- Mental status: confusion to coma
- Pulmonary artery (PA) catheter measurements: decreased CO, decreased SV, increased SVR, low pulmonary artery occlusion pressure (PAOP)
- Organ dysfunction (see Table 13–2)

Laboratory Tests

- Increased serum lactate
- Decreased arterial pH
- Decreased hemoglobin/hematocrit (hemorrhagic hypovolemic shock)
- Hypernatremia
- Elevated serum creatinine (SCr)
- Elevated blood urea nitrogen
- Hyperglycemia

arterial blood gas (ABG) sampling. A bladder catheter should be inserted for ongoing monitoring of urine output. Baseline laboratory tests that should be done immediately include complete blood cell count with differential, serum chemistry profile, liver enzymes, prothrombin and partial thromboplastin times, and serum lactate. A urinalysis and an ABG should also be obtained, and ongoing electrocardiogram (ECG) monitoring should be performed. In addition to restoring circulating blood volume, it is necessary to prevent further losses from the vascular space. This is especially true with hemorrhagic hypovolemic shock where identifying the bleeding site and achievement of hemostasis are critical in the successful resuscitation of the patient. This frequently involves surgical treatment of hemorrhages.

Upon stabilization, placement of a pulmonary artery (PA) catheter may be indicated based on the need for more extensive cardiovascular monitoring than is available from noninvasive measurements such as vital signs, cardiac rhythm, and urine output.[10,11] Key measured parameters obtained from a PA catheter are the pulmonary artery occlusion pressure (PAOP), which is a measure of left ventricular preload, and CO. From the CO values and simultaneous measurement of HR and BP, one can calculate the left ventricular SV and SVR.[11] Placement of a PA catheter should be reserved for patients at high risk of death due to the severity of shock or preexisting medical conditions such as heart failure.[12] An alternative to the PA catheter is placement of a central venous catheter that typically resides in the superior vena cava to monitor central venous pressure (CVP). Although central venous catheters are less expensive and more readily placed, they are not particularly accurate in monitoring effective fluid resuscitation.[11]

▸ *Fluid Therapy*

The use of fluids is the cornerstone of managing hypovolemic shock.[1,2] KEY CONCEPT *Three major therapeutic options are available to clinicians for restoring circulating blood volume: crystalloids (electrolyte-based solutions), colloids (large molecular weight solutions), and blood products.*[13] Blood products are used only in instances involving hemorrhage (or severe preexisting anemia), thus leaving crystalloids and colloids as the mainstay of therapy in all types of hypovolemic shock, along with adjunctive vasopressor support. The aggressiveness of fluid resuscitation (rate and volume) is driven by the severity of the hypovolemic shock and the underlying cause. Warming of all fluids to 37°C (98.6°F) prior to administration is an important consideration to prevent hypothermia, arrhythmias, and coagulopathy because these complications will have a negative impact on the success of the resuscitation effort.[14]

Crystalloids Conventional "balanced" crystalloids are fluids with (a) electrolyte composition that approximates plasma, such as lactated Ringer (LR), or (b) a total calculated osmolality similar to that of plasma (280–295 mOsm/kg or mmol/kg), such

Patient Encounter, Part 1

A 65-year-old woman is admitted to the trauma center after a robbery attempt in which she received two gunshot wounds; one to her right hip and one to her right thigh. The patient cannot reliably communicate with the healthcare team because she is confused and agitated. The initial diagnosis by the trauma team is hypovolemic shock. A physical examination is being performed and blood samples are being sent to the laboratory.

What type of hypovolemic shock does the patient likely have and what is the cause?

What signs and symptoms would you expect to see in this patient with hypovolemic shock?

What laboratory abnormalities might be expected in this patient?

Describe the first nonpharmacologic steps in treating the patient.

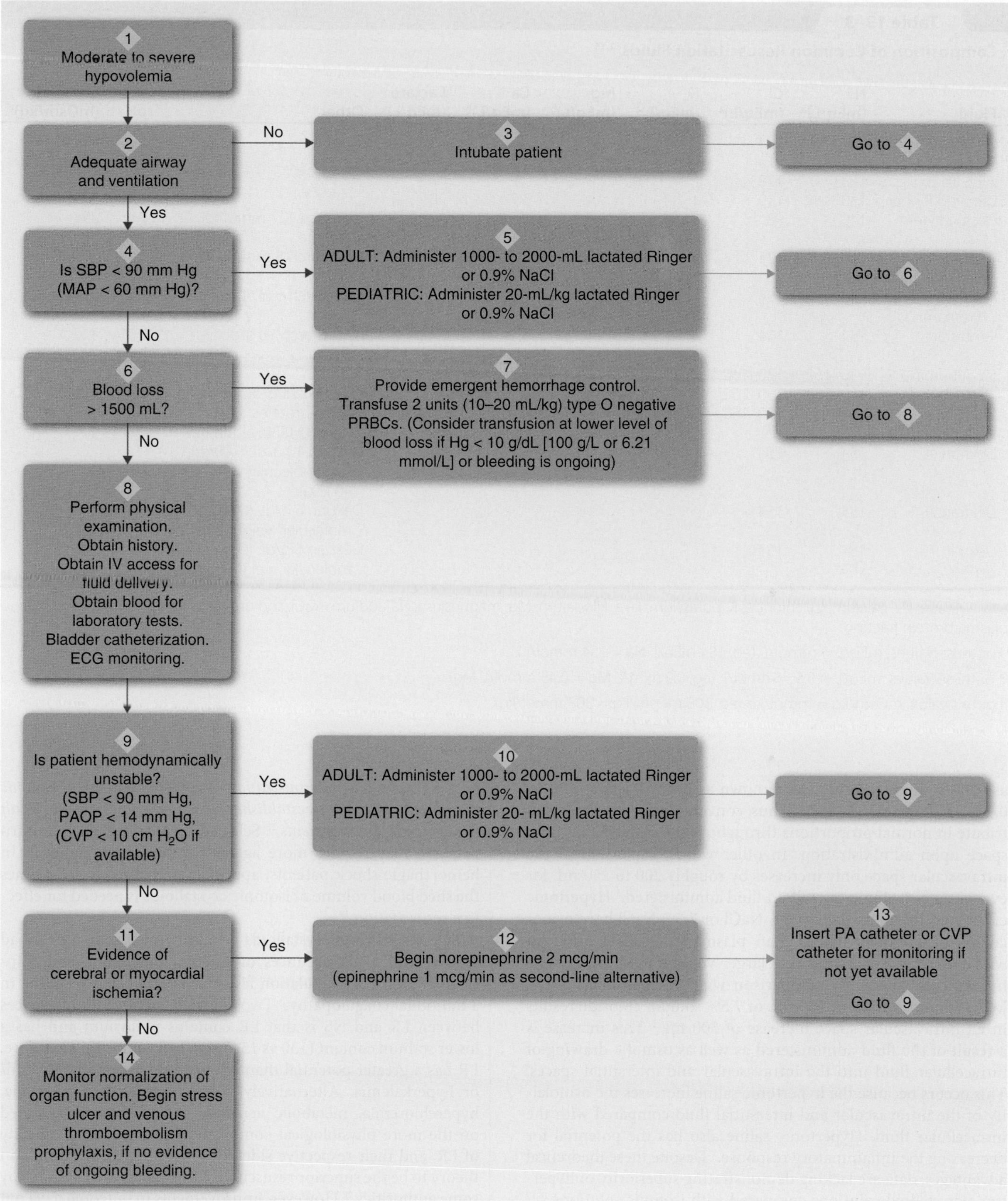

FIGURE 13–3. Treatment algorithm for the management of moderate to severe hypovolemia. (CVP, central venous pressure; ECG, electrocardiogram; Hg, hemoglobin; IV, intravenous; MAP, mean arterial pressure; NaCl, sodium chloride or normal saline; PA, pulmonary artery; PAOP, pulmonary artery occlusion pressure; PRBCs, packed red blood cells; SBP, systolic blood pressure.) Hemoglobin concentration of 10 g/dL is equivalent to 100 g/L or 6.2 mmol/L.

Table 13–3

Composition of Common Resuscitation Fluids[13,15]

Fluid	Na (mEq/L)[a]	Cl (mEq/L)[a]	K (mEq/L)[a]	Mg (mEq/L)[b]	Ca (mEq/L)[b]	Lactate (mEq/L)[a]	Other	pH	Osmolality (mOsm/kg)[c]
0.9% NaCl	154	154						5.0	308
3% NaCl	513	513						5.0	1027
7.5% NaCl	1283	1283						5.0	2567
Lactated Ringer	130	109	4		3	28		6.5	273
Plasma-Lyte A	140	98	5	3			27 mEq/L (27 mmol/L) Acetate	7.4	294
Hetastarch (Hextend)	143	124	3	0.9	5	28	Hetastarch 6 g/dL (60 g/L)	5.9	307
Hetastarch (Hespan)	154	154					Hetastarch 6 g/dL (60 g/L)	5.5	310
Pentastarch	154	154					Pentastarch 10 g/dL (100 g/L)	5.0	326
5% Albumin	130–160	130–160					Albumin 5 g/dL (50 g/L)	6.9	
25% Albumin	130–160	130–160					Albumin 25 g/dL (250 g/L)	6.9	
5% PPF	130–160	130–160	0.25				Plasma proteins 5 g/dL (50 g/L) (88% albumin)	7.0	
Dextran 40	154	154					Dextran 10 g/dL (100 g/L) (avg molecular weight 40 kDa)		
Dextran 70	154	154					Dextran 6 g/dL (60 g/L) (avg molecular weight 70 kDa)	5.5	308
Dextran 75	154	154					Dextran 6 g/dL (60 g/L) (avg molecular weight 75 kDa)	5.5	308

avg, average; Ca, calcium; Cl, chloride; K, potassium; kDa, kilodalton; Mg, magnesium; Na, sodium; NaCl, sodium chloride or normal saline; PPF, plasma protein fraction.

[a]For these values, mEq/L = mmol/L (eg, 154 mEq/L Na = 154 mmol/L).

[b]For these values, mEq/L × 0.5 = mmol/L (eg, 0.9 mEq/L Mg = 0.45 mmol/L Mg).

[c]For this value, mOsm/kg = mmol/kg (eg, 308 mOsm/kg = 308 mmol/kg).

as 0.9% sodium chloride (also known as normal saline [NS] or 0.9% NaCl) (Table 13–3).[13,15] Thus, conventional crystalloids distribute in normal proportions throughout the extracellular fluid space upon administration. In other words, expansion of the intravascular space only increases by roughly 200 to 250 mL for every liter of isotonic crystalloid fluid administered.[5] Hypertonic crystalloid solutions such as 3% NaCl or 7.5% NaCl have osmolalities substantially higher than plasma. The effect observed with these fluids is a relatively larger volume expansion of the intravascular space. By comparison with conventional crystalloids, administration of 250 mL of 7.5% sodium chloride results in an intravascular space increase of 500 mL.[5] This increase is a result of the fluid administered as well as osmotic drawing of intracellular fluid into the intravascular and interstitial spaces. This occurs because the hypertonic saline increases the osmolality of the intravascular and interstitial fluid compared with the intracellular fluid. Hypertonic saline also has the potential for decreasing the inflammatory response.[1] Despite these theoretical advantages, data are lacking demonstrating superiority of hypertonic crystalloid solutions compared with isotonic solutions.[16,17] Crystalloids are generally advocated as the initial resuscitation fluid in hypovolemic shock because of their availability, low cost, and equivalent outcomes compared with colloids.[10] A reasonable initial volume of an isotonic crystalloid (0.9% NaCl or LR) in adult patients is 1000 to 2000 mL administered over the first hour of therapy.[6] Ongoing external or internal bleeding requires more aggressive fluid resuscitation. KEY CONCEPT *In the absence of ongoing blood loss, administration of 2000 to 4000 mL of isotonic crystalloid normally reestablishes baseline vital signs in adult hypovolemic shock patients.*[18] Selected populations, such as burn patients, may require more aggressive fluid resuscitation.[19] In hemorrhagic shock patients, approximately three to four times the shed blood volume of isotonic crystalloids is needed for effective resuscitation.[19]

Side effects from crystalloids primarily involve fluid overload and electrolyte disturbances of sodium, potassium, and chloride.[1] Dilution of coagulation factors can also occur resulting in a dilutional coagulopathy.[5] Two clinically significant differences between LR and NS is that LR contains potassium and has a lower sodium content (130 vs 154 mEq/L or mmol/L). Therefore, LR has a greater potential than NS to cause hyponatremia and/or hyperkalemia. Alternatively, NS can cause hypernatremia, hyperchloremia, metabolic acidosis, and hypokalemia. Based on the more physiological composition and buffering capacity of LR, and their respective side-effect profiles, LR is deemed in theory to be the superior resuscitative fluid compared with NS by some authorities.[20] However, improvements in outcome have not been documented.[21]

Colloids Understanding the effects of colloid administration on circulating blood volume necessitates a review of those physiological forces that determine fluid movement between capillaries and the interstitial space throughout the circulation (Figure 13–4).[5,22] Relative hydrostatic pressure between the capillary lumen and the interstitial space is one of the major

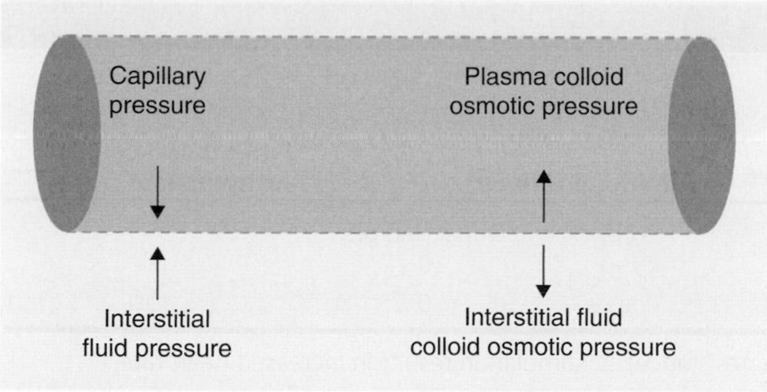

FIGURE 13–4. Operative forces at the capillary membrane tend to move fluid either outward or inward through the capillary membrane. In hypovolemic shock, one therapeutic strategy is the administration of colloids that can sustain and/or draw fluid from the interstitial space by increasing the plasma colloid osmotic pressure. (From Guyton AC, Hall JE. Textbook of Medical Physiology, 8th ed. Philadelphia, PA: Saunders, 1991:174, with permission.)

determinants of net fluid flow in or out of the circulation. The other major determinant is the relative colloid osmotic pressure between the two spaces (ie, oncotic pressure). Administration of exogenous colloids results in an increase in the intravascular colloid osmotic pressure. The effects of colloids on intravascular volume are a consequence of their relatively large molecular size (greater than 30 kDa), limiting their passage across the capillary membrane in large amounts. Alternately stated, colloids can be conceptualized as "sponges" drawing fluid into the intravascular space from the interstitial space. In the case of isosmotic colloids (5% albumin, 6% hetastarch, and dextran products), initial expansion of the intravascular space is essentially 65% to 75% of the volume of colloid administered, accounting for some "leakage" of the colloid from the intravascular space.[5]

KEY CONCEPT *Thus, in contrast to isotonic crystalloid solutions that distribute throughout the extracellular fluid space, the volume of iso-oncotic colloids administered remains relatively confined to the intravascular space.* In the case of hyperoncotic solutions such as 25% albumin, fluid is pulled from the interstitial space into the vasculature, resulting in an increase in the intravascular volume that is much greater than the original volume of the 25% albumin that was administered. Although theoretically attractive, hyperoncotic solutions should not be used for hypovolemic shock because the expansion of the intravascular space is at the expense of depletion of the interstitial space. Exogenous colloids available in the United States include 5% albumin, 25% albumin, 5% plasma protein fraction (PPF), 6% hetastarch, 10% pentastarch, 10% dextran 40, 6% dextran 70, and 6% dextran 75 (see Table 13–3). The first three products are derived from pooled human plasma. Hetastarch and pentastarch are semisynthetic hydroxyethyl starches derived from amylopectin. The dextran products are semisynthetic glucose polymers that vary in terms of the average molecular weight of the polymers. Superiority of one colloid solution over another in terms of efficacy has not been clearly established.[23,24]

For years within the critical care literature, a controversy known as the "colloid versus crystalloid debate" raged over the relative merits of the two types (colloid and crystalloid) of resuscitation fluids. Largely in response to a major trial conducted in 2005 that demonstrated no difference in mortality between patients receiving saline versus albumin,[25] the Food and Drug Administration (FDA) issued a notice to health care providers in May 2005 declaring albumin safe for use in most critically ill patients.[26] However, based on previous data, there does not appear to be a clear-cut overall advantage relative to mortality for either crystalloids or colloids in these patient groups.[26] This was confirmed in a large study known as the CRISTAL (Colloids Versus Crystalloids for the Resuscitation of the Critically Ill) Randomized Trial published in 2013.[27] Thus, most clinicians today prefer using crystalloids based on their availability and inexpensive cost compared with colloids.[19,28] However, in addition to these factors, a major shift in this debate has recently taken place focused on adverse events.

Generally, the major adverse effects associated with colloids are fluid overload, dilutional coagulopathy, and anaphylactoid/anaphylactic reactions.[29] Because of direct effects on the coagulation system with the hydroxyethyl starch and dextran products, they should be used cautiously in hemorrhagic shock patients. This is another reason why crystalloids may be preferred in hemorrhagic shock. Hetastarch can increase serum amylase. More importantly, hetastarch has been associated with an increased risk of acute kidney injury in several recent clinical trials. As such, hydroxyethyl starch products are no longer recommended.[24]

Blood Products KEY CONCEPT *Blood products are indicated in hypovolemic shock patients who have sustained blood losses from hemorrhage exceeding 1500 mL.* This, in fact, is the only setting in which freshly procured whole blood is administered. In virtually all other settings, blood products are given as the individual components of whole blood units, such as packed red blood cells (PRBCs), fresh-frozen plasma (FFP), platelets, cryoprecipitate, and concentrated coagulation factors.[30] This includes ongoing resuscitation of hemorrhagic shock when PRBCs can be transfused to increase oxygen-carrying capacity in concert with crystalloid solutions to increase blood volume. In patients with documented coagulopathies, FFP for global replacement of lost or diluted clotting factors, or platelets for patients with severe thrombocytopenia (less than 20 to 50 × 10^3/mm^3 or 20 to 50 × 10^9/L) should be administered.[31,32] Data suggests that increasing the ratio of FFP to PRBC units may be associated with improved mortality and a reduction in the number of PRBC transfusions in patients requiring multiple transfusions.[33,34] Type O negative blood or "universal donor blood" is given in emergent cases of hemorrhagic shock. Thereafter, blood that has been typed and cross-matched with the recipient's blood is given.

The traditional threshold for PRBC transfusion in hypovolemic shock has been a serum hemoglobin of less than 10 g/dL (100 g/L or 6.2 mmol/L) and hematocrit (Hct) less than 30% (0.30). However, for critically ill patients who have received appropriate fluid resuscitation and have no signs of ongoing bleeding, a more restrictive transfusion threshold of 7 g/dL (70 g/L or 4.34 mmol/L) appears to be safe.[35] Traditional risks from allogeneic blood product administration include hemolytic and nonhemolytic transfusion reactions and transmission of blood-borne infections in contaminated blood. Recent large studies have also shown that transfusions are associated with increased infection and higher mortality, possibly because of adverse immune and inflammatory effects.[30,36] Increased thromboembolic events and mortality have been documented for patients receiving PRBCs stored longer than 28 days.[37] Thus administration of blood products should be restricted whenever possible and used as early as possible following donation.

Table 13–4

Vasopressor Drugs Recommended for Use in Circulatory Shock[1]

Drug	Usual IV Dose	Adrenergic Effects[a]			Potential to Cause Arrhythmias
		α	$β_1$	Dopaminergic	
Norepinephrine	0.5–80 mcg/min	+++	++	0	++
Epinephrine	1–200 mcg/min	+	+++	0	+++

[a]α Stimulation results in arterial vasoconstriction (increased systemic vascular resistance), $β_1$ stimulation results in increased heart rate, increased myocardial contractility. IV, intravenous.

0 = None

\+ = Low

++ = Moderate

+++ = High

► *Pharmacologic Therapy*

Vasopressor is the term used to describe any pharmacologic agent that can induce arterial vasoconstriction through stimulation of the $α_1$-adrenergic receptors. KEY CONCEPT *Although replenishment of intravascular volume is undoubtedly the cornerstone of hypovolemic shock therapy, use of vasopressors may be warranted as a temporary measure in patients with profound hypotension or evidence of organ dysfunction in the early stages of shock.*[2,10] Vasopressors are typically used concurrently with fluid administration after the latter has not resulted in adequate restoration of BP and/or tissue perfusion.[38] Table 13–4 lists those vasopressors recommended for use in the management of hypovolemic shock.[1] Although vasopressor therapy may improve the hemodynamic profile in shock patients, data are lacking that they improve mortality.[39] Furthermore, a study found that early use of vasopressors (ie, phenylephrine, norepinephrine, dopamine, vasopressin) in the resuscitation of patients with hemorrhagic shock may actually be associated with increased mortality.[40] Regardless, data suggest that if vasopressors are used, norepinephrine is preferable to dopamine secondary to increased incidence of arrhythmias associated with the latter agent in the treatment of shock patients.[41,42] Thus norepinephrine should be considered the first-line vasopressor therapy for these patients.[2,39] In addition to dopamine, epinephrine should be considered as a second-line vasopressor in patients with shock because of its association with tachyarrhythmias, impaired abdominal organ (splanchnic) circulation, and hypoglycemia.[2,38] In cases involving concurrent heart failure, an inotropic agent such as dobutamine may be needed, in addition to the use of a vasopressor.[2]

Vasopressors are almost exclusively administered as continuous infusions because of their very short duration of action and the need for close titration of their dose-related effects. Starting doses should be at the lower end of the dosing range followed by rapid titration upward if needed to maintain adequate BP. Monitoring of end-organ function such as adequate urine output should also be used to monitor therapy. Once BP is restored, vasopressors should be weaned and discontinued as soon as possible to avoid any untoward events.[2] The most significant

Patient Encounter, Part 2

PMH: Hypertension and a "bad heart" per the family

Meds: Lisinopril 40 mg by mouth daily; atenolol 25 mg by mouth daily; hydrochlorothiazide 25 mg by mouth daily; enteric-coated aspirin 81 mg by mouth daily

SH: Jehovah's Witness

FH: Noncontributory

PE:

VS: BP 75/37 mm Hg, P 135 beats/min, RR 21 breaths/min, T 36.1°C (97.0°F), Ht 5′4″ (163 cm), Wt 75 kg (165 lb), urine output: none since bladder catheterization 10 minutes ago

Neuro: Confused and agitated upon entering the trauma center. Now with worsening confusion.

Cardiovascular: Heart sounds and ECG normal except for tachycardia

Pulmonary: Normal breath sounds but undergoing tracheal intubation for mechanical ventilation

Abd: WNL

Extremities: Moderate bleeding from two gunshot entrance wounds to right hip and thigh

Pertinent labs: pH 7.21, $Paco_2$ 50 mm Hg (6.65 kPa), Pao_2 70 mm Hg (9.31 kPa), Na 149 mEq/L (149 mmol/L), HCO_3 16 mEq/L (16 mmol/L), lactate 7.0 mg/dL (0.78 mmol/L), SCr 1.8 mg/dL (159 μmol/L), Hct 29% (0.29)

Describe treatment goals for the patient in the next hour.

Describe treatment goals for the patient in the next 24 hours.

Develop a pharmacologic and fluid therapy plan for initial therapy. Defend your selections compared with alternative agents.

Discuss the role in therapy for blood products, sodium bicarbonate, and recombinant factor VIIa in the patient at this time.

Patient Encounter, Part 3

One hour after the initial fluid bolus, the patient's vital signs are BP 80/55 mm Hg, P 120 beats/min, RR 18 breaths/min, urine output: 15 mL in the past hour. Pertinent new labs: lactate 5.1 mg/dL (0.57 mmol/L). She is still weak and confused.

Assess the patient's condition compared with 1 hour ago.

Develop a plan for additional therapy, if any, that you recommend at this time.

Outline a plan for monitoring the patient over the next 24 hours.

systemic adverse events associated with vasopressors are excessive vasoconstriction resulting in decreased organ perfusion and potential to induce arrhythmias (see Table 13–4). Central venous catheters should be used to minimize the risk of local tissue necrosis that can occur with extravasation of peripheral IV catheters.

Hemostatic Agents

The off-label use of the procoagulant recombinant activated factor VII (rFVIIa) as an adjunctive agent to treat uncontrolled hemorrhage has gained popularity in recent years. Regardless, the off-label use of rFVIIa has been criticized based on an increased risk of arterial thromboembolic events in patients, especially patients older than 65 years.[43,44] The optimal dose of rFVIIa in nonhemophilic patients is also unknown. In light of the uncertain efficacy, safety concerns, and its high acquisition costs, the use of rFVIIa is not advocated for patients with refractory hemorrhage. A promising alternative to rVIIa in patients with hemorrhagic shock is tranexamic acid, an antifibrinolytic. A recent study of tranexamic acid in trauma patients with or at risk of significant bleeding demonstrated a decrease in mortality compared with placebo.[45] As such, a recent European guideline recommends the use of tranexamic acid within 3 hours of injury (1 gram IV over 10 minutes then 1 gram over 8 hours) as an adjunctive agent in the management of bleeding trauma patients.[46]

Supportive Care Measures

Lactic acidosis, which typically accompanies hypovolemic shock as a consequence of tissue hypoxia, is best treated by reversal of the underlying cause. Administration of alkalizing agents such as sodium bicarbonate has not been demonstrated to have any beneficial effects and may actually worsen intracellular acidosis.[47] Because GI ischemia is a common complication of hypovolemic shock, prevention of stress-related mucosal disease should be instituted as soon as the patient is stabilized. The most common agents used for stress ulcer prophylaxis are the histamine$_2$-receptor antagonists and proton pump inhibitors. Prevention of thromboembolic events is another secondary consideration in hypovolemic shock patients. This can be accomplished with the use of external devices such as sequential compression devices and/or antithrombotic therapy such as the low-molecular-weight

Patient Care Process

Patient Assessment:

- Review/conduct a medical history to determine the cause of shock to guide pharmacologic and nonpharmacologic therapy.
- Assess airway/ventilator status to determine the need for supplemental oxygen/mechanical ventilation.
- Monitor vital signs and urine output at least every 15 minutes (continuously if possible) to determine shock severity.
- Review pertinent laboratory tests (electrolytes, complete blood count [CBC], coagulation tests, ABG, serum lactate, liver function tests) to help determine shock severity and organ dysfunction.

Therapy Evaluation (assumes the patient has received some initial treatment in the emergency department):

- Evaluate the adequacy of current fluid therapy: appropriateness of venous access to deliver fluid resuscitation, fluid selection, rate of administration and response to therapy, adverse events that may be occurring (eg, pulmonary edema, electrolyte disturbances).
- Evaluate the adequacy of current blood product therapy (if applicable): product selection, dose, adverse events (eg, infusion reactions).
- Evaluate the adequacy of current vasopressor/inotropic therapy (if applicable): drug selection, dose, response to therapy, adverse events (eg, cardiac arrhythmias).

Care Plan Development:

- If SBP is less than 90 mm Hg (MAP less than 60 mm Hg), start aggressive crystalloid IV fluid therapy.
- If required (see Figure 13–3), transfuse PRBCs and provide emergent control of ongoing hemorrhaging.
- If there is evidence of cerebral or myocardial ischemia, begin vasopressor therapy.
- Follow the treatment algorithm described in Figure 13–3.
- During the resuscitation process, match the ongoing selection of IV fluid, blood products, and vasopressors/inotropes to the patient's physiologic needs. Avoid electrolyte disturbances and adverse drug events.
- If a PA catheter is placed, use the resulting data to optimize therapy.
- Consider using tranexamic acid in bleeding trauma patients.

Follow-Up Evaluation:

- Meet appropriate treatment goals for the first hour and first 24 hours of therapy (see Outcome Evaluation).
- Be sure the underlying cause of hypovolemic shock has been addressed (eg, control of bleeding or GI fluid losses).
- Begin supportive care measures such as prophylaxis for stress ulcers and venous thromboembolism.

heparin products or unfractionated heparin. Patients with adrenal insufficiency due to preexisting disease, glucocorticoid use, or critical illness may have refractory hypotension despite resuscitation. Such patients should receive appropriate glucocorticoid replacement therapy (eg, hydrocortisone).

OUTCOME EVALUATION

KEY CONCEPT *Successful treatment of hypovolemic shock is measured by the restoration of BP to baseline values and reversal of associated organ dysfunction.* The likelihood of a successful fluid resuscitation is directly related to the expediency of treatment. Therapy goals include:

- Arterial systolic blood pressure (SBP) greater than 90 mm Hg (MAP greater than 60–75 mm Hg) within 1 hour
- Organ dysfunction reversal evident by increased urine output to greater than 0.5 mL/kg/hour (1.0 mL/kg/hour in pediatrics), return of mental status to baseline, and normalization of skin color and temperature over the first 24 hours
- HR should begin to decrease reciprocally to increases in the intravascular volume within minutes to hours
- Normalization of laboratory measurements expected within hours to days following fluid resuscitation. Specifically, normalization of base deficit and serum lactate is recommended within 24 hours to potentially decrease mortality[48]
- Achievement of PAOP to a goal pressure of 14 to 18 mm Hg occurs (alternatively, CVP 8–15 mm Hg)

Abbreviations Introduced in this Chapter

ABG	Arterial blood gas
ADH	Antidiuretic hormone
ARDS	Acute respiratory distress syndrome
ATP	Adenosine triphosphate
BP	Blood pressure
Ca	Calcium
CBC	Complete blood count
Cl	Chloride
CO	Cardiac output
CRISTAL	Colloids Versus Crystalloids for the Resuscitation of the Critically Ill trial
CVP	Central venous pressure
ECG	Electrocardiogram
ECV	Extracellular volume
FDA	Food and Drug Administration
FFP	Fresh-frozen plasma
GI	Gastrointestinal
Hct	Hematocrit
Hg	Hemoglobin
HR	Heart rate
IV	Intravenous
K	Potassium
LR	Lactated Ringer
MAP	Mean arterial pressure
Mg	Magnesium
MODS	Multiple organ dysfunction syndrome
Na	Sodium
NaCl	Sodium chloride or normal saline
NS	Normal saline
PA	Pulmonary artery
$Paco_2$	Partial pressure of arterial carbon dioxide
Pao_2	Partial pressure of arterial oxygen
PAOP	Pulmonary artery occlusion pressure
PPF	Plasma protein fraction
PRBCs	Packed red blood cells
rFVIIa	Recombinant activated factor VII
SBP	Systolic blood pressure
SCr	Serum creatinine
SV	Stroke volume
SVR	Systemic vascular resistance
VIP	Ventilate, infuse, pump

REFERENCES

1. Todd RS, Turner KL, Moore FA. Shock: General. In: Gabrielli A, Lyon JA, Yu M, eds. Civetta, Taylor, & Kirby's Critical Care. 4th ed. Philadelphia, PA: Wolters Kluwer Lippincott Williams & Wilkins; 2009:813–834.
2. Vincent JL, De Backer D. Circulatory shock. N Engl J Med. 2013;369(18):1726–1734.
3. Braunwald E. Regulation of the circulation. I. N Engl J Med. 1974;290(20):1124–1129.
4. Vallet B, Wiel E, Lebuffe G. Resuscitation from circulatory shock. In: Fink MP, Abraham E, Vincent JL, Kochanek PM, eds. Textbook of Critical Care. 5th ed. Philadelphia: Elsevier Saunders; 2005:905–910.
5. Puyana JC. Resuscitation of hypovolemic shock. In: Fink MP, Abraham E, Vincent JL, Kochanek PM, eds. Textbook of Critical Care. 5th ed. Philadelphia: Elsevier Saunders; 2006:1933–1943.
6. Cinat ME, Hoyt DB. Hemorrhagic Shock. In: Gabrielli A, Lyon JA, Yu M, eds. Civetta, Taylor, & Kirby's Critical Care. Philadelphia, PA: Wolters Kluwer Lippincott Williams & Wilkins; 2009:893–923.
7. Jones AE, Kline JA. Shock. In: Marx JA, Hockberger RS, Walls RM, eds. Rosen's Emergency Medicine: Concepts and Clinical Practice. 6th ed. Philadelphia: Mosby Elsevier; 2006:41–56.
8. Harbrecht BG, Alarcon LH, Peitzman AB. Management of shock. In: Moore EE, Feliciano DV, Mattox KL, eds. Trauma. 5th ed. New York: McGraw-Hill; 2004:201–226.
9. Ciesla DJ, Moore EE, Johnson JL, et al. Multiple organ dysfunction during resuscitation is not postinjury multiple organ failure. Arch Surg. 2004;139(6):590–594.
10. Moore FA, McKinley BA, Moore EE. The next generation in shock resuscitation. Lancet. 2004;363(9425):1988–1996.
11. Rhodes A, Grounds RM, Bennett ED. Hemodynamic monitoring. In: Fink MP, Abraham E, Vincent JL, Kochanek PM, eds. Textbook of Critical Care. 5th ed. Philadelphia: Elsevier Saunders; 2005:735–739.
12. Practice guidelines for pulmonary artery catheterization: An updated report by the American Society of Anesthesiologists Task Force on Pulmonary Artery Catheterization. Anesthesiology. 2003;99(4):988–1014.
13. Myburgh JA, Mythen MG. Resuscitation fluids. N Engl J Med. 2013;369(13):1243–1251.
14. Hoffman GL. Blood and blood components. In: Marx JA, Hockberger RS, Walls RM, eds. Rosen's Emergency Medicine. Concepts and Clinical Practice. 6th ed. Philadelphia: Mosby Elsevier; 2006:56–61.
15. Zaloga GP, Kirby RR, Bernards WC, Layon AJ. Fluids and electrolytes. In: Civetta JM, Taylor RW, Kirby RR, eds. Critical Care. 3rd ed. New York: Lippincott-Raven; 1997:413–441.
16. Patanwala AE, Amini A, Erstad BL. Use of hypertonic saline injection in trauma. Am J Health Syst Pharm. 2010;67(22): 1920–1928.
17. Roberts I, Blackhall K, Alderson P, et al. Human albumin solution for resuscitation and volume expansion in critically ill patients. Cochrane Database Syst Rev. 2011(11):CD001208.
18. Mullins RJ. Management of shock. In: Mattox KL, Feliciano DV, Moore EE, eds. Trauma. 4th ed. New York: McGraw-Hill; 2000:195–232.

19. Shafi S, Kauder DR. Fluid resuscitation and blood replacement in patients with polytrauma. Clin Orthop Relat Res. 2004;(422):37–42.
20. Todd SR, Malinoski D, Muller PJ, Schreiber MA. Lactated Ringer's is superior to normal saline in the resuscitation of uncontrolled hemorrhagic shock. J Trauma. 2007;62(3):636–639.
21. Moore FA, McKinley BA, Moore EE, et al. Inflammation and the Host Response to Injury, a large-scale collaborative project: Patient-oriented research core—standard operating procedures for clinical care. III. Guidelines for shock resuscitation. J Trauma. 2006;61(1):82–89.
22. Guyton AC, Hall JE. Textbook of Medical Physiology. 10th ed. Philadelphia: Saunders; 2000.
23. Bunn F, Alderson P, Hawkins V. Colloid solutions for fluid resuscitation. Cochrane Database Syst Rev. 2003(1):CD001319.
24. Perel P, Roberts I, Ker K. Colloids versus crystalloids for fluid resuscitation in critically ill patients. Cochrane Database Syst Rev. 2013;2:CD000567.
25. Finfer S, Bellomo R, Boyce N, et al. A comparison of albumin and saline for fluid resuscitation in the intensive care unit. N Engl J Med. 2004;350(22):2247–2256.
26. Safety of albumin administration in critically ill patients. Rockville, MD: U.S. Food and Drug Administration 2005 May 16, 2005.
27. Annane D, Siami S, Jaber S, et al. Effects of fluid resuscitation with colloids vs crystalloids on mortality in critically ill patients presenting with hypovolemic shock: The CRISTAL randomized trial. JAMA. 2013;310(17):1809–1817.
28. Perel P, Roberts I. Colloids versus crystalloids for fluid resuscitation in critically ill patients. Cochrane Database Syst Rev. 2007(4):CD000567.
29. Barron ME, Wilkes MM, Navickis RJ. A systematic review of the comparative safety of colloids. Arch Surg. 2004;139(5):552–563.
30. Boucher BA, Hannon TJ. Blood management: A primer for clinicians. Pharmacotherapy. 2007;27(10):1394–1411.
31. Kelley DM. Hypovolemic shock: an overview. Crit Care Nurs. Q 2005;28(1):2–19.
32. Spahn DR, Bouillon B, Cerny V, et al. Management of bleeding and coagulopathy following major trauma: An updated European guideline. Crit Care. 2013;17(2):R76.
33. Maegele M, Lefering R, Paffrath T, et al. Red-blood-cell to plasma ratios transfused during massive transfusion are associated with mortality in severe multiple injury: A retrospective analysis from the Trauma Registry of the Deutsche Gesellschaft für Unfallchirurgie. Vox Sang. 2008;95(2):112–119.
34. Wafaisade A, Maegele M, Lefering R, et al. High plasma to red blood cell ratios are associated with lower mortality rates in patients receiving multiple transfusion (4≤red blood cell units<10) during acute trauma resuscitation. J Trauma. 2011;70(1):81–89.
35. Napolitano LM, Kurek S, Luchette FA, et al. Clinical practice guideline: Red blood cell transfusion in adult trauma and critical care. Crit Care Med. 2009;37(12):3124–3157.
36. Rohde JM, Dimcheff DE, Blumberg N, et al. Health care-associated infection after red blood cell transfusion: A systematic review and meta-analysis. JAMA. 2014;311(13):1317–1326.
37. Spinella PC, Carroll CL, Staff I, et al. Duration of red blood cell storage is associated with increased incidence of deep vein thrombosis and in hospital mortality in patients with traumatic injuries. Crit Care. 2009;13(5):R151.
38. Hollenberg SM. Vasoactive drugs in circulatory shock. Am J Respir Crit Care Med. 2011;183(7):847–855.
39. Havel C, Arrich J, Losert H, et al. Vasopressors for hypotensive shock. Cochrane Database Syst Rev. 2011(5):CD003709.
40. Sperry JL, Minei JP, Frankel HL, et al. Early use of vasopressors after injury: Caution before constriction. J Trauma. 2008;64(1):9–14.
41. De Backer D, Biston P, Devriendt J, et al. Comparison of dopamine and norepinephrine in the treatment of shock. N Engl J Med. 2010;362(9):779–789.
42. Patel GP, Grahe JS, Sperry M, et al. Efficacy and safety of dopamine versus norepinephrine in the management of septic shock. Shock. 2010;33(4):375–380.
43. Levi M, Levy JH, Andersen HF, Truloff D. Safety of recombinant activated factor VII in randomized clinical trials. N Engl J Med. 2010;363(19):1791–1800.
44. O'Connell KA, Wood JJ, Wise RP, et al. Thromboembolic adverse events after use of recombinant human coagulation factor VIIa. JAMA. 2006;295(3):293–298.
45. Shakur H, Roberts I, Bautista R, et al. Effects of tranexamic acid on death, vascular occlusive events, and blood transfusion in trauma patients with significant haemorrhage (CRASH-2): A randomised, placebo-controlled trial. Lancet. 2010;376(9734): 23–32.
46. Rossaint R, Bouillon B, Cerny V, et al. Management of bleeding following major trauma: An updated European guideline. Crit Care. 2010;14(2):R52.
47. Kim HJ, Son YK, An WS. Effect of sodium bicarbonate administration on mortality in patients with lactic acidosis: A retrospective analysis. PLoS One. 2013;8(6):e65283.
48. Tisherman SA, Barie P, Bokhari F, et al. Clinical practice guideline: Endpoints of resuscitation. J Trauma. 2004;57(4):898–912.

14 Asthma

Lori Wilken and Michelle T. Martin

LEARNING OBJECTIVES

Upon completion of the chapter, the reader will be able to:

1. Describe the pathophysiology and clinical presentation of acute and chronic asthma.
2. List the treatment goals for asthma.
3. Identify environmental factors associated with worsening asthma control.
4. Select inhaled drug delivery devices based upon patient characteristics.
5. Evaluate current metered-dose inhaler technique.
6. Recommend a therapeutic plan based upon asthma control and severity.
7. Develop an individualized asthma action plan.

INTRODUCTION

KEY CONCEPT *Asthma is a complex disorder and has been defined as "a heterogeneous disease, usually characterized by chronic airway inflammation."*[1] Airflow limitation results in wheezing, breathlessness, chest tightness, and coughing, particularly at night or early in the morning.[1] Severity of chronic disease ranges from mild intermittent symptoms to a severe and disabling disease. Despite variability in the severity of chronic asthma, all patients with asthma are at risk of acute severe disease. International guidelines emphasize the importance of treating underlying airway inflammation to control asthma and reducing asthma-associated risks.[1–3]

EPIDEMIOLOGY AND ETIOLOGY

KEY CONCEPT *Asthma is the most prevalent chronic disease of childhood, and it causes significant morbidity and mortality in both adults and children.* About 235 million adults and children worldwide have asthma.[4] In the United States, asthma affects 8% of adults (18.7 million) and 9.3% of children (6.8 million).[5] Asthma is the primary diagnosis for 14.2 million physician office visits, 1.8 million emergency department visits, and 3345 deaths annually.[5]

Asthma is also a significant economic burden in the United States, with costs totaling nearly $60 billion annually.[6] Prescription medications are the single largest direct medical expenditure and account for 71% of direct medical costs.[6]

Asthma results from a complex interaction of genetic and environmental factors. There appears to be an inherited component because the presence of asthma in a parent is a strong risk factor for developing asthma in a child. This risk increases when a family history of atopy is also present. The presence of atopy is a strong prognostic factor for continued asthma as an adult.

Environmental exposure also appears to be an important etiologic factor. Although asthma occurs early in life for most patients, those with occupational asthma develop the disease later upon exposure to specific allergens in the workplace. Exposure to secondhand smoke after birth increases the risk of childhood asthma.[7] Adult-onset asthma may be related to **atopy**, nasal polyps, aspirin sensitivity, occupational exposure, or recurrence of childhood asthma.

PATHOPHYSIOLOGY

KEY CONCEPT *Asthma is characterized by airway narrowing and inflammation primarily in medium-sized bronchi.* A key feature of the pathophysiology is airway hyperresponsiveness, which is exaggerated narrowing of the airways in response to a trigger or allergen such as cold air, strong odors, pollen, or dust. Airway narrowing results from contraction of airway smooth muscle, increased mucus secretion, airway edema, and remodeling.[1]

Airway inflammation is initiated by an inhaled allergen or trigger such as dust, pollen, or animal dander inducing a type 2 T-helper CD4$^+$ (T_H2) response. This leads to B-cell production of antigen-specific immunoglobulin E (IgE), proinflammatory cytokines, and chemokines that recruit and activate eosinophils, neutrophils, and alveolar macrophages.[2] Further exposure to the antigen results in cross-linking of cell-bound IgE in mast cells and basophils, causing release of preformed inflammatory mediators such as histamine, cysteinyl leukotrienes, and prostaglandin D_2.[1]

Activation and degranulation of mast cells and basophils result in an early-phase response involving acute bronchoconstriction that lasts approximately 1 hour after allergen exposure. In the late-phase response, activated airway cells release inflammatory cytokines and chemokines, thereby recruiting more inflammatory cells into the lungs. The late-phase response occurs 4 to 6 hours after the initial allergen challenge and results in less intense bronchoconstriction as well as increased airway hyperresponsiveness and airway inflammation.[2]

CLINICAL PRESENTATION AND DIAGNOSIS

See accompanying box for the clinical presentation and diagnosis of asthma. Diagnosis is based on a detailed medical history, physical examination of the upper respiratory tract and skin, and spirometry. The clinician determines if episodic symptoms of airflow obstruction are present, whether airflow obstruction is at least partially reversible, and that alternative diagnoses are excluded.[1-3] Spirometry is required for diagnosing asthma in patients older than 5 years because the medical history and physical examination are not reliable for characterizing the status of lung impairment or excluding other diagnoses.[1-3] Methacholine or histamine bronchoprovocation test is used to clinically evaluate airway hyperresponsiveness.

▸ *Chronic Asthma*

Chronic asthma is classified as either: (a) intermittent asthma or (b) persistent asthma that may be categorized as mild, moderate, or severe. Initial assessment of severity is made at the time of diagnosis, and initial therapy is based on this assessment. Table 14–1 describes the categories of asthma severity in patients younger than 12 years. The assessment of severity is similar in older patients.[2]

KEY CONCEPT *In chronic asthma, initial classification of asthma severity is based on current disease impairment and future risk.* The term *impairment* refers to the frequency and severity of symptoms, use of short-acting β_2-agonists (SABA) for quick relief of symptoms, pulmonary function, and impact on normal activity and quality of life. *Risk* refers to the potential for future severe exacerbations and asthma-related death, progressive loss of lung function (adults) or reduced lung growth (children), and the occurrence of drug-related adverse effects.[2]

▸ *Acute Asthma*

In acute asthma, the severity of an exacerbation does not depend on the classification of the patient's chronic asthma because even patients with intermittent asthma can have life-threatening acute exacerbations. Severity at the time of evaluation can be estimated by signs and symptoms or presenting PEF or FEV_1. The exacerbation is considered *mild* if the patient is only having dyspnea with activity and the PEF is at least 70% of the personal

Clinical Presentation and Diagnosis of Asthma

General Findings

- Severity ranges from normal pulmonary function with symptoms only during acute exacerbations to significantly decreased pulmonary function with continuous symptoms.
- Acute asthma can present rapidly (within 3–6 hours), but deterioration more commonly occurs over a longer period, even days or weeks. Acute asthma can be life threatening, and its severity does not necessarily correspond to severity of the chronic disease.
- Chronic asthma varies from no coughing, shortness of breath, or wheezing to daily coughing, wheezing, and shortness of breath, depending upon severity.
- Family history, social history, precipitating factors, history of exacerbations, and development of symptoms are important components of an asthma diagnosis.

Symptoms

- Patients usually complain of wheezing, shortness of breath, coughing (usually worse at night), and chest tightness.
- Patients may be anxious and agitated. In acute severe asthma, patients may be unable to communicate in complete sentences.
- Mental status changes (eg, confusion, irritability, agitation) may indicate impending respiratory failure.
- The presence of precipitating factors (eg, smoke, mold, or viral illness) worsens symptoms.
- Symptoms usually have a pattern (eg, worse at night, seasonal symptoms).

Signs

- Vital signs may reflect tachypnea, tachycardia, and hypoxemia.
- On inspection, there may be hyperexpansion of the thorax and use of accessory muscles.
- Auscultation of the lungs may detect end-expiratory wheezes in mild exacerbations or wheezing throughout inspiration and expiration in severe exacerbations.
- Bradycardia and absence of wheezing may indicate impending respiratory failure.
- In acute asthma, patients may present with pulsus paradoxus, diaphoresis, and cyanosis.

Laboratory Tests

- Spirometry demonstrates reversible airway obstruction with an FEV_1/FVC (forced expiratory volume in 1 second/forced vital capacity) less than 80% (0.80) and either: (a) an increase in FEV_1 of 12% or 200 mL after receiving a bronchodilator, or (b) an increase of 10% in the predicted FEV_1 after receiving a bronchodilator. Spirometry may be normal if the patient is not symptomatic.
- A complete blood count with differential should be obtained in patients with fever or purulent sputum. The eosinophil count may be elevated, reflecting an allergic component.
- Elevated serum immunoglobulin E (IgE) levels may be present.
- Arterial blood gases (to evaluate Pco_2) should be obtained for patients in severe distress, suspected hypoventilation, or when peak expiratory flow (PEF) or FEV_1 is 30% or less after initial treatment.

Other Diagnostic Tests

- Full pulmonary function tests should be performed at baseline in patients 5 years or older to rule out other disorders
- Pulse oximetry is performed at each visit to assess for hypoxemia.

Table 14–1

Classification of Asthma Severity in Patients by Age[a]

	Components of Severity	Intermittent	Persistent: Mild	Persistent: Moderate	Persistent: Severe
Impairment	Symptoms	2 days/week or less	> 2 days/week but not daily	Daily	Throughout the day
	Nighttime awakenings				
	Ages 0–4	0	1–2 times/month	3–4 times/month	> 1 time/week
	Ages 5 and older	2 times/month or less	3–4 times/month	> 1 time/week but not nightly	Often 7 nights/week
	SABA use for symptoms (not prevention of EIB)	2 days/week or less	> 2 days/week but not > 1 time/day	Daily	Several times/day
	Interference with normal activity	None	Minor limitation	Some limitation	Extremely limited
	Lung function[b] ages 5–11	FEV_1 > 80%, FEV_1/FVC > 85%	FEV_1 > 80%, FEV_1/FVC > 80%	FEV_1 60–80%, FEV_1/FVC 75–80%	FEV_1 < 60%, FEV_1/FVC < 75%
	Lung function[b] ages 12 and older	FEV_1 > 80%, FEV_1/FVC > 85%	FEV_1 > 80%, FEV_1/FVC normal	FEV_1 60–80%, FEV_1/FVC reduced 5%	FEV_1 < 60%, FEV_1/FVC reduced > 5%
Risk	**Exacerbations Requiring Systemic (Oral) Corticosteroids**				
	Ages 0–4	0–1/year	Two or more exacerbations in 6 months, four or more wheezing episodes/year lasting for > 1 day *and* risk factors for persistent asthma		
	Ages 5–11	0–1/year	2/year or more →	→	→
	Ages 12 and older	0–1/year	2/year or more →	→	→
	Recommended step for initiating treatment				
	Ages 0–11	Step 1	Step 2	Step 3, and consider short course of oral corticosteroids	
	Ages 12 and older	Step 1	Step 2	Step 3 or 4	Step 5 or 6

SABA, short-acting β_2-agonist; EIB, exercise-induced bronchospasm.

[a]From NHLBI National Asthma Education and Prevention Program, Expert Panel Report-3. Guidelines for the diagnosis and management of asthma. NIH Publication No. 07-4051. Bethesda, MD: U.S. Department of Health and Human Services, 2007, http://www.ncbi.nlm.nih.gov/books/NBK7232/. See http://www.nhlbi.nih.gov/guidelines/asthma/asthgdln.pdf for adults and children 12 years of age and older.

[b]Normal FEV_1/FVC: ages 8–19 = 85% (0.85); ages 20–39 = 80% (0.80); ages 40–59 = 75% (0.75); ages 60–80 = 70% (0.70).

best value, *moderate* if the dyspnea limits activity and the PEF is 40% to 69% of the personal best, and *severe* with PEF less than 40% and dyspnea interferes with conversation or occurs at rest. When the patient is not able to speak or the personal best PEF is less than 25% of the personal best predicted value, it is a *life-threatening* exacerbation.

TREATMENT OF ASTHMA

Desired Outcomes

▸ *Chronic Asthma*

Therapy for chronic asthma is directed at maintaining long-term control using the least amount of medications and minimizing adverse effects.[1,2] Treatment goals are to: (a) prevent chronic and troublesome symptoms, (b) require infrequent use (2 or fewer days/week) of SABA for quick relief of symptoms, (c) maintain normal or near-normal pulmonary function, (d) maintain normal activity levels, (e) meet patients' and families' expectations of satisfaction with asthma care, (f) prevent exacerbations of asthma and the need for emergency department visits or hospitalizations, (g) prevent progressive loss of lung function, and (h) provide optimal pharmacotherapy with minimal or no adverse effects.

▸ *Acute Asthma*

Acute or worsening asthma can be a life-threatening situation and requires rapid assessment and appropriate intensification of therapy. Mortality associated with asthma exacerbations is usually related to inappropriate assessment of the severity of the exacerbation resulting in insufficient treatment or referral for medical care. The goals of therapy are to: (a) correct significant **hypoxemia**, (b) reverse airflow obstruction rapidly, and (c) reduce the likelihood of exacerbation relapse or recurrence of severe airflow obstruction in the future.[1,2]

Nonpharmacologic Therapy

Nonpharmacologic therapy is incorporated into each step of care, and patient education occurs whenever health care professionals interact with patients. Patient education begins at the time of diagnosis and is tailored to meet individual patient needs. Components of education involve asthma trigger avoidance, proper administration of inhaled medications, and asthma self-management.

▸ *Factors Associated with Worsening Asthma Control*

Major triggers that may worsen asthma control include exposure to pollen, mold, dust mites, cockroaches, pet dander, air pollution, cold air, exercise, strong odors, emotions, tobacco smoke, certain medications, illicit drug use, sulfite-containing foods and beverages, and comorbid conditions (eg, allergic rhinitis, sinusitis, upper respiratory infections, gastroesophageal reflux disease, obesity, and obstructive sleep apnea).

▸ *Trigger Avoidance*

Education on identifying and controlling asthma triggers is critical to providing adequate asthma treatment.[1–3] Environmental controls to reduce the allergen load in the patient's home may reduce asthma symptoms, school absences because of asthma, and unscheduled clinic and emergency visits for asthma.

The normal adult and child immunization schedule is recommended for patients with asthma.[8] A yearly influenza vaccine is recommended for patients 6 months and older with asthma to decrease the risk of complications from influenza.[9] The pneumococcal polysaccharide vaccine (PPSV23) may decrease the risk of pneumococcal disease in patients with asthma and is recommended as a one-time immunization before the age of 65 years and again after age 65. In patients 65 years and older, the pneumococcal conjugated vaccine (PCV13) in conjunction with PPSV23 is recommended to provide broader protection against invasive pneumococcal disease. PCV13 is administered 6 to 12 months prior to giving PPSV23.[10]

Nonselective β-blockers, such as carvedilol, labetalol, nadolol, pindolol, propranolol, and timolol (including ophthalmic preparations) may worsen asthma control. These agents are avoided in patients with asthma unless the benefits of therapy outweigh the risks.[2] For patients with asthma requiring β-blocker therapy, a β_1-selective agent such as metoprolol or atenolol is the best option. Because selectivity is dose related, the lowest effective dose is used.

Patients with aspirin-sensitive asthma are usually adults and often present with the triad of rhinitis, nasal polyps, and asthma. In these patients, acute asthma may occur within minutes of receiving aspirin or nonsteroidal anti-inflammatory drugs (NSAIDs). These patients are advised against using NSAIDs.[2]

Pharmacologic Therapy

Treatment of chronic asthma involves avoidance of triggers known to precipitate or worsen asthma and use of long-term control and quick-relief medications. Long-term control medications include inhaled corticosteroids (ICS), inhaled long-acting β_2-agonists (LABAs), oral theophylline, oral leukotriene receptor antagonists (LTRAs), and omalizumab. In patients with severe asthma, oral corticosteroids (OCS) may be used as a long-term control medication. Quick-relief medications include SABAs, anticholinergics, and short bursts of systemic corticosteroids.

Patient Encounter 1

A 3-year-old boy is seen today by the pediatrician. He has been newly diagnosed with mild persistent asthma based on his symptoms. He currently does not take any medications.

What is the best method of delivery and treatment regimen for this patient's asthma?

What education is required for the method of medication delivery for the quick-relief agent?

Describe the education that you would provide to the patient's parents about using an inhaled corticosteroid.

What is the best way to deliver asthma medication when he is 7 years old?

What education is required for the method of medication delivery you would recommend for a 7-year-old patient?

► *Drug Delivery Devices*

KEY CONCEPT *Direct airway administration of asthma medications through inhalation is the most efficient route and minimizes systemic adverse effects.* Inhaled asthma medications are available in metered-dose inhalers (MDIs), dry powder inhalers (DPIs), soft mist inhalers (SMIs), and nebulized solutions. Selection of the appropriate inhalation device depends on patient characteristics and medication availability (Table 14–2).

Poor inhaler technique results in increased oropharyngeal deposition of the drug, leading to decreased efficacy and increased adverse effects. Figure 14–1 describes the steps for appropriate use of MDIs. Because MDIs are challenging to use correctly, use of valved holding chambers (VHCs) or spacers is recommended with MDIs to decrease the need for coordination of actuation with inhalation, decrease oropharyngeal deposition, and increase pulmonary drug delivery.[11,12]

► *β_2-Adrenergic Agonists*

β_2-Agonists relax airway smooth muscle by directly stimulating β_2-adrenergic receptors in the airway.[13] They also increase mucociliary clearance and stabilize mast cell membranes. Inhaled β_2-agonists are classified as either short-acting (SABA) or long-acting (LABA) based on duration of action. Oral β_2-agonists have increased adverse effects and are not used for asthma treatment.

The early-phase response to antigen in an asthma exacerbation is blocked by pretreatment with inhaled SABAs. The SABAs have significantly better bronchodilating activity in acute asthma than theophylline or anticholinergic agents. Adverse effects of β_2-agonists include tachycardia, tremor, and hypokalemia, which are usually not troublesome with inhaled dosage forms.

Short-Acting Inhaled β_2-Agonists KEY CONCEPT *Inhaled SABAs are the most effective agents for reversing acute airway obstruction caused by bronchoconstriction and are the drugs of choice for treating acute asthma and symptoms of chronic asthma as well as preventing exercise-induced bronchospasm.*[1] Inhaled SABAs have an onset of action of less than 5 minutes and a duration of action of 4 to 6 hours. Using an MDI with a VHC or spacer has faster medication delivery and is as effective as administration by nebulization.

Albuterol (known as salbutamol outside the United States), the most commonly used inhaled SABA, is available as an MDI and solution for nebulization. Levalbuterol, the pure R-enantiomer of albuterol (and referred to as R-salbutamol outside the United States), is available as an MDI and solution for nebulization. Levalbuterol has similar efficacy to albuterol and is purported to have fewer side effects; however, clinical trials have not demonstrated this benefit.[14]

Doses for SABAs are provided in Table 14–3. During an asthma exacerbation, the usual SABA doses are doubled and the regimen changes from as-needed to scheduled use. Scheduled chronic daily dosing of SABAs is not recommended for two reasons. First, the need to use an inhaled SABA is one key indicator of uncontrolled asthma. Therefore, patients are educated to record SABA use. Second, scheduled SABA use decreases the duration of bronchodilation provided by the SABA.

Long-Acting Inhaled β_2-Agonists Salmeterol and formoterol are LABAs that provide up to 12 hours of bronchodilation after a single dose. Because of the long duration of bronchodilation, these agents are useful for patients experiencing nocturnal

Table 14–2

Age Recommendations and Features of Inhalation Devices[2]

Device Type	Recommended Age	Advantages	Disadvantages
Metered-dose inhaler (MDI)	5 years of age and older	• Delivery of medication in < 2 minutes • Portable, durable • Lower medication dose needed vs nebulization	• Technique/coordination may be difficult • Propellant may taste bad or irritate the airways
MDI plus valved-holding chamber (VHC)	If < 4 years old, use VHC with mask; If ≥ 4 years of age, use VHC	• VHC enhances MDI technique • VHC decreases topical side effects of ICS • Albuterol MDI with VHC is as effective as nebulization for asthma exacerbation	• Bulky • Lack of coverage by some insurance plans • Limited testing of MDIs with various VHC, leading to unpredictable results • Potential for increased systemic side effects with inhaled corticosteroids (ICS)
Soft mist inhaler (SMI)	Respimat 18 years of age and older	• No propellant or dry powder • Better lung deposition than MDI and DPI	• Challenging to assemble for first-time use • Coordination of breath and activation required
Jet nebulizer	Any age, preferably infants or elderly	• No coordination required • Oxygen may be delivered simultaneously with medications	• Requires 5–15 minutes to deliver medication • Limited number of medications available for nebulization • Not portable (most require electricity)
Ultrasonic nebulizer	Any age; preferably infants or elderly	• Typically more portable than jet nebulizer • Faster delivery of medications than jet nebulizer	• Heat generated from nebulizer breaks down suspensions for nebulization • Do not use with budesonide suspension for nebulization
Dry powder inhaler (DPI)	Aerolizer 5 years of age and older; Diskus 4 years of age and older; Ellipta 12 years of age and older; Flexhaler 6 years of age and older; Handihaler[a] 18 years old and older; Respiclick 12 years of age and older; Twisthaler age 12 years and older	• Easy to use • Sweet taste • Quick delivery of medication • Amount of lactose filler is insufficient to cause concern in lactose intolerance	• Limited product stability after opening • Optimal delivery of medication in children < 4 years old is not feasible because high inspiratory volume is needed

[a]Not approved for treatment of asthma.

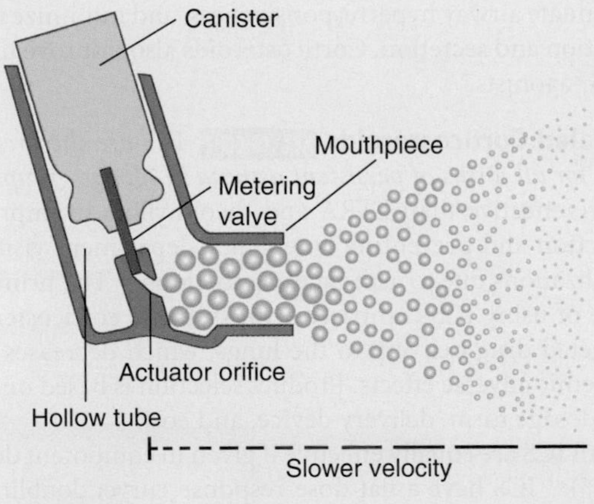

1. Remove the cap and shake the inhaler well.
2. Exhale all air away from the inhaler.
3. Place the mouthpiece into the mouth with lips closed tightly around the inhaler.
4. To deliver a dose, press down on the canister **one time** while inhaling a slow steady breath. A puff or mist of medication is sprayed out of the inhaler into the mouth.
5. Hold your breath for 10 seconds.
6. Exhale.
7. Wait 1 minute if the dose is to be repeated.
8. Recap the inhaler when you are finished.
9. Rinse your mouth with water if the medication is an inhaled corticosteroid.

Comments

- Prime the MDI the first time it is used or if it has not been used in 10 days. Prime the inhaler by spraying four sprays into the air.
- For patients who cannot hold their breath for 10 seconds, instruct them to hold their breath as long as possible.
- Do not immerse the canister of medication in water at any time.
- If a counter is not available on the inhaler, the patient should tally the number of puffs used to determine when the inhaler is empty.

FIGURE 14–1. Proper use of a metered-dose inhaler (MDI). Inhaler image reprinted with permission from Kelly HW, Sorkness CA. Asthma. In: DiPiro JT, Talbert RL, Yee GC, et al, eds. Pharmacotherapy: A Pathophysiologic Approach, 8th ed. New York: McGraw-Hill, 2011. Figure 33–4, 448.

Table 14–3

Usual Dosages for Quick-Relief Medications for Asthma in Home Setting[a,b]

Medications	Dosage Form	Children 0–11 years	Adults and Children 12 Years of Age and Older
Inhaled SABA			
Albuterol	HFA MDI and DPI 90 mcg/inhalation, 200 inhalations/canister	1–2 puffs every 4–6 hours as needed	2 puffs every 4–6 hours as needed
Albuterol	Nebulizer solution 0.63 mg/3 mL, 1.25 mg/3 mL, 2.5 mg/3 mL, 5 mg/mL (0.5%)	0.63–5 mg every 4–6 hours as needed	1.25–5 mg every 4–8 hours as needed
Levalbuterol	HFA (MDI) 45 mcg/puff, 200 puffs/canister	2 puffs every 4–6 hours as needed for ages 5–11 years	2 puffs every 4–6 hours as needed
Levalbuterol	Nebulizer solution 0.31 mg/3 mL, 0.63 mg/3 mL, 1.25 mg/0.5 mL, 1.25 mg/3 mL	0.31–1.25 mg every 6–8 hours as needed	0.63–1.25 mg every 6–8 hours as needed
Systemic Corticosteroids			
Methylprednisolone	2, 4, 6, 8, 16, 32 mg oral tablets	1-2 mg/kg/day by mouth in 2 divided doses for 3-10 days (maximum 60 mg/day)	40–60 mg/day by mouth as single or two divided doses for 3–10 days
Prednisolone	5 mg oral tablets; 5 mg/5 mL and 15 mg/5 mL oral liquid	1–2 mg/kg/day, (maximum 60 mg/day) for 3–10 days	40–60 mg/day by mouth as single or two divided doses for 3–10 days
Prednisone	1, 2.5, 5, 10, 20, 50 mg oral tablets; 5 mg/mL and 5 mg/5 mL oral liquid	1–2 mg/kg/day, (maximum 60 mg/day) for 3–10 days	40–60 mg/day by mouth as single or two divided doses for 3–10 days

DPI, dry powder inhaler; HFA, hydrofluoroalkane; MDI, metered-dose inhaler; SABA, short-acting β_2-agonist.

[a]Dosages are provided for products that have been approved by the US FDA or have sufficient clinical trial safety and efficacy data in the appropriate age ranges to support their use.

[b]Doses are increased in the hospital/emergency department setting.

symptoms. Salmeterol is a partial agonist with an onset of action of approximately 30 minutes. Formoterol is a full agonist that has an onset of action similar to that of albuterol; it is not approved for treatment of acute bronchospasm in the United States, but it is approved for this use in Europe.

LABAs are indicated for chronic treatment of asthma as add-on therapy for patients not controlled on low to medium doses of ICS. Adding an LABA is at least as effective in improving symptoms and decreasing asthma exacerbations as doubling the dose of an ICS or adding an LTRA to ICS.[3,15] Adding an LABA to ICS therapy also reduces the amount of ICS necessary for asthma control.[3]

Although both formoterol and salmeterol are effective as add-on therapy for moderate persistent asthma, LABAs should not be used as monotherapy for chronic asthma. There may be an increased risk of severe asthma exacerbations and asthma-related deaths when LABAs are used alone.[16] Labeling for all drugs containing LABAs includes a black box warning against their use without an ICS. The risk of increased severe asthma exacerbations does not appear to be increased in adults receiving both an LABA and ICS.[17]

Salmeterol and formoterol are available as single-ingredient products and as fixed-ratio combination products containing an ICS (fluticasone propionate/salmeterol, budesonide/formoterol, or mometasone/formoterol). The LABA vilanterol is available in combination with fluticasone furoate for once daily dosing in patients aged 18 or older. Combination products may increase adherence because of the need for fewer inhalers and inhalations. However, they offer less flexibility in dosage adjustment of individual ingredients if that is necessary. Doses used for long-term control of chronic asthma are provided in Table 14–4.

► *Corticosteroids*

Corticosteroids are the most potent anti-inflammatory agents available for asthma treatment and are available in inhaled, oral, and injectable dosage forms. They decrease airway inflammation, attenuate airway hyperresponsiveness, and minimize mucus production and secretion. Corticosteroids also improve the response to β_2-agonists.

Inhaled Corticosteroids KEY CONCEPT *ICS are the preferred therapy for all forms of persistent asthma in all age groups.*[1,2] ICS are more effective than LTRA and theophylline in improving lung function and preventing emergency department visits and hospitalizations due to asthma exacerbations.[1,2] The primary advantage of using ICS compared with systemic corticosteroids is the targeted drug delivery to the lungs, which decreases the risk of systemic adverse effects. Product selection is based on preference for dosage form, delivery device, and cost.

All ICS are equally effective if given in equipotent doses (Table 14–5).[18] ICS have a flat dose-response curve; doubling the dose has a limited additional effect on asthma control.[19] Cigarette smoking decreases the response to ICS, and smokers require higher doses of ICS than nonsmokers.[20] Although some beneficial effect is seen within 12 hours of administration of an ICS, 2 weeks of therapy is necessary to see significant clinical effects. Longer treatment may be necessary to realize the full effects on airway inflammation.

For most delivery devices, the majority of the drug is deposited in the mouth and throat and swallowed. Local adverse effects of ICS include oral candidiasis, cough, and dysphonia. The incidence of local adverse effects can be reduced by using an MDI with a VHC and by having the patient rinse the mouth with

Table 14–4

Usual Doses of Long-Term Control Medications in Asthma[a]

Medication	Dosage Form	Ages 0–11 Years	Adults and Children 12 Years of Age and Older
Inhaled Corticosteroids (see Table 14–5)			
Long-Acting β_2-Agonists			
Salmeterol	DPI 50 mcg/blister	Ages 0–3 years: N/A Ages 4–11 years: One inhalation every 12 hours	One inhalation every 12 hours
Formoterol	DPI 12 mcg/capsule	Ages 0–4 years: N/A Ages 5–11 years: Inhalation of one capsule every 12 hours	Inhalation of one capsule every 12 hours
Leukotriene Modifiers			
Montelukast	4 mg or 5 mg chewable tablets 4 mg granule packets 10 mg tablet	Ages 1–5 years: 4 mg at bedtime Ages 6–11 years: 5 mg at bedtime	Ages 12–14 years: 5 mg at bedtime Ages 15 and older: 10 mg at bedtime
Zafirlukast	10 or 20 mg tablets	Ages 0–6 years: N/A Ages 7–11 years: 10 mg twice daily	20 mg tablet twice daily
Zileuton	600 mg extended-release tablet	N/A	1200 mg twice daily after meals
	600 mg tablet	N/A	600 mg four times daily
Methylxanthines			
Theophylline	100, 200, 300, 400, 450, 600 mg extended-release tablets; 80 mg/15mL solution and elixir; liquids, sustained-release tablets and capsules	Ages < 1 year: [0.2 (age in weeks) + 5] × body weight in kg (in divided doses/day)[b] Ages 1–11 years (< 45 kg): Starting dose 12–14 mg/kg/day (max 300 mg/day) × 3 days, increase to 16 mg/kg/day (max 400 mg/day) × 3 days, then increase to 20 mg/kg/day (max 600 mg/day) Ages 1–11 years (45 kg or greater): Starting dose 300 mg/day (in divided doses) × 3 days, titrate up 400 mg/day × 3 days, then titrate up to usual maximum of 600 mg/day	Starting dose 300 mg/day (in divided doses or daily depending on product) × 3 days, titrate up 400 mg/day × 3 days, then titrate up to usual maximum of 600 mg/day; monitor serum levels
Immunomodulator			
Omalizumab	SC injection, 150 mg/1.2 mL after reconstitution with 1.4 mL sterile water for injection	N/A	150–375 mg SC every 2–4 weeks, depending on body weight and pretreatment serum IgE level. See dosing chart.[c]

DPI, dry powder inhaler; IgE, immunoglobulin E; N/A, safety and efficacy not established; SC, subcutaneously.

[a]Dosages are provided for products that have been approved by the US FDA or have sufficient clinical trial safety and efficacy data in the appropriate age ranges to support their use.

[b]See guidelines for premature infants.

[c]http://www.xolair.com/pdf/dosingtables.pdf.

water and expectorate after using the ICS. Decreasing the dose reduces the incidence of hoarseness.

Systemic absorption occurs via the pulmonary and oral routes. Systemic adverse effects include adrenal suppression, decreased bone mineral density, skin thinning, cataracts, and easy bruising, and occur more frequently with higher ICS doses.[2] Linear growth velocity is reduced by less than half a centimeter per year and height after 1 year of treatment is decreased by less than 1 cm in children treated with low and medium dose ICS.[21,22]

A significant drug interaction causing Cushing syndrome and adrenal insufficiency occurs when potent inhibitors of CYP3A4 (ritonavir, itraconazole, ketoconazole) are administered with high doses of ICS.[18]

Poor adherence to ICS treatment is common and contributes to uncontrolled asthma.[23] The slow onset of action and concerns about side effects are major deterrents to using these highly effective medications.

Considerable variability in response to ICS exists, with up to 40% of patients not responding to ICS. This lack of response may be related to functional glucocorticoid-induced transcript 1 gene (*GLCCI1*) variant in some patients with asthma.[24]

Systemic Corticosteroids Prednisone, prednisolone, and methylprednisolone are the cornerstone of treatment for acute asthma not responding to an SABA (see Table 14–3 for recommended doses).[1,2] The onset of action for systemic corticosteroids is 4 to 12 hours. For this reason, systemic corticosteroids are started early in the course of acute exacerbations. The oral route is preferred in acute asthma; there is no evidence that intravenous corticosteroid administration is more effective. Therapy

Table 14–5

Estimated Comparative Daily Dosages for Inhaled Corticosteroids for Asthma[2,32]

	Low Daily Dose		Medium Daily Dose		High Daily Dose	
Medication	**Ages 0–11 Years**	**Ages 12 Years and Older**	**Ages 0–11 Years**	**Ages 12 Years and Older**	**Ages 0–11 Years**	**Ages 12 Years and Older**
Beclomethasone HFA (MDI) 40 or 80 mcg/puff	40 mcg, 1–2 puffs twice daily or 80 mcg, 1 puff twice daily[a]	80 mcg, 1 puff twice daily	80 mcg, 2 puffs twice daily[a]	80 mcg, 3 puffs twice daily	80 mcg, > 2 puffs twice daily[a]	80 mcg, > 3 puffs twice daily
Budesonide DPI 90 or 180 mcg/inhalation	90 mcg, 1–2 inhalations twice daily or 180 mcg, 1 inhalation twice daily[a]	180 mcg, 1 inhalation twice daily	180 mcg, 2 inhalations twice daily[a]	180 mcg, 2–3 inhalations twice daily	180 mcg, > 2 inhalations twice daily[a]	180 mcg, > 3 inhalations twice daily
Budesonide inhalation suspension for nebulization 0.25 mg/2 mL, 0.5 mg/2 mL, 1 mg/2 mL	Ages 0–4: 0.25 mg once or twice daily; Ages 5–11: 0.25 mg twice daily or 0.5 mg once daily	N/A	Ages 0–4: 0.25–0.5 mg twice daily; Ages 5–11: 0.5 mg twice daily	N/A	Ages 0–4: > 0.5 mg twice daily; Ages 5–11: 1 mg twice daily	N/A
Ciclesonide HFA 80, 160 mcg/puff	80 mcg, 1 puff once or twice daily or 160 mcg, 1 puff daily[b]	160 mcg, 1 puff once or twice daily	80 mcg, > 1–2 puffs twice daily or 160 mcg, 1 puff twice daily[b]	160 mcg, 2 puffs twice daily	160 mcg, > 1 puff twice daily[b]	160 mcg, > 2 puffs twice daily
Flunisolide HFA 80 mcg/puff	80 mcg, 1 puff twice daily[a]	80 mcg, 2 puffs twice daily	80 mcg, 2 puffs twice daily[a]	80 mcg, 3–4 puffs twice daily	80 mcg, 3–4 puffs twice daily[a]	80 mcg, > 4 puffs twice daily
Fluticasone furoate DPI 100 or 200 mcg/inhalation	N/A	100 mcg, 1 inhalation daily	N/A	200 mcg, 1 inhalation daily	N/A	200 mcg, 1 inhalation daily
Fluticasone propionate HFA (MDI) 44, 110, or 220 mcg/puff	44 mcg, 1–2 puffs twice daily	110 mcg, 1 puff twice daily	110 mcg, 1 puff twice daily	110 mcg, 2 puffs twice daily or 220 mcg, 1 puff twice daily	110 mcg, > 1 puff twice daily or 220 mcg, 1 puff twice daily	220 mcg, > 1 puff twice daily
Fluticasone propionate DPI 50, 100, or 250 mcg/inhalation	50 mcg, 1–2 inhalations twice daily or 100 mcg, 1 inhalation twice daily[a]	100 mcg, 1 inhalation twice daily	100 mcg, 2 inhalations twice daily[a]	250 mcg, 1 inhalation twice daily	100 mcg, > 2 inhalations twice daily[a]	250 mcg, > 1 inhalation twice daily
Mometasone DPI 110, 220 mcg/inhalation	110 mcg, 1 inhalation daily[c]	220 mcg, 1 inhalation daily	110 mcg, 1–2 inhalations twice daily or 220 mcg, 1 inhalation twice daily[c]	220 mcg, 1 inhalation twice daily or 2 inhalations daily	110 mcg, > 2 inhalations twice daily or 220 mcg, > 1 inhalation twice daily[c]	220 mcg, > 1–2 inhalations twice daily
Combined ICS/LABA						
Fluticasone/Salmeterol DPI 100/50 mcg, 250/50 mcg, 500/50 mcg; HFA (MDI) 45/21 mcg, 115/21 mcg, 230/21 mcg	100/50 mcg, 1 inhalation twice daily[d]	100/50 mcg, 1 inhalation twice daily or 45/21 mcg, 2 puffs twice daily	100/50 mcg, 1 inhalation twice daily[d]	250/50 mcg, 1 inhalation twice daily or 115/21 mcg, 2 puffs twice daily	100/50 mcg, 1 inhalation twice daily[d]	500/50 mcg, 1 inhalation twice daily or 230/21 mcg, 2 puffs twice daily
Budesonide/Formoterol HFA (MDI) 80/4.5 mcg, 160/4.5 mcg	N/A[b]	80/4.5 mcg, 1 puff twice daily	N/A[b]	160/4.5 mcg, 1 puff twice daily	N/A[b]	160/4.5 mcg, 2 puffs twice daily
Mometasone/Formoterol (MDI)100/5 mcg, 200/5 mcg	N/A[b]	100/5 mcg, 1 puff twice daily	N/A[b]	200/5 mcg, 1 puff twice daily	N/A[b]	200/5 mcg, 2 puffs twice daily

(Continued)

Table 14–5

Estimated Comparative Daily Dosages for Inhaled Corticosteroids for Asthma[2,32] (*Continued*)

	Low Daily Dose		Medium Daily Dose		High Daily Dose	
Medication	Ages 0–11 Years	Ages 12 Years and Older	Ages 0–11 Years	Ages 12 Years and Older	Ages 0–11 Years	Ages 12 Years and Older
Fluticasone furoate/ Vilanterol (DPI) 100/25 mcg, 200/25 mcg	N/A[b]	100/5 mcg, 1 inhalation daily[e]	N/A[b]	100/5 mcg, 1 inhalation daily[e]	N/A[b]	200/5 mcg, 1 inhalation daily[e]

DPI, dry powder inhaler; HFA, hydrofluoroalkane; ICS, inhaled corticosteroid; LABA, long-acting β_2-agonist; MDI, metered-dose inhaler, N/A, safety and efficacy not established.

[a]N/A in children 0–4 years of age.

[b]Not yet FDA approved in children 0–11 years of age.

[c]Doses based on clinical trials. FDA approved in children ages 4–11 years at maximum dose of 110 mcg daily.

[d]Doses based on clinical trials. A maximum of fluticasone/salmeterol 100/50 mcg, 1 inhalation twice daily is approved in children ages 4–11 years without specification of low, medium, or high dosage.

[e]FDA approved for adults 18 years and older.

with systemic corticosteroids is continued until the PEF is 70% or more of the personal best measurement and asthma symptoms are resolved. The duration of therapy usually ranges from 3 to 10 days. Tapering the corticosteroid dose in patients receiving short bursts (up to 10 days) is usually not necessary because any adrenal suppression is transient and rapidly reversible.[2]

Because of serious potential adverse effects, systemic corticosteroids are avoided as long-term controller medication for asthma, if possible. Systemic corticosteroids are only used in patients who have failed other therapies, including immunomodulators. If systemic therapy is necessary, once-daily or every-other-day therapy is used with repeated attempts to decrease the dose or discontinue the drug.

▶ *Anticholinergics*

Anticholinergic agents inhibit the effects of acetylcholine on muscarinic receptors in the airways and protect against cholinergic-mediated bronchoconstriction. The bronchodilating effects of anticholinergic agents are not as pronounced as SABAs in asthma.[1,2]

Ipratropium bromide is available as an MDI and solution for nebulization. Its onset of action is approximately 15 minutes, and the duration of action is 4 to 8 hours. The addition of ipratropium bromide to SABAs during a moderate to severe asthma exacerbation improves pulmonary function and decreases hospitalization rates in both adult and pediatric patients.[25] An SABA combined with ipratropium to increase bronchodilation is only indicated in the emergency department setting.

Tiotropium bromide is a long-acting inhaled anticholinergic available as a DPI and SMI. It has an onset of action of approximately 30 minutes and duration longer than 24 hours. Tiotropium is used (off-label) as a long term controller medication in patients 18 years or older with uncontrolled asthma already taking an ICS or an ICS and LABA combination.[26,27] Tiotropium decreases severe exacerbations, improves lung function, and is steroid sparing. Because of its safety and efficacy profile, tiotropium is the preferred anticholinergic agent for chronic asthma treatment. The newer anticholinergics aclidinium bromide and umeclidinium bromide have less clinical evidence supporting their use in asthma.

Anticholinergic drugs may cause bothersome adverse effects such as blurred vision, dry mouth, and urinary retention. Increased cardiovascular events have been reported for ipratropium but not tiotropium.[28,29]

▶ *Leukotriene Receptor Antagonists*

The LTRAs are anti-inflammatory medications that either inhibit 5-lipoxygenase (zileuton) or competitively antagonize the effects of leukotriene D_4 (montelukast, zafirlukast). These agents improve FEV_1 and decrease asthma symptoms, SABA use, and asthma exacerbations. Although these agents offer the convenience of oral administration, they are significantly less effective than low ICS doses.[2,30] Combining an LTRA with an ICS is not as effective as an ICS plus an LABA but is considered steroid sparing.[1,2] LTRAs are beneficial for asthma patients with allergic rhinitis, aspirin sensitivity, or exercise-induced bronchospasm. See Table 14–4 for dosing.

Montelukast is generally well tolerated with minimal need for monitoring and few drug interactions. Zileuton and zafirlukast are less commonly used because of the risk of hepatotoxicity. Zileuton use requires liver function monitoring prior to use, monthly for 3 months, every 3 months for the first year of use, and periodically thereafter. Zileuton and zafirlukast are metabolized through the CYP 2C9 hepatic pathway and have significant drug interactions. All three agents have reports of neuropsychiatric events, such as sleep disorders, aggressive behavior, and suicidal thoughts.

▶ *Methylxanthines*

Theophylline has anti-inflammatory properties and causes bronchodilation by inhibiting phosphodiesterase and antagonizing adenosine.[31] Its use is limited because of inferior efficacy as a long-term controller medication compared with ICS, a narrow therapeutic index with potentially life-threatening toxicity, and multiple clinically important drug interactions.

Theophylline is primarily metabolized by CYP1A2, CYP2E1, and CYP3A4 and is involved in a large number of disease and drug interactions. Theophylline exhibits nonlinear pharmacokinetics; therefore, serum concentration changes due to dosage adjustments, drug interactions, and hepatic function may not always be predictable.

Target serum theophylline concentrations are 5 to 15 mg/L (28–83 μmol/L); an increased risk of adverse effects outweighs the increased bronchodilation in most patients above 15 mg/L (83 μmol/L).[31] Headache, nausea, vomiting, and insomnia may occur at serum concentrations less than 20 mg/L (111 μmol/L) but are rare when the dose is started low and increased slowly. More serious adverse effects (eg, cardiac arrhythmias, seizures) can occur at higher concentrations. See Table 14–4 for dosing.

▶ *Immunomodulators*

Omalizumab is a recombinant humanized monoclonal anti-IgE antibody that inhibits binding of IgE to receptors on mast cells and basophils, resulting in inhibition of inflammatory mediator release and attenuation of the early- and late-phase allergic response. Omalizumab is indicated for treatment of patients with moderate to severe persistent asthma whose asthma is not controlled by ICS and who have a positive skin test or *in vitro* reactivity to aeroallergens. Omalizumab significantly decreases ICS use, reduces the number and length of exacerbations, and increases asthma-related quality of life.[32]

Omalizumab is given as a subcutaneous injection every 2 to 4 weeks in the office or clinic. The initial dose is based on the patient's weight and baseline total serum IgE concentration (see Table 14–4). Subsequent IgE levels are not monitored.

The most common adverse effects are injection site reactions and include bruising, redness, pain, stinging, itching, and burning. Anaphylactic reactions are rare but may occur at any time after medication administration. Monitoring the patient for an anaphylactic reaction for 2 hours after medication administration is recommended for the first 3 months; thereafter, monitoring time can be reduced to 30 minutes.[33] It is also important to issue a prescription for and provide patient education on the use of subcutaneous epinephrine for an anaphylactic reaction from omalizumab. Omalizumab has been associated with an increased risk of cardiovascular and cerebrovascular events (eg, myocardial infarction, transient ischemic attack, venous thrombosis) and perhaps cancer, but the magnitude of the increased risk is unclear.[34]

Treatment of Chronic Asthma

KEY CONCEPT *The intensity of pharmacotherapy for chronic asthma is based on disease severity for initial therapy and level of control for subsequent therapies.* The least amount of medications necessary to meet the therapeutic goals is used.[2]

The first step in asthma management is evaluating the patient's asthma severity and control (see Table 14–1 for descriptions of asthma severity). Pharmacologic treatment is initiated based on the recommendations for stepwise therapy (Figure 14–2). Treatment recommendations involve three categories based on patient age: (1) children younger than 5 years, (2) children between the ages of 5 and 11 years, and (3) individuals 12 years and older. Therapeutic plans must be individualized.

▶ *Intermittent Asthma*

Patients with intermittent asthma only need SABAs. This asthma classification includes patients with exercise-induced bronchospasm (EIB), seasonal asthma, or asthma symptoms associated with infrequent trigger exposure. Patients pretreat with an SABA prior to exposure to a known trigger, such as exercise.

Exercise is one of the most common precipitants of asthma symptoms. Shortness of breath, wheezing, or chest tightness usually occur during or shortly after vigorous exercise, peak 5 to 10 minutes after stopping the activity, and resolve within 20 to 30 minutes. Warming up prior to exercise and covering the mouth and nose with a scarf or mask during cold weather may prevent exercise-induced asthma. Pretreatment with an SABA 5 to 20 minutes prior to exercise is the treatment of choice and will protect against bronchospasm for 2 to 3 hours. Regular treatment with an ICS or LTRA is recommended if SABA treatment is needed daily for exercise and not working effectively.[35]

▶ *Persistent Chronic Asthma*

Patients with persistent chronic asthma require daily long-term control therapy. ICS are the long-term control medication of choice at all levels of severity (mild, moderate, and severe) and in all age groups.[2] SABAs are prescribed for all patients with asthma for use on an as-needed basis.

After initiating therapy, patients are monitored within 2 to 6 weeks to ensure that asthma control has been achieved. Table 14–6 describes how to assess patients for asthma control. Before increasing therapy, the patient's inhaler technique and

Patient Encounter 2

A 16-year-old girl presents to clinic with exercise-induced bronchoconstriction (EIB). She is concerned because she needs to use her albuterol inhaler before daily basketball practices and sometimes needs additional doses during games. She denies any symptoms at any other times throughout the day.

What alternative to albuterol is available to treat her EIB?

What education about nonpharmacologic measures can improve this patient's EIB?

Patient Encounter 3

A 62-year-old man with moderate persistent asthma since childhood presents to a clinic appointment with his mometasone/formoterol 100 mcg/5 mcg inhaler. He uses the inhaler as needed for wheezing and coughing. He complains of waking up at night coughing and hoarse. When he uses the inhaler, he spaces the inhaler two fingers away from his mouth and then actuates the inhaler twice at one time. He has no other asthma medications. He was in the emergency department 2 months ago with an asthma exacerbation.

What issues is this patient having with his current asthma management?

How will you explain the importance of ICS adherence to the patient?

What other medication should he carry with him at all times?

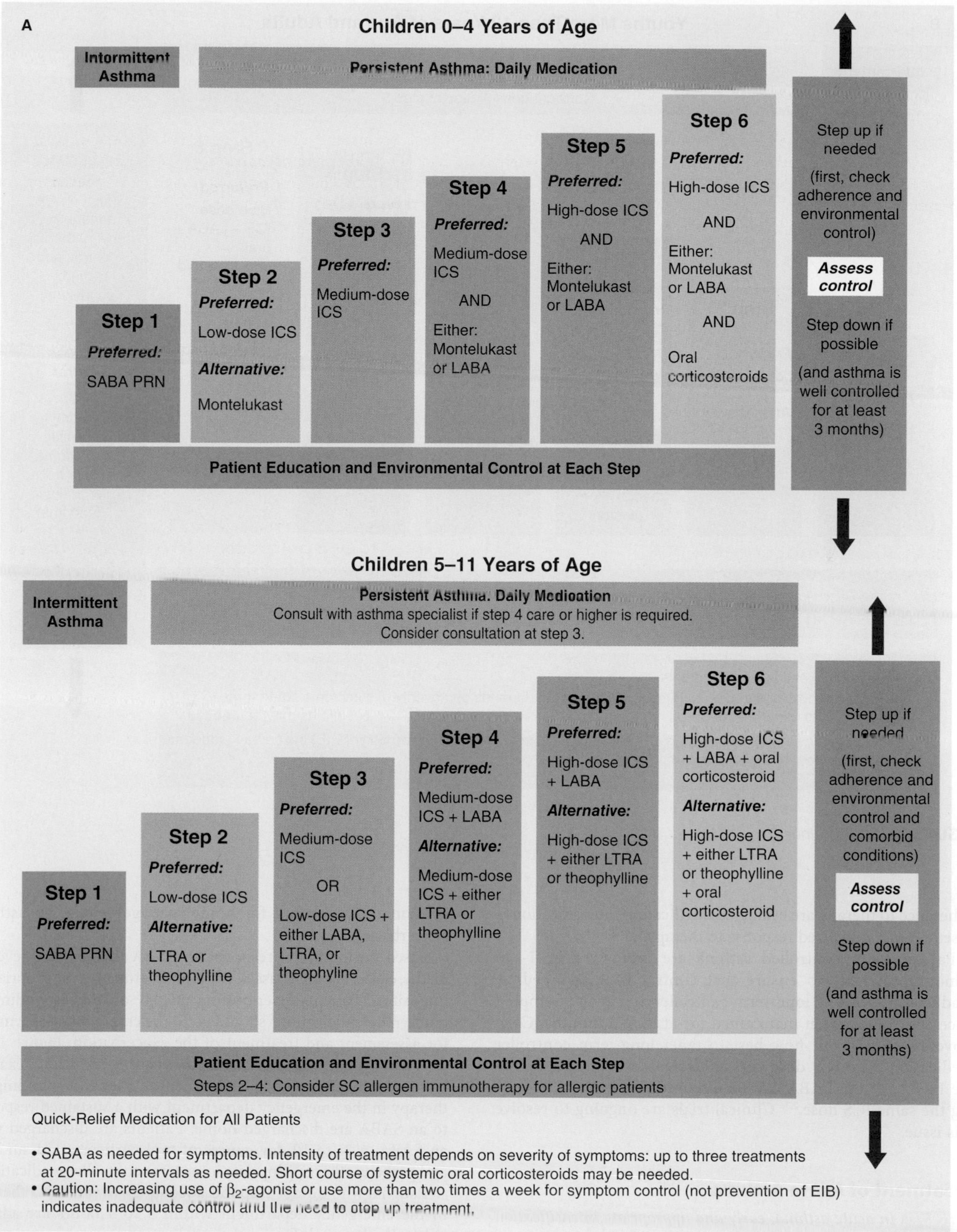

FIGURE 14–2. Stepwise approach for managing asthma in (A) children and (B) adults. (ICS, inhaled corticosteroid; LABA, long-acting β agonist; LTRA, leukotriene receptor antagonist; PRN, as needed; SABA, short-acting β_2-agonist; SC, subcutaneous.)

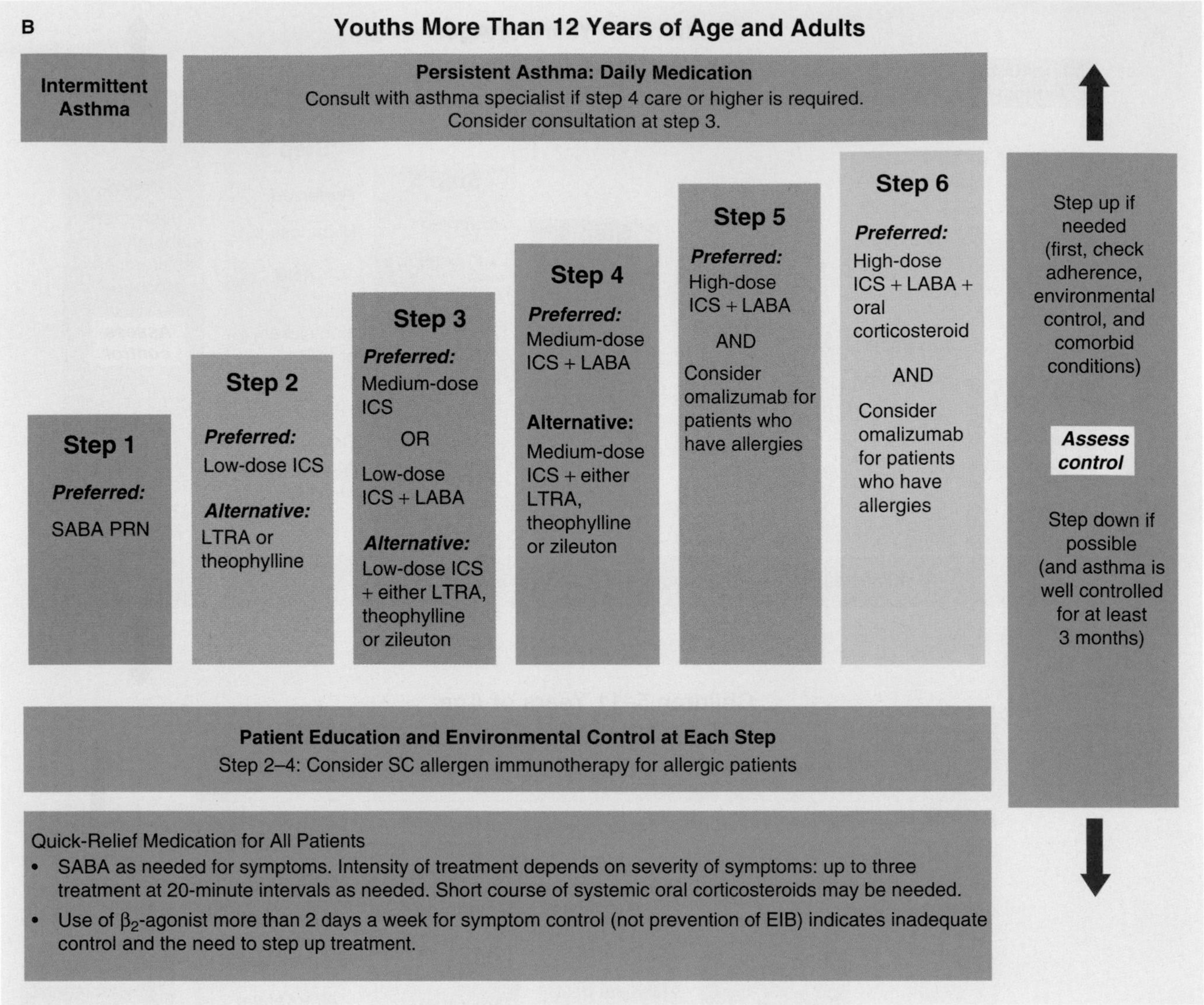

FIGURE 14–2. *(Continued)*

adherence to therapy are evaluated. Medication intensification is based on individualized response to therapy.

Patients with controlled asthma are monitored at 1- to 6-month intervals to ensure that control is maintained. A gradual step-down in long-term controller therapy is attempted once control has been maintained for at least 3 months. Controversy exists about how best to taper long-term controller medication. The ICS dose can be decreased before removing the LABA, or the LABA can be discontinued while maintaining the same ICS dose.[2,36] Clinical trials are ongoing to resolve this issue.

Treatment of Acute Asthma

KEY CONCEPT *In acute asthma, early and appropriate intensification of therapy is important to resolve the exacerbation and prevent relapse and future severe airflow obstruction.* Early and aggressive treatment is necessary for quick resolution.[37]

The optimal treatment of acute asthma depends on the severity of the exacerbation. The patient's condition usually deteriorates over several hours, days, or weeks. Figure 14–3 contains an algorithm for home management of an asthma exacerbation.

Based on the initial response to SABA therapy, the severity of the exacerbation is assessed, and treatment is appropriately intensified. Patients deteriorating quickly or not responding to quick-relief medications should go to the emergency department for assessment and treatment of the exacerbation. Figure 14–4 provides a treatment algorithm for treating an asthma exacerbation in the emergency department. Patients responding to therapy in the emergency department with a sustained response to an SABA are discharged home. Patients are discharged with an SABA, a 3- to 10-day course of oral corticosteroid, an ICS, and perhaps other appropriate long-term controller medications.

Patients who do not respond adequately to intensive therapy in the emergency department within 3 to 4 hours are admitted to the hospital. During hospitalization, oxygen, continuous nebulization of SABA, systemic corticosteroids, and alternative treatments such as magnesium and heliox may be used to treat the exacerbation.

Patients with oxygen saturation less than 90% (0.90; < 95% [0.95] in children, pregnant women, and patients with coexisting

Table 14–6

Assessing Asthma Control and Adjusting Therapy Based on Age[a]

	Components of Control	Well Controlled			Not Well Controlled			Very Poorly Controlled		
		Ages 0–4	Ages 5–11	12 Years and Older	Ages 0–4	Ages 5–11	12 Years and Older	Ages 0–4	Ages 5–11	12 Years and Older
Impairment	Symptoms	2 days/week or less but not > once each day	2 days/week or less	2 days/week or less	> 2 days/week or multiple times on 2 days/week or less	> 2 days/week	> 2 days/week	Throughout the day →		
	Nighttime awakenings	1 time/month or less		2 times/month or less	> 1 time/month	2 times/week or more	1–3 times/week	> 1 time/week	2 times/week or more	4 times/week or more
	SABA use for symptoms (not EIB prevention)	2 days/week or less →			> 2 days/week →			Several times per day →		
	Interference with normal activity	None →			Some limitation →			Extremely limited →		
	FEV_1 or PEFR	N/A	> 80%	> 80% predicted/ personal best	N/A	60%–80%	60%–80% predicted/ personal best	N/A	< 60%	< 60% predicted/ personal best
	FEV_1/FVC	N/A	> 80% (0.80)	> 80% (0.80)	N/A	75%–80% (0.75–0.80)	60%–80% (0.60–0.80)	N/A	< 75% (0.75)	< 60% (0.60)
	Questionnaires: ATAQ, ACQ, ACT	N/A	N/A	0 0.75 or less[a] 20 or more	N/A	N/A	1–2 1.5 or more 16–19	N/A	N/A	3–4 N/A 15 or less
Risk	Exacerbations requiring oral systemic corticosteroids	0–1/year. Consider severity and interval since last exacerbation			2–3/year	2/year or more	2/year or more	> 3/year	2/year or more	2/year or more
	Reduction in lung growth or progressive loss of lung function	N/A	Requires long-term follow-up		N/A	Requires long-term follow-up		N/A	Requires long-term follow-up	
	Treatment-related ADRs	Medication side effects can vary in intensity from none to very troublesome and worrisome. The level of intensity does not correlate with specific levels of control but should be considered in the overall assessment of risk.								
Recommended action for treatment. See Figure 14–4 for treatment steps.		Maintain current step. Follow-up every 1–6 months. Consider step down if well controlled at 3 months.			Step up 1 step. Reevaluate in 2–6 weeks. If ADRs, consider alternative treatment options.			Consider short course of systemic (oral) corticosteroids. Step up 1–2 steps. Reevaluate in 2 weeks. If ADRs, consider alternative treatment options.		

[a]ACQ values of 0.76–1.4 are indeterminate regarding well-controlled asthma.

ACT, Asthma Control Test; ACQ, Asthma Control Questionnaire; ATAQ, Asthma Therapy Assessment Questionnaire; ADR, adverse drug reaction; EIB, exercise-induced bronchospasm; FEV_1, forced expiratory volume in 1 second; FVC, forced vital capacity; N/A, safety and efficacy not established; PEFR, peak expiratory flow rate; SABA, short-acting β_2-agonist.

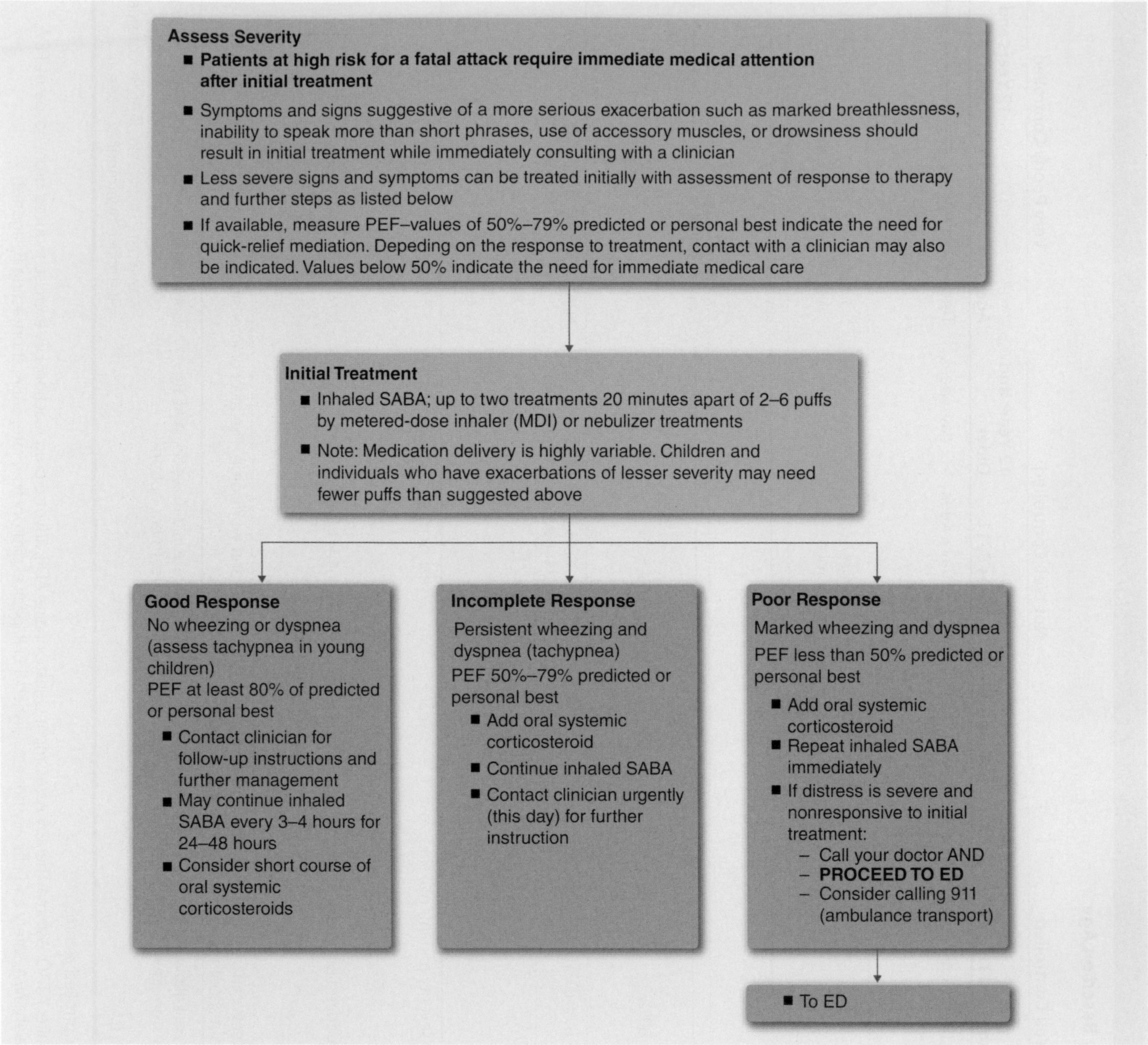

FIGURE 14–3. Management of asthma exacerbations: home treatment. (ED, emergency department; MDI, metered-dose inhaler; PEF, peak expiratory flow; SABA, short-acting β_2-agonist.) (From NHLBI National Asthma Education and Prevention Program, Expert Panel Report-3. Guidelines for the diagnosis and management of asthma. NIH Publication No. 07-4051. Bethesda, MD: U.S. Department of Health and Human Services, 2007, http://www.ncbi.nlm.nih.gov/books/NBK7232/.)

heart disease) receive oxygen with the dose adjusted to keep oxygen saturation above this level. Administration of low oxygen concentrations (< 30% [0.30] of the fraction of inspired oxygen or FiO_2) by nasal cannula or facemask is usually sufficient to reverse hypoxemia in most patients.

Asthma Self-Management

Self-management plans give patients the freedom to adjust therapy based on personal assessment of disease control using a predetermined plan. Written asthma action plans are part of standard care for asthma. Figure 14–5 is an example of an asthma action plan.

The plan includes instructions on daily management and how to recognize and handle worsening asthma.[2] Asthma control is assessed by evaluating symptoms of worsening asthma and/or monitoring PEF. Early signs of deterioration include increasing nocturnal symptoms, increasing use of inhaled SABAs, or symptoms that do not respond to increased use of inhaled SABAs. Providing patients with a prescription for oral corticosteroids to use on an as-needed basis for the initiation of an asthma exacerbation is part of asthma self-management.

Measurement of PEF is considered for patients with moderate to severe persistent asthma, poor perception of worsening asthma or airflow obstruction, and those with an unexplained response to environmental or occupational exposures.[2] PEF measurements are not necessary for a patient to receive an asthma action plan. The plan can be based upon symptoms only. PEF is measured daily in the morning upon waking or when asthma

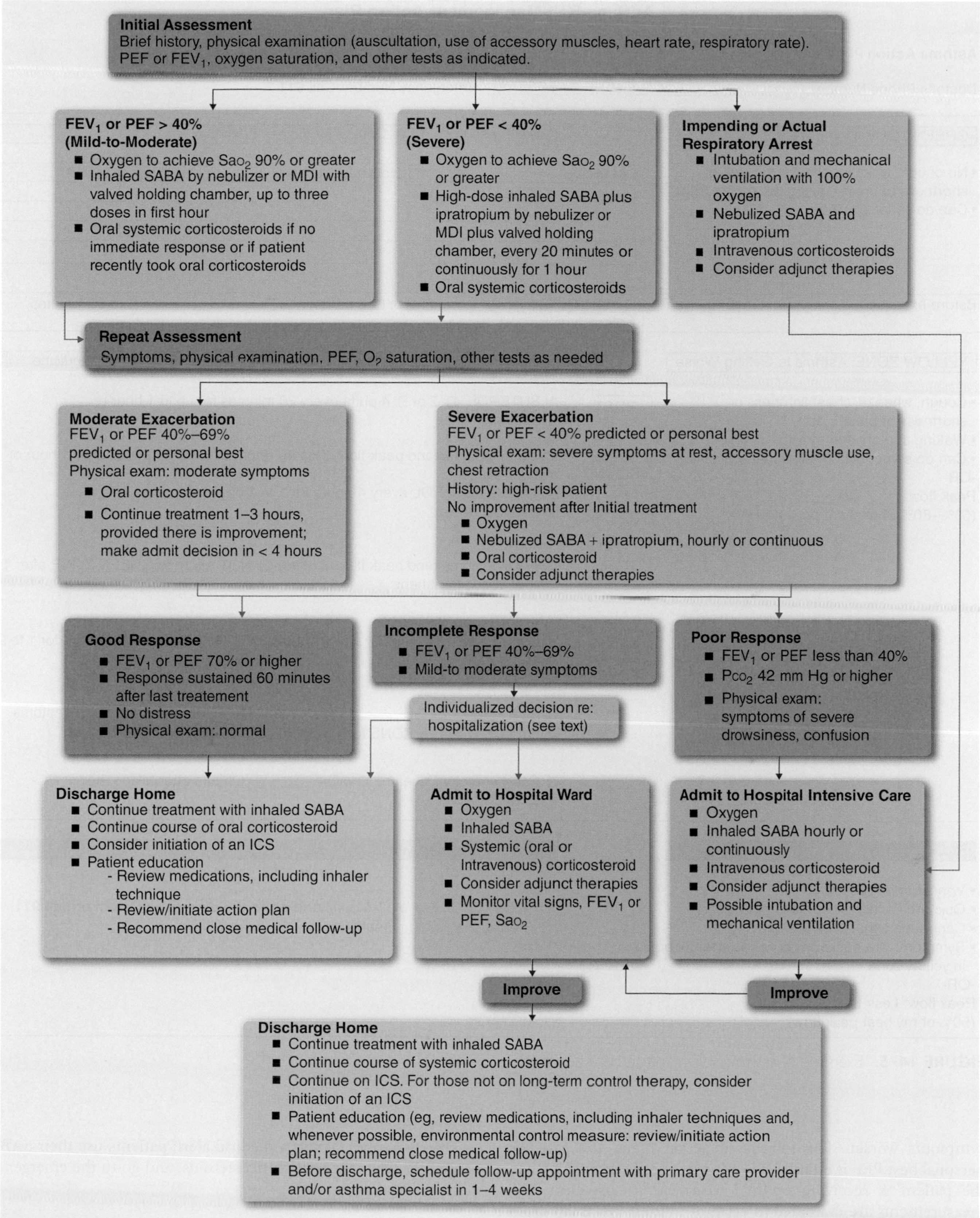

Initial Assessment
Brief history, physical examination (auscultation, use of accessory muscles, heart rate, respiratory rate). PEF or FEV1, oxygen saturation, and other tests as indicated.
FEV1 or PEF > 40% (Mild-to-Moderate)
Oxygen to achieve Sao2 90% or greater
Inhaled SABA by nebulizer or MDI with valved holding chamber, up to three doses in first hour
Oral systemic corticosteroids if no immediate response or if patient recently took oral corticosteroids
FEV1 or PEF < 40% (Severe)
Oxygen to achieve Sao2 90% or greater
High-dose inhaled SABA plus ipratropium by nebulizer or MDI plus valved holding chamber, every 20 minutes or continuously for 1 hour
Oral systemic corticosteroids
Impending or Actual Respiratory Arrest
Intubation and mechanical ventilation with 100% oxygen
Nebulized SABA and ipratropium
Intravenous corticosteroids
Consider adjunct therapies
Repeat Assessment
Symptoms, physical examination, PEF, O2 saturation, other tests as needed
Moderate Exacerbation
FEV1 or PEF 40%–69% predicted or personal best
Physical exam: moderate symptoms
Oral corticosteroid
Continue treatment 1–3 hours, provided there is improvement; make admit decision in < 4 hours
Severe Exacerbation
FEV1 or PEF < 40% predicted or personal best
Physical exam: severe symptoms at rest, accessory muscle use, chest retraction
History: high-risk patient
No improvement after Initial treatment
Oxygen
Nebulized SABA + ipratropium, hourly or continuous
Oral corticosteroid
Consider adjunct therapies
Good Response
FEV1 or PEF 70% or higher
Response sustained 60 minutes after last treatement
No distress
Physical exam: normal
Incomplete Response
FEV1 or PEF 40%–69%
Mild-to moderate symptoms
Individualized decision re: hospitalization (see text)
Poor Response
FEV1 or PEF less than 40%
Pco2 42 mm Hg or higher
Physical exam: symptoms of severe drowsiness, confusion
Discharge Home
Continue treatment with inhaled SABA
Continue course of oral corticosteroid
Consider initiation of an ICS
Patient education
- Review medications, including inhaler technique
- Review/initiate action plan
- Recommend close medical follow-up
Admit to Hospital Ward
Oxygen
Inhaled SABA
Systemic (oral or Intravenous) corticosteroid
Consider adjunct therapies
Monitor vital signs, FEV1 or PEF, Sao2
Admit to Hospital Intensive Care
Oxygen
Inhaled SABA hourly or continuously
Intravenous corticosteroid
Consider adjunct therapies
Possible intubation and mechanical ventilation
Improve
Improve
Discharge Home
Continue treatment with inhaled SABA
Continue course of systemic corticosteroid
Continue on ICS. For those not on long-term control therapy, consider initiation of an ICS
Patient education (eg, review medications, including inhaler techniques and, whenever possible, environmental control measure: review/initiate action plan; recommend close medical follow-up)
Before discharge, schedule follow-up appointment with primary care provider and/or asthma specialist in 1–4 weeks

FIGURE 14–4. Management of asthma exacerbations: emergency department and hospital-based care. (FEV_1, forced expiratory volume in 1 second; ICS, inhaled corticosteroid; MDI, metered-dose inhaler, P_{CO_2}, partial arterial pressure of carbon dioxide; PEF, peak expiratory flow, SABA, short acting β_2-agonist; Sa_{O_2}, oxygen saturation.) (From NHLBI National Asthma Education and Prevention Program, Expert Panel Report-3 [Internet]. Guidelines for the diagnosis and management of asthma. NIH Publication No. 07-4051. Bethesda, MD: U.S. Department of Health and Human Services, 2007. http://www.ncbi.nlm.nih.gov/books/NBK7232/.)

Asthma Self-Management Action Plan

Asthma Action Plan for_______________ Doctor's Name_______________________ Date _____________

Doctor's Phone Number ___________________________________ Emergency Number Call **911**

GREEN ZONE: Doing Well	Take These Long-Term-Control Medicines Each Day		
• No cough, wheeze, chest tightness, or shortness of breath during the day or night • Can do usual activities	Medicine	How much to take	When to take it
Before exercise	☐ ALBUTEROL before exercise	☐ 2 or ☐ 4 puffs	5 to 60 minutes

YELLOW ZONE: Asthma Is Getting Worse

- Cough, wheeze, chest tightness or shortness of breath, or
- Waking at night due to asthma, or
- Can do some, but not all, usual activities

-OR-

Peak flow:______to _____

(50%–80% of my best peak flow)

Add: Quick-Relief Medicine – and keep taking your GREEN ZONE medicine

FIRST → ALBUTEROL ☐ 2 or ☐ 4 puffs every 20 minutes for up to 1 hour or
☐ Nebulizer, once

SECOND → If your symptoms (and peak flow, if used) return to GREEN ZONE after 1 hour of above treatment:
☐ Take ALBUTEROL every 4 hours for 1 to 2 days
☐ Call your doctor

THIRD → If your symptoms (and peak flow, if used) <u>do NOT return to GREEN ZONE</u> after 1 hour of above treatment:

☐ Continue ALBUTEROL ☐ 2 or ☐ 4 puffs or ☐ Nebulizer every 4 hours for 1 to 2 days

☐ Add: PREDNISONE ______ mg per day for 3 to 10 days until your symptoms return to the GREEN ZONE for 1 to 2 days then STOP prednisone

☐ Call the doctor ☐ before ☐ within ________ hours after taking the PREDNISONE

RED ZONE: Medical Alert!

- Very short of breath, or
- Quick-relief medicines have not helped, or
- Cannot do usual activities, or
- Symptoms are same or get worse after 24 hours in yellow zone

-OR-

Peak flow: Less than _____

(50% of my best peak flow)

Go to the Emergency Room or CALL 911

Take:
☐ ALBUTEROL ☐ 4 or ☐ 6 puffs **and go to the emergency room or call 911**
☐ Prednisone _______ mg NOW

FIGURE 14–5. Example of asthma self-management action plan.

symptoms worsen. For PEF-based action plans, the patient's personal best PEF is established over a 2- to 3-week period when the patient is receiving optimal treatment.[2] Subsequent PEF measurements are evaluated in relation to their variability from the patient's best PEF measurement. PEF measurements in the range of 80% to 100% of personal best (green zone) indicate that current therapy is acceptable. A PEF in the range of 50% to 79% of personal best (yellow zone) indicates an impending exacerbation, and therapy is intensified with SABA therapy, possibly oral corticosteroids, and a call to the physician. A PEF less than 50% (red zone) signals a medical alert; patients use their SABA immediately, take oral corticosteroids, and go to the emergency department.

Special Populations

▸ *Pregnancy*

Approximately 4% to 8% of pregnant women are affected by asthma with about one-third experiencing worsening asthma during pregnancy.[38] It is safer for pregnant women to have

Patient Encounter 4

A 5-year-old girl is seen in the emergency department for an asthma exacerbation. She has not seen the doctor in over 1 year, and her parents ran out of refills for her asthma medications. She was previously prescribed fluticasone 44 mcg, one inhalation twice daily and levalbuterol 2 puffs every 4 hours as needed for shortness of breath. Her weight today is 30 pounds (13.6 kg). The physician makes the diagnosis of a moderate asthma exacerbation.

What medication regimen would you recommend for the patient while in the emergency department?

The patient's asthma improves, and she is ready to be discharged home from the emergency department. Her mother informs you that she has not been able to afford the asthma medication from the pharmacy, and that had contributed to the patient not taking her medications. Her insurance provider lists albuterol, beclomethasone, and ciclesonide on its formulary.

Based on this information, what medication regimen would you recommend upon discharge from the emergency department?

Provide the patient and her mother with a written asthma action plan.

What education would you provide to the patient and her parents?

asthma treated with medications than to experience worsening asthma. Uncontrolled asthma is a greater risk to the fetus than asthma medication use. Consequently, asthma exacerbations should be managed aggressively with pharmacotherapy. The stepwise approach to asthma therapy in pregnancy is similar to that for the general population.

Budesonide has the most safety data in humans and is the preferred ICS. However, there are no data indicating that other ICS present increased risk to the mother or fetus. Albuterol is the drug of choice for treating asthma symptoms and exacerbations in pregnancy.

► *Young Children*

Although asthma is the most common disease in children, its diagnosis and monitoring are challenging. Treatment in children 0 to 4 years of age is extrapolated from studies completed in adults and older children. Albuterol and ICS are the treatments of choice in this group. However, use of montelukast is common because it is available in an oral, chewable formulation and is not a corticosteroid. Route of delivery is an important issue. Nebulization treatment is commonly used, and MDI with VHC is becoming more popular due to its decreased time of administration compared with nebulization. Budesonide is the only corticosteroid available in nebulization form and is approved for use in this age group. If young patients are not controlled on as-needed SABA, they should be stepped up to low-dose ICS. LTRA are alternatives to ICS. If the patient continues to be uncontrolled on low-dose ICS, the ICS may be increased to medium dose or an LTRA may be added to the low-dose ICS.[1]

OUTCOME EVALUATION

Chronic Asthma

- Assess onset, duration, and timing of subjective symptoms such as wheezing, shortness of breath, chest tightness, cough, nocturnal awakenings, and activity level. Use validated questionnaires (such as the Asthma Control Test, Asthma

Patient Care Process

Chronic Asthma

Patient Assessment:

- Obtain spirometry or peak flow measurement. For PEF, use the highest reading of three attempts.
- Review previous full pulmonary function tests, CBC, IgE levels, chemistry panel, liver function tests and/or theophylline trough level, if appropriate.
- Auscultate the lungs for wheezing. Examine ears, eyes, nose, and throat. Look in the mouth for signs of oral candidiasis if on ICS.
- Measure height, weight, blood pressure, heart rate, and pulse oximetry.
- Ask about tobacco use and exposure to secondhand smoke (tobacco or marijuana).
- Assess asthma control using validated questionnaires (eg, ACT or c-ACT).
  - Identify asthma attacks since the last visit, including emergency room visits or hospitalizations or use of oral corticosteroid bursts.
  - Ask about SABA use in the past week and identify specific causes for use of the inhaler.
  - Identify the number of missed days of school or work because of asthma.
  - Ask about patient (or caregiver) goals and satisfaction with asthma control.
- Evaluate medication side effects (rapid heart rate, jitteriness, bad taste, cough, dysphonia, lack of efficacy).
- Verify medication adherence (understanding of purpose, cost issues, controller inhaler use, formulary issues, and duplications of therapy).
- Ask the patient to demonstrate his/her inhaler use. Ask when the inhaler is used, how many times in the past week the inhaler was used, and when the inhaler is refilled.
- Perform medication reconciliation identifying new or changes in medications that may worsen asthma or cough, including OTC and herbal products.
- Assess diet and exercise and use of SABA before exercise.
- Identify changes in home, work, or school environment.
- Assess control of gastroesophageal reflux disease (GERD), allergic rhinitis, sleep apnea, anxiety, and depression.
- Review the patient's asthma action plan and use of the plan.

Patient Care Process (*Continued*)

Therapy Evaluation:

- If the patient is not controlled, before adding medications or increasing dosing, make sure the patient is using the current inhalers correctly and is willing to use the inhaler.
- Identify patient preference, ability to pay and insurance coverage for MDI, DPI, SMI, or nebulization. Use pictures and videos of inhalers. (http://use-inhalers.com/)
- Examine the patient's inhaler for the number of doses remaining. Call the dispensing pharmacy to determine fill history of inhalers.
- Discuss rinsing a spitting after ICS use and possibly the need for a spacer to decrease side effects.
- If the patient is controlled and has been on the current regimen for 3 months or longer, consider discontinuing or lowering the dose of controller medications.

Care Plan Development:

- Evaluate risk and impairment; use Figure 14–2 to select step of therapy based on age, Table 14–6 to adjust therapy, and Tables 14–2 to 14–5 to select or adjust doses.
- Provide an updated medication list with indication and use of each inhaler device.
- Provide an updated asthma action plan (Figure 14–5) with medication changes at least yearly.
- Review environmental asthma triggers and avoidance plans.
- Treat oral candidiasis if present.
- Update immunizations.
- Discuss diet and exercise (using SABA prior to exercise if needed).
- Refill all asthma-related medications, including medications to treat allergic rhinitis and GERD.

Follow-Up Evaluation:

- Schedule follow-up physician visits depending on asthma control (2 weeks–6 months).
- Check spirometry yearly.
- Review inhaler technique and use at every visit.
- Update asthma action plan yearly or with each medication change.
- Monitor liver function tests if patient is taking zileuton.
- Obtain IgE levels and allergy skin testing if omalizumab is being considered.

Acute Asthma

Patient Assessment:

- Auscultate the lungs for wheezing. Examine ears, eyes, nose, and throat. Look in the mouth for signs of oral candidiasis if on ICS or OCS.
- Measure peak flow if older than 5 years. Check weight, pulse oximetry, respiratory rate, and pulse.
- Assess for subjective markers of severity of dyspnea (if it occurs only with activity, it limits activity, it occurs at rest and interferes with conversation, or the patient is too dyspneic to speak), and use of accessory muscles in infants.
- Assess medication causes of asthma exacerbation (no asthma medication, improper use, ineffective medication, drug interaction).
- Ask about the frequency of SABA use at home prior to coming into ED and use of oral corticosteroid.
- Determine environmental triggers for asthma exacerbation (viral illness, change in weather, exposure to allergen).
- Perform other tests as appropriate: arterial blood gases, serum electrolytes, chest radiography, CBC, and electrocardiogram to rule out other causes of symptoms.

Therapy Evaluation:

- Evaluate response to SABA after every dose or every 20 minutes by assessing wheezing, dyspnea, chest tightness, and with peak flow measurement, if age appropriate.
- Evaluate response to oral corticosteroid after 4 to 6 hours of administration by examining signs and symptoms of asthma exacerbation.

Care Plan Development:

- Use Table 14–6 to assess control and adjust therapy based on age. Most patients should receive an SABA inhaler, OCS burst, and an ICS.
- Provide education about proper inhaler technique, indication and proper use of medications, and self-titration of medications with worsening asthma.
- Educate about environmental triggers.
- Provide an updated asthma action plan with medication changes, and use this to educate patient and family about appropriate prevention of and response to future asthma exacerbations.

Follow-Up Evaluation:

- Provide a follow-up appointment with the primary care physician within 1 to 4 weeks.
- Evaluate level of asthma control using validated questionnaires and recovery (decrease in symptoms such as wheezing) after the exacerbation.
- Review inhaler use and technique.
- Update asthma action plan.

Therapy Assessment Questionnaire, or Asthma Control Questionnaire) to objectively document control.

- Monitor the use of SABAs. Using an SABA more than twice a week in intermittent asthma may indicate the need to initiate long-term control therapy. Use of more than one canister per month indicates the need to step up long-term control therapy.
- Determine the frequency of patient exacerbations. Frequent exacerbations, unscheduled clinic visits, emergency department visits, and hospitalizations due to asthma may indicate the need to reassess the patient's asthma regimen and environment.
- Measure lung function using office spirometry yearly or after therapeutic changes have been made in patients older than 5 years
- Identify environmental factors triggering asthma exacerbations and provide trigger avoidance recommendations.
- Perform medication reconciliation to identify discrepancies in medications prescribed and used by the patient and to determine drug and disease state interactions.
- Assess the patient's inhaler technique at every visit and always ensure proper technique before stepping up therapy.
- Determine adherence to long-term controller medications. Assess the patient's understanding of the indication for long-term controller medication and identify adverse events, cost issues, and need for refills.
- Review and update the patient's asthma action plan and provide the patient with a written copy of the plan.
- Update the patient's immunization status and provide an annual influenza vaccination.

Acute Asthma

In addition to the outcomes measured for chronic asthma, acute asthma monitoring also includes the following:

- Measure PEF and assess asthma symptoms. The goal PEF measurement is 70% of the patient's personal best peak flow after the first three doses of an inhaled SABA and improved asthma symptoms. Spirometry is not usually conducted in the emergency department.
- Check respiratory rate and measure oxygenation using pulse oximetry and provide oxygen via nasal cannula if needed. The goal oxygen saturation is greater than 90% (0.90) in adults and greater than 95% (0.95) in children, pregnant women, and patients with coexisting cardiovascular disease.
- Obtain a PCO_2 measurement via arterial blood gases in patients with severe asthma exacerbations. An increased PCO_2 indicates the potential for respiratory failure.
- Monitor serum potassium for hypokalemia upon admission and periodically throughout the admission in patients receiving high dose or continuous nebulization of SABA.

Abbreviations Introduced in This Chapter

CYP	Cytochrome P-450 isoenzyme
DPI	Dry powder inhaler
FEV_1	Forced expiratory volume in 1 second
FVC	Forced vital capacity
HFA	Hydrofluoroalkane
ICS	Inhaled corticosteroid
IgE	Immunoglobulin E
LABA	Long-acting β2-agonist
MDI	Metered-dose inhaler
NHLBI	National Heart, Lung, and Blood Institute
NSAID	Nonsteroidal anti-inflammatory drug
PCO_2	Partial arterial pressure of carbon dioxide
PEF	Peak expiratory flow
SABA	Short-acting β_2-agonist
SMI	Soft mist inhaler
TH2	Type 2 T-helper $CD4^+$ cell

REFERENCES

1. Global strategy for asthma management and prevention 2014 (update) [Internet]. http://www.ginasthma.org/local/uploads/files/GINA_Report_2014_Aug12.pdf.
2. NHLBI National Asthma Education and Prevention Program, Expert Panel Report-3 [Internet]. Guidelines for the diagnosis and management of asthma. NIH Publication No. 07-4051. Bethesda, MD: U.S. Department of Health and Human Services, 2007. http://www.ncbi.nlm.nih.gov/books/NBK7232/.
3. British Guideline on the Management of Asthma; A national clinical guideline 2014 (update). British Thoracic Society Scottish Intercollegiate Guidelines Network. [Internet]. https://www.brit-thoracic.org.uk/document-library/clinical-information/asthma/btssign-asthma-guideline-2014/.
4. World Health Organization. Asthma fact sheet No. 307. November 2013. http://www.who.int/mediacentre/factsheets/fs307/en/index.html.
5. CDC Fast Stats: Asthma. July 2014. http://www.cdc.gov/nchs/fastats/asthma.htm.
6. Barnett SBL, Nurmagambetov TA. Control of asthma in the United States: 2002–2007. J Allergy Clin Immunol. 2011;127:145–152.
7. U.S. Department of Health and Human Services. The Health Consequences of Smoking—50 Years of Progress: A Report of the Surgeon General. Atlanta, GA: U.S. Department of Health and Human Services, Centers for Disease Control and Prevention, National Center for Chronic Disease Prevention and Health Promotion, Office on Smoking and Health, 2014. http://www.surgeongeneral.gov/library/reports/50-years-of-progress/full-report.pdf. Accessed Nov. 2, 2014.
8. Centers for Disease Control and Prevention. Lung disease including asthma and adult vaccination. http://www.cdc.gov/vaccines/adults/rec-vac/health-conditions/lung-disease.html.
9. Centers for Disease Control and Prevention. Flu and people with asthma. http://www.cdc.gov/flu/asthma/.
10. Centers for Disease Control and Prevention. Pneumococcal vaccination. http://www.cdc.gov/pneumococcal/vaccination.html#ppsv23.
11. Dolovich MB, Ahrens RC, Hess DR, et al. Device selection and outcomes of aerosol therapy: Evidence-based guidelines. Chest. 2005;127:335–371.
12. Rubin BK. Pediatric aerosol therapy: new devices and new drugs. Respir Care. 2011;56(9):1411–1421.
13. Proskocil BJ, Fryer AD. β_2-agonist and anticholinergic drugs in the treatment of lung disease. Proc Am Thorac Soc. 2005;2:305–310.
14. Kelly HW. Levalbuterol for asthma: A better treatment? Curr Allergy Asthma Rep. 2007;7:310–314.
15. Lemanske RF, Mauger DT, Sorkness CA. Step-up therapy for children with uncontrolled asthma receiving inhaled corticosteroids. N Engl J Med. 2010;362:975–985.

16. Nelson HS, Weiss ST, Bleeker ER, et al, and the Smart Study Group. The salmeterol multicenter asthma research trial: A comparison of usual pharmacotherapy for asthma or usual pharmacotherapy plus salmeterol. Chest. 2006;129:15–26.
17. Bateman E, Neslon H, Bousquet J, et al. Meta-analysis: Effects of adding salmeterol to inhaled corticosteroids on serious asthma-related events. Ann Intern Med. 2008;149:33–42.
18. Kelly HW. Comparison of inhaled corticosteroids: An update. Ann Pharmacother. 2009;43:519–527.
19. Kelly HW. Inhaled corticosteroid dosing: Doubling for nothing? J Allergy Clin Immunol. 2011; 128:278–281.
20. Tomlinson JEM, McMahon AD, Chaudhuri R, et al. Efficacy of low and high dose inhaled corticosteroid in smokers versus non-smokers with mild asthma. Thorax. 2005;60:282–287.
21. Zhang L, Prietsch SOM, Ducharme FM. Inhaled corticosteroids in children with persistent asthma: Effects on growth. Cochrane Database Syst Rev. 2014 Jul 17;7:CD009471. doi: 10.1002/14651858.CD009471.pub2.
22. Pruteanu AI, Chauhan BF, Zhang L, Prietsch SOM, Ducharme FM. Inhaled corticosteroids in children with persistent asthma: Dose-response effects on growth. Cochrane Database Syst Rev. 2014 Jul 17;7:CD009878. doi: 10.1002/14651858.CD009878.pub2.
23. Gamble J, Stevenson M, McClean E, et al. The prevalence of non-adherence in difficult asthma. Am J Respir Crit Care Med. 2009;180:817–822.
24. Tantisira KG, Lasky-Su J, Harada M. Genomewide association between GLCCI1 and response to glucocorticoid therapy in asthma. N Engl J Med. 2011;365:1173–1183.
25. Rodrigo GJ, Castro-Rodrigo JA. Anticholinergics in the treatment of children and adults with acute asthma: A systematic review with meta-analysis. Thorax. 2005;60:740–746.
26. Peters SP, Kunselman SJ, Icitovic N, et al. Tiotropium bromide step-up therapy for adults with uncontrolled asthma. N Engl J Med. 2010;363:1715–1726.
27. Kerstjens HAM, Disse B, Schroder-Babo W, et al. Tiotropium improves lung function in patients with severe uncontrolled asthma: A randomized controlled trial. J Allergy Clin Immunol. 2011;128:308–314.
28. Ogale SS, Lee TL, Au DH, et al. Cardiovascular events associated with ipratropium bromide in COPD. Chest. 2010;137:13–19.
29. Celli B, Decramer M, Leimer I, et al. Cardiovascular safety of tiotropium in patients with COPD. Chest. 2010;137:20–30.
30. Sorkness CA, Lemanske RF Jr, Mauger DT, et al. Long-term comparison of 3 controller regiments for mild-moderate persistent childhood asthma: The pediatric asthma controller trial. J Allergy Clin Immunol. 2007;119:64–72.
31. Barnes PJ. Theophylline. New perspective on an old drug. Am J Respir Crit Care Med. 2003;167:813–818.
32. Busse WW, Morgan WJ, Gergen PJ. Randomized trial of omalizumab (Anti-IgE) for asthma in inner-city children. N Engl J Med. 2011;364:1005–1015.
33. Kim HL, Leigh R, Becker A. Omalizumab: Practical considerations regarding the risk of anaphylaxis. Allergy Asthma Clin Immunol. 2010;6:32–41.
34. U.S. Department of Health and Human Services. U.S. Food and Drug Administration FDA Drug Safety Communication: FDA approves label changes for asthma drug Xolair (omalizumab), including describing slightly higher risk of heart and brain adverse events. September 26, 2014. http://www.fda.gov/Drugs/DrugSafety/ucm414911.htm.
35. Parsons JP, Hallstrand TS, Mastronarde JG, et al. An official American Thoracic Society clinical practice guideline: Exercise-induced bronchoconstriction. Am J Respir Crit Care Med. 2013; 187:1016–1027.
36. Rogers L, Reibman J. Stepping down asthma treatment: How and when. Curr Opin Pulm Med. 2012; 18(1):70–75.
37. Camargo CA Jr, Rachelefsky G, Schatz M. Managing asthma exacerbations in the emergency department: Summary of the National Asthma Education and Prevention Program Expert Panel Report 3 guidelines for the management of asthma exacerbations. Proc Am Thorac Soc. 2009;6(4):357–366.
38. American College of Obstetricians and Gynecologists (ACOG). Asthma in pregnancy. ACOG practice bulletin no. 90. Washington, DC: American College of Obstetricians and Gynecologists, February 2008. http://www.guideline.gov/content.aspx?id=12630.

15 Chronic Obstructive Pulmonary Disease

Tara R. Whetsel and Jon P. Wietholter

LEARNING OBJECTIVES

Upon completion of the chapter, the reader will be able to:

1. Describe the pathophysiology of chronic obstructive pulmonary disease (COPD).
2. Identify signs and symptoms of COPD.
3. List the treatment goals for a patient with COPD.
4. Design an appropriate COPD maintenance treatment regimen based on patient-specific data.
5. Design an appropriate COPD exacerbation treatment regimen based on patient-specific data.
6. Develop a monitoring plan to assess effectiveness and adverse effects of pharmacotherapy for COPD.
7. Formulate an appropriate education plan for a patient with COPD.

INTRODUCTION

Chronic obstructive pulmonary disease (COPD) is a progressive disease characterized by airflow limitation that is not fully reversible. Previous definitions of COPD included chronic bronchitis and emphysema. Chronic bronchitis is defined clinically as a chronic productive cough for at least 3 months in each of two consecutive years in a patient in whom other causes have been excluded.[1] Emphysema is defined pathologically as destruction of alveoli.[1] The major risk factor for both conditions is cigarette smoking, and many patients share characteristics of each one. Therefore, current guidelines focus instead on chronic airflow limitation.

The Global Initiative for Chronic Obstructive Lung Disease (GOLD) is an expert panel of health professionals who developed consensus guidelines for the diagnosis and care of patients with COPD that are updated annually.[1] Clinical practice guidelines for the diagnosis and management of stable COPD have also been published by several medical organizations.[2]

EPIDEMIOLOGY AND ETIOLOGY

COPD is a major cause of morbidity and mortality and a significant cause of disability worldwide. In 2011, 12.7 million US adults were estimated to have COPD.[3] COPD is the third leading cause of death in the United States; in 2010, 134,676 adults died from the disease. Its estimated cost to the United States in 2010 was $49.9 billion, with direct medical costs accounting for $29.5 billion of the total.[3]

COPD is caused by repeated inhalation of noxious particles or gases, most commonly cigarette smoke. Marijuana and other forms of tobacco, including secondhand smoke, are also risk factors.[1] Not all smokers develop clinically significant COPD, which suggests that genetic susceptibility plays a role. The best documented genetic factor is a rare hereditary deficiency of α_1-antitrypsin (AAT). Severe deficiency of this enzyme results in premature and accelerated development of emphysema. Other COPD risk factors include occupational exposure to dusts and chemicals (vapors, irritants, and fumes), biomass smoke inhalation, asthma, bronchial hyperresponsiveness, maternal smoking, childhood asthma, and severe childhood respiratory infections.[4] Environmental air pollution has been implicated as a cause, but its exact role is unclear.

PATHOPHYSIOLOGY

Repeated exposure to noxious particles and gases causes chronic inflammation, resulting in pathologic changes in the central and peripheral airways, lung **parenchyma**, and pulmonary vasculature that lead to obstruction.[1,5,6] An imbalance between **proteinases** and **antiproteinases** in the lungs and oxidative stress are also important in the pathogenesis of COPD (**Figure 15–1**).

Inflammation is present in the lungs of all smokers. It is unclear why only 15% to 30% of smokers develop COPD, but susceptible individuals appear to have an exaggerated inflammatory response.[5,6] KEY CONCEPT *The inflammation of COPD differs from that seen in asthma, so the use of and response to anti-inflammatory medications is different.* The inflammation of asthma is mainly mediated through eosinophils and mast cells. In COPD, the primary inflammatory cells are neutrophils, macrophages, and $CD8^+$ T lymphocytes.[5,6] Activated inflammatory cells release mediators such as interleukin-1, interleukin-8, and tumor necrosis factor-α. Activated neutrophils secrete proteinases such as elastase and proteinase-3. These mediators and proteinases sustain inflammation and damage lung structures.

Proteinases and antiproteinases are part of the normal protective and repair mechanisms in the lungs. An imbalance of proteinase–antiproteinase activity in COPD results from either increased production or activity of destructive proteinases or inactivation or reduced production of protective antiproteinases. AAT (an antiproteinase) inhibits trypsin, elastase, and several

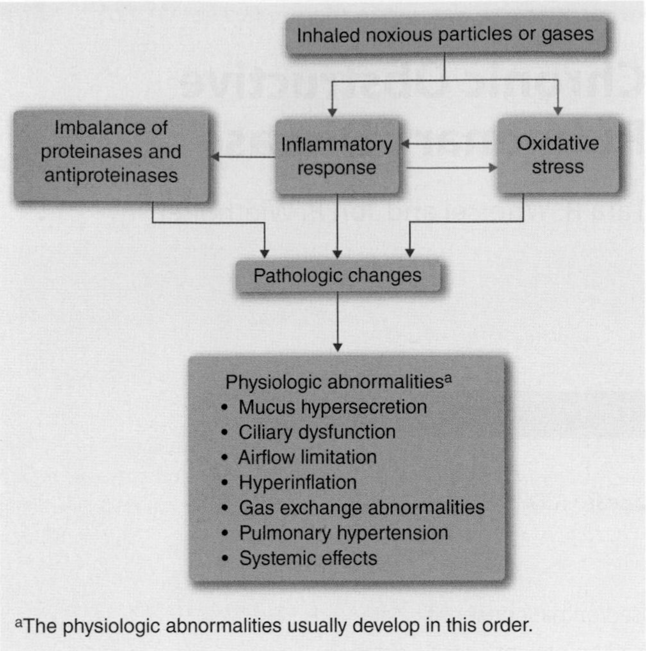

FIGURE 15–1. Pathophysiology of COPD.

other proteolytic enzymes. Deficiency of AAT results in unopposed proteinase activity, which promotes destruction of alveolar walls and lung parenchyma, leading to emphysema.

Oxidative stress occurs from smoke exposure and an increase in activated neutrophils and macrophages. Oxidative stress promotes inflammation and contributes to the proteinase–antiproteinase imbalance by reducing antiproteinase activity. In addition, oxidants constrict airway smooth muscle, contributing to reversible airway narrowing.

In the central airways (the trachea, bronchi, and larger bronchioles), inflammatory cells and mediators stimulate mucus gland hyperplasia and mucus hypersecretion. Mucus hypersecretion and ciliary dysfunction lead to chronic cough and sputum production. The major site of airflow obstruction is the peripheral airways (small bronchi and bronchioles). Narrowing of small airways results from remodeling (thickening of the airway wall caused by disrupted tissue repair), increased mucus, and accumulation of inflammatory debris.[4,5,6] The reduced airway diameter causes increased resistance to airflow. Parenchymal destruction leads to loss of elasticity and structural support resulting in closure of small airways during expiration, further obstructing airflow.

As airflow obstruction worsens, the rate of lung emptying slows and the interval between inspirations does not allow expiration to the relaxation volume of the lungs. This leads to pulmonary hyperinflation, which initially only occurs during exercise but later is also seen at rest. Hyperinflation contributes to the discomfort associated with airflow obstruction by flattening the diaphragm and placing it at a mechanical disadvantage.

In advanced COPD, airflow obstruction, damaged bronchioles and alveoli, and pulmonary vascular abnormalities lead to impaired gas exchange, resulting in hypoxemia and eventually hypercapnia. Hypoxemia is initially present only during exercise but occurs at rest as the disease progresses. Inequality in the ventilation/perfusion ratio (V_A/Q) is the major mechanism underlying hypoxemia. As hypoxemia worsens, the body may increase erythrocyte production in an attempt to increase oxygen delivery to tissues.

Pulmonary hypertension develops late in the course of COPD, usually after development of severe hypoxemia. It is the most common cardiovascular complication of COPD and can result in cor pulmonale, or right-sided heart failure. Progressive loss of skeletal muscle mass in longstanding COPD contributes to exercise limitation and declining health status.

CLINICAL PRESENTATION AND DIAGNOSIS

See accompanying box for the clinical presentation of COPD.

Diagnosis

A suspected diagnosis of COPD should be based on patient symptoms and history of exposure to risk factors. Spirometry is required to confirm the diagnosis, using the ratio of forced expiratory volume in 1 second (FEV_1) to forced vital capacity (FVC). A postbronchodilator FEV_1/FVC ratio less than 70% (0.70) confirms airflow limitation that is not fully reversible.[1,2] Spirometry results can further be used to classify severity of airflow limitation in these patients. The GOLD classification categories of severity based on postbronchodilator FEV_1 are as follows: GOLD 1, Mild = 80% predicted or greater; GOLD 2, Moderate = 50%–79% predicted; GOLD 3, Severe = 30%–49% predicted; GOLD 4, Very Severe = less than 30% predicted.[1] Full pulmonary function tests (PFTs) with lung volumes and diffusion capacity

Clinical Presentation of COPD

General

- Patients are initially asymptomatic. COPD is usually not diagnosed until declining lung function leads to significant symptoms and prompts patients to seek medical care.

Symptoms

- Symptom onset is variable and does not correlate well with severity of airflow limitation measured by FEV_1.[1]
- Initial symptoms include chronic cough (for more than 3 months) that may be intermittent at first, chronic sputum production, and dyspnea on exertion. Patients may complain of a sensation of heaviness in the chest.
- As COPD progresses, dyspnea at rest and/or orthopnea develop, and ability to perform activities of daily living declines.

Signs

- Inspection may reveal use of accessory muscles of respiration (paradoxical movements of the chest and abdomen in a seesaw-type motion), pursed-lips breathing, and hyperinflation of the chest with increased anterior–posterior diameter ("barrel chest").
- On lung auscultation, patients may have distant breath sounds, wheezing, a prolonged expiratory phase, and rhonchi.
- In advanced COPD, signs of hypoxemia may include cyanosis and tachycardia.
- Signs of cor pulmonale include increased pulmonic component of the second heart sound, jugular venous distention (JVD), lower extremity edema, and hepatomegaly.

and arterial blood gases (ABGs) are not necessary to establish the diagnosis or severity of COPD.

Pulse oximetry should be obtained in patients with an FEV_1 less than 35% predicted or with signs or symptoms suggestive of cor pulmonale or respiratory failure.[1] If oxygen saturation is less than 92% (0.92), ABGs should be assessed.[1] Patients may exhibit increased arterial carbon dioxide tension ($Paco_2$) and decreased arterial oxygen tension (Pao_2).

A complete blood count (CBC) may reveal an elevated hematocrit that may exceed 55% (0.55; polycythemia). An AAT level should be obtained in patients less than 45 years old presenting with signs and symptoms consistent with COPD, especially if there is a strong family history of emphysema or limited smoking history/exposure. Chest radiography may show lung hyperinflation and signs of emphysema.

It is important to distinguish COPD from asthma because treatment and prognosis differ. Differentiating factors include age of onset, smoking history, triggers, occupational history, and degree of reversibility measured by prebronchodilator and postbronchodilator spirometry. In some patients, a clear distinction between asthma and COPD is not possible. Management of these patients should be similar to that of asthma.

TREATMENT

Desired Outcomes

The goals of COPD management include: (a) smoking cessation if applicable, (b) reducing symptoms, (c) improving exercise tolerance, (d) minimizing the rate of decline in lung function, (e) maintaining or improving quality of life, and (f) preventing and treating exacerbations.

General Approach to Treatment

KEY CONCEPT *An integrated approach of health maintenance (eg, smoking cessation), drug therapy, and supplemental therapy (eg, oxygen and pulmonary rehabilitation) should be used. Symptom severity and risk of COPD exacerbations can be used to guide therapy decisions.*

The modified Medical Research Council Questionnaire (mMRC) or COPD Assessment Test (CAT) is recommended for symptom assessment. The CAT is preferred because it provides a more comprehensive assessment. It is unnecessary to use both mMRC and CAT. An mMRC grade of 0 or 1 or a CAT score less than 10 indicates fewer symptoms. These patients may be managed with a short-acting inhaled bronchodilator used as needed. Patients with more symptoms will have an mMRC grade of 2 or more or a CAT score of 10 or more. These patients require inhaled long-acting bronchodilators on a scheduled basis.

Risk of future COPD exacerbation can be assessed using spirometric classification or number of exacerbations per year. Patients with a history of two or more exacerbations per year or one or more exacerbation(s) requiring hospitalization are at high risk for future exacerbations. An FEV_1 less than 50% predicted also indicates high risk. Patients at high risk of COPD exacerbations should be treated with medications shown to reduce the frequency of exacerbations. Figure 15–2 provides an overview of the management of stable COPD.

Patient Encounter, Part 1

A 63-year-old man with a past medical history of hypertension, asthma, and tobacco abuse (50 pack–year history) presents to the clinic complaining of shortness of breath with moderate physical activity, a chronic cough of more than 2 years, and difficulty catching his breath while laying down.

What symptoms and/or risk factors does he have that are suggestive of COPD?

What additional information do you need before creating a treatment plan for this patient?

Nonpharmacologic Therapy

▶ Smoking Cessation

KEY CONCEPT *Smoking cessation slows the rate of decline in pulmonary function in patients with COPD.*[7,8] Cessation can also reduce cough and sputum production and decrease airway reactivity. Therefore, it is a critical part of any treatment plan. Unfortunately, achieving and maintaining cessation is a major challenge. A clinical practice guideline from the US Public Health Service recommends a specific action plan depending on the current smoking status and desire to quit (Figure 15–3).[9] Brief interventions are effective and can increase cessation rates significantly. The 5 As and the 5 Rs can be used to guide brief interventions (Table 15–1).

All tobacco users should be assessed for their readiness to quit and appropriate strategies implemented. Those who are ready to quit should be treated with a combination of behavioral and cognitive strategies and pharmacotherapy (refer to Smoking Cessation in Chapter 36). In COPD patients, the likelihood of sustained abstinence is higher with nicotine replacement therapy than with sustained-release bupropion.[10]

▶ Pulmonary Rehabilitation

Pulmonary rehabilitation results in significant and clinically meaningful improvements in dyspnea, exercise capacity, health status, and health care utilization.[11] It should be prescribed for symptomatic patients with an FEV_1 less than 50% predicted.[2] Clinicians may consider pulmonary rehabilitation for symptomatic patients with FEV_1 above 50% predicted, but evidence of benefit is less clear. A comprehensive pulmonary rehabilitation program should include exercise training, smoking cessation, nutrition counseling, and education.

Rehabilitation programs may be conducted in the inpatient, outpatient (most common), or home setting. The minimum length of an effective program is 6 weeks; the longer the program, the more sustained the results.[1,11] It is important for patients to continue with a home exercise program to maintain the benefits gained from the pulmonary rehabilitation program.

▶ Long-Term Oxygen Therapy

Long-term oxygen administration (greater than 15 hours/day) to patients with chronic respiratory failure has been shown to reduce mortality and improve quality of life.[1,2] Oxygen therapy should be initiated in stable patients with COPD who have severe resting hypoxemia as determined by Pao_2 at or below 55 mm Hg (7.3 kPa) or oxygen saturation (Sao_2) at or below 88% (0.88),[1,2] or with evidence of pulmonary hypertension, peripheral edema suggesting congestive heart failure, or polycythemia.[1]

The dual-prong nasal cannula is the standard means of delivering continuous oxygen flow. The goal is to increase the baseline oxygen saturation to at least 90% (0.90) and/or Pao_2 to at least

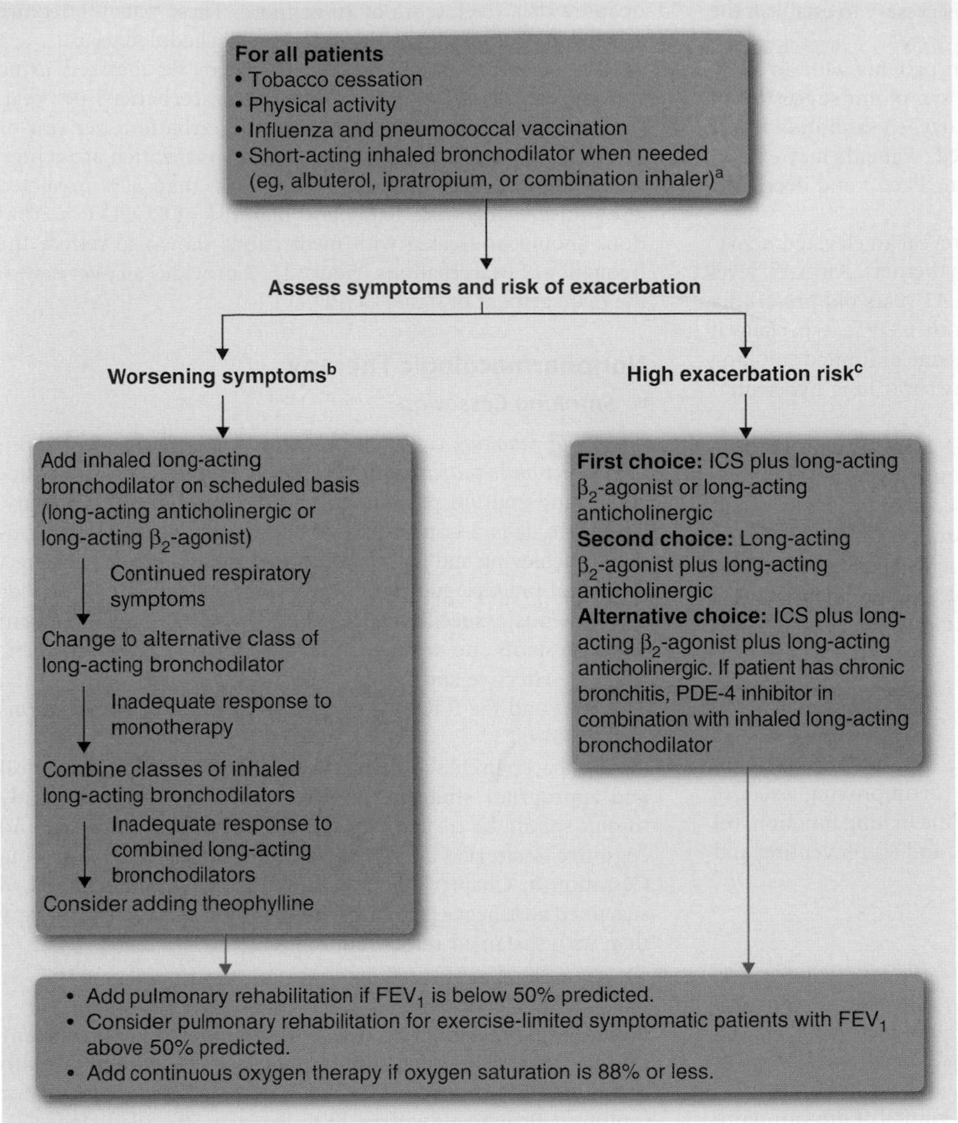

For all patients
• Tobacco cessation
• Physical activity
• Influenza and pneumococcal vaccination
• Short-acting inhaled bronchodilator when needed (eg, albuterol, ipratropium, or combination inhaler)a
Assess symptoms and risk of exacerbation
Worsening symptomsb
High exacerbation riskc
Add inhaled long-acting bronchodilator on scheduled basis (long-acting anticholinergic or long-acting β2-agonist)
Continued respiratory symptoms
Change to alternative class of long-acting bronchodilator
Inadequate response to monotherapy
Combine classes of inhaled long-acting bronchodilators
Inadequate response to combined long-acting bronchodilators
Consider adding theophylline
First choice: ICS plus long-acting β2-agonist or long-acting anticholinergic
Second choice: Long-acting β2-agonist plus long-acting anticholinergic
Alternative choice: ICS plus long-acting β2-agonist plus long-acting anticholinergic. If patient has chronic bronchitis, PDE-4 inhibitor in combination with inhaled long-acting bronchodilator
• Add pulmonary rehabilitation if FEV1 is below 50% predicted.
• Consider pulmonary rehabilitation for exercise-limited symptomatic patients with FEV1 above 50% predicted.
• Add continuous oxygen therapy if oxygen saturation is 88% or less.

FIGURE 15–2. Treatment algorithm for stable COPD.[1,2] (ICS, inhaled corticosteroid; PDE-4, phosphodiesterase-4; FEV_1, forced expiratory volume in 1 second.) [a]GOLD patient category A (low exacerbation risk, fewer symptoms). [b]GOLD patient category B (low exacerbation risk, more symptoms). [c]GOLD patient category C (high exacerbation risk, fewer symptoms) or GOLD patient category D (high exacerbation risk, more symptoms). [d]Albuterol should be used as rescue therapy for patients treated with a long-acting anticholinergic.

60 mm Hg (8.0 kPa), allowing adequate oxygenation of vital organs. The flow rate, expressed as liters per minute (L/min), must be increased during exercise and sleep and can be adjusted based on pulse oximetry. Hypoxemia also worsens during air travel; patients requiring oxygen should generally increase their flow rate by 3 L/min during flight.[1]

Oxygen therapy should be continued indefinitely if it was initiated while the patient was in a stable state (rather than during an acute episode). Withdrawal of oxygen because of improved Pao_2 in such a patient may be detrimental.

► *Surgery*

Bullectomy, lung volume reduction surgery, and lung transplantation are surgical options for very severe COPD. These procedures may result in improved spirometry, lung volumes, exercise capacity, dyspnea, health-related quality of life, and possibly survival. Patient selection is critical because not all patients benefit.

Pharmacologic Therapy of Stable COPD

The medications available for COPD are effective for reducing or relieving symptoms, improving exercise tolerance, reducing the number and severity of exacerbations, and improving quality of life. Evidence that medications slow the rate of decline in lung function or improve mortality is inconclusive.[1,2]

► *Bronchodilators*

KEY CONCEPT *Bronchodilators are the mainstay of treatment for symptomatic COPD. They reduce symptoms and improve exercise tolerance and quality of life.*[1] They can be used as needed for symptoms or on a scheduled basis to prevent or reduce symptoms. Bronchodilator drugs commonly used in COPD include β_2-agonists, anticholinergics, and methylxanthines. The choice depends on availability, individual response, side-effect profile, and preferences. The inhaled route is preferred, but attention must be paid to proper inhaler technique. Long-acting bronchodilators are more expensive than short-acting bronchodilators but are superior on important clinical outcomes, including frequency of exacerbations, degree of dyspnea, and health-related quality of life.[1,12] Monotherapy with long-acting bronchodilators is preferred; combination therapy may be appropriate in symptomatic patients with an FEV_1 less than 60% predicted or in patients with frequent exacerbations, although it is unclear when combination therapy provides added benefit.[2]

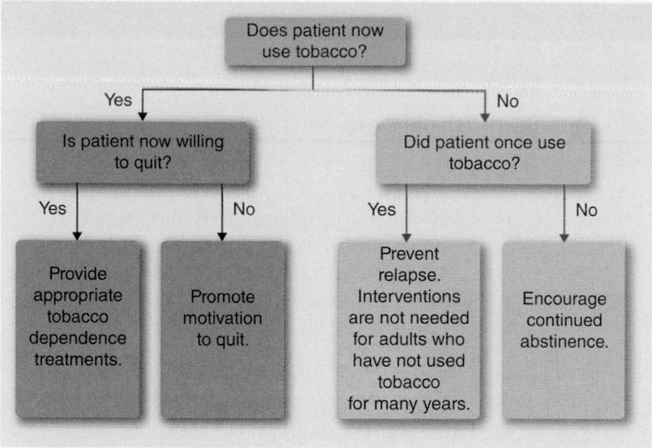

FIGURE 15–3. Algorithm for routine assessment of tobacco use status. (From Fiore MC, Jaén CR, Baker TB, et al. Treating tobacco use and dependence. Clinical Practice Guideline. U.S. Department of Health and Human Services, 2008, http://www.ahrq.gov/professionals/clinicians-providers/guidelines-recommendations/tobacco/clinicians/update/index.html)

β_2-Agonists These agents cause airway smooth muscle relaxation by stimulating adenyl cyclase to increase formation of cyclic adenosine monophosphate (cAMP). They may also improve mucociliary transport. β_2 Agonists are available in inhalation, oral, and parenteral dosage forms; the inhalation route is preferred because of fewer adverse effects.

These drugs are also available in short-acting and long-acting formulations (Table 15–2). The short-acting β_2-agonists include albuterol (known as salbutamol outside the United States), levalbuterol (known as R-salbutamol outside the United States), and terbutaline. They are used as "rescue" therapy for acute symptom relief. Most COPD patients need continuous bronchodilator therapy on a scheduled basis every day. For these patients, short-acting β_2-agonists are inconvenient as maintenance therapy because of the need for frequent dosing.

Long-acting β_2-agonists (LABAs) include salmeterol, formoterol, arformoterol, indacaterol, olodaterol, and vilanterol. Arformoterol is the (*R*,*R*)-isomer of formoterol; both drugs are available for nebulization, providing an alternative for patients with poor inhaler technique. Indacaterol, olodaterol, and vilanterol are long acting, allowing for once daily dosing compared to twice daily dosing for salmeterol, formoterol, and arformoterol. At the time of this writing, vilanterol is only available in combination inhalers (Table 15–3). Some of the LABAs have been shown to decrease COPD exacerbations and improve exercise tolerance, dyspnea, and quality of life.[12,13] Patients treated with LABAs should also have a short-acting β_2-agonist such as albuterol for as-needed use ("rescue" medication) but should be advised to avoid excessive use.

Adverse effects of both long- and short-acting β_2-agonists are dose related and include palpitations, tachycardia, hypokalemia, and tremor. Sleep disturbance may also occur and appears to be worse with higher doses of inhaled LABAs. Increasing doses beyond those clinically recommended is without benefit and could be associated with increased adverse effects.

Table 15–1

Components of Brief Interventions for Tobacco Users

The 5 As for Brief Intervention	
Ask:	Identify and document tobacco-use status for every patient at every visit
Advise:	Urge every tobacco user to quit
Assess:	Is the tobacco user willing to make a quit attempt at this time?
Assist:	Use counseling and pharmacotherapy to help patients willing to make a quit attempt
Arrange:	Schedule follow-up contact, preferably within the first week after the quit date
The 5 Rs to Motivate Smokers Unwilling to Quit at Present	
Relevance:	Tailor advice and discussion to each smoker
Risks:	Help the patient identify potential negative consequences of tobacco use
Rewards:	Help the patient identify the potential benefits of quitting
Roadblocks:	Help the patient identify barriers to quitting
Repetition:	Repeat the motivational message at every visit

Anticholinergics Ipratropium, tiotropium, aclidinium, and umeclidinium are all bromide salts available for inhalation treatment of COPD. They produce bronchodilation by competitively blocking muscarinic receptors in bronchial smooth muscle. They may also decrease mucus secretion, although this effect is variable. Tiotropium and umeclidinium have long half-lives allowing for once-daily dosing. Aclidinium has a slightly faster onset of action than tiotropium but a shorter half-life, requiring twice-daily dosing. Ipratropium has an elimination half-life of about 2 hours, necessitating dosing every 6 to 8 hours. Because of a longer onset of action (within 15 minutes), ipratropium is not usually recommended as a "rescue" medication, particularly in patients tolerating a short-acting β_2-agonist.

Clinical trials with some of these agents have shown decreased symptoms, reduced COPD exacerbations and hospitalizations, and improved quality of life.[14–18] Tiotropium may be more effective than salmeterol for reducing exacerbations in patients with moderate to very severe COPD.[18] Other comparative studies and meta-analyses have found few differences among long-acting anticholinergics and LABAs.[1,2] Patients using anticholinergics as maintenance therapy should be prescribed albuterol as their rescue therapy; ipratropium is not recommended as an alternative to albuterol because of the risk of excessive anticholinergic effects (particularly urinary retention) when combined with long-acting anticholinergics.[19]

Inhaled anticholinergics are well tolerated with the most common adverse effect being dry mouth. Occasional metallic taste has also been reported, most commonly with ipratropium. Other anticholinergic adverse effects include constipation, tachycardia, blurred vision, and precipitation of narrow-angle glaucoma symptoms. Urinary retention could be a problem, especially for patients with concurrent bladder outlet obstruction. Early studies suggested an increased risk of myocardial infarction and cardiovascular death,[20,21] but subsequent large trials of tiotropium powder for inhalation found no increased cardiovascular risk.[15,18] The cardiovascular safety of tiotropium aerosol solution remains controversial, especially in patients with cardiovascular disease or chronic kidney disease.[22] The FDA is requiring a post-marketing clinical trial to evaluate the cardiovascular safety of aclidinium due to its structural similarity to atropine.

Methylxanthines Theophylline is a methylxanthine derivative and nonselective phosphodiesterase inhibitor that increases intracellular cAMP within airway smooth muscle resulting in bronchodilation. It also has anti-inflammatory effects. In patients with COPD, theophylline increases exercise tolerance,

Table 15–2

Maintenance Medications for COPD

	Medication	Onset	Peak	Duration	Usual Dose
Short-Acting β_2-Agonists	**Albuterol**[a]				
	Nebulization	5–8 min	1–2 hours	3–6 hours	2.5 mg every 4–8 hours (max: 30 mg/day)
	Inhalation	5–8 min	0.5–1 hour	3–6 hours	MDI (90 mcg/puff) one to two puffs every 4–6 hours (max: 1080 mcg/day)
	Oral	7–30 min	2–3 hours	6–8 hours ER: 8–12 hours	2–4 mg three to four times a day ER: 4–8 mg every 12 hours (max: 32 mg/day)
	Levalbuterol				
	Nebulization	10–20 min	1.5 hours	5–8 hours	0.63–1.25 mg three times per day, 6–8 hours apart (max: 3.75 mg/day)
	Inhalation	5–10 min	1–1.5 hours	3–6 hours	MDI (45 mcg/puff) one to two puffs every 4–6 hours (max: 540 mcg/day)
	Terbutaline				
	Oral	0.5–2 hours	1–3 hours	6–8 hours	2.5–5 mg three times per day, 6 hours apart[b] (max: 15 mg/day)
Long-Acting β_2-Agonists	**Formoterol**				
	Inhalation	1–3 min	1–3 hours	8–12 hours	Powder (12 mcg/inhalation) one inhalation every 12 hours (max: 24 mcg/day)
	Nebulization	1–3 min	1–3 hours	8–12 hours	20 mcg every 12 hours (max: 40 mcg/day)
	Salmeterol				
	Inhalation	10 min to 1 hour	2–3 hours	12 hours	Powder (50 mcg/inhalation) one inhalation every 12 hours (max: 100 mcg/day)
	Indacaterol				
	Inhalation	5 min	1–4 hours	24 hours	Powder (75 mcg/inhalation) one inhalation every 24 hours (max: 75 mcg/day)
	Olodaterol				
	Inhalation[c]	5 min	—	24 hours	2.5 mcg/inhalation Two inhalations every 24 hours (max: 5 mcg/day)
	Vilanterol				
	Inhalation	15–30 min	1 hour	24 hours	Powder (25 mcg/inhalation) one inhalation every 24 hours (max: 25 mcg/day)
	Arformoterol				
	Nebulization	7–20 min	1–3 hours	12 hours	15 mcg every 12 hours (max: 30 mcg/day)
Short-Acting Anticholinergic	**Ipratropium**				
	Nebulization	15 min	1–2 hours	4–8 hours	500 mcg every 6–8 hours (max: 2,000 mcg/day)
	Inhalation	15 min	1–2 hours	4–8 hours	MDI (18 mcg/puff) two puffs four times/day (max: 216 mcg/day)
Long-Acting Anticholinergic	**Tiotropium**				
	Inhalation	30 min	1–4 hours	24 hours	Powder (18 mcg/inhalation) one inhalation every 24 hours (max: 18 mcg/day)[d] Aerosol solution (2.5 mcg/inhalation) two inhalations every 24 hours (max 5 mcg/day)[d]
	Aclidinium				
	Inhalation	30 min	1–4 hours	12 hours	Powder (400 mcg/inhalation) one inhalation every 12 hours (max: 800 mcg/day)
	Umeclidinium				
	Inhalation	30 min	1–3 hours	24 hours	Powder (62.5 mcg/inhalation) one inhalation every 24 hours (max: 62.5 mcg/day)
Methylxanthine	**Theophylline**				
	Oral	0.5–2 hours	Up to 24 hours, depending on formulation	6–24 hours	400–600 mg/day divided every 6–24 hours based on formulation (max: 800 mg/day) Adjust dose to serum concentrations of 5–15 mcg/mL (5–15 mg/L; 28–83 μmol/L)
Phosphodiesterase-4 Inhibitor	**Roflumilast** Oral	4 wks	—	—	500 mcg daily[e]

(Continued)

Table 15–2

Maintenance Medications for COPD (*Continued*)

	Medication	Onset	Peak	Duration	Usual Dose
Inhaled Corticosteroids	Beclomethasone	1–7 days	1–4 wks		MDI (40, 80 mcg/puff) 40–160 mcg twice a day (max: 640 mcg/day)
	Budesonide	1–7 days	1–2 wks		Powder (90, 180 mcg/inhalation) 180–360 mcg twice a day (max: 1440 mcg/day)
	Ciclesonide	1–7 days	1–4 wks		MDI (80, 160 mcg/puff) 80–320 mcg one or two times per day (max: 640 mcg/day)
	Fluticasone	1–7 days	1–2 wks		MDI (44, 110, 220 mcg/puff) 88–440 mcg twice a day (max: 1760 mcg/day) Powder (50, 100, 250 mcg/inhalation) 100–1000 mcg twice a day (max: 2000 mcg/day)
	Mometasone	1–7 days	1–2 wks		Powder (110, 220 mcg/inhalation) 220–440 mcg one or two times/day (max: 880 mcg/day)

In elderly patients, start with the lowest recommended dose and increase as necessary.

ER, extended-release; MDI, metered-dose inhaler.

[a]Albuterol is known as salbutamol and levalbuterol is known as levosalbutamol (or R-salbutamol) outside the United States.

[b]Not recommended if creatinine clearance (CrCl) less than or equal to 10 mL/min (0.17 mL/s); for CrCl 11 to 50 mL/min (0.18–0.83 mL/s), reduce dose by 50%.

[c]Solution delivered via Respimat device.

[d]Patients with reduced activity in the CYP2D6 pathway (poor metabolizers [PMs]) have higher plasma concentrations than those with normal activity (extensive metabolizers [EMs]); PMs may require lower doses and should be monitored closely for adverse effects.

[e]Not recommended in patients with moderate or severe hepatic impairment.

reduces air trapping, and may reduce exacerbations.[23] Its use is limited due to a narrow therapeutic index, multiple drug interactions, and adverse effects. Theophylline should be reserved for patients who cannot use inhaled medications or who remain symptomatic despite appropriate use of inhaled bronchodilators.

Therapeutic drug monitoring is needed to optimize therapy because of wide interpatient variability. Serum concentrations from 5 to 15 mcg/mL (5–15 mg/L; 28–83 μmol/L) provide adequate clinical response with a greater margin of safety than the previously recommended range of 10 to 20 mcg/mL (10–20 mg/L; 55–111 μmol/L). However, bronchodilatory effects are small when the serum concentration is below 10 mcg/mL (10 mg/L; 55 μmol/L).[23] Multiple factors can alter theophylline clearance including concomitant medications, disease states, tobacco smoke, and marijuana. Chemicals in tobacco smoke induce theophylline metabolism and increase its clearance. Because many patients with COPD are current or past smokers, it is important to assess current tobacco use and adjust

Table 15–3

Combination Inhalers for Management of COPD

Brand Name	Corticosteroid / Anticholinergic	β_2-Agonist	Dosage Strengths	Frequency
Inhaled Corticosteroid/Long-acting β_2-Agonist				
Brand Name	**Corticosteroid**	**β_2-Agonist**	**Dosage Strengths**	**Frequency**
Advair Diskus DPI	Fluticasone propionate	Salmeterol	100, 250, 500 mcg/ 50 mcg	Twice daily
Advair HFA	Fluticasone propionate	Salmeterol	45, 115, 230 mcg/21 mcg	Twice daily
Symbicort	Budesonide	Formoterol	80, 160 mcg/4.5 mcg	Twice daily
Dulera[a]	Mometasone furoate	Formoterol	100, 200 mcg/5 mcg	Twice daily
Breo	Fluticasone furoate	Vilanterol	100 mcg/25 mcg	Daily
Long-acting Anticholinergic/Long-acting β_2-Agonist				
Brand Name	**Anticholinergic**	**β_2-Agonist**	**Dosage Strengths**	**Frequency**
Anoro	Umeclidinium	Vilanterol	62.5 mcg/25 mcg	Daily
Stiolto	Tiotropium	Olodaterol	2.5 mcg/2.5 mcg	Daily
Short-acting Anticholinergic/Short-acting β_2-Agonist				
Brand Name	**Anticholinergic**	**β_2-Agonist**	**Dosage Strengths**	**Frequency**
Combivent	Ipratropium	Albuterol	20 mcg/100 mcg	Four to six times per day

DPI, dry powder inhaler; HFA, hydrofluoroalkane.

[a]Dulera was not FDA approved for management of COPD at the time of this writing.

theophylline dose as needed. The most common adverse effects of theophylline include heartburn, restlessness, insomnia, irritability, tachycardia, and tremor. Dose-related adverse effects include nausea and vomiting, seizures, and arrhythmias.

▶ Corticosteroids

Inhaled corticosteroids improve symptoms, lung function, quality of life, and exacerbation rates in patients with an FEV_1 less than 60%.[1,2] They do not appear to modify the rate of decline in pulmonary function or improve mortality.[1,24]

KEY CONCEPT *Inhaled corticosteroids are recommended for patients with severe and very severe COPD and frequent exacerbations that are not adequately controlled by first-line long-acting bronchodilators.*[1] Monotherapy with inhaled corticosteroids is less effective than combined therapy with an LABA and is therefore not recommended.[1] Combination inhaler devices are convenient and ensure that patients receive both medications (Table 15–3).

The most common adverse effects from inhaled corticosteroids include oropharyngeal candidiasis and hoarse voice. These can be minimized by rinsing the mouth after use and by using a spacer device with metered-dose inhalers (MDIs). Increased bruising, decreased bone density, and increased incidence of pneumonia have also been reported; the clinical importance of these effects remains uncertain.[1,2,24]

Long-term use of oral corticosteroids should be avoided if possible due to an unfavorable risk-to-benefit ratio. The steroid myopathy that can result from long-term use of oral corticosteroids weakens muscles, further decreasing the respiratory drive in patients with advanced disease.

▶ Phosphodiesterase-4 (PDE-4) Inhibitors

Roflumilast is an oral PDE-4 inhibitor approved for prevention of COPD exacerbations in patients with severe COPD associated with chronic bronchitis and a history of exacerbations. PDE-4 inhibitors are believed to reduce inflammation by inhibiting breakdown of cAMP. They do not cause direct bronchodilation. Roflumilast has more frequent adverse events than inhaled LABAs, anticholinergics, and corticosteroids and only a modest benefit in lung function and exacerbation rate.[1,25] It is expensive and has little effect on symptoms or quality of life.[25] Common adverse effects include diarrhea, weight loss, nausea, headache, insomnia, decreased appetite, and abdominal pain; neuropsychiatric effects such as anxiety, depression, and increased suicidality have also been reported. Roflumilast is an option in patients with chronic bronchitis who are not adequately controlled by optimal inhaled medications.[1] It should not be combined with theophylline because both inhibit PDE-4.[23]

▶ Combination Therapy

For patients who remain symptomatic on monotherapy, a combination of bronchodilators can be used.[1,2] Combining long-acting inhaled medications is preferred over short-acting agents or theophylline. Combining an LABA with a long-acting anticholinergic produces a greater change in spirometry than either drug alone.[26,27]

Triple therapy with inhaled corticosteroid, LABA, and long-acting anticholinergic is commonly used in patients who remain symptomatic on dual therapy. Triple therapy appears to improve lung function and quality of life but may not further reduce exacerbations or dyspnea.[28–30] A large, randomized trial found no deleterious effect on exacerbation rates when inhaled fluticasone was withdrawn over 12 weeks from patients with stable, severe COPD treated with tiotropium, salmeterol, and fluticasone.[31] Based on these results, a step-down in therapy by gradually withdrawing the inhaled corticosteroid can be considered in patients with stable COPD. Further studies are needed to determine if the benefits of triple therapy outweigh the increased risk of adverse effects and added cost.

Potential benefits and risks of any combination therapy should be considered on a case-by-case basis. Patients should be monitored closely and therapy should be changed if the combination is not more effective.

▶ Vaccinations

Serious illness and death in COPD patients can be reduced by about 50% with annual influenza vaccination. The optimal time for vaccination is usually from early October through mid-November.

A onetime pneumococcal polysaccharide vaccine (PPSV23) should be administered to all adults with COPD. Patients older than 65 years should be revaccinated if it has been more than 5 years since initial vaccination and they were younger than 65 years at the time. Pneumococcal conjugate vaccine (PCV13) is recommended in all persons 65 years old and older who have not previously received PCV13. PCV13 should be administered first with PPSV23 administered 6 to 12 months later.

▶ α_1-Antitrypsin Augmentation Therapy

Augmentation therapy consists of weekly transfusions of pooled human AAT with the goal of maintaining adequate plasma levels of the enzyme. It is recommended for individuals with AAT deficiency and moderate airflow obstruction (FEV_1 35%–60% predicted).[32] In these patients, augmentation therapy appears to reduce overall mortality and slow decline in FEV_1, although large randomized controlled trials have not been conducted. The benefits of augmentation therapy are unclear in patients with severe (FEV_1 less than 35% predicted) or mild (FEV_1 greater than 60% predicted) airflow obstruction. It is not recommended for individuals with AAT deficiency who do not have lung disease.

▶ Other Pharmacologic Therapies

Leukotriene modifiers (eg, zafirlukast and montelukast) have not been adequately evaluated in COPD patients and are not recommended for routine use. Small short-term studies showed improvement in pulmonary function, dyspnea, and quality of life when leukotriene modifiers were added to inhaled bronchodilator therapy.[33] Additional long-term studies are needed to clarify their role.

N-acetylcysteine has antioxidant and mucolytic activity, but clinical trials have produced conflicting results. One of the largest trials found *N*-acetylcysteine to be ineffective in reducing the decline in lung function and preventing exacerbations.[34] Routine use is not presently recommended.

Prophylaxis with daily oral azithromycin significantly reduced the incidence of acute exacerbations in select subgroups of COPD patients; however, the risks associated with long-term antibiotic use should be further studied before continuous prophylactic use of antibiotics can be routinely recommended.[1,35] Azithromycin may be associated with cardiovascular morbidity and mortality due to prolongation of the QT interval; electrocardiography to assess the QTc interval should be considered prior to starting therapy.[36]

Antitussives are contraindicated in COPD because cough has an important protective role by promoting clearance of secretions. Opioids may be effective for dyspnea in advanced disease and may be used to manage symptoms in terminal patients. Serious adverse effects are possible, so close monitoring is necessary if opioids are used.

Traditionally, β-blockers have been used sparingly or avoided in patients with COPD due to concerns of worsening respiratory status. However, multiple retrospective studies found that β-blocker use may actually be beneficial in COPD patients, possibly due to cardiovascular effects and β_2-receptor upregulation improving the effectiveness of inhaled β_2-agonists. β-Blockers have been associated with reduced mortality and exacerbation rates without negatively impacting pulmonary function even in patients without overt cardiovascular disease.[37–39] Although randomized controlled trials would be preferred to confirm the benefits of β-blockers in COPD, they appear to be safe and can be continued, particularly when used to treat comorbidities such as coronary artery disease and atrial fibrillation. Selective β_1-blockers are preferred, but nonselective agents have also shown benefits.[37,38]

Therapy of COPD Exacerbations

An exacerbation is defined as "an acute event characterized by a worsening of the patient's respiratory symptoms that is beyond normal day-to-day variations and leads to a change in medication."[1] Patients with COPD have on average 1 to 2 exacerbations annually with the frequency increasing with disease progression.[40] Exacerbations negatively impact quality of life, hasten lung function decline, increase health care costs, and increase mortality in patients requiring hospitalization.[1,41] While it is often difficult to discern what causes an exacerbation, many precipitating factors have been identified, including air pollution, interruption of maintenance therapies, and viral and bacterial respiratory tract infections.[1,40] Severity of an exacerbation is defined by clinical presentation, not through spirometry due to the difficulty of administration and interpretation of the results.[1]

The treatment goals for exacerbations are to limit the impact of the current exacerbation while preventing the occurrence of future exacerbations. It is estimated that greater than 80% of exacerbations could be managed on an outpatient basis if evaluated and triaged appropriately.[1] Patients presenting with signs of a severe COPD exacerbation (eg, use of accessory muscles to breathe, cyanosis, peripheral edema) should be admitted to the hospital.[1] Patients with signs and symptoms suggesting a life-threatening exacerbation (eg, mental status changes, worsening respiratory status despite ventilator support, hemodynamic instability) should be admitted for rigorous monitoring in an intensive care unit (ICU).[1]

Starting in 2014, the US Centers for Medicare and Medicaid Services (CMS) will penalize hospitals via reduced reimbursement rates for patients readmitted within 30 days of an initial COPD exacerbation. For this reason, appropriate management including medication reconciliation and patient counseling is necessary both during the exacerbation and upon hospital discharge.[42]

▸ *Nonpharmacologic Management*

Pulse oximetry may be useful for determining whether supplemental oxygen therapy is needed during a COPD exacerbation. If necessary, oxygen should be titrated to a saturation of 88% to

Patient Encounter, Part 2: The Medical History, Physical Examination, and Diagnostic Tests

PMH: Hypertension for 25 years, asthma for 50 years

Allergies: Anaphylaxis to penicillin and cephalexin

SH: Smokes one pack per day; social intake of alcohol (2–3 drinks per week); occasional use of marijuana; no other illicit drug use

FH: Noncontributory

Meds: Carvedilol 6.25 mg twice daily, albuterol MDI one to two puffs every 4 to 6 hours as needed

ROS: (–) fever, chills, or night sweats; (–) skin rash; (–) nasal congestion, drainage; (–) chest pain, paroxysmal nocturnal dyspnea; (+) orthopnea; (+) shortness of breath, cough with clear phlegm; (–) wheezing; (–) hemoptysis; (–) heartburn, reflux symptoms, N/V/D, change in appetite, change in bowel habits; (–) pedal edema

PE:

VS: BP 155/98 mm Hg, P 76 beats/min, RR 23/min, T 35.8°C (96.4°F), Wt 90 kg (198 lb), Ht 72 in. (183 cm), BMI 26.9 kg/m²

HEENT: EOMI; moist mucous membranes; no JVD; no palpably enlarged cervical lymph nodes

Lungs: Clear breath sounds; expiratory phase is diminished; no wheezes or crackles; (+) rhonchi

CV: RRR, normal S_1, S_2; no murmur, gallop, or rub

Abd: Soft, nontender, normoactive bowel sounds, no hepatomegaly

Ext: No cyanosis, edema, or finger clubbing

Pulmonary Function Tests

	Prebronchodilator		Postbronchodilator	
	Actual	% Predicted	Actual	% Predicted
FVC (L)	3.68	80%	3.76	82%
FEV_1 (L)	1.99	55%	2.01	56%
FEV_1/FVC			53% (0.53)	

CXR: Upper lobe bullous emphysema with mild hyperexpansion bilaterally

COPD Assessment Test score: 23

What other laboratory tests may be beneficial in the clinical evaluation of the patient's COPD?

Given this additional information, what is your assessment of the patient's condition?

What nonpharmacologic and pharmacologic alternatives are available for managing this patient's COPD?

With the data provided, create a care plan for managing the patient's COPD.

92% (0.88–0.92).[1] ABGs should be evaluated within an hour after initiation of oxygen to confirm appropriate oxygenation without compensatory carbon dioxide retention or if acute-on-chronic respiratory failure is suspected.[1]

If mechanical ventilation is required, it can be provided by noninvasive (nasal or face mask) or invasive (orotracheal tube or tracheostomy) methods.[1] Noninvasive mechanical ventilation (NIV) improves acute respiratory acidosis and decreases respiratory rate, work of breathing, length of hospital stay, intubation rates, and mortality and should be attempted prior to invasive methods.[1]

► *Pharmacologic Management*

Bronchodilators Administration of a short-acting β_2-agonist with or without ipratropium is considered standard bronchodilator therapy during a COPD exacerbation.[43] Increased doses and/or frequency are often needed during an exacerbation, and an MDI with or without a spacer or a nebulizer can be used. Prior maintenance bronchodilator therapy should be continued during an exacerbation. However, long-acting anticholinergics should be discontinued if ipratropium is used as part of the exacerbation bronchodilator regimen. Intravenous (IV) aminophylline is a second-line therapy used only when patients have failed standard bronchodilator therapy; it is typically reserved for critically ill patients.[1]

At time of discharge, maintenance therapy should include a long-acting anticholinergic or inhaled corticosteroid plus LABA. Other medications found to decrease exacerbation rates can be considered (Figure 15–2).

Corticosteroids Systemic corticosteroids, while not having a defined mortality benefit, have been shown to shorten recovery time, improve lung function, reduce the risk of early relapse, reduce the risk of treatment failure, and hasten symptomatic improvement during COPD exacerbations.[1,44] A 5-day course using 40 mg of oral prednisone or prednisolone is recommended.[1,45] IV corticosteroids should be used only if the oral route is not tolerated because there is no clinical benefit over oral therapy.[1,44] Nebulized budesonide may be used as an alternative but is more expensive and is not recommended over oral or IV corticosteroids during an exacerbation.[1]

Antibiotics Routine use of antibiotics is controversial due to the possibility of nonbacterial causes of COPD exacerbations.[1,46] Approximately 50% of exacerbations are caused by bacterial infections, and there may be benefit to treating most, if not all, COPD exacerbations with antibiotics.[40,47,48] In severe exacerbations (eg, patients in intensive care units), antibiotics reduce short-term mortality and treatment failure rates.[1] Practice guidelines recommend using antibiotics for patients with increased sputum purulence and either increased sputum volume or increased dyspnea, patients with all three of these symptoms, or patients who require mechanical ventilation.[1]

The most common bacterial pathogens isolated during COPD exacerbations are *Haemophilus influenzae, Streptococcus pneumonia, and Moraxella catarrhalis*.[40] Appropriate antibiotic selections in COPD exacerbations are included in Table 15–4. Local resistance patterns should be considered when selecting an antimicrobial regimen.

Other Therapies Patients must be educated on the importance of smoking cessation both during and after an exacerbation. Hospitalized patients with COPD exacerbations should receive thromboprophylaxis due to increased risk of venous thromboembolism.[1] Patients should be evaluated for influenza and pneumococcal immunization status, and those who are not up-to-date should receive either or both vaccines prior to discharge.

Table 15–4

Recommended Antibiotic Therapy in Acute Exacerbations of COPD

Suspected Pathogens Causing COPD Exacerbation	Commonly Used Antibiotics[a]
Haemophilus influenzae *Streptococcus pneumoniae* *Moraxella catarrhalis*	Ampicillin or amoxicillin ± β-lactamase inhibitor Azithromycin or clarithromycin Doxycycline Third-generation cephalosporin Levofloxacin or moxifloxacin
Pseudomonas aeruginosa	Ciprofloxacin[b] or levofloxacin Piperacillin–tazobactam or ticarcillin–clavulanate Cefepime or ceftazidime Meropenem, imipenem–cilistatin, or doripenem Gentamicin, tobramycin, or amikacin[c]
Methicillin-resistant *Staphylococcus aureus* (MRSA)	Vancomycin[d] Linezolid[d]

[a]Refer to local antibiogram to determine which antibiotic selection is most appropriate.

[b]Limited efficacy against *Streptococcus pneumonia*.

[c]Aminoglycosides are not effective against *Streptococcus pneumoniae*.

[d]Not effective against *Haemophilus influenzae* or *Moraxella catarrhalis*.

OUTCOME EVALUATION

- Monitor patients for improvement in symptoms. Ask if there is a difference since starting treatment and if so, is it meaningful to them. Are they less breathless? Can they do more activities and/or sleep better? If treatment response

Patient Encounter, Part 3

Six months after his last clinic appointment, the patient arrives at the local emergency department complaining of significant shortness of breath even while resting, increasing sputum production, and change in sputum color. Upon examination, he is using accessory muscles to breathe and has an oxygen saturation of 87% (0.87). Based on these findings alone, he is diagnosed with a COPD exacerbation and is admitted to the internal medicine ward.

What additional information do you need before creating a treatment plan?

What nonpharmacologic and pharmacologic alternatives are available for this patient?

With the data provided, create a care plan for managing this COPD exacerbation.

Patient Care Process

Patient Assessment:

- Assess the type, frequency, and severity of the patient's symptoms.
- Ask about disease impact on the patient's life, including limitation of activity, missed work, and feelings of depression or anxiety.
- Obtain a thorough history of prescription, nonprescription, and dietary supplement use.
- Use either the CAT (preferred) or mMRC to measure symptomatic impact of COPD.
- Review available FEV_1 information to classify severity of airflow limitation.
- Assess the risk of exacerbations based on grade of airflow limitation, number of exacerbations in previous 12 months, and whether exacerbations resulted in hospitalization.
- Based on symptoms and risk of exacerbations, determine if COPD is adequately treated.
- Assess tobacco use status.

Therapy Evaluation:

- If COPD is not adequately treated, determine what pharmacotherapy is indicated (Figure 15–2).
- If patient is already receiving pharmacotherapy, assess efficacy, safety, inhaler technique, and adherence. Ask patient if there are problems obtaining medications.

Care Plan Development:

- Design a therapeutic plan including lifestyle modifications (eg, smoking cessation) and optimal drug therapy (Figure 15–2). Consider the need for pulmonary rehabilitation, oxygen therapy, and/or surgery.
- Use combination inhalers when appropriate to minimize drug administration burden.
- Provide annual influenza vaccination and one-time pneumococcal vaccination if needed.
- Provide patient education about the disease state and therapeutic plan:
  - What COPD is and its natural course
  - Smoking cessation counseling
  - Role of regular exercise
  - How and when to take medications, importance of adherence, adverse effects and how to minimize them
  - Signs and symptoms of an exacerbation and what to do if one occurs
  - Advanced directives and end-of-life issues for patients with severe disease
- Address any patient concerns about COPD and its management.

Follow-Up Evaluation:

- Follow up every 3 to 6 months to assess effectiveness and safety of therapy. Review smoking status, symptoms, exacerbation frequency and severity, and medication regimen.
- Obtain spirometry annually to assess disease progression.

was inadequate and the patient was using the medication correctly, consider discontinuing the medication and selecting another agent.

- Changes in FEV_1 should not be the main outcome assessed because FEV_1 changes correlate weakly with symptoms, exacerbations, and health-related quality of life. There is no evidence to support routine periodic spirometry after initiation of therapy.[2] The GOLD guidelines recommend annual spirometry to assess decline in lung function.[1]
- The CAT is an eight-item questionnaire that can be used every 2 to 3 months to assess for trends and changes in symptoms and disease impact on daily life.[1] Additionally, higher CAT scores may be predictive of future exacerbations.[49] The test can be accessed at www.catestonline.org.
- The Medical Research Council dyspnea scale can be used to monitor physical limitation due to breathlessness. The scale is simple to administer and correlates well with health status.[50] However, the CAT is preferred because it is more comprehensive.
- Monitor theophylline levels with goal serum concentrations of 5 to 15 mcg/mL (5–15 mg/L; 28–83 μmol/L). Obtain trough levels 1 to 2 weeks after initiation of treatment and after any dosage adjustment. Routine levels are not necessary unless toxicity is suspected or symptoms have worsened.
- Monitor the patient for adverse effects of the medications selected.

Note

After this edition went to press, the FDA approved glycopyrrolate oral inhalation powder, a new long-acting anticholinergic agent, for long-term maintenance treatment of airflow obstruction in patients with COPD. It is available as a single entity inhaler (glycopyrrolate 15.6 mcg per inhalation; Seebri Neohaler) that is dosed twice daily. The FDA also approved a combination product with a long-acting β_2-agonist (glycopyrrolate 15.6 mcg/indacaterol 27.5 mcg per inhalation; Utibron Neohaler), which is also dosed twice daily for the same indication.

Abbreviations Introduced in This Chapter

AAT	α_1-Antitrypsin
ABG	Arterial blood gas
cAMP	Cyclic adenosine monophosphate
CAT	COPD Assessment Test
COPD	Chronic obstructive pulmonary disease
FEV_1	Forced expiratory volume in 1 second
FVC	Forced vital capacity

GOLD	Global Initiative for Chronic Obstructive Lung Disease
LABA	Long-acting β_2-agonists
MDI	Metered-dose inhaler
mMRC	Modified Medical Research Council
NIV	Noninvasive mechanical ventilation
$Paco_2$	Partial pressure of arterial carbon dioxide
Pao_2	Partial pressure of arterial oxygen
PDE-4	Phosphodiesterase-4
PFTs	Pulmonary function tests
Sao_2	Arterial oxygen saturation
V_A/Q	Ventilation/perfusion ratio

REFERENCES

1. GOLD Science Committee. Global strategy for the diagnosis, management, and prevention of chronic obstructive pulmonary disease, updated 2014, www.goldcopd.com.
2. Qaseem A, Wilt TJ, Weinberger, et al. Diagnosis and management of stable chronic obstructive pulmonary disease: A clinical practice guideline update from the American College of Physicians, American College of Chest Physicians, American Thoracic Society, and European Respiratory Society. Ann Intern Med. 2011;155:179–191.
3. American Lung Association. Chronic Obstructive Pulmonary Disease (COPD) Fact Sheet, May 2014, www.lungusa.org.
4. Decramer M, Janssens W, Miravitlles M. Chronic obstructive pulmonary disease. Lancet. 2012;379:1341–1351.
5. Tam A, Sin DD. Pathobiologic mechanisms of chronic obstructive pulmonary disease. Med Clin North Am. 2012;96:681–698.
6. Cosio MG, Saetta M, Agusti A. Immunologic aspects of chronic obstructive pulmonary disease. N Engl J Med. 2009;360: 2445–2454.
7. Anthonisen NR, Connett JE, Murray RP. Smoking and lung function of the lung health study participants after 11 years. Am J Respir Crit Care Med. 2002;166:675–679.
8. Scanlon PD, Connett JE, Waller LA, et al. Smoking cessation and lung function in mild-to-moderate chronic obstructive pulmonary disease. The Lung Health Study. Am J Respir Crit Care Med. 2000;161:381–390.
9. Fiore MC, Jaén CR, Baker TB, et al. Treating tobacco use and dependence. Clinical Practice Guideline. U.S. Department ofHealth and Human Services, 2008, http://www.ahrq.gov/professionals/clinicians-providers/guidelines-recommendations/tobacco/clinicians/update/index.html.
10. Strassmann R, Bausch B, Spaar A, et al. Smoking cessation interventions in COPD: A network meta-analysis of randomised trials. Eur Respir J. 2009;34:634–640.
11. Casaburi R, ZuWallack R. Pulmonary rehabilitation for management of chronic obstructive pulmonary disease. N Engl J Med. 2009;360:1329–1335.
12. Tashkin DP, Fabbri LM. Long-acting beta-agonists in the management of chronic obstructive pulmonary disease: Current and future agents. Respir Res. 2010;11:149, http://respiratory-research.com/content/11/1/149.
13. Koch A, Pizzichini E, Hamilton A, et al. Lung function efficacy and symptomatic benefit of olodaterol once daily delivered via Respimat® versus placebo and formoterol twice daily in patients with GOLD 2-4 COPD: Results from two replicate 48-week studies. Int J Chron Obstruct Pulmon Dis. 2014;9:697–714.
14. Karner C, Chong J, Poole P. Tiotropium versus placebo for chronic obstructive pulmonary disease. Cochrane Database Syst Rev. 2014;7:CD009285.
15. Tashkin DP, Celli B, Senn S, et al. A 4-year trial of tiotropium in chronic obstructive pulmonary disease. N Engl J Med. 2008;359: 1543–1554.
16. Hatipoglu U, Aboussouan LS. Chronic obstructive pulmonary disease: An update for the primary physician. Cleve Clin J Med. 2014;81:373–383.
17. Trivedi R, Richard N, Mehta R, Church A. Umeclidinium in patients with COPD: A randomised, placebo-controlled study. Eur Respir J. 2014;43:72–81.
18. Vogelmeier C, Hederer B, Glaab T, et al. Tiotropium versus salmeterol for the prevention of exacerbations of COPD. N Engl J Med. 2011;364:1093–1103.
19. Stephenson A, Seitz D, Bell CM, et al. Inhaled anticholinergic drug therapy and the risk of acute urinary retention in chronic obstructive pulmonary disease: A population-based study. Arch Intern Med. 2011;171:914–920.
20. Singh S, Loke YK, Furberg CD. Inhaled anticholinergics and risk of major adverse cardiovascular events in patients with chronic obstructive pulmonary disease. JAMA. 2008;300:1439–1450.
21. Lee TA, Pickard AS, Au DH, et al. Risk for death associated with medications for recently diagnosed chronic obstructive pulmonary disease. Ann Intern Med. 2008;149:380–390.
22. Mathioudakis AG, Chatzimavridou-Grigoriadou V, Evangelopoulou E, et al. Comparative mortality risk of tiotropium administered via handihaler or respimat in COPD patients: are they equivalent? Pulm Pharmacol Ther. 2014;28:91–97.
23. Barnes PJ. Theophylline. Am J Respir Crit Care Med. 2013;188: 901–906.
24. Calverley PMA, Anderson JA, Celli B, et al. Salmeterol and fluticasone propionate and survival in chronic obstructive pulmonary disease. N Engl J Med. 2007;356:775–789.
25. Chong J, Leung B, Poole P. Phosphodiesterase 4 inhibitors for chronic obstructive pulmonary disease. Cochrane Database Syst Rev. 2013;11:CD002309.
26. Tashkin DP, Pearle J, Iezzoni D, Varghese ST. Formoterol and tiotropium compared with tiotropium alone for treatment of COPD. COPD. 2009;6:17–25.
27. van Noord JA, Aumann JL, Janssens E, et al. Comparison of tiotropium once daily, formoterol twice daily and both combined once daily in patients with COPD. Eur Respir J. 2005;26:214–222.
28. Welte T, Miravitlles M, Hernandez P, et al. Efficacy and tolerability of budesonide/formoterol added to tiotropium in patients with chronic obstructive pulmonary disease. Am J Respir Crit Care Med. 2009;180:741–750.
29. Aaron SD, Vandemheen KL, Fergusson D, et al. Tiotropium in combination with placebo, salmeterol, or fluticasone-salmeterol for treatment of chronic obstructive pulmonary disease: A randomized trial. Ann Intern Med. 2007;146:545–555.
30. Karner C, Cates CJ. Combination inhaled steroid and long-acting beta$_2$-agonist in addition to tiotropium versus tiotropium or combination alone for chronic obstructive pulmonary disease. Cochrane Database Syst Rev. 2011;3:CD008532.
31. Magnussen H, Disse B, Rodriguez-Roisin R, et al. Withdrawal of inhaled glucocorticoids and exacerbations of COPD. N Engl J Med. 2014;371:1285–1294.
32. Alpha-1 Antitrypsin Deficiency Task Force. American Thoracic Society/European Respiratory Society statement: Standards for the diagnosis and management of individuals with alpha-1 antitrypsin deficiency. Am J Respir Crit Care Med. 2003;168:818–900.
33. Usery JB, Self TH, Muthiah MP, Finch CK. Potential role of leukotriene modifiers in the treatment of chronic obstructive pulmonary disease. Pharmacotherapy. 2008;28:1183–1187.
34. Decramer M, Rutten-van Molken M, Dekhuijzen PNR, et al. Effects of N-acetylcysteine on outcomes in chronic obstructive pulmonary disease (Bronchitis Randomized on NAD Cost-Utility Study, BRONCUS): A randomised placebo-controlled trial. Lancet. 2005;365:1552–1560.
35. Albert RK, Connett J, Bailey WC, et al. Azithromycin for prevention of exacerbations of COPD. N Engl J Med. 2011;365: 689–698.
36. Albert RK, Schuller JL. Macrolide antibiotics and the risk of cardiac arrhythmias. Am J Respir Crit Care Med. 2014;189:1173–1180.

37. Rutten FH, Zuithoff NPA, Hak E, et al. Beta-blockers may reduce mortality and risk of exacerbations in patients with chronic obstructive pulmonary disease. Arch Intern Med. 2010;170: 880–887.
38. Short PM, Lipworth SI, Elder DH, et al. Effect of beta blockers in treatment of chronic obstructive pulmonary disease: A retrospective cohort study. BMJ. 2011;342:d2549. doi: 10.1136/bmj.d2549.
39. Etminan M, Jafari S, Carleton B, FitzGerald JM. Beta-blocker use and COPD mortality: A systematic review and meta-analysis. BMC Pulm Med. 2012;12:48.
40. Sethi S, Murphy TF. Infection in the pathogenesis and course of chronic obstructive pulmonary disease. N Engl J Med. 2008;359: 2355–2365.
41. Punekar YS, Shukla A, Mullerova H. COPD management costs according to the frequency of COPD exacerbations in UK primary care. Int J Chron Obstruct Pulmon Dis. 2014;9:65–73.
42. Feemster LC, Au DH. Penalizing hospitals for chronic obstructive pulmonary disease readmissions. Am J Respir Crit Care Med. 2014;189:634–639.
43. National Institute for Clinical Excellence (NICE). Chronic obstructive pulmonary disease. Management of chronic obstructive pulmonary disease in adults in primary and secondary care. http://www.nice.org.uk/guidance/cg101/resources/guidance-chronic-obstructive-pulmonary-disease-pdf, 2010.
44. Ceviker Y, Sayiner A. Comparison of two systemic steroid regimens for the treatment of COPD exacerbations. Pulm Pharmacol Ther. 2014;27:179–183.
45. Leuppi JD, Schuetz P, Bingisser R, et al. Short-term vs conventional glucocorticoid therapy in acute exacerbations of chronic obstructive pulmonary disease: The REDUCE randomized clinical trial. JAMA. 2013;309:2223–2231.
46. Vollenweider DJ, Jarrett H, Steurer-Stey CA, et al. Antibiotics for exacerbations of chronic obstructive pulmonary disease. Cochrane Database Syst Rev. 2012;12:CD010257.
47. Rothberg MB, Pekow PS, Lahti M, et al. Antibiotic therapy and treatment failure in patients hospitalized for acute exacerbations of chronic obstructive pulmonary disease. JAMA. 2010;303:2035–2042.
48. Stefan MS, Rothberg MB, Shieh MS, et al. Association between antibiotic treatment and outcomes in patients hospitalized with acute exacerbation of COPD treated with systemic steroids. Chest. 2013;143:82–90.
49. Lee SD, Huang MS, Kang J, et al. The COPD assessment test (CAT) assists prediction of COPD exacerbations in high-risk patients. Resp Med. 2014;108:600–608.
50. Bestall JC, Paul EA, Garrod R, et al. Usefulness of the Medical Research Council (MRC) dyspnoea scale as a measure of disability in patients with chronic obstructive pulmonary disease. Thorax. 1999;54:581–586.

16 Cystic Fibrosis

Kimberly J. Novak

LEARNING OBJECTIVES

Upon completion of the chapter, the reader will be able to:

1. Explain the pathophysiology of cystic fibrosis (CF) and its multiorgan system involvement.
2. Describe the common clinical presentation and diagnosis of CF.
3. Consider long-term treatment goals with respect to clinical course and prognosis of CF.
4. Identify nonpharmacologic therapies for CF management.
5. Recommend appropriate pharmacologic therapies for chronic CF management.
6. Design appropriate antibiotic regimens for acute pulmonary exacerbations of CF.
7. Apply pharmacokinetic principles when calculating drug doses in CF patients.
8. Formulate monitoring plans for acute and chronic CF pharmacotherapy.

INTRODUCTION

Cystic fibrosis (CF) is an inherited multiorgan system disorder affecting children and, increasingly, adults. It is the most common life-shortening genetic disease among whites and the major cause of severe chronic lung disease and pancreatic insufficiency in children. Disease generally manifests as mucosal obstruction of exocrine glands caused by defective ion transport within epithelial cells. Due to the array of affected organ systems and complicated medical therapies, appropriate CF treatment necessitates interprofessional team collaboration.

EPIDEMIOLOGY AND ETIOLOGY

In the United States (US), CF most commonly occurs in whites, affecting from 1 in 1900 to 3700 individuals. CF is less common in Hispanics (1 in 9000), African Americans (1 in 15,000), and Asian Americans (1 in 32,000).[1] CF is inherited as an autosomal recessive trait, and approximately 1 in 25 whites are heterozygous carriers. Offspring of a carrier couple (each parent being heterozygous) have a 1 in 4 chance of having the disease (homozygous), a 1 in 2 chance of being a carrier (heterozygous), and a 1 in 4 chance of receiving no trait. The gene mutation is found on the long arm of chromosome 7 and encodes for the CF transmembrane regulator (CFTR) protein, which functions as a chloride channel to transport water and electrolytes. Over 1900 mutations have been described in the CF gene; however, the *F508del* mutation is most common and is present in 70% to 90% of CF patients in the United States.[1–4]

PATHOPHYSIOLOGY

CF is a disease of exocrine gland epithelial cells where CFTR expression is prevalent. Normally, these cells transport chloride through CFTR chloride channels with sodium and water accompanying this flux across the cell membrane (Figure 16–1). CFTR is regulated by protein kinases in response to varying levels of the intracellular second messenger cyclic-3′,5′-adenosine monophosphate (cAMP). CFTR also downregulates the epithelial sodium channel and regulates calcium-activated chloride and potassium channels, and it may function in exocytosis and formation of plasma membrane molecular complexes and proteins important in inflammatory responses.[4] KEY CONCEPT *In CF, the CFTR chloride channel is dysfunctional and usually results in decreased chloride secretion and increased sodium absorption, leading to altered viscosity of fluid excreted by the exocrine glands and mucosal obstruction.*

Pulmonary System

Chronic lung disease leads to death in 90% of patients. KEY CONCEPT *Pulmonary disease is characterized by thick mucus secretions, impaired mucus clearance, chronic airway infection and colonization, obstruction, and an exaggerated neutrophil-dominated inflammatory response.*[1,3] This process leads to air trapping, atelectasis, mucus plugging, bronchiectasis, cystic lesions, pulmonary hypertension, and eventual respiratory failure. Pulmonary function declines approximately 1% to 2% per year; an individual's rate of decline depends on severity of CFTR dysfunction and comorbidities.[1,5] Sinusitis and nasal polyps are also common, and microbial colonization is similar to that of the lungs.

Bacterial pathogens are often acquired in age-dependent sequence. Early infection is most often caused by *Staphylococcus aureus* and nontypeable *Haemophilus influenzae*. *Pseudomonas aeruginosa* infection is the most significant CF pathogen among all age groups. *P. aeruginosa* expresses extracellular toxins that perpetuate lung inflammation. Mucoid strains of *P. aeruginosa* produce an alginate biofilm layer that interferes with antibiotic penetration. Organisms identified later in the disease course

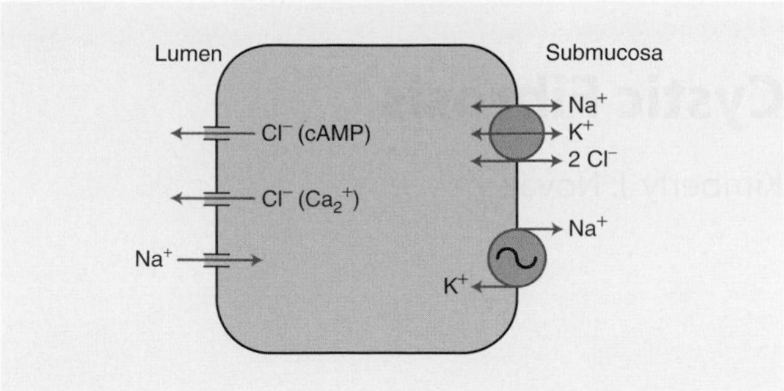

FIGURE 16–1. Electrolyte transport in the airway epithelial cell. (Ca, calcium; cAMP, cyclic-3′, 5′-adenosine monophosphate; Cl, chloride; Na, sodium; K potassium.) (From Milavetz G, Smith JJ. Cystic fibrosis. In: DiPiro JT, Talbert RL, Yee GC, et al., eds. Pharmacotherapy: A Pathophysiologic Approach, 7th ed. New York, NY: McGraw-Hill, 2008:536.)

include *Stenotrophomonas maltophilia*, *Achromobacter xylosoxidans*, *Burkholderia cepacia*, fungi including *Candida* and *Aspergillus* species, and nontuberculous mycobacteria among others.[1,5] Cultured organisms may represent initial infection, chronic colonization, or microbial overgrowth in an acute exacerbation.

Gastrointestinal System

Gastrointestinal (GI) involvement often presents as meconium ileus, small-bowel obstruction shortly after birth due to abnormally thick meconium. Older CF patients may develop distal intestinal obstruction syndrome (DIOS) due to fecal impaction in the terminal ileum and cecum.

Maldigestion due to pancreatic enzyme insufficiency is present in 85% to 90% of CF patients.[6,7] Thick pancreatic secretions and cellular debris obstruct pancreatic ducts and lead to fibrosis. Volume and concentration of pancreatic enzymes and bicarbonate are reduced, leading to maldigestion of fat and protein and subsequent malabsorption of fat-soluble vitamins (A, D, E, and K). Symptoms include abdominal distention, steatorrhea, flatulence, and malnourishment despite voracious appetite. Maldigestion is progressive and may develop later in a previously pancreatic-sufficient patient. Other complications may include GI reflux, dysmotility, salivary dysfunction, intussusception, volvulus, atresia, rectal prolapse, and complications related to corrective surgery for meconium ileus.

Hepatobiliary disease occurs due to bile duct obstruction from abnormal bile composition and flow. Hepatomegaly, splenomegaly, and cholecystitis may be present. Hepatic steatosis may be present due to effects of malnutrition. Progression from cholestasis (impaired bile flow) to cirrhosis, esophageal varices, and portal hypertension takes several years. Many patients are compensated and asymptomatic but may be susceptible to acute decompensation in the event of extrinsic hepatic insult from viruses, medications, or other factors.[8]

Endocrine System

CF-related diabetes (CFRD) occurs in 20% of adolescents and 40% to 50% of adults, disproportionally affecting women. Although it shares characteristics of both type 1 and type 2 diabetes mellitus, CFRD is categorized separately. Reduced functional pancreatic islet cells and increased islet amyloid deposition results in insulin insufficiency, the primary cause of CFRD. Insulin secretion is delayed in response to glucose challenge, and absolute insulin secretion over time is reduced. Some insulin resistance may also be present in CFRD and may fluctuate in relation to infection and inflammation.[9]

Postprandial hyperglycemia is common, but because some basal insulin secretion is maintained, fasting hyperglycemia is less severe and ketosis is rare.[6] Diet, acute and chronic infection, and corticosteroid use lead to fluctuation in glucose tolerance over time.[9] CFRD is associated with greater nutritional failure, increased pulmonary disease, and earlier mortality. Pulmonary function decline and nutritional consequences associated with progressive CFRD may overshadow risks of long-term macrovascular and microvascular complications.

Reproductive System

CF patients often experience delayed puberty. In females, menarche occurs 18 months later than average; menstrual irregularity is common, and fertility is reduced due to increased cervical mucus viscosity. Due to increasing life expectancy, pregnancy is becoming more common; however, outcomes depend on prepartum nutritional and pulmonary status. Almost all males with CF are azoospermic due to congenital absence of the vas deferens with resultant obstruction; however, conception still occurs occasionally. Conception can also occur through application of assisted reproductive technologies.[10]

Musculoskeletal System

Several factors contribute to development of bone disease in CF: (a) malabsorption of vitamins D and K and calcium, (b) poor nutrition and decreased body mass, (c) physical inactivity, (d) corticosteroid therapy, and (e) delayed puberty. Chronic pulmonary infection, through release of inflammatory cytokines, can increase bone resorption and decrease formation. Osteopenia, osteoporosis, pathological fractures, and kyphosis can occur.[11,12] Episodic or chronic arthritis may occur due to immune complex formation in response to chronic inflammation.[5] Digital clubbing is commonly observed and is a marker for hypoxia.

Hematological System

Anemia may be present due to impaired erythropoietin regulation, nutritional factors (vitamin E and iron malabsorption), or chronic inflammation. Increased cytokine production can lead to shortened red blood cell survival, reduced erythropoietin response, and impaired mobilization of iron stores. Additionally, with chronic hypoxia, normal hemoglobin and hematocrit values may represent relative anemia.[13] Increased red blood cell production is a physiological response to hypoxia; however, this response may be blunted in CF and may result in symptoms of anemia despite normal lab values.

Abnormal bleeding or clotting may also be observed as a result of vitamin K malabsorption, antibiotic-associated depletion of GI flora and vitamin K synthesis, reduced coagulation factor synthesis due to liver disease, and/or a procoagulant state due to inflammation.

Integumentary System

Sweat contains abnormally high concentrations of sodium and chloride due to impaired reabsorption within the sweat duct from loss of CFTR channels. Patients are usually asymptomatic (other than a characteristic salty taste to the skin).[3] In rare instances such as hot weather or excessive sweating during physical activity, patients may become dehydrated and experience symptoms of hyponatremia (nausea, headache, lethargy, and confusion).

Clinical Presentation of Cystic Fibrosis

General

- Usually diagnosed in neonates (meconium ileus or newborn screening) or during early childhood. May present later in life due to less severe symptoms or misdiagnosis.

Symptoms

- Pulmonary: Chronic cough, sputum production, decreased exercise tolerance, and recurrent pneumonia and sinusitis. Exacerbations may be marked by increased cough, sputum changes (darker, thicker), **hemoptysis**, dyspnea, and fever.
- GI: Numerous large, foul-smelling loose stools (steatorrhea), flatulence, and abdominal pain. Intestinal obstruction may present as abdominal pain and distention and/or decreased bowel movements.
- Nutritional: Poor weight gain despite voracious appetite and hunger. Dry skin, skin rash, and visual disturbances may be noted in vitamin deficiency.
- CFRD: Weight loss, increased thirst, and more frequent urination.

Signs

- Obstructive airways disease: Tachypnea, dyspnea, **cyanosis**, wheezes, crackles, sternal retractions, digital clubbing, and barrel chest.
- Failure to thrive: Below age-based normal in both height and weight in children; adults may be near/below ideal body weight or have a low body mass index (BMI).
- Salty taste to the skin.
- Hepatobiliary disease: Hepatomegaly, splenomegaly, and prolonged bleeding may occur.
- Recurrent pancreatitis (usually in pancreatic-sufficient patients): Episodic epigastric abdominal pain, persistent vomiting, and fever.

Laboratory Tests

- Leukocytosis with increase in polymorphonuclear (PMN) leukocytes and bands may occur in acute pulmonary exacerbations.
- Maldigestion: Decreased serum levels of fat-soluble vitamins (A, D, E, and K). Decreased vitamin K levels may result in elevated prothrombin time (PT) and international normalized ratio (INR).
- Glucose intolerance: Blood glucose between 140 and 199 mg/dL (7.8–11.0 mmol/L) 2 hours after an oral glucose-tolerance test.
- CFRD: Blood glucose 200 mg/dL (11.1 mmol/L) or higher 2 hours after an oral glucose-tolerance test or fasting hyperglycemia (fasting blood glucose 126 mg/dL [7.0 mmol/L] or more regardless of the postglucose challenge level).
- Hepatobiliary disease: Serum aspartate aminotransferase, alanine aminotransferase, alkaline phosphatase, γ-glutamyltransferase, and bilirubin may be elevated.

Other Tests

- Microbial cultures (sputum, throat, **bronchoalveolar lavage**, or sinus): Isolation of *P. aeruginosa, S. aureus, S. maltophilia,* and other CF-related organisms.
- Pulmonary function tests (PFTs): Decreased forced expiratory volume in 1 second (FEV_1) and forced vital capacity (FVC), typically lower during acute pulmonary exacerbations.
- Chest x-ray or CT scan: Infiltrates, atelectasis, bronchiectasis, and mucus plugging.
- Abdominal x-ray or CT scan: Intestinal obstruction may be manifested as meconium ileus, DIOS, or intussusception. Rectal prolapse may be noted on physical examination.
- Maldigestion: Elevated fecal fat content, reduced pancreatic stool elastase (less than 200 mcg/g of feces).

CLINICAL PRESENTATION AND DIAGNOSIS

See the accompanying box for the clinical presentation of CF.

Diagnosis

Testing for CF is part of required newborn screening panels in all US states in an effort to identify patients prior to symptom development, initiate early treatment, and improve long-term outcomes.[14] A positive newborn screen for CF is not diagnostic (due to false-positive results among CF carriers), nor does a negative screen universally exclude the diagnosis. All "positive screens," as well as individuals presenting with signs and symptoms of CF, are referred to a CF care center for sweat chloride test and genetic evaluation. Diagnosis of CF is based on two separate elevated sweat chloride concentrations of 60 mEq/L (60 mmol/L) or greater obtained through pilocarpine **iontophoresis** ("sweat test"). Genetic testing (CFTR mutation analysis) may be performed to confirm the diagnosis, screen in utero, or detect carrier status. More than 70% of diagnoses are made by 12 months of age, and almost all are made by age 12.[14]

Clinical Course and Prognosis

Clinical course varies because of multiple genetic mutations and the heterogeneous profile of the *F508del* mutation. Some patients develop severe lung disease early in childhood and reach end-stage disease by adolescence, whereas others maintain near-normal lung function into adulthood. Newly diagnosed adults tend to present with chronic respiratory symptoms but usually have milder lung disease, less frequent *Pseudomonas* infection, and less severe pancreatic insufficiency.[6]

Life expectancy has greatly increased from a predicted survival of 16 years of age in 1970 to more than 40 years for patients born in the 1990s.[5,6] According to the Cystic Fibrosis Foundation Registry, nearly half of patients are over 18 years of age.[14]

Patient Encounter, Part 1

A 2-month-old female infant is being evaluated at CF clinic due to an abnormal newborn screen (elevated immunoreactive trypsinogen; one copy of gene mutation *G551D* on initial testing). Sweat chloride testing is performed on bilateral thighs with results reported as follows:

Sample 1: Sweat chloride 88 mEq/L (88 mmol/L)

Sample 2: Sweat chloride 72 mEq/L (72 mmol/L)

Upon parental interview, the infant is a voracious eater and has five to eight loose stools per day that have a creamy appearance. She is mostly breastfed, with some supplemental 20 kcal/ounce (0.67 kcal/mL; 2.8 kJ/mL) infant formula, and she just regained her birth weight of 3.5 kg. Parents also report that she passed her meconium in the newborn nursery on the third day of life after getting a baby laxative.

What information is consistent with a diagnosis of CF?

What are the next steps in the CF diagnostic process?

The parents are overwhelmed with the diagnosis of CF and are very worried about life expectancy. How would you explain the infant's prognosis?

TREATMENT

Desired Outcomes

Therapeutic outcomes in CF care relate to chronic and acute treatment goals. With chronic management, the primary goals are to delay disease progression and optimize quality of life. KEY CONCEPT *Maximizing nutritional status through pancreatic enzyme replacement and vitamin and nutritional supplements is necessary for normal growth and development and for maintaining long-term lung function.* Reduction of airway inflammation and infection and aggressive preventive therapies minimize acute pulmonary exacerbations and delay pulmonary decline. In pulmonary exacerbations, therapy is directed toward reducing acute airway inflammation and obstruction through aggressive airway clearance and antibiotic therapy with a goal of returning lung function to pre-exacerbation levels or greater.

Nonpharmacologic Therapy

▶ *Airway Clearance Therapy*

KEY CONCEPT *Airway clearance therapy is a necessary routine for all CF patients to clear secretions and control infection, even at diagnosis prior to becoming symptomatic.* Waiting until development of a first pulmonary exacerbation or daily symptoms delays benefits and may accelerate pulmonary decline. The traditional form of chest physiotherapy (CPT) is percussion and postural drainage. Areas of the patient's chest, sides, and back are rapidly "clapped" by hand in different patient positions, followed by cough or forced expiration to mobilize secretions. Patients may also be taught autogenic drainage, which consists of deep breathing exercises followed by forced cough.

Several airway clearance devices are also available. Flutter valve devices use oscillating positive expiratory pressure (OPEP) to cause vibratory airflow obstruction and an internal percussive effect to mobilize secretions. Intrapulmonary percussive ventilation (IPV) provides continuous oscillating pressures during inhalation and exhalation. High-frequency chest compression (HFCC) with an inflatable vest that provides external oscillation is most commonly used and often preferred because patients can perform therapy independently from an early age.[6,15]

Effective cough and expectoration of mucus are essential for good clearance technique. Airway clearance therapy is typically performed once or twice daily for maintenance care and is increased to three or four times per day during acute exacerbations.

▶ *Nutrition*

Most CF patients have increased caloric needs due to increased energy expenditure through increased work of breathing, increased basal metabolism, and maldigestion. Prevention of malnutrition requires early patient-specific nutritional intervention. Caloric requirements to promote age-appropriate weight gain or maintenance are typically 110% to 200% of the recommended daily allowance (RDA) for age, gender, and size and increase as disease progresses.[16]

Nutrition in malnourished patients consists of baseline required calories plus additional calories for weight gain. Even with aggressive diet and oral suppl ements, the caloric requirement may not be achieved, and placement of a gastrostomy or jejunostomy tube for nighttime supplemental feeds may be necessary.[6] Patients with refractory malabsorption, CFRD, and/or tube feedings have unique caloric needs. Collaboration with dieticians specially trained in CF nutrition is essential.

Pharmacologic Therapy

▶ *Airway Clearance Therapy*

Airway clearance therapy is usually accompanied by bronchodilator treatment with albuterol (known as salbutamol outside the US) to stimulate mucociliary clearance and prevent bronchospasm associated with therapy (Table 16–1).

A mucolytic agent is administered afterward to reduce sputum viscosity and enhance clearance. Dornase alfa (Pulmozyme) is a recombinant human (rh) DNase that selectively cleaves extracellular DNA released during neutrophil degradation in viscous CF sputum. Nebulization of dornase alfa improves daily pulmonary symptoms and function, reduces pulmonary exacerbations, and improves quality of life.[15,17] Daily dosing is most common, but some patients benefit from twice daily administration.[15] Hypertonic saline for inhalation (HyperSal) 7% or 3.5% is often used as an alternative or add-on mucolytic agent for osmotic effects or sputum induction. It must be preceded by a bronchodilator due to greater incidence of bronchospasm and may not be tolerated by some patients.[15,18] *N*-acetylcysteine is another mucolytic agent, but its unpleasant odor and taste limit patient acceptance.[6]

Some patients with CF also have reactive airways or concurrent asthma and benefit from long-acting β_2-agonists.[6,15,19] Patients with recurrent wheezing or dyspnea who improved with albuterol (salbutamol) should be considered for maintenance asthma therapy, as should patients with bronchodilator-responsive pulmonary function tests (PFTs).

Montelukast, antihistamines, and/or intranasal steroids are used for CF patients with allergic or rhinosinusitis symptoms.

Inhaled corticosteroids may attenuate reactive airways and reduce airway inflammation in some patients; however, clear benefit in CF has not been established.[15,19] Drug delivery to the site of inflammation is limited by mucus plugging, which may limit efficacy. Patients on asthma therapies should administer these medications after airway clearance to optimize drug delivery.

Table 16–1

Common Pulmonary Medications Used in Cystic Fibrosis

Medication	Pediatric Dose	Adult Dose
Albuterol (salbutamol)	2.5 mg nebulized with chest physiotherapy two to four times daily; alternatively, two puffs via metered-dose inhaler may be substituted	2.5 mg nebulized with chest physiotherapy two to four times daily; alternatively, two puffs via metered-dose inhaler may be substituted
Dornase alfa	2.5 mg nebulized once or twice daily	2.5 mg nebulized once or twice daily
Hypertonic saline 7%, 3.5%, or 3%	4 mL nebulized one to four times per day	4 mL nebulized one to four times per day
Azithromycin	Body weight 25–39 kg: 250 mg on Mondays, Wednesdays, and Fridays	Body weight 40 kg or more. 500 mg on Mondays, Wednesdays, and Fridays
Ibuprofen[a]	20–30 mg/kg/dose given twice daily	20–30 mg/kg/dose given twice daily
Ivacaftor [b]	50–150 mg every 12 hours	150 mg every 12 hours

[a]Adjusted to achieve peak serum concentrations of 50 to 100 mcg/mL (243–485 μmol/L). Maintain chronic dosing with same dosage form and manufacturer. Note that therapy is not always continued into adulthood.

[b]Dose may require adjustment in patients with moderate or severe hepatic impairment and/or when coadministered with moderate or strong CYP3A inhibitors.

Long-term systemic corticosteroids reduce airway inflammation and improve lung function. However, beneficial effects diminish upon discontinuation, and concern for long-term adverse effects limits use as maintenance therapy.[19,20] Systemic corticosteroids may be used short term in acute exacerbations or for treatment of allergic response to *Aspergillus* colonization (allergic bronchopulmonary aspergillosis, or ABPA); however, dose and duration of therapy should be minimized.[1,20]

High-dose ibuprofen targeting peak concentrations of 50 to 100 mcg/mL (243–485 μmol/L) has been shown to slow disease progression, particularly in children 5 to 13 years of age with mild lung disease (FEV_1 greater than 60% predicted). At high doses, ibuprofen inhibits the lipoxygenase pathway, reducing neutrophil migration and function as well as release of lysosomal enzymes. At lower concentrations achieved with analgesic dosing, neutrophil migration increases, potentially increasing inflammation.[21,22] A dose of 20 to 30 mg/kg given twice daily is usually needed to attain target levels, but interpatient variability necessitates serum concentration monitoring.[21] Due to monitoring requirements and concerns regarding long-term safety and tolerability, only a few CF centers prescribe high-dose ibuprofen.[1,15]

Azithromycin is a macrolide antibiotic commonly used in CF as an anti-inflammatory agent to improve overall lung function. Proposed mechanisms include interference with *Pseudomonas* alginate biofilm production, bactericidal activity during stationary *Pseudomonas* growth, neutrophil inhibition, interleukin-8 reduction, and reduction in sputum viscosity.[23,24] Due to its long tissue half-life, azithromycin is typically dosed 3 days per week (Monday, Wednesday, and Friday). Alternatively, patients may take 500 or 250 mg either daily or only Monday through Friday, based on the same weight parameters. Patients should have a screening acid-fast bacillus sputum culture prior to initiation and then every 6 months, because isolation of nontuberculous mycobacteria is a contraindication to chronic azithromycin therapy.[19]

Antibiotic Therapy

KEY CONCEPT *Antibiotic therapy is used in three distinct situations: (a) eradication and delay of colonization in early lung disease (treatment of positive cultures regardless of symptoms), (b) suppression of bacterial growth once colonization is present, and (c) reduction of bacterial load in acute exacerbations in an attempt to return lung function to pre-exacerbation levels or greater.*[1] KEY CONCEPT *Antibiotic selection is based on periodic culture and sensitivity data, typically covering all organisms identified during the preceding year. If no culture data are available, empirical antibiotics should cover the most likely organisms for the patient's age group.* Due to altered pharmacokinetics and microorganism resistance, dose optimization is key (Table 16–2).

Oral Antibiotic Therapy Severity of pulmonary symptoms also guides antibiotic selection. For recent-onset or mild symptoms, patients may be treated with outpatient oral and inhaled antibiotics for 14 to 21 days. Oral fluoroquinolones are a mainstay for *P. aeruginosa* treatment in CF, even in children. Despite concerns regarding cartilage and tendon toxicity in young animals, clinical practice has not shown an increased risk in human children.[25] To prevent development of resistance and promote synergy, inhaled tobramycin, aztreonam, or colistin is usually added for double coverage.[1,26] Methicillin-sensitive *S. aureus* (MSSA) may be treated with oral amoxicillin–clavulanic acid, dicloxacillin, first- or second-generation cephalosporins, trimethoprim–sulfamethoxazole, clindamycin, doxycycline, or minocycline, depending on sensitivity. Methicillin-resistant *S. aureus* (MRSA) may be treated with oral trimethoprim–sulfamethoxazole, clindamycin, doxycycline, minocycline, or linezolid. *H. influenzae* often produces β-lactamases but can usually be treated with amoxicillin–clavulanic acid, a cephalosporin, or trimethoprim–sulfamethoxazole. Oral trimethoprim–sulfamethoxazole or minocycline may be used to treat *S. maltophilia*.

Intravenous Antibiotic Therapy For severe infections or patients failing outpatient therapy, IV antibiotic therapy is prescribed for 2 to 3 weeks as inpatient therapy. Some patients may be discharged to finish their IV course or even receive their entire IV course at home. KEY CONCEPT *Typical regimens for severe infections include an antipseudomonal β-lactam plus an aminoglycoside for added synergy and delay of resistance development.*[1,26–28] Cephalosporins tend to be better tolerated and offer the benefit of less frequent administration. Extended-spectrum penicillins have been associated with a higher incidence of allergy. Aztreonam offers little cross-reactivity in penicillin- or cephalosporin-allergic patients; however, it has no gram-positive coverage. Meropenem should be reserved for organisms resistant to all other antibiotics to minimize development of resistance in the carbapenem drug class.

Tobramycin IV is generally the first-line aminoglycoside. Isolates are usually resistant to gentamicin, and amikacin is reserved for tobramycin-resistant strains. Pharmacokinetic targets are listed in Table 16–3. Higher peak serum concentrations are desired to maximize efficacy, whereas lower trough levels reduce risk of toxicity. Once daily dosing targets higher peaks and lower troughs, optimizing the concentration-dependent killing of aminoglycosides (eg, tobramycin 10–15 mg/kg/day or amikacin

Table 16–2

Selected Antibiotic Dosing in Cystic Fibrosis[a]

Antibiotic	Pediatric Dose (mg/kg/day)	Adult Maximum Daily Dose	Interval (hours)
Intravenous			
Tobramycin, gentamicin[b]	10	None	8–24
Amikacin[b]	30	None	8–24
Ceftazidime	150–200	6–8 g	6–8
Cefepime	150	6 g	8
Piperacillin–tazobactam[c]	400	16 g	6
Ticarcillin–clavulanate[c]	400–600	12–18 g	4–6
Meropenem	120	6 g	8
Imipenem–cilastatin[c]	100	2 g	6
Aztreonam	200	8 g	6
Ciprofloxacin	30	1.2 g	8–12
Levofloxacin	10–20	750 mg	12–24
Nafcillin	200	12 g	4–6
Vancomycin[b]	60	None	6–12
Linezolid	30	1.2 g	8–12
Colistin	5–8	480 mg	8
Chloramphenicol[b]	60–80	4 g	6
Oral			
Amoxicillin ± clavulanic acid[c]	90	4 g	12
Dicloxacillin	100	2 g	6
Cephalexin	50–100	4 g	6–8
Trimethoprim–sulfamethoxazole[d]	12–20	1280 mg	6–12
Clindamycin	30	1.8 g	6–8
Ciprofloxacin	40	2 g	12
Levofloxacin	10–20	750 mg	12–24
Minocycline[e]	4	200 mg	12
Linezolid	30	1.2 g	8–12
Inhaled			
Tobramycin	160–600 mg/day	600 mg	12
Aztreonam lysine	225 mg/day	225 mg	8
Colistin	75–150 mg/day	300 mg	12

[a]All doses assume normal renal and hepatic function. Consult a specialized drug reference for dosage adjustment if function is impaired. Dose and/or interval may require adjustment.

[b]Empirical starting doses only. Adjust dose per therapeutic drug monitoring.

[c]Dose based on β-lactam component.

[d]Dose based on trimethoprim component.

[e]Children older than 8 years.

30–45 mg/kg/day).[27] However, time below the minimum inhibitory concentration (MIC) is prolonged with once-daily administration in many children, possibly leading to loss of synergy for a substantial portion of the dosing interval, and may not always be optimal. Once-daily dosing is reasonable for children, adolescents, and adults with longer elimination half-lives in whom the time below the MIC can be minimized. Incorporation of the patient-specific pharmacokinetic history is essential for optimal aminoglycoside dosing. Long-term studies are needed to examine the efficacy and resistance patterns associated with once-daily aminoglycosides in CF patients.[1,26,27]

As with Pseudomonas infections, most other serious gram-negative infections are also treated with combination therapy. *S. maltophilia* is highly resistant and most often treated with trimethoprim–sulfamethoxazole or ticarcillin–clavulanate. There are few therapeutic options for *A. xylosoxidans* and *B. cepacia*.

An oral fluoroquinolone may be substituted for an IV aminoglycoside based on sensitivity data or presence of renal dysfunction and/or ototoxicity. Due to excellent bioavailability, fluoroquinolones, trimethoprim–sulfamethoxazole, doxycycline, minocycline, and linezolid should be used orally for most patients able to take enteral medications. Due to toxicity risk, colistin IV and chloramphenicol IV are reserved for life-threatening, highly resistant infections.

Inpatient treatment of MRSA can consist of IV vancomycin or oral agents as previously described, depending on the severity of infection and concomitant organisms.

Inhaled Antibiotic Therapy Chronic or rotating inhaled antibiotic maintenance therapy may be used to suppress *P. aeruginosa* colonization; however, long-term systemic antibiotics are not recommended due to emergence of resistance.[1,19] Inhaled tobramycin (TOBI, Bethkis) is typically administered to patients 6 years of age and older in alternating 28-day cycles of 300 mg nebulized twice daily, followed by a 28-day washout period to minimize development of resistance. Long-term cyclical administration improves pulmonary function, decreases microbial burden, and reduces hospitalization for IV therapy.[15,29] A dry powder formulation of tobramycin (TOBI Podhaler™, 112 mg inhaled twice daily) can also be used in 28-day on/off cycles with reduced administration time.[30] Due to minimal systemic absorption, pharmacokinetic monitoring is not necessary with normal renal function. Lower doses of nebulized tobramycin solution for injection have been used in younger children, and *Pseudomonas* eradication studies used 300 mg twice daily in children as young as 6 months.[31]

Aztreonam lysine for inhalation (Cayston) is also used for *P. aeruginosa* suppression in 28-day on/off cycles for CF patients 6 years of age and older.[19] A dose of 75 mg three times daily is given via the Altera nebulizer system, a high-efficiency drug delivery device with shorter administration time.[32,33]

Nebulized colistin using the IV formulation may be an option in patients with tobramycin-resistant strains or intolerance to inhaled tobramycin or aztreonam lysine. Pretreatment with albuterol is necessary due to increased risk of bronchoconstriction.[1,6]

Selection of inhaled antibiotics is based on culture data and patient preference. Alternating inhaled antibiotic regimens are sometimes used in patients with more advanced lung disease.[15] Inhaled antibiotics are typically stopped during acute exacerbations requiring IV therapy because drug delivery is reduced with increased sputum production, and concomitant use of IV aminoglycosides may increase risk of toxicity.[26,27]

Pharmacokinetic Considerations KEY CONCEPT *CF patients have larger volumes of distribution for many antibiotics due to an increased ratio of lean body mass to total body mass and lower fat stores. CF patients also have enhanced total body clearance, although the exact mechanism has not been determined; both renal and extrarenal processes have been proposed.*[26]

Because of these pharmacokinetic changes, higher doses of aminoglycosides are needed to achieve target serum levels and adequate tissue penetration.[28] Higher doses of β-lactam antibiotics are also needed to achieve and sustain levels above the MIC. Trimethoprim–sulfamethoxazole displays enhanced renal clearance and hepatic metabolism in the CF population.

Table 16–3

Target Intravenous Antibiotic Serum Concentrations in Cystic Fibrosis

	Traditional Units of Measurement		SI Units of Measurement	
Antibiotic	**Goal Peak[a] (mcg/mL)**	**Goal Trough[b] (mcg/mL)**	**Goal Peak[a] (μmol/L)**	**Goal Trough[b] (μmol/L)**
Tobramycin, gentamicin	10–12[c]	< 1.5[c]	21–26[c]	< 3.2[c]
	20–30[d]	< 1[d]	42–63[d]	< 2.1[d]
Amikacin	30–40[c]	< 5[c]	51–68[c]	< 8.6[c]
	60–90[d]	< 3[d]	103–154[d]	< 5.1[d]
Vancomycin	–[e]	15–20	–[e]	10–14

Note: Values reported in mcg/mL are numerically equivalent to mg/L.

[a]Peaks calculated 30 minutes after end of infusion for aminoglycosides.

[b]Troughs calculated immediately prior to the time the dose is due.

[c]Goals refer to traditional dosing (every 8 or 12 hours). Higher peaks may be targeted with corresponding lower trough concentrations for aminoglycosides based on center practice.

[d]Goals refer to once-daily (high-dose extended interval) dosing.

[e]Not routinely measured.

Fluoroquinolones and vancomycin have fewer pharmacokinetic deviations; however, higher doses are typically needed to attain inhibitory serum and tissue concentrations against CF pathogens.[26]

Although most CF patients have shorter drug half-lives and larger volumes of distribution than non-CF patients, some patients exhibit decreased renal clearance because of concomitant nephrotoxic medications, diabetic nephropathy, or other reasons.

▶ *Gastrointestinal Therapy*

Pancreatic Enzyme Replacement This is the mainstay of GI therapy. Most enzyme products available in the US are formulated as capsules containing enteric-coated microspheres or microtablets that escape enzyme inactivation by gastric acid and promote dissolution in the more alkaline duodenum (Table 16–4). Capsules may be opened and the microbeads swallowed with food (for infants and young children), as long as they are not chewed or mixed with alkaline or hot foods (which denature enzymes). Although products may contain similar enzyme ratios, they are not bioequivalent and cannot be interchanged.[6,34]

Pancreatic enzymes are initiated at 500 to 1000 units/kg/meal of lipase component (because fats are most difficult to digest) with half-doses given for snacks. Enzymes should be taken at the beginning or divided throughout the meal and must be given with any fat-containing snack. Infants are typically started at 1500 to 2500 units of lipase/120 mL of formula or breast milk and may require division of capsule contents via visual estimation to obtain appropriate doses. Pancreatic enzymes cannot be placed in formula bottles due to inability to pass consistently through the nipple slit. Instead, enzyme microbeads are placed on a small dot of infant applesauce (or moistened infant rice cereal) and administered via infant spoon with subsequent nursing or bottle-feeding to facilitate swallowing. The oral mucosa must be examined afterward to ensure that all enzymes are swallowed because remnant microbeads can cause oral erosions (ulcers).

KEY CONCEPT *Titration of pancreatic enzyme doses is based on control of steatorrhea, stool output, and abdominal symptoms.* Infants should have no more than three to four stools per day, whereas older patients should have no more than two to three (children) or one to two (adolescents/adults) well-formed stools per day. Doses are titrated at 2- to 3-week intervals in increments of 150 to 250 units of lipase/kg/meal (or the next easily administered capsule or half-capsule) up to 2500 units/kg/meal. Maximum infant doses are typically 4000 units of lipase/120 mL of formula. Higher doses should be used cautiously due to risk of fibrosing colonopathy.[6,34] Patients responding poorly to maximal doses of one product may benefit from changing to another product and/or addition of a histamine H_2-receptor antagonist

Table 16–4

Common Pancreatic Enzyme Replacement Products

Trade Name	Lipase (Units)	Amylase (Units)	Protease (Units)
CREON 3000	3000	15,000	9500
CREON 6000	6000	30,000	19,000
CREON 12,000	12,000	60,000	38,000
CREON 24,000	24,000	120,000	76,000
CREON 36,000	36,000	180,000	114,000
Pancreaze MT 4[a]	4200	17,500	10,000
Pancreaze MT 10[a]	10,500	43,750	25,000
Pancreaze MT 16[a]	16,800	70,000	40,000
Pancreaze MT 20[a]	21,000	61,000	37,000
Pertzye 8000	8000	30,250	28,750
Pertzye 16,000	16,000	60,500	57,500
Ultresa	13,800	27,600	27,600
Ultresa	20,700	41,400	41,400
Ultresa	23,000	46,000	46,000
Viokace[b]	10,440	39,150	39,150
Viokace[b]	20,880	78,300	78,300
Zenpep 3000	3000	16,000	10,000
Zenpep 5000	5000	27,000	17,000
Zenpep 10,000	10,000	55,000	34,000
Zenpep 15,000	15,000	82,000	51,000
Zenpep 20,000	20,000	109,000	68,000
Zenpep 25,000	25,000	136,000	85,500
Zenpep 40,000	40,000	218,000	136,000

[a] The number after a trade name refers to the approximate number of thousands of units of lipase contained per dosage form.

[b] Nonenteric coated enzyme. Must be given with a gastric acid suppressant. Often administered via feeding tube.

or proton pump inhibitor.[6] Acid suppression may boost the effective enzyme dose, if duodenal pH is not alkaline enough to neutralize residual gastric acid and dissolve enteric coating. Acid suppression also treats concomitant gastroesophageal reflux disease, which is common in CF.[6,7,15,34]

Fat-Soluble Vitamin Supplementation This is usually required in pancreatic insufficiency. Specially formulated products for CF patients (AquADEKs, Vitamax, MVW Complete, Choiceful) are usually sufficient to attain normal serum vitamin levels at a dose of 1 mL daily for infants, one tablet daily for younger children, and one tablet/capsule twice daily for teenagers and adults. Additional supplementation may be needed in uncontrolled malabsorption or for replacement of severe vitamin deficiency based on serum vitamin levels.[6,34] Appetite stimulants such as cyproheptadine may be an option for promoting nutrition and weight gain, but efficacy has not been established.

Liver Disease Ursodiol at 20 mg/kg/day in two divided doses may slow progression of liver disease. It improves bile flow and may displace toxic bile acids that accumulate in a cholestatic liver, stimulate bicarbonate secretion into the bile, offer a cytoprotective effect, and reduce elevated liver enzymes.[6,8]

Intestinal Obstruction Treatment of DIOS consists of enteral administration of polyethylene glycol (PEG) electrolyte solutions. Severe presentations may require surgical resection. Enemas may also be used to facilitate stool clearance. IV fluids are often required to correct dehydration due to vomiting or decreased oral intake. Reevaluation of enzyme adherence and dosing is essential to prevent recurrence, and some patients may require daily PEG administration (MiraLAX).[6]

▸ *CF-Related Diabetes*

Patients with mild CFRD may be managed with carbohydrate modification if nutritional status is optimal. However, most patients present with poor nutrition and weight loss and require more aggressive treatment. KEY CONCEPT *Because CFRD results from insulin insufficiency, exogenous insulin replacement is usually required.* Many patients can be successfully managed by meal coverage with short- or rapid-acting insulin (regular, lispro, or aspart) dosed per carbohydrate counting. Patients with fasting hyperglycemia or patients receiving nighttime tube feedings typically also require longer-acting basal insulin. Regular home glucose monitoring is essential to appropriate therapy. Oral antidiabetic agents have not been studied adequately in CFRD, and routine use is not recommended.[6,9]

▸ *Bone Disease and Arthritis*

CF patients with low bone mineral density and low serum vitamin D levels may improve bone health through supplemental vitamin D analogs beyond those found in standard CF vitamins. For cholecalciferol (or ergocalciferol), a minimum of 400 to 500 IU and 800 to 1000 IU should be taken daily by infants and patients older than 1 year of age, respectively.[11,12,34] Vitamin D concentrations should be measured annually in the winter for evaluation of dosing.[12] Total weekly or biweekly doses of 12,000 IU for children younger than 5 years of age and 50,000 IU for patients 5 years of age and older may be required to achieve target vitamin D concentrations. Supplemental calcium should be provided if 1300 to 1500 mg of elemental calcium intake cannot be achieved through diet.[11,34]

Antiresorptive agents (oral or IV bisphosphonates) may be used to treat adult CF patients with osteoporosis. Remaining upright daily for 30 minutes after dosing may be difficult for patients needing to perform airway clearance therapy, so products offering less frequent dosing should be considered. Pamidronate 30 mg IV every 3 months has been shown to increase bone mineral density in adult CF patients.[11] Androgen replacement may benefit bone health in some male CF patients with documented hypogonadism.[5,11]

> **Patient Encounter, Part 2**
>
> The parents received education about CF and met with the multidisciplinary CF team. Additional laboratory testing was sent to confirm the CF genotype. The team would like to initiate first-line CF therapies because the baby displays symptoms of pancreatic insufficiency (see Part 1). The infant weighs 3.5 kg and is 55 cm long.
>
> *Given this information, what is your assessment of the infant's nutritional status?*
>
> *What are the treatment goals for this patient?*
>
> *What nonpharmacologic therapy should be initiated?*
>
> *What pharmacologic therapy should be initiated?*

Pharmacogenomic Therapy

Since the discovery of the CF gene and the CFTR protein defect, research has focused on gene mutation-specific pharmacologic therapy to correct or modulate dysfunctional CFTR protein. Ivacaftor (Kalydeco, VX-770) is a CFTR potentiator that activates defective CFTR at the cell surface and improves CFTR function in patients with gating mutations. Ivacaftor is indicated for treatment of CF patients 6 years and older who have at least one *G551D* (present in approximately 4% of the CF population in the United States), *G1244E, G1349D, G178R, G551S, S1251N, S1255P, S549N,* or *S549R,* or *R117H* CFTR gene mutation. Ivacaftor treatment (added to standard CF care) is associated with improved lung function (approximately 10% increase in FEV_1), decreased pulmonary exacerbations, weight gain, and increased quality of life.[19,35] Ivacaftor given alone is not effective for patients homozygous for *F508del*.

The ivacaftor dose is 150 mg orally every 12 hours with food containing at least 20 g of fat for patients age six years and older. Patients 2 to 5 years of age should receive 50 mg (<14 kg) or 75 mg (> 14 kg) orally every 12 hours. Dosage must be reduced in moderate to severe hepatic impairment (Child-Pugh Class B or C) and when coadministered with moderate or strong CYP3A inhibitors (eg, azole antifungals, clarithromycin, erythromycin). Use with strong CYP3A inducers (eg, rifampin, rifabutin, phenytoin, phenobarbital, carbamazepine) is contraindicated. Ivacaftor therapy is generally well tolerated, although elevated liver enzymes have been reported; hepatic enzymes should be monitored quarterly in the first year of therapy.

Additional CFTR potentiators targeting other CFTR gene mutations are under investigation. (Note: In July 2015 as this book was going to press, the US Food and Drug Administration approved the combination of lumacaftor 200 mg/ivacaftor 125 mg (Orkambi) to treat CF in patients 12 years and older who are homozygous for the F508del mutation.)

OUTCOME EVALUATION

Pulmonary Function

- Monitor for changes in pulmonary symptoms (cough, sputum production, respiratory rate, and oxygen saturation).

Patient Encounter, Part 3

The infant is now 13 months old (weight: 10 kg) and is brought to a routine CF clinic appointment. Her parents report that she has had a cough productive of yellow sputum for the past week and an intermittent fever of up to 101.1°F (38.4°C). Also, the baby is not interested in eating and has been sleeping more. Vital signs are as follows: BP 84/39 mm Hg, HR 135 beats/min, RR 48/min, T 101.3°F (38.5°C), oxygen saturation 92% (0.92). Review of throat cultures since diagnosis reveals the following organisms:

- *S. aureus:* methicillin-sensitive
- *P. aeruginosa*: sensitive to ceftazidime, cefepime, piperacillin/tazobactam, ticarcillin–clavulanate, aztreonam, meropenem, ciprofloxacin, and tobramycin; resistant to levofloxacin, amikacin, and gentamicin
- *S. maltophilia*: sensitive to trimethoprim–sulfamethoxazole, minocycline, and ticarcillin–clavulanate; resistant to ceftazidime, meropenem, and levofloxacin

The infant has no known drug allergies.

Based on the information available, design an antibiotic regimen for outpatient therapy of this first pulmonary exacerbation.

What antibiotic(s) and dose(s) would you recommend for inpatient therapy?

Develop a monitoring plan to assess antibiotic response.

Symptoms should improve with antibiotics and aggressive airway clearance therapy. PFTs should be markedly increased after 1 week and trend back to pre-exacerbation levels after 2 weeks of therapy. If improvement lags, 3 weeks of therapy may be needed.

- For IV antimicrobial therapy, obtain serum drug levels for aminoglycosides and/or vancomycin and perform pharmacokinetic analysis. Adjust the dose, if needed, according to the targets in **Table 16–3**. Obtain follow-up trough levels and serum creatinine at weekly intervals or sooner if renal function is unstable.

Gastrointestinal Function

- Monitor short- and long-term nutritional status through evaluation of height, weight, and BMI. Ideally, parameters should be near the normals (50th percentile) for non-CF patients.
- Evaluate the patient's stool patterns. Steatorrhea indicates suboptimal enzyme replacement or noncompliance. Infants should have two to three well-formed stools daily, whereas older children and adults may have one or two stools daily.
- Monitor efficacy of vitamin supplementation through yearly serum vitamin levels. Obtain levels more frequently if treating a deficiency.

CF-Related Diabetes

- Monitor morning fasting and 2-hour postprandial blood glucose in patients with CFRD or those taking systemic corticosteroids. Follow A1C levels on an outpatient basis to assess long-term glucose control. Levels may be falsely low in CF due to a shorter red blood cell half-life.

Patient Care Process

Patient Assessment:

- Conduct a history of prescription, nonprescription, and alternative medications. Review drug allergies, especially antibiotics.
- Assess airway clearance methods and pulmonary symptoms. Evaluate for pulmonary exacerbation. Review frequency and quality of cough, sputum production, dyspnea, respiratory rate, oxygen saturations, temperature, and PFT trends.
- Review culture and sensitivity tests over the last 1 to 2 years. Review other available laboratory tests (renal and hepatic function, complete blood count, vitamin levels, blood glucose, A1C).
- Assess nutritional status, weight, height, and BMI trends. Are oral supplements or tube feedings being used?
- Assess GI symptoms: quantity and quality of bowel movements, gastroesophageal reflux, bloating, flatulence, or abdominal pain.

Therapy Evaluation:

- Evaluate medications for effectiveness, drug interactions, and adverse reactions. Are all appropriate maintenance medications prescribed and dosed appropriately for weight and age?
- Assess adherence, including timing of inhaled medications with respect to airway clearance therapies and timing of enzymes and insulin with regard to meals.
- Determine if antibiotics are indicated. Review pharmacokinetic history. What antibiotics were used previously? Was response better to a particular regimen?

Care Plan Development:

- Devise an appropriate IV or oral/inhaled antibiotic regimen for a pulmonary exacerbation. Optimize doses based on pharmacokinetic and pharmacodynamic parameters.
- Optimize maintenance therapies, doses, and schedules that promote efficacy and ease care burden.
- Educate the patient and family, stressing importance of therapy adherence.

Follow-Up Evaluation:

- For antibiotic regimens, evaluate pulmonary symptoms daily if inpatient (every 1 to 2 weeks if outpatient).
- For IV antibiotic regimens, obtain drug levels and perform pharmacokinetic dose adjustments as necessary. Monitor renal function at least weekly. Evaluate fluid intake and urine output daily.
- Assess effectiveness and safety of maintenance therapies at least quarterly.

Abbreviations Introduced in This Chapter

ABPA	Allergic bronchopulmonary aspergillosis
CF	Cystic fibrosis
CFRD	Cystic fibrosis-related diabetes

CFTR	Cystic fibrosis transmembrane regulator
CPT	Chest physiotherapy
DIOS	Distal intestinal obstruction syndrome
FEV_1	Forced expiratory volume in 1 second
FVC	Forced vital capacity
HFCC	High-frequency chest compression
IPV	Intrapulmonary percussive ventilation
MIC	Minimum inhibitory concentration
MRSA	Methicillin-resistant *Staphylococcus aureus*
MSSA	Methicillin-sensitive *Staphylococcus aureus*
OPEP	Oscillating positive expiratory pressure
PEG	Polyethylene glycol
PFT	Pulmonary function test
PMN	Polymorphonuclear
PT	Prothrombin time
RDA	Recommended daily allowance

REFERENCES

1. Gibson RL, Burns JL, Ramsey BW. State of the art: Pathophysiology and management of pulmonary infections in cystic fibrosis. Am J Respir Crit Care Med. 2003;168:918–951.
2. Cystic fibrosis mutation database [Internet]. http://www.genet.sickkids.on.ca/StatisticsPage.html. Accessed August 19, 2014.
3. Davies JC, Ebdon A, Orchard C. Recent advances in the management of cystic fibrosis. Arch Dis Child. 2014;99:1033–1036.
4. Rowe SM, Miller SM, Sorscher EJ. Mechanisms of disease: Cystic fibrosis. N Engl J Med. 2005;352:1992–2001.
5. Quon BS, Aitken ML. Cystic fibrosis: What to expect now in the adult years. Paediatr Respir Rev. 2012;13:206–214.
6. Yankaskas JR, Marshall BC, Sufian JD, et al. Cystic fibrosis adult care consensus conference report. Chest. 2004;125:1S–39S.
7. Li L, Somerset S. Digestive system dysfunction in cystic fibrosis: Challenges for nutrition therapy. Dig Liver Dis. 2014;26:865–874.
8. Debray D, Deirdre K, Houwen R, et al. Best practice guideline for the diagnosis and management of cystic fibrosis-associated liver disease. J Cyst Fibros. 2011;10(2):S29–S36.
9. Moran A, Brunzell C, Cohen RC, et al. Clinical care guidelines for cystic fibrosis related diabetes. Diabetes Care. 2010;33(12):2697–2708.
10. Sueblinvong V, Whittaker LA. Fertility and pregnancy: Common concerns of the aging cystic fibrosis population. Clin Chest Med. 2007;28(2):433–443.
11. Aris RM, Merkel PA, Bachrach LK, et al. Consensus statement: Guide to bone health and disease in cystic fibrosis. J Clin Endocrinol Metab. 2005;90:1888–1896.
12. Tangpricha V, Kelly A, Stephenson A, et al. An update on the screening, diagnosis, management, and treatment of vitamin D deficiency in individuals with cystic fibrosis: Evidence-based recommendations from the Cystic Fibrosis Foundation. J Clin Endocrinol Metab. 2012;97(4):1082–1093.
13. von Drygalski A, Biller J. Anemia in cystic fibrosis: Incidence, mechanisms, and association with pulmonary function and vitamin deficiency. Nutr Clin Pract. 2008;23(5):557–563.
14. Cystic Fibrosis Foundation. Cystic fibrosis foundation patient registry annual data report 2012. Bethesda, MD: Cystic Fibrosis Foundation, 2013. http://www.cff.org/treatments/CareCenterNetwork/PatientRegiPatientReg/. Accessed November 1, 2014.
15. Cohen-Cymberknoh M, Shoseyov D, Kerem E. Managing cystic fibrosis: Strategies that increase life expectancy and improve quality of life. Am J Respir Crit Care Med. 2011;183:1463–1471.
16. Stallings VA, Stark LJ, Robinson KA, et al. Evidence-based practice recommendations for nutrition-related management of children and adults with cystic fibrosis and pancreatic insufficiency: Results of a systematic review. J Am Diet Assoc. 2008;108:832–839.
17. Fuchs HJ, Borowitz DS, Christiansen DH, et al. Effect of aerosolized recombinant human DNase on exacerbations of respiratory symptoms and on pulmonary function in patients with cystic fibrosis. N Engl J Med. 1994;331:637–642.
18. Elkins MR, Robinson M, Rose BR, et al. A controlled trial of long-term inhaled hypertonic saline in patients with cystic fibrosis. N Engl J Med. 2006;354:229–240.
19. Mogayzel PJ, Naureckas ET, Robinson KA, et al. Cystic fibrosis pulmonary guidelines: Chronic medications for maintenance of lung health. Am J Respir Crit Care Med. 2013;187(7):680–689.
20. Nichols DP, Konstan MW, Chmiel JF. Anti-inflammatory therapies for cystic fibrosis-related lung disease. Clinic Rev Allerg Immunol. 2008;35:135–156.
21. Konstan MW, Byard PJ, Hoppel CL, Davis PB. Effect of high-dose ibuprofen in patients with cystic fibrosis. N Engl J Med. 1995;332:848–854.
22. Konstan MW, Krenicky JE, Finney MR, et al. Effect of ibuprofen on neutrophil migration in vivo in cystic fibrosis and healthy subjects. J Pharmacol Exp Ther. 2003;306:1086–1091.
23. Equi A Balfour-Lynn IM, Bush A, Rosenthal AB. Long term azithromycin in children with cystic fibrosis: A randomized, placebo-controlled crossover trial. Lancet. 2002;360:978–984.
24. Saiman L, Marshall BC, Mayer-Hamblett N, et al. Azithromycin in patients with cystic fibrosis chronically infected with *Pseudomonas aeruginosa*: A randomized controlled trial. JAMA. 2003;290:1749–1756.
25. Yee CL, Duffy C, Gerbino PG, et al. Tendon or joint disorders in children after treatment with fluoroquinolones or azithromycin. Pediatr Infect Dis J. 2002;21:525–529.
26. Kirkby S, Novak K, McCoy K. Update on antibiotics for infection control in cystic fibrosis. Expert Rev Anti Infect Ther. 2009;7(8):967–980.
27. Flume PA, Mogayzel PJ, Robinson KA, et al. Cystic fibrosis pulmonary guidelines: Treatment of pulmonary exacerbations. Am J Respir Crit Care Med. 2009;180(9):802–808.
28. Zobell JT, Young DC, Waters CD, et al. Optimization of anti-pseudomonal antibiotics for cystic fibrosis pulmonary exacerbations: VI. Executive summary. Pediatr Pulmonol. 2013;48:525–537.
29. Ramsey BW, Pepe MS, Quan JM, et al. Intermittent administration of inhaled tobramycin in patients with cystic fibrosis. N Engl J Med. 1999; 340:23–30.
30. Lam J, Vaughan S, Parkins MD. Tobramycin inhalation powder (TIP): An efficient treatment strategy for the management of chronic *Pseudomonas aeruginosa* infection in cystic fibrosis. Clin Med Insights Circ Respir Pulm Med. 2013;7:61–77.
31. Ratjen F, Munck A, Kho P, Angyalosi G. Treatment of early *Pseudomonas aeruginosa* infection in patients with cystic fibrosis: The ELITE trial. Thorax. 2010;65(4):289–291.
32. McCoy KS, Quittner AL, Oermann CM, et al. Inhaled aztreonam lysine for chronic airway *Pseudomonas aeruginosa* in cystic fibrosis. Am J Respir Crit Care Med. 2008;178(9):921–928.
33. Kirkby S, Novak K, McCoy. Aztreonam (for inhalation solution) for the treatment of chronic lung infections in patients with cystic fibrosis: An evidence based review. Core Evidence. 2011;6:59–66.
34. Borowitz D, Baker RD, Stallings V. Consensus report on nutrition for pediatric patients with cystic fibrosis. J Pediatr Gastroenterol Nutr. 2002;35(3):246–259.
35. Ramsey BW, Davies J, McElvaney NG, et al. A CFTR potentiator in patients with cystic fibrosis and the G551D mutation. N Engl J Med. 2011;365:1663–1672.

17 Gastroesophageal Reflux Disease

Dianne May and Marie A. Chisholm-Burns

LEARNING OBJECTIVES

Upon completion of the chapter, the reader will be able to:

1. Explain the underlying causes of gastroesophageal reflux disease (GERD).
2. Understand the difference between symptom-based esophageal GERD syndromes and extraesophageal GERD syndromes.
3. Determine which diagnostic tests should be recommended based on the clinical presentation.
4. Identify the desired therapeutic outcomes for patients with GERD.
5. Recommend appropriate nonpharmacologic and pharmacologic interventions for patients with GERD.
6. Formulate a monitoring plan to assess the effectiveness and safety of pharmacotherapy for GERD.
7. Educate patients on appropriate lifestyle modifications and drug therapy issues including compliance, adverse effects, and drug interactions.

INTRODUCTION

Gastroesophageal reflux disease (GERD) is defined as troublesome symptoms and/or complications caused by refluxing of stomach contents into the esophagus.[1,2] To be considered GERD-related, these troublesome symptoms should adversely affect patient well-being.[1] KEY CONCEPT *Esophageal GERD syndromes can be divided into two distinct categories: (a) symptom-based esophageal syndromes and (b) tissue injury-based esophageal syndromes.*[1] Symptom-based esophageal syndrome is associated with troublesome reflux symptoms with or without normal endoscopic findings. Conditions associated with esophageal tissue injury include erosive esophagitis, strictures, Barrett esophagus, and esophageal adenocarcinoma. Erosive esophagitis occurs when the esophagus is repeatedly exposed to refluxed material for prolonged periods. The inflammation that occurs progresses to erosions of the squamous epithelium.

Barrett esophagus is a complication of GERD characterized by replacement of the normal squamous epithelial lining of the esophagus with specialized columnar-type epithelium. Barrett esophagus is more common in male patients with a long history of reflux (greater than 5–10 years), age older than 50 years, and obesity. The presence of Barrett esophagus may be a risk factor for developing adenocarcinoma of the esophagus.

Extraesophageal reflux syndrome involves "atypical" symptoms outside the esophagus, primarily chronic cough, laryngitis, and asthma.[2] Reflux chest pain syndrome may also occur and may be indistinguishable from cardiac chest pain. When extraesophageal manifestations are present, other causes must be excluded before considering a diagnosis of GERD. In addition, atypical symptoms should only be considered GERD-related if a concurrent esophageal GERD syndrome is present.

EPIDEMIOLOGY AND ETIOLOGY

GERD is prevalent in patients of all ages; approximately 18% to 28% of adults in the United States are affected.[3] Although mortality is rare, symptoms can significantly decrease quality of life. There does not appear to be a gender difference in incidence except for its association with pregnancy. Barrett esophagus and esophageal adenocarcinoma occur more frequently in males.[4]

PATHOPHYSIOLOGY

The retrograde movement of acid or other noxious substances from the stomach into the esophagus is a major factor in the development of GERD.[5] Commonly, gastroesophageal reflux is associated with defective lower esophageal sphincter (LES) pressure or function. Problems with other normal mucosal defense mechanisms such as anatomic factors, esophageal clearance, mucosal resistance, gastric emptying, epidermal growth factor, and salivary buffering may also contribute to the development of GERD. Other factors that may promote esophageal damage upon reflux into the esophagus include gastric acid, pepsin, bile acids, and pancreatic enzymes.

Lower Esophageal Sphincter Pressure

The lower esophageal sphincter (LES) is normally in a tonic, contracted state, preventing reflux of gastric material from the stomach. It relaxes on swallowing to permit the free passage of food into the stomach.

Mechanisms by which defective LES pressure may cause gastroesophageal reflux are threefold. First, and probably most important, reflux may occur after spontaneous transient LES relaxations that are not associated with swallowing.[6] Esophageal distention, vomiting, belching, and retching can cause relaxation of the LES. Transient decreases in sphincter pressure are responsible for approximately 40% of the reflux episodes in patients with GERD.[6]

Second, reflux may occur after transient increases in intra-abdominal pressure (stress reflux) such as that occurring during straining, bending over, or a Valsalva maneuver.[5]

Third, the LES may be atonic, thus permitting free reflux. Although transient relaxations are more likely to occur when there is normal LES pressure, the latter two mechanisms are more likely when the LES pressure is decreased by such factors as gastric distention or smoking. Certain foods and medications may worsen esophageal reflux by decreasing LES pressure or by irritating the esophageal mucosa (Table 17–1).[7,8]

Anatomic Factors

Disruption of the normal anatomic barriers by a hiatal hernia was once thought to be a primary cause of gastroesophageal reflux. Presently, the presence of a hiatal hernia is considered to be a separate entity that may or may not be associated with reflux.

Esophageal Clearance

Many patients with GERD produce normal amounts of acid, but the acid produced spends too much time in contact with the esophageal mucosa. Contact time depends on the rate at which the esophagus clears the noxious material, as well as the frequency of reflux.

Swallowing contributes to esophageal clearance by increasing salivary flow. Saliva contains bicarbonate that buffers the residual gastric material on the surface of the esophagus. Saliva production decreases with age, making it more difficult to maintain a neutral intraesophageal pH. Swallowing is also decreased during sleep, which contributes to nocturnal GERD in some patients.

Mucosal Resistance

The esophageal mucosa and submucosa contain mucus-secreting glands that release bicarbonate, which can neutralize acidic refluxate in the esophagus. A decrease in this normal defense mechanism can lead to esophageal erosions.

Gastric Emptying and Increased Abdominal Pressure

Gastric volume is related to the amount of material ingested, rate of gastric secretion and emptying, and amount/frequency of duodenal reflux into the stomach. Delayed gastric emptying can lead to increased gastric volume and contribute to reflux by increasing intragastric pressure. Factors that increase gastric volume and/or decrease gastric emptying, such as smoking and high-fat meals, are often associated with gastroesophageal reflux.

Obesity is an independent risk factor for increased GERD symptoms and complications. Obesity has been linked to GERD because of increased abdominal pressure. Even weight gain in patients with a normal body mass index may cause new-onset GERD symptoms.[2] Morbidly obese patients may also have more transient LES relaxations, incompetent LES, and impaired esophageal motility.[6]

Composition of Refluxate

The composition, pH, and volume of the refluxate are other factors associated with gastroesophageal reflux. Duodenogastric reflux esophagitis, or "alkaline esophagitis," refers to esophagitis induced by the reflux of bilious and pancreatic fluid. The percentage of time that esophageal pH is below 4 is greater for patients with severe GERD.

Table 17–1[7]

Foods and Medications That May Worsen GERD Symptoms

Decreased LES Pressure	
Foods	
Fatty meal/fried foods	Coffee, caffeinated drinks
Carminatives (eg, peppermint)	Garlic
	Onions
Chocolate	Chili peppers
Medications	
Anticholinergics	Ethanol
Barbiturates	Isoproterenol
Benzodiazepines	Nicotine
Caffeine	Nitrates
Dihydropyridine calcium channel blockers	Opioids (eg, morphine)
	Phentolamine
Dopamine	Progesterone
Estrogen	Theophylline
Direct Irritants to the Esophageal Mucosa	
Foods	
Carbonated beverages	Orange juice
Citrus fruits	Spicy foods
Coffee	Tomatoes
Medications	
Aspirin	NSAIDs
Bisphosphonates	Quinidine
Iron	Potassium chloride

GERD, gastroesophageal reflux disease; LES, lower esophageal sphincter; NSAIDs, nonsteroidal anti-inflammatory drugs.

Adapted from May DB, Rao S. Gastroesophageal reflux disease. In: DiPiro JT, et al, eds. Pharmacotherapy: A Pathophysiologic Approach, 9th ed. New York, NY. McGraw-Hill, 2014:457, with permission.

Patient Encounter, Part 1

A 45-year-old Caucasian man presents to your clinic complaining of severe burning in his throat, regurgitation, and difficulty swallowing. He has been self-medicating with over-the-counter omeprazole 20 mg every morning for the last month with no improvement. His weight is 105 kg and his height is 5'11" (180 cm). Drug allergies include ramipril (difficulty breathing, swollen lips).

Are this patient's symptoms consistent with GERD?

Would you classify this patient as having a symptom-based esophageal GERD syndrome, tissue injury-based esophageal GERD syndrome, or an extraesophageal syndrome? Explain.

Would the patient's symptoms be described as typical, atypical, or complicated?

What risk factors does he have that may worsen GERD symptoms?

CLINICAL PRESENTATION AND DIAGNOSIS

KEY CONCEPT *Patients with GERD may display symptoms described as: (a) typical, (b) atypical, or (c) complicated* (see accompanying box Clinical Presentation of GERD).[7,8]

Diagnosis of GERD

The most useful tool in the diagnosis of GERD is the clinical history, including both presenting symptoms and risk factors. KEY CONCEPT *Patients presenting with uncomplicated, typical symptoms of reflux (heartburn and regurgitation) should not receive invasive esophageal evaluation as a first step.* These patients generally benefit from a trial of patient-specific lifestyle modifications and empiric acid-suppressing therapy.[1] A clinical diagnosis of GERD is assumed in patients responding to appropriate therapy. Further diagnostic testing is indicated to: (a) avert misdiagnosis, (b) identify complications, and (c) evaluate empiric treatment failures.

Other diagnostic tests may include endoscopy, ambulatory esophageal reflux monitoring, and manometry. **Endoscopy** is preferred for assessing mucosal injury and to identify complications such as strictures. A mucosal biopsy is taken to identify Barrett esophagus and adenocarcinoma. Endoscopy should also be performed in patients with troublesome dysphagia, unexplained weight loss, epigastric mass, or esophageal GERD syndromes not responding to an empiric trial of twice-daily proton pump inhibitor (PPI).[1]

Ambulatory esophageal reflux monitoring identifies patients with excessive esophageal acid exposure and frequency of reflux episodes. It helps determine whether symptoms are acid related and may be useful in patients not responding to acid suppression therapy. **Manometry** may be beneficial for patients who have failed twice-daily PPIs and have normal endoscopic findings or those contemplating antireflux surgery.

Various methods may be used, including ambulatory **impedance pH monitoring**, catheter pH, or wireless pH monitoring.

TREATMENT

Desired Outcomes

KEY CONCEPT *The goals of treatment of GERD are to alleviate symptoms, decrease the frequency of recurrent disease, promote healing of mucosal injury, and prevent complications.*

Clinical Presentation of GERD

Symptom-Based GERD Syndrome (with/without Esophageal Tissue Injury)

- Typical symptoms: Heartburn, hypersalivation, regurgitation, belching
- Alarm symptoms: Dysphagia, odynophagia, hematemesis (from bleeding esophageal erosions), weight loss
- Extraesophageal presentation: Chronic cough, laryngitis, wheezing (GERD may be a contributing factor in some patients with asthma); noncardiac chest pain

Tissue Injury–Based GERD Syndrome (with/without Esophageal Symptoms)

- Presentation may vary from asymptomatic to alarm symptoms
- Endoscopy may reveal esophagitis, strictures, Barrett esophagus, adenocarcarcinoma of the esophagus

General Approach to Treatment

KEY CONCEPT *Treatment for GERD involves one or more of the following modalities: (a) patient-specific lifestyle changes and patient-directed therapy, (b) pharmacologic intervention primarily with acid-suppressing therapy, or (c) antireflux surgery.* The best initial therapeutic option depends on the frequency and severity of symptoms, degree of esophagitis, and presence of complications (Table 17–2).

KEY CONCEPT *Acid-suppressing therapy is the mainstay of treatment and should be considered for anyone not responding to lifestyle changes and patient-directed therapy after 2 weeks.* The PPIs provide the greatest relief of symptoms and highest rates of healing, especially in patients with erosive disease or moderate to severe symptoms.

Maintenance therapy may be necessary to control symptoms and prevent complications. In patients with GERD refractory to adequate acid suppression, the diagnosis should be confirmed through further diagnostic tests before long-term therapy or surgery are considered.

Nonpharmacologic Therapy

Nonpharmacologic treatment of GERD includes patient-specific lifestyle modifications or surgery.

Patient Encounter, Part 2: Medical History, Physical Examination, and Diagnostic Tests

PMH: Dyslipidemia, type 2 diabetes mellitus, and hypertension for approximately 20 years (all well-controlled with medication)

FH: Noncontributory

SH: Works as a maintenance worker at the local elementary school; lives at home with wife and teenage daughter. Smokes two and a half packs of cigarettes per day

Meds: Metformin 500 mg twice daily, hydrochlorothiazide 12.5 mg once daily, amlodipine 10 mg once daily, atorvastatin 20 mg at bedtime

ROS: (+) Heartburn, regurgitation, difficulty swallowing; (–) chest pain, nausea, vomiting, diarrhea, weight loss, change in appetite, shortness of breath or cough

PE:

VS: BP 125/72 mm Hg, P 82 beats/min, RR 16 breaths/min, T 37°C (98.6°F)

CV: RRR, normal S_1, S_2; no murmurs, rubs, or gallops

Abd: Soft, nontender, nondistended; (+) bowel sounds, (–) hepatosplenomegaly, heme (–) stool

Given this additional information, what factors could be contributing to the patient's GERD symptoms?

Should patient-directed therapy with over-the-counter omeprazole 20 mg orally every morning be continued? Explain.

Does this patient require further diagnostic evaluation based on his clinical presentation? If so, which procedure would you recommend?

What nonpharmacologic and pharmacologic changes would you recommend for his GERD therapy?

Table 17–2

Therapeutic Approach to GERD in Adults

Recommended Treatment Regimen	Comments
Intermittent, Mild Heartburn	
Individualized lifestyle modifications *PLUS* patient-directed therapy with antacids and/or nonprescription-strength H_2RA or nonprescription-strength PPIs: • Magnesium hydroxide/aluminum hydroxide (eg, Maalox) 30 mL as needed or after meals and at bedtime • Antacid/alginic acid (Gaviscon) two tablets or 15 mL after meals and at bedtime • Calcium Carbonate (Tums) 500 mg tablets, two to four tablets as needed OR • Cimetidine (Tagamet HB) 200 mg up to twice daily • Famotidine (Pepcid AC) 10 mg up to twice daily • Nizatidine (Axid AR) 75 mg up to twice daily • Ranitidine (Zantac 75) up to twice daily OR • Esomeprazole (Nexium 24-hour) 22.3 mg once daily • Omeprazole (Prilosec OTC) 20 mg once daily • Omeprazole/Sodium Bicarbonate (Zegerid OTC) 10 mg/1100 mg once daily • Lansoprazole (Prevacid 24-hour) 15 mg once daily	If symptoms unrelieved by lifestyle modifications and nonprescription medications after 2 weeks, refer patient for medical attention
Symptomatic Relief of GERD	
Individualized lifestyle modifications *PLUS* prescription-strength H_2RA for 6–12 weeks or prescription-strength PPIs for 4–8 weeks: • Cimetidine (Tagamet) 400 mg twice daily • Famotidine (Pepcid) 20 mg twice daily • Nizatidine (Axid) 150 mg twice daily • Ranitidine (Zantac) 150 mg twice daily OR • Dexlansoprazole (Dexilant) 30 mg once daily • Esomeprazole (Nexium) 20 mg once daily • Lansoprazole (Prevacid) 15–30 mg once daily • Omeprazole (Prilosec) 20 mg once daily • Omeprazole/sodium bicarbonate (Zegerid) 20 mg once daily • Pantoprazole (Protonix) 40 mg once daily • Rabeprazole (Aciphex) 20 mg once daily	For typical symptoms, treat empirically with prescription-strength acid suppression therapy Mild GERD may be treated effectively with H_2RAs If symptoms recur, consider maintenance therapy Administer PPIs 30–60 minutes before meals
Healing of Erosive Esophagitis or Treatment of Moderate–Severe Symptoms or Complications	
Individualized lifestyle modifications *PLUS* prescription-strength PPIs (up to twice daily) for 4–16 weeks (8 weeks recommended for healing erosive esophagitis): • Dexlansoprazole (Dexilant) 60 mg once daily • Esomeprazole (Nexium) 20–40 mg once daily • Lansoprazole (Prevacid) 30 mg up to twice daily • Omeprazole (Prilosec) 20 mg up to twice daily • Omeprazole/sodium bicarbonate (Zegerid) 20 mg up to twice daily • Pantoprazole (Protonix) 40 mg up to twice daily • Rabeprazole (Aciphex) 20 mg up to twice daily	For extraesophageal or alarm symptoms, obtain endoscopy to evaluate mucosa Administer PPIs 30–60 minutes before meals If symptoms are relieved, consider maintenance therapy Evaluate patients not responding to pharmacologic therapy via manometry and/or ambulatory esophageal reflux monitoring

GERD, gastroesophageal reflux disease; H_2RA, histamine$_2$-receptor antagonist; PPI, proton pump inhibitor.

Adapted from May DB, Rao S. Gastroesophageal reflux disease. In: DiPiro JT, et al, eds. Pharmacotherapy: A Pathophysiologic Approach, 9th ed. New York, NY: McGraw-Hill, 2014:462–463, with permission.

► *Lifestyle Modifications*

Although most patients do not respond to lifestyle changes alone, the importance of maintaining these changes throughout the course of therapy should be discussed. The most beneficial lifestyle changes include: (a) losing weight if overweight or obese and (b) elevating the head of the bed with a foam wedge if symptoms are worse when recumbent. A reduction in body mass index by 3.5 units improves GERD symptoms and decreases need for GERD-related medications.[9] Elevating the head of the bed decreases nocturnal esophageal acid contact time.

Other lifestyle modifications should be considered based on patient circumstances. These might include: (a) eating smaller meals and avoiding meals 3 hours before sleeping, (b) avoiding foods or medications that exacerbate GERD, (c) smoking cessation, and (d) avoiding alcohol. The patient's medication and food histories should be evaluated to identify potential factors that may exacerbate GERD symptoms (Table 17–1).

▶ *Antireflux Surgery or Bariatric Surgery*

KEY CONCEPT *Antireflux surgery, such as Nissen fundoplication, offers an alternative for refractory GERD or when pharmacologic management is undesirable in patients with well-documented GERD.*[1] The goal of surgery is to reestablish the antireflux barrier, to position the LES within the abdomen where it is under positive (intra-abdominal) pressure, and to close any associated hiatal defect. Antireflux surgery provided more symptom control than omeprazole in patients with esophagitis in a 7-year follow-up study.[10] Antireflux surgery may be considered in patients who: (a) are intolerant to pharmacologic treatment; (b) desire surgery despite successful treatment because of lifestyle considerations, such as when daily medication adherence, tolerability, or cost are concerns; (c) have complications of GERD; or (d) have extra-esophageal manifestations.[1,11] The evidence for surgery is not as strong in those who do not respond to PPI therapy.[1,2] Roux-en-Y gastric bypass surgery has been shown to reduce symptoms of GERD in obese patients.[2,12]

Pharmacologic Therapy

▶ *Antacids*

Antacids are an appropriate component of treating mild GERD because they are effective for immediate, symptomatic relief. They are used concurrently with other acid-suppressing therapies. Common antacids include magnesium hydroxide/aluminum hydroxide combination products and those containing calcium carbonate.

Dosage recommendations for antacids vary and range from hourly dosing to administration on an as-needed basis. In general, antacids are short-acting, requiring frequent administration to provide continuous acid neutralization.

Antacids also have significant drug interactions with ferrous sulfate, isoniazid, sulfonylureas, and fluoroquinolones. Antacid drug interactions are influenced by antacid composition, dose, schedule, and formulation. Antacids may cause constipation or diarrhea (depending on the product), acid-base disturbances, and changes in mineral metabolism.

▶ *Histamine$_2$-Receptor Antagonists (H$_2$RAs)*

Cimetidine, famotidine, nizatidine, and ranitidine decrease acid secretion by inhibiting the histamine$_2$-receptors in gastric parietal cells. For symptomatic relief of mild GERD, low-dose nonprescription H$_2$RAs may be beneficial. If patients do not respond to nonprescription treatment after 2 weeks, prescription standard-dose therapy (Table 17–2) is warranted. When given in divided doses, H$_2$RAs provide effective symptomatic relief for patients with mild to moderate GERD, but endoscopic healing rates are lower than with PPIs (about 52% vs 84%).[2] Response to the H$_2$RAs depends on disease severity, dosage regimen, and duration of therapy. Although higher doses may provide higher symptomatic and endoscopic healing rates, limited information exists regarding their safety when given at two to four times the standard dose, and they can be less effective and more costly than once-daily PPIs.

In general, H$_2$RAs are well tolerated and have similar efficacy. The most common adverse effects include headache, fatigue, dizziness and either constipation or diarrhea.

▶ *Proton Pump Inhibitors (PPIs)*

Esomeprazole, lansoprazole, omeprazole, pantoprazole, rabeprazole, and dexlansoprazole block gastric acid secretion by inhibiting gastric H$^+$/K$^+$-adenosine triphosphatase in gastric parietal cells. This produces a profound, long-lasting antisecretory effect capable of maintaining the gastric pH above 4, even during acid surges occurring postprandially.

The PPIs are superior to H$_2$RAs in patients with moderate to severe GERD. This includes not only patients with erosive esophagitis or complicated symptoms (Barrett esophagus or strictures) but also those with symptom-based esophageal syndromes.

A PPI should be given empirically to patients with troublesome GERD symptoms. If the standard once-daily regimen does not eliminate symptoms, then empiric therapy with twice-daily dosing should be given or the patient should be changed to a different PPI. Patients not responding to twice-daily PPI therapy should be considered treatment failures, and further diagnostic evaluation should be performed.[1] Evidence does not support using high-dose PPIs in patients with Barrett esophagus with the sole intent of reducing the risk of progression to dysplasia or cancer.[13]

Because PPIs degrade in acidic environments, they are primarily formulated in delayed-release capsules or tablets. For patients unable to swallow intact capsules, pediatric patients, or those with nasogastric tubes, the contents of the capsule can be mixed in applesauce or placed in orange juice.[14] The acidic juices help maintain the integrity of the enteric-coated pellets until they reach the small intestine.[14] Esomeprazole pellets can be mixed with water prior to delivery through a nasogastric tube.[14] Lansoprazole is available as a delayed-release orally disintegrating tablet. Esomeprazole, omeprazole, lansoprazole, and pantoprazole are also available as oral suspensions.

The only PPI available in an immediate-release formulation is omeprazole combined with sodium bicarbonate (Zegerid). The proposed benefit of this product is fast onset of action and increase in pH provided by sodium bicarbonate, which helps prevent omeprazole degradation in the stomach. Sodium bicarbonate may also stimulate gastrin production, which may activate the proton pumps and optimize omeprazole effectiveness.

Patients taking pantoprazole or rabeprazole should be instructed not to crush, chew, or split the delayed-release tablets. Pantoprazole and esomeprazole are the only PPIs available in an intravenous (IV) formulation. The IV product is not more effective than the oral form and is significantly more expensive.

Most patients should be instructed to take their PPI in the morning, 30 to 60 minutes before breakfast to maximize efficacy, because these agents inhibit only actively secreting proton pumps. Patients with nighttime symptoms may benefit from taking the PPI prior to the evening meal. If a second dose is needed, it should be administered before the evening meal and not at bedtime. Regardless of the time of day, PPIs should be given prior to a meal to gain the most benefit. The exception to this is the immediate-release omeprazole–sodium bicarbonate combination product.

All PPIs can decrease the absorption of medications that require an acidic environment to be absorbed and are all metabolized by the cytochrome P-450 system to some extent. Omeprazole and lansoprazole are metabolized by CYP2C19 enzymes. Concerns have been raised about PPIs used concurrently with clopidogrel, a prodrug that must be converted to its active form by CYP2C19. Inhibition of CYP2C19 by PPIs has been suggested to decrease the effectiveness of clopidogrel and increase the risk of cardiac events. However, a consensus report found little evidence of cardiovascular harm when PPIs were used concurrently with clopidogrel.[15] Omeprazole is the strongest CYP2C19 inhibitor among the PPIs, and therefore most likely to cause problems in patients on clopidogrel. Although generally not of major concern, omeprazole may inhibit the metabolism of CYP2C19 substrates such as diazepam, warfarin, or phenytoin. No interactions with dexlansoprazole, lansoprazole, pantoprazole, or rabeprazole have been seen with CYP2C19 substrates. Esomeprazole does not interact with warfarin or phenytoin. Pantoprazole is metabolized by a cytosolic sulfotransferase and is therefore less likely to have significant drug interactions than other PPIs.

Drug interactions with omeprazole are of particular concern in patients who are "slow metabolizers", which represent a small percentage of the US population. Unfortunately, it is unclear which patients have the polymorphic gene variation that makes them slow metabolizers. Alternatively, patients who are considered rapid metabolizers, which is most common in the Asian population (12%–20%), may not respond as well. This genetic variation among patients may alter the effect of PPIs due to the ability of their enzyme system to metabolize the drug.

The PPIs are generally well tolerated. The most common adverse effects are headache, diarrhea, constipation, and abdominal pain. Short-term use of PPIs has been associated increased risk of community-acquired pneumonia in GERD patients.[2] Potential concerns about long-term use of PPIs include development of enteric infections (eg, *Clostridium difficile)*, vitamin B_{12} deficiency, and hypomagnesemia.[16] There is little evidence of an increased risk of vitamin B12 deficiency. Hypomagnesemia is a rare adverse effect of PPIs, but it can be potentially life threatening. Higher doses and long-term use (greater than 1 year) are most likely to be associated with hypomagnesemia. Periodic monitoring of magnesium concentration is warranted in patients receiving long-term PPI therapy.

Limited data suggest that acid suppression caused by PPIs can inhibit calcium absorption and decrease bone density. There are conflicting data regarding an increased risk of fractures in patients taking PPIs.[17,18] PPIs are not presently contraindicated in patients with osteoporosis despite an FDA advisory suggesting that the odds ratio for hip, wrist, and cervical spine fractures in six studies was higher in patients on long-term or high-dose PPI therapy.[18] Nevertheless, routine bone density studies or calcium supplementation are not warranted based on PPI use alone.[1] Screening and testing for osteoporosis should be performed as recommended for any other patient, regardless of PPI use.

▶ *Prokinetic Agents*

Metoclopramide and bethanechol have inferior efficacy and adverse effect profiles when used for GERD treatment. Consequently, their use is not recommended.

▶ *Mucosal Protectants*

Sucralfate, a nonabsorbable aluminum salt of sucrose octasulfate, has very limited value in the treatment of GERD and is not recommended.

Combination Therapy

Two agents of different therapeutic classes should not be used routinely. Patients not responding to standard H_2RA doses should be switched to a PPI instead of adding a prokinetic agent. Monotherapy with a PPI is not only more effective, but it also improves compliance and is ultimately more cost-effective.

The addition of an H_2RA at bedtime to PPI therapy has been suggested to decrease nocturnal acid breakthrough. Although there may be an immediate effect to control symptoms and maintain the pH greater than 4, tachyphylaxis may quickly develop. If H_2RAs are used at night, it may be preferable to only use them as needed to provide a "drug holiday" that may lessen the occurrence of tachyphylaxis.[2]

Maintenance Therapy

KEY CONCEPT *Many patients with GERD experience relapse if medication is withdrawn, and long-term maintenance treatment may be required.* Candidates for maintenance therapy include patients whose symptoms return once therapy is discontinued or decreased, history of erosive esophagitis, Barrett esophagus, or extraesophageal symptoms (associated with concurrent esophageal GERD syndromes).

The goal of maintenance therapy is to improve quality of life by controlling symptoms and preventing complications. Acid-suppressing therapy should be reduced to the lowest dose that controls symptoms and routinely evaluated to determine if long-term therapy is indicated. This is especially true in light of safety concerns with long-term PPI use.

The H_2RAs may be effective maintenance therapy for patients with mild disease. The PPIs are first choice for maintenance treatment of moderate to severe GERD. A short course of "on-demand" therapy may be appropriate in patients with symptomatic esophageal syndromes without esophagitis when symptom control is the primary outcome of interest.[1] Antacids have the fastest onset and may be used in combination with an H_2RA or PPI for on-demand symptom relief.

Long-term use of higher PPI doses is not indicated unless the patient has complicated symptoms, has erosive esophagitis per endoscopy, or has had further diagnostic evaluation to determine degree and frequency of acid exposure. Antireflux surgery may be a viable alternative to long-term medication use for maintenance therapy in select patients.

Special Populations

▶ *Patients with Extraesophageal GERD*

Therapy for GERD is not beneficial for treating extraesophageal symptoms in patients without a concomitant esophageal GERD syndrome.[1] Chronic cough, laryngitis, and asthma are associated with GERD.[1] Other causes should be excluded before attributing extraesophageal symptoms to GERD. Treatment with twice-daily PPIs for 2 months may be warranted in patients with extraesophageal GERD syndromes.[1] Patients with chest pain should receive twice-daily PPI therapy for 4 weeks after cardiac causes have been excluded. Low response to PPI therapy in patients with noncardiac chest pain may occur when there is no objective evidence of GERD. Extraesophageal symptoms should only be considered GERD-related (and thereby responsive to PPI therapy) if a concurrent esophageal GERD syndrome is present. Manometry or ambulatory esophageal reflux monitoring should be considered in patients who do not respond to PPIs.[1]

Maintenance therapy is generally indicated in patients with extraesophageal GERD syndromes but not with noncardiac chest pain alone.[1]

► Children with GERD

Generally, gastroesophageal reflux (GER) is a normal physiologic process in children that occurs several times per day with no clinical consequence. As with adults, GERD is present when symptoms become troublesome or if complications are present.[19,20]

Regurgitation is common in children and is defined as the effortless and nonprojectile passage of refluxed gastric contents into the pharynx or mouth. This is also known as spitting-up or the "happy spitter," which may occur daily in as many as 50% of infants younger than 3 months.[19] More troublesome symptoms may include vomiting, poor weight gain, sleep disturbances, and refusing to eat.[20]

Reflux episodes are common during transient LES relaxations not related to swallowing because of developmental immaturity of the LES.[19] Other causes include impaired luminal clearance of gastric acid and type of infant formula. Patients with neurologic impairment, obesity, repaired esophageal atresia, congenital esophageal disease, cystic fibrosis, hiatal hernia, repaired achalasia, or lung transplant are at a higher risk for developing GERD.[19]

Lifestyle modifications are emphasized in pediatric patients with uncomplicated GERD. Symptoms usually resolve by 12 to 18 months of life and respond to supportive therapy, including dietary adjustments such as smaller meals, more frequent feedings, or thickened infant formula. However, excessive thickening of infant formula is discouraged. Postural management (eg, positioning the infant in an upright position, especially after meals) may be helpful. Changes in maternal diet such as restricting eggs and milk may be useful in breast-fed infants with GERD symptoms.[20] If lifestyle modifications are not effective, medical therapy may be indicated.

Acid suppression with either an H_2RA or PPI is the mainstay of pharmacologic therapy.[19] Chronic use of antacids or routine use of prokinetics or sucralfate is not recommended. Monotherapy with an H_2RA is commonly used; ranitidine 2 to 4 mg/kg/day IV (or 4–8 mg/kg/day orally) is effective in neonates and pediatric patients. However, chronic use may lead to tachyphylaxis.

The use of PPIs in pediatric patients has increased significantly. The potential overuse of PPIs in infants is of concern. Esomeprazole is indicated for patients 1 month old to less than 1 year old for short-term treatment of erosive esophagitis (up to 6 weeks). The dose ranges from 2.5 to 10 mg depending on weight. It is indicated for healing erosive esophagitis and short-term symptomatic relief of GERD (4–8 weeks) in children more than 1 year old. The approved GERD dose of esomeprazole in children 12 to 17 years old is 20 to 40 mg and 10 to 20 mg in patients 1 to 11 years old.

Safety and effectiveness of lansoprazole has been shown for pediatric patients 1 to 17 years old for short-term treatment of symptomatic GERD and erosive esophagitis. Studies in adolescents (12–17 years old) demonstrated pharmacokinetics similar to those seen in adults. The recommended dose is 15 mg once daily for children weighing 30 kg or less and 30 mg once daily for those weighing more than 30 kg.

The approved GERD dose of omeprazole in children is the same as esomeprazole. Although not approved in pediatric patients younger than 1 year, omeprazole 1 mg/kg/day (given once or twice daily) has been used for esophagitis. The long-term safety of prolonged use in children is unknown, and therefore clinicians must carefully weigh risk versus benefit.[19]

► Patients with Refractory GERD

Refractory GERD may be present in patients not responding to 4 to 8 weeks of twice-daily PPI therapy. Compliance and timing of medication should always be assessed prior to deciding that a patient is refractory to acid-suppressing therapy. Endoscopy is indicated to determine if underlying pathology exists. In addition, patients with esophagitis may have a genotype that renders the PPIs less effective. Because of variability in patient response, consideration may be given to switching to an alternative PPI before increasing to twice-daily PPI in patients not responding to once-daily PPI therapy. Nonreflux-related esophageal causes may include dysmotility syndromes such as achalasia or scleroderma, or eosinophilic esophagitis.[21]

OUTCOME EVALUATION

- Monitor for symptom relief and the presence of complicated symptoms.
- Record the frequency and severity of symptoms by interviewing the patient after 4 to 8 weeks of acid-suppressing therapy. Continued symptoms may indicate the need for long-term maintenance therapy.
- Monitor for adverse drug reactions, drug–drug interactions, and adherence.
- Educate patients about symptoms that suggest the presence of complications requiring immediate medical attention, such as dysphagia or odynophagia.
- Refer patients who present with extraesophageal symptoms to their physician for further diagnostic evaluation.
- Reassess the need for chronic PPI therapy.
- KEY CONCEPT *Review patient profiles for drugs that may aggravate GERD.*

Patient Encounter, Part 3: Monitoring for Safety and Efficacy

The patient returns to your clinic for his annual follow-up appointment. His GERD symptoms are now well controlled, and he is receiving long-term maintenance therapy with lansoprazole 30 mg once daily. He is worried that he may get bone fractures if he stays on the PPI long term.

What would you tell this patient about the effects PPIs may have on risk of bone fractures?

How would you monitor the patient for efficacy outcomes?

How would you monitor the patient for safety outcomes?

How can cultural biases be avoided to make the best treatment decisions for the patient?

Implement a follow-up plan to determine whether the goals have been achieved and adverse effects avoided.

Patient Care Process

Patient Assessment:

- Determine if patient is experiencing any signs and symptoms of GERD.
- Assess symptoms and associated GERD complications to determine if all needed diagnostic evaluations that will influence therapy or monitoring are completed and reviewed.
- Perform a thorough medication history by evaluating use of prescription, nonprescription, and herbal/dietary supplement products to assess products used and which alleviated or increased GERD symptom(s).
- Verify patient medication allergies and intolerances.

Therapy Evaluation:

- Determine if patient-specific lifestyle modifications and/or pharmacologic therapy are indicated.
- Inquire about which treatments have been helpful in the past; assess how much each therapy helped, how well it was tolerated, and how the therapy was accessed.
- If patient is already receiving therapy, evaluate it for possible adverse drug reactions and drug interactions.
- Assess patient adherence and track progression toward established therapeutic goals (ie, tissue healing and/or symptomatic relief).
- Determine the patient's ability to obtain the medication prescribed (eg, available on formulary, covered by insurance, affordable to patient).

Care Plan Development:

- Instruct patient on appropriate individualized lifestyle modifications.
- Recommend appropriate therapy and dose (Table 17–2), aimed at healing esophageal tissue damage and/or improving esophageal symptoms.
- Stress the importance of medication and lifestyle adherence.
- Educate the patient on how and when each medication should be taken.
- Review potential adverse drug reactions and significant drug interactions with the patient.
- Alert the patient to symptoms that should be reported to the health care provider.
- Answer any drug- and disease-related questions that may arise.

Follow-Up Evaluation:

- Monitor for signs or symptoms of complications.
- Assess for improvement in quality-of-life measures and achievement of therapeutic outcomes.
- Recommend appropriate follow-up tests as appropriate (eg, serum magnesium concentration).
- Determine if long-term maintenance treatment is necessary after completion of the initial course of therapy.

Abbreviations Introduced in This Chapter

GERD	Gastroesophageal reflux disease
H_2RA	Histamine$_2$-receptor antagonist
LES	Lower esophageal sphincter
PPI	Proton pump inhibitor

REFERENCES

1. Kahrilas PJ, Shaheen NJ, Vaezi MF, et al. AGA Institute Medical Position Panel. American Gastroenterological Association Medical Position Statement on the management of gastroesophageal reflux disease. Gastroenterology. 2008;135: 1383–1391.
2. Katz PO, Gerson LB, Vela MF. Guidelines for the diagnosis and management of gastroesophageal reflux disease. Am J Gastroenterol. 2013;108:308–328.
3. El-Serag HB, Sweet S, Winchester CC, Dent J. Update on the epidemiology of gastro-oesophageal reflux disease: A systematic review. Gut. 2014;63:871–880.
4. Rubenstein JH, Scheiman JM, Sadeghi S, et al. Esophageal adenocarcinoma incidence in individuals with gastroesophageal reflux: Synthesis and estimates from population studies. Am J Gastroenterol. 2011;106:254–260.
5. Boeckxstaens GEE. Review article: The pathophysiology of gastro-oesophageal reflux disease. Aliment Pharmacol Ther. 2007;26:149–160.
6. Herbella FA, Patti MG. Gastroesophageal reflux disease: From pathophysiology to treatment. World J Gastroenterol. 2010; 16(30): 3745–3749.
7. May DB, Rao SSC. Gastroesophageal reflux disease. In: DiPiro JT, Talbert RL, Yee GC, et al, eds. Pharmacotherapy: A Pathophysiologic Approach, 9th ed. New York, NY: McGraw-Hill, 2014:457–463.
8. Kahrilas PJ. Gastroesophageal reflux disease. N Engl J Med. 2008;359:1700–1707.
9. Ness-Jensen E, Lindam A, Lagergren J, Hveem K. Weight loss and reduction in gastroesophageal reflux. A prospective population-based cohort study: The HUNT study. Am J Gastroenterol. 2013; 108:376–382.
10. Lundell L, Miettinen P, Myrvold HE, et al. Seven-year follow-up of a randomized clinical trial comparing proton-pump inhibition with surgical therapy for reflux oesophagitis. Br J Surg. 2007; 94:198–203.
11. Stefanidis D, Hope WW, Kohn GP, et al. Guidelines for surgical treatment of gastroesophageal reflux disease (GERD). Practice/Clinical Guidelines published on 2/2010 by the Society of American Gastrointestinal and Endoscopic Surgeons (SAGES) [Internet]. http://www.sages.org/publication/id/22/.
12. Gagne DJ, Dovec E, Urbandt JE. Laparoscopic revision of vertical banded gastroplasty to Roux-en-Y gastric bypass: Outcomes of 105 patients. Surg Obes Relat Dis. 2011;7:493–499.
13. American Gastroenterological Association. Medical position statement of the management of Barrett's esophagus. Gastroenterology. 2011;140:1084–1091.
14. Williams NT. Medication administration through enteral feeding tubes. Am J Health Syst Pharm. 2008;65:2347–2357.

15. Abraham NS, Hlatky MA, Antman EM, et al. ACCF/ACG/AHA 2010 Expert consensus document on the concomitant use of proton pump inhibitors and thienopyridines: A focused update of the ACCF/ACG/AHA 2008 expert consensus document on reducing the gastrointestinal risks of antiplatelet therapy and NSAID use: A report of the American College of Cardiology Foundation Task Force on expert consensus documents. Circulation. 2010;122:2619–2633.
16. Thomson ABR, Sauve MD, Kassam N, Kamitakahara H. Safety of the long-term use of proton pump inhibitors. World J Gastroenterol. 2010;16(19):2323–2330.
17. FDA Drug Safety Communication [Internet]. Possible increased risk of fractures of the hip, wrist, and spine with the use of proton pump inhibitors [cited 2010 May 25]. www.fda.gov.
18. FDA Drug Safety Communication [Internet]. Possible increased risk of fractures of the hip, wrist, and spine with the use of proton pump inhibitors. www.fda.gov. Updated March 23, 2011.
19. Vandenplas Y, Rudolph CE, Di Lorenz C, et al. Pediatric gastroesophageal reflux clinical practice guidelines: Joint recommendations of the North American Society for Pediatric Gastroenterology, Hepatology, and Nutrition (NASPGHAN) and the European Society for Pediatric Gastroenterology, Hepatology, and Nutrition (ESPGHAN). J Pediatr Gastroenterol Nutr. 2009;49:498–547.
20. Lightdale Jr, Gremse DA; Section on Gastroenterology, Hepatology, and Nutrition. Gastroesophageal reflux: Management guidance for the pediatrician. Pediatrics. 2013;131(5):e1684–e1695.
21. Dellon ES, Shaheen NJ. Persistent reflux symptoms in the proton pump inhibitor era: The changing face of gastroesophageal reflux disease. Gastroenterology. 2010;139:7–13.

18 Peptic Ulcer Disease

Catherine A. Bourg, Dianne May

LEARNING OBJECTIVES

Upon completion of the chapter, the reader will be able to:

1. Recognize differences between ulcers induced by *Helicobacter pylori*, nonsteroidal anti-inflammatory drugs (NSAIDs), and stress-related mucosal damage (SRMD) in terms of risk factors, pathogenesis, signs and symptoms, clinical course, and prognosis.
2. Identify desired therapeutic outcomes for patients with *H. pylori*–associated ulcers and NSAID-induced ulcers.
3. Identify factors that guide selection of an *H. pylori* eradication regimen and improve adherence with these regimens.
4. Determine the appropriate management for a patient taking a nonselective NSAID who is at high risk for ulcer-related gastrointestinal (GI) complications (eg, GI bleed) or who develops an ulcer.
5. Employ an algorithm for evaluation and treatment of a patient with signs and symptoms suggestive of an *H. pylori*–associated or NSAID-induced ulcer.
6. Given patient-specific information and the prescribed treatment regimen, formulate a monitoring plan for drug therapy either to eradicate *H. pylori* or to treat an active NSAID-induced ulcer or gastrointestinal (GI) complication.

INTRODUCTION

Peptic ulcer disease (PUD) refers to a defect in the gastric or duodenal mucosal wall that extends through the **muscularis mucosa** into the deeper layers of the submucosa.[1] PUD is a significant cause of morbidity and is associated with substantial health care costs.[2,3] Although there are many etiologies of PUD, the three most common are (a) *H. pylori* infection, (b) use of nonsteroidal anti-inflammatory drugs (NSAIDs), and (c) stress-related mucosal damage (SRMD).

Complications of PUD include GI bleeding, perforation, and obstruction. Complications of untreated or undiagnosed *H. pylori* infection include gastric cancer and PUD. This chapter focuses mainly on pharmacotherapy of PUD related to *H. pylori* infection or NSAID use. Prophylaxis of stress-related mucosal damage in hospitalized patients is also discussed briefly.

EPIDEMIOLOGY AND ETIOLOGY

In the United States, PUD affects approximately 4.5 million people annually.[4] The mean direct medical cost (including pharmacy, inpatient, and outpatient costs) was $23,819 per patient per year in one study evaluating workplace absences, short-term medical disability, worker's compensation, and medical and pharmacy claims for six large US employers.[5]

The prevalence of *H. pylori* infection in the United States and Canada is about 30%, whereas the global prevalence is greater than 50%. Factors that influence the incidence and prevalence of *H. pylori* infection include age, ethnicity, sex, geography, and socioeconomic status.

Helicobacter Pylori

H. pylori is usually contracted in the first few years of life and tends to persist indefinitely unless treated. The infection normally resides in the stomach and is transmitted through ingestion of fecal-contaminated water or food. The organism causes **gastritis** in all infected individuals, but fewer than 10% actually develop symptomatic PUD.

Nonsteroidal Anti-Inflammatory Drugs

Chronic NSAID ingestion causes nausea and dyspepsia in nearly half of patients. Peptic ulceration occurs in up to 30% of chronic NSAID (including aspirin) users, with GI bleeding or perforation occurring in 1.5% of patients who develop an ulcer.[2] Ulcer-related complications result in 100,000 hospitalizations and more than 20,000 deaths in the United States each year.[2]

Risk factors for NSAID-induced PUD and complications are presented in Table 18–1. Risk factors are generally additive. Corticosteroid therapy is not an independent risk factor for ulceration but increases PUD risk substantially when combined with NSAID therapy.[6] Whether *H. pylori* infection is a risk factor for NSAID-induced ulcers remains controversial; however, *H. pylori* and NSAIDs act independently to increase ulcer risk and ulcer-related bleeding and also appear to have synergistic effects.[7]

Stress-Related Mucosal Damage

SRMD occurs most frequently in critically ill patients due to mucosal defects caused by gastric mucosal ischemia and intraluminal acid.[8] The ulcers are usually superficial, but SRMD

Table 18–1

Risk Factors for Ulcers and GI Complications Related to NSAID Use

- Age older than 60 years
- Concomitant anticoagulant use
- Preexisting coagulopathy (elevated INR or thrombocytopenia)
- Concomitant corticosteroid or selective serotonin reuptake inhibitor therapy
- Previous PUD or PUD complications (bleeding/perforation)
- Cardiovascular disease and other comorbid conditions
- Multiple NSAID use (eg, low-dose aspirin plus another NSAID)
- Duration of NSAID use (> 1 month)
- High-dose NSAID use
- NSAID-related dyspepsia
- Cigarette smokers

INR, international normalized ratio; NSAID, nonsteroidal anti-inflammatory drug; PUD, peptic ulcer disease.

may also penetrate into the submucosa and cause significant GI bleeding. Physiologically stressful situations that lead to SRMD include sepsis, organ failure, prolonged mechanical ventilation, thermal injury, and surgery. Critical care patients with the specific characteristics listed above are at highest risk.[9]

Zollinger–Ellison Syndrome

Zollinger–Ellison syndrome (ZES) is caused by a gastrin-producing tumor called a gastrinoma. The resulting gastric acid hypersecretion causes diarrhea and malabsorption. Ulcers tend to be numerous and have a high risk of perforation and bleeding.[10] Treatments include surgical resection when feasible and high-dose oral proton pump inhibitor (PPI) therapy.

Other Causative Factors

Cigarette smoking is associated with a higher prevalence of ulcers in *H. pylori*-infected patients.[2] The detrimental effects of smoking on the gastric mucosa may involve increased pepsin secretion, duodenogastric reflux of bile salts, elevated levels of free radicals, and reduced **prostaglandin**-2 (PG_2) production, resulting in decreased mucus and bicarbonate secretion.[11]

Although psychosocial factors such as life stress, personality patterns, and depression may influence PUD prevalence, a clear causal relationship has not been demonstrated.[2]

Dietary factors such as coffee, tea, cola, alcohol, and spicy foods may cause dyspepsia but have not been shown to independently increase PUD risk.

PATHOPHYSIOLOGY

Ulcers related to *H. pylori* infection more commonly affect the duodenum (duodenal ulcers), whereas NSAID-related ulcers more frequently affect the stomach (gastric ulcers) (Figure 18–1). However, ulcers may be found in either location from either cause.[10]

Ulcer formation in the GI tract results from disrupted homeostasis between factors that break down food (eg, gastric acid and pepsin) and those that promote mucosal defense and repair (eg, bicarbonate, mucus secretion, and PGs).

Gastric Acid and Pepsin

Hydrochloric acid and pepsin are the primary substances that cause gastric mucosal damage in PUD. Three different stimuli

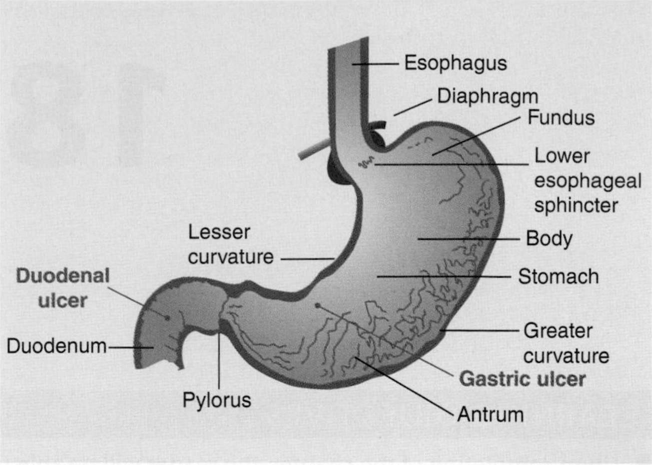

FIGURE 18–1. Anatomic structure of the stomach and duodenum and most common locations of gastric and duodenal ulcers. (From Love B, Thoma MN. Peptic ulcer disease. In: DiPiro JT, Talbert RA, Yee GC, et al, eds. Pharmacotherapy: A Pathophysiologic Approach, 9th ed. New York, NY: McGraw-Hill, 2014 with permission. www.accesspharmacy.com.)

(eg, histamine, acetylcholine, and gastrin) cause acid secretion through interactions with the histaminic, cholinergic, and gastrin receptors on the surface of parietal cells. Gastric acid output occurs in two stages: (a) basal acid output during fasting, and (b) maximal acid output in response to meals. Basal acid secretion follows a circadian cycle and is modulated by the effects of acetylcholine and histamine on parietal cells.[12]

Food increases gastric acid secretion in two ways: (1) vagus nerve stimulation in response to sight, smell, or taste; and (2) stomach distention during the gastric and intestinal phases of acid secretion.

After stimulation by histamine, acetylcholine, and gastrin, acid is secreted by the H^+-K^+-ATPase$^+$ (proton) pump, located on the luminal side of parietal cells. Acid secretion in PUD is usually normal or only slightly elevated. NSAID ingestion does not usually affect acid secretion, whereas *H. pylori* infection often slightly increases acid output.[12]

Pepsinogen released from chief cells in the body of the stomach is converted to pepsin in an acidic environment; pepsin initiates protein digestion and collagen proteolysis and serves as a signal for the release of other digestive enzymes such as gastrin and cholecystokinin.[13] The proteolytic activity of pepsin appears to influence ulcer formation.

Mucosal Defense and Repair

Several normal processes prevent mucosal damage and subsequent ulcer formation. The buffering action of the mucus/phospholipid and bicarbonate barrier shields the gastric epithelial surface from gastric acid.[2] This allows an acidic environment in the gastric lumen but a near neutral pH on the epithelial lining.

PGs inhibit gastric acid secretion and protect gastric mucosa by stimulating mucus, bicarbonate, and phospholipid production. PGs also increase mucosal blood flow and stimulate epithelial cell regeneration.[2] Damage to the mucosal defense system is the primary method by which *H. pylori* and NSAIDs cause peptic ulcers.

▸ *Helicobacter pylori*

H. pylori, a gram-negative rod, is found on the surface of the gastric epithelium. Flagella provide motility that allows the organism to penetrate the mucous gel barrier and infect epithelial cells.[14] Cellular invasion by *H. pylori* is necessary for an active infection. The organism survives in the acidic milieu of the stomach by producing urease, an enzyme that hydrolyzes urea in gastric juice into carbon dioxide and ammonia.[14]

H. pylori may cause gastroduodenal mucosal injury through (a) direct mucosal damage, (b) alterations in host inflammatory responses, and (c) hypergastrinemia and elevated acid secretion.

Nonsteroidal Anti-Inflammatory Drugs

NSAIDs can cause gastric mucosal damage by two mechanisms: (1) direct irritation of the gastric epithelium, and (2) systemic inhibition of endogenous mucosal PG synthesis. Direct irritation occurs because NSAIDs are weak acids. Less acidic agents, such as nonacetylated salicylates, may confer decreased GI toxicity.[15] Direct irritant effects contribute to NSAID-induced gastritis but play a minor role in the development of NSAID-induced PUD.

Systemic inhibition of PG synthesis is the primary means by which NSAIDs cause PUD. NSAID inhibition of PG production by blocking the cyclooxygenase-2 (COX-2) enzyme produces beneficial analgesic and anti-inflammatory effects. However, NSAIDs may also block the COX-1 enzyme, which produces PGs that provide gastroprotection. NSAIDs given parenterally (eg, ketorolac) and rectally (eg, indomethacin) have an incidence of PUD similar to oral NSAIDs. Topical NSAIDs (eg, diclofenac) are unlikely to cause PUD because very low serum concentrations are achieved. The antiplatelet effects of NSAIDs may worsen bleeding complications associated with PUD.

Clinical Presentation of PUD

Symptoms

- Dyspepsia and mild epigastric pain that may be described as burning, gnawing, or aching in character.
- Epigastric pain with duodenal ulcers typically occurs 1 to 3 hours after meals or at night and is often relieved by food.
- Pain with gastric ulcers occurs is often aggravated by food.
- Abdominal pain may be described as burning or a feeling of discomfort.
- Pain severity pain often fluctuates and the character can vary from dull to sharp.
- Patients may also complain of heartburn, belching, bloating, nausea, or vomiting.

Signs

- Weight loss may be associated with nausea and vomiting.
- Complications such as bleeding, perforation, or obstruction may occur.
- Alarm findings include family history of upper GI malignancy, unintentional weight loss, overt GI bleeding, iron deficiency anemia, progressive dysphagia or odynophagia, early satiety, persistent vomiting, palpable mass, or lymphadenopathy.

CLINICAL PRESENTATION AND DIAGNOSIS

Clinical Presentation

See text box for the clinical presentation of PUD. Dyspepsia (upper abdominal discomfort) is found in 10% to 40% of the general population. PUD is found in 5% to 15% of patients with dyspepsia.

PUD can be classified as uncomplicated or complicated. Uncomplicated disease is typically characterized by mild epigastric pain, whereas complicated disease involves acute upper GI complications such as GI bleeding, obstruction, or perforation. Bleeding may be occult or may present as melena or hematemesis. Up to 20% of patients who develop a PUD-related hemorrhage do not have prior symptoms. Gastric outlet obstruction is usually caused by ulcer-related inflammation or scar formation. Patients typically present with early satiety after meals, nausea, vomiting, abdominal pain, and weight loss. Perforation requires emergent surgical intervention, and these patients should not undergo endoscopy.

Diagnosis

Radiologic and/or endoscopic procedures are usually required to document the presence of ulcers. Endoscopic testing is invasive and expensive, but it is indicated in patients older than 55 years with new-onset dyspepsia or any patient with alarming features.[1,16,17] Patients with dyspepsia who are younger than 55 years without alarming features may forego endoscopy but should be tested for *H. pylori* and treated if positive.[1,16,17] Those who test negative for *H. pylori* should be offered a trial (4–8 weeks) of acid suppression therapy or proceed to endoscopy. Persistent dyspepsia despite a trial of acid suppressive therapy warrants upper endoscopy evaluation.[1]

Testing for *H. pylori* infection is indicated in patients with active PUD, history of documented PUD, or gastric mucosa-associated lymphoid tissue (MALT) lymphoma.[17] Diagnostic tests to detect *H. pylori* presence can be either endoscopic or nonendoscopic.[14,17] Endoscopic diagnosis involves extraction of gastric tissue samples that are subsequently tested for *H. pylori*.[17] Histology is the standard identification method, but culture, polymerase chain reaction (PCR), and the rapid urease test can also identify *H. pylori* in tissue samples.[18]

Nonendoscopic testing methods for *H. pylori* include the urea breath test, serologic testing, and stool antigen assay.[14,17] These tests are less invasive and less expensive than endoscopy. The urea breath test is usually first line because of its high sensitivity and specificity and short turnaround time.[18,19] Concomitant acid-suppressive or antibiotic therapy may give false-negative results.[19] The urea breath test can also be used to confirm eradication of *H. pylori* infection.[19]

Serologic testing provides a quick (within 15 minutes) office-based assessment of exposure to *H. pylori*, but it cannot differentiate active infection from previously treated infection; patients can remain seropositive for years after eradication. Serologic testing is also less sensitive and specific than the urea breath test.[14] Serologic testing is recommended in patients with recent or current antibiotic or acid-suppressive therapy.[20]

Stool antigen assays can be useful for initial diagnosis or to confirm *H. pylori* eradication. They have high sensitivity and specificity and are affected less by concomitant medication use.[14] Use of antimicrobial agents within 4 weeks, PPIs within 2 weeks, and histamine-2 receptor antagonists (H_2RAs) within 24 hours of testing can suppress the infection and reduce the sensitivity of testing.[14]

TREATMENT

The treatment selected for PUD depends on the etiology of the ulcer, whether the ulcer is new or recurrent, and whether complications have occurred. Figure 18–2 shows an algorithm for evaluation and treatment of a patient with signs and symptoms suggestive of an *H. pylori*–associated or NSAID-induced ulcer.

Desired Outcomes

The goals of PUD therapy are to resolve symptoms, reduce acid secretion, promote epithelial healing, prevent ulcer-related complications, and prevent ulcer recurrence. For *H. pylori*–related PUD, eradication of *H. pylori* is an additional outcome.

Nonpharmacologic Therapy

▸ *Risk Factor Avoidance*

KEY CONCEPT *Patients with PUD should avoid exposure to factors known to worsen the disease, exacerbate symptoms, or lead to ulcer recurrence.* Patients should be advised to reduce psychological stress and avoid cigarette smoking, alcohol consumption, and NSAID or aspirin use if possible. Patients who require chronic NSAID therapy (eg, for rheumatoid arthritis) may be given prophylaxis with misoprostol or a PPI (see section on prevention of NSAID-induced ulcers).

▸ *Surgery*

The high success rates of medical therapies have reduced the need for surgical procedures. Elective surgeries performed for PUD have decreased by more than 70% since the 1980s mainly due to *H. pylori* eradication.[21] Surgical interventions are generally reserved for complicated or refractory PUD.[6]

For patients with acute GI bleeding, endoscopic hemostasis can be achieved using contact thermal therapy, mechanical therapy using clips, or epinephrine injection followed by either thermal or mechanical therapy.[22] **Angiography** with embolization of

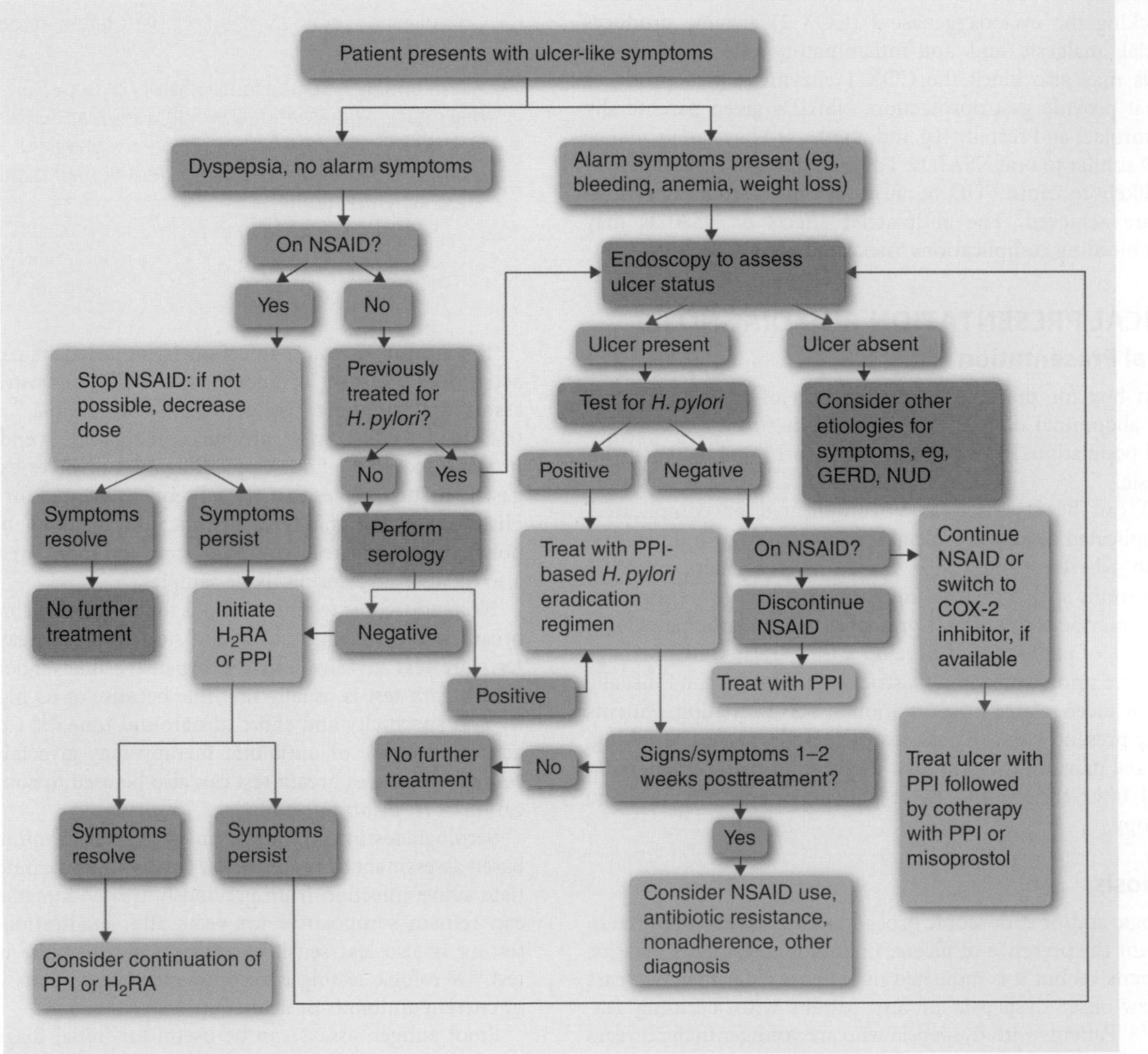

FIGURE 18–2. Guidelines for the evaluation and management of a patient who presents with dyspeptic or ulcer-like symptoms. (COX-2, cyclooxygenase-2; GERD, gastroesophageal reflux disease; H_2RA, H_2-receptor antagonist; NSAID, nonsteroidal antiinflammatory drug; NUD, nonulcer dyspepsia; PPI, proton pump inhibitor.) (From Love B, Thoma MN. Peptic ulcer disease. In: DiPiro JT, Talbert RA, Yee GC, et al, eds. Pharmacotherapy: A Pathophysiologic Approach, 9th ed. New York, NY: McGraw Hill, 2014; with permission. www.accesspharmacy.com.)

bleeding lesions can be used if the bleeding cannot be stopped endoscopically and the patient is either high risk for surgery or not a surgical candidate.[23]

Pharmacologic Therapy

▸ *Treatment of* H. pylori*–Associated Ulcers*

The goal of *H. pylori* therapy is to eradicate the organism using an effective antibiotic-containing regimen. KEY CONCEPT *Reliance on conventional acid-suppressive drug therapy alone as an alternative to H. pylori eradication is inappropriate because it is associated with a higher incidence of ulcer recurrence and ulcer-related complications.* Reinfection rates are generally low after the initial course of therapy as long as the patient was adherent. The selected *H. pylori* regimen should have a per-protocol cure rate of 90% or more or a cure rate based on intention-to-treat analysis of 80% or more.[24] In addition to proven efficacy, the optimal treatment regimen should cause minimal adverse events, have low risk for development of bacterial resistance, and be cost-effective.[14,17]

H. pylori treatment regimens are presented in Table 18–2. KEY CONCEPT *Eradication therapy with a PPI-based three-drug regimen should be considered for all patients who test positive for H. pylori and have an active ulcer or a documented history of either an ulcer or ulcer-related complication. Different antibiotics should be used if a second course of H. pylori eradication therapy is required.* The cure rates of *H. pylori* with H_2RAs in combination with antibiotics are lower than with PPIs.

The first-line regimen should consist of triple drug therapy with a PPI plus clarithromycin and either amoxicillin or metronidazole.[14,25] Amoxicillin should not be used in penicillin-allergic patients, and metronidazole should be avoided if alcohol is going to be consumed. A single daily PPI dose may be less effective than twice-daily dosing when used in a triple-drug regimen. Substitution of one PPI for another is acceptable and does not affect eradication rates. Monotherapy with a single antibiotic or antiulcer agent is not recommended due to high failure rates. In the United States, two-drug regimens consisting of a PPI and a single antibiotic are also not recommended.[26]

The duration of therapy for *H. pylori* eradication is controversial; US guidelines recommend either 10 or 14 days. Compared with 7 days of triple therapy, a 10-day duration increases eradication rates by 4% and 14 days increases eradication rates by 5% to 12%.[20,25] Longer treatment courses may decrease adherence and increase drug costs; ultimately, the most effective eradication regimens still fail in 10% to 20% of patients.[10]

Bismuth-based four-drug regimens have clinical cure rates similar to three-drug PPI-based regimens. Bismuth-based

Table 18–2

Drug Regimens to Eradicate *Helicobacter pylori*[a,b]

Treatment Regimen	Cure Rates[b]
First Line: Three Drugs[c]	
Clarithromycin 500 mg + metronidazole 500 mg + omeprazole 20 mg, each given twice daily	Good to excellent
Clarithromycin 500 mg + amoxicillin 1 g + lansoprazole 30 mg, each given twice daily	Good to excellent
First Line: Four Drugs	
Helidac™ (bismuth subsalicylate 525 mg + metronidazole 250 mg + tetracycline 500 mg, each given four times a day) + ranitidine 150 mg twice daily[c]	Good
Bismuth subsalicylate 525 mg four times a day + metronidazole 250 mg four times a day + tetracycline 500 mg four times a day + PPI twice daily OR ranitidine 150 mg twice daily[d,e]	Good
Pylera™ (bismuth subcitrate potassium 140 mg + metronidazole 125 mg + tetracycline 125 mg) three capsules twice daily + omeprazole 20 mg twice daily × 10 days	Good to excellent
Rescue/Salvage Therapy	
Amoxicillin 1 g + PPI (each given two times daily) + levofloxacin 500 mg daily[c]	Good
Other Proposed Regimens for Rescue/Salvage Therapy[f]	
• Sequential Therapy	
Days 1–5: Amoxicillin 1 g + esomeprazole 40 mg, each given twice daily	Good to excellent
Days 6–10: Clarithromycin 500 mg + metronidazole 500 mg + Esomeprazole 40 mg, each given twice daily	
• Modified Regimen	
Amoxicillin 1 g + standard dose PPI + levofloxacin 250 mg (each given twice daily)[c]	Good
• Concomitant Regimen	
Esomeprazole 40 mg + amoxicillin 1 g + clarithromycin 500 mg + metronidazole 500 mg, each given twice daily × 10 days	Good to excellent

[a]Regimens are based on efficacy for a 14-day treatment duration unless otherwise noted.
[b]Based on cure rates of 80% to 90% = Good; greater than 90% = Excellent.
[c]Given for 10 to 14 days.
[d]Although commercially available, regimens containing H_2RAs are not preferred.
[e]Duration of therapy is 7 to 10 days.
[f]Proposed for patients failing previous therapy.
H_2RA, histamine-2 receptor antagonist; PPI, proton pump inhibitor.

Patient Encounter 1

A 62-year-old man presents with abdominal pain and heartburn that occur two to three times per week. He also reports a 10-pound (4.5-kg) weight loss in the last 6 weeks, despite not dieting or increasing physical activity.

PMH: Hypertension × 5 years

FH: Mother alive at 84 with hypertension, type 2 diabetes; father deceased at 68 following MI

SH: Smokes half pack per day; no alcohol or illicit drug use

Allergies: NKDA

Meds: Lisinopril/hydrochlorothiazide 20/25 mg daily, acetaminophen 500 mg as needed for headache

Based on this patient's clinical presentation, what is the most appropriate course of action to establish a diagnosis?

The patient receives a diagnosis of H. pylori infection based on the diagnostic method recommended. What eradication therapy would you recommend?

The patient completed the course of eradication therapy recommended; however upon completion, he developed hives and difficulty breathing. This was determined to be a penicillin allergy. The patient returns with similar symptoms 3 months later.

What regimen would you recommend for eradication therapy?

regimens usually include a bismuth salt, tetracycline, metronidazole, and an acid suppressing agent (PPI or H_2RA). Bismuth salts promote ulcer healing through antibacterial and mucosal protective effects. Disadvantages of bismuth-based regimens include frequency of administration (four times a day), risk for salicylate toxicity in renal impairment, and bothersome side effects (eg, stool and tongue discoloration, constipation, nausea, vomiting).[10] Therefore, bismuth-based quadruple therapy is usually considered second-line treatment.

Several combination products are available that may increase adherence to the regimen. Pylera (bismuth subcitrate potassium 140 mg, metronidazole 125 mg, and tetracycline 125 mg) combined with omeprazole 20 mg twice daily is as effective as omeprazole–amoxicillin–clarithromycin in eradicating *H. pylori* in patients with duodenal ulcers.[26] The usual dose is three capsules four times daily after meals and at bedtime with 8 oz (237 mL) water for 10 days.

Helidac™ is a package of 14 blister cards with each card containing a single-day supply of bismuth subsalicylate (two 262.4-mg chewable tablets four times daily), metronidazole (250-mg tablet four times daily), and tetracycline (500-mg capsule four times daily). Unlike Pylera™, Helidac™ is not a combination product; all three medications must be taken four times daily for 14 days in combination with an H_2RA rather than a PPI. However, cure rates with H_2RAs are less than with PPIs and are therefore not preferred.[14]

PrevPac™ contains lansoprazole 30 mg, amoxicillin 1 gram, and clarithromycin 500 mg; each agent is dosed twice daily. A study in patients with duodenal ulcer showed comparable eradication rates with 10-day and 14-day regimens. Pylera™, Helidac™, and PrevPac™ are substantially more expensive than the costs of their individual generic and nonprescription components.

Patients may remain infected with *H. pylori* after the initial treatment course because of reinfection, nonadherence, or antimicrobial resistance. Factors associated with decreased adherence include polypharmacy, need for frequent drug administration or long treatment duration, and use of drugs that may cause intolerable side effects. Potential adverse drug effects include taste disturbances (clarithromycin and metronidazole), nausea, vomiting, abdominal pain, and diarrhea. Superinfections with oral thrush or vaginal candidiasis can occur. Alcohol should be avoided during treatment with metronidazole or tinidazole due to the potential for a disulfiram-like reaction.[27]

Preexisting antimicrobial resistance accounts for up to 70% of all treatment failures and is most often related to metronidazole or clarithromycin. Metronidazole-resistant strains are more prevalent in Asia (85%) than North America (40%).[26] Clarithromycin resistance rates are approximately 10% in the United States. Although a threshold of 20% is recommended to differentiate between regions of high and low clarithromycin resistance, triple therapy regimens containing clarithromycin can begin to lose efficacy when resistance is between 7% and 10%.[31] Primary resistance to amoxicillin and tetracycline remains low in both the United States and Europe.[26] Culture and sensitivity studies are not routinely performed with *H. pylori* infection unless a patient has already failed two different treatment regimens.[14,17,20]

Initiation of a second *H. pylori* treatment regimen after failure of initial treatment is usually associated with a lower success rate. Reasons for failure are often the same as those reported with failure of the initial regimen. In these situations, quadruple therapy for 14 days is generally required, and metronidazole or clarithromycin should be replaced by another antibiotic if either one of these agents was used in the initial regimen.[26] If both clarithromycin and metronidazole were used as initial therapy, a regimen consisting of amoxicillin 1 g twice daily, levofloxacin 250 mg twice daily, and a PPI twice daily may be used for 10 to 14 days.[28] Another salvage therapy consisting of amoxicillin 1 g twice daily, rifabutin 150 mg twice daily, and ciprofloxacin 500 mg twice daily for 14 days is also effective, but patients receiving this regimen experienced more adverse effects.[10,29,30]

There is no standard third-line therapy for *H. pylori* treatment. If the patient was adherent with initial treatment, then culture and sensitivity testing should be completed in order to select an antimicrobial regimen with adequate sensitivities.[10,20] Sequential therapy is a possible alternative 10-day regimen that may also be used to treat *H. pylori* infection and consists of using different combinations of antibiotics for 5 days each in addition to a PPI twice daily. Eradication rates are reported to be between 85% and 90%.[31]

Several additional modifications to treatment regimens have been proposed. Modified triple therapy containing levofloxacin may be considered in populations with high clarithromycin resistance; eradication rates range from 72% to 96%. The standard sequential therapy regimen has also been modified by replacing clarithromycin with tetracycline with variable results. Lastly, concomitant four-drug regimens and hybrid (sequential-concomitant) therapy have also been evaluated. One study comparing sequential versus concomitant regimens using a PPI, amoxicillin, clarithromycin, and metronidazole showed similar eradication rates (92.3% and 93%, respectively) and may represent options in the setting of antibiotic resistance.[31,32]

Confirmation of *H. pylori* infection eradication is recommended in patients with a history of *H. pylori*–associated ulcer, MALT lymphoma, resection for early gastric cancer, and patients whose symptoms persist after *H. pylori* treatment for dyspepsia.[14]

Patient Encounter 2

A 52-year-old man presents with persistent epigastric pain and heartburn. His chief complaint today is, "I think my ulcer is back again!"

PMH: Hypertension × 2 years

FH: Mother deceased at age 70, cancer; father alive with hypertension, dyslipidemia

SH: Nonsmoker, 1 to 2 alcoholic beverages three times weekly, no illicit drug use

Allergies: NKDA

Meds: Hydrochlorothiazide 25 mg daily, amlodipine 5 mg daily

The patient previously completed the following courses for *H. pylori* eradication:

- Clarithromycin 500 mg + amoxicillin 1 g + lansoprazole 30 mg, each given twice daily
- Pylera + omeprazole 20 mg twice daily for 10 days

H. pylori recurrence is confirmed with a urea breath test.

Discuss possible reasons for treatment failure in this patient.

What regimen would you recommend for salvage eradication therapy?

Eradication may be confirmed by either the urea breath test or stool antigen testing. Eradication may also be confirmed by endoscopy, but this should only be done when endoscopy is required because it is more expensive and invasive.[14]

▸ *Treatment of NSAID-Induced Ulcers*

Treatment recommendations to heal NSAID-induced ulcers or provide maintenance therapy in patients receiving NSAIDS are shown in Table 18–3. Choice of regimen depends on whether NSAID use is to be continued. NSAIDs should be discontinued and replaced with alternatives (eg, acetaminophen), when possible. For patients who cannot discontinue NSAID therapy, PPIs, H_2RAs, or sucralfate are effective for ulcer healing and to prevent further recurrences.[10] PPIs are usually preferred because they provide more rapid relief of symptoms, have the strongest acid suppression, and heal ulcers more quickly than H_2RAs or sucralfate.[10] Standard doses of H_2RAs effectively heal duodenal ulcers but are minimally effective in gastric ulcers. In ulcers larger than 5 mm, the rate of ulcer healing may be as low as 25% after 8 weeks of therapy with an H_2RA.[7] A PPI provides equivalent efficacy with treatment duration of only 4 weeks. PPI therapy should only be continued for longer than 4 weeks if an ulcer is confirmed to still be present or if the patient develops severe complications from PUD.

▸ *Prevention of NSAID-Induced Ulcers*

Prophylactic regimens against PUD are often required in patients receiving long-term NSAID or aspirin therapy for osteoarthritis, rheumatoid arthritis, or cardioprotection.[33] Misoprostol, H_2RAs, PPIs, and COX-2 selective inhibitors have been evaluated in controlled trials to reduce the risk of NSAID-induced PUD. KEY CONCEPT *In patients at risk for NSAID-induced ulcers, PPIs at standard doses reduce the risk of both gastric and duodenal ulcers as effectively as misoprostol and more effectively than H_2RAs.* In addition, PPIs are generally better tolerated than misoprostol.

Table 18–3
Oral Drug Regimens to Heal Peptic Ulcers or Maintain Ulcer Healing in the Absence of Antibiotic Therapy

Drug	DU or GU Healing (mg/day)	Maintenance of DU or GU Healing (mg/day)
Mucosal Protectant		
Sucralfate	1 g four times a day	1 g four times a day
	2 g two times a day	1–2 g two times a day
H_2-Receptor Antagonists		
Cimetidine	300 mg four times a day 400 mg two times a day 800 mg at bedtime	400–800 mg daily
Famotidine	20 mg two times a day 40 mg at bedtime	20–40 mg daily
Nizatidine	150 mg two times a day 300 mg at bedtime	150–300 mg daily
Ranitidine	150 mg two times a day 300 mg at bedtime	150–300 mg daily
Proton Pump Inhibitors		
Dexlansoprazole	30–60 mg daily	30–60 mg daily
Esomeprazole	20–40 mg daily	20–40 mg daily
Lansoprazole	15–30 mg daily	15–30 mg daily
Omeprazole	20–40 mg daily	20–40 mg daily
Pantoprazole	40 mg daily	40 mg daily
Rabeprazole	20 mg daily	20 mg daily

DU, duodenal ulcer; GU, gastric ulcer.

Misoprostol Misoprostol is a synthetic prostaglandin E1 (PGE_1) analog that exogenously replaces PG stores. It is indicated for reducing the risk of NSAID-induced gastric ulcers in patients at high risk of complications from ulcers (eg, the elderly and patients with concomitant debilitating disease), as well as patients at high risk of developing gastric ulceration, such as patients with a history of ulcers. Misoprostol 200 mcg four times a day reduces ulcer complications by inhibiting acid secretion and promoting mucosal defense.[7] It is superior to H_2RAs for prevention of NSAID-induced ulcers. Misoprostol use is limited by a high frequency of bothersome GI effects such as abdominal pain, flatulence, and diarrhea, and it is contraindicated in pregnancy due to potential abortifacient effects. Arthrotec is a combination product that contains diclofenac (either 50 or 75 mg) and misoprostol 200 mcg in a single tablet.

H_2-Receptor Antagonists The efficacy of H_2RAs (eg, famotidine 40 mg daily) in preventing NSAID-related ulcers varies. Duodenal ulcers appear to respond better than gastric ulcers (the most frequent type of ulcer associated with NSAIDs). Higher doses of H_2RAs (eg, famotidine 40 mg twice daily) may reduce the risk of NSAID-induced gastric and duodenal ulcers, but results from clinical trials are variable.

Duexis™, a prescription combination product containing ibuprofen 800 mg and famotidine 26.6 mg, is indicated for relief of signs and symptoms of rheumatoid arthritis and osteoarthritis and to decrease the risk of developing upper GI ulcers. The recommended dosage is one tablet orally three times daily.

Clinical trials evaluating this agent are 6 months or less in duration and primarily evaluated patients younger than 65 years with no ulcer history.

Proton Pump Inhibitors PPI therapy is more effective than H_2RAs in reducing the risk of nonselective NSAID-related gastric and duodenal ulcers. PPIs are as effective as misoprostol but better tolerated. All PPIs are effective when used in standard doses. In patients who experience a PUD-related bleeding event while taking aspirin but who require continued aspirin therapy, the addition of a PPI reduces the incidence of recurrent GI bleeding.[5] Prevacid NapraPAC™ provides naproxen (either 250, 375, or 500 mg) and lansoprazole 15 mg in individual blister packages. Vimovo™ provides naproxen (either 375 mg or 500 mg) and esomeprazole 20 mg in each tablet.

COX-2 Selective Inhibitors NSAIDs with COX-2 selectivity were developed in an attempt to reduce the incidence of PUD and its complications. KEY CONCEPT *However, selective COX-2 inhibitors are no more effective than the combination of a PPI and a nonselective NSAID in reducing the incidence of ulcers and are associated with a higher incidence of cardiovascular events than traditional nonselective NSAIDs (eg, ischemic stroke).*[10] Celecoxib is the only agent in this class on the market in the United States.

Given the CV risk of COX-2 inhibitors, a nonselective NSAID and a PPI is recommended instead of celecoxib in patients at high risk for NSAID-related PUD.[10,34]

Sucralfate This drug is a negatively charged, nonabsorbable agent that forms a complex by binding with positively charged proteins in exudates, forming a viscous, paste-like adhesive substance that protects the ulcerated area of the gastric mucosa against gastric acid, pepsin, and bile salts.[7,15] Limitations of sucralfate include the need for multiple daily dosing, large tablet size, and interaction with a number of other medications (eg, digoxin and fluoroquinolones).

Adverse effects of sucralfate include constipation, nausea, metallic taste, and the possibility for aluminum toxicity in patients with renal failure. Sucralfate is effective in the treatment of NSAID-related ulcers when the NSAID will be stopped, but it is not recommended for NSAID-related ulcer prophylaxis.

▶ Prevention of Stress-Related Mucosal Damage

Prevention of stress ulcers involves maintaining hemodynamic stability to maximize mesenteric perfusion and pharmacologic suppression of gastric acid production. Stress ulcer prophylaxis is only indicated in intensive care unit (ICU) patients with certain risk factors (see Table 18–4).[8,35] The clinician must weigh the risks and benefits of using acid suppression, especially PPIs, in low-risk patients. PPIs and H_2RAs are the drugs of choice for SUP; however, antacids and sucralfate may be acceptable options in some patients.

▶ Long-Term Maintenance of Ulcer Healing

KEY CONCEPT *Low-dose maintenance therapy with a PPI or H_2RA is only indicated* in patients with severe complications secondary to PUD such as gastric outlet obstruction or patients who need to be on long-term NSAIDs or high-dose corticosteroids and are at high risk for bleeding. Drug regimens and doses for PUD treatment and maintenance are presented in **Table 18–3**.

▶ Treatment of GI Bleeding

The immediate priorities in treating patients with a bleeding peptic ulcer are to achieve IV access, correct fluid losses, and restore hemodynamic stability. Insertion of a nasogastric tube is helpful in initial patient assessment, but the absence of bloody or coffee-ground material does not definitively rule out ongoing or recurrent bleeding; about 15% of patients without bloody nasogastric tube output have a high-risk lesion at endoscopy.[22]

Patients should be started on IV PPI therapy because optimal platelet aggregation, partially inhibited fibrinolysis, and better clot stabilization on the ulcer are achieved when the gastric pH is greater than 6.[36] Intravenous PPI therapy should be continued

Patient Encounter 3

A 68-year-old woman presents with reports of dark, tarry stools for 3 days. She denies coffee-ground emesis or recent weight loss but reports occasional abdominal pain.

PMH: Hypertension × 10 years, type 2 diabetes × 5 years, dyslipidemia × 5 years, osteoarthritis × 3 years

FH: Parents deceased; mother with stroke at age 82, father with MI at age 74; one sister alive at 74 with hypertension, type 2 diabetes, and dyslipidemia

SH: Smokes one pack per day, denies alcohol or illicit drug use

Allergies: NKDA

Meds: Lisinopril 40 mg daily, amlodipine 5 mg daily, metformin 1000 mg twice daily, glipizide 10 mg twice daily, simvastatin 40 mg daily, meloxicam 15 mg twice daily, aspirin 81 mg daily, Tums™ Extra Strength as needed for dyspeptic symptoms

Other: An endoscopy is performed and reveals a duodenal ulcer that is negative for *H. pylori*

What risk factors does this patient have for GI complications related to NSAID use?

Make a recommendation for treatment of this patient's ulcer.

Discuss the use of prophylactic therapy in this patient after the treatment course is completed.

Table 18–4

Appropriate Indications for Stress Ulcer Prophylaxis in Intensive Care Unit Patients[9]

- Mechanical ventilation for longer than 48 hours
- Coagulopathy or hepatic failure (platelet count < 50×10^3/mm^3 (50×10^9/L), INR > 1.5, or aPTT > two times control)
- History of GI ulceration or bleeding within 1 year of admission
- Head trauma or Glasgow Coma Score of 10 or less (or inability to obey simple commands)
- Thermal injuries to more than 35% of body surface area
- Multiple traumas (injury severity score of 16 or greater)
- Partial hepatectomy
- Transplant patients in the ICU perioperatively
- Spinal cord injuries
- Two of the following risk factors: sepsis, ICU stay for more than 1 week, occult bleeding lasting 6 or more days, and use of high-dose corticosteroids (> 250 mg/day of hydrocortisone or equivalent)

GI, gastrointestinal; ICU, intensive care unit; INR, international normalized ratio; aPTT, activated partial thromboplastin time.

Patient Encounter 4

A 55-year-old man is brought to the surgical ICU after emergency surgery following a motor vehicle accident. The physician would like him to remain NPO (nothing by mouth, except for medications) for at least several days until he improves clinically and can sit up in bed.

PMH: Hypertension × 10 years, type 2 diabetes × 5 years

FH: Father with type 2 diabetes

SH: Smokes one pack per day; no alcohol use; no illicit drug use

Allergies: NKDA

Meds: Lisinopril/hydrochlorothiazide 20/25 mg daily, metformin 500 mg twice daily, aspirin 81 mg daily, ibuprofen 800 mg alternating with oxycodone 5 mg/acetaminophen 325 mg two tablets every 8 hours for surgical site pain

Based on this patient's clinical presentation, is he a candidate for stress ulcer prophylaxis?

What pharmacologic therapy would you recommend for this patient?

Two days later, the patient is transferred to a general medicine floor and begins a regular diet that is well tolerated. Ibuprofen has been discontinued, and he is alternating between oxycodone/acetaminophen and acetaminophen alone to relieve incision site pain. He is sitting up in bed and feeling much better. Is this patient still a candidate for stress ulcer prophylaxis?

for 72 hours (because most rebleeding occurs during this time) followed by oral PPI therapy. Three-day PPI infusion therapy has been shown to be as effective as twice-daily IV PPI therapy.[36]

▶ *Treatment of Refractory Ulcers*

Refractory ulcers are defined as ulcers that fail to heal despite 8 to 12 weeks of acid suppressive therapy.[1] The presence of refractory ulcers requires a thorough assessment, including evaluation of medication adherence, extensive counseling and questioning regarding recent over-the-counter and prescription medication use, and testing for *H. pylori* using a different method than previously done if testing was negative. Changing from H_2RA therapy to a PPI should be considered.[15] Other considerations include esophagogastroduodenoscopy (EGD) with biopsy of the ulcer to exclude malignancy, *H. pylori* testing (if not done initially), serum gastrin measurement to exclude ZES, and gastric acid studies. Increasing the starting dose of PPI therapy may heal up to 90% of refractory ulcers after 8 weeks of therapy.[16]

Patient Care Process: Peptic Ulcer Disease

Patient Assessment:

- Based on review of signs and symptoms and assessment of risk factors (Table 18–1), determine whether the patient is experiencing signs or symptoms of PUD.
- Obtain a history of prescription and over-the-counter medications and dietary supplements. Verify patient allergies and intolerances.
- Review available diagnostic tests (eg, serologic testing, urea breath test, stool antigen assay, endoscopy) to determine etiology of peptic ulcer.

Therapy Evaluation:

- If patient is already receiving pharmacotherapy, assess its efficacy, safety, and patient adherence. Are there any significant drug interactions?
- If patient has been diagnosed with a peptic ulcer, determine which course of therapy is indicated.
- Evaluate patient accessibility to medication (eg, formulary status, insurance coverage).

Care Plan Development:

- Recommend an appropriate regimen (Tables 18–2 and 18–3) that will eradicate *H pylori* and/or heal the peptic ulcer.
- Avoid drug classes to which the patient is allergic. Assess the potential for drug interactions, particularly in patients taking regimens containing metronidazole, clarithromycin, and/or cimetidine.
- If the patient has been treated for *H. pylori* previously, recommend different antibiotics if this episode is a result of treatment failure.
- Inform patients about potential adverse drug effects and drug interactions.
- Educate the patient on the importance of adherence to eradication and ulcer healing therapy.
- Identify appropriate lifestyle modifications.

Follow-Up Evaluation:

- Monitor annually for signs and symptoms of complications such as unintentional weight loss or bleeding.
- Evaluate the need for a prophylactic acid suppressive regimen in patients requiring chronic NSAID therapy.
- Assess patient adherence and progress toward efficacy and safety goals.

OUTCOME EVALUATION

- Obtain a baseline complete blood count (CBC). Recheck the CBC if the patient exhibits alarm signs or symptoms.
- Obtain a baseline serum creatinine measurement. Calculate the estimated creatinine clearance and adjust the dose of H_2RAs and sucralfate if needed.
- Obtain a history of symptoms from the patient. Monitor for improvements in pain symptoms (eg, epigastric or abdominal pain) daily.
- Monitor the patient for the development of any alarm signs and symptoms.
- Recommend a follow-up visit if signs and symptoms worsen at any time or do not improve within the defined treatment period.
- Assess for potential drug interactions whenever there is a change in the patient's medications.
- Educate the patient on the importance of adhering to the *H. pylori* eradication regimen.

- Monitor the patient for complications related to antibiotic therapy (eg, diarrhea or oral thrush) during and after completion of *H. pylori* eradication therapy.
- Recommend follow-up care if the patient's signs and symptoms do not improve after completion of *H. pylori* eradication therapy.

Abbreviations Introduced in This Chapter

COX	Cyclooxygenase
CV	Cardiovascular
DU	Duodenal ulcer
EGD	Esophagogastroduodenoscopy
GI	Gastrointestinal
GU	Gastric ulcer
H_2RA	Histamine-2 receptor antagonist
INR	International normalized ratio
MALT	Mucosa-associated lymphoid tissue
NSAID	Nonsteroidal anti-inflammatory drug
NUD	Nonulcer dyspepsia
PG	Prostaglandin
PGE_1	Prostaglandin E_1
PPI	Proton pump inhibitor
PUD	Peptic ulcer disease
SRMD	Stress-related mucosal damage
SUP	Stress ulcer prophylaxis
ZES	Zollinger–Ellison syndrome

REFERENCES

1. Banerjee S, Cash BD, Dominitz JA, et al. The role of endoscopy in the management of patients with peptic ulcer disease. Gastrointest Endosc. 2010;71:663–668.
2. Vakil N. Peptic ulcer disease. In: Feldman M, Friedman LW, Brandt L, eds. Sleisenger and Fordtran's Gastrointestinal and Liver Disease, 9th ed. Philadelphia, PA: Saunders, 2010:861–868.
3. Hunt RH, Xiao SD, Megraud F, et al. World Gastroenterology Organisation Global Guideline: *Helicobacter pylori* in developing countries. J Clin Gastroenterol. 2011;45:383–388.
4. Anand BS, Julian K. Peptic Ulcer Disease. Medscape. http://www.emedicine.medscape.com/article/181753-overview. Accessed August 5, 2014.
5. Joish VN, Donaldson G, Stockdale W, et al. The economic impact of GERD and PUD: Examination of direct and indirect costs using a large integrated employer claims database. Curr Med Res Opin. 2005;21:535–544.
6. Chan FK, Graham DY. Review article: Prevention of non-steroidal anti-inflammatory drug gastrointestinal complications—Review and recommendations based on risk assessment. Aliment Pharmacol Ther. 2004;19:1051–1061.
7. Chan FK, Lau JY. Treatment of peptic ulcer disease. In: Feldman M, Friedman LW, Brandt L, eds. Sleisenger and Fordtran's Gastrointestinal and Liver Disease, 9th ed. Philadelphia, PA: Saunders, 2010:869–886.
8. Quenot JP, Thiery N, Barbar S. When should stress ulcer prophylaxis be used in the ICU? Curr Opin Crit Care. 2009;15:139–143.
9. American Society of Health-System Pharmacists: ASHP Therapeutic Guidelines on Stress Ulcer Prophylaxis. Am J Health Syst Pharm. 1999;56:347–379.
10. Malfertheiner P, Chan F, McColl K. Peptic ulcer disease. Lancet. 2009;374:1449–1461.
11. Zhang L, Ren JW, Wong CCW, et al. Effects of cigarette smoke and its active components on ulcer formation and healing in the gastrointestinal mucosa. Curr Med Chem. 2012;19:63–69.
12. Schubert ML, Kaunitz JD. Gastric secretion. In: Feldman M, Friedman LW, Brandt L, eds. Sleisenger and Fordtran's Gastrointestinal and Liver Disease, 9th ed. Philadelphia, PA: Saunders, 2010:817–832.
13. Semrin MG, Russo MA. Anatomy, Histology, Embryology, and Developmental anomalies of the stomach and duodenum. In: Feldman M, Friedman LW, Brandt L, eds. Sleisenger and Fordtran's Gastrointestinal and Liver Disease, 9th ed. Philadelphia, PA: Saunders, 2010:773–788.
14. McColl KE. *Helicobacter pylori* infection. N Engl J Med. 2010;362:1597–1604.
15. Berardi R, Fugit R. Peptic ulcer disease. In: DiPiro JT, Talbert RL, Yee GC, et al, eds. Pharmacotherapy: A Pathophysiologic Approach, 9th ed. New York, NY: McGraw-Hill, 2014:471–495.
16. Talley NJ. American Gastroenterological Association Medical Position Statement: Evaluation of dyspepsia. Gastroenterology. 2005;129:1753–1755.
17. Chey WD, Wong BCY. American College of Gastroenterology Guideline on the Management of *Helicobacter pylori* Infection. Am J Gastroenterol. 2007;102:1808–1825.
18. Garza Gonzalez E, Perez-Perez GI, Maldonado-Garza HJ, Bosque-Padilla FJ. A Review of Helicobacter pylori diagnosis, treatment, and methods to detect eradication. World J Gastroenterol. 2014;20(6):1438–1449.
19. Anglin R, Yuan Y, Moayyedi P, et al. Risk of upper gastrointestinal bleeding with selective serotonin reuptake inhibitors with or without concurrent nonsteroidal anti-inflammatory use: a systematic review and meta-analysis. Am J Gastroenterol. 2014;109:811–819.
20. Malfertheiner P, Megraud F, O'Morain C, et al. The European Helicobacter Study Group (EHSG). Current concepts in the management of *Helicobacter pylori* infection: The Maastricht III Consensus Report. Gut. 2007;56:772–781.
21. Bertleff MJ, Lange JF. Perforated peptic ulcer disease: A review of history and treatment. Dig Surg. 2010;27:161–169.
22. Gralnek IM, Barkun AN, Bardou M. Management of acute bleeding from a peptic ulcer. N Engl J Med. 2008;359:928–937.
23. Wong TCI, Wong KT, Chiu PWY, et al. A comparison of angiographic embolization with surgery after failed endoscopic hemostasis to bleeding peptic ulcers. Gastrointest Endosc. 2011;73:900–908.
24. Ikenberry SO, Harrison ME, Lichtenstein D, et al. The role of endoscopy in dyspepsia. Gastrointest Endosc. 2007;66: 1071–1075.
25. Fuccio L, Minardi ME, Zagari RM, et al. Meta-analysis: Duration of first-line proton-pump inhibitor based triple therapy for *Helicobacter pylori* eradication. Ann Intern Med. 2007;147:553–562.
26. Peura DA, Crowe SE. *Helicobacter pylori*. In: Feldman M, Friedman LW, Brandt L, eds. Sleisenger and Fordtran's Gastrointestinal and Liver Disease, 9th ed. Philadelphia, PA: Saunders, 2010:833–844.
27. Khoshbaten M, Ghaffarifar S, Imani AJ, Shahnazi T. Effects of early oral feeding on relapse and symptoms of upper gastrointestinal bleeding in peptic ulcer disease. Dig Endosc. 2013;25:125–129.
28. Jodlowski TZ, Lam S, Ashby CR. Emerging therapies for the treatment of *Helicobacter pylori* infections. Ann Pharmacother. 2008;42:1621–1639.
29. Morgan DR, Torres J, Sexton R, et al. Risk of recurrent *Helicobacter pylori* infection 1 year after initial eradication therapy in 7 Latin American communities. JAMA. 2013;309:578–586.
30. Jafri NS, Hornung CA, Howden CW. Meta-analysis: Sequential therapy appears superior to standard therapy for *Helicobacter pylori* infection in patients naive to treatment. Ann Intern Med. 2008;148:923–931.

31. Frederico A, Gravina AG, Miranda A, et al. Eradication of *Helicobacter pylori* infection: Which regimen first? World J Gastroenterol. 2014;20(3):665–672.
32. Wu, DC, Hsu P, Wu JY, et al. Sequential and concomitant therapy with 4 drugs are equally effective for eradication of *H. pylori* infection. Clin Gastroenterol Hepatol. 2010;8(1):36–41.
33. Targownik LE, Metge CJ, Leung S, Chateau DG. The relative efficacies of gastroprotective strategies in chronic users of nonsteroidal anti-inflammatory drugs. Gastroenterology. 2008;134:937–944.
34. Chan FK, Abraham NS, Scheiman JM, et al. Management of patients on nonsteroidal anti-inflammatory drugs: A clinical practice recommendation from the first international working party on gastrointestinal and cardiovascular effects of nonsteroidal anti-inflammatory effects and anti-platelet agents. Am J Gastroenterol. 2008;103:2908–2918.
35. Grube RA, May B. Stress ulcer prophylaxis in hospitalized patients not in intensive care units. Am J Health Syst Pharm. 2007;64:1396–1400.
36. Songür Y, Balkarli A, Acartürk G, Senol A. Comparison of infusion or low-dose proton pump inhibitor treatments in upper gastrointestinal system bleeding. Eur J Intern Med. 2011;22:200–204.

19 Inflammatory Bowel Disease

Brian A. Hemstreet

LEARNING OBJECTIVES

Upon completion of the chapter, the reader will be able to:

1. Characterize the pathophysiologic mechanisms underlying inflammatory bowel disease (IBD).
2. Recognize the signs and symptoms of IBD, including major differences between ulcerative colitis (UC) and Crohn disease (CD).
3. Identify appropriate therapeutic outcomes for patients with IBD.
4. Describe pharmacologic treatment options for patients with acute or chronic symptoms of UC and CD.
5. Create a patient-specific drug treatment plan based on symptoms, severity, and location of UC or CD.
6. Recommend appropriate monitoring parameters and patient education for drug treatments for IBD.

INTRODUCTION

KEY CONCEPT *The term inflammatory bowel disease (IBD) encompasses ulcerative colitis (UC) and Crohn disease (CD). Both disorders are associated with acute and chronic inflammation of the GI tract.* Differences exist between UC and CD with regard to regions of the GI tract that may be affected and the distribution and depth of intestinal inflammation. Patients with IBD may also develop inflammation involving organs other than the GI tract, known as extraintestinal manifestations. Symptoms of IBD are associated with significant morbidity, reduction in quality of life, and costs to the health care system.[1–6]

EPIDEMIOLOGY AND ETIOLOGY

IBD is most common in Western countries such as the United States and Northern Europe. The age of initial presentation is bimodal, with patients typically diagnosed between the ages of 20 to 40 or 60 to 80 years. Approximately 1.4 million Americans have UC or CD. Up to 70,000 new cases of IBD are diagnosed in the United States each year.

Men and women are approximately equally affected by IBD in Western countries.[6] In general, whites are affected more often than blacks, and persons of Jewish descent are also at higher risk. The incidence of IBD is 10 to 40 times greater in individuals with a first-degree relative who has IBD compared with the general population.[4,5,7] A positive family history may be more of a contributing factor for development of CD than UC.[7–9]

ETIOLOGY

The exact cause of IBD is not fully understood. Genetic predisposition, dysregulation of the inflammatory response within the GI tract, and environmental or antigenic factors are thought to be involved.[3,4] The fact that a positive family history is a strong predictor of IBD supports the theory that genetic predisposition may be involved in many cases. Many potential candidate genes have been identified.

An alteration in the inflammatory response regulated by intestinal epithelial cells may also contribute to development of IBD. This may involve inappropriate processing of antigens presented to the GI epithelial cells.[3,4,10,11] The inflammatory response in IBD may be directed at bacteria that normally colonize the GI tract. Products derived from these bacteria may translocate across the mucosal layer of the GI tract and interact with various cells involved in immunologic recognition. The result is T-cell stimulation, excess production of proinflammatory cytokines, and persistent inflammation within the GI tract. Drugs such as nonsteroidal anti-inflammatory drugs (NSAIDs) that disrupt the integrity of the GI mucosa may facilitate mucosal entry of intestinal antigens and lead to IBD flares.[12]

Use of oral contraceptives has been associated with increased development of IBD in some cohort studies, but a strong causal relationship has not been proven.[6,8]

Smoking has protective effects in UC, leading to reductions in disease severity.[6] The opposite is true in CD because smoking may lead to increases in symptoms or worsening of the disease.[6,10]

PATHOPHYSIOLOGY

Ulcerative Colitis

The inflammatory response in UC is propagated by atypical type 2 helper T cells that produce proinflammatory cytokines such as interleukin (IL)-1, IL-6, and tumor necrosis factor-alfa (TNF-α).[4,9] The potential role of environmental factors in development of UC implies that the immune response is directed against an unknown antigen. The findings that development and severity of UC are reduced in patients who smoke, or in those with appendectomies, may support the theory that these factors may somehow modify either the genetic component or phenotypic response to immunologic stimuli.[3,10]

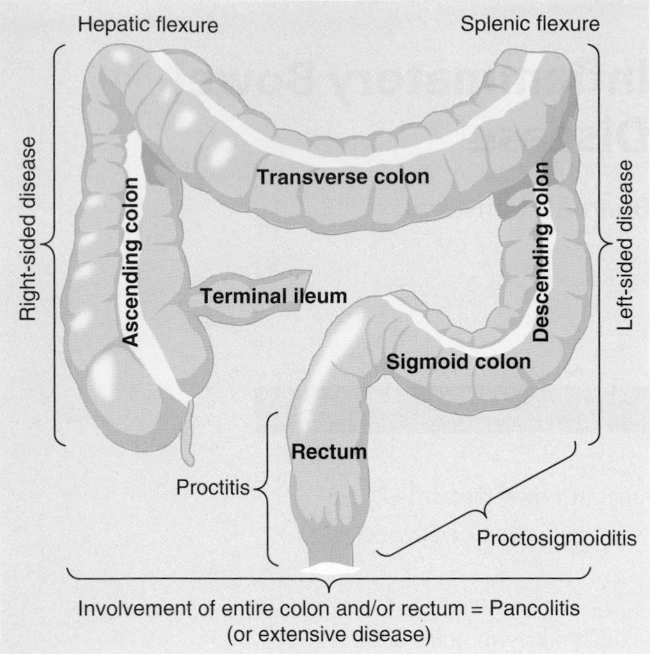

FIGURE 19–1. Major GI landmarks and disease distribution in inflammatory bowel disease.

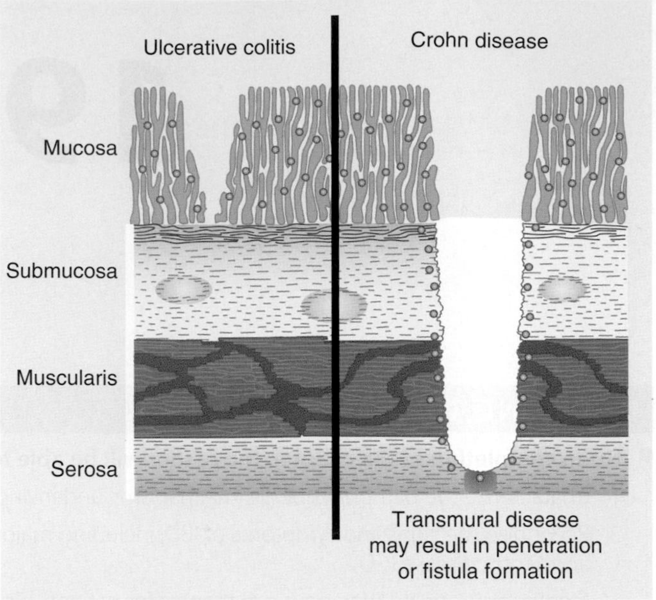

FIGURE 19–2. Depth of disease penetration in ulcerative colitis and Crohn disease.

The inflammatory process within the GI tract is limited to the colon and rectum in patients with UC (Figure 19–1). Most patients with UC have involvement of the rectum (proctitis) or both the rectum and the sigmoid colon (proctosigmoiditis). Inflammation involving the entire colon is referred to as extensive disease or pancolitis. Left-sided (distal) disease, defined as inflammation extending from the rectum to the splenic flexure, occurs in 30% to 40% of patients.[12] A small number of cases of UC involve mild inflammation of the terminal ileum, referred to as "backwash ileitis."

The pattern of inflammation in UC is continuous and confluent throughout the affected areas of the GI tract. The inflammation is superficial and does not typically extend below the submucosal layer of the GI tract (Figure 19–2). Ulceration or erosion of the GI mucosa may be present and varies with disease severity. Formation of crypt abscesses within the mucosal layers of the GI tract is characteristic of UC and may help to distinguish it from CD. Severe inflammation may also result in areas of hypertrophied GI mucosa, which may manifest as pseudopolyps within the colon.[13] The inflammatory response may progress in severity, leading to mucosal friability and significant GI bleeding.

Crohn Disease

As with UC, the immune activation seen in CD involves the release of many proinflammatory cytokines. Cytokines thought to play major roles in CD are derived from T-helper type 1 cells and include interferon-γ, TNF-α, and IL-1, IL-6, IL-8, and IL-12. TNF-α is a major contributor to the inflammatory process in CD.[10,11] Its physiologic effects include activation of macrophages, procoagulant effects in the vascular endothelium, and increased production of matrix metalloproteinases in mucosal cells.[13–15] TNF-α is also thought to induce production of nuclear factor $\kappa\beta$, which stimulates further production of TNF-α and other proinflammatory cytokines.[3,15]

In contrast to UC, the inflammation in CD may affect any part of the entire GI tract from the mouth to the anus. The small intestine is most commonly involved, and the terminal ileum and cecum are almost always affected. Approximately 20% of patients have isolated colonic involvement, whereas inflammation proximal to the small intestine is almost never seen without the presence of small or large intestinal disease.[13]

The pattern of inflammation in CD is discontinuous; areas of inflammation are intermixed with areas of normal GI mucosa, resulting in characteristic "skip lesions." Superficial aphthous ulcers may also develop in the GI mucosa. These ulcers may coalesce into larger linear ulcers, resulting in fissure formation as they increase in depth, giving rise to the characteristic "cobblestone" pattern observed upon examination of the mucosa.

The inflammation may be transmural, penetrating to the muscularis or serosal layers of the GI tract (Figure 19–2). This propensity for transmural involvement may lead to serious complications such as strictures, fistulae, abscesses, and perforation.[13] Although rectal inflammation is typically less common in CD than UC, several types of perianal lesions may be observed including skin tags, hemorrhoids, fissures, anal ulcers, abscesses, and fistulae.[14]

CLINICAL PRESENTATION AND DIAGNOSIS

KEY CONCEPT *Differentiation between UC and CD is based on signs and symptoms as well as characteristic endoscopic findings, including the extent, pattern, and depth of inflammation.* See accompanying box for the clinical presentation of IBD.

Extraintestinal Manifestations and Complications of IBD

KEY CONCEPT *Patients may manifest signs and symptoms of disease in areas outside the GI tract (extraintestinal manifestations).*[5,13] Painful joint complications associated with IBD include sacroiliitis and ankylosing spondylitis. Ocular involvement with episcleritis, uveitis, or iritis may manifest as blurred vision, eye pain, and photophobia. Associated skin findings include pyoderma gangrenosum (papules and vesicles that develop into painful ulcerations) and erythema nodosum (red nodules of varying size typically found on the lower extremities). Nephrolithiasis may

Clinical Presentation of IBD

General

- Patients with UC or CD may present with similar symptoms.
- The onset may be insidious and subacute.
- Some patients present with extraintestinal manifestations before GI symptoms occur.
- It may be impossible to distinguish between UC and CD in approximately 10% of cases. These patients are described as having "indeterminate colitis."

Symptoms

- *Ulcerative colitis*: Diarrhea (bloody, watery, or mucopurulent), rectal bleeding, abdominal pain/cramping, weight loss and malnutrition, tenesmus, constipation (with proctitis)
- *Crohn disease*: Diarrhea (less bloody than UC), rectal bleeding (less than UC), abdominal pain/cramping, weight loss and malnutrition (more common than UC), fatigue/malaise

Signs

- *Ulcerative colitis*: Fever, tachycardia (with severe disease), dehydration, arthritis, hemorrhoids, anal fissures, perirectal abscesses
- *Crohn disease:* Fever, tachycardia (with severe disease), dehydration, arthritis, abdominal mass and tenderness, perianal fissure or fistula

Laboratory Tests

- *Ulcerative colitis*: Leukocytosis, decreased hematocrit/hemoglobin, elevated erythrocyte sedimentation rate (ESR) or C-reactive protein (CRP), positive test for fecal occult blood, (+) perinuclear antineutrophil cytoplasmic antibodies (pANCA; up to 70% of patients)
- *Crohn disease*: Leukocytosis, decreased hematocrit/hemoglobin, elevated ESR or CRP, positive test for fecal occult blood, (+) anti–*Saccharomyces cerevisiae* antibodies (up to 50% of patients), hypoalbuminemia with severe disease

also develop at a higher rate in patients with IBD. Oxalate stones are more common in CD, and uric acid-containing stones are more common in UC.[13]

Liver and biliary manifestations of IBD include increased incidence of gallstone formation in patients with CD and development of sclerosing cholangitis or cholangiocarcinoma in patients with UC. Patients with UC are at increased risk for developing colorectal cancer and should undergo periodic cancer screening. Ongoing inflammation due to active IBD may induce a hypercoagulable state, resulting in higher rates of both arterial and venous thromboembolism, including deep vein thrombosis and pulmonary embolism. Likewise, inflammation and recurrent blood loss may result in chronic anemia. Patients with IBD also have higher rates of osteopenia, osteoporosis, and fractures, which are most strongly associated with use of corticosteroids.[16]

A serious complication of UC is toxic megacolon, defined as dilation of the transverse colon greater than 6 cm (2.4 in). Patients with toxic megacolon typically manifest systemic signs of severe inflammation such as fever, tachycardia, and abdominal distention.[3,13] Surgical intervention, including colonic resection, may be necessary to acutely manage toxic megacolon.

Patients with CD may develop significant weight loss or nutritional deficiencies secondary to malabsorption of nutrients in the small intestine, or as a consequence of multiple small- or large-bowel resections. Common nutritional deficiencies in IBD include vitamin B_{12}, fat-soluble vitamins, zinc, folate, and iron. Malabsorption in children with CD may contribute to significant reductions in growth and development.

Diagnosis

Because patients often present with nonspecific GI symptoms, initial diagnostic evaluation includes methods to characterize the disease and rule out other potential etiologies. This may include stool cultures to examine for infectious causes of diarrhea.

Endoscopic approaches are typically used and may include colonoscopy, proctosigmoidoscopy, or possibly upper GI endoscopy in patients with suspected CD. Endoscopy is useful for determining the disease distribution, pattern and depth of inflammation, and to obtain mucosal biopsy specimens. Supplemental information from imaging procedures, such as computed tomography, abdominal x-ray, abdominal ultrasound, or intestinal barium studies may provide evidence of complications such as obstruction, abscess, perforation, or colonic dilation.[9]

The information derived from diagnostic testing and the patient's medical history and symptoms are used to gauge disease severity. The severity of active UC is generally classified as mild, moderate, severe, or fulminant.[1] Mild UC typically involves up to four bloody or watery stools per day without systemic signs of toxicity or elevation of erythrocyte sedimentation rate (ESR). Moderate disease is classified as more than four stools per day with evidence of systemic toxicity. Severe disease is considered more than six stools per day and evidence of anemia, tachycardia, or an elevated ESR or C-reactive protein (CRP). Lastly, fulminant UC may present as more than 10 stools per day with continuous bleeding, signs of systemic toxicity, abdominal distention or tenderness, colonic dilation, or a requirement for blood transfusion.

A similar classification scheme is used to gauge the severity of active CD.[2] Patients with mild to moderate CD are typically ambulatory and have no evidence of dehydration; systemic toxicity; loss of body weight; or abdominal tenderness, mass, or obstruction. Moderate to severe disease is considered in patients who fail to respond to treatment for mild to moderate disease or those with fever, weight loss, abdominal pain or tenderness, vomiting, intestinal obstruction, or significant anemia. Severe to fulminant CD is classified as the presence of persistent symptoms or evidence of systemic toxicity despite outpatient corticosteroid treatment, or the presence of cachexia, rebound tenderness, intestinal obstruction, or abscess.

TREATMENT

Desired Outcomes

Treatment goals for IBD involve both management of active disease and prevention of disease relapse. KEY CONCEPT *Major treatment goals include alleviation of signs and symptoms and suppression of inflammation during acute episodes and maintenance of remission thereafter*. Addressing active IBD in a timely and appropriate manner may prevent major complications and reduce the need for hospitalization or surgical intervention.

Once control of active disease is obtained, treatment regimens are designed to achieve these long-term goals: (a) maintain remission and prevent disease relapse, (b) improve the patient's quality of life, (c) prevent the need for surgical intervention or hospitalization, (d) manage extraintestinal manifestations, (e) prevent malnutrition, and (f) prevent treatment-associated adverse effects.

General Approach to Treatment

Pharmacologic interventions for IBD are designed to target the underlying inflammatory response. KEY CONCEPT *When designing a drug regimen for treatment of IBD, several factors should be considered, including the patient's symptoms; medical history; current medication use; drug allergies; and extent, location, and severity of disease*. The history may also help identify a family history of IBD or potential exacerbating factors, such as tobacco or NSAID use.

Nonpharmacologic Therapy

No specific dietary restrictions are recommended for patients with IBD, but avoidance of high-residue foods in patients with strictures may help prevent obstruction. Avoidance of excess dietary fat may also be preferred. Nutritional strategies in patients with long-standing IBD may include use of vitamin and mineral supplementation. Administration of vitamin B_{12}, folic acid, fat-soluble vitamins, and iron may be needed to prevent or treat deficiencies. In severe cases, enteral or parenteral nutrition may be needed to achieve adequate caloric intake.

Patients with IBD, particularly those with CD, are also at risk for bone loss. This may be a function of malabsorption of vitamin D or repeated courses of corticosteroids.[16] Risk factors for osteoporosis should be determined, and baseline bone density measurement may be considered.[16] Vitamin D and calcium supplementation should be used in all patients receiving long-term corticosteroids. Oral bisphosphonate therapy may also be considered in patients receiving prolonged courses of corticosteroids or in those with osteopenia or osteoporosis.

Surgical intervention is an option in patients with complications such as fistulae or abscesses, or in patients with medically refractory disease. UC is curable with performance of a total colectomy; patients with UC may opt to have a colectomy to reduce the chance of developing colorectal cancer. Patients with CD may have affected areas of intestine resected. Unfortunately, CD may recur following surgical resection. Repeated surgeries in CD may lead to significant malabsorption of nutrients and drugs consistent with development of short-bowel syndrome.

Pharmacologic Therapy

Several pharmacologic classes are available for acute treatment and maintenance therapy of IBD. Selection of an initial agent for patients with active IBD should be designed to deliver maximum efficacy while minimizing toxicity. Response rates to individual classes of medications for both UC and CD are discussed within the specific treatment section for each disease.

▸ *Symptomatic Interventions*

Patients with active IBD often have severe abdominal pain and diarrhea. Medications used to manage these symptoms may have adverse consequences. Ⓚ *Antidiarrheal medications that reduce GI motility such as loperamide, diphenoxylate/atropine, and codeine should be avoided in patients with active IBD due to the risk of precipitating acute colonic dilation (toxic megacolon).*[13] Drugs with anticholinergic properties, such as hyoscyamine and dicyclomine, are often used to treat intestinal spasm and pain, but these drugs may also reduce GI motility and should generally be avoided in active IBD.

Patients who have had multiple intestinal resections due to CD may have diarrhea related to the inability to reabsorb bile salts. Cholestyramine may improve diarrheal symptoms in this population.[14] NSAIDs should be avoided for pain management because they can worsen IBD symptoms. Opioid analgesics should be used with caution because they may significantly reduce GI motility.

▸ *Aminosalicylates*

The aminosalicylates are among the most commonly used drugs for inducing and maintaining remission in patients with mild to moderate IBD (Table 19–1). These drugs are designed to deliver 5-aminosalicylate (5-ASA, mesalamine) to areas of inflammation within the GI tract. The mechanism of mesalamine is not fully understood, but it appears to have favorable anti-inflammatory effects. The delivery of mesalamine to the affected sites is accomplished by either linking mesalamine to a carrier molecule or altering the formulation to release drug in response to changes in intestinal pH. Topical suppositories and enemas are designed to deliver mesalamine directly to the distal colon and rectum.[7,17–20]

The prototypical aminosalicylate is sulfasalazine, which chemically is mesalamine linked by a diazo bond to the carrier molecule sulfapyridine. This linkage prevents premature absorption of mesalamine in the small intestine. Once sulfasalazine is delivered to the colon, bacterial degradation of the diazo bond frees mesalamine from sulfapyridine. Sulfapyridine is then absorbed and excreted renally while mesalamine acts locally within the GI tract.

Newer mesalamine products utilize nonsulfapyridine methods for drug delivery. Olsalazine consists of two mesalamine molecules linked together, whereas balsalazide uses the inert carrier molecule 4-aminobenzoyl-β-alanine. Both drugs use a diazo bond similar to sulfasalazine. Lialda is a proprietary multimatrix (MMX) mesalamine formulation with a pH-sensitive coat that releases in the terminal ileum, allowing for once-daily dosing.[17]

Patient Encounter 1

A 28-year-old woman presents to the clinic for treatment of UC. A prior colonoscopy revealed disease in the descending colon and rectum. She reports two to four loose stools per day 2 to 3 days per week with intermittent blood and abdominal pain. Her medical provider has determined this episode to be of mild to moderate severity. It is interfering with her daily activities and ability to work and socialize. Her medical history is significant for seasonal allergies. She takes Yaz, loratadine, and naproxen as needed. She reports one-half pack per day tobacco use and social intake of alcohol. She has an allergy to penicillin (hives).

How would you determine what treatment options are most appropriate for this patient?

How would you educate this patient on the appropriate use of her recommended drug therapy for IBD?

Table 19–1

Aminosalicylates for Treatment of IBD

Drug	Trade Names	Formulation	Strengths	Daily Dosage Range (g)	Site of Action
Sulfasalazine	Azulfidine Azulfidine En-tabs	Immediate-release or enteric-coated tablets	500 mg	2–6	Colon
	Sulfazine Sulfazine EC	Suspension	250 mg/5mL		
Mesalamine	Rowasa	Enema	4 g/60 mL	4	Distal left colon and rectum
	Asacol Asacol-HD	Delayed-release resin tablet	400 mg, 800 mg	1.6–4.8	Distal ileum and colon
	Canasa	Rectal suppository	1000 mg	1	Rectum
	Pentasa	Microgranule controlled-release capsule	250 mg	2–4	Small bowel
			500 mg	2–4	Colon
	Lialda	MMX formulated pH-dependent polymer film coated tablet	1.2 g	1.2–4.8	Terminal ileum and colon
	Apriso	Enteric-coated granules in polymer matrix	375 mg	1.5	Colon
Olsalazine	Dipentum	Delayed-release capsule	250 mg	1–3	Colon
Balsalazide	Colazal	Delayed-release capsule	750 mg	2–6.75	Colon
	Giazo	Tablet	1.1 g	2.2–6.6	Colon

MMX, multimatrix.

Apriso contains enteric-coated mesalamine granules also with a polymer matrix for extended release that can be given once daily.

Sulfasalazine is associated with various adverse effects, most of which are thought to be due to the sulfapyridine component. Common dose-related adverse effects include headache, dyspepsia, nausea, vomiting, and fatigue.[20–22] Idiosyncratic effects include bone marrow suppression, reduction in sperm counts in males, hepatitis, and pulmonitis. Hypersensitivity reactions may occur in patients allergic to sulfonamide-containing medications.

Nonsulfapyridine-based aminosalicylates are better tolerated than sulfasalazine. Although the types of adverse effects are similar, they occur much less frequently. However, olsalazine is associated with a higher incidence of secretory diarrhea than other aminosalicylates. These agents can be used safely in patients with a reported sulfonamide allergy, but they are more expensive than generic sulfasalazine.

▶ *Corticosteroids*

Corticosteroids have potent anti-inflammatory properties and are used in active IBD to suppress inflammation rapidly. They may be administered systemically or delivered locally to the site of action (Table 19–2). Corticosteroids usually improve symptoms and disease severity rapidly, but use should be restricted to short-term management of active disease. Long-term systemic corticosteroid use is associated with significant adverse effects, including cataracts, skin atrophy, hypertension, hyperglycemia, adrenal suppression, osteoporosis, increased risk of infection, and delayed growth in children, among others.[20–22]

Budesonide is a high-potency glucocorticoid used in IBD that has low systemic bioavailability when administered orally.[23,24] Oral formulations may release in either the terminal ileum or colon. Compared to traditional corticosteroids, budesonide may reduce long-term adverse effects and can be used for induction therapy.[22–24]

▶ *Immunosuppressants*

Agents targeting the immune response or cytokines involved in IBD are potential treatment options (Table 19–3). Azathioprine and its active metabolite 6-mercaptopurine (6-MP) inhibit purine biosynthesis and reduce IBD-associated GI inflammation. They are most useful for maintaining remission of IBD or reducing the need for long-term use of corticosteroids.[22,24,25–27] Use in active disease is limited by their slow onset of action, which may be as long as 3 to 12 months. Adverse effects associated with azathioprine and 6-MP include hypersensitivity reactions resulting in pancreatitis, fever, rash, hepatitis, and leukopenia.[21,22,25] Patients should be tested for activity of thiopurine methyltransferase (TPMT), the major enzyme responsible for metabolism of azathioprine prior to use. Deficiency or reduced activity of

Table 19–2

Corticosteroids for Treatment of IBD

Drug	Trade Names	Daily Dose
Prednisone	Generic	20–60 mg orally
Prednisolone	Generic	20–60 mg orally
Budesonide	Entocort EC	Induction: 9 mg orally Maintenance: 6 mg orally up to 12 weeks
	Uceris	9 mg daily for up to 8 weeks
Methylprednisolone	Medrol (orally) Solu-Medrol (IV)	15–60 mg orally or IV
Hydrocortisone	Solu-Cortef	300 mg IV in three divided doses
	Cortenema	100 mg rectally at bedtime
	Cortifoam	90 mg rectally once or twice daily
	Anusol-HC	25–50 mg rectally twice daily
	Proctocort	30 mg rectally twice daily

Table 19–3

Immunosuppressant and Biologic Agents for Treatment of IBD

Drug	Trade Name(s)	Dose
Azathioprine	Imuran, Azasan	1.5–2.5 mg/kg/day orally
6-Mercaptopurine	Purinethol, Purixan	1.5–2.5 mg/kg/day orally
Methotrexate	Trexall	15–25 mg weekly (IM/SC/orally)
Cyclosporine	Sandimmune	4 mg/kg/day IV continuous infusion
Infliximab	Remicade	Induction: 5 mg/kg IV at 0, 2, and 6 weeks; 10 mg/kg per dose IV for nonresponders Maintenance: 5 mg/kg IV every 8 weeks
Adalimumab	Humira	Induction: 160 mg SC day 1 (given as four 40-mg injections in 1 day or as two 40-mg injections per day for 2 consecutive days), then 80 mg SC 2 weeks later (day 15) Maintenance: 40 mg SC every other week, starting on day 29 of therapy
Certolizumab	Cimzia	Induction: 400 mg SC initially, then 400 mg SC at 2 and 4 weeks Maintenance: 400 mg SC every 4 weeks if initial response
Golimumab	Simponi	200 mg SC at week 0 and 2; then every 4 weeks
Natalizumab	Tysabri	Induction/maintenance: 300 mg IV every 4 weeks; discontinue by 12 weeks if no response or if unable to withdraw steroids within 6 months
Vedolizumab	Entyvio	300 mg IV at weeks 0, 2, and 6; then every 8 weeks; discontinue if no response at 14 weeks

IM, intramuscular; IV, intravenously; SC, subcutaneously.

TPMT may result in toxicity from azathioprine and 6-MP and may require dose reductions.

Methotrexate is a folate antagonist used primarily for maintaining remission of CD. It may be administered orally, subcutaneously, or IV and may have a steroid-sparing effect in patients with steroid-dependent disease.[6,22,26,27] Long-term methotrexate use may result in serious adverse effects, including hepatotoxicity, pulmonary fibrosis, and bone marrow suppression.

Cyclosporine is a cyclic polypeptide immunosuppressant typically used to prevent organ rejection in transplant patients. Its use in IBD is restricted to patients with fulminant or refractory symptoms in patients with active disease. Significant toxicities associated with cyclosporine are nephrotoxicity, risk of infection, seizures, hypertension, and liver function test abnormalities.[1,22]

► *Biologic Agents*

Several biologic agents targeting TNF-α are used for treatment of IBD (Table 19–3). Reduction in TNF-α activity is associated with improvement in the underlying inflammatory process. Infliximab is a chimeric anti-TNF-α agent (ie, 75% human, 25% mouse), certolizumab is a pegylated antibody fragment, and both adalimumab and golimumab are humanized anti-TNF-α antibodies.

Disadvantages of anti-TNF biologic therapy include the need for parenteral administration, significant drug cost, and the potential for serious adverse effects. Adalimumab, golimumab, and certolizumab are administered subcutaneously, whereas infliximab requires intravenous (IV) infusion. Adverse effects of IV infliximab may include infusion-related reactions such as fever, chest pain, hypotension, and dyspnea. Antibodies may develop to infliximab over time that may reduce its efficacy and predispose patients to development of infusion-related adverse effects.

All TNF-α inhibitors have been associated with reactivation of serious infections, particularly intracellular pathogens such as tuberculosis, as well as hepatitis B.[15,21] Biologic agents should not be used in patients with existing infections, and patients should be screened for latent tuberculosis and viral hepatitis prior to initiating therapy. Exacerbation of heart failure is also a potential adverse effect, so these agents should be avoided in patients with advanced or decompensated heart failure.[15,20,21] Anti-TNF-α agents also carry a risk of developing lymphoma, including a rare form known as hepatosplenic T-cell lymphoma. The risk appears to be highest in younger male patients and those using concomitant azathioprine or 6-MP.[26–28]

Natalizumab and vedolizumab are humanized monoclonal antibodies that antagonize integrin heterodimers, prevent α_4-mediated leukocyte adhesion to adhesion molecules, and prevent migration across the endothelium.[29–31] Natalizumab is associated with development of progressive multifocal leukoencephalopathy (PML). Vedolizumab carries a theoretical risk of PML, but this has not been reported to date. Use of natalizumab and vedolizumab is restricted to patients with who have failed all other therapies, including anti TNF-α *agents*.

► *Other Agents*

Antibiotics have been used in IBD based on the rationale that they may interrupt the inflammatory response directed against endogenous bacterial flora. Metronidazole and ciprofloxacin have been the two most widely studied agents.[1,2,32] Metronidazole may benefit some patients with pouchitis (inflammation of surgically created intestinal pouches) and patients with CD who have had ileal resection or have perianal fistulas. Ciprofloxacin has shown some efficacy in refractory active CD and may be used in combination with metronidazole. Long-term metronidazole use is associated with development of peripheral neuropathy.

Because smoking is associated with reduced UC symptoms, transdermal nicotine has been studied as a potential treatment option. Improvement in mild to moderate UC symptoms may be seen and may be more evident in patients who are ex-smokers.[1,33] Daily doses between 15 and 25 mg appear to be most effective.

Probiotics such as *Lactobacillus acidophilus* or *Bifidobacterium* have been used with the rationale that modification of host flora may alter the inflammatory response. There are minimal data to support use of probiotics in CD.[2] In patients with UC, the probiotic preparation VSL#3 demonstrated efficacy in reducing recurrence of pouchitis in patients with ileal pouch anal anastomosis and may prevent relapse in mild to moderate disease.[1,34]

Treatment of UC

Drug and dosing guidelines based on disease severity and location are presented in Table 19–4. See Figure 19–3 for a treatment algorithm for mild, moderate, severe, and fulminant UC.

► *Mild to Moderate Active UC*

KEY CONCEPT *Treatment of acute episodes of UC is dictated by the severity and extent of disease. First-line therapy of mild to moderate disease involves oral or topical aminosalicylate derivatives or oral budesonide.* Topical mesalamine is superior to both topical corticosteroids and oral aminosalicylates for inducing remission in active mild to moderate UC.[1,35–37] Enemas are appropriate for patients with left-sided disease because the medication will reach the splenic flexure. Suppositories deliver mesalamine up to approximately 20 cm and are most appropriate for treating proctitis.[6,7,35] Oral and topical mesalamine preparations may be used together for maximal effect. Oral mesalamine may also be used for patients who are unwilling or unable to use topical preparations.[35–37]

Topical corticosteroids are usually reserved for patients who do not respond to topical mesalamine.[1,22] Patients should be properly educated regarding appropriate use of topical products, including proper administration and adequate retention in order to maximize efficacy. Oral budesonide may be used as either an alternative or add-on to aminosalicylates in patients with active UC.[24]

For patients with disease extending proximal to the splenic flexure, oral sulfasalazine or any of the oral mesalamine products are considered first-line therapy.[1,6] Doses should provide 4 to 6 g of sulfasalazine or 2.4 g of mesalamine or equivalent.[6] Use of the once-daily formulations may improve patient adherence.[17] Induction of remission may require 4 to 8 weeks of therapy at appropriate treatment doses.

► *Moderate to Severe Active UC*

In moderate to severe UC oral corticosteroids may be used for short-term treatment of patients who are unresponsive to sulfasalazine or mesalamine. Prednisone doses of 40 to 60 mg/day (or equivalent) are recommended.[1,22] Infliximab, adalimumab, and golimumab are effective for patients with moderate to severe disease who are unresponsive to oral therapies. Azathioprine or 6-MP is used for patients unresponsive to corticosteroids or those who become steroid dependent and may be combined with infliximab for increased effectiveness.[37,38] Vedolizumab is generally reserved for patients who fail oral therapies and anti TNF-α agents.[30]

► *Severe or Fulminant UC*

Patients with severe UC symptoms require hospitalization. If the patient is unresponsive to mesalamine and oral corticosteroids, a course of IV corticosteroids should be initiated.[1]

Table 19–4

Treatment Recommendations for UC

Disease Severity and Location	Active Disease	Maintenance of Remission
Mild Disease		
Proctitis	Mesalamine suppository 1 g rectally daily	May reduce suppository frequency to 1 g three times per week
Left-sided disease	Mesalamine enema 1 g rectally daily, *or* Mesalamine 2.4–4.8 g/day or sulfasalazine 4–6 g/day orally	May reduce enema frequency to 1 g every other day, *or* taper to mesalamine 1.6–2.4 g/day or sulfasalazine 2–4 g/day orally
Extensive disease	Mesalamine 2.4–4.8 g/day or sulfasalazine 4–6 g/day orally or Budesonide 9 mg orally once daily	Taper to mesalamine 1.6–2.4 g/day or sulfasalazine 2–4 g/day orally May continue for 8 weeks
Moderate Disease		
Proctitis	Mesalamine suppository 1 g rectally daily; If no response to mesalamine: • Prednisone 40–60 mg/day orally	May reduce suppository frequency to 1 g three times per week; taper prednisone as soon as possible; Consider adding azathioprine or 6-MP 1.5–2.5 mg/kg/day orally
Left-sided disease	Mesalamine enema 1 g rectally at bedtime daily, *or* mesalamine 2.4–4.8 g/day or sulfasalazine 4–6 g/day orally May combine enema and oral therapies	May reduce enema frequency to 1 g three times per week if symptoms permit May reduce dose of oral agents if symptoms permit; consider adding azathioprine or 6-MP 1.5–2.5 mg/kg/day orally
Extensive disease	Mesalamine 2.4–4.8 g/day or sulfasalazine 4–6 g/day orally; or Budesonide 9 mg orally once daily If no response to mesalamine or sulfasalazine: • Prednisone 40–60 mg/day orally; *or* • Infliximab 5 mg/kg IV at weeks 0, 2, and 6 or Adalimumab or golimumab per dosing above	Taper mesalamine to 1.6–2.4 g/day or sulfasalazine 2–4 g/day orally; May continue for 8 weeks If prednisone or infliximab were required: • Taper prednisone as soon as possible; • Give infliximab 5 mg/kg IV every 8 weeks or adalimumab every 2 weeks or golimumab every 4 weeks Consider adding azathioprine or 6-MP 1.5–2.5 mg/kg/day orally
Severe or Fulminant Disease	Hydrocortisone 300 mg IV daily (or equivalent) × 7 days, *or* Infliximab 5 mg/kg IV at weeks 0, 2, and 6 or adalimumab *or* golimumab If no response to IV corticosteroids or infliximab: • Cyclosporine 4 mg/kg/day IV	Change to oral corticosteroid and taper as soon as possible Restart oral mesalamine or sulfasalazine May continue infliximab at maintenance doses of 5 mg/kg every 8 weeks, adalimumab every 2 weeks, golimumab every 4 weeks

6-MP, 6-mercaptopurine.

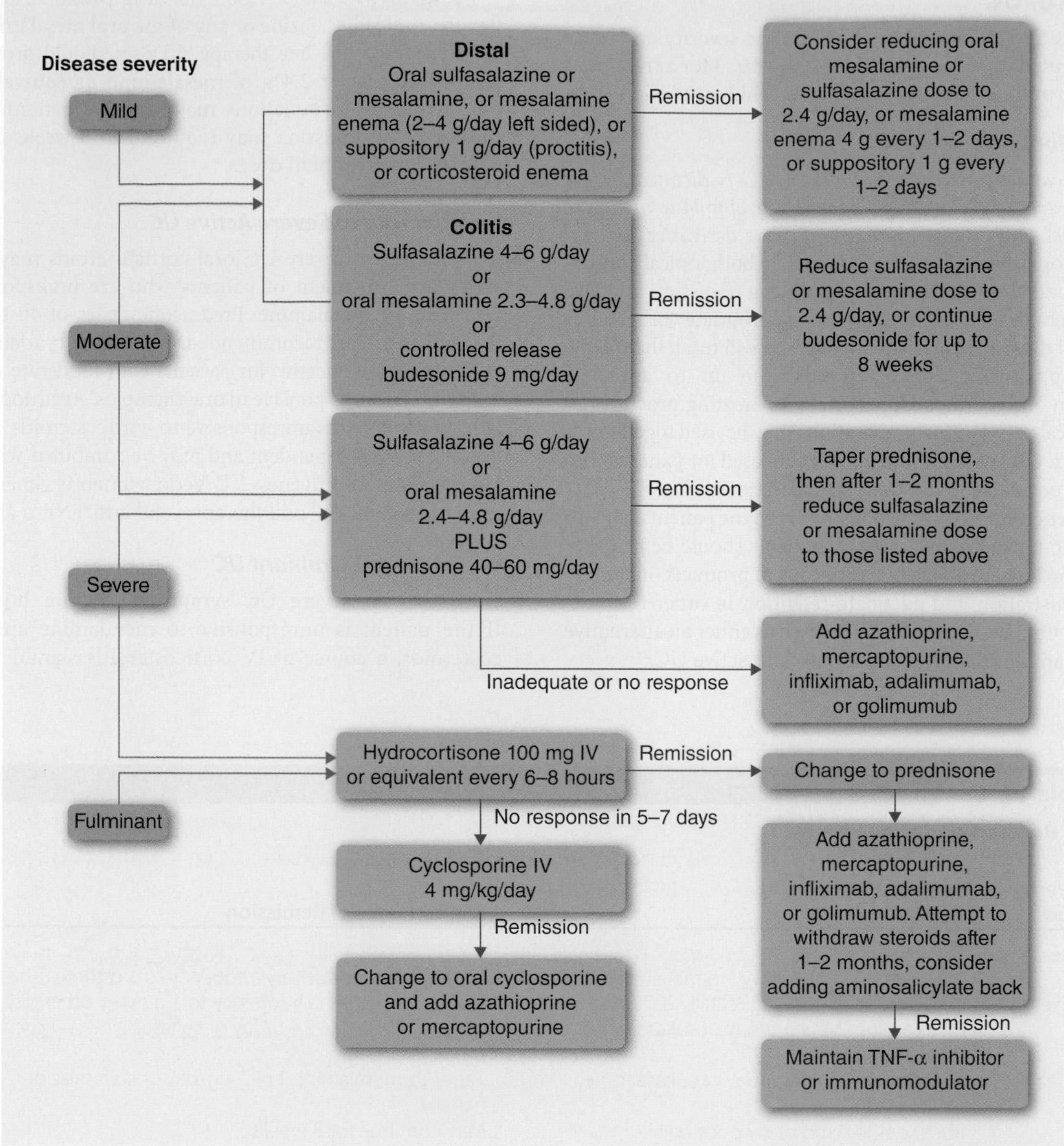

FIGURE 19–3. Treatment approaches for ulcerative colitis. (Adapted from Hemstreet BA. Inflammatory bowel disease. In: DiPiro JT, Talbert RL, Yee GC, et al., eds. Pharmacotherapy: A Pathophysiologic Approach, 9th ed. New York, NY: McGraw-Hill, 2014 with permission. www.accesspharmacy.com.)

Hydrocortisone 300 mg/day IV given in three divided doses or methylprednisolone 60 mg IV once daily for 7 to 10 days are recommended.[1,22] Infliximab and adalimumab are also options for severe UC. Cyclosporine 2 to 4 mg/kg/day given as a continuous IV infusion should be reserved for patients unresponsive to 7 to 10 days of IV corticosteroid therapy.

Patients with fulminant disease are treated similarly, although infliximab, adalimumab, and golimumab are not indicated for this situation. Patients with fulminant UC should be assessed for signs of significant systemic toxicity or colonic dilation, which may require surgical intervention.

► *Maintenance of Remission in UC*

Unfortunately, up to 50% of patients receiving oral therapies and up to 70% of untreated patients relapse within 1 year after achieving remission.[37] For this reason, patients may require maintenance drug therapy indefinitely to preserve remission.

KEY CONCEPT *Maintenance of remission of UC may be achieved with oral or topical aminosalicylates.* In patients with proctitis, mesalamine suppositories 1 g daily may prevent relapse in up to 90% of patients.[1,7,35] Mesalamine enemas are appropriate for left-sided disease and may often be dosed two to three times weekly. Oral mesalamine at lower doses (eg, 1.2–1.6 g/day) may be combined with topical therapies to maintain remission.

Oral sulfasalazine or mesalamine is effective in maintaining remission in patients with more extensive disease.[1,6] Lower daily doses (eg, 2–4 g sulfasalazine or 2–2.4 g mesalamine) may be used for disease maintenance. Oral or topical corticosteroids are not effective for maintaining remission and should be avoided due to the high incidence of adverse effects.

Patient Encounter 2, Part 1

A 32-year-old Hispanic man presents to the gastroenterology clinic for a 1-month follow-up for treatment of CD with complaints of crampy abdominal pain and two to three loose stools 3 to 4 days per week. He reports intermittent nausea and states that "these pills aren't working." He denies vomiting, fever, or chills, and has been using nonprescription loperamide intermittently to treat his diarrhea.

What other pertinent information from the history would be beneficial regarding his current treatment?

How would you classify the severity of this patient's IBD based on the information presented?

What additional information would you obtain prior to recommending drug therapy?

KEY CONCEPT *Immunosuppressants such as azathioprine, 6-MP, infliximab, adalimumab, and golimumab can be used to maintain UC remission in unresponsive patients or those who develop corticosteroid dependency.* Intermittent infliximab, adalimumab, or golimumab dosing may be used to maintain remission and reduce the need for corticosteroids in patients with moderate to severe UC. Combining azathioprine and infliximab may be more effective initially, and patients may be able to be transitioned to azathioprine monotherapy. Vedolizumab may be used last line if indicated if patients had a favorable response to induction therapy.[30] Colectomy is an option for patients with progressive disease who cannot be maintained on drug therapy alone.

▶ Treatment of CD

Drug and dosing guidelines based on disease severity and location are presented in Table 19–5. See Figure 19–4 for a treatment algorithm for mild, moderate, severe, and fulminant CD.

▶ Mild to Moderate Active CD

KEY CONCEPT *Induction of remission of mild to moderate active CD may be accomplished with oral budesonide or possibly aminosalicylates.* Budesonide 9 mg orally once daily for up to 8 weeks may be used for mild to moderate active CD in patients with involvement of the terminal ileum or ascending colon, with success expected in 50% to 69% of patients.[3,22,23,39] Because the formulation releases budesonide in the terminal ileum, it is not effective in reaching sites distal to the ascending colon.[23,39] Conventional oral corticosteroids such as prednisone and methylprednisolone may also be used and may be slightly more effective than budesonide for inducing remission, but they carry a higher risk of adverse effects.[6]

Sulfasalazine or mesalamine products have demonstrated minimal efficacy but may be tried in patients with ileal, ileocolonic, or colonic CD due to their more favorable adverse effect profile when compared to corticosteroids.[2,3,39] Induction of remission may require up to 16 weeks of treatment at full doses.[39]

Metronidazole or ciprofloxacin can be used in patients who do not respond to budesonide or oral aminosalicylates. Response rates of up to 50% are reported, but data are conflicting, and these agents should generally not be considered first-line therapy.[2,3,32,39]

▶ Moderate to Severe Active CD

Patients with moderate to severe active CD may be treated with oral corticosteroids (eg, prednisone 40–60 mg daily). Budesonide

Table 19–5

Treatment Recommendations for CD

Disease Location and Severity	Active Disease	Maintenance of Remission
Mild Disease		
Ileal or ileocolonic	Mesalamine 3.2–4.8 g/day or sulfasalazine 4–6 g/day orally	Taper mesalamine 1.6–2.4 g/day or sulfasalazine 2–4 g/day orally
Ileal ± ascending colon	Budesonide 9 mg daily orally for up to 8 weeks	Taper budesonide to 6 mg daily for up to 3 months
Perianal	Mesalamine 2.4–4.8 g/day or sulfasalazine 4–6 g/day orally May add metronidazole 10–20 mg/kg/day or ciprofloxacin 1 g daily	Taper mesalamine to 1.6–2.4 g/day or sulfasalazine 2–4 g/day orally
Moderate Disease	Same treatment as for mild disease but may consider: • Infliximab *or* adalimumab *or* certolizumab (see Table 19–3 for dosage regimens) *or* • Prednisone 40–60 mg/day orally, *or* • Budesonide 9 mg/day orally for up to 8 weeks • Consider natalizumab or vedolizumab if no response to prior therapies If fistulizing disease, consider: • Infliximab, adalimumab, or certolizumab pegol	Continue aminosalicylate at maintenance dose; If loss of response to infliximab, consider adalimumab Taper prednisone as soon as possible; Taper budesonide to 6 mg daily for 3 months Consider adding azathioprine or 6-MP 1.5–2.5 mg/kg/day orally or methotrexate 12.5–25 mg orally or IM/SC once weekly Consider natalizumab or vedolizumab if no response to previous therapies
Severe or Fulminant Disease	Hydrocortisone 300 mg IV daily (or equivalent) × 7 days, *or* Infliximab (severe or fistulizing disease) 5 mg/kg IV at 0, 2, and 6 weeks • Adalimumab or certolizumab *or* • Consider natalizumab or vedolizumab if no response to prior therapies Consider cyclosporine 4 mg/kg/day for refractory disease	Taper corticosteroid as soon as possible May continue infliximab, adalimumab, certolizumab, or natalizumab (see Table 19–3 for dosage regimens) Consider adding azathioprine or 6-MP 1.5–2.5 mg/kg/day orally or methotrexate 12.5–25 mg orally or IM/SC weekly

6-MP, 6-mercaptopurine; IM, intramuscular; SC, subcutaneous.

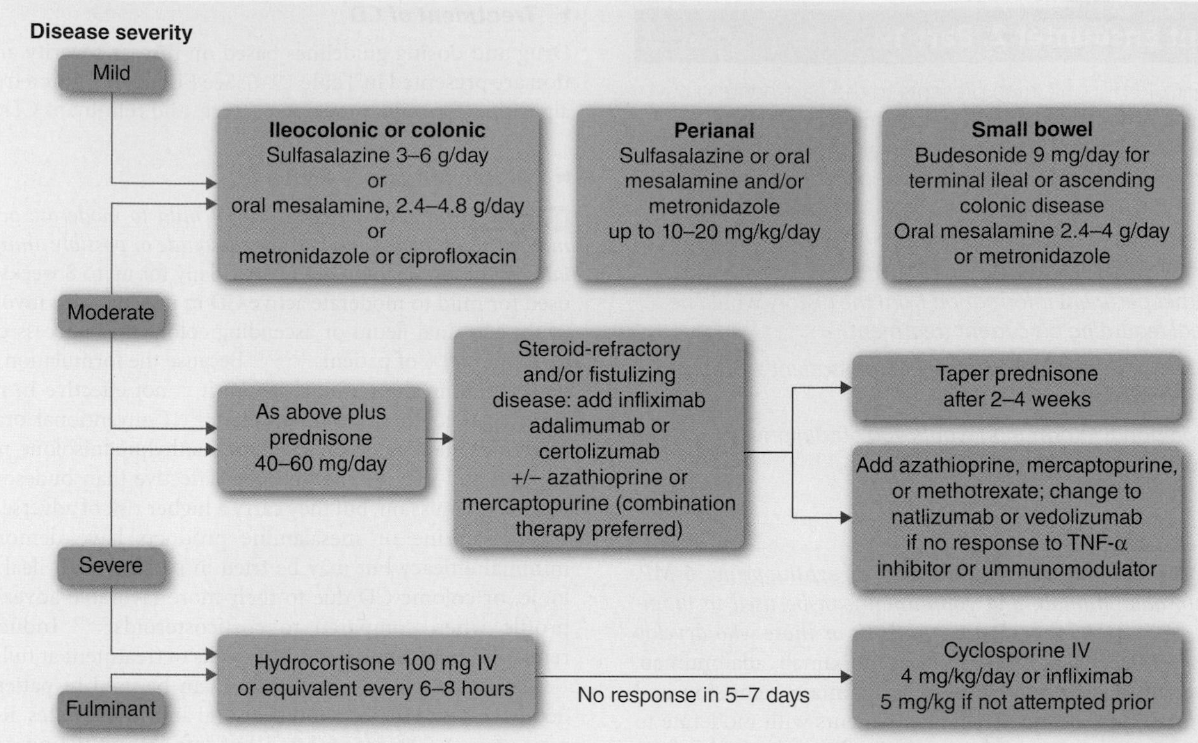

FIGURE 19–4. Treatment approaches for Crohn disease. (Adapted from Hemstreet BA. Inflammatory bowel disease. In: DiPiro JT, Talbert RL, Yee GC, et al., eds. Pharmacotherapy: A Pathophysiologic Approach, 9th ed. New York, NY: McGraw-Hill, 2014 with permission. www.accesspharmacy.com.)

9 mg orally once daily may be used for moderately active CD involving the terminal ileum or ascending colon.

Infliximab is an effective alternative to corticosteroid therapy for patients with moderate to severe CD including patients with fistulizing or perianal disease.[22,23,26,27] Adalimumab or certolizumab may be used in patients with inadequate response to infliximab.[22,23,26,27] Anti TNF-α agents may be combined with azathioprine for enhanced efficacy.[26,27] This combination is superior to either agent alone. Natalizumab or vedolizumab may be used for patients failing oral therapies and anti-TNF-α agents.[29,31]

For patients with perianal fistulae, antibiotics (metronidazole or ciprofloxacin), infliximab, adalimumab, and certolizumab are appropriate treatment options. Complex perianal fistulae may require surgical intervention but may also be amenable to treatment with antibiotics, azathioprine, 6-MP, or anti-TNF-α agents.[15,22,26,27]

▸ *Severe to Fulminant Active CD*

Most patients with severe to fulminant CD require hospitalization for appropriate treatment. Patients should be assessed for possible surgical intervention if abdominal distention, masses, abscess, or obstruction are present. Daily IV doses of corticosteroids equivalent to prednisone 40 to 60 mg are recommended as initial therapy to rapidly suppress severe inflammation.

Although infliximab, adalimumab, or certolizumab may be used in severe active CD, there is no evidence that these agents are effective for fulminant disease. Natalizumab or vedolizumab can be used for severe CD but are reserved for patients failing other available therapies, including TNF-α inhibitors.

Adjunctive therapy with fluid and electrolyte replacement should be initiated. Nutritional support with enteral or parenteral nutrition may be indicated for patients unable to eat for more than 5 to 7 days.[2] Some evidence suggests that enteral nutrition provides anti-inflammatory effects in patients with active CD.[39,40,41]

Limited evidence indicates that cyclosporine, or possibly tacrolimus, may be effective as salvage therapy for patients who fail IV corticosteroid therapy.[2,3,22] Surgical intervention may ultimately be necessary for medically refractory disease.

▸ *Maintenance of Remission in CD*

Patients with CD are at high risk for disease relapse after induction of remission. Within 2 years, up to 80% of patients experience a relapse; therefore, many patients require indefinite maintenance therapy. KEY CONCEPT *Maintenance of remission of CD may be achieved with immunosuppressants (azathioprine, 6-MP, or methotrexate), biologic agents (infliximab, adalimumab, certolizumab pegol, natalizumab, or vedolizumab), and less frequently with oral or topical aminosalicylate derivatives.*

In contrast to their use in UC, sulfasalazine and the newer aminosalicylates are marginally effective in preventing CD relapse in patients with medically induced remission, with success rates of only 10% to 20% at 1 year.[3,39] Despite not being recommended as first-line therapy, aminosalicylates are routinely used to attempt maintenance of remission of CD. Some evidence suggests that aminosalicylates may prevent or delay disease recurrence in patients with surgically induced remisson.[2,39]

The anti-TNF-α agents infliximab, adalimumab, and certolizumab are effective in maintaining remission in CD.[26,27] Azathioprine and 6-MP in oral doses up to 2.5 mg/kg/day have been shown to maintain remission in 45% of patients for up to 5 years.[22,25,26,27] There is evidence to support use of anti-TNF-α combination therapy with azathioprine but less as monotherapy with methotrexate to maintain remission in CD.[26,27] Natalizumab or vedolizumab may be used for maintenance in patients unresponsive to anti-TNF-α agents.[29,31]

Patient Encounter 2, Part 2: Medical History and Physical Examination

PMH: CD diagnosed 1 month ago, GERD

FH: Both parents alive; father has history of CVA and type 2 DM. Mother has a history of MI; brother with type 1 DM

SH: Works in construction; 1 to 2 alcoholic drinks per day; smokes one pack per day

Allergies: Morphine (itching)

Meds: Sulfasalazine 1000 mg orally four times daily, loperamide orally as needed, esomeprazole 20 mg orally once daily

ROS: (+) Diarrhea, abdominal pain, fatigue, fever, thirst

PE:

VS: BP 128/78 mm Hg, P 100 beats/min, RR 18/min, T 37.5°C (99.5°F)

CV: Tachycardia with normal rhythm. No murmurs, rubs, or gallops

HEENT: Dry mucous membranes

Skin: Dry with no evidence of tenting

Abd: Soft, nondistended, moderate diffuse tenderness, (+) bowel sounds, (–) hepatosplenomegaly, (–) masses, heme (+) stool

MS: 5/5 strength in upper and lower extremities; normal ROM

Labs:

Sodium 138 mEq/L (138 mmol/L)
Potassium 3.8 mEq/L (3.8 mmol/L)
Chloride 99 mEq/L (99 mmol/L)
Bicarbonate 27 mEq/L (27 mmol/L)
BUN 17 mg/dL (6.1 mmol/L)
Serum creatinine 1.1 mg/dL (97 μmol/L)
Serum glucose 100 mg/dL (5.6 mmol/L)
Albumin 3.8 g/dL (38 g/L)
ALT 25 IU/L (0.42 μkat/L)
AST 23 IU/L (0.38 μkat/L)
ESR 110 mm/hour
CRP 1.2 mg/dL (12 mg/L)
A1C 6.1% (0.061; 43 mmol/mol Hb)
Hemoglobin 11 g/dL (110 g/L or 6.83 mmol/L)
Hematocrit 34% (0.34)
WBC count $17.0 \times 10^3/mm^3$ ($17.0 \times 10^9/L$)
Platelets $480 \times 10^3/mm^3$ ($480 \times 10^9/L$)

Abdominal x-ray: (–) obstruction, free-air, or colonic dilation

Colonoscopy: Patchy inflammation extending to and involving the terminal ileum with evidence of recent bleeding, (–) polyps or strictures, biopsy taken

Pathology: Evidence of granuloma and PMN infiltration

How is this additional information helpful in determining disease extent and location?

What factors should you consider in choosing appropriate drug therapy for this patient?

What treatment options would you consider at this time?

Systemic or topical corticosteroids should not be used for maintaining remission in patients with CD. Unfortunately, up to 50% of patients treated acutely with corticosteroids become dependent on them to prevent symptoms.[2] Budesonide 6 mg orally once daily may be used in place of conventional corticosteroids for up to 3 months after remission induction in mild to moderate CD or in patients dependent on corticosteroids.[3,23,39]

Treatment of IBD in Special Populations (Table 19–6)

▶ *Elderly Patients*

Approximately 15% of patients with IBD initially develop symptoms after age 65.[42] In general, IBD presents similarly in older patients and younger individuals. Elderly patients may have more comorbid diseases, some of which may make the diagnosis of IBD more difficult. Such conditions include ischemic colitis, diverticular disease, and microscopic colitis. Increased age is also associated with a higher incidence of adenomatous polyps, but the onset of IBD at an advanced age does not appear to increase the risk of developing colorectal cancer. Elderly patients may also use more medications, particularly NSAIDs, which may induce or exacerbate colitis.

Treatment of older patients with IBD is similar to that for younger patients, but special consideration should be given to some of the medications used. Corticosteroids may worsen diabetes, hypertension, heart failure, or osteoporosis. The TNF-α inhibitors should be used cautiously in patients with heart failure and should be avoided in New York Heart Association class III or IV disease. Older patients requiring major surgical interventions may be at higher risk for surgical complications or may not meet eligibility criteria for surgery because of comorbid conditions, age-related organ dysfunction, or reduced functional status.

▶ *Children and Adolescents*

Approximately 50,000 individuals younger than 20 years of age in the United States have IBD, which represents 5% of all IBD patients. CD occurs twice as frequently as UC in children.[43] A major issue in children with IBD is the risk of growth failure secondary to inadequate nutritional intake and corticosteroid therapy. Failure to thrive may be an initial presentation of IBD in this population. Aggressive nutritional interventions may be required to facilitate adequate caloric intake. Chronic corticosteroid therapy may also be associated with reductions in growth and bone demineralization. Using lower doses in patients who are corticosteroid dependent may reduce altered height velocity.[44] Guidelines for management of acute severe UC in children favor methylprednisolone as first-line therapy, with calcineurin inhibitors or infliximab used for unresponsive patients.[45]

The aminosalicylates, azathioprine, 6-MP, and infliximab are all viable options for treatment and maintenance of IBD in pediatric patients. Infliximab is approved for use in the United States for patients 6 to 17 years of age with moderate to severe active CD. Use of immunosuppressive therapy or infliximab may help reduce overall corticosteroid exposure. Adalimumab is also approved for use in patients 6 years of age or older with CD.[46,47] Certolizumab, natalizumab, and vedolizumab are only FDA approved for use in adults with IBD; data in children are limited.[48]

▶ *Pregnant Women*

Inducing and maintaining remission of IBD prior to conception is the optimal approach in women planning to become pregnant. Active IBD may result in prematurity and low birth weight newborns. Thus pregnant women with IBD should be monitored closely, particularly during the third trimester.[49,50]

Table 19–6

Dosing Considerations of IBD Therapies in Special Populations

Therapy	Pediatric Patients	Elderly Patients	Pregnancy[44–46]
Sulfasalazine	Age > 2 years: 40–60 mg/kg/day in 3–6 divided doses; 30 mg/kg/day in 3–6 divided doses for maintenance	No specific changes	Category B Administer folic acid 2 mg daily during prenatal period and pregnancy
Mesalamine	No specific changes; Balsalazide indicated for age > 5 years	No specific changes	Category B (Olsalazine Category C) Generally considered safe and effective
Corticosteroids	No specific changes	No specific changes Elderly patients at high risk for osteoporosis	Older agents not rated Budesonide category C Generally considered safe and effective
TNF-α inhibitors	Infliximab indicated for pediatric patients: 5 mg/kg at 0, 2, and 6 weeks, then every 8 weeks Adalimumab indicated for patients age ≥ 6 or greater: 80 mg (< 40 kg), 40 mg week 2, then 20 mg every other week or 160 mg (> 40 kg) initial followed by 80 mg week 2, then 40 mg every other week	Avoid in patients with heart failure Elderly patients at higher risk for infections	Category B Pregnancy registry for adalimumab via manufacturer
Natalizumab	Dose of 3 mg/kg IV at 0, 4, and 8 weeks reported; data are lacking in children	No specific changes	Category C Report pregnancy to manufacturer's pregnancy registry
Vedolizumab	Not indicated	No specific changes	Category B Manufacturer pregnancy exposure registry
Azathioprine 6-Mercaptopurine	1.5–2 mg/kg/day to start	No specific changes	Category D Accepted as safe Avoid initiating during pregnancy, but continue if patient is already receiving when pregnant
Methotrexate	17 mg/m^2 orally/SC/IM	No specific changes	Category X Contraindicated
Cyclosporine	No specific changes	No specific changes	Category C Use only in refractory patients
Metronidazole	30–50 mg/kg/day divided every 6 hours	No specific changes	Category B Use short courses if possible
Ciprofloxacin	Avoid use	Adjust dose for CrCl < 50 mL/min (0.83 mL/s)	Category C Consider other alternatives

CrCl, creatinine clearance; IM, intramuscular; SC, subcutaneously.

Patients do not need to discontinue drug therapy for IBD once they become pregnant, but certain adjustments may be required.[49,50] The aminosalicylates are considered safe in pregnancy, but sulfasalazine is associated with folate malabsorption. Because pregnancy results in a higher folate requirement, pregnant patients treated with sulfasalazine should be supplemented with folic acid 1 mg orally twice daily.[49]

Corticosteroids may be used for treatment of active disease but not for maintenance of remission. Generally, corticosteroids confer no additional risk on the mother or fetus and are generally well tolerated. Both azathioprine and 6-MP have been used successfully in pregnant patients and appear to carry minimal risk, despite carrying an FDA pregnancy category D rating.[49] Infliximab, adalimumab, golimumab, and certolizumab are all FDA category B drugs and appear to carry minimal risk in pregnant patients.[49] Little is known about excretion of these drugs in breast milk, so benefit versus risk should be considered if they are used during nursing. Natalizumab is a pregnancy category C drug and vedolizumab is category B; both should be used only when other therapies have been exhausted.

Methotrexate is a known abortifacient and carries an FDA category X pregnancy rating. Thus, it is contraindicated during pregnancy. Metronidazole carries a theoretical risk of mutagenicity in humans, but short courses are safe during pregnancy. Prolonged use of metronidazole should be avoided in pregnant patients due to lack of safety data supporting its use.[49] Ciprofloxacin should be avoided in pregnant women.

OUTCOME EVALUATION

- Monitor for improvement of symptoms in patients with active IBD, such as reduction in the number of daily stools, abdominal pain, fever, and heart rate.
- For patients in remission, assure that proper maintenance doses are used and inform the patient to seek medical attention if symptoms recur or worsen.
- Evaluate patients receiving systemic corticosteroid therapy for improvement in symptoms and opportunities to taper or discontinue therapy. For patients using more than 5 mg daily of prednisone for more than 2 months or for steroid-dependent patients consider the following:
  - Central bone mineral density testing to evaluate need for calcium, vitamin D, or bisphosphonate therapy

Patient Care Process

Patient Assessment:

- Evaluate the medical record to determine the extent, location, and severity of IBD.
- Assess for evidence of extraintestinal manifestations or GI complications related to IBD.
- Interview the patient to evaluate the impact on quality of life and to identify psychosocial problems related to the presence of IBD.

Therapy Evaluation:

- Determine if the patient is treatment naive or if they are currently receiving pharmacotherapy.
- Evaluate the patient's current medication doses and adherence to therapy. Identify potential barriers to adherence, such as cost or inability to properly use certain drug formulations.
- Identify adverse effects related to current therapy.

Care Plan Development:

- Based on the current therapy and disease severity and location choose appropriate drug(s) and formulations to target the regions of intestinal inflammation.
- Educate the patient on proper use of drug therapy, including when to expect symptom improvement after initiation of treatment and which signs or symptoms to report that might be adverse drug effects.
- Refer patients to available support groups or IBD organizational resources if they are having difficulty coping with their disease.

Follow-Up Evaluation:

- Depending on disease severity, follow up in 2 to 4 weeks. Earlier telephone follow-up may be required to determine whether the patient is achieving some relief of symptoms.

    - Periodic monitoring of blood glucose, lipids, and blood pressure
    - Evaluation for evidence of Cushingoid features or signs or symptoms of infection

- When considering treatment with azathioprine or 6-MP, obtain baseline complete blood count (CBC), liver function tests, and TPMT activity. These tests, except TPMT, should be monitored closely (every 2–4 weeks) at the start of therapy and then approximately every 3 months during maintenance therapy.
- With azathioprine and 6-MP, monitor for hypersensitivity reactions including severe skin rashes and pancreatitis. Educate the patient regarding signs and symptoms of pancreatitis (nausea, vomiting, and abdominal pain).
- Prior to initiating methotrexate therapy, obtain CBC, serum creatinine, liver function tests, chest x-ray, and pregnancy test (if female). Monitor blood counts weekly for 1 month, then monthly thereafter.
- Prior to initiating infliximab, adalimumab, or certolizumab, obtain a tuberculin skin test to rule out latent tuberculosis, monitor for signs and symptoms of tuberculosis, and measure viral hepatitis serologies. Also monitor patients with a prior history of hepatitis B virus infection for signs of liver disease, such as jaundice. Assure that patients do not have a clinically significant systemic infection or New York Heart Association class III or IV heart failure.
- In patients receiving infliximab, monitor for infusion-related reactions such as hypotension, dyspnea, fever, chills, or chest pain when administering IV doses.
- In patients with fistulae, monitor at every infliximab, adalimumab, golimumab, or certolizumab dosing interval for evidence of fistula closure and overall reduction in the number of fistulae.
- Obtain a magnetic resonance imaging procedure prior to initiation of natalizumab or vedolizumab therapy. Monitor patients for signs of progressive multifocal leukoencephalopathy such as mental status changes, signs of liver disease (eg, jaundice), and hypersensitivity reactions following administration.

Abbreviations Introduced in This Chapter

5-ASA	5-Aminosalicylate
6-MP	6-Mercaptopurine
CD	Crohn disease
CRP	C-reactive protein
ESR	Erythrocyte sedimentation rate
HLA	Human leukocyte antigen
IBD	Inflammatory bowel disease
IL	Interleukin
NSAID	Nonsteroidal anti-inflammatory drug
pANCA	Perinuclear antineutrophil cytoplasmic antibodies
PR	Per rectum
TNF-α	Tumor necrosis factor-α
TPMT	Thiopurine methyltransferase
UC	Ulcerative colitis

REFERENCES

1. Kornbluth A, Sachar DB. Ulcerative practice guidelines in adults: American College of Gastroenterology, Practice Parameters Committee. Am J Gastroenterol. 2010;105:501–523.
2. Lichtenstein GR, Hanauer SB, Sandborn WJ. The Practice Parameters Committee of the American College of Gastroenterology. Management of Crohn's disease in adults. Am J Gastroenterol. 2009;104:465–483.
3. Schirbel A, Fiocchi C. Inflammatory bowel disease: Established and evolving considerations on its etiopathogenesis and therapy. J Dig Dis. 2010;11:266–276.
4. Lakatos PL, Fischer S, Lakatos L, Gal I, Papp J. Current concept on the pathogenesis of inflammatory bowel disease-crosstalk between genetic and microbial factors: Pathogenic bacteria and altered bacterial sensing or changes in mucosal integrity take "toll." World J Gastroenterol. 2006;12(12):1829–1841.

5. Gismera CS, Aladrén BS. Inflammatory bowel diseases: A disease(s) of modern times? Is incidence still increasing? World J Gastroenterol. 2008;14(36):5491–5498.
6. Talley NJ, Abreu MT, Anchkar JP, et al. An evidenced based systematic review on medical therapies for inflammatory bowel disease. Am J Gastroenterol. 2011;106:S2–S25.
7. Lie MR, Kanis SL, Hansen BE, van der Woude CJ. Drug therapies for ulcerative proctitis: Systematic review and meta-analysis. Inflamm Bowel Dis. 2014;20:2157–2178.
8. Sandler RS, Eisen GM. Epidemiology of inflammatory bowel disease. In: Kirsner JB, ed. Inflammatory Bowel Diseases. Philadelphia, PA: Saunders, 2000:89–112.
9. Achkara JP, Duerr R. The expanding universe of inflammatory bowel disease genetics. Curr Opin Gastroenterol. 2008;24: 429–434.
10. Podolsky DK. Inflammatory bowel disease. N Engl J Med. 2002;347:417–429.
11. MacDonald TT, Di Sabatino A, Gordon JN. Immunopathogenesis of Crohn's disease. JPEN J Parenter Enteral Nutr. 2005;29(4 Suppl): S118–S125.
12. Cipolla G, Crema F, Sacco S, et al. Nonsteroidal anti-inflammatory drugs and inflammatory bowel disease: Current perspectives. Pharmacol Res. 2002;46:1–6.
13. Larsen S, Bendtzen K, Nielsen OH. Extraintestinal manifestations of inflammatory bowel disease: Epidemiology, diagnosis, and management. Ann Med. 2010;42(2):97–114.
14. Gecse KB, Bemelman W, Kamm MA, et al. A global consensus on the classification, diagnosis and multidisciplinary treatment of perianal fistulising Crohn's disease. Gut. 2014;63:1381–1392.
15. Ford AC, Sandborn WJ, Khan KJ, et al. Efficacy of biological therapies in inflammatory bowel disease: Systematic review and meta-analysis. Am J Gastroenterol. 2011;106:644–659.
16. American Gastroenterological Association. AGA technical review on osteoporosis in gastrointestinal diseases. Gastroenterology. 2003;124:795–841.
17. Ng SC, Kamm MA. Review article: New drug formulations, chemical entities and therapeutic approaches for the management of ulcerative colitis. Aliment Pharmacol Ther. 2008;28:815–829.
18. Sandborn WJ, Hanauer SB. Systematic review: The pharmacokinetic profiles of oral mesalamine formulations and mesalazine pro-drugs used in the management of ulcerative colitis. Aliment Pharmacol Ther. 2003;17:29–42.
19. Sandborn WJ. Rational selection of oral 5-aminosalicylate formulations and prodrugs for the treatment of ulcerative colitis [editorial]. Am J Gastroenterol. 2002;97(12):2939–2941.
20. Navarro F, Hanauer SB. Treatment of inflammatory bowel disease: Safety and tolerability issues. Am J Gastroenterol. 2003;98(12 Suppl):S18–S23.
21. Pascal J, Valérie P, Felley C, et al. Drug safety in Crohn's disease therapy. Digestion. 2007;76:161–168.
22. American Gastroenterological Association Institute. Technical review on corticosteroids, immunomodulators, and infliximab in inflammatory bowel disease. Gastroenterology. 2006;130: 940–987.
23. Hofer KN. Oral budesonide in the management of Crohn's disease. Ann Pharmacother. 2003;37:1457–1464.
24. Gionchetti P, Pratico C, Rizzello F, et al. The role of Budesonide-MMX in active ulcerative colitis. Expert Rev Gastroenterol Hepatol. 2014:8(3):215–222.
25. Fraser AG, Orchard TR, Jewell DP. The efficacy of azathioprine for the treatment of inflammatory bowel disease: A 30 year review. Gut. 2002;50:485–489.
26. Terdiman JP, Gruss CB, Heidelbaugh JJ, et al. American Gastroenterological Association Institute technical review on the use of thiopurines, methotrexate, and anti-TNF-α biologic drugs for the induction and maintenance of remission in inflammatory Crohn's disease. Gastroenterology. 2013;145:1459–1463.
27. American Gastroenterological Association Institute technical review on the use of thiopurines, methotrexate, and anti-TNF-α biologic drugs for the induction and maintenance of remission in inflammatory Crohn's disease. Gastroenterology. 2013;145: 1464–1478.
28. Akobeng AA, Sandborn WJ, Bickston SJ, et al. Tumor necrosis factor-alpha antagonists twenty years later: What do Cochrane reviews tell us? Inflamm Bowel Dis. 2014;20:2132–2141.
29. Stefanelli T, Malesci A, De La Rue SA, Danese S. Anti-adhesion molecule therapies in inflammatory bowel disease: Touch and go. Autoimmun Rev. 2008;7:364–369.
30. Feagan BG, Rutgeerts P, Sands BE, et al; the GEMINI 1 Study Group. Vedolizumab as induction and maintenance therapy for ulcerative colitis. N Engl J Med. 2013;369(8):699–710.
31. Sandborn WJ, Feagan BG, Rutgeerts, P, et al; the Gemini 2 Study Group. Vedolizumab as induction and maintenance therapy for Crohn's Disease. N Engl J Med. 2013;369(8):711–721.
32. Khan KJ, Ullman TA, Ford AC, et al. Antibiotic therapy in inflammatory bowel disease: A systematic review and meta-analysis. Am J Gastroenterol. 2011;106:661–673.
33. Nikfar S, Ehteshami-Ashar S, Rahimi R, Abdollahi M. Systematic review and meta-analysis of the efficacy and tolerability of nicotine preparations in active ulcerative colitis. Clin Ther. 2010;32:2304–2315.
34. Williams NT. Probiotics. Am J Health Syst Pharm. 2010;67: 449–458.
35. Marshall JK, Irvine EJ. Putting rectal 5-aminosalicylic acid in its place: The role in distal ulcerative colitis. Am J Gastroenterol. 2000;95:1628–1636.
36. Cohen RD, Woseth DM, Thisted RA, Hanauer SB. A meta-analysis and overview of the literature on treatment options for left-sided ulcerative colitis and ulcerative proctitis. Am J Gastroenterol. 2000;95:1263–1276.
37. Brain O, Travis SPL. Therapy of ulcerative colitis: State of the art. Curr Opin Gastroenterol. 2008;24:469–474.
38. Panaccione R, Ghosh, S, Middleton S, et al. Combination therapy with infliximab and azathioprine is superior to monotherapy with either agent in ulcerative colitis. Gastroenterology. 2014; 146(2):392–400.
39. Sandborn WJ, Feagan BG, Lichtenstein GR. Medical management of mild to moderate Crohn's disease: Evidence-based treatment algorithms for induction and maintenance of remission. Drugs. 2007;67(17):2511–2537.
40. Griffiths AM. Enteral nutrition in the management of Crohn's disease. JPEN J Parenter Enteral Nutr. 2005;29(4 Suppl): S108–S117.
41. Sanderson IR, Croft NM. The anti-inflammatory effects of enteral nutrition. JPEN J Parenter Enteral Nutr. 2005;29(4 Suppl): S134–S140.
42. Robertson DJ, Grimm IS. Inflammatory bowel disease in the elderly. Gastroenterol Clin North Am. 2001;30:409–426.
43. Kim SC, Ferry GD. Inflammatory bowel diseases in pediatric and adolescent patients: Clinical, therapeutic, and psychosocial considerations. Gastroenterology. 2004;126:1550–1560.
44. Navarro FA, Hanauer SB, Kirschner BS. Effect of long-term low-dose prednisone on height velocity and disease activity in pediatric and adolescent patients with Crohn's disease. J Pediatr Gastroenterol Nutr. 2007;45:312–318.
45. Turner D, Travis SP, Griffiths AM, et al. Consensus for managing acute severe ulcerative colitis in children: A systematic review and joint statement from ECCP, ESPGHAN, and the Porto IBD Working group of ASPGHAN. Am J Gastroenterol. 2011; 106:574–588.

46. Noe JD, Pfefferkorn M. Short-term response to adalimumab in childhood inflammatory bowel disease. Inflamm Bowel Dis. 2008;14:1683–1687.
47. Wyneski MJ, Green A, Kay M, et al. Safety and efficacy of adalimumab in pediatric patients with Crohn disease. J Pediatr Gastroenterol Nutr. 2008;47:19–25.
48. Hyams JS, Wilson DC, Thomas A, et al. Natalizumab therapy for moderate to severe Crohn disease in adolescents. J Pediatr Gastroenterol Nutr. 2007;44:185–191.
49. Ferrero S, Ragni N. Inflammatory bowel disease: Management issues during pregnancy. Arch Gynecol Obstet. 2004;270:79–85.
50. Dubinsky M, Abraham B, Mahadevan U. Management of the pregnant IBD patient. Inflamm Bowel Dis. 2008;14:1736–1750.

20 Nausea and Vomiting

Sheila Wilhelm and Melissa Lipari

LEARNING OBJECTIVES

Upon completion of the chapter, the reader will be able to:

1. Identify common causes of nausea and vomiting.
2. Describe the pathophysiologic mechanisms of nausea and vomiting.
3. Identify the three stages of nausea and vomiting.
4. Distinguish between simple and complex nausea and vomiting.
5. Create goals for treating nausea and vomiting.
6. Recommend treatment regimens for nausea and vomiting associated with cancer chemotherapy, surgery, pregnancy, or motion sickness.
7. Outline a monitoring plan to evaluate treatment outcomes for nausea and vomiting.

INTRODUCTION

Nausea and vomiting result from complex interactions of the gastrointestinal (GI) system, the vestibular system, and the brain and have a variety of causes. Preventing and treating nausea and vomiting requires pharmacologic and nonpharmacologic measures tailored to individual patients and situations.

EPIDEMIOLOGY AND ETIOLOGY

KEY CONCEPT *Nausea and vomiting are symptoms that can be due to many different causes such as GI, cardiac, neurologic, and endocrine disorders (Table 20–1).*[1,2] Cancer chemotherapy agents are rated according to their emetogenic potential, and antiemetic therapy is prescribed based on these ratings. Radiation therapy can induce nausea and vomiting, especially when it is used to treat abdominal malignancies.[3]

Oral contraceptives, hormone therapy, and opioids can cause nausea and vomiting.[1,4] Some medications, such as digoxin and theophylline, cause nausea and vomiting in a dose-related fashion, which may indicate excessive drug concentrations. Ethanol and other toxins also cause nausea and vomiting.

Postoperative nausea and vomiting (PONV) occurs in 30% of surgical patients overall and in up to 70% of high-risk patients.[5,6] Risk factors for PONV include female sex, history of motion sickness or PONV, nonsmoking status, and use of opioids postoperatively.[6–8] The choice of anesthetic agents and duration of surgery may also contribute to PONV.[5,6,8]

Nausea and vomiting of pregnancy (NVP) affects 70% to 85% of pregnant women, especially early in pregnancy.[9] In up to 2% of pregnancies, this can lead to **hyperemesis gravidarum**, a potentially life-threatening condition of prolonged nausea, vomiting, and resultant malnutrition.[9]

PATHOPHYSIOLOGY

Nausea and vomiting consist of three stages: (1) **nausea**; (2) **retching**; and (3) **vomiting**. Nausea is the subjective feeling of a need to vomit.[1,4] It is often accompanied by autonomic symptoms of pallor, tachycardia, diaphoresis, and salivation. Retching follows nausea and consists of contractions of the diaphragm, abdominal wall, and chest wall and spasmodic breathing against a closed glottis.[1] Retching, which can occur without vomiting, produces the pressure gradient needed for vomiting, although no gastric contents are expelled. Vomiting, or **emesis**, is a reflexive, rapid, and forceful oral expulsion of upper GI contents due to sustained contractions in the abdominal and thoracic musculature.[1]

Specific areas in the brain and GI tract are stimulated when the body is exposed to noxious stimuli or GI irritants: the **chemoreceptor trigger zone (CTZ)** in the area postrema of the fourth ventricle of the brain, the vestibular apparatus, visceral afferents from the GI tract, and the cerebral cortex.[2,4] These in turn stimulate regions of the reticular areas of the medulla within the brain stem. This area is the central vomiting center, which coordinates the impulses sent to the salivation and respiratory centers, and the pharyngeal, GI, and abdominal muscles that lead to vomiting (Figure 20–1).[10]

The CTZ, located outside the blood–brain barrier, is exposed to cerebrospinal fluid and blood.[2] Therefore, it is easily stimulated by uremia, acidosis, and circulating toxins such as chemotherapeutic agents. The CTZ has many 5-hydroxytryptamine (serotonin) type 3 (5-HT_3), neurokinin-1 (NK_1), and dopamine (D_2) receptors.[11] Visceral vagal nerve fibers are rich in 5-HT_3 receptors. They respond to GI distention, mucosal irritation, and infection.

Motion sickness is caused by stimulation of the vestibular system, rich in histaminic (H_1) and muscarinic cholinergic receptors.[12] The cerebral cortex is affected by sensory input such as sights, smells, or emotions that can lead to vomiting. This area is involved in anticipatory nausea and vomiting associated with chemotherapy.

Table 20–1
Causes of Nausea and Vomiting

GI or Intraperitoneal	Cardiac	Neurologic	Other Causes	Therapy Induced	Endocrine/ Metabolic
Obstructing disorders	Cardiomyopathy	Vestibular disease	Bulimia	Cancer chemotherapy	Pregnancy (NVP)
Achalasia	Myocardial infarction	Motion sickness	Anorexia nervosa	Antibiotics	Hyperemesis gravidarum
Enteric infections	Heart failure	Labyrinthitis	Cyclic vomiting syndrome	Antiarrhythmics	Renal disease (uremia)
Appendicitis		Head trauma		Digoxin	Diabetes (ketoacidosis)
Pancreatitis		Migraine headache		Oral hypoglycemics	Thyroid disease
Inflammatory bowel diseases		Increased intracranial pressure		Oral contraceptives	Parathyroid disease
Cholecystitis		Intracranial hemorrhage		Theophylline	Adrenal insufficiency
Hepatitis		Meningitis		Opioids	Hyponatremia
Gastroparesis		Hydrocephalus		Anticonvulsants	Hypercalcemia
Gastroesophageal reflux		Psychogenic causes		Radiation therapy	
Peptic ulcer disease		Self-induced		Ethanol	
Peritonitis		Depression		Toxins	

Nausea and vomiting can be classified as either simple or complex.[13] Simple nausea and vomiting occurs occasionally and is either self-limiting or relieved by minimal therapy. It does not detrimentally affect hydration status, electrolyte balance, or weight. Alternatively, complex nausea and vomiting requires more aggressive therapy because electrolyte imbalances, dehydration, and weight loss may occur.

CLINICAL PRESENTATION AND DIAGNOSIS

Refer to the accompanying box for the clinical presentation and diagnosis of nausea and vomiting.

TREATMENT

Desired Outcomes

The primary goals of treatment are to relieve the symptoms of nausea and vomiting, increase the patient's quality of life, and prevent complications such as dehydration or malnutrition. Drug therapy for nausea and vomiting should be safe, effective, and economical.

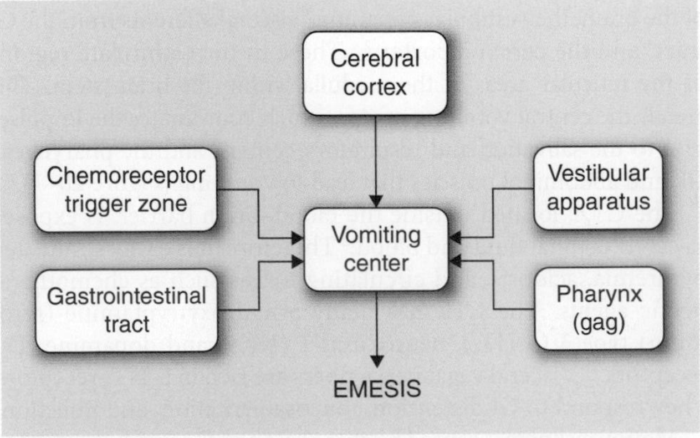

FIGURE 20–1. Primary afferent components to the vomiting center. (From Case 31. In: Toy EC, Loose DS, Tischkau SA, Pillai AS, eds. Case Files™: Pharmacology, 3rd ed. New York, NY: McGraw-Hill; 2014. http://accesspharmacy.mhmedical.com, with permission. Accessed September 07, 2014.)

General Approach to Treatment

KEY CONCEPT *To treat nausea and vomiting most effectively, it is important to first identify and treat the underlying cause.* Profuse or prolonged vomiting can lead to complications of dehydration and metabolic abnormalities. Patients must have adequate hydration

Clinical Presentation and Diagnosis of Nausea and Vomiting

Symptoms

- Patients with nausea often complain of autonomic symptoms such as diaphoresis, disinterest in surroundings, pallor, faintness, and salivation.

Signs

- With complex and prolonged nausea and vomiting, patients may show signs of malnourishment, weight loss, and dehydration (dry mucous membranes, skin tenting, tachycardia, and lack of axillary moisture).

Laboratory Tests

- Dehydration, electrolyte imbalances, and acid–base disturbances may be evident in complex and prolonged nausea and vomiting.
- Dehydration is suggested by elevated blood urea nitrogen (BUN), serum creatinine (SCr), and BUN-to-SCr ratio (20:1 or greater using traditional units of measurement [100:1 or greater using SI units of mmol/L]).
- Calculated fractional excretion of sodium (FeNa) less than 1% (0.01) in patients with compromised baseline renal function and less than 0.2% (0.002) in patients with normal baseline renal function indicates dehydration and reduced renal perfusion.
- Low serum chloride and elevated serum bicarbonate levels indicate metabolic alkalosis.
- Hypokalemia may occur from GI potassium losses and intracellular potassium shifts to compensate for alkalosis.

and electrolyte replacement orally (if tolerated) or IV to prevent and correct these problems. Some pharmacologic treatments work locally in the GI tract, whereas others work in the central nervous system (CNS).[1]

Nonpharmacologic Therapy

KEY CONCEPT *Nonpharmacologic approaches to nausea and vomiting include dietary, physical, and psychological measures.* Dietary management is important when treating NVP due to concern for teratogenic effects with drug therapies.[14] Recommendations include eating frequent, small meals; avoiding spicy or fatty foods; eating high-protein snacks; and eating bland or dry foods the first thing in the morning.[9,14] The dietary supplement ginger (500–1000 mg daily given in three to four divided doses) was effective in NVP in some studies and is recommended in treatment guidelines.[9,14]

Acupressure and electroacupoint stimulation of the P6 (Neiguan) point on the inside of the wrist seem safe and cost-effective; however, efficacy data for treatment of NVP, PONV and motion sickness are conflicting.[9,15,16,17] Hypnosis and psychotherapy are also safe during pregnancy and in situations where adverse drug effects and interactions are a concern.

Pharmacologic Therapy

Table 20–2 contains the names, usual dosages, and common adverse effects of the pharmacologic treatments for nausea and vomiting.[1,3,6,13]

▶ *Anticholinergics (Scopolamine)*

Scopolamine blocks muscarinic receptors in the vestibular system, thereby halting signaling to the CNS. It is effective for preventing and treating motion sickness and has some efficacy in preventing PONV.[18,19] Scopolamine is available as an adhesive transdermal patch that is effective for up to 72 hours after application. This may be beneficial for patients unable to tolerate oral medications or those requiring continuous prevention of motion sickness (eg, passengers on cruise ships). Transdermal scopolamine should be applied 4 hours prior to motion sickness triggers and the evening before surgery if used to prevent PONV. Scopolamine is associated with adverse anticholinergic effects such as sedation, visual disturbances, dry mouth, and dizziness.

▶ *Antihistamines*

Antihistamines are used to prevent and treat nausea and vomiting due to motion sickness, vertigo, or migraine headache.[1,12,20] Their efficacy is presumably due to the high concentration of H_1 and muscarinic cholinergic receptors within the vestibular system. Similarly to scopolamine, first-generation antihistamines cause undesired effects including drowsiness and blurred vision. Cetirizine and fexofenadine, two second-generation antihistamines without CNS depressant properties, were found to be ineffective for treating motion sickness, perhaps because they lack CNS effects.[20]

Some first-generation antihistamines such as diphenhydramine, dimenhydrinate, and meclizine are available without a prescription, making self-treatment convenient. Antihistamines are available in a variety of dosage forms, including oral capsules, tablets, and liquids. Liquid formulations are convenient for children or adults who are unable to swallow solid dosage forms.

▶ *Dopamine Antagonists*

Stimulation of D_2 receptors in the CTZ leads to nausea and vomiting (Figure 20–1). Phenothiazine antiemetics act primarily via a central antidopaminergic mechanism in the CTZ.[1] Phenothiazines used to treat nausea and vomiting include promethazine, prochlorperazine, and chlorpromazine. Availability as oral solids and liquids, rectal suppositories, and parenteral formulations permits use in a variety of settings including severe motion sickness or vertigo, gastritis or gastroenteritis, NVP, PONV, and chemotherapy-induced nausea and vomiting (CINV).[21–23]

Phenothiazines may cause sedation, orthostatic hypotension, and extrapyramidal symptoms (EPS) such as dystonia (involuntary muscle contractions), tardive dyskinesia (irreversible and permanent involuntary movements), and akathisia (motor restlessness or anxiety).[1,24] Chronic phenothiazine use has been associated with EPS, but single doses have also caused these effects.[25]

Droperidol, a butyrophenone, is another centrally acting antidopaminergic agent effective for preventing PONV.[1,5] It may also be used for treating CINV for patients who are intolerant to serotonin receptor antagonists and corticosteroids.[3] Its adverse effects include sedation, agitation, and restlessness. Droperidol carries a US FDA black box warning regarding the potential for QT interval prolongation and cardiac arrhythmias that may result in torsades de pointes and sudden cardiac death.[26] Droperidol should not be used in patients with a prolonged QT interval or in those who are at risk for developing a prolonged QT interval (eg, heart failure, electrolyte abnormalities, or concurrently taking other medications that may prolong the QT interval).[26] A 12-lead electrocardiogram (ECG) is recommended prior to treatment with droperidol.

Haloperidol is another butyrophenone with some antiemetic effects at low doses (0.5–2 mg).[6] It has been explored as an alternative to droperidol.[27]

Metoclopramide and domperidone (not available in the United States) act as D_2-receptor antagonists centrally in the CTZ and peripherally in the GI tract.[1,28] They also display cholinergic activity, which increases lower esophageal sphincter tone and promotes gastric motility. Their antiemetic and prokinetic effects are useful in PONV, CINV, NVP, gastroparesis, and gastroesophageal reflux disease (GERD).[1,3,5,9] Metoclopramide is available in injectable, oral solid, and oral liquid dosage forms, allowing for its use in both hospitalized and ambulatory patients.

Metoclopramide crosses the blood–brain barrier and has centrally mediated adverse effects. Young children and the elderly are especially susceptible to these effects, which include somnolence, reduced mental acuity, anxiety, depression, and EPS and occur in 10% to 20% of patients.[1,29]

Domperidone minimally crosses the blood–brain barrier and is less likely to cause centrally mediated adverse effects.[1,29] It should not be used for patients with underlying long QT interval or for those taking medications that prolong the QT interval. Both metoclopramide and domperidone can cause hyperprolactinemia, galactorrhea, and gynecomastia.

▶ *Corticosteroids*

Oral or IV corticosteroids, especially dexamethasone and methylprednisolone, are used alone or in combination with other antiemetics for preventing and treating PONV, CINV, or radiation-induced nausea and vomiting.[3,6,11,30] Efficacy is thought to be due to release of 5-HT, reduced permeability of the blood–brain barrier, and decreased inflammation.[31] Common adverse effects with short-term use include GI upset, anxiety, insomnia, and hyperglycemia.[3] Because their use is generally of short duration, long-term adverse effects (eg, decreased bone mineral density, diabetes, cataracts) are not usually seen.

Table 20–2

Antiemetic Agents: Usual Doses for Adults and Children and Adverse Effects

Drug	Adult Dosing	Pediatric Dosing	Adverse Effects[a]
Anticholinergics			
Scopolamine	TD: 1.5 mg patch applied 1 or more hours before the procedure, 4 hours prior to motion sickness triggers, repeated every 72 hours as needed	N/A	Most common: Dry mouth, drowsiness, blurred vision Rare: Disorientation, dizziness, hallucinations
Antihistamines			
Cyclizine	Oral: 50 mg every 4–6 hours as needed	Oral: 6–11 years: 25 mg every 6–8 hours as needed (max: three tablets per day)	Most common: Sedation, dry mouth, constipation Less common: Confusion, blurred vision, urinary retention
Dimenhydrinate	Oral: 50–100 mg every 4–6 hours as needed	Oral: 2–6 years, 12.5–25 mg every 6–8 hours not to exceed 75 mg in 24 hours; 6–12 years, 25–50 mg every 6–8 hours, not to exceed 150 mg in 24 hours	
Diphenhydramine	Oral: 25–50 mg every 4–6 hours IV/IM: 10–50 mg every 2–4 hours as needed	Oral/IV/IM: 2–6 years, 6.25 mg every 4–6 hours	
Hydoxyzine	Oral/IV/IM: 25–100 mg every 4–6 hours as needed	Oral: 0.6 mg/kg IM: 0.5–1 mg/kg	
Meclizine	Oral: 12.5–25 mg every 12–24 hours as needed	Oral: ≥ 12 years: use adult dose	
Phenothiazines			
Chlorpromazine	Oral: 10–25 mg every 4–6 hours as needed IV/IM: 25–50 mg every 4–6 hours as needed	Oral: ≥ 6 months, 0.5 mg/kg every 4–6 hours as needed IV/IM: ≥ 6 months, 0.5–1 mg/kg every 6–8 hours	Most common: Sedation, lethargy, skin sensitization Less common: Cardiovascular effects, EPS, cholestatic jaundice, hyperprolactinemia
Prochlorperazine	Oral: 5–10 mg three to four times a day as needed Supp: 25 mg twice daily as needed IV/IM 2.5–10 mg every 3–4 hours as needed	Oral: > 2 years and > 9 kg: 0.4 mg/kg/day or 10 mg/m^2 daily in two to three divided doses Supp: See oral dosing IM: > 2 years and > 9 kg: 0.13 mg/kg	Avoid using in pediatric patients if possible due to sensitivity to adverse effects. If use is considered necessary, employ the lowest effective dose
Promethazine	Oral/IM/IV/Supp: 12.5–25 mg every 4–6 hours as needed	Oral/IM/IV/Supp: ≥ 2 years, 0.25–0.5 mg/kg or 7.5–15 mg/m^2 four to six times daily	
Butyrophenones			
Droperidol	IM/IV: 0.625–2.5 mg every 4–6 hours as needed	IM/IV: 2–12 years: 0.05–0.1 mg/kg (max 2.5 mg) every 4–6 hours as needed	Most common: Sedation, hypotension, tachycardia Less common: EPS, dizziness, increased blood pressure, chills, hallucinations, QT prolongation
Haloperidol	Oral, IM/IV: 0.5–5 mg every 12 hours as needed	N/A	
Benzamides			
Domperidone	Oral: 10–20 mg every 4–8 hours as needed Supp: 30–60 mg every 4–8 hours as needed	Oral: 0.2–0.4 mg/kg every 4–8 hours as needed for CINV prophylaxis Supp: Max daily dose based on weight	Most common: Sedation, restlessness, diarrhea (metoclopramide), agitation, CNS depression Less common: EPS, hypotension, neuroleptic syndrome, supraventricular tachycardia (with IV), QT prolongation, serotonin syndrome (when used with serotonergic agents)
Metoclopramide	PONV: 10–20 mg oral/IV/IM 10 min prior to anesthesia CINV Prophylaxis: 1–2 mg/kg oral/IV every 2–4 hours	N/A	

(Continued)

Table 20–2

Antiemetic Agents: Usual Doses for Adults and Children and Adverse Effects (*Continued*)

Drug	Adult Dosing	Pediatric Dosing	Adverse Effects[a]
Trimethobenzamide	IM: 200 mg two to four times a day as needed	Not recommended	
Corticosteroids			
Dexamethasone	*CINV*: 12–20 mg oral/IV day 1, then 8–12 mg oral/IV daily *PONV*: 4–5 mg oral/IV at induction of anesthesia	*CINV*: 10 mg/m^2 prior to chemotherapy then 5 mg/m^2	Most common: GI upset, anxiety, insomnia Less common: Hyperglycemia, facial flushing, euphoria, perineal itching or burning (with dexamethasone)
Methylprednisolone	125–500 mg oral/IV every 6 hours for total of four doses	N/A	
Cannabinoids			
Dronabinol	Oral: 5–15 mg/m^2 every 2–4 hours as needed	Use adult dose with caution and adjust based on response	Most common: Drowsiness, euphoria, somnolence, vasodilation, vision changes, dysphoria
Nabilone	Oral: 1–2 mg two to three times a day as needed	N/A	Less common: Diarrhea, flushing, tremor, myalgia
Benzodiazepines			
Lorazepam	Oral/IV: 0.5–2 mg prior to chemotherapy	Oral/IV: 2–15 years old: 0.05 mg/kg (up to 2 mg) prior to chemotherapy	Most common: Sedation, amnesia Rare: Respiratory depression, ataxia, blurred vision, hallucinations
Alprazolam	Oral: 0.5–2 mg three times a day prior to chemotherapy	N/A	
Serotonin Antagonists			
Dolasetron	*CINV*: Contraindicated due to dose-dependent QTc prolongation *PONV*: 12.5 mg IV 15 min before end of anesthesia or at onset of N/V or 100 mg po within 2 hours before surgery	*CINV*: Contraindicated due to dose-dependent QTc prolongation *PONV*: 0.35 mg/kg IV (max 12.5 mg) or 1.2 mg/kg po (max 100 mg) within 2 hours before surgery	Most common: Headache, QT prolongation Less common: Constipation, asthenia, somnolence, diarrhea, fever, tremor or twitching, ataxia, lightheadedness, dizziness, nervousness, thirst, muscle pain, warm or flushing sensation on IV administration, serotonin syndrome (with ondansetron when used with serotonergic agents) Rare: Transient elevations in hepatic transaminases Granisetron may be degraded by light. Cover patch application site (eg, with clothing) if risk of exposure to sunlight or sunlamps during use and for 10 days after removal
Granisetron	*CINV*: 10 mcg/kg IV prior to chemotherapy; or 1 mg orally 1 hour before chemotherapy and 1 mg 12 hours after first dose, or 2 mg 1 hour before chemotherapy *PONV*: 1 mg IV before induction of anesthesia or immediately before reversal of anesthesia, or at onset of N/V	*CINV*: 2–16 years: Use adult dosing IV or po regimen *PONV*: Not recommended for pediatric patients	
Granisetron	*CINV*: 1 patch 24–48 hours before chemotherapy; may wear for up to 7 days	N/A	
Ondansetron	*CINV*: Oral: 24 mg single dose prior to chemotherapy, or 8 mg prior to chemotherapy, repeat every 12 hours IV: 0.15 mg/kg, not to exceed 16 mg per dose, for three doses. Give the first dose 30 min prior to chemotherapy. Repeat dose 4 and 8 hours after the first dose *PONV*: 4 mg IV/IM before anesthesia induction or at onset of N/V; 16 mg orally once given 1 hour before anesthesia induction	*CINV*: Oral: 4–11 years, 4 mg 30 min prior to chemotherapy, repeat at 4 and 8 hours and every 8 hours for 1–2 days after chemotherapy completion IV: 6 months to 18 years: 0.15 mg/kg, not to exceed 16 mg per dose, for three doses. Give the first dose 30 min prior to chemotherapy. Repeat dose 4 and 8 hours after the first dose *PONV*: 1 month–12 years: 4 mg IV/IM before anesthesia induction for over 40 kg and 0.1 mg/kg IV for under 40 kg Oral recommendations not available	

(*Continued*)

Table 20–2

Antiemetic Agents: Usual Doses for Adults and Children and Adverse Effects (*Continued*)

Drug	Adult Dosing	Pediatric Dosing	Adverse Effects[a]
Palonosetron	*CINV*: 0.25 mg IV 30 min before chemotherapy; 0.5 mg orally 1 hour before chemotherapy *PONV*: 0.075 mg IV before anesthesia induction	*CINV*: 20 mcg/kg (maximum 1.5 mg) IV 30 min before chemotherapy	
Neurokinin-1 Antagonist			
Aprepitant	*CINV*: 150 mg IV (fosaprepitant) 30 min before chemotherapy on first day of chemotherapy only; or 125 mg orally on day 1, 1 hour prior to chemotherapy followed by 80 mg on days 2 and 3 *PONV*: 40 mg orally 3 hours prior to anesthesia induction	N/A	Most common: Fatigue, hiccups Less common: Dizziness, headache, insomnia Rare: Transient elevations in hepatic transaminases
Netupitant	*CINV*: Netupitant 300 mg plus palonosetron 0.5 mg combination product on day 1, 1 hour prior to chemotherapy	N/A	

CINV, chemotherapy-induced nausea and vomiting; EPS, extrapyramidal symptoms; IM, intramuscularly; Inj, injectable dosage form for IV or IM use; N/A, not available; PONV, postoperative nausea and vomiting; TD, transdermal; Supp, rectal suppository.

[a]Most common, greater than 10%; less common, 1% to 10%; rare, less than 1%. Based on US FDA-approved labeling and generalized to drug class.

► *Cannabinoids*

Cannabinoids have antiemetic and appetite stimulant activity when used alone or in combination with other antiemetics.[32] Oral dronabinol and nabilone are used for preventing and treating refractory CINV.[3,32] Cannabinoids are thought to exert their antiemetic effect centrally, although the exact mechanism of action is unknown.[32] Sedation, euphoria, hypotension, ataxia, dizziness, and vision difficulties can occur.

► *Benzodiazepines*

Benzodiazepines, especially lorazepam, are used to prevent and treat CINV.[3,11,30] Lorazepam is used as an adjunct to antiemetic agents.[3] Sedation and amnesia are common side effects. Respiratory depression can occur with high doses or when other central depressants such as alcohol are used concomitantly.

► *Serotonin Antagonists*

Serotonin is a neurotransmitter synthesized in neurons in the CNS and in enterochromaffin cells of the GI tract. Chemotherapeutic agents release 5-HT, which is a predominant mediator in nausea and vomiting.[33] This increase in 5-HT concentrations stimulates the visceral vagal nerve fibers and CTZ, thereby triggering nausea and vomiting. Selective 5-HT_3 receptor antagonists (ondansetron, granisetron, dolasetron, and palonosetron) prevent and treat nausea and vomiting due to stimulation of these receptors, especially for CINV and PONV.[30,33] These agents are well tolerated; the most common adverse effects are headache, somnolence, diarrhea, and constipation.[3] Dose-related QT changes (including torsades de pointes) have been reported, and ECG monitoring is recommended for patients with risk factors for QT prolongation who will receive ondansetron or dolasetron.[34] Granisetron labeling does not include a recommendation for ECG monitoring, and palonosetron has not been associated with QT prolongation.

Palonosetron is the first 5-HT_3 antagonist to be approved for preventing both acute and delayed CINV.[3] Compared to other 5-HT_3 antagonists, palonosetron has a longer serum half-life (40 hours compared to 4–9 hours) and a higher receptor-binding affinity, which may contribute to its efficacy in preventing delayed CINV.[35] Palonosetron combined with dexamethasone is the 5-HT_3 antagonist of choice for preventing CINV due to moderately emetogenic chemotherapy.[3]

► *Neurokinin-1 Receptor Antagonists*

Substance P is a neurokinin neurotransmitter that binds to neurokinin-1 (NK_1) receptors in the GI tract and the brain and is believed to mediate both acute and delayed nausea and vomiting.[36] Aprepitant was the first NK_1 receptor antagonist antiemetic and is effective for preventing acute and delayed CINV when used with a 5-HT_3 antagonist and a corticosteroid.[36,37] It is also effective for preventing PONV.[6,38] Aprepitant has numerous drug interactions because it is an inhibitor and substrate of the CYP 3A4 metabolic pathway.[38]

Netupitant is the second NK_1 receptor antagonist; it is available only as a combination product with palonosetron (Akynzeo) for preventing acute and delayed CINV following moderately or highly emetogenic chemotherapy.[39–41]

Chemotherapy-Induced Nausea and Vomiting

CINV is classified as: (a) acute (within 24 hours after chemotherapy); (b) delayed (greater than 24 hours after chemotherapy); or (c) anticipatory (prior to chemotherapy when acute or delayed

Table 20–3

Emetogenicity of Chemotherapeutic Agents[3,11,36]

Minimal Emetogenic Potential (< 10% Risk)[a]	Moderate Emetogenic Potential (30%–90% Risk)
Bevacizumab	Azacitidine
Bleomycin	Alemtuzumab
Busulfan	Bendamustine
Cetuximab	Carboplatin
Chlorambucil	Clofarabine
2-Chlorodeoxyadenosine	Cyclophosphamide < 1500 mg/m²
Erlotinib	Cytarabine > 1000 mg/m²
Fludarabine	Daunorubicin[b]
Hydroxyurea	Doxorubicin[b]
Pralatrexate	Epirubicin[b]
Rituximab	Idarubicin[b]
Vinblastine	Ifosfamide
Vincristine	Irinotecan
Vinorelbine	Oxaliplatin
Low Emetogenic Potential (10%–30% Risk)	**High Emetogenic Potential (> 90% Risk)**
Bortezomib	Carmustine
Cabazitaxel	Cisplatin
Catumaxomab	Cyclophosphamide 1500 mg/m² or more
Cytarabine 1 g/m² or less	Dactinomycin
Docetaxel	Dacarbazine
Doxorubicin liposome injection	Lomustine
Etoposide	Mechlorethamine
Fluorouracil	Pentostatin
Gemcitabine	Streptozotocin
Methotrexate	
Mitomycin	
Mitoxantrone	
Paclitaxel	
Panitumumab	
Premetrexed	
Temsirolimus	
Topotecan	
Trastuzumab	

[a]"% risk" is the incidence of emesis without the administration of antiemetics.

[b]Anthracyclines when combined with cyclophosphamide are considered high emetic risk.

Table 20–4

Recommended Drug Regimens for Prevention of CINV Based on Emetogenic Risk[3,11,30,38–41]

Emetogenic Risk	Acute CINV (Day 1)	Delayed CINV (Days 2–4)
Minimal	None	None
Low	Dexamethasone	None
Moderate	Palonosetron[a] + dexamethasone	Dexamethasone (days 2 and 3)
	Alternative regimen: Any 5-HT_3 antagonist + aprepitant[b,c] + dexamethasone	Aprepitant (days 2 and 3)
High (includes AC regimens)	Any 5-HT_3 antagonist + dexamethasone + aprepitant[b,c]	Aprepitant (days 2 and 3) + dexamethasone (days 2–3 or days 2–4)

AC, anthracycline (daunorubicin, doxorubicin, epirubicin, or idarubicin) plus cyclophosphamide; CINV, chemotherapy-induced nausea and vomiting.

[a]If palonosetron is not available, may substitute a first generation 5-HT_3 antagonist, preferably granisetron or ondansetron.

[b]If fosaprepitant 150 mg IV is substituted for oral aprepitant on day 1, subsequent aprepitant doses on days 2 and 3 are not required.

[c]Netupitant/palonosetron combination may be used instead of aprepitant and 5-HT_3 antagonist on day 1 with no subsequent doses required.

nausea and vomiting occurred with previous courses).[3,30] Risk factors for CINV include poor emetic control with prior chemotherapy, female sex, low chronic alcohol intake, and younger age.[30]

Chemotherapeutic agents are classified according to their emetogenic potential (Table 20–3), which aids in predicting CINV.[3,11,36] Risk factors for anticipatory nausea and vomiting include poor prior control of CINV and a history of motion sickness or NVP.[3]

KEY CONCEPT *A combination of antiemetics with different mechanisms of action is recommended to prevent acute CINV for patients receiving moderately or highly emetogenic chemotherapy,* (Table 20–4).[3,11,30] Patients receiving chemotherapeutic agents with low emetogenic potential should receive a corticosteroid as CINV prophylaxis, and those receiving chemotherapy with minimal emetogenic risk do not require prophylaxis.

Delayed nausea and vomiting is more difficult to prevent and treat. It occurs most often with cisplatin- and cyclophosphamide-based regimens, especially if delayed nausea and vomiting occurred with previous chemotherapy courses.[3,30] Patients who had poorly controlled acute CINV in the past are at greatest risk for delayed CINV.[3]

Oral and IV antiemetics can be equally effective for CINV, depending on patient characteristics such as ability to take oral medications, dosage form availability, and cost.[3] Patients undergoing chemotherapy should have antiemetics available to treat breakthrough nausea and vomiting even if prophylactic antiemetics were given.[3,30] A variety of antiemetics may be used, including lorazepam, dexamethasone, methylprednisolone, prochlorperazine, promethazine, metoclopramide, 5-HT_3 antagonists, and dronabinol. If breakthrough CINV occurs despite prophylaxis, treatment with an antiemetic with a different mechanism of action is recommended.

The best strategy for preventing anticipatory nausea and vomiting is to prevent acute and delayed CINV by using the most effective antiemetic regimens based on the emetogenic potential of the chemotherapy and patient factors. CINV should be aggressively prevented with the first cycle of therapy. If anticipatory nausea and vomiting occurs, benzodiazepines and behavioral therapy such as relaxation techniques are recommended.[3,11]

Postoperative Nausea and Vomiting

PONV is a common complication of surgery that can lead to delayed discharge and unanticipated hospitalization.[5] The overall incidence of PONV is 25% to 30%, but it can occur in 70% to 80% of high-risk patients.[5,6,8] Risk factors for PONV include patient factors (female sex, nonsmoking status, and history of PONV or

Patient Encounter 1

A 53-year-old woman with a new diagnosis of node-positive breast cancer is scheduled to begin chemotherapy with doxorubicin 50 mg/m², cyclophosphamide 500 mg/m², and docetaxel 75 mg/m².

PMH: Hypertension, type 2 diabetes mellitus x 2 years

SH: Smokes one pack per day; occasional alcohol use

FH: hypertension, dyslipidemia

Current Meds: Lisinopril 20 mg daily; metformin 1000 mg twice daily

VS: BP 132/82 mmg Hg, HR 80 beats/min, RR 16 breaths/min, T 98.6°F (37.0°C)

Labs: Serum creatinine 0.9 mg/dL (80 μmol/L), serum potassium 3.9 mEq/L (3.9 mmol/L), fasting blood glucose 103 mg/dL (5.7 mmol/L), A1C 7.1% (0.071; 54 mmol/mol Hb)

What is the emetogenic potential of this patient's new chemotherapy regimen?

What type of CINV is this patient at risk of experiencing with her first cycle of chemotherapy?

What treatment options are available for this patient?

motion sickness), anesthetic factors (volatile anesthetics, nitrous oxide, or intraoperative or postoperative opioids), and surgical factors (duration and type of surgery).[5–8]

The first step in preventing PONV is reducing baseline risk factors when appropriate.[5,6] For example, the incidence of PONV may be less with regional anesthesia than general anesthesia, and nonsteroidal anti-inflammatory drugs may cause less PONV than opioid analgesics.

KEY CONCEPT *Some agents should be administered prior to induction of anesthesia (aprepitant, palonosetron, dexamethasone) whereas others are more effective when administered at the end of surgery (droperidol, 5-HT$_3$ receptor antagonists). Scopalomine should be administered the evening prior to surgery or 2 hours prior to surgery.*[1,5,8] Aprepitant prevents PONV, but it is not more effective than other agents and is costly.[6] Combinations of antiemetics are recommended to prevent PONV for high-risk patients.[6] A 5-HT$_3$ antagonist plus droperidol or dexamethasone, or dexamethasone plus droperidol are effective combinations.[5,6] If PONV occurs despite appropriate prophylaxis, it should be treated with an antiemetic from a pharmacologic class not already administered.[6,8] If no prophylaxis was used, a low-dose 5-HT$_3$ antagonist should be used.[6,8]

Nausea and Vomiting of Pregnancy

KEY CONCEPT *Nausea and vomiting affect the majority of pregnant women; the teratogenic potential of the therapy is the primary consideration in drug selection.*[9] Risks and benefits of any therapy must be weighed by the health care professional and the patient.

Pyridoxine (vitamin B$_6$) 10 to 25 mg four times daily alone or in combination with an antihistamine such as doxylamine is often used for NVP.[9,14] A combination product is available (Diclegis) with a recommended dose of two 10 mg/10 mg delayed-release tablets at bedtime. Pyridoxine is well tolerated, but doxylamine and other antihistamines may cause drowsiness.

For more severe NVP, promethazine, metoclopramide, and trimethobenzamide may be effective and have not been associated with teratogenic effects.[9,14] Ondansetron (pregnancy category B) has been used to treat severe NVP; animal data do not indicate a safety concern in pregnancy, but safety and efficacy data in humans for NVP are sparse.

Patient Encounter 2

A 27-year-old healthy woman seeks your advice. She is 10 weeks pregnant and complains of constant nausea, frequent vomiting, and weight loss. She does not smoke or drink alcohol. She has been taking prenatal vitamins since before her pregnancy and has tried avoiding provoking stimuli, eating frequent small meals, and avoiding spicy and fatty foods.

What type of nausea and vomiting is this patient experiencing?

What nonpharmacologic and pharmacologic treatment options may help prevent and treat this patient's nausea and vomiting?

Should this patient seek additional medical attention for her symptoms?

In rare instances (0.5%–2% of pregnancies), NVP progresses to hyperemesis gravidarum.[9] Enteral or parenteral nutrition may be required if weight loss occurs. A corticosteroid such as methylprednisolone may be considered. Because methylprednisolone is associated with oral clefts in the fetus when used during the first trimester, corticosteroids should be reserved as a last resort and should be avoided during the first 10 weeks of gestation.[9,14]

Motion Sickness and Vestibular Disturbances

Nausea and vomiting can be caused by disturbances of the vestibular system in the inner ear because of infection, trauma, neoplasm, or motion.[12] Patients may experience dizziness and vertigo in addition to nausea and vomiting. If a patient is susceptible to motion sickness, preventive measures include minimizing exposure to movement, restricting visual activity, ensuring adequate ventilation, reducing the magnitude of movement, and taking part in distracting activities.[12]

KEY CONCEPT *Because the vestibular system is replete with muscarinic type cholinergic and histaminic (H$_1$) receptors, anticholinergics and antihistamines are the most commonly used agents to prevent and treat motion sickness.* Oral medications should be taken prior to motion exposure to allow time for adequate absorption. Once

Patient Encounter 3

A 29-year-old woman who presents to your practice is planning a 14-day Mediterranean cruise. She does not have a significant past medical history and is taking levonorgestrel 100 mcg–ethinyl estradiol 20 mcg daily for contraception. She has experienced nausea and vomiting during boat rides in the past and is seeking your advice.

What recommendations for nonpharmacologic interventions would you give this patient to help prevent motion sickness?

What are the pharmacologic options for this patient to prevent or treat nausea and vomiting?

What potential adverse effects would you counsel this patient about?

Patient Care Process

Patient Assessment:

- Obtain a thorough patient history including the prescription, nonprescription, and herbal medications being used. Identify any substances that may be causing or worsening nausea and vomiting.
- Identify the underlying cause of the nausea and vomiting and eliminate it if possible.
- Assess the patient to determine whether the nausea and vomiting is simple or complex and whether patient-directed therapy is appropriate.

Therapy Evaluation:

- Determine which treatments for nausea and vomiting have been used in the past and their degree of efficacy.

Care Plan Development:

- Counsel the patient to avoid known triggers.
- Develop a treatment plan with the patient and other health care professionals if appropriate.
- Choose treatments based on the underlying cause of nausea and vomiting, duration and severity of symptoms, comorbid conditions, medication allergies, presence of contraindications, risk of drug–drug interactions, and adverse-effect profiles.
- Use the oral route for mild nausea with minimal or no vomiting. Seek an alternative route (eg, transdermal, rectal, parenteral) if the patient is unable to retain oral medications due to vomiting.
- Provide patient education regarding causes of nausea and vomiting, avoidance of triggers, potential complications, treatment options, medication adverse effects, and when to seek medical attention.
- Educate the patient about nonpharmacologic measures such as stimulus avoidance, dietary changes, acupressure or acupuncture, and psychotherapy.

Follow-Up Evaluation:

- To assess efficacy, ask the patient whether nausea or vomiting is resolving with therapy. Assess whether treatment failure is due to inappropriate medication use or the need for additional or different treatments and proceed accordingly.
- Assess adverse effects by asking the patient what he or she has experienced. Patient observation or examination is also useful for diagnosing adverse effects such as EPS.

nausea and vomiting due to motion sickness occur, oral medication absorption may be unreliable, making the therapies ineffective. Transdermal scopolamine may be helpful for patients who cannot tolerate oral medications or who require treatment for a prolonged period.[18] Drowsiness and reduced mental acuity are the most bothersome side effects of antihistamines and anticholinergics. Visual disturbances, dry mouth, and urinary retention can also occur.

OUTCOME EVALUATION

- The symptoms of simple nausea and vomiting are self-limited or relieved with minimal treatment. Monitor patients for adequate oral intake and alleviation of nausea and vomiting.
- Patients with complex nausea and vomiting may have malnourishment, dehydration, and electrolyte abnormalities.
- If the patient has weight loss, assess whether enteral or parenteral nutrition is needed.
- Assess for dry mucous membranes, skin tenting, tachycardia, and lack of axillary moisture to determine if dehydration is present.
- Obtain blood urea nitrogen (BUN), serum creatinine (SCr), calculated fractional excretion of sodium (FeNa), serum electrolytes, and arterial blood gases.
- Ask patients to rate the severity of nausea.
- Monitor the number and volume of vomiting episodes.
- Ask patients about adverse effects to the antiemetics used. Use this information to assess efficacy and tailor the patient's antiemetic regimen.

Abbreviations Introduced in This Chapter

ASCO	American Society of Clinical Oncology
BUN	Blood urea nitrogen
CINV	Chemotherapy-induced nausea and vomiting
CNS	Central nervous system
CTZ	Chemoreceptor trigger zone
D_2	Dopamine type 2 receptor
EPS	Extrapyramidal symptoms
FeNa	Fractional excretion of sodium
GERD	Gastroesophageal reflux disease
GI	Gastrointestinal
H_1	Histamine type 1 receptor
5-HT_3	5-Hydroxytryptamine (serotonin) type 3 receptors
NK_1	Neurokinin type 1 receptors
NVP	Nausea and vomiting of pregnancy
PONV	Postoperative nausea and vomiting
SCr	Serum creatinine

REFERENCES

1. Quigley EM, Hasler WL, Parkman HP. AGA technical review on nausea and vomiting. Gastroenterology. 2001;120;263–286.
2. Proctor DD. Approach to the patient with gastrointestinal disease. In: Goldman L, Ausiello D, Arend W, et al., eds. Cecil Medicine: Expert Consult (Cecil Textbook of Medicine). 23rd ed. Philadelphia: Saunders; 2007.
3. Basch E, Prestrud AA, Hesketh PJ, et al. Antiemetics: American Society of Clinical Oncology clinical practice guideline update. J Clin Oncol. 2011;29:4189–4198.

4. Chepyala P, Olden KW. Nausea and vomiting. Curr Treat Options Gastroenterol. 2008;11:135–144.
5. Gan TJ, Diemunsch P, Habib AS, et al. Consensus guidelines for the management of postoperative nausea and vomiting. Anesth Analg. 2014;118:85–113.
6. Gan TJ, Meyer TA, Apfel CC, et al. Society for Ambulatory Anesthesia guidelines for the management of postoperative nausea and vomiting. Anesth Analg. 2007;105:1615–1628.
7. Apfel CC, Laara E, Koivuranta M, Greim CA, Roewer N. A simplified risk score for predicting postoperative nausea and vomiting: Conclusions from cross-validations between two centers. Anesthesiology. 1999;91:693–700.
8. Wilhelm SM, Dehoorne-Smith ML, Kale-Pradhan PB. Prevention of postoperative nausea and vomiting. Ann Pharmacother. 2007;41:68–78.
9. ACOG (American College of Obstetrics and Gynecology) Practice Bulletin: Nausea and vomiting of pregnancy. Obstet Gynecol. 2004;103:803–814. Reaffirmed 2009 http://www.guideline.gov/content.aspx?id=10939&search=nausea+vomiting+pregnancy (accessed July 7, 2014).
10. Case 31. In: Toy EC, Loose DS, Tischkau SA, Pillai AS, eds. Case Files™: Pharmacology, 3rd ed. New York, NY: McGraw-Hill; 2014. http://accesspharmacy.mhmedical.com, with permission. Accessed September 07, 2014.
11. Hesketh PJ. Chemotherapy-induced nausea and vomiting. N Engl J Med. 2008;358:2482–2494.
12. Shupak A, Gordon CR. Motion sickness: Advances in pathogenesis, prediction, prevention, and treatment. Aviat Space Environ Med. 2006;77:1213–1223.
13. DiPiro CV, Ignoffo RJ. Nausea and Vomiting. In: DiPiro JT et al, eds. Pharmacotherapy: A Pathophysiologic Approach, 9th ed. New York, NY: McGraw-Hill; 2014. www.accesspharmacy.com. Accessed June 16, 2014.
14. Niebyl JR, Briggs GG. The pharmacologic management of nausea and vomiting of pregnancy. J Fam Pract. 2014;63:S31–S37.
15. Miller KE, Muth ER. Efficacy of acupressure and acustimulation bands for the prevention of motion sickness. Aviat Space Environ Med. 2004;75:227–234.
16. Lee A, Fan LT. Stimulation of the wrist acupuncture point P6 for preventing postoperative nausea and vomiting. Cochrane Database Syst Rev. 2009(2):CD003281. doi: 10.1002/14651858.CD003281.pub3.
17. Spinks A, Wasiak J. Scopolamine (hyoscine) for preventing and treating motion sickness. Cochrane Database Syst Rev. 2011(6):CD002851. doi: 10.1002/14651858.CD002851.pub4.
18. Apfel CC, Zhang K, George E, et al. Transdermal scopolamine for the prevention of postoperative nausea and vomiting: a systematic review and meta-analysis. Clin Ther. 2010;32:1987–2002.
19. Cheung BS, Heskin R, Hofer KD. Failure of cetirizine and fexofenadine to prevent motion sickness. Ann Pharmacother. 2003;37:173–177.
20. Bles W, Bos JE, Kruit H. Motion sickness. Curr Opin Neurol. 2000;13:19–25.
21. Ernst AA, Weiss SJ, Park S, Takakuwa KM, Diercks DB. Prochlorperazine versus promethazine for uncomplicated nausea and vomiting in the emergency department: A randomized, double-blind clinical trial. Ann Emerg Med. 2000;36:89–94.
22. Habib AS, Gan TJ. The effectiveness of rescue antiemetics after failure of prophylaxis with ondansetron or droperidol: A preliminary report. J Clin Anesth. 2005;17:62–65.
23. Olsen JC, Keng JA, Clark JA. Frequency of adverse reactions to prochlorperazine in the ED. Am J Emerg Med. 2000;18:609–611.
24. Collins RW, Jones JB, Walthall JD, et al. Intravenous administration of prochlorperazine by 15-minute infusion versus 2-minute bolus does not affect the incidence of akathisia: A prospective, randomized, controlled trial. Ann Emerg Med. 2001;38:491–496.
25. MedWatch 2001 Safety Information Summaries: Inapsine (Droperidol). http://www.fda.gov/Safety/MedWatch/SafetyInformation/SafetyAlertsforHumanMedicalProducts/ucm173778.htm. Accessed July 22, 2014.
26. Rosow CE, Haspel KL, Smith SE, Grecu L, Bittner EA. Haloperidol versus ondansetron for prophylaxis of postoperative nausea and vomiting. Anesth Analg. 2008;106:1407–1409.
27. Masaoka T, Tack J. Gastroparesis: Current concepts and management. Gut Liver. 2009;3:166–173.
28. Stevens JE, Jone KL, Rayner CK, Horowitz M. Pathophysiology and pharmacotherapy of gastroparesis: Current and future perspectives. Expert Opin Pharmacother. 2013;14:1171–1186.
29. Lohr L. Chemotherapy-induced nausea and vomiting. Cancer J. 2008;14:85–93.
30. Minami M, Endo T, Hirafuji M, et al. Pharmacological aspects of anticancer drug-induced emesis with emphasis on serotonin release and vagal nerve activity. Pharmacol Ther. 2003;99:149–165.
31. Davis M, Maida V, Daeninck P, Pergolizzi J. The emerging role of cannabinoid neuromodulators in symptom management. Support Care Cancer. 2007;15:63–71.
32. Trigg ME, Higa GM. Chemotherapy-induced nausea and vomiting: antiemetic trials that impacted clinical practice. J Oncol Pharm Pract. 2010;16:233–244.
33. Smith HS, Cox LR, Smith EJ. 5-HT3 receptor antagonists for the treatment of nausea/vomiting. Ann Palliat Med. 2012;1:115–120.
34. Affronti ML, Bubalo J. Palonosetron in the management of chemotherapy-induced nausea and vomiting in patients receiving multiple-day chemotherapy. Cancer Manag Res. 2014:6;329–337.
35. Navari RM. Management of chemotherapy-induced nausea and vomiting: focus on newer agents and new uses for older agents. Drugs. 2013;73:249–262.
36. dos Santos LV, Souza FH, Brunetto AT, et al. Neurokinin-1 receptor antagonists for chemotherapy-induced nausea and vomiting: A systematic review. J Natl Cancer Inst. 2012;104:1280–1292.
37. Kovac AL. Update on the management of postoperative nausea and vomiting. Drugs. 2013;73:1525–1547.
38. Ruhlmann CH, Herrstedt J. Safety evaluation of aprepitant for the prevention of chemotherapy-induced nausea and vomiting. Expert Opin Drug Saf. 2011;10:449–462.
39. Gralla RJ, Bosnjak SM, Hontsa A, et al. A phase III study evaluating the safety and efficacy of NEPA, a fixed-dose combination of netupitant and palonosetron, for prevention of chemotherapy-induced nausea and vomiting over repeated cycles of chemotherapy. Ann Oncol. 2014;25(7):1333–1339.
40. Hesketh PJ, Rossi G, Rizzi G, et al. Efficacy and safety of NEPA, an oral combination of netupitant and palonosetron, for prevention of chemotherapy-induced nausea and vomiting following highly emetogenic chemotherapy: A randomized dose-ranging pivotal study. Ann Oncol. 2014;25(7):1340–1346.
41. Aapro M, Rugo H, Rossi G, et al. A randomized phase III study evaluating the efficacy and safety of NEPA, a fixed-dose combination of netupitant and palonosetron, for prevention of chemotherapy-induced nausea and vomiting following moderately emetogenic chemotherapy. Ann Oncol. 2014;25(7):1328–1333.

21 Constipation, Diarrhea, and Irritable Bowel Syndrome

Beverly C. Mims and Clarence E. Curry Jr

LEARNING OBJECTIVES

Upon completion of the chapter, the reader will be able to:

1. Identify the causes of constipation.
2. Compare the features of constipation with those of irritable bowel syndrome with constipation (IBS-C).
3. Recommend lifestyle modifications and pharmacotherapy for treatment of constipation.
4. Distinguish between acute and chronic diarrhea.
5. Compare and contrast diarrhea caused by different infectious agents.
6. Explain how medication use can cause diarrhea.
7. Discuss nonpharmacologic strategies for treating diarrhea.
8. Identify the signs and symptoms of IBS.
9. Contrast IBS with diarrhea (IBS-D) and IBS-C
10. Establish treatment goals for IBS.
11. Evaluate the effectiveness of pharmacotherapy for IBS.

CONSTIPATION

KEY CONCEPT *Constipation, when not associated with symptoms of irritable bowel syndrome (IBS), is a syndrome characterized by infrequent bowel movements (less than 3 stools per week) or difficult passage of stools, hard stools, or a feeling of incomplete evacuation.*[1–3] Occasional constipation usually does not require medical evaluation or treatment.

EPIDEMIOLOGY AND ETIOLOGY

Constipation affects all ages and occurs in approximately 16% of all adults and in one-third of adults age 60 and older.[1,4] Although constipation is rarely life threatening, it results in over 8 million physician visits, 1.1 million hospitalizations, and 5.3 million prescriptions annually.[5–7]

Non-whites, institutionalized elderly, and women are more prone to develop constipation. Some disease states and many medications are associated with constipation.[1,2] Constipation has significant socioeconomic costs and considerable quality-of-life ramifications.[8,9]

PATHOPHYSIOLOGY

Constipation can be due to primary and secondary causes (Table 21–1). Primary or idiopathic constipation is categorized as normal-transit constipation (NTC), slow-transit constipation (STC), or defecatory disorder constipation. In NTC, colonic motility is unchanged and patients experience hard stools despite normal movements. In STC, motility is decreased or caloric intake is inadequate, leading to infrequent, harder, drier stools. Defecatory disorders involve prolonged rectal storage of fecal residue or disorders of evacuation with normal or delayed colonic transit resulting in incomplete expulsion of feces from the rectum. Underlying causes may include inadequate relaxation of muscles or paradoxical contractions of the pelvic diaphragm, perineal membrane and deep perineal pouch (the pelvic floor) and the external anal sphincter during defecation.

Opioid-induced constipation (OIC) is defined as a change from baseline bowel habits after initiating opioid therapy that is characterized by any of the following: reduced bowel movement frequency, development or worsening of straining to pass bowel movements, a sense of incomplete bowel evacuation, or harder stool consistency.[10]

Functional constipation is defined as constantly problematic, infrequent, or seemingly incomplete defecation that does not meet IBS criteria.[4]

CLINICAL PRESENTATION AND DIAGNOSIS

Refer to the accompanying box for the clinical presentation of constipation.

Diagnosis

A complete history (including dietary and hydration habits) should be obtained to evaluate symptoms and confirm the diagnosis. Evaluation of psychosocial status is recommended because constipation may occur in patients who are depressed or in psychosocial distress. Other risk factors include age, terminal illness, travel, pregnancy, and neurological disorders. Family history

Table 21–1

Some Causes of Constipation

Primary Causes	
Normal-transit constipation	
Slow-transit constipation (motility disorders, inadequate caloric intake)	
Defecatory disorders (pelvic floor dysfunction)	
Secondary Causes (Selected)	
Endocrine/metabolic conditions (diabetes mellitus, hypercalcemia, hypokalemia, hypomagnesemia, hypothyroidism, uremia)	
Myopathies (amyloidosis, scleroderma)	
Neurogenic conditions (brain trauma, stroke, Parkinson disease, multiple sclerosis, spinal cord injury or tumor)	
Mechanical obstruction (colon cancer, lesion compression, stricture, rectocele)	
Medications (analgesics, anticholinergics, antidiarrheals, antihistamines, some antipsychotics and antidepressants, aluminum-containing products, calcium channel blockers, calcium-containing products, clonidine, diuretics, iron-containing supplements, ondansetron, phenothiazines)	
Other (autonomic neuropathy, cardiac disease, cognitive impairment, diet, immobility, laxative abuse, postponing urge to defecate, psychiatric conditions)	

should be assessed for presence of inflammatory bowel disease and colon cancer. A full record of prescription medications, over-the-counter products, and dietary supplements is mandatory to identify drug-related causes.

KEY CONCEPT *The diagnosis of constipation is made when two or more of the following diagnostic criteria occur for at least 3 of 6 months:*[1,2] *(a) straining on passage of stools, (b) lumpy or hard stools, (c) sensation of incomplete evacuation, (d) a feeling of anorectal obstruction or blockage, (e) need for manual maneuvers, and (f) fewer* than three defecations per week.[1]

Endoscopic evaluation is required in patients with weight loss, rectal bleeding, or anemia to exclude cancer or strictures, especially in patients older than 50 years. Anorectal examination, manometry, radiography, colonoscopy, and other procedures may be useful in certain circumstances.

In most cases, the physical examination is normal and no underlying cause of constipation is identified. Evaluation may also reveal one or more of the following conditions: (a) IBS with constipation (IBS-C) when there is bloating, abdominal pain, and incomplete defecation; (b) STC with normal pelvic floor function and evidence of slow transit; (c) a defecatory disorder; (d) a combination of IBS-C and STC; (e) organic constipation (mechanical obstruction or adverse drug effect); and (f) secondary constipation (metabolic disorder).[1]

Clinical Presentation of Constipation

Symptoms of Constipation

- Infrequent bowel movements (fewer than three per week; straining; lumpy or hard stools; painful or difficult defecation; bloating; sensation of incomplete evacuation, anorectal obstruction, or blockage; and need for manual maneuvers to facilitate defecations.
- Other complaints may include painful or difficult defecation, bloating, and absence of loose stools.
- Alarm (or red flag) findings include worsening of constipation, sudden change in bowel habits after age 50, blood in the stool, weight loss, family history of colon cancer, anemia, or recent constipation onset without explanation.

Laboratory Tests (To Identify Secondary Causes)

- Thyroid function tests (hypothyroidism)
- Serum calcium (may be increased or decreased)
- Glucose (diabetes mellitus)
- Serum electrolytes (dehydration, volume depletion)
- Urinalysis (dehydration)
- Complete blood count (anemia)

TREATMENT

Desired Outcomes

The primary goals are to: (a) identify underlying causes, (b) treat or remove secondary causes, (c) relieve symptoms, and (d) restore normal bowel function.[1–4]

Nonpharmacologic Therapy

Treatment of constipation depends on the characteristics and severity of symptoms. KEY CONCEPT *In most cases, lifestyle and dietary modifications should be employed prior to use of laxatives.* Each day most persons experience a strong peristaltic wave known as the gastrocolic reflex, and a bowel movement usually follows. The urge to have a bowel movement should not be ignored. Intentionally delaying bowel movements may lead to difficulty in passing stool.

Increased dietary fiber intake or fiber supplementation (total 20–35 g/day) can improve NTC, whereas patients with STC or drug-induced constipation are unlikely to respond to increased fiber. High-fiber foods include beans, whole grains, bran cereals, fresh fruits, and vegetables such as asparagus, brussels sprouts, cabbage, and carrots.

There are two types of fiber: soluble and insoluble. Soluble fiber is dissolved by water and forms a gel that slows digestion. Some sources of soluble fiber include lentils, apples, nuts, flaxseed, and psyllium. Insoluble fiber does not dissolve in water and remains mostly intact as it decreases the time at which food and feces traverse the intestines. Insoluble fiber adds bulk to the diet and helps prevent constipation. Some sources of insoluble fiber include whole wheat, corn bran, couscous, dark leafy green vegetables, and root vegetable skins.

Adequate fluid intake is important, especially in patients with evidence of dehydration; patients should be encouraged to drink when thirsty. The thirst mechanism changes with age; keeping a daily intake diary may assist patients who need to be reminded to drink fluids. Increased exercise may improve symptoms of constipation.[1,2] Limited data exist on the effect of probiotics in constipation.[1]

Biofeedback-aided pelvic floor training may be useful for treatment of defecatory disorders. Patients are guided to demonstrate the ability to coordinate abdominal and pelvic floor motion during evacuation.[1,11]

Surgery may be considered after all other approaches have failed and activities of daily living are compromised. Abdominal colectomy and ileorectal anastomosis may be considered in select patients with slow-transit constipation.[1]

Pharmacologic Therapy

KEY CONCEPT *Oral laxatives are the primary pharmacologic intervention for relief of constipation; several different drug classes are available* (Table 21–2).

▶ *Bulk Producers*

These agents are either naturally derived (psyllium), semisynthetic (polycarbophil), or synthetic (methylcellulose). They act by swelling in intestinal fluid, forming a gel that aids in fecal elimination and promoting peristalsis. They may cause flatulence (less commonly with methylcellulose) and abdominal cramping. Bulk-forming laxatives must be taken with sufficient water (8 oz or 240 mL/dose) to avoid becoming lodged in the esophagus and producing obstruction or worsening constipation. Hypersensitivity reactions may occur and rarely may be manifested as an anaphylactic reaction.

▶ *Hyperosmotics*

These products cause water to enter the lumen of the colon. Lactulose, sorbitol, and glycerin are osmolar sugars. Polyethylene glycol (PEG) 3350 with electrolytes is most useful for acute complete bowel evacuation prior to GI examination. PEG 3350 without electrolytes is useful in patients who are experiencing acute constipation or who have had inadequate response to other agents.[12] Lactulose acidifies colonic contents, increases water content of the gut, and softens the stool. Glycerin causes local irritation and possesses hyperosmotic action. Osmotic agents may cause flatulence, abdominal cramping, and bloating.

Sorbitol and glycerin may be administered rectally but can cause rectal discomfort and irritation. Oral sorbitol may affect blood glucose levels in diabetic patients.

▶ *Lubricants*

Lubricant laxatives coat the stool, allowing it to be expelled more easily. The oily film covering the stool also keeps the stool from losing its water to intestinal reabsorption processes. Oral mineral oil (liquid petrolatum) is a nonprescription heavy oil that should be used with caution, if at all, because it can be aspirated into the lungs and cause lipoid pneumonia. This is of particular concern in the young and elderly. It may also inhibit absorption of fat-soluble vitamins.

▶ *Stimulant Laxatives*

Diphenylmethane derivatives (eg, bisacodyl) and anthraquinones (eg, senna) have a selective action on the nerve plexus of intestinal smooth muscle leading to enhanced motility. Enteric-coated bisacodyl tablets should be swallowed whole to avoid gastric irritation and vomiting. Ingestion should be avoided within 1 to 2 hours of antacids, H_2-receptor antagonists, proton pump inhibitors, and milk. Bisacodyl oral tablets, rectal suppository, and enema products are available. The onset of effect is more rapid with rectal administration. The effects can be harsh (cramping), depending on the dose taken. Castor oil is used less frequently; it is pregnancy category X and is associated with uterine contractions and rupture. Use of castor oil in breastfeeding is considered "possibly unsafe."

▶ *Emollients*

Also known as surfactants and stool softeners, emollients (eg, salts of docusate) act by increasing the surface-wetting action on the stool leading to a softening effect. They reduce friction and make the stool easier to pass. The onset of action of stool

Table 21–2

Dosage Recommendations for Treatment of Constipation

Agent	Adults and Children Ages 12 and Over	Children Ages 6–11 Years
OTC Agents That Cause Softening of Feces in 1–3 Days		
Bulk-forming agents/osmotic laxatives		
Methylcellulose	4–6 g/day	0.45–1.5 g po per dose up to 3 g/day
Polycarbophil	4–6 g po daily	On advice of practitioner
Psyllium	Varies with product	On advice of practitioner
Emollients		
Docusate sodium	50–360 mg po daily	50–100 mg po daily
Docusate calcium	50–360 mg po daily	On advice of practitioner
Docusate potassium	100–300 mg po daily	100 mg po daily
Lactulose	15–30 mL po daily	7.5 mL (5 g) po daily
Sorbitol	30–50 g/day po daily	2 mL/kg (as 70% solution) po daily
Mineral oil	15–30 mL po daily	5–15 mL po daily
OTC Agents That Result in Soft or Semifluid Stool in 6–12 Hours		
Bisacodyl (oral)	5–15 mg po	5–10 mg (0.3 mg/kg) po
Senna	Dose varies with formulation	6–25 mg po once or twice daily
OTC Agents That Cause Watery Evacuation in 1–6 Hours or Less		
Magnesium citrate	120–300 mL po	100–150 mL po
Magnesium hydroxide[a]	30–60 mL po (15–30 mL of concentrate po)	2.5–5 mL po up to four times
Magnesium sulfate[a]	10–30 g po	5–10 g po
Bisacodyl (suppository)	10 mg rectally	5 mg rectally (1/2 suppository)
Polyethylene glycol–electrolyte preparations	Up to 4 L po	Safety and efficacy not established
RX Miscellaneous Agents for Treatment of Constipation		
Linaclotide	145 mcg po once daily	Safety and efficacy not established in patients under age 18; contraindicated in children < 6 years
Lubiprostone	24 mcg po twice daily with food and water	Safety and efficacy not established in children
Methylnaltrexone bromide	Given subcutaneously every other day: 12 mg if 62–114 kg, 8 mg if 38–61 kg; other doses based on weight if outside these parameters	Safety and efficacy not established in children
Naloxegol	25 mg po once daily in the morning on empty stomach	Safety and efficacy not established in children

[a]Magnesium can accumulate in renal dysfunction.

softeners is longer than with most stimulants and may take up to 72 hours. These agents tend to be less effective in treating constipation of long duration.

▶ *Saline Agents*

Salts of sodium, magnesium, and phosphate pull water into the lumen of the intestines resulting in increased enteral pressure. Magnesium and phosphate may accumulate in patients with renal dysfunction. Principal concerns with sodium phosphate derivatives include dehydration, hypernatremia, hyperphosphatemia, acidosis, hypocalcemia, and worsening renal function. Elderly individuals and patients with congestive heart failure and renal dysfunction should be advised to avoid saline agents. Nonprescription oral sodium phosphate solutions are no longer available because of the risk of acute phosphate nephropathy. Prescription oral phosphate products contain a black box warning about use in high-risk patients.

▶ *Intestinal Secretagogues*

Lubiprostone (Amitiza) This oral agent is derived from prostaglandin E_1 and acts locally on intestinal chloride channels to increase intestinal fluid secretion, resulting in increased intestinal motility and passage of stool. It is approved for treatment of chronic idiopathic constipation (CIC) and OIC in adults with chronic noncancer pain.[13,14] Efficacy and safety have not been established for constipation due to methadone (a diphenylheptane opioid derivative) or in children.[15,16] Adverse effects of lubiprostone include dyspnea, nausea, diarrhea, abdominal distention and pain, flatulence, vomiting, and loose stools.[13,14] Nausea may be minimized by taking lubiprostone with food. The capsule should be swallowed whole; it should not be chewed or broken apart. Lubiprostone is classified as pregnancy category C.

Linaclotide (Linzess) The parent compound and its active metabolite activate guanylate cyclase-C (GC-C) act locally by increasing intracellular and extracellular concentrations of cyclic guanosine monophosphate.[17] Cyclic GMP stimulates secretion of chloride and bicarbonate into the intestinal lumen, resulting in increased interstitial fluid and intestinal transit. Linaclotide is indicated for treatment of IBS-C and CIC in adults only.[18,19]

Linaclotide 145 mcg is administered once daily at least 30 minutes before the first meal of the day on an empty stomach (Table 21–3). Loose stools and greater stool frequency may occur after administration with a high-fat breakfast. The capsule should be swallowed whole and not be broken or chewed.[18]

Table 21–3

Selected Drugs and Substances That May Cause Acute Diarrhea

Drugs			
Antibiotics	Hydralazine	Metformin	Sorbitol
Colchicine	Laxatives	Misoprostol	Theophylline
Digitalis	Mannitol	Quinidine	Thyroid products
Dietary Supplements			
St. John's wort	Echinacea	Ginseng	Aloe vera
Poisons			
Arsenic	Cadmium	Mercury	Monosodium glutamate

Adverse effects of linaclotide include diarrhea, headache, fatigue, dehydration, abdominal pain, flatulence, and abdominal distention. Patients should be monitored for fluid and electrolyte loss. Linaclotide is classified as pregnancy category C.[18,19]

▶ *Peripherally Acting μ-opioid Receptor Antagonists (PAMORAs)*

Methylnaltrexone Bromide (Relistor) This agent is a selective antagonist of opioid binding at the μ-opioid receptor and is a quaternary derivative of naltrexone. It inhibits opioid-induced decrease in GI motility and transit time in patients with OIC. Methylnaltrexone bromide is indicated for OIC in patients with advanced illness, receiving palliative care, and who have experienced insufficient response to laxative therapy. Use beyond 4 weeks has not been studied.

The most common side effects are abdominal pain and cramping, flatulence, nausea, dizziness, hyperhidrosis, and diarrhea. Therapy should be discontinued if persistent, severe, or worsening abdominal symptoms occur.[20] It is classified as pregnancy category B.

Naloxegol (Movantik) This is the first orally administered medication approved by the FDA for treatment of OIC in adults with chronic noncancer pain.[21] Naloxegol is a pegylated naloxone molecule. It is classified as a schedule II controlled substance because it is structurally related to noroxymorphone, a metabolite of oxycodone.[22] Naloxegol is effective in patients who have taken opioids for at least 4 weeks. Use beyond 4 weeks has not been studied. Naloxegol is contraindicated in patients with GI obstruction and in patients receiving strong CYP3A4 inhibitors (eg, clarithromycin, itraconazole, ketoconazole) and should be avoided in patients taking moderate CYP3A4 inhibitors (eg, diltiazem, erythromycin, verapamil). Maintenance laxative therapy should be discontinued before starting naloxegol, but it can be resumed if patients have ongoing constipation.

Naloxegol should be administered on an empty stomach at least 1 hour prior to the first meal of the day or 2 hours after the meal. Tablets should be swallowed whole, and patients should be instructed to avoid consumption of grapefruit and grapefruit juice. Concomitant use with other opioid antagonists can result in additive adverse effects and should be avoided. If opioid therapy is discontinued, naloxegol should also be stopped.

Adverse effects of naloxegol include abdominal pain, GI perforation, diarrhea, nausea, flatulence, vomiting and headache. Naloxegol is pregnancy category C.[21–24]

Patients physically dependent on opioids may experience an opioid withdrawal syndrome when given opioid antagonists.[20,24] Postmarketing studies of potential adverse cardiovascular events of naloxegol are expected.[25]

Treatment Recommendations

The conventional effective, safe, and inexpensive modalities (fluid intake; dietary and supplemental fiber; stool softeners; and saline, stimulant, or osmotic laxatives) should be attempted before agents such as secretagogues or PAMORAs are prescribed. μ-Receptor antagonists are indicated only for treatment of OIC.

Patients who are not constipated but need to avoid straining (eg, patients with hemorrhoids, hernia, or myocardial infarction) may benefit from stool softeners or mild laxatives such as PEG 3350.

Pregnant women should be advised to eat regular meals that are balanced among fruits, vegetables, and whole grains and

Patient Encounter 1

A 45-year-old man requests a recommendation for treatment of constipation. Review of his medication profile reveals the following: hydrocodone/acetaminophen 10 mg/325 mg every 4 to 6 hours as needed for pain, clonidine 0.2 mg three times daily and hydrochlorothiazide 25 mg daily for hypertension, simvastatin 20 mg each evening for dyslipidemia, omeprazole 20 mg daily for gastroesophageal reflux disease, and bupropion-SR 150 mg twice daily for smoking cessation.

What general approach to this patient should be employed?

What are the possible contributing causes of his constipation?

What nonpharmacologic and pharmacologic therapies would be appropriate for his condition?

maintain adequate water intake to avoid constipation. Bulk producers and stool softeners (pregnancy category C) are probably safe during pregnancy because they are poorly absorbed. Lactulose and magnesium products are pregnancy category B. Magnesium-based antacids are not classified into pregnancy categories but have minimal absorption and are considered low risk in pregnant women. Long-term use of magnesium citrate should be avoided (pregnancy category B). Laxatives may provide relief for constipation occurring during the postpartum period when the mother is not breastfeeding.

Laxatives should not be given to children younger than 6 years unless prescribed by a physician. Because children may not be able to describe their symptoms well, they should be evaluated by a health care provider before being given a laxative. Evaluation of the patients' ability to recognize and self-report constipation symptoms should be considered. Treating secondary causes may resolve constipation without use of laxatives. As in adults, children benefit from a balanced diet and adequate water intake.

Because many elderly persons experience constipation, laxative use is sometimes viewed as a normal part of daily life. However, oral ingestion of mineral oil can present a particular hazard to bedridden elderly persons because it can lead to pneumonia via inhalation of oil droplets. Lactulose may be a better choice in this situation. Regular use of any laxative that affects fluid and electrolytes may result in significant adverse effects.

Patients with the following conditions should use laxatives only under the supervision of a health care provider: (a) colostomy; (b) diabetes mellitus (some laxatives contain sugars such as dextrose, galactose, and/or sucrose); (c) heart disease (some products contain sodium); (d) kidney disease; and (e) swallowing difficulty (bulk-formers may produce esophageal obstruction).

OUTCOME EVALUATION

- Ask the patient about symptom improvement to determine effectiveness of laxative therapy. Patients should have an increase in stool frequency to three or more well-formed stools per week. Patients should report reduced defecation time or absence of excessive straining.
- When acute overuse or chronic misuse of saline or stimulant laxatives is suspected, electrolyte disturbances should be evaluated (eg, hypokalemia, hypernatremia, hyperphosphatemia, hypocalcemia).
- Some laxatives (eg, bulk producers) contain significant amounts of sodium or sugar and may be unsuitable for salt-restricted or diabetic patients. Monitoring of fluid retention (edema) and blood pressure changes is indicated in patients on sodium-restricted diets. Glucose monitoring may be required in diabetic patients with chronic use. Use of low-sodium or sugar-free products may be indicated.
- Saline laxatives containing magnesium, potassium, or phosphates should be used cautiously in persons with reduced kidney function. Monitor appropriate serum electrolyte concentrations in patients with unstable renal function evidenced by changing serum creatinine or creatinine clearance.
- All laxatives are contraindicated in patients with undiagnosed abdominal pain, nausea, or vomiting. Patients should consult their health care providers if changes in bowel habits persist for more than 14 days or if laxative use for 7 or more days results in no effect.

Patient Care Process for Constipation

Patient Assessment:

- Assess symptoms to determine if patient-directed therapy is appropriate or whether the patient should be evaluated by a physician. Determine type, frequency, and duration of symptoms; presence or absence of abdominal pain; and exclude the presence of alarm symptoms.
- Review available information to determine potential causes and type of constipation. List factors that seem to make it better or worse. Assess dietary habits, fluid intake, and level of physical activity. Use of bowel and medication diary may help identify patterns. Use of the Bristol Stool Form Scale may be considered.

Therapy Evaluation:

- Obtain a thorough history of prescription, nonprescription, and dietary supplement use. Determine what treatments have been helpful in the past, whether the patient is taking any medications that may contribute to constipation, usual diet, and fluid intake. Assess for the presence of adverse drug reactions, drug allergies, and drug interactions.

Care Plan Development:

- Recommend administration of soluble dietary fiber such as psyllium, then an osmotic agent such as PEG, then a magnesium-based or stimulant/stool softener-based product.
- Provide patient education about constipation, dietary modifications, and drug therapy. Consider asking, "Do you take the time to have a bowel movement?"

Follow-Up Evaluation:

- Advise the patient about when to expect onset of relief and that if symptoms continue or worsen to seek further medical attention.
- Develop a plan to assess the effectiveness of laxative use in cases of functional constipation.

DIARRHEA

Like constipation, diarrhea is a symptom of an underlying disorder, not a disease itself. It is characterized by increased stool frequency (usually greater than three times daily), stool weight, liquidity, and decreased consistency of stools compared with an individual's usual pattern. Acute diarrhea is defined as diarrhea lasting for 14 days or less. Diarrhea lasting more than 30 days is called chronic diarrhea. Illness of 15 to 30 days is referred to as persistent diarrhea.

EPIDEMIOLOGY AND ETIOLOGY

Most cases of diarrhea in adults are mild and resolve quickly. Infants and children (especially less than 3 years) are highly susceptible to the dehydrating effect of diarrhea, and its occurrence in this age group should be taken seriously.

Acute Diarrhea

The terms *acute diarrhea* and *acute gastroenteritis* are not synonymous because diarrheal events do not invariably produce enteritis or involve the stomach. Acute diarrhea has many possible causes, but infection is the most common. Infectious diarrhea occurs because of transmission of contaminated food and water via the fecal–oral route.

Viruses cause a large proportion of cases; common culprits include Rotavirus, Norwalk, and adenovirus. Bacterial causes include *Escherichia coli*, *Salmonella* species, *Shigella* species, *Vibrio cholerae,* and *Clostridium difficile*. The term *dysentery* describes some of these bacterial infections when associated with serious occurrences of bloody diarrhea.

Acute diarrheal conditions can also result from parasites and protozoa such as *Entamoeba histolytica*, *Microsporidium*, *Giardia lamblia*, and *Cryptosporidium parvum*. Most of these infectious agents can cause traveler's diarrhea, a common malady afflicting travelers worldwide. It usually occurs during or just after travel following ingestion of fecally contaminated food or water. It has an abrupt onset but usually subsides within 2 to 3 days.

Noninfectious causes of acute diarrhea include drugs and toxins (Table 21–3), laxative abuse, food intolerance, IBS, inflammatory bowel disease, ischemic bowel disease, lactase deficiency, Whipple disease, pernicious anemia, diabetes mellitus, malabsorption, fecal impaction, diverticulosis, and celiac sprue.

Lactose intolerance is responsible for many cases of acute diarrhea, especially in persons of African descent, Asians, and Native Americans. Possible food-related causes include fat substitutes, dairy products, and products containing nonabsorbable carbohydrates.

The diarrhea of IBS is sudden, perhaps watery but likely loose, usually accompanied by urgency, bloating, and abdominal pain often in the morning or immediately following a meal. Inflammatory bowel disease is typically associated with the sudden onset of bloody diarrhea accompanied by urgency, crampy abdominal pain, and fever. Patients who experience bowel ischemia may develop bloody diarrhea, particularly if they progress to shock.

Chronic Diarrhea

Most cases of chronic diarrhea result from functional or inflammatory bowel disorders, endocrine disorders, malabsorption syndromes, and drugs (including laxative abuse). Daily watery stools may not occur with chronic diarrhea. Diarrhea may be either intermittent or continual.

PATHOPHYSIOLOGY

Approximately 9 L (2.4 gallons) of fluid normally traverse the GI tract daily. Of this amount, 2 L represent gastric juice, 1 L is saliva, 1 L is bile, 2 L are pancreatic juice, 1 L is intestinal secretions, and 2 L are ingested. Of the 9 L of fluid presented to the intestine, only about 150 to 200 mL remain in the stool after reabsorptive processes occur.

Any event that increases the amount of fluid retained in the stool may result in diarrhea. Large-stool diarrhea often signifies small intestinal involvement, whereas small-stool diarrhea usually originates in the colon. Diarrhea may be classified according to pathophysiologic mechanisms, including osmotic, secretory, inflammatory, and altered motility.

Osmotic diarrhea results from the intake of unabsorbable, water-soluble solutes in the intestinal lumen leading to water retention. Common causes include lactose intolerance and ingestion of magnesium-containing antacids.

Secretory diarrhea results from increased movement (secretion) of ions into the intestinal lumen, leading to increased intraluminal fluid. Medications, hormones, and toxins may be responsible for secretory activity.

Inflammatory (or exudative) diarrhea results from changes to the intestinal mucosa that damage absorption processes leading to increased proteins and other products in the intestinal lumen with fluid retention. The presence of blood or fecal leukocytes in the stool indicates an inflammatory process. The diarrhea of inflammatory bowel disease fits this classification.

Increased motility results in decreased contact time of ingested food and drink with the intestinal mucosa, leading to reduced reabsorption and increased fluid in the stool. Diarrhea resulting from altered motility is often established after other mechanisms have been excluded. IBS-related diarrhea is due to altered motility.

Diarrhea may be attributed to a single or multiple overlapping mechanisms. For example, malabsorption syndromes and traveler's diarrhea are associated with both secretory and osmotic mechanisms.

Drug-induced diarrhea can occur by several mechanisms. First, water can be drawn into the intestinal lumen osmotically (eg, saline laxatives). Second, the intestinal bacterial ecosystem can be upset leading to emergence of invasive pathologic organisms triggering secretory and inflammatory processes (eg, antibiotic use). Third, altered motility may occur with drugs such as tegaserod maleate. Other drugs produce diarrhea through undetermined mechanisms (eg, procainamide, colchicine). Discontinuation of the offending drug may be the only measure needed to ameliorate diarrhea.

CLINICAL PRESENTATION AND DIAGNOSIS

Refer to the accompanying box for the clinical presentation of diarrhea.

Diagnosis

Patients with diarrhea should be questioned about the onset of symptoms, recent travel, diet, source of water, and medication use. Other important considerations include duration and severity of the diarrhea and the presence of abdominal pain or vomiting; blood in the stool; stool consistency, appearance, and frequency; and weight loss. Although most cases of diarrhea are self-limited, infants, children, elderly persons, and immunocompromised patients are at risk for increased morbidity.

Clinical Presentation of Diarrhea

Signs and Symptoms of Acute Diarrhea

- Acute diarrhea presents abruptly as loose, watery, or semiformed stools.
- Abdominal cramps and tenderness, rectal urgency, nausea, bloating, and fever may be present.
- Patients infected with invasive organisms may have bloody stools and severe abdominal pain.

Laboratory Tests in Acute Diarrhea

- Stool cultures can help identify infectious causes. Methods using real-time polymerase chain reaction shorten the reporting time.
- Stool may be analyzed for mucus, fat, osmolality, fecal leukocytes, and pH. Mucus fragments suggest colonic involvement; fat in the stool suggests malabsorption. Fecal leukocytes are present in inflammatory diarrheas including bacterial infections. Stool pH (normally greater than 6) is decreased by bacterial fermentation processes.
- Assessment of stool volume and electrolytes in large-volume watery stools may identify osmotic or secretory diarrhea.
- CBC and blood chemistries may be helpful when symptoms persist. Findings of anemia, leukocytosis, or neutropenia offer further clues to the underlying cause.

Signs and Symptoms of Chronic Diarrhea

- Presenting symptoms may be severe or mild. Weight loss can be demonstrated, and weakness may be present.
- Dehydration may manifest as decreased urination, dark-colored urine, dry mucous membranes, increased thirst, and tachycardia.

Laboratory Tests in Chronic Diarrhea

- Tests described for acute diarrhea are also useful to diagnose chronic diarrhea; the differential diagnosis is more complicated. Results can help categorize the diarrhea as watery, inflammatory, or fatty, narrowing the focus on a primary disorder.
- Colonoscopy allows visualization, and biopsy of the colon and is preferred when there is blood in the stool or if the patient has acquired immune deficiency syndrome.

Findings on physical examination can assist in determining hydration status and disease severity. The presence of blood in the stool suggests an invasive organism, an inflammatory process, or perhaps a neoplasm. Large-volume stools suggest a small-intestinal disorder, whereas small-volume stools suggest a colon or rectal disorder. Patients with prolonged or severe symptoms may require colonoscopic evaluation to identify the underlying cause.

TREATMENT

Acute diarrhea is generally self limited, lasting 3 to 4 days even without treatment. Most healthy adults with diarrhea do not develop significant dehydration or other complications and can self-medicate symptomatically if necessary. KEY CONCEPT *Dehydration can occur when diarrhea is severe and oral intake is limited, particularly in the elderly and infants.* Other complications of diarrhea resulting from fluid loss include electrolyte disturbances, metabolic acidosis, and cardiovascular collapse.

Children are more susceptible to dehydration (particularly when vomiting occurs) and may require medical attention early in the course, especially if younger than 3 years. Physician intervention is also necessary for elderly patients who are sensitive to fluid loss and electrolyte changes due to concurrent chronic illness.

Patients should undergo medical evaluation in the following circumstances: (a) moderate to severe abdominal tenderness, distention, or cramping; (b) bloody stools; (c) evidence of dehydration (eg, thirst, dry mouth, fatigue, dark-colored urine, infrequent urination, reduced urine, dry skin, reduced skin elasticity, rapid pulse, rapid breathing, muscle cramps, muscle weakness, sunken eyes, or lightheadedness); (d) high fever (38.3°C or 101°F or higher); (e) evidence of weight loss greater than 5% of total body weight; and (f) diarrhea that lasts longer than 48 hours.

Desired Outcomes

The goals of treatment for diarrhea are to relieve symptoms, maintain hydration, treat the underlying cause(s), and maintain nutrition. KEY CONCEPT *The primary treatment of acute diarrhea includes fluid and electrolyte replacement, dietary modifications, and drug therapy.*

Nonpharmacologic Therapy

▶ *Fluid and Electrolytes*

Fluid replacement is not a treatment to relieve diarrhea but rather an attempt to restore fluid balance. In many parts of the world where diarrheal states are frequent and severe, fluid replacement is accomplished using **oral rehydration solution** (ORS), a measured mixture of water, salts, and glucose. The solution recognized by the World Health Organization consists of 75 mEq/L (75 mmol/L) sodium, 75 mmol/L glucose, 65 mEq/L (65 mmol/L) chloride, 20 mEq/L (20 mmol/L) potassium, and 10 mEq/L (3.3 mmol/L) citrate, having a total osmolarity of 245 mOsm/L. A simple solution can be prepared from 1 L water mixed with eight teaspoonfuls of sugar and one teaspoonful of table salt. Some commercial products include Pedialyte, Rehydralyte, and CeraLyte.

Consistent intake of water (perhaps by slowly sipping), along with eating as tolerated, should restore lost fluids and salt for typical diarrhea sufferers. Patients may also replace lost fluid by drinking flat soft drinks such as ginger ale, tea, fruit juice, broth, or soup. Although sports drinks may be used to treat dehydration, caution should be exercised so they are not viewed as a casual panacea. Severe diarrhea may require use of parenteral solutions, and parenteral products should be used if patients are vomiting or unconscious.[26]

▶ *Dietary Modifications*

During an acute diarrheal episode, patients typically eat less as they focus on the diarrhea. Both children and adults should attempt to maintain nutrition because food helps replete lost nutrients and fluid volume. However, food-related fluid may not be sufficient to compensate for diarrheal losses. Some foods may be inappropriate if they irritate the GI tract or if they are implicated as the cause of the diarrhea. Patients with chronic diarrhea may find that increasing bulk in the diet may help (eg, rice, bananas, whole wheat, and bran).

Table 21–4

Pharmacotherapy for Diarrhea

Drug	Usual Oral Dose	Type of Diarrhea
Attapulgite	Adults: 1200–1500 mg after each loose stool. Maximum: 9000 mg in 24 hours Children 6–12 years: 750 mg after each loose stool. Maximum: 4500 mg in 24 hours	Acute and chronic
Calcium polycarbophil	Adults: 1000 mg four times daily or after each loose stool, not to exceed 12 tablets per day Children 6–12 years: 500 mg three times daily Children 3–6 years: 500 mg twice daily	Chronic
Loperamide	Adults: 4 mg initially, then 2 mg after each subsequent loose stool. Maximum: 16 mg in 24 hours Children maximum doses: Age 2–5: 3 mg Age 6–8: 4 mg Age 8–12: 6 mg	Acute and chronic
Diphenoxylate/atropine	Adults: Two tablets (5 mg) initially, then one tablet every 3–4 hours, not to exceed 20 mg in 24 hours Children 2–12 years: Oral solution (avoid tablets) 0.3–0.4 mg/kg/day in divided doses. Do not administer to children younger than 2 years	Acute and chronic
Bismuth subsalicylate	Adults: 30 mL (regular strength) or two tablets, repeated every 30–60 minutes as needed. Maximum: eight doses daily Children: Consumers should speak with a physician before giving to children under 12 years of age	Traveler's and nonspecific acute diarrhea

Pharmacologic Therapy

The goal of drug therapy is to control symptoms, enabling the patient to continue with as normal a routine as possible while avoiding complications (Table 21–4). Most infectious diarrheas are self-limited or curable with anti-infective agents.

▶ *Adsorbents and Bulk Agents*

Attapulgite adsorbs excess fluid in the stool with few adverse effects. Formulations of attapulgite are available in Canada but not within the United States. Calcium polycarbophil is a hydrophilic polyacrylic resin (widely available in the United States) that also works as an adsorbent, binding about 60 times its weight in water and leading to formation of a gel that enhances stool formation. Neither attapulgite nor polycarbophil is systemically absorbed. Calcium polycarbophil is effective in reducing fluid in the stool. However, caution must be exercised because it can also adsorb nutrients and other medications, thereby reducing their benefits. Its administration should be separated from other oral medications by 2 to 3 hours. Psyllium and methylcellulose products may also be used to reduce fluid in the stool and relieve chronic diarrhea.

▶ *Antiperistaltic (Antimotility) Agents*

Antiperistaltic drugs prolong intestinal transit time, thereby reducing the amount of fluid lost in the stool. The two drugs in this category are loperamide HCl (available over-the-counter as Imodium A–D and generically) and diphenoxylate HCl with atropine sulfate (available by prescription as Lomotil and generically). The atropine is included only as an abuse deterrent; when taken in large doses, the unpleasant anticholinergic effects of atropine negate the euphoric effect of diphenoxylate. Both loperamide and diphenoxylate are effective in relieving symptoms of acute noninfectious diarrhea and are safe for most patients experiencing chronic diarrhea. These products should be discontinued in patients whose diarrhea worsens despite therapy.

▶ *Antisecretory Agents*

Bismuth subsalicylate (BSS) is thought to have antisecretory and antimicrobial effects and is used to treat acute diarrhea. Although it passes largely unchanged through the GI tract, the salicylate portion is absorbed in the stomach and small intestine. For this reason, BSS should not be given to people who are allergic to salicylates, including aspirin. Caution should be exercised with regard to the total dose given to patients taking salicylates for other reasons to avoid salicylism. Patients taking BSS should be informed that their stool will turn black.

Octreotide is an antisecretory agent used for severe secretory diarrhea associated with cancer chemotherapy, human immunodeficiency virus, diabetes, gastric resection, and GI tumors. It is administered as a subcutaneous or IV bolus injection in an initial dose of 50 mcg three times daily to assess the patient's

Patient Encounter 2

A 63-year-old woman who works as a kindergarten bus driver and school aide visits an urgent care clinic 1 week after the fall school year begins complaining of fatigue, nausea, vomiting, episodes of mild abdominal pain, and frequent watery stools. She states that she has been thirstier than usual and her saliva has been thick and sticky. She also states that her heart was racing after her evening walk the night before. She was "excited to see her kids again" but she hasn't felt well for the past 2 or 3 days. She stopped drinking an herbal tea she enjoyed that a friend gave her. Her temperature at home last night was 100°F (37.8°C). Other than arthritic knees and elbows, she is healthy and reports no known allergies; she recently began taking vitamin C to "improve resistance to infections."

Assess the likelihood that her diarrhea is due to an invasive microorganism.

Identify which of her symptoms suggest the presence of dehydration.

Discuss potential treatment measures for this woman.

tolerance to GI adverse effects. Possible adverse effects include nausea, bloating, pain at the injection site, and gallstones (with prolonged therapy).

▶ *Probiotics*

Probiotics are dietary supplements containing bacteria (*Lactobacillus* species, *Bifidobacterium* species, and others) that may promote health by enhancing the normal microflora of the GI tract while resisting colonization by potential pathogens. Probiotics can stimulate the immune response and suppress the inflammatory response. Probiotics can be taken in tablets, gummies, capsules, powders, and liquids. The type of product is not as important as the viability and number of organisms present.

Yogurt may provide relief from diarrhea due to lactose intolerance. The *Lactobacillus acidophilus* in yogurt, cottage cheese, and acidophilus milk improve digestion of lactose and may prevent or relieve diarrhea related to lactose deficiency and milk intake. Although lactase is not a probiotic, lactase tablets may also be used to prevent diarrhea in susceptible patients.

▶ *Antiinfectives*

Empiric antibiotic therapy is an appropriate approach to traveler's diarrhea. Eradication of the causal microbe depends on the etiologic agent and its antibiotic sensitivity. Most cases of traveler's diarrhea and other community-acquired infections result from enterotoxigenic (ETEC) or enteropathogenic *E. coli* (EPEC). Routine stool cultures do not identify these strains; primary empiric antibiotic choices include fluoroquinolones such as ciprofloxacin or levofloxacin. Azithromycin may be a feasible option when fluoroquinolone resistance is encountered. Rifaximin can also treat traveler's diarrhea effectively.

Although most cases of infectious diarrhea resolve with therapy, routine antibiotic use may contribute to antimicrobial resistance. Empiric treatment should be considered for other acute infectious diarrhea including those caused by nonhospital-acquired invasive organisms such as *Campylobacter, Salmonella,* and *Shigella* organisms producing moderate to severe fever, **tenesmus**, and bloody stools.

Shiga toxin-producing *E. coli* (STEC) O157 should not be treated with antibiotics or antimotility agents.[27] There is no evidence that antibiotic treatment is helpful, and antibiotic use with *E. coli* 0157 infection may increase the risk of a form of kidney failure called hemolytic-uremic syndrome (HUS).

OUTCOME EVALUATION

- Monitor the patient with diarrhea from the point of first contact until symptoms resolve, keeping in mind that most episodes are self-limiting.
- Question the patient to determine whether symptom resolution occurs within 48 to 72 hours in acute diarrhea.
- Monitor for the maintenance of hydration, particularly when symptoms continue for more than 48 hours. Ask about increased thirst, decreased urination, dark-colored urine, dry mucous membranes, and rapid heartbeat, which suggest dehydration especially when nausea and vomiting are present.
- Monitor for symptom control in patients with chronic diarrhea.
- When antibiotics are used, monitor for completion of the course of therapy.

Patient Care Process for Diarrhea

Patient Assessment:

- Determine symptoms, severity, frequency, and exacerbating factors.
- Assess hydration status.
- Assess symptoms to determine if patient-directed therapy is appropriate or a referral is needed.
- Inquire about recent foreign travel.
- Obtain history of prescription, nonprescription, and dietary supplement use.

Therapy Evaluation:

- Review current therapy as potential cause(s) of diarrhea.
- Determine if any diarrhea treatments have been attempted, including home remedies.
- Refer for medication evaluation if patient is pregnant, breastfeeding, younger than 3 years or older than 70 years, or has multiple medical conditions.

Care Plan Development:

- If home care is recommended, provide clear instructions about how to proceed if symptoms do not improve or new symptoms emerge.
- Discuss the importance of maintaining nutrition by diet modification.
- Educate the patient about: (a) acute and chronic diarrhea causes, (b) possible complications, (c) treatment goals, (d) the medication used to manage diarrhea, and (e) if appropriate, the circumstances when antibiotics are necessary.

Follow-Up Evaluation:

- Although most diarrheal episodes resolve with minimal intervention, individuals with a protracted course should be followed until symptoms have abated or are under control. Pay special attention to the very young, the aged, and those who are medically compromised.

IRRITABLE BOWEL SYNDROME

IBS is a disorder of the GI tract that interferes with the normal functions of the colon. IBS was previously preferred to as **mucous colitis, spastic colon**, irritable colon, or nervous stomach. KEY CONCEPT *IBS is described as a functional disorder, which means that it involves symptoms that cannot be attributed to a specific injury, infection, or other physical problem.* A functional disorder occurs because of altered physiologic processes rather than structural or biochemical defects and may be subject to nervous system influence. IBS is associated with frequent fluctuation in symptoms, loss of productivity, and decreased quality of life.

EPIDEMIOLOGY AND ETIOLOGY

IBS is one of the most common disorders seen in primary care and the most common reason for referral to gastroenterologists. Although between 15% and 20% of Americans suffer from IBS, only about one-quarter of those affected seek medical attention. The associated costs to society are estimated to be billions of dollars,[28] and the recurrent nature of IBS contributes to these costs through missed workdays, inattention on the job, and high consumption of health care services.

In the United States, IBS affects women about twice as often as men. However, this may simply reflect a greater tendency to seek medical care. IBS can occur at any age but is most common between 20 and 50 years; onset beyond age 60 is rare. However, prevalence for older adults is the same as for young persons. Prevalence is similar in whites and African Americans but may be lower in people of Hispanic origin. A genetic link is unproven, but IBS seems more common in certain families.

There is a strong association between emotional distress and IBS. Psychosocial trauma (eg, a history of abuse, recent death of a close relative or friend, or divorce) is more likely to be found in patients presenting with IBS than in the general population. An increased prevalence of psychiatric disorders such as anxiety, depression, personality disorders, and somatization occurs among adults with IBS. Alcohol consumption and smoking have not been shown to be risk factors for developing IBS.[29] However, alcohol may worsen symptoms in affected persons.

Some people show first evidence of IBS after contracting gastroenteritis (sometimes referred to as postinfectious IBS). This has led to speculation about whether infection heightens GI tract susceptibility. Menstrual periods may trigger symptoms in some women.

PATHOPHYSIOLOGY

Enteric nerves control intestinal smooth muscle action and are connected to the brain by the autonomic nervous system. IBS is thought to result from dysregulation of this "brain–gut axis." The enteric nervous system is composed of two ganglionated plexuses that control gut innervation: the submucous plexus (Meissner plexus) and the myenteric plexus (Auerbach plexus). The enteric nervous system and the central nervous system (CNS) are interconnected and interdependent. A number of neurochemicals mediate their function, including serotonin (5-hydroxytryptamine or 5-HT), acetylcholine, substance P, and nitric oxide, among others.

Serotonin is particularly important because the GI tract contains the largest amounts in the body. Two 5-HT receptor subtypes, 5-HT_3 and 5-HT_4, are involved in gut motility, visceral sensitivity, and gut secretion. The 5-HT_3 receptors slow colonic transit and increase fluid absorption, whereas 5-HT_4 receptor stimulation accelerates colonic transit.

Although no single pathologic defect accounts for the pattern of exacerbation and remission in IBS, CNS abnormalities, dysmotility, visceral hypersensitivity, and other factors have been implicated.[30]

The passage of fluids into and out of the colon is regulated by epithelial cells. In IBS, the colonic lining (epithelium) appears to function properly. However, increased movement of the contents in the colon can overwhelm its absorptive capacity. Disturbed intestinal motility appears to be a central feature of IBS, which leads to altered stool consistency. Studies suggest that the colon of IBS sufferers is abnormally sensitive to normal stimuli.[31] Enhanced visceral sensitivity manifests as pain, especially related to gut distention.

Some IBS patients demonstrate sensitivity to common foods such as wheat, beef, pork, soy, and eggs. Evidence suggests that an immune component may be involved in IBS patients who experience bloating and dysmotility-like dyspepsia and that gender specificity exists.[32]

CLINICAL PRESENTATION AND DIAGNOSIS

Refer to the accompanying box for the clinical presentation of IBS.

Diagnosis

KEY CONCEPT *The diagnosis of IBS is made by symptom-based criteria and the exclusion of organic disease.* IBS is diagnosed by obtaining a thorough history to distinguish the characteristic symptoms of IBS from other conditions having similar symptoms. Patients should be questioned about the frequency, consistency, color, and size of stools. Because of the functional nature of IBS, a patient may present with symptoms of upper GI problems such as gastroesophageal reflux disease or with excessive flatulence. Patients should also be questioned about diet to establish any symptom relationship to meals or specifically after consumption of certain foods.

Barium enema, sigmoidoscopy, or colonoscopy may be indicated in the presence of red flag symptoms (fever, weight loss, bleeding, and anemia, persistent severe pain), which often point to a potentially serious non-IBS problem. A barium enema may identify polyps, diverticulosis, tumors, or other abnormalities that might be responsible for the symptoms. Furthermore, barium enema may detect exaggerated haustral contractions, which can impede stool movement and contribute to constipation. Flexible sigmoidoscopy can identify obstructions in the rectum and lower colon, whereas colonoscopy can evaluate the entire colon for organic disease.

The Rome III diagnostic criteria define IBS as occurring when symptoms of recurrent abdominal pain or discomfort exist for at least 3 days/month in the last 3 months associated with two or more of the following: (a) improvement with defecation, (b) onset associated with a change in the frequency of stool, and/or (c) onset associated with a change in the form (appearance) of stool. These criteria should be fulfilled for the previous 3 months with symptom onset at least 6 months prior to diagnosis. The Rome II criteria presume the absence of a structural or biochemical explanation for the symptoms. IBS is unlikely if symptom onset occurs in old age, the disorder has a steady but aggressive course, or the patient experiences frequent awakening because of symptoms.

TREATMENT

Desired Outcomes

KEY CONCEPT *The principal goal of IBS treatment is to reduce or control symptoms.* The treatment strategy is based on: (a) the prevailing symptoms and their severity, (b) the degree of functional impairment, and (c) the presence of psychological components. See Figure 21–1 for a suggested algorithm for management of IBS. A standard treatment regimen is not possible because of the heterogeneous nature of the IBS patient population. Patients suffering from IBS can benefit from clinician support and reassurance.

Nonpharmacologic Therapy

▶ *Diet and Other General Modifications*

Dietary modification is a standard therapeutic modality. Food hypersensitivities and adverse effects have been associated with

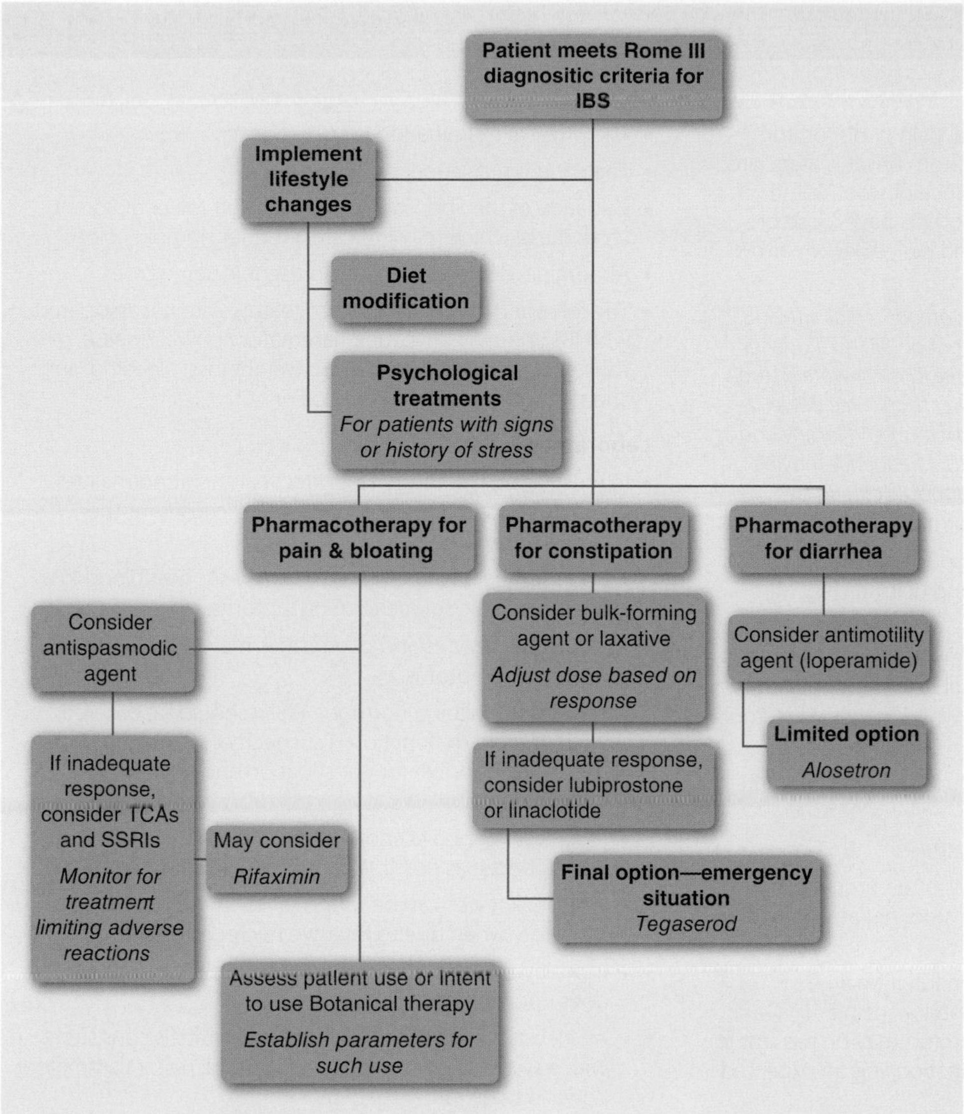

FIGURE 21–1. Algorithm for management of irritable bowel syndrome. IBS, irritable bowel syndrome; SSRI, selective serotonin reuptake inhibitor; TCA, tricyclic antidepressant.

IBS, especially IBS-D. Elimination diets are the most commonly used strategy, usually focusing on milk and dairy products, fructose and sorbitol, wheat, and beef. Flatulence may be controlled by reducing gas-causing foods (beans, celery, onions, prunes, bananas, carrots, and raisins). Response to elimination diets varies widely, but they may be useful in individual patients. Care should be taken to avoid nutritional deficits while attempting to eliminate offending foods.

The low FODMAP (fermentable oligosaccharides, disaccharides, monosaccharides and polyols) diet is said to control IBS symptoms in some patients. FODMAPS are carbohydrates that are poorly absorbed and quickly fermented (by bacterial action). The gas byproduct of the bacterial action is thought to contribute to IBS symptoms.[33]

Probiotics may also be an option for some patients with IBS. *Bifidobacterium infantis* is one product used for its effect in constipation, diarrhea, gaseousness, bloating, and abdominal discomfort. It has not been associated with significant untoward effects.[34] The usual dose is one 4-mg capsule daily.

▶ *Psychological Treatments*

Psychotherapy focused on reducing the influence of the CNS on the gut has been studied. Cognitive behavioral therapy (CBT), dynamic psychotherapy, relaxation therapy, and hypnotherapy have been effective in some patients. However, psychological approaches are not considered replacements for usual care.[35]

Pharmacologic Therapy

▶ *Agents for Pain and Bloating*

Botanicals Peppermint oil is widely advocated; it acts as an antispasmodic agent due to its ability to relax GI smooth muscle. However, it also relaxes the lower esophageal sphincter, which could allow reflux of gastric contents into the esophagus. The usual dose is one to two enteric-coated capsules containing 0.2 mL of peppermint oil two to three times daily. *Matricaria recutita,* known as German chamomile, is also purported to have antispasmodic properties. It is taken most often as a tea up to four times a day. Benzodiazepine, alcohol, and warfarin users should be cautioned against taking this product because it can cause drowsiness, and it contains coumarin derivatives.[36] Primrose oil is used by some patients, but evidence of effectiveness is lacking.

Antispasmodics Dicyclomine and hyoscyamine have been among the most frequently used medications for treating abdominal pain in patients with IBS (Table 21–5). Side effects include

Clinical Presentation of IBS

Symptoms

- Patients report a history of abdominal pain or discomfort that is relieved with defecation. Symptom onset is associated with change in frequency or appearance of stool. Some persons experience hard, dry stools; others have loose or watery stools. Stools may be small and pellet-like or narrow and pencil-like in appearance.
- KEY CONCEPT *Symptoms can typically be categorized as either IBS with diarrhea (IBS-D) or IBS with constipation (IBS-C). Patients with IBS-D usually report more than three loose or watery stools daily. Those with IBS-C usually have fewer than three bowel movements per week; stools are typically hard and lumpy and accompanied by straining. However, stool frequency may be normal in many cases. The Rome III diagnostic criteria (see* ***Diagnosis****) places emphasis on stool form.*
- Some patients report alternating episodes of diarrhea and constipation (IBS with constipation and diarrhea [IBS-M], where M represents mixed).
- Other common symptoms include: (a) feelings of incomplete evacuation, (b) abdominal fullness, (c) bloating, (d) flatulence, (e) passage of clear or white mucus with stool, and (f) occasional fecal incontinence.
- Periods of normal stools and bowel function are punctuated by episodes of sudden symptoms.
- Symptoms are often exacerbated by stress.
- Left lower quadrant abdominal pain is often brought on or made worse by eating. Passage of stool or flatus may provide some relief.
- IBS-C can often be distinguished from functional constipation by the presence of abdominal pain and discomfort. Although pain and discomfort may be present in some patients with functional constipation, it is an expected feature of IBS.
- Patients with IBS may experience comorbidities outside the GI tract such as fibromyalgia, sleep disturbances, headaches, dyspareunia, and temporomandibular joint syndrome.

Signs

- The physical examination is often normal in IBS.
- The patient may appear to be anxious.
- Palpation of the abdomen may reveal left lower quadrant tenderness, which may indicate a tender sigmoid colon.
- Abdominal distention may be present in some cases.
- The following "red flag" or alarm features are *not* associated with IBS and may indicate inflammatory bowel disease, cancer, or other disorders: fever, weight loss, bleeding, and anemia, and persistent severe pain.

Laboratory Tests

- In most cases, laboratory testing reveals no abnormalities, but certain tests can help identify other causes for the patient's symptoms.
  - CBC may identify anemia, which may suggest blood loss and an organic source for GI symptoms.
  - Serum electrolytes and chemistries may indicate metabolic causes of symptoms.
  - Thyroid-stimulating hormone (TSH) should be ordered when thyroid dysfunction is suspected. Hypothyroidism may be responsible for constipation and related symptoms.
  - Stool testing for ova and parasites may identify *C. difficile* and amoebae as possible causes of diarrhea rather than IBS.
  - Fecal leukocytes can be found in inflammatory diarrhea, especially when due to invasive microorganisms.
  - A positive stool guaiac test indicating blood in the GI tract does not support a diagnosis of IBS.
  - An elevated erythrocyte sedimentation rate is consistent with a systemic inflammatory process such as inflammatory bowel disease rather than IBS.
  - Testing for lactase deficiency can confirm the presence of lactose intolerance, which may explain the symptoms.

Patient Encounter 3, Part 1

A recently widowed 33-year-old African-American woman presents to the clinic complaining of headaches, sleep disturbances, cramping abdominal pain, bloating, excessive flatulence, and loose watery stools. When asked to show where her abdomen hurts, she points to both her lower left and lower right abdomen. She indicates that the pain seems to lessen after a bowel movement. Further, she states that the symptoms have become worse over the last month, alternating between episodes of watery stools and hard, dry stools that make it difficult to defecate. During some weeks, her diarrheal episodes cause her to call in sick to work. During other weeks, she can go a couple of days without a single bowel movement. She recently canceled an outing with friends because she was worried about her body "acting up." She was diagnosed with fibromyalgia 7 months ago. Her doctor started pregabalin to treat fibromyalgia. She states that the pregabalin has helped somewhat.

Identify symptoms characteristic of IBS in this patient.

Discuss how this patient fits within the typical epidemiologic profile of patients with IBS.

Patient Encounter 3, Part 2

Upon further questioning, the patient recalls experiencing similar symptoms about 11 years ago when she thought she would have to leave school because of dwindling finances. She did not seek medical attention then because she couldn't afford it. She is a full-time pharmacy technician and recently started studying for the PCAT. Her diet consists mostly of fast food.

PMH: Insomnia, headaches, fibromyalgia

FH: None

SH: Has a glass of wine occasionally with dinner

Meds: Pregabalin 150 mg two times daily for fibromyalgia; melatonin 3 mg one tablet 1 to 2 hours before bedtime as needed for insomnia; ibuprofen 600 mg every 6 hours as needed for headache; loperamide 2 mg as needed for diarrhea; docusate sodium 100 mg as needed for constipation

Allergies: Penicillin (rash, hives, and difficulty breathing after taking amoxicillin at the age of 9)

PE:

General: Well nourished; somewhat anxious and nervous when speaking

VS: BP 135/87 mm Hg; Pulse 86 beats/min; RR 18 breaths/min; T 97.4°F (36.3°C); Ht 5′5″ (165 cm); Wt 148 lbs (67.3 kg)

Integ: Nails are chewed up; skin appears dry and scaly

HEENT: PERRLA, EOMI

Ext: Normal, no swelling

Chest: Clear to A and P bilaterally

CV: RRR

Abd: (+) BS, tender LLQ and LRQ

Rectal: No abnormalities, negative stool guaiac test

Which of this patient's findings are indicative of IBS?

Propose a comprehensive treatment approach to IBS in this patient. Where appropriate, consider the presence and influence of comorbidities.

blurred vision, constipation, urinary retention, and (rarely) psychosis. Although their effectiveness remains unconfirmed, these drugs may deserve a trial in patients with intermittent postprandial pain.[29,37]

Antidepressants Tricyclic antidepressants (TCAs) such as amitriptyline and doxepin have been used with some success for treatment of IBS-related pain. They modulate pain principally through effects on neurotransmitter reuptake, especially norepinephrine and serotonin. Their helpfulness in functional GI disorders seems independent of mood-altering effects normally associated with these agents. Low-dose TCAs (eg, amitriptyline, desipramine, or doxepin 10–25 mg daily) may help patients with IBS who predominantly experience diarrhea or pain. The selective serotonin-reuptake inhibitors (SSRIs) paroxetine, fluoxetine, and sertraline are potentially useful due to the significant effect of serotonin in the gut. SSRIs principally act on 5-HT_1 or 5-HT_2 receptors, but they can also have some effect on gut-predominant 5-HT_3 and 5-HT_4 receptors, perhaps reducing visceral hypersensitivity. They may be beneficial for patients with IBS-C or when

Table 21–5
Pharmacologic Treatments for IBS

Generic Name	Dose
Antispasmodics	
Dicyclomine	10–20 mg po every 4–6 hours as needed
Hyoscyamine	0.125–0.25 po mg or sublingually every 4 hours as needed
Propantheline bromide	15 mg po three times a day (before meals) and 30 mg at bedtime
Clidinium bromide plus chlordiazepoxide HCl	5–10 mg po three to four times a day
Hyoscyamine, scopolamine, atropine, phenobarbital	One to two tablets po three to four times daily
Tricyclic Antidepressants	**In IBS with Diarrhea:**
Amitriptyline	50–150 mg po daily
Doxepin	10–150 mg po daily
Selective Serotonin-Reuptake Inhibitors	**In IBS with Constipation:**
Paroxetine (others can be used)	10–40 mg po daily
Bulk-Forming Laxatives	
Psyllium	2.5–4 g po daily
Methylcellulose	4–6 g po daily
Antimotility Agents	
Loperamide	4 mg po; then 2 mg po after each loose stool; daily maximum: 16 mg
5-HT_3 Receptor Antagonist	
Alosetron[a]	0.5 mg two times a day for 4 weeks; then assess appropriate dose
5-HT_4 Receptor Agonist	
Tegaserod maleate[b]	6 mg po twice daily
Guanylate Cyclase-C (GC-C) Agonist	
Linaclotide	290 mcg orally once daily
Nonabsorbable antibiotic	
Rifaximin	550 mg three times daily for 14 days; patients who experience symptom recurrence can be retreated up to two times with the same dosage regimen.
Mu-Opioid Receptor Agonist	
Eluxadoline	100 mg twice daily with food; 75 mg twice daily is recommended for select patients (eg, hepatic impairment)
Chloride Channel Activator	
Lubiprostone	8 mcg orally twice daily with food and water

[a]Withdrawn from general use; available only under special circumstances.

[b]Withdrawn from general use; available only as emergency treatment.

the patient presents with IBS complicated by a mood disorder.[39] Serotonin–norepinephrine reuptake inhibitors may offer some benefit in IBS patients who also have depression or anxiety accompanied by significant pain.

▸ *Agents for Constipation Predominance*

Bulk Producers These agents may improve stool passage in IBS-C but are unlikely to have a favorable effect on pain or global IBS symptoms.[40] Psyllium may increase flatulence, which may worsen discomfort in some patients. Methylcellulose products are less likely than psyllium to increase gas production. Although fiber-based supplement use is common in IBS-C, methylcellulose may be dose adjusted in diarrhea to increase stool consistency.

Linaclotide (Linzess) This drug is a guanylate cyclase-C (GC-C) agonist indicated for treatment of IBS-C in adults.[40] Linaclotide relieves the abdominal pain, bloating and constipation associated with IBS-C while exhibiting a low tendency for systemic side effects. However, diarrhea may prove troublesome in some patients. Clinical trials have demonstrated improved quality of life in treated patients.[41]

Lubiprostone (Amitiza) This agent is also FDA approved for treatment of IBS-C, but only in women age 18 years and older. Lubiprostone is generally well tolerated in such patients. It is typically given in smaller doses than used in chronic idiopathic constipation. However, as with treatment for constipation, nausea may be an adverse effect that limits use.

Tegaserod Maleate (Zelnorm) This 5-HT_4 receptor agonist was shown to be effective in IBS-C but was withdrawn from the market because of the risk of heart attack, stroke, and unstable angina (heart/chest pain). The FDA can authorize its availability and use for emergency situations only.

▸ *Agents for Diarrhea Predominance*

Eluxadoline (Viberzi) This agent is a mu-opioid receptor agonist that reduces bowel contractions. In July 2015, the FDA approved eluxadoline for treatment of adults with IBS-D. The most common adverse effects are constipation, nausea, and abdominal pain.

Rifaximin (Xifaxan) This is a semisynthetic antibiotic with very low systemic absorption. Research suggests bacterial overgrowth plays a role in producing bloating experienced by some IBS patients. Rifaximin has proven to be better than placebo in relieving bloating, and its lack of absorption reduces the likelihood of adverse effects.[38] In July 2015, the FDA approved rifaximin for treatment of IBS-D in adults.

Loperamide Loperamide stimulates enteric nervous system receptors, inhibiting peristalsis and fluid secretion. It improves stool consistency and reduces the number of stools.[38] Consequently, it is most useful in patients who have diarrhea as a prominent symptom. However, it does not lessen abdominal pain and can occasionally aggravate pain.

Alosetron (Lotronex) Stimulation of 5-HT_3 receptors triggers hypersensitivity and hyperactivity of the large intestine. Alosetron, a selective 5-HT_3 antagonist, blocks these receptors and is indicated for treatment of women with severe IBS-D. To be eligible for treatment, patients should have frequent and severe abdominal pain, frequent bowel urgency or incontinence, and restricted daily activities. Alosetron has been shown to improve overall symptoms and quality of life. It can cause constipation in some patients. Because of an association with ischemic colitis, alosetron can be prescribed only within strict guidelines, including signing of a consent form by both patient and physician. Patients selected for treatment must exhibit severe chronic IBS symptoms and have failed to respond to conventional therapy.

Patient Care Process for IBS

Patient Assessment:

- Determine the type, severity, and frequency of symptoms and possible exacerbating factors.
- Listen attentively to the patient's complaints and reassure the patient to allay fears about invasive disease.
- Obtain a thorough current history of prescription, nonprescription, and dietary supplement use.

Therapy Evaluation:

- Determine if any IBS treatments have been attempted and their effectiveness.
- Establish whether self-care is appropriate or a medical referral is needed.

Care Plan Development:

- Determine whether the patient has received prior education about IBS, lifestyle modifications, drug therapy for IBS, and symptom prevention measures. If necessary:
    - Explain medication use relative to symptom intensity.
    - Describe potential adverse effects.
    - List drugs that may interact with the therapy.

Follow-Up Evaluation:

- IBS management requires a team approach to achieve optimal results. Encourage patients to report every professional interaction since their last encounter to ensure new advice and recommendations given are appropriate.
- Remain aware of red flag symptoms.

OUTCOME EVALUATION

- Monitor for adequate symptom relief. Patients whose pain does not respond to drug therapy may have a psychological comorbid condition requiring psychiatric intervention.
- Monitor for relief of pain if initially present. Monitor IBS-C or IBS-D patients for stool frequency, appearance, and size relative to normal characteristics. As stools normalize, associated symptoms such as bloating and abdominal distention should resolve.
- For IBS-C and IBS-M patients taking bulk producers, monitor for relief of constipation. Hard stools should soften within 72 hours.
- Monitor antidepressant and antispasmodic therapy for relief of abdominal pain.
- Assess 5-HT_4 receptor agonists (tegaserod) for relief of crampy abdominal pain and bloating.
- Monitor linaclotide for treatment-limiting diarrhea in IBS-C.
- Evaluate 5-HT_3 receptor antagonists (alosetron) for relief of abdominal pain and fecal incontinence. Monitor for constipation.
- Expect antimotility agents to reduce stool frequency and control diarrhea within 18 to 36 hours unless severe.

- Monitor CBC, serum electrolytes and chemistries, stool guaiac, and erythrocyte sedimentation rate yearly for changes that might signal an overlapping organic problem.
- Refer for medical evaluation any patient presenting with red flag signs (eg, fever, weight loss, bleeding, anemia, persistent severe pain).

Abbreviations Introduced in This Chapter

BSS	Bismuth subsalicylate
CBT	Cognitive behavioral therapy
CIC	Chronic idiopathic constipation
EPEC	Enteropathogenic *Escherichia coli*
ETEC	Enterotoxigenic *Escherichia coli*
IBS	Irritable bowel syndrome
IBS-C	Irritable bowel syndrome with constipation
IBS-D	Irritable bowel syndrome with diarrhea
IBS-M	Irritable bowel syndrome with constipation and diarrhea (mixed)
NTC	Normal-transit constipation
OIC	Opioid-induced constipation
ORS	Oral rehydration solution
STC	Slow-transit constipation
PAMORA	Peripherally acting μ-opioid receptor antagonist
TCA	Tricyclic antidepressant

REFERENCES

1. Bucharucha AE, Pemberton JH, Locke GR. American Gastroenterological Association technical review on constipation. Gastroenterolgy. 2013;144:218–238.
2. Bucharucha AE, Dorn SD, Lembo A, Pressman A. American Gastrological Association medical position statement on constipation. Gastroenterology. 2013;144:211–217.
3. Drossman DA. The functional gastrointestinal disorders and the Rome III process. Gastroenterology. 2006;130:1377–1390.
4. Longstreth GF, Thompson WG, Chey WD. Functional bowel disorders. Gastroenterology. 2006;130:1480–1491.
5. Everhardt JE, ed. The burden of digestive diseases in the United States. Bethesda, MD: National Institute of Diabetes and Digestive and Kidney Diseases, U.S. Department of Health and Human Services; 2008. NIH Publication 09-6433.
6. Higgins PD, Johanson JF. Epidemiology of constipation in North America: A systematic review. Am J Gastroenterol. 2004;99:750–759.
7. Centers for Disease Control and Prevention, National Center for Health Statistics. Underlying cause of death, detailed mortality, 2012, sorted by diseases of the digestive system (K00–K92). CDC WONDER online database. http://wonder.cdc.gov/. Updated April 19, 2013. Accessed November 4, 2014.
8. Wald A, Scarpignato C, Kamm MA, et al. The burden of constipation on quality of life: Results of a multinational survey. Aliment Pharmacol Ther. 2007;26(2):227–236.
9. Sanchez MIP, Bercik P. Epidemiology and burden of chronic constipation. Can J Gastroenterol. 2011;25(Suppl B):11B–15B.
10. Camilleri M, Drossman DA, Becker G, et al. Emerging treatments in neurogastroenterology: A multidisciplinary working group consensus statement on opioid-induced constipation. Neurogastroenterol Motil. 2014;26:1386–1395.
11. Heymen S, Scarlett Y, Jones K, et al. Randomized, controlled trial shows biofeedback to be superior to alternative treatments for patients with pelvic floor dyssynergia-type constipation. Dis Colon Rectum. 2007;50(4):428–441.
12. Lembo A, Camilleri M. Chronic constipation. N Engl J Med. 2003;349:1360–1368.
13. Johanson JF, Ueno R. Lubiprostone, a locally acting chloride channel activator, in adult patients with chronic constipation: A double blind, placebo-controlled, dose-ranging study to evaluate efficacy and safety. Aliment Pharmacol Ther. 2007; 1351–1361.
14. Drossman DA, Chey WD, Johanson JF, et al. Clinical trial: Lubiprostone in patients with constipation-associated irritable bowel syndrome—results of two randomized, placebo controlled studies. Aliment Pharmacol Ther. 2008;29:329–341.
15. Cuppoletti J, Chakrabarti J, Tewari K, Malinowska DH. Methadone but not morphine inhibits lubiprostone-stimulated Cl^- currents in T84 intestinal cells and recombinant human CIC-2, but not CFTR Cl^- currents. Cell Biochem Biophys. 2013;66:53–63.
16. Brenner DM, Chey WD. An evidence-based review of novel and emerging therapies for constipation in patients taking opioid analgesics. Am J Gastroenterol Suppl. 2014;2(1):38–46.
17. Bryant AP, Busby RW, Bartolini WP, et al. Linaclotide is a potent and selective guanylate cyclase C agonist that elicits pharmacological effects locally in the gastrointestinal tract. Life Sci. 2010;86:760–765.
18. Food and Drug Administration. Center for Drug Evaluation and Research. Approval Package for: Linzess Capsules, 145 mcg and 290 mcg, 2012. http://www.fda.gov/downloads/Drugs/Approval/Review/202811.pdf.Accessed October 30, 2014.
19. Food and Drug Administration. Center for Drug Evaluation and Research. Labeling Revision for: Linzess Capsules, 145 mcg and 290 mcg, 2014. http://www.fda.gov/downloads/Drugs/Approval/Labeling Revision/NDC 202811/S-004.pdf.Accessed October 30, 2014.
20. Portenoy RK, Thomas J, Moehl Boatwright ML, et al. Subcutaneous methylnaltrexone for the treatment of opioid-induced constipation in patients with advanced illness: A double-blind randomized, parallel group, dose-ranging study. J Pain Symptom Manage. 2008:35(5);458–468.
21. Webster L, Dhar S, Eldon M, et al. A phase 2, double-blind, randomized, placebo-controlled, dose-escalation study to evaluate the efficacy, safety, and tolerability of naloxegol in patients with opioid-induced constipation. Pain. 2013: 154:1542–1550.
22. Poulsen JL, Brock C, Olesen AE, et al. Clinical potential of naloxegol in the management of opioid-induced bowel dysfunction. Clin Exp Gastroenterol. 2014:7;345–358.
23. Chey WD, Webster L, Sostek M, et al. Naloxegol for opioid-induced constipation in patients with noncancer Pain. 2014 DOI:10.1056/NEJMMoa1310246. Accessed June 6, 2014.
24. Food and Drug Administration Center for Drug Evaluation and Research. Briefing Document. Anesthetic and Analgesic Drug Products Advisory Committee Meeting report proceedings. June 12, 2014. Food and Drug Administration. Silver Spring, MD.
25. Food and Drug Administration Center for Drug Evaluation and Research. Letter. NDA 204760 September 16, 2014. Food and Drug Administration. Silver Spring, MD. http://www.accessdata.fda.gov/drugsatfda_docs/nda/2014/204760Orig1s000Approv.pdf. Accessed Nov. 9, 2014.
26. Pawlowski SW, Warren CA, Guerrant R. Diagnosis and treatment of acute or persistent diarrhea. Gastroenterology. 2009.136, 1874–1886.
27. Davis TK, McKee R, Schnadower D, Tarr PI. Treatment of Shiga toxin-producing Escherichia coli infections. Infect Dis Clin North Am. 2013;27(3):577–597.
28. Chang JY, Talley NJ. An update on irritable bowel syndrome: from diagnosis to emerging therapies. Curr Opin Gastroenterol. 2011;27:72–78.

29. Cremonini F, Talley NJ. Irritable bowel syndrome: Epidemiology, natural history, health care seeking, and emerging risk factors. Gastroenterol Clin North Am. 2005;34:189–204.
30. Gunnarsson J, Simén M. Peripheral factors in the pathophysiology of irritable bowel syndrome. Dig Liver Dis. 2009;41(1):788–793.
31. Chang JY, Talley NJ. Current and emerging therapies in irritable bowel syndrome: From pathophysiology to treatment. Trends Pharmacol Sci. 2010;31(7):326–334.
32. Cremon C, Gargano L, Morselli-Labate AM, et al. Mucosal immune activation in irritable bowel syndrome: Gender-dependence and association with digestive symptoms. Am J Gastroenterol. 2009;104(2):401–403.
33. Fedewa A, Rao SSC. Dietary fructose intolerance, fructan intolerance and FODMAPs. Curr Gastroenterol Rep. 2014;16:370–378.
34. O'Mahony L, McCarthy J, Kelly P, et al. *Lactobacillus and Bifidobacterium* in irritable bowel syndrome: Symptom responses and relationship to cytokine profiles. Gastroenterology. 2005;128:541–551.
35. Zijdenbos IL, de Wit NJ, van der Heijden GJ, et al. Psychological treatments for the management of irritable bowel syndrome. Cochrane Database Syst Rev. 2009;(1):CD006442.
36. Miller LG. Herbal medicinals: Selected clinical considerations focusing on known or potential drug-herb interactions. Arch Intern Med. 1998;158:2200–2211.
37. Thoua NM, Murray CD. Motility and functional bowel disease: Irritable bowel syndrome. Gastroenterology. 2011;39(4): 214–217.
38. Menees SB, Maneerattannaporn M, Kim HM, Chey WD. The efficacy and safety of rifaximin for irritable bowel syndrome: A systematic review and meta-analysis. Am J Gastroenterol. 2012;107(1):28–35.
39. Schoenfeld P. Efficacy of current drug therapies in irritable bowel syndrome: What works and does not work. Gastroenterol Clin North Am. 2005;34:319–335.
40. Yu SW, Rao SS. Advances in the management of constipation--predominant irritable bowel syndrome: The role of linaclotide. Therap Adv Gastroenterol. 2014;7(5):193–205.
41. Layer P, Stanghelli V. Linaclotide for the management of irritable bowel syndrome with constipation. Aliment Pharmacol Ther. 2014;39(4):371–384.

22 Portal Hypertension and Cirrhosis

Laurajo Ryan

LEARNING OBJECTIVES

Upon completion of the chapter, the reader will be able to:

1. Explain the pathophysiology of cirrhosis and portal hypertension.
2. Identify signs and symptoms of liver disease in a given patient.
3. Identify laboratory abnormalities that result from liver disease and describe the pathophysiology of each abnormality.
4. Describe the consequences associated with decreased hepatic function.
5. Create treatment goals for a patient with portal hypertension and its complications.
6. Evaluate patient history and physical examination findings to determine the etiology of cirrhosis.
7. Recommend a specific treatment regimen for a patient with cirrhosis that includes lifestyle changes, nonpharmacologic therapy, and pharmacologic therapy.

INTRODUCTION

Cirrhosis involves replacement of normal hepatic cells with fibrous scar tissue and progressive deterioration of liver function. Scarring is accompanied by loss of viable hepatocytes, the functional cells of the liver. KEY CONCEPT *Cirrhosis is irreversible and leads to* ***portal hypertension****, which in turn is responsible for the complications of advanced liver disease.* Complications of cirrhosis include ***ascites, spontaneous bacterial peritonitis*** (SBP), ***hepatic encephalopathy*** (HE), ***hepatorenal syndrome*** (HRS), and ***variceal bleeding***.[1] These complications carry high mortality rates and are associated with disease progression.

EPIDEMIOLOGY AND ETIOLOGY

Cirrhosis is the 12th leading cause of death in the United States. It also places an enormous economic and social burden on society from hospitalizations, lost wages, decreased productivity, and emotional strain of the disease on both patients and their families.

Cirrhosis is the result of long-term insult to the liver, and damage usually doesn't become clinically evident until the fourth decade of life. Alcohol ingestion and viral hepatitis C infection are the most common causes of cirrhosis in the United States, whereas hepatitis B accounts for the majority of cases worldwide.[2]

Alcoholic cirrhosis usually develops only after decades of heavy drinking. It develops more quickly in women than men, even after taking body weight into account. Estimates vary, but alcoholic cirrhosis can develop after as few as two to three daily drinks in women and three to four drinks in men, although five to eight daily drinks is more typical.[3] Differences in metabolism may account for this gender disparity; women metabolize less alcohol in the gastrointestinal (GI) tract, allowing delivery of more ethanol (which is directly hepatotoxic) to the liver.[4] Genetic factors also play a role in disease progression; some patients develop cirrhosis with much less cumulative alcohol intake than is typical (either fewer drinks per day or faster disease onset), but others with much greater intake never develop cirrhosis.

Infection with one or more strains of viral hepatitis causes acute, potentially reversible, hepatic inflammation, whereas chronic infection with hepatitis B or C can lead to cirrhosis. Both hepatitis B and C infections are transmitted through IV drug use, but sexual contact is the more common route of hepatitis B transmission.[5] See Chapter 24, Viral Hepatitis, for a complete discussion of infectious hepatitis.

PATHOPHYSIOLOGY

Portal Hypertension and Cirrhosis

The portal vein is the primary vessel leading into the liver; it receives deoxygenated venous blood from the splanchnic bed (intestines, stomach, pancreas, and spleen) at a rate of 1 to 1.5 L/min (Figure 22–1). Portal flow accounts for approximately 75% of blood delivered to the liver, and the hepatic artery provides the remaining 25% in the form of oxygenated blood from the abdominal aorta. Normal portal vein pressure is 5 to 10 mm Hg, and portal hypertension, which is a consequence of increased resistance to hepatic blood flow, occurs when portal pressure exceeds 10 to 12 mm Hg.[6]

Portal hypertension can develop from prehepatic, intrahepatic, or posthepatic damage. This chapter focuses on the most common cause of portal hypertension, which is intrahepatic (sinusoidal) damage. The sinusoids are porous vessels within the liver that surround radiating rows of hepatocytes (Figure 22–2). Sinusoids transport systemic blood that contains ingested substances (eg, food, drugs, toxins) to the hepatocytes. The liver processes the nutrients (carbohydrates, proteins, lipids, vitamins,

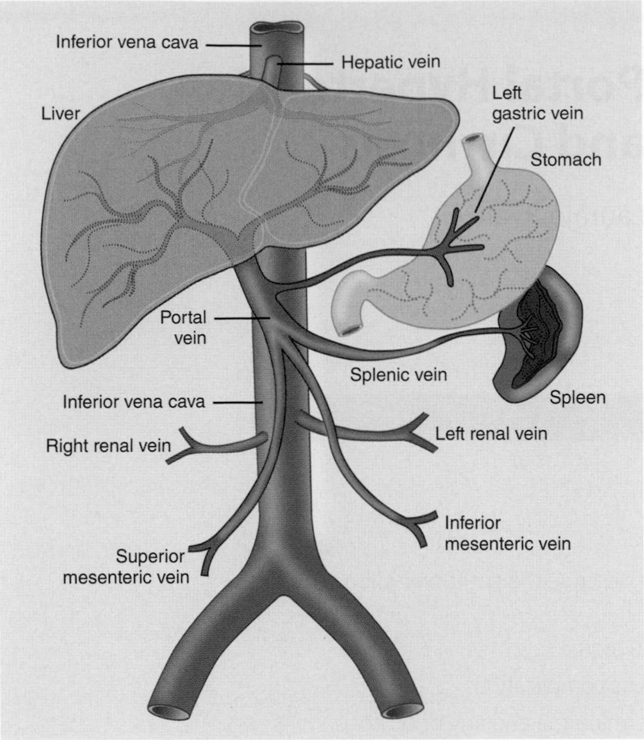

FIGURE 22–1. The portal venous system. (From Sease JM. Portal hypertension and cirrhosis. In: DiPiro JT, Talbert RL, Yee GC, et al., eds. Pharmacotherapy: A Pathophysiologic Approach, 9th ed. New York, NY: McGraw-Hill, 2014. www.accesspharmacy.com, with permission.)

and minerals) for either immediate use or storage, while drugs and toxins are broken down through a variety of metabolic processes.

The progressive destruction of hepatocytes combined with an increase in fibroblasts and connective tissue culminates in cirrhosis. Fibrosis scar tissue nodules modify the basic architecture of the liver, disrupting hepatic blood flow and normal liver function.

Reduced hepatic blood flow significantly alters normal metabolic processes and decreases protein synthesis. Hepatic drug metabolism is reduced, which can result in higher drug concentrations and extended half-life of drugs normally eliminated by the liver, especially those with high first-pass metabolism. Decreased hepatic metabolism can also reduce or delay prodrug activation and cause therapeutic failure. The liver processes metabolic waste products for excretion; in cirrhosis, bilirubin (from the enzymatic breakdown of heme) can accumulate, causing jaundice (yellowing of the skin), scleral icterus (yellowing of the sclera), and tea-colored urine (urinary bilirubin excreted as urobilinogen).

Changes in steroid hormone production, conversion, and handling are prominent features of cirrhosis. These changes manifest as decreased libido, gynecomastia (development of breast tissue in men), testicular atrophy, and feminization in men. Another effect of changes in sex hormone metabolism is development of palmar erythema and spider angiomata (nevi). Spider angiomata are vascular lesions found mainly on the trunk and have a central arteriole (body) surrounded by radiating "legs." When blanched, the lesions fill from the center body outward toward the legs. They are not specific to cirrhosis, but the number and size do correlate with disease severity, and their presence relates to risk of variceal hemorrhage.[7]

Increased intrahepatic resistance to portal blood flow increases pressure on the entire splanchnic bed; an enlarged spleen (splenomegaly) is a common finding in cirrhotic patients. Splenic platelet sequestration secondary to splenomegaly is one of the causes of thrombocytopenia in cirrhotic patients.

Portal hypertension mediates systemic and splanchnic arterial vasodilation by increasing production of nitric oxide and other vasodilators in an attempt to counteract the increased pressure gradient. Nitric oxide causes a fall in systemic arterial pressure; this drop in pressure activates the renin–angiotensin–aldosterone system (RAAS) and the sympathetic nervous system, and increases antidiuretic hormone (ADH, vasopressin) production.[8] These systems are activated in an attempt to maintain arterial blood pressure and renal blood flow by increasing sodium and water retention. The excess sodium and water puts increased pressure on the vascular system. The umbilical vein, which is usually eradicated in infancy, may become patent as a result of the increased pressure and cause prominent dilated veins that are visible on the surface of the abdomen. This phenomenon is called caput medusae because it resembles the head of the mythical Gorgon Medusa.

Ascites

Ascites is the accumulation of fluid in the peritoneal space. It is the most common condition associated with decompensated cirrhosis and indicates a dire prognosis.[9]

The pathophysiology of ascites, portal hypertension, and cirrhosis are interrelated (Figure 22–3). Cirrhotic changes and subsequent decreases in synthetic function lead to decreased albumin production (hypoalbuminemia). Albumin is the primary intravascular protein responsible for maintaining vascular oncotic pressure; low serum albumin levels, elevated hydrostatic pressure, and increased capillary permeability allow fluid to leak from the vascular space into body tissues. This results in ascites, peripheral edema, and fluid in the pulmonary system. Obstruction of hepatic sinusoids and hepatic lymph nodes also allows fluid to seep into the peritoneal cavity, further contributing to ascitic fluid formation.

Lowered effective intravascular volume decreases renal perfusion; the kidney reacts by activating the RAAS, increasing plasma renin activity, aldosterone production, and sodium retention. The subsequent increase in intravascular volume furthers the imbalance of intravascular oncotic pressure, allowing even more fluid to escape to the extravascular spaces, increasing ascites and peripheral edema. Unchecked, these combined effects enable the cycle of portal pressure and ascites to continue, creating a self-perpetuating loop of ascites formation.

Patients with ascites avidly retain sodium and water, not only through elevated aldosterone concentrations (from increased production and decreased clearance), but also through increases in ADH and sympathetic nervous system activation. Patients may become hyponatremic if there is a decrease in free water excretion. This is not a result of too little sodium; it is a dilutional effect. Untreated, this combination of factors can lead to a decrease in renal function and the HRS.[3,8]

Hepatorenal Syndrome

HRS is a decline renal function in the setting of cirrhosis that is not caused by intrinsic renal disease. Type 1 HRS is characterized

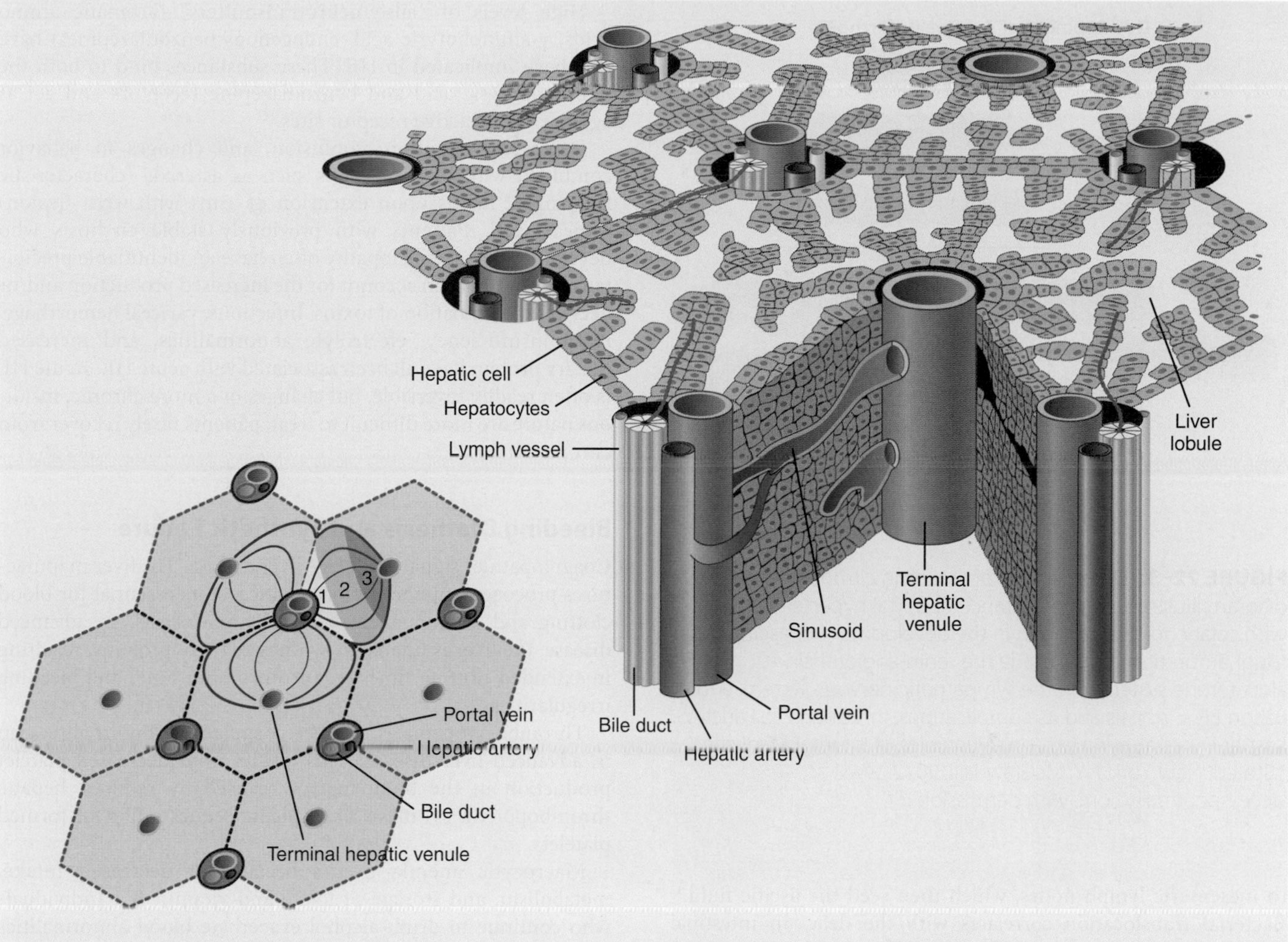

FIGURE 22–2. Relationship of sinusoids to hepatocytes and the venous system. (From Sease JM. Portal hypertension and cirrhosis. In: DiPiro JT, Talbert RL, Yee GC, et al., eds. Pharmacotherapy: A Pathophysiologic Approach, 9th ed. New York, NY: McGraw-Hill, 2014. www.accesspharmacy.com, with permission.)

by rapid deterioration of renal function (acute kidney injury [AKI]) in the presence of decompensated cirrhosis that is not reversible with volume repletion. Untreated it is rapidly fatal with a 50% mortality rate at 14 days. Renal artery vasoconstriction (stimulated by the sympathetic nervous system) and decreased mean arterial pressure (mediated by nitric oxide) decrease renal perfusion and precipitate renal failure. The kidneys attempt to counteract this drop in renal perfusion through RAAS activation. Production of renin stimulates a cascade that causes fluid retention and peripheral vasoconstriction in an attempt to increase renal blood flow. Prostaglandin E_2 and prostacyclin production are increased to stimulate renal vasodilation. HRS develops when these mechanisms are overwhelmed and renal perfusion drops acutely. SBP is a common trigger for HRS, as are nonsteroidal anti-inflammatory drugs (NSAIDs), which precipitate HRS by inhibiting prostaglandin production. Type 2 HRS has similar pathophysiology to type 1 HRS but is characterized by a less acute decline in renal function.

The traditional laboratory parameters used to monitor renal function (serum creatinine, blood urea nitrogen [BUN]) tend to be low in cirrhotic patients because of reduced muscle mass and decreased hepatic urea production, respectively. Because of this, even minor changes in these laboratory test results should be monitored closely; small changes in values may represent large changes in renal function.

Varices

The splanchnic system drains venous blood from the GI tract to the liver. In portal hypertension, there is resistance to drainage from the originating organ; collateral vessels (varices) develop in the esophagus, stomach, and rectum to compensate for the increased blood volume. Varices divert blood meant for hepatic circulation back to the systemic circulation, which decreases clearance of medications and potential toxins through loss of first-pass metabolism. Varices are weak superficial vessels; any additional increase in pressure can cause them to rupture and bleed.[10]

Spontaneous Bacterial Peritonitis (SBP)

SBP is an acute bacterial infection of peritoneal (ascitic) fluid in the absence of intra-abdominal infection or intestinal perforation; up to 30% of patients with ascites develop SBP.[11] The peritoneal cavity is usually a sterile space, and one proposed mechanism of bacterial contamination is translocation of intestinal bacteria

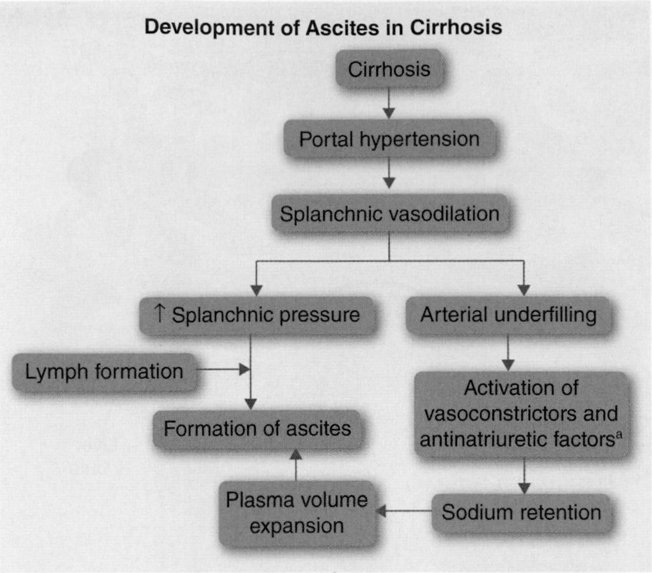

FIGURE 22–3. Development of ascites in cirrhosis. This flow diagram illustrates the importance of portal hypertension with splanchnic vasodilation in the development of ascites. [a]Antinatriuretic factors include the renin-angiotensin-aldosterone system and the sympathetic nervous system. (From Bacon BR. Cirrhosis and its complications. In: Longo DL, Fauci AS, Kasper DL, et al, eds. Harrison's Principles of Internal Medicine, 18th ed. New York, NY: McGraw-Hill, 2012. www.accesspharmacy.com, with permission.)

to mesenteric lymph nodes, which then seed the ascitic fluid.[12] Bacterial translocation correlates with the delay in intestinal transit time and increased intestinal wall permeability observed in cirrhotic patients. Another possible mechanism of SBP is the hematogenous spread of bacteria into the peritoneal space.[13] Low protein ascites (less than 1 g/dL [10 g/L]) is also associated with increased rates of SBP; presumably low protein is correlated to low antibacterial activity.

Enteric gram-negative aerobes (*Escherichia coli*, *Klebsiella pneumoniae*) are the most common bacteria isolated from patients with SBP. The most common gram-positive pathogen is *Streptococcus pneumoniae*.[9] Once a bacterial pathogen is identified, the antimicrobial spectrum should be narrowed; SBP is rarely polymicrobial.

Hepatic Encephalopathy

Numerous factors, many of them poorly understood, are involved in the development of hepatic encephalopathy (HE). In severe hepatic disease, systemic circulation bypasses the liver; substances that are normally hepatically metabolized accumulate in the systemic circulation. These metabolic by-products, especially nitrogenous waste, are neurotoxic.[14]

Ammonia (NH_3) is just one of the toxins implicated in HE. It is a metabolic by-product of protein catabolism; it is also generated by bacteria in the GI tract. In a normally functioning liver, hepatocytes degrade ammonia to form urea, which is renally excreted. In cirrhosis, conversion to urea is reduced and ammonia accumulates, resulting in encephalopathy. Patients with HE commonly have elevated serum ammonia concentrations, but ammonia levels do not correlate with the degree of CNS impairment.[14]

High levels of "false neurotransmitters" (aromatic amino acids, γ-aminobutyric acid, endogenous benzodiazepines) have also been implicated in HE. These substances bind to both the γ-aminobutyric acid and benzodiazepine receptors and act as agonists at the active receptor sites.[14]

Decreased cognition, confusion, and changes in behavior combined with physical signs such as asterixis (characteristic flapping of hands upon extension of arms with wrist flexion) indicate HE. Patients with previously stable cirrhosis who develop acute encephalopathy often have an identifiable precipitating event that can account for the increased production and/or decreased elimination of toxins. Infections, variceal hemorrhage, renal insufficiency, electrolyte abnormalities, and increased dietary protein have all been associated with acute HE. Acute HE is often readily reversible, but changes of a more chronic, insidious nature are more difficult to treat; patients rarely recover from chronic HE.

Bleeding Diathesis and Synthetic Failure

Coagulopathies signal end-stage liver disease. The liver manufactures procoagulant and anticoagulant factors essential for blood clotting and maintenance of blood homeostasis. In advanced disease, the liver is unable to synthesize these proteins, resulting in extended clotting times (eg, prothrombin time) and bleeding irregularities.[15]

Thrombocytopenia is another coagulation abnormality seen in advanced liver disease. This results from decreased platelet production in the bone marrow caused by reduced hepatic thrombopoietin synthesis and splenic sequestration of formed platelets.

Macrocytic anemia occurs because of decreased intake, metabolism, and storage of folate and vitamin B_{12}. Individuals who continue to drink alcohol exacerbate blood abnormalities because ethanol is toxic to bone marrow.

Alcoholic Liver Disease

Alcoholic liver disease progresses through several distinct phases—from fatty liver to alcoholic hepatitis and finally cirrhosis. Changes in metabolism account for the fatty liver, hypertriglyceridemia, and acidemia observed in alcoholic liver disease. Fatty liver and alcoholic hepatitis may be reversible with cessation of alcohol intake. The scarring of cirrhosis is permanent, but maintaining abstinence from alcohol can decrease complications and slow progression to end-stage liver disease.[9] Continuing to drink alcohol speeds the advancement of liver dysfunction and cirrhotic complications.

Ethanol metabolism begins prior to absorption; alcohol dehydrogenase in the gastric mucosa oxidizes a portion of ingested alcohol to acetaldehyde. The remaining alcohol is rapidly absorbed from the GI tract and enters body tissues quite easily due to its high lipid solubility. KEY CONCEPT *Alcohol dehydrogenase oxidizes ethanol in body tissues, primarily the liver, causing inflammation and fibrosis.*[16] High ethanol levels saturate the alcohol dehydrogenase enzyme system. When it is overwhelmed, the microsomal ethanol oxidizing system takes over the detoxification process. This system is an inducible cytochrome P-450 (CYP450) enzyme system; it participates in phase 1 metabolism, and like alcohol dehydrogenase, produces acetaldehyde as its end product.[17] Acetaldehyde exerts direct toxic effects on the liver by damaging hepatocytes, inducing fibrosis, and directly coupling to proteins, interfering with their intended actions.

Less Common Causes of Cirrhosis

Genetics and metabolic risk factors mediate other less common causes of cirrhosis. These diseases vary widely in prevalence, disease progression, and treatment options.

Primary biliary cirrhosis is characterized by progressive inflammatory destruction of the bile ducts. This immune-mediated inflammation of the intrahepatic bile ducts causes remodeling and scarring, resulting in retention of bile in the liver, hepatocellular damage, and cirrhosis. The number of patients affected with primary biliary cirrhosis is difficult to estimate because it is often asymptomatic and people may be diagnosed incidentally during a routine health care visit.

Nonalcoholic fatty liver disease (NAFLD) begins with asymptomatic fatty liver but can progress to cirrhosis. NAFLD is a diagnosis of exclusion; viral, genetic, or environmental causes must be eliminated prior to making this diagnosis. NAFLD is directly related to numerous metabolic abnormalities. Risk factors include diabetes mellitus, dyslipidemia, obesity, insulin resistance, and other conditions associated with increased hepatic fat.[18]

Hereditary hemochromatosis is an autosomal recessive disease that causes increased intestinal iron absorption and subsequent deposition in hepatic, cardiac, and pancreatic tissue. Hepatic iron overload results in fibrosis, hepatic scarring, cirrhosis, and hepatocellular carcinoma. Repeated blood transfusions can also cause hemochromatosis, but this mechanism rarely leads to cirrhosis.

Wilson disease is an autosomal recessive disease that leads to cirrhosis through protein abnormalities. The protein responsible for facilitating copper excretion in the bile is faulty, so copper accumulates in hepatic tissue. High copper levels are toxic to hepatocytes. Fibrosis and cirrhosis may develop in untreated patients. Patients with Wilson disease usually present with symptoms of liver and/or neurologic disease while still in their teens.

A third autosomal recessive genetic disease is α_1-antitrypsin deficiency. Abnormalities in the α_1-antitrypsin protein impair its secretion from the liver. α_1-Antitrypsin deficiency causes cirrhosis in children as well as adults; adults usually have concomitant pulmonary disease such as chronic obstructive pulmonary disease.

CLINICAL PRESENTATION AND DIAGNOSIS

Refer to the accompanying clinical presentation box for the symptoms, signs, and laboratory abnormalities associated with cirrhosis.

Diagnosis of Cirrhosis

In some cases, cirrhosis is diagnosed incidentally before the patient develops symptoms or acute complications, but many patients have decompensated disease at presentation. They may present with variceal bleeding, ascites, SBP, or HE. At diagnosis, patients may have some, all, or none of the laboratory abnormalities and/or signs and symptoms associated with cirrhosis.[19]

Liver biopsy is the only way to definitively diagnose cirrhosis, but this is often deferred in lieu of a presumptive diagnosis. Ultrasound and computed tomography are used routinely; a small nodular liver with increased echogenicity is consistent with cirrhosis. The modified Child–Pugh and Model for End-Stage Liver Disease (MELD) classification systems (Table 22–1) are used to classify disease severity and evaluate the need for transplantation.

Table 22–1

Child–Pugh and MELD Classifications for Determining Severity of Liver Damage

Child–Pugh Classification[a]

Variable	1 Point	2 Points	3 Points
Bilirubin (mg/dL)	< 2	2–3	> 3
(μmol/L)	< 34	34–51	> 51
Albumin (g/dL) (g/L)	> 3.5	2.8–3.5	< 2.8
	> 35	28–35	< 28
Prothrombin time (seconds prolonged) or	1–3	4–6	> 6
INR	< 1.8	1.8–2.3	> 2.3
Ascites	None	Slight	Moderate
Encephalopathy	None	Grade 1–2	Grade 3–4

MELD Classification

The formula for the MELD score is 3.8 × Ln (bilirubin [mg/dL]) + 11.2 × Ln (INR) + 9.6 × Ln (creatinine [mg/dL]) + 6.4 × (etiology: 0 if cholestatic or alcoholic, 1 otherwise).

Using SI units, the MELD score is 3.8 × Ln(bilirubin [μmol/L]/17.1) + 11.2 × Ln(INR) + 9.6 × Ln(creatinine [μmol/L]/88.4) + 6.4 × (etiology: 0 if cholestatic or alcoholic, 1 otherwise).

INR, international normalized ratio; Ln, natural logarithm; MELD, Model for End-Stage Liver Disease.

[a]Class A: 1 to 6 total points; B: 7 to 9 points; C: 10 to 15 points.

From Lucey MR, Brown KA, Everson GT, et al. Minimal criteria for placement of adults on the liver transplant waiting list: A report of a national conference organized by the American Society of Transplant Physicians and the American Association for the Study of Liver Diseases. Liver Transpl Surg 1997;3:628–637; and Kamath PS, Wiesner RH, Malinchoc M, et al. A model to predict survival in patients with end-stage liver disease. Hepatology 2001;33:464–470.

Patients with ascites or known varices are presumed to have portal hypertension. Direct measurements of portal pressure are usually deferred because they require invasive procedures and increase the risk of bleeding.

Diagnosis of Ascites

Ultrasound evaluation may be necessary to detect ascites in obese patients or those with only small amounts of fluid accumulation. Analysis of ascitic fluid obtained during paracentesis provides diagnostic clues to the etiology of the ascites. Diagnostic evaluation should include cell count with differential, albumin, total protein, Gram stain, and bacterial cultures. In patients without an established diagnosis of liver disease, the serum ascites–albumin gradient (SAAG) is used to determine the cause of portal hypertension.[9] SAAG compares serum albumin concentration to ascitic fluid albumin concentration:

$$\text{Alb}_{\text{serum}} - \text{Alb}_{\text{ascites}} = \text{SAAG}$$

A value of 1.1 g/dL (11 g/L) or greater identifies portal hypertension as the cause of the ascites with 97% sensitivity.[9] In portal hypertension, the low albumin in the ascitic fluid balances the oncotic pressure gradient with the hydrostatic pressure gradient of portal hypertension. The differential diagnoses for SAAG values less than 1.1 g/dL (11 g/L) include peritoneal carcinoma, peritoneal infection (tuberculosis, fungal, cytomegalovirus), and nephrotic syndrome. Serum albumin should be measured at the time of paracentesis for an accurate comparison.[9]

Clinical Presentation of Cirrhosis and Complications of Portal Hypertension

General

- Signs and symptoms are specific to the complication the patient is experiencing at the time of presentation.

Symptoms

- Patients with cirrhosis may be asymptomatic until acute complications develop.
- Nonspecific symptoms include anorexia, fatigue, weakness, and changes in libido and sleep patterns. Patients may also experience easy bruising and bleeding from minor injuries.
- Patients with ascites may complain of abdominal pain, nausea, increasing tightness and fullness in the abdomen, shortness of breath, and early satiety.
- Hemorrhage from esophageal or gastric varices may be associated with melena, pallor, fatigue, and weakness from blood loss. Patients often present with nausea, vomiting, and hematemesis.
- Bleeding from rectal varices may present as hematochezia.
- In patients with bleeding varices, digestion of swallowed blood represents a high protein load; this causes nausea and can precipitate symptoms of HE.
- In patients with HE, neurologic changes can be overwhelming or so subtle that they are not clinically apparent except during a targeted clinical evaluation.
- Patients with HE may complain of disruption of sleep patterns and day-to-night inversion; patients have delayed bedtime and wake times, which may progress to complete inversion of the normal diurnal cycle.
- If SBP occurs, symptoms of infection may include fever, chills, abdominal pain, and mental status changes.

Signs

- Nonspecific signs of liver disease include jaundice, scleral icterus, tea-colored urine, bruising, hepatomegaly, splenomegaly, spider angiomata, caput medusae, palmar erythema, gynecomastia, and testicular atrophy.
- Ascites can be detected by increased abdominal girth accompanied by shifting dullness and a fluid wave.
- Signs of variceal bleeding depend on the degree of blood loss and abruptness of onset. Rapid and massive blood loss is more likely to result in hemodynamic instability than slow, steady bleeding.
- Signs of acute bleeding may include pallor, hypotension, tachycardia, mental status changes, and hematemesis.
- Markers of hepatic encephalopathy (HE) include decreased cognition, confusion, changes in behavior, and asterixis.
- Patients with SBP may present with fever, painful tympanic abdomen, and changes in mental status.
- Decreases in clotting factors may manifest as abnormal bruising and bleeding.
- Dupuytren's contracture is a contraction of the palmar fascia that usually affects the fourth and fifth digits. It is not specific to cirrhosis and can also be seen in repetitive use injuries.

Laboratory Abnormalities

- Hepatocellular damage manifests as elevated alanine aminotransferase (ALT) and aspartate aminotransferase (AST). The degree of transaminase elevation does not correlate with the remaining functional metabolic capacity of the liver. An AST level twofold higher than ALT suggests alcoholic liver damage.
- Elevated alkaline phosphatase is nonspecific and may correlate with liver or bone disease; it tends to be elevated in biliary tract disease; γ-glutamyl transferase (GGT) is specific to the bile ducts, and in conjunction with an elevated alkaline phosphatase, suggests hepatic disease. Extremely elevated GGT levels further indicate obstructive biliary disease.
- Increased total, direct, and indirect bilirubin concentrations indicate defects in transport, conjugation, or excretion of bilirubin.
- Lactate dehydrogenase (LDH) is a nonspecific marker of hepatocyte damage; a disproportionate elevation of LDH indicates ischemic injury.
- Thrombocytopenia may occur because of decreased platelet production and splenic sequestration of platelets.
- Anemia (decreased hemoglobin and hematocrit) occurs as a result of variceal bleeding, decreased erythrocyte production, alcohol use, and hypersplenism.
- Elevated prothrombin time (PT) and international normalized ratio (INR) are coagulation derangements that indicate loss of synthetic capacity in the liver and correlate to functional loss of hepatocytes.
- Decreased serum albumin and total protein occur in chronic liver damage due to loss of synthetic capacity within the liver.
- The serum albumin-to-ascites gradient is 1.1 g/dL (11 g/L) or greater caused by portal hypertension.
- Increased blood ammonia concentration is characteristic of HE, but levels do not correlate to degree of impairment.
- Increased serum creatinine signaling a decline in renal function may be seen with hepatorenal syndrome.
- Signs and symptoms of SBP in a patient with cirrhosis and ascites should prompt a diagnostic paracentesis (Figure 22–4). In SBP, there is decreased total serum protein, elevated white blood cell count (with left shift), and the ascitic fluid contains at least 250 cells/mm^3 (250 × 10^6/L) neutrophils. Bacterial culture of ascitic fluid may be positive, but lack of growth does not exclude the diagnosis.

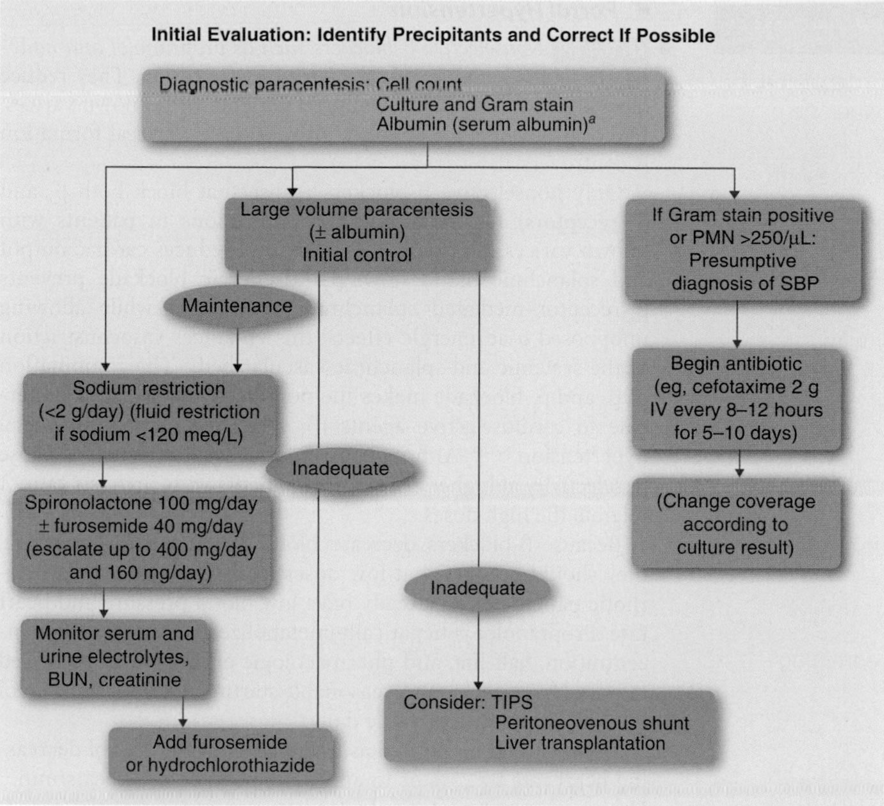

FIGURE 22–4. Approach to the patient with ascites and spontaneous bacterial peritonitis (SBP). (BUN, blood urea nitrogen; Na, sodium; PMN, polymorphonuclear leukocyte; TIPS, transjugular intrahepatic portosystemic shunt.) (From Chung RT, Podolsky DK. Cirrhosis and its complications. In: Kasper DL, Braunwald E, Fauci AS, et al., eds. Harrison's Principles of Internal Medicine, 17th ed. New York, NY: McGraw-Hill, 2005:1858–1869, with permission.) [a]If PMN is greater than 250/μL (250×10^6/L) but culture is negative (culture-negative neutrocytic ascites), begin empiric antibiotics and retap after 48 hours. If culture is positive but PMN less than 250/μL (250×10^6/L), treat as if PMN greater than 250/μL (250×10^6/L) (presumed SBP). If polymicrobial infection exists, exclude SBP.

TREATMENT OF PORTAL HYPERTENSION, CIRRHOSIS, AND COMPLICATIONS

Desired Outcomes

Recognizing and treating the underlying cause of cirrhosis is paramount. KEY CONCEPT *Cirrhosis is irreversible; treatments are directed at limiting disease progression and minimizing complications.* The immediate treatment goals are to stabilize acute complications such as variceal bleeding and prevent SBP. Once life-threatening conditions have stabilized, the focus shifts to preventing complications and further liver damage. The sections that follow concentrate on therapy to prevent and treat cirrhotic complications.

Nonpharmacologic Therapy

Avoiding additional hepatic insult is critical for successful cirrhosis treatment. Lifestyle modifications can limit disease complications and slow further liver damage. The only proven treatment for alcoholic liver disease is immediate cessation of alcohol use. Patients with cirrhosis from causes other than alcohol also benefit from avoiding alcohol consumption. Regardless of the etiology, all cirrhotic patients should abstain from alcohol to prevent further liver damage.

Patients with ascites require dietary sodium restriction. Intake should be limited to less than 800 mg sodium (2 g sodium chloride) per day. More stringent restriction may cause faster mobilization of ascitic fluid, but adherence to such strict limits is very difficult. Ascites usually responds well to sodium restriction accompanied by diuretic therapy.[9]

Medications must be monitored carefully for potential adverse effects. Hepatically metabolized medications may accumulate in patients with liver disease. Little guidance is available on drug dosing in hepatic impairment because these patients have historically been excluded from drug trials. Daily acetaminophen use should not exceed 2 g. Dietary supplements, herbal remedies, and nutraceuticals have not been well studied in hepatic impairment and cannot be recommended.

In patients with variceal bleeding, nasogastric (NG) suction reduces the risk of aspirating stomach contents. Aspiration pneumonia is a major cause of death in patients with variceal bleeding. NG suction can also decrease vomiting by removing blood from the GI tract during acute episodes of variceal bleeding; blood in the GI tract is very nauseating.

Endoscopic band ligation (application of a stricture around the varix) is used to stop acutely bleeding varices. Band ligation is the preferred endoscopic treatment and is effective in stopping acute variceal bleeding in up to 90% of patients.[20] It is also the standard of care for secondary prophylaxis of repeat bleeding in patients with a history of either esophageal or gastric variceal bleeding. Band ligation is best used in conjunction with pharmacologic treatment.[21,22]

During episodes of acute HE, temporary protein restriction to decrease ammonia production can be a useful adjuvant to pharmacologic therapy. Long-term protein restriction in cirrhotic patients is not recommended. Cirrhotic patients are already in a nutritionally deficient state, and prolonged protein restriction will exacerbate the problem.[14]

Hepatitis A and B vaccination is recommended in patients with cirrhosis to prevent additional liver damage from an acute viral infection.[23] Pneumococcal and influenza vaccination may also be appropriate and can reduce hospitalizations.

Shunts are long-term solutions to decrease elevated portal pressure. Shunts divert blood flow through or around the diseased liver, depending on the location and type of shunt employed.

Patient Encounter, Part 1

A 42-year-old man is brought to the emergency department by the police. The patient's family called them when he began to threaten them verbally and physically.

Chief Complaint: Not obtained; patient is combative with incoherent speech

HPI: Per family, patient has been on a "drinking binge" for the past 4 days after losing his job and was abusive when he returned home

PMH: Hypertension × 7 years, hypertriglyceridemia

Drug Allergies: Wife reports a penicillin allergy (unknown reaction)

PSH: Adenoidectomy

SH: Married, lives with his wife and their two children; works in construction; 30-year history of alcohol abuse

FH: Mother with HTN, alcohol abuse and depression; father with type 2 DM

Meds (Outpatient): Metoprolol tartrate; daily NSAID use

ROS: Not obtained; patient refuses to speak to admitting team

PE:

VS: BP 88/68 mm Hg, P 76 beats/min, T 99.1°F (37.3°C), RR 18 breaths/min, oxygen saturation 98% (0.98) on room air, Ht 69" (175 cm), Wt 76 kg, BMI 24.8 kg/m^2

HEENT: PERRL, EOMI, (+) scleral icterus, jaundice

CV: RRR; no murmurs, rubs, or gallops

Chest: CTA bilaterally, mild crackles in right base

Abd: Soft, slightly tender, grossly distended abdomen, distant bowel sounds, hepatosplenomegaly, large ascites

Ext: 2+ pedal pulses, 3+ pitting edema

Based on the current information, what is the most likely cause of his mental status changes?

What signs and symptoms does this patient have that are consistent with cirrhosis?

What risk factors does he have for cirrhosis?

Transjugular intrahepatic portosystemic shunts (TIPS) create a communication pathway between the intrahepatic portal vein and the hepatic vein. TIPS procedures may be preferred over surgically inserted shunts because they are placed through the vascular system rather than through more invasive surgical procedures, but they still carry a risk of bleeding and infection. TIPS placement can improve HRS but is associated with an increased incidence of HE.[14] The increased risk of HE results from decreased detoxification of nitrogenous waste products because the shunt allows blood to evade metabolic processing.

Pharmacologic Therapy

Drug therapy directed at reducing portal hypertension can alleviate symptoms and prevent complications but cannot reverse cirrhosis.

▶ *Portal Hypertension*

KEY CONCEPT *Nonselective β-blockers such as propranolol and nadolol are first-line treatments for portal hypertension.* They reduce bleeding and decrease mortality in patients with known varices. Use of β-blockers for primary prevention of variceal formation is controversial.

Only nonselective β-blockers (those that block both β_1 and β_2 receptors) reduce bleeding complications in patients with known varices. Blockade of β_1 receptors reduces cardiac output and splanchnic blood flow. β_2-Adrenergic blockade prevents β_2-receptor–mediated splanchnic vasodilation while allowing unopposed α-adrenergic effects; this enhances vasoconstriction of the systemic and splanchnic vascular beds. The combination of β_1 and β_2 blockade makes the nonselective β-blockers preferable to cardioselective agents (β_1 selective) in treating portal hypertension.[1,21,24] Although cardioselective β-blockers do lose β_1 selectivity at higher doses, most patients with cirrhosis cannot tolerate the high doses.

Because β-blockers decrease blood pressure and heart rate, they should be started at low doses to increase tolerability; cirrhotic patients often already have low blood pressure and heart rate. Propranolol is hepatically metabolized, so initial drug concentration, half-life, and pharmacologic effects are all increased in portal hypertension. A reasonable starting dose of propranolol is 10 to 20 mg once or twice daily.

Doses should be titrated as tolerated with the goal of decreasing heart rate by 25% or to approximately 55 to 60 beats/min.[21] Heart rate is not an accurate predictor of portal pressure reduction but is the acknowledged surrogate marker of effectiveness because there are no other acceptable alternatives.

Nitrates have been suggested for patients who do not achieve therapeutic goals (heart rate reduction) with β-blocker therapy alone. Nitrates (eg, isosorbide mononitrate), alone and in combination with β-blockers, reduced portal pressure in clinical trials; however, they increase mortality when used alone. Patients treated with combination therapy have significantly more adverse events compared to β-blocker monotherapy.[25,26] Current evidence only supports use of the combination to prevent rebleeding, not for primary prophylaxis. Unfortunately, β-blockers either alone or in combination may be intolerable for many patients with advanced cirrhosis.

▶ *Ascites*

KEY CONCEPT *The goals of treating ascites are to minimize acute discomfort, reequilibrate ascitic fluid, and prevent SBP. Treatment should modify underlying disease pathology; without directed therapy, fluid rapidly reaccumulates.*

Acute discomfort from ascites may be ameliorated by therapeutic paracentesis. Often removing just 1 to 2 L of ascitic fluid provides relief from pain and fullness. Volume resuscitation should be provided for large volume paracentesis; 6 to 8 g of IV albumin should be given per liter of fluid removed. Albumin 25% should be used because it has one-fifth the volume of the 5% product. Large-volume paracentesis without albumin administration can precipitate HRS through decreased perfusion. Albumin has not be shown to be beneficial in hemodynamically stable patients if less than 5 L of fluid is removed.[9]

Diuretics Diuretics are usually required in addition to sodium restriction (see Nonpharmacologic Therapy). KEY CONCEPT *Spironolactone (an aldosterone antagonist) with or without furosemide forms the basis of pharmacologic therapy for ascites. Cirrhosis is*

Patient Encounter, Part 2

Laboratory results for the patient showed the following:

Sodium 123 mEq/L (123 mmol/L)	Albumin 1.7 g/dL (17 g/L)
Potassium 2.9 mEq/L (2.9 mmol/L)	Total bilirubin 3.8 mg/dL (65.0 μmol/L)
Chloride 97 mEq/L (97 mmol/L)	Alk phos 213 IU/L (3.55 μkat/L)
Bicarbonate 17 mEq/L (17 mmol/L)	AST 137 IU/L (2.28 μkat/L)
BUN 8 mg/dL (2.9 mmol/L)	ALT 66 IU/L (1.10 μkat/L)
SCr 0.8 mg/dL (71 μmol/L)	INR 1.8
Glucose 114 mg/dL (6.3 mmol/L)	PT 19 seconds
Hemoglobin 7.6 g/dL (76 g/L; 4.72 mmol/L)	GGT 163 IU/L (2.72 μkat/L)
Hematocrit 23% (0.23)	LDH 187 IU/L (3.12 μkat/L)
WBC $7.2 \times 10^3/mm^3$ ($7.2 \times 10^9/L$)	Serum NH_3 72 mcg/dL (42 μmol/L)
Platelets $82 \times 10^3/mm^3$ ($82 \times 10^9/L$)	Blood alcohol content 0.08 g/dL (17 mmol/L)

Which laboratory values suggest a diagnosis of cirrhosis?

What is the likely cause of the patient's mental status change? Are there other conditions that may have contributed to the mental status change?

What is a likely trigger for his mental status change?

a high aldosterone state; spironolactone counteracts the effects of RAAS activation. In cirrhosis, not only is aldosterone production increased, but its half-life is also prolonged because of decreased hepatic metabolism. Spironolactone also conserves potassium that would otherwise be excreted because of elevated aldosterone levels.

Spironolactone is typically used with a loop diuretic for more potent diuresis. A ratio of 40 mg furosemide (the most commonly used loop diuretic) to 100 mg spironolactone (the most common starting dose for cirrhosis) can usually maintain serum potassium concentrations within the normal range.

Doses should be titrated at intervals of every 3 to 5 days. Because spironolactone is used for its antialdosterone effects, higher doses (up to 400 mg/day) are used in cirrhosis compared to lower doses used to treat heart failure or hypertension. If intolerable side effects such as painful gynecomastia occur with spironolactone, other potassium-sparing diuretics may be used, but clinical trials have not shown equivalent efficacy.[21]

Because ascites equilibrates with vascular fluid at a much slower rate than does peripheral edema, aggressive diuresis is associated with intravascular volume depletion rather than depletion of peritoneal fluid. The maximum amount of ascitic fluid that can be removed through diuresis is approximately 0.5 L/day.[9] Aggressive diuresis should be avoided unless patients have concomitant peripheral edema. These patients may require increasing furosemide doses until they are euvolemic; IV diuretics are often necessary.[21] Diuretic therapy in cirrhosis is typically lifelong.

▸ Varices

Variceal bleeding is common in cirrhotic patients. KEY CONCEPT *During acute variceal hemorrhage, it is crucial to control bleeding, prevent rebleeding, and avoid complications such as SBP.* Acute mortality is approximately 20%, and 1-year mortality is greater than 60% in patients with very elevated portal pressure; patients must be treated aggressively.[27] A treatment algorithm for acute variceal bleeding is depicted in Figure 22–5.

Octreotide (a synthetic somatostatin analog) causes selective vasoconstriction of the splanchnic bed, decreasing portal venous pressure with few serious side effects. The most common octreotide dose is a 50 mcg IV loading dose followed by a 50 mcg/hour continuous IV infusion. Therapy should continue for at least 24 to 72 hours after bleeding has stopped, but the optimal treatment duration has not been defined. Some clinicians continue octreotide for a full 5 days because this is the time frame with highest risk of rebleeding. Octreotide combined with endoscopic therapy results in decreased rebleeding rates and transfusion needs when compared with endoscopic treatment alone.[10]

▸ Spontaneous Bacterial Peritonitis

Prophylactic antibiotic therapy is recommended during acute variceal bleeding to prevent SBP; this is typically initiated with a third-generation cephalosporin. Prophylactic antibiotic therapy reduces in-hospital infections and mortality in patients hospitalized for variceal bleeding.[26]

If SBP is suspected, empiric antibiotic therapy should be initiated with a broad-spectrum antiinfective agent after ascitic fluid collection, pending cultures and susceptibilities (Figure 22–4).[28,29] In the setting of presumed infection, delaying treatment while awaiting laboratory confirmation is inappropriate and may result in death. The initial antibiotic should be an IV third-generation cephalosporin (eg, cefotaxime 2 g every 8 hours, ceftriaxone 1 g every 24 hours). These agents cover the most common gram-negative and gram-positive organisms implicated in SBP, but local resistance patterns must be taken into account when choosing empiric antibiotic therapy. Once a bacterial pathogen has been identified, coverage may be narrowed to an agent that is highly active against that particular organism. SBP is rarely polymicrobial.

SBP is the primary cause of HRS. The risk of renal failure can be reduced with albumin therapy, 1.5 g/kg initially, followed by 1 g/kg on day 3 of SBP therapy.[29]

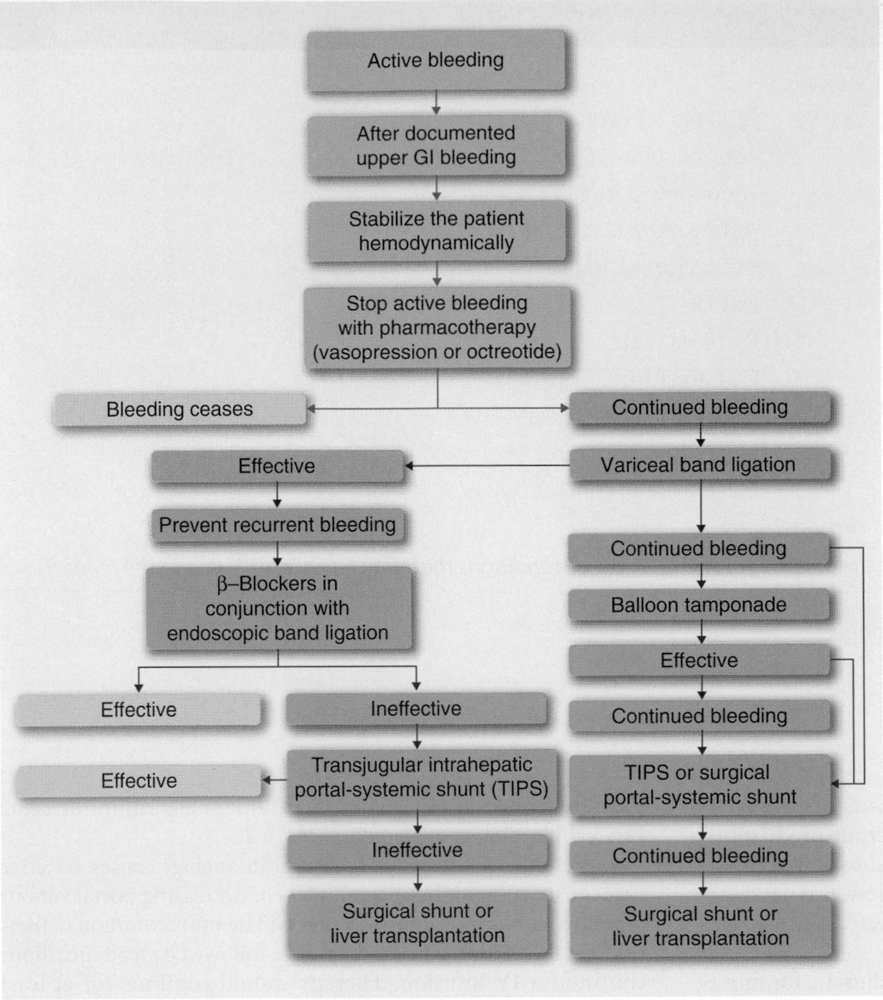

FIGURE 22–5. Treatment algorithm for active GI bleeding resulting from portal hypertension. (Adapted from Schiano TD, Bodenheimer HC. Complications of chronic liver disease. In: Friedman SL, McQuaid KR, Grendell JH, eds. Current Diagnosis and Treatment in Gastroenterology, 2nd ed. New York, NY: McGraw-Hill, 2003:649, with permission.)

KEY CONCEPT *Long-term SBP prophylaxis decreases mortality and is recommended in a select group of patients—those with a history of SBP and low-protein ascites (ascitic fluid albumin less than 1.5 g/dL [15 g/L]) plus one of the following: SCr 1.5 mg/dL (133 μmol/L) or greater, BUN 25 mg/dL (8.9 mmol/L) or greater, serum sodium 130 mEq/L (130 mmol/L) or less, or Child–Pugh score of at least 9, with bilirubin of at least 3 mg/dL (51.3 μmol/L).* Recommended oral regimens include one trimethoprim–sulfamethoxazole double-strength tablet daily or ciprofloxacin 750 mg daily.[9]

▶ *Hepatorenal Syndrome*

HRS is a life-threatening complication of cirrhosis. Targeted treatment increases central venous system volume. Peripheral vasoconstriction redistributes fluid from the periphery to the venous system; fluid is retained in the vascular space by administering albumin (to increase oncotic pressure). The ultimate goal is to increase renal perfusion.

A common regimen involves giving albumin 1 g/kg on day of diagnosis (day 1), followed by 20 to 40 g on subsequent treatment days. This regimen is used in combination with midodrine (an α-agonist) and octreotide. The initial midodrine dose is 7.5 mg orally three times daily; octreotide is administered subcutaneously (as opposed to IV during variceal bleeding) 100 mcg three times daily. Both drugs can be titrated as tolerated to achieve increases in mean arterial pressure of at least 15 mm Hg.

Terlipressin, a vasopressin analog available in Europe, has been used with success in patients with HRS, but it is not currently available in the United States.

▶ *Encephalopathy*

Lactulose KEY CONCEPT *Lactulose is the foundation of pharmacologic therapy to prevent and treat HE. It is a nondigestible synthetic disaccharide laxative; it is hydrolyzed in the gut to an osmotically active compound that draws water into the colon and stimulates defecation.* Lactulose lowers colonic pH, which favors the conversion of ammonia (NH_3) to ammonium (NH_4^+),[30] which cannot cross back from the gut into the systemic circulation because it is ionic. Lactulose is usually initiated at 15 to 30 mL two to three times per day and titrated to a therapeutic goal of two to four soft bowel movements daily.[14]

Antibiotic Therapy Rifaximin is a nonabsorbable antibiotic that decreases urease-producing gut bacteria, decreasing ammonia production. It is used extensively in Europe as first-line therapy for HE. Although rifaximin is both effective and well tolerated, its expense may prohibit long-term use. In the United States it is typically reserved for use as add-on therapy

Patient Encounter, Part 3

While in the ED, the patient was given one unit of packed red blood cells; antibiotics were not initiated due to report of PCN allergy. He was taken for endoscopy, banded in four places, and started on an octreotide infusion. Later in the day, he is awake and oriented to person and year, but not place. He admits to heavy alcohol use since losing his job. He admits to one bout of vomiting that "looked like coffee grounds" and dark tarry stools on and off for "a while."

What pharmacologic and nonpharmacologic interventions are needed to prevent progression of cirrhosis and future decompensation?

after failed lactulose monotherapy. Rifaximin is approved in the United States to prevent recurrences of hepatic encephalopathy at a dose of 550 mg twice daily, but 400 mg three times a day is often used.

Metronidazole and neomycin have also been used to treat hepatic encephalopathy but are not generally recommended because of toxicity; prolonged metronidazole use is associated with peripheral neuropathy, and although neomycin is classified as a nonabsorbable aminoglycoside antibiotic, patients with cirrhosis do have detectable plasma concentrations. The increased absorption is thought to be due to decreased integrity of the intestinal mucosa and may lead to nephrotoxicity. Neomycin should not be used.

Flumazenil Evidence for false transmitters as the cause of encephalopathy has been demonstrated by functional improvement after administering flumazenil (a benzodiazepine antagonist). Unfortunately, long-term benefit has not been demonstrated, and because flumazenil can only be administered parenterally, it is not an appropriate choice for clinical use; flumazenil use is limited to the research setting.

Patient Encounter, Part 4

The next day, the patient's mental status declines; he becomes somnolent and irritable. On physical examination his abdomen is very tender to mild palpation.

VS: BP 68/50 mm Hg, P 102 beats/min, T 101.9°F (38.8°C), RR 18 breaths/min, oxygen saturation 98% (0.98) on room air.

The medical resident suspects SBP and orders a paracentesis. The ascitic fluid shows PMNs 370 cells/μL (370 × 10^6/L), Gram stain negative, SAAG 1.2 g/dL (12 g/L).

Should you wait for the culture results to be sure there is actually an infection before starting antibiotics?

If antibiotics are indicated, what drug(s) and regimen(s) would you recommend?

What additional treatment should he receive?

If SBP is not treated appropriately, what are potential clinical consequences?

Is this patient a candidate for long-term antibiotic prophylaxis?

What are the feasible options for long-term antibiotic prophylaxis?

Patient Care Process for Cirrhosis and its Complications

Patient Assessment:

- Conduct a review of systems and physical examination at each visit to determine if the patient has had progression of complications and if the patient is responding to therapy.
- Assess heart rate and blood pressure for appropriate response to β-blockers.
- Question the patient about adverse effects; hepatically metabolized medications can accumulate and cause side effects.
- Obtain a complete history of alcohol intake and hepatotoxic drug use, including over-the-counter products and dietary supplements.

Therapy Evaluation:

- Ask the patient about adherence to prescribed therapy, dietary restrictions, and cessation of alcohol intake.
- Ask about bleeding, bruising, and fatigue; there is a direct link between loss of synthetic function and disease progression.

Care Plan Development:

- Refer the patient for substance abuse counseling for education about alcohol cessation if appropriate.
- Consider antibiotic prophylaxis for SBP in patients with low-protein ascites or prior SBP.
- Provide lactulose to patients with a history of HE.
- Consider β-blockers in patients with a history of variceal bleeding.

Follow-Up Evaluation:

- At each visit, evaluate the pharmacotherapy regimen for appropriate drug choice and dose, nonprescription drug use, adverse effects, and use of potentially hepatotoxic medications.
- Provide education regarding dietary sodium restriction at each visit; consider referral to a dietician if appropriate.

► *Coagulation Abnormalities*

Vitamin K is essential for hepatic synthesis of coagulation factors. The elevated clotting time that results from decreased protein synthesis is indistinguishable from coagulopathy that is a result of malnutrition or poor intestinal absorption. When given subcutaneously (10 mg for 3 days), Vitamin K_1 (phytonadione) can replete stores and establish if coagulation abnormalities are due to decreased synthetic function alone. It is unusual to completely reverse clotting abnormalities, but most patients experience a decrease in INR, conferring a decreased risk of bleeding. Because cirrhotic patients may have decreased bile production resulting in decreased absorption of fat-soluble vitamins, phytonadione should be given subcutaneously instead of orally to ensure absorption.

OUTCOME EVALUATION

- Reevaluate the pharmacotherapy regimen at each visit to assess adherence, effectiveness, adverse events, and need for drug titration.
- Determine adherence to lifestyle changes such as cessation of ethanol intake and avoidance of over-the-counter medications (particularly NSAIDs and acetaminophen) and dietary supplements that may exacerbate complications of cirrhosis.
- Assess dietary sodium intake by patient food recall. Measure dietary sodium adherence using spot urine sodium-to-potassium ratio to assess appropriate sodium excretion.
- Measure heart rate to assess effectiveness of β-blocker therapy, reduction of 25% from baseline or to 55 to 60 beats/min is desirable. Ask the patient-specific, directed questions regarding adverse effects of β-blockers; inquire about symptoms of orthostatic hypotension (eg, lightheadedness, dizziness, or fainting).
- Evaluate effectiveness of diuretic therapy with regard to ascitic fluid accumulation and development of peripheral edema. Ask the patient-directed questions regarding abdominal girth, fullness, tenderness, and pain. Weigh the patient at each visit, and ask the patient to keep a weight diary. Assess for peripheral edema at each visit.
- Obtain complete blood count (CBC) and PT/INR to assess for anemia, thrombocytopenia, or coagulopathy. Ask about bruising, bleeding, hematemesis, hematochezia, and melena to assess for bleeding.
- Review biopsy reports and laboratory data. Hepatic transaminases and blood ammonia levels do not correlate well with disease progression, but increased coagulation times are markers of loss of synthetic function.
- Evaluate for signs and symptoms of HE. Mental status changes may be subtle; questioning family members or caregivers about confusion or personality changes may reveal mild HE even if the patient is unaware of deficits. In patients taking lactulose therapy, titrate the dose to achieve two to four soft bowel movements daily.

Abbreviations Introduced in This Chapter

ADH	Antidiuretic hormone
ALT	Alanine aminotransferase
AST	Aspartate aminotransferase
BUN	Blood urea nitrogen
CBC	Complete blood count
CYP450	Cytochrome P-450 isoenzyme
GGT	γ-Glutamyl transferase
GI	Gastrointestinal
HE	Hepatic encephalopathy
HRS	Hepatorenal syndrome
INR	International normalized ratio
LDH	Lactate dehydrogenase
MELD	Model for End-Stage Liver Disease
NAFLD	Nonalcoholic fatty liver disease
NG	Nasogastric
NH_3	Ammonia
NH_4^+	Ammonium
NSAID	Nonsteroidal anti-inflammatory drug
PT	Prothrombin time
RAAS	Renin-angiotensin-aldosterone system
SAAG	Serum ascites–albumin gradient
SBP	Spontaneous bacterial peritonitis
TIPS	Transjugular intrahepatic portosystemic shunt

REFERENCES

1. Tsochatzis E, Bosch J, Burroughs A. Liver cirrhosis. Lancet. 2014; 383:1749–1761.
2. National Digestive Diseases Information Clearinghouse. Cirrhosis of the liver. NIH Publication No. 14–1134. Bethesda, MD, 2014.
3. Rehm J, Taylor B, Mohapatra S. Alcohol as a risk factor for liver cirrhosis: a systematic review and meta-analysis. Drug Alcohol Rev. 2010;29:437–445.
4. Soldin O, Mattison D. Sex differences in pharmacokinetics and pharmacodynamics. Clin Pharmacokinet. 2009;48:143–157.
5. Te H, Jensen D. Epidemiology of hepatitis B and C viruses: a global overview. Clin Liver Dis. 2010;14:1–21.
6. De Franchis R, Dell'era A. Invasive and noninvasive methods to diagnose portal hypertension and esophageal varices. Clin Liver Dis. 2014;18:293–302.
7. Berzigotti A, Gilabert R, Abraldes JG, et al. Noninvasive prediction of clinically significant portal hypertension and esophageal varices in patients with compensated liver cirrhosis. Am J Gastroenterol. 2008;103:1159–1167.
8. Afzelius P, Bazeghi N, Bie P, et al. Circulating nitric oxide products do not solely reflect nitric oxide release in cirrhosis and portal hypertension. Liver Int. 2011;31:1381–1387.
9. Runyon BA, AASLD. Introduction to the revised American Association for the Study of Liver Diseases Practice Guideline management of adult patients with ascites due to cirrhosis 2012. Hepatology. 2013; 57:1651-1653.
10. Garcia-Tsao G, Sanyal AJ, Grace ND, et al. Prevention and management of gastroesophageal varices and variceal hemorrhage in cirrhosis. Hepatology. 2007;46:922–938.
11. Rimola A, Garcia-Tsao G, Navasa M, et al. Diagnosis, treatment and prophylaxis of spontaneous bacterial peritonitis: a consensus document. International ascites club. J Hepatol. 2000; 32:142–153.
12. Steed H, Macfarlane GT, Blackett KL, et al. Bacterial translocation in cirrhosis is not caused by an abnormal small bowel gut microbiota. FEMS Immunol Med Microbiol. 2011;63:346–354.
13. Eckmann C, Dryden M, Montravers P. Antimicrobial treatment of "complicated" intra-abdominal infections and the new idsa guidelines - a commentary and an alternative european approach according to clinical definitions. Eur J Med Res. 2011;16:115–126.
14. Vilstrup H, Amodio P, Bajaj J, et al. Hepatic encephalopathy in chronic liver disease: 2014 Practice Guideline by the American Association for the Study of Liver Diseases and the European Association for the Study of the Liver. Hepatology. 2014;60:715–735.
15. Tripodi A, Primignani M, Chantarangkul V, Mannucci PM. Pro-coagulant imbalance in patients with chronic liver disease. J Hepatol. 2010; 53: 586–587.
16. Seth D, Haber PS, Syn W-K, Diehl AM, Day CP. Pathogenesis of alcohol-induced liver disease: Classical concepts and recent advances. J Gastroenterol Hepatol. 2011;26:1089–1105.
17. Sakaguchi S, Takahashi S, Sasaki T, Kumagai T, Nagata K. Progression of alcoholic and non-alcoholic steatohepatitis: Common metabolic aspects of innate immune system and oxidative stress. Drug Metab Pharmacokinet. 2011;26:30–46.

18. Chitturi S, Abeygunasekera S, Farrell GC, et al. NASH and insulin resistance: insulin hypersecretion and specific association with the insulin resistance syndrome. Hepatology. 2002;35:373–379.
19. Bravo AA, Sheth SG, Chopra S. Liver biopsy. N Engl J Med. 2001; 344:495–500.
20. Runyon B, Montano A, Akriviadis E, et al. The serum ascites albumin gradient is superior to the exudate-transudate concept in the differential diagnosis of ascites. Ann Intern Med. 1992; 117:215–220.
21. Sharara A, Rockey D. Gastroesophageal variceal hemorrhage. N Engl J Med. 2001;345:669–681.
22. Lo GH, Lai KH, Cheng JS, et al. Endoscopic variceal ligation plus nadolol and sucralfate compared with ligation alone for the prevention of variceal rebleeding: A prospective, randomized trial. Hepatology. 2000;32:461–465.
23. De La Pena J, Brullet E, Sanchez-Hernandez E, et al. Variceal ligation plus nadolol compared with ligation for prophylaxis of variceal rebleeding: A multicenter trial. Hepatology 2005; 41:572–578.
24. Pagliaro L, D'amico G, Sorensen TI, et al. Prevention of first bleeding in cirrhosis. A meta-analysis of randomized trials of nonsurgical treatment. Ann Intern Med. 1992;117:59–70.
25. De Franchis R. Revising consensus in portal hypertension: Report of the Baveno V consensus workshop on methodology of diagnosis and therapy in portal hypertension. J Hepatol. 2010;53:762–768.
26. Merkel C, Sacerdoti D, Bolognesi M, et al. Hemodynamic evaluation of the addition of isosorbide-5-mononitrate to nadolol in cirrhotic patients with insufficient response to the beta-blocker alone. Hepatology. 1997;26:34–39.
27. Garcia-Tsao G, Bosch J. Management of varices and variceal hemorrhage in cirrhosis. N Engl J Med. 2010;362:823–832.
28. Such J, Runyon B. Spontaneous bacterial peritonitis. Clin Infect Dis. 1998;27:669–674.
29. Salerno F, Navickis R, Wilkes M. Albumin infusion improves outcomes of patients with spontaneous bacterial peritonitis: A meta-analysis of randomized trials. Clin Gastroenterol Hepatol. 2013;11:123–130.
30. Sharkey K, Wallace J. Treatment of disorders of bowel motility and water flux; antiemetics; agents used in biliary and pancreatic disease. In: Brunton L, Lazo J, Parker K, eds. Goodman & Gilman's the Pharmacologic Basis of Therapeutics. New York, NY: McGraw-Hill, 2011:1323–1350.

23 Pancreatitis

Janine E. Then and Heather M. Rouse

LEARNING OBJECTIVES

Upon completion of the chapter, the reader will be able to:

1. Describe the pathophysiology of acute pancreatitis and chronic pancreatitis.
2. Differentiate acute pancreatitis from chronic pancreatitis.
3. Formulate care plans for managing acute and chronic pancreatitis.
4. Choose appropriate pancreatic enzyme supplementation for patients with chronic pancreatitis.

INTRODUCTION

The pancreas is a gland in the abdomen lying in the curvature of the stomach as it empties into the duodenum. It functions primarily as an exocrine gland but also has endocrine function. The exocrine cells of the pancreas are called **acinar cells** that produce and store digestive enzymes that mix with a bicarbonate-rich solution released from duct cells to produce pancreatic juice. This juice is released through the **ampulla of Vater** into the duodenum to aid in digestion and buffer acidic fluid released from the stomach (Figure 23–1).[1]

Pancreatic enzymes are produced and stored as inactive proenzymes within **zymogen** granules to prevent autolysis and digestion of the pancreas. Amylase and lipase are released from the zymogen granules in the active form, whereas the proteolytic enzymes are activated in the duodenum by enterokinase. Enterokinase triggers the conversion of trypsinogen to the active protease **trypsin**, which then activates the other proenzymes to their active enzymes. The pancreas contains a trypsin inhibitor to prevent autolysis.

ACUTE PANCREATITIS

EPIDEMIOLOGY AND ETIOLOGY

KEY CONCEPT *In the Western Hemisphere, acute pancreatitis is caused mainly by ethanol use/abuse and gallstones (**cholelithiasis**).* Ethanol use accounts for about 30% of acute pancreatitis cases and gallstones about 30% to 40% of cases. Other common causes include hypertriglyceridemia, endoscopic retrograde cholangiopancreatography (ERCP), pregnancy, and autodigestion due to early activation of pancreatic enzymes. Numerous medications have been implicated as causes of acute pancreatitis, but other causes should be ruled out before discontinuing a medication indefinitely (Table 23–1).[2,3]

PATHOPHYSIOLOGY

Ethanol abuse may cause precipitation of pancreatic enzymes in pancreatic ducts, leading to chronic inflammation and fibrosis resulting in loss of exocrine function. Ethanol may be directly toxic to the pancreatic cells and may lead to an upregulation of enzymes that produce toxic metabolites leading to further damage.[4] Gallstones can obstruct the ampulla of Vater causing pancreatic enzymes or bile to move in a retrograde fashion into the pancreas. This retrograde movement may be responsible for pancreatic autolysis.[1]

Autolysis of the pancreas can occur when zymogens are activated in the pancreas before being released into the duodenum. Acute pancreatitis can result from the initial injury to the zymogen-producing cells, which is followed by neutrophil, lymphocyte, and macrophage invasion of the pancreas and further activation of enzymes within the pancreas.

Acute pancreatitis can progress to peripancreatic fluid collections in or around the pancreas; they usually require no intervention and resolve spontaneously.[5,6] **Pancreatic pseudocysts** are walled-off fluid collections that form 4 weeks or longer after the onset of acute pancreatitis. Many pseudocysts resolve spontaneously, but some require surgical or percutaneous drainage. Rupture of a pancreatic pseudocyst is a serious complication and can lead to peritonitis and gastrointestinal (GI) bleeding.[5]

Pancreatic enzyme damage may lead to pancreatic necrosis, which is diffuse inflammation of the pancreas containing both necrotic tissue and fluid. KEY CONCEPT *Pancreatic necrosis occurs within the first 2 weeks of acute pancreatitis and affects 10% to 20% of patients.* Infected necrotic fluid collections occur in 16% to 47% of patients, usually due to bacteria normally present in the GI tract (*Escherichia coli*, Enterobacteriaceae, *Staphylococcus aureus*, viridans group streptococci, and anaerobes). Disseminated infection may result from pancreatic necrosis.[5,7] Pancreatic abscess is pancreatic necrosis that is walled-off by granulation tissue and occurs weeks after acute pancreatitis.

CLINICAL PRESENTATION AND DIAGNOSIS

Patients with acute pancreatitis may develop severe local and systemic complications. Multiorgan failure is a poor prognostic indicator. Disease severity can be predicted using the Ranson criteria, Glasgow severity scoring system, Acute Physiology and

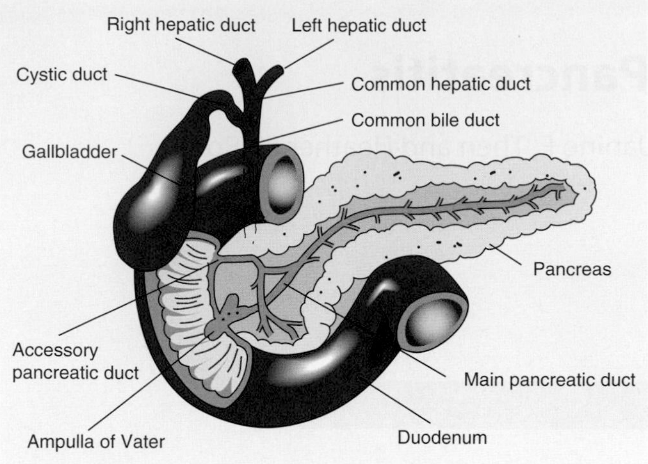

FIGURE 23–1. Anatomical structure of the pancreas and biliary tract. (From Bolesta S, Montgomery PA. Pancreatitis. In: DiPiro JT, Talbert RL, Yee GC, et al., eds. Pharmacotherapy: A Pathophysiologic Approach, 9th ed. New York, NY: McGraw-Hill, 2014; Fig. 25–1, with permission. www.accesspharmacy.com)

Chronic Health Evaluation II (APACHE II), and sequential organ failure assessment (SOFA). Awareness of risk factors for severe disease, including age greater than 55 years, comorbid conditions, laboratory findings, and presence of SIRS, may be more beneficial than scoring systems.[8]

DIAGNOSIS

Diagnosis of acute pancreatitis is based on patient history, signs and symptoms, and laboratory values. The history can identify risk factors for acute pancreatitis, including alcohol abuse and medications. A serum lipase greater than three times the normal limit supports the diagnosis. The serum lipase has greater sensitivity and specificity for acute pancreatitis than does the serum amylase due to its duration of elevation.[9,10] Elevated hepatic enzymes may indicate gallstone pancreatitis, and triglycerides should be checked to rule out hypertriglyceridemia as the cause.[8,10]

Abdominal ultrasound can identify gallstones and sludge in the common bile duct but has limited sensitivity. Computed tomography (CT) may be more useful in staging pancreatitis or identifying complications. ERCP should be used early when patients have concurrent acute cholangitis. Magnetic resonance imaging (MRI) and magnetic resonance cholangiopancreatography (MRCP) are more costly options that can be used to evaluate severity and pancreatic abnormalities.[8,10]

Clinical Presentation of Acute Pancreatitis

Signs and Symptoms

- Sudden upper abdominal pain is the most common symptom.
- Pain may radiate to the back, and ecchymosis may be present in the flank and periumbilical areas.
- Nausea and vomiting are other common symptoms.
- Tachycardia, hypotension, fever, and abdominal distention may be present.

Laboratory Tests

- The serum amylase may be elevated to more than three times the upper limit of normal within the first 12 hours of the onset of acute pancreatitis. The degree of elevation does not correlate with disease severity, and levels may return to normal before the patient presents for care.
- Serum lipase rises within 4 to 8 hours of onset, peaks at 24 hours, and returns to normal within 8 to 14 days.
- Other laboratory abnormalities may include elevated white blood cell (WBC) count, hyperglycemia, hypocalcemia, hyperbilirubinemia, elevated serum lactate dehydrogenase (LDH), and hypertriglyceridemia.

Table 23–1

Selected Medications Associated with Acute Pancreatitis

Cardiovascular: Enalapril, lisinopril, ramipril, losartan, furosemide, hydrochlorothiazide, amiodarone, statins

Anti-infectives: Metronidazole, sulfonamides, tetracycline, tigecycline, pentamidine, isoniazid, lamivudine, didanosine, nelfinavir, interferon/ribavirin

Gastrointestinal: Omeprazole, mesalamine

Neurologic: Valproic acid, clozapine

Hormone Therapy: Conjugated estrogens, tamoxifen

Oncologic: Ifosfamide, cytarabine

Analgesics: Sulindac, salicylates

Other: Propofol, mercaptopurine, azathioprine, corticosteroids, marijuana

TREATMENT

Desired Outcomes

The goals of treatment for acute pancreatitis include: (a) resolution of nausea, vomiting, abdominal pain, and fever; (b) ability to tolerate oral intake; (c) normalization of serum amylase, lipase, and white blood cell (WBC) count; and (d) resolution of abscess, pseudocyst, or fluid collection as measured by CT scan.

Nonpharmacologic Therapy

Many medications can precipitate an attack of acute pancreatitis. If a medication is suspected to be the cause of acute pancreatitis, it should be discontinued and an alternative therapy should be considered.[2,3]

KEY CONCEPT *Therapy of acute pancreatitis is primarily supportive unless a specific etiology is identified (Figure 23–2). Supportive therapy involves fluid repletion, nutrition support, and analgesia.* Patients with acute pancreatitis are administered IV fluids to maintain hydration and blood pressure. Lactated Ringer's solution at a rate of 250 to 500 mL/hour should be used to provide aggressive hydration. The total amount of fluids administered should be based on vital signs and urine output. Fluid requirements should be assessed carefully, especially in patients with concomitant cardiac, renal, and liver disease. Electrolytes such as potassium and magnesium may be added to the infusions if necessary. Hyperglycemia can be managed with insulin-containing IV infusions.[8]

While it is common to discontinue oral feedings during acute pancreatitis, this does not prevent further damage because

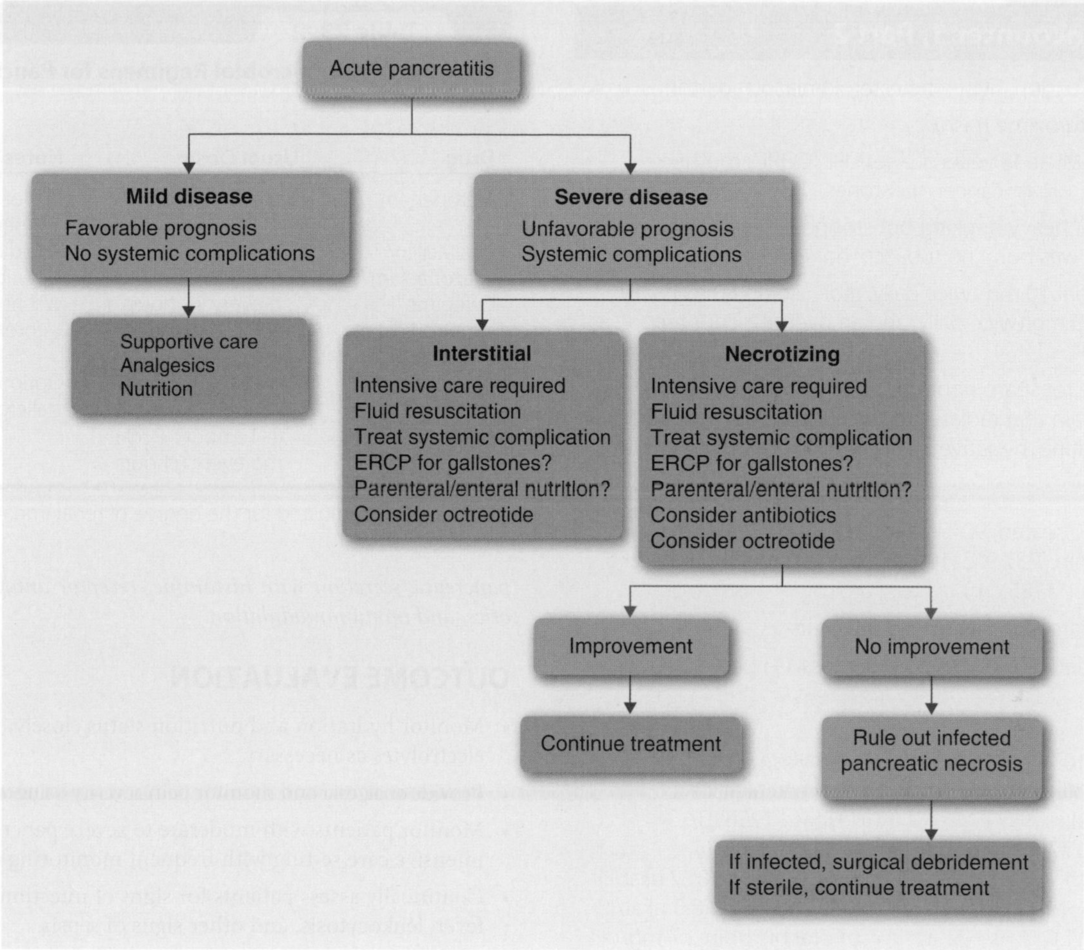

FIGURE 23–2. Algorithm for evaluation and treatment of acute pancreatitis. (ERCP, endoscopic retrograde cholangiopancreatography.) (From Bolesta S, Montgomery PA. Pancreatitis. In: DiPiro JT, Talbert RL, Yee GC, et al., eds. Pharmacotherapy: A Pathophysiologic Approach, 9th ed. New York, NY: McGraw-Hill, 2014; Figure 25–3, with permission.) www.accesspharmacy.com.

secretion of trypsin is already reduced during acute pancreatitis.[7] In mild to moderate pancreatitis, diet should be advanced based on resolution of nausea, vomiting, and pain. In severe pancreatitis, enteral nutrition should be started as early as possible and may include nasogastric or nasojejunal feedings. Early use of enteral nutrition has been shown to decrease surgical interventions and infectious complications. Enteral nutrition is preferred, but if a patient is not meeting caloric goals, it may be supplemented with total parenteral nutrition.[7,8,10,11] If pancreatic necrosis or abscesses are present, surgical or interventional procedures may be necessary.

Patient Encounter 1, Part 1

A 67-year-old man presents to the emergency department with a 2-day history of nausea and vomiting. He also complains of abdominal pain that is unrelieved and persistent. He has not eaten in the past 2 days because food exacerbates the pain. Upon examination, his abdomen is found to be distended.

What information about the patient presentation is consistent with acute pancreatitis?

What tests may be helpful in the diagnosis of acute pancreatitis?

Pharmacologic Therapy

▶ *Analgesics*

Meperidine has historically been the most popular analgesic in acute pancreatitis because it is purported to cause less spasm and resulting pain in the sphincter of Oddi than other opioids. The importance of this has not been confirmed in clinical studies, so patients should be given the most effective analgesic. Hydromorphone, morphine, and fentanyl are reasonable alternatives to meperidine and may be more desirable due to other adverse effects associated with meperidine (see Chapter 34, Pain Management).

▶ *Antibiotics*

Antibiotics do not prevent formation of pancreatic abscess or necrosis when given early in the course of acute pancreatitis.[8,10] Empiric antibiotics are not indicated if the patient has mild disease or a known noninfectious cause. In necrotizing pancreatitis, antibiotics may be appropriate for patients who fail to improve after 1 week or deteriorate. The decision to use antibiotics should be guided by fine needle aspiration whenever possible.[8] If necrosis is confirmed, antibiotics are insufficient as sole therapy;

Patient Encounter 1, Part 2

PMH: Hypertension, hypercholesterolemia, osteoarthritis

Allergies: cefuroxime (rash)

FH: Father—MI at 48 years of age, CHF, COPD; mother—osteoporosis, breast cancer, gallstones

SH: History of heavy drinking but stopped 12 years ago when his first child was born; no tobacco; no recreational drugs

Meds: Enalapril 10 mg twice daily, atorvastatin 80 mg daily, naproxen 500 mg twice daily, and an over-the-counter "stomach pill"

ROS: Positive for sharp right upper quadrant (RUQ) abdominal pain that radiates to the right shoulder and back, nausea, vomiting; negative for substernal chest pain

PE:

VS: BP 105/60 seated, 90/50 standing, P 120 beats/min, RR 22 breaths/min, T 37.9°C (100.2°F), pain score 9/10, Wt 91 kg (200 lb), Ht 6′1″ (185 cm)

CV: Regular rate and rhythm, no murmurs

Abd: Distended, (+) rebound tenderness, (+) bowel sounds, (+) guarding

Labs:

WBC 15.8 × 10^3/mm^3 (15.8 × 10^9/L)	Amylase 90 IU/L (1.50 μkat/L)
Hgb 10.9 g/dL (109 g/L, 6.77 mmol/L)	Lipase 1250 IU/L (20.8 μkat/L)
Hct 30% (0.30)	AST 520 IU/L (8.67 μkat/L)
Platelets 250 × 10^3/ mm^3 (250 × 10^9/L)	ALT 480 IU/L (8.0 μkat/L)
	Total bilirubin 2.7 mg/dL (46.2 μmol/L)
BUN 19 mg/dL (6.8 mmol/L)	LDH 1050 IU/L (17.5 μkat/L)
SCr 1.2 mg/dL (106 μmol/L)	
Glucose 220 mg/dL (12.2 mmol/L)	

Abdominal x-ray and ultrasound: Pending

What clinical signs are consistent with acute pancreatitis?

What additional information is needed at this point?

What treatment(s) would you initiate?

surgical debridement is necessary for cure but may be delayed to allow for the necrosis to become walled off.[6,7,8,10,12] Consideration should be given to discontinuing antibiotics if no source of infection is confirmed.

Infections are usually polymicrobial, so broad-spectrum antibiotics with activity against enteric gram-negative bacilli are appropriate (Table 23–2). Patients may receive long courses of broad-spectrum antibiotics and may develop superinfections with resistant bacteria. Routine use of antifungal agents (eg, fluconazole) is not recommended but may be considered if peritonitis or GI perforation develops due to the presence of fungi such as *Candida albicans* in the GI tract.[8,13]

▶ *Ineffective Therapies*

KEY CONCEPT *Therapies with no proven benefit on morbidity and mortality include reducing pancreatic secretion by administering somatostatin analogues or atropine, reducing gastric acidity and*

Table 23–2

Selected IV Antimicrobial Regimens for Pancreatic Necrosis

Drug	Usual Dose[a]	Notes
Meropenem	1 g every 8 hours	Risk of superinfection
Piperacillin/ tazobactam	3.375–4.5 g every 6–8 hours	Avoid if allergic to penicillin
Cefepime + metronidazole	2 g every 12 hours + 500 mg every 8–12 hours	Will not cover enterococci
Aztreonam + vancomycin + metronidazole	1 g every 8 hours + 15 mg/kg every 8–12 hours + 500 mg every 6 hours	Option for penicillin-allergic patients

[a]Doses must be adjusted for the degree of renal impairment.

pancreatic secretion with histamine$_2$-receptor antagonists, probiotics, and immunomodulation.

OUTCOME EVALUATION

- Monitor hydration and nutrition status closely; replete electrolytes as necessary.
- Provide analgesia and monitor pain severity using validated scales.
- Monitor patients with moderate to severe pancreatitis in an intensive care setting with frequent monitoring of vital signs.
- Continually assess patients for signs of infection, including fever, leukocytosis, and other signs of sepsis.

Patient Care Process for Acute Pancreatitis

Patient Assessment:

- Assess fluid and nutritional status and abdominal pain severity.
- Review laboratory data to determine if lipase and/or amylase are elevated. If triglycerides are elevated, identify potential causes.
- Review imaging results to determine potential causes and extent of pancreatic damage.

Therapy Evaluation:

- Review medication history for potential risk factors for pancreatitis.

Care Plan Development:

- Provide fluid repletion until the patient shows signs of adequate perfusion (monitor blood pressure and urine output).
- Provide analgesia using multimodal therapy.
- Initiate enteral nutrition early; consider parenteral nutrition if enteral nutrition is not tolerated within 1 week.

Follow-Up Evaluation:

- Assess vital signs frequently.
- Provide ongoing monitoring for potential infection.

CHRONIC PANCREATITIS

EPIDEMIOLOGY AND ETIOLOGY

The incidence of chronic pancreatitis (CP) ranges from 3.5 to 10 per 100,000 population. KEY CONCEPT *The most common cause of CP in adults in Western countries is ethanol abuse.* Other causes include genetic predisposition, obstructive disease (secondary to ductal strictures or pseudocysts), autoimmune pancreatitis, abnormal cystic fibrosis transmembrane conductance regulator (CFTR) function as seen in cystic fibrosis (CF) patients, tropical pancreatitis, and idiopathic pancreatitis.[4,14] Cigarette smoking is an independent risk factor for CP.[15]

PATHOPHYSIOLOGY

CP is an inflammatory process that occurs over time leading to impaired endocrine and exocrine function secondary to diffuse scarring and fibrosis. Hypotheses on the pathogenesis of ethanol-induced pancreatitis include: (a) precipitation of secreted pancreatic proteins within small pancreatic ducts leading to acinar atrophy and fibrosis, (b) disruption of acinar cells leading to early activation of digestive enzymes and autodigestive pancreatic injury, and (c) oxidative pancreatic stress caused by toxic metabolites of ethanol.[4,14]

KEY CONCEPT *Long-term sequelae of CP include dietary malabsorption, impaired glucose tolerance, cholangitis, and potential addiction to opioid analgesics.* As pancreatic exocrine function diminishes, patients have decreased ability to absorb lipids and protein with normal dietary intake, leading to weight loss and malnutrition. Fat- or protein-containing stools are common; carbohydrate absorption is usually unaffected.[14] Patients with CP are at risk and should be screened for fat-soluble vitamin deficiencies (A, D, E, and K).[16,17]

CLINICAL PRESENTATION AND DIAGNOSIS

The symptoms, signs, and laboratory abnormalities associated with CP are shown in the accompanying box. Pancreatic biopsy with histologic examination is the gold standard for diagnosis of CP, but it is rarely performed. In the absence of histology, abdominal ultrasound, CT, MRCP, or ERCP can assist in the diagnosis.[4,14]

Clinical Presentation of Chronic Pancreatitis

General

- Presentation of CP can be similar to that of acute pancreatitis.

Symptoms

- Pain is the most common symptom, and it typically starts in the epigastrium and may radiate to the back or scapula. Pain can be sharp or dull, is not relieved by antacids, and can be provoked by ethanol ingestion or a fatty meal.
- Pain may be associated with nausea and vomiting, causing patients to avoid food.
- Weight loss can result from chronic fat and protein malabsorption.

Signs

- Steatorrhea (due to fat malabsorption), malnutrition, and glucose intolerance are often present in advanced CP.
- GI bleeding can result from erosion of intestinal blood vessels by pancreatic enzymes or as a result of thrombosis.
- Chronic obstruction of the common bile duct by the inflamed pancreas can cause icterus, cholangitis, and biliary cirrhosis.

Laboratory Tests

- Glucose intolerance may occur because of chronic destruction of pancreatic endocrine function.
- Serum amylase and lipase concentrations may be normal to slightly elevated in CP and are not particularly useful in the diagnosis.
- The serum bilirubin or alkaline phosphatase may be elevated due to inflammation near the common bile duct.

Patient Encounter 1, Part 3

The patient has now been hospitalized for 10 days with continued pain and food intolerance. This morning his WBC count is elevated at $21.2 \times 10^3/mm^3$ ($21.2 \times 10^9/L$), and he has a temperature of 38.7°C (101.6°F). He is hypotensive with a MAP of 60 mm Hg, and his HR is 115 beats/min. His respiratory rate is 28 breaths/min and SCr is 2.0 mg/dL (177 μmol/L). A CT scan demonstrates pancreatic necrosis, and a fine needle aspiration is performed. His APACHE II score is calculated to be 13.

Based on his APACHE II score of 13, should the patient be considered for transfer to the intensive care unit?

Which microorganisms should empiric antibiotics cover?

What antimicrobials would be appropriate to initiate after cultures are sent?

Besides antibiotics, what other pharmacologic treatments may need to be optimized?

TREATMENT

Desired Outcomes

Goals of pharmacotherapy for CP include: (a) relief of acute and chronic abdominal pain, (b) correction of dietary malabsorption with exogenous pancreatic enzymes, and (c) treatment of endocrine insufficiency and associated diabetes.

▸ *Nonpharmacologic Therapy*

KEY CONCEPT *Avoidance of ethanol, cigarette smoking, and fatty meals can decrease the pain of CP.* Alcohol and cigarette abstainers may have slower disease progression and better response to pain therapy than nonabstainers.[4,14,15] Patients should consume a diet consisting of frequent small low-fat meals (less than 20 g fat/day) or one with medium-chain triglycerides where absorption requires only minimal amounts of pancreatic enzymes.[4,18] Most surgical procedures to reduce inflammation or remove strictures have not been studied in clinical trials and carry a high risk of morbidity and mortality.[4,14]

Pharmacologic Therapy

▸ Analgesics

KEY CONCEPT *Pain management is an important component of therapy and similar to that of acute pancreatitis.* Nonopioid analgesics (eg, acetaminophen, nonsteroidal anti-inflammatory drugs [NSAIDs]) are preferred, but the severe and persistent nature of the pain often requires opioid therapy. Patients can require chronic doses of opioid analgesics, with resulting risk of addiction.[4,19] Patients should also be assessed for neuropathic pain and treated accordingly (eg, tricyclic antidepressants, pregabalin).[19,20] Refer to Chapter 34 (Pain Management) for guidance in selecting an analgesic dose.

▸ Pancreatic Enzymes

Pancreatic enzyme supplements (PES) are indicated in symptomatic patients with steatorrhea. The goal is to deliver exogenous enzyme to the duodenum without causing further GI side effects, risking noncompliance due to the large number of dosage units required, or causing undue medication expense. KEY CONCEPT *Supplementation with pancreatic enzymes may reduce the pain and fatty diarrhea associated with CP.* Common PES contain lipase, amylase, and protease in varying proportions. The half-life of endogenous lipase is based on the presence of its substrates (ie, triglycerides), and therefore dietary fat restriction should be reconsidered when pancreatic enzyme replacement is used.[18,21]

PES products approved by the US Food and Drug Administration are shown in Table 23–3.[22] Enteric-coated products are designed to release enzymes in the alkaline environment (pH greater than 5.5) of the duodenum, thus minimizing enzyme destruction in the stomach. However, in patients with delayed gastric emptying, the efficacy of the enteric-coated PES may be decreased due to early activation of the lipase enzymes. Addition of an H_2-blocker or proton pump inhibitor will decrease stomach acidity, thereby enhancing delivery of the PES to the site of action. The nonenteric-coated PES are deactivated immediately in an acidic environment and therefore must be administered with a proton pump inhibitor.[18,21]

Table 23–3

FDA-Approved Pancreatic Enzyme Supplements

	Enzyme Content (Units)[a]		
Product	**Lipase**	**Amylase**	**Protease**
Creon 3000	3000	15,000	9500
Creon 6000	6000	30,000	19,000
Creon 12,000	12,000	60,000	38,000
Creon 24,000	24,000	76,000	120,000
Creon 36,000	36,000	180,000	114,000
Pancreaze 4200	4200	17,500	10,000
Pancreaze 10,500	10,500	43,750	25,000
Pancreaze 16,800	16,800	70,000	40,000
Pancreaze 21,000	21,000	61,000	37,000
Pancrelipase	5000	27,000	17,000
Zenpep 3000	3000	16,000	10,000
Zenpep 5000	5000	27,000	17,000
Zenpep 10,000	10,000	55,000	34,000
Zenpep 15,000	15,000	82,000	51,000
Zenpep 20,000	20,000	109,000	68,000
Zenpep 25,000	25,000	136,000	85,000
Ultresa 13,800	13,800	27,600	27,600
Ultresa 20,700	20,700	41,400	41,400
Ultresa 23,000	23,000	46,000	46,000
Pertyze[b]	8000	30,250	28,750
Pertyze[b]	16,000	60,500	57,500
Viokace 10,440[c]	10,440	39,150	39,150
Viokace 20,880[c]	20,880	78,300	78,300

[a]All products are porcine derived.

[b]Bicarbonate-buffered enteric-coated microspheres.

[c]Nonenteric-coated tablets; must be administered with a proton pump inhibitor.

Patient Encounter 2

A 53-year-old woman presents to the emergency department complaining of a chronic dull pain in her abdomen for several months that is no longer relieved with over-the-counter analgesics. She has also had light-colored liquid stools for the past month and has lost 10 pounds because of decreased appetite and worsening abdominal pain with meals.

PMH: Hypothyroidism, depression, recurrent acute pancreatitis, bipolar disorder

SH: Consumes a six-pack of beer per day and has a 35 pack–year history of cigarette smoking

Meds: Duloxetine 60 mg daily, levothyroxine 100 mcg every morning, divalproex sodium 500 mg twice daily, and recent use of ibuprofen 400 mg every 4 hours without pain relief

ROS: (+) for RUQ abdominal pain that radiates to her back, decreased appetite, 10-lb (4.5-kg) weight loss and diarrhea for the past month. (–) for chest pain or shortness of breath

PE:

VS: BP 118/67 mm Hg, HR 75 beats/min, RR 15 breaths/min, T 37.1°C (98.8°F), Wt 47.6 kg (105 lb), Ht 5′4″ (163 cm)

Pain Assessment: 6–8 out of 10 (numerical rating scale); currently 8/10 pain. Describes as dull aching pain and tingling, needle-like pain

CV: Regular rate and rhythm, no murmurs

Abd: Distended, (+) rebound tenderness, (+) bowel sounds

Labs:

Amylase 50 IU/L (0.83 μkat/L)	BUN 19 mg/dL (6.8 mmol/L)
Lipase 100 IU/L (1.7 μkat/L)	SCr 0.75 mg/dL (66 μmol/L)
AST 32 IU/L (0.53 μkat/L)	Glucose 248 mg/dL (13.8 mmol/L)
ALT 29 IU/L (0.48 μkat/L)	Triglycerides 180 mg/dL (2.03 mmol/L)

CT Scan Abdomen: Diffuse pancreatic scarring and calcifications

What signs and symptoms are consistent with chronic pancreatitis?

Why are the serum amylase and lipase normal?

What lifestyle modifications would you recommend for this patient?

What, if any, treatment regimens would you initiate, and how would you monitor their effects?

Patient Care Process for Chronic Pancreatitis

Patient Assessment:

- Determine whether the patient is receiving any medications that may cause or exacerbate pancreatitis. Does the patient have a significant alcohol or smoking history?
- Evaluate nutritional status and current diet habits. Evaluate vitamin A, D, E, and K levels, fasting blood glucose, and A1C.
- Ask the patient to describe the pain. What makes the pain worse and what relieves it?

Therapy Evaluation:

- If the patient is already receiving pharmacotherapy, assess efficacy, safety, and patient adherence. Are there any significant drug interactions?

Care Plan Development:

- If there is significant alcohol or smoking history, inform the patient about the need for abstinence and provide appropriate resources to maintain abstinence.
- Refer the patient for nutritional counseling if there is decreased caloric intake, significant weight loss, or signs of malnutrition.
- Initiate PES in patients with steatorrhea. As PES is titrated, patients can reintroduce fats into the diet because PES are more effective in the presence of their substrate.
- Supplement any identified nutritional deficiencies. If the patient has elevated fasting blood glucose or A1C, consider starting antidiabetic therapy (see Chapter 43, Diabetes Mellitus).
- Develop a plan for analgesia to control and prevent pain.

Follow-Up Evaluation:

- Adjust PES dosage based on nutritional status and pain with meals on a monthly basis until adequate control. Once stable doses of PES and analgesia are established, monitor the patient once or twice yearly.
- Evaluate the patient's Vitamin A, D, E, K levels, fasting blood glucose, and A1C annually.
- Reassess analgesia and adjust medication and dosages as indicated.

Pancreatic enzyme supplements should be taken immediately prior to meals and snacks to aid in the absorption and digestion of food. Dosing is based on body weight, clinical symptoms, and stool fat content. A normal starting dose is 500 units/kg/meal of lipase with half of the mealtime dose administered with snacks. Doses of lipase more than 10,000 units/kg/day should be used with caution because they may be associated with colonic stricture and fibrosis.[18,21]

► *Endocrine*

Patients with CP can develop glucose intolerance, but it usually does not progress to overt diabetes mellitus until late in the disease. Fasting blood glucose should be monitored annually, and ensuing diabetes should be treated with insulin. Patients with CP are at increased risk of hypoglycemia due to dysfunction of the pancreatic alpha cells, which are responsible for glucagon secretion.[4,14,23]

► *Other Therapies*

In patients with autoimmune pancreatitis, prednisolone 30 to 40 mg/day tapered over a 3-month period may provide rapid relief of symptoms.[24] Antioxidants such as methionine, ascorbic acid, and selenium may reduce the number of painful days per month in patients with CP.[4,25,26]

OUTCOME EVALUATION

- Monitor pain control and adjust analgesics accordingly.
- Encourage lifestyle modifications such as abstinence from ethanol and cigarettes.
- Counsel patients to monitor for weight gain or loss and fatty stool output as markers of malabsorption.
- Educate patients that adherence with PES is key to improved outcomes.

Abbreviations Introduced in This Chapter

APACHE II	Acute Physiology and Chronic Health Evaluation II
CF	Cystic fibrosis
CFTR	Cystic fibrosis transmembrane conductance regulator
CP	Chronic pancreatitis
CT	Computed tomography
ERCP	Endoscopic retrograde cholangiopancreatography
GI	Gastrointestinal
LDH	lactate dehydrogenase
MAP	Mean arterial pressure
MRCP	Magnetic resonance cholangiopancreatography
MRI	Magnetic resonance imaging
PES	Pancreatic enzyme supplements
RUQ	Right upper quadrant
SOFA	Sequential organ failure assessment
WBC	White blood cell

REFERENCES

1. Hegyi P, Pandol S, Venglovecz V, Rakonczay Z Jr. The acinar-ductal tango in the pathogenesis of acute pancreatitis. Gut. 2011;60:544–552.
2. Nitsche CJ, Jamieson N, Lerch MM, Mayerle JV. Drug induced pancreatitis. Best Pract Res Clin Gastroenterol. 2010;24:143–155.
3. Balani AR, Grendell JH. Drug-induced pancreatitis: incidence, management and prevention. Drug Saf. 2008;31(10):823–837.
4. Braganza JM, Lee SH, McCloy RF, McMahon MJ. Chronic pancreatitis. Lancet. 2011;377:1184–1197.
5. Brun A, Agarwal N, Pitchumoni CS. Fluid collections in and around the pancreas in acute pancreatitis. J Clin Gastroenterol. 2011;45:614–625.

6. Whitehead DA, Gardner TB. Evidence-based management of necrotizing pancreatitis. Curr Treat Options Gastroenterol. 2014;12(3):322–332.
7. Talukdar R, Vege SS. Early management of severe acute pancreatitis. Curr Gastroenterol Rep. 2011;13:123–130.
8. Tenner S, Baillie J, DeWitt J, Vege SS. American College of Gastroenterology Guideline: Management of Acute Pancreatitis. Am J Gastroenterol. 2013;108:1400–1415.
9. Frank B, Gottlieb K. Amylase normal, lipase elevated: is it pancreatitis? A case series and review of the literature. Am J Gastroenterol. 1999;94(2):463–469.
10. Schneider L, Buchler MW, Werner J. Acute pancreatitis with an emphasis on infection. Infect Dis Clin North Am. 2010;24:921–941.
11. Quan H, Wang X, Guo C. A meta-analysis of enteral nutrition and total parenteral nutrition in patients with acute pancreatitis. Gastroenterol Res Pract. 2011;2011:698248.
12. Nicholson LJ. Acute pancreatitis: Should we use antibiotics? Curr Gastroenterol Rep. 2011;13:336–343.
13. Trikudanathan G, Navaneethan U, Vege SS. Intra-abdominal fungal infections complicating acute pancreatitis: A review. Am J Gastroenterol. 2011;106:1188–1192.
14. Witt H, Apte MV, Keim V, Wilson JS. Chronic pancreatitis: Challenges and advances in pathogenesis, genetics, diagnosis and therapy. Gastroenterology. 2007;132:1557–1573.
15. Yadav D, Whitcomb DC. The role of alcohol and smoking in pancreatitis. Nat Rev Gastroenterol Hepatol. 2010;7:131–145.
16. Duggan SN, Smyth ND, O'Sullivan M, et al. The prevalence of malnutrition and fat-soluble vitamin deficiencies in chronic pancreatitis. Nutr Clin Pract. 2014;29(3):348–354.
17. Sikkens EC, Cahen DL, Koch AD, et al. The prevalence of fat-soluble vitamin deficiencies and a decreased bone mass in patients with chronic pancreatitis. Pancreatology. 2013;13(3):238–242.
18. Domínquez-Muňoz JE. Pancreatic exocrine insufficiency: Diagnosis and treatment. J Gastroenterol Hepatol. 2011;26 (suppl 2):12–16.
19. Puylaert M, Kapural L, Van Zundert J, et al. Pain in chronic pancreatitis. Pain Pract 2011;11(5):492–505.
20. Olesen SS, Bouwense SA, Wilder-Smith OH, Van Goor H, Drewes AM. Pregabalin reduces pain in patients with chronic pancreatitis in a randomized, controlled trial. Gastroenterology. 2011;141:536–543.
21. Berry AJ. Pancreatic enzyme replacement therapy during pancreatic insufficiency. Nutr Clin Pract. 2014;29(3):312–321.
22. Giuliano CA, Dehoorne-Smith ML, Kale-Pradhan PB. Pancreatic enzyme products: Digesting the changes. Ann Pharmacother. 2011;45:658–666.
23. Ewald N, Hardt PD. Diagnosis and treatment of diabetes mellitus in chronic pancreatitis. World J Gastroenterol. 2013;19(42):7276–7281.
24. Hirano K, Tada M, Isayama H, et al. Long-term prognosis of autoimmune pancreatitis with and without corticosteroid treatment. Gut. 2007;56(12):1719–1724.
25. Bhardwaj P, Garg PK, Maulik SK, et al. A randomized controlled trial of antioxidant supplementation for pain relief in patients with chronic pancreatitis. Gastroenterology. 2009;136:149–159.
26. Zhou D, Wang W, Cheng X, Wei J, Zheng S. Antioxidant therapy for patients with chronic pancreatitis: A systematic review and meta-analysis. Clin Nutr. 2014. http://dx.doi.org/10.1016/j.clnu.2014.07.003

24 Viral Hepatitis

Juliana Chan

LEARNING OBJECTIVES

Upon completion of the chapter, the reader will be able to:

1. Differentiate the five types of viral hepatitis by epidemiology, etiology, pathophysiology, clinical presentation, and natural history.
2. Identify modes of transmission and risk factors among the major types of viral hepatitis.
3. Evaluate hepatic serologies to understand how the type of hepatitis is diagnosed.
4. Create treatment goals for a patient infected with viral hepatitis.
5. Recommend appropriate pharmacotherapy for prevention of viral hepatitis.
6. Develop a care plan for treatment of chronic viral hepatitis.
7. Formulate a monitoring plan to assess adverse effects of pharmacotherapy for viral hepatitis.

INTRODUCTION

The most common types of viral hepatitis include hepatitis A (HAV), B (HBV), C (HCV), D (HDV), and E (HEV). Acute hepatitis may be associated with all five types of hepatitis and rarely exceeds 6 months in duration. Chronic hepatitis (disease lasting longer than 6 months) is usually associated with hepatitis B, C, and D. KEY CONCEPT *Chronic viral hepatitis may lead to the development of cirrhosis and may result in end-stage liver disease (ESLD) and hepatocellular carcinoma (HCC).* Complications of ESLD include ascites, edema, hepatic encephalopathy, infections (eg, spontaneous bacterial peritonitis), hepatorenal syndrome, and esophageal varices. *Therefore, prevention and treatment of viral hepatitis may prevent ESLD and HCC.*

Viral hepatitis may occur at any age and is the most common cause of liver disease in the world. The true prevalence and incidence may be underreported because most patients are asymptomatic. The epidemiology, etiology, and pathogenesis vary depending on the type of hepatitis and are considered separately below.

EPIDEMIOLOGY AND ETIOLOGY

Hepatitis A

Hepatitis A (HAV) affects 1.4 million people yearly worldwide.[1] The prevalence is highest in economically challenged and underdeveloped countries, including Africa, parts of South America, the Middle East, and Southeast Asia.[2] The decrease in HAV incidence is due to vaccination programs, but outbreaks may still occur, as evidenced in 2013 by a food outbreak with pomegranate seeds affecting 162 people over 10 States in the United States.[3] The number of acute HAV infections and hospitalizations annually have decreased markedly since the introduction of the HAV vaccine in 1995.[4]

HAV is primarily detected in contaminated feces and infects people via the fecal–oral route.[1,2] Outbreaks occur in areas of poor sanitation.[2] About 45% of the reported cases have no identifiable risk factors; individuals at greatest risk of acquiring HAV are listed in Table 24–1.[2]

There are no documented cases of chronic hepatitis A.[2] Death from HAV is rare and mostly associated with fulminant hepatitis; approximately 100 people in the United States die each year from HAV-related causes.[2]

Hepatitis B

Chronic hepatitis B (CHB) is a bloodborne infection affecting about 240 million people worldwide that may lead to cirrhosis and complications of ESLD.[5,6] Globally, more than 780,000 deaths are associated with HBV annually.[6] Despite having an effective vaccine against HBV since 1982, there were 18,800 new HBV infections in 2011 in the United States.[4] Fewer than 1% of individuals in North America and Western Europe are chronically infected, compared with 2% to 5% and 8% to 15% in developing areas such as the Middle East and East Asia, respectively.[2,6]

The highest concentration of the HBV is found in blood and serous fluids.[7] Thus the primary modes of transmission are by blood or body fluids through perinatal, sexual, or percutaneous exposure (see Table 24–1).[7,8] Infants born to mothers who are infected with actively replicating HBV have a 70% to 90% risk of becoming infected.[7] Approximately 16% of the reported cases have no identifiable risk factors.[7,8]

Hepatitis C

Approximately 130 to 185 million people are infected with chronic HCV worldwide, and about 4 million have the disease in the United States.[9,10] The prevalence is higher among non-Hispanic blacks than non-Hispanic whites, and men are more likely to be infected than women.[10] Also, HCV may be categorized based on genotypes, which are geographically specific. There are 6 genotypes (numbered 1–6) and 67 subtypes

Table 24–1

Risk Factors for Acquiring Viral Hepatitis

Hepatitis A	
International travelers to endemic areas (eg, Africa, Asia, and parts of South America)	
Sexual contact with infected persons (eg, men having sex with other men)	
Day care centers or household contacts with people infected with HAV	
IV drug users using unsterilized needles	
Workers involved with nonhuman primates	
Patients with clotting factor disorders	
Hepatitis B and D	
Infants born to infected mothers	
International travelers to endemic areas	
Men having sex with other men	
Individuals with multiple heterosexual partners	
IV drug users using unsterilized needles	
Recipients of blood products	
Household contacts with acute hepatitis B	
Healthcare providers and public safety workers in contact with infected blood	
Residents and staff of facilities for developmentally disabled persons	
Patients undergoing dialysis	
Hepatitis C	
Current or former injection drug users	
Recipients of blood products (clotting factor concentrates made before 1987, blood transfusions or solid organ transplants before July 1992)	
Health care providers in contact with infected needles	
Chronic hemodialysis	
Individuals having multiple sexual partners	
HIV infection	
Perinatal transmission (< 5%)	
Unprofessional body piercing and tattooing	
Person born from 1945 through 1965	
Hepatitis E	
International travelers to endemic areas (eg, parts of Asia, Africa, and Mexico)	
Ingesting foods and drinks contaminated with bodily waste	

(genotypes 1a, 1b, 2a, 3b, etc), with the newest genotype recently identified, genotype 7.[11] Genotype 1 is the most common in the United States, whereas genotype 4 is most common in the Middle East. Approximately 75% of patients with HCV in the United States have genotype 1, and about 15% and 9% have genotypes 2 and 3, respectively.[12] Genotype does not indicate disease severity but is used to determine the duration of therapy and the likelihood of therapeutic response.[13]

Contaminated needles and syringes with or without paraphernalia (eg, containers, filters) used by intravenous drug users (IVDU) are the primary source of HCV transmission. As many as 70% to 90% of IVDUs have HCV infection.[12] The risk of HCV transmission via blood transfusion is very low (0.001% per unit transfused).[13,14] Approximately 10% of individuals with HCV have no identifiable risk factors.[14]

Hepatitis D

Hepatitis D (delta hepatitis) affects approximately 15 to 20 million people worldwide.[15] Areas with the highest prevalence of HDV include the Middle East, parts of Africa and Central Asia, and parts of South America.[15]

HDV infection is unique because it can only occur in people who are also infected with the HBV. The most likely modes of transmitting HDV are similar to those of HBV (see Table 24–1).[15]

Hepatitis E

Hepatitis E is found worldwide, with an estimated 20 million individuals infected annually. About 56,000 deaths occur each year from HEV, primarily in Egypt, East Asia, and South Asia.[16]

Hepatitis E primarily occurs in underdeveloped countries with poor sanitation. The HEV is transmitted mainly by the fecal–oral route (eg, contaminated drinking water).[16]

PATHOPHYSIOLOGY

Hepatitis A

Hepatitis A is a nonenveloped single-stranded RNA virus classified as the *Hepatovirus* genus under the Picornaviridae family.[2] The primary host for the HAV is humans, with hepatic cells as the main site for viral replication. As part of the viral degradation process, the HAV is released into the biliary system causing elevated HAV concentrations in the feces. Hepatitis A infections are usually self-limiting and do not lead to chronic disease; rarely it may result in fulminant hepatitis.[1,2]

Hepatitis B

The hepatitis B virus (known as the Dane particle) belongs to the Hepadnaviridae family.[7] It is a partially double-stranded DNA virus with a phospholipid layer containing hepatitis B surface antigen (HBsAg) that surrounds the nucleocapsid. The nucleocapsid contains the core protein that produces hepatitis B core antigen (HBcAg), which is undetectable in the serum. Hepatocellular injury from HBV is thought to be due to a cytotoxic immune reaction that occurs when HBcAg is expressed on the surface of the hepatic cells. Fortunately, antibodies against hepatitis B core antigen (anti-HBc) are measurable in the blood, where anti-HBc to immunoglobulin M (IgM) indicates active infection and anti-HBc to IgG indicates either chronic infection or possible immunity against HBV.

In most cases viral replication occurs when the hepatitis B envelope antigen (HBeAg) is present and circulating in the blood. The serum HBV DNA concentration is a measure of viral infectivity and quantifies viral replication. Once the hepatitis B infection resolves, antibodies against the hepatitis B envelope (anti-HBe) and antibodies against hepatitis B surface antigen (anti-HBs) develop, and HBV DNA levels become undetectable. However, if these antibodies do not develop, the likelihood of developing CHB increases. This depends primarily on the host's immune system at the time of infection. In immunocompetent individuals, the disease resolves spontaneously and does not lead to further complications. In immunocompromised persons, the HBV is less likely to be eradicated, thus causing persistent infection leading to hepatic cell damage and inflammation.[8]

CHB occurs in less than 5% of patients older than 5 years, whereas the rate is more than 90% in infants born to mothers infected with HBV.[5–7] Approximately 90% of adults infected with the HBV develop anti-HBs, which results in lifelong immunity. About 30% of adults with initial symptoms of HBV present with jaundice or fatigue, and about 0.5% exhibit fulminant hepatitis.[8]

Patient Encounter, Part 1

A 43-year-old white woman presents to the doctor's office for a yearly check-up. Her only complaint is fatigue for the last year, but she feels well with no other complaints. She was in China for a business trip a week ago.

PMH: Mild depression, diet-controlled hypertension

PSH: None

FH: Father with HTN; Mother with NASH. Married with a 12-year-old son

SH: She is in a monogamous relationship. Has never smoked tobacco. Used illicit drugs at age 18. Drinks alcohol socially (drank heavily during teenage years). Professor in business administration at a local university.

Meds: Multivitamin daily, birth control pills

ROS: Complains of irritability and insomnia; no nausea, vomiting, diarrhea, abdominal pain, or anorexia; never experienced an episode of jaundice, pale stools, or tea-colored urine

PE:

VS: BP 132/86 mm Hg, P 80 beats/min, RR 20/minute, T 37.0°C (98.6°F), Wt 76 kg (167.2 lb), Ht 5′9″ (175 cm)

Abd: Soft, nontender, normal liver span; no hepatosplenomegaly, no ascites

The remainder of the examination was within normal limits.

Labs:

Sodium 141 mEq/L (141 mmol/L)
Potassium 4.1 mEq/L (4.1 mmol/L)
Chloride 99 mEq/L (99 mmol/L)
CO_2 21 mEq/L (21 mmol/L)
BUN 20 mg/dL (7.1 mmol/L)
Serum creatinine 1.2 mg/dL (106 μmol/L)
Glucose 122 mg/dL (6.8 mmol/L)
Hemoglobin 14.1 g/dL (141 g/L or 8.74 mmol/L)
Hematocrit 42.1% (0.42)
WBC 5.1 × 10^3/mm^3 (5.1 × 10^9/L)
Platelets 119 × 10^3/mm^3 (119 × 10^9/L)
AST 40 IU/L (0.67 μkat/L)
ALT 42 IU/L (0.70 μkat/L)
Total bilirubin 1.0 mg/dL (17.1 μmol/L)
Albumin 3.6 g/dL (36 g/L)
Alkaline phosphatase 164 IU/L (2.73 μkat/L)
TSH 1.3 μIU/mL (1.3 mIU/L)
Anti-HAV IgM (–)
Anti-HAV IgG (–)
Anti-HBs (+)
HBsAg (–)
HBeAg (–)
Anti-HBc IgG (–)
Anti-HBc IgM (–)
Anti-HBe (–)
Anti-HCV (+)
Genotype 2
HCV RNA 123,750 IU/mL (123,750 kIU/L)

Liver biopsy: Mild inflammation and moderate fibrosis (grade 1, stage 3 disease) consistent with chronic hepatitis C

What information is suggestive of viral hepatitis?

What risk factors does she have for viral hepatitis?

What additional information do you need before creating a treatment plan for this patient?

Hepatitis C

Hepatitis C, first known as non-A, non-B hepatitis, is a bloodborne infection caused by a single-stranded RNA virus belonging to the Flaviviridae family and the *Hepacivirus* genus.[18]

Antibodies against HCV (anti-HCV) in the blood indicate infection. If the infection persists for more than 6 months and viral replication is confirmed by HCV RNA levels, the person has chronic hepatitis C, which occurs in more than 70% of cases.[10,19]

About 15% to 45% of patients have acute hepatitis C that resolves without any further complication.[20] Chronic disease may be due to an ineffective host immune system, with cytotoxic T lymphocytes unable to eradicate the HCV, thereby allowing persistent damage to hepatic cells. The most common risk factors for developing hepatic fibrosis include obesity, diabetes, heavy alcohol use, male sex, and coinfections with HIV or HBV.[20]

Approximately 55% to 85% of chronic cases progress to mild, moderate, or severe hepatitis. Cirrhosis and its complications may take several decades to develop in about 15% to 30% of patients infected with HCV. Once cirrhosis is confirmed, the risk of developing HCC is about 2% to 4% per year.[20]

Hepatitis D

The HDV belongs to the genus *Delta virus* of the Deltaviridae family.[15] The HDV is a defective single-stranded circular RNA virus that requires the presence of HBV for HDV viral replication, causing either coinfection (both hepatitis B and D infection occurring simultaneously) or superinfection (acquiring HDV after having long-standing HBV disease).[15] This occurs because the HDV antigen (HDVAg) is coated by the HBsAg.[15]

Hepatitis E

Hepatitis E is a nonenveloped single-stranded messenger RNA virus of the Hepevirus genus.[16] The HEV is similar to HAV in that the virus is found in contaminated feces, thus infecting people via the fecal–oral route. High HEV levels in the bile often prompt viral shedding in the feces. Hepatitis E infections are usually self-limiting and rarely result in hepatic complications. Chronic hepatitis E occurs rarely and is more likely to occur in immunocompromised individuals (eg, HIV infection) or organ transplant recipients.[16,21]

CLINICAL PRESENTATION AND DIAGNOSIS

See box on the next page for the clinical presentation of viral hepatitis.

Diagnosis of Viral Hepatitis

Diagnosing viral hepatitis may be difficult because most infected individuals are asymptomatic.[2,9,15,16] Because symptoms alone cannot identify the specific type of hepatitis, laboratory serologies must be obtained (Table 24–2). A liver biopsy may be obtained to determine the severity of the liver disease, but this is an invasive test that may be associated with complications such as bleeding and death.[22] Therefore, several patented noninvasive blood tests (FibroTest®, HepaScore®) have been developed that use a panel of serum biomarkers (eg, ALT, AST, platelet count) along with the age and sex of the patient to determine the degree of hepatic fibrosis. These invasive and noninvasive tests are imperfect and are usually only able to identify mild and severe disease. Therefore, it is important to monitor laboratory values over time to assess the severity of liver fibrosis (eg, AST, ALT, serum albumin, platelet counts, prothrombin time/INR).

Clinical Presentation of Viral Hepatitis

Symptoms

- Most patients infected with any type of viral hepatitis have no symptoms.
- Symptomatic patients may experience a flu-like syndrome, fevers, fatigue/malaise, anorexia, nausea, vomiting, diarrhea, dark urine, pale-appearing stools, pruritus, and abdominal pain.

Signs

- Jaundice may be evident in the whites of the eyes (scleral icterus) or skin.
- An enlarged liver (hepatomegaly) and spleen (splenomegaly) may be present.
- In fulminant hepatitis with hepatic encephalopathy, patients may have asterixis and coma.
- In rare instances, extrahepatic symptoms may develop arthritis, postcervical lymphadenopathy, palmar erythema, cryoglobulinemia, and vasculitis.

Laboratory Tests

- See Table 24–2.

▸ *Hepatitis A*

The diagnosis of hepatitis A is made by detecting immunoglobulin antibodies to the capsid proteins of the HAV. Detectability of IgM anti-HAV in the serum indicates acute infection. IgM appears approximately 3 weeks after exposure and becomes undetectable within 6 months. In contrast, IgG anti-HAV appears in the serum at approximately the same time that IgM anti-HAV develops but indicates protection and lifelong immunity against hepatitis A.[2]

▸ *Hepatitis B*

Hepatitis B is diagnosed when HBsAg is detectable in the serum, but HBsAg does not distinguish between acute and chronic HBV. The presence of IgM antibodies to HBcAg indicates active infection. IgG anti-HBc indicates either chronic infection or possible immunity against HBV.[7]

In most cases, detectable HBeAg indicates active viral replication. Measurement of HBV DNA determines viral infectivity and quantifies viral replication. Once HBV viral replication ceases, anti-HBe is detectable in the serum. However, a minority of patients may develop anti-HBe and still have elevated HBV DNA levels because of a mutation in the HBV.[23] Therefore, CHB infections may be differentiated as either HBeAg-positive or HBeAg-negative.[5,23] Hepatitis B serologies are evaluated to assess HBV treatment response and determine whether to vaccinate.

▸ *Hepatitis C*

Hepatitis C is diagnosed by testing for anti-HCV in the serum and confirmed by the presence of HCV RNA. HCV RNA levels quantify viral replication and are used to determine if antiviral treatment for HCV is effective. An HCV genotype should be obtained to determine the likelihood of response to anti-HCV therapy and the duration of treatment required.[24]

▸ *Hepatitis D*

Hepatitis D infection requires the presence of HBV for HDV viral replication. Measuring HDV RNA levels confirms hepatitis D infection and is the most accurate diagnostic test. The presence of IgM anti-HD indicates active disease, and IgG anti-HD also becomes detectable if the infection does not resolve spontaneously. HDV antibodies do not confer immunity.[15]

▸ *Hepatitis E*

Diagnosis of acute hepatitis E is based on the presence of IgM anti-HEV. IgG anti-HEV emerges when the HEV infection resolves.[16] A blood test for HEV RNA levels is available but is used primarily in clinical trials.

PREVENTION AND TREATMENT OF VIRAL HEPATITIS

Desired Outcomes

Treatment outcomes for viral hepatitis are to (a) prevent the spread of infection, (b) prevent and treat symptoms, (c) suppress viral replication, (d) normalize hepatic aminotransferases, (e) improve liver histology, and (f) decrease morbidity and mortality by preventing cirrhosis, HCC, and ESLD.

For hepatitis B, additional treatment goals include seroconversion or loss of HBsAg, and seroconversion or loss of HBeAg. An additional goal for chronic hepatitis C is achieving undetectable HCV RNA for at least 12 weeks after completing hepatitis C therapy, known as achieving a sustained virologic response (SVR).

General Approach

Managing viral hepatitis involves both prevention and treatment. Prevention of hepatitis A and B (and indirectly for hepatitis D) can be achieved with immune globulin or vaccines. KEY CONCEPT *Acute viral hepatitis is primarily managed with supportive care.* Mild to moderate symptoms rarely require hospitalization, but hospital admission is recommended in individuals experiencing significant nausea, vomiting, diarrhea, and encephalopathy. Liver transplantation may be required in rare instances if fulminant hepatitis develops. Treatment is available for chronic HBV, HCV, and HDV.

Hepatitis A Prevention

KEY CONCEPT *Good personal hygiene and proper disposal of sanitary waste are required to prevent HAV fecal–oral transmission.*[1,2] This includes frequent hand washing with soap and water after using the bathroom and prior to eating meals. Drinking bottled water and avoiding fruits, vegetables, and raw shellfish harvested from sewage-contaminated water may minimize the risk of becoming infected with the HAV.

Individuals at risk of acquiring HAV (see Table 24–1) should receive serum immune globulin (IG) and/or the hepatitis A vaccine.[2,25]

▸ *Immune Globulin*

Immune globulin is a solution containing antibodies from sterilized pooled human plasma that provides passive immunization against HAV.[2] IG is available as an IV (IGIV) or intramuscular (IGIM) formulation, but only IGIM is used for prevention of HAV. IGIM does not confer lifelong immunity but is effective in providing pre- and postexposure prophylaxis against HAV.[2]

IGIM should be injected into a deltoid or gluteal muscle. It does not affect the immune response of inactivated or live-virus vaccines; however, administrating live vaccines concomitantly with IGIM may decrease the immune response significantly.[2]

Preexposure Prophylaxis IGIM administration is indicated for individuals at high risk of acquiring the HAV who (a) are younger than 12 months, (b) elect not to receive the hepatitis A

Table 24–2

Interpretation of Viral Hepatitis Serology Panels

Type	Laboratory Test	Result	Interpretation of Panel
Hepatitis A	IgM anti-HAV IgG anti-HAV	Negative Negative	Susceptible to infection
	IgM anti-HAV IgG anti-HAV	Positive Positive	Acutely infected Immune due to either natural infection or HAV vaccine
Hepatitis B[a]	HBsAg anti-HBc anti-HBs	Negative Negative Negative	Susceptible to infection
	HBsAg anti-HBc anti-HBs	Negative Positive Positive	Immune due to natural infection
	HBsAg anti-HBc anti-HBs	Negative Negative Positive	Immune due to hepatitis B vaccination
	HBsAg anti-HBc IgM anti-HBc anti-HBs	Positive Positive Positive Negative	Acutely infected
	HBsAg anti-HBc IgM anti-HBc anti-HBs	Positive Positive Negative Negative	Chronically infected
	HBsAg anti-HBc Anti-HBs	Negative Positive Negative	Four interpretations possible: (a) Resolved infection (most common); (b) false-positive anti-HBc, thus susceptible, (c) low-level chronic infection; (d) resolving acute infection
Hepatitis C	anti-HCV	Negative	Susceptible to infection
	anti-HCV	Positive	Acutely or chronically infected
Hepatitis D[b]	IgM anti-HDV HDVAg HBsAg HBeAg anti-HBc	Positive Positive Positive Positive Positive	Acute HBV-HDV coinfection
Hepatitis E	IgM anti-HEV IgG anti-HEV	Negative Negative	Susceptible to infection
	IgM anti-HEV	Positive	Acutely infected
	IgG anti-HEV	Positive	Immune due to natural infection

anti-HAV, hepatitis A antibody; anti-HBc, hepatitis B core antibody; anti-HBs, hepatitis B surface antibody; HBsAg, hepatitis B surface antigen; anti-HCV, hepatitis C antibody; anti-HDV, hepatitis D antibody; anti-HEV, hepatitis E antibody; HAV, hepatitis A virus; HBV, hepatitis B virus; HDV, hepatitis D virus; HDVAg, hepatitis D antigen; IgG, immunoglobulin G; IgM, immunoglobulin M.

[a]Centers for Disease Control and Prevention. Hepatology [Internet]. http://www.cdc.gov/hepatitis/HBV/PDFs/SerologicChartv8.pdf.

[b]Hepatitis D should be suspected in those who have HBsAg positivity. Hepatitis D may present as either coinfection where both HDV and HBV serologies appear simultaneously, whereas for superinfection, HBV has been present for some time and later HDV develops.

vaccine, or (c) cannot receive the hepatitis A vaccine (eg, because of allergic reaction). Because active immunity takes several weeks to develop, travelers who are older than 40 years, are immunocompromised, or have chronic liver disease or other chronic medical conditions who plan to depart for endemic areas within 2 weeks *and* have not received the hepatitis A vaccine should receive IGIM. If the duration of travel is less than 3 months, a dose of IGIM 0.02 mL/kg and hepatitis A vaccine may be administered at the same time but given in different injection sites.[2,25] If travel duration is expected to be longer than 2 months, IGIM 0.06 mL/kg should be administered to provide immunity for up to 5 months. If protection is required beyond 5 months, readministration of IGIM is recommended.[2,25]

Postexposure Prophylaxis Individuals in contact with people infected with acute HAV (see Table 24–1) may be candidates for postexposure prophylaxis. IGIM is recommended for individuals younger than 12 months or older than 40 years of age, immunocompromised, diagnosed with chronic liver disease, or have contraindications to the hepatitis A vaccine.[2,25]

The risk of infection may be decreased by 90% if IGIM 0.02 mL/kg is given within 2 weeks of being exposed to the HAV. IGIM may still be beneficial if given more than 2 weeks after exposure to a known case of HAV.[2,25]

Table 24–3

Recommended Intramuscular Doses of Hepatitis A Vaccines[a]

Product	Recipient Age (years)	Dose (Units)	Volume (mL)	No. of Doses	Schedule (months)
VAQTA	1–18	25	0.5	2	0, 6–18
	19 or more	50	1	2	0, 6–18
HAVRIX	1–18	720 ELISA	0.5	2	0, 6–12
	19 or more	1440 ELISA	1	2	0, 6–12

ELISA, enzyme-linked immunosorbent assay.

[a]Centers for Disease Control and Prevention. Hepatitis A FAQs for Health Professionals [Internet]. http://www.cdc.gov/hepatitis/HAV/HAVfaq.htm#vaccine.

▸ *Hepatitis A Vaccine*

Persons at risk of acquiring HAV should receive the hepatitis A vaccine to provide pre- and postexposure prophylaxis. Two inactivated hepatitis A vaccines are available in the United States, HAVRIX and VAQTA. The recommended dosing regimen is to administer two injections 6 months apart (at months 0 and 6).[2,25] These vaccines are considered interchangeable, and doses depend on age (Table 24–3).[2]

Efficacy is defined by measuring antibody response. Protective levels are considered to be greater than 20 mIU/mL (20 IU/L) for HAVRIX and greater than 10 mIU/mL (10 IU/L) for VAQTA. Within 4 weeks of administration of the first vaccine dose, more than 95% of adults and 97% of children and adolescents develop protective antibody concentrations. All recipients receiving the second dose in clinical trials had 100% antibody coverage; therefore, postvaccination measurement of antibody response is not required.[2]

For preexposure prophylaxis, the hepatitis A vaccine is recommended for travelers to endemic hepatitis A countries. It should be administered to healthy travelers 40 years of age and younger regardless of the scheduled dates for departure. This recommendation does not apply to adults older than 40 years or immunocompromised persons; these individuals should receive both the hepatitis A vaccine and IGIM (0.02 mL/kg) if travel will occur in less than 2 weeks.[25]

For postexposure prophylaxis, the hepatitis A vaccine is effective in preventing clinical infection in healthy individuals between 12 months and 40 years of age when administered within 14 days after exposure.[25] Individuals outside these age ranges or with significant comorbid conditions should receive IGIM rather than the hepatitis A vaccine because this population has not been studied.[25]

The hepatitis A vaccine may provide effective immunity for about 25 and 14 to 20 years in adults and children, respectively.[26] The most common and often self-limiting adverse effects in adults include injection site reactions (eg, tenderness, pain, and warmth), headaches, fatigue and flu-like symptoms. Infants and children may have feeding disturbances. Local reactions may be minimized by using an appropriate needle length based on the person's age and size and by administering it intramuscularly in the deltoid muscle. Hepatitis A vaccine given during pregnancy has not been evaluated in clinical trials. Because both brands of vaccine are made from inactivated HAV, the risk of developing fetal complications should be minimal.[26]

Hepatitis B Prevention

KEY CONCEPT *Individuals may minimize their risk of acquiring the HBV by avoiding contaminated blood products and high-risk behavior (see* Table 24–1*) and by receiving the hepatitis B vaccine.*[7] Screening pregnant women for HBV and providing universal hepatitis B vaccinations to all newborns is effective in preventing hepatitis B infections.[27] In some cases, postexposure prophylaxis with hepatitis B immune globulin (HBIG) may be recommended to prevent the development of acute infection and complications associated with HBV.

▸ *Hepatitis B Immune Globulin*

Hepatitis B immune globulin (HBIG) is a sterile solution containing antibodies prepared from pooled human plasma that has a high concentration of anti-HBs. A single dose of HBIG 0.06 mL/kg is effective in providing passive immunization in preventing CHB infections.[7] HBIG should only be administered intramuscularly.

The most common side effects of HBIG include erythema at the injection site, headaches, myalgia, fatigue, urticaria, nausea, and vomiting. Serious adverse effects are rare and may include liver function test abnormalities, arthralgias, and anaphylactic reactions. HBIG should be used with caution in individuals who have experienced hypersensitivity reactions to immune globulin or have immunoglobulin A deficiency. Concomitant administration of HBIG and live vaccines should be avoided because the efficacy of the immunization may decrease significantly.

▸ *Hepatitis B Vaccine*

Two hepatitis B vaccines are available in the United States-Recombivax HB and Engerix-B. KEY CONCEPT *Persons at high risk (see* Table 24–1*) of acquiring the HBV should be vaccinated with the hepatitis B vaccine at months 0, 1, and 6.* The hepatitis B vaccine dose depends on the person's age (Table 24–4).

The hepatitis B vaccine is also indicated for postexposure prophylaxis to prevent CHB. Individuals exposed to HBV should receive the hepatitis B vaccine with or without HBIG, preferably within 24 hours of exposure based on the source of exposure and the vaccination status of the exposed person (Table 24–5).[7] Postexposure prophylaxis for perinatal exposure depends on several factors, including maternal HBsAg status and the newborn's weight (Table 24–6).[27]

For optimal response, the hepatitis B vaccine should be administered intramuscularly (into the anterolateral thigh region in neonates and infants and into the deltoid region in older children and adults) and not IV or intradermally. Intragluteal IM injections should be avoided because they may result in lower rates of immunity.[7,27]

The hepatitis B vaccine is effective when antibody concentrations are greater than 10 mIU/mL (10 IU/L), but postvaccination antibody testing is not routinely recommended because most

Table 24–4

Recommended Intramuscular Dosing Regimens for Hepatitis B Vaccines*

Product	Patient Categories	Dose (mcg)	Volume (mL)	No. of Doses	Schedule (months)
Recombivax HB	0–19 years of age	5	0.5	3	0, 1, 6
	11–15 years of age[a]	10	1	2	1, 4–6
	≥ 20 years of age	10	1	3	0, 1, 6
	Hemodialysis[b] < 20 years of age	5	0.5	3	0, 1, 6
	Hemodialysis ≥ 20 years of age	40	1	3	0, 1, 6
Engerix-B	0–19 years of age	10	0.5	3	0, 1, 6
	≥ 20 years of age	20	1	3	0, 1, 6
	Hemodialysis[b] < 20 years of age	10	0.5	3	0, 1, 6
	Hemodialysis ≥ 20 years of age	40[c]	2	4	0, 1, 2, 6

[a]Adolescents 11 through 15 years of age may receive either the 5-mcg three-dose pediatric formulation or a 10-mcg two-dose regimen using the adult formulation.

[b]Higher doses might be more immunogenic, but no specific recommendations have been made.

[c]Two 1.0-mL doses administered at one site.

*Centers for Disease Control and Prevention. Hepatitis B FAQs for Health Professionals [Internet]. http://www.cdc.gov/hepatitis/HBV/HBVfaq.htm#vaccFAQ

Table 24–5

Recommendations for Prophylaxis after Exposure to the Hepatitis B Virus

	Treatment to Administer If Serology Test of Source Person Is:	
Exposed Person's Vaccination Status	**HBsAg-Positive**	**Unknown HBsAg Status**
Unvaccinated	HBIG × 1 and initiate HB vaccine series	Initiate HB vaccine series
Previously vaccinated[a]	Administer HB vaccine booster dose	No treatment

HB, hepatitis B; HBsAg, hepatitis B surface antigen; HBIG, hepatitis B immune globulin.

[a]A person who has written documentation of a complete hepatitis B vaccine series and did not receive postvaccination testing.

Table 24–6

Recommendations for Hepatitis B Prophylaxis to Prevent Perinatal Transmission

	Mother's HBsAg Status		
Treatment	**Positive**	**Negative**	**Unknown**
HBIG[a]	Given within 12 hours of birth	None	Test HBsAg. If positive, give within 7 days; if negative, give none
AND			
Hepatitis B vaccine[b]			
Dose 1	Within 12 hours of birth	Based on infant's weight[c]	Within 12 hours of birth
Dose 2	At month 1–2	At month 1–2	At month 1–2
Dose 3[d]	At month 6	At month 6–18	At month 6

[a]0.5 mL intramuscularly in a different site from vaccine.

[b]See Table 24–4 for appropriate hepatitis B vaccine dose.

[c]Full-term infants who are medically stable and weigh 2000 g or more born to HBsAg-negative mothers should receive the hepatitis B vaccine before hospital discharge. Preterm infants weighing less than 2000 g born to HBsAg-negative mothers should receive the first dose of hepatitis B vaccine 1 month after birth or at hospital discharge.

[d]The final dose in the vaccine series should not be administered before age 24 weeks (164 days).

From Mast FF, Margolis HS, Fiore AE, et al. A comprehensive immunization strategy to eliminate transmission of hepatitis B virus infection in the United States: Recommendations of the Advisory Committee on Immunization Practices (ACIP) part 1: Immunization of infants, children, and adolescents. MMWR Recomm Rep 2005; 54(RR-16):1–31.

people completing the vaccination series obtain adequately antibody levels. It may be advisable to determine if immunity has been achieved in some populations (eg, infants born to HBsAg-positive mothers, health care workers at high risk of contacting HBV-infected blood, immunocompromised patients).[28]

Effective immunity may last for more than 20 years in healthy individuals. However, patients with poor immune systems may have an anamnestic response that requires titers to be checked periodically with booster doses given.[27]

The most frequent adverse effects are local injection site reactions, flu-like symptoms, dizziness, and irritability. Anaphylaxis, serum sickness–like hypersensitivity syndrome, chronic fatigue syndrome, and neurologic diseases (leukoencephalitis, optic neuritis, and transverse myelitis) have been reported rarely.[7] Hepatitis B vaccine is not contraindicated during pregnancy.[7]

► Hepatitis A and B Combination Vaccine

KEY CONCEPT *Twinrix, a vaccine that combines both inactivated HAV and HBV, is approved for immunizing individuals older than 18 years who are at risk for HAV and HBV infections.*[27,29] A 1-mL dose of Twinrix should be administered at months 0, 1, and 6. Twinrix may also be given in an accelerated dosing regimen at day 0, 7, 21 to 30, with a fourth dose at month 12.[29] The accelerated schedule is intended for patients who start the vaccination series but are unable to complete the standard three-dose schedule in time to develop adequate immunity before embarking on travel that will put them at risk of exposure to hepatitis A and B. The side-effect profile of Twinrix is similar to giving each vaccine separately.

Chronic Hepatitis B Treatment

The American Association for the Study of Liver Diseases (AASLD) guidelines state that patients with HBeAg-positive CHB (also known as wild-type CHB) with persistently elevated ALT (more than two times the upper limit of normal) and elevated HBV DNA levels greater than 20,000 IU/mL (20,000 kIU/L) require treatment to delay progression to cirrhosis and prevent the development of ESLD.[30] Similar treatment criteria apply to patients infected with HBeAg-negative CHB (also known as precore mutant or promoter mutant) with the exception of HBV DNA levels; therapy should be initiated when viral levels are greater than 2000 IU/mL (2000 kIU/L).[30]

The primary treatment endpoint is to suppress HBV replication to achieve undetectable serum levels. Additionally, the ideal treatment should induce a biochemical response (decrease or normalize ALT levels) and histological response (decrease liver inflammation documented by liver biopsy scores).[30]

KEY CONCEPT *The drug of choice for CHB depends on the patient's past medical history, ALT, HBV DNA level, HBeAg status, severity of liver disease, and history of previous HBV therapy.* The safety and efficacy profile of the medication and the likelihood of developing drug resistance should also be considered. There are seven approved HBV agents: two formulations of interferon alfa and five nucleoside/nucleotide analogs.

Entecavir and tenofovir are recommended as first-line therapy due to profound HBV DNA suppression and minimal resistance.[30] Pegylated interferon-α_{2a} is also considered a first-line agent for HBV with compensated liver disease because it lacks drug resistance.

Adefovir is second line to tenofovir because adefovir is less potent in suppressing HBV replication. Lamivudine is no longer recommended due to a high rate of resistance.[23,30] Patients currently on adefovir or lamivudine and responding to treatment should continue with the regimen. However, if there is inadequate virologic response or drug resistance develops, adding or switching to a more potent HBV agent should be considered. The role of telbivudine in HBV therapy is limited due to its intermediate rate of resistance.[23,30]

For all oral HBV agents, patients should be monitored for lactic acidosis and severe hepatomegaly because some cases have been fatal. Additionally, hepatic function tests should be carefully monitored if treatment is to be discontinued, because severe acute exacerbations of hepatitis have been reported. Dosage adjustments are required in patients with renal dysfunction for all oral HBV regimens. With all oral HBV agents, HIV resistance may develop if given as monotherapy; therefore, patients should be tested for HIV infection prior to starting a single anti-HBV agent. Patients coinfected with HIV and HBV should concomitantly receive highly active antiretroviral therapy (HAART) with an HBV agent. Each HBV agent is described briefly in the sections that follow.

► Interferon and Pegylated Interferon

Interferon-α_{2b} and pegylated interferon-α_{2a} are the only interferon therapies approved for HBV. Pegylated interferon is interferon attached to a polyethylene glycol molecule that increases the half-life of the drug, thereby allowing once-weekly dosing versus thrice-weekly administration of unmodified interferon. Interferon is effective in suppressing, and in some cases ceasing, viral replication without inducing resistance.[30] Approximately one-third of HBeAg-positive patients achieve HBeAg seroconversion after 48 weeks of pegylated interferon therapy.[23,30] HBeAg-negative hepatitis B may require at least 48 weeks of pegylated interferon to attain undetectable HBV DNA levels.[23] Factors associated with a greater chance of HBeAg seroconversion include low baseline HBV DNA concentrations and high pretreatment ALT levels.[23]

Pegylated interferon is well tolerated with similar or better efficacy than unmodified interferon; thus, the once-weekly formulation is recommended for CHB.[30] The approved dose of pegylated interferon-α_{2a} (Pegasys) for HBeAg-positive CHB is 180 mcg subcutaneously once weekly for 48 weeks. The same dose is recommended for HBeAg-negative CHB; however, the duration of therapy may be more than 48 weeks to increase sustained responses.[23,30]

Even though the advantages of interferon or pegylated interferon include a finite duration of treatment, lack of resistance, and possible HBsAg loss or seroconversion (development of anti-HBs), there are several significant disadvantages. These include the need for subcutaneous injections and a pronounced adverse-effect profile that may require dosage reductions or treatment discontinuation.

Most patients experience flu-like symptoms (fevers, chills, rigors, and myalgias). These symptoms may be mild to moderate in severity and usually occur with the first injection and diminish with continued treatment. These symptoms may be minimized by premedication with acetaminophen or nonsteroidal anti-inflammatory drugs. Self-administering pegylated interferon prior to bedtime can help patients sleep through the symptoms. Psychiatric adverse effects occur frequently and may include irritability, depression, and, rarely, suicidal ideation which may require antidepressants or anxiolytics. Patients with severe symptoms including suicidal ideation should discontinue treatment immediately.[19,34]

Approximately 35% of patients develop an ALT flare when treated with interferon. Increase in ALT levels has been associated with a positive response but may lead to hepatic decompensation, which can be fatal. Therefore, only patients with compensated liver disease and stable medical comorbidities should be considered for treatment with any formulation of interferon.

▶ *Entecavir*

Entecavir (Baraclude) is a guanosine nucleoside analog approved for children (greater than 2 years of age) and adults with either HBeAg-positive, HBeAg-negative, or lamivudine-resistant CHB.[23,30] Resistance rates are low (1%–2%) in lamivudine-naive patients treated with entecavir for up to 5 years. For patients previously treated with lamivudine and switched to entecavir, the resistance rate is approximately 28% at 1 year and up to 50% at 5 years.[23,30,31]

The dose of entecavir is 0.5 mg once daily for patients 16 years or older with compensated liver disease and naïve to lamivudine therapy. Entecavir 1 mg once daily is recommended for lamivudine or telbivudine resistance or decompensated liver disease. Entecavir should be given on an empty stomach (at least 2 hours after or 2 hours before a meal). The side-effect profile of entecavir is similar to lamivudine and adefovir dipivoxil.

▶ *Tenofovir Disoproxil Fumarate*

Tenofovir disoproxil fumarate (Viread) is an acyclic adenine nucleotide reverse transcriptase inhibitor that is similar in structure to adefovir dipivoxil. Tenofovir inhibits HIV and HBV replication and is indicated for children more than 2 years of age and adults with either HBeAg-positive or HBeAg-negative CHB and/or HIV when prescribed with other HAART therapies. Tenofovir is preferred over adefovir for CHB because of greater effectiveness in inhibiting HBV replication and lack of resistance.[32] Patients developing resistance to lamivudine, entecavir, or adefovir may benefit from tenofovir.[30,32]

The dose of tenofovir is 300 mg orally once daily taken on an empty stomach. Tenofovir is well tolerated with adverse effects similar to other HBV oral agents. Several case reports have implicated tenofovir in causing nephrotoxicity and Fanconi's syndrome.[30,32] Decreased bone mineral density and osteomalacia have been reported in HIV patients receiving tenofovir. It would be prudent to monitor creatinine clearance, phosphate levels, liver function tests, and bone mineral density prior to initiating treatment and during therapy.

▶ *Adefovir Dipivoxil*

Adefovir dipivoxil (Hepsera) is a prodrug of adefovir, an adenosine nucleotide analog that inhibits DNA polymerase, indicated for CHB in patients older than 12 years. Resistance to adefovir is minimal for the first few years of treatment but increases to approximately 30% after 5 years of therapy.[30]

The dose of adefovir is 10 mg once daily taken with or without food. The most common side effects include asthenia, abdominal pain, diarrhea, dyspepsia, headaches, nausea, and flatulence. Adefovir is associated with nephrotoxicity at higher doses (30 mg/day). Renal function should be monitored during treatment in all patients, especially those with preexisting or risk factors for renal impairment.

▶ *Lamivudine*

Lamivudine (Epivir-HBV) is an oral synthetic cytosine nucleoside analog with antiviral effects against HIV and HBV. Lamivudine is effective in suppressing HBV replication, normalizing ALT levels, and improving liver histology. Patients may have a similar or a superior response in achieving these endpoints when compared with interferon or pegylated interferon. Prolonged lamivudine therapy (up to 5 years) may be needed to sustain seroconversion, but this leads to lamivudine resistance as high as 60% to 70% at 5 years.[30] Due to the high rate of resistance, lamivudine is no longer recommended as first-line therapy for CHB.[30]

The adult dose of lamivudine is 100 mg orally once daily for CHB without HIV coinfection. Lamivudine 3 mg/kg once daily up to a maximum dose of 100 mg is approved for pediatric patients (2–17 years of age). It may be taken with or without food.

Adverse effects are minimal and include fatigue, diarrhea, nausea, vomiting, and headaches. ALT levels should be monitored because a two- to threefold increase may be observed. ALT should be monitored closely when therapy is discontinued because increased levels may indicate a flare in disease activity leading to liver failure.

▶ *Telbivudine*

Telbivudine (Tyzeka) is an L-nucleoside analog that inhibits HBV replication. It is indicated for patients 16 years or older with HBeAg-positive or HBeAg-negative CHB. Telbivudine offers a slightly more effective reduction in HBV DNA levels and normalization of aminotransferases than lamivudine. Telbivudine resistance is lower than lamivudine, but rates are significant with continued treatment. Also, there is a higher rate of telbivudine treatment failure in patients who have lamivudine resistance.[30] Telbivudine is not highly recommended but may be considered if adefovir or tenofovir resistance is present.

The dose of telbivudine is 600 mg orally once daily with or without food. Adverse effects are similar to other HBV oral agents. Patients should also be monitored for signs and symptoms of myopathy characterized by elevated creatine kinase levels and muscle weakness.[33] Peripheral neuropathy has also occurred, mostly in patients who were treated concomitantly with pegylated interferon.[30] ALT and AST levels may become elevated while on treatment at rates similar to lamivudine.

Hepatitis C Prevention

Avoiding high-risk behaviors such as sharing needles among IV drug users is the primary means of avoiding infection with the HCV. The risk of acquiring HCV through a blood transfusion is 1 in 2 million since 1992, when widespread screening of blood products and universal precautions took effect. It has been estimated that more than 75% of individual infected with the HCV were born during the baby boomer population; therefore, the CDC now recommends that all people born between 1945 and 1965 be tested at least once in their lifetime for HCV. Currently, there are no vaccines available to prevent HCV, but several are under development.[18] Therefore, high-risk individuals (see Table 24–1) should be tested for HCV because most people are asymptomatic and unaware they are infected.[20]

Chronic Hepatitis C Treatment

Treatment for HCV has revolutionized over the past decade, with efficacy rates well above 90% compared to 50% to 80% prior to 2011. The primary goal of HCV treatment is to achieve a sustained virologic response (SVR), also known as a "virological cure," which is defined as achieving undetectable HCV RNA levels at 12 weeks or longer after treatment completion. Normalization of liver function tests and improvement of histology are additional treatment outcomes, but more importantly the goal is to prevent the progression and development of cirrhosis, HCC, and ESLD.[19,20] Patients with advanced disease and cirrhosis achieving SVR are not free of developing liver complications; therefore, initiating HCV treatment early is important.

Patient Encounter, Part 2: Creating a Care Plan

Based on the information presented, create a care plan for this patient's hepatitis. Your plan should include:

(a) a statement of the drug-related needs and/or problems;

(b) the goals of therapy;

(c) a patient-specific detailed therapeutic plan;

(d) a follow-up plan to determine whether the goals have been achieved; and

(e) a follow-up plan to identify potential adverse effects of therapy.

KEY CONCEPT *Treatment for chronic hepatitis C depends on the patient's past medical history, previous HCV treatment history, severity of liver disease, and HCV genotype.* The most important predictor of response to therapy is the hepatitis C genotype.[19,24]

▶ *Interferon/Pegylated Interferon and Ribavirin*

Interferon was first approved for chronic HCV but is no longer recommended because less than 10% of patients with genotype 1 and only about 30% with genotype 2 or 3 achieve an SVR.[19] Pegylated interferon-α_{2a} (Pegasys) and pegylated interferon-α_{2b} (PEG-Intron) have extended half-lives allowing for once-weekly administration compared to thrice weekly with unpegylated interferon. The SVR rates to pegylated interferon can be increased from 25% to 40% to 45% to 55% by adding ribavirin, a synthetic guanosine analog that inhibits viral polymerase. From 2002 to 2011, pegylated interferon plus ribavirin was considered standard-of-care for HCV.[19] The HCV dosing regimens that include pegylated interferon and ribavirin are listed in Table 24–7.

As described in the previous section on chronic hepatitis B treatment, interferon has frequent and sometimes severe adverse effects. In addition, up to 35% of patients treated with pegylated interferon plus ribavirin require either a dosage reduction or drug discontinuation due to hematologic complications (thrombocytopenia, neutropenia, anemia).[35,36] Pegylated interferon should either be reduced in dosage or discontinued if thrombocytopenia or neutropenia develops. Ribavirin causes a dose-related hemolytic anemia that may require dosage reductions or discontinuation.[37] Adjunctive therapies have been used, including granulocyte colony-stimulating factor for neutropenia and epoetin alfa or darbepoetin for anemia.[19]

Because ribavirin can be teratogenic and embryocidal, all women of childbearing age and men who are able to father a child must use two forms of contraception during HCV therapy containing ribavirin and for 6 months after treatment.

▶ *Direct-Acting Antiviral Agents—First Generation*

Since 2011, a new category of drugs for HCV known as direct-acting antivirals (DAAs) have emerged. The first-generation DAAs approved were the protease inhibitors boceprevir and telaprevir, which are now no longer commercially available in the United States. These agents have resulted in higher SVR rates

Table 24–7

Recommended and Alternative Treatment Regimens, Dosing, and Duration for Treatment-Naïve Patients with HCV[a]

Genotype	Recommended	Alternative	Not Recommended[b]
1a[c]	LDV/SOF × 12 wks[d] PTV + RTV + OBV + DSV + R × 12 or 24 wks[e] SOF + SMV +/− R × 12 or 24 wks[e]	None	P+R ± TVR or BOC or SMV or SOF × 12 to 48 wks SOF + R × 24 wks
1b[c]	LDV/SOF × 12 wks[d] PTV + RTV + OBV + DSV × 12 wks for no cirrhosis PTV + RTV + OBV + DSV + R × 12 wks for cirrhosis SOF + SMV × 12 wks for no cirrhosis SOF + SMV × 24 wks for cirrhosis	None	P+R ± TVR or BOC or SMV or SOF × 12 to 48 wks SOF + R × 24 wks
2	SOF + R × 12 wks	None	P + R ± TVR or BOC or LDV
3	SOF + R × 24 wks	SOF + P + R × 12 wks	P + R ± TVR or BOC or SMV
4	LDV/SOF × 12 wks PTV + RTV + OBV + DSV + R × 12 wks SOF + R × 24 wks	SOF + P + R × 12 wks SOF + SMV ± R × 12 wks	P + R ± TVR or BOC or SMV
5	SOF + P + R × 12 wks	P + R × 48 wks	P + R ± TVR or BOC or SMV
6	LDV/SOF × 12 wks	SOF + P + R × 12 wks	P ± R ± TVR or BOC

BOC, boceprevir; DAA, direct-acting antiretroviral; DSV, dasabuvir; IFN, Interferon; LDV/SOF, ledipasvir and sofosbuvir; OMB, Ombitasvir; P, pegylated interferon[f]; PTV, paritaprevir; R, ribavirin[g]; RTV, Ritonavir; SMV, simeprevir; SOF, sofosbuvir; TVR, telaprevir; wks, weeks.

[a]Refer to ref. 24, www.hcvguidelines.org for dosing recommendations for patients with renal impairment (CrCl less than 30 mL/min [0.5 mL/s]).

[b]Monotherapy with P, R, or a DAA is not recommended for any genotype.

[c]Options listed are similar in efficacy, regimen choice may be based on potential drug interaction profile.

[d]Treatment duration dependent on prior HCV treatment history, cirrhosis status, and baseline viral load.

[e]Treatment duration is dependent on cirrhosis status.

[f]If using pegylated interferon-α2a (Pegasys) dose is 180 mcg weekly, or pegylated Interferon-α2b (PEG-Intron) 1.5 mcg/kg; both must be renally adjusted base on CrCl.

[g]Weight-based ribavirin (1000 mg [<75 kg] to 1200 mg [>75 kg]), must be renally adjusted base on CrCl.

of 63% to 66% when coadministered with pegylated interferon and ribavirin compared to about 50% with pegylated interferon and ribavirin alone.[38,39] Despite higher SVR rates, first-generation DDAs are no longer recommended due significant adverse effects, (ie, blood dyscrasias, dermatological effects), increased pill burden (11–22 pills daily), complicated dosing regimens, significant and multiple drug interactions, and increased rates of viral resistance.[24]

▸ *Direct-Acting Antiviral Agents—Second Generation*

Drug development for HCV continues to evolve, resulting in higher SVR rates (well above 90%), fewer adverse effects, and shorter treatment durations with less complex regimens compared to pegylated interferon and ribavirin with or without a first-generation DAA. In late 2013, simeprevir and sofosbuvir were approved. Please see www.hcvguidelines.org for the most up-to-date HCV treatment recommendations.[24]

***Simeprevir* (Olysio)** This agent is an NS3/4A serine protease inhibitor indicated only for HCV genotype 1 compensated liver disease, including cirrhosis. Simeprevir must be administered with pegylated interferon and ribavirin to minimize the risk of developing drug resistance. The simeprevir triple therapy SVR rate varies depending on the patient's genotype 1 subtype. The overall SVR rates in the registry trial, QUEST-1 and QUEST-2, were about 80% for triple therapy. However, when subgroup analysis was performed between genotype 1a compare to genotype 1b, the SVR rates were 24% to 43% versus 78% to 84%, respectively.[24,30,41] The lower SVR rate with genotype 1a may be due to the baseline presence of NS3 Q80K polymorphism, a naturally occurring variation of the HCV virus.[42] Therefore, baseline screening for NS3 Q80K polymorphism is highly recommended if simeprevir is being considered for HCV genotype 1a disease; if positive for the polymorphism, then an alternative HCV therapy should be used. Currently, triple therapy with simeprevir, pegylated interferon, and ribavirin is not recommended for HCV genotype 1a or 1b disease due to its adverse effect profile, drug–drug interactions, long treatment duration, and lower SVR rates compare to newer interferon-free HCV oral regimens.

Sofosbuvir (Sovaldi) This is the first agent of the NS5B polymerase inhibitor class approved for treatment of HCV genotypes 1, 2, 3, and 4; it also has efficacy in genotypes 5 and 6.[45] The overall SVR rates for genotype 1 is approximately 90% when receiving sofosbuvir, ribavirin, and pegylated interferon.[24] The dose of sofosbuvir is 400 mg daily with or without food for 12 to 24 weeks.

Sofosbuvir is also indicated for patients with HCC waiting for a liver transplant and for patients coinfected with HIV and HCV, regardless of genotype.[24]

Oral sofosbuvir in combination with ribavirin is the first interferon-free regimen approved for genotypes 2 and 3. SVR rates for genotype 2 with 12 weeks of ribavirin and sofosbuvir is 90% to 97%. SVR rates for genotype 3 with 12 weeks of sofosbuvir and ribavirin (56%) were less than with 24 weeks of pegylated interferon and ribavirin (63%), suggesting that genotype 3 is more difficult to treat.[24] Given this information, the recommended treatment duration with sofosbuvir and ribavirin for genotype 3 is 24 weeks, resulting in SVR rates of about 80% to 85%.[45]

Triple therapy with sofosbuvir is well tolerated with minimal adverse effects beyond what is seen with pegylated interferon and ribavirin, but it is no longer recommended for genotype 1 disease.[24,45] Sofosbuvir has fewer drug interactions than other protease inhibitors; however, some may be significant because sofosbuvir is a substrate of intestinal P-glycoprotein. Agents that should be avoided with sofosbuvir include St. John's wort, certain anticonvulsants (carbamazepine, phenytoin), some HIV protease inhibitors (tipranavir/ritonavir) and some antimycobacterials (rifampin).

Simeprevir* and *Sofosbuvir This FDA-approved regimen given for 12 weeks may be considered for genotype 1 treatment-naïve or treatment-experienced patients without cirrhosis. The same regimen is also approved for 24 weeks for patients with cirrhosis who are treatment naïve or treatment experienced. Patients with minimal or advanced liver disease who were either naïve or null responders to pegylated interferon and ribavirin who received sofosbuvir and simeprevir with or without ribavirin achieved an SVR 12 weeks after treatment ended (SVR-12) greater than 93%. Patients with HCV genotype 1a who were positive for the Q80K polymorphism should not preclude them from this combination as relapse rates were low; however, it is important to know that the COSMO trial evaluating these HCV treatment regimens included a small sample size of 167 divided in four treatment groups (simeprevir and sofosbuvir with or without ribavirin treated for either 12 or 24 weeks). This treatment regimen is well tolerated with minimal side effects with additional adverse effects that may be experienced when administered with ribavirin.[24]

Sofosbuvir and Ledipasvir (Harvoni) This is the first fixed-dose combination (FDC) tablet and the first FDA-approved all-oral HCV regimen that does not require administration with interferon or ribavirin. Ledipasvir has a different mechanism of action than sofosbuvir; it inhibits the HCV NS5A protein, which is required for viral replication. The product is indicated for chronic HCV genotype 1 infection in adults. Adverse effects are minimal, and drug interactions are similar to those receiving sofosbuvir alone. The dose is one tablet (sofosbuvir 400 mg/ledipasvir 90 mg) daily (with or without food) for 8, 12, or 24 weeks depending on prior HCV treatment history, cirrhosis status, and baseline viral load.

Ombitasvir, Paritaprevir, Ritonavir, and Dasabuvir (Viekira Pak) This fixed-dose combination product is the second FDA-approved all-oral HCV regimen that does not require administration with interferon but may be administered with or without ribavirin. The drugs have different mechanisms of action to inhibit HCV viral replication. Ombitasvir is a NS5A inhibitor, paritaprevir is a NS3/4A protease inhibitor, and dasabuvir is a nonnucleoside NS5B polymerase inhibitor with ritonavir, a CYP3A inhibitor. The product is indicated for chronic HCV genotype 1a and 1b infection and has an SVR rate between 90% and 99%.

The combination is also indicated for patients who are coinfected with HIV and HCV or liver transplant recipients with normal liver function and mild fibrosis. The product is not recommended for patients with decompensated liver disease. The duration of treatment and the decision to add ribavirin are based on genotype subtype and whether cirrhosis is present.

This treatment is well tolerated with minimal side effects; however, additional adverse effects may occur if given with ribavirin.[24] Drug–drug interactions may be significant with drugs metabolized via the CYP3A and/or CYP2C8 metabolic pathway.

The recommended dosage of the combination product is two tablets daily in the morning with food (each containing ombitasvir 12.5 mg, paritaprevir 75 mg, and ritonavir 50 mg) plus one tablet containing dasabuvir 250 mg twice daily (morning and evening) with food. Weight-based ribavirin may be recommended if the patient has cirrhosis or has genotype 1a infection or is not naïve to HCV therapy.[24]

► ***Cost of HCV Treatment***

The new generation of HCV agents is associated with improved SVR rates and side-effect profiles. However, their cost may affect whether patients receive treatment. The wholesale acquisition price for sofosbuvir in the United States is $1000 per day, or $84,000 to $168,000 for a 12- or 24-week treatment regimen, excluding the cost of other coadministered medications. The cost for a 28-day supply of simeprevir is $22,120, excluding other drugs given concomitantly. If the combination of simeprevir and sofosbuvir is prescribed, the cost is well over $150,000 for a 12-week course. The combination tablet Harvoni (sofosbuvir/ledipasvir) has a wholesale price of about $94,500 for a 12-week treatment course. The Viekira Pak containing ombitasvir, paritaprevir, ritonavir, and dasabuvir has a wholesale acquisition cost of $83,320 to $167,640 for 12 or 24 weeks of treatment, respectively. In an ideal world, all patients infected with HCV would be treated. The unfortunate reality is that the high cost of newer HCV regimens strains health care resources, making it infeasible to treat everyone. The AASLD and World Health Organization (WHO) recommend that patients be prioritized based on liver disease severity. Individuals with advanced fibrosis (Stage F3) and cirrhosis (Stage F4) should be first priority. If resources are available, patients with mild (Stage F1) or moderate disease (Stage F2) should also receive treatment.[20,24]

Hepatitis D Prevention and Treatment

Hepatitis D infection is possible only if the patient is also infected with HBV; therefore, hepatitis B vaccination can indirectly prevent hepatitis D infections. The recommended treatment for HDV is pegylated interferon for 48 to 72 weeks.[15] First-line oral agents for treating HBV infections (eg, tenofovir) may be considered in patients coinfected with HDV and HBV if HBV DNA levels are high. Monotherapy with nucleoside/nucleotide analogs is ineffective in reducing HDV DNA levels but may decrease hepatitis B viral loads.[15]

Patient Encounter, Part 3

The patient received treatment for hepatitis C for 4 weeks, and the following laboratory test results have just been obtained:

Sodium 138 mEq/L (138 mmol/L)	WBC 4.1 × 10^3/mm^3 (4.1 × 10^9/L)
Potassium 4.0 mEq/L (4.0 mmol/L)	Platelets 114 × 10^3/mm^3 (114 × 10^9/L)
Chloride 98 mEq/L (98 mmol/L)	AST 41 IU/L (0.68 μkat/L)
CO_2 19 mEq/L (19 mmol/L)	ALT 32 IU/L (0.53 μkat/L)
BUN 21 mg/dL (7.5 mmol/L)	Total bilirubin 1.7 mg/dL (29.1 μmol/L)
Serum creatinine 1.0 mg/dL (88 μmol/L)	Albumin 3.6 g/dL (36 g/L)
Glucose 103 mg/dL (5.7 mmol/L)	Alkaline phosphatase 168 IU/L (2.80 μkat/L)
Hemoglobin 9.8 g/dL (98 g/L or 6.08 mmol/L)	HCV RNA level: undetectable
Hematocrit 29.6% (0.296)	

What questions should you ask the patient?

What action should you take to treat any complaints the patient may have?

What action should you take based on the patient's week 4 HCV RNA level?

Hepatitis E Prevention and Treatment

Because hepatitis E is transmitted via the fecal–oral route, good personal hygiene and proper disposal of sanitary waste are the most effective ways to prevent viral acquisition. There are no commercially available vaccines in the United States to prevent hepatitis E. However, a hepatitis E vaccine has been licensed in China since 2011 and may become available for countries with high HEV infection incidence rates.[16]

OUTCOME EVALUATION

Monitoring for efficacy in patients treated for chronic hepatitis B or C includes evaluating aminotransferase levels and hepatitis B or C viral levels and serologies.

Hepatitis B

- Obtain an ALT at baseline and then every 3 to 6 months during hepatitis B treatment.
- Monitor HBV DNA levels every 3 to 6 months to determine treatment response.
- Monitor HBeAg and anti-HBe every 6 months to determine if seroconversion to anti-HBe occurred or HBeAg was lost in HBeAg-positive CHB patients.[30]
- Monitor HBsAg every 6 to 12 months to determine if HBsAg was lost or anti-HBs developed in CHB HBeAg-negative patients with persistently undetectable serum HBV DNA levels.[30]
- Reevaluate at month 6 and either switch or add a more potent hepatitis B antiviral agent to the current hepatitis B regimen if the HBV DNA level has not decreased by 2 logs after 6 months of therapy.[30]
- Continue treatment in CHB HBeAg-positive patients until HBeAg seroconversion has been attained along with undetectable HBV DNA levels. Once anti-HBe appears, complete an additional 6 months of hepatitis B therapy.[30]
- Continue treatment in CHB HBeAg-negative patients until HBsAg is lost.[30]
- Monitor closely for hepatitis flare and viral relapse when discontinuing hepatitis B therapy.
- Obtain a CBC with differential every 4 weeks and thyroid-stimulating hormone (TSH) and fasting lipid panel every 12 weeks when receiving pegylated interferon therapy for hepatitis B.[30]
- Monitor serum creatinine for nephrotoxicity at baseline and every 12 weeks for patients receiving tenofovir or adefovir.
- Monitor creatine kinase at baseline and periodically (eg, every 12 weeks) for patients taking telbivudine because muscle weakness and myopathy have occurred.[23,30]

Hepatitis C

- Sustained virologic response (SVR) is defined as having an undetectable HCV RNA level at least 3 months posttreatment; this is the ultimate goal of HCV therapy and indicates a virological cure.[24]

Patient Encounter, Part 4

The patient has now been treated for a total of 12 weeks and the HCV RNA level is undetectable.

What action should you take based on the week 12 HCV RNA level?

What other information should you counsel the patient about in addition to the side effects associated with the hepatitis C therapy?

- End of treatment response (ETR or EOT) is defined as having undetectable HCV RNA levels at the end of treatment.
- Biochemical response is defined as normalization of ALT; monitor ALT levels every 4 weeks.
- Histologic response is defined as improving inflammation and fibrosis as documented by liver biopsy scores.
- Check the HCV RNA level per HCV guideline recommendations to determine the effectiveness of the HCV therapy and discontinue treatment if the HCV RNA has not decreased or become undetectable at certain time points.[24,38]

Patient Encounter, Part 5

The patient's husband was recently tested for viral hepatitis and found to be positive for hepatitis B. His only past medical history is mild depression and diabetes. He has not had any surgeries. He is taking metformin and no other over-the-counter drugs, or dietary supplements.

All laboratory test results are normal except for the following:

AST 93 IU/L (1.55 μkat/L)	HBeAg (–)
ALT 102 IU/L (1.70 μkat/L)	Anti-HB cIgG (+)
Anti-HAV IgM (–)	Anti-HBc IgM (–)
Anti-HAV IgG (+)	Anti-HBe (–),
Anti-HBs (–)	Anti-HCV (–)
HBsAg (+)	HBV DNA 3,108,514 IU/mL (3,108,514 kIU/L)

Based on the information presented:

(a) what additional information do you need before creating a treatment plan for this patient?

(b) create a detailed therapeutic care plan for the patient;

(c) discuss adverse effects to monitor;

(d) discuss a follow-up plan to determine whether the treatment goals have been achieved.

Patient Care Process

Patient Assessment:

- Evaluate patient social history and risk factors for acquiring viral hepatitis (see Table 24–1).
- Obtain past medical history focusing on psychiatric, cardiac, endocrine, and renal disorders. Is any disease present that may worsen the liver condition or be a contraindication to treatment?
- Conduct a medication (prescription, over-the-counter drugs, dietary supplements) to identify drug-interactions or drug-induced liver toxicity.
- Obtain a vaccination history to determine which vaccines have been given or need to be administered.
- Review laboratory tests to determine severity of liver disease. Review hepatitis serologies to determine if vaccination is needed (see Tables 24–3 and 24–4).
- Review the liver biopsy report, if available, to determine severity of liver damage and assess the need for treatment.

Therapy Evaluation:

- Determine if treatment is indicated by reviewing laboratory values, liver serologies, and liver biopsy report (if available).
- If patient does not have advanced disease or cirrhosis that qualifies for therapy, have patient return every 3 to 6 months to monitor health condition and laboratory tests
- If patient qualifies for treatment, assess for uncontrolled medical conditions, and if present, treat or refer to an appropriate medical specialty for evaluation (eg, HIV, diabetes, thyroid disease, tuberculosis).
- Assess current medications before initiating hepatitis therapy to identify potential drug–drug interactions and ensure that doses are appropriate based on organ function.
- If the patient is already receiving hepatitis treatment when referred for continuity of care, evaluate past medical history for unstable medical conditions, abnormal laboratory values, and medications with potential for drug interactions or adherence problems.

Care Plan Development:

- Refer to AASLD HBV guidelines for CHB treatment recommendations.
- Refer to www.hcvguidelines.org for HCV treatment guidelines.
- Work with Specialty Pharmacy to ensure that medications are covered and continued without disruption in treatment.
- Encourage adherence to hepatitis treatment regimens.
- Obtain pregnancy test and educate women of childbearing potential and men who are able to father a child to use two forms of contraception during and for 6 months after ribavirin base therapies.

Follow-Up Evaluation:

- At each visit for patients on treatment, review the medication list, assess for medication adverse effects and drug interactions, and review laboratory tests to assess efficacy and toxicity.
- Use adjunctive therapies (eg, growth factors) as appropriate to treat medication side effects.

(Continued)

Patient Care Process (Continued)

- Confirm adherence and number of missed doses to minimize drug resistance.
- Follow laboratory test results every week to every 2 weeks upon initiating treatment and once stable, then monthly to every 3 months.
- If viral level is undetectable post 3 or 6 months of HCV therapy, then educate the patient that reinfection may occur.
- If viral level is undetectable for an HBV patient, then educate that treatment duration may last for years.

- Monitor WBC, ANC, and platelets either weekly or biweekly during the first month of therapy and monthly thereafter if stable while on pegylated interferon.
- Monitor hemoglobin levels weekly or biweekly during the first month and monthly thereafter if stable while on ribavirin.
- Monitor for fatigue, shortness of breath, and chest pain and dermatological complications while on ribavirin; if significant complaints, discontinue treatment.
- Monitor TSH and fasting lipid panel every 12 weeks while receiving pegylated interferon.
- Monitor serum creatinine in patients receiving ribavirin to detect renal insufficiency that may result in ribavirin accumulation and toxicity (eg, hemolytic anemia).
- Conduct a thorough medication reconciliation of prescription, over-the-counter, and dietary and herbal supplements prior and during HCV therapy, especially if prescribed a DAA.
- Monitor total bilirubin concentrations every 2 to 4 weeks while on simeprevir, and perhaps more often if the patient is cirrhotic or has decompensated liver disease.

Abbreviations Introduced in This Chapter

ALT	Alanine aminotransferase
ANC	Absolute neutrophil count
Anti-HAV	Hepatitis A virus antibody
Anti-HBc	Hepatitis B core antibody
Anti-HBe	Hepatitis B envelope antibody
Anti-HBs	Hepatitis B surface antibody
Anti-HCV	Hepatitis C antibody
Anti-HDV	Hepatitis D antibody
Anti-HEV	Hepatitis E antibody
AST	Aspartate aminotransferase
CHB	Chronic hepatitis B infection
CrCl	Creatinine clearance
DAA	Direct acting antiretroviral
ETR	End of treatment response
ESLD	End-stage liver disease
HAV	Hepatitis A virus
HBcAg	Hepatitis B core antigen
HBeAg	Hepatitis B envelope antigen
HBIG	Hepatitis B immunoglobulin
HBsAg	Hepatitis B surface antigen
HBV	Hepatitis B virus
HBV DNA	Hepatitis B deoxyribonucleic acid
HCV	Hepatitis C virus
HCV RNA	Hepatitis C virus ribonucleic acid
HDV	Hepatitis D virus
HDVAg	Hepatitis D antigen
HDV RNA	Hepatitis D virus ribonucleic acid
HEV	Hepatitis E virus
IgG	Immunoglobulin G
IgG anti-HD	IgG antibodies to hepatitis D virus antigen
IgM	Immunoglobulin M
IgM anti-HD	IgM antibodies to hepatitis D virus antigen
IG	Immune globulin
IGIM	Immune globulin for intramuscular administration
IGIV	Immune globulin for IV administration
MMR	Measles, mumps, rubella vaccine
PCR	Polymerase chain reaction
RVR	Rapid virologic response
SVR	Sustained virologic response

REFERENCES

1. World Health Organization. Hepatitis A Fact Sheet. http://www.who.int/mediacentre/factsheets/fs328/en/. Accessed June 28, 2014.
2. Centers for Disease Control and Prevention. Hepatitis A. Epidemiology and Prevention of Vaccine-Preventable Diseases. Atkinson W, Wolfe S, Hamborsky J, eds. 12th ed., second printing. Washington DC: Public Health Foundation, 2012. http://www.cdc.gov/vaccines/pubs/pinkbook/hepa.html. Accessed July 31, 2014.
3. Centers for Disease Control and Prevention (CDC). Multistate outbreak of hepatitis A virus infections linked to pomegranate seeds from Turkey. http://www.cdc.gov/hepatitis/Outbreaks/2013/A1b-03-31/index.html. Accessed June 28, 2014.
4. Surveillance for acute viral hepatitis—United States, 2011. [Internet] http://www.cdc.gov/hepatitis/Statistics/2011Surveillance/Commentary.htm. Accessed June 28, 2014.
5. McMahon BJ. Chronic hepatitis B virus infection. Med Clin North Am 2014;98(1):39–54.
6. World Health Organization. Hepatitis B Fact Sheet. http://www.who.int/mediacentre/factsheets/fs204/en/. Acessed June 28, 2014.
7. Centers for Disease Control and Prevention. Hepatitis B. Epidemiology and Prevention of Vaccine-Preventable Diseases. Atkinson W, Wolfe S, Hamborsky J, eds. 12th ed., second printing. Washington DC: Public Health Foundation, 2012. http://www.cdc.gov/vaccines/pubs/pinkbook/hepb.html. Accessed July 31, 2014.
8. Mast EE, Weinbaum CM, Fiore AE, et al. A comprehensive immunization strategy to eliminate transmission of hepatitis B virus infection in the U.S.: Recommendations of the Advisory Committee on Immunization Practices (ACIP) Part II: Immunization of adults. MMWR Recomm Rep. 2006;55(RR-16):1–33.
9. World Health Organization. Hepatitis C Fact Sheet. http://www.who.int/mediacentre/factsheets/fs164/en/. Accessed June 29, 2014.
10. Thomas DL. Global control of hepatitis C: where challenge meets opportunity. Nat Med. 2013;19(7):850–858.
11. Smith DB, Bukh J, Kuiken C, et al. Expanded classification of hepatitis C virus into 7 genotypes and 67 subtypes: Updated criteria and genotype assignment web resource. Hepatology. 2014;59(1):318–327.
12. Nainan OV, Alter MJ, Kruszon-Moran D, et al. Hepatitis C virus genotypes and viral concentrations in participants of a general

population survey in the United States. Gastroenterology. 2006;131(2):478–484.
13. Centers for Disease Control and Prevention. Hepatitis C FAQs for Health Professionals. http://www.cdc.gov/hepatitis/HCV/index.htm. Accessed June 29, 2014.
14. Centers for Disease Control and Prevention. Recommendations for prevention and control of hepatitis C virus (HCV) infection and HCV-related chronic disease. MMWR Recomm Rep. 1998; 47(RR-19):1–39.
15. Alves C, Branco C, Cunha C. Hepatitis delta virus: a peculiar virus. Adv Virol. 2013;2013:560105.
16. World Health Organization. Hepatitis E Fact Sheet. http://www.who.int/mediacentre/factsheets/fs280/en/. Accessed June 29, 2014.
17. Chisari FV, Isogawa M, Wieland SF. Pathogenesis of hepatitis B virus infection. Pathol Biol. 2010;58(4):258–266.
18. Zingaretti C, De Francesco R, Abrignani S. Why is it so difficult to develop a hepatitis C virus preventive vaccine? Clin Microbiol Infect. 2014;20 Suppl 5:103–1099.
19. Ghany MG, Strader DB, Thomas DL, Seeff LB. Diagnosis, management, and treatment of hepatitis C: An update. Hepatology. 2009;49(4):1335–1374.
20. World Health Organization. Guidelines for the screening, care, and treatment of persons with hepatitis C infection. April 2014. http://apps.who.int/iris/bitstream/10665/111747/1/9789241548755_eng.pdf?ua=1. Accessed July 31, 2014.
21. Wang Y, Metselaar HJ, Peppelenbosch MP, Pan Q. Chronic hepatitis E in solid-organ transplantation: the key implications of immunosuppressants. Curr Opin Infect Dis. 2014;27(4):303–308.
22. Castera L. Noninvasive methods to assess liver disease in patients with hepatitis B or C. Gastroenterology. 2012;142(6):1293–1302.
23. Trépo C, Chan HL, Lok A. Hepatitis B virus infection. Lancet 2014 Jun 18. pii: S0140-6736(14)60220-60228.
24. AASLD/IDSA/IAS–USA. Recommendations for testing, managing, and treating hepatitis C. http://www.hcvguidelines.org. Accessed December 28, 2014.
25. Centers for Disease Control and Prevention (CDC). Update: Prevention of hepatitis A after exposure to hepatitis A virus and in international travelers. Updated recommendations of the Advisory Committee on Immunization Practices (ACIP). MMWR Morb Mortal Wkly Rep. 2007;56(41):1080–1084.
26. Centers for Disease Control and Prevention. Hepatitis A FAQs for Health Professionals. http://www.cdc.gov/hepatitis/HAV/HAVfaq.htm#vaccine. Accessed July 8, 2014.
27. Mast EE, Margolis HS, Fiore AE, et al. A comprehensive immunization strategy to eliminate transmission of hepatitis B virus infection in the United States: Recommendations of the Advisory Committee on Immunization Practices (ACIP) Part 1: Immunization of infants, children, and adolescents. MMWR Recomm Rep. 2005;54(RR-16):1–31.
28. Centers for Disease Control and Prevention. Hepatitis B FAQs for Health Professionals. http://www.cdc.gov/hepatitis/HBV/HBVfaq.htm#vaccFAQ. Accessed July 8, 2014.
29. Notice to Readers: FDA Approval of an Alternate Dosing Schedule for a Combined Hepatitis A and B Vaccine (Twinrix). MMWR Recomm Rep. 2007;56(40):1057.
30. Lok AS, McMahon BJ. Chronic hepatitis B: Update 2009. Hepatology 2009:1–36. http://www.aasld.org/practiceguidelines/documents/bookmarked%20practice%20guidelines/chronic_hep_b_update_2009%208_24_2009.pdf. Accessed July 9, 2014.
31. Lee JH, Cho Y, Lee DH, et al. Prior exposure to lamivudine increases entecavir resistance risk in chronic hepatitis B Patients without detectable lamivudine resistance. Antimicrob Agents Chemother. 2014;58(3):1730–1737.
32. Marcellin P, Gane E, Buti M, et al. Regression of cirrhosis during treatment with tenofovir disoproxil fumarate for chronic hepatitis B: A 5-year open-label follow-up study. Lancet. 2013;381(9865):468–475.
33. Lai CL, Gane E, Liaw YF, Hsu CW, et al. Telbivudine versus lamivudine in patients with chronic hepatitis B. N Engl J Med. 2007;357(25):2576–2588.
34. Chan J. Hepatitis C. Dis Mon. 2014;60(5):201–212.
35. Sulkowski MS, Cooper C, Hunyady B, et al. Management of adverse effects of Peg-IFN and ribavirin therapy for hepatitis C. Nat Rev Gastroenterol Hepatol. 2011;8(4):212–223.
36. Negro F. Adverse effects of drugs in the treatment of viral hepatitis. Best Pract Res Clin Gastroenterol. 2010;(2):183–192.
37. McHutchison JG, Manns MP, Brown RS Jr, et al. Strategies for managing anemia in hepatitis C patients undergoing antiviral therapy. Am J Gastroenterol. 2007;102(4):880–809.
38. Ghany MG, Nelson DR, Strader DB, et al. An update on treatment of genotype 1 chronic hepatitis C virus infection: 2011 practice guideline by the American Association for the Study of Liver Diseases. Hepatology. 2011;54(4):1433–1444.
39. Rong L, Dahari H, Ribeiro RM, Perelson AS. Rapid emergence of protease inhibitor resistance in hepatitis C virus. Sci Transl Med. 2010;2(30):30ra32.
40. Jacobson IM, Dore GJ, Foster GR, et al. Simeprevir with pegylated interferon alfa 2a plus ribavirin in treatment-naive patients with chronic hepatitis C virus genotype 1 infection (QUEST-1): a phase 3, randomised, double-blind, placebo-controlled trial. Lancet. 2014 Jun 3. pii: S0140-6736(14)60494-3.
41. Manns M, Marcellin P, Poordad F, et al. Simeprevir with pegylated interferon alfa 2a or 2b plus ribavirin in treatment-naive patients with chronic hepatitis C virus genotype 1 infection (QUEST-2): A randomised, double-blind, placebo-controlled phase 3 trial. Lancet. 2014 Jun 3. pii: S0140-6736(14)60538-9.
42. Lenz O, Verbinnen T, Lin TI, et al. In vitro resistance profile of the hepatitis C virus NS3/4A protease inhibitor TMC435. Antimicrob Agents Chemother. 2010;54(5):1878–1887.
43. Pawlotsky JM. New hepatitis C therapies: The toolbox, strategies, and challenges. Gastroenterology. 2014;146(5):1176–1192.
44. You DM, Pockros PJ. Simeprevir for the treatment of chronic hepatitis C. Expert Opin Pharmacother. 2013;14(18):2581–2589.
45. Koff RS. Review article: The efficacy and safety of sofosbuvir, a novel, oral nucleotide NS5B polymerase inhibitor, in the treatment of chronic hepatitis C virus infection. Aliment Pharmacol Ther. 2014;39(5):478–487.

25 Acute Kidney Injury

Mary K. Stamatakis

LEARNING OBJECTIVES

Upon completion of the chapter, the reader will be able to:

1. Assess a patient's kidney function based on clinical presentation, laboratory results, and urinary indices.
2. Identify pharmacotherapeutic outcomes and endpoints of therapy in a patient with acute kidney injury (AKI).
3. Apply knowledge of the pathophysiology of AKI to the development of a treatment plan.
4. Design a diuretic regimen to treat volume overload in AKI.
5. Develop strategies to minimize the occurrence of drug and radiocontrast-induced AKI.
6. Monitor and evaluate the safety and efficacy of the therapeutic plan.

INTRODUCTION

Acute kidney injury (AKI) is a potentially life-threatening syndrome that occurs primarily in hospitalized patients and frequently complicates the course of critically ill patients. It is characterized by a rapid decrease in glomerular filtration rate (GFR) and the resultant accumulation of nitrogenous waste products (eg, creatinine), with or without a decrease in urine output.

The term AKI has replaced the term *acute renal failure* (ARF) because it more completely encompasses the entire spectrum of acute injury to the kidney, from mild changes in kidney function to end-stage kidney disease requiring renal replacement therapy (RRT). Furthermore, the definition of ARF was inconsistent in the literature.[1] Efforts to standardize the definition of ARF led to a change in terminology to AKI and development of a consensus definition.

KEY CONCEPT *AKI is defined as an increase in serum creatinine (SCr) of at least 0.3 mg/dL (27 μmol/L) within 48 hours, a 50% increase in baseline SCr within 7 days, or a urine output of less than 0.5 mL/kg/hour for at least 6 hours.* Only one criterion needs to be met for diagnosis of AKI.[2]

EPIDEMIOLOGY AND ETIOLOGY

Approximately 5% to 7% of all hospitalized patients develop AKI. AKI is 5 to 10 times more prevalent in the hospital setting than in the community setting.[3] About 5% to 20% of critically ill patients develop AKI,[3] and 30% to 40% of survivors progress to chronic kidney disease (CKD).[4] Despite improvements in the medical care of individuals with AKI, mortality generally exceeds 15% for patients in general wards to 50% for ICU patients.[5]

PATHOPHYSIOLOGY

There are three categories of AKI: prerenal, intrinsic, and postrenal AKI. The pathophysiologic mechanisms differ for each of the categories.

Prerenal AKI

Prerenal AKI occurs in approximately 10% to 25% of patients diagnosed with AKI and is characterized by reduced blood delivery to the kidney. A common cause is intravascular volume depletion due to conditions such as hemorrhage, dehydration, or GI fluid losses. Early volume restoration can prevent progression and improve recovery because no structural damage to the kidney has occurred.[6] Conditions of reduced cardiac output (eg, congestive heart failure [CHF], myocardial infarction) and hypotension can also reduce renal blood flow, resulting in decreased glomerular perfusion and prerenal AKI. With a mild to moderate decrease in renal blood flow, intraglomerular pressure is maintained by dilation of afferent arterioles (arteries supplying blood to the glomerulus), constriction of efferent arterioles (arteries removing blood from the glomerulus), and redistribution of renal blood flow to the oxygen-sensitive renal medulla.

Drugs may cause a functional AKI when they interfere with these autoregulatory mechanisms. Nonsteroidal anti-inflammatory drugs (NSAIDs) impair prostaglandin-mediated dilation of afferent arterioles. Angiotensin-converting enzyme (ACE) inhibitors and angiotensin receptor blockers (ARBs) inhibit angiotensin II–mediated efferent arteriole vasoconstriction and cause prerenal AKI in 6% to 38% of treated patients.[6] The calcineurin inhibitors cyclosporine and tacrolimus, particularly in high doses, are potent renal vasoconstrictors. All these agents can reduce intraglomerular pressure, with a resultant decrease in GFR. Prompt discontinuation of the offending drug can often return kidney function to normal.

Other causes of prerenal AKI are renovascular obstruction (eg, renal artery stenosis), hyperviscosity syndromes (eg, multiple myeloma), and systemic vasoconstriction (eg, hepatorenal syndrome).

Intrinsic AKI

Intrinsic renal failure is caused by diseases that can affect the structure of the nephron, such as the tubules, glomerulus, interstitium, or blood vessels. Acute tubular necrosis (ATN) is a term that is often used synonymously with intrinsic AKI, but ATN relates more specifically to a pathophysiologic condition resulting from toxic (eg, aminoglycosides, contrast agents, amphotericin B) or ischemic insult to the kidney. ATN accounts for 50% of all cases of AKI.[7] Glomerular, interstitial, and blood vessel diseases may also lead to intrinsic AKI but occur with a much lower incidence. Examples include glomerulonephritis, systemic lupus erythematosus, interstitial nephritis, and vasculitis. In addition, prerenal AKI can progress to intrinsic AKI if the underlying condition is not promptly corrected.

Postrenal AKI

Postrenal AKI is due to obstruction of urinary outflow. Causes include benign prostatic hypertrophy, pelvic tumors, and precipitation of renal calculi.[7] Rapid resolution of postrenal AKI without structural damage to the kidney can occur if the underlying obstruction is corrected. Postrenal AKI accounts for less than 10% of cases of AKI.

CLINICAL PRESENTATION AND DIAGNOSIS

The definition and categorization of AKI has evolved over the past decade. The first AKI classification system was *RIFLE*, which stands for Risk, Injury, Failure, Loss, and End stage. It categorizes patients into stages based on change in SCr or GFR from baseline, or decreased urine output.[8] RIFLE includes three stages of severity and two outcome categories.

After development of the *RIFLE* criteria, the Acute Kidney Injury Network (AKIN) modified the *RIFLE* definition and staging for AKI. The AKIN staging system is based on changes in SCr (and not GFR) and uses three stages (stages 1 to 3); Stage 1 also includes an absolute increase in SCr of 0.3 mg/dL (27 μmol/L) or greater.[9] This highlights the association of even small increases in SCr concentration with morbidity and mortality, making early detection critical. It also categorizes all patients receiving RRT as stage 3.[10] Studies have validated both RIFLE and AKIN criteria in identifying hospitalized patients at risk of mortality associated with AKI.[11,12] A merging of the RIFLE and AKIN classification of AKI is advocated by the 2012 Kidney Disease: Improving Global Outcomes (KDIGO) Clinical Practice Guidelines for Acute Kidney Injury (Table 25–1).[2]

Decreased urine output may be a more sensitive marker than increases in SCr in early AKI; however, decreased urine output is not universally present in AKI. Oliguria and anuria are defined as daily urine outputs of less than 400 and 50 mL, respectively. Reduced urine output is associated with increased mortality and may represent a more severe form of AKI. Nonoliguric AKI is defined as urine output greater than 400 mL/day. It may still represent severe AKI but is associated with better patient outcomes.[13]

Frequent monitoring of a patient's SCr and blood urea nitrogen (BUN) and comparison to baseline can indicate if a patient's kidney function is worsening or improving. BUN is a less sensitive marker for evaluation of AKI. Urea is a product of amino acid metabolism. While urea is eliminated via GFR, it also undergoes reabsorption in the proximal tubule and is urine flow dependent. Increased urea reabsorption occurs when urine flow to the kidney is decreased. Thus, in prerenal AKI, an elevated BUN in relationship to SCr occurs and may assist in the diagnosis of prerenal AKI. Additionally, BUN production can be increased due to extrarenal factors such as increased dietary protein or absorption of blood from a gastrointestinal bleed.

Although some clinical and laboratory findings assist in the general diagnosis of AKI, others are used to differentiate among prerenal, intrinsic, and postrenal AKI. For example, patients with prerenal AKI typically demonstrate enhanced sodium reabsorption, which is reflected by a low urine sodium concentration and a low fractional excretion of sodium. Urine is typically more concentrated with prerenal AKI, and there is a higher urine osmolality and urine-to-plasma creatinine ratio compared with intrinsic and postrenal AKI.

Other factors, such as symptoms, laboratory test results, urinary indices, and results of diagnostic procedures, aid in the diagnosis and assessment of disease severity.

TREATMENT

Desired Outcomes

A primary goal in the care of patients with AKI is ameliorating identifiable underlying causes of AKI such as hypovolemia, nephrotoxic drugs, or ureter obstruction. Prerenal and postrenal AKI can be reversed if the underlying problem is promptly identified and corrected, whereas treatment of intrinsic renal failure is more supportive in nature. For patients with prerenal AKI, isotonic crystalloids such as 0.9% normal saline are used for expansion of intravascular volume and return to a state of proper fluid balance (euvolemia).[14] In addition to fluids, vasopressors (ie, norepinephrine, dopamine, vasopressin) may be needed in patients with septic shock to treat prerenal AKI. There is no sufficient data to support one agent as superior over another;

Table 25–1

Staging System for AKI

Stage	Serum Creatinine	Percentage Serum Creatinine Increase from Baseline	Urine Output	Need for Renal Replacement Therapy
1	≥ 0.3 mg/dL (27 μmol/L) increase from baseline	150%–199% (1.5- to 1.9-fold)	< 0.5 ml/kg/hour for 6–12 hours	No
2	—	200–299% (2- to 2.9-fold)	< 0.5 ml/kg/hour for ≥ 12 hours	No
3	Increase to ≥ 4 mg/dL (354 μmol/L)	≥ 300% (> 3-fold)	< 0.3 ml/kg/hour for ≥ 24 hours or anuria for ≥ 12 hours	Initiation of renal replacement therapy indicates stage 3 regardless of serum creatinine or urine output

Based on the KDIGO staging system for AKI. Only one of the three criteria needs to be met in order to qualify for the higher stage.

Clinical Presentation and Diagnosis of AKI

Signs and Symptoms of AKI

- Peripheral edema
- Weight gain
- Nausea, vomiting, diarrhea, anorexia
- Mental status changes
- Fatigue
- Shortness of breath
- Pruritus
- Volume depletion (prerenal AKI)
- Weight loss (prerenal AKI)
- Anuria alternating with polyuria (postrenal AKI)
- Colicky abdominal pain radiating from flank to groin (postrenal AKI)

Physical Examination Findings

- Increased blood pressure
- Jugular venous distention (JVD)
- Pulmonary edema
- Rales
- Asterixis
- Pericardial or pleural friction rub
- Hypotension or orthostatic hypotension (prerenal AKI)
- Rash (intrinsic AKI due to acute interstitial nephritis)
- Bladder distention (postrenal bladder outlet obstruction)
- Prostatic enlargement (postrenal AKI)

Laboratory Tests

- Elevated SCr (reference range approximately 0.6–1.2 mg/dL [53–106 μmol/L])
- Elevated BUN (reference range approximately 8 to 25 mg/dL [2.9–8.9 mmol/L])
- BUN-to-creatinine ratio greater than 20:1 for units of mg/dL (prerenal AKI); less than 20:1 for units of mg/dL (intrinsic or postrenal AKI)
- Hyperkalemia
- Metabolic acidosis

Urinalysis

- Sediment
  - Scant or bland (prerenal or postrenal AKI)
  - Brown, muddy granular casts (intrinsic ATN)
  - Proteinuria (glomerulonephritis or allergic interstitial nephritis)
  - Eosinophiluria (acute interstitial nephritis)
  - Hematuria or red blood cell casts (glomerular disease or bleeding in urinary tract)
  - WBCs or casts (acute interstitial nephritis or severe pyelonephritis)

Urinary Indices	Prerenal AKI	Intrinsic and Postrenal AKI
Urine osmolality (solute concentration in the urine in mOsm/kg or mmol/kg)	> 500	< 350
Urine sodium concentration (mEq/L or mmol/L)	< 20	> 40
Specific gravity	> 1.020	< 1.015
Urine-to-plasma creatinine ratio	> 40:1	< 20:1
Fractional excretion of sodium (FENa)	< 1%	> 1%

$$\text{Fractional excretion of sodium (FENa)} = 100 \times \frac{\left(\begin{array}{c}\text{Urinary sodium concentration} \times \\ \text{Plasma creatinine concentration}\end{array}\right)}{\left(\begin{array}{c}\text{Plasma sodium concentration} \times \\ \text{Plasma creatinine concentration}\end{array}\right)}$$

FENa is a measure of the percentage of sodium excreted by the kidney. A FENa less than 1% may indicate prerenal AKI because it represents the response of the kidney to decreased renal perfusion by decreasing sodium excretion. Loop diuretics such as furosemide enhance sodium excretion and increase FENa, confounding the interpretation of the test.

Common Diagnostic Procedures

- Urinary catheterization (used to rule out urethral obstruction. A catheter is inserted into the bladder; increased urine output may occur with postrenal obstruction.)
- Renal ultrasound (uses sound waves to assess size, position, and abnormalities of the kidney. Can assist in the differentiation between AKI [normal-sized kidneys] and CKD [small kidneys]. Can also show obstruction of the urinary tract which is indicative of postrenal AKI.)
- Computed tomography (provides similar information as renal ultrasound but with greater spatial resolution; assists in the diagnosis of masses, stones, and pyelonephritis.)
- Magnetic resonance imaging (Uses strong magnetic fields and radio waves to form images of the kidney; used as an alternative to computed tomography scanning to avoid contrast.)
- Renal angiography (shows blood flow through the kidney; IV contrast dye is administered and narrowing of the vasculature can be seen in conditions such as renal artery stenosis and renal vein thrombosis.)
- Retrograde pyelography (injection of contrast dye into the ureters to localize the site of urinary tract obstruction.)
- Kidney biopsy (collection of a kidney tissue sample for microscopic evaluation; may aid in the diagnosis of glomerular and interstitial diseases.)

however, greater adverse events have been reported with dopamine compared to norepinephrine.[15] KEY CONCEPT *However, there is no evidence that drug therapy hastens patient recovery, decreases length of hospitalization, or improves survival in AKI.*

Pharmacologic Therapy

► *Loop Diuretics*

Most studies evaluating loop diuretics (furosemide, bumetanide, torsemide, and ethacrynic acid) for prevention or treatment of AKI demonstrate improved urine output but no effect on survival or need for dialysis. There are some reports that loop diuretics may worsen kidney function and may be due in part to preload reduction that results in renal vasoconstriction.[16] Thus, loop diuretics should be reserved for the treatment of volume overload and should not be given to prevent AKI or hasten recovery of kidney function in euvolemic or hypovolemic individuals.[17]

Loop diuretics are all equally effective when given in equivalent doses. Therefore, selection is based on the side-effect profile, cost, and pharmacokinetic differences. Ototoxicity is a well-established side effect of furosemide and ethacrynic acid that occurs rarely with bumetanide and torsemide. For furosemide, the risk of ototoxicity is greater when administered by the IV route at a rate exceeding 4 mg/min.

The incidence of ototoxicity is higher for ethacrynic acid compared with the other loop diuretics. However, ethacrynic acid is the only loop diuretic that does not contain a sulfonamide moiety and its use has been recommended in individuals with a sulfa allergy. However, there is very weak evidence of cross-allergenicity between sulfa-containing antibiotics and diuretics.[18] With its high incidence of ototoxicity, ethacrynic acid is not recommended.

There are several pharmacokinetic differences among loop diuretics. About 85% of furosemide is excreted unchanged by the kidney.[19] In contrast, liver metabolism accounts for 50% and 80% of the elimination of bumetanide and torsemide, respectively.[19] The bioavailability of both torsemide and bumetanide is higher than for furosemide with an IV-to-oral ratio of 1:1. The bioavailability of oral furosemide is approximately 50% to 65%.[20] Thus, the IV-to-oral ratio for furosemide is about 1:2.

The pharmacodynamic characteristics of loop diuretics are similar when equivalent doses are administered. Loop diuretics exert their effect from the luminal (urinary) side of the tubule. Substances that interfere with the secretion of loop diuretics, such as endogenous organic acids that accumulate in kidney disease, competitively inhibit secretion of loop diuretics into the lumen of the tubules. Therefore, large doses of loop diuretics are often necessary in kidney disease to ensure that adequate drug reaches the nephron lumen. Loop diuretics also have a ceiling effect where maximal natriuresis occurs.[19] Thus, very large doses of furosemide (eg, 1 g) are not necessary and may unnecessarily increase the risk of ototoxicity.

Several adaptive mechanisms by the kidney limit effectiveness of loop diuretic therapy. As the concentration of diuretic in the loop of Henle decreases, postdiuretic sodium retention can occur. This effect can be minimized by decreasing the dosage interval (ie, dosing more frequently) or by administering a continuous infusion.[21]

Prolonged administration of loop diuretics can lead to a second type of diuretic resistance. Hypertrophy of distal convoluted tubule cells can occur secondary to enhanced delivery of sodium to the distal tubule.[19] Subsequently, increased sodium chloride absorption occurs in the distal tubule, which diminishes the effect of the loop diuretic on overall sodium excretion. Addition of a distal convoluted tubule diuretic, such as metolazone or hydrochlorothiazide, to a loop diuretic can result in a synergistic increase in urine output. There are no data to support greater efficacy of one distal convoluted tubule diuretic over another. It is common practice to administer the distal convoluted tubule diuretic 30 to 60 minutes prior to the loop diuretic in an attempt to inhibit sodium reabsorption at the distal convoluted tubule before it is inundated with sodium from the loop of Henle. However, the effectiveness of this strategy has not been studied.

A usual starting dose of IV furosemide for treatment of AKI is 40 mg (Figure 25–1). Reasonable starting doses for bumetanide and torsemide are 1 and 20 mg, respectively.[19] Efficacy of diuretic administration can be determined by comparison of a patient's hourly fluid balance. Other methods to minimize volume overload, such as fluid restriction and concentration of IV medications, should be initiated as needed. If urine output does not increase to about 1 mL/kg/hour, the dosage can be increased to a maximum of 160 to 200 mg of furosemide or its equivalent (see Figure 25–1).[20] Dosing frequency is based on the patient's response, the ability to restrict sodium intake, and the duration of action of the diuretic. Other methods to improve diuresis can be initiated sequentially, such as (a) shortening the dosage interval, (b) adding hydrochlorothiazide or metolazone, and (c) switching to a continuous infusion loop diuretic. In patients with a CrCl of 25 mL/min (0.42 mL/s) or higher, furosemide at a dose of 10 mg/hour would be a reasonable initial infusion rate.[16] A rate of 20 mg/hour would be reasonable in patients with a CrCl less than 25 mL/min (0.42 mL/s).[16] Continuous infusion loop diuretics

Patient Encounter, Part 1

A 63-year-old woman presents to the clinic with complaints of weakness and nausea. She has a past medical history of stage 2 chronic kidney disease with proteinuria (baseline SCr 1.0 mg/dL [88 μmol/L]), gout, hypertension, and chronic back pain. Her estimated GFR is 65 mL/min/1.73 m^2. She reports having nausea, vomiting, and a low-grade fever last week. Her grandson had similar symptoms, and she did not seek treatment. Her fever resolved with naproxen, but she still feels weak and nauseated. She states that she feels like she is "holding on to water" even though she takes her "water pill." Her weight is usually about 143 pounds (65 kg), and today she weighs 149 lbs (67.6 kg). Upon preliminary examination, she was found to have 2+ pitting edema, BP 160/94, and crackles on auscultation.

Meds: Fexofenadine 180 mg orally once daily; Enalapril 5 mg orally once daily; furosemide 40 mg orally once daily; atorvastatin 10 mg orally daily; metformin 500 mg orally twice daily; glyburide 5 mg orally daily; metoprolol 25 mg orally twice daily; allopurinol 300 mg orally daily; naproxen 220 mg as needed for arthritis pain and fever

What signs and symptoms suggest acute kidney injury (AKI)?

What risk factors does she have for developing AKI?

What additional laboratory information do you need to fully assess the patient?

What questions would you ask her regarding her pharmacotherapy?

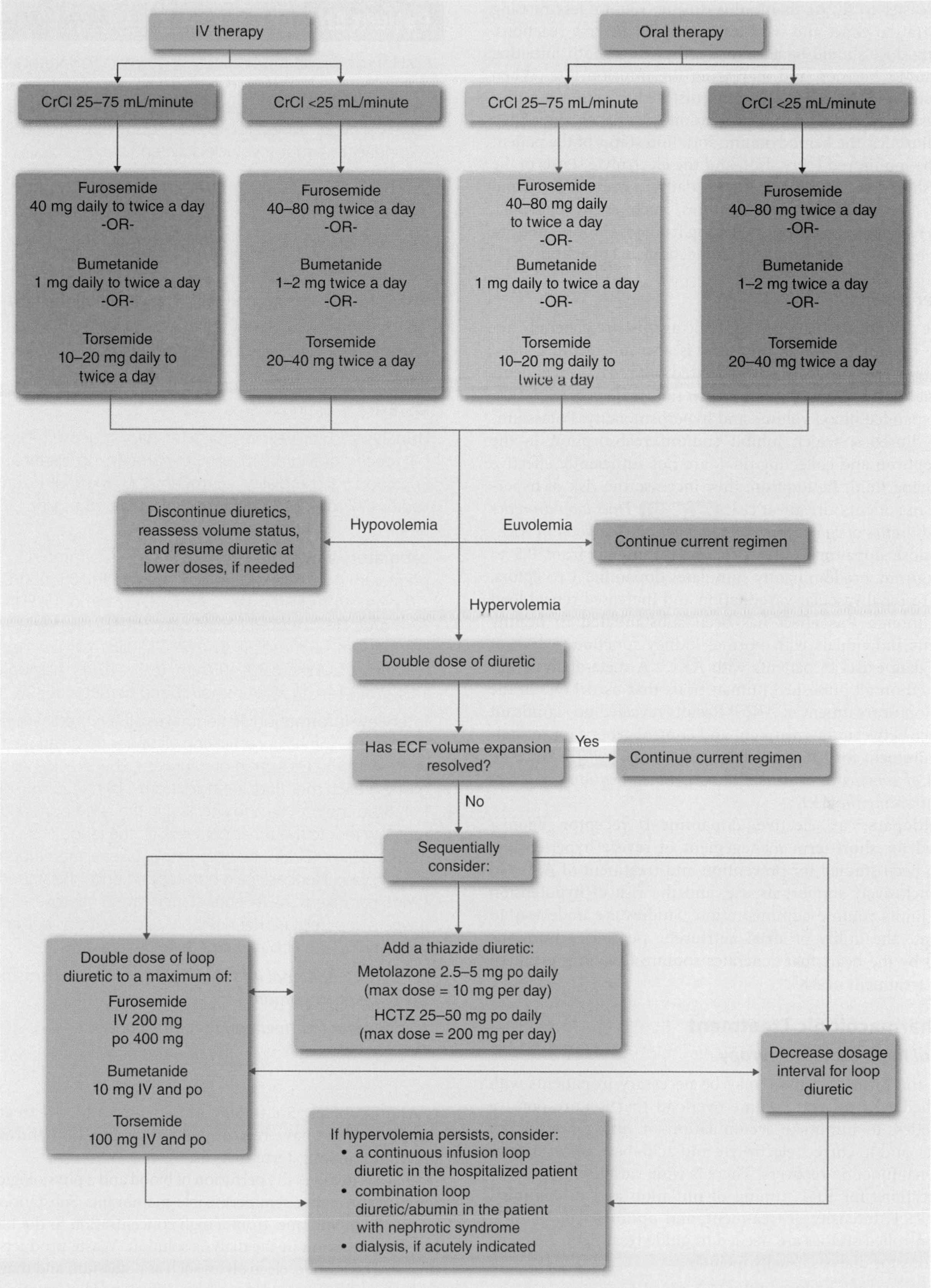

FIGURE 25–1. Algorithm for treatment of extracellular fluid expansion. (CrCl, creatinine clearance; ECF, extracellular fluid; HCTZ, hydrochlorothiazide; po, oral.)

may be easier to titrate than bolus dosing, require less nursing administration time, and may lead to fewer adverse reactions. A loading dose should be administered prior to both initiating a continuous infusion and increasing the infusion rate. When high doses of loop diuretics are administered or with a continuous infusion, particularly in combination with distal convoluted tubule diuretics, the hemodynamic and fluid status of the patient should be monitored every shift, and the electrolyte status of the patient should be monitored at least daily to prevent profound diuresis and electrolyte abnormalities, such as hypokalemia. Patients will not benefit from switching from one loop diuretic to another because of the similarity in mechanisms of action.

▶ *Other Agents*

Thiazide diuretics, when used as single agents, are generally not effective for fluid removal. Mannitol is also not recommended for treating volume overload associated with AKI. In patients with renal dysfunction, mannitol excretion is decreased, resulting in expanded blood volume and hyperosmolality. Potassium-sparing diuretics, which inhibit sodium reabsorption in the distal nephron and collecting duct, are not sufficiently effective in removing fluid. In addition, they increase the risk of hyperkalemia in patients already at risk. KEY CONCEPT *Thus loop diuretics are the diuretics of choice for managing volume overload in AKI.*

Low-dose dopamine (LDD), in doses ranging from 0.5 to 3 mcg/kg/min, predominantly stimulates dopamine-1 receptors, leading to renal vascular vasodilation and increased renal blood flow. Although this effect has been substantiated in healthy euvolemic individuals with normal kidney function, a lack of efficacy data exists in patients with AKI.[22] A meta-analysis was performed on all published human trials that used LDD in the prevention or treatment of AKI.[23] Results revealed no significant difference between the treatment and control groups for mortality, requirement for RRT, or adverse effects. KEY CONCEPT *Based on the lack of conclusive evidence, there is no indication for use of LDD in treating the AKI.*

Fenoldopam, a selective dopamine-1 receptor agonist approved for short-term management of severe hypertension, has also been studied for prevention and treatment of AKI. No data conclusively support its use, and the risk of hypotension further limits routine administration. Studies are underway to investigate the utility of atrial natriuretic peptide, a hormone secreted by the heart that generates sodium loss, in prevention or early treatment of AKI.

Patient Encounter, Part 2

PMH: Type 2 diabetes mellitus for 10 years (laboratory test results from 3 months ago: A1C = 7.4% [0.074; 57 mmol/mol hemoglobin], SCr 1.0 mg/dL [88 μmol/L]); dyslipidemia for 10 years; hypertension for 10 years; gout; episodic back pain secondary to a motor vehicle accident

FH: Father with history of type 2 diabetes and chronic kidney disease; mother with history of hypertension

SH: No smoking, no alcohol use

PE:

VS: BP 160/94 mm Hg, pulse 85 beats/min, RR 22 breaths/min, T 37.6°C, Wt 67.6 kg (149 lb), Ht 5′7″ (170 cm)

Chest: Basilar crackles, inspiratory wheezes

CV: RRR, S_1, S_2 normal

MS/Ext: 2 + pitting edema

Urinalysis: Color, yellow; character, hazy; glucose (–); ketones (–); specific gravity 1.010; pH 5; (+) protein; no bacteria; nitrite (–); blood (–); osmolality 325 mOsm/L (325 mmol/L); urinary sodium 77 mEq/L (77 mmol/L); creatinine 25 mg/dL (2210 μmol/L)

Laboratory Values: Sodium 136 mEq/L (136 mmol/L), potassium 4.2 mEq/L (4.2 mmol/L), chloride 105 mEq/L (105 mmol/L), bicarbonate 22 mEq/L (22 mmol/L), BUN 32 mg/dL (11.4 mmol/L), SCr 1.6 mg/dL (141 μmol/L), magnesium 1.6 mg/dL (0.66 mmol/L), glucose 120 mg/dL (6.7 mmol/L), WBC 6.9 × 10^3/mm^3 (6.9 × 10^9/L), hemoglobin 14.4 g/dL (144 g/L; 8.94 mmol/L), and hematocrit 42% (0.42)

Interview Information: Patient takes all her medications as prescribed. She has been taking all of her medications for years, with the exception of naproxen. She checks her fasting glucose each morning. It ranges from 110 to 125 mg/dL (6.1–6.9 mmol/L). She also checks it in the afternoons and it runs low four to five times per week (in the range of 60–70 mg/dL [3.3–3.9 mmol/L]). She occasionally takes acetaminophen (once a week) for back pain but stopped once she started taking naproxen. She recently started taking naproxen 3 or 4 weeks ago because her neighbor told her it was better for pain. She takes it about two or three times a day

Given this additional information, what is your assessment of the patient's condition?

Identify your treatment goals for the patient.

Nonpharmacologic Treatment

▶ *Renal Replacement Therapy*

RRT in the form of dialysis may be necessary in patients with established AKI to treat volume overload that is unresponsive to diuretics, to minimize accumulation of nitrogenous waste products, and to correct electrolyte and acid–base abnormalities while renal function recovers. There is wide variation in practice on indications for RRT, timing of initiation and discontinuation of RRT, intensity of treatment, and optimal type of RRT. Well-controlled studies are needed to guide treatment. Absolute indications for dialysis usually include:

- BUN greater than 100 mg/dL (35.7 mmol/L)
- Potassium greater than 6 mEq/L (6 mmol/L)
- Magnesium greater than 9.7 mg/dL (4.0 mmol/L)
- Metabolic acidosis with a pH less than 7.15
- Diuretic-resistant fluid overload[24]

Approximately 5% to 30% of patients with AKI treated with dialysis will not have recovery of kidney function and will need to remain on long-term dialysis.

Dialysis involves the perfusion of blood and a physiologic dialysis solution through a semipermeable membrane. Substances diffuse across the membrane, from a high concentration in the blood to a low concentration in the dialysis solution. Waste products such as urea and creatinine, electrolytes such as potassium and magnesium, and some drugs are removed by diffusion. Hydrostatic pressure differences result in convection and ultrafiltration and removal of water and some larger molecular weight substances from the body. Two types of dialysis modalities are commonly used in AKI: intermittent hemodialysis (IHD) and continuous renal replacement therapy (CRRT). IHD is a higher efficiency form of dialysis where both diffusion and ultrafiltration/convection occur and that is provided for several hours a day at a variable frequency (usually daily or three to five times per week). CRRT is a pump-driven form of dialysis that provides slow fluid and solute removal on a continuous 24-hour basis. Examples of CRRT include:

- continuous venovenous hemofiltration (CVVH)
- continuous venovenous hemodialysis (CVVHD)
- continuous venovenous hemodiafiltration (CVVHDF)

The primary advantage of CRRT is hemodynamic stability and better volume control, particularly in patients who are unable to tolerate rapid fluid removal. The primary disadvantages associated with CRRT are continuous nursing requirements, continuous anticoagulation, frequent clotting of the dialyzer, patient immobility, and increased cost. There is no conclusive evidence that one type of dialysis is preferred over another in terms of mortality and recovery of renal function. Thus, selection of CRRT over IHD is often governed by the critical illness of the patient and by the comfort level of the institution with one particular type of dialysis.[25] Mortality in critically ill patients receiving CRRT is 40% to 53%.[25,26]

▶ *Supportive Therapy*

Supportive therapy in AKI includes adequate nutrition, correction of electrolyte and acid–base abnormalities (particularly hyperkalemia and metabolic acidosis), fluid management, and correction of any hematologic abnormalities. Because AKI can be associated with multiorgan failure, treatment may include the medical management of infections, cardiovascular and GI conditions, and respiratory failure.

PREVENTION OF ACUTE RENAL FAILURE

KEY CONCEPT *Identifying patients at high risk for development of AKI and implementing preventive methods to decrease its occurrence or severity is critically important.*

Avoidance

The best preventive measure for AKI, especially in individuals at high risk, is to avoid medications that are known to precipitate AKI. Nephrotoxicity is a significant side effect of aminoglycosides, ACE inhibitors, ARBs, amphotericin B, NSAIDs, cyclosporine, tacrolimus, and radiographic contrast agents.[6] Unfortunately, an effective, non-nephrotoxic alternative may not always be appropriate for a given patient, and the risks and benefits of selecting a drug with nephrotoxic potential must be considered. For example, serious gram-negative infections may require double antibiotic coverage and aminoglycoside coverage may be necessary based on culture and sensitivity reports. In situations such as this, monitoring of aminoglycoside drug concentrations is warranted.

Drug-Induced AKI

▶ *Aminoglycosides*

Aminoglycosides (gentamicin, tobramycin, and amikacin) cause nonoliguric intrinsic AKI in about 10% to 25% of treated patients.[27] Injury is due to binding of aminoglycosides to proximal tubular cells in the renal cortex, and subsequent cellular uptake and cell death. In addition, aminoglycosides cause renal vasoconstriction and mesangial contraction.[28] In clinical practice, all aminoglycosides have comparable nephrotoxicity; thus similar precautions should be used for all of the agents. High cumulative drug exposure increases the incidence of aminoglycoside-induced AKI. Additional risk factors include a prolonged course of aminoglycoside therapy (typically after 7 to 10 days of therapy), preexisting CKD, increased age, and concurrent administration of other nephrotoxic drugs. If feasible, alternative antibiotics should be selected in individuals who are at high risk for developing AKI.

Methods to minimize drug exposure with conventional dosing (multiple doses per day) include maintaining trough concentrations less than 2 mcg/mL (2 mg/L; 4.2 μmol/L) for gentamicin and tobramycin and less than 10 mcg/mL (10 mg/L; 17.1 μmol/L) for amikacin, minimizing length of therapy, and avoiding repeated courses of aminoglycosides. Concurrent exposure to other nephrotoxic medications and dehydration may also worsen AKI. There is conflicting evidence as to whether the combination of vancomycin and an aminoglycoside has a higher incidence of AKI than aminoglycoside therapy alone. Aminoglycoside-induced AKI is usually reversible upon drug discontinuation; however, dialysis may be needed in some individuals while kidney function improves.

Extended-interval (eg, once daily) dosing is another method to minimize toxicity. The goal of extended-interval dosing is to provide greater efficacy against the microorganism with a lower incidence of nephrotoxicity. Aminoglycosides demonstrate concentration-dependent killing and a prolonged postantibiotic effect.[27] Extended-interval aminoglycoside dosing reduces the incidence of nephrotoxicity by providing high transient concentrations of drug that saturate proximal tubule uptake sites. Once saturated, the remaining aminoglycoside molecules pass through the proximal tubule and are excreted in the urine.[29] Thus, less drug is available for cellular uptake during a 24-hour period. Extended-interval aminoglycoside dosing is as effective as conventional dosing and is not more nephrotoxic; some studies have shown it to be less nephrotoxic than conventional dosing. Aminoglycosides can also cause hearing loss and/or vestibular toxicity, although the incidence of ototoxicity appears to be similar with extended-dosing and conventional dosing. Prolonged exposure to the drug, repeated courses of therapy, and concurrent use of other ototoxic drugs increase ototoxicity. Extended-interval dosing is not recommended in patients with preexisting kidney disease, conditions where high concentrations are not needed (eg, urinary tract infections), hyperdynamic patients who may demonstrate increased drug clearance (eg, burn patients), and others where you would suspect altered pharmacokinetics or increased risk of ototoxicity.

▶ *Amphotericin B*

The reported incidence of amphotericin B–induced AKI varies widely in the literature, from about 30% to as high as 80% of patients treated with the conventional desoxycholate formulation.[29] Nephrotoxicity is due to renal arterial vasoconstriction and distal renal tubule cell damage. Risk factors for development of AKI include high daily dosage, large cumulative dose (greater than 2 to 3 g), preexisting kidney dysfunction, dehydration, and concomitant use of other nephrotoxic drugs. Tubular abnormalities manifesting as hypomagnesemia and hypokalemia often occur within the first 2 weeks of treatment, followed by the overt development of AKI.

Three lipid-based formulations of amphotericin B have been developed in an attempt to improve efficacy and limit toxicity, particularly nephrotoxicity: amphotericin B lipid complex, amphotericin B colloidal dispersion, and liposomal amphotericin B. The range of nephrotoxicity reported is 15% to 25% for these formulations. The mechanism for decreased nephrotoxicity has not been completely elucidated, but it is thought to be due to preferential delivery of amphotericin B to the site of infection, with less affinity for the kidney.[31] Costs for liposomal formulations are significantly higher than for the conventional formulation; thus, lipid-based formulations are typically recommended for individuals with risk factors for AKI. Administration of IV normal saline may also attenuate nephrotoxicity associated with amphotericin B.

Whether there are significant differences in nephrotoxicity between the three lipid-based formulations remains unclear. In a recent meta-analysis of eight studies evaluating the nephrotoxicity of liposomal amphotericin B compared with amphotericin B lipid complex, nephrotoxicity was generally similar.[32] However, large prospective studies comparing the incidence of nephrotoxicity among liposomal formulations are needed to definitively ascertain differences in nephrotoxicity.

▶ *Radiocontrast Agents*

Radiocontrast agents are administered during radiologic studies and are associated with a well-documented risk of contrast-induced AKI (CI-AKI). Although definitions have been variable in the literature, CI-AKI is frequently defined as a rise in SCr of at least 0.5 mg/dL (44 μmol/L) or a 25% increase in Scr within 48 hours of contrast administration. Patients at risk for developing CI-AKI include patients with a GFR less than 60 mL/min (1.0 mL/s), diabetes, dehydration, age more than 65 years, concomitant nephrotoxic drug administration, and higher dose of contrast dye.[33] The risk increases as GFR decreases and patients with CKD and another comorbidity (eg, diabetes or dehydration) are at a significantly higher risk.

Contrast agents are water soluble, triiodinated, benzoic acid salts. The mechanism of nephrotoxicity is not fully understood; however, direct tubular toxicity, renal ischemia, and tubular obstruction have been implicated.[34] Diatrizoate and metrizoate are ionic, high osmolar contrast agents. Iohexol, iopamidol, ioversol, and iopromide are nonionic, low osmolar agents. The incidence of nephrotoxicity with ionic and nonionic agents is similar in patients at low risk for developing AKI; however, in high-risk patients, nephrotoxicity is significantly greater when high ionic, high osmolar contrast agents are used. The cost of nonionic agents is approximately 10-fold higher, which may limit their routine use to high risk patients.

Therapeutic measures to decrease the incidence of CI-AKI include extracellular volume expansion, limiting the amount of contrast administered, and use of nonionic contrast agents. Treatment with oral acetylcysteine has produced mixed results. Theophylline, fenoldopam, loop diuretics, mannitol, dopamine, and calcium antagonists have no effect or may worsen AKI. The antioxidant ascorbic acid has produced variable results and is not likely to have a beneficial effect.[35]

The most effective therapeutic maneuver to decrease the incidence of CI-AKI is extracellular volume expansion.[36] Either isotonic sodium chloride or sodium bicarbonate may attenuate the intrarenal and direct tubulotoxic effects, and dilute the contrast agent in the kidney tubules. Sodium bicarbonate may have the added benefit of alkalinizing renal tubule fluid, which is thought to reduce the formation of oxygen-free radicals. There is no standard dosage regimen for either fluid. A common regimen is IV isotonic sodium chloride (1 mL/kg of body weight/hour) administered for 12 hours before and 12 hours after the procedure. Urine output of more than 150 mL/hour has been associated with a reduced incidence of AKI.[37] Sodium bicarbonate at a rate of 3 mL/kg/hour (154 mEq/L [154 mmol/L]) for 1 hour before the procedure, and 1 mL/kg/hour for 6 hours postcontrast has been administered.[38] Although some studies comparing sodium chloride to sodium bicarbonate have demonstrated a lower incidence of CI-AKI with sodium bicarbonate,[39] others have not.[40] The recommendation of the KDIGO Clinical Practice Guidelines workgroup is that either agent can be selected until more consistent benefits are realized.[2] Fluid should be administered cautiously to patients with CHF, left ventricular dysfunction, and significant renal dysfunction.

Because production of reactive oxygen species has been implicated in the pathophysiology of CI-AKI, prophylactic administration of the antioxidant acetylcysteine has been investigated. A plethora of studies evaluating the efficacy of oral acetylcysteine have been conducted with mixed results; 7 of 11 meta-analyses indicates a benefit of acetylcysteine in CI-AKI.[41] The studies were varied in terms of study population, sample size, definition of contrast nephropathy, type of contrast agent used, hydration, and formulation and dosage of acetylcysteine administered, thus making collective interpretation of the results difficult. Acetylcysteine is routinely used in many hospitals due to its low cost and safe side-effect profile at low oral doses, although data are not conclusive that it prevents development of AKI or alters patient outcomes such as mortality, need for dialysis, and length of hospitalization.

Doses of acetylcysteine in clinical studies ranged from 600 to 1200 mg orally every 12 hours for 2 days, with the first one or two doses administered prior to the contrast procedure. The KDIGO Clinical Practice Guidelines suggest that oral acetylcysteine can be used in combination with IV fluids in patients at risk for CI-AKI.[5(2)] It is not considered a replacement for adequate hydration, which remains the standard of care for prevention of CI-AKI.

▶ *Cyclosporine and Tacrolimus*

The calcineurin inhibitors cyclosporine and tacrolimus are administered as part of immunosuppressive regimens in kidney, liver, heart, lung, and bone marrow transplant recipients. They are also used in autoimmune disorders such as psoriasis and multiple sclerosis. The pathophysiologic mechanism for AKI is renal vascular vasoconstriction.[42] It often occurs within the first 6 to 12 months of treatment and can be reversible with dose reduction or drug discontinuation. Risk factors include high dose, elevated trough blood concentrations, increased age, and concomitant therapy with other nephrotoxic drugs.[42] Cyclosporine and tacrolimus are extensively metabolized by the liver through the cytochrome P450 3A4 pathway; drugs that inhibit their metabolism (eg, erythromycin, clarithromycin, fluconazole, ketoconazole, verapamil, diltiazem, nicardipine) can increase plasma concentrations of cyclosporine and tacrolimus and precipitate AKI.

Because AKI is dose dependent, careful monitoring of cyclosporine or tacrolimus trough concentrations can minimize its occurrence; however, AKI can still occur with normal or low blood concentrations. In addition, there is some evidence that calcium channel blockers have a renoprotective effect through dilation of the afferent arterioles and are often used preferentially as antihypertensive agents in kidney transplant recipients. However, the dosage of calcineurin inhibitors would need to be reduced to avoid high plasma concentrations.

It is often difficult to differentiate AKI from acute rejection in the kidney transplant recipient because both conditions may present with similar symptoms and physical examination findings. However, fever and graft tenderness are more likely to occur with rejection, whereas neurotoxicity is more likely to occur with cyclosporine or tacrolimus toxicity. Kidney biopsy is often needed to confirm the diagnosis of rejection.

▸ *ACE Inhibitors and ARBs*

In instances of decreased renal blood flow (eg, kidney disease, renal artery stenosis), production of angiotensin II increases, resulting in efferent arteriole vasoconstriction and maintenance of glomerular capillary pressure and GFR. ACE inhibitors and ARBs decrease angiotensin II synthesis, thereby dilating efferent arterioles and decreasing glomerular capillary pressure and GFR.[30]

When initiating therapy with an ACE inhibitor or ARB, a modest increase in SCr should be anticipated within the first week of starting therapy.[32(30)] However, large increases (greater than 30% increase in SCr above baseline) that do not plateau after several weeks of therapy suggest AKI, and the drug should be discontinued.[30] Risk factors for developing AKI are preexisting renal dysfunction, severe atherosclerotic renal artery stenosis, volume depletion, and severe CHF. Discontinuation of the drug usually results in the return of renal function to baseline. Initiating therapy with low doses of a short-acting agent such as captopril is recommended for patients at risk of developing AKI. If tolerated, patients can later be converted to a longer-acting agent.

▸ *Nonsteroidal Anti-Inflammatory Drugs*

NSAIDs (eg, ibuprofen, naproxen, sulindac) can cause prerenal AKI through inhibition of prostaglandin-mediated renal vasodilation. Risk factors are similar to those of ACE inhibitors and ARBs. Additional risk factors include hepatic disease with ascites, systemic lupus erythematosus, and advanced age. Concurrent use of NSAIDS in patients on diuretics and ACE inhibitors or ARBs result in an increased risk of AKI, particularly within the first 30 days of coadministration.[43]

The onset of AKI is often within days of initiating therapy, and patients typically present with oliguria. It is usually reversible with drug discontinuation. Agents that preferentially inhibit cyclooxygenase-2 pose a similar risk as traditional nonselective NSAIDs.[30]

▸ *Other Drugs*

Other drugs commonly implicated in causing AKI include acyclovir, adefovir, carboplatin, cidofovir, cisplatin, foscarnet, ganciclovir, indinavir, methotrexate, pentamidine, ritonavir, sulfinpyrazone, and tenofovir.[44]

Patient Encounter, Part 3

The patient is admitted to the hospital for treatment of AKI. Based on the information available, create a care plan for this patient's AKI and provide overall recommendations for her drug therapy. The plan should include (a) a statement of the drug related needs and/or problems, (b) a patient-specific detailed therapeutic plan, and (c) monitoring parameters to assess efficacy and safety.

OUTCOME EVALUATION

Goals of therapy are to maintain a state of euvolemia with good urine output (at least 1 mL/kg/hour), to return SCr to baseline, and to correct electrolyte and acid-base abnormalities. In addition, appropriate drug dosages based on kidney function and avoidance of nephrotoxic drugs are goals of therapy. Assess vital signs, weight, fluid intake, urine output, BUN, creatinine, and electrolytes daily in unstable patients.

DRUG DOSING CONSIDERATIONS IN AKI

The most accurate reflection of overall kidney function is GFR. Defined as the volume of plasma filtered across the glomerulus per unit time, GFR correlates with the excretory, endocrine and metabolic functions of the kidney. **Creatinine clearance** (CrCl) is routinely used as an estimate of GFR in patients with normal kidney function or with CKD for purposes of drug dosing; however, equations to estimate CrCl (eg, Cockcroft and Gault) and GFR (eg, Modification of Diet in Renal Disease [MDRD]) are not accurate or reliable in AKI, particularly in critically ill patients.[45] They tend to overestimate CrCl and GFR when kidney function is worsening.[46] Use of Cockcroft–Gault equation should be limited to instances when SCr is at steady state, with no more than a 10 to 15% change in SCr within 24 hours.

In instances where kidney function is fluctuating, several equations (Jelliffe, Brater, Chiou) have been developed to assess unstable kidney function. These equations estimate CrCl by considering the change in SCr over a specified time period (Table 25–2, Jelliffe equation.)[47] Although they are more mathematically difficult to calculate, they take into consideration a change in SCr compared with an equation that only includes a single creatinine concentration. It should be noted that these methods have not been validated, and drug dosage adjustments based on CrCl estimates from these formulas in patients with AKI have not been evaluated.

Determining the optimal dose of drugs in AKI is challenging. A variety of factors influence drug dosing, such as (1) alterations in drug pharmacokinetics that occur during AKI, (2) difficulties in accurately quantifying kidney function in AKI, (3) the influence of intermittent or continuous RRT on drug clearance, and (4) challenges in interpreting information from the literature and applying it to a specific patient. Table 25–3 provides a more complete list of different considerations when dosing medications in patients with AKI.

For drugs with a narrow therapeutic window, serum drug concentration monitoring may be available to guide drug dosing. If therapeutic drug monitoring is not available, dosing based on an estimated CrCl is recommended, with frequent reassessment of kidney function and evaluation of the patient's status to assess efficacy and adverse effects of therapy. Selection of a drug with hepatic elimination rather than renal excretion is a reasonable alternative, if possible.

In critically ill septic patients, interpatient variability in pharmacokinetics renders dosing of antibiotics difficult. Underdosing a critically ill patient may be a greater risk than potential adverse effects attributed to higher plasma concentrations, particularly with antibiotics such as β-lactams, quinolones, and carbepenems, where therapeutic drug monitoring is not available.[48] Thus, the risk of undertreatment of the infection needs to be balanced with the risk of adverse effects from the antibiotic.

Table 25–2

Jelliffe Equation for Changing Renal Function[47]

Males	
E^{ss} = IBW ([29.3 – 0.203 [age]])	E^{SS} = steady-state creatinine excretion
$E^{ss} = E^{ss}$ (1.035 – 0.0337 [SCr])	Δt = time in days between measurement of SCr_1 and SCr_2
$E^{corr} = E^{SS}_{corr} - \frac{(4 \times IBW \times [SCr_2 - SCr_1])}{\Delta t}$	IBW = ideal body weight, kg
CrCl (mL/min/1.73 m^2) = E/([14.4][SCr])	Age, years
Females	
E^{ss} = IBW ([25.1 – 0.175 [(age)])	E^{SS}_{corr} = corrected steady-state creatinine excretion
$E^{ss} = E^{ss}$(1.035 – 0.0337 [SCr])	SCr_1 = first serum creatinine concentration
$E^{corr} = E^{SS}_{corr} - \frac{(4 \times IBW \times [SCr_2 - SCr_1])}{\Delta t}$	SCr_2 = second serum creatinine concentration
CrCl (mL/min/1.73 m^2) = E/([14.4][SCr])	E = creatinine excretion

CrCl, creatinine clearance. For conversion of mg/dL to μmol/L creatinine multiply by 88.4.

DRUG DOSING CONSIDERATIONS IN DIALYSIS

Dialysis membranes are classified as low flux or high flux. Low flux membranes are typically made from cellulose or cuprophane and have a relatively small pore size, whereas high flux membranes, made of synthetic substances such as polysulfone and polyamide, have a pore size that is considerably larger. Pore size of the dialysis membrane governs drug removal. For low flux membranes, drugs with a molecular weight less than 1000 Da are removed. With high flux membranes that have larger pore sizes, drugs in the range of 10,000 to 20,000 Da can be removed by diffusion of the molecules from the blood and into the dialysis solution. With hemofiltration, larger molecules are removed up to the molecular weight cutoff of the hemofilters, usually about 40,000 Da.

In additional to molecular weight, three additional characteristics of a drug govern removal during dialysis: percentage of drug eliminated by the kidney, volume of distribution, and protein binding. For example, removal during CRRT is greater when renal clearance accounts for 30% or more of total body clearance of the drug, volume of distribution is less than 1 L/kg, and protein binding is less than 50% because dialysis cannot remove protein-bound drugs.[49] Other factors that affect drug clearance include type of RRT (ie, IHD, CVVH, CVVHD); characteristics of the dialysis membrane; and blood, ultrafiltrate, and dialysis flow rates. In general, drug removal is greatest with CVVHDF, followed by CVVH and then IHD.[50]

Drug information references provide drug dosing recommendations in IHD and CRRT; however, they must be interpreted cautiously due to the variability in dialysis techniques used.

Table 25–3

Drug Dosing Considerations in AKI

Alteration in drug pharmacokinetics	• Increase in volume of distribution due to fluid retention may occur. • Reduction in excretion of both drugs and metabolites eliminated by the kidney. • Nonrenal clearance of some drugs may be reduced.
Difficulty in quantifying an accurate assessment of kidney function in AKI	• Cockcroft-Gault and MDRD equations are not meant for AKI population; equations are based on a single SCr. • SCr as a marker for kidney function is influenced by nonrenal factors (such as nutritional status and liver function). • Equations to estimate kidney function in cases of changing kidney function have not been well studied.
AKI patients undergoing dialysis	• Different types of dialysis modalities results in differences in drug removal (eg, IHD vs. CRRT). • Differences in intensity of dialysis dose may affect drug removal (eg, length of dialysis treatment, blood and dialysate flow rate). • Populations studied in the literature are likely to be different than the specific patient being treated (eg, different types of dialysis, length of treatment).
Textbook dosing and literature recommendations	• Studies in patients with AKI are sparse. • Many drug information recommendations on dosing are based on the manufacturer's original pharmacokinetics information, often in patients with chronic kidney disease. • Most drug dosing guidelines were developed prior to standardization of SCr measurements between laboratory tests; thus today's SCr measurements are 5% to 10% higher than those reported prior to 2010.[49] • There is growing support for incorporation of the MDRD equation in future pharmacokinetic studies and to guide drug dosing, although use of this equation is limited to chronic kidney disease.

MDRD, Modification of Diet in Renal Disease equation; SCr, serum creatinine.

The Patient Care Process

Patient Assessment

- Assess kidney function by evaluating a patient's signs and symptoms, laboratory test results, and urinary indices.
- Obtain a thorough and accurate drug history including the use of nonprescription drugs such as NSAIDs.

Therapy Evaluation

- Determine if drug therapy may be contributing to AKI. Consider not only drugs that can directly cause AKI (eg, aminoglycosides, amphotericin B, NSAIDs, cyclosporine, tacrolimus, ACE inhibitors, and ARBs) but also drugs that can predispose a patient to nephrotoxicity or prerenal AKI (ie, diuretics and antihypertensive agents).
- Determine if any drugs need to be discontinued, or alternative drugs selected, to prevent worsening of kidney function.
- Determine if any drugs undergo significant kidney elimination or if drugs require specific monitoring in patients with kidney disease.

Care Plan Development

- Adjust drug dosages based on estimated kidney function or evidence of adverse drug reactions or interactions.
- Provide supportive therapy, including adequate nutrition, correction of electrolyte and acid–base abnormalities (particularly hyperkalemia and metabolic acidosis), fluid management, and correction of any hematologic abnormalities.
- Implement preventative strategies to decrease the risk of AKI, such as administration of saline with contrast dye

Follow-Up Evaluation

- Monitor the patient's weight, urine output, electrolytes (such as potassium), and blood pressure to assess efficacy of the diuretic regimen.
- Monitor SCr to evaluate whether kidney function is worsening or improving.

Abbreviations Introduced In This Chapter

ACE	Angiotensin-converting enzyme
AKI	Acute kidney injury
AKIN	Acute Kidney Injury Network
ARB	Angiotensin receptor blocker
ARF	Acute renal failure
ATN	Acute tubular necrosis
BUN	Blood urea nitrogen
CHF	Congestive heart failure
CI-AKI	Contrast-induced acute kidney injury
CKD	Chronic kidney disease
CrCl	Creatinine clearance
CRRT	Continuous renal replacement therapy
CVVH	Continuous venovenous hemofiltration
CVVHD	Continuous venovenous hemodialysis
CVVHDF	Continuous venovenous hemodiafiltration
FENa	Fractional excretion of sodium
GFR	Glomerular filtration rate
IHD	Intermittent hemodialysis
KDIGO	Kidney Disease: Improving Global Outcomes
JVD	Jugular venous distention
LDD	Low-dose dopamine
MDRD	Modification of Diet in Renal Disease
NSAIDs	Nonsteroidal anti-inflammatory drugs
RIFLE	Risk, Injury, Failure, Loss, End stage
RRT	Renal replacement therapy
SCr	Serum creatinine

REFERENCES

1. Bellomo R, Kellum JA, Ronco C. Defining and classifying acute renal failure: from advocacy to consensus and validation of the RIFLE criteria. Intensive Care Med. 2007;33:409–413.
2. Acute Kidney Injury Work Group. KDIGO Clinical Practice Guideline for Acute Kidney Injury. Kidney Int. 2012;2:1–138.
3. Yong K, Dogra G, Boudville N, Pinder M, Lim W. Acute kidney injury: Controversies revisited. Int J Nephrol. 2011:762634.
4. Goldberg R, Dennen P. Long-term outcomes of acute kidney injury. Adv Chronic Kidney Dis. 2008;15:297–307.
5. Ympa YP, Sakr Y, Reinhart K, et al. Has mortality from acute renal failure decreased? A systematic review of the literature. Am J Med. 2005;118:827–832.
6. Himmelfarb J, Joannidis M, Molitoris B, et al. Evaluation and initial management of acute kidney injury. Clin J Am Soc Nephrol. 2008;3:962–967.
7. Lameire N, van Biesen W, Vanholder R. Acute renal failure. Lancet 2005;365:417–430.
8. Kellum JA. Acute kidney injury. Crit Care Med. 2008;36: S141–S145.
9. Mehta RL, Kellum JA, Shah SV, et al. Acute Kidney Injury Network: Report of an initiative to improve outcomes in acute kidney injury. Crit Care. 2007;11:R31.
10. Singbartl K, Kellum JA. AKI in the ICU: Definition, epidemiology, risk stratification, and outcomes. Kidney Int. 2012;81:819–825.
11. Joannidis M, Metnitz B, Bauer P, et al. Acute kidney injury in critically ill patients classified by AKIN versus RIFLE using the SAPS 3 database. Intensive Care Med. 2009;35:1692–1702.
12. Thomas ME, Blaine C, Dawnay A, et al. The definition of acute kidney injury and its use in practice. Kidney Int. 2015;87:62–73.
13. Bellomo R, Kellum JA, Ronco C. Defining acute renal failure: Physiologic principles. Intensive Care Med. 2004;30:33–37.
14. Finfer S, Bellomo R, Boyce N, et al. A comparison of albumin and saline for fluid resuscitation in the intensive care unit. N Engl J Med. 2004;350:2247–2256.
15. De Backer D, Biston P, Devriendt J, et al. Comparison of dopamine and norepinephrine in the treatment of shock. N Engl J Med. 2010;362:779–789.
16. Bagshaw SM, Bellomo R, Kellum JA. Oliguria, volume overload, and loop diuretics. Crit Care Med. 2008;36:S172–S178.
17. Bellomo R, Kellum JA, Ronco C. Acute kidney injury. Lancet. 2012:380:756–766.
18. Wulf NR, Matuszewski KA. Sulfonamide cross-reactivity: Is there evidence to support broad cross-allergenicity? Am J Health-Syst Pharm. 2013:70:1483–1494.
19. Brater DC. Update in diuretic therapy: Clinical pharmacology. Semin Nephrol. 2011;31:483–494.
20. Wargo KA, Banta WM. A comprehensive review of the loop diuretics: Should furosemide be first line? Ann Pharmacother. 2009;43: 1836–1847.
21. Asare K. Management of loop diuretic resistance in the intensive care unit. Am J Health Syst Pharm. 2009;66:1635–1640.

22. Bellomo R, Chapman M, Finfer S, et al. Low-dose dopamine in patients with early renal dysfunction: A placebo-controlled randomized trial. Australian and New Zealand Intensive Care Society (ANZICS) Clinical Trials Group. Lancet. 2000;356: 2139–2143.
23. Friedrich JO, Adhikari N, Herridge MS, et al. Meta-analysis: Low-dose dopamine increases urine output but does not prevent renal dysfunction or death. Ann Intern Med. 2005;142:510–524.
24. Gibney N, Burdmann EA, Bunchman T, et al. Timing of initiation and discontinuation of renal replacement therapy in AKI: Unanswered key questions. Clin J Am Soc Nephrol. 2008; 3:876–880.
25. Bellomo R, Cass A, Cole L, et al. The RENAL Replacement Therapy Study Investigators. N Engl J Med. 2009;361:1627–1638.
26. Palevsky PM, Hongyuan J, O'Connor TZ, et al. The VA/NIH Acute Renal Failure Trial Network. N Engl J Med. 2008;359:7–20.
27. Pagkalis S, Mantadakis E, Mavros MN, Ammari C, Falagas ME. Pharmacological considerations for the proper clinical use of aminoglycosides. Drugs. 2011;71:2277–2294.
28. Lopez-Novoa JM, Quiros Y, Vicente L, Morales AI, Lopez-Hernandez J. New insights into the mechanism of aminoglycoside nephrotoxicity: An integrative point of view. Kidney Int. 2011: 79:33–45.
29. Sadfar A, Ma J, Saliba F, et al. Drug-induced nephrotoxicity caused by amphotericin B lipid complex and liposomal amphotericin B. Medicine. 2010;89:236–244.
30. Pannu N, Nadim M. An overview of drug-induced acute kidney injury. Crit Care Med. 2008;36:S216–S223.
31. Saliba F, Dupont B. Renal impairment and amphotericin B formulations in patients with invasive fungal infections. Med Mycol. 2008;46:97–112.
32. Moen MD, Lyseng-Williamson KA, Scott LJ. Liposomal amphotericin B: A review of its use as empirical therapy in febrile neutropenia and in the treatment of invasive fungal infections. Drugs. 2009;69:361–392.
33. Seeliger E, Sendeski M, Rihal CS, Persson PB. Contrast-induced kidney injury: mechanisms, risk factors, and prevention. Eur Heart J. 2012:33:2007–2015.
34. McCullough PA, Soman SS. Contrast-induced nephropathy. Crit Care Clin. 2005;21:261–280.
35. Boscheri A, Weinbrenner C, Botzek B, et al. Failure of ascorbic acid to prevent contrast-media induced nephropathy in patients with renal dysfunction. Clin Nephrol. 2007;68:279–286.
36. Solomon R, Werner C, Mann D, et al. Effects of saline, mannitol, and furosemide on acute decreases in renal function by radiocontrast agents. N Eng J Med. 1994;331:1416–1420.
37. Stevens MA, McCullough PA, Tobin KJ, et al. A prospective randomized trial of prevention measures in patients at high risk for contrast nephroapthy: Results of the P.R.I.N.C.E. Study. Prevention of Radiocontrast Induced Nephropathy Clinical Evaluation. J Am Coll Cardiol. 1999;33:403–411.
38. Maioli M, Toso A, Leoncini M, et al. Sodium bicarbonate versus saline for the prevention of contrast-induced nephropathy in patients with renal dysfunction undergoing coronary angiography or intervention. J Am Coll Cardiol. 2008;52:599–604.
39. Briguori C, Airoldi F, D'Andrea D, et al. Renal insufficiency following Contrast Media Administration Trial (REMEDIAL). A randomized comparison of three preventative strategies. Circulation. 2007;115:1211–1217.
40. Brar SS, Shen AY, Jorgensen MB, et al. Sodium bicarbonate vs sodium chloride for the prevention of contrast medium-induced nephropathy in patients undergoing coronary angiography. JAMA. 2008;300:1038–1046.
41. Fishbane S. N-acetylcysteine in the prevention of contast-induced nephropathy. Clin J Am Soc Nephrol. 2008;3:281–287.
42. De Mattos AM, Olyaei AJ, Bennett WM. Nephrotoxicity of immuno-suppressive drugs: Long-term consequences and challenges for the future. Am J Kidney Dis. 2000;35:333–346.
43. Lapi F, Azoulay L, Yin H, et al. Concurrent use of diuretics, angiotensive converting enzyme inhibitors, and angiotensive receptor blockers with non-steroidal anti-inflammatory drugs and risk of acute kidney injury: Nested case-control study. BMJ. 2013;346:e8525.
44. Izzedine H, Launay-Vacher V, Deray G. Antiviral drug-induced nephropathy. Am J Kidney Dis. 2005;45:804–817.
45. Bragadottir G, Redfors B, Ricksten SE. Assessing glomerular filtration rate (GFR) in critically ill patients with acute kidney injury—true GFR versus urinary creatinine clearance and estimating equations. Crit Care. 2013;17:R108.
46. Bouchard J, Macedo E, Soroko S, et al. Comparison of methods for estimating glomerular filtration rate in critically ill patients with acute kidney injury. Nephrol Dial Transplant. 2010;25:102–107.
47. Jelliffe R. Estimation of creatinine clearance in patients with unstable renal function, without a urine specimen. Am J Nephrol. 2002;22:320–324.
48. Blot S, Lipman J, Roberts DM, Roberts JA. The influence of acute kidney injury on antimicrobial dosing in critically ill patients: are dose reductions always necessary? Diagn Microbiol. Infect Dis 2014;79:77–84.
49. Susla GM. The impact of continuous renal replacement therapy on drug therapy. Clin Pharmacol Ther. 2009;86:562–565.
50. Pea F. Viale P, Pavan F, Furlanut M. Pharmacokinetic considerations for antimicrobial therapy in patients receiving replacement therapy. Clin Pharmacokinet. 2007;46:997–1038.

26 Chronic and End-Stage Renal Disease

Kristine S. Schonder

LEARNING OBJECTIVES

Upon completion of the chapter, the reader will be able to:

1. List the risk factors for development and progression of chronic kidney disease (CKD).
2. Explain the mechanisms associated with progression of CKD.
3. Outline the desired outcomes for treatment of CKD.
4. Develop a therapeutic approach to slow progression of CKD, including lifestyle modifications and pharmacologic therapies.
5. Identify specific consequences associated with CKD.
6. Design an appropriate therapeutic approach for specific consequences associated with CKD.
7. Recommend an appropriate monitoring plan to assess the effectiveness of pharmacotherapy for CKD and specific consequences.
8. Educate patients with CKD about the disease state, the specific consequences, lifestyle modifications, and pharmacologic therapies used for treatment of CKD.

INTRODUCTION

The kidney is made up of approximately 2 million **nephrons** that are responsible for filtering, reabsorbing, and excreting solutes and water. The kidney has three primary functions: excretory (excrete fluid, electrolytes, and solutes); metabolic (metabolize vitamin D and some drugs, such as insulin and some β-lactams); and endocrine (produce erythropoietin). As the number of functioning nephrons declines, the primary functions of the kidney that are affected include:

- Production and secretion of **erythropoietin**
- Activation of vitamin D
- Regulation of fluid and electrolyte balance
- Regulation of acid–base balance

Chronic kidney disease (CKD) is defined as abnormalities in the structure or function of the kidney, present for 3 months or more, with implications for health.[1] Markers of structural abnormalities include **albuminuria** (30 mg/24 hours or more or an albumin: **creatinine** ratio (ACR) of more than 30 mg/g [or 3.5 mg/mmol for female and 2.5 mg/mmol for male but varies between different guidelines and location]); hematuria or casts in urine sediment; electrolyte and other abnormalities caused by renal tubular disorders; abnormalities detected by histology or imaging; or history of kidney transplantation. Functional abnormalities are indicated by a decline in **glomerular filtration rate** (GFR) less than 60 mL/min/1.73m^2 (0.58 mL/s/m^2). Generally, CKD is a progressive decline in kidney function (number of functioning nephrons) that occurs over several months to years. A rapid decline in kidney function over days to weeks is known as acute kidney injury (AKI), which is discussed in Chapter 25.

Because the decline in kidney function in CKD is often irreversible, treatment of CKD is aimed at slowing the progression to end-stage kidney disease (ESKD).

EPIDEMIOLOGY AND ETIOLOGY

KEY CONCEPT *The Kidney Disease: Improving Global Outcomes (KDIGO) CKD Work Group developed a classification system for CKD.[1] The staging system defines the stages of CKD based on cause, GFR category and albumin category, as outlined in* ***Tables 26–1*** *and* ***26–2***. The previous classification system for CKD was developed by the National Kidney Foundation's Kidney Disease Outcomes Quality Initiative (KDOQI), which used only the GFR to determine the stage of CKD.[3] Most of the literature and guidelines refer to the KDOQI staging system. Table 26–1 correlates the KDIGO and KDOQI systems and both will be referred to throughout the chapter.

The United States Renal Data System (USRDS), using data from the National Health and Nutrition Examination Survey (NHANES), estimates the prevalence of CKD in the United States is 13.6%, corresponding to nearly 44 million people.[3] CKD is more common in people older than 60 years and African Americans. Diabetes increases the risk of developing CKD by more than 3-fold and hypertension increases the risk more than twice than those who do not have either disease.[3]

KEY CONCEPT *CKD is a progressive disease that eventually leads to ESKD.* The prevalence of ESKD has increased nearly 11-fold since 1980 to almost 634,000 people in 2012 with over 114,000 new cases of ESKD diagnosed in 2014.[3] The prevalence of ESKD is related to ethnicity, affecting 3.5 times more African Americans, 1.6 times more Native Americans, and 1.5 more Hispanics as whites.[3]

Table 26–1

GFR Categories in CKD

GFR Category	GFR (mL/min/1.73 m²)[1]	Terms	KDOQI Category[2]
G1	≥ 90	Normal or high (with kidney damage)	Stage 1
G2	60–89	Mildly decreased (with kidney damage)	Stage 2
G3a	45–59	Mildly to moderately decreased	Stage 3
G3b	30–44	Moderately to severely decreased	Stage 3
G4	15–29	Severely decreased	Stage 4
G5	< 15	Kidney failure	Stage 5 (ESRD, if requiring dialysis)

[1]Multiply by 0.00963 to convert to units of mL/s/m².

CKD, chronic kidney disease; GFR, glomerular filtration rate.

Adapted from Table 29–1 in Chapter 29: Chronic Kidney Disease. In Pharmacotherapy: A Pathophysiologic Approach, 9th Ed. 2014. McGraw-Hill.

Identifying risk factors for CKD is difficult because CKD progresses slowly and is often not diagnosed until late in the disease. Risk factors identified for CKD are classified into three categories (see Table 26–3):

- **Susceptibility factors** are associated with an increased risk of developing CKD but are not directly proven to cause CKD. These factors are generally not modifiable by pharmacologic therapy or lifestyle modifications.
- **Initiation factors** directly cause CKD. These factors are modifiable by pharmacologic therapy.
- **Progression factors** result in a faster decline in kidney function and cause worsening of CKD. These factors may also be modified by pharmacologic therapy or lifestyle modifications to slow the progression of CKD.

Susceptibility Factors

Susceptibility factors can be used to identify targets for CKD screening programs. For example, older patients, those with low kidney mass or birth weight, and those with a family history of kidney disease should be routinely screened for CKD. Minority and low socioeconomic communities may be targets for more widespread CKD screening programs. Other factors, such as hyperlipidemia, are not directly proven to cause CKD but can be modified by drug therapies.

▶ *Hyperlipidemia*

Patients with CKD have a higher prevalence of dyslipidemia compared with the general population. More than 81% of patients with a GFR less than 60 mL/min/1.73 m² (0.58 mL/s/m²) had hyperlipidemia.[3] The dyslipidemia in CKD is manifested primarily as elevated triglycerides and lipoprotein(a) levels, and decreased high-density lipoprotein cholesterol (HDL-C) levels. Total cholesterol and low-density lipoprotein cholesterol (LDL-C) levels generally remain within normal limits.[4] Kidney disease alters lipid metabolism, allowing lipoproteins to remain in circulation longer.[4] In contrast, patients with nephrotic syndrome, characterized by urine protein rates that exceed 3 g/24 hours, often have elevated total cholesterol and LDL-C. Nephrotic syndrome may be associated with increased hepatic lipid production and decreased LDL-receptor activity.[5] Dyslipidemia can promote kidney injury and subsequent progression of CKD. Endothelial dysfunction results from inflammation and monocyte activation, whereas deposition of lipids results in glomerulosclerosis and glomerular mesangium dysfunction.[4]

Initiation Factors

The three most common causes of CKD in the United States are diabetes mellitus (DM), hypertension, and glomerulonephritis. Together these account for more than 75% of CKD cases (37% for diabetes, 25% for hypertension, and 14% for glomerulonephritis).[3] These are discussed in further detail in the following sections. Other causes of CKD include polycystic kidney disease, Wegener granulomatosis, vascular diseases, human immunodeficiency virus (HIV) nephropathy, and AKI.

▶ *Diabetes*

DM is the most common cause of CKD, causing 37% of all ESKD, which is an increase from 15% in 1995.[3] The risk of developing diabetic kidney disease (DKD) associated with DM

Table 26–2

Albumin Categories in CKD

Category	AER (mg/24 hours)	ACR (Approximate Equivalent) (mg/mmol)[a]	ACR (Approximate Equivalent) (mg/g)	Terms
A1	< 30	< 3.4	< 30	Normal to mildly decreased
A2	30–300	3.4–34	30–300	Moderately increased
A3	> 300	> 34	> 300	Severely increased[b]

ACR, albumin-to-creatinine ratio; AER, albumin excretion rate; CKD, chronic kidney disease.

[a]Actual cutoffs vary between different guidelines and locations. Sex-specific cutoffs are often used with lower cutoffs for males compared with females.

[b]Including nephrotic syndrome (albumin excretion usually > 2200 mg/24 hours [ACR > 2200 mg/g; > 250 mg/mmol]).

Table 26–3

Risk Factors Associated with CKD

Susceptibility
• Advanced age
• Reduced kidney mass
• Low birth weight
• Racial/ethnic minority
• Family history of kidney disease
• Low income or education
• Systemic inflammation
• Dyslipidemia
Initiation
• Diabetes mellitus
• Hypertension
• Autoimmune disease
• Polycystic kidney disease
• Drug toxicity
• Urinary tract abnormalities (infections, obstruction, stones)
Progression
• Hyperglycemia: Poor blood glucose control (in patients with diabetes)
• Hypertension: Elevated blood pressure
• Proteinuria
• Tobacco smoking

is closely linked to hyperglycemia and is similar for both type 1 and type 2. The prevalence of albuminuria is 25% to 40% in patients with type 1 DM after 15 to 25 years[6] and 43% in patients with type 2 DM.[7]

► *Hypertension*

The second most common cause of CKD is hypertension.[3] It is more difficult to determine the true risk of developing CKD in patients with hypertension because the two are so closely linked, with CKD also being a cause of hypertension. The prevalence of hypertension is correlated with the degree of kidney dysfunction (decreased GFR) with 36% of patients with CKD Stage 1, 48% of patients with CKD Stage 2, and 85% of patients with CKD Stage 3 presenting with hypertension.[8] The risk of developing ESKD increases with the degree of hypertension and is linked to both systolic and diastolic blood pressure.[8]

► *Glomerulonephritis*

The term *glomerulonephritis* includes many specific diseases that can affect glomerular function. These include such diseases as IgA nephropathy and glomerulonephritis associated with systemic lupus erythematosus and streptococcal disease, among many others. The etiologic and pathophysiologic features of glomerular diseases vary with the specific disease, making it difficult to extrapolate the risk for progression of CKD in patients affected by glomerular diseases. Certain glomerular diseases are known to rapidly progress to ESKD; others progress more slowly or may be reversible.

Progression Factors

Progression factors can be used as predictors of CKD. The most important predictors of CKD include proteinuria, elevated blood pressure, hyperglycemia, and AKI. Tobacco smoking also plays a role in progression of CKD.

► *Proteinuria*

The presence of protein in the urine is a marker of glomerular dysfunction and some tubulointerstitial diseases. The degree of proteinuria correlates with the risk for progression of CKD.[9] The effects of proteinuria appear to be worse with milder stages of CKD. Compared with patients with no proteinuria, proteinuric patients with Stage 3 CKD are 15 times more likely to double serum creatinine; patients with Stage 4 CKD are 8 times more likely to double serum creatinine.[9] The mechanisms by which proteinuria potentiates CKD are discussed later. Albuminuria (greater than 30 mg albumin excreted per day) is also linked with vascular injury and increased cardiovascular mortality.[7]

► *Elevated Blood Pressure*

Systemic blood pressure correlates with glomerular pressure, and elevations in both systemic blood pressure and glomerular pressure contribute to glomerular damage. The rate of GFR decline is related to elevated systolic blood pressure and mean arterial pressure. The decline in GFR is estimated to be 14 mL/min/year (0.23 mL/s/year) in patients with diabetes with a sustained systolic blood pressure of 180 mm Hg. Conversely, the decline in GFR decreases to 2 mL/min/y (0.03 mL/s/year) with a systolic blood pressure of 135 mm Hg.[10]

► *Elevated Blood Glucose*

The reaction between glucose and protein in the blood produces advanced glycation end products (AGEs), which are metabolized in the proximal tubules. Hyperglycemia increases the synthesis of AGEs, which affects glomerular, tubular, and vascular function in the kidney. AGEs are known to affect podocyte activity, the epithelial cells responsible for filtering blood in the glomerulus, which contributes to proteinuria, and, in turn, damages tubules.[11]

► *Acute Kidney Injury*

Nephron damage that results from AKI increases the risk of developing CKD, even if renal function recovers.[12] The most predictive risk factor of whether patients will develop CKD is the severity of AKI. Severe AKI is associated with a 28-fold increased risk of developing CKD, but even mild AKI is associated with a 2-fold increased risk. Older age also increases the risk of developing CKD after AKI. The cause of AKI may also affect the risk of CKD.[12]

PATHOPHYSIOLOGY

A number of factors can cause initial damage to the kidney. The resulting sequelae, however, follow a common pathway that promotes progression of CKD and results in irreversible damage leading to ESKD (Figure 26–1).

Regardless of the initial cause of kidney damage, the result is a decrease in the number of functioning nephrons. The remaining nephrons hypertrophy to increase glomerular filtration and tubular function, both reabsorption and secretion, in an attempt to compensate for the loss of kidney function. Initially, these adaptive changes preserve many of the clinical parameters of kidney function, including creatinine and electrolyte excretion. However, as time progresses, angiotensin II is required to maintain the hyperfiltration state of the functioning nephrons. Angiotensin II is a potent vasoconstrictor of both the afferent and efferent arterioles but has a preferential effect to constrict the efferent arteriole, thereby increasing the pressure in the glomerular capillaries. Increased glomerular capillary pressure expands the pores in the glomerular basement membrane, altering the

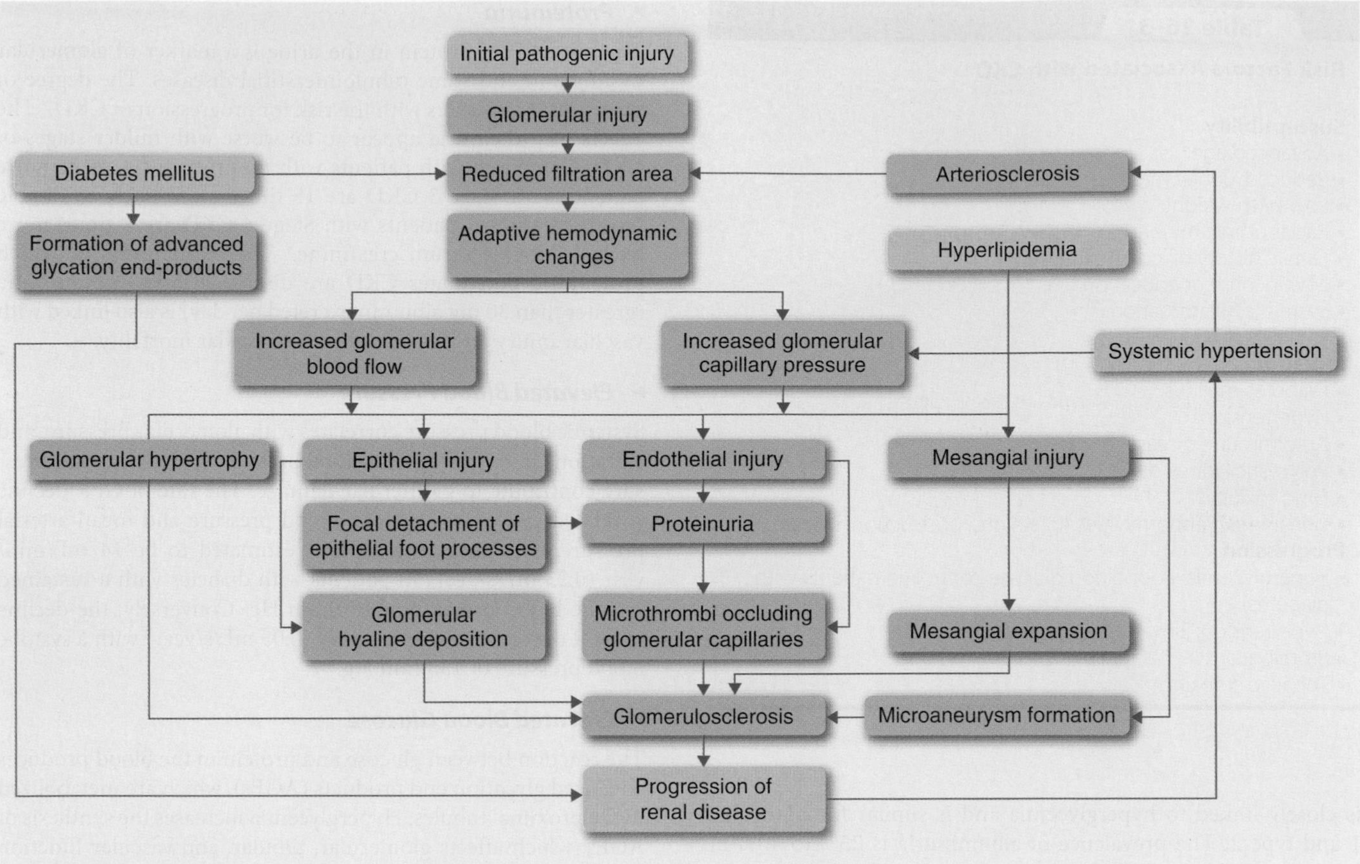

FIGURE 26–1. Proposed mechanisms for progression of kidney disease. (From Hudson JQ, Wazny LD. Chronic kidney disease. In: DiPiro JT, Talbert RL, Yee GC, et al., eds. Pharmacotherapy: A Pathophysiologic Approach, 9th ed. New York, NY: McGraw-Hill Education, 2014:636, with permission.)

size-selective barrier and allowing proteins to be filtered through the glomerulus.[13]

Proteinuria increases nephron loss through various complex mechanisms. Filtered proteins are reabsorbed in the renal tubules, which activates the tubular cells to produce inflammatory and vasoactive cytokines and triggers complement activation. These cytokines cause interstitial damage and scarring in the renal tubules, leading to damage and loss of more nephrons. Ultimately, the process leads to progressive loss of nephrons to the point where the number of remaining functioning nephrons is too small to maintain clinical stability, and kidney function declines.

ASSESSMENT

Because CKD often presents without symptoms, assessment for CKD relies on appropriate screening strategies in all patients with risk factors for developing CKD. Evaluation for CKD and the subsequent treatment strategies depend on the diagnosis, comorbid conditions, severity and complications of disease, and risk factors for the progression of CKD. KEY CONCEPT *Early treatment of CKD and the associated complications of CKD are the most important factors to decrease morbidity and mortality associated with CKD.* Screening for CKD should be performed in all people with an increased risk for developing CKD, including patients with DM, hypertension, genitourinary abnormalities, autoimmune disease, increased age, a family history of kidney disease, or following AKI. Assessment for CKD includes measurement of SCr, urinalysis, blood pressure, serum electrolytes, and/or imaging studies.

A key part of CKD assessment is analysis for proteinuria, which is the primary marker of structural kidney damage, even in patients with normal GFR. Protein excretion can be assessed by measuring urine albumin-to-creatinine ration (ACR), urine protein-to-creatinine ratio, or urinalysis with a reagent strip test.[3] A urinary protein excretion of 30 mg/day or more or an ACR or 30mg/g (or 3.5 mg/mmol for female and 2.5 mg/mmol for male but varies between different guidelines and locations) or more on a random untimed urine sample is considered to be significant in the context of CKD.[1] Albuminuria should be assessed with GFR at least annually in people with CKD. Assessment of protein excretion is particularly important in patients with DM, even without CKD. Screening for albumin excretion should be performed 5 years after the diagnosis of type 1 DM and at the time of diagnosis of type 2 DM.[14]

Complications

KEY CONCEPT *The decline in kidney function is associated with a number of complications, which are discussed later in the chapter, including:*

- *Hypertension*
- *Fluid and electrolyte disorders*
- *Anemia*
- *Metabolic bone disease*

TREATMENT

Desired Outcomes

The primary goal is to slow and prevent the progression of CKD to prevent a cardiovascular event, CKD complications and the need for kidney replacement therapy. This requires early identification of patients at risk for CKD to initiate interventions early in the course of the disease.

Nonpharmacologic Therapy

▶ *Nutritional Management*

Reduction in dietary protein intake has been shown to slow the progression of kidney disease.[15] Protein intake should be lowered to 0.8 g/kg/day in adults with diabetes or people with a GFR less than 30 ml/min/1.73 m^2 (0.29 mL/s/m^2) who are not on **dialysis**. Protein intake should not exceed 1.3 mg/kg/day in any adult with CKD.[1] However, protein restriction must be balanced with the risk of malnutrition in patients with CKD. In particular, patients on dialysis are at risk for nutritional abnormalities, which can lead to increased rates of hospitalization and death.[16] Malnutrition is common in patients with ESKD for various reasons, including decreased appetite, protein catabolism due to protein losses in the urine, and nutrient losses through dialysis. For this reason, patients receiving dialysis should maintain protein intake of 1.2 g/kg/day and maintain a caloric intake of 30 to 35 kcal/kg (125–147 kJ/kg) of ideal body weight.[16]

Limiting salt intake to less than 2 g (90 mmol) of sodium per day (equivalent to 5 g sodium chloride) will help to control blood pressure and reduce water retention in CKD. Patients with CKD should be encouraged to increase physical activity, with a goal of at least 30 minutes five times per week, to achieve a healthy weight, with a goal BMI of 20 to 25.[1]

Pharmacologic Therapy

▶ *CKD with Diabetes*

Figure 26–2 outlines the management of patients with CKD and DM. The target glycated hemoglobin level (HbA1c) should be less than 7.0% (0.07; 53 mmol/mol Hgb) for patients with DM to decrease the incidence of albuminuria in patients with and without documented DKD.[1,14] This generally involves intensive insulin therapy for type 1 DM or insulin-dependent type 2 DM or optimizing doses of oral hypoglycemic agents in patients with non-insulin-dependent type 2 DM. However, glycemic control should be balanced with the risk of hypoglycemia, especially in patients with CKD and DM with comorbidities.[1]

KEY CONCEPT *Angiotensin-converting enzyme inhibitors (ACEI) and angiotensin receptor blockers (ARBs) are the antihypertensive agents of choice in patients with CKD with an albumin excretion rate (AER) of 30 mg/day or more because of their greater effect on lowering proteinuria, compared with other antihypertensive agents.* ACEIs and ARBs should be started at a low dose and

Clinical Presentation and Diagnosis of CKD

General

The development of CKD is usually subtle in onset, often with no noticeable symptoms.

Symptoms

Stages 1 and 2 CKD are generally asymptomatic.

Stages 3 and 4 CKD may be associated with minimal symptoms.

Stage 5 CKD can be associated with pruritus, dysgeusia, nausea, vomiting, constipation, muscle pain, fatigue, and bleeding abnormalities.

Signs

Cardiovascular: Worsening hypertension, edema, dyslipidemia, left ventricular hypertrophy, electrocardiographic changes, and chronic heart failure.

Musculoskeletal: Cramping.

Neuropsychiatric: Depression, anxiety, impaired mental cognition.

Gastrointestinal (GI): Gastroesophageal reflux disease, GI bleeding, and abdominal distention.

Genitourinary: Changes in urine volume and consistency, "foaming" of urine (indicative of proteinuria), and sexual dysfunction.

Laboratory Tests

Stages 1 and 2 CKD: **Blood urea nitrogen** (BUN) and serum creatinine (SCr) are generally within normal limits, despite mildly decreased GFR.

Stages 3, 4, and 5 CKD: Increased BUN and SCr; decreased GFR.

Advanced stages: Increased potassium, phosphorus, and magnesium; decreased bicarbonate (metabolic acidosis); calcium levels are generally low in earlier stages of CKD and may be elevated in Stage 5 CKD, secondary to the use of calcium-containing phosphate binders.

Decreased albumin, if inadequate nutrition intake in advanced stages.

Decreased red blood cell (RBC) count, hemoglobin (Hgb), and hematocrit (Hct); Decreased iron stores (iron level, total iron binding capacity [TIBC], serum ferritin level, and transferrin saturation [TSat]). Erythropoietin levels are not routinely monitored and are generally normal to low. Urine positive for albumin or protein.

Increased parathyroid hormone (PTH) level; decreased vitamin D levels (Stages 4 or 5 CKD).

Stool may be Hemoccult-positive if GI bleeding occurs from uremia.

Other Diagnostic Tests

Structural abnormalities of kidney may be present on diagnostic examinations.

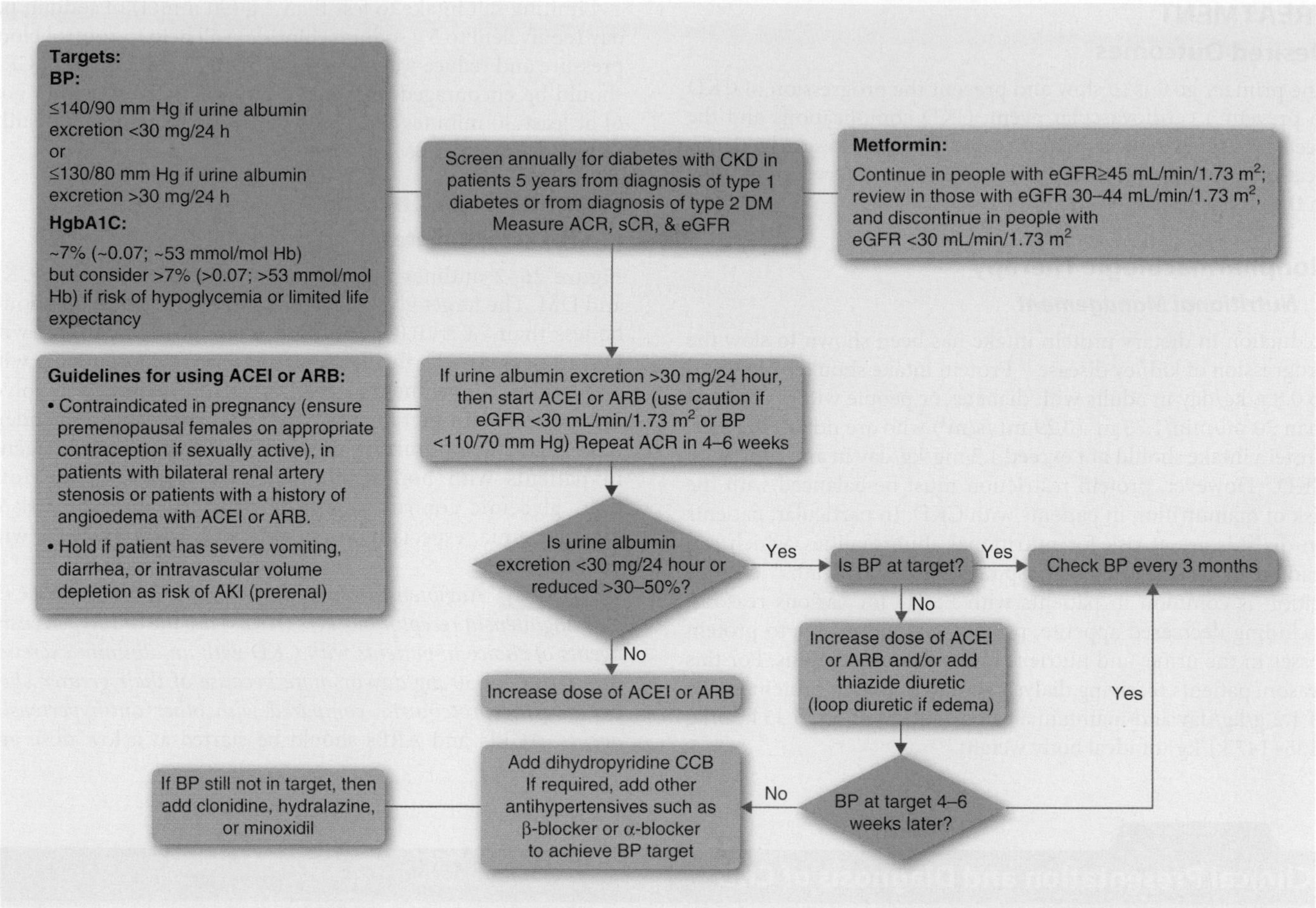

Targets:
BP:
≤140/90 mm Hg if urine albumin excretion <30 mg/24 h
or
≤130/80 mm Hg if urine albumin excretion >30 mg/24 h
HgbA1C:
~7% (~0.07; ~53 mmol/mol Hb) but consider >7% (>0.07; >53 mmol/mol Hb) if risk of hypoglycemia or limited life expectancy
Screen annually for diabetes with CKD in patients 5 years from diagnosis of type 1 diabetes or from diagnosis of type 2 DM Measure ACR, sCR, & eGFR
Metformin:
Continue in people with eGFR≥45 mL/min/1.73 m²; review in those with eGFR 30–44 mL/min/1.73 m², and discontinue in people with eGFR <30 mL/min/1.73 m²
Guidelines for using ACEI or ARB:
• Contraindicated in pregnancy (ensure premenopausal females on appropriate contraception if sexually active), in patients with bilateral renal artery stenosis or patients with a history of angioedema with ACEI or ARB.
• Hold if patient has severe vomiting, diarrhea, or intravascular volume depletion as risk of AKI (prerenal)
If urine albumin excretion >30 mg/24 hour, then start ACEI or ARB (use caution if eGFR <30 mL/min/1.73 m² or BP <110/70 mm Hg) Repeat ACR in 4–6 weeks
Is urine albumin excretion <30 mg/24 hour or reduced >30–50%?
Yes
Is BP at target?
Yes
Check BP every 3 months
No
Increase dose of ACEI or ARB and/or add thiazide diuretic (loop diuretic if edema)
Yes
No
Increase dose of ACEI or ARB
BP at target 4–6 weeks later?
No
Add dihydropyridine CCB If required, add other antihypertensives such as β-blocker or α-blocker to achieve BP target
If BP still not in target, then add clonidine, hydralazine, or minoxidil

FIGURE 26–2. Algorithm for management of CKD with DM. Management is based on urine albumin excretion, target blood pressure, and GFR. (ACE-I, angiotensin-converting enzyme inhibitor; ACR, albumin-to-creatinine ratio; ARB, angiotensin receptor blocker; BP, blood pressure; CCB, calcium channel blocker; eGFR, estimated glomerular filtration rate; HgbA$_{1C}$, hemogloblin A$_{1C}$; sCR, serum creatinine.) (From Hudson JQ, Wazny LD. Chronic kidney disease. In: DiPiro JT, Talbert RL, Yee GC, et al., eds. Pharmacotherapy: A Pathophysiologic Approach, 9th ed. New York, NY: McGraw-Hill Education, 2014:642, with permission.)

the dose should be titrated upward slowly to minimize the risk of AKI (see Chapter 25). Ideally, the dose of ACEIs and ARBs should be increased to achieve a 30% to 50% reduction in urinary albumin excretion, but this may be limited by side effects, such as hyperkalemia, in patients with CKD.

► *Optimal Blood Pressure Control*

Reductions in blood pressure are associated with a decrease in proteinuria, leading to a decrease in the rate of progression of kidney disease. Figure 26–3 outlines the management of blood pressure in patients with CKD. Blood pressure goals for patients with CKD are dependent on the degree of urinary albumin excretion. The KDIGO guidelines recommend that patients with CKD who have an AER less than 30 mg/day should achieve a blood pressure target of less than or equal to 140/90 mm Hg. If AER is 30 mg/day or greater, the blood pressure goal is less than or equal to 130/80 mm Hg.[17] The first-line antihypertensive agents for patients with an AER of 30 mg/day or more are ACEIs or ARBs, because of their ability to also lower protein excretion.

In patients with Stage 5 CKD who are receiving hemodialysis, cardiovascular mortality is affected by blood pressure both before and after hemodialysis.[18] A systolic blood pressure greater than 160 mm Hg and diastolic blood pressure greater than 90 mm Hg after hemodialysis are independently associated with an increased risk of cardiovascular mortality (hazard ratio [HR]: 1.2 for each).[18] Similarly, a systolic blood pressure less than 120 mm Hg or diastolic blood pressure less than 60 mm Hg before hemodialysis is associated with a higher risk of cardiovascular mortality (HR: 1.1 and 1.3, respectively [p less than 0.05 for each]); the same systolic or diastolic blood pressure at the end of hemodialysis is associated with a comparable risk (HR 1.1 and 1.2, respectively [p less than 0.05 for each]).[18] However, there are no consensus guidelines on the optimal blood pressure goals before or after hemodialysis. Newer evidence suggests that blood pressure on nonhemodialysis days may be a more appropriate measure, and correlates better with cardiovascular outcomes.[19]

Because hypertension and kidney dysfunction are linked, blood pressure control can be more difficult to attain in patients with CKD compared with patients with normal kidney function. All antihypertensive agents have similar effects on reducing blood pressure. However, two or more agents are generally required to achieve the blood pressure goal of less than 140/90 mm Hg or 130/80 mm Hg in CKD patients.[17] Timing of blood pressure medications may also be important. One study suggests

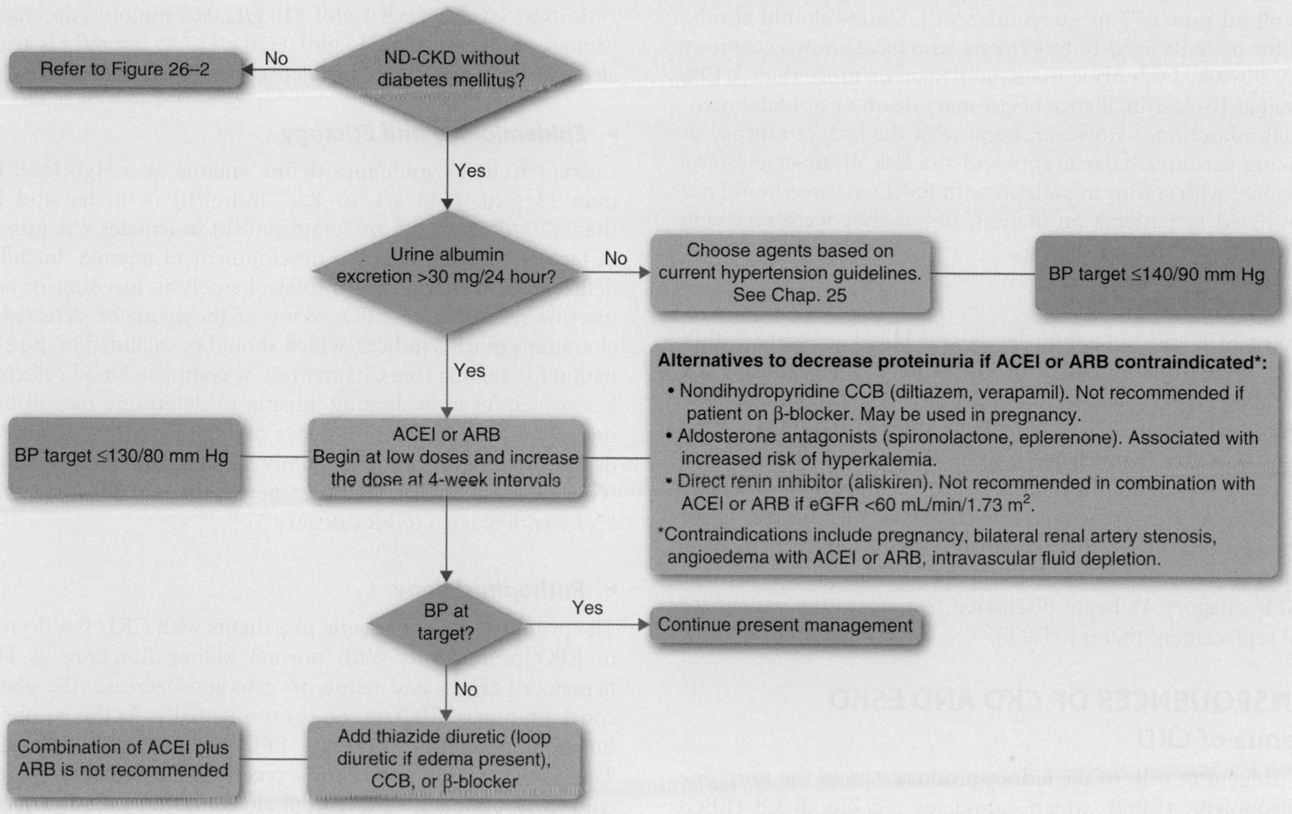

FIGURE 26–3. Algorithm for management of hypertension in CKD. Management is based on urine albumin excretion and target blood pressure. (ACE-I, angiotensin-converting enzyme inhibitor; ARB, angiotensin receptor blocker; BP, blood pressure; CCB, calcium channel blocker; eGFR, estimated glomerular filtration rate; ND-CKD, non-dialysis chronic kidney disease.) (From Hudson JQ, Wazny LD. Chronic kidney disease. In: DiPiro JT, Talbert RL, Yee GC, et al., eds. Pharmacotherapy: A Pathophysiologic Approach, 9th ed. New York, NY: McGraw-Hill Education, 2014:643, with permission.)

that administration of at least one antihypertensive medication at bedtime decreased cardiovascular risk by 14% in patients with CKD compared with taking all antihypertensive medications in the morning.[20]

▸ *Reduction in Proteinuria*

Reduction of proteinuria within the first year of therapy predicts long-term renal and cardiovascular prognosis.[21] The ability of antihypertensive agents to reduce protein excretion differs. ACEIs and ARBs decrease glomerular capillary pressure and volume because of their effects on angiotensin II. This, in turn, reduces the amount of protein filtered through the glomerulus, independent of the reduction in blood pressure,[21] which ultimately decreases the progression of CKD. The ability of ACEIs and ARBs to reduce proteinuria is greater than that of other antihypertensives, up to 35% to 40%,[21] making ACEIs and ARBs the antihypertensive agents of choice for all patients with CKD with an AER of 30 mg/day or more, unless contraindicated. Combining ACEIs and ARBs should be done with caution. Although it has been demonstrated that combination therapy leads to greater reductions in protein excretion,[22] this also leads to faster progression of CKD.[23]

The nondihydropyridine calcium channel blockers (CCBs) have been shown to also decrease protein excretion in patients with and without diabetes,[24] but the reduction in proteinuria appears to be related to the reductions in blood pressure. The maximal effect of nondihydropyridine CCBs on proteinuria is seen with a blood pressure reduction to less than 130/80 mm Hg, and no additional benefit is seen with increased doses. Dihydropyridine CCBs, however, do not have the same effects on protein excretion. In fact, dihydropyridine CCBs may worsen protein excretion, despite similar reductions in blood pressure as nondihydropyridine CCBs.[24]

▸ *Hyperlipidemia Treatment*

Hyperlipidemia plays a role in the development of cardiovascular disease (CVD) in patients with CKD. The primary goal of treatment of dyslipidemias is to decrease the risk of atherosclerotic CVD. A secondary goal in patients with CKD is to reduce proteinuria and decline in kidney function. Treatment of hyperlipidemia in patients with CKD has been demonstrated to increase GFR by 1 mL/min/year (0.016 mL/s/year) of treatment with antihyperlipidemic agents.[7]

Because data do not support the use of LDL-C levels to guide treatment of hyperlipidemia, the KDIGO guidelines recommend starting statins for all patients with non-dialysis-dependent CKD aged 50 years and older, regardless of GFR category.[25] Ezetimibe should be considered when GFR is less than 60 ml/min/1.73 m² (0.58 mL/s/m²). Statins should also be used for patients aged 18 to 49 years who have known coronary artery disease, DM, prior ischemic stroke, or more than a 10% estimated 10-year incidence of coronary death or nonfatal myocardial infarction.[25] However, because of the lack of efficacy in reducing cardiovascular events and the risk of adverse effects associated with statins in patients with ESKD, statins should not be initiated in patients on dialysis, unless they were receiving statins prior to starting dialysis.[25]

Outcome Evaluation

Monitor SCr and potassium levels and blood pressure within 1 week after initiating ACEI or ARB therapy. Discontinue the medication and switch to another agent if a sudden increase in SCr greater than 30% occurs, hyperkalemia develops, or the patient becomes hypotensive. Titrate the dose of the ACEI or ARB every 1 to 3 months to effect using the maximum tolerable dose. If blood pressure is not reduced to goal, add another agent to the regimen. Refer the patient to a nephrologist to manage complications associated with CKD. As CKD progresses to Stage 4 (GFR category 4), begin discussion to prepare the patient for renal replacement therapy (RRT).

CONSEQUENCES OF CKD AND ESKD

Anemia of CKD

The progenitor cells of the kidney produce 90% of the hormone erythropoietin (EPO), which stimulates red blood cell (RBC) production. KEY CONCEPT *Reduction in the number of functioning nephrons decreases renal production of EPO, which is the primary cause of anemia in patients with CKD. The development of anemia of CKD results in decreased oxygen delivery and utilization, leading to increased cardiac output and left ventricular hypertrophy (LVH), which increase the cardiovascular risk and mortality in patients with CKD.* Each 1 g/dL (10 g/L; 0.62 mmol/L) decrease in hemoglobin (Hgb) below 12 g/dL (120 g/L; 7.45 mmol/L) is associated with a 5% increase in the relative risk (RR) of mortality.[26]

▸ Epidemiology and Etiology

Current KDIGO guidelines define anemia as a Hgb level less than 13 g/dL (130 g/L or 8.07 mmol/L) in males and less than 12 g/dL (120 g/L or 7.45 mmol/L) in females.[27] A number of factors contribute to the development of anemia, including deficiencies in vitamin B_{12} or folate, hemolysis, bleeding, or bone marrow resistance to EPO. Many of these can be detected by alterations in RBC indices, which should be included in the evaluation for anemia (see Chapter 66). A complete blood cell count is also helpful in evaluating anemia to determine overall bone marrow function. The prevalence of anemia correlates with the degree of kidney dysfunction. Only 8.4% of patients with Stage 1 (GFR category 1) have anemia, whereas the number increases to 53.4% with Stage 5 (GFR category 5).[28]

▸ Pathophysiology

The primary cause of anemia in patients with CKD is a decrease in EPO production. With normal kidney function, as Hgb, hematocrit (Hct), and tissue oxygenation decrease, the plasma concentration of EPO increases exponentially. As the number of functioning nephrons decrease, EPO production also decreases. Thus, as Hgb, Hct, and tissue oxygenation decrease in patients with CKD, plasma EPO levels remain constant within the normal range but low relative to the degree of hypoxia present. The result is a normochromic, normocytic anemia.

Several other factors contribute to the development of anemia in patients with CKD. Uremia, the accumulation of toxins that results from declining kidney function, decreases the lifespan of

Patient Encounter 1

A 52-year-old Caucasian man presents to the clinic for a routine checkup. He has no complaints today, but needs a refill for his insulin.

PMH: Diabetes mellitus, diagnosed 3 years ago; hypothyroidism; hypertension

SH: He is unemployed; he smokes 2 ppd; stopped drinking alcohol 5 years ago after a bout of pancreatitis; reports a remote history of marijuana use in the past in his 20s

Meds: Insulin glargine 30 units SC daily; levothyroxine 75 mcg orally daily; omeprazole 20 mg orally twice daily; metoprolol succinate 25 mg orally daily

ROS: Unremarkable

PE:

VS: BP 152/99 mm Hg, P 85 beats/min, T 98.8°F (37.1°C), Ht 6′ (183 cm), Wt 167 lb (75.8 kg)

CV: RRR, normal S_1, S_2; no murmurs, rubs or gallops; lungs clear

Abd: No organomegaly, bruits or tenderness, (+) bowel sounds; heme (−) stool

Exts: Trace pedal edema bilaterally; decreased sensation in feet to light touch; no lesions

Labs (Fasting): Sodium 141 mEq/L (141 mmol/L); potassium 4.0 mEq/L (4.0 mmol/L); chloride 99 mEq/L (99 mmol/L); carbon dioxide 26 mEq/L (26 mmol/L); blood urea nitrogen (BUN) 26 mg/dL (9.3 mmol/L); serum creatinine (SCr) 1.6 mg/dL (141 μmol/L); glucose 148 mg/dL (8.2 mmol/L); total cholesterol 254 mg/dL (6.57 mmol/L); low-density lipoprotein cholesterol (LDL-C) 164 mg/dL (4.24 mmol/L); high-density lipoprotein cholesterol (HDL-C) 30 mg/dL (0.78 mmol/L); triglycerides 300 mg/dL (3.39 mmol/L); $hemoglobin_{A1c}$ (Hb_{A1c}) 8.4% (0.084; 68 mmol/mol Hgb); urine albumin: creatinine 45 mg/g creatinine (5.1 mg/mmol creatinine)

What risk factors does the patient have for the development of CKD?

What signs and symptoms are consistent with CKD?

How would you classify his CKD?

What lifestyle modifications would you recommend for this patient with CKD?

What pharmacologic alternatives are available for this patient for treatment of CKD?

Clinical Presentation and Diagnosis of Anemia of CKD

General

Anemia of CKD generally presents with fatigue and decreased quality of life.

Symptoms

Anemia of CKD is associated with symptoms of cold intolerance, shortness of breath, and decreased exercise capacity.

Signs

Cardiovascular: Left ventricular hypertrophy, ECG changes, congestive heart failure.

Neurologic: Impaired mental cognition.

Genitourinary: Sexual dysfunction.

Laboratory Tests

Decreased RBC count, Hgb, and Hct.

Decreased serum iron level, TSat and serum ferritin, and increased TIBC.

RBCs from a normal of 120 days to as low as 60 days in patients with Stage 5 CKD. Iron deficiency and blood loss from regular laboratory testing and hemodialysis also contribute to the development of anemia in patients with CKD.

▶ *Treatment*

Patients with CKD should be evaluated for anemia when the GFR falls below 60 mL/min (1.0 mL/s) or if the SCr rises above 2 mg/dL (177 μmol/L). An anemia workup should be performed if the Hgb is less than 13 g/dL (130 g/L or 8.07 mmol/L) in males or less than 12 g/dL (120 g/L or 7.45 mmol/L) in females. The workup for anemia should rule out other potential causes for anemia (see Chapter 66). Abnormalities found during the anemia workup should be corrected before initiating erythropoiesis-stimulating agents (ESAs), particularly iron deficiency, because iron is an essential component of RBC production. If Hgb is below 10 g/dL (100 g/L or 6.21 mmol/L) when all other causes of anemia have been corrected, EPO deficiency should be assumed. EPO levels are not routinely measured and have little clinical significance in monitoring progression and treatment of anemia in patients with CKD.

Nonpharmacologic Therapy Approximately 1 to 2 mg of iron is absorbed daily from the diet. This small amount is generally not adequate to preserve adequate iron stores to promote RBC production in patients with CKD-related anemia. RBC transfusions have been used in the past as the primary means to maintain Hgb and Hct levels in patients with anemia of CKD. This treatment is still utilized today in patients with severe anemia or contraindications to ESAs, but it is considered a third-line therapy for chronic anemia of CKD.

Pharmacologic Therapy The first-line treatment for anemia of CKD involves replacement of iron stores with iron supplements. When iron supplementation alone is not sufficient to increase Hgb levels, ESAs are necessary to replace erythropoietin. ESAs are synthetic formulations of EPO produced by recombinant human DNA technology. Use of ESAs increases the iron demand for RBC production and iron deficiency is common, requiring iron supplementation to correct and maintain adequate iron stores to promote RBC production. The approach to the management of anemia of CKD with iron supplementation and ESAs is illustrated in Figure 26–4.

Iron Supplementation. Use of ESAs can lead to iron deficiency if iron stores are not adequately maintained. Iron supplementation should be considered when:

- Serum ferritin levels greater than 500 ng/mL (500 mcg/L; 1124 pmol/L)
- Transferrin saturation (TSat): greater than 30% (0.30).[27]

Serum ferritin is an acute phase reactant that may become elevated with inflammation and infection. Thus when serum ferritin

Patient Encounter 2, Part 1

A 42-year-old Caucasian woman with a history of lupus nephritis presents to your clinic for a routine checkup. She complains of getting fatigued easily at work. She works as a secretary at a busy law office and notes that she is not able to keep up with her work. She notes that she feels winded when she walks even short distances.

PMH: systemic lupus erythematosus; seizure disorder

Current Meds: Lisinopril 20 mg orally daily; furosemide 20 mg orally daily; levetiracetam 250 mg orally twice daily

ROS: Skin pale in color; fatigue daily throughout the day with minimal exertion; otherwise unremarkable

PE:

VS: BP 97/62 mm Hg, P 94 beats/min, T 97.5°F (36.4°C), Ht 5′ (152 cm), Wt 110 lb (49.9 kg)

CV: RRR, normal S_1, S_2

Abd: No organomegaly, bruits or tenderness; (+) bowel sounds; heme (–) stool

Ext: 2+ pedal edema bilaterally

Labs: Sodium 136 mEq/L (136 mmol/L); potassium 3.9 mEq/L (3.9 mmol/L); chloride 104 mEq/L (104 mmol/L); carbon dioxide 23 mEq/L (23 mmol/L); BUN 34 mg/dL (12.1 mmol/L); SCr 3 mg/dL (265 μmol/L); glucose 70 mg/dL (3.9 mmol/L); white blood cell (WBC) count 5.3×10^3 cells/mm^3 (5.3×10^9/L); red blood cell (RBC) count 3.1×10^6 cells/mm^3 (3.1×10^{12}/L); hemoglobin (Hgb) 9.1 g/dL (91 g/L; 5.65 mmol/L); hematocrit 27% (0.27); platelets 428×10^3 cells/mm^3 (428×10^9/L)

What signs and symptoms are consistent with anemia of CKD?

What additional information could you request to determine other causes of anemia in this patient?

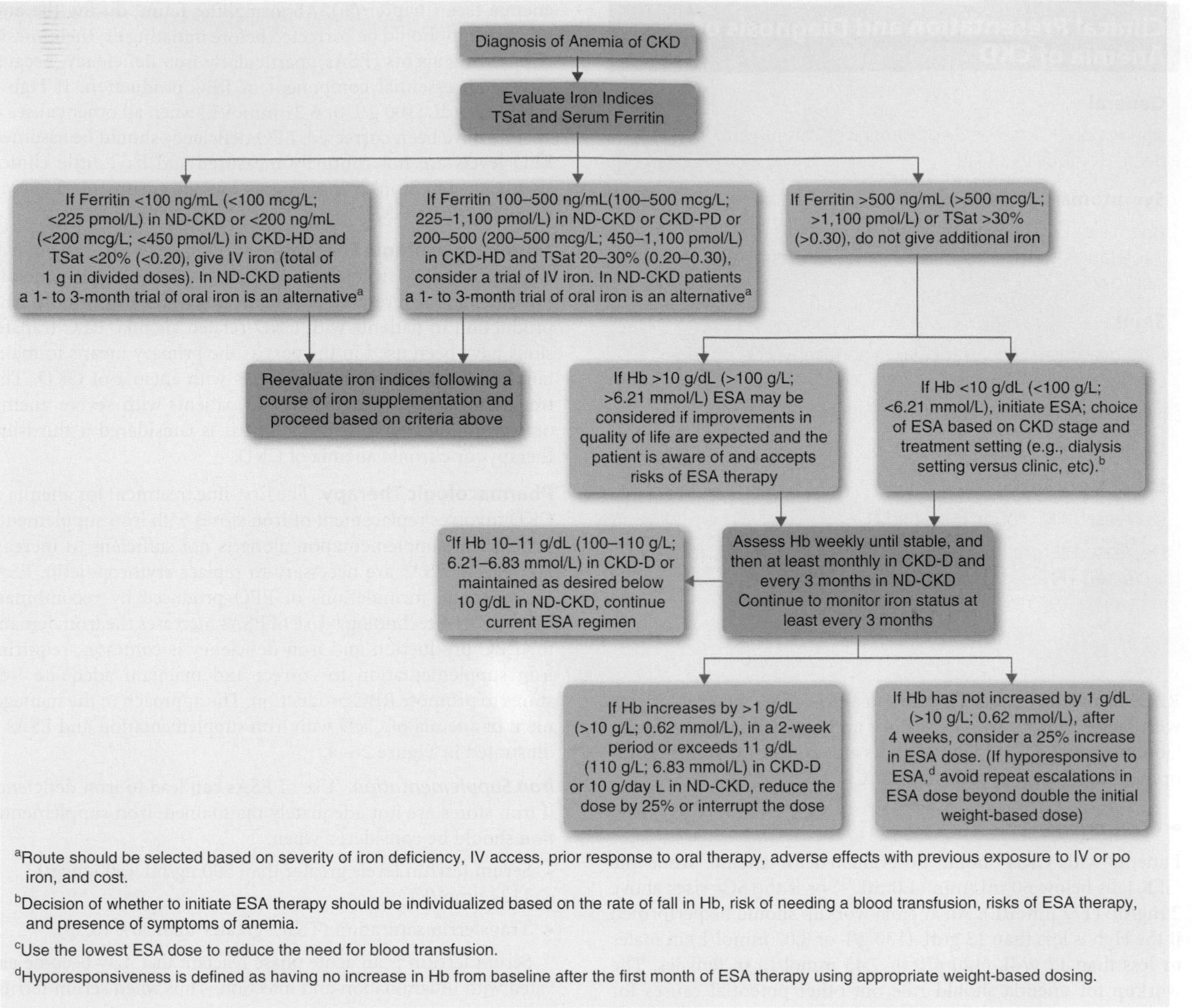

FIGURE 26–4. Algorithm for management of anemia of CKD. (CKD-HD, chronic kidney disease receiving hemodialysis; ESA, erythropoiesis-stimulating agent; Hgb, hemoglobin; ND-CKD, chronic kidney disease not receiving dialysis; SC, subcutaneous; TSat, transferrin saturation.) (From Hudson JQ, Wazny LD. Chronic kidney disease. In: DiPiro JT, Talbert RL, Yee GC, et al., eds. Pharmacotherapy: A Pathophysiologic Approach, 9th ed. New York, NY: McGraw-Hill Education, 2014:651, with permission.)

is normal or elevated in conjunction with TSat levels less than 30% (0.30), treatment should be based on the clinical picture of the patient. Iron supplementation may be indicated if Hgb levels are below the goal level, but avoided if the patient is infected.

Oral iron supplements are generally less costly than IV supplements and are generally the first-line treatment for iron supplementation for patients with CKD not receiving hemodialysis. When administering iron by the oral route, 200 mg of elemental iron should be delivered daily in divided doses to increase or maintain adequate iron stores.[27]

When oral iron is not effective to increase iron stores or for patients receiving hemodialysis, IV iron should be administered. Table 26–4 lists the FDA-approved doses of the currently available IV iron products. Patients receiving hemodialysis have ongoing blood losses with each hemodialysis session, which can lead to iron losses of 1 to 2 g/year. For hemodialysis, IV iron may be administered episodically based on routine surveillance of iron stores as a total of 1 g of IV iron, administered in small sequential doses to replete iron stores. An alternative method to administer IV iron is to give smaller maintenance doses of iron weekly or with each dialysis session (eg, iron dextran or iron sucrose 20 to 100 mg/week; sodium ferric gluconate 62.5 to 125 mg/week). The latter approach of giving smaller maintenance doses may result in lower cumulative doses of iron and lower doses of ESAs.[27] Ferric carboxymaltose is a new IV iron replacement product approved for two doses separated by 7 days of 750 mg each for patients weighing at least 50 kg or 15 mg/kg/dose for patients under 50 kg.

IV iron preparations are equally effective in increasing iron stores. Anaphylaxis may occur with all IV preparations, but most notably with iron dextran, which can also cause delayed reactions, such as arthralgias and myalgias. A test dose of 25-mg

Table 26–4

IV Iron Products

Iron Formulation (Product)	FDA-Approved Indications	FDA-Approved Dosing	Warnings	Dose Ranges[a]	How Supplied
Iron dextran (INFeD, Dexferrum)	Patients with iron deficiency in whom oral iron is unsatisfactory	IV push: 100 mg over 2 minutes (25 mg test dose required)	Black box (risk of anaphylactic reactions)	25–1000 mg	2-mL vials containing 50-mg elemental iron per mL
Ferric gluconate (Ferrlecit, Sodium ferric gluconate)	Adult and pediatric HD patients ≥ 6 years of age receiving ESA therapy	IV push (adult): 125 mg over 10 minutes IV infusion (adult): 125 mg in 100 mL of 0.9% NaCl over 60 minutes IV infusion (pediatric): 1.5 mg/kg in 25 mL of 0.9% NaCl over 60 minutes; maximum dose 125 mg	General	6.25–1000 mg	5-mL ampules containing 62.5-mg elemental iron (12.5 mg/mL)
Iron sucrose (Venofer)	HD patients with CKD receiving ESA therapy	IV push: 100 mg over 2–5 minutes IV infusion: 100 mg in maximum of 100 mL of 0.9% NaCl over 15 minutes	General	25–1000 mg	5-mL single-dose vials containing 100-mg elemental iron (20 mg/mL)
	Non-dialysis-CKD patients receiving or not receiving ESA therapy	IV push: 200 mg over 2–5 minutes on five different occasions within 14-day period			
	PD patients receiving ESA therapy	IV infusion: 2 infusions 14 days apart, of 300 mg in maximum of 250 mL of 0.9% NaCl over 1.5 hour, followed by 1 infusion 14 days later, of 400 mg in maximum of 250 mL of 0.9% NaCl over 2.5 hours			
Ferumoxytol (Feraheme)	Adults with iron-deficiency anemia associated with CKD	IV: 510 mg (17 mL) as a single dose, followed by a second 510-mg dose 3–8 days after the initial dose (rate of 1 mL or 30 mg/s)	General	1020 mg (two doses of 510 mg separated by 3–8 days)	17-mL vials containing 510 mg (30 mg/mL)
Ferric carboxymaltose (Injectafer)	Adults with non-dialysis dependent CKD	IV push: 750 mg over 10 minutes IV infusion: 750 mg in 100–250 mL of 0.9% NaCl over at least 15 minutes	General	1500 mg (two doses of 750 mg separated by at least 7 days)	15-mL vials containing 750-mg elemental iron

CKD, chronic kidney disease; ESA, erythropoietin-stimulating agent; HD, hemodialysis; PD, peritoneal dialysis.

[a]Small dosing ranges (eg, 25–100 mg/week) generally used for maintenance regimens. Larger doses (eg, 1 g) should be administered in divided doses.

iron dextran should be administered 30 minutes before the full dose to monitor for potential anaphylactic reactions, although anaphylactic reactions can occur in patients who safely received prior doses of iron dextran. A test dose is not require for the newer iron preparations, sodium ferric gluconate, iron sucrose, ferumoxytol, and ferric carboxymaltose because they are associated with fewer severe reactions and a much lower risk of anaphylaxis, making them the first-line agents in CKD. The most common side effects seen with these preparations include hypotension, flushing, nausea, and injection site reactions.

After administering a 1 g course of IV iron, iron status should be monitored to determine the effectiveness of the treatment. Serum ferritin and TSat should be monitored no sooner than 1 week after the last dose of IV iron. If Hgb does not increase after a course of IV iron or serum ferritin is not greater than 500 ng/mL (500 mcg/L; 1124 pmol/L) and TSat greater than 30% (0.30), an additional 1 g of IV iron may be administered, based on the clinical situation.

Erythropoiesis-Stimulating Agents. ESAs may be considered if Hgb levels remain persistently low to improve symptoms of anemia. In patients not receiving dialysis, the decision to initiate ESAs should be based on the rate of Hgb decline, prior response to anemia treatment, risks associated with ESAs and the patient's symptoms. The KDIGO guidelines recommend considering initiating ESAs when Hgb is less than 10 g/dL (100 g/L or 6.21 mmol/L).[27]

However, the target for Hgb is unclear because use of ESAs to increase Hgb levels beyond 12 g/dL (120 g/L or 7.45 mmol/L) is associated with increased mortality.[29,30] The ESAs currently available in the United States are as follows:

- Epoetin alfa (distributed as Epogen and Procrit)
- Darbepoetin alfa (Aranesp)

Epoetin α and epoetin β, which is available outside the United States, have the same biological activity as endogenous EPO. Darbepoetin alfa differs from epoetin alfa by the addition of carbohydrate side chains that increase the half-life of darbepoetin alfa compared with epoetin alfa and endogenous EPO, allowing for less frequent dosing than that of epoetin alfa. All ESAs are equivalent in their efficacy and have a similar adverse-effect profile.

The most common adverse effect seen with ESAs is increased blood pressure, which may require antihypertensive agents to control blood pressure. Caution should be used when initiating an ESA in patients with very high blood pressures (greater than 180/100 mm Hg). If blood pressures are refractory to antihypertensive agents, ESAs may need to be withheld. Seizures and pure red cell aplasia have also been reported in patients initiating ESA therapy.

Subcutaneous (SC) administration of ESA produces a more predictable and sustained response than IV administration, and it is therefore the preferred route of administration for both agents. IV administration is often utilized in patients who have established IV access or are receiving hemodialysis. Starting doses of ESAs depend on the Hgb level, the target Hgb level, the rate of Hgb increase, and clinical circumstances.[27] The initial increase in Hgb should be 1 to 2 g/dL (10–20 g/L or 0.62–1.24 mmol/L) per month. The recommended starting dose of epoetin alfa is 50 to 100 units/kg/dose administered SC or IV two to three times weekly; the starting dose of darbepoetin alfa is 0.45 mcg/kg administered SC or IV once weekly (Table 26–5).

When prescribing ESAs, clinicians should not attempt to target "normal" Hgb levels (ie, greater than 13 g/dL [130 g/L or 8.07 mmol/L] in males; greater than 12 g/dL [120 g/L or 7.45 mmol/L] in females). Several clinical trials have demonstrated that targeting Hgb levels greater than 13 g/dL (130 g/L or 8.07 mmol/L) resulted in more cardiovascular complications or death, compared with target Hgb levels less than 11 g/dL (110 g/L or 6.83 mmol/L), with little or no benefit on the quality of life.[29,30] Although not completely understood, the increased mortality is postulated to result from increased blood viscosity, which can trigger platelet activity, and hemoconcentration, which occurs when large amounts of fluid are removed during hemodialysis.[30] A third mechanism may relate to relative unphysiological concentrations of EPO that are achieved with intermittent dosing of ESAs, which may promote inflammation or thrombosis.[30]

Further studies are needed to evaluate the appropriate target level for Hgb. Nonetheless, based on these findings, the US FDA recommended addition of a black box warning to the product information for all ESAs indicating the maximum target Hgb should not exceed 11 g/dL (110 g/L or 6.83 mmol/L) and requires a medication guide be given to patients who are receiving ESAs.

▶ *Outcome Evaluation*

Evaluate Hgb monthly when ESA therapy is initiated or the dose is adjusted to ensure Hgb does not exceed 11.5 g/dL (115 g/L or 7.14 mmol/L).[27] The ESA dose can increase monthly if Hgb is below goal. Once a stable Hgb is attained, evaluate Hgb every 3 months thereafter. While the patient is receiving ESA therapy, monitor iron stores at least every 3 months or more frequently when initiating or increasing the dose of ESAs, when monitoring response to a course of IV therapy, or when blood loss or other circumstances that may lead to depletion of iron stores occur.[28] When the goal Hgb is reached, monitor iron stores every 3 months. Serum ferritin and TSat should be monitored no sooner than 1 week after the last dose of IV iron is administered.

CKD-Mineral and Bone Disorder and Secondary Hyperparathyroidism

▶ *Epidemiology and Etiology*

Increases in parathyroid hormone (PTH) occur early as kidney function begins to decline. The actions of PTH on bone turnover lead to CKD-mineral and bone disorders (CKD-MBD). The majority of patients with GFR categories 3–5 have CKD-MBD.[31] The type of bone disease can vary based on the degree of bone turnover. High bone turnover, known as osteitis fibrosa cystica, is generally mediated by high levels of PTH. Adynamic bone disease, characterized by low bone turnover, is now the most common form of bone disease, which may be related to excessive

Table 26–5

Estimated Starting Doses of Darbepoetin Alfa Based on Previous Epoetin Alfa Dose

Previous Epoetin Alfa Dose (units/week)	Weekly Darbepoetin Alfa Dose (mcg/week)
Less than 2500	6.25
2500–4999	12.5
5000–10,999	25
11,000–17,999	40
18,000 33,999	60
34,000–59,999	100
60,000–89,999	150
90,000 or more	200

Patient Encounter 2, Part 2

The patient returns to your clinic in 1 week and states that her symptoms have not changed. She is asking about the results of her laboratory studies.

Labs: WBC 5.9 × 10^3 cells/mm^3 (5.9 × 10^9/L); RBC 2.9 × 10^6 cells/mm^3 (2.9 × 10^{12}/L); Hgb 8.9 g/dL (89 g/L; 5.52 mmol/L); hematocrit 26% (0.26); mean corpuscular volume (MCV) 84 fL; mean corpuscular hemoglobin concentration (MCHC) 29 g/dL (290 g/L); platelets 415 × 10^3 cells/mm^3 (415 × 10^9/L); iron 31 mcg/dL (5.5 μmol/L); total iron binding capacity (TIBC) 490 mcg/dL (87.7 μmol/L); ferritin 42 ng/mL (42 mcg/L; 94 pmol/L); transferrin saturation (TSat) 14% (0.14); stool guaiac negative × 3

What treatment would you recommend for this patient for treatment of anemia?

How would you evaluate the effectiveness of treatment of anemia?

suppression of PTH.[32] The development of CKD-MBD can dramatically affect morbidity in patients with CKD.

► Pathophysiology

As kidney function declines in patients with CKD, decreased phosphorus excretion disrupts the balance of calcium and phosphorus homeostasis. Decreased vitamin D activation in the kidney also decreases calcium absorption from the gastrointestinal (GI) tract. Fibroblast growth factor 23 (FGF-23) is a hormone produced by osteocytes and osteoblasts that is stimulated by increased phosphate and calcitriol. In CKD, elevated phosphate concentrations increase expression of FGF-23, which promotes phosphorus excretion and downregulates vitamin D activation in the kidney.[32] Each of these stimulates the parathyroid glands. KEY CONCEPT *The parathyroid glands release PTH in response to decreased serum calcium and increased serum phosphorus levels. The actions of PTH include the following:*

- Increasing calcium resorption from bone
- Increasing calcium reabsorption from the proximal tubules in the kidney
- Decreasing phosphorus reabsorption in the proximal tubules in the kidney
- Stimulating activation of vitamin D by 1-α-hydroxylase to calcitriol (1,25-dihydroxyvitmin D_3) to promote calcium absorption in the GI tract and increased calcium mobilization from bone

All these actions are directed at increasing serum calcium levels and decreasing serum phosphorus levels, although the activity of calcitriol also increases phosphorus absorption in the GI tract and mobilization from the bone, which can worsen hyperphosphatemia. Calcitriol also decreases PTH levels through a negative feedback loop. These measures are sufficient to correct serum calcium levels in the earlier stages of CKD.

As kidney function continues to decline and the GFR falls less than 30 mL/min/1.73 m² (0.29 mL/s/m²), phosphorus excretion continues to decrease and calcitriol production decreases,[32] causing PTH levels to begin to rise significantly, leading to **secondary hyperparathyroidism** (sHPT). The excessive production of PTH leads to hyperplasia of the parathyroid glands, which decreases the sensitivity of the parathyroid glands to serum calcium levels and calcitriol feedback, further promoting sHPT.

The most dramatic consequence of sHPT is alterations in bone turnover and the development of **renal osteodystrophy** (ROD). Other complications of CKD can also promote ROD. Metabolic acidosis decreases bone formation by reducing hydroxyapatite solubility, inhibiting osteoblast activity, stimulating osteoclast activity, and reducing the sensitivity of the parathyroid gland to serum calcium levels.[33] Excessive aluminum levels cause aluminum uptake into bone in place of calcium, weakening the bone structure. The pathogenesis of sHPT and CKD-MBD are depicted in Figure 26–5.

► Treatment

General Approach KEY CONCEPT Diagnosis and management of bone disease in CKD is based on corrected serum levels of calcium and phosphorus, and intact PTH levels (iPTH).[31] In general, calcium, phosphorus, and PTH levels should be maintained in the normal range for all stages of CKD. For patients receiving dialysis, it is often difficult to achieve normal serum levels for these parameters. Attempts should be made to

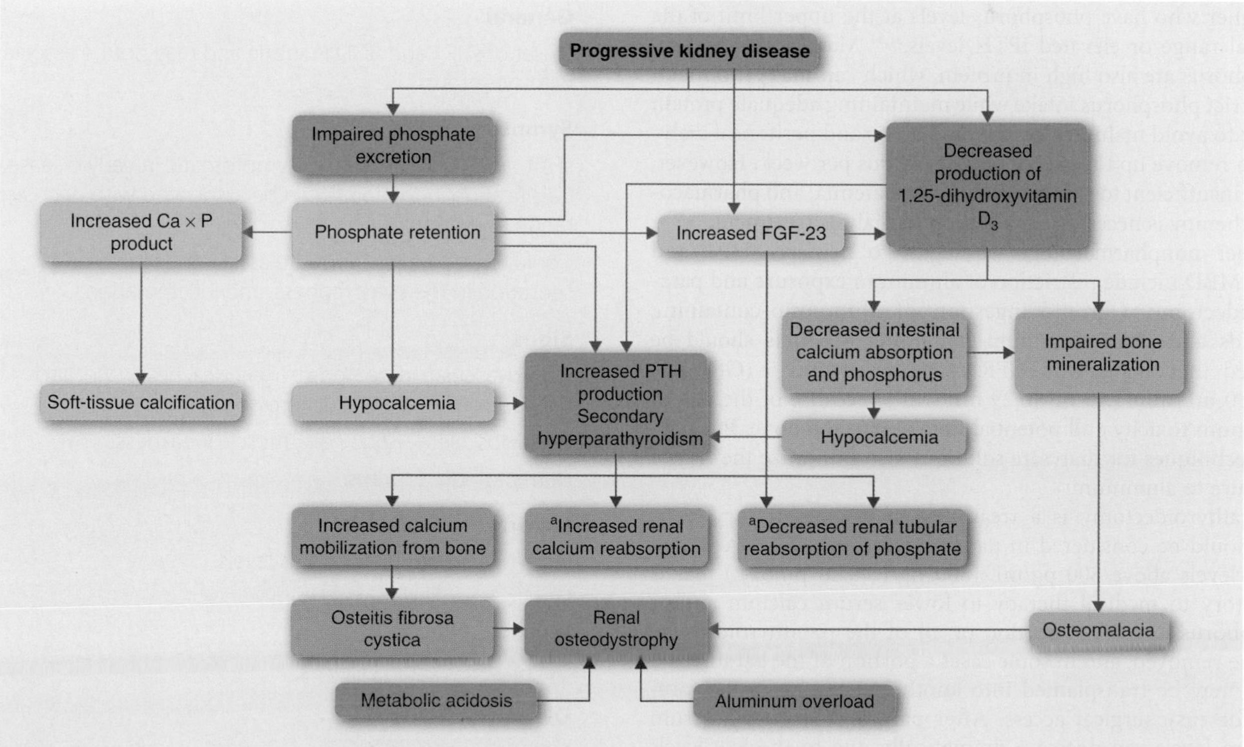

FIGURE 26–5. Pathogenesis of CKD-MBD and renal osteodystrophy.ªThese adaptations are lost as kidney failure progresses. (From Hudson JQ, Wazny LD. Chronic kidney disease. In: DiPiro JT, Talbert RL, Yee GC, et al., eds. Pharmacotherapy: A Pathophysiologic Approach, 9th ed. New York, NY: McGraw-Hill Education, 2014:638, with permission.)

Table 26–6

Target Levels for Calcium, Phosphorus, and Intact PTH

Parameter	GFR Categories 3a and 3b (Stage 3)	GFR Category 4 (Stage 4)	GFR Category 5 (Stage 5)
Corrected Calcium	"Normal range"	"Normal range"	8.4–9.5 mg/dL (2.10–2.38 mmol/L)[a,b]
Phosphorus	"Normal range"	"Normal range"	3.5–5 mg/dL (1.13–1.62 mmol/L)[a,b]
Intact PTH[a,c]	35–70 pg/mL[d] (3.7–7.5 pmol/L)	70–100 pg/mL (7.5–10.7 pmol/L)	150–300 pg/mL (16.0–32.1 pmol/L)

Ca–P, calcium–phosphorus product; GFR, glomerular filtration rate; PTH, parathyroid hormone.

[a]Based on KDOQI guidelines (Nigwekar SU, Bhan I, Thadhani R. Ergocalciferol and cholecalciferol in CKD. Am J Kidney Dis. 2011;60[1]:139–156).

[b] KDIGO guidelines recommend "normal range."

[c]KDIGO guidelines recommend two to nine times normal.

[d]Units of pg/mL are equivalent to ng/L.

maintain calcium and phosphorus levels as close to normal as possible, but levels slightly above the normal range are acceptable in most cases. Target ranges for the various parameters are listed in Table 26–6.

The primary target for treatment is control of serum phosphorus levels because this is the initial parameter that disrupts homeostasis. However, serum phosphorus can be difficult to control, particularly in the latter stages of CKD. Management of sHPT often requires supplemental treatment with vitamin D analogs or cinacalcet in addition to phosphorus management.

Nonpharmacologic Therapy The first-line treatment for the management of hyperphosphatemia is dietary phosphorus restriction to 800 to 1000 mg/day in patients with Stage 3 CKD or higher who have phosphorus levels at the upper limit of the normal range or elevated iPTH levels.[31,34] Many foods high in phosphorus are also high in protein, which can make it difficult to restrict phosphorus intake while maintaining adequate protein intake to avoid malnutrition. Hemodialysis and peritoneal dialysis can remove up to 2 to 3 g of phosphorus per week. However, this is insufficient to control hyperphosphatemia, and pharmacologic therapy is necessary in addition to dialysis treatment.

Other nonpharmacologic strategies to manage sHPT and CKD-MBD include restriction of aluminum exposure and parathyroidectomy. Chronic ingestion of aluminum-containing antacids and other aluminum-containing products should be avoided in patients with GFR categories 4 and 5 (GFR less than 30 mL/min/1.73 m^2 [0.29 mL/s/m^2]) because of the risk of aluminum toxicity and potential uptake into the bone. Purification techniques for dialysate solutions also minimize the risk of exposure to aluminum.

Parathyroidectomy is a treatment of last resort for sHPT, but should be considered in patients with persistently elevated iPTH levels above 800 pg/mL (800 ng/L; 85.6 pmol/L) that is refractory to medical therapy to lower serum calcium and/or phosphorus levels.[31] A portion or all of the parathyroid tissue may be removed, and in some cases a portion of the parathyroid tissue may be transplanted into another site, usually the forearm for easy surgical access. After parathyroidectomy, serum calcium levels can decrease dramatically due to the low levels of PTH after the parathyroid tissue is removed, which decreases intestinal calcium absorption and bone resorption. Therefore, serum ionized calcium levels should be monitored frequently (every 4–6 hours for the first 48–72 hours) in patients receiving a parathyroidectomy. Calcium supplementation is usually necessary, administered IV initially, then orally (with vitamin D supplementation) once normal calcium levels are attained for several weeks to months after the procedure.

Clinical Presentation and Diagnosis of sHPT and ROD

General

Onset of sHPT and ROD is subtle and may not be associated with symptoms.

Symptoms

sHPT and ROD are usually asymptomatic in early disease. Calcification in the joints can be associated with decreased range of motion.

Conjunctival calcifications are associated with a gritty sensation in the eyes, redness, and inflammation.

Signs

Cardiovascular: Increased stroke index, heart rate, and diastolic and mean arterial pressures.

Musculoskeletal: Bone pain, muscle weakness.

Dermatologic: Pruritus.

Laboratory Tests

Increased serum phosphorus levels.

Low to normal serum calcium levels.

Increased PTH levels.

Decreased vitamin D levels.

Diagnostic Tests

Radiographic studies show calcium–phosphate deposits in joints and/or cardiovascular system.
Bone biopsy of the iliac crest (not routinely performed).

Pharmacologic Therapy

Phosphate-Binding Agents. When serum phosphorus levels cannot be controlled by restriction of dietary intake, phosphate-binding agents are used to bind dietary phosphate in the GI tract to form an insoluble complex that is excreted in the feces. Phosphorus absorption is decreased, thereby decreasing serum phosphorus levels. The drugs used for binding dietary phosphate are listed in Table 26–7. These agents should be administered with each meal and can be tailored to the amount of phosphorus that is typically ingested during each meal. For example, patients can take a smaller dose with smaller meals or snacks, and a larger dose with larger meals. Although phosphate binders are not FDA approved for patients with CKD who are not receiving dialysis, they are used clinically when phosphorus levels are elevated, regardless of the GFR category.

Calcium-based phosphate binders, including calcium carbonate and calcium acetate, are effective in decreasing serum phosphate levels, as well as in increasing serum calcium levels. Calcium acetate binds more phosphorus than the carbonate salt, making it a more potent agent for binding dietary phosphate. Calcium citrate is usually not used as a phosphate-binding agent because the citrate salt can increase aluminum absorption. The calcium-containing phosphate binders also aid in the correction of metabolic acidosis, another complication of kidney failure. Calcium-based phosphate binders should not be used if serum calcium levels are near the upper end of the normal range or are elevated, if arterial calcifications are present, or if the patient has adynamic bone disease.[31] The dose of calcium-based phosphate binders should not provide more than 1500 mg of elemental calcium per day, and the total elemental calcium intake per day should not exceed 2000 mg, including medication and dietary intake.[34] The most common adverse effects of calcium-containing phosphate binders are constipation and hypercalcemia.

Aluminum- and magnesium-containing phosphate-binding agents are not recommended for chronic use in patients with CKD to avoid aluminum and magnesium accumulation. Aluminum-containing agents may be used for a short course of therapy (less than 4 weeks) if phosphorus levels are significantly elevated greater than 7 mg/dL (2.26 mmol/L), but should be replaced by other phosphate-binding agents after no more than 4 weeks. Excessive aluminum levels lead to aluminum intoxication, causing neurotoxicity that can manifest as encephalopathy or dementia, bone disease, and anemia. In addition to the risk of magnesium accumulation, the use of magnesium-containing agents is also limited by the GI side effects, primarily diarrhea.

Sevelamer, lanthanum, and iron-based phosphate binders do not contain calcium, magnesium, or aluminum. These agents are particularly useful in patients with hyperphosphatemia who have elevated serum calcium levels or who have vascular or soft tissue calcifications. Sevelamer is a cationic polymer that is not systemically absorbed and binds to phosphate in the GI tract, and it prevents absorption and promotes excretion of phosphate through the GI tract via the feces. Sevelamer has an added benefit of reducing LDL-C by up to 30% and increasing HDL-C levels.[34] The most common side effects of sevelamer are GI complaints, including nausea, constipation, and diarrhea. The cost of sevelamer is significantly higher compared with calcium-containing phosphate binders, which often makes sevelamer a second-line agent for controlling phosphorus levels. However, some studies demonstrate that sevelamer may decrease mortality in patients receiving hemodialysis compared with calcium-containing phosphate binders, primarily by decreasing the occurrence of calcifications in the coronary arteries.[31] Sevelamer may lower FGF-23 levels, which can negatively impact renal phosphate excretion.[35] Sevelamer carbonate may have added benefit to aid in the correction of metabolic acidosis.

Lanthanum is a naturally occurring trivalent rare earth element (atomic number 57). Lanthanum carbonate quickly dissociates in the acidic environment of the stomach, where the lanthanum ion binds to dietary phosphorus, forming an insoluble compound that is excreted in the feces. Lanthanum has been shown to be as effective as other phosphate binders and may improve bone turnover, compared with calcium-containing products.[31] Side effects of lanthanum include nausea, peripheral edema, and myalgias.

Sucroferric oxyhydroxide and ferric citrate are iron-based phosphate binders that lower phosphate levels. Sucroferric oxyhydroxide is an insoluble form of iron that binds to phosphate in the GI tract and has been shown to be as effective as other phosphate binders with a lower pill burden.[36] Ferric citrate also lowers phosphate as effectively as other phosphate binders and can also increase serum ferritin and TSAT levels.[36] The major side effects associated with both products are GI side effects, namely diarrhea. Sucroferric oxyhydroxide cannot be taken with levothyroxine and must be taken 1 hour after doxycycline and alendronate. This product was not studied in patients on peritoneal dialysis, with significant liver or GI disease, or following major GI surgery.[36]

Vitamin D Therapy. Vitamin D regulates many processes in the body, including calcium and phosphorus absorption from the GI tract and kidney, PTH secretion, maintaining muscle, cardiovascular, immune and brain function, and glucose control. Vitamin D is activated in various tissues, with the liver and kidney being primary sites. In CKD, a decrease in renal metabolism of vitamin D decreases circulating concentrations of the activated form of vitamin D, calcitriol (1,25-dihydroxyvitamin D) and its precursor 25-hydroxyvitamin D. Vitamin D deficiency becomes evident as early as Stage 2 (GFR category 2).[37] PTH levels rise as early as Stage 3 (GFR category 3) as a result of low calcitriol concentrations.

Exogenous vitamin D compounds that mimic the activity of calcitriol act directly on the parathyroid gland to decrease PTH secretion by upregulation of the vitamin D receptor in the parathyroid gland, which decreases parathyroid gland hyperplasia and PTH synthesis and secretion. This is particularly useful when reduction of serum phosphorus levels does not sufficiently reduce PTH levels.

Vitamin D supplementation (Table 26–8) can be used to lower serum PTH levels in patients with CKD. Ergocalciferol and cholecalciferol have been shown to be effective in lowering PTH secretion in patients with Stage 3 CKD[31] and are useful in later stages of CKD to maintain adequate 25-hydroxyvitamin D levels for extrarenal functions. In Stages 4 and 5 (GFR categories 4 and 5), activated vitamin D analogs must be used to decrease PTH secretion. Synthetic calcitriol has the same biologic activity as endogenous calcitriol. Doxercalciferol (1-α-hydroxyvitamin D_2) is another vitamin D analog that is hydroxylated in the liver to 1,25-dihydroxyvitamin D_2, which has the same biologic activity as calcitriol. Both calcitriol and doxercalciferol upregulate vitamin D receptors in the intestines, which increases calcium and phosphorus absorption, increasing the risk of hypercalcemia and hyperphosphatemia. It is important that serum calcium and phosphorus levels are within the normal range for the stage of CKD prior to starting either of these therapies. Paricalcitol (19-nor-1,25-dihydroxyvitamin D_2) is a vitamin D analog that has equal efficacy to calcitriol but may cause less

Table 26–7

Phosphate-Binding Agents Used to Treat Hyperphosphatemia in CKD

Compound	Trade Name	Dosage Form	Compound Content (mg)	Elemental Calcium Content (mg)	Starting Dose	Comments
Calcium carbonate (40% elemental calcium)	Tums	Chewable tablet	500, 750, 1000, 1250	200, 300, 400, 500	0.5–1 g (elemental calcium) three times a day with meals	First-line agent; dissolution characteristics and phosphorus-binding effect may vary from product to product; try to limit daily intake of elemental calcium to 1500 mg/day
	Oscal-500	Tablet	1250	500		
	Caltrate 600	Tablet	1500	600		
	Nephro Calci	Tablet	1500	600		
	LiquiCal	Liquid gelcap	1200	480		
	Calci-Chew	Chewable tablet	1250	500		Approximately 39 mg phosphorus bound per 1 g calcium carbonate
Calcium acetate (25% elemental calcium)	PhosLo Phoslyra	Capsule, Tablet Solution	667 667/5 mL	167	0.5–1 g (elemental calcium) three times a day with meals	First-line agent; comparable efficacy to calcium carbonate with one-half the dose of elemental calcium; do not exceed 1500 mg elemental calcium intake per day Approximately 45 mg phosphorus bound per 1 g calcium acetate By prescription only
Sevelamer HCl	Renagel	Tablet	400, 800	—	800 mg three times a day with meals	First-line agent; lowers LDL-C
Sevelamer carbonate	Renvela	Tablet, Powder for suspension	800			More expensive than calcium products; preferred in patients at risk for extraskeletal calcification May require large doses to control phosphorus levels
Lanthanum	Fosrenol	Chewable tablet	500, 750, 1000	—	750–1500 mg three times a day with meals	Second-line agent; more expensive than calcium products; preferred in patients at risk for extraskeletal calcification Most patients require 1500–3000 mg/day to control phosphorus
Aluminum hydroxide	AlternaGel Amphojel	Suspension	Various	—	300–600 mg three times a day with meals	Third-line agents; do not use concurrently with citrate-containing products Reserve for short-term use (4 weeks) in patients with hyperphosphatemia not responding to other binders
Magnesium carbonate/calcium carbonate	MagneBind 400	Tablet	400 mg (elemental magnesium)	80	400 mg three times a day with meals	Third-line agent; Same as for calcium carbonate and magnesium carbonate
Sucroferric oxyhydroxide	Velphoro	Chewable tablet	500	—	500 mg three times a day with meals	Do not use with levothyroxine; separate from doxycycline and alendronate by 1 hour
Ferric citrate	Auryxia	Tablet	1000	—	2000 mg (2 tablets) three times a day with meals	Maximum dose is 12 tablets per day Each tablet provides 210 mg elemental iron

CKD, chronic kidney disease; LDL-C, low-density lipoprotein cholesterol.

Table 26–8

Available Treatments for Secondary Hyperparathyroidism

Generic Name	Trade Name	Dosage Range	Dosage Forms	Frequency of Administration
Vitamin D precursor				
Ergocalciferol	Vitamin D_2	400–50,000 IU	By mouth	Daily (doses of 400–2000 IU)
Cholecalciferol	Vitamin D_3			Weekly or monthly for higher doses (50,000 IU)
Active Vitamin D				
Calcitriol	Calcijex	0.5–5 mcg	Intravenous	Three times per week
	Rocaltrol	0.25–5 mcg	By mouth	Daily, every other day, or three times per week
Vitamin D analogs				
Paricalcitol	Zemplar	1–4 mcg	By mouth	Daily or three times per week
		2.5–15 mcg	Intravenous	Three times per week
Doxercalciferol	Hectorol	5–20 mcg	By mouth	Daily or three times per week
		2-8 mcg	Intravenous	Three times per week
Calcimimetics				
Cinacalcet	Sensipar	30–180 mg	By mouth	Daily

hypercalcemia. Alfacalcidol (1-α-hydroxyvitamin D_3), falecalcitriol, and 22-oxacalcitriol (maxacalcitol) are only available outside the United States.

Calcimimetics Cinacalcet is a calcimimetic that increases the sensitivity of receptors on the parathyroid gland to serum calcium levels to reduce PTH secretion, but has no effect on intestinal absorption of calcium or phosphorus, and may even lower serum calcium levels.[31] Thus, cinacalcet is beneficial for patients with elevated PTH levels who have increased calcium or phosphorus levels or cannot use vitamin D therapy. Cinacalcet should also be used with caution in patients with seizure disorders because low serum calcium levels can lower the seizure threshold.

▶ *Outcome Evaluation*

Monitor serum calcium and phosphorus levels regularly in patients receiving phosphate-binding agents. When initiating therapy, monitor serum levels every 1 to 4 weeks, depending on the severity of hyperphosphatemia. Titrate doses of phosphate binders to achieve the target levels of serum calcium and phosphorus and iPTH (see Table 26–6). Once target levels are achieved, monitor serum calcium and phosphorus levels every 1 to 3 months. Monitor intact PTH levels monthly while initiating vitamin D therapy, then every 3 months once stable iPTH levels are achieved. When starting or increasing the dose of cinacalcet, monitor serum calcium and phosphorus levels within 1 week; iPTH levels should be monitored within 1 to 4 weeks. Once target levels are achieved, decrease monitoring to every 3 months.

Impaired Electrolyte and Acid–Base Homeostasis

The kidney is responsible for regulating homeostasis for sodium, potassium, water, and acid base. Reductions in the number of functioning nephrons decrease glomerular filtration regulation of electrolytes and acid secretion.

▶ *Pathophysiology*

As the number of functioning nephrons decreases, the remaining nephrons are able to increase excretion of sodium, water, potassium, and hydrogen ions. However, this is limited and as the number of functioning nephrons decreases as CKD progresses, total excretion of electrolytes and fluid eventually decreases.

Sodium and water balance is maintained by natriuretic peptides, namely atrial natriuretic peptide (ANP), which increases sodium excretion in the kidneys.[38] The relative increase in sodium excretion by a smaller number of functioning nephrons results in an osmotic diuresis that promotes water excretion,

Patient Encounter 3

A 61-year-old African American woman with a history of hypertension presents to your clinic for a routine follow-up. He has no complaints at this time.

PMH: Hypertension, diagnosed 25 years ago; hyperlipidemia

Current Meds: Aspirin 81 mg orally daily; atorvastatin 10 mg orally daily; carvedilol 25 mg orally twice daily; hydralazine 50 mg orally daily; lisinopril 40 mg orally daily; nifedipine ER 90 mg orally daily

ROS: Unremarkable

PE:

VS: BP 146/94 mm Hg, P 70 beats/min, T 96.3°F (35.7°C), Ht 5′9″ (175 cm), Wt 177 lb (80.3 kg)

CV: RRR, normal S_1, S_2

Abd: No organomegaly, bruits, tenderness; (+) bowel sounds; heme (–) stool

Ext: 1+ edema bilaterally

Labs: Sodium 136 mEq/L (136 mmol/L); potassium 5.7 mEq/L (5.7 mmol/L); chloride 99 mEq/L (99 mmol/L); carbon dioxide 17 mEq/L (17 mmol/L); BUN 36 mg/dL (12.9 mmol/L urea); SCr 3.0 mg/dL (265 μmol/L); glucose 113 mg/dL (6.3 mmol/L); calcium 8.4 mg/dL (2.10 mmol/L); phosphate 6.9 mg/dL (2.23 mmol/L); albumin 3.1 g/dL (31 g/L); intact parathyroid hormone (iPTH) 410 pg/mL (410 ng/L; 43.9 pmol/L); WBC 5.2×10^3 cells/mm^3 (5.2×10^9/L); RBC 4.2×10^6 cells/mm^3 (4.2×10^{12}/L); Hgb 9.4 g/dL (94 g/L; 5.83 mmol/L); Hct 28% (0.28); platelets 412×10^3 cells/mm^3 (412×10^9/L)

What signs are consistent with CKD mineral and bone disorder (MBD)?

What treatment would you recommend for CKD-MBD?

but impairs the ability of the kidneys to concentrate and dilute urine. Thus, urine becomes fixed at an osmolality close to that of the plasma, approximately 300 mOsm/kg (300 mmol/kg), and presents as nocturia. Sodium and fluid retention increases intravascular volume and raises systemic blood pressure, which can present as early as Stage 3 CKD.[38]

Potassium excretion occurs in both the distal tubules of the kidney and in the GI tract, which is mediated by aldosterone stimulation. Aldosterone increases in response to rising serum potassium, which then increases potassium excretion in both the functioning nephrons and GI tract. This maintains serum potassium concentrations within the normal range through GFR categories 1 to 4 CKD. Hyperkalemia begins to develop when GFR falls below 20% of normal, when the number of functioning nephrons and renal potassium secretion is so low that the capacity of the GI tract to excrete potassium has been exceeded.[39]

Medications can increase the risk of hyperkalemia in patients with CKD, including ACE-I and ARBs, used for the treatment of proteinuria and hypertension. Potassium-sparing diuretics, used for the treatment of edema and chronic heart failure, can also exacerbate the development of hyperkalemia, and they should be used with caution in patients with Stage 3 CKD (GFR category 3) or higher.

Hydrogen ions are excreted at the same rate of production by the kidney via buffers in the urine created by ammonia generation and phosphate excretion to maintain the pH of body fluids within a very narrow range. As kidney function declines, bicarbonate reabsorption is maintained, but hydrogen excretion is decreased because the ability of the kidney to generate ammonia is impaired. The positive hydrogen balance leads to metabolic acidosis, which is characterized by a serum bicarbonate level of 15 to 20 mEq/L (15–20 mmol/L), and an elevated anion gap greater than 17 mEq/L (17 mmol/L), resulting in a pH less than 7.35. Metabolic acidosis generally presents when the GFR declines below 25 mL/min/1.73 m^2 (0.24 mL/s/m^2).[36]

Metabolic acidosis contributes to various complications associated with CKD. Metabolic acidosis can directly cause bone disease, particularly in children, and contribute significantly to the bone disease induced by secondary hyperparathyroidism, as discussed previously. Metabolic acidosis also decreases hepatic albumin synthesis, which contributes to hypoalbuminemia and muscle wasting. Furthermore, metabolic acidosis can accelerate progression of CKD by causing tubular injury. Reversal of metabolic acidosis has been demonstrated to decrease progression of CKD, improve bone disease, and increase serum albumin concentrations.[36]

Clinical Presentation and Diagnosis of Electrolyte and Acid–Base Abnormalities

General

Alterations in sodium and water balance in CKD manifests as increased edema.

Hyperkalemia is generally asymptomatic in patients with CKD until serum potassium levels are greater than 5.5 mEq/L (5.5 mmol/L), when cardiac abnormalities present.

Metabolic acidosis is generally asymptomatic in patients with CKD.

Symptoms

Nocturia can present in Stage 3 CKD.

Edema generally presents in Stage 4 CKD or later.

Mild hyperkalemia and metabolic acidosis are generally not associated with overt symptoms.

Symptoms of hyperkalemia generally appear when GFR falls below 20 ml/min/1.73m^2 (0.19 ml/s/m^2), such as muscle weakness, fatigue, nausea, and paresthesias.

Symptoms of chronic metabolic acidosis present as bone abnormalities and growth retardation in children.

Signs

Cardiovascular:

- Sodium: Worsening hypertension, edema.
- Potassium: ECG changes (peaked T waves, widened QRS complex, loss of P wave).

Genitourinary: Sodium abnormalities result in change in urine volume and consistency.

Laboratory Tests

Sodium: Increased blood pressure; sodium levels remain within the normal range; urine osmolality is generally fixed at 300 mOsm/kg (300 mmol/kg).

Potassium: Increased serum potassium levels.

Metabolic acidosis: Decreased serum bicarbonate levels (CO_2); decreased pH.

▶ *Treatment*

Nonpharmacologic treatment The kidney is unable to adjust to abrupt changes in sodium and potassium intake in patients with severe CKD. Electrolyte disorders resulting from an acute increase in intake can be more severe and prolonged.

Sodium and Water. Patients should be advised to refrain from adding salt to their diet but should not restrict sodium intake. Changes in sodium intake should occur slowly over a period of several days to allow adequate time for the kidney to adjust urinary sodium content. Sodium restriction produces a negative sodium balance, which causes fluid excretion to restore sodium balance. The resulting volume contraction can decrease perfusion of the kidney and hasten the decline in GFR. Saline-containing IV solutions should be used cautiously in patients with CKD because the salt load may precipitate volume overload.

Fluid restriction is generally unnecessary as long as sodium intake is controlled. The thirst mechanism remains intact in CKD to maintain total body water and plasma osmolality near normal levels. Fluid intake should be maintained at the rate of urine output to replace urine losses, usually fixed at approximately 2 L/day as urine concentrating ability is lost. Significant increases in free water intake orally or IV can precipitate volume overload and hyponatremia. Patients with Stage 5 CKD require RRT to maintain normal volume status. Fluid intake is often limited in patients receiving hemodialysis to prevent fluid overload between dialysis sessions.

Diuretic therapy is often necessary to prevent volume overload in patients with CKD in those who still produce urine. When GFR falls below 30 ml/min/1.73 m^2 (0.29 mL/s/m^2), thiazide diuretics alone may not be effective in reducing fluid retention.[17] Loop diuretics are most frequently used to increase sodium and water excretion. As CKD progresses, higher doses, as much as 80 to 1000 mg/day of furosemide, or continuous infusion of loop diuretics may be needed, or combination therapy with loop and thiazide diuretics to increase sodium and water excretion.[17]

Potassium. Patients who develop hyperkalemia should restrict dietary intake of potassium to 50 to 80 mEq (50–80 mmol) per day. Potassium concentrations can also be altered in the dialysate for patients receiving hemodialysis and peritoneal dialysis to manage hyperkalemia. Because GI excretion of potassium plays a large role in potassium homeostasis in patients with Stage 5 CKD, a good bowel regimen is essential to minimize constipation. Severe hyperkalemia is most effectively managed by hemodialysis.

Acute hyperkalemia can be managed medically until dialysis can be initiated. Diuretics, sodium polystyrene sulfonate, and fludrocortisone are useful in the management of hyperkalemia in patients with CKD. Acute hyperkalemia that results in cardiac abnormalities can be managed with calcium, insulin and dextrose. The management of hyperkalemia is discussed in more detail in Chapter 27.

Metabolic Acidosis. Pharmacologic therapy with sodium bicarbonate or citrate/citric acid preparations may be needed in patients with Stage 3 CKD (GFR category 3) or higher to replenish body stores of bicarbonate. Calcium carbonate and calcium acetate, used to bind phosphorus in sHPT, also aid in increasing serum bicarbonate levels, in conjunction with other agents.

Sodium bicarbonate tablets are administered in increments of 325- and 650-mg tablets. A 650-mg tablet of sodium bicarbonate contains 7.7 mEq (7.7 mmol) each of sodium and bicarbonate. Sodium retention associated with sodium bicarbonate can cause volume overload, which can exacerbate hypertension and chronic heart failure. Patient tolerability of sodium bicarbonate is low because of carbon dioxide production in the GI tract that occurs during dissolution.

Solutions that contain sodium citrate/citric acid (Shohl's solution and Bicitra) provide 1 mEq/L (1 mmol/L) each of sodium and bicarbonate. Polycitra is a sodium/potassium citrate solution that provides 2 mEq/L (2 mmol/L) of bicarbonate but contains 1 mEq/L (1 mmol/L) each of sodium and potassium, which can promote hyperkalemia in patients with severe CKD. The citrate portion of these preparations is metabolized in the liver to bicarbonate; the citric acid portion is metabolized to CO_2 and water, increasing tolerability compared with sodium bicarbonate. Sodium retention is also decreased with these preparations. However, these products are liquid preparations, which may not be palatable to some patients. Citrate can also promote aluminum intoxication by augmenting aluminum absorption in the GI tract.

When determining the dose of bicarbonate replacement, the goal for therapy is to achieve a normal serum bicarbonate level of 24 mEq/L (24 mmol/L). The dose is usually determined by calculating the base deficit: (0.5 L/kg × [body weight]) × ([normal CO_2] [measured CO_2]). Because of the risk of volume overload resulting from the sodium load administered with bicarbonate replacement, the total base deficit should be administered over several days. Once the goal serum bicarbonate level is attained, a maintenance dose of bicarbonate is necessary and should be titrated to maintain serum bicarbonate levels. Altering bicarbonate levels in the dialysate fluid in patients receiving dialysis may assist with the treatment of metabolic acidosis, although pharmacologic therapy may still be required.

▸ *Outcome Evaluation*

Monitor serum electrolytes and arterial blood gases regularly. Monitor edema after initiation of diuretic therapy. Monitor fluid intake to ensure obligatory losses are being met and avoid dehydration. If adequate diuresis is not attained with a single agent, consider combination therapy with another diuretic. In patients with cardiac abnormalities due to elevated potassium levels, monitor ECG continuously until serum potassium levels drop below 5 mEq/L (5 mmol/L) or cardiac abnormalities resolve. Evaluate serum potassium and glucose levels within 1 hour in patients who receive insulin and dextrose therapy. Evaluate serum potassium levels within 2 to 4 hours after treatment with SPS or diuretics. Repeat doses of diuretics or SPS if necessary until serum potassium levels fall below 5 mEq/L (5 mmol/L). Monitor blood pressure and serum potassium levels in 1 week in patients who receive fludrocortisone. Correct metabolic acidosis slowly to prevent the development of metabolic alkalosis or other electrolyte abnormalities.

RENAL REPLACEMENT THERAPY

Patients who progress to ESKD require RRT. The modalities that are used for RRT are dialysis, including hemodialysis (HD) and peritoneal dialysis (PD), and kidney transplantation. The United States Renal Data Service (USRDS) reported that the number of patients with ESKD was 636,905, with 114,813 new cases diagnosed in 201.[3] Kidney transplantation is the preferred method of RRT, owing to improved patient survival. The expected life expectancy of patients with ESKD is only 25% of the general population, while patients with a transplant have a life expectancy that approaches 75% to 80% of the general population.[3] However, organ availability limits the number of patients who can receive a kidney transplant. Only 2.5% of patients with newly diagnosed ESKD receive kidney transplants each year.[3] Therefore, the most common form of RRT is dialysis, accounting for 70% of all patients with ESKD.[3] The principles and complications associated with dialysis are discussed later. Chapter 55 discusses the principles of kidney transplantation.

Indications for Dialysis

KEY CONCEPT *Planning for dialysis should begin when GFR falls less than 30 mL/min/1.73 m² (0.29 mL/s/m²) (Stage 4; GFR category 4),[1] when progression to ESKD is inevitable, to allow time to educate the patient and family on the treatment modalities and establish the appropriate access for the modality of choice.* Ideally, initiation of dialysis should be done at a point when the patient is ready to undergo treatment, rather than when the patient is in emergent need of dialysis.

Initiation of dialysis depends on the patient's clinical status and not based solely on laboratory values. Symptoms that may indicate the need for dialysis include persistent anorexia, nausea, vomiting, fatigue, and pruritus. Other criteria that indicate the need for dialysis include declining nutritional status, declining serum albumin levels, uncontrolled hypertension, and volume overload, which may manifest as chronic heart failure, and electrolyte abnormalities, particularly hyperkalemia. **Blood urea nitrogen** (BUN) and SCr levels may be used as a guide for the initiation of dialysis, but they should not be the absolute

Table 26–9

Advantages and Disadvantages of Hemodialysis

Advantages

1. Higher solute clearance allows intermittent treatment
2. Parameters of adequacy of dialysis are better defined and therefore underdialysis can be detected early
3. The technique's failure rate is low
4. Even though intermittent heparinization is required, hemostasis parameters are better corrected with hemodialysis than peritoneal dialysis
5. In-center hemodialysis enables closer monitoring of the patient

Disadvantages

1. Requires multiple visits each week to the hemodialysis center, which translates into loss of control by the patient
2. Dysequilibrium, dialysis, hypotension, and muscle cramps are common. May require months before patient adjusts to hemodialysis
3. Infections in hemodialysis patients may be related to the choice of membranes; the complement-activating membranes are more deleterious
4. Vascular access is frequently associated with infection and thrombosis
5. Decline of residual renal function is more rapid compared with peritoneal dialysis

From Sowinski KM, Churchwell MD, Decker BS. Hemodialysis and peritoneal dialysis. In: DiPiro JT, Talbert RL, Yee GC, et al., eds. Pharmacotherapy: A Pathophysiologic Approach, 9th ed. New York, NY: McGraw-Hill, 2014:666, with permission.

Table 26–10

Advantages and Disadvantages of Peritoneal Dialysis

Advantages

1. More hemodynamic stability (blood pressure) due to slow ultrafiltration rate
2. Increased clearance of larger solutes, which may explain good clinical status in spite of lower urea clearance
3. Better preservation of residual renal function
4. Convenient intraperitoneal route of administration of drugs such as antibiotics and insulin
5. Suitable for elderly and very young patients who may not tolerate hemodialysis well
6. Freedom from the "machine" gives the patient a sense of independence (for continuous ambulatory peritoneal dialysis)
7. Less blood loss and iron deficiency, resulting in easier management of anemia or reduced requirements for erythropoietin and parenteral iron
8. No systemic heparinization requirement
9. Subcutaneous versus IV erythropoietin or darbepoetin is usual, which may reduce overall doses and be more physiologic

Disadvantages

1. Protein and amino acid losses through the peritoneum and reduced appetite owing to continuous glucose load and sense of abdominal fullness predispose to malnutrition
2. Risk of peritonitis
3. Catheter malfunction, and exit site and tunnel infection
4. Inadequate ultrafiltration and solute dialysis in patients with a large body size, unless large volumes and frequent exchanges are employed
5. Patient burnout and high rate of technique failure
6. Risk of obesity with excessive glucose absorption
7. Mechanical problems such as hernias, dialysate leaks, hemorrhoids, or back pain may occur
8. Extensive abdominal surgery may preclude peritoneal dialysis
9. No convenient access for IV iron administration

From Sowinski KM, Churchwell MD, Decker BS. Hemodialysis and peritoneal dialysis. In: DiPiro JT, Talbert RL, Yee GC, et al., eds. Pharmacotherapy: A Pathophysiologic Approach, 9th ed. New York, NY: McGraw-Hill, 2014:667, with permission.

indicator. Dialysis is initiated in most patients after the GFR falls below 15 mL/min/1.73 m^2 (0.14 mL/s/m^2).[1] Patients should determine which modality of dialysis to use based on their own preferences. Advantages and disadvantages of hemodialysis and peritoneal dialysis are listed in Tables 26–9 and 26–10, respectively.

The goals of dialysis are to remove toxic metabolites to decrease uremic symptoms, correct electrolyte abnormalities, restore acid–base status, and maintain volume status to ultimately improve quality of life and decrease the morbidity and mortality associated with ESKD.

Hemodialysis

Hemodialysis is the most common method of RRT, initiated in 91% of US patients with newly diagnosed ESKD each year, with a total of 408,711 patients receiving HD in 2012.[3] Home HD is becoming increasingly more popular, but most patients continue to receive HD from a dialysis center.

▸ *Principles of Hemodialysis*

KEY CONCEPT *Hemodialysis involves the exposure of blood to a semipermeable membrane (dialyzer) against which a physiologic solution (dialysate) is flowing (Figure 26–6).* The dialyzer is composed of thousands of capillary fibers made up of the semipermeable membrane, which are enclosed in the dialyzer, to increase the surface area of blood exposure to maximize the efficiency of removing substances. The dialysate is composed of purified water and electrolytes, and it is run through the dialyzer countercurrent to the blood on the other side of the semipermeable membrane. The process allows for the removal of several substances from the bloodstream, including water, urea, creatinine, electrolytes, uremic toxins, and drugs. Sterilization is not required for dialysate because the membrane prevents bacteria from entering into the bloodstream. However, if the membrane ruptures during hemodialysis, infection becomes a major concern for the patient.

Three types of membranes used for dialysis are classified by the size of the pores and the ability to remove solutes from the bloodstream:

- Conventional (standard) membranes have small pores, which limit solute removal to relatively small molecules, such as creatinine and urea.
- High-efficiency membranes also have small pores but have a higher surface area that increases removal of small molecules, such as water, urea, and creatinine from the blood.
- High-flux membranes have larger pores that allow for the removal of substances with higher molecular-weight, including some drugs, such as vancomycin, than conventional membranes.

Three primary processes are utilized for the removal of substances from the blood:

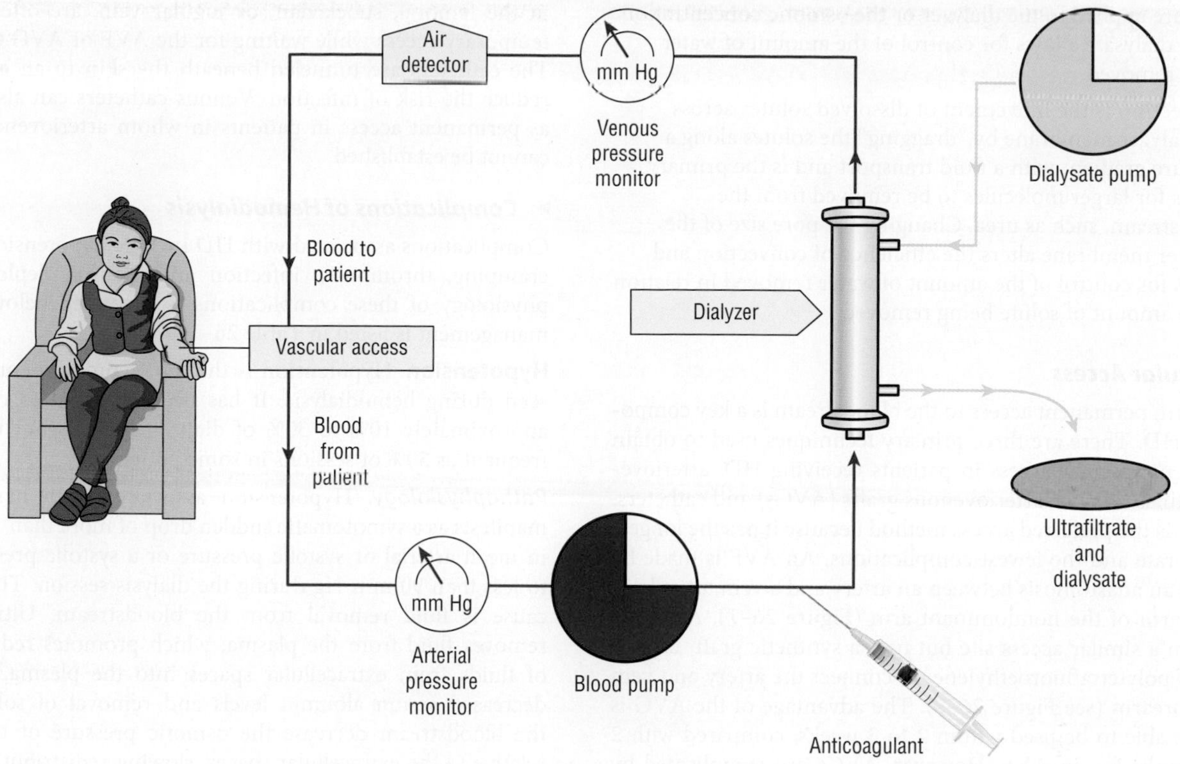

FIGURE 26–6. In hemodialysis, the patient's blood is pumped to the dialyzer at a rate of 300 to 600 mL/min. An anticoagulant (usually heparin) is administered to prevent clotting in the dialyzer. The dialysate is pumped at the rate of 500 to 1000 mL/min through the dialyzer countercurrent to the flow of blood. The rate of fluid removal from the patient is controlled by adjusting the pressure in the dialysate compartment. (From Sowinski KM, Churchwell MD, Decker BS. Hemodialysis and peritoneal dialysis. In: DiPiro JT, Talbert RL, Yee GC, et al., eds. Pharmacotherapy: A Pathophysiologic Approach, 9th ed. New York, NY: McGraw-Hill, 2014:669, with permission.)

- **Diffusion** is the movement of a solute across the dialyzer membrane from an area of higher concentration (usually the blood) to a lower concentration (usually the dialysate). This process removes small molecules from the bloodstream, such as electrolytes. At times, solutes can be added to the dialysate that are diffused into the bloodstream. Changing the composition of the dialysate allows for control of the amount of electrolytes that are being removed.
- **Ultrafiltration** is the movement of solvent (plasma water) across the dialyzer membrane by applying hydrostatic or osmotic pressure, and it is the primary means for removing water from the bloodstream. Changing the hydrostatic

Patient Encounter 4, Part 1

A 35-year-old Caucasian man with a history of IgA nephropathy presents to the clinic with complaints that he "feels awful." He hasn't felt like eating for several weeks and has lost 15 lb (6.8 kg) in the last 3 months.

PMH: IgA nephropathy; depression; hypertension; hyperlipidemia

Current Meds: Bupropion 150 mg orally daily; cinacalcet 30 mg orally daily; escitalapram 10 mg orally daily; hydralazine 50 mg orally three times daily; labetalol 200 mg orally twice daily; calcium acetate 1334 mg orally three times daily with meals; pravastatin 40 mg orally daily

ROS: Lethargic male in mild distress

PE:

VS: BP 178/108 mm Hg, P 86 beats/min, T 97.2°F (36.2°C), Ht 5'10" (178 cm), Wt 186 lb (84.4 kg)

CV: RRR, normal S_1, S_2, present

Lungs: Crackles at bases; mild inspiratory wheezes

Ext: 4+ bilateral lower extremity edema present to mid-thigh

Labs: Sodium 138 mEq/L (138 mmol/L); potassium 6.3 mEq/L (6.3 mmol/L); chloride 106 mEq/L (106 mmol/L); carbon dioxide 15 mEq/L (15 mmol/L); BUN 42 mg/dL (15.0 mmol/L); SCr 4.2 mg/dL (371 μmol/L); glucose 62 mg/dL (3.4 mmol/L); calcium 9.8 mg/dL (2.45 mmol/L); phosphate 5.6 mg/dL (1.81 mmol/L); iPTH 315 pg/mL (315 ng/L; 33.7 pmol/L); WBC 6.8×10^3 cells/mm^3 (6.8×10^9/L); RBC 4.0×10^6 cells/mm^3 (4.0×10^{12}/L); Hgb 10.4 g/dL (104 g/L; 6.46 mmol/L); Hct 30% (0.30); platelets 278×10^3 cells/mm^3 (278×10^9/L)

What indications does the patient have for dialysis?

What alternatives for renal replacement therapy exist for the patient?

What are the advantages and disadvantages of each modality for renal replacement?

pressure applied to the dialyzer or the osmotic concentration of the dialysate allows for control of the amount of water being removed.

- Convection is the movement of dissolved solutes across the dialyzer membrane by "dragging" the solutes along a pressure gradient with a fluid transport and is the primary means for larger molecules to be removed from the bloodstream, such as urea. Changing the pore size of the dialyzer membrane alters the efficiency of convection and allows for control of the amount of water removed in relation to the amount of solute being removed.

▶ *Vascular Access*

Long-term permanent access to the bloodstream is a key component of HD. There are three primary techniques used to obtain permanent vascular access in patients receiving HD: arteriovenous fistulas (AVFs), arteriovenous grafts (AVGs) and catheters. An AVF is the preferred access method because it has the longest survival rate and the fewest complications. An AVF is made by creating an anastomosis between an artery and a vein, usually in the forearm of the nondominant arm (Figure 26–7). An AVG results in a similar access site but uses a synthetic graft, usually made of polytetrafluoroethylene, to connect the artery and vein in the forearm (see Figure 26–7). The advantage of the AVG is that it is able to be used within 2 to 3 weeks, compared with 2 to 3 months for an AVF. However, AVGs are complicated by stenosis, thrombosis, and infections, which lead to a shorter survival time of the graft. Double-lumen venous catheters, placed in the femoral, subclavian, or jugular vein, are often used as temporary access while waiting for the AVF or AVG to mature. The catheters are tunneled beneath the skin to an exit site to reduce the risk of infection. Venous catheters can also be used as permanent access in patients in whom arteriovenous access cannot be established.

▶ *Complications of Hemodialysis*

Complications associated with HD include hypotension, muscle cramping, thrombosis, infection and vitamin depletion. The physiology of these complications is described below and the management is listed in Table 26–11.

Hypotension Hypotension is the most common complication seen during hemodialysis. It has been reported to occur with approximately 10% to 30% of dialysis sessions but may be as frequent as 50% of sessions in some patients.[40]

Pathophysiology. Hypotension associated with hemodialysis manifests as a symptomatic sudden drop of more than 30 mm Hg in mean arterial or systolic pressure or a systolic pressure drop to less than 90 mm Hg during the dialysis session. The primary cause is fluid removal from the bloodstream. Ultrafiltration removes fluid from the plasma, which promotes redistribution of fluids from extracellular spaces into the plasma. However, decreased serum albumin levels and removal of solutes from the bloodstream decrease the osmotic pressure of the plasma relative to the extracellular spaces, slowing redistribution during hemodialysis. The decreased plasma volume causes hypotension. Other factors that can contribute to hypotension include

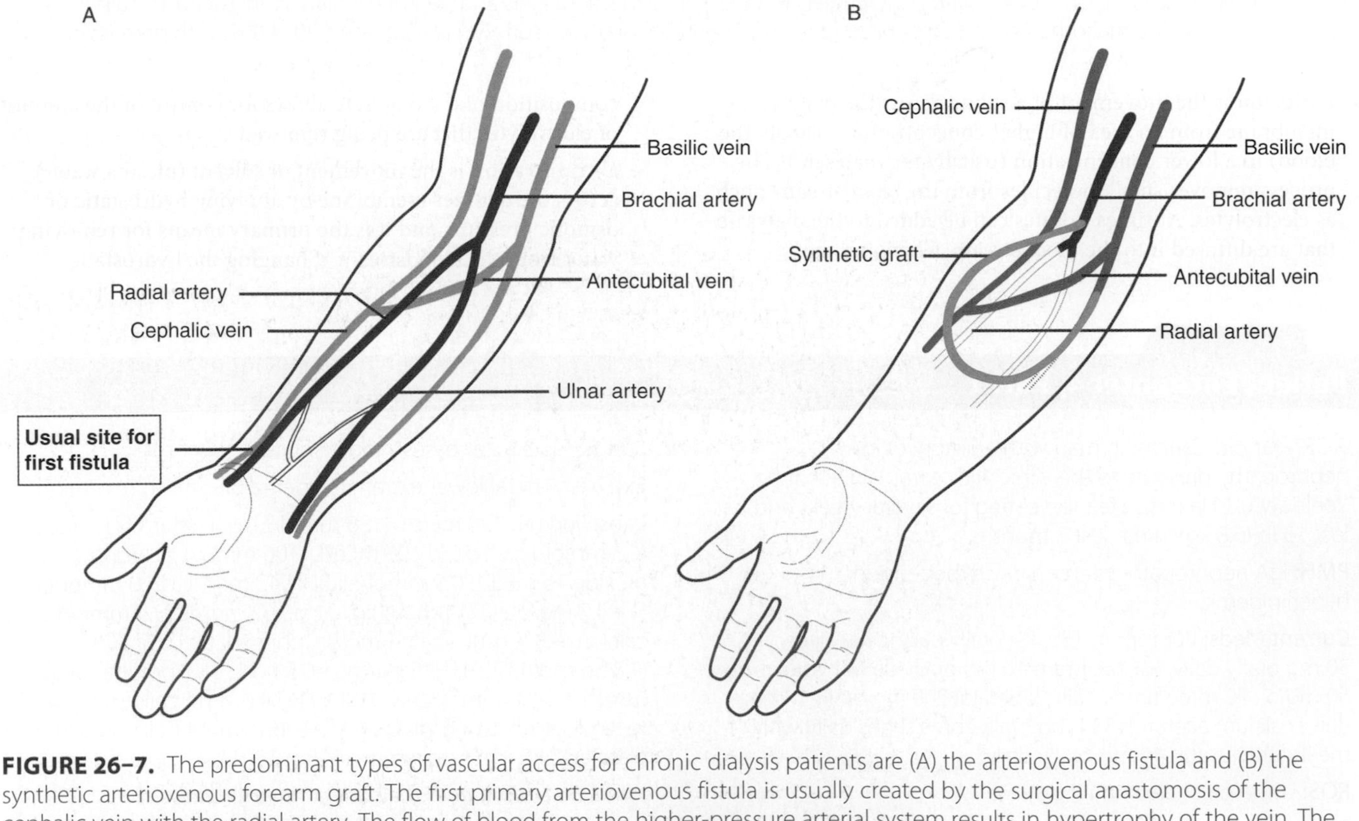

FIGURE 26–7. The predominant types of vascular access for chronic dialysis patients are (A) the arteriovenous fistula and (B) the synthetic arteriovenous forearm graft. The first primary arteriovenous fistula is usually created by the surgical anastomosis of the cephalic vein with the radial artery. The flow of blood from the higher-pressure arterial system results in hypertrophy of the vein. The most common AV graft (depicted in green) is between the brachial artery and the basilic or cephalic vein. The flow of blood may be diminished in the radial and ulnar arteries because it preferentially flows into the low pressure graft. (From Sowinski KM, Churchwell MD, Decker BS. Hemodialysis and peritoneal dialysis. In: DiPiro JT, Talbert RL, Yee GC, et al., eds. Pharmacotherapy: A Pathophysiologic Approach, 9th ed. New York, NY: McGraw-Hill, 2014:668, with permission.)

Table 26–11

Management of Complications Associated with Hemodialysis

Hypotension	Acute treatment	Place in Trendelenburg position (head lower than feet) Normal saline 100–200 mL Hypertonic saline (23.4%) 10–20 mL Mannitol 12.5 g
	Prevention	Accurate determination of "dry weight" Midodrine 2.5–10 mg 30 minutes prior to HD Other options with limited evidence: Levocarnitine 20 mg/kg IV after HD Sertraline 50–100 mg daily Fludrocortisone 0.1 mg before HD
Muscle Cramps	Acute treatment	Normal saline 100–200 mL Hypertonic saline (23.4%) 10–20 mL Dextrose 50% 50 mL (for nondiabetic patients)
	Prevention	Decrease ultrafiltration rate Accurate determination of "dry weight" Stretching exercises, massage, flexing, compression devices Vitamin E 400 IU daily
Central Venous Catheter Thrombosis	Acute treatment	Normal saline flush Alteplase 2 mg/2 mL per catheter lumen port Reteplase 0.4 units/0.4 mL per catheter lumen port
	Prevention	Heparin lock (1000–10,000 units/1 mL) Sodium citrate 4% lock
Vitamin Depletion	Prevention	Multivitamin B complex with vitamin C supplement

antihypertensive medications prior to HD, a target "dry weight" (the target weight after HD session is complete) that is too low, diastolic or autonomic dysfunction, low dialysate calcium or sodium, high dialysate temperature, or ingesting meals prior to or during HD.

Risk factors that may increase the potential for hypotension include elderly age, diabetes, autonomic neuropathy, uremia, and cardiac disease.[40] The symptoms associated with hypotension during dialysis include dizziness, nausea, vomiting, sweating, and chest pain.

Muscle Cramps Muscle cramps can occur with up to 20% of dialysis sessions.[40] The cause is often related to excessive ultrafiltration, which causes hypoperfusion of the muscles. Other contributing factors to the development of muscle cramps include hypotension and electrolyte and acid–base imbalances that occur during hemodialysis sessions.

Thrombosis Thrombosis associated with hemodialysis most commonly occurs in patients with venous catheter access for dialysis and is a common cause of catheter failure. However, thrombosis can occur in synthetic grafts and less frequently in AV fistulas.

Infection Infections are an important cause of morbidity and mortality in patients receiving hemodialysis. The cause of infection is usually related to organisms found on the skin, namely *Staphylococcus epidermidis* and *Staphylococcus aureus*. Methicillin-resistant *S. aureus* (MRSA) is a common cause of infections in patients receiving hemodialysis. Other organisms have also been found to cause access-related infections. The greatest risk to patients receiving hemodialysis is the development of bacteremia. As with thrombosis, venous catheters are most commonly infected, followed by synthetic AV grafts, and finally AV fistulas.

Blood cultures should be obtained for any patient receiving hemodialysis who develops a fever. Nonpharmacologic management of infections involves preventive measures with sterile technique, proper disinfection, and minimizing the use and duration of venous catheters for hemodialysis access.

Pharmacologic management of infections should cover the gram-positive organisms that most frequently cause access-related infections. Patients who have positive blood cultures should receive treatment tailored to the organism isolated. Preventive measures for access-related infections include mupirocin at the exit site and povidone-iodine ointment. The recommendations of the National Kidney Foundation (NKF) for treatment of infections associated with hemodialysis are listed in Table 26–12.

Table 26–12

Management of Hemodialysis Access Infections[41]

AV Fistula	Treat as subacute bacterial endocarditis for 6 weeks Initial antibiotic choice should always cover gram-positive organisms (eg, vancomycin 20 mg/kg IV with serum concentration monitoring or cefazolin 20 mg/kg IV three times per week) Gram-negative coverage is indicated for patients with diabetes, HIV infection, prosthetic valves, or those receiving immunosuppressive agents (gentamicin 2 mg/kg IV with serum concentration monitoring)
Synthetic Grafts (AVG)	
Local infection	Empiric antibiotic coverage for gram-positive, gram-negative, and *Enterococcus* (eg, gentamicin plus vancomycin, then individualize after culture results become available); continue for 2–4 weeks
Extensive infection	Antibiotics as above plus total resection
Access < 1 month old	Antibiotics as above plus removal of the graft
Tunneled Cuffed Catheters (Internal Jugular, Subclavian)	
Infection localized to catheter exit site	No drainage: topical antibiotics (eg, mupirocin ointment) Drainage present: Gram-positive coverage (eg, cefazolin 20 mg/kg IV three times a week)
Bacteremia with or without systemic signs or symptoms	Gram-positive coverage as above If stable and asymptomatic, change catheter and provide culture-specific antibiotic coverage for a minimum of 3 weeks

AV, arteriovenous.

Vitamin Depletion Water-soluble vitamins removed by HD contribute to malnutrition and vitamin deficiency syndromes. Patients receiving HD often require replacement of water-soluble vitamins to prevent adverse effects. The vitamins that may require replacement are ascorbic acid, thiamine, biotin, folic acid, riboflavin, and pyridoxine. Patients receiving HD should receive a multivitamin B complex with vitamin C supplement, but they should not take supplements that include fat-soluble vitamins, such as vitamins A, E, or K, which can accumulate in patients with kidney failure.

Peritoneal Dialysis

Peritoneal dialysis is initiated in 6% of patients with newly diagnosed ESKD each year. Currently, 40,631 patients were receiving PD dialysis in 2012.[3] Peritoneal dialysis is associated with improved survival compared with hemodialysis.[3] Peritoneal dialysis preserves residual renal function, which improves cardiovascular stability and may account for the improved survival. Thus PD may be the preferred method of dialysis in patients with residual renal function.

▶ *Principles of Peritoneal Dialysis*

PD utilizes similar principles as hemodialysis in that blood is exposed to a semipermeable membrane against which a physiologic solution is placed. In the case of PD, however, the semipermeable membrane is the peritoneal membrane, and a sterile dialysate is instilled into the peritoneal cavity. The peritoneal membrane is composed of a continuous single layer of mesothelial cells that covers the abdominal and pelvic walls on one side of the peritoneal cavity, and the visceral organs including the GI tract, liver, spleen, and diaphragm on the other side. The mesothelial cells are covered by microvilli that increase the surface area of the peritoneal membrane to approximate body surface area (1–2 m^2). Blood vessels that supply the abdominal organs, muscle, and mesentery serve as the blood component of the system.

The gaps between the mesothelial cells allow for large solutes to pass through into the bloodstream. Both the interstitium and endothelial cells of the blood vessels provide resistance to limit the solute size that is removed from the blood. Diffusion is the most important component of solute transport in PD, which is enhanced by the large surface area and volume of dialysate, as well as contact time with the peritoneal membrane. Ultrafiltration is achieved in PD by creating an osmotic pressure gradient between the dialysate and the blood. Traditionally, glucose has been used to create the osmotic gradient, but the solutions are not biocompatible with the peritoneal membrane, resulting in cytotoxicity of the cells. More recently, polymeric glucose derivatives such as icodextrin have been used to create a colloid-driven osmosis that results in ultrafiltration and convection of solute removal.

In PD, prewarmed dialysate is instilled into the peritoneal cavity where it "dwells" for a specified length of time (usually one to several hours, depending on the type of PD) to adequately clear metabolic waste products and excess fluids and electrolytes. At the end of the dwell time, the dialysate is drained and replaced with fresh dialysate. The continuous nature of PD provides for a more physiologic removal of waste products from the bloodstream, which mimics endogenous kidney function by decreasing the fluctuations seen in serum concentrations of the waste products. Similarly, water is removed at a more constant rate, lessening the fluctuations in intravascular fluid balance and providing for more hemodynamic stability.

Patient Encounter 4, Part 2

The patient returns to the dialysis clinic 6 months later for his follow-up after starting peritoneal dialysis. He states that his dialysate was cloudy yesterday evening.

PE:

VS: BP 145/88 mm Hg, P 78 beats/min, T 101.4 F (38.6° C), Wt 178 lb (80.7 kg)

Abd: Erythema and tenderness at the catheter site

What organisms are most likely to cause his peritonitis?

What empiric antibiotic treatment is recommended?

Several types of PD are used:

- Continuous ambulatory peritoneal dialysis (CAPD) is the most common. The patient exchanges 1 to 3 L of dialysate every 4 to 6 hours throughout the day with a longer dwell time overnight.
- Automated peritoneal dialysis (APD) procedures involve the use of a cycler machine that performs sequential exchanges overnight while the patient is sleeping.
- Continuous cycling PD (CCPD) performs three to five exchanges throughout the night. The final exchange remains in the peritoneal cavity to dwell for the duration of the day.
- Nightly intermittent PD (NIPD) performs six to eight exchanges throughout the night. The final exchange of dialysate is drained in the morning, and the peritoneal cavity remains empty throughout the day.
- Nocturnal tidal PD (NTPD) is similar to NIPD, with the exception that only a portion of the dialysate is exchanged throughout the night. The final exchange is drained in the morning, and the peritoneal cavity remains empty throughout the day.

▶ *Peritoneal Access*

Access to the peritoneal cavity requires placement of an indwelling catheter with the distal end of the catheter resting in the peritoneal cavity. The central portion of the catheter is generally tunneled under the abdominal wall and subcutaneous tissue where it is held in place by cuffs that provide stability and mechanical support to the catheter. The proximal portion of the catheter exits the abdomen near the umbilicus (Figure 26–8). Several types of indwelling catheters are available; the most common is the Tenckhoff catheter. Placement and handling of the catheter during PD exchanges requires a sterile environment to minimize the risk of infectious complications.

▶ *Complications of Peritoneal Dialysis*

Complications associated with PD include mechanical problems related to the PD catheter, metabolic problems associated with the components of the dialysate fluid, damage to the peritoneal membrane, and infections (Table 26–13). Strategies to manage infectious complications of PD are discussed below.

Peritonitis Peritonitis is a leading cause of morbidity in PD patients, which often leads to loss of the catheter and subsequent change to HD as the treatment modality. However, recent advances with connectors used during instillation and drainage

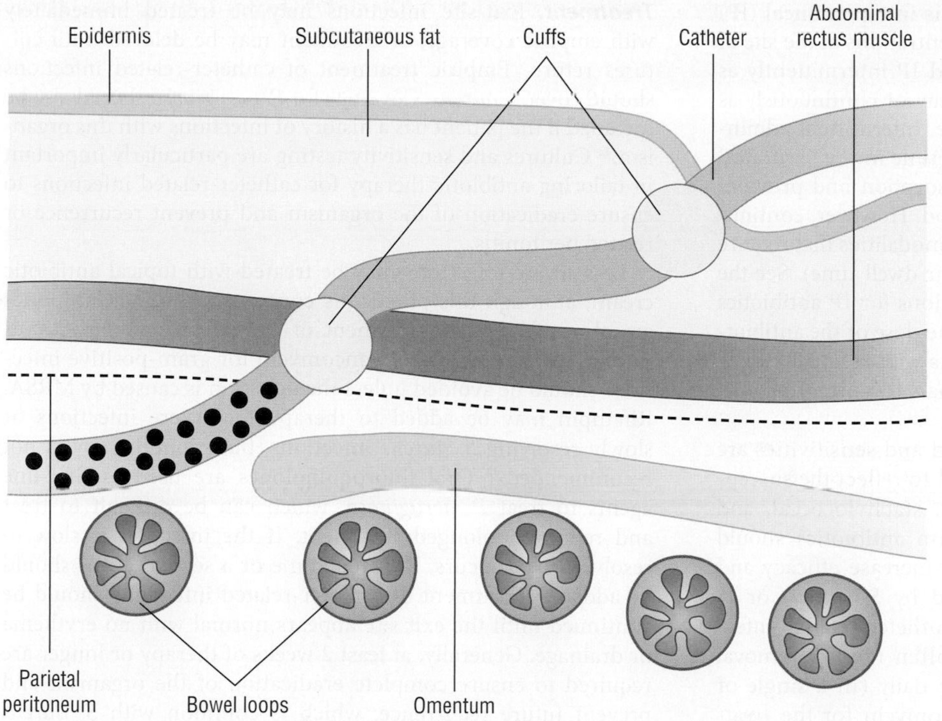

FIGURE 26–8. Diagram of the placement of a peritoneal dialysis catheter through the abdominal wall into the peritoneal cavity. (From Sowinski KM, Churchwell MD, Decker BS. Hemodialysis and peritoneal dialysis. In: DiPiro JT, Talbert RL, Yee GC, et al., eds. Pharmacotherapy: A Pathophysiologic Approach, 9th ed. New York, NY: McGraw-Hill, 2014:675, with permission.)

Table 26–13

Common Complications During Peritoneal Dialysis

Mechanical Complications
Kinking in catheter
Catheter migration
Catheter adherence to peritoneal tissue
Excessive movement of catheter at exit site
Peritoneal Damage
Alterations in permeability of the peritoneal membrane
Sclerosis of the peritoneal membrane
Pain
Impingement of the catheter tip on visceral organs
Instillation pain
• Rapid inflow of dialysate
• Acidic pH of dialysate
• Chemical irritation from dialysate additives (eg, antibiotics)
• Low dialysate temperature
Infections
Peritonitis
Exit-site infections
Tunnel infections
Metabolic Complications
Exacerbation of diabetes mellitus from glucose load
Fluid overload
• Exacerbation of chronic heart failure
• Edema
• Pulmonary congestion
Electrolyte abnormalities
Malnutrition
• Albumin and amino acid loss
• Muscle wasting
• Increased adipose tissue
• Fibrin formation in dialysate
Weight gain

of dialysate and delivery systems have dramatically decreased the incidence of peritonitis. Peritonitis can be caused by chemical irritation or microorganisms.

Pathophysiology. Gram-positive organisms, namely *S. epidermidis*, are the most common cause of peritonitis. Other pathologic organisms include *S. aureus*, streptococcal species, enterococcus species, gram-negative organisms including *Escherichia coli* and *Pseudomonas* species, and fungal organisms. Peritonitis should be presumed if cloudy fluid is drained from the peritoneal cavity and the fluid should be evaluated by cultures. Antibiotic treatment should be initiated immediately, until cell counts and cultures prove otherwise.[42] Patients with peritonitis may also complain of abdominal pain, although pain may be absent in some cases.

Treatment. The International Society of Peritoneal Dialysis (ISPD) revised the recommendations for the treatment of PD-related infections in 2010.[42] Drug selection for empirical treatment of peritonitis should cover both gram-positive and gram-negative organisms specific to the dialysis center and be based on the protocols and sensitivity patterns of organisms known to cause peritonitis, as well as the history of infections in the patient. First-generation cephalosporins, such as cefazolin, or vancomycin are recommended for empirical coverage of gram-positive organisms. Appropriate coverage for gram-negative organisms includes third- or fourth-generation cephalosporins, such as ceftazidime or cefepime, or aminoglycosides. Alternatives for gram-negative coverage include oral fluoroquinolones. An example of an appropriate empiric treatment for peritonitis includes cefazolin in combination with ceftazidime, cefepime, or an aminoglycoside. If the patient has a cephalosporin allergy, vancomycin in combination with an aminoglycoside is an alternative empirical treatment.[42] It should be noted that aminoglycosides can decrease residual renal function in patients receiving peritoneal dialysis.

The preferred route of administration is intraperitoneal (IP) rather than IV to achieve maximum concentrations at the site of infection. Antibiotics can be administered IP intermittently as a single large dose in one exchange per day or continuously as multiple smaller doses with each exchange. Intermittent administration requires at least 6 hours of dwell time in the peritoneal cavity to allow for adequate systemic absorption and provides adequate levels to cover the 24-hour period. However, continuous administration is better suited for PD modalities that require more frequent exchanges (less than 6-hour dwell time). See the ISPD guidelines for dosing recommendations for IP antibiotics in CAPD and automated PD patients.[42] The dose of the antibiotics should be increased by 25% for patients with residual kidney function who are able to produce more than 100-mL urine output per day.

Once the organism has been identified and sensitivities are known, drug selection should be adjusted to reflect the susceptibilities of the organism. Streptococcal, staphylococcal, and enterococcal species sensitive to β-lactam antibiotics should be treated with continuous IP dosing to increase efficacy and minimize resistance.[42] Peritonitis caused by *S. aureus* or *P. aeruginosa* are often associated with catheter-related infections, which are difficult to treat and often require removal of the catheter. Rifampin 600 mg orally daily (in a single or divided dose) may be added to IP vancomycin for the treatment of methicillin-resistant *S. aureus* (MRSA) but should be limited to duration of 1 week to minimize the development of resistance. Two antibiotics are required for treatment of *P. aeruginosa* peritonitis.[42] If multiple organisms are cultured, treatment should cover all of the organisms, including anaerobic organisms, and the patient should be evaluated for other intra-abdominal pathologies.[42]

Peritonitis caused by fungal organisms is associated with mortality in 25% of patients,[42] which can be reduced by removing the catheter after fungal organisms are identified. Empirical treatment should include IP amphotericin B and flucytosine.[42] Although IP amphotericin administration is associated with chemical irritation and pain, penetration of amphotericin into the peritoneal cavity is poor with IV administration. Fluconazole, voriconazole, or caspofungin may be suitable alternatives, depending on culture results.

Catheter-Related Infections Catheter-related infections generally occur at the exit site or the portion of the catheter that is tunneled in the subcutaneous tissue. Previous infections increase the risk and incidence of catheter-related infections.

Pathophysiology. The major pathologic organisms responsible for causing catheter-related infections are *S. aureus* and *P. aeruginosa*. These organisms also cause the most serious catheter-related infections. *S. epidermidis* is found in less than 20% of catheter-related infections. Other organisms include diphtheroids, anaerobic bacteria, *Legionella*, and fungi.[42]

Exit-site infections present with purulent drainage at the site. Erythema may or may not be present with an exit-site infection. Tunnel infections are generally extensions of exit-site infections and rarely occur alone. Symptoms of a tunnel infection may include tenderness, edema, and erythema over the tunnel pathway but are often asymptomatic. Ultrasound can be used to detect tunnel infections in asymptomatic patients. Exit-site infections caused by *S. aureus* and *P. aeruginosa* often spread to tunnel infections and are the most common causes of catheter-infection–related peritonitis.

Treatment. Exit-site infections may be treated immediately with empiric coverage, or treatment may be delayed until cultures return. Empiric treatment of catheter-related infections should cover *S. aureus*. Coverage for *P. aeruginosa* should also be included if the patient has a history of infections with this organism.[42] Cultures and sensitivity testing are particularly important in tailoring antibiotic therapy for catheter-related infections to ensure eradication of the organism and prevent recurrence or related peritonitis.

Less severe infections may be treated with topical antibiotic cream, although this practice is controversial. Oral antibiotics are also effective for treatment of catheter-related infections. Empiric or routine use of vancomycin for gram-positive infections should be avoided unless the infection is caused by MRSA. Rifampin may be added to therapy for severe infections or slowly resolving *S. aureus* infections, but monotherapy is not recommended.[42] Oral fluoroquinolones are used as first-line agents to treat *P. aeruginosa*, which can be difficult to treat and require prolonged treatment. If the infection is slow to resolve or if it recurs, IP ceftazidime or a second agent should be added.[42] Treatment of catheter-related infections should be continued until the exit site appears normal with no erythema or drainage. Generally, at least 2 weeks of therapy or longer are required to ensure complete eradication of the organism and prevent future recurrence, which is common with *S. aureus* and *P. aeruginosa*. Infections that do not resolve may require replacement of the PD catheter. Catheter-related infections that present in conjunction with or progress to peritonitis with the same organism require removal of the PD catheter until the peritonitis is resolved.[42]

Prophylaxis of Peritonitis and Catheter-Related Infections Prevention of peritonitis and catheter-related infections starts when the catheter is placed. The exit site should be properly cared for until it is well healed before it can be used for PD. Patients should receive proper instructions for care of the catheter during this time period, which can last up to 2 weeks. Patients should also be instructed on the proper techniques to use for dialysate exchanges to minimize the risk of infections during exchanges, which is the most common cause of peritonitis.

Intranasal *S. aureus* increases the risk of *S. aureus* exit-site infections, tunnel infections, peritonitis, and subsequent catheter loss.[43] Several measures have been used to decrease the risk of peritonitis caused by *S. aureus*, including mupirocin cream or ointment applied daily around the exit site, intranasal mupirocin cream twice daily for 5 days each month, or rifampin 300 mg orally twice daily for 5 days, repeated every 3 months.[42,43] Mupirocin use is preferred over rifampin to prevent the development of resistance to rifampin, although mupirocin resistance has also been reported.[42] Other measures that have been used to decrease both *S. aureus* and *P. aeruginosa* infections include gentamicin cream applied twice daily and ciprofloxacin otic solution applied daily to the exit site.[42]

Outcome Evaluation Clinical improvement should be seen within 48 hours of initiating treatment for peritonitis or catheter-related infections. Perform daily inspections of peritoneal fluid or the exit site to determine clinical improvement. Peritoneal fluid should become clear with improvement of peritonitis and erythema, and discharge should remit with improvement of catheter-related infections. If no improvement is seen within 48 hours, obtain additional cultures and cell counts to determine the appropriate alterations in therapy.

Patient Care Process: Chronic Kidney Disease

Patient Assessment:

- Determine if the patient should be evaluated for CKD. Does the patient have any risk factors for CKD? (see Table 26–3)
- Review medical and medication history. Does the patient have any concomitant diseases such as diabetes or hypertension that should be treated to prevent the progression of CKD? (see Table 26–3) Is the patient taking any medications that may contribute to kidney dysfunction?
- Review available laboratory tests to determine the staging of CKD (see Tables 26–1 and 26–2) and whether complications associated with CKD are present.

Therapy Evaluation:

- For DM, evaluate glucose and blood pressure control (see Figure 26–2).
- If proteinuria is present, determine if an ACE-I or ARB is appropriate for the patient. (see Figure 26–3).
- If anemia is present, determine other factors may be contributing to anemia of CKD (see Figure 26–4).
- If the patient has electrolyte or mineral imbalances, determine if medical therapy is necessary (see Figure 26–5).
- If the patient is already receiving pharmacotherapy, assess efficacy, safety, and patient adherence.
- For dialysis, determine if any dialysis complications are present (Tables 26–11, 26–12, and 26–13).

Care Plan Development:

- Select appropriate medical treatment to slow progression of CKD (see Figures 26–2 and 26–3).
- Select appropriate medical treatments to control complications of CKD, including anemia (see Figure 26–4, Tables 26–4 and 26–5); mineral and bone diseases (see Figure 26–5, Tables 26–7 and 26–8); and electrolyte imbalances.
- Ensure that all of the patient's medications are adjusted appropriately for his/her level of kidney function.
- Educate the patient on dietary and lifestyle changes to limit progression of CKD and manage electrolyte and mineral imbalances.
- Stress the importance of adherence with the treatments for CKD and associated complications, including lifestyle modifications and medications. Recommend a therapeutic regimen that is easy for the patient to accomplish.

Follow-Up Evaluation:

- Monitor serum creatinine and urine protein excretion at least annually in patients at risk for CKD.
- Monitor electrolyte and mineral levels and blood counts every 3 to 6 months or more frequently if patient requires treatment.

Abbreviations Introduced in This Chapter

2,3-DPG	2,3-Diphosphoglycerate
ACE-I	Angiotensin-converting enzyme inhibitor
AGE	Advanced glycation end-product
AKI	Acute kidney injury
APD	Automated peritoneal dialysis
ARB	Angiotensin receptor blocker
AVF	Arteriovenous fistula
AVG	Arteriovenous graft
BUN	Blood urea nitrogen
Ca–P	Calcium–phosphorus product
CAPD	Continuous ambulatory peritoneal dialysis
CCPD	Continuous cycling peritoneal dialysis
CHD	Coronary heart disease
CKD	Chronic kidney disease
CKD-MBD	Chronic kidney disease mineral and bone disease
CVD	Cardiovascular disease
DDAVP	Desmopressin
DKD	Diabetic kidney disease
DM	Diabetes mellitus
ECG	Electrocardiogram
EPO	Erythropoietin
ESA	Erythropoiesis-stimulating agent
FE_K	Fractional excretion of potassium
FE_{Na}	Fractional excretion of sodium
GFR	Glomerular filtration rate
GI	Gastrointestinal
HbA_{1c}	Hemoglobin A_{1c}
Hct	Hematocrit
HD	Hemodialysis
HDL-C	High-density lipoprotein cholesterol
Hgb	Hemoglobin
HMG-CoA	3-Hydroxy-3-methylglutaryl coenzyme A
IP	Intraperitoneal
iPTH	Intact parathyroid hormone
ISPD	International Society of Peritoneal Dialysis
KDIGO	Kidney Disease: Improving Global Outcomes
LDL-C	Low-density lipoprotein cholesterol
LVH	Left ventricular hypertrophy
MCHC	Mean corpuscular hemoglobin concentration
MCV	Mean corpuscular volume
MDRD	Modification of Diet in Renal Disease (study)
MRSA	Methicillin-resistant *Staphylococcus aureus*
NIPD	Nightly intermittent peritoneal dialysis
NKF	National Kidney Foundation
NKF-K/DOQI	National Kidney Foundation-Dialysis Outcome Quality Initiative
NTPD	Nocturnal tidal peritoneal dialysis
PD	Peritoneal dialysis
PTH	Parathyroid hormone
RBC	Red blood cell
ROD	Renal osteodystrophy
RRT	Renal replacement therapy
SC	Subcutaneous
SCr	Serum creatinine
sHPT	Secondary hyperparathyroidism
SPS	Sodium polystyrene sulfonate
TIBC	Total iron binding capacity
TSat	Transferrin saturation
USRDS	United States Renal Data Service

REFERENCES

1. Kidney Disease: Improving Global Outcomes (KDIGO) CKD Work Group. KDIGO 2012 Clinical Practice Guideline for the Evaluation and Management of Chronic Kidney Disease. Kidney Int Suppl. 2013;3:1–150.
2. National Kidney Foundation. K/DOQI clnical practice guidelines for chronic kidney disease: Evaluation, classification, and stratification. AM J Kidney Dis. 2002;39:S1–S266.
3. U.S. Renal Data System (USRDS). USRDS 2014 annual data report: An overview of the epidemiology of kidney disease in the United States. *National Institutes of Health, National Institute of Diabetes and Digestive and Kidney Diseases.* Bethesda, MD, 2014.
4. Attman PO, Samuelsson O. Dyslipidemia of kidney disease. Curr Opin Lipidol. 2009;20(4):293–299.
5. Tsimihodimos V, Dounousi E, Siamopoulos KC. Dyslipidemia in chronic kidney disease: An approach to pathogenesis and treatment. Am J Nephrol. 2008;28(6):958–973.
6. Steinke JM. The natural progression of kidney injury in young type 1 diabetic patients. Curr Diab Rep. 2009;9(6):473–479.
7. Kalaitzidis R, Bakris G. Pathogenesis and treatment of microalbuminuria in patients with diabetes: The road ahead. J Clin Hypertens. 2009;11(11):636–643.
8. Telda FM, Brar A, Browne R, Brown C. Hypertension in chronic kidney disease: navigating the evidence. Int J Hypertens. 2011; 2011:132405. doi: 10.4061/2011/132405.
9. Hemmelgarn BR, Manns, BJ, Lloyd A, et al. Relation between kidney function, proteinuria, and adverse outcomes. JAMA. 2010;303(5):423–429.
10. Bakris GL. A practical approach to achieving recommended blood pressure goals in diabetic patients. Arch Int Med. 2001;161:2661–2667.
11. D.Agati V, Schmidt AM. RAGE and the pathogenesis of chronic kidney disease. Nat Rev Nephrol. 2010;6:352–360.
12. Heung M, Chawla LS. Predicting progression to chronic kidney disease after recovery from acute kidney injury. Curr Opin Nephrol Hypertens 2012;21(6):628–634.
13. López-Novoa J, Martínez-Salgado C, Rodríguez-Peña AB, Hernández FJL. Common pathophysiological mechanisms of chronic kidney disease: Therapeutic perspectives. Pharmacol Ther. 2010;128(1):61–81.
14. National Kidney Foundation. KDOQI clinical practice guidelines and clinical practice recommendations for diabetes and chronic kidney disease. Am J Kidney Dis. 2007;49(2 Suppl 2):S12–S154.
15. Fouque D, Aparicio M. Eleven reasons to control the protein intake of patients with chronic kidney disease. Nat Clin Pract Nephrol. 2007;3(7):383–392.
16. Ikizler TA, Cano NJ, Franch H, et al. Prevention and treatment of protein energy wasting in chronic kidney disease patients: A consensus statement by the International Society of Renal Nutrition and Metabolism. Kidney Int. 2013;84(6):1096–1107.
17. Kidney Disease: Improving Global Outcomes (KDIGO) Blood Pressure Work Group. KDIGO Clinical Practice Guideline for the Management of Blood Pressure in Chronic Kidney Disease. Kidney Int Suppl. 2012;2:337–414.
18. Robinson BM, Tong L, Zhang J, et al. Blood pressure levels and mortality risk among hemodialysis patients in the Dialysis Outcomes and Practice Patterns Study. Kidney Int. 2012; 82(5):570–580.
19. Agarwal R. Blood pressure and mortality among hemodialysis patients. Hypertension. 2010;55:762–768.
20. Hermida RC, Ayala DE, Mojón A, Fernández JR. Bedtime dosing of antihypertensive medications reduces cardiovascular risk in CKD. J Am Soc Nephrol. 2011;22(12):2313–2321.
21. Bakris GL. Slowing nephropathy progression: Focus on proteinuria reduction. Clin J Am Soc Nephrol. 2008;3 (Suppl):S3–S10.
22. Acri M, Erdem Y. Dual blockade of the renin-angiotensin system for cardiorenal protection: An update. Am J Kidney Dis. 2009;53(2):332–345.
23. Mann JFE, Schmieder RE, McQueen M, et al. Renal outcomes with telmisartan, ramipril, or both, in people at high vascular risk (the ONTARGET study): A multicenter, randomized, double-blind, controlled trial. Lancet. 2008;372:547–553.
24. Kalaitzidis RG, Bakris GL. Should proteinuria reduction be the criterion for antihypertensive drug selection for patients with kidney disease? Curr Opin Nephrol. 2009;18:386–391.
25. Kidney Disease: Improving Global Outcomes (KDIGO) Lipid Work Group. KDIGO Clinical Practice Guideline for Lipid Management in Chronic Kidney Disease. Kidney Int Suppl. 2013; 3:259–305.
26. Hörl WH. Anaemia management and mortality risk in chronic kidney disease. Nat Rev Nephrol. 2013;9:291–301.
27. Kidney Disease: Improving Global Outcomes. KDIGO clinical practice guideline for anemia in chronic kidney disease. Kidney Int Suppl. 2012;2(4):279–335.
28. Stauffer ME, Fan T (2014) Prevalence of Anemia in Chronic Kidney Disease in the United States. PLoS ONE. 9(1): e84943. doi:10.1371/journal.pone.0084943.
29. Drueke TB, Loctelli F, Clyne N, et al. Normalization of hemoglobin level in patients with chronic kidney disease and anemia. N Engl J Med. 2006;335(20):2071–2084.
30. Singh AK. What is causing the mortality in treating the anemia of chronic kidney disease: Erythropoietin dose or hemoglobin level? Curr Opin Nephrol Hypertens. 2010;19(5):420–424.
31. KDIGO clinical practice guideline for the diagnosis, evaluation, prevention, and treatment of chronic kidney disease-mineral and bone disorder (CKD-MBD). Kidney Int. 2009;76 (Suppl 113):S1–S130.
32. Saliba W, El-Haddad B. Secondary hyperparathyroidism: Pathophysiology and treatment. J Am Board Fam Med. 2009; 22(5):574–581.
33. Kraut JA, Madias NE. Consequences and therapy of the metabolic acidosis of chronic kidney disease. Pediatr Nephrol. 2011;26:19–28.
34. National Kidney Foundation. K/DOQI clinical practice guidelines for bone metabolism and disease in chronic kidney disease. Am J Kidney Dis. 2003;42(Suppl 3):S1–S202.
35. Ketteler M, Biggar PH. Use of phosphate binders in chronic kidney disease. Curr Opin Nephrol Hypertens. 2013;22;413–420.
36. Nastou D, Fernández-Fernández B, Elewa U, et al. Next-generation phosphate binders: focus on iron-based binders. Drugs 2014;74:863–877.
37. Nigwekar SU, Bhan I, Thadhani R. Ergocalciferol and cholecalciferol in CKD. Am J Kidney Dis. 2011;60(1):139–156.
38. Shemin D, Dworkin LD. Sodium balance in renal failure. Curr Opin Nephrol Hyperten. 1997;6(2):128–132.
39. Musso CG. Potassium metabolism in patients with chronic kidney disease (CKD), part I: Patients not on dialysis (stages 3–4). Int Urol Nephrol. 2004;36:465–468.
40. Davenport A. Intradialytic complications during hemodialysis. Hemodial Int. 2006;10(2):162–167.
41. KDIGO clinical practice guidelines and clinical practice recommendations recommendations for 2006 updates: Hemodialysis adequacy, peritoneal dialysis adequacy and vascular access. Am J Kidney Dis 2006;48 (Suppl 1) :S1–S322.
42. Li PKT, Szeto CC, Piraino B, et al. ISPD guidelines/recommendations: Peritoneal dialysis-related infections recommendations: 2010 update. Perit Dial Int. 2010;30(4):393–423.
43. Piraino B, Bernardini J, Brown E, et al. ISPD position statement on reducing the risks of peritoneal dialysis-related infections. Perit Dial Int. 2011;31(6):614–630.

27 Fluids and Electrolytes

Mark A. Malesker and Lee E. Morrow

LEARNING OBJECTIVES

Upon completion of the chapter, the reader will be able to:

1. Estimate the volumes of various body fluid compartments.
2. Calculate the daily maintenance fluid requirement for patients given their weight and gender.
3. Differentiate among currently available fluids for volume resuscitation.
4. Identify the electrolytes primarily found in the extracellular and intracellular fluid compartments.
5. Describe the unique relationship between serum sodium concentration and total body water (TBW).
6. Review the etiology, clinical presentation, and management for disorders of sodium, potassium, calcium, phosphorus, and magnesium.

BODY FLUID COMPARTMENTS

A thorough understanding of the fundamentals of fluid and electrolyte homeostasis is essential given the frequency with which clinical disturbances are seen and the profound effects these disturbances can have on various aspects of patient care. However, the interplay of body fluids, serum electrolytes, and clinical monitoring is complex, and a thorough command of these issues is a challenging task even for advanced practitioners.[1] Practitioners must be familiar with the key concepts of body compartment volumes, calculation of daily fluid requirements, and the various types of fluid available for replacement. The management of disorders of sodium, potassium, calcium, phosphorus, and magnesium integrates these concepts with issues of dose recognition and patient safety.

The most fundamental concept to grasp is an assessment of total body water (TBW), which is directly related to body weight. KEY CONCEPT *TBW constitutes approximately 50% of lean body weight in healthy females and 60% of lean body weight in males. For clinical purposes, most clinicians generalize that total body water accounts for 60% of lean body weight in adults, regardless of gender.* The percentage of TBW decreases as body fat increases and/or with age (75%–85% of body weight is water for newborns). Unless the patient is obese (body weight greater than 120% of ideal body weight [IBW]), clinicians typically use a patient's actual body weight when calculating TBW.[2] In obese patients, it is customary to estimate TBW using lean body weight or IBW as calculated by the Devine–Devine method: males' lean body weight = 50 kg + (2.3 kg/in. × [height in inches − 60]) and females' lean body weight = 45.5 kg + (2.3 kg/in. × [height in inches − 60]).[3–5] Note that 1 kg is equivalent to 2.2 lb, 1 inch is equivalent to 2.54 cm, and 1 L of water weighs 1 kg (2.2 lb).

The intracellular fluid (ICF) represents the water contained within cells and is rich in electrolytes such as potassium, magnesium, phosphates, and proteins. KEY CONCEPT *The ICF is approximately two-thirds of TBW regardless of gender.* For a 70-kg person, this would mean that the TBW is 42 L and the ICF is approximately 28 L. Note that ICF represents approximately 40% of total body weight.

The extracellular fluid (ECF) is the fluid outside the cell and is rich in sodium, chloride, and bicarbonate. KEY CONCEPT *The ECF is approximately one-third of TBW (14 L in a 70-kg person) and is subdivided into two compartments: the interstitial fluid and the intravascular fluid.* The interstitial fluid represents the fluid occupying the spaces between cells and is about 25% of TBW (10.5 L in a 70-kg person). The intravascular fluid (also known as plasma) represents the fluid within the blood vessels and is about 8% of TBW (3.4 L in a 70-kg person). Because the exact percentages are cumbersome to recall, many clinicians accept that the ECF represents roughly 20% of body weight (regardless of gender) with 15% in the interstitial space and 5% in the intravascular space.[6] Note that serum electrolytes are routinely measured from the ECF.

The transcellular fluid includes the viscous components of the peritoneum, pleural space, and pericardium, as well as the cerebrospinal fluid, joint space fluid, and the GI digestive juices. Although the transcellular fluid normally accounts for about 1% of TBW, this amount can increase significantly during various illnesses favoring fluid collection in one of these spaces (eg, pleural effusions or ascites in the peritoneum). The accumulation of fluid in the transcellular space is often referred to as "third spacing." To review the calculations of the body fluid compartments in a representative patient, see Patient Encounter 1.

Fluid balance is assessed by several means each of which has its limitations. Blood pressure (BP) measurements estimate fluid status relative to the amount of blood volume pumped by the heart but are affected by cardiac function and vascular pliability. Patients with significant volume deficiency may appear hypotensive, but this is a late finding that may require greater than 20% of TBW to be lost. Patients with significant volume excess may appear edematous; however, third spacing may hide this finding

Patient Encounter 1: Body Fluid Compartments

Calculate the total body water, ICF, and ECF in a 75 kg man.

Patient Encounter 2: Fluid Requirements

Calculate the daily fluid requirement for an 80 kg adult man.

until late in the course as well. The physical examination can indicate the presence of fluid deficits (dry mucous membranes) and fluid excess (peripheral edema, coarse breath sounds). More invasive assessments would include the use of an arterial catheter, a pulmonary artery catheter to measure left ventricular function and fluid status, and a central venous catheter that measures fluid status and right ventricular function. However, the correlation between these measured pressures and their associated volume is an area of debate.

To maintain fluid balance, the total amount of fluid gained throughout the day (input, or "ins") must equal the total amount of fluid lost (output, or "outs"). Although most forms of the body's input and output can be measured, several cannot. For a normal adult on an average diet, ingested fluids are easily measured and average 1400 mL/day. Other fluid inputs, such as those from ingested foods and the water by-product of oxidation, are not directly measurable. Fluid outputs such as urinary and stool losses are also easily measured and referred to as sensible losses. Other sources of fluid loss, such as evaporation of fluid through the skin and/or lungs, are not readily measured and are called insensible losses. Table 27–1 shows the estimated ins and outs (I&Os) for a healthy 68-kg (150-lb) man.[6] The measurable I&Os are routinely measured in hospitalized patients and are used to estimate total fluid balance for each 24-hour period. It is important to realize that in hospitalized patients, multiple other forms of fluid loss must be considered. These include losses from enteric suctioning (most commonly, nasogastric [NG] tubes), from surgical drains (eg, chest tubes, nephrostomy tubes, and pancreatic drains), via fistulous tracts, and enhanced evaporative losses (burns and fever).

TBW depletion (often referred to as "dehydration") is typically a gradual, chronic problem. Because TBW depletion represents a loss of hypotonic fluid (proportionally more water is lost than sodium) from all body compartments, a primary disturbance of osmolality is usually seen. The signs and symptoms of TBW depletion include CNS disturbances (mental status changes, seizures, and coma), excessive thirst, dry mucous membranes, decreased skin turgor, elevated serum sodium, increased plasma osmolality, concentrated urine, and acute weight loss. Common causes of TBW depletion include insufficient oral intake, excessive insensible losses, diabetes insipidus, excessive osmotic diuresis, and impaired renal concentrating mechanisms. Elderly long-term care residents are frequently admitted to the acute care hospital with TBW depletion secondary to lack of adequate oral intake, often with concurrent excessive insensible losses.

The volume of fluid required to correct TBW depletion equals the basal fluid requirement plus ongoing exceptional losses plus the fluid deficit. Basal daily fluid requirements are calculated using the formulas in Table 27–2. For an adult, this represents 1500 mL/day for the first 20 kg of body weight plus 20 mL/day for each additional kilogram. The volume of replacement fluids required for a given patient (the fluid deficit) can be estimated by the acute weight change in the patient (1 kg = 1 L of fluid). Because the precise weight change is not typically known, it is often calculated as follows: fluid deficit = normal TBW – present TBW. Normal TBW is estimated based on the patient's weight using the formulas in Table 27–2, and the present TBW is estimated based on the patient's current body weight. The choice of fluids used for replacement is guided by the presence of concurrent electrolyte abnormalities. The adequacy of replacement is guided by each patient's objective response to fluid replacement (improved skin turgor, adequate urine output, normalization of heart rate, BP, etc).

Once TBW has been restored, the volume of "maintenance" fluid equals the basal fluid requirement plus ongoing exceptional losses. If the pathophysiologic process leading to TBW depletion has not been identified and corrected (or accounted for in the calculation of maintenance fluid requirements), TBW depletion will quickly recur. To review the concepts involved in the calculation of replacement fluids for a representative patient, see Patient Encounter 2.

Compared with TBW depletion, ECF depletion tends to occur acutely. In this setting, rapid and aggressive fluid replacement is required to maintain adequate organ perfusion. Because ECF depletion is generally due to the loss of isotonic fluid (proportional losses of sodium and water), major disturbances of plasma osmolality are not common. ECF depletion manifests clinically as signs and symptoms associated with decreased tissue perfusion: dizziness, orthostasis, tachycardia, decreased urine output, increased hematocrit, decreased central venous pressure, and/or hypovolemic shock. Common causes of ECF depletion include external fluid losses (burns, hemorrhage, diuresis, GI losses, and adrenal insufficiency) and third spacing of fluids (septic shock, anaphylactic shock, or abdominal ascites).

In clinical practice, the most commonly encountered problem is depletion of TBW and ECF. Accordingly, the fluid resuscitation strategy should address both of these compartments. As these

Table 27–1

Approximate I&Os for a Healthy 68-kg (150-lb) Man

Input	mL/day	Output	mL/day
Ingested fluid[a]	1400	Urine[a]	1500
Fluid in food	850	Skin losses	500
Water of oxidation	350	Respiratory tract losses	400
		Stool	200
Total	2600	Total	2600

[a]Readily quantifiable.

Table 27–2

Useful Calculations for the Estimation of Patient Maintenance Fluid Requirements

Neonate (1–10 kg) = 100 mL/kg
Child (10–20 kg) = 1000 mL + 50 mL for each kilogram > 10
Adult (> 20 kg) = 1500 mL + 20 mL for each kilogram > 20

compartments are repleted, serum electrolytes must be monitored closely as discussed in subsequent sections of this chapter.

THERAPEUTIC FLUIDS

Crystalloids

KEY CONCEPT *Therapeutic IV fluids include crystalloid solutions and colloidal solutions.* Crystalloids are composed of water and electrolytes, all of which pass freely through semipermeable membranes and remain in the intravascular space for shorter periods of time. As such, these solutions are very useful for correcting electrolyte imbalances but result in smaller hemodynamic changes for a given unit of volume.

Crystalloids can be classified further according to their tonicity. Isotonic solutions (ie, normal saline or 0.9% sodium chloride [NaCl]) have a tonicity equal to that of the ICF (approximately 310 mEq/L or 310 mmol/L) and do not shift the distribution of water between the ECF and the ICF. Because hypertonic solutions (eg, hypertonic saline or 3% NaCl) have greater tonicity than the ICF (greater than 376 mEq/L or 376 mmol/L), they draw water from the ICF into the ECF. In contrast, hypotonic solutions (eg, 0.45% NaCl) have less tonicity than the ICF (less than 250 mEq/L or 250 mmol/L) leading to osmotic pressure gradient that favors shifts of water from the ECF into the ICF. The tonicity, electrolyte content, and glucose content of selected fluids are shown in Table 27–3.

The tonicity of crystalloid solutions is directly related to their sodium concentration. The most commonly used crystalloids include normal saline, dextrose/half-normal saline, hypertonic saline, and lactated Ringer's solution. Excessive administration of any fluid replacement therapy, regardless of tonicity, can lead to fluid overload, particularly in patients with cardiac or renal insufficiency. Glucose is often added to hypotonic crystalloids in amounts that result in isotonic fluids (D_5W, D5½NS, and D5¼NS). These solutions are often used as maintenance fluids to provide basal amounts of calories and water.

▶ *Normal Saline (0.9% NaCl or NS)*

Normal saline is an isotonic fluid composed of water, sodium, and chloride. It provides primarily ECF replacement and can be used for virtually any cause of TBW depletion. Common uses of normal saline include perioperative fluid administration; volume resuscitation of shock, sepsis, hemorrhage, or burn patients; fluid challenges in hypotensive or oliguric patients; and hyponatremia. Normal saline can also be used to treat metabolic alkalosis (also known as contraction alkalosis). Large volumes of normal saline can cause a hyperchloremic metabolic acidosis.

▶ *Half-Normal Saline (0.45% NaCl or ½ NS)*

Half-normal saline is a hypotonic fluid that provides free water in relative excess when compared with the sodium concentration. This crystalloid is typically used to treat patients who are hypertonic due to primary depletion of the ECF. Because half-normal saline is hypotonic, serum sodium must be closely monitored during administration.

▶ *5% Dextrose/Half-Normal Saline (D5 ½ NS)*

D5 ½ NS is a hypotonic fluid that is commonly used as a maintenance fluid. This crystalloid is typically used once fluids deficits have been corrected with normal saline or lactated Ringer's solution. Because half-normal saline is hypotonic, serum sodium must be closely monitored during administration.

Table 27–3

Electrolyte and Dextrose Content of Selected Crystalloid Fluids

IV Solution	Osmolarity (mOsm or mmol)	Dextrose (g/L) mmol/L	Sodium (mEq/L) mmol/L	Potassium (mEq/L) mmol/L	Calcium (mEq/L) mmol/L	Chloride (mEq/L) mmol/L	Lactate (mEq/L) mmol/L
D5%	250	50 2.78					
D10%	505	100 5.55					
0.9% NaCl	308		154			154	
0.45% NaCl	154		77			77	
3% NaCl	1025		512			512	
D5% and 0.45% NaCl	405	50 2.78	77			77	
D5% and 0.2% NaCl	329	50 2.78	34			34	
Ringer's injection	310		147	4	5 2.5	156	
Lactated Ringer's solution	274		130	4	3 1.5	109	28
Lactated Ringer's solution and D5%	525	50 2.78	130	4	3 1.5	109	28

D, dextrose; NaCl, sodium chloride.

▶ *Hypertonic Saline (3% NaCl)*

Hypertonic saline is obviously hypertonic and provides a significant sodium load to the intravascular space. This solution is used very infrequently given the potential to cause significant shifts in the water balance between the ECF and the ICF. It is typically used to treat patients with severe hyponatremia who have symptoms attributable to low serum sodium. Hypertonic saline in concentrations of 7.5% to 23.4% has been used to acutely lower intracranial pressure in the setting of traumatic brain injury and stroke. The literature is inconsistent for the optimal hypertonic concentration, dosing, timing of replacement, and goals for use in this population. Serum sodium and neurologic status must be very closely monitored whenever given.

▶ *Ringer's Lactate*

This isotonic volume expander contains sodium, potassium, chloride, and lactate in concentrations that approximate the fluid and electrolyte composition of the blood. Ringer's lactate (also known as "Lactated Ringers," or LR) provides ECF replacement and is most often used in the perioperative setting and for patients with lower GI fluid losses, burns, or dehydration. The lactate component of LR works as a buffer to increase the pH. Accordingly, large volumes of LR may cause iatrogenic metabolic alkalosis. Because patients with significant liver disease are unable to metabolize lactate sufficiently, LR administration in this population may lead to accumulation of lactate with iatrogenic lactic acidosis.

▶ *5% Dextrose in Water (D_5W)*

D_5W solution is a combination of free water and dextrose that provides a modest amount of calories but no electrolytes. Although it is technically isotonic, it acts as a hypotonic solution in the body. It is commonly used to treat severe hypernatremia. D_5W is also used in small volumes (100 mL) to dilute many IV medications or at a low infusion rate (10–15 mL/hour) to "keep the vein open" (KVO) for IV medications.

Colloids

In contrast to crystalloids, colloids do not dissolve into a true solution and therefore do not pass readily across semipermeable membranes. As such, colloids effectively remain in the intravascular space and increase the oncotic pressure of the plasma. This effectively shifts fluid from the interstitial compartment to the intravascular compartment. In clinical practice, these theoretical benefits are generally short lived (given metabolism of colloidal proteins/sugars), and for most patients there is little therapeutic advantage of colloids over crystalloids or vice versa. Examples of colloids include 5% albumin, 25% albumin, the dextrans, hetastarch, and fresh-frozen plasma (FFP). Because each of these agents contains a substance (proteins and complex sugars) that will ultimately be metabolized, the oncotic agent will be ultimately lost and only the remaining hypotonic fluid delivery agent will remain. As such, use of large volumes of colloidal agents is more likely to induce fluid overload compared with crystalloids. Although smaller volumes of colloids have equal efficacy as larger volumes of crystalloids, they generally must be infused more slowly. Often the net result is that the time to clinical benefit is the same regardless of which class of fluid is utilized. For example, 500 mL of normal saline is required to increase the systolic BP to the same degree as seen with approximately 250 mL of 5% albumin; however, the normal saline can be administered twice as fast.

▶ *Albumin*

Albumin is a protein derived from fractionating human plasma. Because albumin infusion is expensive and may be associated with adverse events, it should be used for acute volume expansion and *not* as a supplemental source of protein calories. Historically, albumin was used indiscriminately in the intensive care unit until anecdotal publications suggested that albumin may cause immunosuppression. However, the Saline Versus Albumin Fluid Evaluation (SAFE) trial randomized nearly 7000 hypovolemic patients to either albumin or normal saline therapy and found that the mortality for those who received albumin was the same as for those who received normal saline.[7] A subsequent post hoc analysis reported that patients with traumatic brain injury had higher mortality rates when given albumin for fluid resuscitation. These conflicting findings highlight the controversy and confusion surrounding the use of human albumin versus normal saline therapy for resuscitation of critically ill patients.[8–9] In 1818 patients with severe sepsis, albumin replacement with crystalloids as compared to crystalloids alone did not improve the rate of survival at 28 and 90 days.[10]

Based on limited availability, health systems and hospitals have had to define the appropriate albumin indications for their patients and ration albumin accordingly. Evidence-based indications for albumin include plasmapheresis/apheresis, large-volume paracentesis (greater than 4 L removed), hypotension in hemodialysis, and the need for aggressive diuresis in hypoalbuminemic hypotensive patients. Inappropriate uses of albumin include nutritional supplementation, impending hepatorenal syndrome, pancreatitis, alteration of drug pharmacokinetics, or acute normovolemic hemodilution in surgery. Practitioners can keep up with medication shortages by checking the American Society of Health-System Pharmacists (ASHP) Web site—www.ashp.org.

▶ *Hydroxyethyl Starch Solutions and Dextran*

While albumin is the most commonly used colloid, the other available products are not without their own risks and benefits. Hydroxyetyl starch solutions (HES) include Hetastarch (various manufacturers) and Voluven, Hospira, contain 6% starch and 0.9% NaCl. Hextend, Hospira, is a comparable plasma expander that contains 6% hetastarch in lactated electrolyte solution. HES products have no oxygen-carrying capacity and are administered intravenously as plasma expanders. Limitations of these products include acquisition cost, hypersensitivity reactions, and bleeding. Dosing should be reduced in the presence of renal dysfunction. Recent clinical data linking HES solutions with an increased risk of mortality and renal injury requiring renal replacement therapy in critically ill patients prompted the FDA to issue a MedWatch safety communication in November 2013. FDA concluded these solutions should not be used in critically ill patients, including sepsis and those admitted to the intensive care unit, and a boxed warning to highlight the risk of mortality and severe renal injury is warranted. A list of recommendations for patients and health care providers to consider before use of HES solutions can be found on the FDA website. (http://www.fda.gov/Safety/MedWatch/)

Low-molecular-weight dextran (various manufacturers) and high-molecular-weight dextran (various manufacturers) are polysaccharide plasma expanders. Anaphylactic reactions and prolonged bleeding times have limited the use of these products. Potential mechanisms of colloid solution-induced bleeding include platelet inhibition or possible dilution of clotting factors via infusion of a large-volume colloid solution.

A recent Cochrane review regarding the use of colloids versus crystalloids for fluid resuscitation in critically ill patients found no evidence from randomized clinical trials that resuscitation with colloids reduces the risk of death in patients with trauma, burns or following surgery. Additionally, the use of HES might be associated with mortality and given the lack of survival benefit and increased expense over crystalloids the continued of use of colloids is limited.[11]

Fluid Management Strategies

Classic indications for IV fluid include maintenance of BP, restoring the ICF volume, replacing ongoing renal or insensible losses when oral intake is inadequate, and the need for glucose as a fuel for the brain.[12] Although large volumes of fluid are given during the resuscitation of most trauma patients, a recent analysis reported uncertainty about the use of early large-volume fluid replacement in patients with active bleeding, calling into question our understanding of the need for fluids in various patient populations.[13]

When determining the appropriate fluid to be utilized, it is important to first determine the type of fluid problem (TBW vs ECF depletion), and start therapy accordingly. For patients demonstrating signs of impaired tissue perfusion, the immediate therapeutic goal is to increase the intravascular volume and restore tissue perfusion. The standard therapy is normal saline given at 150 to 500 mL/hour (for adult patients) until perfusion is optimized. Although LR is a therapeutic alternative, lactic acidosis may arise with massive or prolonged infusions. LR has less chloride content versus normal saline (109 mEq/L [109 mmol/L] vs 154 mEq/L [154 mmol/L]) and has the advantage of use when large volumes of normal saline produce acidosis during fluid resuscitation. In severe cases, a colloid or blood transfusion may be indicated to increase oncotic pressure within the vascular space. Once euvolemia is achieved, patients may be switched to a more hypotonic maintenance solution (D5½ NS or 0.45% NaCl) at a rate that delivers estimated daily needs.

The clinical scenario and the severity of the volume abnormality dictate monitoring parameters during fluid replacement therapy. These may include the subjective sense of thirst, mental status, skin turgor, orthostatic vital signs, pulse rate, weight changes, blood chemistries, fluid input and output, central venous pressure, pulmonary capillary wedge pressure, and cardiac output. Fluid replacement requires particular caution in patient populations at risk of fluid overload, such as those with renal failure, cardiac failure, hepatic failure, or the elderly. Other complications of parenteral fluid therapy include IV site infiltration, infection, phlebitis, thrombophlebitis, and extravasation.

In summary, common settings for fluid resuscitation include hypovolemic patients (eg, sepsis or pneumonia), hypervolemic patients (eg, congestive heart failure [CHF], cirrhosis, or renal failure), euvolemic patients who are unable to take oral fluids in proportion to insensible losses (eg, the perioperative period), and patients with electrolyte abnormalities (see below).

ELECTROLYTES

Normally, the number of anions (negatively charged ions) and cations (positively charged ions) in each fluid compartment are equal. Cell membranes play the critical role of maintaining distinct ICF and ECF spaces, which are biochemically distinct. Serum electrolyte measurements reflect the stores of ECF electrolytes rather than that of ICF electrolytes. Table 27–4 lists the chief cations and anions along with their normal concentrations in the ECF and ICF. The principal cations are sodium, potassium, calcium, and magnesium; the key anions are chloride, bicarbonate, and phosphate. In the ECF, sodium is the most common cation and chloride is the most abundant anion; in the ICF, potassium is the primary cation and phosphate is the main anion. Normal serum electrolyte values are listed in Table 27–5.

Table 27–4

Normal Cation and Anion Concentrations in the ECF and ICF

	ECF		ICF	
Ion Species	Plasma (mEq/L [mmol/L])	Interstitial Fluid (mEq/L [mmol/L])	Ion Species	mEq/L [mmol/L]
Cations			Cations	
Na^+	142 [142]	144 [144]	K^+	135 [135]
K^+	4 [4]	4 [4]	Mg^{2+}	43 [21.5]
Ca^{2+}	5 [2.5]	2.5 [1.25]		
Mg^{2+}	3 [1.5]	1.5 [0.75]		
Total	154 [150]	152 [150]	Total	178 [156.5]
Anions			Anions	
Cl^-	103 [103]	114 [114]	PO_4^{2-}	90 [45]
HCO_3^-	27 [27]	30 [30]	Protein	70 [70]
PO_4^{2-}	2 [1]	2 [1]	SO_4^{2-}	18 [9]
SO_4^{2-}	1 [0.5]	1 [0.5]		
Organic acid	5 [5]	5 [5]		
Protein	16 [16]	0		
Total	154 [152.5]	152 [150.5]	Total	178 [124]

ECF, extracellular fluid; ICF, intracellular fluid.

Osmolality is a measure of the number of osmotically active particles per unit of solution, independent of the weight or nature of the particle. Equimolar concentrations of all substances in the undissociated state exert the same osmotic pressure. Although the normal serum osmolality is 280 to 300 mOsm/kg (280–300 mmol/kg), multiple scenarios exist where this value becomes markedly abnormal. KEY CONCEPT *The calculated serum osmolality helps determine deviations in TBW content.* As such, it is often useful to calculate the serum osmolality as follows:

Serum **osmolality** (mOsm/kg) =
2 (Na mEq/L) + (glucose [mg/dL])/18 + (BUN [mg/dL])/2.8.

Serum osmolality using SI units (mmol/kg) =
2 (Na mmol/L) + (glucose mmol/L) + (BUN mmol/L)/2.8.

Table 27–5

Normal Ranges for Serum Electrolyte Concentrations

Sodium	135–145 mEq/L or 135–145 mmol/L
Potassium	3.5–5.0 mEq/L or 3.5–5.0 mmol/L
Chloride	98–106 mEq/L or 98–106 mmol/L
Bicarbonate	21–30 mEq/L or 21–30 mmol/L
Magnesium	1.4–2.2 mEq/L or 0.7–1.1 mmol/L
Calcium:	
Total	4.4–5.2 mEq/L (9–10.5 mg/dL) or 2.2–2.6 mmol/L
Ionized	2.2–2.8 mEq/L (4.5–5.6 mg/dL) or 1.1–1.4 mmol/L
Phosphorus	3–4.5 mg/dL (1.0–1.5 mmol/L)

Patient Encounter 3: Calculate the Plasma Osmolality

A 50-year-old homeless man is brought to the emergency department staggering and smelling like beer. Rapid respiration, tachycardia, and a BP of 90/60 mm Hg were noted. The sodium is 140 mEq/L (140 mmol/L), potassium 3.6 mEq/L (3.6 mmol/L), chloride 100 mEq/L (100 mmol/L), bicarbonate 12 mEq/L (12 mmol/L), glucose 200 mg/dL (11.1 mmol/L), and BUN 28 mg/dL (10.0 mmol/L). The measured osmolarity is 360 mOsm/kg (360 mmol/kg).

Calculate the osmolality.

Calculate the osmolar gap.

What is the likely cause of an increased gap in this patient?

Because the body regulates water to maintain osmolality, deviations in serum osmolality are used to estimate TBW stores. Water moves freely across all cell membranes, making serum osmolality an accurate reflection of the osmolality within all body compartments. An increase in osmolality is equated with a loss of water greater than the loss of solute (TBW depletion). A decrease in serum osmolality is seen when water is retained in excess of solute (CHF or hepatic cirrhosis). The difference between the measured serum osmolality and the calculated serum osmolality, using the equation just stated, is referred to as the **osmolar gap**. Under normal circumstances the osmolar gap should be 10 mOsm/kg (10 mmol/kg) or less. An increased osmolar gap suggests the presence of a small osmotically active agent and is most commonly seen with the ingestion of alcohols (ethanol, methanol, ethylene glycol, or isopropyl alcohol) or medications such as mannitol or lorazepam. Patient Encounter 3 illustrates the utility of serum osmolality in a clinical setting.

Many of the electrolyte disturbances discussed in the remainder of this chapter represent medical emergencies that call for aggressive interventions including the use of concentrated electrolytes. It is very difficult to immediately reverse the effects of concentrated electrolytes when they are administered improperly, and these solutions are a frequent source of medical errors with significant potential for patient harm. KEY CONCEPT *As such, The Joint Commission recommends that concentrated electrolyte solutions (KCl, potassium phosphate, and NaCl greater than 0.9%) be removed from patient care areas.* Hospitals should keep concentrated electrolytes in patient care areas only when patient safety necessitates their immediate use and precautions are used to prevent inadvertent administration. Collaborative cooperation among pharmacists, nurses, and physicians is essential. In addition, The Joint Commission recommends standardizing and limiting the number of drug concentrations available in each institution and the use of ready-to-administer dosage forms so as to further reduce the risk of medication errors and improve outcomes.[14]

Sodium

The body's normal daily sodium requirement is 1.0 to 1.5 mEq/kg (1.0–1.5 mmol/kg) (80–130 mEq [80–130 mmol]) to maintain a normal serum sodium concentration of 135 to 145 mEq/L (135–145 mmol/L). Sodium is the predominant cation of the ECF and largely determines ECF volume. Sodium is also the primary factor in establishing the osmotic pressure relationship between the ICF and ECF. All body fluids are in osmotic equilibrium, and changes in serum sodium concentration are associated with shifts of water into and out of body fluid compartments. When sodium is added to the intravascular fluid compartment, fluid is pulled intravascularly from the interstitial fluid and the ICF until osmotic balance is restored. As such, a patient's measured sodium concentration should *not* be viewed as an index of sodium need because this parameter reflects the balance between total body sodium content and TBW. Disturbances in the sodium concentration most often represent disturbances of TBW. Sodium imbalances cannot be properly assessed without first assessing body fluid status.

KEY CONCEPT *Hyponatremia is the most common electrolyte disorder in hospitalized patients and defined as a serum sodium concentration below 135 mEq/L (135 mmol/L).* Clinical signs and symptoms appear at concentrations below 120 mEq/L (120 mmol/L) and typically consist of irritability, mental slowing, unstable gait/falls fatigue, headache, and nausea. With profound hyponatremia (less than 110 mEq/L [110 mmol/L]), confusion, seizures, stupor/coma, and respiratory arrest may be seen. Clinical practice guidelines regarding the diagnosis and treatment of hyponatremia have recently been published. Hyponatremia can be classified based upon serum sodium concentration, rate of development, symptom severity, serum osmolality, and volume status.[15] Because therapy is also influenced by volume status, hyponatremia is further defined as (a) hypertonic hyponatremia, (b) hypotonic hyponatremia with an increased ECF volume, (c) hypotonic hyponatremia with a normal ECF volume, and (d) hypotonic hyponatremia with a decreased ECF volume.[16]

Hypertonic hyponatremia is usually associated with significant hyperglycemia. Glucose is an osmotically active agent that leads to an increase in TBW with little change in total body sodium. For every 60 mg/dL (3.3 mmol/L) increase in serum glucose above 200 mg/dL (11.1 mmol/L), the sodium concentration is expected to decrease by approximately 1 mEq/L (1 mmol/L). Appropriate treatment of the hyperglycemia will return the serum sodium concentration to normal.[15]

Hypotonic hyponatremia with an increase in ECF (hypervolemic hyponatremia) is also known as dilutional hyponatremia. In this scenario, patients have an excess of total body sodium and TBW; however, the excess in TBW is greater than the excess in total body sodium. Common causes include CHF, hepatic cirrhosis, and nephrotic syndrome. Treatment includes sodium and fluid restriction in conjunction with treatment of the underlying disorder, for example, salt and water restrictions are used in the setting of CHF along with loop diuretics, angiotensin-converting enzyme inhibitors, and spironolactone.

In hypotonic hyponatremia with a normal ECF volume (euvolemic hyponatremia), patients have an excess of TBW with relatively normal sodium content. In essence, there is a presence of excess free water. This is most frequently seen in patients with the syndrome of inappropriate antidiuretic hormone secretion (SIADH). Common causes of SIADH include carcinomas (eg, lung or pancreas), pulmonary disorders (eg, pneumonias or tuberculosis), CNS disorders (eg, meningitis, stroke, tumor, or trauma), and medications (eg, sulfonylureas, antineoplastic agents, barbiturates, morphine, antipsychotics, tricyclic antidepressants, nonsteroidal anti-inflammatory agents, selective serotonin reuptake inhibitors, dopamine agonists, and general anesthetics). These medications stimulate the release of antidiuretic hormone (ADH) from the pituitary gland resulting in water retention and dilution of the body's sodium stores.

Short-term treatment of euvolemic hyponatremia includes fluid restriction, isotonic normal saline, hypertonic saline, or conivaptan. Initial treatment generally consists of fluid restriction alone. Hypertonic saline is used only when the sodium concentration is less than 110 mEq/L (110 mmol/L) and/or severe symptoms (eg, seizures) are present. Given the limitations associated with these treatment strategies (unpredictable therapeutic effects and side effects), the arginine vasopressin antagonist conivaptan (Vaprisol, Astellas Pharma) was developed for short-term treatment of euvolemic hyponatremia. While conivaptan can also be used to manage hypervolemic hyponatremia in hospitalized patients, it should not be used for hypovolemic hyponatremia. Conivaptan is dosed 20 mg IV over 30 minutes, followed by a 20-mg continuous infusion over 24 hours for up to 4 days.

Long-term treatment options for euvolemic hyponatremia include fluid restriction, demeclocycline, loop diuretics, saline, lithium, urea, and tolvaptan. Demeclocycline (available as generic) is dosed at 600 to 1200 mg/day, takes days before clinical effect is realized, and can cause nephrotoxicity. Lithium (various generics) also has a slow onset of action and is limited by CNS side effects, GI disturbances, and cardiotoxicity. Furosemide (various generics) or other loop diuretics allow relaxation of fluid restriction but can cause significant volume depletion and electrolyte disturbances, and it has the potential for ototoxicity. No specific USP formulation exists for urea and poor palatability, and side effects limits it use. Tolvaptan (Samsca, Otsuka) is an oral alternative to IV conivaptan. This product is indicated for treatment of clinically significant hypervolemic and euvolemic hyponatremia (sodium less than 125 mEq/L [125 mmol/L]) or less marked hyponatremia that is symptomatic and has resisted correction with fluid restriction. Patients with CHF, cirrhosis, and SIADH would be candidates for long-term use. Tolvaptan has a boxed warning for initiation of treatment in a hospital setting because of the need for close sodium monitoring. The initial dose is 15 mg orally daily and may be titrated up to a max of 60 mg. Concurrent use with potent CYP 3A4 inhibitors should be avoided: ketoconazole (available as generic), clarithromycin (available as generic), ritonavir (Norvir, Abbott), diltiazem (available as generic), verapamil (available as generic), fluconazole (available as generic), and grapefruit juice.

In hypotonic hyponatremia with a decreased ECF volume (hypovolemic hyponatremia), patients usually have a deficit of both total body sodium and TBW, but the sodium deficit exceeds the TBW deficit. Common causes include diuretic use, profuse sweating, wound drainage, burns, GI losses (vomiting or diarrhea), hypoadrenalism (low cortisol and low aldosterone), and renal tubular acidosis. Treatment includes the administration of sodium to correct the sodium deficit and water to correct the TBW deficit. The sodium deficit can be calculated with the following equation[2]:

Sodium deficit (mEq or mmol) = (TBW [in liters]) (desired Na^+ concentration [mEq/L or mmol/L] – current Na^+ concentration).

Although both water and sodium are required in this instance, sodium needs to be provided in excess of water to fully correct this abnormality. As such, hypertonic saline (3% NaCl) is often used. One can estimate the change in serum sodium concentration after 1 L of 3% NaCl infusion using the following equation[16]:

Change in serum Na^+ (mEq/L or mmol/L) = (infusate Na^+ – serum Na^+)/(TBW + 1).

In this formula, TBW is increased by 1 to account for the addition of the liter of 3% NaCl. Patient Encounters 4 and 5 illustrate the concepts of calculating and correcting the sodium deficit.

Patient Encounter 4: Calculation of Sodium Deficit

Calculate the sodium deficit for an 80 kg man with a serum sodium of 121 mEq/L (121 mmol/L).

Depending on the severity of the hyponatremia and acuity of onset, 0.9%, 3%, or 5% NaCl can be utilized. Most patients can be adequately managed with normal saline rehydration, which is generally the safest agent. Hypertonic saline (3% or 5% NaCl) is generally reserved for patients with severe hyponatremia (less than 120 mEq/L [120 mmol/L]) accompanied by coma, seizures, or high urinary sodium losses. Roughly one-third of the sodium deficit can be replaced over the first 12 hours as long as the replacement rate is less than 0.5 mEq/hour (0.5 mmol/hour). The remaining two-thirds of the deficit can be administered over the ensuing days. Overly aggressive correction of symptomatic hyponatremia (greater than 12 mEq/L [12 mmol/L]) can result in central pontine myelinolysis.[17] Given the potential for irreversible neurologic damage if untreated or if improperly treated, acute hyponatremia is an urgent condition that should be promptly treated with careful attention to monitoring serial sodium values and adjusting therapeutic infusions accordingly.[18]

Hypernatremia is a serum sodium concentration greater than 145 mEq/L (145 mmol/L) and can occur in the absence of a sodium deficit (pure water loss) or in its presence (hypotonic fluid loss).[19] The signs and symptoms of hypernatremia manifest with a serum sodium concentration greater than 160 mEq/L (160 mmol/L) and are usually the same as those found in TBW depletion: thirst, mental slowing, and dry mucous membranes. Signs and symptoms become more profound as hypernatremia worsens, with the patient eventually demonstrating confusion, hallucinations, acute weight loss, decreased skin turgor, intracranial bleeding, and/or coma. Many coexisting disorders and medications may complicate the diagnosis.

The classic causes of hypernatremia are associated with TBW depletion. These include dehydration from loss of hypotonic fluid from the respiratory tract or skin, decreased water intake, osmotic diuresis (eg, mannitol, available as generic), and diabetes insipidus (eg, decreased ADH; phenytoin, available as generic; lithium, available as generic). Hypernatremia in hospitalized patients occurs secondary to inappropriate fluid management in patients at risk for increased free water losses and impaired thirst or restricted water intake.[20] Iatrogenic hypernatremia is occasionally caused by the administration of excessive hypertonic saline. Treatment of hypernatremia includes calculation of the TBW deficit followed by the administration of hypotonic fluids as previously described. The fluid volume should be replaced over 48 to 72 hours depending on the severity of symptoms and the degree of hypertonicity.[21] For asymptomatic patients, the rate of correction should not exceed 0.5 mEq/L/hour (0.5 mmol/L/hour).

Patient Encounter 5: Estimate the Anticipated Change in Serum Sodium

Estimate the anticipated change in serum sodium concentration after the infusion of 1 L of 3% NaCl in an 80 kg man with a serum sodium of 121 mEq/L (121 mmol/L).

Patient Encounter 6: Calculate Water Deficit

Calculate the water deficit in a 78 kg man with a serum sodium of 157 mEq/L (157 mmol/L).

Table 27–6

Potassium Content in Various Potassium Salt Preparations

Potassium Salt	mEq/g (mmol/g)
Potassium gluconate[a]	4.3
Potassium citrate[a]	9.8
Potassium bicarbonate[a]	10.0
Potassium acetate[a]	10.2
Potassium chloride[b]	13.4

[a]Favored for hypokalemia and concurrent acidosis.
[b]Favored for hypokalemia and concurrent alkalosis.

One rule of thumb is to replace half the calculated TBW deficit over 12 to 24 hours and the other half of the deficit over the next 24 to 48 hours.[2,19] Excessively rapid correction of hypernatremia may lead to cerebral edema and death. Patient Encounters 6 and 7 reinforce the concepts of calculating TBW deficit and expected changes in serum sodium concentration with therapy.

Potassium

The body's normal daily potassium requirement is 0.5 to 1 mEq/kg (0.5–1 mmol/kg) or 40 to 80 mEq (40–80 mmol) to maintain a serum potassium concentration of 3.5 to 5 mEq/L (3.5–5 mmol/L). Potassium is the most abundant cation in the ICF, balancing the sodium contained in the ECF and maintaining electroneutrality of bodily fluids. Because the majority of potassium is intracellular, serum potassium concentration is not a good measure of total body potassium; however, clinical manifestations of potassium disorders correlate well with serum potassium. The acid–base balance of the body affects serum potassium concentrations: hyperkalemia is routinely seen in patients with decreased pH (acidosis). Potassium regulation is primarily under the control of the kidneys with excess dietary potassium being excreted in the urine. Although mild abnormalities of serum potassium are considered a nuisance, severe hyperkalemia or hypokalemia can be life threatening.[22–24]

Hypokalemia (serum potassium less than 3.5 mEq/L [3.5 mmol/L]) is a common clinical problem. While generally asymptomatic, signs and symptoms of hypokalemia include cramps, muscle weakness, polyuria, electrocardiogram (ECG) changes (flattened T waves and presence of U waves), and cardiac arrhythmias (bradycardia, heart block, atrial flutter, premature ventricular contractions, and ventricular fibrillation). Causes of hypokalemia include GI losses (vomiting, diarrhea, or NG tube suction), renal losses (high aldosterone and low magnesium), inadequate potassium intake (in IV fluids or oral), or alkalosis. Many medications can precipitate hypokalemia. β_2-agonists (eg, albuterol, available as generic) and insulin (multiple product formulations) lower potassium via cellular redistribution. The use of loop diuretics (furosemide, Lasix, also available as generic), thiazide diuretics (hydrochlorothiazide, available as generic), high-dose antibiotics (penicillin, available as generic), and corticosteroids (prednisone, available as generic) cause renal potassium wasting. In addition, amphotericin B (available as generic), cisplatin (available as generic), and foscarnet (available as generic) can also produce hypokalemia secondary to depletion of magnesium. Hypomagnesemia diminishes intracellular potassium concentration and produces potassium wasting. Given the potential for significant morbidity and mortality, serum potassium concentrations should be monitored closely for patients with known (or suspected) hypokalemia.[2,24,25] Hypokalemia is a risk factor for digitalis toxicity.

Each 1 mEq/L (1 mmol/L) fall in serum potassium (ie, from 4 to 3 mEq/L [4 to 3 mmol/L]) represents a loss of approximately 200 mEq (200 mmol) of potassium in the adult. However, when the serum potassium is below 3 mEq/L (3 mmol/L), each 1 mEq/L (1 mmol/L) fall in serum potassium represents a 200 to 400 mEq (200–400 mmol) reduction in serum concentration in the adult patient. Potassium repletion should be guided by close monitoring of serial serum concentrations instead of using empirically chosen amounts. Of the five potassium salts available, potassium acetate (10.2 mEq/K^+/g or 10.2 mmol/K^+/g) and KCl (13.4 mEq/K^+/g or 13.4 mmol/K^+/g) are the most commonly used forms. When hypokalemia occurs in the setting of alkalosis, KCl is the preferred agent; in acidosis, potassium should be provided in the form of acetate, citrate, bicarbonate, or gluconate salt. Table 27–6 outlines the potassium content of each potassium salt preparation, and Table 27–7 lists each of the oral potassium replacement products. Potassium acetate and chloride are available for IV infusions as premixed solutions. The usual dose of these agents is 10 to 20 mEq (10–20 mmol) diluted in 100 mL of normal saline.[2,25,26]

Moderate hypokalemia is defined as a serum potassium of 2.5 to 3.5 mEq/L (2.5–3.5 mmol/L) without ECG changes. In

Table 27–7

Oral Potassium Replacement Products

Product	Salt	Strength[a]
Extended/controlled-release tablets	Chloride	8 mEq (600 mg)
		10 mEq (750 mg)
		15 mEq (1125 mg)
		20 mEq (1500 mg)
Effervescent tablets	Chloride and bicarbonate	10 mEq 20 mEq
		25 mEq
		50 mEq
Liquid	Chloride	20 mEq/15 mL (10%)
		40 mEq/15 mL (20%)
Powder packets	Chloride	
		20 mEq
		25 mEq

[a]For potassium, 1 mEq = 1 mmol.

Patient Encounter 7: Calculate the Anticipated Change in Serum Sodium

Calculate the anticipated change in serum sodium concentration after IV infusion of 1 L of 5% dextrose in a 78 kg man with a serum sodium of 157 mEq/L (157 mmol/L).

this setting, potassium replacement can usually be given orally at a dose of 40 to 120 mEq/day (40–20 mmol/day). Anecdotally, oral potassium supplementation (see Table 27–7) is often more effective in repleting moderate hypokalemia. For patients with an ongoing source of potassium loss, chronic replacement therapy should be considered. The potassium deficit is a rough approximation of the amount of potassium needed to be replaced and can be estimated as follows:

Potassium deficit (mEq or mmol/L) =
(4.0 – current serum potassium) × 100

Severe hypokalemia is defined as a serum potassium less than 2.5 mEq/L (2.5 mmol/L) or hypokalemia of any magnitude that is associated with ECG changes (eg, flattening of T wave or elevation of U wave) and cardiac arrhythmias. In these situations, IV replacement should be initiated urgently. KEY CONCEPT *Potassium infusion at rates exceeding 10 mEq/hour (10 mmol/hour) requires cardiac monitoring given the potential for cardiac arrhythmias.* Although the maximally concentrated solution for potassium replacement is 80 mEq/L (80 mmol/L), the maximum infusion rate is 40 mEq/hour (40 mmol/hour) and must be administered via a central line. Table 27–8 outlines current IV potassium replacement guidelines.

Caution must be exercised when repleting potassium with IV agents given possible vein irritation and/or thrombophlebitis. The risk of these complications is minimized by using less concentrated solutions and by giving infusions via central access if possible. Administration of potassium in vehicles containing glucose is discouraged because glucose facilitates the intracellular movement of potassium. Posttherapy improvements in serum potassium may be transient, and continuous monitoring is required. Patients with low serum magnesium will have exaggerated potassium losses from the kidneys and GI tract leading to refractory hypokalemia. In this situation, the magnesium deficit must be corrected in order to successfully treat the concurrent potassium deficiency. In the hypokalemic patient with concurrent acidosis, potassium is often given as the acetate salt, given that acetate is metabolized to bicarbonate. In the patient with depleted phosphorus and potassium, therapy with potassium phosphate is the natural choice.[22,27,28]

Hyperkalemia is defined as a serum potassium concentration greater than 5 mEq/L (5 mmol/L). Manifestations of hyperkalemia include muscle weakness, paresthesias, hypotension, ECG changes (eg, peaked T waves, shortened QT intervals, and wide QRS complexes), cardiac arrhythmias, and a decreased pH. Causes of hyperkalemia fall into three broad categories: (a) increased potassium intake, (b) decreased potassium excretion, and (c) potassium release from the intracellular space.

Increased potassium intake results from excessive dietary potassium (salt substitutes), excess potassium in IV fluids, and other select medications (potassium-sparing diuretics, cyclosporine [available as generic], angiotensin-converting enzyme inhibitors, nonsteroidal anti-inflammatory agents, pentamidine [available as generic], unfractionated heparin, and low-molecular-weight heparins). Decreased potassium excretion results from acute renal failure, chronic renal failure, or Addison disease. Excess potassium release from cells results from tissue breakdown (surgery, trauma, hemolysis, or rhabdomyolysis), blood transfusions, and metabolic acidosis.

In addition to discontinuing all potassium supplements, potassium-sparing medications, and potassium-rich salt substitutes, management of hyperkalemia addresses three concurrent strategies: (a) agents to antagonize the proarrhythmic effects of hyperkalemia, (b) agents to drive potassium into the intracellular space and acutely lower the serum potassium, and (c) agents that will definitively (but more gradually) lower the total body potassium content.[29] If the serum potassium concentration is greater than 7 mEq/L (7 mmol/L) and/or ECG changes are present, IV calcium is provided to stabilize the myocardium. Depending on the acuity of the situation, 1 g of calcium chloride (13.5 mEq or 6.75 mmol) is administered by direct injection or diluted in 50 mL of D_5W and delivered IV over 15 minutes. Clinical effects are seen within 1 to 2 minutes of infusion and persist for 10 to 30 minutes. Repeat doses may be administered as necessary. Because most patients with clinically significant hyperkalemia receive multiple boluses of calcium directed by ECG findings, iatrogenic hypercalcemia is a potential complication of hyperkalemia treatment. As such, total calcium concentration is commonly checked with each potassium concentration measurement. Ionized calcium measurements should be obtained in patients who have comorbid conditions that would lead to inconsistency between total serum calcium and free calcium (abnormal albumin, protein, or immunoglobulin concentrations).

Dextrose and insulin (with or without sodium bicarbonate) are typically given at the time of calcium therapy in order to redistribute potassium into the intracellular space. Dextrose 50% (25 g in 50 mL) can be given by slow IV push over 5 minutes or dextrose 10% with 20 units of regular insulin can be given by continuous IV infusion over 1 to 2 hours. The onset of action for this combination is 30 minutes; the duration of clinical effects is 2 to 6 hours. High-dose inhaled β_2-agonists (eg, albuterol, available as generic) may also be used to acutely drive potassium into the intracellular space.

It is critically important to recognize that the treatments of hyperkalemia discussed thus far are transient, temporizing measures. They are intended to provide time to institute definitive therapy aimed at removing excess potassium from the body. Agents that increase potassium excretion from the body include sodium polystyrene sulfonate (Kayexalate, available as generic), loop diuretics, and hemodialysis or hemofiltration (used only in patients with renal failure). Sodium polystyrene sulfonate can be given orally, via NG tube, or as a rectal retention enema and is dosed at 15 to 60 g in four divided doses per day. In September 2009, MedWatch issued a safety alert that cases of colonic necrosis and other serious GI-adverse events (bleeding, ischemic colitis, perforation) had been reported in association with Kayexalate use. The majority of these cases reported the concurrent use of sorbitol. Concurrent administration of sorbitol is no longer recommended. Medication safety alerts are available at www.fda.gov/MedWatch.

Table 27–8

Recommended Potassium Dosage/Infusion Rate

Clinical Scenario	Maximum Infusion Rate[a]	Maximum Concentration[a]	Maximum 24-Hour Dose[a]
$K^+ > 2.5$ mEq/L *and* No ECG changes of hypokalemia	10 mEq/hour	40 mEq/L	200 mEq
$K^+ < 2.5$ mEq/L *or* ECG changes of hypokalemia	40 mEq/hour	80 mEq/L	400 mEq

[a]For potassium, 1 mEq = 1 mmol.

Calcium

More than 99% of total body calcium is found in bone; the remaining less than 1% is in the ECF and ICF. Calcium plays a critical role in the transmission of nerve impulses, skeletal muscle contraction, myocardial contractions, maintenance of normal cellular permeability, and the formation of bones and teeth. There is a reciprocal relationship between the serum calcium concentration (normally 8.6–10.2 mg/dL [2.15–2.55 mmol/L]) and the serum phosphate concentration that is regulated by a complex interaction between parathyroid hormone, vitamin D, and calcitonin. About one-half of the serum calcium is bound to plasma proteins; the other half is free ionized calcium. Given that the serum calcium has significant protein binding, the serum calcium measurement must be corrected in patients who have low albumin concentrations (the major serum protein). The most commonly used formula adds 0.8 mg/dL (0.2 mmol/L) of calcium for each gram of albumin deficiency as follows:

Corrected [Ca mg/dL] =
Measured [Ca mg/dL]
+ [0.8 × (4–measured albumin g/dL)][30–32]
Corrected [Ca mmol/L] =
Measured [Ca mmol/L]
+ [0.02 × (40–measured albumin g/L)]

Hypocalcemia is caused by inadequate intake (vitamin deficiency, poor dietary calcium sources, alcoholism) or excessive losses (hypoparathyroidism, renal failure, alkalosis, pancreatitis). Clinical manifestations of hypocalcemia are seen with total serum concentrations less than 6.5 mg/dL (1.63 mmol/L) or an ionized calcium less than 1.12 mmol/L and include tetany, circumoral tingling, muscle spasms, hypoactive reflexes, anxiety, hallucinations, hypotension, myocardial infarction, seizures, lethargy, stupor, and **Trousseau's sign** or **Chvostek's sign**.[24,33] Trousseau's sign is elicited by inflating a BP cuff on the patient's upper arm, whereby hypocalcemic patients will experience tetany of the wrist and hand as evidenced by thumb adduction, wrist flexion, and metacarpophalangeal joint flexion. Chvostek sign is elicited by tapping on the proximal distribution of the facial nerve (adjacent to the ear). This will produce a brief spasm of the upper lip, eye, nose, or face in hypocalcemic patients. Ionized calcium concentrations are typically used to assess calcium status in the critically ill patient.

Causes of hypocalcemia include hypoparathyroidism, hypomagnesemia, alcoholism, hyperphosphatemia, blood product infusion (due to chelation by the citrate buffers), chronic renal failure, vitamin D deficiency, acute pancreatitis, alkalosis, and hypoalbuminemia. In the setting of hypocalcemia, magnesium concentration should be checked and corrected if low. Given that hypocalcemia may be caused by hypomagnesemia, clinicians should be aware that the serum calcium concentrations may not normalize until serum magnesium is replaced. Medications that cause hypocalcemia include phosphate replacement products, loop diuretics, phenytoin (Dilantin, available as generic), phenobarbital (available as generic), corticosteroids, aminoglycoside antibiotics, and acetazolamide (available as generic).[34–36]

Oral calcium replacement products include calcium carbonate (Os-Cal, GlaxoSmithKline and various generics; Tums, GlaxoSmithKline and various generics) and calcium citrate (Citracal, Mission Bayer and various generics). IV calcium replacement products include calcium gluconate and calcium chloride (both products available as generic). KEY CONCEPT *Calcium gluconate is preferred for peripheral use because it is less irritating to the veins; it may also be given intramuscularly.* Each 10 mL of a 10% calcium gluconate solution provides 90 mg (4.5 mEq or 2.25 mmol) of elemental calcium. KEY CONCEPT *Calcium chloride is associated with more venous irritation and extravasation and is generally reserved for administration via central line.* Each 10 mL of a 10% calcium chloride solution contains 270 mg (13.5 mEq or 6.75 mmol) of elemental calcium. IV calcium products are given as a slow push or added to 500 to 1000 mL of 0.9% normal saline for slow infusion.[33,36] In addition to hypocalcemia, IV calcium may also be used for massive blood transfusions, calcium channel blocker overdose, and emergent hyperkalemia and hypermagnesemia.

For acute symptomatic hypocalcemia, 200 to 300 mg of elemental calcium is administered IV and repeated until symptoms are fully controlled. This is achieved by infusing 1 g of calcium chloride or 2 to 3 g of calcium gluconate at a rate no faster than 30 to 60 mg of elemental calcium per minute. More rapid administration is associated with hypotension, bradycardia, or cardiac asystole. Total calcium concentration is commonly monitored in critically ill patients. Under normal circumstances, about half of calcium is loosely bound to serum proteins while the other half is free. Total calcium concentration measures bound and free calcium. Ionized calcium measures free calcium only. Under usual circumstances, a normal calcium concentration implies a normal free ionized calcium concentration. Ionized calcium should be obtained in patients with comorbid conditions that would lead to inconsistency between total calcium and free serum calcium (abnormal albumin, protein, or immunoglobulin concentrations). For chronic asymptomatic hypocalcemia, oral calcium supplements are given at doses of 2 to 4 g/day of elemental calcium. Many patients with calcium deficiency have concurrent vitamin D deficiency that must also be corrected in order to restore calcium homeostasis.[2,33,37]

Hypercalcemia is defined as a calcium concentration greater than 10.2 mg/dL (2.55 mmol/L). It may be categorized as mild if total serum calcium is 10.3 to 12 mg/dL (2.58–3.00 mmol/L), moderate if total serum calcium is 12.1 to 13 mg/dL (3.03–3.25 mmol/L), or severe when serum concentration is greater than 13 mg/dL (3.25 mmol/L). Causes of hypercalcemia include hyperparathyroidism, malignancy, Paget disease, Addison disease, granulomatous diseases (eg, tuberculosis, sarcoidosis, or histoplasmosis), hyperthyroidism, immobilization, multiple bony fractures, acidosis, and milk-alkali syndrome. Multiple medications cause hypercalcemia and include thiazide diuretics, estrogens, lithium (available as generic), tamoxifen (Nolvadex, available as generic), vitamin A, vitamin D, and calcium supplements.[2,33,36,37]

Because the severity of symptoms and the absolute serum concentration are poorly correlated in some patients, institution of therapy should be dictated by the clinical scenario. All patients with hypercalcemia should be treated with aggressive rehydration: normal saline at 200 to 300 mL/hour is a routine initial fluid prescription. For patients with mild hypercalcemia, hydration alone may provide adequate therapy. The moderate and severe forms of hypercalcemia are more likely to have significant manifestations and require prompt initiation of additional therapy. These patients may present with anorexia, confusion, and/or cardiac manifestations (bradycardia and arrhythmias with ECG changes). Total calcium concentrations greater than 13 mg/dL (3.25 mmol/L) are particularly worrisome because these concentrations can unexpectedly precipitate acute renal failure, ventricular arrhythmias, and sudden death.

Table 27–9

Selected Treatment Options for the Management of Hypercalcemia

Therapy	Dose	Onset	Duration	Efficacy[a]
Normal saline	3–6 L/day	Hours	Hours	1–2 mg/dL (0.25–0.50 mmol/L)
Furosemide (Lasix, available as generic)	80–160 mg/day	Hours	Hours	1–2 mg/dL (0.25–0.50 mmol/L)
Hydrocortisone (available as generic)	200 mg/day	Hours	Days	Mild/unpredictable
Calcitonin (Miacalcin, Novartis)	4–8 units/kg	Hours	Hours	1–2 mg/dL (0.25–0.50 mmol/L)
Pamidronate (Aredia, available as generic)	30–90 mg/week	Days	1–4 weeks	1–5 mg/dL(0.25–1.25 mmol/L)
Zoledronic acid (Zometa, Novartis)	4–8 mg	Days	Weeks	1–5 mg/dL (0.25–1.25 mmol/L
Gallium (Ganite, Genta Inc.)	200 mg/m^2	Days	Days to weeks	1–5 mg/dL (0.25–1.25 mmol/L)

[a]Expected decrease in serum Ca^{2+}.

Once fluid administration has repleted the ECF, forced diuresis (with associated calcium loss) can be initiated with a loop diuretic. For this approach to be successful, normal kidney function is required. In renal failure patients, the alternative therapy is emergent hemodialysis. Other treatment options include bisphosphonates (zoledronic acid [Zometa, Novartis], pamidronate [Aredia, available as generic]), hydrocortisone (available as generic), calcitonin, and gallium. Given their efficacy and favorable side-effect profile, bisphosphonates are typically the agents of choice. Table 27–9 outlines the treatment options for hypercalcemia, including time to onset of effect, duration of effect, and efficacy.[2,33,34,37]

Phosphorus

Phosphorus is primarily found in the bone (80%–85%) and ICF (15%–20%): the remaining less than 1% is found in the ECF. Note that phosphorus is the major anion within the cells. Given this distribution, serum phosphate concentration does not accurately reflect total body phosphorus stores. Phosphorus is expressed in milligrams (mg) or millimoles (mmol), not as milliequivalents (mEq). Because phosphorus is the source of phosphate for adenosine triphosphate (ATP) and phospholipid synthesis, manifestations of phosphorus imbalance are variable.

Dietary intake, parathyroid hormone levels, and renal function are the major determinants of the serum phosphorus concentration, which is normally 2.7 to 4.5 mg/dL (0.87–1.45 mmol/L).[2,33,39,40] Hypophosphatemia is defined by a serum phosphorus concentration less than 2.5 mg/dL (0.81 mmol/L); severe hypophosphatemia occurs when the phosphorus concentration is less than 1 mg/dL (0.32 mmol/L). Hypophosphatemia can be caused by increased distribution to the ICF (hyperglycemia, insulin therapy, or malnourishment), decreased absorption (starvation, excessive use of phosphorus-binding antacids, vitamin D deficiency, diarrhea, or laxative abuse) or increased renal loss (diuretic use, diabetic ketoacidosis, alcohol abuse, hyperparathyroidism, or burns).[35,37] KEY CONCEPT *Severe hypophosphatemia can result in impaired diaphragmatic contractility and acute respiratory failure.* Medications that cause hypophosphatemia include diuretics (acetazolamide [Diamox, available as generic], furosemide [Lasix, available as generic], hydrochlorothiazide [HydroDIURIL, available as generic]), sucralfate (Carafate, available as generic), corticosteroids, cisplatin (available as generic), antacids (aluminum carbonate, calcium carbonate, and magnesium oxide [antacids all available as generic]), foscarnet (available as generic), phenytoin (Dilantin, available as generic), phenobarbital (available as generic), and phosphate binders (sevelamer [Renvela, Genzyme Corp.], and calcium acetate [PhosLo, available as generic]).

Signs and symptoms of hypophosphatemia include paresthesias, muscle weakness, myalgias, bone pain, anorexia, nausea, vomiting, red blood cell breakdown (hemolysis), acute respiratory failure, seizures, and coma.[37,41] For mild hypophosphatemia, patients should be encouraged to eat a high-phosphorus diet, including eggs, nuts, whole grains, meat, fish, poultry, and milk products. For moderate hypophosphatemia (1–2.5 mg/dL, 0.32–0.81 mmol/L), oral supplementation of 1.5 to 2 g/day (30–60 mmol/day) is usually adequate. Diarrhea may be a dose-limiting side effect with oral phosphate replacement products.

Injectable phosphate products are reserved for patients with severe hypophosphatemia or those in the intensive care unit.[42] The available agents are provided as sodium or potassium salts; however, unless concurrent hypokalemia is present, sodium phosphate is usually used. Empirically, for a mild serum phosphorus deficiency (2.3–3.0 mg/dL, 0.74–0.97 mmol/L), the corresponding IV phosphorus dose is 0.32 mmol/kg; for a moderate deficiency of serum phosphorus 1.6 to 2.2 mg/dL (0.52–0.71 mmol/L), the replacement dose is 0.64 mmol/kg; and the dose is 1 mmol/kg when the serum phosphorus is less than 1.5 mg/dL (0.48 mmol/L).[36] IV phosphorus preparations are usually infused over 4 to 12 hours. Table 27–10 compares the available phosphate replacement products.

Hyperphosphatemia is defined by a serum phosphorus concentration greater than 4.5 mg/dL (1.45 mmol/L). The manifestations of hyperphosphatemia are similar to findings of hypocalcemia (see earlier), and include paresthesias, ECG changes (prolonged QT interval and prolonged ST segment), and metastatic calcifications. Causes of hyperphosphatemia include impaired phosphorus excretion (hypoparathyroidism or renal failure), redistribution of phosphorus to the ECF (acid–base imbalance, rhabdomyolysis, muscle necrosis, or tumor lysis during chemotherapy), and increased phosphorus intake (various medications).[37] Medications that can cause hyperphosphatemia include enemas containing phosphorus (eg, Fleet, Fleet), laxatives containing phosphate or phosphorus, parenteral or oral supplements (eg, K-Phos Neutral, Beach), vitamin D supplements, and the bisphosphonates (eg, pamidronate, various manufacturers).[43]

Hyperphosphatemia is generally benign and rarely needs aggressive therapy. Dietary restriction of phosphate and protein is effective for most minor elevations. Phosphate binders such as aluminum-based antacids, calcium carbonate, calcium acetate (PhosLo, available as generic), sevelamer hydrochloride (Renagel, Genzyme), sevelamer carbonate (Renvela, Genzyme, Global), and lanthanum carbonate (Fosrenol, Shire) may be necessary for some patients (typically those with chronic renal failure).[49] Sucroferric oxyhydroxide (Velphoro, Fresenius Medical Care)

Table 27–10

Phosphate Replacement Products

Product	Route	$mgPO_4^-$	$mmolPO_4^-$	mEq (mmol) Na^+	mEq (mmmol) K^+
Potassium phosphate (KPO_4/mL), available as generic	IV	94	3	0	4.4
Sodium phosphate ($NaPO_4$/mL), available as generic	IV	94	3	4	0
Phos-NaK packets, Cypress	Oral	250	8	7.2	7
K-Phos Neutral tablets, Beach	Oral	250	8	13.1	1.4
Uro-KP-Neutral tablets, Star	Oral	250	8	10.9	1.27
K-Phos Original tablets, Beach	Oral	114	3.7	—	3.7

and ferric citrate (Auryxia, Keryx Biopharmaceuticals) are iron-based phosphate binders. If patients exhibit findings of hypocalcemia (tetany), IV calcium should be administered empirically.

Magnesium

The body's normal daily magnesium requirement is 300 to 350 mg/day to maintain a serum magnesium concentration of 1.5 to 2.4 mEq/L (0.75–1.20 mmol/L). Because magnesium is the second most abundant ICF cation, serum concentrations are a relatively poor measure of total body stores. Magnesium catalyzes and/or activates more than 300 enzymes, provides neuromuscular stability, and is involved in myocardial contraction. Magnesium is generally not part of standard chemistry panels and therefore must be ordered separately.[2,33,43-45]

Hypomagnesemia is defined as a serum magnesium less than 1.5 mEq/L (0.75 mmol/L) and is most frequently seen in the intensive care and postoperative settings. Hypomagnesemia results from inadequate intake (alcoholism, dietary restriction, or inadequate magnesium in total parenteral nutrition [TPN]), inadequate absorption (steatorrhea, cancer, malabsorption syndromes, or excess calcium or phosphorus in the GI tract), excessive GI loss of magnesium (diarrhea, laxative abuse, NG tube suctioning, or acute pancreatitis), or excessive urinary loss of magnesium (primary hyperaldosteronism, certain medications, diabetic ketoacidosis, and renal disorders). Hypomagnesemia often occurs in the setting of hypokalemia and hypocalcemia. Clinicians should evaluate the magnesium concentration in these patients and correct if low. In order for calcium and potassium concentrations to normalize, magnesium supplementation is often required. Medications that potentially can cause hypomagnesemia include aminoglycoside antibiotics, amphotericin B (available as generic), cisplatin (available as generic), insulin, cyclosporine (available as generic), loop diuretics, and thiazide diuretics. There is also a strong correlation between hypokalemia and hypomagnesemia.[37,38,43,46] Clinicians should be alerted that the long-term use of proton pump inhibitors may be associated with unexplained hypomagnesemia, with subsequent hypokalemia or hypocalcemia.

The findings of hypomagnesemia include muscle weakness, cramps, agitation, confusion, tremor, seizures, ECG changes (increased PR interval, prolonged QRS complex, and increased QT interval), findings of hypocalcemia (see earlier), refractory hypokalemia (see earlier), metabolic alkalosis, and digoxin toxicity.[43,47,48]

Asymptomatic mild magnesium deficiencies (1.0–1.5 mEq/L) (0.50–0.75 mmol/L) can be managed with increased oral intake of magnesium-containing foods or with oral supplementation. Magnesium oxide (Mag-Ox, Blaine Pharmaceuticals and various manufacturers) 400-mg tablets contain 241 mg (20 mEq or 10 mmol) of magnesium, and magnesium chloride hexahydrate tablets (Slow-Mag, Purdue) contains 64 mg of elemental magnesium. Diarrhea is often a dose-limiting side effect of oral supplementation. Severely deficient patients (less than 1.0 mEq/L) (0.50 mmol/L) and all deficient critically ill patients should be managed with IV magnesium sulfate. Ten milliliters of a 10% magnesium sulfate solution contains 1 g of magnesium, which is equivalent to 98 mg (8.12 mEq or 4.06 mmol) of elemental magnesium. IV magnesium supplementation may also be used in the setting of status asthmaticus, premature labor, and torsade de pointes. In May 2013, the FDA released a drug safety communication recommending against the prolonged use of magnesium sulfate to stop preterm labor due to bone changes in exposed babies. Administration of magnesium sulfate injection to pregnant women longer than 5 to 7 days may lead to low calcium levels and bone fractures in the developing baby or fetus. (http://www.fda.gov/Safety/MedWatch/) Magnesium concentrations need to be monitored closely in these patients. **KEY CONCEPT** *Because magnesium concentration does not correlate well with total body magnesium stores, magnesium is often administered empirically to critically ill patients.*[2,33]

The most common causes of hypermagnesemia are renal failure, often in conjunction with magnesium-containing medications (cathartics, antacids, or magnesium supplements), and lithium therapy (available as generic). Hypermagnesemia is defined as a serum magnesium concentration greater than 2.4 mEq/L (1.20 mmol/L). Mild hypermagnesemia is present if the serum magnesium concentration is between 2.5 and 4 mEq/L (1.25–2.00 mmol/L) and manifests as nausea, vomiting, cutaneous vasodilation, and bradycardia. Moderate hypermagnesemia is present if the serum magnesium concentration is between 4 and 12 mEq/L (2–6 mmol/L) and may manifest with hyporeflexia, weakness, somnolence, hypotension, and ECG changes (increased QRS interval). Severe hypermagnesemia is present if the serum magnesium concentration is greater than 13 mEq/L (6.5 mmol/L) and can manifest as muscle paralysis, complete heart block, asystole, respiratory failure, refractory hypotension, and death.[2,50]

All patients with hypermagnesemia should have all magnesium supplements or magnesium-containing medications discontinued.[2,33] Iatrogenic hypermagnesemia has been observed after IV magnesium therapy for refractory asthma or preeclampsia. Mild hypermagnesemia and moderate hypermagnesemia without cardiac findings can be treated with normal saline infusion and furosemide therapy (assuming the patient has normal

Patient Encounter 8: Putting It All Together

ND, a 77-year-old male nursing home resident, is admitted to the hospital with a 3-day history of altered mental status. The patient was unable to give a history or review of systems. On physical examination, the vital signs revealed a BP of 100/60 mm Hg, pulse 110 beats/min, respirations 14 breaths/min, and a temperature of 38.3°C (101°F). Rales and dullness to percussion were noted at the posterior right base. The cardiac examination was significant for tachycardia. No edema was present. Laboratory studies included sodium 160 mEq/L (160 mmol/L), potassium 4.6 mEq/L (4.6 mmol/L), chloride 120 mEq/L (120 mmol/L), bicarbonate 30 mEq/L (30 mmol/L), glucose 104 mg/dL (5.8 mmol/L), BUN 34 mg/dL (12.1 mmol/L), and creatinine 2.2 mg/dL (194 μmol/L). The CBC was within normal limits. Chest x-ray indicated a right lower lobe pneumonia. The patient is 5′ 10″ (178 cm) tall and currently weighs 72.7 kg (160 lb). His normal weight is 77.3 kg (170 lb).

What are the likely causes for the increased sodium concentration in this patient?

Calculate the TBW, ICF, and ECF for this patient.

Calculate ND's fluid deficit if one is present.

In the next 24 hours, the medical team wants to replace 50% of the fluid deficit plus an extra 240 mL to account for increased insensible losses in addition to the patient's maintenance needs. Using the equation (1500 mL + 20 mL for each kilogram greater than 20 kg), calculate the rate of fluid administration for the total fluids needed in this 24-hour period and over the next 48 hours.

Calculate ND's daily maintenance fluids.

Calculate ND's fluid administration rate for the first 24 hours (hospital day 1).

Calculate ND's fluids for the subsequent 48 hours (hospital days 2 and 3) if the goal is to replete the remaining fluid deficit during that time.

What type of fluid should be used to treat ND's fluid disorder?

renal function). Moderate hypermagnesemia with cardiac irritability and severe hypermagnesemia require concurrent IV calcium gluconate to reverse the neuromuscular and cardiovascular effects. Calcium gluconate given at typical doses of 1 to 2 g IV will have transient effects and can be repeated as clinically indicated. Hemodialysis may be necessary for those with severely compromised renal function.

CONCLUSION

Because disturbances in fluid balance are routinely encountered in clinical medicine, it is essential to have a thorough understanding of body fluid compartments and the therapeutic use of fluids. Similarly, disturbances in serum sodium, potassium, calcium, phosphorus, and magnesium are ubiquitous and must be mastered by all clinicians. Dysregulation of fluid and/or electrolyte status has serious implications regarding the concepts of drug absorption, volumes of distribution, and toxicity. Similarly, many medications can disrupt fluid and/or electrolyte balance as an unintended consequence.

Abbreviations Introduced in This Chapter

ADH	Antidiuretic hormone
ASHP	American Society of Health-System Pharmacists
ATP	Adenosine triphosphate
BP	Blood pressure
BUN	Blood urea nitrogen
Ca^{+}	Calcium
CHF	Congestive heart failure
Cl	Chloride
D_5W	Dextrose 5% water
ECF	Extracellular fluid
ECG	Electrocardiogram
FFP	Fresh-frozen plasma
IBW	Ideal body weight
ICF	Intracellular fluid
I&Os	Ins and outs
JCAHO	Joint Commission on Accreditation of Healthcare Organizations
K^{+}	Potassium
KPO^{4}	Potassium phosphate
KVO	Keep the vein open
LR	Lactated Ringer (solution)
Mg^{++}	Magnesium
Na^{+}	Sodium
NaCl	Sodium chloride
$NaPO_4$	Sodium phosphate
NG	Nasogastric
NS	Normal saline
SI	Standardized international units
SIADH	Syndrome of inappropriate antidiuretic hormone secretion
TBW	Total body water
TPN	Total parenteral nutrition

REFERENCES

1. Faber MD, Kupin WL, Heilig CW, Narins RG. Common fluid–electrolyte and acid–base problems in the intensive care unit: Selected issues. Semin Nephrol. 1994;14:8–22.
2. Kraft MD, Btaiche IF, Sacks GS, Kudsk KA. Treatment of electrolyte disorders in adult patients in the intensive care unit. Am J Health Syst Pharm. 2005;62:1663–1682.
3. Faubel S, Topf J. The Fluid Electrolyte and Acid–Base Companion. San Diego, CA: Alert and Oriented Publishing, 1999.
4. Chenevey B. Overview of fluids and electrolytes. Nurs Clin North Am. 1987;22:749–759.
5. Devine BJ. Gentamicin therapy. Drug Intell Clin Pharm. 1974;7:650–655.
6. Rose BD, Post TW. Clinical Physiology of Acid–Base and Electrolyte Disorders, 5th ed. New York, NY: McGraw Hill, 2001.
7. The SAFE Study Investigators. A comparison of albumin and saline for fluid resuscitation in the intensive care unit. N Engl J Med. 2004;350:2247–2256.
8. The Albumin Reviewers (Alderson P, Bunn F, Lefebvre C, Li Wan Po A, Li L, Roberts I, Schlerhout G. Human albumin solution for resuscitation and volume expansion in critically ill patients. Cochrane Database Syst Rev. 2004:CD001208.
9. Weil MH, Tang W. Albumin versus crystalloid solutions for the critically ill and injured. Crit Care Med. 2004;32:2154–2155.
10. Caironi P, Tognoni G, Masson S, et al. Albumin replacement in patients with severe sepsis or shock. N Engl J Med. 2014 Apr 10;370(15):1412–1421.
11. Perel P, Roberts I, Ker K Colloids versus crystalloids for fluid resuscitation in critically ill patients. Cochrane Database Syst Rev. 2013 Feb 28;2:CD000567.

12. Shafiee MAS, Bohn D, Hoorn EJ, Halperin ML. How to select optimal maintenance intravenous therapy. QJ Med. 2003;96:601–610.
13. Kwan I, Bunn F, Roberts I, on behalf of the WHO Pre-Hospital Trauma Care Steering Committee. Timing and volume of fluid administration for patients with bleeding. Cochrane Database Syst Rev. 2003: CD002245.
14. The Joint Commission [Internet]. Oakbrook Terrace (IL): The Joint Commission; c2012 [updated 2012 Feb 1; cited 2012 Feb 2]. Available from: http://www.jointcommission.org.
15. Spasovski G, Vanholder R, Allolio B, et al. Clinical practice guideline on diagnosis and treatment of hyponatremia. Intensive Care Med 2014;40:320–331.
16. Adrigoue H, Madias NE. Hyponatremia. N Engl J Med. 2000;342:1581–1589.
17. Sterns RH. The treatment of hyponatremia: First, do no harm. Am J Med. 1990;88:557–560.
18. Cluitmans FHM, Meinders AE. Management of severe hyponatremia: Rapid or slow correction? Am J Med. 1990;88:161–166.
19. Adrogue HJ, Madias NE. Hypernatremia. N Engl J Med. 2000;342:1493–1499.
20. Palevsky PM, Bhagrath R, Greenberg A. Hypernatremia in hospitalized patients. Ann Intern Med. 1996;124:197–203.
21. Kang SK, Kim W, Oh MS. Pathogenesis and treatment of hypernatremia. Nephron. 2002;92(Suppl 1):14–17.
22. Mandal AK. Hypokalemia and hyperkalemia. Med Clin North Am. 1997;81:611–639.
23. Halperin ML. Potassium. Lancet. 1998;352:135–140.
24. Body JJ, Bouillon R. Emergencies of calcium homeostasis. Rev Endocr Metab Disord. 2003;4:167–175.
25. Gennari FJ. Hypokalemia. N Engl J Med. 1998;339:451–458.
26. Hamil RJ, Robinson LM, Wexler HR, Moote C. Efficacy and safety of potassium infusion therapy in hypokalemic critically ill patients. Crit Care Med. 1991;19:694–699.
27. Kruge JA, Carlson RW. Rapid correction of hypokalemia using concentrated intravenous potassium chloride infusions. Arch Intern Med. 1990;150:613–617.
28. Cohn JN, Kowey PR, Whelton PK, Prisant M. New guidelines for potassium replacement in clinical practice. Arch Intern Med. 2000;160:2429–2436.
29. Williams ME. Hyperkalemia. Crit Care Clin. 1991;7:155–174.
30. Carroll MF, Schade DS. A practical approach to hypercalcemia. Am Fam Physician. 2003;67:1959–1966.
31. Bushinsky DA, Monk RD. Calcium. Lancet. 1998;352:305–311.
32. Zaloga GP. Hypocalcemia in critically ill patients. Crit Care Med. 1992;20:251–262.
33. Metheny NM. Fluid and Electrolyte Balance: Nursing Considerations, 4th ed. New York, NY: Lippincott, 2000.
34. Davidson TG. Conventional treatment of hypercalcemia of malignancy. Am J Health-Syst Pharm. 2001;58(Suppl 3):S8–S15.
35. Weisinger JR, Bellorin-Font E. Magnesium and phosphorous. Lancet. 1998;352:391–396.
36. Brown KA, Dickerson RN, Morgan LM, Alexander KH, Minard G, Brown RO. A new graduated regimen for phosphorous replacement in patients receiving nutritional support. J Parenteral Enteral Nutr. 2006;30:209–214.
37. Just the Facts: Fluids and Electrolytes. Philadelphia, PA: Lippincott Williams & Wilkins, 2005.
38. Bilezikian JP. Clinical review 51. Management of hypercalcemia. J Clin Endocrinol Metab. 1993;77:1445–1449.
39. Knochel JP. The pathophysiology and clinical characteristics of severe hypophosphatemia. Arch Intern Med. 1977;137:203–220.
40. Stoff JS. Phosphate homeostasis and hypophosphatemia. Am J Med. 1982;72:489–495.
41. Aubier M, Murciano D, Lecocguic Y, et al. Effect of hypophosphatemia on diaphragmatic contractility in patients with acute respiratory failure. N Engl J Med. 1985;313:420–424.
42. Perreault MM, Ostron NI, Tiemey MG. Efficacy and safety of intravenous phosphate replacement in critically ill patients. Ann Pharmacother. 1997;31:683–688.
43. Kee JL, Paulanka BJ, Purnell LD. Fluids and Electrolytes with Clinical Applications. A Programmed Approach, 7th ed. Clifton Park, NY: Delmar Learning, 2000.
44. Oster JR, Epstein M. Management of magnesium depletion. Am J Nephrol. 1988;8:349–354.
45. Al-Ghamdi SMG, Cameron EC, Sutton AL. Magnesium deficiency: Pathophysiologic and clinical overview. Am J Kidney Dis. 1994;24:737–752.
46. Salem M, Munoz R, Chernow B. Hypomagnesemia in critical illness: A common and clinically important problem. Crit Care Clin. 1991;7:225–252.
47. Zalman SA. Hypomagnesemia. J Am Soc Nephol. 1999: 10:1616–1622.
48. Dube L, Granry JC. The therapeutic use of magnesium in anesthesiology, intensive care and emergency medicine: A review. Can J Anesth. 2003;50:732–746.
49. Schucker JJ, Ward KE. Hyperphosphatemia and phosphate buffers. Am J Health-Syst Pharm. 2005;62:2355–2361.
50. Van Hook JW. Hypermagnesemia. Crit Care Clin. 1991;7:215–223.

28 Acid–Base Disturbances

Lee E. Morrow and Mark A. Malesker

LEARNING OBJECTIVES

Upon completion of the chapter, the reader will be able to:

1. Compare and contrast the four primary acid–base disturbances within the human body.
2. Apply simple formulas in a systematic manner to determine the etiology of simple acid–base disturbances and the adequacy of compensation.
3. Integrate the supplemental concepts of the anion gap and the excess gap to further assess for complex acid–base disturbances.
4. Discuss the most common clinical causes for each primary acid–base abnormality.
5. Describe the potential clinical complications of altered acid–base homeostasis.
6. Propose an appropriate treatment plan for patients with deranged acid–base physiology.

Given its reputation for complexity and the need to memorize innumerable formulas, acid–base analysis intimidates many health care providers. In reality, acid–base disorders always obey well-defined biochemical and physiological principles. The pH determines a patient's acid–base status and an assessment of the bicarbonate (HCO_3^-) and arterial carbon dioxide ($Paco_2$) values identifies the underlying process. Rigorous use of a systematic approach to arterial blood gases increases the likelihood that derangements in acid–base physiology are recognized and correctly interpreted. This chapter outlines a clinically useful approach to acid–base abnormalities and then applies this approach in a series of increasingly complex clinical scenarios.

Disturbances of acid–base equilibrium occur in a wide variety of illnesses and are among the most frequently encountered disorders in critical care medicine. The importance of a thorough command of this content cannot be overstated given that acid–base disorders are remarkably common and may result in significant morbidity and mortality. Although severe derangements may affect virtually any organ system, the most serious clinical effects are cardiovascular (arrhythmias, impaired contractility), neurologic (coma, seizures), pulmonary (dyspnea, impaired oxygen delivery, respiratory fatigue, respiratory failure), and/or renal (hypokalemia). Changes in acid–base status also affect multiple aspects of pharmacokinetics (clearance, protein binding) and pharmacodynamics.

ACID–BASE HOMEOSTASIS

Acid–base homeostasis is responsible for maintaining blood hydrogen ion concentration [H^+] near normal despite the daily acidic and/or alkaline loads derived from the intake and metabolism of foods. Acid–base status is traditionally represented in terms of pH, the negative logarithm of [H^+]. Because [H^+] is equal to 24 times the ratio of $Paco_2$ to HCO_3^-, the pH can be altered by a change in either the bicarbonate concentration or the dissolved carbon dioxide. A critically important concept is that [H^+] depends only on the *ratio* of $Paco_2$ to HCO_3^- and not the absolute amount of either. As such, a normal $Paco_2$ or HCO_3^- alone does not guarantee that the pH will be normal. Conversely, a normal pH does not imply that either the $Paco_2$ or HCO_3^- will be normal.[1]

KEY CONCEPT *Acid–base homeostasis is tightly regulated by the complex, but predictable, interactions of the kidneys, the lungs, and various buffer systems. The kidneys control serum HCO_3^- concentration through the excretion or reabsorption of filtered HCO_3^-, the excretion of metabolic acids, and synthesis of new HCO_3^-. The lungs control arterial carbon dioxide (CO_2) concentrations through changes in the depth and/or rate of respiration.* The net result is tight regulation of the blood pH by these three distinct mechanisms working in harmony: extracellular bicarbonate and intracellular protein buffering systems; pulmonary regulation of $Paco_2$, effectively allowing carbonic acid to be eliminated by the lungs as CO_2; and renal reclamation or excretion of HCO_3^- and excretion of acids such as ammonium.

Because the kidneys excrete less than 1% of the estimated 13,000 mEq (13,000 mmol) of H^+ ions generated in an average day, renal failure can be present for prolonged periods before life-threatening imbalances occur. Conversely, cessation of breathing for minutes results in profound acid–base disturbances.[1]

The best way to assess a patient's acid–base status is to review the results of an arterial blood gas (ABG) specimen. Blood gas analyzers directly measure the pH and $Paco_2$, while the HCO_3^- value is calculated using the Henderson–Hasselbalch equation. A more direct measure of serum HCO_3^- is obtained by measuring the total venous carbon dioxide (tCO_2). Because dissolved carbon dioxide is almost exclusively in the form of HCO_3^-, tCO_2 is essentially equivalent to the measured serum HCO_3^- concentration.

This value (HCO_3^-) is routinely reported on basic chemistry panels. In the remainder of this chapter, the pH and $Paco_2$ values should be assumed to come from an ABG while HCO_3^- values should be considered to be measured serum concentrations.

BASIC PATHOPHYSIOLOGY

Under normal circumstances, the arterial pH is tightly regulated between 7.35 and 7.45. **Acidemia** is an abnormally low arterial blood pH (less than 7.35) while **acidosis** is a pathologic process that acidifies body fluids. Similarly, **alkalemia** is an abnormally high arterial blood pH (greater than 7.45) while **alkalosis** is a pathologic process that alkalinizes body fluids. As such, although a patient can simultaneously have acidosis *and* alkalosis, the end result will be acidemia *or* alkalemia.

Changes in the arterial pH are driven by changes in the $Paco_2$ and/or the serum HCO_3^-. Carbon dioxide is a volatile acid regulated by the depth and rate of respiration. Because CO_2 can be either "blown off" or "retained" by the respiratory system, it is referred to as being under respiratory control. KEY CONCEPT *Respiratory acidosis and alkalosis result from primary disturbances in the arterial CO_2 concentration. Metabolic compensation of respiratory disturbances is a slow process, often requiring days for the serum HCO_3^- to reach the steady state.* KEY CONCEPT *Respiratory acidosis is caused by respiratory insufficiency resulting in an increased arterial CO_2 concentration. The compensation for respiratory acidosis (if present for prolonged periods) is an increase in serum HCO_3^-.* KEY CONCEPT *Respiratory alkalosis is caused by hyperventilation resulting in a decreased arterial CO_2 concentration. The compensation for respiratory alkalosis (if present for prolonged periods) is a decrease in serum HCO_3^-.*

A respiratory acid–base disorder is a pH disturbance caused by pathologic alterations of the respiratory system or its CNS control. Such an alteration may result in the accumulation of $Paco_2$ beyond normal limits (more than 45 mm Hg or 6.0 kPa), a situation termed *respiratory acidosis*, or it may result in the loss of $Paco_2$ beyond normal limits (less than 35 mm Hg or 4.7 kPa), a condition termed *respiratory alkalosis*. Variations in respiratory rate and/or depth allow the lungs to achieve changes in the $Paco_2$ very quickly (within minutes).

Bicarbonate is a base regulated by renal metabolism via the enzyme carbonic anhydrase. As such, HCO_3^- is often referred to as being under metabolic control. KEY CONCEPT *Metabolic acidosis and alkalosis result from primary disturbances in the serum HCO_3^- concentration. Respiratory compensation of metabolic disturbances begins within minutes and is complete within 12 hours.* KEY CONCEPT *Metabolic acidosis is characterized by a decrease in serum HCO_3^-. The anion gap is used to narrow the differential diagnosis because metabolic acidosis may be caused by addition of acids (increased anion gap) or loss of HCO_3^- (normal anion gap). The compensation for metabolic acidosis is an increase in ventilation with a decrease in arterial CO_2.* KEY CONCEPT *Metabolic alkalosis is characterized by an increase in serum HCO_3^-. This disorder requires loss of fluid that is low in HCO_3^- from the body or addition of HCO_3^- to the body. The compensation for metabolic alkalosis is a decrease in ventilation with an increase in arterial CO_2.*

A metabolic acid-base disorder is a pH disturbance caused by derangement of the pathways responsible for maintaining a normal HCO_3^- concentration. This may result in a pathologic accumulation of HCO_3^- (greater than 26 mEq/L [26 mmol/L]), a condition termed *metabolic alkalosis*, or it may result in the loss of HCO_3^- beyond normal (less than 22 mEq/L [22 mmol/L]), a condition termed *metabolic acidosis*. In contrast to the lungs' rapid effects on CO_2, the kidneys change the HCO_3^- very slowly (hours to days).

Respiratory and metabolic derangements can occur in isolation or in combination. If a patient has an isolated primary acid–base disorder that is not accompanied by another primary acid–base disorder, a **simple (uncomplicated) disorder** is present. The most common clinical disturbances are **simple acid–base disorders**. If two or three primary acid–base disorders are simultaneously present, the patient has a **mixed (complicated) disorder**. More complex clinical situations lead to mixed acid–base disturbances. Because CO_2 is a volatile acid, it can rapidly be changed by the respiratory system. If a respiratory acid–base disturbance is present for minutes to hours, it is considered an **acute disorder**, while if it is present for days or longer it is considered a **chronic disorder**. By definition, the metabolic machinery that regulates HCO_3^- results in slow changes, and all metabolic disorders are chronic.

Changes that follow the primary disorder and attempt to restore the blood pH to normal are referred to as compensatory changes. It should be stressed that compensation never normalizes the pH. Because all metabolic acid–base disorders are chronic and the normal respiratory system can quickly alter the $Paco_2$, essentially all metabolic disorders are accompanied by some degree of respiratory compensation.[2,3] Similarly, chronic respiratory acid–base disorders are typically accompanied by attempts at metabolic compensation.[4,5] However, with acute respiratory acid–base disorders there is insufficient time for the metabolic pathways to compensate significantly.[6] As such, acute respiratory derangements are essentially uncompensated.

The amount of compensation (metabolic or respiratory) can be reliably predicted based on the degree of derangement in the primary disorder. Table 28–1 outlines the simple acid–base disorders and provides formulas for calculating the expected compensatory responses.[7] Although it is not mandatory to memorize these

Table 28–1

The Six Simple Acid–Base Disorders

Type of Disorder	pH	$Paco_2$[a]	HCO_3^-
1. Metabolic acidosis	↓	Decreased[b] $Paco_2 = (1.5 \times HCO_3^-) + 8$	Decreased[c]
2. Metabolic alkalosis	↑	Increased[b] $Paco_2 = (0.9 \times HCO_3^-) + 15$	Increased[c]
3. Acute respiratory acidosis	↓	Increased[c]	Approximately normal $\Delta HCO_3^- = 0.1 \times \Delta Paco_2$[a]
4. Chronic respiratory acidosis	↓	Increased[c]	Increased[d] $\Delta HCO_3^- = 0.35 \times \Delta Paco_2$[a]
5. Acute respiratory alkalosis	↑	Decreased[c]	Approximately normal $\Delta HCO_3^- = 0.2 \times \Delta Paco_2$[a]
6. Chronic respiratory alkalosis	↑	Decreased[c]	Decreased[d] $\Delta HCO_3^- = 0.4 \times \Delta Paco_2$[a]

[a]$Paco_2$ in mm Hg. Multiply $Paco_2$ in mm Hg by 0.133 to convert to kPa.

[b]Respiratory compensation: If inappropriate, see Table 28–2.

[c]Primary disorder.

[d]Metabolic compensation: If inappropriate, see Table 28–2.

Table 28–2

Diagnosis of Concurrent Acid–Base Disturbances When Compensation Is Inappropriate

Primary Acid–Base Disturbance	Assessment of Compensation	Concurrent Acid–Base Disturbance
Metabolic acidosis	$Paco_2$ too low[a]	Respiratory alkalosis
	$Paco_2$ too high[a]	Respiratory acidosis
Metabolic alkalosis	$Paco_2$ too low[a]	Respiratory alkalosis
	$Paco_2$ too high[a]	Respiratory acidosis
Respiratory acidosis	HCO_3^- too low[b]	Metabolic acidosis
	HCO_3^- too high[b]	Metabolic alkalosis
Respiratory alkalosis	HCO_3^- too low[b]	Metabolic acidosis
	HCO_3^- too high[b]	Metabolic alkalosis

[a]Measured $Paco_2$ more than 4 mm Hg (0.5 kPa) from the calculated value.

[b]Measured HCO_3^- more than 2 mEq/L (2 mmol/L) from the calculated value.

formulas in order to interpret acid–base problems, they can be helpful tools. If the measured values differ markedly from the calculated values (the measured serum HCO_3^- is greater than 2 mEq/L [2 mmol/L] from the calculated value or the measured $Paco_2$ is greater than 4 mm Hg [0.5 kPa] from the calculated value), a second acid–base disorder is present as outlined in Table 28–2.

APPLICATION OF BASIC PATHOPHYSIOLOGY

When given an ABG for interpretation, it is essential to use an approach that is focused yet comprehensive.[8] An algorithm illustrating this concept is shown in Figure 28–1. Using this algorithm, Step 1 is to identify all abnormalities in the pH, $Paco_2$, and/or HCO_3^- and then decide which abnormal values are primary and which are compensatory. This is best done by initially looking at the pH. Whichever side of 7.40 the pH is on, the process that caused it to shift to that side is the primary abnormality. If the arterial pH is lower than 7.40 (acidemia), an elevated $Paco_2$ (greater than 45 mm Hg or 6.0 kPa, respiratory acidosis) or a lowered HCO_3^- (less than 22 mEq/L [22 mmol/L], metabolic acidosis) would be the primary abnormality. If the arterial pH is higher than 7.40 (alkalemia), a decreased $Paco_2$ (less than 35 mm Hg or 4.7 kPa, respiratory alkalosis) or an increased HCO_3^- (greater than 26 mEq/L [26 mmol/L], metabolic alkalosis) would be the primary abnormality. Once the primary disorder is established, step 2 is to apply the formulas from Table 28–1 to assess whether compensation is appropriate and to look for concurrent processes.[7]

An alternative to a diagnostic algorithm is use of a graphic nomogram.[9] Nomograms are plots of the pH, $Paco_2$, and HCO_3^- that allow the user to rapidly determine whether arterial blood gas values are consistent with one of the six simple primary acid–base disturbances. Although nomograms are commonly used to identify acid–base disturbances in clinical practice, only individuals who fully comprehend the fundamental concepts of acid–base assessment should use these tools. Also, appreciate that nomograms have limited utility when dealing with complex acid–base derangements.

Acid–base disturbances are always manifestations of underlying clinical disorders. It is useful to specifically define the primary acid–base abnormality because each disorder is caused by a limited number of disease processes. Establishing the specific disease process responsible for the observed acid–base disorder is clinically important because treatment of a given disorder will only be accomplished by correcting the underlying disease process.

ADVANCED PATHOPHYSIOLOGY

The concepts in this section are used to further expand on steps 3 and 4 of the diagnostic algorithm shown in Figure 28–1. Under normal circumstances the serum is in the isoelectric state. This means that the positively charged entities reported in a standard chemistry panel (cations: sodium and potassium) should be exactly balanced by the negatively charged entities (anions: chloride and bicarbonate). However, this relationship is consistently incorrect because the measured cations are higher than the measured anions by 10 to 12 mEq/L (10–12 mmol/L). This discrepancy results from the presence of unmeasured anions (eg, circulating proteins, phosphates, and sulfates). This apparent difference in charges, the serum anion gap, is calculated as follows:

$$\text{Anion gap} = Na^+ - (Cl^- + HCO_3^-)$$

Because the serum potassium content is relatively small and is very tightly regulated, it is generally omitted from the calculation.[10]

It is important to realize that the serum HCO_3^- concentration may be affected by the presence of unmeasured endogenous acids (lactic acid or ketoacids). Bicarbonate will attempt to buffer these acids, resulting in a 1 mEq (1 mmol) loss of serum HCO_3^- for each 1 mEq (1 mmol) of acid titrated. Because the cation side of the equation is not affected by this transaction, the loss of serum HCO_3^- results in an increase in the calculated anion gap. Identification of an increased anion gap is very important because a limited number of clinical scenarios lead to this unique acid–base disorder. A mnemonic to recall the differential diagnosis for an anion gap acidosis is shown in Table 28–3. The concept of the increased anion gap is applied later in Patient Encounters 6 through 10.

Step 3 in Figure 28–1 suggests that any time an ABG is analyzed, it is wise to concurrently inspect the serum chemistry values and to calculate the anion gap. The body does not generate an anion gap to compensate for a primary disorder. As such, if the calculated anion gap exceeds 12 mEq/L (12 mmol/L), there is a primary metabolic acidosis regardless of the pH or the serum HCO_3^- concentration. The anion gap may be artificially lowered by decreased serum albumin, multiple myeloma, lithium intoxication, or a profound increase in the serum potassium, calcium, or magnesium.[11]

Step 4 in Figure 28–1 shows how calculation of the anion gap also facilitates determination of the **excess gap** or the degree to which the calculated anion gap exceeds the normal anion gap. The excess gap is calculated as follows:

$$\begin{aligned}\text{Excess gap} &= \text{calculated anion gap} - \text{normal anion gap}\\ &= [Na^+ - (Cl^- + HCO_3^-)] - 12\end{aligned}$$

The excess gap represents the amount of HCO_3^- that has been lost due to buffering unmeasured cations. The excess gap can be added back to the measured HCO_3^- to determine what the patient's HCO_3^- would be if these endogenous acids were not present. This is a very valuable tool that can be used in narrowing the differential diagnosis of certain acid–base disorders as well as in uncovering occult or mixed acid–base disorders.

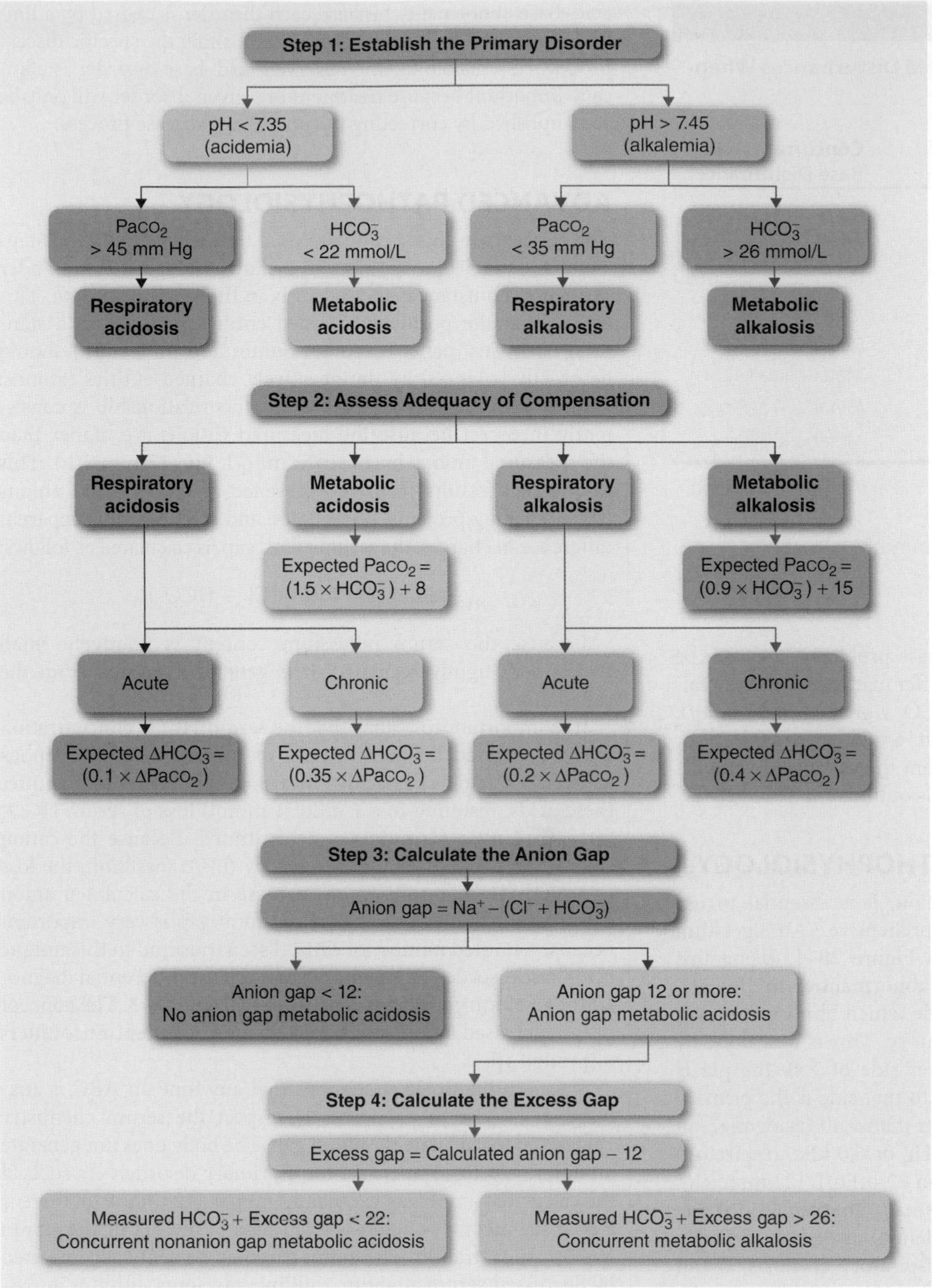

FIGURE 28–1. An algorithmic approach to acid–base disorders. Normal values: pH 7.35 to 7.45, $Paco_2$ 35 to 45 mm Hg (4.7–6.0 kPa), HCO_3^- 22 to 26 mEq/L (26 mmol/L), anion gap less than 12 mEq/L (12 mmol/L). Note that $Paco_2$ should be in millimeters of mercury to use the equations in the figure. (Cl^-, chloride ion; HCO_3^-, bicarbonate; Na^+, sodium ion; $Paco_2$, partial pressure of arterial carbon dioxide.)

In summary, the approach to assessment of acid–base status involves four key steps as outlined in Figure 28–1: step 1 = initial inspection of the pH, $Paco_2$, and HCO_3^-; step 2 = assessment of the adequacy of compensation; step 3 = calculation of the anion gap; and step 4 = calculation of the excess gap.

ETIOLOGY AND TREATMENT

KEY CONCEPT *Arterial blood gases, serum electrolytes, physical examination findings, the clinical history, and the patient's recent medications must be reviewed in order to establish the etiology of a given acid–base disturbance.* Tables 28–4 through 28–7 outline the most commonly encountered causes for each of the primary acid–base disorders. The therapeutic approach to each of these acid–base derangements should emphasize a search for the cause, as opposed to immediate attempts to normalize the pH.

KEY CONCEPT *It is critical to treat the underlying causative process to effectively resolve most observed acid–base disorders. However, supportive treatment of the pH and electrolytes is often needed until the underlying disease state is improved.*[12,13]

All patients with significant disturbances in their acid–base status require continuous cardiovascular and hemodynamic monitoring. Because frequent assessment of the patient's response to treatment is critical, an arterial line is often placed to minimize patient discomfort with serial ABG collections. If the anion gap was initially abnormal, serial chemistries should be followed to ensure that the anion gap resolves with treatment. Specific treatment decisions depend on the underlying pathophysiologic state

Patient Encounters 1 Through 5: Application of Basic Pathophysiology

Case Study 1

An unconscious 19-year-old man is brought to the emergency department by friends who state that the patient took a handful of pain pills at a college dorm "pill party." The patient's ABG has a pH of 7.16, $Paco_2$ of 70 (9.3 kPa), and HCO_3^- of 27 mEq/L (27 mmol/L).

What is the primary acid–base disorder?

Has compensation occurred?

Given the clinical history, what is the most likely explanation for the ABG findings?

Case Study 2

The next patient is a 59-year-old man undergoing lung transplant evaluation for advanced emphysema. An ABG drawn during the transplant workup shows a pH of 7.34, a $Paco_2$ of 70 mm Hg (9.3 kPa), and an HCO_3^- of 35 mEq/L (35 mmol/L).

What is the primary acid–base disorder?

Has compensation occurred?

Given the clinical history, what is the most likely explanation for the ABG findings?

Case Study 3

A healthy 24-year-old pharmacy student is having an ABG drawn as part of her clinical pulmonary rotation. Her ABG shows a pH of 7.50, a $Paco_2$ of 29 mm Hg (3.9 kPa), and an HCO_3^- of 22 mEq/L (22 mmol/L).

What is the primary acid–base disorder?

Has compensation occurred?

Given the clinical history, what is the most likely explanation for the ABG findings?

Case Study 4

This 62-year-old woman with hyperlipidemia has experienced multiple myocardial infarctions resulting in ischemic cardiomyopathy and congestive heart failure. She requires daily furosemide (Lasix) therapy to remain euvolemic. An ABG was drawn for increasing dyspnea and shows the following: pH of 7.50, a $Paco_2$ of 47 mm Hg (6.3 kPa), and an HCO_3^- of 36 mEq/L (36 mmol/L).

What is the primary acid–base disorder?

Has compensation occurred?

Given the clinical history, what is the most likely explanation for the ABG findings?

Case Study 5

The final patient in this section is a 46-year-old woman with chronic renal insufficiency who is being hospitalized for *Clostridium difficile*-associated diarrhea. Her ABG shows a pH of 7.20, a $Paco_2$ of 20 mm Hg (2.7 kPa), and an HCO_3^- of 8 mEq/L (8 mmol/L).

What is the primary acid–base disorder?

Has compensation occurred?

Given the clinical history, what is the most likely explanation for the ABG findings?

(eg, dialysis for renal failure, insulin for diabetic ketoacidosis, or improving tissue perfusion and oxygenation for lactic acidosis).

Metabolic Acidosis

Metabolic acidosis is characterized by a reduced arterial pH, a primary decrease in the HCO_3^- concentration, and a compensatory reduction in the $Paco_2$. The etiologies of metabolic acidosis are divided into those that lead to an increase in the anion gap and those associated with a normal anion gap and are listed in Table 28–4. Although there are numerous mnemonics to recall the differential diagnosis of the metabolic acidosis, two simple ones are shown in Table 28–3. High anion gap metabolic acidosis is most frequently caused by lactic acidosis, ketoacidosis, and/or renal failure. Although there is considerable variation, the largest anion gaps are caused by ketoacidosis, lactic acidosis, and methanol or ethylene glycol ingestion.[14]

Symptoms of metabolic acidosis are attributable to changes in cardiovascular, musculoskeletal, neurologic, or pulmonary functioning. Respiratory compensation requires marked increases in minute ventilation and may lead to dyspnea, respiratory fatigue, and respiratory failure. Acidemia predisposes to ventricular arrhythmias and reduces cardiac contractility, each of which can result in pulmonary edema and/or systemic hypotension.[15] Neurologic symptoms range from lethargy to coma and are usually proportional to the severity of the pH derangement. Chronic metabolic acidosis leads to a variety of musculoskeletal problems, including impaired growth, rickets, osteomalacia, or osteopenia. These changes are believed to be caused by the release of calcium and phosphate during bone buffering of excess H^+ ions.

As previously discussed, in anion gap metabolic acidosis, the isoelectric state is maintained because unmeasured anions are present. With a *normal* anion gap metabolic acidosis, the isoelectric state is maintained by an increase in the measured chloride. Because of this, normal anion gap metabolic acidosis is often referred to as hyperchloremic acidosis.

Table 28–3

Mnemonics for the Differential Diagnoses of Metabolic Acidosis

Elevated Anion Gap[a]	Normal Anion Gap[a]
M—Methanol, metformin	U—Ureteral diversion
U—Uremia	S—Saline infusion
D—Diabetic (or alcoholic) ketoacidosis	E—Exogenous acid
	D—Diarrhea
P—Paraldehyde, phenformin	C—Carbonic anhydrase inhibitors
I—Isoniazid, iron	
L—Lactic acidosis	A—Adrenal insufficiency
E—Ethylene glycol, ethanol	R—Renal tubular acidosis
S—Salicylates	

[a]Anion gap = serum sodium concentration − (serum chloride concentration + serum bicarbonate concentration). Under normal circumstances, the anion gap should be 10 mEq/L (10 mmol/L) or less.

Table 28–4

Common Causes of Metabolic Acidosis

Elevated Anion Gap[a]	Normal Anion Gap[a]
Intoxications	Bowel fistula
Methanol	Diarrhea
Ethylene glycol	Dilutional acidosis
Salicylates	Drugs
Paraldehyde	Acetazolamide[b]
Isoniazid	Ammonium chloride[b]
Ketoacidosis	Amphotericin B[b]
Diabetic	Arginine hydrochloride[c]
Ethanol	Cholestyramine[b]
Starvation	Hydrochloric acid[b]
Lactic acidosis	Lithium[b]
Carbon monoxide poisoning	Parenteral nutrition[b]
Drugs	Topiramate[b]
IV lorazepam (due to vehicle)[c]	Zonisamide[b]
Metformin[b]	Lead poisoning
Nitroprusside (due to cyanide accumulation)[b]	Renal tubular acidosis
Nucleoside reverse transcriptase inhibitors[b]	Surgical drains
Propofol[c]	Ureteral diversion
Seizures	Villous adenomas (some)
Severe hypoxemia	
Shock	
Renal failure	

[a]Anion gap = serum sodium concentration – (serum chloride concentration + serum bicarbonate concentration). Under normal circumstances, the anion gap should be 10 mEq/L (10 mmol/L) or less.

[b]May be observed with therapeutic doses or overdoses.

[c]Typically observed only with overdoses.

In patients with a normal anion gap metabolic acidosis, it is often helpful to calculate the urine anion gap (UAG).[16] The UAG is calculated as follows:

$$UAG = (\text{Urine Na}^+ + \text{Urine K}^+) - \text{Urine Cl}^-$$

The normal UAG ranges from 0 to 5 mEq/L (0–5 mmol/L) and represents the presence of unmeasured urinary anions. In metabolic acidosis, the excretion of NH_4^+ and concurrent Cl^- should increase markedly if renal acidification capacity is intact. This results in UAG values from −20 to −50 mEq/L (−20 to −50 mmol/L). This occurs because the urinary Cl^- concentration now markedly exceeds the urinary Na^+ and K^+ concentrations. Diagnoses consistent with an excessively negative UAG include proximal (type 2) renal tubular acidosis, diarrhea, or administration of acetazolamide or hydrochloric acid (HCl). Excessively positive values of the UAG suggest a distal (type 1) renal tubular acidosis.

In order to effectively treat metabolic acidosis, the *causative process* must be identified and treated.[17] The precise role of adjunctive therapy with sodium bicarbonate ($NaHCO_3$) is not universally agreed upon. However, most practitioners accept that $NaHCO_3$ is indicated when renal dysfunction precludes adequate regeneration of HCO_3^- or when severe acidemia (pH less than 7.15) is present. The metabolic acidosis seen with lactic acidosis and ketoacidosis generally resolves with therapy targeted at the underlying cause, and $NaHCO_3$ may be unnecessary regardless of the pH. The metabolic acidosis of renal failure, renal tubular acidosis, or intoxication with ethylene glycol, methanol, or salicylates is much more likely to require $NaHCO_3$ therapy.

If $NaHCO_3$ is used, the plasma HCO_3^- should not be corrected entirely. Instead, aim at increasing HCO_3^- above an absolute value of 10 mEq/L (10 mmol/L). The total HCO_3^- deficit can be calculated from the current bicarbonate concentration ($HCO^-_{3\,curr}$), the desired bicarbonate concentration ($HCO^-_{3\,post}$), and the body weight (in kilograms) as follows:

$$HCO_3^- \text{ deficit} = [(2.4/HCO^-_{3\,curr}) + 0.4] \times \text{weight} \times (HCO^-_{3\,curr} - HCO^-_{3\,post})$$

No more than half of the calculated HCO_3^- deficit should be given initially to avoid volume overload, hypernatremia, hyperosmolarity, overshoot alkalemia, hypocalcemia and/or hypokalemia. The calculated HCO_3^- deficit reflects only the present situation and does not account for ongoing H^+ production and HCO_3^- loss. When giving HCO_3^- therapy, serial blood gases are needed to monitor therapy.

Another option for patients with severe acidemia is tromethamine (THAM).[18] This inert amino alcohol buffers acids and CO_2 through its amine ($-NH_2$) moiety:

$$THAM - NH_2 + H^+ = THAM - NH_3^+$$

$$THAM - NH_2 + H_2O + CO_2 = THAM - NH_3^+ + HCO_3^-$$

Protonated THAM (with Cl^- or HCO_3^-) is excreted in the urine at a rate that is slightly higher than creatinine clearance. As such, THAM augments the buffering capacity of the blood without generating excess CO_2. THAM is less effective in patients with renal failure, and toxicities may include hyperkalemia, hypoglycemia, and possible respiratory depression. THAM is particularly useful in patients with volume overload because it does not contain sodium.

THAM is often administered as an empiric dose of 18 g (150 mEq [150 mmol]) in 500-mL water via slow IV infusion. Additional infusions are given as dictated by the severity and progression of acidosis.

Chronic metabolic acidosis can successfully be managed using potassium citrate/citric acid (Polycitra-K, Cytra-K) or sodium citrate/citric acid (Bicitra, Oracit).

Metabolic Alkalosis

Metabolic alkalosis is characterized by an increased arterial pH, a primary increase in the HCO_3^- concentration, and a compensatory increase in the $Paco_2$. Patients will always hypoventilate to compensate for metabolic alkalosis—even if it results in profound hypoxemia. For a metabolic alkalosis to persist, there must concurrently be a process that elevates serum HCO_3^- concentration (gastric or renal loss of acids) and another that impairs renal HCO_3^- excretion (hypovolemia, hypokalemia, or mineralocorticoid excess). The etiologies of metabolic alkalosis are listed in Table 28–5.

Patients with metabolic alkalosis rarely have symptoms attributable to alkalemia. Rather, complaints are usually related to volume depletion (muscle cramps, positional dizziness, weakness) or to hypokalemia (muscle weakness, polyuria, polydipsia).

In order to effectively treat metabolic alkalosis, the *causative process* must be identified and treated. The major causes of metabolic alkalosis are often readily apparent after carefully reviewing the patient's history and medication list. In hospitalized patients, always look for administration of compounds such as citrate in blood products and acetate in parenteral nutrition that can raise the HCO_3^- concentration. If the etiology of the metabolic

Patient Encounters 6 through 10: Application of Advanced Pathophysiology

Case Study 6

A 31-year-old man with severe cognitive impairment is admitted to the intensive care unit after ingesting an unknown quantity of aspirin tablets. His presenting laboratory test results show a pH of 7.50, a $Paco_2$ of 20 mm Hg (2.7 kPa), an HCO_3^- of 16 mEq/L (16 mmol/L), a sodium concentration of 140 mEq/L (140 mmol/L), and a chloride level of 103 mEq/L (103 mmol/L).

What is the primary acid–base disorder?

Is there a mixed disorder?

Given the clinical history, what is the most likely explanation for the ABG findings?

Case Study 7

A 56-year-old man is brought to the emergency room by his family. He has not felt well for the past week and did not attend his regular hemodialysis sessions. He began vomiting 36 hours ago but refused medical evaluation. When family members found him unresponsive this morning, they sought medical attention. Laboratory analyses show: pH of 7.40, $Paco_2$ of 40 mm Hg (5.3 kPa), HCO_3^- of 24 mEq/L (24 mmol/L), sodium concentration of 145 mEq/L (145 mmol/L), and chloride level of 100 mEq/L (100 mmol/L).

What is the primary acid–base disorder?

Is there a mixed disorder?

Given the clinical history, what is the most likely explanation for the ABG findings?

Case Study 8

A 56-year-old woman is brought to the emergency room by rescue squad after several complaints were called in to 911 for a "profoundly intoxicated" individual in a city park. Shortly after arrival in the emergency room she has several episodes of emesis with witnessed aspiration. She is transferred to the ICU where she develops progressive hypoxia during the ensuing hours. Following elective intubation her blood work shows a pH of 7.50, a $Paco_2$ of 20 mm Hg (2.7 kPa), an HCO_3^- of 15 mEq/L (15 mmol/L), a sodium concentration of 145 mEq/L (145 mmol/L), and a chloride level of 100 mEq/L (100 mmol/L).

What is the primary acid–base disorder?

Is there a mixed disorder?

Given the clinical history, what is the most likely explanation for the ABG findings?

Case Study 9

A 69-year-old insulin-dependent diabetic man is being evaluated for unresponsiveness. His wife says he had "stomach flu" for several days with frequent bouts of emesis. She thinks he has stopped taking his insulin since he hasn't been eating. He became somnolent yesterday and she called an ambulance when she noticed his breathing was very slow and shallow. The blood work drawn prior to urgent intubation shows a pH of 7.10, a $Paco_2$ of 50 mm Hg (6.7 kPa), an HCO_3^- of 15 mEq/L (15 mmol/L), a sodium concentration of 145 mEq/L (145 mmol/L), and a chloride level of 100 mEq/L (100 mmol/L).

What is the primary acid–base disorder?

Is there a mixed disorder?

Given the clinical history, what is the most likely explanation for the ABG findings?

Case Study 10

The final patient is a 23-year-old woman who was admitted 6 hours ago for diabetic ketoacidosis. With appropriate therapy, her hyperglycemia has improved and her serum ketones are clearing. Because she continues to feel poorly, repeat blood work is obtained. Studies show a pH of 7.15, a $Paco_2$ of 15 mm Hg (2.0 kPa), an HCO_3^- of 5 mEq/L (5 mmol/L), a sodium concentration of 140 mEq/L (140 mmol/L), and a chloride level of 110 mEq/L (110 mmol/L).

What is the primary acid–base disorder?

Is there a mixed disorder?

Given the clinical history, what is the most likely explanation for the ABG findings?

alkalosis is still unclear, measurement of the urinary chloride may be useful. Some processes leading to metabolic alkalosis (vomiting, nasogastric suction losses, factitious diarrhea) will have low urinary Cl^- concentrations (less than 25 mEq/L [25 mmol/L]) and are likely to respond to administration of saline. Other causes (diuretics, hypokalemia, and mineralocorticoid excess) will have higher urinary Cl^- concentrations (greater than 40 mEq/L [40 mmol/L]) and are less likely to correct with saline infusion.

In general, contributing factors such as diuretics, nasogastric suction, and corticosteroids should be discontinued if possible. Any fluid deficits should be treated with IV normal saline. Again, patients with metabolic alkalosis and high urine Cl^- (while relatively uncommon) are generally resistant to saline loading. Potassium supplementation should always be given if it is also deficient.

In patients with mild or moderate alkalosis who require ongoing diuresis but have rising HCO_3^- concentrations, the carbonic anhydrase inhibitor acetazolamide can be used to reduce the HCO_3^- concentration. Acetazolamide is typically dosed at 250 mg every 6 to 12 hours as needed to maintain the pH in a clinically acceptable range. This agent results in gradual changes in the serum HCO_3^- and is not used to acutely correct a patient's acid–base status. If alkalosis is profound and potentially life threatening (due to seizures or ventricular tachyarrhythmias), hemodialysis or transient HCl infusion can be considered. The hydrogen ion deficit (in milliequivalents or millimoles) can be estimated from the current bicarbonate concentration (HCO^-_{3curr}), the desired bicarbonate concentration (HCO^-_{3post}), and the body weight (in kilograms) as follows:

$$H^+ \text{ deficit} = 0.4 \times \text{weight} \times (HCO^-_{3curr} - HCO^-_{3post})$$

After estimating the H^+ deficit, 0.1 to 0.2 N hydrochloric acid (HCl) is infused at 20 to 50 mEq/hour (20–50 mmol/hour) into a central vein. Arterial pH must be monitored at least hourly and the infusion stopped as soon as clinically feasible. Ammonium chloride and arginine hydrochloride, agents that result in the formation of HCl, are not commonly prescribed because they may lead to significant toxicity. Ammonium chloride may cause accumulation of ammonia leading to encephalopathy while arginine

Table 28–5

Common Causes of Metabolic Alkalosis

Urine Cl^- < 10 mEq/L (10 mmol/L)	Urine Cl^- > 10 mEq/L (10 mmol/L)
Alkali administration	Drugs[a]
IV bicarbonate therapy	Corticosteroid therapy
Oral alkali therapy	Diuretics
Parenteral nutrition with acetate	Hypokalemia
"Contraction alkalosis" postdiuretic use	Mineralocorticoid excess
Decreased chloride intake	Hyperaldosteronism
Loss of gastric acid	Bartter syndrome
Vomiting	Cushing syndrome
Nasogastric suction	
Posthypercapnia	
Villous adenomas (some)	

[a]May be observed with therapeutic doses or overdoses.

hydrochloride can induce life-threatening hyperkalemia through unclear mechanisms.

Respiratory Acidosis

Respiratory acidosis is characterized by a reduced arterial pH, a primary increase in the arterial $Paco_2$ and, when present for sufficient time, a compensatory rise in the HCO_3^- concentration. Because increased CO_2 is a potent respiratory stimulus, respiratory acidosis represents ventilatory failure or impaired central control of ventilation as opposed to an increase in CO_2 production. As such, most patients will have hypoxemia in addition to hypercapnia. The most common etiologies of respiratory acidosis are listed in Table 28–6.

Table 28–6

Common Causes of Respiratory Acidosis

CNS disease	Pneumonia
Brainstem lesions	Pneumonitis
Central sleep apnea	Pulmonary edema
Infection	Restrictive lung disease
Intracranial hypertension	Ascites
Trauma	Chest wall disorder
Tumor	Fibrothorax
Vascular	Kyphoscoliosis
Drugs[a]	Obesity
Aminoglycosides	Pleural effusion
Anesthetics	Pneumoconiosis
β-Blockers	Pneumothorax
Botulism toxin	Progressive systemic sclerosis
Hypnotics	Pulmonary fibrosis
Narcotics	Spinal arthritis
Neuromuscular blocking agents	Smoke inhalation
Organophosphates	Upper airway obstruction
Sedatives	Foreign body
Neuromuscular disease	Laryngospasm
Guillain-Barré syndrome	Obstructive sleep apnea
Muscular dystrophy	Others
Myasthenia gravis	Abdominal distention
Polymyositis	Altered metabolic rate
Pulmonary disease	Congestive heart failure
Lower airway obstruction	Hypokalemia
Chronic obstructive pulmonary disease	Hypothyroidism
Foreign body	Inadequate mechanical ventilation
Status asthmaticus	

[a]May be observed with therapeutic doses or overdoses.

Severe, acute respiratory acidosis produces a variety of neurologic abnormalities. Initially these include headache, blurred vision, restlessness, and anxiety. These may progress to tremors, asterixis, somnolence, and/or delirium. If untreated, terminal manifestations include peripheral vasodilation leading to hypotension and cardiac arrhythmias. Chronic respiratory acidosis is typically associated with cor pulmonale and peripheral edema.

In order to effectively treat respiratory acidosis, the *causative process* must be identified and treated. If a cause is identified, specific therapy should be started. This may include naloxone for opiate-induced hypoventilation or bronchodilator therapy for acute bronchospasm. Because respiratory acidosis represents ventilatory failure, an increase in alveolar ventilation is required. This can often be achieved by controlling the underlying disease (eg, bronchodilators and corticosteroids in asthma) and/or physically augmenting ventilation.

Although their precise role and mechanisms of action are unclear, agents such as medroxyprogesterone, theophylline, and doxapram stimulate respiration and have been used to treat mild to moderate respiratory acidosis. Moderate or severe respiratory acidosis requires assisted ventilation. This can be provided to spontaneously breathing patients via bilevel positive airway pressure (BiPAP) delivered via a tight-fitting mask or by intubation followed by mechanical ventilation. In mechanically ventilated patients, respiratory acidosis is treated by increasing the minute ventilation. This is achieved by increasing the respiratory rate and/or tidal volume.

As with the treatment of metabolic acidosis, the role of $NaHCO_3$ therapy is not well defined for respiratory acidosis. Realize that administration of $NaHCO_3$ can paradoxically result in increased CO_2 generation ($HCO_3^- + H^+ \rightarrow H_2CO_3 + CO_2$) and worsened acidemia. Careful monitoring of the pH is required if $NaHCO_3$ therapy is started for this indication. The use of tromethamine in respiratory acidosis (see Metabolic Acidosis section earlier) has unproven safety and benefit.

The goals of therapy in patients with chronic respiratory acidosis are to maintain oxygenation and to improve alveolar ventilation if possible. Because of the presence of metabolic compensation, it is usually not necessary to treat the pH, even in patients with severe hypercapnia. Although the specific treatment varies with the underlying disease, excessive oxygen and sedatives should be avoided because they can worsen CO_2 retention.

Respiratory Alkalosis

Respiratory alkalosis is characterized by an increased arterial pH, a primary decrease in the arterial $Paco_2$ and, when present for sufficient time, a compensatory fall in the HCO_3^- concentration. Respiratory alkalosis represents hyperventilation and is remarkably common. The most common etiologies of respiratory alkalosis are listed in Table 28–7 and range from benign (anxiety) to life threatening (pulmonary embolism). Some causes of hyperventilation and respiratory acidosis are remarkably common (hypoxemia or anemia).

The symptoms produced by respiratory alkalosis result from increased irritability of the central and peripheral nervous

Table 28–7

Common Causes of Respiratory Alkalosis

CNS disease	Pulmonary disease
Infection	Early restrictive lung disease
Trauma	Infection
Tumor	Pneumothorax
Vascular	Pulmonary edema
Drug or toxin induced[a]	Pulmonary embolism
Catecholamines	Tissue hypoxia
Doxapram	Burn injury
Methylphenidate	Excessive mechanical ventilation
Methylxanthines	Fever
Nicotine	Hepatic failure
Progesterone	Hypoxemia
Salicylates	Pain
Psychiatric disease	Postmetabolic acidosis
Anxiety	Pregnancy
Hyperventilation	Severe anemia
Hysteria	Thyrotoxicosis
Panic disorder	

[a]May be observed with therapeutic doses or overdoses.

systems. These include light-headedness, altered consciousness, distal extremity paresthesias, circumoral paresthesia, cramps, carpopedal spasms, and syncope. Various supraventricular and ventricular cardiac arrhythmias may occur in extreme cases, particularly in critically ill patients. An additional finding in many patients with severe respiratory alkalosis is hypophosphatemia, reflecting a shift of phosphate from the extracellular space into the cells. Chronic respiratory alkalosis is generally asymptomatic.

It is imperative to identify serious causes of respiratory alkalosis and institute effective treatment. In spontaneously breathing patients, respiratory alkalosis is typically only mild or moderate in severity and no specific therapy is indicated. Severe alkalosis generally represents respiratory alkalosis imposed on metabolic alkalosis and may improve with sedation or rebreathing maneuvers (rebreathing mask, paper bag). Patients receiving mechanical ventilation are treated with reduced minute ventilation achieved by decreasing the respiratory rate and/or tidal volume. If the alkalosis persists in the ventilated patient, high-level sedation or paralysis is effective.

SUMMARY

Acid–base disturbances are common clinical problems that are not difficult to analyze if approached in a consistent manner. The pH, $Paco_2$, and HCO_3^- should be inspected to identify all abnormal values. This should lead to an assessment of which deviations represent the primary abnormality and which represent compensatory changes. The serum electrolytes should always be used to calculate the anion gap. In cases in which the anion gap is increased, the excess anion gap should be added back to the measured HCO_3^-. The anion gap and the excess gap are useful tools that can identify hidden disorders. This rigorous assessment of the patient's acid–base status, incorporated with the available clinical data, increases the likelihood that the clinician will successfully determine the cause of each identified disorder. Although supportive therapy is often required for profound acid–base disturbances, definitive therapy must target the underlying process that has led to the observed derangements.

Patient Care Process

Patient Assessment:

- Based upon physical examination, review of systems, and laboratory data, determine whether the patient is experiencing manifestations of an acid-base disorder
- Determine whether pH is consistent with acidosis or alkalosis
- Check for laboratory validity (determine whether CO_2 and HCO_3^- are consistent with the pH)
- Review the history to see if there are any clues to the cause of the disorder
- Determine whether the primary disorder is of respiratory or metabolic origin
  - Alkalemia
    - Respiratory alkalosis if CO_2 less than 40 mm Hg (5.3 kPa)
    - Metabolic alkalosis if HCO_3 greater than 26 mm Hg (3.3 kPa)
  - Acidemia
    - Respiratory acidosis if CO_2 greater than 40 mmHg (5.3 kPa)
    - Metabolic acidosis if HCO_3 less than 22 mmHg (3.3 kPa)
- Calculate compensatory response (determine whether mixed acid–base disorder)
- Calculate the anion gap
- Consider additional laboratory tests to further differentiate the cause of the disorder

Therapy Evaluation:

- If the patient demonstrates an acid–base disorder, determine whether pharmacotherapy is indicated
- If the patient has received pharmacotherapy to correct acid–base disorder, assess efficacy, safety, and patient response
- Determine if any medications on the patient profile are contributing to the existing acid–base disorder

Care Plan Development:

- Urgently correct any life-threatening acid–base disorder
- Assess the underlying etiology of the altered pH and intervene accordingly
- Ensure drug doses are optimal to correct the acid base disorder

Follow-Up Evaluation:

- Review medical history, physical examination findings, blood gas result, and laboratory tests

Abbreviations Introduced In This Chapter

ABG	Arterial blood gas
BiPAP	Bilevel positive airway pressure
Cl^-	Chloride ion
CO2	Carbon dioxide
Δ(delta)	Change
H^+	Hydrogen ion
HCl	Hydrochloric acid

HCO_3^-	Bicarbonate
HCO^-_{3corr}	Current bicarbonate
HCO^-_{3post}	Post-therapy bicarbonate
Hg	Mercury
K^+	Potassium ion
Na^+	Sodium ion
$NaHCO_3$	Sodium bicarbonate
NH_2	Terminal amine group
NH_4^+	Ammonium
pH	Logarithm of the hydrogen ion concentration
$Paco_2$	Partial pressure of arterial carbon dioxide
tCO_2	Total venous carbon dioxide
THAM	Tromethamine
UAG	Urine anion gap

REFERENCES

1. Rose BD, Post TW. Clinical Physiology of Acid–Base and Electrolyte Disorders, 5th ed. New York, NY: McGraw-Hill, 2001:299.
2. Schlichtig R, Grogono A, Severinghaus J. Human $Paco_2$ and standard base excess for compensation of acid–base imbalances. Crit Care Med. 1998;26:1173–1179.
3. Pierce NF, Fedson DS, Brigham KL, et al. The ventilatory response to acute base deficit in humans. Time course during development and correction of metabolic acidosis. Ann Intern Med. 1970;72:633–640.
4. Javaheri S, Kazemi H. Metabolic alkalosis and hypoventilation in humans. Am Rev Respir Dis. 1987;136:1011–1016.
5. Polak A, Haynie GD, Hays RM, Schwartz WB. Effects of chronic hypercapnia on electrolyte and acid–base equilibrium. J Clin Invest. 1961;40:1223–1237.
6. Gennari FJ, Goldstein MB, Schwartz WB. The nature of the renal adaptation to chronic hypocapnia. J Clin Invest. 1972; 51:1722–1730.
7. van Ypersele de Striho C, Brasseur L, de Coninck JD. The "carbon dioxide response curve" for chronic hypercapnia in man. N Engl J Med. 1966;275:117–122.
8. Haber RJ. A practical approach to acid–base disorders. West J Med. 1991;155:146–151.
9. Arbus GS. An in-vivo acid–base nomogram for clinical use. Can Med Assoc J. 1973;109:291–293.
10. Narins R. Clinical Disorders of Fluid and Electrolyte Metabolism, 5th ed. New York, NY: McGraw-Hill, 1994:778.
11. Goodkin DA, Gollapudi GK, Narins RG. The role of the anion gap in detecting and managing mixed metabolic acid–base disorders. Clin Endocrinol Metab. 1984;13:333–349.
12. Adrogué HJ, Madias NE. Management of life-threatening acid–base disorders. First of two parts. N Engl J Med. 1998;338:26–34.
13. Adrogué HJ, Madias NE. Management of life-threatening acid–base disorders. Second of two parts. N Engl J Med. 1998;338:107–111.
14. Abelow B. Understanding Acid–Base. Baltimore, MD: Williams & Wilkins, 1998:229.
15. Kearns T, Wolfson A. Metabolic acidosis. Emerg Med Clin North Am. 1989;7:823–835.
16. Batlle DC, Hizon M, Cohen E, Gutterman C, Gupta R. The use of the urinary anion gap in the diagnosis of hyperchloremic metabolic acidosis. N Engl J Med. 1988;318:594–599.
17. Hood FL, Tannen RL. Protection of acid–base balance by pH regulation of acid production. N Engl J Med. 1998;339:819–826.
18. Chernow B, ed. The Pharmacologic Approach to the Critically Ill Patient, 3rd ed. Baltimore, MD: Williams & Wilkins, 1994:965.

29 Alzheimer Disease

Megan J. Ehret and Kevin W. Chamberlin

LEARNING OBJECTIVES

Upon completion of the chapter, the reader will be able to:

1. Describe the epidemiology of Alzheimer disease (AD) and its effects on society.
2. Describe the pathophysiology, including genetic and environmental factors that may be associated with AD.
3. Detail the clinical presentation of the typical patient with AD.
4. Describe the clinical course of the disease and typical patient outcomes.
5. Explain how nonpharmacologic therapy is combined with pharmacologic therapy for patients with AD.
6. Recognize and recommend treatment options for disease-specific symptoms as well as behavioral/noncognitive symptoms associated with AD.
7. Educate patients and/or caregivers about the expected outcomes for patients with AD, and provide contact information for support/advocacy agencies.

INTRODUCTION

KEY CONCEPT *Alzheimer disease (AD) is characterized by progressive cognitive decline including memory loss, disorientation, and impaired judgment and learning.* It is primarily diagnosed by exclusion of other potential causes for dementias. There is no single symptom unique to AD; therefore, diagnosis relies on a thorough patient history. The exact pathophysiologic mechanism underlying AD is not entirely known, although certain genetic and environmental factors may be associated with the disease. There is no cure for AD; however, drug treatment can slow symptom progression.

Family members of AD patients are profoundly affected by the increased dependence of their loved ones as the disease progresses. Referral to an advocacy organization, such as the Alzheimer Association, can provide early education and social support of both the patient and family. The Alzheimer Association has developed a list of common warning signs, which include memory loss, difficulty planning and doing usual tasks, disorientation, difficulty with visual images, problems with word finding, misplacing things, impaired judgment, social withdrawal, and changes in mood.[1]

EPIDEMIOLOGY AND ETIOLOGY

AD is the most common type of dementia, affecting an estimated 5.2 million Americans in 2011.[2] It is the sixth leading cause of death across all age groups in the United States and the fifth leading cause of death for individuals 65 years of age and older.[2] Various classifications of dementia include dementia of the Alzheimer type, vascular dementia, and dementia due to human immunodeficiency virus (HIV) disease, head trauma, Parkinson disease, Huntington disease, Pick disease, or Creutzfeldt-Jakob disease.[3] This chapter addresses only dementia of the Alzheimer type.

The prevalence of AD increases with age. Of those affected, one in nine are 65 years of age or older, and 1/3 are 85 years of age or older.[2] It is projected that by the year 2050, there will be a threefold increase in prevalence, yielding potentially 13.8 million AD patients due to a population increase in persons older than 65 years.[2] Additionally, total spending for AD is projected to increase from $214 billion in 2014 to over $1.2 trillion in 2050.[4] Furthermore, AD costs paid by Medicare and Medicaid in 2050 will have increased from 2010 by more than 600% and 400%, respectively.[4] The severity of AD also correlates with increasing age and is classified as mild, moderate, or severe. Other risk factors for AD include family history, female gender, and vascular risk factors such as diabetes, hypertension, heart disease, and current smoking.[5] It is unknown how other factors such as environment contribute and interact with the genetic predisposition for AD.

The mean survival time of persons with AD is reported to be approximately 6 years from the onset of symptoms. However, age at diagnosis, severity of AD, and other medical conditions affect survival time.[6] Although AD does not directly cause death, it is associated with an increase in various risk factors that often contribute to death, such as senility, sepsis, stroke, pneumonia, dehydration, and decubitus ulcers.

The etiology of AD is unknown, however, genetic factors may contribute to errors in protein synthesis resulting in the formation of abnormal proteins involved in pathogenesis.[7] Early onset, which is defined as AD prior to age 60, accounts for approximately 1% of all AD. This type is usually familial and follows an autosomal dominant pattern in approximately 50% of cases of early-onset AD. Mutations in three genes, presenilin 1 on chromosome 14, amyloid precursor protein (APP) on chromosome 21, and presenilin 2 on chromosome 1, lead to an increase in the accumulation of amyloid beta (Aβ) in the brain, resulting in oxidative stress, neuronal destruction, and the clinical syndrome of AD.[8,9]

The genetic basis for the more common late-onset AD appears more complex. Genetic susceptibility is more sporadic, and it may be more dependent on environmental factors.[7] The apolipoprotein E (apo E) gene on chromosome 19 has been identified as a strong risk factor for late-onset AD. There are three variants of apo E; however, carriers of two or more of the apo E4 allele have an earlier onset of AD (~ 6 years earlier) compared with noncarriers.[7] Only 50% of AD patients have the apo E4 allele, thus indicating it is only a susceptibility marker.

PATHOPHYSIOLOGY

KEY CONCEPT *Pathologic hallmarks of the disease in the brain include neurofibrillary tangles and neuritic plaques (senile plaques) made up of various proteins that result in a shortage of the neurotransmitter acetylcholine (Ach).* These are primarily located in brain regions involved in learning, memory, and emotional behaviors such as the cerebral cortex, hippocampus, basal forebrain, and amygdala.[10]

Tangles

Neurofibrillary tangles (NFTs) are intracellular and consist of abnormally phosphorylated tau (τ) protein, which is involved in microtubule assembly. NFTs interfere with neuronal function, resulting in cell damage, and their presence has been correlated with the severity of dementia.[11] Unfortunately, NFTs are insoluble even after the cell dies, and they cannot be removed once established, thus prevention is key. The neurons that provide most of the cholinergic innervation to the cortex are most prominently affected.[12]

Plaques

Neuritic or senile plaques are extracellular protein deposits of β-amyloid protein, which are central to the pathogenesis of AD.[10] The β-amyloid protein is present in a nontoxic, soluble form in human brains. In AD, conformational changes occur that render it insoluble and cause it to deposit into amorphous diffuse plaques associated with dystrophic neuritis.[13] Over time, these deposits become compacted into plaques, and the β-amyloid protein becomes fibrillar and neurotoxic. Inflammation occurs secondary to clusters of astrocytes and microglia surrounding these plaques.

Acetylcholine

In AD, the plaques and tangles damage Ach pathways, leading to a shortage of Ach, resulting in learning and memory impairment.[14] The loss of Ach activity correlates with the severity of AD. The basis of pharmacologic treatment of AD has been to improve cholinergic neurotransmission in the brain. Blocking acetylcholinesterase, the enzyme that degrades Ach in the synaptic cleft, leads to an increased level of Ach with a goal of stabilizing neurotransmission.[14]

Glutamate

Glutamate is the primary excitatory neurotransmitter in the central nervous system; it is involved in memory, learning, and neuronal plasticity. It affects cognition through facilitation of connections with cholinergic neurons in the cerebral cortex and basal forebrain.[15] In AD, one type of glutamate receptor, *N*-methyl-D-aspartate (NMDA), is less prevalent than normal. There also appears to be overactivation of unregulated glutamate signaling. This results in a rise in calcium ions that induces secondary cascades, which lead to neuronal death and an increased production of APP.[14] The increased production of APP is associated with higher rates of plaque development and hyperphosphorylation of τ protein.[15]

Cholesterol

Increased cholesterol concentrations have been associated with AD. The cholesterol increases β-amyloid protein synthesis, which can lead to plaque formation.[14] Also, the apo E4 allele is thought to be involved in cholesterol metabolism and is associated with higher cholesterol levels.[14]

Estrogen

Estrogen appears to have properties that protect against memory loss associated with normal aging. Estrogen may block β-amyloid protein production and even trigger nerve growth in cholinergic nerve terminals.[16] Estrogen also helps prevent oxidative cell damage.[16] Despite this, the Women's Health Initiative Memory Study reported that hormone replacement therapy with either estrogen alone or estrogen plus medroxyprogesterone resulted in negative effects on memory.[17]

CLINICAL PRESENTATION AND DIAGNOSIS

KEY CONCEPT *The diagnosis of AD is established following an extensive history and physical examination, and by ruling out other*

Clinical Presentation and Diagnosis of Alzheimer Disease

General

The diagnosis of AD, is primarily one of exclusion, but medical and psychiatric history, neurological examination, interview of caregivers and family members, and laboratory and imaging data also have a role.

Signs and Symptoms

- Cognitive: memory loss, problems with language, disorientation to time and place, poor or decreased judgment, problems with learning and abstract thinking, misplacing things
- Noncognitive: Changes in mood or behavior, changes in personality, or loss of initiative
- Functional: Difficulty performing familiar tasks

Laboratory Tests

- MRI or CT to measure changes in brain size and volume and rule out stroke, brain tumor, or cerebral edema.
- Tests to exclude possible causes of dementia: depression screen, vitamin B_{12} levels, thyroid function tests (thyroid-stimulating hormone and free triiodothyronine and thyroxine), complete blood count, and chemistry panel.[18]
- Other diagnostic tests to consider for differential diagnosis: erythrocyte sedimentation rate, urinalysis, toxicology, chest x-ray, heavy metal screen, HIV testing, CSF examination, electroencephalography, and neuropsychological tests such as the Folstein Mini Mental State Examination.

Table 29–1

***DSM-5* Diagnostic Criteria for Major Neurocognitive Disorders**

A. Evidence of significant cognitive decline from a previous level of performance in one or more cognitive domains (complex attention, executive function, learning and memory, language, perceptual-motor, or social cognition) based on:
   1. Concern of the individual, a knowledgeable informant, or the clinician that there has been a significant decline in cognitive function and
   2. A substantial impairment in cognitive performance, preferably documented by standardized neuropsychological testing or, in its absence, another quantified clinical assessment

B. Cognitive deficits interfere with independence in everyday activities

C. Cognitive deficits do not occur exclusively in the contest of delirium

D. Cognitive deficits are not better explained by another mental disorder

Data from American Psychiatric Association. Diagnostic and Statistical Manual of Mental Disorders, 5th ed, Washington, DC: American Psychiatric Association;2013:602–603, with permission.

potential causes of dementia. There are no biological markers other than those pathophysiological changes found at autopsy that can confirm AD, although the development of in vivo plaque detection methods may change this.

AD is a progressive disease that, over time, affects multiple areas of cognition. The American Psychiatric Association recently updated the criteria for AD in the *Diagnostic and Statistical Manual* (*DSM-5*). See Tables 29–1, 29–2, and 29–3 for full criteria.[3]

Table 29–2

***DSM-5* Diagnostic Criteria for Mild Neurocognitive Disorder**

A. Evidence of modest cognitive decline from a previous level of performance in one or more cognitive domains (complex attention, executive function, learning and memory, language, perceptual-motor, or social cognition) based on:
   1. Concern of the individual, a knowledgeable informant, or the clinician that there has been a mild decline in cognitive function and
   2. A modest impairment in cognitive performance, preferably documented by standardized neuropsychological testing, or in its absence, another quantified clinical assessment

B. Cognitive deficits do not interfere with capacity for independence in everyday activities

C. Cognitive deficits do not occur exclusively in the context of delirium

D. Cognitive deficits are not better explained by another mental disorder

Data from American Psychiatric Association. Diagnostic and Statistical Manual of Mental Disorders, 5th ed, Washington, DC: American Psychiatric Association;2013;605; with permission.

Table 29–3

***DSM-5* Diagnostic Criteria for Major or Mild Neurocognitive Disorder Due to Alzheimer Disease**

A. Criteria are met for major or mild neurocognitive disorder

B. Insidious onset and gradual progression of impairment in one or more cognitive domains (for major neurocognitive disorder, at least two domains must be impaired)

C. Criteria are met for either probable or possible Alzheimer disease as follows:

   For Major Neurocognitive Disorder:

   Probable Alzheimer disease is diagnosed if either of the following is present; otherwise possible Alzheimer disease should be diagnosed.
   1. Evidence of a causative Alzheimer disease genetic mutation from family history or genetic testing
   2. All three of the following are present:
      a. Clear evidence of decline in memory and learning and at least one other cognitive domain
      b. Steadily progressive gradual decline in cognition, without extended plateaus
      c. No evidence of mixed etiology

   For Mild Neurocognitive Disorder:

   Probable Alzheimer disease: diagnosed if there is evidence of a causative Alzheimer disease genetic mutation from either genetic testing or family history

   Possible Alzheimer disease: diagnosed if there is no evidence of a causative Alzheimer disease genetic mutation from either genetic testing or family history, and all three of the following are present:
   1. Clear evidence of decline in memory and learning
   2. Steadily progressive, gradual decline in cognition, without extended plateaus
   3. No evidence of mixed etiology

D. Disturbance is not better explained by cerebrovascular disease, another neurodegenerative disease, the effects of a substance, or another mental, neurological, or systematic disorder

Data from American Psychiatric Association. Diagnostic and Statistical Manual of Mental Disorders, 5th ed, Washington, DC: American Psychiatric Association;2013;611; with permission.

TREATMENT

Desired Outcomes

There are four agents approved for the treatment of AD, but none are curative or known to directly reverse the disease process.

KEY CONCEPT *Treatment is focused on delaying disease progression and preservation of functioning as long as possible.* Secondary goals include treating psychiatric and behavioral symptoms that may occur during the course of the disease.

General Approach to Treatment

KEY CONCEPT *The current gold standard of treatment for cognitive symptoms includes pharmacologic management with a* **cholinesterase (ChE) inhibitor** and/or an **NMDA antagonist**. Donepezil, rivastigmine, and galantamine are three ChEs used for cognitive symptoms. The first ChE approved for AD was tacrine; however, it is no longer available in the United States. Its use was limited due to its propensity for hepatotoxicity, difficult titration schedule, four times daily dosing, poor bioavailability, and troublesome incidence of nausea, diarrhea, and urinary incontinence. The only NMDA antagonist is memantine. Psychiatric and behavioral

Table 29–4

Basic Principles in the Management of Patients with AD

- Using a gentle, calm approach to the patient
- Giving reassurance when needed
- Empathizing with the patient's concerns
- Using distraction and redirection
- Maintaining daily routines
- Providing a safe environment
- Providing daytime activities
- Avoiding overstimulation
- Using familiar decorative items in the living area
- Bringing abrupt declines in function and the appearance of new symptoms to professional attention

Table 29–5

Treatment Algorithm for Cognitive Symptoms of AD

1. Patient diagnosed with AD
2. Assess all comorbid medical disorders and drug therapies that may affect cognition
3. Rule out comorbid depression
4. Evaluate for pharmacotherapy based on illness stage
   a) Mild AD: Cholinesterase inhibitor
   b) Moderate to severe AD: Cholinesterase inhibitor, memantine, or combination cholinesterase inhibitor and memantine
3. Deteriorating Mini Mental State Exam (MMSE) score
   > 2–4 points after 1 year: Change to a different cholinesterase inhibitor
4. Stable MMSE: Continue regimen

symptoms that occur during the course of the disease should be treated as they occur.

Essential elements in the treatment of AD include education, communication, and planning with the patient's family/caregiver. Treatment options, legal and financial decisions, and course of the illness should be discussed with the patient and family members. In this regard, the clinician's emphasis should be on helping to maintain a therapeutic living environment while minimizing the burden of care resulting from the disease.

Nonpharmacologic Therapy

The life of a patient with AD must become progressively more simple and structured as the disease progresses, and the caregiver must learn to keep requests and demands on the patient simple. Basic principles in the treatment of patients with AD are shown in Table 29–4.

Pharmacologic Therapy

► *Conventional Pharmacologic Treatment for Cognitive Symptoms*

ChE Inhibitors (Donepezil, Rivastigmine, and Galantamine)

The ChE inhibitors are FDA approved for the treatment of AD. Guidelines recommend the use of ChE inhibitors as a valuable treatment for AD and the use of memantine for moderate to severe AD.[18] The few head-to-head studies comparing the ChE Inhibitors conclude there are no major differences in clinical outcomes, so the selection of one ChE over another should be based on differences in mechanisms of action, adverse reactions, and titration schedules.[19]

Treatment should begin as early as possible after diagnosis.[20] Table 29–5 provides a recommended treatment algorithm. Patients should be switched to another ChE inhibitor from their initial ChE inhibitor if they show an initial lack of efficacy, initially respond but then lose clinical benefit, or experience safety/tolerability issues. This switch should not be attempted until the patient has been on a maximally tolerated dose for 3 to 6 months. The switch should also be based on realistic expectations of the patient and/or caregiver.[21] ChE inhibitor therapy should be discontinued in patients who experience poor tolerance or adherence, who do not improve after 6 months at optimal dosing, who fail attempts at monotherapy with at least two agents or combination therapy, who continue to deteriorate at the pretreatment rate, who have dramatic clinical deterioration following initiation of treatment, or who deteriorate to the point where there is no significant effect on quality of life. Patients with a Mini Mental State Exam (MMSE) score less than 10 may also benefit from discontinuation of medication; however, this has not been substantially proven in clinical studies.[22]

Donepezil

Donepezil is a piperidine ChE inhibitor that reversibly and noncompetitively inhibits centrally active acetylcholinesterase.[23] A dose of 10 mg/day has demonstrated efficacy in patients with either mild to moderate or moderate to severe forms of AD. A 23-mg dose of donepezil is also approved for patients with moderate to severe disease. The 23-mg dose showed a small improvement in cognitive symptoms compared to the 10 mg/day dose; however, there was no improvement in overall functioning, and there was a higher incidence of adverse effects.[24] Table 29–6 describes dosing strategies for all of the approved agents for AD. The most frequent adverse effects are mild to moderate gastrointestinal symptoms. Others include headache, dizziness, syncope, bradycardia, and muscle weakness. Table 29–7 compares their major side effects.[23,25–28]

Only a small number of drug interactions have been reported with donepezil. In vitro studies show a low rate of binding of donepezil to cytochrome P450 (CYP)3A4 or 2D6. Whether donepezil has the potential for enzyme induction is unknown. Monitoring for increased peripheral side effects is advised when adding a CYP2D6 or 3A3/4 inhibitor to donepezil treatment. Also, inducers of CYP2D6 and 3A4 could increase the rate of elimination of donepezil.[23]

Rivastigmine

Rivastigmine, approved for the treatment of mild to moderate AD, has central activity for both acetylcholinesterase and butyrylcholinesterase.[28] Acetylcholinesterase is found in two forms: globular 4 and globular 1. In postmortem studies, globular 4 is significantly depleted, whereas globular 1 is still abundant. Thus, blocking metabolism of globular 1 may lead to higher concentrations of Ach. Rivastigmine has higher activity at globular 1 than at globular 4. Theoretically, this may be advantageous because rivastigmine prevents the degradation of Ach via the acetylcholinesterase globular 1 pathways over the course of the disease, compared with the other ChE inhibitors.

The dual inhibition of acetylcholinesterase and butyrylcholinesterase may lead to broader efficacy. As acetylcholinesterase activity decreases with disease progression, the acetylcholinesterase-selective agents may lose their effect, whereas the dual inhibitors may still be effective due to the added inhibition of

Table 29–6

Dosing Strategies for Cognitive Agents

	Donepezil (Aricept)	Rivastigmine (Exelon)	Galantamine (Razadyne)	Memantine (Namenda)[a]
Starting dose	5 mg daily in the evening	1.5 mg twice daily or 4.6 mg/24 hour applied daily (patch)	4 mg twice daily or 8 mg daily in the morning	5 mg daily or 7 mg daily (ER formulation)
Maintenance dose	5–23 mg daily	3–6 mg twice daily or 9.5 mg/24 hour applied daily (patch)	8–12 mg twice daily or 16–24 mg daily	10 mg twice daily or 28 mg daily (ER formulation)
Time between dose adjustments	4–6 weeks between 5 and 10 mg increment; 3 months between 10 and 23 mg increment	2 weeks for oral and 4 weeks for patch	4 weeks	1 week
Dosage adjustments for renal or hepatic impairment	None	Moderate to severe renal impairment, mild to moderate hepatic impairment, or low body weight (< 50 kg): consider maximum dose of 4.6 mg/24 hour	Do not exceed 16 mg for moderately impaired hepatic or renal function; do not administer in severe renal or hepatic impairment	Severe renal impairment: target maintenance dose of 5 mg twice daily or 14 mg daily

[a]As of August 15, 2014, Forest Pharmaceuticals, Inc. plans to discontinue the sale of all configurations of Namenda. They will continue to sell oral solution of Namenda as well as once-daily Namenda XR. Namzaric, a fixed-dose combination of extended-release memantine and donepezil, (14/10 mg and 28/10 mg) was recently approved.

Eisai. Aricept (donepezil hydrochloride) [product information]. Teaneck, NJ: Author, 2013.

Novartis. Exelon (rivastigmine tartrate) [product information]. East Hanover, NJ: Author, 2013.

Ortho McNeil Neurologics. Razadyne ER/Razadyne (galantamine hydrobromide) [product information]. Titusville, NJ: Author, 2013.

Forest Pharmaceutica, Inc. Namenda (memantine hydrochloride) [product information]. St. Louis, MO: Author, 2013.

Forest Pharmaceutica, Inc. Namenda XR (memantine hydrochloride) extended release [product information]. St. Louis, MO: Author, 2013.

Table 29–7

Adverse Effects for Currently Approved Medications for Alzheimer Disease[a]

Adverse Event	Donepezil 5–10 mg/day (%) (*n* = 747)	Donepezil 23 mg/day (%) (*n* = 963)	Rivastigmine 6–12 mg/day (%) (*n* = 1189)	Galantamine IR 16–24 mg/day (%) (*n* = 1040)	Memantine IR 5–20 mg/day (%) (*n* = 940)	Memantine XR 28 mg/day (%) (*n* = 341)
Nausea	11	12	47	24	NR	NR
Vomiting	5	9	31	13	3	2
Diarrhea	10	8	19	9	NR	5
Headache	10	4	17	8	6	6
Dizziness	8	5	21	9	7	5
Muscle cramps	6	NR	NR	NR	NR	NR
Insomnia	9	3	9	5	NR	NR
Fatigue	5	2	9	5	2	3
Anorexia	4	5	17	9	NR	NR
Depression	3	NR	6	7	NR	3
Abnormal dreams	3	NR	NR	NR	NR	NR
Weight decrease	3	5	3	7	NR	NR
Abdominal pain	NR	NR	13	5	NR	2
Rhinitis	NR	NR	4	4	NR	NR

NR, not reported.

[a]Caution is urged in making comparisons between drugs based on these data because different clinical trials often collect adverse event data using different methodologies.

Eisai. Aricept (donepezil hydrochloride) [product information]. Teaneck, NJ: Author, 2013.

Novartis. Exelon (rivastigmine tartrate) [product information]. East Hanover, NJ: Author, 2013.

Ortho McNeil Neurologics. Razadyne ER/Razadyne (galantamine hydrobromide) [product information]. Titusville, NJ: Author, 2013.

Forest Pharmaceutica, Inc. Namenda (memantine hydrochloride) [product information]. St. Louis, MO: Author, 2013.

Forest Pharmaceutica, Inc. Namenda XR (memantine hydrochloride) extended release [product information]. St. Louis, MO: Author, 2013.

butyrylcholinesterase. However, this has not been demonstrated clinically.

Rivastigmine is available as an oral formulation and as a patch. When switching from the oral formulation to the patch, if the patient is taking less than 6 mg/day orally, the 4.6 mg/24 hour patch is recommended. If the patient is taking 6 to 12 mg/day orally, the 9.5 mg/24 hour patch is recommended. The first patch should be applied on the day following the last oral dose.[25]

Cholinergic side effects are common, but they are usually well tolerated if the recommended dosing schedule is followed. If side effects cause intolerance, several doses can be held, then dosing can be restarted at the same or next lower dose. Drugs that induce or inhibit CYP450 metabolism are not expected to alter rivastigmine metabolism.[25]

Galantamine

Galantamine, approved for the treatment of mild to moderate AD, is a ChE inhibitor, which elevates Ach in the cerebral cortex.[26] It also modulates the nicotinic Ach receptors to increase Ach release from surviving presynaptic nerve terminals. It may also increase glutamate and serotonin levels, but whether this brings additional benefit is unknown.

CYP3A4 and 2D6 are the major metabolizing enzymes, and pharmacokinetic studies with inhibitors of these enzymes have shown increased galantamine concentrations or reductions in clearance. Similar to donepezil, if inhibitors are given concurrently with galantamine, monitoring for increased cholinergic side effects should be done.[26]

NMDA Receptor Antagonist

Memantine is a noncompetitive antagonist of the NMDA type of glutamate receptors, which are located throughout the brain. It regulates activity throughout the brain by controlling the amount of calcium that enters the nerve cell, a process essential for establishing an environment required for information storage. Overstimulation of the NMDA receptor by excessive glutamate allows too much calcium into the cell, disrupting information processing. Blocking NMDA receptors with memantine may protect neurons from the effects of excessive glutamate without disrupting normal neurotransmission.[27,28]

Memantine is approved to treat moderate to severe AD. It can be given as monotherapy or in combination with ChE inhibitors. Memantine is not indicated for mild AD, and current evidence does not support its use in mild AD.[29] The 28-mg memantine extended release has not been compared with the immediate-release formulation; thus it is unknown if the 28 mg/day dose of memantine is more effective than the traditional 20 mg/day maximum. Adverse reactions associated with memantine include constipation, confusion, dizziness, headache, coughing, and hypertension. Closer monitoring should be done if memantine is given concurrently with a ChE inhibitor.

In vitro studies have shown that memantine produces minimal inhibition of CYP450 enzymes CYP1A2, 2A6, 2C9, 2D6, 2E1, and 3A4, and that no pharmacokinetic interactions with drugs metabolized by these enzymes should be expected.[27,28]

Future Therapies

KEY CONCEPT *Future therapies for AD may include disease-modifying therapies.* Current investigations involving the amyloid hypothesis are evaluating various compounds in the secondary prevention of AD. Mechanisms by which these compounds are thought to work include[8]:

Patient Encounter, Part 1

A man presents at the clinic with his 73-year-old mother complaining that his mother's memory is worsening. He complains that his mother is continuing to forget things, including paying the bills and emptying the cat's litter box. Three months ago she was started on galantamine 8 mg daily, which was titrated to 16 mg daily. Her son organizes a weekly pillbox and helps administer the medications. The son asks if there is anything else his mother could take to help her memory.

What education points about Alzheimer disease would you provide to the son?

Where would you recommend the son find more information about Alzheimer disease?

How would you address the son's question regarding the pharmacologic management of his mother's Alzheimer disease?

- Reducing levels of brain Aβ or manipulating its configuration
- Targeting τ proteins
- Targeting inflammatory approaches
- Addressing insulin resistance in the brain

Recent studies of bapineuzumab and solanezumab, humanized monoclonal antibody targeting the Aβ, failed to demonstrate a significant change in the Alzheimer Disease Assessment Scale (ADAS-cog11) in phase 3 clinical trials.[30,31]

Nonconventional Pharmacologic Treatment

Many other nonconventional treatments have historically been used as adjunctive treatments of AD. Vitamin E was previously recommended because of its antioxidant properties, but a meta-analysis suggested that greater than 400 IU/day should be avoided due to an increased all-cause mortality.[32] Currently, vitamin E is not recommended for the treatment of AD. Estrogen has been investigated for use in AD, but it was associated with an increased risk of dementia. For nonsteroidal anti-inflammatory drugs (NSAIDs) there is a lack of convincing data supporting efficacy, and gastritis, GI bleeds, and increased cardiovascular events are associated with their use. They are not recommended for treatment or prevention of AD at this time.[33] Statins (3-hydroxy-3-methylglutaryl-CoA reductase inhibitors) should be reserved for those who have other indications for their use.[34] Until Ginkgo biloba has a more standardized manufacturing process and its long-term safety and efficacy are established, it should be recommended with caution.[35] The medical food caprylidene (AC-1202, Axona) is a medium chain triglyceride approved for the dietary management of metabolic processes associated with mild to moderate AD.[36] Reduced neuronal metabolism of glucose has been associated with AD. Ketone bodies can potentially be used as an alternative energy source for AD patients.[36] Caprylidene is converted by the liver into the ketone body β-hydroxybutyrate (BHB). BHB crosses the blood–brain barrier and can be utilized by neurons as a potential energy source to generate ATP and increase pools of acetylcholine. Caprylidene requires a prescription and is supplied in 40-g powder packets. One packet can be mixed with 4 to 8 ounces of liquid (~120–240 mL) and dosed once daily after a meal. The most common side effects are mild

GI disturbances including nausea, diarrhea, flatulence, and dyspepsia.[37]

Treatment of Behavioral Symptoms

KEY CONCEPT *Treatment of behavioral symptoms should begin with nonpharmacologic treatments but may also include antipsychotic agents and/or antidepressants.* Nonpharmacologic recommendations for treatment include[38]:

- Music
- Videotapes of family members
- Audiotapes of the voices of caregivers
- Walking and light exercise
- Sensory stimulation and relaxation

Antipsychotics are frequently used for neuropsychiatric symptoms associated with AD. A recent meta-analysis concluded that only 17% to 18% of dementia patients demonstrated treatment response to atypical antipsychotics.[39] A double-blind, placebo-controlled trial of olanzapine, quetiapine, or risperidone for the treatment of psychosis, aggression, or agitation in patients with AD showed that adverse effects offset the benefits in the efficacy of atypical antipsychotics.[40]

In April 2005, the FDA issued a statement requiring black-box warnings on all antipsychotics stating that elderly people with dementia-related psychosis treated with an antipsychotic are at an increased risk of death compared with those treated with placebo. Fifteen of 17 trials investigating olanzapine, aripiprazole, quetiapine, and risperidone in elderly demented patients with behavioral disorders showed an increase in mortality compared with the placebo-treated groups (1.6–1.7 times increased risk of death). Causes for these deaths were heart-related events (heart failure and sudden death) and infections (mostly pneumonia).

The antipsychotics are not approved for the treatment of elderly patients with dementia-related psychosis. Therefore, it is important to individually assess and balance the risk versus benefit of antipsychotic use in this population.

Depressive symptoms occur in as many as 50% of patients with AD and can be difficult to differentiate from symptoms of dementia, so symptoms of depression should be documented for several weeks prior to initiating therapy for depression with AD.[8] The selective serotonin reuptake inhibitors (SSRIs) are most commonly used based on their side-effect profile and evidence of efficacy.[8] Indications for the use of antidepressants include depression characterized by poor appetite, insomnia, hopelessness, anhedonia, withdrawal, suicidal thoughts, and agitation. A recent trial suggested a lack of benefit of sertraline and mirtazapine compared with placebo and an increased risk of adverse effects.[41]

Other miscellaneous therapies for AD include benzodiazepines for anxiety, agitation, and aggression. However, their routine use is not advised.[8] Additionally, benzodiazepines are associated with an increase in falls leading to the potential for hip fractures in the elderly.[42] Mood stabilizer anticonvulsants, carbamazepine, valproic acid, or gabapentin may be used as alternatives, but the current evidence is conflicting.[43] Buspirone has shown benefit in treating agitation and aggression in a limited number of patients with minimal adverse effects.[44,45] In open-label and controlled studies, selegiline decreased anxiety, depression, and agitation.[46,47] Finally, trazodone has been shown to decrease insomnia, agitation, and dysphoria, and it has been used to treat sundowning in AD patients. Table 29–8 provides dosing strategies for the noncognitive symptoms of AD.[48]

Patient Encounter, Part 2

The patient returns to the clinic in 6 months. She has been receiving 24 mg/day of galantamine. Her memory symptoms have slowed in their decline, but recently she has been agitated at bedtime and talking to her deceased sister. The son is particularly concerned about the symptoms and wants to know what he could do to help. The patient's record is as follows:

PMH: Diabetes mellitus since age 51, it was well controlled until last year when she became confused about when to take her medication; hypertension treated for 23 years and well controlled; has been hypotensive on a few occasions recently during physicals; osteopenia, last bone mineral density test 12 months ago (T-score = – 1.2); on therapy; hypercholesterolemia, last cholesterol panel 12 months ago showed well-controlled levels in normal range; on therapy

FH: Father died of myocardial infarction at age 76; mother died of breast cancer at age 79

SH: Lives with wheelchair-bound husband; son lives across street and checks in daily; denies drinking alcohol or smoking

Meds: Metformin 1000 mg orally twice daily; insulin glargine 18 units subcutaneously at bedtime; hydrochlorothiazide 12.5 mg orally once daily in the morning; lisinopril 20 mg orally once daily in the morning; calcium carbonate and vitamin D 600 mg/200 international units orally twice daily with lunch and dinner; pravastatin 20 mg orally once daily with dinner; galantamine 24 mg daily in the morning

ROS: (+) Weight loss of 6.3 kg (14 lb) since last visit; (-) N/V/D, change in appetite, heartburn, chest pain, or shortness of breath

PE:

VS: BP 111/72 mm Hg supine, P 79 beats/min, RR 16 breaths/min, T 37°C (98.6°F)

Gen: Poorly groomed, thin woman looks stated age

Neuro: Folstein Mini-Mental State Exam score 18/30; disoriented to month, date, and day of week, clinic name and floor; poor registration with impaired attention and short-term memory; good language skills but problems with commands

CT Scan: Mild-to-moderate generalized cerebral atrophy

What do you recommend with regard to her current galantamine treatment?

What nonpharmacologic and pharmacologic interventions could be recommended for the agitation and psychosis?

GENOMICS

KEY CONCEPT *Therapeutic response in AD is genotype specific, depending on the genes associated with pathogenesis and/or genes responsible for drug metabolism.* Apo E-4/4 carriers tend to show a faster disease progression and a poorer therapeutic response to all available treatments than any other polymorphic variants associated with AD. CYP450 enzyme extensive and intermediate metabolizers are the best responders to pharmacotherapy, while poor and ultrarapid metabolizers are the worst responders. The pharmacogenetic response in AD may depend on interaction of

Table 29–8

Medications Used for Noncognitive Symptoms of Dementia

Drugs	Starting Dose (mg)	Maintenance Dose in Dementia (mg/day)	Dosing Adjustment for Hepatic Impairment (mg)	Dosing Adjustment for Renal Impairment (mg)	Target Symptoms
Antipsychotics					
Aripiprazole	10–15	30 (maximum)	None needed	None needed	Psychosis: hallucinations, delusions, suspiciousness Disruptive behaviors: agitation, aggression
Olanzapine	2.5	5–10	None needed	None needed	
Quetiapine	25	100–400	Lower starting dose and longer titration schedule to effective dose based on response and tolerability	None needed	
Risperidone	0.25	0.5–2	Lower starting dose and longer titration schedule to effective dose based on response and tolerability	Lower starting dose and longer titration schedule to effective dose based on response and tolerability	
Antidepressants					
Citalopram	10	10–20	20 mg/day maximum; may increase only in nonresponsive patients	Mild to moderate impairment: none needed	Depression: poor appetite, insomnia, hopelessness, anhedonia, withdrawal, suicidal thoughts, agitation, anxiety
Escitalopram	5	10 (maximum)	10 mg/day maximum	Mild to moderate impairment: none needed	
Fluoxetine	5	10–20	A lower dose or less frequent schedule is recommended	None needed	
Paroxetine	10	10–40	10 mg/day; may increase by 10 mg/day at intervals of at least 1 week	10 mg/day; may increase by 10 mg/day at intervals of at least 1 week	
Sertraline	12.5	150 (maximum)	Lower or less frequent doses should be used	None needed	
Mirtazapine	15	15–50	Caution should be used	Caution should be used	
Trazodone	25	75–150	None needed	None needed	
Anticonvulsants					
Carbamazepine	100	300–600	Should not be used in aggravated liver dysfunction or active liver disease	None needed	Agitation or aggression
Valproic acid	125	500–1500	Should not be administered	None needed	

Adapted from Slattum PW, Peron EP, Massey-Hill A. Alzheimer's disease. In: Dipiro JT, Talbert RL, Yee GC, et al, eds. Pharmacotherapy: A Pathophysiologic Approach. 9th ed. New York, NY: McGraw-Hill;2014:828, with permission.

genes involved in drug metabolism and genes associated with AD pathogenesis.[49]

OUTCOME EVALUATION

- The success of therapy is measured by the degree to which the care plan decreases the pretreatment rate of cognitive deterioration, preserves the patients' functioning, and treats psychiatric and behavioral symptoms. The primary outcome measure is thus subjective information from the patient and the caregiver, although the MMSE can be a helpful tool. There are no physical examination or laboratory parameters to evaluate the success of therapy.

Patient Encounter, Part 3

The patient returns to the clinic for follow-up 1 year later. Her son states her memory has continued getting worse. Her current MMSE is 16/30. The addition of olanzapine 2.5 mg at bedtime helped with her agitation. Her son would like to know if there are any other choices to help treat his mom.

What changes to the patient's current medications would you recommend?

Patient Care Process

Patient Assessment:

- Assess the frequency and duration of cognitive and noncognitive symptoms. Could the patient be depressed?
- Review any available diagnostic data from the medical and psychiatric history including interviews from family, neuropsychologic testing, and other labs. (ie, MRI, CT, vitamin deficiencies, thyroid function tests, complete blood counts, and chemistry panel)
- Obtain a thorough history of prescription, nonprescription, and natural drug product use. Is the patient taking any medications that could contribute to cognitive changes in the elderly?

Therapy Evaluation:

- If needed, provide patients and caregivers information about lifestyle modification, and refer them to support when needed.
- Assess the current regimen for appropriateness, effectiveness, adverse effects, drug interactions, appropriate dosing, and medication adherence (see Table 29–7).

Care Plan Development:

- Be a resource and give continuous support to the patient and caregivers throughout the long course of the disease.
- Select an appropriate ChE inhibitor to avoid drug–drug interactions and adverse effects and in consideration of cost and patient preference (see Tables 29–6 and 29–8).
- Develop a plan to monitor cognitive response to treatment over time.
- Select appropriate medications for behavior symptoms if lifestyle modifications do not achieve goals (see Table 29–8).
- Educate patient and caregivers on what to expect from pharmacotherapy.

Follow-Up Evaluation:

- Follow up at needed intervals to assess effectiveness and safety of therapy. Review medical history and physical exam findings, lab tests, and results of other diagnostic tests.
- Monitor pharmacotherapy initiation (see Table 29–6), and regularly evaluate the patient for the presence of adverse drug reactions, drug allergies, drug–drug and drug–disease interactions, and adherence.
- If symptoms progress, consider stopping/switching the ChE inhibitor. Switch if there is initial lack of efficacy, loss of clinical benefit, or if poor tolerability develops. Discontinue if there is poor adherence, 6 months with no clinical improvement, or if there is continued deterioration at pretreatment rates.
- Continue to offer support to the patient and caregiver.

- Develop a plan to assess the effectiveness of the ChE inhibitor in slowing the deterioration of cognitive functioning after an appropriate interval (every 3–6 months).
- Assess improvement in quality-of-life measures such as ability to function independently and for slowing of memory deterioration (every 3–6 months).
- Evaluate the patient for the presence of adverse drug reactions, drug allergies, and drug interactions at appropriate intervals (soon after drug initiation or change and every 3–6 months).

CONCLUSION

AD is a progressive deterioration of cognitive abilities usually with behavioral disturbances and personality changes in the later stages of the disease. In an effort to help prepare patients and their caregivers for the inevitable, the Alzheimer Association has developed ten quick tips on "Living with Alzheimer disease" and they can also provide many resources for patients and caregivers.[50] Access the association at:

Alzheimer Association
Contact Center: 1-800-272-3900
TDD access: 1.312.335.8882
Website: www.alz.org
E-mail: info@alz.org
National office: 225 N. Michigan Ave., Fl. 17
Chicago, IL 60601-7633

Abbreviations Introduced in This Chapter

Ach	Acetylcholine
Aβ	Amyloid beta
AD	Alzheimer disease
apo E	Apolipoprotein E
APP	Amyloid precursor protein
BHB	β-Hydroxybutyrate
ChE	Cholinesterase
CYP	Cytochrome P450
DSM-5	*Diagnostic and Statistical Manual of Mental Disorders*, 5th edition
MMSE	Mini Mental State Examination
NMDA	*N*-Methyl-D-aspartate
NFTs	Neurofibrillary Tangles
NSAID	Nonsteroidal anti-inflammatory drug
SSRI	Selective serotonin reuptake inhibitor
τ	Tau protein

REFERENCES

1. Alzheimer's Association [Internet], [cited 2014 May 28]. http://www.alz.org/alzheimers_disease_ 10_signs_of_alzheimers.asp.
2. Hebert LE, Weuve J, Scherr PA, Evans DA. Alzheimer Disease in the United States (2010-2050) estimated using the 2010 census. Neurology. 2013;80(19):1778–1783.

3. American Psychiatric Association. Diagnostic and Statistical Manual of Mental Disorders. 5th ed. Washington, DC: American Psychiatric Association; 2013:591–643.
4. Unpublished tabulations based on data from Medicare current beneficiary survey for 2008. Prepared under contract by Julie Brown, M.D., M.P.H, Dartmouth Institute for Health Policy and Critical Care, Dartmouth Medical School; November 2011.
5. Luchsinger JA, Reitz C, Honig LS, et al. Aggregation of vascular risk factors and risk of incident Alzheimer disease. Neurology. 2005;65:545–551.
6. Ganguli M, Dodge HH, Shen C, et al. Alzheimer disease and mortality. Arch Neurol. 2005;62:779–784.
7. Kamboh MI. Molecular genetics of late-onset Alzheimer's disease. Ann Hum Genet. 2004;68:381–404.
8. Haas C. Strategies, development, and pitfalls of therapeutic options for AD. J Alzheimers Dis. 2012;28:241–281.
9. Golanski E, Hulas-Bigoszewskak, Sieruta M, et al. Earlier onset of Alzheimer's disease: risk polymorphisms within PRNP, PRND, CYP46, and APOE genes. J Alzheimers Dis. 2009;17:359–368.
10. Mattson MP. Pathways towards and away from Alzheimer's disease. Nature. 2004;430:631–639.
11. APA Working Group on Alzheimer's Disease and other Dementias; Rabins PV, Blacker D, et al. American Psychiatric Association practice guideline for the treatment of patients with Alzheimer's disease and other dementias. 2nd ed. Am J Psychiatry. 2007;164:5–56.
12. Cacabelos R, Fernandez-Novoa L, Lombardi V, et al. Molecular genetics of Alzheimer's disease and aging. Methods Find Exp Clin Pharmacol. 2005;27:1–573.
13. Yankner BA, Lu T. Amyloid beta-protein toxicity and the pathogenesis of Alzheimer's disease. J Biol Chem. 2009; 284: 4755–4759.
14. Pietrzik C, Behl C. Concepts for the treatment of Alzheimer's disease: Molecular mechanisms and clinical application. Int J Exp Pathol. 2005;86:173–185.
15. Mishizen-Eberz AJ, Rissman RA, Carter TL, et al. Biochemical molecular studies of NMDA receptor subunits NR1/2A/2B in hippocampal subregions throughout progression of Alzheimer's disease pathology. Neurobiol Dis. 2004;15:80–92.
16. Gonzalez C, Diaz F, Alonso A. Neuroprotective effects of estrogens: Cross-talk between estrogen and intracellular insulin signaling. Infect Disord Drug Targets. 2008;8:65–67.
17. Shumaker SA, Legault C, Kuller L, et al. Conjugated equine estrogens and incidence of probable dementia and mild cognitive impairment in postmenopausal women (Women's Health Initiative Memory Study). JAMA. 2004;291:2947–2958.
18. Alexopoulos GS, Jeste DV, Chung H, et al. The expert consensus guideline series. Treatment of dementia and its behavioral disturbances. Introduction: Methods, commentary, and summary. Postgrad Med. 2005;No:6–22.
19. Birks J. Cholinesterase inhibitors for Alzheimer's disease. Cochrane Database Syst Rev. 2006:CD005593.
20. Hogan DB, Bailey P, Black S, et al. Diagnosis and treatment of dementia: 5. Nonpharmacologic and pharmacologic therapy for mild to moderate dementia. CMAJ. 2008;179:1019–1026.
21. Gauthier S, Emre M, Farlow MR, et al. Strategies for continued successful treatment of Alzheimer's disease: Switching cholinesterase inhibitors. Curr Med Res Opin. 2003;19(8): 707–714.
22. Hogan DB. Progress update: Pharmacological treatment of Alzheimer's disease. Neuropsychiatr Dis Treat. 2007;3:569–578.
23. Eisai. Aricept (donepezil hydrochloride) [product information]. Teaneck, NJ: Author, 2013.
24. Farlow MR, Salloway S, Atriot PN, et al. Effectiveness and tolerability of high dose (23 mg/d) versus standard-dose (10 mg/d) donepezil in moderate to severe Alzheimer's disease: A 24-week, randomized, double-blind study. Clin Ther. 2010; 32:1234–1251.
25. Novartis. Exelon (rivastigmine tartrate) [product information]. East Hanover, NJ: Author, 2013.
26. Ortho-McNeil Neurologics. Razadyne ER/Razadyne (galantamine hydrobromide) [product information]. Titusville, NJ: Author, 2013.
27. Forest Pharmaceutica, Inc. Namenda (memantine hydrochloride) [product information]. St. Louis, MO: Author, 2013.
28. Forest Pharmaceutica, Inc. Namenda XR (memantine hydrochloride) extended release [product information]. St. Louis, MO: Author, 2013.
29. Schneider LS, Dogerman KS, Higgins JP, et al. Lack of evidence for the efficacy of memantine in mild Alzheimer's disease. Arch Neurol. 2011;68:991–998.
30. Doody RS, Thomas, RG, Farlow M, et al. Phase 3 trials of solanezumab for mild-to-moderate Alzheimer's disease. NEJM. 2014;370:311–321.
31. Salloway S, Sperling R, Fox NC, et al. Two phase 3 trials of bapineuzumab in mild-to-moderate Alzheimer's disease. NEJM. 2014;370:322–333.
32. Miller ER, Pastor-Barriuso R, Dalal D, et al. Meta-analysis: High-dosage vitamin E supplementation may increase all-cause mortality. Ann Intern Med. 2005;142:37–46.
33. Aisen PS, Schafer KA, Grundman M, et al. Effects of rofecoxib or naproxen versus placebo on Alzheimer's disease progression. JAMA. 2003;289:2819–2826.
34. Cooper JL. Dietary lipids in the etiology of Alzheimer's disease. Drugs Aging. 2003;20:399–418.
35. Dekosky ST, Williamson JD, Fitzpatrick AL, et al. Ginkgo biloba for prevention of dementia: A randomized controlled trial. JAMA. 2008;300:2253–2262.
36. Shan RC. Medical foods for Alzheimer's disease. Drugs Aging. 2011;28:421–428.
37. Accera. Axona (caprylidene) [product information]. Bloomfield, CO: Author, 2012.
38. Cummings J. Drug therapy: Alzheimer's disease. N Engl J Med. 2004;351:56–67.
39. Schneider LS, Dagerman K, Insel PS. Efficacy and adverse effects of atypical antipsychotics for dementia. Meta-analysis of randomized, placebo-controlled trials. Am J Geriatr Psychiatry. 2006;14:191–210.
40. Schneider LS, Tariot PN, Dagerman KS, et al. Effectiveness of atypical antipsychotic drugs in patients with Alzheimer's disease. N Engl J Med. 2006;355:1525–1538.
41. Banerjee S, Hellier J, Dewey M, et al. Sertraline or mirtazapine for depression in dementia (HTA-SADD): A randomized, multicentre, double-blind, placebo-controlled trial. Lancet. 2011;378:403–411.
42. Allain H, Bentue-Ferrer D, Polard E, et al. Postural instability and consequent falls and hip fractures associated with use of hypnotics in the elderly: A comparative review. Drugs Aging. 2005; 22:749–765.
43. Passmore MJ, Gardner DM, Polak Y, et al. Alternatives to atypical antipsychotics for the management of dementia-related agitation. Drugs Aging. 2008;25:381–398.
44. Sakuye KM, Camp CJ, Ford PA. Effects of buspirone on agitation associated with dementia. Am J Geriatr Psychol. 1993;1: 82–84.
45. Hermann N, Eryavec G. Buspirone in the management of agitation and aggression associated with dementia. Am J Geriatr Psychol. 1993;1:249–253.
46. Tariot PN, Cohen RM, Sunderland T, et al. L-deprenyl in Alzheimer's disease. Arch Gen Psychol. 1987;44:427–433.

47. Schneider LS, Pollock VE, Zemansky MF, et al. A pilot study of low dose L-deprenyl in Alzheimer's disease. J Geriatr Psychol Neurol. 1991;4:143–148.
48. Slattum PW, Peron EP, Massey-Hill A. Alzheimer's disease. In. Dipiro JT, Talbert RL, Yee GC, et al, eds. Pharmacotherapy: A Pathophysiologic Approach. 9th ed. New York, NY: McGraw-Hill; 2014:828.
49. Cacabelos R. Pharmacogenomics and therapeutic prospects in dementia. Eur Arch Psychiatry Clin Neurosci. 2008;258:28–47.
50. Alzheimer's Association. If you have Alzheimer's disease [Internet], [cited 2014 May 28]. www.alz.org/national/documents/brochure_ifyouhave_earlystage.pdf.

30 Multiple Sclerosis

Melody Ryan

LEARNING OBJECTIVES

Upon completion of the chapter, the reader will be able to:

1. Identify risk factors for multiple sclerosis (MS).
2. Describe pathophysiologic findings of MS.
3. Distinguish between forms of MS based on patient presentation and disease course.
4. Compare and contrast MS disease-modifying treatment choices for a given patient.
5. Determine appropriate symptomatic treatment choices for a given patient.
6. Develop a monitoring plan for a patient placed on specific medications.

INTRODUCTION

Multiple sclerosis (MS) is an inflammatory disease of the central nervous system (CNS), variable in symptoms and presentation. *Multiple* describes the number of CNS lesions, and *sclerosis* refers to the demyelinated lesions, today called plaques.

EPIDEMIOLOGY AND ETIOLOGY

Epidemiology

Approximately 2.3 million people worldwide have MS.[1] Diagnosis usually occurs between 20 and 50 years, affecting twice as many women as men.[1] Whites and people of northern European heritage are more likely to develop MS; prevalence decreases with decrease in latitude.[1,2] Risk factors include family history of MS, autoimmune diseases, or migraine; personal history of autoimmune diseases or migraine; and, in women, cigarette smoke exposure.

Etiology

▶ *Inheritance Theory*

Family members of MS patients have a 5% risk; monozygotic twins have a concordance rate of 25% to 30%.[2] Genetics cannot fully explain the etiology of MS because only a small proportion of patients report a family member with MS; however, genetic risks may explain up to 35% of cases.[3]

▶ *Environment Theory*

Epstein-Barr virus is thought to be a possible infectious etiologic agent.[3] Infection cannot fully explain MS because there is a high rate of seropositivity in the population, but MS is much less common. Other environmental theories involve decreased patient or maternal vitamin D serum concentrations or high sodium consumption.[2,3]

PATHOPHYSIOLOGY

While the causative agent of MS is unclear, the result is the development of an autoimmune disorder with areas of CNS inflammation and degeneration.

Inflammation

An unknown antigen presented by the major histocompatibility complex (MHC) class II molecules causes T-cells to become autoreactive (Figure 30–1). Autoreactive T-cells enter lymphatic tissues to expand. Upon a signal involving sphingosine-1-phosphate, T-cells reenter the circulation.[4] Once activated, T-cells attach to upregulated adhesion molecules and produce matrix metalloproteinases (MMP) that cause blood–brain barrier breakdown. In the CNS, T-cells come into contact with antigen-presenting cells and proliferate. The T-helper cells differentiate into proinflammatory T-helper-1 cells (Th1 cells) and anti-inflammatory T-helper-2 cells (Th2 cells).[4] Th1 cells secrete cytokines that enhance macrophage and microglial cells that attack **myelin**.[4]

B-cells cross damaged sections of the blood–brain barrier where autoreactive T-cells trigger B-cells to form myelin autoantibodies. B-cell antibodies also initiate the complement cascade, causing myelin degradation.[4] These inflammatory processes probably cause relapses.[4] All current MS therapies are targeted toward preventing or slowing the inflammatory processes.

Degeneration

Axonal injury and transection disrupts nerve signals. Growing evidence suggests cytotoxic T-cells cause axonal injury as early as 2 weeks after diagnosis and throughout the disease.[4] Axonal loss is likely responsible for MS progression.[4]

CLINICAL PRESENTATION AND DIAGNOSIS

Clinical Course

KEY CONCEPT *MS is classified into relapsing and progressive disease (Figure 30–2).*[7] These categories are subclassifed according to disease activity and progression. Clinically isolated syndrome (CIS) is a first clinical presentation for which the criteria of dissemination in time has not been met to diagnose MS.[7]

Relapsing-remitting MS is the most common form (85%), developing into progressive form in 50% of patients within

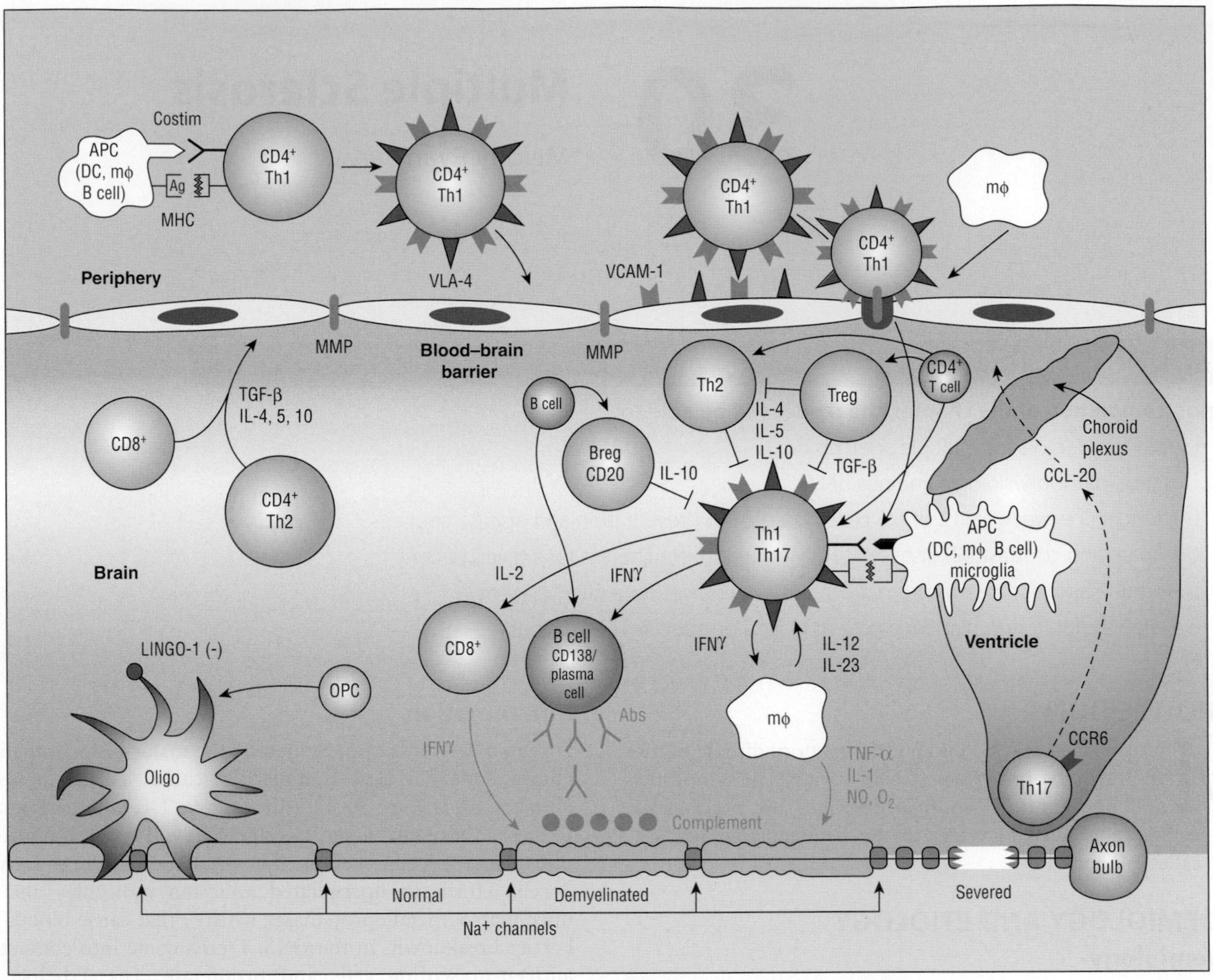

FIGURE 30–1. Autoimmune theory of the pathogenesis of MS. In MS, the immunogenic cells tend to be more myelin-reactive, and these T-cells produce cytokines mimicking a Th1-mediated proinflammatory reaction. T-helper cells (CD4+) appear to be key initiators of myelin destruction in MS. These autoreactive CD4+ cells, especially of the Th1 subtype, are activated in the periphery, perhaps following a viral infection. The activation of T- and B-cells requires two signals. The first signal is the interaction between MHC and antigen presenting cell (APC) (macrophage, dendritic cell, B-cell). The second signal consists of the binding between B7 on the APC and CD28 on the T-cell for T-cell activation. Similarly, CD40 expressed on APCs and CD40L expressed on T-cells interaction to signal the proliferation of B-cells within the blood-brain barrier following the entry of T-cells. The T-cells in the periphery express adhesion molecules on their surfaces that allow them to attach and roll along the endothelial cells that constitute the blood-brain barrier. The activated T-cells also produce MMP that help to create openings in the blood–brain barrier, allowing entry of the activated T-cells past the blood–brain barrier and into the CNS. Once inside the CNS, the T cells produce proinflammatory cytokines, especially interleukins (ILs) 1, 2, 12, 17, and 23, tumor necrosis factor-α (TNF-α), and interferon-γ (INF-γ), which further create openings in the blood–brain barrier, allowing entry of B-cells, complement, macrophages, and antibodies. The T-cells also interact within the CNS with the resident microglia, astrocytes, and macrophages, further enhancing production of proinflammatory cytokines and other potential mediators of CNS damage, including reactive oxygen intermediates and nitric oxide. The role of modulating, or downregulating, cytokines such as IL-4, IL-5, IL-10, and transforming growth factor-β (TGF-β) also has been described. These cytokines are the products of CD4+, CD8+, and Th1-cells. New pathogenic mechanisms involve, but are not limited to, receptor-ligand–mediated T-cell entry via choroid plexus (CCR6-CCL20 axis), coupling of key receptor-ligands for inhibition of myelination/demyelination (LINGO-1/NOGO66/p75, or TROY complex, Jagged-Notch signaling). (AG, antigens; APC, antigen-presenting cell; DC, dendrite cell; IgG, immunoglobulin G; Mφ, macrophage; Na^+, sodium ion; MMP, matrix metalloproteinases; MHC, major histocompatibility complex; OPC, oligodendrocyte precursor cell; VLA, very late antigen; VCAM, vascular cell adhesion molecule.) (From Bainbridge JL, Miravalle A, Corboy JR. Multiple sclerosis. In: DiPiro JT, Talbert RL, Yee GC, et al, eds. Pharmacotherapy: A Pathophysiologic Approach. 9th ed. New York, NY: McGraw-Hill; 2014:835–854, with permission.)

Clinical Presentation of MS[5,6]

MS symptoms depend on the location of lesions within the CNS. Myelin increases the speed of nerve impulse transmission; demyelination slows the speed. No impulses can be transmitted if the axon is transected. The primary symptoms of MS are caused by this delay or cessation of impulses. Secondary symptoms of MS result from the primary symptoms.

Primary Symptoms	Frequency of Occurrence (%)	Related Secondary Symptoms
Urinary symptoms	70	
Incontinence		Decubitus ulcers
Urinary retention		Urinary tract infections
Spasticity	70–80	Falls, care difficulties, pain, gait problems
Visual symptoms		
Optic neuritis	70	Falls, care difficulties
Bowel symptoms	39–73	
Incontinence		Decubitus ulcers
Constipation		Pain
Depression	50	Suicide
Anxiety	36	
Cognitive deficits	43–70	Decline in work or social performance, care difficulties
Fatigue	92	Effects on employment and social roles
Uhthoff phenomenon	80	
Sexual dysfunction		
Erectile dysfunction	50–90	
Female sexual dysfunction	40–85	
Tremor	80	Inability to perform activities of daily living
Pain	86	
Trigeminal neuralgia		
Lhermitte sign		
Dysesthetic pain	14–29	
Impaired gait	64	

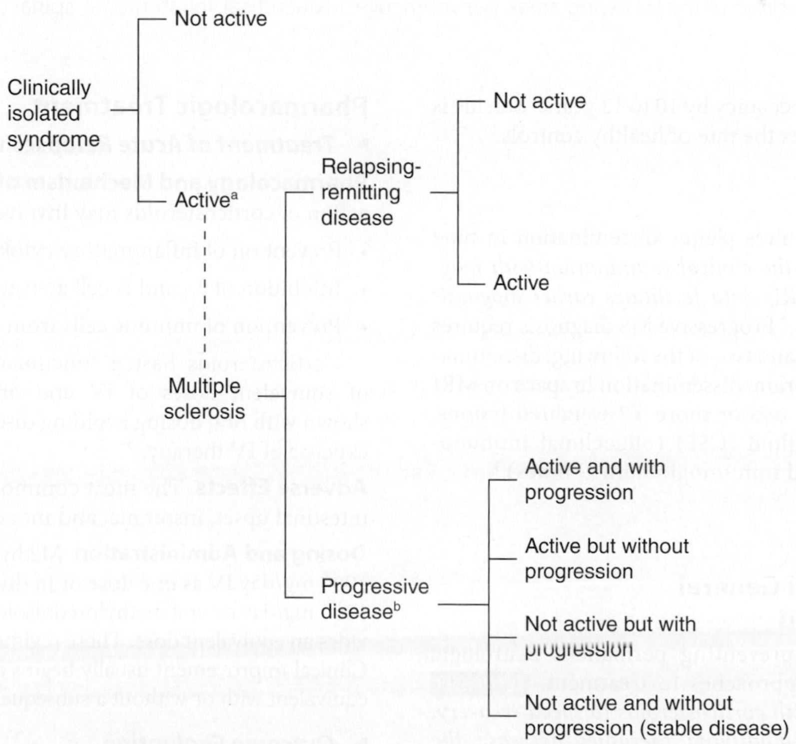

FIGURE 30–2. Clinical Patterns of Multiple Sclerosis.[7] [a]Clinically isolated syndrome, if active, may fulfill multiple sclerosis diagnostic criteria. [b]Progressive disease may be primary progressive with progressive accumulation of disability from onset or secondary progressive with progressive accumulation of disability after initial relapsing course.

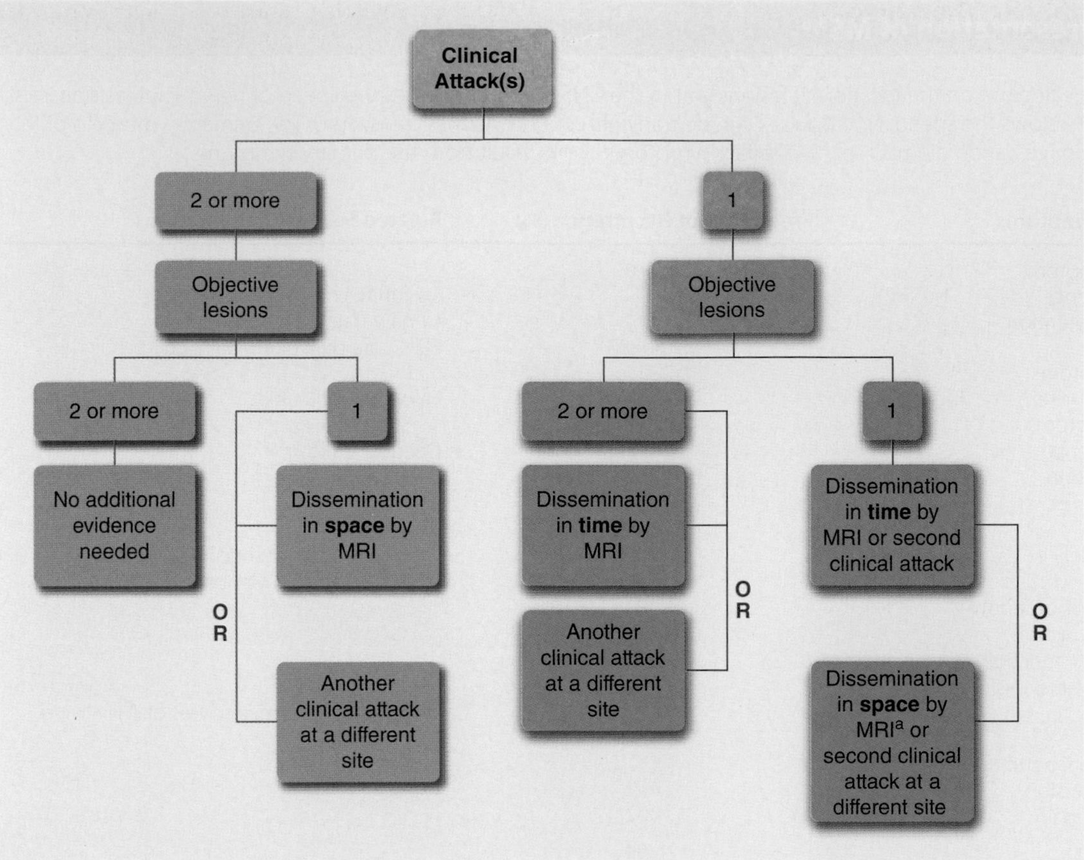

FIGURE 30–3. McDonald diagnostic criteria for MS.[9] An attack is defined as a patient-reported or objectively observed event typical of an acute inflammatory demyelinating event in the CNS with a duration of at least 24 hours in the absence of fever or infection. MRI evidence of dissemination over time is a new T2-weighted lesion after the initial clinical event or the simultaneous presence of asymptomatic gadolinium-enhancing and nonenhancing lesions at any time. [a]Dissemination in space by MRI evidence of one or more T2-weighted lesions in at least two of the following areas: periventricular, juxtacortical, infratentorial, spinal cord.

10 years.[1] MS reduces life expectancy by 10 to 12 years.[8] Suicide is high in MS patients, 7.5 times the rate of healthy controls.[8]

Diagnosis

Relapsing MS diagnosis requires plaque dissemination in time and space. KEY CONCEPT *Using the clinical examination with magnetic resonance imaging (MRI) data facilitates earlier diagnosis and treatment* (Figure 30–3).[9] Progressive MS diagnosis requires 1 year of disease progression and two of the following: dissemination in space on MRI of the brain, dissemination in space on MRI in the spinal cord based on two or more T2-weighted lesions, and positive cerebrospinal fluid (CSF) (oligoclonal immunoglobulin G bands or elevated immunoglobulin G index).[9]

TREATMENT

Desired Outcomes and General Approach to Treatment

The goal of treatment is preventing permanent neurologic damage. There are three approaches to treatment. KEY CONCEPT *First, treat acute relapses with corticosteroids to speed recovery.* KEY CONCEPT *Second, disease-modifying therapies decrease the number of relapses, prevent permanent neurologic damage, and prevent disability.* KEY CONCEPT *Third, symptomatic treatments minimize quality of life impact of MS.*

Pharmacologic Treatment

▶ *Treatment of Acute Relapses with Corticosteroids*

Pharmacology and Mechanism of Action The mechanism of action of corticosteroids may involve:

- Prevention of inflammatory cytokine activation
- Inhibition of T- and B-cell activation
- Prevention of immune cells from entering the CNS[10]

Corticosteroids hasten functional recovery.[10] Equal efficacy of equivalent doses of IV and oral dosage forms has been shown with oral dosing avoiding discomfort, inconvenience, and expense of IV therapy.[10]

Adverse Effects The most common adverse effects are gastrointestinal upset, insomnia, and mood disturbance.[10]

Dosing and Administration Methylprednisolone is given 500 to 1000 mg/day IV as one dose or in divided doses. Oral prednisone 1250 mg/day or oral methylprednisolone 1000 to 1250 mg/day provides an equivalent dose. These regimens are given for 3 to 7 days.[10] Clinical improvement usually begins during treatment. Recovery is equivalent with or without a subsequent oral corticosteroid taper.[11]

▶ *Outcome Evaluation*

- Monitor for symptom improvement
- Educate regarding adverse effects

Disease-Modifying Therapies

Agents indicated for MS are shown in Table 30–1. These immunomodulators reduce annualized relapse rates 30% to 70%.[12–25] No agents are approved for primary progressive MS; however, the available disease-modifying therapies may be effective in patients with progressive disease who have relapses.

▸ β-Interferons

Pharmacology and Mechanism of Action The following mechanisms of action are thought to be important:

- Decrease in T-cell activation, decreasing cytokine secretion
- Prevention of upregulation of adhesion molecules on activated T-cells, limiting T-cells access to the CNS
- Suppression of MMPs, maintaining the integrity of the blood–brain barrier
- Decrease in microglial proliferation, preserving myelin
- Promotion of formation of Th2 cells rather than Th1 cells, decreasing inflammation
- Increase in neural growth factor production, assisting in repair of the CNS[12,26]

Efficacy in Patients with Relapsing Remitting MS β-Interferons reduce relapses by about one-third versus placebo.[12] CIS treatment resulted in fewer patients developing clinically definite MS compared with placebo.[12]

Efficacy in Patients with Secondary Progressive MS Who Experience Relapses β-Interferons reduce the risk of relapses, but do not slow progression.[13] Treatment is most effective if clinical relapses or MRI inflammatory activity is present.[13]

Adverse Effects Adverse effects are common with β-interferons (**Tables 30–1 and** 30–2). Flu-like symptoms (fever, fatigue, muscle aches, malaise, and chills) begin a few hours postinjection and dissipate within 8 to 24 hours.[14] Injection site reactions range from redness to necrosis. There are preventive and treatment measures for these reactions (Table 30–3). Because of conflicting data, it is difficult to determine if β-interferons cause depression.[15]

Tests for Responsiveness Some patients do not respond to β-interferons; it may be possible to identify nonresponders by determining the type I interferon signature. Patients who have increased expression of the type I interferon gene (interferon^{high}) have more proinflammatory effects. Interferon^{high} patients are less likely to respond to β-interferons than interferon^{low} patients.[26] Antibodies to β-interferons can reduce effect.[12] Neutralizing antibodies develop 6 to 18 months after initiation. Neutralizing antibodies can form against any β-interferon and are cross-reactive.[12] Neutralizing antibodies may disappear even during continued treatment. There are no standardized recommendations for neutralizing antibody testing.[12]

Patient Encounter, Part 1

A 23-year-old white woman visits the emergency department today with complaints of loss of visual acuity in her left eye with some eye pain that developed over several hours. She has never experienced symptoms like this previously. She has been generally healthy and is up to date on her vaccinations. She has moved to your area to attend university. Before that, she lived in Maine her entire life.

What information is suggestive of multiple sclerosis (MS)?

What risk factors does she have for MS?

What additional information or testing would assist in making the diagnosis of MS?

What treatment could be provided to the patient for the current acute event?

▸ Glatiramer Acetate

Pharmacology and Mechanism of Action Glatiramer acetate's mechanism of action is unknown; the following properties are observed:

- Binds to MHC class II, blocking the activation of T-cells
- Activates Th2 cells, preventing inflammation
- Activated Th2 cells secrete brain-derived neurotrophic factor, which may be neuroprotective[17]

Efficacy Glatiramer acetate reduces relapses by 28% compared with placebo, but does not prevent sustained progression of MS.[18] It is used in CIS to prevent conversion to clinically definite MS.[17]

Adverse Effects Patients report injection site reactions (see Table 30–2). Icing the injection site preinjection and postinjection and/or topical anesthetics improve these reactions. If a systemic reaction (flushing, chest tightness, palpitations, anxiety, and shortness of breath) occurs, it is usually within 30 minutes of the injection; recurrence is infrequent. Doses may be reduced by 75% for the week following the reaction, then increased by 25% per week to the full dose.[14]

▸ Issues with Self-Injected Disease-Modifying Therapies

Adherence KEY CONCEPT *Adherence to injectable medications is a significant problem*, with 22% to 59% discontinuation. Realistic therapy expectations, higher educational levels, and higher self-efficacy improve adherence; depression and cognitive problems lower adherence.[19]

Patient Education Refer to Table 30–4 for patient self-injection education.

▸ Teriflunomide

Pharmacology and Mechanism of Action Teriflunomide's mechanism of action may include:

- Cytostatic effect on rapidly dividing B- and T-cells by inhibiting dihydro-orotate dehydrogenase
- Inhibiting T-cell activation, entry to the CNS, and secretion of proinflammatory cytokines[20]

Pharmacokinetics Half-life of teriflunomide is 2 weeks; taking 3 months to achieve steady-state concentrations. Metabolized by the liver, it is contraindicated in hepatic failure. Teriflunomide inhibits CYP2C8 and induces CYP1A2 and CYP2C9. It undergoes significant enterohepatic circulation; its half-life is substantially reduced by cholestyramine.

Efficacy Teriflunomide reduces relapse rate and progression of disease for relapsing forms of MS.[20] It also prevents CIS from converting to clinically definite MS.[21]

Adverse Effects Teriflunomide is generally well tolerated. If patients develop liver injury, teriflunomide must be stopped and accelerated elimination undertaken. Patients should be screened for tuberculosis prior to initiating therapy.[20]

Table 30–1

Comparison of Disease-Modifying Therapies

Drug	Dose	Route	Frequency	Selected Adverse Effects
Dimethyl fumarate (Tecfidera)	240 mg	By mouth	Twice daily	Flushing 30% Gastrointestinal effects 25% Leucopenia/lymphopenia 4%–10%
Fingolimod (Gilenya)	0.5 mg	By mouth	Daily	Headache 25% Increased aspartate aminotransferase/alanine aminotransferase 14% Influenza viral infections 13% Diarrhea 12% Cough 10% Bradycardia 4% Lymphopenia 4%
Glatiramer acetate (Copaxone)	20 mg 40 mg	SQ SQ	Daily Three times per week	Injection site reaction 90% Systemic reaction 15% Alopecia 61% Menstrual disorders 61% Urinary tract infection 32% Amenorrhea 25% Leukopenia 19% γ-Glutamyl transferase increase 15%
Peginterferon β-1a (Plegridy)	125 mcg	SQ	Every 2 weeks	Injection site reactions 62% Flu-like symptoms 47%
Interferon β-1a (Avonex)	30 mcg	IM	Weekly	Flu-like symptoms 61% Anemia 8%
Interferon β-1a (Rebif)	44 mcg	SQ	Three times per week	Flu-like symptoms 28% Injection site reactions 66% Leukopenia 22% Increased aspartate aminotransferase/alanine aminotransferase 17%–27%
Interferon β-1b (Betaseron, Extavia)	0.25 mg	SQ	Every other day	Flu-like symptoms 60%–76% Injection site reactions 50%–85% Asthenia 49% Menstrual disorder 17% Leukopenia 10%–16% Increased aspartate aminotransferase/alanine aminotransferase 4%–19%
Mitoxantrone (Novantrone)	12 mg/m² up to 140 mg/m² (maximum lifetime dose)	IV	Every 3 months	Nausea 76% Arrhythmia 3%–18% Cardiotoxicity 2.7% Alopecia 61% Menstrual disorders 61% Urinary tract infection 32% Amenorrhea 25% Leukopenia 19% γ-Glutamyl transferase increase 15%
Natalizumab (Tysabri)	300 mg	IV	Every 4 weeks	Headache 38% Fatigue 27% Arthralgia 19% Urinary tract infection 20% Hypersensitivity reaction < 1% Progressive multifocal leukoencephalopathy 0.13%
Teriflunomide (Aubagio)	7 or 14 mg	By mouth	Daily	Increased alanine aminotransferase 12%–14% Alopecia 10%–13% Diarrhea 15%–18%

Rommer PS, Zettl UK, Kieseier B, et al. Requirements for safety monitoring of approved multiple sclerosis therapies: an overview. Clin Exper Immunol. 2013;175:397–407.

Galetta SL, Markowitz C. U.S. FDA-approved disease-modifying treatments for multiple sclerosis: Review of adverse effect profiles. CNS Drugs. 2005;29:239–252.

Calabresi PA, Kieseier BC, Arnold DL, et al. Pegylated interferon beta-1a for relapsing-remitting multiple sclerosis (ADVANCE): a randomized, phase 3, double-blind study. Lancet Neurol. 2014;13:657–665.

Table 30–2

Monitoring Disease-Modifying Therapies

Therapy	Tests	Frequency
β-Interferons	CBC, bilirubin, electrolytes, AST, ALT, γ-glutamyl transferase, alkaline phosphatase	Baseline, 1, 3, and 6 months; then every 3 months
	Thyroid function tests	Baseline and every 6 months in patients with a history of thyroid dysfunction
	EDSS, MSFC, neurologic history and examination	Every 3 months during the first year of therapy; then every 6 months
Dimethyl fumarate	CBC	Baseline
	EDSS, MSFC, neurologic history and examination	Every 3 months during the first year of therapy; then every 6 months
Glatiramer acetate (Copaxone)	EDSS, MSFC, neurologic history and examination	Every 3 months during the first year of therapy; then every 6 months
Mitoxantrone (Novantrone)	CBC, bilirubin, AST, ALT, alkaline phosphatase, pregnancy test	Before each infusion
	Electrocardiogram	Baseline and prior to each infusion
	Echocardiogram or MUGA scan	Baseline; prior to each infusion, and yearly after stopping mitoxantrone
	EDSS, MSFC, neurologic history and examination	Every 3 months during the first year of therapy; then every 6 months
Natalizumab	EDSS, MSFC, neurologic history and examination	Baseline; every 3 months during the first year of therapy; then every 6 months
	HIV, CBC, AST, ALT, MRI	Baseline; repeat MRI at 6 months; then yearly
	MRI, CSF examination for JC virus	Periodically and at onset of new neurologic symptoms not suggestive of MS
	Preinfusion patient checklist	Prior to every infusion
	Status report and reauthorization questionnaire	Every 6 months
Fingolimod	Varicella zoster immunity evaluation and/or vaccination and FEV_1 (full pulmonary function testing if patient has history of asthma or COPD), pregnancy test	Baseline
	CBC, ALT, AST, bilirubin	Baseline and every 6 months
	Pulse and blood pressure	Baseline; observe in clinical area for 6 hours after initial dose with hourly monitoring
	Ophthalmology evaluation	Baseline; 3–4 months; then as needed
	Dermatologic evaluation	Baseline; then as needed
	Electrocardiogram	Baseline and 6 hours after initial dose
	EDSS, MSFC, neurologic history and examination	Every 3 months during the first year of therapy; then every 6 months
Teriflunomide	CBC, screen for tuberculosis, pregnancy testing	Baseline
	ALT, AST, bilirubin	Baseline and monthly for first 6 months
	Blood pressure	Baseline; then periodically
	EDSS, MSFC, neurologic history and examination	Every 3 months during the first year of therapy; then every 6 months

Rudick RA, Goelz SE. Beta-interferon for multiple sclerosis. Exp Cell Res. 2011;317:1301–1311.

Rommer PS, Zettl UK, Kieseier B, et al. Requirements for safety monitoring of approved multiple sclerosis therapies: an overview. Clin Exper Immunol. 2013;175:397–407.

Galetta SL, Markowitz C. U.S. FDA-approved disease-modifying treatments for multiple sclerosis: Review of adverse effect profiles. CNS Drugs. 2005;29:239–252.

Scott LJ. Glatiramer acetate: a review of its use in patients with relapsing-remitting multiple sclerosis and in delaying the onset of clinically definite multiple sclerosis. CNS Drugs. 2013;27:971–988.

LaMantia L, Munari LM, Lovati R. Glatiramer acetate for multiple sclerosis. Cochrane Database Syst Rev. 2010;5: CD004678. DOI: 10.1002/14651858.CD004678.pub2.

Brunetti L, Wagner ML, Maroney M, Ryan M. Teriflunomide for the treatment of relapsing multiple sclerosis: a review of clinical data. Ann Pharmacother. 2013;47:1153–1160.

Linker RA, Gold R. Dimethyl fumarate for treatment of multiple sclerosis: mechanism of action, effectiveness, and side effects. Curr Neurol Neurosci Rep. 2013;13:394.

Willis MA, Cohen JA. Fingolimod therapy for multiple sclerosis. Semin Neurol. 2013;33:37–44.

Hoepner R, Faissner S, Salmen A, et al. Efficacy and side effects of natalizumab therapy in patients with multiple sclerosis. J Cent Nerv Syst Dis. 2014;6:1–49.

Martinelli Boneschi F, Vacchi L, et al. Mitoxantrone for multiple sclerosis. Cochrane Database Syst Rev. 2013;5:CD002127. DOI: 10.1002/14651858.CD002127.pub3.

Table 30–3

Prevention or Treatment Strategies for β- Interferon Adverse Effects

Flu-Like Symptoms	Injection Site Reaction	Laboratory Abnormalities[a]
Inject dose in the evening	Bring medication to room temperature	Hemoglobin < 9.4 g/dL (94 g/L or 5.8 mmol/L)
Begin at ¼–½ dose for 2 weeks of treatment; then increase to a full dose	Ice injection site before and after injection Rotate injection sites	White blood cells < 3 × 10^3/mm^3 (3 × 10^9/L) Absolute neutrophil count < 1.5 × 10^3/mm^3 (1.5 × 10^9/L)
Use ibuprofen 200 mg before and 6 and 12 hours after injection	Inject in areas with more subcutaneous fat (buttocks or abdomen)	Platelets < 75 × 10^3/mm^3 (75 × 10^9/L) Bilirubin > 2.5 × baseline
Alternatives to ibuprofen include acetaminophen, prednisone taper, and pentoxifylline	Use an autoinjection device If severe, use hydrocortisone 1% cream on the site If necrotic: temporarily discontinue; consult dermatologist; do not use topical corticosteroids	AST/ALT > 5 × baseline Alkaline phosphatase > 5 × baseline

ALT, alanine aminotransferase; AST, aspartate aminotransferase.

[a]At these threshold values, β-interferon should be temporarily discontinued and laboratory values monitored.

Rommer PS, Zettl UK, Kieseier B, et al. Requirements for safety monitoring of approved multiple sclerosis therapies: an overview. Clin Exper Immunol. 2013;175:397–407.

Galetta SL, Markowitz C. U.S. FDA-approved disease-modifying treatments for multiple sclerosis: Review of adverse effect profiles. CNS Drugs. 2005;29:239–252.

▸ *Dimethyl Fumarate*

Pharmacology and Mechanism of Action Dimethyl fumarate is thought to treat MS in the following ways:

- Shift cytokine production from a proinflammatory state to an anti-inflammatory state
- Prevent macrophage entry into the CNS by an unknown mechanism
- Stabilization of transcription factor nuclear (erythroid-derived 2) related factor which may reduce oxidative stress[22]

Efficacy Dimethyl fumarate reduced relapses approximately 50%. It slowed MS progression in some studies.[22]

Adverse Effects Dimethyl fumarate causes a transient, dose-dependent flushing sometimes with itching. Likely due to histamine release, incidence decreases after the first month and may be improved by slower dose titration, administration with food, and/or H2-blocking antihistamines.[22] Gastrointestinal adverse effects may be lessened with a slow dose increase and administration with food.[22]

▸ *Fingolimod*

Pharmacology and Mechanism of Action Fingolimod is a sphingosine 1-phosphate receptor modulator. It retains T-cells in lymphoid tissues, depleting peripheral blood and CNS lymphocytes. Fingolimod also binds to sphingosine 1-phospate receptors in the brain where may reduce inflammatory cytokines.[23]

Pharmacokinetics Fingolimod is highly protein bound with a long half-life of 8 to 9 days (steady-state concentrations achieved in 1-2 months).[23]

Efficacy Treatment reduced the annualized relapse rate to 0.18 compared with 0.40 for placebo. It also slowed MS progression.[23]

Adverse Effects Fingolimod reduces circulating lymphocytes by about 75%; infections and malignancies are concerns.[23] Sphingosine 1-phosphate receptors elsewhere in the body are associated with first-dose bradycardia, macular edema, and reduced forced vital capacity.[23] Fingolimod is contraindicated in patients with myocardial infarctions, unstable angina, stroke, transient ischemic attacks, or some types of congestive heart failure within the past 6 months or in patients with many types of atrioventricular block, prolonged QT interval, or who are taking class Ia or III antiarrhythmic medicines.[23] Extensive monitoring is required at baseline and for the first dose; monitoring must be repeated if therapy is interrupted.[23]

Table 30–4

Patient Education for Self-Injection

Keep all nonrefrigerated supplies together and out of the reach of children and pets
If refrigerated, allow medication to warm to room temperature
Wash hands thoroughly
Choose injection site, rotating among sites
Ice area to be injected for no more than 15 minutes, if desired
Clean injection site thoroughly with alcohol or soap and water
Administer injection
Ice injection site for no more than 15 minutes after injection, if desired

▸ *Natalizumab*

Pharmacology and Mechanism of Action Natalizumab is a α_4-integrin antagonist; its postulated mechanism of action follows:

- Binds to $\alpha_4\beta_1$ and $\alpha_4\beta_7$ integrins, preventing lymphocyte migration into the CNS and inflammation
- Inhibits binding of α_4-positive leukocytes to fibronectin and osteopontin, decreasing the activation of leukocytes already within the CNS[24]

Efficacy Treatment with natalizumab reduced relapses by 68% at 1 year and disability by 42% at 2 years versus placebo.[24]

Adverse Effects Hypersensitivity reactions (itching, dizziness, fever, rash, hypotension, dyspnea, chest pain, and anaphylaxis) have been observed, usually within 2 hours of administration. If hypersensitivity occurs, natalizumab is discontinued. A separate infusion reaction (headache, dizziness, fatigue, nausea, sweats, and rigors) may occur within 2 hours of dosing.[14] Histamine

1 and 2 receptor blockers can be used to prevent these symptoms, and discontinuation is not required. A serious, but rare, adverse effect is progressive multifocal leukoencephalopathy (PML). PML, caused by the JC polyomavirus virus, is rapidly progressive and often results in death or permanent disability. Though most associated with natalizumab, it has been reported in two patients treated with dimethyl fumarate.[14] Specific recommendations are to test for JC virus, avoid natalizumab in immunocompromised patients; carefully assess for immune compromise in patients previously treated with immunosuppression, radiation therapy, or chemotherapy; use only as monotherapy, and carefully monitor patients.[14] Risk of PML increases with increased infusions.[14] Vigilance is paramount because PML can mimic symptoms associated with MS.[24]

Due to this risk, natalizumab is distributed through a restricted program. KEY CONCEPT These concerns lead to the recommendation that *natalizumab be reserved for patients with rapidly advancing disease who have failed other therapies.*

Antinatalizumab antibodies develop in 9% to 12% of patients. If patients have antibodies 6 months after start of therapy, relapse rates and disability increase; antibody development is also associated with hypersensitivity reactions.[24]

▶ *Mitoxantrone*

Pharmacology and Mechanism of Action Mitoxantrone is an anthracenedione antineoplastic; the mechanisms of action important for MS include:

- Causes apoptosis in T-cells and APCs, preventing initial T-cell activation
- Inhibits DNA and RNA synthesis, decreasing proliferation of T cells, B cells, and macrophages
- Decreases cytokine release, preventing inflammation
- Inhibits macrophages, preventing myelin degradation[25]

Efficacy Mitoxantrone is indicated for secondary-progressive MS, progressive-relapsing MS, and for patients with worsening relapsing-remitting MS. It reduces the relapse rate and attack-related MRI outcome measures and MS progression.[25] KEY CONCEPT *Because of its potential for significant toxicities, mitoxantrone is reserved for patients with rapidly advancing disease who have failed other therapies.*

Adverse Effects Bluish discoloration of the sclera and urine lasts 24 hours or more postinfusion.[14] Transient leukopenia and neutropenia are common. Amenorrhea may be permanent.[25]

Cardiotoxicity is a serious adverse effect. Mitoxantrone should not be used in patients with baseline cardiomyopathy, even if asymptomatic. Cyclooxygenase-2 inhibitors potentially worsen cardiac toxicity and should be avoided.[25] Maximum lifetime dose of mitoxantrone is 140 mg/m^2.

Acute myelogenous leukemia occurred in 0.07% of mitoxantrone-treated patients, appearing within 2 to 4 years of initiating mitoxantrone and responsive to standard therapy.[25]

Dosing and Administration Mitoxantrone is infused intravenously over 30 minutes to reduce cardiotoxicity.[25] In standard dosing regimens, mitoxantrone is administered every 3 months. Some centers have used mitoxantrone as induction therapy in patients with very active MS. With this strategy, mitoxantrone either at usual or slightly higher dose is given for a short period of time. This treatment may be followed by β-interferon or glatiramer acetate. These regimens have been effective at reducing relapses and progression in small numbers of patients.[27]

▶ *Other Therapy Considerations*

Pregnancy Because MS affects many women of childbearing age, the teratogenic effects of medications is concerning. Women generally experience a decrease in relapses during the second and third trimesters of pregnancy with an increase in the first 3 months postpartum.[28] Although none of the disease modifying therapies is recommended for use during pregnancy, data from pregnancy registries demonstrate no adverse outcomes with interferon β, glatiramer acetate, and natalizumab.[28] Fetal risk is unknown for dimethyl fumarate. Sphingosine 1-phosphate receptors are important in fetal formation, thus fingolimod should be discontinued for at least 2 months before conception to allow for its elimination. Mitoxantrone and teriflunomide are contraindicated during pregnancy and teriflunomide is contraindicated for men who have sexual intercourse with women who may become pregnant.[28] Because of the long half-life of teriflunomide, accelerated elimination is recommended for women who wish to become pregnant.[28]

Vaccinations Patients taking teriflunomide, mitoxantrone, or fingolimod should not receive attenuated live virus vaccines.[20,24,29] Vaccines may be less effective while on fingolimod, and vaccines should be held for 4 to 6 weeks after a mitoxantrone dose.[20,24]

Choosing Therapy KEY CONCEPT *There is no consensus on the best medication for initial therapy.* Figure 30–4 suggests a treatment approach.

▶ *Outcome Evaluation*

- Assess symptom changes periodically.
- In β-interferon-treated patients with frequent relapses, test for neutralizing antibodies.
- Monitor medication-specific adverse effects (see Tables 30–1 and 30–3).
- Assess adherence.

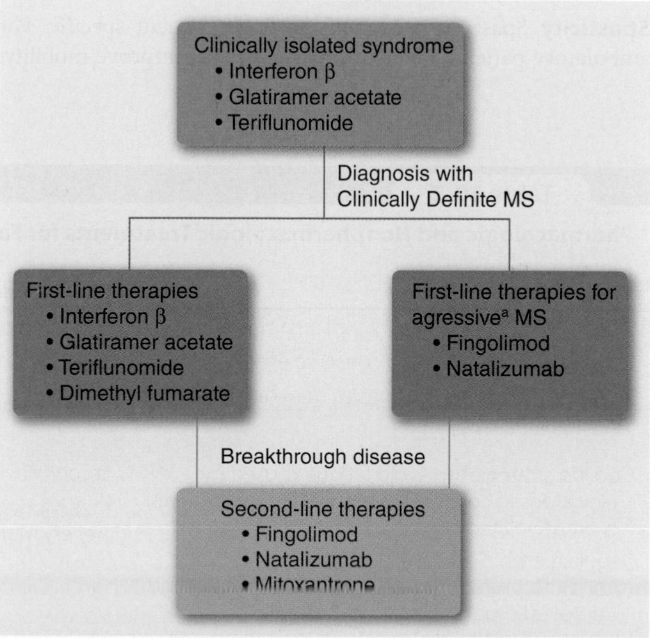

FIGURE 30–4. Treatment algorithm for CIS and relapsing-remitting MS.[30] [a]A definition of aggressive multiple sclerosis has been proposed as follows: two or more relapses in the preceding year and two or more gadolinium-enhancing lesions on brain MRI scans or a significant T2 lesion burden.[31]

Patient Encounter, Part 2

PMH: None

FH: No family history of MS. Both parents alive and well. No siblings

SH: Graduate student in economics. Single. She does not smoke, drink alcohol, or use illicit drugs

Allergies: NKDA

Meds: None

ROS: (–) N/V/D, HA, SOB, chest pain, cough

PE:

VS: 126/74, P 70, RR 18, T 38°C (100.4°F)

Skin: Warm, dry

HEENT: Left pupillary response to light is sluggish, decreased visual acuity left eye

CV: RRR, normal S1 and S2, no m/r/g

Chest: CTA

Abd: Soft, NT/ND

Neuro: A & O × 3; CN II-XII intact, end point nystagmus on lateral gaze bilaterally

Motor: mild weakness in right arm, poor finger-to-nose left upper extremity

Labs: WNL

Imaging: T2-weighted MRI shows a gadolinium-enhancing T2-weighted lesion on the left optic nerve and two nonenhancing T2-weighted white matter lesions near the cortex (juxtacortical region)

Given this additional information, what is your assessment of the patient's condition?

Identify your treatment goals for this patient.

What pharmacologic alternatives are available for her?

What counseling points will you give the patient for administration of the chosen therapy?

▶ *Symptomatic Therapies*

Symptoms most unique to MS are fatigue, spasticity, impaired ambulation, and pseudobulbar affect. Treatment of other important symptoms such as urinary incontinence, pain, depression, cognitive impairment, and sexual dysfunction is addressed elsewhere in this text.

Fatigue There are nonpharmacologic and pharmacologic strategies for coping with fatigue (Table 30–5). Medicines should be reviewed to identify possible contributors to fatigue. Pharmacologic management of fatigue includes amantadine or stimulants; however, efficacy evidence is limited.[32]

Spasticity Spasticity treatment goals are patient specific. For ambulatory patients, reducing spasticity may improve mobility. For bed-bound patients, treating spasticity may relieve pain and facilitate care. Physical therapy is a nonpharmacologic treatment for spasticity.[33]

KEY CONCEPT *MS patients must be treated with agents specific for upper motor neuron spasticity (Table 30–6).*[33] MS spasticity is classified as focal or generalized. If the spasticity involves only one muscle group, it is focal and may benefit from botulinum toxin administration.[33] Systemic medications are used for generalized spasticity. No conclusion can be reached regarding efficacy superiority of one agent.[33]

Impaired Ambulation Nonpharmacological treatment includes assistive devices, physical therapy, and/or exercise. Extended-release dalfampridine is indicated for improvement in walking speed.

Table 30–5

Pharmacologic and Nonpharmacologic Treatments for Fatigue

Nonpharmacologic	Pharmacologic	Renal Dosing
Appropriate rest-to-activity ratio	*First-line therapy:*	
Use of assistive devices to conserve energy	Amantadine 100 mg orally every morning and early afternoon	CrCl 30–50 mL/min (0.50–0.84 mL/s): 100 mg/day
Environmental modifications to make activities more energy efficient		CrCl 15–29 mL/min (0.25–0.49 mL/s): 100 mg every other day
		CrCl < 15 mL/min (0.25 mL/s): 200 mg every 7 days
Cooling strategies to avoid fatigue caused by elevations in core body temperature due to heat, exercise-related exertion, and fever	*Second-line therapy:* Methylphenidate 10–20 mg every morning and noon	
Regular aerobic exercise, geared to the person's ability, to promote cardiovascular health, strength, improved mood, and reduce fatigue		
Progressive resistance training of lower limb muscles		
Stress management techniques		

CrCl, creatinine clearance.

From Asano M, Finlayson ML. Meta-analysis of three different types of fatigue management interventions for people with multiple sclerosis: exercise, education, and medication. Mult Scler Int. 2014;2014:798285.

Table 30–6

Comparison of Antispasticity Agents

Place in Therapy	Medication	Mechanism of Action	Dose
First line	Baclofen	Presynaptic and postsynaptic γ-aminobutyric acid type B receptor agonist	5 mg orally three times daily; increase by 5 mg/dose every 3 days to a maximum of 80 mg/day *Renal dysfunction:* Dose reduction may be necessary
	Tizanidine	Centrally acting α_2-receptor agonist	2 mg orally three times daily; increase gradually by 2 mg at each dose with 1–4 days between dose increases to a maximum of 36 mg/day *Hepatic and renal dysfunction:* Dose reduction may be necessary
Second line	Dantrolene	Direct inhibitor of muscle contraction by decreasing the release of calcium from skeletal muscle sarcoplasmic reticulum	25 mg orally daily; increase to 25 mg three to four times daily; then increase by 25 mg every 4–7 days to a maximum of 400 mg/day
	Diazepam	γ-aminobutyric acid agonist	2–10 mg orally three to four times daily *Cirrhosis:* Reduce dose by 50%
Third-line	Intrathecal baclofen	Presynaptic and postsynaptic γ-aminobutyric acid type B receptor agonist	Titrated individually; usual range: 62–749 mcg/day
Focal spasticity	Botulinum toxin	Prevents release of acetylcholine in the neuromuscular junction	Individualized

Data from Gold R, Oreja-Guevera C. Advances in the management of multiple sclerosis spasticity: multiple sclerosis spasticity guidelines. Expert Rev Neurother. 2013;13(Suppl 12):55–59.

Patient Encounter, Part 3

The patient begins therapy with teriflunomide 14 mg orally daily. She does very well with no relapses and minimal adverse effects for 2 years during which time she marries. At her next neurology appointment, she states that she would like to begin a family in the next 6 months. She also reports that she is having episodes of unexpected crying, but she does not endorse symptoms of depression. She is diagnosed with pseudobulbar affect.

How will you respond to her interest in becoming pregnant?

What treatment will you recommend for her MS?

What treatment should you consider for pseudobulbar affect?

The Patient Care Process

Patient Assessment:

- Based on physical exam and review of systems, determine whether patient is experiencing a MS exacerbation currently. Determine presence of any symptoms such as urinary incontinence.
- Review the medical history and MRI findings. Does the patient have CIS? Does patient have aggressive MS (see Figure 30–4)? Is patient pregnant? Does patient want to become pregnant?
- Conduct a medication history (including prescription and nonprescription medications). Has patient been treated with any MS medications or immunosuppressants previously? Is patient experiencing adverse effects?
- Review available laboratory tests, especially leucocytes and liver function tests.

Therapy Evaluation:

- If patient is already receiving disease-modifying or symptomatic pharmacotherapy, assess efficacy, safety, and patient adherence. Are there any significant drug interactions?
- Determine if patient has prescription coverage or if recommended agents are included on patient's insurance formulary. If necessary, obtain prior authorizations.

Care Plan Development:

- Treat any relapses with IV or oral corticosteroids.
- Work with patient to select therapy, considering:
  - Route of administration
  - Frequency of administration
  - Adverse-effect profile and other concerns (eg, neutralizing antibodies)
  - Cost, including preauthorization needs for patient's insurance.
- Obtain required baseline laboratory studies (see Table 30–5).
- Educate patient regarding self-injection, if necessary (see Table 30–4), and adherence.
- Initiate needed symptomatic treatments.
- Address any concerns about MS and its management.

(Continued)

The Patient Care Process (*Continued*)

- Refer patient to the National MS Society for information, newsletters, and local support groups (www.nationalmssociety.org).
- Instruct patient to contact clinician for any sudden symptom changes suggestive of relapse.

Follow-Up Evaluation:

- Monitor patient for efficacy and adverse effects of disease-modifying and symptomatic therapies every 3 months for the first year and every 6 months thereafter and as required for therapy (see Tables 30–2 and 30–5).
- Obtain MRI annually or more frequently as dictated by symptoms and selected therapy.
- Assess adherence with medications at each visit.

This potassium channel blocker prolongs action potentials, improving conduction in demyelinated neurons.[34] Not all patients respond; response can be assessed at 2 months.[34] Urinary tract infections, insomnia, dizziness, headache, nausea, asthenia, back pain, and balance disorder all occur frequently with dalfampridine.[34] Seizures are an uncommon adverse effect; patients with seizure disorders should not receive dalfampridine.[34]

Pseudobulbar Affect Ten percent of patients with MS develop pseudobulbar affect, characterized by inappropriate laughing or crying and causing social isolation.[35] Dextromethorphan prevents the release of excitatory neurotransmitters. Low-dose quinidine blocks first-pass metabolism of dextromethorphan and increases serum concentrations. A 49% decrease in episodes was seen with treatment.[35]

▶ *Outcome Evaluation*

- Assess improvement/recurrence of symptoms.
- Monitor adverse effects of medications.
- Monitor adherence.

Abbreviations Introduced in This Chapter

ALT	Alanine aminotransferase
APC	Antigen-presenting cell
AST	Aspartate aminotransferase
CBC	Complete blood count
CIS	Clinically isolated syndrome
CNS	Central nervous system
COPD	Chronic obstructive pulmonary disease
CrCl	Creatinine clearance
CSF	Cerebrospinal fluid
DC	Dendrite cell
ECG	Electrocardiogram
EDSS	Expanded Disability Status Scale
FEV_1	Forced expiratory volume in 1 second
HIV	Human immunodeficiency virus
IgG	Immunoglobulin G
IL	Interleukin
INF	Interferon
MHC	Major histocompatibility complex
MMP	Matrix metalloproteinase
Mφ	Macrophage
MRI	Magnetic resonance imaging
MS	Multiple sclerosis
MSFC	Multiple Sclerosis Functional Composite
MUGA	Multiple-gated acquisition
OPC	Oligodendrocyte precursor cell
PML	Progressive multifocal leukoencephalopathy
TGF	Transforming growth factor
Th1	T-helper-1 cells
Th2	T-helper-2 cells
TNF	Tumor necrosis factor
VCAM	Vascular cell adhesion molecule
VLA	Very late antigen

REFERENCES

1. National Multiple Sclerosis Society. Who gets MS? (epidemiology). [Internet] http://www.nationalmssociety.org/What-is-MS/Who-Gets-MS. Accessed August 15, 2014.
2. Huynh JL, Casaccia P. Epigenetic mechanisms in multiple sclerosis: Implications for pathogenesis and treatment. Lancet Neurol. 2013;12:195–206.
3. Hauser SL, Chan JR, Oksenberg JR. Multiple sclerosis: prospects and promise. Ann Neurology. 2013;75:317–327.
4. Aktas O, Kieseier B, Hartung HP. Neuroprotection, regeneration and immunomodulation: Broadening the therapeutic repertoire in multiple sclerosis. Trends Neurosci. 2010;33:140–152.
5. Smakoff LM, Goodman AD. Symptomatic management in multiple sclerosis. Neurol Clin. 2011;29:449–463.
6. Toosy AT, Mason DF, Miller DH. Optic neuritis. Lancet Neurol. 2014;13:83–99.
7. Lublin FD, Reingold SC, Cohen JA, et al. Defining the clinical course of multiple sclerosis. The 2013 revisions. Neurol. 2014;83:278–286.
8. Hurwitz BJ. Analysis of current multiple sclerosis registries. Neurology. 2011;76 (Suppl 1):S7–S13.
9. Polman CH, Reingold SC, Banwell B, et al. Diagnostic criteria for multiple sclerosis: 2010 revisions to the McDonald criteria. Ann Neurol. 2011;69:292–302.
10. Burton JM, O'Connor PSW, Hohol M, Beyene J. Oral versus intravenous steroids for treatment of relapses in multiple sclerosis (review). Cochrane Database Syst Rev. 2012; 12:1–66.
11. Perumal JS, Caon C, Hreha S, et al. Oral prednisone taper following intravenous steroids fails to improve disability or recovery from relapses in multiple sclerosis. Eur J Neurol. 2008;15: 677–680.
12. Rudick RA, Goelz SE. Beta-interferon for multiple sclerosis. Exp Cell Res. 2011;317:1301–1311.

13. La Mantia L, Vacchi L, De Pietrantonj C, et al. Interferon beta for secondary progressive multiple sclerosis. Cochrane Database Syst Rev. 2012:1–60.
14. Rommer PS, Zettl UK, Kieseier B, et al. Requirements for safety monitoring of approved multiple sclerosis therapies: An overview. Clin Exper Immunol. 2013;175:397–407.
15. Galetta SL, Markowitz C. U.S. FDA-approved disease-modifying treatments for multiple sclerosis: Review of adverse effect profiles. CNS Drugs. 2005;29:239–252.
16. Calabresi PA, Kieseier BC, Arnold DL, et al. Pegylated interferon beta-1a for relapsing-remitting multiple sclerosis (ADVANCE): A randomized, phase 3, double-blind study. Lancet Neurol. 2014;13:657–665.
17. Scott LJ. Glatiramer acetate: A review of its use in patients with relapsing-remitting multiple sclerosis and in delaying the onset of clinically definite multiple sclerosis. CNS Drugs. 2013;27: 971–988
18. LaMantia L, Munari LM, Lovati R. Glatiramer acetate for multiple sclerosis. Cochrane Database Syst Rev. 2010;5: CD004678. DOI: 10.1002/14651858.CD004678.pub2.
19. Menzin J, Caon C, Nichols C, et al. Narrative review of the literature on adherence to disease-modifying therapies among patients with multiple sclerosis. J Manag Care Pharm. 2013;19: S24–S40.
20. Brunetti L, Wagner ML, Maroney M, Ryan M. Teriflunomide for the treatment of relapsing multiple sclerosis: A review of clinical data. Ann Pharmacother. 2013;47:1153–1160.
21. Miller A, Wolinski J, Kappos L, et al. TOPIC main outcomes: efficacy and safety of once-daily oral teriflunomide in patients with clinically isolated syndrome [abstract]. Mult Scler J. 2013; 19(Suppl 1):22.
22. Linker RA, Gold R. Dimethyl fumarate for treatment of multiple sclerosis: mechanism of action, effectiveness, and side effects. Curr Neurol Neurosci Rep. 2013;13:394.
23. Willis MA, Cohen JA. Fingolimod therapy for multiple sclerosis. Semin Neurol. 2013;33:37–44.
24. Hoepner R, Faissner S, Salmen A, et al. Efficacy and side effects of natalizumab therapy in patients with multiple sclerosis. J Cent Nerv Syst Dis. 2014;6:1–49.
25. Martinelli Boneschi F, Vacchi L, et al. Mitoxantrone for multiple sclerosis. Cochrane Database Syst Rev. 2013;5:CD002127. DOI: 10.1002/14651858.CD002127.pub3.
26. Verweij CL, Vosslamber S. Relevance of the type I interferon signature in multiple sclerosis towards a personalized medicine approach for interferon-beta therapy. Discov Med. 2013;15:51–60.
27. Edan G, Le Page E. Induction therapy for patients with multiple sclerosis: Why? When? How? CNS Drugs. 2013;27:403–409.
28. Houtchens M. Multiple sclerosis and pregnancy. Clin Obstet Gynecol. 2013;56:342–349.
29. Pelligrino P, Carnovale C, Perrone V, et al. Efficacy of vaccination against influenza in patients with multiple sclerosis: The role of concomitant therapies. Vaccine. 2014;32:4730–4735.
30. Sorensen PS. New management algorithms in multiple sclerosis. Curr Opin. 2014;27:246–259.
31. Perumal J, Gauthier S, Nealson N, Vartanian. A practice definition of aggressive onset multiple sclerosis [abstract]. Mult Scler J. 2012;18 (Suppl 4):55–277.
32. Asano M, Finlayson ML. Meta-analysis of three different types of fatigue management interventions for people with multiple sclerosis: Exercise, education, and medication. Mult Scler Int. 2014;2014:798285.
33. Gold R, Oreja-Guevera C. Advances in the management of multiple sclerosis spasticity: Multiple sclerosis spasticity guidelines. Expert Rev Neurother. 2013;13(Suppl 12).55–59.
34. Bethoux F. Gait disorders in multiple sclerosis. Continuum. 2013;19:1007–1032.
35. Schoedel KA, Morrow SA, Sellers EM. Evaluating the safety and efficacy of quinidine/dextromethorphan in the treatment of pseudobulbar affect. Neuropsychiatr Dis Treat. 2014;10: 1161–1174.

31 Epilepsy

Timothy E. Welty and Edward Faught

LEARNING OBJECTIVES

Upon completion of the chapter, the reader will be able to:

1. Describe the epidemiology and social impact of epilepsy.
2. Define terminology related to epilepsy, including seizure, convulsion, and epilepsy.
3. Describe the basic pathophysiology of seizures and epilepsy.
4. Differentiate and classify seizure types given a description of the clinical presentation of the seizure and electroencephalogram.
5. Identify key therapeutic decision points and therapeutic goals in the treatment of epilepsy.
6. Discuss nonpharmacologic treatments for epilepsy.
7. Recommend an appropriate pharmacotherapeutic regimen with monitoring parameters for the treatment of epilepsy.
8. Devise a plan for switching a patient from one antiepileptic regimen to a different regimen.
9. Manage potential drug interactions with antiepileptic drugs.
10. Determine when and how to discontinue antiepileptic drug therapy.
11. Educate a patient or caregiver on epilepsy and pharmacotherapy for this disorder.

EPIDEMIOLOGY, SOCIAL IMPACT, AND ETIOLOGY

Epidemiology

Epilepsy is a disorder that afflicts approximately 2 million individuals in the United States, with an age-adjusted prevalence of approximately 4 to 7 cases per 1000 persons.[1] The incidence of epilepsy in the United States is estimated at 35 to 75 cases per 100,000 persons per year.[2,3] In developing countries, the incidence is higher at 100 to 190 cases per 100,000 persons per year. About 8% of the US population will experience a **seizure** during their lifetime. New-onset seizures occur most frequently in infants younger than 1 year of age and in adults after age 55.[4]

Social Impact

Epilepsy has a profound impact on a patient's life. Due to restrictions on driving in all states, individuals who have recently had a seizure face major impediments to engaging in simple activities[5] Fifty percent of patients with epilepsy report cognitive and learning difficulties.[6,7] Transportation and educational difficulties combine with persistent seizures to cause unemployment or underemployment, and as a result, problems with paying for health care. Additionally, the social stigma of embarrassment or injury due to seizures in public results in isolation of the patient.

Patients with epilepsy often depend on caregivers to assist with medications, transportation, and ensuring the patient's safety, so they should be informed about treatments and managing seizures.

Etiology

In approximately 80% of patients with epilepsy, the underlying etiology is unknown.[8] The most common causes of epilepsy are head trauma and stroke. Developmental and identifiable genetic defects cause about 5% of cases. Genetic causes are presumed in up to 25% of patients, but are often unproven. Brain tumors, central nervous system (CNS) infections, and neurodegenerative diseases are other common causes. Human immunodeficiency virus infection and neurocysticercosis infection are also important causes.

Isolated seizures can be caused by stroke, CNS trauma, CNS infections, metabolic disturbances (eg, hyponatremia, hypoglycemia), and hypoxia. If these causes of seizures are not corrected, they may lead to the development of epilepsy. Drugs commonly associated with causing seizures are tramadol, bupropion, theophylline, some antidepressants, some antipsychotics, amphetamines, cocaine, imipenem, lithium, excessive doses of penicillins or cephalosporins, and sympathomimetics or stimulants.

PATHOPHYSIOLOGY

Seizures

Regardless of the underlying etiology, all seizures involve a sudden electrical disturbance of the cerebral cortex. A population of neurons fires rapidly and repetitively for seconds to minutes. Cortical electrical discharges become excessively rapid, rhythmic, and synchronous. This phenomenon is presumably related to an excess of excitatory neurotransmitter action, a failure of inhibitory neurotransmitter action, or a combination of the two. In individual patients, it is usually impossible to identify which neurochemical factors are responsible.

Neurotransmitters

The major excitatory neurotransmitter is glutamate.[9] When glutamate is released from a presynaptic neuron, it attaches to receptors on the postsynaptic neuron. The result is opening of membrane channels to allow sodium or calcium to flow into the postsynaptic neuron, depolarizing it and transmitting the excitatory signal.[10] Many antiepileptic drugs (AED) (eg, phenytoin, carbamazepine, lamotrigine) work by interfering with this mechanism, blocking the release of glutamate or by blocking sodium or calcium channels.[11] At usual doses, these drugs typically do not block normal neuronal signaling, only the excessively rapid firing characteristic of seizures, usually not affecting normal brain function.

The major inhibitory neurotransmitter is *γ-aminobutyric acid* (GABA). It attaches to neuronal membranes and opens chloride channels. When chloride flows into the neuron, it becomes hyperpolarized and less excitable. This mechanism is probably critical for suppressing seizure activity. Barbiturates and benzodiazepines primarily act to enhance the action of GABA.

Cortical function is modulated by many other neurotransmitters, but their role in the action of AEDs is poorly understood.

Neuronal Mechanisms

Seizures originate in a group of neurons with abnormal electrical behavior, presumably due to an imbalance of neurotransmitter function.[12] In individual neurons, firing is excessively prolonged and repetitive. Instead of firing a single action potential, these neurons stay depolarized too long, firing many action potentials. This long, abnormal depolarization is called a *paroxysmal depolarizing shift (PDS).*

Excessive electrical discharges can spread to adjacent neurons or distant ones connected by fiber tracts. The seizure spreads to other areas of the brain, by recruiting neurons into uncontrolled firing patterns. Recruited neurons may not be abnormal, but are diverted from their normal functioning to participate in the excessive discharges. The area of spread determines the clinical manifestations of the seizure.

Nearly all seizures stop spontaneously, because brain inhibitory mechanisms overcome the abnormal excitation.

Epilepsy

Epilepsy is the tendency to have recurrent, unprovoked seizures. A recent statement by the International League Against Epilepsy (ILAE) recommends that this definition include persons with a single seizure, if they have at least a 70% chance of having another seizure. Practically, this defines two populations of patients who should be treated, and implies a permanent change in cortical function, rendering neurons more likely to participate in a seizure discharge. This process is called epileptogenesis, and the exact way in which it occurs is unknown. A process called kindling is considered similar to epileptogenesis in humans, and occurs in animals after prolonged, intermittent electrical brain stimulation.

Epilepsy may develop days, months, or years after a brain insult. It may be that a small group of abnormal neurons causes adjacent or connected normal neurons to gradually become abnormal. When a network of abnormal neurons becomes sufficiently large, it is capable of sustaining an excessive firing pattern for at least several seconds: a seizure. This hyperexcitable network of neurons is the seizure focus.

If the change in cortical electrical characteristics is permanent, why do seizures not occur all the time? This is probably because the occurrence of an individual seizure depends on an interplay of environmental and internal brain factors that intermittently result in loss of the normal mechanisms that control abnormal neuronal firing. Some causes of seizures are sleep loss and fatigue, but it is impossible to determine what triggers a specific seizure.

Epilepsy may remain stable, decrease in severity, or worsen over time. Repeated seizures may cause further damage to the cortex and loss of neurons, especially inhibitory neurons. Reorganization of connections between groups of neurons may strengthen excitatory connections and weaken inhibitory connections.

There are many reasons for controlling seizures completely. Epilepsy is associated with an increased mortality rate, from injuries with seizures or sudden death.[13] Early control of epileptic seizures may reduce the possibility of permanent changes in brain function, although this hypothesis is unproven.

Genetic Factors

Patients with seizures may be concerned that their children or other family members will inherit epilepsy. Patients with acquired causes of seizures, such as head trauma or stroke, will not transmit epilepsy. Some patients may have inherited epilepsy. Most of these individuals have primary generalized epilepsy, and develop seizures during childhood.[14,15] However, the hereditary tendency is weak. Complex inheritance patterns are usually seen, indicating the likely involvement of several abnormal genes or other factors for seizures to occur in offspring. Most patients can be reassured that their children and siblings are unlikely to develop epilepsy.

SEIZURE CLASSIFICATION AND PRESENTATION

General Principles

Careful diagnosis and identification of seizure types is essential to proper treatment of epilepsy. Numerous schemes and descriptions of seizures exist, but the ILAE has established the currently accepted standard for classifying epileptic seizures (Figure 31–1) and epilepsies or epilepsy syndromes (Table 31–1).[16,17] Classification of epileptic seizures is based on electroencephalographic (EEG) findings combined with the clinical symptoms or semiology of the seizure events. Clinical presentation of seizures varies widely depending on the region and amount of brain involved in the seizure.

Primary Generalized Seizures

If the entire cerebral cortex is involved in the seizure from the onset, the seizure is classified as primary generalized. This category is now referred to as "genetic generalized seizures," the apparent cause of most of these syndromes. Types of primary generalized seizures are: Tonic-clonic, Absence, Myoclonic, and Atonic.

Partial Seizures

When the seizure begins in a localized area of the brain, it is defined as partial. There are three types of partial seizures in the current classification system (see Figure 31–1): Simple, Complex, and Secondarily generalized.

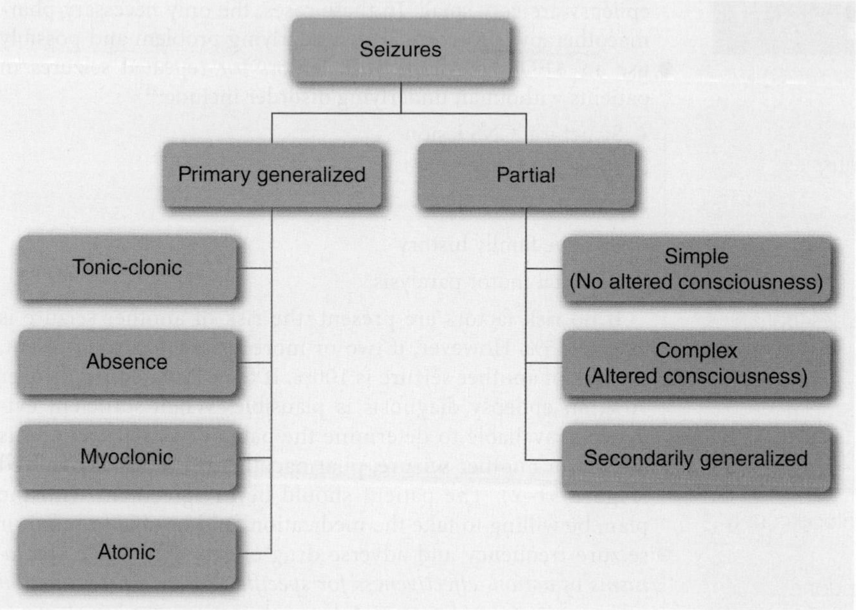

FIGURE 31–1. International League Against Epilepsy seizure classification.

Epilepsy Syndromes

Classification of epilepsies and epilepsy syndromes is helpful in determining appropriate pharmacotherapy. This classification scheme is based on the type of seizures and the presumed cause: **Idiopathic (Genetic) epilepsies, Symptomatic epilepsies,** and **Cryptogenic (Cause Unknown) epilepsies.**

A complete description of a patient's epilepsy should include the seizure type with the epilepsy or syndrome type (eg, idiopathic, symptomatic, cryptogenic).

Table 31–1

ILAE Classification Scheme for Epilepsies and Epilepsy Syndromes

I. Localization-related (focal, local, partial) epilepsies and epileptic syndromes
  A. Idiopathic with age-related onset
    1. Benign childhood epilepsy with centrotemporal spikes
    2. Childhood epilepsy with occipital paroxysms
  B. Symptomatic
II. Generalized epilepsies and epileptic syndromes
  A. Idiopathic and age-related onset
    1. Benign neonatal epilepsy
    2. Childhood absence epilepsy (pyknolepsy)
    3. Juvenile myoclonic epilepsy (impulsive petit mal)
    4. Juvenile absence epilepsy with generalized tonic-clonic seizure on awakening
  B. Secondary (idiopathic or symptomatic)
    1. West syndrome (infantile spasms)
    2. Lennox-Gastaut syndrome
  C. Symptomatic
    1. Nonspecific etiology (early myoclonic encephalopathy)
    2. Specific syndromes (epileptic seizures that may complicate many diseases, eg, Ramsay-Hunt syndrome, Unverricht disease)

Data from Commission on Classification and Terminology of the International League Against Epilepsy. Proposal for revised classification of epilepsies and epileptic syndromes. Epilepsia. 1989;30:389–399.

Commonly encountered epilepsy syndromes are: **Juvenile myoclonic epilepsy (JME), Lennox-Gastaut syndrome (LGS), Mesial temporal lobe epilepsy (MTLE), and Infantile spasms (West's Syndrome).**

Other Classifications

A new ILAE classification system improves the description of the seizure type and epilepsy, and will be finalized soon.[18,19] The scheme involves five axes:

Axis 1: Description of the seizure event
Axis 2: Epileptic seizure type or types
Axis 3: Any syndrome type
Axis 4: Etiology when known
Axis 5: Degree of impairment by the epilepsy

The new system replaces "partial seizures" with "focal seizures", "idiopathic epilepsies" with "genetic epilepsies", and "cryptogenic epilepsies" with "epilepsies of unknown cause."

DIAGNOSIS

A correct and accurate diagnosis is essential prior to starting pharmacotherapy. KEY CONCEPT *A distinction between a single seizure and epilepsy should be made, and other seizure-like disorders (eg, syncope, psychogenic, nonepileptic events, anxiety attacks, cardiac arrhythmias, hypoglycemia, transient ischemic attacks, tics, and complicated migraine headaches) should be ruled out.* Seizures are typically brief spells, lasting less than 5 minutes. However, prolonged seizures lasting greater than or equal to 5 minutes or occurring one after another without recovery in between are status epilepticus, which requires immediate medical attention (Chapter 32).

A proper diagnostic workup of a patient presenting with seizures includes the following elements:

- Complete neurologic examination
- EEG
- Laboratory tests (complete blood count [CBC], liver function tests [LFTs], serum chemistry)
- Neuroimaging (preferably **magnetic resonance imaging [MRI]**)

Clinical Presentation and Diagnosis

Presentation

- Episodes of sudden and brief loss of consciousness
- Episodes of uncontrolled jerking of groups of muscles
- Sudden unexplained falls
- Sudden and brief episodes of confusion

Diagnosis

- Thorough clinical history, including a complete description of the episodes
- Complete neurological physical examination
- Imaging of the brain: preferably a MRI, but a computerized tomogram (CT) of the brain may be used in absence of a MRI
- Laboratory tests: serum electrolytes, complete blood count, renal function, and liver function
- Electroencephalogram (EEG) recording: may be done with special techniques, including hyperventilation and photostimulation. Sleep deprivation may also be used
- Video-electroencephalogram (VEEG)

Many of the tests are done to rule out other causes of seizures (eg, infection, electrolyte imbalance), and in most patients will be normal. Often the EEG appears normal between seizures.[20] Sleep deprivation, photic stimulation, prolonged (greater than 20 minutes) EEG recording, and 24-hour EEG monitoring with video correlation can be done to capture seizure or seizure-like activity on the EEG.

TREATMENT

Desired Outcomes

The ultimate outcome goal for any patient with epilepsy is elimination of all seizures without adverse effects of the treatment. An effective treatment plan allows the patient to pursue a normal lifestyle with complete control of seizures. The treatment should enable the patient to drive, perform well in school, hold a reasonable job, and function effectively in the family and community. However, 30% to 50% of patients are not able to fully achieve these outcomes. In these cases, the goal of therapy is to provide a tolerable balance between reduced seizure severity and/or frequency and medication adverse effects, enabling the individual to have a lifestyle as nearly normal as possible.

General Approach to Treatment

Once it is concluded that the patient has seizures, the type of seizure and epilepsy syndrome, if any, must be determined.

KEY CONCEPT *Selection of appropriate pharmacotherapy depends on distinguishing, identifying, and understanding different seizure types.* Without an accurate classification of the seizure type, it is possible to select a medication that is ineffective or even harmful to the patient.

KEY CONCEPT *Prior to starting pharmacologic therapy, it is essential to determine the risk of having a subsequent seizure.* If there is an underlying treatable cause, such as hyponatremia or a CNS infection, the risks of another seizure and the development of epilepsy are very small. In these cases, the only necessary pharmacotherapy is to correct the underlying problem and possibly use an AED short-term. Risk factors for repeated seizures in patients without an underlying disorder include:[21]

- Structural CNS lesion
- Abnormal EEG
- Partial seizure type
- Positive family history
- Postictal motor paralysis

If no risk factors are present, the risk of another seizure is 10% to 15%. However, if two or more risk factors are present, the risk of another seizure is 100%. If the estimated risk is over 70%, an epilepsy diagnosis is plausible. When sufficient evidence is available to determine the patient has seizures and is at risk for another seizure, pharmacotherapy is usually started (Figure 31–2). The patient should be in agreement with the plan, be willing to take the medication, and be able to monitor seizure frequency and adverse drug effects. KEY CONCEPT *Mechanisms of action, effectiveness for specific seizure types, common adverse effects, and potential drug interactions are key elements in selecting a medication.* Other patient factors such as gender, concomitant drugs, age, economic factors, and lifestyle also need to be considered.

Nonpharmacologic Therapy

Nonpharmacologic treatments for epilepsy are available. For some patients, surgery is the treatment approach with the greatest probability of eliminating seizures.[22] The most common surgical approach for epilepsy is temporal lobectomy. When the seizure focus can be localized and it is in a region of the brain that is not too close to critical areas, such as those responsible for speech or muscle control, surgical removal of the focus can result in 80% to 90% of patients becoming seizure free. According to a National Institutes of Health Consensus Conference, three criteria should be met for patients to be candidates for surgery.[23] Other surgical procedures that are less likely to make a patient seizure free include corpus callosotomy and extratemporal lesion removal.

Vagal nerve stimulation is another nonpharmacologic approach to treating all types of seizures.[24] An unit that generates an intermittent electrical current is placed under the skin in the chest. A wire is tunneled under the skin to the left vagus nerve in the neck and delivers a small electrical stimulus to the vagus nerve. Additional stimulations can be initiated by swiping a magnet over the device located in the chest. This treatment is essentially equivalent to starting a new medication with regard to efficacy, with fewer than 10% of refractory patients becoming seizure free. Vagal nerve stimulation is usually reserved for patients who do not respond to several drugs and are not surgical candidates. Finally, a deep brain stimulation device has been approved for individuals with seizures refractory to other treatments. Some AED therapy is usually continued in patients with devices.

Another nonpharmacologic treatment is the ketogenic diet.[25] This diet produces a keto-acidotic state through the elimination of nearly all carbohydrates. The diet consists of dietary fats (eg, butter, heavy cream, fatty meats) and protein with no added sugar. Daily urinalysis for ketones is performed to ensure the patient remains in ketosis. Any inadvertent consumption of sugar results in the diet needing to be reinitiated. Pharmacists must be vigilant in maintaining the diet, by determining the sugar or carbohydrate content of medications the patient is taking.

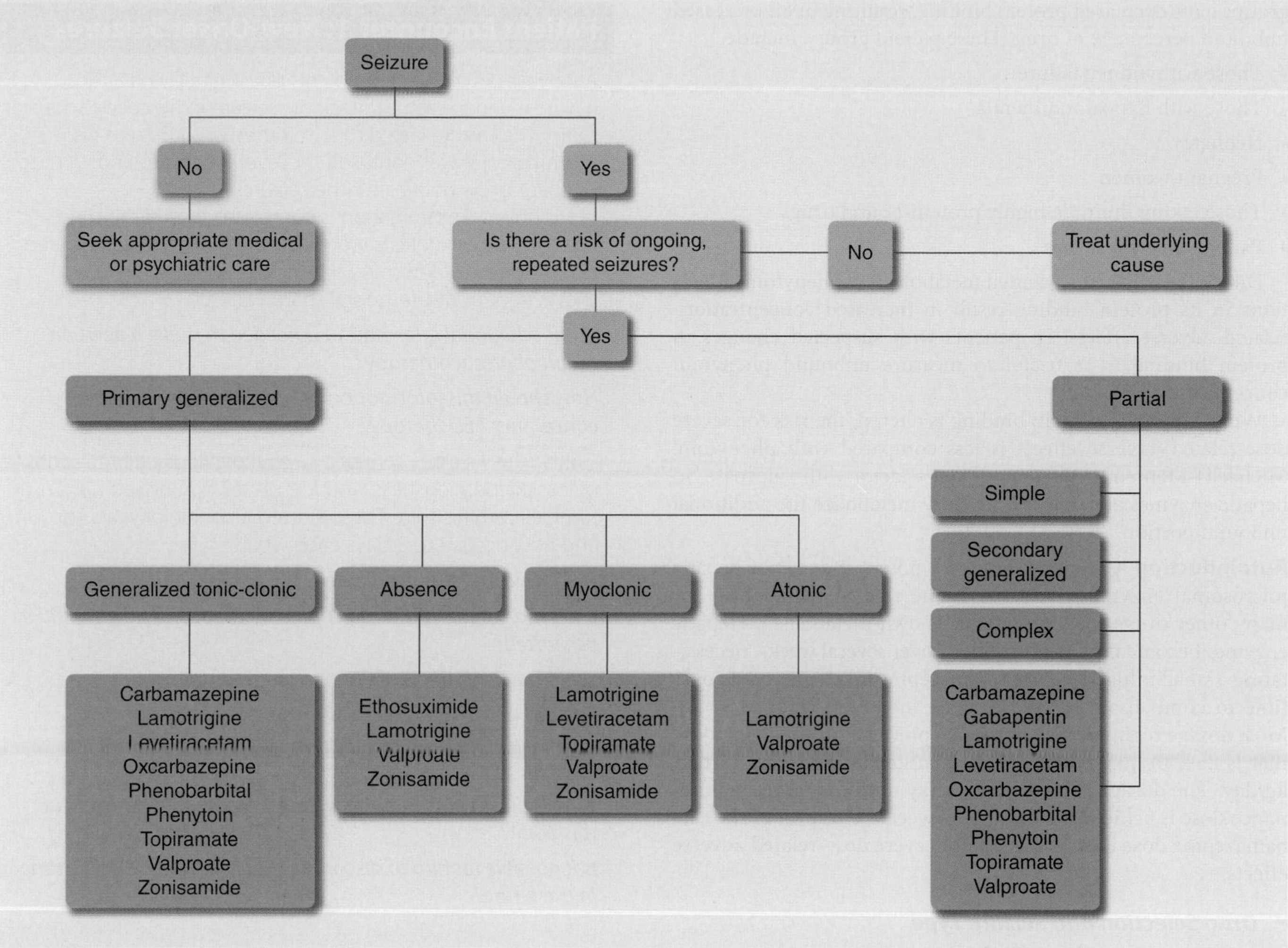

FIGURE 31–2. Treatment algorithm for seizures.

This diet is typically used only in children with difficult-to-control seizures. In certain patients the diet can be extremely effective, resulting in complete seizure control and reduction of AEDs. However, it is difficult to maintain, and palatability of the diet, growth retardation, and hypercholesterolemia are concerns.

Pharmacologic Therapy

▶ *Special Considerations*

Use of AEDs presents some unique challenges.[26]

Michaelis-Menten Metabolism Phenytoin metabolism is capacity limited. Michaelis-Menten pharmacokinetics occurs when the maximum capacity of hepatic enzymes to metabolize the drug is reached, and this may occur within the normal dose range. The clinical significance is that small changes in doses result in large changes in serum concentrations. Too large a dose change may result in concentration-related toxicity or breakthrough seizures. Individual differences in metabolism, result in a different relationship between dose and serum concentrations. These differences can be defined only by careful use of serum concentration and dosing data. There are numerous schemes for determining appropriate dosage adjustments of phenytoin, but for routine clinical practice, dosage adjustments for adults with normal protein binding of phenytoin and a steady-state serum concentration can be made using the following plan:

- For serum concentrations less than 7 mcg/mL (mg/L; 28 μmol/L), the total daily dose is increased by 100 mg.
- For serum concentrations of 7 to 12 mcg/mL (mg/L; 28–48 μmol/L), the total daily dose is increased by 50 mg.
- For serum concentrations more than 12 mcg/mL (mg/L; 48 μmol/L), the total daily dose is increased by no more than 30 mg.[27]

Protein Binding Some AEDs, especially phenytoin and valproate, are highly bound to plasma proteins. When interpreting a reported concentration for these drugs, it is important to remember the value represents the total (ie, bound and unbound) concentration in the blood. Because of differences in the metabolism of these drugs, the clinical effects of altered protein binding are different.

Normally, 88% to 92% of phenytoin is bound to plasma protein, leaving 8% to 12% as unbound. The unbound component produces the clinical effect in the CNS, produces dose-related side effects in the CNS and at other sites, distributes to other peripheral sites, and gets metabolized. Certain patient groups have decreased protein binding, resulting in an increased unbound percentage of drug. These patient groups include:

- Those with kidney failure
- Those with hypoalbuminemia
- Neonates
- Pregnant women
- Those taking multiple highly protein-bound drugs
- Patients in critical care

Due to the Michaelis-Menten metabolism of phenytoin, alterations in its protein binding result in increased concentration-related adverse effects. In patients with suspected changes in protein binding, it is useful to measure unbound phenytoin concentrations.

When valproate protein binding is altered, the risk for severe dose-related adverse effects is less compared with phenytoin. Michaelis-Menten metabolism is not a factor with valproate, so hepatic enzymes are able to efficiently metabolize the additional unbound portion.

Autoinduction Carbamazepine is a potent inducer of hepatic microsomal enzymes. It increases the rate of metabolism for many other drugs, and the rate of its own metabolism. Hepatic enzymes become maximally induced over several weeks, necessitating a small initial dose of carbamazepine that is increased over time to compensate for the enzyme induction (Figure 31–3). Most dosage regimens for carbamazepine call for a starting dose that is 25% to 30% of the typical maintenance dose of 15 mg/kg/day. The dosage is increased weekly until the target maintenance dose is achieved within 3 to 4 weeks. Titration of the carbamazepine dose lessens the risk for severe dose-related adverse effects.

Patient Encounter 1: New-Onset Seizures

A 22-year-old man is seen by his physician 4 days after having a generalized tonic-clonic seizure in his college dorm room. The seizure lasted for 5 minutes, according to his roommate. He was confused for several minutes and went to sleep for a few hours after the seizure.

His physical examination is completely normal, and no focal neurologic deficits were observed. An MRI was ordered and reported as right mesial temporal sclerosis. An EEG shows right fronto-temporal sharp waves.

What additional information is needed to make a decision about pharmacotherapy?

How should this information be used to make choices concerning AED therapy?

During the visit, he mentions several previous brief episodes of loss of consciousness, and friends tell him his left hand fumbles with his shirt. These started a couple of years ago and now occur 2 to 3 days each week.

Is pharmacotherapy indicated?

If it is indicated, what drug should be used, and how should it be started?

What adverse effects are important to monitor?

Three months later he is doing well. He reports no generalized tonic-clonic seizures, and the brief spells are reduced to about 2 per month.

What adjustments in pharmacotherapy should be made at this point?

Is it possible for him to discontinue AED therapy at some time in the future?

▸ Drug Selection and Seizure Type

The key to selecting effective pharmacotherapy is to base the decision on the seizure type. Several consensus treatment guidelines from the Scottish Intercollegiate Guidelines Network (SIGN), the National Institute for Clinical Excellence in the United Kingdom (NICE), the American Academy of Neurology (AAN), and ILAE all link seizure type to the selection of pharmacotherapy (Table 31–2).[28–30] While the guidelines make recommendations for specific drugs to be used in certain seizure types, the consensus recommendations use only high-quality data available from the medical literature. In many cases, a recommendation is not made due to lack of sufficient data for an evidence-based decision. Therefore, a drug may not appear in a guideline because insufficient data was available at the time the guideline was developed. Absence of a recommendation does not mean the drug is ineffective for a specific seizure type. For example, according to the AAN Practice Parameter, topiramate is useful as monotherapy for primary generalized tonic-clonic seizures, but insufficient evidence was available at the time of guideline development to make any recommendation regarding gabapentin, lamotrigine, oxcarbazepine, tiagabine, levetiracetam, or zonisamide.[31]

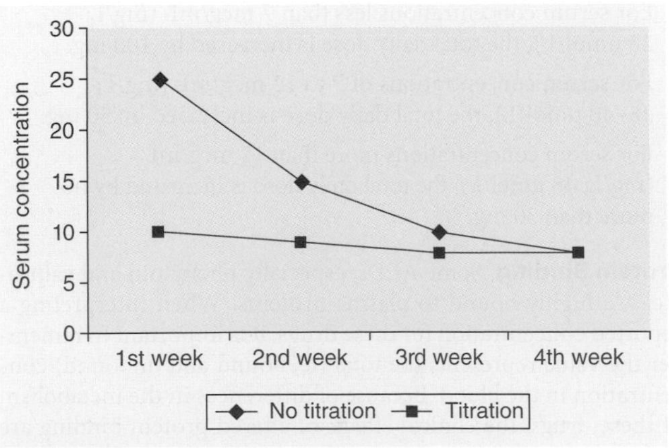

FIGURE 31–3. Carbamazepine serum concentrations with a titration schedule compared to initiation with no titration. Concentrations are expressed in mcg/mL. Conversion of carbamazepine concentrations to μmol/L requires multiplying by 4.23.

Outside of the evidence-based guidelines, other pharmacologic treatments are commonly used or avoided. For initial treatment of absence seizures, ethosuximide and valproate are used. In absence and myoclonic seizures, carbamazepine, oxcarbazepine, gabapentin, tiagabine, and pregabalin should be avoided due to association with worsening of these seizure types.

KEY CONCEPT *Antiepileptic drug therapy should usually be initiated carefully using a titration schedule to minimize adverse events.* Moderate target doses are chosen until the patient's response can be further evaluated in the clinic. If seizures continue, the dose is increased gradually until the patient becomes seizure free or adverse effects appear. For some drugs like lamotrigine, specific titration guidelines are established by the manufacturer.

Treatment of refractory seizures (ie, unresponsive to at least two first-line AEDs) is somewhat different. Combinations of drugs may be useful in patients with difficult to control seizures. All AEDs, except ethosuximide, are effective in combination therapy for partial seizures.

▸ *Complications of Pharmacotherapy*

Adverse effects of AEDs are frequently dose limiting or cause a drug to be discontinued. Two types of adverse effects occur with AEDs: serum concentration-related and idiosyncratic (Table 31–3). Concentration-related adverse effects happen with increasing frequency and severity as the dose or serum concentration of a drug is increased. Common concentration-related adverse effects include sedation, ataxia, and diplopia. Adverse effects are considered one of the AED selection criteria. For example, if a patient has a job that requires mental alertness, it is best to choose an AED that is less likely to cause sedation (eg, lamotrigine).

Idiosyncratic adverse effects are not dose or concentration related and almost always result in the AED being discontinued. Rash is the most common of these. Severe skin, hepatic, or hematological reactions occur rarely, but are potentially

Table 31–2

Evidence-Based Guidelines for Initial Monotherapy Treatment of Epilepsy

Seizure Type	AAN	SIGN	NICE	ILAE
Primary generalized tonic-clonic	Carbamazepine[a] Lamotrigine[a] Oxcarbazepine[a] Phenobarbital[a] Phenytoin[a] Topiramate[a] Valproate[a]	Lamotrigine Valproate	Carbamazepine Lamotrigine Valproate *Adjunctive:* Clobazam Lamotrigine Levetiracetam Topiramate Valproate	*Adults:* Carbamazepine[c] Lamotrigine[c] Oxcarbazepine[c] Phenobarbital[c] Phenytoin[c] Topiramate Valproate[c] *Children:* Carbamazepine[c] Phenobarbital[c] Topiramate[c] Valproate[c]
Absence	Lamotrigine (children)	Ethosuximide Lamotrigine Valproate	Ethosuximide Lamotrigine Valproate *Alternatives:* Clobazam Clonazepam Levetiracetam Topiramate Zonisamide	*Children:* Ethosuximide[c] Lamotrigine[c] Valproate[c]
Myoclonic	Not mentioned	Lamotrigine Valproate	Levetiracetam Topiramate Valproate *Alternative:* Clobazam Clonazepam Zonismaide Piracetam[b]	Clonazepam[d] Lamotrigine[d] Levetiracetam[d] Topiramate[d] Valproate[d] Zonisamide[d]
Tonic	Not mentioned	Not mentioned	Lamotrigine Valproate *Second-line:* Clobazam Clonazepam Levetiracetam Topiramate	Not mentioned
Atonic	Not mentioned	Not mentioned	Valproate *Alternatives:* Lamotrigine Topiramate Rufinamide	Not mentioned

(*Continued*)

Table 31–2

Evidence-Based Guidelines for Initial Monotherapy Treatment of Epilepsy (*Continued*)

Seizure Type	AAN	SIGN	NICE	ILAE
Partial with or without secondary generalization	Carbamazepine Gabapentin Lamotrigine Oxcarbazepine Phenobarbital Phenytoin Topiramate Valproate	Phenytoin Carbamazepine Valproate Lamotrigine Oxcarbazepine	Carbamazepine Lamotrigine Oxcarbazepine Valproate Topiramate *Second-line:* Clobazam Gabapentin Levetiracetam Phenytoin Tiagabine	*Adults*: Carbamazepine[e] Phenytoin[e] Valproate[c] Gabapentin[c] Lamotrigine[c] Oxcarbazepine[c] Phenobarbital[c] Topiramate[c] Vigabatrin[c] *Children*: Oxcarbazepine[e] Carbamazepine[c] Phenobarbital[c] Phenytoin[c] Topiramate[c] Valproate[c] Lamotrigine[c] Vigabatrin[c] *Elderly*: Lamotrigine[e] Gabapentin[e] Carbamazepine[c] Topiramate[c] Valproate[c]

AAN, American Academy of Neurology; ILAE, International League Against Epilepsy; NICE, National Institute for Clinical Excellence in the United Kingdom; SIGN, Scottish Intercollegiate Guidelines Network.

[a]Based on data from newly diagnosed epilepsy patients of multiple seizure types.

[b]Not currently available in the United States.

[c]Possibly effective.

[d]Probably effective.

[e]Proven effective.

Privitera MD. Clinical rules for phenytoin dosing. Ann Pharmacother. 1993;27(10):1169–1173.

Scottish Intercollegiate Guidelines Network. Diagnosis and management of epilepsy in adults [Internet], [cited 2011 Oct 10]. http://www.sign.ac.uk/pdf/sign70.pdf.

National Institute for Clinical Excellence. The epilepsies: The diagnosis and management of the epilepsies in children and adults in primary and secondary care [Internet], [cited 2014 Sep 15]. http:// http://www.nice.org.uk/guidance/CG137/chapter/Introduction.

French JA, Kanner AM, Bautista J, et al. Efficacy and tolerability of the new antiepileptic drugs I: Treatment of new onset epilepsy report of the Therapeutics and Technology Assessment Subcommittee and Quality Standards Subcommittee of the American Academy of Neurology and the American Epilepsy Society. Neurology. 2005;62:1252–1260.

life-threatening. The AED should be discontinued immediately when these reactions occur. Carbamazepine, phenytoin, phenobarbital, valproate, lamotrigine, oxcarbazepine, and felbamate are most likely to cause reactions. There is a possibility of cross-reactivity for these adverse effects, especially for carbamazepine, phenytoin, phenobarbital, and oxcarbazepine. It is estimated that 15% to 25% of patients who have an idiosyncratic reaction to one drug will have a similar reaction to the other drugs.

► *Chronic Adverse Effects*

Because AEDs are administered for long periods of time, adverse effects due to prolonged drug exposure are of concern. Some chronic adverse effects associated with AEDs include peripheral neuropathy and cerebellar atrophy. Other chronic adverse effects are extensions of acute adverse effects, for example, weight gain.

Osteoporosis is a major chronic adverse effect of several drugs.[32,33] Carbamazepine, phenytoin, phenobarbital, oxcarbazepine, and valproate decrease bone mineral density, after 6 months of treatment. The risk of osteoporosis due to chronic AED use is comparable to the risk with chronic use of glucocorticosteroids. Patients taking carbamazepine, oxcarbazepine, phenytoin, phenobarbital, or valproate more than 6 months should take supplemental calcium and vitamin D. Routine monitoring for osteoporosis should be performed every 2 years, and patients should be instructed on ways to protect themselves from fractures.

Table 31–3

Characteristics of Common AEDs

Drug	Mechanism of Action	Dose	Pharmacokinetic Parameters	Usual Serum Concentration Range	Dose-Related Adverse Effects	Idiosyncratic Adverse Effects
Carbamazepine (Tegretol, Tegretol XR, Carbatrol, generic)	Fast sodium channel inactivation	*Loading dose:* Not recommended due to excessive dose-related toxicity *Maintenance dose:* Titrate dosage to target over 3–4 weeks Adults: 10–20 mg/kg/day as a divided dose Children: 20–30 mg/kg/day as a divided dose	*Half-life:* 10–25 hours with chronic dosing *Apparent volume of distribution:* 0.8–1.9 L/kg *Protein binding:* 67%–81% *Primary elimination route:* Hepatic	4–12 mcg/mL (mg/L; 17–51 μmol/L)	Diplopia, drowsiness, nausea, sedation	Aplastic anemia, hyponatremia, leucopenia, osteoporosis, rash
Clobazam (Onfi)	Enhance GABA	Weight < 30 kg, start 5 mg/day, titrate to 20 mg/day in two divided doses Weight > 30 kg start 10 mg/day, titrate to 40 mg/day in two divided doses	*Half-life:* 10–50 hours *Apparent volume of distribution:* ~0.9 L/kg *Protein binding:* ~90% *Primary elimination route:* Hepatic; metabolized to active metabolite that is further metabolized by CYP 2C19	Not established	Sedation somnolence lethargy pyrexia irritability drooling aggression	
Clonazepam (Klonopin, generic)	Enhance GABA activity	*Loading dose:* Not recommended due to increased adverse effects *Maintenance dose:* Initiate at 0.5 mg one to three times daily, titrate dose to effectiveness, usually 3–5 mg daily in two or three divided doses	*Half-life:* 30–40 hours *Apparent volume of distribution:* 3.2 L/kg *Protein binding:* 47%–80% *Primary elimination route:* Hepatic	Not established	Ataxia, memory impairment, sedation, slowed thinking	
Ethosuximide (Zarontin, generic)	Modulate calcium channels	*Loading dose:* Not recommended due to increased adverse effects *Maintenance dose:* Initiate at 250 mg twice daily and titrate to 500–1000 mg twice daily	*Half-life:* 60 hours *Apparent volume of distribution:* 0.6–0.7 L/kg *Protein binding:* None *Primary elimination route:* Hepatic	40–100 mcg/mL (mg/L; 283–708 μmol/L)	Ataxia, sedation	Hepatotoxicity, neutropenia, rash

(Continued)

Table 31–3

Characteristics of Common AEDs (*Continued*)

Drug	Mechanism of Action	Dose	Pharmacokinetic Parameters	Usual Serum Concentration Range	Dose-Related Adverse Effects	Idiosyncratic Adverse Effects
Felbamate (Felbatol)	Inhibit glutamate activity	*Loading dose:* Not recommended due to increased adverse effects *Maintenance dose:* 1200–3600 mg/day in three or four divided doses	*Half-life:* Monotherapy: 20 hours Concurrent enzyme inducers: 11–16 hours *Apparent volume of distribution:* 0.7–0.8 L/kg *Protein binding:* 25%–35% *Primary elimination route:* Hepatic	Not established	Anxiety, insomnia, nausea	Anorexia, aplastic anemia, headache, hepatotoxicity, weight loss
Gabapentin (Neurontin, generic)	Modulate calcium channels and enhance GABA activity	*Loading dose:* Not recommended due to short half-life *Maintenance dose:* 900–3600 mg/day in three or four divided doses (doses up to 10,000 mg/day have been tolerated)	*Half-life:* 5–7 hours (proportional to creatinine clearance) *Apparent volume of distribution:* 0.6–0.8 L/kg *Protein binding:* < 10% *Primary elimination route:* Renal	Not established	Drowsiness, sedation	Peripheral edema, weight gain
Lacosamide (Vimpat)	Slow sodium channel inactivation; modulate collapsin response; mediator protein-2	*Loading dose:* Data unavailable *Maintenance dose:* 200–400 mg/day; Start at 100 mg/day in two divided doses and titrate upward according to response	*Half-life:* Approximately 13 hours *Volume of distribution:* 0.6 L/kg *Protein binding:* < 15% *Primary elimination route:* 40% renal 60% hepatic	Not established	Ataxia, dizziness, diplopia, headache, nausea, vomiting	PR interval prolongation
Lamotrigine (Lamictal, Lamictal XR, generic)	Fast sodium channel inactivation	*Loading dose:* Not recommended due to increased risk of rash *Maintenance dose:* 150–800 mg/day in 2 or 3 divided doses. Doses should be initiated and titrated according to the manufacturer's recommendations to reduce the risk of rash	*Half-life:* Monotherapy: 24 hours Concurrent enzyme inducers: 12–15 hours Concurrent enzyme inhibitors: 55–60 hours *Apparent volume of distribution:* 1.1 L/kg *Protein binding:* 55% *Primary elimination route:* Hepatic	Not established	Ataxia, drowsiness, headache, insomnia, sedation	Rash

Levetiracetam (Keppra, Keppra XR, generic)	Modulate synaptic vesicle protein	*Loading dose:* Not recommended due to excessive adverse effects *Maintenance dose:* 1000–3000 mg/day. Start at 1000 mg/day and titrated upward as indicated by response	*Half-life:* 6–8 hours *Apparent volume of distribution:* 0.5–0.7 L/kg *Protein binding:* < 10% *Primary elimination route:* 70% renal 30% hepatic	Not established	Somnolence, dizziness	Depression
Oxcarbazepine (Trileptal, generic)	Fast sodium channel inactivation	*Loading dose:* Not recommended due to excessive adverse effects *Maintenance dose:* 600–1200 mg/day. Start at 300 mg twice daily and titrated upward as indicated by response	*Half-life:* Parent drug Approximately 2 hours; 10-monohydroxy *Metabolite* Approximately 9 hours *Apparent volume of distribution:* 0.5–0.7 L/kg *Protein binding:* 40% *Primary elimination route:* Hepatic	Not established	Diplopia, dizziness, somnolence	Hyponatremia, 25–30% cross-sensitivity in patients with hypersensitivity to carbamazepine
Phenobarbital (Luminal, generic)	Fast sodium channel inactivation	*Loading dose:* 10–20 mg/kg as single or divided IV infusion or orally in divided doses over 24–48 hours *Maintenance dose:* Adults: 1–4 mg/kg/day as a single or divided dose Children: 3–6 mg/kg/day as divided dose Neonates: 1–3 mg/kg/day as divided dose	*Half-life:* Adults: 49–120 hours Children: 37–73 hours Neonates: approximately 115 hours *Volume of distribution:* 0.7–1 L/kg *Protein binding:* Approximately 50% *Primary elimination route:* Hepatic	15–40 mcg/mL (mg/L; 65–172 μmol/L)	Ataxia, drowsiness, sedation	Attention deficit, cognitive impairment, hyperactivity, osteoporosis, passive-aggressive behavior

(Continued)

Table 31–3

Characteristics of Common AEDs (*Continued*)

Drug	Mechanism of Action	Dose	Pharmacokinetic Parameters	Usual Serum Concentration Range	Dose-Related Adverse Effects	Idiosyncratic Adverse Effects
Phenytoin (Dilantin, generic)	Fast sodium channel inactivation	*Loading dose:* Adults: 15–20 mg/kg single IV dose or divided oral dose Infants younger than 3 months: 10–15 mg/kg single IV dose Neonates: 15–20 mg/kg single IV dose *Maintenance dose:* Adults: 5–7 mg/kg/day, as single or divided dose Children: 6–15 mg/kg/day, as divided dose Neonates: 3–8 mg/kg/day, as divided dose	*Half-life:* Follows capacity-limited or Michaelis-Menten pharmacokinetics. Half-life increases as the dose and serum concentration increases. *Volume of distribution:* Adults: 0.7 L/kg Children: 0.8 L/kg Neonates: 1.2 L/kg *Protein binding:* Adults, children: 88%–92% Neonates: 65% *Primary elimination route:* Hepatic	10–20 mcg/mL (mg/L; 40–79 μmol/L) total concentration 1–2 mcg/mL (mg/L; 4–8 μmol/L) unbound concentration	Ataxia, diplopia, drowsiness, sedation	Anemia, gingival hyperplasia, hirsutism, lymphadenopathy, osteoporosis, rash
Pregabalin (Lyrica)	Modulate calcium channels	*Loading dose:* Not recommended due to increased adverse effects *Maintenance dose:* Initiate at 150 mg/day in two or three divided doses and titrate to a maximum dose of 600 mg/day	*Half-life:* 6.3 hours, proportional to creatinine clearance *Apparent volume of distribution:* 0.5 L/kg *Protein binding:* Negligible *Primary elimination route:* Renal	Not established	Ataxia, blurred vision, dizziness, dry mouth, somnolence	Edema, weight gain
Rufinamide (Banzel)	Unknown, may enhance inactivation of sodium channels	*Loading dose:* Data unavailable *Maintenance dose:* Children: 45 mg/kg/day or 3200 mg/day; start at 10 mg/kg/day in two divided doses and titrate upward according to response Adults: 3200 mg/day; start at 400–800 mg/day in two divided doses and titrate upward according to response	*Half-life:* 6–10 hours *Apparent volume of distribution:* Approximately 0.7 L/kg, varies with dose *Protein binding:* 34% (27% to albumin) *Primary elimination route:* Hepatic	Not established	Dizziness, fatigue, headache, nausea, somnolence, vomiting	

Tiagabine (Gabitril, generic)	Enhance GABA activity	*Loading dose:* Not recommended due to excessive adverse effects *Maintenance dose:* 32–56 mg/day in four divided doses. Doses should be titrated upward over 6 weeks, starting at 4 mg/day	*Half-life:* Monotherapy: 7–9 hours Concurrent enzyme inducers 2.5–4.5 hours *Apparent volume of distribution:* 0.6–0.8 L/kg *Protein binding:* 96% *Primary elimination route:* Hepatic	Not established	Dizziness, somnolence, irritability, slowed thinking	
Topiramate (Topamax, generic)	Fast sodium channel inactivation, inhibit glutamate activity, enhance GABA activity	*Loading dose:* Not recommended due to excessive adverse effects *Maintenance dose:* 100–400 mg/day in two or three divided doses. Doses should be started at 25–50 mg/day and gradually titrated upward over 3–6 weeks to avoid excessive adverse effects	*Half-life:* Monotherapy: 21 hours Concurrent enzyme inducers: 11–16 hours *Apparent volume of distribution:* 0.55–0.8 L/kg *Protein binding:* 13%–17% *Primary elimination route:* 60% renal 40% hepatic	Not established	Ataxia, dizziness, drowsiness, slowed thinking	Acute glaucoma, metabolic acidosis, oligohidrosis, paresthesia, renal calculi, weight loss
Valproic acid/ divalproex sodium (Depakene, Depakote, Depakote ER, generic)	Fast sodium channel inactivation	*Loading dose:* 20–40 mg/kg *Maintenance dose:* Adults: 15–45 mg/kg/day in two to four divided doses Children: 5–60 mg/kg/day in two to four divided doses	*Half-life:* Adults: 8–15 hours Children: 4–15 hours Infants younger than 2 months: 65 hours *Volume of distribution:* 0.1–0.5 L/kg *Protein binding:* 90% (decreases with increasing serum concentrations) *Primary elimination route:* Hepatic	50–100 mcg/mL (mg/L; 346–693 μmol/L) Children may require concentrations up to 150 mcg/mL (mg/L; 1040 μmol/L)	Drowsiness, nausea, sedation, tremor	Hepatotoxicity, osteoporosis, pancreatitis, weight gain

(Continued)

Table 31–3

Characteristics of Common AEDs (*Continued*)

Drug	Mechanism of Action	Dose	Pharmacokinetic Parameters	Usual Serum Concentration Range	Dose-Related Adverse Effects	Idiosyncratic Adverse Effects
Vigabatrin (Sabril)	Inhibits GABA transaminase	*Children:* 1 month–2 years: 50 mg/kg/day in two divided doses *Adults:* Initiate at 1000 mg/day in two divided doses, titrate up to 3000 mg/day *Renal failure:* CrCl 50–80 mL/min (0.83-1.33 mL/s), decrease dose by 25%; CrCl 30–50 mL/min (0.50–0.83 mL/s), decrease dose by 50%; CrCl 10–30 mL/min (0.17–0.50 mL/s), decrease dose by 75%	*Half-life:* 7.5 hours, proportional to creatinine clearance *Volume of distribution:* 1.1 L/kg *Protein binding:* negligible *Primary route of elimination:* Renal	Not established	Convulsion, dizziness, headache, nasopharyngitis, somnolence, weight gain	Vision loss and blindness
Zonisamide (Zonegran, generic)	Modulate sodium and calcium channels	*Loading dose:* Not recommended due to excessive adverse effects *Maintenance dose:* 100–600 mg/day; start at 100 mg/day and titrated upward as indicated by response	*Half-life:* Approximately 63 hours *Apparent volume of distribution:* 1.45 L/kg *Protein binding:* 40% *Primary elimination route:* Hepatic	Not established	Dizziness, somnolence	Metabolic acidosis, oligohidrosis, paresthesia, renal calculi

GABA, γ-aminobutyric acid.

Nordli DR, DeVivo DC. The ketogenic diet. In: Wyllie E, ed. The Treatment of Epilepsy. 4th ed. Philadelphia, PA: Lippincott Williams & Wilkins; 2006.

Schmidt D, Loscher W. Uncontrolled epilepsy following discontinuation of antiepileptic drugs in seizure-free patients: A review of current clinical experience. Acta Neurol Scand. 2005;111(5):291–300.

Bailer M. The pharmacokinetics and interactions of new antiepileptic drugs: An overview. Ther Drug Monit. 2005;27(6):722–726.

Patient Encounter 2: Managing Chronic Adverse Reactions

A 41-year-old woman with complex partial seizures has been treated with phenytoin 400 mg/day for 20 years. Her seizures are well controlled on this regimen, and she works as a pharmaceutical sales representative. She expresses concern about taking the phenytoin for so long.

What chronic adverse effects are important to monitor in this patient?

How should monitoring for these adverse effects be done?

What measures can be taken to prevent these adverse effects?

▸ Practical Issues

Comorbid Disease States Patients with epilepsy often have comorbid disease states. Care must be taken when treating comorbid conditions, as numerous drugs can interact with AED. These interactions necessitate close monitoring for changes in efficacy or increased toxicity, and dosage changes of other drugs may be necessary when an AED is added or removed. Patients with headaches need special attention in the selection of an AED. Agents known to prevent headache (eg, valproate and topiramate) may be preferred, and agents associated with increased headaches (eg, lamotrigine and felbamate) may be secondary or tertiary alternatives.

Depression is common in patients with epilepsy. Approximately 30% have symptoms of major depression at some point.[34] Patients with epilepsy should be routinely assessed for signs of depression, and treatment initiated if necessary. Most AEDs can exacerbate depression, and patients should be warned to watch for mood changes. Some AEDs (eg, lamotrigine, carbamazepine, oxcarbazepine) may be useful in treating depression. If treatment for depression is necessary, an agent that is unlikely to increase seizures and does not interact with AEDs should be chosen. However, treatment with an appropriate antidepressant should not be withheld because of a small risk of increasing seizure frequency.

Switching Drugs Changing from one AED to another can be a complex process. If the first drug is stopped too abruptly, breakthrough seizures may occur. KEY CONCEPT *Changes in AED regimens should be done in a stepwise fashion, keeping in mind drug interactions that may be present and may necessitate dosage changes in concomitant drugs.* Typically the new drug is started at a low initial dose and gradually increased over several weeks. Once the new drug is at a minimally effective dose, the drug to be discontinued is gradually tapered while the dose of the new drug continues to be increased to the target dose. During a transition between drugs, patients should be cautioned about the possibility of increased seizures or adverse reactions.

Stopping Therapy Epilepsy is generally considered to be a lifelong disorder requiring ongoing treatment. However, some patients who are seizure free may desire to discontinue their medications.[35] Patients who become seizure free following surgery for epilepsy may have medications slowly tapered starting 2 years after surgery. Many patients will choose to stay on at least one medication, following successful surgery, to ensure they remain seizure free. KEY CONCEPT *Discontinuation of AEDs should be done gradually, only after the patient has been seizure free for 2 to 5 years and with careful consideration of factors predictive of seizure recurrence.*[36] They are:

- No seizures for 2 to 5 years
- Normal neurologic examination
- Normal intelligence quotient
- Single type of partial or generalized seizure
- Normal EEG with treatment

Individuals who fulfill all of these criteria have a 61% chance of remaining seizure free after AEDs are discontinued. Additionally, there is a direct relationship between the duration of seizure freedom with medications and the chance of remaining seizure free after medications are withdrawn. Withdrawal of AEDs is done slowly, usually with a tapering dose over at least 1 to 3 months.

▸ Dosing

Dosing of AEDs is determined by general guidelines and response of the patient. Serum concentrations may be helpful in benchmarking a specific response. Therapeutic ranges that are often quoted are broad guidelines for dosing, but should never replace careful evaluation of the patient's response.

▸ Drug Interactions

AEDs are associated with many different drug interactions.[37–39] Most interactions occur due to alterations in absorption, metabolism, and protein binding. Tube feedings and antacids are known to reduce the absorption of phenytoin and carbamazepine. Phenytoin, carbamazepine, and phenobarbital are potent inducers of various CYP450 isoenzymes, increasing the clearance of other drugs metabolized through these pathways (Table 31–4). In contrast, valproate is a CYP450 and UDP-glucuronosyltransferase (UGT) isoenzyme inhibitor and reduces the clearance of some drugs. Phenytoin and valproate are highly protein bound and can be displaced when taken together or with other highly protein-bound drugs. For example, when phenytoin and valproate are taken together, there may be increased dose-related adverse effects within several hours of dosing. This can be avoided by staggering doses or giving smaller doses more frequently during the day. Whenever a change in a medication regimen occurs, drug interactions should be considered and appropriate adjustments in dose of AEDs made.

▸ Special Populations

KEY CONCEPT *Children and women with epilepsy have unique problems related to the use of AEDs.* In children, developmental changes occur rapidly, and metabolic rates are greater than those seen in adults. When treating a child, it is imperative to control seizures as quickly as possible to avoid interference with development of the brain and cognition. AED doses are increased rapidly, and frequent changes in the regimen are made to maximize seizure control. Due to rapid metabolic rates seen in children, doses of AEDs are typically higher on a milligram per kilogram basis compared with adults, and serum concentrations are used more extensively to help ensure an adequate trial of a drug has been given.

For women, the treatment of epilepsy poses challenges, including teratogenicity, breastfeeding, interactions between AEDs and hormonal contraceptives, and reduced fertility.[40,41] Recommendations are developed for managing women of childbearing potential and who are pregnant (Table 31–5). Several AEDs

Table 31–4

Cytochrome P450 and AED Interactions

Enzyme	Substrate	Common Inducers	Common Inhibitors
CYP 1A2	Carbamazepine	Carbamazepine Phenytoin Phenobarbital Rifampin	Cimetidine Ciprofloxacin Erythromycin Clarithromycin
CYP 2C9	Phenobarbital[a] Phenytoin[a] Carbamazepine Valproate	Carbamazepine Phenytoin Phenobarbital Rifampin	Amiodarone Cimetidine Fluconazole Valproate
CYP 2C19	Phenobarbital Phenytoin Valproate Lacosamide		Felbamate Ticlopidine Topiramate Zonisamide
CYP 2D6	Zonisamide	Carbamazepine	
CYP 3A4	Carbamazepine[a] Tiagabine[a] Zonisamide[a]	Carbamazepine Phenytoin Phenobarbital Rifampin	Amiodarone Erythromycin Ketoconazole
Uridine diphosphate glucuronyl-transferase	Lamotrigine[a] Carbamazepine Valproate	Lamotrigine Phenobarbital Phenytoin Hormonal contraceptives	Valproate

[a]Primary route of metabolism.

Perucea E. Clinically relevant drug interactions with antiepileptic drugs. Br J Clin Pharmacol. 2006;61(3):246–255.

Bailer M. The pharmacokinetics and interactions of new antiepileptic drugs: An overview. Ther Drug Monit. 2005;27(6):722–726.

Anderson GD. Pharmacogenetic and enzyme induction/inhibition properties of antiepileptic drugs. Neurology. 2004;63(10 Suppl 4):53–58.

are implicated in causing birth defects.[42] Neural tube defects (eg, spina bifida, microcephaly, anencephaly) are associated most commonly with valproate and possibly carbamazepine. Additionally, valproate is associated with impaired cognitive development in children born to women taking valproate during pregnancy. It is best to avoid the use of valproate, if possible, in women of childbearing potential. All women of childbearing potential who take AEDs should take 1 to 4 mg daily of supplemental folic acid to reduce the risk of birth defects. Many AEDs are excreted in breast milk. However, infants were exposed to higher concentrations of AED in utero, so it is unclear if drugs in breast milk are harmful to the child. Decisions about breastfeeding are made on an individual basis.

Many AEDs induce hepatic microsomal enzyme systems and reduce the effectiveness of hormonal contraceptives. Women taking AEDs that may reduce the effectiveness of hormonal contraceptives should also use other forms of birth control. In contrast to these interactions, hormonal contraceptives induce glucuronidation of lamotrigine and valproate, and cause reductions in serum concentrations of these drugs during days of the cycle when hormones are taken; serum concentrations increase during days when hormones are not taken. Serum concentrations

Patient Encounter 3: Birth Control

A 21-year-old woman comes to clinic to discuss birth control. She is currently taking oxcarbazepine 1200 mg/day for complex partial seizures. Her seizures are well controlled, except for two seizures in the last year when she missed doses due to not getting refills on time. Otherwise she is in good health.

What advice should be given regarding birth control?

What impact will oxcarbazepine have on hormonal contraceptives?

What AEDs should generally be avoided in women of childbearing potential?

What additional medications or supplements should be considered?

Table 31–5

Management of AEDs During Pregnancy

Give supplemental folic acid 1–4 mg daily to all women of childbearing potential
Use monotherapy whenever possible
Use lowest doses that control seizures
Continue pharmacotherapy that best controls seizures prior to pregnancy
Monitor AED serum concentrations at start of pregnancy and monthly thereafter
Adjust AED doses to maintain baseline serum concentrations
Administer supplemental vitamin K during eighth month of pregnancy to women receiving enzyme-inducing AEDs
Monitor postpartum AED serum concentrations to guide adjustments of drug doses

Patient Encounter 4: Seizures in Older Adults

An 80-year-old man has experienced spells where he is briefly unresponsive and has slight movements of his right hand. He has no recollection of these episodes. He has a history of atrial fibrillation and hypertension. His MRI and EEG are reported to be normal.

Should pharmacotherapy be started in this patient?

If pharmacotherapy is started, what AED is preferable?

How should efficacy and toxicity be monitored in this patient?

of many AEDs, drop during pregnancy, and dose increases based on frequent serum concentration monitoring is necessary. Due to induction or inhibition of sex hormone metabolism and changes in binding of hormones to sex hormone binding globulin, some AEDs reduce fertility. Valproate has been associated with a drug-induced polycystic ovarian syndrome. Women who experience difficulties with fertility should seek the advice of health care professionals with expertise in fertility.

KEY CONCEPT *Older adults have the highest incidence of newly diagnosed epilepsy and face unique challenges in treatment.* The highest incidence of seizures and epilepsy is in individuals older than 65 years. Cerebrovascular disease, tumors, trauma, and neurodegenerative diseases are the primary causes of epilepsy in this age group. Diagnosis of epilepsy in older adults is difficult. This is due to the subtle symptoms of seizures, often compromised memory in the elderly, and the fact that many elderly live alone. Carbamazepine, lamotrigine, and gabapentin have been studied in older adults, and all are effective in controlling seizures.[43–45] Fewer adverse events occur with lamotrigine and gabapentin. Elderly patients are more sensitive to adverse events, so smaller doses tend to be used in this age group.

OUTCOME EVALUATION

KEY CONCEPT *Patients receiving AEDs for seizures should have regular monitoring for seizure frequency, seizure patterns, acute adverse effects, chronic adverse effects, comorbid conditions, and possible drug interactions.*

Efficacy

- Seizure counts are the standard way to evaluate the efficacy of treatment.
- Encourage patients to keep a seizure calendar that notes the time and day a seizure occurs and the type of seizure. Compare seizure counts on a monthly basis to determine the level of seizure control.

Toxicity

- Monitor acute toxicity of AEDs at every clinic visit.
- Question patients about common adverse effects of the AEDs they are receiving. Weigh the impact of acute adverse effects against the extent of seizure control. If it is determined, the adverse effects negatively impact the patient more than the extent of seizure control benefits the patient, adjust the therapeutic regimen. Continuously monitor chronic adverse effects of AEDs.

Comorbid Conditions

Routinely evaluate patients for signs and symptoms of depression.

Patient Care Process

Patient Assessment:

- Based on the description of a patient's spells, neurological examination, laboratory testing, EEG findings, and MRI, determine if the patient actually has seizures and is at risk for future seizures.
- Review the patient's medical history. For women, determine the potential for pregnancy.
- Take a medication history, including prescription medication, over-the-counter medication, and herbal supplement use.
- Identify allergies.
- Determine frequency of seizures.

Therapy Evaluation:

- Is the patient receiving medications that could cause seizures?
- Is the patient receiving treatment for seizures?
- Identify potential drug interactions between medications the patient may be currently taking and possible AEDs to be started.
- Identify lifestyle factors that will impact choice of AEDs.
- Determine insurance coverage for AEDs.

Care Plan Development:

- Determine the desired seizure outcomes for the patient.
- Select an AED taking into account seizure type, potential drug interactions, adverse effects of AEDs, and lifestyle factors.
- Design a dose titration plan that minimizes the risk for adverse effects.
- Educate the patient and caregivers on epilepsy, safety factors, including driving regulations, importance of adherence, dose titration schedule, and appropriate use of medications.
- For women of childbearing potential discuss interactions with hormonal contraception, risk of birth defects, and use of supplemental folic acid.
- Provide a seizure diary for recording the frequency and types of seizure events.

Follow-Up Evaluation:

- Schedule the patient to return to clinic every 2 to 4 months until stable, then schedule clinic visits every 6 to 12 months.
- Evaluate the seizure diary for changes in seizure frequency or types of seizure events.
- Identify idiosyncratic adverse effects in patients initiating a new AED.
- Identify dose-related adverse effects. Also identify psychological adverse effects, such as depression or anxiety.
- Monitor bone density at baseline and every 2 years for patients receiving phenobarbital, phenytoin, carbamazepine, oxcarbazepine, and valproate.
- Check AED serum concentrations, especially in children, pregnant women, and women immediately postpartum.
- Adjust medication doses for newly identified drug interactions.

Abbreviations Introduced in This Chapter

AAN	American Academy of Neurology
AED	Antiepileptic drug
CNS	Central Nervous System
EEG	Electroencephalograph
GABA	γ-aminobutyric acid
ILAE	International League Against Epilepsy
JME	Juvenile myoclonic epilepsy
LFTs	Liver function tests
LGS	Lennox-Gastaut syndrome
MRI	Magnetic resonance imaging
MTLE	Mesial temporal lobe epilepsy
NICE	National Institute for Clinical Excellence in the United Kingdom
PDS	Paroxysmal depolarizing shift
SIGN	Scottish Intercollegiate Guidelines Network

REFERENCES

1. Hauser WA, Kurland LT. The epidemiology of epilepsy in Rochester, Minnesota, 1935 through 1967. Epilepsia. 1975;16: 143–161.
2. Annegers JF, Hauswer WA, Eleveback LR. Remission of seizures and relapse in patients with epilepsy. Epilepsia. 1979;20:729–737.
3. Shamansky SL, Glaser GH. Socioeconomic characteristics of childhood seizure disorders in the New Haven area: An epidemiologic study. Epilepsia. 1979;20:457–474.
4. Jallon P, Samdja D, Cabre P, et al. Epileptic seizures epilepsy and risk factors: Experiences with an investigation in Martinique. Epimart Group. Rev Neurol (Paris). 1998;154:408–411.
5. Epilepsy Foundation. Driver information by state [Internet], [cited 2011 Oct 10]. http://www.epilepsyfoundation.org/living/wellness/transportation/drivinglaws.etm.
6. Elger CE, Helmstaedter C, Kurthen M. Chronic epilepsy and cognition. Lancet Neurol. 2004;3(11):663–672.
7. Epilepsy Foundation. Education [Internet], [cited 2011 Oct 10]. http://www.epilepsyfoundation.org/answerplace/Social/education/.
8. Jallon P, Loiseau P, Loiseau J. Newly diagnosed unprovoked epileptic seizures: Presentation at diagnosis in the CAROLE study. Epilepsia. 2001;42:464–475.
9. Najm I, Möddel G, Janigro D. Mechanisms of epileptogenesis and experimental models of seizures. In: Wyllie E, ed. The Treatment of Epilepsy. 4th ed. Philadelphia, PA: Lippincott Williams & Wilkins; 2006.
10. Jones SW. Basic cellular neurophysiology. In: Wyllie E, ed. The Treatment of Epilepsy. 4th ed. Philadelphia, PA: Lippincott Williams & Wilkins; 2006.
11. Czapinski P, Blaszczyk B, Czuczwar SJ. Mechanisms of action of antiepileptic drugs. Curr Top Med Chem. 2005;5(1):3–14.
12. Abrous DN, Koehl M, Le Moal M. Adult neurogenesis: From precursors to network and physiology. Physiology. 2005;85(2): 523–569.
13. Gaitatzis A, Sander JW. The mortality of epilepsy revisited. Epileptic Disord. 2004;6:3–13.
14. Panayiotopoulos CP. Idiopathic generalized epilepsies: A review and modern approach. Epilepsia. 2005;46(Suppl 9):1–6.
15. Wong M. Advances in the pathophysiology of developmental epilepsies. Semin Pediatr Neurol. 2005;12:72–87.
16. Commission on Classification and Terminology of the International League Against Epilepsy. Proposal for revised clinical and electroencephalographic classification of epileptic seizures. Epilepsia. 1981;22:489–501.
17. Commission on Classification and Terminology of the International League Against Epilepsy. Proposal for revised classification of epilepsies and epileptic syndromes. Epilepsia. 1989;30:389–399.
18. Fisher RS, van Emde Boas W, Blume W, et al. Epileptic seizures and epilepsy: Definitions proposed by the International League Against Epilepsy (ILAE) and the International Bureau for Epilepsy (IBE). Epilepsia. 2005;46(4):470–472.
19. Engel J Jr. A proposed diagnostic scheme for people with epileptic seizures and with epilepsy: Report of the ILAE Task Force on Classification and Terminology. Epilepsia. 2001;42: 796–803.
20. Smith SJ. EEG in the diagnosis, classification, and management of patients with epilepsy. J Neurol Neurosurg Psychiatry. 2005;76(Suppl 2):ii2–ii7.
21. Hauser WA, Rich SS, Annegers JF, et al. Seizure recurrence after a first unprovoked seizure: An extended follow-up. Neurology. 1990;40:1163–1170.
22. Lachhwani DK, Wyllie E. Outcome and complications of epilepsy surgery. In: Wyllie E, ed. The Treatment of Epilepsy. 4th ed. Philadelphia, PA: Lippincott Williams & Wilkins; 2006.
23. National Institute of Neurological Disorders and Stroke. Surgical treatment of epilepsy. Proceedings of a Consensus Conference. March 19–21, 1990. Epilepsy Res. 1992;5(Suppl):1–250.
24. Wheless JW. Vagus nerve stimulation therapy. In: Wyllie E, ed. The Treatment of Epilepsy. 4th ed. Philadelphia, PA: Lippincott Williams & Wilkins; 2006.
25. Nordli DR, DeVivo DC. The ketogenic diet. In: Wyllie E, ed. The Treatment of Epilepsy. 4th ed. Philadelphia, PA: Lippincott Williams & Wilkins; 2006.
26. Perruca E. An introduction to antiepileptic drugs. Epilepsia. 2005;46(Suppl 4):31–37.
27. Privitera MD. Clinical rules for phenytoin dosing. Ann Pharmacother. 1993;27(10):1169–1173.
28. Scottish Intercollegiate Guidelines Network. Diagnosis and management of epilepsy in adults [Internet], [cited 2011 Oct 10]. http://www.sign.ac.uk/pdf/sign70.pdf.
29. National Institute for Clinical Excellence. The epilepsies: The diagnosis and management of the epilepsies in children and adults in primary and secondary care [Internet], [cited 2014 Sep 15]. http://http://www.nice.org.uk/guidance/CG137/chapter/Introduction.
30. French JA, Kanner AM, Bautista J, et al. Efficacy and tolerability of the new antiepileptic drugs I: Treatment of new onset epilepsy report of the Therapeutics and Technology Assessment Subcommittee and Quality Standards Subcommittee of the American Academy of Neurology and the American Epilepsy Society. Neurology. 2005;62:1252–1260.
31. French JA, Kanner AM, Bautista J, et.al. Efficacy and tolerability of the new antiepileptic drugs II: Treatment of refractory epilepsy report of the Therapeutics and Technology Assessment Subcommittee and Quality Standards Subcommittee of the American Academy of Neurology and the American Epilepsy Society. Neurology. 2005;62:1261–1273.
32. Vestergaard P. Epilepsy, osteoporosis and fracture risk—A meta-analysis. Acta Neurol Scand. 2005;112:227–286.
33. Koppel BS, Harden CL, Nikolov BG, Labar DR. An analysis of lifetime fractures in women with epilepsy. Acta Neurol Scand. 2005;111(4):225–228.
34. Harden CL, Goldstein MA. Mood disorders in patients with epilepsy: Epidemiology and management. CNS Drugs. 2002;16:291–302.
35. Schmidt D, Loscher W. Uncontrolled epilepsy following discontinuation of antiepileptic drugs in seizure-free patients: A review of current clinical experience. Acta Neurol Scand. 2005;111(5):291–300.
36. Tsur VG, O'Dell C, Shinnar S. Initiation and discontinuation of antiepileptic drugs. In: Wyllie E, ed. The Treatment of Epilepsy. 4th ed. Philadelphia, PA: Lippincott Williams & Wilkins; 2006.
37. Perucea E. Clinically relevant drug interactions with antiepileptic drugs. Br J Clin Pharmacol. 2006;61(3):246–255.

38. Bailer M. The pharmacokinetics and interactions of new antiepileptic drugs: An overview. Ther Drug Monit. 2005;27(6): 722–726.
39. Anderson GD. Pharmacogenetic and enzyme induction/inhibition properties of antiepileptic drugs. Neurology. 2004;63(10 Suppl 4): 53–58.
40. Crawford P. Best practice guidelines for the management of women with epilepsy. Epilepsia. 2005;46(Suppl 9):117–124.
41. Foldvary-Schaefer N, Morrel MJ. Epilepsy in women: The biological basis for the female experience. Cleve Clin J Med. 2004;71(Suppl 2): S1–S8.
42. Artama M, Auvinen A, Raudaskoski T, et al. Antiepileptic drug use of women with epilepsy and congenital malformations in offspring. Neurology. 2005;64(11):1874–1878.
43. Brodie MJ. Overstall, PW, Giorgi L. Multicentre, double-blind, randomized, comparison between lamotrigine and carbamazepine in elderly patients with newly diagnosed epilepsy. Epilepsy Res. 1999;37:81–87.
44. Rowan AJ, Ramsay RE, Collins JF, et.al. New onset geriatric epilepsy, a randomized study of gabapentin, lamotrigine, and carbamazepine. Neurology. 2005;64:1868–1873.
45. Saetre E, Peruccad, E, Isojärvi J, et.al. An international multicenter randomized double-blind controlled trial of lamotrigine and sustained-release carbamazepine in the treatment of newly diagnosed epilepsy in the elderly. Epilepsia. 2007;48:1292–1302.

32 Status Epilepticus

Eljim P. Tesoro and Gretchen M. Brophy

LEARNING OBJECTIVES

Upon completion of the chapter, the reader will be able to:

1. Describe the pathophysiology of status epilepticus.
2. Explain the urgency of diagnosis and treatment of status epilepticus.
3. Recognize the signs and symptoms of status epilepticus.
4. Identify the treatment goals for a patient in status epilepticus.
5. Formulate an initial treatment strategy for a patient in generalized convulsive status epilepticus.
6. Compare the pharmacotherapeutic options for refractory status epilepticus.
7. Describe adverse drug events associated with the pharmacotherapy of status epilepticus.
8. Recommend monitoring parameters for a patient in status epilepticus.

INTRODUCTION

KEY CONCEPT *Status epilepticus (SE) is a neurologic emergency that can lead to permanent brain damage or death.* KEY CONCEPT *SE is defined as continuous seizure activity lasting more than 5 minutes or two or more seizures without complete recovery of consciousness.*[1] Refractory status epilepticus (RSE) is unresponsive to emergent (first-line) or urgent (second-line) therapy.

SE can present as nonconvulsive status epilepticus (NCSE) or generalized convulsive status epilepticus (GCSE). NCSE is characterized by persistent impaired consciousness without clinical seizure activity and is diagnosed with **electroencephalography** (EEG). GCSE is characterized by full-body motor seizures and involves the entire brain.

EPIDEMIOLOGY AND ETIOLOGY

The incidence of SE in the United States is 12.5/100,000/year, with an in-hospital mortality rate of 9.2%,[2] and an estimated annual direct cost for inpatient admissions of $4 billion.[3] It occurs most frequently in males, African Americans, children, and the elderly.

KEY CONCEPT *It is important to evaluate etiologies of SE for timely and optimal seizure control.* Causes of SE include metabolic disturbances (eg, hyponatremia, hypernatremia, hyperkalemia, hypocalcemia, hypomagnesemia, hypoglycemia); central nervous system (CNS) disorders, infections, injuries; **hypoxia**; drug toxicity (eg, theophylline, isoniazid, cyclosporine, cocaine). Chronic causes of SE include preexisting **epilepsy**, chronic alcoholism (withdrawal seizures), CNS tumors, and strokes.[4] In epileptics, the common causes of SE are anticonvulsant withdrawal or subtherapeutic levels.

PATHOPHYSIOLOGY

Status epilepticus occurs when the brain fails to stop isolated seizures, due to a mismatch of neurotransmitters. **Glutamate**, the primary excitatory neurotransmitter, stimulates postsynaptic *N*-methyl-D-aspartate (NMDA) receptors, causing neuronal depolarization. Sustained depolarization causes neuronal injury and death.[5] The primary inhibitory neurotransmitter, **γ-aminobutyric** acid (GABA), opposes excitation by stimulating $GABA_A$ receptors, producing hyperpolarization and inhibition of the postsynaptic cell membrane. GABA-mediated inhibition diminishes with continuous seizure activity, causing a decreased response to GABA-receptor agonists.[6] Seizures lasting more than 30 minutes cause significant injury and neuronal loss because of excessive electrical activity and cerebral metabolic demand. Decreased $GABA_A$-receptor response and increasing neuronal injury with prolongation of seizure activity necessitates rapid control of SE.

Systemic changes appear in two phases during SE. Phase I occurs during the first 30 minutes, and phase II occurs after 30 to 60 minutes.[7]

Phase I

During phase I, autonomic activity increases, resulting in hypertension, tachycardia, hyperglycemia, hyperthermia, sweating, and salivation. Cerebral blood flow increases to preserve oxygen supply to the brain. Increases in sympathetic and parasympathetic stimulation with muscle hypoxia can cause ventricular arrhythmias, severe acidosis, and rhabdomyolysis which can lead to hypotension, shock, hyperkalemia, and acute kidney injury.

Patient Encounter 1, Part 1

A 79-year-old woman with a history of hypertension, diabetes, and arthritis was admitted with traumatic subdural hematoma after sustaining a fall down a flight of stairs in her home. She underwent surgery 2 days ago to evacuate the hematoma and is currently recovering in the ICU. She was started on fosphenytoin for seizure prophylaxis upon admission along with her home medications. She has only one peripheral IV line and has very poor vascular access. Her nurse reports that a few minutes ago she was alert and awake, but now she is unarousable and is having jerky, convulsive movements on both sides of her body. The doctor evaluates her and the jerky activity stops, but then starts again about 1 minute later. She never regained consciousness between these episodes. Her diagnosis is status epilepticus. Ht 165 cm (5′5″), Wt 133 kg (293 lbs).

What initial assessments should be performed?

What are some possible etiologies for her seizure?

What nonpharmacologic interventions need to be performed at this time?

Phase II

After 30 to 60 minutes of continuous seizure activity, loss of cerebral autoregulation, decreased cerebral blood flow, increased intracranial pressure, and systemic hypotension occur. Cerebral metabolic demand remains high; however, the body is unable to compensate, resulting in hypoglycemia, hyperthermia, respiratory failure, hypoxia, respiratory and metabolic acidosis, hyperkalemia, hyponatremia, and uremia. Motor activity may not be clinically evident during prolonged seizures, but electrical activity may still exist (ie, NCSE) requiring prompt recognition and aggressive treatment.

CLINICAL PRESENTATION AND DIAGNOSIS

History

KEY CONCEPT *When a patient presents with seizures, a thorough history is needed to determine the type and duration of previous seizure activity. This will help guide therapy and clarify necessary laboratory and diagnostic tests.* A diagnosis of SE can be made when a patient with a history of repeated seizures and impaired consciousness has a seizure witnessed by a health care professional. However, emergent treatment should not be delayed if seizure activity is suspected based on reports from the patient's family or emergency response personnel.

Physical Examination

Once seizures are controlled, a neurologic exam should evaluate the level of consciousness (coma, lethargy, or somnolence), motor function and reflexes (rhythmic contractions, rigidity, spasms, or posturing), and pupillary response. A physical exam can identify secondary injuries.

Clinical Symptoms

Patients with SE usually present with generalized, convulsive, tonic-clonic seizures. They may also be hypertensive, tachycardic, febrile, and diaphoretic which resolve after seizure termination. A loss of bowel or bladder function, respiratory compromise, and nystagmus may also be observed. When seizure activity exceeds 30 to 60 minutes, muscle contractions may no longer be visible, necessitating an EEG to diagnosis SE. Twitching of the face, hands, or feet may be seen in these comatose patients with prolonged seizures.

Clinical Presentation of Status Epilepticus

General

The patient may present with or without clinically noticeable seizure activity.

Symptoms

- Impaired consciousness ranging from lethargy to coma
- Disorientation after cessation of GCSE
- Pain from associated injuries (eg, tongue lacerations, dislocated shoulder, head trauma, facial trauma)

Signs

Phase I:	Phase II (greater than 30 minutes of SE):
Generalized convulsions	Respiratory failure with pulmonary edema
Hypertension, tachycardia	Cardiac failure (arrhythmias, shock)
Fever and sweating	Hypotension
Muscle contractions, spasms	Hyperthermia
Respiratory compromise	Rhabdomyolysis and multiorgan failure
Incontinence	

Laboratory Tests

- Hyperglycemia (phase I) and hypoglycemia (phase II) can occur
- Hyponatremia, hypernatremia, hyperkalemia, hypocalcemia, hypomagnesemia, and hypoglycemia can cause SE
- The white blood cell (WBC) count may slightly increase
- Abnormal arterial blood gases (ABGs) due to hypoxia and respiratory or metabolic acidosis
- Elevated serum creatinine will be present in renal failure patients
- Myoglobinuria can occur in patients with continuous seizures

Diagnostic Tests

EEG to confirm seizure activity

CT or MRI may reveal mass lesions or hemorrhage

Laboratory Parameters

KEY CONCEPT *It is important to obtain a serum chemistry profile to help identify possible causes of SE, such as* hypoglycemia, hyponatremia or hypernatremia, hypomagnesemia, and hypocalcemia; patients with renal and liver failure are at high risk as well. In febrile patients with elevated white blood count (WBC) counts, active infections should be considered and treated appropriately. Cultures from the blood, cerebrospinal fluid (CSF), respiratory tract, and urine should be collected once seizures are controlled. Computed tomography (CT) or magnetic resonance imaging (MRI) can rule out CNS abscesses, bleeding, or tumors, all of which may be a source of seizures. Order a blood alcohol level and urine toxicology screen to determine if SE is caused by alcohol withdrawal, illicit drug use, or a drug overdose. Serum drug levels should be obtained in an overdose situation to rule out toxicity. KEY CONCEPT *Knowing the cause of SE will guide initial antiepileptic therapy and increase the probability of seizure termination.*

In patients taking antiepileptic drugs (AEDs), a baseline serum concentration is useful to determine if the concentration is below the desired range and whether a loading dose (LD) is needed. Albumin levels, renal and liver function tests should also be utilized to assess therapy.

Hypoxia and respiratory or metabolic acidosis are common in patients with SE. Pulse oximetry and arterial blood gas (ABG) measurements are used to assess pulmonary status and determine if airway protection or supplemental oxygen is needed. Metabolic acidosis may resolve on its own without treatment after termination of clinical seizure activity.

Diagnostic Tests

EEG is required to identify SE in a comatose patient. Continuous EEG monitoring should be used in patients who remain unconscious after initial antiepileptic treatment, those receiving long-acting paralytic agents, or those requiring prolonged RSE therapy. Treatment should not be delayed while awaiting EEG results. CT and MRI scans are useful to identify traumatic injury, mass lesions, or evidence of infection as the cause of SE.

TREATMENT

Desired Outcomes

KEY CONCEPT *The goal of therapy is to terminate physical and electroencephalographic evidence of seizures, prevent recurrence, and minimize adverse drug events.* Poor outcomes are associated with prolonged SE and refractory SE.[8] Complications of SE should also be treated.

General Approach

The initial approach to SE involves removing the patient from harmful surroundings and ensuring maintenance of airway, breathing, and circulation. Benzodiazepines are the preferred initial drugs to stop acute seizure activity (emergent therapy), followed by an AED (urgent therapy) for suppression of seizures. Medications are given intravenously (IV) for immediate onset of action, but if IV access is not available, select medications may be given rectally, intramuscularly (IM), buccally, or nasally. After seizures stop, clinicians must identify and treat underlying causes of the seizures, such as toxins, hypoglycemia, or brain injury. Patients with known seizure disorders should be evaluated for abrupt cessation of their medications, noncompliance, or drug interactions. Recent guidelines provide treatment algorithms for SE.[1,9]

Nonpharmacologic Treatment

Oxygen administration or intubation for mechanical ventilation should be performed in cases of hypoxia, and temperature management should be considered for febrile seizures. Specialists in neurology or epileptology should be consulted as appropriate. Admission to an intensive care unit (ICU) allows for aggressive treatment and monitoring.

Pharmacologic Treatment

▶ *Initial Treatment*

Hypoglycemia-induced SE is treated with IV dextrose. IV thiamine is given to alcoholics prior to administering any dextrose-containing solutions to prevent encephalopathy.

Patient Encounter 1, Part 2

Physical examination and a review of her chart and recent laboratory studies reveal the following additional information about this patient:

PE:

VS: BP 178/92 mm Hg, pulse 109 beats/min, RR 26 breaths/min, T 39.0°C (102.2°F)

CNS: Unresponsive, unarousable

CV: Sinus tachycardia; normal S1, S2; no murmurs, rubs, gallops

Pulm: Tachypneic; oxygen saturation 88% (0.88) on room air; no rhonchi, wheezes, rales

Abd: Deferred

Exts: Rhythmic tonic-clonic movements of all extremities

GU: Incontinent of urine and stool

HEENT: Persistent upward gaze

Current Meds: Fosphenytoin 100 mg PE IV every 8 hours; famotidine 20 mg IV every 12 hours; metoprolol 50 mg by mouth every 12 hours; insulin glargine 25 units subcutaneous at bedtime; insulin aspart 5 units subcutaneous with meals; acetaminophen/hydrocodone 325 mg/5 mg tablet by mouth every 4 hours as needed for pain; morphine 2 mg IVP every 2 hours as needed for pain

Labs: Sodium 132 mEq/L (132 mmol/L); potassium 4.1 mEq/L (4.1 mmol/L); phenytoin 2.7 mcg/mL (11 μmol/L); albumin 3.5 g/dL (35 g/L); chloride 105 mEq/L (105 mmol/L); carbon dioxide 12 mEq/L (12 mmol/L); blood urea nitrogen 10 mg/dL (3.6 mmol/L); serum creatinine 0.9 mg/dL (80 μmol/L); glucose 54 mg/dL (3.0 mmol/L); WBC 15 × 10^3/mm^3 (15 × 10^9/L); hemoglobin 9.6 g/dL (96 g/L or 5.96 mmol/L); hematocrit 28% (0.28 volume fraction); platelets 235 × 10^3/mm^3 (235 × 10^9/L); prothrombin time 12 seconds; international normalized ratio 1.1; activated partial thromboplastin time 28 seconds

What is your assessment of the cause of this patient's condition?

What pharmacologic interventions need to be performed at this time?

Identify your goals of therapy for this patient.

What therapies must be instituted next?

▶ *Benzodiazepines*

KEY CONCEPT *Initial or emergent drug therapy begins with IV administration of a benzodiazepine. This class of agents is highly effective in terminating seizures.*[10,11] *Intravenous bolus doses of diazepam, lorazepam, and midazolam have been used in SE because of their rapid effects on GABA receptors. Lorazepam is the preferred agent of most clinicians.* When treating patients on chronic benzodiazepine therapy, consider using higher doses to overcome tolerance. Diazepam and lorazepam should be diluted 1:1 with normal saline before parenteral administration via peripheral veins to avoid vascular irritation from the propylene glycol diluent.

Diazepam Being extremely lipophilic, diazepam penetrates the CNS quickly, but rapidly redistributes into body fat and muscle.

This results in a rapid decline in CNS levels and early recurrence of seizures. Doses can be given every 5 minutes until seizure activity stops or toxicities are seen (eg, respiratory depression). Diazepam can be administered as a rectal gel enabling non-medical personnel to provide timely therapy at home or in public areas.[12] IM administration of diazepam is not recommended because of erratic absorption.

Lorazepam Less lipophilic than diazepam, lorazepam has a longer redistribution half-life, resulting in longer duration of action and decreased need for repeated doses. Both lorazepam and diazepam are effective in stopping seizures,[13] but lorazepam is currently preferred due to a longer duration of action. It can be redosed every 5 to 10 minutes (up to a maximum cumulative dose of 8 mg) until seizure activity stops or side effects such as respiratory depression occur. IM administration is not preferred due to slow and unpredictable absorption.

Midazolam Midazolam is water-soluble and can be administered intramuscularly,[14] buccally,[15,16] and nasally.[17,18] Compared to diazepam and lorazepam, it has less respiratory and cardiovascular side effects. Its short half-life requires that it be redosed frequently or administered as a continuous IV infusion. Liquid or injectable formulations can be given buccally or intranasally (0.3 mg/kg) in pediatric patients. Rapid breathing and increased secretions can interfere with nasal administration. A recent study in adults and children showed that IM midazolam was as safe and effective as IV lorazepam for prehospital termination of seizures.[18]

► *Anticonvulsants*

KEY CONCEPT *After administering the first dose of benzodiazepine, an AED such as phenytoin, valproate sodium, or phenobarbital should be started to prevent further seizures (urgent therapy).* AEDs must not be given as first-line therapy since they are infused relatively slowly to avoid adverse effects, delaying their onset of action. If the underlying cause of the seizures has been corrected (eg, hypoglycemia) and seizure activity has ceased, an AED may be unnecessary. This may be reasonable when patients become alert and oriented or if an EEG confirms absence of seizure activity.

After the AED LD is administered, maintenance doses should be initiated to ensure that therapeutic levels are sustained. Chronic and idiosyncratic side effects and potential drug interactions should be considered if the patient continues AED therapy. Drugs should be adjusted for any hepatic or renal dysfunction. Table 32–1 summarizes the doses used in SE, and Table 32–2 is an example algorithm for treatment of patients in SE.

Phenytoin The most widely used AED for urgent treatment of SE is phenytoin, which is available in its original form or as a prodrug, fosphenytoin. LDs must be modified in patients already taking phenytoin with subtherapeutic levels in order to avoid toxic serum concentrations. Doses are infused no faster than 50 mg/minute due to risks of hypotension or arrhythmias. Continuous monitoring of ECG and blood pressure is recommended. Maintenance doses can be started 12 hours after the LD. Phenytoin should not be infused with other medications because of stability concerns (it is soluble in propylene glycol and compatible only in 0.9% sodium chloride solutions). It should not be given IM due to its alkalinity. Extravasation of phenytoin can cause local tissue discoloration, edema, pain, and sometimes necrosis (purple glove syndrome). Oral loading is not recommended in SE due to the limitations of single dose absorption (ie, doses greater than 400 mg are not fully absorbed) and delayed peak concentrations when given orally. Obese patients require larger LDs due to a larger volume of distribution (V_d).[19] A dosing weight (DW) can be calculated using total body weight (TBW) and ideal body weight (IBW): DW = IBW + 1.33(TBW-IBW). V_d can be calculated as follows: V_d = 0.7 L/kg X DW (in kg). A LD can then be calculated using Vd and a target concentration: LD = C_{target} X V_d.

Fosphenytoin Fosphenytoin is a water-soluble, phosphoester prodrug that is rapidly converted to phenytoin in the body. It is compatible with most IV solutions. It is dosed in phenytoin equivalents (PE), and it can be infused up to 150 mg PE/minute. Although it has fewer cardiovascular side effects than phenytoin, clinicians should continuously monitor blood pressure, ECG, and heart rate. Maintenance doses can be started 12 hours after the LD. Paresthesias, especially around the lips and groin are common, but typically resolve within a few minutes and should not necessitate stopping the infusion. If a postload serum level is desired, it should be obtained 2 hours after an IV load.

Phenobarbital If phenytoin or fosphenytoin fails to prevent seizure recurrence, phenobarbital can be considered. However, emerging evidence suggests that phenobarbital may not be effective if SE persists despite benzodiazepines and phenytoin. This may be due to progressive resistance of the $GABA_A$ receptor, where barbiturates also act.[20] Adverse reactions of phenobarbital include sedation, hypotension, and respiratory depression; therefore, patients receiving a rapid IV LD of phenobarbital should have hemodynamic monitoring and be mechanically ventilated if at high risk of respiratory compromise. Its long half-life makes it a popular agent for both acute treatment and chronic maintenance therapy or as adjunct therapy to prevent withdrawal seizures when weaning refractory SE patients off pentobarbital infusions.

Valproate Sodium Although valproate sodium is not Food and Drug Administration (FDA)-approved for SE, it has been used IV in various types of SE including generalized tonic-clonic, myoclonic, and NCSE.[21] It is particularly useful in patients with

Patient Encounter 2, Part 1

A 19-year-old man admitted for two reported episodes of intermittent jerking in his left arm that were witnessed by his mother this morning. He is nonresponsive at the time of these episodes and does not remember anything during that period of time. He does not take any medications and has no allergies to medications. One week ago, he was seen in the emergency department as he was confused and having difficulties walking after being hit in the head with a soccer ball during a tournament. At that time, a CT scan of his head showed no hemorrhage, and he was diagnosed with having a mild traumatic brain injury. Today while the nurse is taking his vital signs, he becomes confused and then unarousable with jerky movements on the left side of his body. His diagnosis is status epilepticus after this seizure activity does not stop over the next 5 minutes.

VS: BP 111/75 mm Hg, HR 108 beats/min, RR 21 breaths/min, T 37.0°C (98.6°F), Wt 82 kg (180 lb), Ht 185 cm (6′1″)

What is the most likely cause of this patient's SE?

What possible treatment options exist at this time?

How would you optimize this patient's outcome?

Table 32–1

Medications Used in Adult Status Epilepticus

Drug Name (Brand Name)	Loading Dose and RSE Maintenance Dose (If Applicable)	Administration Rate	Therapeutic Level	Side Effects	Comments
Diazepam (Valium)	0.15 mg/kg (up to 10 mg per dose); may repeat in 5 minutes	5 mg/min (IVP)	N/A	Hypotension, respiratory depression	Rapid redistribution rate; can be given rectally
Lorazepam (Ativan)	0.1 mg/kg (up to 4 mg per dose); repeat in 5–10 minutes	2 mg/min (IVP)	N/A	Hypotension, respiratory depression	May be longer acting than diazepam
Midazolam (Versed)	0.2 mg/kg IM up to 10 mg per dose RSE: 0.2 mg/kg (2 mg/min) IV then 0.05–2 mg/kg/hour		N/A	Sedation, respiratory depression	Can also be given buccally, intranasally
Phenytoin (Dilantin)	20 mg/kg	Up to 50 mg/min	Total phenytoin level: 10–20 mcg/mL (mg/L; 40–79 μmol/L) Free phenytoin level: 1–2 mcg/mL (mg/L; 4–8 μmol/L)	Arrhythmias, hypotension,	Hypotension, especially in older adults
Fosphenytoin (Cerebyx)	20 mg PE/kg	Up to 150 mg PE/min	Total phenytoin level: 10–20 mcg/mL (mg/L; 40–79 μmol/L) Free phenytoin level: 1–2 mcg/mL (mg/L; 4–8 μmol/L)	Paresthesias, hypotension	Less CV side effects than phenytoin
Phenobarbital (Luminal)	20 mg/kg	50–100 mg/min	15–40 mcg/mL (mg/L; 65–172 μmol/L)	Hypotension, sedation, respiratory depression	Long-acting
Valproate sodium (Depacon)	20–40 mg/kg	3–6 mg/kg/min	50–150 mcg/mL (mg/L; 347–1040 μmol/L)		Less CV side effects than phenytoin
Lacosamide (Vimpat)	200–400 mg IV	Over 15 minutes		PR prolongation, hypotension	
Topiramate (Topamax)	200–400 mg NG/PO every 6 hours		2–20 mcg/mL (mg/L; 6–59 μmol/L)	Metabolic acidosis	
Propofol (Diprivan)	Bolus: 1–2 mg/kg RSE: 30–250 mcg/kg/min	Approximately 40 mg every 10 seconds	N/A (typically titrated to EEG)	Hypotension, respiratory depression, PRIS	Requires mechanical intubation; high lipid load (increased calories);
Pentobarbital (Nembutal)	Bolus: 10–15 mg/kg RSE: 0.5–4 mg/kg/hour	Up to 50 mg/min	10–20 mcg/mL (mg/L; 44–89 μmol/L) (typically titrated to EEG)	Hypotension, respiratory depression, cardiac depression, infection, ileus	Requires mechanical intubation, vasopressors, hemodynamic monitoring
Ketamine	RSE: 0.5–4.5 mg/kg IV bolus, then infusion up to 5 mg/kg/hour		N/A	Hypertension, arrhythmias	Has been associated with cerebral atrophy

CV, cardiovascular; EEG, electroencephalogram; IM, intramuscular; IVP, intravenous push; N/A, not applicable; NG, nasogastric; PE, phenytoin equivalents; PO, by mouth; PRIS, propofol-related infusion syndrome

cardiorespiratory compromise and/or those allergic to phenytoin and phenobarbital.[22]

Treatment of Refractory Status Epilepticus

KEY CONCEPT *Seizure activity unresponsive to emergent and urgent therapy is considered RSE.*[23] Refractory SE can occur in up to 30% of patients with SE and has a mortality rate approaching 50%. Patients in RSE are unlikely to regain independent function, even if seizures are controlled. Clinical signs may become subtle and an EEG may be required to detect ongoing seizure activity. KEY CONCEPT *Even SE patients without clinical signs of seizing are at risk for brain damage or even death.*

Optimal therapy for RSE is undetermined.[24] Clinicians must aggressively investigate and treat possible causes including infection, tumors, drugs or toxins, metabolic disorders, liver failure, or fever. In general, patients with RSE are managed in an ICU where hemodynamic and respiratory support and frequent monitoring are available. Continuous EEG monitoring is essential and should not be delayed. Any AEDs initiated before treatment for RSE should be continued, and their serum levels optimized to

Table 32–2

Algorithm for Treatment of Status Epilepticus in Adult

Time (minutes)	Assessment/Monitoring	Treatment
0	Vital signs (HR, RR, BP, T) Assess airway Monitor cardiac function (ECG) Pulse oximeter Check blood glucose Check laboratory tests: complete blood count, serum chemistries, liver function tests, arterial blood gas, blood cultures, serum anticonvulsant levels, urine drug/alcohol screen	Stabilize airway (intubate if necessary) Administer oxygen Secure IV access and start fluids Give IV thiamine (100 mg), then IV dextrose (50 mL of 50% solution) if hypoglycemic
0–10	Vital signs Physical exam Patient history including medications (prescription, OTC, and herbals)	Lorazepam 0.1 mg/kg (maximum 4 mg) IVP at 2 mg/min (may repeat in 5–10 minutes to maximum of 8 mg if no response) If no IV access, can give: diazepam 10 mg PR (may repeat in 10 minutes if no response); midazolam 0.2 mg/kg IM (maximum 10 mg; may repeat in 10 minutes if no response) AED may not be necessary if underlying cause is corrected and seizures have ceased
10–20	Vital signs Review laboratory results and correct any underlying abnormalities CT scan (if seizures controlled)	Phenytoin 15–20 mg/kg IV at a maximum rate of 50 mg/min (or fosphenytoin 15–20 mg PE/kg IV at a maximum rate of 150 mg PE/min) In patients allergic to phenytoin, give valproate sodium 20 mg/kg IV at a maximum rate of 6 mg/kg/min Treat for possible infection
20–30	Vital signs Consult neurologist/epileptologist Consider admission to ICU Consider EEG	If seizures continue: additional phenytoin bolus 5–10 mg/kg (or fosphenytoin 5–10 mg PE/kg) **OR** start phenobarbital at 20 mg/kg IV at a maximum rate of 100 mg/min **OR** start valproate sodium 20 mg/kg IV at a maximum rate of 6 mg/kg/min in patients who are not intubated
> 30–60 *refractory status epilepticus*	Vital signs Transfer to ICU Obtain EEG Consider MRI when controlled	Midazolam 0.2 mg/kg IV bolus followed by 0.05–2 mg/kg/hour CI **OR** propofol 1 mg/kg bolus followed by 30–250 mcg/kg/min CI **OR** pentobarbital 10–15 mg/kg bolus over 1–2 hours followed by 0.5–4 mg/kg/hour Consider intubation and/or vasopressor support if needed Optimize AED levels: repeat boluses of phenobarbital 10 mg/kg **OR** valproate sodium 20 mg/kg at 6 mg/kg/min max

BP, blood pressure; CI, continuous infusion; CT, computed tomography; ECG, electrocardiogram; EEG, electroencephalograph; HR, heart rate; ICU, intensive care unit; IV, intravenous; IVP, intravenous push; OTC, over the counter; MRI, magnetic resonance imaging; PE, phenytoin equivalents; PR, per rectum; RR, respiratory rate; T, temperature.

Patient Encounter 2, Part 2

Over the next hour, he is treated with your recommendations for emergent and urgent treatment of SE as above. His jerky movements have stopped, but he remains comatose.

VS: BP 110/72 mm Hg, HR 101 beats/min, RR 12 breaths/min, T 37.1°C (98.8°F)

A continuous EEG is started and reveals the patient is currently in SE

What is your assessment of the patient's condition at this time?

What is your recommendation for further nonpharmacologic and pharmacologic therapy?

How would you optimize his outcome?

prevent breakthrough or withdrawal seizures. KEY CONCEPT *Treatment of RSE consists of intensive monitoring, supportive care, and a continuous intravenous infusion of midazolam, propofol, or pentobarbital to suppress clinical and EEG evidence of seizures (Tables 32–1 and 32–3).*[25] These agents are typically titrated to achieve "burst suppression" on the EEG, although no strong evidence exists to support this practice. Patients should be intubated and mechanically ventilated before initiating treatment for RSE. Seizure control per EEG should be maintained for 24 to 48 hours before considering tapering therapy. Consultation with neurologists or epileptologists is highly recommended.

► *Midazolam*

Midazolam infusions must be adjusted, especially in patients with renal impairment, as the active metabolite can accumulate.[26] Breakthrough seizures are common with midazolam infusions and usually respond to boluses and a 20% increase in infusion

Table 32–3

Medications Used in Pediatric Status Epilepticus

Drug	Dose	Comments
Diazepam (Valium injection, Diastat rectal gel)	IV: 0.2–0.3 mg/kg over 2–5 minutes	Maximum dose in children < 5 years: 5 mg Maximum dose in children > 5 years: 15 mg
	PR: 2–5 years: 0.5 mg/kg 6–11 years: 0.3 mg/kg > 12 years: 0.2 mg/kg	A second rectal dose can be given 4–12 hours after the first dose if necessary
Lorazepam (Ativan)	0.05–0.1 mg/kg IV over 2–4 minutes	May redose twice in 10–15 minutes if necessary
Midazolam (Versed)	0.2 mg/kg IV bolus followed by 0.05–0.6 mg/kg/hour continuous infusion	Bolus dose may also be given intranasally, buccally, or intramuscularly
Phenytoin (Dilantin)	15–20 mg/kg IV at 1–3 mg/kg/min *max*	
Fosphenytoin (Cerebyx)	15–20 mg PE/kg IV at 3 mg PE/kg/min *max*	
Phenobarbital (Luminal)	15–20 mg/kg IV at 100 mg/min *max*	
Valproate sodium (Depacon)	15–20 mg/kg IV at 1.5–3 mg/kg/min	May have fewer cardiovascular side effects than other agents
Propofol (Diprivan)		Not recommended due to adverse events (eg, propofol-related infusion syndrome)
Pentobarbital (Nembutal)	10–15 mg/kg IV over 1–2 hours followed by continuous infusion at 1 mg/kg/hour	Titrated to EEG

PR, per rectum; EEG, electroencephalograph; IV, intravenous; PE phenytoin equivalent.

rate. Despite this, tachyphylaxis can occur, and patients should be switched to another agent if seizures continue.

▸ *Propofol*

LDs of the anesthetic propofol can be given every 3 to 5 minutes until clinical response, after which an infusion can be initiated. Propofol causes hypotension, especially with LDs; therefore, some clinicians avoid LDs and quickly titrate with a continuous infusion. Long-term, high-dose (greater than 80 mcg/kg/min) propofol infusions are associated with rhabdomyolysis, acidosis, and cardiac arrhythmias (propofol-related infusion syndrome), especially in children.[27] It has a very short serum half-life and should be tapered off slowly to avoid withdrawal seizures. Propofol infusions are a source of calories (1 kcal/mL [4.2 kJ/mL]), so nutrition requirements have to be adjusted accordingly.

▸ *Pentobarbital*

Barbiturate infusions are reported to be highly effective in treating RSE,[28] but they cause significant hypotension, myocardial and respiratory depression, ileus, and infections. Therefore, patients require mechanical ventilation and invasive hemodynamic monitoring. Patients often require IV vasopressor therapy and total parenteral nutrition. Barbiturates are beneficial in decreasing elevated intracranial pressure (ICP).

A meta-analysis reported a lower incidence of treatment failure with pentobarbital (3%) compared to midazolam (21%) or propofol (20%), although the risk of hypotension requiring vasopressor therapy was higher with pentobarbital.[28] This relative efficacy for pentobarbital must be considered together with its complications when determining which agent to use. Patients who fail midazolam and/or propofol should be switched to pentobarbital.

▸ *Levetiracetam*

Although not FDA-approved for SE, levetiracetam does not have the cardiopulmonary, hepatic, and sedative side effects seen with the other agents; nor does it have potentially harmful drug interactions. Both IV[29] and oral[30] formulations have been used in RSE patients as add-on therapy with some success, although it is unclear if levetiracetam would be effective as monotherapy.[31] LDs up to 2000 mg over 15 to 30 minutes in the critically ill have been given with very little toxicity.[32]

▸ *Other Agents*

Ketamine,[33] topiramate, and inhaled anesthetics have also been used for RSE. Ketamine is an NMDA receptor antagonist that has been given orally[34] and intravenously[35] for RSE in children. Topiramate is an oral AED with multiple mechanisms of action in RSE. The oral dose in adults ranges from 300 to 1600 mg/day.[36] Children have also been administered topiramate at a starting dose of 2 to 3 mg/kg/day and titrated to a maintenance dose of 5 to 6 mg/kg/day.[16] Topiramate can induce metabolic acidosis, requiring careful monitoring. The inhaled anesthetics, desflurane and isoflurane,[37] require special equipment for administration in an ICU. Lacosamide, an enhancer of slow inhibition of sodium channels, has limited drug interactions.[38] It has been used orally[39] and intravenously[40] in the setting of refractory partial SE.

Special Populations

Certain patients require special considerations due to their altered metabolism, unique volume of distribution, or increased risk for side effects.[41] Although many of these patients are excluded from clinical trials in SE, the standard algorithm for SE still applies in terms of immediate care, assessment, and drugs (see Table 32–2).

▸ *Pediatrics*

The treatment approach for SE in children is similar to that in adults with a few exceptions (see Table 32–3). The doses are also weight-based but are typically higher than those used in adults due to faster hepatic clearance. Timely IV access in children may be difficult, so alternate routes of administration have been used, including intranasal, buccal, rectal, and IM. Early administration of benzodiazepines and reduced time to hospital admission are important in decreasing prolonged seizures.[42]

▶ *Geriatrics*

Older adults are often vulnerable because of multiple disease states and polypharmacy. Seizures in older adults often arise from metabolic disorders, drug interactions, or incorrect dosing of medications in patients with impaired renal and hepatic function and decreased protein binding. Clinicians treating older adult patients with SE should investigate drug- and disease state–induced causes, since treating these etiologies alone may terminate seizures. Acute treatment with benzodiazepines and AEDs is no different in older adults, but they may experience more profound sedative and cardiorespiratory side effects. Phenytoin and fosphenytoin LDs should be carefully calculated in older adults whose weights may be overestimated, and who may not tolerate high doses. They should also be infused more slowly to minimize hypotension and arrhythmias. Phenobarbital may cause respiratory depression earlier in older adults, especially after benzodiazepines. Clinicians should consider using smaller doses and evaluate for renal and hepatic insufficiency if repeated doses are to be given.

▶ *Pregnancy*

The main concern in the treatment of pregnant females in SE is the safety of the fetus which is at risk of hypoxia during periods of prolonged seizures. Although many drugs used in SE are teratogenic, clinicians should still use them acutely to stop seizures, but consider alternative agents for maintenance therapy.[43] The volume of distribution and clearance of many drugs are increased during pregnancy, and this must be considered when calculating doses.

OUTCOME EVALUATION

Start pharmacologic treatment as soon as possible.

- First-line (emergent) treatment for SE should halt seizure activity within minutes of administration.
- In patients who are unarousable following treatment, confirm termination of seizures with an EEG.
- Perform a physical exam and evaluation of the patient's laboratory results to help determine if the cause or complications of seizure activity are being appropriately treated.

Once seizure activity has ceased and the patient has stabilized, review the patient's therapeutic regimen.

- Evaluate and monitor serum trough concentrations of AEDs with defined target ranges to determine patient-specific therapeutic goals.
- In patients with RSE on multiple AEDs, slowly decrease the dose of one drug at a time while continuing to evaluate the patient for seizure activity.
- Continue to monitor AED serum trough concentrations approximately every 3 to 5 days until the AEDs have reached steady-state concentrations.
- Monitor for signs of drug toxicity and seizures until drug concentrations have stabilized.
- Closely evaluate medication profiles, and change drugs or doses to minimize any drug interactions, if possible.

Patient Care Process

Patient Assessment:

- Based on physical exam and review of systems, determine whether the patient is in SE.
- Obtain a medical history to elucidate precipitating factors. Does the patient have epilepsy?
- Review laboratory data, including any recent anticonvulsant levels. Is there evidence of alcohol or illicit drug use?
- Review vital signs, oxygen saturation, and point of care glucose testing.

Therapy Evaluation:

- Correct reversible causes of status epilepticus. Is the patient hypoxic, hypoglycemic or hyponatremic? If the patient is taking anticonvulsants, are the patient's serum levels therapeutic? Is the patient taking illicit or toxic substances?
- Determine whether patient has cardiovascular or respiratory compromise.
- If the patient is taking anticonvulsants, assess efficacy, safety, and adherence.
- Identify and address drug interactions.
- If a patient has an anticonvulsant allergy or a genetic predisposition that increases adverse reactions, identify alternative agents.

Care Plan Development:

- Conduct a thorough medication history, including prescription, nonprescription, and alternative drugs as well as herbal/dietary supplement use. Does the patient take anticonvulsants? Is the patient adherent? Does the patient have any allergies?
- Provide therapeutic doses of emergent and urgent therapies within the appropriate time frame (see Tables 32–1 and 32–2). Is the patient a child or older adult? Is the patient obese or pregnant?
- Identify drug interactions with current drug therapy and adjust as needed.
- Obtain expertise of neurologist or epileptologist when appropriate.

Follow-up Evaluation:

- Determine if physical seizures have stopped and the patient regains consciousness. If not, consider continuous EEG monitoring for at least 24 to 48 hours to identify possible nonconvulsive SE.
- Obtain serum anticonvulsant levels at steady state; sooner if patient continues to have seizures. Obtain trough concentrations when possible.

Abbreviations Introduced in This Chapter

ABG	Arterial blood gas
AED	Antiepileptic drug
CNS	Central nervous system
CSF	Cerebrospinal fluid
CT	Computerized tomography

ECG	Electrocardiogram
EEG	Electroencephalography
GABA	γ-aminobutyric acid
GCSE	Generalized convulsive status epilepticus
ICP	Intracranial pressure
ICU	Intensive care unit
IM	Intramuscular
IV	Intravenous
LD	Loading dose
MRI	Magnetic resonance imaging
NCSE	Nonconvulsive status epilepticus
NMDA	*N*-methyl-D-aspartate
PE	Phenytoin equivalent
RSE	Refractory status epilepticus
SE	Status epilepticus
WBC	White blood cell

REFERENCES

1. Brophy GM, Bell R, Claassen J, et al. Guidelines for the evaluation and management of status epilepticus. Neurocrit Care. 2012;17: 3–23.
2. Dham BS, Hunter K, Rincon F. The epidemiology of status epilepticus in the United States. Neurocrit Care. 2014;20:476–483.
3. Penberthy LT, Towne A, Garnett LK, et al. Estimating the economic burden of status epilepticus to the health care system. Seizure. 2005;14:46–51.
4. Lowenstein DH, Alldredge BK. Status epilepticus. N Engl J Med. 1998;338:970–9766.
5. Wu YW, Shek DW, Garcia PA, et al. Incidence and mortality of generalized convulsive status epilepticus in California. Neurology. 2002;58:1070–1076.
6. Chen JW, Naylor DE, Wasterlain CG. Advances in the pathophysiology of status epilepticus. Acta Neurol Scand Suppl. 2007;186:7–15.
7. Huff JS, Fountain NB. Pathophysiology and definitions of seizures and status epilepticus. Emerg Med Clin North Am. 2011;29:1–13.
8. Legriel S, Azoulay E, Resche-Rigon M, et al. Functional outcome after convulsive status epilepticus. Crit Care Med. 2010;38: 2295–303.
9. Hirsch LJ, Gaspard N. Status epilepticus. Continuum (Minneap Minn). 2013;19:767–794.
10. Treiman DM, Meyers PD, Walton NY, et al. A comparison of four treatments for generalized convulsive status epilepticus. Veterans Affairs Status Epilepticus Cooperative Study Group. N Engl J Med. 1998;339:792–798.
11. Alldredge BK, Gelb AM, Isaacs SM, et al. A comparison of lorazepam, diazepam, and placebo for the treatment of out-of-hospital status epilepticus. N Engl J Med. 2001;345:631–637.
12. Fitzgerald BJ, Okos AJ, Miller JW. Treatment of out-of-hospital status epilepticus with diazepam rectal gel. Seizure. 2003;12: 52–55.
13. Cock HR, Schapira AH. A comparison of lorazepam and diazepam as initial therapy in convulsive status epilepticus. QJM. 2002;95:225–231.
14. Towne AR, DeLorenzo RJ. Use of intramuscular midazolam for status epilepticus. J Emerg Med. 1999;17:323–328.
15. Scott RC, Besag FM, Boyd SG, et al. Buccal absorption of midazolam: pharmacokinetics and EEG pharmacodynamics. Epilepsia. 1998;39:290–294.
16. Kahriman M, Minecan D, Kutluay E, et al. Efficacy of topiramate in children with refractory status epilepticus. Epilepsia. 2003;44: 1353–1356.
17. Knoester PD, Jonker DM, Van Der Hoeven RT, et al. Pharmacokinetics and pharmacodynamics of midazolam administered as a concentrated intranasal spray. A study in healthy volunteers. Br J Clin Pharmacol. 2002;53: 501–507.
18. Silbergleit R, Durkalski, V., Lowenstein, D, et al; NETT Investigators. Intramuscular versus intravenous therapy for prehospital status epilepticus. N Engl J Med. 2012;366:591–600.
19. Abernethy DR, Greenblatt DJ. Phenytoin disposition in obesity. Determination of loading dose. Arch Neurol. 1985;42(5): 468–471.
20. Mazarati AM, Baldwin RA, Sankar R, Wasterlain CG. Time-dependent decrease in the effectiveness of antiepileptic drugs during the course of self-sustaining status epilepticus. Brain Res. 1998;814:179–185.
21. Limdi NA, Shimpi AV, Faught E, et al. Efficacy of rapid IV administration of valproic acid for status epilepticus. Neurology. 2005;64:353–355.
22. Alvarez V, Januel JM, Burnand B, Rossetti AO. Second-line status epilepticus treatment: comparison of phenytoin, valproate, and levetiracetam. Epilepsia. 2011;52:1292–1296.
23. Mayer SA, Claassen J, Lokin J, et al. Refractory status epilepticus: Frequency, risk factors, and impact on outcome. Arch Neurol. 2002;59:205–210.
24. Holtkamp M. Treatment strategies for refractory status epilepticus. Curr Opin Crit Care. 2011;17:94–100.
25. Shorvon S. Super-refractory status epilepticus: An approach to therapy in this difficult clinical situation. Epilepsia. 2011;52(Suppl 8): 53–56.
26. Naritoku DK, Sinha S. Prolongation of midazolam half life after sustained infusion for status epilepticus. Neurology. 2000;54: 1366–1368.
27. Iyer VN, Hoel R, Rabinstein AA. Propofol infusion syndrome in patients with refractory status epilepticus: An 11-year clinical experience. Crit Care Med. 2009;37:3024–3030.
28. Claassen J, Hirsch LJ, Emerson RG, Mayer SA. Treatment of refractory status epilepticus with pentobarbital, propofol, or midazolam: A systematic review. Epilepsia. 2002;43:146–153.
29. Moddel G, Bunten S, Dobis C, et al. Intravenous levetiracetam: A new treatment alternative for refractory status epilepticus. J Neurol Neurosurg Psychiatry. 2009;80:689–692.
30. Patel NC, Landan IR, Levin J, et al. The use of levetiracetam in refractory status epilepticus. Seizure. 2006;15:137–141.
31. Knake S, Gruener J, Hattemer K, et al. Intravenous levetiracetam in the treatment of benzodiazepine refractory status epilepticus. J Neurol Neurosurg Psychiatry. 2008;79:588–589.
32. Ruegg S, Naegelin Y, Hardmeier M, et al. Intravenous levetiracetam: Treatment experience with the first 50 critically ill patients. Epilepsy Behav. 2008;12:477–480.
33. Zeiler FA, Teitelbaum J, Gillman LM, West M. NMDA antagonists for refractory seizures. Neurocrit Care. 2014;20:502–513.
34. Mewasingh LD, Sekhara T, Aeby A, et al. Oral ketamine in paediatric non-convulsive status epilepticus. Seizure. 2003;12: 483–489.
35. Sheth RD, Gidal BE. Refractory status epilepticus: Response to ketamine. Neurology. 1998;51:1765–1766.
36. Towne AR, Garnett LK, Waterhouse EJ, et al. The use of topiramate in refractory status epilepticus. Neurology. 2003;60:332–334.
37. Mirsattari SM, Sharpe MD, Young GB. Treatment of refractory status epilepticus with inhalational anesthetic agents isoflurane and desflurane. Arch Neurol. 2004;61:1254–1259.
38. Kellinghaus C, Berning S, Immisch I, et al. Intravenous lacosamide for treatment of status epilepticus. Acta Neurol Scand. 2011;123: 137–141.
39. Tilz C, Resch R, Hofer T, Eggers C. Successful treatment for refractory convulsive status epilepticus by non-parenteral lacosamide. Epilepsia. 2010;51:316–317.

40. Goodwin H, Hinson HE, Shermock KM, et al. The use of lacosamide in refractory status epilepticus. Neurocrit Care. 2011; 14: 348–353.
41. Leppik IE. Treatment of epilepsy in 3 specialized populations. Am J Manag Care. 2001;7:S221–S226.
42. Chin RF, Neville BG, Peckham C, et al. Treatment of community-onset, childhood convulsive status epilepticus: A prospective, population-based study. Lancet Neurol. 2008;7:696–703.
43. Molgaard-Nielsen D, Hviid A. Newer-generation antiepileptic drugs and the risk of major birth defects. JAMA. 2011;305: 1996–2002.*S*

33 Parkinson Disease

Thomas R. Smith and Mary L. Wagner

LEARNING OBJECTIVES

Upon completion of the chapter, the reader will be able to:

1. Describe the pathophysiology of Parkinson disease (PD) related to neurotransmitter involvement and targets for drug therapy in the brain.
2. Recognize the cardinal motor symptoms of PD and determine a patient's clinical status and disease progression based on the Movement Disorder Society Unified Parkinson Disease Rating Scale (MDS UPDRS).
3. For a patient initiating therapy for PD, recommend appropriate drug therapy and construct patient-specific treatment goals.
4. Recognize and recommend appropriate treatment for nonmotor symptoms.
5. Formulate a plan to minimize patient "off-time" and maximize "on time" including timing, dosage, and frequency of medications.
6. Recognize and treat various motor complications that develop as PD progresses.
7. Construct appropriate patient counseling regarding medications and lifestyle modifications for a patient with PD.
8. Develop a monitoring plan to assess effectiveness and adverse effects of treatment.

INTRODUCTION

KEY CONCEPT *Parkinson disease (PD) is a slow, progressive neurodegenerative disease of the extrapyramidal motor system.* Dopamine neurons in the **substantia nigra** are primarily affected, and degeneration of these neurons causes a disruption in the ability to generate body movements. Cardinal features of PD include tremor at rest, rigidity, **akinesia/bradykinesia**, and postural instability. There is no cure, and treatment is aimed at controlling symptoms and slowing disease progression.

EPIDEMIOLOGY AND ETIOLOGY

PD affects approximately 1 million Americans, and a lifetime risk of developing the disease is 1.5%. Median age of onset is 60 years, but about 10% of people with PD are younger than 45 years. The average duration of time from diagnosis to death is about 15 years. Approximately 15% of patients with PD have a first-degree relative with the disease.[1,2]

The etiology of neuron degeneration in PD remains unknown, but aging has been implicated as a primary risk factor. Other explanations for the cell death may include oxidative stress, mitochondrial dysfunction, increased concentrations of excitotoxic amino acids and inflammatory cytokines, immune system disorders, trophic factor deficiency, signal-mediated **apoptosis**, and environmental toxins. Conditions that may promote oxidative stress include increased monoamine oxidase-B (MAO-B) metabolism or decreased glutathione clearance of free radicals.[2–5]

Genetic mutations such as those in *LRRK2* have been linked to PD, and particular mutations may predict early versus late onset of the disease.[2,3] A combination of inducers of cell death and genetic mutations may be at play in the development of PD.[2] In PD pigmented cells in the substantia nigra that make and store dopamine are lost. When patients are diagnosed, they have lost 50% to 60% of their dopamine neurons located here, and the remaining neurons elsewhere in the central nervous system (CNS) may be dysfunctional. Neurons have lost about 80% of their activity in the striatum at the onset of PD. Cortical **Lewy bodies** along with Lewy neurites in various CNS locations as well as the GI system may explain some of the nonmotor symptoms of PD.[2,4,5]

PATHOPHYSIOLOGY

The extrapyramidal motor system controls muscle movement through pathways and nerve tracts that connect the cerebral cortex, **basal ganglia**, thalamus, cerebellum, reticular formation, and spinal neurons. Patients with PD lose dopamine neurons in the substantia nigra, located in the midbrain within the brainstem. The substantia nigra sends nerve fibers to the corpus striatum, which is part of the basal ganglia in the cerebrum. The corpus striatum is made up of the caudate nucleus and the lentiform nuclei that consist of the pallidum (globus pallidus) and putamen (Figure 33–1). As dopamine neurons die, dopamine-relayed messages cannot communicate to other motor centers of the brain, and patients develop motor symptoms. A variety

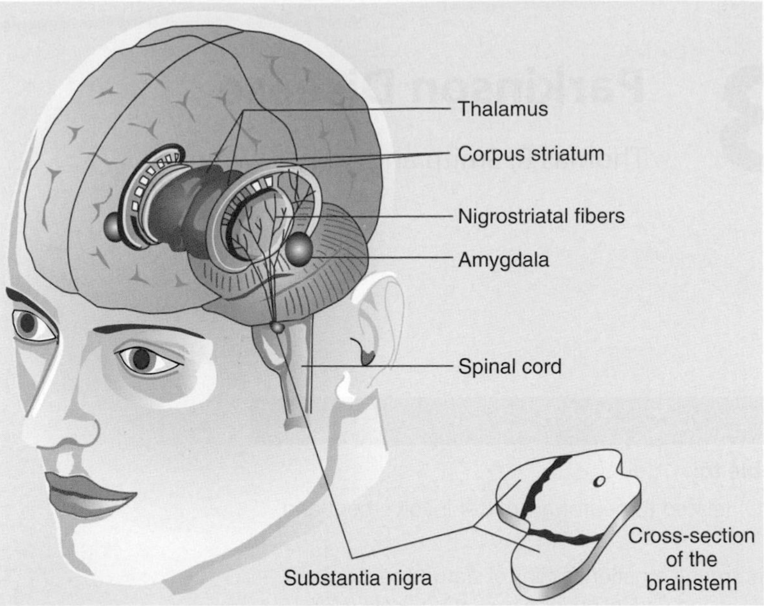

FIGURE 33–1. Anatomy of the extrapyramidal system. The extrapyramidal motor system controls muscle movement through a system of pathways and nerve tracts that connect the cerebral cortex, basal ganglia, thalamus, cerebellum, reticular formation, and spinal neurons. Patients with PD have a loss of dopamine neurons in the substantia nigra in the brainstem that leads to depletion of dopamine in the corpus striatum. The corpus striatum is made up of the caudate nucleus and the lentiform nuclei that are made up of the putamen and the globus pallidus.

of neurotransmitters are active in the basal ganglia, and their concentrations decrease with degeneration. These changes may explain some of the nonmotor symptoms seen in PD.[2,5,6] For example, loss of dopamine and norepinephrine neurons in the limbic system is associated with depression and anxiety, while loss of these neurotransmitters along with acetylcholine and serotonin in the limbic system and other regions is associated with cognitive impairment.[7]

Clinical Presentation of PD

Patients with PD display both motor and nonmotor symptoms. The nonmotor symptoms may precede the motor symptoms.

Motor Symptoms (Mnemonic TRAP)

T = Tremor at rest ("pill rolling")

R = Rigidity (stiffness and cogwheel rigidity)

A = Akinesia or bradykinesia

P = Postural instability and gait abnormalities

Nonmotor Symptoms (Mnemonic SOAP)

S = Sleep disturbances (insomnia, REM sleep behavioral disorder, restless legs syndrome [RLS])

O = Other miscellaneous symptoms (problems with nausea, fatigue, speech, pain, dysesthesias, vision, seborrhea)

A = Autonomic symptoms (drooling, constipation, sexual dysfunction, urinary problems, sweating, orthostatic hypotension, dysphagia)

P = Psychological symptoms (anxiety, psychosis, cognitive impairment, depression)

Response Fluctuations (Mnemonic MAD)

M = Motor fluctuations (delayed peak, wearing off, random off, freezing)

A = Akathisia

D = Dyskinesias (eg, chorea, dystonia, diphasic dyskinesia)

Patient Encounter, Part 1: Initial Visit—Medical History

A 68-year-old woman with a 5-year history of PD, comes in for an initial visit at the movement disorder clinic due to complaints of worsening symptoms. She was last seen 6 months ago by her family doctor where her UPDRS score was 40 (while on). The only change made to her medications at that time was the addition of prochlorperazine for nausea. Since her last visit, she has noticed a tremor in both hands instead of only her left hand as it was previously. During her off periods, she says her muscles are "stiff as a board," and she moves very slowly and has trouble maintaining balance occasionally. This affects her in the kitchen preparing food, and she is unable to walk her dog, an activity she enjoys that also provides her exercise. She reports a history of constipation that is somewhat improved from increased dietary fiber. Recently, she has had to use the restroom more often at night which disrupts her sleep.

Identify this patient's motor and nonmotor symptoms of PD.

What additional information would you collect before creating this patient's treatment plan?

The disease may begin in the autonomic system, olfactory system, or vagus nerve in the lower brainstem and then spread to the upper brainstem and cerebral hemisphere affecting dopamine pathways later in the course of disease progression.[2] It is essential to rule out drug-induced pseudoparkinsonism. Offending agents include drugs that deplete dopamine such as antipsychotics, metoclopramide, and certain antiemetics such as prochlorperazine. Removing the offending agent generally resolves symptoms.[1,8]

CLINICAL PRESENTATION AND DIAGNOSIS

The diagnosis of PD is based substantially on signs and symptoms rather than diagnostic tests or imaging. A single-photon emission computed tomography scan in conjunction with DaTscan, a radiopharmaceutical contrast agent, may help differentiate PD from other disorders such as essential tremor, but not from similar Parkinson-plus syndromes such as multiple system atrophy or progressive nuclear palsy.[9] Therefore, a thorough patient history and detailed description of symptom onset is essential in making an accurate diagnosis.

Motor Symptoms

KEY CONCEPT *PD is a slow, progressive neurodegenerative disease of the extrapyramidal motor system with classic motor symptoms of tremor, rigidity, akinesia/bradykinesia, and postural/gait instability (TRAP).*

The onset of PD is gradual, and impairment of movement may go unnoticed initially. Tremor occurs during rest and disappears with purposeful movement. The hand tremor can appear as if the patient is rolling a pill between his or her fingers. Patients usually describe rigidity as stiffness, and muscles often display uniform resistance on examination. Cogwheel rigidity is found when the examiner extends or flexes the patient's extremities and feels rhythmical jerking as if hitting a series of teeth on the rim of a wheel. Bradykinesia is defined as hesitancy in movement initiation, slowness in movement performance, or rapid fatiguing during movement. Patients may have a decrease in automatic movements, such as eye blinking, **hypomimia**, or a decrease in arm swing while walking. Postural instability results from the loss of reflexes necessary to maintain balance when ambulating. Stooped posture resulting in unsteadiness is common. Gait abnormalities may include slow shuffling, leg dragging, **festination**, propulsion, retropulsion, or freezing. Rigidity and bradykinesia may make handwriting difficult as evidenced by **micrographia**.[2,10–14]

Nonmotor Symptoms

Nonmotor symptoms associated with PD may precede the onset of motor symptoms by many years. These commonly include sleep disturbances, autonomic impairment, psychological disturbances, and others such as **anosmia** or sensory disturbances. Nonmotor symptoms may be a result of PD itself or medications.[2,6,10,15–21]

Speech problems may manifest as **hypophonia**, slurring, monotone speech, rapid speech, or stammering. Visual problems such as difficulty reading, double vision, decreased blinking, and burning or itchy eyes are the result of impairment of the ocular mucles.[2,6,10–14]

Because the autonomic nervous system is disturbed in PD, orthostatic hypotension, gastrointestinal (GI), urinary, sexual, and dermatologic symptoms are common. Orthostatic hypotension may cause dizziness, lightheadedness, fainting upon standing, or fall-related injuries. GI symptoms include constipation and **dysphagia**. Swallowing difficulties may lead to weight loss, **sialorrhea**, and aspiration.[15,17] Genitourinary symptoms include incontinence, urgency, and frequency. Symptoms may worsen at night, causing nocturia. Sexual dysfunction manifests as decreased libido or inability to achieve orgasm in both sexes and erectile or ejaculatory dysfunction in men. Dermatologic symptoms include sweating and intolerance to temperature changes.[2,6,10,15,17]

Psychological symptoms—psychosis, dementia, impaired **cognitive function**, depression, and anxiety—may occur during the natural course of PD, during symptom exacerbation, or as adverse effects from medications. Psychosis occurs in nearly 30% of PD patients and may include vivid dreams, hallucinations, paranoia, and delusions. Psychosis is rarely seen in untreated patients. Dementia and depression occur frequently with the latter likely due to abnormalities in dopamine and serotonin activity. Some features of PD, such as decreased facial expression and bradykinesia, may make the diagnosis of depression more difficult. Often comorbid with depression, anxiety has been noted in up to 66% of patients with motor fluctuations.[2,7,15,18–20]

Sleep disorders occur commonly and may be due to loss of neuronal functioning or medication adverse effects. Excessive daytime sleepiness, insomnia, and abnormal sleep events, such as rapid eye movement (REM) sleep behavior disorder (RBD) may occur.[10,15,16]

Motor Complications

Motor complications occur with disease progression as dopamine reserves are depleted and as a complication of treatment, particularly with levodopa. Motor complications include **delayed peak response**, early and unpredictable "wearing off," freezing, and **dyskinesias**. Dyskinesias include **chorea** and **dystonia**. Risk factors for developing motor complications include younger age at diagnosis, high dosage of levodopa, and longer duration and severity of disease. Wearing off can be conceptualized as the therapeutic window of levodopa narrowing over time. The therapeutic window is defined as the minimum effective concentration of levodopa required to control PD symptoms ("on" without dyskinesia) and the maximum concentration before experiencing side effects from too much levodopa ("on" with dyskinesia). Although the plasma half-life of levodopa is 1.5 to 2 hours, the therapeutic effect in early PD lasts about 5 hours, and the patient experiences no dyskinesias. This is due to supplemental dopamine production in the CNS. As PD progresses, this endogenous supply is decreased, the therapeutic window narrows, and each dose of levodopa acts unpredictably, with the therapeutic effect lasting only 2 to 3 hours. Dyskinesias become more likely to occur during the on state.[5,21,22]

KEY CONCEPT *The most useful diagnostic tool is the clinical history, including both presenting symptoms and associated risk factors. The Movement Disorder Society modified the previous Unified Parkinson Disease Rating Scale (MDS UPDRS), and it can be used to describe total symptom burden, track disease progression, and assess treatment efficacy.* This clinician and patient rated scale has four parts that can be used individually or in combination. It evaluates nonmotor symptoms associated with PD, activities of daily living (ADL), motor symptoms, and complications of therapy. Each symptom is given a numerical score from 0 to 4 (none to severe). It takes about 30 minutes to complete, so it may not be collected in its entirety at each visit.[23]

TREATMENT

Desired Outcomes

KEY CONCEPT *The goals of treatment include:*

- *maintaining patient independence, ADL, and quality of life (QOL)*
- *minimizing the development of response fluctuations*
- *limiting medication-related adverse effects*

General Approach to Treatment

KEY CONCEPT *Treatment of PD is categorized into three types: (1) lifestyle changes, nutrition, and exercise; (2) pharmacologic intervention, primarily with drugs that enhance dopamine concentrations; and (3) surgical treatments for those who fail pharmacologic interventions.*

Initial treatment depends on the patient's age, risk of adverse effects, degree of physical impairment, and readiness to initiate therapy. Initiating therapy with levodopa may be more beneficial for mobility than starting with a MAO-B inhibitor or dopamine agonists.[24]

The 2002 American Academy of Neurology guidelines and 2006 European National Institute for Health and Clinical Excellence guidelines suggest that symptomatic treatment should be delayed until the patient experiences functional disability.[25,26] Some data, however, suggest that earlier treatment may delay the progression of disease. In support of this, some clinicians note that progression of symptoms occurs most rapidly around the time of diagnosis and in early PD, and slows later in the disease.[27,28] However, studies examining this have design flaws and inconsistent results.[12,14] Until current clinical practice guidelines are revised, one must weigh the pros and cons of delaying pharmacotherapy or starting medications early on an individual patient basis.[25]

Patient Encounter, Part 2: Initial Visit—Physical Examination and Diagnostic Tests

Chief Complaint: Increased tremor, rigidity, and slowness, postural instability

PMH: Constipation for greater than 10 years

SH: Retired. Lives with husband and has two children. Denies alcohol use. Denies smoking

Meds: Carbidopa/levodopa 10 mg/100 mg orally—two tablets at 7 AM, one tablet at noon, and one tablet at 7 PM; prochlorperazine 10 mg orally three times a day

ROS: (–) Agitation, depression, or psychosis; reports nausea, denies vomiting, diarrhea, HA, dizziness, or pain

PE:

Gen: Flat affect, looks older than stated age, speaks softly and often difficult to hear, slow, shuffling gait

VS: BP: sitting 125/80 mm Hg, standing 105/70 mm Hg; P 65 beats/min, RR 18/min, Wt 59 kg (130 lb), Ht 165 cm (65 in)

HEENT: Decreased eye blinking and facial expression, CN II-XII intact, PERRLA, TMs intact

CV: RRR, normal S1, S2; no murmurs, rubs, gallop

Abd: Soft, nontender, nondistended; (+) bowel sounds, no hepatosplenomegaly

Skin: Normal

Exts: Mild tremor in both hands and feet. Cogwheel rigidity bilateral elbows, no edema

Neuro: Slow, shuffling gait, sensory function intact, normal muscle strength, normal reflexes, alert, mental status examination normal

Rating Scales: Mini Mental Status Exam (MMSE) = Normal 29/30; UPDRS = 50 while "on"

Labs: Normal metabolic profile and CBC

Given this additional information, what is your assessment of the patient's condition?

Identify treatment goals for the patient.

Describe nonpharmacologic and pharmacologic treatments that are available for the patient.

Nonpharmacologic Therapy

► *Lifestyle Modifications*

Nonpharmacologic therapy, including education and lifestyle modifications such as exercise, should be started early and continued throughout treatment for PD. These treatments may improve ADLs, gait, balance, and mental health. The most common interventions include maintaining good nutrition, physical condition, and social interactions.[1,10]. Coordinated care with an optometrist/ophthalmologist, dentist, dietician, physical therapists, speech therapist, and social worker is needed to maximize patient outcomes. Each of these specialists plays a specific role in the treatment team (Table 33–1).[30]

Surgery

As patients develop inadequate control of motor symptoms despite medical treatment, surgery with deep brain stimulation (DBS) may be considered. This procedure electrically stimulates the subthalamic nucleus or globus pallidus interna. DBS may significantly reduce motor symptoms and complications and improve QOL compared to medication management. Trials indicate that targeting the subthalamic nucleus is preferred when a decrease in PD medication use is desired while targeting the globus pallidus may be better suited when dyskinesias are present.[31,32] These surgeries are not without risk and are generally

Table 33–1

Specialist Care for Patients with PD

Provider	Reason for Referral
Dentist	PD medications may decrease saliva flow and increase the risk of dental caries
Dietician	Recommend appropriate caloric intake, meal selection, and protein consumption which may: • improve constipation and nausea • decrease weight loss and aspiration • minimize erratic drug absorption
Speech therapist	Improved swallowing, articulation, and force of speech
Physical therapy	Improve strength, activity, sleep quality and reduce fall risk May provide neuroprotection
Occupational therapist	Educate on adaptive environment of home, specialized clothing, and personal training to evaluate and maximize: • Independence • Safety • ADLs • Handwriting • Driving ability • Use of communication software
Social worker	Arrange for community assistance programs Increase engagement in family activities, and minimize conflict through family counseling

Nutt JG, Wooten GF. Diagnosis and initial management of Parkinson's disease. N Engl J Med. 2005;353:1021–1027.[1]

Anonymous. Drugs for Parkinson's disease. Treat Guidel Med Lett. 2011;9(101):1–6.[29]

utilized after complications with or poor response to medication management.

Pharmacologic Therapy

KEY CONCEPT *Drug therapy is aimed at enhancing dopaminergic activity in the substantia nigra. The best time to initiate dopaminergic therapy is controversial and patient specific.* Medications help minimize motor symptoms, and improve QOL and ADLs, but they are not curative (Table 33–2).[1,2,33,34] PD patients with optimal treatment have greater mortality and morbidity than the general population.[1]

KEY CONCEPT *Choice of pharmacologic agent should be individualized based on patient-specific parameters, and dose frequency should be scheduled based on individual response to maximize "on time" and minimize "off time".*

Pharmacologic options for PD include anticholinergics (Ach), amantadine, MAO-B inhibitors, dopamine agonists, levodopa/carbidopa, and catechol-*O*-methyltransferase (COMT) inhibitors. Because most pharmacologic treatments in PD aim to avoid degeneration of the dopaminergic nigrostriatal pathway, it is essential to understand how all drugs may affect dopamine concentrations (Figure 33–2). The American Academy of Neurology and the Movement Disorder Society determined that it is reasonable to start treatment with either levodopa or a dopamine agonist.[11–15]

Choice of agent varies based on clinical experience and patient preference. Starting with a dopamine agonist may help to delay the onset of dyskinesias and the on and off fluctuations seen with long-term levodopa use. However, this approach may result in less motor benefit and greater risk of hallucinations or somnolence. Levodopa results in greater motor improvement and should be used as initial therapy in the elderly (greater than 75 years) and in those with cognitive impairment.[28] Data are insufficient to recommend initiating treatment with combined levodopa and a dopamine agonist. Initiating treatment with anticholinergic medications, amantadine, or MAO-B inhibitors is recommended only for patients who have mild symptoms because they are not as effective as dopamine agonists or levodopa.[1,2,11–15,33,34]

Medications should be started at the lowest dose and increased gradually based on symptoms (see Table 33–2). Adjust dose timing, frequency, or both based on the patient's report of "on

Table 33–2

Dosing of Medications Used to Treat PD

Generic Name (Trade Name)	Initial Dose	Titration and Maintenance Dose	Available Formulations	Hepatic or Renal Adjustments
Levodopa Formulations				
Levodopa with carbidopa (Sinemet)	Half tablet (100 mg LD, 25 mg CD) twice daily for 1 week, then half tablet three times daily	Increase by half tablet daily every week; usual MD is 300–2000 mg daily; because the duration of LD is 2–3 hours, patients may require doses every 2 hours.	Parcopa—orally disinteg rating LD Duodopa—Portable pump that continuously delivers LD and carbidopa via a duodenal tube—in phase III trials in the US Stalevo—CD/LD/Entacapone tablet	
Sinemet CR	One tablet (100 mg LD, 25 mg CD) two to three times daily	Increase to 200 mg LD tablet two to four times daily; usual MD is 200–2200 mg daily.	Sustained-release tablet	
Rytary (extended-release levodopa with carbidopa)	In levodopa naïve patients: 23.75 mg/95 mg taken orally three times a day for the first 3 days	On the fourth day of treatment, the dosage may be increased to 36.25 mg/145 mg taken three times a day. Individual doses may be increased and doses may be given up to five times a day based on individual response; patients previously on immediate release levodopa should follow recommended conversions.	Extended-release capsule	
Dopamine Agonists				
Apomorphine (Apokyn)	Start an antiemetic for 3 days; then give apomorphine 2 mg SC injection (1 mg if outpatient) while monitoring blood pressure	Increase by 1–2 mg every ≥ 2 hours; usual MD is 2–6 mg three to five times daily for off periods.	Subcutaneous solution	Reduce initial dose to 1 mg in mild to moderate renal failure.
Bromocriptine (Parlodel)	1.25 mg twice daily	Increase by 2.5 mg daily every 14 to 28 days.	Capsule, tablet	Dosing adjustments may be necessary with hepatic impairment.

(continued)

Table 33–2

Dosing of Medications Used to Treat PD (*Continued*)

Generic Name (Trade Name)	Initial Dose	Titration and Maintenance Dose	Available Formulations	Hepatic or Renal Adjustments
Pramipexole (Mirapex)	0.125 mg three times daily	Increase about weekly by 0.375–0.75 mg/day to a MD of 0.5–1.5 mg three times daily.	Tablet	Dosage reduction needed in creatinine clearance < 50 mL/min (0.83 mL/s).
Mirapex ER	0.375 mg once daily	Increase up to 0.75 mg/day after a minimum of 5 days. Dose may then be increased in increments of 0.75 mg/day no more frequently than every 5–7 days.	Extended-release tablet	
Ropinirole (Requip)	0.25 mg three times daily	Increase about weekly by 0.75–1.5 mg daily to a MD dose of 3–9 mg three times daily. Then may increase by 3 mg/day on a weekly basis to a maximum of 24 mg/day.	Tablet	
Requip XL	2 mg once daily for 1–2 weeks	Increase by 2 mg/day in 1-week intervals; maximum dose is 24 mg/day.	Extended-release tablet	
Rotigotine (Neupro)	2 mg patch once daily for early-stage PD; 4 mg patch for advanced-stage PD	Increase by 2 mg/24 hours on a weekly basis.	Patch	
MAOIs				
Selegiline (Eldepryl)	5 mg in the morning	If symptoms continue, add 5 mg at noon; 5 mg daily may be as clinically effective as 10 mg daily with fewer side effects.	Tablet, capsule	Use is not recommended for creatinine clearance < 30 mL/min (0.50 mL/s) or severe hepatic impairment.
Selegiline ODT (Zelapar)	1.25 mg once daily	If symptoms continue after 6 weeks, increase dose to 2.5 mg every morning. Avoid food or liquid for 5 minutes before or after the dose.	Dispersable tablet	
Rasagiline (Azilect)	If used with levodopa, 0.5 mg daily	If symptoms continue, increase to 1 mg daily.	Tablet	Use 0.5 mg/day in mild hepatic impairment. Do not use in moderate to severe impairment.
COMT Inhibitors				
Tolcapone (Tasmar)	100 mg with first Sinemet dose once daily	If symptoms continue, increase to 2 and then 3 times daily, then to 200 mg each dose; usual MD is 100–200 mg three times daily.	Tablet	Do not use in patients with active liver disease or SGPT/ALT or SGOT/AST > the upper limit of normal.
Entacapone (Comtan)	200 mg tab with each Sinemet dose	Usual MD is 200 mg three to four times daily (up to eight tablets per day).	Tablet	Decrease dose by 50% with hepatic impairment.
Others				
Amantadine (Symmetrel)	100 mg daily at breakfast	After 1 week, add 100 mg daily; usual MD is 200–300 mg daily with last dose in afternoons.	Capsule, tablet, oral syrup	Decrease dose for creatinine clearance < 80 mL/min (1.33 mL/s)
Benztropine (Cogentin)	0.5 to 1 mg at bedtime	Assess if dose is adequate and titrate by 0.5 mg increments at 5- to 6-day intervals to a maximum of 6 mg if necessary.	Tablet, solution for injection	

Ach, acetylcholine; CD, carbidopa; COMT, catechol-*O*-methyltransferase; DA, dopamine; LD, levodopa; MAO, monoamine oxidase; MD, maintenance dose; NMDA, *N*-methyl-D-aspartate.

Data from Refs. 1, 2, 33, 34, and 35.

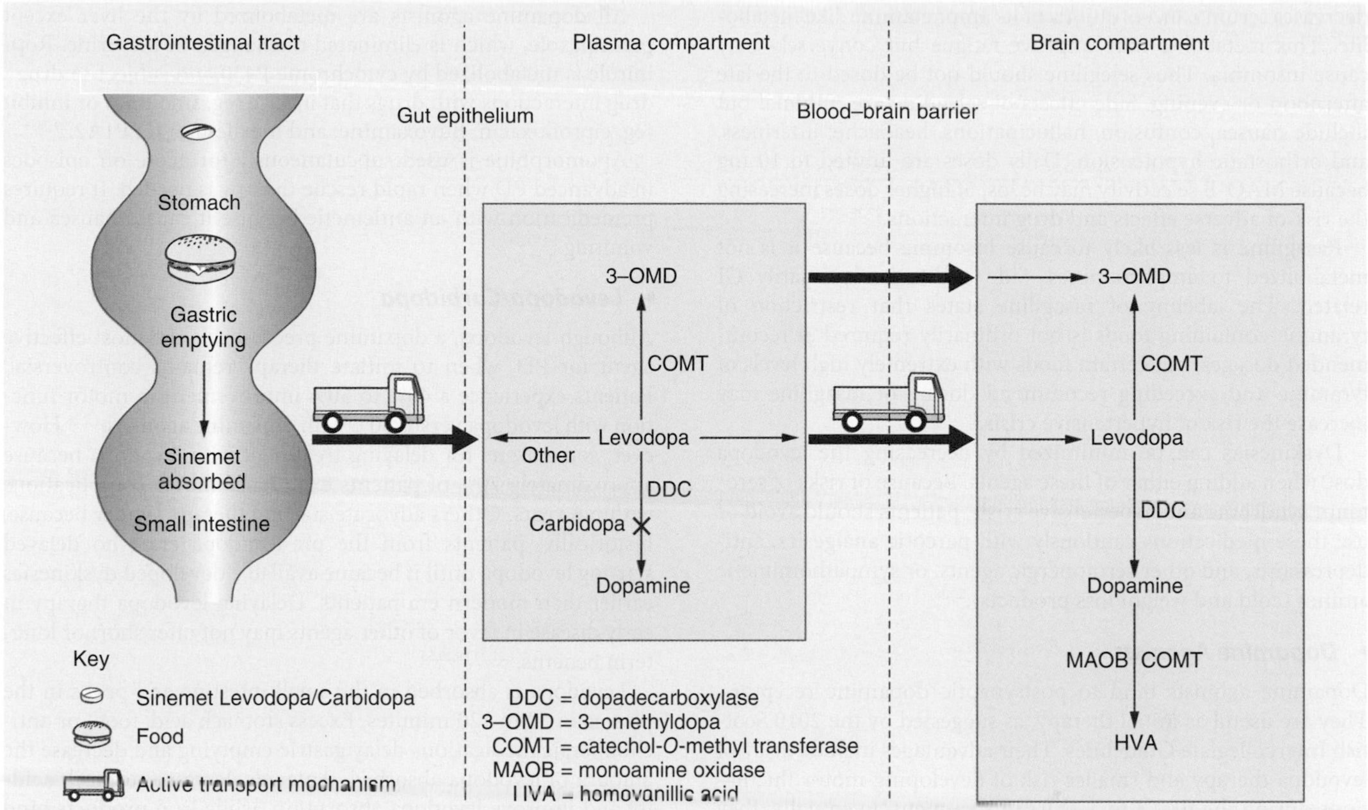

FIGURE 33–2. Levodopa absorption and metabolism. Levodopa is absorbed in the small intestine and distributed into the plasma and brain compartments by an active transport mechanism. Levodopa is metabolized by dopa decarboxylase, monoamine oxidase, and catechol-*O*-methyltransferase. Carbidopa does not cross the blood–brain barrier. Large neutral amino acids in food compete with levodopa for intestinal absorption (transport across gut endothelium to plasma). They also compete for transport into the brain (plasma compartment to brain compartment). Food and Ach delay gastric emptying resulting in levodopa degradation in the stomach and a decreased amount of levodopa absorbed. If the interaction becomes a problem, administer levodopa 30 minutes before or 60 minutes after meals.

time" duration and wearing off symptoms. Dyskinesias related to dopamine concentrations can be managed by decreasing the dose, frequency, or use of medications that may enhance dopamine concentrations. If a dopaminergic medication is to be discontinued, it should be decreased gradually and the patient monitored for worsening of symptoms.

▶ Anticholinergics

Anticholinergics (Ach) block acetylcholine, decreasing the acetylcholine to dopamine concentration ratio. They minimize resting tremor and drooling, but are not as effective as other agents for rigidity, bradykinesia, and gait problems. Side effects include dry mouth, blurred vision, constipation, cognitive impairment, hallucinations, urinary retention, orthostatic hypotension, temperature sensitivity, and sedation. They are usually avoided or used with caution in patients older than 70 years because of an increased risk of cognitive impairment.[1,2,10,29,33] Ach should be discontinued gradually to avoid withdrawal effects or worsening of symptoms. Additionally, Achs may be associated with an increased incidence of amyloid plaques and neurofibrillary tangles in patients with PD. There is concern that this may translate to an increased risk of Alzheimer disease.[36] Ach decrease gastric motility, which may delay gastric emptying and lead to erratic and decreased levodopa absorption.[37]

▶ Amantadine

Amantadine is an *N*-methyl-D-aspartate (NMDA)-receptor antagonist that blocks glutamate transmission, promotes dopamine release, and blocks acetylcholine. It improves PD symptoms in mildly affected patients and may reduce dyskinesia severity and duration.[22,38,39] Patients who develop tolerance to amantadine's effects may benefit from a drug holiday through a gradual taper to discontinuation to minimize withdrawal effects. Side effects include nausea, dizziness, **livedo reticularis**, peripheral edema, orthostatic hypotension, hallucinations, restlessness, anticholinergic effects, and insomnia. It should be avoided in the elderly who cannot tolerate its anticholinergic effects.[29,33,39]

▶ MAO-B Inhibitors

Selegiline and rasagiline selectively and irreversibly block MAO-B metabolism of dopamine in the brain. They may provide a mild symptomatic benefit for patients who choose to delay dopaminergic medications, and they reduce off time when added to levodopa therapy.[10-13,39] Combining selegiline or rasagiline with levodopa in early treatment may delay motor complications.[22,27,40]

Both rasagiline and selegiline are thought to be neuroprotective, but there is no evidence to validate this.[41]

Selegiline is available in an orally disintegrating tablet designed to avoid first-pass metabolism. This improves bioavailability and decreases serum concentrations of its amphetamine-like metabolite. This metabolite may improve fatigue but conversely may cause insomnia. Thus selegiline should not be dosed in the late afternoon or evening. Side effects of selegiline are minimal but include nausea, confusion, hallucinations, headache, jitteriness, and orthostatic hypotension. Daily doses are limited to 10 mg because MAO-B selectivity may be lost at higher doses increasing the risk of adverse effects and drug interactions.[27,28]

Rasagiline is less likely to cause insomnia because it is not metabolized to amphetamines. Side effects are primarily GI related. The labeling of rasagiline states that restriction of tyramine-containing foods is not ordinarily required at recommended dosages, but certain foods with extremely high levels of tyramine and exceeding recommend dosing of rasagiline may increase the risk of hypertensive crisis.[40]

Dyskinesias can be minimized by decreasing the levodopa dose when adding either of these agents. Because of risks of serotonin syndrome and hypertensive crisis, patients should avoid or use these medications cautiously with narcotic analgesics, antidepressants, and other serotonergic agents, or sympathomimetic amines (cold and weight loss products).[27,28]

▶ *Dopamine Agonists*

Dopamine agonists bind to postsynaptic dopamine receptors. They are useful as initial therapy, as suggested by the 2010 Scottish Intercollegiate Guidelines. Their advantages include delay of levodopa therapy and smaller risk of developing motor fluctuations during the first 4 to 5 years of treatment. Eventually, they inadequately control the patient's symptoms, and levodopa will need to be started. In advanced disease, they can be added to levodopa to minimize response fluctuations, decrease off time, improve wearing-off symptoms, allow a reduction in levodopa dose, and improve ADLs.[1,2,11,13,34,42]

Dopamine agonists include the ergot derivatives (bromocriptine) and the nonergot derivatives (rotigotine, pramipexole, ropinirole, and apomorphine). Generally, the nonergot agents are chosen first over bromocriptine due to a more favorable adverse effect profile and stronger evidence of efficacy.[43] If patients fail one dopamine agonist, another can be tried. Although not well established, it appears that bromocriptine 30 mg, ropinirole 15 mg, and pramipexole 4.5 mg are equivalent, and this relationship can be a guide when switching agents. Rotigotine is available as a once-daily skin patch which minimizes pulsatile dopaminergic stimulation.[1,28,29,33,38]

Common side effects include nausea, vomiting, sedation (highest with apomorphine), pedal edema, orthostatic hypotension (highest with pramipexole) and psychiatric effects that are greater than with levodopa (nightmares, confusion, and hallucinations). Uncommon ergot side effects include painful reddish discoloration of the skin over the shins and pleuropulmonary, retroperitoneal, and cardiac fibrosis.[1,29,33,38] Patients' therapy may be complicated by the dopamine dysregulation syndrome (DDS). This includes an addictive pattern of dopamine agonist use, complex stereotyped behavior known as **punding**, and impulse control disorders (ICDs) such as gambling or compulsive shopping. Reducing or eliminating the agonist usually resolves these problems.[44]

Dopamine agonists may cause excessive daytime sleepiness in 50% of PD patients. Sudden sleep attacks may occur and are potentially dangerous if occurring during certain activities such as driving. Modafinil and other agents to promote wakefulness may be used for daytime sleepiness, but use for sleep attacks remains controversial.[32,45]

All dopamine agonists are metabolized by the liver except pramipexole, which is eliminated unchanged in the urine. Ropinirole is metabolized by cytochrome P450 and subject to drug–drug interactions with drugs that induce (eg, smoking) or inhibit (eg, ciprofloxacin, fluvoxamine, and mexiletine) CYP1A2.[29,33]

Apomorphine is used subcutaneously for acute off episodes in advanced PD when rapid rescue therapy is needed. It requires premedication with an antiemetic because it causes nausea and vomiting.[29,33,38]

▶ *Levodopa/Carbidopa*

Although levodopa, a dopamine precursor, is the most effective agent for PD, when to initiate therapy remains controversial. Patients experience a 40% to 50% improvement in motor function with levodopa versus 30% with dopamine agonists.[1,2,28] However, some argue for delaying treatment with levodopa because approximately 70% of patients experience motor complications within 6 years. Others advocate starting therapy sooner because, historically, patients from the pre-levodopa era who delayed starting levodopa until it became available developed dyskinesias earlier than modern era patients. Delaying levodopa therapy in early disease in favor of other agents may not offer short or long-term benefits.[1,21,24,28,29,33]

Levodopa is absorbed in the small intestine and peaks in the plasma in 30 to 120 minutes. Excess stomach acid, food, or anticholinergic medications delay gastric emptying and decrease the amount of levodopa absorbed. Antacids decrease stomach acidity and improve levodopa absorption, while iron products bind levodopa and may reduce its absorption. Levodopa absorption requires active transport by a large neutral amino acid transporter protein (see Figure 33–2). Amino acids in food compete for this transport mechanism. Thus, in advanced disease, avoidance of protein-rich meals in relationship to levodopa doses may be helpful.[1,28,29,33]

Controlled-release (CR) formulations act longer than immediate-release tablets but are absorbed slower. This results in a delayed onset (45–60 minutes) compared with the standard formulation (15–30 minutes); thus patients may require immediate-release tablets or even a liquid formulation when they want a quicker onset of effect, such as with the first morning dose. Because of reduced bioavailability, the total daily dose of CR preparations should be increased by 30%. In early 2015, an extended-release formulation of levodopa (Rytary) was approved. Doses are not directly interchangeable with other levodopa preparations. Its ideal place in therapy is yet to be determined.[1,28,29,33]

Converting patients from oral formulations to enteral or duodenal levodopa administration reduces motor fluctuations and improves UPDRS scores. The levodopa/carbidopa combination can be administered directly to the duodenum via a small tube. This formulation is marketed under the trade name Duodopa in Europe and Canada, but it is unavailable in the United States. It is reserved for advanced PD with severe motor fluctuations.[46]

Levodopa is usually administered as a combination product with carbidopa, a dopa-decarboxylase inhibitor, which decreases the peripheral conversion of levodopa to dopamine. This allows for lower levodopa doses and minimizes levodopa peripheral side effects, eg, nausea, vomiting, anorexia, and hypotension. Carbidopa does not cross the blood–brain barrier and does not interfere with levodopa conversion in the brain. Generally 75 to 100 mg daily of carbidopa is required to adequately block peripheral dopa-decarboxylase. Higher doses of carbidopa may reduce nausea when initiating levodopa.[1,28,28,33]

Initial levodopa side effects include orthostatic hypotension, dizziness, anorexia, nausea, vomiting, and discoloration of urine/sweat. Most of these effects can be minimized by taking levodopa with food and by slowly titrating the dose. Side effects that develop later in therapy include dyskinesias, sleep attacks, impulse control disorders, and psychiatric effects (confusion, hallucinations, nightmares, and altered behavior). Dyskinesias caused by adding other PD drugs to levodopa may be improved by decreasing the levodopa dose.[1,28,29,33]

Because Levodopa is short acting, it has a greater risk of causing end of dose wearing off periods that require medication adjustments. Patients with severe dyskinesias and off periods may achieve more constant blood concentrations (lower peak and higher trough concentrations) with a liquid formulation of levodopa with carbidopa compounded from tablets. This may allow for more precise dosing and improvements in motor symptoms and complications.[28,29,33,46]

► *Catechol-O-Methyltransferase (COMT) Inhibitors*

Inhibitors of COMT, an enzyme that catalyzes levodopa to 3-omethyldopa, are added to levodopa/carbidopa to increase levodopa concentrations, extend its half-life, and decrease wearing off time. Using the COMT inhibitors entacapone or tolcapone may allow for a decrease in daily levodopa dose while increasing on time by 1 to 2 hours. Side effects include diarrhea (worse with tolcapone), nausea, vomiting, anorexia, dyskinesias, urine discoloration, daytime sleepiness, sleep attacks, orthostatic hypotension, and hallucinations. Dyskinesias should improve with a decrease in the levodopa dose.[28,29,33]

Tolcapone should be used only in patients who do not tolerate or respond to entacapone due to its hepatic safety profile. Serum liver function tests should be monitored at baseline, every 2 to 4 weeks for 6 months, and then periodically for the remainder of therapy. Patients who fail to show symptomatic benefit after 3 weeks should discontinue tolcapone.[28,33,34]

► *Herbs and Supplements*

There is very little support for using creatine, gingko, ginseng, green tea, ginger, yohimbine, or St. John's wort in patients with PD.

Patients should eat a balanced diet and consider a multivitamin with minerals, but supplementation with specific vitamins is generally unceccesary.[9]

TREATMENT OF NONMOTOR SYMPTOMS

KEY CONCEPT *Treatment of nonmotor symptoms should be based on whether they are exacerbated by an off state or might be related to other neurotransmitter dysfunction.*

The treatment of nonmotor symptoms, such as psychological conditions, sleep disorders, and autonomic dysfunction, should include both pharmacologic and nonpharmacologic approaches. Patients should be supported to maintain ADLs, a positive self-image, family communication, and a safe environment.

Psychological Symptoms

Psychological symptoms and psychosis are potential problems in PD patients. When psychological changes are suspected, potential causes to rule out include infections, metabolic changes, electrolyte disturbances, or toxic exposures.

► *Depression*

Depression is extremely common in patients with PD, affecting 40% or more of patients, and it often precedes the disease. Brain catecholamine changes and serotonin dysregulation contribute to depression associated with PD. Although evidence supports efficacy of tricyclic antidepressants in this population, their adverse effect profile limits their use. Alternatively, selective serotonin reuptake inhibitors may be considered because of their increased tolerability. Pramipexole may also improve depression.[19] Antidepressants are also useful for the treatment of anxiety disorders. Because off periods can both precipitate anxiety and worsen depression, therapy should be adjusted to maximize on periods.[2,7,8,15,18]

► *Dementia*

Dementia occurs in approximately 80% of patients with PD 20 years after diagnosis, and decreased cholinergic neurotransmission is implicated. Cholinesterase inhibitors may be effective, but the efficacy of memantine is unclear.[2,15,18–20,38]

► *Psychosis*

First treat any underlying medical causes for psychosis (infections, electrolyte disturbances). Then gradually decrease and stop low-efficacy PD medications. Antipsychotics should be used cautiously in patients with PD because they may worsen motor symptoms and may increase the risk of death in patients with concurrent dementia. However, if reducing PD medication compromises motor control or does not improve psychosis, low-dose quetiapine (12.5–200 mg) at bedtime may improve psychosis and is preferred with close monitoring for long-term metabolic side effects. Clozapine is also recommended but requires stringent monitoring (see Chapter 37).[2,15,16–20]

Sleep Problems

Sleep problems and fatigue are common in PD and may be due to medications, uncontrolled PD symptoms, or other causes such as nocturia, sleep attacks during the day, depression, RBD, or restless legs syndrome (RLS). Instruction on good sleep hygiene, improvement in nighttime PD symptoms, or cognitive behavioral therapy may help.[7,15,16]

The rotigotine patch may improve early morning motor function and overall quality of sleep.[47]

Amantadine and selegiline may worsen insomnia, selegiline and tricyclic antidepressants may worsen REM sleep, and some antidepressants and antipsychotics may worsen RLS. Melatonin may improve patient perception of sleep, but this has not been fully validated. Levodopa/carbidopa reduces nighttime periodic leg movements; while data regarding nonergot dopamine agonists are lacking in patients with PD. When iron is used for RLS, it may decrease the absorption of levodopa and increase constipation. A nighttime dose of a COMT inhibitor may improve RLS.[2,6,16]

Autonomic and Other Problems

Drooling may be accompanied by speech problems and dysphagia. Ach, botulinum toxin injections, and sublingual atropine can decrease drooling. Nausea improves if PD medications are taken with meals and with antiemetic therapy (eg, domperidone or trimethobenzamide).

Sexual dysfunction or urinary problems may require further evaluation. Adjustment of PD therapy to increase on time, removal of drugs that decrease sexual response, and pharmacologic therapy (eg, sildenafil) may improve sexual dysfunction. Studies of sexual dysfunction in women with PD are lacking.

Patients with urinary frequency may find a bedside urinal and a decrease in evening fluid intake helpful. Improvement in PD symptom control can decrease urinary frequency, but worsening symptoms may require catheterization or pharmacologic measures (eg, oxybutynin, tolterodine, propantheline, imipramine, hyoscyamine, or nocturnal intranasal desmopressin).

Anticholinergic drugs can cause urinary retention and constipation. Constipation can be improved by increased fluid intake, a fiber-rich diet, probiotics, and physical activity. Stool softeners, osmotic or bulk-forming laxatives, glycerin suppositories, or enemas may help, while cathartic laxatives should be avoided.

Dyskinesia-related sweating may respond to PD therapy adjustment or β-blockers.

Treating orthostasis includes the removal of offending drugs (eg, tricyclic antidepressants, PD medications, alcohol, and antihypertensives) increasing carbidopa doses, increased salt or fluids to the diet, compression stockings, fludrocortisone, indomethacin, or midodrine. Droxidopa, a norepinephrine synthetic precursor, was recently approved for treating orthostatic hypotension associated with PD.[38]

Seborrhea usually responds to over-the-counter dandruff shampoos or topical steroids.[2,6,10,17]

Treatment of Response Fluctuations

KEY CONCEPT *As the disease progresses, most patients develop response fluctuations. Treatment is based on capitalizing on the pharmacokinetic and pharmacodynamic properties of PD medications.*

Treatment includes adjusting or adding medications to maximize the patient's on time, minimizing the time on with dyskinesia, and minimizing off time (Table 33–3). Use various dosage plans to minimize suboptimal or delayed peak levodopa concentrations by adding longer acting medications to minimize wearing-off periods, adding or adjusting medications to stop an unpredicted off period, and providing treatments that decrease freezing episodes. Treatment plans also involve adjusting or adding medications to decrease chorea, dystonia, **diphasic dyskinesias, or akathisia**. Patients should schedule activities when they are on. An extra dose of medication carried with them when they are away from home in case their medication wears off is also adviseable.[2,7,12,14,22]

Patient Encounter, Part 3: First Follow-up Visit 3 Months Later

The patient returns for a follow-up visit 3 months after adjustments were made to her therapy. At her last appointment, ropinirole was added and prochlorperazine was removed. Since then, she reports improvement in her ability to cook and can go for longer walks. She feels that she has less tremor and stiffness throughout the day with no off periods. However, about an hour after she takes her morning dose of carbidopa/levodopa with ropinirole, her husband describes movements consistent with chorea. Additionally, her husband reports that she sometimes sees faces in the shadows at night. She also reports feeling dizzy and lightheaded when standing quickly from sitting in a chair and has fallen. She is more physically active with improved PD symptoms. She is taking polyethylene glycol one time per week with five to seven bowel movements per week. Her nighttime urgency to urinate is decreased with a reduction in fluids and her nausea has improved with a change to carbidopa/levodopa 25 mg/100 mg tablets.

UPDRS 40 (on)

Create a problem list and provide an assessment of each problem.

Considering the goals of therapy, treatment options, and your assessment of each of the problems, create a care plan for each problem.

Patient Encounter, Part 4: Second Follow-up Visit 3 Months Later

The patient comes in for a follow-up visit with no new complaints. At her last visit 3 months ago, ropinirole was removed, and her daily Sinemet dose was increased to cover the afternoon off period that had previously been treated with ropinirole. Since then she reports a similar level of functioning with minimal off time and no dyskinesias. She denies any auditory or visual hallucinations or vivid dreams. She denies feeling dizzy when standing and does not report any more falls. She has joined an exercise class at the senior center. She continues to have five to seven bowel movements per week.

UPDRS 40 (on)

Meds: Carbidopa/levodopa 25 mg/100 mg orally—two tablets at 7 AM, one tablet at 11:30 AM, one tablet at 4 PM, and one tablet at 9 PM; polyethylene glycol (MiraLAX) 17 g/scoop. One scoop in 4 to 8 oz (120–240 mL) of liquid, one to two times per week as needed for constipation

If her psychosis had continued and was determined to be a nonmotor symptom of PD rather than an adverse effect of her dopaminergic therapy, what options might you consider?

If this patient's dyskinesias in the morning continued despite removal of the dopamine agonist, what options might you consider?

Were therapeutic goals achieved in this patient after discontinuation of her dopamine agonist and adjustment of her carbidopa/levodopa?

How would you counsel a patient who has been on PD medications and is initiating an atypical antipsychotic such as quetiapine?

If a patient was unable to speak due to disease progression, what would be the advantages and disadvantages of having a significant other communicate for the patient?

OUTCOME EVALUATION

KEY CONCEPT *Patient monitoring involves a regular systematic evaluation of efficacy and adverse events, referral to appropriate specialists, and patient education.* Evaluate the clinical outcomes of treatment over time by assessing the change in the UPDRS from baseline. Instruct patients to record daily the amount of on and off time to guide medication adjustment. Patients with PD have an increased risk for falls. Assess fall risk and implement appropriate safety measures to prevent falls. Scales assessing QOL, depression, anxiety, and sleep disorders are useful to track progression.

Table 33–3

Management of Motor Complications in Advanced PD

I. Motor Fluctuations

A. Suboptimal or delayed peak response

Nonpharmacologic Approaches	Drugs to Alter Formulation or Dose	Drugs to Add
Take Sinemet on an empty stomach Decrease dietary protein and fat around the delayed dose Minimize constipation Asses for *Helicobacter pylori* infection	Use Parcopa, crush Sinemet, or make liquid Sinemet Substitute standard Sinemet for some of the Sinemet CR Withdraw drugs with anticholinergic properties	Intermittent subcutaneous apomorphine

B. Optimal peak but early wearing off

Nonpharmacologic Approaches	Drugs to Alter Formulation or Dose	Drugs to Add
	Decrease dose and increase frequency of standard Sinemet Substitute Sinemet CR for some of the standard Sinemet	Dopamine agonist MAO-B inhibitor Amantadine COMT inhibitor

C. Optimal peak but unpredictable offs

Nonpharmacologic Approaches	Drugs to Alter Formulation or Dose	Drugs to Add
Adjust time of medications with meals and avoid high-protein meals or redistribute the amount of protein in diet Deep brain stimulation procedure	Substitute or add rapid-dissolving tablet or liquid Sinemet Switch to a different dopamine agonist if already on one Consider continuous infusion of levodopa or apomorphine	COMT inhibitor Dopamine agonist if not using one

D. Freezing

Nonpharmacologic Approaches	Drugs to Alter Formulation or Dose	Drugs to Add
Gait modifications (use visual cues such as walkover lines, tapping, rhythmic commands, rocking; use rolling walker) Physical therapy	Due to the difficulty in directly treating this complication, adjust current medications based on other PD symptoms. Guide changes based on the following: • On freezing, reduce dopamine medications, inject botulinum toxin • Off freezing, increase Sinemet dose or add dopamine agonists	If present, treat anxiety with pharmacologic agents

II. Dyskinesias

Nonpharmacologic Approaches	Drugs to Alter Formulation or Dose	Drugs to Add
Chorea Deep-brain stimulation	*Chorea* Decrease risk of occurrence by lowering Sinemet dose when adding other PD medications Evaluate the value of adjunctive PD medications and discontinue if motor complications outweigh benefit Adjust levodopa formulation, dose, or frequency	*Chorea* Amantadine Propranolol Fluoxetine Buspirone Clozapine
Off period dystonia in the early morning (eg, foot cramping) No recommendations	*Off period dystonia in the early morning (eg, foot cramping)* Add or change short acting to long acting formulations (Sinemet CR, ropinirole XL, pramipexole ER, or rotigotine patch) at bedtime if having nighttime offs Change morning Sinemet CR dose to immediate-release with or without CR	*Off period dystonia in the early morning (eg, foot cramping)* Lithium Baclofen Selective denervation with botulinum toxin
Diphasic dyskinesia Deep-brain stimulation	*Diphasic dyskinesia* Change controlled-release preparations to immediate release; consider liquid Sinemet Increase Sinemet dose and frequency	*Diphasic dyskinesia* Dopamine agonist Amantadine COMT inhibitor

III. Akathisia

Nonpharmacologic Approaches	Drugs to Alter Formulation or Dose	Drugs to Add
No recommendations	Evaluate if due to antidepressant or antipsychotic and decrease dose or change drug	Benzodiazepine Propranolol Dopamine agonist Gabapentin

From Refs. 2, 12, 21, and 22.

Patient Care Process

Patient Assessment:

- Based on reported symptoms and physical exam, document type of symptoms, frequency, and exacerbating factors (clinical presentation table).
- Review diagnostic data and determine if symptoms are adequately controlled or if PD treatment-related complications exist. How does the current UPDRS score compare to previous measurements? Is there evidence of motor fluctuations or dyskinesias?
- Obtain a medication history. What treatments have been helpful? Is the patient taking any medications that may worsen PD symptoms?

Therapy Evaluation:

- Determine if therapy for motor symptoms of PD are maximizing on time and should be maintained or require adjustment.
- Evaluate for polypharmacy. Is this necessary or can medications be removed?
- Review nonmotor symptoms and evaluate if they are adequately treated. Have QOL measures improved?
- Assess the complete PD pharmacologic profile for efficacy, drug or diet interactions, adverse drug reactions, and adherence.

Care Plan Development:

- Educate the patient about lifestyle modifications that will improve symptoms and sustain independence.
- Recommend a therapeutic regimen that is easy for the patient to follow.
- Provide instruction on how to use medications, and allow the patient to adjust medications for fluctuations in response.
- Refer the patient and family members to further information such as books and websites (eg, http://www.apdaparkinson.org; http://www.parkinson.org). Provide information concerning local PD support groups when available.

Follow-Up Evaluation

- Assess the patient's symptoms and disease progression through the UPDRS and QOL measures periodically. This interval will vary depending on symptom control, stage of illness, and changes to therapy.
- Follow up at least every 6 to 12 months (or earlier) and determine when symptoms are controlled, if the patient is experiencing any drug interactions or adverse reactions, and provide patient education on medications and nonpharmacologic options as appropriate.

Abbreviations Introduced in This Chapter

Ach	Anticholinergics
ADLs	Activities of daily living
COMT	Catechol-*O*-methyltransferase
CR	Controlled-release
DBS	Deep brain stimulation
DDS	Dopamine dysregulation syndrome
GI	Gastrointestinal
ICD	Impulse control disorder
MAO	Monoamine oxidase
NMDA	*N*-methyl-D-aspartate
PD	Parkinson disease
QOL	Quality of life
RBD	Rapid eye movement sleep behavior disorder
RLS	Restless legs syndrome
TRAP	Tremor, rigidity, akinesia/bradykinesia, postural/gait instability
UPDRS	Unified Parkinson Disease Rating Scale

REFERENCES

1. Nutt JG, Wooten GF. Diagnosis and initial management of Parkinson's disease. N Engl J Med. 2005;353:1021–1027.
2. Lees AJ, Hardy J, Revesz T. Parkinson's disease. Lancet. 2009;373(9680):2055–2066. Review. Erratum in: Lancet. 2009; 374(9691):684.
3. Tanner CM, Ross GW, Jewell SA, et al. Occupation and risk of parkinsonism: A multicenter case-control study. Arch Neurol. 2009;66(9):1106–1113.
4. Suchowersky O, Gronseth G, Perlmutter J, et al; Quality Standards Subcommittee of the American Academy of Neurology. Practice parameter: Neuroprotective strategies and alternative therapies for Parkinson disease (an evidence-based review): Report of the Quality Standards Subcommittee of the American Academy of Neurology. Neurology. 2006;66:976–982. Erratum in: Neurology. 2006;67(2):299.
5. Goetz CG. Hypokinetic Movement Disorders. In: Textbook of Clinical Neurology [Internet]. 3rd ed. Philadelphia, PA: Saunders; 2007:Chap.16 [cited 2011 Oct 10]. http://www.mdconsult.com. (last accessed August 15, 2014).
6. Truong DD, Bhidayasiri R, Wolters E. Management of nonmotor symptoms in advanced Parkinson disease. J Neurol Sci. 2008;266:216–228.
7. Blonder LX, Slevin JT. Emotional dysfunction in Parkinson's disease. Behav Neuro. 2011;24(3):201–217.
8. Susatia F, Fernandez HH. Drug-induced parkinsonism. Curr Treat Options Neurol. 2009;11(3):162–169.
9. Fernandez HH. Updates in the medical management of Parkinson disease. Clev Clin J Med. 2012;79(1):28–35.
10. Weiner WJ, Shulman LM, Lang AE. Parkinson's Disease: A Complete Guide for Patients and Families. 3rd ed. Baltimore, MD: John Hopkins University Press; 2013.
11. Horstink M, Tolosa E, Bonuccelli U, et al; European Federation of Neurological Societies; Movement Disorder Society-European Section. Review of the therapeutic management of Parkinson's disease. Report of a joint task force of the European Federation of Neurological Societies and the Movement Disorder Society-European Section. Part I: Early (uncomplicated) Parkinson's disease. Eur J Neurol. 2006;13(11):1170–1185.
12. Horstink M, Tolosa E, Bonuccelli U, et al; European Federation of Neurological Societies; Movement Disorder Society-European Section. Review of the therapeutic management of Parkinson's

disease. Report of a joint task force of the European Federation of Neurological Societies (EFNS) and the Movement Disorder Society-European Section (MDS-ES). Part II: Late (complicated) Parkinson's disease. Eur J Neurol. 2006;13(11):1186–1202.
13. Oertel WH, Berardelli A, Bloem BR. Early (uncomplicated) Parkinson's disease. In: Gilhus NE, Barnes MP, Brainin M, eds. European Handbook of Neurological Management. Vol. 1. 2nd ed. Blackwell, 2011:217–236.
14. Oertel WH, Berardelli A, Bloem BR. Late (uncomplicated) Parkinson's disease. In: Gilhus NE, Barnes MP, Brainin M, eds. European Handbook of Neurological Management. Vol. 1. 2nd ed. Blackwell, 2011:237–267.
15. Zesiewicz TA, Sullivan KL, Arnulf I, et al; Quality Standards Subcommittee of the American Academy of Neurology. Practice parameter: Treatment of nonmotor symptoms of Parkinson disease: Report of the Quality Standards Subcommittee of the American Academy of Neurology. Neurology. 2010;74(11): 924–931.
16. Jahan I, Hauser RA, Sullivan KL, et al. Sleep disorders in Parkinson's disease. Neuropsychiatr Dis Treat. 2009;5:535–540.
17. Pfeiffer RF. Autonomic dysfunction in Parkinson's disease. Expert Rev Neurother. 2012;12(6)697–706.
18. Aarsland D, Marsh L, Schrag A. Neuropsychiatric symptoms in Parkinson's disease. Mov Disord. 2009;24:15:2175–2186.
19. Bakay S, Bechet S, Barjona A, et al. Dementia in Parkinson's disease: Risk factors, diagnosis and treatment. Rev Med Liege. 2011;66(2):75–81.
20. Burn DJ. The treatment of cognitive impairment associated with Parkinson's disease. Brain Pathol. 2010,20(3):672–678.
21. Bhidayasiri R, Truong DD. Motor complications in Parkinson disease: Clinical manifestations and management. J Neurol Sci. 2008;266:204–215.
22. Gottwald MD, Aminoff MJ. Therapies for dopaminergic-induced dyskinesias in Parkinson disease. Ann Neurol. 2011;69(6):919–927.
23. Goetz CG, Tilley BC, Shaftman SR, et al. Movement Disorder Society-Sponsored Revision of the Unified Parkinson's Disease Rating Scale (MDS-UPDRS): Scale Presentation and Clinimetric Testing Results. Mov Disord. 2008;23(15):2129–2170.
24. PD Med Collaborative Group. Long-term effectiveness of dopamine agonists and monoamine oxidase B inhibitors compared with levodopa as initial treatment for Parkinson's disease (PD MED): A large, open-label, pragmatic randomised trial. Lancet. 2014;384(9949):1196–205.
25. Miyasaki JM, Martin W, Suchowersky O, et al. Practice parameter: Initiation of treatment for Parkinson's disease: An evidence-based review. Report of the Quality Standards Subcommittee of the American Academy of Neurology. Neurology. 2002;58: 11–17.
26. National Collaborating Centre for Chronic Conditions. Parkinson's disease: National Clinical Guideline for Management in Primary and Secondary Care [Internet]. London, UK: Royal College of Physicians; 2006 [cited 2011 Oct 10]. http://www.ncbi.nlm.nih.gov/books/NBK48513/ (last accessed September 1, 2014).
27. Clarke CE, Patel S, Ives N, et al. Should treatment for Parkinson's disease start immediately on diagnosis or delayed until functional disability develops? Mov Disord. 2011;26(7):1187–1193.
28. Olanow CW, Stern MB, Sethi K. The scientific and clinical basis for the treatment of Parkinson's disease. Neurology. 2009;72 (21 Suppl 4):S1–S136.
29. Anonymous. Drugs for Parkinson's disease. Treat Guidel Med Lett. 2011;9(101):1–6.
30. Keus SHJ, Bloem BR, Hendriks EJM, et al. Evidence-based analysis of physical therapy in Parkinson's disease with recommendations for practice and research. Mov Disord. 2007;22:451–460.
31. Williams NR, Okun MS. Deep Brain Simulation (DBS) at the interface of neurology and psychiatry. J Clin Invest. 2013;123(11):4546–4556.
32. Gazewood JD, Richards DR, Clebak, K. Parkinson Disease: An Update. Am Fam Physician. 2013;87(4):267–273.
33. Chen JJ, Swope DM. Pharmacotherapy for Parkinson's disease. Pharmacotherapy. 2007;27(12 Pt2):S161–S173.
34. Scottish Intercollegiate Guidelines Network (SIGN). Diagnosis and pharmacological management of Parkinson's disease. A national clinical guideline [Internet]. Edinburgh, UK: Scottish Intercollegiate Guidelines Network (SIGN); 2010 Jan. 61 p. (SIGN publication; no. 113), [cited 2011 Oct 10]. www.sign.ac.uk/pdf/sign113.pdf (last accessed September 15, 2014).
35. Lexicomp Online®, Lexi-Drugs®, Hudson, Ohio: Lexi-Comp, Inc.; January 29, 2015 (last accessed October 20, 2014).
36. Langmead CJ, Watson J, Reavill C. Muscarinic acetylcholine receptors as CNS drug targets. Pharmacol Ther. 2008;117(2): 232–243.
37. Heetun ZS, Quigley E. Gastroparesis and Parkinson's disease: A systematic review. Parkinsonism Relat Disord. 2012; 18:443–440.
38. Connolly BS, Lang AE. Pharmacological Treatment of Parkinson Disease: A Review. JAMA. 2014;311(16):1670–1683.
39. Product information. Symmetrel (amantadine). Chadds Ford, PA. Endo Pharmaceuticals, January 2009.
40. Fernandez HH, Chen JJ. Monoamine oxidase-B inhibition in the treatment of Parkinson's disease. Pharmacotherapy. 2007;27 (12 Pt 2):S174–S185.
41. Ahlskog JE, Uitti RJ. Rasagiline, Parkinson neuroprotection, and delayed-start trials: Still no satisfaction? Neurology. 2010;74(14):1143–1148.
42. Hauser RA. Early pharmacologic treatment in Parkinson's disease. Am J Manag Care. 2010;(16 Suppl Implications):S100–S107.
43. Perez-Lloret S, Rascol O. Dopamine receptor agonists for the treatment of early or advanced Parkinson's disease. CNS Drugs. 2012;24(11):941–968.
44. Voon V, Gao J, Brezing C, et al. Dopamine agonists and risk: Impulse control disorders in Parkinson's disease. Brain. 2011;134(Pt 5):1438–1446.
45. Knie B, Mitra MT, Logishetty K, Chaudhuri KR. Excessive daytime sleepiness in patients with Parkinson's disease. CNS Drugs. 2011;25(3):203–212.
46. Antonini A, Chaudhuri KR, Martinez-Martin P, et al. Oral and infusion levodopa-based strategies for managing motor complications in patients with Parkinson's disease. CNS Drugs. 2010;24(2):119–129.
47. Trenkwalder C, Kies B, Rudzinska M, et al; Recover Study Group. Rotigotine effects on early morning motor function and sleep in Parkinson's disease: A double-blind, randomized, placebo-controlled study (RECOVER). Mov Disord. 2011;26(1):90–99.

34 Pain Management

Christine Karabin O'Neil

LEARNING OBJECTIVES

Upon completion of the chapter, the reader will be able to:

1. Identify characteristics of the types of pain: nociceptive, inflammatory, neuropathic, and functional.
2. Explain the mechanisms involved in pain transmission.
3. Select an appropriate method of pain assessment.
4. Recommend an appropriate choice of analgesic, dose, and monitoring plan for a patient based on type and severity of pain and other patient-specific parameters.
5. Perform calculations involving equianalgesic doses, conversion of one opioid to another, rescue doses, and conversion to a continuous infusion.
6. Educate patients and caregivers about effective pain management, dealing with chronic pain, and the use of nonpharmacologic measures.

INTRODUCTION

Pain is defined by the International Association for the Study of Pain (IASP) as "an unpleasant sensory and emotional experience associated with actual or potential tissue damage, or described in terms of such damage."[1] KEY CONCEPT *Pain is an unpleasant subjective experience that is the net effect of a complex interaction of the ascending and descending neurons involving biochemical, physiologic, psychological, and neocortical processes.* Pain can affect all areas of a person's life including sleep, thought, emotion, and activities of daily living. Because there are no reliable objective markers for pain, the patient is the only person who can describe the intensity and quality of their pain.

Pain is the most common symptom prompting patients to seek medical attention and is reported by more than 80% of individuals who visit their primary care provider.[2] Despite the frequency of pain symptoms, individuals often do not obtain satisfactory relief of pain. This has led to initiatives in health care to make pain the fifth vital sign, thus making pain assessment equal in importance to obtaining a patient's temperature, pulse, blood pressure, and respiratory rate.

EPIDEMIOLOGY AND ETIOLOGY

Prevalence of Pain

Most people experience pain at some time in their lives, and pain is a symptom of a variety of diseases. Thus identifying the exact prevalence of pain is a difficult task. According to the American Pain Foundation, more than 76 million people in the United States suffer from chronic pain, and an additional 25 million experience acute pain from injury or surgery.[2]

Prevalence rates for a variety of different types of pain have been described. Approximately one-fourth of US adults reported having low back pain lasting at least 1 day in the past 3 months.[3] Migraine affects more than 28 million Americans, and 78% of Americans experience a tension headache during their lifetime.[4] Pain resulting from fibromyalgia affects 10 million Americans.[5] Pain ranges in prevalence from 14% to 100% among cancer patients.[6] The prevalence of neuropathic pain is unknown because of the lack of epidemiologic studies. Current estimates suggest that approximately 1.5% of the population in the United States might be affected by **neuropathic pain**.[7] Approximately 25% to 50% of all pain clinic visits are related to neuropathic pain.[8] Central neuropathic pain is estimated to occur in 2% to 8% of all stroke patients.[9]

The elderly, defined as people 65 years and older, bear a significant burden of pain, and pain continues to be underrecognized and undertreated in this population. The prevalence of pain in people older than 60 years is twice that in those younger than 60 years.[10] Studies suggest that 25% to 50% of community-dwelling elderly suffer pain. Pain is quite common among nursing home residents. It is estimated that pain in 45% to 80% of nursing home patients contributes to functional impairment and a decreased quality of life.[11]

The financial impact of pain is considered to be significant. The American Productivity Audit of the US workforce, conducted from 2001 to 2002, revealed that the cost of lost productivity due to arthritis, back pain, headache, and other musculoskeletal pain was approximately $61.2 billion per year.[12]

Undertreatment of Pain

Despite the growing emphasis on pain management, pain often remains undertreated and continues to be a problem in hospitals, long-term care facilities, and the community. In one series of reports, 50% of seriously ill hospitalized patients reported pain; however, 15% were dissatisfied with pain control, and some remained in pain after hospitalization.[13,14]

Misconceptions about pain management, both from patients and health care providers, are among the most common causes of analgesic failure. Concerns about opiate misuse, abuse, and diversion also contribute to less than optimal pain management and cause providers to exercise caution when prescribing opiates for pain. Misunderstandings about the terms **addiction, physical dependence, tolerance,** and **pseudoaddiction** are additional obstacles to optimal pain management.

Patients might present barriers to pain management by not reporting pain symptoms because of fear of becoming addicted or because of cultural beliefs. Elderly patients might not report pain for a variety of reasons including belief that pain is something they must live with, fear of consequences (eg, hospitalization, loss of independence), or fear that the pain might be forecasting impending illness, inability to understand terminology used by health care providers, or a belief that showing pain is unacceptable behavior.

PATHOPHYSIOLOGY

Types of Pain

Several distinct types of pain have been described, for example, nociceptive, inflammatory, neuropathic, and functional.[15] Nociceptive pain is a transient pain in response to a noxious stimulus at **nociceptors** that are located in cutaneous tissue, bone, muscle, connective tissue, vessels, and viscera. Nociceptors are classified as thermal, chemical, or mechanical. The nociceptive system extends from the receptors in the periphery to the spinal cord, brainstem, to the cerebral cortex where pain sensation is perceived. This system is a key physiologic function that prevents further tissue damage due to the body's autonomic withdrawal reflex. When tissue damage occurs despite the nociceptive defense system, inflammatory pain ensues. The body now changes focus from protecting against painful stimuli to protecting the injured tissue. The inflammatory response contributes to pain hypersensitivity that serves to prevent contact or movement of the injured part until healing is complete, thus reducing further damage.

Neuropathic pain is defined as spontaneous pain and hypersensitivity to pain associated with damage to or pathologic changes in the peripheral nervous system as in painful diabetic peripheral neuropathy (DPN), adult immune deficiency syndrome (AIDS), polyneuropathy, postherpetic neuralgia (PHN), or in the central nervous system (CNS), which occurs with spinal cord injury, multiple sclerosis, and stroke. Functional pain, a relatively newer concept, is pain sensitivity due to an abnormal processing or functioning of the CNS in response to normal stimuli. Several conditions considered to have this abnormal sensitivity or hyperresponsiveness include fibromyalgia and irritable bowel syndrome.

Mechanisms of Pain

► *Pain Transmission*

The mechanisms of nociceptive pain are well defined and provide a foundation for the understanding of other types of pain.[16] Following nociceptor stimulation, tissue injury causes the release of substances (bradykinin, serotonin, potassium, histamine, prostaglandins, and substance P) that might further sensitize and/or activate nociceptors. Nociceptor activation produces action potentials (transduction) that are transmitted along myelinated Aδ-fibers and unmyelinated C-fibers to the spinal cord. The Aδ-fibers are responsible for first, fast, sharp pain and release excitatory amino acids that activate α-amino-3-hydroxy-5-methylisoxazole-4-propionic acid (AMPA) receptors in the dorsal horn. The C-fibers produce second pain, which is described as dull, aching, burning, and diffuse. These nerve fibers synapse in the dorsal horn of the spinal cord, where several neurotransmitters are released including glutamate, substance P, and calcitonin gene-related peptide. Transmission of pain signals continues along the spinal cord to the thalamus, which serves as the pain relay center, and eventually to the cortical regions of the brain where pain is perceived.

► *Pain Modulation*

Modulation of pain (inhibition of nociceptive impulses) can occur by a number of processes. Based on the gate-control theory, pain modulation might occur at the level of the dorsal horn.[17] Because the brain can process only a limited number of signals at one time, other sensory stimuli at nociceptors might alter pain perception. This theory supports the effectiveness of counterirritants and transcutaneous electrical nerve stimulation (TENS) in pain management. Pain modulation can occur through several other complex processes. The endogenous opiate system consists of endorphins (enkephalins, dynorphins, and β-endorphins) that interact with μ-, δ-, and κ-receptors throughout the CNS to inhibit pain impulses and alter perception. The CNS also includes inhibitory descending pathways from the brain that can attenuate pain transmission in the dorsal horn. Neurotransmitters involved in this descending system include endogenous opioids, serotonin, norepinephrine, γ-aminobutyric acid (GABA), and neurotensin. The perception of pain involves not only nociceptive stimulation but physiologic and emotional input that contributes to the perception of pain. Consequently, cognitive behavioral treatments such as distraction, relaxation, and guided imagery can reduce pain perception by altering pain processing in the cortex.

► *Peripheral Sensitization, Central Sensitization, and Windup*

Under normal conditions, a balance generally exists between excitatory and inhibitory neurotransmission. Changes in this balance can occur both peripherally and centrally, resulting in exaggerated responses and sensitization, such as that observed in inflammatory, neuropathic, or functional chronic pain. Pain in these settings might occur spontaneously without any stimulus or might be evoked by a stimulus. Evoked pain might arise from a stimulus that normally does not cause pain (**allodynia**) such as a light touch in neuropathic pain. **Hyperalgesia**, an exaggerated and/or prolonged pain response to a stimulus that normally causes pain, can also occur as a result of increased sensitivity in the CNS.

During normal pain transmission, the AMPA receptors are activated, but the *N*-methyl-D-aspartate (NMDA) receptor is blocked by magnesium.[16] Repeated nerve depolarization causes release of the magnesium block, allowing the influx of calcium and sodium, and results in excessive excitability and amplification of signals. Continued input from C-fibers and subsequent increases in substance P and glutamate causes the activation of the NMDA receptor, a process referred to as windup. Windup increases the number and responsiveness of neurons in the dorsal horn irrespective of the input from the periphery. Recruitment of neurons not normally involved in pain transmission or spread occurs, leading to allodynia, hyperalgesia, and spread to uninjured tissues.[18] The windup phenomenon supports the observation that untreated acute pain can lead to chronic pain and the belief that pain processes are plastic and not static.

CLINICAL PRESENTATION AND DIAGNOSIS

Classification of Pain

Pain has always been described as a symptom. However, recent advances in the understanding of neural mechanisms have demonstrated that unrelieved pain might lead to changes in the nervous system known as neural plasticity. Because these changes reflect a process that influences a physiologic response, pain, particularly chronic pain, might be considered a disease unto itself.

Pain can be divided into two broad categories: acute and chronic pain. Acute pain is also referred to as adaptive pain because it serves to protect the individual from further injury or promote healing.[17] However, chronic pain has been called maladaptive, a pathologic function of the nervous system or pain as a disease.

► *Acute Pain*

Acute pain is pain that occurs as a result of injury or surgery and is usually self-limited, subsiding when the injury heals. Untreated acute pain can produce physiologic symptoms including tachypnea, tachycardia, and increased sympathetic nervous system activity, such as pallor, diaphoresis, and pupil dilation. Furthermore, poorly treated pain can cause psychological stress and compromise the immune system due to the release of endogenous corticosteroids. Somatic acute pain arises from injury to skin, bone, joint, muscle, and connective tissue, and it is generally localized to the site of injury. Visceral pain involves injury to nerves on internal organs (eg, intestines, liver) and can present as diffuse, poorly differentiated, and often referred pain. Acute pain should be treated aggressively, even before the diagnosis is established, except in conditions of head or abdominal injury where pain might assist in the differential diagnosis.

► *Chronic Pain*

Chronic pain persists beyond the expected normal time for healing and serves no useful physiologic purpose. Chronic pain might be nociceptive, inflammatory, neuropathic, or functional in origin; however, all forms share some common characteristics. Chronic pain can be intermittent or persistent, or both. Physiologic responses observed in acute pain are often absent in chronic pain; however, other symptoms might predominate. The four main effects of chronic pain include (a) effects on the physical function, (b) psychological changes, (c) social consequences, and (d) societal consequences. Effects of chronic pain on physical function include impaired activities of daily living and sleep disturbances. Psychological components of chronic pain might include depression, anxiety, anger, and loss of self-esteem. As a result of physical and psychological changes, social consequences might ensue, such as changes in relationships with friends and family, intimacy, and isolation. Management of chronic pain should be multimodal and might involve cognitive interventions, physical manipulations, pharmacologic agents, surgical intervention, and regional or spinal anesthesia.

Chronic Malignant Pain Chronic malignant pain is associated with a progressive disease that is usually life threatening such as cancer, AIDS, progressive neurologic diseases, end-stage organ failure, and dementia.[19] The goal is pain alleviation and prevention, often through a systematic and stepwise approach. Tolerance, dependence, and addiction are often not a concern due to the terminal nature of the illness.

Chronic Nonmalignant Pain Pain not associated with a life-threatening disease and lasting more than 6 months beyond the healing period is referred to as chronic nonmalignant pain. Pain associated with low back pain, osteoarthritis, previous bone fractures, peripheral vascular disease, genitourinary infection, rheumatoid arthritis, and coronary heart disease is considered nonmalignant. The numerous causes of this type of chronic pain make treatment complex and involves a multidisciplinary approach. Treatment is initially conservative but might involve the use of more potent analgesics including opiates in psychologically healthy patients.[20]

Neuropathic Pain Neuropathic pain is considered to be a type of chronic nonmalignant pain involving disease of the central and peripheral nervous systems. Neuropathic pain might be broadly categorized as peripheral or central in nature. Examples of neuropathic pain include PHN, which is pain associated with acute herpetic neuralgia or an acute shingles outbreak. Peripheral or polyneuropathic pain is associated with the distal polyneuropathies of diabetes, human immunodeficiency virus (HIV), and chemotherapeutic agents. Types of **central pain** include central stroke pain, trigeminal neuralgia, and a complex of syndromes known as complex regional pain syndrome (CRPS). CRPS includes both reflex sympathetic dystrophy and **causalgia**, both of which are neuropathic pain associated with abnormal functioning of the autonomic nervous system.

The symptoms of neuropathic pain are characterized as tingling, burning, shooting, stabbing, electric shock–like quality, or radiating pain. The patient might describe either a constant dull throbbing or burning pain, or an intermittent pain that is stabbing or shooting. Damage to the peripheral nerves might frequently be referred to the body region innervated by those nerves.

Clinical Presentation and Diagnosis of Pain

General

Patients may be in acute distress (acute pain) or have no signs or symptoms of suffering (chronic pain).

Symptoms

Pain is described based on the following characteristics: onset, duration, location, quality, severity, and intensity. Other symptoms may include anxiety, depression, fatigue, anger, fear, and insomnia.

Signs

Acute pain may cause hypertension, tachycardia, diaphoresis, mydriasis, and pallor.

Diagnosis

The patient is the only person who can describe the intensity and quality of their pain. There are no laboratory tests that can diagnose pain.

Pain Assessment

Effective pain management begins with a thorough and accurate assessment of the patient. Even though pain is a common presenting complaint, lack of regular assessment and reassessment of pain remains a problem and contributes to the undertreatment of pain.[21]

▶ *Pain Assessment Guidelines/Regulations for Specific Practice Settings*

Screening for pain should be a part of a routine assessment, which has led several organizations such as the Veterans Health Administration (VHA) and the American Pain Society (APS) to declare pain as the fifth vital sign. Many states have adopted a bill of rights for patients in pain. In 2001, the Joint Commission on Accreditation of Health Care Organizations (JCAHO) incorporated pain as the fifth vital sign in its accreditation standards.[22] According to the JCAHO, patients have a right to appropriate assessment and management of their pain and education regarding their pain. KEY CONCEPT *Following initial assessment of pain, reassessment should be done as needed based on medication choice and the clinical situation.*

▶ *Methods of Pain Assessment*

A patient-oriented approach to pain is essential, and methods do not differ greatly from those used in other medical conditions. A comprehensive history (medical, family, and psychological) and physical are necessary to evaluate underlying disease processes for the source of pain and other factors contributing to the pain.[18] A thorough assessment of the characteristics of the pain should be completed, including questions about the pain (onset, duration, location, quality, severity, and intensity), pain relief efforts, and efficacy and side effects of current and past treatments for pain. A common mnemonic for pain assessment is PQRST (Palliative/precipitating, Quality, Radiation, Severity, and Time).[23] Some clinicians have suggested the addition of U ("you") to this mnemonic.[24] During the pain interview, the impact of the pain on the patient's functional status, behavior, and psychological states should also be assessed. Evaluation of psychological status is especially important in patients with chronic pain because depression and other affective disorders might be common comorbid conditions. A history of drug and alcohol use should be elicited due to the potential for addiction in patients who take opiates or other pain medications with a potential for abuse. Other conditions, such as renal or hepatic dysfunction, diabetes, and conditions that affect bowel function, can influence therapy choices and goals. A discussion of the patient's expectations and goals with respect to pain management (level of pain relief, functional status, and quality of life) should also be part of any pain interview.

▶ *Pain Assessment Tools*

Pain, particularly acute pain, might be accompanied by physiologic signs and symptoms, but there are no reliable objective markers for pain. Many tools have been designed for assessing the severity of pain including rating scales and multidimensional pain assessment tools.

Rating scales provide a simple way to classify the intensity of pain, and they should be selected based on the patient's ability to communicate (Figure 34–1).[25] Numeric scales are widely used and ask patients to rate their pain on a scale of 0 to 10, with 0 indicating no pain and 10 being the worst pain possible. Using this type of scale, 1 to 3 is considered mild pain, 4 to 6 is moderate pain, and 7 to 10 is severe pain. The visual analog scale (VAS) is similar to the numerical scale in that it requires patients to place a mark on a 10-cm line where one end is no pain, and the worst possible pain is on the other end. For patients who have difficulty assigning a number to their pain, a categorical scale might be an option to communicate the intensity of the pain experience. Examples of this include a simple descriptive list of words and the Wong–Baker FACES of Pain Rating Scale.[26]

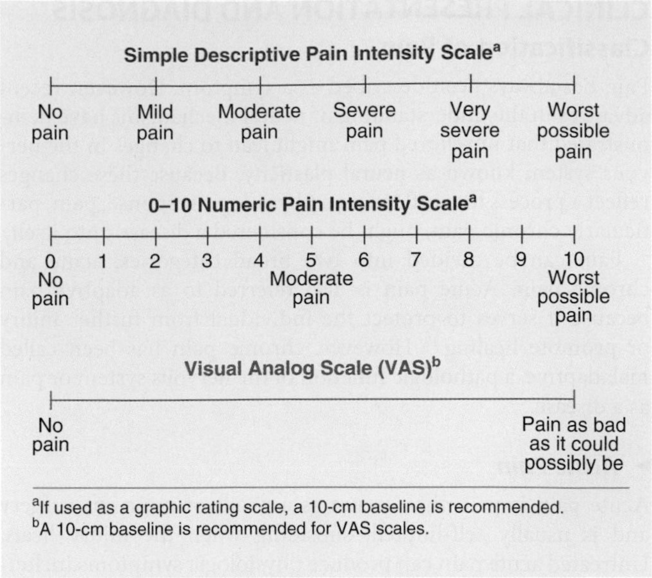

FIGURE 34–1. Pain rating scales. (From U.S. Department of Health and Human Services, Agency for Health Care Policy and Research. Clinical practice guideline, cancer pain management. Rockville, MD: AHCPR; 1994 [cited 2014 Nov 6]. http://www.ncbi.nlm.nih.gov/books/bookres.fcgi/hstat6/f37_capcf4.gif.)

Multidimensional assessment tools obtain information about the pain and impact on quality of life, but they are often more time consuming to complete. Examples of these types of tools include the Initial Pain Assessment Tool, Brief Pain Inventory, McGill Pain Questionnaire, the Neuropathic Pain Scale, and the Oswestry Disability Index.[27–31]

▶ *Pain Assessment in Challenging Populations*

Children Pain interviews can be conducted with children as young as 3 or 4 years of age; however, communication might be limited by vocabulary.[32] Terms familiar to children such as *hurt, owie,* or *boo boo* might be used to describe pain. The VAS is best used with children older than 7 years. Other scales based on numbers of objects (eg, pokers chips), increasing color intensity, or faces of pain might be helpful for children between 4 and 7 years of age. In children younger than 3 to 4 years, behavioral or physiologic measures, such as pulse or respiratory rate, might be more appropriate. Pain assessment in newborns and infants relies on behavioral observation for such clues as vocalizations (crying and fussing), facial expressions, body movements (flailing of limbs and pulling legs in), withdrawal, and change in eating and sleeping habits.[33] Preschool children experiencing pain might become clingy, lose motor and verbal skills, and start to deny pain because treatment might be linked to discomfort or punishment. School-age children might exhibit aggressiveness, nightmares, anxiety, and withdrawal when in pain; adolescents might respond to pain with oppositional behavior and depression.

Elderly Most of the previously discussed pain scales can be used in older persons who are cognitively intact or with mild dementia. The pain thermometer and FACES of pain have been studied in older persons. In persons with moderate to severe dementia or those who are nonverbal, observation of pain behaviors, such as guarding or grimacing, provides an alternative for pain assessment. The Pain Assessment in Advanced Dementia (PAINAD)

Patient Encounter, Part 1

HPI: A 68-year-old woman who fell on a banana peel while vacationing at the lake sustained an ankle fracture. She is to undergo repair with pin placement

PMH: Hypertension for 18 years; diabetes type 2 for 13 years

FH: Mother had osteoporosis; father had diabetes

SH: Lives with husband; has two grown children

Meds: Lisinopril 20 mg daily, metformin 500 mg three times daily

Pain Assessment: Patient rates pain as 8 on a scale of 0 to 10

Based on the type of injury, what type of pain is this patient likely to experience?

What type of pain management regimen would you recommend in the postoperative period? Explain your answer.

tool might be used to quantify signs of pain and involves observing the older adult for 15 minutes for breathing, negative vocalizations, facial expression, body language, and consolability.[34] Regardless of which pain assessment tool is used, the practitioner should first determine if the patient understands the concept of the scale to ensure reliability of the instrument.

TREATMENT

Desired Outcomes

Prevention, reduction, and/or elimination of pain are important goals for the treatment of acute pain. With chronic pain, elimination of pain might not be possible, and goals might focus on improvement or maintenance of functional capacity and quality of life.

General Approach to Treatment

KEY CONCEPT *Effective treatment involves an evaluation of the cause, duration, and intensity of the pain, and selection of an appropriate treatment modality for the pain situation.* Depending on the type of pain, treatment might involve pharmacologic and nonpharmacologic therapy or both. General principles for the pharmacologic management of pain are listed in the section "Patient Care Process." Two common approaches to the selection of treatment are based on severity of pain and the mechanism responsible for the pain (Figure 34–2). Clinical practice guidelines for pain management are available from the APS, the Agency for Healthcare Research and Quality (AHRQ), the American Geriatrics Society (AGS), and the American Society of Anesthesiologists (ASA).

▶ *Selection of Agent Based on Severity of Pain*

KEY CONCEPT *Whenever possible, the least potent oral analgesic should be selected.* Guidelines for the selection of therapeutic agents based on pain intensity are derived from the World Health Organization (WHO) analgesic ladder for the management of cancer pain (Table 34–1).[35] Mild to moderate pain is generally treated with nonopioid analgesics. Combinations of medium-potency opioids and acetaminophen (APAP) or nonsteroidal anti-inflammatory drugs (NSAIDs) are often used for moderate pain. Potent opioids are recommended for severe pain. Throughout this progression, adjuvant medications are added, as needed, to manage side effects and to augment analgesia. While these guidelines can be useful for initial therapy, the clinical situation (type of pain), cost, pharmacokinetic profile of available drugs, and patient-specific factors (age, concomitant illnesses,

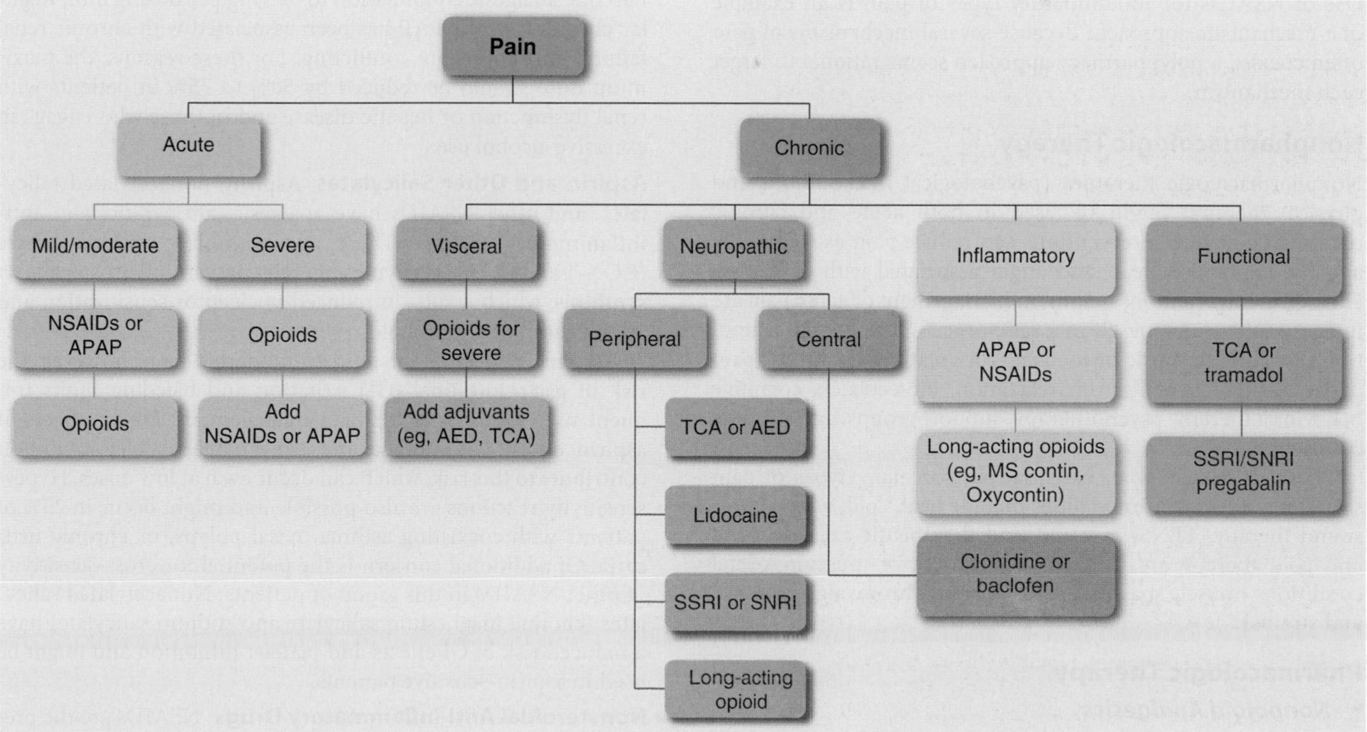

FIGURE 34–2. Pain algorithm. (AED, antiepileptic drugs; APAP, acetaminophen; MS, morphine sulfate; NSAIDs, nonsteroidal anti-inflammatory drugs; SNRI, serotonin norepinephrine reuptake inhibitors; SSRI, selective serotonin reuptake inhibitors; TCA, tricyclic antidepressants.)

Table 34–1

Selection of Analgesics Based on Intensity of Pain

Pain Intensity	Corresponding Numerical Rating	WHO Therapeutic Recommendations	Examples of Initial Therapy	Comments
Mild	1–3/10	Nonopioid analgesic; regular scheduled dosing	Acetaminophen 1000 mg every 6 hours; ibuprofen 600 mg every 6 hours	Consider adding an adjunct or using an alternate regimen if pain is not reduced in 1–2 days
Moderate	4–6/10	Add an opioid to the nonopioid for moderate pain; regular scheduled dosing	Acetaminophen 325 mg + codeine 60 mg every 4 hours; acetaminophen 325 mg + oxycodone 5 mg every 4 hours	Consider step-up therapy if pain is not relieved by two or more different drugs
Severe	7–10/10	Switch to a high-potency opioid; regular scheduled dosing	Morphine 10 mg every 4 hours; or hydromorphone 4 mg every 4 hours	

Data from Refs. 35, 36, and 39.

previous response, and other medications) must also be considered. Pain medications might also be used in the absence of pain in anticipation of a painful event such as surgery to minimize peripheral and central sensitization.

▸ *Mechanistic Approach to Therapy*

Current analgesic therapy is aimed at controlling or blunting pain symptoms. However, diverse mechanisms contributing to the various types of pain continue to be further elucidated. An understanding of these new mechanisms of pain transmission might lead to improvement in pain management as pharmacologic management of pain becomes more mechanism specific. Use of NSAIDs for inflammatory types of pain is an example of a mechanistic approach. Because several mechanisms of pain often coexist, a polypharmacy approach seems rational to target each mechanism.

Nonpharmacologic Therapy

Nonpharmacologic therapies (psychological interventions and physical therapy) might be used in both acute and chronic pain. Psychological interventions can reduce pain as well as the anxiety, depression, fear, and anger associated with pain. Psychological interventions helpful in management of acute pain are imagery (picturing oneself in a safe, peaceful place) and distraction (listening to music or focusing on breathing). Chronic pain patients might benefit from relaxation, biofeedback, cognitive behavioral therapy, psychotherapy, support groups, and spiritual counseling.

Physical therapy is an essential part of many types of pain situations. Treatment modalities include heat, cold, water, ultrasound therapy, TENS, massage, and therapeutic exercise. Heat and cold therapy are utilized in a variety of musculoskeletal conditions (muscle spasms, low back pain, fibromyalgia, sprains, and strains).

Pharmacologic Therapy

▸ *Nonopioid Analgesics*

Acetaminophen APAP, an analgesic and antipyretic, is often selected as initial therapy for mild to moderate pain and is considered first line in several pain situations such as low back pain and osteoarthritis.[36] Mechanistically, APAP is believed to inhibit prostaglandin synthesis in the CNS and block pain impulses in the periphery. APAP is well tolerated at usual doses and has few clinically significant drug interactions except causing increased hypoprothrombinemic response to warfarin in patients receiving APAP doses of more than 2000 mg/day. The maximum recommended dose for patients with normal renal and hepatic function is 4000 mg/day. Hepatotoxicity has been reported with excessive use and overdose, and the risk of this adverse effect increases in those with hepatitis or chronic alcohol use, as well as those who binge drink or are in a fasting state. Due to concerns of unintentional overuse and hepatoxicity, the FDA requires warning labels on OTC APAP products and limited the APAP component of narcotic analgesic combination to 325 mg per dosing unit. Regular chronic use of APAP has been associated with chronic renal failure, but reports are conflicting. For these reasons, the maximum dose should be reduced by 50% to 75% in patients with renal dysfunction or hepatic disease and in those who engage in excessive alcohol use.

Aspirin and Other Salicylates Aspirin, nonacetylated salicylates, and other NSAIDs have analgesic, antipyretic, and anti-inflammatory actions. These agents inhibit cyclooxygenase (COX-1 and COX-2) enzymes, thereby preventing prostaglandin synthesis, which results in reduced nociceptor sensitization and an increased pain threshold.

Aspirin is effective for mild to moderate pain; however, the risk of gastrointestinal (GI) irritation and bleeding limits frequent use of this drug for pain management. Direct effects of aspirin on the GI mucosa and irreversible platelet inhibition contribute to this risk, which can occur even at low doses. Hypersensitivity reactions are also possible and might occur in 25% of patients with coexisting asthma, nasal polyps, or chronic urticaria. Of additional concern is the potential for cross-sensitivity of other NSAIDs in this group of patients. Nonacetylated salicylates (choline magnesium salicylate and sodium salicylate) have a reduced risk of GI effects and platelet inhibition and might be used in aspirin-sensitive patients.

Nonsteroidal Anti-inflammatory Drugs NSAIDs are the preferred agents for mild to moderate pain in situations that are mediated by prostaglandins (rheumatoid arthritis, menstrual cramps, and postsurgical pain) and in the management of pain from bony metastasis, but they are of minimal use in neuropathic pain.

NSAIDs provide analgesia equal to or better than that of aspirin or APAP combined with codeine, and they are very effective for inflammatory pain and pain associated with bone metastasis.[16] These agents are classified by their chemical structures (fenamates, acetic acids, propionic acids, pyranocarboxylic acids, pyrrolizine carboxylic acids, and COX-2 inhibitors). Although only some members of this class have approval for treatment of pain, it is likely that all of them have similar analgesic effects. All members of this class appear to be equally effective, but there is great intrapatient variability in response. After an adequate trial of 2 to 3 weeks with a particular oral agent, it is reasonable to switch to another member of the class. Ketorolac and ibuprofen are available in parenteral and oral dosage forms; unlike other NSAIDs, ketorolac's duration of use is limited to 5 days. NSAIDs demonstrate a flat-dose response curve, with higher doses producing no greater efficacy than moderate doses but resulting in an increased incidence of adverse effects (GI irritation, hepatic dysfunction, renal insufficiency, platelet inhibition, sodium retention, and CNS dysfunction).

Patients at increased risk of NSAID-induced GI adverse effects (eg, dyspepsia, peptic ulcer formation, and bleeding) include the elderly, those with peptic ulcer disease, coagulopathy, and patients receiving high doses of concurrent corticosteroids. Nephrotoxicity is more common in the elderly, patients with creatinine clearance values less than 50 mL/min (0.84 mL/s), and those with volume depletion or on diuretic therapy. NSAIDs should be used with caution in patients with reduced cardiac output due to sodium retention and in patients receiving antihypertensives, warfarin, and lithium.

NSAIDs are classified as nonselective (they inhibit COX-1 and COX-2) or selective (inhibit only COX-2) based on degree of COX inhibition. COX-2 inhibition is responsible for anti-inflammatory effects, whereas COX-1 inhibition contributes to increased GI and renal toxicity associated with nonselective agents. Because the antiplatelet effect of nonselective NSAIDs is reversible, concurrent use might reduce the cardioprotective effect of aspirin due to competitive inhibition of COX-1. For this reason, administration of aspirin prior to the NSAID is recommended.[37] A boxed warning highlighting the potential for increased risk of cardiovascular events and GI bleeding is now required for all prescription nonselective NSAIDs and celecoxib. Stronger warnings about these adverse events are also required on nonprescription NSAIDs. When a NSAID is needed in a patient with cardiovascular risk, the benefits of therapy must outweigh the risks, and the lowest effective dose of the NSAID is recommended.[38]

▸ *Opioid Analgesics*

Opioids are considered the agents of choice for the treatment of severe acute pain and moderate to severe pain associated with cancer.[39] For chronic pain, use of long-term opioids has increased dramatically, however, evidence on the benefits, risk of abuse, and potential harm of long-term use of opioids in chronic pain is limited.[40] Opioids are classified by their activity at the receptor site, usual pain intensity treated, and duration of action (short acting versus long acting).

Selection and Dosing The opioids exert their analgesic efficacy by stimulating opioid receptors (μ, κ, and δ) in the CNS. There is a wide variety of potencies among the opioids, with some used for moderate pain (codeine, hydrocodone, tramadol, and partial agonists) and others reserved for severe pain (morphine and hydromorphone). Pure agonists (morphine) bind to μ-receptors to produce analgesia that increases with dose without a ceiling effect. Pure agonists are divided into three chemical classes: phenanthrenes or morphine-like, phenyl piperidine or meperidine-like, and diphenyl heptane or methadone-like. Partial agonists/antagonists (butorphanol, pentazocine, and nalbuphine) partially stimulate the μ-receptor and antagonize the κ-receptors. This activity results in reduced analgesic efficacy with a ceiling dose, reduced side effects at the μ-receptor, psychotomimetic side effects due to κ-receptor antagonism, and possible withdrawal symptoms in patients who are dependent on pure agonists.

Selection of the agent and route depend on individual patient-related factors including severity of pain, individual perceptions, weight, age, opioid tolerance, and concomitant disease (renal or hepatic dysfunction). Because pure agonists are pharmacologically similar, choice of agent might be also guided by pharmacokinetic parameters and other drug characteristics. Hepatic impairment can decrease the metabolism of most opioids, particularly methadone, meperidine, and pentazocine. Furthermore, the clearance of meperidine and morphine and their metabolites is reduced in renal dysfunction.

Table 34–2 provides a summary of opiate options, but several drugs warrant further discussion. Normeperidine, the active metabolite of meperidine, can produce tremors, myoclonus, delirium, and seizures. Due to the potential for accumulation of normeperidine, meperidine should not be used in the elderly, those with renal impairment, in patients using patient-controlled analgesia (PCA) devices, or for more than 1 to 2 days of intermittent dosing. Methadone is unique among the opiates because it has several mechanisms (μ-agonist, NMDA-receptor antagonist, and inhibition of reuptake of serotonin and norepinephrine). The long-half of methadone (30 hours) permits extended dosing

Table 34–2

Equianalgesic Doses of Selected Opioids

Opioid (Brand Name)	Dose Equianalgesic to 10 mg of Parenteral Morphine (mg): Parenteral (mg)	Oral (mg)
Mild to Moderate Pain		
Codeine (generic, various)	120	200
Hydrocodone (Vicodin, Lorcet)	N/A	30
Oxycodone (OxyContin, OxyFAST, Oxy IR)	N/A	20
Meperidine (Demerol)	100	400
Moderate to Severe Pain		
Morphine (Roxanol, MS Contin, Kadian, Avinza)	10	30
Hydromorphone (Dilaudid)	1.5	7.5
Oxymorphone (Opana, Opana SR, Numorphan)	1	N/A
Levorphanol (Levo-Dromoran)	2	4
Fentanyl (Duragesic)	0.1–0.2	N/A[a]
Methadone (Dolophine)	10[b]	3–5[b]

[a]Transdermal: 100 mcg/hour = 2–4 mg/hour of IV morphine.

[b]Dosage calculations when converting from morphine to methadone are not linear. The equianalgesic dose of methadone will decrease progressively as the morphine equivalents increase (Table 34–4).

Data from Refs. 24, 39, 42, and 43

intervals; however, the potential for accumulation with repeated dosing often results in challenging dose conversion and concerns for respiratory depression. Another safety concern with methadone involves risk of arrhythmia secondary to QT prolongation. Tramadol is a synthetic opioid with a dual mechanism of action (μ-agonist and inhibition of serotonin and norepinephrine reuptake) and efficacy and safety similar to that of equianalgesic doses of codeine plus APAP. Tramadol has been evaluated in several types of neuropathic pain and might have a role in the treatment of chronic pain. Tramadol is associated with an increased risk of seizures in patients with a seizure disorder, those at risk for seizures, and those taking medications that can lower the seizure threshold. Doses greater than 500 mg have also been associated with seizures. The use of tramadol with other serotonergic drugs (eg, selective serotonin reuptake inhibitors [SSRIs]) might precipitate serotonin syndrome. Although originally thought not to be habit forming, dependence can occur with tramadol.

About 70% of individuals will experience significant analgesia from 10 mg/70 kg of body weight of IV morphine or its equivalent.[16] For severe pain in opiate-naive patients, a usual starting dose is 5 to 10 mg of IV morphine every 4 hours. In the initial stages of severe pain, medication should be given around the clock. Rescue doses should be made available for breakthrough pain in doses equivalent to 10% to 20% of the total daily opioid requirement and administered every 2 to 6 hours if needed. Alternatively, one-sixth of the total daily dose or one-third of the 12-hourly dose might be used. Scheduled doses should be titrated based on the degree of pain. One method involves adjustment of the maintenance dose based on the total 24-hour rescue dose requirement. Alternatively, utilizing dose escalation, doses could be increased by 50% to 100% or 30% to 50% of the current dose, for those in severe and moderate pain, respectively. Once pain relief is achieved, and if treatment is necessary for more than a few days, conversion to a controlled-release or long-acting opioid should be made with an equal amount of agent. Several sustained-release products are available containing morphine, oxycodone, and fentanyl. Some clinicians will reduce the total daily dose of the long-acting dosage form by 25% when initiating a sustained-release product to reduce the likelihood of oversedation. The dose of a pure agonist is limited only by tolerability to side effects. Tolerance might develop to analgesic effects, necessitating increasing doses to achieve the same level of pain relief. Physical dependence will occur with the long-term use of opioids. However, addiction or psychological dependence is unlikely in legitimate pain patients unless there are predisposing risk factors. Pain patients who are undertreated might appear to be drug seeking (pseudoaddiction); however, effective pain management resolves the behaviors. When opioids are used for chronic pain, use of informed consent for chronic opioid therapy, medication management agreements, or pain contracts might be appropriate to monitor the use (prescribing and dispensing) of controlled substances.

Opioids are administered by a variety of routes, including oral (tablet and liquid), sublingual, rectal, transdermal, transmucosal, IV, subcutaneous, and intraspinal. Although the oral and transdermal routes are most common, the method of administration is based on patient needs (severity of pain) and characteristics (swallowing difficulty and preference). Oral opioids have an onset of effect of 45 minutes, so IV or subcutaneous administration might be preferred if more rapid relief is desired. Intramuscular (IM) injections are not recommended because of pain at the injection site and wide fluctuations in drug absorption and peak plasma concentrations achieved. More invasive routes of administration such as PCA and intraspinal (epidural and intrathecal) are primarily used postoperatively but might also be used in refractory chronic pain situations. PCA delivers a self-administered dose via an infusion pump with a preprogrammed dose, minimum dosing interval, and a maximum hourly dose. Morphine, fentanyl, and hydromorphone are commonly administered via PCA pumps by the IV route but less frequently by the subcutaneous or epidural route.

Epidural analgesia is frequently used for lower extremity procedures and pain (eg, knee surgery, labor pain, and some abdominal procedures). Intermittent bolus or continuous infusion of preservative-free opioids (morphine, hydromorphone, or fentanyl) and local anesthetics (bupivacaine) might be used for epidural analgesia. Opiates given by this route might cause pruritus that is relieved by naloxone. Adverse effects including respiratory depression, hypotension, and urinary retention might occur. When epidural routes are used in narcotic-dependent patients, systemic analgesics must also be used to prevent withdrawal because the opioid is not absorbed and remains in the epidural space. Doses of opioids used in epidural analgesia are 10 times less than IV doses, and intrathecal doses are 10 times less than epidural doses (ie, 10 mg of IV morphine is equivalent to 1 mg epidural morphine and 0.1 mg of intrathecally administered morphine).[38]

Combination Analgesics Combinations of opioids and nonopioids often result in enhanced analgesia and lower dose of each. Combination analgesics are frequently used in moderate pain. However, in severe pain, the nonopioid component reaches maximum dosage, and thus the usefulness of nonopioids in this situation is limited. Additionally, the combination products are short acting and often not suitable for chronic therapy. Single agents offer greater dosing flexibility than combination products.

Opioid Allergy True narcotic allergies are rare and should not be confused with pruritus associated with opiate use. Cross-sensitivity between morphine-like, meperidine-like, and methadone-like agents is unlikely. Therefore, when an individual is allergic to one drug in a chemical class of opioids, it is reasonable to select an agent in another chemical class. For the purpose of drug selection in patients with allergies, mixed agonists/antagonists should be treated as morphine-like agents.

Tapering of Opioids Tapering of opioids might be necessary once the painful situation has resolved in patients receiving doses greater than 160 mg/day of oral morphine (or the equivalent) or in those with prolonged opioid use. In these situations, the dose should be reduced by 15% to 20% each day to avoid withdrawal symptoms.

Managing Opioid Side Effects and Drug Interactions Side effects common to all opioids include sedation, hallucinations, constipation, nausea and vomiting, urinary retention, myoclonus, and respiratory depression. Table 34–3 shows management strategies for side effects. The most frequent side effects are sedation, nausea, and constipation. Sedation and nausea are common when initiating therapy and when increasing doses. Tolerance to respiratory depression develops rapidly with repeated doses, and respiratory depression is rarely a clinically significant problem in pain patients even those with respiratory impairment. Constipation is a significant adverse effect to which tolerance does develop, and prophylaxis with stimulant laxatives (eg, senna or bisacodyl) and stool softeners such as docusate is recommended.

Table 34–3
Managing Opioid Side Effects

Adverse Effects	Drug Treatment/Management
Excessive sedation	Reduce dose by 25% or increase dosing interval
Constipation	Casanthranol-docusate one capsule at bedtime or twice daily; senna one to two tablets at bedtime or twice daily; bisacodyl 5–10 mg daily plus docusate 100 mg twice daily; polyethylene glycol 3350 17 grams daily; methylnaltrexone 0.15 mg/kg SQ every other day; naloxegol 12.5–25 mg daily
Nausea and vomiting	Prevention: Hydroxyzine 25–100 mg (po/IM) every 4–6 hours as needed; diphenhydramine 25–50 mg (po/IM) every 6 hours as needed; ondansetron 4 mg IV or 16 mg po Treatment: Prochlorperazine 5–10 mg (po/IM) every 3–4 hours as needed or 25 mg PR twice daily; ondansetron 4–8 mg IV every 8 hours as needed
Gastroparesis	Metoclopramide 10 mg (po/IV) every 6–8 hours
Vertigo	Meclizine 12.5–25 mg po every 6 hours as needed
Urticaria/itching	Hydroxyzine 25–100 mg (po/IM) every 4–6 hours as needed; diphenhydramine 25–50 mg (po/IM) every 6 hours as needed
Respiratory depression	Mild: Reduce dose by 25% Moderate to severe: Naloxone 0.4–2 mg IV every 2–3 minutes (up to 10 mg) for complete reversal; 0.1–0.2 mg IV every 2–3 minutes until desired reversal for partial reversal; may need to repeat in 1–2 hours depending on narcotic half-life
CNS irritability	Discontinue opioid; treat with benzodiazepine

IM, intramuscular; po, orally; PR, per rectum.
Data from Refs. 25, 39, and 42.

Codeine, hydrocodone, morphine, methadone, and oxycodone are substrates of the cytochrome P450 (CYP) enzyme: CYP2D6.[41] Inhibition of CYP2D6 results in decreased analgesia of codeine and hydrocodone due to decreased conversion to the active metabolites (eg, morphine and hydromorphone, respectively) and increased effects of morphine, methadone, and oxycodone. Methadone is also a substrate of CYP3A4, and its metabolism is increased by phenytoin and decreased by cimetidine. CNS depressants might potentiate the sedative effects of opiates.

Opioid Rotation Opioid rotation is the switch from one opioid to another to achieve a better balance between analgesia and treatment-limiting adverse effects. This practice is often used when escalating doses (greater than 1 g morphine/day) become ineffective. In some settings, opioid rotation is used routinely to prevent the development of analgesic tolerance.[42]

Equianalgesic Dosing of Opioid Analgesics Conversion from one dosage form to another or from one opioid to another might be necessary in situations such as ineffective pain control, emergence of side effects, change in patient status, and in formulary restrictions. KEY CONCEPT *Equianalgesic doses should be used when converting from one opioid to another.* Clinicians should be familiar with the equianalgesic dosing and conversion strategies to avoid analgesic failure. Opioid potency is compared using a reference standard of 10 mg parenteral morphine. Switching from one dosage form to another of the same opioid (ie, IV to oral) is relatively simple. The current total daily dose is calculated and the total of the new dosage form is determined using a ratio of the equianalgesic doses. This result is then adjusted based on the usual dosing frequency of the new form. When converting to a sustained-release form of the same opioid, the oral dosage may be reduced by 25% to avoid initial sedation; however, the specific product literature should also be consulted.

The first step in an opioid rotation is to calculate the patient's total daily dose of opioid based on the regularly scheduled dose and the total amount of rescue dose needed in 24 hours. This total is then converted to morphine-dosing equivalents using equianalgesic doses (see Table 34–2). The total daily morphine dose is then used to calculate the daily dose of the new opioid using dosing equivalents from an equianalgesic table. Because cross-tolerance may not be complete between opioids, some references suggest that the calculated equianalgesic dose be reduced by 25% to 50%.[39] If the opioid switch is due to uncontrolled pain, a dosage reduction may not be needed. The calculated equianalgesic dose may need to be reduced more in the medically frail and when converting to methadone.[43,44] Methadone appears to be much more potent than once believed, and morphine-to-methadone ratios vary according to the total dose of morphine taken at the time of making the conversion to methadone (Table 34–4).[45,46] Conversion to methadone is a complex process, and several different strategies have been proposed including a switch of the entire dose in 1 day or a gradual conversion over 3 days.

Patient Encounter, Part 2

Following surgery she was placed on morphine patient-controlled analgesia (PCA). She has been using 55 mg of morphine/24 hours with adequate pain control; however, she has developed redness and itching on her neck that is believed to be due to the morphine.

Current Meds: Morphine PCA; lisinopril 20 mg daily; metformin 500 mg three times daily; lovenox 30 mg subcutaneously daily, until ambulating. She will be discharged to a skilled nursing facility for rehabilitation therapy.

The physician would like to convert her to a combination preparation of hydrocodone and APAP.

What dosing regimen would you suggest?

Recommend a monitoring plan for this patient.

How would you assess pain response?

The patient is concerned about the redness and itching she developed while on morphine. What other interventions or education may be necessary at this time?

▸ *Adjuvant Agents for Chronic Pain*

The role of NSAIDs and opioids in chronic nonmalignant pain has been discussed; however, a review of adjuvant agents for

Table 34–4

Methadone Dose Conversions

Total Daily Dose of Oral Morphine	Morphine:Methadone Factor
< 100 mg	3:1 3 mg morphine:1 mg methadone
101–300 mg	5:1
301–600 mg	10:1
601–800 mg	12:1
801–1000 mg	15:1
> 1000 mg	20:1

Data from Gazelle G, Fine PG. Fast fact and concepts #75. Methadone for the treatment of pain. End-of-life Physician Education Resource Center [Internet], [cited 2014 Aug 31]. http://www.eperc.mcw.edu/EPERC/FastFactsIndex/ff_075.htm, with permission.

Table 34–5

Selected Adjuvant Analgesics and Suggested Dosing

Agent	Dosing Guidelines	FDA-Approved Indication
Amitriptyline (Elavil)	10–25 mg at bedtime with weekly increments to a target dose of 25–150 mg of amitriptyline or an equivalent dose of another TCA	
Duloxetine (Cymbalta)	DPN: 60 mg daily Fibromyalgia: 30 mg daily, may be increased to a target dose of 60 mg/day	DPN, fibromyalgia
Gabapentin (Neurontin)	Initially, 300 mg three times a day up to a maximum of 3600 mg daily, in divided doses[a]	PHN
Pregabalin (Lyrica)	DPN: Initially, 50 mg three times a day; may be increased to 100 mg three times a day within 1 week based on efficacy and tolerability[a] PHN: Initially 75 mg twice a day or 50 mg three times a day; may be increased to 100 mg three times a day within 1 week based on efficacy and tolerability[a] Fibromyalgia: Initially 75 mg twice a day, increase after 1 week to 300 mg to 450 mg/day (in divided doses every 12 hours)	DPN, PHN, and fibromyalgia
Lidocaine 5% (Lidoderm patch)	Up to three patches may be applied directly over the painful site once daily; patches are applied using a regimen of 12 hours on and 12 hours off	PHN

DPN, diabetic peripheral neuropathy; PHN, postherpetic neuralgia; TCA, tricyclic antidepressant.

[a]Dosing for creatinine clearance of ≥ 60 mL/min (1.0 mL/s).

Data from Refs. 47–50.

chronic pain, particularly neuropathic pain, is warranted. Adjuvant analgesics are drugs that have indications other than pain but are useful as monotherapy or in combination with nonopioids and opioids. Common adjuvants include antiepileptic drugs (AEDs), antidepressants, antiarrhythmic drugs, local anesthetics, topical agents (eg, capsaicin), and a variety of other drugs (eg, NMDA antagonists, clonidine, and muscle relaxants).

There is little consensus on the optimal management of neuropathic pain because much of the evidence for treatment effectiveness consists of anecdotal reports or poorly designed trials. Published guidelines have been suggested for the general management of neuropathic pain.[47] Suggestions for first-line therapy include gabapentin or pregabalin, transdermal lidocaine, or tricyclic antidepressants (TCAs) (Table 34–5).[47–50] Newer antidepressants, such as the SSRIs, have fewer side effects but appear to be less effective than the TCAs for neuropathic pain. However, serotonin-norepinephrine reuptake inhibitors (SNRIs), (eg, duloxetine and venlafaxine) have been used successfully for painful DPN. A stepwise approach is suggested for managing the patient with neuropathic pain beginning with the least invasive, effective therapeutic choice and proceeding to the rational use of multiple drug regimens (see Figure 34–2). Choice of agent might also depend on dosing frequency and comorbidities. Data on combination therapy are lacking, and the use of combined treatment is empirical based on the additive therapeutic benefit. Scheduled medication regimens instead of "as-needed" dosing should be used when treating chronic pain, and the effectiveness of therapy should be reassessed regularly. If patients are managed on a multiple drug regimen and changes are indicated, changing only one drug at a time is suggested. Topical agents (eg, capsaicin) might be added to a regimen to reduce the oral medication load, particularly if adverse effects are a problem or if pain is not relieved.

Patient Encounter, Part 3

She was discharged to a skilled nursing facility and is receiving physical therapy and occupational therapy 6 days each week.

Current Meds: Lisinopril 20 mg daily; metformin 500 mg three times daily; lovenox 30 mg subcutaneously daily, until ambulating; hydrocodone/acetaminophen 5/325 mg every 6 hours as needed for pain

Pain Assessment: Patient reports pain of 7 out of 10; worse with movement

Physical therapy notes indicate patient is unable to complete therapy goals due to complaints of pain

Based on this information, what would you recommend as the consultant pharmacist to optimize pain control?

▸ *Complementary and Alternative Medicine*

Complementary and alternative medicine (CAM) is a term used to encompass a variety of therapies (eg, acupuncture, chiropractic, botanical and nonbotanical dietary supplements, and homeopathy). Painful conditions are among the most common reasons

Patient Encounter, Part 4

The patient has been at the skilled nursing facility for 3 weeks and is making progress toward rehabilitation goals. She is walking with a walker almost 200 ft (61 m); however, she complains that her feet feel "very heavy" and feel like pins and needles. As a result, she requests to rest several times during her therapy sessions. During unit rounds, her therapist inquires whether her previous pain medication should be reordered.

Pain Assessment: 0 out of 10

Current Meds: Lisinopril 20 mg daily; metformin 500 mg three times daily; lovenox 30 mg subcutaneously daily, until ambulating 200 ft

What additional recommendations would you have at this time regarding pain management?

Are there any other therapeutic issues that should be addressed?

individuals seek relief from CAM. A variety of dietary supplements have been suggested for painful conditions such as S-adenosylmethionine (SAM-e), ginger, fish oil, feverfew, γ-linoleic acid, glucosamine, and chondroitin. Of these, glucosamine and chondroitin are the most popular and have the most evidence supporting their efficacy. Glucosamine in doses of 1500 mg/day has been shown to be effective in reducing the pain of osteoarthritis by fostering repair of cartilage, and it is recommended by the Osteoarthritis Research Society International (OARSI).[36]

Patient Care Process

Patient Assessment:

- Identify the source of pain.
- Assess the level of pain using a pain intensity scale.
- Review the medical and medication history.

Therapy Evaluation:

- If patient is already receiving drug therapy, assess efficacy, side effects, adherence, and drug interactions.
- Determine if patient has insurance coverage for prescription medications.

Care Plan Development:

- Base the initial choice of analgesic on the severity and type of pain, as well as on the patient's medical condition and concurrent medications.
- Select the least potent oral analgesic that provides adequate pain relief and causes the fewest side effects.
- Avoid excessive sedation.
- Adjust the route of administration if the patient is unable to take oral medications.
- Use equianalgesic doses as a guide when switching opioids.
- Use a dosing schedule versus as-needed dosing.

Follow-up Evaluation:

- Assess the patient for analgesic effectiveness and for side effects at each visit or more frequently, depending on the acuity of the patient's condition
- Titrate the dose to one that achieves an adequate level of pain control.

OUTCOME EVALUATION

Routine pain assessment is essential for evaluating outcomes of therapy. For example, pain goals for acute pain might include "pain scale less than 3." Functional goals such as "be able to play a game with grandchildren," or "be able to knit again" may be appropriate for chronic pain. Assess patients periodically, depending on the method of analgesia and pain condition, for achievement of pain goals. Evaluate the patient for the presence of adverse drug reactions, drug allergies, and drug interactions.

Abbreviations Introduced in This Chapter

AED	Antiepileptic drug
AGS	American Geriatrics Society
AHRQ	Agency for Healthcare Research and Quality
AIDS	Autoimmune deficiency syndrome
AMPA	α-amino-3-hydroxy-5-methylisoxazole-4-propionic acid
APAP	Acetaminophen
APS	American Pain Society
ASA	American Society of Anesthesiologists
CAM	Complementary and alternative medicine
CNS	Central nervous system
COX	Cyclooxygenase
CRPS	Complex regional pain syndrome
CYP	Cytochrome P450 enzyme
DPN	Cytochrome P450 enzyme
GABA	γ-Aminobutyric acid
HIV	Human immunodeficiency virus
IASP	International Association for the Study of Pain
IM	Intramuscular
JCAHO	Joint Commission on Accreditation of Healthcare Organizations
NMDA	*N*-methyl-D-aspartate
NSAID	Nonsteroidal anti-inflammatory drug
OARSI	Osteoarthritis Research Society International
PAINAD	Pain Assessment in Advanced Dementia (tool)
PCA	Patient-controlled analgesia
PHN	Postherpetic neuralgia
PQRST	Palliative/precipitating, Quality, Radiation, Severity, and Time
SAM-e	*S*-adenosylmethionine
SNRI	Serotonin-norepinephrine reuptake inhibitor
SSRI	Selective serotonin reuptake inhibitor
TCA	Tricyclic antidepressant
TENS	Transcutaneous electrical nerve stimulation
VAS	Visual analog scale
VHA	Veterans Health Administration
WHO	World Health Organization

REFERENCES

1. International Association for the Study of Pain. IASP Taxonomy [Internet], [cited 2014 Nov 6]. http://www.iasp-pain.org/AM/Template.cfm?Section=Pain_Defi...isplay.cfm&ContentID=1728.
2. American Pain Foundation. Pain Facts and Figures [Internet], [cited 2014 Nov 6]. http://www.painfoundation.org/media/resources/pain-facts-figures.html.

3. Deyo RA, Mirza SK, Martin BL. Back pain prevalence and visit rates: Estimates from U.S. national surveys, 2002. Spine. 2006;31: 2724–2727.
4. National Headache Foundation. Common headache conditions: Migraine and tension-type headache [Internet], [cited 2014 Nov 6]. http://www.headaches.org/educational_modules/np_modules/p1_1a.html.
5. National Fibromyalgia Association. Prevalence [Internet], [cited 2014 Nov 6]. http://www.fmaware.org/site/PageServera6cc.html?pagename=fibromyalgia_affected.
6. Christo PJ, Mazloomdoost D. Cancer pain and analgesia. Ann N Y Acad Sci. 2008;1138:278–298.
7. Dieleman JP, Kerklaan J, Huygen FJ, et al. Incidence rates and treatment of neuropathic pain conditions in the general population. Pain. 2008;137:681–688.
8. Wallace MS. Diagnosis and treatment of neuropathic pain. Curr Opin Anaesthesiol. 2005;18:548–554.
9. Sadosky A, McDermott AM, Brandenburg NA, Strauss M. A review of the epidemiology of painful diabetic peripheral neuropathy, postherpetic neuralgia, and less commonly studied neuropathic pain conditions. Pain Pract. 2008;8:45–56.
10. American Geriatrics Society Panel on the Pharmacological Management of Persistent Pain in Older Persons. Pharmacological management of persistent pain in older persons. J Am Geriatr Soc. 2009;57:1331–1346.
11. Ferrell BA. The management of pain in long-term care. Clin J Pain. 2004;20:240–243.
12. Stewart WF, Ricci JA, Chee E, et al. Lost productivity time and cost due to common pain conditions in the US workforce. JAMA. 2003;290:2443–2454.
13. Desbiens NA, Wu AW, Broste SK, et al. Pain and satisfaction with pain control in seriously ill hospitalized adults: Findings from the SUPPORT research investigations. Crit Care Med. 1996;24: 1953–1961.
14. Desbiens NA, Wu AW. Pain and suffering in seriously ill hospitalized patients. J Am Geriatr Soc. 2000;48:S183–S186.
15. Woolf CJ. Pain: Moving from symptom control toward mechanism-specific pharmacologic management. Ann Intern Med. 2004;140: 441–451.
16. Kral LA, Ghafoor VL. Pain and its management. In: Allredge BK, Corelli RL, Ernst ME, et al, eds. Applied Therapeutics: The Clinical Use of Drugs. 10th ed. Philadelphia, PA: Lippincott Williams & Wilkins; 2012:112-147.-40.
17. Renn CL, Doresy SG. The physiology and processing of pain. A review. AACN Clin Issues. 2005;16:277–290.
18. Heinricher MM, Tavares I, Leith JL, Lumb BM. Descending control of nociception: Specificity, recruitment and plasticity. Brain Res Rev. 2009;60:214–225.
19. Ashburn MA, Lipman AG. Pain in society. In: Lipman AG, ed. Pain Management for Primary Care Clinicians. Bethesda, MD: American Society of Health-System Pharmacists; 2004:1–12.
20. Noble M, Tregear SJ, Treadwell JR, Schoelles K. Long-term opioid therapy for chronic noncancer pain: A systematic review and meta-analysis of efficacy and safety. J Pain Symptom Manage. 2008;35:214–228.
21. Curtiss CP, McKee AL. Assessment of the person with pain. In: Lipman AG, ed. Pain Management for Primary Care Clinicians. Bethesda, MD: American Society of Health-System Pharmacists; 2004:27–42.
22. Joint Commission on Accreditation of Healthcare Organizations. Pain assessment and management: An organizational approach. Oakbrook Terrace, IL: JCAHO; 2000:1–6.
23. Twycross RG. Pain and analgesics. Curr Med Res Opin. 1978;5: 497–505.
24. Gammaitoni AR, Fine P, Alvarez N, et al. Clinical application of opioid equianalgesic data. Clin J Pain. 2003;19:286–297.
25. U.S. Department of Health and Human Services, Agency for Health Care Policy and Research. Clinical practice guideline, cancer pain management. Rockville, MD: AHCPR, 1994 [Internet], [cited 2014 Nov 6]. http://www.ncbi.nlm.nih.gov/books/bookres.fcgi/hstat6/f37_capcf4.gif.
26. Wong D, Baker C. Pain in children: Comparison of assessment scales. Pediatr Nurs. 1988;14:9–17.
27. Brief Pain Inventory [Internet], [cited 2014 Nov 6]. http://www.mdanderson.org/education-and-research/departments-programs-and-labs/departments-and-divisions/symptom-research/symptom-assessment-tools/bpilong.pdf.
28. Initial Pain Assessment Tool [Internet], [cited 2014 Nov 6]. http://www.partnersagainstpain.com/printouts/A7012AF4.pdf.
29. Melzack R. The McGill Pain Questionnaire. From description to measurement. Anesthesiology. 2005;103:199–202.
30. Galer BS, Jensen MP. Development and preliminary validation of a pain measure specific to neuropathic pain: The Neuropathic Pain Scale. Neurology. 1997;48:332–338.
31. Oswestry Disability Index [Internet], [cited 2014 Nov6]. Available from http://thepainsource.com/wp-content/uploads/2010/12/Oswestry-Disability-Questionnaire.pdf.
32. American Academy of Pediatrics. Committee on Psychosocial Aspects of Child and Family Health; Task Force on Pain in Infant, Children, and Adolescents. The assessment and management of acute pain in infants, children, and adolescents. Pediatrics. 2001; 108:793–797.
33. Chiaretti A, Pierri F, Valentini P, et al. Current practice and recent advances in pediatric pain management. Eur Rev Med Pharmacol Sci. 2013;17(Suppl1):112–126.
34. Warden V, Hurley AC, Volicer L. Development and psychometric evaluation of the Pain Assessment in Advanced Dementia (PAINAD) scale. J Am Med Dir Assoc. 2003;4:9–15.
35. World Health Organization. WHO's pain ladder [Internet], [cited 2014 Nov 6]. http://www.who.int/cancer/palliative/painladder/en/.
36. Zhang W, Moskowitz RW, Nuki G, et al. OARSI recommendations for the management of hip and knee osteoarthritis, Part II: OARSI evidence-based, expert consensus guidelines. Osteoarthritis Cartilage. 2008;16:137–162.
37. Kurth T, Glynn RJ, Walker AM, et al. Inhibition of clinical benefits of aspirin on first myocardial infarction by nonsteroidal anti-inflammatory drugs. Circulation. 2003;108:1191–1195.
38. Moore RA, Derry S, McQuay HJ. Cyclo-oxygenase 2-selective inhibitors and nonsteroidal anti-inflammatory drugs: Balancing gastrointestinal and cardiovascular risk. BMC Musculoskelet Disord. 2007;8:73.
39. American Pain Society. Principles of Analgesic Use in the Treatment of Acute Pain and Cancer Pain. 5th ed. Glenview, IL: American Pain Society; 2003:13–41.
40. Agency for Healthcare Research and Quality. The effectiveness and risks of long-term opioid treatment of chronic pain[Internet], [cited 2014 Nov 6]. http://www.ahrq.gov/research/findings/evidence-based-reports/opoidstp.html.
41. Armstrong SC, Wynn GH, Sandson NB. Pharmacokinetic drug interactions of synthetic opiate analgesics. Psychosomatics. 2009;50:169–176.
42. Cleary JF. The pharmacologic management of cancer pain. J Palliat Med. 2007;10:1369–1394.
43. Ripamonti C, Groff L, Brunelli C, et al. Switching from morphine to oral methadone in treating cancer pain: What is the equianalgesic dose ratio? J Clin Oncol. 1998;16:3216–3221.
44. Mancini I, Lossignol D, Body JJ. Opioid switch to oral methadone in cancer pain. Curr Opin Oncol. 2000;12:308–313.

45. Ripamonti C, Bianchi M. The use of methadone for cancer pain. Hematol Oncol Clin North Am. 2002;16:543–555.
46. Gazelle G, Fine PG. Fast fact and concepts #75. Methadone for the treatment of pain. End-of-life Physician Education Resource Center [Internet], [cited 2014 Nov 6]. http://www.eperc.mcw.edu/EPERC/FastFactsIndex/ff_075.htm.
47. Hurley RW, Adams MCB, Benzon HT. Neuropathic pain: Treatment guidelines and updates. Curr Opin Anesthesiol. 2013;26:580–587.
48. Freynhagen R, Bennett MI. Diagnosis and management of neuropathic pain. BMJ. 2009;339:b3002.
49. Zin CS, Nissen LM, Smith MT, et al. An update on the pharmacological management of post-herpetic neuralgia and painful diabetic neuropathy. CNS Drugs. 2008;22:417–442.
50. Dworkin RH, O'Connor AB, Backonja M, et al. Pharmacologic management of neuropathic pain: Evidence-based recommendations. Pain. 2007;132:237–251.

35 Headache

Joshua W. Fleming, Leigh Ann Ross, and
Brendan S. Ross

LEARNING OBJECTIVES

Upon completion of the chapter, the reader will be able to:

1. Differentiate types of headache syndromes based on clinical features.
2. Recommend nonpharmacologic measures for headache treatment and prevention.
3. Determine when the pharmacologic treatment of headache is indicated.
4. Construct individualized treatment regimens for the acute and chronic management of headache syndromes.
5. Monitor headache treatment to ensure its safety, tolerability, and efficacy.

INTRODUCTION

Headache is a common medical complaint with approximately 47% of the adult population experiencing at least one headache per year.[1] KEY CONCEPT *Even when persistent or recurrent, headaches are usually a benign primary condition; secondary headaches are caused by an underlying medical disorder and may be medical emergencies.* Primary headache syndromes are the focus of this chapter. Patients may seek headache care from multiple providers. All clinicians should be familiar with the various types of headache, clinical indicators suggesting the need for urgent medical attention or specialist referral, and nonpharmacologic and pharmacologic options for treatment. KEY CONCEPT *The International Headache Society (IHS) classifies primary headaches as migraine, tension-type, or cluster and other trigeminal autonomic cephalalgias.*[2]

EPIDEMIOLOGY OF HEADACHE DISORDERS

Migraine Headache

Migraine is a primary headache disorder with an estimated 3-month prevalence rate in the United States of 16.6% to 22.7%, based on data from multiple general health surveillance studies.[3] Prevalence of migraine depends on age, gender, and income. In children and adolescents onset typically begins at age 7.9 years for males and 10.9 years for females.[4] In adults, prevalence is much higher in women (17.1%) than men (6.1%), and occur most often between 30 and 49 years of age.[5] The difference in gender distribution is thought to be due to hormonal differences. In households with an annual income greater than $90,000, migraine prevalence is much lower (13.6% women; 4.2% men) than in households with an annual income less than $22,500 (20.1% women; 8.8% men).[5]

Tension-Type Headache

KEY CONCEPT *Tension-Type Headache (TTH) is the most common primary headache disorder and can be further divided into episodic or chronic.*[2] TTHs are underrepresented in clinical practice because most patients do not present for care.[6] The term *TTH* is used to describe all headache syndromes in which sensitization to pericranial **nociception**, noxious stimuli, is the most significant factor in the pathogenesis of pain.[7] Overall prevalence of TTH is approximately 86%, and incidence is more common in women than men. Episodic TTH is the most common type followed by frequent episodic TTH, and finally chronic TTH. Incidence of TTH increases until approximately age 40, then incidence begins to slowly decline.[6] Environmental factors, as opposed to genetic predisposition, play a central role in the development of TTH. The mean frequency of attacks is 3 days per month in episodic disorders; chronic TTH is defined as 15 or more attacks in a 1-month period.[2]

Cluster Headache and Other Trigeminal Autonomic Cephalalgias

Cluster headache disorders are uncommon and severe primary headache syndromes.[2] In the most recent studies the lifetime prevalence is estimated to be 124 per 100,000.[8] Unlike migraine and TTH, cluster headaches are more frequently found in men. Onset most commonly occurs between 20 and 40 years.[2] A genetic predisposition is apparent, although affected individuals often provide the additional history of tobacco use, caffeine intake, and alcohol abuse.[8] Attacks consist of debilitating, unilateral head pains that occur in series lasting up to months at a time but may abate for extended periods, resulting in months or years between occurrences. In rare instances, cluster headache can be a chronic disorder without remission.[2]

ETIOLOGY AND PATHOPHYSIOLOGY OF HEADACHE DISORDERS

Migraine Headache

The exact mechanism by which migraines produce headache remains obscure, but the belief that only vascular changes are responsible for the pain is no longer accepted.[9] The vascular hypothesis suggested that intracerebral vasoconstriction led to neural ischemia, which was followed by reflex extracranial vasodilation and pain. Negative neuroimaging evidence for such vascular changes and the effectiveness of medications with no vascular properties make this contention untenable.[7] A neuronal etiology has emerged as the leading mechanism for the development of migraine pain.[10] It is believed that depressed neuronal electrical activity spreads across the brain, producing transitory neural dysfunction.[11] Headache pain is likely due to compensatory overactivity in the trigeminovascular system of the brain. Activation of trigeminal sensory nerves leads to the release of vasoactive neuropeptides (eg, calcitonin gene-related peptide [CGRP], neurokinin A, substance P) that produce a sterile inflammatory response around vascular structures in the brain, provoking the sensation of pain.[10] Continued sensitization of CNS sensory neurons can potentiate and intensify headache pain as an attack progresses.[11] Bioamine pathways projecting from the brainstem regulate activity within the trigeminovascular system. The pathogenesis of migraine is most likely due to an imbalance in the modulation of nociception and blood vessel tone by serotonergic and noradrenergic neurons.[10]

Tension-Type Headache

The pathophysiologic mechanisms producing TTHs are not clearly understood and are likely multifactorial. However, central sensitization to peripheral nociceptive input arising from the pericranial myofascia is the leading hypothesis. The belief that sustained muscle contraction is solely responsible for generating the pain cannot be supported. Muscle tenderness is prominent in this syndrome, but it only reflects a heightened sensitivity to pain. TTH pain is believed to arise by disturbances in the muscles and tissues of the head being misinterpreted due to disordered CNS pain processing.[12]

Cluster Headache and Other Trigeminal Autonomic Cephalalgias

Cluster headache is one of a group of disorders referred to as trigeminal autonomic cephalalgias.[13] This autonomic nervous system dysfunction is characterized by sympathetic underactivity coupled with parasympathetic activation. Similar to migraine, the pain of a cluster headache is believed to be the result of vasoactive neuropeptide release and neurogenic inflammation. The exact cause of trigeminal activation in this intermittently manifest syndrome is unclear.[14] One hypothesis is that hypothalamic dysfunction, occasioned by diurnal or seasonal changes in neurohumoral balance, are responsible for headache periodicity.[7] Serotonin affects neuronal activity in the hypothalamus and trigeminal system and may play a role in the pathophysiology of cluster headache. The precipitation of cluster headache by high-altitude exposure also implicates hypoxemia in the pathogenesis of trigeminal autonomic cephalalgias.[15]

CLINICAL PRESENTATION AND DIAGNOSIS OF HEADACHES

Migraine Headache

Migraine presents as a recurrent headache that is severe enough to interfere with daily functioning. KEY CONCEPT *Migraine headaches are classified as migraine with aura and migraine without aura.*[2] Aura is defined as a transient focal neurologic symptom that can occur prior to or during an attack. These typically present as wavy lines or spots, but can also present as a scotoma.[2] The IHS outlines diagnostic criteria that differentiate migraine with and without aura. Migraines can be triggered by changes in behavior, environment, diet, and hormone levels. Migraines can additionally be triggered by intake of tyramine, aspartame, monosodium glutamate, and nitrites.[16] Migraines occurring 15 or more days per month for a 3-month period or longer, without the overuse of analgesic medications, are classified as chronic migraines.[2] Severe and debilitating migraine pain lasting more than 72 hours is termed status migrainosus.[2]

Clinical Presentation and Diagnosis of Migraine without Aura

Patients experiencing "migraine without aura" may display the following headache symptoms and characteristics:

Two or more of the following are present:

1. Pain interrupts or worsens with physical activity
2. Unilateral pain
3. Pulsating pain
4. Moderate to severe pain intensity

One or more of the following are present during headache:

1. Nausea/vomiting
2. Photophobia and phonophobia

Duration: 4 to 72 hours (treated or not treated)

Criteria for diagnosis: Five or more attacks fulfilling above criteria are necessary

Laboratory assessments that may be helpful in excluding medical comorbidities: Complete blood count (CBC), chemistry panel, thyroid function tests (TFTs), erythrocyte sedimentation rate (ESR)

Clinical Presentation and Diagnosis of Migraine with Aura

Patients experiencing "migraine with aura" may display the following headache symptoms and characteristics:

One or more of the following present with no motor weakness:

1. Visual
2. Sensory
3. Speech and/or language
4. Motor
5. Brainstem
6. Retinal

Two or more of the following:

1. At least one aura symptom that spreads gradually over at least 5 minutes
2. Individual aura symptoms last 5 to 60 minutes
3. At least one aura symptom is unilateral
4. The aura is accompanied or followed by a headache within 60 minutes

Criteria for diagnosis: Two or more attacks fulfilling above criteria are necessary

Clinical Presentation and Diagnosis of Tension-Type Headache

Patients experiencing TTH may display the following headache symptoms and characteristics:

Two or more of the following present and are not aggravated by routine physical activity:

1. Bilateral pain
2. Nonpulsating pain
3. Mild or moderate pain intensity

Both of the following:

1. No nausea or vomiting (anorexia possible)
2. Either photophobia or phonophobia (not both)

Duration: 30 minutes to 7 days

Criteria for diagnosis: 10 or more attacks fulfilling above criteria occurring on average less than 1 day per month are necessary

Tension-Type Headache

TTH pain differs from migraine pain in that it is usually reported to be mild to moderate in severity, nonpulsating, and bilateral.[6] The pain is described by sufferers as a band-like tightness or pressure around the head. No transient neurologic deficits are noted, and systemic symptoms are rare. TTHs occurring more than 15 days per month for more than 3 months, without evidence medication overuse, would be classified as chronic TTH.[2]

Cluster Headache

Pain associated with cluster headache differs from migraine and TTH in that it is severe, intermittent, and short in duration.[7] Headaches typically occur at night, but attacks may occur multiple times per day.[14] The pain is usually unilateral, but, unlike migraine, it is not described as pulsatile.[7] Aura is not a feature, and pain intensity peaks early after onset, although it may persist for hours.[7] The headache is described as explosive and excruciating. A constellation of features, ascribed to parasympathetic overactivity, can be seen, such as ipsilateral conjunctival injection and lacrimation, rhinorrhea, and sweating.[14] Cluster headache patients tend to become excited and restless during attacks, rather than seeking quiet and solitude as in migraine.[13]

Clinical Presentation and Diagnosis of Cluster Headache

Patients experiencing "cluster headache" may display the following headache symptoms and characteristics:

At least one or more of the following symptoms:

1. Lacrimation
2. Nasal congestion and/or rhinorrhea
3. Eyelid edema
4. Forehead or facial sweating/flushing
5. Sensation of fullness in the ear
6. Miosis and/or ptosis

Or a sense of restlessness or agitation

Duration of pain: 15–180 minutes (untreated)

Frequency of attacks: One every other day and/or up to 8 per day for more than half the time the disorder is active (may have long periods when headaches are inactive)

Criteria for diagnosis: Five or more attacks fulfilling the above criteria

Patient Encounter, Part 1

A 34-year-old woman complains of "almost monthly" headaches around the time of menstruation. She states that the pain is so severe that she has to stay home from work and lie down in a darkened room. She describes her pain as sharp, unilateral, and pulsating. She reports that she can tell when it is about to begin because she can see "floaters" then her peripheral vision begins to fade. She reports using OTC pain relievers to help ease the pain, but she has not had any success thus far.

What type of headache is the patient most likely experiencing?

What characteristics of the headache support this diagnosis?

What are possible causes or triggers of headache in this patient?

What additional information is needed to formulate a treatment plan?

TREATMENT OF HEADACHE DISORDERS

Desired Outcomes

The most important goal of acute headache management is pain relief. KEY CONCEPT *The short-term treatment goal of migraine is to achieve rapid pain relief to allow the patient to resume normal activities. The long-term goal of therapy is to prevent headache recurrences and to diminish headache severity.*[17] Similarly, the goal of TTH care is to lessen headache pain, whereas the long-term goal is to avoid analgesic overuse and dependence.[18] The short-term therapeutic goal in cluster headache is to achieve rapid pain relief. Prophylactic therapy may be necessary to obtain the intermediate-term outcome of reducing the frequency and severity of headaches within a periodic cluster series, as well as to achieve the long-term goal of delaying or eliminating recurrent periods.[19]

General Approach to Treatment

First-line pharmacologic agents include nonsteroidal and opiate analgesics, and serotonin-receptor agonists (triptans).[17] KEY CONCEPT *Pharmacologic treatment of acute headache should be started early to abort the intensification of pain and to improve response to therapy.* The long-term management of headache syndromes focuses on lifestyle modification and other nonpharmacologic therapeutic options; if headaches are severe and frequent, then prophylactic pharmacologic therapy is needed.[17] KEY CONCEPT *Several clinical markers, so-called red flags, have been identified that warrant urgent physician referral and further diagnostic evaluation* (Table 35–1).[20]

Nonpharmacologic Therapy

The successful management of headache disorders depends on comprehensive patient education. Recording headache frequency, duration, severity, possible triggers, and medication

Table 35–1

Headache "Red Flags" Indicating Need for Urgent Medical Evaluation

New-onset sudden and/or severe pain
Stereotyped pain pattern worsens
Systemic signs (eg, fever, weight loss, or accelerated hypertension)
Focal neurologic symptoms (ie, other than typical visual or sensory aura)
Papilledema
Cough-, exertion-, or Valsalva-triggered headache
Pregnancy or postpartum state
Patients with cancer, human immunodeficiency virus (HIV), and other infectious and immunodeficiency disorders
Seizures

Adapted from Refs. 15 and 20.

response in a "headache diary" provides beneficial information for the patient regarding headache precipitants and useful insights for the clinician selecting appropriate management strategies.[21] To prevent future occurrences, exposure to headache triggers (Table 35–2) should be limited.[15] In the acute setting, environmental control can lessen the severity of an attack, so patients may benefit from resting in a dark, quiet area.[22] Behavioral interventions, such as biofeedback, relaxation therapy, and cognitive-behavioral training, are effective and can be recommended for headache prevention. Headache sufferers may also benefit from stress management training.[15] Acupuncture has yielded inconsistent benefits in clinical trials.[23] Although the response is variable, headache patients should be advised to moderate alcohol use and curtail tobacco abuse.[19] All such nonpharmacologic therapies may be useful in augmenting pharmacologic response.

Table 35–2

Migraine Triggers

Behavioral:
Fatigue
Menstruation or menopause
Sleep excess or deficit
Stress
Vigorous physical activity

Environmental:
Flickering lights
High altitude
Loud noises
Strong smells
Tobacco smoke
Weather changes

Food:
Alcohol
Caffeine intake or withdrawal
Chocolate
Citrus fruits, bananas, figs, raisins
Dairy products
Fermented or pickled products

Food Containing:
Monosodium glutamate (MSG): Asian food, seasoned salt
Nitrites: processed meats
Saccharin/aspartame: diet soda or diet food
Sulfites: shrimp
Tyramine: cheese, wine, organ meats
Yeast: breads

Medications:
Cimetidine
Estrogen or oral contraceptives
Indomethacin
Nifedipine
Nitrates
Reserpine
Theophylline
Withdrawal due to overuse of analgesics, benzodiazepines, decongestants, or ergotamines

Adapted from Refs. 15 and 16.

Patient Encounter, Part 2: Medical History, Physical Examination, and Diagnostic Tests

PMH: Hypertension (HTN)

FH: Father living, age 67 years: HTN, diabetes mellitus; mother living, age 62 years: migraine headaches; two sisters in good health

SH: Recently divorced; medical lab technician; former smoker; "social" alcohol intake (one to two mixed drinks on weekends), three to four cups of coffee per day

Meds: Hydrochlorothiazide/triamterene 50/25 mg orally per day; ibuprofen 200 mg, two tablets orally every 4 to 6 hours as needed for headache

ROS: Headache, moderate-severe intensity, sensitivity to light; no dizziness; no chest pain or palpitations; no shortness of breath with exertion; no weakness or joint discomfort

PE:

VS: BP 143/81, P 91, RR 18, T 37.0°C (98.6°F) oral

HEENT: No papilledema, neck tender without stiffness

CV: RRR, normal S1, S2, S4 gallop, no MR

Chest: CTA

Abd: Benign, bowel sounds positive

Neuro: Nonfocal

Labs: CBC and chemistry panel within normal limits

What is your assessment of this patient's condition?

What medical comorbidities or drug therapies may be contributing to her distress?

Identify treatment goals for this patient.

What nonpharmacologic options are needed at present, and what options are appropriate in the long term?

What pharmacologic therapy would you recommend in the acute setting?

Does this patient require long-term pharmacologic prophylaxis against recurrent headaches?

Pharmacologic Therapy

▶ *Migraine*

Analgesics, such as nonsteroidal anti-inflammatory drugs (NSAIDs) and acetaminophen, with or without an opioid, are the initial pharmacologic option for the acute management of migraine headache especially when severity is mild to moderate. If these analgesics prove to be ineffective, and when headaches are severe, then migraine-specific medications, such as triptans, are administered.[17] Early abortive treatment should be the rule. If the orally administered route is selected for medication administration, then larger doses than otherwise required to produce pain relief may need to be provided, due to the enteric stasis and poor drug absorption accompanying migraine attacks. Intranasal, parenteral, and rectal administration can circumvent this complication.[17]

Clinical trial evidence supports many NSAID medications in the acute treatment of migraines with and without aura.[24] Acetaminophen alone or in proprietary combinations with aspirin, opioids, caffeine, or butalbital is also effective.[25]

The triptans are considered specific therapies in that they target the pathophysiology underlying migraine.[17] Triptans inhibit neurotransmission in the trigeminal complex and activate serotonin 1B/1D pathways in the brainstem, which modulate nociception. They also decrease the release of vasoactive neuropeptides leading to vascular reactivity and pain.[26] The triptans are available in intranasal, subcutaneous, and oral dosage forms. The available agents differ in their dosing and pharmacokinetic properties, but all are effective treatments to abort or diminish migraine headache (Table 35–3).[27] Patient responses can be variable; if a patient does not respond to one agent, then another is selected before a patient is prematurely labeled as triptan-unresponsive.[28] The initial severity of headache correlates with symptomatic response; thus administration should be prompt. Relief is usually experienced within 2 to 4 hours. Treatment delay may lead to decreased analgesia through the development of refractory central pain sensitization. Efficacy tends to be dose related, although adverse effects are less so.[29] These medications are well tolerated; the most common side effects are dizziness, a sensation of warmth, chest fullness, and nausea. Rarely, ischemic vascular events may be precipitated by the potential vasoconstrictive nature of these drugs.[30] An initial dose under direct practitioner supervision is indicated for patients at increased cardiovascular risk. Triptans are avoided in patients with migraine associated with neurologic focality, a history of previous stroke, poorly controlled hypertension, or unstable angina. Triptans are relatively contraindicated for routine use in pregnancy.[22] Triptans should not be used with concurrent ergotamine administration.[30]

Ergotamine derivatives produce salutary effects on serotonin receptors similar to triptans. They also impact adrenergic and dopaminergic receptors. Ergotamine tartrate and dihydroergotamine (DHE) are the most commonly used agents.[17] The latter is not available in an oral dosage form. Analgesic onset is within 4 hours, although additional dosing is required if an acceptable

Table 35–3

Comparison of Serotonin Receptor Agonists (Triptans)

Medication (Brand Name)	Dosage Forms	Strength (mg)	Usual Dosage (mg)	May Repeat (hours)	Hepatic and Renal Dosing Considerations (mg)	Potential Drug Interactions
Almotriptan (Axert)	Oral tablets	6.25 12.5	6.25–12.5	2	HI and Severe RI: 6.25 starting dose and ≤ 12.5	Ergot derivatives Substrate: CYP 3A4, CYP 2D6
Eletriptan (Relpax)	Oral tablets	20 40	20–40	2	Severe HI: Not recommended	Ergot derivatives Substrate: CYP 3A4, CYP 2D6
Frovatriptan (Frova)	Oral tablets	2.5	2.5	2	Severe HI: Use caution	Ergot derivatives Substrate: CYP 1A2
Naratriptan (Amerge)	Oral tablets	1 2.5	2.5	4	Mild-mod RI or HI: Do not exceed 2.5; Severe RI (< 15 mL/min [0.25 mL/s]): Do not administer	Ergot derivatives Substrate: CYP (various)
Rizatriptan (Maxalt and Maxalt MLT)	Oral tablets Disintegrating tablets	5 10	5–10	2	None identified	Ergot derivatives MAO-A inhibitors
Sumatriptan (Imitrex)	Oral tablets Subcutaneous injection Nasal spray	25, 50, 100 4,6 5, 20/spray	50 6 5–20	2 1 2	Mild-mod HI: Oral dose not to exceed 50; Severe HI: contraindicated	Ergot derivatives MAO-A inhibitors
Sumatriptan/ Naproxen sodium (Treximet)	Oral tablets Nasal spray	85/500 5, 20/spray	85/500 5–20	12 2	RI (CLcr < 30 mL/min [0.50 mL/s]): Not recommended; Mild to Severe HI: Contraindicated	Ergot derivatives MAO-A inhibitors
Zolmitriptan (Zomig and Zomig-ZMT)	Oral tablets Disintegrating tablets Nasal spray	2.5, 5 2.5, 5 2.5, 5/spray	2.5 1.25–2.5 2.5	2 2 2	CLcr 5–25 mL/min (0.08–0.42 mL/s): Clearance reduced by 25%, use caution. Mod-Severe HI: Not recommended	Ergot derivatives MAO-A inhibitors Substrate: CYP 1A2

CLcr, creatinine clearance; CYP, cytochrome P450 enzyme; HI, hepatic impairment; MAO-A, monoamine oxidase type A; RI, renal impairment.
Adapted from Refs. 15 and 31–38.

response is not achieved. When dosed parenterally, these drugs are usually provided with an antiemetic due to their potential to worsen the nausea associated with migraine. Metoclopramide and chlorpromazine are the drugs of choice in such instances. Intranasal DHE can be self-administered to abort an attack.[17] The outpatient use of subcutaneous ergotamines is limited by the lack of a prefilled syringe form. The same cautions associated with triptan use are also applicable to ergot use in patients at risk for vascular events.

The choice of initial therapy for acute migraine attacks is a subject of debate among specialists. Some believe that nonspecific analgesics should be used first line, whereas others believe migraine-specific drugs should be the choice for patients with severe pain or a history of significant disability.[39] A stepped-care approach within attacks from less to more specific drugs is usually recommended. Once a history of headache refractory to common analgesics is established, triptans should be used as initial therapy.[17] Selection of initial headache treatment is important in reducing the incidence of medication-overuse headache (MOH). This occurs when patients use ergotamines, triptans, opioids, or other combinations for more than 10 days per month. This can also be considered in patients who are using nonspecific analgesics for more than 15 days per month.[40] In patients who present to the hospital with intractable pain, IV metoclopramide supplemented with DHE may be needed. Oral medications in this setting are not used because nausea and vomiting limit their bioavailability.[17] Migraine patients with frequent and severe attacks are candidates for prophylactic treatment.[41]

▶ *Tension-Type Headache*

Most individuals who experience episodic TTHs will not seek medical attention.[2] Instead, they will find relief with the use of widely available OTC analgesics. Acetaminophen products and NSAIDs are commonly utilized. An individual patient may benefit from topical analgesics (eg, ice packs) or physical manipulation (eg, massage) during an acute attack, but the evidence supporting nonpharmacologic therapies is inconsistent.[7] Relaxation techniques can often reduce headache frequency and severity. When pain is unrelieved, prescription-strength NSAID use is required, or the combination of acetaminophen with an opioid analgesic may be necessary. The frequent use of these more potent analgesics should be limited, so that the development of dependency is prevented. As described above, MOH can occur with frequent use of analgesics for TTH. For patients experiencing frequent TTH, prophylactic treatment should be considered.[40]

▶ *Cluster Headache*

Cluster headache responds to many of the treatment modalities used in acute migraine; however, initial prophylactic therapy is required to limit the frequency of recurrent headaches within a periodic series. A therapy specific to cluster headaches is the administration of high-flow-rate oxygen: 100% at 5 to 10 L/min by nonrebreather face mask for approximately 15 minutes.[42] If the pain is not aborted, retreatment is indicated. No long-term side effects are seen with short-term oxygen use. If oxygen therapy is not wholly effective, then drugs are useful adjunctive therapy. Drug therapy is also used when supplemental oxygen is not readily available. The triptan class is safe and effective. Intranasal or subcutaneous sumatriptan as well as intranasal zolmitriptan has demonstrated efficacy in decreasing cluster headache pain.[43] Oral triptans are also effective, but their delayed onset of action may limit their applicability in acute cluster headache treatment.[26] Cluster headache is rapid in onset and achieves peak intensity quickly, but it can be of short duration. Oral agents may have utility in limiting the recurrence of cluster attacks. Intranasal, intramuscular, or IV ergotamine agents are an alternative to triptan use.[7] Repeated dosing may break a cluster series. For those patients in whom triptans and ergotamine derivatives are contraindicated due to ischemic vascular disease, octreotide may be helpful to relieve pain.[43] Octreotide is a somatostatin analogue that has a short half-life and may be administered subcutaneously. Unlike the other abortive agents, it has no vasoconstrictive effects; the most prominent treatment emergent adverse effect is gastrointestinal (GI) upset. Glucocorticoids, provided IV and later tapered orally, are effective when cluster headache attacks are not satisfactorily controlled.[14]

Pharmacologic Therapy for Headache Prophylaxis

KEY CONCEPT *Prophylaxis for headache disorders is indicated if headaches are frequent or severe, if significant disability occurs, if pain-relieving medications are used frequently, or if adverse events occur with acute therapies.*[17]

▶ *Migraine Prophylaxis*

Migraine headaches that are severe, frequent, or lead to significant disability require long-term medication therapy. Prophylactic therapy is also recommended for migraines associated with neurologic focality because it may prevent permanent disability.[17] Although multiple medication classes have garnered Food and Drug Administration (FDA) labeling for migraine prevention, there is no consensus on the best initial therapy (Table 35–4).[41] KEY CONCEPT *The choice of pharmacologic agent is individually tailored to patient tolerability and medical comorbidities.*

Table 35–4

Medications for Prophylaxis of Migraines

Medication (Brand Name)	Usual Dosage (mg/day)	Main Adverse Effects
Antiepileptics:		
Topiramate (Topamax)[a]	50–200	Paresthesias, dizziness, fatigue, nausea
Valproic acid (Depakene)[a]	500–1500	
Divalproex sodium (Depakote)[a]	500–1500	
β-Blockers:		
Atenolol (Tenormin)[b]	50–200	
Metoprolol (Lopressor)[a]	50–200	Fatigue, exercise intolerance
Nadolol (Corgard)[b]	20–160	
Propranolol (Inderal)[a]	80–240	
Timolol (Blocadren)[a]	20–30	
Antidepressants:		
Amitriptyline (Elavil)[a]	10–150	Weight gain, dry mouth, sedation
Venlafaxine (Effexor)[a]	37.5–150	

[a]Level A: Established efficacy.
[b]Level B: Probably effective.
Data from Refs. 17 and 39.

The β-blockers have long been a mainstay in migraine prevention, and many have been proven to be effective in improving patient symptoms. Cautious dosage titration is advised for those patients who do not have other indications for β-blocker use. Comorbid reactive airway disease is a relative contraindication to β-blocker prophylaxis, and patients with cardiac conduction disturbances should be closely monitored. Calcium channel antagonists are often used when patients cannot tolerate β-blockers. None of the calcium channel blockers carry an FDA indication, and their efficacy is considered to be variable. Angiotensin receptor blockers (ARBs) and angiotensin converting enzyme inhibitors (ACEIs) have been evaluated for migraine prevention, but only two, lisinopril and candesartan, have shown possible efficacy.[41]

Low-dose amitriptyline or other tricyclic antidepressants (TCAs) are of proven efficacy in migraine prevention.[41] Due to sedation, these medications are commonly administered at night. Later generation TCAs (eg, nortriptyline) or heterocyclic compounds (eg, trazodone) have fewer dose-limiting adverse effects than the TCAs, especially anticholinergic effects (eg, dry mouth, constipation, and urinary retention), but efficacy has been variable with these agents. Selective serotonin reuptake inhibitors (SSRIs) and serotonin norepinephrine reuptake inhibitors (SNRIs) have been evaluated for migraine prevention, but thus far, only venlafaxine has demonstrated probable efficacy. Caution is advised when using a serotenergic antidepressant and a triptan concurrently, as the combination may rarely precipitate serotonin syndrome, a serious and potentially life-threatening drug–drug interaction that presents clinically with confusion, GI upset, symptomatic blood pressure (BP) changes, and muscle rigidity.[17]

The antiepileptics valproic acid and topiramate are approved for migraine prophylaxis. In patients whose migraine headaches are believed to be related to trigeminal neuralgia, carbamazepine is used as prevention for both disorders.[41] The precise mechanism of action of these agents is unclear, but enhancement of γ-aminobutyric acid (GABA) neuroinhibition and modulation of the neuroexcitatory amino acid glutamate is likely.[44] Divalproex sodium doses are gradually titrated to 1000 mg/day; topiramate is titrated to a maximum of 100 mg twice per day. At these doses, serum drug level monitoring is infrequently needed. These medications are as effective as propranolol at reducing the frequency and severity of migraines and are preferred for prevention in patients intolerant to β-blockers.[45] Topiramate is especially useful in patients who have metabolic syndrome, diabetes, and dyslipidemia because it is unlikely to cause weight gain often seen with valproic acid. Patients prescribed topiramate should be advised to stay well hydrated to prevent dysgeusia, disordered taste, and more seriously, hyperthermia.[46]

Methysergide is an ergotamine derivative that impacts central serotonin balance. Inflammatory fibrosis is a rare but serious, adverse reaction associated with the prolonged use of methysergide. Retroperitoneal fibrosis, pulmonary fibrosis, or fibrosis in cardiac tissue can occur. These conditions may resolve upon drug withdrawal, but cardiac valvular damage can be irreversible. Some experts believe it is the best choice for refractory migraine with frequent attacks, but due to its significant adverse effect profile, it is not marketed in the United States.[47]

Given that migraines can be triggered by changes in hormonal balance, it is not surprising that some women have migraines around the time of menstruation. Often, these migraines can be prevented by starting NSAIDs prior to the beginning of menstruation. Triptans can be tried in patients unresponsive to NSAIDs. Three triptans have been shown to be effective in preventing menstrual migraines. Frovatriptan, naratriptan, and zolmitriptan can be considered, and should be started 2 to 3 days prior to the beginning of menstruation.[41]

OnabotulinumtoxinA has received FDA approval for the treatment of chronic migraine, but the evidence supporting its use is conflicting. In 2008, the American Academy of Neurology conducted an evidence review, and concluded that OnabotulinumtoxinA was probably ineffective for the prevention of migraines.[48] In the PREEMPT 1 and PREEMPT 2 trials, there was a statistically significant reduction in the number of headache days per month when compared to placebo, but the absolute difference between the two groups was only 1.8 days.[49,50]

While evidence is limited, some complementary alternative therapies can be considered for migraine prophylaxis. Petasites (butterbur) has been associated with a potential 60% reduction in number of headaches experienced over a 1-month period when compared to placebo. Studies for riboflavin have been mixed, with some older studies supporting its use for migraine prevention, but some newer studies have failed to show efficacy. Finally, MIG-99 (feverfew) has also shown possible efficacy with very limited trial evidence.[24]

▶ Tension-Type Headache Prophylaxis

The prevention of chronic TTHs uses the same pharmacologic strategies as for migraine prophylaxis. TCAs are a mainstay of chronic therapy. The efficacy of serotonergic agonists remains in question. Although there is little need for muscle relaxants (eg, methocarbamol) in the treatment of acute TTH, they are often provided as a preventive intervention.[7] Combination prophylactic therapies may be needed to wean patients from daily analgesic abuse. Stress reduction techniques may be particularly effective in this setting.

▶ Cluster Headache Prophylaxis

The calcium channel blocker verapamil is the mainstay of cluster attack prevention and chronic prophylaxis.[7] Within an attack period, it is dosed at 240 to 360 mg/day. Higher doses may be necessary to stave off recurrent cluster periods. Beneficial effects may be appreciated after 1 week of treatment, but 4 to 6 weeks is usually needed. Adverse effects include smooth muscle relaxation with the subsequent exacerbation of gastroesophageal reflux and the development of constipation. Caution should be exercised in patients with myocardial disease because verapamil is an inotropic and chronotropic cardiac suppressant.[7] Pharmacokinetic drug–drug interactions must be considered, as verapamil is a potent inhibitor of oxidative metabolism through cytochrome P450 (CYP) enzyme 3A4. Eletriptan is a CYP 3A4 substrate and should not be administered concurrently with verapamil.[7,28] Lithium is another effective therapy to reduce headache frequency in a cluster series and to limit recurrences.[14] The dose administered should be individualized to achieve a low serum concentration (0.4–0.8 mEq/L [mmol/L]). Dose adjustments in the setting of renal disease or congestive heart failure are required.[7] Lithium is contraindicated in patients concurrently prescribed thiazide diuretics and ACEIs or ARBs. Patient persistence with long-term lithium therapy may be hindered by the emergence of tremor, GI distress, and lethargy. Verapamil and lithium doses can be lowered when used in combination with ergotamine. If possible, bedtime dosing is recommended, given the nocturnal predilection of cluster headache attacks.[13]

Patient Encounter, Part 3: Creating a Care Plan

Based on the information presented, create a care plan for the acute and chronic management of this patient's headache. Your plan should include:

A statement of the drug-related needs and/or problems.

The goals of therapy.

A detailed, patient-specific therapeutic plan.

A monitoring plan to determine whether the goals have been achieved and adverse effects avoided.

SPECIAL POPULATIONS

Migraine Headache in Children and Adolescents

Migraine headaches are common in children, and their prevalence increases in the adolescent years.[51,52] The diagnosis and evaluation of headaches is especially difficult in children, given their decreased ability to articulate symptoms. Treatment presents another challenge because medications used for headache management in adults have not been fully evaluated for efficacy and safety in children. Consensus panel recommendations identify ibuprofen as effective and acetaminophen as probably effective in the acute treatment of headache in patients older than 6 years.[4] Aspirin use is avoided due to the risk of precipitating Reye syndrome. Antiemetic therapy can be used alone or in combination with analgesics; promethazine is usually prescribed, as it is less prone to cause extrapyramidal reactions than other antiemetics. For adolescents older than 12, triptans are effective and are beneficial for abortive migraine therapy.[4] Medication prophylaxis for migraines in children and adolescents is understudied. The data are conflicting, and no consensus recommendation for the use of preventive drug therapy exists.[4] Nonpharmacologic interventions and trigger identification and avoidance are advised.

Pregnancy

Headaches are more common in women than in men. Fluctuations in estrogen levels are believed to account for this gender discrepancy. Headaches are common in pregnancy. TTHs predominate; migraine attacks may increase in frequency, but more usually frequency decreases during pregnancy.[53] Recommendations for headache care during pregnancy are based on limited evidence and are largely anecdotal. Because headaches are not associated with fetal harm, reflexive pharmacologic therapy should be avoided and drug treatment choices considered carefully. Standard nonpharmacologic therapies are often sufficient. Acetaminophen is safe for the pregnant woman and her fetus.[53] NSAIDs are avoided late in the third trimester to prevent detrimental prostaglandin alterations leading to premature ductus arteriosus closure. Opioids are second-line agents and should not to be used chronically because they can lead to dependence in the mother and to acute withdrawal in the infant after birth.[53] Centrally acting antiemetic agents are safe and may be useful as adjunctive agents. Corticosteroids may be needed for intractable headache relief. Prednisone and methylprednisone are preferred, as they are metabolized in the placenta and do not expose the fetus. In pregnant women with migraine, vasoconstrictive agents

Patient Care Process

KEY CONCEPT *Individualized treatment regimens for headache disorders are based on: headache type, pattern of occurrence, response to therapy, medication tolerability, and comorbid medical conditions.*

Patient Assessment:

- Assess the patient complaint to yield a detailed description of the headache and to determine if immediate referral for emergency or specialist care is necessary.
- Obtain a complete medical and social history to identify any potential drug–disease interactions or social factors that may influence treatment choices.
- Obtain a family medical history, focusing on headache or mental health disorders in first-degree relatives.
- Complete a review of systems and physical examination to identify causes or complications of headache.
- Determine the type of headache disorder and rule out acute complications.

Therapy Evaluation:

- Identify medication allergies, and obtain a thorough history of nonprescription and prescription drug use to identify potential drug–drug interactions that may arise when selecting acute and prophylactic headache treatment.
- If patient is already receiving pharmacotherapy, assess for appropriateness and efficacy.

Care Plan Development:

- Recommend appropriate pharmacologic therapy to abort headache based on type, patient characteristics, current medication profile, and comorbid conditions.
- When selecting new agents for acute management or for prophylaxis, ensure that the medication is financially accessible.
- Educate the patient on the administration, maximum dosage, and anticipated adverse effects of the prescribed medication, and advise the patient when to seek emergency medical attention.
- Instruct the patient to keep a headache diary to assess therapeutic response.
- Educate on the potential for medication overuse headache.

Follow-Up Evaluation:

- Follow-up should be scheduled within 4 weeks of starting any new medications for headache to assess efficacy.
- As patient becomes more aware of headache symptoms and appropriate agents are on board for prevention and treatment of headache, follow-up can become less frequent (ie, 3–6 months).

such as triptans are relatively contraindicated, even though maternal registry data reveal little teratogenicity. If triptans are considered for acute migraine treatment, sumatriptan, naratriptan, and rizatriptan have the greatest evidence of safe use during pregnancy.[53] Ergot compounds are strictly avoided because they may precipitate uterine contractions and placental ischemia leading to hypoxemia in the fetus. Migraine prophylaxis is considered cautiously because β-blockers and calcium channel antagonists may lead to maternal hypotension and diminished placental blood flow or fetal bradycardia.[53] Antiepileptic drug use in this setting has not been sufficiently studied to allow definitive recommendations.

Outcome Evaluation

Monitoring for therapeutic response is an important part of headache management. In acute management, monitor patients for the pain improvement within 2 to 4 hours and for normal functioning within 3 to 4 hours of treatment initiation. If pain control has not been achieved, additional therapy may be needed for a therapeutic effect. With chronic management for headache prevention, monitor overall headache status every several weeks to months for improvement. A slow decrease in headache frequency is anticipated over this time. Encourage patients to track progress in a headache diary to assist in monitoring improvements in frequency and severity of headaches and corresponding disability. Clinicians monitor attack frequency to determine therapeutic response, seeking a 50% or greater reduction over the course of treatment. Monitoring for adverse effects is central to successful treatment. For acute management, monitor for GI effects from analgesics such as NSAIDs or octreotide, vasoconstrictive symptoms from triptans, and nausea and vascular problems from ergotamine derivatives. Monitor those taking beta blockers for reactive airway disease and cardiac conduction disturbances. Monitor those taking TCAs for sedation and anticholinergic effects such as dry mouth, constipation, and urinary retention. Monitor those taking topiramate for dysguesia, disordered taste, or hyperthermia. Monitor patients taking calcium channel blockers for gastroesophageal reflux symptoms and constipation, and monitor those taking lithium for tremor, GI distress, and lethargy. To ensure optimal headache management, in acute treatment and prophylactic therapy, monitor regimens both for therapeutic outcomes and adverse events, which may impact quality of life and medication adherence.

Abbreviations Introduced in This Chapter

ACEI	Angiotensin-converting enzyme inhibitor
ARB	Angiotensin receptor blocker
BP	Blood pressure
CGRP	Calcitonin gene-related peptide
CTA	Clear to auscultation
CYP	Cytochrome P450 isoenzyme system
DHE	Dihydroergotamine
FDA	Food and Drug Administration
GABA	γ-aminobutyric acid
HTN	Hypertension
IHS	International Headache Society
MAO-A	Monoamine oxidase type A
MOH	Medication overuse headache
MR	Murmur, rub
NSAID	Nonsteroidal anti-inflammatory drug
OTC	Over the counter
RR	Respiratory rate
SNRI	Serotonin-norepinephrine reuptake inhibitor
SSRI	Selective serotonin reuptake inhibitor
TCA	Tricyclic antidepressant
TTH	Tension-type headache

REFERENCES

1. Fact sheet: Headache disorders [Internet]. World Health Organization; 2012 [cited 2014 Aug 22]. http://www.who.int/mediacentre/factsheets/fs277/en/. Accessed December 13, 2014.
2. Headache Classification Subcommittee of the International Headache Society. The International Classification of Headache Disorders, 3rd edition (beta version). Cephalalgia. 2013;33:629–808.
3. Smitherman TA, Burch R, Sheikh H, Loder E. Lipton RB, Bigal ME, Diamond M, et al. The prevalence, impact, treatment of migraine and severe headaches in the United States: A review of statistics from national surveillance studies. Headache. 2013;53:427–436.
4. Lewis D, Ashwal S, Hershey A, et al. Practice parameter: Pharmacological treatment of migraine headache in children and adolescents: Report of the American Academy of Neurology Quality Standards Subcommittee of the Practice Committee of the Child Neurology Society. Neurology. 2004;63:2215–2224.
5. Lipton RB, Bigal ME, Diamond M, et al. Migraine prevalence, disease burden, and the need for preventative therapy. Neurology. 2007;68:343–349.
6. Russell MB, Levi N, Benth JS, and Fenger K. Tension-type headache in adolescents and adults: A population based study of 33,764 twins. Eur J Epidemiol. 2006;21:153–160.
7. Silberstein SD, Lipton RB, Goadsby PJ. Headache in Clinical Practice. London, UK: Martin Dunitz; 2002:21–33,69–128.
8. Broner SW and Cohen JM. Epidemiology of cluster headache. Curr Pain Headache Rep. 2009 Apr;13(2):141–146.
9. Goadsby PJ, Lipton RB, Ferrari MD. Migraine—current understanding and treatment. N Engl J Med. 2002;346:257–270.
10. Hargreaves RJ, Shepheard SL. Pathophysiology of migraine: New insights. Can J Neurol Sci. 1999;26(Suppl 3):S12–S19.
11. Edvinsson L. On migraine pathophysiology. In: Edvinsson OL, ed. Migraine and Headache Pathophysiology. London, UK: Martin Dunitz; 1999:3–15.
12. Jenson R. Pathophysiological mechanisms of tension-type headache: A review of epidemiological and experimental studies. Cephalalgia. 1999;19:602–621.
13. Matharu MS, Boes CJ, Goadsby PJ. Management of trigeminal autonomic cephalalgias and hemicrania continua. Drugs. 2003;63:1637–1677.
14. Bahra A, May A, Goadsby PJ. Cluster headache: A prospective clinical study with diagnostic implications. Neurology. 2002;58:354–361.
15. Minor DS, Wofford MR. Chapter 45. Headache Disorders. In: DiPiro JT, Talbert RL, Yee GC, et al eds. Pharmacotherapy: A Pathophysiologic Approach, 9th ed. New York, NY: McGraw-Hill; 2014:943–958.
16. Martin VT, Behbehani MM. Toward a rational understanding of migraine trigger factors. Med Clin North Am. 2001 Jul;85:911–941.
17. Silberstein SD. Practice parameter: Evidence-based guidelines for migraine headache (an evidence-based review). Neurology. 2000;55:754–763.
18. Silberstein SD, Goadsby PJ, Lipton RB. Management of migraine: An algorithmic approach. Neurology. 2000;55 (Suppl 2):S46–S52.

19. Biondi D, Mendes P. Treatment of primary headache: Cluster headache. In: Standards of Care for Headache Diagnosis and Treatment. Chicago, IL: National Headache Foundation; 2004:59–72.
20. Lipton RB, Bigal ME, Steiner TJ, et al. Classification of primary headaches. Neurology. 2004;63:427–435.
21. Silberstein SD, Goadsby PJ. Migraine: Preventive treatment. Cephalalgia. 2002;22:491–512.
22. del Rio MS, Silberstein SD. How to pick optimal acute treatment for migraine headache. Curr Pain Headache Rep. 2001;5:170–178.
23. Evans RW. A rational approach to the management of chronic migraine. Headache. 2013;53:168–176.
24. Holland S, Silberstein SD, Freitag F, et al. Evidence based guideline update: NSAIDs and other complementary treatments for episodic migraine prevention in adults: Report of the Quality Standards Subcommittee of the American Academy of Neurology and the American Headache Society. Neurology. 2012;78:1346–1353.
25. Snow V, Weiss K, Wall EM, Mottur-Pilson C. Pharmacologic management of acute attacks of migraine and prevention of migraine headache. Ann Intern Med. 2002;137:840–849.
26. Bahra A, Gawel MJ, Hardebo JE, et al. Oral zolmitriptan is effective in the acute treatment of cluster headache. Neurology. 2000;54:291–296.
27. Ferrari MD, Roon KI, Lipton RB, Goadsby PJ. Oral triptans (serotonin 5-HT1B/1D agonists) in acute migraine treatment: A meta-analysis of 53 trials. Lancet. 2001;358:1558–1575.
28. Pringsheim T, Gawel M. Triptans: Are they all the same? Curr Pain Headache Rep. 2002;6:140–146.
29. Deleu D, Hanssens Y. Current and emerging second-generation triptans in acute migraine therapy: A comparative review. J Clin Pharmacol. 2000;40:687–700.
30. Ferrari MD. Migraine. Lancet. 1998;351:1043–1051.
31. Axert [package insert]. Titusville, NJ: Janssen Pharmaceuticals; 2013.
32. Relpax [package insert]. New York, NY: Pfizer; 2013.
33. Frova [package insert]. Malern, PA: Endo Pharmaceuticals; 2013.
34. Amerge [package insert]. Research Triangle Park, NC: GlaxoSmithKline; 2013.
35. Maxalt [package insert]. Whitehouse Station, NJ: Merck & Co., Inc.; 2013.
36. Imitrex [package insert]. Research Triangle Park, NC: GlaxoSmithKline; 2013.
37. Treximet [package insert]. Research Triangle Park, NC: GlaxoSmithKline; 2012.
38. Zomig [package insert]. Hayward, CA: Impax Laboratories, Inc.; 2012.39.
39. Dahlof CGH. Current concepts of migraine and its treatment. Neurology. 1999;14:67–77.
40. Munksgaard SB, Jensen RH. Medication overuse headache. Headache. 2014 Jul;54:1251–1257.
41. Silberstein SD, Holland S, Freitag F, et al. Evidence-based guideline update: Pharmacologic treatment for episodic migraine prevention in adults: Report of the Quality Subcommittee of the American Academy of Neurology and the American Headache Society. Neurology. 2012;78:1337–1345.
42. Rozen TD. High oxygen flow rates for cluster headache. Neurology. 2004;63(3):593.
43. Tyagi A, Matharu M. Evidence base for the medical treatments used in cluster headache. Curr Pain Headache Rep. 2009;13:168–178.
44. Cutrer FM. Antiepileptic drugs: How they work in headache. Headache. 2001;41(Suppl):S3–S10.
45. Bigal ME, Krymchantowski AV, Rapoport AM. New developments in migraine prophylaxis. Expert Opin Pharmacother. 2003;4: 433–443.
46. Topamax [package insert]. Titusville, NJ: Janssen Pharmaceuticals; 2014.
47. Silberstein SD. Methysergide. Cephalalgia. 1998;18:421–435.
48. Naumann M, So Y, Argoff CE, et al. Assessment: Botulinum neurotoxin in the treatment of autonomic disorders and pain (an evidence based review): Report of the Therapeutics and Technology Assessment Subcommittee of the American Academy of Neurology. Neurology. 2008;70:1707–1714.
49. Aurora SK, Dodlick DW, Turkel CC, et al. OnabotulinumtoxinA for treatment of chronic migraine: Results from the double-blind, randomized, placebo-controlled phase of the PREEMPT 1 trial. Cephalalgia. 2010;30:793–803.
50. Diener HC, Dodlick DW, Aurora SK, et al. OnabotulinumtoxinA for treatment of chronic migraine: Results from the double-blind, randomized, placebo-controlled phase of the PREEMPT 2 trial. Cephalalgia. 2010;30:804–814.
51. Lipton RB, Stewart WF, Diamond S, et al. Prevalence and burden of migraine in the United States: Data from the American Migraine Study II. Headache. 2001;41:646–657.
52. Loder E. Menstrual migraine: Timing is everything. Neurology. 2004;63:202.
53. MacGregor EA. Headache in pregnancy. Neurol Clin. 2012;30: 835–866.

36 Substance-Related Disorders

Christian J. Teter and Devon A. Sherwood

LEARNING OBJECTIVES

Upon completion of the chapter, the reader will be able to:

1. Identify the prevalence of use for commonly used substances (ie, alcohol, opioids, central nervous system [CNS] stimulants, cannabinoids, and nicotine) in the US population.
2. Explain the commonalities of action of abused substances on the reward system in the brain.
3. Identify the typical signs and symptoms of intoxication and withdrawal associated with the use of alcohol, opioids, CNS stimulants, cannabinoids, and nicotine.
4. Determine the appropriate treatment measures to produce a desired outcome after episodes of intoxication and withdrawal.
5. Determine when a patient meets criteria for substance use disorder.
6. Choose specific pharmacotherapeutic options based on patient-specific factors.
7. Recommend a comprehensive medication treatment and monitoring program to help maintain recovery and prevent relapse to substance use.

INTRODUCTION

Substance use disorders are highly prevalent worldwide. In the United States (U.S.), historically, tolerance of substance use and abuse has been cyclical. For example, cocaine was first isolated from coca leaves in 1860. Its use was advocated by many in the medical establishment until around the mid-1890s when it became evident chronic use might be addictive in some individuals and could have deleterious physiologic effects. Its use decreased after restriction of prescribing and dispensing in the early 20th century. In the 1980s, a smokeable formulation of cocaine (ie, crack) became available, and cocaine use again became epidemic. This historically cyclic nature of substance abuse is common to many substances of abuse.

KEY CONCEPT *Pharmacotherapy has a role in treatment of some substance-related disorders, including intoxication, withdrawal, and/or long-term relapse prevention. These substances include alcohol, opioids, central nervous system (CNS) stimulants, cannabinoids (CB), and nicotine. This chapter focuses on pharmacotherapy for these common substance-related disorders.* Although other substances are misused (eg, prescription sedatives and tranquilizers), those are not the focus of this chapter.

EPIDEMIOLOGY AND ETIOLOGY

The US federal government annually conducts the National Survey on Drug Use and Health (NSDUH) using a representative sample of persons aged 12 years or older to determine the prevalence of licit and illicit drug use.[1] In 2012, more than half (52.1%; 135.5 million) of Americans reported being a current (ie, past month) alcohol drinker. At least once in the 30 days prior to the survey, about one-quarter of Americans (23.0%; 59.7 million) reported binge drinking (ie, 5+ drinks), and 6.5% (17.0 million) reported heavy drinking (ie, binge drinking on 5+ occasions). Approximately one-quarter (26.7%; 69.5 million) were current users of tobacco products, with young adults aged 18 to 25 reporting the highest rates of current tobacco product use (38.1%). Regarding illicit drug use, 9.2% of the US population (23.9 million) reported current illicit drug use, with nonmedical psychotherapeutics being second only to marijuana (Figure 36–1). In 2012, there were 2.9 million illicit drug initiates, with marijuana being the first drug used in a majority of cases (65.6%). Notably, 1.4 million (roughly one-half of the entire drug initiate sample) first-time marijuana users were under the age of 18. Approximately one-quarter nonmedically used a psychotherapeutic as their first illicit drug (ie, 17.0% with pain relievers, 4.1% with tranquilizers, 3.6% with stimulants, and 1.3% with sedatives).[1] The NSDUH findings indicate that substance use is wide ranging; peaks at 18 to 25 years of age; and consists of a significant number of individuals using prescription medications nonmedically, which is a relatively new and growing public health concern.

Reward Pathway

KEY CONCEPT *Virtually all abused substances appear to activate the same brain reward pathway, which is highlighted by dopaminergic neurotransmission arising in the ventral tegmental area (VTA) and projecting to the nucleus accumbens (NA) and prefrontal cortex (PFC).*

Figure 36–2 depicts the mesocorticolimbic dopamine pathway. Key components are dopamine (DA) projections from the VTA to the NA and to the PFC.[2,3] Many studies support that this

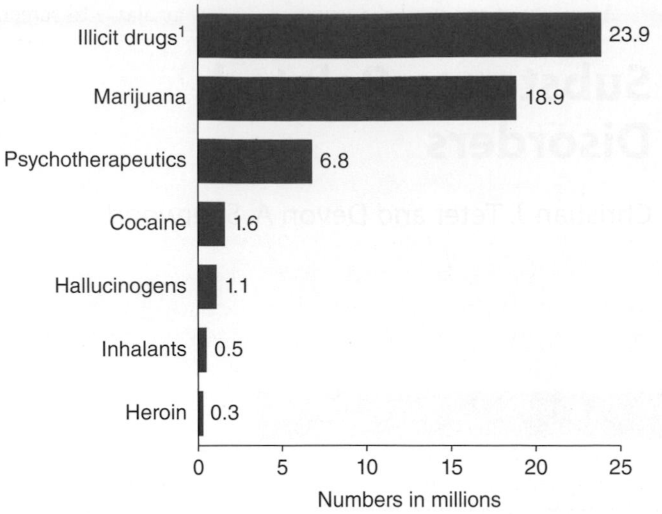

FIGURE 36–1. Past-month illicit drug use among the US population in 2012. [a]Illicit drug use includes a wide variety of substances such as marijuana or hashish, cocaine (including crack), heroin, hallucinogens, inhalants, or prescription-type psychotherapeutics used nonmedically. (Data and figure in the public domain from Substance Abuse and Mental Health Services Administration, Results from the 2012 National Survey on Drug Use and Health: Summary of National Findings, NSDUH Series H-46, HHS Publication No. [SMA] 13-4795. Rockville, MD: Substance Abuse and Mental Health Services Administration, 2013.)

mesolimbic DA system is involved in natural rewards and drug reinforcement[4]; however, there is also evidence that dopamine-independent reinforcement exists.[5] In any case, abused drugs generally produce pleasant effects considered desirable by the user. The initial hedonic experiences secondary to use of drugs appear to be primarily attributable to activation of primary reward circuits in the brain. These same reward circuits operate under normal circumstances to reinforce activities that promote survival, such as consuming food and water, social affiliation, or sexual activity. However, these systems appear to be disrupted after drug use in susceptible individuals.

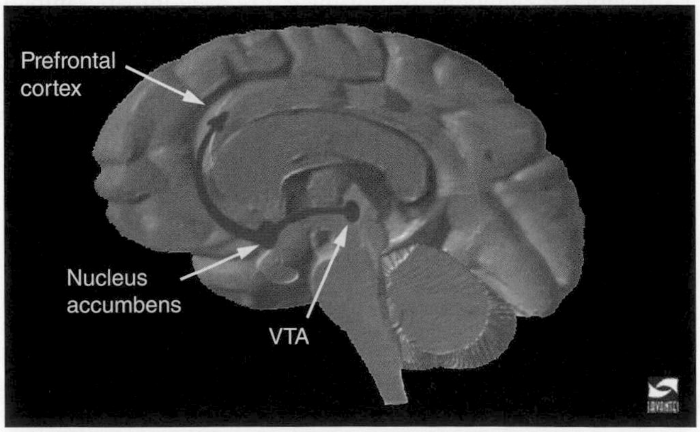

FIGURE 36–2. The mesocorticolimbic dopaminergic pathway (ie, the "reward pathway") VTA, ventral tegmental area. (Data from The Neurobiology of Drug Addiction [Internet]. http://www.drugabuse.gov/publications/teaching-packets/neurobiology-drug-addiction/section-i-introduction-to-brain.)

Although most individuals experience pleasant effects, not everyone abuses these drugs or becomes dependent on them. Why some persons abuse drugs while most do not relates to complex genetic, environmental, and cultural factors.

PATHOPHYSIOLOGY

Neuronal Adaptation

KEY CONCEPT *Although activation of reward pathways explains the pleasurable sensations associated with acute substance use, chronic use (which may result in substance-related disorders) may be related to neuroadaptive effects within the brain.*

A recent review by two preeminent researchers in the addiction sciences describes the addiction cycle moving past acute rewarding effects of substances of abuse and into other important processes.[5] They describe three phases of the addiction cycle: (a) binge/intoxication, (b) withdrawal/negative affect, and (c) preoccupation/anticipation. Binge/intoxication refers to the acute rewarding effects of drugs of abuse and the corresponding CNS circuitry. However, chronic use of substances leads to neuroadaptations in the brain and associated symptoms; more specifically, chronic drug abuse appears to cause a generalized decrease in DA neurotransmission. Additionally, with chronic drug use, release of corticotropin-releasing factor (CRF) is increased, indicating an activation of central stress pathways. In phase 3, other neurotransmitter systems (ie, beyond DA) are postulated to be involved. For example, elevated CRF, norepinephrine, and glutamate may exist in the "extended amygdala" during prolonged abstinence. Perhaps these changes lead to a long-term need to use substances to relieve unpleasant symptoms, such as stress.[5] Multiple factors are associated with an increased risk of relapse, including the availability of the abused drug, an increase in psychological stressors, and a triggering of cues such as seeing a white powder or going to a location where drugs were previously attained or used. These factors may trigger residual adaptive changes (eg, elevated glutamatergic activity) that occurred during the period of drug addiction.

Patient Encounter 1

A 38-year-old man is being seen in the outpatient clinic for long-term substance use and a recent relapse to oxycodone. The patient has been treated with buprenorphine for close to one year with periods of stability. However, each time there is an attempt at tapering off buprenorphine, the patient experiences intense dysphoria causing him to relapse to oxycodone use. His buprenorphine treatment has been discontinued for approximately three weeks. Recently, he has come to realize that he is reluctant to return home because his girlfriend is still actively using opioids for recreational purposes. However, he states that he is committed to finally "shaking his habit and putting in the work to stay clean."

What is the most immediate action to be taken regarding this man's treatment?

After acute detoxification, how can he be helped to maintain abstinence, and is there a medication that offers advantages over other first-line options?

CLINICAL PRESENTATION AND DIAGNOSIS

KEY CONCEPT *Individuals with a pattern of chronic use of commonly abused substances should be assessed to determine if they meet the Diagnostic and Statistical Manual of Mental Disorders, fifth edition (DSM-5) criteria for substance related disorders.*[6] Most notably, in cases of addiction, there is a loss of control over substance use or use has become compulsive. Criteria for substance use disorders from the *DSM-5* are listed in Table 36–1.[6] Consistent with the *DSM-5*, the remainder of this chapter is organized by pharmacologic class and discusses intoxication, withdrawal, and substance use disorders for each class (except tobacco use disorders, which do not have a *DSM-5* intoxication criteria set).

Table 36–1

***DSM-5* Criteria for Diagnosis of Substance Use Disorders**

A problematic pattern of substance use leading to clinically significant impairment or distress; manifested by at least two of the following, occurring within a 12-month period:

1. Substance often taken in larger amounts or over longer period than intended.
2. Persistent desire or unsuccessful efforts to cut down or control substance use.
3. Great deal of time spent in activities necessary to obtain substance, use the substance, or recover from its effects.
4. Craving or a strong desire or urge to use the substance.
5. Recurrent substance use resulting in failure to fulfill major role obligations at work, school, or home.
6. Continued substance use despite having persistent or recurrent social or interpersonal problems caused or exacerbated by the effects of substance.
7. Important social, occupational, or recreational activities are given up or reduced because of substance use.
8. Recurrent substance use in situations in which it is physically hazardous.
9. Substance use is continued despite knowledge of having a persistent or recurrent physical or psychological problem likely to have been caused or exacerbated by the substance.
10. Tolerance, as defined by either of the following:
    a. Need for markedly increased amounts of substance to achieve intoxication or desired effect.
    b. Markedly diminished effect with continued use of same amount of substance.
11. Withdrawal, as manifested by either of the following:
    a. Characteristic withdrawal syndrome for the substance (refer to Criteria A and B of the *DSM-5* criteria set for substance withdrawal).
    b. Substance (or closely related substance) is taken to relieve or avoid withdrawal symptoms.

Specify[a] current severity:

Mild: Presence of two to three symptoms.

Moderate: Presence of four to five symptoms.

Severe: Presence of six or more symptoms.

Data from the American Psychiatric Association. Diagnostic and Statistical Manual of Mental Disorders. 5th ed. Arlington, VA: American Psychiatric Association, 2013; with permission.

[a]Additional specifiers (eg, early vs sustained remission) and substance-specific notes (eg, taking opioid under medical supervision) are included in the *DSM-5*.

A variety of standardized instruments are available to screen for and assess the various stages of substance use and its consequences, such as withdrawal symptoms and functional impairment (Table 36–2).[7–10] The Addiction Severity Index (ASI) is the gold-standard instrument that assesses seven problem areas associated with substance use, such as medical status and psychiatric status, in addition to measures of alcohol and drug use.

Intoxication Signs and Symptoms

Intoxication caused by most substances is described in the *DSM-5* as clinically significant, problematic behavioral, or psychological changes to the user, which are caused by the physiological effects of the substance. These changes are seen during or shortly after use of the substance. Euphoria or experiencing a pleasurable sensation are effects of most drugs of abuse.[11] Other signs and symptoms are specific to the particular drug or drug class involved. Table 36–3 lists the psychological/behavioral and physiologic effects of intoxication from selected substances.[6,12–15]

Withdrawal Signs and Symptoms

Although most abused drugs can cause some degree of physiologic dependence, the severity of withdrawal varies considerably among these drugs. Table 36–4 lists common withdrawal symptoms seen upon abstinence from drug use.[6,12–16] Typically, withdrawal symptoms are opposite of acute effects of the drug. For example, although alcohol is a CNS depressant, signs and symptoms of withdrawal signify a hyperalert physiologic response.

TREATMENT OF SUBSTANCE USE DISORDER

OVERALL THEORY OF USE OF PHARMACOLOGIC AGENTS TO TREAT SUBSTANCE-RELATED DISORDERS

Unlike some medical diseases, substance use disorders cannot be cured with medications alone. However, we can sometimes alleviate the effects of drug intoxication, attenuate adverse effects of withdrawal, or somewhat decrease craving and likelihood of relapse to substance abuse. For example, pleasurable and intoxicating effects of opioids appear to be caused by their action as

Patient Encounter 2

A 43-year-old woman with a history of hypertension presents to your clinic for follow-up evaluation of her blood pressure. During the visit, you discover that she admits to drinking a bottle of wine each evening despite her uncontrolled hypertension. She states that her drinking has "crept up" on her over the years and that she finds a bottle of red wine helps to "take the edge off." The patient states that her strong urges to drink wine at times causes her concern. Notably, she reports experiencing headaches, which she attributes to the combination of red wine and her poor blood pressure management.

What information would suggest this patient might have an alcohol use disorder?

Are there any standardized instruments that you can recommend to screen for an alcohol use disorder?

Table 36–2

Commonly Used Instruments for Assessing Patients with Substance Use Disorders

Instrument	Purpose	Values and Interpretation
Addiction Severity Index (ASI) Assessment tool (past 30 days or lifetime) for various substances	Semistructured interview that addresses seven problem areas: medical status, employment and support, alcohol use, drug use, legal status, family and social status, and psychiatric status Questions include frequency, duration, and severity of problems	Patient and interviewer ratings included Interviewer severity ratings of "need for additional treatment" + composite scores to measure severity Scoring completed by a technician or computerized scoring and interpretation Composite score normative data from nationally representative sample of treatment programs is available for those seeking to compare a patient's ASI data with national data (http://www.tresearch.org); otherwise, comparisons with previous (eg, baseline) composite scores are useful
Alcohol Use Disorders Identification Test (AUDIT) Screening tool	Evaluates quantity and frequency of drinking; physiologic dependence on alcohol; harmful use Clinician administered	10 items (scores 0–40) Score of 8 or above identifies heavy drinkers and those with possible alcohol use disorders "Zones" of interventions based on scores
CAGE C = Cut down A = Angry/annoyed G = Guilty E = Eye opener Screening tool	Used to identify the presence of problematic drinking No training necessary; clinician or self-administered	Four items Score of 2 or more is positive and suggests problem drinking Positive screen prompts the need for further assessment
Clinical Institute for Withdrawal Assessment–Alcohol, Revised (CIWA-Ar) Assessment tool	Gold standard alcohol withdrawal assessment; used as part of symptom-triggered approach Clinician administered	10 items; maximum score = 67 < 10: mild w/d 10–18: moderate w/d Greater than 18: severe w/d Monitor scores over time; 8 to 10 or greater (depending on institutional protocols or co-occurring conditions) indicate need for medication
Clinical Opiate Withdrawal Scale (COWS) Assessment tool	Used to follow the course of withdrawal symptoms and effectiveness of medication regimens Clinician administered	11 items; scoring 0 (asymptomatic) to 4 or 5 (severely symptomatic) for each item based on intensity of signs and symptoms Total score (sum of 11 items): 5–12: Mild 13–24: Moderate 25–36: Moderately severe Greater than 36: Severe withdrawal Monitor scores over time (lower score implies less opioid withdrawal severity); higher scores may indicate need for medication; no standard cut-off exists
Fagerström Test for Nicotine Dependence	Assesses extent of nicotine tolerance, dependence, and craving; contains six questions; higher scores may predict greater difficulty in quitting	Total scoring for dependence: 0–2: Very low 3–4: Low 5: Moderate 6–7: High 8–10: Very high

Data from Refs. 7 to 10.

w/d, withdrawal.

agonists on μ-receptors of the opioid neurotransmitter system. Competitive μ-opioid antagonists such as naloxone and naltrexone acutely reverse many opioid effects, including symptoms of intoxication. To date, we do not have specific antagonists for most other substances. Similarly, reversal of withdrawal syndromes caused by abused substances is not always possible. One pharmacologic solution for reversing withdrawal symptoms, most commonly used by substance dependent individuals, is to readminister the drug that caused the physiologic dependence. The more commonly used treatment method is to administer a medication that has some cross-dependence with the abused drug but has fewer reinforcing effects and a more predictable pharmacokinetic profile. For example, benzodiazepines are used for the withdrawal of ethanol. Although benzodiazepines can cause physiologic dependence, they are rated as less desirable than ethanol by substance abusers, cause fewer long-term adverse health effects than ethanol, and are easier to manage medically. Regarding longer term medication management, an example is maintaining an opioid-addicted individual on a regimen of medically managed, orally administered opioids (ie, substitution therapy) compared with more dangerous illicit opioid use. Regardless of the specific pharmacotherapy chosen,

Table 36–3

Signs and Symptoms of Drug Intoxication for Select Substances

Drug	Behavioral Effects	Physiologic Effects
Ethanol	Changes in mood and behavior, inappropriate aggressive or sexual behavior, giddiness or verbally loud, impaired judgment; possibly progressing to somnolence and coma as the blood level increases	Blood levels 0.02%–0.1% (20–100 mg/dL or 4.3–21.7 mmol/L): Euphoria, feeling of well-being, disinhibition, slight impairment (eg, reaction time) Blood levels 0.1%–0.2% (100–200 mg/dL or 21.7–43.4 mmol/L): Significant impairment (eg, balance, speech, vision and hearing, reaction times), dysphoria Blood levels 0.2%–0.3% (200–300 mg/dL or 43.4–65.1 mmol/L): Marked ataxia, mental confusion, and nausea and vomiting Blood levels 0.3%–0.4% (300–400 mg/dL or 65.1–86.8 mmol/L): Severe dysarthria, amnesia, hypothermia Blood levels > 0.4% (400 mg/dL or 86.8 mmol/L): Alcoholic coma, decreased respiration or respiratory arrest; aspiration of gastric contents or airway obstruction caused by flaccid tongue, drop in blood pressure and body temperature
Opioids	Drowsiness, sedation, slurred speech, impaired memory and attention, psychomotor retardation	Nausea, vomiting, respiratory depression (dose-related), stupor, coma, constipation common in chronic users, itching, miosis, hypothermia, bradycardia
CNS stimulants	Elated mood, hypervigilance, anxiety or panic, impaired judgment, violence to others or self, paranoia or psychosis with delusions and hallucinations (generally tactile or auditory, rarely visual), increased motor activity, compulsive or stereotyped behavior (eg, skin picking)	Neurologic/Neuromuscular: mydriasis, headache, tremor, hyperreflexia, muscle twitching, flushing, hyperthermia or cold sweats, rhabdomyolysis (possibly resulting in renal failure), muscular weakness, dyskinesias, seizures, coma Cardiovascular: increased pulse and blood pressure, peripheral vasoconstriction, arrhythmias, myocardial infarction, cerebral hemorrhage GI: Nausea, vomiting, weight loss
Cannabinoids	Euphoria, impaired motor coordination, anxiety, impaired judgment, social withdrawal	Tachycardia (can exceed 20 beats/min increases), dry mouth, conjunctival injection, increased appetite

CNS, central nervous system; GI, gastrointestinal.

Data from Refs. 6 and 12 to 15.

Table 36–4

Signs and Symptoms of Drug Withdrawal for Select Substances

Drug	Timeline	Symptoms
Ethanol	As ethanol levels decrease:	
	Early symptoms	Tremor, nausea, vomiting, tachycardia (> 110 beats/min), hypertension (> 140/90 mm Hg), headache, vivid dreams, insomnia
	Peak (24 hours)	Seizure-activity (usually one or two grand mal type but can be numerous and possibly fatal)
	72–96 hours	Delirium tremens
	Onset at any time	Hallucinations, usually visual
Opioids	For shorter acting opioids (eg, heroin, morphine, oxycodone) withdrawal may begin within 6–24 hours after last dose and last for about 1 week; with longer acting opioids (eg, methadone) it may take up to 2–4 days for withdrawal to emerge, and it will last longer	GI: Nausea, vomiting, diarrhea, dehydration Neurologic or psychological: irritability, restlessness, yawning, tremulousness, twitching Cardiovascular: Increased heart rate and blood pressure Musculoskeletal: Chills, increased body temperature, piloerection, rhinorrhea Ocular: Lacrimation, mydriasis
CNS stimulants	**Stage 1:** Immediately following binge	Stimulant craving, intense dysphoria, depression, anxiety, agitation
	Stage 2: Within 1–4 hours	Desire for sleep, dysphoria continues
	Stage 3: Days 3–4	Hypersomnia, increased appetite, craving may dissipate but return later
Cannabinoids	Withdrawal symptoms onset typically within 24–72 hours; peak within 1 week	Severity reflects degree and duration of cannabinoid use; symptoms include irritability, nervousness, anxiety, sleep abnormalities, restlessness, depressed mood, headache, tremors, sweating, chills
Nicotine	Begins within 24 hours of cessation; may persist	Severity reflects degree and duration of nicotine use; symptoms include anxiety, irritability, frustration, anger, craving, difficulty concentrating, decreased heart rate, and increased appetite

CNS, central nervous system; GI, gastrointestinal.

Data from Refs. 6 and 12 to 16.

medications should always be used as adjuncts to a comprehensive psychosocial approach.

TREATMENT OF INTOXICATION SYNDROMES

KEY CONCEPT *The treatment goals for acute intoxication of ethanol, opioids, CNS stimulants, and cannabinoids include (a) management of psychological/psychiatric manifestations of intoxication, such as aggression, hostility, and psychosis and (b) management of medical manifestations of intoxication, such as respiratory depression, hyperthermia, hypertension, cardiac arrhythmias, and stroke.* In all cases of substance intoxication that requires medical intervention, referral to and participation in substance abuse treatment is desirable.

Alcohol Intoxication

Desired outcomes are appropriate management of medical problems, prevention of harmful behaviors, and stabilization of mood. Most cases of mild to moderate intoxication with alcohol, including cases with blood alcohol concentrations (BACs) at lower limits of legal intoxication, do not require formal treatment. Providing a safe environment and reassurance until alcohol effects have worn off is sufficient in most cases. Initially, BACs may continue to rise if gastrointestinal (GI) absorption is still occurring. Otherwise, BACs generally decrease at a rate of 15 to 20 mg/dL (0.015%–0.02% or 3.3–4.3 mmol/L) per hour. See Table 36–3 for physiologic effects of alcohol, in nontolerant individuals, at various BACs. It is important to note that tolerant individuals may not show the same level of symptoms at a given BAC as nontolerant individuals.

At more severe levels of intoxication, confusion, stupor, coma, and death may occur. Clinicians must rule out other causes of these serious adverse events, because alcohol-intoxicated individuals commonly combine alcohol with other substances, sustain head or other injuries, and have vitamin deficiencies and electrolyte abnormalities. If consciousness is impaired, then thiamine should be given intravenously (IV) or intramuscularly (IM) at 100 mg/day for at least 3 days. If hypoglycemia is suspected, then thiamine administration should precede administration of glucose-containing fluids to prevent precipitation of acute Wernicke's syndrome (see Alcohol Withdrawal section). Patients may also develop adverse interactions between alcohol and prescribed medications including disulfiram. See Table 36–5 for drug–drug interactions associated with abused substances.[17,18]

Behaviorally, patients may insist on driving, become physically aggressive and agitated, or otherwise become a danger to themselves or others. Indeed, most suicidal behaviors among alcohol-dependent individuals occur while they are intoxicated. Antipsychotics may lower the seizure threshold and are best avoided. However, in some instances, agitation may require treatment with an antipsychotic (eg, haloperidol 5–10 mg by mouth every 2–4 hours or olanzapine 10 mg given IM with repeated doses at least 2 hours apart). Sedation with benzodiazepines has been used, but in the presence of alcohol, respiratory depression can be dangerous or even fatal.

There are no medications that can fully reverse the effects of alcohol intoxication. Caffeine and other stimulants are neither indicated nor considered a viable option to make driving safe.

Opioid Intoxication

The word *opioid* refers to the class of medications and substances that exert their action through the opioid system. Opioids encompass a wide range of substances, including naturally occurring (eg, morphine) and synthetic (eg, oxycodone) substances.

Patients who are acutely intoxicated with an opioid usually present with miosis, euphoria, slow breathing, slow heart rate, low blood pressure, and constipation. Seizures may occur with certain agents, such as meperidine (Demerol). It is critically important to monitor patients carefully to avoid cardiac and respiratory depression and death from opioid overdose. One strategy is to reverse intoxication using naloxone (Narcan) 0.4 to 2 mg IV every 2 to 3 minutes up to 10 mg; the IM or subcutaneous (SC) route may be used if IV access is not available. Because naloxone is shorter acting than most abused opioids, it may need to be readministered at periodic intervals; otherwise, patients could lapse into cardiopulmonary arrest after a symptom-free interval of reversed intoxication. In addition, naloxone can induce withdrawal symptoms in opioid-dependent patients, so patients may awaken feeling distressed and agitated. It should be noted that buprenorphine intoxication may be more difficult to reverse.[19]

It is critically important to secure the airway and ensure breathing in cases of opioid overdose. In some cases, intubation and manual or mechanical ventilation might be required to avoid oxygen desaturation leading to brain hypoxia or anoxia and brain damage or death.

Recently, new opportunities for "take-home" naloxone have emerged in the United States. For example, naloxone hydrochloride injection (Evzio) was Food and Drug Administration (FDA)-approved for this purpose.[20] It is too early to determine the public health impact of this approach for treatment of opioid overdoses.

Stimulant (Cocaine and Amphetamines) Intoxication

Desired outcomes of stimulant intoxication treatment are appropriate management of medical and psychiatric problems. Medical problems include hyperthermia, hypertension, cardiac arrhythmias, stroke, and seizures. Some medical problems are related to route of administration, such as nosebleeds with intranasal administration and infections with IV administration. Psychiatric effects include anxiety, irritability, aggression, and psychosis.

Notably, stimulant intoxication is the only stimulant use disorder for which specific pharmacotherapy has demonstrated effectiveness. Recommended medications in acute settings include benzodiazepines, aspirin, nitroglycerin, nitroprusside, and phentolamine.[21] The American Heart Association guidelines indicate that acute use of β-blockers is not recommended and may lead to worsening cocaine-related chest pain (caused by coronary vasoconstriction) and hypertension secondary to unopposed alpha activity.

Cocaine is short acting, and a single benzodiazepine sedative-hypnotic may be sufficient treatment for anxiety reactions. Depending on the half-life of the benzodiazepine, one or more sequential doses may be required for longer acting amphetamine intoxication. Antipsychotics are indicated when psychosis is present, and psychosis usually responds quite rapidly in the absence of other co-occurring psychiatric disorders.

Cannabinoid (Marijuana, etc) Intoxication

There are no established treatment recommendations for CB intoxication. Symptomatic treatment (eg, tachycardia, anxiety, paranoia, and psychosis) is the commonly used approach. The exception is potent synthetic cannabinoids, which may require aggressive benzodiazepine treatment for intense symptoms of anxiety or psychosis. These intense psychiatric symptoms have been theorized to result either from the potent full-agonist cannabinoids that are used to prepare them, or possibly due to the

Table 36–5

Clinically Relevant Drug Interactions with Substances or Medications Used to Treat Substance Use Disorders

Drug	Interacting Drug	Type of Interaction and Appropriate Action
Amphetamines (including dextro- and methamphetamine)	MAOIs (phenelzine, selegiline, tranylcypromine, possibly linezolid)	Pharmacodynamic interaction resulting in an increased blood pressure; possibly resulting in hypertensive emergency or stroke; **AVOID** this drug combination
	Sodium bicarbonate	Sodium bicarbonate increases renal tubular reabsorption of amphetamine, resulting in prolonged amphetamine elimination half-life; closely monitor this combination
Bupropion	MAOIs	Neurotoxicity; **AVOID** this drug combination
	Substances that lower seizure threshold	Alcohol (*withdrawal*); **AVOID** bupropion in patients at risk for experiencing alcohol withdrawal
Buprenorphine	Atazanavir	Combination of buprenorphine + atazanavir (without ritonavir) results in both lower atazanavir levels and greater buprenorphine exposure; **AVOID** this bidirectional-interacting drug combination
	Conivaptan	Conivaptan is a potent CYP3A4 inhibitor; manufacturer recommends its use be **avoided** with medications metabolized by CYP3A4
	CYP3A4 inhibitors (in addition to specific medications listed)	May raise buprenorphine levels; monitor for greater than expected buprenorphine effects
Cannabinoids	Drugs that elevate heart rate: anticholinergics, caffeine, stimulants	Clinically significant elevations in heart rate may occur; AVOID combination
Cigarette smoking	Clozapine and olanzapine	Cigarette smoking induces CYP1A2, increasing metabolism of clozapine; may need to increase clozapine dose when patient begins to smoke or decrease clozapine dose if smoking is stopped
	Theophylline	Theophylline is CYP1A2 substrate; may need to increase theophylline dose when patient begins to smoke or decrease the theophylline dose if smoking is stopped
Disulfiram	Alcohol-containing solutions (variety of medications)	Disulfiram reaction; **AVOID** combination
	Metronidazole	Combination of disulfiram and metronidazole has lead to CNS effects (eg, psychosis); **AVOID** combination
	Benzodiazepines (including alprazolam, diazepam, flurazepam, triazolam)	Disulfiram (weakly) inhibits CYP enzymes 1A2, 2C9, and 3A4; many benzodiazepines are metabolized via these pathways; lorazepam, temazepam, and oxazepam are primarily conjugated to inactive products and are reasonable alternatives Otherwise, if benzodiazepines are combined with disulfiram, the pharmacologic effect may be greater than expected, and the dose of benzodiazepine may need to be lowered
	Cocaine	Disulfiram decreases clearance of cocaine from the body; may see increased or prolonged cocaine effects with combination
	Phenytoin	Disulfiram decreases metabolism of phenytoin, resulting in higher phenytoin levels; phenytoin dose may need to be reduced; because phenytoin undergoes nonlinear metabolism, it is difficult to predict magnitude of increase in blood levels that could be seen; best to avoid this interaction if possible
Ethanol (alcohol)	Acetaminophen	Chronic ethanol use increases risk of hepatotoxicity when acetaminophen is used in high doses
	Bupropion	Abrupt *discontinuation* of alcohol with continued bupropion use may lower seizure threshold; combination should be **avoided** in those at risk for seizure activity (eg, alcoholics with cooccurring depressive symptoms)
	Cefamandole, cefoperazone, cefotetan, and moxalactam, metronidazole	Disulfiram-type reaction may occur when these anti-infectives are combined with alcohol; reaction includes flushing, diaphoresis, tachycardia, headache, and increases in blood pressure; **AVOID** alcohol if these drugs are used
	Cycloserine	Neurotoxicity (specifically seizure risk) may be enhanced with combination of alcohol and cycloserine; **AVOID** combination
	Didanosine	Risk for pancreatitis may be increased with combination of alcohol and didanosine; **AVOID** combination
	Methotrexate	Hepatotoxicity is a higher risk when methotrexate is given to those who chronically drink large amounts of alcohol; **AVOID** methotrexate in this group if possible; otherwise monitor LFTs
	MAOIs	Ethanol **DOES NOT** interact with MAOIs; however, tyramine may be a component of some aged alcoholic drinks, such as red wines or tap beers; if reaction occurs, hypertension and a pounding headache are most likely symptoms; usually white wine is tolerable (in moderation) and most widely available domestic canned beers do not contain significant amounts of tyramine
	Tapentadol	Combination of alcohol and *extended-release* tapentadol may result in increased maximum serum concentrations of tapentadol; **AVOID** this drug combination

(*Continued*)

Table 36–5

Clinically Relevant Drug Interactions with Substances or Medications Used to Treat Substance Use Disorders (*Continued*)

Drug	Interacting Drug	Type of Interaction and Appropriate Action
Methadone	Carbamazepine	Carbamazepine is potent inducer of CYP3A4 and methadone is primarily metabolized via CYP3A4; if carbamazepine is added to drug regimen containing methadone, the methadone dose will probably need to be adjusted upward to avoid withdrawal
	Conivaptan	Conivaptan is a potent inhibitor of CYP3A4; manufacturer recommends its use be AVOIDED in medications metabolized by CYP3A4
	CYP3A4 inhibitors (in addition to specific medications listed)	Methadone serum concentrations may be increased when combined with potent CYP3A4 inhibitors; methadone dose adjustment should be based on clinical judgment, but a decrease of dose may be necessary
	Didanosine	Methadone decreases the amount of didanosine that is orally absorbed; therapeutic monitoring of didanosine effects are recommended, and doses may need to be increased
	Efavirenz	This HIV drug is a CYP3A4 inducer; efavirenz decreases methadone blood levels and has precipitated withdrawal in opioid-dependent individuals; may need to increase methadone dose
	MAOIs	Potential serotonin syndrome when MAOIs are combined with methadone; transdermal selegiline lists co-treatment with methadone as a CONTRAINDICATION
	Nevirapine	Nevirapine is an HIV drug that is a CYP3A4 inducer; in a small sample, nevirapine caused a 50% reduction in methadone blood levels, resulting in complaints of methadone withdrawal symptoms in patients receiving methadone maintenance; may need to increase methadone dose in patients who have nevirapine added to their drug regimen
	QTc-prolonging drugs or medications	Medications that prolong the QT interval (eg, ziprasidone) should be AVOIDED with methadone coadministration when possible because of potential additive QT-prolonging effects
	Stavudine	Methadone decreases the amount of stavudine (a reverse transcriptase inhibitor) by about 25%. Although this may not be clinically significant in some cases, the clinician should be aware of the possibility of this interaction
	St. John's wort	This herbal remedy may induce CYP3A4; the certainty of an interaction probably rests on the specific preparation being used, but caution dictates that this herbal product should be avoided in those receiving methadone treatment; withdrawal symptoms have been noted in patients taking methadone maintenance who have added St. John's wort to their drug regimen
	Tamoxifen	Methadone may inhibit the formation of important active tamoxifen metabolites (eg, endoxifen), and therapeutic monitoring is recommended
	Zidovudine	Methadone increases the blood level of this anti-HIV drug, probably via methadone inhibition of both metabolic and renal clearance of zidovudine; may need to decrease zidovudine dose to avoid toxicity
Naltrexone	Opioid-based pain medications	Blockade of pain relief; use nonopioid treatment approaches (eg, NSAIDs); refer to Special Dosing Considerations within Alcohol Use Disorder section

CYP, cytochrome P450 isoenzyme; LFT, liver function test; MAOI, monoamine oxidase inhibitor.

Caution should always be exercised when combinations of medications with similar pharmacologic properties are used (eg, additive CNS depression associated with coingestion of alcohol and nonmedical use of prescription opioids).

Data from Refs. 17 and 18.

lack of cannabidiol in these synthetic products. Cannabidiol has been associated with antipsychotic effects.[22]

TREATMENT OF WITHDRAWAL SYNDROMES

KEY CONCEPT *The treatment goals for withdrawal from ethanol, opioids, CNS stimulants, and cannabinoids include (a) a determination if pharmacologic treatment of withdrawal symptoms is necessary, (b) management of other medical manifestations, and (c) referral to the appropriate program for long-term substance abuse treatment.* The desired outcomes in the treatment of withdrawal syndromes are to ensure patient safety, comfort, and successful transition from treatment of withdrawal to longer-term maintenance. Referral to specialized treatment for substance use disorders is strongly recommended after treatment of withdrawal syndromes. Achieving a drug-free state by detoxification and then rehabilitation with a focus on total abstinence is the ideal outcome.

Alcohol Withdrawal

Alcohol withdrawal syndromes have two distinct presentations (ie, uncomplicated and complicated), which differ in terms of their pharmacologic treatment and need for hospitalization.

▸ *Uncomplicated Alcohol Withdrawal*

This is the most commonly observed syndrome, and as the name denotes, is not complicated by seizures, **delirium tremens (DTs)**, or hallucinosis. Symptoms are typically rated using a validated scale such as the Clinical Institute Withdrawal Assessment–Alcohol, Revised (CIWA-Ar) (see Table 36–2). The recommended CIWA-Ar threshold score for treating uncomplicated alcohol withdrawal with medications on an outpatient basis is 8 to 10. For patients who score greater than or equal to 15, inpatient treatment should be considered. Patients who score 20 or higher on the CIWA-Ar should always be treated with medication. The risks of not treating high-scoring patients with medications are seizures and DTs, and those with a prior history of seizures or DTs have increased risk for subsequent episodes. There is some evidence for "kindling" during successive episodes of alcohol withdrawal, such that symptom severity and complications increase with additional withdrawal episodes. Therefore, with a history of seizures or DTs, the lower range of 8 to 10 is recommended, and hospitalization is safer than outpatient detoxification.

Benzodiazepines are the treatment of choice for uncomplicated alcohol withdrawal.[10,12] Anticonvulsants have been used to treat uncomplicated withdrawal (particularly carbamazepine and sodium valproate); however, they are not as well studied and are less commonly used. The most commonly used benzodiazepines are lorazepam, diazepam, and chlordiazepoxide. They differ in three major ways: (a) their pharmacokinetic properties, (b) the available routes for their administration, and (c) the rapidity of their onset of action due to the rate of GI absorption and rate of crossing the blood–brain barrier. Benzodiazepines are often given in one of two ways: (1) Symptom-triggered approach, or (2) loading dose strategy. Typically, adjunctive "as needed" medications are used as well.

Benzodiazepines can be administered using a symptom-triggered approach when withdrawal signs and symptoms are present.[23] Medication (eg, lorazepam) is administered every hour when the CIWA-Ar is greater than or equal to eight. For example, the shorter-acting agent lorazepam is given at the recommended 1 to 2 mg dose. The CIWA-Ar is repeated hourly after each administration during the first 24 hours until the patient is comfortably sedated. Due to a short half-life, dosing of lorazepam on subsequent days may be needed, and risk of seizures may possibly (although not definitively proven) be higher.

Longer-acting agents (eg, diazepam, chlordiazepoxide) are often used via the loading dose strategy in which larger doses are given initially followed by a taper over 3–5 days. The long half-lives of these drugs and their active metabolites usually provide a natural taper without further drug administration. This approach may be accompanied by as needed short-acting benzodiazepine doses for breakthrough alcohol withdrawal symptoms. The loading dose strategy is especially useful in the hospital, where patients can be medically monitored throughout the day. Diazepam may be "preferred" to chlordiazepoxide, given its less variable pharmacokinetic profile (eg, fewer active metabolites, narrower range for time to maximum concentration) and a faster onset of action (ie, quickly enters the CNS due to high lipophilicity).

Special Dosing Considerations In contrast to chlordiazepoxide and diazepam, lorazepam is not metabolized into active compounds in the liver. It is excreted by the kidneys after glucuronidation. This is important because many alcohol dependent patients have compromised liver function. Therefore, when treatment is initiated before results of liver function tests (LFTs) are known, lorazepam may be preferred. Patients with liver disease may still be treated with diazepam or chlordiazepoxide at lower doses.

Diazepam is more lipophilic than lorazepam or chlordiazepoxide, resulting in quicker GI absorption and passage across the blood–brain barrier, making it valuable in an inpatient setting, especially to prevent seizures. However, a faster onset of action may be associated with feeling high (ie, "euphoria") and is a treatment disadvantage.

American Psychiatric Association (APA) Guidelines recommend thiamine be given routinely to patients being treated for moderate to severe alcohol use disorders to treat or prevent adverse neurologic symptoms.[12] However, according to a recent Cochrane Review, there are inadequate data from randomized, controlled trials regarding the most efficacious thiamine dose, frequency, and route of administration to prevent or treat Wernicke's syndrome associated with alcohol use disorders.[24] APA Guidelines recommend thiamine 50 to 100 mg per day given IV or IM, although some guidelines recommend higher doses (eg, thiamine 300 mg/day for low risk patients).[12,25] It is particularly important that administration of thiamine (essential for proper energy utilization by the CNS) precedes administration of glucose-containing IV fluids, which can help prevent an acute exacerbation of Wernicke's syndrome.

▶ *Complicated Alcohol Withdrawal*

Alcohol Withdrawal Seizures Alcohol withdrawal seizures, a medical emergency, should be treated in an inpatient setting. Withdrawal seizures are usually few in number and generalized. Although binge drinking and alcohol withdrawal can lead to status epilepticus, the occurrence of focal seizures or status epilepticus may also suggest another etiology. Management consists of keeping the airway open and preventing self-injury during convulsions. Benzodiazepines are the treatment of choice. IV diazepam 5 to 10 mg is preferred to terminate a seizure in progress if IV access is available. Dose may be repeated in 5 minutes if seizures persist. Alternatively, lorazepam 4 mg may be given IM followed by insertion of an IV line when convulsive movements have subsided. In the event of a recurrent seizure, lorazepam 2 mg IV may be administered if the patient received IM lorazepam. IM use of diazepam or chlordiazepoxide should be avoided because of erratic absorption that complicates the timing of subsequent doses and can result in delayed oversedation. IV benzodiazepines may depress respiration, so they should be administered only when and where advanced cardiopulmonary support is available. When the patient can take medication orally, then treatment may continue using the symptom-triggered or loading dose procedure. Electrolyte imbalances can contribute to seizures and should be corrected if they exist. For example, it may be advisable to administer magnesium in addition to benzodiazepine treatment. Phenytoin should be avoided for preventing or treating alcohol-related seizures as no data demonstrate efficacy.[26]

Alcohol Withdrawal Delirium (Delirium Tremens) Delirium tremens is a medical emergency necessitating hospitalization to prevent death. DTs are characterized by hallucinations, delirium, severe agitation, fever, elevation of blood pressure and heart rate, and possible cardiac arrhythmias. Parenterally administered benzodiazepines are the treatment of choice.[23] The antipsychotic haloperidol is given for severe agitation unresponsive to benzodiazepine therapy. Evidence does not support use of an antipsychotic as single agent.[27] Furthermore, newer generation antipsychotic agents have not been studied for treatment of DTs. Thiamine should be given according to the same guidelines described above.

Opioid Withdrawal

It is rare to die from withdrawal from opioids alone; however, underlying medical complications (eg, hypertension) and recent myocardial infarction increase risk of complications and death. Therefore, it is important to manage and stabilize any medical issues and then determine if hospitalization is appropriate. Patients with underlying medical problems should be evaluated for possible triage to an inpatient detoxification program to be followed up with either inpatient or outpatient substance abuse treatment. Rapid referral for substance abuse treatment can introduce patients to the concept of recovery while they still vividly remember negative consequences from using substances. Withdrawal from opioids is commonly described by patients as resembling "a bad case of the flu." Symptoms include nausea; vomiting; diarrhea; anxiety; headaches; mydriasis; rhinorrhea; lacrimation; muscle, bone, and joint pain; piloerection; yawning; fever; increased heart rate; and hypertension.

Use of clinical withdrawal scales (see Table 36–2), such as the Clinical Opiate Withdrawal Scale (COWS), provide high interrater reliability and clinical utility given objective measurement of withdrawal severity. The full items contained in the COWS instrument (*along with many other substance use disorder [SUD] instruments*) can be obtained free-of-charge from the Substance Abuse and Mental Health Services Administration (SAMHSA).[9] The baseline score assists in deciding whether to treat pharmacologically or to observe. As withdrawal scores become larger (eg, COWS scores five or greater), opioid substitution or a "symptoms-based approach" may be indicated. In severe withdrawal, either buprenorphine (ie, partial μ-opioid agonist) or methadone (ie, full μ-opioid agonist) are recommended for detoxification. Methadone is the gold-standard μ-opioid agonist for treating opioid use disorders, but under current US law, methadone detoxification requires referral to a federally approved methadone detoxification program. The two pharmacologic options for treatment of opioid withdrawal in regular clinical settings are opioid substitution with buprenorphine and symptomatic treatment (discussed in the following paragraphs).

▶ *Opioid Substitution*

Treatment with a μ-opioid agonist is accomplished with either buprenorphine or methadone. Methadone can be used for opioid detoxification and long-term relapse prevention, particularly among heavy opioid users. However, given extensive medical use restrictions (eg, used only in federally approved opioid treatment programs; OTP) and wide availability of methadone detoxification regimens, this chapter focuses on buprenorphine.

Buprenorphine is a partial agonist at μ-opioid receptors that is available in multiple formulations in the United States with varying pharmacokinetic profiles. For example, buprenorphine in combination with naloxone is available via sublingual tablet, sublingual film, and buccal film. Certain formulations (eg, sublingual film) may have greater buprenorphine bioavailability, and hence lower dosage requirements, compared to sublingual tablets. Buprenorphine plus naloxone is the recommended formulation (over buprenorphine alone) unless the patient is pregnant or hypersensitive to naloxone, in which case buprenorphine alone is appropriate. Opioid antagonists, such as naloxone, have been associated with severe negative outcomes among pregnant women (eg, spontaneous abortion) and should be avoided in this population. Naloxone was added to the Suboxone formulation to secure FDA approval in the United States. Naloxone is poorly absorbed via sublingual or buccal routes, but blocks opioid receptors if injected, thus minimizing diversion to the street for IV use.

To initiate buprenorphine induction, a patient has to be in moderate or severe withdrawal, and the last opioid use should be at least 12 to 24 hours earlier, depending on the half-life of the opioid used (longer half-life, longer a clinician should wait before initiating buprenorphine induction). Otherwise, buprenorphine likely will induce withdrawal because it has high affinity for μ-receptors, and it will displace other full μ-opioid agonists. Buprenorphine can be initiated following a protocol such as the example in Table 36–6 to titrate the dosing.[9] When a final dose is established, there are generally two treatment approaches, depending on many factors such as patient preference. A maintenance dose can be prescribed or the dose can be tapered down gradually to zero within 1 to 2 weeks (a 25% reduction per day is a general rule of thumb).

Table 36–6

Sample Regimen[a] for Buprenorphine Induction Treatment of Opioid Withdrawal and Long-Term Relapse Prevention

Day	Buprenorphine Sublingual/Buccal Dosage
1	2 mg every 2 hours (maximum, 8 mg on first day)
2	Start with total day 1 dose; additional 2–4 mg every 2 hours (maximum, 16 mg)
3+	Start with total day 2 dose; additional 2–4 mg every 2 hours (maximum, 32 mg)
4–5	Maintain on dose required to alleviate withdrawal symptoms[b]

[a]For withdrawal from any opioid.

[b]Patient will likely be transitioned to long-term maintenance dose indefinitely.

Data from Center for Substance Abuse Treatment. Clinical Guidelines for the Use of Buprenorphine in the Treatment of Opioid Addiction. Treatment Improvement Protocol (TIP) Series 40. DHHS Publication no. (SMA) 04–3939. Rockville, MD: Substance Abuse and Mental Health Services Administration; 2004.

▶ *Symptoms-Based Treatment*

Symptomatic treatment focuses on minimizing withdrawal symptoms to help patients be comfortable. Symptom-specific medications, as shown in Table 36–7, are often used as adjunct

Table 36–7

A "Symptoms-Based" Treatment Approach for Opioid Withdrawal

Following medications are used for symptoms that cause distress and includes use of any single or combination of two or more of the following agents, depending on symptoms reported:

1. Insomnia: Diphenhydramine 50–100 mg, trazodone 75–200 mg, or hydroxyzine 25–50 mg at bedtime
2. Headache, muscle aches, and pain: Acetaminophen 500 mg–1 g every 6 hours, ibuprofen 600 mg by mouth every 8 hours, or naproxen 600 mg by mouth every 12 hours
3. Noradrenergic hyperactivity: Clonidine (Catapres) 0.1–0.2 mg every 6–8 hours; maximum dosage not to exceed 1.2 mg in 24 hours
4. Abdominal cramps: Dicyclomine 10–20 mg every 6 hours
5. Constipation: Milk of magnesia at 30 mL daily
6. Diarrhea: Bismuth subcarbonate 30 mL can be given every 2 to 3 hours

Data from Refs. 9 and 12.

medication with opioid substitution.[9,12] Clonidine is one of the primary nonopioid medications used during withdrawal to decrease the excessive noradrenergic symptoms (eg, sweating) of opioid withdrawal. However, use of clonidine requires close monitoring of blood pressure; it should be held if systolic blood pressure is below 90 mm Hg or diastolic blood pressure is below 60 mm Hg. Compared with opioid substitution, clonidine does not help other withdrawal symptoms, such as craving.[12]

▶ *General Patient Guidelines for Outpatient Opioid Detoxification*

Patient safety is the highest priority. The first step is to educate patients about the course of withdrawal. Symptoms peak at around 5 to 7 days and may last up to 2 weeks, depending on half-life of the opioid being used before detoxification. Patients should be advised regarding the side effects of medications used to detoxify. There is an overdose potential if clonidine is mixed with opioids, other CNS sedatives, or antihypertensives. Risk of these adverse events needs to be balanced with potential benefits. Side effects of buprenorphine include constipation, sedation, and headaches. Potential for serious overdose exists when buprenorphine is mixed with benzodiazepines or other sedative–hypnotics.

Risk of developing physiologic tolerance to buprenorphine is high if used for prolonged periods. In this case, buprenorphine should be slowly tapered to discontinuation. Withdrawal from buprenorphine is generally easier and less severe than withdrawal from a pure agonist, such as methadone. However, there is concern regarding a subset of patients who have difficulty stopping buprenorphine treatment. This has prompted federal research into the issue (see www.clinicaltrials.gov regarding ongoing studies). The duration of buprenorphine treatment is specific to each individual's needs and resources, and difficulty in tapering the medication to discontinuation complicates this decision further.

Patients often think all they need is detoxification, but this is not accurate. Positive outcomes are tied to successful rehabilitation and acquiring recovery skills after detoxification. This goal can be accomplished by either achieving detoxification on-site during rehabilitation or by quick and seamless transition from detoxification to a rehabilitation program. The more time that elapses between the two modalities, the greater the likelihood of treatment failure and drug relapse.

Stimulant (Cocaine, Amphetamines) Withdrawal

Cocaine and amphetamine withdrawal are grouped together because their symptom profiles as described in *DSM-5*[6] are similar, and the physiologic basis of their withdrawal syndromes involves the DA neurotransmitter system. Stimulants of this group also include methylphenidate, but not nicotine and caffeine, which have different neurophysiologic mechanisms of action. Major adverse complications of stimulant withdrawal are profound depression with suicidal thoughts, and the primary goal of treatment is to prevent suicide. Therefore, unless suicidality warrants hospitalization, stimulant withdrawal can be treated in outpatient settings with psychological support and reassurance with an emphasis on patient safety. A number of medications have been studied to alleviate symptoms of stimulant withdrawal and the intense craving that may accompany it, but inconsistent results preclude any recommendations for their routine use. Patients with stimulant use disorders should be referred for substance abuse treatment because of high risk for continued use either during or immediately following stimulant withdrawal.

Cannabinoid (Marijuana, Hashish) Withdrawal

Symptoms of cannabinoid withdrawal are primarily behavioral. For example, significant anxiety may accompany cannabinoid withdrawal, which can lead many individuals to resume substance use. This is particularly problematic following heavy and prolonged cannabinoid use. Management of withdrawal focuses on these behavioral symptoms, as there are no FDA approved medications specifically targeted at cannabinoid withdrawal.

GENERAL APPROACH TO THE TREATMENT OF SUBSTANCE USE DISORDERS

KEY CONCEPT *A multimodal and comprehensive approach is preferred when treating individuals with substance use disorders given the heterogeneous nature of addiction. Pharmacologic treatment is always adjunctive to psychosocial therapy.* Steps to be taken in the management of addiction are similar for all substances, and are highlighted in the Patient Care Process.[12]

Comorbid psychiatric conditions such as anxiety, depression, insomnia, pain, and continued smoking should be addressed. All these conditions increase risk of relapse to drug use. Although complete abstinence may be desirable in many patients, decreasing substance use and negative consequences may be sufficient in certain cases (ie, "harm reduction" concept)."

Nonpharmacologic Therapy

Although pharmacologic agents may help prevent relapse, psychotherapy should be the core therapeutic intervention. Psychotherapy typically addresses one or more of the following tasks:

- Motivation enhancement to stop or reduce drug use
- Coping skills education
- Providing alternative reinforcement
- Managing painful affect (eg, dysphoria)
- Enhancing social support and interpersonal functioning

A thorough review of these psychosocial approaches is beyond the scope of this chapter and are available elsewhere.[12] However, a few of the commonly used techniques are cognitive-behavioral therapy (CBT), motivational-enhancement therapy (MET), and other behavioral therapies (eg, community reinforcement).

Pharmacologic Therapy

▶ *Maintenance Treatment*

KEY CONCEPT *Certain pharmacologic agents have been shown to be helpful for long-term maintenance in patients with substance use disorders. Typically, these medications exert their effects by one of the following theorized mechanisms: (a) drug substitution therapy with an agonist, (b) blocking drug effects with an antagonist, and (c) miscellaneous relapse prevention medications with indirect mechanisms of action.* Medications from each of these categories are discussed in greater detail in the following paragraphs for alcohol, opioid, cannabinoid, stimulant, and tobacco use disorders.

▶ *Alcohol Use Disorder*

The three FDA-approved medications to treat alcohol use disorders are naltrexone (oral and depot), acamprosate, and disulfiram. Naltrexone and acamprosate are generally considered first-line agents as evidenced by their "grade A" efficacy rating in the seminal paper by Garbutt et al.[28] However, in motivated patients, disulfiram is another reasonable option.[29]

Naltrexone Naltrexone is a competitive opioid antagonist that decreases alcohol intake in both animals and humans. Evidence suggests that it both decreases craving for alcohol and alcohol-induced euphoria (ie, reduces positive reinforcement of drinking). Numerous controlled trials and meta-analyses have demonstrated that naltrexone is more efficacious than placebo for a variety of drinking measures.[12] One meta-analysis that included more than 20 controlled trials demonstrated naltrexone significantly decreased relapse risk compared with placebo.[30] Reported predictors of naltrexone efficacy include family history of alcoholism, genetic differences in opioid alleles, drinking problems at early age, and high levels of craving.[12,31] In a landmark study assessing efficacy of behavioral treatment, medication management, and their combinations for treatment of alcohol dependence, naltrexone was associated with a higher percent days abstinent.[32] An oversimplified interpretation of this complex study suggests that naltrexone was effective (eg, percent days abstinent), but that acamprosate was not associated with any treatment advantage.[32]

Naltrexone is available in both oral and sustained-release injections. Usual oral dose of naltrexone is 50 mg/day, with a range from 25 to 100 mg. The 25-mg dose is commonly given initially as a test dose and then increased to 50 mg/day as tolerated. Adherence to naltrexone strongly affects drinking outcomes; therefore, a sustained-release IM injection of naltrexone has been marketed. A 380-mg monthly injection of naltrexone (Vivitrol) resulted in significantly greater reductions in heavy drinking days compared with placebo injection.[33]

Most common naltrexone side effects are nausea, vomiting, headache, insomnia, and nervousness. Injectable naltrexone is associated with injection site pain or reactions. Because naltrexone can precipitate withdrawal in patients dependent on opioids, the first dose should be withheld 7 to 10 days after last opioid use and given only when urine drug screen for opioids is negative. Naltrexone can be hepatotoxic, albeit typically not at oral doses less than 250 mg/day or at recommended injectable dose of 380 mg/mo. Baseline and periodic LFTs are recommended.

Drug Interactions Naltrexone can block effects of opioid receptor agonists, rendering them therapeutically ineffective (see Table 36–5). Given that opioid agonists are a mainstay of pain management, alternative pain treatment (eg, conscious sedation) may be required in patients receiving naltrexone maintenance.

Special Dosing Considerations It is important for patients taking naltrexone to carry a pocket warning card or wear a warning bracelet because, in the event that emergency treatment is needed, they will be insensitive to opioid analgesia unless potentially toxic doses are administered. Patients need to be warned of the potential for opioid overdose under two conditions. First, dosing with opioids to reverse opioid insensitivity (ie, naltrexone's competitive blockade of opioid receptors) requires high doses of opioids that can cause respiratory depression and death. Second, chronic opioid antagonist therapy may cause patients to become hypersensitive to opioids after stopping naltrexone, thereby increasing risk of respiratory depression and death when opioids are used.

Acamprosate Acamprosate appears to be a glutamatergic antagonist and may have GABA-ergic effects.[3] Alcohol use acutely inhibits glutamatergic function. During acute and post-acute alcohol withdrawal, increased activity of the glutamate system is caused by upregulation of receptors combined with absence of alcohol-related inhibition. Thus, acamprosate may correct glutamate/GABA imbalances that occur following chronic alcohol use (eg, reduce negative reinforcement associated with craving and withdrawal).

Generally, trials assessing efficacy of acamprosate have shown mixed results. This may be partly attributable to differences in research methodologies, such as varying levels of abstinence required in trials before acamprosate initiation.[12] Notably, in the landmark Combining Medications and Behavioral Interventions for Alcoholism (COMBINE) study mentioned earlier, acamprosate appeared to offer no treatment advantage,[32] but a meta-analysis of randomized control trials suggests it is more efficacious than placebo.[34] Another recent meta-analysis suggests that acamprosate may be more effective at maintaining abstinence, but naltrexone may more effectively prevent full relapse to heavy drinking in nonabstinent individuals.[35] Despite the variable methodologies and results, there appear to be sufficient evidence that acamprosate is more effective than placebo, although differences may be modest.

The dose of acamprosate is 666 mg orally three times daily. It is not metabolized by the liver and is excreted unchanged by the kidneys. Consequently, it is contraindicated in patients with severe renal impairment (creatinine clearance less than or equal to 30 mL/min [0.50 mL/s]), and dose reduction is necessary when creatinine clearance is between 30 and 50 mL/min (0.50 and 0.83 mL/s). Most common acamprosate side effects are GI, including nausea and diarrhea. CNS adverse effects include insomnia, anxiety, and depressive symptoms.

Disulfiram Disulfiram irreversibly blocks the enzyme aldehyde dehydrogenase (ALDH), a step in the metabolism of alcohol. This results in increased blood levels of the toxic metabolite acetaldehyde. As acetaldehyde levels increase, patients experience the disulfiram-ethanol reaction (decreased blood pressure, increased heart rate, chest pain, palpitations, dizziness, flushing, sweating, weakness, nausea and vomiting, headache, shortness of breath, blurred vision, and syncope). Symptom severity increases with amount of alcohol consumed, and emergency treatment may be warranted. Psychologically, disulfiram works through aversion, and drinking is avoided to prevent the aversive disulfiram–ethanol reaction. Efficacy of disulfiram is directly dependent on medication adherence,[36] and more recent reports advocate that disulfiram can be highly effective when procedures for enhancing adherence are used.[29]

The usual starting dose of disulfiram is 250 mg/day orally (can be started at 500 mg/day for first 1 to 2 weeks), and the range is 125 to 500 mg/day. Compared with 250 mg/day, the larger dose is recommended if a patient does not experience a disulfiram–ethanol reaction after alcohol consumption, and the smaller dose is given when intolerable side effects are experienced at higher doses. Dosing begins only after the BAC is zero (usually 12–24 hours after the last drink) and after the patient understands the consequences of the disulfiram–ethanol reaction.

Disulfiram is contraindicated in patients with cardiovascular or cerebrovascular disease or in combination with antihypertensive medications because the cardiovascular effects of the disulfiram–alcohol reaction could be fatal in such patients. Most common disulfiram side effects are rash, drowsiness, a metallic or garlic-like taste, and headache. If drowsiness occurs, dose may be lowered or given at night. Other less common, but concerning, adverse effects include neuropathies and hepatoxicity. Given the serious nature of these adverse effects, baseline and periodic monitoring is recommended. If serum levels of alanine aminotransferase (ALT) or aspartate aminotransferase (AST) are greater than three times the upper limit of normal values, then disulfiram should be withheld and testing repeated every 1 to 2 weeks until normal. When LFTs return to normal range, they may be repeated every 1 to 6 months. It is advisable to follow LFTs and clinical symptoms until resolution has been confirmed.[37] Although elevated LFTs may signal disulfiram-induced hepatotoxicity, it is also likely the patient was nonadherent to treatment and resumed drinking, ultimately leading to hepatotoxicity. Another uncommon side effect of disulfiram is psychosis, which has been reported in doses exceeding 500 mg/day, especially in predisposed patients. This may be related to disulfiram's ability to inhibit dopamine β-hydroxylase, resulting in increased dopamine activity. Nevertheless, alcohol-dependent patients with schizophrenia and other cooccurring mental disorders have received disulfiram at usual therapeutic doses without difficulties.[38]

Drug Interactions The disulfiram–ethanol interaction serves as disulfiram's mechanism of action. Depending on dose of disulfiram, sensitivity to disulfiram, amount of alcohol consumed, and metabolism, patients may be at risk for an adverse interaction with alcohol for 2 to 14 days after stopping disulfiram (5 days on average) and should be warned accordingly. See Table 36–5 for relevant interactions that occur with disulfiram (particularly with metronidazole).

Medication Selection See Table 36–8 for patient-specific factors that can guide medication selection for alcohol use disorders.[37] Universally accepted treatment algorithms for the treatment of alcohol use disorders are lacking.

Patient Encounter 3

A 19-year-old woman was transferred to the cardiology unit from the emergency department (ED) after she called 911 claiming that she had chest pain and that her heart was racing. This in turn caused her significant anxiety. Upon arrival in the ED, it was noted that her heart rate was 130 beats/min in a resting position. She was in otherwise good physical condition with no previous cardiac history, although her eyes appeared extremely red and hazy. After a comprehensive urine toxicology analysis was positive for cannabinoids, she admitted that she had used "K2" at a party. She said she almost never uses illegal drugs. However, she was told "K2" could "help her anxiety" (diagnosed with generalized anxiety disorder at age 15 years), which has worsened since starting college. The treatment plan is to address the patient's substance use and anxiety disorder after the acute cardiac issues are resolved.

What physical signs and symptoms does she manifest that are consistent with cannabinoid intoxication?

What is the most appropriate pharmacotherapy for this patient's acute substance use condition?

▸ *Opioid Use Disorders*

After conclusion of withdrawal, patients may not feel their usual selves for some time and could relapse to using opioids, just to "feel normal." Long-term use of opioids results in brain changes,

Table 36–8

Alcohol Use Disorder Medication Decision Grid

Pretreatment Indicator	Acamprosate (Campral)	Disulfiram (Antabuse)	Oral Naltrexone (ReVia)	Injectable Naltrexone (Vivitrol)
Renal failure	X	A	A	A
Significant liver disease	A	C	C	C
Coronary artery disease	A	C	A	A
Chronic pain	A	A	C	C
Current opioid use	A	A	X	X
Psychosis	A	C	A	A
Unwilling or unable to sustain total abstinence	A	X	A	A
Risk factors for poor medication adherence	C	C	C	A
Diabetes	A	C	A	A
Obesity that precludes IM injection	A	A	A	X
Family history of AUDs	A	A	+	+
Bleeding or other coagulation disorders	A	A	A	C
High level of craving	A	A	+	+
Opioid dependence in remission	A	A	+	+
History of postacute withdrawal syndrome	+	A	A	A
Cognitive impairment	A	X	A	A

+ = particularly appropriate; A = appropriate to use; C = use with caution; X = contraindicated.

AUD, alcohol use disorder; IM, intramuscular.

Data from Center for Substance Abuse Treatment. Incorporating Alcohol Pharmacotherapies into Medical Practice. Treatment Improvement Protocol (TIP) Series 49. HHS Publication No. (SMA) 09-4380. Rockville, MD: Substance Abuse and Mental Health Services Administration; 2009.

and the brain might not readily return to its prior homeostasis. The goal of treatment is to encourage stability, both in the body and in the patient's life. If an individual is not successful in quitting opioids (eg, because of withdrawal symptoms or postacute craving), then maintenance treatment should be considered.

Opioid Agonists **The time-honored opioid agonist treatment for opioid use disorders is methadone maintenance. However, methadone maintenance can be provided only in federally approved OTPs. The other first-line agent, which will be the focus of this chapter, is buprenorphine maintenance.**

The more widely available office-based opioid treatment (OBOT) exclusively uses buprenorphine, a partial μ-agonist (typically in same medication formulation with naloxone).[9] Under provisions of the Drug Addiction Treatment Act of 2000, physicians may prescribe buprenorphine in their office if they meet predetermined requirements (eg, training) and become qualified providers. When these criteria are met, they obtain an "X" on their Drug Enforcement Administration (DEA) number.[9]

The effective maintenance dose of buprenorphine (with or without naloxone) is usually between 8 and 16 mg/day, with maximum reported efficacy at 64 mg/day. Patients receiving buprenorphine maintenance should sign a treatment contract requiring full adherence, financial responsibility for treatment, adherence to office policies, respectful behavior to staff, and agreement to provide random urine samples for drug screens. Patients should bring their prescribed medication for pill counts at every visit. In the event of OBOT failure, the alternative to buprenorphine maintenance is referral to an OTP for methadone administration.

In 2010, the injectable formulation of naltrexone was approved for prevention of opioid relapse following successful opioid detoxification. However, its place in the long-term treatment of opioid use disorders remains to be established. Please refer to alcohol use disorder section for additional naltrexone drug information. Chronic naltrexone use may complicate the risk of overdose with full opioid agonists as described above.

Although there are no treatment algorithms to guide medication selection, there are protocols for some medications that assist with dosing and titration. For example, **the extensive buprenorphine treatment protocol available from SAMHSA provides guidelines on how to dose buprenorphine from induction to maintenance treatment.[9]** Of note, **findings from a recent Cochrane meta-analysis indicate that methadone may offer an advantage over buprenorphine for select treatment outcomes (eg, retention in treatment).[39]** Therefore, **there may be circumstances under which referral to methadone maintenance remains the best option.**

▶ *Cannabinoid Use Disorders*

There are no proven pharmacotherapies for treatment of cannabinoid use disorders. Pharmacotherapy trials have emerged in the literature[40–42], but it is too soon to evaluate the role of medications for the treatment of cannabinoid use disorders.

▶ *Stimulant Use Disorders*

There are no proven pharmacotherapies for treatment of stimulant use disorders. However, the APA Practice Guidelines mention three medications as possible treatment options for CNS stimulant use disorders when combined with psychosocial approaches (ie, after psychosocial approaches alone have failed). These medications include topiramate, disulfiram, and modafinil. For example, disulfiram shows some promise in randomized, controlled trials possibly due to its inhibition of dopamine β-hydroxylase enzyme that converts DA to norepinephrine (NE) in the brain. The resulting increase in DA levels may counter DA deficiency states that are believed to underlie cocaine withdrawal and craving.[12]

▶ *Tobacco Cessation*

Nonpharmacologic Behavioral treatment delivered by a variety of clinicians (eg, physician, psychologist, nurse, pharmacist, and dentist) increases abstinence rates. The five As should be applied by all clinicians.[16]

- Ask if they smoke.
- Advise to quit.
- Assess motivation for change.
- Assist if willing to change.
- Arrange for follow-up.

Smoking cessation counseling should be provided to all smokers, and those interested should be assisted to achieve cessation. It is now a standard of practice for clinicians to screen for smoking and provide all smokers with brief advice and assistance with appropriate medications to quit or provide referral to specialized services when needed.

Pharmacologic According to the seminal tobacco use clinical practice guideline,[16] there are seven first-line medications available to treat nicotine use disorders (**Table 36–9**).[43]

Symptomatic detoxification and maintenance for tobacco use disorders is achieved with any single or combination of the currently available nicotine replacement therapies (NRTs).[16] Similar to opioid agonists, these NRTs act as substitution therapy with a safer alternative. NRT is generally considered safe with one notable exception: Given the pregnancy category D assigned to NRT, the decision to use NRT for pregnant women must be made on a case-by-case basis. According to clinical practice guidelines, pregnant smokers should be encouraged to quit smoking without use of medication.[16] Given the various NRT products that are efficacious at treating tobacco use disorders, choice of specific NRT depends on other factors, such as patient preference.[12]

First-line non-nicotine medications proven beneficial for treating tobacco use disorders are bupropion and varenicline. The sustained-release form of the antidepressant bupropion (Zyban) was approved by the FDA for treatment of tobacco use disorders. Bupropion blocks reuptake of DA and NE, and it appears that one of its metabolites is a nicotinic antagonist.[3] These mechanisms may help explain how bupropion acts to reduce nicotine reinforcement, withdrawal, and craving.

Varenicline (Chantix) is a $\alpha_4\beta_2$ nicotinic acetylcholine (nACh) partial agonist.[3] Varenicline decreases withdrawal and craving and prevents reinforcing effects of nicotine if the patient relapses. It is at least as effective as bupropion in clinical trials. Both bupropion and varenicline have been associated with severe psychiatric disturbances when used for smoking cessation.[44,45]

As shown in **Table 36–10**, various NRTs, bupropion, and varenicline increase abstinence rates at 6 months compared to placebo.[16] Furthermore, combining the nicotine patch with ad libitum nicotine gum provides the highest likelihood of abstinence at 6 months. The single agent (ie, monotherapy) with the highest odds of maintaining abstinence is varenicline (2 mg/day dose).[16,43]

Table 36–9

First-Line Medications for Treatment of Tobacco Use Disorders

Medication	Dosing and Administration	Adverse Effects
Nicotine patch (7, 14, and 21 mg)	One patch per day on a hairless area of body between the waist and neck; rotate patch site ≥ 10 cigarettes/day: 21 mg × 4 weeks, 14 mg × 2–4 weeks, 7 mg × 2–4 weeks < 10 cigarettes/day: 14 mg × 4 weeks, 7 mg × 4 weeks Duration: 8–12 weeks	Local skin reactions, insomnia, vivid dreams, headache May apply hydrocortisone or triamcinolone to ameliorate skin reactions Warnings and Precautions: Pregnancy category D CV risks: Recent (< 2 weeks) MI, arrhythmias, unstable angina
Nicotine gum (2 or 4 mg)	One piece every 1–2 hours (maximum, 24 pieces/day); chew and "park" Use 2-mg dose if 25 cigarettes/day or less and the 4-mg dose if 25 cigarettes/day or more or chewing tobacco Do not eat or drink (except water) 15 minutes before or during use Duration: 12 weeks (or as needed)	Sore mouth, hiccups, stomachache, dyspepsia, insomnia Avoid chewing (ie, should "park" the gum in cheek) and limit swallowing excess saliva to avoid GI problems Warnings and Precautions: Pregnancy category D CV risks: Recent (< 2 weeks) MI, arrhythmias, unstable angina
Nicotine lozenge (2 or 4 mg)	Use 2-mg dose for first cigarette 30 minutes or more after waking or 4-mg dose for first cigarette < 30 minutes after waking Weeks 1–6: 1 every 1–2 hours; weeks 7–9: 1 every 2–4 hours, weeks 10–12: 1 every 4–8 hours Do not eat or drink 15 minutes before or during use Maximum is 20 lozenges per day; use one lozenge at a time Duration: 3 to 6 months	Hiccups, cough, heartburn, nausea, headache, insomnia Avoid chewing (ie, should "park" the lozenge in cheek) and limit swallowing excess saliva to avoid GI problems Warnings and Precautions: Pregnancy category (not evaluated) CV risks: Recent (< 2 weeks) MI, arrhythmias, unstable angina
Nicotine nasal spray (0.5 mg delivered to each nostril)	One "dose" = 1 squirt/nostril One to two doses/hour (8–40 doses per day; maximum, five doses per hour) Do not inhale Duration: 3 to 6 months; taper (see dependence risk)	Nasal irritation, nasal congestion, changes in smell Warnings and Precautions: Pregnancy category D CV risks: Recent (< 2 weeks) MI, arrhythmias, unstable angina Avoid in persons with reactive airway disease Dependence (risk is higher)
Nicotine inhaler (4 mg in each cartridge)	Use 6–16 cartridges per day Inhale (ie, "puff") 80 times/cartridge Do not eat or drink 15 minutes before or during use; puff lightly and do not inhale into lungs (avoid coughing); avoid cold temperatures Duration: Up to 6 months; taper	Mouth and throat irritation (improves with use), cough, rhinitis, sneezing, headache Warnings and Precautions: Pregnancy category D CV risks: Recent (< 2 weeks) MI, arrhythmias, unstable angina
Bupropion	Initial dosing: 150 mg once daily × 3 days Maintenance dosing: 150 mg twice daily Should initiate at least 1 week before target quit date; efficacy of maintenance at 300 mg/day has been shown up to 6 months May be combined with NRT	US Boxed Warning(s): Serious neuropsychiatric events (eg, mood disturbances) when used for smoking cessation
Varenicline	Initial dosing: Days 1–3: 0.5 mg once daily Days 4–7: 0.5 mg twice daily Maintenance dosing: Day 8 and after: 1 mg twice daily Renal dosing (CrCl < 30 mL/min [< 0.50 mL/s]): Requires lower doses; 0.5 mg once daily with a maximum of 0.5 mg twice daily Initiate varenicline at least 1 week before target quit date or begin varenicline dosing and then quit smoking between days 8 and 35	CNS: Insomnia, headache, abnormal dreams GI: Dose-related nausea US Boxed Warning: Serious neuropsychiatric events (depression, suicidal thoughts, and suicide) have been reported with varenicline use

CNS, central nervous system; CrCl, creatinine clearance; CV, cardiovascular; GI, gastrointestinal; NRT, nicotine replacement therapy; MI, myocardial infarction.

Data from Teter CJ. Substance Use Disorders. 2012 Board Certified Psychiatric Pharmacist (BCPP) Examination Review and Recertification Course. Lincoln, NE: College of Psychiatric & Neurologic Pharmacists; 2012.

Table 36–10

Six-Month PostQuit Smoking Abstinence Rates and Associated Odds Ratios[a]

Medication	Abstinence Rate (%)	Odds Ratio (95% CI)
Placebo	13.8	1.0
NRTs		
Nicotine gum (6–14 weeks)	19.0	1.5 (1.2–1.7)
Nicotine patch (6–14 weeks)	23.4	1.9 (1.7–2.2)
Nicotine gum (> 14 weeks)	26.1	2.2 (1.5–3.2)
Nicotine patch (> 14 weeks)	23.7	1.9 (1.7–2.3)
Non-NRTs		
Bupropion SR	24.2	2.0 (1.8–2.2)
Varenicline (1 mg/day)	25.4	2.1 (1.5–3.0)
Varenicline (2 mg/day)	33.2	3.1 (2.5–3.8)
Combination Strategies		
Patch (>14 weeks) + ad lib gum or spray	36.5	3.6 (2.5–5.2)
Patch + bupropion SR	28.9	2.5 (1.9–3.4)

[a]Meta-analysis; 83 studies included.

CI, confidence interval; NRT, nicotine replacement therapy; SR, sustained release.

Data from Refs. 16 and 43.

OUTCOME EVALUATION

KEY CONCEPT *A major component of successful treatment of substance use disorders is to monitor use of medications and identify a mechanism for long-term support of sobriety that might be appropriate for a specific individual such as AA, or recovery programs for professionals such as doctors, nurses, and pharmacists.*

To determine immediate treatment outcomes for patients with intoxication and withdrawal syndromes, evaluate parameters such as blood pressure, heart rate, respirations, and body temperature, as well as mental state. Choose from a number of validated and standardized rating scales to monitor the responsiveness of withdrawal syndromes to medical treatment. To determine the overall effectiveness of your health system for the treatment of substance related disorders, monitor outcomes using sentinel events such as the rates of cardiopulmonary arrest, seizures, discharges against medical advice, patient violence, and use of physical restraints. The ultimate goal should be to enable the transition of patients to formal substance use treatment when indicated.

Important outcome indicators to evaluate postintoxication and/or postwithdrawal treatment can be divided into three major groups: decreased consumption of substances, decreased problems associated with substance use, and improved psychosocial functioning. When complete abstinence has not been achieved, quantify the consumption of substances using quantity–frequency measures, rates of abstinence, and time to first relapse as determined by interviews and self-report and by biological markers such as urine and blood tests. The Addiction Severity Index (see Table 36–2) can be used to assess alcohol and drug-related problems in various domains, and provides a more comprehensive picture of the substance user's life.

KEY CONCEPT *Clinicians must be familiar with "essential" resources, many of which are in the public domain.* Table 36–11 provides a list of these resources along with website addresses. These websites provide information useful for clinical management, research, teaching, and policy development purposes.

Table 36–11

Essential Substance Use Disorder Treatment Resources[a]

Source	Website	Example Highlight
American Psychiatric Association (APA)	www.psych.org	Practice Guidelines (*evidence-based treatment recommendations*)
American Society of Addiction Medicine (ASAM)	www.asam.org	Principles of Addiction Medicine (*gold-standard addiction textbook*)
National Institute on Alcohol Abuse and Alcoholism (NIAAA)	www.niaaa.nih.gov	Alcohol Research & Health (*peer-reviewed journal*)
National Institute on Drug Abuse (NIDA)	www.drugabuse.gov	Education Resources (*downloadable teaching slides; see Figure 36–2 in this chapter, for example*)
Substance Abuse and Mental Health Services Administration (SAMHSA)	www.samhsa.gov	National Survey on Drug Use and Health (NSDUH) (*national, representative alcohol and drug use survey*)
		Treatment Improvement Protocols (TIPs) (*evidence-based treatment recommendations*)

[a]There is a great deal of information from these resources, some of which is available in the public domain and may be used without permission. For example, the Treatment Improvement Protocols are comprehensive documents that can be accessed (free of charge) via the internet.

Patient Care Process

Patient Assessment:

- Evaluate patient's history and symptoms to determine if substance intoxication, withdrawal, or longer-term substance use disorder are likely (see Tables 36–1, 36–3, and 36–4).
- Conduct mental (eg, Mini-Mental Status Exam) and physical examination (eg, vital signs).
  - More detailed or substance-specific mental/physical examination may be required depending on presentation.

Therapy Evaluation:

- Assess medication adherence among patients receiving pharmacotherapy; substance use disorders are major risk factors for medication nonadherence.
- Assess all pharmacotherapy for effectiveness, safety, and drug interactions.

Care Plan Development:

- If substance *intoxication* is likely scenario:
  - Management of intoxication is typically supportive; most important goal is to maintain cardiopulmonary function. If consciousness is impaired, obtain blood chemistries to help identify causative substance and rule out other etiologies.
- Observe patient until intoxication has resolved for safety of patient and others.
- If substance *withdrawal* is the likely scenario:
  - Select appropriate withdrawal severity instrument to help guide medication use (see Table 36–2).
  - Severe symptoms (eg, alcohol withdrawal seizures) should be treated in the inpatient setting.
- Achieving long-term recovery: consider medication management as *adjunct* to psychosocial approaches.

KEY CONCEPT Follow-Up Evaluation:

- Regularly assess effectiveness and safety of therapy and emphasize importance of adherence to the treatment plan.
- Encourage patient to consider long-term treatment for substance use, especially after multiple episodes of intoxication or withdrawal.
  - Improved coping skills, functioning, and relapse prevention are key goals during long-term treatment.

Abbreviations Introduced in This Chapter

AA	Alcoholics Anonymous
ALDH	Aldehyde dehydrogenase
ALT	Alanine aminotransferase
APA	American Psychiatric Association
ASI	Addiction Severity Index
AST	Aspartate aminotransferase
AUDIT	Alcohol Use Disorders Identification Test
BAC	Blood alcohol concentration
CB	Cannabinoid
CBT	Cognitive-behavioral therapy
CIWA-Ar	Clinical Institute Withdrawal Assessment–Alcohol, Revised
CNS	Central nervous system
COWS	Clinical Opiate Withdrawal Scale
CRF	Corticotropin-releasing factor
DA	Dopamine
DEA	Drug Enforcement Administration
DSM-5	*Diagnostic and Statistical Manual of Mental Disorders,* 5th edition
DTs	Delirium tremens
ED	Emergency department
FDA	Food and Drug Administration
GABA	γ-aminobutyric acid
GI	Gastrointestinal
IM	Intramuscular
IV	Intravenous
LFT	Liver function test
MET	Motivational enhancement therapy
NA	Nucleus accumbens
nACh	Nicotinic acetylcholine
NE	Norepinephrine
NMDA	*N*-methyl-D-aspartate
NRT	Nicotine replacement therapy
NSDUH	National Survey on Drug Use and Health
OBOT	Office-based opioid treatment
OTP	Opioid Treatment Program
PFC	Prefrontal cortex
SAMHSA	Substance Abuse and Mental Health Services Administration
SC	Subcutaneous
SUD	Substance use disorder
VTA	Ventral tegmental area

REFERENCES

1. Substance Abuse and Mental Health Services Administration, Results from the 2012 National Survey on Drug Use and Health: Summary of National Findings, NSDUH Series H-46, HHS Publication No. (SMA) 13-4795. Rockville, MD: Substance Abuse and Mental Health Services Administration, 2013.
2. National Institute on Drug Abuse [Internet]. The Neurobiology of Drug Addiction [last accessed and cited 2015 Jan 12]. http://www.drugabuse.gov/publications/teaching-packets/neurobiology-drug-addiction/section-i-introduction-to-brain.
3. Stahl SM. Stahl's Essential Psychopharmacology: Neuroscientific Basis and Practical Applications. New York: Cambridge University Press; 2008.
4. Dobrin CV, Roberts DCS. The anatomy of addiction. In: Ries RK, Fiellin DA, Miller SC, Saitz R, eds. Principles of Addiction Medicine, 4th ed. Philadelphia, PA: Lippincott Williams & Wilkins, 2009:27–38.
5. Koob GF, Volkow ND. Neurocircuitry of addiction. Neuropsychopharmacology. 2010;35(1):217–238.
6. American Psychiatric Association. Diagnostic and Statistical Manual of Mental Disorders. 5th ed. Arlington, VA: American Psychiatric Association; 2013.
7. Rush AJ, First MB, Blacker D, eds. Handbook of Psychiatric Measures. 2nd ed. Arlington, VA: American Psychiatric Publishing; 2008.

8. Addiction Severity Index (ASI) [Internet]. Philadelphia (PA): Treatment Research Institute [last accessed and cited 2015 Jan 12]. http://www.tresearch.org.
9. Center for Substance Abuse Treatment. Clinical Guidelines for the Use of Buprenorphine in the Treatment of Opioid Addiction. Treatment Improvement Protocol (TIP) Series 40. DHHS Publication no. (SMA) 04-3939. Rockville, MD: Substance Abuse and Mental Health Services Administration; 2004.
10. Center for Substance Abuse Treatment. Detoxification and Substance Abuse Treatment. Treatment Improvement Protocol (TIP) Series 45. DHHS Publication No. (SMA) 06-4131. Rockville, MD: Substance Abuse and Mental Health Services Administration; 2006.
11. Volkow ND, Li T-K. Drug addiction: The neurobiology of behavior gone awry. In: Ries RK, Fiellin DA, Miller SC, Saitz R, eds. Principles of Addiction Medicine. 4th ed. Philadelphia, PA: Lippincott Williams & Wilkins; 2009:3–12.
12. American Psychiatric Association. Practice Guideline for the Treatment of Patients with Substance Use Disorders, 2nd ed. Arlington, VA: American Psychiatric Association, 2006.
13. Mayo-Smith MF. Management of alcohol intoxication and withdrawal. In: Ries RK, Fiellin DA, Miller SC, Saitz R, eds. Principles of Addiction Medicine. 4th ed. Philadelphia, PA: Lippincott Williams & Wilkins; 2009:559–572.
14. Tetrault JM, O'Connor PG. Management of opioid intoxication and withdrawal. In: Ries RK, Fiellin DA, Miller SC, Saitz R, eds. Principles of Addiction Medicine. 4th ed. Philadelphia, PA: Lippincott Williams & Wilkins; 2009:589–606.
15. Wilkins JN, Danovitch I, Gorelick DA. Management of stimulant, hallucinogen, marijuana, phencyclidine, and club drug intoxication and withdrawal. In: Ries RK, Fiellin DA, Miller SC, Saitz R, eds. Principles of Addiction Medicine. 4th ed. Philadelphia, PA: Lippincott Williams & Wilkins; 2009:607–628.
16. Fiore MC, Jaén CR, Baker TB, et al. Treating tobacco use and dependence: 2008 Update. Clinical Practice Guideline. Rockville, MD: U.S. Department of Health and Human Services. Public Health Service, 2008.
17. Lexi-Comp Online [Internet]. Hudson, OH: Lexi-Comp; 2015 [last accessed and cited January 12, 2015 from institutional university access database; https://online-lexi-com.une.idm.oclc.org/lco/action/home?siteid=1].
18. Clinical Pharmacology [Internet]. Tampa (FL): Elsevier/Gold Standard; 2015 [last accessed and cited January 12, 2015 from institutional university access database; http://www.clinicalpharmacology-ip.com.une.idm.oclc.org/default.aspx].
19. Sarton E, Teppema L, Dahan A. Naloxone reversal of opioid-induced respiratory depression with special emphasis on the partial agonist/antagonist buprenorphine. Adv Exp Med Biol. 2008;605:486–491.
20. Evzio Prescribing Information. Manufactured for Kaleo, Inc., Richmond, VA 23219. Issued: 4/2014.
21. McCord J, Jneid H, Hollander JE, et al. Management of cocaine-associated chest pain and myocardial infarction: A scientific statement from the American Heart Association Acute Cardiac Care Committee of the Council on Clinical Cardiology. Circulation. 2008;117:1897–1907.
22. Borgelt LM, Franson KL, Nussbaum AM, Wang GS. The pharmacologic and clinical effects of medical cannabis. Pharmacotherapy. 2013;33(2):195–209.
23. Daeppen JB, Gache P, Landry U, et al. Symptom-triggered vs fixed-schedule doses of benzodiazepine for alcohol withdrawal: A randomized treatment trial. Arch Intern Med. 2002;162:1117–1121.
24. Day E, Bentham P, Callaghan R, et al. Thiamine for Wernicke-Korsakoff syndrome in people at risk from alcohol abuse. Cochrane Database Syst Rev. 2004;(1):CD004033.
25. Lingford-Hughes AR, Welch S, Nutt DJ. Evidence-based guidelines for the pharmacological management of substance misuse, addiction and comorbidity: Recommendations from the British Association for Psychopharmacology. J Psychopharmacol. 2004;18:293–335.
26. Blondell RD. Ambulatory detoxification of patients with alcohol dependence. Am Fam Physician. 2005;71(3):495–502.
27. Mayo-Smith MF, Beecher LH, Fischer TL, et al. Management of alcohol withdrawal delirium. An evidence-based practice guideline. Arch Intern Med. 2004;164:1405–1412.
28. Garbutt JC, West SL, Carey TS, et al. Pharmacological treatment of alcohol dependence: A review of the evidence. JAMA. 1999;281:1318–1325.
29. Fuller RK, Gordis E. Does disulfiram have a role in alcoholism treatment today? Addiction. 2004;99:21–24.
30. Srisurapanont M, Jarusuraisin N. Naltrexone for the treatment of alcoholism: A meta-analysis of randomized controlled trials. Int J Neuropsychopharmacol. 2005;8:267–280.
31. Rubio G, Ponce G, Rodriguez-Jimenez R, et al. Clinical predictors of response to naltrexone in alcoholic patients: Who benefits most from treatment with naltrexone? Alcohol Alcohol. 2005;40:227–233.
32. Anton R, O'Malley SS, Ciraulo DA, et al, for the COMBINE Study Research Group. Combined pharmacotherapies and behavioral interventions for alcohol dependence. The COMBINE Study: A randomized controlled trial. JAMA. 2006;295:2003–2017.
33. Garbutt JC, Kranzler HR, O'Malley SS, et al. Efficacy and tolerability of long-acting injectable naltrexone for alcohol dependence: A randomized controlled trial. JAMA. 2005;293:1617–1625.
34. Mann K, Lehert P, Morgan MY. The efficacy of acamprosate in the maintenance of abstinence in alcohol-dependent individuals: Results of a meta-analysis. Alcohol Clin Exp Res. 2004;28:51–63.
35. Rösner S, Leucht S, Ehert P, Soyka M. Acamprosate supports abstinence, naltrexone prevents excessive drinking: Evidence from a meta-analysis with unreported outcomes. J Psychopharmacol. 2008;22:11–23.
36. Fuller RK, Branchey L, Brightwell DR, et al. Disulfiram treatment of alcoholism. A Veterans Administration cooperative study. JAMA. 1986;256:1449–1455.
37. Center for Substance Abuse Treatment. Incorporating Alcohol Pharmacotherapies into Medical Practice. Treatment Improvement Protocol (TIP) Series 49. HHS Publication No. (SMA) 09-4380. Rockville, MD: Substance Abuse and Mental Health Services Administration; 2009.
38. Petrakis IL, Poling J, Levinson C, et al. Naltrexone and disulfiram in patients with alcohol dependence and comorbid psychiatric disorders. Biol Psychiatry. 2005;57:1128–1137.
39. Mattick RP, Kimber J, Breen C, Davoli M. Buprenorphine maintenance versus placebo or methadone maintenance for opioid dependence. Cochrane Database Syst Rev. 2008;(3):CD002207.
40. Gray KM, Carpenter MJ, Baker NL, et al. A double-blind randomized controlled trial of N-acetylcysteine in cannabis-dependent adolescents. Am J Psychiatry. 2012;169(8):805–812.
41. McRae AL, Brady KT, Carter RE. Buspirone for treatment of marijuana dependence: A pilot study. Am J Addict. 2006;15(5):404.
42. Levin FR, Mariani JJ, Brooks DJ, et al. Dronabinol for the treatment of cannabis dependence: A randomized, double-blind, placebo-controlled trial. Drug Alcohol Depend. 2011;116(1–3):142–150.
43. Teter CJ. Substance Use Disorders. 2012 Board Certified Psychiatric Pharmacist (BCPP) Examination Review and Recertification Course. Lincoln, NE: College of Psychiatric and Neurologic Pharmacists, 2012, pp. 661–709.
44. U.S. Food and Drug Administration. Drug Safety Newsletter Volume 2, Number 1, 2009.
45. U.S. Food and Drug Administration [Internet]. Varenicline (marketed as Chantix) Information [last accessed and cited January 12, 2015]. http://www.fda.gov/Drugs/DrugSafety/PostmarketDrugSafetyInformationforPatientsandProviders/ucm106540.htm.

37 Schizophrenia

Deanna L. Kelly, Elaine Weiner, and
Heidi J. Wehring

LEARNING OBJECTIVES

Upon completion of the chapter, the reader will be able to:

1. Recognize signs and symptoms of schizophrenia and be able to distinguish among positive, negative, and cognitive impairments associated with the illness.
2. Explain pathophysiologic mechanisms that are thought to underlie schizophrenia.
3. Identify treatment goals for a patient with schizophrenia.
4. Recommend appropriate antipsychotic medications based on patient-specific data.
5. Compare side-effect profiles of individual antipsychotics.
6. Educate patients and families about schizophrenia, treatments, and the importance of adherence to antipsychotic treatment.
7. Describe components of a monitoring plan to assess the effectiveness and safety of antipsychotic medications.

INTRODUCTION

In most cases, schizophrenia is a devastating, chronically debilitating disorder. It may be thought of as a clinical syndrome, with many possible pathophysiological pathways that ultimately manifest with psychotic symptoms, including hallucinations, delusions, and disordered thinking. Commonly, these symptoms are accompanied by cognitive impairment (abnormalities in thinking, reasoning, attention, memory, and perception), impaired insight and judgment, and negative symptoms including loss of motivation (avolition), loss of emotional range (restricted affect), and a decrease in spontaneous speech (poverty of speech). Cognitive impairments and negative symptoms account for much of the poor social and functional outcomes. Schizophrenia is the fourth leading cause of disability among adults and is associated with substantially lower rates of employment, marriage, and independent living compared with population norms. However, earlier diagnosis, treatment, and advances in research and newer treatment developments have led to better outcomes.

EPIDEMIOLOGY AND ETIOLOGY

Approximately 1% of the world population suffers from schizophrenia, with symptoms typically presenting in late adolescence or early adulthood.[1] Prevalence is equal in men and women, but symptoms appear earlier in men with first hospitalization typically occurring at 15 to 24 years compared to 25 to 34 years.

The etiology of schizophrenia remains unknown. A genetic basis is supported by the fact that first-degree relatives of patients with schizophrenia carry a 10% risk of developing the disorder, and when both parents have the diagnosis, the risk to their offspring is 40%. For monozygotic twins, the concordance rate is about 50%. Many genes have been weakly associated with the development of schizophrenia; however, there is probably no single "schizophrenia gene." Research continues to explore candidate genes, loci, and copy number variants, hoping to better understand the genetic contribution.[2] Possibly, when a genetic liability is present, environmental stimuli may trigger expression of the illness. Some data suggest intrauterine exposure to significant stress, viral or bacterial infections may be a risk factor; however, more research is needed.

PATHOPHYSIOLOGY

The dopamine hypothesis, the oldest pathophysiologic theory, proposes that psychosis is caused by excessive dopamine in the brain. This hypothesis followed the discovery that chlorpromazine, the first antipsychotic medication, was a postsynaptic dopamine antagonist. Drugs that cause an increase in dopamine (eg, cocaine and amphetamines) worsen or cause psychotic symptoms, and drugs that decrease dopamine (eg, antipsychotics) improve psychotic symptoms. However, data reveal a more complicated picture with both hyperdopaminergic and hypodopaminergic brain regions in schizophrenia. Hypodopaminergic activity in the prefrontal lobe is thought to relate to the core negative symptoms. Thus, a more modern reworking of the dopamine hypothesis is the "dysregulation hypothesis," which takes these findings into account.[3] It is possible, however, that the hypothesized dopamine abnormalities may represent changes occurring secondary to other pathophysiologic abnormalities. Other implicated neurotransmitter systems include a combined dysfunction of the dopamine and glutamate neurotransmitter systems.[4] It is hypothesized that glutamate, possibly through malfunctioning *N*-methyl-D-aspartate (NMDA) receptors, impacts dopaminergic activity in

Patient Encounter, Part 1

A 23-year-old single man presents to the clinic with his mother with an approximately 1-year history of being fearful in public and continuously hearing voices of "famous people" talking with him and giving him advice. He was psychiatrically hospitalized following an episode of hypothyroidism during his sophomore year in college. Following that, 1 year ago, he withdrew from college, as he was having difficulty concentrating, and he was struggling academically. He was employed briefly as a waiter, but he felt he was not able to concentrate there as well. He also felt that the stress of working with many people made his fears worse. He lives with his mother. His parents are divorced, and he does not see his father, as he feels fearful and harshly criticized by him. He has given consent for his mother to be involved in his treatment, and during her interview, she states that his father will be of "no use," as he is "from a culture that doesn't believe in mental illness." She worries that her son spends too much time in his room and that he no longer does the activities he used to enjoy, such as listening to music and going to movies. The patient states he "doesn't really miss" doing these things, and he doesn't want to be pressured to do them. His mother also worries that he has strange eating habits and that his sleep is "off"—up at night and sleeping too much during the day.

What diagnoses are suggested by this presentation?

What additional information would help to clarify the diagnosis and why?

Should the patient's parents be involved in his care?

the mesolimbic and mesocortical pathways. NMDA antagonists such as phencyclidine (PCP) and ketamine can elicit a state resembling schizophrenia, including positive and negative symptoms and cognitive impairments. There is speculation regarding a role for serotonin receptor antagonism in antipsychotic efficacy[5] because many second-generation antipsychotics (SGAs) are active at serotonin receptors. However, a compelling pathophysiologic theory relating to dopamine and serotonin receptor affinities does not yet exist. It is notable that to date, antipsychotics without any primary or secondary dopamine-modulating properties have been ineffective for the treatment of positive symptoms of schizophrenia.

CLINICAL PRESENTATION AND DIAGNOSIS

In addition to the positive, negative, and cognitive symptoms of schizophrenia, people with schizophrenia may appear uncooperative, suspicious, hostile, anxious, or aggressive. Psychotic and depressive symptoms may lead to poor hygiene and impaired self-care. Sleep and appetite are often disturbed, and they often have difficulty living independently, forming close relationships with others, and initiating or maintaining employment. Comorbid medical disorders, such as type 2 diabetes and chronic obstructive pulmonary disease, are prevalent in people with schizophrenia because of sedentary lifestyles, poor dietary habits, obesity, or cigarette smoking. Approximately 60% of people with schizophrenia smoke, and approximately 50% use illicit drugs and alcohol.[6]

KEY CONCEPT *A diagnosis of schizophrenia is made clinically because there are no psychological assessments, brain imaging, or laboratory examinations that confirm the diagnosis.*

The diagnosis is made by ruling out other causes of psychosis and meeting specified diagnostic criteria. When present, a family history of mental illness supports the diagnosis. The commonly accepted diagnostic criteria for schizophrenia are from the *Diagnostic and Statistical Manual of Mental Disorders*, 5th edition (*DSM-5*)[7](Table 37–1).

KEY CONCEPT *Patients presenting with odd behaviors, illogical thought processes, fixed false beliefs, and hallucinations should be comprehensively assessed to rule out other diagnoses or contributing factors.*[8,9]

At minimum, patients with psychosis should have a medical workup at the time of admission to rule out other diagnoses or contributing factors. Often, people with psychosis are poor historians and the gathering of collateral information is necessary. Comorbid substance abuse, medical illnesses, and psychosocial stressors, often confound the diagnosis.

COURSE AND PROGNOSIS

Treatment of schizophrenia is often associated with poor long-term outcomes, however, some people can achieve remission. Typically there are intermittent acute psychotic episodes with a downward decline in psychosocial functioning. Though many of the more dramatic and acute symptoms may fade with time, severe residual symptoms may persist. Involvement with law enforcement is fairly common for vagrancy, loitering, and disturbing the peace. Life expectancy is shortened primarily because of suicide, cardiovascular disease, accidents, and compromised self-care. Lifetime risk of suicide for people with schizophrenia is 5% to 10%.[10] Persistent compliance with a tolerable drug regimen improves prognosis, while relapse without medication exceeds 50% in the year following noncompliance.

The onset of schizophrenia can be rapid with acute psychosis presenting as the first symptom, or onset can be insidious with negative symptoms and social impairments predating psychosis by many years. Whether insidious or acute, the period around the diagnosis is difficult for patients, families, and clinicians. Patients may hide symptoms from family and friends and isolate themselves from social support networks. Gradual development of psychosis and the misunderstanding of symptoms can delay diagnosis and treatment. Recent data suggest that people treated early in their illness may have a better prognosis. Therefore, the first challenge of optimal therapy is to initiate treatment closer to the onset of psychosis.

TREATMENT

Desired Outcomes

KEY CONCEPT *The goals of treatment are to reduce symptomatology and psychotic relapses and to improve functional and social outcomes.*[9] Patients should receive comprehensive treatment as early as possible. In the past, the primary treatment goal was to decrease positive symptoms and associated hostile and aggressive behaviors. Newer approaches also focus on functional and social outcomes. Though antipsychotic medications may improve combativeness, hostility, sleep, and appetite, other aspects of the illness are less responsive to treatment. Improvements in negative symptoms, cognitive functioning, social skills, and judgment generally require adjunctive treatments and a longer period to improve.

Clinical Presentation of Schizophrenia

General

Schizophrenia is a chronic disorder of thought and affect, causing significantly impaired vocational and interpersonal function. Onset is usually preceded by gradual social withdrawal, diminished interests, changes in appearance and hygiene, changes in cognition, and bizarre or odd behaviors. The clinical presentation of a person with schizophrenia is extremely varied.

Symptoms

Psychotic symptoms (positive symptoms):

- Hallucinations (distortions or exaggeration of perception)
  - Most frequently auditory, can also be visual, olfactory, gustatory, and tactile.
  - Can be voices or thoughts that feel distinct from the person's mind.
  - Voices may be threatening or commanding (eg, commanding the person to perform a particular action).
- Delusions (fixed false beliefs)
  - Beliefs despite invalidating evidence
  - May be bizarre in nature
  - Often paranoid in nature which may cause suspiciousness
- Thought disorder (illogical thought and speech)
  - Loosening of associations
  - Tangentiality
  - Thought blocking
  - Concreteness
  - Circumstantiality
  - Perseveration
  - Thinking and speech may be incomprehensible and illogical

Negative symptoms:

- Impoverished speech and thinking
- Lack of social drive (avolition)
- Flatness of emotional expression
- Apathy
- May be primary or occur secondarily to medication side effects, mood disorder, environmental understimulation, or demoralization
- The best strategy for differentiating primary from secondary negative symptoms is to observe for their persistence over time despite efforts at resolving the other causes

Cognitive impairments (diminished function in the following):

- Attention
- Processing speed
- Verbal, visual memory, and working memory
- Problem solving
- There is a loss of, on average, one standard deviation of preillness IQ, with the average IQ between 80 and 84.

Laboratory and Other Diagnostic Assessments

- An initial psychotic work up includes a thorough neurologic, medical and laboratory evaluation to rule out other causes
  - Electrolytes
  - Blood urea nitrogen
  - Serum creatinine
  - Urinalysis
  - Liver and thyroid function profile
  - Syphilis serology
  - Serum pregnancy test
  - Urine toxicology

General Approach to Treatment

The concept of recovery has become an increasingly prominent treatment goal. Treatment planning increasingly includes providing recovery-oriented services to people with schizophrenia. A range of nonpharmacologic interventions are now part of the long-term strategy to improve functioning. Implementation of evidence-based practice and prescribing behaviors, has led to the use of interventions that promote a remission or recovery attitude.[11–13] Moreover, recent attempts to improve and measure patient satisfaction have fostered patient empowerment and hope. Despite these conceptual advances and treatment improvements, many patients still fail to receive comprehensive care, and long-term outcomes remain poor.

KEY CONCEPT *The cornerstone of treatment is antipsychotic medications, and most patients with schizophrenia relapse when not medicated.* Treatment with antipsychotic medications should begin as soon as psychotic symptoms are recognized. Most patients are on lifelong antipsychotic medication because nonadherence and discontinuation are associated with high relapse rates. Often, adjunctive medications may also be necessary for specific symptoms or comorbid diagnoses. If other symptoms are present, such as depression and anxiety, these symptoms should be aggressively treated. Psychosocial treatments are also often used concomitantly.

Antipsychotic Treatment

Historically, only first-generation antipsychotics (FGAs; typical antipsychotics) were available, but since 1990, the SGAs (ie, atypical antipsychotics) have been marketed in the United States. These agents include risperidone, olanzapine, quetiapine, ziprasidone, aripiprazole, paliperidone, iloperidone, asenapine, lurasidone, and clozapine. Clozapine, the prototype SGA, is reserved as second-line therapy because of its unusual side-effect profile (see below).

KEY CONCEPT *Compared with the FGAs, the SGAs are associated with a lower risk of motor side effects (tremor, stiffness, restlessness, and dyskinesia).*

With the introduction of SGAs, the use of FGAs has progressively decreased, and FGAs have less than 10% market share of the antipsychotics used for schizophrenia. This decline occurred

Table 37–1

Diagnostic Criteria for Schizophrenia

A. Two (or more) of the following, each present for a significant portion of time during a 1-month period (or less if successfully treated). At least one of these must be 1, 2, or 3:
   1. Delusions
   2. Hallucinations
   3. Disorganized speech (eg, frequent derailment or incoherence)
   4. Grossly disorganized or catatonic behavior
   5. Negative symptoms (ie, diminished emotional expression or avolition)

B. For a significant portion of the time since the onset of the disturbance, level of functioning in one or more major areas, such as work, interpersonal relations, or self-care, is markedly below the level achieved before onset (or when onset is in childhood or adolescence, there is a failure to achieve expected level of interpersonal, academic, or occupational functioning).

C. Continuous signs of the disturbance persist for at least 6 months. This 6-month period must include at least 1 month of symptoms (or less if successfully treated) that meets Criterion A (ie, active-phase symptoms) and may include periods of prodromal or residual symptoms. During these prodromal or residual periods, the signs of disturbance may be manifested by only negative symptoms or by two or more symptoms listed in Criterion A present in an attenuated form (eg, odd beliefs, unusual perceptual experiences).

D. Schizoaffective disorder and depressive or bipolar disorder with psychotic features have been ruled out because either (1) no major depressive or manic episodes have occurred concurrently with the active-phase symptoms or (2) if mood episodes have occurred during active-phase symptoms, they have been present for a minority of the total duration of the active and residual periods of the illness

E. The disturbance is not attributable to the physiological effects of a substance (eg, drug of abuse or medication) or another medical condition

F. If there is a history of autism spectrum disorder or communication disorder of childhood onset, the additional diagnosis of schizophrenia is made only if prominent delusions or hallucinations, in addition to the other required symptoms of schizophrenia, are also present for at least 1 month (or less if successfully treated)

Reproduced with permission from the American Psychiatric Association. Diagnostic and Statistical Manual of Mental Disorders. 5th ed. Washington, DC: American Psychiatric Association; 2013.

Patient Encounter, Part 2

PPH: The patient was seen for his first ever mental health appointment by a psychologist in his late teens, when he had family therapy with his father to address relationship issues. He has started to see that psychologist again, following his first psychiatric hospitalization. His toxicology screens have been negative for alcohol and drugs of abuse.

PMH: He was first psychiatrically hospitalized following an episode of hypothyroidism during his sophomore year in college, but his symptoms continued even when his thyroid disease was stabilized. He has no other medical illness, history of head trauma, or seizure disorder.

SH: His parents divorced in a contentious custody battle, when he was in grade school. Prior to his sophomore year in college, he had no academic or social problems. He used alcohol periodically in college but denies using since leaving college. He denies ever using marijuana or other substances of abuse. He has held several part time jobs from the ages of 18 to 23 years, the last of which was as a waiter. He has no health insurance.

FH: His grandfather had an alcohol problem, and his great uncle has a history of psychiatric hospitalization, though the specific circumstances are unknown. His mother and aunt reportedly have depression.

Mental Status Examination

Appearance: Appears somewhat disheveled, dressed in dirty clothes, and hair looks like it has not been washed or brushed for several days. No abnormal movements. Poor eye contact.

Speech: Quiet and somewhat monotonous

Mood: Nervous. He denies feeling depressed, down, or blue.

Affect: Guarded and mildly anxious with restricted range. He denies feeling sad, guilty, hopeless, or helpless.

Thought content: He is an adequate historian but has a tendency to leave out detail. He hears the voices of famous Hollywood movie stars and pop music artists. Intermittently, he hears his dad's voice saying critical things. Sometimes, he feels that others know his thoughts. He denies suicidal or homicidal thoughts.

Thought processes: Vague and sometimes illogical.

Cognition: Grossly intact.

Insight and judgment: Impaired at this time. He is not sure he has a mental illness, as he continues to think his problems are related to his thyroid illness.

Given this additional information, how has your differential diagnosis changed?

What medications would you consider to be first-line options, and why?

What are the goals of initial treatment?

because of the touted better side-effect profile and other possible benefits of SGAs in nonpyshcotic domains of the illness. However, a large landmark study (the Clinical Antipsychotics Trials of Intervention Effectiveness; CATIE trial; *n* greater than 1400) examined the effectiveness of SGAs relative to a midpotency FGA, perphenazine. The study revealed that the FGA was equal to the SGAs for the primary endpoint of time to discontinuation of medication.[14] SGAs have historically been much more expensive than the FGAs; however risperidone, olanzapine, quetiapine, ziprasidone, aripiprazole, and clozapine are now available in generic formulations. In conclusion, when selecting an antipsychotic, the risk-to-benefit profile becomes fundamental and the varying side-effect profiles must be considered.

Second-Generation (Atypical) Antipsychotics

FGAs exert most of their effects through dopamine-receptor blockade at the dopamine$_2$ (D_2) receptor. SGAs have greater affinity for serotonin receptors than for dopamine receptors. Despite heterogeneous receptor binding, the efficacy among the SGAs is similar.[14] Additionally, recent data for SGAs and FGAs (lower doses) document similar overall efficacy with an effect size for acute treatment of 0.30 to 0.60 for most antipsychotics.[15] These findings have led to a modest resurgence of FGA use. Only clozapine, however, has demonstrated superior efficacy and that is in treatment-resistant patients. An important distinction of the SGAs is their lower propensity to cause extrapyramidal symptoms (EPSs) and tardive dyskinesia (TD). TD risk with SGAs is 1.5% annually in adults (less than 54 years of age) compared to approximately a 5% annual risk with FGA treatment.[16]

KEY CONCEPT *The SGAs are heterogeneous with regard to side-effect profiles. Many SGAs carry an increased risk for weight gain and for the development of glucose and lipid abnormalities; therefore, careful monitoring is essential.* Dosing and comparative side effects of SGA are shown in Tables 37–2 and 37–3.

► Risperidone

Risperidone, a benzisoxazole derivative, was the initial first-line oral SGA to become available generically. It has high binding affinity to both serotonin 2_A (5-HT_{2A}) and D_2 receptors and binds to α_1 and α_2 receptors, with very little blockade of cholinergic receptors.[17] Risperidone is also approved for relapse prevention and is associated with significantly lower relapse rates than long-term haloperidol treatment.[18] At doses less than or equal to 6 mg/day, EPSs are low, although higher doses are associated with a greater incidence of EPS. Risperidone use causes serum prolactin elevations similar to or greater than FGAs. Elevated prolactin levels can, but do not always, lead to amenorrhea, galactorrhea, gynecomastia, and sexual dysfunction. Mild to moderate weight gain and mild elevations in serum lipids and glucose may occur. However, patients chronically treated with other antipsychotics may experience a decline in cholesterol and triglyceride levels when changed to risperidone monotherapy.[14]

► Olanzapine

Olanzapine has greater affinity for 5-HT_{2A} than for D_2 receptors. It also has affinity at the binding sites of D_4, D_3, 5-HT_3, 5-HT_6, α_1-adrenergic, muscarinic$_{1-5}$ (M_{1-5}), and histamine$_1$ (H_1) receptors.[19] In the CATIE trial, olanzapine was associated with the longest time to treatment discontinuation,[14] suggesting it may differ from the other SGAs in effectiveness. Olanzapine has a low rate of EPS and causes slight, transient prolactin elevations. Olanzapine causes significant weight gain across the dosage range, similar to that seen with clozapine and greater than that observed with the other SGAs. Olanzapine is also associated with hypertriglyceridemia, increased fasting glucose, and new-onset type 2 diabetes (ie, metabolic syndrome). Among the first-line SGAs, it is associated with the greatest elevations in these metabolic parameters.[14]

► Quetiapine

Quetiapine, structurally related to clozapine and olanzapine, has high affinity for 5-HT_{2A} receptors and lower affinity for D_2 and D_1 receptors. It has some affinity for α_1, α_2, and H_1 receptors but very little for muscarinic receptors. Quetiapine may be beneficial for anxiety and depression. Motor side effects and prolactin elevations are uncommon. Orthostasis occurred in 4% of subjects in clinical trials. Sedation is generally transient. Mild weight gain and minor elevations in triglycerides can occur. Use of quetiapine with agents that can prolong the QTc interval or in patients with prolonged QTc should be avoided.

► Ziprasidone

Ziprasidone was developed to block D_2 receptors but also to bind with greater affinity to central 5-HT_{2A} receptors. It has a binding affinity ratio of 11:1 for 5-HT_{2A}:D_2 receptors. It has a relatively high affinity for 5-HT_{2C}, 5-HT_{1D}, α_1-adrenergic, and D_1 receptors.[20] It should be taken with food. Liability for EPS, weight gain, and lipid elevations is low but does occur. Ziprasidone causes some prolongation of the QTc interval in adults. However, overdose data and pharmacokinetic interaction data show little evidence that significant QTc prolongation occurs. Use of ziprasidone with agents that can prolong the QTc interval or in patients with existing diseases associated with prolonged QTc should be avoided.

► Aripiprazole

Aripiprazole is a dopamine modulator, with both antagonist and agonist activity at the D_2 receptor. It is the only D_2 partial agonist available for the treatment of schizophrenia. The goal was to have an agent that functions as an antagonist in hyperdopaminergic states and as an agonist in hypodopaminergic states. Aripiprazole is also a partial agonist at 5-HT_{1A} receptors, an antagonist at 5-HT_{2A} receptors, and has affinity for D_3 receptors. Additionally, it has moderate affinity for α_1 and H_1 receptors with no appreciable affinity for the M_1 receptor.[21] In CYP2D6-poor metabolizers start dosing with one-half the usual dose with adjustment to clinical efficacy. Give one-quarter the usual dose if given concomitantly with a CYP3A4 inhibitor. Sedation, nausea, and vomiting are the most often seen side effects. Elevations in weight, lipids, and glucose are generally negligible, and it does not usually cause elevations in serum prolactin. In fact, patients switched to aripiprazole from other antipsychotic agents may experience decreases in prolactin.

► Paliperidone

Paliperidone is the 9-hydroxy (9-OH) metabolite of risperidone. The efficacy of risperidone and paliperidone are similar. Receptor binding affinity is also similar between the two agents, with paliperidone having a greater affinity at 5-HT_{2A} compared with D_2 receptors. Unlike many other antipsychotic medications, paliperidone is mostly excreted unchanged, a potential advantage in patients with liver impairment. Patients should be told to expect to see the shell of the tablet in the stool because it may not dissolve in the digestive tract.[22] Side effects of paliperidone are expected to be similar to those of risperidone, including the potential for dose-related EPS and prolactin elevation.[22]

Table 37–2

Second-Generation (Atypical) Antipsychotics

Second-Generation Antipsychotic	Usual Starting and Target Dose (mg/day) (Schizophrenia)	Maximum Dose Likely to Be Beneficial (mg/day)	Available Dosage Forms
Aripiprazole (Abilify)	Initial: 10–15 Target: 15–30	30	• 2-, 5-, 10-, 15-, 20-, and 30-mg tablets • 1-mg/mL oral solution • 10- and 15-mg Abilify Discmelt orally disintegrating tablets • IM 9.75 mg/1.3 mL • Abilify Maintena extended-release 300- and 400-mg vial powder for suspension long acting injection
Asenapine (Saphris)	Initial: 5 twice daily Target: 10–20 total daily dose	10–20	• 5- and 10-mg sublingual tablets
Clozapine (Clozaril, Fazaclo, Versacloz, also available generically)	Initial: 12.5–25/day Target: 300–450	500–800	• 25-, 50-, 100-, and 200-mg tablets • FazaClo (orally disintegrating tablets) 12.5-, 25-, 100-, 150-, 200-mg • Versacloz (oral suspension) 50 mg/mL
Iloperidone (Fanapt)	Initial: 1 twice daily Target: 12–24 total daily dose	24	• 1-, 2-, 4-, 6-, 8-, 10-, 12-mg tablets
Lurasidone (Latuda)	Initial: 40 Target: 40–160	160	• 20-, 40-, 60-, 80-, 120 mg tablets
Olanzapine (Zyprexa, also available generically)	Initial: 2.5-10 Target: up to ~20	30–40[a]	• 2.5-, 5-, 7.5-, 10-, 15-, and 20-mg tablets • Zyprexa Zydis (orally disintegrating tablets) 5, 10, 15, and 20 mg • IM 10 mg vial (after reconstitution, ~5 mg/mL) • Zyprexa Relprevv 210-, 300-, and 405-mg/vial powder for suspension long-acting injection
Paliperidone (Invega)	Initial: 6 Target: 6–12	6–12	• 1.5-, 3-, 6-, and 9-mg tablets • Invega Sustenna 39-, 78-, 117-, 156-, 234-mg prefilled syringes
Quetiapine (Seroquel, also available generically)	**Regular release** Initial: 25 twice daily Target: 300–750 **Extended release** Initial: 300 Target 400–800	800	• 25-, 50-, 100-, 200-, 300-, and 400-mg tablets • Seroquel XR (extended-release tablets) 50-, 150-, 200-, 300-, and 400-mg tablets
Risperidone (Risperdal, also available generically)	Initial: 1–2 Target: 4–6	6–8	• 0.25-, 0.5-, 1-, 2-, 3-, and 4-mg tablets • 1 mg/mL (30 mL) solution • Risperdal M-tab (orally disintegrating tablets) 0.5-, 1-, 2-, 3-, and 4-mg tablets • Risperdal Consta long-acting injectable 12.5-, 25-, 37.5-, and 50-mg vial/kit
Ziprasidone (Geodon, also available generically)	Initial: 20 twice daily Target: 120–160 total daily dose	160–240[a]	• 20-, 40-, 60-, and 80-mg capsules • IM 20 mg/mL

[a]Outside product labeling guidelines.

IM, intramuscular.

Table 37–3

Comparative Side Effects Among the SGAs and Haloperidol

Side Effect	Cloz	Risp[a]	Olan	Quet	Zip	Ari	Ilo	Asen	Lur	Hal
Anticholinergic side effects	+++	±	++ (Higher doses)	+	±	±	±	+	±	±
EPS at clinical doses	+	+	±	±	±	±	+	+	+	++
Dose-dependent EPS	0	++	+	0	+	±	+	+	+	+++
Orthostatic hypotension	+++	++	+	++	+	+	++	+	+	++
Prolactin elevation	0	+++	+	±	+	0	+	±	±	+
QTc prolongation	+	±	±	+	+	±	+	+	+	±
Sedation	+++	+	+	++	+	+	++	+	+	+
Seizures	++	±	±	±	±	±	±	±	±	±
Weight gain	+++	++	+++	++	+	+	+	+	+	±
Glucose dysregulation	++	+	++	+	±	±	±	±	±	±
Lipid abnormalities	+++	+	+++	++	±	±	±	±	±	±

Cloz, clozapine; Risp, risperidone; Olan, olanzapine; Quet, quetiapine; Zip, ziprasidone; Ari, aripiprazole; Ilo, iloperidone; Asen, asenapine; Lur, lurasidone; Hal, haloperidol.

[a]Side effects similar for paliperidone.

0, absent; ±, minimal; +, mild or low risk; ++, moderate; +++, severe; EPS, extrapyramidal side effects; SGA, second-generation antipsychotic.

▸ *Iloperidone*

Iloperidone is indicated for acute treatment of adults with schizophrenia. It exhibits high affinity for $5HT_{2a}$, dopamine D_2, and D_3 receptors and acts as an antagonist at these, as well as at the $5HT_{1a}$ and norepinephrine α_1/α_{2c} receptors. Doses must be titrated because of the risk of orthostatic hypotension, and dosing should be reduced by half in CYP2D6 poor metabolizers. Common adverse reactions include dizziness, dry mouth, fatigue, orthostatic hypotension, tachycardia, and weight gain. Dizziness, tachycardia, and weight gain were twice as common with higher dose (20–24 mg total daily dose) versus lower doses (10–16 mg total daily dose).[23] Use of iloperidone with agents that can prolong the QTc interval or in patients with diseases that are associated with prolonged QTc should be avoided.

▸ *Asenapine*

Asenapine is approved for the acute treatment of schizophrenia in adults. Its mechanism of action is thought to be its antagonistic activity at $5HT_{2a}$ and D_2 receptors. It also exhibits a high affinity for other serotonergic and dopaminergic receptors, as well as α_1- and α_2-adrenergic receptors and H_1-receptors. Asenapine tablets must be placed under the tongue and allowed to dissolve completely; tablets should not be chewed or swallowed. Patients should not drink or eat for 10 minutes after administration. No added benefit was seen with doses above 10 mg twice daily, but adverse effects increase. Common adverse effects include somnolence, dizziness, and akathisia. It has shown little effect on metabolic parameters and weight change. Labeling for asenapine was modified to address rare occurrence of hypersensitivity reactions, including anaphylaxis and angioedema.[24]

▸ *Lurasidone*

Lurasidone antagonizes D_2 and $5HT_{2A}$ receptors. It also has moderate affinity as an antagonist at α_{2C}, is a partial agonist at $5HT_{1A}$, and is an antagonist at α_{2A}-receptors. Lurasidone should be taken with food. Adverse reactions reported in at least 5% of patients (and at least twice the placebo rate) include somnolence, akathisia, nausea, parkinsonism, and agitation. Lurasidone has shown only a small effect on body weight and causes minimal changes in other metabolic parameters.[24]

First-Generation (Typical) Antipsychotics

The FGAs are high-affinity D_2-receptor antagonists. During chronic treatment, they block 65% to 80% of D_2 receptors in the striatum and other dopamine tracts in the brain.[25] Clinical response is generally associated with 60% D_2-receptor blockade, while 70% and 80% are associated with hyperprolactinemia and EPS, respectively. During the 1990s, SGAs began to replace FGAs as first-line therapy.

Patient Encounter, Part 3

The patient is taking risperidone, following an unsuccessful trial of aripiprazole titrated up to 20 mg. He has been titrated up to 6 mg/day of risperidone, and his sleep pattern has normalized. He is also less preoccupied by his auditory hallucinations and the feeling that he has a relationship with famous movie stars. He is pleased that he has been able to stay out of the hospital for the last month but is anxious that he will need to be hospitalized again. Sure enough, when he comes in for his next appointment, he is anxious, as his father's voice is saying critical things to him. He is vague regarding his medication compliance. He is upset that he has gained weight on the medication. His mother, who is with him at the appointment, cannot vouch for his taking his medications and does not want to begin monitoring them, as she is worried they will get into power struggles over it. The possibility of hospitalization is discussed, but neither want hospitalization, and because he is not assessed to be a danger to self or others, his care provider does not force the issue and suggests, instead, the use of a long-acting intramuscular form of antipsychotic medication. Using an IM, they can all be sure that he is getting his medication regularly.

How would a clinician discuss the advantages of taking a long-acting intramuscular mediation?

What drug choices would the patient have for a long-acting antipsychotic, and how would you help him make the choice?

Table 37–4

First-Generation (Typical) Antipsychotics[a]

Class	Agent (Brand Name)	Dosage Range (mg/day)	Chlorpromazine Equivalents (mg)	Available Formulations
Butyrophenone	Haloperidol (Haldol)	5–30	2	T, LC, I
Dibenzoxazepine	Loxapine (Loxitane, Adasuve)	25–100	10	C, IP
Diphenylbutylpiperidine	Pimozide (Orap)	1–10	1–2	T
Phenothiazines	Chlorpromazine (Thorazine)	300–800	100	T, LC, I, R
	Fluphenazine (Prolixin)	2–40	2	T, L, I
	Perphenazine (Trilafon)	8–64	10	T, LC
	Thioridazine (Mellaril)	300–800	100	T, LC
	Trifluoperazine (Stelazine)	15–30	5	T
Thioxanthenes	Thiothixene (Navane)	5–40	4	C

[a]Low-potency antipsychotics include thioridazine, mesoridazine, and chlorpromazine. High-potency antipsychotics include haloperidol, fluphenazine, thiothixene, and pimozide.

C, capsule; C-SR, controlled or sustained release; I, injection; L, liquid solution, elixir, or suspension; LC, liquid concentrate; R, rectal suppository; T, tablet; IP, inhalation powder.

Doses for FGAs are frequently given as **chlorpromazine equivalents**, which are defined as the FGA equipotent dose with 100 mg of chlorpromazine. The target dose recommendation for acute psychosis is 400 to 600 chlorpromazine equivalents unless the patient's history indicates that dose may not be tolerated. Generally, maintenance therapy is 300 to 600 chlorpromazine equivalents daily. Dosing and available dosage forms are shown in Table 37–4. All FGAs are equally efficacious when studied in equipotent doses in groups of patients. However, an individual patient may not respond equally to each antipsychotic. Selection of a particular antipsychotic is based on patient variables, such as the need to avoid certain side effects or drug–drug interactions or previous patient or family history of response.

▸ *Decanoates*

Long-acting, depot preparations are available for two FGAs (fluphenazine decanoate and haloperidol decanoate) in the United States. These compounds are esterified antipsychotics in sesame seed oil for deep intramuscular (IM) injection. Patients should be exposed to the oral form of the drug first to ensure tolerability. With initial dosing of haloperidol decanoate, concomitant oral supplementation may be temporarily necessary while the drug accumulates, as steady state is achieved after four to five dosing intervals. Fluphenazine decanoate is dosed at 1- to 3-week intervals, but haloperidol decanoate is usually dosed once a month. Conversion from oral to depot dosing and maintenance dosing recommendations are shown in Table 37–5. Generally, 12.5 mg (0.5 mL) of fluphenazine decanoate given every 2 weeks is approximately equivalent to 10 mg/day of fluphenazine orally. A maintenance haloperidol decanoate dose of 150 mg every 4 weeks is approximately equivalent to 10 mg/day of oral haloperidol. Initial decanoate injections should be preceded by a small test dose.

Side Effects of the First-Generation Antipsychotics

In general, the low-potency FGA agents are less likely to cause EPS than the high-potency agents. (See Table 37–4) Of note, high potency and midpotency agents may cause less EPS than once believed and were similar to SGAs in the CATIE trial.[14]

The FGAs are commonly associated with EPS (including akathisia [motor or subjective restlessness], dystonia [muscle spasm], and pseudoparkinsonism [akinesia, tremor, and rigidity]) caused by dopamine antagonism in the nigrostriatal pathways. Akathisia, the most common motor side effect of FGAs occurs in 20% to 40% of people. Roughly half of the cases of akathisia present within 1 month of antipsychotic initiation, though it may present within 5 to 10 days after the first dose or after an increase in dosage. Younger people and those taking high doses of high-potency antipsychotics are at greater risk for development of akathisia.

Acute dystonic reactions are abrupt in onset and are usually seen within 24 to 96 hours after a first dose or increase in dosage. Characteristic signs and symptoms include abnormal positioning or spasm of the muscles of the head, neck, limbs, or trunk. Dystonia may occur in 10% to 20% of patients. There is higher risk for dystonia in young male patients and those taking high-potency FGAs.

Pseudoparkinsonism may be present in 30% to 60% of people treated with FGAs. The onset of symptoms is usually within 1 to 2 weeks after dose initiation or dose increase. Risk factors include older age, female gender, high doses, and possibly those with depressive symptoms.[26]

TD is a movement disorder characterized by abnormal choreiform (rapid, objectively purposeless, irregular, and spontaneous) and athetoid (slow and irregular) movements beginning late in relation to initiation of antipsychotic therapy. It usually develops over several months or after at least 3 months of cumulative exposure to antipsychotics. Severity can range from mild and barely noticeable to severe, causing interference with ambulation. Visible TD symptoms may stigmatize persons taking antipsychotics. The estimated average prevalence of TD is 20% in patients given FGAs with a range of 13% to 36%. The incidence of new cases per treatment year with FGAs is approximately 5%.[27] TD is reversible in one-third to half of cases with the cessation of the antipsychotic.[28] When antipsychotics are tapered or discontinued, there is typically an transient worsening of abnormal movements. Risk factors for TD include older age; longer duration of antipsychotic treatment; and presence of EPS, substance abuse, and mood

Table 37–5

Antipsychotic Dosing of Long-Acting Preparations

Drug	Starting Dose	Maintenance Dose	Comments
Aripiprazole long-acting injection (Abilify Maintena)	400 mg monthly and 14 consecutive days of concurrent oral aripiprazole (10–20 mg) or current oral antipsychotic after first injection	400 mg monthly	Establish tolerability with oral agent first Dosage adjustments for CYP2D6 poor metabolizers, and in persons who take strong CYP2D6 or 3A4 inhibitors; recommend to avoid use if strong 3A4 inducer
Haloperidol decanoate	20 × oral haloperidol daily dose; in the elderly use 10–15 × oral haloperidol daily dose; Generally 100–450 mg/mo Initial dose should not exceed 100 mg regardless of previous dose requirements (if > 100 mg, give 3–7 days apart)	10–15 × oral haloperidol daily dose, generally 50–300 mg/mo	With initial dosing, oral supplementation may temporarily be necessary; deep IM injection generally with 21-gauge needle; maximum volume per injection site should not exceed 3 mL Available in 50 and 100 mg/mL (5-mL vials and 1-mL ampules)
Fluphenazine decanoate	1.2 × oral fluphenazine daily dose; generally 12.5–mg/2–3 weeks	Based on starting dose and clinical response Generally 12.5–25 mg dosed at 2–4-week intervals (may be up to 6 weeks in some cases)	Can be administered IM or SC; 21-gauge needle, must be dry Should not exceed 100 mg; when dosing above 50 mg, should increase in increments of 12.5 mg Available in 25 mg/mL (5-mL vials)
Olanzapine (Zyprexa Relprevv)	**To target oral 10 mg/day dose:** Either 210 mg/2 week or 405 mg/4 week during first 8 weeks **To target oral 15 mg/day dose:** 300 mg/2 week for first 8 weeks **To target 20 mg/day oral dose:** 300 mg/2 week	**To target oral 10 mg/day dose:** after 8 weeks, give 150 mg/2 week or 300 mg/4 week **To target oral 15 mg/day dose:** after 8 weeks, 210 mg/2 week or 405 mg/4 week **To target 20 mg/day oral dose:** continue with 300 mg/2 week	Gluteal injection, 19-gauge needle Do not confuse with rapid-acting IM injection Must reconstitute with included diluent Measure amount to inject from vial (there will be remaining suspension in vial) Zyprexa Relprevv Patient Care Program: 3-hour observation period; patient must be accompanied to destination No refrigeration needed, use within 24 hours, or immediately once suspension is in syringe
Paliperidone (Invega Sustenna)	Initiate with 234 mg on day 1 and 156 mg 1 week later, both in deltoid muscle	Recommended monthly maintenance dose is 117 mg (range, 39–234 mg)	First two doses must be given in the deltoid muscle; after that, monthly doses given in either the deltoid or gluteal muscle; available as 39-, 78-, 117-, 156-, and 234-mg prefilled syringes
Risperidone long-acting injection (Risperdal Consta)	25 mg every 2 weeks	25–50 mg every 2 weeks	Previous antipsychotics should be continued for 3 weeks after initial dose of risperidone long-acting injection Recommended to establish tolerability with oral risperidone prior to initiation of long-acting injection Available in 12.5-, 25-, 37.5-, and 50-mg vial/kit; must use needle supplied with kit, administer IM

IM, intramuscular; SC, subcutaneous.

disorders. SGAs have a lower risk of TD than FGAs. New-onset TD incidence is approximately 0.8% per year with SGA treatment versus 5.4% per year for FGAs.[16] A subsequent review of studies reports a smaller difference in incidence of TD between agents (3.9% for SGAs and 5.5% for FGAs).[29]

Neuroleptic malignant syndrome (NMS), a life-threatening emergency characterized by severe muscular rigidity, autonomic instability, and altered consciousness, can occur uncommonly with all FGAs and may also occur with SGAs. Rapid dose escalation, use of high-potency FGAs at higher doses, and younger patients have a higher risk of NMS. When NMS is diagnosed or suspected, antipsychotics should be discontinued and supportive, symptomatic treatment begun (eg, antipyretics, cooling blanket, intravenous fluids, oxygen, monitoring of liver enzymes, and complete blood cell count). Dopamine agonists (eg, bromocriptine) should be considered in moderate to severe cases.

Table 37–6

Side Effects of First-Generation Antipsychotics

	EPS	Sedation	Anticholinergic Side Effects	Cardiovascular Side Effects	Seizure Effects/QTc Prolongation
Chlorpromazine	++	++++	+++	++++	++
Thioridazine	++	++++	++++	++++	+++
Loxapine	+++	+++	++	+++	+
Trifluoperazine	+++	++	++	++	+
Perphenazine	+++	++	++	++	+
Thiothixene	+++	++	++	++	+
Fluphenazine	++++	++	++	++	+
Haloperidol	++++	+	+	+	+

+, very low; ++, low; +++, moderate; ++++, high; EPS, extrapyramidal side effects.

Dermatologic side effects, photosensitivity, and cataracts may occur with the phenothiazine FGAs. Sedation is mediated by H_1-receptor antagonism; anticholinergic side effects (constipation, blurred vision, dry mouth, and urinary retention) are caused from M_1-receptor antagonism; and α_1-receptor blockade is associated with orthostatic hypotension and tachycardia (Table 37–6). QTc prolongation may occur with the lower potency FGAs, and thioridazine has a black-box warning for QTc prolongation.

Treatment Guidelines and Algorithms

A widely accepted treatment algorithm in the United States is the Texas Implementation of Medication Algorithms (TIMA), developed by a national panel of experts and updated in 2008.[30] Algorithms go beyond guidelines, providing a framework for clinical decision making. According to the TIMA schizophrenia algorithm, the SGAs (except clozapine) should be used as first-line treatment. Choice of SGA is guided by side-effect profiles and patient clinical characteristics. Treatment with a given drug should be continued for 4 to 6 weeks to assess response. If only partial response or nonresponse is noted, a trial of a second SGA should be initiated (Figure 37–1). Other similar guidelines include the APA Practice Guidelines for Schizophrenia,[8] the Expert Consensus Guideline Series,[9] and the 2009 Schizophrenia Patient Outcomes Research Team (PORT) Treatment Recommendations.[31] In contrast to the TIMA guidelines, the PORT recommends use of either FGAs or SGAs as first-line therapy.

Treatment Adherence

Estimates of nonadherence to antipsychotics range from approximately 24% to 88% with a mean of approximately 50%. Subjects who are nonadherent have about a fourfold greater risk of a relapse than those who are adherent[32]. Neurocognitive deficits and paranoid symptoms may hamper adherence, and identification of nonadherence by caretakers and providers can be challenging. Antipsychotic side effects such as EPS, weight gain, and sexual dysfunction are also major contributing factors to treatment nonadherence. Other factors include delusions, substance abuse, and negative symptoms.[33] For patients who have relapsed several times because of nonadherence, have a history of dangerous behavior, or risk a significant loss of social or vocational gains when relapsed, treatment with long-acting formulations should be encouraged. Risperidone, paliperidone, olanzapine, and aripiprazole are available as long-acting injectable formulations. In general, oral tolerability of these agents should be ensured prior to initiating long-acting injection. Dosing and other information about these formulations is shown in Table 37–5.

Special Populations

▶ *Dosing in Renal and Hepatic Impairment*

Table 37–7 shows dosing guidance on specific antipsychotic medications.

▶ *Children and Adolescents*

Around 10% to 30% of patients with schizophrenia have psychotic symptoms before their 18th birthday. The diagnosis of schizophrenia in children and adolescents is often challenging, and the differential diagnosis includes autistic spectrum disorders, attention-deficit/hyperactivity disorder, and language or communication disorders. The existence of prominent hallucinations or delusions helps make the diagnosis because they are not prominent in other disorders. Fifty-four percent to 90% of patients developing schizophrenia before age 18 years have premorbid abnormalities such as withdrawal, odd traits, and isolation.[34]

Treatment for psychotic children and adolescents ideally is intensive, comprehensive, and structured. Day treatment, hospitalization, or long-term residential treatment may be necessary. Pharmacologic treatment is indicated if psychotic symptoms cause significant impairments or interfere with other interventions. Children and adolescents are more vulnerable to EPS, particularly dystonias, than are adults. Because of concerns about EPS and TD in children and adolescents, it is recommended that antipsychotic therapy be initiated with SGAs. Aripiprazole, risperidone, quetiapine, olanzapine, and paliperidone are approved by the Food and Drug Administration (FDA) for the treatment of schizophrenia in pediatric and adolescent populations. Initiation and target dosing is lower for adolescents than adults.

Agents with significant sedative and anticholinergic side effects are not preferred because they can interfere with thinking, thus impairing school performance. Compared with adults, children and adolescents tend to gain more weight when taking these agents. Young patients should be started on lower doses than adults and should be titrated at a slower rate. Side effects should be monitored closely initially and throughout therapy.

▶ *Elderly*

Psychotic symptoms in late life (after 65 years of age) generally result from an ongoing chronic illness; however, a small

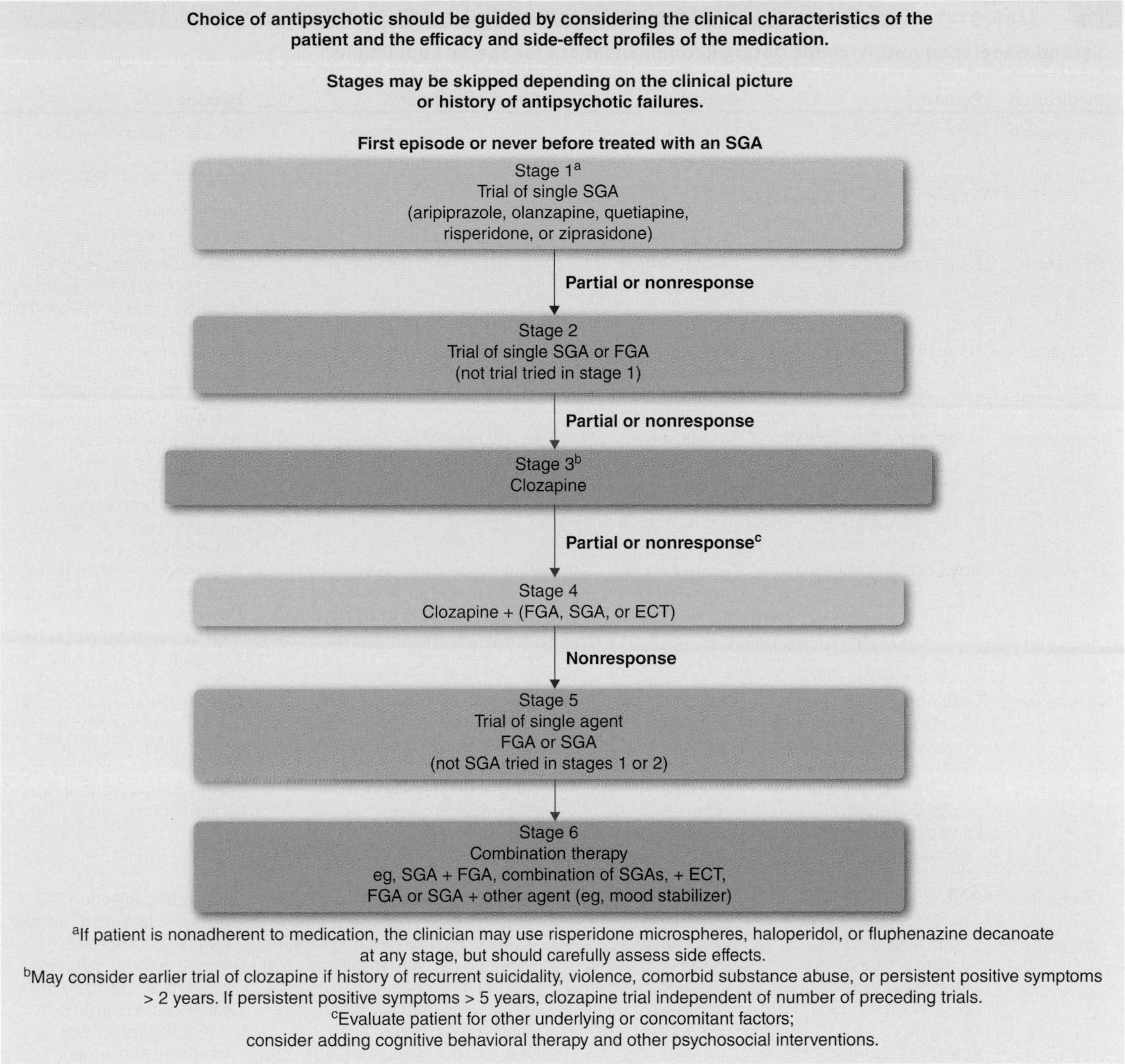
Choice of antipsychotic should be guided by considering the clinical characteristics of the patient and the efficacy and side-effect profiles of the medication.
Stages may be skipped depending on the clinical picture or history of antipsychotic failures.
First episode or never before treated with an SGA
Stage 1a
Trial of single SGA
(aripiprazole, olanzapine, quetiapine, risperidone, or ziprasidone)
Partial or nonresponse
Stage 2
Trial of single SGA or FGA
(not trial tried in stage 1)
Partial or nonresponse
Stage 3b
Clozapine
Partial or nonresponsec
Stage 4
Clozapine + (FGA, SGA, or ECT)
Nonresponse
Stage 5
Trial of single agent
FGA or SGA
(not SGA tried in stages 1 or 2)
Stage 6
Combination therapy
eg, SGA + FGA, combination of SGAs, + ECT,
FGA or SGA + other agent (eg, mood stabilizer)
aIf patient is nonadherent to medication, the clinician may use risperidone microspheres, haloperidol, or fluphenazine decanoate at any stage, but should carefully assess side effects.
bMay consider earlier trial of clozapine if history of recurrent suicidality, violence, comorbid substance abuse, or persistent positive symptoms > 2 years. If persistent positive symptoms > 5 years, clozapine trial independent of number of preceding trials.
cEvaluate patient for other underlying or concomitant factors;
consider adding cognitive behavioral therapy and other psychosocial interventions.

FIGURE 37–1. Texas Implementation of Medication Algorithms (TIMA) algorithm for antipsychotic treatment in schizophrenia. Choice of antipsychotic should be guided by considering the clinical characteristics of the patient and the efficacy and side effect profiles of the medication. Any stage may be skipped depending on the clinical picture or history of antipsychotic failures. (ECT, electroconvulsive therapy; FGA, first-generation antipsychotic; SGA, second-generation antipsychotic.) (Adapted from the Texas Department of State Health Services, with permission.)

percentage of patients develop psychotic symptoms de novo, defined as late-life schizophrenia. However, other illnesses with psychotic symptoms are common in this population; approximately one-third of patients with Alzheimer disease, Parkinson disease, and vascular dementia experience psychotic symptoms.

Antipsychotics can be safe and effective for the treatment of schizophrenia in the elderly, if used at lower doses than those commonly used in younger adults. Older adults are particularly vulnerable to the side effects of the FGAs. Pseudoparkinsonism reportedly occurs in more than 50% of elderly patients receiving these agents, and the cumulative annual incidence of TD in middle-aged and elderly patients is greater than 25%. Limited data suggest the risk of TD to be approximately 4% with the SGA and the likelihood of reversing this condition diminishes with age.[35]

Orthostasis, estimated to occur in 5% to 30% of geriatric patients, is a major contributing factor to falls that often lead to injuries and loss of independence. Low-potency antipsychotics and clozapine are more likely to cause significant orthostasis. Antipsychotics may cause or worsen anticholinergic effects, including constipation, dry mouth, urinary retention, and cognitive impairment. Greater antipsychotic-associated impairment

Table 37–7

Second-Generation Antipsychotic Dosing Recommendations for Special Populations

Medication	Pediatric	Geriatric	Renal Impairment	Hepatic
Aripiprazole	Ages 13–17 years (schizophrenia): Initiate 2 mg every day, increasing to 5 mg daily after 2 days and target of 10 mg after several days, 30 mg/day maximum	No oral adjustment necessary	No adjustment necessary	No adjustment necessary
Asenapine	No pediatric FDA indication	No adjustment necessary	No adjustments necessary	No adjustment necessary for mild to moderate impairment, but use not recommended in severe impairment
Clozapine	No pediatric FDA indication	Experience is limited; low dose and slow titration	Adjustments may be necessary with significant impairment; no specific recommendations available	Adjustments may be necessary with significant impairment; no specific recommendations available
Iloperidone	No pediatric FDA indication	No adjustment necessary	No adjustment information provided, but unlikely necessary	No adjustment needed for mild impairment; exercise caution with moderate impairment; not recommended for severe impairment
Lurasidone	No pediatric FDA indication	No adjustment required	With moderate to severe renal impairment, recommended starting dose 20 mg daily; do not exceed 80 mg daily	With moderate impairment, initial dose 20 mg daily; max dose 80 mg daily With severe impairment, initial dose 20 mg daily, max dose 40 mg daily
Olanzapine	**Oral:** Ages 13–17 years (schizophrenia): Initial dose, 2.5–5 mg orally every day with target dose of 10 mg/day; maximum dose, 20 mg/day **Long-acting injection:** Not approved in children	**Oral:** 5 mg/day, if escalation needed use caution **Long-acting injection:** Consider starting dose of 150 mg every 4 weeks for elderly or debilitated patients	**Oral:** In renal impairment, no adjustment usually necessary; however, consider a lower initial dose of 5 mg/day **Long-acting injection:** No information given	**Oral:** No dosage adjustment noted in prescribing information except in combination with fluoxetine **Long-acting injection:** No information given
Paliperidone	**Oral:** Ages 12–17 years (schizophrenia) Dose by body weight: < 51 kg, initiate 3 mg/day oral, increase at increments of > 5 days; maximum, 6 mg/day At least 51 kg, initiate at 3 mg/day, increase at increments of > 5 days, maximum of 12 mg/day	**Oral:** For patients with normal renal function, no adjustment is required, but if renal impairment guidance is available	**Long-acting injection:** CrCl 50–79 mL/min (0.83–1.32 mL/s); initiate with 156 mg IM day 1, 117 mg IM 1 week later, with maintenance at 78 mg IM monthly CrCl < 50 mL/min (0.83 mL/s): Use not recommended **Oral:** CrCl 50–79 mL/min (0.83–1.32 mL/s): 3 mg once daily initiation, maximum 6 mg/day CrCl between 10 and 49 mL/min (0.17–0.82 mL/s): 1.5 mg once daily initiation; maximum, 3 mg/day CrCl < 10 mL/min (0.17 mL/s): Use is not recommended	**Long-acting injection:** No dosage adjustment needed for mild or moderate impairment; no guidance given for severe impairment **Oral:** No dose adjustment is required for mild or moderate impairment
Quetiapine	**Regular-release tablets:** Indicated for schizophrenia (ages 13–17 years): Initiate 25 mg twice daily; recommended target dose 400–800 mg/day; maximum, 800 mg/day **Extended-release tablets:** Initiate 50 mg/day; recommended target dose 400-800 mg	**Regular-release tablets:** Slower dose escalation and a lower target dose **Extended-release tablets:** Initiate at 50 mg/day and increase at 50-mg/day increments based on response or tolerance	No dosing recommendations for renal dysfunction	**Regular-release tablets:** Lower starting dose (25 mg) and slower titration may be needed **Extended-release tablets:** Should be initiated with 50 mg/day, increasing in 50-mg/day increments

(Continued)

Table 37–7

Second-Generation Antipsychotic Dosing Recommendations for Special Populations (*Continued*)

Medication	Pediatric	Geriatric	Renal Impairment	Hepatic
Risperidone	**Oral:** Pediatric ages 13 years and older (schizophrenia): Initiate at 0.5 mg orally daily, adjusting at intervals of at least 24 hours and in increments of 0.5–1 mg/day as tolerated Recommended target dose, 3 mg/day	**Long-acting IM:** Initial dose, 25 mg IM every 2 weeks with a 3-week oral crossover; may consider 12.5 mg starting dose **Oral:** Initiate at 0.5 mg twice daily; may increase by 0.5 mg twice daily, increases above 1.5 mg twice daily done at intervals of at least 1 week	**Long-acting IM:** Patients with renal impairment should receive titrated doses of oral risperidone before initiation of IM (more detail in prescribing information) **Oral:** Recommended initial dose in CrCl < 30 ml/min (0.50 mL/s), 0.5 mg twice daily; dose may be increased by 0.5 mg twice daily, but increases above 1.5 mg twice daily should be done at intervals of at least 1 week. Clearance of risperidone is decreased by 60% in patients with moderate-to-severe renal disease (CrCl < 60 ml/min [1.0 mL/s])	**Long-acting IM:** Titrate with oral risperidone (see renal dosing) **Oral:** Recommended initiation in Child-Pugh Class C (see renal dosing)
Ziprasidone	No pediatric indication	No official adjustment recommended; consider starting at lower end of the dosage range	**Oral doses:** No adjustment necessary for mild to moderate renal impairment **IM doses:** Use with caution because of cyclodextrin sodium excipient	No adjustment necessary for mild to moderate hepatic impairment; however, caution is warranted

CrCl, creatinine clearance; FDA, Food and Drug Administration; IM, intramuscular.

in cognitive functioning may occur in the elderly compared to younger adults. In the elderly, this can lead to decreased independence, a very problematic issue. As a result of data showing a statistically significant increase in mortality in elderly dementia patients taking SGAs, a black-box warning was added to the manufacturer's information for all antipsychotics. Patients and families should be informed of this risk before using these agents in patients with dementia. Dosing in the elderly is initiated lower, and titration is slower than in younger adults. Maximum doses are often half of adult doses (see Table 37–7).

▸ *Dually Diagnosed Patients*

Estimates of the proportion of schizophrenia patients abusing alcohol and/or illicit drugs range from 40% to 60%.[36] Generally, the most common drugs of abuse are cannabis, cocaine, and alcohol. Substance use often worsens the clinical course and complicates treatment. Dually diagnosed patients are more likely to be nonadherent with treatment. They have a poorer response rate to the FGAs, more severe psychosis, and higher rates of relapse and rehospitalization than patients who are not abusing substances. EPS may occur more frequently in substance-abusing patients, and alcohol use is a risk factor for developing TD. SGAs are effective in this population, and they may cause a reduction in the use of drugs and alcohol.[37]

▸ *Treatment-Resistant Patients*

For 20% to 30% of people with schizophrenia, drug treatment is ineffective. A standard definition of treatment resistance is persistent positive symptoms despite treatment with at least two different antipsychotics given at adequate doses (a dose equivalent to at least 600 mg of chlorpromazine) for an adequate duration (4–6 weeks). In addition, patients must have a moderately severe illness as defined by rating instruments, and have a persistence of illness for at least 5 years.[38] These patients are often highly symptomatic and require extensive periods of hospitalization.

Clozapine Clozapine remains the only drug with proven superior efficacy in treatment-resistant patients, and it is the only drug approved for treatment-resistant schizophrenia,[15] with response rates of 30% to 50% in treatment-resistant patients. It is efficacious after nonresponse to other SGAs, in partially responsive patients and patients who have had a poor response to other medication for years. According to published guidelines and recommendations, clozapine should be considered after two failed antipsychotic trials but may be considered sooner if the individual patient situation warrants.[32] Additionally, it has a beneficial effect for aggression and suicidality and is FDA approved for treatment of suicidal behavior in people with psychosis.[39]

It is unknown which pharmacologic properties account for clozapine's superior efficacy. Clozapine has a low affinity for D_2 receptors, blocks D_1 receptors, and is a 5-HT_{2A} antagonist.

Clozapine's use is limited by the regulatory requirements resulting from the risk for agranulocytosis (0.86%–1% of patients), which is a rare but potentially life-threatening side effect. The required long-term hematologic monitoring (Table 37–8) can be a barrier for both patients and care providers. Other rare side effects include seizures and myocarditis. Other common unpleasant side effects include sedation, dizziness, constipation, enuresis, weight gain, and hypersalivation.

The optimal plasma level of clozapine is a minimum trough level of 300 to 350 ng/mL (300–350 mcg/L; 0.92–1.07 μmol/L; or 918–1071 nmol/L), usually corresponding to a daily dose of 200 to 400 mg, although dosage must be individualized. Males and smokers tend to require higher does to achieve the targeted blood level due to more rapid metabolism.

Table 37–8

Monitoring of White Blood Cell Count and Absolute Neutrophil Count During Clozapine Treatment

	Hematologic Values	Frequency of WBC and ANC Monitoring
Before clozapine initiation	Recommended levels: WBC ≥ $3.5 \times 10^3/mm^3$ ($3.5 \times 10^9/L$) and ANC ≥ $2 \times 10^3/mm^3$ ($2 \times 10^9/L$) No history of a myeloproliferative disorder or clozapine-induced agranulocytosis	
Initiation to 6 months	WBC ≥ $3.5 \times 10^3/mm^3$ ($3.5 \times 10^9/L$) and ANC ≥ $2 \times 10^3/mm^3$ ($2 \times 10^9/L$)	Weekly for 6 months
6–12 months	WBC ≥ $3.5 \times 10^3/mm^3$ ($3.5 \times 10^9/L$) and ANC ≥ $2 \times 10^3/mm^3$ ($2 \times 10^9/L$)	Every 2 weeks for 6 months
After 12 months of therapy	WBC ≥ $3.5 \times 10^3/mm^3$ ($3.5 \times 10^9/L$) and ANC ≥ $2 \times 10^3/mm^3$ ($2 \times 10^9/L$)	Every 4 weeks
Whenever clozapine is discontinued		Weekly for at least 4 weeks from day of discontinuation
Mild leukopenia or granulocytopenia	WBC value lies between $3 \times 10^3/mm^3$ ($3 \times 10^9/L$) and $3.5 \times 10^3/mm^3$ ($3.5 \times 10^9/L$) or ANC lies between $1.5 \times 10^3/mm^3$ ($1.5 \times 10^9/L$) and $2 \times 10^3/mm^3$ ($2 \times 10^9/L$)	Twice weekly until returned to recommended levels
Moderate leukopenia or granulocytopenia	WBC value lies between $2 \times 10^3/mm^3$ ($2 \times 10^9/L$) and $3 \times 10^3/mm^3$ ($3 \times 10^9/L$) or ANC value lies between $1 \times 10^3/mm^3$ ($1 \times 10^9/L$) and $1.5 \times 10^3/mm^3$ ($1.5 \times 10^9/L$)	Interrupt therapy; monitor daily until WBC > $3 \times 10^3/mm^3$ ($3 \times 10^9/L$) and ANC > $1.5 \times 10^3/mm^3$ ($1.5 \times 10^9/L$); then twice weekly until back to recommended levels
Severe leukopenia or granulocytopenia or agranulocytosis	WBC < $2 \times 10^3/mm^3$ ($2 \times 10^9/L$) or ANC < $1 \times 10^3/mm^3$ ($1 \times 10^9/L$) ANC ≤ $0.5 \times 10^3/mm^3$ ($0.5 \times 10^9/L$) (agranulocytosis)	Discontinue treatment and do not rechallenge; monitor daily until WBC > $3 \times 10^3/mm^3$ ($3 \times 10^9/L$) and ANC > $1.5 \times 10^3/mm^3$ ($1.5 \times 10^9/L$); then twice weekly until back to recommended levels

ANC, absolute neutrophil count; WBC, white blood cell count.

▶ *Acutely Psychotic Patients*

Psychiatric emergencies occur in emergency departments, psychiatric units, medical facilities, and outpatient settings. Although verbal interventions are recommended as initial management, most psychiatric emergencies require both pharmacologic and psychological interventions. Safe and effective IM formulations are available for a number of FGAs and three SGAs (aripiprazole, ziprasidone, and olanzapine). These IM SGAs are now recommended as first-line therapy in agitated schizophrenia patients; however, IM benzodiazepines, most often lorazepam with or without concomitant oral antipsychotics are also used. Concomitant IM olanzapine and benzodiazepines may cause cardiorespiratory depression and should be avoided if possible. High doses of FGAs, termed *rapid neuroleptization*, are no longer recommended.

Patient Encounter, Part 4

He is initially reluctant to get "a shot" but finally agrees, as he also does not want to get into power struggles with his mother about whether or not he is taking his medication. His clinician encourages him to exercise regularly and eat a healthy diet that is low in carbohydrates.

Over the next several months, he is more stable on the long-acting intramuscular form of risperidone, and he has not gained further weight. His eating habits are normal. He is less anxious, and his sleep is better. He is still, at times, preoccupied with the "Hollywood stars," and at times, the voice he hears of his father is upsetting to him, particularly when he is falling asleep at night. After 6 months of treatment, his clinician notices slight mouth movements that could be early tardive dyskinesia. After discussion of the risks and benefits, the patient agrees to a trial of clozapine. In a separate phone call to his mom, his clinician reviews the pros and cons of the clozapine trial.

Why is his clinician considering a clozapine trial?

What are the rare serious side effects of clozapine versus the common manageable side effects?

▶ *Pregnancy and Lactation*

When to use antipsychotics in pregnancy and during lactation remains a complicated decision based on a careful analysis of risks and benefits. Women with schizophrenia, even those who are unmedicated, have a significantly greater risk of obstetrical compilations (eg, stillbirth, infant death, preterm delivery, low infant birth weight, and infants who are small for gestational age).

Women who have a psychotic relapse during pregnancy are at greatest risk for birth complications.[40] Because psychotic relapse may be more detrimental than antipsychotic treatment to both the mother and baby, antipsychotics are often continued during pregnancy. Women taking antipsychotics who become pregnant should not discontinue them without consulting their health care professionals.

Essentially all antipsychotic medications are distributed to the placenta. Both FGAs and SGAs may be associated with an increased risk of neonatal complications. High-potency FGAs have a low risk for congenital abnormalities; however, limb defects and dyskinesias are reported.[41] Low-potency phenothiazine antipsychotics may increase the risk of congenital abnormalities when used in the first trimester. There appears to be little risk associated with first-line SGAs.[42] Long-term neurobehavioral studies of children exposed to SGAs in utero have not yet been done, however, and certain FGA agents may be preferred in drug-naïve pregnant patients because of availability of more reproductive safety data. If pregnancy occurs during antipsychotic treatment, however, continuation of previous therapy is preferred. On the basis of available data, each case should be weighed individually.

A labeling change for antipsychotic medications has been implemented by the FDA to address the potential risk for EPS and symptoms of withdrawal in newborns whose mothers were treated with antipsychotics in the third trimester. Withdrawal symptoms may include agitation, abnormal muscle tone (increased or decreased), tremor, sleepiness, and difficulty in breathing or feeding, which may last for hours to days after delivery. In some newborns, specific treatment for withdrawal is not needed, whereas in others, longer hospital stays may be required.

Although SGAs are excreted in breast milk, most case reports document a low frequency of deleterious effects on the infant. Women taking prolactin sparing SGAs (SGAs other than risperidone and paliperidone) may have enhanced fertility compared with women taking other antipsychotics because they are less likely to be anovulotory. Therefore, women of childbearing potential taking antipsychotics must be educated about birth control.

Pharmacokinetics

All antipsychotics are, at least to some extent, metabolized by hepatic CYP450 metabolic enzymes to water-soluble compounds that are excreted by the kidneys (Table 37–9). Unlike the other antipsychotics, ziprasidone is mostly metabolized by aldehyde oxidase, a metabolic system independent of the CYP450 system. Paliperidone, the 9-OH metabolite of risperidone, is mostly excreted unchanged in the urine, although up to one-third may be metabolized. The transmembrane energy-dependent efflux transporter P-glycoprotein may limit the ability of drugs to penetrate the blood–brain barrier and therefore impact pharmacologic activity in the brain.[43] Antipsychotics currently known to use this pathway include perphenazine, haloperidol, fluphenazine, quetiapine, risperidone, and olanzapine.[44]

Additive side effects may occur with combined drug therapies, and a few clinically significant drug interactions are notable (see Table 37–9). Cigarette smoking decreases serum concentrations of clozapine and olanzapine by induction of CYP1A2. Although antipsychotics are highly protein bound, protein-binding interactions are generally not clinically significant. Absorption of most antipsychotics is not affected by food, with the exception of lurasidone and ziprasidone. The mean maximum concentration of lurasidone increases threefold when administered with food, and ziprasidone's absorption is increased by 60% to 70% when given with meals.

Ziprasidone, iloperidone, and quetiapine have potential to prolong the QTc interval. Using them with other agents that prolong the QTc interval should be undertaken with caution. These other agents include, but are not limited to, quinidine, sotalol, chlorpromazine, droperidol, mesoridazine, pimozide, thioridazine, gatifloxacin, halofantrine, mefloquine, moxifloxacin, and pentamidine. Combining higher doses of ziprasidone, iloperidone or quetiapine with ketoconazole or erythromycin should be undertaken cautiously.

Table 37–9

Metabolism and Drug Interactions with Antipsychotics

Antipsychotic	Major Metabolic Pathways	Other Metabolic Pathways	Increase Antipsychotic Concentrations	Decrease Antipsychotic Concentrations
Aripiprazole	CYP 3A4	CYP 2D6	Fluvoxamine, ketoconazole	Carbamazepine
Asenapine	Glucuronidation by UGT1A4 and CYP 1A2	CYP 3A4, CYP 2D6	Fluvoxamine	
Chlorpromazine	CYP 2D6	CYP 1A2, CYP 3A4		
Clozapine	CYP 1A2	CYP 3A4, CYP 2D6, CYP 2C19, CYP 2C9	Fluvoxamine, ciprofloxacin, paroxetine	Cigarette smoking
Fluphenazine	CYP 2D6		Paroxetine	
Haloperidol	CYP 2D6, CYP 3A4	CYP 1A2	Fluvoxamine, fluoxetine, ketoconazole	Carbamazepine
Iloperidone	CYP 2D6, CYP 3A4	1A2, 2E1	Ketoconazole, fluoxetine, paroxetine	
Loxapine	CYP 1A2, CYP 2D6, CYP 3A4			
Lurasidone	CYP 3A4		Ketoconazole, diltiazem	Rifampin
Olanzapine	CYP 1A2, Glucuronidation by UGT1A4	CYP 2D6	Fluvoxamine, ciprofloxacin, paroxetine	Cigarette smoking
Paliperidone	CYP 2D6, CYP 3A4 (in vitro, but limited role in vivo)		Divalproex sodium, paroxetine	Carbamazepine (via increased renal elimination)
Perphenazine	CYP 2D6		Fluvoxamine, fluoxetine, paroxetine	
Pimozide	CYP 3A4	CYP 1A2	Strong CYP 2D6 inhibitors, CYP 3A4 inhibitors	CYP 3A4 inducers
Quetiapine	CYP 3A4	2D6	Fluvoxamine, ketoconazole	Carbamazepine
Risperidone	CYP 2D6	3A4	Fluoxetine, paroxetine	Carbamazepine
Thioridazine	CYP 2D6	2C19	Fluvoxamine	Cigarette smoking
Thiothixene	CYP 1A2		CYP 1A2 inhibitors	CYP 1A2 inducers
Trifluoperazine	CYP 1A2		CYP 1A2 inhibitors	CYP 1A2 inducers
Ziprasidone	Aldehyde oxidase	CYP 1A2, CYP 3A4	Fluvoxamine, ketoconazole	Carbamazepine

CYP450, cytochrome P450 isoenzyme.

Added pharmacodynamic effects are possible when combining antipsychotics with others drugs that can cause sedation, hypotension, anticholinergic symptoms, and weight gain or metabolic abnormalities.

Adjunct Treatments

The judicious use of pharmacologic therapies other than antipsychotics is often necessary for the treatment of motor side effects, anxiety, depression, mood elevation, and possibly residual psychotic symptoms. Anticholinergic medications (eg, benztropine, 1 to 2 mg two times daily; trihexyphenidyl, 1 to 3 mg three times daily; and diphenhydramine, 25 to 50 mg two times daily) are used to treat EPS. They may be prescribed prophylactically with high-D_2-binding agents or in patients at risk for EPS or for treatment of EPS. β-Blockers (eg, propranolol 30–120 mg/day) are sometimes effective for patients who develop akathisia. In some situations, such as on an inpatient unit, the concomitant use of benzodiazepines (eg, lorazepam 1–3 mg/day) with the SGAs may be necessary for agitation or insomnia.

Antidepressants may be useful for patients with schizophrenia who have depressive symptoms. Because suicide and depression are linked, aggressive treatment is necessary when depression is present. The selective serotonin reuptake inhibitors (SSRIs) are the preferred agents, but they may inhibit the CYP450 enzymes, thus raising plasma concentrations of clozapine, olanzapine, and haloperidol. Mood stabilizers, such as lithium and the anticonvulsants, have long been used adjunctively with the antipsychotics to treat the affective component of schizoaffective disorder.

Approximately 30% of treatment-resistant patients given clozapine do not respond, and another 30% have only a partial response. Limited treatment options are available for these patients. A number of augmentation strategies have been tried, including FGAs, SGAs, mood stabilizers (eg, lithium, valproate, and topiramate), minocycline, antidepressants, transcranial magnetic stimulation (TMS) and electroconvulsive therapy (ECT). Though controlled trial results are mixed, some data support the adjunctive use of risperidone, lamotrigine, or aripiprazole in clozapine-treated patients.[45]

Psychosocial Treatment

KEY CONCEPT *Psychosocial support helps improve functional outcomes.* Residual symptoms often persist such as avolition, isolation, and impaired social functioning, limiting participation in social, vocational, and educational endeavors. Psychosocial interventions, as adjuncts to pharmacotherapy, are designed to improve psychosocial functioning, self-esteem, and life satisfaction. These treatments are mainly used as targeted treatments for social and cognitive impairments.[13] In the United States, psychosocial treatments are less standardized than in Europe, but their use is on the rise. There are much data to support family education in decreasing relapse rates and vocational support to improve vocational outcomes. A few of the best-supported and most promising approaches to psychosocial rehabilitation are social skills training (SST), cognitive behavioral therapy (CBT), acceptance commitment therapy, and cognitive remediation (CR). In addition, Assertive Community Treatment (ACT) and Medical Home care models may improve outcomes.[13]

Patient Education

KEY CONCEPT *Education of the patient and family regarding the benefits and risks of antipsychotic medications and the importance of treatment adherence must be ongoing and integrated into pharmacologic management.* Medication management discussions offer an opportunity to provide illness and treatment education including the nature and course of schizophrenia, and can serve as a time to hear the patient's life goals. Key considerations include:

- Involve families in the education and treatment plans because family psychoeducation may decrease relapse, improve symptomatology, and enhance psychosocial and family outcomes.[46]
- Be clear that there is no cure for schizophrenia and that medication can be effective to decrease and improve many symptoms.
- Explain common and rare but dangerous side effects.
- Stress the importance of medication and treatment adherence for improving long-term outcomes.
- Decision making on the best course of treatment should be a shared process.

> **Patient Encounter, Part 5**
>
> Over the next 6 months, the patient becomes less preoccupied with his psychotic thoughts, though they do not resolve completely. He feels somewhat sad and anxious about the future, unsure of his goals, and preoccupied with all the time he "has wasted being crazy." He continues to be socially withdrawn, not sure how to react to others when they ask him what he has been doing over the last 2 years and what he is doing now. He doesn't know how to interact with his old friends, as they often meet in bars, and he does not feel comfortable there.
>
> *What are the possible underlying causes of his current mental state?*
>
> *How might the clinician consider addressing his concerns?*

OUTCOME EVALUATION

Developing a good working alliance with the patient is essential. In the absence of a solid therapeutic relationship, patients are frequently reluctant to share their beliefs, personal experiences, and life goals.

Symptom Monitoring

Many assessments are available to objectively rate positive and negative symptoms, level of function, and life satisfaction. The most commonly used scales include:

- Positive and Negative Symptom Scale (PANSS)
- Brief Psychiatric Rating Scale (BPRS)
- Clinical Global Impression (CGI) Scale

Using these scales on a regular basis, particularly when switching medications or changing doses, is a more reliable means of monitoring symptoms. Symptom assessments cannot capture the full range of possible improvements, but they can be useful in deciding whether a medication is having substantial benefit.

Side-Effect Monitoring

KEY CONCEPT *Regularly monitor for side effects and overall health status.*[47,48] Perform orthostatic blood pressure measurements before initiating antipsychotics and regularly throughout treatment. Ask about impaired menstruation, libido, and sexual performance

Table 37–10

Monitoring Protocol for Patients on Second-Generation Antipsychotics

	Baseline	4 Weeks	8 Weeks	12 Weeks	Quarterly	Annually	Every 5 Years
Personal or family history[a]	X					X	
Weight	X	X	X	X	X		
Waist circumference	X					X	
Blood pressure	X			X		X	
Fasting plasma glucose	X			X		X	
Fasting plasma lipids	X			X			X

[a]Of obesity, diabetes, dyslipidemia, hypertension, or cardiovascular disease.
Data from Refs. 49 and 50, with permission (50).

regularly. Encourage patients to have annual eye examinations because several antipsychotic medications have been associated with the premature development of cataracts. At baseline check body weight, fasting glucose, glycated hemoglobin, and lipid profile, and repeat these measurements 4 months after initiation of medication and then yearly.[49,50] For patients at higher risk of developing diabetes and those who gain weight, check body weight more often (Table 37–10). Perform baseline electrocardiography for patients with preexisting cardiovascular disease or risk for arrhythmia. With clozapine therapy, there is a risk for the development of agranulocytosis, which is greatest in the first 6 months of treatment. Required monitoring of white blood cell counts is described in Table 37–8.

Commonly used rating scales to monitor for EPS include the Simpson Angus Scale (SAS) and the Extrapyramidal Symptom Rating Scale (ESRS). Akathisia is commonly monitored by the Barnes Akathisia Scale (BAS). The emergence of dyskinesias could represent the emergence of TD. Monitor patients on SGAs for TD at least annually, and patients taking FGAs at each visit. The most commonly used instrument to measure these symptoms is the Abnormal Involuntary Movement Scale (AIMS).

Patient Care Process

Patient Assessment:

- Review the patient's chief complaint, presenting symptoms, and history, including family psychiatric history. Assess organization of thoughts and range of affect. Assess presence of mood disturbance, likelihood of harm to self or others, and presence of hallucination, paranoia and/or delusions of control.
- Assess medical records, including laboratory and imaging studies, to rule out medical causes of psychosis.
- Obtain collateral information from family, past medical records and other providers to help clarify the history.
- Elicit the patient's housing arrangements, social and vocational goals.

Therapy Evaluation:

- Assess current treatments and outcomes of prior treatments.
- Select an antipsychotic based on the side-effect profile that is most appropriate and acceptable to the patient.
- Consider collaboration with other professionals or family members.
- Consider how income and insurance coverage might influence pharmacotherapy choice.

Care Plan Development:

- Collaboratively, develop a treatment plan that addresses medication adherence and healthy lifestyle goals, including substance and cigarette use.
- Communicate that treatment plan adherence will enhance the likelihood of meeting goals.
- Devise a plan to optimize compliance.
- Educate the patient and, with patient consent, their family about the illness, medication treatments, possible side effects, and goals of treatment.
- Enlist adjunctive treatments, including psychosocial therapies to optimize outcomes.

Follow-up Evaluation:

- Schedule appointments more frequently initially to assess effectiveness, adverse drug reactions, drug interactions, and allergies.
- Assess the need for adjunctive therapies to enhance progress toward goals.
- Monitor appropriate laboratory measures to prevent or minimize adverse effects, including metabolic abnormalities.
- Assess for emergence of new target symptoms.
- Optimize dosing and consider clozapine if criteria are met for treatment resistance.

Abbreviations Introduced in This Chapter

5-HT	Serotonin
ACT	Assertive Community Treatment
AIMS	Abnormal Involuntary Movement Scale
ANC	Absolute neutrophil count
BAS	Barnes Akathisia Scale
BPRS	Brief Psychiatric Rating Scale
CATIE	Clinical Antipsychotics Trials of Intervention Effectiveness
CBT	Cognitive behavioral therapy
CGI	Clinical Global Impression Scale
CR	Cognitive remediation
CYP450	Cytochrome P450 isoenzyme
D	Dopamine
DSM-5	*Diagnostic and Statistical Manual of Mental Disorders*, 5th edition
ECT	Electroconvulsive therapy
EPS	Extrapyramidal side effects
ESRS	Extrapyramidal Symptom Rating Scale
FDA	Food and Drug Administration
FGA	First-generation antipsychotic
H	Histamine
IM	Intramuscular
M	Muscarinic
NMDA	*N*-methyl-D-aspartate
NMS	Neuroleptic malignant syndrome
PANSS	Positive and Negative Symptom Scale
PCP	Phencyclidine
PORT	Schizophrenia Patient Outcomes Research Team
QTc	Corrected QT interval
SAS	Simpson Angus Scale
SGA	Second-generation antipsychotic
SSRI	Selective serotonin reuptake inhibitor
SST	Social skills training
TD	Tardive dyskinesia
TIMA	Texas Implementation of Medication Algorithms
TMS	Transcranial magnetic stimulation
WBC	White blood cell

REFERENCES

1. Schultz SK, Andreasen NC. Schizophrenia. Lancet. 1999;353(9162): 1425–1430.
2. Kim Y, Zerwas S, Trace SE, Sullivan PF. Schizophrenia genetics: Where next? Schizophr Bull. 2011;37(3):456–463.
3. Abi-Dargham A. Do we still believe in the dopamine hypothesis? New data bring new evidence. Int J Neuropsychopharmacol. 2004;7(Suppl 1):S1–S5.
4. Javitt DC. Glutamate and schizophrenia: Phencyclidine, N-methyl-D-aspartate receptors, and dopamine-glutamate interactions. Int Rev Neurobiol. 2007;78:69–108.
5. Meltzer HY, Massey BW. The role of serotonin receptors in the action of atypical antipsychotic drugs. Curr Opin Pharmacol. 2011;11(1):59–67.
6. Goff DC, Cather C, Evins AE, et al. Medical morbidity and mortality in schizophrenia: Guidelines for psychiatrists. J Clin Psychiatry. 2005;66(2):183–194.
7. American Psychiatric Association. Diagnostic and Statistical Manual of Mental Disorders. 5th ed. Washington, DC: American Psychiatric Association; 2013.
8. American Psychiatric Association. Practice guidelines for the treatment of patients with schizophrenia. Am J Psychiatry. 2004;161(2 Suppl):1–56.
9. The expert consensus guideline series: Treatment of schizophrenia. J Clin Psychiatry. 1996;57(Suppl 12B):31.
10. Hor K, Taylor M. Suicide and schizophrenia: A systematic review of rates and risk factors. J Psychopharmacol. 2010;24(4 Suppl): 81–90.
11. Casey DE. Long-term treatment goals: Enhancing healthy outcomes. CNS Spectr. 2003;8(11 Suppl 2):26–28.
12. Resnick SG, Fontana A, Lehman AF, Rosenheck RA. An empirical conceptualization of the recovery orientation. Schizophr Res. 2005;75(1):119–128.
13. Dixon LB, Dickerson F, Bellack AS, et al. The 2009 schizophrenia PORT psychosocial treatment recommendations and summary statements. Schizophr Bull. 2010;36(1):48–70.
14. Lieberman JA, Stroup TS, McEvoy JP, et al. For the Clinical Antipsychotic Trials of Intervention Effectiveness (CATIE) Investigators. Effectiveness of antipsychotic drugs in people with chronic schizophrenia. N Engl J Med. 2005;353(12):1209–1223.
15. Leucht S, Cipriani A, Spineli L, et al. Comparative efficacy and tolerability of 15 antipsychotic drugs in schizophrenia: A multiple-treatments meta-analysis. Lancet. 2013;382:951–962.
16. Correll CU, Leucht S, Kane JM. Lower risk for tardive dyskinesia associated with second-generation antipsychotics: A systematic review of 1-year studies. Am J Psychiatry. 2004;161(3):414–425.
17. Schotte A, Janssen PFM, Gommeren W, et al. Risperidone compared with new and reference antipsychotic drugs: In vitro and in vivo receptor binding. Psychopharmacology. 1996;124(1–2):57–73.
18. Csernansky JG, Mahmoud R, Brenner R, Risperidone-USA-79 Study Group. A comparison of risperidone and haloperidol for the prevention of relapse in patients with schizophrenia. N Engl J Med. 2002;346(1):16–22.
19. Richelson E. Receptor pharmacology of neuroleptics: relation to clinical effects. J Clin Psychiatry. 1999;60(Suppl 10):5–14.
20. Seeger TF, Seymour PA, Schmidt AW, et al. Ziprasidone (CP-88,059): A new antipsychotic with combined dopamine and serotonin receptor antagonist activity. J Pharmacol Exp Ther. 1995;275(1):101–113.
21. Shapiro DA, Renock S, Arrington E, et al. Aripiprazole, a novel atypical antipsychotic drug with a unique and robust pharmacology. Neuropsychopharmacology. 2003;28(8):1400–1411.
22. Dolder C, Nelson M, Deyo Z. Paliperidone for schizophrenia. Am J Health Syst Pharm. 2008;65(5):403–413.
23. Arif SA, Mitchell MM. Iloperidone: A new drug for the treatment of schizophrenia. Am J Health Syst Pharm. 2011;68:301–308.
24. Citrome L. Iloperidone, asenapine, and lurasidone: A brief overview of 3 new second generation antipsychotics. Postgrad Med. 2011;123(2):153–162.
25. Kapur S, Seeman P. Does fast dissociation from the dopamine d(2) receptor explain the action of atypical antipsychotics? A new hypothesis. Am J Psychiatry. 2001;158(3):360–369.
26. Wirshing WC. Movement disorders associated with neuroleptic treatment. J Clin Psychiatry. 2001;62(Suppl 21):15–18.
27. Margolese HC, Chouinard G, Kolivakis TT, et al. Tardive dyskinesia in the era of typical and atypical antipsychotics. Part 2: Incidence and management strategies in patients with schizophrenia. Can J Psychiatry. 2005;50(11):703–714.
28. van Harten PN, Tenback DE. Tardive dyskinesia: Clinical presentation and treatment. Int Rev Neurobiol. 2011;98:187–210.
29. Correll CU, Schenk EM. Tardive dyskinesia and new antipsychotics. Curr Opin Psychiatry. 2008;21:151–156.

30. Moore TA, Buchanan RW, Buckley PF, et al. The Texas Medication Algorithm Project antipsychotic algorithm for schizophrenia: 2006 update. J Clin Psychiatry. 2007; 68(11):1751–1762.
31. Buchanan RW, Kreyenbuhl J, Kelly DL, et al. The 2009 schizophrenia PORT psychopharmacological treatment recommendations and summary statements. Schizophr Bull. 2010;36(1):71–93.
32. Byerly MJ, Nakonezny PA, Lescouflair E. Antipsychotic medication adherence in schizophrenia. Psychiatr Clin North Am. 2007;30(3):437–452.
33. Ascher-Svanum H, Zhu B, Faries D, et al. A prospective study of risk factors for nonadherence with antipsychotic medication in the treatment of schizophrenia. J Clin Psychiatry. 2006;67(7):1114–1123.
34. Remschmidt H. Early-onset schizophrenia as a progressive-deteriorating developmental disorder: Evidence from child psychiatry. J Neural Transm. 2002;109:101–117.
35. Jeste DV, Caligiuri MP, Paulsen JS, et al. Risk of tardive dyskinesia in older patients. A prospective longitudinal study of 266 outpatients. Arch Gen Psychiatry. 1995; 52:756–765.
36. Lubman DI, King JA, Castle DJ. Treating comorbid substance use disorders in schizophrenia. Int Rev Psychiatry. 2010;22(2):191–201.
37. Wobrock T, Soyka M. Wobrock T, Soyka M. Pharmacotherapy of schizophrenia with comorbid substance use disorder—reviewing the evidence and clinical research. Prog Neuropsychopharmacol Biol Psychiatry. 2008;32(6):1375–1385.
38. Conley RR, Kelly DL. Management of treatment resistance in schizophrenia. Biol Psychiatry. 2001;50(11):898–911.
39. Meltzer HY. Suicide in schizophrenia, clozapine and adoption of evidence based medicine. J Clin Psychiatry. 2005;60(Suppl 12): 47–50.
40. Nilsson E, Hultman CM, Cnattinguis S, et al. Schizophrenia and offspring's risk for adverse pregnancy outcomes and infant death. Br J Psychiatry. 2008;193:311–315.
41. Diav-Citrin O, Schechtman S, Ornoy S, et al. Safety of haloperidol and penfluridol in pregnancy: A multicenter, prospective, controlled study. J Clin Psychiatry. 2005;66(3):317–322.
42. Gentile S. Antipsychotic therapy during early and late pregnancy. A systematic review. Schizophr Bull. 2010;36(3):518–544.
43. Wang JS, Taylor R, Ruan Y, et al. Olanzapine penetration into brain is greater in transgenic Abcb1a P-glycoprotein-deficient mice and FVB1 (wild type) animals. Neuropsychopharmacology. 2004;29(3):551–557.
44. Sandson NB, Armstrong SC, Cozza KL. An overview of psychotropic drug-drug interactions. Psychosomatics. 2005;46(5):464–494.
45. Torrey EF, Davis JM. Adjunct treatments for schizophrenia and bipolar disorder: What to try when you are out of ideas. Clin Schizophr Relat Psychoses. 2012;5(4):208–216.
46. Murray-Swank AB, Dixon L. Family psychoeducation as evidence-based practice. CNS Spect. 2004;9(12):905–912.
47. Marder SR, Essock SM, Miller AL, et al. The Mount Sinai conference on the pharmacotherapy of schizophrenia. Schizophr Bull. 2002;28(1):5–16.
48. Marder SR, Essock SM, Miller AL, et al. Physical health monitoring of patients with schizophrenia. Am J Psychiatry. 2004;161(8):1334–1349.
49. American Diabetes Association; American Psychiatric Association; American Association of Clinical Endocrinologists; North American Association for the Study of Obesity. Consensus development conference on antipsychotic drugs and obesity and diabetes. Diabetes Care. 2004;27(2):596–601.
50. Love RC, Mackowick M, Carpenter D, Burks EJ. Expert consensus-based medication-use evaluation criteria for atypical antipsychotic drugs. Am J Health Syst Pharm. 2003;60:2455–2470.

38 Major Depressive Disorder

Cherry W. Jackson and Marshall E. Cates

LEARNING OBJECTIVES

Upon completion of this chapter, the reader will be able to:

1. Explain the etiology and pathophysiology of major depressive disorder (MDD).
2. Identify the signs and symptoms of MDD.
3. Outline the treatment goals for a patient with MDD.
4. Recommend pharmacotherapy given a specific patient with MDD.
5. Develop a monitoring plan for a specific patient with MDD which includes the assessment of efficacy as well as toxicity.
6. Predict, prevent, identify, and resolve potential drug-related problems.
7. Educate patients and caregivers on the proper use of antidepressant therapy.

INTRODUCTION

Major depression is a common, seriously disabling, disorder nonresponsive to volitional efforts to feel better. Individuals with major depressive disorder (MDD) experience pervasive symptoms affecting mood, thinking, physical health, work, and relationships. Suicide often results when MDD is inadequately diagnosed and treated.[1]

Over and under detection of MDD is an important consideration. Primary care providers have become increasingly involved in the management of MDD. Studies show that over detection of MDD can outnumber missed cases.[1] Antidepressants account for 15 of the top 200 prescriptions drugs dispensed in the United States.[2] Inadequate treatment remains a serious concern.[3]

Patient Encounter, Part 1

A 62-year-old man with diabetes, hypertension, and recently diagnosed Parkinson disease presents to the psychiatry clinic. He complains of depressed mood, poor sleep, and appetite. He has lost 25 pounds (11.4 kg) in the last 2 months. He also has been isolating himself from other people, and has had crying spells. He says that he has been thinking about committing suicide, but he does not have a specific plan.

What symptoms of MDD does he have?

What medical or psychiatric issues could be contributing to his symptoms?

What additional information do you need to know before creating a treatment plan for this patient?

EPIDEMIOLOGY AND ETIOLOGY

The lifetime and 12-month prevalence estimates for MDD are 16.2% and 6.6%, respectively.[4] Women are twice as likely as men to experience MDD. The average age of onset is in the mid-twenties; many patients with MDD have comorbid psychiatric disorders, especially anxiety and substance abuse disorders.[5]

According to the World Health Organization (WHO), depression is the leading cause of disability (based on years lived with disability) and the fourth leading cause of the global burden of disease.[6]

Symptoms of depression are due to a change in the brain neurotransmitters, norepinephrine (NE), serotonin (5-HT), and dopamine (DA).

PATHOPHYSIOLOGY

The cause of MDD is unknown but is probably multifactorial. Multiple theories abound, and practitioners suggest that development of depression likely involves a complex interaction of genetic predisposition, psychological stressors, and underlying pathophysiology. There are no currently accepted unifying theories to adequately explain the pathophysiology of depression.

Genetics

First-degree relatives of MDD patients are about three times more likely to develop MDD compared with controls. Adoption and twin studies also suggest aggregation of MDD is due to genetic influences.[7] Major depression has been associated with four different genes. They include polymorphisms in the glucocorticoid receptor gene NR3C1, the monoamine oxidase A gene, the gene for glycogen synthase kinase-3β, and a group-2 metabotropic glutamate receptor gene (GRM3).[8]

Stress

Major life stressors do not always cause depression. Nevertheless, there is an undeniable association between life stressors and depression, and there appears to be a significant causative interaction between life stressors and genetic predisposition. Although acute stressors may precipitate depression, chronic stressors cause longer episodes and are more likely to lead to relapse and recurrence.[9]

Biogenic Amine and Receptor Hypotheses

KEY CONCEPT *The primary hypothesis is the biogenic amine hypothesis which states that a deficit of NE, DA, or 5-HT at the synapse is the cause of depression.* Support for this hypothesis is that existing antidepressants increase synaptic monoamine concentrations (see Pharmacologic Therapy). One argument against this hypothesis is that patients with depression do not always have decreased monoamine levels. Additionally, monoamine levels are altered within hours of initiating antidepressant therapy, but response is delayed by 2 to 4 weeks or more.

The receptor hypothesis suggests that depression is related to abnormal functioning of neurotransmitter receptors. In this hypothesis, chronic administration of antidepressants alters receptor sensitivity causing desensitization or down regulation of β-adrenergic and 5-HT receptors leading to therapeutic response. Importantly, the time required for changes in receptor sensitivity correlates with antidepressant onset.[10] These hypotheses are clearly oversimplifications of the pathophysiology of depression. MDD probably involves a complex dysregulation of monoamine systems that modulate and are modulated by other neurobiological systems.

Other Neurobiological Hypotheses

At least three categories of peripheral hormones are associated with the pathophysiology of depression. They include (1) neurotrophic and other growth factors including brain derived neurotrophic factor (BDNF), vascular endothelial growth factor (VEGF), and insulin-like growth factor, (2) proinflammatory cytokines including interleukin-1β, interleukin-6, and tumor necrosis factor-α; and (3) the hypothalamic pituitary axis (HPA).[8]

Proinflammatory cytokines are increased in individuals with MDD, and antidepressants suppress the synthesis of these cytokines. HPA axis regulation is impaired in depression, and antidepressants can attenuate the neuroendocrine response. BDNF is decreased in patients with MDD, and antidepressants reverse this response.[8]

CLINICAL PRESENTATION AND DIAGNOSIS

The diagnosis of a major depressive episode (MDE) requires the presence of five depressive symptoms for a minimum of 2 weeks that cause clinically significant effects.[5] The diagnosis of MDD is based on the presence of one or more MDEs during a person's lifetime (Table 38–1).[5]

Table 38–1

Clinical Presentation of Depression: Diagnostic Criteria for Major Depressive Episode

At least five of the following symptoms have been present during the same 2-week period and represent a change from previous functioning.

- Depressed mood[a]
- Markedly diminished interest or pleasure in usual activities[a]
- Increase of decrease in appetite or weight
- Increase or decrease in amount of sleep
- Increase or decrease in psychomotor activity
- Fatigue or loss of energy
- Feelings of worthlessness or guilt
- Diminished ability to think, concentrate, or make decisions
- Recurrent thoughts of death, suicidal ideation, or suicide attempt

The symptoms cause clinically significant distress or impairment in functioning.

The symptoms are not due to the direct physiologic effects of a substance or medical condition.

[a]One of these two symptoms must be present.

Data from American Psychiatric Association. Major Depressive Disorders. Diagnostic and Statistical Manual of Mental Disorders. 5th ed. Washington, DC: American Psychiatric Association; 2013: 160–168.

Differential Diagnosis

MDEs also occur in bipolar disorder. Individuals with bipolar disorder also experience hypomanic, manic, or mixed episodes (see Chapter 39) during the course of their illness, but individuals with MDD do not.[5]

The anxiety, personality, and substance use disorders are frequently associated with MDD. Several chronic medical conditions have strong correlations with MDD. MDD is associated with a 65% increased risk of diabetes in elderly patients.[11] MDD is also strongly correlated with coronary artery disease. Other medical disorders associated with depression include hypothyroidism, cancer, anemia, infections, electrolyte disturbances, folate deficiency, neurologic disorders, and cardiovascular and respiratory disease.[5] Identification and treatment of MDD in patients with chronic medical conditions is important. Inadequate recognition and treatment of depression may increase the mortality associated with these medical disorders.[11] Use of central nervous system (CNS) depressants such as alcohol, benzodiazepines, or narcotics, is associated with an increased incidence of depression.[12] Some drugs that cause depressive symptoms include corticosteroids, contraceptives, levetiracetam, topiramate, vigabatrin, gonadotropin-releasing hormone agonists, interferon-α, interleukin-2, varenicline, mefloquine, isotretinoin, propranolol, clonidine, methyldopa, reserpine, and sotalol.[13]

Persistent depressive disorder (dysthymia) is a chronic form of depression that must be differentiated from MDD. Many symptoms of dysthymia are similar to those of MDD, but they are chronic and milder. Symptoms must be present for at least 2 years and may include sleep and appetite disturbances, lack of energy, poor self-image, and difficulty making decisions. Individuals with dysthymia are more likely to develop MDD than the general population, and when this occurs it is called "double depression."[4]

COURSE AND PROGNOSIS

Symptoms of a major depressive episode usually develop gradually over days to weeks, but mild depressive and anxiety symptoms may last weeks to months before onset of the full syndrome. Untreated, MDEs last 6 months or more, but a minority of individuals experience chronic episodes that last at least 2 years. Approximately two-thirds of patients recover and return to normal mood, but one-third have only a partial **remission**.[4]

The course of MDD varies markedly between patients. KEY CONCEPT *It is not uncommon for a patient to experience only a single MDE, but most patients with MDD experience multiple episodes.* The number of prior episodes predicts the likelihood of developing subsequent episodes. A patient experiencing a third MDE has a 90% chance of having a fourth one. MDD has a high mortality rate because approximately 15% of patients ultimately complete suicide.[4]

TREATMENT

Desired Outcomes

The goal of therapy for patients with MDD is resolution of depressive symptoms, return to **euthymia**, and prevention of relapse and recurrence of symptoms. KEY CONCEPT *One extremely important goal is prevention of suicide attempts.* Other desired outcomes include improving quality of life including normalization of functioning in areas such as work and relationships, minimization of adverse effects, and reduction of health care costs.

Patient Encounter, Part 2: Medical History, Physical Examination, and Diagnostic Tests

The workup reveals:

PMH: Multiple medical problems including insulin-dependent diabetes mellitus, hypertension, and recently diagnosed Parkinson disease. He is followed by a primary care physician

PPH: He has multiple psychiatric hospitalizations with the last being 2 years prior to this admission. He has a diagnosis of major depressive episode (MDE). He has also been hospitalized three times for substance abuse. His drug of choice is alcohol

FH: Mother had diabetes mellitus and MDD, died at age 58; father had a history of alcoholism and died at age 78; brother is a recovering alcoholic

SH: Worked as a movie director. Found out that he had Parkinson disease 2 months ago. Last drink of alcohol was 6 months ago, before his last hospitalization. He denies smoking or illicit substances

Current Meds: Sertraline 100 mg daily; trazodone 100 mg at bedtime; nicardipine 20 mg three times daily; novulin 70/30 56 units in the morning, 15 units in the evening; carbidopa/levodopa 25/100 three times daily

ROS: Decreased sleep; decreased appetite; weight loss; all others noncontributory

PE:

VS: Ht 5'11"(180 cm) Wt 183 lbs. (83.2 kg), weight loss of 25 lbs (11.4 kg) over past 8 weeks

MSE: Depressed mood, decreased sleep, decreased appetite, isolation, positive suicidal ideation without plan

Labs: Within normal limits. Urine drug screen—negative

Given this additional information, what is your assessment of the patient's condition?

Does he have risk factors for depression?

Identify treatment goals for the patient.

What nonpharmacologic and pharmacologic alternatives are available for this patient?

Nonpharmacologic Therapy

Evidence supports efficacy of interpersonal and cognitive-behavioral therapy in the treatment of MDD. Psychotherapy alone is an initial treatment option for mild to moderate depression, and it may be useful combined with pharmacotherapy for the treatment of severe depression. This combination can be more effective than either treatment alone in severe or recurrent MDD. Combination treatment may be helpful for patients with psychosocial stressors, interpersonal difficulties, or comorbid personality disorders.[14]

Electroconvulsive therapy (ECT) is a highly efficacious and safe treatment alternative for MDD. The response rate is about 80% to 90%, and it exceeds 50% for patients who have failed pharmacotherapy.[15] ECT may be beneficial for MDD that is complicated with psychotic features, severe suicidality, refusal to eat, pregnancy, or contraindication or nonresponse to pharmacotherapy.[15] Six to 12 treatments are typically necessary with response occurring in 10 to 14 days. When ECT is discontinued, antidepressants are initiated to help maintain response. Side effects after ECT include temporary confusion, retrograde and anterograde amnesia.[14]

Light therapy is an alternative treatment for depression associated with seasonal (eg, winter) exacerbations. Side effects include eye strain, headache, insomnia, and hypomania.[16]

Vagus nerve stimulation (VNS), which was approved by the Food and Drug Administration (FDA) in 2005, may be used for treatment-resistant depression. A pulse generator is surgically implanted under the skin of the left chest, and an electrical lead connects the generator to the left vagus nerve which sends signals to the brain. This therapy is used along with pharmacotherapy and ECT.[17] Adverse effects of VNS include alterations in patients' voice, coughing, pharyngitis, sore throat, hoarseness, headache, nausea, vomiting, dyspnea, and paresthesia.[17]

Transcranial magnetic stimulation is a noninvasive and well-tolerated procedure that is FDA approved for use after one failed trial of an antidepressant.[18] Physical exercise may reduce depressive symptoms, but well-controlled studies are needed to verify this.[19]

Pharmacologic Therapy

Individual antidepressants, even those within the same class, have important pharmacologic differences (Tables 38–2 and 38–3).[10,20] Monoamine oxidase inhibitors (MAOIs) inhibit the enzyme responsible for the breakdown of 5-HT, NE, and DA. There are two main forms of MAO: While both MAO-A and MAO-B have receptors in the brain, MAO-A has more receptors in the gut, and MAO-B is primarily found in the brain. Inhibition of MAO-A impacts the breakdown of 5-HT, dopamine, epinephrine, and NE. MAO-B is primarily involved in the inhibition of DA and phenethylamine. Dietary restrictions are necessary for MAO-A inhibitors, but not usually for MAO-B inhibitors. The tricyclic antidepressants (TCAs) possess both serotonin reuptake inhibition (SRI) and norepinephrine reuptake inhibition (NRI) properties, but they also block other receptors, including α_1-adrenergic, histamine-1, and muscarinic cholinergic receptors, which contribute to side effects, not efficacy. The primary action of the specific serotonin reuptake inhibitors (SSRIs) is SRI. Bupropion is a NE and DA reuptake inhibitor (NDRI). Venlafaxine, desvenlafaxine, and duloxetine are 5-HT and NE

Table 38–2

Primary Pharmacologic Actions[a] of Antidepressants[8,10]

Action	MAOIs	TCAs	SSRIs	Bupropion	SNRI's	Vilaz	Traz	Nefaz	Mirtaz	Vorti
Monoamine oxidase inhibition	X									
Serotonin reuptake inhibition		X	X		X	X	X	X		X
Norepinephrine reuptake inhibition		X		X	X					
Dopamine reuptake inhibition				X						
α_2-Adrenergic receptor blockade									X	
Serotonin $_{1A}$ receptor agonist										X
Serotonin$_{1A}$ receptor partial agonist						X				
Serotonin $_{1B}$ receptor partial agonist										X
Serotonin$_{2A}$ receptor blockade							X	X	X	
Serotonin $_{2C}$ receptor blockade							X	X	X	
Serotonin$_3$ receptor blockade									X	X
Serotonin$_7$ receptor blockade										X
α_1-Adrenergic receptor blockade		X					X	X		
Histamine-1 receptor blockade		X					X		X	
Muscarinic cholinergic receptor blockade		X								

[a]See text for discussion of more secondary pharmacologic actions.

MAOI, monoamine oxidase inhibitor; SNRI, serotonin norepinephrine reuptake inhibitor; SSRI, selective serotonin reuptake inhibitor; TCA, tricyclic antidepressant; Vilaz, vilazodone; Traz, trazodone; Mirtaz, mirtazapine; Vorti, vortioxetine.

Table 38–3

Efficacy and Adverse Effect Profile Based on Pharmacology

Pharmacologic Action	Result
SRI	Antidepressant and antianxiety efficacy (via interaction of 5-HT at 5-HT$_{1A}$ receptors)
	Anxiety, insomnia, sexual dysfunction (via interaction of 5-HT at 5-HT$_{2A}$ receptors)
	Anxiety, anorexia (via interaction of 5-HT$_{2C}$ receptors)
	Nausea, GI problems (via interaction of 5-HT at 5-HT$_3$ receptors)
NRI	Antidepressant efficacy
	Tremor, tachycardia, sweating, jitteriness, increased blood pressure
Dopamine reuptake inhibition	Antidepressant efficacy, euphoria, psychomotor activation, aggravation of psychosis
α_2-Adrenergic receptor blockade	Increase in serotonergic and noradrenergic activity-see actions of SRI and NRI above
Serotonin$_{1A}$receptor agonist	Antianxiety, antidepressant augmentation, decreased blood pressure,
Serotonin $_{1A}$ partial agonism	Antianxiety, antidepressant augmentation, decreased blood pressure, decreased heart rate
Serotonin$_{2A}$ receptor blockade	Antianxiety efficacy
	Increased REM sleep; decreased sexual dysfunction
Serotonin$_{2C}$ receptor blockade	Antianxiety efficacy
	Increased appetite or weight gain
Serotonin$_3$ receptor blockade	Antinauseant, decreased GI problems
Serotonin$_7$ receptor blockade	Antidepressant, modulates glutamate
α_1-Adrenergic receptor blockade	Orthostatic hypotension, dizziness, reflex tachycardia
Histamine-1 receptor blockade	Sedation, weight gain
Muscarinic cholinergic receptor blockade	Dry mouth, blurred vision, constipation, urinary hesitancy, sinus tachycardia, memory problems

GI, gastrointestinal; NRI, norepinephrine reuptake inhibition; REM, rapid eye movement; SRI, serotonin reuptake inhibition.

Data from Refs. 8 and 10.

reuptake inhibitors (SNRIs) and weak inhibitors of DA reuptake. Compared with venlafaxine and desvenlafaxine, which have primarily SRI activity, duloxetine has more balanced SRI and NRI activities and has a higher affinity for reuptake sites. Nefazodone and trazodone are 5-HT antagonists. Their SRI activity is not as pronounced as that of the SSRIs, but they potently block 5-HT_{2A} receptors, which allow more 5-HT to interact at postsynaptic 5-HT_{1A} sites. In addition, trazodone blocks histaminergic and α-adrenergic receptors, and nefazodone possesses weak NRI and α-adrenergic blocking properties. Vilazodone, a combination of an SRI and a partial agonist at 5-HT_{1A} receptors, is thought to reduce negative feedback on endogenous serotonin receptors which may improve the medications antidepressant effect.[21] Vortioxetine is an agonist/antagonist/partial agonist at various 5-HT receptors. Vortioxetine has affinity for β-adrenergic receptors which may be associated with side effects and histaminic and acetylcholinergic receptors which may have an effect on memory.[22] Finally, mirtazapine is a noradrenergic and specific serotonergic antidepressant. It blocks presynaptic α_2 autoreceptors on noradrenergic neurons and heteroreceptors on serotonergic neurons, resulting in increases in NE and 5-HT synaptic concentrations. Mirtazapine also blocks postsynaptic serotonergic receptors and histamine-1 receptors.[10]

Complementary and Alternative Treatments

St. John's wort (hypericum perforatum) is an herbal medication that has shown efficacy in mild to moderate depression, but minimal efficacy for moderate to severe depression.[19] It has mild MAO-inhibiting properties. Many patients believe that herbal medications are devoid of adverse effects and drug interactions; however, St. John's wort can cause gastrointestinal (GI) irritation, headache, fatigue, and nervousness, and it triggers drug interactions through induction of CYP3A4 enzymes, and potentially other mechanisms.[23] The safety and efficacy of St. John's wort combined with standard antidepressant medications remains unknown.

S-adenosyl methionine (SAM-e), a naturally occurring compound in the body, tends to be lower in people with major depression. Treatment with SAM-e increases blood levels of both S-adenosyl methionine and hydroxyindolacetic acid. It is sold as a nutritional supplement and lacks the standardization of medications that are FDA approved.[24]

Low folate levels are associated with a greater risk of depression or a lack of response to antidepressants. Because folic acid prevents neural tube defects in pregnancy and causes few to no adverse effects, it can be used in doses of 0.4 to 1 mg/day to improve the efficacy of the antidepressants.[25]

Low doses of omega-3 fatty acids (eicosapentaenoic, docosahexaenoic acid, or both) have been used adjunctively for major depression. More study is needed to establish their role.[26]

Adverse Effects

The adverse effects of the antidepressants are often a function of their underlying pharmacologic profiles (see Table 38–3). The TCAs cause sedative, anticholinergic, and cardiovascular adverse effects. Although common, they can also be serious in some cases. The tertiary amines (eg, amitriptyline, imipramine) are more sedative and anticholinergic than the secondary amines (eg, desipramine, nortriptyline). The TCAs have a quinidine-like effect on the heart, which makes them toxic in overdose. The average lethal dose in a young adult is 30 mg/kg, which is typically less than a 1-month supply.[20]

The adverse effect profile of the SSRIs includes sexual dysfunction (eg, delayed or absent orgasms), CNS stimulation (eg, nervousness and insomnia), and GI disturbances (eg, nausea and diarrhea).[20,27] KEY CONCEPT *Sexual dysfunction, common and challenging to manage, often leads to noncompliance.*[28] Various strategies to deal with antidepressant induced sexual function include waiting for symptoms to subside, reducing the dosage, permitting periodic "drug holidays," prescribing adjunctive therapy, and switching antidepressants.[27] However, waiting for symptoms to subside usually does not work, because sexual dysfunction may very well persist throughout the duration of therapy. Reducing the dose and using drug holidays may weaken the antidepressant effects. Thus, clinicians often prescribe adjunctive therapy such as dopaminergic drugs (eg, bupropion, amantadine), 5-HT_2 antagonists (cyproheptadine, nefazodone), and phosphodiesterase inhibitors (eg, sildenafil) or simply switch to antidepressants with less likelihood of causing these effects, such as bupropion, mirtazapine, or nefazodone.[27]

Bupropion causes insomnia, nightmares, decreased appetite, anxiety, and tremors, but the most concerning adverse effect are seizures. Because of the risk for seizures, patients with a CNS lesion, history of seizures, head trauma, or bulimia should not receive the drug. The daily dose of bupropion should not exceed 450 mg/day (immediate release and extended release), and any single dose of the immediate-release formulation should not exceed 150 mg. The maximum dose of sustained release is 200 mg twice daily. Insomnia and/or nightmares often respond to moving the last daily dose from bedtime to late afternoon.[29]

The adverse effects of the SNRIs are similar to those of the SSRIs. Nausea can be troublesome with venlafaxine and desvenlafaxine, which sometimes necessitates using lower starting doses and giving the medication with food. A dose-related elevation in blood pressure can occur at higher doses, and blood pressure monitoring should be conducted for patients receiving venlafaxine or desvenlafaxine. Duloxetine should not be prescribed to patients with moderate to heavy alcohol use or evidence of chronic liver disease owing to the potential for hepatic injury.[30]

Trazodone causes sedation, and it is used more often as an adjunct with other antidepressants for sleep than as an antidepressant. Priapism is a rare but serious adverse effect in men taking trazodone. It is less likely with nefazodone because it has a weaker effect at α-adrenergic receptors and a balancing of adrenergic effects owing to weak NRI activity. Unfortunately, nefazodone has been associated with development of fatal hepatotoxicity, which has led to a black-box warning and significant reduction in its use. It has been discontinued in some countries.[27]

Mirtazapine can cause sedation and weight gain by blocking histamine-1 receptors. Despite being partially a serotonergic drug, it rarely causes serotonergic-related adverse effects because it also blocks the various postsynaptic 5-HT receptors. Although it carries a bolded warning for neutropenia owing to a handful of cases reported during clinical trials, it is questionable whether neutropenia is more problematic with mirtazapine than other antidepressants.[31]

The relative incidence of adverse effects among the newer antidepressants is shown in Table 38–4.

Pharmacokinetic Parameters

Pharmacokinetic parameters of the newer antidepressants are shown in Table 38–5. Several antidepressants are not highly protein bound, the most notable of these are venlafaxine and desvenlafaxine. The elimination half-lives of nefazodone and venlafaxine are relatively short compared with the other agents.

Table 38–4

Relative Incidence of Adverse Effects of Newer Antidepressants

Drug	Sedation	Activation	Weight Gain	Weight Loss	GI Upset	Sexual Dysfunction
Bupropion	+	++++	+	++	+++	+
Citalopram	+	+	+	+	++++	++++
Desvenlafaxine	++	+++	+	+	++++	++++
Fluoxetine	+	++++	+	+	++++	++++
Mirtazapine	+++	+	++	+	+	+
Nefazodone	++	+	+	+	++	+
Paroxetine	++	++	+	+	++++	++++
Sertraline	+	+++	+	+	++++	++++
Venlafaxine	++	+++	+	+	++++	++++
Vilazodone	+	+	+	+	++++	+
Vortioxetine	+	+	+	+	++++	+

+, minimal; ++, low; +++, moderate; ++++, high; GI, gastrointestinal.

Data from Refs. 8, 10, and 27.

Conversely, fluoxetine has a very long half-life (ie, 5–9 days) with chronic dosing, and its active metabolite (norfluoxetine) has an even longer half-life. Because of this, a 5-week washout of fluoxetine is required before starting an MAOI. A 2-week washout is generally considered sufficient for other SSRIs. Sertraline and citalopram also have active metabolites, but these metabolites (desmethylsertraline and desmethylcitalopram, respectively) are only about one-eighth as potent as the parent compounds for SRI activity.[31,32,33]

Drug Interactions

Antidepressant drug interactions can be pharmacokinetic or pharmacodynamic. The usual pharmacodynamic drug interactions involve the "dirty receptors" blocked by some antidepressants. TCAs can cause significant additive effects with other drugs that cause sedation, hypotension, or anticholinergic effects. Similarly, trazodone and mirtazapine can interact with other drugs that cause hypotensive and sedative effects. By far, the most concerning pharmacodynamic interactions are hypertensive crisis and serotonin syndrome, which are both life-threatening. Hypertensive crisis is characterized by sharply elevated blood pressure, occipital headache, stiff or sore neck, nausea, vomiting, and sweating. It may result during MAOI therapy if the patient takes a sympathomimetic drug, such as ephedrine, pseudoephedrine, phenylephrine, phenylpropanolamine, or stimulants such as amphetamines or methylphenidate or if the patient consumes

Table 38–5

Pharmacokinetic Parameters of Newer Antidepressants

Drug	Protein Binding(%)	Elimination Half-Life (hours)	Active Metabolite(s)	Cytochrome P450	
				Substrate	Inhibitor
Bupropion	84	10–21	Yes	2B6	2D6 (+)
Citalopram	80	33	Yes	2C19	2D6 (+)
Desvenlafaxine	30	7.5	No	2D6	2D6 (+)
Duloxetine	90	9–19	No	1A2, 2D6	2D6 (+++)
Escitalopram	56	27–32	No	2C19	2D6 (+)
Fluoxetine	94	4–6 days with chronic dosing 4–16 days (active metabolite)	Yes	2D6	2C (++) 2D6 (++++) 3A4 (+)
Fluvoxamine	77	15–26	No	1A2, 2D6	1A2 (++++), 2C (++) 3A4 (+++)
Mirtazapine	85	20–40	No	1A2, 2D6, 3A4	None
Nefazodone	99	2–4	Yes	None	3A4 (++++)
Paroxetine	95	21	No	2D6	2D6 (++++)
Selegiline	99	1.2–2	Yes	None	None
Sertraline	98	27	Yes	None	2C (++), 2D6 (+), 3A4 (+)
Venlafaxine	27	5	Yes	2D6	2D6 (+)
Vilazodone	99	25	No	3A4	2C8 (+), 2C19(++), 2D6(++)
Vortioxctine	98	66	No	2D6	None

++++, high; +++, moderate; ++, low; +, very low; 0, absent.

Data from Refs. 8 and 10.

foods rich in tyramine, such as tap beers, aged cheeses, fava beans, yeast extracts, liver, dry sausage, sauerkraut, or tofu.[34] There are extensive lists of foods and drinks that are not permitted during therapy with MAOIs, and these should always be provided to patients. Because many over-the-counter (OTC) products contain sympathomimetics, patients should always be told to consult with their pharmacist or other clinician before using these drugs. Serotonin syndrome is characterized by confusion, restlessness, fever, abnormal muscle movements, hyperreflexia, sweating, diarrhea, and shivering. It may result when a serotonergic agent is added to any other serotonergic agent, but the MAOIs are strongly associated with severe cases of serotonin syndrome. Serotonin syndrome is complicated by (a) an unawareness by clinicians of the diagnosis and (b) the fact that many implicated drugs are not serotonergic in nature, such as dextromethorphan, meperidine, tramadol, linezolid, triptans, and methylene blue.[34]

Many antidepressants inhibit cytochrome P450 isoenzymes, elevating plasma levels of substrates for those isoenzymes and potentially leading to adverse effects or toxicity (see Table 38–5).[31]

Dosing

Antidepressant dosing is summarized in Table 38–6.[12,20] The extended release formulation of venlafaxine and bupropion allow for once daily dosing. The delayed-release capsule of fluoxetine can be given weekly, which can be started 7 days after the last regular-release capsule or tablet. Selegiline is available as a transdermal patch, and a dose of 6 mg/24 hours can be used without the usual dietary restrictions associated with MAOI use, although patients on the higher doses (9 and 12 mg/24 hours) should follow usual dietary restrictions. Liquid dosage forms and disintegrating tablets of various antidepressants are ideal for patients who have difficulty swallowing tablets or capsules and those who may attempt to "cheek" their medication.

The starting dose is the usual therapeutic dose for most SSRIs, desvenlafaxine, duloxetine, and mirtazapine, but there is usually a need for at least some upward titration of venlafaxine, vilazodone, vortioxetine, bupropion, and nefazodone. An advantage of TCAs is that plasma levels may be used to help guide dosing, especially for those that have well-defined therapeutic plasma level ranges, including nortriptyline (50–150 ng/mL [mcg/L; 190–570 nmol/L]), desipramine (100–160 ng/mL [mcg/L; 375–601 nmol/L]), amitriptyline (75–175 ng/mL [mcg/L; 270–631 nmol/L]), and imipramine (200–300 ng/mL [mcg/L; 713–1070 nmol/L]).

Efficacy of Pharmacotherapy

KEY CONCEPT *Each antidepressant has a response rate of approximately 60% to 80%, and no antidepressant medication or class has been reliably shown to be more efficacious than another.*[20] MAOIs may be the most effective medication for atypical depression, but MAOI use continues to wane because of adverse effects, dietary and drug restrictions, and the possibility of fatal drug interactions.[20] There is some evidence that dual-action antidepressants, such as TCAs and SNRIs, may be more effective in patients with severe depression than the single action drugs such as the SSRIs,[20] but the more general assertion that multiple mechanisms of action confer efficacy advantages is controversial.[35]

Selection of Medication

Figure 38–1 depicts a well-known algorithm for the treatment of nonpsychotic MDD-the Texas Medication Algorithm Project (TMAP).[36] Notable aspects of this algorithm include the preferential use of newer antidepressants in the earlier stages of treatment and sequential trials of antidepressant monotherapy prior to the use of combination therapy (see Managing Partial Response or Nonresponse.) Patients undergoing treatment guided by this algorithm fared better than those who received treatment not guided by the algorithm over a 1-year period. Antipsychotics should be combined with antidepressants in cases of depression with psychotic features.[37]

Various factors must be taken into account when selecting antidepressant therapy for a particular patient. The most reliable predictor of response is the patient's history of response (eg, efficacy, side effects, and overall satisfaction) to antidepressants. To a lesser extent, the history of a first-degree relative's response to antidepressants may be used to predict a patient's response. Adverse effect profiles should be considered, because compliance is influenced by tolerability. The patient is the best source of information regarding acceptability of adverse effects. Patients should be educated about how to deal with side effects (eg, using chewing gum, hard candy, or ice chips for dry mouth). The clinician must anticipate and be vigilant for potential drug–drug interactions and drug-disease interactions. For instance, a patient with a seizure disorder would be an inappropriate candidate for bupropion therapy. The presence of comorbid psychiatric conditions can suggest the best antidepressant to choose. For example, an SSRI can treat both MDD and panic disorder, obviating the need for two separate medications. Fluvoxamine, an SSRI, is marketed for obsessive compulsive disorder, although it also treats depression. The potential for accidental or intentional overdose and affordability of the medication also influence drug selection.[20]

Time Course of Response

Antidepressants do not produce an immediate clinical response. Improvement in physical symptoms such as sleep, appetite, and energy, can occur within the first or second week of treatment. Although a meta-analysis suggests earlier effects of antidepressant treatment, KEY CONCEPT *it is widely accepted that approximately 2 to 4 weeks of treatment is required before improvement is seen in emotional symptoms such as sadness and anhedonia. As long as 6 to 8 weeks may be required to see full antidepressant effects.*[20,31]

Managing Partial or No Response

Approximately one-third of patients with MDD do not respond satisfactorily to their first antidepressant medication.[37] In such cases, the clinician must evaluate the adequacy of antidepressant therapy, including dosage, duration, patient compliance, verification of the patient's diagnosis, and reconsideration of clinical factors that could be impeding successful therapy, such as concurrent medical conditions (eg, thyroid disorder), comorbid psychiatric conditions (eg, alcohol abuse), and psychosocial issues (eg, marital stress).[38]

A series of reports from the Sequenced Treatment Alternatives to Relieve Depression (STAR*D) trial revealed that remission is associated with a better overall prognosis than improvement alone. STAR*D also established that in patients with a greater level of nonresponse to treatment, clinicians are less likely to push the patient to achieve remission, and in addition, those patients with the greatest levels of nonresponse had the highest rates of relapse. STAR*D established some successful treatment recommendations.[39] For patients experiencing a partial response, extending the medication trial and/

Table 38–6

Dosing of Antidepressants in Adults

Generic Name	Brand Name	Generic	Initial Dose (mg/day)	Usual Dosing Range (mg/day)	Usual Dosage Schedule	Renal Dosing Adjustment	Hepatic Dosing Adjustment
MAOIs							
Phenelzine	Nardil	Yes	15–30	15–90	Twice daily	None	None
Selegiline	Emsam	No	6	6–12	Once daily	None	None
Tranylcypromine	Parnate	Yes	10–20	30–60	Twice daily	None	None
Isocarboxazid	Marplan	No	10–20	40–60 mg	Twice daily	None	None
TCAs and Tetracyclics							
Amitriptyline	Elavil[a]	Yes	25–50	100–300	Once or twice daily	Nondialyzable	Use with caution
Amoxapine	Asendin[a]	Yes	25–50	100–400	Once to twice daily	None	None
Clomipramine	Anafranil	Yes	25	100–250	Once daily	Use with caution	None
Desipramine	Norpramin	Yes	25–50	100–300	Once or twice daily	None	Use with caution
Doxepin	Sinequan[a]	Yes	25–50	100–300	Once or twice daily	Use with caution	Use a lower dose
Imipramine	Tofranil	Yes	25–50	100–300	Once daily	Use with caution	None
Maprotiline	Ludiomil[a]	Yes	50–75	100–225	Once to twice daily	None	None
Nortriptyline	Pamelor	Yes	25	50–150	Once daily	Use with caution	Use a lower dose
Protriptyline	Vivactil	No	5–10	15–60	Once daily	Use with caution	Use with caution
Trimipramine	Surmontil	Yes	25–50	100–300	Once or twice daily	Use with caution	Use with caution
SSRIs							
Citalopram	Celexa	Yes	20	20–40[b]	Once daily	No adjustment for clcr > 20 mL/min (0.33 mL/s); for clcr < 20 mL/min (0.33 mL/s), use with caution	20 mg/day maximum; may increase to 40 mg in nonresponders
Escitalopram	Lexapro	Yes	10	10–20	Once daily	No adjustment for clcr > 20 mL/min (0.33 mL/s); for clcr < 20 mL/min (0.33 mL/s), use with caution	10 mg/day
Fluoxetine	Prozac	Yes	10–20	20–80	Once daily	None	Use lower or less frequent dosing
	Prozac weekly	Yes	90	90	Once weekly	None	Use lower or less frequent dosing
Fluvoxamine	Luvox	Yes	50	50–300	Twice daily	None	Reduce dose
	Luvox CR	Yes	100	100–300	Once daily	None	Reduce dose
Paroxetine	Paxil	Yes	10–20	20–50	Once daily	In ClCr < 30 mL/min (0.50 mL/s) 10 mg/day increase weekly to a dose of 40 mg/day or less	Severe impairment, 10 mg daily; increase weekly to dose of 40 mg/day
	Paxil CR	Yes	12.5–25	25–62.5	Once daily	In ClCr < 30 mL/min (0.50 mL/s), 12.5 mg daily initially; may increase weekly to a dose of 50 mg/day or less	Severe impairment, 12.5 mg daily, increase weekly to dose of 40 mg/day or less
Sertraline	Zoloft	Yes	25–50	50–200	Once daily	None	Use a lower dose
NDRI							
Bupropion	Wellbutrin	Yes	150–200	300–450[c]	Twice to thrice daily	Consider lower dose	75 mg/day
	Wellbutrin SR	Yes	150	300–400[c]	Twice daily	Consider lower dose	100 mg/day or 150 mg every other day
	Wellbutrin XL	Yes	150	300–450[c]	Once daily	Consider lower dose	150 mg every other day

(*Continued*)

Table 38–6

Dosing of Antidepressants in Adults (*Continued*)

Generic Name	Brand Name	Generic	Initial Dose (mg/day)	Usual Dosing Range (mg/day)	Usual Dosage Schedule	Renal Dosing Adjustment	Hepatic Dosing Adjustment
SNRIs							
Desvenlafaxine	Pristiq	No	50	50–100	Once daily	ClCr 30–50 mL/min (0.50 – 0.83 mL/s), 50 mg maximum daily dose, ClCr < 30 mL/min (0.50 mL/s), 50 mg every other day	50 mg/day, 100 mg/day maximum
Duloxetine	Cymbalta	Yes	40–60	40–60	Once to twice daily	Use lower dose, not recommended for ClCr < 30 mL/min (0.50 mL/s)	Not recommended
Venlafaxine	Effexor	Yes	37.5–75	75–375	Once, twice or three times daily	Reduce dose 25%–50%	Reduce dose by 50%
	Effexor XR	Yes	37.5–75	75–225	Once daily	Reduce dose 25%–50%	Reduce dose by 50%
Levomilnacipran	Fetzima	No	20 mg	40–120 mg	Once daily	CrCl < 60 mL/min (1.0 mL/s), 80 mg/day maximum dose; CrCl < 30 mL/min (0.50 mL/s), 40 mg/day maximum dose	None
SARIs							
Nefazodone	Serzone[a]	Yes	100–200	300–600	Twice daily	Use with caution	Discontinue if ALT/AST is more than three times normal
Trazodone	Desyrel[a]	Yes	50–150	200 600	Twice daily	Use with caution	Use with caution
	Oleptro	No	150	150–375	Daily	Use with caution	Use with caution
NaSSA							
Mirtazapine	Remeron	Yes	15	15–45	Once daily	ClCr < 40 mL/min (0.67 mL/s), 30% decreased clearance ClCr < 10 mL/min (0.17 mL/s), 50% decreased clearance	Clearance decreased by 30%; monitor closely
SRI/5-HT$_{1A}$							
Vilazodone	Viibryd[c]	No	10	20–40	Once daily	None	Use with caution
Vortioxetine	Brintellix	No	10	20	Once daily	None	None

[a]Brand no longer available in the United States.

[b]Maximum dose is 40 mg/day.

[c]Upper limit of this range is the maximum dose.

ALT, alanine aminotransferase; AST, aspartate aminotransferase; MAOI, ClCr, creatinine clearance; monoamine oxidase inhibitor; NaSSA, noradrenergic and specific serotonergic antidepressant; NDRI, norepinephrine and dopamine reuptake inhibitor; SARI, serotonin antagonist and reuptake inhibitor; SNRI, serotonin and norepinephrine reuptake inhibitor; SSRI, selective serotonin reuptake inhibitor; SRI/5-HT$_{2A}$, partial agonist-serotonin reuptake inhibitor/serotonin$_{2A}$ partial agonist; TCA, tricyclic antidepressant.

Data from Refs. 12, 19, 21, 33, and 39.

or using higher doses within the recommended dosage range may be helpful. Another option is augmentation therapy, ie, adding another medication that generally is not used as an antidepressant, such as, lithium, buspirone, or triiodothyronine.[40] Second-generationantipsychotics, aripiprazole, and the extended-release formulation of quetiapine, are approved by the FDA for augmenting partial response to antidepressants.[41] Whereas efficacy has been suggested for dopaminergic drugs (eg, pramipexole) and psychostimulants (eg, methylphenidate), various other medications such as anticonvulsants (eg, valproic acid), modafanil, and estrogen have anecdotal evidence supporting their use as augmenting agents. A third option is combination therapy, whereby another antidepressant, typically from a different pharmacologic class is added to the first

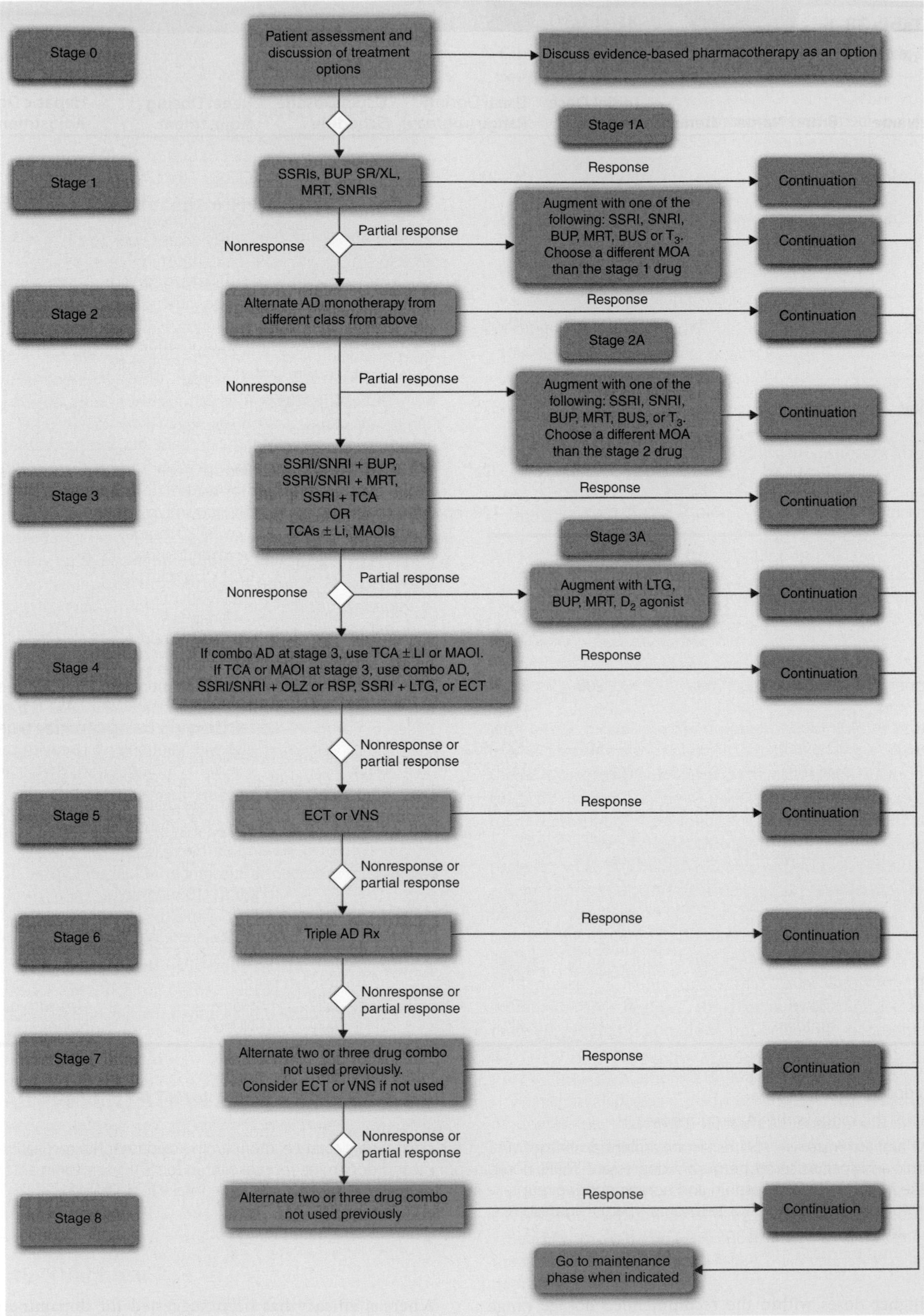

FIGURE 38–1. Strategies for the treatment of nonpsychotic major depression. (AD, antidepressant; BUP, bupropion; BUS, buspirone; ECT, electroconvulsive therapy; Li, lithium; T_3, liothyronine; LTG, lamotrigine; MAOI, monoamine oxidase inhibitor; MOA, mechanism of action; MRT, mirtazapine; OLZ, olanzapine; RSP, risperidone; Rx, prescription; SNRI, serotonin and norepinephrine reuptake inhibitor; SSRI, selective serotonin reuptake inhibitor; TCA, tricyclic antidepressant; VNS vagus nerve stimulation.) Redrawn with permission from the Texas Medication Algorithm Project.[35]

antidepressant.[42] Examples include combining bupropion and SSRIs or combining TCAs and SSRIs.

Switching to a different antidepressant is a common strategy for patients who have had no response to initial antidepressant therapy, but also is acceptable in cases of partial response. Relative to augmentation or combination therapy, advantages of switching include improved compliance, decreased costs, and less concern over drug–drug interactions. Disadvantages include loss of time, and loss of any improvement seen with the initial drug.[43] When switching from one antidepressant to another, clinicians may choose to stay within the same class (eg, sertraline to fluoxetine) or go outside of the class (eg, paroxetine to venlafaxine). The olanzapine-fluoxetine combination medication Symbyax has been approved for treatment-resistant depression.[43]

Nonpharmacologic interventions in cases of treatment nonresponse include adding or changing to psychotherapy or initiating ECT.

Duration of Therapy

Treatment of MDD encompasses three phases: acute, continuation, and maintenance **(Figure 38–2)**[10] The goal of antidepressant therapy is remission of MDE symptoms. This acute phase of treatment typically lasts 6 to 12 weeks. KEY CONCEPT *Because the typical MDE lasts 6 months or longer, if antidepressant therapy is interrupted after the acute phase, the patient may relapse into a depressive episode. When treating the first depressive episode, antidepressants must be given for an additional 4 to 9 months in the continuation phase to prevent relapse.*

Maintenance treatment takes place after the normal course of a MDE to prevent recurrence, which is the development of future episodes. This phase can last for years, or for a lifetime. Although patients who have a MDE should receive acute and continuation treatment, not all of them require maintenance treatment, because not all patients experience multiple major depressive episodes. In some patients with multiple episodes, many years may separate the episodes. Therefore, the clinician must consider various factors in determining whether an individual requires maintenance treatment. A major factor is the number of prior episodes experienced by the patient. The more prior episodes experienced, the higher the risk for future episodes. After three or more MDEs, patients are generally given lifelong maintenance treatment because of the high (ie, 90%) chance of experiencing additional episodes. Other factors to consider are the severity of previous episodes, if suicide attempts were made, whether psychotic features were present, and patient preference. The dose of the antidepressant required in the acute phase of treatment should be sustained during the continuation and maintenance phases.

Discontinuation of Therapy

When discontinuing therapy, it is best to gradually taper the antidepressant for two reasons. First, almost all antidepressants can produce withdrawal syndromes if discontinued abruptly or tapered too rapidly, especially antidepressants with shorter half-lives (eg, venlafaxine, paroxetine, and fluvoxamine).[37] Withdrawal syndromes can cause sleep disturbances, anxiety, fatigue, mood changes, malaise, GI disturbances, and a host of other symptoms which often are confused with depressive relapse or recurrence.[37] In general, a tapering schedule involving a small dosage decrement (eg, paroxetine 5 mg) every 3 to 5 days should prevent significant withdrawal symptoms.[36] Second, depressive symptoms may return on taper or discontinuation of the antidepressant. So, if the medication is gradually tapered, then early signs of depression can be countered with a return to the original dosage and a potentially quicker response.[37] Depending on the patient's illness and the clinical circumstances, tapering of the antidepressant can be extended for weeks or even months because of the concern over relapse or recurrence.

Special Considerations

▸ *Pregnant or Breastfeeding Patients*

Depression is quite common in pregnancy, especially for women with a history of recurrent depression. Both maternal and fetal well-being must be considered when weighing risks and benefits of antidepressant therapy during pregnancy. While somewhat controversial, the prescribing information for paroxetine was changed to reflect findings of an increased risk of congenital malformations, particularly atrial and ventricular septal defects, in infants born to women taking the drug during the first trimester. Sertraline and citalopram have also been associated with septal heart defects when taken during the first trimester. In addition, the incidence of having a baby with a septal heart defect was four times higher for mothers taking more than one SSRI in the first trimester. More recent studies have questioned these results.[43]

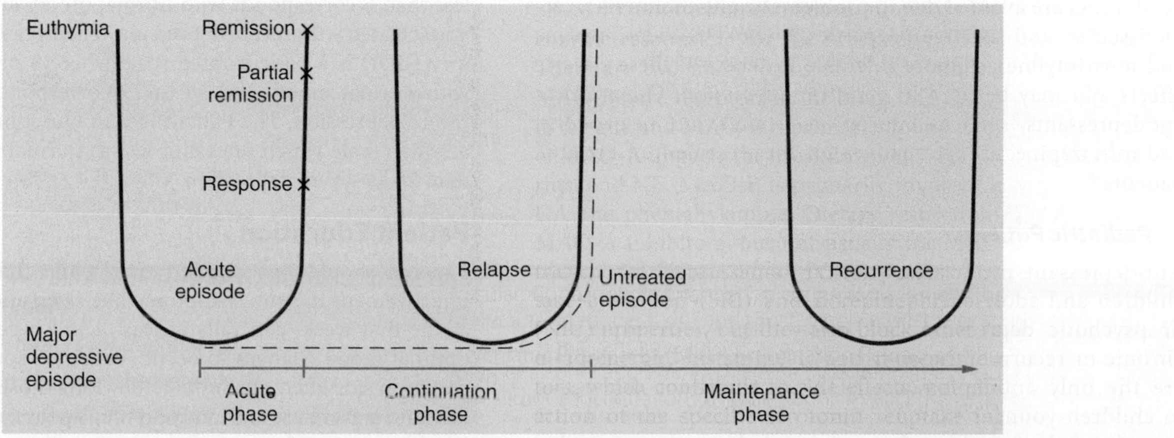

FIGURE 38–2. The course of depression and phases of treatment. Data from Refs. 10 and 19.

Patient Encounter, Part 3: Creating a Care Plan

On the basis of information presented, create a care plan. Your plan should include:

(a) A statement of the drug-related needs and/or problems.

(b) The goals of therapy.

(c) A patient-specific detailed therapeutic plan.

(d) A plan for follow-up to determine whether the goals have been achieved.

Antidepressants are reported to occasionally cause perinatal sequelae, such as poor neonatal adaptation, respiratory distress, feeding problems, and jitteriness. Data on the long-term effects of in utero antidepressant exposure are limited. Sertraline, fluoxetine, citalopram, and the TCAs have the greatest reproductive safety data and should be considered first-line treatments when pharmacotherapy is indicated.[44]

There is some drug exposure to the infant from nursing mothers who are taking antidepressants. Although there have been rare anecdotal reports of adverse effects (ie, respiratory depression and seizure-like episodes) in infants exposed to antidepressants through breast milk, no rigorous study has confirmed this, and it is generally accepted that the benefits of breastfeeding outweigh the risks to the infant posed by antidepressant exposure.[44,45] However, the decision needs to be made on an individual basis.

► *Geriatric Patients*

Depression in older adults is under recognized and undertreated.[46] Although not uncommon in community samples, MDD is prevalent among those living in long-term care facilities. Barriers to recognition of geriatric depression include "masked" presentations, that is complaints of physical symptoms (eg, pain and GI problems) instead of mood symptoms, the frequent presence of medical illnesses, and the overlap of mood and cognitive symptoms with those of dementia.[46] Age-related pharmacokinetic and pharmacodynamics changes cause geriatric patients to be more sensitive to antidepressant medications. Thus, lower starting doses of antidepressants and slow upward titrations as tolerated are recommended for geriatric patients.[46] The SSRIs are chosen frequently for geriatric depression because of their overall favorable adverse effect profiles and low toxicity; most TCAs are avoided due to problematic anticholinergic, cardiovascular, and sedative properties.[46] The TCAs desipramine and nortriptyline are more tolerable in terms of these adverse effects and may be used in geriatric depression. Other newer antidepressants, such as bupropion, venlafaxine, nefazodone, and mirtazapine, are alternatives for the treatment of geriatric patients.[46]

► *Pediatric Patients*

Antidepressant medications appear to be useful for certain children and adolescents, particularly those who have severe or psychotic depression, fail psychotherapy, or experience chronic or recurrent depression. Fluoxetine and escitalopram are the only antidepressants FDA approved for depression in children younger than 18 years.[47] The SSRIs generally are considered the initial antidepressants of choice, but comorbid conditions may favor alternative agents. "Behavioral activation" can occur with the SSRIs, including such symptoms as impulsivity, silliness, daring conduct, and agitation.[45] Desipramine must be used with caution in this population because of several reports of sudden death, and baseline and follow-up electrocardiography is warranted when using desipramine in pediatric patients.

The FDA warns that antidepressants increase the risk of suicidality (ie, suicidal thinking and behavior) in children and young adults. A large analysis of clinical trials showed the risk of such events was 4% for antidepressants versus 2% for placebo, although no completed suicides occurred in the trials. Because antidepressants carry a black-box warning regarding suicidality, medication guides must be distributed with each prescription or refill of antidepressants. KEY CONCEPT *Pediatric patients and young adults should be observed closely for suicidality, worsened depression, agitation, irritability, and unusual changes in behavior, especially during the initial few months of therapy and at times of dosage changes. Furthermore, families and caregivers should be advised to monitor patients for such symptoms.*[48]

► *Suicidal Patients*

The FDA has determined that in addition to children and adolescents, there is an increased risk of suicidality in patients between the ages of 18 and 24 years. Similar monitoring for suicidality and clinical worsening that is mandated for pediatric patients should also be followed for these young adult patients.[49]

Whereas the TCAs and MAOIs have narrow therapeutic indices, the SSRIs, SNRIs, nefazodone, and mirtazapine have wide therapeutic indices.

Patient Counseling

Major counseling points are outlined in Table 38–7. KEY CONCEPT *Lack of patient understanding concerning optimal antidepressant therapy frequently leads to partial or noncompliance with therapy, thus the primary purpose of antidepressant counseling is to enhance compliance and improve outcomes.*[50]

OUTCOME EVALUATION

Symptom Assessment

The patient interview should assess response of target symptoms. Rating scales are useful in this regard. The Hamilton Depression Scale (HAM-D) is a 17-item, clinician administered scale where less than 6 corresponds with normal mood, and greater than 25 is associated with severe depression. The Beck Depression Inventory (BDI) is a patient-rated scale where 9 or less is associated with normal mood, and 20 to 29 corresponds to moderate to severe depression. The Patient Health Questionnaire (PHQ-9) is a 9-item scale which rates 4 or less as normal mood and greater than 20 as severe depression.

Patient Education

Patients should be educated that while they may see some improvement in some symptoms like sleep and appetite as early as the first week, generally at least 4 to 8 weeks is required for optimal mood changes to occur. Patients should also recognize common side effects including, how long those side effects might last, and if there are any simple remedies for treatment (eg, using ice chips or sugarless gum for a dry mouth).

Table 38–7
Patient Counseling

Counseling Point	Clinical Rationale
Mechanism of action—The medication works by affecting certain chemicals in the brain	Patient may feel that depression is a character weakness or personality flaw instead of a biological disorder
Lack of addiction potential—Although the medication affects certain chemicals in the brain, it is not addicting	Patient may worry that because the antidepressant is psychoactive, it must be addicting
Need for routine use—The medication will only work if it is taken as prescribed every day	Patient may try taking the medication on an as-needed basis
Delayed onset of action—It may take several weeks to see significant improvement in symptoms	Patient may prematurely discontinue therapy before the onset of beneficial effects
Prolonged duration of therapy—The medication should be taken for at least 6–12 months; do not discontinue it without consulting with the prescriber	Patient may prematurely discontinue therapy after symptoms have remitted, which could lead to relapse or recurrence
Adverse effects—Mention common and expected adverse effects as well as what to do if they occur	Patient may be more likely to discontinue therapy and distrust the prescriber if adverse effects occur without forewarning
Avoidance of alcohol and CNS depressants—Use of alcohol or other CNS depressants could cause worsened depression and additive adverse effects with the medicine	Patient may be unaware of the possible consequences of drinking alcohol or taking other drugs with antidepressants
Risk of suicidality—Be alert to symptoms of worsening depression and suicidality	Patient may become suicidal or have suicidal thinking while taking the antidepressant

CNS, central nervous system.
Data from Refs. 19 and 50.

Monitoring Adverse Effects

Evaluation for suicidal ideation should be a part of every patient visit. Patients can be taught to manage side effects such as sedation, constipation, and dry mouth. Potential side effects such as weight gain and sexual dysfunction should be discussed with the patient and monitored at each visit. Venlafaxine may increase blood pressure, and patients should have their blood pressure checked at each visit. Patients with cardiovascular risk factors or over the age of 40 should have an electrocardiogram (ECG) completed prior to initiating a TCA. Patients taking TCAs such as amitriptyline, imipramine, nortriptyline, or desipramine should have antidepressant serum levels checked if overdose, side effects, or nonadherence is an issue. Patients should be monitored for serotonin syndrome if they are taking two or more serotonergic medications.

Patient Care Process

Patient Assessment:

- Determine if the patient is experiencing symptoms of depression.
- Review the medical history. Does the patient have any medical problems that might cause the current symptoms?
- Conduct a medication history (including prescriptions, OTC medications, and dietary supplements) to identify possible causes of depression.
- Review available laboratory tests, especially thyroid function tests, renal and hepatic function.

Therapy Evaluation:

- Determine if antidepressant therapy is needed.
- Evaluate past history of depression treatment, including response and adverse effects.
- Assess efficacy, safety, and adherence to current pharmacotherapy.
- Ensure that the patient can afford and access prescribed medications.

Care Plan Development:

- Choose lifestyle modifications and antidepressant therapy that are safe and effective.
- Determine if the drug dosage is optimal for treatment. Take an algorithmic approach to treatment (see Figure 38–1).
- Address patient concerns.
- Discuss with the patient the importance of medication adherence and lifestyle modifications.

Follow-up Evaluation:

- Follow-up to assess effectiveness and safety of therapy.
- Monitor the patient every 3 to 6 months to assess for return of symptoms. Determine if patient is experiencing any adverse effects or drug interactions.

Abbreviations Introduced in This Chapter

BDI	Beck Depression Inventory
BDNF	Brain derived neurotrophic factor
CNS	Central nervous system
DA	Dopamine
DSM-5	*Diagnostic and Statistical Manual of Mental Disorders,* 5th edition
ECG	Electrocardiogram
ECT	Electroconvulsive therapy
FDA	Food and Drug Administration
GI	Gastrointestinal
HAM-D	Hamilton Depression Scale
HPA	Hypothalamic pituitary axis
5-HT	Serotonin
MAOI	Monoamine oxidase inhibitor
MDD	Major depressive disorder
MDE	Major depressive episode
NaSSA	Noradrenergic and specific serotonergic antidepressant
NDRI	Norepinephrine and dopamine reuptake inhibitor
NE	Norepinephrine
NRI	Norepinephrine Reuptake Inhibitor
PHQ-9	Patient Health Questionairre-9
SAM-e	S-adenosyl methionine
SARI	Serotonin antagonist and reuptake inhibitor
SNRI	Serotonin and norepinephrine reuptake inhibitor
SRI	Serotonin reuptake inhibition
SSRI	Selective serotonin reuptake inhibitor
STAR*D	Sequenced Treatment Alternatives to Relieve Depression
TCA	Tricyclic antidepressant
TMAP	Texas Medication Algorithm Project
VEGF	Vascular endothelial growth factor
VNS	Vagus nerve stimulation
WHO	World Health Organization

REFERENCES

1. Mitchell AJ, Vaze A, Rao S. Clinical diagnosis of depression in primary care: A meta-analysis. Lancet. 2009;374:609–619.
2. Bartholow M. Top 200 drugs of 2012. Pharmacy Times. 2013;79 (7):42–44.
3. Hasin DS, Goodwin RD, Stinson FS, et al. Epidemiology of major depressive disorder. Arch Gen Psychiatry. 2005;62:1097–1106.
4. Kessler RC, Angermeyer M, Anthony JC, et al. Lifetime prevalence and age-of-onset distributions of mental disorders in the World Health Organization's World Mental Health Survey Initiative. World Psychiatry. 2007;6(3):168–176.
5. American Psychiatric Association. Major Depressive Disorders. Diagnostic and Statistical Manual of Mental Disorders. 5th ed. Washington, DC: American Psychiatric Association; 2013: 160–168.
6. World Health Organization. Depression 2012. http://www.who.int/mediacentre/factsheets/fs369/en/. Accessed August 25, 2014.
7. Levinson DF. The genetics of depression: A review. Biol Psychiatry. 2006;60:84–92.
8. Kupfer DJ, Frank E, Phillips ML. Major depressive disorder: New clinical, neurobiological and treatment perspectives. Lancet. 2012;379:1045–1055.
9. Muscatell KA, Slavich GM, Monroe SM, et al. Stressful life events, chronic difficulties, and the symptoms of clinical depression. J Nerv Ment Dis. 2009;197:154–160.
10. Stahl SM. Antidepressants. Essential Psychopharmacology: Neuroscientific Basis and Practical Applications. 4th ed. New York: Cambridge University Press. 2013:135–295.
11. Goldberg G. The detection and treatment of depression in the physically ill. World Psychiatry. 2010;9:16–20.
12. Narasimhan M, Raynor JD, Jones AB. Depression in the medically ill: Diagnostic and therapeutic implications. Curr Psychiatry Rep. 2008;10:272–279.
13. Patten SB, Barbui C. Drug-induced depression: A systemic review to inform clinical practice. Psycho Psychosom. 2004; 73:207–215.
14. Cuijpers P, Dekker J, Hollon SD, Andersson G. Adding psychotherapy to pharmacotherapy in the treatment of depressive disorders in adults: A meta-analysis. J Clin Psychiatry. 2009; 70:1219–1229.
15. Bolwig TG. Neuroimaging and electroconvulsive therapy. J ECT. 2014;30(2):138–142.
16. Lam RW, Levitt AJ, Levitan RD, et al. The Can-SAD study: A randomized controlled trial of the effectiveness of light therapy and fluoxetine in patients with winter seasonal affective disorder. Am J Psychiatry. 2006;163:805–812.
17. VNS therapy system. http://www.fda.gov/cdrh/mda/docs/p970003s050.html. Accessed August 30, 2014.
18. George MS, Post RM. Daily left prefrontal repetitive transcranial magnetic stimulation for acute treatment of medication resistant depression. Am J Psychiatry. 2011; 168:356–364.
19. Practice guideline for the treatment of patients with major depressive disorder. 3rd ed. http://www.psych.org/guidelines/mdd2010. Accessed August 15, 2014.
20. Sussman N, Thase ME. Selecting a first-line antidepressant: New analysis. Primary Psychiatry. 2009;16:19–22.
21. Allergan Pharmaceuticals, Inc. Manufacturer's Information. St. Louis, MO; Viibryd 2015.
22. Bang-Andersen B, Ruhland T, Jørgensen M, et al. Discovery of 1-[2-(2,4-dimethylphenylsulfanyl)phenyl]piperazine (Lu AA21004): a novel multimodal compound for the treatment of major depressive disorder. J Med Chemistry. 2011;54(9):3206–3221.
23. Sarris, J. St. John's wort for the treatment of psychiatric disorders. Psychiatr Clin North Am. 2013;36(1):65–72.
24. Carpenter DJ. St. John's wort and S-adenosyl methionine as "natural" alternatives to conventional antidepressants in the era of the suicidality boxed warning: What is the evidence for clinically relevant benefit? Alternative medicine review. J Clin Ther. 2011; 16(1):17–39.
25. Bedson E, Bell D, Carr D, et al. Folate Augmentation of Treatment–Evaluation for Depression (FolATED): Randomized trial and economic evaluation. Health Technol Assess. 2014;18:48.
26. Appleton KM, Perry R, Sallis HM, et al. Omega-3 fatty acids for depression in adults. Cochrane Database of Systematic Reviews 2014, Issue 5. Art No:CD004692. DOI:10.1002/14651858.CD004692.pub3.
27. Crawford AA, Lewis S, Nutt D, et al. Adverse effects from antidepressant treatment: Randomized controlled trial of 601 depressed individuals. Psychopharmacology. 2014;231(15) 2921–2931.
28. Kennedy SH, Rizvi S. Sexual dysfunction, depression, and the impact of antidepressants. J Clin Psychopharmacol. 2009;29: 157–164.
29. Furukawa TA, Ogawa Y, Takeshima N, et al. Bupropion versus other antidepressive agents for depression. Cochrane Database of Systematic Reviews 2014, Issue 3. Art No:CD011036. DOI:10.1002/14651858.CD011036.
30. Baghai TC, Zirngibl C, Heckel B, et al. Individualized pharmacological treatment of depressive disorders state of the art and recent developments. J Depress Anxiety. 3(154):2167–2180.

31. Schellander R, Donnerer J. Antidepressants: Clinically relevant drug interactions to be considered. Int J Exp Clin Pharmacol. 2010;96:203–215.
32. Boyce RD, Handler SM, Karp JF, et al. Age related changes in antidepressant pharmacokinetics and potential drug-drug interactions: A comparison of evidence-based literature and package insert information. Am J Geriatr Pharmacother. 2012; 10(2):139–150.
33. Mandnoli R, Mercolini L, Raggi MA. Evaluation of the pharmacokinetics, safety and clinical efficacy of sertraline. Expert Opin Drug Metab Toxicol. 2013;9(11):1495–1505.
34. Tao R, Rudacille M, Zhang G, Ma Z. Changes in intensity of serotonin syndrome caused by adverse interaction between monoamine oxidase inhibitors and serotonin reuptake blockers. Neuropsychopharmacology. 2014;39(8):1996–2007.
35. Burke WJ. Selective versus multi-transmitter antidepressants: Are two mechanisms better than one? J Clin Psychiatry. 2004; 65(Suppl 4):37–45.
36. Texas Medication Algorithm Project-nonpsychotic depression algorithm. http://www.dshs.state.tx.us/mhprograms/disclaimer.shtm. Accessed August 1, 2014.
37. Trivedi MH, Rush AJ, Crismon ML, et al. Clinical results for patients with major depressive disorder in the Texas Medication Algorithm Project. Arch Gen Psychiatry. 2004;61:669–680.
38. Posternak MA, Zimmerman M. Is there a delay in the antidepressant effect? a meta-analysis. J Clin Psychiatry. 2005; 66:148–158.
39. Trivedi M, Fava M, Marangell LB. Use of treatment algorithms for depression. J Clin Psychiatry. 2006;67:1458–1465.
40. Rush JA. STAR*D: What have we learned? Am J Psychiatry. 2007;164:201–204.
41. Wen XJ, Wang LM, Liu ZL, et al. Meta-analysis on the efficacy and tolerability of the augmentation of antidepressants with atypical antipsychotics in patients with major depressive disorder. 2014. Braz J Med Bio Res. 2014;47(7):605–616.
42. McIntyre RS, Filteau MJ, Martin L, et al. Treatment-resistant depression: Definitions, review of the evidence, and algorithmic approach. J Affect Disord. 2014;156:1–7.
43. Slomski A. Antidepressants in pregnancy don't lead to cardiac defects in infants. JAMA. 2014;312(4):327.
44. Boyce P, Galbally M, Snellen M, Buist, A. Pharmacological management of major depression in pregnancy. Psychopharmacology and Pregnancy 2014;67–85. DOI:10.1007/978-3-642-54562-7_6. Springer-Verlag Berlin Heidelberg.
45. Gentile S. The use of contemporary antidepressants during breastfeeding: A proposal for a specific safety index. Drug Safety. 2007;30:107–121.
46. Mukai Y, Rajesh R, Tampi MD. Treatment of depression in the elderly: A review of the recent literature on the efficacy of single- versus dual action antidepressants. Clin Ther. 2009; 31:945–961.
47. Ryan ND. Treatment of depression in children and adolescents. Lancet. 2005;366:933–940.
48. FDA public health advisory-suicidality in children and adolescents being treated with antidepressant medications. http://www.fda.gov/drug/cder/antidepressants/SSRIPHA200410.htm. Accessed August 10, 2014.
49. FDA Public health advisory-antidepressant use in children, adolescents and adults. http://www.fda.gov/drugs/drug safety. information by drug class.UMC096274. Accessed August 25, 2014.
50. Bollini P, Pampallona S, Kupelnick B, et al. Improving compliance in depression. A systematic review of narrative reviews. Clin Pharm Ther. 2006;31:253–260.

39 Bipolar Disorder

Brian L. Crabtree and Lydia E. Weisser

LEARNING OBJECTIVES

Upon completion of the chapter, the reader will be able to:

1. Explain the pathophysiologic mechanisms underlying bipolar disorder.
2. Recognize the symptoms of a manic episode and depressive episode in patients with bipolar disorder.
3. Identify common comorbidities of bipolar disorder.
4. Recognize the *Diagnostic and Statistical Manual of Mental Disorders,* 5th edition, criteria for bipolar disorder as well as the subtypes of bipolar I disorder, bipolar II disorder, and cyclothymic disorder.
5. List the desired therapeutic outcomes for patients with bipolar disorder.
6. Explain the use of drugs as first-line therapy in bipolar disorder, including appropriate dosing, expected therapeutic effects, potential adverse effects, and important drug–drug interactions.
7. Recommend individualized drug therapy for acute treatment and relapse prevention based on patient-specific data.
8. Recommend monitoring methods for assessment of therapeutic and adverse effects of drugs used in the treatment of bipolar disorder.
9. Recommend treatment approaches for special populations of patients with bipolar disorder, including pediatric patients, geriatric patients, and pregnant patients.
10. Educate patients with bipolar disorder about their illness, drug therapy required for effective treatment, and the importance of adherence.

INTRODUCTION

Bipolar disorder is characterized by one or more episodes of mania or **hypomania**, often with a history of one or more major depressive episodes.[1] It is chronic, with relapses and remissions. Mood episodes can be manic, depressed, or mixed. They can be separated by periods of long stability or cycle rapidly. They occur with or without psychosis. Disability and other consequences (eg, increased risk of suicide) can be devastating to patients and families. Correct and early diagnosis and treatment are essential to prevent complications and maximize response to treatment.

EPIDEMIOLOGY AND ETIOLOGY

Epidemiology

Bipolar disorders are categorized into bipolar I disorder, bipolar II disorder, and other specified and unspecified bipolar and related disorders. Bipolar I disorder is characterized by one or more manic or **mixed mood episodes.** Bipolar II disorder is characterized by one or more major depressive episodes and at least one hypomanic episode. Hypomania is an abnormally and persistently elevated, expansive, or irritable mood but not of sufficient severity to cause significant impairment and does not require hospitalization. The lifetime prevalence of bipolar I disorder is estimated at 0.6%. The lifetime prevalence of bipolar II disorder is about 0.4%. When including the entire spectrum of bipolar disorders, the prevalence is approximately 3%.[2]

Bipolar I disorder affects men and women equally. Bipolar II is more common in women. Rapid cycling and mixed mood episodes occur more in women. In all, 78% to 85% of individuals with bipolar disorder report having another *Diagnostic and Statistical Manual*, 5th edition (*DSM-5*), diagnosis during their lifetime. The most common comorbid conditions are anxiety, substance abuse, and impulse control disorders. Medical comorbidities are common.[2]

The mean age of onset is 20 years, although onset may occur in early childhood to the mid-40s.[1] If onset occurs after age 60, it is probably due to medical causes. An early onset is associated with greater comorbidities, more mood episodes, a greater proportion of days depressed, and greater lifetime risk of suicide attempts compared with later onset. Substance abuse and anxiety disorders are more common in patients with early onset. Patients with bipolar disorder have higher rates of suicidal thoughts, attempts, and completed suicides than the general population.

Etiology

The precise etiology is unknown. Thought to be genetically based, bipolar disorder is influenced by a variety of factors that may enhance gene expression. These include trauma, environmental factors, anatomical abnormalities, and exposure to chemicals or drugs.[3,4]

Patient Encounter, Part 1

Chief Complaint: "My family thinks there is something wrong with me."

HPI: Joan is a 20-year-old college student who is brought by her family following spring break. The patient states she has only come for the appointment because her family insisted and was concerned because she was "not acting like myself." She denies any physical problems except mild hypertension and recently underwent a complete physical examination by her primary care physician. Screening laboratory studies including metabolic profile, complete blood count, thyroid function, B12 and folate, electrocardiogram, and chest x-ray were generally unremarkable except for an elevated BUN of 24 mg/dL (8.6 mmol/L) and elevated serum creatinine of 2.1 mg/dL (186 μmol/L). Joan was subsequently referred to a psychiatrist for further evaluation.

Joan is a single, well-nourished, well-developed African American woman appearing her stated age. She is attired in a low-cut blouse and short skirt, very high heels, and is wearing bright lipstick, false eyelashes, purple eye shadow, and an excessive amount of perfume. She seems to have difficulty maintaining an appropriate social distance during the interview and is at times flirtatious and somewhat seductive. Her speech is rapid and difficult to interrupt, and she is quite distractible. Joan says she feels "fantastic" and has lost 8 lb (3.6 kg) over the past 2 weeks without making a conscious effort. She states she is very energetic and enjoyed partying with her friends over spring break, getting approximately 1 to 2 hours of sleep each night but feeling fine the following day. Although Joan has been an excellent student in the past, her grades this semester have been slipping, as she has found it difficult to complete assignments and is now in danger of failing. She states she is not concerned about her classes as she is considering going to New York to become a model. Although Joan has always been a good money manager, recently she has gone on extensive shopping sprees, buying clothing and jewelry she cannot afford.

What diagnoses are suggested by this patient's presentation?

What additional information is needed to clarify the diagnosis?

PATHOPHYSIOLOGY

Neurochemical

The pathophysiology remains incompletely understood. Imaging techniques such as positron emission tomography (PET) scans and functional magnetic resonance imaging (fMRI) are used to elucidate the cause. Historically, research focused on neurotransmitters such as norepinephrine (NE), dopamine (DA), and serotonin. One hypothesis is that bipolar disorder is caused by an imbalance of cholinergic and catecholaminergic activity. Serotonin is suggested to modulate catecholamines. Dysregulation of this relationship could cause mood disturbance. A variety of neurotransmitters are involved that interact with multiple neurochemical and neuroanatomic pathways.[3] The pathophysiology is also hypothesized from the mechanisms of lithium and other drugs. Lithium, valproate, and carbamazepine all have similar effects on neuronal growth that are reversible by inositol, supporting a hypothesis that bipolar disorder may be related to inositol disturbance.[5] Brain-derived neurotrophic factor (BDNF) may play a role in bipolar disorder. Serum BDNF is low in mania and improves with treatment.[6]

Genetic

Results of family studies suggest a genetic basis.[4] Lifetime risk of bipolar disorder in relatives of a bipolar patient is 40% to 70% for a monozygotic twin and 5% to 10% for other first-degree relatives.

CLINICAL PRESENTATION AND DIAGNOSIS

Diagnosis of Bipolar Disorder

KEY CONCEPT *Patients presenting with depressive or elevated mood features and a history of abnormal or unusual mood swings should be assessed for bipolar disorder.* Bipolar disorder is categorized into four subtypes: bipolar I (periods of major depressive, manic, and/or mixed episodes); bipolar II (periods of major depression and hypomania), cyclothymic disorder (periods of hypomanic episodes and depressive episodes that do not meet all criteria for diagnosis of a major depressive episode), and other specified and unspecified bipolar and related disorders. The defining feature of bipolar disorder is one or more manic or hypomanic episodes in addition to depressive episodes that are not caused by a medical condition, substance abuse, or other psychiatric disorder.[1]

Initial and subsequent episodes are mostly depressive.[7] Studies show bipolar I patients spend about 32% of weeks with depressive symptoms compared with 9% of weeks with manic or hypomanic symptoms.[8] Patients with bipolar II disorder spend 50% of weeks symptomatic for depression and only 1% with hypomania.[9] Because patients may present with depression and spend more time depressed than with mood elevation, bipolar disorder is often misdiagnosed or underdiagnosed. It is helpful to use a screening tool such as the mood disorder questionnaire.[10]

DSM-5 criteria for the diagnosis of bipolar disorder are summarized in **Table 39–1.**

▶ *Bipolar I Disorder*

The diagnosis of bipolar I disorder requires at least one episode of mania for at least 1 week with a persistently elevated, expansive, or irritable mood with related symptoms of decreased need for sleep, excessive energy, racing thoughts, a propensity to be involved in high-risk activities, and excessive talkativeness.[1] Bipolar I depression can be misdiagnosed as major depressive disorder (MDD); therefore, it is essential to rule out past episodes of hypomania or mania. If bipolar depression is mistaken for MDD and the patient is treated with antidepressants, it can precipitate a manic episode or induce rapid cycling.

▶ *Bipolar II Disorder*

The distinguishing feature of bipolar II disorder is a current or past hypomanic episode and a current or past major depressive episode. Irritability and anger are common. There cannot have been a prior full-manic episode.[1]

▶ *Cyclothymic Disorder*

Cyclothymic disorder is a chronic mood disturbance lasting at least 2 years (1 year in children and adolescents) and characterized

Table 39–1

Evaluation of and Diagnostic Criteria for Mood Episodes

Diagnostic workup depends on clinical presentation and findings		• Mental status examination • Psychiatric, medical, and medication history • Physical and neurologic examination • Basic laboratory tests: CBC, blood chemistry screen, thyroid function, urinalysis, urine drug screen • Psychological testing • Brain imaging: MRI and fMRI; alternative: CT, PET • Lumbar puncture • Electroencephalogram
Diagnosis episode	**Impairment of functioning or need for hospitalization[a]**	***DSM-5* criteria[b]**
Major depressive	Yes	Greater than or equal to 2-week period of either depressed mood or loss of interest or pleasure in normal activities, associated with at least five of the following symptoms: • Depressed, sad mood (adults); can be irritable mood in children • Decreased interest and pleasure in normal activities • Decreased appetite, weight loss • Insomnia or hypersomnia • Psychomotor retardation or agitation • Decreased energy or fatigue • Feelings of guilt or worthlessness • Impaired concentration and decision making • Suicidal thoughts or attempts
Manic	Yes	Greater than or equal to 1-week period of abnormal and persistently elevated mood (expansive or irritable), associated with at least three of the following symptoms (four if the mood is only irritable): • Inflated self-esteem (grandiosity) • Racing thoughts (FOI) • Distractible (poor attention) • Increased activity (either socially, at work, or sexually) or increased motor activity or agitation • Excessive involvement in activities that are pleasurable but have a high risk for serious consequences (buying sprees, sexual indiscretions, poor judgment in business ventures)
Hypomanic	No	At least 4 days of abnormal and persistently elevated mood (expansive or irritable); associated with at least three of the following symptoms (four if the mood is only irritable): • Inflated self-esteem (grandiosity) • Decreased need for sleep • Increased talking (pressure of speech) • Racing thoughts (FOI) • Increased activity (either socially, at work, or sexually) or increased motor activity or agitation • Excessive involvement in activities that are pleasurable but have a high risk for serious consequences (buying sprees, sexual indiscretions, poor judgment in business ventures)
Mixed	Yes	Criteria for both a major depressive episode and manic episode (except for duration) occur nearly every day for at least a 1-week period
Rapid cycling	Yes	At least four mood episodes (depressive, manic, mixed, or hypomanic) in 12 months

FOI, flight of ideas.

[a]Impairment in social or occupational functioning; need for hospitalization because of potential self-harm, harm to others, or psychotic symptoms.

[b]The disorder is not caused by a medical condition (eg, hypothyroidism) or substance-induced disorder (eg, antidepressant treatment, medications, electroconvulsive therapy).

Data from American Psychiatric Association. Diagnostic and Statistical Manual of Mental Disorders. 5th ed. Washington, DC: American Psychiatric Press; 2013 and Drayton SJ, Pelic CM. Bipolar disorder. In: DiPiro JT, Talbert RL, Yee GC, et al, eds. Pharmacotherapy. A Pathophysiologic Approach. 9th ed. New York, NY: McGraw-Hill. 2014; 1067–1081.

Patient Encounter, Part 2: Medical History, Physical Exam, Laboratory Exam

Your interview reveals the following information:

PMH: No known medical problems except a history of hypertension marginally controlled by hydrochlorothiazide 50 mg/day. Joan also admits to being treated for chlamydia last year

PPH: Noncontributory

FH: Parents alive and well. The patient's maternal grandmother was hospitalized several times at the state psychiatric hospital for treatment of unspecified mental illness in the remote past. A maternal aunt committed suicide 5 years ago. The patient's father is a recovering alcoholic who regularly attends AA. The patient has one brother and sister in good health

SH: Joan admits to numerous sexual partners beginning at the age of 18 when she first went away to college. She states none of her relationships has lasted more than a few weeks, although she would like to eventually get married. She is presently majoring in mathematics and previously aspired to be a high school teacher; however, she has failing grades in most of her classes this semester. Her roommates have complained about her coming in late at night and have also complained about Joan's use of drugs in their apartment. Joan admits to partying several nights each week as well as more on weekends

SUH: The patient denies use of tobacco products, hallucinogens, amphetamines, opioids, benzodiazepines, or intravenous drugs. She does admit to smoking marijuana on a daily basis, has experimented with cocaine in the past, and drinks heavily on the weekends. She does not drink coffee but consumes several cans of caffeinated soda each day. She denies use of vitamins or herbal supplements

Meds: Hydrochlorothiazide 50 mg by mouth daily

ROS: Decreased appetite with recent 8 lb (3.6 kg) weight loss, decreased need for sleep, increased energy, distractibility, pressured speech, hypersexuality. LMP 2 weeks ago

PE:

VS: BP 150/90, P 94, RR 18, T 98.7°F (37.1°C)

HEENT: PERRLA. Extraocular movements intact. Nares patent. Ear canals patent and eardrums easily visualized. Neck supple without JVD, bruits, or lymphadenopathy. Thyroid smooth, symmetric and nontender

CV: Heart with regular rate and rhythm; no murmurs, gallops or rubs

Abdomen: Soft, nontender, without organomegaly or masses. Positive bowel sounds in all four quadrants

Exts: Without clubbing, cyanosis, or edema. Peripheral pulses full and equal bilaterally

CN: II-XII intact

Labs: Urine drugs screen + for THC; HIV negative; serum β-HCG negative

Considering this additional information, what is the most likely diagnosis?

by mood swings that include periods of hypomanic symptoms that do not meet the criteria for a hypomanic episode and depressive symptoms that do not meet the criteria for a major depressive episode. Hypomanic symptoms include inflated self-esteem or **grandiosity** (nondelusional), decreased need for sleep, pressured speech, **flight of ideas (FOI)**, distractibility, and increased involvement in goal-directed activities, not causing severe impairment or requiring hospitalization. Psychotic features are not present.[1]

▶ *Suicide*

Patients with bipolar disorder have high risk of suicide. Factors that increase risk are early age at onset, high number of depressive episodes, comorbid alcohol abuse, personal history of antidepressant-induced mania, and family history of suicidal behavior. About one-third of individuals with bipolar disorder report a previous attempt.[11] One of five attempts is fatal, in contrast to one of 10 to one of 20 in the general population.

▶ *Differential Diagnosis*

Schizophrenia and bipolar disorder share certain symptoms, including psychosis in some patients. The prominence of mood symptoms and the history of mood episodes distinguish bipolar disorder and schizophrenia. In addition, psychosis of schizophrenia occurs in the absence of prominent mood symptoms. Schizoaffective disorder may also be considered when developing a differential diagnosis. Schizoaffective disorder is characterized by a period of illness during which there is a major depressive episode or a manic episode, concurrent with symptoms that meet criterion A for schizophrenia (eg, delusions, hallucinations, disorganized speech, grossly disorganized or catatonic behavior, and/or negative symptoms such as affective flattening, alogia, or avolition). During the same period of illness, there have been delusions or hallucinations for at least 2 weeks in the absence of prominent mood symptoms.[1]

Personality disorders are inflexible and maladaptive patterns of behavior that deviate markedly from expectations of society beginning in adolescence or early adulthood.[1] Personality disorders and bipolar disorder may be comorbid, and patients with personality disorders may have mood symptoms. The two diagnoses are distinguished by the predominance of mood symptoms and the episodic course of bipolar disorder in contrast to the stability and persistence of the behavioral patterns of personality disorders.

▶ *Comorbid Psychiatric and Medical Conditions*

Lifetime prevalence rates of comorbidity with bipolar disorder are as high as 58%.[2] Comorbidities, especially substance abuse, make establishing a diagnosis more difficult and complicate treatment. Comorbidities also place the patient at risk for a poorer outcome, high rates of suicidality, onset of depression, and higher costs of treatment.[1] Psychiatric comorbidities include:

- Personality disorders
- Alcohol and substance abuse or dependence
- Anxiety disorders
- Panic disorder

Clinical Presentation and Diagnosis

Patients presenting with depressive or elevated mood features and a history of abnormal or unusual mood swings should be assessed for bipolar disorder.

General

The patient may present in a hypomanic, manic, depressed, or mixed state and may or may not be in acute distress.

Symptoms

Mood and Affect:

- Mood elevation
- Expansive mood
- Irritable mood
- Depression
- Hopelessness
- Suicidality

Physical and Behavioral:

- Agitation
- Impulsivity
- Aggression
- Rapid, pressured speech
- Insomnia (sometimes for days or weeks)
- Hypersexuality
- Increased physical energy
- Inflated self-esteem, boasting, grandiosity
- Heightened interest in pleasurable activities with a high risk of negative consequences (eg, spending sprees, promiscuity)
- Fatigue
- Hypersomnia

Thought Processes, Content, and Perceptions:

- Racing thoughts, FOI, distractibility
- Delusions of grandeur, ideas of reference, persecution, wealth, religion

Psychosocial

- Substance use
- Disrupted relationships
- Job loss

Laboratory and Other Diagnostic Assessments

KEY CONCEPT *The diagnosis of bipolar disorder is made based on clinical presentation, a careful diagnostic interview, and a review of the history. There are no laboratory examinations, brain imaging studies, or other procedures that confirm the diagnosis, but such testing can be done to rule out other medical diagnoses.*

- Urinalysis with culture, urine drug toxicology, thyroid function, and complete blood count in elderly patients to rule out infection and anemia
- Mood disorder questionnaire, completed by the patient, asks about common symptoms of bipolar disorder, problems caused by the symptoms, and family history in a "yes" or "no" answer format. It is then scored by the clinician

Suicidality risk is increased in the presence of:

- Substance abuse
- Prior suicide attempts and lethality of attempts
- Access to a means of suicide
- Command hallucinations or psychosis
- Severe anxiety
- Family history of attempted or completed suicide

Data from Refs. 1 and 3.

FOI, flight of ideas.

- Obsessive-compulsive disorder
- Social phobia
- Eating disorders
- Attention-deficit/hyperactivity disorder

Medical comorbidities include:

- Migraine
- Multiple sclerosis
- Cushing syndrome
- Brain tumor
- Head trauma

Patient Encounter, Part 3: Creating a Care Plan

Based on all information presented, create a care plan for this patient's bipolar disorder. Your plan should include (a) a statement of the drug-related needs or problems, (b) the goals of therapy, (c) a patient-specific therapeutic plan, and (d) a plan for follow-up to assess therapeutic response and adverse effects.

TREATMENT

Desired Outcomes

KEY CONCEPT *Goals of treatment are to reduce symptoms, induce remission, prevent relapse, improve patient functioning, and minimize adverse effects of drug therapy.*

General Approach to Treatment

Treatment guidelines for manic and depressive episodes of bipolar disorder are included in Table 39–2.

Table 39–2

Guidelines for the Acute Treatment of Mood Episodes in Patients with Bipolar I Disorder

Acute Manic or Mixed Episode		**Acute Depressive Episode**	
General guidelines Assess for secondary causes of mania or mixed states (eg, alcohol or drug use) Taper off antidepressants, stimulants, and caffeine if possible Treat substance abuse Encourage good nutrition (with regular protein and essential fatty acid intake), exercise, adequate sleep, stress reduction, and psychosocial therapy		General guidelines Assess for secondary causes of depression (eg, alcohol or drug use) Taper off antipsychotics, benzodiazepines or sedative-hypnotic agents if possible Treat substance abuse Encourage good nutrition (with regular protein and essential fatty acid intake), exercise, adequate sleep, stress reduction, and psychosocial therapy	
Hypomania	**Mania**	**Mild to Moderate Depressive Episode**	**Severe Depressive Episode**
First, optimize current mood stabilizer or initiate mood-stabilizing medication: lithium,[a] valproate,[a] or carbamazepine.[a] Consider adding a benzodiazepine (lorazepam or clonazepam) for short-term adjunctive treatment of agitation or insomnia if needed	First, two- or three-drug combinations: lithium or valproate plus a benzodiazepine (lorazepam or clonazepam) for short-term adjunctive treatment of agitation or insomnia; lorazepam is recommended for catatonia. If psychosis is present, initiate atypical antipsychotic in combination with above	First, initiate and/or optimize mood-stabilizing medication: lithium[a], lurasidone, olanzapine/fluoxetine, quetiapine, or lamotrigtine[b]	First, two- or three-drug combinations: lithium,[a] lurasidone, quetiapine, olanzapine/fluoxetine, or lamotrigine[b] plus an antidepressant[c]; lithium plus lamotrigine
Alternative medication treatment options: carbamazepine[a]; If patient does not respond or tolerate, consider atypical antipsychotic (eg, olanzapine, quetiapine, risperidone) or oxcarbazepine	Alternative medication treatment options: carbamazepine[a]; If patient does not respond or tolerate, consider oxcarbazepine	Alternative anticonvulsants: valproate,[a] carbamazepine,[a] or oxcarbazepine	Alternative anticonvulsants: valproate;[a] carbamazepine,[a] or oxcarbazepine Second, if response is inadequate, consider adding an atypical antipsychotic (quetiapine, lurasidone) to mood stabilizer Third, if response is inadequate, consider a three-drug combination:
Second, if response is inadequate, consider a two-drug combination: • Lithium[a] plus an anticonvulsant or an atypical antipsychotic • Anticonvulsant plus an anticonvulsant or atypical antipsychotic	Second, if response is inadequate, consider a three-drug combination: • Lithium plus antipsychotic plus an antidepressant • Anticonvulsant plus an anticonvulsant plus an atypical antipsychotic Third, if response is inadequate consider ECT for mania with psychosis or catatonia[a]; or add clozapine for treatment-refractory illness		• Lithium plus lamotrigine[b] plus an an antidepressant • Lithium[a] plus an anticonvulsant plus an atypical antipsychotic Fourth, if response is inadequate, consider ECT for treatment-refractory illness and depression with psychosis or catatonia[d]

ECT, electroconvulsive therapy; MAOI, manoamine oxidase inhibitor; SNRI, serotonin-norepinephrine reuptake inhibitor; SSRI, selective serotonin reuptake inhibitor; TCA, tricyclic antidepressant.

[a]Use standard therapeutic serum concentration ranges if clinically indicated; if partial response or breakthrough episode, adjust dose to achieve higher serum concentrations without causing intolerable adverse effects; valproate is preferred over lithium for mixed episodes and rapid cycling; lithium and/or lamotrigine is preferred over valproate for bipolar depression.

[b]Lamotrigine is not approved for the acute treatment of depression, and the dose must be started low and slowly titrated to decrease adverse effects if used for maintenance therapy of bipolar I disorder. A drug interaction and a severe dermatologic rash can occur when lamotrigine is combined with valproate (ie, lamotrigine doses must be halved from standard dosing titration).

[c]Antidepressant monotherapy is not recommended for bipolar depression. Bupropion, SSRIs (eg, citalopram, escitalopram, or sertraline), and SNRIs (eg, venlafaxine) have shown good efficacy and fewer adverse effects in the treatment of unipolar depression; MAOIs and TCAs have more adverse effects (eg, weight gain) and can have a higher risk of causing antidepressant-induced mania; fluoxetine, fluvoxamine, nefazodone, and paroxetine inhibit liver metabolism and should be used with caution in patients on concomitant medications that require cytochrome P450 clearance; paroxetine and venlafaxine have a higher risk for a discontinuation syndrome.

[d]ECT is used for severe mania or depression during pregnancy and for mixed episodes; prior to treatment, anticonvulsants, lithium, benzodiazepines should be tapered off to maximize therapy and minimize adverse effects.

Data from Refs. 14 and 38.

Table 39–3

Secondary Causes of Mania

General Medical Conditions	
Alzheimer disease	
Cerebral infarction	
Cerebral tumors	
Closed head injury	
Cushing syndrome	
Hemodialysis	
Hepatic encephalopathy	
Huntington disease	
Hyperthyroidism	
Ictal or postictal mania	
Multiple sclerosis	
Neurosyphilis	
Systemic lupus erythematosus	
Vitamin B deficiency	
Medications	
Corticosteroids	
Diltiazem	
Levodopa	
Oral contraceptives	
Zidovudine	
Illicit Substances	
Anabolic steroids	
Hallucinogens	
Stimulants (cocaine, amphetamines)	

Data from Drayton SJ, Pelic CM. Bipolar disorder. In: DiPiro JT, Talbert RL, Yee GC, et al, eds. Pharmacotherapy: A Pathophysiologic Approach. 9th ed. New York, NY: McGraw-Hill. 2014;1067–1081.

Although it is a goal of treatment, not all patients achieve remission. The mainstay of drug therapy has been mood-stabilizing drugs but research based on multiple treatments indicates antipsychotic drugs, both first-generation (FGAs) and second-generation (SGAs), may be more effective for acute mania.[15] Antipsychotic drugs may be used as monotherapy or adjunctively with mood-stabilizing drugs. A person entering treatment for a first mood episode in bipolar disorder must have a complete assessment and careful diagnosis to rule out nonpsychiatric causes. A variety of conditions can cause similar symptoms (Table 39–3). Because early and accurate diagnosis is essential to maximizing response to treatment, pharmacologic and nonpharmacologic therapy should begin as soon as possible. Treatment is often lifelong. Comorbid conditions should also be addressed.

▸ *Suicidality Risk*

Patients should be assessed for potential for violence and harm to others. Friends or family can be asked to remove the home guns, caustic chemicals, medications, and objects that patients might use to harm themselves or others. Risk factors for suicide include severity of depression, feelings of hopelessness, comorbid personality disorder, and a history of a previous suicide attempt.[11]

▸ *Nonpharmacologic Therapy*

KEY CONCEPT *Interpersonal, family, or group psychotherapy with a qualified therapist or clinician assists individuals with bipolar disorder to improve functional outcomes and may help treat or prevent mood episodes,* establish a daily routine and sleep schedule, and improve interpersonal relationships.[12]

Cognitive-behavioral therapy (CBT) is a type of psychotherapy that stresses the importance of recognizing patterns of cognition (thought) and how thoughts influence subsequent feelings and behaviors. Other people, situations, and events external to the individual are not seen as the sources of thoughts and behaviors. With CBT, patients are taught self-management skills to change negative thoughts even if external circumstances do not change.

Electroconvulsive therapy (ECT) is the application of electrical impulses to the brain for the treatment of severe depression, mixed states, psychotic depression, and treatment refractory mania. It also may be used in pregnant women who cannot take carbamazepine, lithium, or divalproex.

Education for patients, families, and groups about chronicity of bipolar disorder and self-management through sleep hygiene, nutrition, exercise, stress reduction, and abstinence from alcohol or drugs is critical to success. The development of a crisis intervention plan is essential.

▸ *Pharmacologic Therapy*

KEY CONCEPT *The primary treatment modality for manic episodes is mood-stabilizing agents or antipsychotic drugs, often in combination.*[13,14]

Mood-stabilizing drugs are first-line treatments and include lithium, divalproex, carbamazepine, and lamotrigine. The SGAs, including risperidone, olanzapine, quetiapine, ziprasidone, aripiprazole, lurasidone, and asenapine, are approved for treatment of acute mania. Lithium, lamotrigine, aripiprazole, olanzapine, and quetiapine are approved for maintenance therapy. Quetiapine's maintenance therapy indication in bipolar I disorder is adjunctive with lithium or divalproex. Drugs used with less research support and without Food and Drug Administration (FDA) approval include topiramate and oxcarbazepine. Benzodiazepines are used adjunctively for mania.

KEY CONCEPT *The primary treatment for depressive episodes in bipolar disorder is mood-stabilizing agents or certain antipsychotics.*

Among antipsychotic drugs, quetiapine as monotherapy, lurasidone as monotherapy or adjunctive to lithium or divalproex, and olanzapine in combination with fluoxetine are approved. Antidepressants can be used but along with a mood stabilizer to reduce risk of a mood switch to mania and after the patient has failed to respond adequately to mood-stabilizing therapy. Evidence of efficacy of antidepressant drugs in bipolar depression is considered controversial.[13,15] Combinations of two mood-stabilizing drugs or a mood-stabilizing drug and either an antipsychotic or antidepressant drug are common, especially in acute mood episodes.

KEY CONCEPT *The primary treatment for relapse prevention is mood-stabilizing agents, often combined with antipsychotic drugs.* Aripiprazole, olanzapine, and quetiapine are approved for maintenance therapy.

Table 39–4 includes a summary of current drug therapy for bipolar disorder. An algorithm for treatment of bipolar mania is shown in Table 39–2.

▸ *Mood-Stabilizing Drugs*

The optimal mood-stabilizing drug is effective in treatment of acute mania and acute bipolar depression and in prevention of manic relapse and bipolar depression relapse. All currently approved mood-stabilizing drugs have demonstrated efficacy over placebo for one or more of these areas, but there are differences among them with regard to specific patient populations. The choice of treatment is dictated by patient characteristics and history. Few studies systematically compare mood stabilizers with each other. Efficacy of individual agents in placebo-controlled trials is similar. Lithium and divalproex are first-choice drugs for the classic presentation of bipolar disorder.

Table 39–4

Product Formulation, Dose, and Clinical Use of Agents Used in Treatment of Bipolar Disorder

Generic Name	Brand Names	Formulations	Dosages	Clinical Use	Dosage Adjustment in Renal or Hepatic Impairment
Lithium Salts					
FDA approved in bipolar disorder					
Lithium carbonate	Lithobid	ER tablets: 300 mg	900–2400 mg/day once daily or in two to four divided doses, preferably with meals. There is wide variation in the dosage needed to achieve therapeutic response and 12-hour serum lithium concentration (ie, 0.6–1.2 mEq/L (mmol/L) for maintenance therapy and 1.0–1.5 mEq/L (mmol/L) for acute mood episodes taken 12 hours after last dose). Single daily dosing is effective and causes fewer renal effects	Monotherapy or in combination with other drugs for the acute treatment of mania and for maintenance treatment	Reduce starting dosage by at least 50% in renal impairment
	Generic	ER tablets: 450 mg			
	Generic	ER tablets: 300 mg			
	Generic	Tablet: 300 mg			
		Capsules: 150, 300, 600 mg			
Lithium citrate	Generic	300 mg (8 mmol)/5 mL			
Anticonvulsants					
FDA approved for use in bipolar disorder					
Carbamazepine	Equetro (only the Equetro brand is FDA approved for bipolar disorder)	Capsules: 100 mg, 200 mg, 300 mg SR; may open capsule but do not crush or chew beads; take with food	Start at 100–200 mg bid; increase by 200 mg every 3–4 days to 200–1800 mg/day in two to four divided doses	Monotherapy or in combination with other drugs for the acute treatment of mania or mixed episodes for bipolar I disorder	Reduce starting dosage by at least half or avoid in hepatic impairment
		Tablets: 200 mg	Target serum concentration is 4–12 mcg/mL (17–51 μmol/L)		
	Tegretol, generic	Chewable tablet: 100 mg			
	Tegretol XR	Suspension: 100 mg/5 mL			
	Carbatrol	ER tablets: 100, 200, 400 mg			
		ER capsules: 100, 200, 300 mg			
Divalproex sodium	Depakote, generic	Enteric-coated, delayed-release tablets: 125, 250, 500 mg	750–3000 mg/day (20–60 mg/kg/day) in two to three divided doses for delayed-release divalproex or valproic acid	Monotherapy or in combination with other drugs for the acute treatment of mania. Although commonly used for relapse prevention, maintenance treatment is not FDA approved	Reduce starting dosage by half or avoid in hepatic impairment
	Depakote ER	Sprinkles: 125 mg	ER divalproex may be given once daily		
		ER tablets: 250, 500 mg	A loading dose of 20–30 mg/kg/day can be given, then 20 mg/kg/day and titrated to a serum concentration of 50–125 mcg/mL (347–866 μmol/L)		
Valproic acid	Depakene, generic	Capsules: 250 mg			
Valproic acid syrup	Depakene, generic	250 mg/5 mL			
Lamotrigine	Lamictal, generic	Tablets: 25, 100, 150, 200 mg	50–400 mg/day in divided doses. Dosage should be slowly increased by following prescribing information. If divalproex is added to lamotrigine, the lamotrigine dosage should be reduced by half	Monotherapy or in combination with other drugs for maintenance treatment	
		Chewable tablets: 2, 5, 25 mg			
		Orally disintegrating tablets: 25, 50, 100, 200 mg			
	Lamictal XR (not FDA approved for bipolar disorder)	ER tablets: 25, 50, 100, 200 mg			

Anticonvulsants and Other Drugs Not FDA Approved for Use in Bipolar Disorder				
Clonazepam	Klonopin, generic	Tablets: 0.5, 1, 2 mg Wafers: 0.125, 0.25, 0.5, 1, 2 mg	0.5–20 mg/day in divided doses or one dose at bedtime Dosage should be slowly adjusted up and down according to response and adverse effects	Use in combination with other drugs for the acute treatment of mania or mixed episodes
Lorazepam	Ativan, generic	Tablets: 0.5, 1, 2 mg Oral solution: 2 mg/mL Injection: 2, 4 mg/mL	2–10 mg/day in divided doses or one dose at bedtime Dosage should be slowly adjusted up and down according to response and adverse effects	
Oxcarbazepine	Trileptal, generic	Tablets: 150, 300, 600 mg Suspension: 300 mg/5 mL	300–1200 mg/day in two divided doses Doses should be slowly adjusted up and down according to response and adverse effects (eg, 150–300 mg twice daily and increase by 300–600 mg/day at weekly intervals)	May cause fewer adverse drug–drug interactions than carbamazepine, but causes more gastrointestinal side effects and hyponatremia. Evidence is limited regarding efficacy
Atypical Antipsychotics				
FDA approved for bipolar disorder				
Aripiprazole	Abilify Abilify Discmelt	Tablets: 2, 5, 10, 15, 20, 30 mg Oral solution: 5 mg/5 mL Tablets, orally disintegrating: 10, 15 mg	10–30 mg/day once daily	Use as monotherapy or in combination with lithium or valproate for the acute treatment of mania or mixed states for bipolar I disorder and prevention of manic relapse
Asenapine	Saphris	Sublingual tablets: 5, 10 mg	5–20 mg/day in two divided doses. Must be held under the tongue until dissolved completely, not chewed or swallowed, with no food or liquid for 10 minutes after administering	Use as monotherapy or in combination with lithium or valproate for the acute treatment of mania or mixed states of bipolar I disorder
Lurasidone	Latuda	Tablets: 20, 40, 60, 80, 120 mg	20–120 mg once daily	Use as monotherapy or in combination with lithium or valproate for depression of bipolar I disorder
Olanzapine	Zyprexa, generic Zyprexa Zydis	Tablets: 2.5, 5, 7.5, 10, 15, 20 mg Tablets, orally disintegrating: 5, 10, 15, 20 mg	5–20 mg/day in one or two doses	Used as monotherapy or in combination with lithium or valproate for acute treatment of mania or mixed states for bipolar I disorder and prevention of manic relapse. Used in combination with fluoxetine (OFC) for treatment of bipolar depression
Olanzapine/Fluoxetine combination (OFC)	Symbyax	Capsules: 3/25, 6/25, 6/50, 12/25, 12/50 mg		
Quetiapine	Seroquel Seroquel XR	Tablets: 25, 50, 100, 200, 300, 400 mg ER tablets: 50, 150, 200, 300, 400 mg	50–800 mg/day in divided doses or once daily when stabilized	Used as monotherapy or in combination with lithium or divalproex for acute treatment of mania, mixed states for bipolar I disorder, and depression of bipolar I and bipolar II disorder. Used adjunctively with lithium or divalproex for relapse prevention of bipolar mania and depression
Risperidone	Risperdal, generic Risperdal M-Tabs Risperdal Consta	Tablets: 0.25, 0.5, 1, 2, 3, 4 mg Oral solution: 1 mg/mL Tablets, orally disintegrating: 0.5, 1, 2, 3, 4 mg Long-acting injectable: 12.5, 25, 37.5, 50 mg	0.5–6 mg/day in one or two doses	Used as monotherapy or adjunctively with lithium or divalproex for acute mania or mixed episodes of bipolar I disorder
Ziprasidone	Geodon	Capsules: 20, 40, 60, 80 mg	40–160 mg/day in divided doses	Used as monotherapy or adjunctively with lithium or divalproex for acute mania or mixed episodes of bipolar I disorder

DIVALPROEX, divalproex; ER, extended release; FDA, Food and Drug Administration; SR, sustained release; OFC, olanzapine-fluoxetine combination.
Data from Refs. 13–15, 20–22, 24, 27–29, and 38.

Lithium Lithium, the first approved mood-stabilizing drug, remains a first-line agent and sets the standard for efficacy against which other drugs are measured. It is antimanic, prevents relapse, and has modest efficacy for acute bipolar depression. One of the oldest drugs used for psychiatric illness, research continues to support its use.[15] In most studies, lithium's efficacy is equivalent to that of anticonvulsant mood stabilizers and SGAs. It is most effective for patients with few previous episodes, symptom-free interepisode remission, and a family history of bipolar disorder with good response to lithium. Evidence suggests genetic phenotypes that are more responsive to lithium.[16] However, patients with rapid cycling are less responsive to lithium than to other mood-stabilizing drugs such as divalproex. Additionally, its efficacy for bipolar depression is less robust than for mania.[15] It may also be less effective in mixed mood episodes (symptoms of mania and depression occurring simultaneously).

Evidence shows lithium's effect on suicidal behavior is superior to that of other mood-stabilizing drugs.[17] Lithium reduces the risk of deliberate self-harm or suicide by 70%.

Mechanism of Action Lithium's mechanism of action is not well understood and is multimodal. Possibilities include altered ion transport, effects on neurotransmitter signaling, blocking adenyl cyclase, effects on inositol, neuroprotection or increased BDNF, and inhibition of second messenger systems.[18]

Dosing and Monitoring Lithium is usually initiated at a dosage of 600 to 900 mg/day. Although it is commonly given in a divided dosage, once-daily dosing is recommended, especially with sustained-release formulations. Once-daily dosing can improve adherence and reduce renal side effects. Lithium has a narrow therapeutic index, meaning the toxic dosage is not much greater than the therapeutic dosage. Lithium requires regular serum concentration monitoring as a guide to titration and to minimize adverse effects. At least weekly monitoring is recommended until stabilized; then the frequency can be decreased. Well-maintained patients who tolerate lithium without difficulty can be monitored by serum concentration as infrequently as twice yearly. The dosage is titrated to achieve a serum lithium concentration of 0.6 to 1.4 mEq/L (mmol/L). Higher serum concentrations are required to treat an acute episode than to prevent relapse. Serum lithium above 0.8 mEq/L (mmol/L) may be more effective at preventing relapse than lower serum concentrations. The suggested therapeutic serum concentration range is based on a 12-hour postdose sample collection, usually a morning trough in patients taking more than one dose per day. At least 2 weeks at a suggested therapeutic serum concentration is required for an adequate trial. Table 39–5 shows pharmacokinetic parameters and desired serum concentrations of mood-stabilizing drugs. It is common for lithium to be combined with other mood stabilizers or antipsychotics to achieve more complete remission.

Adverse Effects The most common adverse effects are gastrointestinal (GI) upset, tremor, and polyuria,[19] which are dose related. Nausea, dyspepsia, and diarrhea are minimized by coadministration with food, use of the sustained-release formulation, and giving smaller doses more frequently to reduce the amount of drug in the GI tract. Tremor is present in up to 50% of patients. In addition to these approaches, low-dose β-blockers, such as propranolol 20 to 60 mg/day, reduces tremor.

Lithium impairs the kidney's ability to concentrate urine because of its inhibitory effect on vasopressin. This causes an increase in urine volume and frequency of urination and an increase in thirst. Polyuria and polydipsia occur in up to 70% of patients. A severe form of polyuria, when urine volume exceeds 3 L/day, is termed lithium-induced nephrogenic diabetes insipidus. It can be treated with hydrochlorothiazide or amiloride. If the former is used, the lithium dosage should be reduced by 33% to 50% to account for the drug–drug interaction that increases serum lithium and causes toxicity. Long-term lithium has been associated with structural kidney changes, such as glomerular sclerosis or tubular atrophy. Once-daily dosing of lithium is less likely to cause renal adverse effects than divided-daily dosing.

Lithium is concentrated in the thyroid gland and can impair thyroid hormone synthesis. Although goiter is uncommon, as many as 30% of patients develop at least transiently elevated thyroid-stimulating hormone. Lithium-induced hypothyroidism is not usually an indication to discontinue the drug. Patients can be supplemented with levothyroxine.

Other common adverse effects include poor concentration, acneiform rash, alopecia, worsening of psoriasis, weight gain, metallic taste, impaired glucose regulation, and benign leukocytosis. Lithium causes a flattening of the T wave of the electrocardiogram (ECG), considered benign and not clinically significant. Less commonly, it can cause or worsen arrhythmias.[19]

Lithium and other mood-stabilizing drugs require baseline and routine laboratory monitoring to help determine medical appropriateness for initiation of therapy and monitoring of adverse effects. Guidelines for such monitoring are outlined in Table 39–6.

Acute lithium toxicity, which occurs at serum concentrations over 2 mEq/L (mmol/L), can be severe and life threatening, necessitating emergency treatment. Symptoms include severe vomiting and diarrhea, deterioration in motor coordination, including coarse tremor, ataxia, and dysarthria, and impaired cognition. In its most severe form, seizures, cardiac arrhythmias, coma, and kidney damage are reported. Treatment includes discontinuation of lithium, IV fluids to correct fluid and electrolyte imbalance, and osmotic diuresis or hemodialysis. In case of overdose, gastric lavage is indicated. Clinical symptoms continue after the serum concentration is lowered because clearance from the central nervous system (CNS) is slower than from serum. Factors predisposing to lithium toxicity include fluid and sodium loss from hot weather or exercise or drug interactions that increase serum lithium.[19]

Drug Interactions Drug interactions involving lithium are common. Because lithium is not metabolized or protein bound, it is not associated with metabolic drug interactions that occur with other mood-stabilizing drugs. Common and significant drug interactions involve thiazide diuretics, nonsteroidal anti-inflammatory drugs, and angiotensin-converting enzyme (ACE) inhibitor drugs. If a diuretic must be used with lithium and a thiazide is not required, loop diuretics such as furosemide are less likely to increase lithium retention. The ACE inhibitors and angiotensin receptor blockers (ARB) can abruptly increase serum lithium with the potential of acute toxicity, even after months of no change in serum lithium. This combination is strongly discouraged.[19]

Divalproex Sodium and Valproic Acid Divalproex sodium is composed of sodium valproate and valproic acid. The delayed-release and extended-release formulations are converted in the intestine into valproic acid (VPA), which is systemically absorbed. It is FDA approved for treatment of the manic phase of bipolar disorder. It is equal in efficacy to lithium and some other drugs for bipolar mania. It has utility in bipolar disorder with rapid cycling, mixed mood features, and substance abuse comorbidity. Although not FDA approved for relapse prevention, studies support its use, and it is widely prescribed for maintenance therapy. Divalproex can be used as monotherapy or in combination with lithium or an antipsychotic.[13]

Table 39–5

Pharmacokinetics and Therapeutic Serum Concentrations of Lithium and Anticonvulsants Used in the Treatment of Bipolar Disorder

	Lithium	Carbamazepine	Oxcarbazepine	Divalproex (DIVALPROEX) Sodium/Valproic Acid (VPA)	Lamotrigine
Gastrointestinal Absorption					
Regular release	Rapid: 95%–100% within 1–6 hours	Slow and erratic: 85%–90%	Slow and complete: 100%	Rapid and complete (VPA)	Rapid: 98%
Syrup, suspension, solution	Faster rate of absorption: 100%	Faster rate of absorption	Unknown	Faster rate of absorption than tablets	NA
ER/enteric-coated tablets	Delayed absorption: 60%–90%	Delayed absorption: 89% of the suspension; and less than regular-release tablets	NA	Delayed absorption with delayed-release tablets; valproate is rapidly converted to VPA in the intestine and then is rapidly and almost completely absorbed from the GI tract ER bioavailability is approximately 15% less than delayed release	Delayed absorption but not significantly different from regular release
Delay in absorption by food	Yes	No; reports of increased rate of absorption with fatty meals (ER capsule)	No	Yes; food slows the rate of absorption but not the extent for DIVALPROEX	Bioavailability not affected by food
Time to reach peak serum concentrations	0.5–3 hours (regular-release) 4–12 hours (ER) 0.25–1 hour (oral solution)	4–5 hours (regular-release); 1.5 hours (suspension); 3–12 hours (ER tablets); 4.1–7.7 hours (ER capsules); higher peak concentrations with chewable tablets	4.5 hours (range of 3–13 hours)	1–4 hours (VPA) 3–5 hours (DIVALPROEX single dose) 7–14 hours (DIVALPROEX ER multiple dosing)	1–4 hours (regular release), 4–6 hours (ER)
Distribution					
Volume of distribution	Initial: 0.3–0.4 L/kg Steady state: 0.7–1 L/kg	0.6–2 L/kg (adults)	10-monohydroxy metabolite: 49 L/kg	11 L/1.73 m^2 (total valproate); 92 L/1.73 m^2 (free valproate)	0.9–1.3 L/kg
Crosses the placenta	Yes; pregnancy risk category: D Risk of cardiac defects: 0.1%–0.5%	Yes; pregnancy risk category: D	Yes; pregnancy risk category: C	Yes; pregnancy risk category: D Risk of neural tube defects: 1%–5%	Yes; pregnancy risk category: C
Crosses into breast milk	Yes; 35%–50% of mother's serum concentration; breastfeeding not recommended	Yes; ratio of concentration in breast milk to plasma is 0.4 for drug and 0.5 for epoxide metabolite; considered compatible with breastfeeding	Yes; both drug and active metabolite; breastfeeding not recommended	Yes; considered compatible with breastfeeding	Yes; breastfeeding not recommended
Protein binding	No	75%–90%	40% of active metabolite	80%–90% (dose dependent)	55%

(Continued)

Table 39–5

Pharmacokinetics and Therapeutic Serum Concentrations of Lithium and Anticonvulsants Used in the Treatment of Bipolar Disorder (*Continued*)

	Lithium	Carbamazepine	Oxcarbazepine	Divalproex (DIVALPROEX) Sodium/Valproic Acid (VPA)	Lamotrigine
Renal clearance	Yes; 10–40 mL/min with 90%–98% of dose excreted in urine; 80% of lithium that is filtered by the renal glomeruli is reabsorbed	Yes; 1%–3% excreted unchanged in urine	Yes; 95% excreted in the urine; < 1% excreted unchanged	Yes; 30%–50% excreted as glucuronide conjugate; < 3% excreted unchanged	Yes; 94% excreted as glucuronide conjugate
Metabolism					
Hepatic metabolism	No	Yes; oxidation and hydroxylation; induces liver enzymes to increase its own metabolism and metabolism of other drugs	Yes; oxidation and conjugation	Yes; oxidation and glucuronide conjugation	Yes; glucuronic acid conjugation induces its own metabolism in normal volunteers
Metabolites	No	Yes; 10, 11-epoxide (active)	Yes; 10-monohydroxy metabolite (active)	Yes (not active)	No
Kinetics	First-order	First-order after initial enzyme induction phase	First-order	First-order	First-order
Half-life ($t_{1/2}$)	18–27 hours (adult); > 36 hours (elderly or patients with renal impairment)	Half-life decreases over time due to autoinduction: 25–65 hours (initial) 12–17 hours (adult multiple dosing) 8–14 hours (children multiple dosing)	2 hours (parent) 9 hours (metabolite)	5–20 hours (adults)	25 hours; increases to 59 hours with concomitant VPA therapy
Cytochrome P450 (CYP450) isoenzyme					
CYP450 substrate	No	2C8 and 3A3/4	Unknown	2C19	Unknown
CYP450 inhibitor	No	No	2C19	2C9, 2D6, and 3A3/4	Unknown
CYP450 inducer	No	1A2, 2C9/10, and 3A3/4	3A3/4	No	Unknown
Therapeutic Serum/Plasma Concentrations					
	1–1.5 mEq/L (mmol/L): for adult, acute mania 0.4–0.6 mEq/L (mmol/L): for elderly or medically ill patients 0.6–1.2 mEq/L (mmol/L): for adult, maintenance; ranges based on 12-hour postdose sample collection	4–12 mcg/mL (17–51 μmol/L): for adult, acute mania and maintenance 4–8 mcg/mL (17–34 μmol/L): for elderly or medically ill	No established therapeutic range; 12–30 mcg/mL (47–118 μmol/L) for 10-hydroxy metabolite based on epilepsy trials	50–125 mcg/mL (347–866 μmol/L): adult, acute mania and maintenance 40–75 mcg/mL (277–520 μmol/L) : elderly or medically ill	No established therapeutic range: 4–20 mcg/mL (16–78 μmol/L) based on epilepsy trials

ER, extended release; GI, gastrointestinal; NA, not applicable.

Data from Refs. 19–22 and 24.

Mechanism of Action. The mechanism is not well understood. It is known to affect ion transport and enhance activity of γ-aminobutyric acid (GABA). Similar to lithium, it has possible neuroprotective effects through enhancement of BDNF.[18]

Dosing and Monitoring. Divalproex is initiated at 500 to 1000 mg/day, but studies indicate a therapeutic serum VPA concentration can be reached more quickly through a loading dose approach of 20 to 30 mg/kg/day. Using this approach, patients may respond with a significant reduction in symptoms within the first few days of treatment. The dosage is then titrated according to response, tolerability, and serum concentration. The most often referenced desired VPA serum concentration is 50 to 125 mcg/mL (347–866 μmoles/L), but it is not unusual for patients to require more than 100 mcg/mL (693 μmoles/L) for optimal efficacy.

Table 39–6

Guidelines for Baseline and Routine Laboratory Tests and Monitoring for Agents Used in the Treatment of Bipolar Disorder

	Baseline: Physical Examination and General Chemistry[a]	Hematologic Tests[b]		Metabolic Tests[c]		Liver Function Tests[d]		Renal Function Tests[e]		Thyroid Function Tests[f]		Serum Electrolytes[g]		Dermatologic[h]	
	Baseline	Baseline	6–12 Months	Baseline	6–12 Months	Baseline	6–12 Months	Baseline	6–12 Months	Baseline	6–12 Months	Baseline	6–12 Months	Baseline	3–6 Months
SGAs[i]	X			X	X										
Carbamazepine[j]	X	X	X			X	X	X				X	X	X	X
Lamotrigine[k]	X													X	X
Lithium[l]	X	X	X	X	X			X	X	X	X	X	X	X	X
Oxcarbazepine[m]	X											X	X	X	X
Valproate[n]	X	X	X	X	X	X	X							X	X

[a]Screen for drug abuse and serum pregnancy.

[b]CBC with differential and platelets.

[c]Fasting glucose, serum lipids, weight.

[d]Lactate dehydrogenase, aspartate aminotransferase, alanine aminotransferase, total bilirubin, alkaline phosphatase.

[e]Serum creatinine, blood urea nitrogen, urinalysis, urine osmolality, specific gravity.

[f]Triiodothyronine, total thyroxine, thyroxine uptake, and thyroid-stimulating hormone.

[g]Serum sodium.

[h]Rashes, hair thinning, alopecia.

[i]Atypical antipsychotic: Monitor for increased appetite with weight gain (primarily in patients with initial low or normal body mass index); monitor closely if rapid or significant weight gain occurs during early therapy; cases of hyperlipidemia and diabetes reported.

[j]Carbamazepine: Manufacturer recommends CBC and platelets (and possibly reticulocyte counts and serum iron) at baseline, and that subsequent monitoring be individualized by the clinician (eg, CBC, platelet counts, and liver function tests every 2 weeks during the first 2 months of treatment, then every 3 months if normal). Monitor more closely if patient exhibits hematologic or hepatic abnormalities or if the patient is receiving a myelotoxic drug; discontinue if platelets are less than 100,000/mm^3 (100 × 10^9/L), if WBC is less than 3000/mm^3 (3 × 10^9/L) or if there is evidence of bone marrow suppression or liver dysfunction. Serum electrolyte levels should be monitored in the elderly or those at risk for hyponatremia. Carbamazepine interferes with some pregnancy tests.

[k]Lamotrigine: If renal or hepatic impairment, monitor closely and adjust dosage according to manufacturer's guidelines. Serious dermatologic reactions have occurred within 2 to 8 weeks of initiating treatment and are more likely to occur in patients receiving concomitant valproate, with rapid dose escalation, or using doses exceeding the recommended titration schedule.

[l]Lithium: Obtain baseline ECG for patients older than 40 years or if preexisting cardiac disease (benign, reversible T-wave depression can occur). Renal function tests should be obtained every 2 to 3 months during the first 6 months, then every 6 to 12 months; if impaired renal function, monitor 24-hour urine volume and creatinine every 3 months; if urine volume more than 3 L/day, monitor urinalysis, osmolality, and specific gravity every 3 months. Thyroid function tests should be obtained once or twice during the first 6 months, then every 6 to 12 months; monitor for signs and symptoms of hypothyroidism; if supplemental thyroid therapy is required, monitor thyroid function tests and adjust thyroid dose every 1 to 2 months until thyroid function indices are within normal range, then monitor every 3 to 6 months.

[m]Oxcarbazepine: Hyponatremia (serum sodium concentrations less than 125 mEq/L [mmol/L]) has been reported and occurs more frequently during the first 3 months of therapy; serum sodium concentrations should be monitored in patients receiving drugs that lower serum sodium concentrations (eg, diuretics or drugs that cause inappropriate antidiuretic hormone secretion) or in patients with symptoms of hyponatremia (eg, confusion, headache, lethargy, and malaise). Hypersensitivity reactions have occurred in approximately 25% to 30% of patients with a history of carbamazepine hypersensitivity and requires immediate discontinuation.

[n]Valproate: Weight gain reported in patients with low or normal body mass index. Monitor platelets and liver function during first 3 to 6 months if evidence of increased bruising or bleeding. Monitor closely if patients exhibit hematologic or hepatic abnormalities or in patients receiving drugs that affect coagulation, such as aspirin or warfarin; discontinue if platelets are less than 100,000/mm^3/L (100 × 10^9/L) or if prolonged bleeding time. Pancreatitis, hyperammonemic encephalopathy, polycystic ovary syndrome, increased testosterone, and menstrual irregularities have been reported; not recommended during first trimester of pregnancy due to risk of neural tube defects.

Data from Refs. 14 and 38.

Some patients require high milligram dosages in order to reach a desired serum concentration. The suggested serum concentration range is based on trough values. Serum concentration monitoring is recommended at least every 2 weeks until stabilized, then less frequently. The extended-release formulation can be taken once daily (see Table 39–4). If the extended-release formulation is administered at night, a morning blood sampling is a peak, not a trough. The drug should be given in the morning so that blood sampling the following morning would be a trough value and more easily interpreted if the typical blood sampling time is in the morning. The systemic bioavailability of extended-release divalproex is about 15% less than that of the delayed-release formulation. Patients who have difficulty swallowing large tablets can use the sprinkle formulation. The immediate-release formulation, either capsules or syrup, is given three or four times per day.[20]

Adverse Effects. The most common adverse effects are GI (loss of appetite, nausea, dyspepsia, diarrhea), tremor, and drowsiness. GI distress can be reduced by coadministration with food. The delayed-release and extended-release formulations are less likely to cause gastric distress than immediate-release valproic acid. Dosage reduction can reduce all of the common side effects. As with lithium, a low-dose β-blocker may alleviate tremor. Weight gain is common, occurring in up to 50% of patients.[20]

Other less common adverse effects include alopecia or a change in hair color or texture. Hair loss can be minimized by supplementation with a vitamin containing selenium and zinc. Polycystic ovarian syndrome associated with increased androgen production is reported. Thrombocytopenia is common, and the platelet count should be monitored periodically. It is a dose-related adverse effect and usually asymptomatic, but the drug is usually stopped if the platelet count is less than $100 \times 10^3/mm^3$ ($100 \times 10^9/L$). More rare are hepatic toxicity and pancreatitis, which are not always dose related. Severe GI symptoms of hepatic or pancreatic toxicity include vomiting, pain, and loss of appetite. When these occur, the patient should be evaluated for possible hepatitis or pancreatitis. Divalproex has a wide therapeutic index. Acute toxicity for high dosages or overdosage is not life threatening.

Drug Interactions. Drug interactions involving divalproex are common. It is a weak inhibitor of some drug metabolizing liver enzymes and can affect metabolism of other drugs. These include other anticonvulsants and antidepressants. The interaction between divalproex and lamotrigine is significant. The risk of a dangerous rash caused by lamotrigine is increased when given concurrently with divalproex. When lamotrigine is added to divalproex, the initial lamotrigine dosage should be one-half the typical starting dosage, and lamotrigine should be titrated more slowly than usual. When divalproex is added to lamotrigine, the lamotrigine dosage should be reduced by 50%.[21] Conversely, the metabolism of divalproex can be increased by enzyme-inducing drugs such as carbamazepine and phenytoin, but divalproex may simultaneously slow metabolism of the other agents.[20]

Carbamazepine Although long used as a mood-stabilizer, only the extended-release formulation is FDA approved for treatment of bipolar disorder. Although it has efficacy for mood stabilization, it is less desirable as a first-line agent because of safety and drug interactions. It is reserved for patients who fail to respond to lithium or for patients with rapid cycling or mixed bipolar disorder. Carbamazepine can be used as monotherapy or in combination with lithium or an antipsychotic drug.[22]

Mechanism of Action. The mechanism of action of carbamazepine is not well understood. It blocks ion channels and inhibits sustained repetitive neuronal excitation, but whether this explains its efficacy as a mood stabilizer is not known.[22]

Dosing and Monitoring. Carbamazepine is initiated at 400 to 600 mg/day. The sustained-release formulation can be given in two divided doses. In addition to a formulation that is completely sustained release, an additional extended-release formulation contains a matrix of 25% immediate-release, 40% extended-release, and 35% enteric-release beads.[22] The suggested therapeutic serum concentration is 4 to 12 mcg/mL (17-51 μmol/L). As with divalproex, some patients require high dosages to achieve a desired serum concentration and therapeutic effect. The dosage can be increased by 200 to 400 mg/day as often as every 2 to 4 days. Serum concentration monitoring is suggested at least every 2 weeks until stabilized.[22]

Adverse Effects. The most common adverse effects are drowsiness, dizziness, ataxia, lethargy, and confusion. At mildly toxic levels, it causes diplopia and dysarthria. These can be minimized through dosage adjustments, use of sustained-release formulations, and giving more of the drug late in the day. GI upset is common. Carbamazepine has an antidiuretic effect similar to the syndrome of inappropriate antidiuretic hormone secretion and can cause hyponatremia. Mild elevations in liver enzymes can occur, but hepatitis is less common. Mild, dose-related leukopenia is not unusual and not an indication for discontinuation. More serious blood count abnormalities such as aplastic anemia and agranulocytosis are rare but life threatening.[22] Suggested baseline and routine laboratory monitoring are reviewed in Table 39–6.

Drug Interactions. Carbamazepine induces hepatic metabolism of many drugs, including other anticonvulsants, antipsychotics, some antidepressants, oral contraceptives, and antiretroviral agents. Carbamazepine is an autoinducer (ie, it induces its own metabolism). The dosage may require an increase after 1 month or so of therapy because of this effect. Conversely, the metabolism of carbamazepine can be slowed by enzyme inhibiting drugs such as some antidepressants; macrolide antibiotics, including erythromycin and clarithromycin; azole antifungal drugs, including ketoconazole and itraconazole; and grapefruit juice. Carbamazepine should not be given concurrently with clozapine because of the additive risk of agranulocytosis.[23]

Lamotrigine Lamotrigine is effective for maintenance treatment of bipolar disorder. It is more effective for depression relapse prevention than for mania relapse prevention. Its primary limitation as an acute treatment is the time required for titration to an effective dosage. In addition to maintenance monotherapy, it is sometimes used in combination with lithium or divalproex, although combination with divalproex increases the risk of rash, and lamotrigine dosage adjustment is required.[21]

Mechanism of Action. The mechanism of action of lamotrigine appears to involve blockage of ion channels and effects on glutamate transmission, although the precise mechanism is not clear.[21]

Dosing and Monitoring. Lamotrigine is initiated at 25 mg/day for 1 to 2 weeks, then increased in a dose-doubling manner every 1 to 2 weeks to a target of 200 to 400 mg/day. If lamotrigine is added to divalproex, the starting dosage is 25 mg every other day with a slower titration to reduce risk of rash. If divalproex is added to lamotrigine, the lamotrigine dosage should be reduced by 50% for the same reason. If lamotrigine therapy is interrupted for more than a few days, it should be restarted at the initial dosage and retitrated. Serum concentration monitoring is not recommended.[21]

Adverse Effects. The adverse effect of greatest significance is a maculopapular rash, occurring in up to 10% of patients.[21] Although usually benign and temporary, some rashes can progress to life-threatening Stevens-Johnson syndrome. The risk of rash is greater with a rapid dosage titration and when given concurrently with divalproex or other metabolic enzyme inhibitors. The risk is minimal when the dosage titration schedule is slow. Other side effects include dizziness, drowsiness, headache, blurred vision, and nausea. In contrast to other mood-stabilizing drugs such as lithium and divalproex, lamotrigine does not significantly influence body weight.

Drug Interactions. The mechanisms of drug–drug interactions involving lamotrigine are unclear. Lamotrigine's primary route of metabolism is conjugative glucuronidation, although it is known to exhibit metabolic autoinduction. It is not significantly metabolized by CYP P450 enzymes. It does not affect drug metabolizing hepatic enzymes. Divalproex slows the rate of elimination of lamotrigine by about half, necessitating dosage reduction. Conversely, carbamazepine increases the rate of lamotrigine metabolism. Upward adjustment in dosage may be needed.[21]

Oxcarbazepine Oxcarbazepine is an analogue of carbamazepine, developed as an anticonvulsant. An advantage over carbamazepine is that routine monitoring of hematology profiles and serum concentrations is not indicated because it is less likely to cause hematologic abnormalities.[24] Additionally, drug interactions are less significant, although it is a mild inducer of certain metabolic pathways. Vigilance for drug interactions is needed, especially with oral contraceptives. Oxcarbazepine appears in the most recent treatment algorithms for bipolar disorder,[13] but clinical trial data are limited.[13]

Adverse Effects. Adverse effects include drowsiness, dizziness, GI upset, and hyponatremia, the latter two of which may be more likely than with carbamazepine.[24]

Others High-potency benzodiazepine agents such as clonazepam and lorazepam are used as adjunctive therapy, especially during acute mania, to reduce anxiety and improve sleep.[26] As complementary or alternative medicines gain wider usage, omega-3 fatty acids have been used in mood disorders, but do not appear in treatment guidelines.

▶ *Antipsychotic Drugs*

First-generation antipsychotics such as chlorpromazine and haloperidol have long been used in the treatment of acute mania. SGA drugs, including aripiprazole, asenapine, olanzapine, quetiapine, risperidone, and ziprasidone, are approved for the treatment of bipolar mania or mixed mood episodes as monotherapy or in combination with mood stabilizers.[13] Aripiprazole, olanzapine, and quetiapine are approved for maintenance therapy for prevention of manic relapse. The combination of olanzapine and fluoxetine is approved for treatment of acute bipolar depression. Quetiapine is approved as monotherapy for acute bipolar depression and as adjunctive therapy with lithium or divalproex for prevention of bipolar depression relapse. Lurasidone is approved as monotherapy and as adjunctive therapy with lithium or divalproex for acute bipolar depression. Approval of antipsychotic drugs in patients with bipolar disorder applies without regard to presence of psychosis. In comparative studies, SGAs are equivalent or superior in efficacy to lithium and divalproex for treatment of acute mania. Treatment guidelines include antipsychotic drugs as first-line therapy.[13] The combination of mood stabilizers and antipsychotics is more likely to achieve remission than monotherapy. Quetiapine data in relapse prevention of both manic and bipolar depression episodes favored combination therapy over mood-stabilizer monotherapy.[27]

The mechanisms of action, usual dosages, pharmacokinetics, adverse effects, and drug interactions involving antipsychotic drugs are discussed in detail in the chapter on schizophrenia. Dosages in bipolar disorder are similar to those used in schizophrenia. Higher dosages are often required to treat an acute episode. The recommended dosage of aripiprazole for bipolar disorder is 20 to 30 mg/day, somewhat higher than the average dosage used in schizophrenia.[28] The recommended dosage for quetiapine in treatment of acute bipolar depression is 300 mg/day, less than the 600 mg/day recommended in acute mania.[29]

SGAs are less likely than FGAs to cause neurologic side effects, especially movement abnormalities. SGAs are more likely to cause metabolic side effects, such as weight gain, glucose dysregulation, and dyslipidemia.[30] Among SGAs approved for treatment of bipolar disorder, olanzapine is most likely to cause metabolic side effects. Asenapine, lurasidone, quetiapine, and risperidone cause less metabolic effects than olanzapine. Aripiprazole, lurasidone, and ziprasidone are least associated with effects on weight, glucose, and lipids.

▶ *Antidepressants*

Treatment of depressive episodes in patients with bipolar disorder presents a particular challenge because of risk of a drug-induced mood switch to mania. The FDA requires the product label of all antidepressants to contain language about the potential risk of inducing a mood switch to mania. Most research shows no advantage for adjunctive antidepressant use compared with mood-stabilizer therapy alone.[13,15] Treatment guidelines and current FDA approvals indicate lithium and quetiapine as first-line therapy.[13] The approval of lurasidone for acute bipolar depression is recent, thus it is not widely included in first-line recommendations. When usual treatment fails, evidence supports use of antidepressants.[13,15]

Guidelines agree that when antidepressants are used, they should be combined with a mood stabilizer to reduce risk of mood switch. The question of which antidepressant drugs are less likely to cause a mood switch is not resolved, but tricyclic antidepressants are thought to carry greater risk. A comparison of venlafaxine, sertraline, and bupropion as adjunctive therapy to a mood stabilizer showed venlafaxine with highest risk of a mood switch to mania or hypomania and bupropion with the least.[31]

Special Populations

Assessment and management by appropriate psychiatric specialists is important for special populations, such as pediatric, geriatric, and pregnant patients.

▶ *Pediatrics*

Evidence regarding treatment of bipolar disorder in children and adolescents is more limited than in adults. Children and adolescents are sensitive to medication side effects, including metabolic side effects of SGAs. With these caveats, evidence supports use of mood stabilizers and SGAs in children and adolescents with bipolar disorder. Lithium is FDA approved for treatment of bipolar disorder in children and adolescents as young as age 12. Aripiprazole, olanzapine, quetiapine, and risperidone are FDA approved in children and adolescents as young as age 10.[13,32]

Initial dosages in the pediatric population are lower than in adults. Metabolic elimination rates of many drugs are increased in children, so they may actually require higher dosages on a weight-adjusted basis. Dosages are titrated carefully according to response and tolerability.

Children and adolescents are especially likely to experience weight gain from SGAs.[33] Cognitive toxicity, manifested as confusion, memory or concentration impairment, or impaired learning, is difficult to detect and is a consideration in the pediatric population so that intellectual and educational development is not hindered.

For comorbid bipolar disorder and attention-deficit/hyperactivity disorder when stimulant therapy is indicated, treatment of mania is recommended before starting the stimulant to avoid exacerbation of mood symptoms.

► *Geriatrics*

Treatment of older adults with bipolar disorder requires care because of increased risks associated with medical conditions and drug–drug interactions.[34] General medical conditions, including endocrine, metabolic, or infectious diseases, can mimic mood disorders. Patients should be evaluated for such medical illnesses that cause or worsen mood symptoms. As physiologic systems change with aging, elimination of drugs is slowed. Examples are slowed renal elimination of lithium and slowed hepatic metabolism of carbamazepine and valproic acid. As a result, dosages required for therapeutic effect are lower in geriatric patients. Also, changes in membrane permeability increase risk of CNS side effects. Increased frequency of patient monitoring is required, including serum drug concentration monitoring.

Vigilance for drug–drug interactions is required because of more medications prescribed to older adults and enhanced sensitivity to adverse effects. Pharmacokinetic interactions include metabolic enzyme induction or inhibition and protein binding displacement interactions (eg, divalproex and warfarin). Pharmacodynamic interactions include additive sedation and cognitive toxicity, which increases risk of falls and other impairments.

► *Pregnancy and Postpartum*

Treatment of bipolar disorder during pregnancy is fraught with controversy and conflicting recommendations. The key issue is the relative risk of teratogenicity with drug use during pregnancy versus risk of bipolar relapse without treatment with consequent harm to both patient and fetus. Therapeutic judgments depend on the history of the patient and whether the pregnancy is planned or unplanned. Treatment is best managed when pregnancy is planned. Clinicians should discuss the issue with every patient with bipolar disorder who is of childbearing potential. A pregnancy test should be obtained before initiating therapy. For a patient with severe illness, a history of multiple mood episodes, rapid cycling, or suicide attempts, discontinuing treatment, even for a planned pregnancy, is unwise. For a patient with a remote history of a single mood episode with subsequent long stability and contemplating pregnancy, the answer is less clear. Patients should be provided clear and reliable information about risks versus benefits of stopping or continuing therapy so they can make an informed decision. Patients who decide to discontinue medication before pregnancy should taper medication slowly.[13,35]

Lithium administration during the first trimester is associated with Ebstein anomaly, a downward displacement of the tricuspid valve. Although more likely to occur in children of patients who took lithium during pregnancy, the absolute risk is small, around 0.1%. Pharmacokinetic handling of lithium changes as pregnancy progresses. Renal lithium clearance increases, which requires a dosage increase to maintain a therapeutic serum concentration. It is advisable to decrease or discontinue lithium at term or onset of labor to avoid toxicity postpartum when there is a large reduction in fluid volume.[36]

Lithium can cause hypotonicity and cyanosis in the neonate, termed the "floppy baby" syndrome. Most data indicate normal neurobehavioral development when these symptoms resolve. Lithium is readily transferred via breast milk. Breastfeeding is not advised for patients taking lithium.[19]

Valproic acid and carbamazepine are human teratogens. Neural tube defects such as spina bifida occur in up to 9% of infants exposed during the first trimester. The risk of neural tube defects is related to exposure during the third and fourth weeks of gestation. As such, women with unplanned pregnancies may not know they are pregnant until after the risk of exposure has occurred. Carbamazepine can cause fetal vitamin K deficiency. Vitamin K is important for facial growth and for clotting factors. The risk of facial abnormalities is increased with carbamazepine and VPA, and neonatal bleeding is increased in infants of mothers who are treated with carbamazepine during pregnancy.[37,38]

Fewer data are available on other anticonvulsant mood-stabilizing drugs. Lamotrigine may be associated with an increased risk of oral clefts.[37,38]

The FGAs have been available for many years, and more data are available on their use in pregnancy compared with SGAs, but guidelines for bipolar disorder do not otherwise support FGAs as an initial choice.

Use of antidepressant drugs during pregnancy is discussed in the chapter on depression.

OUTCOME EVALUATION

Assessment of Therapeutic Effects

Effective interviewing skills and a therapeutic relationship with the patient are essential to assessing response. Understand the particular symptom profile and needs of individual patients. These are the primary therapeutic monitoring parameters. In addition to clinical interview, some clinicians use symptom rating scales such as the Young Mania Rating Scale (YMRS) for mania and the Hamilton Depression Rating Scale (Ham-D, discussed in the chapter on depression). The YMRS is composed of 11 items based on a patient's perception over the preceding 48 hours. Adjunctive information is obtained from clinical observations. The scale takes about 15 to 30 minutes to administer.[39]

Patient Encounter, Part 4: Outcome Evaluation

After an initial assessment, including evaluation of potential suicidality, support systems, and need for inpatient versus outpatient treatment, Joan was hospitalized briefly and then followed in the community on medication as well as psychotherapy. Joan has discontinued her use of alcohol and is now attending Alcoholics Anonymous meetings along with her father. She has also stopped smoking marijuana. Her school performance has returned to normal, and her grades are improving. Joan has responded well to treatment with divalproex 500 mg by mouth twice daily. Recent serum valproic acid levels have stabilized at 80 mcg/mL (554 μmol/L). She now returns to the clinic for routine follow-up. Joan initially complained about mild headaches and nausea which have subsequently resolved, and she has tolerated the divalproex well. However, she now asks how long she must take this medication since she is feeling completely well.

How would you assess therapeutic and adverse effects of treatment for this patient?

How would you educate the patient regarding the need for continued maintenance treatment?

Patient Care Process

Patient Assessment:

- Assess the patient's symptoms and review the history. Review the family history, including the history of response to treatment by family members.
- Obtain an initial medical evaluation to rule out other causes of mood episodes.
- Evaluate physiologic parameters that may influence pharmacokinetics.

Therapy Evaluation:

- Obtain a thorough medication use history, including present and past prescription and nonprescription drugs, the patient's self-assessment of response and side-effects, alcohol, tobacco, caffeine, illicit substances, herbal products, dietary supplements, allergies, and adherence.
- Assess potential drug–disease, drug–drug, and drug–food interactions.

Care Plan Development:

- Develop a plan for monitoring therapeutic outcomes, focusing on the individual symptom profile and level of function of the patient. Include a plan for dosage adjustments or alternate therapy if the patient fails to respond adequately. Include serum drug concentration monitoring as appropriate.
- Develop a monitoring plan for drug side effects. Include measures to prevent side effects as well as management if they occur. Include appropriate laboratory measures.
- Determine the role of nonpharmacologic therapy and how it is to be integrated with drug therapy.
- Educate the patient on the nature of bipolar disorder, its treatment, and what to expect with regard to response and side effects, and stress the need for adherence to treatment even when feeling well.
- Encourage a healthy lifestyle, including eliminating or stopping substance abuse, smoking cessation, and encouraging proper nutrition and exercise.

Follow-Up Evaluation:

- See the patient daily if hospitalized or weekly if an outpatient to assess efficacy and safety until stabilized. Utilize the clinical interview, physical exam, and lab tests.
- Once stabilized, follow up at decreased frequency, every 3 to 6 months. Use the same parameters and check for new drugs or drug-drug interactions.

Check serum concentrations of mood-stabilizing drugs as a guide to dosage adjustment for optimal efficacy. The frequency of follow-up visits depends on response, tolerability, and adherence.

Assessment of Adverse Effects

Adverse effects cause more nonadherence than any other factor. Monitor patients regularly for adverse effects and health status, especially because mood stabilizers and antipsychotics commonly cause metabolic side effects such as weight gain. Repeat laboratory tests for renal and thyroid function for patients taking lithium and hematology and liver function for patients taking carbamazepine or divalproex. Annual measurement of serum lipase is advisable for patients taking divalproex. More specific discussion of metabolic side effect monitoring of patients taking SGAs is provided in the chapter on schizophrenia.

Patient Education

KEY CONCEPT *Education of the patient regarding benefits and risks of drug therapy and the importance of adherence to treatment must be integrated into pharmacologic management.* This is important because responsiveness to treatment declines as the number of mood episodes increases. Discuss the nature and chronic course of bipolar disorder and risks of repeated relapses. Help patients understand treatment is not a cure but that many patients enjoy symptom-free or nearly symptom-free function. Make it clear that long-term recovery is dependent on adherence to pharmacologic and nonpharmacologic treatment. Explain the purpose of medication, common side effects to expect, and how to respond to side effects. Provide the patient and family with written information about indications, benefits, and side effects. Discuss less frequent but more dangerous side effects of drugs, and give written instructions on seeking medical attention immediately should they occur.

Abbreviations Introduced in This Chapter

5-HT	5-hydroxytryptamine
Abd	Abdomen
ACE	Angiotensin-converting enzyme
ARB	Angiotensin receptor blocker
BDNF	Brain-derived neurotrophic factor
BP	Blood pressure
CBC	Complete blood count
CBT	Cognitive-behavioral therapy
CN	Cranial nerve
CNS	Central nervous system
DA	Dopamine
DSM-5	*Diagnostic and Statistical Manual of Mental Disorders*, 5th edition
ECG	Electrocardiogram
ECT	Electroconvulsive therapy
Exts	Extremities
FDA	Food and Drug Administration
FGA	First-generation antipsychotic
fMRI	Functional magnetic resonance imaging
FOI	Flight of ideas
GABA	γ-aminobutyric acid
GI	Gastrointestinal
Ham-D	Hamilton Depression Rating Scale
β-HCG	Beta-human chorionic gonadotropin
HIV	Human immunodeficiency virus
JVD	Jugular venous distention
LMP	Last menstrual period
MDD	Major depressive disorder
MRI	Magnetic resonance imaging
NE	Norepinephrine
P	Pulse

PERRLA	Pupils equal round and reactive to light and accommodation
PET	Positron emission tomography
RR	Respiration rate
SGA	Second-generation antipsychotic
T	Temperature
THC	Tetrahydrocannabinol, psychoactive Substance in marijuana
VPA	Valproic acid
YMRS	Young Mania Rating Scale

REFERENCES

1. American Psychiatric Association. Diagnostic and Statistical Manual of Mental Disorders. 5th ed. Washington, DC: American Psychiatric Press; 2013.
2. Merikangas KR, Jin R, He JP, et al. Prevalence and correlates of bipolar spectrum disorder in the world mental health survey initiative. Arch Gen Psychiatry. 2011;68:241–251.
3. Thase ME. Mood disorders: Neurobiology. In: Sadock BJ, Sadock VA, Ruiz P, eds. Kaplan and Sadock's Comprehensive Textbook of Psychiatry. 9th ed. Philadelphia, PA: Lippincott Williams & Wilkins; 2009:1664–1674.
4. Kerner B. Genetics of bipolar disorder. Appl Clin Genet. 2014; 7:33–42.
5. Serretti A, Drago A, De Ronchi D. Lithium pharmacodynamics and pharmacogenetics: Focus on inositol mono phosphatase (IMPase), inositol poliphosphatase (IPPase) and glycogen sinthase kinase 3 beta (GSK-3 beta). Curr Med Chem. 2009;16: 1917–1948.
6. Hashimoto K. Brain-derived neurotrophic factor as a biomarker for mood disorders: An historical overview and future directions. Psychiatry Clin Neurosci. 2010;64:341–357.
7. Perugi G, Micheli C, Akiskal HS, et al. Polarity of the first episode, clinical characteristics, and course of manic depressive illness: A systematic retrospective investigation of 320 bipolar I patients. Compr Psychiatry. 2000;41:13–18.
8. Judd LL, Akiskal HS, Schettler PJ, et al. The long-term natural history of the weekly symptomatic status of bipolar I disorder. Arch Gen Psychiatry. 2002;59:530–537.
9. Judd LL, Akiskal HS, Schettler PJ, et al. A prospective investigation of the natural history of the long-term weekly symptomatic status of bipolar II disorder. Arch Gen Psychiatry. 2003;60: 261–269.
10. Hirschfeld RM, Holzer C, Calabrese JR, et al. Validity of the mood disorder questionnaire: A general population study. Am J Psychiatry. 2003;160:178–180.
11. Novick DM, Swartz HA, Frank E. Suicide attempts in bipolar I and bipolar II disorder: A review and meta-analysis of the evidence. Bipolar Disord. 2010;12:1–9.
12. Hollon SD, Ponniah K. A review of empirically supported psychological therapies for mood disorders in adults. Depress Anxiety. 2010;27:891–932.
13. Yatham LN, Kennedy SH, Parikh SV, et al. Canadian Network for Mood and Anxiety Treatments (CANMAT) and International Society for Bipolar Disorders (ISBD) collaborative update on CANMAT guidelines for the management of patients with bipolar disorder: Update 2013. Bipolar Disord. 2013;15:1–44.
14. Cipriani A, Barbui C, Salanti G, et al. Comparative efficacy and acceptability of antimanic drugs in acute mania: A multiple-treatments meta-analysis. Lancet. 2011;378:1306–1315.
15. Sidor MM, Macqueen GM. An update on antidepressant use in bipolar depression. Curr Psychiatry Rep. 2012;14:696–704.
16. Severino G, Squassina A, Costa M, et al. Pharmacogenomics of bipolar disorder. Pharmacogenomics. 2013;14:655–674.
17. Cipriani A, Hawton K, Stockton S, et al. Lithium in the prevention of suicide in mood disorders: Updated systematic review and meta-analysis. BMJ. 2013;346:f3646.
18. Meyer JM. Chapter 16. Pharmacotherapy of psychosis and mania. In: Brunton LL, Chabner BA, Knollmann BC, eds. Goodman & Gilman's The Pharmacological Basis of Therapeutics, 12th ed. New York, NY: McGraw-Hill; 2011; 417–456.
19. Lithium carbonate package insert. Columbus, OH:Roxane Laboratories, 2011.
20. Depakote (divalproex sodium) package insert. North Chicago, IL: Abbott Laboratories, 2014.
21. Lamictal (lamotrigine) package insert. Research Triangle Park, NC: GlaxoSmithKline, 2014.
22. Equetro (carbamazepine extended-release) package insert. Parsippany, NJ: Validus Pharmaceuticals, 2012.
23. Flanagan RJ, Dunk L. Haematological toxicity of drugs used in psychiatry. Hum Psychopharmacol. 2008;23:27–41.
24. Trileptal (oxcarbazepine) package insert. East Hanover, NJ: Novartis Pharmaceuticals, 2014.
25. Vasudev A, Macritchie K, Vasudev K, et al. Oxcarbazepine for acute affective episodes in bipolar disorder. Cochrane Database Syst Rev. 2011;(12):CD004857.
26. Nardi AE, Perna G. Clonazepam in the treatment of psychiatric disorders: An update. Int Clin Psychopharmacol. 2006;21:131–142.
27. Vieta E, Suppes T, Ekholm B, et al. Long-term efficacy of quetiapine in combination with lithium or divalproex on mixed symptoms in bipolar I disorder. J Affect Disord. 2012;142:36–44.
28. Aripiprazole package insert. Tokyo: Otsuka Pharmaceutical. Tokyo, Otsuka Pharmaceutical, 2014.
29. Seroquel XR package insert. Wilmington, DE: AstraZeneca Pharmaceuticals, 2013.
30. American Diabetes Association, American Psychiatric Association, American Association of Clinical Endocrinologists, North American Association for the Study of Obesity. Consensus development conference on antipsychotic drugs and obesity and diabetes. Diabetes Care. 2004;27:596–601.
31. Leverich GS, Altshuler LL, Frye MA, et al. Risk of switch in mood polarity to hypomania or mania in patients with bipolar depression during acute and continuation trials of venlafaxine, sertraline, and bupropion as adjuncts to mood stabilizers. Am J Psychiatry. 2006;163:232–239.
32. Thomas T, Stansifer L, Findling RL. Psychopharmacology of pediatric bipolar disorders in children and adolescents. Pediatr Clin North Am. 2011;58:173–187.
33. Pringsheim T, Lam D, Ching H, et al. Metabolic and neurological complications of second-generation antipsychotic use in children: A systematic review and meta-analysis of randomized controlled trials. Drug Saf. 2011;34:651–668.
34. Lala SV, Sajatovic M. Medical and psychiatric comorbidities among elderly individuals with bipolar disorder: A literature review. J Geriatr Psychiatry Neurol. 2012;25:20–25.
35. Yonkers KA, Vigod S, Ross LE. Diagnosis, pathophysiology, and management of mood disorders in pregnant and postpartum women. Obstet Gynecol. 2011;117:961–977.
36. Deligiannidis KM, Byatt N, Freeman MP. Pharmacotherapy for mood disorders in pregnancy. A review of pharmacokinetic changes and clinical recommendations for therapeutic drug monitoring. J Clin Psychopharmacol. 2014;34:244–255.
37. Wlodarczyk BJ, Palacios AM, George TM, et al. Antiepileptic drugs and pregnancy outcomes. Am J Med Genet A. 2012;158A:2071–2090.
38. Drayton SJ, Pelic CM. Bipolar disorder. In: DiPiro JT, Talbert RL, Yee GC, et al, eds. Pharmacotherapy: A Pathophysiologic Approach. 9th ed. New York, NY: McGraw-Hill. 2014;1067–1081.
39. Young RC, Biggs JT, Ziegler VE, et al. A rating scale for mania: Reliability, validity and sensitivity. Br J Psychiatry. 1978; 133:429–435.

40 Generalized Anxiety Disorder, Panic Disorder, and Social Anxiety Disorder

Sheila R Botts, Sallie Charles, and Douglas A Newton

LEARNING OBJECTIVES

Upon completion of the chapter, the reader will be able to:

1. Describe pathophysiology of generalized anxiety, panic, and social anxiety disorders (SAD).
2. List common presenting symptoms of generalized anxiety, panic, and SAD.
3. Identify the desired therapeutic outcomes for patients with generalized anxiety, panic, and SAD.
4. Discuss appropriate lifestyle modifications and over-the-counter medication use in these patients.
5. Recommend psychotherapy and pharmacotherapy interventions for patients with generalized anxiety, panic, and SAD.
6. Develop a monitoring plan for anxiety patients placed on specific medications.
7. Educate patients about their disease state and appropriate lifestyle modifications, as well as psychotherapy and pharmacotherapy for effective treatment.

INTRODUCTION

Anxiety disorders are among the most frequent mental disorders encountered by clinicians. All anxiety disorders share features of fear and anxiety that differ from developmentally normative fear or anxiety by being excessive, persistent, and resulting in behavioral disturbances.

Anxiety disorders are often missed or attributed incorrectly to other medical illnesses, and most patients are treated inadequately.[1] The burden of diagnosis usually falls to primary care clinicians, to whom most patients present in the context of other complaints. Untreated anxiety disorders may result in increased health care utilization, morbidity and mortality, and a poorer quality of life.

EPIDEMIOLOGY AND ETIOLOGY

Epidemiology

▶ *Prevalence*

The lifetime prevalence of anxiety disorders collectively is 28.8% with specific phobia (12.5%) and social anxiety disorder (SAD) (12.1%) being the most common.[2,3] Data from the National Comorbidity Survey, Revised (NCS-R) estimate the lifetime prevalence of generalized anxiety disorder (GAD) for those 18 years of age and older to be 5.7%, and rates for panic disorder (PD), 4.7%.[3,4]

Anxiety disorders are more prevalent among women than men(2:1).[2] Prevalence rates across the anxiety spectrum increase from the younger age group (18–29 years) to older age groups (30–44 and 45–59 years); however, rates are substantially lower for those older than age 59 years.[3]

▶ *Course of Illness*

PD and GAD have a median age of onset of 24 and 31 years, respectively, whereas SAD develops earlier (median age 13 years).[3] Although GAD and PD may not manifest fully until adulthood, as many as half of adult anxiety patients report subthreshold symptoms during childhood.[5]

Anxiety disorders are chronic, and symptoms tend to wax and wane, with fewer than one-third of patients experiencing spontaneous symptom **remission**.[6] The risk for relapse and recurrence of symptoms is also high for anxiety disorders. In a 12-year follow-up study of anxiety disorder patients, recurrence rates ranged from 58% of PD and GAD patients to 39% of SAD patients.[7]

Remission, if achieved with treatment, is most likely to occur within the first 2 years of an index episode.[6] Similarly, the highest rates of relapse are within the same timeframe. This suggests that many patients need ongoing maintenance treatment. Rates of remission and relapse do not appear to vary by sex[6]; however, one study reported that women with PD without agoraphobia were three times more likely than men to relapse. Patients with anxiety disorders spend a significant portion of time "being ill" during a particular episode, ranging from 41% to 80% of the time.[7] Anxiety disorders are associated with impaired psychosocial functioning and a compromised quality of life.[8] Appropriate treatment improves overall quality of life and psychosocial functioning.[8]

▶ *Comorbidity*

More than 90% of individuals with an anxiety disorder have a lifetime history of one or more other psychiatric disorders.[9] Depression is the most common comorbidity, followed by alcohol and substance use disorders, as well as other co-occurring anxiety disorders, especially GAD and PD.[9] Generally, the onset of SAD and GAD symptoms precedes major depressive disorder (MDD), but there is an equal chance of PD onset before, during, or after MDD. Comorbid psychiatric illness is associated with lower rates of remission and higher rates of relapse. Both disorders must be treated appropriately.

Etiology

Both genetic and psychosocial factors appear to play a role in the initiation and expression of anxiety disorders.[10] Documentation of moderate genetic risk has been identified for all anxiety disorders, although conflicting data exist. No definitive gene or set of genes has been identified as causative for a specific anxiety disorder. Additionally, it is unclear if anxiety disorders share common genetic risk factors. Genetic overlap may exist between GAD and PD and, to a lesser extent, SAD.[10]

Genetics may create a vulnerable phenotype for an anxiety disorder, and an individual's life stressors and means of coping with the stress may play a role in precipitation and continued expression of the anxiety disorder.[11] Some researchers believe that stressful life events may have a strong role in the onset of anxiety disorders, especially in GAD and PD.[10] It has been reported that those experiencing one or more negative life events have a threefold increased chance of developing GAD.[2] Similar findings have been reported with PD.[11]

PATHOPHYSIOLOGY

The thalamus and amygdala are important in the generation of a normal fear response and play a central role in most anxiety disorders (**Figure 40–1**). The thalamus provides the first real processing region to organize sensory data obtained from the environment. It passes information to higher cortical centers for finer processing and to the amygdala for rapid assessment of highly charged emotional information. The amygdala provides emotional valence or the emotional importance of the information. This helps the organism to act quickly on ambiguous but vital events. The cortex then performs a more detailed analysis and sends updates to the amygdala for comparison and any needed course corrections, thus enabling a decision on a course of action.

Anxiety becomes an anxiety disorder when the fear-response system leads to maladaptive behavior or distress. Anxiety can become independent of stimuli as in PD, be associated with benign stimuli as in phobias, or continue beyond the stimulus duration as in GAD.

Direct and indirect connections to the reticular activating system (RAS), a region spanning the medulla, pons, and midbrain, help to regulate arousal, vigilance, and fear. These connections are modulated by serotonin (5-HT) and norepinephrine (NE), which have their primary origins in the RAS.[12] The amygdala sends projections to the hypothalamus, thus influencing the autonomic nervous system to affect heart rate, blood pressure, and stress-associated changes. It also influences the **hypothalamic–pituitary–adrenal** (HPA) **axis**, leading to a cascade of stress hormones.[13] One such hormone is cortisol, which, if elevated for prolonged periods, can damage the brain and other organs.

Noradrenergic System

Norepinephrine-producing cells reside primarily in a region of the brain called the **locus ceruleus** (LC). Increased activity in this region is associated with an increase in arousal, anxiety, and panic. Drugs such as yohimbine that increase activity in the LC can be anxiogenic; drugs that decrease activity in the LC appear to improve anxiety. Furthermore, dysregulation of this region is implicated by elevated levels of NE or its metabolites in subjects with GAD, PD, and specific phobias.[13]

Serotonergic System

The **raphe nuclei** and the resident cell bodies of 5-HT-producing neurons have a complicated role related to anxiety symptoms. Activity of 5-HT cells in the raphe nuclei over time inhibits firing of noradrenergic cells in the LC. Other influences include their ability to regulate cells in the prefrontal cortex and amygdala.

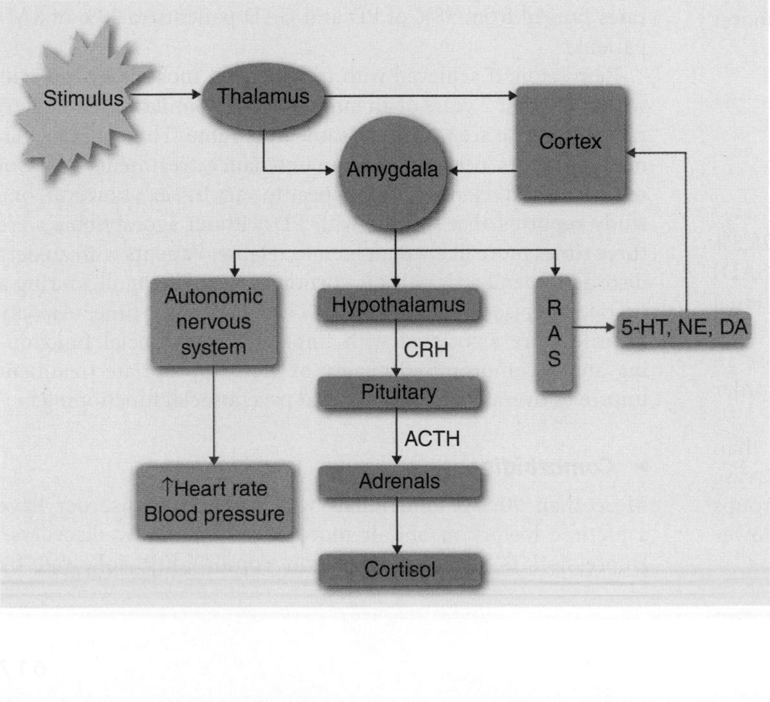

FIGURE 40–1. Neurocircuitry and key neurotransmitters involved in mediating anxiety disorders. (ACTH, adrenocorticotrophic hormone; CRH, corticotropin-releasing hormone; DA, dopamine; 5-HT, serotonin; NE, norepinephrine; RAS, reticular activating system.)

Perhaps the strongest evidence for the involvement of the serotonergic system is the success of serotonin reuptake inhibitors in treatment of anxiety disorders.[13]

γ-Aminobutyric Acid

γ-Aminobutyric acid (GABA) plays a complex role as an inhibitor neurotransmitter with nonspecific effects. GABA-ergic drugs reduce anxiety, but the lack of a specific target for their effect leads to multiple undesirable effects. Current research is focused on defining receptor subtypes that may allow for greater specificity in targeting anxiety symptoms.[14]

Hypothalamic–Pituitary–Adrenal Axis

The HPA axis provides a critical mechanism for regulation of the stress response and its effects on the brain and other organ systems. Several important hormones, including corticotropin releasing hormone and cortisol, are involved in this pathway. These hormones regulate the effects of anxiety on the body and provide positive feedback to the brain.[13] A cycle of anxiety and sensitization by such feedback could, if unchecked, result in escalation of symptoms. Neuropeptides may provide one mechanism to balance positive and negative feedback, helping to minimize such escalation.

Neuropeptides

Several neuropeptides(eg, neuropeptide Y [NPY], substance P, and cholecystokinin) are under investigation for their role in anxiety disorders. NPY appears to reduce the effect of stress hormones and inhibit activity of the LC. Both mechanisms may contribute to the anxiolytic properties seen experimentally. Substance P may have anxiolytic and antidepressant properties partly because of its effects on corticotropin-releasing hormone.[15]

Patient Encounter 1, Part 1

A 24-year-old woman presents to the primary care clinic with complaints of fatigue, joint pain, insomnia, irritability, and daily headaches. She admits to having one to two drinks at night to help with her sleep and "turn her mind off". She states she panicked at the beginning of her economics exam and ran from the room. She states she is overwhelmed with her coursework in an MBA program, and her relationship with her boyfriend has been tumultuous over the past several months. Her medical history is positive for depression and migraine headaches.

Meds: Topiramate 50 mg/day

What manifestations described above are suggestive of an anxiety disorder?

What additional information do you need to establish a diagnosis and develop a treatment plan?

What other diagnoses should be considered in your differential diagnosis?

Could her medication be contributing to her symptoms?

Clinical Presentation and Diagnosis of GAD

General

Onset is typically in early adulthood. Anxiety emerges and dissipates more gradually than in PD. Laboratory evaluation usually is reserved for later onset, atypical presentation, or poor response to treatment.

Symptoms[2]

- Excessive anxiety or worry involving multiple events or activities occurring more days than not for at least 6 months
- Difficulty controlling worry
- Anxiety and worry associated with at least three of the following:
  - Restlessness
  - Easily fatigued
  - Poor concentration or mind going blank
  - Irritability
  - Muscle tension
  - Insomnia or unsatisfying sleep
- The anxiety or worry causes significant distress or functional impairment and is NOT attributable to another substance, medical, or psychiatric condition

Differential Diagnosis

Rule out underlying medical or psychiatric disorders and medications that may cause anxiety (Tables 40–1 and 40–2)

Table 40–1

Medical Conditions That Can Cause Anxiety

Psychiatric Disorders
Mood disorders, hypochondriasis, personality disorders, alcohol or substance abuse, alcohol or substance withdrawal, other anxiety disorders

Neurologic Disorders
CVA, seizure disorders, dementia, stroke, migraine, encephalitis, vestibular dysfunction

Cardiovascular Disorders
Angina, arrhythmias, congestive heart failure, mitral valve prolapse, myocardial infarction

Endocrine and Metabolic Disorders
Hypothyroidism or hyperthyroidism, hypoglycemia, Cushing disease, Addison disease, pheochromocytoma, hyperadrenocorticism, hyponatremia, hyperkalemia, vitamin B_{12} deficiency

Respiratory Disorders
Asthma, COPD, pulmonary embolism, pneumonia, hyperventilation

Other
Carcinoid syndrome, anemias, SLE

COPD, chronic obstructive pulmonary disease; CVA, cerebrovascular accident; SLE, systemic lupus erythematosus.

Data from Refs. 2 and 16.

Table 40–2

Medications Associated with Anxiety Symptoms

Category	Examples
Anticonvulsants	Carbamazepine, ethosuximide
Antidepressants	Bupropion, SSRIs, SNRIs, TCAs
Antihypertensives	Felodipine
Antimicrobials	Cephalosporins, ofloxacin, isoniazid
Antiparkinson drugs	Levodopa
Bronchodilators	Albuterol, isoproterenol, theophylline
Corticosteroids	Prednisone, methylprednisolone
Decongestants	Pseudoephedrine, phenylephrine
Herbals	Ma huang, St. John's wort, ginseng, guarana, belladonna
NSAIDs	Ibuprofen, indomethacin
Stimulants	Amphetamines, caffeine, cocaine, methylphenidate
Thyroid hormones	Levothyroxine
Toxicity	Anticholinergics, antihistamines, digoxin
Withdrawal of CNS depressants (abrupt)	Alcohol, barbiturates, benzodiazepines

CNS, central nervous system; SNRI serotonin norepinephrine reuptake inhibitor; SSRI, selective serotonin reuptake inhibitor; TCA, tricyclic antidepressant; NSAID, non-steroidal anti-inflammatory drug.

Data from Refs. 2, 16, and 17.

TREATMENT: GENERALIZED ANXIETY DISORDER

Desired Outcomes

KEY CONCEPT *The goals of therapy for GAD are to acutely reduce the severity and duration of anxiety symptoms and restore overall functioning. The long-term goal is to achieve and maintain remission.* With a positive response to treatment, comorbid depressive symptoms should be minimized.

General Approach to Treatment

Patients with GAD may be managed with psychotherapy, pharmacotherapy, or both. Treatment should be individualized based on symptom severity, comorbid illnesses, medical status, age, and patient preference. Patients with severe symptoms resulting in functional impairment should receive antianxiety medication.

Nonpharmacologic Therapy

Nonpharmacologic therapy includes psychoeducation, exercise, stress management, and psychotherapy. Psychoeducation should provide information on GAD and its management. Patients should be instructed to avoid stimulating agents, eg, caffeine, decongestants, diet pills, and excessive alcohol use. Regular exercise is also recommended. Cognitive-behavioral therapy (CBT) is the most effective psychological therapy for GAD patients. It helps patients to recognize and alter patterns of distorted thinking and dysfunctional behavior. Treatment gains with CBT may be maintained for up to 1 year.[18] CBT may be delivered in individual or group settings.[19] Computerized CBT offered over the Internet is effective and may offer an alternative to face-to-face therapy for patients with access barriers.[20] The effect sizes of trials with CBT are comparable to those of pharmacologic therapies. A recent trial in children with GAD suggests the combination of CBT and medication is superior to either treatment alone.[21]

Patient Encounter 1, Part 2

After a medical workup, she was diagnosed with GAD and unspecified depressive disorder.

PMH: Depression, Migraine

FH: Mother treated for depression; father, alcohol dependence

SH: One to two drinks per night; lives with boyfriend

Meds: Topiramate 50 mg/day

What are first-line treatment options for this patient?

What factors should be considered in selecting the patient's treatment?

What is the role of benzodiazepines for this patient?

How should the patient be monitored when receiving an antidepressant?

Pharmacologic Therapy

Antidepressants, benzodiazepines, pregabalin, buspirone, hydroxyzine, and the second-generation antipsychotics (SGAs) have controlled clinical trial data supporting their use in GAD. KEY CONCEPT *Antidepressants are the drugs of choice for chronic GAD because of a tolerable side-effect profile; no risk for dependency; and efficacy in common comorbid conditions, including depression, panic, obsessive-compulsive disorder (OCD), and SAD.* Benzodiazepines remain the most effective and commonly used treatment for short-term management of anxiety when immediate relief of symptoms is desired. They are also recommended for intermittent or adjunctive use during GAD exacerbation or for sleep disturbance during the initiation of antidepressant treatment.[18] Buspirone and pregabalin are alternative agents for patients with GAD without depression. Hydroxyzine is usually adjunctive and is less desirable for long-term treatment because of side effects, eg, sedation and anticholinergic effects.

Patients with GAD should be treated to symptom remission. Although supporting data are lacking, recent guidelines recommend continuing treatment for 1 year.[18,19,22,23] Continuation of antidepressant therapy after acute response significantly decreases the risk of relapse (odds ratio, 0.2 [0.15–0.26]).[22] An algorithm for the pharmacologic management of GAD is shown in Figure 40–2.

► *Antidepressants*

Antidepressants (Table 40–3) reduce the psychic symptoms (eg, worry and apprehension) of anxiety with a modest effect on autonomic or somatic symptoms (eg, tremor, rapid heart rate, and/or sweating). All antidepressants evaluated provide a similar degree of anxiety reduction. The onset of antianxiety effect is delayed 2 to 4 weeks. Selective serotonin reuptake inhibitors (SSRIs) or serotonin-norepinephrine reuptake inhibitors (SNRIs) are usually preferred over tricyclic antidepressants (TCAs) because of improved safety and tolerability. Selection of a specific antidepressant generally is based on history of prior response, side effect and drug interaction profile (see Chapter 38), cost, or formulary availability.

Antidepressants modulate synaptic 5-HT, NE, and/or dopamine (DA) reuptake and receptor-activated neuronal signal transduction. These intracellular changes modify the expression of genes and proteins important in stress response (eg, glucocorticoid

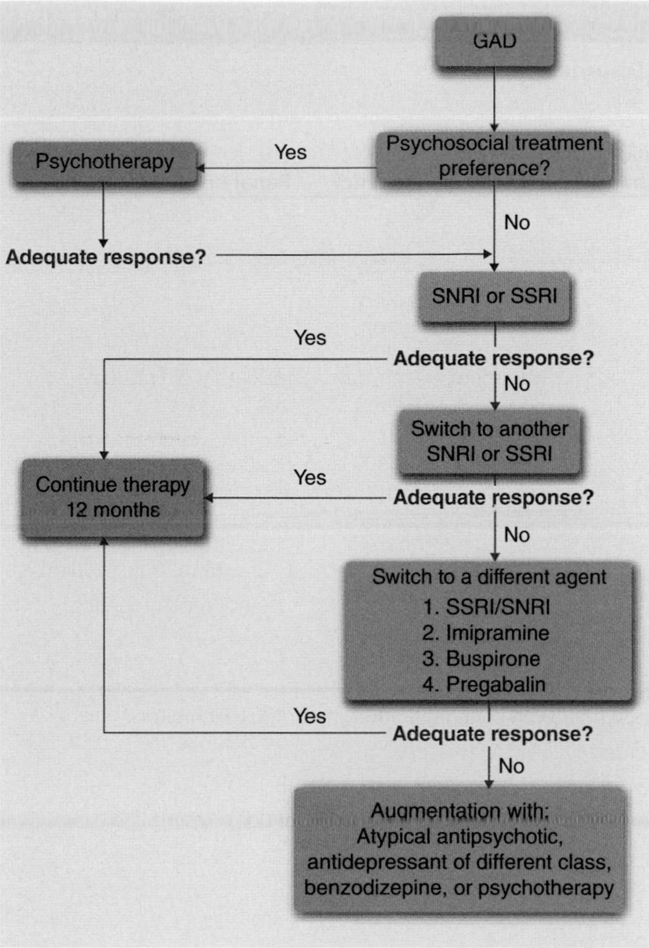

FIGURE 40–2. Treatment algorithm for generalized anxiety disorder. (BZ, benzodiazepine; SNRI, serotonin-norepinephrine reuptake inhibitor; SSRI, selective serotonin reuptake inhibitor.) Data from Refs. 17, 18, 23.

receptors, brain-derived neurotrophic factor, corticotropin-releasing hormone).[24] Activation of these "stress-adapting" pathways may improve both somatic and psychic symptoms of anxiety.[24]

Serotonin Norepinephrine Reuptake Inhibitors Venlafaxine and duloxetine are approved by the Food and Drug Administration (FDA) for the treatment of GAD. They alleviate anxiety with and without depression and have improved tolerability over TCAs. Venlafaxine is effective at doses 75 to 225 mg/day and maintains response with extended treatment.[18] It is also effective for GAD in children and adolescents.[19] The most common side effects reported in patients with GAD are nausea, somnolence, dry mouth, dizziness, sweating, constipation, and anorexia.[18,25]

Duloxetine is similarly effective and tolerated as venlafaxine.[25] For patients with concurrent pain syndromes, duloxetine has been found to improve anxiety, pain, and functional impairment more than placebo.[26] Newer SNRIs, milnacipran, levomilnacipran, and vortioxetine have not been evaluated in the treatment of GAD.

Selective Serotonin Reuptake Inhibitors The SSRIs paroxetine, escitalopram, and sertraline have been shown to be significantly more effective than placebo in reducing anxiety symptoms in adults with GAD. Response rates range from 56% to 68% during acute treatment, with remission achieved in approximately one-third of patients.[27–30] Common side effects include somnolence, headache, nausea, dry mouth (paroxetine), diarrhea (sertraline), sweating (sertraline), decreased libido, ejaculation disorder, anorgasmia, and asthenia.

SSRI therapy is better tolerated than TCAs, and tolerability is similar to that of venlafaxine. Citalopram is efficacious in the treatment of GAD in the elderly.[31] The SSRIs, sertraline, fluoxetine, and fluvoxamine have demonstrated benefits in children and adolescents with GAD and are the preferred pharmacologic treatment in this population.[19]

Tricyclic Antidepressants Imipramine treatment of GAD results in a higher rate of remission of anxiety symptoms than treatment with trazodone or diazepam.[18] Both antidepressants were more effective than diazepam or placebo in reducing psychic symptoms of anxiety. TCA use is limited by bothersome adverse effects (eg, sedation, orthostatic hypotension, anticholinergic effects, and weight gain). TCAs have a narrow therapeutic index and are lethal in overdose because of atrioventricular block.

Novel Antidepressants Mirtazapine, an α-2 adrenergic antagonist and postsynaptic serotonin (5-HT_2, 5-HT_3) receptor antagonist, is an effective antidepressant but has not been extensively evaluated in anxiety disorders. One open-label study found 12-week treatment of GAD with mirtazapine 30 mg to be efficacious and well tolerated.[18] It is not associated with sexual dysfunction, but does have a propensity to cause sedation and weight gain. Bupropion, a dopamine and norepinephrine reuptake-inhibitor, lacks the common antidepressant side effects of weight gain and sexual dysfunction. Bupropion has not been studied or used extensively in anxiety disorders owing to its stimulating effects that would be expected to worsen anxiety symptoms. However, a small controlled trial comparing bupropion XL with escitalopram found bupropion to have comparable anxiolytic efficacy and tolerability.[18] Vilazodone, a SSRI, and 5-HT 1A receptor partial agonist has not been evaluated in anxiety disorders.

▸ *Benzodiazepines*

KEY CONCEPT *Benzodiazepines are recommended for acute treatment of GAD when short-term relief is needed, as an adjunct during initiation of antidepressant therapy, or to improve sleep.*[18] Benzodiazepine treatment results in a significant improvement in 65% to 75% of GAD patients, and most of the improvement occurs in the initial 2 weeks.[18] They are more effective for somatic symptoms than psychic symptoms. Major benzodiazepine disadvantages are lack of effectiveness for depression; risk for dependency and abuse; and potential interdose rebound anxiety, especially with short-acting benzodiazepines. They should be avoided in older adults and patients with current or past chemical dependency.

Benzodiazepines enhance transmission of the inhibitory neurotransmitter GABA through interaction with the $GABA_A$-receptor complex.[17,18] Only 7 of the 13 currently marketed benzodiazepines are approved by the FDA for the treatment of anxiety disorders (Table 40–4). All benzodiazepines are expected to provide equivalent benefit when given in comparable doses. They differ substantially in their pharmacokinetic properties and potency for the $GABA_A$-receptor.

Benzodiazepines are metabolized by hepatic oxidation (cytochrome P450 3A4) and glucuronide conjugation. Because lorazepam and oxazepam bypass hepatic oxidation and are conjugated only, they are preferred agents for patients with reduced hepatic function secondary to aging or disease (eg, cirrhosis; hepatitis B or C from intravenous drug use). Many benzodiazepines are metabolized to long-acting metabolites (see Table 40–4) that

Table 40–3

Antidepressants Used in the Treatment of Generalized Anxiety Disorder

Medication Class	Recommended Starting Dose (mg/day)	Usual Therapeutic Dosage Range (mg/day)	Hepatic Insufficiency	Renal Insufficiency
SSRIs				
Citalopram[a] (Celexa)	20	20–40	Maximum, 20 mg/day	
Escitalopram[b] (Lexapro)	10	10–20	Maximum, 10 mg/day	
Fluoxetine (Prozac)	20	20–80	Titrate with caution	
Fluvoxamine (Luvox)	50	100–300	Titrate with caution	
Paroxetine (Paxil)	20	20–50	Titrate with caution	
Paroxetine CR (Paxil CR)	25	25–62.5	Maximum, 50 mg/day	Maximum, 50 mg/day
Sertraline (Zoloft)	50–100	50–200	Reduce dose	
SNRIs				
Venlafaxine XR[b] (Effexor XR)	75	75–225	Reduce dose by 50%	Reduce dose 25%–50%
Desvenlafaxine (Pristiq)	50	50–100	Maximum, 100 mg/day	Maximun, 50 mg/day; CrCl < 30 mL/min (0.50 mL/s), dose once every other day
Duloxetine[c] (Cymbalta)	30	60–120	Use not recommended	CrCl < 30 mL/min (0.50 mL/s) Use not recommended[b]
TCAs				
Imipramine (Tofranil)	50–75	75–200	Titrate with caution	

[a]Maximum daily dose of citalopram is 20 mg/day when used in the elderly or when given concomitantly with CYP2C19 inhibitors.

[b]Food and Drug Administration approved for use in generalized anxiety disorder.

[c]Duloxetine use is not recommended in severe renal impairment (creatinine clearance < 30 mL/min [< 0.50 mL/s])

SNRI, serotonin and norepinephrine reuptake inhibitor; SSRI, selective serotonin reuptake inhibitor; TCA, tricyclic antidepressant.

Data from Refs. 17 and 32.

Table 40–4

Comparison of the Benzodiazepines

Drug Name (Brand Name) *Active Metabolites*	Time to Peak Concentration (hours)	Half-Life Range (hours)	Approved Dosage Range (mg/day)	Dose Equivalent (mg)
Alprazolam[a,b] (Xanax)	1–2	12–15	1–4 (GAD) 1–10 (PD)	0.5
Chlordiazepoxide[a] (Librium)	1–4	5–30	25–100	10
Desmethylchlordiazepoxide		18		
Demoxepam		14–95		
Desmethyldiazepam		40–120		
Oxazepam		5–15		
Clonazepam[b] (Klonopin)	1–4	18–50	1–4	0.25
Clorazepate[a] (Tranzene)	1–2		7.5–60	7.5
Desmethyldiazepam		40–120		
Oxazepam		5–15		
Diazepam[a] (Valium)	0.5–2	20–80	2–40	5
Desmethyldiazepam		40–120[c]		
Temazepam		8–15		
Oxazepam		5–15		
Lorazepam[a] (Ativan)	2–4	10–20	0.5–10	0.75–1
Oxazepam[a] (Serax)	2–4	5–15	30–120	15

[a]Food and Drug Administration (FDA) approved for use in generalized anxiety disorder.

[b]FDA approved for use in panic disorder.

[c]CYP2C19 genetic polymorphisms resulting in little or no enzyme activity are present in 15% to 20% of Asians and 3% to 5% of blacks and whites, resulting in reduced clearance of desmethyldiazepam.[34]

Data from Refs. 32 and 33.

Table 40–5

Pharmacokinetic Drug Interactions with Benzodiazepines

Drug	Effect
Alcohol (chronic)	Increased CL of BZs
Carbamazepine	Increased CL of alprazolam
Cimetidine	Decreased CL of alprazolam, diazepam, chlordiazepoxide, and clorazepate and increased $t_{1/2}$
Disulfiram	Decreased CL of alprazolam and diazepam
Erythromycin	Decreased CL of alprazolam
Fluoxetine	Decreased CL of alprazolam and diazepam
Fluvoxamine	Decreased CL of alprazolam and prolonged $t_{1/2}$
Itraconazole	Potentially decreased CL of alprazolam and diazepam
Ketoconazole	Potentially decreased CL of alprazolam
Nefazodone	Decreased CL of alprazolam, AUC doubled, and $t_{1/2}$ prolonged
Omeprazole	Decreased CL of diazepam
Oral contraceptives	Increased free concentration of chlordiazepoxide and slightly decreased CL; decreased CL and increased $t_{1/2}$ of diazepam and alprazolam
Paroxetine	Decreased CL of alprazolam
Phenobarbital	Increased CL of clonazepam and reduced $t_{1/2}$
Phenytoin	Increased CL of clonazepam and reduced $t_{1/2}$
Probenecid	Decreased CL of lorazepam and prolonged $t_{1/2}$
Propranolol	Decreased CL of diazepam and prolonged $t_{1/2}$
Ranitidine	Decreased absorption of diazepam
Rifampin	Increased metabolism of diazepam
Theophylline	Decreased alprazolam concentrations
Valproate	Decreased CL of lorazepam

AUC, area under the plasma concentration time curve; BZ, benzodiazepine; CL, clearance; $t_{1/2}$, elimination half-life.

Adapted from Kirkwood CK, Melton ST. Anxiety disorders: I. Generalized anxiety, panic and social anxiety disorders. In: DiPiro JT, Talbert RL, Yee GC, et al., eds. Pharmacotherapy: A Pathophysiologic Approach. 7th ed. New York: McGraw-Hill, 2008:1169, with permission.

provide long-lasting anxiety relief. Drugs that either inhibit or induce CYP450 isozymes or glucuronidation can cause drug interactions (Table 40–5).

The most common side effects of benzodiazepine therapy include central nervous system (CNS) depressive effects (eg, drowsiness, sedation, psychomotor impairment, and ataxia) and cognitive effects (eg, poor recall and anterograde amnesia). Anterograde amnesia is more likely with high-potency benzodiazepines such as alprazolam.[35] Some patients also may be disinhibited and experience confusion, irritability, aggression, and excitement.[17,18] Discontinuation of benzodiazepines may be associated with withdrawal, rebound anxiety, and a high rate of relapse. Higher doses of benzodiazepines and a longer duration of therapy increase the severity of withdrawal and risk of seizures after abrupt or rapid discontinuation. Patients should be tapered rather than discontinued abruptly from benzodiazepine therapy to avoid withdrawal symptoms. The duration of the taper should increase with extended duration of benzodiazepine therapy.[17,18] For example, patients on benzodiazepine therapy for 2 to 6 months should be tapered over 2 to 8 weeks, but patients receiving 12 months of treatment should be tapered over 2 to 4 months. A general approach to the taper is to reduce the dose by 25% every 5 to 7 days until reaching half the original dose and then decreasing by 10% to 12% per week until discontinued. Patients should expect minor withdrawal symptoms and discomfort even when tapering. Rebound symptoms (eg, return of original symptoms at increased intensity) are transient. The patient should be educated that rebound anxiety is not a relapse. Relapse or recurrence of anxiety may occur in as many as 50% of patients discontinuing benzodiazepine treatment.[17,18] It is unclear if this relapse rate represents an inferiority of benzodiazepines or supports the chronic nature of GAD.

▶ *Pregabalin*

Pregabalin is a calcium channel modulator, and its anxiolytic properties are attributed to its selective binding to the α-2-delta subunit of voltage-gated calcium channels. In a 4-week controlled trial versus alprazolam and placebo, pregabalin was effective for both somatic and psychic symptoms of anxiety with onset of effect similar to that of alprazolam.[36] Compared with venlafaxine and placebo, pregabalin was safe, well tolerated, and efficacious in GAD, and results were seen 1 week sooner than with venlafaxine.[37] Pregabalin reduced the risk of relapse versus placebo in a 26-week relapse prevention trial.[38] It has a short elimination half-life and must be dosed two to three times daily. It is excreted renally with a low risk of drug–drug interactions. Pregabalin is a schedule V controlled substance owing to a propensity to cause euphoria, and it may cause withdrawal symptoms if discontinued abruptly. It should be used cautiously in patients with a current or past history of substance abuse. It is not beneficial for depression or other anxiety disorders.

▶ *Alternative Agents*

Hydroxyzine, buspirone, and SGAs are alternative agents. Hydroxyzine may be effective for acute reduction of somatic symptoms of anxiety[18] but not for psychic features of anxiety, depression, or other common comorbid anxiety disorders. Buspirone, a 5-HT_{1A} partial agonist, is thought to exert its anxiolytic effects by reducing presynaptic 5-HT firing.[39] Unlike benzodiazepines, it does not have abuse potential, cause withdrawal reactions, or potentiate alcohol and sedative-hypnotic effects. It has a gradual onset of action (ie, 2 weeks) and does not provide immediate anxiety relief. Data are inconsistent regarding its efficacy in chronic GAD or GAD with comorbid depression.[18]

It may be less effective in patients who have been treated previously (4 weeks–5 years) with benzodiazepines.[18]

Buspirone should be initiated at 7.5 mg twice daily and titrated in 5-mg/day increments (every 2–3 days) to a usual target dose of 20 to 30 mg/day.[18,39] The maximum daily dose is considered to be 60 mg/day. Buspirone is well tolerated and does not cause sedation. The most common side effects include dizziness, nausea, and headaches. Drugs that inhibit CYP3A4 (eg, verapamil, diltiazem, itraconazole, fluvoxamine, and erythromycin) can increase buspirone levels. Enzyme inducers (eg, rifampin) can reduce buspirone levels significantly. Buspirone may increase blood pressure when coadministered with a monoamine oxidase inhibitor (MAOI).

Clinical Presentation and Diagnosis of PD

General

Typically presents in late adolescence or early adulthood. Onset in older adults raises suspicion of a relationship to medical disorders or substance use. Laboratory evaluation must be driven by history and physical examination.

Symptoms[2]

Recurrent, unexpected panic attacks. A panic attack is an abrupt surge of intense fear or discomfort peaking within minutes, and with four or more of the following symptoms:

- Palpitations or rapid heart rate
- Sweating
- Trembling or shaking
- Sensation of shortness of breath or smothering
- Feeling of choking
- Chest pain or discomfort
- Nausea or abdominal distress
- Feeling dizzy or lightheaded
- Chills or hot flushes
- Paresthesias
- Derealization or depersonalization
- Fear of dying
- Fear of losing control or "going crazy"

At least one of the attacks has been followed by 1 month or more of one or both:

- Persistent concern or worry about additional attacks
- Significant maladaptive change in behavior related to the attacks (eg, avoidance)

Differential Diagnosis

Rule out underlying medical or psychiatric disorders and medications that may cause anxiety (see Tables 40–1 and 40–2).

Laboratory Evaluation

- Urine drug screen
- Basic metabolic panel ($HgbA_{1C}$)look at guideline
- Thyroid-stimulating hormone
- Electrocardiogram

The SGAs, quetiapine, olanzapine, and risperidone have demonstrated benefit in GAD. In three large placebo controlled trials, quetiapine in daily doses of 50 to 300 mg resulted in 26% greater likelihood of treatment response (effect size, ~0.3).[40] Quetiapine had similar outcomes to paroxetine 20 mg/day and escitalopram 10 mg/day.[40] Risperidone and olanzapine may improve treatment outcomes in patients with inadequate response to initial pharmacotherapy.[18] SGAs are associated with a risk of weight gain, sedation, fatigue, and extrapyramidal symptoms in anxiety patients.

Outcome Evaluation

Assess patients for improvement of anxiety symptoms and return to baseline occupational, social, and interpersonal functioning. With effective treatment, patients should have no or minimal symptoms of anxiety or depression. With initiation of drug therapy, evaluate patients frequently for tolerability and response. Monitor for suicidal ideation and behaviors for children, adolescents, and young adults (24 years of age or less) initiated on antidepressants.[41] Increase the dose in patients exhibiting a partial response after 2 to 4 weeks on an antidepressant or 2 weeks on a benzodiazepine. Individualize the duration of treatment as some patients require up to 1 year of treatment.[18]

TREATMENT: PANIC DISORDER

Desired Outcomes

The main objectives of treatment are to reduce the severity and frequency of panic attacks, reduce anticipatory anxiety and agoraphobic behavior, and minimize symptoms of depression or other comorbid disorders.[42] The long-term goal is to achieve and sustain remission and restore overall functioning.

General Approach to Treatment

Treatment options include medication, psychotherapy, or a combination of both. In some cases, pharmacotherapy will follow psychotherapy treatments when full response is not realized. Patients with panic symptoms without agoraphobia may respond to pharmacotherapy alone. Agoraphobic symptoms generally take longer to respond than panic symptoms. KEY CONCEPT *The acute*

Patient Encounter 2

A 14-year-old Hispanic female presents to the pediatric clinic, accompanied by her mother, with complaints of nausea, bloating, and stomach pain. Her mother reports that she is having difficulty adjusting to her new high school and teachers. Mother states "she's always been shy and doesn't like change, and this time she is having significant difficulty adjusting". She has missed 4 days of school over the past 3 weeks with complaints of nausea and stomach pain. She is required to participate in a drama production at the school next week and she is refusing.

Her medical history is positive for ADHD

Meds: methylphenidate ER (24 hour) 36 mg/day

Her medical workup is noncontributory, and she is diagnosed with SAD

What treatment options should be considered for AD?

What are the benefits of using pharmacotherapy versus psychotherapy versus both?

phase of PD treatment lasts about 12 weeks and should markedly reduce or eliminate panic attacks and minimize anticipatory anxiety and phobic avoidance. Treatment should be continued to prevent relapse for an additional 12 to 18 months before attempting discontinuation.[44] For patients who relapse after discontinuation, therapy should be resumed.[42]

Nonpharmacologic Therapy

Patients with PD should avoid stimulant agents (eg, decongestants, diet pills, and caffeine) that may precipitate a panic attack. CBT generally includes psychoeducation, self-monitoring, countering anxious beliefs, exposure to fear cues, and modification of anxiety-maintaining behaviors.[18,42] Exposure therapy is useful for patients with phobic avoidance. CBT is considered a first-line treatment of PD, with efficacy similar to that of pharmacotherapy. Some studies suggest lower risk of relapse after CBT versus drug therapy.[42] In a trial of PD with or without agoraphobia, SSRI plus CBT was more effective than either therapy alone after 9 months of treatment.[43]

Pharmacologic Therapy

Patients with PD may be treated with TCAs, SSRIs, SNRIs, or MAOIs, as well as benzodiazepines[18,42] (**Table 40–6**) with similar effectiveness, but SSRIs have become the treatment of choice. Benzodiazepines often are used concomitantly with antidepressants, especially early in treatment, or as monotherapy to acutely reduce panic symptoms. Benzodiazepines are not preferred for long-term treatment but may be used when patients fail several antidepressant trials.[18,42] PD patients with comorbid depression should be treated with an antidepressant. An algorithm for pharmacologic management of PD appears in **Figure 40–3**.

▶ *Antidepressants*

Antidepressants typically require 4 weeks for onset of antipanic effect, with optimal response at 6 to 12 weeks. Reduction of anticipatory anxiety and phobic avoidance generally follows improvement in panic symptoms. KEY CONCEPT *PD patients are more likely to experience stimulant-like side effects of antidepressants than patients with major depression. Antidepressants should be initiated at lower doses (see* Table 40–6*) in PD patients than in depressed patients.* Target doses are similar to those used for depression. KEY CONCEPT *Antidepressants should be tapered when treatment is discontinued to avoid withdrawal symptoms, including irritability, dizziness, headache, and dysphoria.*

Tricyclic Antidepressants Treatment with imipramine, leaves 45% to 70% of patients panic free. Desipramine and clomipramine are also effective. However, TCAs are considered second- or third-line pharmacotherapy because of poorer tolerability and toxicity on overdose.[18,42] TCAs are associated with a higher rate of treatment discontinuation than SSRIs.[42] PD patients taking TCAs may experience anticholinergic effects, orthostatic hypotension, sweating, sleep disturbances, dizziness, fatigue, sexual dysfunction, and weight gain. Stimulant-like side effects occur in up to 40% of patients.[42]

Selective Serotonin Reuptake Inhibitors SSRIs are the drugs of choice for patients with PD. All SSRIs have demonstrated effectiveness in controlled trials, with 60% to 80% of patients

Table 40–6

Antidepressants Used in the Treatment of Panic Disorder[18,23,42]

Medication Class	Recommended Starting Dose (mg/day)	Usual Therapeutic Dosage Range (mg/day)	Advantages	Disadvantages
SSRIs/SNRIs			**SSRIs (in general)**	**SSRIs (in general)**
Citalopram	10	20–40	Antidepressant activity; antianxiety activity; single daily dosing (all but fluvoxamine); low toxicity; available in generic	Activation; delayed onset of action; may precipitate mania; sexual side effects; GI side effects
Escitalopram	5–10	10–20		
Fluoxetine[a]	5–10	20–60		
Fluvoxamine	25	100–300		
Paroxetine[a]	10	20–60		
Sertraline[a]	25	50–200		
Venlafaxine XR[a]	37.5	75–225		
TCAs			**TCAs (in general)**	**TCAs (in general)**
Clomipramine	25 mg (twice a day)	75–250	Established efficacy; available in generic	Activation; sedation; anticholinergic effects; cardiovascular effects; delayed onset of action; may precipitate mania; sexual side effects; toxic in overdose; weight gain
Imipramine[a]	10–25	75–250		
MAOI				
Phenelzine	15	45–90	Antidepressant effects; available in generic	Dietary restrictions; drug interactions; weight gain; orthostasis; may precipitate mania

[a] Food and Drug Administration approved for use in panic disorder.

GI, gastrointestinal; MAOI, monoamine oxidase inhibitor; SSRI, selective serotonin reuptake inhibitor; TCA, tricyclic antidepressant.

Data from Refs. 18, 23, and 40.

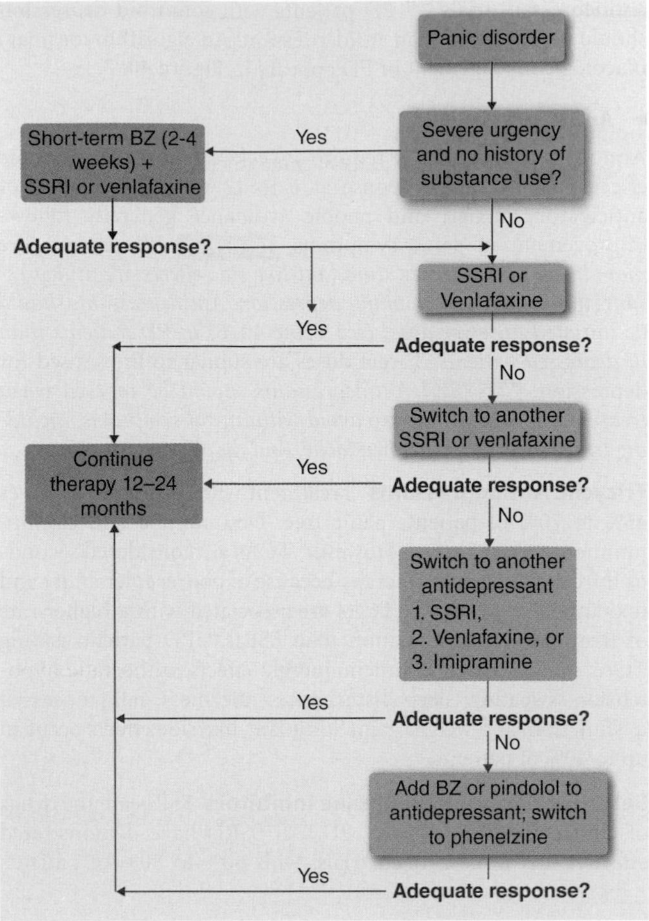

FIGURE 40–3. Algorithm for the pharmacotherapy of panic disorder. BZ, benzodiazepine; SSRI, selective serotonin reuptake inhibitor. (Adapted from Young AS, Klap R, Sherbourne CD, Wells KB. The quality of care for depressive and anxiety disorders in the United States. Arch Gen Psychiatry. 2001;58:55–61 and Bruce SE, Yonkers SE, Otto MW, et al. Influence of psychiatric comorbidity on recovery and recurrence in generalized anxiety disorder, social phobia, and panic disorder: A 12-year prospective study. Am J Psychiatry. 2005;162:1179–1187, with permission.)

achieving a panic-free state.[18,40] With similar efficacy reported and no trials comparing different SSRIs, drug selection generally is based on pharmacokinetics, drug interactions, side effects, and cost differences (see Chapter 38). The most common side effects of SSRIs include headaches, irritability, nausea and other gastrointestinal complaints, insomnia, sexual dysfunction, increased anxiety, drowsiness, and tremor.[42]

Serotonin Norepinephrine Reuptake Inhibitors Venlafaxine, in dosages of 75 to 225 mg/day, reduced panic and anticipatory anxiety in short-term controlled trials and prevented relapse with extended treatment over 6 months.[42,44] The most common side effects include anorexia, dry mouth, constipation, somnolence, tremor, abnormal ejaculation, and sweating. There is insufficient evidence to support the use of other SNRIs.

Monoamine Oxidase Inhibitors MAOIs have not been evaluated systematically for treatment of PD under the current diagnostic classification and generally are reserved for patients who are refractory to other treatments.[42] They have significant side effects that limit adherence. Additionally, patients must adhere to dietary restriction of tyramine and avoid sympathomimetic drugs to avoid hypertensive crisis (see Chapter 38).

The reversible inhibitors of monoamine oxidase (RIMAs) (brofaromine and meclobemide,[unavailable in the United States]) have been studied with mixed results.[18,42]

Other Antidepressants There is insufficient evidence to support the use of bupropion, trazodone, nefazodone, or mirtazapine for treatment of PD.[18,42]

► *Benzodiazepines*

Benzodiazepines are effective antipanic agents with significant effects on anticipatory anxiety and phobic behaviors. Alprazolam, the benzodiazepine most studied, is associated with significant panic reduction after 1 week of therapy (eg, 55%–75% panic free).[42,45] Benzodiazepines achieve outcomes similar to antidepressants over extended treatment, but benzodiazepine-treated patients

Clinical Presentation and Diagnosis of SAD

General

Individuals have marked fear or anxiety about one or more social situations where they are exposed to possible scrutiny or negative evaluation (eg, common social interactions, conversation, eating, drinking or performing). SAD differs from specific phobia, in which the fear and anxiety are limited to a particular object or situation (eg, insects, heights, public transportation). In children, the anxiety must be present in peer settings, not just in interactions with adults.

Symptoms[2]

- The individual fears acting in a way or showing anxiety that will be negatively evaluated (ie, humiliating or embarrassing or lead to rejection or offend others)
- Social situations almost always provoke fear or anxiety and are avoided or endured with intense fear or anxiety. Children may express fear or anxiety by crying, tantrums, freezing, clinging or failing to speak in social situations.

The fear or anxiety is

- out of proportion to the actual threat posed by the social situation;
- persistent, typically lasting for 6 months or more;
- causes clinically significant distress or impairment in social, occupational, or other area of functioning;
- not attributable to physiological effects of a substance or another medical condition; and
- not better explained by the symptoms of another mental disorder (eg, panic disorder, body dysmorphic disorder, or autism spectrum disorder)

Differential Diagnosis

Rule out underlying medical or psychiatric disorders and medications that may cause anxiety (see Tables 40–1 and 40–2).

Laboratory Evaluation

Laboratory investigation is of limited value and should be pursued only in context of other history or physical examination findings.

are more likely to relapse when the drugs are discontinued.[42] The risk for dependence and withdrawal and lack of efficacy for depression are significant concerns for long-term treatment of patients with PD. There is no evidence that tolerance to therapeutic effect occurs. Patients with PD experience greater rebound anxiety and relapse when discontinuing benzodiazepines than do patients with GAD. Tapering should be done at a slower rate and over a more extended period of time than with other anxiety disorders.[18,42]

KEY CONCEPT *The dose of benzodiazepine required for improvement generally is higher than that used in other anxiety disorders,* and this may explain why high-potency agents such as alprazolam and clonazepam generally are preferred. Lorazepam and diazepam, when given in equivalent doses, produce similar treatment benefits.[18,42] Doses should be titrated to response (see Table 40–4). The use of extended-release alprazolam or clonazepam may minimize breakthrough panic symptoms that are sometimes observed with immediate-release alprazolam.[45]

The most common side effects of benzodiazepines are sedation, fatigue, and cognitive impairment.[42] Benzodiazepines should be avoided in patients with current or past substance abuse or dependence or sleep apnea. Additionally, caution should be used in older adults because they have more pronounced psychomotor and cognitive side effects.

▸ *β-Blockers*

Pindolol 25 mg three times a day is an effective adjunctive treatment with an SSRI.[42] Propranolol 120 to 240 mg/day has been found equivalent to alprazolam in reduction of panic attacks.[42] β-blockers are not expected to reduce psychic anxiety or avoidance behavior. Additionally, heart rate and blood pressure reduction are dose-related adverse events that may limit use.

Outcome Evaluation

Assess patients for symptom improvement frequently (eg, weekly) during the first 4 weeks of therapy. With effective therapy, patients should experience significant reductions in the frequency and intensity of panic attacks, anticipatory anxiety, and phobic avoidance with resumption of normal activities. Rating scales, such as the Panic Disorder Symptom Scale (PDSS) can be useful in measuring symptom change over time. Assess patients for co-morbidities (eg, depression) as well as suicidal ideation. Alter the therapy of patients who do not achieve a significant reduction in panic symptoms after 6 to 8 weeks on an adequate dose of antidepressant or 3 weeks on a benzodiazepine. Regularly evaluate patients for adverse effects and medication adherence, and educate them about appropriate expectations of drug therapy.

When significant response to drug therapy is achieved, continue treatment for at least 1 year. Evaluate for symptom relapse and adverse effects that may emerge with continued treatment (eg, weight gain and sexual dysfunction). During drug discontinuation, monitor frequently for withdrawal, rebound anxiety, and relapse.

TREATMENT: SOCIAL ANXIETY DISORDER

Desired Outcomes

SAD is a chronic disorder that begins in adolescence and occurs with significant functional impairment and high rates of comorbidity. The goal of acute treatment is to reduce physiologic symptoms of anxiety, fear of social situations, and phobic behaviors. Patients with comorbid depression should have a significant reduction in depressive symptoms. The long-term goal is to restore social functioning and improve the patient's quality of life.

General Approach to Treatment

Patients with SAD may be managed with pharmacotherapy or psychotherapy. There is insufficient evidence to recommend one treatment over the other, and data are lacking on the benefits of combining treatment modalities. Children with SAD should be offered psychotherapy first.[46] Pharmacotherapy often is the first choice of treatment owing to relative greater access and reduced cost compared with psychotherapy.[46] Many patients will not achieve a full response.

Nonpharmacologic Therapy

Patient education on disease course, treatment options, and expectations is essential. Support groups may be beneficial for some patients. CBT targets avoidance-learning and negative-thinking patterns associated with social anxiety. CBT is effective for reducing anxiety and phobic avoidance and leads to a greater likelihood of maintaining response after treatment discontinuation than does pharmacotherapy.[46]

Pharmacologic Therapy

Several pharmacologic agents have demonstrated effectiveness in SAD, including the SSRIs, venlafaxine, phenelzine, RIMAs, benzodiazepines, gabapentin, and pregabalin. KEY CONCEPT *SSRIs are considered the drugs of choice based on their tolerability and efficacy for SAD and comorbid depression if present.* KEY CONCEPT *The onset of response for antidepressants may be as long as 8 to 12 weeks.*[18,47] *Patients responding to medication should be continued on treatment for at least 1 year.* Many patients relapse when medication is discontinued, and there are no clear predictive factors for who will maintain response.[47] Some patients may elect more long-term treatment owing to fear of relapse. A suggested treatment algorithm is shown in Figure 40–4.

▸ *Selective Serotonin Reuptake Inhibitors and Venlafaxine*

The efficacy of paroxetine, sertraline, escitalopram, fluvoxamine, and venlafaxine was established in large controlled trials.[18,47,48] SSRIs and SNRIs improve social anxiety and phobic avoidance and reduce overall disability. Approximately 50% of patients achieve response during acute treatment. Limited data support the effectiveness of citalopram and fluoxetine in SAD.[47,49]

The initial dose of SSRI is similar to that used in depression. Patients should be titrated as tolerated to response. Many patients require maximum recommended daily doses. Patients with comorbid PD should be started on lower doses (see Table 40–6). When discontinuing SSRIs, the dose should be tapered slowly to avoid withdrawal symptoms. Relapse rates may be as high as 50%, and patients should be monitored closely for several weeks.[46,47] Side effects of SSRIs in SAD are similar to those seen in depression and include nausea, sexual dysfunction, somnolence, and sweating.

Venlafaxine extended release, in doses of 75 to 225 mg/day, has similar efficacy to SSRIs.[18] Doses should be tapered slowly when discontinuing. Common side effects are anorexia, dry mouth, nausea, insomnia, and sexual dysfunction.

▸ *Monoamine Oxidase Inhibitors and Reversible Inhibitors of Monoamine Oxidase*

Phenelzine, effective in 64% to 69% of SAD patients,[47] is generally reserved for treatment-refractory patients owing to dietary restrictions,[49] drug interactions, and side effects. The RIMAs brofaramine and meclobemide are also effective.

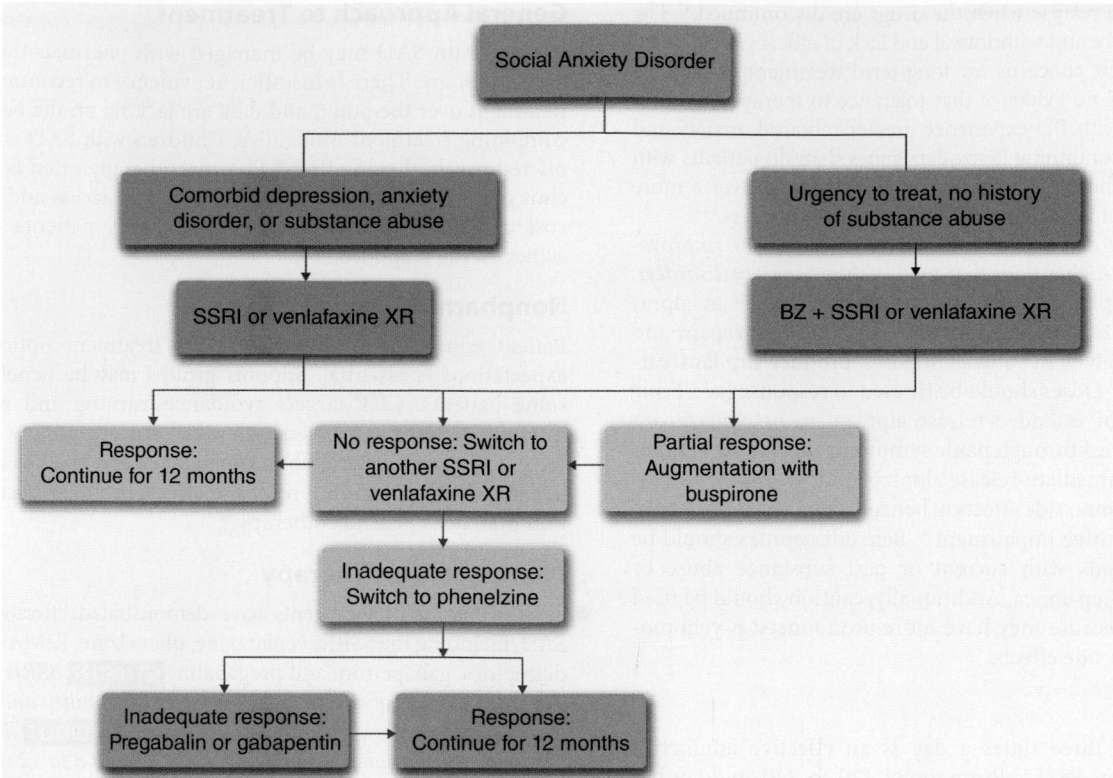

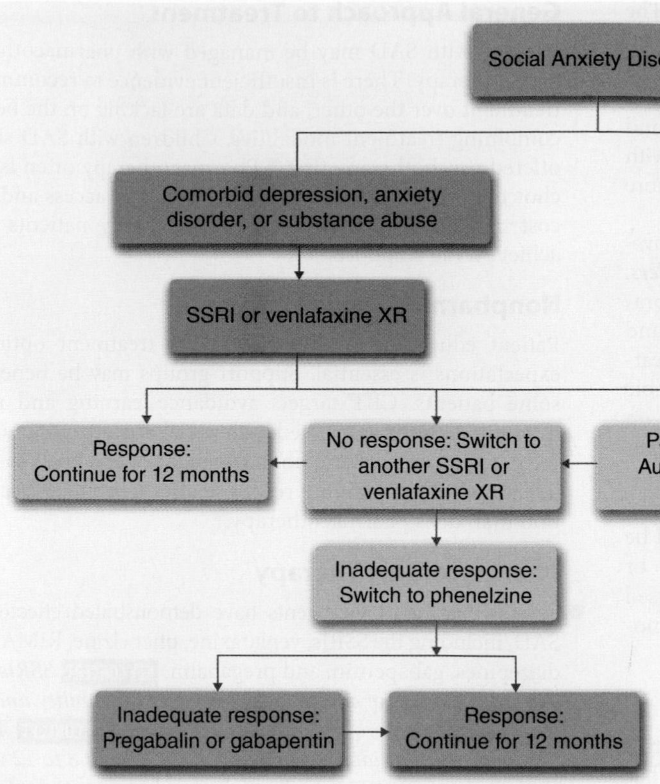

FIGURE 40–4. Algorithm for the pharmacotherapy of social anxiety disorder. BZ, benzodiazepine; SSRI, selective serotonin reuptake inhibitor. (Adapted from Melton ST, Kirkwood CK. Anxiety disorders I: Generalized anxiety, panic and social anxiety disorders. In: DiPiro JT, Talbert RL, Yee GC, et al, eds. Pharmacotherapy: A Pathophysiologic Approach. 8th ed. New York: McGraw-Hill; 2011:1209–1227, with permission.)

Patient Care Process

Patient Assessment:

- Based on clinical presentation and mental status exam, determine whether the patient is experiencing symptoms of sufficient intensity and duration to warrant treatment. Is there functional impairment?
- Based on physical exam and review of systems, does the patient have another condition causing anxiety?
- Determine if the patient has another psychiatric condition, such as depression or a substance use disorder? Is the patient experiencing suicidal ideation?
- Conduct a medication history (including prescriptions, over-the-counter (OTC) medications, and dietary supplements) to identify possible causes of anxiety/panic. Does the patient have any drug allergies? Is the patient experiencing side effects from therapy?

Therapy Evaluation:

- Determine whether treatment for the anxiety disorder is needed and if pharmacotherapy is preferred over behavioral interventions based on symptom severity and previous treatment and response.
- If patient is already receiving pharmacotherapy, assess efficacy, safety, and patient adherence. Are there any significant drug interactions?

Care Plan Development:

- Select lifestyle modifications and antianxiety therapy that are likely to be effective and safe. Used shared decision making for selection of behavioral and pharmacotherapy intervention(s). Consider comorbid conditions when selecting initial agent.
- Address any patient concerns about anxiety and its management.
- Discuss importance of medication adherence and lifestyle modifications.

Follow-up Evaluation:

- Follow-up at monthly intervals or more frequently during acute treatment to assess effectiveness and tolerability.
- Use appropriate rating scales to assess symptom change over time.
- Once anxiety is controlled and baseline function restored, determine the appropriateness of treatment beyond 1 year based on the patient's previous treatment, comorbidities, and ongoing environmental stressors.

▸ *Alternative Agents*

Benzodiazepines Benzodiazepines are used commonly in SAD; however, limited data support their use. Clonazepam was shown effective for social anxiety, fear, and phobic avoidance, and it reduced social and work disability during acute treatment.[47] Long-term treatment is not desirable for many SAD patients because of the risk of withdrawal and difficulty with discontinuation, cognitive side effects, and lack of effect on depressive symptoms. Benzodiazepines may be useful for acute relief of physiologic symptoms of anxiety when used concomitantly with antidepressants or psychotherapy. Benzodiazepines are contraindicated in SAD patients with current or past alcohol or substance abuse.

Anticonvulsants Gabapentin and pregabalin, structurally similar anticonvulsants, have each demonstrated modest benefit in a randomized, placebo controlled trial.[18,50] Gabapentin was titrated to a maximum dose of 3600 mg/day and pregabalin to 600 mg/day. While both medications have good tolerability, they should be considered for patients with inadequate response to SSRI/SNRIs.

β-Blockers β-blockers decrease the physiologic symptoms of anxiety and are useful for reducing performance anxiety. Propranolol or atenolol should be administered 1 hour before a performance situation. β-blockers are not useful in SAD.[47]

Outcome Evaluation

KEY CONCEPT *Pharmacotherapy for patients with SAD should lead to improvement in anxiety and fear, functionality, and overall well-being.*[18] Many patients will experience significant improvement in symptoms but may not achieve full remission. Monitor patients weekly during acute treatment (eg, initiation and titration of pharmacotherapy) and monthly once stabilized. Inquire about adverse effects, SAD symptoms, suicidal ideation, and symptoms of comorbid psychiatric conditions at each visit. Ask patients to keep a diary to record fears, anxiety levels, and behaviors in social situations.[18] Administer the Leibowitz Social Anxiety Scale (LSAS) to rate SAD severity and change, and the Social Phobia Inventory can be used as a "self-assessment" tool. Counsel patients on appropriate expectations of pharmacotherapy in SAD, including gradual onset of effect and the need for extended treatment of at least 6 months following response.

Abbreviations Introduced in This Chapter

CBT	Cognitive-behavioral therapy
CNS	Central nervous system
DA	Dopamine
FDA	Food and Drug Administration
GABA	γ-aminobutyric acid
GAD	Generalized anxiety disorder
HPA	Hypothalamic-pituitary-adrenal
5-HT	Serotonin
LC	Locus ceruleus
LSAS	Liebowitz Social Anxiety Scale
MAOI	Monoamine oxidase inhibitor
MDD	Major depressive disorder
NCS-R	National Comorbidity Survey, Revised
NE	Norepinephrine
NPY	Neuropeptide Y
OCD	Obsessive-compulsive disorder
OTC	Over-the-counter
PD	Panic disorder
PDSS	Panic Disorder Symptom Scale
RAS	Reticular activating system
RIMA	Reversible inhibitors of monoamine oxidase A
SAD	Social anxiety disorder
SGA	Second-generation antipsychotic
SNRI	Serotonin-norepinephrine reuptake inhibitor
SSRI	Selective serotonin reuptake inhibitor
TCA	Tricyclic antidepressant

REFERENCES

1. Young AS, Klap R, Sherbourne CD, Wells KB. The quality of care for depressive and anxiety disorders in the United States. Arch Gen Psychiatry. 2001;58:55–61.
2. American Psychiatric Association. Diagnostic and Statistical Manual of Mental Disorders, 5th ed. Arlington, VA: American Psychiatric Association, 2013. Web. [access date August 26, 2014]. dsm.psychiatryonline.org.
3. Kessler RC, Berglund P, Demler O, et al. Lifetime prevalence and age-of-onset distributions of the DSM-IV disorders in the National Comorbidity Survey Replication. Arch Gen Psychiatry. 2005A;62:593–602.
4. Kessler RC, Chiu WT, Demler O, et al. Prevalence, severity, and comorbidity of 12-month DSM-IV disorders in the National Comorbidity Survey Replication. Arch Gen Psychiatry. 2005;62:617–627.
5. Pollack MH. The pharmacotherapy of panic disorder. J Clin Psychiatry 2005;66(Suppl 4):23–27.
6. Yonkers KA, Bruce SE, Dyck IR, Keller MB. Chronicity, relapse, and illness-course of panic disorder, social phobia, and generalized anxiety disorder: Findings in men and women from 8 years of follow-up. Depress Anxiety. 2003;17:173–179.
7. Bruce SE, Yonkers SE, Otto MW, et al. Influence of psychiatric comorbidity on recovery and recurrence in generalized anxiety disorder, social phobia, and panic disorder: A 12-year prospective study. Am J Psychiatry. 2005;162:1179–1187.
8. Cramer V, Torgersen S, Kringlen E. Quality of life and anxiety disorders: A population study. J Nerv Ment Dis. 2005;193:196–202.
9. Kaufman J, Charney D. Comorbidity of mood and anxiety disorders. Depress Anxiety. 2000;12(Suppl 1):69–76.
10. Hettema JM, Prescott CA, Myers JM, et al. The structure of genetic and environmental risk factors for anxiety disorders in men and women. Arch Gen Psychiatry. 2005;62:182–189.
11. Ninan PT, Dunlop BW. Neurobiology and etiology of panic disorder. J Clin Psychiatry. 2005;66(Suppl 4):3–7.
12. Pierii JN, Lewis DA. Functional neuroanatomy. In: Sadock BJ, Sadock VA, eds. Kaplan & Sadock's Comprehensive Textbook of Psychiatry. 8th ed. Philadelphia, PA: Lippincott Williams & Wilkins; 2005:3–32.
13. Gould TD, Gray NA, Manji HK. Cellular neurobiology of severe mood and anxiety disorders: Implications for development of novel therapeutics. In: Charney DS, ed. Molecular Neurobiology for the Clinician (Review of Psychiatry Series. Vol. 22. No. 3; Oldham JM, Riba MB, series, eds). Washington, DC: American Psychiatric Publishing; 2003:123–200.
14. Plata-Salaman CR, Shank RP, Smith-Swintosky VL. Amino acids as neurotransmitters. In: Sadock BJ, Sadock VA, eds. Kaplan & Sadock's Comprehensive Textbook of Psychiatry. 8th ed. Philadelphia, PA: Lippincott Williams & Wilkins, 2005:60–72.
15. Young LJ, Owens MJ, Nemeroff CB. Neuropeptides: biology, regulation, and role in neuropsychiatric disorders. In: Sadock BJ, Sadock VA, eds. Kaplan & Sadock's Comprehensive Textbook of Psychiatry. 8th ed. Philadelphia, PA: Lippincott Williams & Wilkins; 2005:3–32.

16. House A, Stark D. Anxiety in medical patients. BMJ. 2002;325:207–209.
17. Melton ST, Kirkwood CK. Anxiety Disorders I: Generalized Anxiety, Panic, and Social Anxiety Disorders. Dipiro JT, Talbert RL, Yee GC, et al, eds. Pharmacotherapy: A Pathophysiologic Approach. 9th ed. New York: McGraw-Hill; 2014:717–732.
18. Bandelow B, Zohar J, Hollander E, et al. World Federation of Societies of Biological Psychiatry (WFSBP) Guidelines for the pharmacological treatment of anxiety, obsessive-compulsive and posttraumatic stress disorders—first revision. World J Biol Psychiatry. 2008;9:248–312.
19. Practice Parameter for the Assessment and treatment of children and adolescents with anxiety disorders. J Am Acad Child Adolesc Psychiatry. 2007;46(2):267–283.
20. Andrews G, Cuijpers P, Craske MG, et al. Computer therapy for anxiety and depressive disorders is effective, acceptable, and practical health care: A meta-analysis. PLoS One. 2010;5(10):e13196.
21. Walkup JT, Albano AM, Piacentini J, et al. Cognitive behavioral therapy, sertraline or a combination in childhood anxiety. N Engl J Med. 2008;359(26):2753–2766.
22. Donovan MR, Glue P, Kolluri S, and Emir B. Comparative efficacy of antidepressants in preventing relapse in anxiety disorders: A meta-analysis. J Affective Disord. 2010;123:9–16.
23. Davidson JR, Zhang W, Connor KM, et al. Review: A psychopharmacological treatment algorithm for generalised anxiety disorder (GAD). J Psychopharmacol. 2010;24:3.
24. Shelton RC, Brown LL. Mechanisms of action in the treatment of anxiety. J Clin Psychiatry. 2001;62(Suppl 12):10–15.
25. Allgulander C, Nutt D, Detke M, et al. A non-inferiority comparison of duloxetine and venlafaxine in the treatment of adult patients with generalized anxiety disorder. J Psychopharmacol. 2008;22(4):417–425.
26. Hartford JT, Endicott J, Kornstein SG, et al. Implications of pain in generalized anxiety disorder: Efficacy of duloxetine. Prim Care Companion J Clin Psychiatry. 2008;10(3):197–204.
27. Rickels K, Zaninelli R, McCafferty J, et al. Paroxetine treatment of generalized anxiety disorder: A double-blind, placebo-controlled study. Am J Psychiatry. 2003;160:749–756.
28. Stocchi F, Nordera G, Jokinen R, et al. Efficacy and tolerability of paroxetine for the long-term treatment of generalized anxiety disorder (GAD). J Clin Psychiatry. 2003;64(3):250–258.
29. Davidson JR, Bose A, Korotzer A, Zheng H. Escitalopram in the treatment of generalized anxiety disorder: Double-blind, placebo-controlled, flexible-dose study. Depress Anxiety. 2004;19(4):234–240.
30. Allgulander C, Dahl AA, Austin C, et al. Efficacy of sertraline in a 12-week trial for generalized anxiety disorder. Am J Psychiatry. 2004;161(9):1642–1649.
31. Lenze EJ, Mulsant BH, Shear MK, et al. Efficacy and tolerability of citalopram in the treatment of late-life anxiety disorders: Results from an 8-week randomized, placebo-controlled trial. Am J Psychiatry. 2005;162(1):146–150.
32. Micromedex Healthcare Series. Drugdex Evaluations. © 1974–2012 Thomson Reuters.
33. Chouinard G. Issues in the clinical use of benzodiazepines: Potency, withdrawal, and rebound. J Clin Psychiatry. 2004;65 (Suppl 5):7–12.
34. US Food and Drug Administration [online]. [cited 2011 Oct 10]. http://www.fda.gov/Drugs/ScienceResearch/ResearchAreas/Pharmacogenetics/ucm083378.htm. Accessed February 7, 2012.
35. Longo LP, Johnson B. Benzodiazepines: Side effects, abuse risk and alternatives (addiction part 1). Am Fam Physician. 2000;61:2121–2128.
36. Rickels K, Pollack MH, Feltner DE, et al. Pregabalin for the treatment of generalized anxiety disorder: A 4-week, multicenter, double-blind, placebo-controlled trial of pregabalin and alprazolam. Arch Gen Psychiatry. 2005;62:1022–1030.
37. Montgomery SA, Tobias K, Zornberg GL, et al. Pregabalin and venlafaxine improve symptoms of generalised anxiety disorder. Evid Based Ment Health. 2007;10:23.
38. Feltner D, Wittchen HU, Kavoussi R, et al. Long-term efficacy of pregabalin in generalized anxiety disorder. Int Clin Psychopharmacol. 2008;23:18–28.
39. Chessick CA, Allen MH, Thase M, et al. Azapirones for generalized anxiety disorder. Cochrane Database Syst Rev. 2006;(3):CD006115.
40. Maher AR, Maglione M, Bagley S, et al. Efficacy and comparative effectiveness of atypical antipsychotic medications for off-label uses in adults: A systematic review and meta-analysis. JAMA. 2011;306(12):1359–1369.
41. Bridge JA, Iyengar S, Salary CB, et al. Clinical response and risk for reported suicidal ideation and suicide attempts in pediatric antidepressant treatment: A meta-analysis of randomized controlled trials. JAMA. 2007;297:1683–1696.
42. Stein MB, Goin MK, Pollack MH, et al. Practice Guideline for the Treatment of Patients with Panic Disorder. 2nd ed. Washington, DC: American Psychiatric Association; 2009. [cited 2011 Oct 10]. Available from http://www.psychiatryonline.com/content.aspx?aID=58560. Accessed September 12, 2011.
43. van Apeldoorn FJ, van Hout WJ, Mersch PP, et al. Is a combined therapy more effective than either CBT or SSRI alone? Results of a multicenter trial on panic disorder with or without agoraphobia. Acta Psychiatr Scand. 2008;117(4):260–270.
44. Ferguson JM, Khan A, Mangano R, et al. Relapse prevention of panic disorder in adult outpatient responders to treatment with venlafaxine extended release. J Clin Psychiatry. 2007;68(1):58–68.
45. Rickels K. Alprazolam extended release in panic disorder. Expert Opin Pharmacother. 2004;5(7):1599–1611.
46. National institute for Health and Care Excellence. Social Anxiety Disorder: Recognition, assessment and treatment. NICE Clinical Guideline 159, May 2013. http://guidance.nice.org.uk/CG159 Accessed 9/10/2014.
47. Blanc C, Bragdon LB, Schneier R, Liebowitz MR. The evidence-based pharmacotherapy of social anxiety disorder. Int J Neuropsychopharmacol. 2013;16(1):235–249.
48. deMenezes GB, Coutinho ESF, Fontenelle LF, et al. Second-generation antidepressants in social anxiety disorder: Meta-analysis of controlled clinical trials. Psychopharmacology. 2011;215:1–11.
49. Gardner DM, Shulman KI, Walker SE, Tailor SA. The making of a user friendly MAOI diet. J Clin Psychiatry. 1996;57(3):99–104.
50. Schneier FR. Social anxiety disorder. N Engl J Med. 2006;355:1029–1036.

41 Sleep Disorders

John M. Dopp and Bradley G. Phillips

LEARNING OBJECTIVES

Upon completion of the chapter, the reader will be able to:

1. List the sequelae of undiagnosed or untreated sleep disorders and appreciate the importance of successful treatment of sleep disorders.
2. State the incidence and prevalence of sleep disorders.
3. Describe the pathophysiology and characteristic features of the sleep disorders covered in this chapter, including insomnia, narcolepsy, restless legs syndrome (RLS), obstructive sleep apnea (OSA), and parasomnias.
4. Assess patient sleep complaints, conduct sleep histories, and evaluate sleep studies to recognize daytime and nighttime symptoms and characteristics of common sleep disorders.
5. Recommend and optimize appropriate sleep hygiene and nonpharmacologic therapies for the management and prevention of sleep disorders.
6. Recommend and optimize appropriate pharmacotherapy for sleep disorders.
7. Describe the components of the patient care process to implement and assess safety and efficacy of pharmacotherapy for common sleep disorders.
8. Educate patients about preventive behavior, appropriate lifestyle modifications, and drug therapy required for effective treatment and control of sleep disorders.

INTRODUCTION

Individuals with normal sleep patterns sleep up to one-third of their lives and spend more time sleeping than in any other single activity. Despite this, our understanding of the full purpose of sleep and the mechanisms regulating sleep homeostasis remains incomplete. Sleep is necessary to enable one to maintain wakefulness and good health. Disruption of normal sleep is a major cause of societal morbidity, lost productivity, and reduced quality of life.[1] Sleep disturbances may contribute to the development and progression of comorbid medical conditions.[1]

Sleep is governed and paced by the suprachiasmic nucleus in the brain that regulates circadian rhythm. Environmental cues and amount of previous sleep also influence sleep on a daily basis. There are two main types of sleep: **rapid eye movement (REM) sleep**, during which eye movements and dreaming occur but the body is mostly paralyzed, and **non–rapid eye movement (NREM) sleep**, which consists of four substages (stages 1–4). Stage 1 serves as a transition between wake and sleep. Most of the time asleep is spent in stage 2 NREM sleep. Stages 3 and 4 sleep often are grouped together and referred to as *deep sleep*, or *delta sleep*, because prominent delta waves are seen on the electroencephalogram (EEG) during these sleep stages.

EPIDEMIOLOGY AND ETIOLOGY

Approximately 50% of adults will report a sleep complaint over the course of their lives.[2] In general, sleep disturbances increase with age, and each disorder may have gender differences. The full extent and impact of disordered sleep on our society are not known because many patients' sleep disorders remain undiagnosed. Normal sleep, by definition, is "a reversible behavioral state of perceptual disengagement from and unresponsiveness to the environment."[3] Individuals with sleep disorders exhibit or complain about consequent symptoms (eg, daytime sleepiness) or a bed partner often observes hallmark characteristics of the sleep disorder. Insomnia, RLS, and sleep-related breathing disorders are the most common sleep disorders.

Insomnia

The prevalence of insomnia increases with age and is nearly 1.5 times greater in women than in men. Approximately one-third of patients older than age 65 years have persistent insomnia.[4,5] About 10% of adults experience chronic insomnia, and slightly more experience short-term insomnia. KEY CONCEPT *Insomnia is most frequently a symptom or manifestation of an underlying disorder (comorbid or secondary insomnia) but may occur in the absence of contributing factors (primary insomnia).* Forty percent of patients with psychiatric conditions have accompanying insomnia.[6] Secondary insomnia may be triggered by acute stress and resolve when the stress resolves. Numerous coexisting medical conditions, such as pain, thyroid abnormalities, asthma, and gastroesophageal reflux, and medications, including selective serotonin reuptake inhibitors (SSRIs), steroids, stimulants, and β-agonists, can cause insomnia.

Narcolepsy

Although difficult to estimate, the prevalence of narcolepsy is between 0.03% and 0.06%.[7] Significant differences have been reported for various ethnic groups. Narcolepsy has a higher prevalence in Japanese and a lower prevalence in Israeli populations.[8,9] **Cataplexy** is not required for diagnosis; however, between 50% and 80% of patients with narcolepsy have accompanying cataplexy.[10]

Restless Legs Syndrome

RLS occurs in 6% to 12% of the population.[11,12] Prevalence increases with age and in various medical conditions, such as end-stage renal disease, pregnancy, and iron deficiency.[13] RLS appears to be more common in women than in men and has a genetic link in a majority of patients.[14]

Obstructive Sleep Apnea

OSA affects 4% of middle-aged white men and 2% of middle-aged white women.[15] In women, the frequency increases after menopause. Prevalence is the same or higher in African Americans and lower in Asian populations. The risk for OSA increases with age and obesity. Individuals with OSA experience repetitive upper airway collapse during sleep, which decreases or stops airflow, with subsequent arousal from sleep to resume breathing. Severity is determined by **nocturnal polysomnography** (NPSG) or home sleep study and is graded by the number of episodes of apnea (total cessation of airflow) and hypopnea (partial airway closure with blood oxygen desaturation) experienced during sleep. Severity is expressed as the **respiratory disturbance index** (RDI), quantified in events per hour.

Parasomnias

NREM **parasomnias** have variable prevalence rates depending on patient age and comorbid diagnoses. Sleep talking, bruxism, sleepwalking, sleep terrors, and enuresis occur more frequently in childhood than in adulthood. Nightmares appear to occur with similar frequency in adults and children. REM-sleep behavior disorder (RBD), an REM-sleep parasomnia, has a reported prevalence of 0.5%, is more common in elderly men, and frequently is associated with concomitant neurologic conditions.[16]

PATHOPHYSIOLOGY

Although the neurophysiology of sleep is complex, certain neurotransmitters promote sleep and wakefulness in different areas of the central nervous system (CNS). Whereas serotonin is thought to control NREM sleep, cholinergic and adrenergic transmitters mediate REM sleep. Dopamine, norepinephrine, **hypocretin**, substance P, and histamine all play a role in wakefulness. Perturbations of various neurotransmitters are responsible for some sleep disorders and explain why various treatments are beneficial.

Insomnia

There is no single pathophysiologic explanation for the manifestations of insomnia. Current hypotheses focus on a combination of possible models that incorporate physiologic, cognitive, and cortical arousal. Most models focus on hyperarousal and its interference with the initiation or maintenance of sleep.

Narcolepsy

The onset of narcolepsy–cataplexy is typically in adolescence, suggesting that the disease may require environmental influence to develop. Currently, it is believed that narcolepsy results from autoimmune insult to the CNS because it is associated with human leukocyte antigen (major histocompatibility complex) DQB10602 and DQ1A1*0102.[17,18] Concentrations of hypocretin (a wake-promoting neuropeptide) in the cerebrospinal fluid of patients with narcolepsy are reduced significantly, suggesting that the autoimmune attack is against hypocretin-producing cells in the hypothalamus.[19]

Restless Legs Syndrome and Periodic Limb Movements of Sleep

RLS is a neurologic medical condition characterized by an irresistible desire to move the limbs. It is thought that these abnormal sensations are a result of iron deficiency in the brain and iron-handling abnormalities in the CNS. Iron and H-ferritin concentrations, along with transferrin receptor and iron transporter numbers, are reduced in the substantia nigra of patients with RLS.[20] These iron abnormalities lead to dysfunction of dopaminergic transmission in the substantia nigra. Recently, it has been suggested that local hypoxia in the legs may contribute to pathophysiology of RLS.[21]

Obstructive Sleep Apnea

At least 20 muscles and soft tissue structures control patency of the upper airway. Patients with OSA may have differences in upper airway muscle activity during sleep and may have smaller airways, predisposing them to upper airway collapse and consequent apneic episodes during sleep. The inability of the upper airway to contend with factors that promote collapse, including fat deposition in the neck, negative pressure in the airway during inspiration, and a smaller lower jawbone, also may play a role in the pathogenesis of OSA.

Poor sleep architecture and fragmented sleep secondary to OSA can cause excessive daytime sleepiness (EDS) and neurocognitive deficits. These sequelae can affect quality of life and work performance and may be linked to occupational and motor vehicle accidents. OSA is also associated with systemic disease such as hypertension, heart failure, and stroke.[22,23] OSA is likely an independent risk factor for the development of hypertension.[24] Furthermore, when hypertension is present, it is often resistant to antihypertensive therapy. Patients with sleep apnea often are obese and may be predisposed to weight gain. Hence, obesity may further contribute to cardiovascular disease in this patient population.

Several factors suggest an association between OSA and systemic disease. Breathing against a closed upper airway during sleep causes intermittent and repetitive episodes of hypoxemia and hypercapnia, dramatic changes in intrathoracic pressure, and activation of the sympathetic nervous system. These responses can produce acute hemodynamic and humoral responses. Blood pressure can increase to 220/120 mm Hg with each apneic episode.[25]

Parasomnias

The pathogenesis of parasomnias (eg, sleepwalking, enuresis, sleep talking) is variable poorly described, and involves state dissociation, whereby two states of being overlap simultaneously. For example, abnormal activation of the central pattern generator of the spinal cord that produces motor movements is hypothesized to underlie sleepwalking behavior. In RBD, active

Clinical Presentation and Diagnosis

KEY CONCEPT *Patients with sleep complaints should have a careful sleep history performed to assess their possible sleep disorder in order to guide diagnostic and therapeutic decisions.*

Daytime symptoms and associated characteristics: EDS is the primary symptom described by patients with sleep disorders. It is usually described as not waking up refreshed in the morning or falling asleep or fighting the urge to sleep during the day despite a night of sleep. Other daytime characteristics of sleep disorders include:

- Irritability, fatigue, or depression
- Confusion or impaired performance at work or school
- Cataplexy
- Hypertension

Nighttime sleep complaints: Depending on the sleep disorder, patients may exhibit or experience various nocturnal complaints during sleep. Some complaints can be uncovered by clinical history alone (eg, hallucinations, RLS, snoring), but others can be diagnosed during sleep studies (eg, OSA, nighttime awakenings, somnambulism, PLMS, etc). Frequent complaints include:

- Inability to fall asleep, nighttime awakenings
- Sleep walking (somnambulism), sleep talking (somniloquy)
- Cessation of breathing (apnea), snoring
- Sleep paralysis or hallucinations when waking or falling asleep
- Restlessness (PLMS or RLS)

inhibition of motor activity in the perilocus coeruleus region is lost, resulting in loss of paralysis and dream enactment.

CLINICAL PRESENTATION AND DIAGNOSIS

KEY CONCEPT *Although the clinical history guides diagnosis and therapy, only NPSG, home sleep studies, and/or multiple sleep latency tests (MSLTs) can definitively diagnose and guide therapy for OSA, narcolepsy, and periodic limb movements of sleep (PLMS).* All patients presenting with sleep complaints should have a thorough interview and history to inventory their sleep habits and sleep hygiene.

Insomnia

Insomnia is often characterized by difficulty falling asleep, frequent nocturnal awakenings, early morning awakenings, and nonrestorative sleep, which may result in daytime impairments in concentration and school or work performance. In comorbid (secondary) insomnia, social factors (eg, family difficulties, bereavement), medications (eg, antidepressants, β-agonists, corticosteroids, decongestants), and coexisting medical or psychiatric conditions (eg, depression, bipolar disorder) may help to explain difficulties in initiating and maintaining sleep. Insomnia duration may be described as transient (less than 1 week), acute (1–4 weeks), or chronic (greater than 1 month) in duration.

Narcolepsy

The hallmark of narcolepsy is EDS and the need for periods of sleep during the day. Patients with narcolepsy may experience repeated nighttime awakenings, terrifying dreams, and difficulty falling asleep. They frequently experience abnormal manifestations of REM sleep, including hallucinations and sleep paralysis that occur on falling asleep and/or awakening. Cataplexy is a weakness or loss of skeletal muscle tone in the jaw, legs, or arms that is elicited by emotion (eg, anger, surprise, laughter, or sadness).

Obstructive Sleep Apnea

Common characteristics of OSA include snoring, choking, gasping for air, nocturnal reflux symptoms, and morning headaches. A bed partner or roommate may observe these symptoms and witness apneic episodes where the patient stops breathing. Patients with large neck sizes (greater than 45 cm [~18 in] neck circumference) and a body mass index (BMI) of 30 kg/m^2 or greater are at higher risk for OSA.

Periodic Limb Movements of Sleep and Restless Legs Syndrome

Although RLS symptoms can vary, patients commonly report creepy-crawly, burning, tingling, or achy feelings in the legs or arms. These sensations create a desire to move the limbs and may produce motor restlessness. Symptoms are worse in the evening and are worse or exclusively present at rest, with temporary relief with movement. Symptoms also can occur during sleep and often lead to semirhythmic PLMS. PLMS are objective findings during NPSG recorded by leg electrodes. PLMS are present in most patients with RLS but can occur independently.

Parasomnias

Parasomnias are characterized by undesirable physical or behavioral phenomena that occur during sleep (eg, sleepwalking, sleep eating, sleep talking, bruxism [grinding of teeth], enuresis, night terrors, and RBD). People with RBD act out their dreams during sleep, often in a violent manner.

Circadian Rhythm Disorders

The most common circadian rhythm disorders (CRDs) include jet lag, shift-work sleep disruption, delayed sleep-phase disorder, and advanced sleep-phase disorder. Jet lag occurs when a person travels across time zones, and the external environmental time is mismatched with the internal circadian clock. Delayed and advanced sleep-phase disorders occur when bed and wake times are delayed or advanced (by 3 or more hours) compared with socially prescribed bed and wake times.

Sleep Diagnostics

Complete NPSG is the "gold standard" for diagnosing and identifying sleep-disordered breathing, PLMS, parasomnias, and nocturnal sleep irregularities related to narcolepsy. Sleep is observed and monitored in a controlled setting using an EEG, electrooculography, electromyography, electrocardiography, air thermistors, abdominal and thoracic strain belts, and an oxygen saturation monitor. This setup records sleep onset, arousals, sleep stages, eye movements, leg and jaw movements, heart rhythm, airflow, respiratory effort, and oxygen desaturations. Home sleep studies are increasingly used to diagnose sleep apnea due to their reduced cost and increased patient convenience. These devices typically measure nasal airflow, respiratory effort, oxygen saturation, and heart rate to determine if a patient experiences apnea/hypopnea episodes.

The MSLT is a commonly performed test to assess daytime sleepiness. During the MSLT, the patient attempts to take a 20-minute nap every 2 hours during the day beginning 2 hours after morning awakening (after a normal night's sleep) to evaluate physiologic sleepiness. The patient is instructed not to resist the urge to fall asleep. Sleep latency of less than 5 or 6 minutes is considered pathologically sleepy. The occurrence of an REM onset period during two naps with short sleep latency is indicative of a diagnosis of narcolepsy.

TREATMENT

Desired Outcomes

KEY CONCEPT *Treatment goals vary among different sleep disorders but generally include restoration of normal sleep patterns, elimination of daytime sequelae, improved quality of life, and prevention of complications and adverse effects from therapy.*

General Approach to Treatment

Nonpharmacologic interventions for insomnia are outlined in Table 41–1. Sleep hygiene should be reinforced in all patients, and behavioral, cognitive, and stimulus-control interventions are used mainly for patients with insomnia-type complaints. Both pharmacologic and nonpharmacologic therapies are effective at improving sleep and reducing insomnia complaints. An algorithm for the initial assessment and first treatment step of EDS is provided in Figure 41–1.

Insomnia

KEY CONCEPT *Early treatment of insomnia may prevent the development of persistent psychophysiologic insomnia.* The ideal hypnotic drug would be effective at reducing sleep latency, increasing total sleep time, and would be free of unwanted side effects. KEY CONCEPT *Benzodiazepine receptor agonists (BZDRAs) (including traditional benzodiazepines, zolpidem, zaleplon, and eszopiclone) and ramelteon are approved by the Food and Drug Administration (FDA) for the treatment of insomnia and are first-line therapies.*[2,26,27] Pharmacologic treatment of insomnia is recommended for transient and acute insomnia. Long-term use of hypnotics is not contraindicated unless the patient has another contraindication to their use. Eszopiclone is the only sedative hypnotic approved by the FDA for chronic use up to 6 months.[28] Although not first-line agents for insomnia, sedating antidepressants are also commonly prescribed.

Table 41–1

Nonpharmacologic Therapies for Insomnia

Sleep Hygiene
- Keep a regular sleep schedule.
- Exercise frequently but not immediately before bedtime.
- Avoid alcohol and stimulants (caffeine, nicotine) in the late afternoon and evening.
- Maintain a comfortable sleeping environment that is dark, quiet, and free of intrusions.
- Avoid consuming large quantities of food or liquids immediately before bedtime.

Stimulus Control
- Go to bed only when sleepy.
- Avoid daytime naps.
- If you cannot sleep, get out of bed and go to another room—only return to your bed when you feel the need to sleep.
- Bed is for sleep and intimacy only (no eating or watching TV in bed).
- Always wake up at the same time each day.

Relaxation Training
- Reduce somatic arousal (muscle relaxation).
- Reduce mental arousal (eg, attention-focusing procedures, imagery training, meditation).
- Use biofeedback (visual or auditory feedback to reduce tension).

Cognitive Therapy
- Alter beliefs, attitudes, and expectations about sleep.

▶ *Benzodiazepine Receptor Agonists*

Pharmacokinetic differences between the eight BZDRAs help to guide selection, depending on patient considerations and specific sleep complaints (Table 41–2). These agents occupy the benzodiazepine site on the γ-aminobutyric acid (GABA) type A receptor complex, resulting in opening of chloride channels that facilitate GABA inhibition and promote sleepiness.[33] BZDRAs have become the first-line agents for treating insomnia and sleep-maintenance problems. They are all efficacious, have wide therapeutic indices, and have a low incidence of abuse.[26,28,29]

Patients should be instructed to take BZDRAs at bedtime and avoid activities requiring alertness after ingestion. Although BZDRAs generally are well tolerated and have good safety profiles, mild to moderate side effects can occur, and precautions are warranted.

Precautions and Safety The most common side effects associated with BZDRAs include residual sedation into the waking hours after sleep, grogginess, and psychomotor impairment.[30] Selection of a hypnotic with a duration of action matching the patient's budgeted sleep time can help minimize the risk of residual sedation. BZDRAs should be initiated at low doses, and agents with active metabolites (see Table 41–2) should be avoided in elderly patients. BZDRAs may cause anterograde amnesia, defined as memory loss of activities and interactions after ingestion of the drug. All sedatives can cause anterograde amnesia, and higher doses increase the extent of amnesia.[31,32]

On discontinuation of hypnotic BZDRAs, patients may experience rebound insomnia that may last for a few nights. Rebound insomnia occurs more frequently after discontinuation of shorter duration BZDRAs compared with longer duration BZDRAs. Intermittent hypnotic therapy with the lowest dose possible reduces the likelihood of tolerance, dependence, and withdrawal when therapy is stopped. Patients should be counseled that rebound insomnia is not necessarily a return of their original symptoms, and it may take a few nights for rebound symptoms to subside. In general, eszopiclone, zaleplon, and zolpidem appear to be associated with lower risk of tolerance, rebound insomnia, and withdrawal than traditional benzodiazepines.

▶ *Sedating Antidepressants*

Sedating antidepressants (eg, trazodone, amitriptyline, mirtazapine, nefazodone, doxepin) are commonly used for insomnia and may be an appealing option in patients with concomitant depression. However, at the doses frequently used for sleep, only mirtazapine exhibits significant antidepressant activity. Furthermore, quality clinical studies demonstrating efficacy for insomnia are lacking. Side effects from antidepressants can be frequent, including carryover sedation, grogginess, anticholinergic effects, and weight gain. Tricyclic antidepressants (TCAs) should be used with caution in the elderly and patients with cardiovascular and hepatic impairment. Mirtazapine can cause daytime sedation, dizziness, and weight gain, and trazodone can

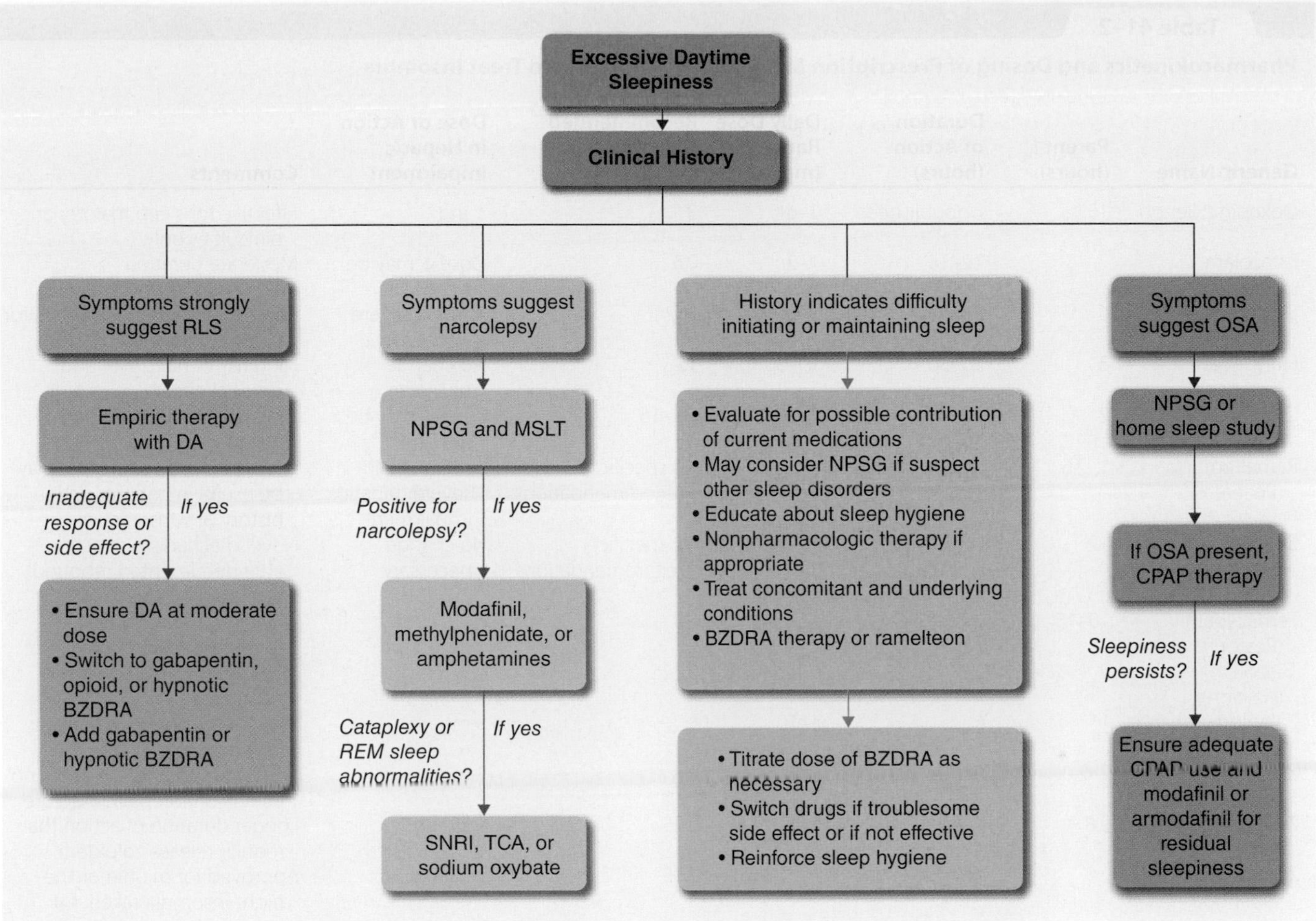

FIGURE 41–1. Primary assessment and initial treatment for complaint of excessive daytime sleepiness. BZDRA, benzodiazepine receptor agonist; CPAP, continuous positive airway pressure; DA, dopamine agonist; MSLT, multiple sleep latency test; OSA, obstructive sleep apnea; RLS, restless legs syndrome; SNRI, serotonin and norepinephrine reuptake inhibitor; NPSG, nocturnal polysomnography; TCA, tricyclic antidepressant.

cause hypotension and dizziness and should be used with caution in patients with heart disease or hypertension and those taking cardiovascular agents.[33,34] Doxepin is approved for treatment of sleep maintenance insomnia in low doses (3–6 mg).

▶ *Over-the-Counter and Other Miscellaneous Agents*

Over-the-counter antihistamines such as diphenhydramine are frequently used (usual doses, 25–50 mg) for difficulty sleeping. Diphenhydramine is approved by the FDA for the treatment of insomnia and can be effective at reducing sleep latency and increasing sleep time.[35] However, diphenhydramine produces undesirable anticholinergic effects and carryover sedation that limit its use, especially in the elderly. Valerian root is an herb that has inconsistent effects on sleep but may reduce sleep latency and increase efficiency at commonly used doses of 400 to 900 mg valerian extract. Ramelteon, a melatonin receptor agonist, is indicated for insomnia characterized by difficulty with sleep onset. Ramelteon is not a controlled substance and can be a viable option for patients with a history of substance abuse. It has documented efficacy treating sleep onset difficulties in those with mild to moderate chronic obstructive pulmonary disease and OSA.[36-38] Suvorexant (an orexin receptor antagonist) was recently approved for treatment of insomnia. It is the first medication that turns off wakefulness mechanisms instead of stimulating pathways that induce sleepiness. Suvorexant is indicated for both difficulty initiating and maintaining sleep, and like BZDRAs, it is classified as a schedule IV controlled substance.[39]

Narcolepsy

Therapy for narcolepsy involves two key principles: (a) treatment of EDS with scheduled naps and CNS stimulants and (b) suppression of cataplexy and REM-sleep abnormalities with aminergic signaling

Patient Encounter, Part 1

An 18-year-old woman with a history of asthma comes to your clinic complaining of excessive daytime sleepiness, disrupted nighttime sleep, and strange weakness when she is surprised. She reports that she falls asleep relatively easily during the day if given a chance. She takes ethinyl estradiol/norethindrone 35 mcg/1 mg, albuterol MDI two puffs as needed shortness of breath, and fluticasone MDI 100 mcg two puffs twice a day.

What sleep disorders do her symptoms suggest?

What additional information do you need to know in your assessment of this patient?

Table 41–2

Pharmacokinetics and Dosing of Prescription Medications[a] Approved to Treat Insomnia

Generic Name	Parent $t_{1/2}$ (hours)	Duration of Action (hours)	Daily Dose Range (mg)	Recommended Daily Dose in Elderly (mg)[b]	Dose or Action in Hepatic Impairment	Comments
Doxepin (Silenor)	15.3	Unpublished[c]	3–6	3	3 mg	Effective for sleep maintenance difficulties only
Estazolam (Prosom)	2	12–15	1–2	0.5	Dose ↓ may be needed	Moderate duration
Eszopiclone (Lunesta)	6	8	2–3	1–2	1 mg in severe impairment	Can be used up to 6 months for chronic insomnia
Flurazepam (Dalmane)	8	10–30	15–30	15	No change necessary	High risk of hangover and residual effects
Quazepam (Doral)	2	25–41	7.5–15	7.5–15	Dose ↓ may be needed	High risk of hangover and residual effects
Ramelteon (Rozerem)	1–2.6	Unpublished[c]	8	No specific recommendations	Do not use in severe hepatic impairment	Noncontrolled substance; may be useful in patients with a history of substance abuse
Suvorexant (Belsomra)	12	Unpublished[c]	10–20	No specific recommendations	No change necessary	Novel mechanism of action—little documented rebound upon discontinuation
Temazepam (Restoril)	10–15	7	7.5–30	7.5	No change necessary	Moderate duration, well tolerated, inexpensive
Triazolam (Halcion)	2	6–7	0.125–0.25	0.125	0.125 mg	Short acting; little residual hangover
Zaleplon (Sonata)	1	6	5–10	5	5 mg	Short acting; only for difficulty falling asleep
Zolpidem (Ambien)	2–2.6	6–8	5–10[d]	5	5 mg	Short to moderate duration; no effects on sleep architecture
Zolpidem CR (Ambien CR)	2.8	7–8	6.25–12.5[d]	6.25	6.25 mg	Longer duration of action than regular release zolpidem
Zolpidem sublingual (Intermezzo)	2.5	< 4	1.75–3.5[d]	1.75	1.75 mg	Approved for middle-of-the-night insomnia taken > 4 hours before awakening

[a]In 2007, the Food and Drug Administration required additional information added to the safety labeling of sedative–hypnotic drugs concerning potential risks, including severe allergic reactions and complex sleep-related behaviors, which may include sleep driving. Sleep driving is defined as driving while not fully awake after ingestion of a sedative–hypnotic product with no memory of the event.

[b]If a dosing range is displayed, the first dose listed should be the starting dose.

[c]Data not available.

[d]For zolpidem, recommended dose for women is 5 mg, 6.25 mg for zolpidem CR, and 1.75 mg for sublingual zolpidem.

Adapted, with permission, from DiPiro JT, Talbert RL, Yee GC, et al (eds). Pharmacotherapy: A Pathophysiologic Approach. 9th ed. New York: McGraw-Hill; 2014:1118.

drugs. Modafinil (Provigil), armodafinil (Nuvigil), methylphenidate, and amphetamines are effective FDA-approved drugs for the treatment of EDS with narcolepsy.[40] Modafinil and armodafinil (the active R-isomer of modafinil) are Schedule IV medications, and these drugs may have fewer peripheral and cardiovascular effects than traditional stimulants. Selegiline, a selective monoamine oxidase B enzyme inhibitor, is metabolized to amphetamines and can reduce daytime sleepiness. In an individual patient, one wake-promoting agent may work better than another, and if the first drug selected is not successful at adequate doses, a trial with another agent should be attempted. KEY CONCEPT *Treatment of EDS in narcolepsy and other sleep disorders may require sustained- and immediate-release stimulants to promote wakefulness throughout the day and at key times that require alertness.* One potential treatment regimen includes a sustained-release stimulant preparation first thing in the morning and again at noon followed by an immediate-release stimulant preparation as needed in the late afternoon or before driving to maintain wakefulness. One advantage of traditional CNS stimulants over modafinil is their ability to help control cataplexy and REM-sleep abnormalities.

Traditional CNS stimulants have the potential to increase blood pressure and heart rate when used long term. In addition, excessive CNS stimulation can cause tremors and tics and can carry over into evening hours, disrupting normal nighttime sleep. Caution should be used in patients with underlying cardiovascular or cerebrovascular disease and in patients with a history of seizures because stimulants may lower the seizure threshold.

▶ *Cataplexy*

Traditionally, aminergic signaling antidepressants have been used effectively to control symptoms of cataplexy, sleep paralysis, and other REM-sleep manifestations of narcolepsy.[40] These include TCAs and certain selective serotonin and serotonin/norepinephrine reuptake inhibitors (SSRIs and SNRIs). Clomipramine, protriptyline, imipramine, venlafaxine, and fluoxetine are the agents that have been used most frequently. In addition, low-dose selegiline

Patient Encounter, Part 2: Medical History, Physical Examination, and Diagnostic Test

The patient undergoes further workup for her sleep complaint, which includes an overnight sleep study (in-lab) and a daytime nap study (MSLT).

PMH: Asthma × 8 years

FH: Noncontributory

SH: College freshman, has never smoked, does not drink alcohol

Meds: Ethinyl estradiol/norethindrone 35 mcg/1 mg, albuterol MDI two puffs Q 4–6 hours as needed, fluticasone MDI two puffs twice a day

ROS: (+) daytime sleepiness (Epworth sleepiness score: 18 out of 24); (–) symptoms of RLS

PE:

VS: BP 122/68, P 72, RR 16, T 37°C (98.6°F); BMI 21 kg/m^2

Labs: TSH 1.6 μIU/mL (mIU/L)

Overnight Polysomnogram: Bedtime at 10 PM; awake at 7 AM. No snoring or apneas observed, shortened REM sleep latency (15 minutes), frequent awakenings (13), 63 minutes awake after sleep onset.

- RDI 1 events/hour
- No significant leg movements

MSLT Test: Mean sleep latency = 3.5 minutes, 2 out of 5 sleep-onset REM periods

Given this additional information, summarize the patient's diagnosis.

Identify your treatment goals and therapy recommendations for the patient.

What nonpharmacologic and pharmacologic alternatives are available for this patient if the prescribed therapy is not successful or not tolerated?

may be effective at reducing cataplexy. Although not approved by the FDA for treatment of cataplexy, these drugs suppress REM sleep and have been the mainstay of anticataplectic therapy for years. Sodium oxybate, a potent sedative with a very short duration of action, is FDA approved for the treatment of narcolepsy with cataplexy. Its mechanism of action is not entirely known. Two doses per night are taken, one at bedtime and one follow-up dose taken 2½ to 4 hours later. Sodium oxybate is tightly regulated and is available from only one central pharmacy because of its high abuse potential.

Restless Legs Syndrome

KEY CONCEPT *RLS treatment involves suppression of abnormal sensations and leg movements and consolidation of sleep. Dopaminergic and sedative–hypnotic medications are prescribed commonly.* Dopamine agonists (DAs) successfully treat RLS symptoms and offer many advantages over levodopa–carbidopa, including longer half-lives to cover overnight symptoms, flexible dosing, and a reduced incidence of symptom augmentation. Up to 80% of patients who take levodopa–carbidopa eventually will experience symptom augmentation: RLS symptoms appear earlier in the day, previously unaffected body parts become involved, duration of relief gets shorter, and higher doses of medication are required to control symptoms.[41] Augmentation may be reduced by use of longer-duration DAs.[42] Ropinirole (Requip), pramipexole (Mirapex), and rotigotine (Neupro) are FDA approved for the treatment of RLS and are available in sustained-release products.[43] Gabapentin is an effective treatment for RLS, particularly in patients with painful symptoms.[44] The gabapentin prodrug (gabapentin enacarbil) is FDA approved for RLS at a recommended dose of 600 mg taken with food at about 5 pm.[45] BZDRAs such as temazepam, clonazepam, zolpidem, and zaleplon reduce arousals in patients with RLS.[46] Their main benefit is derived from improving sleep continuity in patients with RLS, particularly as adjunct treatment with other pharmacologic therapies. Opioids are effective in some patients with RLS symptoms, with oxycodone, hydrocodone, and codeine being used most frequently. For both BZDRAs and opioids, caution should be used in the elderly, in patients who are at risk for sleep apnea, and in patients with a history of substance abuse. Low iron levels frequently exacerbate RLS symptoms. Iron supplementation should be prescribed in patients who are iron deficient. Iron supplementation in patients with serum ferritin concentrations of less than 50 to 75 mcg/L (ng/mL; 112–169 pmol/L) improves RLS symptoms. Medications frequently used for RLS are shown in **Table 41–3**.

Obstructive Sleep Apnea

KEY CONCEPT *The main therapy for OSA is nasal* ***continuous positive airway pressure*** *(CPAP) therapy,* which alleviates sleep-disordered breathing by producing a positive pressure column in the upper airway using room air. A flexible tube connects the CPAP machine to a mask that covers the nose. CPAP therapy has a favorable impact on blood pressure and attenuates some of the potential hemodynamic and neurohumoral responses that may link OSA to systemic disease.

Not all individuals tolerate CPAP therapy, in part because it requires wearing a mask during sleep, and therapy can dry and irritate the upper airway. In some individuals, these barriers for adherence may be lessened or eliminated by properly fitting the mask, adding humidity to therapy, or using bilevel positive airway pressure (BiPAP) or auto titrating continuous positive airway pressure (AutoPAP) therapy. BiPAP therapy applies a variable pressure into the airway during the inspiratory phase of respiration but, unlike CPAP, reduces the applied pressure during the expiratory phase. AutoPAP machines are set for a pressure range and individualizes the pressure based on breath-to-breath analysis of the necessary pressure to keep the airway open.

Obesity can worsen sleep apnea, and weight management should be implemented for all overweight patients with OSA. In obese patients with mild OSA, weight loss alone can be effective, and studies have reported reduced severity of OSA with gastric stapling. For patients who cannot tolerate CPAP, oral appliances can be used to advance the lower jawbone and to keep the tongue forward to enlarge the upper airway. For individuals who have OSA only when on their backs during sleep, positional therapies may be effective. Surgical therapy (uvulopalatopharyngoplasty) is not a first-line option because of its invasiveness and relatively low long-term effectiveness.

There is no drug therapy for OSA. Drug therapy for symptoms of OSA may be considered in selected patients. Modafinil and armodafinil are wake-promoting medications that are approved by the FDA to treat residual daytime sleepiness despite CPAP therapy. Initiation of these medications should be attempted only after patients are using optimal CPAP therapy to alleviate

Table 41–3

Frequently Used Medications for Restless Legs Syndrome

Generic Name (Brand Name)	Half-Life (Hours)	Dose Range (mg/day)[a]	Potential Side Effect or Disadvantage
Dopaminergic Agents[b]			
Levodopa–carbidopa (Sinemet)	1.5–2	100–200 of levodopa	Nausea or vomiting; high incidence of symptom augmentation
Pramipexole (Mirapex)	8–12[c]	0.125–0.5	Nausea or vomiting; risk of compulsive behaviors[d]
Ropinirole (Requip)	6[e]	0.25–3	Nausea or vomiting; risk of compulsive behaviors[d]
Rotigotine (Neupro)	5–7	1–3	Application site reactions with patch
Anticonvulsants			
Gabapentin (Neurontin, Horizant)	5–7[c]	300–3600	Dizziness, ataxia
Pregabalin (Lyrica)	5–6.5	50–300	Weight gain, daytime sedation
Hypnotic Agents			
Clonazepam (Klonopin)	30–40	0.5–2	Tolerance, carryover sedation
Temazepam (Restoril)	10–15	7.5–30	Tolerance, carryover sedation
Zolpidem (Ambien)	2–2.6[e]	5–10	Tolerance
Zaleplon (Sonata)	1[e]	5–10	Tolerance; may not last entire night
Opioids			
Hydrocodone	3.8–4.5[e]	5–10	Constipation, nausea, sedation
Codeine	2.5–3.5[e]	30–60	Constipation, nausea, sedation
Methadone	22[e]	5–20	Constipation, nausea, sedation
Oxycodone	3.2–12[c,e]	5–30	Constipation, nausea, sedation

[a]Usual range; all medications (other than dopaminergic agents) are dosed at bedtime.

[b]Dopaminergic agents are frequently given at bedtime or 2 hours before bedtime or the anticipated onset of RLS symptoms.

[c]May be longer in patients with renal dysfunction.

[d]Compulsive behaviors such as gambling, shopping, sexual behaviors, and eating have been reported in patients taking dopamine agonists.

[e]May be longer in patients with hepatic dysfunction.

Data from Earley CJ. Restless legs syndrome. N Engl J Med. 2003;348:2103–2109.

sleep-disordered breathing. The need for treating residual sleepiness in this population is not clear because it may not be related to the OSA and is similar to sleepiness in the general population.[47] OSA should always be considered and evaluated in hypertensive patients who are resistant to therapy.

Parasomnias

NREM parasomnias usually do not require treatment. If needed, low-dose BZDRAs such as clonazepam can be prescribed for bothersome episodes. Clonazepam reduces the amount of sleep time spent in stages 3 and 4 of NREM sleep, when most NREM parasomnias occur. For treating RBD, clonazepam 0.5 to 2 mg at bedtime is the drug of choice, although melatonin 3 to 12 mg at bedtime also may be effective. Patients with RBD also should have dangerous objects removed from the bedroom and environmental accommodations made to reduce the chance of injury from breakthrough episodes.

Circadian Rhythm Disorders

Melatonin, 0.5 to 5 mg taken at appropriate target bedtimes for east or west travel, is the drug of choice for jet lag. Melatonin significantly reduces jet lag and shortens sleep latency in travelers.[48] Hypnotic agents with relatively short durations of action (3–5 hours) may also be used to sustain sleep during the initial adaptation to the new time zone.

Drug–Disease and Drug–Drug Interactions

KEY CONCEPT *It is important to review medication profiles for drugs that may aggravate sleep disorders. Patients should be monitored for adverse drug reactions and potential drug–drug interactions and assessed for treatment adherence.* Pharmacotherapy for sleep disorders should be individualized. Often medications can treat several concomitant sleep disorders. Conversely, drug therapy may be effective for one sleep disorder and exacerbate another. For example, antidepressants may alleviate depressive symptoms but exacerbate symptoms of RLS. Medications that

Patient Encounter, Part 3: Modifying the Treatment Plan

The patient returns to the clinic 3 months later. The physician previously diagnosed her with narcolepsy and cataplexy. She received a prescription for methylphenidate 20-mg tablets and was instructed to take one tablet twice daily (7 AM and noon). She reports today that the methylphenidate has made her feel more awake and slightly reduced her cataplexy. She still is somewhat sleepy during the day and has cataplexy more often than she would like. Her Epworth Sleepiness Scale (ESS) score today is 13 out of 24. She would like a medication that lasts longer and provides better control of her cataplexy.

Based on the information presented, recommend therapy for the patient.

What narcolepsy medications would you not want to use for this patient?

What medication-related precautions would you want to counsel the patient on?

Patient Care Process

Patient Assessment:

- Perform a detailed history of prescription, nonprescription, and complementary or alternative medication use.
- Based on patient nighttime and daytime complaints and bed partner report, determine the suspected sleep problem and its consequences.
- Review objective and subjective data regarding sleepiness, nighttime sleep quality, and limb movements, sleep disordered breathing, and parasomnias.
- Evaluate concomitant sleep and medical conditions that influence therapy decisions.

Therapy Evaluation:

- Evaluate effectiveness, safety, adherence, and side effects of therapy.
- Determine whether the patient has insurance coverage for prescribed medications.

Care Plan Development:

- For treatment of insomnia, try to ensure the lowest possible doses are prescribed and used for the shortest time period possible.
- If patient complaints are not entirely improved, consider increasing dose or adding a complementary agent.
- Ensure sleep hygiene (see Table 41–1) and drug therapy are appropriate for each sleep complaint.
- Determine if medication doses are optimal for treatment of various sleep disorders (see Tables 41–2 and 41–3).
- For insomnia select medications whose duration of action matches the timing of the difficulty sleeping (eg, difficulty initiating or maintaining sleep).

Follow-up Evaluation:

- Evaluate improvement in the specific sleep complaint (eg, how has therapy affected sleep latency or sleep maintenance?).
- Monitor daytime sleepiness, sleep diaries, and diaries of sleep events (PLMS, hallucinations, snoring, apneas, etc) and monitor cataplexy and other daytime symptoms to determine if therapy is effective.
- Make appropriate changes to therapy to address inadequately controlled symptoms and reported adverse effects.

block dopaminergic transmission may worsen RLS symptoms. Alcohol and CNS depressants, including opiates, sedatives, and muscle relaxants, can worsen OSA, even in small doses, by reducing respiratory drive and relaxing the upper airway muscles responsible for maintaining patency. CNS depressants should be avoided, and if they are necessary, they should not be administered before sleep. Drug therapy for sleep disorders should be patient specific, and careful consideration should be given to coexisting diseases, concomitant medications, and potential drug–drug and drug–disease interactions to optimize patient care and treatment.

OUTCOME EVALUATION

● Evaluate whether the treatment plan restored normal sleep patterns, reduced daytime sequelae, and improved quality of life without causing adverse effects. Schedule patients for follow-up within 3 weeks for insomnia and within 3 months for other sleep disorders. Perform a detailed clinical history to determine the patient's perception of treatment progress and symptoms along with medication effectiveness and side effects.

Instruct patients to keep sleep diaries (number of hours, number of awakenings, and worsening or improved sleep) and daytime symptoms, along with documentation of episodes such as cataplexy or RBD. Increase medication to effective doses, and if necessary, start additional therapy to control symptoms. Patients with sleep disorders should experience relief of symptoms the first night of drug therapy but may not receive maximal benefit (effect on daytime symptoms) for a few weeks. Perform a detailed history of prescription, nonprescription, and complementary or alternative medications and review the patient's sleep diary, daytime symptoms, and nonpharmacologic therapies on a regular basis.

Abbreviations Introduced in This Chapter

AutoPAP	Auto-titrating continuous positive airway pressure
BiPAP	Bilevel positive airway pressure
BMI	Body mass index
BZDRA	Benzodiazepine receptor agonist
CNS	Central nervous system
CPAP	Continuous positive airway pressure
CRD	Circadian rhythm disorder
DA	Dopamine agonist
EDS	Excessive daytime sleepiness
EEG	Electroencephalogram
ESS	Epworth Sleepiness Scale
FDA	Food and Drug Administration
GABA	γ-Aminobutyric acid
MSLT	Multiple sleep latency test
MWT	Maintenance of wakefulness test
NPSG	Nocturnal polysomnography
NREM	Non–rapid eye movement
OSA	Obstructive sleep apnea
PLMS	Periodic limb movements of sleep
RBD	REM-sleep behavior disorder
RDI	Respiratory disturbance index
REM	Rapid eye movement
RLS	Restless legs syndrome
SNRI	Serotonin/norepinephrine reuptake inhibitor
SSRI	Selective serotonin reuptake inhibitor
TCA	Tricyclic antidepressant

REFERENCES

1. Malow B. Approach to the patient with disordered sleep. In: Kryger M, Roth T, Dement W, eds. Principles and Practice of Sleep Medicine. 5th ed. St. Louis: Elsevier Saunders; 2011:641–646.
2. NIH State-of-the-Science Conference Statement on Manifestations and Management of Chronic Insomnia in Adults [online]. 2005, [cited 2011 Oct 10]. http://consensus.nih.gov/2005/insomnia.htm Accessed December 22, 2104.
3. Carskadon MA, Dement WC. Normal human sleep: An overview. In: Kryger M, Roth T, Dement W, eds. Principles and Practice of Sleep Medicine. 5th ed. St. Louis: Elsevier Saunders; 2011:16–26.
4. Roth T. Insomnia: Definition, prevalence, etiology, and consequences. J Clin Sleep Med. 2007;15(5 Suppl):S7–S10.

5. Kim K, Uchiyama M, Okawa M, et al. An epidemiological study of insomnia among the Japanese general population. Sleep. 2000;23: 41–47.
6. McCall WV. A psychiatric perspective on insomnia. J Clin Psychiatry. 2001;62(Suppl 10):27–32.
7. Silber MH, Krahn LE, Olson EJ, et al. The epidemiology of narcolepsy in Olmsted County, Minnesota: A population-based study. Sleep. 2002;25:197–202.
8. Tashiro T, Kambayashi T, Hishikawa Y. An epidemiological study of narcolepsy in Japanese. Proceedings of the 4th International Symposium on Narcolepsy. Tokyo, Japan. June 16–17, 1994:13.
9. Lavie P, Peled R. Narcolepsy is a rare disease in Israel. Sleep. 1987;10:608–609.
10. Mignot E, Hayduk R, Black J, et al. HLA DQB1*0602 is associated with cataplexy in 509 narcoleptic patients. Sleep. 1997;20:1012–1020.
11. Berger K, Kurth T. RLS epidemiology—frequencies, risk factors and methods in population studies. Mov Disord. 2007;22(Suppl):S420–S423.
12. Phillips B, Young T, Finn L, et al. Epidemiology of restless legs symptoms in adults. Arch Intern Med. 2000;160:2137–2141.
13. Lee KA, Zaffke ME, Baratte-Beebe K. Restless legs syndrome and sleep disturbance during pregnancy: The role of folate and iron. J Womens Health Gend Based Med. 2001;10:335–341.
14. Bonati MT, Ferini-Strambi L, Aridon P, et al. Autosomal dominant restless legs syndrome maps on chromosome 14q. Brain. 2003;126:1485–1492.
15. Young T, Palta M, Dempsey J, et al. The occurrence of sleep-disordered breathing among middle-aged adults. N Engl J Med. 1993;328:1230–1235.
16. Ohayon MM, Caulet M, Priest RG. Violent behavior during sleep. J Clin Psychiatry. 1997;58:369–376.
17. Mignot E, Lin X, Arrigoni J, et al. DQB10602 and DQA1*0102(DQ1) are better markers than DR2 for narcolepsy in Caucasian and black Americans. Sleep. 1994;17:S60–S67.
18. Mignot E, Kimura A, Lattermann A, et al. Extensive HLA class II studies in 58 non-DRB1*15(DR2) narcoleptic patients with cataplexy. Tissue Antigens. 1997;49:329–341.
19. Nishino S, Ripley B, Overeem S, et al. Hypocretin (orexin) deficiency in human narcolepsy. Lancet. 2000;355:39–40.
20. Connor JR, Boyer PJ, Menzies SL, et al. Neuropathological examination suggests impaired brain iron acquisition in restless legs syndrome. Neurology. 2003;61:304–309.
21. Salminen AV, Rimpila V, Polo O. Peripheral hypoxia in restless legs syndrome (Willis-Ekbom disease). Neurology. 2014;82:1856–1861.
22. Somers VK, White DP, Amin R, et al. Sleep apnea and cardiovascular disease: An American Heart Association/American College of Cardiology Foundation Scientific Statement from the American Heart Association Council for High Blood Pressure Research Professional Education Committee, Council on Clinical Cardiology, Stroke Council, and Council on Cardiovascular Nursing. In collaboration with the National Heart, Lung, and Blood Institute, National Center on Sleep Disorders Research (National Institutes of Health). Circulation. 2008;118:1080–1111.
23. Sahlin C, Sandberg O, Gustafson Y, et al. Obstructive sleep apnea is a risk factor for death in patients with stroke. Arch Intern Med. 2008;168:297–301.
24. Peppard PE, Young T, Palta M, et al. Prospective study of the association between sleep-disordered breathing and hypertension. N Engl J Med. 2000;342:1378–1384.
25. Somers VK, Dyken ME, Clary MP, et al. Sympathetic neural mechanisms in obstructive sleep apnea. J Clin Invest. 1995;96:1897–1904.
26. Buscemi N, Vandermeer B, Friesen C, et al. The efficacy and safety of drug treatments for chronic insomnia in adults: A meta-analysis of RCTs. J Gen Intern Med. 2007;22:1335–1350.
27. Schutte-Rodin S, Broch L, Buysse D, et al. Clinical guideline for the evaluation and management of chronic insomnia in adults. J Clin Sleep Med. 2008;4:487–504.
28. Krystal AD, Walsh JK, Laska E, et al. Sustained efficacy of eszopiclone over 6 months of nightly treatment: Results of a randomized, double-blind, placebo-controlled study in adults with chronic insomnia. Sleep. 2003;26:793–799.
29. Becker WC, Fiellin DA, Desai RA. Non-medical use, abuse and dependence on sedatives and tranquilizers among U.S. adults: Psychiatric and socio-demographic correlates. Drug Alcohol Depend. 2007;90:280–287.
30. Roth T, Roehrs T. Issues in the use of benzodiazepine therapy. J Clin Psychiatry. 1992;53(Suppl):S14–S18.
31. Roth T, Roehrs TA, Stepanski EJ, et al. Hypnotics and behavior. Am J Med. 1990(Suppl);8:S43–S46.
32. Greenblatt D, Harmatz JS, Shapiro L, et al. Sensitivity to triazolam in elderly. N Engl J Med. 1991;324:1691–1698.
33. Golden RN, Dawkins K, Nicholas L. Trazodone and nefazodone. In: Schatzberg A, Nemeroff CB, eds. The American Psychiatric Textbook of Psychopharmacology. Washington, DC: American Psychiatric Publishing; 2004:315–325.
34. Bucknall C, Brooks D, Curry PV, et al. Mianserin and trazodone for cardiac patients with depression. Eur J Clin Pharmacol. 1988;33:565–569.
35. Kudo Y, Kurihara M. Clinical evaluation of diphenhydramine hydrochloride for the treatment of insomnia in psychiatric patients. J Clin Pharmacol. 1990;30:1041–1048.
36. Johnson MW, Suess PE, Griffiths RR. A novel hypnotic lacking abuse liability and sedative adverse effects. Arch Gen Psychiatry. 2006;63:1149–1157.
37. Kryger M, Roth T, Wang-Weigand S, et al. The effects of ramelteon on respiration during sleep in subjects with moderate to severe chronic obstructive pulmonary disease. Sleep Breath. 2009;13:79–84.
38. Kryger M, Wang-Weigand S, Roth T. Safety of ramelteon in individuals with mild to moderate obstructive sleep apnea. Sleep Breath. 2007;11:159–164.
39. Product Information: Belsomra, (suvorexant). Whitehouse Station, NJ: Merck & Co., Inc., 8/2014.
40. Morganthaler TI, Kapur VK, Brown T, et al. Practice parameters for the treatment of narcolepsy and other hypersomnias of central origin an American Academy of Sleep Medicine Report. Sleep. 2007;30: 1705–1711.
41. Earley CJ, Allen RP. Pergolide and carbidopa/levodopa treatment of the restless legs syndrome and periodic leg movements in sleep in a consecutive series of patients. Sleep. 1996;19:801–810.
42. Benes H, Garcia-Borreguero D, Ferini-Strambi L, et al. Augmentation in the treatment of restless legs syndrome with transdermal rotigotine. Sleep Med. 2012;13:589–597.
43. Aurora RN, Kristo DA, Bista SR, et al. The treatment of restless legs syndrome and periodic limb movement disorder in adults– an update for 2012: Practice parameters with an evidence-based systematic review and meta-analyses: An American Academy of Sleep Medicine Clinical Practice Guideline. Sleep. 2012;35:1039–1062.
44. Garcia-Borreguero D, Larrosa O, de la Llave Y, et al. Treatment of restless legs syndrome with gabapentin: A double-blind, cross-over study. Neurology. 2002;59:1573–1579.
45. Product Information: Horizant, gabapentin enacarbil. Research Triangle Park, NC: GlaxoSmithKline Pharmaceuticals, 2011.
46. Earley CJ. Restless legs syndrome. N Engl J Med. 2003; 348:2103–2109.
47. Stradling JR, Smith D, Crosby J. Post-CPAP sleepiness—a specific syndrome? J Sleep Res. 2007;16:436–438.
48. Herxheimer A, Petrie KJ. Melatonin for the prevention and treatment of jet lag. Cochrane Database Syst Rev. 2005;(4):CD001520.

42 Attention-Deficit/ Hyperactivity Disorder

Kevin W. Cleveland and John Erramouspe

LEARNING OBJECTIVES

Upon completion of the chapter, the reader will be able to:

1. Explain accepted criteria necessary for the diagnosis of attention-deficit/hyperactivity disorder (ADHD).
2. Recommend a therapeutic plan, including drug selection, initial doses, dosage forms, and monitoring parameters, for a patient with ADHD.
3. Differentiate among the available pharmacologic agents used for ADHD with respect to pharmacology and pharmaceutical formulation.
4. Recommend second-line and/or adjunctive agents that can be effective alternatives in the treatment of ADHD when stimulant therapy is less than adequate.
5. Address potential cost–benefit issues associated with pharmacotherapy of ADHD.
6. Recommend strategies for minimizing adverse effects of ADHD medications.

Attention-deficit/hyperactivity disorder is characterized by a persistent pattern of inattention and/or hyperactivity-impulsivity. It can have a severe impact on a patient's ability to function in both academic and social environments. Early diagnosis and appropriate treatment are essential to compensate for areas of deficit.

EPIDEMIOLOGY AND ETIOLOGY

KEY CONCEPT *This disorder usually begins by 3 years of age but must occur before 12 years of age to meet current diagnostic criteria.* In the United States, ADHD is the most common neurobehavioral disorder that affects children.[1–4] ADHD has been estimated to occur in 4.3% to 9.5% of school-aged children.[4,5] ADHD occurs more than twice as often in school-aged boys than girls.[5]

Although ADHD generally is considered a childhood disorder, symptoms can persist into adolescence and adulthood. The prevalence of adult ADHD is estimated to be 2.5 %; however, 60% of adults with ADHD have symptoms that manifested in childhood.[6,7,8] Furthermore, problems associated with ADHD (eg, social, marital, academic, career, anxiety, depression, smoking, and substance abuse problems) increase with the transition of patients into adulthood.

PATHOPHYSIOLOGY

KEY CONCEPT *The exact pathologic cause of ADHD has not been identified.* ADHD is generally thought of as a disorder of self-regulation or **response inhibition**. Patients who meet the criteria for ADHD have difficulty maintaining self-control, resisting distractions, and concentrating on ideas.[4,9,10] Furthermore, children with ADHD often alternate between inattentiveness to monotonous tasks and overexcitement. Multiple brain studies have failed to elucidate any pathophysiologic basis for ADHD.

KEY CONCEPT *Dysfunction of the neurotransmitters norepinephrine and dopamine is thought to be key in the pathology of ADHD.* Whereas norepinephrine is responsible for maintaining alertness and attention, dopamine is responsible for regulating learning, motivation, goal setting, and memory. Both of these neurotransmitters predominate in the frontal subcortical system, an area of the brain responsible for maintaining attention and memory. Genetics appears to play a role because a child who has a parent with ADHD has a 50% chance of developing ADHD. An association has been made between the development of ADHD and fetal alcohol syndrome, lead poisoning, maternal smoking, and hypoxia.[4,10]

CLINICAL PRESENTATION AND DIAGNOSIS

KEY CONCEPT *ADHD is rarely encountered without comorbid conditions and often is undiagnosed.* Between 50% and 60% of patients with ADHD will have one or more comorbidities (eg, learning disabilities, oppositional defiant, conduct, anxiety, or depressive disorders).[2] It is important to identify and appropriately treat coexisting conditions in patients with ADHD.

According to newer diagnostic and treatment guidelines, all patients 4 to 18 years of age presenting with inattention, hyperactivity, impulsivity, academic, and/or behavioral problems should be evaluated for ADHD. Additional information about behavior in various settings should be gathered from the patient, family, and teachers, or supervisors. The age of onset, frequency, severity, and duration of symptoms should be documented.[6,11]

The most useful diagnostic criteria for ADHD is the *Diagnostic and Statistical Manual of Mental Disorders*, 5th edition (*DSM-5*).[6] The *DSM-5* defines three presentations of ADHD: (a) predominately inattentive, (b) predominantly hyperactive impulsive; and (c) combined, in which both inattentive and hyperactive or impulsive symptoms are evident.[11] Neuroimaging, electroencephalograms, and continuous performance examinations are investigational and not used clinically for diagnosis. It is recommended that parents and teachers complete a standardized rating scale based on the *DSM-5* criteria.[6] These rating scales are not by themselves diagnostic but are diagnostic aids when added to a careful history and interview.[12]

Although ADHD is considered a childhood disorder, signs and symptoms persist into adolescence in 40% to 80% of cases and into adulthood in approximately 60% of cases.[1,7] Adult ADHD is difficult to assess, and diagnosis is always suspect in patients failing to display clear symptoms before 12 years of age.[10,11] Untreated adults with ADHD have higher rates of psychopathology, substance abuse, social dysfunction, and occupational underachievement than adults without ADHD.

TREATMENT

Desired Outcomes

KEY CONCEPT *The primary therapeutic objectives in ADHD are to improve behavior and increase attention or response inhibition; secondary goals of treatment are to:*

- Improve relationships with family, teachers, and peers
- Decrease disruptive behavior in academic and social settings
- Improve academic performance
- Increase independence in activities
- Minimize undesirable adverse effects of therapy

> **Clinical Presentation and Diagnosis of ADHD**
>
> **General**
>
> Patients with ADHD can present with inattention, hyperactivity–impulsivity, or both. ADHD is typically encountered with comorbid conditions.
>
> **Symptoms**
>
> - Inattentive type: difficulty paying attention to details in school, work, and social activities; difficulty completing tasks that require a lot of mental effort; easily distracted; forgetful
> - Hyperactive–impulsive type: difficulty sitting still, fidgets; has trouble playing quietly and waiting turns; frequently interrupts
> - Combined: exhibits both inattention and hyperactivity–impulsivity
>
> **Diagnostic Criteria**
>
> - Must exhibit 6 of 9 symptoms before 12 years of age that persist for at least 6 months
> - Symptoms must be present in two or more settings and adversely affect functioning in social situations, school, or work
> - Must meet the diagnostic criteria in *DSM-5* for ADHD
> - Symptoms cannot be better explained by another mental disorder (eg, autism)

Nonpharmacologic (Behavioral) Therapy

Behavioral therapy can be useful; however, it is generally not recommended as first-line monotherapy except in preschool-aged children (4–5 years of age).[6,11] KEY CONCEPT *Several studies have demonstrated that treatment with medication alone is superior to behavioral intervention alone in improving attention. However, behavioral therapy in combination with stimulant therapy is better at improving oppositional and aggressive behaviors.*[13] Behavioral modification involves training parents, teachers, and caregivers to change the physical and social environment and establish a reward or consequence system.[10,11] Success of behavioral modifications depends on the cooperation and involvement of the patient's parents and teachers.

Pharmacologic Therapy

The proposed mechanism of ADHD pharmacotherapy is to modulate neurotransmitter function in order to improve academic and social functioning. Pharmacologic therapy can be divided into two categories—stimulants and nonstimulants. Stimulants include methylphenidate, dexmethylphenidate, dextroamphetamine–amphetamine (amphetamine salts), dextroamphetamine, and lisdexamfetamine, and nonstimulant medications include atomoxetine, bupropion, clonidine, and guanfacine.

▶ *Stimulants*

KEY CONCEPT *Psychostimulants (eg, methylphenidate and dextroamphetamine with or without amphetamine) are the most effective agents in treating ADHD. Following diagnosis of ADHD, a stimulant medication should be considered first-line therapy in patients 6 years of age or older.* In preschool-aged children, methylphenidate can be added to the patient's treatment if behavioral

> **Patient Encounter, Part 1**
>
> The single mother of a rowdy 8-year-old boy comes to your clinic. The mother is upset due to a recent altercation with her grandfather over her son's behavior. Her grandfather claims her son swears, is careless, violent, and has destructive tendencies such as pulling and flicking the hair and head of other family members, especially his 5-year-old brother. She had been living with her parents in an effort to save money since she has a minimum wage job as a room cleaner for a local motel, but recently she has moved her two sons and herself to their own apartment. During the visit, her son is easily distracted, all over the examination room investigating and getting into everything. He even launches a paper airplane twice during the visit which hits both his mother and you. His performance at school on the few assignments he has completed has consistently been failing. During his physical education class, he frequently pushes and shoves others in order to not have to wait for his turn. On two occasions, he has been sent home from school for unruly behavior.
>
> ***Which of the patient's symptoms are suggestive of ADHD?***
>
> ***What other comorbid conditions should the child be evaluated for before starting therapy for ADHD?***
>
> ***What other information do you need to assess for ADHD?***
>
> ***What help or suggestions could you offer to his parents?***

modification monotherapy is not sufficient in managing ADHD symptoms.[10] Stimulants are safe and effective and have a response rate of 70% to 90%.[3,11,14] Generally, a trial of at least 3 months on a stimulant is appropriate, and this includes dose titration to response while balancing side effects.[8,10,11] KEY CONCEPT *If treatment with the first stimulant formulation fails, it is recommended to switch to a different stimulant formulation.*[6,10] For example, if the patient was started on methylphenidate but could not tolerate the side effects, switching to dextroamphetamine with or without amphetamine is appropriate. Most patients who fail one stimulant will respond to an alternative stimulant.[10,11] KEY CONCEPT *If the patient fails two adequate trials of different stimulant medications, a third stimulant formulation or second-line nonstimulant such as bupropion, atomoxetine, guanfacine, or clonidine can be considered.* The diagnosis of ADHD should be revalidated as well.

Stimulants theoretically exert their primary effect by blocking the reuptake of dopamine and norepinephrine. They have been shown to decrease fidgeting and finger tapping, increase on-task classroom behavior and positive interactions at home and in social environments, and ameliorate conduct and anxiety disorders.[14]

Stimulants should be initiated at recommended starting doses and titrated up with a consistent dosing schedule to the appropriate response while minimizing side effects (Table 42–1). Generally, stimulants should not be used in patients who have glaucoma, severe hypertension or cardiovascular disease, hyperthyroidism, severe anxiety, or previous illicit or stimulant drug abuse. Stimulants can be used, albeit cautiously, in patients with seizure disorders, Tourette syndrome, and motor tics.[14]

Stimulant drug formulations can be divided into short-, intermediate-, and extended-acting preparations (see Table 42–1). Initial response to short-acting stimulant formulations (eg, methylphenidate and dextroamphetamine) is seen within 30 minutes and can last for 4 to 6 hours.[6,10,14] Thus short-acting stimulant formulations must frequently be dosed at least twice daily, increasing the chance of missed doses and noncompliance. Patients using any stimulant formulation, but especially short-acting formulations, can experience a rebound effect of ADHD symptoms as the stimulant wears off.[14]

Most intermediate-acting stimulants release the medication in a slow, continuous fashion without any early release (except Dexedrine Spansules). The onset of action for this category of stimulants (typically 60–90 minutes) may be inadequate for some patients. Some practitioners prescribe a short-acting stimulant concurrently with an intermediate-acting stimulant to curtail the delay in onset of action of the intermediate-acting stimulant. However, this practice can increase patient copay costs.

To minimize rebound symptoms associated with short-acting formulations and still achieve early stimulant release, extended-acting formulations with rapid onsets have been developed. These formulations have an early release of medication and deliver a delayed release of stimulant in either a pulsed (Adderall XR, Focalin XR, Metadate CD, Quillivant XR and Ritalin LA) or continuous manner (Concerta). Formulations available as capsules contain coated beads that can be opened and sprinkled on semisolid food. Concerta tablets have an immediate-release overcoat and an oral osmotic controlled-release that delivers methylphenidate in an extended manner. Patients should be counseled that the empty tablet shell of Concerta can be seen in the stool.

Two extended-acting stimulants, Daytrana and Vyvanse, have slower onsets of action than the other extended-acting stimulants with a rapid release. Daytrana transdermal patches are to be applied for only 9 hours per day and have a delayed onset of 2 hours, and their effects persist for 3 hours after being removed. Some patients report skin sensitization and irritation. Vyvanse is a prodrug that is hydrolyzed to its active form, dextroamphetamine, after oral ingestion. Inhalation or injection abuse potential is minimized because of impeded hydrolysis by these routes. Onset of action for Vyvanse has been reported to be 2 hours.[15]

Adverse effects of stimulants can be generalized to the whole class (Table 42–2). Most side effects can be managed by changing the dosing routine (ie, giving with food, dividing daily dose, or giving the dose earlier in the day). Serious side effects (eg, hallucinations and abnormal movements) require discontinuation of medication.[6,10,14] To avoid potential drug–food interactions and absorption issues, stimulants should be given 30 to 60 minutes before eating.

Growth suppression or delay is a major concern for parents of children taking stimulants. Growth delay appears to be transient and to resolve by midadolescence, but more data are needed to resolve this issue. Another concern is risk of substance abuse with stimulant use. A diagnosis of ADHD alone increases the risk of substance abuse in adolescents and adults. However, stimulant use has not been shown to further increase this risk but actually may decrease this risk, provided ADHD is treated adequately.[16]

The choice of ADHD medication should be made based on the patient's condition, prescriber's familiarity with the medications, ease of administration, and cost. Stimulants should be used as first-line agents in most ADHD patients, although studies in groups of patients have shown no clear advantage of one stimulant over another.[17]

▶ *Nonstimulants*

Atomoxetine Atomoxetine is approved for the treatment of ADHD in both children and adults. In clinical studies, it demonstrated superior efficacy over placebo and either equivalent efficacy compared with a suboptimal immediate-release methylphenidate dose or inferior to Concerta.[18–23] KEY CONCEPT *Atomoxetine may be used as a second- or third-line medication for ADHD.*

Atomoxetine selectively inhibits the reuptake of adrenergic neurotransmitters, principally norepinephrine.[18–21] Atomoxetine is metabolized through the cytochrome P450 (CYP) 2D6 pathway. Concurrent use of certain antidepressants (ie, fluoxetine, paroxetine) may inhibit this enzyme and necessitate slower dose titration of atomoxetine. Approximately 5% to 10% of the population are CYP2D6 poor metabolizers, and atomoxetine's half-life is increased significantly in this population.[24] The recommended dosing for atomoxetine depends on patient weight and is given once or twice daily[24] (see Table 42–1). In poor metabolizers, atomoxetine should be dosed once daily at 25% to 50% of the dose typically used in normal metabolizers.[24] The maximum therapeutic effect of atomoxetine may take up to 4 weeks, significantly longer than with stimulants. Common side effects of atomoxetine are similar to those of stimulants. Some studies have reported an increase in blood pressure and heart rate.[19–21] It can slow growth rate and cause weight loss; thus, height and weight should be monitored routinely in children[19–21] (see Table 42–2). Atomoxetine's labeling includes warnings about severe hepatotoxicity and increased association with suicidal thinking.

Atomoxetine can be given once daily in many patients. It appears to lack any abuse potential and is not a controlled substance.[25] One big disadvantage of atomoxetine is cost compared with other ADHD medications (Table 42–3).

Table 42–1

Selected Medications for ADHD[a]

Drug, Generic (Brand Name)	Initial Dose	Titration Schedule Increments	Typical Dosing Range (Maximum Dose)
Stimulants			
Short Acting			
Methylphenidate[b] (Methylin, Ritalin)	5 mg twice daily	5–10 mg/day in weekly intervals	5–20 mg two to three times daily (60 mg/day)
Dexmethylphenidate[b] (Focalin)	2.5 mg twice daily	2.5–5 mg/day in weekly intervals	5–10 mg twice daily (20 mg/day)
Dextroamphetamine[b] (Dexedrine)	2.5–5 mg every morning	2.5–5 mg/day in weekly intervals	5–20 mg twice daily (40 mg/day)
Intermediate Acting			
Methylphenidate[b] (Ritalin SR, Metadate ER, Methylin ER)	10 mg once daily	10 mg/day in weekly intervals	20–40 mg daily in the morning (60 mg/day)
Dextroamphetamine–amphetamine[b] (Adderall)	2.5–5 mg once to twice daily	2.5–5 mg/day in weekly intervals	10–30 mg every morning or 5–20 mg twice daily (40 mg/day)
Dextroamphetamine[b] (Dexedrine Spansule)	5 mg every morning	5 mg/day in weekly intervals	5–30 mg daily or 5–15 mg twice daily (40 mg/day)
Extended Acting			
Methylphenidate[b]			
(Concerta)	18 mg every morning	9–18 mg/day in weekly intervals	18–54 mg every morning (54 mg/day in children)
(Metadate CD)	20 mg every morning	10–20 mg/day in weekly intervals	20–40 mg daily in the morning (60 mg/day)
(Ritalin LA)	20 mg every morning	10 mg/day in weekly intervals	20–40 mg daily in the morning (60 mg/day)
(Quillivant XR)[c]	20 mg every morning	10-20 mg/day in weekly intervals	20-40 mg daily in the morning (60 mg/day)
Dextroamphetamine/amphetamine[b] (Adderall XR)	5–10 mg every morning (children); 20 mg once daily (adults)	5–10 mg/day in weekly intervals	10–30 mg every morning or 5–15 mg twice daily (30 mg/day, children) (60 mg/day, adult)
Dexmethylphenidate[b] (Focalin XR)	5 mg every morning (children); 10 mg every morning (adults)	5 mg/day in weekly intervals	10–20 mg daily in the morning (20 mg/day)
Lisdexamfetamine[b] (Vyvanse)	30 mg every morning (children and adults)	10–20 mg/day in weekly intervals	30–70 mg daily in the morning (70 mg/day)
Nonstimulants			
Atomoxetine[b,d] (Strattera)	≤ 70 kg: 0.5 mg/kg/day divided once to twice daily	To target dose of 1.2 mg/kg/day after 3 days	40–60 mg/day (1.4 mg/kg or 100 mg/day, whichever is less)
	> 70 kg: 40 mg once daily	40 mg/day after 3 days (may ↑ to total of 100 mg/day after 2–3 weeks)	40–80 mg/day divided once to twice daily (100 mg/day)
Clonidine (Catapres)	0.05 mg once daily	0.05 mg/day every 3–7 days	0.1 mg 1 to 4 times daily (0.4 mg/day)
(Kapvay)[b]	0.1 mg at bedtime	0.1 mg/day in weekly intervals	0.1–0.2 mg twice daily (0.4 mg/day)
Guanfacine (Tenex)	0.5 mg at bedtime	0.5 mg every 3–14 days	1.5–3 mg/day divided into 2–3 doses (4 mg/day)
(Intuniv)[b]	1 mg once daily	No more than 1 mg/week	1–4 mg daily (4 mg/day)
Bupropion (Wellbutrin, Wellbutrin SR, Wellbutrin XL)	3 mg/kg/day for 7 days (children); 150 mg once daily of SR or XL (adults)	3 mg/kg/day in weekly intervals (children); increase 150–300 mg/day in weekly intervals (adults)	6 mg/kg/day or 400 mg/day—whichever is smaller (children); 150–450 mg/day (400 mg/day SR; 450 mg/day XL—adults)

[a]Pediatric dosing except when adult dosing specified.

[b]Approved by the US FDA for the treatment of ADHD.

[c]Oral extended-release suspension.

[d]Dose adjustment required in patients with hepatic insufficiency.

CD, extended release (biphasic immediate release with extended release); ER, extended release; LA, long acting; SR, sustained release; XL, extended release.

Table 42–2

Patient Monitoring and Management of Selected Adverse Effects of ADHD Medications

Drug	Adverse Effects	Management	Monitoring
Stimulants			
Methylphenidate dexmethylphenidate dextroamphetamine with or without amphetamine lisdexamfetamine	GI upset, nausea, decreased appetite, potential growth delay	Administer after breakfast and lunch Encourage high-calorie meals/beverages and snacks after dinner Divide dose Change to shorter-acting stimulant Discontinue on weekends and during holidays	Height, weight, blood pressure, pulse ECG if warranted Eating and sleeping patterns Evaluate every 2–4 weeks until stable dose is achieved; then evaluate every 3 months
	Insomnia	Move dose(s) earlier in the day and discontinue later day dose if problem persists Change to a shorter-acting stimulant Consider adjunct hypnotic (eg, melatonin) or alternate medication (eg, guanfacine, bupropion)	
	Headache	Decrease dose Change to longer-acting stimulant or nonstimulant (eg, atomoxetine) Consider analgesic (eg, acetaminophen)	
	Irritability, dysphoria, agitation	Early onset (peak related): Decrease dose or change to longer-acting stimulant Late onset (withdrawal related): Change to longer-acting stimulant Evaluate for comorbidity and treat if present	
	Tics	Decrease dose Change to a different stimulant or a nonstimulant (eg, guanfacine, atomoxetine) Add an antipsychotic (eg, risperidone)	
Nonstimulants			
Atomoxetine	Increased blood pressure and pulse, nausea, vomiting, fatigue, and insomnia	Decrease dose or change to another medication (eg, guanfacine, bupropion)	Same as above but with baseline and routine liver function tests for hepatotoxicity
	Hepatotoxicity, suicidal thoughts	Discontinue or change to another medication	
Clonidine and guanfacine	Sedation	Decrease dose Administer closer to bedtime	Same as above
Bupropion	GI upset, restlessness, sleep disturbances, tremor	Decrease dose or change to another medication (eg, guanfacine)	Height, weight, blood pressure, pulse every month
	Tics, rash, seizures	discontinue medication	Eating and sleeping patterns

ECG, electrocardiography; GI, gastointestinal.

Because of the high cost, lack of long-term efficacy data, and few comparison studies with stimulants, atomoxetine should be advocated only if the patient has failed or is intolerant to stimulant therapy.

Bupropion Bupropion is a monocyclic antidepressant that weakly inhibits the reuptake of norepinephrine and dopamine. It is effective for symptoms of ADHD in children, and preliminary results suggest it may be as effective as methylphenidate.[26,27] Similar results have been shown in adults.[26] Bupropion is well tolerated with minimal side effects (eg, insomnia, headache, nausea, and tremor) which typically disappear with continuation of therapy and with slow titration of dose. Bupropion can worsen tics and movement disorders. It is a rational choice in an ADHD patient with comorbid depression.[26] However, seizures have been associated with bupropion doses greater than 6 mg/kg/day.[28] Seizures related to high doses can be minimized by reducing the dose or switching to a longer-acting formulation. Bupropion can increase the risk of suicidal ideation and is contraindicated in patients with seizure and eating disorders.

Clonidine and Guanfacine Clonidine and guanfacine are central α_2-adrenergic agonists that inhibit the release of norepinephrine presynaptically. Both of these agents are less effective than stimulants in treating ADHD but typically are used as adjuncts to stimulants to control disruptive or aggressive behavior and alleviate insomnia.[29] The effects of immediate-release guanfacine typically last 3 to 4 hours longer than immediate-release clonidine, and the drug requires less frequent dosing. Extended-release formulations of guanfacine (Intuniv) and clonidine

Table 42–3

Cost[a] of 30-Day Supply of Selected ADHD Medication Regimens

Medications	Regimens	Cost[a]
Short-Acting Rapid-Onset Stimulants		
Methylphenidate		
Generic	5-, 10-, or 20-mg tablet twice daily	$
Dexmethylphenidate		
Generic	2.5-mg tablet twice daily	$
Generic	5- or 10-mg tablet twice daily	$$
Dextroamphetamine		
Generic	5-mg tablet twice daily	$
Intermediate-Acting Slower-Onset Stimulants		
Methylphenidate		
Methylin ER	10- or 20-mg ER tablet daily	$
Dextroamphetamine[b]		
Generic	10-, or 15-mg capsule daily	$$$$
Dextroamphetamine/amphetamine		
Generic	5-, 7.5-, 10-, 12.5-, 15-, 20-, or 30-mg tablet daily	$
Extended-Acting Rapid-Onset Stimulants		
Methylphenidate		
Concerta (brand & generics)[b]	18-, 27-, 36-, or 54-mg tablet daily	$$$$
Metadate CD (brand & generics)[c]	10-, 20-, or 30-mg capsule daily	$$$$
Ritalin LA (brand & generics)[c]	10-, 20-mg capsule daily	$$$$
Quillivant XR[c]	10, 20, 25, or 30 mg of suspension daily	$$$$
Dextroamphetamine/amphetamine		
Adderall XR (brand and generics)	5-, 10-, 15-, 20-, 25-, or 30-mg capsule daily	$$$$
Dexmethylphenidate		
Focalin XR (brand & generics)[c]	5-, 10-, 15-, 20-, 25-, 30-, 35-, or 40-mg capsule daily	$$$$
Extended-Acting Slower-Onset Stimulants		
Lisdexamfetamine		
Vyvanse	20-, 30-, 40-, 50-, 60-, or 70-mg capsule daily	$$$$
Nonstimulants		
Atomoxetine		
Strattera	10-, 18-, 25-, 40-, 60-, 80-, or 100-mg capsule daily	$$$$
Clonidine		
Generic	0.1-, 0.2-, or 0.3-mg tablet twice daily	$
Kapvay	0.1- or 0.2-mg tablet twice daily	$$$$
Guanfacine		
Generic	1- or 2-mg tablet twice daily	$
Intuniv	1-, 2-, 3-, or 4-mg tablet daily	$$$$
Bupropion		
Generic	75-mg tablet twice daily	$
Generic	150-mg SR tablet twice daily	$
Generic	200-mg SR tablet twice daily	$$
Generic	150-mg XL tablet daily	$

[a]Cost based on brand regimen specified without a dispensing fee or discount for a 30-day supply. (From PrescriptionBlueBook.com or various online State Maximum Allowable Costs [SMAC].)

[b]Ascending release (early then gradual/continuous).

[c]Bimodal release (early then late; mimics twice daily dosing of shorter-acting stimulant counterpart).

$, less than $40; $$, $40–$79; $$$, $80–$120; $$$$, greater than $120.

CD, controlled release (biphasic immediate release with extended release); ER, extended release; LA, long-acting; SR, sustain release; XL, extended release.

(Kapvay) were developed to minimize dosing frequency and improve treatment of anger, hostility, and irritability in patients with ADHD. Similar to other nonstimulants, these two dosage forms can also be used in patients who are intolerant to stimulants. However, use of these dosage forms is limited because of a lack of comparative trials to stimulants and high cost. Common side effects with clonidine and guanfacine are low blood pressure and sedation. Sedation generally subsides after 2 to 3 weeks of therapy.[29,30] Rarely, severe side effects such as bradycardia, rebound hypertension, irregular heart beats, and sudden death have been reported.

Pharmacoeconomic and Treatment Adherence Considerations

Annual health care costs of patients with ADHD are more than double those of patients without ADHD.[31,32] The financial burden of ADHD is attributed to the direct cost of pharmacotherapy, office visits, diagnostic measurements, therapy monitoring, and indirect costs (eg, lost work time and productivity). When selecting a treatment, the cost burden to the patient's family should be considered. Short-acting stimulants may be more cost effective in many patients compared with longer-acting stimulant formulations (see Table 42–3), but in certain circumstances, longer-acting stimulant formulations may provide a greater benefit owing to increased adherence to the medication and prolonged control of symptoms of ADHD. All intermediate-acting and various extended-acting (Concerta, Ritalin LA, Metadate CD, Focalin XR, and Adderall XR) stimulant formulations are now available as generic products, making them potentially more affordable. In addition, some nonstimulant ADHD medications (eg, bupropion and immediate-release α_2-adrenergic agonists) appear to be less costly than many stimulant formulations; however, these agents have not been consistently proven to have superior efficacy over stimulants. Decisions on selection of specific ADHD medications should not be based solely on cost but also on efficacy and safety along with adherence to the prescribed regimen.

OUTCOME EVALUATION

Carefully document core ADHD symptoms at baseline to provide a reference point from which to evaluate effectiveness of treatment. Improvement in individualized patient outcomes are desired, such as (a) family and social relationships, (b) disruptive behavior, (c) completing required tasks, (d) self-motivation, (e) appearance, and (f) self-esteem. Elicit evaluations of the patient's behavior from family, school, and social environments in order to assess these outcomes. Using standardized rating scales (eg, Conners Rating Scales—Revised, Brown Attention-Deficit Disorder Scale, and Inattentive-Overactive with Aggression [IOWA] Conners Scale) in both children and adults with ADHD helps to minimize variability in evaluation.[33] After initiation of pharmacotherapy, evaluate every 2 to 4 weeks to determine efficacy of treatment and potential effects on height, weight, pulse, and blood pressure. Use physical examinations or liver function tests as appropriate to monitor for adverse effects. In children being considered for ADHD pharmacotherapy, obtain baseline electrocardiograms (ECGs) when known or suspected cardiac disease exists or the clinician judges it necessary.[34–36] Typically,

Patient Encounter Part 2: Additional Historical and Physical Examination Findings

Wt: 25.7 kg (56.5 lb)

Allergies: None known

Ht: 3'10" (119 cm)

BP: 99/59 mm Hg

P: 92 beats/min

The family does not qualify for medical assistance, and they can hardly afford their monthly expenses

What stimulants and nonstimulants are available that might control this child's symptoms?

Which ADHD medications should you be concerned about using?

What medications will maximize efficacy, facilitate adherence, minimize potential side effects, and offer an acceptable cost?

What baseline assessment do you need before starting stimulant therapy?

What are important counseling points to discuss with the parents before starting any ADHD medication?

Patient Care Process

Patient Assessment:

- Suspected ADHD: evaluate patient for signs and symptoms of hyperactivity-impusivity and/or inattentiveness.
- Utilize patient symptoms and parent-teacher evaluation to determine if the patient meets the *DSM-5* criteria for ADHD.
- Perform a complete medical history, home assessment, physical, and neurological examination. Include blood pressure, pulse, and height and weight measurements. A baseline ECGs may be obtained in children when known or suspected cardiac disease exists. What is the patient's age?

Therapy Evaluation:

- Evaluate current and past medications for effectiveness and side effects. Does the patient have clear indications or any contraindications for therapy?
- Evaluate the cost effectiveness/burden of current therapy and the patient's ability to remain adherent to therapy.
- Assess for adherence and drug interactions.

Care Plan Development:

- If patient is younger than 6 years, initiate behavioral modification therapy before starting low dose methylphenidate (see Table 42–1). Start older patients on low-dose stimulant therapy (see Table 42–1).
- Continuously stress the importance of adherence.
- Consider switching to a different stimulant formulation if initial stimulant is not effective (see Table 42–1).
- A trial of at least two stimulants should be attempted before a nonstimulant is considered.
- Reevaluate the diagnosis if all treatment attempts fail.
- Educate the patient's parents and/or caregivers that behavioral therapy is not as effective as stimulant therapy and about the growth delay and substance abuse risks with stimulants.

Follow-up Evaluation:

- Perform a general physical examination yearly and monitor blood pressure quarterly in adults.
- Evaluate for improvement in behavioral modification therapy patients every 3 months. Obtain information from parent/teacher rating scales.
- Measure effectiveness and safety (side effect profile) of stimulant therapy monthly for the first 3 months. Has the patient's behavior improved? Is the patient experiencing any adverse effects?

Review medical history and obtain height, weight, heart rate, and blood pressure at each visit.

therapeutic benefits will be seen within days of initiating stimulants and within 1 or 2 months of starting bupropion and atomoxetine. When a maintenance dose has been achieved, schedule follow-up visits every 3 months. At these visits, assess height and weight, and screen for possible adverse drug effects. If a patient has failed to respond to multiple agents, reevaluate for other possible causes of behavior dysfunction. Counsel patients and their families that treatment generally is long term. Typically, appropriately treated patients learn to better control their ADHD symptoms as adults.

Abbreviations Introduced in This Chapter

ADHD	Attention deficit hyperactivity disorder
CYP	Cytochrome P450
DSM-5	*Diagnostic and Statistical Manual of Mental Disorders*, 5th edition, Text Revision
ECG	Electrocardiogram
IOWA	Inattentive Overactive with Aggression

REFERENCES

1. Wolraich ML, Wibbelsman CJ, Brown TE, et al. Attention-deficit/hyperactivity disorder among adolescents: a review of the diagnosis, treatment, and clinical implications. Pediatrics. 2005;115(6):1734–1746.
2. Ryan-Krause P. Attention deficit hyperactivity disorder: Part I. J Pediatr Health Care. 2010;24(3):194–198.
3. Pastor PN, Reuben CA. Diagnosis of attention deficit hyperactivity disorder and learning disability: United States, 2004-2006. National Center for Health Statistics. Vital Health Stat. 2008;10(237).
4. Biederman J, Faraone S. Attention-deficit hyperactivity disorder. Lancet. 2005;366:237–248.
5. Centers for Disease Control and Prevention. Increasing prevalence of parent-reported attention-deficit/hyperactivity disorder among children - United States, 2003 and 2007. MMWR Morb Mortal Wkly Rep. 2010;59(44):1439–1443.
6. American Psychiatric Association. Diagnostic and Statistical Manual of Mental Disorders. Fifth edition (DSM-5). Washington, DC: American Psychiatric Press; 2013.
7. Feldman HM, Reiff MI. Clinical practice. Attention deficit-hyperactivity disorder in children and adolescents. N Engl J Med. 2014;370(9):838–846.
8. Elliott H. Attention deficit hyperactivity disorder in adults: a guide for the primary care physician. South Med J. 2002;95:736–742.
9. Voeller KKS. Attention-deficit hyperactivity disorder (ADHD). J Child Neurol. 2004;19:798–814.
10. Institute for Clinical Systems Improvement (ICSI). Health care guideline: diagnosis and management of attention deficit hyperactivity disorder in primary care for school-age children and adolescents, 9th ed. Bldoominton, MN: Institute for Clinical Systems Improvement. March 2012, [cited 2014 Sept 01]. https://www.icsi.org/%5Fasset/60nzr5/ADHD-Interactive0312.pdf. Accessed Sep 1, 2014.
11. Subcommittee on Attention-Deficit/Hyperactivity Disorder; Steering Committee on Quality Improvement and Management, Wolraich M, Brown L, Brown RT, et al. ADHD: Clinical practice guideline for the diagnosis, evaluation, and treatment of attention-deficit/hyperactivity disorder in children and adolescents. Pediatrics. 2011;128(5):1007–1022.
12. Pliszka S. AACAP Work Group on Quality Issues. Practice parameter for the assessment and treatment of children and adolescents with attention-deficit/hyperactivity disorder. J Am Acad Child Adolesc Psychiatry. 2007;46:894–921.
13. MTA Cooperative Group. A 14-month randomized clinical trial of treatment strategies for attention-deficit/hyperactivity disorder. Arch Gen Psychiatry. 1999;56(12):1073–1086.
14. Greenhill LL, Pliszka S, Dulcan MK, et al. Practice parameter for the use of stimulant medications in the treatment of children, adolescents, and adults. J Am Acad Child Adolesc Psychiatry. 2002;41(Suppl 2): S26–S49.
15. Biederman J, Boellner SW, Childress A, et al. Lisdexamfetamine dimesylate and mixed amphetamine salts extended-release in children with ADHD: a double-blind, placebo-controlled, crossover analog classroom study. Biol Psychiatry. 2007;62:970–976.
16. Wilens TE, Faraone SV, Biederman J, et al. Does stimulant therapy of attention-deficit/hyperactivity disorder beget later substance abuse? A meta-analytic review of the literature. Pediatrics. 2003;111:179–185.
17. Brown RT, Amler RW, Freeman WS, et al. Treatment of attention-deficit/hyperactivity disorder: overview of the evidence. Pediatrics. 2005;115:749–757.
18. Michelson D, Faries D, Wernicke J, et al. Atomoxetine in the treatment of children and adolescents with attention-deficit/hyperactivity disorder: a randomized, placebo-controlled, dose-response study. Pediatrics. 2001;108(5):E83.
19. Kratochvil CJ, Heiligenstein JH, Dittmann R, et al. Atomoxetine and methylphenidate treatment in children with ADHD: a prospective, randomized, open-label trial. J Am Acad Child Adolesc Psychiatry. 2002;41(7):776–784.
20. Michelson D, Allen AJ, Busner J, et al. Once-daily atomoxetine treatment for children and adolescents with attention deficit hyperactivity disorder: A randomized, placebo-controlled study. Am J Psychiatry. 2002;159:1896–1901.
21. Biederman J, Heiligenstein JH, Faries DE, et al. Efficacy of atomoxetine versus placebo in school-age girls with attention-deficit/hyperactivity disorder. Pediatrics. 2002;110(6):E75.
22. Newcorn JH, Kratochvil CJ, Allen AJ, et al. Atomoxetine and osmotically released methylphenidate for the treatment of attention deficit hyperactivity disorder: Acute comparison and differential response. Am J Psychiatry. 2008;165(6):721–730.
23. Wang Y, Zheng Y, Du Y, et al. Atomoxetine versus methylphenidate in paediatric outpatients with attention deficit hyperactivity disorder: A randomized, double-blind comparison trial. Aust N Z J Psychiatry. 2007;41(3):222–230.
24. Belle DJ, Ernest S, Sauer J, et al. Effect of potent CYP2D6 inhibition by paroxetine on atomoxetine pharmacokinetics. J Clin Pharmacol. 2002;42:1219–1227.
25. Heil SH, Holmes HW, Bickel WK, et al. Comparison of the subjective physiological, and psychomotor effects of atomoxetine and methylphenidate in light drug users. Drug Alcohol Depend. 2002;67(2):149–156.
26. Maneeton N, Maneeton B, Intaprasert S, Woottiluk P. A systematic review of randomized controlled trials of bupropion versus methylphenidate in the treatment of attention-deficit/hyperactivity disorder. Neuropsychiatr Dis Treat. 2014;10:1439–1449.
27. Wilens TE, Spencer TJ, Biederman J, et al. A controlled clinical trial of bupropion for attention deficit hyperactivity disorder in adults. Am J Psychiatry. 2001;158:282–288.
28. Tallian K. Pharmacotherapy of ADHD. In: Schumock G, Brundage D, Chapman M, et al., eds. Pharmacotherapy Self-Assessment Program, 5th ed. Pediatrics II. Kansas City, MO: American College of Clinical Pharmacy, 2006:275–297.
29. Scrahill L. Alpha-2 adrenergic agonists in children with inattention, hyperactivity and impulsiveness. CNS Drugs. 2009;23 (Suppl 1):43–49.
30. Connor DF, Findling RL, Kollins SH, et al. Effects of guanfacine extended release on oppositional symptoms in children aged 6-12

years with attention-deficit hyperactivity disorder and oppositional symptoms: a randomized double-blind, placebo-controlled trial. CNS Drugs. 2010;24(9):755–768.
31. Matza LS, Paramore C, Prasad M. A review of the economic burden of ADHD. Cost Eff Resour Alloc. 2005;3:5.
32. Birnbaum HG, Kessler RC, Lowe SW, et al. Costs of attention deficit-hyperactivity disorder (ADHD) in the U.S.: Excess costs of persons with ADHD and their family members in 2000. Curr Med Res Opin. 2005;21(2):195–205.
33. Collett BR, Ohan JL, Myers KM. Ten-year review of rating scales. V: Scales assessing attention-deficit/hyperactivity disorder. J Am Acad Child Adolesc Psychiatry. 2003;42(9):1015–1037.
34. Vetter VL, Elia J, Erickson C, et al. Cardiovascular monitoring of children and adolescents with heart disease receiving medications for Attention Deficit/Hyperactivity Disorder: A scientific statement from the American Heart Association Council on Cardiovascular Disease in the Young Congenital Cardiac Defects Committee and the Council on Cardiovascular Nursing. Circulation. 2008;117:2407–2423.
35. Perrin JM, Friedman RA, Knilans TK, et al. Cardiovascular monitoring and stimulant drugs for Attention-Deficit/Hyperactivity Disorder. Pediatrics 2008;122:451–453.
36. ECGs before stimulants in children. Med Lett Drugs Ther. 2008;50(1291):60.

43 Diabetes Mellitus

Julie Sease and Kayce Shealy

LEARNING OBJECTIVES

Upon completion of the chapter, the reader will be able to:

1. Discuss the incidence and economic impact of diabetes.
2. Distinguish clinical differences in type 1, type 2, and gestational diabetes.
3. List screening and diagnostic criteria for diabetes.
4. Discuss therapeutic goals for blood glucose and blood pressure for a patient with diabetes.
5. Recommend nonpharmacologic therapies, including meal planning and physical activity, for patients with diabetes.
6. Compare oral agents used in treating diabetes by their mechanisms of action, time of action, side effects, contraindications, and effectiveness.
7. Select appropriate insulin therapy based on onset, peak, and duration of action.
8. Discuss the signs, symptoms, and treatment of hypoglycemia.
9. Define *diabetic ketoacidosis* and discuss treatment goals.
10. Develop a comprehensive therapeutic monitoring plan for a patient with diabetes based on patient-specific factors.

INTRODUCTION

KEY CONCEPT *Diabetes mellitus (DM) describes a group of chronic metabolic disorders characterized by hyperglycemia that may result in long-term microvascular and neuropathic complications. These complications contribute to diabetes being the leading cause of (a) new cases of blindness among adults, (b) end-stage renal disease, and (c) nontraumatic lower limb amputations. Macrovascular complications (coronary artery disease, peripheral vascular disease, and stroke) are also associated with DM.*

EPIDEMIOLOGY AND ETIOLOGY

DM affects an estimated 29.1 million persons in the United States, or 9.3% of the population.[1] Although an estimated 21 million persons have been diagnosed, another 8.1 million have DM but are unaware they have the disease. The total financial impact of DM in 2012 was approximately $245 billion, with direct medical costs equaling $176 billion (2.3 times higher than what expenditures would be in the absence of diabetes) and indirect costs secondary to disability, work loss, and premature mortality equaling $69 billion.

DM is characterized by a complete lack of insulin, a relative lack of insulin, or insulin resistance as well as disorders of other hormones. These defects result in an inability to use glucose for energy. The increasing prevalence of DM is partly caused by three influences: lifestyle, ethnicity, and age.

Lifestyle

A sedentary lifestyle coupled with greater consumption of high-fat, high-carbohydrate foods, and larger portion sizes have resulted in increasing rates of persons being obese. Current estimates indicate that 34.9% of the US population is obese when obesity is defined as a body mass index (BMI) of greater than 30 kg/m^2.[2] In a 2008 survey, the Centers for Disease Control and Prevention (CDC) found that 25.4% of American adults spent none of their free time being physically active.[3]

Ethnicity

In addition to current lifestyle trends and increased body weight, certain ethnic groups are at a disproportionately high risk for developing DM. The risk of diabetes is 18% higher among Asian Americans, 68% higher among Hispanics, and 74% higher among non-Hispanic Blacks compared with non-Hispanic White adults.[1] New cases of DM are diagnosed at a higher rate among United States minority populations than in non-Hispanic Whites.

Age

The third factor contributing to the increased prevalence of type 2 DM (T2DM) is age. In 2012, 11.2 million people in the United States who were 65 years of age or older had diabetes compared with only 208,000 younger than age 20 years.[1] As the population ages, the incidence of T2DM is expected to increase.

KEY CONCEPT *Type 1 DM (T1DM) is usually diagnosed before age 30 years but can develop at any age. Autoimmune destruction of the β cells causes insulin deficiency. T2DM accounts for approximately 90% to 95% of all diagnosed cases of DM, is progressive in its development, and is often preceded by an increased risk for diabetes (previously known as prediabetes). A combination of insulin deficiency, insulin resistance, and other hormonal irregularities, primarily involving glucagon, are key problems with T2DM. The majority of people with T2DM are overweight, and an increasing number of cases in children have been observed.*

T1DM is an autoimmune disease in which insulin-producing β cells in the pancreas are destroyed, leaving the individual insulin deficient.[4] Individuals with T1DM may develop islet cell antibodies, insulin autoantibodies, glutamic acid decarboxylase autoantibodies, protein tyrosine phosphatase autoantibodies, or zinc transporter protein autoantibodies, though most laboratories do not have reliably sensitive or specific assays to measure all five. As more β cells are destroyed, glucose metabolism becomes compromised because of reduced insulin release after a glucose load. At the time of diagnosis of T1DM, it is commonly believed that most patients have an 80% to 95% loss of β-cell function.[5] The remaining β-cell function at diagnosis creates a "honeymoon period" during which smaller amounts of insulin are required to control glucose levels. After this, remaining β-cell function is lost, and patients become completely insulin deficient and require more exogenous insulin.

Latent autoimmune diabetes in adults (LADA), slow-onset type 1, or type 1.5 DM, is a form of autoimmune T1DM that occurs in individuals older than the usual age of T1DM onset.[6] Patients often are mistakenly thought to have T2DM because the person is older and may respond initially to treatment with oral blood glucose–lowering agents. These patients do not have insulin resistance, but antibodies are present in the blood that are known to destroy pancreatic β cells. C-peptide, a surrogate marker for insulin secretion, may be used to establish or verify a diagnosis of T1DM.[4] When C-peptide levels are drawn, a simultaneous blood glucose level should also be taken.

Categories of increased risk for diabetes (commonly referred to as prediabetes) include impaired fasting glucose (IFG), impaired glucose tolerance (IGT), or hemoglobin A_{1c} (A_{1c}) between 5.7% and 6.4% (0.057 and 0.064; 39 and 46 mmol/mol hemoglobin [Hgb]).[7] IFG is defined as having a fasting blood glucose (FBG) level between 100 and 125 mg/dL (5.6 and 6.9 mmol/L). IGT is defined by a postprandial blood glucose level between 140 and 199 mg/dL (7.8 and 11.0 mmol/L). The development of IFG, IGT, or A_{1c} between 5.7% and 6.4% (0.057 and 0.064; 39 and 46 mmol/mol) places the individual at high risk of eventually developing diabetes.

T2DM is usually slow and progressive in its development. Risk factors for T2DM include:

- First-degree family history of DM (ie, parents or siblings)
- Overweight or obese
- Habitual physical inactivity
- Race or ethnicity (Native American, Latino or Hispanic American, Asian American, African American, and Pacific Islanders)
- Previously identified IFG, IGT, or A_{1c} between 5.7% and 6.4% (0.057 and 0.064 or 39 and 46 mmol/mol Hgb)
- Hypertension (greater than or equal to 140/90 mm Hg or on therapy for hypertension)
- High-density lipoprotein (HDL) cholesterol less than 35 mg/dL (0.91 mmol/L) and/or a triglyceride level greater than 250 mg/dL (2.83 mmol/L)
- History of gestational diabetes or delivery of a baby weighing greater than 4 kg (9 lb)
- History of cardiovascular disease
- History of polycystic ovarian syndrome
- Other conditions associated with insulin resistance (eg, acanthosis nigricans)

Gestational diabetes mellitus (GDM) is defined as glucose intolerance in women during pregnancy. Clinical detection of and therapy for GDM are important because blood sugar control produces significant reductions in adverse maternal, fetal, and neonatal outcomes.

Diabetes from other causes includes genetic defects in β-cell function, genetic defects in insulin action, diseases of the exocrine pancreas such as cystic fibrosis, and drug- or chemical-induced diabetes. Drugs that may cause increased blood glucose include glucocorticoids, pentamidine, nicotinic acid, β-adrenergic agonists, thiazides, phenytoin, clozapine, olanzapine, and γ-interferon.[8] Although the use of these medications is not contraindicated in persons with DM, caution and awareness of the effects on blood glucose should be taken into account when managing these patients.

PATHOPHYSIOLOGY

Normal Carbohydrate Metabolism

The body's main fuel source is glucose. Cells metabolize glucose completely through glycolysis and the Krebs cycle, producing adenosine triphosphate (ATP) as energy.[9] Glucose is stored in the liver and muscles as glycogen. Glycogenolysis converts stored glycogen back to glucose.[10] Glucose also may be stored in adipose tissue, which may subsequently undergo lipolysis yielding free fatty acids.[9] In the fasting state, free fatty acids supply much of the energy needs for the body except for the central nervous system, which requires glucose to function normally.[10] Proteins also can be converted to glucose through gluconeogenesis.[9] Homeostasis is achieved through a balance of the metabolism of glucose, free fatty acids, and amino acids to maintain a blood glucose level sufficient to provide an uninterrupted supply of glucose to the brain.[10]

Insulin and glucagon are produced in the pancreas by cells in the islets of Langerhans. β cells make up 70% to 90% of the islets and produce insulin and amylin, whereas α cells produce glucagon.[9] The main function of insulin is to decrease blood glucose levels. Glucagon, along with other counterregulatory hormones such as growth factor, cortisol, and epinephrine, increases blood glucose levels.[10] Although blood glucose levels vary, the opposing actions of insulin and glucagon, along with the counterregulatory hormones, normally maintain fasting values between 79 and 99 mg/dL (4.4–5.5 mmol/L).

► *Normal Insulin Action*

Fasting insulin levels in the circulation average from 43 to 186 pmol/L (6–26 μIU/mL).[9] After food is consumed, blood glucose levels rise, and the insulin-secretion response occurs in two phases. An initial burst, known as *first phase insulin response*, lasts approximately 5 to 10 minutes and serves to suppress hepatic glucose production and cause insulin-mediated glucose disposal in adipose tissue. This bolus of insulin minimizes hyperglycemia during meals and during the postprandial period.

The *second phase of insulin response* is characterized by a gradual increase in insulin secretion, which lasts 60 to 120 minutes and stimulates glucose uptake by peripheral insulin-dependent tissues, namely muscle. Slower release of insulin allows the body to respond to the new glucose entering from digestion while maintaining blood glucose levels.

Amylin is a naturally occurring hormone that is cosecreted from β cells with insulin. People with diabetes have either a relative or complete lack of amylin. Amylin has three major mechanisms of action: suppression of postmeal glucagon secretion; regulation of the rate of gastric emptying from the stomach to the small intestine, which increases satiety; and regulation of plasma glucose concentrations in the bloodstream.

▶ *Impaired Insulin Secretion*

A pancreas with normal β-cell function is able to adjust insulin production to maintain normal blood glucose levels.[10] In T2DM, more insulin is secreted to maintain normal blood glucose levels until eventually the pancreas can no longer produce sufficient insulin.[9] The resulting hyperglycemia is enhanced by extremely high insulin resistance, pancreatic burnout in which β cells lose functional capacity, or both. Impaired β-cell function results in a reduced ability to produce a first-phase insulin response sufficient to signal the liver to stop producing glucose after a meal.[11] Over time, patients with T2DM experience progressive β-cell death and many require exogenous insulin to maintain blood glucose control.

▶ *Insulin Resistance*

Insulin resistance is the primary factor that differentiates T2DM from other forms of diabetes. Insulin resistance may be present for several years prior to the diagnosis of DM and can continue to progress throughout the course of the disease.[9] Resistance to insulin occurs in adipose tissue, skeletal muscle and the liver.[8] Insulin resistance in the liver poses a double threat because the liver becomes nonresponsive to insulin for glucose uptake, and hepatic production of glucose after a meal does not cease, leading to elevated fasting and postmeal blood glucose levels.

▶ *Metabolic Syndrome*

Insulin resistance has been associated with a number of other cardiovascular risks, including abdominal obesity, hypertension, dyslipidemia, hypercoagulation, and hyperinsulinemia.[12] The clustering of these risk factors has been termed **metabolic syndrome**. Criteria defining the metabolic syndrome as established by the International Diabetes Federation are summarized in Table 43–1.[12] Patients having these additional risk factors have been found to be at much higher cardiovascular risk than would be expected from the individual components of the syndrome.

▶ *Incretin Effect*

When nutrients enter the stomach and intestines, incretin hormones are released, which stimulate insulin secretion.[13] This so-called **incretin effect** is mediated by two hormones, glucagon-like peptide-1 (GLP-1) and glucose-dependent insulinotropic peptide (GIP), with GLP-1 being studied the most. GLP-1 is secreted by the L cells of the ileum and colon primarily, and GIP is secreted by the K cells. GLP-1 secretion is caused by endocrine and neural signals started when nutrients enter the gastrointestinal (GI) tract. Within minutes of food ingestion, GLP-1 levels rise rapidly. A glucose-dependent release of insulin occurs, and the dipeptidyl peptidase-4 (DPP-4) enzyme cleaves GLP-1 rapidly to an inactive metabolite. Much of the research on glucose-lowering products involves prolonging the action of GLP-1. Other glucose-lowering effects of GLP-1 include suppression of glucagon, slowing gastric emptying, and increasing satiety.

Table 43–1

Five Components of Metabolic Syndrome[12]

Risk Factor	Defining Level
1. Abdominal obesity	
• Men	Waist circumference > 102 cm (40 in)[a]
• Women	Waist circumference > 88 cm (35 in)[a]
2. Triglycerides	≥ 150 mg/dL (1.70 mmol/L)
3. HDL cholesterol	
• Men	< 40 mg/dL (1.03 mmol/L)
• Women	< 50 mg/dL (1.29 mmol/L)
4. Blood pressure	≥ 130/85 mm Hg
5. Fasting glucose	≥ 100 mg/dL (5.6 mmol/L)

Individuals having at least three of the five above criteria meet the diagnostic criteria for metabolic syndrome. HDL, high-density lipoprotein.

[a]These values are most likely to continue being used clinically in the United States, though the International Diabetes Federation advocates for use of waist circumference measurements based on ethnic group.

CLINICAL PRESENTATION AND DIAGNOSIS

Screening

Currently, the American Diabetes Association (ADA) recommends routine screening for T2DM every 3 years in all adults starting at 45 years of age.[7] Testing for T2DM should be considered, regardless of age, in adults who have a BMI greater than or equal to 25 kg/m² (or BMI greater than or equal to 23 kg/m² for

Clinical Presentation and Diagnosis of Diabetes Mellitus

Characteristic	T1DM	T2DM
Usual age of onset	Childhood or adolescence	Adult
Speed of onset	Abrupt	Gradual
Family history	Negative	Positive
Body type	Thin	Obese or history of obesity
Metabolic syndrome	No	Often
Autoantibodies	Present	Rare
Symptoms	Polyuria, polydipsia, polyphagia, rapid weight loss	Asymptomatic
Ketones at diagnosis	Present	Uncommon
Acute complications	Diabetic ketoacidosis (DKA)	Rare
Microvascular complications at diagnosis	Rare	Common
Macrovascular complications at or before diagnosis	Rare	Common

Table 43–2

American Diabetes Association Screening Recommendations for Diabetes[7]

Asymptomatic Type 1

The ADA does not recommend screening for T1DM because of the low incidence in the general population and due to the acute presentation of symptoms

Asymptomatic Type 2

1. The ADA recommends screening for T2DM every 3 years in all adults beginning at 45 years of age, particularly in those with a BMI ≥ 25 kg/m^2 (or BMI ≥ 23 kg/m^2 for Asian Americans)
2. Testing should be considered for persons younger than 45 years of age or more frequently in individuals who are overweight (BMI ≥ 25 kg/m^2 (for the general population and ≥ 23 kg/m^2 for Asian Americans) and have additional risk factors:
   - Habitually inactive
   - First-degree relative with diabetes
   - Member of a high-risk ethnic population (eg, African American, Latino, Native American, Asian American, Pacific Islander)
   - Delivered a baby weighing > 4.1 kg (9 lb) or previous diagnosis of GDM
   - Hypertensive (≥ 140/90 mm Hg)
   - HDL cholesterol level less than 35 mg/dL (0.91 mmol/L) and/or triglyceride level > 250 mg/dL (2.83 mmol/L)
   - Polycystic ovary syndrome
   - Previous IGT or IFG
   - Other clinical conditions associated with insulin resistance (eg, acanthosis nigricans)
   - History of cardiovascular disease

Type 2 in Children and Adolescents

Criteria:

- Overweight (BMI > 85th percentile for age and sex, weight for height > 85th percentile, or weight > 120% of ideal for height)

Plus any two of the following risk factors:

- Family history of T2DM in first- or second-degree relatives
- Race or ethnicity (Native American, African American, Latino or Hispanic American, Asian American, Pacific Islander)
- Signs of insulin resistance or conditions associated with insulin resistance (acanthosis nigricans, hypertension, dyslipidemia, or polycystic ovary disease)
- Maternal history of diabetes or GDM during child's gestation

Age of initiation

Age 10 years or at onset of puberty, if puberty occurs at a younger age

Frequency of testing:

Every 3 years

Test method: FPG or OGTT possibly more suitable than A_{1c}

Gestational diabetes

1. Screen for undiagnosed T2DM at first prenatal visit in those with risk factors using standard criteria
2. All women should be screened with an OGTT between weeks 24 and 28 of gestation

A_{1c}, hemoglobin A_{1c}; ADA, American Diabetes Association; BMI, body mass index; FPG, fasting plasma glucose; GDM, gestational diabetes mellitus; HDL, high-density lipoprotein; IFG, impaired fasting glucose; IGT, impaired glucose tolerance; OGTT, oral glucose tolerance test; T1DM, type 1 diabetes mellitus; T2DM, type 2 diabetes mellitus.

Asian Americans) and one or more additional risk factors. The ADA does not currently recommend widespread screening for T1DM, although measurement of islet autoantibodies may be appropriate for high-risk individuals, including those who have relatives with T1DM. See Table 43–2[7] for complete screening guidelines.

Gestational Diabetes

All pregnant women who have risk factors for T2DM should be screened for undiagnosed T2DM at their first prenatal visit using standard diagnostic criteria. Any woman found to have diabetes at that early point in pregnancy is considered to have T2DM, not GDM. All other pregnant women, not currently known to have DM should be screened for GDM. Two possible strategies exist for GDM screening. They are a "one-step" 2-hour 75-gram oral glucose tolerance test (OGTT) and a "two-step" process which includes a 1-hour 50-gram nonfasting screen followed by a 3-hour 100-gram OGTT for those with a 1-hour screening glucose of greater than or equal to 140 mg/dL (7.8 mmol/L). The diagnostic criteria for the "one-step" 2-hour 75-gram OGTT are listed in Table 43–3.[7] Any woman diagnosed with GDM should be retested at 6 to 12 weeks postpartum using the OGTT with nonpregnant diagnostic criteria.

Table 43–3

Diagnosis of Gestational Diabetes Mellitus With a 75-g Glucose Load[7]

	Plasma Glucose	
Time	**mg/dL**	**mmol/L**
75-g glucose load		
Fasting	92 or more	5.1 or more
1 hour	180 or more	10.0 or more
2 hours	153 or more	8.5 or more

A positive diagnosis of diabetes is made when any of the listed glucose values are exceeded. The test should be done in the morning after an 8-hour fast.

Note: these values are based on American Diabetes Association guidelines.

Table 43–4

ADA Criteria for Diagnosis of Diabetes[7]

Symptoms of diabetes plus a casual plasma glucose concentration ≥ 200 mg/dL (11.1 mmol/L). *Casual* is defined as any time of day without regard to time since the last meal. The classic symptoms of diabetes include polyuria, polydipsia, and unexplained weight loss.

or

FPG ≥ 126 mg/dL (7.0 mmol/L). *Fasting* is defined as no caloric intake for at least 8 hours.

or

Two-hour postload glucose ≥ 200 mg/dL (11.1 mmol/L) during an OGTT. The test should be performed as described by the WHO using a glucose load containing the equivalent of 75 g of anhydrous glucose dissolved in water.

or

A_{1c} ≥ 6.5% (0.065; 48 mmol/mol Hgb). The test should be performed in a laboratory using a method that is NGSP certified to the DCCT assay.

ADA, American Diabetes Association; A_{1c}, hemoglobin A_{1c}; DCCT, Diabetes Control and Complications Trial; FPG, fasting plasma glucose; Hgb, hemoglobin; NGSP, National Glycohemoglobin Standardization Program; OGTT, oral glucose tolerance test; WHO, World Health Organization.

In the absence of unequivocal hyperglycemia, these criteria should be confirmed by repeat testing on a different day. The OGTT is not recommended for routine clinical use.

Diagnostic Criteria

The diagnosis of DM includes glycemic outcomes exceeding threshold values with one of three testing options (Table 43–4).[7] Confirmation of abnormal values must be made on a subsequent day for diagnosis unless unequivocal symptoms of hyperglycemia exist, such as polydipsia, polyuria, and polyphagia. Either A_{1c}, fasting plasma glucose (FPG), or OGTT are appropriate tests for detecting DM.

The ADA categorizes patients demonstrating A_{1c} between 5.7% and 6.4% (0.057 and 0.064 or 39 and 46 mmol/mol Hgb), IFG, or IGT as having increased risk for future diabetes. The categorization thresholds of glucose status for FPG determination and the OGTT are listed in Table 43–5.[7] IFG and IGT may coexist or may be identified independently. FPG level represents hepatic glucose production during the fasting state, whereas postprandial glucose levels in the OGTT may reflect glucose uptake in peripheral tissues, insulin sensitivity, or a decreased first-phase insulin response. The OGTT identifies people with either IFG or IGT and therefore potentially more people at increased risk for DM and cardiovascular disease. The OGTT is a more cumbersome test to perform than either the A_{1c} or FPG; however, the efficacy of interventions for primary prevention of T2DM have been demonstrated among patients with IGT, not among those with IFG or specific A_{1c} levels.

Table 43–5

ADA Categorization of Glucose Status[7]

	mg/dL	mmol/L
FPG		
• Normal	< 100	< 5.6
• IFG (prediabetes)	100–125	5.6–6.9
• Diabetes	≥ 126	≥ 7.0
2-hour postload plasma glucose (OGTT)		
• Normal	< 140	< 7.8
• IGT (prediabetes)	140–199	7.8–11.0
• Diabetes	≥ 200	≥ 11.1

ADA, American Diabetes Association; FPG, fasting plasma glucose, IFG, impaired fasting glucose; IGT, impaired glucose tolerance; OGTT, oral glucose tolerance test.

Patient Encounter, Part 1

A 42-year-old African American woman presents to her physician for a follow-up appointment for her recent pregnancy. Upon questioning, she states that she was diagnosed with gestational diabetes during the pregnancy, and that two of her previous three children weighed greater than 9 pounds (~4 kg) at birth. She is currently 12 weeks postpartum and is without complaint.

PMH: Allergic rhinitis, gestational diabetes

FH: Father has diabetes, hypertension, and a history of myocardial infarction at age 54 years; mother has diabetes and a history of stroke at age 70 years; brother has hypercholesterolemia

SH: Smokes half pack per day for 10 years, but quit during her pregnancy; denies alcohol or illicit drug use; denies physical activity

Allergies: Sulfa and penicillin

Meds: Fluticasone nasal spray, one spray each nostril daily

VS: BP 114/85 mm Hg, P 82 beats/min, RR 20 breaths/min, T 37°C (98.6°F), Ht 5′3″ (160 cm), Wt 165 lb (75 kg)

ROS: (+) Fatigue, (–) N/V/D, HA, SOB, chest pain

What risk factors does this patient have for diabetes?

Which type of diabetes do her characteristics suggest?

What additional information is needed to diagnose this patient with diabetes?

TREATMENT

Goals of Therapy

KEY CONCEPT *DM treatment goals include reducing, controlling, and managing long-term microvascular, macrovascular, and neuropathic complications; preserving β-cell function; preventing acute complications from high blood glucose levels; minimizing hypoglycemic episodes; and maintaining the patient's overall quality of life. To achieve the majority of these goals, near-normal blood glucose levels are fundamental; thus, glycemic control remains a primary objective in diabetes management.* Two landmark trials, the Diabetes Control and Complications Trial (DCCT)[14] and the United Kingdom Prospective Diabetes Study (UKPDS),[15] showed that lowering blood glucose levels decreased the risk of developing chronic complications. A near-normal blood glucose level can be achieved with appropriate patient education, lifestyle modification, and medications.

Proper care of DM requires goal setting and assessment for glycemic control, self-monitoring of blood glucose (SMBG), monitoring of blood pressure and lipid levels, regular monitoring for the development of complications, dietary and exercise lifestyle modifications, and proper medication use. The complexity of proper DM self-care principles has a dramatic impact on a patient's lifestyle and requires a highly disciplined and dedicated person to maintain long-term control.

▸ Setting and Assessing Glycemic Targets

KEY CONCEPT *Patients and clinicians can evaluate disease state control of the patient's diabetes by monitoring daily blood glucose values, A_{1c} or estimated average glucose (eAG) values, and blood pressure.* SMBG enables patients to obtain their current blood glucose level at any time easily and relatively inexpensively. The A_{1c} test provides a weighted-mean blood glucose level from approximately the previous 3 months.

Self-Monitoring of Blood Glucose SMBG is the standard method for routinely checking blood glucose levels. Each reading provides a point-in-time evaluation of glucose control that can vary widely depending on numerous factors, including food, exercise, stress, and time of day.

By examining multiple individual points of data, patterns of control can be established. Therapy can be evaluated from these patterns, and adjustments can be made to improve overall blood glucose control. The ADA premeal plasma glucose goals are 80 to 130 mg/dL (4.4–7.2 mmol/L) and peak postprandial plasma glucose goals are less than 180 mg/dL (10.0 mmol/L).[7] The American Association of Clinical Endocrinologists (AACE) supports tighter SMBG controls, with premeal goals of less than 110 mg/dL (6.1 mmol/L) and peak postmeal goals of less than 140 mg/dL (7.8 mmol/L).[16] For patients using multiple daily insulin injections or insulin pump therapy, SMBG may need to be performed six to eight times per day.[7] The optimal frequency of testing in patients using less frequent insulin injections, noninsulin therapies, or medical nutrition therapy (MNT) is less clear. Each patient should be educated regarding how often and when to perform SMBG, and these measurements should be evaluated and used by both the patient and his or her health care providers to help the patient gain and maintain blood glucose control.

Typically, in SMBG, a drop of blood from the fingertip is placed on a test strip that is then read by a blood glucose monitor. Recent technological advancements have decreased the blood sample size required to as small as 0.3 μL, provided the capability of alternate-site testing (abdomen, arm, leg, palm), and allowed for the delivery of readings in as few as 5 seconds. Many SMBG devices can download or transfer information to a computer program that can summarize and produce graphs of the data. Identifying patterns in the patient's blood glucose data can aid practitioners in modifying treatment for better glucose control. Specific therapy adjustments can be made for patterns found at certain times of the day, on certain days, or with large day-to-day variances.

In choosing a glucose meter for a patient, several additional factors may aid in the best selection for the patient. Larger display areas or units with audible instructions and results may be better suited for older individuals and those with visual impairment. Patients with arthritis or other conditions that decrease dexterity may prefer larger meters with little or no handling of glucose strips. Younger patients or busy professionals may prefer smaller meters with features such as faster results, larger memories, reminder alarms, and downloading capabilities. Continuous glucose sensors are now available that work with or independently of insulin pumps. These monitors provide blood glucose readings, primarily through interstitial fluid (ISF). A small sterile disposable glucose-sensing device called a sensor is inserted into the subcutaneous tissues. This sensor measures the change in glucose in ISF and sends the information to a monitor, which stores the results.

Hemoglobin A_{1c} Glucose interacts spontaneously with Hgb in red blood cells to form glycated derivatives. The most prevalent derivative is A_{1c}. Greater amounts of glycation occur when blood glucose levels increase. Because Hgb has a life span of approximately 3 months, levels of A_{1c} provide a marker reflecting the average glucose levels over this timeframe.[7] The ADA goal for persons with DM is less than 7% (0.07; 53 mmol/mol Hgb), whereas the AACE supports a goal of less than or equal to 6.5% (0.065; 48 mmol/mol Hgb).[7,16] Testing A_{1c} levels should occur at least twice a year for patients who are meeting treatment goals and four times per year for patients not meeting goals or those who have had recent changes in therapy.

Estimated Average Glucose The eAG is used to correlate A_{1c} values with readings that patients obtain from their home glucose monitors.[7] The equation to convert from A_{1c} to eAG is: eAG (mg/dL) = 28.7 × A_{1c} − 46.7 (or eAG [mmol/L] = 1.59 × A_{1c} − 2.59 for A_{1c} expressed as a percentage).[17] The goal eAG is 154 mg/dL (8.5 mmol/L), which corresponds with an A_{1c} of less than 7% (0.07; 53 mmol/mol Hgb).

Ketone Monitoring Urine and blood ketone testing is important in people with T1DM, in pregnancy with preexisting diabetes, and in GDM. People with T2DM may have positive ketones and develop diabetic ketoacidosis (DKA) if they are ill.

The presence of ketones may indicate a lack of insulin or ketoacidosis, a condition that requires immediate medical attention. When there is a lack of insulin, peripheral tissues cannot take up and store glucose. This causes the body to think it is starving, and because of excessive lipolysis, ketones, primarily β-hydroxybutyric acid and acetoacetic acid, are produced as byproducts of free fatty acid metabolism in the liver. Glucose and ketones are osmotically active, and when an excessive amount of ketones is formed, the body gets rid of them through urine, leading to dehydration. Patients with T1DM should test for ketones during acute illness or stress or when blood glucose levels are consistently elevated above 300 mg/dL (16.7 mmol/L). This commonly occurs when insulin is omitted or when diabetes is poorly controlled due to nonadherence, illness, or other reasons. Women with preexisting diabetes before pregnancy or with GDM should check ketones using their first morning urine sample or when any symptoms of ketoacidosis such as nausea, vomiting, or abdominal pain are present. Blood ketone testing methods that quantify β-hydroxybutyric acid, the predominant ketone body, are available and are the preferred way to diagnose and monitor ketoacidosis. Home tests for β-hydroxybutyric acid are available. The specific treatment of DKA may include rehydration, correction of electrolyte imbalances, and insulin administration.

▸ Blood Pressure and Monitoring for Complications

The ADA standards of medical care address many of the common comorbid conditions, as well as complications that result from the progression of DM. Table 43–6 presents goals for blood pressure measurements and monitoring parameters for complications associated with diabetes.[7]

General Approach to Therapy

▸ Type 1 Diabetes Mellitus

Treatment of T1DM requires providing exogenous insulin to replace the endogenous loss of insulin from the nonfunctional pancreas. Ideally, insulin therapy mimics normal insulin physiology. The basal-bolus approach attempts to reproduce basal

Table 43–6

ADA Recommended Goals of Therapy[7]

Area	Goals
Glycemia	
A_{1c}	< 7% (0.07; 53 mmol/mol Hgb) Evaluate every 3 months until in goal; then every 6 months
eAG	< 154 mg/dL (8.6 mmol/L)
Preprandial plasma glucose	80–130 mg/dL (4.4–7.2 mmol/L)
Peak postprandial plasma glucose[a]	< 180 mg/dL (10.0 mmol/L)
Blood Pressure	< 140/90 mm Hg Evaluate at every visit
Lipids	Evaluate at diagnosis and/or age 40, then every 1–2 years thereafter
Monitoring for Complications	
Eyes	Dilated eye exam yearly
Feet	Feet should be examined at every visit
Urinary microalbumin	Yearly

A_{1c}, hemoglobin A_{1c}; ADA, American Diabetes Association; eAG, estimated average glucose; Hgb, hemoglobin.

[a]Peak postprandial glucose measurements should be made 1 to 2 hours after the beginning of the meal.

insulin response using intermediate- or long-acting insulin, whereas short- or rapid-acting insulin replicates bolus release of insulin physiologically seen around a meal in nondiabetics. A number of different regimens have been used through the years to more closely follow natural insulin patterns. As a rule, basal insulin makes up approximately 50% of the total daily dose. The remaining half is provided with bolus doses around three daily meals.

Exact doses are individualized to the patient and the amount of food consumed. T1DM patients frequently are started on about 0.6 unit/kg/day, and then doses are titrated until glycemic goals are reached. Most people with T1DM use between 0.6 and 1 unit/kg/day.

Currently, the most advanced form of insulin delivery is the insulin pump, also referred to as continuous subcutaneous insulin infusion (CSII). See Figure 43–1. Using rapid-acting insulin only, these pumps are programmed to provide a slow release of small amounts of insulin as the basal portion of therapy, and larger boluses of insulin are injected by the patient to account for the consumption of food. Pramlintide, a synthetic analog of the naturally occurring hormone amylin, is another injectable blood glucose–lowering medication that can be used in people with T1DM or in people with T2DM using insulin for treatment.

▶ *Type 2 Diabetes Mellitus*

Treatment of patients with T2DM has changed dramatically over the past decade with the addition of a number of new drugs and recommendations to maintain tighter glycemic control.[16,18,19] However, lifestyle modifications including education, nutrition, and exercise are paramount to managing the disease successfully.

▶ *Gestational Diabetes*

An individualized meal plan consisting of three meals and three snacks per day is commonly recommended in GDM. Preventing ketosis, promoting adequate growth of the fetus, maintaining satisfactory blood glucose levels, and preventing nausea and other undesired GI side effects are desired goals in these patients. An abundance of glucose causes excessive insulin production by the fetus, which if left uncontrolled, can lead to the development of an abnormally large fetus. Infant hypoglycemia at delivery, hyperbilirubinemia, and complications associated with delivery of a large baby also may occur when blood glucose levels are not controlled adequately. Insulin should be used when blood glucose levels are not maintained adequately by diet and physical activity. Insulin detemir, insulin aspart, lispro, and regular insulin carry Category B safety ratings.

Nonpharmacologic Therapy

▶ *Medical Nutrition Therapy*

MNT is considered an integral component of diabetes management and diabetes self-management education. People with DM

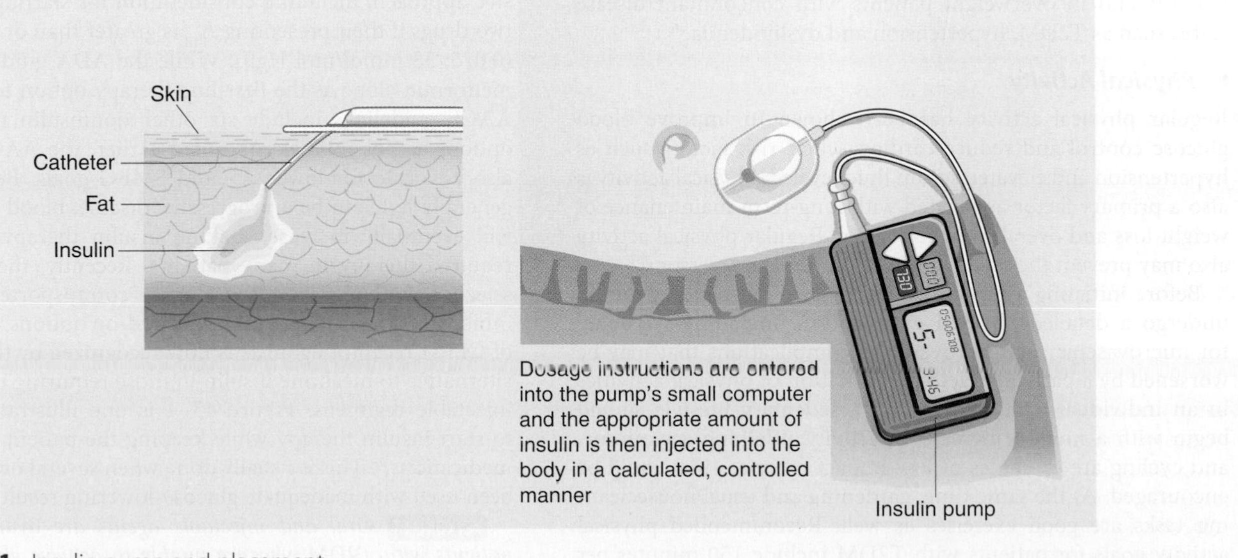
Skin
Catheter
Fat
Insulin
Dosage instructions are entered into the pump's small computer and the appropriate amount of insulin is then injected into the body in a calculated, controlled manner
Insulin pump

FIGURE 43–1. Insulin pump and placement.

should receive individualized MNT, preferably by a registered dietitian. MNT should be provided as an ongoing dialog customized to take into account cultural, lifestyle, and financial considerations.

The primary focus of MNT for patients with T1DM is matching optimal insulin dosing to carbohydrate consumption. In T2DM, the primary focus is portion control and controlling blood glucose, blood pressure, and lipids through individualizing limits of carbohydrates, saturated fats, sodium, and calories. Carbohydrates are the primary contributor to postmeal glucose levels. The percentages of fat, protein, and carbohydrate included in each meal should be individualized based on the specific goals of each patient.[7]

▶ *Dietary Supplements*

There is insufficient evidence of efficacy for improved blood glucose control for any individual herb or supplement.[7] Herbs and supplements commonly touted to improve glucose control include chromium, magnesium, vitamin D, and cinnamon. Patients will inquire about and use dietary supplements. It is important that clinicians respect the patient's health beliefs, address their questions and concerns, and educate them on the differences between dietary supplements and prescribed therapies.

▶ *Weight Management*

Moderate weight loss in patients with T2DM has been shown to reduce cardiovascular risk, as well as delay or prevent the onset of DM in those with prediabetes.[7,20] The recommended primary approach to weight loss is therapeutic lifestyle change (TLC), which integrates a 7% reduction in body weight and an increase in physical activity.[7] A slow but progressive weight loss of 0.45 to 0.91 kg (1–2 lb) per week is preferred.[21] Although individual target caloric goals should be set, a general rule for weight loss diets is that they should supply at least 1000 to 1200 kcal/day (about 4200–5000 kJ/day) for women and 1200 to 1600 kcal/day (about 5000–6700 kJ/day) for men. Gastric reduction surgeries (gastric banding or procedures that bypass, transpose, or resect portions of the small intestine), when used as a part of a comprehensive approach to weight loss, are recommended for consideration in patients with T2DM and a BMI that exceeds 35 kg/m^2.[7] Two drug therapy options were recently approved, lorcaserin and phentermine/topiramate extended release, to aid weight loss in obese patients and in overweight patients with concomitant disease states such as T2DM, hypertension and dyslipidemia.[16]

▶ *Physical Activity*

Regular physical activity has been shown to improve blood glucose control and reduce cardiovascular risk factors such as hypertension and elevated serum lipid levels.[20] Physical activity is also a primary factor associated with long-term maintenance of weight loss and overall weight control. Regular physical activity also may prevent the onset of T2DM in high-risk persons.

Before initiating a physical activity program, patients should undergo a detailed physical examination, including screening for microvascular or macrovascular complications that may be worsened by a particular activity. Initiation of physical activities in an individual with a history of a sedentary lifestyle should begin with a modest increase in activity. Walking, swimming, and cycling are examples of low-impact exercises that could be encouraged. At the same time, gardening and usual housecleaning tasks are good exercises as well. Recommended physical activity goals for patients with T2DM include 150 minutes per week of moderate to vigorous aerobic exercise spread out during at least 3 days of the week with no more than two consecutive days between bouts of aerobic activity and moderate to vigorous resistance training at least 2 to 3 days per week.[7]

▶ *Psychological Assessment and Care*

Mental health and social state have been shown to have an impact on a patient's ability to carry out DM management care tasks.[7] Clinicians should incorporate psychological assessment and treatment into routine care. The ADA guidelines recommend ongoing psychological screening, including determining the patient's attitudes regarding DM; expectations of medical management and outcomes; mood and affect; general and diabetes-related quality of life; and financial, social, and emotional resources. Patients demonstrating poor self-management should be screened for diabetes-related distress, depression, anxiety, an eating disorder, and/or cognitive impairment.

▶ *Immunizations*

Influenza and pneumonia are common preventable infectious diseases that increase mortality and morbidity in persons with chronic diseases, including DM. Yearly influenza vaccinations, commonly called flu shots, are recommended for all patients with DM 6 months of age or older.[7] Pneumococcal vaccination with the polysaccharide vaccine 23 is also recommended for patients with DM who are 2 years of age or older as a one-time vaccination. Adults aged greater than or equal to 65 years of age who have not previously been vaccinated should receive the pneumococcal conjugate vaccine 13 followed by the polysaccharide vaccine 6 to 12 months later. Adults who have received the polysaccharide vaccine should receive the conjugate vaccine after greater than or equal to 12 months. The hepatitis B vaccine series should also be administered as per the CDC's recommendations in patients with diabetes.

Pharmacotherapy

Figures 43–2 and 43–3 summarize treatment algorithms for T2DM.[16,18] While similar, these treatment algorithms differ in that, at this time, the ADA guidelines do not advocate for the use of several treatment options that the AACE guidelines include; namely, colesevelam, α-glucosidase inhibitors, and bromocriptine. Also, the AACE guidelines take a more aggressive approach, including consideration for starting a patient on two drugs if their presenting A_{1c} is greater than or equal to 7.5% (0.075; 58 mmol/mol Hgb). While the ADA guidelines include metformin alone as the first-line therapy option for T2DM, the AACE guidelines include six other noninsulin initial therapy options as possibilities. As noted earlier, the AACE guidelines also advocate for lower A_{1c} and SMBG goals. Because T2DM generally tends to be a progressive disease, blood glucose levels will eventually increase, making insulin therapy the eventual required therapy in many patients. Recently, the ADA added selective sodium-dependent glucose cotransporter-2 (SGLT-2) inhibitors as second and third line add-on options.[7] The addition of GLP-1 receptor agonists is now recognized by the ADA as an alternative to mealtime insulin in those requiring more complex injectable regimens. Figure 43–4 is one illustration of a way to start insulin therapy while keeping the patient on some oral medications.[19] This is usually done when several oral agents have been used with inadequate glucose-lowering results.

KEY CONCEPT *Oral and injectable agents are available to treat patients with T2DM who are unable to achieve glycemic control*

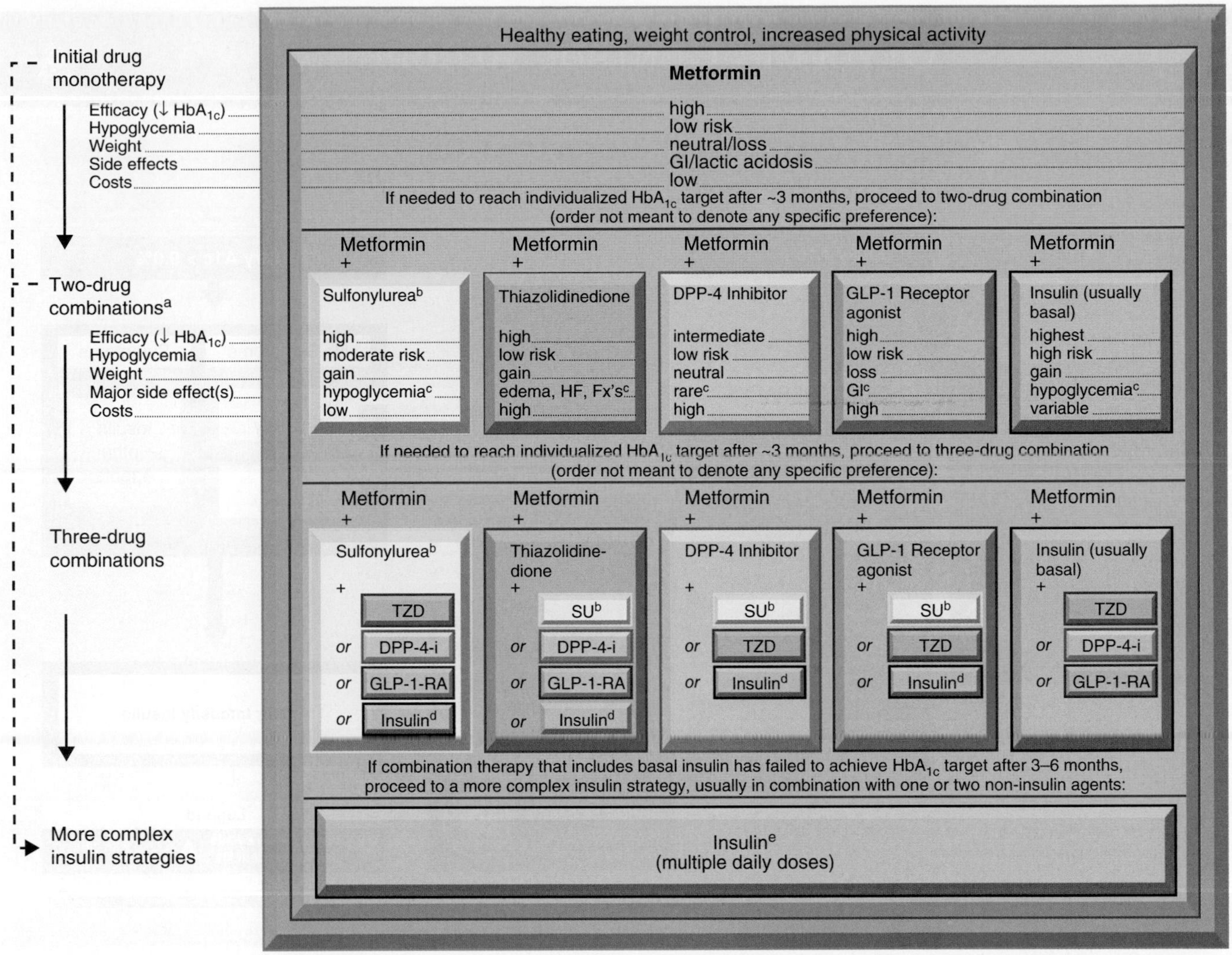

FIGURE 43–2. Patient centered approach to antihyperglycemic therapy in type 2 diabetes as per the American Diabetes Association/European Association for the Study of Diabetes. Begin with lifestyle changes and add metformin monotherapy at, or soon after, diagnosis. If HbA_{1c} target is not achieved after 3 months, consider one of five treatment options combined with metformin: a SU, TZD, DPP-4 i, GLP-1 RA, or basal insulin. Choice is based on patient and drug characteristics. [a]Consider beginning at this stage in patients with HbA_{1c} greater than 9% (0.09; 75 mmol/mol Hgb). [b]Consider meglitinides in patients with irregular meal schedules or who develop postprandial hypoglycemia on sulfonylureas. [c]Consider additional potential adverse effects. [d]Usually a basal insulin in combination with noninsulin agents. [e]Some noninsulin agents may be continued with insulin. Consider beginning at this stage if patient presents with glucose greater than 300 mg/dL (16.7 mmol/L). (DPP-4, dipeptidyl peptidase-4; DPP-4 i, dipeptidyl peptidase-4 inhibitor; Fx, fractures; GI, gastrointestinal; GLP-1, glucagon-like peptide-1; GLP-1 RA, glucagon-like peptide-1 receptor agonist; HbA_{1c}, hemoglobin A_{1c}; HF, heart failure; SU, sulfonylurea; TZD, thiazolidinedione.) (From Inzucchi SE, Bergenstal RM, Buse JB, et al. Management of hyperglycemia in type 2 diabetes: A patient-centered approach. Diabetes Care. 2012;35:1364–1379, with permission.)

through meal planning and physical activity. Table 43–7[16,18,22] lists the oral agents and Table 43–8 lists each noninsulin drug class with site of action and mechanism of action. The various classes of blood glucose–lowering agents target different organs and have different mechanisms of action. Each of these agents may be used individually or in combination with other medications that target different organs for synergistic effects. In addition to single agent products, there are many combination products marketed as well.

▸ *Sulfonylureas*

Sulfonylureas enhance insulin secretion by blocking ATP-sensitive potassium channels in the cell membranes of pancreatic β cells. This action results in membrane depolarization, allowing an influx of calcium to cause the translocation of secretory granules of insulin to the cell surface, and enhances insulin secretion in a non–glucose-dependent manner. Insulin is then transported through the portal vein to the liver, suppressing hepatic glucose production. These drugs are classified as being either first- or second-generation agents. Both classes of sulfonylureas are equally effective when given at equipotent doses. Today, the vast majority of patients receiving a sulfonylurea are prescribed a second-generation agent.

All sulfonylureas undergo hepatic biotransformation, with most agents being metabolized by the cytochrome P450 2C9 pathway. The first-generation sulfonylureas are more likely to cause drug interactions than second-generation agents. All sulfonylureas, except tolbutamide, require a dosage adjustment or are

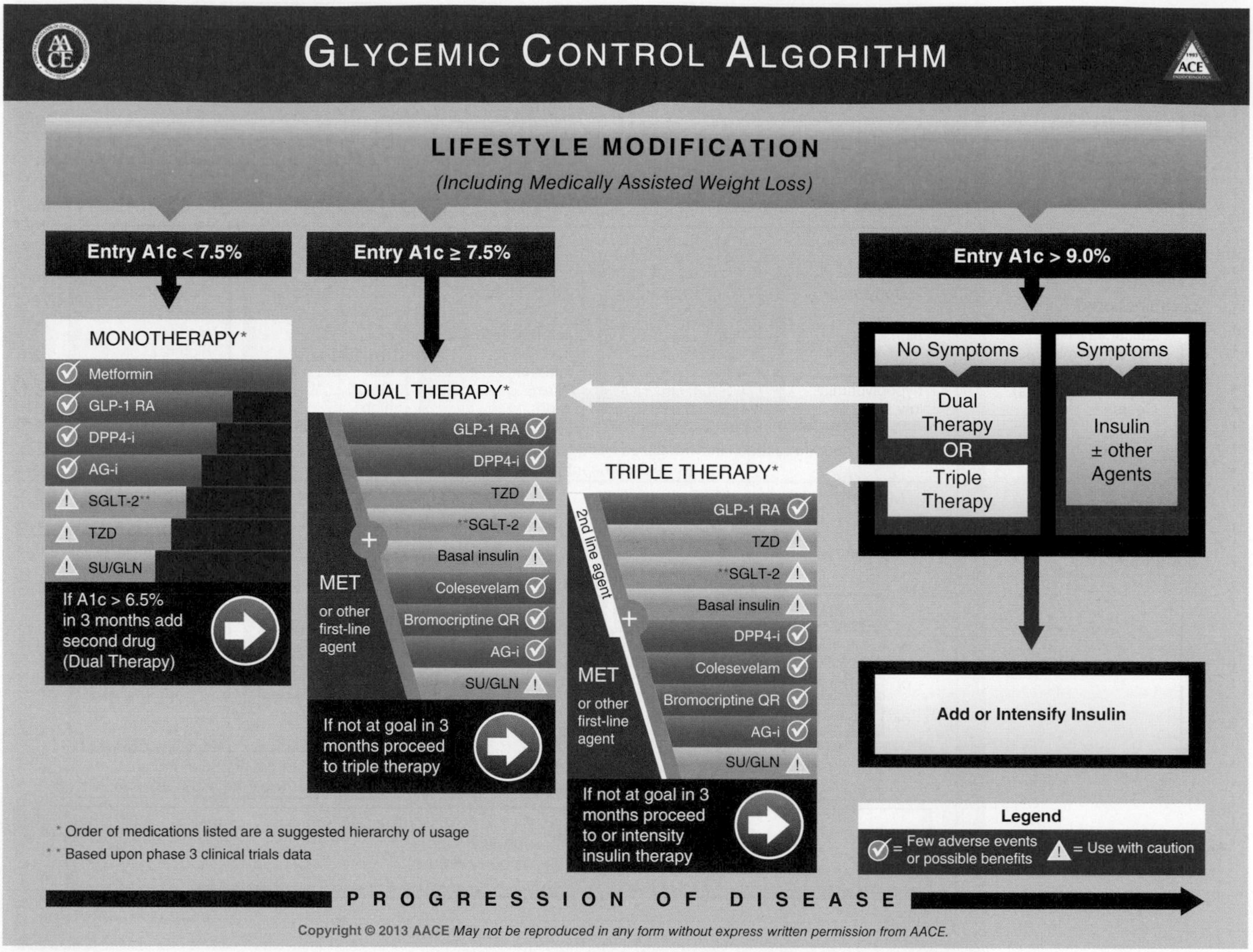

FIGURE 43–3. Algorithm for the metabolic management of type 2 diabetes as per AACE. (AACE, American Association of Clinical Endocrinologists; A_{1c}, hemoglobin A_{1c}; AG-i, alpha glucosidase inhibitor; DPP4-i, dipeptidyl peptidase-4 inhibitor; GLN, meglitinides; GLP-1 RA, glucagon-like peptide-1 receptor agonist; MET, metformin; QR, quick release; SGLT-2, sodium-dependent glucose cotransporter-2; SU, sulfonylurea; TZD, thiazolidinedione.) (From Garber AJ, Abrahamson MJ, Barzilay JI, et al. American Association of Clinical Endocrinologists' comprehensive diabetes management algorithm 2013 consensus statement. Endocr Pract. 2013;19[Suppl 1]: 1–48, with permission.)

not recommended in renal impairment.[22] In elderly patients or those with compromised renal or hepatic function, lower starting dosages are necessary.

Sulfonylureas' blood glucose–lowering effects can be observed in both fasting and postprandial levels. Monotherapy with these agents generally produces a 1.5% to 2% (0.015–0.02 or 17–22 mmol/mol Hgb) decline in A_{1c} concentrations and a 60 to 70 mg/dL (3.3–3.9 mmol/L) reduction in FBG levels.[8] Secondary failure with these drugs occurs as a result of continued pancreatic β-cell destruction. One limitation of sulfonylurea therapy is the inability of these products to stimulate insulin release from β cells at extremely high glucose levels, a phenomenon called glucose toxicity. Common adverse effects include hypoglycemia and weight gain. There may be some cross-sensitivity in patients with sulfa allergy.

▸ *Nonsulfonylurea Secretagogues (Glinides)*

Although producing the same effect as sulfonylureas, nonsulfonylurea secretagogues, also referred to as meglitinides, have a much shorter onset and duration of action. Meglitinides produce a pharmacologic effect by interacting with ATP-sensitive potassium channels on the β cells; however, this binding is to a receptor adjacent to those to which sulfonylureas bind.

The primary benefit of nonsulfonylurea secretagogues is in reducing postmeal glucose levels. These agents have demonstrated a reduction in A_{1c} levels between 0.8% and 1% (0.008 and 0.01; 9–11 mmol/mol Hgb).[8] Because they have a rapid onset and short duration of action, they are to be taken 15 to 30 minutes before a meal.

▸ *Biguanides*

The only biguanide approved by the Food and Drug Administration (FDA) and currently available in the United States is metformin. This agent is thought to lower blood glucose by decreasing hepatic glucose production and increasing insulin sensitivity in both hepatic and peripheral muscle tissues; however, the exact mechanism of action remains unknown. It has been shown to reduce A_{1c} levels by 1.5% to 2% (0.015–0.02; 17–22 mmol/mol

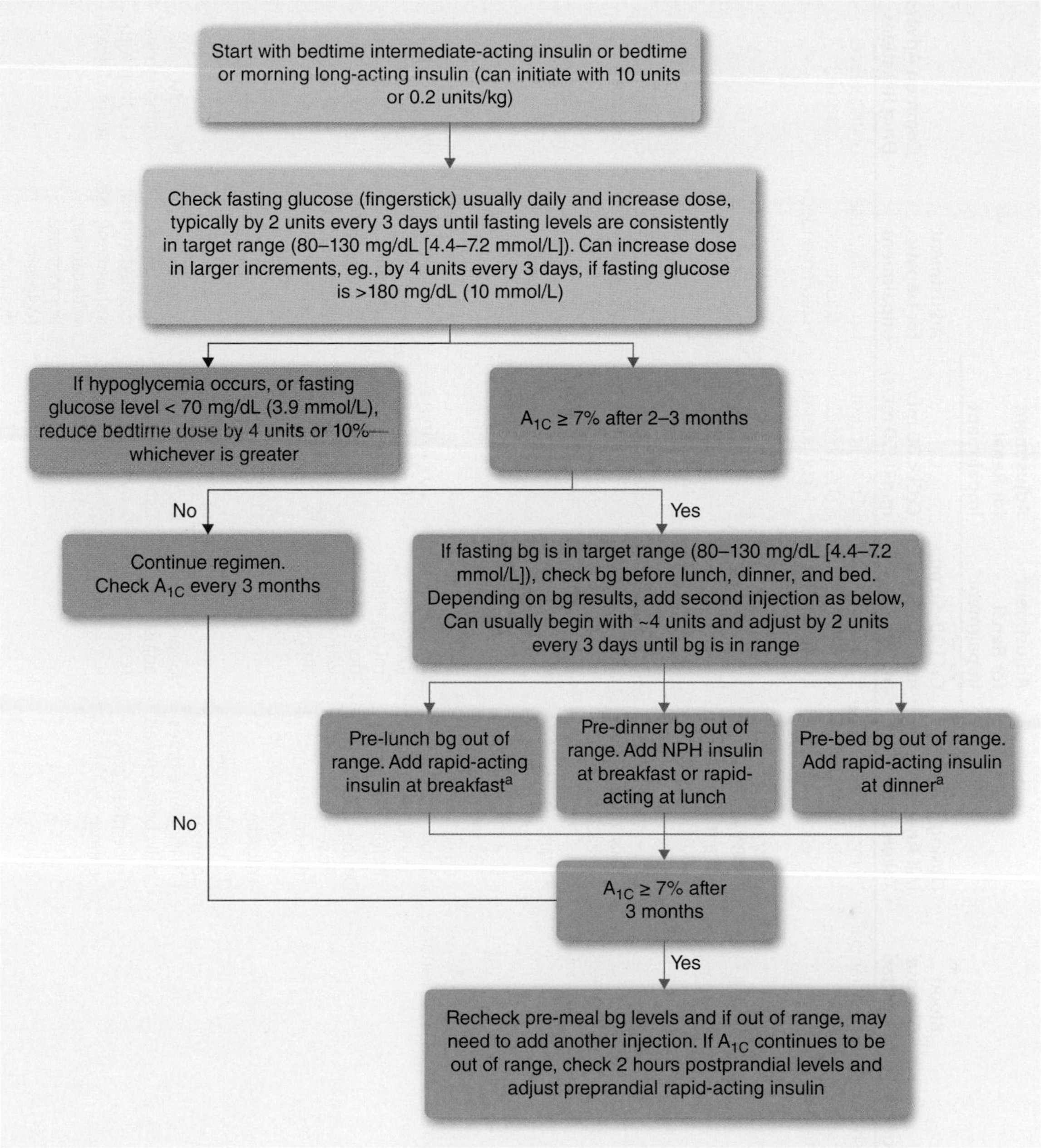

FIGURE 43–4. Initiation and adjustment of insulin regimens. Insulin regimens should be designed taking lifestyle and meal schedule into account. The algorithm can only provide basic guidelines for initiation and adjustment of insulin. [a]Premixed insulins not recommended during adjustment of doses; however, they can be used conveniently, usually before breakfast and/or dinner, if proportion of rapid- and intermediate-acting insulins is similar to the fixed proportions available. A_{1c} of 7% is equivalent to 0.07 or 53 mmol/mol Hgb. (A_{1c}, hemoglobin A_{1c}; bg, blood glucose; NPH, neutral protamine Hagedorn.) (From Nathan DM, Buse JB, Davidson MB, et al. Medical management of hyperglycemia in type 2 diabetes: A consensus algorithm for the initiation and adjustment of therapy: A consensus statement from the American Diabetes Association and the European Association for the Study of Diabetes. Diabetes Care. 2009;32:193–203, with permission.)

Hgb) and FPG levels by 60 to 80 mg/dL (3.3–4.4 mmol/L) when used as monotherapy.[8] Unlike the sulfonylureas, metformin retains the ability to reduce fasting glucose levels when they are over 300 mg/dL (16.7 mmol/L). Metformin does not affect insulin release from β cells of the pancreas, so hypoglycemia is not a common side effect.[22]

Metformin significantly reduced all-cause mortality and the risk of stroke in overweight patients with T2DM compared with intensive therapy with sulfonylurea or insulin in the UKPDS.[23] It also reduced diabetes-related death and myocardial infarction compared with a conventional therapy arm. Given that metformin is the only oral antihyperglycemic medication proven to reduce mortality and is available generically, metformin is considered foundational therapy along with lifestyle modification for T2DM and is often used in combination with other antihyperglycemics for synergistic effects.[7]

Table 43–7

Oral Agents for the Treatment of T2DM[16,18,22]

Drug Class	Drugs: Trade	Drugs: Generic/ Commercially Available	Target Area	Blood Glucose Affected	Dosing Strategy (All Agents Are Taken Orally)	Adjustment for Renal Impairment: CrCl 30–50 mL/min (0.50–0.83 mL/s)	Adjustment for Renal Impairment: CrCl < 30 mL/min (0.50 mL/s)	Adjustment for Hepatic Impairment	Common Adverse Drug Reactions
α-Glucosidase Inhibitors	Precose	Acarbose/Y	Brush border of small intestine	Postprandial	25 mg three times daily with first bite of each main meal Advance at 4–8 week intervals to a maximum of 100 mg three times daily	SCr > 2 mg/dL (177 μmol/L): Not recommended	SCr > 2 mg/dL (177 μmol/L): Not recommended	No specific dose adjustment recommended	GI (flatulence, diarrhea)
	Glyset	Miglitol/N			25 mg three times daily with first bite of each main meal Advance at 4–8 week intervals to a maximum of 100 mg three times daily	SCr > 2 mg/dL (177 μmol/L): Not recommended	SCr > 2 mg/dL (177 μmol/L): Not recommended	No adjustment necessary	GI (flatulence, diarrhea)
Meglitinides (should not be used in combination with other insulin secretagogues)	Prandin	Repaglinide/N	Pancreas	Postprandial	0.5 mg 15–30 minutes before each meal Double preprandial dose every 7 days to a maximum of 4 mg/dose or 16 mg/day (To be taken only if eating)	20–40 mL/min (0.33–0.67 mL/s): Initial dose: 0.5 mg with careful titration	< 20 mL/min (0.33 mL/s): Not studied	Use conservative initial and maintenance doses and use longer intervals between dose adjustments	Hypoglycemia (although less risk than with sulfonylureas)
	Starlix	Nateglinide/Y			120 mg three times daily before meals (To be taken only if eating)	No specific dose adjustment recommended	Use with caution in severe dysfunction	No dose adjustment needed in mild impairment; use with caution in moderate to severe dysfunction	Hypoglycemia (although less risk than with sulfonylureas)

Second-generation sulfonylureas	Micronase	Glyburide/Y	Pancreas	Fasting and postprandial	.5–3 mg/day with breakfast Increase by 1.5 mg weekly to a maximum of 12 mg/day	Not recommended	Not recommended	Use conservative dosing and avoid in severe disease	Hypoglycemia, weight gain
	DiaBeta	Glyburide/Y			2.5–5 mg/day with breakfast Increase by 2.5 mg weekly to a maximum of 20 mg/day	Not recommended	Not recommended	Use conservative dosing and avoid in severe disease	Hypoglycemia, weight gain
	Glucotrol	Glipizide/Y			5 mg/day 30 minutes before a meal Increase by 5 mg weekly to a maximum of 40 mg/day; divide dose if > 15 mg/day	No specific dose adjustment recommended	No specific dose adjustment recommended	Initial dose: 2.5 mg/day	Hypoglycemia, weight gain
	Glucotrol XL	Glipizide ER/Y			5 mg once daily before a meal Increase by 5 mg weekly to a maximum of 20 mg/day	No specific dose adjustment recommended	No specific dose adjustment recommended	No specific dose adjustment recommended	Hypoglycemia, weight gain
	Amaryl	Glimeperide/Y			1–2 mg with breakfast Increase by 2 mg every 1–2 weeks to a maximum of 8 mg/day	No specific dose adjustment recommended	< 22 mL/min (0.37 mL/s): Initial starting dose should be 1 mg	No specific dose adjustment recommended	Hypoglycemia, weight gain
Biguanides	Glucophage Fortamet Riomet	Metformin/Y	Liver	Fasting and postprandial	500 mg/day to twice daily with meals Advance weekly to a maximum of 2000–2550 mg/day	Avoid	Avoid	Avoid	GI (diarrhea, abdominal pain)
	Glucophage ER, Glumetza	Metformin, ER/Y			500–1000 mg/day; dose may be increased by 500 mg weekly to a maximum of 2000 mg/day				

(Continued)

Table 43–7

Oral Agents for the Treatment of T2DM[16,18,22] (*Continued*)

	Drugs					Adjustment for Renal Impairment	Adjustment for Renal Impairment		
Drug Class	Trade	Generic/ Commercially Available	Target Area	Blood Glucose Affected	Dosing Strategy (All Agents Are Taken Orally)	CrCl 30–50 mL/ min (0.50–0.83 mL/s)	CrCl < 30 mL/ min (0.50 mL/s)	Adjustment for Hepatic Impairment	Common Adverse Drug Reactions
Thiazolidinediones	Actos	Pioglitazone/N	Peripheral tissue	Fasting and postprandial	15–30 mg/day Increase after 12 weeks to a maximum of 45 mg/day	No adjustment necessary	No adjustment necessary	Clearance lower in Child-Pugh grade B/C; do not start if transaminases > 2.5 × ULN and discontinue if ALT rises to and remains at more than three times ULN	Weight gain
Dipeptidyl peptidase-4 inhibitors	Januvia	Sitagliptin/N	GI tract (increases GLP-1)	Fasting and postprandial	100 mg/day	50 mg once daily	25 mg once daily	Child-Pugh score 7–9: No dosage adjustment necessary Child Pugh score > 9: Not studied	Upper respiratory, diarrhea
	Onglyza	Saxagliptin/N			2.5 or 5 mg/daily	2.5 mg once daily	2.5 mg once daily	No dose adjustment necessary	UTI, headache
	Tradjenta	Linagliptin/N			5 mg/day	No dose adjustment necessary	No dose adjustment necessary	No dose adjustment necessary	Headache, arthralgia, nasopharyngitis
	Nesina	Alogliptin/N			25 mg/day	> 30 mL/min (0.50 mL/s) but < 60 mL/min (1 mL/s): 12.5 mg/ day	> 15 mL/min (0.25 mL/s) but < 30 mL/min (0.50 mL/s): 6.25 mg/ day < 15 mL/min (0.25 mL/s): 6.25 mg/ day	No dose adjustment necessary Child Pugh score > 9: Not studied	Headache, increased ALT greater than three times ULN, nasopharyngitis, upper respiratory

Selective sodium-dependent glucose cotransporter-2 inhibitor	Invokana	Canagliflozin/N	Kidney	Fasting and postprandial	100 mg/day in the morning; may increase to 300 mg/day	> 45 mL/min (0.75 mL/s) but < 60 mL/min (1.0 mL/s): 100 mg/day 30 mL/min (0.50 mL/s) to 45 mL/min (0.75 mL/s): not recommended	< 30 mL/min (0.50 mL/s): contraindicated	Mild to moderate: no adjustment necessary Severe: not recommended	Hyperkalemia, genitourinary infection, hypovolemia, renal insufficiency, hypotension
	Farxiga	Dapagliflozin/N			5 mg/day in the morning; may increase to 10 mg/day	< 60 mL/min (1.0 mL/s): not recommended	< 30 mL/min (0.50 mL/s): contraindicated	Mild to moderate: No adjustment necessary Severe: not studied	Genitourinary infection, hypovolemia/hypotension, dysuria, polyuria, dyslipidemia, mild hypoglycemia, nasopharyngitis
	Jardiance	Empagliflozin/N			10 mg/day in the morning; may increase to 25 mg/day	Not yet available	Not yet available	Not yet available	Genitourinary infection, hypovolemia/hypotension, dysuria, polyuria, mild hypoglycemia
Dopamine receptor agonist	Cycloset	Bromocriptine mesylate/N	Hypothalamus	Postprandial	0.8 mg once daily within 2 hours of waking; may increase in weekly intervals to 4.8 mg once daily	No dose adjustment necessary	No dose adjustment necessary	No specific dose adjustment recommended, although adjustment may be necessary because of extensive hepatic metabolism	Nausea, headache
Bile acid sequestrant	Welchol	Colesevelam/N	Intestinal lumen	Fasting	1.875 g twice daily or 3.75 g once daily	No dose adjustment necessary	No dose adjustment necessary	No dose adjustment necessary	Constipation

ALT, alanine aminotransferase; CrCl, creatinine clearance; ER, extended release; GI, gastrointestinal; GLP-1, glucagon-like peptide-1; SCr, serum creatinine; T2DM, type 2 diabetes mellitus; ULN, upper limit of normal; UTI, urinary tract infection.

Table 43–8

Site and Mechanism of Action for Noninsulin Agents

Site of Action	Drug Class	Mechanism of Action
Pancreas	Sulfonylureas	Enhances insulin secretion
	Nonsulfonylurea secretagogues	Enhances insulin secretion
	GLP-1 agonists	Enhances insulin secretion and suppresses glucagon secretion
	Pramlintide	Suppresses glucagon secretion
Liver	Biguanide	Decreases hepatic glucose production and increases insulin sensitivity
	Thiazolidinedione	Increases insulin sensitivity
Muscle	Biguanide	Increases insulin sensitivity
	Thiazolidinedione	Increases insulin sensitivity
Adipose tissue	Thiazolidinedione	Increases insulin sensitivity
Intestines	GLP-1 agonists	Increases satiety and regulates gastric emptying
	Pramlintide	Increases satiety and regulates gastric emptying
	Dipeptidyl peptidase-4 inhibitors	Increases endogenous GLP-1
	α-Glucosidase inhibitors	Delays absorption of carbohydrates
Kidney	SGLT-2 inhibitors	Inhibits glucose reabsorption in the kidney's proximal tubule

GLP-1, glucagon-like peptide-1; SGLT-2, sodium-dependent glucose cotransporter-2.

Per US labeling, metformin is contraindicated in patients with abnormal creatinine clearance for any cause and in patients with a serum creatinine level greater than or equal to 1.4 mg/dL (124 μmol/L) in women and 1.5 mg/dL (133 μmol/L) in men.[22] It should not be initiated in patients 80 years of age or older unless normal renal function has been established. Additionally, therapy with metformin should be withheld in patients undergoing surgery or radiographic procedures in which a nephrotoxic dye is used. Therapy should be withheld the day of the radiographic procedure, and renal function should be assessed 48 hours after the procedure. If renal function is normal, therapy may be resumed.

Primary side effects associated with metformin therapy are GI in nature, including decreased appetite, nausea, and diarrhea. These side effects can be minimized through slow titration of the dose and often subside within 2 weeks.[19] Interference with vitamin B_{12} absorption has also been reported.[8] Metformin is thought to inhibit mitochondrial oxidation of lactic acid, thereby increasing the chance of lactic acidosis, a condition which rarely occurs. Patients at greatest risk for developing lactic acidosis include those with renal impairment and those who are of advanced age.[22] Metformin should be withheld promptly in cases of hypoxemia, sepsis, or dehydration. Patients should avoid consumption of excessive amounts of alcohol while taking metformin, and use of the drug should be avoided in patients with liver disease.

▸ *Thiazolidinediones*

Thiazolidinediones (TZDs) are known to increase insulin sensitivity by stimulating peroxisome proliferator-activated receptor gamma (PPAR-γ) which increases insulin sensitivity and decreases plasma fatty acids. As monotherapy, TZDs reduce FPG levels by around 60 to 70 mg/dL (3.3–3.9 mmol/L), and the effect on A_{1c} is an up to 1.5% (0.015; 17 mmol/mol Hgb) reduction.[8] The onset of action for TZDs is delayed for several weeks and may require up to 12 weeks before maximum effects are observed.

Both pioglitazone and rosiglitazone minimally increase HDL cholesterol, 2.4 to 5.2 mg/dL (0.06–0.13 mmol/L) on average.[24] Pioglitazone has been shown to decrease serum triglycerides (TG) 51.9 mg/dL (0.59 mmol/L) on average, but an increase in TG has been observed with rosiglitazone. Low-density lipoprotein (LDL) cholesterol concentrations increase by 12.3 mg/dL (0.32 mmol/L) and 21.3 mg/dL (0.55 mmol/L) on average with pioglitazone and rosiglitazone, respectively.

The TZDs may produce fluid retention and edema. Thus, these drugs are contraindicated in situations in which an increased fluid volume is detrimental such as heart failure. Fluid retention appears to be dose related and increases when combined with insulin therapy.

A few cases of hepatotoxicity have been reported with rosiglitazone and pioglitazone. Patients with a baseline elevated alanine aminotransferase (ALT) level should be started on TZD therapy with caution. Therapy should be stopped if ALT levels exceed three times the upper limit of normal while on therapy and remain there, especially if the patient's total bilirubin is also elevated.[8]

Increased rates of upper and lower limb fractures are known to occur with TZD therapy. Premenopausal anovulatory women may begin to ovulate on TZD therapy, and therefore counseling regarding this should be provided to all women capable of becoming pregnant. A slight increased risk for bladder cancer has been noted with pioglitazone therapy, especially among men and smokers.

A 2007 meta-analysis conducted by Nissen and colleagues reported a significantly greater risk of myocardial infarction with rosiglitazone compared with other oral agents.[25] A subsequent prospective study found rosiglitazone use to be associated with a nonsignificant increase in myocardial infarction risk and a nonsignificant reduction in stroke, but a trend toward increased cardiovascular risk in those patients with a history of ischemic heart disease.[26] In May 2011, the FDA chose to restrict access and distribution of rosiglitazone to the Avandia-Rosiglitazone Medicines Access Program.[22] Following receipt of subsequent data that showed the risk of heart attack with rosiglitazone was not increased as compared with metformin and sulfonylureas, the FDA lifted their restrictions on the drug in November 2013.

▸ *α-Glucosidase Inhibitors*

Acarbose and miglitol are α-glucosidase inhibitors which compete with the enzymes of the small intestines that break down complex carbohydrates. These drugs delay absorption of carbohydrates and reduce postprandial blood glucose concentrations as much as 40 to 50 mg/dL (2.2 to 2.8 mmol/L); however, A_{1c} reductions range only from 0.3% to 1% (0.003–0.01; 3–11 mmol/mol Hgb).[8] High incidences of GI side effects, including flatulence (42%–74%), abdominal discomfort (12%–19%), and diarrhea (29%–31%), have limited their use.[22] Low initial doses followed by gradual titration may minimize GI side effects.

The α-glucosidase inhibitors are contraindicated in patients with chronic intestinal diseases including inflammatory bowel disease. In addition, neither drug in this class is recommended for patients with a serum creatinine greater than 2 mg/dL (177 μmol/L).[8]

▸ Dipeptidyl Peptidase-4 Inhibitors (Gliptins)

The dipeptidyl peptidase-4 (DPP-4) inhibitors (sitagliptin, saxagliptin, linagliptin, and alogliptin) are approved as adjunct to diet and exercise to improve glycemic control in adults with T2DM. They lower blood glucose concentrations by inhibiting DPP-4, the enzyme that degrades endogenous GLP-1, thereby increasing the amount of endogenous GLP-1. The blood glucose–lowering effect of the gliptins is primarily on postprandial levels. Typical A_{1c} reductions are 0.7% to 1% (0.007–0.01; 8–11 mmol/mol Hgb).[8] Common adverse effects include headache and nasopharyngitis. Hypoglycemia is not a common adverse effect with these agents because insulin secretion results from GLP-1 activation caused by meal-related glucose detection and not from direct pancreatic β-cell stimulation. Acute pancreatitis, including hemorrhagic and necrotizing pancreatitis, has been reported in patients taking glipitins.[22]

▸ Selective Sodium-Dependent Glucose Cotransporter-2 (SGLT-2) Inhibitors

Canagliflozin, dapagliflozin, and empagliflozin, SGLT-2 inhibitors, are approved as adjunct to diet and exercise to improve glycemic control in adults with T2DM. The SGLT-2 receptor is responsible for 90% of the active glucose reabsorption of the kidney's proximal tubule.[8] By inhibiting this receptor, glucose reabsorption is decreased. Glucose passes into the urine, serum glucose is lowered and modest weight loss is promoted. Typical A_{1c} reductions are 0.7% to 1.3% (0.007–0.013; 8–14.3 mmol/mol Hgb).[22] Possible adverse reactions include urinary tract infections, genital mycotic infections, increased urination, hypotension, and increased serum creatinine.

▸ Central-Acting Dopamine Agonist

A quick release formulation of the central-acting dopamine agonist, bromocriptine, is approved for the treatment of T2DM. The mechanism of action for how bromocriptine regulates glycemic control is unknown, but data indicate that bromocriptine administered in the morning improves insulin sensitivity, and this is likely a result of its affect on dopamine oscillations.[8] When used to treat patients with T2DM, bromocriptine should be taken 2 hours after waking in the morning with food.[22] A modest A_{1c} reduction of 0.3% to 0.6% (0.003–0.006; 3–7 mmol/mol Hgb) can be expected from this drug.[8] Main side effects include rhinitis, dizziness, asthenia, headache, sinusitis, constipation, and nausea. Contraindications include syncopal migraine and women who are nursing.[22]

▸ Bile Acid Sequestrants

Colesevelam is the only bile acid sequestrant currently approved as an adjunctive therapy to improve glycemic control in conjunction with diet, exercise, and insulin or oral agents for the treatment of T2DM. It acts on the intestinal lumen to bind bile acid, but the drug's exact mechanism that results in plasma glucose lowering is unknown. An A_{1c} reduction of approximately 0.4% (0.004; 5 mmol/mol Hgb) and a FPG reduction of about 5 to 10 mg/dL (0.3–0.6 mmol/L) can be expected when colesevelam is added.[8] Common adverse effects include constipation and dyspepsia. Drug–drug interactions are possible because of absorption and can be particularly important in patients who are taking levothyroxine, glyburide, oral contraceptives, phenytoin, warfarin, and digoxin. These medications should not be taken together, and they should be separated by at least 4 hours before dosing colesevelam. Malabsorption of fat-soluble vitamins (A, D, E, and K) is also a concern.

▸ Insulin

Insulin is the one agent that can be used in all types of DM and has no specific maximum dose, meaning it can be titrated to suit each individual patient's needs. KEY CONCEPT *Insulin is the primary treatment to lower blood glucose levels for patients with T1DM, and injected amylin can be added to decrease fluctuations in blood glucose levels.* An insulin treatment algorithm for T2DM is found in Figure 43–2.[19]

Insulin can be divided into two main classes, basal and bolus, based on their length of action to mimic endogenous insulin physiology. Most formulations are available as U-100, indicating a concentration of 100 unit/mL. Insulin is typically refrigerated, though most vials are good for 28 days at room temperature.[22] Specific details of insulin products are listed in Table 43–9.[22,27]

The most common route of administration for insulin is subcutaneous injection using a syringe or pen device. Patients should be educated to rotate their injection sites to minimize lipohypertrophy, a buildup of fat that decreases or prevents proper insulin absorption. Additionally, patients should understand that the absorption rate may vary among injection sites (abdomen, thigh, arm, and buttocks) because of differences in blood flow, with absorption occurring fastest in the abdomen and slowest in the buttocks.

Insulin syringes are distinguished according to the syringe capacity, syringe markings, and needle gauge and length. Insulin pens are self-contained systems of insulin delivery. The primary advantage of the pen system is the patient does not have to draw up the dose from the insulin vial. Both insulin syringes and pens are now available with shorter needles (4–6 mm, compared to traditional lengths of 8–12.7 mm) which do not require the patient to pinch up their skin before injecting. With the no pinch technique, the needle is injected straight in at a 90-degree angle until flush with the skin. However, these products require a 10 second count to allow enough time for the insulin to be injected. This technique makes injections easier, especially the traditionally more difficult sites such as arms and buttocks.

Bolus Insulins

Regular Insulin. Regular insulin is unmodified crystalline insulin commonly referred to as natural or human insulin. It is a clear solution that has a relatively short onset and duration of action and is designed to cover insulin response to meals. On subcutaneous injection, regular insulin forms small aggregates called hexamers that undergo conversion to dimers followed by monomers before systemic absorption can occur. Patients should be counseled to inject regular insulin subcutaneously 30 minutes before consuming a meal. Regular insulin is the only insulin that can be administered intravenously (IV).

Rapid-Acting Insulin. Three rapid-acting injectable insulins have been approved in the United States: aspart, glulisine, and lispro. Substitution of one or two amino acids in regular insulin results in the unique pharmacokinetic properties characteristic of these agents. The onset of action of injectable rapid-acting insulins varies from 15 to 30 minutes, with peak effects occurring one to two hours after administration and is dosed before

Table 43–9

Insulin Agents for the Treatment of T1DM and T2DM[22,27,28]

Generic Name (Insulin)	Brand/Rx Status	Manufacturer	Strength	Onset (minutes)	Peak (hours)	Duration (hours)	Administration Options
Rapid-Acting Insulin							
Lispro	Humalog/Rx	Eli Lilly	U-100	15–30	0.5–2.5	3–4	SC; 10-mL vial, 3-mL cartridge, and disposable pen
Aspart	Novolog/Rx	Novo-Nordisk	U-100	15–30	1–3	3–5	SC; 10-mL vial, 3-mL cartridge, and disposable pen
Glulisine	Apidra/Rx	Aventis	U-100	15–30	1–2	3–4	SC; 10-mL vial, 3-mL cartridge, and disposable pen
Recombinant human insulin regular	Afrezza/Rx	MannKind	Not applicable	12–15	1	2.5–3	Inh; Technosphere insulin particles for oral inhalation
Short-Acting Insulin							
Regular	Humulin R/OTC	Eli Lilly	U-100, U-500	30–60	2–3	3–6	IV, SC; U-100 10-mL vial; U-500 20-mL vial
	Novolin R/OTC	Novo-Nordisk	U-100				IV, SC; 10-mL vial, 3-mL cartridge, 3-mL *Innolet*
Intermediate-Acting Insulin							
Neutral protamine Hagedorn	Humulin N/OTC	Eli Lilly	U-100	2–4 hours	4–6	8–12	SC; 10-mL vial, 3-mL cartridge
	Novolin N/OTC	Novo-Nordisk	U-100				SC; 10-mL vial, 3-mL cartridge, 3-mL *InnoLet*
Long-Acting Insulin							
Glargine	Lantus/Rx	Sanofi-Aventis	U-100	4–5 hours	Flat	22–24	SC; 10-mL vial, 3-mL cartridge for *Opticlik* (available in SoloSTAR disposable pen)
	Toujeo/Rx		U-300				SC;1.5-mL SoloSTAR disposable pen
Detemir	Levemir/Rx	Novo-Nordisk	U-100	3–4 hours	Flat	Up to 24	SC; 10-mL vial, 3-mL cartridge, 3-mL *Innolet*, 3-mL disposable *FlexPen*
Combination Insulin Products							
Neutral protamine Hagedorn and regular	Humulin 70/30/ OTC	Eli Lilly	U-100	30–60	1.5–16	10–16	SC: 10-mL vial, 3-mL disposable pen
	Novolin 70/30/ OTC	Novo-Nordisk	U-100	30–60	2–12	10–16	SC; 10-mL vial, 3-mL cartridge, 3-mL *Innolet*
	Humulin 50/50/ OTC	Eli Lilly	U-100	30–60	2–5.5	10–16	SC; 10-mL vial
Neutral protamine lispro and lispro	Humalog Mix 75/25/Rx	Eli Lilly	U-100	15–30	1–6.5	15–18	SC; 10-mL vial, 3-mL disposable pen
Neutral protamine aspart and aspart	Novolog Mix 70/30/Rx	Novo-Nordisk	U-100	15–30	1–4	Up to 24	SC; 10-mL vial, 3-mL cartridge, 3-mL disposable *FlexPen*

Inh, inhalation; IV, intravenous; OTC, over-the-counter; Rx, prescription required; SC, subcutaneous; T1DM, type 1 diabetes mellitus; T2DM, type 2 diabetes mellitus.

or with meals. An inhaled rapid-acting insulin was also recently approved. Its peak effect is expected to occur around 15 to 20 minutes following a dose with a duration of action of only two to three hours.[28]

Basal Insulins

Intermediate-Duration Insulin. Neutral Protamine Hagedorn, better known as NPH insulin, is prepared by a process in which protamine is conjugated with regular insulin, rendering a product with a delayed onset but extended duration of action, and is designed to cover insulin requirements in between meals and/or overnight. With the advent of the long-acting insulins, NPH insulin use has declined because of (a) an inability to predict accurately when peak effects occur and (b) a duration of action of less than 24 hours. Additionally, protamine is a foreign protein that may increase the possibility of an allergic reaction.

NPH insulin can be mixed with regular insulin and used immediately or stored for future use. NPH insulin can be mixed with either aspart or lispro insulins, but it must be injected immediately after mixing. Whenever mixing insulin products with NPH insulin, the shorter acting insulin should be drawn into the syringe first.

Long-Duration Insulin. Glargine and detemir are designed as once-daily-dosing basal insulins which provide a relatively constant insulin concentration over 24 hours.[22,27] Insulin glargine differs from regular insulin by three amino acids, resulting in a low solubility at physiologic pH. The clear solution is supplied at a pH of 4, which precipitates on subcutaneous administration. Detemir binds to albumin in the plasma, which gives it sustained action. Neither glargine nor detemir can be administered IV or mixed with other insulin products. Although detemir is recommended for dosing in the evening if being used as a once-daily dose, it stands to reason that both glargine and detemir could be administered irrespective of meals or time of day. Another long-duration insulin, insulin degludec, developed to offer an even more consistent insulin concentration throughout the day, is currently under FDA review.

Combination Insulin Products. A number of combination insulin products are available commercially. NPH is available in combinations of 70/30 (70% NPH and 30% regular insulin) and 50/50 (50% NPH and 50% regular insulin). Two short-acting insulin analog mixtures are also available. Humalog mix 75/25 contains 75% insulin lispro protamine suspension and 25% insulin lispro. Novolog mix 70/30 contains 70% insulin aspart protamine suspension and 30% insulin aspart. The lispro and aspart insulin protamine suspensions were developed specifically for these mixture products and are not commercially available separately.

▶ *Insulin Pump Therapy*

Insulin pump therapy consists of a programmable infusion device that allows for basal infusion of insulin 24 hours daily (see Figure 43–1), as well as bolus administration before meals and snacks. Regular or rapid-acting insulin is delivered from a reservoir either by infusion set tubing or through a small canula. Most pump infusion sets are inserted in the abdomen, arm, or other infusion site by a small needle. Most patients prefer insertion in abdominal tissue because this site provides optimal insulin absorption. Infusion sets should be changed every 2 to 3 days to reduce the possibility of infection.

Patients use a carbohydrate-to-insulin ratio to determine how many units of insulin are required. More specifically, an individual's ratio is calculated to determine how many units of the specific insulin being used in the pump "covers" for a certain amount of carbohydrates to be ingested at a particular meal. The 450 rule (for regular insulin) or the 500 rule (for rapid-acting insulin) is commonly used. To calculate the ratio using the 500 rule, the patient would divide 500 by his or her total daily dose of insulin. Once this ratio is determined, patients can eat more or fewer carbohydrates at a given meal and adjust the bolus dose accordingly.

In addition to mealtime boluses, correction doses based on premeal glucose readings are also used. The amount of additional insulin for the correction is based on either the 1500 rule for regular insulin or the 1800 rule for rapid-acting insulin. If using rapid-acting insulin, divide 1800 by the patient's total daily insulin dose. The resulting value will represent the reduction in glucose (mg/dL) produced by one unit of insulin. The correction dose would be given in addition to the bolus dose needed based on the patient's carbohydrate-to-insulin ratio and the amount of carbohydrates present in the meal he or she is about to consume.

Insulin pump therapy may be used to lower blood glucose levels in any type of DM; however, patients with T1DM are the most likely candidates to use these devices. Use of an insulin pump may improve blood glucose control, reduce wide fluctuations in blood glucose levels, and allow individuals to have more flexibility in timing and content of meals and exercise schedules.

▶ *Noninsulin Injectable Agents*

Glucagon-Like Peptide 1 Agonists Exenatide, liraglutide, albiglutide, and dulaglutide are indicated for the treatment of T2DM to improve glycemic control. These agents are part of the group of drugs known as incretins (Table 43–10).[8,22,29]

GLP-1 agonists lower blood glucose levels by: (a) producing glucose-dependent insulin secretion; (b) reducing postmeal glucagon secretion, which decreases postmeal glucose output; (c) increasing satiety which decreases food intake; and (d) regulating gastric emptying, which allows nutrients to be absorbed into the circulation more smoothly. Typical A_{1c} reductions vary between GLP-1 agonists. Exenatide immediate release lowers A_{1c} around 0.9% (0.009; 10 mmol/mol Hgb), exenatide extended-release lowers A_{1c} around 1.6% (0.016; 18 mmol/mol Hgb), liraglutide reduces A_{1c} around 1.1% (0.011; 12 mmol/mol Hgb), and albiglutide reduces A_{1c} around 0.78% (0.0078; 8.8 mmol/mol Hgb).[8,30] GLP-1 agonists typically produce moderate weight loss of around 1 to 3 kg (2.2–6.6 lbs) depending on the drug chosen.[8] Exenatide is eliminated renally and is not recommended in patients with a creatinine clearance of less than 30 mL/min (0.50 mL/s).[22] No specific dose adjustments are recommended for liraglutide or albiglutide in renal impairment. An increased risk of hypoglycemia occurs when GLP-1 agonists are used in combination with a sulfonylurea or insulin.[8] The main side effects of GLP-1 agonist therapy include nausea, vomiting, and diarrhea. These GI adverse effects tend to lessen over time. GLP-1 agonists have been associated with cases of acute pancreatitis. Any patient presenting with symptoms of acute pancreatitis, including abdominal pain, nausea, and vomiting, should have GLP-1 agonist therapy discontinued until pancreatitis can be ruled out. Albiglutide, liraglutide, exenatide extended-release, and dulaglutide packagings contain a black-box warning about thyroid C-cell tumors.[22] They are contraindicated in patients with a personal or family history of medullary thyroid cancer and in those with a history of multiple endocrine tumors.

Amylin Pramlintide acetate is a synthetic analog of human amylin, which is a naturally occurring neuroendocrine peptide that is cosecreted with insulin by the β cells of the pancreas in response to food. Amylin secretion is very low or completely deficient in patients with T1DM and lower than normal in patients with T2DM who require insulin. Pramlintide slows gastric emptying without altering absorption of nutrients, suppresses glucagon secretion, and leads to a reduction in food intake by increasing satiety. By slowing gastric emptying, the normal initial postmeal spike in blood glucose is reduced.

Pramlintide is given by subcutaneous injection before meals to lower postprandial blood glucose elevations in patients with types 1 or 2 DM. Pramlintide generally results in an additional A_{1c} reduction of 0.4% to 0.5% (0.004–0.005; 5–6 mmol/mol Hgb) and an average weight loss of 1 to 2 kg (2.2–4.4 lb).[8] Hypoglycemia, nausea, and vomiting are the most common side effects encountered with pramlintide therapy, although pramlintide itself does not produce hypoglycemia. To decrease the risk of hypoglycemia, doses of short-acting, rapid-acting, or premixed insulins should be reduced by 30% to 50% before pramlintide is initiated. Primarily, the kidneys metabolize pramlintide, but dosage adjustments in liver or kidney impairment are not required.

Table 43–10

Noninsulin Injectable Agents for the Treatment of Diabetes[8,22,29]

Generic Name (Brand)	Type of Diabetes	Dosage Strengths[a]	Starting Dosage	Doses/Day	Titration Interval	Maximum Dose	Time to Effect (minutes)	Comments and Cautions
Pramlintide[b] (Symlin)	T1DM	15, 30, 45, 60 mcg	15 mcg	3	3–7 days	60 mcg	20	Take just before major meals; reduce insulin by 50% Maintenance dose 30–60 mcg
	T2DM	60, 120 mcg	60 mcg	3	3–7 days	120 mcg	20	Side effects: Hypoglycemia, nausea, vomiting Available in SymlinPen 60 and 120
Exenatide[b] (Byetta, Bydureon)	T2DM	Immediate-release: 5 mcg, 10 mcg; extended-release: 2 mg	Immediate-release: 5 mcg, extended-release: 2 mg	Immediate-release: 2, extended-release: N/A; once-weekly	Immediate-release: 1 month, extended-release: N/A	Immediate-release: 10 mcg, extended-release: 2 mg	Immediate-release: 15–30	Inject immediate-release formulation 15–20 minutes before two meals of the day with 6 hours separating the meals; prefilled disposable pen; may delay absorption of oral drugs; separate doses by 1 hour Extended-release formulation can be administered regardless of meals Side effects: Nausea, vomiting, diarrhea, increased hypoglycemia with sulfonylureas
Liraglutide[b] (Victoza)	T2DM	6 mg/3 mL pen	0.6 mg	1	1 week	1.8 mg	Not applicable	Can be dosed at any time of day regardless of meals; may delay absorption of oral drugs; separate doses by 1 hour Side effects: Nausea, vomiting, increased hypoglycemia with sulfonylureas
Albiglutide[b] (Tanzeum)	T2DM	30 mg single-dose pen; 50-mg single-dose pen	30 mg	N/A; once weekly	6 weeks	50 mg	Not applicable	If missed dose occurs within 3 days of the regularly scheduled dose, dose should be administered at that time. If missed dose occurs more than 3 days past scheduled dose, wait until next regularly scheduled dose to administer next dose Side effects: upper respiratory infection, diarrhea, nausea, injection site reaction
Dulaglutide[b] (Trulicity)	T2DM	0.75 mg single-dose pen and prefilled syringe; 1.5-mg single-dose pen and prefilled syringe	0.75 mg	N/A; once weekly	Not specified	1.5 mg	Not applicable	If missed dose occurs within 3 days of the regularly scheduled dose, dose should be administered at that time. If missed dose occurs more than 3 days past scheduled dose, wait until next regularly scheduled dose to administer next dose Side effects: nausea, diarrhea, vomiting, abdominal pain, decreased appetite, dyspepsia, fatigue.

[a]Pramlintide supplied as 0.6 mg/mL in 5-mL vials. Exenatide immediate-release supplied as 250 mcg/mL, 1.2 mL for the 5-mcg prefilled pen, and 2.4 mL for the 10-mcg per dose prefilled pen. Exenatide extended-release supplied as 2 mg sterile powder plus 0.65 mL diluent in single use trays. Liraglutide supplied in 6 mg/3 mL prefilled pen, which can be dialed to the desired dose of 0.6, 1.2, or 1.8 mg. Albiglutide supplied in a 30-mg and a 50-mg single-dose pen. Dulaglutide supplied in a 0.75-mg and 1.5-mg single-dose pen and prefilled syringe.

[b]Generic not available in United States.

T1DM, type 1 diabetes mellitus; T2DM, type 2 diabetes mellitus

Pramlintide has the potential to delay the absorption of orally administered medications. When rapid absorption is needed for the efficacy of an agent, pramlintide should be administered 1 hour after or 3 hours before the drug. Pramlintide should not be used in patients receiving medications that alter GI motility. A disposable pen formulation is now on the market and available as SymlinPen 60 for patients with T1DM and SymlinPen 120 for people with T2DM.

Treatment of Concomitant Conditions

► *Cardiovascular Health*

Cardiovascular disease is the major cause of morbidity and mortality for patients with DM. Interventions targeting smoking cessation, blood pressure control, lipid management, antiplatelet therapy, and lifestyle changes (including diet and exercise) can reduce the risk of cardiovascular events and should be considered as important as glycemic control in the management of a patient with DM. All patients with a history of cardiovascular disease should be prescribed aspirin 75 to 162 mg/day as a secondary prevention strategy.[7] For those with aspirin allergy, another antiplatelet option such as clopidogrel 75 mg/day should be used. The ADA currently recommends that antiplatelet therapy should also be considered for patients with DM and no history of heart disease if that patient's risk of cardiovascular event is calculated to be greater than 10% over 10 years. This includes most men older than 50 years of age and most women older than 60 years of age who have at least one additional cardiovascular risk factor.

The results of a number of trials, including the Action to Control Cardiovascular Risk in Diabetes (ACCORD),[31] Action in Diabetes and Vascular Disease (ADVANCE),[32] and Veterans Affairs Diabetes Trial (VADT,)[33] taken together with long-term follow-up information from the UKPDS[34] and DCCT [35,36] trials, have been used to formulate conclusions regarding the effect of glucose lowering on cardiovascular health. Those conclusions are: (1) short-term (3–5 years) intensive glycemic control does not improve the risk of macrovascular complications in patients with long-standing T2DM; and (2) a decrease in macrovascular risk from improved glycemic control may take more than a decade to be realized. Because of the results of these trials, the A_{1c} goal used for most patients with T2DM is less than 7% (0.07; 53 mmol/mol Hgb), whereas a goal of less than or equal to 6.5% (0.065; 48 mmol/mol Hgb) may be used for otherwise healthy individuals who are thought to be early in the course of their diabetes.[7,16] More relaxed A_{1c} targets may be employed for those patients who are older, have numerous medical conditions limiting their life expectancy, are at increased risk for hypoglycemia, or who have had T2DM for a long period of time.

► *Dyslipidemia*

The 2013 American College of Cardiology/American Heart Association Guideline on the Treatment of Blood Cholesterol to Reduce Atherosclerotic Cardiovascular Risk in Adults recommends statin therapy be considered if a patient falls into one of four statin benefit groups.[37] The groups are:

1. Patients with clinical atherosclerotic cardiovascular disease (ASCVD);
2. Patients with no prior history of ASCVD but a LDL level of 190 mg/dL (4.91 mmol/L) or higher;
3. Patients with diabetes and no history of clinical ASCVD who are between the ages of 40 and 75 years with a LDL level between 70 and 189 mg/dL (1.81 and 4.89 mmol/L); and
4. Patients ages 40 to 75 years with no prior history of ASCVD or diabetes who have a LDL level between 70 and 189 mg/dL (1.81 and 4.89 mmol/L)and a 10-year estimated ASCVD risk of 7.5% or higher.

Severe hypertriglyceridemia may warrant therapy with niacin, a fibrate, and/or fish oil. Although it was common practice in the past to add niacin or a fibrate onto statin therapy to augment triglyceride and HDL once LDL goals were met, cardiovascular outcome benefit has not been proven when these drugs are added to statin therapy over statin therapy alone.[38,39] Refer to Chapter 12, Dyslipidemias, for more information on managing cardiovascular risk through the optimal use of antihyperlipidemic therapies.

► *Hypertension*

KEY CONCEPT *Uncontrolled blood pressure plays a major role in the development of macrovascular events as well as microvascular complications, including retinopathy and nephropathy, in patients with DM. The ADA recommends that systolic blood pressure goals for patients with DM be individualized but generally set at less than 140 mm Hg.[7] The diastolic blood pressure goal for patients with DM is less than 90 mm Hg.* In addition, there are several general principles regarding the treatment of hypertension in diabetes patients. Angiotensin-converting enzyme (ACE) inhibitors or angiotensin II receptor blockers are recommended as initial therapy because of their beneficial effects on renal function. It can be expected that most patients will require more than one agent to reach blood pressure goal. Renal function and serum potassium levels should be monitored closely in all patients taking an ACE inhibitor, angiotensin II receptor blocker, and/or diuretic. ACE inhibitors and angiotensin II receptor blockers are contraindicated in patients who are pregnant and in those with bilateral renal artery stenosis.

Patient Encounter, Part 2: Follow-Up Visit

The patient returns a week later with results from her fasting blood work. The physician also requests a fasting glucose, A_{1C} and vitals at today's visit. The results are listed below.

VS: BP 122/76 mm Hg, P 70 beats/min, RR 19 breaths/min, T 38°C (100°F)

A_{1c} (today): 8.2% (0.082; 66 mmol/mol Hgb)

FPG (today): 189 mg/dL (10.5 mmol/L)

Labs (2 days ago): Na 136 mEq/L (136 mmol/L); K 3.6 mEq/L (3.6 mmol/L); Cl 98 mEq/L (98 mmol/L); CO_2 24 mEq/L (24 mmol/L); BUN 15 mg/dL (5.4 mmol/L); SCr 0.9 mg/dL (80 μmol/L); Glu 172 mg/dL (9.5 mmol/L)

The patient is diagnosed with type 2 diabetes. Identify the goals of treatment for this patient.

What nonpharmacologic alternatives are available for this patient for her diabetes?

What are the three general categories of pharmacologic alternatives used to lower blood glucose?

What is the most appropriate initial therapy for this patient in regards to her diabetes?

What additional interventions are recommended for this patient today?

▶ Human Immunodeficiency Virus (HIV) and Acquired Immune Deficiency Syndrome (AIDS)

Patients with risk factors for diabetes are more likely to develop diabetes when exposed to highly active antiretroviral therapy.[40] Universal screening of all HIV patients for diabetes is controversial, but most clinicians support screening for those with risk factors, especially if those risk factors include positive family history and central adiposity. Disturbances in glucose homeostasis are a known side effect of protease inhibitor therapy. Indinavir and ritonavir block insulin-mediated glucose disposal, causing insulin resistance, but amprenavir and atazanzvir have no effect on this pathway. Indinavir also increases hepatic glucose production and release and causes insulin to lose its ability to suppress hepatic glucose production. Nelfinavir, lopinavir, and saquinavir cause a 25% reduction in β-cell function, reducing first-phase insulin release. Drug selection for treating protease inhibitor–induced hyperglycemia should address the mechanism behind the adverse effect. Protease inhibitor therapy avoidance should be considered in patients with preexisting glucose abnormalities and in those with a first-degree relative with diabetes. Metformin should be used with caution in patients taking the nucleoside reverse transcriptase inhibitors stavudine, zidovudine, and didanosine because of an increased risk for lactic acidemia.

▶ Antipsychotic Drug Therapy

An association has been recognized between second-generation antipsychotics and the development of diabetes.[41] Risk seems to be highest with clozapine and olanzapine, but data are conflicting for risperidone and quetiapine. Aripiprazole and ziprasione have not, as of yet, shown an increased risk for diabetes with their use. Nutrition and physical activity counseling is recommended for all patients with mental illness who are overweight or obese, especially if they are beginning second-generation antipsychotic therapy. After therapy initiation, the patient's weight should be assessed at weeks 4, 8, and 12 and then every 3 months. In the event of weight gain greater than or equal to 5% of the patient's baseline weight, a therapeutic adjustment should be considered. For patients who develop worsening glycemia or dyslipidemia while on antipsychotic therapy, it is recommended that a switch to a second-generation antipsychotic with less weight gain or diabetes potential be considered.

Treatment of Acute Complications

▶ Hypoglycemia

Hypoglycemia, or low blood sugar, can be defined clinically as a blood glucose level of less than or equal to 70 mg/dL (3.9 mmol/L).[42] Individuals with DM can experience symptoms of hypoglycemia at varying blood glucose levels. Those with uncontrolled glucose can experience pseudohypoglycemia which is when symptoms of hypoglycemia occur even at normal glucose levels. Those with recent low blood glucose levels may have no symptoms even at glucose values below the hypoglycemia threshold and, therefore, patients with recurrent hypoglycemia may benefit from a period of more relaxed glycemic targets.[7] Typical symptoms of hypoglycemia include shakiness, sweating, fatigue, hunger, headaches, and confusion.

Common causes of hypoglycemia include delayed or inadequate amounts of food intake, especially carbohydrates, excessive doses of medications (eg, sulfonylureas and insulin), exercising when insulin doses are reaching peak effect, or inadequately adjusted drug therapy in patients with impaired renal or hepatic function. Patients experiencing symptoms of hypoglycemia should check their blood glucose level, consume 15 g of carbohydrate, wait 15 minutes for symptom resolution, and retest.[42] Examples of acceptable treatments may include a small box of raisins, 4 oz (~120 mL) of orange juice, 8 oz (~240 mL) of skim milk, or three to six glucose tablets. In patients receiving an α-glucosidase inhibitor in combination with a sulfonylurea or insulin, hypoglycemia should be treated with glucose tablets or skim milk owing to the mechanism of action of the α-glucosidase inhibitors. For patients with hypoglycemia experiencing a loss of consciousness, a glucagon emergency kit should be administered by the intramuscular or subcutaneous route. It is important to contact emergency medical personnel in this particular situation. The patient should be rolled onto his or her side to prevent aspiration because many patients receiving the glucagon injection vomit.

▶ Diabetic Ketoacidosis

Diabetic ketoacidosis is a reversible but potentially life-threatening medical emergency that results from a relative or absolute deficiency in insulin. Without insulin, the body cannot use glucose as an energy source and must obtain energy via lipolysis. This process produces ketones and leads to acidosis. Although DKA occurs frequently in young patients with T1DM on initial presentation, it can occur in adults as well. Often, precipitating factors such as infection, omission, or inadequate administration of insulin can cause DKA. Signs and symptoms develop rapidly within 1 day or so and commonly include fruity or acetone breath; nausea; vomiting; dehydration; polydipsia; polyuria; and deep, rapid breathing.

Hallmark diagnostic criteria for DKA include hyperglycemia (greater than 250 mg/dL [13.9 mmol/L]), ketosis (anion gap greater than 12 mEq/L [12 mmol/L]), and acidosis (arterial pH less than or equal to 7.3).[43] Typical fluid deficit is 5 to 7 L or more, and major deficits of serum sodium and potassium are common.

The severity of DKA depends on the magnitude of the decrease in arterial pH, serum bicarbonate levels, and the mental state rather than the magnitude of the hyperglycemia. Treatment goals of DKA consist of reversing the underlying metabolic abnormalities, rehydrating the patient, and normalizing the serum glucose. Fluid replacement with normal saline at 1 to 1.5 L/hour for the first hour is recommended to rehydrate the patient and to ensure the kidneys are perfused.

Potassium and other electrolytes are supplemented as indicated by laboratory assessment. The use of sodium bicarbonate in DKA is controversial and generally only recommended when the pH is less than 7. Regular insulin at 0.1 unit/kg/hour by continuous IV infusion is the preferred treatment in DKA to regain metabolic control rapidly. When plasma glucose values drop below 250 mg/dL (13.9 mmol/L), dextrose 5% should be added to the IV fluids. During the recovery period, it is recommended to continue administering insulin and to allow patients to eat as soon as possible. Dietary carbohydrates combined with insulin assist in the clearance of ketones. See Table 43–11 for the management of DKA.[43]

▶ Hyperosmolar Hyperglycemic State

Hyperosmolar hyperglycemic state (HHS) is a life-threatening condition similar to DKA that also arises from inadequate

Patient Encounter, Part 3: Follow-Up

The patient returns in 3 months for a follow-up visit. She brings her blood glucose readings from the past week for review in addition to more fasting blood work. Blood glucose readings are in units of mg/dL (mmol/L). Her most recent medication list is below. There are no changes to her health record from previous visits.

Allergies: Sulfa and penicillin

Meds: Fluticasone nasal spray, one spray each nostril daily if needed during allergy season; metformin 1000 mg by mouth twice daily

VS: BP 154/96 mm Hg, P 78 beats/min, RR 18 breaths/min, T 37°C (98.6°F)

Labs: Total cholesterol 240 mg/dL (6.21 mmol/L); HDL 41 mg/dL (1.06 mmol/L); LDL 163 mg/dL (4.22 mmol/L); TG 183 mg/dL (2.07 mmol/L); AST 28 U/L (0.47 μKat/L); ALT 31 U/L (0.52 μKat/L)

Day	FPG	PPG
Monday	118 (6.5)	168 (9.3)
Tuesday	122 (6.8)	187 (10.4)
Wednesday	134 (7.4)	140 (7.8)
Thursday	110 (6.1)	244 (13.5)
Friday	98 (5.4)	257 (14.3)
Saturday	128 (7.1)	297 (16.5)
Sunday	116 (6.4)	240 (13.3)

Are this patient's blood glucose levels within target? What pattern seems to be established?

Which classes of antidiabetic drugs act in a manner that would specifically correct the undesirable glucose pattern?

Based on the information available from this encounter and previous encounters, develop a care plan for this patient. The plan should include (a) identification and assessment of all drug-related needs and/or problems, (b) a detailed therapeutic plan to address each need and problem, and (c) monitoring parameters to assess safety and efficacy.

insulin, but HHS occurs primarily in older patients with T2DM. DKA and HHS also differ in that HHS lacks the ketonemia and acidosis associated with DKA. Patients with hyperglycemia and dehydration lasting several days to weeks are at the greatest risk of developing HHS. Infection, silent myocardial infarction, cerebrovascular accident, mesenteric ischemia, acute pancreatitis, and the use of medications that affect carbohydrate metabolism including steroids and thiazide diuretics are known precipitating causes of HHS. Two main diagnostic criteria for HHS are a plasma glucose value of greater than 600 mg/dL (33.3 mmol/L) and a serum osmolality of greater than 320 mOsm/kg (320 mmol/kg).[43] The extreme hyperglycemia and large fluid deficits resulting from osmotic diuresis are major challenges to overcome with this condition. Similar to DKA, the treatment of HHS consists of aggressive rehydration, correction of electrolyte imbalances, and continuous insulin infusion to normalize serum glucose. Blood glucose levels should be reduced gradually to minimize the risk of cerebral edema.

Table 43–11

Management of Diabetic Ketoacidosis[41]

1. Confirm diagnosis (increased plasma glucose, positive serum ketones, metabolic acidosis).
2. Admit to hospital; intensive care setting may be necessary for frequent monitoring or if pH < 7 or unconscious.
3. Asses serum electrolytes (K^+, Na^+, Mg^{2+}, Cl^-, bicarbonate, phosphate), acid–base status—pH, HCO^-_3, Pco_2, β-hydroxybutyrate, and renal function (creatinine, urine output).
4. Replace fluids: 0.9% saline 1 L/hour over first 1–3 hours; subsequently, 0.45% saline at 4–14 mL/kg/hour; change to 5% dextrose with 0.45% saline when plasma glucose reaches 250 mg/dL (13.9 mmol/L).
5. Administer regular insulin: IV (0.15 U/kg bolus followed by 0.1 unit/kg/hour infusion); check glucose hourly and double insulin infusion until glucose level falls at steady hourly rate of 50–70 mg/dL (2.8–3.9 mmol/L). Alternatively, could use SC or IM routes, although dosing regimen different. If initial serum potassium is less than 3.3 mEq/L (3.3 mmol/L), do not administer insulin until the potassium is corrected to > 3.3 mEq/L (3.3 mmol/L).
6. Assess patient: What precipitated the episode (eg, nonadherence, infection, trauma, infarction, cocaine)? Initiate appropriate workup for precipitating event (cultures, chest x-ray, ECG).
7. Measure chemistry (especially K^+, bicarbonate, phosphate and anion gap) every 2–4 hours until stable.
8. Replace K^+: If K^+ is < 3.3 mEq/L (3.3 mmol/L), hold insulin and give 40 mEq (40 mmol) of K^+ per liter of IV fluid. If K^+ is > 5 mEq/L (5 mmol/L), do not give K^+ but check level every 2 hours. When K^+ > 3.3 mEq/L (3.3 mmol/L) but < 5 mEq/L (5.5 mmol/L), ECG normal, urine flow and normal creatinine documented, administer 20–30 mEq/L (20–30 mmol/L) of IV fluid to maintain K^+ at 4–5 mEq/L (4–5 mmol/L).
9. Continue above until patient is stable, glucose goal is 150–250 mg/dL (8.3–13.9 mmol/L), and acidosis is resolved. Insulin infusion may be decreased to 0.05–0.1 unit/kg/hour.
10. Administer intermediate- or long-acting insulin as soon as patient is eating. Allow for overlap in insulin infusion and subcutaneous insulin injection.

Cl, chloride; ECG, electrocardiogram; HCO_3, serum bicarbonate; IM, intramuscular; IV, intravenous; K, potassium; Mg, magnesium; Na, sodium; Pco_2, partial pressure of carbon dioxide in the arterial blood; SC, subcutaneous.

Treatment of Long-Term Complications

▸ *Retinopathy*

Diabetic retinopathy occurs when the microvasculature that supplies blood to the retina becomes damaged. This damage permits leakage of blood components through the vessel walls. Diabetic retinopathy is the leading cause of blindness in adults 20 to 74 years of age in the United States.[7] The risk of retinopathy is increased in patients with long-standing DM, chronic hyperglycemia, hypertension, and nephropathy. Other eye disorders, including glaucoma and cataracts, are more likely to occur in patients with diabetes as well.

The ADA recommends that patients with T2DM receive a dilated eye examination at the time of diagnosis by an ophthalmologist or optometrist.[7] Examinations should begin within 5 years of diagnosis of T1DM. Once one or more normal examinations occur, the dilated eye exam is recommended to be repeated at least every two years. But, in patients with documented retinopathy, an annual dilated eye exam is recommended. Glucose and blood pressure control are the best strategies for decreasing the risk and slowing the progression of retinopathy.

▸ Neuropathy

KEY CONCEPT *Peripheral neuropathy is a possible complication of diabetes. The most common types of peripheral neuropathy include chronic sensorimotor distal peripheral neuropathy, which can cause pain, tingling, and numbness in the feet and hands, and autonomic neuropathy, which can lead to hypotension, gastroparesis, sexual dysfunction, and autonomic failure in response to hypoglycemia.*[7] Two drugs, pregabalin and duloxetine, have been approved for the relief of distal peripheral neuropathy pain. A number of other drugs are also sometimes used including venlafaxine, amitriptyline, valproate, and opioids.

▸ Microalbuminuria and Nephropathy

DM is a leading contributor to end-stage renal disease. Early evidence of nephropathy is the presence of albumin in the urine. Therefore, as the disease progresses, larger amounts of protein spill into the urine. The ADA recommends urine protein tests annually in T2DM patients.[7] For patients with T1DM, annual urine protein testing should begin 5 years after the diagnosis of diabetes. The most common form of screening for protein in the urine is a random collection for measurement of the urine albumin-to-creatinine ratio. The desirable value is less than 30 mcg of albumin per milligram of creatinine (3.4 mg/mmol creatinine). The terms microalbuminuria and macroalbuminuria are being replaced by the term "persistent albuminuria," with the level of albuminuria further defined as either being between 30 and less than 299 mcg of albumin per milligram of creatinine (3.4–34 mg/mmol creatinine; previously referred to as microalbuminuria) or greater than or equal to 300 mcg of albumin per milligram of creatinine (greater than or equal to 34 mg/mmol creatinine; previously known as macroalbuminuria).

Glycemic control and blood pressure control are primary measures for the prevention of progression of nephropathy. ACE inhibitors and angiotensin II receptor blockers prevent the progression of renal disease in patients with T2DM. Treatment of advanced nephropathy includes dialysis and kidney transplantation.

▸ Foot Ulcers

KEY CONCEPT *Lower extremity amputations are one of the most feared and disabling sequelae of long-term uncontrolled DM. A foot ulcer is an open sore that develops and penetrates to the subcutaneous tissues. Complications of the feet develop primarily as a result of peripheral vascular disease, neuropathies, and foot deformations.*

Peripheral arterial disease causes ischemia to the lower limbs. This decreased blood flow deprives the tissues of oxygen and nutrients and impairs the ability of the immune system to function adequately. Symptoms of peripheral arterial disease include intermittent claudication, cold feet, pain at rest, and loss of hair on the feet and toes. Smoking cessation is the single most important treatment for peripheral arterial disease. In addition, exercising by walking to the point of pain and then resting and resuming can be a vital therapy to maintain or improve the symptoms of peripheral arterial disease. Pharmacologic intervention with antiplatelet therapy (aspirin 160–325 mg/day or clopidogrel 75 mg/day) is indicated in patients with peripheral arterial disease.[44] For those that remain symptomatic, cilostazol 100 mg twice daily may be useful to improve blood flow and reduce the symptoms of peripheral vascular disease.

Neuropathies play a large part in the development of foot ulcers. Loss of sensation in the feet allows trauma to go unnoticed. Autonomic neuropathy can cause changes in blood flow, perspiration, skin hydration, and possibly, bone composition of the foot. Motor neuropathy can lead to muscle atrophy, resulting in weakness and changes in the shape of the foot. To prevent foot complications, the ADA recommends daily visual examination of the feet and a foot check performed at every physician visit.[7] Sensory testing with a 10-gauge monofilament can detect areas of neuropathy. Treatment consists of glycemic control, preventing infection, debriding dead tissues, applying dressings, treating edema, and limiting ambulation. Additionally, diabetics should wear properly fitted, cushioned footwear and padded socks.

Special Situations

▸ Hospitalized Care

The NICE-SUGAR (intensive versus conventional glucose in critically ill patients) trial compared intensive (81–108 mg/dL [4.5–6.0 mmol/L]) with conventional (less than 180 mg/dL [10.0 mmol/L]) glucose control using IV insulin in intensive care unit patients.[45] At 90 days, intensively controlled patients had an increased absolute risk of death. Significantly more hypoglycemia was observed in the intensively controlled group.

Current recommendations call for critically ill patients to be started on IV insulin therapy at a threshold of 180 mg/dL (10.0 mmol/L).[7] A goal range of 140 to 180 mg/dL (7.8–10.0 mmol/L) is recommended for the majority of patients. More stringent goals may be considered for selected critically ill patients, but only if hypoglycemia can be avoided. Scheduled subcutaneous insulin regimens with basal, nutritional, and correction components are recommended for patients who are not critically ill. Goals of less than 140 mg/dL (7.8 mmol/L) for fasting glucose and less than 180 mg/dL (10.0 mmol/L) for random glucose are recommended for noncritically ill patients.

▸ Sick Days

Patients should monitor their blood glucose levels more frequently during sick days because it is common for illness to increase blood glucose values.[46] Patients with T1DM should check their glucose and urine for ketones every 4 hours when sick. Patients with T2DM may also need to check for ketones when their blood glucose levels are greater than 300 mg/dL (16.7 mmol/L). Patients should continue to take their medications while sick. T1DM patients may require additional insulin coverage, and some with T2DM who are currently on oral medication regimens may require insulin during an acute illness. Patients should be advised to maintain their normal caloric and carbohydrate intake while ill as well as to drink plenty of noncaloric beverages to avoid dehydration. When having difficulty eating a normal diet, patients may be advised to use nondiet beverages, sports drinks, broths, crackers, soups, and nondiet gelatins to provide normal caloric and carbohydrate intake and avoid hypoglycemia. With proper management, patients can decrease their chance of illness-induced hospitalization, particularly DKA and HHS.

Patient Encounter, Part 4: Insulin Therapy

The patient returns to the office for her annual checkup. It has been 5 years since she was first diagnosed with diabetes. Her updated information is below. Her past medical and family histories are unchanged. She states that she has been adherent to medications and lifestyle changes. She complains that she has burning and tingling constantly in both of her feet.

SH: Smokes half pack cigarettes per day for 15 years; drinks bottle of wine on the weekends; denies illicit drug use

Allergies: Sulfa and penicillin

Meds: Lisinopril 20 mg by mouth once daily; atorvastatin 20 mg by mouth once daily; fluticasone nasal spray, one spray each nostril daily if needed during allergy season; metformin 1000 mg by mouth twice daily; liraglutide 1.2 mg subcutaneously once daily; multivitamin by mouth once daily

Meal History: Has been consuming approximately 30 to 45 g of carbohydrates per meal three times a day; saturated fat is limited to 12 g/day, and sodium is 2000 mg/day

Physical Activity: Was walking 4 or 5 days per week for 30 minutes at moderate intensity but has not done so recently due to tingling in feet

VS: BP 135/82 mm Hg, P 85 beats/min, RR 20 breaths/min, T 38°C (100°F), Ht 5′3″ (160 cm), Wt 155 lb (70.5 kg)

Labs: Na 139 mEq/L (139 mmol/L); K 5 mEq/L (5 mmol/L); Cl 103 mEq/L (103 mmol/L); CO_2 23 mEq/L (23 mmol/L); BUN 16 mg/dL (5.7 mmol/L); SCr 0.9 mg/dL (80 μmol/L); FPG 180 mg/dL (10.0 mmol/L); A_{1c} 9.7% (0.097; 83 mmol/mol Hgb); AST 28 U/L (0.47 μKat/L); ALT 31 U/L (0.52 μKat/L)

- Fasting lipid profile:
  - Total cholesterol: 202 mg/dL (5.22 mmol/L)
  - LDL: 108 mg/dL (2.79 mmol/L)
  - HDL: 43 mg/dL (1.11 mmol/L)
  - TG: 205 mg/dL (2.32 mmol/L)

What additional pharmacologic options are available for this patient to lower her blood glucose to goal?

Which insulin and starting dose would be most appropriate for this patient?

What additional medications, screenings, labs, and/or referrals are recommended for the patient at this point?

What is an important lifestyle modification this patient still needs to make?

Patient Care Process

Patient Assessment:

- Assess patient for development or progression of DM and complications (see Tables 43–4 and 43–5).
- Evaluate SMBG for glycemic control, including FPG and postprandial levels (see Table 43–6).
  - Are the blood glucose values too high or low?
  - Are there specific times of day or specific days not in control?
  - Is hypoglycemia occurring?
- Review laboratory data for attainment of goals (see Table 43–6). What goals are not being met? What tests or referrals to other health care team members are needed?
- Assess patient for quality-of-life measures such as physical, psychological, and social functioning and well-being.

Therapy Evaluation:

- Perform medication history of prescription, over-the-counter, and herbal product use.
- Are there any medication problems, including presence of adverse drug reactions, drug allergies, and drug interactions?
- If patient is already receiving treatment for DM, has he/she been adherent to recommended lifestyle modifications and drug therapies? Is the patient having difficulty affording their therapies?
- Determine if patient has prescription coverage.
- Is the patient taking medications that may affect glucose control?

Care Plan Development:

- Recommend appropriate therapy and develop a plan to assess effectiveness (see Tables 43–7, 43–9, and 43–10).
- Stress adherence to prescribed lifestyle and medication regimen.
- Provide education on diabetes, lifestyle modifications, appropriate monitoring, and drug therapy:
  - Causes of DM complications and how to prevent them.
  - How diet and exercise can affect diabetes.
  - How to perform SMBG and what to do with the results.
  - When to take medications and what to expect, including adverse effects.
  - What warning sign(s) should be reported to the physician.

Follow-up Evaluation:

- Set follow up for SMBG and tolerability/presence of adverse effects based on therapy chosen.
- Follow up A_{1c} every 3 months until patient reaches goal, then every 6 months. See Table 43–6 for other monitoring parameters and frequency.

OUTCOME EVALUATION

- The success of therapy for DM is measured by the ability of the patient to manage his or her disease appropriately between health care provider visits.
- Appropriate therapy necessitates adequate patient education about the disease, development of a meal plan to which patients can comply, and integration of a regular exercise program.
- Patient care plans should include a number of daily evaluations to be performed by the patient, such as examining the feet for any sores, cuts, or abrasions; checking the skin for dryness to prevent cracking and chafing; and monitoring blood glucose values as directed. Weekly appraisals of weight and blood pressure are also advised.
- Until A_{1c} levels are at goal, quarterly visits with the patient's primary health care provider are recommended. Table 43–6 summarizes the specific ADA goals for therapy. The practitioner should review SMBG data and a current A_{1c} level for progress and address any therapeutic or educational issues.
- At a minimum, yearly laboratory evaluation of serum lipids, urinary microalbumin, and serum creatinine should be performed.

Abbreviations Introduced in This Chapter

A_{1c}	Hemoglobin A_{1c}
AACE	American Association of Clinical Endocrinologists
ACCORD	Action to Control Cardiovascular Risk in Diabetes
ACE	Angiotensin-converting enzyme
ADA	American Diabetes Association
ADVANCE	Action in Diabetes and Vascular Disease
AG-i	Alpha glucosidase inhibitor
AIDS	Acquired immune deficiency syndrome
ALT	Alanine aminotransferase
ASCVD	Atherosclerotic cardiovascular disease
ATP	Adenosine triphosphate
bg	Blood glucose
BMI	Body mass index
BUN	Blood urea nitrogen
CDC	Centers for Disease Control and Prevention
Cl	Chloride
CrCl	Creatinine clearance
CSII	Continuous subcutaneous insulin infusion
DCCT	Diabetes Control and Complications Trial
DKA	Diabetic ketoacidosis
DM	Diabetes mellitus
DPP-4	Dipeptidyl peptidase-4
DPP-4-i	Dipeptidyl peptidase-4 inhibitor
eAG	Estimated average glucose
ECG	Electrocardiogram
ER	Extended release
FBG	Fasting blood glucose
FDA	Food and Drug Administration
FPG	Fasting plasma glucose
Fx	Fracture
GDM	Gestational diabetes mellitus
GI	Gastrointestinal
GIP	Glucose-dependent insulinotropic peptide
GLN	Meglitinide
GLP-1	Glucagon-like peptide-1
GLP-1-RA	Glucagon-like peptide-1 receptor agonist
Hgb	Hemoglobin
HbA_{1c}	Hemoglobin A_{1c}
HCO_3	Serum bicarbonate
HDL	High-density lipoprotein
HF	Heart failure
HHS	Hyperosmolar hyperglycemic state
HIV	Human immunodeficiency virus
IFG	Impaired fasting glucose
IGT	Impaired glucose tolerance
IM	Intramuscular
Inh	Inhalation
ISF	Interstitial fluid
IV	Intravenous
K	Potassium
LADA	Latent autoimmune diabetes in adults
LDL	Low-density lipoprotein cholesterol
MET	Metformin
Mg	Magnesium
MNT	Medical nutrition therapy
Na	Sodium
NGSP	National Glycohemoglobin Standardization Program
NICE-SUGAR	Intensive versus conventional glucose control in critically ill patients
NPH	Neutral protamine Hagedorn
OGTT	Oral glucose tolerance test
OTC	Over-the-counter
Pco_2	Partial pressure of carbon dioxide in arterial blood
PPAR-γ	Proxisome proliferator activated receptor gamma
PPG	Postprandial glucose
QR	Quick release
Rx	Prescription
SC	Subcutaneous
SCr	Serum creatinine
SGLT-2	Sodium-dependent glucose cotransporter-2
SMBG	Self-monitoring of blood glucose
SU	Sulfonyurea
T1DM	Type 1 diabetes mellitus
T2DM	Type 2 diabetes mellitus
TG	Triglycerides
TLC	Therapeutic lifestyle change
TZD	Thiazolidinedione
UKPDS	United Kingdom Prospective Diabetes Study
ULN	Upper limit of normal
UTI	Urinary tract infection
VADT	Veterans Affairs Diabetes Trial
WHO	World Health Organization

REFERENCES

1. Centers for Disease Control and Prevention. National Diabetes Statistics Report, 2014 [Internet]. U.S. Department of Health and Human Services; 2014 [cited 2014 Jul 15]. http://www.cdc.gov/diabetes/pubs/statsreport14/national-diabetes-report-web.pdf. Accessed July 15, 2014.
2. Ogden CL, Carroll MD, Kit BK, Flegal KM. Prevalence of obesity among adults: United States, 2011-2012 [Internet]. NCHS data brief, no 131. Hyattsville, MD: National Center for Health Statistics; 2013 [cited 2014 Jul 15]. http://www.cdc.gov/nchs/data/databriefs/db131.htm#definitions. Accessed July 15, 2014.
3. Centers for Disease Control and Prevention. Highest rates of leisure-time physical inactivity in Appalachia and South [Internet]. U.S. Department of Health and Human Services, 2011 [cited 2014 Jul 15]. http://www.cdc.gov/media/releases/2011/p0216_physicalinactivity.html. Accessed July 15, 2014.

4. Chiang JL, Kirkman MS, Laffel LMB, et al. Type 1 diabetes through the life span: A position statement of the American Diabetes Association. Diabetes Care. 2014;37:2034–2054.
5. Klinke DJ. Extent of beta cell destruction is important but insufficient to predict the onset of type 1 diabetes mellitus. PLoS One. 2008;3(1):e1374.
6. Tuomi T, Santoro N, Caprio S, Cai M, Weng J, Groop L. The many faces of diabetes: A disease with increasing heterogeneity. Lancet. 2014;383:1084–1094.
7. American Diabetes Association. Standards of medical care in diabetes—2015. Diabetes Care. 2015;38(Suppl 1):S4–S93.
8. Triplitt CL, Repas T, and Alvarez CA. Diabetes mellitus. In: DiPiro JT, Talbert RL, Yee GC, Matzke GR, Wells BG, and Posey LM, eds. Pharmacotherapy: A Pathophysiologic Approach. 9th ed. New York: McGraw-Hill; 2014:1143–1189.
9. Molina PE. Endocrine pancreas. In: Endocrine Physiology. 4th ed. New York: McGraw-Hill; 2013:163–186.
10. Powers AC, D'Alessio D. Endocrine pancreas and pharmacotherapy of diabetes mellitus and hypoglycemia. In: Brunton L, Chabner B, Knollman B, eds. Goodman and Gillman's The Pharmacological Basis of Therapeutics. 12th ed. New York: McGraw Hill; 2011: 1237–1274.
11. Virally M, Blickle JF, Girard J, Halimi S, Simon D, and Guillausseau PJ. Type 2 diabetes mellitus: Epidemiology, pathophysiology, unmet needs and therapeutical perspectives. Diabetes and Metab. 33;2007:231–244.
12. Alberti K, Zimmet P, Shaw J: Metabolic syndrome—a new world–wide definition. A consensus statement from the international diabetes federation. Diabet Med. 2006,23:469–480.
13. Cernea S, Raz I. Therapy in the early stage: Incretins. Diabetes Care. 2011;34(Suppl 2):S264–S271.
14. The Diabetes Control and Complications Trial Research Group. The effect of intensive treatment of diabetes on the development and progression of long-term complications in insulin-dependent diabetes mellitus. N Engl J Med. 1993;329(14):977–986.
15. UK Prospective Diabetes Study (UKPDS) Group. Intensive blood-glucose control with sulfonylureas or insulin compared with conventional treatment and risk of complications in patients with type 2 diabetes (UKPDS 33). Lancet. 1998;352(9131): 837–853.
16. Garber AJ, Abrahamson MJ, Barzilay JI, et al. American association of clinical endocrinologists' comprehensive diabetes management algorithm 2013 consensus statement. Endocr Pract. 2013;19(Suppl 1):1–48.
17. Nathan D, Kuenen J, Borg R, et al. For the A1c Derived Average Glucose (ADAG) study group. Translating the A1c assay into estimated average glucose values. Diabetes Care. 2008;31:1473–1478.
18. Inzucchi SE, Bergenstal RM, Buse JB, et al. Management of hyperglycemia in type 2 diabetes: A patient-centered approach. Diabetes Care. 2012;35:1364–1379.
19. Nathan DM, Buse JB, Davidson MB, et al. Medical management of hyperglycemia in type 2 diabetes: A consensus algorithm for the initiation and adjustment of therapy: A consensus statement from the American Diabetes Association and the European Association for the Study of Diabetes. Diabetes Care. 2009;32:193–203.
20. American College of Sports Medicine and American Diabetes Association. Exercise and type 2 diabetes. Med Sci Sports Exerc. 2010; 42:2282–2303.
21. Rodbard HW, Davidson JA, Garber AJ, et al. Statement by an American Association of Clinical Endocrinologists/American College of Endocrinology consensus panel on type 2 diabetes mellitus: An algorithm for glycemic control. Endocrine Pract. 2009;15:540–559.
22. Lexicomp Online. Hudson, OH: Lexi-Comp, Inc; 2014. http://online.lexi.com/crlsql/servlet/crlonline. Accessed August 25, 2014.
23. UK Prospective Diabetes Study (UKPDS) Group. Effect of intensive blood-glucose control with metformin on complications in overweight patients with type 2 diabetes (UKPDS 34). Lancet. 1998;352:854–865.
24. Blake EW, Sease JM. Effect of diabetes medications on cardiovascular risk and surrogate markers in patients with type 2 diabetes. J Pharm Technol. 2009;25:24–36.
25. Nissen SE, Wolski K. The effect of rosiglitazone on the risk of myocardial infarction and death from cardiovascular causes. N Eng J Med. 2007;356:1–15.
26. Home PD, Pocock SJ, Beck-Nielsen H, et al. Rosiglitazone evaluated for cardiovascular outcomes in oral agent combination therapy for type 2 diabetes (RECORD): A multicentre, randomised, open-label trial. Lancet. 2009;373:2125–2135.
27. Facts & Comparisons eAnswers. Indianapolis, IN: Clinical Drug Information, LLC; 2014. http://online.factsandcomparisons.com/login.aspx?url=/index.aspx&qs=. Accessed August 30, 2014.
28. Doheny K. Inhaled insulin: What to tell patients [Internet]. Medscape Pharmacists; July 1, 2014. [cited 2014 August 30]. http://www.medscape.com/viewarticle/827637?src=rss#1.
29. Russell S. Incretin-based therapies for type 2 diabetes mellitus: a review of direct comparisons of efficacy, safety and patient satisfaction. Int J Clin Pharm. 2013;35:159–172.
30. Pratley RE, Nauck MA, Barnett AH, et al, for the HARMONY 7 Study Group. Once-weekly albiglutide versus once-daily liraglutide in patients with type 2 diabetes inadequately controlled on oral drugs (HARMONY 7): A randomised, open-label, multicentre, noninferiority phase 3 study. Lancet Diabetes Endocrinol. 2014;2:289–297.
31. The Action to Control Cardiovascular Risk in Diabetes Study Group. Effects of intensive glucose lowering in type 2 diabetes. N Engl J Med. 2008;358:2545–2559.
32. The ADVANCE Collaborative Group. Intensive blood glucose control and vascular outcomes in patients with type 2 diabetes. N Engl J Med. 2008;358:2560–2572.
33. Duckworth W, Abraira C, Mortiz T, et al. Glucose control and vascular complications in veterans with type 2 diabetes. N Engl J Med. 2009;360:1–11.
34. Holman RR, Paul SK, Bethel MA, et al. 10-year follow-up of intensive glucose control in type 2 diabetes. N Engl J Med. 2008;359:1577–1589.
35. EDIC Writing Group. Sustained effect of intensive treatment of type 1 diabetes mellitus on developments and progression of diabetic neuropathy: The Epidemiology of Diabetes Interventions and Complications Study. JAMA. 2003;290;2159–2167.
36. DCCT/EDIC Study Research Group. Intensive diabetes treatment and cardiovascular disease in patients with type 1 diabetes. N Engl J Med. 2005;353:2643–2653.
37. Stone NJ, Robinson J, Lichtenstein AH, et al. 2013 ACC/AHA guideline on the treatment of blood cholesterol to reduce atherosclerotic cardiovascular risk in adults: a report of the American College of Cardiology/American Heart Association task force on practice guidelines. Circulation. 2014;129: S1–S45.
38. Keech A, Simes RJ, Barter P, et al. Effects of long-term fenofibrate therapy on cardiovascular events in 9795 people with type 2 diabetes mellitus (the FIELD study): Randomised controlled trial. Lancet. 2005;366:1849–1861.
39. AIM-HIGH Investigators. Niacin in patients with low HDL cholesterol levels receiving intensive statin therapy. N Engl J Med. 2011;365:2255–2267.
40. Spollett GR. Hyperglycemia in HIV/AIDS. Diabetes Spectr. 2006;19:163–166.

41. American Diabetes Association, American Psychiatric Association, American Association of Clinical Endocrinologists, and North American Association for the Study of Obesity. Consensus development conference on antipsychotic drugs and obesity and diabetes. Diabetes Care. 2004;27:596–601.
42. Seaquist ER, Anderson J, Childs B, et al. Hypoglycemia and diabetes: a report of a workgroup of the American Diabetes Association and the Endocrine Society. Diabetes Care. 2013;36: 1384–1395.
43. Kitabachi AE, Upierrez GE, Miles JM, and Fisher JN. Hyperglycemic crises in adult patients with diabetes. Diabetes Care. 2009;32:1335–1343.
44. Alonso-Coello P, Bellmunt S, McGorrian C, et al. Antithrombotic therapy in peripheral artery disease. Antithrombotic therapy and prevention of thrombosis, 9th ed: American College of Chest Physicians Evidence-Based Clinical Practice Guidelines. Chest 2012;141(2)(Suppl):e669S–e690S.
45. Cook D, Dodek P, Henderson WR, et al. Intensive versus conventional glucose control in critically ill patients. N Engl J Med. 2009;360:1283–1297.
46. American Diabetes Association. When you're sick [Internet]. American Diabetes Association; 2014 [cited 2014 September 5]. http://www.diabetes.org/living-with-diabetes/treatment-and-care/whos-on-your-health-care-team/when-youre-sick.html. Accessed September 5, 2014.

44 Thyroid Disorders

Michael D. Katz

LEARNING OBJECTIVES

Upon completion of the chapter, the reader will be able to:

1. Discuss the prevalence of common thyroid disorders, including mild and overt hypothyroidism and hyperthyroidism.
2. Explain the major components of the hypothalamic–pituitary–thyroid axis and interaction among these components.
3. Discuss the relationship between serum thyroid-stimulating hormone (TSH) levels and primary thyroid disease, and the advantages for use of TSH levels over other tests such as serum T_4 (thyroxine) and T_3 (triiodothyronine) levels.
4. Identify typical signs and symptoms of hypothyroidism and the consequences of suboptimal treatment.
5. Describe clinical use of levothyroxine (LT_4) in the treatment of hypothyroidism.
6. Discuss the issues regarding LT_4 product bioequivalence and reasons for maintaining patients on the same product.
7. Describe the management of hypothyroidism and hyperthyroidism in pregnant women.
8. Identify typical signs and symptoms of Graves disease and consequences of inadequate treatment.
9. Discuss the pharmacotherapy of Graves disease, including advantages and disadvantages of antithyroid drugs versus radioactive iodine, adverse effects, and patient monitoring.
10. Describe the potential effects of selected drugs, including amiodarone, lithium interferon-α, and tyrosine kinase inhibitors on thyroid function.

INTRODUCTION

Thyroid disorders are common. More than 2 billion people, or 38% of the world's population, have iodine deficiency, resulting in 74 million people with **goiters**. Although overt iodine deficiency is not a significant problem in developed countries, a number of common thyroid conditions exist. The most common are **hypothyroidism** and **hyperthyroidism**, which often require long-term pharmacotherapy. Undetected or improperly treated thyroid disease can result in long-term adverse sequelae, including increased mortality. It is important that clinicians are aware of the prevalence of thyroid disorders, methods of identifying thyroid disorders, and appropriate therapy. This chapter focuses on the most common pharmacologically treated thyroid disorders.

EPIDEMIOLOGY OF THYROID DISEASE

Among 4392 people 12 years of age and older in a sample representing the geographic and ethnic distribution of the US population, hypothyroidism was found in 3.7% (3.4% mild) and hyperthyroidism in 0.5%.[1] The prevalence of hypothyroidism was higher in older age groups and in whites and Hispanics; blacks had a lower prevalence of hypothyroidism. The prevalence of hypothyroidism correlated with age. Compared with the total population, people aged 50 to 79 years had an almost twofold higher prevalence, and those aged 80 years and older had a fivefold higher prevalence. Pregnant women also had a higher prevalence of hypothyroidism. The Colorado Thyroid Health Survey assessed thyroid function in 25,862 subjects attending a health fair.[2] Overall prevalence of an abnormal TSH level was 11.7% of the study population, with 9.4% hypothyroid (9% subclinical) and 2.2% hyperthyroid (2.1% subclinical). Of the 916 subjects taking thyroid medication, 60% were **euthyroid**, with an equal distribution between subclinical hypothyroidism and hyperthyroidism. The National Health and Nutrition Examination Survey (NHANES) study also found that many patients receiving thyroid medications had an abnormal TSH level. These findings imply that many patients who are receiving thyroid medications are not being managed successfully.

THYROID HORMONE PHYSIOLOGY AND BIOSYNTHESIS[1]

KEY CONCEPT *The thyroid gland is the largest endocrine gland in the body, residing in the neck anterior to the trachea between the cricoid cartilage and suprasternal notch. The thyroid gland produces two biologically active hormones, thyroxine (T_4) and triiodothyronine (T_3).* Thyroid hormones are essential for proper fetal growth and development, particularly of the central nervous system (CNS). After delivery, the primary role of thyroid hormone is in regulation of energy metabolism. These hormones can affect the function of virtually every organ in the body. KEY CONCEPT *The parafollicular C cells of the thyroid gland produce calcitonin.* The function of calcitonin and its therapeutic use are discussed in other chapters in this book.

T_4 and T_3 are produced by the **organification** of iodine in the thyroid gland. Iodine is actively transported into the thyroid follicular cells. This inorganic iodine is oxidized by **thyroid peroxidase** and covalently bound to tyrosine residues of **thyroglobulin**. These iodinated tyrosine residues, monoiodotyrosine and diiodotyrosine, couple to form T_4 and T_3. Eighty percent of thyroid hormone is synthesized as T_4 and is stored in the thyroid bound to thyroglobulin. Thyroid hormones are released from the gland when needed, primarily under the influence of TSH (thyrotropin from the anterior pituitary). T_4 and T_3 are transported in the blood by three proteins, 70% bound to thyroid-binding globulin (TBG), 15% to transthyretin (thyroid-binding prealbumin), and 15% to albumin. T_4 is 99.97% protein bound, and T_3 is 99.7% protein bound, with only the unbound or free fractions physiologically active. The high degree of protein binding results in a long half-life of these hormones: approximately 7 to 10 days for T_4 and 24 hours for T_3.

Most of the physiologic activity of thyroid hormones is from the actions of T_3. T_4 can be thought of primarily as a prohormone. Eighty percent of needed T_3 is derived from conversion of T_4 to T_3 in peripheral tissue under the influence of tissue deiodinases. These deiodinases allow end organs to produce the amount of T_3 needed to control local metabolic functions. These enzymes also catabolize T_3 and T_4 to biologically inactive metabolites.

The production and release of thyroid hormones are regulated by the hypothalamic–pituitary–thyroid axis (**Figure 44–1**). Hypothalamic thyrotropin-releasing hormone (TRH) stimulates the release of TSH when there are physiologically inadequate levels of thyroid hormones. TSH promotes production and release of thyroid hormones. As circulating thyroid hormone levels rise to needed levels, negative feedback results in decreased release of TSH and TRH. Release of TRH is also inhibited by somatostatin and its analogs, and release of TSH can also be inhibited by dopamine, dopamine agonists, and high levels of glucocorticoids.

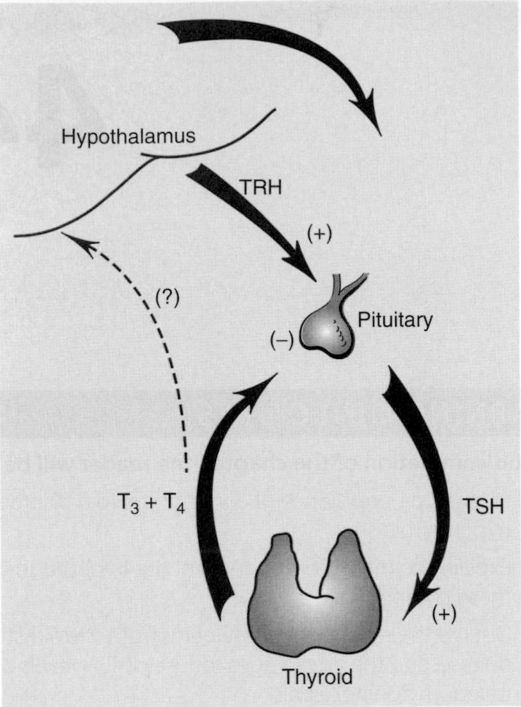

FIGURE 44–1. Hypothalamic–pituitary–thyroid axis. Thyrotropin-releasing hormone (TRH) is synthesized in the neurons within the paraventricular nucleus of the hypothalamus. TRH is released into the hypothalamic–pituitary portal circulation and carried to the pituitary, where it activates the pituitary to synthesize and release thyrotropin (TSH). TSH activates the thyroid to stimulate the synthesis and secretion of thyroxine (T_4) and triiodothyronine (T_3). T_4 and T_3 inhibit TSH secretion, closing the feedback loop. Negative feedback from T_4 and T_3 to hypothalamic TRH is less certain, hence the question mark.

SPECTRUM OF THYROID DISEASE

There are two general modes of presentation for thyroid disorders: changes in the size or shape of the gland and changes in secretion of hormone from the gland. In some cases, structural changes can result in changes in hormone secretion. Thyroid nodules and goiters in euthyroid patients are common problems. Patients with a goiter who are biochemically euthyroid often require no specific pharmacotherapy unless the goiter is caused by iodine deficiency. In developing countries, iodized salt is the primary therapy in treating goiter. Thyroid nodules, seen in 4% to 7% of adults, may be malignant or may autonomously secrete thyroid hormones. A discussion of thyroid nodules is beyond the scope of this chapter; however, thyroid cancer is discussed briefly in the context of levothyroxine (LT_4) suppressive therapy. Refer to other resources for a more extensive review of thyroid cancer management.

Changes in hormone secretion, often due to an underlying inflammatory disorder (thyroiditis), can result in hormone deficiency or excess. Although patients with overt hypothyroidism and hyperthyroidism may have dramatic signs and symptoms, most patients have subtle signs and symptoms that progress slowly over time. The availability of sensitive and specific biochemical tests for diagnosis of thyroid hormone disorders has facilitated screening and earlier case-finding and diagnosis, including in those with mild or subclinical thyroid disorders. Screening of newborns for congenital hypothyroidism has reduced the incidence of mental retardation and neonatal hypothyroidism (**cretinism**) dramatically in the United States. However, congenital hypothyroidism owing to iodine deficiency remains a significant worldwide public health problem.

PATIENT ASSESSMENT AND MONITORING

Assessment of patients for thyroid disorders entails a history and physical examination. In many patients with mild or subclinical thyroid disease, there may be an absence of specific signs and symptoms, and physical examination findings may be normal. Various diagnostic tests can be used, including serum thyroid hormone(s), TSH, thyroid antibody levels, and imaging techniques (**Table 44–1**). Laboratory assessment of patients with suspected thyroid disorders must be based on the continuum of disease from subclinical or mild to overt (**Figure 44–2**).

TSH Levels

KEY CONCEPT *In most patients with thyroid hormone disorders, measurement of a serum TSH level is adequate for initial screening and diagnosis of hypothyroidism and hyperthyroidism. Serum free thyroxine*

Table 44–1

Selected Thyroid Tests for Adults

Test	Reference Range	Comments
TSH	0.5–4.5 mIU/L (μIU/mL)	Gold standard; may be lowered by dopamine, dopamine agonists, glucocorticoids, octreotide, recovery from severe nonthyroidal illness
FT_4	0.7–1.9 ng/dL (9.0–24.5 pmol/L)	May be normal in mild thyroid disease
Anti-TPOAb, Anti-TGAb	Variable[a]	Present in autoimmune hypothyroidism; predicts more rapid progression from subclinical to overt hypothyroidism
TSI (TSHR-SAb)	Undetectable	Confirms Graves disease

Anti-TPOAb, antithyroid peroxidase antibody; FT_4, free T_4 (thyroxine); Anti-TGAb, antithyroglobulin antibodies; TSH, thyroid-stimulating hormone; TSHR-SAb, TSH receptor-stimulating antibodies; TSI, thyroid-stimulating immunoglobulin

[a]Anti-TPOAb reference ranges are highly variable from one laboratory to another depending on the method used. Results greater than the upper cutoff are considered abnormal and are consistent with increased risk for autoimmune thyroid disease.

(FT_4) and triiodothyronine (FT_3) levels may be helpful in distinguishing mild (subclinical) thyroid disease from overt disease. TSH for most patients being treated for thyroid disorders should be the mean normal value of 1.5 milli international units/L (mIU/L) or 1.5 micro international units/mL (μIU/mL) (target range, 0.5–4 mIU/L or μIU/mL), although patients must be individually titrated based on resolution of signs and symptoms as well as biochemical tests. Target TSH may be different in the elderly and in patients being treated with LT_4 for thyroid cancer.

TSH is a highly sensitive bioassay of the thyroid axis. A twofold change in serum-free T_4 levels will result in a 100-fold change in TSH levels. This biologic magnification by TSH allows it to be used in early diagnosis as well as in closely titrating therapy in hypothyroidism and hyperthyroidism. In patients with primary hypothyroidism or hyperthyroidism resulting from gland dysfunction, there is an inverse relationship between the TSH level and thyroid function. High TSH signifies hypothyroidism (or iatrogenic underreplacement), and low TSH signifies hyperthyroidism (or iatrogenic overreplacement). There is controversy regarding the normal or laboratory reference ranges for TSH.[3] NHANES showed the mean TSH level in a normal population was 1.46 mIU/L (μIU/mL) (clinical laboratories use either unit of measurement, usually expressed as mIU/L or μIU/mL), but the values were not normally distributed. Although most laboratories quote the upper limit of normal for TSH between 4 and 5 mIU/L (μIU/mL), 95% of subjects had a TSH level of between 0.5 and 2.5 mIU/L (μIU/mL). The population of subjects whose TSH level was 2.5 to 4.5 mIU/L (μIU/mL) may have had mild hypothyroidism, or the non-normal distribution may reflect different normal ranges in a heterogeneous (age, sex, race) population. The mean normal TSH appears to be higher in the elderly with no clinical evidence of hypothyroidism,[4] and there is some evidence that normal TSH ranges are sex and ethnicity specific.[1] The target TSH for most patients being treated for thyroid disorders is not the same as the reference range. Ideally, TSH should be the mean normal value of 1.5 mIU/L (μIU/mL; target range, 0.5–4 mIU/L or μIU/mL).[3] The upper limit of the target range may be higher in the elderly. Therapy may be titrated within the target TSH range to maximally improve patient signs and symptoms without causing adverse effects of overtreatment or undertreatment.

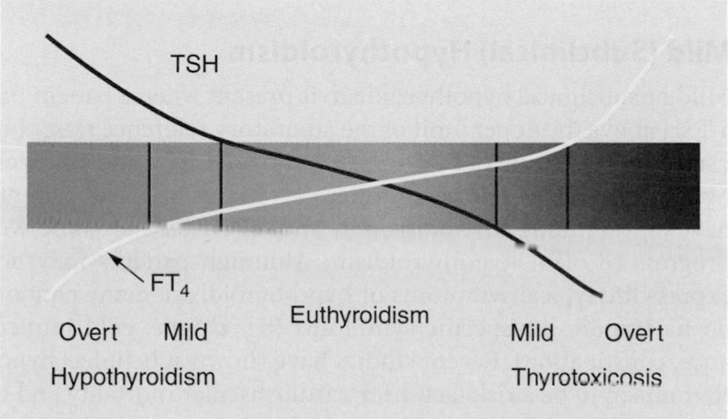

FIGURE 44–2. The continuum of thyroid disorders. (FT_4, free T_4; TSH, thyroid-stimulating hormone.)

Serum T_4 and T_3 Levels

Serum T_4 and T_3 levels are used commonly to assess thyroid function. Older screening tests of thyroid function measure total serum T_4 or T_3 levels. Because of the high degree of protein binding of these hormones, the free fraction can be altered by changes in the levels of binding proteins or the degree of protein binding. Since a number of factors can alter protein binding, these older assays are very insensitive and should no longer be used routinely even with protein-binding adjustment factors such as the free T_4 index. Free or unbound T_4 (FT_4) and T_3 (FT_3) assays are readily available and are more sensitive in identifying thyroid dysfunction than the older total assays.[4] However, patients with mild hypothyroidism or hyperthyroidism have normal FT_4 levels despite abnormal TSH levels.

Other Diagnostic Tests

Global tests of thyroid gland function can be performed to assess the rate of hormone synthesis. The radioactive iodine uptake (RAIU) is elevated in those with hyperthyroidism and can aid in identifying **thyrotoxicosis** owing to nonthyroid gland sources. Radionuclide thyroid scans are used in the evaluation of thyroid nodules. Because many thyroid disorders are autoimmune, measurement of various serum antithyroid antibodies can be performed. Antithyroid peroxidase antibodies (anti-TPOAb) and antithyroglobulin antibodies (anti-TGAb) are present in many patients with hypothyroidism. Most patients with Graves disease have TSH receptor-stimulating antibodies (TSHR-SAb) as well as elevated anti-TPOAb and antimicrosomal antibodies.

HYPOTHYROIDISM

Hypothyroidism is the most common clinical disorder of thyroid function. It is the clinical syndrome that results from inadequate secretion of thyroid hormones from the thyroid gland. The vast majority of hypothyroid patients have primary gland failure, but occasional patients have pituitary or hypothalamic failure. Most studies define hypothyroidism based on a serum TSH level above the upper limit of the laboratory reference range. In adults, 1.4% of women and 0.1% of men are biochemically hypothyroid. However, incidence is highly age dependent. In the Colorado Thyroid Health Study, by age 64 years, 12% of women and 5% of men were hypothyroid, and in the over 74 years age group, incidence in men approached that of women.[2] Most epidemiologic studies of hypothyroidism in the elderly show a prevalence of 6% to 12%.[4] There is a strong correlation between the presence of anti-TPOAb or anti-TGAb and the risk of developing hypothyroidism. In patients with subclinical hypothyroidism and positive anti-TPOAb, 5% per year will progress to overt hypothyroidism.[5] Other risk factors for development of hypothyroidism include the postpartum state, family history of autoimmune thyroid disorders, a previous history of head and neck or thyroid surgery, head and neck irradiation, other autoimmune endocrine disorders such as type 1 diabetes and Addison disease, other nonendocrine autoimmune diseases such as celiac disease and pernicious anemia, history of treatment for hyperthyroidism, treatment with amiodarone or lithium, and an iodine-deficient diet.[3,6]

Screening for Hypothyroidism

Because prevalence of hypothyroidism is high in certain populations, screening may be useful. Screening for hypothyroidism in women older than age 35 years may be cost-effective, though some organizations recommend screening of adults after age 50 or 60 years.[7] Others advocate a case-finding approach, defined as performing a TSH determination in patients based on risk factors or presence of signs and symptoms.[3]

Causes of Hypothyroidism

The most common causes of hypothyroidism are listed in Table 44–2.[3,8–11] Up to 90% of patients with autoimmune thyroiditis (**Hashimoto disease**) have circulating anti-TPOAbs. The autoimmune inflammatory response results in a lymphocytic infiltration of the thyroid gland and its eventual destruction.

Iatrogenic hypothyroidism can occur after thyroid irradiation or surgery and excessive doses of antithyroid drugs. Several drugs can cause hypothyroidism, including iodine-containing drugs such as amiodarone and iodinated radiocontrast media, lithium, interferon-α, multikinase and tyrosine kinase inhibitors (imatinib, sunitinib, sorafenib), *p*-aminosalicylic acid, ethionamide, sulfonylureas, valproic acid and other antiepileptic drugs, and aminoglutethimide.[3,11,12] Iodine deficiency is a common worldwide cause of hypothyroidism, including congenital hypothyroidism in newborns. Patients with hypothalamic or pituitary disease often have other signs of pituitary disease, such as hypogonadism, and their TSH levels are low.

Table 44–2

Common Causes of Hypothyroidism[3,8–11]

Primary Hypothyroidism
Autoimmune thyroiditis (Hashimoto disease)
Iatrogenic (irradiation, surgery)
Drugs (amiodarone, radiocontrast media, lithium, interferon-α, tyrosine kinase inhibitors)
Silent thyroiditis (including postpartum)
Iodine deficiency and excess

Secondary Hypothyroidism
Pituitary disease
Hypothalamic disease

Clinical Presentation and Diagnosis of Hypothyroidism[3,6,8–10]

Symptoms

Fatigue	Cold intolerance
Lethargy	Hoarseness
Sleepiness	Dry skin
Mental impairment	Decreased perspiration
Depression	Decreased appetite
Weight gain	Constipation
Menstrual disturbances	Arthralgia
Paresthesia	

Signs

Slow movements	Dry skin
Slow speech	Nonpitting edema (myxedema)
Hoarseness	Hyporeflexia
Bradycardia	Delayed relaxation of reflexes

Screening/Diagnosis

- A TSH level of 4.5 to 10 mIU/L (μIU/mL) may constitute mild or subclinical hypothyroidism.
- A TSH level greater than 10 mIU/L (μIU/mL) signifies overt hypothyroidism.
- The free T_4 level will be normal (0.7–1.9 ng/dL or 9.0–24.5 pmol/L) in mild or subclinical hypothyroidism and low (less than 0.7 ng/dL or 9.0 pmol/L) in patients with obvious signs and/or symptoms.

Signs and Symptoms of Hypothyroidism

KEY CONCEPT *Hypothyroidism can affect virtually any tissue or organ in the body. The most common symptoms, such as fatigue, lethargy, sleepiness, cold intolerance, and dry skin, are nonspecific and can be seen with many other disorders. The classic overt signs, such as myxedema and delayed deep tendon reflexes, are seen uncommonly now because more patients are screened or seek medical attention earlier. Patients with mild (also known as subclinical) hypothyroidism may have subtle symptoms that progress so slowly that they are not noticed easily by the patient or family. The lack of overt or specific signs and symptoms emphasizes the importance of using serum TSH level to identify patients with hypothyroidism.*

Mild (Subclinical) Hypothyroidism

Mild or subclinical hypothyroidism is present when a patient has a TSH above the upper limit of the laboratory reference range but usually below 10 mIU/L or μIU/mL, normal FT_4, and no overt hypothyroid signs and symptoms.[4,13,14] Many of these patients have autoimmune thyroiditis and anti-TPOAbs and some will progress to overt hypothyroidism. Although patients may not express the typical symptoms of hypothyroidism, many patients do have mild, nonspecific symptoms (eg, fatigue, cold intolerance, constipation). Recent studies have shown subclinical hypothyroidism to be a risk factor for cardiovascular mortality and to be associated with decreased myocardial contractility, decreased exercise tolerance, elevated low-density lipoprotein (LDL) cholesterol, and neuropsychiatric symptoms.[13–16]

Sequelae of Hypothyroidism

Hypothyroidism is a chronic disease that may result in significant long-term sequelae. Hypercholesterolemia is associated with hypothyroidism, increasing the long-term risk of cardiovascular disease and cardiovascular mortality. Between 4% and 14% of patients with hypercholesterolemia are found to be hypothyroid. The Colorado Thyroid Health Study showed a direct correlation between degree of TSH elevation and rise in serum cholesterol.[2] Hypothyroidism also may result in increased systemic vascular resistance, decreased cardiac output, and increased diastolic blood pressure. Hypothyroidism can cause significant neuropsychiatric problems, including a dementia-like state in the elderly that is reversible with LT_4 therapy. Maternal hypothyroidism can have dire consequences for developing fetuses. Fetuses are almost completely dependent on maternal thyroid hormones during the first trimester, a time crucial for development of the CNS. Inadequately treated maternal hypothyroidism results in increased risk of miscarriage and developmental impairment in the child.[17]

Myxedema coma is seen in advanced hypothyroidism. These patients develop CNS depression, respiratory depression, cardiovascular instability, and fluid and electrolyte disturbances. Myxedema coma often is triggered by an underlying acute medical condition such as infection, stroke, trauma, or administration of CNS depressant drugs.

Treatment of Hypothyroidism

KEY CONCEPT *There are three major goals in the treatment of hypothyroidism: replace the missing hormones, relieve signs and symptoms, and achieve a stable biochemical euthyroid state.* Although these goals should not be difficult to achieve, 20% to 40% of treated patients are not receiving optimal pharmacotherapy.

▸ *Thyroid Hormone Products*

A number of thyroid hormone products are marketed in the United States (Table 44–3). These products include synthetic LT_4 and T_3, combinations of synthetic LT_4 and T_3, and animal-derived products. KEY CONCEPT *Despite the availability of a wide array of thyroid hormone products, it is clear that synthetic LT_4 is the treatment of choice for almost all patients with hypothyroidism.*[3] *LT_4 mimics the normal physiology of the thyroid gland, which secretes mostly T_4 as a prohormone. Peripheral tissues convert T_4 to T_3 as needed based on metabolic demands. If T_3 is used to treat hypothyroidism, the peripheral tissues lose their ability to control local metabolic rates. LT_4 also has distinct pharmacokinetic advantages over T_3. With a 7- to 10-day half-life, LT_4 provides a very smooth dose-response curve with little peak and trough effect. In a small number of patients who have impairment of conversion of T_4 to T_3, addition of T_3 may be warranted.* T_3, with a 24-hour half-life, provides a significant peak and trough effect, and many patients have symptoms of thyrotoxicosis after each dose is administered. The use of compounded T_3 products that have not been approved by the Food and Drug Administration (FDA) or dietary supplements marketed for "thyroid health" should be strongly discouraged. For patients who have difficulty adhering to a once-daily regimen, a once-weekly LT_4 regimen is safe and effective.[3]

Animal-derived products such as desiccated thyroid are obtained from pig thyroid and have various degrees of purity. These products contain both LT_4 and T_3, but the amount of T_3 is much higher (T_4:T_3 = 4:1) than what would be found in the human thyroid gland (T_4:T_3 = 14:1). With the desiccated thyroid products, there are concerns about standardizing the amount of hormone and lot-to-lot variability. Although some patients want to use desiccated thyroid because it is "natural," the products are in no way natural for humans. With the strong evidence supporting the safety and efficacy of LT_4 in the treatment of hypothyroidism, there is no rationale for the use of these animal-derived products. Patients who are being treated with these agents should be strongly encouraged to switch to synthetic LT_4. Additionally, patients should be encouraged to not purchase thyroid hormone- or iodine-containing products from health food stores or internet sites.

Several studies have been published that evaluate use of LT_4 and T_3 combinations in ratios that mimic human physiology.

Table 44–3

Thyroid Preparations

Drug (Brand Name)	Content	Relative Dose	Comments
Levothyroxine, (Synthroid, Levoxyl, Unithroid), other brands, and generics	Synthetic LT_4; 25-, 50-, 75-, 88-, 100-, 112-, 125-, 137-, 150-, 175-, 200-, and 300-mcg tablets; 100-, 200-, and 500-mcg vial for injection	60 mcg	Gold standard for treating hypothyroidism; products not therapeutically equivalent; full replacement dose, 1–1.6 mcg/kg/day; when switching from animal product, lower calculated daily dose by 25–50 mcg; IV form rarely needed
Liothyronine (Cytomel)	Synthetic T_3; 5-, 25-, and 50-mcg tablets	15 mcg	Rarely needed in treatment of hypothyroidism; rapid absorption and pharmacologic effect; increased toxicity versus LT_4; no outcome benefit to combining with LT_4
Thyroid (desiccated) USP (Armour, others)	Desiccated pork thyroid glands; contains T_3 and T_4; 15-, 16.25-, 30-, 32.5-, 48.75-, 60-, 65-, 90-, 97.5-, 120-, 130-, 162.5-, 180-, 195-, 240-, 260-, 300-, and 325-mg tablets	65 mg	Nonphysiologic T_4:T_3 ratio; unpredictable hormone content and stability; T_3 content may cause toxicity; no role in modern therapy
Liotrix (Thyrolar)	Synthetic T_4, T_3 in fixed 4:1 ratio; ¼-, ½-, 1-, 2-, 3-strength tablets	12.5/50 mcg T_3:T_4 (1 strength)	Nonphysiologic T_4:T_3 ratio; T_3 content may cause toxicity; no role in modern therapy

IV, intravenous; LT_4, levothyroxine; T_3, triiodothyronine; T_4, thyroxine.

A meta-analysis of randomized, controlled clinical trials comparing LT_4 and T_3 combinations with LT_4 monotherapy show no outcome benefit with combination therapy.[18] Except in rare circumstances (eg, patients with impaired T_4-to-T_3 conversion as evidenced by adequate LT_4 dose, continued symptoms and low FT_3 level), there is no rationale for using combinations of LT_4 and T_3 to treat hypothyroidism.

▶ Bioequivalence and LT_4 Product Selection

LT_4 products have a long history of bioavailability problems.[3,19] Over the years, LT_4 bioavailability has increased, so maintenance doses today are significantly lower than those seen before the early 1980s. Currently, the average bioavailability of LT_4 products is about 80%. Because of long-standing concerns about LT_4 bioequivalence and because LT_4 products had never undergone formal approval by the FDA under the 1938 Food, Drug, and Cosmetics Act, the FDA mandated that all manufacturers of LT_4 products submit an Abbreviated New Drug Application (ANDA) to keep their products on the US market after 2001.[20] Products approved under this process would have to comply with FDA manufacturing and bioequivalence standards. This action has resulted in many changes in the United States LT_4 market, as well as renewed interest in LT_4 bioequivalence. Since 2001, a variety of brand and generic products have been approved by the FDA. Some marketed products carry AB ratings (bioequivalence) to certain other products, using a complex AB1, AB2, AB3, and AB4 system.[21]

For many years, there have been concerns regarding the FDA bioequivalence methodology for LT_4 products. FDA bioequivalence standards allow a −20% to +25% variance in single-dose pharmacokinetic parameters between the test and reference products. Many people believe this degree of allowed variance is not appropriate for a narrow-therapeutic-index (NTI) drug such as LT_4. Furthermore, there are unique challenges to performing bioequivalence studies with an endogenous hormone such as LT_4. Because these single-dose pharmacokinetic studies are done in healthy volunteers, the pharmacokinetic data are a combination of endogenous and exogenous LT_4. Seventy percent of the area under the curve (AUC) in these studies consists of the subjects' endogenous T_4. Blakesley and colleagues showed the standard FDA bioequivalence methodology would rate 600-, 450-, and 400-mcg LT_4 doses as bioequivalent.[22] This study also showed that mathematically removing the subjects' endogenous T_4 level (baseline correction) improves the sensitivity of the analysis. Based on these data, since 2003, the FDA has required that LT_4 bioequivalence data undergo baseline correction. Although this method has improved the ability to identify large differences in LT_4 bioequivalence, small but clinically significant differences will not be identified. In 2008, the FDA adopted stricter criteria for LT_4 tablet shelf-life potency (95%–105% of stated potency vs standard 90%–110%), which may reduce the intrapatient variability seen during long-term LT_4 therapy.

More important than bioequivalence is the therapeutic equivalence of LT_4 products. Will patients have the same outcomes if bioequivalent products are used? A study by Dong and colleagues helps to answer this question.[23] Twenty-two well-controlled hypothyroid women were randomly switched to the same dose of four different products every 6 weeks. Nonbaseline corrected bioequivalence data showed these products to be bioequivalent. However, as each product switch occurred, more of the subjects had an abnormal TSH level.[24] By the end of the third product switch, 52% had an abnormal TSH level. This is strong evidence that LT_4 products are not therapeutically equivalent even if they are rated as bioequivalent by the FDA.

Evidence does exist that small differences in LT_4 dose can result in large changes in TSH. In one study, when the daily dose was reduced by 25 mcg, 78% had an elevated TSH level.[25] When the daily dose was increased by 25 mcg, 55% had a low TSH level. Clearly, differences in LT_4 dose or bioavailability within the FDA-allowed variance for bioequivalent products can cause significant changes in TSH.

KEY CONCEPT *There is no evidence that one LT_4 product is better than another. However, given the evidence that these products do have differences in bioavailability, patients should be maintained on the same LT_4 product. Given the generic substitution regulations of most states, this is best accomplished by prescribing a brand-name product or otherwise ensuring the product remains constant and not allowing substitution.* Although practitioners are pressured by insurance companies and employers to substitute LT_4 products as a cost-saving measure, such switching is not in the best interest of the patient and should not be allowed. If patients are switched to a different product, the prescriber should be notified, and a TSH determination should be done in 6 to 8 weeks to allow dose retitration. The economic impact of retitration must be considered when formularies are changed to reduce drug acquisition cost.

▶ Therapeutic Use of LT_4

LT_4 replacement is indicated for patients with overt hypothyroidism.[3,6,8–10] However, the need for treatment is controversial in patients with mild or subclinical disease. There are no prospective clinical trials that show an outcome benefit with treating these patients. A retrospective study from the United Kingdom showed that LT_4 therapy in patients with mild hypothyroidism reduced ischemic heart disease events in patients 70 years and younger.[26] In patients without symptoms who have underlying heart disease, high cardiovascular risk, goiter, positive anti-TPOAb and/or are infertile or pregnant, LT_4 replacement should be considered.[3,27] Patients with mild or subclinical hypothyroidism do not need to be started on the full LT_4 replacement dose because they still have some endogenous hormone production. Start these patients on 25 to 50 mcg/day and titrate every 6 to 8 weeks based on TSH levels. Over time, it is likely the LT_4 dose will need to be increased slowly as the patient's thyroid gland loses residual function.

In patients younger than age 65 years with overt hypothyroidism, the average LT_4 replacement dose is 1.6 mcg/kg/day (use ideal body weight in obese patients[3]). However, there is wide interpatient variability in the optimal replacement dose, so individual dose titration is necessary. If there is no history of cardiac disease, these patients may be started on the full replacement dose.

The full replacement dose in patients older than age 75 years is lower, about 1 mcg/kg/day.[4,5] In the elderly, the starting dose should be 25 to 50 mcg/day, and the dose should then be titrated to the target TSH value. In patients with ischemic heart disease, start with 12.5 to 25 mcg/day and slowly titrate. If the patient develops angina or other forms of myocardial ischemia, lower the dose and titrate more slowly. At the start of therapy and with each change in dose, recheck the TSH in 6- to 8-week intervals. If the TSH is not in the target range (0.5–4 mIU/L or μIU/mL), change the dose by 10% to 20% and then recheck the TSH 6 to 8 weeks later. As the dose is titrated, assess the patient's symptoms. Many patients will improve quickly, and younger patients will feel best if the TSH is titrated to low-normal to middle-normal levels (0.5–1.5 mIU/L or μIU/mL).

Patient Encounter 1, Part 1

A 36-year-old woman comes to the clinic complaining of fatigue, lethargy, heavy periods, dry skin, and constipation for the past 6 months. She thought it was because she was "working too hard and was not eating right," but the symptoms have not improved despite her primary care provider giving her a vitamin with iron. She noticed a 2.5-kg (5.5-lb) weight gain over the past 4 months. Her friend gave her some sertraline, but she did not take it. She takes no medications other than a hormonal contraceptive, occasional acetaminophen for headache and MiraLAX for constipation. Her vital signs and physical examination, including her most recent pelvic examination findings several months ago, are normal.

Labs

Serum Cholesterol: 205 mg/dL (5.30 mmol/L; normal, less than 200 mg/dL, or 5.17 mmol/L); LDL cholesterol 96 mg/dL (2.48 mmol/L; normal less than 130 mg/dL or 3.36 mmol/L)

TSH: 7.8 mIU/L (μIU/mL; reference range, 0.5–4.5 mIU/L or μIU/mL)

Free T_4: 0.96 ng/dL (12.4 pmol/L; reference range, 0.7–1.9 ng/dL, or 9.0–24.5 pmol/L)

PE:

VS: Wt 68 kg (150 lb); Ht 5′5″ (165 cm); BMI 25 kg/m²

Should the patient receive LT_4 therapy? Why or why not?

If you feel treatment is indicated, what initial dose of LT_4 would you choose?

If you feel treatment is not indicated, how would you monitor the patient?

What would you tell the patient regarding the significance of her symptoms, elevated TSH level, and risk versus benefits of LT_4 therapy?

▶ Risks of Overtreatment and Undertreatment

Patients receiving LT_4 therapy who are not maintained in a euthyroid state are at risk for long-term adverse sequelae. In general, overtreatment and a suppressed TSH are more common than undertreatment with an elevated TSH.[27] Patients with long-term overtreatment are at higher risk for atrial fibrillation and other cardiovascular morbidities, depression or mental status changes, and osteoporosis. Elderly patients being treated with LT_4 have a dose-related risk of fractures even if the TSH is not suppressed below normal values.[28] Although studies have not defined a specific TSH target range for the elderly, these patients should receive close monitoring and dose adjustments to prevent overtreatment. Patients who are undertreated are at higher risk for hypercholesterolemia and other cardiovascular problems, depression or mental status changes, and obstetric complications.

▶ Alterations In LT_4 Dose Requirements

A number of factors can alter LT_4 dose requirements (Table 44–4), including time of administration and drug–drug and drug–food interactions.[3,9] LT_4 has the greatest and most consistent bioavailability when taken in the evening on an empty stomach.[29] The most common cause of increased dose requirement is coadministration of LT_4 with calcium or iron supplements (including prenatal vitamins). Counsel patients that they should take the LT_4 dose at least 2 hours before or 6 hours after the calcium or iron dose. The most common cause of decreased dose requirement is aging.

Table 44–4

Factors That Alter LT_4 Dose Requirements[3,9]

Increased Dose Requirement	Decreased Dose Requirement
Decreased LT_4 Absorption	Aging
Malabsorption syndromes	Delivery of pregnancy
Drugs or Diet	Withdrawal of interacting substance
Bile acid binders	
Caffeine	
Calcium	
Charcoal	
Chromium picolinate	
Ciprofloxacin	
Fiber	
Grapefruit juice	
H_2-blockers	
Iron	
Malabsorption syndromes	
Oral bisphosphonates	
Orlistat	
Phosphate binders (sevelamer, aluminum)	
Proton pump inhibitors	
Sodium polystyrene sulfonate	
Soy	
Sucralfate	
Tube feeding	
Increased TBG	
Cirrhosis	
Estrogen therapy	
Hereditary	
Pregnancy	
Tamoxifen, raloxifene therapy	
Increased Clearance	
Carbamazepine	
Growth hormone	
Nevirapine	
Oxcarbazepine	
Phenobarbital	
Phenytoin	
Primidone	
Quetiapine	
Rifampin	
Sertraline	
Stavudine	
Tyrosine kinase inhibitors	
Valproic acid	
Impaired Deiodination	
Amiodarone	
Mechanism Unknown	
Critical illness	

LT_4, levothyroxine; TBG, thyroxine-binding globulin.

Table 44–5

Monitoring LT_4 Therapy

- Serum TSH
  - Every 6–12 months or if change in clinical status
  - 6–8 weeks after any dose or product change
  - As soon as possible in pregnancy; then monthly
- Same product prescribed and dispensed with every refill
- Watch for mg/mcg dosing errors
- Assess patient's understanding of disease, therapy, and need for adherence and tight control
- Assess for signs and symptoms of over- and undertreatment
- Identify potential interactions between LT_4, and foods and/or drugs

LT_4, levothyroxine; TSH, thyroid-stimulating hormone.

▶ *Patient Monitoring*

Patients on stable LT_4 therapy do not need frequent monitoring. In most patients, measuring TSH every 6 to 12 months along with an assessment of clinical status is adequate (Table 44–5). If the patient's clinical status changes (eg, pregnancy), more frequent monitoring may be necessary. LT_4 prescriptions should be written as microgram doses to avoid potential errors when written as milligram doses.

Patient education is an important component of care. Treatment adherence rates (at least 80% of doses taken) in hypothyroid patients are 68%, slightly less than adherence rates seen in hypertensive patients.[30] Educate patients about the benefits of proper therapy, importance of adherence, consistency in time and method of administration, and importance of receiving a consistent LT_4 product. Some patients take excessive amounts of LT_4 in an effort to "feel better" or as a weight loss treatment. Explain to patients that excessive amounts of LT_4 will not improve symptoms more than therapeutic doses, can cause serious problems, and is not an effective treatment for obesity.

▶ *Special Populations and Conditions*

Hypothyroidism and Pregnancy Hypothyroidism during pregnancy has a variety of maternal and fetal adverse effects.[3,17,31] During pregnancy, β-human chorionic gonadotropin (β-hCG) acts as a TSH receptor agonist, increasing the amount of thyroid hormone available for fetal growth and development.

Maternal hypothyroidism results in an increased rate of miscarriage and decreased intellectual capacity of the child. Endocrinologists recommend a TSH measurement as soon as the pregnancy is confirmed. Most hypothyroid women who become pregnant will quickly need an increased dose of LT_4, typically 20% to 50% above the prepregnancy dose.[31] The increased dose should be maintained throughout the pregnancy, with monthly TSH monitoring to keep the TSH in the middle- to low-normal range. After delivery, the LT_4 dose usually can be reduced to prepregnancy levels, although patients with preexisting autoimmune thyroiditis may have increased postpartum dose requirements. Because prenatal vitamins contain significant amounts of calcium and iron, remind these patients to take the LT_4 dose at least 2 hours before or 6 hours after the vitamin.

Children Congenital hypothyroidism is uncommon in the United States, and all newborns in the United States undergo screening with a TSH level. As soon as the hypothyroid state is identified, the newborn should receive the full LT_4 replacement dose. The replacement dose of LT_4 in children is age dependent. In newborns, the usual dose is 10 to 17 mcg/kg/day. LT_4 tablets may be crushed and mixed with breast milk or formula, but it is best to administer LT_4 to infants and children on an empty stomach.[32] Serum FT_4 levels (target, 1.6–2.2 ng/dL or 20.6–28.3 pmol/L) are used for dose titration in infants because the TSH level may not respond to treatment as it does in older children and adults. By 6 months of age, the required dose is reduced to 5 to 7 mcg/kg/day, and from ages 1 to 10 years, the dose is 3 to 6 mcg/kg/day. After age 12 years, adult doses can be given.

Myxedema Coma This is a life-threatening condition owing to severe, long-standing hypothyroidism and has a mortality rate of 60% to 70%. These patients are given 300 to 500 mcg LT_4 intravenously initially, using caution in patients with underlying cardiac disease. Although administration of T_3 would provide a more rapid onset of action, there is no evidence that T_3 improves outcomes in patients with myxedema coma. Historically, glucocorticoids, such as hydrocortisone 50 to 100 mg every 6 hours, are administered owing to concern about simultaneous adrenal insufficiency. Although there is no strong evidence for an outcome benefit, the use of glucocorticoids is reasonable because such treatment may be lifesaving, and the risks of a short course of corticosteroids at this dose are low. As patients improve, the LT_4 dose can be given orally in a typical full replacement dose.

Patient Encounter 1, Part 2

One year later, the patient comes to you for routine follow-up stating that she has felt progressively worse since her last visit. She feels more fatigued, and gained 4 more kg and her periods are even heavier now (which she ascribes to stopping her contraceptive). Several months ago she elected to "go natural," and stopped taking all medications except for supplements purchased at a health food store. Her most recent TSH determination, obtained 2 days ago, was 12.8 mIU/L (μIU/mL; reference range, 0.5–4.5 mIU/L or μIU/mL).

Why is LT_4 therapy indicated now?

What would you recommend regarding her LT_4 dose and monitoring?

What instructions would you give the patient regarding her LT_4 therapy?

HYPERTHYROIDISM AND THYROTOXICOSIS

Hyperthyroidism is much less common than hypothyroidism. Refer to the Epidemiology of Thyroid Disease section.

Causes of Thyrotoxicosis and Hyperthyroidism

Hyperthyroidism is related to excess thyroid hormone secreted by the thyroid gland. Thyrotoxicosis is any syndrome caused by excess thyroid hormone and can be related to excess hormone production (hyperthyroidism). The common causes of thyrotoxicosis are shown in Table 44–6.[33–35] Graves disease is the most common cause of hyperthyroidism. Thyrotoxicosis in the elderly is more likely caused by toxic thyroid nodules or multinodular goiter than by Graves disease. Excessive intake of thyroid hormone may be caused by overtreatment with prescribed therapy or as a self-remedy for obesity, as thyroid hormones can be obtained easily without a prescription from health food stores or internet sources.

Patient Care Process: Hypothyroidism

Patient Assessment:

- Evaluate for signs and symptoms of hypothyroidism (see Clinical Presentation and Diagnosis of Hypothyroidism). As signs and symptoms of hypothyroidism are nonspecific, clinicians should have a high index of suspicion in higher risk patients including women and the elderly.
- Use serum TSH to identify patients with hypothyroidism (see Clinical Presentation and Diagnosis of Hypothyroidism), and check TSH in pregnant women as soon as pregnancy is determined.

Therapy Evaluation:

- If patient has been or is already receiving pharmacotherapy to treat thyroid disease, assess efficacy, safety, LT_4 product received (eg, any recent changes in product) and patient adherence. Are there any significant drug interactions?
- If patient is not at desired TSH level and not on therapy, determine if pharmacotherapy is indicated.

Care Plan Development:

- Provide synthetic LT_4 replacement to patients with overt hypothyroidism.
- Consider replacement therapy in patients with TSH level of greater than 4.5 but less than 10 mIU/L (μIU/mL) who have nonspecific or subtle symptoms (eg, mild fatigue, lethargy), an elevated cholesterol level, underlying heart disease, or positive anti-TPOAbs.
- Patients with mild hypothyroidism may be started at 25 to 50 mcg/day of LT_4.
- Patients with overt hypothyroidism who are older than 12 and younger than 65 years and do not have cardiac disease may receive the calculated full replacement LT_4 dose of 1.6 mcg/kg/day (based on ideal body weight if obese).
- Elderly patients or those with cardiac disease should be started at a lower LT_4 dose (eg, 12.5–25 mcg/day).
- Provide a brand-name LT_4 product, and do not allow product switches. If the product is switched, check TSH in 6 weeks and retitrate the dose.
- Provide LT_4 prescriptions as microgram, not milligram, doses to avoid errors.
- Make sure patients understand importance of adherence and risks of overuse and underuse of LT_4.
- In pregnant patients, expect to increase LT_4 dose early in first trimester. Maintain TSH in low to middle normal range. After delivery, consider reducing LT_4 dose to prepregnancy level, if appropriate.

Follow-up Evaluation:

- Measure serum TSH 6 to 8 weeks after starting or after any dose change. If TSH level is not in target range, alter dose by 10% to 20% increments. Target TSH for patients on LT_4 replacement therapy for hypothyroidism is 0.5 to 2.5 mIU/L (μIU/mL). Younger patients often feel best at a TSH level in the low- to middle-normal range (ie, 0.5–1.5 mIU/L or μIU/mL).
- Check TSH every 6 to 12 months in stable patients receiving LT_4 replacement.
- Monitor for drug interactions, such as LT_4 absorption problems caused by calcium and iron.
- At each visit, assess for signs and symptoms of overtreatment and undertreatment.
- In pregnant patients, check TSH monthly.

Table 44–6

Causes of Thyrotoxicosis[33–35]

Primary Hyperthyroidism	
Graves disease	
Toxic multinodular goiter	
Toxic adenoma	
Thyroid cancer	
Struma ovarii	
Iodine excess (including radiocontrast, amiodarone)	
Thyrotoxicosis without Hyperthyroidism	
Subacute thyroiditis	
Silent (painless) thyroiditis	
Excess thyroid hormone intake (thyrotoxicosis factitia)	
Drug-induced (amiodarone, iodine, lithium, interferons)	
Secondary Hyperthyroidism	
TSH-secreting pituitary tumors	
Trophoblastic (hCG-secreting) tumors	
Gestational thyrotoxicosis	

hCG, human chorionic gonadotropin; TSH, thyroid-stimulating hormone.

Clinical Manifestations of Thyrotoxicosis

Many of the signs and symptoms seem to be related to autonomic hyperactivity. The clinical manifestations of hyperthyroidism may be subtle and slowly progressive. Screening of patients for thyroid disease may identify patients with subclinical or mild thyrotoxicosis. Patients may seek medical attention only after a long period of thyrotoxicosis or owing to an acute complication such as atrial fibrillation. Clinical manifestations of thyrotoxicosis in the elderly may be blunted or atypical. These patients may present only with atrial fibrillation, depression, or altered mental status or cognition.

Mild (Subclinical) Hyperthyroidism

Mild (subclinical) hyperthyroidism is defined as a low TSH level with a normal FT_4 level.[13,26] Although there may be few or no symptoms in these patients, there are several areas of concern.[14,33] Some patients progress to overt thyrotoxicosis. Patients with subclinical hyperthyroidism have been shown to experience long-term cardiovascular[33,36] and bone sequelae.[37] Mild hyperthyroidism appears to increase cardiovascular morbidity and mortality.[36] Prolonged subclinical thyrotoxicosis speeds

Clinical Presentation and Diagnosis of Hyperthyroidism[33-35]

Symptoms

- Nervousness
- Fatigue
- Weakness
- Increased perspiration
- Heat intolerance
- Tremor
- Hyperactivity, irritability
- Palpitations
- Appetite change (usually increased)
- Weight change (usually weight loss)
- Menstrual disturbances (often oligomenorrhea)
- Diarrhea

Signs

- Hyperactivity
- Tachycardia
- Atrial fibrillation (especially in elderly adults)
- Hyperreflexia
- Warm, moist skin
- Ophthalmopathy, dermopathy (Graves disease)
- Goiter
- Muscle weakness

Screening/Diagnosis

- Low TSH level (less than 0.5 mIU/L or μIU/mL) signifies thyrotoxicosis.
- FT_4 is elevated in overt hyperthyroidism but may be normal in mild hyperthyroidism.
- Increased radioiodine uptake in the thyroid indicates increased hormone production by the thyroid gland.
- Almost all patients with Graves disease will have positive TSHR-SAbs and positive anti-TPOAbs.

the loss of bone mineral density and increases fracture rates in postmenopausal women.[33,37] Treatment of patients with mild hyperthyroidism is controversial but should be considered in patients with TSH levels less than 0.1 mIU/L (μIU/mL), Graves disease, postmenopausal women, and patients with underlying cardiovascular disease.[33] Patients who do not have a fully suppressed (below the lower limit of detection) TSH or other risk factors for hyperthyroid complications (eg, osteoporosis, cardiac arrhythmias) may just undergo observation, with TSH testing every 6 months to identify progression of the hyperthyroid state.

Graves Disease

Graves disease is an autoimmune syndrome that includes hyperthyroidism, diffuse thyroid enlargement, **exophthalmos** and other eye findings, and skin findings.[33-35] The prevalence of Graves disease in the United States is approximately 0.4% in women and 0.1% in men. The peak age of incidence is 20 to 49 years, with a second peak after 80 years of age. Hyperthyroidism results from the production of TSHR-SAbs in at least 80% of patients with clinical Graves disease. These antibodies have TSH agonist activity, thereby stimulating hormone synthesis and release. These antibodies cross-react with orbital and fibroblastic tissue, resulting in ophthalmopathy and dermopathy. Although the underlying cause of Graves disease is not known, heredity seems to play a role. Subclinical Graves disease may become acutely overt in the presence of iodine excess, infection, stress, parturition, smoking, and lithium and cytokine therapy.

Several features of Graves disease are distinct from other forms of thyrotoxicosis. Clinically apparent ophthalmopathic changes are seen in 20% to 40% of patients[34,35,38] and include exophthalmos, **proptosis, chemosis, conjunctival injection**, and periorbital edema. Eyelid retraction causes a typical staring or startled appearance (**Figure 44–3**). Patients may complain of vague eye discomfort and excess tearing. In severe cases, the eyelids are unable to close completely, resulting in corneal damage. In very severe cases, the optic nerve can be compressed, resulting in permanent vision loss. All patients with suspected or known Graves disease must be evaluated and monitored by an ophthalmologist. Treatment of the underlying hyperthyroid state often, but not always, improves the ophthalmopathy.

Dermopathy occurs in 5% to 10% of patients with Graves disease and usually is associated with severe ophthalmopathy. Skin findings include hyperpigmented, nonpitting induration of the skin, typically over the pretibial area (pretibial myxedema), the dorsa of the feet, and the shoulder areas. **Clubbing** of the digits (thyroid acropachy) is associated with long-standing thyrotoxicosis.

Treatment of Hyperthyroidism

Treatment of thyrotoxicosis caused by hyperthyroidism is similar regardless of the underlying cause.[33-35] KEY CONCEPT *The goals of treating hyperthyroidism are to relieve signs and symptoms, reduce thyroid hormone production to normal levels and achieve biochemical euthyroidism, and prevent long-term adverse sequelae.*

▸ *β-Blockers*

Because many of the manifestations of hyperthyroidism appear to be mediated by the β-adrenergic system, β-adrenergic blockers are used to rapidly relieve palpitations, tremor, anxiety, and heat intolerance. Because β-blockers do not reduce the synthesis of thyroid hormones, they are used only until more specific antithyroid therapy is effective. Because nonselective agents can impair the conversion of T_4 to T_3, propranolol and nadolol are preferred. An initial propranolol dose of 20 to 40 mg four times daily should be titrated to relieve signs (target resting heart rate less than 90 beats/min) and symptoms. β-Blockers should not be used in patients with decompensated heart failure or asthma. A more β-1 specific blocker (eg, metoprolol, atenolol) may be used when a relative contraindication to a β-blocker exists; however, when an absolute contraindication to β-blockers exists, clonidine, verapamil or diltiazem may be used for rate control.

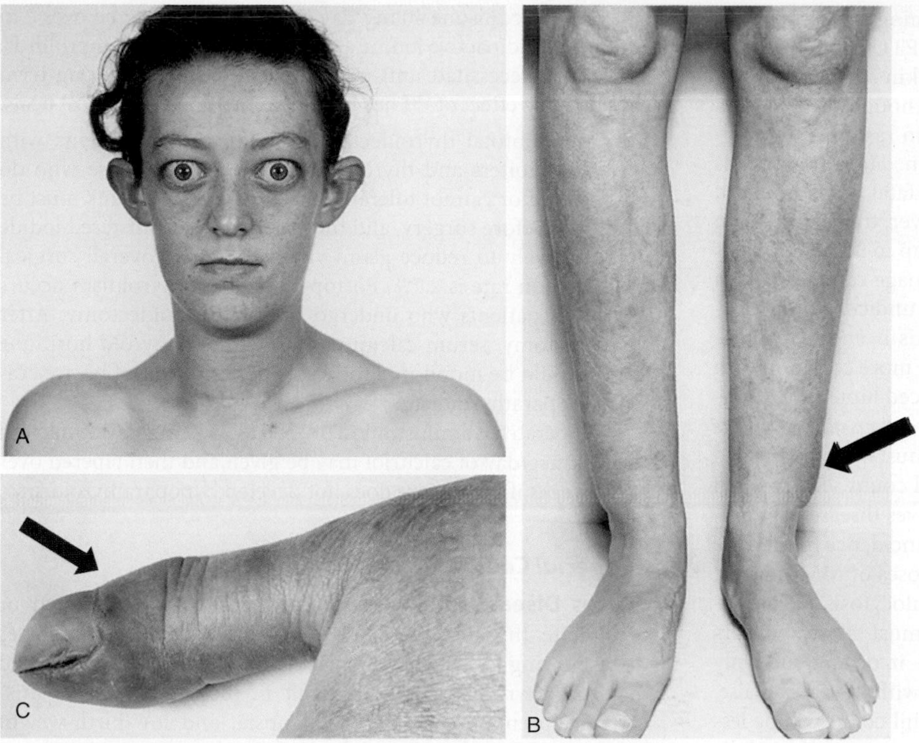

FIGURE 44–3. Features of Graves disease. (**A**) Facial appearance: exophthalmos, eyelid retraction, periorbital edema, and proptosis. (**B**) Thyroid dermopathy over lateral aspects of the shins (*arrow*). (**C**) Thyroid clubbing or acropachy (*arrow*). (From Jameson JL, Weetman AP. Disorders of the thyroid gland. In: Kasper DL, Braunwald E, Fauci AS, et al, eds. Harrison's Principles of Internal Medicine. 16th ed. New York: McGraw-Hill; 2004:2114.)

▸ *Methods to Reduce Thyroid Hormone Synthesis*

Excess production of thyroid hormone can be reduced in four ways: iodides, antithyroid drugs, radioactive iodine, and surgery.

Iodide Large doses of iodide inhibit the synthesis and release of thyroid hormones. Serum T_4 levels may be reduced within 24 hours, and the effects may last for 2 to 3 weeks. Iodides are used most commonly in Graves disease patients before surgery and to quickly reduce hormone release in patients with thyroid storm. Potassium iodide is administered either as a saturated solution (SSKI) that contains 38 mg iodide per drop or as Lugol solution, which contains 6.3 mg iodide per drop. The typical starting dose is 120 to 400 mg/day. Iodide therapy should start 7 to 14 days before surgery. Iodide should not be given before radioactive iodine treatment because the iodide will inhibit concentration of the radioactivity in the thyroid. Iodides also are used to protect the thyroid from radioactive iodine fallout after a nuclear accident or attack. Daily administration of 30 to 100 mg iodide markedly reduces thyroid gland uptake of radioactive iodine. The most frequent toxic effects with iodide therapy are hypersensitivity reactions, "iodism" (characterized by palpitations, depression, weight loss, and pustular skin eruptions), and gynecomastia.

Antithyroid Drugs The thionamide agents propylthiouracil (PTU) and methimazole (MMI) are used in the United States to treat hyperthyroidism.[39] Carbimazole, an MMI prodrug, is used in some countries (10 mg carbimazole = 6 mg MMI). These drugs inhibit thyroid hormone synthesis by interfering with thyroid peroxidase–mediated iodination of tyrosine residues in thyroglobulin. PTU has the added effect of inhibiting the conversion of T_4 to T_3. The thionamides also have immunosuppressant effects. In patients with Graves disease treated with thionamides, TSHR-SAb levels and other immune mediators decrease over time. Both drugs are well absorbed from the gastrointestinal (GI) tract. PTU has a half-life of 1 to 2.5 hours, whereas the half-life of MMI is 6 to 9 hours.

Antithyroid drugs are used as primary therapy for Graves disease or as preparative therapy before surgery or radioactive iodine administration. The decision to use antithyroid drugs as primary therapy must be weighed against the risks and benefits of radioiodine or surgery. Patient preference must be considered.

In most patients, there is no clear efficacy advantage of one thionamide over the other, but in the United States, MMI use has increased dramatically since the mid-1990s in lieu of PTU.[40] Although PTU has the advantage of inhibiting T_4-to-T_3 conversion, MMI can be given as a single daily dose and may have a better overall safety profile, particularly less hepatotoxicity. MMI is preferred to normalize thyroid function before radioactive iodine therapy, although both thionamides increase the failure rate of radioactive iodine therapy.[41] The usual starting dose of MMI is 10 to 20 mg/day, and the usual starting dose of PTU is 50 to 150 mg three times daily. Thyroid hormone levels drop in 2 to 3 weeks, and after 6 weeks, 90% of patients with Graves disease will be euthyroid. Thyroid function testing should be performed every 4 to 6 weeks until stable. After the patient becomes euthyroid, the antithyroid drug dose often can be decreased (5–10 mg/day MMI, 100–200 mg/day PTU) to maintain the euthyroid state. Excessive doses of antithyroid drugs will result in hypothyroidism.

Remission of Graves disease occurs in 40% to 60% of patients after 1 to 2 years of therapy. Antithyroid therapy may be stopped or tapered after 12 to 24 months. Relapse usually occurs in the first 3 to 6 months after stopping antithyroid therapy. Levels of TSHR-SAb after a course of treatment may have predictive value for the risk of relapse in that antibody-positive patients almost always relapse. However, antibody-negative patients also may relapse after therapy is stopped. About 75% of women in remission who become pregnant will have a postpartum relapse. When therapy is discontinued, a therapeutic strategy should be in place in the event of relapse. Many patients will opt for radioactive iodine as a long-term solution.

Antithyroid drugs are associated with an overall low rate of adverse effects, although serious adverse effects can occur. In

2010, the FDA released a new boxed warning on severe liver injury with PTU.[42] The warning states that PTU should only be used in patients who cannot tolerate MMI. Skin rash, arthralgias, and GI upset are seen in 5% of patients. Although the drug can be continued in the presence of a minor skin rash, the development of arthralgia warrants discontinuation. Hepatotoxicity is an uncommon but potentially serious or fatal adverse effect, occurring in 0.1% to 0.2% of patients. However, transient rises in aminotransferase enzyme levels are seen in up to 30% of patients treated with PTU. Severe hepatocellular damage can occur from PTU, whereas MMI can cause cholestatic jaundice. Antineutrophil cytoplasmic antibody (ANCA) vasculitis is another potentially serious but uncommon reaction that is more common with PTU, and patients may develop a drug-induced lupus syndrome.

KEY CONCEPT *Agranulocytosis is one of the most serious adverse effects of antithyroid drug therapy.* Agranulocytosis must be distinguished from a transient decrease in white blood cell count seen in up to 12% of adults and 25% of children with Graves disease. Agranulocytosis occurs in 0.3% of patients, and the incidence may be the same with PTU and MMI therapy. Lower doses of MMI may be associated with a lower incidence of agranulocytosis.[33] Agranulocytosis, thought to be autoimmune, almost always occurs within the first 3 months of therapy, and it occurs suddenly and unpredictably. Patients will present with fever, malaise, and a sore throat, and the absolute neutrophil count will be less than 1000/mm^3 (1×10^9/L). Patients may develop sepsis and die rapidly. If agranulocytosis occurs, discontinue the antithyroid drug immediately, administer broad-spectrum antibiotics if the patient is febrile, and consider administration of filgrastim. The white blood cell count should recover in 1 or 2 weeks. Patients who develop agranulocytosis should not be switched to another thionamide drug. Monitoring for agranulocytosis is controversial owing to its sudden and unpredictable nature. Most do not recommend routine monitoring of the complete blood count (CBC), although early detection could improve patient outcomes. Patients initiating thionamide therapy must be informed about the signs and symptoms of agranulocytosis and other serious side effects. Patients should be counseled to report signs and symptoms suggestive of infection, such as fever and sore throat lasting more than 2 or 3 days, bruising, pruritic rash, jaundice, dark urine, arthralgias, abdominal pain, nausea, or fatigue.

Radioactive Iodine Radioactive iodine, typically ^{131}I, produces thyroid ablation without surgery. ^{131}I is well absorbed after oral administration. The iodine is concentrated in the thyroid gland and has a half-life of 8 days. Over a period of weeks, thyroid cells that have taken up the ^{131}I begin to develop abnormalities and necrosis. Eventually, thyroid cells are destroyed, and hormone production is reduced. After a single dose, 40% to 70% of patients will be euthyroid in 6 to 8 weeks, and 80% will be cured. In most patients, hypothyroidism will develop, and long-term LT_4 replacement will be necessary. Because ^{131}I has a slow onset of action, most patients are treated initially with β-blockers and antithyroid drugs to prevent ^{131}I-induced thyroid storm. MMI is the preferred agent before the administration of ^{131}I. MMI is discontinued 3 to 5 days before the administration of ^{131}I and is restarted 3 to 7 days later. MMI is then slowly tapered over the next 4 to 6 weeks as thyroid function normalizes. β-Blockers can be continued during ^{131}I therapy. The dose of ^{131}I is based on the estimated weight of the patient's thyroid gland (typical dose, 10–15 mCi [370–555 MBq]). Radioactive iodine therapy is contraindicated during pregnancy and breastfeeding. Radioactive iodine therapy may acutely worsen Graves ophthalmopathy. Patients with prominent eye disease may be started on prednisone 40 mg/day, with the dose tapered over 2 to 3 months. Radioactive iodine also may cause a painful thyroiditis, which may necessitate anti-inflammatory therapy. No long-term carcinogenic effect of ^{131}I has been demonstrated in clinical trials.

Surgery Subtotal thyroidectomy is indicated in patients with very large goiters and thyroid malignancies and those who do not respond or cannot tolerate other therapies. Patients must be euthyroid before surgery, and they are often administered iodide preoperatively to reduce gland vascularity. The overall surgical complication rate is 2.7%. Postoperative hypothyroidism occurs in 10% of patients who undergo subtotal thyroidectomy. After thyroidectomy, serum calcium and intact parathyroid hormone levels should be monitored for early identification of postoperative hypoparathyroidism.

Postoperative administration of 1250 to 2500 mg/day of calcium and 0.5 mcg/day of calcitriol may be given and then tapered over 1 to 2 weeks if the patient does not develop hypoparathyroidism.

▶ *Special Conditions and Populations*

Graves Disease and Pregnancy Pregnancy may worsen or precipitate thyrotoxicosis in women with underlying Graves disease owing to the TSH agonist effect of β-hCG.[31,43] Untreated maternal thyrotoxicosis may result in increased rates of miscarriage, premature delivery, eclampsia, and low-birth-weight infants. Fetal and neonatal hyperthyroidism may occur as a result of transplacental passage of TSHR-SAbs. Because radioactive iodine is contraindicated and surgery is best avoided during pregnancy, most patients are treated with antithyroid drugs. PTU is considered the treatment of choice, particularly in the first trimester. While MMI is thought to have greater teratogenic potential versus PTU, the relative safety of these medications in pregnancy is not clear.[44] Patients receiving prepregnancy MMI should be switched to PTU as soon as the pregnancy is confirmed. The lowest possible dose of PTU to maintain maternal euthyroidism should be used. Given the potential maternal adverse effects of PTU (eg, hepatotoxicity), it may be preferable to switch from PTU to MMI for the second and third trimesters.[42] Antithyroid therapy in excessive doses may suppress fetal thyroid function. Although PTU and MMI are found in breast milk, nursing mothers should be switched to MMI after delivery because of the risk of hepatotoxicity from PTU in the mother and infant.

Pediatric Hyperthyroidism β-Blockers are administered to children who are symptomatic or have a heart rate greater than 100 beats/min.[33] MMI is the preferred antithyroid drug therapy in children at a dose of 0.2 to 0.5 mg/kg/day.[33] Once a euthyroid state is achieved, the MMI dose can be reduced by 50% or more to maintain euthyroidism. As in adults, antithyroid drugs are administered to children with Graves disease for 1 to 2 years. If remission does not occur in that time, long-term antithyroid drug therapy, radioactive iodine, or surgical therapy is offered. Long-term studies with ^{131}I use in children show no increased risk of thyroid cancer or leukemia.

Thyroid Storm Thyroid storm is a life-threatening condition caused by severe thyrotoxicosis.[33,45] Signs and symptoms include high fever, tachycardia, tachypnea, dehydration, delirium, coma, and GI disturbances. Thyroid storm is precipitated in a previously hyperthyroid patient by infection, trauma, surgery, radioactive iodine treatment, and sudden withdrawal from antithyroid drugs. Patients are treated with a short-acting β-blocker such as intravenous (IV) esmolol, IV or oral iodide, and large doses of

Patient Encounter 2

A 19-year-old woman comes to the clinic stating, "I'm so jumpy and sweaty and hungry, and I'm losing weight. I think I'm losing my mind. What is wrong with me?" She first noticed these symptoms 3 months ago, and they have worsened steadily. She feels anxious for no reason and has trouble sleeping. She has noticed that her appetite has increased, although she has lost about 2 kg (4.4 lb) over the past 3 months. Sometimes she can feel her heart beating in her chest, but she denies chest pain or syncope. Her only medications are a vitamin product, occasional naproxen for headaches, and a hormonal contraceptive. She thinks that her mother had some kind of thyroid problem when she was pregnant with her.

PE:

VS: Pulse 122 beats/min, BP 106/71 mm Hg, RR 12 breaths/min, T 37.8°C (100.1°F)

HEENT: Diffusely enlarged thyroid; mild exophthalmos

CV: Tachycardic, RRR

Exts: Fine tremor

Skin: Warm, moist, and soft

ECG: Sinus tachycardia

Labs: Electrolytes, CBC normal. TSH less than 0.1 mIU/L (μIU/mL; reference range 0.5–2.5 mIU/L or μIU/mL); FT_4 4.2 ng/dL (54.1 pmol/L; reference range 0.7–1.9 ng/dL, or 9.0–24.5 pmol/L); + TSHR-SAbs

What therapeutic options exist for this patient's Graves disease?

What pharmacotherapy would you recommend? What if she were pregnant?

How would you initiate and titrate therapy?

What would you tell the patient regarding the cause of her signs and symptoms, significance of her abnormal thyroid function tests, and therapeutic options?

PTU (500–1000 mg load; then 250 mg every 4 hours) or MMI (60–80 mg/day). Supportive care with acetaminophen to suppress fever, fluid and electrolyte management, and antiarrhythmic agents are important components of therapy. IV hydrocortisone 300 mg initially and then 100 mg every 8 hours is used often because of the potential presence of adrenal insufficiency.

NONTHYROIDAL ILLNESS (EUTHYROID SICK SYNDROME)

A number of changes in the hypothalamic–pituitary–thyroid axis occur during acute illness.[46] These changes are termed *nonthyroidal illness* or *euthyroid sick syndrome*. The type and degree of abnormalities depend on the severity of illness. Mild to moderate

Patient Care Process: Hyperthyroidism

Patient Assessment:

- A low or undetectable TSH level identifies thyrotoxicosis. See Clinical Presentation and Diagnosis of Hyperthyroidism.
- Via a diagnostic assessment, identify the underlying cause. (eg, presence of eye and/or skin findings and presence of TSHR-SAbs may be used to identify Graves disease).

Therapy Evaluation:

- If patient has been or is currently receiving pharmacotherapy to treat hyperthyroidism, assess efficacy, safety, and patient adherence. Are there any significant drug interactions?
- If patient is not at desired TSH level, determine if pharmacotherapy is indicated.

Care Plan Development:

- Treat severe or troublesome autonomic signs and symptoms with a nonselective β-blocker such as propranolol 20 to 40 mg four times daily. Titrate β-blocker dose based on signs and symptoms.
- Consider reducing excess thyroid hormone production with an antithyroid drug and/or radioactive iodine. If radioactive iodine is given, make sure that antithyroid drugs are stopped 4 to 6 days before treatment.
- MMI is the antithyroid drug of choice in most patients.
- Refer patients with Graves disease to an ophthalmologist for assessment and monitoring.
- Treat pregnant hyperthyroid women with PTU.
- Address any patient concerns regarding therapy.

Follow-up Evaluation:

- Monitor patients on antithyroid drugs for signs and symptoms of adverse effects. For example,
  - After baseline CBC with differential and liver profile, repeat CBC when patient has a febrile illness and repeat liver panel if signs or symptoms of hepatotoxicity occur (some recommend routine monitoring during the first 6 months of therapy).
  - Assess any skin rash or development of arthralgias.
- Antithyroid drugs have a delayed effect. After 2 to 4 weeks of therapy, adjust the dose if TSH is not in target range (0.5–2.5 mIU/L or μIU/mL). When patient is euthyroid, consider reducing dose of antithyroid drug to avoid hypothyroidism.
- Consider stopping antithyroid therapy in patients with Graves disease after 12 to 18 months to see if remission has occurred.
- Several months after radioactive iodine, expect that the patient will require permanent LT_4 replacement; thus, evaluate for such.

medical illness, surgery, or starvation causes a decrease in serum T_3 levels owing to decreased peripheral conversion of T_4 to T_3. The reduced T_3 levels do not correlate with ultimate mortality and are thought to be an adaptive response to stress. Patients with more severe illness, especially those in the intensive care unit, frequently have reduced total T_4 levels, although FT_4 levels often are normal. In critically ill patients, there is a correlation between degree of serum T_4 reduction and mortality. In most acutely ill patients who are euthyroid, TSH level is normal. However, administration of dopamine, octreotide, or high doses of glucocorticoids can reduce TSH levels. During recovery from acute illness, the TSH level may become modestly elevated to renormalize serum T_4 levels. During this time, thyroid function tests may be misinterpreted to indicate hypothyroidism. Despite the sometimes very low T_4 levels, there is no evidence that LT_4 administration has any survival benefit.[47] Patients with possible thyroid abnormalities during acute illness should be evaluated by an endocrinologist.

THYROID CANCER AND LT_4 SUPPRESSION

KEY CONCEPT *The growth and spread of thyroid carcinoma are stimulated by TSH. An important component of thyroid carcinoma management is the use of LT_4 to suppress TSH secretion. Early in therapy, patients receive the lowest LT_4 dose sufficient to fully suppress TSH to undetectable levels. Controlled trials show that suppressive LT_4 therapy reduces tumor growth and improves survival.* These patients are purposefully "overtreated" with LT_4, sometimes to a fully suppressed TSH level, and rendered subclinically or mildly hyperthyroid. Postmenopausal women should receive aggressive osteoporosis therapy to prevent LT_4-induced bone loss. Other thyrotoxic complications, such as atrial fibrillation, should be monitored and managed appropriately.

DRUG-INDUCED THYROID ABNORMALITIES

Drugs can affect thyroid function in a number of ways.[3,11] The effects of drugs on thyroid hormone protein binding, LT_4 absorption, and metabolism have been discussed previously. Several commonly used medications can alter thyroid hormone secretion.

Amiodarone

Amiodarone is a commonly prescribed antiarrhythmic drug that contains two iodide atoms, constituting 38% of its mass.[48] Each 200-mg dose of amiodarone provides 75 mg of iodide. Amiodarone deiodination releases about 6 mg of free iodine daily, 20 to 40 times more than the average daily intake of iodine in the United States. Amiodarone blocks conversion of T_4 to T_3, inhibits entry of T_3 into cells, and decreases T_3 receptor binding. Amiodarone causes rapid reduction in serum T_3 levels, increases free and total T_4 levels, and increases TSH level. After 3 months of therapy, TSH levels usually return to normal, although the serum T_3 and T_4 level changes may remain. Most of these patients are euthyroid because the FT_3 levels are in the low-normal range.

Amiodarone can frequently cause thyroid abnormalities in previously euthyroid patients. In a study of amiodarone treatment of persistent atrial fibrillation, 25.8% of patients developed subclinical hypothyroidism, and 5% developed overt hypothyroidism.[49] Hyperthyroidism occurred in 5.3%. Thyroid abnormalities, when they occurred, were seen within 6 months of initiation of amiodarone therapy in almost all patients. Amiodarone-induced hypothyroidism is more common in iodine-sufficient areas of the world. Patients with underlying autoimmune thyroiditis are much more likely to develop amiodarone-induced hypothyroidism. Amiodarone-induced hypothyroidism occurs most commonly within the first year of therapy. If amiodarone cannot be discontinued, LT_4 therapy will be effective in most patients. If amiodarone can be stopped, thyroid function will return to normal in 2 to 4 months.

Amiodarone is more likely to cause thyrotoxicosis in iodine-deficient areas. Type 1 amiodarone-induced thyrotoxicosis is caused by iodine excess and typically occurs in patients with preexisting multinodular goiter or subclinical Graves disease. Type 2 amiodarone-induced thyrotoxicosis is a destructive thyroiditis that occurs in patients with no underlying thyroid disease. Amiodarone-induced thyrotoxicosis is more common in men. Because amiodarone has β-blocking activity, palpitations and tachycardia may be absent. In type 1 thyrotoxicosis, amiodarone should be discontinued. If amiodarone therapy cannot be stopped, larger doses of antithyroid drugs may be needed to control thyrotoxicosis. In type 2 thyroiditis, stopping amiodarone may not be necessary because spontaneous resolution may occur. Prednisone 40 to 60 mg/day will quickly improve thyrotoxic symptoms. Prednisone may be tapered after 1 to 2 months of therapy.

KEY CONCEPT *Patients receiving amiodarone must receive monitoring for thyroid abnormalities. Baseline measurements of serum TSH, FT_4, FT_3, anti-TPOAbs, and TSHR-SAbs should be performed. TSH, FT_4, and FT_3 should be checked 3 months after initiation of amiodarone and then a TSH at least every 3 to 6 months.*

Lithium

Lithium is associated with hypothyroidism in up to 34% of patients, and hypothyroidism may occur after years of therapy.[50] Lithium appears to inhibit thyroid hormone synthesis and secretion. Patients with underlying autoimmune thyroiditis are more likely to develop lithium-induced hypothyroidism. Patients may require LT_4 replacement even if lithium is discontinued.

Interferon-α

Interferon-α causes hypothyroidism in up to 39% of patients being treated for hepatitis C infection.[3,11] Patients may develop a transient thyroiditis with hyperthyroidism before becoming hypothyroid. The hypothyroidism may be transient as well. Asians and patients with preexisting anti-TPOAbs are more likely to develop interferon-induced hypothyroidism. The mechanism of interferon-induced hypothyroidism is not known. If LT_4 replacement is initiated, it should be stopped after 6 months to reevaluate the need for replacement therapy.

Tyrosine Kinase Inhibitors

Tyrosine kinase inhibitors (TKIs) are targeted antineoplastic agents used in several types of malignancies, including thyroid cancer.[12] Several TKIs have significant effects on thyroid function, both in previously hypothyroid patients on LT_4 replacement and in previously euthyroid patients. Imatinib has been shown to cause a fourfold increase in TSH levels in patients being treated for thyroid cancer. Sunitinib and sorafenib have been associated with primary hypothyroidism in 20% to 40% of treated patients. Some sorafenib patients developed mild hyperthyroidism before becoming hypothyroid. Patients receiving TKI therapy should have baseline and periodic thyroid function monitoring.

OUTCOME EVALUATION

- Desired outcomes include relieving signs and symptoms and achieving a euthyroid state.

- Success of therapy for thyroid disorders must be based not only on short-term improvement of the patient's clinical status and abnormal laboratory values but also on achievement of a long-term, stable euthyroid state. Maintaining TSH level in the normal range improves symptoms and reduces the risk of long-term complications.
- Because pharmacotherapy often is lifelong, especially in patients with hypothyroidism, patients must undergo periodic monitoring to avoid long-term complications. In hypothyroid patients, such monitoring may involve simply asking the patient about signs and symptoms and a yearly measurement of TSH level.
- Any change in the patient's clinical status, such as a new pregnancy or a major change in body weight, necessitates a reevaluation of therapy. Patients at high risk for complications, such as pregnant women, the elderly, and patients with underlying cardiac disease, must be monitored more closely.
- Patients should be educated and periodically reminded about the importance of adherence and long-term tight control, the need for periodic clinical and laboratory monitoring, and the importance of staying on one LT_4 product.
- In hyperthyroid patients, the method of achieving desired outcomes may change over time with the use of antithyroid drugs versus radioactive iodine.
- Patients who receive antithyroid drugs must be monitored for adverse drug events such as hepatotoxicity and agranulocytosis.
- Patients who receive radioactive iodine must be monitored for development of hypothyroidism.
- In patients with thyroid cancer, the desired outcomes with LT_4 therapy often are different from those in hypothyroid patients. LT_4 doses sufficient to suppress tumor growth may result in a suppressed TSH and mild hyperthyroidism. These patients must be monitored closely for complications of the mild hyperthyroid state, such as bone mineral loss and development of atrial fibrillation.

Abbreviations Introduced in This Chapter

ANCA	Antineutrophil cytoplasmic antibody
ANDA	Abbreviated New Drug Application
Anti-TGAb	Antithyroglobulin antibody
Anti-TPOAb	Antithyroid peroxidase antibody
AUC	Area under the (time-concentration) curve
β-hCG	β-Human chorionic gonadotropin
CBC	Complete blood count
CNS	Central nervous system
FDA	Food and Drug Administration
FT_3	Free T_3
FT_4	Free T_4
GI	Gastrointestinal
hCG	Human chorionic gonadotropin
IV	Intravenous
LDL	Low-density lipoprotein
LT_4	Levothyroxine
MMI	Methimazole
NHANES	National Health and Nutrition Examination Survey
NTI	Narrow therapeutic index
PTU	Propylthiouracil
RAIU	Radioactive iodine uptake
SSKI	Saturated solution of potassium iodide
T_3	Triiodothyronine
T_4	Thyroxine
TBG	Thyroxine-binding globulin
TKI	Tyrosine kinase inhibitor
TRH	Thyrotropin-releasing hormone
TSH	Thyroid-stimulating hormone (thyrotropin)
TSHR-Sab	Thyroid-stimulating hormone receptor-stimulating antibodies
TSI	Thyroid-stimulating immunoglobulin

REFERENCES

1. Aoki Y, Belin RM, Clickner R, et al. Serum TSH and total T_4 in the United States population and their association with participant characteristics: National Health and Nutrition Examination Survey (NHANES 1999–2002). Thyroid. 2007;17:1211–1223.
2. Canaris GJ, Manowitz NR, Mayor G, Ridgeway EC. The Colorado thyroid disease prevalence study. Arch Intern Med. 2000;160:526–534.
3. Garber JR, Cobin RH, Gharib H, Hennessey JV, et al. Clinical practice guidelines for hypothyroidism in adults: Cosponsored by the American Association of Clinical Endocrinologists and the American Thyroid Association. Thyroid. 2012;22:1200–1235.
4. Surks MI, Hollowell JG. Age-specific distribution of serum thyrotropin and antithyroid antibodies in the US population: Implications for the prevalence of subclinical hypothyroidism. J Clin Endocrinol Metab. 2007;92:4575–4582.
5. Vanderpump MPJ, Tunbridge WMG, French JM, et al. The incidence of thyroid disorders in the community: A twenty year follow-up of the Whickham survey. Clin Endocrinol (Oxf). 1995;43:55–69.
6. Devdhar M, Ousman YH, Burman KD. Hypothyroidism. Endocrinol Metab Clin North Am. 2007;36:595–615.
7. Danese MD, Powe NR, Sawin CT, Ladenson PW. Screening for mild thyroid failure at the periodic health examination. A decision and cost-effectiveness analysis. JAMA. 1996;276:285–292.
8. Gaitonde DY, Rowley KD, Sweeney LB. Hypothyroidism: An update. Am Fam Physician. 2012;86:244–251.
9. Khandelwal D, Tandon N. Overt and subclinical hypothyroidism: Who to treat and how. Drugs. 2012;72:17–33.
10. McDermott MT. In the clinic. Hypothyroidism. Ann Intern Med. 2009;151(11):ITC61.
11. Barbesino G. Drugs affecting thyroid function. Thyroid. 2010;20:763–770.
12. Lai ECC, Yang YHK, Lin SJ, Hseih CY. Use of antiepileptic drugs and risk of hypothyroidism. Pharmacoepidemiol Drug Safety. 2012;22:1071–1079.
13. Cooper DS, Biondi B. Subclinical thyroid disease. Lancet. 2012;379:1142–1154
14. Singh S, Duggal J, Molnar J, et al. Impact of subclinical thyroid disorders on coronary heart disease, cardiovascular and all-cause mortality: A meta-analysis. Int J Cardiol. 2008;125:41–48.
15. Ochs N, Auer R, Bauer DC, et al. Meta-analysis: subclinical thyroid dysfunction and the risk for coronary heart disease and mortality. Ann Intern Med. 2008;148:832–845.
16. Biondi B, Cooper DS. The clinical significance of subclinical thyroid dysfunction. Endocrine Rev. 2008;29:76–131.
17. Yazbeck CF, Sullivan SD. Thyroid disorders during pregnancy. Med Clin N Amer. 2012;96:235–256.
18. Grozinsky-Glasberg S, Fraser A, Nahshoni E, et al. Thyroxine-triiodothyronine combination therapy versus thyroxine monotherapy for clinical hypothyroidism: Meta-analysis of randomized controlled trials. J Clin Endocrinol Metab. 2006; 91:2592–2599.
19. Hennessey JV. Levothyroxine a new drug? Since when? How could that be? Thyroid. 2003;13:279–282.

20. U.S. Department of Health and Human Services, Food and Drug Administration Center for Drug Evaluation and Research Guidance for Industry. Levothyroxine Sodium Products Enforcement of August 14, 2001 Compliance Date and Submission of New Applications [online]. http://www.fda.gov/downloads/drugs/guidancecomplianceregulatoryinformation/guidances/ucm079807.pdf. Accessed September 28, 2014.
21. Food and Drug Administration Center for Drug Evaluation and Research Electronic Orange Book. Approved Drug Products with Therapeutic Equivalence Evaluations [online]. http://www.accessdata.fda.gov/scripts/cder/ob/docs/queryai.cfm. Accessed September 28, 2014.
22. Blakesley V, Awni W, Locke C, Ludden T, et al. Are bioequivalence studies of levothyroxine sodium formulations in euthyroid volunteers reliable? Thyroid. 2004;14:191–200.
23. Dong BJ, Hauck WW, Gambertoglio JG, Gee L, et al. Bioequivalence of generic and brand-name levothyroxine products in the treatment of hypothyroidism. JAMA. 1997;277:1205–1213.
24. Mayor GH, Orlando T, Kurtz NM. Limitations of levothyroxine bioequivalence evaluation: an analysis of an attempted study. Am J Ther. 1995;2:417–432.
25. Carr D, McLeod DT, Parry G, Thornes HM. Fine adjustment of thyroxine replacement dosage: comparison of the thyrotrophin releasing hormone test using a sensitive thyrotrophin assay with measurement of free thyroid hormones and clinical assessment. Clin Endocrinol. 1988;28:325–333.
26. Helfand M, Crapo LM. Monitoring therapy in patients taking levothyroxine. Ann Intern Med. 1990;113:450–454.
27. Garg A, Vanderpump MPJ. Subclinical thyroid disease. Brit Med Bull. 2013;107:101–116.
28. Turner MR, Camacho X, Fischer HD, et al. Levothyroxine dose and risk of fractures in older adults: Nested case-control study. BMJ. 2011;342:d2238.
29. Bolk N, Visser TJ, Nijman J, et al. Effects of evening vs morning levothyroxine intake: a randomized double-blind crossover trial. Arch Intern Med. 2010;170:1996–2003.
30. Briesacher BA, Andrade SE, Fouayzi H, Chan A. Comparison of drug adherence rates among patients with seven different medical conditions. Pharmacotherapy. 2008;28:437–443.
31. Abalovich M, Amino N, Barbour LA, et al. Management of thyroid dysfunction during pregnancy and postpartum: An Endocrine Society Clinical Practice Guideline. J Clin Endocrinol Metab. 2007;92(Suppl):S1–S47.
32. Zeitler P, Solberg P. Food and levothyroxine administration in infants and children. J Pediatr. 2010;157:13–15.
33. Bahn RS, Burch HB, Cooper DS, et al. Hyperthyroidism and other causes of thyrotoxicosis: Management guidelines of the American Thyroid Association and American Association of Clinical Endocrinologists. Thyroid. 2011;21:593–646.
34. Seigel SC, Hodak SP. Thyrotoxicosis. Med Clin N Amer. 2012;96:175–201.
35. Franklyn JA, Boelaert K. Thyrotoxicosis. Lancet. 2012;379:1155–1166.
36. Collet TH, Gussekloo J, Bauer DC, et al. Subclinical hyperthyroidism and the risk of coronary heart disease and mortality. Arch Int Med. 2012;172:799–809.
37. Wirth CD, Blum MR, da Costa BR, et al. Subclinical thyroid dysfunction and the risk for fractures: A systematic review and meta-analysis. Ann Int Med. 2014; 161:189–199.
38. Stan MN, Garrity JA, Bahn RS. The evaluation and treatment of Graves ophthalmopathy. Med Clin N Amer. 2012;96:311–328.
39. Cooper DS. Drug therapy: Antithyroid drugs. New Engl J Med. 2005;352:905–917.
40. Emiliano AB, Governale L, Parks M, Cooper DS. Shifts in propylthiouracil and methimazole prescribing practices: antithyroid drug use in the United States from 1991 to 2008. J Clin Endocrinol Metab. 2010;95:2227–2233.
41. Walker MA, Briel M, Chrit-Crain M, et al. Effects of antithyroid drugs on radioiodine treatment: Systematic review and meta-analysis of randomized controlled trials. BMJ. 2007;335:1–7.
42. U.S. Food and Drug Administration FDA drug safety communication: New boxed warning on severe liver injury with propylthiouracil [online]. [cited 2011 Oct 10]. http://www.fda.gov/Drugs/DrugSafety/PostmarketDrugSafetyInformationforPatientsandProviders/ucm209023.htm. Accessed September 28, 2014.
43. Marx H, Amin P, Lazarus JH. Hyperthyroidism and pregnancy. BMJ. 2008;336:663–667.
44. Rivkees SA. Propylthiouracil versis methimazole during pregnancy: An evolving tale of difficult choices. J Clin Endocrinol Metab. 2013;98:4332–4335.
45. Klubol-Gwiezdzinska J, Wartofsky L. Thyroid emergencies. Med Clin N Amer. 2012;96:385–403.
46. Pappa TA, Apostolos G, Veganakis MA. The nonthyroidal illness syndrome in the non-critically ill patient. Eur J Clin Invest. 2011;41:212–220.
47. Kaptein EM, Sanchez A, Beale E, Chan LS. Thyroid hormone therapy for postoperative nonthyroidal illness: A systematic review and synthesis. J Clin Endocrinol Metab. 2010;95:4526–4534.
48. Padmanabhan H. Amiodarone and thyroid dysfunction. South Med J. 2010;103:922–930.
49. Batcher EL, Tang C, Singh BN, et al. Thyroid function abnormalities during amiodarone therapy for persistent atrial fibrillation. Am J Med. 2007;120:880–885.
50. Lazarus JH. Lithium and thyroid. Best Pract Res Clin Endocrinol Metab. 2009;23:723–733.

45 Adrenal Gland Disorders

Devra K. Dang, Judy T. Chen, Frank Pucino, Jr, and Karim Anton Calis

LEARNING OBJECTIVES

Upon completion of the chapter, the reader will be able to:

1. Explain the regulation and physiologic roles of hormones produced by the adrenal glands.
2. Recognize the clinical presentation of adrenal insufficiency.
3. Describe the pharmacologic management of acute and chronic adrenal insufficiency.
4. Recommend therapy monitoring parameters for adrenal insufficiency.
5. Recognize the clinical presentation of Cushing syndrome and the physiologic consequences of cortisol excess.
6. Describe the pharmacologic and nonpharmacologic management of Cushing syndrome.
7. Recommend strategies to prevent the development of hypercortisolism and hypocortisolism.
8. Recommend therapy monitoring parameters for Cushing syndrome.

INTRODUCTION

The adrenal glands are important in the synthesis and regulation of key human hormones. They play a crucial role in water and electrolyte homeostasis, as well as regulation of blood pressure, carbohydrate and fat metabolism, physiologic response to stress, and sexual development and differentiation. This chapter focuses on pharmacologic and nonpharmacologic management of the two most common conditions associated with adrenal gland dysfunction: glucocorticoid insufficiency (eg, Addison disease) and glucocorticoid excess (Cushing syndrome). Other adrenal disorders such as **congenital adrenal hyperplasia**, **pheochromocytoma**, hypoaldosteronism, and hyperaldosteronism are beyond the scope of this chapter.

PHYSIOLOGY, ANATOMY, AND BIOCHEMISTRY OF THE ADRENAL GLAND

The adrenal gland is located on the upper segment of the kidney. It consists of an outer cortex and an inner medulla. The adrenal medulla secretes the catecholamines epinephrine (also called adrenaline) and norepinephrine (also called noradrenaline), which are involved in the regulation of the sympathetic nervous system. The adrenal cortex consists of three histologically distinct zones: the outer zona glomerulosa, the zona fasciculata, and an innermost layer called the zona reticularis. Each zone is responsible for production of different hormones (Figure 45–1).[1]

The zona glomerulosa is responsible for the production of the mineralocorticoids **aldosterone**, 18-hydroxy-corticosterone, corticosterone, and deoxycorticosterone. Aldosterone promotes renal sodium retention and potassium excretion. Its synthesis and release are regulated by renin in response to decreased vascular volume and renal perfusion. Adrenal aldosterone production is regulated by the **renin-angiotensin-aldosterone system**.

The zona fasciculata is the middle layer and produces the glucocorticoid hormone cortisol. **Cortisol** is responsible for maintaining homeostasis of carbohydrate, protein, and fat metabolism. Its secretion follows a circadian rhythm, generally beginning to rise at approximately 3 to 4 AM and peaking around 6 to 8 AM. Thereafter, cortisol levels decrease throughout the day, approach 50% of the peak value by 4 PM, and reach their nadir around midnight.[2] The normal rate of cortisol production is approximately 8 to 15 mg/day.[3] Cortisol plays a key role in the body's response to stress. Its production increases markedly during physiologic stress, such as during acute illness, surgery, or trauma. In addition, certain conditions such as alcoholism, depression, anxiety disorder, obsessive-compulsive disorder, poorly controlled diabetes, morbid obesity, starvation, anorexia nervosa, and chronic renal failure are associated with increased cortisol levels. High total cortisol levels are also observed in the presence of increased cortisol binding globulin (the carrier protein for 80% of circulating cortisol molecules), which is seen in pregnancy or other high-estrogen states (eg, exogenous estrogen administration).[2] Cortisol is converted in the liver to an inactive metabolite known as cortisone.

The zona reticularis produces the androgens androstenedione, dehydroepiandrosterone (DHEA), and the sulfated form of dehydroepiandrosterone (DHEA-S). Only a small amount of testosterone and estrogen is produced in the adrenal glands. Androstenedione and DHEA are converted in the periphery, largely to testosterone and estrogen.

Adrenal hormone production is controlled by the hypothalamus and pituitary. **Corticotropin-releasing hormone** (CRH) is secreted by the hypothalamus and stimulates secretion of **adrenocorticotropic hormone** (ACTH; also known as corticotropin) from the anterior pituitary. ACTH in turn stimulates the adrenal cortex to produce cortisol. When sufficient or excessive cortisol

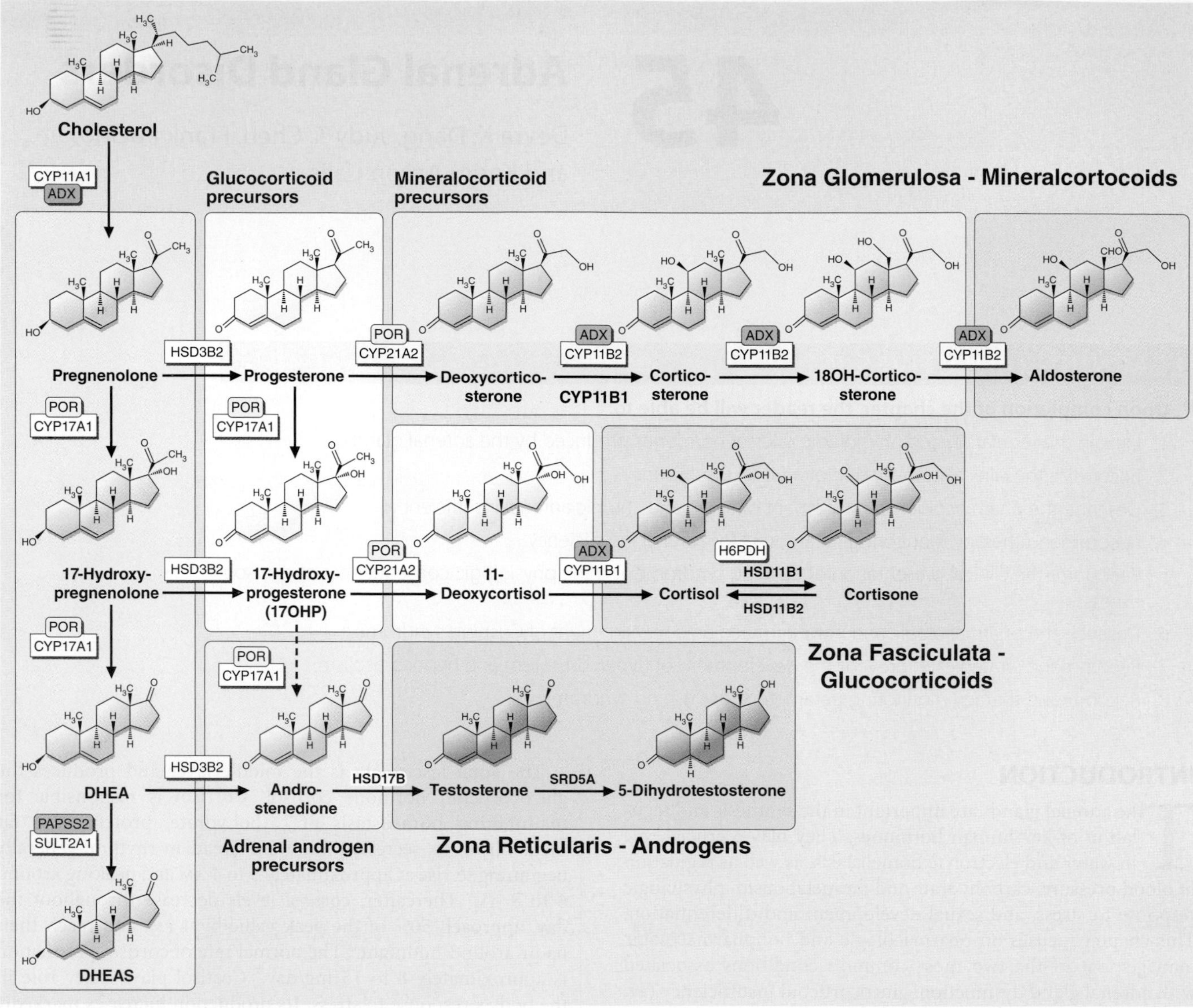

FIGURE 45–1. The adrenal cortex consists of three histologically distinct zones: the outer zona glomerulosa, the middle zona fasciculata, and an innermost layer called the zona reticularis. Each zone is responsible for production of different hormones. The zona glomerulosa is responsible for the production of mineralocorticoids such as aldosterone. The zona fasciculata produces cortisol and the zona reticularis produces androgens. ADX, adrenodoxin; CYP11A1, side chain cleavage enzyme; CYP17A1, 17-α-hydroxylase/17,20 lyase; CYP21A2, 21-hydroxylase; CYP11B1, 11-β-hydroxylase; CYP11B2, aldosterone synthase; DHEA, dehydroepiandrosterone; DHEAS, dehydroepiandrosterone sulfate; H6PDH, hexose-6-phosphate dehydrogenase; HSD11B1, 11-β-hydroxysteroid dehydrogenase type 1; HSD11B2, 11-β-hydroxysteroid dehydrogenase type 2; HSD3B2, 3-β-hydroxysteroid dehydrogenase type 2; HSD17B, 17-β-hydroxysteroid dehydrogenase; PAPSS2, PAPS synthase type 2; POR, P450 oxidoreductase; SRD5A, 5-α-reductase; SULT2A1, DHEA sulfotransferase. Adapted, with permission, from Arlt W. Disorders of the adrenal cortex. In: Longo DL, Fauci AS, Kasper DL, et al., eds. Harrison's Principles of Internal Medicine. New York: McGraw-Hill, 2011.

levels are reached, a negative feedback is exerted on the secretion of CRH and ACTH, thereby decreasing overall cortisol production. The control of adrenal androgen synthesis also follows a similar negative feedback mechanism. Figure 46–1 depicts hormonal regulation with the hypothalamic-pituitary-adrenal (HPA) axis.

ADRENAL INSUFFICIENCY

Epidemiology and Etiology

Adrenal insufficiency generally refers to the inability of the adrenal glands to produce adequate amounts of cortisol for normal physiologic functioning or in times of stress. The condition is usually classified as primary, secondary, or tertiary, depending on the etiology (Table 45–1).[2,4–7] The estimated prevalence of primary adrenal insufficiency and secondary adrenal insufficiency is approximately 60 to 143 and 150 to 280 cases per 1 million persons, respectively. Whereas primary adrenal insufficiency is usually diagnosed in the third to fifth decade of life, secondary adrenal insufficiency is commonly detected during the sixth decade.[2,8] Adrenal insufficiency is more prevalent in women than in men, with a ratio of 2.6:1.[2] Chronic adrenal insufficiency is rare.

Table 45–1

Etiologies of Adrenal Insufficiency[2,4–7]

Primary Adrenal Insufficiency (Addison disease)

- Autoimmune—accounts for 70%–90% of all cases of primary adrenal insufficiency
- Infectious or granulomatous diseases
  - Cytomegalovirus
  - Fungal (histoplasmosis, coccidioidomycosis, cryptococcosis, *Blastomyces dermatitidis* infection)
  - HIV (human immunodeficiency virus), AIDS (acquired immunodeficiency syndrome)
    - Mycobacterial, cytomegaloviral, *Pneumocystic jiroveci*, and *Toxoplasma gondii* infection
  - Sarcoidosis
  - Tuberculosis
- Bilateral adrenal hemorrhage or infarction—usually due to anticoagulant therapy, coagulopathy, thromboembolic disease, or meningococcal infection. Causes acute adrenal insufficiency
- Adrenalectomy
- Adrenoleukodystrophy (in men)
- Adrenomyeloneuropathy
- Infiltrative disorders: amyloidosis, hemochromatosis
- Genetic causes
  - Congenital adrenal hyperplasia
  - Familial glucocorticoid deficiency and hypoplasia
- Metastatic malignancy

Secondary Adrenal Insufficiency

- Cushing syndrome
- Panhypopituitarism
- Pituitary tumor
- Transsphenoidal pituitary microsurgery
- Pituitary irradiation
- Traumatic brain injury

Tertiary Adrenal Insufficiency

- Hypothalamic dysfunction

Drug-induced (most common cause of secondary and tertiary adrenal insufficiency)

- Chronic glucocorticoid administration at supraphysiologic doses
- Steroidogenesis inhibitors
- Megestrol acetate—has glucocorticoid-like activity
- Mifepristone (RU 486)—antagonizes glucocorticoid receptors
- Tyrosine kinase inhibitors
- Inducers of CYP450 enzymes that increase cortisol metabolism (2B1, 2B2, 3A4)

CYP450, cytochrome P-450

Pathophysiology

Primary adrenal insufficiency, also known as Addison disease, occurs when the adrenal glands are unable to produce cortisol. It occurs from destruction of the adrenal cortex, usually from an autoimmune process. In general, the clinical manifestations are observed when destruction of the cortex exceeds 90%.[6] KEY CONCEPT Signs and symptoms of adrenal insufficiency reflect the disturbance of normal physiologic carbohydrate, fat, and protein homeostasis caused by inadequate cortisol production and inadequate cortisol action. Primary adrenal insufficiency usually develops gradually. Patients may remain asymptomatic in the early stages with signs and symptoms present only during times of physiologic stress. Persistent signs and symptoms of hypocortisolism typically occur with disease progression. Additionally,

Clinical Presentation and Diagnosis of Chronic Adrenal Insufficiency[2,5,6,8]

General

- Symptoms develop gradually, especially in the early stages, may be vague, and mimic other medical conditions.
- Patients with autoimmune adrenal insufficiency may have other autoimmune disorders such as type 1 diabetes mellitus or autoimmune thyroiditis.

Symptoms (Percent Prevalence)

- Weakness and fatigue (99%)
- Anorexia, nausea, and diarrhea (56%–90%); may range from mild to severe with vomiting and abdominal pain
- Hypoglycemia may occur
- Amenorrhea may occur
- Salt craving occurs in approximately 22% with Addison disease due to aldosterone deficiency

Signs

- Weight loss (97%)
- Hypotension (less than 110/70 mm Hg) and orthostasis (87%)
- Dehydration, hypovolemia, and hyperkalemia (in primary adrenal insufficiency only) due to aldosterone deficiency.
- Hyponatremia and hypochloridemia levels due to aldosterone deficiency. Hyponatremia can also be present in secondary insufficiency due to cortisol deficiency and increased antidiuretic hormone secretion leading to subsequent water retention.
- Increased serum blood urea nitrogen and creatinine due to dehydration.
- Hyperpigmentation of skin and mucous membranes (92%). Usually observed around creases, pressure areas, areolas, genitalia, and new scars. Dark freckles and patches of vitiligo may be present. Hyperpigmentation, due to increased ACTH levels, occurs in most patients with primary but not secondary or tertiary insufficiency.
- Personality changes (irritability and restlessness) due to cortisol deficiency.
- Loss of axillary and pubic hair in women due to decreased androgen production.
- Blood count abnormalities (normocytic, normochromic anemia, relative lymphocytosis, neutrophilia, eosinophilia) due to cortisol and androgen deficiency.

Laboratory Tests (see Table 45–2[1,5,9,10])

- Decreased basal and stress-induced cortisol levels.
- Decreased aldosterone level (in primary insufficiency only).
- Lack of increase in cortisol and aldosterone level after ACTH stimulation.

Other Diagnostic Tests

- Computed tomography (CT) scan or magnetic resonance imaging (MRI) of the adrenal glands, pituitary, and/or hypothalamus can aid in determining etiology.
- Presence of antiadrenal antibodies is suggestive of an autoimmune etiology.

Table 45–2

Tests for Diagnosing Adrenal Insufficiency[1,2,5,10]

Test	Procedure	Rationale	Finding in Adrenal Insufficiency	Comments
Screening and Diagnostic Tests for Adrenal Insufficiency				
Unstimulated serum cortisol measurement	Measure serum cortisol at 6–8 AM	Serum cortisol level peaks in the early morning	Serum cortisol < 3 mcg/dL (83 nmol/L)	• Evaluate result in context of those from other test(s) • Can be performed in conjunction with the rapid ACTH stimulation test (measure baseline serum cortisol before administering 250 mcg of cosyntropin)
Rapid ACTH stimulation test (also called cosyntropin stimulation test)	Measure serum cortisol 30–60 minutes after administering cosyntropin 250 mcg IM or IV	Increased cortisol secretion in normal individuals in response to ACTH stimulation but not in adrenal insufficiency	Serum cortisol concentration < 18–20 mcg/dL (497–552 nmol/L)	• Used as gold standard test for diagnosing primary adrenal insufficiency • False negative results may occur if ACTH deficiency is of recent onset (< 1 month) • If measured serum cortisol concentration is low, measure plasma ACTH, aldosterone, and renin concentrations to differentiate between primary and secondary or tertiary adrenal insufficiency (see below) • A normal response does not exclude mild secondary adrenal insufficiency or recent onset ACTH deficiency. Additional testing (eg, insulin tolerance or metyrapone test) may be required
Insulin tolerance test (insulin-induced hypoglycemia test)	Administer insulin IV to induce hypoglycemia then measure serum cortisol during symptomatic hypoglycemia (confirm that blood glucose is < 40 mg/dL [2.2 mmol/L])	Evaluates ability of entire HPA axis to respond to stress (hypoglycemia)	Serum cortisol concentration < 18 mcg/dL (497 nmol/L) is indicative of secondary adrenal insufficiency	• If the result of the rapid ACTH stimulation test is normal, either this or the overnight metyrapone test is still needed to evaluate for secondary adrenal insufficiency. The insulin tolerance test is considered the gold standard • Contraindicated in patients with a seizure history, older than 60 years, or with cardiovascular or cerebrovascular disease • Requires close medical supervision • Contraindicated in adrenal crisis and primary adrenal insufficiency
Overnight metyrapone test	Administer metyrapone at midnight then measure serum cortisol at 8 AM the next day	Metyrapone inhibits cortisol synthesis. Its administration leads to rise in levels of ACTH and the precursor of cortisol, 11-deoxycortisol. Patients with adrenal insufficiency do not exhibit this	Normal response is a decrease in serum cortisol to < 5 mcg/dL (138 nmol/L) and an increase in 11-deoxycortisol to > 7 mcg/dL (202 nmol/L). Response not seen in secondary adrenal insufficiency	• Distinguishes between normal individuals and patients with secondary adrenal insufficiency • Contraindicated in adrenal crisis and primary adrenal insufficiency
Tests for Differential Diagnosis of Primary, Secondary, and Tertiary Adrenal Insufficiency				
Plasma ACTH concentration	Measure plasma ACTH	In primary adrenal insufficiency, hypocortisolism leads to elevated plasma ACTH concentration via positive HPA axis feedback	• Primary adrenal insufficiency: elevated plasma ACTH. • Secondary or tertiary adrenal insufficiency: plasma ACTH low or inappropriately normal	• Evaluate result of test in combination with those from the plasma aldosterone and plasma renin tests

(Continued)

Table 45–2

Tests for Diagnosing Adrenal Insufficiency[1,2,5,10] (*Continued*)

Test	Procedure	Rationale	Finding in Adrenal Insufficiency	Comments
Plasma aldosterone concentration	Measure plasma aldosterone from same blood samples as those used in ACTH stimulation test	Patients with primary adrenal insufficiency may experience a reduction in aldosterone production	• Primary adrenal insufficiency: low plasma aldosterone • Secondary or tertiary adrenal insufficiency: aldosterone concentration is usually normal (≥ 5 ng/dL [139 pmol/L])	• Evaluate result of test in combination with those from plasma ACTH and plasma renin tests
Plasma renin concentration or activity	Measure plasma renin concentration or activity	Mineralocorticoid deficiency occurs in primary adrenal insufficiency but is usually not present in secondary or tertiary adrenal insufficiency	• Primary adrenal insufficiency: elevated plasma renin • Secondary or tertiary adrenal insufficiency: plasma renin concentration or activity is usually normal	• Evaluate result of test in combination with those from plasma ACTH and plasma aldosterone concentration tests

ACTH, adrenocorticotropic hormone or corticotropin; HPA, hypothalamic-pituitary-adrenal; IM, intramuscularly; IV, intravenously

primary adrenal insufficiency may be accompanied by a reduction in aldosterone and androgen production.

Secondary adrenal insufficiency occurs as a result of pituitary gland dysfunction, whereby decreased production and secretion of ACTH leads to a decrease in cortisol synthesis. Tertiary adrenal insufficiency is a disorder of the hypothalamus that results in decreased production and release of CRH, which in turn decreases pituitary ACTH production and release. In contrast to Addison disease, aldosterone production is unaffected in the secondary and tertiary forms of the disease. Chronic adrenal insufficiency often has a good prognosis if diagnosed early and treated appropriately.

Acute adrenal insufficiency (ie, adrenal crisis) results from the body's inability to sufficiently increase endogenous cortisol during periods of excessive physiologic stress. Adrenal crisis can occur when patients with chronic adrenal insufficiency do not receive adequate glucocorticoid replacement during stressful conditions such as those experienced during surgery, infection, fever, acute illness, invasive medical procedures, or trauma. Acute adrenal insufficiency can also result from bilateral adrenal infarction due to hemorrhage, embolus, sepsis, or adrenal vein thrombosis. Patients who are critically ill may also experience impaired HPA axis function, with an overall prevalence rate of 10% to 20%, and as high as 60% in those experiencing septic

Clinical Presentation and Diagnosis of Acute Adrenal Insufficiency (Adrenal Crisis)[2,6,8]

General

- Onset of symptoms is acute and precipitated by excessive physiologic stress or abrupt discontinuation of supraphysiologic doses of chronic glucocorticoid.

Symptoms

- Severe weakness and fatigue
- Abdominal or flank pain

Signs

- Severe dehydration leading to hypotension and shock (circulatory collapse). Hypovolemia may not be responsive to intravenous (IV) hydration and may require the use of vasopressors.
- Tachycardia
- Nausea, vomiting
- Fever
- Confusion
- Hypoglycemia
- Laboratory abnormalities are similar to those observed in chronic adrenal insufficiency.

Laboratory Tests

- The unstimulated serum cortisol and rapid ACTH stimulation tests are useful in diagnosis (see Table 45–2). The insulin tolerance test is contraindicated due to preexisting hypoglycemia. The metyrapone test is also contraindicated since metyrapone inhibits cortisol production.

Note: Due to the life-threatening nature of this condition, empiric treatment should be started before laboratory confirmation in patients who present with the clinical picture of acute adrenal crisis.

shock. These patients are also at risk for the life-threatening consequences of an adrenal crisis. To better recognize this condition, the term *critical illness–related corticosteroid insufficiency* was coined by the American College of Critical Care Medicine Task Force.[9] Additionally, abrupt discontinuation or rapid tapering of glucocorticoids, given chronically in supraphysiologic doses, may lead to adrenal crisis. This condition results from prolonged suppression of the HPA axis and subsequent adrenal gland atrophy and hypocortisolemia. Other drugs associated with adrenal insufficiency include those that inhibit production (eg, ketoconazole) or increase metabolism (eg, the cytochrome P-450 3A4 inducer rifampin) of cortisol.[6] Regardless of the etiology, patients experiencing an adrenal crisis require immediate glucocorticoid treatment since manifestations such as circulatory collapse can lead to life-threatening sequelae.

Treatment and Outcome Evaluation

▸ *Chronic Adrenal Insufficiency*

The general goals of treatment are to manage symptoms and prevent development of adrenal crisis. KEY CONCEPT *Lifelong glucocorticoid replacement therapy may be necessary for patients with adrenal insufficiency, and mineralocorticoid replacement therapy is usually required for those with Addison disease.* Glucocorticoids with sufficient mineralocorticoid activity are generally required. However, the addition of a potent mineralocorticoid such as fludrocortisone, along with adequate salt intake, is sometimes needed to prevent sodium loss, hyperkalemia, and intravascular volume depletion. Mineralocorticoid supplementation typically is not indicated for the treatment of secondary or tertiary adrenal insufficiency because aldosterone production is often unaffected. Moreover, patients with secondary or tertiary adrenal insufficiency may only require replacement therapy until the HPA axis recovers. Hydrocortisone is often prescribed because it most closely resembles endogenous cortisol with its relatively high mineralocorticoid activity and short half-life, and allows the design of regimens that simulate the normal circadian cycle.[5] Other glucocorticoids, however, can be used. Table 45–3 lists the pharmacologic characteristics of commonly used glucocorticoids.[11]

Because patients with primary adrenal insufficiency can experience DHEA deficiency, DHEA replacement has also been tried. Several small clinical studies, consisting mostly of women, suggest that treatment with DHEA can improve mood and fatigue and provide a general sense of well-being.[12–14] However, a recent meta-analysis of 10 studies found that DHEA use in women only slightly improved health-related quality of life and depression but did not affect anxiety or sexual well-being; it concluded that the totality of available data does not support routine supplementation with DHEA.[15] The use of DHEA remains controversial and requires further study. Management strategies for chronic adrenal insufficiency are outlined below:[2,4,5,8,16]

- For the treatment of primary adrenal insufficiency (Addison disease) in adults, 15–25 mg/day of oral hydrocortisone is typically administered in two divided doses, with two-thirds of the dose given in the morning upon awakening to mimic the early morning rise in endogenous cortisol, and the remaining one-third of the dose given in the late afternoon to avoid insomnia and allow for the lowest concentration in the blood at around midnight. Hydrocortisone may also be given in three doses but this may decrease adherence. The longer-acting glucocorticoids (eg, prednisone, dexamethasone) may provide a more prolonged clinical response thereby avoiding symptom recurrence that can occur at the end of the dosing interval with short-acting agents such as hydrocortisone. Longer-acting agents also may improve adherence in some patients. Monitor the patient's weight, blood pressure, and serum electrolytes along with symptom resolution and general well-being; adjust dosages accordingly as needed. Doses of hydrocortisone, dexamethasone, prednisone, and other glucocorticoids may need to be increased or decreased in patients taking cytochrome P-450 (CYP450) 3A4 inducers or inhibitors, respectively. Monitor for adverse drug reactions related to glucocorticoid administration. Glucocorticoid therapy at physiologic replacement doses should not lead to development of Cushing syndrome;

Table 45–3

Pharmacologic Characteristics of Major Corticosteroids[11]

Corticosteroid	Glucocorticoid (Anti-Inflammatory) Potency	Mineralocorticoid (Sodium-Retaining) Potency	Duration of Action[a]	Equivalent Dose (mg)[b]
Glucocorticoid				
Cortisol	1	1	S	20
Cortisone	0.8	0.8	S	25
Prednisone	4	0.8	I	5
Prednisolone	4	0.8	I	5
Methylprednisolone	5	0.5	I	4
Triamcinolone	5	0	I	4
Betamethasone	25	0	L	0.75
Dexamethasone	25	0	L	0.75
Mineralocorticoid				
Fludrocortisone	10	125	I	[c]

[a]S, short (ie, 8–12 hour biological $t_{1/2}$); I, intermediate (ie, 12–36 hour biological $t_{1/2}$); L, long (ie, 36–72 hour biological $t_{1/2}$).

[b]These dose relationships apply only to oral or intravenous administration, as glucocorticoid potencies may differ greatly following intramuscular or intraarticular administration.

[c]This agent is not used for glucocorticoid effects.

Adapted, with permission, from Shimmer BP, Funder JW. ACTH, adrenal steroids, and pharmacology of the adrenal cortex. In: Brunton LL, Chabner BA, Knollmann BC, eds. Pharmacological Basis of Therapeutics, 12th ed. New York: McGraw-Hill, 2011: Figure 42–2.

Patient Encounter 1, Part 1: Presentation and Medical History

A 48-year-old woman presents to the primary care clinic with complaints of fatigue and asking for a prescription for "vitamin injections." She states that she has been feeling very tired for the past year. Upon further questioning, she also complains of dizziness, especially with positional changes, and intermittent nausea, abdominal pain, and diarrhea.

PMH: Tuberculosis—completed treatment course; history of candidal vulvovaginitis; depression

FH: Mother with type 1 diabetes

SH: Denies smoking, alcohol use or illicit drug use

Current Meds: Sertraline 100 mg once daily; loperamide 2 mg as needed for diarrhea (nonprescription)

PE:

VS: Sitting BP 106/68 mm Hg, P 74 beats/min, standing BP 96/68 mm Hg, RR 14 breaths/min, Wt 130 pounds (59 kg)—5 pound (2.3 kg) loss in last 6 months, Ht 5′2″(157 cm)

Skin: Hyperpigmentation in creases of palms

CV: RRR, normal S_1, S_2; no murmurs, rubs, or gallops

Labs (fasting): Serum electrolytes: sodium 133 mEq/L (133 mmol/L), potassium 5.2 mEq/L (5.2 mmol/L), chloride 98 mEq/L (98 mmol/L), bicarb 30 mEq/L (30 mmol/L), blood urea nitrogen (BUN) 25 mg/dL (8.9 mmol/L), serum creatinine 1.2 mg/dL (106 μmol/L), glucose 60 mg/dL (3.3 mmol/L).

Which signs or symptoms of adrenal insufficiency does the patient exhibit?

Does her presentation offer any clues as to etiology or classification of adrenal insufficiency?

Which tests would be most useful for determining etiology and confirming diagnosis of adrenal insufficiency?

however, careful monitoring should still be performed, and the smallest effective dose used. Educate patients regarding the need for increased glucocorticoid dosage during excessive physiologic stress. In addition, administer oral fludrocortisone at a daily dose of approximately 0.05 to 0.2 mg in the morning. Monitor for resolution of hypotension, dizziness, dehydration, hyponatremia, and hyperkalemia; and increase the dose if needed. Conversely, consider decreasing the dose if adverse reactions from mineralocorticoid administration such as hypertension, hypokalemia, fluid retention, and other significant adverse events occur. In patients receiving hydrocortisone, it should be noted that this drug also possesses mineralocorticoid activity. All patients with Addison disease should also maintain adequate sodium intake. Lastly, although controversial, consider giving DHEA 25–50 mg/day (in the morning) to female patients who do not experience an improvement in mood and well-being even with adequate glucocorticoid and mineralocorticoid replacement. In these patients, monitor serum DHEA-S (aim for the middle range of normal levels in healthy young people) and free testosterone level.

- Patients with secondary and tertiary adrenal insufficiency are treated with oral hydrocortisone or a longer-acting glucocorticoid as described for primary adrenal insufficiency. However, patients with secondary and tertiary adrenal insufficiency may require a lower dose. Some patients (eg, patients with drug-induced adrenal insufficiency or adrenal insufficiency following treatment for Cushing syndrome) will only require glucocorticoid replacement temporarily, which can be discontinued after recovery of the HPA axis. Monitor for progression of the underlying etiology of adrenal insufficiency. Fludrocortisone therapy is generally not needed.

Patient Encounter 1, Part 2: Treatment

After appropriate laboratory and diagnostic tests are performed, the patient is diagnosed with Addison disease.

How should her chronic primary adrenal insufficiency be treated?

What monitoring parameters (therapeutic and toxic) should be implemented?

► Acute Adrenal Insufficiency

KEY CONCEPT *During an acute adrenal crisis, the immediate treatment goals are to correct volume depletion, manage hypoglycemia, and provide glucocorticoid replacement.* Volume depletion and hypoglycemia can be corrected by giving large volumes (~ 2–3 L) of IV normal saline and 5% dextrose solution.[2] Glucocorticoid replacement can be accomplished by administering IV hydrocortisone, starting at a dose of 100 mg every 6 hours for 24 hours, decreasing to 50 mg every 6 hours on the second day after achieving hemodynamic stability, and thereafter be tapered to a lower maintenance dose by the fourth or fifth day and fludrocortisone can be added if needed. The dose can be increased to 200 to 400 mg/day if complications.[2] For the treatment of patients with critical illness-related corticosteroid insufficiency, see the 2008 consensus statements from the American College of Critical Care Medicine Task Force.[9]

KEY CONCEPT *Patients with known adrenal insufficiency should be educated about the need for additional glucocorticoid replacement and prompt medical attention during periods of physiologic stress.* Although the dosage of glucocorticoid is generally individualized, a common recommendation is to double the maintenance dose of hydrocortisone if the patient experiences fever or undergoes invasive dental or diagnostic procedures.[5] Patients who experience vomiting or diarrhea may not adequately absorb oral glucocorticoids and may benefit from parenteral therapy until symptoms resolve. Prior to surgery, additional glucocorticoid replacement (higher dose and parenteral route) must be given to prevent adrenal crisis. The dose and protocol varies depending

Patient Care Process: Adrenal Insufficiency

Patient Assessment:

- Evaluate for typical clinical manifestations of chronic or acute adrenal insufficiency. Clinical presentation can differentiate between chronic primary and secondary/tertiary adrenal insufficiency.
- Review medical and medication history to determine if the patient has any etiologies of adrenal insufficiency.
- Perform the rapid ACTH stimulation test to assess for presence of adrenal insufficiency (see Table 45–2).
- After diagnosis is confirmed, perform further testing to differentiate between primary, secondary, and tertiary adrenal insufficiency (see Table 45–2).

Therapy Evaluation:

- Determine whether patient will require mineralocorticoid replacement therapy in addition to glucocorticoid supplementation.

Care Plan Development:

- In patients presenting with acute adrenal crisis not previously diagnosed with adrenal insufficiency, immediate treatment with injectable hydrocortisone and IV saline and dextrose solutions should be initiated prior to confirmation of diagnosis because of the life-threatening nature of this condition. Determine and correct the underlying cause of the acute adrenal crisis (eg, infection).
- In patients with chronic adrenal insufficiency, devise a strategy to give supplemental doses of glucocorticoid when varying degrees of physiologic stress are experienced (eg, minor infection, pending surgery). Monitor patient for signs of an acute adrenal crisis and develop a plan to treat this emergency condition.
- Educate both patient and family members/caregiver regarding:
  - Causes of adrenal insufficiency, including drug-induced etiologies.
  - How to recognize clinical manifestations.
  - How to prevent an acute adrenal crisis: adhere to therapy; do not abruptly stop glucocorticoid treatment; increase glucocorticoid dose during different severity levels of physiologic stress including childbirth.
  - When to self-administer parenteral glucocorticoid and seek emergency care.
  - Need to notify all health care providers of condition.
  - Wearing or carrying a medical alert (eg, bracelet, card).
  - Dietary and pharmacologic therapy, including duration of treatment and potential adverse consequences of glucocorticoid and mineralocorticoid replacement.

Follow-Up Evaluation:

- Monitor for adequacy of treatment and adverse reactions from glucocorticoid and/or mineralocorticoid therapy.
- Determine duration of treatment for patients with secondary and tertiary adrenal insufficiency.

on the type of surgery (eg, larger doses for major surgery compared to minor surgery).

HYPERCORTISOLISM (CUSHING SYNDROME)

Epidemiology and Etiology

Cushing syndrome refers to the pathophysiologic changes associated with exposure to supraphysiologic cortisol concentrations (endogenous hypercortisolism) or pharmacologic doses of glucocorticoids (exogenous hypercortisolism). Cushing syndrome from endogenous causes is a rare condition, with an estimated incidence of two to five cases per 1 million persons per year.[17] Patients receiving chronic supraphysiologic doses of glucocorticoids, such as those with rheumatologic disorders, are at high risk of developing Cushing syndrome.

Pathophysiology

Cushing syndrome can be classified as ACTH-dependent or ACTH-independent (**Table 45–4**).[1,18–20] ACTH-dependent Cushing syndrome results from ACTH-secreting (or rarely CRH-secreting) **adenomas**. The term *Cushing disease* refers specifically to Cushing syndrome from an ACTH-secreting pituitary adenoma. ACTH-independent Cushing syndrome is due either to excessive cortisol secretion by the adrenal glands (independent of ACTH stimulation) or to exogenous glucocorticoid administration. The plasma ACTH concentration is elevated in ACTH-dependent conditions but not in ACTH-independent conditions because elevated cortisol concentrations suppress pituitary ACTH secretion via negative feedback. ACTH and cortisol concentrations are elevated episodically in ACTH-dependent

Table 45–4

Etiologies of Cushing Syndrome[2,18–20]

ACTH-Dependent

- ACTH-secreting pituitary tumor (Cushing *disease*)—70% of endogenous cases
- ACTH-secreting nonpituitary tumors (ectopic ACTH syndrome)—15% of endogenous cases; usually from small cell lung carcinoma and bronchial carcinoids; also from pheochromocytoma, or from thymus, pancreatic, ovarian, or thyroid tumor. The tumor is usually disseminated (difficult to localize).
- CRH-secreting nonpituitary tumors (ectopic CRH syndrome)—rare

ACTH-Independent—15% of endogenous cases

- Unilateral adrenal adenoma
- Adrenal carcinoma
- Bilateral nodular adrenal hyperplasia—rare (< 1%)

Drug-Induced Cushing Syndrome (ACTH-independent)—most common cause of Cushing syndrome

- Prescription glucocorticoid preparations (most routes of administration)
- Nonprescription and herbal products with glucocorticoid activity (eg, nonprescription anti-itch products with hydrocortisone, herbal products with magnolia bark or those claiming to contain adrenal cortex extracts or other by-products)
- Other drugs with glucocorticoid activity (eg, megestrol acetate, medroxyprogesterone)

ACTH, adrenocorticotropic hormone or corticotropin; CRH, corticotropin-releasing hormone

Clinical Presentation and Diagnosis of Cushing Syndrome[2,17,18,24]

General

- Onset of signs and symptoms range from gradual to rapid, depending on etiology.
- Differential diagnoses include diabetes mellitus and the metabolic syndrome because these conditions share several similar characteristics with Cushing syndrome (eg, obesity, hypertension, hyperlipidemia, hyperglycemia, and insulin resistance). In women, the presentations of hirsutism, menstrual abnormalities, and insulin resistance are similar to those of polycystic ovary syndrome. Cushing syndrome can be differentiated from these conditions by identifying the classic signs and symptoms described below.
- True Cushing syndrome also must be distinguished from other conditions that share some clinical presentations (as well as elevated plasma cortisol concentrations) such as depression, anxiety disorder, obsessive-compulsive disorder, alcoholism, obesity, uncontrolled diabetes, eating disorders, and physiologic stress—the so-called pseudo-Cushing states.

Signs and Symptoms (Percent Prevalence)

General appearance

- Weight gain and obesity, manifesting as truncal obesity (90%)
- Rounded and puffy face ("moon facies") (75%)
- Dorsocervical ("buffalo hump") and supraclavicular fat accumulation
- Hirsutism (75%)

Skin changes from atrophy of dermis and connective tissue

- Thin skin
- Facial plethora (70%)
- Skin striae ("stretch marks" that are usually red or purple in appearance and greater than 1 cm) (50%)—not common in patients older than 40 years of age
- Acne (35%)
- Easy bruising (40%)
- Hyperpigmentation—typically with ectopic ACTH syndrome

Metabolic

- Hyperglycemia that can range from impaired glucose tolerance (75%) to diabetes mellitus (20%–50%)
- Hyperlipidemia (70%)
- Polyuria (30%)
- Kidney stones (15%–50%)
- Hypokalemic alkalosis (from mineralocorticoid effect of cortisol)

Cardiovascular

- Hypertension (from mineralocorticoid effect of cortisol) (85%)
- Peripheral edema

Genitourinary

- Menstrual irregularities (typically amenorrhea) (70%)
- Erectile dysfunction (85%)

Other

- Psychiatric changes such as depression, emotional lability, psychosis, euphoria, anxiety, and decreased cognition (85%)
- Sleep disturbances
- Osteopenia (80%) and osteoporosis—usually affecting trabecular bone
- Linear growth impairment in children
- Proximal muscle weakness (65%)
- Avascular necrosis (more common in iatrogenic cases)
- Glaucoma, cataracts
- Impaired wound healing and susceptibility to opportunistic infections
- Hypothyroidism

Laboratory tests

- Diagnosis is often complex and generally requires the involvement of endocrinologists and specialized testing centers.
- Initial screening tests are listed in Table 45–5.[2,24] Typically, a combination of two screening tests is used to establish the preliminary diagnosis.
- After the diagnosis is confirmed, additional tests (eg, midnight serum cortisol or combined dexamethasone suppression plus CRH test) can be performed to determine the etiology or rule out false positive/negative results.

Other diagnostic tests

Imaging studies and inferior petrosal sinus sampling may be needed to distinguish between pituitary, ectopic, and adrenal tumors.

disease due to random hypersecretion of ACTH.[6] In general, patients with Cushing syndrome due to endogenous or exogenous glucocorticoid excess present with similar clinical manifestations. However, patients with ectopic ACTH syndrome may not exhibit the typical signs and symptoms of hypercortisolism due to the acute onset nature of the underlying disease process.[2]

Cushing disease and adrenal **carcinomas** cause adrenal androgen hypersecretion in high enough concentrations to result in signs of androgen excess such as acne, menstrual irregularities, and **hirsutism**, and cause **virilization** in women.[6] Drug-induced Cushing syndrome from glucocorticoid administration occurs most commonly in patients receiving oral therapy, but other routes such as inhalation, dermal, nasal, and intraarticular have also been implicated.[18] Over-the-counter products, including dietary supplements, should also be evaluated since they may contain corticosteroids. Drug-induced Cushing syndrome has been reported with the use of Chinese herbal products adulterated with corticosteroids.[21,22] The risk of glucocorticoid-induced Cushing syndrome appears to increase with higher doses and/or longer treatment durations.[18]

Left untreated, patients with Cushing syndrome may experience severe complications of hypercortisolism, resulting in up to a nearly four-fold increase in mortality.[23] Mortality in patients with Cushing is mostly attributed to cardiovascular disease.

Table 45–5

First-Line Screening Tests in Patients with Characteristics of Cushing Syndrome[2,24]

Test	Test Procedure and Measurement	Rationale	Typical Finding in Cushing Syndrome	Comments
24-hour urinary free cortisol	Collect urine over 24 hours and measure unbound cortisol excreted by kidneys	Urinary cortisol is elevated in hypercortisolic states	Elevated urinary free cortisol (value depends on the assay used)	• Easy to perform but should not be used alone since sensitivity and specificity depend on assay used • To exclude periodic hypercortisolism, two or more samples should be obtained (with urinary creatinine measurement to assess completeness of collection) • Distinguishes the effects of Cushing syndrome (elevation) from obesity (no elevation). However, false positive in other pseudo-Cushing states, physiologic stress, if fluid intake ≥ 5 L/day, or taking carbamazepine or fenofibrate (if measured by HPLC) • False negative if moderate to severe renal function, or subclinical hypercortisolism
Overnight dexamethasone suppression test (DST)	Give 1 mg oral dexamethasone at 11 PM, then measure plasma cortisol at 8–9 AM the next morning	Dexamethasone administration suppresses morning plasma cortisol in normal individuals	Plasma cortisol < 1.8 μg/dL (50 nmol/L) is not suggestive of Cushing syndrome	• Simple to perform and inexpensive • Can be used in conjunction with, or instead of, the urinary free cortisol test • False positive if pseudo-Cushing states, physiologic stress, pregnancy, estrogen treatment (including contraceptives), uremia, taking inducers of dexamethasone metabolism (phenytoin, alcohol, etc), or decreased dexamethasone absorption • False negative if subclinical hypercortisolism, slow metabolism of dexamethasone (eg, CYP3A4 inhibitors), or liver or renal impairment • In pseudo-Cushing states, the 48-hour 2-mg DST (administer 0.5 mg dexamethasone every 6 hours for 48 hours then measure serum cortisol at 8 or 9 AM after the last dose) is preferred
Late-night salivary cortisol	Collect salivary cortisol concentration at 11 PM	Loss of circadian rhythm of cortisol secretion (no nadir at night) in Cushing syndrome but not in pseudo-Cushing states	Elevated late-night salivary cortisol	• Easiest screening test to perform (sample can be collected at home by patient) • To exclude periodic hypercortisolism, two or more samples (on two separate evenings) should be obtained • False positive possible with cigarette smoking, chewing tobacco, licorice ingestion, in pseudo-Cushing states • Adjust collection time in shift workers and others with bedtime significantly after midnight

CYP, cytochrome P-450; HPLC, high-performance liquid chromatography

Hypertension, hyperglycemia, and hyperlipidemia are common findings and can be associated with cardiac hypertrophy, atherosclerosis, and hypercoagulability. Osteopenia, osteoporosis, and increased fractures also have been reported.[23] Prevention and management of these conditions are discussed elsewhere in this text. Children may experience linear growth retardation from reduced growth hormone secretion and inhibition of epiphyseal cartilage development in long bones.[17,23]

Treatment

The goal of treatment in patients with Cushing syndrome is reversal of hypercortisolism and management of the associated comorbidities, including the potential for long-term sequelae such as cardiac hypertrophy. KEY CONCEPT *Surgical resection is considered the treatment of choice for Cushing syndrome from endogenous causes if the tumor can be localized and if there are no contraindications.* The treatment of choice for Cushing syndrome from exogenous causes is gradual discontinuation of the offending agent.

▸ Nonpharmacologic Therapy

Transsphenoidal pituitary microsurgery is the treatment of choice for Cushing disease. Removal of the pituitary tumor can bring about complete remission or cure in 78% to 97% of cases. HPA axis suppression associated with chronic hypercortisolism can result in prolonged adrenal insufficiency lasting for months after surgery and requiring exogenous glucocorticoid administration. Pituitary irradiation or bilateral adrenalectomy is usually reserved for patients who are not surgical candidates or for those who relapse or do not achieve complete remission following pituitary surgery. Because the response to pituitary irradiation can be delayed (several months to years), concomitant treatment with cortisol-lowering medication may be necessary. Bilateral adrenalectomy is also used for management of adrenal carcinoma and in patients with poorly controlled ectopic Cushing disease in whom the ACTH-producing lesion cannot be localized. Bilateral laparoscopic adrenalectomy achieves an immediate and total remission (nearly 100% cure rate), but these patients will require lifelong glucocorticoid and mineralocorticoid supplementation.[7,25] Nelson syndrome may develop in nearly 20% to 50% of patients who undergo bilateral adrenalectomy without pituitary irradiation. This condition presumably results from persistent hypersecretion of ACTH by the intact pituitary adenoma, which continues to grow because of the loss of feedback inhibition by cortisol. Treatment of Nelson syndrome may involve pituitary irradiation or surgery.[6]

The treatment of choice in patients with adrenal adenomas is unilateral laparoscopic adrenalectomy. These patients require glucocorticoid supplementation during and after surgery due to atrophy of the contralateral adrenal gland and suppression of the HPA axis. Glucocorticoid therapy is continued until recovery of the remaining adrenal gland is achieved. Patients with adrenal carcinomas have a poor prognosis, with a 5-year survival of 20% to 58%, because of the advanced nature of the condition (metastatic disease). Surgical resection to reduce tumor burden and size, pharmacologic therapy, or bilateral laparoscopic adrenalectomy are the treatment options commonly utilized to manage this condition.[2,7]

▸ Pharmacologic Therapy

KEY CONCEPT *Pharmacotherapy is indicated when the ectopic ACTH-secreting tumor cannot be localized; to control hypercortisolism to prepare for surgery; and in patients who: (1) are not surgical candidates; (2) have failed surgery or had a relapse after surgery; or (3) have Cushing disease awaiting the onset of effect of pituitary radiation.*[26] The drugs used are classified according to their mechanism and site of action (Table 45–6[25–31]). The most widely used therapeutic class is the adrenal steroidogenesis inhibitors, which can improve hypercortisolism by inhibiting enzymes involved in the biosynthesis of cortisol.[26] Because of their potential to cause adrenal suppression, temporary glucocorticoid replacement, and in some cases mineralocorticoid supplementation, may be needed during and after treatment.

KEY CONCEPT *In drug-induced Cushing syndrome, discontinuation of the offending agent is the best management option. However, abrupt withdrawal of the glucocorticoid can result in adrenal insufficiency or exacerbation of the underlying disease.*[18] KEY CONCEPT *Glucocorticoid doses less than 7.5 mg/day of prednisone or its equivalent for less than 3 weeks generally would not be expected to lead to suppression of the HPA axis.*[3,7] However, in patients receiving pharmacologic doses of glucocorticoids for prolonged periods, gradual tapering to near physiologic levels (5–7.5 mg/day of prednisone or its equivalent) should precede drug discontinuation. Administration of a short-acting glucocorticoid in the morning and use of alternate-day dosing may reduce the risk of adrenal suppression. Testing of the HPA axis may be useful in assessing adrenal reserve. In some cases, supplemental glucocorticoid administration during excessive physiologic stress may be needed for up to 1 year after glucocorticoid discontinuation.[18] Table 45–7 lists strategies to prevent the development of hypercortisolism and hypocortisolism.

Outcome Evaluation

- Monitor patients receiving surgical, medical, or radiation therapy for resolution of the clinical manifestations of hypercortisolism. Symptoms often improve immediately after surgery and soon after initiation of drug therapy. However, it may take months for symptoms to resolve following radiation therapy.
- Monitor for normalization of serum cortisol concentrations.
- Patient Care Process discusses additional evaluation strategies.

Patient Encounter 2

A 61-year-old man presents to a clinical pharmacist for diabetes education. He was recently diagnosed with type 2 diabetes. He also has a diagnosis of hypertension, atrial fibrillation, dyslipidemia, chronic obstructive pulmonary disease (COPD), and depression. He complains of thirst, polyuria, and fatigue. Physical exam reveals an obese (BMI 37 kg/m^2) gentleman with truncal obesity, dorsocervical fat, several small bruises on abdomen and extremities, and facial plethora. His current medications include metformin, lisinopril, hydrochlorothiazide, warfarin, atorvastatin, fluticasone/salmeterol, tiotropium, albuterol, and fluoxetine. He has been treated several times this year with high-dose prednisone therapy for frequent COPD exacerbations. The clinical pharmacist suggests evaluation for possible Cushing syndrome.

Which findings are suggestive of Cushing syndrome?

Aside from Cushing syndrome, what are some major differential diagnoses for clinical presentation?

The patient is diagnosed with drug-induced Cushing syndrome after evaluation and diagnostic testing by the endocrinologist. What patient education points should be provided?

Table 45–6

Pharmacologic Treatments for Cushing Syndrome[25–31]

Drug	Mechanism of Action	Dosage[a]: Initial, Usual, Maximum, Dosing Adjustment for Renal and/or Hepatic Failure	Common and/or Major Adverse Reactions	Comment
Inhibitors of Adrenal Steroidogenesis				
Ketoconazole[b] (oral administration)	Inhibits several CYP450 enzymes including 17,20-lyase, 17-hydroxylase, and 11β-hydroxylase. Also inhibits cholesterol synthesis	*Adults*: 200 mg twice daily; 400–800 mg/day in two divided doses; NTE 1,200 mg/day in two to three divided doses Extensively metabolized by liver and dosing adjustment should be considered in severe liver disease. Dosing adjustment not needed in renal disease	Generally well tolerated. Symptoms of adrenal insufficiency (eg, nausea, vomiting, decreased appetite, fatigue) Gynecomastia, decreased libido, and impotence (due to inhibition of testosterone synthesis) Hepatotoxicity	• Effective in a majority of causes; rapid clinical improvement seen • Monitor efficacy with urinary cortisol • Monitor liver transaminases for hepatotoxicity • Useful in women with hirsutism and patients with hyperlipidemia • Requires gastric acidicity for dissolution and absorption therefore not useful in patients with achlorhydria and those taking proton pump inhibitors or round-the-clock antacids or histamine-2 receptor blockers • Is a CYP3A4 substrate and a strong CYP3A4 inhibitor. Also has other CYP450 interaction potential. Coadministration with certain medications can lead to QT prolongation and dysrhythmia
Metyrapone[b] (oral administration)	Inhibits 11β-hydroxylase. Also suppresses aldosterone synthesis	*Adults*: 750 mg/day; 500–4000 mg/day in four divided doses; NTE 6 g/day Dosages in special populations (liver and kidney disease, elderly patients) have not been established	Generally well-tolerated Hirsutism, acne, adrenal insufficiency, GI intolerance, rash, hypokalemia, edema, hypertension	• Used in Cushing disease, ectopic ACTH syndrome, and adrenal carcinoma • Also used as a test to diagnose adrenal insufficiency
Etomidate[b] (intravenous infusion administration)	Inhibits 17,20-lyase, 17-hydroxylase, and 11β-hydroxylase	*Adults*: Limited clinical experience, 0.2–0.4 mg/kg/hour Extensively metabolized in the liver to inactive metabolites. Because of changes in protein binding, dosing adjustment may be needed in kidney and liver disease	Injection site pain, nausea, vomiting, myoclonus, hypotension	• Is a general anesthetic • Generally reserved for patients with more severe symptoms and in emergency settings
Adrenolytic Agent				
Mitotane (oral administration)	Inhibits steroidogenesis at lower doses and is adrenolytic at higher doses. Inhibits 11β-hydroxylase and cholesterol side-chain cleavage. Reduces aldosterone synthesis	*Adults*: for adrenal carcinoma: 2 to 6 g/day in three to four divided doses; 9–10 g/day in three to four divided doses; NTE 18–19 g/day in three to four divided doses; for other types of Cushing syndrome: 0.5 g at bedtime; 1–2 g/day; NTE 2–3 g/day, (usual/max)—give ½ the dose at bedtime to minimize nausea. Elderly patients may require a dose decrease Primarily metabolized by the liver and dosing adjustment may be needed in liver disease	GI intolerance (high incidence), fatigue, dizziness, somnolence, gynecomastia Hyperlipidemia requiring lipid-lowering treatment Adrenal insufficiency requiring glucocorticoid replacement therapy	• FDA-approved for treatment of inoperable adrenal cortical carcinoma. Can be used in other types of Cushing syndrome • Efficacy takes several weeks • Lower rate of relapse when used with pituitary radiation. Also enables lower doses and therefore lower rate of adverse reactions • Hypocortisolism (if occurs) may persist several weeks/months after discontinuation as drug is stored in fatty tissues • Strong inducer of CYP3A4

Peripheral Glucocorticoid Antagonist				
Mifepristone (RU 486) (oral administration)	Antagonizes glucocorticoid receptors	*Adults*: 300 mg once daily; NTE 1200 mg once daily (but only up to 20 mg/kg/day) Maximum 300 mg/day with concomitant strong CYP450 inhibitors Do not exceed 600 mg/day in renal impairment or mild-to-moderate hepatic impairment. Do not use in severe hepatic impairment	Nausea, fatigue, headache, hypokalemia, arthralgia, vomiting, peripheral edema, hypertension, dizziness, decreased appetite, endometrial hypertrophy, prolonged QT interval. Has abortifacient and embryotoxic properties	• FDA-approved for control of hyperglycemia secondary to hypercortisolism in adult patients with endogenous Cushing syndrome who have type 2 diabetes mellitus or glucose intolerance and have failed surgery or are not candidates for surgery • Increases cortisol and ACTH levels via antagonism of negative feedback of ACTH secretion • Requires cautious use since limited clinical experiences and cannot use cortisol or ACTH levels to monitor efficacy of treatment • Quicker effectiveness compared to other drug treatment options • Is a CYP3A4 substrate. Also inhibits CYP3A and has other CYP450 interaction potential
Somatostatin Analog				
Pasireotide (subcutaneous injection)	Binds to somatostatin receptor subtype 5 overexpressed in corticotroph tumor cells resulting in inhibition of ACTH secretion	*Adults*: 0.6 mg or 0.9 mg twice daily; 0.3–0.9 mg twice daily; NTE 0.9 mg twice daily. Consider lower initial dose in the elderly Moderate hepatic impairment (Child Pugh B): initial 0.3 mg twice a day, maximum 0.6 mg twice a day. Avoid in severe hepatic impairment (Child Pugh C). No dosage adjustment needed in renal impairment	Hyperglycemia, GI pain, nausea, diarrhea, headache, fatigue, bradycardia, QT prolongation, liver test elevations, cholelithiasis, pituitary hormone (other than ACTH) inhibition	• FDA-approved for treatment of adult patients with Cushing disease for whom pituitary surgery is not an option or has not been curative • Measure response based on 24-hour urinary free cortisol level and/or improvement in signs and symptoms

[a]Dosing guidelines (including age ranges) and safety for children have not been definitively established.

[b]These medications do not have FDA-approved indications for the treatment of Cushing syndrome in either adults or children.

ACTH, adrenocorticotropic hormone or corticotropin; CYP, cytochrome P-450; FDA, Food and Drug Administration; GI, gastrointestinal; NTE, not to exceed.

Table 45–7

Principles of Glucocorticoid Administration to Avoid Hypercortisolism or Hypocortisolism

To Prevent Hypercortisolism and Development of Cushing Syndrome

- Give the lowest glucocorticoid dose that will manage the disease being treated and for the shortest possible duration
- If feasible, give glucocorticoid via administration routes that minimize systemic absorption (such as inhalation or dermal)
- If feasible, administer glucocorticoid treatment every other day (calculate the total 48-hour dose and give as a single dose of intermediate-acting glucocorticoid in the morning)[6]
- Avoid concurrent administration of drugs that can inhibit glucocorticoid metabolism

To Prevent Hypocortisolism and Development of Adrenal Insufficiency or Adrenal Crisis

- If the patient requires discontinuation from chronic treatment with supraphysiologic doses of glucocorticoid, the following discontinuation protocol can be used:[6]
  - Gradually taper the dose to approximately 20 mg of prednisone or equivalent per day, given in the morning, and then
  - Change glucocorticoid to every other day administration, in the morning
  - Stop the glucocorticoid when the equivalent physiologic dose is reached (20 mg/day of hydrocortisone or 5–7.5 mg/day of prednisone or equivalent)
  - Understand that recovery of the HPA axis may take up to a year after glucocorticoid discontinuation during which the patient may require supplementation therapy during periods of physiologic stress
- Evaluate patients at risk for adrenal insufficiency as a result of treatment(s) of Cushing syndrome and initiate glucocorticoid and mineralocorticoid replacement therapy as appropriate
- Avoid concurrent administration of drugs that can induce glucocorticoid metabolism
- Educate patients about:
  - The need for replacement or supplemental glucocorticoid and mineralocorticoid therapy
  - How to administer parenteral glucocorticoid if unable to immediately access medical care during an emergency
  - Need to wear or carry medical identification regarding condition (eg, card, bracelet)

HPA, hypothalamic-pituitary-adrenal

Patient Care Process: Cushing Syndrome

Patient Assessment:

- Perform a comprehensive examination, including a thorough medical history and history of all medications and herbal or dietary supplements.
- Determine if Cushing syndrome is drug induced.
- Establish diagnosis and etiology based on diagnostic testing.

Therapy Evaluation:

- Evaluate patient for appropriateness of surgery, radiation, and/or pharmacologic therapy depending on etiology.

Care Plan Development:

- Attempt to taper glucocorticoid if etiology is exogenous administration.
- If endogenous Cushing syndrome, determine if patient is an appropriate candidate for surgical resection of the tumor or has contraindications to surgical resection such as advanced disease (metastatic adrenal carcinoma).
- Assess response and complications associated with surgery including:[25]
  - Measuring plasma cortisol postsurgery to determine if the patient displays persistent hypercortisolism (surgical treatment failure) or hypocortisolism (adrenal insufficiency requiring steroid replacement therapy).
  - In patients demonstrating hypocortisolism:
    i. Monitor for signs and symptoms of glucocorticoid withdrawal (headache, fatigue, malaise, myalgia).
    ii. Monitor for signs and symptoms of adrenal insufficiency and develop a treatment plan.
    iii. Monitor morning cortisol or response to ACTH stimulation every 3 to 6 months to assess for HPA axis recovery. Discontinue glucocorticoid replacement therapy when cortisol concentrations are greater than 19 mcg/dL (524 nmol/L) on either test.
    iv. Monitor cortisol, ACTH, low-dose dexamethasone suppression, or other tests to assess for risk of relapse of hypercortisolism.
- If surgical resection does not achieve satisfactory disease control or is not indicated, evaluate the patient for pituitary radiation or bilateral adrenalectomy with concomitant pituitary radiation.
- Monitor patients treated with surgery or pituitary radiation for development of pituitary hormone deficiency.
- Evaluate patients with adrenal adenomas for unilateral adrenalectomy.
  - Give glucocorticoid and mineralocorticoid replacement (permanently in the case of bilateral adrenalectomy).
- Provide patient education regarding:
  - Causes of Cushing syndrome, including drug-induced etiologies
  - How to recognize the clinical manifestations
  - Possible sequelae of Cushing syndrome

Patient Care Process: Cushing Syndrome (*Continued*)

- How to reduce the modifiable cardiovascular and metabolic complications
- Advantages and disadvantages of potential treatment options including possible adverse consequences
- Need for glucocorticoid and mineralocorticoid replacement after treatment, if appropriate
- Importance of adherence to therapy

Follow-Up Evaluation:

- Monitor for response to therapy, need for dose adjustments, and presence of adverse drug reactions.
- Once disease control is achieved, continue to monitor biochemical markers and patient for development of complications of Cushing syndrome, as relapse may occur.

Abbreviation Introduced in This Chapter

ACTH	Adrenocorticotropic hormone or corticotropin
AIDS	Acquired immunodeficiency syndrome
BUN	Blood urea nitrogen
CRH	Corticotropin-releasing hormone
COPD	Chronic obstructive pulmonary disease
CT	Computed tomography
CYP450	Cytochrome P-450
DHEA	Dehydroepiandrosterone
DHEA-S	Sulfated form of dehydroepiandrosterone
DST	Dexamethasone suppression test
FDA	Food and Drug Administration
GI	Gastrointestinal
HIV	Human immunodeficiency virus
HPA	Hypothalamic-pituitary-adrenal
HPLC	High performance liquid chromatography
IM	Intramuscular
IV	Intravenous or intravenously
MRI	Magnetic resonance imaging

REFERENCES

1. Arlt W. Disorders of the adrenal cortex. In: Longo D, Fauci A, Kasper DL, Hauser S, Jameson JL, Loscalzo J, eds. Harrison's Principles of Internal Medicine. New York: McGraw-Hill, 2011.
2. Carroll TB, Aron DC, Findling JW, Tyrrell JB. Glucocorticoids and adrenal androgens. In: Gardner DG, Shoback D, eds. Basic and Clinical Endocrinology, 9th ed. New York: McGraw-Hill, 2011. Available at http://www.accessmedicine.com/content.aspx?aID=8403322. Accessed October 2, 2014.
3. Cooper MS, Stewart PM. Corticosteroid insufficiency in acutely ill patients. N Engl J Med. 2003;348:727–734.
4. Charmandari E, Nicolaides NC, Chrousos GP. Adrenal insufficiency. Lancet. 2014;383:2152–2167.
5. Salvatori R. Adrenal insufficiency. JAMA. 2005;294:2481–2488.
6. Williams GH, Dluhy RG. Disorders of the adrenal cortex. In: Kasper DL, Braunwald E, Fauci A, Hauser S, Longo D, Jameson JL, eds. Harrison's Principles of Internal Medicine. New York City: McGraw-Hill, 2005.
7. Young WF, Jr., Thompson GB. Laparoscopic adrenalectomy for patients who have Cushing's syndrome. Endocrinol Metab Clin North Am. 2005;34:489–499, xi.
8. Arlt W, Allolio B. Adrenal insufficiency. Lancet. 2003;361:1881–1893.
9. Marik PE, Pastores SM, Annane D, et al. Recommendations for the diagnosis and management of corticosteroid insufficiency in critically ill adult patients: consensus statements from an international task force by the American College of Critical Care Medicine. Crit Care Med. 2008;36:1937–1949.
10. Javorsky BR, Aron DC, Findling JW, Tyrrell JB. Hypothalamus and pituitary gland. In: Gardner DG, Shoback D, eds. Basic and Clinical Endocrinology. New York: Lange Medical Books/McGraw-Hill, 2011. Available at http://www.accessmedicine.com/content.aspx?aID=8403322. Accessed October 2, 2014.
11. Shimmer BP, Funder JW. ACTH, adrenal steroids, and pharmacology of the adrenal cortex. In: Brunton LL, Chabner BA, Knollmann BC, eds. Pharmacological Basis of Therapeutics, 12th ed. New York: McGraw-Hill, 2011. Available at http://accessmedicine.mhmedical.com.online.uchc.edu/ViewLarge.aspx?figid=41278558. Accessed November 1, 2014.
12. Gurnell EM, Hunt PJ, Curran SE, et al. Long-term DHEA replacement in primary adrenal insufficiency: a randomized, controlled trial. J Clin Endocrinol Metab. 2008;93:400–409.
13. Hunt PJ, Gurnell EM, Huppert FA, et al. Improvement in mood and fatigue after dehydroepiandrosterone replacement in Addison's disease in a randomized, double blind trial. J Clin Endocrinol Metab. 2000;85:4650–4656.
14. Johannsson G, Burman P, Wiren L, et al. Low dose dehydroepiandrosterone affects behavior in hypopituitary androgen-deficient women: a placebo-controlled trial. J Clin Endocrinol Metab. 2002;87:2046–2052.
15. Alkatib AA, Cosma M, Elamin MB, et al. A systematic review and meta-analysis of randomized placebo-controlled trials of DHEA treatment effects on quality of life in women with adrenal insufficiency. J Clin Endocrinol Metab. 2009;94:3676–3681.
16. Husebye ES, Allolio B, Arlt W, et al. Consensus statement on the diagnosis, treatment and follow-up of patients with primary adrenal insufficiency. J Intern Med. 2014;275:104–115.
17. Findling JW, Raff H. Screening and diagnosis of Cushing's syndrome. Endocrinol Metab Clin North Am. 2005;34:385–402, ix–x.
18. Hopkins RL, Leinung MC. Exogenous Cushing's syndrome and glucocorticoid withdrawal. Endocrinol Metab Clin North Am. 2005;34:371–384, ix.
19. Lacroix A, Bourdeau I. Bilateral adrenal Cushing's syndrome: macronodular adrenal hyperplasia and primary pigmented nodular adrenocortical disease. Endocrinol Metab Clin North Am. 2005;34:441–458, x.
20. Raff H, Findling JW. A physiologic approach to diagnosis of the Cushing syndrome. Ann Intern Med. 2003;138:980–991.
21. Goldman JA, Myerson G. Chinese herbal medicine: camouflaged prescription antiinflammatory drugs, corticosteroids, and lead. Arthritis Rheum. 1991;34:1207.
22. Keane FM, Munn SE, du Vivier AW, Taylor NF, Higgins EM. Analysis of Chinese herbal creams prescribed for dermatological conditions. BMJ. 1999;318:563–564.

23. Arnaldi G, Angeli A, Atkinson AB, et al. Diagnosis and complications of Cushing's syndrome: a consensus statement. J Clin Endocrinol Metab. 2003;88:5593–5602.
24. Nieman LK, Biller BM, Findling JW, et al. The diagnosis of Cushing's syndrome: an Endocrine Society Clinical Practice Guideline. J Clin Endocrinol Metab. 2008;93:1526–1540.
25. Utz AL, Swearingen B, Biller BM. Pituitary surgery and postoperative management in Cushing's disease. Endocrinol Metab Clin North Am. 2005;34:459–478, xi.
26. Nieman LK. Medical therapy of hypercortisolism (Cushing's syndrome). In: UpToDate, Lacroix A (Ed), UpToDate, Waltham, MA. (Accessed on August 20, 2014).
27. Package insert. Korlym (mifepristone). Menlo Park, CA: Corcept Therapeutics Incorporated; 2013 June.
28. Package insert. Lysodren (mitotane). Princeton, NJ: Bristol-Myers Squibb; 2013 November.
29. Package insert. Signifor (pasireotide). Stein, Switzerland: Novartis Pharma Stein AG; 2012 December.
30. Chu JW, Matthias DF, Belanoff J, Schatzberg A, Hoffman AR, Feldman D. Successful long-term treatment of refractory Cushing's disease with high-dose mifepristone (RU 486). J Clin Endocrinol Metab. 2001;86:3568–3573.
31. Sonino N, Boscaro M. Medical therapy for Cushing's disease. Endocrinol Metab Clin. 1999;28:211–22.

46 Pituitary Gland Disorders

Judy T. Chen, Devra K. Dang, Frank Pucino, Jr, and Karim Anton Calis

LEARNING OBJECTIVES

Upon completion of the chapter, the reader will be able to:

1. List the mediators and primary effects of pituitary hormones.
2. Identify clinical features of patients with acromegaly.
3. Discuss the role of surgery and radiation therapy for patients with acromegaly.
4. Select appropriate pharmacotherapy for patients with acromegaly based on patient-specific factors.
5. Identify clinical features of children and adults with growth hormone (GH) deficiency and select appropriate pharmacotherapy for these patients.
6. Recommend monitoring parameters necessary to assess therapeutic outcomes and adverse effects in patients receiving GH therapy.
7. List common etiologies of hyperprolactinemia.
8. Identify clinical features of patients with hyperprolactinemia.
9. Select appropriate pharmacologic and nonpharmacologic treatments for patients with hyperprolactinemia based on patient-specific factors.

PHYSIOLOGY OF THE PITUITARY GLAND

The pituitary, referred to as the "master gland," is a small endocrine gland located at the base of the brain and is responsible for the regulation of many other endocrine glands and body systems. Growth, development, metabolism, reproduction, and stress homeostasis are among the functions influenced by the pituitary. Functionally, the gland consists of two distinct sections: the anterior pituitary lobe and the posterior pituitary lobe. The pituitary receives neural and hormonal input from the inferior hypothalamus via blood vessels and neurons.

The posterior pituitary is innervated by nervous stimulation from the hypothalamus, resulting in the release of specific hormones to exert direct tissue effects. The hypothalamus synthesizes two hormones, oxytocin and vasopressin. These hormones are stored and released from the posterior pituitary lobe. The anterior pituitary lobe is under the control of several releasing and inhibiting hormones secreted from the hypothalamus via a portal vein system. It synthesizes and secretes six major hormones. **Figure 46–1** summarizes the physiologic mediators and effects of each of these hormones.

Hormonal Feedback Regulatory Systems

The hypothalamus is responsible for the synthesis and release of hormones that regulate the pituitary gland. Stimulation or inhibition of the pituitary hormones elicits a specific cascade of responses in peripheral target glands. In response, these glands secrete hormones that exert a **negative feedback** on other hormones in the hypothalamic–pituitary axis (see Figure 46–1). This negative feedback serves to maintain body system homeostasis. In general, high circulating hormone concentrations inhibit the release of hypothalamic and anterior pituitary hormones.

Damage and destruction of the pituitary gland may result in secondary hypothyroidism, **hypogonadism**, adrenal insufficiency, growth hormone (GH) deficiency, hypoprolactinemia, or **panhypopituitarism**. A tumor (adenoma) located in the pituitary gland may result in excess secretion of a hormone or may physically compress the gland and suppress adequate hormone release. The type, location, and size of a pituitary tumor often determine a patient's clinical presentation. This chapter discusses the pathophysiology and role of pharmacotherapy in the treatment of **acromegaly**, GH deficiency, and **hyperprolactinemia**. The following hormones are discussed elsewhere in this textbook: adrenocorticotropic hormone (ACTH), thyroid-stimulating hormone (TSH), luteinizing hormone (LH), follicle-stimulating hormone (FSH), antidiuretic hormone (or vasopressin; ADH), and oxytocin.

GROWTH HORMONE (SOMATOTROPIN)

Somatotropin or GH, the most abundant hormone produced by the anterior pituitary lobe, is regulated primarily by the hypothalamic–pituitary axis. The hypothalamus releases growth hormone–releasing hormone (GHRH) to stimulate GH synthesis and secretion, whereas somatostatin inhibits it.[1] Release of GH into the circulation stimulates the liver and other peripheral target tissues to produce insulin-like growth factors (IGFs). These IGFs are the peripheral GH targets. There are two types of IGFs, **IGF-I** and IGF-II. IGF-I is responsible for growth of bone and other tissues, whereas IGF-II is primarily responsible for regulating fetal growth. High concentrations of IGF-I inhibit

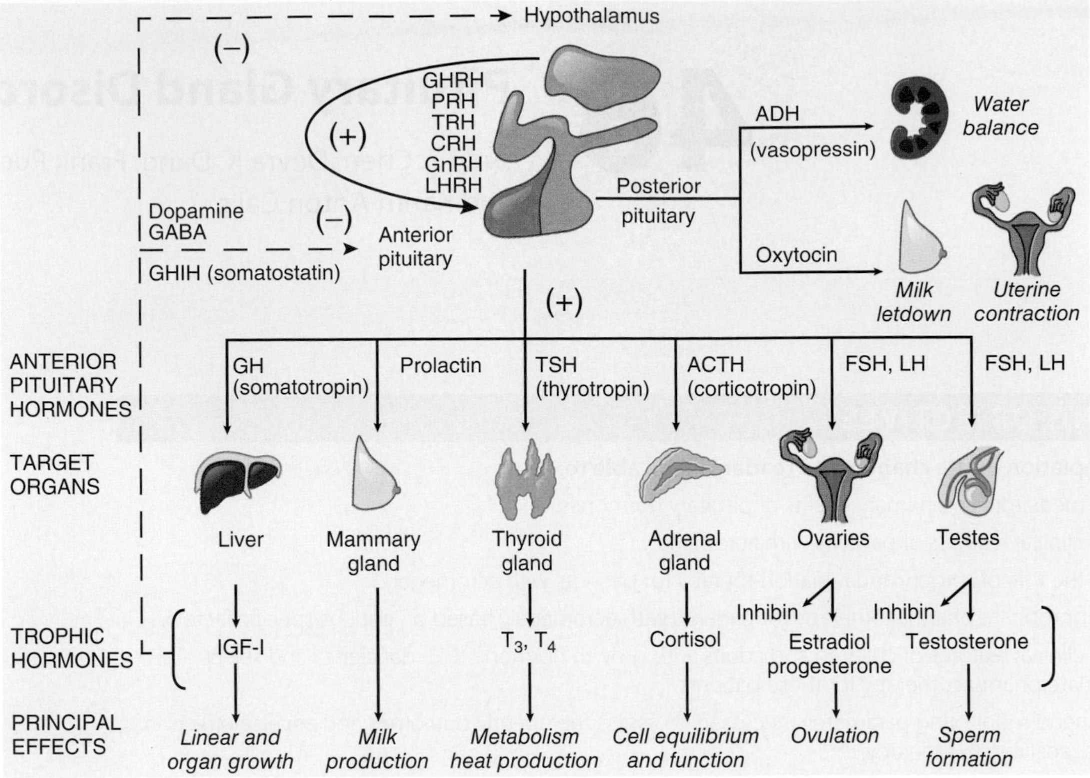

FIGURE 46–1. Hypothalamic–pituitary–target-organ axis. The hypothalamic hormones regulate the biosynthesis and release of eight pituitary hormones. Stimulation of each of these pituitary hormones produces and releases trophic hormones from their associated target organs to exert their principal effects. These trophic hormones regulate the activity of endocrine glands. Subsequently, increased serum concentration of the trophic hormones released from the target organs can inhibit both the hypothalamus and the anterior pituitary gland to maintain homeostasis (negative feedback). Inhibin is produced by the testes in men and the ovaries in women during pregnancy. Inhibin directly inhibits pituitary production of follicle-stimulating hormone (FSH) through a negative feedback mechanism. Melanocyte-stimulating hormone (MSH) produced by the anterior pituitary is not illustrated in the figure. (–), inhibit; (+), stimulate; ACTH, adrenocorticotropic hormone (corticotropin); ADH, antidiuretic hormone (vasopressin); CRH, corticotropin-releasing hormone; FSH, follicle-stimulating hormone; GABA, γ-aminobutyric acid; GH, growth hormone (somatotropin); GHIH, growth hormone–inhibiting hormone (somatostatin); GHRH, growth hormone–releasing hormone; GnRH, gonadotropin-releasing hormone; IGF-I, insulin-like growth factor-I; LH, luteinizing hormone; LHRH, luteinizing hormone–releasing hormone; PRH, prolactin-releasing hormone; T_3, triiodothyronine; T_4, thyroxine; TRH, thyrotropin-releasing hormone; TSH, thyroid-stimulating hormone (thyrotropin).

GH secretion through somatostatin, thereby inhibiting GHRH secretion at the hypothalamus.[1] The hypothalamus also may stimulate the release of somatostatin to inhibit GH secretion. The effects of IGF-I in peripheral tissues are both GH dependent and GH independent.[2] GH is an anabolic hormone with direct "anti-insulin" metabolic effects. By stimulating protein synthesis and shifting the body's energy source from carbohydrates to fats, GH promotes a diabetic state (Table 46–1).[2] GH controls somatic growth and has a critical role in the development of normal skeletal muscle, myocardial muscle, and bone.

In healthy individuals, GH is secreted in a pulsatile manner with several short bursts occurring mostly during the night. The amount of GH secretion fluctuates throughout a person's lifetime. Secretion of GH is lowest during infancy, increases during childhood, peaks during adolescence, and then declines gradually during the middle years.[1] These changes are parallel to an age-related decline in lean muscle mass and bone mineral density.

Growth Hormone Excess

► *Epidemiology and Etiology*

Acromegaly affects both genders equally, and the average age of presentation is 44 years. Approximately 40 to 125 people per 1 million are affected, with an estimated annual incidence of three to four cases per 1 million people.[3] In more than 95% of cases, overproduction of GH is caused by a benign pituitary adenoma, whereas malignant adenomas are rare. Most pituitary adenomas occur spontaneously as a result of a sporadic genetic mutation acquired during life. Depending on tumor size, pituitary adenomas

Table 46–1

Effects of Growth Hormone[2]

	Effect(s)
Lipid metabolism	Increases breakdown of fat (lipolysis) Increases circulating fatty acid concentrations Increases lean body mass
Protein metabolism	Increases muscle mass
Carbohydrate metabolism	Decreases glucose utilization Increases insulin resistance Hyperglycemia Increases hepatic glucose output

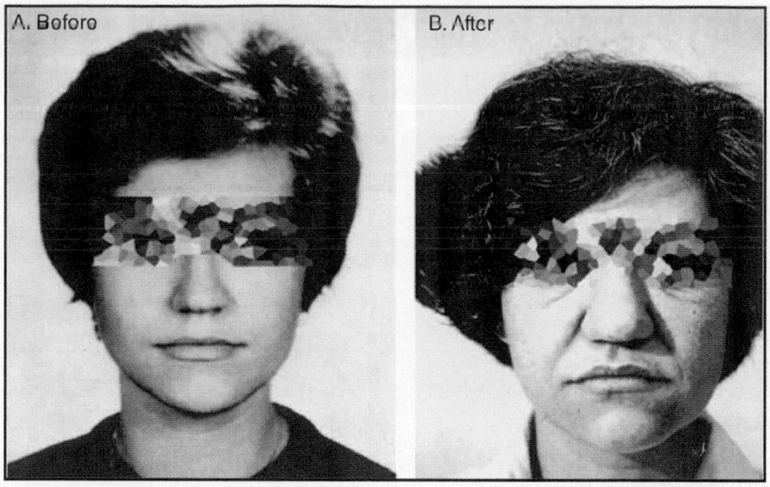

FIGURE 46–2. Before and after photographs of a patient with acromegaly. Compare the photographs (**A**) before the onset of acromegaly and (**B**) after approximately 20 years when the diagnosis was well established. Notice the coarsening of facial features, with an enlarged nose, lips, and forehead.

are classified as: (a) microadenomas if they are 10 mm or less in diameter; or (b) macroadenomas if they are greater than 10 mm. Although these tumors can produce GH, they more commonly secrete GHRH, resulting in excessive GH and IGF-I production.

▸ *Pathophysiology*

Acromegaly is a rare disorder that manifests gradually over time and typically occurs after fusion of the epiphyses (growth plates) of the long bones.[3] The facial and hand features of an acromegalic patient are depicted in Figures 46–2 and 46–3. **Gigantism** refers to GH excess that occurs during childhood before epiphyseal closure and results in excessive linear growth. Because the signs and symptoms of acromegaly are insidious, diagnosis of this disorder is often delayed for up to 10 years after the initial presentation of symptoms.[3] Therefore, it is important for practitioners to be vigilant in identifying this disease in the early stages.

Diagnosis of acromegaly is based on both clinical and biochemical findings. Because GH fluctuates throughout the day, a single random measurement is never a reliable diagnostic tool to evaluate GH excess.[1] GH is suppressed after administration of a 75-g oral glucose challenge because postprandial hyperglycemia inhibits secretion of GH. Therefore, measurement of serum GH secretion in response to an oral glucose tolerance test (OGTT) is the primary biochemical test for diagnosing acromegaly. If the nadir GH concentration is greater than 0.4 ng/mL (0.4 mcg/L; 18 pmol/L) during the test or the random GH concentration is greater than 1 ng/mL (1 mcg/L; 45 pmol/L), the patient is diagnosed with acromegaly.[4] In addition to clinical presentation, an elevated IGF-I serum concentration helps to confirm the diagnosis. IGF-I concentrations are often represented as age- and sex matched population values.[4] They are relatively stable and correlate positively with mean GH concentrations,[1] thus making elevations in IGF-I concentrations an ideal and reliable biochemical marker to monitor disease activity and response to therapy.[3,4]

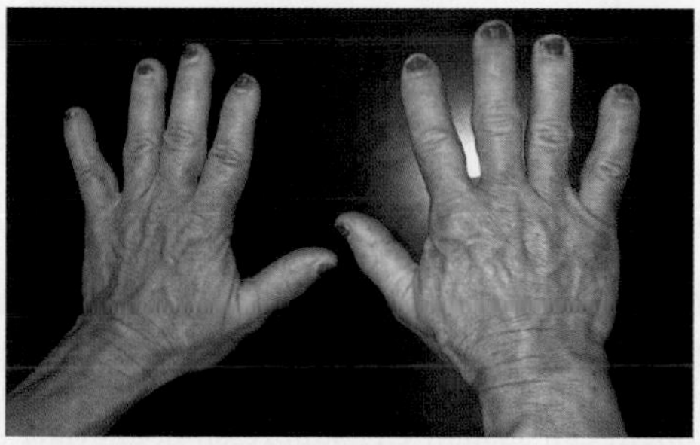

FIGURE 46–3. Photograph of hands from a patient with acromegaly. Soft tissue swelling and enlargement of the hand in a woman with acromegaly resulting in increased ring and glove size.

▸ *Acromegaly Treatment*

Desired Outcomes Patients with untreated acromegaly experience a two- to three-fold increase in mortality rate primarily because of cardiovascular and pulmonary diseases.[6] KEY CONCEPT *Prolonged exposure to elevated GH and IGF-I can lead to serious complications in patients with acromegaly. Aggressively manage comorbid conditions such as hypertension, diabetes, dysrhythmias, coronary artery disease, and heart failure to prevent cardiovascular, pulmonary, metabolic, respiratory, and neuropathic complications.*[4] Normalization of GH and IGF-I concentrations lowers the mortality risk and may improve overall life expectancy. The goals of therapy are as follows[3,7]:

- Reduce fasting morning GH and IGF-I concentrations as close to normal as possible
- Reduce tumor size to relieve tumor mass effect
- Prevent tumor recurrence
- Preserve normal pituitary function
- Improve clinical signs and symptoms
- Alleviate significant morbidities
- Reduce mortality rates to those of the general population

Surgical Treatment According to the American Association of Clinical Endocrinologists (AACE) treatment guidelines for acromegaly, KEY CONCEPT *surgical resection of the pituitary tumor through* transsphenoidal pituitary microsurgery *is the treatment of choice for most patients with GH-producing pituitary adenomas.*[3] When performed by experienced surgeons, approximately 80% of patients with microadenomas and fewer than 50% of patients with macroadenomas achieve biochemical control.[3] Complete

Clinical Presentation and Diagnosis of Acromegaly[3–5]

General

The patient will experience slow development of soft tissue overgrowth affecting many body systems. Signs and symptoms may progress gradually over 7 to 10 years.

Symptoms

- Headache and compromised visual function (loss of peripheral vision and blurred vision) caused by the actual tumor mass and its close proximity to the optic structures
- Weakness, low blood sugar, or weight loss caused by disruption of adrenal function (ie, ACTH deficiency) by effect of tumor mass on the pituitary
- Fatigue and weight gain caused by disruption of thyroid function (ie, TSH deficiency) by effect of tumor mass on the pituitary
- Absence of regular menstrual periods (amenorrhea), impotence, and decreased libido caused by disruption of the gonadotropin secretion (ie, LH and FSH)
- Excessive sweating, joint pain, nerve pain, and abnormal neurologic sensations (paresthesias) related to elevated GH and IGF-I concentrations

Signs

- Coarsening of facial features
- Increased hand volume
- Increased ring and shoe size
- Increased spacing between teeth
- Increased acne or oily skin
- Enlarged tongue
- Deepening of voice
- Thick, irregular, and patchy skin discoloration
- Enlarged nose, lips, and forehead (frontal bossing)
- Abnormal protrusion of the mandible (prognathia) and bite abnormalities
- Inappropriate secretion of breast milk (galactorrhea)
- Abnormal enlargement of various organs (organomegaly) such as liver, spleen, and heart
- Carpal tunnel syndrome caused by nerve compression from the swollen tissue

Laboratory Tests

- Random GH concentration greater than 1 ng/mL (1 mcg/L; 45 pmol/L) or nadir GH concentration greater than 0.4 ng/mL (0.4 mcg/L; 18 pmol/L) after an OGTT and elevated IGF-I concentration compared with age-matched control values.
- Loss of other hormonal functions caused by tumor mass compression of the anterior pituitary.
- Measure prolactin concentration in all patients because prolactin cosecretion is common.
- Glucose intolerance may be present in up to 50% of patients.

Additional Clinical Sequelae

- Cardiovascular diseases: hypertension, coronary heart disease, cardiomyopathy, left ventricular hypertrophy, and arrhythmia.
- Osteoarthritis and joint damage develop in up to 75% of patients.
- Respiratory disorders and sleep apnea occur in up to 70% of patients.
- Type 2 diabetes mellitus develops in 56% of patients.
- Increased risk for the development of esophageal, colon, and stomach cancer.

Other Diagnostic Tests

- Perform magnetic resonance imaging (MRI) examination of the pituitary to locate the tumor and validate the diagnosis.
- Obtain serum prolactin concentrations to assess for hyperprolactinemia and hypopituitarism.
- Without obvious pituitary tumor but proven acromegaly, measurement of GHRH may be helpful to detect ectopic tumors.

Adapted from Jordan JK, Sheehan AH, Yanovski JA, Calis KA. Pituitary gland disorders. In: Dipiro JT, Talbert RL, Yee GC, et al, eds. Pharmacotherapy. A Pathophysiologic Approach. 9th ed. New York: McGraw-Hill; 2014:1237–1252.

resection of a macroadenoma may be difficult if the tumor has already invaded the surrounding nerves and tissues. In such cases, debulking of the tumor along with adjunctive radiation and/or pharmacotherapy may improve treatment outcome. Infrequent surgical complications include meningitis, serious visual impairment, cerebrospinal fluid leakage, diabetes insipidus, and permanent hypopituitarism.[3] Relative contraindications to surgery include patient frailty, acromegaly-associated comorbidities, and medically unstable conditions such as airway difficulties, severe hypertension, or uncontrolled diabetes.

Pharmacologic Therapy Pharmacologic therapy is often necessary for patients in whom surgery is not an option (Figure 46–4).[7] Somatostatin analogs, GH receptor antagonists, and dopamine agonists are the primary pharmacologic therapies used for the management of acromegaly (Table 46–2).[3,7,8] Pharmacologic therapy avoids hypopituitarism and other surgical risks.

Somatostatin Analog (GH-Inhibiting Hormone) KEY CONCEPT *Somatostatin analogs are the mainstay of pharmacotherapy for the treatment of acromegaly when surgery is not appropriate, or as an adjuvant therapy until patients achieve a sustained response to radiation therapy.*[7] These agents mimic endogenous somatostatins and bind to somatostatin receptors in the pituitary to cause potent inhibition of GH, insulin, and glucagon secretion. Long-term treatment can sustain GH suppression, alleviate soft tissue manifestations, and reduce tumor size. Use of the first-generation somatostatin analog octreotide is limited by its extremely short duration of action, which necessitates frequent injections of

Patient Encounter 1, Part 1: Acromegaly: Medical History and Clinical Presentation

A 61-year-old Caucasian woman has not seen her primary care provider for years prior due to financial issues and now complains of a sore on her abdomen, frequent headaches, and seeing "red and blue spots" in her vision. The patient has noticeably large facial features, and manly arms, hands, and legs. She states, "I used to have those beautiful piano fingers until I reached my teens!" She had always believed her masculine features were due to growing up with five brothers.

PMH: Uncontrolled hypertension for 4 years; recently diagnosed type 2 diabetes mellitus

FH: Positive for diabetes in patient's mother and five brothers

Allergies: NKDA

SH: Unemployed and uninsured, cleans 60+ hallways at her apartment to cover rent and utility; recently quit smoking

Meds: Lisinopril/hydrochlorothiazide 20/12.5 mg once daily; metformin 1000 mg twice daily; insulin glargine 20 units once daily; aspirin 81 mg once daily

Based on the information available, what signs and symptoms are suggestive of acromegaly?

What comorbidities are present in the patient as result of untreated acromegaly?

What diagnostic tests should be performed to confirm the patient's diagnosis of acromegaly?

at least three times per day. The long-acting preparations of octreotide and lanreotide are considered the cornerstone of therapy because of improved patient adherence and acceptability. Somatostatin analogs modestly reduce pituitary tumor size in more than half of the patients with acromegaly.[9] Their efficacy and safety have been demonstrated in long-term studies (up to 9 years with octreotide and 4 years with lanreotide).[10–12] Overall, the somatostatin analogs normalize GH and IGF-I concentrations in 56% and 55% of patients, respectively.[10] The efficacy of lanreotide autogel is comparable to that of depot formulations of lanreotide and octreotide in achieving clinical and biochemical control.[3,10] Because somatostatin analogs can achieve substantial relief of clinical symptoms with significant reduction in tumor size,[13] it is important to monitor patients for tumor recurrence if treatment is discontinued.[3] It is not yet

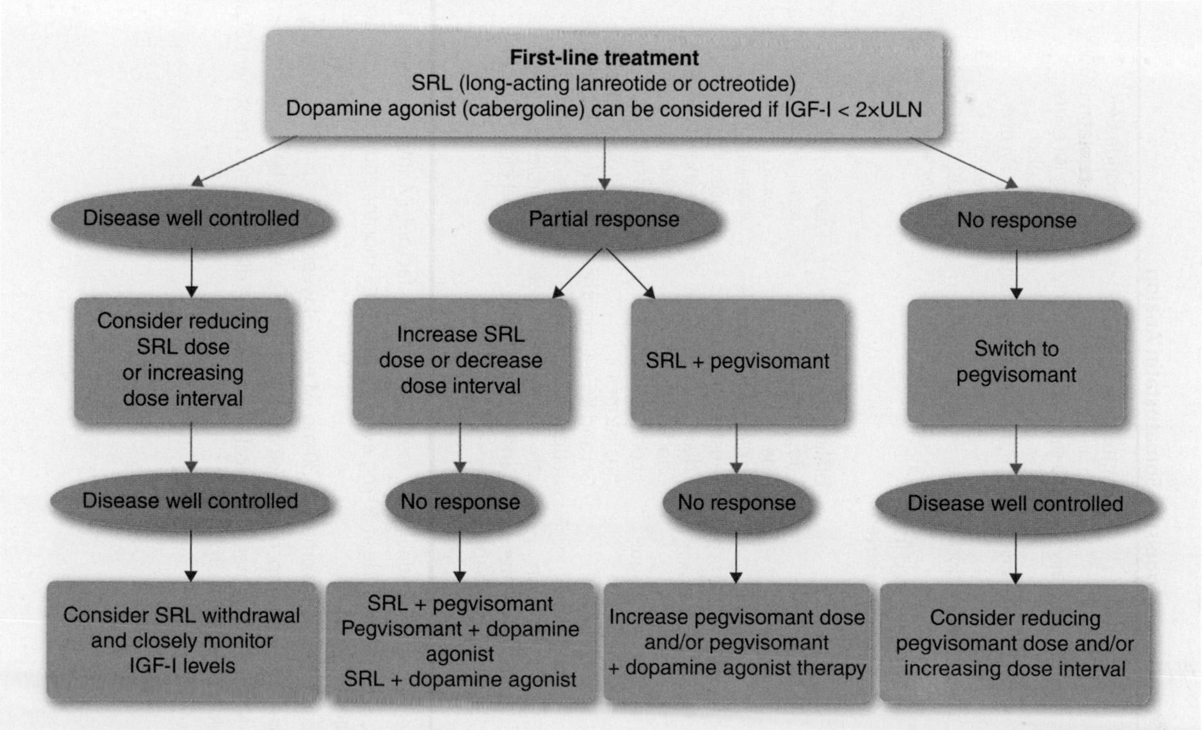

FIGURE 46–4. Medical management of patients with acromegaly.[7] A proposed algorithm for the medical management of acromegaly after surgery or as primary treatment strategy when surgery is inappropriate. Radiation therapy as rescue therapy has not been considered in this algorithm because its use is usually determined by a multidisciplinary management team. IGF-I, insulin-like growth factor I; SRL, somatostatin receptor ligan; ULN, upper limit of normal. (Reprinted by permission from Macmillan Publishers Ltd: Nature Publishing Group, Giustina A, Chanson P, Kleinberg D, et al. Expert consensus document: A consensus on the medical treatment of acromegaly. Nat Rev Endocrinol. 2014;10:243–248.)

Table 46-2

Comparison of Various Drugs for Treatment of Acromegaly[3,7,8]

Drug Class	Dopamine Agonist	Somatostatin Analog				GH Receptor Antagonist
Medication	Cabergoline	Octreotide (Sandostatin)	Octreotide LAR (Sandostatin LAR)	Lanreotide SR	Lanreotide Autogel (Somatuline Depot)	Pegvisomant (Somavert)
Starting dose	1 mg/week orally	50 mcg SC thrice daily	20 mg IM every 4 weeks	60 mg IM every 2 weeks	90 mg deep SC every 4 weeks[a]	10 mg SC daily after initial loading dose of 40 mg
Maximal dose	4 mg/week orally	200 mcg SC thrice daily	40 mg IM every 4 weeks[b]	120 mg IM every 7 days	120 mg deep SC every 4 weeks	40 mg SC daily[c]
Dosage in hepatic insufficiency	Dosage reduction may be recommended for patients with severe hepatic failure	—	Cirrhosis: 10 mg IM every 4 weeks	Dosage reduction may be necessary; no guidelines available	Moderate to severe impairment: starting dose 60 mg every 4 weeks	Discontinue therapy if liver function tests are elevated at least five times the upper limit of normal or transaminase at least three times upper limit of normal with any increase in serum total bilirubin
Dosage in renal failure	None	Dialysis dependent: adjustment may be necessary; no guidelines available	Dialysis-dependent renal impairment: 10 mg IM every 4 weeks	Dosage reduction may be necessary; no guidelines available	Moderate to severe impairment: starting dose, 60 mg every 4 weeks	None
Side effects	Nausea, GI cramps, headache, drowsiness, dizziness, fatigue	Nausea, GI cramps, diarrhea, flatulence, abdominal pain, constipation, gallstones	Nausea, GI cramps, diarrhea, flatulence, abdominal pain, constipation, gallstones	Nausea, GI cramps, diarrhea, flatulence, abdominal pain, constipation, gallstones	Nausea, GI cramps, diarrhea, flatulence, abdominal pain, constipation, gallstones	Headache, fatigue, GI cramps, abnormal liver enzymes, injection site reactions, sweating
Monitoring suggestions	GH, IGF-I, and prolactin concentration 4–6 weeks after each dose change	GH and IGF-I 3 months after dose change, thyroid function tests and blood glucose	GH and IGF-I 3 months after dose change, thyroid function tests and blood glucose	GH and IGF-I 3 months after dose change, thyroid function tests and blood glucose	GH and IGF-I 3 months after dose change, thyroid function tests and blood glucose	Liver function tests (serum transaminase, total bilirubin, alkaline phosphatase) monthly for 6 months, quarterly for next 6 months, then biannually for the next year; MRI every 6 months; IGF-I (not GH) after first year, then yearly

GH, growth hormone; GI, gastrointestinal; IGF-I, insulin-like growth factor-I; IM, intramuscularly; LAR, long-acting release; MRI, magnetic resonance imaging; SC, subcutaneously; SR, slow-release.

[a]In the United States, initiate lanreotide at 90 mg every 28 days for 3 months and then titrate accordingly based on patient response. Different labeled dosing guidelines exist for the United Kingdom and Canada.

[b]Product labeling recommends a maximum of 30 mg IM every 4 weeks.

[c]Alternative dose administration protocol of twice a week or once a week has been used.[3]

Adapted from AACE Medical Guidelines for Clinical Practice for the diagnosis and treatment of acromegaly. Endocr Pract. 2004;10:213–225 by permission of publisher, American Association of Clinical Endocrinologists (AACE) Corp.

known whether use of somatostatin analogs before surgery has additional benefits over surgery alone.[3]

Somatostatin analogs are generally well tolerated. Transient gastrointestinal (GI) disturbances are common but usually subside within the first 3 months of therapy. Somatostatin analogs inhibit gallbladder contractility and decrease bile secretion; therefore, their major adverse effect is development of biliary sludge and asymptomatic gallstones (cholelithiasis). Cholelithiasis typically occurs in patients treated for 12 months or longer and is unrelated to age, gender, or dose. Somatostatin analog-induced gallstones are generally asymptomatic, and prophylactic therapy is usually not needed.[6] Additionally, somatostatin analogs may alter the balance of counterregulatory hormones (ie, glucagon, insulin, and GH), resulting in either hypoglycemia or hyperglycemia. Octreotide also may suppress pituitary release of TSH, leading to decreased thyroid hormone secretion and subsequent hypothyroidism in 12% of treated patients. Close monitoring of thyroid function and glucose metabolism is recommended. Sinus bradycardia, conduction abnormalities, and arrhythmias have been reported with octreotide and lanreotide. Because of the potential adverse effects of the somatostatin analogs, concomitant use with insulin, oral hypoglycemic agents, β-blockers, or calcium channel blockers may require careful dosage adjustment. Somatostatin analogs may also alter the bioavailability and elimination of cyclosporine, and monitoring of cyclosporine serum concentration is necessary.

GH-Receptor Antagonist The advent of a GH-receptor antagonist represents a novel approach to the treatment of acromegaly. Pegvisomant is the only genetically engineered GH-receptor antagonist that blocks the action of GH. Pegvisomant is indicated for treatment of acromegaly in patients who have an inadequate response to surgery or radiation therapy. The effects of pegvisomant work independently of tumor characteristics, somatostatin, and dopamine receptors. Long-term safety and efficacy of pegvisomant (up to 5 years) from an ongoing postmarketing surveillance registry (ACROSTUDY) suggest a reasonable benefit/risk balance.[14] In patients who were relatively unresponsive to other medical or surgical therapies, normal IGF-I concentrations were achieved in 63% of the patients treated with pegvisomant (mean dose of 18 mg/day)[14] and in 69% to 100% of patients treated with pegvisomant and somatostatin analog therapy.[15–17] Pegvisomant therapy may have favorable effects on glucose tolerance (the body's ability to metabolize glucose) and insulin sensitivity (capacity of cells to respond to insulin). However, use of pegvisomant is associated with significant dose-dependent increases in GH despite declining IGF-I concentrations. The dose-dependent increase in GH is troubling because it has been suggested that persistent elevation of GH concentration may be indicative of tumor growth. Although the incidence of pituitary tumor enlargement is low (3.2%), careful monitoring with periodic imaging scans is nonetheless warranted, especially when administering pegvisomant to patients at risk for visual damage from large tumors that may impinge on the optic chiasm.[14] KEY CONCEPT *Pegvisomant is recommended in patients who have inadequate response to somatostatin analogs, or as an adjuvant for patients who have only a partial response to somatostatin analogs.*[3,7] The long-term use of pegvisomant appears to be well tolerated with a low incidence of adverse effects, including self-limiting injection-site reactions (2.2%) and elevated liver enzymes (2.5%).[14] Although elevations of liver enzymes often are self-limiting and not associated with symptoms,[3] hepatotoxicity has been reported in clinical trials, particularly in diabetic patients receiving combined pegvisomant and somatostatin analogs.[17,18] Therefore, serum transaminases, total bilirubin, and alkaline phosphatase should be assessed before initiating therapy and periodically thereafter. Use caution when administering pegvisomant to patients with elevated liver function tests, and therapy should be discontinued in patients who present with clinical signs and symptoms of hepatic injury.

Dopamine Agonists Dopamine is one of the neurotransmitters that can increase GH secretion in healthy adults. However, dopamine agonists administered to patients with acromegaly exert the opposite effect and suppress GH release from the tumor. The first dopamine agonist used for acromegaly, bromocriptine, achieved normal IGF-I concentrations in fewer than 10% of patients.[6] The large doses of bromocriptine required to achieve the desired response are often associated with dose-limiting toxicity such as GI discomfort and orthostatic hypotension. Cabergoline, a selective long-acting dopamine agonist with improved tolerability, can effectively reduce GH and IGF-I concentrations in approximately 40% of patients.[3] Acromegalic patients with coexisting hyperprolactinemia achieve a more favorable response to cabergoline.[3] Although orally administered dopamine agonists are the least expensive medical therapy for managing acromegaly, the major disadvantage is their relative lack of efficacy compared with existing therapeutic options. KEY CONCEPT *Cabergoline may be considered for patients with modest elevation of GH and IGF-I concentrations less than two times the upper limit of normal. It may also be used as adjunctive therapy in patients unresponsive to monotherapy with somatostatin analogs or pegvisomant.*[7] Although cardiac valvular abnormalities have been observed in patients using higher doses of cabergoline for Parkinson disease, similar findings have not been reported in patients with acromegaly.[3,19] Nonetheless, echocardiographic monitoring for potential cardiac abnormalities is warranted for patients who require prolonged, high-dose cabergoline therapy.

Radiation Therapy Radiation therapy is an important adjunctive therapy in patients with residual GH excess after surgery or pharmacologic therapy. Treatment involves the use of radiation to destroy rapidly growing tumor cells, and often results in a reduction in tumor size. A major complication of radiation therapy is hypopituitarism, requiring lifelong hormone replacement.[3] There is also the potential for optic nerve damage if the pituitary tumor is near the optic tracts. Radiation therapy may take 10 to 20 years before its full effects become evident.[3] Owing to this delay in onset of effectiveness, pharmacologic therapy with a somatostatin analog often is indicated as bridge therapy.[3] Men and women who desire to have children should be warned that pituitary irradiation therapy may impair fertility because of subsequent gonadotropin deficiency.[3]

▶ *Outcome Evaluation*

- Lifelong biochemical assessment is critical for determining therapeutic outcomes. Although some patients may experience a rapid decline in GH concentrations after surgery, stabilization of IGF-I concentrations usually occurs 3 months after surgery but rarely may be delayed for up to 12 months. Fully assess pituitary function 2 to 3 months after surgery.[3] Monitor GH and IGF-I concentrations every 3 to 6 months postoperatively to assess treatment response.[3] Obtain IGF-I concentrations annually in all postsurgical patients to monitor for potential pituitary tumor recurrence.[3]
- Assess MRI 3 to 4 months after surgery and 3 to 6 months after starting medical therapy.[20] Because up to 10% of pituitary tumors may recur within 15 years after surgery,[21] continual postoperative monitoring is recommended.

- For patients treated with somatostatin analogs, assess baseline fasting blood glucose, thyroid function tests, and heart rate. Thereafter, periodically monitor patients for adverse reactions such as GI disturbances, glucose intolerance, signs and symptoms of thyroid abnormalities, bradycardia, and arrhythmias in patients receiving long-term somatostatin analogs. Reevaluate IGF-I and GH concentrations at 3-month intervals to determine therapeutic response and inquire about symptoms of gallbladder disease (eg, intermittent pain in the upper right abdomen) during follow-up appointments.[3] If normalization of GH and IGF-I concentrations are not fully achieved after 1 year, perform MRI 6 months later and annually thereafter to monitor tumor mass.[3]
- For patients treated with a GH receptor antagonist, GH concentrations are not measured because pegvisomant is a modified GH molecule that is detected in commercial GH assays, resulting in falsely elevated GH concentrations. Therefore, monitor IGF-I concentrations to assess response to pegvisomant therapy. After appropriate dose titration, monitor IGF-I concentrations every 6 months.[3] Concern for tumor growth requires careful monitoring of tumor size; therefore, perform MRI every 6 months during the first year of therapy and annually thereafter.[3] Because of the potential for hepatotoxicity with pegvisomant therapy, it is mandatory to monitor liver enzymes prior to initiation of therapy, monthly during the first 6 months, quarterly for the next 6 months, and then biannually thereafter.[3] More frequent monitoring of liver enzymes is warranted in patients with elevated liver enzymes at baseline.[3]
- For patients receiving dopamine agonists, the maximal suppression of GH and IGF-I concentrations may take up to 3 months to achieve. After stable control of biochemical markers is achieved with dopamine agonists or somatostatin analogs, monitor GH and IGF-I concentrations annually.[3]
- With conventional multidose radiation therapy, the most rapid decline in GH serum concentrations occurs within the first 2 years; monitor GH concentrations at the second year and annually thereafter.[3,21] Patients who receive single-dose radiation therapy should be evaluated at 6-month intervals because response is observed earlier. Repeatedly assess pituitary function over the years after radiation therapy.[3]

Growth Hormone Deficiency

► *Epidemiology and Etiology*

In the United States, GH deficiency affects approximately 50,000 adults, with around 6000 new cases diagnosed annually.[22] Approximately 10,000 to 15,000 children have growth failure owing to GH deficiency. Children may present with GH deficiency at any time during their developmental stages. The evaluation for GH deficiency in a child of short stature should be deferred until appropriate exclusion of other identifiable causes of growth failure, such as hypothyroidism, chronic illness, malnutrition, genetic syndromes, and skeletal disorders, has occurred. Several medications, such as somatostatin analogs, gonadotropin-releasing hormone (GnRH) agonists, methoxamine, phentolamine, isoproterenol, glucocorticoids, cimetidine, methylphenidate, and amphetamine derivatives, may induce GH insufficiency.[23]

► *Pathophysiology*

GH deficiency exists when GH is absent or produced in inadequate amounts. GH deficiency may be congenital, acquired, or result from disruption of the hypothalamus–pituitary axis. GH deficiency may be an isolated condition or occasionally be accompanied by another endocrine disorder (eg, panhypopituitarism). Because GH is frequently undetectable with random sampling, a stimulation or provocative test usually is performed to confirm the diagnosis. The gold standard for diagnosis of

Patient Encounter 1, Part 2: Acromegaly: Physical Examination and Diagnostic Tests

PE:

VS: BP 162/116 mm Hg, P 112 beats/min, RR 18 breaths/min, T 36.8°C (98.3°F), Ht 168 cm (5′6″), Wt 72 kg (159 lbs), BMI 25.8 kg/m^2

ROS: (+) HA, (+) deepening of voice

HEENT: Visual field defects; head is elongated with bony prominence of the forehead, nose, and lower jaw; large fleshy nose

CV: RRR, normal S_1 and S_2; no murmurs, rubs, or gallops, (–) chest pain, palpitation, orthopnea, and leg swelling

Pulm: (–) SOB, (–) cough

GI: (–) Nausea, vomiting, and abdominal pain

Abd: Soft, nontender, nondistended; (+) bowel sounds, (–) hepatosplenomegaly

Skin: Skin lesion healing

Neuro: A & O x 3. Normal reflexes

Psychiatric: Normal mood and affect. Spacy, sweet, but needs extra help understanding instructions

Available Labs: Electrolytes and renal function are within normal limits. Fasting blood glucose concentration is 346 mg/dL (19.2 mmol/L), $HgbA_{1c}$ is 11.9% (0.119; 107 mmol/mol), (+) microalbuminuria. GH concentration 1 hour after an OGTT is 83.6 ng/mL (83.6 mcg/L; 3779 pmol/L). Elevated IGF-I concentration at 998 ng/mL (998 mcg/L; 131 nmol/L). TSH is slightly low at 0.33 μU/mL (0.33 mU/L) and FT_4 is within normal range at 1.1 ng/dL (14.2 pmol/L)

MRI: (+) 12 mm benign pituitary adenoma extending toward the optic chiasm; no invasion into the cavernous sinus

If the patient is unwilling to undergo surgery, what pharmacologic treatment options are available for her?

Given that she is currently uninsured without a source of income, what factors need to be considered when choosing a pharmacologic treatment option?

Provide monitoring parameters to assess efficacy and safety to the patient starting on octreotide long-acting release.

Patient Care Process: Acromegaly

Patient Assessment:

- Assess the patient's clinical signs and symptoms to determine the severity of acromegaly.
- Review the biochemical disease markers to assess the severity of acromegaly.
- Review the available diagnostic data to determine pituitary tumor size and location.
- Determine if the patient has a coexisting prolactin secreting tumor and if the tumor extends toward the optic chiasm or if it is continuous on the optic tracts.

Therapy Evaluation:

- Assess presence of acromegaly complications. Identify any significant comorbidities associated with acromegaly that require immediate treatment or early diagnosis.
- Determine treatment options the patient has tried in the past.
- Evaluate patient for presence of surgical contraindications to transsphenoidal microsurgery. Determine if the patient is able or willing to undergo surgical intervention.
- If surgical intervention does not achieve satisfactory disease control, select subsequent appropriate pharmacologic therapy based on patient-specific factors (see Figure 46–4). Be sure to consider if the patient has any contraindications or allergies to therapies (see Table 46–2).

Care Plan Development:

- Assess patient's response and complications to surgical intervention. Measure both GH and IGF-I concentrations.
- Determine if selected drug doses are optimal (see Table 46–2). Consider if the patient's therapy requires any dose adjustments.
- Provide patient education regarding disease state, and nondrug and drug therapy:
  - Possible complications of acromegaly
  - How to reduce the modifiable cardiovascular and metabolic risk factors
  - Potential effectiveness and disadvantages of existing treatment options
  - Importance of adherence to therapy
  - Potential adverse effects
- Evaluate patient for presence of adverse drug reactions and drug interactions.

Follow-up Evaluation:

- Assess biochemical markers annually once disease control is achieved.
- Routinely assess acromegaly complications; include blood pressure, glucose tolerance, fasting lipid profile, cardiac evaluations (if clinically indicated), colonoscopy, dual-energy x-ray absorptiometry (DEXA) scan (hypogonadal only), evaluation of residual pituitary function, and sleep apnea.

adults with GH deficiency is the insulin tolerance test (ITT), with glucagon as an alternative if GHRH is unavailable.[24] Adults exhibiting a peak GH concentration of less than 5.1 ng/mL (5.1 mcg/L; 230 pmol/L) after two ITT simulation tests would warrant treatment.[24] In prepubertal children, measurement of IGF-I concentrations may be useful in evaluating GH deficiency.[25] The diagnosis of GH deficiency in children is further supported if height is more than two standard deviations below

Clinical Presentation and Diagnosis of Growth Hormone Deficiency in Children[5,22]

General

The patient will have a physical height that is greater than two standard deviations below the population mean for a given age and gender.

Signs

- The patient will present with reduced growth velocity and delayed skeletal maturation.
- Children with GH-deficient or GH-insufficient short stature also may present with abdominal obesity, prominence of the forehead, and immaturity of the face.

Laboratory Tests

- Patients will exhibit a peak GH concentration of less than 10 ng/mL (10 mcg/L; 452 pmol/L) after a GH stimulation test.
- Reduced IGF-I concentration also may be present.
- Because GH deficiency may be accompanied by the loss of other pituitary hormones, hypoglycemia, and hypothyroidism also may be noted.

Other Diagnostic Tests

- Perform MRI or computed tomography (CT) scan of the hypothalamic–pituitary region to detect structural or developmental anomaly.
- Perform radiography of the left wrist and hand for children older than 1 year of age to estimate bone age (knee and ankle for children younger than 1 year of age).

Adapted from Jordan JK, Sheehan AH, Yanovski JA, Calis KA. Pituitary gland disorders. In: Dipiro JT, Talbert RL, Yee GC, et al, eds. Pharmacotherapy. A Pathophysiologic Approach. 9th ed. New York: McGraw-Hill; 2014:1237–1252.

Clinical Presentation and Diagnosis of Growth Hormone Deficiency in Adults[24,26,27,31,34]

General

The patient likely will have a history of childhood-onset GH deficiency; hypothalamic or pituitary disorder; or the presence of three or four other pituitary hormone deficiencies caused by head trauma, tumor, infiltrative diseases, surgery, or radiation therapy.

Symptoms

- Reduced strength and exercise capacity
- Defective sweating
- Psychological problems
- Low self-esteem
- Depression
- Fatigue or listlessness
- Sleep disturbance
- Anxiety
- Social isolation
- Emotional lability and impaired self-control
- Poor marital and socioeconomic performance

Signs

- Increased fat mass (especially abdominal obesity)
- Reduced lean body mass
- Reduced muscle strength
- Reduced exercise performance
- Thin, dry skin; cool peripheries; poor venous access
- Depressed affect, labile emotions
- Impaired cardiac function as evidenced by abnormal echocardiography or stress test results

Laboratory Tests

- Patients will exhibit a peak GH concentration of less than 5.1 ng/mL (5.1 mcg/L; 231 pmol/L) after a GH stimulation test. Insulin tolerance test (ITT) is the gold standard stimulation test. Low or low-normal IGF-I concentration also may be present. Presence of three or more pituitary hormone deficiencies with a low IGF-I concentration do not require further stimulation test.
- Increased low-density lipoprotein cholesterol, total cholesterol, triglycerides; decreased high-density lipoprotein cholesterol.
- Reduced bone mineral density associated with an increased risk of fracture.
- Increased insulin resistance and prevalence of impaired glucose tolerance.
- GH deficiency may be accompanied by the loss of other pituitary hormones.

the population mean (age- and sex-matched).[22] Failure of linear growth is an almost universal presenting feature of childhood GH deficiency.

Childhood GH deficiency may or may not continue into adulthood. Most adults with GH deficiency have overt pituitary disease and present with nonspecific clinical disorders distinct from pediatric GH deficiency. Adult GH deficiency presumably is associated with an increased risk of death from cardiovascular diseases.[24]

▶ *Treatment*

Desired Outcomes The goal of treatment for GH deficiency is to correct associated clinical symptoms.[22] In children, prompt diagnosis and early initiation of treatment are important to maximize final adult height. In adults, the goal is to achieve normal physiologic GH concentrations in an attempt to reverse metabolic, functional, and psychological abnormalities.[24,26]

Pharmacologic Therapy KEY CONCEPT *Recombinant GH therapy is the main pharmacologic treatment for GH deficiency in both children and adults.* It promotes skeletal, visceral, and general body growth; stimulates protein anabolism; and affects bone, fat, and mineral metabolism (see Table 46–1).[2] GH therapy requires subcutaneous or intramuscular administrations. Because two-thirds of GH secretion normally occurs during sleep, it is recommended to administer GH injections in the evening.[27] Many preparations of synthetic GH (somatropin) are available with a variety of injection devices to make administration more appealing and easier. Tev-Tropin is only approved for use in children, and other somatropin products such as Nutropin AQ, Humatrope, Norditropin, Genotropin, Omnitrope, and Saizen are approved in both children and adults.

KEY CONCEPT *Although comparative trials have not been conducted to date, recombinant GH products appear to have similar efficacy for treating GH deficiency as long as the regimen follows currently approved guidelines.* GH secretion decreases with age; therefore, older adults with GH deficiency often require substantially lower replacement doses than younger individuals. The optimal therapeutic approach is to initiate GH therapy at lower doses and titrate according to clinical response, adverse effects, and IGF-I concentrations.[28,29] Table 46–3 lists the recommended GH replacement doses for children and adults.[29,30] Conventional weight-based regimens are not recommended in adults due to lack of evidence supporting higher dosages in heavier individuals and greater potential for adverse effects.[24,26,31] Maintenance doses may be lower with chronic GH therapy.[32] For elderly patients, lower GH replacement doses often are adequate because of increased GH sensitivity.[26,28,29] Women with intact hypothalamic–pituitary–gonadal axis or on estrogen therapy (or oral contraceptives) generally require a higher GH dose than men due to decreased GH concentrations associated with estrogen.[28,29] Carefully monitor patients requiring replacement therapy with estrogens, thyroid hormones, or glucocorticoids because of potential interactions with GH therapy.[26] The potency of GH products is generally expressed as 3 international units (IU or mU) per 1 milligram of protein.[24] Selection of an injection device depends on patient preference due to lack of differences in clinical outcomes among the various injection systems.[29,30]

Table 46–3

Dose Recommendation for Growth Hormone Deficiency in Children and Adults[29,30]

	Growth Hormone Replacement Dose	Dose Titration
Children[30]	Dosing Range	• Evaluate every 3–6 months based on height and height velocity. • Monitor IGF-I and IGFBP-3 yearly. • Monitor TSH and T_4 for hypothyroidism. • Reduce dose if serum IGF-I concentration is substantially above normal after 2 years of therapy.
Prepubertal children	25–50 mcg/kg/day	
Adolescents	25–100 mcg/kg/day	
Adults[29]	Starting Dose	• Increase dose by 0.1–0.2 mg/day based on clinical response, serum IGF-I concentrations, and side effects at 1- to 2-month intervals. Longer time intervals and smaller dose titration may be necessary in older adults.
Age < 30 years	0.4–0.5 mg/day[a]	
Age 30–60 years	0.2–0.3 mg/day	
Age > 60 years	0.1–0.2 mg/day	
Diabetes or glucose intolerance (overweight, obese, or history of gestational diabetes)	0.1–0.2 mg/day	
Hepatic impairment	—	• Clearance may be reduced in patients with severe hepatic dysfunction; specific dosing suggestions are not available.
Renal impairment	—	• Patients with chronic renal failure tend to have decreased clearance; specific dosing suggestions are not available.

[a]Might require a higher dose for patients transitioning from pediatric treatment.

IGFBP-3, insulin-like growth factor-bind protein 3; IGF-I, insulin-like growth factor-I; T_4, thyroxine; TSH, thyroid-stimulating hormone.

Evidence has suggested that GH treatment in GH-deficient children can increase short-term growth and improve final adult height.[22] Beneficial effects of GH therapy in adults with GH deficiency have been demonstrated to normalize body composition and metabolic process; improve cardiac risk profile, bone mineral density, quality of life, and psychological well-being; and increase muscle strength and exercise capacity.[24,33] The available data on cardiovascular and metabolic benefits of long-term GH replacement therapy in adults are inconsistent and additional research is needed to adequately assess the risks and benefits of long-term GH replacement.[33] Overall, reduction in mortality with GH therapy remains to be established.

Practitioners should begin GH therapy as soon as possible to optimize long-term growth, especially for young children in whom GH deficiency is complicated by fasting hypoglycemia.[22] Selection of the optimal GH replacement dose will need to be individualized depending on response, financial resources, and product availability. Although the appropriate time to discontinue therapy remains controversial in childhood GH deficiency, it is reasonable to continue GH replacement until the child has reached satisfactory adult height, achieved documented epiphyseal closure, or failed to respond to therapy.[22] Management of the transition between pediatric and adult GH replacement remains a challenge because limited data are available. The secretion of GH during adolescence is normally lower than during puberty but higher than during adulthood. Therefore, for patients in a transition phase who may be restarting GH therapy, the initial dose for an adolescent is approximately the average of the pediatric dose required for growth and the adult dose.[29] Starting GH therapy at a low dose and gradually titrating upward may decrease the potential for adverse effects. The optimal duration of treatment with GH therapy remains unclear, but lifelong therapy may be required. However, GH replacement should be discontinued if therapeutic benefit is not achieved after 2 years of therapy.[29]

In both children and adults, treatment with GH may mask underlying central hypothyroidism and adrenal insufficiency.[35] Treatment with GH also may induce insulin resistance and lead to the development of glucose intolerance in patients with preexisting risk factors. Adults are more susceptible to dose-related adverse effects of GH-induced symptoms, such as edema, arthralgia, myalgia, and carpal tunnel syndrome, which may necessitate dose reductions in up to 40% of adults.

Children treated with GH replacement therapy rarely experience significant adverse effects. Benign increases in intracranial pressure related to GH therapy may manifest as headaches, visual changes, or altered concentrations of consciousness. This condition is generally reversible upon discontinuation of treatment. Often, GH therapy can be restarted with smaller doses without symptom recurrence. Presently, there is no compelling evidence that GH replacement therapy is associated with an increased risk of leukemia, solid tumor, or tumor recurrence.[22,26,29] GH replacement therapy is contraindicated in all patients with active malignancy.[29] However, in children with a history of malignancies, it would be prudent to wait for a 1-year tumor-free period (5 years for adults) before initiating GH therapy.[22] Any patients treated for a prior malignancy may be at risk for a second malignancy and should be monitored carefully for tumor recurrence.[22] Because deaths have been reported with use of GH in children with Prader-Willi syndrome who are severely obese or suffer from respiratory impairments, use of GH is contraindicated in these individuals. Evidence from the long-term surveillance study, Safety and Appropriateness of Growth hormone treatments in Europe (SAGhE), remains inconclusive regarding GH therapy and its risk of increased morbidity. Therefore, further surveillance monitoring is warranted.[36]

▶ *Outcome Evaluation*

- Children with GH deficiency should be evaluated by a pediatric endocrinologist every 3 to 6 months. Monitor for an increase in height and change in height velocity to assess response to GH therapy.[22,30] Every effort should be made

Patient Care Process: GH Deficiency in Children

Patient Assessment:

- Assess the child's growth characteristics and compare the physical height with a population standard (eg, Centers for Disease Control and Prevention Growth Charts).
- Obtain a thorough history and physical examination that may indicate the possible presence of GH deficiency.
- Exclude other identifiable causes of growth failure.
- Perform imaging tests of the hypothalamic–pituitary region to detect structural or developmental anomalies.
- Perform radiography of the wrist and hand to estimate bone age.
- Perform a provocative test to measure GH and IGF-I concentrations.

Therapy Evaluation:

- Determine if GH therapy is indicated. Make sure the child does not have any contraindications to GH therapy.
- Determine whether patient has prescription coverage.

Care Plan Development:

- Initiate GH replacement therapy based on patient preference (see Table 46–3).
- Assess response (increase in height and change in height velocity) and adverse effects of GH replacement therapy. Make dosage adjustments when appropriate.
- Provide patient education regarding disease state and drug therapy. Discuss with child and parents:
  - GH deficiency
  - Potential effectiveness and disadvantages of existing GH replacement therapy
  - Importance of adherence to therapy
  - Potential for adverse effects or need for lifelong replacement.

Follow-up Evaluation:

- Continue GH replacement therapy until child reaches satisfactory adult height, achieves documented epiphyseal closure, or fails to respond to treatment.
- Review and retest the child using adult GH deficiency diagnostic criteria when the child reaches final adult height.

to maximize height before the onset of puberty. After final adult height is reached and GH is discontinued for at least 1 month, retest and reevaluate the patient using the adult GH-deficiency diagnostic criteria.[24,29,30]

- Although GH and IGF-I concentrations do not always correlate with growth response, measure IGF-I concentrations yearly to assess adherence to therapy and patient response. If the IGF-I concentrations are substantially above the normal range 2 years after GH replacement therapy, the dose should be reduced.[30] IGF-I concentration may be used as a guide to gradually reduce replacement dose after epiphyseal closure.
- Routine monitoring of fasting lipid profile, bone mineral density, and body composition in children is not typically required during GH replacement but should be done before and after discontinuation of therapy.[22,30]

Patient Care Process: GH Deficiency in Adults

Patient Assessment:

- Assess the patient's clinical signs and symptoms to determine the severity of GH deficiency.
- Perform a provocative test to measure GH concentrations.
- Evaluate the patient for the presence of metabolic abnormalities and cardiovascular and fracture risks.

Therapy Evaluation:

- Determine if GH therapy is indicated. Make sure the patient does not have any contraindications to GH therapy.
- Determine whether patient has prescription coverage.

Care Plan Development:

- Initiate GH replacement therapy based on patient preference and characteristics (see Table 46–3)
- Assess the efficacy and adverse effects of GH therapy and consider if the patient's therapy requires any dose adjustments based on IGF-I concentration, patient response, and adverse effects
- Provide patient education regarding disease state and drug therapy:
  - Possible complications of GH deficiency
  - How to reduce the modifiable cardiovascular and metabolic risk factors
  - Potential disadvantages and effectiveness of existing GH replacement therapy
  - Importance of adherence to therapy
  - Potential for adverse effects or need for lifelong replacement

Follow-up Evaluation:

- Monitor for improvement of metabolic, cardiovascular, bone mineral density, and body composition parameters to assess response to GH therapy

- In adults, measurement of serum IGF-I, along with careful clinical evaluation, appears to be the most reliable way to assess the appropriateness of the GH dose. Measure IGF-I serum concentrations 1 to 2 months during dose titration and semiannually thereafter.[24]
- Continuously monitor for dose-related adverse effects such as edema, arthralgia, myalgia, and carpal tunnel syndrome.
- Evaluate psychological well-being.
- Assess patients' bone mineral density every 2 to 3 years.[29]
- When maintenance therapy is achieved, assess body composition (body mass index [BMI], waist circumference, waist-to-hip ratio), metabolic status (fasting glucose concentration, free thyroxine serum, hemoglobin A_{1c}), cardiac risk factors (eg, fasting lipid profile), hypothalamic–pituitary–adrenal axis function (eg, morning serum cortisol response to ACTH stimulation), and testosterone concentrations at 6- to 12- month intervals.[26,29]

PROLACTIN

Prolactin is an essential hormone for normal production of breast milk after childbirth. It also plays a pivotal role in a variety of reproductive functions. Prolactin is regulated primarily by the hypothalamus–pituitary axis and secreted solely by the lactotroph cells of the anterior pituitary gland. Under normal conditions, secretion of prolactin is predominantly under inhibitory control by dopamine. Increases of hypothalamic thyrotropin-releasing hormone in primary hypothyroidism can stimulate the release of prolactin.

Hyperprolactinemia

► *Epidemiology and Etiology*

Hyperprolactinemia affects women of reproductive age more than men. Although this disorder occurs in less than 1% of the general population, the estimated prevalence in women with reproductive disorders is as high as 15% to 43%.[37] The etiologies of hyperprolactinemia are presented in Table 46–4.[5,23,37–40] Any medications that antagonize dopamine or stimulate prolactin release can induce hyperprolactinemia.[5,23,37,38] Therefore, it is important to exclude medication-induced hyperprolactinemia from other common causes such as pregnancy, primary hypothyroidism, benign prolactin-secreting pituitary adenoma (prolactinoma), and renal insufficiency. Prolactinomas are the most common pituitary tumors. They are classified as microprolactinomas if they are less than 10 mm in diameter and as macroprolactinomas if they are 10 mm or larger in diameter.[38] In general, microprolactinomas rarely increase in size, but macroprolactinomas have the potential to enlarge and invade the surrounding tissues.[41]

► *Pathophysiology*

Hyperprolactinemia is a condition of elevated serum prolactin. It is the most common endocrine disorder of the hypothalamic–pituitary axis. High prolactin concentrations inhibit the release of gonadotropin-releasing hormone by the hypothalamus and subsequently suppress secretion of LH and FSH from the anterior pituitary (see Figure 46–1). High prolactin concentrations result in reduced gonadal hormone concentrations, often leading to reproductive dysfunction and galactorrhea (inappropriate breast milk production).

In combination with clinical symptoms, one or more serum prolactin concentrations greater than 25 ng/mL (25 mcg/L; 1087 pmol/L) will confirm the diagnosis of hyperprolactinemia in women.[39] A number of physiologic factors such as eating, exercise, and stress can transiently elevate prolactin concentrations.[5] Therefore, prolactin measurements should be obtained at rest, preferably in the morning under fasting conditions.[37] If an intravenous line is present or planned, it is prudent to wait at least 2 hours after line insertion before measuring serum prolactin to decrease detecting transient physiologic increases in prolactin concentration.[5,23,37–40] Although medication-induced hyperprolactinemia is typically associated with prolactin concentrations

Table 46–4

Causes of Hyperprolactinemia[5,23,37–40]

Physiologic Causes
Pregnancy
Stress (including exercise and hypoglycemia)
Breast stimulation
Breastfeeding
Coitus
Sleep
Meal
Increased prolactin production
Ovarian: Polycystic Ovarian Syndrome
Oophorectomy (removal of an ovary)
Pituitary tumors
Adenomas
Microprolactinoma (< 10 mm diameter)
Macroprolactinoma (≥ 10 mm diameter)
Hypothalamic stalk interruption (prevent dopamine from reaching the pituitary)
Hypophysitis (inflammation)
Ectopic tumors
Hypothalamic Prolactin Stimulation
Primary hypothyroidism
Adrenal insufficiency
Reduced Prolactin Elimination
Chronic renal failure
Hepatic cirrhosis
Neurogenic Causes
Chest wall injury (eg, surgery, herpes zoster)
Spinal cord lesions
Abnormal Molecules
Macroprolactinemia
Medications
Dopamine antagonists: antipsychotics[a], phenothiazines, metoclopramide, domperidone
Dopamine-depleting agents: reserpine, α-methyldopa
Prolactin stimulators: serotonin reuptake inhibitors, dexfenfluramine, estrogens, progestins, antiandrogens, gonadotropin-releasing hormone analogs, benzodiazepines, tricyclic antidepressants, monoamine oxidase inhibitors, protease inhibitors, $histamine_2$ receptor antagonists
Other: isoniazid, cocaine, opioids, verapamil
Seizures
Idiopathic (Unknown)

[a]Atypicals (olanzapine and clozapine) other than risperidone may cause an early but transient elevation in prolactin.[32]

Adapted in part, with permission, from Jordan JK, Sheehan AH, Yanovski JA, Calis KA. Pituitary gland disorders. In: Dipiro JT, Talbert RL, Yee GC, et al, eds. Pharmacotherapy. A Pathophysiologic Approach. 9th ed. New York: McGraw-Hill; 2014:1237–1252.

Clinical Presentation and Diagnosis of Hyperprolactinemia[5,38–40]

General

Hyperprolactinemia most commonly affects women of reproductive age and is very rare in men.

Signs and Symptoms

Premenopausal women

- Headache and compromised or loss of vision caused by the prolactin-secreting tumor and its close proximity to the optic structures.
- Clinical presentation is associated with the degree of prolactin elevation:
  - Prolactin greater than 100 ng/mL (100 mcg/L; 4348 pmol/L): hypogonadism, galactorrhea, and amenorrhea
  - Prolactin 51 to 75 ng/mL (51–75 mcg/L; 2217–3261 pmol/L): oligomenorrhea (infrequent menstruation)
  - Prolactin 31 to 50 ng/mL (31–50 mcg/L; 1348–2174 pmol/L): decreased libido and infertility
- Increased body weight may be associated with a prolactin-secreting pituitary tumor.
- The degree of hypogonadism generally is proportionate to the degree of prolactin elevation.
- Excessive hair growth (hirsutism) and acne also may be present owing to relative androgen excess compared with low estrogen concentrations.

Men

- Decreased libido, decreased energy, erectile dysfunction, impotence, decreased sperm production, infertility, gynecomastia, and rarely, galactorrhea.
- Impotence is unresponsive to treatment and is associated with reduced muscle mass, loss of pubic hair, and osteoporosis.

Laboratory Tests

- Prolactin serum concentrations at rest will be greater than 20 ng/mL (20 mcg/L; 870 pmol/L) in men or 25 ng/mL (25 mcg/L; 1087 pmol/L) in women with at least three measurements.
- Obtain β-human chorionic gonadotropin (β-hCG) concentration to exclude pregnancy.
- Obtain TSH concentration to exclude primary hypothyroidism.
- Obtain blood urea nitrogen and serum creatinine tests to exclude renal failure.

Other Diagnostic Tests

- Perform MRI to locate the tumor, exclude a pseudo-prolactinoma, and validate the diagnosis.
- Consider a bone mineral density test in patients with long-term hypogonadism.

Additional Clinical Sequelae

- The prolonged suppression of estrogen in premenopausal women with hyperprolactinemia leads to decreases in bone mineral density and significant risk for the development of osteoporosis.
- Risk for ischemic heart disease may be increased with untreated hyperprolactinemia.

Adapted, with permission, from Jordan JK, Sheehan AH, Yanovski JA, Calis KA. Pituitary gland disorders. In: Dipiro JT, Talbert RL, Yee GC, et al, eds. Pharmacotherapy. A Pathophysiologic Approach. 9th ed. New York: McGraw-Hill; 2014:1237–1252.

of 25 to 100 ng/mL (25–100 mcg/L; 1087–4348 pmol/L), metoclopramide, risperidone, and phenothiazines have been associated with concentrations greater than 200 ng/mL (200 mcg/L; 8696 pmol/L). However, prolactin concentrations greater than 500 ng/mL (500 mcg/L; 21739 pmol/L) are almost always associated with the presence of a macroprolactinoma.[39]

▸ *Treatment*

Desired Outcomes Because hyperprolactinemia is often associated with hypogonadism, the goals for management of hyperprolactinemia are as follows[39,40]:

- Normalize prolactin concentration
- Restore normal gonadal function and fertility
- Prevent development of osteoporosis
- If a pituitary tumor is present:
  - Ablate or reduce tumor size to relieve tumor mass effect
  - Preserve normal pituitary function
  - Prevent progression of pituitary tumor or hypothalamic disease

General Approaches to Treatment Management of drug-induced hyperprolactinemia is to discontinue the offending agent, if clinically feasible, and replace it with an appropriate alternative that does not cause hyperprolactinemia.[39] When the offending agent cannot be discontinued, cautious use of hormone replacement, biphosphonate therapy, or dopamine agonists may be considered depending on the patient's clinical circumstances.[23] Treatment options for the management of hyperprolactinemia include: (a) clinical observation, (b) pharmacologic therapy with dopamine agonists, (c) transsphenoidal pituitary adenomectomy, and (d) radiation therapy. Clinical observation and close monitoring are justifiable in patients with asymptomatic elevation of prolactin.[39] KEY CONCEPT *Dopamine agonists are the first-line treatment of choice for all patients with symptomatic hyperprolactinemia; transsphenoidal surgery and radiation therapy are reserved for patients who are resistant to or severely intolerant of pharmacologic therapy.*[39] However, in patients with underlying psychiatric symptoms, use of dopamine agonists in addition to an antipsychotic therapy may exacerbate the underlying psychosis and should be used with caution in consultation with a mental health clinician.[23]

Pharmacologic Therapy Dopamine is the principal neurotransmitter responsible for the inhibition of prolactin secretion from the anterior pituitary. Thus, dopamine agonists are the main pharmacologic therapy used for management of hyperprolactinemia. Treatment with dopamine agonists has proven to be extremely effective in normalizing serum prolactin concentration, restoring gonadal function, decreasing tumor size, and improving visual fields.[39,42] Patients with macroprolactinomas generally require a higher dose to normalize prolactin concentrations compared with patients with microprolactinomas.[43]

Two dopamine agonists—bromocriptine and cabergoline—are used for the management of hyperprolactinemia (Table 46–5).[37,44] Because these two dopamine agonists are ergot derivatives, they are contraindicated in combination with potent cytochrome P-450 subfamily IIIA polypeptide 4 (CYP3A4) inhibitors, including protease inhibitors, azole antifungals, and some macrolide antibiotics. Furthermore, ergot derivatives can cause constriction of peripheral and cranial blood vessels. These medications are also contraindicated in patients with uncontrolled hypertension, severe ischemic heart disease, or peripheral vascular disorders.

Bromocriptine Bromocriptine directly binds to the D_2 dopamine receptors. It normalizes prolactin concentration in 68% of patients and reduces tumor size in 62% of patients.[42] Treatment with bromocriptine may also restore menses and fertility in women and improve testosterone secretion, sperm count and erectile function in men. It may also improve visual field defects associated with macroadenomas.[42] Adverse effects such as nausea, dizziness, and orthostatic hypotension often limit 5% to 10% of patients from continuing treatment. To reduce risk of adverse effects and improve patient adherence, bromocriptine may be initiated at a low dose at bedtime.[11] Slowly titrate up to the optimal therapeutic dose because most adverse effects subside with continual treatment. In women, if the adverse GI effects are not tolerable, bromocriptine can be administered vaginally at a reduced dose (2.5 mg/day).[45] Owing to its short half-life of only 6 hours, bromocriptine must be administered in divided doses, which may compromise patient adherence.

Cabergoline Cabergoline has a higher affinity for D_2 dopamine receptors than bromocriptine and possesses a long half-life, allowing for once- or twice-weekly administration. Cabergoline appears to be better tolerated than bromocriptine, and may be more effective in normalizing prolactin concentrations and restoring menses.[46] It is also effective in treating hyperprolactinemia in patients who are resistant to or intolerant of bromocriptine and in men and women with microprolactinomas and macroprolactinomas.[39,46] Given its favorable safety and efficacy profile and ease of administration, cabergoline has replaced bromocriptine as first-line therapy for the management of hyperprolactinemia.[39] Withdrawal of pergolide from the US market due to increased risk for valvular heart disease raised concerns about the safety of cabergoline. However, to date, cabergoline use in patients with hyperprolactinemia[47] or prolactinoma[48] has not been associated with clinically significant valvular heart disease.

Nonpharmacologic Therapy In a small number of patients who have failed or are intolerant of dopamine agonists, transsphenoidal adenomectomy may be necessary.[39] Surgical treatment is also considered in patients with nonprolactin-secreting tumors or macroprolactinomas that jeopardize the optic chiasm.[43] Nonetheless, surgical intervention does not reliably lead to long-term cure and may cause permanent complications.[40,42] Radiation therapy is reserved for failures of both pharmacologic therapy and surgery.[39] However, normalization of prolactin concentration with radiation therapy may take 20 years to show full benefit, and radiation-induced hypopituitarism may require lifelong hormone replacement.

▸ *Management of Hyperprolactinemia in Pregnancy*

Most women with hyperprolactinemia require dopamine agonist therapy to achieve regular ovulatory cycles and pregnancy. Because restoration of the ovulatory cycle may occur immediately after initiation of therapy, it is necessary to caution patients regarding their potential to become pregnant and ensure adequate contraception when beginning therapy.[43]

Overall, there is reassuring evidence that bromocriptine use during pregnancy does not increase fetal malformations, spontaneous abortions, preterm deliveries, or multiple births.[39,49] Although experience during pregnancy is limited, cabergoline does not appear to be teratogenic.[49] Despite these data, continuation of dopamine agonists during pregnancy is generally not recommended. KEY CONCEPT *Women who become pregnant while taking a dopamine agonist should discontinue treatment to minimize fetal exposure.*[39] *Because cabergoline has a prolonged*

Table 46–5

Comparison of Dopamine Agonists for Treatment of Hyperprolactemia[37,44]

	Bromocriptine (Parlodel)	Cabergoline
Starting dose	0.625–1.25 mg/day at bedtime	0.5 mg/week or 0.25 mg twice/week
Titrating dose	1.25 mg increments at 1-week interval	0.5 mg increment at 4-week intervals
Usually effective dose	2.5–15 mg/day	1–2 mg/week
Maximal dose	40 mg/day	4.5 mg/week
Dosing frequency	Two to three divided doses per day	Once or twice weekly
Dosage in hepatic insufficiency	May be required in acute hepatitis or cirrhosis; no guidelines are available	Dose reductions may be recommended for patients with severe hepatic failure (Child-Pugh scores of 10 or higher)
Dosage in renal failure	None	None
Adverse effects	Dizziness, headache, syncope, nausea, vomiting, GI cramps, orthostatic hypotension, nasal congestion	Similar but orthostatic hypotension less common
Cost	Moderately expensive	More expensive

GI, gastrointestinal.

Patient Encounter 2: Hyperprolactinemia: Medical History, Physical Examination, and Diagnostic Tests

A 30-year-old woman presented to primary care clinic 6 months ago with complaints of infrequent menstruation and infertility. Since she started treatment for hyperprolactinemia 5 months ago, she was excited to see return of her regular menses for several months until she realized her last menstrual period was 4 weeks ago.

PMH: None

FM: Mother has hypertension, father with high cholesterol

SH: Married, dental assistant; sexually active (occasional use of condoms)

Meds: Prenatal vitamin one tablet daily; cabergoline 1 mg tablet weekly; acetaminophen 325 mg one to two tablets as needed for menstrual cramps

ROS: Negative, other than in history of present illness

PE:

HEENT: Ophthalmic examination reveals normal visual acuity and fields. (–) goiter

VS: BP 120/65 mm Hg, P 80 beats/min, RR 19 breaths/min, T 37.1°C (98.8°F)

CV: RRR, normal S1, S2; no murmurs, rubs, or gallops

Breasts: (–) Galactorrhea with no abnormalities

Abd: Soft, nontender, nondistended; (+) bowel sounds; (–) hepatosplenomegaly

Rectal: Heme (–) stool

Labs: Electrolytes, renal and thyroid function, β-human chorionic gonadotropin (β-hCG) elevated at 6500 mIU/mL (6500 U/L)

Prolactin: Elevated prolactin at 89 ng/mL (89 mcg/L; 3870 pmol/L) 6 months ago; prolactin at 26 ng/ml (26 mcg/L; 1130 pmol/L) today

Imaging: MRI revealed a 5 mm pituitary tumor (6 months ago)

What signs and symptoms were suggestive of hyperprolactinemia in the patient?

What nonpharmacologic and pharmacologic treatment options are available for her at this time?

half-life, women who plan to become pregnant should discontinue the drug at least 1 month before planned conception.[44]

Microadenomas rarely cause complications during pregnancy. However, untreated macroprolactinomas carry about a 31% risk of tumor enlargement and potentially can jeopardize vision.[39] Therefore, monitor female patients with macroprolactinomas closely for the development of headache and visual impairments. Baseline and routine visual field examinations are essential. Evidence of abnormal visual fields may indicate tumor growth and should be followed by an MRI. If tumors enlarge, bromocriptine is the preferred choice over cabergoline because of greater experience with this drug during pregnancy.[39,49]

Patient Care Process: Hyperprolactinemia

Patient Assessment:

- Assess the patient's clinical signs and symptoms of hyperprolactinemia.
- Review the available diagnostic data to determine severity and exclude other common causes of hyperprolactinemia (see Table 46–4).
- Obtain a thorough medication history to exclude medication-induced hyperprolactinemia (see Table 46–4).

Therapy Evaluation:

- Determine the patient's plan regarding pregnancy because this influences treatment selection.
- Determine if drug therapy is indicated. Make sure the patient does not have any contraindications or allergies to drug therapies.
- Determine whether patient has prescription coverage.

Care Plan Development:

- Initiate the appropriate dopamine agonist at the lowest effective dose for management of hyperprolactinemia (see Table 46–5)
- Provide patient education regarding disease state, and nondrug and drug therapy:
    - Risk factors associated with hyperprolactinemia
    - Potential disadvantages, safety and effectiveness of existing dopamine agonist therapy
    - Potential disadvantages, safety and effectiveness of surgery and radiation treatment
    - Importance of adherence to therapy
    - Potential for adverse effects or long-term complications

Follow-up Evaluation:

- Assess response and adverse effects of dopamine agonists. When appropriate, be sure to make dose adjustments (see Table 46–5).
- If the prolactin concentration remains normal for 2 years, reassess the need to continue treatment.

▸ *Outcome Evaluation*

- Assess patients for tolerability to dopamine agonists.
- Monitor clinical symptoms associated with hyperprolactinemia every month for the first 3 months to assess therapeutic efficacy and assist with dose titration.
- Evaluate the patient for symptoms, such as headache, visual disturbances, menstrual cycles in women, and sexual function in men, to assess clinical response to therapy.[39]
- When the prolactin concentration is normalized and clinical symptoms of hyperprolactinemia have resolved, monitor prolactin concentration every 6 to 12 months.[40]
- If the prolactin concentration is well controlled with dopamine agonist therapy for 2 years with significant tumor reduction, gradually taper therapy to the lowest effective dose or consider discontinuing therapy.[39] Check prolactin concentration after each dose reduction.
- If the prolactin concentrations remain unchanged for 1 year at the reduced dose, dopamine agonist therapy may be discontinued.
- It is essential to monitor prolactin concentration every 6 months or annually to detect the possibility of permanent remission of pituitary disease.[40]
- The need to continue dopamine agonists in postmenopausal women with microprolactinomas must be reassessed because these patients have a higher probability of maintaining normal prolactin concentrations after treatment is discontinued.[38]
- In patients with macroprolactinomas, monitor visual field at baseline and repeat the test 1 month after initiation of a dopamine agonist.
- Repeat the MRI in 1 year after initiating therapy or in 3 months in patient with macroprolactinoma or if an increase in symptoms or rise in prolactin concentration suggests the presence of tumor growth.[39]
- Discontinuation of therapy in patients with macroprolactinomas usually leads to tumor regrowth and recurrence of hyperprolactinemia. This decision warrants careful consideration.

Abbreviations Introduced in This chapter

AACE	American Association of Clinical Endocrinologists
ACTH	Adrenocorticotropic hormone or corticotropin
ADH	Antidiuretic hormone or vasopressin
β-hCG	β-Human chorionic gonadotropin
BMI	Body mass index
CRH	Corticotropin-releasing hormone
CT	Computed tomography
CYP3A4	Cytochrome P-450 subfamily IIIA polypeptide 4
DEXA	Dual-energy x-ray absorptiometry
FSH	Follicle-stimulating hormone
FT_4	Free T_4
GABA	γ-Aminobutyric acid
GH	Growth hormone or somatotropin
GHIH	Growth hormone–inhibiting hormone or somatostatin
GHRH	Growth hormone–releasing hormone
GI	Gastrointestinal
GnRH	Gonadotropin-releasing hormone
$HgbA_{1c}$	Glycated hemoglobin A_{1c}
IGF	Insulin-like growth factor
IGF-I	Insulin-like growth factor-I
IGF-II	Insulin-like growth factor-II
IGFBP-3	Insulin-like growth factor-bind protein-3
IM	Intramuscular
ITT	Insulin tolerance test
LAR	Long-acting release
LH	Luteinizing hormone
LHRH	Luteinizing hormone–releasing hormone
MRI	Magnetic resonance imaging
MSH	Melanocyte-stimulating hormone
OGTT	Oral glucose tolerance test
PRH	Prolactin-releasing hormone
SAGhE	Safety and Appropriateness of Growth hormone treatments in Europe
SC	Subcutaneous
SR	Slow release
SRL	Somatostatin receptor ligan
T_3	Triiodothyronine
T_4	Thyroxine
TRH	Thyrotropin-releasing hormone
TSH	Thyroid-stimulating hormone or thyrotropin
ULN	Upper limit of normal

REFERENCES

1. Muller EE, Locatelli V, Cocchi D. Neuroendocrine control of growth hormone secretion. Physiol Rev. 1999;79:511–607.
2. Le Roith D, Bondy C, Yakar S, et al. The somatomedin hypothesis: 2001. Endocr Rev. 2001;22:53–74.
3. Katznelson L, Atkinson JL, Cook DM, et al. American Association of Clinical Endocrinologists medical guidelines for clinical practice for the diagnosis and treatment of acromegaly—2011 update. Endocr Pract. 2011;17 Suppl 4:1–44.
4. Melmed S, Casanueva FF, Klibanski A, et al. A consensus on the diagnosis and treatment of acromegaly complications. Pituitary. 2013;16:294–302.
5. Jordan JK, Sheehan AH, Yanovski JA, Calis KA. Pituitary Gland Disorders. In: DiPiro JT, Talbert RL, Yee GC, et al, eds. Pharmacotherapy: A Pathophysiologic Approach. 9th ed. New York City: McGraw-Hill; 2014:1237–1252.
6. Jallad RS, Bronstein MD. The place of medical treatment of acromegaly: Current status and perspectives. Expert Opin Pharmacother. 2013;14:1001–1015.
7. Giustina A, Chanson P, Kleinberg D, et al. Expert consensus document: A consensus on the medical treatment of acromegaly. Nat Rev Endocrinol 2014;10:243–248.
8. AACE Medical Guidelines for Clinical Practice for the diagnosis and treatment of acromegaly. Endocr Pract. 2004;10:213–225.
9. Giustina A, Mazziotti G, Torri V, et al. Meta-analysis on the effects of octreotide on tumor mass in acromegaly. PLoS One. 2012;7:e36411.
10. Carmichael JD, Bonert VS, Nuno M, et al. Acromegaly clinical trial methodology impact on reported biochemical efficacy rates of somatostatin receptor ligand treatments: a meta-analysis. J Clin Endocrinol Metab. 2014;99:1825–1833.
11. Cozzi R, Montini M, Attanasio R, et al. Primary treatment of acromegaly with octreotide LAR: A long-term (up to nine years) prospective study of its efficacy in the control of disease activity and tumor shrinkage. J Clin Endocrinol Metab. 2006;91: 1397–1403.
12. Ronchi CL, Varca V, Beck-Peccoz P, et al. Comparison between six-year therapy with long-acting somatostatin analogs and successful surgery in acromegaly: Effects on cardiovascular risk factors. J Clin Endocrinol Metab. 2006;91:121–128.

13. Caron PJ, Bevan JS, Petersenn S, et al. Tumor shrinkage with lanreotide Autogel 120 mg as primary therapy in acromegaly: Results of a prospective multicenter clinical trial. J Clin Endocrinol Metab. 2014;99:1282–1290.
14. van der Lely AJ, Biller BM, Brue T, et al. Long-term safety of pegvisomant in patients with acromegaly: Comprehensive review of 1288 subjects in ACROSTUDY. J Clin Endocrinol Metab. 2012;97:1589–1597.
15. Feenstra J, de Herder WW, ten Have SM, et al. Combined therapy with somatostatin analogues and weekly pegvisomant in active acromegaly. Lancet. 2005;365:1644–1646.
16. Jorgensen JO, Feldt-Rasmussen U, Frystyk J, et al. Cotreatment of acromegaly with a somatostatin analog and a growth hormone receptor antagonist. J Clin Endocrinol Metab. 2005;90: 5627–5631.
17. Neggers SJ, van Aken MO, Janssen JA, et al. Long-term efficacy and safety of combined treatment of somatostatin analogs and pegvisomant in acromegaly. J Clin Endocrinol Metab. 2007;92: 4598–4601.
18. Neggers SJ, de Herder WW, Janssen JA, et al. Combined treatment for acromegaly with long-acting somatostatin analogs and pegvisomant: Long-term safety for up to 4.5 years (median 2.2 years) of follow-up in 86 patients. Eur J Endocrinol. 2009; 160:529–533.
19. Maione L, Garcia C, Bouchachi A, et al. No evidence of a detrimental effect of cabergoline therapy on cardiac valves in patients with acromegaly. J Clin Endocrinol Metab. 2012;97: E1714–E1719.
20. Giustina A, Chanson P, Bronstein MD, et al. A consensus on criteria for cure of acromegaly. J Clin Endocrinol Metab. 2010; 95:3141–3148.
21. Biochemical assessment and long-term monitoring in patients with acromegaly: Statement from a joint consensus conference of the Growth Hormone Research Society and the Pituitary Society. J Clin Endocrinol Metab. 2004;89:3099–3102.
22. Gharib H, Cook DM, Saenger PH, et al. American Association of Clinical Endocrinologists medical guidelines for clinical practice for growth hormone use in adults and children—2003 update. Endocr Pract. 2003;9:64–76.
23. Gums JG, Anderson SD. Hypothalamic, pituitary, and adrenal disorders. In: Tisdale JE, Miller DA, eds. Drug-Induced Diseases: Prevention, Detection, and Management. 2nd ed. Bethesda, Maryland: American Society of Health-System Pharmacists; 2010:605–628.
24. Molitch ME, Clemmons DR, Malozowski S, et al. Evaluation and treatment of adult growth hormone deficiency: An Endocrine Society clinical practice guideline. J Clin Endocrinol Metab. 2011;96:1587–1609.
25. Federico G, Street ME, Maghnie M, et al. Assessment of serum IGF-I concentrations in the diagnosis of isolated childhood-onset GH deficiency: A proposal of the Italian Society for Pediatric Endocrinology and Diabetes (SIEDP/ISPED). J Endocrinol Invest. 2006;29:732–737.
26. Ho KK. Consensus guidelines for the diagnosis and treatment of adults with GH deficiency II: A statement of the GH Research Society in association with the European Society for Pediatric Endocrinology, Lawson Wilkins Society, European Society of Endocrinology, Japan Endocrine Society, and Endocrine Society of Australia. Eur J Endocrinol. 2007;157:695–700.
27. Cummings DE, Merriam GR. Growth hormone therapy in adults. Annu Rev Med. 2003;54:513–533.
28. Gasco V, Prodam F, Grottoli S, et al. GH therapy in adult GH deficiency: A review of treatment schedules and the evidence for low starting doses. Eur J Endocrinol. 2013;168:R55–R66.
29. Cook DM, Yuen KC, Biller BM, et al. American Association of Clinical Endocrinologists medical guidelines for clinical practice for growth hormone use in growth hormone-deficient adults and transition patients - 2009 update. Endocr Pract. 2009;15 Suppl 2:1–29.
30. Wilson TA, Rose SR, Cohen P, et al. Update of guidelines for the use of growth hormone in children: The Lawson Wilkins Pediatric Endocrinology Society Drug and Therapeutics Committee. J Pediatr. 2003;143:415–421.
31. Nilsson AG, Svensson J, Johannsson G. Management of growth hormone deficiency in adults. Growth Horm IGF Res. 2007;17:441–462.
32. Gotherstrom G, Bengtsson BA, Bosaeus I, et al. A 10-year, prospective study of the metabolic effects of growth hormone replacement in adults. J Clin Endocrinol Metab. 2007;92: 1442–1445.
33. Appelman-Dijkstra NM, Claessen KM, Roelfsema F, et al. Long-term effects of recombinant human GH replacement in adults with GH deficiency: A systematic review. Eur J Endocrinol. 2013;169:R1–R14.
34. Casanueva FF, Castro AI, Micic D, et al. New guidelines for the diagnosis of growth hormone deficiency in adults. Horm Res. 2009;71 Suppl 1:112–115.
35. Filipsson H, Johannsson G. GH replacement in adults: interactions with other pituitary hormone deficiencies and replacement therapies. Eur J Endocrinol. 2009;161 Suppl 1:S85–S95.
36. Rosenfeld RG, Cohen P, Robison LL, et al. Long-term surveillance of growth hormone therapy. J Clin Endocrinol Metab. 2012; 97:68–72.
37. Crosignani PG. Current treatment issues in female hyperprolactinaemia. Eur J Obstet Gynecol Reprod Biol. 2006; 125: 152–164.
38. Brue T, Delemer B. Diagnosis and management of hyperprolactinemia: Expert consensus—French Society of Endocrinology. Ann Endocrinol. 2007;68:58–64.
39. Melmed S, Casanueva FF, Hoffman AR, et al. Diagnosis and treatment of hyperprolactinemia: An Endocrine Society clinical practice guideline. J Clin Endocrinol Metab. 2011;96: 273–288.
40. Serri O, Chik CL, Ur E, Ezzat S. Diagnosis and management of hyperprolactinemia. CMAJ. 2003;169:575–581.
41. Faje A, Nachtigall L. Current treatment options for hyperprolactinemia. Expert Opin Pharmacother. 2013;14: 1611–1625.
42. Wang AT, Mullan RJ, Lane MA, et al. Treatment of hyperprolactinemia: A systematic review and meta-analysis. Syst Rev. 2012;1:33.
43. Mann WA. Treatment for prolactinomas and hyperprolactinaemia: A lifetime approach. Eur J Clin Invest. 2011;41: 334–342.
44. Bankowski BJ, Zacur HA. Dopamine agonist therapy for hyperprolactinemia. Clin Obstet Gynecol. 2003;46:349–362.
45. Darwish AM, Farah E, Gadallah WA, Mohammad, II. Superiority of newly developed vaginal suppositories over vaginal use of commercial bromocriptine tablets: A randomized controlled clinical trial. Reprod Sci. 2007;14:280–285.
46. dos Santos Nunes V, El Dib R, Boguszewski CL, Nogueira CR. Cabergoline versus bromocriptine in the treatment of hyperprolactinemia: A systematic review of randomized controlled trials and meta-analysis. Pituitary. 2011;14:259–265.
47. Steffensen C, Maegbaek ML, Laurberg P, et al. Heart valve disease among patients with hyperprolactinemia: A nationwide population-based cohort study. J Clin Endocrinol Metab. 2012;97:1629–1634.
48. Auriemma RS, Pivonello R, Perone Y, et al. Safety of long-term treatment with cabergoline on cardiac valve disease in patients with prolactinomas. Eur J Endocrinol. 2013;169:359–366.
49. Molitch ME. Prolactinoma in pregnancy. Best Pract Res Clin Endocrinol Metab. 2011;25:885–896.

47 Pregnancy and Lactation: Therapeutic Considerations

Ema Ferreira, Évelyne Rey, Caroline Morin, and Katherine Theriault

LEARNING OBJECTIVES

Upon completion of the chapter, the reader will be able to:

1. Explain the principles of embryology and teratology.
2. Identify known teratogens and drugs of concern during lactation.
3. Compare the main sources of drug information relevant to pregnancy and lactation.
4. Evaluate the risks of a drug when taken during pregnancy or lactation.
5. Apply a systematic approach to counseling on the use of drugs during pregnancy and lactation.
6. Recommend the appropriate dose of folic acid to prevent congenital anomalies.
7. Describe physiologic changes during pregnancy and their impact on pharmacokinetics.
8. Choose an appropriate treatment for common conditions in a pregnant or lactating woman.

EPIDEMIOLOGY AND ETIOLOGY

Medication Use During Pregnancy

Most women take at least one medication during their pregnancy (average number of two to four, vitamins and minerals excluded).[1] The most common types of medications used include vitamins and minerals, allergy medication, analgesics, antacids, antibiotics, antiemetics, laxatives, asthma medication, cold and flu remedies, levothyroxine, and progesterone.[1,2]

The safety profile of some medications taken during pregnancy is difficult to assess making it difficult to balance risks and benefits of treatment.

▸ *Background Risks of Anomalies in Pregnancy*

Table 47–1 describes the baseline risks of congenital anomalies and some obstetrical complications observed in the general population—essential information to evaluate risks associated with medication use and to counsel pregnant women.

▸ *Causes of Congenital Anomalies*

KEY CONCEPT *Although the risk of drug-induced teratogenicity is of concern, the actual risk of birth defects from most drug exposures is small.* Medications are associated with less than 1% of all congenital anomalies, although they may play a more important role through interaction with genetic factors. KEY CONCEPT *Health professionals should know which medications have teratogenic risk.* It is important to evaluate and manage drug use in pregnant women and women planning a pregnancy.

Other causes of anomalies include genetic causes in 25 % of cases (inherited disease, gene mutation, chromosomal disorder), maternal infections (1%), maternal conditions (1%–3%; eg, pregestational diabetes), multifactorial heredity (23%–50%), and unknown causes (34%–43%).[5] Theoretical concerns regarding paternal exposure to genotoxic medication are reported, but currently no medication taken by a man has been proven teratogenic.[6]

PATHOPHYSIOLOGY

Age of Pregnancy

The age of pregnancy can be defined as gestational or postconceptional age (PCA).[6] *Gestational age* (GA) is the term used in clinical practice. It is calculated from the first day of the last menstruation or by ultrasound dating.

PCA, calculated from the day of conception, is 14 days shorter than GA if the menstrual cycle is 28 days. Some references in the field of teratology and embryology refer to PCA to describe stages of pregnancy.

Principles of Embryology

Pregnancy can be divided into three development phases: implantation and predifferentiation, organogenesis (or embryogenesis), and fetogenesis. Table 47–2 describes these phases and possible drug effects if taken during these phases, and Figure 47–1 illustrates the critical periods of human in utero development. KEY CONCEPT *The risk of birth defects is usually higher during organogenesis.*

▸ *Teratogens*

A teratogen is an exogenous agent that can modify normal embryonic or fetal development.[5] Teratogenicity can manifest as structural anomalies, functional deficit, cancer, growth retardation, neurologic impairment, or death (spontaneous abortion, stillbirth).

In utero exposure to medication at the end of the pregnancy can also lead to transient neonatal complications, such as withdrawal or side effects (eg, opioids, selective serotonin reuptake inhibitors, antipsychotics, lithium).[6–8]

Patient Encounter, Part 1

A 30-year-old woman comes to your office after a positive urine pregnancy test. You collect the following data:

Estimated Gestational Age: 5 weeks, regular menstrual cycles of 28 days

PMH: Bipolar disorder, hypothyroidism, one spontaneous abortion

FH: Diabetes, hypothyroidism, hypercholesterolemia

SH: Unemployed; cigarettes, one-half pack daily; no alcohol or illicit substances

Meds: Lithium 900 mg orally at bedtime; quetiapine 50 mg orally at bedtime; levothyroxine 50 mcg orally in the morning; all discontinued 1 week ago

Allergy: Dust mites

ROS: Morning nausea; tiredness

VS: Wt 198 lb (90 kg)/Ht 63 in (160 cm), BP 110/72 mm Hg, P 70 beats/min, RR 12 breaths/min; slight enlargement of thyroid

How will you confirm gestational age?

What prenatal work up would you perform at this time?

What is the appropriate counseling at this time?

What are the risks of drugs taken in the first weeks of pregnancy? What resources will you use to find the appropriate information?

What do you recommend for her pharmacologic treatment?

Although we use the term *teratogen* in this chapter, we agree with some authors who prefer to use instead *teratogenic exposure. Teratogenic exposure* considers level (dose) and timing of exposure during pregnancy to determine whether it could lead to a higher risk of a specific malformation.[9]

Criteria have been proposed to determine whether a causal relationship between congenital anomalies and a medication is plausible (teratogenic effect).[9] Exposure to the medication must have happened during the critical period of development of the organ for which a malformation is noticed (see Figure 47–1). Also, a pattern of anomaly or a specific syndrome must be present, and the observed effects must be reproducible in at least two studies conducted in different populations. A rare anomaly associated with a rare exposure is also indicative of a teratogenic effect (eg, ear anomalies and isotretinoin).

Other criteria, listed below, are considered (the probability of finding an association increases with the number of criteria):

- Strength of the association
- Same effects observed in animal studies
- Biological plausibility based on pharmacologic effect
- Higher incidence of the anomaly in the population with the period of use of the medication (eg, thalidomide and limb anomalies)
- Dose–response relationship

With these criteria, there are approximately 30 medications or classes of medications that are considered teratogens (Table 47–3). Drugs not on this list are not necessarily safe to use during pregnancy. We must be careful not to interpret a lack of data as an absence of risk. If a medication is on this list, it does not mean that it is contraindicated during pregnancy. Severity and occurrence of malformations vary from one agent to another; some are always contraindicated, but some others can be used when benefits outweigh potential risks.

Some medications associated with a higher risk of malformation are not included in Table 47–3 since they do not meet all the teratogenicity criteria. For example, benzodiazepines (oral cleft), lamotrigine and topiramate (oral clefts), paroxetine (cardiac septal anomalies), pseudoephedrine (gastroschisis).

Table 47–1

Occurrence of Some Obstetrical Complications and Risk of Congenital Anomalies in the General Population

	Risk of Occurrence in Population (%)
Spontaneous abortion/miscarriage (pregnancy loss that occurs after the pregnancy is known and before 20 weeks of GA; risk increases with higher maternal age)	10–15
Congenital anomalies (percentage of live births):	
• Minor malformations	14
• Major malformations at birth	3
• Major malformations at 2 years old	6
Preterm birth (< 37 completed weeks gestation)*	11.5
Low birth weight (< 2500 g)[a]	8.0

[a]United States data from 2012

GA, gestational age.

Data from Refs. 3, 4, and 5.

RISK EVALUATION

Desired Outcomes

The goal of drug use during pregnancy and lactation is to treat maternal or fetal conditions effectively when necessary while minimizing risk to the developing embryo/fetus or the neonate.

Medication and Pregnancy

▶ *Data Published on Medication Safety During Pregnancy*

Classical randomized controlled trials are usually not available to evaluate the safety of medications used during pregnancy and lactation. Most available data on drug safety during pregnancy come from postmarketing reports.

Animal studies, now mandatory before marketing a medication, can identify high-risk medications and prevent congenital anomalies. However, they must be interpreted with great caution because of many limitations; the major ones are that different species do not share the same pharmacodynamics and pharmacokinetics for the same medication, and usually much higher doses than those used in clinical settings are tested.[11]

Case reports and case series provide the first published data on the use of medications during pregnancy. A causal relationship between a single case report and an anomaly cannot usually be established unless a rare anomaly is repeatedly associated with the use of a specific medication.

Cohort studies and company registries seek to compare the risks observed after exposure to a medication with the risk observed in a control group or in the general population. When

Table 47–2

Phases of Embryonic and Fetal Development

Phase of Development	Stage of Pregnancy[a]	Development Description	Potential Complications
Implantation and predifferentiation (all-or-none period)	0–14 days after conception (14–28 days after LMP)	Very little contact between the blastocyst and the mother's blood Cells are pluripotent, capacity to repair a damage remains Cells are fragile at this moment. If too many are destroyed, a miscarriage will occur before the pregnancy is detected	Spontaneous abortion; Even if stopped during this period, long half-life drugs could cause organogenesis problems
Organogenesis (embryogenesis)	From day 14 until the 9th week after conception (From day 28 until the 11th week after LMP)	Organs are formed; most critical period for structural anomalies Organs are formed at different times; different period of sensitivity for each organ Refer to Figure 47–1 for the time frame of organ formation	Major or minor structural anomalies; Spontaneous abortion
Fetogenesis	After the organogenesis and until birth	The fetus grows Organs begin to function (eg, glomerular filtration) Active cell growth, proliferation, and migration (eg, CNS)	Fetal growth retardation; functional deficit (eg, renal insufficiency), neurologic impairment; spontaneous abortion, stillbirth;neonatal complications

[a]Stage of pregnancy based on a menstrual cycle of 28 days
LMP, last menstrual period; CNS, central nervous system
Data from Refs. 5 and 6.

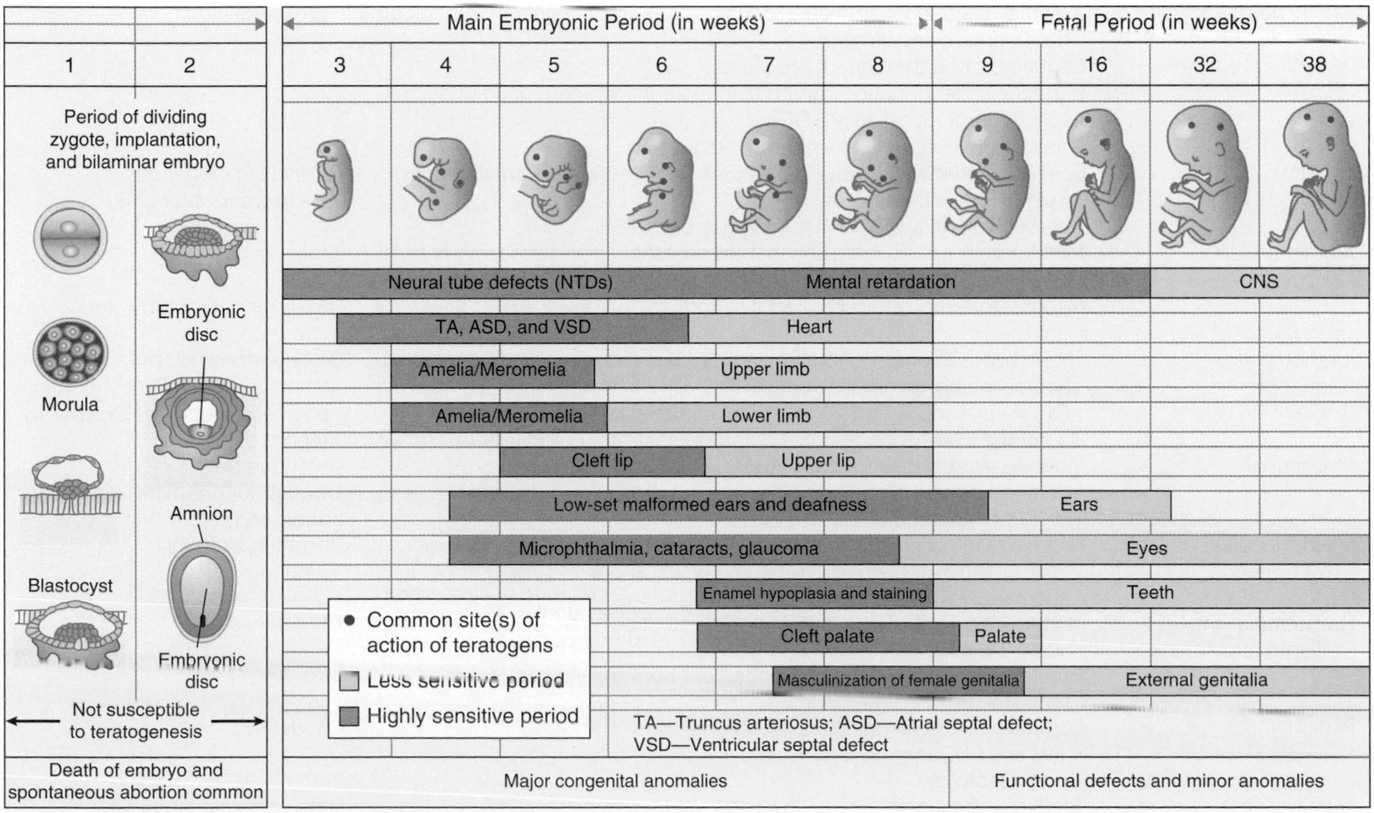

FIGURE 47–1. Embryonic and fetal development. The horizontal bars represent potential sensitivity to teratogens. The colored areas represent the more critical times. Embryonic period is in postconceptional weeks. (Reprinted with permission from Moore KL. The Developing Human. New York: Elsevier, p. 976: copyright 1974.)

Table 47–3

Medications with Proven Teratogenic Effects in Humans

Drug or Drug Class	Teratogenic Effects	Critical Period[a]
Alkylating agents	Malformations of many different organs	Organogenesis
Amiodarone	Transitory hypothyroidism (17%, goiter in some cases) or transitory hyperthyroidism	From 12th week after LMP
Androgens (danazol, testosterone)	Masculinization of genital organs in female fetus	From 9th week after LMP
Angiotensin converting enzyme inhibitors	Renal failure, anuria, oligohydramnios, pulmonary hypoplasia, intrauterine growth restriction, limbs contracture, skull hypoplasia	After the first trimester
Angiotensin II receptor antagonists	Contraindicated after first trimester	
Anticonvulsants (first generation) • Carbamazepine • Phenytoin • Phenobarbital • Valproic acid, divalproex	NTDs (carbamazepine and valproic acid); oral cleft, skeletal, urogenital, craniofacial, digital, and cardiac malformations; microcephalia Major malformations: 5%–10% depending on the agent used (10%–15% for valproic acid). Valproic acid: abnormal neurologic development	Organogenesis for structural anomalies Valproic acid : whole pregnancy for neurologic impairment
Corticosteroids (systemic)	Oral cleft (risk of 3–4/1000 vs 1/1000 in general population)	Organogenesis (most critical period for palate formation between 8 and 11 weeks after LMP)
Diethylstilbestrol	Girls: Cervical or vaginal adenocarcinoma, incidence about 1/1000 exposures. Structural genital anomalies (eg, of cervix, vagina) Boys: Genital anomalies, spermatogenesis anomalies	First and second trimesters
Fluconazole high doses	Skeletal and craniofacial malformations, cleft palate, cardiac anomaly (with chronic dose > 400 mg/day; not reported with 150-mg single dose)	Not defined, but cases are reported where exposure was for most parts of pregnancy
Iodine (supraphysiologic dosage)	Hypothyroidism, goiter	From 12th week after LMP
Isotretinoin, acitretin, and high dose of vitamin A (> 10,000 IU/day)	Spontaneous abortion, CNS, skull, eyes and ears malformations, micrognathia, oral cleft, cardiac malformations, thymus anomalies, mental retardation: estimated at 25%–30% (may be higher for neurologic development impairment) Contraindicated throughout pregnancy Isotretinoin: discontinue 1 month before pregnancy, prescribed under a special program called iPLEDGE Acitretin: discontinue 3 years before pregnancy	Organogenesis (risk of teratogenic effect after organogenesis not excluded)
Lithium	Cardiac malformations: risk of 0.9%–6.8% (higher risks from small studies) (compare to a baseline risk of ~1%) Includes Ebstein's anomaly: risk estimated at 0.05%–0.1%	Cardiac organogenesis (5–10 weeks after LMP)
Methimazole/ propylthiouracil	Methimazole: aplasia cutis, choanal atresia, esophageal atresia, minor facial anomalies, growth delay; risk probably low Methimazole/propylthiouracil: fetal hypothyroidism in 1%–5% of newborns, goiter	Organogenesis Second and third trimesters
Methotrexate, aminopterine	Spontaneous abortion, CNS and cranial malformations (large fontanelles, hydrocephalia, incomplete cranial ossification, craniosynostosis), oral cleft, ear, skeletal and limb malformations, mental retardation Do not use in pregnancy; stop 1 to 3 months before pregnancy	Organogenesis (between 6 and 8 weeks after LMP for structural anomalies but some exceptions reported)
Misoprostol	Moebius syndrome ± limb anomalies ± CNS anomalies Abortion, preterm birth	Organogenesis Throughout pregnancy for abortion/preterm birth
Mycophenolate mofetil, mycophenolic acid	Anomalies including ear anomalies (with or without ear canal), oral cleft, micrognathia; ophtalmic, cardiac and digital anomalies (risk of structural anomalies estimated from 20%–25%); spontaneous abortion (30%–50%)	Uncertain, probably organogenesis
Nonsteroidal anti-inflammatory drugs	In utero closure of ductus arteriosus (constriction is rare before 27 weeks, 50%–70% at 32 weeks (GA) and neonatal pulmonary hypertension Renal toxicity possible after prolonged use from second half of second trimester	Third trimester
Penicillamine	Cutis laxa Joints and CNS anomalies Risk probably low	Not defined
Tetracyclines	Teeth discoloration	From 16 weeks after LMP

(Continued)

Table 47–3

Medications with Proven Teratogenic Effects in Humans (*Continued*)

Drug or Drug Class	Teratogenic Effects	Critical Period[a]
Thalidomide	Limb anomalies (amelia, phocomelia) Cardiac, urogenital, gastrointestinal, and ear malformations Risk of 20%–50 % Prescribed under a special program called STEPS (System for Thalidomide Education and Prescribing Safety)	34–50 days after LMP
Trimethoprim	Cardiac and urogenital malformations, neural tube defects, oral cleft; overall risk probably < 6%	Organogenesis
Warfarin/acenocoumarol	Before 6 weeks: no higher risk of anomaly Taken between 6 and 12 weeks: nasal hypoplasia, epiphysis dysplasia, vertebral malformations, rarely ophtalmic anomalies, scoliosis, hearing loss; overall risk estimated between 6% and 10%. After 12 weeks after LMP: more rarely, heterogeneous CNS anomalies	Between weeks 6 and 12 after LMP

[a]Stages of pregnancy in this table are calculated after last menstrual period (gestational age) and not after conception to be more clinically useful.

CNS, central nervous system; LMP, last menstrual period; NTD, neural tube defect.

Data from Refs. 6, 7, 9, and 10.

studying structural anomalies, it is important to select women exposed to medication during organogenesis. Cohort studies usually are not powerful enough to assess the risk associated with rare anomalies. When a signal of association between an anomaly and a drug exposure is observed, a case-control study, which has more power to detect rare anomalies, can be conducted to clarify the relationship. When several studies have been published using very similar methodologies, meta-analyses can be conducted to yield higher statistical power.[11]

▸ *Sources of Information on the Use of Drugs During Pregnancy and Lactation*

Some specialized information sources provide data on the use of medications during pregnancy and lactation (Table 47–4).

The 1979 Food and Drug Administration (FDA) regulations establishing pregnancy categories for drugs (A, B, C, D, and X) are well known to health care providers. This categorization has long been criticized by experts who recommend instead relying on other information sources.[12] They assert that the categories are too simplistic, can lead to a risk misperception, and do not take into account important information such as expected incidence, severity of anomalies, degree of risk, gestational timing of exposure, and route of administration.[12] In May 2008, the FDA proposed that the categories be removed and replaced by a short statement including description and risk of fetal defects, sources of data (animal or human), comparison with population baseline risk of birth defects, and the relationship with the dosage. An equivalent section for drug use during lactation will be inserted.[12] This new regulation is in the process of being implemented. Meanwhile, clinicians should rely on other information sources to evaluate the risk of a medication during pregnancy.

▸ *Communication of Information*

Communication of data on medication use during pregnancy can be challenging[13]:

- Data may be limited or contradictory.
- Taking medications during pregnancy is a source of anxiety.
- Pregnant women tend to overestimate their risk of an anomaly associated with medication use and to underestimate their risk associated with undertreating their condition.
- Most people do not properly understand numbers and probability.

The objective is to give precise data that will help the patient make an informed decision for her health and the health of her

Table 47–4

Examples of Sources of Information on Drug Use in Pregnancy and Lactation

Books

- Briggs GG, Freeman RK, Yaffe SJ. Drugs in Pregnancy and Lactation: A Reference Guide to Fetal and Neonatal Risk, 10th ed. Philadelphia: Lippincott Williams & Wilkins, 2014.
- Schaefer C, Peters PWJ, Miller RK. Drugs During Pregnancy and Lactation, Treatment Options and Risk Assessment, 3rd ed. Amsterdam: Elsevier, 2014.
- Hale TW. Medications and Mother's Milk, 16th ed. Amarillo, TX: Hale Publishing, L.P., 2014.

Databases

- Reprotox: www.reprotox.org
- Teris: http://depts.washington.edu/terisweb/teris/

Websites/Applications

- www.mothertobaby.org
- www.motherisk.org
- www.marchofdimes.com
- www.cdc.gov
- www.fda.gov
- www.pubmed.com
- List of pregnancy registries: http://www.fda.gov/scienceresearch/specialtopics/womenshealthresearch/
- Lactmed: http://toxnet.nlm.nih.gov/cgi-bin/sis/htmlgen?LACT

Teratology Information Service

- Organization of Teratology Information Specialists (OTIS): Go to *www.mothertobaby.org* to find your local Teratogen Information Service, or call National Toll-Free Number: (866) 626-6847

baby. Unconfirmed hypotheses should not be communicated. Information should include a well-grounded assessment of risks, including baseline risks in the general population, risks associated with the medication, and risks of not treating the disease during pregnancy.[11]

When discussing numbers (eg, percentages, probabilities), some tips to facilitate effective risk communication are[13]:

- Use absolute risks instead of relative risks.
- Use negatively and positively framed information at the same time (eg, 3% chance of having a malformed child; 97% chance of having a normal child).
- Use the same denominator when discussing probabilities.

Finally, to determine a woman's risk of birth defects, obtain good medical, obstetrical, and pharmacotherapeutic histories (including over-the-counter medications and natural health products) and take into account exposures to alcohol, tobacco, and other recreational drugs.[13]

▶ *Preconception Care*

Adverse pregnancy outcomes, including prematurity, low birth weight, and birth defects, are major health concerns. One contributing factor to adverse outcomes is the late start in prenatal care, which can delay the identification and modification of risk factors that can affect pregnancy outcomes. Strategies to improve pregnancy outcomes include identifying and treating nutritional deficiencies and disorders, taking folic acid, avoiding alcohol and substance abuse, smoking cessation, optimizing the management of chronic illnesses and genetic disorders (eg, diabetes, epilepsy, hypertension, maternal phenylketonuria), screening for infections (eg, human immunodeficiency virus, sexually transmitted infections), appropriate vaccination, pregnancy planning, and reaching a healthy weight.[14]

▶ *Folic Acid*

Approximately 1 in every 1000 pregnancies is affected by a neural tube defect (NTD).[15] Data indicate that multivitamins containing folic acid reduce NTD and other congenital anomalies including oral clefts and cardiovascular, limb, and urinary malformations.[16] KEY CONCEPT *All women of childbearing age should be counseled on the appropriate dose of folic acid to prevent congenital anomalies.* The American College of Obstetricians and Gynecologists (ACOG) and the US Preventive Services Task Force recommend that all women of childbearing age take 0.4 to 0.8 mg of folic acid daily, beginning 1 month before pregnancy and through the first 2 to 3 months.[15] Women at higher risk of NTD (eg, previous child or a first-, second-, or third-degree relative with a NTD, those with prepregnancy diabetes, those with epilepsy taking carbamazepine or valproic acid) should take 4 mg of folic acid per day.[15]

▶ *Iron Supplements*

Anemia during pregnancy is defined as a hemoglobin level less than 11 g/dL (110 g/L; 6.83 mmol/L) during the first and third trimesters and less than 10.5 g/dL (105 g/L; 6.52 mmol/L) during the second trimester.[17] Maternal symptoms of anemia include fatigue, palpitations, and decreased resistance to exercise and infections. Fetal risks are prematurity, low birth weight, and perinatal death. All pregnant women should be screened for anemia, and those with iron deficiency should be treated with oral iron preparations in addition to prenatal vitamins.[17] Iron supplementation decreases the prevalence of maternal anemia at delivery. It is unclear whether supplementing nonanemic pregnant women will improve perinatal outcomes.[17]

▶ *Impact of Physiologic Changes During Pregnancy on Pharmacokinetics*

Absorption Drug absorption is affected in several ways during pregnancy. Decreased gastrointestinal transit can delay drug peak effect, prolonging the time of contact of drugs with the intestinal mucosa, and possibly enhancing absorption of certain drugs. Higher gastric pH may affect absorption of weak bases or acids. Skin, tissue, and lung absorption might also be increased by physiologic changes during pregnancy.[18]

Distribution Volume of distribution increases for most drugs during pregnancy due to plasma volume expansion and the presence of amniotic fluid, the placenta, and the fetus. This results in a decrease in maximal concentrations of drugs. In addition, hypoalbuminemia and decreased protein binding increases free fraction of some medications.[18]

Metabolism During pregnancy, the activity of some isoenzymes is increased (eg, CYP3A4, CYP2A6, CYP2D6, CYP2C9), while activity of others is decreased (eg, CYP1A2, CYP2C19). Net impact on drug effect is unpredictable since there is a wide interindividual variability, and some drugs are metabolized by several isoenzymes.[18]

Renal Elimination Renal blood flow and glomerular filtration increase significantly during pregnancy. The impact of this is more important for drugs that are eliminated in the urine which results in a decrease in their half-lives.

Table 47–5 shows clinical recommendations based on pharmacokinetic changes during pregnancy for several drugs.[6,18]

Medication and Lactation

According to the 2012 policy statement from the American Academy of Pediatrics (AAP), mothers should breast-feed exclusively for 6 months and continue for 1 year if possible. Approximately 75% of mothers initiate breast-feeding at birth. However, exclusive breast-feeding drops to 17% at 6 months, as many new mothers supplement breast-feeding with other foods or quit entirely by this point.[19]

▶ *Drug Transfer into Breast Milk*

To study drug effects, breast-fed infant's serum drug levels could be measured to evaluate safety; however, these data are often unavailable. In most instances, the approximate quantity of drug ingested by the breast-fed infant is estimated using published measured drug concentrations in breast milk. With these data, the percentage of pediatric dose or the relative infant dose (percentage of weight-adjusted maternal dose) can be calculated, assuming an average of 150 mL/kg/day of milk ingested by a breast-fed infant.

Percentage of pediatric dosage =

$$\left(\frac{\text{Quantity of medication taken from milk by the baby (mg/kg/day)}}{\text{Usual initial daily pediatric dose (mg/kg/day)}}\right)\times 100$$

Weight adjusted maternal dose or relative infant dose =

$$\left(\frac{\text{Quantity of medication taken from milk by the baby (mg/kg/day)}}{\text{Maternal dose adjusted by weight (mg/kg/day)}}\right)\times 100$$

In the latter equation, maternal dose refers to the dose used by patients in the published study or case report, not to the dose of your actual patient.

Table 47–5

Altered Pharmacokinetics During Pregnancy: Clinical Implications and Management

Drugs	Pharmacokinetic Changes	Recommendations and Monitoring
Aminoglycosides	$\uparrow V_d$, $\uparrow$Cl, $\downarrow t_{1/2}$	Monitor peaks and troughs; increase doses if necessary
Antiretrovirals	Variable Cl and C_{max}	Monitor clinical response; drug levels can be useful to adjust some drug dosages
Caffeine	$\uparrow t_{1/2}$ $\downarrow$Cl (T_1, T_2, T_3)	Risk of more frequent and prolonged side effects; decrease caffeine consumption
Carbamazepine	$\uparrow$Cl $\downarrow t_{1/2}$	Measure free fraction (preferably); increase dose according to clinical response and levels
Digoxin	$\uparrow$Cl $\downarrow C_{max}$	Follow plasma levels; adjust according to clinical response and plasma levels; increase doses if necessary; to treat fetal disease, higher doses might be required; digoxin-like immunoreactive substance might alter levels
Fluoxetine and other SSRIs	$\uparrow$Cl (T_3)	Increase dose according to clinical response; consider decreasing dose after delivery
Heparin	$\uparrow$Cl (T_1, T_2, T_3)	Consider increasing frequency of administration
LMWH		If necessary, follow anti-Xa levels
Lamotrigine	$\uparrow$Cl (T_1, T_2, T_3)	For epilepsy: Measure drug levels at least every trimester; increase dose according to clinical response and levels; return to prepregnancy dose after delivery
Levothyroxine (T4)	$\downarrow$ff	Increase dose at the beginning of pregnancy; follow TSH levels at least every trimester; return to prepregnancy dose after delivery
Lithium	$\uparrow$Cl (T_1, T_2, T_3) $\downarrow t_{1/2}$	Measure drug levels at least every trimester and monthly in T3; increase dose according to levels if necessary; return to prepregnancy dose after delivery
Nicotine	$\downarrow t_{1/2}$ $\uparrow$Cl (T_2, T_3)	Higher doses might be required (smoking cessation) at T2 and T3; however, increased transdermal absorption might lead to higher nicotine plasma levels
Nifedipine	$\uparrow$Cl (T_3)	Monitor clinical effect; increase doses/frequency of administration if necessary
Phenytoin	$\downarrow C_{total}$, ff $\uparrow$Cl (T_3) $\downarrow t_{1/2}$	Measure free fraction; increase dose according to clinical response and levels
Valproic acid	$\downarrow C_{total}$ $\uparrow$ff	Measure free fraction if prepregnancy reference level is available; dose will remain the same in most cases. Increase dose according to clinical response and levels

$\uparrow$, increase; $\downarrow$, decrease; $\leftrightarrow$, unchanged; C_{max}, maximum serum concentration; Cl, clearance; ff, free fraction; T, trimester; $t_{1/2}$, elimination half-life; LMWH, low-molecular-weight heparin; C_{total}, total concentration; SSRI: selective serotonin reuptake inhibitor.

Data from Refs. 6 and 18.

Usually, a percentage of less than 10% of the pediatric dose or, when a pediatric dose is not available, a percentage of less than 10% of weight adjusted maternal dose, is acceptable in full-term healthy infants unless a drug has a toxic side effect profile.[20]

▶ *Drug Pharmacokinetics*

If clinical data are unavailable on drug transfer into breast milk, choose drugs that are highly protein bound, have a high molecular weight, have a short half-life, have no active metabolites, and are well tolerated by children.[20]

▶ *Drugs of Concern During Breast-Feeding*

KEY CONCEPT *Most drugs are safe during breast-feeding.* However, some drugs are of concern and require a more thorough assessment by the clinician (Table 47–6). One should also consider additive side effects of medication for the baby when the mother is taking several medications.

CONDITIONS PREVALENT IN PREGNANCY AND LACTATION

KEY CONCEPT *When possible, treat conditions occurring during pregnancy with nonpharmacologic treatments instead of drug therapy.*

KEY CONCEPT *Evaluate the need for treatment, including benefits and risks. Avoid treatments that do not show evidence of benefit or that can be delayed until after pregnancy or breast-feeding.*

For chronic diseases, please refer to the relevant chapter where you will find considerations during pregnancy under "Special populations".

Nausea and Vomiting of Pregnancy (NVP)

As many as 85% of pregnant women suffer from nausea or vomiting.[23] Nonpharmacologic measures, such as lifestyle (rest, avoidance of nausea triggers) and dietary changes (small and frequent meals, fluid restriction during meals, avoiding spicy or fatty foods, consuming crackers upon rising) should be used as first-line management. Acupuncture and acupressure also can be helpful.[23]

The combination of pyridoxine and doxylamine is the first-line pharmacologic treatment of NVP. When this combination is insufficient, other drugs such as metoclopramide, diphenhydramine, or ondansetron can be prescribed (Table 47–7).[24]

Pain

Pregnant or lactating women experience pain from preexisting conditions or from temporary pathologies (eg, vaso-occlusive crisis in sickle cell disease, fibromas, migraine, etc)

The general principles of treatment are[6,7,25]:

- Maximize nonpharmacological measures
- Acetaminophen is the safest analgesic during pregnancy
- If medications are required, avoid nonsteroidal anti-inflammatory drugs (NSAIDs) during the third trimester, and use them with caution otherwise

Table 47–6

Drugs of Concern During Breast-Feeding

Drug or Class	Comments
Drugs that can decrease the breast milk production	
Clomiphene	Has been used to suppress lactation
Ergot derivatives (bromocriptine, cabergoline, ergotamine)	Have been used to suppress lactation
Estrogens	Hormonal contraceptives with ethinylestradiol should be delayed for 4–6 weeks following delivery
Pseudoephedrine	Do not use in women with low milk production; a few doses will probably not have significant effect
Drugs for which use during breast-feeding may expose the neonate to a significant quantity and may necessitate a strict follow-up	
β-blocking agents (acebutolol, atenolol, sotalol)	Neonatal β-blockade reported Concern for acebutolol, atenolol and sotalol, but other β-blocking agents such as metoprolol, propranolol and labetalol are safe
Amiodarone	May accumulate because of long half-life; possible neonatal thyroid and cardiovascular toxicity
Antineoplastics	Neonatal myelosuppression possible
Chloramphenicol	Severe side effects reported when used to treat babies (blood dyscrasia, grey baby syndrome)
Ergotamine	Symptoms of ergotism (vomiting and diarrhea) reported
Illicit drugs	Unknown contents and effects
Lamotrigine	A breast-fed infant could have blood concentrations between 10% and 50% of maternal blood concentrations (can be in therapeutic range for babies). More than 100 breast-fed babies followed with rare side effects reported including apnea attributed to excessive sedation (n = 1), hepatotoxicity (n = 1) and a few cases of nonsevere or unrelated rashes. Monitor for CNS side effects (sedation, hypotonia, weight gain, and poor sucking) and rash.
Lithium	Up to 50% of maternal serum levels have been measured in infants; cases of infant toxicity (lethargy, cyanosis, electrocardiogram anomalies, dysthyroidia, tremors) have been reported. Monitor infant serum lithium, creatinine, urea, and TSH levels every 4 to 12 weeks and other side effects (jittery, feeding problems, signs of dehydration).
Phenobarbital/primidone	Drowsiness and reduced weight gain reported. Up to 25% of a pediatric dose can be ingested via breast milk. Monitor for CNS side effects (sedation, hypotonia, weight gain, and poor sucking).
Radioactive iodine-131	No breast-feeding for days to weeks to achieve nonsignificant radiation levels (long radioactive half-life). Monitor radioactive levels in milk before allowing breast-feeding.
Tetracyclines	Chronic use may lead to dental staining or decreased epiphyseal bone growth.

Data from Refs. 6, 7, and 20.

- Opiates are not associated with a higher risk of malformations. However, close neonatal monitoring is necessary due to possible withdrawal if opiates are taken regularly near delivery. Limited data exist for some opiates during the first trimester, eg, for fentanyl and tramadol
- There is a lack of information for some medications (eg, pregabalin)
- For migraine, triptan use remains controversial. Sumatriptan has not been associated with a higher risk of birth defects. It can be used but not routinely.

Urinary Tract Infections

Urinary tract infections during pregnancy, including asymptomatic disease, increase the risk of hypertension, low birth weight, and preterm delivery.[5]

Asymptomatic bacteriuria and cystitis cause acute pyelonephritis more often in pregnancy than in nonpregnant women.[26] Acute pyelonephritis may lead to septic shock and adult respiratory distress syndrome and should be treated aggressively with intravenous antibiotics. Outpatient treatment with intramuscular therapy alone or followed by oral treatment is feasible for some women (eg, stable and pregnancy less than 24 weeks).[26] Treatment reduces pregnancy complications.[26–28]

Antimicrobial therapy should target *Escherichia coli* infection and should vary according to local bacterial resistance (see Table 47–7).[26] Avoid trimethoprim-sulfamethoxazole during organogenesis (congenital malformations) and near term (theoretical risk of neonatal jaundice).[7] Quinolones should be reserved for resistant infections due to theoretical concerns of arthropathy.[7]

Repeat urine culture 10 to 14 days after completion of acute pyelonephritis therapy and monthly thereafter. After completion of the acute episode of pyelonephritis, recommend suppressive therapy prophylaxis for the remainder of the pregnancy and for 4 to 6 weeks after delivery (See Table 47-7).[26]

Preterm Labor

Preterm birth, especially before 32 weeks of pregnancy, is the major cause of short- and long-term neonatal mortality and morbidity. The underlying pathophysiologic conditions are diverse, and most are unknown. There is wide variation in management, diagnosis, and treatment of preterm labor across the world.

► *Antenatal Corticosteroids*

The most beneficial intervention in preterm labor is administration of antepartum corticosteroids. Provide a single course of antenatal corticosteroids to women at risk of preterm delivery within 7 days between 24 and 34 weeks' gestation (see Table 47–7).[29] This approach decreases the incidence and severity of neonatal respiratory distress syndrome, intraventricular hemorrhage, necrotizing enterocolitis, and death.[29] Current data do not support the use of repeated courses of corticosteroids (see Table 47–7).[30]

► *Tocolytic Agents*

Tocolytic therapy is used when preterm labor occurs before 33.6 weeks to delay delivery in order to complete a course of corticosteroids and allow transfer of the mother to a center with neonatal intensive care facilities. Tocolytics include magnesium sulfate, β-mimetics (terbutaline), prostaglandin inhibitors (indomethacin), oxytocin receptors blockers (atosiban), and calcium channel blockers (nifedipine) (see Table 47–7).[30] All these agents are effective in delaying delivery by 48 hours. Data indicate that

Clinical Confirmation and Associated Problems of Pregnancy and Lactation

Confirmation of Pregnancy

Positive urine or blood human chorionic gonadotropin followed by positive ultrasound, fetal heart sounds, and/or fetal movement.

Pregnancy Dating and Gestational Age

Calculated from the first day of the last menstrual period.

An ultrasound between 10+0 and 13+6 weeks determines gestational age based on crown-rump length and identifies multiple pregnancies.

Due dates typically are estimated at 40 weeks of gestation; however, infants delivered between 37 and 42 weeks are considered full term.

Pregnancy Symptoms

First trimester : Menstrual spotting, missed menses, fatigue, breast tenderness, increased urination, mood swings, nausea/vomiting, headache, heartburn, constipation

Second trimester : Frequent urination, heartburn, constipation, dry skin, edema, linea nigra, melasma

Third trimester : Backache, edema, shortness of breath, insomnia

Routine Pregnancy Visits

In a normal, uncomplicated pregnancy, visits should occur monthly until 28 weeks of gestation, every 2 to 3 weeks from 28 to 36 weeks of gestation, and then weekly until delivery.

Assess for each of the following at each visit:

- Blood pressure
- Weight
- Urine protein (dipstick)
- Uterine size
- Fetal heart rate
- Fetal movement

Routine Lab Testing for Normal Pregnancies (First Trimester Unless Otherwise Indicated)

- Hemoglobin and hematocrit for anemia (repeated at 26–32 weeks)
- Blood type, Rh, red blood cell antibody screening
- Human immunodeficiency virus
- Venereal Disease Research Laboratory (VDRL) slide test for syphilis
- Rubella immunity
- Varicella immunity
- Hepatitis B surface antigen
- Urinalysis with culture for bacteriuria
- Gonorrhea and chlamydia
- Cervical cytology
- Screens for Down syndrome and neural tube defects (between 11 and 20 weeks)
- Gestational diabetes screening (at 24–28 weeks)
- Group B Streptococcus screening (at 35–37 weeks)
- Women at high risk for these conditions should be tested at the first visit:
  - Hypothyroidism
  - Type 2 diabetes
  - Sickle cell disease or thalassemia
  - Hepatitis C
  - Tuberculosis
  - Bacterial vaginosis

Selected Problems Experienced During Pregnancy or Lactation

Hyperemesis gravidarum. Severe, persistent nausea and vomiting during pregnancy accompanied by dehydration, electrolyte disturbance, ketonuria, and weight loss.

Urinary tract infection. Bacteriuria often asymptomatic in pregnancy. Diagnosed by positive urine culture.

Bacterial vaginosis. Clinically diagnosed by presence of three of the following (Amsel criteria):

- White, homogenous, noninflammatory discharge
- Clue cells on microscopic examination
- Vaginal pH greater than 4.5
- A fishy odor before or after addition of 10% potassium hydroxide (ie, "whiff" test)

Vulvovaginal candidiasis. Typical symptoms include vaginal itching and whitish discharge.

Sexually transmitted infections: Refer to Table 47–8.

Preterm labor. Onset of uterine contractions and cervical modification which may lead to delivery prior to 37 weeks of gestation.

Preterm premature rupture of the membranes. Rupture of the amniotic membranes before 37 weeks and before active labor.

Abruptio placentae. Sudden detachment of the placenta presenting with uterine bleeding, abdominal pain with or without maternal and fetal hemodynamic compromise.

Group B streptococcus colonization. Diagnosed by positive culture on vaginal and rectal swab.

Gestational diabetes. See Chapter 43.

Gestational hypertension. Asymptomatic or presence of neurologic, hepatic, or cardiovascular symptoms. Check for proteinuria.

Mastitis. Characterized by localized redness, tenderness, and warmth on one breast accompanied by fever and flulike symptoms. Although uncommon, symptoms also may be bilateral.

Breast candidiasis. Typical symptoms include nipple pain, itching, burning, and/or breast pain that persist after feeding.

Refs. 21 and 22.

Table 47–7

Medication Dosing Recommendations During Pregnancy and Lactation

Drug	Dosage	Comments
Micronutrients and Vitamins		
Folic acid	0.4–0.8 mg po daily	Dosage necessary to reach RDA: 0.6 mg (pregnancy), 0.5 mg (breast-feeding)
	4 mg po daily	For women at higher risk of having a child with NTD
Iron	60–200 mg (elemental iron) po per day (divided doses if > 60 mg)	Doses to treat iron-deficiency anemia
Nausea and Vomiting		
Diphenhydramine or dimenhydrinate	25–50 mg po four times daily as needed	
Doxylamine	12.5 mg po three to four times daily as needed	
Pyridoxine	25 mg po three times daily as needed	
Doxylamine + pyridoxine (Diclegis)	Two pills at bedtime, one pill in the morning and one pill in the afternoon (one to eight pills daily)	Delayed-release combination of doxylamine and pyridoxine
Metoclopramide	5–15 mg po three to four times daily as needed	
Ondansetron	4–8 mg po three times daily as needed	
Urinary Tract Infections		
Asymptomatic bacteriuria and uncomplicated acute cystitis		
Nitrofurantoin	100 mg po four times daily for 3 to 7 days 100 mg po twice daily (macrocrystalline) for 3 to 7 days	
Cephalexin	250–500 mg po four times daily for 3 to 7 days	
Amoxicillin	500 mg po three times daily for 3 to 7 days	Check for local resistance before prescribing
Acute pyelonephritis		
Ampicillin + gentamicin	1–2 g IV every 6 hours + 1.5 mg/kg/dose IV every 8 hours	Switch to oral antibiotic after 48 hours afebrile and treat for a total of 10 to 14 days, for example: • Cephalexin 500 mg po four times daily • Cefprozil 500 mg po twice daily • Amoxicillin clavulanate 875/125 mg po twice daily
Cefazolin	1–2 g IV every 8 hours	
Cefuroxime	0.75–1.5 g IV every 8 hours	
Ceftriaxone	1–2 g IV or IM every 24 hours	
Prophylaxis		
Nitrofurantoin	50–100 mg po at bedtime	Start after the end of the treatment for pyelonephritis and continue until 4 to 6 weeks after delivery
Cephalexin	250 mg po at bedtime	Nitrofurantoin should be preferred to prevent resistance to cephalosporins.
Fetal Lung Maturation		
Betamethasone	12 mg IM every 24 hours for two doses	A single rescue course may be considered after at least 2 weeks of treatment if gestational age is < 32 6/7 weeks and the woman is likely to give birth within the next week.
Dexamethasone	6 mg IM or IV every 12 hours for four doses	
Tocolytic agents		
Nifedipine (short acting)	30 mg oral load (divided over at least 1 hour), then 10–20 mg every 4–6 hours for 48 hours	Maternal adverse reactions include headache, flushing, dizziness, transient hypotension, and maternal pulmonary edema.
Magnesium sulfate	4–6 g IV bolus over 20 minutes, Then 2–3 g/hour IV drip	Contraindicated in women with myasthenia gravis. Maternal pulmonary edema and cardiac arrest have been reported. Benign side effects include flushing, headache, and nausea.
Indomethacin	50–100 mg oral load, then 25–50 mg po every 6 hours for 48 hours	Avoid in women with a history of renal or hepatic impairment, aspirin or nonsteroidal anti-inflammatory drug (NSAID) allergy, peptic ulcer disease, other bleeding disorders, or after 32 weeks of pregnancy. Reports of increased risk of maternal postpartum hemorrhage, and neonatal complications (eg, premature closure of the ductus arteriosus, renal insufficiency and, if delivery close to NSAID administration, pharmacologic treatment ineffectiveness for patent ductus arteriosus, necrotizing enterocolitis, bronchopulmonary dysplasia, and intraventricular hemorrhage) are worrisome.

(Continued)

Table 47–7

Medication Dosing Recommendations During Pregnancy and Lactation (*Continued*)

Drug	Dosage	Comments
Magnesium sulfate For neuroprotection or prevention of eclampsia.	4 g IV bolus over 20 minutes, then 1 g/hour IV drip	Contraindicated in women with myasthenia gravis. Maternal pulmonary edema and cardiac arrest have been reported. Benign side effects include flushing, headache, and nausea. Treatment limited to 24 hours for neuroprotection.
Premature Rupture of Membranes		
Ampicillin	2 g IV every 6 hours for 48 hours followed by amoxicillin	Ampicillin/amoxicillin are used with erythromycin
Amoxicillin	250 mg po three times daily for 5 days	Ampicillin/amoxicillin are used with erythromycin
Erythromycin base	250 mg IV every 6 hours for 48 hours followed by 333 mg three times daily for 5 days	Ampicillin/amoxicillin are used with erythromycin
Preterm Labor Prevention		
17-α-hydroxyprogesterone	250 mg IM each week	
Progesterone (micronized)	100 mg intravaginally daily or 90 mg (8% gel) (previous preterm delivery) 200 mg intravaginally daily (short cervix)	Start at 16–20 weeks' gestation if previous preterm delivery and at 22 to 26 weeks if short cervix
Group B Streptococcus		
Penicillin G	5 million units IV initially, then 2.5–3 million units IV every 4 hours until delivery	First choice
Ampicillin	2 g IV initially, then 1 g IV every 4 hours until delivery	
Cefazolin	2 g IV initially, then 1 g IV every 8 hours until delivery	
Clindamycin	900 mg IV every 8 hours until delivery	Only if isolate proven sensitive to clindamycin and erythromycin, or sensitive to clindamycin and testing for inducible clindamycin resistance is negative
Vancomycin	1 g IV every 12 hours until delivery	If other options are inappropriate
Cervical ripening		
Misoprostol	25 mcg (1/4 of 100 mcg tablet) vaginally every 3–6 hours	Check for uterine tachysystole with or without fetal heart rate changes
Dinoprostone	0.5 mg gel in cervical canal every 6 hours up to 1.5 mg/24 hours	Do not used if previous uterine surgery including cesarean section
	10 mg extended-release vaginal insert in posterior fornix	Check for uterine tachysystole with or without fetal heart rate changes
Induction of labor		
Misoprostol	25 mcg (one-fourth of 100-mcg tablet) vaginally every 3–6 hours	Check for uterine tachysystole with or without fetal heart rate changes
Oxytocin	0.5–6 mU/min with 1–6 mU/min increases every 15–40 minutes according to contractions	Check for uterine tachysystole and water intoxication
Postpartum hemorrhage treatment		
Oxytocin	10 units IM or 5 units push or 20–40 units in 1 L if IV fluid	Use normal saline or lactated Ringer. Cautious with bolus in women with cardiac disease
Carbetocin	100 mcg IM or IV over 1 minute	
Methylergonovine	0.2 mg IM or IV every 2–4 hours up to five doses	Do not use in hypertensive women
Carboprost tromethamine	0.25 mg IM every 15–90 min up to eight doses	Use with caution in asthmatic women
Dinoprostone	20 mg vaginal suppository every 2 hours	
Misoprostol	400–800 mcg po or 800–1000 mcg rectally once	
Tranexamic acid	10–15 mg/kg IV over 20 minutes	
Hyperthyroidism		
Methimazole	5–10 mg po once or twice daily	Second and third trimesters
Propylthiouracil	50–100 mg po one to three times daily	First trimester. Risk of hepatotoxicity.
Severe Hypertension		
Labetalol	Start with 10–20 mg IV over 2 minutes; repeated 20–80 mg every 15–30 minutes (300 mg total dose) Or 1–2 mg/min IV drip	Not for asthmatic women. May cause fetal bradycardia
Nifedipine (short acting)	5–10 mg po; could be repeated after 30 minutes	Maternal adverse reactions include headache, flushing, dizziness, hypotension, tachycardia, and maternal pulmonary edema.
Hydralazine	5 mg IV or IM; repeated 5–10 mg IV every 30 minutes (20 mg IV and 30 mg total dose) Or 0.5–10 mg/hour IV drip	May cause tachycardia, headaches, hypotension

(*Continued*)

Table 47–7

Medication Dosing Recommendations During Pregnancy and Lactation (*Continued*)

Drug	Dosage	Comments
Nonsevere Hypertension		
First choices		
Methyldopa	250–500 mg po two to four times daily	May cause orthostatic hypotension, drowsiness, depression, hemolytic anemia, positive antibodies antinuclear
Labetalol	100–400 mg po two to four times daily	Not for asthmatic women. May cause hypotension, tiredness, headaches, hepatotoxicity
Nifedipine extended release	20–60 mg po one to two times daily	May cause tachycardia, headaches, edema, hypotension
Second choices		
Hydralazine	10–50 mg po two to four times daily with methyldopa or labetalol	May cause tachycardia, headaches, hypotension, lupus-like syndrome
Metoprolol	25–100 mg po two times daily	Not for asthmatic women; may cause fetal bradycardia, hypotension
Clonidine	0.05–0.2 mg po (maximum: 0.8 mg daily)	May cause hypotension, drowsiness
Hydrochlorothiazide	12.5–50 mg po once daily	May cause hypokalemia, dehydration
Bacterial Vaginosis		
Metronidazole	250 mg po three times daily for 7 days or 500 mg orally twice a day for 7 days 0.75% vaginal gel, once or twice daily for 5 days	Safe in all trimesters
Clindamycin	300 mg po twice daily for 7 days 2 % cream, 5 g intravaginally at bedtime for 7 days 100-mg ovules intravaginally at bedtime for 3 days bedtime for 7 days (breast-feeding)	For metronidazole and clindamycin, use oral formulation during pregnancy and intravaginal formulation during breast-feeding
Vulvovaginal Candidiasis: refer to chapter 83		
6–7 days treatments for intravaginal antifungical azoles are recommended during pregnancy to prevent recurrent episodes; shorter courses are appropriate during breast-feeding		
Mastitis		
Outpatient Treatment		
Dicloxacillin	500 mg po four times daily	Treat for 10–14 days
Cephalexin	500 mg po four times daily	
Amoxicillin 875 mg + 125-mg clavulanate	One tablet po twice daily	
Inpatient Treatment for More Severe Cases		
Oxacillin	2 g IV every 4 hours	Treat IV for 24–48 hours until afebrile then continue with outpatient treatment
Nafcillin	2 g IV every 4 hours	
Clindamycin	600–900 mg IV every 8 hours	
Vancomycin	1 g IV every 8–12 hours	If MRSA suspected or proven
Breast Candidiasis		
Mother		
Clotrimazole, miconazole, or nystatin	Topical cream	After each feeding and for 1 week after symptoms have resolved. Also treat infant even if asymptomatic
Fluconazole	200–400 mg po for one dose followed by 100–200 mg po daily	If topical treatment not efficacious, add fluconazole; use until 1 week after symptoms have resolved (minimum of 2 weeks of treatment). Also treat infant even if asymptomatic.
Infant		
Nystatin oral solution	100,000–200,000 units (1–2 mL) to be swabbed into infant's mouth four times daily, after feedings	
Clotrimazole or miconazole topical cream	Apply in a thin layer in infant's mouth four times daily, after feedings	
Other Treatments for Candidiasis		
Gentian violet 0.5%–1% solution	To be swabbed into infant's mouth once daily for 5 days before a feeding	To be used if other options fail. Can stain clothes and skin If nipples or mouth are not violet after application and the feeding, reapply the treatment

MRSA, methicillin-resistant *Staphylococcus aureus*; NTD, neural tube defect; po, orally; RDA, recommended daily allowance.

Data from Refs. 6, 10, 15, 17, 21, 25–31, and 33–49.

indomethacin and nifedipine have the highest probability of delaying delivery and improving neonatal and maternal outcomes.[32] Combined tocolytics or prolonged or repeated tocolytic therapy may increase fetal risk without evidence of efficacy.[31]

The FDA has advised against the use of terbutaline for tocolysis due to the risk of serious side effects including increased heart rate, transient hyperglycemia, hypokalemia, cardiac arrhythmias, pulmonary edema, and myocardial ischemia.[31]

▶ *Neuroprotection*

Magnesium sulfate given to women at imminent risk of preterm delivery up to 33.6 weeks gestation decreases the incidence of death, cerebral palsy, and gross motor dysfunction. (see Table 47–7).[33]

▶ *Antibiotics*

In the presence of preterm premature rupture of membranes (PPROM), 2 days of parenteral ampicillin/erythromycin followed by 5 days of oral amoxicillin and erythromycin are associated with a delay of delivery and reduction in maternal and neonatal morbidity (see Table 47–7).[34]

▶ *Progesterone*

Progesterone is used to prevent preterm birth in women with previous preterm delivery and may also be used in women with a sonographic short cervix.[35,36]

Group B *Streptococcus* Infection

Ten percent to 30% of pregnant women are colonized by group B streptococcus (GBS) at term. Maternal transmission of GBS during delivery can cause neonatal sepsis and death. Antibiotic therapy is effective in reducing the incidence of early-onset neonatal GBS infection when administered to high-risk groups including women with GBS vaginal/rectal colonization, GBS bacteriuria in the current pregnancy, and those who previously delivered a neonate with GBS disease.[37]

All women should be screened for GBS colonization using a vaginal-rectal swab between 35 and 37 weeks of gestation unless they had a proven GBS bacteriuria during the current pregnancy or a previous neonate with GBS disease. If treatment is indicated, it should be started at the time of membrane rupture or onset of labor, whichever comes first and continued until delivery (see Table 47–7). All women with unknown GBS status should be treated if labor or PPROM occur before 37 weeks. Intravenous penicillin G or ampicillin, or if penicillin-allergic, cefazolin (non-anaphylactic allergy) or clindamycin (anaphylaxis to penicillin) can be used. To use clindamycin, sensitivity to both clindamycin and erythromycin should be proven, or if resistant to erythromycin, testing for clindamycin inducible resistance must be negative. If resistance to either of these is present, vancomycin should be administered.[37]

Neonates should be monitored for signs and symptoms of sepsis for 48 hours after birth. If present, a full diagnostic workup should be initiated and empirical antibiotic therapy started.[38]

Induction of Labor

Several mechanical and pharmacological methods of cervical ripening can be used. Mechanical methods include hygroscopic dilator, Foley catheter, and extraamniotic saline infusion.[39,40]

Pharmacological methods include the administration of prostaglandin E1 (eg, misoprostol) and E2 (eg, dinoprostone). Misoprostol is less expensive, more stable at room temperature, has a higher 24-hour delivery rate, and requires less oxytocin than dinoprostone, but it is associated with more uterine tachysystole.[39] Prostaglandins should not be used in women with a previous caesarean section due to the increased risk of uterine rupture.[40]

When the cervix is deemed favorable, nonpharmacological options for producing contractions are membranes sweeping, nipple stimulation, and amniotomy. Membrane sweeping and breast stimulation are effective in inducing labour within 48 to 72 hours.[39] Amniotomy is more effective when oxytocin is added early after the intervention.[39]

Oxytocin is the most frequently used pharmacological method of labor induction.[39] Active management of labor with oxytocin is associated with more deliveries within 24 hours; however, it increases the use of epidural and the rate of caesarean sections.[39,40] A rare but serious complication of high cumulative dose of oxytocin is water intoxication due to its antidiuretic action.[40] Oral misoprostol is also effective for labor induction but not licensed in the United States for this use.

Postpartum Hemorrhage

Postpartum hemorrhage is generally defined as blood loss greater than 500 mL after vaginal delivery or 1000 mL following a caesarean section.[41] Uterine atony accounts for up to 80% of primary postpartum hemorrhage, but vaginal or cervical trauma, retained placenta, and coagulopathies are also implicated. Supportive measures should be implemented, and the most likely cause of bleeding should be identified and corrected.

Oxytocin and carbetocin (long-acting analog of oxytocin) can prevent excessive blood loss associated with delivery and caesarian section. If this fails, use uterotonics, eg, methylergonovine, carboprost tromethamine, dinoprostone, and misoprostol, which are effective in the treatment of postpartum hemorrhage secondary to uterine atony, used separately or in combination.[42] Methylergonovine should not be administered to hypertensive women. Carboprost tromethamine should be used with caution in asthmatic women.[41] As a last resort, tranexamic acid, an antifibrinolytic agent can be used.[42] Surgical management ranging from uterine tamponade to hysterectomy is used in unresponsive postpartum hemorrhages.[41]

Thyroid Disorders

Notice that the thyroxine-stimulating hormone (TSH) reference range is lower in pregnancy, 0.1 to 2.5 μIU/mL (0.1–2.5 mIU/L) in the first trimester and 0.3 to 3.0 μIU/mL (0.3–3.0 mIU/L) thereafter. Transient gestational hypothyroidism or hyperthyroidism can occur and have adverse effects on the pregnancy and the fetus/neonate, even if subclinical.[43]

Universal screening of thyroid disorders (TSH or thyroid peroxidase antibody) in pregnancy is debated.[43] Subclinical hypothyroidism should be treated, although there are no solid data on the impact of thyroid replacement therapy on maternal and neonatal morbidity, especially in women without thyroid peroxidase antibodies.[43]

Gestational hyperthyroidism associated with hyperemesis gravidarum is self-remitting and does not require antithyroid treatment. In maternal hyperthyroidism, propylthiouracil is used in the first trimester (methimazole is associated with fetal malformations) and methimazole is used thereafter (propylthiouracil is associated with an increased risk of hepatotoxicity) (see Table 47–7).[43] Close fetal and neonatal monitoring is necessary to detect signs of hypothyroidism (induced by antithyroid drugs) or hyperthyroidism (induced by maternal thyroid-stimulating antibodies).

TSH level should be evaluated 6 to 12 weeks after delivery in all women with thyroid disorders during pregnancy. Thyroid replacement drugs and antithyroid drugs can be used during lactation.[20]

Hypertension

Both preexisting (chronic) and gestational hypertension increase the risk of maternal and perinatal morbidity and mortality. Women with preeclampsia, a syndrome generated by endothelial dysfunction, may present with seizures (eclampsia), neurologic, hepatic, and renal or coagulation complications, as well as fetal death and intrauterine growth restriction. Delivery is the only treatment for preeclampsia. Intravenous magnesium sulfate is used to prevent eclampsia (see Table 47–7).[33–44]

During pregnancy, severe hypertension (systolic blood pressure greater than or equal to 160 mm Hg or a diastolic blood pressure greater than or equal to 110 mm Hg) is an emergency and should be treated aggressively, but a limited number of drugs can be used (see Table 47–7). Methyldopa, labetalol, and nifedipine are accepted as first-line treatments for nonsevere hypertension, however, the blood pressure level at which they should be used is debated. Caution is advised with atenolol (intrauterine growth restriction). Angiotensin-converting enzyme inhibitors, angiotensin II receptor antagonists, or renin inhibitors (fetopathy) are contraindicated.[44]

In high-risk women, to prevent preeclampsia, initiate early in pregnancy, low-dose aspirin (75–160 mg daily). Also, if low dietary intake, start calcium supplements (1–2 g/day).[44]

See all women with hypertensive disorders 6 to 12 weeks after delivery to measure blood pressure and proteinuria, assess cardiovascular risk markers, and counsel them on healthy diet, lifestyle modification, future pregnancy, and risk of cardiovascular diseases.

Anticoagulation

The risk of thromboembolic events is increased during pregnancy and even more during the postpartum. Anticoagulation is required in some women, even if they were not anticoagulated before pregnancy.[7,10]

Low-molecular-weight heparins are preferred over unfractionated heparin due to a favorable pharmacokinetic profile. Both are safe during pregnancy and lactation. Doses should be specific to the underlying condition.

Warfarin is associated with fetal malformations when used between 6 and 12 weeks of pregnancy and with fetal and maternal bleeding when used during the third trimester and delivery (see Table 47–3).[7,10] However, it could be used by some women with prosthetic heart valves in the second trimester and early third trimester, as valve thrombosis has been reported with heparin therapy.[10] Warfarin and heparins are safe for use during lactation.[20]

Bacterial Vaginosis

Bacterial vaginosis is associated with PPROM, chorioamnionitis, preterm birth, and postpartum endometritis.[45] Treatment is recommended in all symptomatic women and in asymptomatic women at high risk for preterm delivery, although the treatment has not been shown to reduce the risk of delivery before 37 weeks. The Centers for Disease Control and Prevention (CDC) recommends oral metronidazole or oral clindamycin for the treatment of bacterial vaginosis in pregnant women (see Table 47–7).[45]

Culture should be performed 1 month after completion of therapy since the cure rate is approximately 70%.[45]

Vulvovaginal Candidiasis

Only symptomatic vulvovaginal candidiasis should be treated in pregnant or lactating women (see Table 47–7).[45]

Sexually Transmitted Infections

Table 47–8 presents the management of sexually transmitted infections during pregnancy and lactation, associated risks, and recommended follow-up.[45,46] Treatment of all recent sexual partners is mandatory.

Enhancement of Lactation

Optimization of breast-feeding techniques is the first-line strategy for decreased lactation. No drug is currently approved by the FDA for lactation enhancement, but dopamine antagonists, metoclopramide, and domperidone (not available in the United States), which increase prolactin levels are used for this purpose.[47] Metoclopramide's maternal side effects include fatigue, irritability, headache, and extrapyramidal symptoms. Very few side effects in the infant have been reported. Domperidone has been associated with abnormal heart rhythm and sudden cardiac

Patient Encounter, Part 2

At 28 weeks of pregnancy, the patient is admitted for acute pyelonephritis and back pain. Blood glucose levels are between 100 and 160 mg/dL (5.6 and 8.9 mmol/L). Urine culture reports the presence of *E. coli* and group B Streptococcus.

Meds: Lithium 600 mg orally in the morning and at bedtime; quetiapine 100 mg orally at bedtime; levothyroxine 75 mcg orally daily; insulin NPH 10 units subcutaneously at bedtime; insulin aspart 10 units subcutaneously before breakfast

What treatment do you recommend at this time?

Patient Encounter, Part 3

At 35 weeks' gestation, the patient is admitted for preterm labor.

Meds: Lithium 600 mg orally in the morning and at bedtime; quetiapine 100 mg orally at bedtime; levothyroxine 75 mcg orally in the morning; insulin NPH 16 units subcutaneously at bedtime; Insulin aspart 20 units subcutaneously before breakfast

Will you recommend a tocolytic agent?

If labor progresses, what special care should be provided?

Patient Encounter, Part 4

After 10 hours of labor, the patient delivers vaginally a 5.6 lb (2.55 kg) baby. She plans to breast-feed.

What treatment plan do you recommend after delivery?

What surveillance do you suggest for the newborn/baby?

Can she breast-feed while taking her medications?

Table 47–8

Management of Sexually Transmitted Infections During Pregnancy and Lactation

	Indications for Treatment	Associated Risks During Pregnancy	When to Repeat Testing During Pregnancy	Other
Chlamydia trachomatis	All women with a positive test, even if asymptomatic	Preterm labor; neonatal infection	Third trimester: < 25 years of age, those at increased risk of infection or if first screening positive	Repeat testing 3–4 weeks after therapy
Treatment	Azithromycin 1 g po once Amoxicillin 500 mg po three times daily for 7 days Erythromycin base 500 mg po four times daily for 7 days or 250 mg po four times daily for 14 days Doxycycline 100 mg po twice daily for 7 days only during lactation (discoloration of teeth if used after 16 weeks of gestational age).			
Gonorrhea	All women with a positive test, even if asymptomatic	Preterm labor; neonatal infection	Third trimester: (or 3–6 months after first trimester) if first screening positive or if at risk of reinfection	Repeat testing 1 week after treatment if cefixime or azithromycin used. Repeat 3 weeks after therapy otherwise
Treatment (uncomplicated infection,(pharynx, cervix, urethra, rectum)	First choice : ceftriaxone 250 mg IM once + azithromycin 1 g po once Second choice during breast-feeding : ceftriaxone 250 mg intramuscularly once + doxycycline 100 mg po twice daily for 7 days. Do not use doxycycline during pregnancy Azithromycin 2 g po once for cephalosporin-allergic patients.			
Genital Herpes Simplex	Active lesions; disseminated; Starting at 36 weeks: prevention of recurrence at term	Neonatal infection, especially if acquired near time of delivery (30%–50%)		Cesarean section if active genital lesions at delivery; evaluate newborn for herpes infection
Treatment	**First episode:** *Acyclovir:* 400 mg po three times daily for 7–10 days, or 200 mg five times daily for 7–10 days *Valacyclovir:* 1000 mg po twice daily for 10 days **Recurrent episodes:** *Acyclovir:* 400 mg po three times daily for 5 days, or 800 mg twice daily for 5 days, or 800 mg three times daily for 2 days *Valacyclovir:* 500 mg po twice daily for 3 days **Suppressive therapy:** start at 36 weeks of gestation (or earlier if at risk of preterm delivery) until delivery *Acyclovir:* 400 mg po three times daily *Valacyclovir:* 500 mg po twice daily			
Syphilis	All women with confirmed positive serology	In utero fetal and neonatal infection; congenital malformations	At 28–32 weeks and at delivery if at risk of reinfection, if untested before, if positive serology in the first trimester, or if was previous stillborn at more than 20 weeks	Therapy is efficacious to treat the fetus and to prevent transmission; be aware of Jarisch-Herxheimer reaction; fetal evaluation should include ultrasounds.
Treatment	Desensitize penicillin-allergic patients Primary, secondary, or early latent: Benzathine penicillin G 2.4 million units IM once Late latent or of unknown duration or tertiary: Benzathine penicillin G 2.4 million units IM three times at 1-week interval Neurosyphilis: Aqueous crystalline penicillin G 3–4 million units IV six times daily for 10–14 days or Procaine penicillin 2.4 million units IV daily + probenecid 500 mg four times daily			
Trichomoniasis	Symptomatic women	PPROM, preterm birth, low birth weight; neonatal infection		Therapy does not decrease perinatal mortality
Treatment	Metronidazole 2 g po for one dose. Lactation: consider holding breast-feeding for 12 hours (most important for premature or very young infants).			

po, orally; PPROM, preterm premature rupture of membranes.

Data from Refs. 45 and 46.

Patient Care Process

Patient Assessment:

- Complete medical history including obstetrical history.
- Inquire about changes in disorders evolution and last follow-up with the treating physician.
- Conduct medication history (past/current treatments, compliance, efficacy, and safety).
- Verify immunization status.
- Assess for pregnancy signs and symptoms.
- Perform physical examination.
- Evaluate nutritional status and socioeconomic environment.
- Perform first trimester routine lab testing.
- Order serum drug levels.

Therapy Evaluation:

- Evaluate the need for continuing medication (benefits and risks for mother and fetus).
- Assess efficacy, safety, and patient adherence, and screen for drug interactions.
- Evaluate whether safer and more effective alternative medications are available.

Care Plan Development:

- Avoid treatments without evidence of benefit or that can be delayed until after pregnancy and breast-feeding.
- Address patient concerns (risks of medication, risks of relapse if condition is untreated, prescription coverage and access to care).
- Treat pregnancy symptoms (eg, nausea) if they are bothersome or interfering with other pathologies (eg, diabetes).
- When possible, treat pregnancy conditions with nonpharmacologic treatments instead of drug therapy.
- Recommend appropriate folic acid and multivitamins.
- Provide prenatal counseling regarding lifestyle modifications (healthy diet, exercise, avoidance of tobacco, alcohol, and illicit or unnecessary drugs).
- Encourage breast-feeding. If maternal drug therapy is required during breast-feeding, choose drugs with the best safety profile. Communicate information to all other health care professionals to ensure continuing of care.

Follow-Up Evaluation:

- Follow up at each prenatal visit or more frequently to assess compliance, effectiveness, and safety of treatment.
- Review and repeat assessments as necessary.
- Monitor infants for birth defects, developmental delays, or unusual reactions, and report suspected drug-related reactions to the FDA or pharmaceutical companies.

death; caution is advised when prescribing it with other drugs that prolong the QT interval or that inhibit its metabolism or for women with underlying cardiac conditions.[48]

Mastitis

Bacterial mastitis, seen typically within the first 6 weeks of breast-feeding, is characterized by localized signs of inflammation and engorgement. Fever, shivering, and malaise can also occur. The most commonly encountered bacteria are *Staphylococcus aureus* (including methicillin-resistant), followed by *Streptococcus, Staphylococcus epidermidis*, and *E. coli*.[49]

Cold or warm compresses and more frequent breast-feeding or breast pumping, should be encouraged. Antibiotics (see Table 47–7) and analgesics (eg, acetaminophen, NSAIDs) can be used to relieve pain.[20,49] If a breast abscess is suspected, ultrasound should be performed before surgical drainage.

Breast Candidiasis

Candidiasis presents with severe and persistent nipple pain, which may throb and radiate to the breasts and back. Pain is usually more intense during and immediately after breast-feeding. The breast-fed infant can be symptomatic or asymptomatic. *Candida albicans* is the most commonly found species. It is recommended to breast-feed more frequently than usual for a shorter period of time. Milk does not have to be discarded; however, clothes and towels in contact with breasts and the baby's mouth should be washed in hot water. Antifungal treatment must be given to the mother and the baby simultaneously (see Table 47–7). If no improvement is seen within 24 to 48 hours, treatment should be reevaluated. Analgesics (eg, acetaminophen, NSAIDs) can be used.[49]

Abbreviations Introduced in This Chapter

AAP	American Academy of Paediatrics
ACOG	American College of Obstetricians and Gynecologists
CDC	Centers for Disease Control and Prevention
CNS	Central nervous system
GA	Gestational age
GBS	Group B Streptococcus
LMP	Last menstrual period
NSAID	Nonsteroidal anti-inflammatory drug
NTD	Neural tube defect
OTIS	Organization of Teratology Information Specialists
PCA	Postconceptional age
PPROM	Preterm Premature Rupture of Membranes
STEPS	System for Thalidomide Education and Prescribing Safety
T4	Levothyroxine
TSH	Thyroxine-stimulating hormone
VDRL	Venereal Disease Research Laboratory

REFERENCES

1. Mitchell AA, Gilboa SM, Werler MM, et al. Medication use during pregnancy, with particular focus on prescription drugs: 1976-2008. Am J Obstet Gynecol. 2011;205:51.e1–e8.
2. Thorpe PG, Gilboa SM, Hernandez-Diaz S, et al. Medications in the first trimester of pregnancy: most common exposure and critical gaps in understanding fetal risk. Pharmacoepidemiol Drug Saf. 2013;22(9):1013–1018.
3. Marchofdimes.Pregnancyloss[Internet].http://www.marchofdimes.com/loss/miscarriage.aspx (last accessed July 31 2014).

4. National Center for Health Statistics. Final natality data [Internet]. www.marchofdimes.com/peristats (last accessed July 31, 2014).
5. Moore KL, Persaud TVN, Torchia MG. The developing human—clinically oriented embryology. 9th ed. Philadelphia, PA: Elsevier Saunders, 2013, p. 540.
6. Ferreira E, Martin E, Morin C, ed. Grossesse et allaitement: guide thérapeutique. 2nd ed. Montreal: Éditions du CHU Ste-Justine, 2013, p. 1183.
7. Briggs GG, Freeman RK, Yaffe SJ, eds. Drugs in pregnancy and lactation: a reference guide to fetal and neonatal risk. 9th ed. Philadelphia, PA: Lippincott Williams & Wilkins, 2011, p. 1703.
8. Hudak ML, Tan RC. The Committee on Drugs and The Committee on Fetus and Newborn. Neonatal Drug Withdrawal. Pediatrics 2012;129:e540–e560.
9. Obican S, Scialli AR. Teratogenic exposures. Am J Med Genet C Semin Med Genet. 2011;157:150–169.
10. Bates SM, Greer IA, Middeldorp S, et al. VTE, thrombophilia, antithrombotic therapy, and pregnancy: Antithrombotic Therapy and Prevention of Thrombosis, 9th ed: American College of Chest Physicians Evidence-Based Clinical Practice Guidelines. Chest. 2012;141(2 Suppl):e691S–e736S.
11. Friedman JM. How do we know if an exposure is actually teratogenic in humans? Am J Med Genet C Semin Med Genet. 2011;157:170–174.
12. Kweder SL. Drugs and biologics in pregnancy and breastfeeding: FDA in the 21st century. Birth Defects Res A Clin Mol Teratol. 2008;82; 605–609.
13. Conover EA, Polifka JE. The art and science of teratogen risk communication. Am J Med Genet C Semin Med Genet. 2011; 157:227–233.
14. World Health Organization. Meeting to Develop a Global Consensus on Preconception Care to Reduce Maternal and Childhood Mortality and Morbidity 2013. www.who.int. (last accessed July 18, 2014).
15. US Preventive Services Task Force. Folic Acid for the Prevention of Neural Tube Defects: U.S. Preventive Services Task Force Recommendation Statement. Ann Intern Med. 2009;150:626–631.
16. Goh YI, Koren G. Folic acid in pregnancy and fetal outcomes. J Obstet Gynaecol. 2008;28:3–13.
17. ACOG Practice Bulletin No. 95: Anemia in pregnancy. Obstet Gynecol. 2008;112:201–207.
18. Costantine MM. Physiologic and pharmacokinetic changes in pregnancy. Frontiers in Pharmacology 2014;5:1–5.
19. Eidelman AI, Schanler RJ. Breastfeeding and the use of human milk. Pediatrics. 2012;129:e827–e841.
20. Hale TW, Rowe HE. Medications and Mother's Milk, 16th ed. Amarillo, TX: Hale Publishing, 2014, p. 1275.
21. National Institute for Health and Clinical Excellence. Antenatal Care. NICE clinical guideline 62. March 2008, modified 2010. http://www.nice.org.uk/guidance/cg62/resources/guidance-antenatal-care-pdf (last accessed July 31, 2014).
22. American Academy of Pediatrics and American College of Obstetricians and Gynecologists: Guidelines for perinatal care, 7th ed. Elk Grove Village, IL: AAP. 2012, p. 593.
23. ACOG Practice Bulletin: Nausea and vomiting of pregnancy. Obstet Gynecol. 2004;103:803–814.
24. Madjunkova S, Maltepe C, Koren G. The delayed-release combination of doxylamine and pyridoxine (Diclegis®/Diclectin®) for the treatment of nausea and vomiting of pregnancy. Pediatr Drugs. 2014;16:199–211.
25. Worthington I, Pringsheim T, Gawel MJ, et al. Pharmacological acute migraine treatment strategies: choosing the right drug for a specific patient. Can J Neurol Sci. 2013;40(5 Suppl 3):S1–S80.
26. Jolley JA, Wing DA. Pyelonephritis in pregnancy: an update on treatment options for optimal outcomes. Drugs. 2010;70: 1643–1655.
27. Smaill FM, Vazquez JC. Antibiotics for asymptomatic bacteriuria in pregnancy. Cochrane Database of Systematic Reviews 2015, Issue 8. Art. No.: CD000490. DOI: 10.1002/14651858.CD000490.pub3.
28. Vazquez JC, Abalos E. Treatments for symptomatic urinary tract infections during pregnancy. Cochrane Database of Systematic Reviews 2011, Issue 1. Art. No.: CD002256. DOI: 10.1002/14651858.CD002256.pub2.
29. ACOG Committee Opinion No. 475: Antenatal corticosteroid therapy for fetal maturation. Obstet Gynecol. 2011;117:422–424.
30. Crowther CA, McKinlay CJ, Middleton P, Harding JE. Repeat doses of prenatal corticosteroids for women at risk of preterm birth for improving neonatal health outcomes. Cochrane Database Syst Rev. 2011:CD003935.
31. ACOG practice bulletin. Management of preterm labor. Number 127. Obstet Gynecol. 2012;119:1308–1317.
32. Haas DM, Caldwell DM, Kirkpatrick P, et al. Tocolytic therapy for preterm delivery: systematic review and network meta-analysis. BMJ. 2012:345:e6226.
33. ACOG Committee Opinion No. 573: Magnesium Sulfate Use in Obstetrics. Obstet Gynecol. 2013;122:727–728.
34. ACOG Practice bulletin No. 139: premature rupture of membranes. Obstet Gynecol. 2013;122(4):918–930.
35. ACOG Committee Opinion No. 419. American College of Obstetricians and Gynecologists. Use of progesterone to reduce preterm birth. Obstet Gynecol. 2008;112:963–965.
36. Norwitz ER, Caughey AB. Progesterone supplementation and the prevention of preterm birth. Rev Obstet Gynecol. 2011;4(2):60–72 doi:10.3909/riog0163
37. ACOG Committee Opinion No. 485: Prevention of early-onset group B streptococcal disease in newborns. Obstet Gynecol. 2011;117:1019–1027.
38. Verani JR, McGee L, Schrag SJ. Prevention of perinatal group B streptococcal disease—revised guidelines from CDC, 2010. MMWR Recomm Rep. 2010;59:1–36.
39. ACOG Practice Bulletin No. 107. Induction of labor. Obstet Gynecol. 2009;114(2 Pt 1):386–397.
40. Leduc L, Biringer A, Lee L, et al. Induction of labour. J Obstet Gynaecol Can. 2013;35:S1–S15.
41. ACOG Committee on Practice Bulletins. ACOG Practice Bulletin No. 76. Postpartum haemorrhage. Obstet Gynecol. 2006;108:10-39-47.
42. Mousa HA, Blum J, Abou El Senoun G, et al. Treatment for primary postpartum haemorrhage. Cochrane Database Syst Rev. 2014; No. 2 DOI: 10.1002/14651858.CD003249.pub3.
43. De Groot L, Abalovich M, Alexander EK, et al. Management of thyroid dysfunction during pregnancy and postpartum: an Endocrine Society clinical practice guideline. J Clin Endocrinol Metab. 2012;97:2543–2565.
44. ACOG Executive Summary. Hypertension in pregnancy. Obstet Gynecol. 2013;122:1122–1131.
45. Workowski KA, Berman S. Sexually transmitted diseases treatment guidelines, 2010. MMWR Recomm Rep. 2010;59:1–110.
46. CDC, Update to CDC's Sexually Transmitted Diseases Treatment Guidelines, 2010: Oral Cephalosporins No Longer a Recommended Treatment for Gonococcal Infections. MMWR Morb Mortal Wkly Rep, August 10, 2012 / 61(31);590–594.
47. ABM Clinical Protocol #9: Use of galactogogues in initiating or augmenting the rate of maternal milk secretion (First Revision January 2011). Breastfeed Med. 2011;6:41–49.
48. Bozzo P, Koren G. Health Canada advisory on domperiodone: should I avoid prescribing domperidone to women to increase milk production? Can Fam Phys. 2014;58:952–953.
49. Amir LH. Managing common breastfeeding problems in the community. BMJ. 2014;348:g2954.

48 Contraception

Julia M. Koehler and Kathleen B. Haynes

LEARNING OBJECTIVES

Upon completion of the chapter, the reader will be able to:

1. Discuss the physiology of the female reproductive system.
2. Compare the efficacy of oral contraceptives with that of other methods of contraception.
3. State the mechanism of action of hormonal contraceptives.
4. Discuss risks associated with the use of contraceptives, and state absolute and relative contraindications to their use.
5. List side effects associated with the use of various contraceptives, and recommend strategies for minimizing or eliminating such side effects.
6. Describe advantages and disadvantages of various contraceptives, including oral and nonoral formulations.
7. Cite important drug interactions that may occur with oral contraceptives.
8. Provide appropriate patient education regarding the important differences between various barrier methods of contraception.
9. Discuss how emergency contraception may be employed to prevent unintended pregnancy.
10. Provide appropriate patient education regarding the use of oral contraceptives, and recommend and discuss the use of nonoral contraceptives when appropriate.

INTRODUCTION

Historically, the 1950s was an important time in the control of human fertility. It was during that decade that the first combination oral contraceptives (COCs) were developed. Shortly after the discovery that the exogenous administration of hormones such as progesterone successfully blocked ovulation, the use of hormonal steroids quickly became the most popular method of contraception worldwide. COCs are the most commonly used reversible form of contraception in the United States today, with an estimated 10.6 million women users.[1] Studies of women of childbearing age in the United States estimate that 62% are currently using a contraceptive method.[1] Since the introduction of oral contraceptives, many additional contraceptive forms have been developed and are available for use in the United States, including transdermal systems, transvaginal systems, and intrauterine devices (IUDs). These additional forms of contraception offer women effective and potentially more convenient alternatives to oral contraceptives.

EPIDEMIOLOGY

According to the National Survey of Family Growth, approximately 6.58 million pregnancies occur annually in the United States.[2] It is estimated that nearly half of all pregnancies that occur each year in the United States are unintended.[2,3] Contributing to the risk of unintended pregnancy is the fact that approximately 11% of all women who are at risk of becoming pregnant do not use any form of contraception.[1] In addition, many women who do use contraceptives use their chosen method of contraception imperfectly, and this also increases the risk of unintended pregnancy. For patients with certain medical conditions, such as epilepsy, hypertension, ischemic heart disease, sickle cell disease, lupus, or thromboembolic mutations, unintended pregnancy can further increase the risk for adverse health events.[4] The provision of appropriate and adequate instruction to patients regarding how to use contraceptive methods effectively is essential in order to reduce the risk of unintended pregnancy and, for some women, the associated increase in risk for adverse health-related events.

Exposure to sexually transmitted infections (STIs) is also a concern for women who are sexually active. It is estimated that 20 million people in the United States become newly infected annually with an STI.[5] Given that not all methods of contraception protect the user against STIs, the provision of proper patient education by health care professionals regarding this risk is absolutely essential.

PHYSIOLOGY

The female menstrual cycle is divided into four functional phases: follicular, ovulatory, luteal, and menstrual.[3] The follicular phase begins the cycle, and ovulation generally occurs around day 14. The luteal phase then begins and continues until menstruation occurs.[3] The menstrual cycle is regulated by a negative-feedback

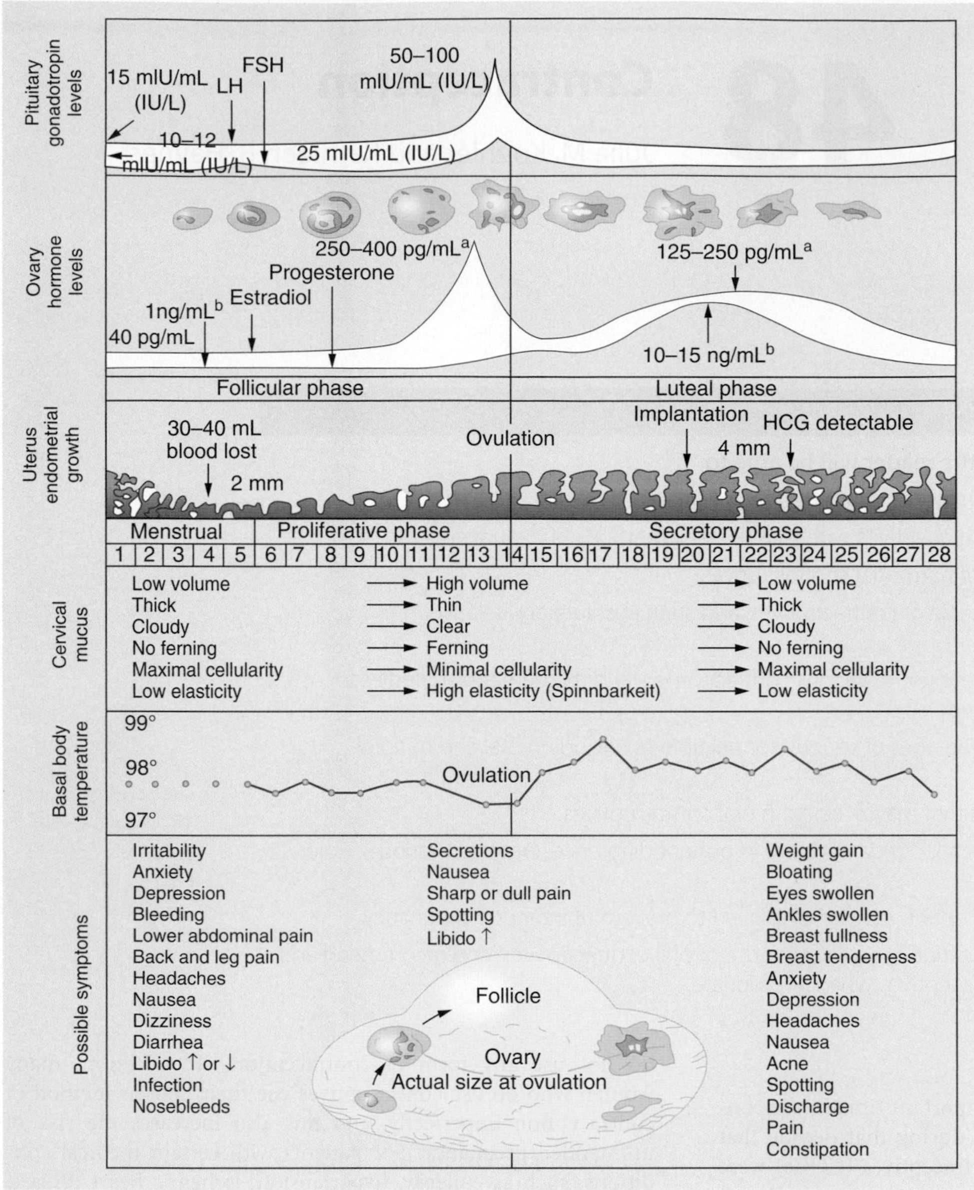

FIGURE 48–1. Menstrual cycle events. [a]Estradiol: 40 pg/mL = 147 pmol/L; 250 to 400 pg/mL = 918 to 1468 pmol/L; 125 to 250 pg/mL = 459 to 918 pmol/L. [b]Progesterone: 1 ng/mL = 3 nmol/L; 10 to 15 ng/mL = 32 to 48 nmol/L. (Adapted with permission from Shulman LP. The menstrual cycle. In: Hatcher RA, Trussel J, Nelson AL, Cates W Jr, Kowal D, Policar M. Contraceptive Technology, 20th rev. ed. New York: Ardent Media, 2011:29–44.)

hormone loop between the hypothalamus, anterior pituitary gland, and ovaries[3] (Figure 48–1).

Initially, the hypothalamus releases gonadotropin-releasing hormone (GnRH), which stimulates the anterior pituitary to produce follicle-stimulating hormone (FSH) and luteinizing hormone (LH). The levels of FSH and LH released vary depending on the phase of the menstrual cycle. Just prior to ovulation, FSH and LH both are at their peak levels. The FSH helps to promote growth of the follicle in preparation for ovulation by causing granulosa cells lining the follicle to grow and produce estrogen. LH promotes androgen production by theca cells in the follicle, promotes ovulation and oocyte maturation, and converts granulosa cells to cells that secrete progesterone after ovulation.

Conception is most likely to occur when viable sperm are present in the upper region of the reproductive tract at the time of ovulation. Fertilization occurs when a spermatozoan penetrates an ovum. Approximately 6 to 8 days after ovulation, attachment of the early embryo to the lining of the uterine cavity—implantation—occurs.

PREVENTION OF PREGNANCY: CONTRACEPTIVES AND DEVICES

Goals of Contraception/Desired Outcome

The most common goal of contraception is the prevention of pregnancy. However, some patients use contraceptive methods for other benefits, such as menstrual cycle regulation, reduction of premenstrual symptoms, or treatment of acne.

Choice of Contraceptives: Important Considerations

When helping a patient with contraceptive selection, the most important goal is finding an option the patient is comfortable with and the clinician feels is beneficial for the patient. It is imperative to explain the side effects, safety concerns, and noncontraceptive benefits of each alternative to the patient so that she may make an informed decision. Fertility goals vary for each patient. It must be determined whether the goal is to postpone conception, space out the next pregnancy, or avoid further pregnancy altogether. Also, a clinician must understand the patient's desire to have or not have a regular bleeding pattern, because many contraceptives will affect menses.

As discussed later in this chapter, contraindications exist for various forms of contraception. Patients must be evaluated by a health care professional to rule out medical contraindications to certain contraceptives. The physical examination also allows health care professionals to identify other medical concerns, such as hypertension or liver disease, that need to be considered when selecting an appropriate contraceptive agent. Clinicians also should review family history for potential risks with certain forms of birth control.

Sexual behavior of the female must be determined to understand the risk for STIs. Women not in a monogamous relationship must consider their risk of STIs as a factor in their contraceptive decision. Some barrier methods protect against STIs, but hormonal contraceptives do not prevent STIs if used alone.

Personal preference plays a large role when determining the best contraceptive option. For instance, if a woman is not interested in using a method that interrupts sexual activity, then a diaphragm would be an inappropriate choice. Preference of the sexual partner may also be important. Certain agents such as male condoms require the male partner to play an active role in contraception.

Cost may also be an issue for patients. Insurance may not cover all forms of contraception, and patients may have to bear the entire cost for certain options.

Efficacy of Contraceptives

The unintended pregnancy rate for women who do not use any form of contraception is unknown. Therefore, it is difficult to determine the true efficacy of contraceptives in preventing unwanted pregnancy. Table 48–1 shows the percentage of women who experience unintended pregnancy within 1 year of contraceptive use with ongoing sexual activity.[3]

Table 48–1

Unintended Pregnancy Rates

Method	Percentage of Women Experiencing Unintended Pregnancy Within First Year of Use: Typical Use[a]	Perfect Use[b]	Percentage of Women Continuing Use at 1 Year[c]
No method	85	85	
Spermicides	28	18	42
Withdrawal	22	4	46
Fertility awareness–based methods	24		47
Standard days method		5	
Two-day method		4	
Ovulation method		3	
Symptothermal method		0.4	
Sponge			
Parous women	24	20	
Nulliparous women	12	9	
Diaphragm	12	6	57
Condom			
Female	21	5	41
Male	18	2	43
Combination pill and mini-pill	9	0.3	67
Ortho Evra patch	9	0.3	67
NuvaRing	9	0.3	67
Depo-Provera	6	0.2	56
IUD			
ParaGard (copper T)	0.8	0.6	78
Mirena (LNG-IUS)	0.2	0.2	80
Implanon	0.05	0.05	84
Nexplanon	0.05	0.05	84
Female sterilization	0.5	0.5	100
Male sterilization	0.15	0.1	100

[a]Among typical couples who initiate use of a method (not necessarily for the first time), the percentage who experience an accidental pregnancy during the first year if they do not stop use for any other reason. Estimates of the probability of pregnancy during the first year of typical use for spermicides, withdrawal, periodic abstinence, the diaphragm, the male condom, the pill, and Depo-Provera are taken from the 1995 National Survey of Family Growth corrected for underreporting of abortion.

[b]Among couples who initiate use of a method (not necessarily for the first time) and who use it *perfectly* (both consistently and correctly), the percentage who experience an accidental pregnancy during the first year if they do not stop use for any other reason.

[c]Among couples attempting to avoid pregnancy, the percentage who continue to use a method for 1 year.

Adapted from Trussel J, Guthrie KA. Choosing a contraceptive: Efficacy, safety, and personal considerations. In: Hatcher RA, Trussel J, Nelson AL, Cates W Jr, Kowal D, Policar M. Contraceptive Technology, 20th rev. ed. New York: Ardent Media, 2011:45–74, with permission.

Oral Contraceptives (Combination)

COCs contain a synthetic estrogen and one of several steroids with progestational activity. Most oral contraceptives contain one of three types of estrogen: ethinyl estradiol (EE), which is pharmacologically active; mestranol, which is converted by the liver to EE; or estradiol valerate, which is metabolized to estradiol and valeric acid. Many different progestins are found in the various oral contraceptives. These include norethindrone, norethindrone acetate, ethynodiol diacetate, norgestrel, levonorgestrel, desogestrel, norgestimate, drospirenone, and dienogest.

The primary mechanism by which COCs prevent pregnancy is through inhibition of ovulation. FSH and LH regulate the production of estrogen and progesterone by the ovaries. Secretion of estrogen and progesterone by the ovaries occurs in a cyclic manner, which determines the regular hormonal changes that occur in the uterus, vagina, and cervix associated with the menstrual cycle. Cyclic changes in the levels of estrogen and progesterone in the blood, together with FSH and LH, modulate the development of ova and the occurrence of ovulation. The estrogen component of COCs is most active in inhibiting FSH release.[3] However, at sufficiently high doses, estrogens also may cause inhibition of LH release. In low-dose COCs, the progestin component causes suppression of LH.[3] Ovulation is prevented by this suppression of the midcycle surge of both FSH and LH[3] and mimics the physiologic changes that occur during pregnancy.

Although suppression of FSH and LH is the primary mechanism by which COCs prevent ovulation, there are other mechanisms by which these hormones work to prevent pregnancy. Other mechanisms include reduced penetration of the egg by sperm, reduced implantation of fertilized eggs, thickening of cervical mucus to prevent sperm penetration into the upper genital tract, and slowed tubal motility, which may delay transport of sperm.[3] Thus, in addition to inhibiting ovulation, COCs induce changes in the cervical mucus and endometrium that make sperm transport and implantation of the embryo unlikely.[3]

Table 48–2 contains a partial listing of the many oral contraceptives available in the United States.[6] Since the mid-1960s, EE has been the primary estrogen used in most COCs. However, the amount of EE used in COCs has decreased progressively since that time, and most now contain 35 mcg or less of EE. In

Table 48–2

Some Available Contraceptives

Estrogen (mcg/tablet)	Progestin (mg/tablet)	Examples of Brand Names
Monophasic Preparations		
EE (20)	Norethindrone acetate (1)	Junel 1/20, Junel Fe 1/20, Larin Fe 1/20, Loestrin 21 1/20, Loestrin Fe 1/20, Microgestin 1/20, Microgestin Fe 1/20, Minastrin 24 Fe
EE (20)	Levonorgestrel (0.09)	Amethyst
EE (20)	Levonorgestrel (0.1)	Lessina, Lutera, Orsythia, Aviane, Falmina, Sronyx
EE (20)	Drospirenone (3)	Yaz, Beyaz[a], Loryna, Gianvi, Vestura
EE (20)	Desogestrel (0.15)	Azurette
EE (25)	Norethindrone (0.8)	Generess Fe
EE (30)	Desogestrel (0.15)	Apri, Desogen, Ortho-Cept, Reclipsen
EE (30)	Levonorgestrel (0.15)	Altavera, Kurvelo, Levora, Marlissa, Nordette, Portia
EE (30)	Drospirenone (3)	Ocella, Safyral[a], Syeda, Yasmin, Zarah
EE (30)	Norgestrel (0.3)	Cryselle, Elinest, Lo/Ovral-28, Low-Ogestrel
EE (30)	Norethindrone acetate (1.5)	Junel 1.5/30, Junel Fe 1.5/30, Larin Fe 1.5/30, Loestrin 21 1.5/30, Loestrin Fe 1.5/30, Microgestin 1.5/30, Microgestin Fe 1.5/30
EE (35)	Norgestimate (0.25)	Mono-Linyah, MonoNessa, Ortho-Cyclen, Previfem, Sprintec
EE (35)	Norethindrone (0.4)	Balziva, Briellyn, Femcon Fe, Ovcon-35, Philith, Zenchant, Zenchant Fe, Zeosa
EE (35)	Norethindrone (0.5)	Brevicon, Modicon, Necon 0.5/35, Nortrel 0.5/35, Wera
EE (35)	Norethindrone (1)	Alyacen 1/35, Cyclafem 1/35, Dasetta 1/35, Necon 1/35, Norinyl 1/35, Nortrel 1/35, Ortho-Novum 1/35, Pirmella 1/35
EE (35)	Ethynodiol diacetate (1)	Kelnor, Zovia 1/35
EE (50)	Norgestrel (0.5)	Ogestrel
EE (50)	Ethynodiol diacetate (1)	Zovia 1/50
Mestranol (50)	Norethindrone (1)	Necon 1/50, Norinyl 1/50
Biphasic Preparations		
EE (10)	Norethindrone acetate (1,0)	Lo Loestrin Fe[b]
EE (20,0,10)	Desogestrel (0.15)	Kariva[b], Mircette[b], Pimtrea[b], Viorele[b]
EE (35)	Norethindrone (0.5,1)	Necon 10/11
Triphasic Preparations		
EE (20,30,35)	Northindrone acetate (1)	Estrostep Fe, Tilia Fe
EE (30,40,30)	Levonorgestrel (0.05,0.075,0.125)	Enpresse, Myzilra, Triphasil, Trivora
EE (35)	Norgestimate (0.18,0.215,0.25)	Ortho Tri-Cyclen, Tri-Estarylla, Tri-Linyah, Tri-Nessa, Tri-Previfem, Tri-Sprintec
EE (35)	Norethindrone (0.5,1,0.5)	Aranelle, Leena, Tri-Norinyl
EE (35)	Norethindrone (0.5,0.75,1)	Alyacen 7/7/7, Cyclafem 7/7/7, Dasetta 7/7/7, Necon 7/7/7, Nortrel 7/7/7, Ortho-Novum 7/7/7, Pirmella 7/7/7
EE (25)	Norgestimate (0.18,0.215,0.25)	Ortho Tri-Cyclen Lo
EE (25)	Desogestrel (0.1,0.125,0.15)	Caziant, Cyclessa, Velivet
Quadriphasic Preparations		
Estradiol valerate (3,2,2,1)	Dienogest (0,2,3,0)	Natazia
Extended Cycle Preparations		
EE (20)	Levonorgestrel (0.09)	Lybrel
EE (20)	Levonorgestrel (0.1)	Amethia Lo, Camrese Lo
EE (30)	Levonorgestrel (0.15)	Amethia, Camrese, Daysee, Introvale, Jolessa, Quasense, Seasonale
EE (20,25,30,10)	Levonorgestrel (0.15,0)	Quartette
EE (20,10)	Levonorgestrel (0.1)	LoSeasonique
EE (30,10)	Levonorgestrel (0.15)	Seasonique
Progestin-Only Preparations		
None	Norethindrone (0.35)	Camila, Errin, Heather, Jencycla, Jolivette, Nora-BE, Nor-QD, Ortho Micronor

EE, ethinyl estradiol

[a]Each tablet also contains 451 mcg of levomefolate calcium

[b]Some references may classify as monophasic since the variation in hormone content does not occur during the first three weeks of the pill pack.

Data compiled in part from Anonymous. Choice of contraceptives: Treatment Guidelines from The Medical Letter. Med Lett. 2010;8:89–96.

addition, to reduce side effects and improve tolerability associated with oral contraceptive use, new progestins and different routes of administration have been explored. In an attempt to minimize the undesirable androgenic side effects associated with the progestins of COCs, the original synthetic progestins were modified to create "third generation" progestins (eg, desogestrel and norgestimate), and newer progestins with antiandrogenic properties (eg, drospirenone) have been discovered. Overall, the synthetic progestins found in today's COCs are extremely potent in their ability to inhibit ovulation and prevent pregnancy.

COCs are available in monophasic, biphasic, triphasic, and quadriphasic preparations. Monophasic preparations contain fixed doses of estrogen and progestin in each active pill. Although all four preparations contain both estrogens and progestins, biphasic, triphasic, and quadriphasic preparations contain varying proportions of one or both hormones during the pill cycle. These preparations were introduced to reduce a patient's cumulative exposure to progestins, as well as to mimic more closely the hormonal changes of the menstrual cycle. However, there is no evidence to suggest that the multiphasic preparations offer any significant clinical advantage over monophasic pills.[6]

Most traditional COCs are packaged as 21/7 cycles (ie, 21 days of active pills and 7 days of placebo). However, newer regimens offer either fewer hormone-free days per traditional, 28-day pill cycle or extended (or in some cases continuous) cycles, which may allow for fewer withdrawal bleeds per year and fewer menstrual-related side effects (eg, menstrual pain, bloating, headaches) for some women.

▶ *Noncontraceptive Benefits of Combination Oral Contraceptives*

In addition to preventing pregnancy, there are several noncontraceptive benefits associated with the use of COCs.

Reduction in the Risk of Endometrial Cancer The risk of endometrial cancer among women who have used oral contraceptives for at least 1 year is approximately 40% less and for at least 10 years is approximately 80% less than the risk in women who have never used oral contraceptives.[3,7] There is additional evidence to suggest this benefit is detectable within 1 year of use, and the reduced risk may persist for up to 20 years following discontinuation of oral contraceptives.[3,8]

Reduction in the Risk of Ovarian Cancer When compared with women who have never used oral contraceptives, women who have used oral contraceptives for up to 4 years are 30% less likely to develop ovarian cancer. There is also additional evidence to suggest that the longer the duration of oral contraceptive use, the greater the reduction in the risk of ovarian cancer. Women who have taken oral contraceptives for 5 to 11 years are 60% less likely to develop ovarian cancer, and women who have taken oral contraceptives for more than 12 years are 80% less likely to develop ovarian cancer than those who have never used oral contraceptives. As with the reduced risk of endometrial cancer, there is evidence to suggest the reduced risk of ovarian cancer may persist for years following discontinuation of oral contraceptives.[9,10]

Improved Regulation of Menstruation and Reduction in the Risk of Anemia Women who take oral contraceptives typically experience more regular menstrual cycles. In general, oral contraceptive use is associated with less cramping and dysmenorrhea.[3,6] Also, women who take oral contraceptives have a smaller volume of menstruum and experience fewer days of menstruation each month and consequently experience less blood loss with each menstrual period.[3,11] Some studies suggest that oral contraceptive use decreases overall monthly menstrual flow by 60% or more and conserves hemoglobin and ferritin levels, which may be particularly beneficial in women who are anemic or at risk for anemia.[3] In addition, some COC formulations contain iron, which may also minimize the risk for anemia (See **Unique Oral Contraceptives** section.)

Reduction in the Risk of Fetal Neural Tube Defects While COCs are not 100% effective at preventing pregnancy, it is possible that a woman may conceive while taking a COC. In addition, many women may become pregnant very soon after discontinuing a COC. In order to decrease the risk of neural tube defects in the fetuses associated with such pregnancies, COC formulations that contain a source of folate in every pill are also available.[3]

Relief from Symptoms Associated with Premenstrual Dysphoric Disorder COCs have been widely used for the treatment of premenstrual dysphoric disorder (PMDD). Current evidence suggests that these agents are most effective at targeting the physical symptoms associated with the disorder and less effective in treating mood-related symptoms.[12] Although multiphasic COCs have been used effectively in the treatment of PMDD, monophasic preparations may yield fewer mood swings and are generally easier to manage. Yaz, which contains the progestin, drospirenone, carries an FDA-approved indication for PMDD.[6]

Relief of Benign Breast Disease Women who use oral contraceptives are less likely to develop benign breast cysts or fibroadenomas and are less likely to experience progression of such conditions.[3,6]

Prevention of Ovarian Cysts Because oral contraceptives suppress ovarian stimulation, women who take them are less likely to develop ovarian cysts.[6]

Decrease in Symptoms Related to Endometriosis COC use has been linked to a decreased incidence of symptomatic endometriosis. In women who suffer from endometriosis, the extended-cycle COCs may provide the most effective relief from menstrual pain by reducing the total number of painful episodes per year.[3]

Improvement in Acne Control All COCs can improve acne by increasing the quantity of sex hormone–binding globulin and thereby decreasing free testosterone concentrations.[6] Third-generation progestins, such as desogestrel and norgestimate, are believed to have less androgenic activity compared with older progestins, and drospirenone is considered to be antiandrogenic.[6] However, it is not clear that COCs containing any of these progestins confer any advantage over other COCs with respect to their ability to improve acne control. Ortho Tri-Cyclen (EE and norgestimate), Estrostep Fe (EE and norethindrone acetate), Yaz, and Beyaz (EE and drospirenone) each carry an FDA-approved indication for the treatment of acne.[3,6]

▶ *Potential Risks of Combination Oral Contraceptives*

Although there are many noncontraceptive benefits associated with the use of COCs, their use is not without risk or potential for adverse effects.

Sexually Transmitted Infections Because the use of COCs may decrease the use of selected barrier contraceptive methods (eg, latex condoms) that do protect against STIs, one of the most common potential risks associated with the use of oral contraceptives is the increased risk of acquiring an STI.[4]

Cardiovascular Events and Hypertension A World Health Organization (WHO) collaborative study found that high-dose

(50 mcg or more of EE) oral contraceptive users with uncontrolled hypertension have an increased risk of experiencing a myocardial infarction or stroke.[6,13] In this study, women who had the lowest risk for experiencing a myocardial infarction or stroke were those who did not smoke, took low-dose oral contraceptives, and had their blood pressure checked prior to beginning oral contraceptives.[14–16] Hypertension secondary to oral contraceptive use is thought to occur in up to 3% of women and is believed to be attributed to the effect that estrogens and progestins can have on aldosterone activity.[3] Given this and the risk for cardiovascular events, women should have their blood pressure checked prior to initiating oral contraceptives, as well as periodically throughout oral contraceptive use. If significant elevations in blood pressure are noted, oral contraceptives should be discontinued. Estrogen-containing contraceptives are not recommended for smokers who are 35 years of age or older, for women with hypertension (especially if untreated), or for women who experience migraine headaches (especially those with focal neurologic symptoms).[4,6]

Venous Thromboembolism It is believed that the estrogen component of COCs stimulates enhanced hepatic production of clotting factors. COCs have been associated with a two- to threefold increase in the risk of venous thromboembolism compared with women who do not use oral contraceptives.[6] Contraceptive users at greatest risk for the development of venous thromboembolism include those who are obese, smoke, have hypertension, have diabetes complicated by end-organ damage, are immobile, have experienced recent trauma or surgery, or have a history of prior thromboembolism. It is important to note, however, that the increase in risk of venous thromboembolism in oral contraceptive users is lower than that associated with pregnancy and the postpartum period.[6,17] Newer, less androgenic progestins, such as desogestrel and drospirenone, have been reported to be associated with a higher risk of venous thromboembolism.[18–21] Currently available studies validating this risk have produced conflicting results. Two studies published in 2011 reported a two- to three-fold greater risk of venous thromboembolic events in women using oral contraceptives containing drospirenone when compared with women using levonorgestrel-containing contraceptives.[22,23] However, the results of the International Active Surveillance Study of Women Taking Oral Contraceptives, published in 2014, demonstrated similar rates of venous and arterial thromboembolism in women taking COCs containing drosperinone, levonorgesterol, or other progestins.[24] In general, progestin-only contraceptives are preferred for women who are at increased risk of cardiovascular or thromboembolic complications, including women with a prior history of thromboembolic disease.[4,6]

Gallbladder Disease In women with preexisting gallstones, low-dose estrogen-containing oral contraceptives may enhance the potential for the development of symptomatic gallbladder disease and may worsen existing gallbladder disease.[3,4] Although this risk has not been demonstrated with the use of higher-dose oral contraceptives, COCs containing estrogen should be used with caution in patients with a history of gallbladder disease.

Hepatic Tumors Although the use of oral contraceptives is not associated with an increased risk for the development of hepatocellular carcinoma, long-term use of high-dose oral contraceptives has been associated with the development of benign liver tumors.[3] Because even benign liver tumors may pose significant risk to the patient, oral contraceptives should be discontinued if liver enlargement is noted on physical examination. In cases of hepatoma (malignancy), the use of COCs is contraindicated.[4]

Patient Encounter, Part 1

A 22-year-old nulliparous woman, presents to your clinic requesting information on contraception. She specifically inquires about options that allow for fewer or no menstrual periods. You begin to take a history and determine that the patient is currently sexually active and is not using any method of birth control. She weighs 135 lb(61.4 kg), is 64 in (163 cm) tall, and has a blood pressure of 108/70 mm Hg. She has no history of smoking. She has migraines without aura, for which she takes propranolol. On further questioning, you discover that she has a positive family history of breast cancer (both her mother and maternal aunt), but no personal history. As you discuss various contraceptive options with the patient, it is clear that she has a preference for an oral contraceptive agent.

What additional information do you need to know before recommending a contraceptive for this patient?

Based on the information provided by the patient, what oral contraceptive agent would you recommend for the patient and why?

What education would you provide to this patient regarding risks associated with oral contraceptive use?

Cervical Cancer There appears to be an increased risk for the development of cervical cancer among long-term users of oral contraceptives.[3] It is uncertain whether this increase in risk is directly attributed to the use of oral contraceptives. Data suggest that oral contraceptive users tend to have more sexual partners and use condoms less frequently, and as a result, this may increase their susceptibility to infection with human papilloma virus (HPV), a known risk factor for cervical cancer.

KEY CONCEPT *Absolute and relative contraindications to the use of oral contraceptives are listed in* **Table 48–3**.[3,4,25]

▶ Adverse Effects of Oral Contraceptives and Their Management

As with all medications, there are potential adverse effects with COCs. KEY CONCEPT *Many side effects can be minimized or avoided by adjusting the estrogen and/or progestin content of the oral contraceptive.* It is also important to individualize the selection of oral contraceptives, because some women are at increased risk for potentially serious side effects.

Common complaints with COCs include headaches, nausea, vomiting, **mastalgia**, and weight gain; although studies have shown a similar percentage of patients taking placebo experience these side effects.[26] Given that oral contraceptives often are discontinued owing to side effects, proper counseling before initiation of COCs is necessary.

Between 30% and 50% of women complain of breakthrough bleeding or spotting when oral contraceptives are initiated. These side effects tend to resolve by the third or fourth cycle.[3] Before changing formulations, other more serious causes of bleeding or spotting, such as pregnancy, infection, and poor absorption of the oral contraceptive owing to drug interaction or GI problems, should be ruled out. Once these causes have been ruled out, the timing of the spotting must be determined in order to adjust the formulation appropriately.

Table 48–3

Contraindications to the Use of Combined Oral Contraceptives (COCs)

Absolute Contraindications
History of thromboembolic disease
History of stroke (or current cerebrovascular disease)
History of (or current) coronary artery disease, ischemic heart disease, or peripheral vascular disease
History of carcinoma of the breast (known or suspected)
History of any estrogen-dependent neoplasm (known or suspected)
Undiagnosed abnormal uterine or vaginal bleeding
Pregnancy (known or suspected)
Heavy smoking (defined as 15 cigarettes or more per day) by women who are 35 years of age or older
History of hepatic tumors (benign or malignant)
Active liver disease
Migraine headaches with focal neurologic symptoms
Postpartum (during the first 21 days, as well as during days 21 through 42 in women with additional risk factors for thromboembolism, including age ≥ 35 years, history of previous venous thromboembolism, preeclampsia, recent cesarean delivery, obesity, and smoking)
Relative Contraindications
Smoking (< 15 cigarettes per day) at any age
Migraine headache disorder without focal neurologic symptoms
Hypertension (NOTE: WHO considers health risk posed by COC use to be "unacceptable" when either systolic blood pressure 160 mm Hg or more, or diastolic blood pressure 90 mm Hg or more)
Fibroid tumors of the uterus
Breast-feeding
Diabetes mellitus
Family history of dyslipidemia
Sickle cell disease
Active gallbladder disease
Age > 50 years
Elective major surgery requiring immobilization (planned in the next 4 weeks)

Data from Refs. 3, 4, and 25.

The most common side effects and ways to adjust therapy to minimize these side effects are listed in Table 48–4.[1,3,6,27,28]

As highlighted in Table 48–4, many of the side effects of COCs may be minimized by adjusting the estrogen or progestin content of the preparation. However, although low-dose COCs may cause fewer side effects, it is important to note that in the event that doses are missed, such COCs may be more likely to result in contraceptive failure.

Progestin-Only Pills

For women unable to take estrogen-containing oral contraceptives, there is an alternative: oral contraceptives containing only the progestin, norethindrone. These agents are slightly less effective than COCs but have other advantages over COCs. Progestin-only products have not shown the same thromboembolic risk as estrogen-containing products. Therefore, women at increased risk for or with a history of thromboembolism may be good candidates for progestin-only oral contraceptives. Also, these products can minimize menses, and many women have **amenorrhea** after six to nine cycles. These products have also been found safe to use in women who are nursing, so they are a viable option for women who breast-feed and desire hormonal contraception. In such patients, it should not be initiated until 6 weeks postpartum. Spotting does not subside in some women, and this is a common cause for discontinuation. These products should be taken at the same time every day, and there is no pill-free or hormone-free period.

Unique Oral Contraceptives

Along with varying doses of estrogen and different progestins, there are also formulation modifications that may benefit various patient situations. In the United States, these formulations include products such as Lo-Loestrin Fe; Amethia, Camrese, Daysee, Introvale, and Seasonale; Amethia Lo and Camrese Lo; Seasonique and Lo Seasonique; Yasmin, Yaz, and Beyaz; Ortho Tri-Cyclen and Estrostep Fe; Kariva, Mircette, Pimtrea, and Viorele; Ovcon 35; Lybrel; Natazia; and Quartette. Each of these products may show benefit in certain women owing to their unique characteristics.

Lo-Loestrin Fe (norethindrone/EE) contains a low-dose estrogen, a high amount of progestin, and medium androgenic activity. Similar to other low-dose estrogen COCs, Lo-Loestrin Fe may offer a smaller margin of error when pills are missed but provide the potential advantage of fewer estrogen-related side effects (eg, nausea and breast tenderness). Unlike the typical 28-pill packs that contain 21 active tablets and seven placebo tablets, Lo-Loestrin Fe contains 24 combination hormone tablets, two estrogen-only tablets, and two placebo (iron-only) tablets. This product provides a shorter hormone-free interval and may allow for shorter menstrual periods and fewer menstrual-related symptoms, such as menstrual-related headaches, menorrhagia, and anemia.

Amethia, Camrese, Daysee, Introvale, Jolessa, and Seasonale, (levonorgestrel/EE) are each monophasic combinations that are packaged as a 91-day treatment cycles with 84 active tablets that are taken consecutively followed by seven placebo tablets. The extended cycle length of these products allows for one menstrual cycle per "season," or four per year. This type of formulation may be appealing to women with perimenstrual side effects or those at higher risk for anemia with menstrual bleeding. These products may improve anxiety, headache, fluid retention, dysmenorrhea, breast tenderness, bloating, and menstrual migraines. However, in the SEA 301 clinical trial comparing the efficacy of Seasonale with that of an equivalent-dosage 28-day cycle regimen, 7.7% versus 1.8% of women discontinued prematurely for unacceptable bleeding.[30] The risk of intermenstrual bleeding and/or spotting may be higher for patients taking these extended-cycle combinations than for patients taking typical 28-day-regimen COCs.

Seasonique and Lo Seasonique (levonorgestrel/EE) are also extended cycle preparations that are similar to those mentioned earlier, but instead these preparations contain seven tablets with low-dose estrogen rather than placebo. Menstruation-related problems that may improve with Seasonique or Lo Seasonique include menstrual-related headaches, menorrhagia, and anemia. In addition, endometriosis-related menstrual pain may be relieved by providing a continuous regimen without a pill-free interval.[31]

Yasmin and Yaz (drospirenone/EE) are unique oral contraceptives that contain the progestin drospirenone. This hormone not only has antiandrogenic properties, but also showed antimineralocorticoid activity in preclinical trials. It has a unique application in young women who experience problems associated with producing too much androgen. Drospirenone is a spironolactone analog, and the 3-mg dose available in COC preparations has antimineralocorticoid activity equal to 25 mg of spironolactone. It can affect the sodium and water balance in the body, although it has not shown superior efficacy for side

Table 48–4

Management of Adverse Effects of Oral Contraceptives

Adverse Effect	Cause	Adjustment	Notes
Spotting/bleeding before finishing active pills	Insufficient progestin	Monophasic with increased progestin or triphasic with increasing progestin[3]	
Continued bleeding after menses	Insufficient estrogen	Increase estrogen or triphasic with lower early progestin[3]	
Midcycle bleeding	Difficult to determine	Increase estrogen and progestin[1]	
Increased breakthrough bleeding in general	Insufficient estrogen	Increase estrogen or triphasic formulation	Will increase amount of withdrawal bleeding during menses
Acne, PMDD, **hirsutism**	Progestin with higher androgenicity (eg, norgestrel, levonorgestrel)	Switch to progestin with lower androgenicity such as norgestimate, norethindrone or drospirenone[6]	
Nausea, vomiting	Related to estrogen	Take at bedtime or with food; decrease estrogen or switch to a progestin-only product	Symptoms often resolve in 1–3 months
Constipation, bloating, distention	Related to progestin	Decrease progestin[1]	Symptoms often resolve in 1–3 months
Headache	Must be evaluated because of warning sign for stroke – monitor blood pressure	If determined to not be serious, but still troublesome consider:[3] a. Discontinue oral contraceptive b. Decrease estrogen c. Decrease progestin d. Eliminate pill-free interval for 2–3 cycles (when headaches occur during pill-free interval)	Discontinue oral contraceptive immediately if any neurologic symptoms or blurred vision
Decrease in libido, decreased vaginal lubrication[27]	Insufficient estrogen	Increase estrogen or consider vaginal hormonal ring (NuvaRing)[3]	Feelings of depression may coincide
Dyslipidemia in general	Progestin with higher androgenicity (eg, norgestrel, levonorgestrel)	Switch to progestin with lower androgenicity such as norgestimate, norethindrone or drospirenone[6]	Obtain a baseline lipid panel in women with risk factors for dyslipidemia – smoking, hypertension, family history of heart disease
Triglycerides > 350 mg/dL (3.96 mmol/L)	Related to estrogen	Decrease estrogen to 20–25 mcg or a progestin-only formulation[3]	
Mastalgia	Related to estrogen	Decrease estrogen[28] or switch to an extended cycle formulation (see Unique Oral Contraceptives, later) if it occurs prior to menses	
Weight gain, fluid retention	Excess estrogen[29] and progestin with higher androgenicity (eg, norgestrel, levonorgestrel)	Decrease estrogen and switch to progestin with lower androgenicity such as norgestimate, norethindrone or drospirenone[3]	
Visual changes or disturbances with contact lenses	Related to estrogen	Use saline eye drops	Referral to ophthalmology if eye drops do not help
Melasma, chloasma	Related to estrogen stimulation of melanocyte production	Consider progestin-only product and use of sunscreen[3]	Women with darker pigmentation are more susceptible; melasma may not be completely reversible on discontinuation

Data from Refs. 1, 3, 6, and 27–29.

effects such as bloating compared with other oral contraceptives. Caution should be used in women with chronic conditions or in women taking other medications that may affect serum potassium. Yaz (drospirenone/EE) is an extended-cycle preparation that contains a low-dose estrogen and antimineralocorticoid and antiandrogenic activity. Yaz also contains 24 rather than 21 active tablets and four rather than seven placebo tablets, allowing for shorter menstrual periods and fewer menstrual-related symptoms, such as menstrual-related headaches, menorrhagia, and anemia.

In 2003, the FDA Advisory Committee for Reproductive Health Drugs recommended the development of a COC tablet containing folic acid in order to minimize the risk of neural tube defects in cases of contraceptive failure. Beyaz and Safyral, which were FDA approved in 2010, are combination tablets containing drospirenone and EE (like Yaz and Yasmin) and 451 mcg of levomefolate calcium, the primary metabolite of folic acid. Similar to Yaz, Beyaz is an extended-cycle preparation, which may allow for shorter menstrual periods and fewer menstrual-related symptoms.

In addition to the prevention of pregnancy, Yaz, Beyaz, Ortho Tri-Cyclen (norgestimate/EE), and Estrostep Fe (norethindrone acetate/EE) each carry an approved indication for treatment of moderate acne vulgaris in females 15 years of age or older desiring contraception who have not responded adequately to conventional antiacne medication. This can help clinicians to streamline medications by serving dual purposes.

Mircette, Kariva, Pimtrea, and Viorele (desogestrel/EE) have a unique dosing schedule. After the usual 21 active tablets, there are only two tablets with inert ingredients. The last five tablets in the package have 10 mcg of EE. In theory, this may minimize bleeding during the menstrual cycle, although the clinical significance of this dosing schedule has not been established. With each of these products, it is important to counsel patients to complete the entire pack and not to discard the last 7 days of medication.

Another unique formulation is a chewable tablet available to women who have difficulty swallowing medications. Ovcon 35 (norethindrone/EE) has all 28 tablets in chewable form and has added spearmint flavoring.

Lybrel (levonorgestrel/EE) was the first continuous-cycle COC approved by the FDA. Active pills are taken every day throughout the year with no pill free interval. The major advantage of this product is elimination of menstrual periods, resulting in improvement in or elimination of menstrual-related symptoms. The most bothersome side effect associated with Lybrel is a high incidence of spotting and breakthrough bleeding during the initial months of use. It appears as though the incidence of breakthrough bleeding with Lybrel decreases with continued use.

Natazia was approved by the FDA in 2010 and is a quadriphasic COC containing estradiol valerate and the progestin, dienogest. Estradiol valerate is metabolized endogenously to estradiol, and dienogest is a strong progestin with antiandrogenic activity. Natazia provides a unique estrogen step-down/progestin step-up regimen, and like Mircette, Kariva, Pimtrea, and Viorele, this COC offers the advantage of a shorter hormone-free interval. This results in fewer days of withdrawal bleeding and may help with menstrual-related headaches.

Finally, Quartette (levonorgestrel/EE), an extended-cycle, quadriphasic preparation approved by the FDA in 2013, contains increasing doses of EE throughout the 91-day pill period. The increasing dose of EE is intended to reduce the rate of breakthrough bleeding or spotting.

Patient Encounter, Part 2: Adverse Effects

After 3 months of taking LoSeasonique, she returns to your clinic complaining of breakthrough bleeding during her sixth week of active pills. She reports no change or increase in frequency of her migraine headaches, and her blood pressure is 110/72 mm Hg. She is frustrated with the breakthrough bleeding and wants to explore other contraceptive options.

What are some potential causes of the breakthrough bleeding that the patient has been experiencing?

What strategy would you recommend to eliminate or minimize the potential adverse effects experienced by the patient?

Drug Interactions with Oral Contraceptives

EE is metabolized in the liver primarily via cytochrome P-450 (CYP450) 3A4. When reviewing drug interactions of oral contraceptives, KEY CONCEPT *clinicians should be aware of the many drugs that may potentially interact with contraceptives—especially those that may reduce the effectiveness of contraceptives.* Refer to Table 48–5 for a list of some of the most common drug interactions seen with oral contraceptives.[3,32,33]

Nonoral Hormonal Contraceptives

KEY CONCEPT *As an alternative to oral contraceptive pills, which must be taken daily in order to reliably prevent pregnancy, nonoral contraceptives in the form of transdermal, transvaginal, and injectable preparations are available and offer patients safe and effective alternatives to the pills for prevention of pregnancy. These formulations also do not require daily administration, making them more convenient than the pill formulations.*

Ortho-Evra is a transdermal patch that contains both an estrogen (20 mcg of EE) and a progestin (150 mcg of norelgestromin). A new patch is applied to the abdomen, buttocks, upper torso, or upper (outer) arm once weekly for 3 weeks, followed by seven patch-free days.[6] Although some women have noted irregular bleeding during the first two cycles of patch use, the patch has been demonstrated to provide similar menstrual cycle control and contraceptive efficacy to that of COCs.[34] It is important to note, however, that higher contraceptive failure rates are seen when the patch is used in women weighing more than 90 kg (about 200 lb).[6,34] Further, manufacturer prescriber information indicates that women who take Ortho-Evra are exposed to approximately 60% more estrogen than women who take COCs with 35 mcg of estrogen.[35] Although the clinical significance of this is not well defined, studies have suggested a link between the use of the patch and an increased risk for venous thromboembolism. A slightly higher reported incidence of breast discomfort and local skin irritation has also been reported with the patch.[6,36]

NuvaRing is a unique transvaginal delivery system that provides 15 mcg of EE and 120 mcg of etonogestrel for the prevention of ovulation. NuvaRing is inserted into the vagina on or before day 5 of the menstrual cycle and is removed from the vagina 3 weeks later.[6] Seven days after the ring is removed, a new ring should be inserted. In clinical trials, NuvaRing demonstrated comparable efficacy and cycle control to COCs as well as a similar side-effect profile.[6,37] NuvaRing should not be removed during intercourse.

Depo-Provera is a progestin-only, injectable contraceptive that contains depot medroxyprogesterone acetate. Depo-Provera is administered intramuscularly as a 150-mg injection once every 3 months. An advantage of Depo-Provera is that it provides an estrogen-free method of contraception either for women in whom estrogens are contraindicated or for women who cannot tolerate estrogen-containing preparations. Depo-Provera is extremely effective in preventing pregnancy. However, the incidence of menstrual irregularities (including amenorrhea) and weight gain appears to be much greater than that seen with COCs. The use of Depo-Provera also has been demonstrated to result in significant loss of bone mineral density (BMD).[38] Although the effect is known to be reversible following product discontinuation, a black-box warning within the product labeling cautions against the risk of potentially irreversible BMD loss

Table 48–5

Commonly Seen Drug Interactions With COCs

Medication	Mechanism	Clinical Effect
Anticonvulsants (carbamazepine, oxcarbazepine, phenytoin, phenobarbital, primidone, topiramate, and felbamate)	Increase metabolism of COCs via induction of various cytochrome P-450 enzymes	Decrease efficacy of COCs (EE doses < 35 mcg are not recommended in women on these medications)
Benzodiazepines (alprazolam)	COCs may inhibit oxidative metabolism	Increase side effects of benzodiazepines
Bosentan	Increase metabolism of COCs via induction of cytochrome P-450 3A4 enzyme	Decrease efficacy of COCs
Colesevelam	Reduce absorption of COCs by nonspecific binding with colesevelam	Decrease efficacy of COCs
Corticosteroids (hydrocortisone, methylprednisolone, prednisone)	COCs may inhibit metabolism of corticosteroids	Increase side effects of corticosteroids
Griseofulvin	Increase metabolism of COCs	Decrease efficacy of COCs; backup method of contraception is recommended
Lamotrigine	COCs increase metabolism of lamotrigine via induction of glucuronidation	Decrease efficacy of lamotrigine; dose adjustment may be necessary
Modafinil	Increase metabolism of COCs	Decrease efficacy of COCs; alternative method of contraception is recommended
Penicillins (amoxicillin, ampicillin); tetracyclines (doxycycline, minocycline, tetracycline)	Broad-spectrum antibiotics may alter intestinal flora, reducing enterohepatic circulation of estrogen metabolites; although the drop in estrogen levels has been shown to be only statistically significant, rather than clinically significant;	Decrease efficacy of COCs; backup barrier method of contraception is controversial[a]
Non-nucleoside reverse transcriptase inhibitors (delavirdine, efavirenz, nevirapine, rilpivirine)	Increase metabolism of COCs	Decrease efficacy of COCs; alternative method of contraception is recommended with efavirenz and nevirapine
Protease inhibitors (amprenavir, atazanavir, boceprevir, darunavir, fosamprenavir, indinavir, nelfinavir, ritonavir, saquinavir, simeprevir, telaprevir, tipranavir)	Increase or decrease in metabolism of COCs	Decrease efficacy of COCs or increase side effects of COCs; alternative method of contraception is recommended with nelfinavir and ritonavir
Rifampin, rifabutin	Increase metabolism of COCs	Decrease efficacy of COCs; backup method of contraception is recommended
Selegiline	COCs decrease metabolism of selegiline	Increase side effects of selegiline; may adjust dose of selegiline if needed
St. John's wort	Increase metabolism of COCs via induction of various cytochrome P-450 enzymes	Decrease efficacy of COCs; avoid use with COCs
Theophylline	COCs decrease theophylline clearance by 34% and increase half-life by 33%	Increase side effects of theophylline

[a]Although package inserts warn of this potential interaction, no scientific literature exists to support that concomitant antibiotics and COCs is associated with contraceptive failure.[33]

Data from Refs. 1, 32, and 33.

associated with long-term use (eg, greater than 2 years) of the injectable product. Although the extended duration of activity of this product may offer women the advantage of less frequent administration, it is important to note that on discontinuation of Depo-Provera, the return of fertility can be delayed by approximately 10 to 12 months (range 4–31 months).[6]

Depo-SubQ Provera 104 is also an injectable contraceptive product that contains only progestin (depot medroxyprogesterone acetate). This product differs from Depo-Provera in that it is given subcutaneously rather than intramuscularly, and it contains only 104 mg of medroxyprogesterone acetate (~30% less hormone) administered every 3 months for the prevention of pregnancy. Clinical trials have demonstrated that the subcutaneous formulation of depot medroxyprogesterone acetate is as effective as the intramuscular formulation in the prevention of pregnancy.[39] This product carries the same warning in its package labeling regarding possible effects on BMD as Depo-Provera.

Long-Acting Reversible Contraception

The currently available products for long-term reversible contraception (LARC) are listed in Table 48–6. Surveys have shown that LARC has the highest satisfaction rate among patients using reversible contraceptives, and use within the United States is on the rise.[1]

Although the mechanism of action for IUDs is not completely understood, several theories have been suggested. The original theory is that the presence of a foreign body in the uterus causes an inflammatory response that interferes with implantation. It is believed that copper-containing IUDs may interfere with sperm transport and fertilization and prevent implantation. Progestin-containing implantable contraceptives can have direct effects on the uterus, such as thickening of cervical mucus and alterations to the endometrial lining.[52] Paragard T 380A does not prevent ovulation, although the other LARCs can because they are progestin-containing products.

Table 48–6
Long-Acting Reversible Contraception

Product	Ingredient	Dosage Form	Duration
Mirena	Levonorgestrel	Intrauterine device	Up to 5 years
Skyla	Levonorgestrel	Intrauterine device	Up to 3 years
ParaGard T 380A	Copper	Intrauterine device	Up to 10 years
Implanon	Etonorgestrel	Implantable device	Up to 3 years
Nexplanon	Etonorgestrel	Implantable device	Up to 3 years

Data from Refs. 52–55.

It is important to evaluate a patient to determine whether she is an appropriate candidate for an implantable contraceptive. IUDs are recommended for women who are in a monogamous relationship, are at low risk for acquiring STIs, have no history of pelvic inflammatory disease (PID), and no history or risk of ectopic pregnancy. Contraindications to the use of progestin-containing LARC products include (a) known or suspected pregnancy, (b) hepatic tumors or active liver disease, (c) undiagnosed abnormal genital bleeding, (d) known or suspected carcinoma of the breast or personal history of breast cancer, (e) history of thrombosis or thromboembolic disorders, and (f) hypersensitivity to any components of the products. There are also multiple additional contraindications to IUD use. Evaluation of the patient is essential because IUDs cannot be used in the following situations: (a) anatomically abnormal or distorted uterine cavity, (b) acute PID or history of PID unless there has been a subsequent intrauterine pregnancy (c) postpartum endometritis or infected abortion in the past 3 months, (d) known or suspected uterine or cervical malignancy, (e) untreated acute cervicitis, (f) previously inserted IUD still in place, (g) increased susceptibility to pelvic infections, and (h) Wilson disease (Paragard T 380A only).

The most common adverse effects are abdominal/pelvic cramping, abnormal uterine bleeding, and expulsion of the device. Other side effects seen are ectopic pregnancy, sepsis, PID, embedment of the device, uterine or cervical perforation, and ovarian cysts.

Nonpharmacologic Contraceptive Methods

▸ Barrier Contraceptives

As an alternative to hormonal contraceptives, several barrier contraceptive options are available for the prevention of pregnancy. Although barrier contraceptives are associated with far fewer adverse effects compared with hormonal contraceptives, their efficacy is highly user-dependent. Overall, compared with both hormonal contraceptives and IUDs, barrier contraceptives are associated with much higher unintended pregnancy rates[6] (see Table 48–1).

Diaphragms and Cervical Caps Diaphragms and cervical caps are dome-shaped rubber caps that are placed over the cervix to provide barrier protection during intercourse. Both diaphragms and cervical caps require fitting by a health care professional, and they must be refitted in the event of weight gain or weight loss. Diaphragms or cervical caps typically can be placed over the cervix as much as 6 hours prior to intercourse. They must be left in place for at least 6 hours after intercourse before they can be removed. Diaphragms should not be left in place longer than 24 hours, and smaller cervical caps should not be left in place longer than 48 hours owing to the risk of toxic shock syndrome (TSS). Diaphragms and cervical caps are used along with spermicides to prevent pregnancy. When sexual intercourse is repeated with the diaphragm, reapplication of the spermicide is necessary. However, when sexual intercourse is repeated with a cervical cap, reapplication of the spermicide typically is not necessary.[6] Whether or not diaphragms or cervical caps provide adequate protection against STIs remains unclear.[40]

Spermicides Nonoxynol-9, a surfactant that destroys the cell membranes of sperm, is the most commonly used spermicide in the United States.[3,6] Nonoxynol-9 is available in a variety of forms, including a cream, foam, film, gel, suppository, and tablet. Spermicides may be used alone, with a barrier method, or adjunctively with other forms of contraceptives to provide additional protection against unwanted pregnancy.[3] To be used most effectively, spermicides must be placed in the vagina not more than 1 hour prior to sexual intercourse, and they must come in contact with the cervix.[6] Although the efficacy of spermicides depends largely on how consistently and correctly they are used, their efficacy is enhanced when they are used in combination with a barrier contraceptive device.[40] Clinical trials assessing the ability of spermicides to protect against STIs have failed to produce positive results.[3] Further, there exists some evidence to suggest that frequent use of spermicides actually may increase risk for acquisition of human immunodeficiency virus (HIV) secondary to vaginal mucosal tissue breakdown, which may allow a portal of entry for the virus.[6] In December 2007, the FDA issued a statement requiring manufacturers of nonoxynol-9 products to include a warning on the product label indicating that the spermicide does not provide protection against infection from HIV or other STIs.

Condoms Condoms, which are available for both male and female use, act as physical barriers to prevent sperm from coming into contact with ova.[3] Condoms are easy to use, available without a prescription, and inexpensive. Most condoms are made of latex. When used correctly, condoms can be very effective in prevention of unwanted pregnancy.[41] Condoms should be stored in a cool, dry place, away from exposure to direct sunlight. When stored improperly or when used with oil-based lubricants, however, latex condoms can break during intercourse, increasing the risk of pregnancy.[6] For latex-sensitive individuals, condoms made from lamb intestine ("natural membrane" condoms) and synthetic polyurethane condoms are available. Unlike latex condoms, condoms made from lamb intestine contain small pores that may permit the passage of viruses and therefore do not provide adequate protection against STIs.[3] KEY CONCEPT *Both latex and synthetic condoms can provide some protection against many STIs. Data from one meta-analysis suggested that HIV transmission can be reduced by as much as 90% when condoms are consistently used.[42] This is in contrast to hormonal contraceptives (oral, transdermal, or vaginal), IUDs, and most other barrier contraceptives, which do not protect against STIs.* Relative to male condoms,

Patient Encounter, Part 3: Missed Doses

The patient calls your clinic in a panic today because she forgot to take her oral contraceptive for the past 3 days, beginning the third week of active pills. Three days have elapsed since she took her last active pill, and she reports having had unprotected sexual intercourse last night. The patient is very concerned about her risk of pregnancy and is interested to learn more about emergency contraception and what her options are.

Given this patient's reported imperfect use of her oral contraceptive, what information can you provide to the patient regarding her risk of pregnancy?

What additional education should be provided to the patient regarding her risk of STIs related to unprotected intercourse?

Provide appropriate patient education regarding the use of various forms of emergency contraception, in the event she decides to use EC.

female condoms may offer even better protection against STIs because they provide more extensive barrier coverage of external genitalia, including the labia and the base of the penis.[3] It is important to note that the male and female condoms are not recommended to be used together because they may adhere to one another, causing displacement of one or both condoms.[3]

Sponge The Today sponge is a small, pillow-shaped polyurethane sponge impregnated with nonoxynol-9.[40] It is an over-the-counter barrier contraceptive that has been shown to be generally less effective at preventing pregnancy than diaphragms.[42] The sponge is moistened with water and then is inserted and placed over the cervix for up to 6 hours prior to sexual intercourse. The sponge then is left in place for at least 6 hours following intercourse.[3] Although the sponge maintains efficacy for 24 hours (even if intercourse is repeated), as with diaphragms, the sponge should be removed after 24 hours owing to the risk of TSS.[6]

▸ *Fertility Awareness–Based Methods*

Fertility awareness–based methods (natural methods) represent another nonpharmacologic means of pregnancy prevention. Although failure rates of such methods can be high, some couples still prefer these types of approaches. Fertility awareness–based methods depend on the ability of the couple to identify the woman's "fertile window," or the period of time in which pregnancy is most likely to occur as a result of sexual intercourse.[3] During the fertile window, the couple practices abstinence, or avoidance of intercourse, in order to prevent pregnancy. In some cases, rather than practicing abstinence during the fertile period, some couples may prefer to employ barrier methods or spermicides as a means of preventing pregnancy rather than to avoid intercourse altogether.[6] In order to identify the fertile window, a number of different fertility awareness–based methods may be tried. The calendar (rhythm) method involves counting the days in the menstrual cycle and then using a mathematical equation to determine the fertile window.[3] The temperature method involves monitoring changes in the woman's basal body temperature using a basal thermometer.[3] The cervical mucus (or Billings ovulation) method involves observing changes in the characteristics of cervical secretions throughout the cycle.[3] Around ovulation, the mucus becomes watery. The symptothermal method, which is considered to be the most difficult to learn but potentially the most effective, is a combination of both the temperature method and the cervical mucus method.[6] In general, fertility awareness–based methods are not recommended for women who have irregular menstrual cycles or who have difficulty interpreting their fertility signs correctly.[3]

Emergency Contraception

Emergency contraception (EC) is used to prevent pregnancy after known or suspected unprotected sexual intercourse. There are five FDA-approved oral agents available for use as EC, with availability from over the counter to prescription only access. The product known as ella (ulipristal acetate), a progesterone-receptor agonist/antagonist, can delay follicular rupture if taken just before ovulation and may cause endometrial changes to interfere with implantation. The available products are listed in the Table 48–7 along with information on availability and correct dosage. It is important to note that EC is more effective the earlier it is used after unprotected intercourse. Common side effects include headache, nausea, abdominal pain, dysmenorrhea, fatigue, and dizziness. If severe abdominal pain occurs, patients should be referred to their health care provider for evaluation of risk of an ectopic pregnancy. Patients should also contact their health care provider if their menstrual cycle is more than 1 week late after taking EC.

Table 48–7
Emergency Contraception

Product	Where stocked	Availability	Ingredient	Dose	When taken
Plan B One-Step	Over the counter	All ages with no identification required	Levonorgestrel	1.5 mg	Within 72 hours of unprotected sex
Next Choice One Dose	Behind the counter	Over the counter for 17 years and older; prescription required for 16 years and younger	Levonorgestrel	1.5 mg	Within 72 hours of unprotected sex
My Way	Behind the counter	Over the counter for 17 years and older; prescription required for 16 years and younger	Levonorgestrel	1.5 mg	Within 72 hours of unprotected sex
Levonorgestrel	Behind the counter	Over the counter for 17 years and older; prescription required for 16 years and younger	Levonorgestrel	0.75 mg (two tablets for a total of 1.5 mg)	Both tablets within 72 hours of unprotected sex
ella	Behind the counter	Only as a prescription	Ulipristal acetate	30 mg	Within 120 hours of unprotected sex

Patient Care Process

Patient Assessment:

- Determine goals related to contraceptive use (pregnancy prevention, menstrual regulation, control of acne?).
- Based on physical exam findings, as well as medical, social (ie, smoking) and family history, determine if patient qualifies for hormonal contraceptives. Rule out pregnancy, and evaluate patient's risk for STIs.
- Conduct thorough medication history to identify potential for drug interactions.

Therapy Evaluation:

- At follow-up visits, assess blood pressure, weight, and menstrual patterns for changes from baseline.
- Assess tolerability of and adherence to the prescribed contraceptive method.
- Assess safety by using the pneumonics, "ACHES" for hormonal contraceptives, and "PAINS" for IUDs:

ACHES -

A = Abdominal pain
C = Chest pain
H = Headaches (especially if associated with focal neurologic symptoms)
E = Eye problems (blurred vision, ocular pain, visual changes)
S = Severe leg pain

- Also monitor for missed periods, signs of pregnancy, appearance of jaundice, and/or severe mood changes.

PAINS -

P = Period late
A = Abdominal pain, pain with intercourse
I = Infection, abnormal/odorous vaginal discharge
N = Not feeling well, fever, chills
S = String (missing, shorter, longer)

Care Plan Development:

- Select a contraceptive option that the patient is comfortable with, that is likely to achieve the patient's desired goal(s), and is not contraindicated.
- Educate regarding the potential for side effects, safety risks, drug interactions, and any noncontraceptive benefits that may result for the chosen method.
- Determine the patient's sexual behavior and evaluate whether the contraceptive method will impact the risk for STIs.
- Evaluate insurance coverage/cost factors.

Follow-up Evaluation:

- Instruct the patient to consult a health care professional upon noticing or experiencing any warning signs.
- Stress the importance of adherence (especially if prevention of pregnancy is desired).
- Educate on what to do in the event of missed doses.

OUTCOME EVALUATION

Side effects of contraceptives tend to occur in the first few months of therapy. Thus schedule a follow-up visit 3 to 6 months after initiating a new contraceptive. Yearly checkups usually are sufficient for patients who are doing well on a particular product.[3] At each follow-up visit, assess blood pressure, headache frequency, and menstrual bleeding patterns, as well as compliance with the prescribed regimen. Strict adherence to the prescribed hormonal contraceptive regimen is essential for effective prevention of unintended pregnancy. KEY CONCEPT *When a contraceptive dose is missed, the risk of accidental pregnancy may be increased. Depending on how many doses were missed, the contraceptive formulation being used, and the phase of the cycle during which doses were missed, counseling regarding the use of additional methods of contraception may be warranted.*

Abbreviations Introduced in This Chapter

BMD	Bone mineral density
COC	Combined oral contraceptive
CYP450	Cytochrome P-450
EC	Emergency contraception
EE	Ethinyl estradiol
FSH	Follicle-stimulating hormone
GnRH	Gonadotropin-releasing hormone
HIV	Human immunodeficiency virus
HPV	Human papilloma virus
IUD	Intrauterine device
LARC	Long-acting reversible contraception
LH	Luteinizing hormone
PID	Pelvic inflammatory disease
PMDD	Premenstrual dysphoric disorder
STI	Sexually transmitted infection
TSS	Toxic shock syndrome
WHO	World Health Organization

REFERENCES

1. Jones J, Mosher W, Daniels K. Current contraceptive use in the United States, 2006-2010, and changes in patterns of use since 1995. Natl Health Stat Rep; No. 60. Hyattsville, MD; National Center for Health Statistics, 2012.
2. Ventura SJ, Cutrin SC, Abma JC, Henshaw SK. Estimated pregnancy rates and rates of pregnancy outcomes for the United States, 1990-2008. Natl Vital Stat Rep 2012 Jun 20;60(7):1–21.
3. Hatcher RA, Trussel J, Nelson AL, et al. Contraceptive Technology, 20th rev. ed. New York: Ardent Media, 2011.
4. Centers for Disease Control and Prevention. U.S. Medical Eligibility Criteria for Contraceptive Use, 2010. MMWR Recomm Rep 2010; 59:1–86.
5. Centers for Disease Control and Prevention (CDC) [Internet]. Sexually transmitted disease: Surveillance 2012. http://www.cdc.gov/std/stats.

6. Anonymous. Choice of contraceptives. Treat Guide Med Lett. 2010;8:89–96.
7. Lurie G, Thompson P, McDuffie KE, et al. Association of estrogen and progestin potency of oral contraceptives with ovarian carcinoma risk. Obstet Gynecol. 2007;109:597–607.
8. Maxwell GL, Schildkraut JM, Calingaert B, et al. Progestin and estrogen: Potency of combination oral contraceptives and endometrial cancer risk. Gynecol Oncol. 2006;103:535–540.
9. Ness RB, Grisso JA, Klapper J, et al. for the SHARE Study Group. Risk of ovarian cancer in relation to estrogen and progestin dose and use characteristics of oral contraceptives. Steroid hormones and reproduction. Am J Epidemiol. 2000;152:233–241.
10. Schildkraut JM, Calingaert B, Marchbanks PA, et al. Impact of progestin and estrogen potency in oral contraceptives on ovarian cancer risk. J Natl Cancer Inst. 2002;94:32–38.
11. Iyer V, Farquhar C, Jepson R. Oral contraceptive pills for heavy menstrual bleeding. Cochrane Database Syst Rev. 2000;2:CD000154.
12. Kroll R, Rapkin AJ. Treatment of premenstrual disorders. J Reprod Med. 2006;51:359–370.
13. Tanis BC, van den Bosch MA, Kemmeren JM, et al. Oral contraceptives and the risk of myocardial infarction. Arch Intern Med. 2001;161:1065–1070.
14. Schwingl PJ, Ory HW, Visness CM. Estimates of the risk of cardiovascular death attributable to low-dose oral contraceptives in the United States. Am J Obstet Gynecol. 1999;180:241–249.
15. Chang CL, Donaghy M, Poulter N. Migraine and stroke in young women: Case-control study. The World Health Organization Collaborative Study of Cardiovascular Disease and Steroid Hormone Contraception. BMJ. 1999;318:13–18.
16. Curtis KM, Chrisman CE, Peterson HB, WHO Programme for Mapping Best Practices in Reproductive Health. Contraception for women in selected circumstances. Obstet Gynecol. 2002;99: 1100–1112.
17. Heit JA, Kobbervig CE, James AH, et al. Trends in the incidence of venous thromboembolism during pregnancy or postpartum: A 30 year population-based study. Ann Intern Med. 2005;143: 697–706.
18. Hennessy S, Berlin JA, Kinman JL, et al. Risk of venous thromboembolism from oral contraceptives containing gestodene and desogestrel versus levonorgestrel: A meta-analysis and formal sensitivity analysis. Contraception. 2001;64:125–133.
19. Kemmeren JM, Algra A, Grobbee DE. Third generation oral contraceptives and risk of venous thrombosis: Meta-analysis. BMJ. 2001;323:131–134.
20. van Hylckama Vlieg A, Helmerhorst FM, Vandenbroucke JP, et al. The venous thrombotic risk of oral contraceptives, effects of oestrogen dose and progestin type: Results of the MEGA case-control study. BMJ. 2009;339:b2921.
21. Lidegaard Ø, Løkkegaard E, Svendsen AL, et al. Hormonal contraception and risk of venous thromboembolism: national follow-up study. BMJ. 2009;339:b2890.
22. Parkin L, Sharples K, Hernandez RK, et al. Risk of venous thromboembolism in users of oral contraceptives containing drospirenone or levonorgestrel: nested case-control study based on UK General Practice Research Database. BMJ. 2011;340:d2139.
23. Jick SS, Hernandez RK. Risk of non-fatal venous thrombo-embolism in women using oral contraceptives containing drospirenone compared with women using oral contraceptives containing levonorgestrel: case-control study using United States claims data. BMJ. 2011;340:d2151.
24. Dinger J, Bardenheuer K, Heinemann K. Cardiovascular and general safety of a 24-day regimen of drospirenone-containing combined oral contraceptives: final results from the International Active Surveillance Study of Women Taking Oral Contraceptives. Contraception. 2014;89:253.
25. Centers for Disease Control and Prevention (CDC). Update to CDC's U.S. Medical Eligibility Criteria for Contraceptive Use, 2010: revised recommendations for the use of contraceptive methods during the postpartum period. MMWR Morb Mortal Wkly Rep. 2011;60:878.
26. Grimes DA, Schulz KF. Nonspecific side effects of oral contraceptives: nocebo or noise? Contraception. 2011:83:5–9.
27. Graham CA, Ramos R, Bancroft J, et al. The effects of steroidal contraceptives on the well-being and sexuality of women: a double-blind, placebo-controlled, two-centre study of combined and progestogen-only methods. Contraception. 1995;52:363–369.
28. Rosenberg MJ, Meyers A, Roy V. Efficacy, cycle control, and side effects of low- and lower-dose oral contraceptives: a randomized trial of 20 micrograms and 35 micrograms estrogen preparations. Contraception. 1999;60:321–329.
29. Burkman RT, Fisher AC, LaGuardia KD. Effects of low-dose oral contraceptives on body weight: results of a randomized study of up to 13 cycles of use. J Rep Med. 2007:52:1030–1034.
30. Duramed Pharmaceuticals. Product information for Seasonale. Pomona, NY: Duramed Pharmaceuticals, 2003.
31. Vercellini P, Frontino G, De Giorgi O, et al. Continuous use of an oral contraceptive for endometriosis-associated recurrent dysmenorrhea that does not respond to a cyclic pill regimen. Fertil Steril. 2003;80:560–563.
32. Tom W. Oral contraceptive drug interactions. Pharmacist's Letter/Prescriber's Letter 2005;21:210903.
33. Toh S, Mitchell AA, Anderka M. Antibiotics and oral contraceptive failure: a case-crossover study. Contraception. 2011;83:418–425.
34. Anonymous. Ortho Evra—A contraceptive patch. Med Lett Drugs Ther. 2002;1122:8.
35. Anonymous. An update on Ortho Evra and the risk of thromboembolism. Pharmacist's Letter/Prescribers Letter 2005; 21:211202.
36. Smallwood GH, Meador ML, Lenihan JP, et al. for the Ortho Evra/Evra 002 Study Group. Efficacy and safety of a transdermal contraceptive system. Obstet Gynecol. 2001;98:799–805.
37. Dieben TO, Roumen FJ, Apter D. Efficacy, cycle control, and user acceptability of a novel combined contraceptive vaginal ring. Obstet Gynecol. 2002;100:585–593.
38. Westhoff C. Bone mineral density and DMPA. J Reprod Med. 2002;47:795–799.
39. Toh YC, Jain J, Rahnny MH, et al. Suppression of ovulation by a new subcutaneous depot medroxyprogesterone acetate (104 mg/0.65 mL) contraceptive formulation in Asian women. Clin Ther. 2004;26:1845–1854.
40. Moench TR, Chipato T, Padian NS. Preventing disease by protecting the cervix: The unexplored promise of internal vaginal barrier devices. AIDS. 2001;15:1595–1602.
41. Davis KR, Weller SC. The effectiveness of condoms in reducing heterosexual transmission of HIV. Fam Plann Perspect. 1999;31:272–279.
42. Kuyoh MA, Toroitich-Ruto C, Grimes DA, et al. Sponge versus diaphragm for contraception: A Cochrane review. Contraception. 2003;67:15–18.

49 Menstruation-Related Disorders

Jacqueline M. Klootwyk and Elena M. Umland

LEARNING OBJECTIVES

Upon completion of the chapter, the reader will be able to:

1. Describe the underlying etiology and pathophysiology of **dysmenorrhea**, amenorrhea, anovulatory bleeding, and **menorrhagia** and how they relate to selecting effective treatment modalities.
2. Describe the clinical presentation of dysmenorrhea, amenorrhea, anovulatory bleeding, and menorrhagia.
3. Recommend appropriate nonpharmacologic and pharmacologic interventions for patients with dysmenorrhea, amenorrhea, anovulatory bleeding, and menorrhagia.
4. Identify the desired therapeutic outcomes for patients with dysmenorrhea, amenorrhea, anovulatory bleeding, and menorrhagia.
5. Design a monitoring plan to assess the effectiveness and adverse effects of pharmacotherapy for dysmenorrhea, amenorrhea, anovulatory bleeding, and menorrhagia.

INTRODUCTION

The most common menstruation-related disorders include dysmenorrhea, amenorrhea, anovulatory bleeding, and menorrhagia. These disorders negatively affect quality of life, reproductive health, work productivity, and may lead to adverse long-term health consequences, such as osteoporosis or polycystic ovarian syndrome.

DYSMENORRHEA

Dysmenorrhea is pelvic pain, generally described as cramping, that occurs during or just prior to menstruation. Primary dysmenorrhea is pain in the setting of normal pelvic anatomy and physiology, whereas secondary dysmenorrhea is associated with underlying pelvic pathology.[1]

Epidemiology and Etiology

Rates of dysmenorrhea range from 16% to 90%.[2] Around 8% to 15% percent of women with dysmenorrhea report limited daily activities or missed days in work or school.[1,3] Risk factors for dysmenorrhea include irregular or heavy menses, age less than 30, menarche prior to age 12, body mass index (BMI) less than 20 kg/m^2, history of sterilization or sexual abuse, and smoking.[1,2] Causes of secondary dysmenorrhea may include endometriosis, pelvic inflammatory disease, uterine or cervical polyps, and uterine fibroids.[1,4,5]

Pathophysiology

KEY CONCEPT *In primary dysmenorrhea, elevated arachidonic acid levels in the menstrual fluid lead to increased concentrations of prostaglandins and leukotrienes in the uterus.* This induces uterine contractions, stimulating pain fibers, reducing uterine blood flow, and causing uterine hypoxia.[1,3,4]

Treatment

▸ *Desired Outcomes*

Desired treatment outcomes (Figure 49–1) are relief of pelvic pain, improved quality of life, and fewer lost days at school and work.

▸ *Nonpharmacologic Therapy*

Nonpharmacologic interventions which diminish dysmenorrhea symptoms include topical heat therapy, regular exercise, transcutaneous electric nerve stimulation (TENS), and acupuncture.[1,3,5] In addition, a low-fat vegetarian diet has been shown to lessen the intensity and duration of dysmenorrhea.[5]

▸ *Pharmacologic Therapy*

Medication management options are summarized in Table 49–1.

Nonsteroidal Anti-inflammatory Drugs (NSAIDs) KEY CONCEPT *NSAIDs are the treatment of choice for dysmenorrhea. By inhibiting prostaglandin production, they exert analgesic properties, decrease uterine contractions, and reduce menstrual blood flow.* Choice of one agent over another is based on cost, convenience, and patient preference.[1–4] Most commonly used agents are naproxen and ibuprofen.

Treatment with an NSAID should begin 1 to 2 days prior to the start of menses or at the onset of dysmenorrhea and continued for 2 to 3 days or until pain resolves.[1] A loading dose (twice the usual single dose) is recommended, followed by the usually recommended dose.[1,2,5] For patients in whom NSAIDs are contraindicated, combination hormonal contraceptives should be considered.[1,4]

Combination Hormonal Contraceptives (CHCs) CHCs improve mild to severe dysmenorrhea by inhibiting the

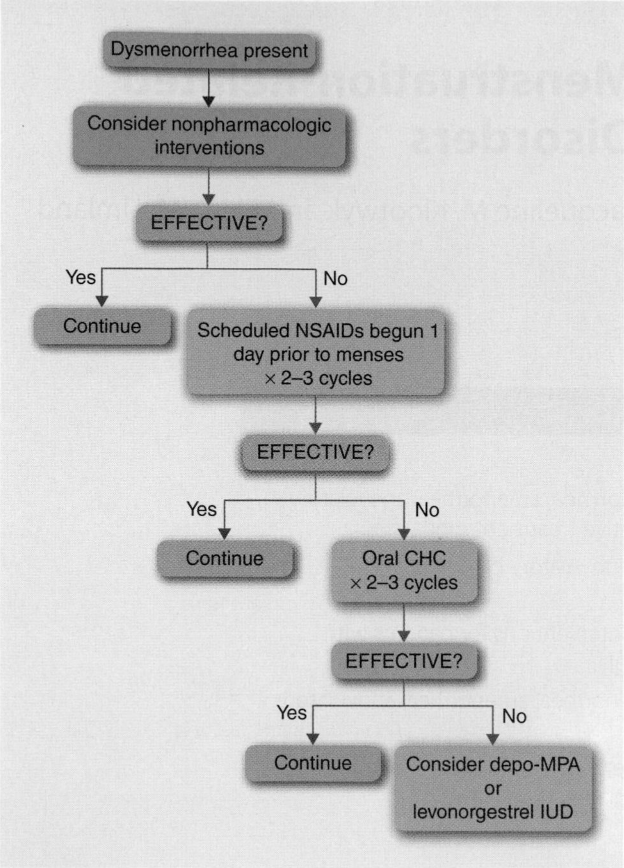

FIGURE 49–1. Treatment algorithm for dysmenorrhea. (CHC, combination hormonal contraceptive; IUD, intrauterine device; MPA, medroxyprogesterone acetate; NSAID, nonsteroidal anti-inflammatory drug.)

Patient Encounter 1, Part 1

A 22-year-old white woman presents to her physician reporting severe pelvic pain and cramping during menses that results in 1 to 2 missed work days each menstrual cycle. Her last menstrual cycle was 9 days ago, and she had her first menstrual cycle at age 11. She is sexually active with one partner and has had 5 sexual partners in the past. Of note, she has a history or Chlamydia in the past. She has been using acetaminophen or ibuprofen as needed for pain and is a current smoker. She does not follow a diet or exercise regimen.

What risk factors does this patient have for primary dysmenorrhea?

What risk factors does the patient have for secondary dysmenorrhea?

proliferation of endometrial tissue and ovulation, thereby reducing prostaglandin secretion and menstrual blood volume.[1,3–5] Two to three months of therapy are required to achieve the full effect.[1] Both standard (28-day) and extended cycle (91-day) therapies are effective for primary dysmenorrhea.[1,2] Extended cycle regimens are considered first line for dysmenorrhea due to endometriosis.[2] Additional benefits include contraception and improving acne.[5] Although monophasic formulations are purported to be more efficacious for this indication, evidence supporting this is limited.[16] If no response occurs after 3 months of therapy, the patient should be evaluated for secondary causes.[1,5]

Progestin-only Hormonal Contraceptives These agents diminish dysmenorrhea by reducing or eliminating menses over time, thus eliminating prostaglandin release.[5] Three agents are available: depot medroxyprogesterone acetate, etonogestrel implant, and levonorgestrel-releasing intrauterine system.

Observational data show a reduction in dysmenorrhea from 60% to 29% with levonorgestrel-releasing intrauterine device (IUD) therapy for 3 years.[5] Although data are limited, this is an option for dysmenorrhea management.[16]

Dysmenorrhea in Adolescents

Dysmenorrhea is reported in 60% to 90% of adolescent females.[1] It is the most common reason for adolescents to miss school or work. One study showed that most young females are treating pelvic pain with nonpharmacologic therapies, while other studies showed that many either do not know to use NSAIDs or use subtherapeutic doses.[5] Treatment in adolescents includes any of the therapies previously discussed. Although NSAIDs and oral CHCs are most common, levonorgestrel IUD use is also an option.[16] KEY CONCEPT *The American College of Obstetricians and Gynecologists (ACOG) states that any woman, including adolescents (regardless of parity) at low risk of sexually transmitted diseases and thus pelvic inflammatory disease, is a good candidate for IUD use.*[17,18]

AMENORRHEA

Amenorrhea is the absence of menses. **Primary amenorrhea** occurs prior to age 15 in the presence of normal secondary sexual development or within 5 years of **thelarche** (if occurring before age 10).[19,20] **Secondary amenorrhea** is the absence of menses for three cycles or 6 months in a previously menstruating woman.[6]

Clinical Presentation and Diagnosis of Dysmenorrhea

General

- Acute distress may be present depending on the severity of menstrual pain.

Symptoms

- Crampy pelvic pain (lasting 1–3 days) beginning shortly before or at menses onset. Associated symptoms may include nausea, vomiting, diarrhea, hypertension, and/or tachycardia.

Laboratory Tests

- Sexually active females should receive a pelvic examination to screen for sexually transmitted diseases.
- Gonorrhea, chlamydia cultures or PCR, wet mount.

Other Diagnostic Tests

- Pelvic ultrasound may be used to identify anatomic abnormalities (eg, masses/lesions), ovarian cysts, or endometriomas.

Table 49–1

Therapeutic Agents for Selected Menstrual Disorders

Specific Menstrual Disorders(s)	Agent(s)	Dose Recommended	Common Adverse Effects
Amenorrhea (primary or secondary)	CEE[a]	0.625–1.25 mg by mouth daily on cycle days 1–26[6]	Thromboembolism, breast enlargement, breast tenderness, bloating, nausea, GI upset, headache, peripheral edema
	Ethinyl estradiol patch[a]	50–100 mcg/24 hours[6]	
	Oral CHC[a]	30–40 mcg formulations	
Amenorrhea (secondary)	Oral medroxyprogesterone acetate[a]	10 mg by mouth on cycle days 14–26[6]	Edema, anorexia, depression, insomnia, weight gain or loss, elevated total and LDL cholesterol, may reduce HDL cholesterol
Amenorrhea (hyperprolactinemia)	Bromocriptine	2.5 mg by mouth two to three times daily[7]	Hypotension, nausea, constipation, anorexia, Raynaud phenomenon
Anovulatory bleeding	Oral CHC[a]	Optimal dose unknown[8] For acute bleeding, product containing 35 mcg ethinyl estradiol; take one tablet by mouth three times daily × 1 week; then one tablet by mouth daily × 3 weeks.[8]	As noted above for CEE, ethinyl estradiol, and oral CHC (progesterone side effects with the CHC depend on agent chosen)
	Oral medroxyprogesterone acetate[a]	For acute bleeding, 20 mg by mouth three times daily × 1 week; then 20 mg by mouth once daily × 3 weeks.[8]	As noted above for oral medroxyprogesterone acetate
Dysmenorrhea	Oral CHC[9,a]	< 35 mcg formulations + norgestrel or levonorgestrel[11]; use of extended-cycle formulations are beneficial for this indication	As noted above for CEE, ethinyl estradiol, and oral CHC (progesterone side effects with the CHC depend on agent chosen)
	Depot medroxyprogesterone acetate[a]	150 mg intramuscularly every 12 weeks	Irregular menses, amenorrhea
	Levonorgestrel IUD[12,a]	20 mcg released daily	Irregular menses, amenorrhea
	NSAIDs—any are acceptable; the most commonly studied/ cited are included in this table[1–4,9]	Diclofenac 50 mg by mouth three times daily[b]	GI upset, stomach ulcer, nausea, vomiting, heartburn, indigestion, rash, dizziness
		Ibuprofen 800 mg by mouth three times daily[a]	
		Mefenamic acid 500 mg by mouth as a loading dose, then 250 mg by mouth up to four times daily as needed[b]	
		Naproxen 550-mg loading dose by mouth started 1–2 days prior to menses, followed by 275 mg by mouth every 6–12 hours as needed[c]	
		Treatment should begin 1–2 days prior to the expected onset of menses	
Menorrhagia	Oral CHC[a]	Optimal dose unknown	As noted above
	Levonorgestrel IUD[a]	20 mcg released daily	As noted above
	Medroxyprogesterone acetate (oral)[a]	5–10 mg by mouth on days 5–26 of the cycle *or* during the luteal phase[10]	As noted above
	NSAIDs	Doses as recommended for above; therapy should be initiated with the onset of menses[10]	As noted above
	Tranexamic acid	1300 mg (650 mg × 2) by mouth three times days × 5 days[8,11,44,45]	Fatigue, abdominal, back, or muscle pain
PCOS-related amenorrhea and/or anovulatory bleeding	Clomiphene[5]	50 mg by mouth daily × 5 days starting 3–5 days after the start of menses; doses up to 100 mg by mouth daily have been used in significantly obese patients	Hot flashes, ovarian enlargement, thromboembolism, blurred vision, breast discomfort
	Depot medroxyprogesterone acetate[a]	150 mg intramuscularly every 12 weeks	As noted above
	Letrozole	2.5–7.5 mg by mouth cycle days 3–7[12]	Hot flashes, fatigue, dizziness, edema

(Continued)

Table 49–1

Therapeutic Agents for Selected Menstrual Disorders (*Continued*)

Specific Menstrual Disorders(s)	Agent(s)	Dose Recommended	Common Adverse Effects
	Medroxyprogesterone acetate (oral)[a]	10 mg by mouth × 10 days[13]	As noted above
	Metformin[a]	1500–2000 mg by mouth daily in 2–3 divided dose[a,d]	Anorexia, nausea, vomiting, diarrhea, flatulence, lactic acidosis

CEE, conjugated equine estrogen; CHC, combination hormonal contraceptive; HDL, high-density lipoprotein; IUD, intrauterine device; LDL, low-density lipoprotein.

[a]Use is contraindicated in patients with severe hepatic impairment.

[b]Not recommended in patients with severe renal impairment.

[c]Use is contraindicated with creatinine clearance less than 30 mL/min (0.5 mL/s).

[d]Contraindicated in males with serum creatinine more than 1.5 mg/dL (133 μmol/L); females with serum creatinine more than 1.4 mg/dL (124 μmol/L); caution with creatinine clearance less than 60 mL/min (1 mL/s).

[e]Contraindicated in patients with active liver disease or if transaminases more than 2.5 times upper limit of normal at baseline, discontinue therapy if ALT is more than three times upper limit of normal.

Data from Refs. 1, 2, 5–15, 44, 45.

Epidemiology and Etiology

KEY CONCEPT *Unrecognized pregnancy is the most common cause of amenorrhea, therefore, a urine pregnancy test should be one of the first steps in evaluating amenorrhea.* Amenorrhea not related to pregnancy, lactation, or menopause occurs in 3% to 4% of women.[20] Additional causes of secondary amenorrhea include polycystic ovarian syndrome (PCOS), hypothalamic suppression, hyperprolactinemia, or primary ovarian insufficiency.[6]

Pathophysiology

In the diagnosis and management of amenorrhea, the uterus, ovaries, anterior pituitary, and hypothalamus should be considered (**Figure 49–2**). Normal menstrual cycle physiology depends on hormonal interactions involving the hypothalamus, anterior pituitary gland, ovary, and endometrium (**Figure 49–3**).[5,6,21] **Table 49–2** shows causative condition(s) and the organ system(s) involved in the pathophysiology of amenorrhea. Amenorrhea is a potential side effect from using low-dose or extended oral CHCs and depot medroxyprogesterone acetate.[6,26] Many women experience delayed return of menses after CHC discontinuation. If spontaneous resolution of amenorrhea does not occur within 3 to 6 months following CHC discontinuation, evaluation for other conditions should be considered (eg, PCOS).

Patient Encounter 1, Part 2

Additional workup reveals:

PMH: asthma

PSH: none

FH: Mother and father are alive and well. She has two younger siblings (ages 17 and 12) who are alive and well.

SH: (+) smoking; (–) drug use; (+) alcohol use (2–4 drinks per week)

Meds: Fluticasone 110 mcg 2 puffs twice daily and albuterol 90 mcg 2 puffs prn SOB

Past Gynecologic Hx: Menarche at age 11; never pregnant; (+) sexual activity; 6 sexual partners; (+) history of Chlamydia; (+) history of painful menses beginning at age 12; (+) heavy menstrual flow; menstrual cycle 26 to 28 days.

ROS: (–) fatigue; (–) headaches; (+) mild acne on face and chest; (+) moderate to severe pelvic pain with menses

PE:

General: Thin-appearing white woman, in no acute distress

VS: BP 116/64, P 74, RR 14, Wt 128 lbs (58.2 kg), Ht 5′4″ (163 cm), BMI: 22 kg/m^2

HEENT: (–) hirsutism

Breasts: (–) galactorrhea

Pelvic examination: normal appearance of external genitalia and vagina, cervix without lesions, uterus midposition without masses, adnexa without masses

Labs: (–)hCG

Given this information, what is your assessment of this patient's condition?

Identify the treatment goals for this patient.

What nonpharmacologic and pharmacologic therapies are recommended for this patient?

What monitoring parameters are necessary to employ in assessing efficacy and safety of the therapeutic options?

Clinical Presentation and Diagnosis of Amenorrhea

General

- Concerns about cessation of menses and fertility implications
- Not generally in acute distress

Symptoms

- Cessation of menses
- Possible reports of infertility, vaginal dryness, decreased libido

Signs

- Absence of menses by age 15 in the presence of normal secondary sexual development or within 5 years of thelarche (if occurs before age 10).
- Recent significant weight loss or gain
- Presence of acne, hirsutism, hair loss, or acanthosis nigricans may suggest androgen excess.

Laboratory Tests

- Pregnancy test
- TSH
- Prolactin
- If PCOS is suspected, consider free or total testosterone, 17-hydroxyprogesterone, fasting glucose, and fasting lipid panel.
- If premature ovarian failure is suspected, consider follicle-stimulating hormone (FSH) and luteinizing hormone (LH) measurements.

Other Diagnostic Tests

- Progesterone challenge
- Pelvic ultrasound to evaluate for polycystic ovaries

Treatment

▸ *Desired Outcomes*

Treatment goals include restoring the normal menstrual cycle, preserving bone density, preventing bone loss, improving quality of life, and restoring ovulation, thus improving fertility. Amenorrhea attributable to hypoestrogenism (eg, premature ovarian insufficiency) can cause hot flashes and dyspareunia. In prepubertal females, the absence of secondary sexual characteristics and menarche may occur.[6]

▸ *Nonpharmacologic Therapy*

Nonpharmacologic therapy for amenorrhea depends on the underlying cause. Amenorrhea secondary to undernutrition or anorexia may respond to weight gain and psychotherapy.[20] If excessive exercise is the culprit, exercise reduction is recommended.[6]

▸ *Pharmacologic Therapy*

Estrogen/Progestin Replacement Therapy KEY CONCEPT *For most conditions associated with primary or secondary amenorrhea, estrogen treatment is recommended. To minimize risk of endometrial hyperplasia and cancer, progestin should also be given to women with an intact uterus.* Estrogen's role is to reduce osteoporosis risk, stimulate and maintain secondary sexual characteristics, and improve quality of life.[14,20] Table 49–1 lists the types and doses of estrogen and progestin therapy for amenorrhea.

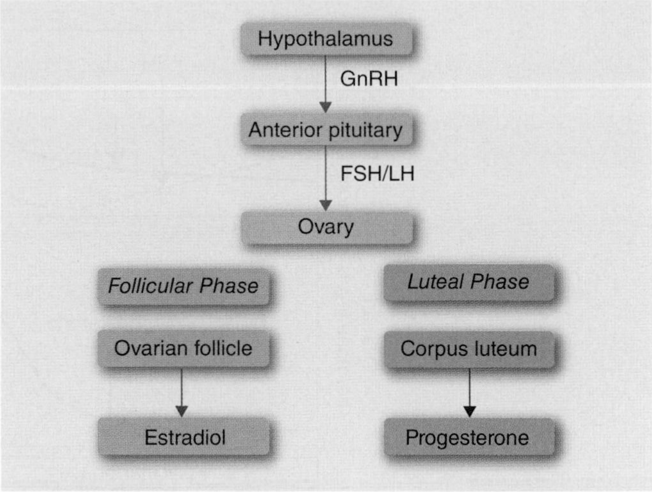

FIGURE 49–2. Summary of normal menstrual cycle. (FSH, follicle-stimulating hormone; GnRH, gonadotropin-releasing hormone; LH, luteinizing hormone.)

Dopamine Agonists In women with hyperprolactinemia who desire conception, dopamine agonists are an option. Dopamine agonists reduce prolactin levels and resolve amenorrhea. Additionally, they restore ovulation in 80% to 90% of women.[27] The most commonly studied agents are bromocriptine and cabergoline.[7,27]

Progestins Progestins have long been used to induce withdrawal bleeding in women with secondary amenorrhea. Efficacy varies depending on the formulation used. Withdrawal bleeding occurs with intramuscularly injected progesterone and oral medroxyprogesterone acetate in 70% and 95% of patients, respectively.[28] The usual dose of medroxyprogesterone acetate is 10 mg orally once daily for 7 to 10 days.[6]

Insulin-Sensitizing Agents Amenorrhea related to anovulation and PCOS may respond to insulin sensitizing agents.[13] Using metformin for this purpose is discussed in the anovulatory bleeding section.

All patients experiencing amenorrhea should follow a diet rich in calcium and vitamin D to support bone health. Supplemental calcium and vitamin D (1200 mg/800 International Units per day) should be recommended for patients with inadequate dietary consumption.[6] Figure 49–4 illustrates treatment recommendations for amenorrhea.[6]

Amenorrhea in Adolescents

Adolescence is when peak bone mass is achieved. The cause of amenorrhea and appropriate treatment must be identified promptly in this population because hypoestrogenism contributes negatively to bone development.[20] Estrogen replacement, typically via a CHC, is important. Although recent data suggest that CHCs and depot medroxyprogesterone acetate may reduce bone mineral density (BMD) for short term, their long-term effects on fractures are unknown. These negative BMD effects

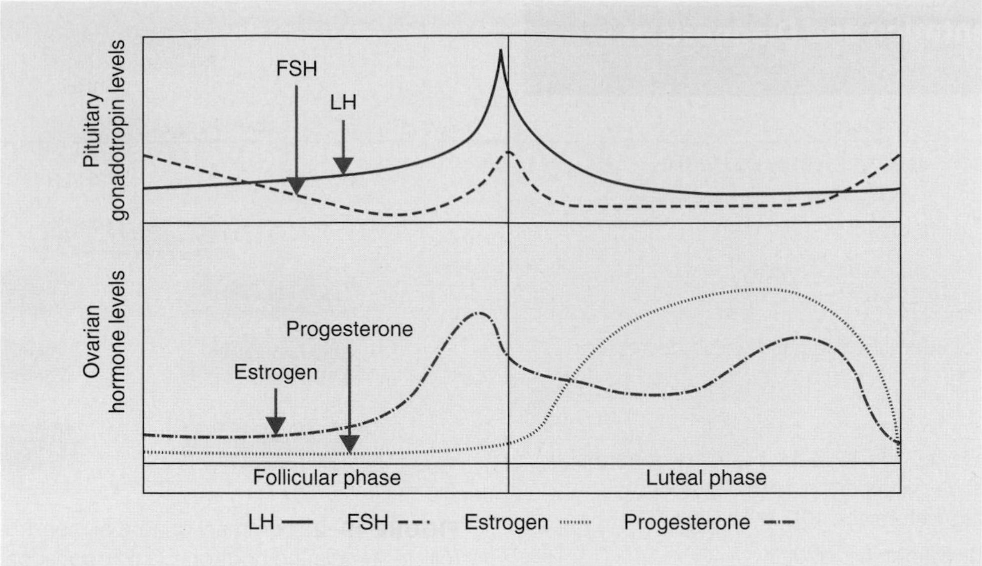

FIGURE 49–3. Hormonal fluctuations with the normal menstrual cycle. (FSH, follicle-stimulating hormone; LH, luteinizing hormone.) (Data from Umland EM, Weinstein LC, Buchanan E. Menstruation- related disorders (Chapter 89). In: Pharmacotherapy: A Pathophysiologic Approach, 8th ed. New York, NY: McGraw-Hill, 2011, with permission.)

appear to be reversible; therefore, CHCs are recommended in the adolescent population.[29] Ensuring adequate dietary or supplemental calcium and vitamin D intake in this population is imperative.

ANOVULATORY BLEEDING

Anovulatory uterine bleeding (AUB) is irregular menstrual bleeding from the endometrium ranging from light spotting to heavy blood flow.[30] KEY CONCEPT *It includes noncyclic menstrual bleeding due to ovulatory dysfunction (AUB-O), including anovulation or oligo-ovulation.[24] AUB-O is secondary to the effects of unopposed estrogen and does not include bleeding owing to an anatomic lesion of the uterus.* AUB is a diagnosis of exclusion and includes PCOS, which typically presents with irregular menstrual bleeding, hirsutism, obesity, and/or infertility.[13]

Epidemiology and Etiology

Anovulatory uterine bleeding is the most common form of noncyclic uterine bleeding.[30] Medical care is often pursued to regulate menstrual cycles or improve fertility. All women of reproductive age should have a pregnancy test when presenting with irregular menstrual bleeding. Anovulation results from dysfunction at any level of the hypothalamic-pituitary-ovarian (HPO) axis which can be due to physiologic life stages such as adolescence, perimenopause, pregnancy, and lactation or pathologic causes (see Table 49–2).[19,24]

During adolescence, ovulatory menstrual cycles may not be regular for 12 to 18 months after menarche.[24,30] Ovulation frequency is related to the age at and time since menarche.[19] In the year following menarche, the feedback mechanism in the HPO axis may be immature, and the luteinizing hormone (LH) surge needed for ovulation fails to occur.[30] During perimenopause, anovulatory cycles occur due to declining quality and quantity of ovarian follicles. As ovarian function declines, estrogen secretion continues, and progesterone secretion decreases. Chronic anovulatory cycles and unopposed estrogen secretion lead to endometrial proliferation and increased risk of polyps, endometrial hyperplasia, and endometrial carcinoma.[24]

Anovulation also occurs at any time during the reproductive years due to a pathologic cause. The most common causes of nonphysiologic ovulatory dysfunction are PCOS, hypothalamic amenorrhea, hyperprolactinemia, and premature ovarian failure. PCOS, responsible for 55% to 91% of ovulatory dysfunction cases, occurs in approximately 7% of women.[13,24]

Pathophysiology

A normal ovulatory cycle includes follicular development, ovulation, corpus luteum development, and luteolysis. During the cycle, the endometrium proliferates and undergoes secretory changes and desquamation. This is influenced by estrogen alone, then by estrogen and progesterone, and culminates with estrogen and progesterone withdrawal. Progesterone stops endometrial growth and stimulates endometrial differentiation. In anovulatory women, a corpus luteum is not formed, and the ovary does not secrete progesterone. Without progesterone, there is no endometrial desquamation or differentiation. Chronic unopposed estrogen causes endometrial proliferation. The endometrium becomes vascular and fragile, resulting in noncyclic menstrual bleeding. The endometrium may also become hyperplastic and progress to a precancerous state, increasing the woman's risk of endometrial cancer (see Table 49–2).[1]

The most common pathologic cause of anovulation is PCOS. Two sets of closely related criteria have been developed. The Rotterdam criteria identify PCOS as a syndrome of ovarian dysfunction diagnosed when two of the following characteristics exist: (a) oligoanovulation or anovulation; (b) clinical signs (hirsutism, acne) or laboratory evidence of hyperandrogenism (total testosterone and sex hormone-binding globulin); and (c) polycystic ovary morphology on ultrasound.[13,31] The Androgen Excess and PCOS Society (AE-PCOS) defines PCOS as hyperandrogenism (clinical or biochemical), ovarian dysfunction

Table 49–2

Pathophysiology of Selected Menstrual Bleeding Disorders[1,6,13,19,22–25]

Organ System	Condition	Pathophysiology/Laboratory Findings
Amenorrhea[1,6,22]		
Uterus	Asherman syndrome	Postcurettage/postsurgical uterine adhesions
	Congenital uterine abnormalities	Abnormal uterine development
Ovaries	Turner syndrome	Lack of ovarian follicles
	Gonadal dysgenesis	Other genetic anomalies
	Premature ovarian failure	Early loss of follicles
	Chemotherapy/radiation	Gonadal toxins
Anterior pituitary	Pituitary prolactin-secreting adenoma	↑ Prolactin suppresses HPO axis
	Hypothyroidism	TRH causing ↑ prolactin, other abnormalities
	Medications—antipsychotics, verapamil	↑ Prolactin suppresses HPO axis
Hypothalamus	"Functional" hypothalamic amenorrhea	↓ Pulsatile GnRH secretion in the absence of other abnormalities
	Disordered eating	↓ Pulsatile GnRH secretion, ↓ FSH and LH secondary to weight loss
	Exercise	↓ Pulsatile GnRH secretion, ↓ FSH and LH secondary to low body fat
	Anovulation/PCOS	Asynchronous gonadotropin and estrogen production, abnormal endometrial growth
Anovulatory Bleeding[1,13,23,24]		
Physiologic causes	Adolescence	Immature hypothalamic-pituitary-ovarian axis: no LH surge
	Perimenopause	Declining ovarian function
Pathologic causes	Hyperandrogenic anovulation (PCOS, congenital adrenal hyperplasia, androgen-producing tumors)	Hyperandrogenism: high testosterone, high LH, hyperinsulinemia, and insulin resistance
	Hypothalamic dysfunction (physical or emotional stress, exercise, weight loss, anorexia nervosa)	Suppression of pulsatile GnRH secretion and estrogen deficiency: low LH, low FSH
	Hyperprolactinemia (pituitary gland tumor, psychiatric medications)	High prolactin
	Hypothyroidism	High TSH
	Premature ovarian failure	High FSH
Menorrhagia[25]		
Hematologic	von Willebrand disease	Factor VII defect causing impaired platelet adhesion and increased bleeding time
	Idiopathic thrombocytopenic purpura	Decrease in circulating platelets—can be acute or chronic
Hepatic	Cirrhosis	Decreased estrogen metabolism, underlying coagulopathy
Endocrine	Hypothyroidism	Alterations in HPO axis
Uterine	Fibroids	Alteration of endometrium, changes in uterine contractility
	Adenomyosis	Alteration of endometrium, changes in uterine contractility
	Endometrial polyps	Alteration of endometrium
	Gynecologic cancers	Various dysplastic alterations of endometrium, uterus, cervix

↑, high; ↓, low; FSH, follicle-stimulating hormone; GnRH, gonadotropin-releasing hormone; HPO, hypothalamic-pituitary-ovarian axis; LH, luteinizing hormone; PCOS, polycystic ovary syndrome; TRH, thyrotropin-releasing hormone; TSH, thyroid-stimulating hormone.

(oligoanovulation or polycystic ovaries) and the exclusion of other causes of androgen excess.[32] No gene or environmental substance appears to cause PCOS.[13] However, familial clustering of PCOS cases suggests that genetics play a role. Insulin resistance, hyperandrogenism, and changes in gonadotropins also influence PCOS development. The underlying cause for increased androgens is unknown.[32,33]

Recently, discussion regarding the link to cardiovascular disease has been emphasized. PCOS is associated with two to five times increased risk of developing type 2 diabetes.[13] In women with PCOS, approximately 60% to 80% have impaired glucose tolerance (IGT).[34] Additionally, in obese women with PCOS, IGT prevalence increases to 95%, and 70% have dyslipidemia.[13,34] Women with PCOS should be screened for IGT, diabetes, hypertension, and dyslipidemia.[13] If any present, there is an increased risk of cardiovascular events.[34,35]

Treatment

▸ *Desired Outcomes*

The desired outcomes of therapy are to stop acute bleeding, prevent future episodes of noncyclic bleeding, decrease long-term complications of anovulation (eg, osteopenia and infertility), and improve overall quality of life.[24]

▸ *Nonpharmacologic Therapy*

Nonpharmacologic treatment options depend on the underlying cause. For all women with PCOS, weight loss may be beneficial. In overweight or obese women, a 5% reduction in weight has been associated with resumption of menses, improved pregnancy rates, and decreased hirsutism, glucose, and lipid levels.[13] In women who have completed childbearing or who have failed medical management, endometrial ablation or resection, and

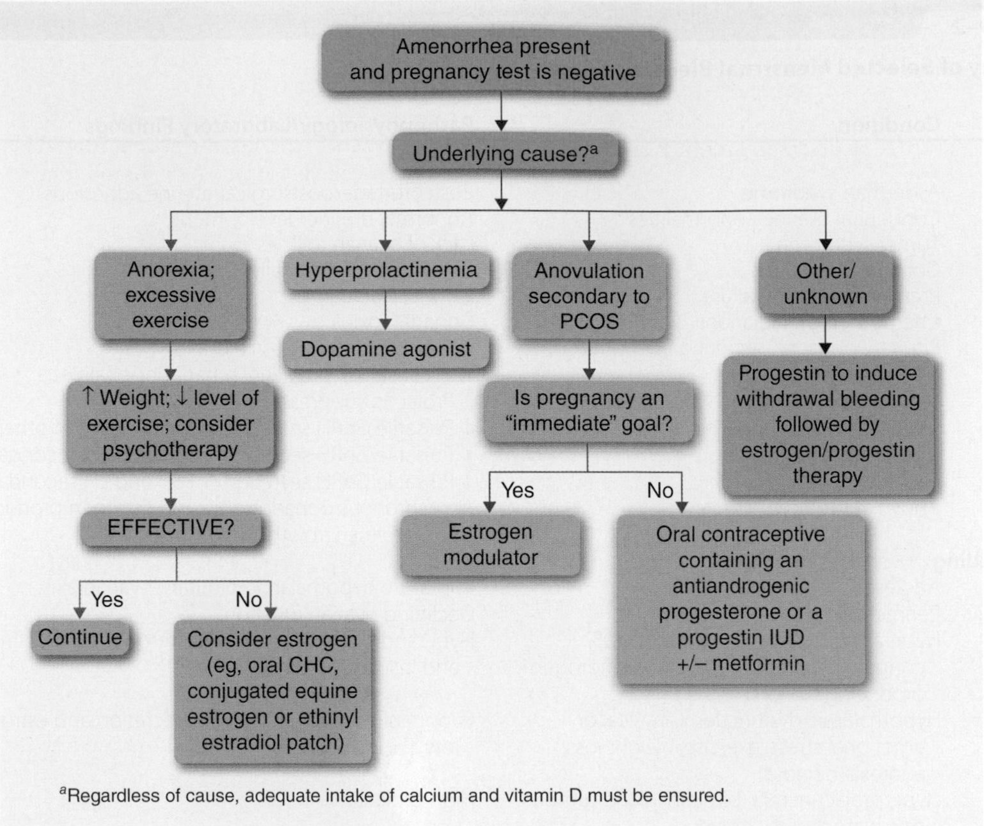

FIGURE 49–4. Treatment algorithm for amenorrhea. (CHC, combination hormonal contraceptive; IUD, intrauterine device; PCOS, polycystic ovarian syndrome.)

hysterectomy are surgical options. The preferred procedure is unclear. For short term, it appears that ablation or resection results in less morbidity and shorter recovery periods.[36] However, a significant number of these women eventually undergo hysterectomy within 5 years.[24]

Clinical Presentation and Diagnosis of Anovulatory Bleeding

General

- Acute distress may or may not be present

Symptoms

- Irregular, heavy, or prolonged vaginal bleeding, perimenopausal symptoms (hot flashes, etc)

Signs

- Acne, hirsutism, obesity

Laboratory Tests

- If suspect PCOS, consider free or total testosterone, fasting glucose, fasting lipid panel.
- If suspect perimenopause, FSH.

Other Diagnostic Tests

- Pelvic ultrasound to evaluate for polycystic ovaries

▶ *Pharmacologic Therapy*

Table 49–1 summarizes therapeutic agents and doses.

Estrogen Estrogen is the recommended treatment for managing acute bleeding episodes. It promotes endometrial growth and stabilization.[24] Given as a CHC, it has averted emergency surgery in 95% of patients.[8] It should then be continued to prevent recurrent anovulatory bleeding. Long-term therapy with a CHC reduces the risk of endometrial cancer compared to unopposed estrogen therapy.[6] CHCs suppress ovarian hormones and adrenal androgen production and indirectly increase sex hormone–binding globulin (SHBG). This, in turn, binds and reduces circulating androgen.[13,24,37] For women with high androgen levels and related signs (eg, hirsutism, acne), low-dose CHCs (35 mcg or less ethinyl estradiol) are the treatment of choice.[24] A CHC containing drospirenone, which has a greater impact on increasing SHBG and antiandrogenic effects, could be considered.[33] However, to date there is no consensus regarding the best CHC choice for treating PCOS.[13]

Medroxyprogesterone Acetate Depot and intermittent oral medroxyprogesterone acetate suppresses pituitary gonadotropins and circulating androgens in women with PCOS.[13] Furthermore, cyclic progesterone may benefit women older than 40 years with anovulatory bleeding.[24] Similar to the use of CHCs, oral medroxyprogesterone acetate has averted emergency surgeries in 100% of patients with acute uterine bleeding justifying immediate medical attention.[8]

Estrogen Modulators If the goal is to induce ovulation, the treatment of choice is clomiphene citrate. It is approximately

Patient Encounter 2

A 40-year-old woman presents to your office for a routine gynecologic examination. She entered menarche at the age of 12. Her last menstrual period was 3 months ago. Her periods are often irregular and occur about every 2 to 3 months. All previous Pap smears have been normal, and there is no history of sexually transmitted infections. She has had one sexual partner whom she is married to. She had one successful pregnancy that took "several years" and three courses of clomiphene due to "follicles" on her ovaries. Her PMH is significant for diabetes and hypertension for which she takes metformin 1000 mg by mouth twice daily and lisinopril 10 mg by mouth once daily. She is married and is not using any form of contraception. She notes that they have decided not to continue to try to have children. On examination, she is an overweight female with mild hirutism.

Labs: Urine HCG negative, free testosterone 100 ng/dL (3.47 nmol/L) (elevated), TSH 2.1 μIU/mL (2.1 mIU/L) (within normal limits), prolactin 9 ng/mL (9 mcg/L [391 pmol/L]) (within normal limits), fasting glucose 120 mg/dL (6.7 mmol/L). Fasting lipid panel: total cholesterol 181 mg/dL (4.68 mmol/L), HDL cholesterol 58 mg/dL (1.50 mmol/L), triglycerides 65 mg/dL (0.73 mmol/L), LDL cholesterol 110 mg/dL (2.84 mmol/L)

Pelvic ultrasound: 17 follicles in right ovary, 13 follicles in left ovary, increased ovarian volume of 12 mL

What anovulatory disorder is most likely present?

What signs/symptoms support this conclusion?

What pharmacologic therapies are recommended for this patient?

three times more effective than metformin at achieving live births.[13] Limited data have shown that adding metformin to clomiphene citrate may be more effective in increasing pregnancy rates, especially in obese women with PCOS who are resistant to clomiphene citrate monotherapy.[13,33,38] Treatment with clomiphene citrate is commonly recommended following withdrawal bleeding induction with oral medroxyprogesterone acetate, 10 mg/day for 10 days.

Recent data have shown beneficial effects with the use of letrozole to improve fertility. In a large trial, when compared to clomiphene citrate, letrozole had a statistically higher live birth rate with a similar adverse effect profile. Additional trials are needed to support this finding.[12,33]

Insulin-sensitizing Agents Metformin improves insulin sensitivity and is recommended in women who cannot tolerate CHC and have IGT or type-2 diabetes mellitus.[33] KEY CONCEPT *In patients with PCOS, it is associated with reduced circulating androgen concentrations, increased ovulation rates, and improved glucose tolerance. Additionally, metformin may decrease cardiovascular risk and promote weight loss.*[13] These improvements are attributed to the SHBG increase that occurs via increased insulin sensitivity. Notably, metformin, a pregnancy category B agent, is not recommended as monotherapy to improve ovulation and fertility. Thiazolidinediones are no longer recommended due to a poor risk-benefit ratio.[33]

Anovulatory Bleeding in Adolescents

Anovulatory cycles are common in the perimenarchal years. Ovulation typically is established a year or more following menarche. When anovulatory bleeding occurs in this population, it may be excessive. Thus, the patient should be evaluated for blood dyscrasias, including von Willebrand disease, prothrombin deficiency, and idiopathic thrombocytopenia purpura.[24,25]

In adolescents, blood dyscrasias should be treated. Acute, severe bleeding is managed with high-dose estrogen. Low-dose CHCs (35 mcg or less ethinyl estradiol) are the treatment of choice in adolescents with chronic anovulation.[24] If obesity is present, lifestyle changes are also recommended first line, and if IGT or metabolic syndrome is present, metformin can be recommended.[33]

MENORRHAGIA

Menorrhagia describes prolonged menstrual bleeding (lasting greater than 7 days) or cyclic, heavy menstrual bleeding (HMB; greater than 80 mL per cycle).[23,30,39] It is difficult to quantify menstrual blood loss in clinical practice. Many women with less than 80 mL of blood loss seek medical attention with concerns of containment flow problems, unpredictable heavy flow, reduced quality of life, and other dysmenorrhea symptoms.[39]

Epidemiology and Etiology

Menorrhagia rates in healthy women range from 9% to 14%, but can be as high as 30%.[23,39] KEY CONCEPT *Causes of menorrhagia can be*

Clinical Presentation and Diagnosis of Menorrhagia

General

- Acute distress may or may not be present

Symptoms

- Reports of heavy/prolonged menstrual flow.
- Fatigue and light-headedness in the case of severe blood loss.
- Dysmenorrhea may be an accompanying symptom

Signs

- Orthostasis, tachycardia, and pallor may be noted, especially with significant acute blood loss.

Laboratory Tests

- Complete blood count (CBC) and ferritin levels; hemoglobin and hematocrit results may be low.
- If the history dictates, testing may be done to identify coagulation disorder(s) as a cause.

Other Diagnostic Tests

- Pelvic ultrasound
- Pelvic magnetic resonance imaging (MRI)
- Pap smear
- Endometrial biopsy
- Hysteroscopy
- Sonohysterogram

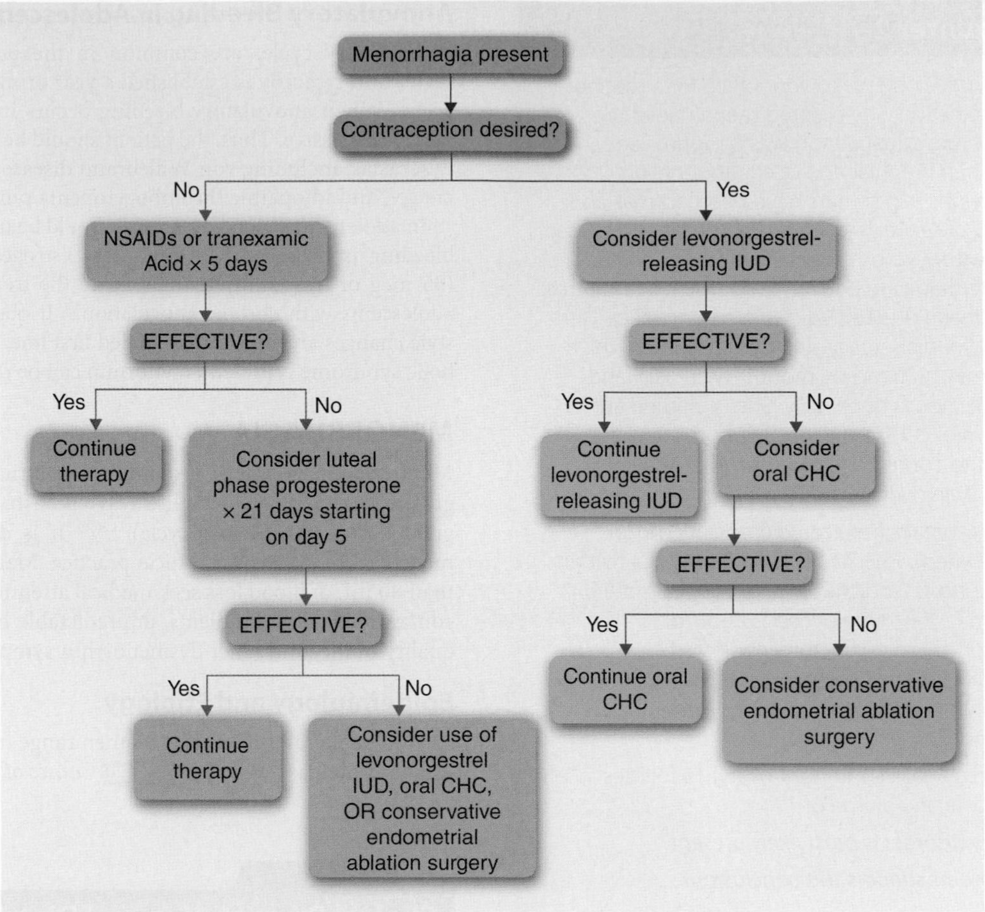

FIGURE 49–5. Treatment algorithm for menorrhagia. (CHC, combination hormonal contraceptive; IUD, intrauterine device; NSAID, nonsteroidal anti-inflammatory drug.)

divided into systemic disorders and reproductive tract abnormalities. KEY CONCEPT *Intrauterine pregnancy, ectopic pregnancy, and miscarriage are at the top of the differential diagnosis list for any woman presenting with heavy menses.* Additionally, genital tract malignancies and infections may present with abnormal bleeding.[23] Systemic disorders include coagulation dysfunction such as von Willebrand disease and platelet function disorders.[23,25,30] Hypothyroidism is also associated with heavy menses. Specific reproductive tract causes of menorrhagia are more common in older childbearing women, and they include fibroids, adenomyosis, endometrial polyps, and gynecologic malignancies.[30]

Pathophysiology

Table 49–2 describes the pathophysiology of menorrhagia and specific conditions resulting in menorrhagia.

Treatment

▸ *Desired Outcomes*

Goals of therapy are to reduce menstrual blood flow, reduce risk of anemia, improve quality of life, and defer the need for surgical intervention. Treatment recommendations are outlined in Table 49–1 and Figure 49–5.

▸ *Nonpharmacologic Therapy*

Surgical interventions are reserved for patients nonresponsive to pharmacologic treatment and include endometrial ablation and hysterectomy.[36]

▸ *Pharmacologic Therapy*

Nonsteroidal Anti-inflammatory Drugs (NSAIDs) NSAIDs are first-line treatments for menorrhagia associated with ovulatory cycles.[37] They are taken only during menses, and a 20% to 35% reduction in blood loss is reported in 75% of treated women.[10,37] KEY CONCEPT *This reduction is directly proportional to*

Patient Encounter 3

A 14-year-old girl presents to her physician reporting moderate pelvic pain and cramping during menses. She also notes that her menses are "heavy" and require a change in tampon every 3–4 hours. Her last menstrual cycle was 12 days ago, and she had her first menstrual cycle at age 12. She is not sexually active. She does not take any routine medications. She is on the high school volleyball team.

Identify the treatment goals for this patient's menorrhagia.

What diagnostic tests should be considered?

What pharmacologic therapies are recommended for this patient?

What monitoring parameters are recommended to assess efficacy and safety of the therapeutic options?

Table 49–3

Expected Outcome Measures for Selected Menstrual Bleeding Disorders[19,23–26,39]

Menstrual Disorder	Expected Outcome Measures
Amenorrhea	*Efficacy:* Normal breast development (especially primary amenorrhea in adolescents); BMD preservation/ improvement; return of menses. *Time to relief/effect:* Menses should occur within 1–2 months of therapy.
Anovulatory bleeding	*Efficacy:* Alleviation of acute bleeding when present; ovulation and subsequent pregnancy in women desiring this; reduced risk of developing the long-term complications of PCOS (eg, diabetes and cardiovascular disease); improved quality of life. *Time to relief/effect:* The acute treatment of heavy bleeding should reduce bleeding within 10 days of therapy onset; return of ovulation may require several months of therapy; when oral CHCs are used, abnormal bleeding control can be expected within 1–2 treatment cycles.
Dysmenorrhea	*Efficacy:* Reduction in menses-related pelvic pain; reduction in time lost from work/school; improved quality of life. *Time to relief/effect:* Improvement in pain may be observed within hours of NSAID therapy; improvement with other options such as oral CHCs may be observed after a full 1–3 cycles of use.
Menorrhagia	*Efficacy:* Decline in amount of blood loss with menses (monitor a decline in the number of times feminine hygiene products such as pads and tampons require changing during menses); increase in hemoglobin/ hematocrit if anemia was present as because of menorrhagia. *Time to relief/effect:* A decline in menstrual blood loss should be realized within 1–2 cycles of therapy initiation.

BMD, bone mineral density; CHCs, combination hormonal contraceptives; NSAID, nonsteroidal anti-inflammatory drug; PCOS, polycystic ovary syndrome.

the amount of pretreatment blood loss.[10] They may also improve dysmenorrhea.

Combination Hormonal Contraceptives CHCs are beneficial to women with menorrhagia who do not desire pregnancy. A 40% to 50% reduction in menstrual blood loss is reported in 68% of menorrhagia patients treated with oral CHCs containing greater than or equal to 35 mcg estradiol.[10,16] Continuous and extended cycle options may also reduce the number of menstrual cycles.[16] As with NSAIDs, KEY CONCEPT *the reduction in blood loss is proportional to pretreatment blood loss.*

Progestins Menorrhagia may also be treated with the levonorgestrel-releasing IUD, which consistently reduces menstrual flow by 75% to 95%, and after 12 months, 20% to 80% of women experience amenorrhea.[10,16,17,37,40] When compared with endometrial ablation, the levonorgestrel IUD causes similar reductions in menstrual blood loss after 6, 12, and 24 months.[41]

Patient Care Process

Patient Assessment:

- Based on physical examination, history, and review of systems, additional work-up may be necessary (eg, amenorrhea, menorrhagia, AUB, or PMDD).
- Document symptoms.
- Conduct a medication history. Have any treatments helped in the past?
- Review the medical history and laboratory data. Does the patient have any complications, such as symptoms of anemia in patients presenting with menorrhagia or difficulty conceiving in women with amenorrhea or anovulatory bleeding?
- Review available diagnostic data to determine hormonal, reproductive, and pregnancy status. Does the patient need a pregnancy test?

Therapy Evaluation:

- Is current pharmacotherapy safe and effective; is dosing appropriate?
- Is the patient adherent to current therapy?
- Does the patient have prescription insurance coverage?

Care Plan Development:

- Educate the patient on lifestyle modifications that will improve symptoms and prevent complications.
- Select pharmacotherapy, if indicated, that is safe and effective.
- Determine whether long-term maintenance treatment is necessary.
- Address any patient concerns on quality of life (physical, psychological, and social functioning) and infertility.
- Discuss the importance of adherence to medication management and lifestyle modifications.

Follow-up Evaluation:

- Develop a plan to assess effectiveness and safety of pharmacotherapy.
- Assess improvement in quality of life and well-being
- Review medical history, physical examination findings, laboratory and diagnostic tests.
- Evaluate for adverse drug reactions, drug allergies, and drug interactions.

Compared with hysterectomy, it leads to similar rates of satisfaction and improved quality of life.[10,42]

Cyclic progestin therapy, either during the luteal phase or for 21 days of the menstrual cycle, reduces menstrual blood loss.[10] The levonorgestrel IUD is more effective than oral norethindrone administered cyclically.[16] In a small open-label study, the levonorgestrel IUD resulted in a greater menstrual blood loss reduction and number of lost days at work or school compared with oral CHCs.[43] Oral progestin therapy is considered a third-line option.[10]

Tranexamic Acid Tranexamic acid reduces plasmin activity and tissue plasminogen activator.[10,44] While an immediate-release product has been available for a long time, a modified-release product has recently become available. It has better gastrointestinal tolerability and gives women another non-hormonal option to manage menorrhagia.[44,45] Additionally, it can be recommended for women with von Willebrand disease.

Menorrhagia in Adolescents

Up to 50% of adolescents with menorrhagia have been shown to have a bleeding disorder, most commonly von Willebrand disease or platelet dysfunction.[25] Although von Willebrand disease has a 1% to 2% incidence in the general population, it is estimated that 5% to 36% of adolescents presenting with heavy menses have this disorder.[25,26] Platelet function disorders exist in 2% to 44% of adolescents with menorrhagia.[25]

OUTCOME EVALUATION

Treatment success for menstruation-related disorders is measured by the degree to which treatment (a) relieves or reverses symptoms, (b) prevents or reverses complications (eg, osteoporosis, anemia, and infertility), and (c) causes minimal adverse effects. Resumption of regular menstrual cycles with minimal premenstrual or dysmenorrhea symptoms should occur. Depending on the desire for conception and related therapy, these cycles may be ovulatory or anovulatory.

Assess treatment effectiveness in reinstating normal menstrual cycles with minimal adverse effects after an appropriate treatment interval (1–2 months). Assess improvement in well-being and quality-of-life (eg, physical, psychological, and social functioning). Evaluate the patient for adverse drug reactions (see Table 49–1), drug allergies, and drug interactions. Table 49–3 lists the expected outcome measures for each discussed menstruation-related disorder.

Abbreviations Introduced in This chapter

ACOG	American College of Obstetricians and Gynecologists
AUB	Anovulatory uterine bleeding
BMD	Bone mineral density
BMI	Body mass index
CBC	Complete blood count
CEE	Conjugated equine estrogen
CHC	Combination hormonal contraceptive
FSH	Follicle-stimulating hormone
GI	Gastrointestinal
GnRH	Gonadotropin-releasing hormone
HCG	Human chorionic gonadotropin
HMB	Heavy menstrual bleeding
HPO	Hypothalamic-pituitary-ovarian
IGT	Impaired glucose tolerance
IUD	Intrauterine device
LH	Luteinizing hormone
MPA	Medroxyprogesterone acetate
MRI	Magnetic resonance imaging
NSAID	Nonsteroidal anti-inflammatory drug
OC	Oral contraceptive
PCOS	Polycystic ovarian syndrome
PID	Pelvic inflammatory disease
SHBG	Sex hormone–binding globulin
TENS	Transcutaneous electrical nerve stimulation

REFERENCES

1. Fritz MA, Speroff L. Clinical Gynecologic Endocrinology and Infertility, 8th ed. Philadelphia, PA: Lippincott Williams & Wilkins, 2010: 567–589.
2. Osayande AS, Mehulic S. Diagnosis and Initial Management of Dysmenorrhea. Am Fam Physician. 2014;89(5):341–346.
3. Morrow C, Naumburg EH. Dysmenorrhea. Prim Care Clin Office Pract. 2009;36:19–32.
4. Lentz GM. Primary and secondary dysmenorrhea, premenstrual syndrome, and premenstrual dysphoric disorder: Etiology, diagnosis, management. In: Lentz GM, ed. Comprehensive Gynecology, 6th ed. Philadelphia, PA: Mosby Elsevier, 2013:791–803.
5. Harel Z. Dysmenorrhea in adolescents. Ann NY Acad Sci. 2008;1135:185–195. doi: 10.1196/annals.1429.007.
6. Klein DA, Poth MA. Amenorrhea: an Approach to Diagnosis and Management. Am Fam Physician. 2013;87(11):781–788.
7. Wang AT, Mullan RJ, Lane MA, et al. Treatment of hyperprolactinemia: a systematic review and meta-analysis. Systematic Reviews. 2012;1:33.
8. Hartmann KE, Jerome RN, Lindegren ML, et al. Primary Care Management of Abnormal Uterine Bleeding. Comparative Effectiveness Review No. 96. (Prepared by the Vanderbilt Evidence-based Practice Center under Contract No. 290-2007-10065 I.) AHRQ Publication No. 13-EHC025-EF. Rockville, MD: Agency for Healthcare Research and Quality. March 2013.
9. Wong CL, Garquhar C, Roberts H, Proctor M. Oral contraceptive pill for primary dysmenorrhoea. Cochrane Database Syst Rev. 2009;4:CD002120.
10. Fraser IS, Porte RJ, Kouides PA, Lukes AS. A benefit-risk review of systemic haemostatic agents: part 2: in excessive or heavy menstrual bleeding. Drug Saf. 2008;31(4):275–282.
11. Sweet MG, Schmidt-Dalton TA, Weiss PM. Evaluation and Management of Abnormal Uterine Bleeding in Premenopausal Women. Am Fam Physician. 2012;85(1):35–43.
12. Legro RS, Brzyski RG, Diamond MP, et al. Letrozole versus Clomiphene for Infertility in the Polycystic Ovary Syndrome. N Engl J Med. 2014;371:119-29. DOI: 10.1056/NEJMoa1313517
13. Polycystic ovary syndrome. ACOG Practice Bulletin No. 108. American College of Obstetricians and Gynecologists. Obstet Gynecol. 2009(Reaffirmed 2013); 114:936–949.
14. Lobo RA. Primary and secondary amenorrhea and precocious puberty: etiology, diagnostic evaluation, management. In: Lentz G, ed. Comprehensive Gynecology, 6th ed. Philadelphia, PA: Mosby Elsevier, 2013:815–836.
15. Lexi-Comp Online. Hudson, OH: Lexi-Comp, Inc., 2014.
16. Noncontraceptive uses of hormonal contraceptives. ACOG Practice Bulletin No. 110. American College of Obstetricians and Gynecologists. Obstet Gynecol. 2010(reaffirmed 2014);115: 206–18.
17. Long-Acting Reversible Contraception: implants and Intrauterine Devices. ACOG Practice Bulletin No. 121. American College of Obstetricians and Gynecologists. Obstet Gynecol. 2011(Reaffirmed 2013);118:184–195.

18. U.S. medical eligibility criteria for contraceptive use, 2010. Centers for Disease Control and Prevention (CDC). MMWR Recomm Rep. 2010;59(RR-4):1–86.
19. Menstruation in girls and adolescents: using the menstrual cycle as a vital sign. ACOG Committee Opinion No. 349. American Academy of Pediatrics; American College of Obstetricians and Gynecologists. Obstet Gynecol. 2006(Reaffirmed 2009);108: 1323–1328.
20. Current evaluation of amenorrhea. The Practice Committee of the American Society for Reproductive Medicine. Fertil Steril. 2008;90:S219–S225.
21. Umland EM, Klootwyk JM. Menstruation-related disorders (Chapter 63). In: Pharmacotherapy: A Pathophysiologic Approach, 9th ed. New York, NY: McGraw-Hill, 2014.
22. Deligeoroglou E, Athanasopoulos N, Tsimaris P, et al. Evaluation and management of adolescent amenorrhea. Ann NY Acad Sci. 2010;1205:23–32.
23. Lobo RA. Abnormal uterine bleeding: Ovulatory and anovulatory dysfunctional uterine bleeding, management of acute and chronic excessive bleeding. In: Lentz GM, ed. Comprehensive Gynecology, 6th ed. Philadelphia, PA: Mosby Elsevier, 2013: 808–814.
24. Management of Anovulatory Bleeding Associated with Ovulatory Dysfunction. ACOG Practice Bulletin No. 136 (2013). American College of Obstetricians and Gynecologists. Obstet Gynecol. 2013;122:176–85.
25. Boswell HB. The adolescent with menorrhagia: why, who, and how to evaluate for a bleeding disorder. J Pediatr Adolesc Gynecol. 2011;24(4):228–230.
26. Adams Hillard PJ. Menstruation in Adolescents What's Normal, What's Not. Ann NY Acad Sci 2008;1135:29–35.
27. Majumdar A, Mangal NS. Hyperprolactinemia. J Hum Reprod Sci. 2013 Jul-Sep;6(3):168–175.
28. Simon JA. Progestogens in the treatment of secondary amenorrhea. J Reprod Med. 1999;44:185–189.
29. Tolaymat LL, Kaunitz AM. Use of hormonal contraception in adolescents: skeletal health issues. Curr Opin Obstet Gynecol. 2009;21(5):396–401.
30. Fritz MA, Speroff L. Clinical Gynecologic Endocrinology and Infertility, 8th ed. Philadelphia, PA: Lippincott Williams & Wilkins; 2010:591–619.
31. Rotterdam ESHRE/ASRM-Sponsored PCOS Consensus Workshop Group. Revised 2003 consensus on diagnostic criteria and long-term health risks related to polycystic ovary syndrome. Fertil Steril. 2004;81(1):19–25.
32. Azziz R, Carmina E, Dewailly D, et al. Task Force on the Phenotype of the Polycystic Ovary Syndrome of The Androgen Excess and PCOS Society. The Androgen Excess and PCOS Society criteria for the polycystic ovary syndrome: the complete task force report. Fertil Steril. 2009;91:456–488.
33. Legro RS, Arslanian SA, Ehrmann DA. Diagnosis and Treatment of Polycystic Ovary Syndrome: an Endocrine Society Clinical Practice Guideline. J Clin Endocrinol Metab. 2013;98:4565–4592.
34. Wild RA, Carmina E, Diamanti-Kandarakis E, et al. Assessment of cardiovascular risk and prevention of cardiovascular disease in women with the polycystic ovary syndrome: a consensus statement by the Androgen Excess and Polycystic Ovary Syndrome (AE-PCOS) Society. J Clin Endocrinol Metab. 2010; 95(5):2038–2049.
35. Fauser BC, Tarlatzis BC, Rebar RW, et al. Consensus on women's health aspects of polycystic ovary syndrome PCOS): the Amsterdam ESHRE/ASRM-Sponsored 3rd PCOS Consensus Workshop Group. Fertil Steril. 2012;97:28–38.
36. Munro MG, Dickersin K, Clark MA, et al. The Surgical Treatments Outcomes Project for Dysfunctional Uterine Bleeding: summary of an Agency for Health Research and Quality-sponsored randomized trial of endometrial ablation versus hysterectomy for women with heavy menstrual bleeding. Menopause. 2011;18(4):445–452.
37. Casablanca Y. Management of dysfunctional uterine bleeding. Obstet Gynecol Clin N Am. 2008;35:219–234.
38. Khorram O, Helliwell JP, Katz S, et al. Two weeks of metformin improves clomiphene citrate-induced ovulation and metabolic profiles in women with polycystic ovary syndrome. Fertil Steril. 2006;85(5):1448–1451.
39. Matteson KA, Boardman LA, Munro MG, Clark MA. Abmormal uterine bleeding: a review of patient-based outcome measures. Fertil Steril. 2009;92(1): 205–216.
40. Reid PC, Virtanen-Kari S. Randomized comparative trial of levonorgestrel intrauterine system and mefenamic acid for the treatment of idiopathic menorrhagia: a multiple analysis using total menstrual fluid loss, menstrual blood loss and pictorial blood loss assessment charts. Br J Obstet Gynecol. 2005; 112:1121–1125.
41. Kaunitz AM, Meredith S, Inki P, et al. Levonorgestrel-releasing intrauterine system and endometrial ablation in heavy menstrual bleeding: a systematic review and meta-analysis. Obstet Gynecol. 2009;113:1104–1116.
42. Kim M, Seong SJ. Clinical applications of levonorgestrel-releasing intrauterine system to gynecologic diseases. Obstet Gynecol Sci. 2013;56(2):67–75.
43. Shaaban MM, Zekherah MS, El-Nashar SA, Sayed GH. Levonorgestrel-releasing intrauterine system compared to low dose combined oral contraceptive pills for idiopathic menorrhagia: a randomized clinical trial. Contraception. 2011;83:48–45.
44. Kost A, Pitney C. Tranexamic Acid (Lysteda) for Cyclic Heavy Menstrual Bleeding. Am Fam Physician. 2011 Oct 15;84(8): 883–886.
45. Hrometz SL. Oral modified-release tranexamic acid for heavy menstrual bleeding. Ann Pharmacotherapy. 2012;46(7-8):1047–53.

50 Hormone Therapy in Menopause

Nicole S. Culhane and Kelly R. Ragucci

LEARNING OBJECTIVES

Upon completion of the chapter, the reader will be able to:

1. Explain the physiologic changes associated with menopause.
2. Identify the signs and symptoms associated with menopause.
3. Determine the desired therapeutic outcomes for a patient taking hormone therapy (HT).
4. Explain how to evaluate a patient for the appropriate use of HT.
5. Recommend nonpharmacologic therapy for menopausal symptoms.
6. List the adverse effects of and contraindications to HT.
7. Differentiate between topical and systemic forms of HT.
8. Explain the risks and benefits associated with HT.
9. Educate a patient regarding the proper use and potential adverse effects of HT.
10. Describe the monitoring parameters for a patient taking HT.
11. Describe the circumstances under which nonhormonal therapies for menopausal symptoms should be considered.

INTRODUCTION

Menopause is the permanent cessation of menses following the loss of ovarian follicular activity. The diagnosis of menopause is primarily a clinical one and is made after a woman experiences amenorrhea for 12 consecutive months. The loss of ovarian follicular activity leads to an increase in follicle-stimulating hormone (FSH), which, on laboratory examination, may help to confirm the diagnosis.

The role of hormone therapy (HT) has changed dramatically over the years. HT has long been prescribed for relief of menopausal symptoms and, until recent years, has been purported to protect women from coronary heart disease (CHD). The reason behind recommending HT in postmenopausal women revolved around a simple theory: If the hormones lost during menopause were replaced through drug therapy, women would be protected from both menopausal symptoms and chronic diseases that often follow after a woman experiences menopause. Recent studies have disproved this theory.

In 1996, the United States Preventive Services Task Force first published its recommendations that not all postmenopausal women should be prescribed HT, but that therapy should be individualized based on risk factors. This recommendation was further supported with publication of the Heart and Estrogen/Progestin Replacement Study (HERS) in 1998, which demonstrated that women who had established CHD were at an increased risk of experiencing a myocardial infarction within the first year of HT use compared with a similar group of women without CHD risk factors. As a result, the authors concluded that HT should not be recommended for the secondary prevention of CHD.[1] Then, in 2002, the Women's Health Initiative (WHI) study was published. This trial demonstrated that HT was not protective against CHD but rather could increase the risk in women with underlying CHD risk factors. The risk of breast cancer was also increased after a woman was on combination estrogen and progestogen for approximately 3 years. It should be noted that this was not the case with estrogen alone. As a result of this study, the US Food and Drug Administration (FDA) issued a statement that HT, in general, should not be initiated or continued for the primary prevention of CHD.[2]

This series of trials led to dramatic changes in how HT is prescribed and greater understanding of the associated risks. HT, once thought of as a cure-all for menopausal symptoms, is now a therapy that should be used primarily to reduce the frequency and severity of moderate to severe **vasomotor symptoms** associated with menopause in women without risk factors for CHD or breast cancer. The changes that have occurred over the years in the use of HT further support the importance of evidence-based practice and judicious medication use.

EPIDEMIOLOGY AND ETIOLOGY

Menopause is a period of time marked by loss of ovarian follicular activity, inadequate estradiol production, and the subsequent cessation of menses. The median age for a woman to experience menopause is 52 years. However, women who have undergone a total abdominal hysterectomy with bilateral salpingo-oophorectomy (surgical menopause) generally experience menopause earlier compared with women who experience natural menopause. Some other factors that may be associated with early menopause include low body weight, increased menstrual cycle length, nulliparity, and smoking. Smokers generally experience menopause approximately 2 years earlier than nonsmokers.[3]

The usual transitional period prior to menopause, known as perimenopause or the *climacteric*, is a period when hormonal and biologic changes begin to occur. These changes may begin 2 to 8 years prior to menopause and eventually lead to irregular menstrual cycles, an increase in cycle interval, and a decrease in cycle length. During this time, women also may experience physical symptoms similar to menopausal symptoms, which may require treatment depending on symptom severity.[3]

Because the perimenopausal and postmenopausal periods are marked by many biologic and endocrinologic changes, women should inform their health care provider when they experience any signs and symptoms in order to discuss the most appropriate therapeutic approach.

Patient Encounter, Part 1

A 52-year-old woman with a history of hypertension, hyperlipidemia, and hypothyroidism presents to the clinic complaining of hot flashes, vaginal dryness, and insomnia. She states that she experiences approximately four hot flashes per day and is awakened from sleep at least two to three times a week in a "pool of sweat" requiring her to change her clothes and bed linens. Her symptoms began about 6 months ago, and over that time, they have worsened to the point where they have become very bothersome. On questioning, she states her last menstrual period was 18 months ago.

Which of the patient's symptoms and past medical history are consistent with menopause?

What additional information do you need to know in order to make an appropriate therapeutic plan for this patient?

PHYSIOLOGY

Reproductive physiology is regulated primarily by the hypothalamic–pituitary–ovarian axis. The hypothalamus secretes gonadotropin-releasing hormone (GnRH), which stimulates the anterior pituitary to secrete FSH and luteinizing hormone (LH). FSH and LH regulate ovarian function and stimulate the ovary to produce sex steroids. All these hormones are influenced by a negative-feedback system and will increase or decrease based on the levels of estradiol and progesterone.

The physiologic changes that occur during the perimenopausal and menopausal periods are caused by the decrease and eventual loss of ovarian follicular activity. As women age, the number of ovarian follicles decreases, and the remaining follicles require higher levels of FSH for maturation and ovulation. During perimenopause, anovulatory cycles are more likely, and the lack of progesterone production leads to irregular and unpredictable menses. During menopause, FSH concentrations increase 10- to 15-fold, LH concentrations increase fivefold, and levels of circulating estradiol decrease by more than 90%.[4]

KEY CONCEPT *Common symptoms of menopause include vasomotor symptoms (hot flashes, night sweats), vulvovaginal atrophy, vaginal dryness, and dyspareunia. Women less commonly may experience mood swings, depression, insomnia, arthralgia, myalgia, urinary frequency, and decreased libido.* Menopausal symptoms tend to be more severe in women who undergo surgical menopause compared with natural menopause because of the more rapid decline in estrogen concentrations.[3] Women who seek medical treatment should undergo laboratory evaluation to rule out other conditions that may present with similar symptoms, such as abnormal thyroid function or pituitary adenoma. Once symptoms have been evaluated and other conditions have been excluded, HT may be considered.

Clinical Presentation and Diagnosis of Menopause

Menopausal Symptoms

- Vasomotor symptoms (hot flashes, night sweats)
- Irregular menses
- Episodic amenorrhea
- Sleep disturbances
- Mood swings
- Vaginal dryness, dyspareunia
- Depression

Less Common Symptoms

- Fatigue
- Irritability
- Migraine
- Arthralgia
- Myalgia
- Decreased libido

Diagnosis

- Amenorrhea for 1 year
- FSH greater than 40 mIU/mL (40 IU/L)
- Fivefold increase in LH

TREATMENT

Desired Outcomes

KEY CONCEPT *HT remains the most effective treatment for vasomotor symptoms and vulvovaginal atrophy and can be considered, especially for women experiencing moderate to severe symptoms.* The goals of treatment are to alleviate or reduce menopausal symptoms and to improve the patient's quality of life (QOL) while minimizing adverse effects of therapy. The appropriate route of administration should be chosen based on individual patient symptoms, and therapy should be continued at the lowest dose for the shortest duration consistent with treatment goals for each patient.

General Approach to Treatment

There are a number of national and international guidelines and consensus statements available on the management of menopause.[5–9] The most current guidelines should always be consulted before making pharmacotherapeutic recommendations for women. Women suffering from vasomotor symptoms should attempt lifestyle or behavioral modifications before seeking medical treatment. Women who seek medical treatment usually suffer from symptoms that diminish their QOL, such as multiple hot flashes per day or week, sleep disturbances, vaginal dryness, or mood swings. HT should be considered for these women but is not the most appropriate choice for all women. KEY CONCEPT. *Women should receive a thorough history and physical examination, including assessing for CHD and breast cancer risk factors and contraindications, before HT is considered. They should be informed of the risks and the benefits of HT and encouraged to be involved in the decision-making process. If a woman does not have any contraindications to HT, including CHD or significant CHD risk factors, and also does not have a personal history of breast cancer, HT could be an appropriate therapy option* (Figure 50–1). Women who have undergone a hysterectomy need only be prescribed estrogen. A progestogen should be added to the estrogen only for women with an intact uterus. Alternative and nonhormonal treatment options are available for women who are not candidates for HT, but they have limited effectiveness and may also have adverse effects.

Nonpharmacologic Therapy

Nonpharmacologic therapies for menopause-related symptoms have not been studied in large randomized trials, and evidence of benefit is not well documented. Due to the minimal adverse effects of these interventions, patients should try lifestyle or behavioral modifications before and in addition to pharmacologic therapy. The most common nonpharmacologic interventions for vasomotor symptoms include the following[3,12,13]:

- Smoking cessation
- Limit alcohol and caffeine
- Limit hot beverages (eg, coffee/tea, soups)
- Limit spicy foods
- Keep cool, and dress in layers
- Stress reduction (eg, meditation, relaxation exercises)
- Increase exercise
- Paced respiration

Exercise demonstrated an improvement in QOL but did not improve vasomotor symptoms. Paced respiration, a form of deep, slow breathing, improved vasomotor symptoms in a small group of patients.

Dyspareunia may result from vaginal dryness. Water-based lubricants may provide relief for several hours after application. Moisturizers may provide relief for a longer period of time and potentially can prevent infections by maintaining the acidic environment in the vagina. Both these treatments require frequent application.

A decline in estrogen concentrations also may be associated with urinary stress incontinence. Kegel exercises are recommended as a first-line intervention for stress incontinence, although pharmacologic therapy also may be necessary. Kegel exercises strengthen the pelvic floor muscles and help to keep the urethral sphincter from relaxing at inappropriate times, such as when lifting heavy objects, coughing, or sneezing. These exercises have no adverse effects, take little time, may be done inconspicuously, and when done correctly, may help to restore normal urine flow.

Patient Encounter, Part 2: Medical History, Physical Examination, and Diagnostic Tests

The workup reveals the following additional information:

PMH: Hypertension since age 45, currently controlled; hyperlipidemia, currently controlled; hypothyroidism since age 25, but symptoms indicative of worsening control; hysterectomy in 2010.

FH: Father: Alive with HTN and CHD (MI at age 60). Mother: Alive with hypothyroidism, HTN, and GERD. Siblings: Two sisters alive and well, menopausal with hx of hot flashes.

SH: Occupation: Nurse; nonsmoker; drinks one to two glasses of red wine with dinner on the weekends; denies illicit drug use.

Meds: Lisinopril/HCTZ 20/12.5 mg once daily; simvastatin 40 mg at bedtime; Synthroid 0.075 mg by mouth once daily; multivitamin by mouth once daily.

ROS: (+) hot flashes, night sweats, vaginal dryness and itching; (+) insomnia, bowel changes, 5-lb weight loss since last visit 6 months ago.

PE:

VS: BP 128/78, P 92, RR 16, T 37.0°C (98.6°F), Wt 74.5 kg (164 lb)

HEENT: WNL

Neck: Supple; no bruits, no adenopathy, no thyromegaly.

Breasts: Supple; no masses

CV: RRR, normal S_1 and S_2; no murmurs, rubs, or gallops

Abd: Soft, nontender, nondistended; (+) BS, no masses

Genitourinary: Pelvic examination normal except (+) mucosal atrophy; (+) hysterectomy

Labs:

FSH: 76 mIU/mL (76 IU/L)

TSH: 0.3 μIU/mL (0.3 mIU/L)

Chem-7: Na 135 mEq/L (135 mmol/L), K 4.5 mEq/L (4.5 mmol/L), Cl 109 mEq/L (109 mmol/L), CO_2 25 mEq/L (25 mmol/L), BUN 9 mg/dL (3.2 mmol/L), SCr 0.9 mg/dL (80 μmol/L), Glucose 98 mg/dL (5.4 mmol/L)

CBC: Hgb 13 g/dL (130 g/L or 8.06 mmol/L), Hct 39% (0.39 volume fraction), WBC 5.5 × 10^3/mm^3 (5.5 × 10^9/L), platelets 234 × 10^3/mm^3(234 × 10^9/L)

Fasting lipid levels: TC 200 mg/dL (5.17 mmol/L), low-density lipoprotein (LDL) 126 mg/dL (3.26 mmol/L), high-density lipoprotein (HDL) 50 mg/dL (1.30 mmol/L), Triglycerides (TG) 115 mg/dL (1.30 mmol/L)

Assess the patient's condition based on this additional information.

What are the goals of treatment for this patient?

Assess the patient's risk factors for heart disease and breast cancer.

Recommend nonpharmacologic and pharmacologic treatment for this patient. Justify your recommendations.

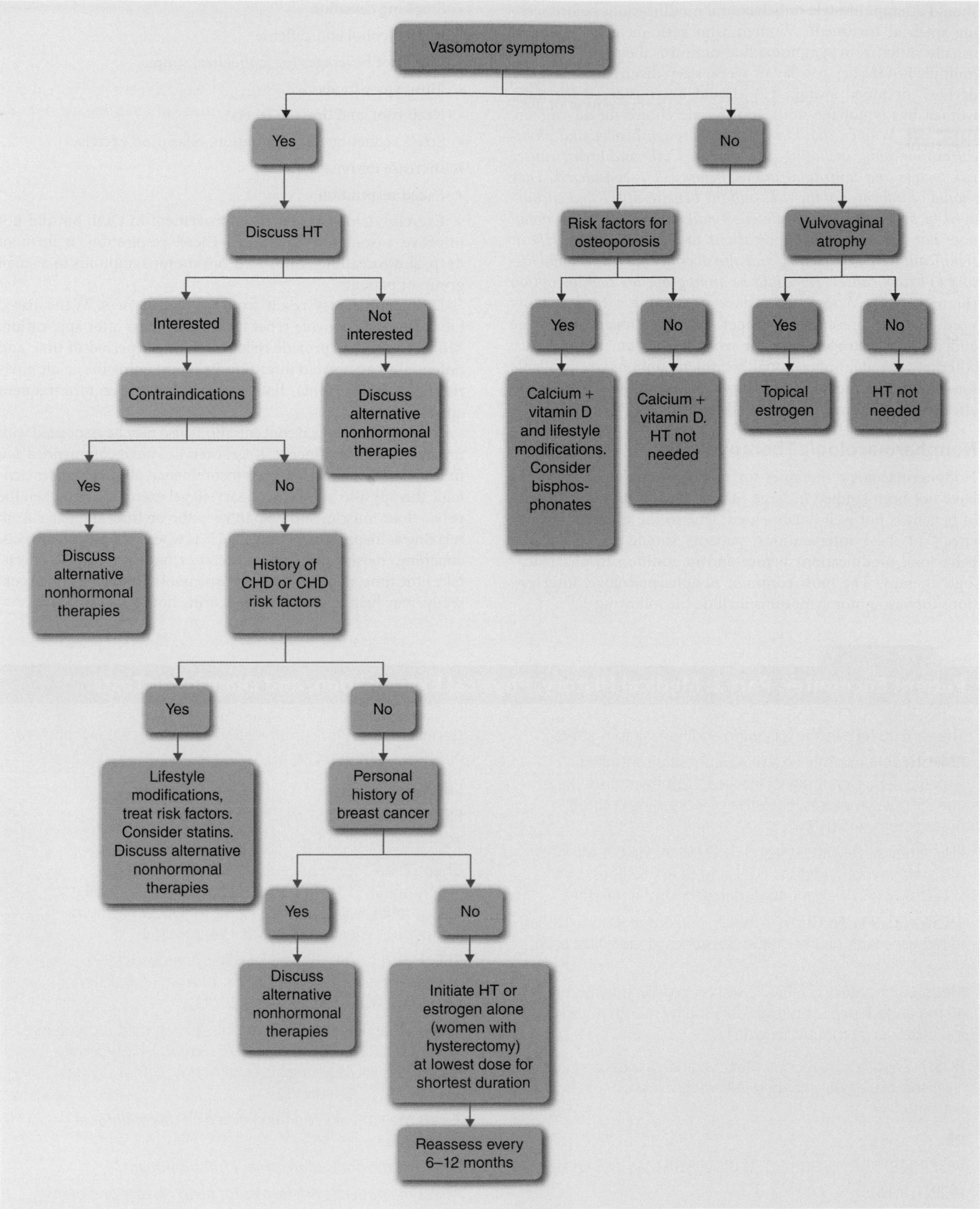

FIGURE 50–1. Treatment algorithm for postmenopausal women.[2,10,11] (CHD, coronary heart disease; HT, hormone therapy.)

Pharmacologic Therapy

▶ Estrogens

Estrogen is indicated for the treatment of moderate to severe vasomotor symptoms and vulvovaginal atrophy associated with menopause. In addition, it is indicated for the prevention of postmenopausal osteoporosis in women with significant risk; however, it is recommended that nonestrogen medications be used long-term. KEY CONCEPT *Oral or transdermal estrogen products should be prescribed at the lowest effective dose and for the shortest duration possible to provide relief of vasomotor symptoms. Topical vaginal products in the form of creams, tablets, or rings should be prescribed for women exclusively experiencing vulvovaginal atrophy.*

Many systemically administered estrogen products are available in the United States. Transdermal estrogen preparations are also available and usually are prescribed for patients who experience adverse effects, elevated triglycerides (TG), or liver function abnormalities while taking an oral product. Although there have been no randomized controlled trials (RCTs) published, one case control study suggests that transdermal preparations have a lower incidence of venous thromboembolism (VTE) than oral preparations.[5,14]

▶ Progestogens

KEY CONCEPT *Women who have an intact uterus should be prescribed a progestogen in addition to estrogen in order to decrease the risk of endometrial hyperplasia and endometrial cancer.*[5] Progestogens should be prescribed for at least 12 to 14 days of the month and often are prescribed continuously. Even low doses of oral estrogen therapy, as well as high dose vaginal preparations, require daily or intermittent administration of a progestogen in order to provide endometrial protection. Table 50–1 lists estrogen and progestogen preparations and dosages.

▶ Adverse Effects

Therapy with estrogen with or without a progestogen should be initiated at the lowest dose in order to minimize adverse effects. Because the adverse effects of these preparations can be similar, it may be difficult to assess whether the estrogen or the progestogen is the cause. Changing preparations, particularly the progestogen, or changing the method of administration may help to alleviate adverse effects. Table 50–2 lists the adverse effects that may be associated with estrogen and progestogen preparations.

▶ Contraindications

HT should not be prescribed to women with a history of or active thromboembolic disease, breast cancer or estrogen-dependent neoplasm, pregnancy, liver disease, or undiagnosed vaginal bleeding. It also should not be used for the prevention or treatment of cardiovascular disease, cerebrovascular disease, or dementia.[3]

▶ Methods of Administration

Cyclic Estrogen and Progestogen Estrogen is administered daily, and progestogen is administered for 12 to 14 days of the month. The disadvantage of this method of administration is the return of monthly menses in approximately 90% of women 1 to 2 days following the last progestogen dose. Women may view this scheduled bleeding as an advantage to this method of administration as it limits spotting or soiling of undergarments.

Continuous Combined Estrogen and Progestogen Estrogen and progestogen are administered daily and result in endometrial atrophy. Therefore, women do not experience a withdrawal bleed but may experience unanticipated breakthrough bleeding or spotting during the month. Although this may sound more appealing than a withdrawal bleed, women may view the unpredictable bleeding or spotting as a disadvantage to this type of administration. If bleeding persists beyond 6 to 12 months, women should seek medical attention to rule out endometrial hypertrophy or carcinoma.

▶ Low-Dose HT

There is an increasing body of evidence proving the effectiveness of low-dose HT regimens in the management of menopausal symptoms. Several trials demonstrated that lower doses of conjugated equine estrogen (CEE) ± medroxyprogesterone acetate (MPA) (CEE 0.45 mg or 0.3 mg ± MPA 2.5 mg or 1.5 mg) decreased hot flashes comparable with standard HT, improved vulvovaginal atrophy, increased bone mineral density (BMD) at the spine and hip, and provided sufficient endometrial protection.[17–20] Currently, no data are available on the effects of low-dose HT on the incidence of VTE, breast cancer, or CHD. Although many women have switched to low-dose HT, time will tell if lower doses translate into lower risks.

▶ Bioidentical HT

Bioidentical hormones are exogenous hormones that are identical to those produced in a woman's body (eg, estradiol, estrone, estriol, and progesterone). They are either commercially manufactured or chemically compounded in pharmacies into formulations such as topical creams, gels, and suppositories. The commercially manufactured prescription products are subject to regulation by the FDA and have been tested for potency, purity, efficacy, and safety (see Table 50–1). Conversely, pharmacist-compounded formulations are not subject to the same regulations and therefore, the efficacy and safety may be questionable. Often women view bioidentical hormones, particularly the pharmacist-compounded formulations, as "natural" and assume these formulations are safer than currently marketed prescription hormone products. Women may feel more comfortable using compounded products that are formulated based on individual hormone levels; however, due to a lack of regulation, these products may potentially cause more harm than benefit. In addition, pharmacist-compounded formulations can result in higher costs, because they are generally not covered by third-party payers. There is little evidence comparing the safety and efficacy of conventional HT to prescription bioidentical HT, and thus the same risks and benefits should be assumed.[5,21]

▶ Benefits of HT

Vasomotor Symptoms HT remains the most effective treatment for vasomotor symptoms, and systemic HT should be considered only in women experiencing these symptoms. Benefits must outweigh risks, and decisions should be made only after careful consideration by the woman and her health care provider. If it is decided to use HT, it should be prescribed at the lowest dose that relieves or reduces menopausal symptoms and should be recommended only for short-term use (generally less than 5 years). Women should be reassessed every 6 to 12 months, and discontinuation of therapy should be considered.

Vulvovaginal Atrophy Approximately 50% of postmenopausal women experience vulvovaginal atrophy and seek medical attention. Vulvovaginal atrophy is associated with vaginal dryness and dyspareunia and also may be associated with recurrent urinary tract infections, urethritis, and urinary urgency and frequency.

Table 50–1

Estrogen and Progestogen Formulations and Dosages[10,15,16]

Product	Available Strengths	Common Dosages
Oral estrogens		
CEE (Premarin)	0.3-1.25 mg	0.3-0.625 mg/day
Synthetic conjugated estrogens (Cenestin; Enjuvia)	0.3-1.25 mg	0.3-0.625 mg/day
Esterified estrogens (Menest)	0.3-2.5 mg	0.3-0.625 mg/day
Estradiol (Estrace[a])	0.5-2 mg	0.5-1 mg/day
Estropipate (Ogen[a])	0.625-2.5 mg	0.625 mg/day
Transdermal estrogens		
Estradiol patch (Alora, Climara, Vivelle Dot)	0.025-0.1 mg/24 hour	0.025-0.05 mg, changed weekly (Climara) or changed twice weekly
(Minivelle)	0.0375-0.1 mg/24 hour	Twice weekly
(Menostar[b])	14 mcg/24 hour	14 mcg once weekly
Estradiol gel		
(Elestrin, Estrogel Divigel)	0.06% 0.1%	0.87 g/day; 1.25 g/day 0.25, 0.5, 1 mg packets/day
Estradiol spray (Evamist)	1.53 mg/actuation	Once daily
Topical estrogens		
Vaginal creams		
CEE (Premarin)	0.625 mg/g	0.5-2 g/day
Estradiol (Estrace)	0.01% estradiol	1 g one to three times/week
Vaginal rings		
Estradiol (Estring; Femring)	0.0075 mg/24 hour; 0.05-0.1 mg/24 hour	1 ring every 3 months
Vaginal tablet		
Estradiol (Vagifem)	10 mcg estradiol	One tablet twice weekly
Emulsions		
Estradiol (Estrasorb)	0.25%	3.84 g applied daily
Progestogens[c,d]		
MPA (Provera)	2.5-10 mg	
Micronized progesterone (Prometrium) Norethindrone acetate (Aygestin)	100-200 mg 0.25-1 mg	
Combination products		
Oral		
CEE + MPA (Prempro; Premphase)	0.3/1.5 mg-0.625/5 mg;	0.3-0.625/2.5-5 mg/day
Conjugated estrogens + bazedoxifene (Duavee)	0.625/5 mg 0.45 mg/20 mg	One tablet daily
Estradiol + norethindrone (Activella)	0.5/0.1 mg-1/0.5 mg	One tablet daily
Estradiol + drospirenone (Angeliq)	0.5/0.25 mg-1/0.5 mg	One tablet daily
Ethynyl estradiol + norethindrone (FemHRT)	2.5 mcg/0.5 mg	One tablet daily
Estradiol + norgestimate (Prefest)	1/0.09 mg	One tablet daily
Esterified estrogens + Methyltestosterone (Covaryx, Covaryx HS)	1.25/2.5 mg; 0.625/1.25 mg	One tablet daily
Transdermal		
Estradiol + norethindrone (Combipatch)	0.05/0.14-0.05/0.25 mg/24 hour	Apply one patch twice weekly
Estradiol + levonorgestrel (Climara Pro)	0.045/0.015 mg/24 hour	Apply one patch once weekly

CEE, conjugated equine estrogens; MPA, medroxyprogesterone acetate.

[a]FDA-approved commercially available biodentical product.

[b]Indicated for the prevention of postmenopausal osteoporosis only.

[c]May be administered cyclically or continuously.

[d]Dose varies based on daily or weekly administration.

Topical vaginal preparations generally should be prescribed as first-line therapy unless the patient is also experiencing vasomotor symptoms. Local vaginal estrogen has demonstrated increased efficacy over systemic estrogen and generally does not require supplementation with a progestogen in women with an intact uterus using low or ultralow doses.[5] Women using regular or high doses of topical estrogen products may require intermittent treatment with a progestogen. Although few data are available on the appropriate progestogen dose, some data indicate that 10 days every 12 weeks may be sufficient to prevent endometrial hyperplasia.[22] Estradiol in the form of a vaginal tablet or a ring is not significantly absorbed systemically and may be used safely in a woman with contraindications to estrogen therapy and symptoms of vulvovaginal atrophy.[5]

Osteoporosis Prevention Postmenopausal osteoporosis is a condition that affects millions of women. Fractures, particularly hip fractures, are associated with a high incidence of morbidity and mortality and decreased QOL. Before the WHI study, only observational data were available regarding the association of HT and the reduction of fractures. The WHI was the first RCT that

Table 50–2

Adverse Effects of Estrogens and Progestogens[4,10,15,16]

Estrogens
Common adverse effects
Nausea
Headache
Bloating
Breast tenderness
Bleeding
Serious adverse effects
Coronary heart disease
Stroke
Venous thromboembolism
Breast cancer
Gallbladder disease
Progestogens
Common adverse effects
Nausea
Headache
Weight gain
Bleeding
Irritability
Depression
Serious adverse effects
Venous thromboembolism
Decreased bone mineral density

demonstrated a reduction in total fractures, including the hip, spine, and wrist.[2,23]

KEY CONCEPT *Because HT should be maintained only for the short term, traditional therapies such as bisphosphonates should be considered as first-line therapy for the prevention of postmenopausal osteoporosis, in addition to appropriate doses of calcium and vitamin D.* Because of the associated risks, HT should not be prescribed solely for the prevention of osteoporosis.

Risks of HT

Cardiovascular Disease CHD is the leading cause of death among women in the United States. Retrospective data indicated that HT was associated with a decrease in risk of CHD by 30% to 50%.[24] However, the results of RCTs demonstrate that HT does not prevent or treat CHD in women and that it actually may cause an increase in CHD events. The HERS was the first RCT conducted in women with established CHD. This trial demonstrated an increased incidence of CHD events within the first year of treatment with HT and an increased risk of VTE and gallbladder disease. There was a trend of decreasing incidence of CHD death in years 3 to 5 that prompted a discontinuation of the study.[1] A follow-up HERS II trial also showed no difference in CHD events after 2.7 years.[25] The WHI was the first RCT conducted in women without established CHD. Women aged 50 to 79 years with an intact uterus were assigned to receive HT (CEE 0.625 mg + MPA 2.5 mg) daily for 8.5 years. The trial was stopped after only 5.2 years owing to an increased incidence of invasive breast cancer in women taking HT compared with those taking placebo. The WHI demonstrated an increased risk of CHD with HT compared with placebo (approximately six more cases of CHD per 10,000 women years). There also was an increased risk of stroke with HT compared with placebo (approximately seven more cases of stroke per 10,000 women years).[26,27]

The estrogen-alone arm of the WHI, which included women aged 50 to 79 years with a history of hysterectomy, continued for another 1.6 years (average follow-up 6.8 years). This arm of the study did not demonstrate an increased risk of CHD compared with placebo. However, there was an increased risk of stroke with estrogen-alone compared with placebo (approximately 12 more strokes for every 10,000 women treated per year with estrogen therapy).[24] Women who initiated HT 10 or more years after menopause tended to have an increased cardiovascular risk compared with women who initiated therapy within 10 years of menopause.[28,29]

These trials demonstrate that HT should not be prescribed for the prevention of CHD or in patients with preexisting CHD. It is important to note that the average age of women included in the HERS and the WHI trials was 67 and 63 years, respectively, and they started HT a mean of 10 years after menopause. Therefore, these trials were unable to assess the true risk in younger, potentially healthier women with fewer cardiovascular risk factors.[24]

Breast Cancer Breast cancer is the most common cancer in women in the United States. Observational data indicated an association between HT and breast cancer risk. The WHI was the first RCT to demonstrate an increased risk of invasive breast cancer among women taking HT. There were eight more cases of invasive breast cancer for every 10,000 women treated per year with HT.[2,30] The increase in risk did correlate with increased age of the women, and the risk appears to be greater in those who initiate therapy within 5 years of the start of menopause. These results are overall supported by results from a follow-up study of the WHI. During approximately 11 years of follow-up, there was a significant increase in invasive breast cancer cases with combination HT compared with placebo. There were also more deaths from breast cancer and deaths overall with combination therapy than with placebo.[31] It should be noted that any increase in risk for breast cancer appears to dissipate over 2 to 3 years after HT is discontinued.[5,32] Whether HT is associated with an increased risk for breast cancer recurrence is still questionable.

Breast cancer was not increased in the estrogen-alone arm of the WHI.[24] These data point to a possible link of progestogen with breast cancer risk. Whether or not the risk differs between continuous and sequential use of progestogens is questionable. Some evidence suggests that sequential use may be safer than taking progestogen each day.[5,33]

The Million Women Study, a prospective cohort study evaluating over one million women in the United Kingdom, demonstrated an increased risk of breast cancer and breast cancer mortality in women aged 50 to 64. Breast cancer risk increased in current users in both the estrogen and progestogen arm and the estrogen only arm of the study, and the risks increased with longer duration of use.[34]

Women with a personal history of breast cancer and possibly even a strong family history of breast cancer should avoid the use of HT and could consider alternative or nonhormonal therapies for the treatment of vasomotor symptoms.

Venous Thromboembolism The WHI demonstrated an increased risk for VTE with HT compared with placebo (approximately 18 more cases of venous thromboembolic events for every 10,000 women treated per year with HT).[2] The risk for deep vein thrombosis was also increased in the estrogen-alone arm of the WHI, but pulmonary embolism was not increased significantly.[24] The risk of thromboembolism may be dose related, and the oral route of administration is associated with a higher risk compared with the transdermal route.[14]

KEY CONCEPT *In summary, combined estrogen plus progestogen should not be used for the prevention of chronic diseases because it increases the risk of CHD, stroke, breast cancer, and VTE. However, rates of fracture were reduced with combined hormonal treatment.*

► *Other Effects of HT*

QOL and Cognition Although women generally consider QOL measures when deciding whether to use HT, the effects of HT on overall QOL have been inconsistent. HT did not demonstrate a clinically meaningful effect on QOL; however, women taking HT did have a small improvement in sleep disturbances, physical functioning, and bodily pain after 1 year of therapy.[35] Results from the HERS demonstrated that HT did improve emotional measures such as depressive symptoms, but only if women suffered from flushing at trial entry.[36]

Observational studies suggested a potential benefit of HT on cognitive functioning and dementia. However, the Women's Health Initiative Memory Study (WHIMS), conducted in postmenopausal women aged 65 years or older, failed to demonstrate an improvement in cognitive function and demonstrated a dementia rate, including Alzheimer disease, two times greater compared with placebo.[37,38] The estrogen-alone arm of the WHIMS also demonstrated similar results.[39,40]

KEY CONCEPT *HT improves overall well-being and mood in women with vasomotor symptoms, but it has not demonstrated an improvement in QOL in women without vasomotor symptoms.*

► *Discontinuation of HT*

KEY CONCEPT *When treating moderate to severe postmenopausal symptoms, the benefit-to-risk ratio appears to be best when HT is started close to the time of menopause. Therapy should be tapered before discontinuation in order to limit the recurrence of hot flashes.* Although vasomotor symptoms in most women will subside within 4 years, approximately 10% of women continue to experience symptoms that interfere with their QOL. Literature suggests that one of every four women needs to be reinitiated on HT due to persistent and bothersome symptoms.[41]

Limited evidence is available to guide health care providers regarding the least disruptive way to taper HT. Slowly discontinuing HT over 3 to 6 months may be associated with less risk of symptom return. Tapering HT may be done by a dose taper or day taper. The dose taper involves decreasing the dose of estrogen over several weeks to months and monitoring closely for symptom return. If symptoms recur, the next reduction in dose should not occur until symptoms resolve or stabilize on the current dose. The day taper involves decreasing the number of days of the week that a woman takes the HT dose, for example, decreasing a daily dose of 0.3 mg estrogen to 0.3 mg estrogen 5 days a week. Again, if symptoms recur, continue on the current dose until symptoms resolve or stabilize before trying a subsequent decrease. These tapering regimens have not been studied in clinical trials and may not prove to be beneficial in individual women.[41]

Patient Encounter, Part 3: Creating a Care Plan

Based on the information presented, create a care plan for this patient's hot flashes and vaginal dryness. The plan should include:

(a) A statement identifying the problem and its severity

(b) Goals of therapy

(c) A therapeutic plan based on individual patient-specific factors

(d) Subjective and objective monitoring parameters

(e) A follow-up evaluation to assess for adverse effects and adherence and to determine whether the goals of therapy have been achieved

Patient Encounter, Part 4

The patient has been in good health for the past 7 years. She reports adherence with her medications, a healthy diet and exercise routine, and her medical conditions are controlled. However, 1 month ago she was diagnosed with stage 2 breast cancer following a routine mammogram. She is concerned that her hormone therapy may have caused the breast cancer.

Educate the patient regarding the risk of breast cancer and hormone therapy.

► *Nonhormonal and Alternative Treatments*

KEY CONCEPT *Since publication of the WHI study, there has been an increase in the use of alternative and nonhormonal therapies for the management of menopausal symptoms, particularly for women with CHD and/or breast cancer risk factors. A wide range of therapies, both prescription and herbal, have been studied with limited success.*

A variety of nonhormonal and alternative therapies (Table 50–3) have been studied for symptomatic management of vasomotor symptoms.[42,43] The limited and often conflicting evidence demonstrates that these agents are only modestly effective and also have associated adverse effects. It should be noted that randomized, placebo-controlled trials of these alternative therapies have not established safety and efficacy for prevention or treatment of menopausal symptoms.

SSRIs and venlafaxine are theorized to reduce the frequency of hot flashes by increasing serotonin in the central nervous system and by decreasing LH. Of the SSRIs, paroxetine has the most published data demonstrating a reduction in hot flashes while treating other symptomatic complaints such as depression and anxiety.[45] Other SSRIs such as fluoxetine, citalopram, and sertraline may also be effective. These antidepressant medications offer a reasonable option for women who are unwilling to or cannot take hormonal therapies, particularly those who suffer from depression or anxiety.

Phytoestrogens are plant sterols that are structurally similar to human and animal estrogen. Soy protein is a common source of phytoestrogens.[42,43] There are differences among classes of phytoestrogens and biologic potencies vary, making it difficult to recommend specific dosing. The most commonly studied phytoestrogen is the isoflavone class. Because the effect of phytoestrogens on breast cancer and other female-related cancers is unknown, these products should not be considered in women with a history of estrogen-dependent cancers. After reviewing hundreds of studies, the North American Menopause Society (NAMS) determined that soy-based isoflavones are modestly effective in relieving menopausal symptoms.[46] The efficacy of

Table 50–3

Nonhormonal Therapies for Menopause[42–48]

Drug	Brand Name	Initial Dose	Usual Dose Range	Comments
Venlafaxine[a,b]	Effexor, Effexor XR	37.5 mg	37.5–150 mg/day	Potential adverse effects include nausea, HA, somnolence, dizziness, insomnia, hypertension, xerostomia constipation, diaphoresis, weakness
Paroxetine, Paroxetine CR	Brisdelle, Paxil, Paxil CR, Pexeva	7.5–10 mg (12.5 mg CR)	7.5–20 mg/day	Potential adverse effects include nausea, somnolence, insomnia, HA, dizziness, xerostomia, constipation, diarrhea, weakness, diaphoresis
Clonidine	Catapres, Catapres IIS, Kapvay	0.1 mg/day	0.1–0.4 mg/day	Potential adverse effects include drowsiness, dizziness, hypotension, dry mouth
Gabapentin[a]	Gralise, Neurontin	300 mg at bedtime	900 mg/day, divided in three daily doses (up to 2400 mg/day)	Potential adverse effects include somnolence and dizziness (can decrease with gradual increase in dosing)
Phytoestrogens (isoflavones)		Products and dosages vary	60–90 mg isoflavone	Best data of complementary treatments. Limited adverse effects
Black cohosh				Long-term effects are unknown (concern of liver toxicity in long term). Should not be generally recommended for vasomotor symptoms
Dong quai, red clover leaf, kava				Have not been shown to be effective and should generally not be recommended for vasomotor symptoms

[a]Dosage adjustments recommended in patients with renal impairment.

[b]Dosage adjustment recommended in patients with hepatic impairment.

isoflavones on bone, cognitive improvement, and cardiovascular health has not been proven.

Black cohosh has been one of the most studied alternative therapies for vasomotor symptoms, but it has not demonstrated a substantial benefit over placebo. The mechanism of action, safety profile, drug–drug interactions, and adverse effects of black cohosh remain unknown. However, there have been case reports of hepatotoxicity with its use.[43,47] In non–placebo-controlled trials conducted for 6 months or less, black cohosh demonstrated small reductions in vasomotor symptoms.[42,43,45] Caution should be exercised when considering the use of this product, and it is not recommended for more than a 6-month period of time. Other alternative treatments that have been utilized include dong quai, red clover leaf, and kava. These have not been shown to be effective in the treatment of menopausal symptoms and may have significant adverse effects.[48]

Gabapentin and clonidine have also been studied for the management of menopausal symptoms. In RCTs, gabapentin at doses of 900 mg/day demonstrated significant reductions in severity and frequency of hot flashes compared with placebo. Clonidine has been studied in several small RCTs at doses of 0.1 to 0.4 mg/day and has demonstrated statistically significant reductions in hot flashes.[45] Overall, alternative and nonhormonal therapies are less effective in treating vasomotor symptoms than HT but do offer another option for women experiencing menopausal symptoms who cannot or are unwilling to take HT. SSRIs and phytoestrogens have the best evidence for efficacy. However, women should weigh the benefits and risks of all therapies, and discuss these options with their health care providers.

OUTCOME EVALUATION

Evaluating the outcomes of any therapy for menopausal symptoms focuses primarily on the woman's report of symptom resolution. Ask women to report the resolution or reduction of hot flashes, night sweats, and vaginal dryness and any improvement or change in sleep patterns. Also ask women taking hormonal therapies to report any breakthrough bleeding or spotting. If abnormal or heavy bleeding occurs, refer the woman to her primary care provider. Monitor subjective parameters such as adverse effects and adherence to the therapy regimen. In addition, monitor objective parameters, including blood pressure, at every outpatient visit; encourage yearly clinical breast examinations, mammograms, lipid panel, and thyroid-stimulating hormone (TSH) determination, particularly for women with hypothyroidism on thyroid therapy, and conduct a BMD test every 2 to 5 years as indicated. Also perform endometrial studies, as necessary, in women with undiagnosed vaginal bleeding. Lastly, evaluate the patient's overall QOL. Because the management of menopause is largely symptomatic, it is important to document symptoms at the beginning of therapy and monitor symptom improvement and potential adverse effects at each visit. Frequent follow-up, proper monitoring, and education will help to ensure that the woman achieves optimal results from any therapy chosen to treat menopausal symptoms.

Patient Encounter, Part 5

It has been 6 months since this patient completed chemotherapy and radiation for breast cancer. She presents to her PCP for follow up with a chief complaint of recurrent hot flashes. She also complains of recurrent vaginal dryness but denies insomnia.

Recommend the most appropriate therapy for her recurrent hot flashes and vaginal dryness.

Patient Care Process

Patient Assessment:

- Obtain a thorough medication history, including the use of over-the-counter and herbal products.
- Rule out other medical conditions that could be contributing to symptoms and manage those conditions prior to initiating therapy for symptoms.
- Evaluate for the presence of vasomotor symptoms and document findings.

Therapy Evaluation:

- If the patient is experiencing bothersome vasomotor symptoms, consider the use of HT only after assessing for risk factors for heart disease and breast cancer.
- If vasomotor symptoms are tolerable and/or the patient has risk factors for heart disease and/or breast cancer, consider alternative, nonhormonal treatments for vasomotor symptoms.

Care Plan Development:

- Discuss lifestyle or behavioral interventions that may help to alleviate vasomotor symptoms.
- Discuss methods of HT administration, and decide in conjunction with the health care provider which one will work best for her.
- Recommend the appropriate dose of HT, and use the lowest effective dose for the shortest duration of time.
- Discuss proper administration, potential adverse effects, and expectations of HT.
- Discuss the importance of adhering to the medication regimen.

Follow-Up Evaluation:

- Monitor for a reduction in vasomotor symptoms, vaginal dryness, and improvement in sleep. Also monitor for breakthrough bleeding and spotting, adverse effects of HT, and improvement in QOL.
- Monitor the following objective parameters: blood pressure at every outpatient visit, yearly lipoprotein panels, yearly breast examinations and mammograms, yearly TSH determinations, and endometrial studies in women with undiagnosed vaginal bleeding.
- Assess symptoms every 6 to 12 months, and consider tapering the HT dose and discontinuing treatment after 5 years. If vasomotor symptoms return, determine whether a longer tapering schedule is warranted or if long-term treatment is necessary. If treatment beyond 5 years is necessary, consider switching to a nonhormonal product.

Abbreviations Introduced in This Chapter

BMD	Bone mineral density
CEE	Conjugated equine estrogen
CHD	Coronary heart disease
FDA	US Food and Drug Administration
FSH	Follicle-stimulating hormone
GnRH	Gonadotropin-releasing hormone
HDL	High-density lipoprotein
HERS	Heart and Estrogen/Progestin Replacement Study
HOPE	Women's Health, Osteoporosis, Progestin/Estrogen trial
HT	Hormone therapy
LDL	Low-density lipoprotein
LH	Luteinizing hormone
MPA	Medroxyprogesterone acetate
NAMS	North American Menopause Society
NNTH	Number needed to treat to harm
QOL	Quality of life
PCP	Primary care provider
RCT	Randomized controlled trial
SSRI	Selective serotonin reuptake inhibitor
TG	Triglycerides
TSH	Thyroid-stimulating hormone
VTE	Venous thromboembolism
WHI	Women's Health Initiative
WHIMS	Women's Health Initiative Memory Study

REFERENCES

1. Hulley S, Grady D, Bush T, et al. Randomized trial of estrogen plus progestin for secondary prevention of coronary heart disease in postmenopausal women. Heart and Estrogen/progestin Replacement Study (HERS) Research Group. JAMA. 1998;280(7):605–613.
2. Rossouw JE, Anderson GL, Prentice RL, et al. Risks and benefits of estrogen plus progestin in healthy postmenopausal women: Principal results from the Women's Health Initiative randomized controlled trial. JAMA. 2002;288(3):321–333.
3. Nelson HD. Menopause. Lancet. 2008;371:760–770.
4. Burger HG. The endocrinology of the menopause. J Steroid Biochem Mol Biol. 1999;69(1–6):31–35.
5. The 2012 hormone therapy position statement of the North American Menopause Society. Menopause. 2012;19:257–271.
6. The North American Menopause Society. Management of postmenopausal osteoporosis: 2010 position statement of The North American Menopause Society. Menopause. 2010;17:25–54.
7. The North American Menopause Society. Treatment of menopause associated vasomotor symptoms: Position statement of The North American Menopause Society. Menopause. 2004; 11(1):11–33.
8. Santen RJ, Allred DC, Ardoin SP, et al. Postmenopausal hormone therapy: An endocrine society scientific statement. J Clin Endocrinol Metab. 2010;95(Suppl 1):S1–S66.
9. The Writing Group on behalf of the Workshop Consensus Group. Aging, menopause, cardiovascular disease and HRT. Climacteric. 2009;12:368–377.
10. Kalantaridou SN, Dang DK, Calis KA. Hormone therapy in women. In: Dipiro, JT, Talbert RL, Yee, GC et al, eds. Pharmacotherapy: A Pathophysiologic Approach, 9th ed. New York: McGraw-Hill, 2014:1315–1336.
11. Rymer J, Wilson R, Ballard K. Making decisions about hormone replacement therapy. BMJ. 2003;326(7384):322–326.
12. McKee J, Warber SL. Integrative therapies for menopause. South Med J. 2005;98(3):319–326.
13. Sikon A, Thacker HL. Treatment options for menopausal hot flashes. Cleve Clin J Med. 2004;71(7):578–582.

14. Canonico M, Oger E, Plu-Bureau G, et al. Hormone therapy and venous thromboembolism among postmenopausal women: impact of the route of estrogen administration and progestogens: The ESTHER Study. Circulation. 2007;115:840–845.
15. Estrogens. In: Lexi-Drugs [Internet]. Hudson, OH: Lexicomp, Inc. Updated 2014, July 22.
16. Medroxyprogestrone acetate. In: Drugdex [Internet]. Greenwood Village, CO: Truven Health Analytics, Inc. Updated 2014, Aug 25.
17. Archer DF, Dorin M, Lewis V, et al. Effects of lower doses of conjugated equine estrogens and medroxyprogesterone acetate on endometrial bleeding. Fertil Steril. 2001;75(6):1080–1087.
18. Lindsay R, Gallagher JC, Kleerekoper M, et al. Effect of lower doses of conjugated equine estrogens with and without medroxyprogesterone acetate on bone in early postmenopausal women. JAMA. 2002;287:2668–2676.
19. Pickar JH, Yeh I, Wheeler JE, et al. Endometrial effects of lower doses of conjugated equine estrogens and medroxyprogesterone acetate. Fertil Steril. 2001;76(1):25–31.
20. Utian WH, Shoupe D, Bachmann G, et al. Relief of vasomotor symptoms and vaginal atrophy with lower doses of conjugated equine estrogens and medroxyprogesterone acetate. Fertil Steril. 2001;75(6): 1065–1079.
21. Bioidential hormones. The Endocrine Society position statement. 2006. http://www.menopause.org/bioidenticalHT_Endosoc.pdf. Accessed January 12, 2012.
22. Davis S. Hormone replacement therapy. Indications, benefits and risk. Aust Fam Physician. 1999;28(5):437–445.
23. Cauley JA, Robbins J, Chen Z, et al. Effects of estrogen plus progestin on risk of fracture and bone mineral density: The Women's Health Initiative randomized trial. JAMA. 2003; 290(13):1729–1738.
24. Anderson GL, Limacher M, Assaf AR, et al. Effects of conjugated equine estrogen in postmenopausal women with hysterectomy: The Women's Health Initiative randomized controlled trial. JAMA. 2004;291(14):1701–1712.
25. Grady D, Herrington D, Bittner V, et al. Cardiovascular disease outcomes during 6.8 years of hormone therapy: Heart and Estrogen/Progestin Replacement Study followup (HERS II). JAMA. 2002;288(1): 49–57.
26. Manson JE, Hsia J, Johnson K, et al. Estrogen plus progestin and the risk of coronary heart disease. N Engl J Med. 2003; 349: 523–534.
27. Wassertheil-Smoller S, Hendrix SL, Limacher M, et al. Effect of estrogen plus progestin on stroke in postmenopausal women: The women's health initiative: A randomized trial. JAMA. 2003; 289:2673–2684.
28. Rossouw JE, Prentice RL, Manson JE, et al. Postmenopausal hormone therapy and risk of cardiovascular disease by age and years since menopause. JAMA. 2007;297:1465–1477.
29. Toh S, Hernández-Díaz S, Logan R, et al. Coronary heart disease in postmenopausal recipients of estrogen plus progestin therapy: Does the increased risk ever disappear? A randomized trial. Ann Intern Med. 2010;152:211–217.
30. Chlebowski RT, Hendrix SL, Langer RD, et al. Influence of estrogen plus progestin on breast cancer and mammography in healthy postmenopausal women: The women's health initiative randomized trial. JAMA. 2003;289:3243–3253.
31. Chlebowski RT, Anderson GL, Gass M, et al. Estrogen plus progestin and breast cancer incidence and mortality in postmenopausal women. JAMA. 2010;304:1684–1692.
32. Calle EE, Feigelson HS, Hildebrand JS, et al. Postmenopausal hormone use and breast cancer associations differ by hormone regimen and histologic subtype. Cancer. 2009;115:936–945.
33. Saxena T, Lee E, Henderson KD, et al. Menopausal hormone therapy and subsequent risk of specific invasive breast cancer subtypes in the California Teachers Study. Cancer Epidemiol Biomarkers Prev. 2010;19:2366–2378.
34. Million Women Study Collaborators. Breast cancer and hormone-replacement therapy in the Million Women Study. Lancet. 2003;362:419–427.
35. Hays J, Ockene JK, Brunner RL, et al. Effects of estrogen plus progestin on health-related quality of life. N Engl J Med. 2003;348(19):1839–1854.
36. Hlatky MA, Boothroyd D, Vittinghoff E, et al. Quality-of-life and depressive symptoms in postmenopausal women after receiving hormone therapy: Results from the Heart and Estrogen/Progestin Replacement Study (HERS) trial. JAMA. 2002;287(5):591–597.
37. Rapp SR, Espeland MA, Shumaker SA, et al. Effect of estrogen plus progestin on global cognitive function in postmenopausal women: The Women's Health Initiative Memory Study: A randomized controlled trial. JAMA. 2003;289(20):2663–2672.
38. Shumaker SA, Legault C, Rapp SR, et al. Estrogen plus progestin and the incidence of dementia and mild cognitive impairment in postmenopausal women: The Women's Health Initiative Memory Study: A randomized controlled trial. JAMA. 2003;289(20):2651–2662.
39. Espeland MA, Rapp SR, Shumaker SA, et al. Conjugated equine estrogens and global cognitive function in postmenopausal women: Women's Health Initiative Memory Study. JAMA. 2004; 291(24):2959–2968.
40. Shumaker SA, Legault C, Kuller L, et al. Conjugated equine estrogens and incidence of probable dementia and mild cognitive impairment in postmenopausal women: Women's Health Initiative Memory Study. JAMA. 2004;291(24):2947–2958.
41. Grady D. A 60 year old woman trying to discontinue hormone replacement therapy. JAMA. 2002;287(16):2130–2137.
42. Nelson HD, Vesco KK, Haney E, et al. Nonhormonal therapies for menopausal hot flashes: Systematic review and meta-analysis. JAMA. 2006;295:2057–2071.
43. Newton KM, Reed SD, LaCroix AZ, et al. Treatment of vasomotor symptoms of menopause with black cohosh, multibotanicals, soy, hormone therapy or placebo: A randomized trial. Ann Intern Med. 2006;145(12):869–879.
44. PL Detail-Document, Postmenopausal Hormone Therapy. Pharmacist's Letter/Prescriber's Letter. March 2014. Accessed August 14, 2014.
45. Cheema D, Coomarasamy A, El-Toukhy T. Non-hormonal therapy of postmenopausal vasomotor symptoms: A structured evidence-based review. Arch Gynecol Obstet. 2007;276(5): 463–469.
46. NAMS 2011 Isoflavones Report. The role of soy isoflavones in menopausal health: Report of the North American Menopause Society. Menopause. 2011;18:732–753.
47. Lontos S, Jones RM, Angus PW, et al. Acute liver failure associated with the use of herbal preparations containing black cohosh. Med J Aust. 2003;179(7):390–391.
48. Nedrow A, Miller J, Walker M, et al. Complementary and alternative therapies for the management of menopause-related symptoms: a systematic evidence review. Arch Intern Med. 2006; 166;1453–1465.

51 Erectile Dysfunction

Cara Liday

LEARNING OBJECTIVES

Upon completion of the chapter, the reader will be able to:

1. Explain the pathophysiology of **erectile dysfunction** (ED).
2. Recognize risk factors and medications associated with the development of ED.
3. Identify the goals of therapy when treating ED.
4. Describe current nonpharmacologic and pharmacologic options for treating ED, and determine an appropriate first- and second-line therapy for a specific patient.
5. Identify patients with significant cardiovascular risk and recommend an appropriate treatment approach for their ED.
6. Compare and contrast the benefits and risks for the current phosphodiesterase (PDE) inhibitors.
7. Assess reasons for PDE failure and determine an optimal approach to improve treatment efficacy.

INTRODUCTION

Erectile dysfunction (ED) is defined as the persistent inability to achieve or maintain an erection sufficient for sexual intercourse. ED is the most prominent sexual problem in men, and it can lead to lower quality of life and self-esteem.[1] Patients may also develop **libido** or ejaculatory disorders, but these are not considered ED.

EPIDEMIOLOGY AND ETIOLOGY

ED increases with age. Few men report erection problems before age 50, but ED increases to 20% to 40% in men aged 60 to 69 years and 50% to 100% in men older than 70 years.[2] The increase in incidence could be due to physiologic changes that occur with aging, the onset of chronic disease states associated with ED, increased medication use, lifestyle factors, or a combination of the above.

PATHOPHYSIOLOGY

The penis consists of three components, two dorsolateral corpora cavernosa and a ventral corpus spongiosum that surrounds the penile urethra and distally forms the glans penis.

Sympathetic and parasympathetic nerves innervate the penis. In the flaccid state, arterial and corporal smooth muscles are tonically contracted, and a balance exists between blood flow into and out of the corpora. With sexual stimulation, nerve impulses from the brain travel down the spinal cord triggering a reduction in sympathetic tone and an increase in parasympathetic activity. This leads to an increased production of nitric oxide (NO). NO enhances the activity of guanylate cyclase, which results in increased production of cyclic guanosine monophosphate (cGMP). Vasoactive peptide and prostaglandins E_1 and E_2 stimulate increased production of cyclic adenosine monophosphate (cAMP). Both cAMP and cGMP reduce calcium concentrations within smooth muscle cells of the penile arteries and the sinusoidal spaces, leading to smooth muscle relaxation and increased blood flow. As the spaces become engorged, intracavernosal pressure increases, subtunical venules are compressed by the tunica albuginea, and the penis becomes rigid and elongated (**Figure 51–1**).

Detumescence occurs with sympathetic discharge after ejaculation. Sympathetic activity induces smooth muscle contraction of arterioles and vascular spaces leading to a reduction in blood inflow, decompression of the sinusoidal spaces, and enhanced outflow.

Testosterone also plays a significant albeit complex role in erectile function. In addition to stabilization of intracavernosal levels of NO synthase, the enzyme responsible for triggering the NO cascade, testosterone is responsible for much of a man's libido. Interestingly, some patients with low or borderline-low serum concentrations will have normal erectile function, whereas those with adequate levels may have dysfunction.

Normal penile erections are complex events that require the full function of the vascular, neurologic, hormonal and psychogenic systems. Anything that affects the function of these systems may lead to ED. KEY CONCEPT *ED can be classified as organic, psychogenic, or a mixture of these.* Organic dysfunction includes abnormalities in the vascular, hormonal, or neurologic systems or may be medication-induced (**Tables 51–1** and **51–2**). It is estimated that 25% of ED cases are due to medications.[5] Note that many of the risk factors for ED are the same as those for cardiovascular (CV) disease, including hypertension, diabetes, dyslipidemia, smoking, obesity, metabolic syndrome, and sedentary behavior.[4] In many patients, ED is the first indication of the endothelial dysfunction associated with CV disease, with two-thirds of patients with coronary artery disease having symptoms of ED before the onset of coronary symptoms.[5] The presence of ED risk factors

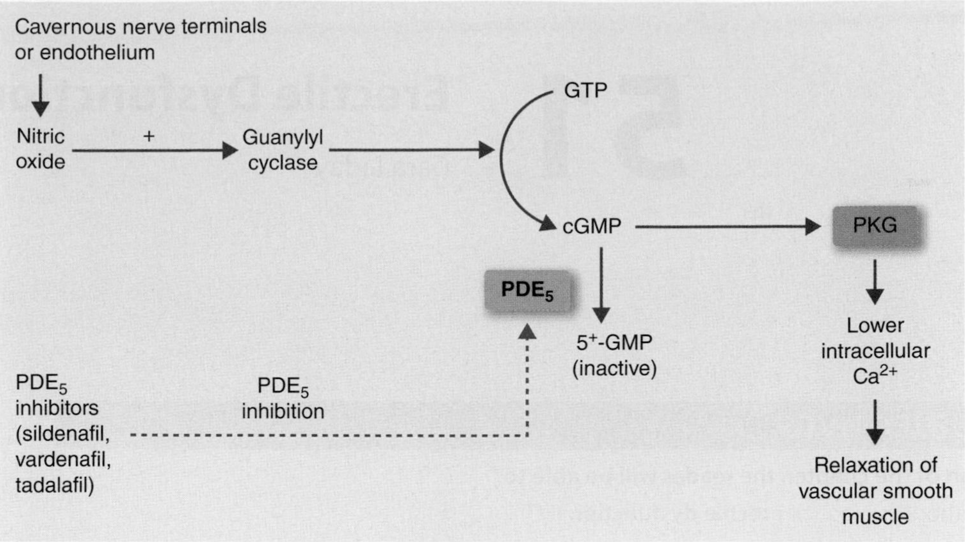

FIGURE 51–1. Mechanism of erection and sites of action of various treatment modalities for erectile dysfunction (ED). Penile erection is achieved through relaxation of smooth muscle cells lining arterial vessels and sinusoidal spaces in the corpora cavernosa, which leads to increased arterial inflow and pressure, decreased venous outflow, and increased intracavernosal pressure. Smooth muscle relaxation is mediated by intracellular generation of cyclic guanosine monophosphate (cGMP) from guanosine triphosphate (GTP) via activation of guanylate cyclase by nitric oxide. Treatment modalities for ED include oral phosphodiesterase type 5 (PDE-5) inhibitors, which inhibit the breakdown of cGMP, and local vasoactive agents. Nitric oxide–cGMP signaling in cavernous smooth muscle. (cGMP, cycle guanosine monophosphate; GTP, guanosine triphosphate; PDE_5, phosphodiesterase 5; PKG, protein kinase G.) (Reproduced, with permission, from Setter SM, Iltz JL, Fincham JE, Campbell RK, Baker DE. Phosphodiesterase 5 inhibitors for erectile dysfunction. Ann Pharmacother. 2005;39(7-8):1286–1295.)

leads to the assumption that the patient has organic dysfunction. Most commonly, medical conditions that impair arterial flow into or out of the erectile tissue or affect the innervation will be strongly associated with ED. Patients with diabetes mellitus have exceptionally high rates of ED as a result of vascular disease and neuropathy. Additionally, a relationship has been found between

Table 51–1

Factors Associated with ED[1,4,11]

Chronic Medical Conditions
Hypertension
Diabetes mellitus
BPH
Coronary and peripheral vascular disease
Neurologic disorders (eg, Parkinson disease and multiple sclerosis)
Endocrine disorders (hypogonadism, pituitary, adrenal, and thyroid disorders)
Psychiatric disorders
Dyslipidemia
Renal failure
Liver disease
Penile disease (Peyronie disease or anatomic abnormalities)
Surgical Procedures
Perineal or vascular surgeries
Radical prostatectomy
Lifestyle
Smoking
Excessive alcohol consumption
Obesity
Poor overall health and reduced physical activity
Trauma
Pelvic fractures or surgeries
Spinal cord or brain injuries

Table 51–2

Medication Classes Associated with ED[3,4,5]

Antihypertensives
β-Blockers (excluding nebivolol)
Thiazide diuretics
Centrally acting agents (clonidine, methyldopa, and reserpine)
Spironolactone
α-Blockers
CNS Depressants
Opioid analgesics
Benzodiazepines
Hypnotics
Lipid Medications
Gemfibrozil
HMG-CoA reductase inhibitors
Antidepressants/Antipsychotics
Tricyclic antidepressants
Monoamine oxidase inhibitors
Selective serotonin reuptake inhibitors/serotonin-norepinephrine reuptake inhibitors
Anticonvulsants
Carbamazepine
Phenytoin
Gastrointestinal Agents
Histamine 2-receptor antagonists
Proton pump inhibitors
Antiandrogens and Hormones
5α-Reductase inhibitors
Progesterone and estrogen
Corticosteroids
Recreational Drugs
Ethanol
Cocaine
Marijuana
Opiates

Clinical Presentation and Diagnosis

Possible Signs and Symptoms

- Embarrassment
- Anxiousness
- Anger
- Marital difficulties
- Low self-confidence or morale; depression
- Full inability to achieve erections
- Ability to achieve partial erections, but not suitable for intercourse
- Erections sufficient for intercourse, but early detumescence
- The problem may have a slow or acute onset, or may wax and wane

Diagnosis

ED may be the presenting symptom of other chronic disease states.

The following should be performed to determine areas that can cause or exacerbate ED and to assess the patient's ability to safely perform intercourse.

- Medical history with emphasis on cardiovascular and psychiatric disorders, diabetes, trauma, and surgical procedures
- Social history including nutrition and history of smoking, recreational drug use, exercise, and alcohol consumption
- Medication history including prescription, nonprescription, and dietary supplements

Physical Examination

- Review for hypogonadism (gynecomastia, testicular atrophy, reduced body hair, increase in body fat)
- Digital rectal examination to determine whether prostate is enlarged
- Vital signs
- Abnormalities of the penis or impaired vasculature and nerve function to the penis

Labs

- Fasting glucose or HbA_{1c}
- Serum testosterone if signs of hypogonadism
- Fasting lipid panel
- Further cardiac testing if warranted

Determine Severity

- Use an abridged, five-item version of the International Index of Erectile Dysfunction (IIEF-5) as a diagnostic tool.[20]
- How do you rate your confidence that you could get and keep an erection?
- When you had erections with sexual stimulation, how often were your erections hard enough for penetration?
- During sexual intercourse, how often were you able to maintain your erection after you had penetrated (entered) your partner?
- During sexual intercourse, how difficult was it to maintain your erection to completion of intercourse?
- When you attempted sexual intercourse, how often was it satisfactory for you?
- Questions scored 1 to 5, very low to very high, respectively. Score of 21 or less indicates ED likely.

low testosterone levels and an increased incidence of metabolic syndrome and type 2 diabetes.[6]

Psychogenic dysfunction occurs if a patient does not respond to psychological arousal. Common causes include performance anxiety, strained relationships, lack of sexual arousability, and overt psychiatric disorders such as depression and schizophrenia.[7] KEY CONCEPT *Many patients may initially have organic dysfunction, but develop a psychogenic component as they try to cope with their inability to achieve an erection.*[1]

CLINICAL PRESENTATION AND DIAGNOSIS OF ED

The introduction of oral medications and direct-to-consumer advertising has made patients feel more comfortable approaching practitioners for treatment advice. Despite this, some patients may only discuss their dysfunction when questioned directly by their provider or if their partner initiates the interaction.

TREATMENT

Desired Outcomes

ED is not a life-threatening condition, but if left untreated, it can be associated with depression, loss of self-esteem, poor self-image, and marital discord.[8] The primary goal of therapy is achievement of erections suitable for intercourse and improvement in patient and partner quality of life. Additionally, the ideal therapy should have minimal side effects, be convenient to administer, have a quick onset of action, and have few or no drug interactions.[9]

General Approach to Treatment

KEY CONCEPT *Before initiating treatment for ED, a physical examination and thorough medical, social, and medication histories with emphasis on cardiac disease must be taken to assess for ability to safely perform sexual activity and to assess for possible drug interactions.* In patients with intermediate or high cardiovascular risk, additional testing should occur to determine whether sexual activity is safe.

KEY CONCEPT *Treatment options for ED include medical devices, pharmacologic treatments, lifestyle modifications, surgery, and psychotherapy. Reversible causes of ED should be identified first and treated appropriately.*

KEY CONCEPT *When determining the best treatment for an individual, the role of the clinician is to inform the patient and his partner of all available options while understanding his medical history, desires, and goals.* KEY CONCEPT *The choice of treatment is primarily left up to the couple, but most often treatment is initiated with the least invasive options such as oral phosphodiesterase (PDE) inhibitors and vacuum erection devices (VEDs).* Ultimately, the choice of therapy should be individualized, taking into account patient and partner preferences, concomitant disease states, response, administration route, cost, tolerability, and safety. Common drug treatment regimens for ED are listed in Table 51–3.

▸ Nonpharmacologic Therapy

Lifestyle Modifications Lifestyle modifications should always be addressed in the management of ED. A healthy diet, increase in regular physical activity, and weight loss are associated with higher International Index of Erectile Function (IIEF) scores and an improvement in erectile function.[10] The clinician should also recommend smoking cessation, reduction in excessive alcohol intake, and discontinuation of illicit drug use.

Psychotherapy Psychotherapy is an appropriate treatment approach for patients with psychogenic or mixed dysfunction. Counseling may include simple sex education and improved partner communication in addition to cognitive and behavioral therapy.[1] Psychotherapy may help relieve anxiety and eliminate unrealistic expectations.[11] Effectiveness is not well documented for organic dysfunction unless combined with pharmacotherapy.

Patient Encounter 1, Part 1

A 68-year-old man with type 2 diabetes, hypertension, chronic kidney disease, and dyslipidemia returns to your clinic for follow-up on his chronic disease states. When reviewing his history, he describes problems with his erections as well as an increase in nocturnal urination and dribbling when voiding. After further questioning, you determine that his erectile dysfunction has progressively gotten worse over the last year. He is quite emotional and states that the problem is distressing and has caused significant marital discord. He wonders about "those ads on television" suggesting a pill.

Based on the available information, how would you classify his erectile dysfunction (ED)?

What additional information do you need before establishing an appropriate treatment regimen and determining his ability to safely perform intercourse?

Table 51–3

Common Drug Treatment Regimens for ED

Route of Administration	Generic Name	Brand Name	Typical Dosing Range[a]	Maximum Dosing Frequency
Oral	Sildenafil	Viagra	25–100 mg 1 hour prior to intercourse	Once daily
	Tadalafil	Cialis	5–20 mg 30 minutes prior to intercourse or daily dose of 2.5–5 mg	Once daily
	Vardenafil	Levitra, Staxyn	5–20 mg 1 hour prior to intercourse	Once daily
	Avanafil	Stendra	100–200 mg 30 minutes prior to intercourse	Once daily
Intracavernosal	Alprostadil	Caverject, Caverject Impulse, Edex	1.25–60 mcg 5–20 minutes prior to intercourse[b]	3 times weekly, 24 hours between injections
Intraurethral	Alprostadil	MUSE	125–1000 mcg 5–10 minutes prior to intercourse[b]	2 times daily
Testosterone Supplementation				
Intramuscular	Testosterone cypionate	Depo-Testosterone	50–400 mg every 2–4 weeks	Once weekly
	Testosterone enanthate	Delatestryl	50–400 mg every 2–4 weeks	Once weekly
Topical	Testosterone patch	Androderm	2–4 mg/day applied to back, abdomen, upper arms, or thighs	Once daily
	Testosterone gel	AndroGel 1%, Testim, Vogelxo	5–10 g gel per day (50–100 mg testosterone) to shoulders, upper arms, abdomen (AndroGel 1% only)	Once daily
		AndroGel 1.62%	40.5–81 mg/day to shoulders or upper arms	Once daily
		Natesto	11 mg every 8 hours (2 pump actuations, 1 per nostril)	3 times daily
		Fortesta	10–70 mg/day to thigh	Once daily
	Testosterone solution	Axiron	30–120 mg/day to axilla	Once daily
Buccal	Testosterone	Striant	30 mg every 12 hours to gum region above incisor; rotate to alternate sides with each dose	2 times daily
Subcutaneous implantable pellet	Testosterone	Testopel	150–450 mg (150 mg for every 25 mg testosterone propionate required weekly)	Every 3–6 months

MUSE, medicated urethral system for erection.

[a]Use the lowest effective dose to limit adverse effects.

[b]Initial dose must be titrated in physician's office.

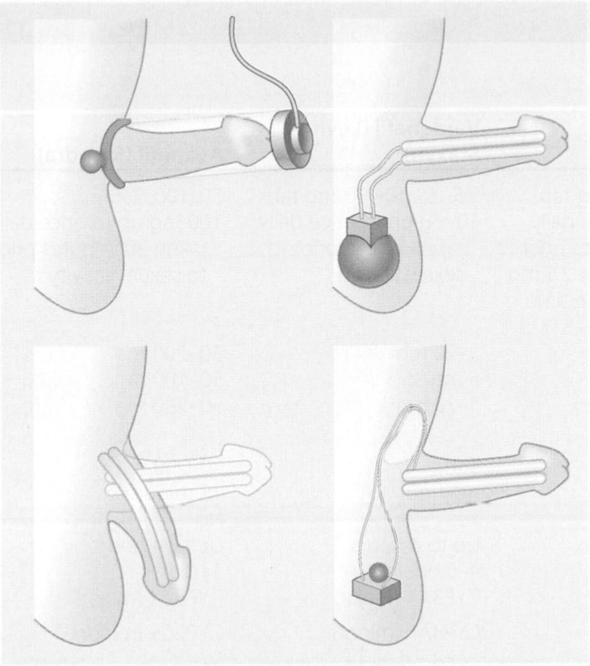

FIGURE 51–2. Available devices and prostheses used to treat ED. (From Wagner G, Saenz de Tejada I. Update on male erectile dysfunction. BMJ 1998;316:678–682.)

Vacuum Erection Devices Vacuum erection devices (VEDs) induce erections by creating a vacuum around the penis; the negative pressure draws blood into the penis by passively dilating arteries and engorging the corpora. The erection is maintained with a constriction band placed at the base of the penis to reduce venous outflow (Figure 51–2). VEDs may be used as often as desired, but it is recommended that the constriction band not be left in place longer than 30 minutes at a time.

Onset of action is slow, which limits spontaneity. In addition, patients and partners may complain of a cold, lifeless, discolored penis that has a hinge-like feel. Painful ejaculation or inability to ejaculate are additional adverse effects. VEDs are relatively contraindicated in persons with sickle cell disease and should be used with caution in those on oral anticoagulants or who have bleeding disorders due to the increased possibility of priapism.

VEDs are highly effective treatment modalities for ED and are considered a first- or second-line therapy. Efficacy rates are as high as 90% in obtaining an erection sufficient for coitus. Although satisfaction rates are as high as 94%, the discontinuation rate after 2 years is close to 50%.[12,13] A double pumping technique in which the vacuum is applied for a 1 to 2 minutes, removed, then reapplied for another 3 to 4 minutes may improve comfort levels and rigidity. Higher efficacy rates can also be achieved by combining VEDs with other therapies. VEDs are generally more acceptable to older patients in stable relationships and with infrequent sexual encounters.[13]

Prostheses Penile prostheses are semirigid malleable or inflatable rods, which are inserted surgically into the corpus cavernosa (see Figure 51–2). The malleable rods are rigid at all times, but may be bent into position by the patient when desired. The inflatable prostheses remain flaccid until the pump within the scrotum moves fluid from a reservoir to the cylinders within the penis. Detumescence is achieved when the fluid is then transferred back to the reservoir by activating a release button.

Patient satisfaction rates can be as high as 100%, with partner satisfaction rates slightly lower, but prostheses are the most invasive treatment available so are considered last-line therapy.[12] Infection occurs in 1% to 3% of first-time prostheses.[12] Semirigid malleable rods may interfere with urination, are difficult to conceal, and have a higher likelihood of erosion.[14]

▸ *Pharmacologic Therapy*

Phosphodiesterase Type 5 Inhibitors Avanafil, sildenafil, tadalafil, and vardenafil act by selectively inhibiting phosphodiesterase (PDE) type 5, which is responsible for degradation of cGMP. With prolonged cGMP activity, smooth muscle relaxation is induced, leading to an erection (see Figure 51–1). However, the PDE inhibitors are only effective in the presence of sexual stimulation to drive the NO/cGMP system, making them facilitators of an erection, not initiators.

KEY CONCEPT *Effectiveness of the four available PDE inhibitors is essentially comparable, but differences exist in onset, duration of action, absorption with a fatty meal and, to a small degree, incidence of side effects and drug interactions* (Table 51–4). Review of available data for each individual agent shows a 60% to 75% response rate depending on the dose of agent used and the etiology of dysfunction.[1,4,11] Response rates tend to be lower in patients with radical prostatectomy as well as those with diabetes, severe nerve damage, or severe vascular disease.[15] Although efficacy rates appear to be similar between agents, there are some data to suggest that continuation rates are higher and patient preference greater with tadalafil.[16] The PDE inhibitors are considered first-line therapies due to high efficacy rates, convenience of dosing, and minimal severe adverse effects.

The most dramatic difference among the four agents is tadalafil's extended duration of action (18 hours), earning it the nickname "the weekender drug." All are approved for as-needed dosing. Tadalafil has also been approved for use as a daily medication at a lower dose (2.5–5 mg) than the as-needed dose with similar efficacy.

The most common side effects experienced with PDE inhibitors include headache, facial flushing, nasal congestion, dyspepsia, myalgia, back pain, and, rarely, priapism. Vardenafil and sildenafil may also cause blurred vision, difficulty in discriminating blue from green, bluish tones in vision, or difficulty seeing in dim light due to cross-reactivity with PDE 6 in the retina. Labeling for all PDE inhibitors includes a warning about rare nonarteritic ischemic optic neuropathy (NAION) in which blood flow is blocked to the optic nerve. If patients experience sudden or decreased vision loss, they should call a health care provider immediately. PDE inhibitors have also been associated with acute hearing impairment although a causal relationship has not been established.[1]

Due to the coexistence of ED and coronary artery disease, a management approach was developed to give recommendations for the use of PDE inhibitors as well as to determine the safety of intercourse in patients with CV disease[17] (Table 51–5). In addition to the inherent risk of renewing sexual activity, PDE inhibitors can lead to significant hypotension. Patients taking organic nitrates are at highest risk, as these drugs potentiate the drop in blood pressure. All four PDE inhibitors are absolutely contraindicated in patients taking any form of nitrate, whether scheduled or sublingual for acute situations. Additionally, caution should be used when combining a PDE inhibitor with α-blockers. Vardenafil contains a precautionary statement about the possibility of QT prolongation. Drug interactions and cautions vary slightly between agents and are described in Table 51–4.

Table 51–4

Comparison of PDE Inhibitors

	Sildenafil (Viagra)	Tadalafil (Cialis)	Vardenafil (Levitra, Staxyn)	Avanafil (Stendra)
Available strengths	25-, 50-, 100-mg tabs	2.5-, 5-, 10-, 20-mg tabs	2.5-, 5-, 10-, 20-mg tabs	50, 100, 200 mg
Initial dosage in healthy adults	50 mg up to once daily taken 1 hour prior to sexual activity	10 mg up to once daily taken 30 minutes prior to sexual activity or 2.5 mg daily at the same time each day	10 mg up to once daily taken 1 hour prior to sexual activity	100 mg up to once daily taken 30 minutes prior to sexual activity
Dosing range for healthy adults	25–100 mg	5–20 mg	5–20 mg	50–200 mg
Dosage in the elderly	25 mg	5–10 mg	5 mg	50–100 mg
Dosage in renal impairment	50 mg (moderate[a]) 25 mg (severe[b])	10 mg (moderate[a]) 5 mg (severe[b])	5–20 mg[c]	50–200 mg[c]
Dosage in hepatic impairment	25 mg	10 mg[c]	5 mg[c]	50–200 mg[c]
Time to onset	30 minutes	15 minutes	< 1 hour	15 minutes
Onset delayed by high-fat meal?	Yes	No	Yes	No
Duration of effect	Up to 4 hours	Up to 36 hours	Up to 4 hours	Up to 4 hours
Half-life	3–4 hours	18 hours	4–5 hours	5 hours
Metabolism	CYP3A4 (major) CYP2C9 (minor)	CYP3A4	CYP3A4 (major) CYP3A5 (minor) CYP2C (minor)	CYP3A4 (major) CYP2C9 (minor)
Clinically relevant drug interactions	Nitrates, protease inhibitors, azole antifungals, erythromycin	Nitrates, α_1-blockers[d], azole antifungals, erythromycin	Nitrates, antiarrhythmic agents[e], α_1-blockers[d], erythromycin	Nitrates, azole antifungals, erythromycin, α_1-blockers[d] grapefruit, protease inhibitors

CYP, cytochrome P-450 isoenzyme.

[a]Moderate renal impairment = creatinine clearance (CrCl) 31 to 50 mL/min (0.51–0.83 mL/s).

[b]Severe renal impairment = CrCl less than 30 mL/min (0.50 mL/s).

[c]Mild to moderate only—contraindicated in severe disease.

[d]Selective α_1-blockers (such as alfuzosin, silodosin, and tamsulosin) are appropriate in combination. If nonselective, initiate with lowest dose possible.

[e]Vardenafil can cause QT-interval prolongation; this effect in combination with certain antiarrhythmic agents can lead to life-threatening arrhythmias.

Up to a third of patients will not respond to therapy with PDE inhibitors. To achieve the greatest effect, patients must be fully informed of onset and duration of effect, impact of high-fat meals, the need for sexual stimulation, and explanation that a single trial is not adequate are all necessary counseling points. It is estimated that six to eight attempts with a medication and specific dose may be needed before successful intercourse results.[4]

Alprostadil Alprostadil is a prostaglandin E_1 analog that induces an erection by stimulating adenyl cyclase, leading to increased cAMP, smooth muscle relaxation, rapid arterial inflow, and increased penile rigidity. Alprostadil is available as an intracavernosal injection (Caverject or Edex) or a transurethral suppository (MUSE, medicated urethral system for erection), with the injectable dose showing greater efficacy (Figure 51–3).[4,5] Both forms of alprostadil are considered more invasive than oral medications or VEDs and are therefore second-line therapies.

MUSE consists of a urethral pellet of alprostadil with an applicator. Onset of action is within 5 to 10 minutes and it is effective for 30 to 60 minutes. Initial dose titration should occur in a physician's office to ensure correct dose and prevent adverse events. Success rates in clinical trials are between 43% and 69%, but typical use has resulted in less successful results in postmarketing studies.[12,18] Aching in the penis, testicles, legs, and perineum; warmth or burning sensation in the urethra, minor urethral bleeding or spotting, priapism, and light-headedness are all possible adverse effects. In addition, partners may experience burning or itching, and use is contraindicated with a pregnant partner unless using a condom.

Intraurethral alprostadil injection is the more effective route and is the only FDA-approved injection for ED. The onset of action is similar to transurethral alprostadil, but duration varies with dose and must be titrated in a physician's office to achieve an erection lasting no more than 1 hour. Injections should be performed into one side directly into the corpus cavernosum, and then the penis should be massaged to distribute the drug to both corpora. Education is extremely important with intracavernosal injections. Patients must be adequately informed of technique, expectations, side effects, and when to seek help. Intracavernosal injections are effective in up to 80% of patients, but side effects, lack of spontaneity, and fear of needles limit their

Table 51–5

Recommendations of the Second Princeton Consensus Conference for Cardiovascular Risk Stratification of Patients Being Considered for PDE Inhibitor Therapy

Risk Category	Description of Patients' Conditions	Management Approach
Low risk	Has asymptomatic CV disease with less than three risk factors for CV disease Has well-controlled hypertension Has mild, stable angina Has mild congestive heart failure (NYHA Class I) Has mild valvular heart disease Had a myocardial infarction more than 8 weeks ago	Patient can be started on PDE inhibitor
Intermediate risk	Has three or more risk factors for CV disease Has mild or moderate, stable angina Had a recent myocardial infarction or stroke within the past 2–8 weeks Has moderate congestive heart failure (NYHA Class III) History of stroke, transient ischemic attack, or peripheral artery disease	Patient should undergo complete CV workup and treadmill stress test to determine tolerance to increased myocardial energy consumption associated with increased sexual activity. Reclassify in low or high risk category
High risk	Has unstable or refractory angina, despite treatment Has uncontrolled hypertension Has severe congestive heart failure (NYHA Class IV) Had a recent myocardial infarction or stroke within the past 2 weeks Has moderate or severe valvular heart disease Has high-risk cardiac arrhythmias Has obstructive hypertrophic cardiomyopathy	PDE inhibitor is contraindicated; sexual intercourse should be deferred

CV, cardiovascular; NYHA, New York Heart Association; PDE, phosphodiesterase.

From Lee M. Erectile dysfunction. In: Dipiro JT, Talbert RL, Yee GC, et al, eds. Pharmacotherapy: A Pathophysiologic Approach. 9th ed. New York: McGraw-Hill; 2014:1337–1360.

Patient Encounter 1, Part 2

PMH: Type 2 diabetes for 15 years; not controlled due to his stressful profession; he often works late, eats on the run, and has no time for exercise. Chronic kidney disease stage 3. Hypertension for 8 years, currently controlled. Dyslipidemia for 8 years, currently controlled

SH: Works long hours as a business executive; drinks alcohol only occasionally; has a 20-pack per year smoking history

Meds: Metformin 1000 mg orally twice daily; metoprolol XL 50 mg orally once daily; hydrochlorothiazide 25 mg once daily; simvastatin 40 mg orally once daily

ROS: (–) Morning, nocturnal, or spontaneous erections suitable for intercourse; (+) nocturia, urgency, incomplete bladder emptying, dribbling; (–) symptoms of prostatitis; (–) chest pain or anginal symptoms; (+) significant life stressors; (+) mild pain in feet

PE:

VS: BP 135/78, P 85, RR 18, Wt 249 lb (113 kg), Ht 70 in (178 cm)

CV: Normal examination

Genital/Rectal: Normal scrotum and testicles w/o masses; penis without discharge or curvature; DRE reveals enlarged prostate

Labs: lipid panel: total cholesterol, LDL, HDL, triglycerides at goal; HbA_{1c} 8% (0.08; 64 mmol/mol Hgb), total testosterone 700 ng/dL (24 nmol/L), PSA 1.2 ng/ml (1.2 mcg/L), BUN 25 mg/dL (8.9 mmol/L); SCr 1.7 mg/dL (150 μmol/L)

Given this additional information, what are his risk factors for ED?

Identify treatment goals for this patient.

Perform a cardiovascular risk assessment to determine risk.

What pharmacologic and nonpharmacologic alternatives are available for this patient?

Which of the available options will be your treatments of choice based on concomitant disease states and medications, degree of invasiveness, side effects, ease of use, and side-effect profile?

What are the safety and efficacy monitoring parameters for the chosen treatment?

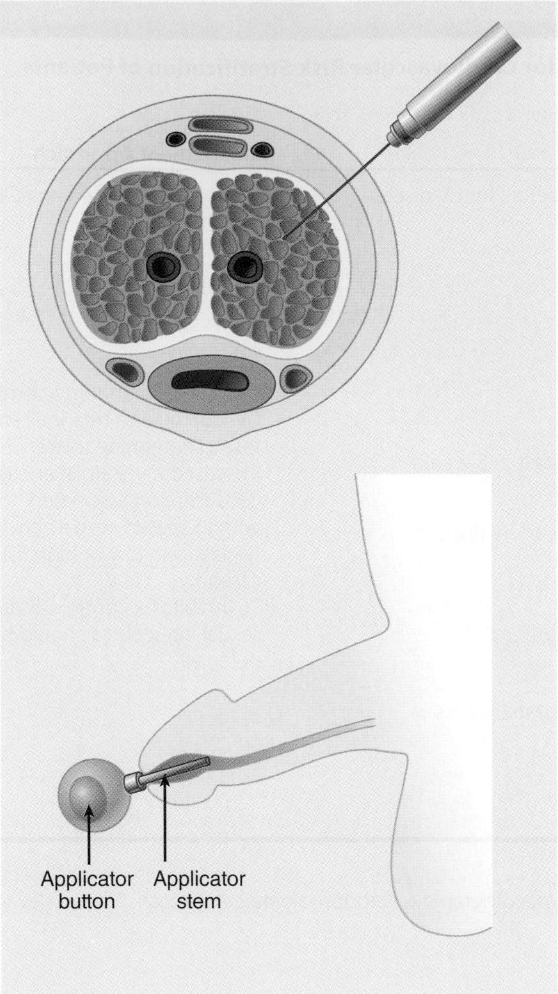

FIGURE 51–3. Intraurethral and intracavernosal administration of alprostadil. (From Wagner G, Saenz de Tejada I. Update on male erectile dysfunction. BMJ 1998;316:678–682.)

widespread use as first-line therapy, and therefore this therapy is most appropriate for patients in long-term stable relationships.[1,4] Adverse effects include pain with injection, bleeding or bruising at the injection site, fibrosis, or priapism. Use with caution in patients with sickle cell disease, those on anticoagulants, or those who have bleeding disorders, due to an increased risk of priapism and bleeding.

Testosterone Supplementation KEY CONCEPT *Androgens are important for general sexual function and libido, but testosterone supplementation is only indicated in patients with documented low serum testosterone levels.* In patients with **hypogonadism**, testosterone replacement is the initial treatment of choice, as it corrects decreased libido, fatigue, muscle loss, sleep disturbances, and depressed mood. However, testosterone is contraindicated in patients with prostate cancer, erythrocytosis, uncontrolled heart failure or sleep apnea.

Testosterone supplementation may improve ED symptoms, but is not universally effective. Initial supplementation should occur for 3 months with reevaluation and the addition of an another ED therapy if needed at that time. Dosage forms include intramuscular, an implanted pellet, topical patches or gel, and a buccal tablet.

Injectable testosterone cypionate and enanthate offer the most inexpensive replacement option. There are several drawbacks associated with parenteral testosterone, including the need to administer deep intramuscular injections every 2 to 4 weeks. Concentrations of hormone are well above physiologic values within the first few days, and then decline and eventually dip below physiologic levels prior to the next dose. These changes in concentration may lead to mood swings and a reduced sense of well-being.[19] Implantable subcutaneous testosterone pellets are a longer-acting and convenient alternative which are placed every 3 to 6 months.

Treatment with topical products is attractive to patients due to convenience, but they tend to be more expensive than the injections. Testosterone patches and gels are administered daily and result in serum levels within the physiologic range during the 24-hour dosing period.[19] Care must be taken with the use of the gel to prevent transfer of testosterone to children and females by washing hands thoroughly, allowing the site to dry, and covering immediately. Newer formulations for the axilla and thigh may reduce this risk. The most common side effects of topical testosterone are dermatologic reactions.

Oral testosterone products are also available for supplementation. Unfortunately, testosterone has poor oral bioavailability and undergoes extensive first-pass metabolism. Alkylated derivatives such as methyltestosterone and fluoxymesterone have been formulated, but this modification makes them considerably more hepatotoxic and therefore undesirable.

An alternative to the oral route is the buccal mucoadhesive system. This system adheres to the inside of the mouth and testosterone is absorbed through the oral mucosa and delivered to the systemic circulation with no first-pass effect. Side effects unique to this dosage form include oral irritation, bitter taste, and gum edema.

General side effects of testosterone include gynecomastia, dyslipidemia, polycythemia, and acne. Weight gain, hypertension, edema, and exacerbations of heart failure also occur due to sodium retention. Before initiating testosterone,

Patient Encounter 2

A 62-year-old man with a history of hypertension, prostatectomy 1 year ago, and recent diagnosis of ED. When in the office for a routine follow-up, he states the pill recently prescribed for his ED is not "doing the trick" so he has not been using it. He also complains that he is tired all the time, does not have much of a libido anymore, and is gaining weight.

Meds: losartan/hydrochlorothiazide 50/25 mg orally once daily, vardenafil 5 mg orally as needed

ROS: (–) Morning, nocturnal, or spontaneous erections suitable for intercourse; (–) nocturia, or urgency

PE:

VS: BP 132/74, P 82, Wt 214 lb (97 kg), Ht 75 in (191 cm)

Labs: Lipid panel, complete metabolic panel within normal limits

Based on the information provided, what is your assessment of the patient's ED?

What should be recommended as the next step in treatment of his ED?

Patient Care Process

Patient Assessment:

- Assess the patient's specific symptoms to determine the type of dysfunction.
- Ask specific questions related to onset and frequency of dysfunction, and status of sexual relationships and assess severity with the IIEF-5 questionnaire.
- Perform complete histories, physical examination and laboratory tests (see Tables 51–1 and 51–2).
- Assess cardiovascular risk (see Table 51–5).

Therapy Evaluation:

- PDE inhibitors are first-line treatment unless contraindicated, not tolerated, or ineffective.
- If patient already receiving treatment, assess efficacy, safety, and patient adherence.

Care Plan Development:

- If possible, discontinue medications that may cause or worsen ED.
- Initiate PDE inhibitor or patient treatment of choice and provide education regarding:
  - ED
  - Lifestyle
  - Treatment of associated disease states
  - Drug therapy—mechanisms of action and adverse effects
  - Device technique

Follow-up Evaluation:

- Follow-up in 4 to 6 weeks or more frequently to assess effectiveness and safety of therapy including specific warning signs (eg, vision changes, fibrosis, pain, priapism, or hypotension).
- Reeducate on lifestyle, associated disease states, expectations, and methods for increasing efficacy with therapy.
- Increase dosage, switch to alternate therapy, or add alternate therapy if needed.

the patient should undergo evaluation for benign prostatic hypertrophy and prostate cancer. Routine follow-up includes yearly prostate-specific antigen, digital rectal examination, and hemoglobin and liver function, in addition to assessment of response.

OUTCOME EVALUATION

Successful therapy for ED results in an increase in erections suitable for intercourse and, most importantly, in an improvement in the patient's quality of life. Ideally, the therapy chosen is free of significant adverse effects, discomfort, and inconvenience. Laboratory evaluation and a physical examination are not necessary for evaluation of effectiveness but may be necessary for adverse event monitoring.

Evaluate satisfaction and effectiveness after a 4-week trial. Some therapies will require multiple visits over the long term to determine the correct dose and to detect adverse effects. If the initial therapy is not effective, the patient must be further evaluated to determine whether the initial assessment of comorbid disease states, type of dysfunction, and patient goals were appropriate. After providing further education and determination of realistic goals, providers may then increase the dose of medication, switch to another therapy, or add a therapy if indicated.

Abbreviations Introduced in This Chapter

cAMP	Cyclic adenosine monophosphate
cGMP	Cyclic guanosine monophosphate
ED	Erectile dysfunction
IIEF	International Index of Erectile Function
MUSE	Medicated urethral system for erection
NAION	Non-arteritic ischemic optic neuropathy
PDE	Phosphodiesterase
VED	Vacuum erection device

REFERENCES

1. McMahon CG. Erectile dysfunction. Intern Med J. 2014;44:18–26.
2. Lewis RW, Fugl-Meyer KS, Corona G, et al. Definitions/epidemiology/risk factors for sexual dysfunction. J Sex Med. 2010;7:1598–1607.
3. Setter SM, Iltz JL, Fincham JE, et al. Phosphodiesterase 5 inhibitors for erectile dysfunction. Ann Pharmacother. 2005;39(7–8):1286–1295.
4. Shamloul R, Ghanem H. Erectile dysfunction. Lancet. 2013;381:153–165.
5. McVary KT. Erectile dysfunction. N Engl J Med. 2007;357:2472–2481.
6. Shabsigh R, Arver S, Channer KS, et al. The triad of erectile dysfunction, hypogonadism and the metabolic syndrome. Int J Clin Pract. 2008;62:791–798.
7. Deveci S, O'Brien K, Ahmed A, et al. Can the International Index of Erectile Function distinguish between organic and psychogenic erectile function? BJU Int. 2008;102:354–356.
8. DiMeo PJ. Psychosocial and relationship issues in men with erectile dysfunction. Urol Nurs. 2006;26:442–446.
9. Mikhail N. Management of erectile dysfunction by the primary care physician. Clev Clin J Med. 2005;293–294, 296–297, 301–305.
10. Gupta BP, Murad MH, Clifton MM, et al. The effect of lifestyle modification and cardiovascular risk factor reduction on erectile dysfunction. Arch Intern Med. 2011;171:1797–1803.
11. Gareri P, Castagna A, Francomano D, et al. Erectile dysfunction in the elderly: An old widespread issue with novel treatment perspectives. Int J Endo. 2014;2014:1–15.
12. Hatzimouratidis K, Eardley I, Giuliano F, et al. Guidelines on male sexual dysfunction: Erectile dysfunction and premature ejaculation: Uroweb 2014. http://www.uroweb.org/gls/pdf/14 male sexual dysfunction_LR.pdf. Accessed August 15, 2014.
13. Yuan J, Hoang AN, Romero CA, et al. Vacuum therapy in erectile dysfunction: Science and clinical evidence. Int J Impot Res. 2010;22:211–219.
14. Brant WO, Bella AJ, Lue TF. Treatment options for erectile dysfunction. Endocrinol Metab Clin N Am. 2007;36:465–479.

15. De Tejada IS. Therapeutic strategies for optimizing PDE-5 inhibitor therapy in patients with erectile dysfunction considered difficult or challenging to treat. Int J Impot Res. 2004;16(Suppl 1): S40–S42.
16. Morales AM, Casillas M, Turbi C. Patients' preference in the treatment of erectile dysfunction. Int J Impot Res. 2011;23:1–8.
17. Nehra A, Jackson G, Miner M, et al. The Princeton III consensus recommendations for the management of erectile dysfunction and cardiovascular disease. Mayo Clin Proc. 2012;87:766–778.
18. American Urological Association Guideline on the Management of Erectile Dysfunction: Diagnosis and Treatment Recommendations; updated 2006. http://www.auanet.org/content/guidelines-and-quality-care/clinical-guidelines.cfm?sub=ed. Accessed August 15, 2014.
19. Traish AM, Miner MM, Morgentaler A, Zitzmann M. Testosterone deficiency. Am J Med. 2011;124:578–587.
20. Rosen RC, Cappelleri JC, Smith MD, et al. Development and evaluation of an abridged, 5-item version of the International Index of Erectile Dysfunction (IIEF-5) as a diagnostic tool for erectile dysfunction. IntJ Impot Res. 1999;11:319–326.
21. Wagner G, Saenz de Tejada I. Update on male erectile dysfunction. BMJ. 1998;316:678–682.
22. Lee M. Erectile dysfunction. In: Dipiro JT, Talbert RL, Yee GC, et al, eds. Pharmacotherapy: A Pathophysiologic Approach. 9th ed. New York: McGraw-Hill; 2014:1337–1360.

52 Benign Prostatic Hyperplasia

Mary Lee and Roohollah Sharifi

LEARNING OBJECTIVES

Upon completion of the chapter, the reader will be able to:

1. Explain the pathophysiologic mechanisms underlying the symptoms and signs of benign prostatic hyperplasia (BPH).
2. Recognize the symptoms and signs of BPH in individual patients.
3. List the desired treatment outcomes for a patient with BPH.
4. Identify factors that guide selection of a particular *α*-adrenergic antagonist for an individual patient.
5. Compare and contrast *α*-adrenergic antagonists versus 5*α*-reductase inhibitors in terms of mechanism of action, treatment outcomes, adverse effects, and interactions when used for management of BPH.
6. Describe the indications, advantages, and disadvantages of various combination drug regimens for BPH that include an α-adrenergic antagonist, 5α-reductase inhibitor, anticholinergic agent, tadalafil, or mirabegron.
7. Describe the indications for surgical intervention of BPH.
8. Formulate a monitoring plan for a patient on a given drug treatment regimen based on patient-specific information.
9. Formulate appropriate counseling information for patients receiving drug treatment for BPH.

INTRODUCTION

The prostate is an organ, which is of the shape and size of a horse chestnut, that encircles the portion of the proximal posterior urethra that is located at the base of the urinary bladder. The prostate produces secretions, which are part of the ejaculate.

Benign prostatic hyperplasia (BPH) is the most common benign neoplasm in males who are at least 40 years of age. BPH can produce lower urinary tract symptoms (LUTS) that are consistent with impaired emptying of urine from and defective storage of urine in the bladder. Medications are a common mode of treatment to reduce symptoms and/or delay complications of BPH. For this reason, clinicians should be knowledgeable about the medical management of this disease.

EPIDEMIOLOGY AND ETIOLOGY

BPH is present as histologic disease in many elderly males. The prevalence increases with advancing patient age. However, of patients with microscopic BPH disease, only about 50% of patients develop an enlarged prostate on digital palpation and 25% of patients exhibit clinical voiding symptoms.[1,2] It is estimated that 8% of males 40 years of age, increasing to 35% of men 60 to 69 years of age, have voiding symptoms consistent with BPH, and 20% to 30% of all male patients who live to the age of 80 years will require a **prostatectomy** for severe voiding symptoms of BPH.[2]

Two chief etiologic factors for BPH include advanced patient age and the stimulatory effect of androgens.

- Prior to 40 years of age, the prostate in the adult male stays the same size, approximately 15 to 20 g. However, in males who have reached 40 years of age, the prostate undergoes a growth spurt, which continues as the male advances in age. Enlargement of the prostate can result in clinically symptomatic BPH.
- The testes and adrenal glands produce 90% and 10%, respectively, of circulating testosterone. Testosterone enters prostate cells, where predominantly Type II 5*α*-reductase converts testosterone to dihydrotestosterone, which combines with a cytoplasmic receptor. The complex enters the nucleus and induces changes in protein synthesis that promote glandular tissue growth of the prostate. Thus 5*α*-reductase inhibitors (eg, finasteride and dutasteride) directly interfere with one of the major etiologic factors of BPH.
- The prostate is composed of two types of tissue: (a) glandular or epithelial tissue, which produces prostatic secretions, including prostate-specific antigen (PSA), and (b) muscle or stromal tissue, which can contract around the urethra and bladder outlet when stimulated. Whereas androgens stimulate glandular tissue growth, androgens have no direct effect on stromal tissue. Stromal tissue growth may be stimulated by estrogen. Because testosterone is converted to estrogen in peripheral tissues in males, testosterone may be

associated indirectly with stromal hyperplasia. Stromal tissue is innervated by α_{1A}-receptors. When stimulated, prostatic stroma contracts around the urethra, narrowing the urethra and causing obstructive voiding symptoms.

PATHOPHYSIOLOGY

KEY CONCEPT *LUTS and signs of BPH are due to static, dynamic, and/or detrusor factors.* The static factor refers to anatomic obstruction of the bladder neck caused by an enlarged prostate gland. As the gland grows around the urethra, the prostate occludes the urethral lumen. The dynamic factor refers to excessive stimulation of α_{1A}-adrenergic receptors in the smooth muscle of the prostate, urethra, and bladder neck, which results in smooth muscle contraction. This reduces the caliber of the urethral lumen. The detrusor factor refers to bladder detrusor muscle hypertrophy in response to prolonged bladder outlet obstruction. To further explain, detrusor muscle fibers undergo hypertrophy so that the bladder can generate higher pressure to overcome bladder outlet obstruction and empty urine from the bladder. The hypertrophic detrusor muscle becomes irritable, contracting abnormally in response to small amounts of urine in the bladder. If obstruction is not treated, the bladder muscle will decompensate and be unable to empty completely; the postvoid residual urine volume (PVR) will increase.

In an enlarged gland, the epithelial/stromal tissue ratio is 1:5.[3] Androgens stimulate epithelial, but not stromal tissue hyperplasia. Hence, androgen antagonism does not induce a complete reduction in prostate size to normal. This explains one of the limitations of the clinical effect of 5α-reductase inhibitors.

Stromal tissue is the primary locus of α_1-adrenergic receptors in the prostate. An estimated 98% of the α-adrenergic receptors in the prostate are found in prostatic stromal tissue. Of the α_1-receptors found in the prostate, 70% of them are of the α_{1A}-subtype and the remainder are of the α_{1B} and α_{1D} subtypes.[4] This explains why α-adrenergic antagonists are effective for managing symptoms of BPH.

Symptoms of BPH are classified as obstructive or irritative. Obstructive symptoms result from failure of the urinary bladder to empty urine when the bladder is full. The patient will complain of a decreased force of the urinary stream, urinary hesitation, dribbling, intermittency, a sensation that the bladder is not empty even after voiding, and straining to empty the bladder. Irritative symptoms, including urinary frequency, nocturia, and urgency, result from the failure of the urinary bladder to store urine until the bladder is full.[1] The natural history of untreated BPH is unclear in patients with mild symptoms. It is estimated that up to 38% of untreated men with mild symptoms will have symptom improvement over a 2.5- to 5-year period.[5] It may be that such patients attribute their symptoms to aging, grow tolerant of their symptoms, or adopt behavioral changes in their lifestyle that minimize their voiding symptoms. On the other hand, a significant portion of patients with mild symptoms will likely experience disease progression. Patients with moderate to severe symptoms can experience a decreased quality of life as daily activities are adjusted because of lower urinary tract voiding symptoms. Also, such patients may develop complications of BPH, which include acute refractory urinary retention, renal failure, urinary tract infection, urinary incontinence, bladder stones, large bladder diverticuli, and recurrent gross hematuria. Predictors of disease progression include an enlarged prostate of at least 30 g (1.05 oz) or PSA of 1.4 ng/mL (1.4 mcg/L) or greater.[6,7] Finally, erectile dysfunction commonly develops in patients with BPH. Effective treatment of BPH symptoms often improves sexual function without initiating specific treatment for erectile dysfunction.[8]

Patient Encounter 1

A 65-year-old man with an AUA Symptom Score of 7, urinary hesitancy, a slow urinary stream, urinary frequency, and nocturia present to clinic. He wakes up two times every night to void. A DRE reveals a prostate of 25 g (0.9 oz). His PSA is 1.4 ng/mL (1.4 mcg/L). A urinary flow rate is 10 mL/s and PVR is 0 mL.

What stage of BPH does this patient have?

How should the patient be managed?

TREATMENT

Desired Outcomes[6,7]

- KEY CONCEPT *Reducing or eliminating obstructive and irritative voiding symptoms.* Drug treatment with an α-adrenergic antagonist or 5α-reductase inhibitor is expected to decrease the American Urological Association (AUA) Symptom Score by 30% to 50% (or at least by three or more points), improve peak and mean urinary flow rate by 1 to 3 mL/s, and decrease postvoid residual urine volume (PVR) to normal (less than 50 mL total) when compared with pretreatment baseline values. The AUA Symptom Score may not correlate with response to therapy.
- Slowing disease progression. When compared with baseline, symptoms and serum blood urea nitrogen (BUN) and creatinine should improve, stabilize, or decrease to the normal range with treatment.
- Preventing disease complications and reducing the need for surgical intervention.
- Avoiding or minimizing adverse treatment effects.
- Providing economical therapy.
- Maintaining or improving quality of life.

General Approach to Treatment

Until recently, the principal approach to treatment focused on reducing BPH symptoms (**Figure 52–1**, **Tables 52–1**, **52–2**, and 52–3). However, treatment should also slow disease progression and decrease complications of BPH.[9]

KEY CONCEPT *For patients with mild symptoms (AUA Symptom Score of 7 or less) that the patient does not consider to be bothersome, watchful waiting is a reasonable approach to treatment.* The patient is instructed to schedule return visits to the clinician every 6 to 12 months. At each visit, the patient's symptoms are reassessed using the AUA Symptom Scoring Index, and results are compared with baseline (see Table 52–1). In addition, the patient is educated about implementing nonpharmacologic measures to reduce voiding symptoms (see section on Nonpharmacologic Therapy) and avoiding factors that worsen obstructive and irritative voiding symptoms (**Table 52–4**). The digital rectal examination (DRE) is repeated annually. If the patient's symptoms are unchanged, then watchful waiting is continued. If the patient's symptoms worsen, then specific treatment is initiated.[7] Watchful waiting is effective in approximately 65% of patients after 5 years.[9]

Clinical Presentation and Diagnosis of BPH

General

Patients may or may not be in acute distress. In early stages of disease, the patient may complain of obstructive voiding symptoms. If untreated, the disease may progress and the patient may complain of irritative voiding symptoms or acute urinary retention, which is painful due to maximal distention of the urinary bladder. Also, the patient may be symptomatic of disease complications, including urosepsis, pyelonephritis, cystitis, or overflow urinary incontinence.

Symptoms

Patients may complain of obstructive voiding symptoms (eg, urinary hesitancy, decreased force of urinary stream, straining to void, incomplete bladder emptying, dribbling, and intermittency) and/or irritative voiding symptoms (eg, urinary frequency, nocturia, and urgency). Severity of symptoms should be assessed by the patient using a standardized instrument (eg, the American Urological Association [AUA] Symptom Scoring Index; Table 52–1). However, it is important to recognize that a patient's perception of the bothersomeness of his voiding symptoms may not match with the AUA Symptom Score. In this case, after thorough evaluation of the signs and complications of BPH disease, if present, the physician and patient should discuss the bothersomeness of the patient's symptoms and decide together on the most appropriate course of treatment for the patient.[1,7] Lower urinary tract symptoms (LUTS) is a term that refers to the collection of obstructive and irritative voiding symptoms characteristic of, but not specific for, BPH. That is, other urologic diseases (eg, urinary tract infection, prostate cancer, prostatitis, or neurogenic bladder) can also cause LUTS.

Signs

- Enlarged prostate on digital rectal examination (DRE); check for prostate nodules or induration, which would suggest prostate cancer instead of BPH as the cause of the patient's voiding symptoms
- Distended urinary bladder
- Rule out **meatal stenosis** or urethral stricture, which could cause voiding symptoms similar to LUTS
- Check anal sphincter tone as an indirect assessment of peripheral innervation to the detrusor muscle of the bladder

Complications of Untreated BPH

Upper and lower urinary tract infection, urosepsis, urinary incontinence refractory urinary retention, chronic renal failure, bladder diverticula, bladder stones, or recurrent gross hematuria.

Medical History

- Check the patient's general health, including previous surgery, presence of diabetes mellitus, or medications that may cause or worsen voiding symptoms.
- Have the patient provide a diary of his voiding pattern for the past week: date and time of each voiding, volume voided, and whether or not the patient had urinary leakage during the day.

Laboratory Tests

- Serum PSA: The combination of PSA and DRE of the prostate can be used to screen for prostate cancer, which could also cause an enlarged prostate. Also, PSA is a surrogate marker for an enlarged prostate due to BPH. A PSA greater than 1.5 ng/mL (1.5 mcg/L) suggests that a patient has a prostate volume greater than 30 cm^3 (30 g or 1.05 oz).[7]
- Urinalysis to rule out infection as a cause of the patient's voiding symptoms; also check urinalysis for microscopic hematuria, which typically accompanies BPH.
- Plasma blood urea nitrogen (BUN) and serum creatinine may be increased as a result of long-standing bladder outlet obstruction. These tests are not routinely performed but rather are reserved for those patients in whom renal dysfunction is suspected.

Other Diagnostic Tests (Table 52–2)

- Decreased peak and mean urinary flow rate (less than 10–15 mL/s) on uroflowmetry; decreased urinary flow rate is not specific for BPH; it can also be due to other urologic disorders (eg, urethral stricture, meatal stenosis, or **bladder hypotonicity**).
- Increased postvoid residual urine volume (PVR) (greater than 50 mL)
- DRE to check for an enlarged prostate (greater than 15–20 g [0.5–0.7 oz]).
- A focused neurological examination to check the integrity of innervation to the urinary bladder (that is responsible for bladder emptying).
- Transurethral cystoscopy reveals an enlarged prostate, which decreases urethral lumen caliber; information from this procedure helps the surgeon decide on the best surgical approach.
- Transrectal ultrasound of the prostate; a transrectal probe is inserted to evaluate prostate size and best surgical approach.
- Transrectal prostate needle biopsy to be done if the patient has areas of nodularity or induration on DRE; tissue biopsy can document the presence of prostate cancer, which can also cause enlargement of the prostate.
- IV pyelogram (IVP) will show retention of radiocontrast in the bladder if the patient has bladder outlet obstruction due to an enlarged prostate; this is only indicated in patients with recurrent hematuria, recurrent urinary tract infection, renal insufficiency, and urolithiasis.
- Filling cystometry provides information on bladder capacity, detrusor contractility, and the presence of uninhibited bladder contractions, which could also cause LUTS.

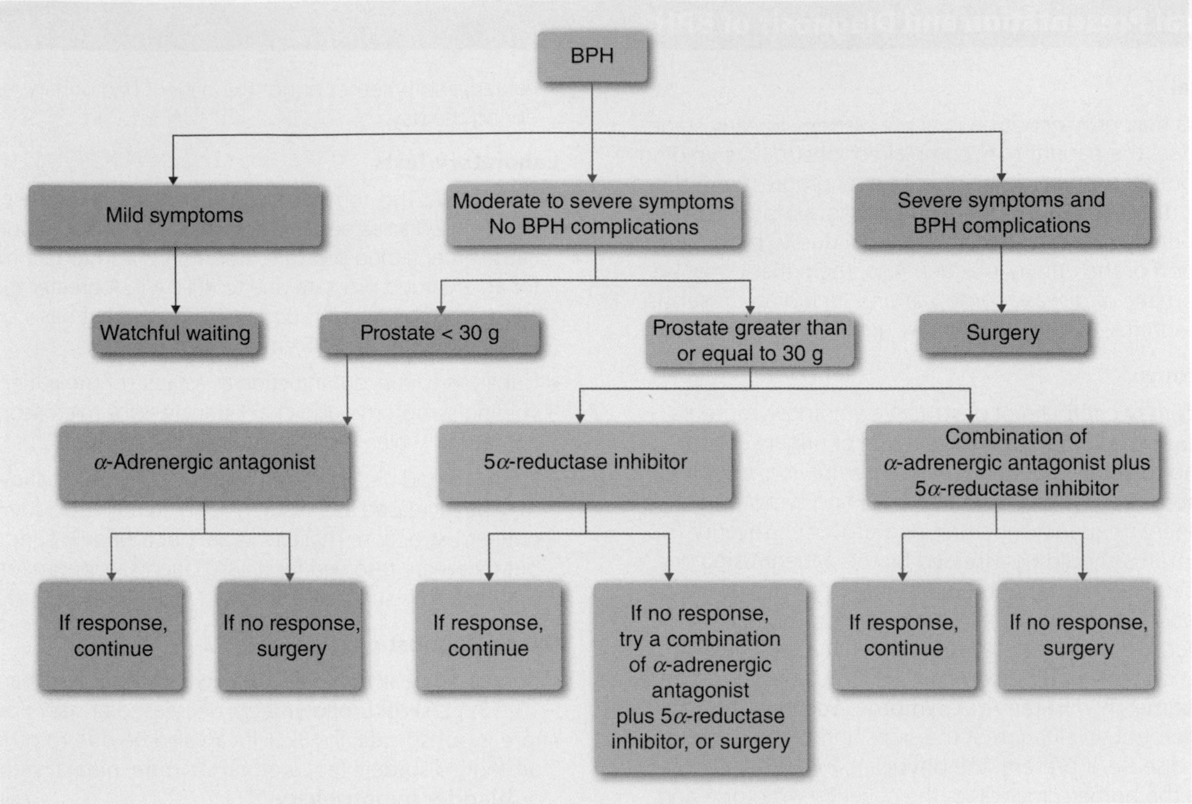

FIGURE 52–1. Algorithm for selection of treatment for BPH based on symptom severity and presence of disease complications.

Table 52–1

Questions to Determine the AUA Symptom Score

Directions for the patient: The patient should be asked to respond to each question based on the absence or presence of symptoms over the past month. For each question, the patient can respond using a 1–5 scale, where 0 = not at all or none; 1 = less than 1 time in 5; 2 = less than half of the time; 3 = about half of the time; 4 = more than half of the time; and 5 = almost always

Directions for the clinician: After the patient completes the questionnaire, the scores for individual items should be tallied for a final score. Scores of 0–7 = mild symptoms; scores of 8–19 = moderate symptoms; scores more than 20 = severe symptoms

Questions to Assess Obstructive Voiding Symptoms

1. How often have you had a sensation of not emptying your bladder completely after you finished urinating?
2. How often have you found you stopped and started again several times when you urinated?
3. How often have you had a weak urinary stream?
4. How often have you had to push or strain to begin urinating?

Questions to Assess Irritative Voiding Symptoms

5. How often have you found it difficult to postpone urination?
6. How often have you had to urinate again < 2 hours after you finished urinating?
7. How many times did you most typically get up to urinate from the time you went to bed at night until the time you got up in the morning?

Data from AUA Practice Guidelines Committee. AUA guideline on the management of benign prostatic hyperplasia (2010). www.auanet.org/content/guidelines-and-quality care/clinical-guidelines.cfm?sub=bph. Last accessed July 7, 2014.

KEY CONCEPT *For patients with moderate to severe symptoms and no complications of BPH, the patient is usually offered drug treatment first. α-Adrenergic antagonists are preferred over 5α-reductase inhibitors because the former have a faster onset of action (days to a few weeks) and improve symptoms independent of prostate size.* α-Adrenergic antagonists are preferred for patients with lower urinary tract voiding symptoms, who also have small prostates (less than 30 cm^3 [approximately 30 g or 1.05 oz]).

5α-Reductase inhibitors have a delayed onset of action (ie, peak effect may be delayed for up to 6 months) and are most effective in patients with moderate LUTS and larger size prostate glands (greater than 30 g or 1.05 oz). Drug treatment must be continued as long as the patient responds (Table 52–5).[7,10]

KEY CONCEPT *Combinations of medications to treat moderate or severe symptoms of BPH are more expensive and can cause more adverse effects than single drug treatment. Therefore, combination medication regimens are reserved for patients who have specific symptoms that do not respond to an adequate trial of single drug treatment or patients who are at high risk of developing complications of BPH.* Refer to the section on Combination Therapy for a detailed description of various regimens and their advantages and disadvantages.

KEY CONCEPT *For patients who are at risk of disease progression (ie, those with large prostates [greater than 30 g or 1.05 oz]), have moderate-severe symptoms that are not responsive to drug treatment, or have complications of BPH disease, surgery is indicated.*[7] Although it is potentially curative, surgery can result in significant morbidity, including erectile dysfunction, retrograde ejaculation, urethral stricture, urinary incontinence, bleeding, or urinary tract infection. The gold standard is prostatectomy, which can be performed transurethrally using electrocautery or

Table 52–2

Objective Tests Used to Assess the Severity and Complications of BPH

Test	How the Test Is Performed	Normal Test Result	Test Result in Patients with BPH
DRE of the prostate	Prostate is palpated through the rectal mucosa; the physician inserts an index finger into the patient's rectum	Prostate is soft, symmetric, mobile; size is 15–20 g (0.5–0.7 oz)	Prostate is enlarged, > 20 g (0.7 oz); no areas of induration or nodularity
Peak and mean urinary flow rate	Patient drinks water until bladder is full; patient empties bladder; volume of urine output and time to empty the bladder are measured; the flow rate (mL/s) is calculated	Peak and mean urinary flow rate are at least 10 mL/s	Peak and mean urinary flow rates are < 10 mL/s
PVR	Measurement of urine left in the bladder after the patient has tried to empty out his bladder; assessed by urethral catheterization or ultrasonography	PVR should be 0 mL	PVR > 50 mL is a significant amount of retained urine; this is associated with recurrent urinary tract infection
Urinalysis	Midstream urine is analyzed microscopically for white blood cells and bacteria	Urine should have no white cells or bacteria in it	Urine with white blood cells and bacteria is suggestive of inflammation and infection; if positive, urine is sent for bacteriologic culture
Prostate needle biopsy	Transrectally, a biopsy needle is inserted into the prostate; tissue core is sent to a pathologist for analysis	A normal prostate should have no evidence of BPH or prostate cancer	The biopsy is consistent with BPH
PSA	Blood test for this chemical, which is secreted by the prostate	< 4 ng/mL (4 mcg/L)	A PSA > 1.5 ng/mL (1.5 mcg/L) is a surrogate marker for an enlarged prostate > 30 g (1.05 oz)

DRE, digital rectal examination; PVR, postvoid residual urine volume; PSA, prostate-specific antigen.

as an open surgical procedure, which can be performed suprapubically or retropubically. A transurethral prostatectomy is typically reserved for prostates of intermediate size (30 g [1.05 oz] to 80 g [2.83 oz]), whereas an open prostatectomy is used for very large prostates (greater than 80 g [2.83 oz]) or when the patient has BPH and other associated urologic disorders, for example, large bladder stones or bladder diverticula, that can be surgically treated at the same time.[7] The newer bipolar technique for performing a TURP, which uses saline irrigating solution, has reduced the incidence of dilutional hyponatremia, a common adverse effect of the older monopolar technique, which uses glycine or sterile water irrigating solution. The outcomes of prostatectomy include an almost immediate improvement of LUTS, an increase of peak urinary flow rate by 6 to 15 mL/s, and a PVR decrease of 30 to 80 mL.

To minimize complications of prostatectomy or in patients who are taking anticoagulants, minimally invasive surgical procedures, such as transurethral incision of the prostate, transurethral needle ablation, transurethral microwave thermotherapy or transurethral laser ablation, are options.[12–14] A

Table 52–3

Staging the Severity of BPH Based on AUA Symptom Score and Example Signs of Disease

	AUA Symptom Score	Signs of Disease
Mild	≤ 7	Enlarged prostate on DRE, peak urinary flow rate ≤ 10 mL/s
Moderate	8–19	All of the above, PVR > 50 mL, irritative symptoms
Severe	≥ 20	All of the above plus one or more complications of BPH

AUA, American Urological Association; BPH, benign prostatic hyperplasia; DRE, digital rectal examination; PVR, postvoid residual urine volume.

The AUA Symptom Score focuses on seven items (incomplete emptying, frequency, intermittency, urgency, weak stream, straining, and nocturia) and asks that the patient quantify the severity of each complaint on a scale of 0 to 5. Thus the score can range from 0 to 35. A decrease in score of 3 points or more is considered a clinically significant improvement.

Table 52–4

Drugs That Can Cause Irritative or Obstructive Voiding Symptoms

Pharmacologic Class	Example Drugs	Mechanism of Effect
Androgens	Testosterone	Stimulate prostate enlargement
α-Adrenergic agonists	Phenylephrine, pseudoephedrine	Stimulate contraction of prostatic and bladder neck smooth muscle
Anticholinergic agents	Antihistamines, phenothiazines, tricyclic antidepressants, antiparkinsonian agents	Block bladder detrusor muscle contraction, thereby impairing bladder emptying
Caffeine	Caffeine	Acts like a diuretic
Diuretics	Thiazides diuretics, loop diuretics	Produce polyuria
Sedatives	Benzodiazepines, ethanol	Can cause functional incontinence

Table 52–5

Comparison of α-Adrenergic Antagonists, 5α-Reductase Inhibitors, Anticholinergic Agents, and Tadalafil for Treatment of BPH

Characteristic	α-Adrenergic Antagonists	5α-Reductase Inhibitors	Anticholinergic Agents	Tadalafil
Relaxes prostatic smooth muscle	Yes	No	No	Yes
Reduces size of enlarged prostate	No	Yes	No	No
Useful in patients with enlarged prostates	Yes (works independent of the size of the prostate)	Yes	Yes	Yes
Efficacy in relieving voiding symptoms and improving flow rate	++	+	+, irritative symptoms	+
Reduces the frequency of BPH-related complications	No	Yes	No	No
Reduces the frequency of BPH-related surgery	No	Yes	No	No
Frequency of daily dosing	Once or twice daily, depending on the agent and the dosage formulation	Once daily	Once or twice daily, depending on the agent	Once daily
Requirement for up-titration of dose	Yes (for terazosin and doxazosin immediate-release); no (for alfuzosin or silodosin; possibly for doxazosin extended-release and tamsulosin)	No	Yes, depending on the agent	No
Peak onset of action	Days to 6 weeks, depending on need for dose titration	6 months	Days	Days
Decreases PSA	No	Yes	No	No
Cardiovascular adverse effects	Yes, hypotension	No	Yes, tachycardia	Yes, hypotension
Drug-induced sexual dysfunction	Ejaculation disorders	Decreased libido, erectile dysfunction, ejaculation disorders	Yes, erectile dysfunction	No

PSA, prostate-specific antigen.

variety of ablative laser energy sources are used to vaporize tissue: holmium, potassium-titanyl-phosphate (KTP or green light), or diode. The choice of energy source is largely determined by the surgeon's level of training, the patient's anatomy, and potential risks for the patient.[11] The potential advantages of minimally invasive surgical procedures include less blood loss, shorter periods of catheterization postoperatively, and the ability to complete the procedure on an outpatient basis. However, minimally invasive surgical procedures are associated with a higher reoperation rate than a prostatectomy. Drug treatment is used in patients with severe disease when the patient refuses surgery or when the patient is not a surgical candidate because of concomitant diseases.

Nonpharmacologic Therapy (Behavioral Modification)

To reduce nocturia, patients should be instructed to stop drinking fluids 3 or 4 hours before going to bed and then void before going to sleep. During the day, timed voidings every 2 to 3 hours and use of double voiding help to empty urine from the bladder. Patients should avoid excessive caffeine and alcohol intake, because these may cause urinary frequency. Patients should avoid taking nonprescription medications that can worsen obstructive voiding symptoms (eg, antihistamines or decongestants) (see Table 52–4). In addition, toilet mapping (knowing the location of toilets on the way to and from various destinations) may help reassure the patient that he can still continue with many of his routine daily activities despite having LUTS. Patients are also advised to lose weight, if overweight. Because testosterone is converted to estrogen in adipose tissue, an alteration in the testosterone:estrogen ratio occurs in overweight men, similar to that which occurs in elderly males, which may contribute to the development of BPH.[17]

Although a variety of herbal agents are used for symptomatic management, including pygeum (African plum), secale cereale (rye pollen), serenoa repens, and hypoxis rooperi (South African star grass), objective evidence of efficacy is lacking.[15,16]

Pharmacologic Therapy

► *α-Adrenergic Antagonist Monotherapy*[17]

KEY CONCEPT *α-Adrenergic antagonists reduce the dynamic factor causing BPH symptoms. These drugs competitively antagonize α-adrenergic receptors, thereby causing relaxation of the bladder neck, prostatic urethra, and prostate smooth muscle.*[7,17] A secondary mechanism of action may be that α-adrenergic antagonists induce prostatic apoptosis,[18] which suggests that these agents may cause some shrinkage of an enlarged prostate.

All α-adrenergic antagonists are considered equally effective in relieving symptoms.[7,17] See Table 52-6 In various clinical trials, 30% to 80% of patients experience improvement in AUA Symptom Score by 30% to 45%, and 20% to 40% of patients experience urinary flow rate increases of 2 to 3 mL/s. The onset of action is

Table 52–6

Comparison of Pharmacologic Properties of α-Adrenergic Antagonists

	Terazosin	Doxazosin	Alfuzosin	Tamsulosin	Silodosin
Brand name	Hytrin	Cardura	Uroxatral	Flomax	Rapaflo
Generation	Second	Second	Second	Third	Third
Uroselective	No	No	Functionally (Clinically)	Pharmacologically	Pharmacologically
Need for up-titration	Yes	Yes (with immediate-release); possibly (with extended-release)	No	Minimal	No
Daily oral dose (mg)	5–20	2–8, immediate-release; 4–8, extended-release	10	0.4–0.8; (0.8 mg/day dose has not consistently produced clinical improvement over 0.4 mg/day)	8
Recommended dose reduction in patients with renal dysfunction	None needed	None needed	Manufacturer recommends caution in patients with severe renal insufficiency. No specific dosing recommendations provided	If creatinine clearance > 10 mL/min (0.17 mL/s), none needed. Tamsulosin has not been studied in patients with creatinine clearance < 10 mL/min (0.17 mL/s)	If creatinine clearance 30–50 mL/min (0.50–0.83 mL/s), use 4 mg/day. Contraindicated in patients with creatinine clearance < 30 mL/min (0.50 mL/s)
Recommended dose reduction in patients with hepatic dysfunction	Manufacturer provides no specific recommendation. Terazosin should be used cautiously as it undergoes extensive hepatic metabolism	Manufacturer provides no specific recommendation. Doxazosin should be used cautiously as it undergoes extensive hepatic metabolism	Contraindicated in patients with moderate/ severe hepatic impairment. Alfuzosin should be used cautiously in patients with mild hepatic impairment	Patients with mild/ moderate hepatic impairment require no dosage adjustment. Tamsulosin has not been studied in patients with severe hepatic impairment	Patients with mild/ moderate hepatic impairment require no dosage adjustment. Contraindicated in patients with severe hepatic impairment
Best time to take doses	At bedtime	Immediate-release: anytime during the day; however, it is typically given at bedtime Extended-release: anytime during the day	After meals for best oral absorption	On an empty stomach for best oral absorption. If taken 30 minutes after a meal, as recommended by the manufacturer, extent of absorption is reduced, thereby further reducing the potential for hypotensive adverse effects	Take with a meal, which decreases extent of absorption. Theoretically, this would help decrease hypotensive adverse effects
Half-life (hours)	12	22	5	10	13
Formulation	Immediate-release	Immediate-release and extended-release	Extended-release	Modified-release	Immediate-release
Cardiovascular adverse effects	++	++	+	0 to +	0 to +
Ejaculation disorders	+	+	+	++	++
Rhinitis	+	+	+	+	+
Malaise	+	+	+	+	+

+, minimal; ++ moderate.

days to weeks, depending on the need for titration of the dose from a subtherapeutic starting dose to a therapeutic maintenance dose. An adequate clinical trial is considered to be at least 1 to 2 weeks of continuous treatment at a full maintenance dose with any of these agents.[7] Durable responses have been demonstrated for up to 10 years with doxazosin.[19] However, some patients will develop disease progression despite treatment. α-Adrenergic antagonists are hepatically metabolized. Therefore, in patients with significant hepatic dysfunction, these drugs should be used in the lowest possible dose. With the exception of silodosin, these drugs do not require dosage modification in patients with renal dysfunction.

These agents can be differentiated by their adverse effect profile. The most common dose-limiting adverse effects are hypotension and syncope, which are more common with immediate-release terazosin and doxazosin, less frequent with extended-release doxazosin and alfuzosin, and least frequent with pharmacologically uroselective α_{1A}-adrenergic antagonists—tamsulosin and silodosin.[20] Combined use with antihypertensives, diuretics, or phosphodiesterase type 5 inhibitors can lead to additive blood pressure–lowering effects; however, this appears to be less of a problem with tamsulosin and silodosin.[7,21]

α-Adrenergic antagonists can be distinguished by several characteristics:

- *Uroselectivity*. Pharmacologic uroselectivity refers to preferential inhibition of α_{1A}-receptors, which predominate in the prostatic stroma, prostatic urethra, and bladder neck, and α_{1D}-receptors, which predominate in the bladder detrusor muscle.[17] Pharmacologically uroselective α_{1A}-adrenergic antagonists have the potential to produce less hypotension, because they have a lower propensity to antagonize α_{1B}-adrenergic receptors in the peripheral vasculature. Tamsulosin and silodosin are the only commercially available α_{1A}-adrenergic antagonists with pharmacologic uroselectivity.[21] In contrast, despite the potential of inhibiting α-adrenergic receptors in both the prostate and peripheral vasculature, functionally uroselective α-adrenergic antagonists in usually prescribed doses produce effective relaxation of prostatic smooth muscle with minimal vascular vasodilation. Thus blood pressure–lowering effects are mild or absent. The only functionally uroselective α-adrenergic antagonist is alfuzosin extended-release tablets.[22]
- KEY CONCEPT *Both pharmacologically and functionally uroselective agents appear to be clinically uroselective, in that they improve BPH symptoms with a low potential to cause cardiovascular adverse effects in humans.*[17] They are preferred in patients who usually have low blood pressure or those taking multiple antihypertensives.[22,23]

  Pharmacologic and functional uroselectivity are dose-related phenomena. Large daily doses of tamsulosin, silodosin, or alfuzosin may cause loss of uroselectivity, with resultant hypotension and dizziness in some patients.[23]

  Despite the blood-pressure lowering property of α-adrenergic antagonists, they are not recommended to be used alone to treat patients with both BPH and essential hypertension. In the ALLHAT study[24], where doxazosin was compared with other agents for treatment of essential hypertension, doxazosin was associated with a higher incidence of congestive heart failure. Therefore, in patients with both hypertension and moderate to severe LUTS, it is recommended that an appropriate antihypertensive be added to an α-adrenergic antagonist.
- *Need for up-titration of daily dose*. Up-titration is required for immediate-release terazosin and doxazosin. It is minimally required for extended-release doxazosin and tamsulosin. It is not required for extended-release alfuzosin or silodosin. The need for up-titration with a particular α-adrenergic antagonist delays its peak onset of action and the time when the patient can experience maximal clinical benefit.
- *Plasma half-life*. α-Adrenergic antagonists with short plasma half-lives (eg, prazosin) require multiple doses during the day. This is challenging for most patients, and thus prazosin is not recommended for BPH.[7]
- *Dosage formulation*. Immediate-release formulations of terazosin and doxazosin are quickly absorbed and produce high peak plasma levels. Modified- or extended-release formulations of doxazosin, alfuzosin, and tamsulosin produce lower peak levels, but more sustained therapeutic plasma levels, than immediate-release formulations and have less potential for producing hypotensive episodes. This allows for initiation of treatment with a therapeutic dose, a shorter time to peak onset of clinical effects, and once daily dosing.[17,22]
- *Adverse effects*. Hypotensive adverse effects of α-adrenergic antagonists can range from asymptomatic blood pressure reductions to dizziness and syncope. This adverse effect occurs in approximately 2% to 14% of treated patients and is most commonly associated with immediate-release terazosin and doxazosin; is less commonly associated with extended-release alfuzosin and extended-release doxazosin; and least commonly associated with tamsulosin and silodosin.[7,22]
  To minimize first-dose syncope from terazosin and doxazosin immediate-release, a slow up-titration from a subtherapeutic dose of 1 mg/day to a therapeutic dose is essential. The first dose should be given at bedtime so that the patient can sleep through the peak serum concentration of the drug when the adverse effect is most likely to occur. A 3- to 7-day interval between each dosage increase should be allowed, and the patient should be maintained on the lowest effective dose of an α-adrenergic antagonist. If the patient is noncompliant with his regimen or he skips or interrupts treatment, the α-adrenergic antagonist should be restarted using the usual starting dose and then retitrated up. He should not be instructed to simply double up on missed doses or resume treatment with his currently prescribed daily dose, as this can lead to significant hypotension or syncope.

Ejaculation disorders, including delayed, absent and retrograde ejaculation, occur with all adrenergic antagonists. This is largely thought to be due to pharmacologic blockade of peripheral α-adrenergic receptors at the bladder neck (ie, the bladder neck is unable to close during ejaculation in the presence of α-adrenergic blockade), however, a central nervous system mechanism of action cannot be discounted.[25] The incidence appears to be dose-related and highest with daily doses of tamsulosin 0.8 mg and silodosin 8 mg, occurring in up to 26% and 28% of treated patients, respectively. Ejaculation disorders generally do not necessitate discontinuation of treatment, except in younger patients. Although this adverse effect may decrease the patient's satisfaction with the quality of sexual intercourse, ejaculation disorders are not harmful to the patient.

Rhinitis and malaise occur with α-adrenergic antagonists and are an extension of the pharmacologic blockade of α-adrenergic receptors in the vasculature of the nasal mucosa and in the central nervous system, respectively. Tolerance often develops to these adverse effects and they rarely require discontinuation of treatment. Avoid use of topical or oral decongestants, as these may exacerbate obstructive voiding symptoms. Cautious use of antihistamines with anticholinergic adverse effects is also recommended in patients with severe BPH and large PVR's, as these drugs may cause acute urinary retention in patients with an obstructed bladder neck.

Floppy iris or small pupil syndrome has been reported with α-adrenergic antagonists, most often with selective α_{1A} adrenergic antagonists.[7,26] In response to tamsulosin, the iris dilator muscle relaxes and the pupil constricts. As a result, when the α-adrenergic antagonist–treated patient undergoes cataract surgery, the iris can become flaccid, floppy, or billows out. This plus the pupillary constriction interfere with the surgical procedure and increase the risk of intraoperative and postoperative complications. A patient who plans to undergo cataract surgery is advised to inform his ophthalmologist that he is taking an α-adrenergic antagonist. Although the drug will not need to be held or discontinued, the ophthalmologist can plan to use certain surgical techniques, for example, iris hooks or iris expansion rings, to deal with the drug's effect on the iris dilator muscle.[27,28] Likewise, prior to initiating an α-adrenergic antagonist, a patient who needs cataract surgery should have this ophthalmologic procedure performed first, if possible.[7]

- *Potential for drug interactions.* Hypotensive adverse effects of terazosin and doxazosin can be additive with those of diuretics, antihypertensives, and phosphodiesterase type 5 inhibitors (eg, sildenafil). In patients at greatest risk for hypotension, or in those patients who tolerate hypotension poorly, including those with poorly controlled coronary artery disease or severe orthostatic hypotension, tamsulosin or silodosin appear to be the safest choice.[22,26,29] In patients who cannot tolerate any α-adrenergic antagonist, a 5α-reductase inhibitor or prostatectomy could be considered, particularly if the prostate is enlarged and greater than 30 g (1.05 oz). When initiating sildenafil, tadalafil, or vardenafil, patients who are taking α-adrenergic antagonists should be stabilized first on a fixed dose of the α-adrenergic antagonist, and then patients should be started on the lowest effective dose of phosphodiesterase inhibitor to minimize the likelihood of hypotensive effects.

Patient Encounter 2

A 64-year-old man who has essential hypertension and has been taking valsartan 160 mg and hydrochlorothiazide 12.5 mg orally every day for the past 2 years presents to the clinic. The patient tolerates this regimen well, and his blood pressure is now 140/80 mm Hg. However, he was recently diagnosed with moderate LUTS, and he began tamsulosin 0.4 mg by mouth daily. Over the course of several weeks, he was titrated up to 0.8 mg daily. Although the patient has experienced significant improvement in his obstructive voiding symptoms, he also complains of dizziness, lightheadedness, and periodically feels like fainting.

How should this patient be managed?

▶ 5α-Reductase Inhibitor Monotherapy

KEY CONCEPT *5α-Reductase inhibitors reduce the static factor, which results in shrinkage of an enlarged prostate by approximately 20% to 25% after 6 months. They do so by inhibiting 5α-reductase, which is responsible for intraprostatic conversion of testosterone to dihydrotestosterone, the active androgen that stimulates prostate tissue growth.* Two subtypes of 5α-reductase, Type I and II, are present in the prostate; the majority is the Type II isoenzyme.[7] Finasteride is a selective Type II isoenzyme inhibitor, whereas dutasteride is a nonselective inhibitor of both Type I and Type II isoenzymes. When compared with finasteride, dutasteride produces a faster and more complete inhibition of 5α-reductase in prostate cells. However, no difference in clinical efficacy or adverse effects has been demonstrated between these two agents.[7,30] Thus finasteride and dutasteride are considered therapeutically equivalent (Table 52–7).

Table 52–7
Comparison of Pharmacologic Properties of 5α-Reductase Inhibitors

	Finasteride	Dutasteride
Brand name	Proscar	Avodart
Subtype inhibition of the 5α-reductase enzyme	Type II	Types I and II
Percentage of inhibition of serum dihydrotestosterone level	70–76	90–95
Percentage of patients with reduction in serum dihydrotestosterone	49	> 85
Time to peak onset of reduction in serum dihydrotestosterone level	6 months	1 month
Percentage of inhibition of intraprostatic dihydrotestosterone	85–90	> 95
Half-life	6.2 hours	3–5 hours
Daily dosage (mg)	5	0.5
Recommended dose reduction in patients with renal dysfunction	None needed	None needed
Recommended dose reduction in patients with hepatic dysfunction	Manufacturer provides no specific recommendation. Finasteride should be used cautiously as it undergoes extensive hepatic metabolism	Manufacturer provides no specific recommendation. Dutasteride should be used cautiously as it undergoes extensive hepatic metabolism

From Keam SJ, Scott LJ. Dutasteride: A review of its use in the management of prostate disorders. Drugs 2008;68:463–485.

With regard to their use for the symptomatic treatment of BPH, finasteride and dutasteride are considered equally effective in relieving LUTS by 15% to 30% in 30% to 70% of patients and increasing the urinary flow rate by 1 to 2 mL/s, which is less improvement than that seen with α-adrenergic antagonists.[7,30,31] A minimum of 6 months is required to evaluate the effectiveness of treatment. This is a disadvantage in patients with moderate to severe symptoms, as it will take that long to determine whether the drug is or is not effective. Durable responses have been demonstrated in responding patients treated up to 6 years with finasteride and 4 years with dutasteride.[32,33] Unlike α-adrenergic antagonists, 5α-reductase inhibitors are used to prevent BPH-related complications and disease progression. Finasteride has been shown to reduce both the incidence of acute urinary retention by 57% and the need for prostate surgery by 55% in patients with significantly enlarged prostate glands (greater than 40 g [1.4 oz]).[34,35] These agents are hepatically metabolized. No specific recommendations for dosage modification are currently available in patients with significant hepatic dysfunction; however, due to the drug's specificity for its enzyme target, it is unlikely that any dosage adjustment will be required. No dosage adjustment is needed in patients with renal impairment. Adverse effects include decreased libido, erectile dysfunction, and ejaculation disorders, which may persist after the drug is stopped, and gynecomastia and breast tenderness. When used to prevent prostate cancer, these agents reduce the incidence of prostate cancer by 25%, but are suspected to increase the risk of developing moderate to high grade cancer, if prostate cancer does develop.[36,37] Serum testosterone levels increase by 10% to 20% in treated patients; however, the clinical significance of this is not clear at this time.[7] Drug interactions are uncommon. These drugs decrease serum levels of PSA by approximately 50%. Therefore, to preserve the usefulness of this laboratory test as a diagnostic and monitoring tool, it is recommended that prescribers obtain a baseline PSA prior to the start of treatment and repeat it at least annually during treatment. A significantly elevated PSA in treated patients suggests that the patient is not compliant with his prescribed 5α-reductase inhibitor regimen or is an indicator for further diagnostic workup for prostate cancer. Exposure to 5α-reductase inhibitors is contraindicated in pregnant females, as the drugs may cause feminization of a male fetus. Pregnant females should not handle these drugs unless they are wearing gloves.

► *Combination Therapy*

KEY CONCEPT *A combination of an α-adrenergic antagonist and 5α-reductase inhibitor may be considered in symptomatic patients who do not respond to an adequate trial of monotherapy or in those at high risk of BPH complications, that is, those with an enlarged prostate of at least 30 g (1.05 oz).*[7,11,30] *In such patients, combination therapy will relieve voiding symptoms and also may reduce the risk of developing BPH-related complications and reduce the need for prostatectomy by 67% after 4 years.*[34,35] The Reduce Trial compared dutasteride, tamsulosin, and the combination of dutasteride and tamsulosin. Results showed that patients treated with the combination had greater symptom improvement after 9 months and less disease progression at 4 years than patients treated with single drug therapy.[38] Because combination therapy is more expensive and associated with the array of adverse effects associated with each drug in the combination, clinicians should discuss the advantages and disadvantages of such a treatment regimen with the patient before a final decision is made (see Table 52-5).[7,30] A commercially available combination formulation of dutasteride 0.5 mg and tamsulosin 0.4 mg may be convenient for some patients.

To streamline and reduce the cost of treatment regimens, it has been suggested that the α-adrenergic antagonist may be discontinued after the first 6 to 12 months of combination therapy in patients with moderate LUTS. However, in patients with severe LUTS and an enlarged prostate gland, the combination regimen should be continued as long as the patients are responding.[39]

Another enhancement to BPH symptom management is the addition of an anticholinergic agent (eg, tolterodine) to an α-adrenergic antagonist with or without a 5α-reductase inhibitor. The rationale for the anticholinergic agent is that irritative symptoms (eg, urinary urgency and frequency) are thought to be due to hyperreactive bladder detrusor muscle contraction, which can be ameliorated by blockade of M_2 and M_3 muscarinic receptors.[40–43] Also, α_{1D}-adrenergic receptors in the detrusor muscle, which cause muscle contraction when stimulated, can be blocked by α-adrenergic antagonists. An α-adrenergic antagonist may decrease involuntary bladder muscle contraction and increase the bladder's compliance. Thus, the combination may have an additive pharmacologic effect on relieving irritative voiding symptoms.[43] A recent meta-analysis documenting the addition of an anticholinergic agent to an α-adrenergic antagonist produced significant irritative symptom improvement, more than what was observed with the α-adrenergic antagonist alone.[43] No cases of urinary retention were reported. If irritative symptoms do not improve after starting an anticholinergic agent, up-titrating the dose or switching to another anticholinergic agent may be helpful. Patients at the highest risk of anticholinergic agent-induced acute urinary retention include those with a high postvoid residual urine volume (250 mL or more). Thus anticholinergic agents should be used precautiously in these patients. Finally, the medication profile of patients should be checked for overall anticholinergic burden, which increases the likelihood of anticholinergic adverse effects, including dry mouth, tachycardia, constipation, confusion, and drowsiness.

Once daily dosing of tadalafil is approved for treatment of LUTS. It may be prescribed alone,[44] or along with an α-adrenergic antagonist[45] or 5α-reductase inhibitor.[46] Its mechanism may be due to relaxation of smooth muscle of the urethra, prostate, and bladder, which is mediated by inhibiting the Rho/Rhokinase pathway. This inhibits the proliferation and contraction of prostatic smooth muscle, or enhances the action of nitric oxide.[8,47] Tadalafil is comparable to α-adrenergic antagonists in relieving LUTS and decreasing the AUA Symptom Score by 3.8 points after 12 weeks; however, it does not increase urinary flow rate or reduce PVR.[48] Because tadalafil is expensive, the best candidates for treatment are those with BPH and erectile

Patient Encounter 3

A 66-year-old man with severe obstructive voiding symptoms of BPH presents to the clinic. A DRE reveals a prostate of 45 g (1.6 oz) and a PSA of 1.8 ng/mL (1.8 mcg/L). He is started on dutasteride 0.5 mg daily by mouth. After 3 months, the patient complains that his symptoms have not significantly improved.

Explain why the patient has not responded to treatment.

Identify an alternative treatment regimen for this patient.

Table 52–8

Summary of Adverse Effects of α-Adrenergic Antagonists, 5α-Reductase Inhibitors, Anticholinergic Agents, and Tadalafil and Management Suggestions

Drug Class	Adverse Reaction	Management Suggestion
α-Adrenergic antagonist	Hypotension	Start with lowest effective dose, give doses at bedtime, and slowly up-titrate at 0.5- to 1-week intervals to a full therapeutic dose, if using immediate-release terazosin or doxazosin. Use tamsulosin, silodosin, extended-release doxazosin, or alfuzosin, as alternatives to immediate-release products, particularly in patients taking other antihypertensives.
	Malaise	Educate the patient that this is a common adverse effect; tolerance may develop to malaise. Usually does not require discontinuation of treatment.
	Rhinitis	Educate the patient that this is a common adverse effect; tolerance may develop to rhinitis. Usually does not require discontinuation of treatment.
	Ejaculation disorders	Educate the patient that this is a common adverse effect and it is not harmful.
5α-Reductase inhibitor	Gynecomastia	Educate the patient that this may be bothersome, but not harmful.
	Decreased libido	If the patient is sexually active, sexual counseling may be helpful. May be reversible despite continued use of the 5α-reductase inhibitor.
	Erectile dysfunction	The addition of sildenafil or another erectogenic drug may be helpful. May be reversible despite continued use of the 5α-reductase inhibitor.
	Ejaculation disorders	Educate the patient that this may occur but it is not harmful. May be reversible despite continued use of the 5α-reductase inhibitor.
Anticholinergic agent	Dry mouth	Educate the patient that this is a common adverse effect. If drinking fluids and sucking on sugarless hard candy are not effective, the physician may switch to another agent in the same class or possibly reduce the daily dose.
	Constipation	This is a common adverse effect. Educate the patient to drink plenty of fluids and eat a high fiber diet.
	Confusion, drowsiness	If this occurs, the physician may switch to another agent in the same class with less potential to cross the blood brain barrier, eg, trospium.
	Acute urinary retention	Do not use anticholinergic agents in patients with a PVR > 250 mL as they are high risk of developing this adverse effect, which is a urologic emergency.
	Increased risk of heat stroke	By decreasing perspiration, patients who are in hot climates and who do not have access to air conditioning, are at risk of heat stroke. Use of anticholinergic agents in elderly who are exposed to these conditions should be avoided.
Tadalafil	Headache	Educate the patient that this is a common adverse effect. It is usually mild, temporary, and does not require treatment. If necessary, a low dose of acetaminophen is usually effective.
	Dizziness	Educate the patient that this is a common adverse effect and does not require treatment. If the patient is taking other blood pressure lowering medications, stabilize blood pressure on these medications before starting tadalafil.
	Dyspepsia	Heartburn-like symptoms may occur. Usually, it is mild and does not require treatment.
	Back pain or myalgia	This occurs more often with tadalafil than with the other phosphodiesterase inhibitors. It usually resolves once the drug is stopped. If not severe, tadalafil may be continued as the adverse effect may resolve with continued tadalafil use.

dysfunction, or those patients with LUTS that is not responsive to α-adrenergic agonists. The usual recommended dose is 5 mg by mouth daily; the dose should be reduced to 2.5 mg daily if the creatinine clearance is 30 to 50 mL/min (0.50–0.83 mL/s). Tadalafil should be avoided if the creatinine clearance is less than 30 mL/min (0.50 mL/s). Tadalafil is contraindicated in patients on nitrates by any route of administration; patients with unstable angina, uncontrolled or high-risk arrhythmias, persistent hypotension, poorly controlled hypertension, or New York Heart Association Classification IV congestive heart failure; or patients who have had a myocardial infarction within the past 2 weeks.[49] Common adverse effects include headache, dizziness, dyspepsia, back pain, and myalgia (Table 52–8).

Mirabegron is a β_3-adrenergic agonist. When it stimulates beta$_3$ adrenergic receptors in the urinary bladder detrusor muscle, mirabegron reduces irritative voiding symptoms and improves urine storage in the bladder.[11] Although not FDA approved for this indication, mirabegron is an alternative to an anticholinergic agent in patients who poorly tolerate anticholinergic adverse effects or whose irritative voiding symptoms do not respond to an anticholinergic agent. Mirabegron is typically added to an α-adrenergic agonist.[50] The usual dose is 50 mg by mouth daily; reduce the dose to 25 mg daily if the creatinine clearance is 15 to 29 mL/min (0.25–0.49 mL/s).

Patient Encounter 4

A 67-year-old man presents with severe LUTS. His prostate gland is estimated to be 40 cm^3 (40 g or 1.4 oz) in size and his PSA is 3 ng/mL (3 mcg/L). The patient also suffers from recurrent urinary tract infection and persistent gross hematuria. The patient's peak urinary flow rate is 5 mL/s and PVR is 200 cm^3 (200 mL). The patient's AUA Symptom Score is 25. The patient prefers medical management for his BPH. He asks if tadalafil would be a good choice for him.

Is tadalafil a good choice? If not, what is the best treatment option for this patient?

Mirabegron should be avoided if the creatinine clearance is less than 15 mL/min (0.25 mL/s). Common adverse effects of mirabegon include headache, hypertension, tachycardia, constipation, and nasopharyngitis.

OUTCOME EVALUATION

KEY CONCEPT *Once the peak effects of drug treatment are expected to occur, monitor the drug for effectiveness. This is approximately 1 month after the start of an α-adrenergic antagonist and 3 and 6 months after the start of a 5α-reductase inhibitor.* Assess symptom improvement using the AUA Symptom Scoring Index. A reduction in symptom score by a minimum of 3 points is anticipated with symptom improvement. However, it should be noted that the AUA Symptom Score may not match the patient's perception of the bothersomeness of his voiding symptoms. If the patient perceives his symptoms as bothersome, independent of the AUA Symptom Score, consideration should be given to modifying the patient's treatment regimen. Similarly, a patient may regard his symptoms as not bothersome even though the AUA symptom score is high. In this case, the physician should objectively assess symptoms at baseline and during treatment by performing a repeat uroflowmetry, which can detect an improvement in peak and mean urinary flow rate, and checking for a reduction in PVR and the absence of complications of BPH. If the patient shows a response to treatment, instruct the patient to continue the drug regimen and have the patient return at 6-month intervals for monitoring. If the patient shows an inadequate response to treatment, the dose of α-adrenergic antagonist can be increased (except for extended-release alfuzosin and silodosin) until the patient's symptoms improve or until the patient experiences adverse drug effects.

For the α-adrenergic antagonists, the severity of hypotensive-related adverse effects, which may manifest as dizziness or syncope, may require a dosage reduction or a slower up-titration of immediate-release terazosin or doxazosin, or halting the up-titration of the α-adrenergic antagonist. If the patient develops adverse effects at this dose, the drug should be discontinued. Other adverse effects of α-adrenergic antagonists are nasal congestion, malaise, headache, and ejaculation disorders. None of

The Patient Care Process

Patient Assessment:

- Based on the patient's chief complaint and review of systems, determine whether the patient is experiencing LUTS.
- Review the medical history and physical examination. Does the patient have a history of BPH? Does he have an enlarged prostate? Does he have a history of complications of BPH, for example, recurrent urinary tract infection, gross hematuria, acute urinary retention, and so on. Have various tests been performed to establish the severity of BPH (Table 52–2)?
- Conduct a medication history (including prescription and over the counter medications, and dietary supplements) that could be contributing to his voiding symptoms (Table 52–4). Does the patient have any drug allergies? Is the patient receiving treatment for LUTS (Table 52–5)? If yes, when was the treatment started and has the patient completed an adequate clinical trial? Is the patient experiencing adverse effects from therapy (Table 52–8)?
- Review available laboratory tests, especially serum electrolytes, renal function, and urinalysis.
- Assess the severity of the patient's LUTS by having the patient complete the AUA Symptom Scoring Index (Table 52–3).

Therapy Evaluation:

- If the patient is already receiving medications for LUTS, assess the efficacy, safety, and patient adherence. Are there any significant drug interactions?
- If the patient needs to be started on drug therapy, ensure that the patient has moderate or severe LUTS, check prostate size, and check patient for any contraindications or precautions for various treatments. Is the patient at risk of BPH progression? Does the patient prefer medical or surgical treatment of BPH?
- Determine whether the patient has prescription coverage or whether recommended agents are included on the institution's formulary.

Care Plan Development:

- Institute nonpharmacologic therapies to minimize LUTS.
- Institute appropriate medication treatment for moderate or severe LUTS.
- Determine whether drug dose is optimal (Table 52–6 and 52–7).
- Address any patient concerns about LUTS, BPH, and management.
- Discuss importance of medication adherence and nonpharmacologic therapies to control LUTS.

Follow-Up Evaluation:

- After starting an α-adrenergic antagonist, assess effectiveness and safety of therapy in 1 month, and then at 6 months. At each visit, repeat AUA Symptoms Scoring Index, check for disease progression, repeat urinary flow rate and PVR and for adverse effects of treatment. As long as the patient continues to respond and tolerates the medication well, repeat all assessments at yearly intervals thereafter.
- After starting a 5α-reductase inhibitor, assess effectiveness and safety of therapy at the end of the third and sixth month.

At each visit, repeat AUA Symptoms Scoring Index, check for disease progression, repeat urinary flow rate and PVR and for adverse effects of treatment. As long as the patient continues to respond and tolerates the medication well, repeat all assessments at yearly intervals thereafter.

these generally require discontinuation of treatment, and these often improve as treatment continues. For the 5α-reductase inhibitors, the most bothersome adverse effects are decreased libido, erectile dysfunction, and ejaculation disorders. In sexually active males, erectile dysfunction may be improved with erectogenic drugs; however, this adverse effect may necessitate discontinuation of treatment.

During continuing treatment of BPH, the patient should undergo an annual repeat PSA and DRE. A rising PSA level suggests that the patient has worsening BPH, new-onset prostate cancer, or that the patient is noncompliant with his regimen of 5α-reductase inhibitor. An abnormal DRE suggestive of prostate cancer would reveal a nodule or area of induration on the prostate. In such a case, a prostate biopsy is required to rule out prostate cancer.

Drug treatment failures may result from a variety of factors. Initial failure to respond to α-adrenergic antagonists occurs in 20% to 70% of treated patients. It is likely in these patients that the static factor may predominate as the cause of symptoms in these patients. In these patients, adding a 5α-reductase inhibitor may be helpful. Initial failure to respond to 5α-reductase inhibitors occurs in 30% to 70% of treated patients. It is likely that the dynamic factor may predominate as the cause of symptoms in these patients. In these patients, switching to or adding an α-adrenergic antagonist may be helpful. In contrast, drug treatment failures after an initial good response to drug therapy will likely be an indication of progressive BPH disease. In such patients, modifying the drug regimen or surgical intervention may be indicated.

Table 52–8 summarizes the adverse effects of the agents used to treat BPH and includes management suggestions for these situations.

Abbreviations Introduced in This Chapter

AUA	American Urological Association
BPH	Benign prostatic hyperplasia
BUN	Blood urea nitrogen
DRE	Digital rectal examination
IVP	Intravenous pyelogram
LUTS	Lower urinary tract symptoms
PSA	Prostate specific antigen
PVR	Postvoid residual urine volume
TURP	Transurethral resection of the prostate

REFERENCES

1. Thorner DA, Weiss JP. Benign prostatic hyperplasia: Symptoms, symptom scores, and outcome measures. Urol Clin North Am. 2009;36:417–429.
2. Berry SJ, Coffey DS, Walsh PC, et al. The development of human benign prostatic hyperplasia with age. J Urol. 1984;132:474–479.
3. Shapiro E, Becich MJ, Hartanö V, et al. The relative proportion of stromal and epithelial hyperplasia as related to the development of clinical BPH. J Urol. 1992;147:1293–1297.
4. Pool JL, Kirby RS. Clinical significance of α_1-adrenoceptor selectivity in the management of benign prostatic hyperplasia. Int Urol Nephrol. 2001;33:407–412.
5. Isaacs JT. Importance of the natural history of benign prostatic hyperplasia in the evaluation of pharmacologic intervention. Prostate 1990; 3(suppl):1–7.
6. Wilt TJ, Down JN. Benign prostatic hyperplasia. Part 2-management. BMJ. 2008;336:206–210.
7. AUA Practice Guidelines Committee. AUA guideline on the management of benign prostatic hyperplasia (2010). www.auanet.org/content/guidelines-and-quality care/clinical-guidelines.cfm?sub=bph. Last accessed July 30, 2014.
8. Mirone V, Sessa A, Giuliano F, et al. Current benign prostatic hyperplasia treatment: Impact on sexual function and management of related sexual adverse effects. Int J Clin Pract. 2011;65:1005–1013.
9. Flanigan RC, Reda DJ, Wasson JH, et al. 5-year outcomes of surgical resection and watchful waiting for men with moderately symptomatic BPH: A department of Veterans Affairs cooperative study. J Urol. 1998;160:12–16.
10. Lin VC, Liao C, Kuo H. Progression of lower urinary tract symptoms after discontinuation of 1 medication from 2-year combined alpha blocker and 5-alpha-reductase inhibitor therapy for benign prostatic hyperplasia in men-a randomized multicenter study. Urology. 2014;83:416–421.
11. Cohen SA, Parsons JK. Combination pharmacological therapies for the management of benign prostatic hyperplasia. Drugs Aging. 2012;29:275–284.
12. Djavan B, Eckersberger E, Johannes Handl M, et al. Durability and retreatment rates of minimally invasive-treatments of benign prostatic hyperplasia: A cross-analysis of the literature. Can J Urol. 2010;17:5249–5254.
13. Oelke M, Bachmann A, Descazeaud A, et al. EAU guidelines on the treatment and follow-up of non-neurogenic male lower urinary tract symptoms including benign prostatic obstruction. Eur Urol. 2013;64:118–140.
14. Lourenco T, Pickard R, Vale L, et al. Minimally invasive treatments of benign prostatic enlargement: Systematic review of randomized controlled trials. BMJ. 2008 Oct 3;337:a1662. doi:10.1136/bmj.a1662.
15. Dedhia RC, Vary KT. Phytotherapy for lower urinary tract symptoms secondary to benign prostatic hyperplasia. J Urol. 2006;179:2119–2125.
16. Macdonald R, Tacklind JW, Rutks I, et al. Serenoa repens monotherapy for benign prostatic hyperplasia (BPH): an updated Cochrane systemic review. BJU Int. 2012;109:1756–61.
17. Lepor H, Kazzazi A, Djavan B. α-Blockers for benign prostatic hyperplasia: The new era. Curr Opin Urol. 2012;22:7–15.
18. Liao CH, Guh JH, Chueh SC. Anti-angiogenic effects and mechanism of prazosin. Prostate. 2011;71:976–984.
19. Dutkiewicz S. Long term treatment with doxazosin in men with benign prostatic hyperplasia: 10 year follow up. Intern Urol Nephrol. 2004;36:169–173.
20. Kaplan SA, Neutel J. Vasodilatory factors in treatment of older men with symptomatic benign prostatic hyperplasia. Urology. 2006;67:225–231.
21. Rossi M, Roumequere T. Silodosin in the treatment of benign prostatic hyperplasia. Drug Des Dev Ther. 2010;4:291–297.
22. Lepor H, Kazzazi A, Djavan B. α-Blockers for benign prostatic hyperplasia: The new era. Curr Opin Urol. 2012;22:7–15.
23. Bird ST, Delaney JA, Brophy JM, et al. Tamsulosin treatment for benign prostatic hyperplasia and risk of severe hypotension in men aged 40-85 years in the United States" risk window analyses using between and within patient methodology. BMJ. 2013 Nov 5;347:f6320. Doi:10.1136/bmj.f6320.
24. Davis BR, Cutler JA, Gordon DJ, et al, for the ALLHAT Research Group. Rationale and design for the antihypertensive and lipid lowering treatment to prevent heart attack trial (ALLHAT). Am J Hypertens. 1996;9:342–360.
25. Hellstrom WJ, Sikka SC. Effects of acute treatment with tamsulosin versus alfuzosin on ejaculatory function in normal volunteers. J Urol. 2007;177:1587–1588.

26. Strittmatter F, Gratzke C, Stief CG, et al. Current pharmacological treatment options for male lower urinary tract symptoms. Expert Opin Pharmacother. 2013;14:1043–1054.
27. Friedman AH. Tamsulosin and the intraoperative floppy iris syndrome. JAMA. 2009;301:2044–2045.
28. Bell CM, Hatch WV, Fischer HD, et al. Association between tamsulosin and serious ophthalmic adverse events in older men following cataract surgery. JAMA. 2009;301:1991–1996.
29. Nieminen T, Tammela TLJ, Koobi T, et al. The effects of tamsulosin and sildenafil in separate and combined regimens on detailed hemodynamics in patients with benign prostatic enlargement. J Urol. 2006;176:2551–2556.
30. Roehrborn CG. Male lower urinary tract symptoms (LUTS) and benign prostatic hyperplasia (BPH). Med Clin North Am. 2011;95:87–100.
31. Wu C, Kappor A. Dutasteride for the treatment of benign prostatic hyperplasia. Expert Opin Pharmacother. 2013;141:1399–1408.
32. Roehrborn CG, Bruskewitz R, Nickel JC, et al. Sustained decrease in incidence of acute urinary retention and surgery with finasteride for 6 years in men with benign prostatic hyperplasia. J Urol. 2004;171:1194–1198.
33. Roehrborn CG, Marks LS, Fenter T, et al. Efficacy and safety of dutasteride in the four-year treatment of men with benign prostatic hyperplasia. Urology. 2004;63:709–715.
34. McConnell JD, Roehrborn CG, Bautista OM, et al. The long term effect of doxazosin, finasteride, and combination therapy on the clinical progression of benign prostatic hyperplasia. N Engl J Med. 2003;349:2389–2398.
35. Roehrborn CG, Siami P, Barkin J, et al. The effects of combination therapy with dutasteride and tamsulosin on clinical outcomes in men with symptomatic benign prostatic hyperplasia: 4 year results from the CombAT study. Eur Urol. 2010;57:123–131.
36. Thompson IM, Goodman PJ, Tangen CM, et al. The influence of finasteride on the development of prostate cancer. N Engl J Med. 2003;349:215–224.
37. Andriole GI, Bostwick DG, Brawley OW, et al. Effect of dutasteride on the risk of prostate cancer. N Engl J Med. 2010;362:1192–202.
38. Roehrborn CG, Nickel JC, Andriole GL, et al. Dutasteride improves outcomes of benign prostatic hyperplasia when evaluated for prostate cancer risk reduction: Secondary analysis of the Reduction of dutasteride of prostate cancer events (REDUCE) Trial. Urology. 2011;78:641–646.
39. Barkin J, Guimaraes M, Jacobi G, et al. Alpha-blocker therapy can be withdrawn in the majority of men following initial combination therapy with the dual 5-alpha reductase inhibitor dutasteride. Eur Urol. 2003;44:461–466.
40. Rovner ES, Kreder K, Sussman DO, et al. Effect of tolterodine extended release with or without tamsulosin on measures of urgency and patient reported outcomes in men with lower urinary tract symptoms. J Urol. 2008;180:1034–1041.
41. Andersson KE. Antimuscarinic mechanisms and the overactive detrusor: An update. Eur Urol. 2011;59:377–386.
42. Oelke M, Baard J, Wijkstra H, et al. Age and bladder outlet obstruction are independently associated with detrusor overactivity in patients with benign prostatic hyperplasia. Eur Urol. 2008;54:419–426.
43. Filson CP, Hollingsworth JM, Clemens JQ et al. The efficacy and safety of combined therapy with α-blockers and anticholinergics for men with benign prostatic hyperplasia: A meta-analysis. J Urol. 2013;190:2153–2160.
44. Dong Y, Shi Z, Wang G, et al. Efficacy and safety of tadalafil monotherapy for lower urinary tract symptoms secondary to benign prostatic hyperplasia: A meta-analysis. Urol Int. 2013;91:10–18.
45. Gacci M, Corona G, Salvi M, et al. A systematic review and meta-analysis on the use of phosphodiesterase 5 inhibitors alone or in combination with α-blockers for lower urinary tract symptoms due to benign prostatic hyperplasia. Eur Urol. 2012;61:994–1003.
46. Casabe A, Roehrborn C, DaPozzo LF, et al. Efficacy and safety of the coadministration of tadalafil once daily with finasteride for 6 months in men with lower urinary tract symptoms and prostatic enlargement secondary to benign prostatic hyperplasia. J Urol. 2014;191:727–733.
47. Lythgoe C, Vary KT. The use of PDE-5 inhibitors in the treatment of lower urinary tract symptoms due to benign prostatic hyperplasia. Curr Urol Rep. 2013;14:585–594.
48. Curran MP. Tadalafil in the treatment of signs and symptoms of benign prostatic hyperplasia with or without erectile dysfunction. Drugs aging. 2012;29:771–781.
49. Nehra A, Jackson G, Miner M, et al. The Princeton III Consensus recommendations for the management of erectile dysfunction and cardiovascular disease. Mayo Clin Proc. 2012;87:766–778.
50. Otsuki H, Kosaka T, Nakamura K, et al. β_3 adrenoceptor agonist mirabegron is effective for overactive bladder that is unresponsive to antimuscarinic treatment or is related to benign prostatic hyperplasia in men. Int Urol Nephrol. 2013;45:53–60.

53 Urinary Incontinence and Pediatric Enuresis

Sum Lam

LEARNING OBJECTIVES

Upon completion of the chapter, the reader will be able to:

1. Explain the pathophysiology of the major types of urinary incontinence (UI): urge, stress, overflow, and functional.
2. Recognize the signs and symptoms of the major types of UI in individual patients.
3. List the treatment goals for a patient with UI.
4. Compare and contrast available therapeutic agents for managing UI; identify factors that guide drug selection for an individual patient.
5. Formulate a monitoring plan and provide patient counseling for a patient on a given treatment regimen based on patient-specific information.
6. Explain the pathophysiology of pediatric enuresis.
7. List treatment goals; compare and contrast available therapeutic agents for managing pediatric enuresis.
8. Formulate a patient-specific monitoring plan and implement patient counseling for a patient on a given treatment regimen.
9. Describe nonpharmacologic treatment approaches for pediatric enuresis.

URINARY INCONTINENCE

INTRODUCTION

Urinary incontinence (UI) is defined as the complaint of involuntary leakage of urine.[1] It is often associated with other bothersome lower urinary tract symptoms such as urgency, increased daytime frequency, and **nocturia**. Despite its prevalence across the lifespan and in both sexes, it remains an underreported health problem that can negatively impact an individual's quality of life. Patients with UI may sense a loss of self-control, independence and self-esteem, and often modify their activities for fear of an "accident." Patients with UI may also suffer from other consequences, including perineal dermatitis and infections, pressure ulcers, urinary tract infections (UTIs) and falls. In the United States, the estimated national cost of urge urinary incontinence (UUI) in 2007 was $66 billion, with projected costs of $76 billion in 2015 and $83 billion in 2020.[2]

EPIDEMIOLOGY AND ETIOLOGY

The true prevalence of UI is unclear because of varying definitions of UI and reporting bias.[3]

- About 44% of noninstitutionalized persons aged 65 and older reported UI[4]
- 7% to 37% of women aged 20 to 39 report some degree of UI
- 9% to 39% of women age 60 and over report daily UI
- 11 to 34% among older men report some degree of UI
- 2 to 11% of older men reporting daily UI
- In the noninstitutionalized setting, more than 50% of elderly women and more than 25% of elderly men reported UI
- 46% of short-term and 76% of long-term nursing home residents report UI[4]

UI can result from abnormalities within (intrinsic to) and outside of (extrinsic to) the urinary tract. Within the urinary tract, abnormalities may occur in the urethra (including the bladder outlet and urinary sphincters), the bladder, or a combination of both structures. Focusing on abnormalities in these two structures, a simple classification scheme emerges for all but the rarest intrinsic causes of UI. KEY CONCEPT *Accurate diagnosis and classification of UI type is critical to the selection of appropriate drug therapy.*

PATHOPHYSIOLOGY

Stress Urinary Incontinence[5]

Stress urinary incontinence (SUI) occurs most frequently in women and is related to the underactivity of urethra and/or urethral sphincters, leading to inadequate resistance to impede urine flow from the bladder. SUI occurs when intra-abdominal pressure is elevated by exertional activities like exercise, running, lifting, coughing, and sneezing. SUI is usually episodic, associated with small volume leakage and rarely causes nocturia or **enuresis**. The etiology for urethral underactivity is not

Patient Encounter 1, Part 1

A 62-year-old Asian woman presents to the clinic with the chief complaint of "not being able to make it to the toilet in time." Every day she experiences a strong, sudden urge to urinate which is difficult to postpone. She makes about 10 trips to a bathroom while awake on a daily basis and gets up twice each night to urinate. She reports no clothes-wetting accidents so far, but is fearful of the embarrassment, especially when she is in the public. Because of the urinary condition, she has given up shopping in large malls, which was her favorite pastime. She also avoided several social and family events in the past month. She states that "life would be so much better if I don't need to run for the bathroom." She denies any urinary leakage when she coughs, laughs, or exercises. Her PVR is less than10 mL. She is diagnosed with overactive bladder without urinary incontinence.

List symptoms that are consistent with her diagnosis.

What additional information do you need to know before creating a treatment plan for this patient?

completely understood, although the loss of the trophic effects of estrogen on the uroepithelium at menopause is thought to be important. The peak of SUI prevalence in the perimenopausal years supports this hypothesis. Clearly established risk factors for SUI include the following:

- Pregnancy (increased risk with increased parity)
- Childbirth (vaginal delivery)
- Menopause
- Cognitive impairment
- Obesity
- Increasing age

SUI is exceedingly rare in males unless the sphincter mechanism is compromised by surgery or trauma. The most common surgeries predisposing to SUI in males are radical prostatectomy for prostate cancer and transurethral resection of the prostate for benign prostatic hyperplasia (BPH).

Urge Urinary Incontinence[5]

UUI is related to the overactivity of detrusor muscle in the bladder, which contracts inappropriately during the filling (urinary storage) phase and generates urgency, or a compelling desire to void which is difficult to defer. The bladder contractions are due to the stimulation of muscarinic cholinergic receptors, especially M2 and M3 subtypes. UUI is associated with large volume leakage, sometimes complete bladder emptying, nocturia and enuresis; thus UUI may disrupt sleep. Overactive bladder (OAB) is a symptom syndrome with or without associated UUI.[6]

Most women with UUI or OAB have no identifiable causes (idiopathic), while in men similar symptoms are associated with benign prostatic hyperplasia (See Chapter 52). Overactivity may be myogenic and/or neurogenic. Clearly established risk factors for UUI include:

- Older age
- Neurologic disorders (eg, stroke, Parkinson disease, multiple sclerosis, and spinal cord injury)
- Bladder outlet obstruction (eg, benign or malignant prostatic enlargement or hyperplasia)
- Hysterectomy
- Recurrent UTIs

Overflow Urinary Incontinence[5]

Overflow urinary incontinence (OUI) is a less common form of UI in men or women. It is related to urethral overactivity and/or bladder underactivity. In short, the bladder is filled to capacity at all times but cannot empty, causing urine to leak out episodically. If caused by bladder underactivity, the progressively weakened detrusor muscle eventually loses the ability to voluntarily contract, which lead to incomplete voiding and large residual urinary volume after micturition. Both myogenic and neurogenic factors have been associated with impaired bladder contractility that leads to OUI. Common neurogenic factors are diabetes, lower spinal cord injury, multiple sclerosis, or radical pelvic surgery.

If due to urethral overactivity, incomplete bladder emptying occurs because the resistance of the urethra and/or sphincters cannot be overcome by detrusor contractility. In men, this most frequently occurs in cases of long-term chronic bladder outlet obstruction due to BPH, prostate cancer, or abdominal-pelvic surgeries. In women, urethral overactivity is rare, but may result from cystocele formation or surgical overcorrection for SUI. In both genders, systemic neurologic diseases such as multiple sclerosis or spinal cord injury may be the etiology.

Functional UI[5]

Functional UI is generally caused by extrinsic factors to the urinary tract, such as:

- Immobility (due to pain, physical limitations)
- Inadequate or delayed access to toileting facilities
- Neurologic impairment (Parkinson disease, multiple sclerosis, spinal cord injury, stroke, apathy due to depression)
- UTIs
- Postmenopausal atrophic urethritis and/or vaginitis
- Diabetes mellitus (glucosuria leading to polyuria)
- Diabetes insipidus (polyuria due to decreased antidiuretic hormone [ADH])

Clinical Presentation of Stress Urinary Incontinence (SUI) Related to Urethral Underactivity[5]

General

Usually occurs during activities like exercise, running, lifting, coughing, or sneezing; much more common in females.

Symptoms

Urine leakage volume is proportional to activity level; not associated with nocturia. No SUI with physical inactivity, especially when supine. May develop urgency and frequency as a compensatory mechanism (or independently as a separate component of bladder overactivity).

Diagnostic Tests

Observation of urethral meatus (opening) while patient coughs or strains.

Clinical Presentation of Urge Urinary Incontinence (UUI) Related to Bladder Overactivity[5]

General

If sensory input from the lower urinary tract is absent, may have bladder overactivity and urine leakage without urgency. Patient with overactive bladder (OAB) may not have UUI.

Symptoms

Patients with OAB typically present with symptoms of urgency, frequency (8 or more micturitions in 24 hours), nocturia (one or more awakening per night to void) with or without UUI.

Diagnostic Tests

Urodynamic studies are the gold standard for diagnosis. Urinary tract infection must be ruled out by urinalysis and urine culture.

Clinical Presentation of Overflow Urinary Incontinence (OUI) Related to Urethral Overactivity and/or Bladder Underactivity[5]

General

Rare type of UI in both genders. Urehral overactivity is usually due to prostatic enlargement (males) or cystocele formation or surgical overcorrection for SUI (females). Bladder underactivity is usually due to a weakened detrusor muscle.

Symptoms

Lower abdominal fullness, hesitancy, straining to void, decreased force of stream, interrupted stream, sense of incomplete bladder emptying. May have urinary frequency and urgency, as well as abdominal pain if acute urinary retention occurs.

Signs

Increased postvoid residual urine volume.

- Pelvic malignancy (extrinsic pressure on urinary tract structures causing obstruction)
- Constipation or fecal impaction
- Congenital malformations of the urinary tract system

Mixed and Drug-Induced UI[5]

Mixed urinary incontinence (MUI) occurs when two or more types of UI coexist in a given patient, which may lead to diagnostic and therapeutic difficulties. Patients may experience worsening of symptom due to the opposing effects of treatments indicated for specific and different types of UI.

KEY CONCEPT *Many medications can influence the lower urinary tract system, and can precipitate or aggravate existing voiding dysfunction that leads to UI* (Table 53–1).

CLINICAL PRESENTATION AND DIAGNOSIS

Guidelines are available for the assessment and diagnosis of UI or OAB.[6–8] In general, obtaining a complete medical history and performing a targeted physical examination are essential to correctly classify the type(s) of UI. The degree of annoyance perceived by the patient due to urinary symptoms must be assessed, although it may not correlate well with quantitative tests such as symptom frequency/severity, use of absorbent products, and postvoid residual (PVR) urine volume (Table 53-2). Major components of the physical examination include the following:[5]

- Abdominal examination for distended bladder, organomegaly, and masses
- Neurologic evaluation of perineum and lower extremities to evaluate lumbosacral nerve function (includes digital rectal

Table 53–1

Medications Influencing Lower Urinary Tract Function

Medication	Effect
Diuretics	Polyuria, frequency, urgency
α-Adrenoceptor antagonists	Urethral relaxation: may relieve obstruction in males, induces/worsens SUI in females
α-Adrenoceptor agonists	Urethral constriction: aggravates obstruction in males (may cause urinary retention), potential SUI treatment in females
Calcium channel blockers (dihydropyridines)	Urethral constriction (may cause urinary retention), especially in males
Opioid analgesics	Impaired bladder contractility (may cause urinary retention)
Sedative-hypnotics	Functional UI due to immobility, delirium, sedation
Psychotherapeutics with anticholinergic properties; anticholinergics	Urinary retention due to impaired bladder contractility or potential UUI treatment
TCAs	Combination of anticholinergic and α-adrenoceptor blocking activities can lead to unpredictable effects on UI
Ethanol	Polyuria and frequency (via effects on ADH), functional UI (delirium, sedation), urgency
ACEIs	Cough leading to SUI (ARBs do not induce cough)
Cyclophosphamide	Hemorrhagic cystitis due to acrolein metabolite (prevent with MESNA)

ACEIs, angiotensin-converting enzyme inhibitors; ADH, antidiuretic hormone (or vasopressin); ARB, angiotensin II receptor blocker; MESNA, sodium 2-mercaptoethanesulfonate; SUI, stress urinary incontinence; TCA, tricyclic antidepressant; UI, urinary incontinence; UUI, urge urinary incontinence.

Table 53–2

Items to Address during Diagnostic Evaluation of UI

Item	Comments
Urine Leakage	
Use of absorbent products	Type(s), quantity, times of day worn
Urine leakage per episode	Dribbling, small or large volumes, intermittently; Consistent or varied quantities
Precipitants	Physical activity, excessive fluid intake, drug(s)
Times of day	Daytime/nighttime/both
Symptoms	
Urgency	Frequency, severity, duration from urge onset to micturition
Frequency	Daytime/nighttime/both, how often
Nocturia	How often, proportion associated with UI
Obstructive symptoms	Type(s) (hesitancy, strain to void, decreased force of stream, start and stop stream, sense of incomplete emptying), severity
Lower abdominal fullness	Frequency, severity
Comorbidities	
Current medication use	See Table 53–1. Remember CAMs, OTCs
Evidence of preexisting or new-onset:	
Diabetes mellitus	
Metastatic or genitourinary malignancy	
Multiple sclerosis or other neurologic disease	
CNS disease above the pons	Usually UUI
Spinal cord injury	UUI or OUI, depending on level and degree of completeness of injury
Recent nongenitourinary surgery	Functional UI
Previous local surgery/radiation	Prostate surgery, lower abdominal cavity surgery (direct injury versus denervation), radiation (direct injury)
Gynecologic history	Childbirth (vaginal versus cesarean section), prior gynecologic surgery, hormonal status (pre- versus peri- versus postmenopausal)
Pelvic floor disease	Constipation, diarrhea, fecal incontinence, dyspareunia, sexual dysfunction, pelvic pain
UTI	Dysuria, CVA tenderness, frequency
Gross hematuria	Possible bladder or other genitourinary cancer

CAM, complementary and alternative medications; CVA, costovertebral angle; OTC, over-the-counter; OUI, overflow urinary incontinence; UTI, urinary tract infection; UUI, urge urinary incontinence.

examination to check rectal tone, reflexes, ability to perform a voluntary pelvic muscle contraction in females; size and surface quality of prostate in males)

- Pelvic examination in women for evidence of prolapse of bladder, small bowel, rectum, or uterus, or signs of estrogen deficiency
- Genital/prostate exam in men
- Urinalysis, PVR urine volume
- Direct observation of urethral meatus (opening) when patient coughs/strains (urine spurt consistent with SUI) (cough stress test)
- Perineal examination for skin maceration, redness, breakdown, ulceration, and evidence of fungal skin infection
- Optional: voiding diary, assessment of incontinence severity[9] (Table 53–3), quality-of-life measures

TREATMENT

Desired and realistic treatment outcomes should be individualized and discussed with each patient. KEY CONCEPT *The treatment goals for UI may change with time, often requires reaching a compromise between efficacy and tolerability of drug therapy.*

Desired Outcomes

- Restoration of continence
- Reduction of the number of UI episodes (daytime and nighttime) and nocturia
- Prevention or delaying of complications associated with UI (eg, pressure ulcers, skin conditions)
- Minimization of adverse effects and costs related to treatment
- Improvement in quality of life

Nonpharmacologic Treatment

At the primary care level, nonsurgical, nonpharmacologic intervention constitutes the chief approach to the management of UI. It has no adverse reactions, is minimally invasive, and can be utilized adjunctively with other treatment modalities. KEY CONCEPT *Nonpharmacologic treatment gives at least an additive effect in efficacy when combined with drug therapy, and can allow the use of lower drug doses.* It is ideal for patients who fit the following scenarios:

- Medically unfit for surgery
- Planning for pregnancies/childbirths, which can compromise the long-term results of certain types of continence surgery

Table 53–3

Overactive Bladder Symptom Score (OABSS)

Question	Symptom	Score	Frequency Over the Past
1	How many times do you typically urinate from waking in the morning until going to bed in the evening?	0	7 or less
		1	8–14
		2	15 or more
2	How many times do you typically wake up to urinate from going to sleep at night until waking in the morning?	0	0
		1	1
		2	2
		3	3 or more
3	How often do you have a sudden compelling desire to urinate, which is difficult to postpone?	0	Not at all
		1	Less than once week
		2	Once a week or more
		3	About once a day
		4	2–4 times a day
		5	5 times a day or more
4	How often do you leak urine because you cannot postpone the sudden desire to urinate?	0	Not at all
		1	Less than once week
		2	Once a week or more
		3	About once a day
		4	2–4 times a day
		5	5 times a day or more
	Sum of OABSS scores ______		

The sampling period is usually defined as "the past week" but, depending on the usage, it can be amended to, for example, "the past 3 days" or "the past month." Whatever the case, it is necessary to specify the sampling period.

Diagnostic criteria for OAB are "an urgency score for Question 3 of 2 or greater, and an OABSS of 3 or greater." OABSS may also be used for assessing the severity of OAB: a total score of 5 or less (mild), 6 to 11 (moderate), and 12 or more (severe).

- Having OUI whose condition is not amenable to surgical or drug treatment
- Avoiding drug therapy or surgery due to safety concern or patient preference

These approaches include lifestyle/behavioral modifications, fluid management, scheduled voiding regimens, pelvic floor muscle rehabilitation (PFMR), external neuromodulation, anti-incontinence devices, acupuncture, and supportive interventions.[3,5] Many of these are best utilized through attendance at multidisciplinary UI clinics staffed by specialized healthcare providers. Of note, weight loss of 5% to 10% in overweight or obese women has an efficacy similar to that of other nonpharmacologic treatments for treating SUI.

Bladder training and prompted voiding improves symptoms of UUI and MUI. PFMR is an effective treatment for adult women with SUI and MUI.[8] Combination therapy with PFMR plus behavioral training achieved better outcomes than drug therapy in women with UUI.[10] Also, this combination treatment was the only nonpharmacologic treatment that renders true objective evidence of restoring continence.[11] However, these methods require motivation from patients. Medical conditions, such as cognitive dysfunction, may interfere with active participation and compromise efficacy. Regular follow-up is important for monitoring outcomes and for providing reassurance and support. Lifestyle/behavioral interventions should be continued during drug therapy in patients with UI, even if the results have not fully achieved the desired outcomes.

External neuromodulation may include nonimplantable electrical stimulation, percutaneous tibial nerve stimulation, or extracorporeal magnetic stimulation. This treatment option is typically prescribed when traditional PFMR has failed. Anti-incontinence devices, such as bed alarms, catheters, pessaries, penile clamps, and external collection devices, are reserved for special situations depending on patient's symptoms, cognition, mobility status, and overall health status. Supportive interventions such as physical therapy may be beneficial for patients with muscle weakness and slow gait that hinder their reach to the toilet in a timely manner. Last, absorbent products provide greater patient confidence in dealing with unpredictable urine loss.[5]

Surgery is rarely an initial treatment for UI; only considered in patients with significantly bothersome symptoms, and when nonsurgical options are undesired or ineffective. Surgery is not as helpful for bladder underactivity but can be used to manage urethral overactivity due to BPH and bladder outlet obstruction (via endoscopic incision using a cystoscope). It is most effective for SUI by stabilizing the urethra and bladder neck and/or augmenting urethral resistance. Common approaches are injection of periurethral bulking agents and midurethral sling procedure. In males, SUI is best treated by implanting an artificial urinary sphincter.[5]

Posterior tibial nerve stimulation is an office-based percutaneous treatment for UUI or OAB. Therapy consists of weekly 30-minute treatments with a needle placed posterior to the medial malleolus of the ankle over the course of 3 months. Efficacy appears similar to or slightly better than oral pharmacotherapy.[5]

Surgical treatment for UUI generally consists of implantation of a sacral nerve stimulator (neuromodulation) or endoscopic

Patient Encounter 1, Part 2: Medical History, Physical Examination, and Diagnostic Tests

PMH: Hypertension, dyslipidemia, seasonal allergy

FH: Noncontributory

SH: Retired high school teacher; now volunteers as a story teller at a local daycare center. Widowed and lives alone. Two married daughters (ages 30 and 32 years) live in the neighborhood. Denies tobacco or alcohol use; drinks five cups of coffee in the morning and two cups of herbal tea at bedtime

All: NKDA

Meds: Lisinopril 10 mg once daily; simvastatin 20 mg once daily; OTC allergy meds as needed for itchy eyes

ROS: Alert, sociable, and pleasant. (–) UI or recent history of UTIs; (+) nocturia; dysuria, lower abdominal fullness, or decreased force of stream

PE:

Gen: Postmenopausal woman with mild kyphosis; NAD

VS: BP 140/80 mm Hg, HR 75 beats/min, RR 18 breaths/min, T 98.3°F (36.8°C), Wt 63 kg, Ht 5′5″ (165 cm)

HEENT: PERRLA; EOMI, TMs WNL

Neck/LN: Supple w/o LAD or masses

Lungs/Thorax: CTA

CV: RRR w/o murmurs, rubs, gallops

Abd: soft, NT/ND w/o masses; (+) BS; bladder not palpable

GU: WNL; no atrophic vaginitis or uterine prolapse

MS/Ext: WNL, no edema

Neuro: DTRs 2+, CN II–XII intact

Labs: Na 135 mEq/L (134 mmol/L); K 4.0 mEq/L (4.0 mmol/L); Cl 100 mEq/L (100 mmol/L); CO_2 22 mEq/L (22 mmol/L); BUN 9 mg/dL (3.2 mmol/L); SCr 1.0 mg/dL (88 μmol/L); Fasting glucose 90 mg/dL(5.0 mmol/L); Hb 12 g/dL (120 g/L; 7.45 mmol/L); Hct 37% (0.37); Plts 300,000/mm^3 (300 × 10^9/L); WBC 6.1 × 10^3/mm^3 (6.1 × 10^9/L) with normal differential

LFTs within normal limits

UA not indicated

Given this additional information, what is your assessment of the patient's condition?

What are the goals of pharmacotherapy for this patient?

What nonpharmacologic and pharmacologic alternatives are available to the patient?

office based injection of botulinum toxin A directly into the smooth or striated muscle.[5] The injections are performed in the office generally with local anesthesia. The duration of effect of the toxin is about 4 to 8 months after which repeat injection is necessary to maintain effect. Intravesical (bladder) botulinum toxin A injections increased bladder capacity/compliance and improved quality of life in patients with refractory OAB.[5]

Patients with UUI and an elevated PVR urine volume may require intermittent self-catheterization along with frequent voiding between catheterizations. Surgical placement of a suprapubic catheter may be necessary in cases when intermittent catheterization is not possible. Catheterization can be combined with pharmacologic treatment for symptom relief.[5]

Pharmacologic Treatment

The ideal treatment agent must have clinical efficacy, minimal side effects, minimal drug–drug/drug–disease interactions, convenient administration, and low cost. KEY CONCEPT *Patient characteristics (eg, age, comorbidities, concurrent drug therapies, and ability to adhere to the prescribed regimen) can influence drug therapy selection.*[5] Although a recent systematic review has shed light on the comparative data on newer agents,[12,13] selection of an initial agent should be based on patient individual characteristics.

▶ *Urge Urinary Incontinence*

Anticholinergic/Antimuscarinic Antimuscarinic agents are the first-line pharmacologic treatment for UUI or OAB (Table 53–4).[6] They are effective in suppressing premature detrusor contractions, enhancing bladder storage, and relieving symptoms. When used with or without bladder training, these agents improved symptoms and quality of life in patients with UUI or OAB; however, they restore continence in less than 15% of patients and reduce episodes of incontinence by only 0.5 to 1 episodes per day.[12,14,15] They are considered equally effective based on statistical superiority over placebo or active controls.

All antimuscarinic agents have similar contraindications and precautions, including urinary retention, gastric retention, and uncontrolled narrow-angle glaucoma.[5] Older immediate release (IR) agents, such as oxybutynin and tolterodine, have been associated with higher rates of dry mouth, constipation, headache, dyspepsia, dry eyes, cognitive impairment, tachycardia, and urinary retention (Table 53–5). Older patients are especially susceptible to these adverse events. Significant dry mouth can be associated with dental caries, ill-fitting dentures, and swallowing difficulty. Chewing sugarless gum or use of saliva substitutes can help to alleviate dry mouth.

Orthostatic hypotension and sedation can be particularly troublesome to patients with cognitive impairment or at risk for falls. Issues with tolerability and multiple daily dose administration associated with IR products may jeopardize medication adherence and can prevent dose titration to achieve optimal clinical response. Thus, these IR products are not preferred in patients with functional limitations and/or those who are already taking complicated drug regimens. Nevertheless, adverse events are not universal and the severity varies with individuals. Older agents, when initiated at the lowest possible doses and gradually titrated, are reasonable to consider in patients where a long-acting product is undesirable.

Extended-release (ER) agents (oxybutynin XL, tolterodine LA, trospium ER, darifenacin ER, fesoterodine ER) cause less dry mouth compared with IR products.[5,7,15] These products cannot be chewed, crushed, or divided, and must be swallowed whole. Oxybutynin transdermal patch and topical gel are alternatives for patients who cannot take or tolerate oral drugs; they have lower rates of dry mouth but are associated with application site

Table 53–4

Approved Drugs for the Management of UUI

Parameter	Oxybutynin	Tolterodine	Trospium Chloride	Solifenacin	Darifenacin	Fesoterodine	Mirabegron
Dosage forms	IR tablets, solution SR-ER tablets, SR-TD patch, topical gel	IR tablets SR-LA capsules	IR tablets ER tablets	IR tablets	ER tablets	ER tablets	ER tablets
Dosing	IR: 2.5–5 mg 2–4 times daily (pediatrics 0.3–0.5 mg/kg/day in three doses) SR (oral): 5–30 mg once daily (pediatrics:0.3–0.5 mg/kg/day) SR (TD): 3.9 mg/day patch applied twice weekly; available over-the-counter SR (gel): 1 sachet (100 mg) applied once daily	IR: 1 or 2 mg twice daily (pediatrics: 1 mg twice daily) ER: 2 or 4 mg once daily (pediatrics: 2 mg once daily)	IR: 20 mg twice daily ER: 60 mg once daily	5–10 mg once daily	7.5–15 mg once daily	4–8 mg once daily	25 mg once daily, then 50 mg once daily after 8 weeks
Kinetics	Active metabolite (N-desethyl) Not altered in renal or hepatic disease or advanced age	Active metabolite (5-hydroxymethyl) Polymorphic metabolism (CYP 2D6) Not altered in advanced age. Significantly altered in hepatic disease (decreased CL in cirrhosis) and renal disease (decreased CL)	Food: decreased BA by 70%–80% Significantly altered in renal disease (decreased CL) but not in hepatic disease or advanced age	Metabolized via CYP 3A4 but only one active metabolite (4-hydroxy) Significantly altered in severe renal impairment, moderate hepatic impairment (Child-Pugh B), and advanced age (decreased CL in all)	Complex metabolism (polymorphic CYP 2D6, CYP 3A4) Not altered in advanced age, renal impairment, mild hepatic impairment (Child-Pugh A) Significantly altered in moderate hepatic impairment (Child-Pugh B) (decreased CL)	Prodrug (for 5-hydroxmethyl tolterodine) Inactive metabolites Not altered in advanced age Significantly altered in renal disease (decreased CL) and moderate hepatic impairment (Child-Pugh B) (decreased CL)	Terminal elimination half-life 50 hours Moderate inhibitor of CYP 2D6
Contraindications and precautions	Use with caution if CYP 3A4 inhibitors are also being taken (decreased oxybutynin CL)	Reduce dose 50% in those taking CYP 3A4 inhibitor(s) or with hepatic cirrhosis or with CrCl less than 30 mL/min (0.50 mL/s) Antacid-SR (oral) prep, interaction (dose-dumping) (not seen with PPIs)	Give on empty stomach Decrease dose 50% when CrCl < 30 mL/min (0.50 mL/s) and use IR formulation	Do not exceed 5 mg/day if CrCl < 30 mL/min (0.50 mL/s), patient has moderate hepatic impairment, or patient is taking CYP 3A4 inhibitor(s) If severe hepatic impairment, do not use	Do not exceed 7.5 mg/day if patient is taking potent CYP 3A4 inhibitor(s) Use caution if patient is taking moderate CYP 3A4 inhibitor(s) or CYP 3A4 or 2D6 substrate(s) Do not chew, divide, or crush the ER tablets	Do not exceed 4 mg/day if CrCl less than 30 mL/min (0.50 mL/s) or patient is taking potent CYP 3A4 inhibitor(s) If severe hepatic impairment, do not use	Limit dose to 25 mg once daily if severe renal impairment or moderate hepatic disease Avoid in end-stage renal disease or severe hepatic impairment, or more BP 180/110 mmHg Monitor for increased BP and urinary retention

BA, bioavailability; BP, blood pressure; CL, total body clearance; CrCl, creatinine clearance; TD, transdermal; ER, extended release; IR, immediate release; LA, long acting; PPIs, proton pump inhibitors; SR, sustained release.

Patient Encounter 1, Part 3: Creating a Care Plan

Patient prefers to try a drug that is least likely to cause dry mouth. She is willing to try topical agents.

Based on the information presented, create a care plan for this patient's OAB. Your plan should include:

(a) A statement of the drug-related needs and/or problems

(b) The goals of therapy

(c) A patient-specific detailed therapeutic plan, including patient counseling to enhance medication adherence, ensure successful therapy, and minimize adverse effects

(d) A plan for follow-up to evaluate therapeutic outcome and drug tolerability

reactions. Rotation of application sites can be helpful to minimize the side effects.

Patients receiving any antimuscarinic agent should be informed about sedation as a possible side effect and warned against operating heavy machinery, such as driving, especially during the initial phase of therapy. Patients with existing cognitive dysfunction or difficulty with balance should be monitored closely for mental status changes and risk for falls. Older individuals are more prone to have constipation of age-related physiologic changes and the increased likelihood of receiving other medications that may exacerbate constipation. Patients should be advised to contact their physician if they experience severe abdominal pain or become constipated for 3 or more days. An important drug–drug interaction to avoid is the concurrent use of acetylcholinesterase inhibitors, which are used to treat dementia (antagonism) and any other anticholinergic agents (increase side effects).[16]

KEY CONCEPT *Antimuscarinic agents should be initiated at the lowest possible dose and gradually titrated upward based on clinical response; not to exceed the maximum recommended doses.* A trial of at least 4 weeks is required to evaluate its efficacy. Consider switching to another agent if the patient reports intolerable side effects or inadequate symptom relief despite optimized dose.

Mirabegron Mirabegron is a β_3-adrenergic agonist approved in June 2012 for the treatment of OAB with UUI. Like antimuscarinic agents, it reduces urinary frequency and incontinence episodes by less than one per day and is also considered the first-line drug therapy for OAB (see Table 53–4).[6,17] It increases bladder capacity by relaxing the detrusor smooth muscle during the storage phase of the urinary bladder fill-void cycle. It requires 4 to 8 weeks of therapy for optimal efficacy.[17]

Mirabegron is available in ER tablets, and should be swallowed whole without chewing, dividing, or crushing. Most commonly reported adverse reactions were hypertension (7%–11%), nasopharyngitis (4%), urinary tract infection (3%–6%) and headache (3%–4%). Patient should be monitored for increased blood pressure and urinary retention, particularly in patients with bladder outlet obstruction or those who are taking anticholinergic drugs.[5] Currently, there is no direct comparison of mirabegron and antimuscarinics for efficacy or tolerability.

Older Agents[5] Tricyclic antidepressants (TCA), such as desipramine, nortriptyline, imipramine, and doxepin, are generally no more effective than oxybutynin IR. They may cause potentially serious adverse effects (eg, orthostatic hypotension, cardiac conduction abnormalities, dizziness, and confusion); thus should be limited to individuals who have one or more indicated comorbidities (eg, depression or neuropathic pain); patients with MUI (because of their effect of decreasing bladder contractility and increasing outlet resistance); and possibly those with nocturnal incontinence associated with altered sleep patterns. Propantheline, flavoxate, dicyclomine, and hyoscyamine are not recommended due to lack of efficacy and/or significant adverse effects.[5]

▶ *Stress Urinary Incontinence*

The goal of pharmacologic therapy of urethral underactivity is to improve the urethral closure mechanism:

- Stimulating α-adrenoceptors in the smooth muscle of the proximal urethra and bladder neck
- Enhancing the supportive structures underlying the urethral mucosa
- Enhancing the positive effects of serotonin and norepinephrine in the afferent and efferent pathways of the micturition reflex

Table 53–5

Adverse Event Incidence Rates with Approved Drugs for Bladder Overactivity[a]

Drug	Dry Mouth (%)	Constipation (%)	Dizziness (%)	Vision Disturbance (%)
Oxybutynin IR	71	15	17	10
Oxybutynin XL	61	13	6	14
Oxybutynin TDS	7	3	NR	3
Oxybutynin gel	10	1	3	3
Tolterodine	35	7	5	3
Tolterodine LA	23	6	2	4
Trospium chloride IR	20	10	NR	1
Trospium chloride XR	11	9	NR	2
Solifenacin	20	9	2	5
Darifenacin	24	18	2	2
Fesoterodine	27	5	NR	3
Mirabegron ER	3	3	3	NR

IR, immediate-release; LA, long acting; NR, not reported; TDS, transdermal system; XL, extended-release; XR, extended-release.

[a]All values constitute mean data, predominantly using product information from the manufacturers.

In generally, there is no role for pharmacologic therapy in SUI in men resulting from surgery or trauma.[18] Initial data, however, suggest a possible role for duloxetine added to PFMR in males status postradical prostatectomy, at least over the first 4 to 6 months.[19] Unlike UUI, SUI in women is frequently curable by surgery, thus obviating years of drug therapy that may not provide adequate symptom relief. Surgery (tension-free vaginal tape sling) is a more cost-effective therapy of SUI than duloxetine in women failing PFMR.[20]

Estrogens[5] KEY CONCEPT *Vaginally administered estrogen plays a limited role in managing SUI unless local signs of estrogen deficiency (eg, atrophic urethritis or vaginitis) are present.* Estrogen products are believed to work by a trophic effect on uroepithelial cells and underlying collagenous subcutaneous tissue, enhancement of local microcirculation by increasing the number of periurethral blood vessels, and enhancement of the number and/or sensitivity of α-adrenoceptors.

Since 1940s, estrogens administered by various routes (oral, transdermal, and local) have been used to manage SUI although recent trials showed them to be no better than placebo. Actually, oral hormone replacement therapy increases the risk of new-onset UI (SUI, UUI, MUI) while carrying numerous short- and long-term risks, including mastodynia (pain in the breast), uterine bleeding, nausea, thromboembolism, cardiac/cerebrovascular ischemic events, and breast/endometrial cancer.[11,21] In contrast, local estrogens (estriol [not available in the US] tablets, conjugated equine estrogen cream, estradiol rings, pessaries) have demonstrated subjective improvement in SUI and UI in general.[21,22] Thus, clinicians may consider only locally administered estrogen products for SUI while monitor for individual response (Table 53–6).

α-Adrenoceptor Agonists[5] Phenylpropanolamine, ephedrine and pseudoephedrine have been used alone or with estrogen for mild and moderate SUI. However, recent data showed that they are not better than placebo or PFMR.[21] Phenylpropanolamine has been removed from the market in the United States due to associated risk of ischemic stroke. However, clinicians should be aware that it can still be purchased via the Internet and should discourage its use. Ephedrine, although still available by prescription, should not be used for SUI due to toxicity and lack of efficacy data. The major impediment to using α-adrenoceptor agonists is the extensive list of contraindications (see Table 53–6). Side effects of pseudoephedrine, an over-the-counter drug, include hypertension, headache, dry mouth, nausea, insomnia, and restlessness.

Duloxetine This selective serotonin-norepinephrine reuptake inhibitor can be used for SUI in the United States. It enhances central serotonergic and adrenergic tone, which is involved in ascending and descending control of urethral smooth muscle and the internal urinary sphincter, and thereby enhances urethral and urinary sphincter smooth muscle tone during the filling phase.[23–25] Recent review shows that it slightly improved incontinence,[11] and may give greater benefit when combined with PFMT.[26] Preliminary results suggest that it may also benefit incontinence and quality of life in men with SUI after radical prostatectomy.[26]

The use of duloxetine in SUI is complicated by intolerability (eg, high rates of nausea), numerous precautions or contraindications, cytochrome P450 (CYP) drug–drug interactions, and possibility of withdrawal symptoms if abruptly discontinued.[23] Duloxetine discontinuation rate at 1 year is as high as 66%, with two-thirds of discontinuations related to adverse events and one-third for lack of efficacy.[27] The most common adverse events reported with duloxetine for SUI were nausea (up to 46%), headache (up to 27%), constipation (up to 27%), dry mouth (up to 22%), and insomnia (up to 14%). Overall, adherence to long-term duloxetine therapy is poor due to adverse events and lack of efficacy.[28]

The usual dosage is 40 to 80 mg/day (in one or two doses) for 12 weeks. Gradual dose titration (starting from 20 mg once daily for at least 1 week, then titrate no shorter than weekly interval) may help to reduce the risks of nausea, dizziness, and premature therapy cessation. Similarly, taper the dose to avoid withdrawal symptoms if duloxetine is discontinued. Dose reduction of 50% for 2 weeks before discontinuation or slow tapering over 4 to 6 months is reasonable. If intolerable withdrawal symptoms occur following a dose reduction, consider resuming the previously prescribed dose and/or decrease dose at a more gradual rate.

▶ *Overflow Incontinence[5]*

There is no established effective pharmacologic therapy for OUI due to bladder underactivity (atonic bladder). A trial of bethanechol (25–50 mg three or four times daily) may be reasonable if contraindications do not exist. Bethanechol is a cholinomimetic that has uncertain efficacy but is associated with bothersome and potentially life-threatening side effects (muscle and abdominal cramping, hypersalivation, diarrhea, and bronchospasm), particularly in patient with preexisting conditions. α-Adrenoceptor antagonists, such as silodosin, prazosin, terazosin, doxazosin, tamsulosin, and alfuzosin, may be beneficial for OUI by relaxing the bladder outflow tract and hence reducing outflow resistance. If pharmacologic therapy fails, intermittent urethral catheterization by the patient or caregiver three or four times per day is recommended. Less satisfactory alternatives include indwelling urethral or suprapubic catheters or urinary diversion. In OUI due to obstruction, such as BPH, the goal of treatment is to relieve the obstruction.

▶ *Mixed Urinary Incontinence*

MUI is usually a combination of UUI plus SUI with one dominant component. It accounts for one-third of UI cases in women. A reasonable management approach is a combination of lifestyle/behavioral modifications and PFMR with pharmacotherapy appropriate to the dominant type of UI. For instance, antimuscarinics can be offered in UUI-predominant cases, whereas duloxetine, local estrogen, and α-adrenoceptor agonists in SUI-predominant cases. In some cases, the less dominant form of UI may respond, but usually not to a degree that is considered adequate by the patient. Most experts feel that SUI-predominant MUI is best treated initially using the nonpharmacologic approach plus surgery for SUI. Unfortunately, these patients with MUI are expected to have a lower success rates with surgery compared to those with pure SUI. The urge component may get better, stay the same, or get worse after surgery. Unfortunately, there is no a priori way to predict the response in a given individual.[29,30]

OUTCOME EVALUATION

- Monitor the patient for symptom relief. Have the treatment achieved the desired outcomes jointly developed by the health care team and the patient/caregiver? If so, to what

Table 53–6

Drugs Used for SUI[a]

Parameter	Estrogens	Pseudoephedrine	Duloxetine
Dosage forms	Avoid systemic (parenteral, oral, TD); use vaginal: tablet, cream, intravaginal ring	Tablets, solution	DR capsules
Dosing	Estradiol 25-mcg vaginal tablets (insert one PV daily for 14 days, then one PV twice weekly) Estradiol vaginal cream (0.1 mg/g) (2–4 g daily PV for 1–2 weeks; then 1 g PV daily or less frequently) CEE vaginal cream (0.625 mg/gm) (0.5–2 g daily PV; consider 3 weeks on, 1 week off; may be able to decrease frequency of use over time) Estradiol 2-, 12.4-, 24.8-mg vaginal rings (1 ring PV every 3 months)	15–60 mg three times daily	40–80 mg/day in one or two doses for 12 weeks (titrate and taper dosage)
Kinetics	Use local route to minimize systemic BA and side effects Estradiol less likely to be absorbed; CEE 1 mg or more daily sufficiently absorbed to cause systemic side effects	Less than 1% of dose is metabolized (inactive metabolites) Primarily renal elimination of unchanged drug Would not expect hepatic impairment to have an effect (no data) Expect significant effect if renal impairment and no effect if advanced age (beyond decreased CrCl with age) (no data)	Extensive metabolism via CYP 2D6 and 1A2 (inactive metabolites) Not altered in advanced age, mild to moderate renal impairment (CrCl 31–80 mL/min [0.51–1.34 mL/s]), mild hepatic impairment (Child-Pugh A) Significantly altered in severe renal disease (CrCl < 30 mL/min [< 0.50 mL/s]) and moderate hepatic impairment (Child-Pugh B)
Contraindications/ precautions	Contraindications include known or suspected breast or endometrial cancer Abnormal genitourinary bleeding of unknown etiology Active thromboembolism (or history of TE associated with previous estrogen use)	Contraindications include hypertension, tachyarrhythmias, coronary artery disease, MI, cor pulmonale, hyperthyroidism, renal failure, narrow-angle glaucoma	Multiple drug–drug interactions possible with CYP 2D6 and 1A2 substrates/inhibitors Avoid if CrCl < 30 mL/min (0.50 mL/s) and in all patients with hepatic disease Can raise BP Do not discontinue abruptly (withdrawal syndrome) Suicide risk even in patients without psychiatric disease Avoid in uncontrolled narrow-angle glaucoma (causes mydriasis) Hepatotoxic; avoid in alcoholics even if signs/symptoms of hepatic disease are absent

BA, bioavailability; BP, blood pressure; CEE, conjugated equine estrogens; CrCl, creatinine clearance; CYP, cytochrome P-450; DR, delayed-release; MI, myocardial infarction; PV, per vagina; TD, transdermal; TE, thromboembolism.

[a]None of these agents are FDA approved for treatment of SUI. Duloxetine is approved in Europe only.

degree? Inspect the daily diary completed by the patient/caregiver and quantitate the clinical response (eg, number of micturitions, number of incontinence episodes, and pad use) since the last visit. If a diary has not been used, ask the patient how many incontinence pads have been used and how they have been doing in terms of "accidents" since the last visit. If appropriate, administer a short-form instrument to measure the impact of symptoms, including quality of life. Compare the findings with previous results.

- Ask patients about adverse effects of drug therapy using a nonleading approach. Ask the patient/caregiver to judge their severity and what measures, if any, they have used to alleviate. Assess medication adherence (ask patient/caregiver about missed doses or do a pill count if the prescription containers are available at the visit).
- The balance of clinical response and tolerability should guide whether the drug dosage is increased, decreased, or left unchanged. Consider stopping/tapering off the regimen and initiate another drug option if bothersome adverse effects compromise patient safety and/or medication adherence.

Patient Care Process: Urinary Incontinence

Patient Assessment:

- Identify urinary symptoms and assess their severity. Assess changes in quality of life (physical, psychological, social functioning, and well-being). Identify exacerbating factors and UI complications. Determine whether a referral to specialized professionals is required.
- Review concurrent medical conditions and assess whether or not urinary symptoms could be disease-related.
- Obtain a thorough medication history, including use of prescription, nonprescription, and complementary/alternative drug products. Assess whether or not urinary symptoms could be drug induced (see Table 53–1). Determine if any current or previous treatments are helpful for UI.
- Include the patient and caregiver to set realistic goals of therapy. In cognitively intact elderly patients, focus communications to elicit the preferences of the patient, not those of potential proxies.

Therapy Evaluation:

- Evaluate the appropriateness of treatment regimen (drug choice, dosage, administration) for his or her type(s) of UI.
- Evaluate the patient for medication adherence, drug-related adverse events, allergies, and drug interactions with concomitant medications or disease states.

Care Plan Development:

- Educate the patient on lifestyle modifications that may improve symptoms: smoking cessation (for patients with cough-induced SUI), weight reduction (for those patients with SUI and UUI), prevention of constipation in patients at risk, caffeine reduction, and modification of diet and fluid intake. Note the timing and quantity of fluid intake, as well as possibility of avoiding foods or beverages that worsen UI.
- Provide patient education regarding the disease state, lifestyle modifications, and drug therapy (see Table 53–4).
- Causes of UI and possible complications:
  - Lifestyle modifications
  - Timing of medication intake
  - Potential adverse events
  - Potential drug–drug or drug–disease interactions
  - Importance of treatment adherence

Follow-up Evaluation:

- Monitor for patient response in 1 or 2 weeks after therapy initiation.
- Develop a plan to assess efficacy after a minimum of 4 weeks.

PEDIATRIC ENURESIS

INTRODUCTION

UI is a common problem in children, and treatment is unnecessary in children younger than 5 years, in whom spontaneous cure is likely. Pediatric enuresis (also called "intermittent nocturnal incontinence" or "nocturnal incontinence") is a condition, which can present alone or coexist with other disorders in children and adolescents. It is defined as discrete episodes of UI during sleep in children at least 5 years old.[31–33] Common terms associated with enuresis are as follows:

- Monosymptomatic enuresis: Enuresis in children without any other lower urinary tract symptoms and without a history of bladder dysfunction
  - Primary enuresis: A process wherein the patient has never been consistently dry throughout the night
  - Secondary enuresis: A process wherein the patient has resumed wetting after a period of dryness of at least 6 months in duration
- Nonmonosymptomatic enuresis: Enuresis in children with other lower urinary tract symptoms (eg, urgency, frequency, daytime incontinence, genital or lower urinary tract pain)[32,33]

Enuresis is not a benign disorder that children will just "grow out of." The emotional and developmental damage produced by enuresis may be more significant to the child than the enuresis itself. Emotional and/or physical abuse of the child by adult caregivers can lead to secondary problems such as chronic anxiety, low self-esteem, and delayed developmental milestones (attending camp, "sleepovers" at the homes of friends, etc).

EPIDEMIOLOGY AND ETIOLOGY

Five to seven million children and adolescents in the United States suffer from nocturnal enuresis. With each year of maturity, the percentage of bed-wetters declines by 15%. Primary enuresis is twice as common as secondary enuresis, which is present in 15% to 25% of bed-wetters.[34] In the enuretic population, 80% to 85% are monosymptomatic, 5% to 10% are nonmonosymptomatic, and less than 5% have an organic cause. Every year about 15% of those suffering from primary monosymptomatic nocturnal enuresis have spontaneous resolution without treatment.[34,35] The prevalence of enuresis is as follows:

- At age 5: 15% to 25%
- At age 12: 8% (boys) and 4% (girls)
- Adolescents: 1% to 3%

The etiology of enuresis is poorly understood, but there is a clear genetic link. Loci for enuresis have been located on chromosomes 5, 12, 13, and 22. The incidence in children from families with both parents had enuresis as children reaches as high as 77%, compared to 44% in whom from families with one parent had enuresis as a child, and 14% in whom from families with no members with enuresis. Sleep disorders are not considered major contributors, with the exception of sleep apnea. Enuresis occurs in all sleep stages in proportion to the time spent in each stage. However, a small proportion of individuals are not aroused from sleep by bladder distention and have uninhibited bladder contractions preceding enuresis.[34]

Patient Encounter 2, Part 1

An 8-year-old girl is brought into your clinic by her mother seeking advice regarding the child's "failure to keep dry at night" which occurs 3 to 4 nights weekly. The mother asks for an over-the-counter medication to help the child. After interviewing the child and mother separately, you determine that the child has had dryness for 1 year at the age of 6, and has resumed wetting 8 months ago. The onset of bedwetting coincides with the settlement of her parents' acrimonious divorce.

What additional information do you need to know before creating a treatment plan for this child?

PATHOPHYSIOLOGY

There are potentially treatable organic causes of enuresis (Table 53–7). Vast majority of children with enuresis have normal urodynamics, including functional bladder capacity, or maximum voided volume. Expected bladder capacity can be estimated by this formula: $(30 + [30 \times \text{age}])$ mL.

In some children, there appears to be a relationship between developmental immaturity in motor and language milestones and enuresis, but the mechanism is unknown. There is evidence that affected individuals have an attenuated vasopressin circadian rhythm (more significant in girls) with lower vasopressin plasma concentrations.[36] Other contributors include detrusor over-activity at night, increased threshold for arousal, and taking certain drugs (eg, lithium, clozapine, risperidone, valproic acid, selective serotonin reuptake inhibitors, and theophylline). Interestingly, caffeine ingestion does not correlate with enuresis.[37] In a minority of cases, psychological factors (eg, divorce of parents, school trauma, sexual abuse, or hospitalization) are clearly contributory to secondary enuresis. In very rare cases, severely dysfunctional families may neglect to properly toilet train the children.

TREATMENT

Desired Outcomes

- Reduction in the number of enuresis episodes and restoration of continence[32]
  - Partial response: a 50% to 89% decrease
  - Response: 90% or more decrease
  - Full response: a 100% decrease or less than 1 symptom occurrence monthly
- Prevention of relapse (greater than 1 symptom recurrence monthly) and maintenance of treatment success[32]
  - Continued success: No relapse in 6 months after the interruption of treatment
  - Complete success: No relapse in 2 years after the interruption of treatment
- Prevention or minimization of disease complications (delay in childhood developmental milestones, adverse psychological effects on the child/caregivers)
- Minimization of adverse effects and costs related to treatment
- Improvement in the quality of life of the child and caregivers

Table 53–7

Major Potentially Treatable Organic Causes of Enuresis

Potentially Treatable by Surgery
- Ectopic ureter
- Lower UTI (correct congenital anomalies)
- Neurogenic bladder
- Bladder calculus (stone) or foreign body
- Obstructive sleep apnea

Potentially Treatable by Drugs
- UTI
- Diabetes mellitus
- Diabetes insipidus
- Fecal impaction
- Constipation

UTI, urinary tract infection.

Clinical Presentation and Diagnosis: Pediatric Enuresis

Proper assessment of the child or adolescent with enuresis should explore every aspect of UI, especially the genitourinary and nervous systems. The minimum assessment should include[33,38,39]:

- Interview of child and parent(s), being sensitive to the emotional consequences of the enuresis.
- Direct physical examination, looking for enlarged adenoids/tonsils, bladder distention, fecal impaction, abnormal genitalia, spinal cord anomalies, and abnormal neurologic signs (look for an organic cause amenable to surgery or drugs; see Table 53–7).
- Obtain urinalysis for glucose, protein, WBC, or leukocyte esterase; obtain urinalysis and urine culture if symptoms of UTI are present.
- A 7 or more day diary of wet and dry nights prior to intervention is useful to monitor the response to treatment.
- Nonmonosymptomatic enuresis may require a more elaborate workup, including voiding cystourethrogram, renal and/or bladder ultrasound, urodynamics, and sleep studies.

General Approach to Treatment

Treatment is guided by the findings of the patient assessment. A referral to urologists is needed in cases of daytime wetting, abnormal voiding (eg, unusual posturing, discomfort, straining, poor stream), history of recurrent UTIs, and abnormalities of the genitalia. Crisis intervention strategies and individual and/or family psychotherapy are recommended in the rare circumstance of a true psychological cause.

Guidelines for the evaluation and management of nocturnal enuresis have been developed.[33,38,39] Management of primary monosymptomatic nocturnal enuresis in children may involve one or a combination of interventions. The management of secondary nocturnal enuresis focuses on addressing the underlying stressor. However, most children with secondary enuresis have

Patient Encounter 2, Part 2

PMH: Unremarkable pregnancy/delivery. Developmental milestones WNL

Immunization: Up to date

FH, SH: Acrimonious divorce of parents about 1 year ago

Meds: None

ROS: (+) nocturnal incontinence 3 or 4 nights per week; no daytime incontinence; (–) vaginal itching, UTIs, urgency, frequency, dysuria, lower abdominal fullness, or other lower urinary track symptoms; no signs of constipation or fecal impaction

PE:

VS: BP 90/65 mm Hg, P 72 beats/min, RR 16 breaths/min, T 37.0°C (98.6°F)

Resp: WNL

CV: WNL

Abd: Soft, nontender, nondistended; (+) bowel sounds; bladder not palpable

Neuro: WNL (gross sensory, motor, reflexes)

GU, Rectal: Deferred

Labs. Urinalysis WNL

Given this additional information, what is your assessment of this patient's condition?

What are the goals of pharmacotherapy for this patient?

What nonpharmacologic and pharmacologic interventions are appropriate for the child?

What initial treatment would you suggest?

no identifiable causes and are treated in the same manner. The algorithm within the NICE guideline (Figure 53–1) is inclusive of the most potentially useful treatments and distinguishes approaches based on the child's age, maturity, and abilities; the frequency of enuresis; and the motivation and needs of the family.[39]

Initial management with education and motivational/behavioral therapy (Table 53–8) should be utilized for 3 to 6 months, provided that the patient and family are sufficiently motivated.[35] More active intervention (eg, enuresis alarm, pharmacologic treatment) is warranted if initial management fails or provides inadequate response. KEY CONCEPT *Enuresis alarms are the most effective long-term therapy, but desmopressin is effective in the short-term (eg, for sleepovers or camp attendance).* KEY CONCEPT *Pharmacotherapy is most valuable in patients who have difficulty in adhering to nonpharmacologic therapy or in those who fail to achieve desired outcomes with nonpharmacologic therapy.*

▶ Nonpharmacologic Treatment

The standard first-line therapy demands for commitment from the child and/or caregiver (see Table 53–8). It involves education about the condition, fluid/diet modification, journal keeping, and behavioral or motivational therapy.[35,40] Motivational therapy allows about 25% of children to achieve 14 consecutive dry nights and 70% of them at least a partial response. About 5% of children experience more than 2 wet nights in 2 weeks. If motivational therapy fails to lead to improvement after 3 to 6 months, active interventions, such as enuresis alarms (Table 53–9) or desmopressin, may be added.[35]

Enuresis alarms are indicated for motivated families and children with frequent enuresis of more than twice per week. They conditioned the child to learn to wake or inhibit bladder contraction in response to the physiologic conditions present before wetting. They are the most effective ways of controlling nocturnal enuresis and preventing relapse, and may be used in children younger than 7 years. They are more effective than TCAs for pediatric enuresis.[41] Alarm therapy can be an effective add-on in patients who are partial- or nonresponders to drug therapy alone. Similarly, drug therapy can be added in patients who achieved suboptimal results from nonpharmacologic therapy alone.[42,43]

Use of enuresis alarms does not provide rapid or short-term improvement, and requires the child be able to wake to sound or touch. Approximately 30% of patients discontinue enuresis alarms for various reasons, including skin irritation, disturbance of other family members, and/or failure to wake the child.[35] Adverse effects of alarms include alarm failure, false alarms, failure to wake the child, disruption of other family members, and lack of adherence because of difficulty using the alarm.[41]

Efficacy may be assessed within 1 to 2 weeks of initiating alarm therapy. Treatment should be continued if the child demonstrates early signs of response. It often requires 3 to 6 months to achieve a minimum of 14 consecutive dry nights. After 3 months of therapy, if the child has achieved at least some response, alarm therapy should be continued.[35,39] If no improvement is seen in 3 months, alternative interventions should be considered. However, enuresis alarm can be reinitiated for relapses.[35]

Measures that do not help or are of questionable value in pediatric enuresis include the following:[44]

- Bladder stretching exercises (done by delaying voiding despite the urge to do so)
- Hypnotherapy
- Dietary changes
- Desensitization to allergens
- Acupuncture
- Chiropractic

▶ Pharmacologic Treatment

Desmopressin (DDAVP)[35,45] A synthetic analogue of vasopressin, desmopressin was first studied in enuresis in the 1970s. It is indicated for nocturnal enuresis in children at least 6 years of age who do not respond to initial management (see Table 53–8), or as an alternative for alarm therapy. It is most effective in children with nocturnal polyuria (nocturnal urine production greater than 130% of expected bladder capacity for age) and normal functional bladder capacity (maximum voided volume greater than 70% of expected bladder capacity for age). It decreases the number of wet nights per week by about one night. About 30% of children become full responders while on the drug, but 60% to 70% of them experience relapses.[35]

KEY CONCEPT *Desmopressin is the drug of choice in pediatric enuresis.* In many countries the enuresis indication has been removed for nasal desmopressin due to higher risk for hyponatremic seizure. Oral desmopressin is an ideal agent for rapid-onset, short-term use (camp attendance or "sleepovers"). To aim for long-term benefit, consider a trial for at least 3 to 6 months. Regular tablets may be started at 0.2 mg (one tablet) 1 hour

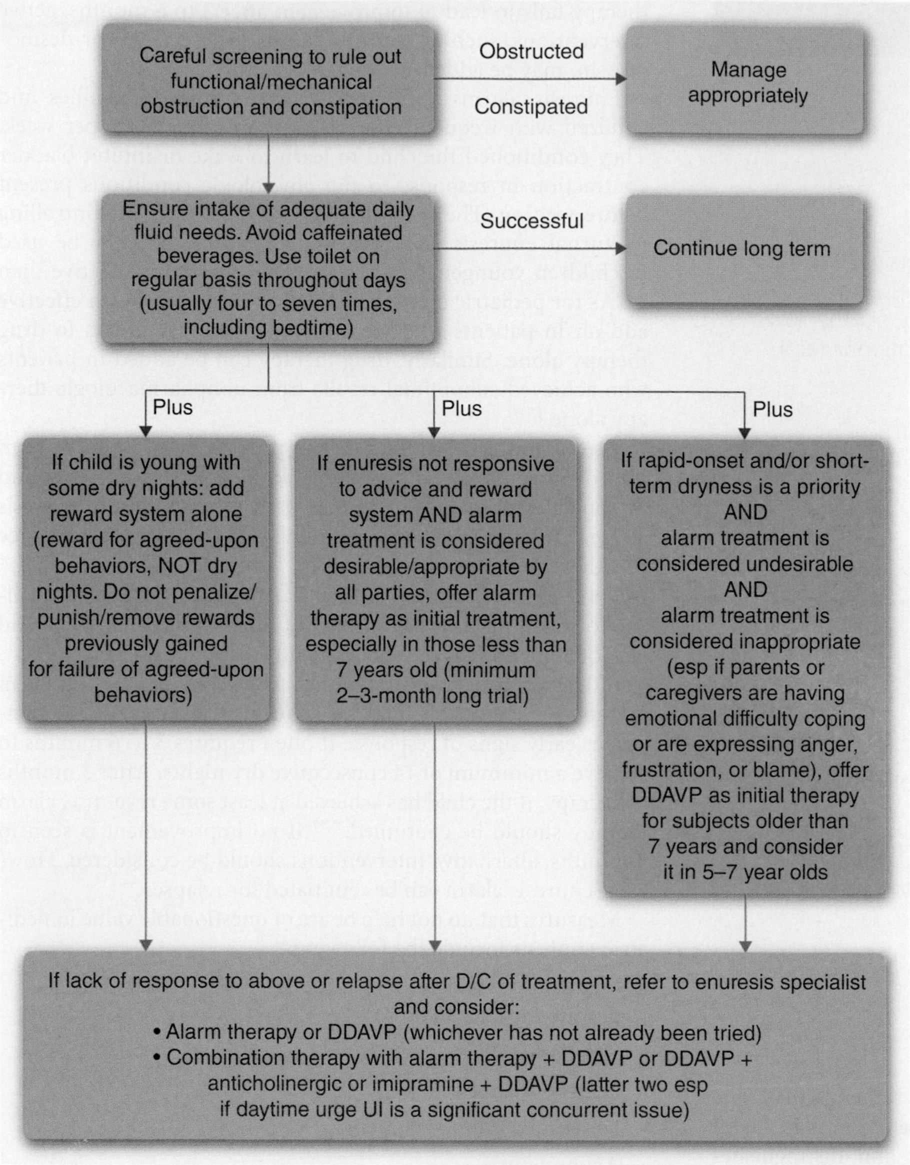

FIGURE 53–1. Enuresis treatment protocol. (D/C, discontinuation; DDAVP, desmopressin; UI, urinary incontinence.) (Modified from Nunes VD, O'Flynn N, Evans J, Sawyer L; Guideline Development Group. Management of bedwetting in children and young people: Summary of NICE guidance. BMJ. 2010;341:c5399.)

Table 53–8

Initial Management of Pediatric Enuresis

Education and Advice to Children and Caregivers

- Enuresis is common; it occurs at least once per week in up to 25% of 5 year olds; enuresis resolves on its own in the majority of children.
- Enuresis is the fault of neither the child nor the caregivers; children should not be punished for bedwetting.
- Reduce the impact of bedwetting by using bed protection and washable/disposable products; using room deodorizers; thoroughly washing the child before dressing; and using emollients to prevent chafing.
- Keeping a calendar of wet and dry nights helps to determine the effect of interventions.
- The child should attempt to void regularly during the day and just before going to bed (a total of four to seven times); if the child wakes at night, the caregivers should take him/her to the toilet.
- Avoid high-sugar and caffeine-based drinks, particularly in the evening hours.
- Concentrate daily fluid intake in the morning and early afternoon. Restrict fluid and solute intake during the evening. A recommendation is to drink 40 % of their total daily fluid in the morning (7 AM to 12 PM), 40 % in the afternoon (12 PM to 5 PM), and only 20 % in the evening (after 5 PM).
- Discourage routine use of diapers and pull-ups, except when the child is sleeping away from home.

Motivational Therapy

- Motivational therapy is a good first-line therapy for nocturnal enuresis in younger children between the ages of 5 to 7 years who do not wet the bed every night.
- Motivate the child by keeping a record of progress and receive rewards for accomplished agreed-upon behavior, such as going to the toilet before bedtime. For example, a sticker on a calendar for each dry night, a book for seven consecutive dry nights, etc. Do not use penalties (ie, removal of previously gained rewards).

Table 53–9

Behavioral Treatments for Enuresis

Lifting	Procedure wherein the caregiver takes the child to the toilet at regular intervals during the night to urinate without fully awakening him or her
Night awakening	Procedure wherein the caregiver fully awakens the child to void shortly before he or she would usually have wet the bed; once the child is consistently dry, the frequency of awakening drops or (for single awakenings) the time of awakening is gradually moved to earlier in the night (ie, closer to bedtime) until the child is dry when awakened 1 hour after going to bed
Alarm	An alarm device and a moisture-sensitive sensor are used in combination, with the sensor being placed under the sheets, or more commonly, attached to the child's pajamas or underwear near the urethra. The arousal devise is usually an auditory alarm and/or a vibrating belt or pager
Overlearning	This is commenced at a minimum of 2 weeks after the alarm has rendered the child dry; the child drinks 500 mL (about 16 oz) during the hour before going to bed; alarm use is continued until he or she is dry for 14 consecutive nights with the extra fluid intake; is used to reduce relapse rates seen with alarm use alone
Dry-bed training	This begins with an intensive first night of training that involves increased fluid consumption, hourly awakenings, praise when the bed is dry at hourly awakenings, and, when the alarm goes off, a mild reprimand and cleanliness training (child changes wet clothes and bed linens, remakes the bed, resets the alarm); before going to bed and after each wetting, the child engages in 20 practice trials of appropriate toileting (ie, positive practice): for each practice trial, the child lies in bed, counts to 50, arises and attempts to urinate in the toilet, then returns to bed; on subsequent nights, child is woken only once, usually about 3 hours after the child has gone to bed; after a dry night, the night awakening moves up 30 minutes earlier; it is discontinued when it is scheduled to occur 1 hour after bedtime; after 7 consecutive dry nights, the alarm is discontinued, but is reinstated if two episodes of wetting occur in a 1-week period

before bedtime; if needed after 10 to 14 days, may increase dose to the maximum dose of 0.4 mg. Sublingual tablets of 120 mcg are available in Canada may be given 30 to 60 minutes before bedtime; if needed after 10 to 14 days, may increase dose to the maximum dose of 240 mcg.[33,35]

The most serious complication of desmopressin therapy is water intoxication with dilutional hyponatremia and seizures. This occurs most frequently with the nasal formulation. Electrolyte monitoring in patients taking the oral formulation is recommended if comorbidities may exacerbate renal or electrolyte complications. To reduce the risk of water intoxication, children should drink no more than 8 oz (240 mL) of fluid from 1 hour before to 8 hours after administration of desmopressin. Treatment should be interrupted during episodes of fluid and/or electrolyte imbalance (eg, fever, recurrent vomiting or diarrhea, vigorous exercise, or other conditions associated with increased water consumption).[35]

Treatment response should be assessed within 1 to 2 weeks. If signs of response are present, desmopressin should be continued for 3 months. If enuresis improves or remits, the family and child can determine whether to use desmopressin every night or just for special occasions, such as sleepovers. When it is administered daily, desmopressin should be withheld for 1 week every 3 months to determine whether continued use is necessary.[35]

Lack of response to desmopressin may be due to reduced nocturnal bladder capacity (the most common reason for unresponsiveness) or persistent nocturnal polyuria (related to increased fluid intake in the evening, increased nocturnal solute excretion) or suboptimal dosing. To minimize relapses, daily desmopressin should be tapered over at least 2 weeks using one-half of the effective doses or giving the effective dose every other day for 2 weeks before discontinuation.[35]

Diuretics play a minor role in the treatment of enuresis for most patients. However, in cases of presumed desmopressin resistance that leads to poor response to usual doses or symptom deterioration after established positive response, oral furosemide 0.5 mg/kg in the early morning may be helpful. Furosemide works by reversing the abnormal circadian rhythm of renal tubular sodium handling, which is common in individuals with enuresis. In a study with 12 children with desmopressin-resistant enuresis, adding furosemide appeared beneficial in 75% of study subjects.[46]

Imipramine[47] Imipramine was first used in the treatment of enuresis in the 1960s. It is considered as the third-line option for monosymptomatic enuresis and may be used in children who have failed alarm therapy and desmopressin. Its mechanism of action is unclear but anticholinergic and antispasmodic effects may increase plasma ADH concentrations. About 50% of patients may respond to treatment and can expect approximately one less wet night per week. Although trials involving other TCAs have been performed over the years, there is insufficient evidence to assess their relative efficacy compared with imipramine.

Treatment with imipramine is associated with a reduction of approximately 1 wet night per week and relapse rates after cessation as high as 50%. The usual initial dose is 10 to 25 mg at bedtime and may be increased by 25 mg if there is no response after 1 week. On average, the bedtime dose is 25 mg for children 5 to 8 years of age and 50 mg for older children. The dose should not exceed 50 mg in children between 6 and 12 years of age and 75 mg in children age 12 or older.[35]

About 25% of children treated with TCAs experience gastrointestinal symptoms. About 5% of children experience neurologic side effects including nervousness, personality change, or sleep disturbances. Clinicians should monitor for the possibility of increased suicidality, particularly in children and young adults with preexisting depressive symptoms.[35] The most serious adverse effects of TCAs are cardiac conduction disturbances and myocardial depression, particularly in cases of overdose. Therefore, safer options should be considered before starting any TCA for pediatric enuresis.[33,35]

Anticholinergics Monotherapy with anticholinergic drugs is ineffective in treating monosymptomatic nocturnal enuresis. These agents should be used only if the child has nocturnal enuresis and daytime incontinence (see Urinary Incontinence). In this case, anticholinergic therapy may be used in combination with desmopressin to increase bladder capacity during sleep.[35]

The usual initial dose of oxybutynin is 5 mg, tolterodine 2 mg, or 0.4 mg/kg propiverine (not available in the United States) at bedtime, titrate upward based on clinical response; the maximal therapeutic effects can be seen within 2 months or sometimes much earlier.[33] Children should be monitored for major adverse events, such as urinary retention (may lead to urinary tract infections), constipation (worsens urinary tract dysfunction) and decreased saliva secretion.

Other Drugs Various medications, such as indomethacin, phenmetrazine, amphetamine sulfate, ephedrine, atropine, furosemide, diclofenac, and chlorprothixene have been tried in the treatment of nocturnal enuresis. Data suggest that indomethacin, diclofenac, and diazepam are superior to placebo, but not better than desmopressin.[47] Current guidelines do not recommend any of these agents for pediatric enuresis.

▸ *Comparison of Therapies*

Multiple meta-analyses have been conducted to compare treatments for enuresis, although most trials enrolled a small number of subjects and were of poor methodological quality.[45,47–49] Overall, data suggest that use of enuresis alarms is the most effective nonpharmacologic method. The initial rate for success (less than 1 wet night per month) is 66%, with 45% long-term success rate after discontinuation (vs 1% with no treatment). Alarm therapy is at least as effective as desmopressin, but with a significantly lower relapse rates (46% vs 60%–70% for desmopressin).[50] Combining enuresis alarms and other behavioral therapy further reduces relapse rates. There is inadequate data to compare the various commercial brands of alarms available to consumers.

▸ *Treatment of Relapse*

A relapse is defined by more than 1 wet night per month after a period of dryness.[32] When it occurs, reinitiate the intervention which was previously effective (see Figure 53–1). For children with multiple recurrences after discontinuation of desmopressin, gradual dose tapering of desmopressin may be helpful. Combination alarm and desmopressin therapy may be beneficial for children who have more than one recurrence following successful treatment with an alarm.[45] Management of therapy-resistant monosymptomatic nocturnal enuresis may include periodic new trials of the enuresis alarm with or without desmopressin, desmopressin alone, or a trial of imipramine.[35]

Nonresponders experience less than 50% improvement in symptoms despite active interventions.[32] When motivated children and families do not respond to at least 3-month therapy of enuresis alarm and/or desmopressin, referral to a specialty clinic (eg, developmental-behavioral pediatrician, pediatric urologist) may be warranted.[35]

OUTCOME EVALUATION

- Monitor the patient for symptom relief. Has the treatment plan achieved the desired outcomes jointly developed by the health care team, the patient, and parents/guardians? If so, to what degree? Evaluate the daily diary completed by the patient or parents/guardians since the last clinic visit and

Patient Care Process: Pediatric Enuresis

Patient Assessment:

- Assess the patient's symptoms. Determine whether the child should be referred to a specialty clinic. Assess whether there are any exacerbating factors or enuresis related complications.
- Review past medical history and available diagnostic data. Are there any potentially treatable organic causes of enuresis (see Table 53–7)?
- Obtain a thorough medication history, including use of prescription, nonprescription, and complementary/alternative drug products. Could any of them contributing to enuresis (see Table 53–1)? Determine which, if any, treatments in the past had been helpful.
- Establish realistic treatment goals with the involvement of the child and caregiver.

Therapy Evaluation:

- If patient is already receiving nonpharmacological interventions and/or drug therapy, assess treatment choice, drug dosing, efficacy, side effect, adherence, etc.
- Have the child and caregiver given the current treatment plan an adequate duration of trial? How is the child responding to current treatment plan?

Care Plan Development:

- Educate the patient and/or caregiver on pediatric enuresis, lifestyle modifications, and motivational therapy (see Table 53–8). The patient and/or caregiver should be referred to local enuresis clinics (if available) for training in behavioral treatments, such as use of enuresis alarms (see Table 53–9). May follow treatment algorithms from current guidelines (see Figure 53–1).
  - Evaluate the patient for adverse events, allergies, and interactions (drug–drug and drug–disease) and adherence.
  - Provide the patient and/or caregiver with education regarding drug therapy (timing of drug administration, side effects, potential drug–drug interactions, etc).

Follow-Up Evaluation:

- Evaluate treatment response in 1 to 2 weeks after therapy initiation.
- Allow at least 3 months to assess efficacy of treatment.

quantitate the clinical response (the number of dry nights per week, the number of nights with two or more enuresis episodes). If a diary has not been used, elicit from the patient and caregiver the clinical response since last visit.

- Elicit adverse events of therapy, including severity, using a nonleading manner. Ask the patient or parents/guardians what measures, if any, were used to alleviate adverse effects. Assess therapy adherence.
- The balance of clinical response, tolerability, and burden on the caregiver will determine the approach to management. As most nonpharmacologic approaches are "all or none" and drug titration is limited by the maximum recommended dose, clinicians may consider changing therapy if clinical results are inadequate over an adequate trial period.
- Refer patients with refractory enuresis to a health care professional who specializes in the management of bedwetting.

ACKNOWLEDGMENT

The author and editors wish to acknowledge and thank Dr. David Guay, the primary author of this chapter in the first, second and third editions of this book.

Abbreviations Introduced in This Chapter

ADH	Antidiuretic hormone
BPH	Benign prostatic hyperplasia
CYP	Cytochrome P450
DDAVP	Desmopressin
DHIC	Detrusor hyperactivity with impaired contractility
ER	Extended release
IR	Immediate release
MUI	Mixed urinary incontinence
OAB	Overactive bladder
OUI	Overflow urinary incontinence
PFMR	Pelvic floor muscle rehabilitation
PVR	Postvoid residual
SUI	Stress urinary incontinence
TCA	Tricyclic antidepressant
UI	Urinary incontinence
US	United States
UTI	Urinary tract infection
UUI	Urge urinary incontinence

REFERENCES

1. Abrams P, Cardozo L, Fall M, et al. The standardization of terminology of lower urinary tract function: Report from the standardization sub-committee of the International Continence Society. Neurourol Urodyn. 2002;21:167–178.
2. Coyne Ks, Wein A, Nicholson S, et al. Economic burden of urgency urinary incontinence in the United Staes: A systematic review. J Manag Care Pharm. 2014;20:130–140.
3. Buckley BS, Lapitan MC; Epidemiology Committee of the Fourth International Consultation on Incontinence. Prevalence of urinary incontinence in men, women, and children-current evidence: Findings of the Fourth International Consultation on Incontinence. Urology. 2010;76:265.
4. Gorina Y, Schappert S, Bercovitz A, et al. Prevalence of incontinence among older Americans. National Center for Health Statistics. Vital Health Stat. 3(36). 2014.
5. Rovner ES, Wyman J, Lam S. Urinary Incontinence. In: DiPiro J, Talbert R, Yee G, Matzke G, Wells BG, Posey LM, eds. Pharmacotherapy: A Pathophysiologic Approach. 9th ed. New York: McGraw-Hill; 2014:1377–1396.
6. Gormley EA, Lightner DJ, Burgio KL, et al. Diagnosis and treatment of overactive bladder (Non-neurogenic) in adults: AUA/SUFU Guideline. American Urological Association. 2014.
7. Lucas MG, Bedretdinova D, Bosch JLHR, et al. Guidelines on urinary incontinence. European Association of Urology. 2013.
8. American College of Obstetricians and Gynecologists. Urinary incontinence in women. Washington DC: American College of Obstetricians and Gynecologists; 2009.
9. Homma Y, Yoshida M, Seki N, et al. Symptom assessment tool for overactive bladder syndrome—overactive bladder symptom score. Urology. 2006; 68:318–323.
10. Kafri R, Shames J, Raz M, et al. Rehabilitation versus drug therapy for urge urinary incontinence: Long-term outcomes. Int Urogynecol J Pelvic Floor Dyfunet. 2008;19:47–52.
11. Shamliyan TA, Kane RL, Wyman J, et al. Systematic review: Randomized, controlled trials of nonsurgical treatments for urinary incontinence in women. Ann Intern Med. 2008;148: 459–473.
12. Shamliyan T, Wyman JF, Ramakrishnan R, Sainfort F, Kane RL. Benefits and harms of pharmacologic treatment for urinary incontinence in women: A systematic review. Ann Intern Med. 2012 19;156(12):861–874, W301–W310.
13. Meek PD, Evang SD, Tadrous M, Roux-Lirange D. Overactive bladder drugs and constipation: A meta-analysis of randomized, placebo-controlled trials. Dig Dis Sci. 2011;56:7–18.
14. Rai BP, Cody JD, Alhasso A, Stewart L. Anticholinergic drugs versus non-drug active therapies for non-neurogenic overactive bladder syndrome in adults. Cochrane Database Syst Rev. 2012:CD003193.
15. Novara G, Balfano A, Secco S, et al. A systematic review and meta-analysis of randomized controlled trials with antimuscarinic drugs for overactive bladder. Eur Urol. 2008;54:740–763.
16. Sink KM, Thomas J 3rd, Xu H, et al. Dual use of bladder anticholinergics and cholinesterase inhibitors: Long-term functional and cognitive outcomes. J Am Geriatr Soc. 2008;56: 847–853.
17. Bridgeman MB, Friia NJ, Taft C, Shah M. Mirabegron: β_3-adrenergic receptor agonist for the treatment of overactive bladder. Ann Pharmacother. 2013;47:1029–1038.
18. Peyromaure M, Ravery V, Boccon-Gibod L. The management of stress urinary incontinence after radical prostatectomy. BJU Int. 2002;90:155–161.
19. Filcamo MT, LiMarzi V, DelPopolo G, et al. Pharmacologic treatment in postprostatectomy stress urinary incontinence. Eur Urol. 2007;51:1559–1564.
20. Jacklin P, Duckett J, Renganathan A. Analytic model comparing the cost utility of TVT versus duloxetine in women with stress urinary incontinence. Int Urogynnecol J. 2010; 21:977–984.
21. Cody JD, Jacobs ML, Richardson K, Moehrer B, Hextall A. Oestrogen therapy for urinary incontinence in post-menopausal women. Cochrane Database Syst Rev. 2012;10:DC001405.
22. Ewiles AA, Althally F. Topical vaginal estrogen therapy in managing postmenopausal urinary symptoom: A reality or a gimmick? Climacteric. 2010;13:405–418.
23. Guay DRP. Duloxetine. The first therapy licensed for stress urinary incontinence. Am J Geriatr Pharmacother. 2005;3:25–38.
24. Fraser MO, Chancellor MB. Neural control of the urethra and development of pharmacotherapy for stress urinary incontinence. BJU Int. 2003;91:743–748.
25. Burgard EC, Fraser MO, Thor KB. Serotonergic modulation of bladder afferent pathways. Urology. 2003;62(Suppl 1):10–15.
26. Cornu JN, Merlet B, Ciofu C, et al. Duloxetine for mild to moderate postprostatectomy incontinence: Preliminary

results of a randomised, placebo-controlled trial. Eur Urol. 2011;59(1):148–154.
27. Duckett JR, Vella M, Kavalakuntla G, et al. Tolerability and efficacy of duloxetine in a nontrial situation. BJOG. 2007;114:543–547.
28. Bump RC, Voss S, Beardsworth A, et al. Long-term efficacy of duloxetine in women with stress urinary incontinence. Br J Urol Int. 2008;102:214–218.
29. Khullar V, Cardozo L, Dmochowski R. Mixed incontinence: Current evidence and future perspectives. Neurourol Urodyn. 2010;29:618–622.
30. Murray S, Lemack GE. Overactive bladder and mixed incontinence. Curr Urol Rep. 2010;11:385–392.
31. Tekgul S, Riedmiller H, Dogan HS, et al. Guidelines on paediatric urology. Arnhem, The Netherlands: European Association of Urology, European Society for Paediatric Urology 2013:126.
32. Nevéus T, von Gontard A, Hoebeke P, et al. The standardization of terminology of lower urinary tract function in children and adolescents: Report from the Standardisation Committee of the International Children's Continence Society (ICCS) J Urol. 2006;176:314–324.
33. Neveus T, Eggert P, Evans J, et al. Evaluation and treatment for monosymptomatic enuresis: A standardization document from the International Children's Continence Society. J Urol. 2010;183:441–447.
34. Thiedke CC. Nocturnal enuresis. Am Fam Physician. 2003;67 (7):1499–1506.
35. Tu ND, Baskin LS, Nocturnal enuresis in children: Management. UpToDate. Updated August 13, 2014.
36. Rittig S, Schaumberg HL, Siggaard C, et al. The circadian effect in plasma vasopressin and urine output is related to desmopressin response and enuresis status in children with nocturnal enuresis. J Urol. 2008;179:2389–2395.
37. Warzak WJ, Evans S, Floress MT, Gross AC, Stoolman S. Caffeine consumption in young children. J Pediatr. 2011;158:508–509.
38. Paediatric Society New Zealand. Noctural enuresis "Bedwetting," 2005.
39. Nunes VD, O'Flynn N, Evans J, Sawyer L; Guideline Development Group. Management of bedwetting in children and young people: Summary of NICE guidance. BMJ. 2010; 341:c5399.
40. Blum NJ. Nocturnal enuresis: Behavioral treatments. Urol Clin North Am. 2004;31:499–507.
41. Glazener CM, Evans JH, Peto RE. Alarm interventions for nocturnal enuresis in children. Cochrane Database Syst Rev. 2005:CD002911.
42. Vogt M, Lehnert T, Till H, Rolle U. Evaluation of different modes of combined therapy in children with monosymptomatic nocturnal enuresis. BJU Intern. 2010;105:1456–1459.
43. Kwak KW, Park KH, Baek M. The efficacy of enuresis alarm treatment in pharmacotherapy-resistant nocturnal enuresis. Urology. 2011;77:200–204.
44. Huang T, Shu X, Huang YS, Cheuk DK. Complementary and miscellaneous interventions for nocturnal enuresis in children. Cochrane Database Syst Rev. 2011:CD005230.
45. Glazener CM, Evans JH. Desmopressin for nocturnal enuresis in children. Cochrane Database Syst Rev. 2009:CD002112.
46. DeGuchtenaere A, Vande Walle C, Van Sintjan P, et al. Desmopressin resistant nocturnal polyuria may benefit from furosemide therapy administered in the morning. J Urol. 2007;178:2635–2639.
47. Glazener CM, Evans JH, Peto RE. Tricyclic and related drugs for nocturnal enuresis in children. Cochrane Database Syst Rev. 2003;(3):CD002117.
48. Deshpande AV, Caldwell PH, Sureshkumar P. Drugs for nocturnal enuresis in children (other than desmopressin and tricyclics). Cochrane Database Syst Rev. 2012;12:CD002238.
49. Caldwell PH, Nankivell G, Sureshkumar P. Simple behavioural interventions for nocturnal enuresis in children. Cochrane Database Syst Rev. 2013;(2):CD003637.
50. Kwak KW, Lee YS, Park KH, Baek M. Efficacy of desmopressin and enuresis alarm as first and second line treatment for primary monosymptomatic nocturnal enuresis: Prospective randomized crossover study. J Urol. 2010;184:2521–2526.

54 Allergic and Pseudoallergic Drug Reactions

J. Russell May and Dennis Ownby

LEARNING OBJECTIVES

Upon completion of the chapter, the reader will be able to:

1. Describe the potential incidence of allergic and pseudoallergic reactions and why it is difficult to obtain accurate numbers.
2. Describe the Gell and Coombs categories of reactions.
3. Identify the classes of drugs most commonly associated with allergic and pseudoallergic reactions.
4. Recommend specific treatment for a patient experiencing anaphylaxis.
5. Recommend an approach to drug selection in patients with multiple drug allergies.
6. Describe drug desensitization procedures for selected drugs.

INTRODUCTION

Allergic and pseudoallergic drug reactions are reported together. They are rarely confirmed by testing, making statistical analysis imprecise, with both over-reporting and under-reporting. KEY CONCEPT *Approximately 5% to 10% of adverse drug reactions are allergic or immunologic; however, allergic and pseudoallergic reactions represent 24% of reported adverse drug reactions in hospitalized patients.*[1,2] *These reactions are costly and cause considerable morbidity and mortality.* Between 10% and 20% of hospitalized patients incur drug reactions (7% in the general population), with about one-third possibly due to hypersensitivity; however, most of these reactions are not reported, especially in pediatrics.[1,3,4] Patients experiencing an allergic drug reaction in the hospital have increased costs of $275 to $600 million annually.[5] This financial burden can occur due to several reasons, including increased indirect cost of (a) time and lost labor; (b) use of more costly alternative medications; and (c) treatment failures. Outpatient rates are not well studied and are much harder to collect. Relying on a patient's history without an attempt to verify the relationships between drugs taken and symptoms experienced results in confusion. Health care professionals and patients use the term "drug allergy" in such a general way that it is not medically useful and, further, perpetuates a level of fear and concern in the public and in medical practice that is inappropriate and costly. This same confusion and anxiety sometimes lead medical personnel to ignore or forget "drug allergy" with potentially catastrophic results. Clearly, an understanding of how allergic and pseudoallergic reactions occur and how they might be managed or prevented is important to health care professionals and their patients.

PATHOPHYSIOLOGY

Drug allergies are immune responses resulting from different mechanisms of immunologic recognition and activation, and reactions are produced by multiple physiologic pathways. This produces a confusing spectrum of clinical pictures and complex pathophysiologic mechanisms. The Gell and Coombs classification has been used for decades and still provides a framework for thinking about mechanisms of immunologic drug reactions, as shown in Table 54–1.[6,7]

However, as knowledge has advanced, the immune mechanisms active in most drug reactions have been found to be more complex and interrelated than suggested by the Gell and Coombs classification.[8] The complexity and unpredictability of most immune-mediated drug reactions combined with the lack of appropriate animal models have hindered a better understanding of the mechanisms of these reactions. However, even with these shortcomings, the classification remains the most commonly used method for attempting to describe drug reactions resulting from hypersensitivity. KEY CONCEPT *Immediate or Type I reactions are those allergic reactions mediated by IgE antibodies specific to the drug; Type II reactions are cytotoxic reactions mediated by drug-specific IgG or IgM antibodies; Type III reactions result from immune complexes circulating in the serum; and Type IV reactions are mediated by cellular mechanisms. Type IV reactions are further subdivided into Type IVa involving recruitment of monocytes, Type IVb with predominately eosinophils, Type IVc composed of* CD4+ *or* CD8+ *T cells, and Type IVd showing neutrophils.*[9]

Immune Mechanisms

The immune mechanisms involved in drug allergies are quite complex.[10] Immune recognition of non-self material is predominantly controlled by specific receptors on the surface of T-cells during interactions with cells specialized for presenting antigens to T-cells. The antigen presenting cells must concomitantly provide a second signal in addition to the antigen to activate the T-cell. If a second signal is not provided, the T-cell becomes nonresponsive or anergic. The second signal controls the type of immune response that will be initiated by the T-cell.

Table 54–1

Reaction Classification, Clinical Symptoms, and Potential Causative Drugs[6,7]

Gell and Coombs Classification	Immune Response	Clinical Symptoms	Potential Causative Drugs[a]
Type I	IgE	Anaphylaxis, urticaria	β-Lactam antibiotics: penicillins (primarily), cephalosporins, carbapenems Non–β-lactam antibiotics: sulfonamides, vancomycin Others: insulins, heparin
Type II	IgG	Hemolytic anemia, thrombocytopenia	Quinidine, methyldopa, penicillins, heparin
Type III	IgG, IgM	Vasculitis, serum sickness, lupus	Penicillins, sulfonamides, radiocontrast agents, phenytoin, minocycline
Type IV			β-Lactam antibiotics, sulfonamides, phenytoin
IVa	Th1 cytokines	Tuberculin reaction eczema	See text for examples
IVb[b]	Th2 cytokines	Maculopapular and bullous exanthema	
IVc[b]	Cytotoxic T cells (CD4 and CD8)	Same as IVb, also eczema, pustular exanthema	
IVd	T cells (IL-8)	Pustular exanthema	

[a]These drugs represent a list of causative agents. Many drugs can cause these reactions.

[b]IVb and IVc reactions may combine to produce erythema multiforme, Stevens-Johnson syndrome, and toxic epidermal necroylsis.

Ig, Immunoglobulin.

Depending on the exposure to antigens and the cytokines involved, naïve T-helper cells (CD4+ T cells) can differentiate into at least five types of effector-helper cells: Type 1 effector helper T cells (Th1), Th2, Th17, Th9, and Th22. Each of these subsets of T cells appears to have a unique regulatory element, pattern of cytokine production, and function. Th1 responses are typically associated with activation of T-cells to induce B-cell immunoglobulin G (IgG) antibody production and to provide direct T-cell recruitment of cells to kill cells infected with viruses or intracellular bacteria. Th2 immune responses typically lead to IgE production and immediate allergic-type reactions. Th17 responses are varied but usually highly inflammatory and important in the clearance of extracellular bacterial and fungal infections. Th17 cells have also been found to be involved in a variety of autoimmune disorders such as psoriasis, rheumatoid arthritis, and inflammatory bowel disease. Th9 cells promote tissue inflammation and cause mucous production but do not have suppressor functions. Th22 cells produce abundant quantities of interleukin 22 (IL-22) and are important in various inflammatory diseases of the skin.

Antigens

The immune system normally is not capable of recognizing small molecules. This fact has resulted in several hypotheses concerning how drugs can elicit an immune response.[10] The first widely accepted hypothesis was the haptenation hypothesis. This hypothesis states that the drug becomes covalently bound to a normal "self" protein and the combination of the drug bound to the protein is large enough to be recognized as foreign by the immune system, leading to an immune response.[10] Another hypothesis is the pro-hapten hypothesis which states that a non-reactive drug becomes chemically reactive during metabolism and then covalently binds to self-proteins. An example of this is sulfamethoxazole which is metabolized to sulfamethoxazole-nitroso which is highly reactive. Another hypothesis is the pharmacologic interaction (p-i) hypothesis which states that the drug (or metabolite) directly binds to the T-cell receptor, initiating an immune response. In this case, T-cells are directly activated, despite not interacting with antigen presenting cells.

As suggested by several of these hypotheses, the metabolism of the drug often plays a critical role. The fact that many drugs are primarily metabolized in the liver helps to explain why the liver is often involved in adverse drug reactions. It has also been recognized that skin keratinocytes are a site of drug metabolism. This discovery helps explain why the skin is involved in many forms of reactions elicited by different drugs.[11] Indeed some of the most common of the life-threatening drug reactions are predominately cutaneous, including Stevens-Johnson syndrome (SJS), toxic epidermal necrolysis (TEN), and drug reaction with eosinophilia and systemic symptoms (DRESS) or drug-induced hypersensitivity syndrome (DIHS).[12]

Pseudoallergic Drug Reactions

KEY CONCEPT *Reactions that clinically resemble allergic reactions but lack an immune basis are referred to as "pseudoallergic." They include almost the entire range of immediate hypersensitivity clinical patterns. Pseudoallergic reactions range in significance from the alarming but trivial anxiety or vasovagal reactions caused by local dental anesthetics to sometimes fatal reactions to ionic radiocontrast media.*

Pseudoallergic reactions are important in patient counseling and management considerations. They represent common biological functions such as direct histamine [H] release by vancomycin or opiates, whereas immunologic (allergic) reactions are based on the structure of the drug. Even a mild drug allergy may carry significant potential for anaphylaxis on readministration. In contrast, pseudoallergic reactions tend to remain constant whether mild or severe and are dose related.

Pseudoallergic reactions, then, are reactions where the components of the immune system are used in exactly the same way, but without the "learning" response by T cells and generally without the much greater danger that true immunologic sensitization implies. Pseudoallergic reactions may be thought of as a subtype

Clinical Presentation and Diagnosis of Allergic and Pseudoallergic Drug Reactions

The clinical presentation of a patient experiencing an allergic reaction varies greatly. The primary reactions are as follows:

Anaphylaxis

Anaphylaxis is an acute life-threatening allergic reaction. Signs and symptoms involve the skin (eg, pruritus, urticaria), respiratory tract (eg, dyspnea, wheezing), gastrointestinal tract (eg, nausea, cramping), and cardiovascular system (eg, hypotension, tachycardia). Onset is usually within 30 minutes, but can be as long as 2 hours. Treatment must begin immediately. Anaphylaxis may recur 6 to 8 hours after exposure, so patients should be observed for at least 12 hours.

Cytotoxic Reactions

These reactions usually take the form of hemolytic anemia, thrombocytopenia, granulocytopenia, or agranulocytosis.

Immune Complex Reactions

These reactions usually involve a serum sickness-like syndrome (eg, arthralgias, fever, malaise, and urticaria) that typically develops 7 to 14 days after exposure to the causative antigen.

Dermatologic Reactions

Rashes may range from mild to life-threatening.

- *Urticaria*: These are itchy, raised, swollen areas on the skin. Also known as hives.
- *Maculopapular rash*: A rash that contains both macules and papules. A macule is a flat, discolored area of the skin, and a papule is a small raised bump. A maculopapular rash is usually a large area that is red and has small bumps.
- *Erythema multiforme*: A rash characterized by papular (small raised bump) or vesicular lesions (blisters) and reddening or discoloration of the skin, often in concentric zones about the lesion.
- *Stevens-Johnson syndrome*: A severe expression of erythema multiforme (also known as erythema multiforme major). It typically involves the skin and the mucous membranes, with the potential for severe morbidity and even death.
- *Toxic epidermal necrolysis*: A life-threatening skin disorder characterized by blistering and peeling of the top layer of skin.

of idiopathic reactions, rather than an activation of the patient's immune system. The pathophysiology of pseudoallergic reactions is generally unknown, but indicators of immune activation are not seen when they occur.

PROBLEMATIC DRUG CLASSES AND TREATMENT OPTIONS

The first priority is to avoid doing serious harm by administering a drug the patient cannot tolerate. We can generally establish the likelihood of a relationship between the suspected drug and observed reaction, and also whether it is likely to be an immune or idiopathic reaction by examining the time course and specific signs and symptoms as precisely and objectively as possible. Reevaluating the patient's physical findings and laboratory values (taking into account preexisting diseases) allows further clarification of the need to change treatments and add therapy for the reaction itself.

Reviewing the original indications for the treatment that caused the reaction is important. For example, in many respiratory illnesses, a prescribed antibiotic may be unnecessary. If the disease persists and indications for some treatment are established, alternatives must be sought, either by adjusting dose or administration rate, finding an effective and unrelated alternative medication, or desensitizing the patient to the original drug.

When adverse drug reactions occur, the health care provider should carefully describe all aspects of the reaction and assess the potential for it to reoccur. Many patients have frightening associations of the term "allergy" with severe and unpredictable anaphylaxis. It is difficult to undo fears created by injudiciously labeling a patient as allergic in the medical record. Labeling a person "allergic" may hamper future medical care, as the patient may refuse treatment or fail to adhere to medication regimens. If the original reaction is clearly documented, health care providers can appropriately counsel patients about any true dangers.

Anaphylaxis is a true medical emergency and must be treated promptly. Otherwise, managing allergic reactions begins with stopping the offending agent. Understanding the allergic reaction and potential for cross-allergenicity between similar drugs will assist in selecting an alternative medication. Desensitization is a management option if the patient truly needs the medication and alternative drugs are not available. Although any drug may cause an allergic or pseudoallergic reaction, several drugs and drug classes are strongly associated with such reactions (Table 54–2). These classes will be discussed individually.

β-Lactam Antibiotics

Hypersensitivity reactions with β-lactam antibiotics, especially penicillin, may encompass any of the Types I through IV Gell-Coombs classifications. The most common reactions are maculopapular and urticarial eruptions.[13] Although rare (less than 0.05%), anaphylactic reactions to penicillins cause the greatest concern, because they are responsible for the majority of all drug-induced anaphylaxis deaths in patients, accounting for 75% of all anaphylaxis cases in the United States.[6,14] The treatment of anaphylaxis is given in Table 54–3.[15]

The health care professional is faced with a difficult task when approaching a patient who claims a history of penicillin allergy. Although as many as 12% of hospital patients state they have an allergy to penicillin, about 90% will have negative skins tests.[16] Table 54–4 shows the traditional protocol for penicillin skin testing.[17] This test only evaluates IgE-mediated reactions. A patient with a history of other serious reactions such as erythema multiforme, Stevens-Johnson syndrome, or toxic epidermal necrolysis should not receive penicillins and should not be tested.

KEY CONCEPT *Penicillins and cephalosporins both have a β-lactam ring joined to an S-containing ring structure (penicillins: a thiazolidine ring; cephalosporins: a dihydrothiazine ring). The extent of cross-allergenicity appears to be relatively low, with an estimate of approximately 4%.*[18] *Cross-allergenicity is less likely with newer*

Table 54–2

Problematic Drug Classes

β-Lactam antibiotics
Sulfonamide antibiotics
Aspirin and nonsteroidal anti-inflammatory drugs
Radiocontrast media
Opiates
Cancer chemotherapy
Insulin
Anticonvulsants

generation cephalosporins compared with the first-generation agents. Anaphylactic reactions to cephalosporins are rare, with a predicted range of 0.0001% to 0.1%. Minor skin reactions including urticaria, exanthems, and pruritus are the most common allergic reactions with cephalosporins, showing severe reactions less often than with penicillins.[19]

For other β-lactam agents, the recommendations are fairly straightforward. Carbapenems should be considered potentially cross-reactive with penicillins and used with caution.[20] Monobactams (eg, aztreonam) do not cross-react with any β-lactam drugs except ceftazidime because they share an identical R-group side chain.

Table 54–3

Pharmacologic Management of Anaphylactic Reactions

Immediate Intervention

Epinephrine 1:1000 (1 mg/mL)

- Adults: Give 0.2–0.5 mg IM, repeat every 5 minutes as needed
- Pediatrics: 0.01 mg/kg (maximum 0.3 mg) IM, repeat every 5 minutes as needed

Subsequent Interventions

Normal saline infusion

- Adults: 1–2 L at a rate of 5–10 mL/kg in the first 5 minutes, followed by slow infusion
- Pediatrics: up to 30 mL/kg in the first hour

Epinephrine infusion

If patient is NOT responding to epinephrine injections and volume resuscitation:

- Adults: epinephrine infusion (1 mg in 250 mL D_5W): 1–4 mcg/min, titrating based on clinical response or side effects
- Pediatrics: epinephrine infusion (0.6 × body weight (in kg) = number of mg diluted to a total of 100 mL normal saline: 1 mL/hour delivers 0.1 mcg/kg/min

Other Considerations After Epinephrine and Fluids

Diphenhydramine

- Adults: 25–50 mg IV or IM
- Pediatrics: 1–1.25 mg/kg (maximum of 300 mg/24 hour)

Ranitidine

- Adults: 50 mg in D_5W 20 mL IV over 5 minutes
- Pediatrics: 1 mg/kg (up to 50 mg) in D_5W 20 mL IV over 5 minutes

Inhaled β-agonist (bronchospasm resistant to epinephrine)

- 2–5 mg in 3 mL of normal saline, nebulized, repeat as needed

Dopamine (hypotension refractory to fluids and epinephrine)

- 2–20 mcg/kg/min titrated to maintain systolic blood pressure > 90 mm Hg

Hydrocortisone (severe or prolonged anaphylaxis)

- Adults: 250 mg IV (prednisone 20 mg can be given orally in mild cases)
- Pediatrics: 2.5–10 mg/kg/24 hours

D_5W, dextrose 5% in water; IM, intramuscularly; IV, intravenous.

Adapted from Lieberman P, Nicklas RA, Oppenheimer J, et al. The diagnosis and management of anaphylaxis practice parameter:2010 update. J Allergy Clin Immunol. 2010;126:477–480.

Table 54–4

Procedure for Performing Penicillin Skin Testing

A. Percutaneous (Prick) Skin Testing

Materials	Volume
Pre-Pen 6 × 10⁶ M	1 Drop
Penicillin G 10,000 Units/mL	1 Drop
β-Lactam drug 3 mg/mL	1 Drop
0.03% albumin-saline control	1 Drop
Histamine control (1 mg/mL)	1 Drop

1. Place a drop of each test material on the volar surface of the forearm.
2. Prick the skin with a sharp needle inserted through the drop at a 45° angle, gently tenting the skin in an upward motion.
3. Interpret skin responses after 15 minutes.
4. A wheal at least 2 × 2 mm with erythema is considered positive.
5. If the prick test is nonreactive, proceed to the intradermal test.
6. If the histamine control is nonreactive, the test is considered uninterpretable.

B. Intradermal Skin Testing

Materials	Volume
Pre-Pen 6 × 10⁶ M	0.02 mL
Penicillin G 10,000 Units/mL	0.02 mL
β-Lactam drug 3 mg/mL	0.02 mL
0.03% albumin-saline control	0.02 mL
Histamine control (0.1 mg/mL)	0.02 mL

1. Inject 0.02–0.03 mL of each test material intradermally (amount sufficient to produce a small bleb).
2. Interpret skin responses after 15 minutes.
3. A wheal at least 6 × 6 mm with erythema and at least 3 mm greater than the negative control is considered positive.
4. If the histamine control is nonreactive, the test is considered uninterpretable.

Antihistamines may blunt the response and cause false-negative reactions.

Adapted from Sullivan TJ. Current Therapy in Allergy. St. Louis, MO: Mosby; 1985:57–61.

Sulfonamide Antibiotics

Sulfonamides are compounds that contain a sulfonamide moiety (ie, SO_2NH_2). This group includes sulfonamide antibiotics (sulfonylarylamines), and nonarylamine sulfonamides such as furosemide, thiazide diuretics, sulfonylureas, and celecoxib. The sulfonamide antibiotics contain an aromatic amine at the N4 position and a substituted ring at the N1 position. Allergists generally agree that most, but not all, patients allergic to antimicrobial sulfonamides will tolerate nonarylamine sulfonamides.[21] Predisposition to allergic reactions is a more likely reason than cross-reactivity between these differing molecules.[22] The term "sulfa allergy" should not be used as it can be confusing to patients and health care providers. The sulfonamide antibiotics are significant because they account for the largest percentage of antibiotic-induced toxic epidermal necrolysis and Stevens-Johnson syndrome cases.[23]

Patient Encounter 1

A 72-year-old man with weight of 137 lb (62 kg) was admitted to a general medicine unit 9 days ago for an upper gastrointestinal bleed. Overnight, he spiked a fever of 104°F (40.0°C) and now has difficulty breathing. A preliminary diagnosis of hospital-acquired pneumonia is made. The medical record states the patient indicated on admission that he does not remember if he has any drug allergies. A combination of piperacillin/tazobactam and vancomycin is ordered. About 10 minutes after the start of the piperacillin/tazobactam infusion, the patient appears agitated and is having greater difficulty breathing. A family member hits the nurse call button.

What type of allergic reaction is the patient most likely having?

What is the first drug (dose and schedule) that should be administered?

What subsequent interventions may be necessary in this patient?

KEY CONCEPT *Reactions to sulfonamide antibiotics, ranging from mild (most common) to life-threatening (rare), occur in 2% to 4% of healthy patients, with rates as high as 65% in patients with acquired immunodeficiency syndrome (AIDS).*[24] Anaphylaxis or **anaphylactoid** reactions almost always occur within 30 minutes but may be up to 90 minutes after exposure, most commonly after parenteral administration. Isolated **angioedema** or urticaria can occur within minutes to days. Serum sickness occurs within 1 to 2 weeks. Fixed drug eruptions (lesions) occur within a half hour to 8 hours. These lesions resolve within 2 to 3 weeks after drug removal. The more severe conditions of Stevens-Johnson syndrome and toxic epidermal necrolysis tend to occur 1 to 2 weeks after initiation of therapy. Because trimethoprim-sulfamethoxazole is the drug of choice for patients with *Pneumocystis jiroveci* pneumonia, desensitization may be necessary. A history of Stevens-Johnson syndrome or toxic epidermal necrolysis is an absolute contraindication for the desensitization procedure.

Patients with Multiple Antibiotic Allergies

Dealing with patients who claim to have multiple antibiotic allergies can be challenging. Combining knowledge of cross-allergenicity with a careful assessment of patient history may be helpful in designing an antimicrobial regimen. Table 54–5 outlines a series of questions that can be useful in developing an effective treatment plan.[25] If available and indicated, skin testing may be useful to complete the puzzle. Often with careful assessment, an antibiotic of choice may be used when the patient's initial history would have ruled it out. Based on data gathered, the patient's record should reflect antibiotics safe to use if needed, antibiotics to be avoided, and antibiotics that can be used only after desensitization. Although Table 54–5 was designed with antibiotics in mind, it can be modified for multiple allergy situations.

Aspirin and Nonsteroidal Anti-Inflammatory Drugs

Aspirin and the nonsteroidal anti-inflammatory drugs (NSAIDs) can induce allergic and pseudoallergic reactions. Because these drugs are so widely used, with much over-the-counter use, the health care professional must have a basic understanding of the types of reactions that can occur and how to prevent them. Three types of reactions occur: bronchospasm with rhinoconjunctivitis, urticaria/angioedema, and anaphylaxis. Remember that patients with gastric discomfort or bruising from these agents may describe themselves as being allergic; however, these are not allergic or pseudoallergic reactions.

Two specific conditions—aspirin-exacerbated respiratory disease (AERD) and chronic idiopathic urticaria—are important because they are commonly seen. AERD may include asthma, rhinitis with nasal polyps, and aspirin sensitivity.[26] Upon exposure to aspirin or an NSAID, patients with AERD experience rhinorrhea, nasal congestion, conjunctivitis, laryngospasm, and asthma. Chronic idiopathic urticaria may also be seen with aspirin or NSAID-induced pseudoallergic reactions.[27] Patients with a history of chronic idiopathic urticaria are likely to see a flare of urticaria if aspirin or a cyclooxygenase (COX)-1 inhibiting NSAID is given. Cross-reactions between aspirin and older COX-1 inhibiting NSAIDs exist in patients with AERD and chronic idiopathic urticaria. Even though product warning labels for COX-2 inhibitors state these agents should not be used in these two conditions, there are no reports of cross-reactivity in AERD and only rare reports in chronic idiopathic urticaria.[28]

KEY CONCEPT *IgE-mediated urticarial/angioedema reactions and anaphylaxis are associated with aspirin and NSAIDs. Urticaria is the most common form of an IgE-mediated reaction. However, most reactions are the result of metabolic idiosyncrasies, such as*

Table 54–5
Multiple Antibiotic Allergies: Obtaining Background Information

For **each** antibiotic to which the patient claims to be allergic, gather the following information:
- What type of infection was being treated?
- Have you ever received the drug without experiencing a reaction?
- How many times have you received the drug and experienced a reaction?
- What was the drug dose and route of administration with the last reaction?
- How many doses did you take before the onset of the last reaction?
- How many doses did you take after the last reaction?
- Can you describe the adverse reaction?
- What was the duration of the reaction?
- What treatment was given for the reaction?
- Was there any permanent damage?

For **each** antibiotic the patient has received and does not claim allergy, gather the following information:
- What was the last type of infection being treated?
- What was the drug dose and route of administration?
- Have you received this drug more than once without reactions?

Other information to be gathered:
- Have you had adverse reactions to any other drugs? If so, give dates and describe the reaction.
- Document any risk factors for allergic reactions such as chronic urticaria, liver or kidney disease, HIV (human immunodeficiency virus), or any other immune deficiencies.

Adapted from Macy E. Multiple antibiotic allergy syndrome. Immunol Allergy Clin North Am 2004;24:533–543.

aspirin-induced respiratory disease which may produce severe and even fatal bronchospasm. This class is second only to β-lactams in causing anaphylaxis. Most reactions in this class are due to a complex metabolic pattern which causes increasingly recurrent and severe nasal polyps and often refractory asthma. The metabolic problem is constant once it emerges, accounting for the persistence and difficulty of these clinical problems. The metabolic problem is also capable of causing severe, sometimes fatal, acute reactions to aspirin or many if not all other NSAIDs. Rare reports of non–cross-reactive severe reactions suggest possible specific IgE-mediated reactions to individual NSAIDs, and there are some occurrences of urticaria related to NSAIDs as well. Because aspirin therapy is highly beneficial in primary and secondary prevention in coronary artery disease (CAD), aspirin desensitization should be considered in patients who have had reactions to aspirin. Desensitization is contraindicated in patients who have experienced an aspirin-induced anaphylactoid reaction, hypotension, tachypnea, or altered consciousness. Alternate agents must be used. A comprehensive approach to aspirin-sensitive patients with CAD has been described.[29]

Radiocontrast Media

KEY CONCEPT *Radiocontrast media may cause serious, immediate pseudoallergic reactions such as urticaria/angioedema, bronchospasm, shock, and death. These reactions have been reduced with the introduction of nonionic, lower osmolality products.* Because a small percentage of patients who have reacted previously to radiocontrast media will react if reexposed, several steps (listed below) should be taken to prevent reactions in these patients. These steps should also be followed in patients with high-risk factors: asthmatic patients, patients on β-blockers, and patients with cardiovascular disease.[5] The steps are as follows:

- Determine whether the study is essential.
- Be sure the patient understands the risks.
- Ensure adequate hydration.
- Use nonionic, lower osmolar agents.
- Pretreat with prednisone 50 mg orally 13, 7, and 1 hour(s) before the procedure and diphenhydramine 50 mg orally 1 hour before the procedure.

Delayed reactions with these agents occur in 1% to 3% of patients.[30] Although reactions are occasionally severe, most are mild and manifest as maculopapular rashes, fixed eruptions, erythema multiforme, and urticarial eruptions.

Opiates

KEY CONCEPT *Opiates (morphine, meperidine, codeine, hydrocodone, and others) stimulate mast cell release directly, resulting in pruritus and urticaria with occasional mild wheezing. Though these reactions are not allergic, many patients state they are "allergic" to one or more of the opiates. Pretreatment with an antihistamine may reduce these pseudoallergic reactions which are rarely, if ever, life-threatening.*[6] Avoiding other mast cell degranulating medications while patients require opiates also reduces the chances of frightening and uncomfortable reactions. Patients may state they are allergic if they have experienced gastrointestinal upset, a common side effect to opiates, with previous exposures. Obtaining a thorough history from the patient will prove useful. If a more serious reaction has occurred, a non-narcotic analgesic should be selected.

Patient Encounter 2

A 20-year-old woman is admitted to the hospital for treatment of a painful wound infection on her thigh. She has a history of hypertension, controlled with lisinopril, and periodic insomnia treated with over-the-counter medications. She is a nonsmoker and reports having one to two glasses of wine per week. Blood and wound cultures were obtained. Before initiating antibiotic therapy, you obtain her drug allergy history. She lists allergies to penicillin, vancomycin, clindamycin, and codeine. The reactions are described as follows:

Penicillin: When receiving penicillin for a sore throat as a teenager, she could not breathe and received an epinephrine injection from her physician.

Vancomycin: When receiving this drug for a previous wound infection several years ago, she developed a red rash on her upper body around her neck and shoulders. It went away a few hours later but came back the next time they infused the drug. Someone suggested that the nurse should infuse the drug slower on the next dose and the rash did not return. The patient states that she does not want to experience that allergy again.

Clindamycin: Several years ago she received a prescription for clindamycin solution. The patient states that it tasted so bad it caused her to throw up, so she must be allergic to it.

Codeine: The patient received a prescription for acetaminophen and codeine the previous summer. The patient says she took it around the clock and it helped the pain. However, she developed constipation and had to take a laxative for a week.

Based on the patient's allergy history, which if any, of the antibiotics listed above could she safely receive?

Can the patient receive an opiate analgesic to relieve the pain from her wound?

Cancer Chemotherapy

Hypersensitivity reactions have occurred with all chemotherapy agents. Reactions are most common with the taxanes, platinum compounds, asparaginases, and epipodophyllotoxins.[13] Reactions range from mild (flushing and rashes) to severe (dyspnea, bronchospasm, urticaria, and hypotension). IgE-mediated Type I reactions are the most common. To reduce the risk, patients are routinely premedicated with corticosteroids and H_1- and H_2-receptor antagonists. The platinum compounds have produced anemia, probably via a cytotoxic immunologic mechanism.

Insulin

Insulin is one of a very few medications that is itself a whole protein and can induce IgE sensitivity directly. This can result in anaphylaxis. Adverse reactions to insulin also include erythema, pruritus, and indurations, which are usually transient and may be injection site related.[31] For sensitivity reactions, treatment options include dexamethasone or desensitization. If the reaction is injection site related, a change in delivery system (ie, insulin pump or inhaled insulin) may be helpful.

Anticonvulsants

A wide range of hypersensitivity reactions, ranging from mild maculopapular skin eruptions to severe life-threatening reactions, can occur with anticonvulsants.[32] Aromatic anticonvulsants, primarily phenytoin, carbamazepine, phenobarbital, and primidone as well as some of the newer agents (lamotrigine, oxcarbazepine, felbamate, and zonisamide) can cause a life-threatening syndrome with symptoms including fever, a maculopapular rash, and evidence of systemic organ involvement. The rash may be mild at first but can progress to exfoliative dermatitis, erythema multiforme, Stevens-Johnson syndrome, or toxic epidermal necrolysis. This syndrome is known as anticonvulsant hypersensitivity syndrome (AHS) or drug rash with eosinophilia and systemic symptoms (DRESS). The causative agent should be withdrawn immediately. Cross-sensitivity among aromatic anticonvulsant drugs ranges between 40% and 80%.[33] If a patient is hypersensitive to an aromatic anticonvulsant, a nonaromatic agent (ethosuximide, gabapentin, levetiracetam, topiramate, lacosamide, and valproic acid) or the benzodiazepines may be useful.[33]

Drug Desensitization

Drug desensitization may be undertaken for some drugs in the absence of useful alternative medications. The risk of severe systemic reactions and anaphylaxis associated with desensitization must be compared with the risk of not treating the patient. A thorough evaluation should establish that the drug probably caused the reaction by an allergic mechanism. Because of the dangers involved with drug desensitization, an expert review of the patient's indication for the drug should be conducted. Consider the possibility that the patient does not really need the drug.

KEY CONCEPT *Desensitization is a potentially life-threatening procedure and requires continuous monitoring in a hospital setting, with suitable access to emergency treatment and intubation if required. It should only be undertaken under the direction of a physician with suitable training and experience. In such hands, desensitization may present less risk than treatment failure with a less effective alternative medication.*

The possibility of readministering a suspected drug may be safely tested by gradual dose escalation in some cases, and there are certainly many more patients who are harmed by inappropriately withholding medications than there are those who suffer significant harm from testing and desensitization.[34]

Only Type I IgE-mediated allergy may be treated by classical desensitization. Desensitization may occur within hours to several weeks, unlike specific immunotherapy injections for inhalant allergy (ie, "allergy shots," which may take months of therapy before a patient realizes any benefit and years to complete). The mechanism of drug desensitization is poorly understood but produces temporary drug-specific tolerance of the offending drug. Any interruption of therapy of 24 hours or more requires full repeat desensitization, and abrupt significant increases of dosage have been reported to break through the tolerance with some drugs.

The desensitization process probably involves either: (a) cross-linking small subthreshold numbers of bound IgE molecules gradually depleting mast cells of their mediators, or (b) binding of the IgE by monomers or hapten-protein entities that cannot cross-link the antibody. The low doses used at the beginning of all protocols would provide small amounts of antigen, favoring these mechanisms. Both drug-specific IgE and IgG serum concentrations increase after successful desensitization, but skin test positivity generally decreases.[35]

Patient Encounter 3

A 62-year-old man is visiting his new primary care physician for follow-up after being hospitalized for a myocardial infarction 10 days ago. The patient's father and older brother died from myocardial infarctions when they were in their late 60s. The patient saw a television commercial touting the benefits of aspirin in preventing heart attacks and wants to start taking it immediately. Upon review of the patient's medical record, his new physician notices that the patient was previously diagnosed with an aspirin allergy. His reaction was primarily a moderate urticaria.

Does this patient's potential benefit of aspirin therapy outweigh the risk when considering his history of allergy?

What course of action would you recommend for this patient?

Oral and intravenous (IV) protocols are available for most drugs in this category, with the oral route producing somewhat milder reactions, but the IV route providing more precision in dosing. IV administration can also be used in unresponsive patients for whom the oral route is not feasible. Protocols generally begin at about 1% of the therapeutic dose and increase in intervals defined by the patient's reaction and the distribution and metabolism of the drug itself. Half-$\log_{10}$ dose increases (about threefold) are often tolerated.

Penicillin desensitization is the most common drug desensitization protocol. It is required for penicillin-allergic patients when penicillin is clearly the only treatment option, for example, when syphilis is present in pregnancy. Protocols have been adopted for most antibiotics. Specific procedures for oral and IV penicillin desensitization have been developed.[36]

Aspirin desensitization is useful in diseases for which low-level antiplatelet action is needed and in the care of patients with aspirin sensitivity and intractable nasal polyps. Lysine aspirin availability in Europe allows desensitization by inhalation at greatly reduced risk. New procedures utilizing ketorolac as a nasal topical application may allow similar reduction of risk in the United States.[37] As with all desensitizations, constant daily administration must be maintained once the desired dose is reached. Several aspirin desensitization protocols have been described in the literature.[38,39]

All desensitization procedures are expected to produce mild symptoms in the patient at some point, and the patient must be made to understand this before doses are started. Mild sensitivity to the drug still remains, and large dose increases as well as missing doses should be avoided. Late complications, such as urticaria, may occur with Type I desensitization, and serum sickness or hemolytic anemia may also occur with high-dose therapy in allergic, desensitized patients.

Some regimens are designed for outpatient administration over much longer time periods and have been used, for example, with allopurinol dermal reactions. Such late-onset morbilliform reactions, sometimes overlapping with erythema multiforme minor, are difficult to evaluate, because it is often unclear to what extent the patients were at risk for a recurrent reaction.

Severe life-threatening reactions not mediated by IgE, such as Stevens-Johnson syndrome and toxic epidermal necrolysis, are absolute contraindications to testing, desensitization attempts, and readministration.

Patient Care Process

Patient Assessment:

- Based on the medication history, physical examination, and review of systems, determine the likelihood of the reaction being a drug-related problem. See Clinical Presentation and Diagnosis of Allergic and Pseudoallergic Drug Reactions. Tables 54–1 and 54–2 may also be helpful.
- Use questions given in Table 54–5 to establish the nature of the reaction and the likelihood it was caused by the suspected drug. For nonantibiotics, the first question regarding infection type is not needed.
- If appropriate, see Table 54–4 for procedures for performing penicillin skin testing.

Therapy Evaluation:

- Document the reaction, in detail, in the patient's medical record.
- Recommend an alternative choice if the prescribed drug is contraindicated, and develop a plan to assess safety and effectiveness.
- Consult with health care professionals trained in desensitization if the patient has a true allergy and no acceptable alternative medication is available.

Care Plan Development:

- If reaction is anaphylactic in nature, see Table 54–3.
- The offending drug should be discontinued.
- The treatment goal is relief of symptoms. For mild symptoms such as rash or itching, an antihistamine such as diphenhydramine may be used. For wheezing, bronchodilators such as albuterol may be helpful.
- Recommend an alternative option for the contraindicated drug, or if no alternative is available, consult with health care professional regarding desensitization.
- Educate the patient about the allergy or pseudoallergy so they are able to work with health care providers to avoid the reaction in the future.

Follow-up Evaluation:

- Follow-up daily or more often, if necessary, to assure resolution of the reaction and optimal response to the alternate therapy.

OUTCOME EVALUATION

To successfully treat a patient with a drug allergy or pseudoallergy, several goals must be accomplished:

- If a reaction occurs, it must be identified and managed quickly.
- The patient should be educated about the reaction.
- True drug contraindications should be avoided if possible.
- Patients should receive the medications they need or a suitable alternative. If this is not possible due to an allergy, desensitization should be considered.
- Patients should always be monitored for adverse drug reactions.

Abbreviations Introduced in This Chapter

AERD	Aspirin-exacerbated respiratory disease
AHS	Anticonvulsant hypersensitivity syndrome
AIDS	Acquired immunodeficiency syndrome
CAD	Coronary artery disease
COX	Cyclooxygenase
D_5W	Dextrose 5% in water
DIHS	Drug-induced hypersensitivity syndrome
DRESS	Drug reaction with eosinophilia and systemic symptoms
H (H_1, H_2)	Histamine
HIV	Human immunodeficiency virus
Ig	Immunoglobulin (followed by the specific type of immunoglobulin: E, G, or M)
IL	Interleukin
IM	Intramuscular
IV	Intravenous
NSAIDs	Nonsteroidal anti-inflammatory drugs
p-i	Pharmacologic interaction
SJS	Stevens-Johnson syndrome
TEN	Toxic epidermal necrolysis
Th	T-helper cell

REFERENCES

1. Lazarou J, Pomeranz BH, Corey PN. Incidence of adverse drug reactions in hospitalized patients. A meta-analysis of prospective studies. JAMA. 1998;269:1200–1205.
2. American Academy of Allergy Asthma and Immunology [Internet]. Allergy statistics: Drug allergy [cited 2014 September 15]. *http://www.aaaai.org/about-the-aaaai/newsroom/allergy-statistics.aspx#Drug_Allergy.* Accessed August 27, 2015.
3. Gomes ER, Demoly P. Epidemiology of hypersensitivity reactions. Curr Opin Allergy Clin Immunol. 2005;5(4):309–316.
4. Impicciatore P, Choonara I, Clarkson A, et al. Incidence of adverse drug reactions in paediatric in/out patients: A systematic review and meta-analysis of prospective studies. Br J Clin Pharmacol. 2001;52:77–83.
5. Adkinson NF, Essayan D, Gruchalla R, et al. Task force report: Future research needs for the prevention and management of immune-mediated drug hypersensitivity reactions. J Allergy Clin Immunol. 2002;109(3):S461–S478.
6. Anon, Part 1: Executive summary of disease management of drug hypersensitivity: A practice parameter. Ann Allergy Asthma Immunol. 1999;83:665–700.
7. Pichler WJ. Delayed drug hypersensitivity reactions. Ann Intern Med. 2003;139:683–690.
8. Uetrecht J, Naisbitt DJ. Idiosyncratuc adverse drug reactions: Current concepts. Pharmacol Rev. 2013;65:779–808.
9. Khan DA, Solensky R. Drug allergy. J Allergy Clin Immunol. 2010;125:S126–S137.
10. Pilger WJ, Naisbitt DJ, Park BK. Immune pathomechanism of drug hypersensitivity reactions. J Allergy Clin Immunol. 2011;127:S74–S81.

11. Paquet P, Delvenne P, Pierard GE. Drug interactions with normal and TEN epidermal keratinocytes. Curr Drug Saf. 2012;7:352–356.
12. Phillips EJ, Chung WH, Mockenhaupt M, et al. Drug hypersensitivity: Pharmacogenetics and clinical syndromes. J Allergy Clin Immunol. 2011;127:S60–S66.
13. Gruchalla RS. Allergic disorders. J Allergy Clin Immunol. 2003;111(2):S548–S559.
14. Neugut A, Ghatak A, Miller R. Anaphylaxis in the United States: an investigation into its epidemiology. Arch Intern Med. 2001;161:15–21.
15. Lieberman P, Nicklas RA, Oppenheimer J, et al. The diagnosis and management of anaphylaxis practice parameter: 2010 update. J Allergy Clin Immunol. 2010; 126:477–80.
16. Thethi AK, Van Dellen RG. Dilemmas and controversies in penicillin allergy. Immunol Allergy Clin North Am. 2004;24: 445–461.
17. Sullivan TJ. Current Therapy in Allergy. St. Louis, MO: Mosby; 1985:57–61.
18. Kelkar PS, Li JT. Cephalosporin allergy. N Engl J Med. 2001;345:804–809.
19. Madaan A, Li JT. Cephalosporin allergy. Immunol Allergy Clin North Am. 2004;24:463–476.
20. Kula B, Djordjevic G, Robinson JL. A systematic review: Can one prescribe carbapenems to patients with IgE-mediated allergy to penicillins or cephalosporins. Clin Infectious Dis. 2014;59:1113–1122.
21. Dibbin DA, Montanaro A. Allergies to sulfonamide antibiotics and sulfur-containing drugs. Ann Allergy Asthma Immunol. 2008;100:91–100.
22. Strom BL, Schinnar R, Apter AJ, et al. Absence of cross-reactivity between sulfonamide antibiotics and sulfonamide nonantibiotics. N Engl J Med. 2003;349(17):1628–1635.
23. Slatore CG, Tilles SA. Sulfonamide hypersensitivity. Immunol Allergy Clin North Am. 2004;24:477–490.
24. Greenberger PA. Drug allergy. J Allergy Clin Immunol. 2006; 117:S464–S470
25. Macy E. Multiple antibiotic allergy syndrome. Immunol Allergy Clin North Am. 2004;24:533–543.
26. Sanchez-Borges M. NSAID hypersensitivity. Med Clin N Am. 2010;94:853–864.
27. Sanchez-Borges M, Caprilles-Hulett A, Caballero-Fonesca F. Cutaneous reactions to aspirin and NSAIDs. Clin Rev Allergy Immunol. 2003;24:125–135.
28. Stevenson DD. Aspirin and NSAID sensitivity. Immunol Allergy Clin North Am. 2004;24:491–505.
29. Ramanuja S, Breall JA, Kalaria VG. Approach to "Aspirin allergy" in cardiovascular patients. Circulation. 2004;110:e1–e4.
30. Christiansen C. X-ray contrast media—An overview. Toxicology. 2005;209:185–187.
31. Richardson T, Kerr D. Skin-related complications of insulin therapy: Epidemiology and emerging management strategies. Am J Clin Dermatol. 2003;4(10):661–667.
32. Behi E, Shorvon S. Antiepileptic drugs and the immune system. Epilepsia. 2011;52 (Suppl 3):40–44.
33. Bohan KH, Mansuri TF, Wilson NM. Anticonvulsant hypersensitivity syndrome: Implications for pharmaceutical care. Pharmacotherapy. 2007;27(10):1425–1439.
34. Adkinson NF Jr. Drug allergy. In: Middleton's Allergy: Principles & Practice. 6th ed. Philadelphia, PA: Mosby; 2003:1690.
35. Schmitz-Schumann M, Juhl E, Costabel U. Analgesic asthma-provocation challenge with acetylsalicylic acid. Atemw Lungenkrkh Jahrgang. 1985;10:479–485.
36. Weiss ME, Adkinson NF. Diagnostic testing for drug hypersensitivity. Immunol Allerg Clin North Am. 1998;18: 731–734.
37. White A, Bigby T, Stevenson D. Intranasal ketorolac challenge for the diagnosis of aspirin exacerbated respiratory disease. Ann Allergy Asthma Immunol. 2006;97:190–195.
38. Melillo G, Balzano G, Bianco S, et al. Report of the INTERASMA Working Group on Standardization of Inhalation Provocation Tests in Aspirin-induced Asthma. Oral and inhalation provocation tests for the diagnosis of aspirin-induced asthma. Allergy. 2001;56(9):899–911.
39. Stevenson DD, Simon R, Sensitivity to aspirin and non-steroidal anti-inflammatory drugs. In: Middleton E, Reed CE, Ellis EF, et al., eds. Allergy Principles and Practice. St. Louis, MO: Mosby; 1998:1225.

55 Solid Organ Transplantation

Steven Gabardi, Spencer T. Martin, and
Ali J. Olyaei

LEARNING OBJECTIVES

Upon completion of the chapter, the reader will be able to:

1. Describe the reasons for solid organ transplantation.
2. Differentiate between the functions of cell-mediated and humoral immunity and how they relate to organ transplant.
3. Describe the roles of antigen-presenting cells in initiating the immune response.
4. Compare and contrast the types of rejection including hyperacute, acute, chronic, and humoral rejection.
5. Define the terms "host–graft adaptation" and "tolerance," paying close attention to their differences.
6. Discuss the desired therapeutic outcomes and appropriate pharmacotherapy utilized to avoid allograft rejection.
7. Compare and contrast currently available immunosuppressive agents in terms of mechanisms of action, adverse events, and drug–drug interactions.
8. Develop a therapeutic drug-monitoring plan to assess effectiveness and adverse events of the immunosuppressive drugs.
9. Design an appropriate therapeutic regimen for the management of immunosuppressive drug complications based on patient-specific information.
10. Write appropriate patient education instructions and identify methods to improve patient adherence following transplantation.

INTRODUCTION

The earliest recorded attempts at organ transplant date back thousands of years.[1] More than a few apocryphal descriptions exist from ancient Egypt, China, India, and Rome describing experimentation with transplantation. However, it was not until the early 1900s that French surgeon, Alexis Carrel, pioneered the art of surgical techniques for transplantation.[1] Together with Charles Guthrie, Carrel experimented in artery and vein transplantation. Using revolutionary methods in **anastomosis** operations and suturing techniques, Carrel laid the groundwork for modern transplant surgery. He was one of the first to identify the dilemma of rejection, an issue that remained insurmountable for nearly half a century.[1]

Prior to the work of Alexis Carrel, malnourishment was the prevailing theory regarding the mechanism of **allograft** rejection.[1] However, in 1910, Carrel noted that tissue damage in the transplanted organ was likely caused by multiple, circulating biological factors. It was not until the late 1940s with the work of Peter Medawar that transplant immunology became more understood. Medawar was able to define the immunologic nature of rejection using skin allografts. In addition, George Snell observed that grafts shared between inbred animals were accepted but were rejected when transplanted between animals of different strains.[1]

The seminal work by early transplant researchers eventually led to the concept of histocompatibility.[1] Histocompatibility describes the process by which polymorphic genes encode cell membrane antigens that serve as targets for immune response, even within a species. Further research in transplant immunobiology led to a more accurate understanding of the alloimmune response.[1]

Joseph Murray performed the first successful organ transplant in 1954.[1] It was a kidney transplant between identical twins. This was a success in large part because no immunosuppression was necessary due to the fact that donor and recipient were genetically identical. Murray's success laid the groundwork for modern-day transplantation.

EPIDEMIOLOGY AND ETIOLOGY

Heart

Nearly 6 million Americans are afflicted with heart failure. Cardiac transplantation is the treatment of choice for patients with severe end-stage heart failure. Candidates for cardiac transplantation generally present with New York Heart Association (NYHA) class III or IV symptoms and have an ejection fraction of less than 20% (0.20). The general indications for cardiac transplantation include rapidly declining cardiac function, requirement of intravenous (IV) inotropes, and having a projected 1-year mortality rate of greater than 75%. Mechanical support with an implantable left ventricular assist device may be appropriate as bridge therapy while patients await a viable organ.[1] Most heart transplants are **orthotopic**; however, in certain situations, **heterotopic** cardiac transplants have been performed. There were 2655 heart transplant procedures done in the United States in 2014.[2] Indications for heart transplant include:

- Cardiomyopathy (ie, dilated myopathy, hypertrophic cardiomyopathy, restrictive myopathy)
- Congenital heart disease
- Coronary artery disease
- Valvular heart disease

Intestine

An intestine transplant may involve the use of an entire intestine or shortened segment. Most intestine transplants completed in the United States involve the transplant of the full organ and are often performed in conjunction with liver transplantation. Although most intestine transplants involve organs harvested from a deceased donor, recent advances in the field have made it possible for living donor intestinal segment transplants. There were 139 intestine transplants (138 deceased donors and 1 living donor) done in 2014.[2] Reasons for intestine transplant include:

- Functional bowel problems (ie, Hirschsprung disease, neuronal intestinal dysplasia, pseudoobstruction, protein-losing enteropathy, microvillous inclusion disease)
- Short gut syndrome (ie, intestinal atresia, necrotizing enterocolitis, intestinal volvulus, massive resection secondary to inflammatory bowel disease, tumors, mesenteric thrombosis)

Kidneys

More than 26 million Americans have chronic kidney disease (CKD), with another 20 million more considered to be at increased risk for kidney disease. End-stage renal disease (ESRD) only constitutes a small portion of those patients with CKD, with more than 640,000 patients diagnosed throughout the United States as of 2012. However, the ESRD population continues to increase. All patients with ESRD should be considered for renal transplantation if they are healthy enough to undergo the surgery.

Most kidney transplants are heterotopic, where the kidney is implanted above the pelvic bone and attached to the patient's iliac artery and vein. The ureter of the transplant kidney is attached directly to the recipient's bladder or native ureter. The native kidneys are usually not removed, and data have shown that under most circumstances, removal of the native kidneys does not influence patient survival (ie, survival of the transplant patient, without regard to function or survival of the allograft) and **allograft survival**.[1] There were 17,108 (11,570 deceased donors and 5,538 living donors) kidney transplants performed in 2014.[2] Reasons for kidney transplant include:

- Congenital, familial, and metabolic disorders (ie, congenital obstructive uropathy, Fabry disease, medullary cystic disease, nephrolithiasis)
- Diabetes mellitus (DM)
- Glomerular diseases (ie, antiglomerular basement membrane disease, focal segmental glomerular sclerosis, IgA nephropathy, hemolytic uremic syndrome, systemic lupus erythematosus, Alport syndrome, amyloidosis, membranous nephropathy, Goodpasture syndrome)
- Hypertension
- Neoplasm (ie, renal cell carcinoma, Wilms tumor)
- Polycystic kidney disease
- Renovascular disease
- Tubular and interstitial diseases (ie, analgesic nephropathy, drug-induced nephritis, oxalate nephropathy, radiation nephritis, acute tubular necrosis, sarcoidosis)

Liver

A liver transplant may involve the use of the entire organ or a segment. The majority of cases involve utilizing the full organ. In recent years, segmental transplants have been conducted using living donors. This procedure requires donation of the left hepatic lobe, which accounts for nearly 60% of the overall liver mass. This type of procedure is possible because the liver can regenerate; therefore, both the donor and recipient, in theory, will have normal liver function shortly after the transplant procedure. There were 6729 (6449 deceased donors and 280 partial lobe-living donors) liver transplants done in 2014.[2] Reasons for liver transplant include:

- Acute hepatic necrosis (ie, chronic or acute hepatitis B or C)
- Biliary atresia
- Cholestatic liver disease/cirrhosis (ie, primary biliary cirrhosis)
- Metabolic disease (ie, Wilson disease, primary oxalosis)
- Neoplasms (ie, hepatoma, cholangiocarcinoma, hepatoblastoma, bile duct cancer)
- Noncholestatic cirrhosis (ie, alcoholic cirrhosis, postnecrotic cirrhosis, drug-induced cirrhosis)

Lungs

Lung transplants may involve deceased donation of two lungs or a single lung. More recently, lobar transplants from blood group–compatible living donors have been performed for a small segment of the population. Most of the lobar transplants have been performed on cystic fibrosis patients. On rare occasions, a simultaneous heart–lung transplant occurs. This type of procedure is reserved for patients with severe pulmonary and cardiac disease. There were 1925 (all deceased donors) lung transplants and 24 simultaneous heart–lung transplant procedures done in 2014.[2] Reasons for lung transplant include:

- α-1-Antitrypsin deficiency
- Congenital disease (ie, Eisenmenger syndrome)
- Cystic fibrosis
- Emphysema/chronic obstructive pulmonary disease
- Idiopathic pulmonary fibrosis
- Primary pulmonary hypertension

Pancreas

The exact nationwide prevalence of all diseases of the pancreas has not been fully quantified; however DM, both types 1 and 2, affects nearly 21 million people in the United States. Some people suffering from DM may also be afflicted with ESRD. A small percentage of these patients undergo a simultaneous pancreas-kidney (SPK) transplant, which may be accomplished using organs from deceased or living donors. Transplant of a pancreas may involve either the entire organ or a pancreas segment. Currently, whole-organ transplant is the most common procedure, with a portion of the duodenum often transplanted along with the pancreas. Living donors are often the source of segmental transplants. In recent years, isolation and transplantation of β-islet cells alone have been completed. Islet transplantation is intended to treat organ dysfunction by replacing nonfunctioning islet cells with new ones. Islet transplants are still considered experimental, and long-term benefit and/or risk of this procedure needs to be studied extensively. Future success of islet cell transplantation is dependent on identifying a nontoxic immunosuppressive combination. There were 245 pancreas transplants and 709 SPK procedures done in 2014.[2] Reasons for pancreas transplants include:

- DM (ie, type 1 and 2, DM secondary to chronic pancreatitis or cystic fibrosis)
- Pancreatic cancer

PATHOPHYSIOLOGY

Major Histocompatibility Complex

The primary target of the immune response after organ transplant is the major histocompatibility complex (MHC).[1,3] The MHC is a region of highly polymorphic genes located on the short arm of chromosome 6. The human MHC is referred to as human leukocyte antigen (HLA). HLA is a set of glycoproteins expressed on the surface of most cells. These proteins are involved in immune recognition, which is the discrimination of self from nonself, but are also the principal antigenic determinants of allograft rejection.[1,3]

The HLA have been classified into two major groups, class I and II:

- Class I: expressed on the surfaces of all nucleated cells and recognized by $CD8^+$ cells (ie, cytotoxic T cells).
  - The three subclasses of MHC class I are HLA-A, HLA-B, and HLA-C.
- Class II: expressed solely on the surfaces of antigen-presenting cells (APCs). The APCs serve to stimulate $CD4^+$ cells (ie, helper T cells).
  - The three subclasses of MHC class II are HLA-DP, HLA-DQ, and HLA-DR.

T and B Lymphocytes

Lymphocytes are one of five kinds of white blood cells. Mature lymphocytes are astonishingly diverse in their functions. The most abundant of the lymphocytes are T lymphocytes (ie, T cells) and B lymphocytes (ie, B cells).

► T Lymphocytes

KEY CONCEPT *T cells play a major role in the cell-mediated immune response.* These cells are produced in the bone marrow, but mature in the thymus, hence the abbreviation "T." There are three recognized subclasses of T cells: cytotoxic T cells, helper T cells, and regulatory T cells:

- Cytotoxic T cells ($CD8^+$) promote target cell destruction by activating cellular apoptosis or killing the target cell via the release of cytotoxic proteins.
- Helper T cells ($CD4^+$) are the great communicators of the immune response. Once activated, they proliferate and secrete cytokines that regulate effector cell function. Some helper T cells secrete cytokines that recruit cytotoxic T cells, B cells, or APCs, whereas others secrete cytokines that turn off the immune response.
- Regulatory T cells, or suppressor T cells, suppress the activation of an immune response.

► B Lymphocytes

B cells play a large role in the humoral immune response. In humans, B cells are produced and mature in the bone marrow. The human body produces several types of B cells. Each B cell is unique, with a distinctive cell surface receptor protein that binds to only one particular antigen. Once B cells encounter their antigen and receive a cytokine signal from helper T cells, they can further differentiate into one of two cells, plasma cells or memory B cells. Plasma cells secrete antibodies that induce the destruction of target antigens through complement recruitment and/or opsonization. Memory B cells play an important role in long-term immunity, as they are capable of rapidly responding to subsequent exposures to their target antigen.

Antigen-Presenting Cells

KEY CONCEPT *An APC is a cell that displays a foreign antigen complexed with MHC on its cell surface.* Its major responsibility is to present these foreign antigens to T cells. T cells can identify this complex using their T-cell receptors (TCRs). There are three main types of APCs: dendritic cells (DCs), macrophages, and activated B cells. DCs are present in tissues that are in contact with the environment, such as skin and the lining of the nose, lungs, stomach, and intestines. They are responsible for phagocytosis. After which, they express the foreign antigen on their cell surface and then migrate to lymphoid tissues to interact with T and B cells to initiate the immune response. Macrophages' main role is removal of pathogens and necrotic debris. However, like DCs, macrophages also phagocytize antigens. The first time an antigen is encountered, the DCs and macrophages act as the primary APCs. However, if the same antigen is encountered again, memory B cells become the most important APC because they initiate the immune response quickly after antigen presentation. It appears that both the DCs and macrophages have the most activity in terms of allorecognition.

Allorecognition

KEY CONCEPT *Recognition of the antigens displayed by the transplanted organ (alloantigens) is the prime event that initiates the immune response against the allograft.* There are currently two accepted pathways for allorecognition:

- Direct pathway: Donor APCs migrate out of the allograft into the recipient's lymph nodes and present donor MHC molecules to the recipient's T cells.
- Indirect pathway: Recipient APCs migrate into the graft and phagocytize alloantigens. The recipient's APCs present donor MHC molecules to the recipient T cells in lymph nodes.

T-Cell Activation

KEY CONCEPT *Whether it is by direct or indirect pathways, in order for a T cell to become activated against the allograft, two interactions or signals must take place between the APCs and the recipient's T cells*[1,3]:

- Signal 1 is the interaction of the TCR with the foreign antigens presented by APCs.

Table 55–1

Organ-Specific Signs and Symptoms of an Acute Rejection Episode[1]

Organ	Clinical Symptoms	Laboratory Signs
Heart	Fever, lethargy, weakness, SOB, DOE, hypotension, tachycardia, atrial flutter, ventricular arrhythmias	Leukocytosis, biopsy positive for mononuclear infiltrates
Kidney	Fever, graft tenderness, decreased urine output, malaise, hypertension, weight gain, edema	Increased SCr, BUN, leukocytosis, biopsy positive for lymphocytic infiltration
Intestine	Fever and GI symptoms (ie, bloating, cramping, diarrhea, increased stomal output)	There are no reliable biochemical markers for intestine transplant rejection, but biopsies may be helpful
Liver	Fever, lethargy, change in color or quantity of bile in patients with biliary T-tube, graft tenderness and swelling, back pain, anorexia, ileus, tachycardia, jaundice, ascites, encephalopathy	Abnormal LFTs, increased bilirubin, alkaline phosphate, transaminases, biopsy positive for mononuclear cell infiltrate with evidence of tissue damage
Lung	Fever, impaired gas exchange, SOB, malaise, anxiety	Decreased FEV, infiltrate on CXR, biopsy positive for lymphocytic infiltration
Pancreas	Fever, graft tenderness and swelling, abdominal pain, ileus, and malaise	Increased FBS, leukocytosis, decreased human C-peptide and urinary amylase levels

BUN, blood urea nitrogen; CXR, chest x-ray; DOE, dyspnea on exertion; FBS, fasting blood sugar; FEV, forced expiratory volume; GI, gastrointestinal; LFTs, liver function tests; SCr, serum creatinine; SOB, shortness of breath.

- Signal 2 is an interaction between one of several costimulatory receptors and paired ligands on the cell surfaces of the APCs and T cells, respectively. Both interactions must occur simultaneously as Signal 1 in the absence of Signal 2 induces T-cell anergy.
- Once activated, T cells undergo clonal expansion under the influence of cytokines, specifically interleukin-2 (IL-2). These steps elicit an antidonor T-cell response that results in graft destruction.

Mechanisms of Acute Rejection

After activation, cytotoxic T cells emerge from lymphoid organs to infiltrate the graft and trigger the immune response. These cells induce graft destruction via two mechanisms: (a) secretion of cytotoxic proteins (ie, perforin, granzyme) and (b) induction of cellular apoptosis through interaction. Besides the cytotoxic T cells, several other cell lines may play a role in allograft destruction, including B cells, granulocytes, and natural killer cells.

Types of Rejection

► *Hyperacute Rejection*

Hyperacute rejection is an immediate recipient immune response against the allograft due to the presence of preformed recipient antibodies directed against the donor's HLA. This type of reaction generally occurs within minutes of transplantation. The organ must be removed immediately to prevent severe systemic responses. In the case of cardiac or lung transplantation in which the organ cannot be promptly removed, short-term mechanical circulatory support is required until an alternative organ becomes available. Those patients at highest risk for hyperacute rejection include any patients that have preformed HLA or ABO blood group antibodies, including patients with a history of previous organ transplant or multiple blood transfusions, as well as women who have had children. Hyperacute rejection has been largely eliminated due to routine pretransplant surveillance testing.

► *Acute Rejection*

Acute rejection is a cell-mediated process that generally occurs early posttransplant; however, it can occur at any time after transplant. This reaction is mediated through alloreactive T cells, as discussed above. Organ-specific signs and symptoms of acute rejection can be seen in Table 55–1.[1]

► *Antibody-Mediated Rejection*

Antibody-mediated rejection (AMR) is the process of creating graft-specific antibodies.[4] This type of rejection occurs less frequently than cell-mediated acute rejection. Histologic findings are similar to those of hyperacute rejection, but the severity of rejection is usually less with AMR. AMR is generally characterized by deposition of immunoglobulins and complement in allograft tissues. However, AMR may be diagnosed without the presence of complement. Treatment for this type of rejection is not well defined; however, several reports have shown that treatments such as plasmapheresis, immunoglobulin therapy, rituximab, bortezomib, or eculizumab may be effective.[4]

► *Chronic Rejection*

Chronic rejection has traditionally been thought of as a slow, insidious form of acute rejection, resulting in worsening organ function over time. The exact immunologic processes of chronic rejection are poorly understood; however, many believe that both the cell-mediated and humoral immune systems and drug-induced toxicities play a vital role in its development. Currently, retransplantation is the only effective treatment option.[1,3]

► *Host–Graft Adaptation*

The term "host–graft adaptation" describes the decreased immune response against the allograft over time.[1,3] This phenomenon is evident by the reduced incidence of acute rejection episodes seen months after transplantation. In theory, host–graft adaptation is thought to be secondary to a weakened T-cell response to donor antigens while patients receive maintenance immunosuppression.[1,3]

Tolerance

Tolerance is the process that allows organ-specific antigens to be accepted as self.[1] This would mean the immune system would cease to respond to the allograft and immunosuppressive medications would not be required. Immune tolerance has been achieved in the lab, but has yet to be successfully accomplished in humans.[1]

Immunologic Barriers to Transplantation

One of the more common barriers to successful transplantation is the presence of preformed HLA antibodies or ABO blood group incompatibility.[4] In cases in which these antibodies exist, if they are not adequately removed prior to transplant, they are likely to result in AMR and poor graft survival. To improve outcomes, assessment of pretransplant immune risk factors plays an important role in the prevention of immune-mediated allograft injuries. The introduction of pretransplant cross-matching and the use of ABO-compatible donors has largely eliminated hyperacute rejection episodes. However, these immunologic barriers are present in several potential recipients with willing organ donors, and patients are left to wait for a deceased donor or undergo pretransplant immunomodulation in an attempt to prevent these antibodies from affecting the allograft.[4]

▸ *ABO Incompatibility*

The expanding deceased donor waiting list encouraged some centers to evaluate the use of ABO desensitization protocols in order to transplant patients with ESRD that had willing but ABO-incompatible donors.[4] The desensitization protocol most commonly used in the United States involves reducing ABO antibody titers through plasmapheresis with IV immune globulin (IVIG). Use of plasma exchange to achieve an ABO antibody titer of less than 1:8 to 1:32 has resulted in long-term renal transplant results that are comparable to those of ABO-compatible transplants, despite an incidence of acute AMR that approaches 10% to 30%.[4]

▸ *HLA Sensitization*

Evaluation of the presence or absence of alloantibodies and T-cell activities to HLA antigens plays a significant role in individualization of immunosuppression.[4] A patient's degree of sensitization is often reported as the percentage of panel-reactive antibodies (PRA), which is an estimate of the likelihood of a positive crossmatch to a pool of potential donors. Advancement in HLA antibody screening and identification through flow cytometry or solid-phase multiplex platforms has overcome many of the issues stemming from older methods of PRA calculations. Patients are considered to be highly sensitized to HLA if they have a PRA of greater than or equal to 80%, making them less likely to receive a deceased donor organ. Patients with higher PRAs and preformed antibodies have poorer long-term allograft survival. Although PRA is a sensitive test and has predictive value, lymphocytes directly obtained from the donor is a superior method of immune monitoring. The assay is aimed to detect the presence of antibodies directed against the HLA antigens of the donor. In this setting, the presence of donor-specific antibodies (DSA) is identified. In one study, allograft survival was significantly lower in patients with DSA.[5] Thus detecting DSA and the presence of high PRA may indicate the need to enhance immunosuppression to improve posttransplant outcomes and allograft survival.[4]

Like ABO incompatibilities, it is possible to desensitize patients against a willing donor despite the presence of DSA or those awaiting a deceased donor transplant with a broad array of preformed anti-HLA antibodies (PRA greater than or equal to 30%).[4] There are two general protocols used for HLA desensitization: high-dose IVIG and low-dose IVIG with plasmapheresis. Despite the relatively high degree of AMR seen in desensitized patients, this population of patients has acceptable short term patient and allograft survival. Unfortunately, the long-term results for graft and patient outcomes using either of these two protocols are unknown.[4]

TREATMENT

Desired Outcome

KEY CONCEPT *The major focus of pharmacotherapy in transplantation is to achieve long-term patient and allograft survival.*[1,3,5,6] Short-term outcomes (eg, acute rejection rates, 1-year graft survival) have improved significantly since the first successful transplant due to an improved understanding of the immune system and enhancements in surgical techniques, organ procurement, immunosuppression, and posttransplant care. Despite the success in improving short-term outcomes, the frequency of graft loss remains higher than desired.[1,3,5,6]

It is imperative that transplant practitioners be aware of the specific advantages and disadvantages of the available immunosuppressants, as well as their adverse reactions and drug–drug interaction (DDI) profiles. There are generally three stages of medical immunosuppression: (a) induction therapy, (b) maintenance therapy, and (c) treatment of rejection. KEY CONCEPT *Overall, the immunosuppressive regimens utilize multiple medications working on different targets of the immune system.* Please refer to Table 55–2 for a list of all available immunosuppressive agents.[1,5,6]

Immunosuppressive Therapies—Induction Therapy

KEY CONCEPT *The goal of induction therapy is to provide a high level of immunosuppression in the early posttransplant period, when the risk of acute rejection is highest.*[5] This stage of immunosuppression is initiated intraoperatively and is concluded within the first 1 to 10 days after transplantation. Antibody induction therapy is not a mandatory stage of recipient immunosuppression and is typically predicated on immunologic risk. However, since acute rejection is a major concern in solid organ transplant recipients and its impact on chronic rejection is undeniable, induction therapy is often considered essential in some organs to optimize outcomes.[5]

▸ *Goals of Induction Therapy*

KEY CONCEPT *First, the induction agents are highly immunosuppressive, allowing for significant reductions in acute rejection and improved 1-year graft survival.*[5] Second, due to their unique pharmacologic effect, these agents are often considered essential in patients at high risk for poor short-term outcomes, such as patients with preformed antibodies, history of previous transplants, multiple HLA mismatches, or transplantation of organs with prolonged cold ischemic time, or from expanded-criteria donors. Specifically in renal transplantation, induction therapy plays an important role in preventing early-onset calcineurin inhibitor (CNI)–induced nephrotoxicity. With induction therapy, CNI initiation can be delayed until the graft regains some degree of function. Induction therapy is imperative when employing corticosteroid sparing or avoidance protocols.[5]

The improved short-term outcomes gained from induction therapy come with a degree of risk.[5] By using these highly immunosuppressive agents, particularly the antilymphocyte antibodies (ALA; the antithymocyte antibodies and alemtuzumab), the ability to mount a cell-mediated immune response is significantly reduced, which increases the risk of opportunistic infections and malignancy. Cytokine release syndrome is a common

Table 55–2

Currently Available Immunosuppressive Agents[1,5,6]

Generic Name (Brand Name)	Common Dosage	Common Adverse Effects
Induction Therapy Agents		
Alemtuzumab (Campath)	20–30 mg × 1–2 doses	Flu-like symptoms, chills, rigors, fever, rash, myelosuppression
Antithymocyte globulin equine (ATGAM)	15 mg/kg IV × 3–14 days	Flu-like symptoms, chills, rigors, fever, rash, myelosuppression
Antithymocyte globulin rabbit (Thymoglobulin)	1.5 mg/kg IV × 3–14 days	Flu-like symptoms, chills, rigors, fever, rash, myelosuppression
Basiliximab (Simulect)	20 mg IV × 2 doses	None reported compared to placebo
Maintenance Immunosuppressants		
Cyclosporine (Sandimmune, Neoral, Gengraf)	4–5 mg/kg by mouth twice a day	Neurotoxicity, gingival hyperplasia, hirsutism, hypertension, hyperlipidemia, glucose intolerance, nephrotoxicity, electrolyte abnormalities
Tacrolimus (Prograf, Astagraf XL, Envarsus XR)	0.05–0.075 mg/kg by mouth twice a day or once daily if using Astagraf XL or Envarsus XR	Neurotoxicity, alopecia, hypertension, hyperlipidemia, glucose intolerance, nephrotoxicity, electrolyte abnormalities
Azathioprine (Imuran)	1–2.5 mg/kg by mouth once a day	Myelosuppression, GI disturbances, pancreatitis
Mycophenolate mofetil (CellCept)	0.5–1.5 gm by mouth twice a day	Myelosuppression, GI disturbances
Enteric-coated MPA (Myfortic)	720 mg by mouth twice a day	Myelosuppression, GI disturbances
Sirolimus (Rapamune)	1–10 mg by mouth once a day	Hypertriglyceridemia, myelosuppression, mouth sores, hypercholesterolemia, GI disturbances, impaired wound healing, proteinuria, lymphocele, pneumonitis
Everolimus (Zortress)	0.75 mg by mouth twice daily	Hypertriglyceridemia, myelosuppression, mouth sores, hypercholesterolemia, GI disturbances, impaired wound healing, proteinuria, lymphocele, pneumonitis
Prednisone (Deltasone)	Maintenance: 2.5–20 mg by mouth once a day	Mood disturbances, psychosis, cataracts, hypertension, fluid retention, peptic ulcers, osteoporosis, muscle weakness, impaired wound healing, glucose intolerance, weight gain, hyperlipidemia
Belatacept (Nulojix)	10 mg/kg on postop days 1 and 4 10 mg/kg at the end of postop weeks 2, 4, 8, and 12 5 mg/kg at the end of postop week 16 and every 4 weeks thereafter	GI disturbances, electrolyte abnormalities, headache

GI, gastrointestinal; IV, intravenous; MPA, mycophenolic acid.

complication of T-cell depleting agents and may require premedications before infusions.[5]

▸ *Currently Available Induction Therapies*

Basiliximab Basiliximab is a chimeric monoclonal antibody that acts as an IL-2 receptor antagonist.[5,7] These receptors are present on almost all activated T cells. Basiliximab inhibits IL-2–mediated activation of lymphocytes, which is an important step in T-cell clonal expansion.

The dose of basiliximab is 20 mg IV given 2 hours prior to the transplant, followed by a second 20-mg dose on postoperative day 4.[5,7] This dosing schedule can be used for both children greater than or equal to 35 kg (77 lb) and adults. Two 10 mg doses with the same dosing schedule should be used for children less than 35 kg (77 lb). There are no specific dosage adjustments needed in renal or hepatic impairment.[5,7]

The incidence of all adverse reactions with basiliximab was similar to placebo in trials. There are no reported DDIs with basiliximab.[5,7]

Antithymocyte Globulin Equine Antithymocyte globulin equine (e-ATG) is a polyclonal antibody that contains antibodies against several T-cell surface markers. After binding to T cells, e-ATG promotes cellular depletion through opsonization and complement-mediated T-cell lysis.[5,7] The common dosing strategy for e-ATG when used for induction therapy is 10 to 30 mg/kg/day IV for 3 to 14 days.[5,7]

After T-cell lysis there is a cytokine release. Due to this phenomenon, e-ATG is associated with several adverse reactions.[5,7] The most common of these include fever (63%), chills (43.2%), headache (34.6%), back pain (43.2%), nausea (28.4%), diarrhea (32.1%), dizziness (24.7%), malaise (3.7%), leukopenia (29.6%), and thrombocytopenia (44.4%). The overall incidence of opportunistic infections is 27.2%, with cytomegalovirus (CMV) disease occurring in 11.1% of patients. There are currently no reported pharmacokinetic DDIs with this agent.[5,7]

Antithymocyte Globulin Rabbit Antithymocyte globulin rabbit (r-ATG) is also a polyclonal antibody that induces T-cell clearance, but more importantly, it alters T-cell activation, homing, and cytotoxic activities.[7] Compared with e-ATG, r-ATG causes less cell lysis. It is also believed that r-ATG plays a role in inducing T-cell apoptosis. This agent is typically dosed at 1.5 mg/kg/day and is usually administered for 3 to 10 days after transplantation.[5] Many renal transplant centers aim to initiate the first dose intraoperatively to reduce organ reperfusion injury.[8]

Adverse reactions are common and may include fever (63.4%), chills (57.3%), headache (40.2%), nausea (36.6%), diarrhea (36.6%), malaise (13.4%), dizziness (8.5%), leukopenia (57.3%), thrombocytopenia (36.6%), and generalized pain (46.3%).[9,10,13] The incidence of infection is 36.6%, with CMV disease occurring in 13.4% of patients. There are no reported DDIs with the use of r-ATG at this time.[5,7]

Alemtuzumab Alemtuzumab is a recombinant DNA-derived monoclonal antibody that binds to CD52, which is present on most B and T lymphocytes, macrophages and natural killer (NK) cells, and a subpopulation of granulocytes.[5,7] After complexing with the CD52 cell surface marker, alemtuzumab induces an antibody-dependent cell lysis. This agent produces a rapid and extensive lymphocyte depletion that may take several months to years to return to pretransplant levels. Although it is not Food and Drug Administration (FDA) approved for use in organ transplantation, studies have demonstrated a dose of 30 mg IV or SC at the time of transplant to be effective in preventing acute rejection.[5]

Alemtuzumab has been associated with serious adverse reactions that include anemia (47%), neutropenia (70%), thrombocytopenia (52%), headache (24%), dysesthesias (15%), dizziness (12%), nausea (54%), vomiting (41%), diarrhea (22%), infusion-related reactions (15% to 89%), and infection (37%; CMV viremia occurred in 15% of patients).[7] The FDA recommends that premedication with acetaminophen and oral antihistamines is advisable to reduce the incidence of infusion-related reactions.[5]

Comparative Efficacy—Induction Therapy Agents Improvements in short-term outcomes gained from the use of induction therapies cannot be denied. However, despite these advances, use of induction therapy has not impacted long-term allograft function or survival. There are a few studies that help to delineate the ideal induction therapy agent. Studies comparing r-ATG and e-ATG show that r-ATG is more effective in lowering acute rejection rates and improving 1-, 5- and 10-year allograft outcomes.[9–11] Conversely, a study evaluating the use of basiliximab versus r-ATG demonstrated similar short-term efficacy between both groups.[12] However, other analyses of these two agents demonstrated similar results for allograft and patient survival, but a benefit for r-ATG in lowering incidence of acute allograft rejection.[13,14] A more recent analysis showed that alemtuzumab improved transplant outcomes when compared with basiliximab in patients with a low immunologic risk, and similar outcomes compared to r-ATG in patients with high immunologic risk.[15] When choosing an agent for induction therapy, one must weigh the risks versus benefits. Overall, the ALAs are considered to be most effective, but are associated with a higher incidence of infectious disease and malignancy.[5]

Immunosuppressive Therapies—Maintenance Therapy

The goals of maintenance immunosuppression are to prevent rejection and optimize patient and graft survival.[6] Antirejection medications require careful selection and dose titration to balance the risks of rejection with those of toxicities.

Common maintenance immunosuppressive agents can be divided into five classes:

- Calcineurin inhibitors (CNI; cyclosporine and tacrolimus)
- Antiproliferatives (azathioprine and the mycophenolic acid [MPA] derivatives)
- Target of rapamycin (ToR) inhibitors (sirolimus and everolimus)
- Corticosteroids
- Costimulatory blockade (belatacept)

Maintenance immunosuppression is generally achieved by combining two or more medications from the different classes, specifically targeting unique components of the immune response.[6] Please refer to Figure 55–1 for a schematic representation of these different drug mechanisms and Figure 55–2 for an example protocol for administration of immunosuppressive medications posttransplant. This method of medication selection also minimizes toxicities by choosing agents with different adverse event profiles. Immunosuppressive regimens vary between organ types and transplant centers, but most often include a CNI with an adjuvant agent, plus or minus corticosteroids. Selection of an immunosuppressive regimen should be

Patient Encounter Part 1

HPI: A 59-year-old woman presents to your transplant center for a living unrelated renal transplant.

PMH: ESRD secondary to diabetes mellitus type 2; obesity (she has lost weight in order to get her BMI less than 35 to be approved for renal transplantation); hypertension; hyperlipidemia; insomnia; gout (has had three episodes of gout in the past 12 months); secondary hyperparathyroidism

FH: Father died from a heart attack 3 years ago; mother is alive and living with a history of breast cancer

SH: Does not work due to poor health, but was formerly a dental hygienist. She admits to social alcohol use (one or two drinks per week) and denies any tobacco and IV drug use

Admission Meds: Diltiazem ER 120 mg by mouth once a day; irbesartan 100 mg by mouth once a day; furosemide 20 mg by mouth twice a day; atorvastatin 20 mg by mouth once a day; zolpidem 10 mg by mouth once a day at bedtime; calcitriol 0.25 mg by mouth once a day; sevelamer carbonate 1600 mg with each meal and 800 mg with each snack; Epo 4000 units IV every hemodialysis session; insulin glargine 22 units administered in the evening; insulin aspart 4 units with each meal and a sliding scale (dependent on blood sugars)

Allergies: Sulfa—hives

Labs: CMV serostatus: donor is CMV IgG positive; CMV serostatus: recipient is CMV IgG negative; EBV serostatus: donor is EBV IgG positive, EBV serostatus: recipient is EBV IgG negative

Identify your treatment goals for this patient.

Create a plan for induction therapy (ie, would you recommend induction therapy, and if so, which agent?).

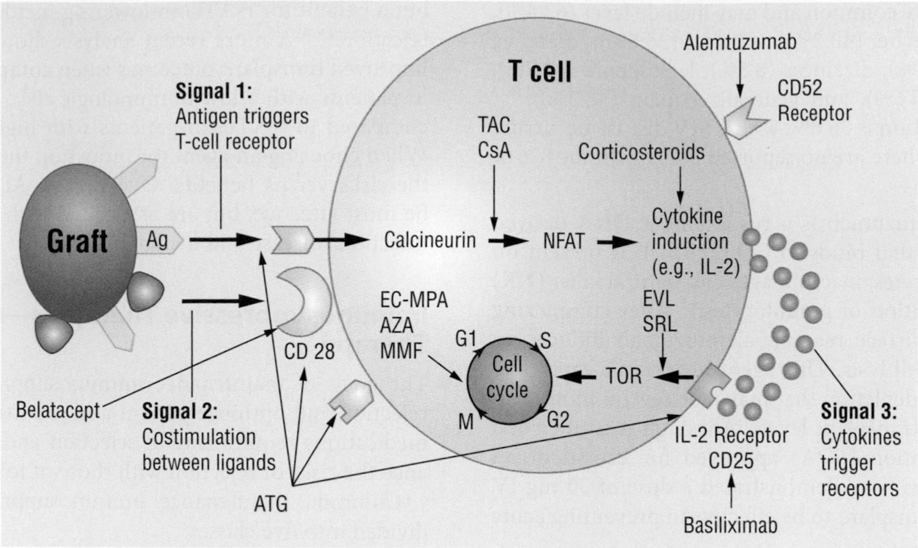

FIGURE 55–1. Identification of the sites of action of the various immunosuppressive medications. Allograft recognition through Signal 1 occurs when the antigen-major histocompatibility complex (MHC) molecule is recognized by the T-cell receptor (TCR). A costimulatory signal, Signal 2, initiates signal transduction with activation of second messengers, one of which is calcineurin. Together, Signal 1 and Signal 2 activate calcineurin phosphatase, which removes phosphates from the nuclear factors, allowing them to enter the nucleus, with a subsequent increase in interleukin-2 (IL-2) gene transcription. Signal 3 occurs with the interaction of IL-2, with the IL-2 receptor on the cell membrane surface. This culminates in a signal that passes through the mammalian target of rapamycin (ToR) and induces cell proliferation and production of cytokines specific to the T cell. (ATG, antithymocyte globulin; AZA, azathioprine; CsA, cyclosporine; EC-MPA, enteric-coated mycophenolic acid; EVL, everolimus; MMF, mycophenolate mofetil; NFAT, nuclear factors; SRL, sirolimus; TAC, tacrolimus.)

patient-specific, and one must take into account the patient's comorbidities, medication regimens, and preferences.[6]

► *Calcineurin Inhibitors*

KEY CONCEPT *Cyclosporine and tacrolimus belong to a class of immunosuppressants called calcineurin inhibitors. These agents are considered to be the cornerstone of modern immunosuppressive protocols.* The CNIs work by complexing with cytoplasmic proteins (cyclosporine with cyclophilin and tacrolimus with FK binding protein-12).[6,7] These complexes inhibit calcineurin phosphatase, which results in reduced IL-2 gene transcription and a reduction in IL-2 synthesis. This diminishes T-cell activation.[6,7]

Cyclosporine Cyclosporine USP was first approved in 1983, but was associated with a variable oral absorption. The development of a newer formulation, cyclosporine microemulsion USP (ie, modified), introduced in 1994, allowed for a more consistent drug exposure due to a more reliable pharmacokinetic profile.[1] Cyclosporine modified is the formulation of choice for most transplant centers utilizing cyclosporine due to the previously mentioned benefit. The two formulations are not interchangeable.[6]

The usual oral adult dose of cyclosporine ranges from 3 to 7 mg/kg/day in two divided doses.[7] The appropriate selection of the starting dose depends on the organ type, the patient's comorbidities, and other concomitant immunosuppressive agents utilized. Cyclosporine modified is available as 25-mg and 100-mg capsules and an oral solution. An IV formulation of conventional cyclosporine is also available. When converting a patient from oral to IV, the dosage should be reduced to approximately one-third of the total daily oral dose.[7]

Cyclosporine whole-blood trough concentrations (C_0) have traditionally been obtained to help monitor for efficacy and safety. Therapeutic C_0 may range from 50 to 400 ng/mL (50–400 mcg/L or 42–333 nmol/L). Target levels should be individualized for each patient, usually depending on the organ transplanted, patient's condition, method of assay (liquid chromatography coupled to tandem mass spectrometry [LC-MS/MS], monoclonal, polyclonal), and time since transplantation.[6] Newer studies suggest that monitoring of concentrations at 2 hours postdose (C_2) correlates better with toxicity and efficacy when compared with C_0.[16]

Tacrolimus Tacrolimus is the second CNI and was approved in 1997. Oral starting doses of tacrolimus range from 0.1 to 0.2 mg/kg/day in two divided doses. Tacrolimus is available in 0.5-, 1-, and 5-mg capsules and as an injectable.[7] Two once daily tacrolimus formulations are also available. Tacrolimus C_0 should be monitored and maintained between 5 and 15 ng/mL (5 and 15 mcg/L or 6 and 18 nmol/L), again depending on the transplanted organ, patient's condition, and time since transplant.[6]

The tacrolimus IV formulation is usually avoided due to the risk of anaphylaxis, because of its castor oil component, and nephrotoxicity.[6] Doses for IV administration are recommended to start at 0.01 mg/kg/day. In an effort to avoid IV tacrolimus, many transplant centers utilize sublingual (SL) tacrolimus in their patients unable to receive the medication by mouth.[6]

Adverse Drug Reactions KEY CONCEPT *One of the major disadvantages of the CNIs is their ability to cause nephrotoxicity.* Acute nephrotoxicity has been correlated with high doses and is usually reversible.[7] Chronic CNI toxicity, however, is typically irreversible and is linked to chronic drug exposure. Table 55–3 expands on the more common calcineurin inhibitor–associated adverse events.[1,6]

Comparative Efficacy—Calcineurin Inhibitors Even though cyclosporine and tacrolimus are both CNIs, there are several

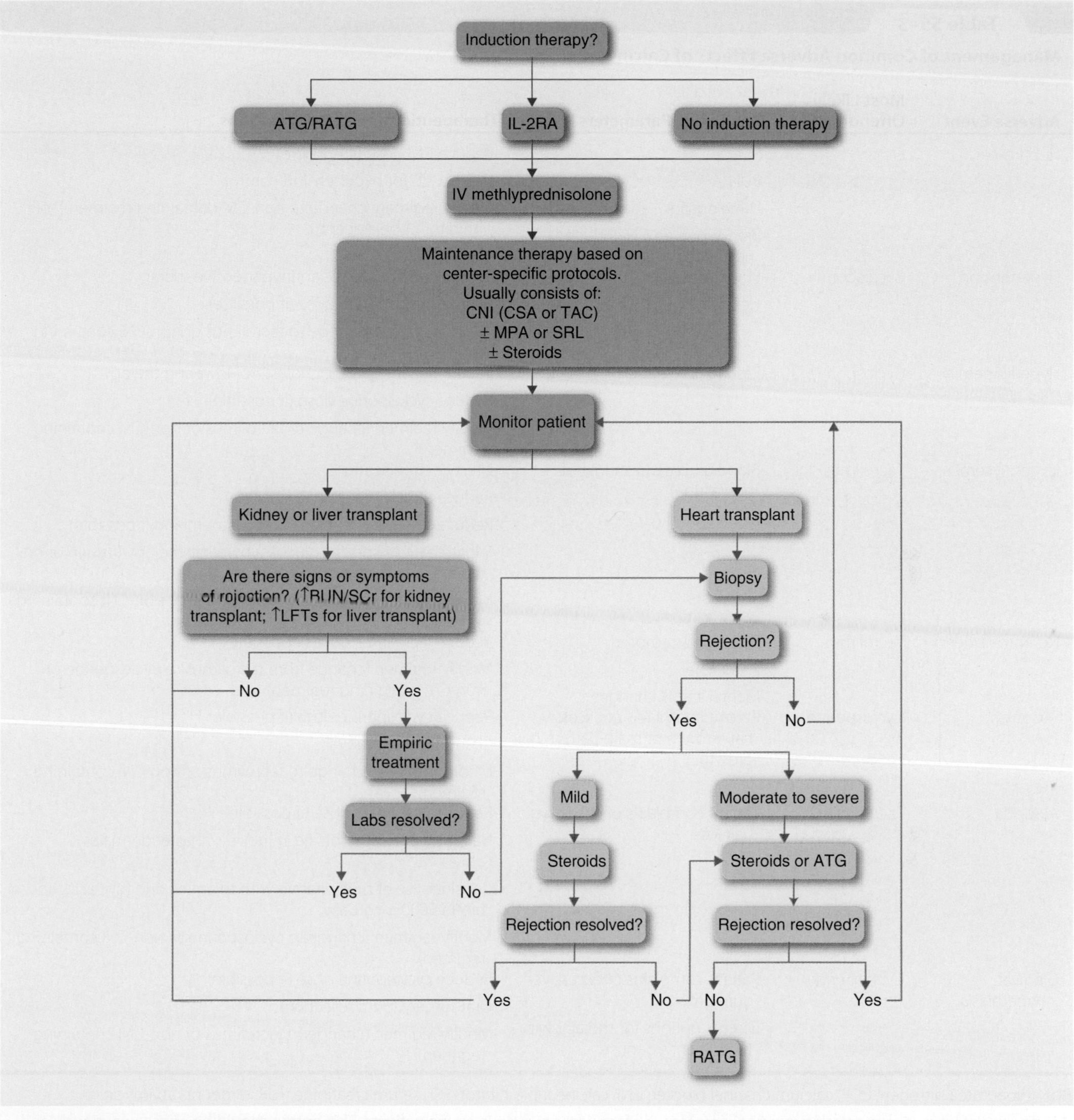

FIGURE 55–2. Example protocol of immunosuppressive medication use in organ transplantation.[a] Center-specific protocols may use rabbit antithymocyte immunoglobulin (RATG), an interleukin-2 receptor antagonist (IL-2RA), or no induction therapy. In any situation, patients receive IV methylprednisone prior to, during, or immediately following the transplant operation. The patient then will begin the maintenance immunosuppressive regimen. The center-specific protocol will specify which calcineurin inhibitor (cyclosporine or tacrolimus) is used in combination with mycophenolate mofetil or sirolimus, with or without steroids. Patients then are monitored for signs and symptoms of rejection. If rejection is suspected, a biopsy can be done for definitive diagnosis, or the patient may be treated empirically for rejection. Empirical treatment generally involves administration of corticosteroids. If signs and symptoms of rejection are resolved with empirical therapy, the patient will continue to be monitored according to the center-specific protocol. If rejection is confirmed by biopsy, treatment may be based on the severity of rejection. High-dose corticosteroids are used most frequently for mild to moderate rejection. RATG can be used for moderate to severe rejections or steroid-resistant rejections. [a]Protocols and algorithms may differ across transplant centers. (ATG, antithymocyte globulin; BUN, blood urea nitrogen; CNI, calcineurin inhibitor; CSA, cyclosporine; IV, intravenous; LFT, liver function test; MPA, mycophenolic acid; SCr, serum creatinine; SRL, sirolimus; TAC, tacrolimus.) (From Schonder KS, Johnson HJ. Solid Organ Transplantation. In: DiPiro JT, Talbert RL, Yee GC, et al., eds. Pharmacotherapy: A Pathophysiologic Approach. 9th ed. New York: McGraw-Hill; 2014:1419.)

Table 55–3

Management of Common Adverse Effects of Calcineurin Inhibitors[1,6]

Adverse Event	Most Likely Offending CNI	Monitoring Parameters	Therapeutic Management Options
Nephrotoxicity	Either	-SCr -BUN -Urine output -Biopsy-proven CNI-induced nephrotoxicity	-Reduce CNI dose (if possible) -Use of CCB for hypertension control -Modify regimen (change to non-CNI containing regimen [ToR inhibitor or belatacept])[a]
Hypertension[b]	Cyclosporine	-Blood pressure -Heart rate	-Initiate patient-specific antihypertensive therapy -Reduce cyclosporine dose (if possible) -Modify regimen (change to tacrolimus or non-CNI containing regimen)[a]
Hyperlipidemia[b]	Cyclosporine	-Fasting lipid panel	-Initiate patient-specific cholesterol-lowering therapy -Reduce cyclosporine dose (if possible) -Modify regimen (change to tacrolimus or non-CNI containing regimen)[a]
Hyperglycemia[c]	Tacrolimus	-Blood glucose (fasting and nonfasting) -Hemoglobin A1c	-Lifestyle modifications -Reduce tacrolimus dose (if possible) -Reduce steroids (if patient is taking them and if possible) -Initiate patient-specific glucose-lowering therapy (insulin or oral therapy) -Modify regimen (change to cyclosporine or non-CNI containing regimen)[a]
Neurotoxicities[c]	Tacrolimus	-Fine hand tremor -Headache -Mental status changes	-Reduce tacrolimus dose (if possible) -Modify regimen (change from tacrolimus to cyclosporine or non-CNI containing regimen)[a]
Hirsutism	Cyclosporine	-Patient complains of excessive hair growth or male-pattern hair growth	-Reduce cyclosporine dose (if possible) -Cosmetic hair removal -Modify regimen (change to tacrolimus or non-CNI containing regimen)[a]
Alopecia	Tacrolimus	-Patient complains of excessive hair loss	-Reduce tacrolimus dose (if possible) -Hair growth treatments (ie, minoxidil, finasteride-males only) -Consider use of multivitamin with thiamine and folic acid, and/or biotin 5000 mcg daily -Modify regimen (change to cyclosporine or non-CNI containing regimen)[a]
Gingival Hyperplasia	Cyclosporine	-Patient complains of excessive gum growth -Discuss options for therapy with the patient's dentist	-Reduce cyclosporine dose (if possible) -Oral surgery (gum resection) -Modify regimen (change to tacrolimus or non-CNI containing regimen)[a]

BUN, blood urea nitrogen; CCB, calcium channel blocker; CNI, calcineurin inhibitor; SCr, serum creatinine; ToR, target of rapamycin.

[a]Modifying the immunosuppressive regimen increases risk for rejection, even in stable patients. This option should be chosen cautiously and be implemented with proper monitoring and follow-up.

[b]Tacrolimus is also associated with hypertension and hyperlipidemia, but to a much lower extent compared to cyclosporine.

[c]Cyclosporine is also associated with hyperglycemia and neurotoxicities, but to a much lower extent compared to tacrolimus.

differences between the two. A meta-analysis comprised of 30 trials and 4102 patients comparing cyclosporine to tacrolimus in kidney transplantation, showed tacrolimus was associated with significantly lower risk of allograft loss at 6 months and lower rates of acute rejection at 1 year.[17] Tacrolimus is the primary CNI in many transplant centers, due in large part to a more favorable adverse reaction profile.[6]

► *Antiproliferatives*

These agents are considered to be adjuvant to the CNIs or ToR inhibitors.[6]

Azathioprine Azathioprine was approved in 1968 as an adjunct immunosuppressant in renal transplant. It is available in oral and IV dosage forms.[7] Prior to the advent of cyclosporine, the combination of azathioprine and corticosteroids was the mainstay of immunosuppressive therapy. Over the past 10 years, the use of azathioprine declined markedly due to the superiority of the MPA derivatives. KEY CONCEPT *Azathioprine is a prodrug for 6-mercaptopurine (6-MP), a purine analog. 6-MP acts as an antimetabolite and inhibits DNA replication with a resultant reduction in T-cell proliferation.*[6] *The typical oral dose of azathioprine for organ transplantation is 1 to 5 mg/kg once a day.*[7] Dose reductions due to severely impaired renal function may be necessary since 6-MP and its metabolites are renally eliminated.[7] Trough concentrations of 6-MP are not monitored; however, most clinicians often monitor for signs of myelosuppression. KEY CONCEPT *Myelosuppression (mainly leukopenia and thrombocytopenia) is a frequent, dose-dependent and dose-limiting complication (greater than 50% of patients) that often prompts dose reductions.*[7] *Other common adverse events include hepatotoxicity (2%–10%) and adverse gastrointestinal (GI) events (10%–15%; mostly nausea and vomiting). Importantly, pancreatitis and venoocclusive disease of the liver occur in less than 1% of patients following chronic azathioprine therapy.*[7]

Mycophenolic Acid Derivatives Mycophenolate mofetil was approved in 1995 and enteric-coated MPA in 2004. Both agents are considered adjunctive immunosuppressants.[6] KEY CONCEPT *Both mycophenolate mofetil and enteric-coated MPA are prodrugs for MPA.* MPA acts by inhibiting inosine monophosphate dehydrogenase, a vital enzyme in the de novo pathway of purine synthesis. Inhibition of this enzyme prevents the proliferation of most cells that are dependent on the de novo pathway for purine synthesis, including T and B cells.[6]

Mycophenolate mofetil is available in 250-mg and 500-mg capsules, an oral suspension (100 mg/mL; in cherry syrup), and as an injectable.[7] The recommended starting dose of mycophenolate mofetil is 1000 to 1500 mg given twice daily. The conversion between oral and IV mycophenolate mofetil is 1:1. Enteric-coated MPA is available in 180-mg and 360-mg tablets. The appropriate equimolar conversion between mycophenolate mofetil and enteric-coated MPA is 1000 mg of mycophenolate mofetil to 720 mg of enteric-coated MPA.[6] The recommended starting dose of enteric-coated MPA is 720 mg given twice daily. Conversion of mycophenolate mofetil to enteric-coated MPA has been proven safe. MPA C_0 can be monitored; however, it is not routinely recommended.[6]

KEY CONCEPT *The most common adverse events associated with these agents are GI (18%–54%; diarrhea, nausea, vomiting, and gastritis) and myelosuppression (20%–40%).*[7] Despite its enteric coating, enteric-coated MPA has the same degree of GI adverse events as mycophenolate mofetil.[6,18] However, recent data suggest there is a benefit in converting patients with documented mycophenolate-induced GI disease from mycophenolate mofetil to enteric-coated MPA.[19]

Comparative Efficacy—Antiproliferatives Due to the results of several studies, the MPA derivatives have replaced azathioprine as the primary antiproliferative agent.[6] The MPA derivatives are generally considered to provide a more specific immunosuppressive effect compared with azathioprine. Mycophenolate mofetil and enteric-coated MPA have similar safety and efficacy data in renal transplant recipients.[18] The decision to choose one agent over another is a purely practitioner-dependent preference.

▶ Target of Rapamycin Inhibitors

Sirolimus KEY CONCEPT *Sirolimus inhibits T-cell activation and proliferation by binding to and inhibiting the activation of the mammalian ToR, which suppresses cellular response to IL-2 and other cytokines (ie, IL-4, IL-15).*[6,7,20] Studies have shown that sirolimus may be used safely and effectively concomitantly with either cyclosporine or tacrolimus instead of an antiproliferative.[21] Sirolimus can also be used as an alternative agent for patients who do not tolerate CNIs due to nephrotoxicity or other adverse events.[6] KEY CONCEPT *At this time, the most exciting data for sirolimus point to its ability to prevent long-term allograft dysfunction when used as a substitute for the CNIs in renal transplant recipients.*[20]

Sirolimus is available in 0.5-mg, 1-mg, and 2-mg tablets and a 1-mg/mL oral solution. Although some may elect not to do a loading dose, the package insert indicates the current approved dosing regimen for sirolimus is a 6-mg loading dose followed by a 2-mg/day maintenance dose.[7] Use of a sirolimus loading dose of 5 to 15 mg/day for 1 to 3 days will allow for a more rapid achievement of adequate immunosuppression.[7] Maintenance doses of sirolimus usually range from 1 to 10 mg/day given once daily. Sirolimus blood C_0 should be maintained between 3 and 10 ng/mL (3 and 10 mcg/L or 3 and 11 nmol/L), depending on the institution-specific protocols.[6] Of note, sirolimus has a half-life of approximately 62 hours, which means that it will not reach steady state after dosage changes for several days.[7]

KEY CONCEPT *The most common adverse events reported with sirolimus are leukopenia (20%), thrombocytopenia (13%–30%), and hyperlipidemia (38%–57%).*[7] Other adverse effects include delayed wound healing, anemia, diarrhea, arthralgias, rash, proteinuria, pneumonitis, and mouth ulcers. KEY CONCEPT *One analysis suggests that use of sirolimus in kidney transplant recipients can reduce cardiovascular risk compared with CNI-based regimens.*[22] Sirolimus has a black-box warning in newly transplanted liver and lung recipients, due to severe and potentially life-threatening adverse events.[7] The long-term use of sirolimus in these populations may be appropriate, but not in the initial posttransplant period (ie, 3–6 months posttransplant).

Everolimus Everolimus is a derivative of sirolimus and has the same mechanism of action.[7,23] Everolimus is only indicated for prevention of rejection in low- to moderate-risk renal and liver transplant recipients. This agent is available in 0.25-mg, 0.5-mg, and 0.75-mg tablets. The recommended starting dose of everolimus is 0.75 to 1 mg twice daily without the need for a loading dose. Maintenance everolimus doses should be maximized to achieve a C_0 goal of 3 to 8 ng/mL (3–8 mcg/L or 3–8 nmol/L).[7,23] With a significantly shorter half-life compared with sirolimus, everolimus steady-state can be reached within 4 to 6 days. KEY CONCEPT *The adverse event profile of everolimus is similar to that of sirolimus.*[7,23]

▶ Corticosteroids

Traditional triple-therapy immunosuppressive regimens have consisted of a primary agent (ie, CNI, ToR inhibitor, belatacept), an antiproliferative and corticosteroids.[6] Many renal transplant protocols have focused on corticosteroid sparing or avoidance. Avoidance or sparing of corticosteroids has been supported in the literature, although more studies are needed to help better characterize which patients should follow these protocols.[6,24] A typical taper includes a bolus of IV methylprednisolone 100 to 500 mg at the time of transplant, then tapered over days to months, depending on the type of organ, to a maintenance dose of prednisone 5 to 10 mg/day. Although most centers still use low-dose steroids for immunologically high-risk patients and nonrenal transplant patients, a number of renal transplant programs have developed an immunosuppression protocol that completely withdraws corticosteroids at some point posttransplantation.[6] Therapeutic drug monitoring of corticosteroids is not employed. KEY CONCEPT *Corticosteroids are associated with a variety of metabolic toxicities.* The most common adverse events have been summarized in Table 55–4.[1,6]

KEY CONCEPT *Corticosteroids have various effects on immune and inflammatory responses, although their exact mechanism of immunosuppression is not fully understood.* It is believed that high doses are directly lymphotoxic, and lower doses act by inhibiting the production of various cytokines that are necessary to amplify the immune response.[6,7]

The most commonly used corticosteroids are methylprednisolone (IV and oral) and prednisone (oral), although prednisolone and dexamethasone have also been shown to be effective for organ transplantation. Corticosteroid doses vary by center-specific protocols, organ type, and patient characteristics.

► Costimulatory Pathway Blocker

Belatacept KEY CONCEPT *Belatacept was approved in 2011 as the first IV biologic maintenance immunosuppressive agent in transplant.*[25] *Belatacept blocks CD80 and CD86 ligands, found on APCs.*[7] The CD80 and CD86 proteins are responsible for stimulating CD28 on inactive T cells, an essential costimulatory interaction (Signal 2). As detailed earlier in this chapter, Signal 1 without a complementary Signal 2 induces T-cell anergy.[25] Studies have shown that in combination with mycophenolate and corticosteroids, belatacept may be used in place of CNIs; demonstrating similar patient and allograft survival compared to a cyclosporine-based regimen.[26,27] KEY CONCEPT *Belatacept improved renal function; however, the incidence of acute rejection was significantly higher.* Belatacept was also associated with improvements in blood pressure and lipid levels.[25]

Belatacept is available in a 250-mg vial that requires reconstitution prior to administration.[7] The recommended dosing regimen for belatacept is 10 mg/kg on the day of transplantation, followed by an additional dose 4 days later, and again at the end of weeks 2, 4, 8, and 12, posttransplant. Beginning at the end of week 16 posttransplant, belatacept is dosed at 5 mg/kg every 4 weeks thereafter.[7,25] Belatacept requires access to an infusion center/suite, or a home infusion service to ensure appropriate administration.

The most common adverse effects associated with belatacept are infectious (urinary tract infection, 37%; upper respiratory infection, 15%), GI (diarrhea, 39%; constipation, 33%; nausea, 24%, vomiting, 22%), metabolic (hyperkalemia, 20%; hypokalemia 21%), and central nervous system (CNS; headache, 21%) complications.[7] Other adverse effects include peripheral edema, anemia, leukopenia, hypotension, arthralgia, and insomnia.[25] KEY CONCEPT *Belatacept has a black-box warning for increased risk of posttransplant lymphoproliferative disorders (PTLD). Due to this risk, it is recommended that belatacept only be used in patients with a proven preexisting immunity to Epstein-Barr virus (EBV).* This black-box warning has also led to the inclusion of a communication plan as part of a belatacept risk evaluation and mitigation strategy to warn practitioners that belatacept use in EBV-naive or unequivocal patients is contraindicated. An additional black-box warning advises against use of belatacept in liver transplant patients due to an increased risk of allograft loss and patient death.[7,25]

Table 55–4
Common Adverse Events Associated with Corticosteroids[1,6]

Body System	Adverse Event
Cardiovascular	Hyperlipidemia Hypertension
Central nervous system	Anxiety Insomnia Mood changes Psychosis
Dermatologic	Acne Diaphoresis Ecchymosis Hirsutism Impaired wound healing Petechiae Thin skin
Endocrine/metabolic	Cushing syndrome Hyperglycemia Sodium and water retention
Gastrointestinal	Gastritis Increased appetite Nausea, vomiting, diarrhea Peptic ulcers
Hematologic	Leukocytosis
Neuromuscular/skeletal	Arthralgia Impaired growth Osteoporosis Skeletal muscle weakness
Ocular	Cataracts Glaucoma
Respiratory	Epistaxis

Immunosuppressive Therapies—Treatment of Acute Rejection Episodes

Acute rejection is generally treated with a course of high-dose methylprednisolone (250 to 1000 mg/day IV for 3 days), which is usually sufficient to ameliorate the episode. If the acute rejection episode is resistant to the initial course of steroids, a second course may be administered or the patient may begin therapy with r-ATG (1.5 mg/kg/day for 4 to 14 days).[28] Cellular rejection refractory to these treatments is rare and is likely due to underlying causes such as an antibody-mediated component or other diagnosis. Treatments of refractory acute rejection may include alemtuzumab, IVIG, high-dose tacrolimus, or organ irradiation.

Immunosuppressive Therapies—Managing Highly Sensitized Patients and Antibody-Mediated Rejection Episodes

The presence of preformed antibodies, high PRA, and DSA are major barriers to successful transplantation.[4] This is true mainly because traditional immunosuppressants do not significantly affect the humoral immune system and are ineffective at management of AMR, which is a leading cause of allograft loss in kidney and heart transplant recipients. Without some form of intervention, antibody formation and rejection can significantly impact morbidity and mortality. Two major strategies are used for reduction of DSA pretransplant: (a) high-dose IVIG and (b) plasmapheresis plus low-dose IVIG. Each approach has advantages and disadvantages.[4]

In plasmapheresis or plasma exchange, patients' plasma is removed and replaced with albumin or fresh-frozen plasma.[4] Plasmapheresis produces a rapid reduction of preformed antibodies and allows transplantation to occur. The purpose of IVIG administration is to decrease anti-HLA alloantibody synthesis. The other mechanisms of IVIG are inhibition of complement-mediated injury, reduced B-cell proliferation and NK cells, and a decrease in phagocytosis. Most patients require four to five plasmapheresis sessions with IVIG to remove DSA. In patients at risk for bleeding, the use of albumin should be limited, and fresh-frozen plasma or a combination of both agents should be considered.[4]

In patients who develop AMR posttransplant, there are limited therapeutic options, none of which are FDA-approved. The potential options include plasmapheresis and IVIG, rituximab, bortezomib, and/or eculizumab.[4] All of these agents have an effect on humoral immunity, which may provide benefit to patients with AMR. The mechanisms of plasmapheresis and IVIG were discussed earlier in this chapter.[4]

Rituximab is a chimeric monoclonal anti-CD20 antibody targeting B cells.[4,7] This agent directly inhibits B-cell proliferation and induces cellular apoptosis through complement-mediated antibody-dependent cellular cytotoxicity. In an analysis of AMR treatment, the use of rituximab in conjunction with plasmapheresis/IVIG resulted in improved 3-year graft survival (92% vs 50%) and significantly reduced DSA at 3 months compared with high-dose IVIG alone.[29] Unfortunately, plasma cells lack CD20 and are unaffected by rituximab. However, rituximab may play an important role in reducing memory B-cell response. Overall, it appears that rituximab may provide beneficial effects in managing AMR when used in combination with other therapies.[4]

Bortezomib is a proteasome inhibitor indicated for treatment of multiple myeloma.[4,7] It works by inducing cell-cycle arrest and apoptosis of plasma cells. Desensitization and treatment protocols using bortezomib have utilized doses of 1.3 mg/m^2 from one to four cycles. Acute hepatic dysfunction has rarely been reported; thus, bortezomib should be used cautiously in patients with moderate-to-severe hepatic impairment. Bortezomib has also been associated with significant myelosuppression and peripheral neuropathy. Bortezomib has been used in combination with plasmapheresis and IVIG or rituximab. The reported outcomes of these cases demonstrate graft survival rates of 85% to 100%. Anti-HLA antibodies are decreased by 50% within two weeks of therapy and remain suppressed for up to 5 months.[30,31] Bortezomib also seems effective in AMR refractory to plasmapheresis and IVIG.[4]

Eculizumab is a humanized monoclonal antibody directed against complement protein C5.[4,7] It inhibits the cleavage to C5a and C5b, thus preventing the generation of the membrane attack complex (MAC) and reducing antibody-dependent cell lysis. Eculizumab carries a FDA boxed warning of meningococcal infection. Meningococcal vaccination is recommended 14 days prior to eculizumab, but meningococcal infections have been reported even in vaccinated patients. There are only a few case reports demonstrating eculizumab's efficacy for treating AMR, showing fast improvement of renal function observed within a week after eculizumab use.[4]

Maintenance Immunosuppressive Therapies—Common Drug–Drug Interactions

KEY CONCEPT *As the number of medications a patient takes increases, so does the potential for DDIs.* Disease severity, patient age, and organ dysfunction are all risk factors for DDIs. In general, DDIs are either pharmacokinetic or pharmacodynamic interactions:

- Pharmacokinetic interactions result when one drug alters the absorption, distribution, metabolism, or elimination of another drug.
- Pharmacodynamic interactions include additive, synergistic, or antagonistic interactions that can affect efficacy or toxicity.

▶ *Pharmacokinetic Interactions*

Pharmacokinetic DDIs pose a major dilemma with the maintenance immunosuppressants. Pharmacokinetic interactions can either result in: (1) increased concentrations of one or more agents, with an increased risk for drug-induced toxicities or (2) lowered (ie, subtherapeutic) drug concentrations, possibly leading to allograft rejection. These interactions can be seen during drug absorption, distribution, metabolism, and elimination.

Interactions of Absorption Gut metabolism, modifications in active transport, and changes in intestinal motility and chelation interactions alter absorption of the immunosuppressants. Active transporters (ie, P-glycoprotein [P-gp]) are present in the gut, brain, liver and kidneys and play an important role in DDIs. P-gp provides a biological barrier, eliminating xenobiotics that may accumulate in these organ systems, thereby having a significant impact on the absorption and distribution of many medications. P-gp affects the absorption of the CNIs and ToR inhibitors. Medications that inhibit or induce the activity of P-gp have a significant impact on bioavailability of some of the immunosuppressive agents. For example, P-gp inhibitors, such as verapamil or quinidine, increase concentrations of cyclosporine, tacrolimus, sirolimus, and everolimus due to reduced P-gp-dependent drug elimination from the systemic circulation.[7]

There is a prominent interaction between the prokinetic agents and the CNIs seen through changes in intestinal motility. Metoclopramide increases the absorption of cyclosporine and tacrolimus by enhancing gastric motility and emptying, resulting in increased CNI concentrations.[7]

Most of the interactions with mycophenolate mofetil and enteric-coated MPA result in reductions in intestinal absorption. Proton pump inhibitors decrease the oral absorption of mycophenolate mofetil, but not enteric-coated MPA.[7] Divalent and trivalent cations (ie, aluminum, magnesium, calcium) decrease MPA absorption through chelation. These agents should be administered at least 1 hour before or 2 hours after MPA. Of note, iron does not appear to interact with the MPA preparations. The clinical implications of these DDIs are unknown, but reductions in MPA exposure can theoretically increase the rejection risk.

Interactions of Distribution Interactions of distribution occur most often with highly protein bound drugs.[7] MPA is the only highly protein bound (97%) maintenance immunosuppressant with an interaction of distribution. Concomitant administration of MPA with salicylates increases MPA free concentrations. The adverse sequelae of this interaction are unknown. Drug interaction studies have not been conducted with MPA derivatives and other highly protein bound drugs.

Interactions of Metabolism Oxidative metabolism by cytochrome P-450 (CYP) isozymes is the primary method of xenobiotic metabolism. The CNIs and ToR inhibitors are substrates of the CYP3A isozyme system. Most CYP-mediated metabolism takes place in the liver; however, CYP is also expressed in the intestine, lungs, kidneys, and brain. Being CYP3A substrates, it would be anticipated that cyclosporine, tacrolimus, sirolimus, and everolimus would all experience similar DDI with known substrates, inhibitors, and inducers of the CYP3A isozyme system.[6] Table 55–5 details the clinically relevant DDIs that occur with the calcineurin and ToR inhibitors due to inhibition or induction of the CYP isozyme system.[7]

Given how extensive some immunosuppressant DDIs are, in some cases empiric dose changes are necessitated when

Table 55–5

Potential Drug–Drug Interactions with the Calcineurin Inhibitors and Target of Rapamycin Inhibitors Mediated Through the Cytochrome P-450 System 3A (CYP3A4) Isozyme[7]

Substrates[a]		Inducers[b]	Inhibitors[c]
Alfentanil	Loratadine	Carbamazepine	Boceprevir
Alprazolam	Lovastatin	Dexamethasone	Cimetidine
Amiodarone	Nevirapine	Etravirine	Clarithromycin
Amlodipine	Nicardipine	Ethosuximide	Clotrimazole
Atorvastatin	Nifedipine	Isoniazid	Delavirdine
Boceprevir	Omeprazole	Nevirapine	Diltiazem
Cilostazol	Paclitaxel	Phenobarbital	Erythromycin
Cisapride	Propafenone	Phenytoin	Fluconazole
Chlorpromazine	Progesterone	Prednisone	Fluoxetine
Clonazepam	Quetiapine	Rifabutin	Fluvoxamine
Cocaine	Quinidine	Rifampin	Grapefruit juice
Cortisol	Rilpivirine	Rilpivirine	Indinavir
Cyclophosphamide	Rivaroxaban	St. John's wort	Itraconazole
Dantrolene	Sertraline		Ketoconazole
Dapsone	Simvastatin		Miconazole
Diazepam	Tamoxifen		Nefazodone
Disopyramide	Testosterone		Nelfinavir
Enalapril	Tolvaptan		Posaconazole
Estradiol	Triazolam		Rilpivirine
Estrogen	Vandetanib		Ritonavir
Etoposide	Venlafaxine		Saquinavir
Everolimus	Vinblastine		Telapravir
Felodipine	Warfarin		Troleandomycin
Flutamide	Zolpidem		Verapamil
Lidocaine			Voriconazole
			Zafirlukast

[a]Substrates of the CYP3A4 isozyme will compete with cyclosporine, tacrolimus, and sirolimus for metabolism; therefore, concentrations of both medications will be increased (usually by ≤ 20%).

[b]Inducers of the CYP3A4 isozyme will enhance the metabolism of cyclosporine, tacrolimus, and sirolimus; therefore, concentrations of these medications will be decreased.

[c]Inhibitors of the CYP3A4 isozyme will decrease the metabolism of cyclosporine, tacrolimus, and sirolimus; therefore, concentrations of these medications will be increased.

coadministration with an interacting medication cannot be avoided. For example, it is recommended to reduce tacrolimus doses by one-third in patients initiating voriconazole. Some clinicians utilize interactions of metabolism to reduce the dose of an immunosuppressant, such as using diltiazem to treat hypertension, which also helps reduce tacrolimus doses and decrease pill burden.

Not all metabolic DDIs occur through the CYP system. Azathioprine has a considerable interaction with allopurinol and febuxostat that is mediated through the inhibition of xanthine oxidase, which is the enzyme responsible for metabolizing 6-MP to 6-thiouricate.[7] Combining these agents can result in 6-MP accumulation and severe myelosuppression. It is recommended that concomitant therapy with azathioprine and allopurinol or febuxostat be avoided, but if necessary, azathioprine doses must be empirically reduced by 75%.[7]

Interactions of Elimination Mycophenolate is metabolized to MPA-glucuronide (MPAG) via hepatic glucuronosyltransferase, and then excreted in bile for gut elimination.[7] Deconjugation of MPAG to MPA by intestinal flora results in continued MPA absorption several hours after its administration. Some medications (ie, cyclosporine, bile-acid sequestrants) interfere with the biliary excretion of MPAG; thereby, eliminating MPA reabsorption in the intestines and lowering the MPA area under the curve (AUC).[7] In this type of interaction, separation of doses is ineffective; therefore, proper patient monitoring is warranted.

▸ *Pharmacodynamic Interactions*

In addition to the numerous pharmacokinetic interactions seen with the maintenance immunosuppressants, there also exists the possibility for pharmacodynamic interactions. Pharmacodynamic interactions are the backbone of modern immunosuppressive therapies that employ multiple medications with different mechanisms of action resulting in additive immunosuppression. Unfortunately, pharmacodynamic interactions can also be problematic, such as when medications with similar adverse events are used concomitantly. For example, nephrotoxic agents, such as amphotericin B, aminoglycosides, and nonsteroidal anti-inflammatory drugs may potentiate the nephrotoxic effects of the calcineurin inhibitors.[7] The use of myelosuppressive agents, such as sulfamethoxazole-trimethoprim and valganciclovir, could enhance the myelosuppressive effects of induction therapy and the maintenance immunosuppressants.[7]

In addition to reviewing prescription medications, it is essential to question patients about the use of nonprescription agents and dietary supplements, as these products also have the potential for significant interactions, through methods discussed above. Some examples of this are St. John's wort inducing the

Patient Encounter Part 2

Identify your treatment goals for the patient in terms of maintenance immunosuppressants.

Create a plan for maintenance therapy for the patient, making sure to compare and contrast the pros and cons of the different maintenance immunosuppressants.

Identify the need to continue the patient's pretransplant medications, and identify any potential DDIs that may exist with the addition of the maintenance immunosuppressants and the medications that the patient is currently taking.

metabolism of CNIs and ToR inhibitors, and willow bark having the potential to worsen CNI-induced nephrotoxicity.

Immunosuppressive Therapies—Management of Immunosuppressive Drug Complications

▸ Opportunistic Infections

KEY CONCEPT *Organ transplant recipients are at increased risk of infectious diseases, which are a chief cause of early morbidity and mortality.*[32] The prevalence of posttransplant infection depends on many factors, including clinical risk factors, environmental exposures, and the degree of immunosuppression. Anti-infectives are universally prescribed in this population, and their use can be split into three different categories:

- Prophylaxis: antimicrobials given to prevent infection
- Empiric: preemptive therapy given based on clinical suspicion of an infection
- Treatment: antimicrobials given to manage a documented infection

Posttransplant infections generally occur in a standard pattern; therefore, prevention is a key management strategy.[32] The information in this section is designed to highlight prophylaxis options routinely used in organ transplant recipients. Please refer to Table 55–6 for a list of agents used for the prevention of *Pneumocystis jiroveci* pneumonia and CMV disease.[33,34]

***Pneumocystis jiroveci* Pneumonia** KEY CONCEPT *Without prophylaxis, P. jiroveci pneumonia occurs in 5% to 15% of transplant recipients.*[33] Antipneumocystis prophylaxis is enormously helpful and is generally used in all organ transplant recipients. The duration of prophylaxis is usually 6 to 12 months after transplant, but may be prolonged in highly immunosuppressed patients (ie, active CMV disease, treatment for rejection) or liver or

Table 55–6

Prophylactic Options for *Pneumocystis jiroveci* Pneumonia and CMV[33,34]

Medication	Dosing	Common Adverse Events
Antipneumocystis Prophylaxis		
Sulfamethoxazole-trimethoprim (Bactrim, Septra, SMZ-TMP, cotrimoxazole)	One SS tablet by mouth once a day[a] One DS tablet by mouth once a day[a] One DS tablet by mouth every M/W/F[a]	Hyperkalemia Myelosuppression Nephrotoxicity Neutropenia Photosensitivity Rash
Pentamidine (NebuPent)	300 mg inhaled every 3–4 weeks	Bronchospasm Cough Hypoglycemia or hyperglycemia
Dapsone (Avlosulfon)	50–100 mg tablet by mouth once a day	Hepatotoxicity Myelosuppression Nephritis
Atovaquone (Mepron)	1500 mg suspension by mouth once a day	Elevated liver transaminases Nausea Rash
Antivirals		
Valganciclovir (Valcyte)	450–900 mg by mouth once a day[a]	Stomach upset (8%–41%) Myelosuppression (2%–27%) Headache (9%–22%)
Ganciclovir (Cytovene)	5 mg/kg IV every day; or 1000 mg by mouth three times a day[a]	Stomach upset (13%–40%) Myelosuppression (5%–40%) Rash (10%–15%)
Valacyclovir (Valtrex)	1–2 g by mouth four times a day[a]	Stomach upset (1%–15%) Myelosuppression (< 1%) Headache (14%–35%)
CMV hyperimmune globulin (CytoGam) and polyvalent IVIG	The maximum recommended total dosage per infusion is 150 mg/kg beginning within 72 hours of transplantation Follow-up doses and time intervals depend on the type of organ transplanted	Stomach upset (1%–6%) Fevers and chills (1%–6%) Flushing (1%–6%)

CMV, cytomegalovirus; DS, double-strength (800 mg SMZ, 160 mg TMP); IVIG, intravenous immune globulin; IV, intravenous; M/W/F, Monday, Wednesday, and Friday; SS, single-strength (400 mg SMZ, 80 mg TMP); SMZ, sulfamethoxazole; TMP, trimethoprim.

[a]Dose adjustment required in renal insufficiency.

lung recipients. Sulfamethoxazole-trimethoprim is the preferred agent for prophylaxis. One of its major advantages is its broad spectrum of activity. Not only is it effective against *Pneumocystis*, but it also has activity against *Toxoplasma* and other common bacterial infections. Patients who have sulfa allergies, glucose-6 phosphate dehydrogenase (G6PD) deficiency, or are intolerant of sulfamethoxazole-trimethoprim should be given one of the second-line treatments. Unfortunately, the second-line agents are antiparasitics and have no meaningful activity against common bacteria. These agents include dapsone, atovaquone, and pentamidine.[33]

Cytomegalovirus CMV is a concerning opportunistic pathogen in transplantation due to its association with poor outcomes.[34] CMV infection is present in 30% to 97% of the general population, but CMV disease is typically restricted to immunocompromised hosts. The risk of CMV disease is highest among CMV-naive recipients who receive a CMV-positive organ (donor+/recipient–). Other factors that augment the risk of CMV disease include organ type (lung and pancreas recipients are highest risk) and immunosuppressive agents (ALA use increases risk). CMV disease characteristically occurs within the first 3 to 6 months posttransplantation, but delayed onset disease has been seen in patients receiving antiviral prophylaxis. Patients with CMV infection may present with flu-like symptoms, including fever, chills, aches, malaise, and fatigue. CMV infection may result in more profound symptoms in the immunosuppressed patient, including leukopenia, thrombocytopenia, and organ dysfunction.[34]

KEY CONCEPT *Several antivirals have proven effective in preventing and treating CMV.*[34] Valacyclovir and valganciclovir, prodrugs of acyclovir and ganciclovir, respectively, have improved bioavailability compared with their parent compounds and offer the advantage of less frequent dosing. CMV prophylaxis is typically continued for the first 200 days, or longer, after transplantation. Although valganciclovir and IV ganciclovir are considered the prophylaxis agents of choice in most organ transplant recipients, national guidelines allow for consideration of prophylaxis with CMV hyperimmune globulin in heart and lung transplant populations. Both IV ganciclovir and oral valganciclovir may be used for preemptive therapy or for treatment of established CMV disease.[34] The adverse events are similar among these agents and include myelosuppression and GI effects.[7]

Fungal Infections Fungal infections are an important cause of morbidity and mortality in solid organ transplant recipients.[35] Immunologic (ie, immunosuppressants, CMV infection), anatomic (ie, tissue ischemia and damage), and surgical (ie, duration of surgery, transfusion requirements) factors contribute to the risk for invasive fungal infections. Mucocutaneous candidiasis (ie, oral thrush, esophagitis) is associated with corticosteroids and ALA. KEY CONCEPT *Oral nystatin or clotrimazole troches are effective prophylactic options for the prevention of thrush.* However, clotrimazole inhibits the CYP3A system in the gut and can alter immunosuppressive levels.[7] The use of systemic antifungal prophylaxis, such as oral fluconazole, is controversial due to the potential for DDIs and the risk of developing resistance. The American Society of Transplantation has recommended antifungal prophylaxis in liver, lung, intestine, and pancreas transplantation.[36,37] The choice of agents depends on the fungal risk in that particular population. For example, liver, intestine, and pancreas transplant recipients are at high risk for candidiasis; therefore, the use of medications that cover *Candida* spp. is crucial, such as the triazoles (ie, fluconazole, itraconazole) or echinocandins (ie, caspofungin, micafungin, anidulafungin). Lung transplant recipients are at high risk for aspergillosis; therefore, it is imperative to use antifungal prophylaxis that covers *Aspergillus* spp., such as the echinocandins, polyenes (ie, amphotericin B, lipid-based amphotericin B products) or new generation triazoles (ie, voriconazole, posaconazole).[36,37]

Polyomavirus One infection complication seen only in renal transplant recipients is polyomavirus. In humans, there are two known pathologic polyoma strains, BK and JC. These viruses are rarely associated with disease in immunocompetent individuals. During periods of immunosuppression, the virus is reactivated and can be associated with significant morbidity.[38]

In renal transplant recipients, the major diseases caused by BK virus (BKV) are tubulointerstitial nephritis and ureteral stenosis.[38] Polyomavirus-associated nephropathy (PyVAN) presents with evidence of allograft dysfunction, resulting in either an asymptomatic acute or slowly progressive rise in serum creatinine concentrations. Some studies have reported that PyVAN may affect up to 10% of renal transplant recipients, frequently resulting in permanent renal dysfunction or allograft loss.[38]

Currently, treatment options for BKV are limited, and management recommendations are generally focused on reductions in immunosuppression. There is a lack of a directed antiviral intervention; however, some centers have utilized IVIG, cidofovir, leflunomide, and the fluoroquinolone antibiotics to manage BKV infections. All of these agents have been reported to provide some benefit in managing BKV in anecdotal cases.[38]

Vaccination Vaccination is one of the most effective means of preventing infection and related complications.[39] However, there is a valid concern that solid organ transplant recipients may mount an inadequate response to vaccination due to immunosuppression. Required vaccinations should be administered prior to transplantation so that an appropriate antibody response can develop (Table 55–7).[39] If this strategy is pursued, the earlier a vaccine is administered, the more effective it may be, as end-stage organ failure can also contribute to a decreased immune response.[39]

In general, the weakest response to vaccine is within the first 6 months posttransplantation due to the intense level of immunosuppression during this period.[39] Vaccination within 6 months of transplant may be considered on a case-by-case basis in those patients who are at high risk of developing infection. Use of inactive vaccines is preferred in transplant recipients due to the relative risk of infection associated with live vaccines. Health care workers and family members who are in close contact with transplant recipients and have received a live vaccine should consider use of respiratory masks for at least 7 days after vaccination and adhere to strict oral and hand hygiene.[39]

▸ *Hypertension*

KEY CONCEPT *Cardiovascular disease has been identified as the leading cause of death in organ transplant recipients.*[40] Posttransplant hypertension is associated with increased cardiac morbidity and patient mortality in transplant patients and is also an independent risk factor for allograft dysfunction. Based on all of the available posttransplant morbidity and mortality data, it is imperative that posttransplant hypertension be identified and managed appropriately.[40]

There are several mechanisms responsible for posttransplant hypertension including renal dysfunction, increased sensitivity to endothelin-1 and angiotensin, increased density of glucocorticoid receptors in the vascular smooth muscle, and decreased

Table 55–7

Recommended Vaccinations Pre- and Posttransplant[39]

Vaccine	Administration: Before SOT	After SOT	Additional Information
Hepatitis A	X		Immunize as soon as possible during course of disease
Hepatitis B	X		Immunize as soon as possible during course of disease (before transplant, administer 40 mcg dose in a series of three to four doses)
Herpes Zoster	X		Live[a] virus, administer ≥ 14 days before immunosuppressant agents are initiated (experts advise 1 month before)
Human Papilloma Virus	X		Recommended for females aged 9–26, no recommendations for SOT
Influenza	X	X	Annual vaccination with inactivated intramuscular formulation recommended before and after SOT
Measles-Rubella	X		Live[a] virus, administer to patients who are seronegative, *before* transplant, or in women of childbearing age for prevention of congenital rubella syndrome
Pneumococcal	X	X	23-valent polysaccharide vaccine should be given once before transplant and boosters at 3 and 5 years after initial dose
Tetanus/Diptheria	X		TDaP booster indicated for < 65 years old (may be given ≤ 2 years after last TDaP booster in SOT patients)
Varicella	X		Live[a] virus, administer to patients who are seronegative, *before* transplant

TDaP, tetanus, diphtheria, and pertussis.

[a]All live vaccines are contraindicated post solid organ transplant (SOT), as they can cause serious infection.

Live vaccines:

Bacillus Calmette-Guerin

Herpes zoster

Live intranasal attenuated influenza

Live oral typhoid

Measles rubella

Vaccinia (smallpox)

Varicella

production of vasodilatory prostaglandins.[40] However, one of the most easily recognized causes of posttransplant hypertension is the use of corticosteroids and CNIs. Corticosteroids cause sodium and water retention, thus increasing blood pressure, whereas CNIs reduce glomerular filtration rate and renal blood flow, increase systemic and intrarenal vascular resistance, promote sodium retention, reduce concentrations of systemic vasodilators (ie, prostacyclin, nitric oxide), and increase concentrations of thromboxanes. Compared with cyclosporine, tacrolimus displays significantly less severe hypertension, and patients taking tacrolimus require significantly fewer antihypertensive medications after transplant.[40]

Treatment KEY CONCEPT *Controlling hypertension after transplant is essential in preventing cardiac morbidity and mortality and prolonging graft survival.* The target blood pressure in transplant recipients should be less than 130/80 mm Hg.[40] This goal blood pressure may not be suitable for all patients. Note: national guidelines for treating hypertension in the general population are often followed, despite their lack of transplant recommendations. Refer to Chapter 5, *Hypertension*, for additional information.

Patient Encounter Part 3

Identify your treatment goals for the patient in terms of antimicrobial prophylaxis.

Create a plan for her antimicrobial prophylaxis, making sure to compare and contrast the pros and cons of the different agents in this patient.

Lifestyle Modifications To achieve a goal blood pressure, lifestyle modifications including diet, exercise, sodium restriction, and smoking cessation are recommended.[40] Unfortunately, lifestyle modifications alone are often inadequate in high-risk populations, and antihypertensive medications are usually initiated early after transplant.[40]

Immunosuppressive Regimen Modification Because tacrolimus has shown the propensity to cause less severe hypertension compared to cyclosporine, conversion from cyclosporine-based immunosuppression to tacrolimus-based immunosuppression may be one way to reduce the severity of hypertension in transplant recipients. KEY CONCEPT *Conversion to a ToR inhibitor or belatacept, which are not associated with hypertension, may also be an alternative to the CNIs in patients with difficult-to-treat hypertension.* Corticosteroid taper or withdrawal are effective strategies for lowering blood pressure, but are not warranted in all clinical situations.[40]

Antihypertensive Agents There is no single class of antihypertensive medications recognized as the ideal agent. Numerous factors must be considered when determining appropriate treatment for a patient, including the safety and efficacy data of available agents, patient-specific comorbidities, and medication cost.[40] A large majority of patients often require multiple medications to achieve goal blood pressure, and combination therapy is regarded as an appropriate first-line therapy.[40]

β-Blockers and thiazide diuretics have proven benefits in reducing cardiovascular disease–associated morbidity and mortality.[40] Tolerability permitting, these agents are to be considered first-line therapies in most transplant recipients. The angiotensin-converting enzyme (ACE) inhibitors and angiotensin receptor blockers (ARB) have definite benefits in patients with nephropathy and are believed to have renoprotective effects in most patients. However, due to their ability to cause an initial increase in serum creatinine, these agents should be used cautiously when combined with the CNIs. The dihydropyridine calcium channel blockers have demonstrated an ability to reverse nephrotoxicity associated with cyclosporine and tacrolimus. The addition of diltiazem to patients' regimens after cardiac transplant has also been shown to retard progression of cardiac allograft vasculopathy. In general, antihypertensive therapy should focus on agents with proven benefits in reducing the progression of cardiovascular disease and must be tailored to a patient's needs.[40]

▸ Hyperlipidemia

KEY CONCEPT *Hyperlipidemia is seen in as high as 60% of transplant patients.*[41] As a result of elevated cholesterol levels, transplant recipients are not only at increased risk of atherosclerotic events, but also allograft vasculopathy. Hyperlipidemia, along with other types of cardiovascular disease, is now one of the primary causes of morbidity and mortality in long-term transplant survivors.[41]

Elevated cholesterol levels in transplant patients are due to age, genetic disposition, renal dysfunction, DM, proteinuria, body weight, and immunosuppressive therapy. Many of the immunosuppressive agents can produce elevations in serum lipid levels.[41]

Treatment KEY CONCEPT *Lowering cholesterol has shown to significantly decrease severe rejection and transplant vasculopathy and improve 1-year survival in heart transplant recipients.*[42] Although these results cannot be extrapolated to other transplant populations, they do demonstrate the potential benefits of aggressive cholesterol lowering in organ transplant recipients. Due to high prevalence of cardiovascular disease among organ transplant recipients, most practitioners consider these patients to be high risk for lipid lowering. Many guidelines state a target calculated low-density lipoprotein cholesterol (LDL-C) level of less than 100 mg/dL (2.59 mmol/L) in high-risk patients.[41] Note: national guidelines for treating hyperlipidemia in the general population are often followed, despite their lack of transplant recommendations. Refer to Chapter 12, *Dyslipidemias*, for additional information.

Lifestyle Modifications Generally, lowering cholesterol in patients begins with therapeutic lifestyle changes. These changes are initiated either alone or in conjunction with lipid-lowering drug therapy, depending on baseline cholesterol levels and other risk factors. Therapeutic lifestyle changes entail a reduction in saturated fat and cholesterol intake and an increase in moderate physical activity.[43] As with hypertension, lifestyle modifications alone rarely allow a patient to achieve a goal LDL-C level. Modification of the immunosuppressive regimen and use of cholesterol-lowering medications are often warranted in this population.[41]

Immunosuppressive Regimen Modifications Tacrolimus has shown the propensity to cause less severe hyperlipidemia when compared with cyclosporine. Conversion from cyclosporine-based immunosuppression to tacrolimus-based immunosuppression may be one way to counteract this disease in transplant recipients. Also, the ToR inhibitors have been associated with significant changes in lipids and triglycerides; therefore, conversion from a ToR inhibitor to a CNI or belatacept may be warranted in patients receiving ToR inhibitor therapy with resistant dyslipidemia.[41]

In past studies, steroid withdrawal in renal transplant patients did demonstrate moderate reductions in total cholesterol and LDL cholesterol; unfortunately, a decrease in high-density lipoprotein (HDL) levels were also noted.[41]

Cholesterol-Lowering Agents 3-Hydroxy-3-methylglutaryl coenzyme A (HMG-CoA) reductase inhibitors, or statins, are considered first-line therapy for hyperlipidemia in the general population.[41] However, there is some uncertainty about the pathogenesis of cardiovascular disease in transplant recipients and whether statin therapy will have similar effectiveness in organ transplant recipients. Statins have shown definite advantages when used in heart transplantation, including a reduction in LDL-C and major adverse cardiac events (MACE), as well as an apparent cardioprotective effect. In renal transplant recipients, statins lower LDL-C levels and reduce the incidence of some cardiac events; however, the ability to lower MACE has not been seen in this population. Despite these mixed results, statins are still considered the primary therapeutic option for hyperlipidemia in organ transplant recipients.[41] When choosing a statin for management of hyperlipidemia in the transplant patient, a focus on potential DDIs is warranted. It is recommended that doses of atorvastatin not exceed 10 mg daily when taken with cyclosporine due to an increased risk of myopathy and rhabdomyolysis. Use of cyclosporine in conjunction with simvastatin is considered a contraindication due to the risk of skeletal muscle effects.[41]

Fibric acid derivatives are an excellent choice for lowering triglycerides, but are not as effective as statins at lowering LDL-C.[41] These agents play a role in conjunction with statins in patients with both elevated cholesterol and triglycerides. Nicotinic acid is very effective at improving the lipid panel, with excellent results in lowering LDL-C, as well as increasing HDL. However, patient tolerability is a concern with this agent. The bile acid sequestrants should be avoided in transplant recipients due to their high incidence of GI adverse events, as well as their propensity for pharmacokinetic DDIs with MPA. Ezetimibe has proven safe and effective in lowering LDL-C in renal transplant recipients. Future studies are needed to establish ideal regimens involving the antihyperlipidemic and immunosuppressive medications to decrease morbidity and mortality and ultimately prevent cardiovascular events.[41]

▸ New-Onset DM After Transplantation

KEY CONCEPT *New-onset DM after transplantation (NODAT) is a serious complication that is often underestimated by transplant practitioners.*[44] Kasiske and colleagues attempted to quantify the cumulative incidence of NODAT in renal transplant recipients and found that 8.3% of patients developed NODAT at 3 months posttransplant, 12.9% at 12 months, and 22.3% at 36 months.[45] Even more alarming is that recent studies have revealed an overwhelming prevalence of impaired glucose tolerance, which is also accepted as a risk factor for long-term morbidity and mortality. NODAT is associated with a 22% higher risk of mortality. Patients with NODAT are also more likely to suffer acute rejection episodes and infectious complications than patients without NODAT.[44]

Prevention KEY CONCEPT *NODAT prevention mainly consists of identifying patients at risk before transplant and controlling modifiable risk factors both before and after transplantation.*[44] The major modifiable risk factors are choice of immunosuppressive therapy and body mass index (BMI). For example:

- Immunosuppressive medications: Steroid minimization and possibly withdrawal are effective strategies for preventing NODAT. Also, patients with worsening blood glucose who are receiving tacrolimus may benefit from conversion to cyclosporine or belatacept.[44]
- Body mass index: A reduction in body weight is recommended in obese patients prior to transplant to lower their NODAT risks.[44]

Treatment KEY CONCEPT *Lifestyle modifications are recommended in patients who have developed or those who are at increased risk of developing NODAT.*[44] Insulin therapy and oral hypoglycemic agents are often utilized in those patients in whom lifestyle modifications alone have not controlled blood glucose. Please refer to Chapter 43, *Diabetes Mellitus*, for proper instruction on choosing the appropriate treatment regimens in patients with DM.

▶ Neoplasia

Cancer Screening in Transplant Patients Transplant recipients are at increased risk for malignancies (Table 55–8).[46,48] The risk of developing Kaposi sarcoma following transplantation is over 200 times that in the general population. In addition, the risk of nonmelanocytic and melanocytic skin cancer is 10 to 20 times higher compared with the nontransplanted population. Transplant recipients are at greatest risk for the types of cancers associated with viral infections, such as PTLD, cervical, and vulvovaginal cancers. Solid organ tumors like colorectal and lung cancers are two to three times higher in transplant recipients when compared with the general population. The American Cancer Society and American Transplant Society recommend cancer screening for most adults who have undergone transplantation (Table 55–9).[46,48] Although clinical research has not yet proven that potential benefits of testing outweigh the harms of testing in transplant recipients, most believe that transplant recipients should be tested and screened very closely.[46]

Table 55–8

Overall Risk of Different Types of Cancer in Transplant Patients[46,48]

Cancer	Cumulative Incidence (/100,000)	Male	Female
Kaposi sarcoma	140	17.4	62
Kidney/ureter	1010	14.1	14.6
Lymphoma	80	6.9	29.1
Bladder	126	1.6	3.6
Esophagus	70	2.4	2.8
Cervix	180	–	5.7
Liver	220	4.2	4.5
Melanoma	320	6.9	5.2
Lung/bronchus/ trachea	690	2.3	3.6
Colorectal	510	1.6	2.8
Breast	1050	4	1.1
Prostate	1740	1.6	–

Skin Cancer Skin cancer remains the most common malignancy after transplantation. The incidence of these types of cancers increases with time posttransplant, with one study showing a prevalence rate of 35% among patients within 10 years after transplant. Also, skin cancers in transplant recipients tend to grow more rapidly and are more likely to metastasize.[46]

The most common risk factors for skin cancer development after transplant include increased age; excessive ultraviolet (UV) light exposure; high degree of immunosuppression; Fitzpatrick skin types I, II, and III; history of skin cancers; and infection by human papillomavirus.[46] KEY CONCEPT *Many believe that ToR inhibitors in place of CNIs in transplant recipients can reduce the risk of nonmelanoma skin carcinomas.*[47]

Transplant practitioners must be vigilant about educating their patients about excessive exposure to the sun.[46] Patients should be warned about the risk of skin cancer and be advised on simple methods to limit risk:

- Wear protective clothing (ie, long-sleeved shirts, pants, dark-colored clothing)
- Use of sunscreen, sun protection factor (SPF) 30 or higher, daily to all sun-exposed skin

▶ Posttransplant Lymphoproliferative Disorders

KEY CONCEPT *PTLDs are a major complication following organ transplantation.*[46] Large series of case reports have demonstrated the incidence of PTLD is 1% for renal patients, 1.8% for cardiac patients, 2.2% for liver patients, and 9.4% for heart–lung patients. The risk of developing non-Hodgkin lymphoma is nearly 50-fold higher in organ transplant recipients compared with the general population. Another risk factor is the presence of EBV. Lymphomas are the most common form of PTLD.[46,48]

The incidence of disease depends on certain factors that include the type of organ transplanted, age of the transplant recipient, type and degree of immunosuppression, and exposure to EBV. The mortality rate in these patients is 50%, with most patients dying shortly after diagnosis. It has also been demonstrated that the risk of developing PTLD is greater in EBV seronegative patients.[46,48] Belatacept has been approved with a black box warning outlining an increased risk of PTLD, especially of the CNS. Patients who are EBV seronegative or have an unknown immunity to EBV should not receive belatacept. Also, immunosuppressive regimens utilizing the ALAs have been proven to increase the risk of PTLD.[46,48]

Treatment KEY CONCEPT *Treatment for PTLD is still controversial; however, the most common treatment options include reduction of immunosuppression, chemotherapy, and anti–B cell monoclonal antibodies.*[46,48] PTLD continues to be a long-term complication of prolonged immunosuppression. Current treatment options are all associated with certain risks. Prevention is the most effective treatment for PTLD. A better understanding of the disease process and the risk factors involved with the development of PTLD will aid in the prophylaxis and treatment of this disorder.[46,48]

▶ Pregnancy

Females of childbearing age who do not wish to become pregnant after transplantation require adequate education on preferred forms of birth control.[49] The optimal method of birth control in this patient population is the barrier method (eg condom, diaphragm). Use of intrauterine devices and progestin-based oral contraceptives are controversial, and associated risks must be considered prior to initiating therapy. Intrauterine devices may be less effective in the setting of immunosuppression and

Table 55–9

Cancer Screening Recommendations in Transplant Patients[46,48]

Cancer Type	General Populations	Transplant Populations
Breast	Mammography every 1–2 years for all women ≥ 50 years old. Clinical breast exam every 3 years in women 20–39 years old, yearly after age 40. Monthly self-exam.	Mammography every 1–2 years for all women ≥ 50 years old. May undergo screening between 40 and 49 years old but no evidence for or against screening in this age group.
Cervical	Annual Pap smear and pelvic exam once sexually active; after three or more tests with normal results, may decrease frequency of exams.	Annual Pap smear and pelvic exam once sexually active.
Colorectal	Annual FOBT plus flexible sigmoidoscopy every 5 years for all patients ≥ 50 years old or colonoscopy and DRE every 10 years.	Annual FOBT plus flexible sigmoidoscopy every 5 years for all transplant patients ≥ 50 years old.
Prostate	Annual DRE and PSA for men ≥ 50 years old with 10-year life expectancy or younger men at high risk.	Annual DRE and PSA measurement in all males ≥ 50 years old.
Hepatocellular	Not recommended for average-risk individuals. α-Fetoprotein and ultrasound every 6 months in high-risk patients (no firm supporting data).	α-Fetoprotein and ultrasound every 6 months in high-risk patients (no firm supporting data).
Skin	Skin exam every 3 years between ages 20 and 40, annually thereafter.	Monthly self-exam. Total body skin exam every 6–12 months by dermatologists.
Renal	Insufficient evidence to support routine screening.	No firm recommendations. Regular ultrasound of native kidneys.
Lung	Insufficient evidence to support routine screening.	No firm recommendations.
Ovarian	Insufficient evidence to support routine screening.	No firm recommendations.
Testicular	Insufficient evidence to support routine screening.	No firm recommendations.
Endometrial	Insufficient evidence to support routine screening.	No firm recommendations

DRE, digital rectal exam; FOBT, fecal occult blood test; PSA, prostate-specific antigen.

predispose patients to an increased risk of infection. Progestin-based contraceptives are considered a less effective form of birth control, but may be a safe option in those patients without hypertension.[49]

Female patients considering pregnancy after transplantation should be educated extensively regarding the potential impact of pregnancy on renal function and the risks that transplantation and medical immunosuppression may present to a fetus.[49] Risks to the infant include premature birth (50%) and intrauterine growth restriction (20%), which may result in death or long-term complications, including cerebral palsy, blindness, deafness, and learning deficiencies. Patients hoping to become pregnant should wait at least 1 year after transplantation to ensure reconstitution of gonadal function posttransplant, as well as demonstrate a 1-year freedom from acute rejection.[49]

Understanding the associated risk of immunosuppressives while pregnant is paramount considering their ability to cross the placenta as well as enter breast milk.[49] Tacrolimus and cyclosporine, both Pregnancy Category C, are the backbone of immunosuppressive therapy and have been used safely and effectively in pregnancy posttransplant for decades. Side effects associated with CNIs such as hypertension, diabetes, and nephrotoxicity should be monitored closely in the pregnant population. The ToR inhibitors are also Pregnancy Category C and have not been associated with fetal malformation but should be used cautiously in pregnant patients. Corticosteroids, pregnancy category B, are recognized to be relatively safe and have been used extensively in pregnancy after transplantation. However, they carry a risk of premature membrane rupture and newborn adrenal insufficiency. More common side effects associated with corticosteroids that may cause complications in pregnancy include hypertension, diabetes, weight gain, and poor wound healing. Due to teratogenic effects in animal studies, azathioprine is considered Pregnancy Category D; however, it has been used extensively as an antimetabolite in pregnant transplant patients without extensive evidence of harm to the fetus. 6-Mercaptopurine has not been shown to cross the placental barrier.[49]

Currently, the MPA derivatives, both Pregnancy Category D, are not considered optimal immunosuppressive agents for patients who become pregnant, and alternative therapies should be pursued.[49] These agents have a FDA-approved risk evaluation and minimization strategy to help minimize fetal exposure to MPA, prevent unplanned pregnancies in patients using MPA, collect data on MPA use in pregnancy via the Mycophenolate Pregnancy Registry, and educate patients about the risks associated with the use of this medication. A less teratogenic antimetabolite, azathioprine, should be substituted for mycophenolate mofetil or enteric-coated MPA in patients who plan on becoming pregnant. The safety of ALAs and rituximab in transplantation has yet to be fully determined; however, IVIG has been widely used without any documented adverse events. Newly available immunosuppressives, belatacept and everolimus, are pregnancy category C but are not recommended for use in pregnant patients due to inadequate human data.[49]

▶ *Immunosuppressant Therapy Adherence*

Transplant recipients require strict adherence to their medication regimens to ensure optimal outcomes. Nonadherence

Patient Encounter Part 4

The patient continues to have her posttransplant care at your renal transplant ambulatory care clinic. She returns to your clinic 1 month after the transplant:

Labs: Na 147 mEq/L (147 mmol/L); K 4.5 mEq/L (4.5 mmol/L); Cl 198 mEq/L (198 mmol/L); CO_2 21 mEq/L (21 mmol/L); BUN 18 mg/dL (6.4 mmol/L); SCr 0.8 mg/dL (71 μmol/L); glucose 198 mg/dL (11.0 mmol/L); lipid panel: TC = 301 mg/dL (7.78 mmol/L), direct LDL = 147 mg/dL (3.80 mmol/L), HDL = 47 mg/dL (1.22 mmol/L), TG = 522 mg/dL (5.90 mmol/L); uric acid 9.6 mg/dL (571 μmol/L); tacrolimus 9.7 ng/mL (9.7 mcg/L or 12.0 nmol/L)

VS: BP 155/90 mm Hg (158/88 mm Hg repeated using manual method), HR 80 beats/min

Meds: Tacrolimus XL 10 mg by mouth once a day; mycophenolate mofetil 1000 mg by mouth twice a day; prednisone—no longer taking as it was completely withdrawn on postoperative day 11; atovaquone 1500 mg by mouth once a day; valganciclovir 900 mg by mouth once a day; atorvastatin 20 mg by mouth once a day; metoprolol XL 100 mg by mouth once a day; amlodipine 5 mg by mouth once a day; zolpidem 10 mg by mouth once a day at bedtime as needed; insulin glargine 32 units administered in the evening; insulin aspart 8 units with each meal and a sliding scale (dependent on blood sugars)

Identify why the patient is taking each agent listed.

What are some treatment options for her elevated blood pressure?

What are some treatment options for her elevated cholesterol?

What are some treatment options for her elevated uric acid?

Design a monitoring plan for the patient's therapy.

Patient Care Process

Early Management of Transplant Recipients

Patient Assessment:

- Review all available diagnostic and laboratory data, and patient history and comorbidities to evaluate patient as a transplant recipient.

Therapy Evaluation:

- Evaluate medications currently being used by patient that will be continued posttransplant such as drugs to treat concomitant disease states (eg, hypertension, DM, dyslipidemia).
- For medications that are likely to be continued posttransplant, assess efficacy, safety, and patient adherence. Are there any significant drug interactions?

Care Plan Development:

- Propose an immunosuppressive regimen following transplantation, including:
  - Induction therapy (see Table 55–2):
    - Based on the type of organ being transplanted, recipient's history and donor characteristics, determine if the patient requires induction therapy.
    - If you decide to use induction therapy, assess for appropriate drug choice, dose, and duration of therapy.
  - Maintenance immunosuppressive agents (see Tables 55–2, 55–3, 55–4, and 55–5, and Figure 55–2):
    - Assess for appropriate choice, dose, and duration of therapy.
- Antimicrobial prophylaxis (see Table 55–6):
  - Assess suitability of chosen prophylactic agents (eg, drug allergies, CMV donor and recipient serostatus, need for antifungal prophylaxis).
- Medications used for comorbidities:
  - Assess appropriate selection of these medications for pharmacokinetic and pharmacodynamic DDIs, need, efficacy, and side effects.
- Determine if patient has insurance coverage and what agents are on formulary.
- Develop patient-specific short-term and long-term therapeutic goals.
- Provide patient education regarding the organ transplant, complications associated with transplantation, need for lifestyle modifications to reduce risk of complications (eg, wear sunscreen, low-sodium diet), and drug therapy (including importance of adherence to therapeutic regimen and insurance/payer information).
- Assess the need for therapeutic drug monitoring of any of the immunosuppressants.
- General therapeutic monitoring parameters based on organ transplanted and toxic monitoring parameters for medications prescribed.
- Continually evaluate the patient for presence of adverse drug reactions, drug allergies, or DDIs.

Follow-Up Evaluation (Outpatient Transplant Clinic):

- Obtain a thorough history of prescription, nonprescription, and complementary and alternative medication use.
- Monitor the patient's maintenance immunosuppression.
  - Assess for appropriate dose and duration of therapy.
- Assess for new or worsening disease states such as hypertension, DM, or dyslipidemia.
- Antimicrobial prophylaxis:
  - Does the patient need continued prophylaxis therapy?
  - When do you stop prophylaxis?

(Continued)

Patient Care Process (*Continued*)

- Medications used for comorbidities:
  - Assess appropriate selection of these medications for pharmacokinetic and pharmacodynamic DDIs, need, and efficacy.
  - Assess whether new medications are needed for existing comorbidities or new diagnoses.
- Reassess your patient-specific short-term and long-term therapeutic goals.
- Continue with patient education in regard to the complications associated with transplantation, the need for lifestyle modifications to reduce risk of complications (eg, wear sunscreen, low-sodium diet), and drug therapy.
- Reemphasize the importance of adherence with therapeutic regimen.
- Assess improvement in quality-of-life measures such as physical, psychological, and social functioning, and well-being.

in this population can be attributed to the complexity of the regimens coupled with the variability in drug dosing, need for therapeutic drug monitoring, avoidance of potential DDIs, infectious risks, and drug toxicities. The incidence of nonadherence to immunosuppressant therapy in the first year posttransplant has been estimated to be as high as 23%.[50] This is especially alarming when one considers that 35% of all graft failures can be directly attributed to nonadherence. Risk factors associated with immunosuppressant therapy nonadherence include a history of substance abuse, personality disorders, and lack of social support. The role of the pharmacist in educating patients on the importance of their medication regimens and stressing the need for adherence is paramount in optimizing both patient and allograft survival after transplantation. Previous reports have suggested that intervention by a pharmacist posttransplant improves adherence.[50]

OUTCOME EVALUATION

- Successful outcomes in solid organ transplantation are generally measured in terms of several separate end points: (a) preventing rejection, (b) preventing immunosuppressive drug complications, and (c) improving long-term survival.
- The short-term goals revolve around reducing the incidence of acute rejection episodes and attaining a high graft survival rate. By accomplishing these goals, transplant clinicians hope to attain good allograft function to allow for an improved quality of life. These goals can be achieved through the appropriate use of medical immunosuppression and scrutinizing over the therapeutic and toxic monitoring parameters associated with each medication employed. In addition, transplant recipients should be monitored for adverse drug reactions, DDIs, and adherence with their therapeutic regimen.
- The long-term goals after organ transplant are to maximize the functionality of the allograft and prevent the complications of immunosuppression, which lead to improved patient survival. Clinicians must play multiple roles in the long-term care of transplant recipients, as not only must the patient be followed from an immunologic perspective, but practitioners must be focused on identifying and treating the adverse sequelae associated with lifelong immunosuppression including cardiovascular disease, malignancy, infection, and osteoporosis, among others. Again, limiting drug misadventures and ensuring adherence with the therapeutic regimen are important and should be stressed.

Abbreviations Introduced in This Chapter

6-MP	6-Mercaptopurine
ACE	Angiotensin-converting enzyme
ALA	Antilymphocyte antibodies
AMR	Antibody-mediated rejection
APC	Antigen-presenting cell
ARB	Angiotensin receptor blocker
ATG	Antithymocyte globulin
AUC	Area under the curve
AZA	Azathioprine
BKV	BK virus
BMI	Body mass index
BUN	Blood urea nitrogen
C_0	Trough concentration
C_2	Drug concentration 2 hours postdose
CCB	Calcium channel blocker
$CD4^+$	Helper T cells
$CD8^+$	Cytotoxic T cells
CKD	Chronic kidney disease
CMV	Cytomegalovirus
CNI	Calcineurin inhibitor
CNS	Central nervous system
CSA	Cyclosporine
CXR	Chest x-ray
CYP	Cytochrome P-450 system
CYP3A	Cytochrome P-450 system 3A isozyme
DC	Dendritic cell
DDI	Drug–drug interaction
DM	Diabetes mellitus
DOE	Dyspnea on exertion
DRE	Digital rectal exam
DS	Double strength
DSA	Donor-specific antibody
e-ATG	Antithymocyte globulin equine
EBV	Epstein-Barr virus
EC	Enteric-coated
ESRD	End-stage renal disease
EVL	Everolimus
FBS	Fasting blood sugar
FDA	Food and Drug Administration
FEV	Forced expiratory volume
FOBT	Fecal occult blood test
G6PD	Glucose-6-phosphate-dehydrogenase
GI	Gastrointestinal
HDL	High-density lipoprotein
HLA	Human leukocyte antigen
HMG-CoA	3-Hydroxy-3-methylglutaryl coenzyme A
IgG	Immunoglobulin G
IL-2	Interleukin-2

IL-2RA	Interleukin-2 receptor antagonist
IV	Intravenous
IVIG	Intravenous immune globulin
LC-MS/MS	Liquid chromatography coupled tandem mass spectrometry
LDL-C	Low-density lipoprotein cholesterol
LFT	Liver function test
MAC	Membrane attack complex
MACE	Major adverse cardiac events
MHC	Major histocompatibility complex
MMF	Mycophenolate mofetil
MPA	Mycophenolic acid
MPAG	MPA-glucorinide
NFAT (NFAT-P)	Nuclear factors
NK	Natural killer
NODAT	New-onset diabetes mellitus after transplantation
NYHA	New York Heart Association
P-gp	P-glycoprotein
PRA	Panel-reactive antibodies
PSA	prostate-specific antigen
PTLD	Posttransplant lymphoproliferative disorders
PyVAN	Polyomavirus-associated nephropathy
r-ATG (RATG)	Antithymocyte globulin rabbit
SCr	Serum creatinine
SL	Sublingual
SMZ-TMP	Sulfamethoxazole-trimethoprim
SOB	Shortness of breath
SOT	Solid organ transplant
SPF	Sun protection factor
SPK	Simultaneous pancreas-kidney
SRL	Sirolimus
SS	Single strength
TAC	Tacrolimus
TC	Total cholesterol
TCR	T cell receptor
TDaP	Tetanus, diphtheria, and pertussis
TG	Triglycerides
ToR	Target of rapamycin
UV	Ultraviolet

REFERENCES

1. Danovitch G. Handbook of Kidney Transplantation, 5th ed. Lippincott, Williams & Wilkins; 2009.
2. The Organ Procurement and Transplantation Network (OPTN). http://optn.transplant.hrsa.gov/data/. Updated August 2015. Accessed August 24, 2015.
3. Halloran PF. Immunosuppressive drugs for kidney transplantation. N Engl J Med. 2004;351:2715–2729.
4. Kim M, Martin ST, Townsend KR, Gabardi S. Antibody-mediated rejection in kidney transplantation: A review of pathophysiology, diagnosis, and treatment options. Pharmacotherapy. 2014;34:733–744.
5. Gabardi S, Martin ST, Roberts KL, Grafals M. Induction immunosuppressive therapies in renal transplantation. Am J Health Syst Pharm. 2011;68:211–218.
6. Lee RA, Gabardi S. Current trends in immunosuppressive therapies for renal transplant recipients. Am J Health Syst Pharm. 2012;69:1961–1975.
7. Micromedex® Healthcare Series, (electronic version). Greenwood Village, Colorado, USA: Thomson Healthcare, Inc.; 2014.
8. Goggins WC, Pascual MA, Powelson JA, et al. A prospective, randomized, clinical trial of intraoperative versus postoperative Thymoglobulin in adult cadaveric renal transplant recipients. Transplantation. 2003;76:798–802.
9. Brennan DC, Flavin K, Lowell JA, et al. A randomized, double-blinded comparison of Thymoglobulin versus Atgam for induction immunosuppressive therapy in adult renal transplant recipients. Transplantation. 1999;67:1011–1018.
10. Hardinger KL, Schnitzler MA, Miller B, et al. Five-year follow up of thymoglobulin versus ATGAM induction in adult renal transplantation. Transplantation. 2004;78:136–141.
11. Hardinger KL, Rhee S, Buchanan P, et al. A prospective, randomized, double-blinded comparison of thymoglobulin versus Atgam for induction immunosuppressive therapy: 10-year results. Transplantation 2008;86:947–952.
12. Lebranchu Y, Bridoux F, Buchler M, et al. Immunoprophylaxis with basiliximab compared with antithymocyte globulin in renal transplant patients receiving MMF-containing triple therapy. Am J Transplant. 2002;2:48–56.
13. Brennan DC, Daller JA, Lake KD, Cibrik D, Del Castillo D. Rabbit antithymocyte globulin versus basiliximab in renal transplantation. N Engl J Med. 2006;355:1967–1977.
14. Martin ST, Roberts KL, Malek SK, et al. Induction treatment with rabbit antithymocyte globulin versus basiliximab in renal transplant recipients with planned early steroid withdrawal. Pharmacotherapy. 2011;31:566–573.
15. Hanaway MJ, Woodle ES, Mulgaonkar S, et al. Alemtuzumab induction in renal transplantation. N Engl J Med. 2011;364:1909–1919.
16. Citterio F, Scata MC, Romagnoli J, Nanni G, Castagneto M. Results of a three-year prospective study of C2 monitoring in long-term renal transplant recipients receiving cyclosporine microemulsion. Transplantation. 2005;79:802–806.
17. Webster AC, Woodroffe RC, Taylor RS, Chapman JR, Craig JC. Tacrolimus versus ciclosporin as primary immunosuppression for kidney transplant recipients: Meta-analysis and meta-regression of randomised trial data. BMJ. 2005;331:810.
18. Gabardi S, Tran JL, Clarkson MR. Enteric-coated mycophenolate sodium. Ann Pharmacother. 2003;37:1685–1693.
19. Reinke P, Budde K, Hugo C, et al. Reduction of gastrointestinal complications in renal graft recipients after conversion from mycophenolate mofetil to enteric-coated mycophenolate sodium. Transplant Proc. 2011;43:1641–1646.
20. Ponticelli C. The pros and the cons of mTOR inhibitors in kidney transplantation. Expert Rev Clin Immunol. 2014;10(2):295–305.
21. MacDonald AS. A worldwide, phase III, randomized, controlled, safety and efficacy study of a sirolimus/cyclosporine regimen for prevention of acute rejection in recipients of primary mismatched renal allografts. Transplantation. 2001;71:271–280.
22. Joannides R, Monteil C, de Ligny BH, et al. Immunosuppressant regimen based on sirolimus decreases aortic stiffness in renal transplant recipients in comparison to cyclosporine. Am J Transplant. 2011;11:2414–2422.
23. Gabardi S, Baroletti SA. Everolimus: A proliferation signal inhibitor with clinical applications in organ transplantation, oncology, and cardiology. Pharmacotherapy. 2010;30:1044–1056.
24. Woodle ES, First MR, Pirsch J, Shihab F, Gaber AO, Van Veldhuisen P. A prospective, randomized, double-blind, placebo-controlled multicenter trial comparing early (7 day) corticosteroid cessation versus long-term, low-dose corticosteroid therapy. Ann Surg. 2008;248:564–577.
25. Martin ST, Tichy EM, Gabardi S. Belatacept: A novel biologic for maintenance immunosuppression after renal transplantation. Pharmacotherapy. 2011;31:394–407
26. Vincenti F, Charpentier B, Vanrenterghem Y, et al. A phase III study of belatacept-based immunosuppression regimens versus cyclosporine in renal transplant recipients (BENEFIT study). Am J Transplant. 2010;10:535–546.
27. Durrbach A, Pestana JM, Pearson T, et al. A phase III study of belatacept versus cyclosporine in kidney transplants

from extended criteria donors (BENEFIT-EXT study). Am J Transplant. 2010;10:547–557.
28. Webster AC, Pankhurst T, Rinaldi F, Chapman JR, Craig JC. Monoclonal and polyclonal antibody therapy for treating acute rejection in kidney transplant recipients: A systematic review of randomized trial data. Transplantation. 2006;81:953–965.
29. Stegall MD, Gloor J, Winters JL, Moore SB, Degoey S. A comparison of plasmapheresis versus high-dose IVIG desensitization in renal allograft recipients with high levels of donor specific alloantibody. Am J Transplant. 2006;6:346–351.
30. Everly MJ, Everly JJ, Susskind B, et al. Bortezomib provides effective therapy for antibody- and cell-mediated acute rejection. Transplantation. 2008;86:1754–1761.
31. Walsh RC, Brailey P, Girnita A, et al. Early and late acute antibody-mediated rejection differ immunologically and in response to proteasome inhibition. Transplantation. 2011;91:1218–1226.
32. Green M. Introduction: Infections in solid organ transplantation. Am J Transplant. 2013;13 Suppl 4:3–8.
33. Martin SI, Fishman JA. Pneumocystis pneumonia in solid organ transplantation. Am J Transplant. 2013;13 Suppl 4:272–279.
34. Razonable RR, Humar A. Cytomegalovirus in solid organ transplantation. Am J Transplant. 2013;13 Suppl 4:93–106.
35. Gabardi S, Kubiak DW, Chandraker AK, Tullius SG. Invasive fungal infections and antifungal therapies in solid organ transplant recipients. Transpl Int. 2007;20:993–1015.
36. Silveira FP, Kusne S. Candida infections in solid organ transplantation. Am J Transplant. 2013;13 Suppl 4:220–227.
37. Singh N, Husain S. Aspergillosis in solid organ transplantation. Am J Transplant. 2013;13 Suppl 4:228–241.
38. Hirsch HH, Randhawa P. BK polyomavirus in solid organ transplantation. Am J Transplant. 2013;13 Suppl 4:179–188.
39. Danziger-Isakov L, Kumar D. Vaccination in solid organ transplantation. Am J Transplant. 2013;13 Suppl 4:311–317.
40. Dunn BL, Teusink AC, Taber DJ, Hemstreet BA, Uber LA, Weimert NA. Management of hypertension in renal transplant patients: A comprehensive review of nonpharmacologic and pharmacologic treatment strategies. Ann Pharmacother. 2010;44:1259–1270.
41. Riella LV, Gabardi S, Chandraker A. Dyslipidemia and its therapeutic challenges in renal transplantation. Am J Transplant. 2012;12:1975–1982.
42. Kobashigawa JA, Katznelson S, Laks H, et al. Effect of pravastatin on outcomes after cardiac transplantation. N Engl J Med. 1995;333:621–627.
43. Riella LV, Safa K, Yagan J, et al. Long-term outcomes of kidney transplantation across a positive complement-dependent cytotoxicity crossmatch. Transplantation. 2014;97:1247–1252.
44. Rakel A, Karelis AD. New-onset diabetes after transplantation: Risk factors and clinical impact. Diabetes Metab. 2011;37:1–14.
45. Kasiske BL, Snyder JJ, Gilbertson D, Matas AJ. Diabetes mellitus after kidney transplantation in the United States. Am J Transplant. 2003;3:178–185.
46. Asch WS, Bia MJ. Oncologic issues and kidney transplantation: A review of frequency, mortality, and screening. Adv Chronic Kidney Dis. 2014;21:106–113.
47. Schena FP, Pascoe MD, Alberu J, et al. Conversion from calcineurin inhibitors to sirolimus maintenance therapy in renal allograft recipients: 24-month efficacy and safety results from the CONVERT trial. Transplantation. 2009;87:233–242.
48. Gottschalk S, Rooney CM, Heslop HE. Post-transplant lymphoproliferative disorders. Annu Rev Med. 2005;56:29–44.
49. Josephson MA, McKay DB. Women and transplantation: Fertility, sexuality, pregnancy, contraception. Adv Chronic Kidney Dis. 2013;20:433–440.
50. Dew MA, DiMartini AF, De Vito Dabbs A, et al. Rates and risk factors for nonadherence to the medical regimen after adult solid organ transplantation. Transplantation. 2007;83:858–873.

56 Osteoporosis

Beth Bryles Phillips and Princy A. Pathickal

LEARNING OBJECTIVES

Upon completion of the chapter, the reader will be able to:

1. Explain the association between osteoporosis and morbidity and mortality.
2. Identify risk factors that predispose patients to osteoporosis.
3. Describe the pathogenesis of fractures.
4. List the criteria for diagnosis of osteoporosis.
5. Recommend appropriate lifestyle modifications to prevent bone loss.
6. Compare and contrast the effect of available treatment options on reduction of fracture risk.
7. Recommend an appropriate treatment regimen for a patient with osteoporosis and develop a monitoring plan for the selected regimen.
8. Educate patients on osteoporosis and drug treatment, including appropriate use, administration, and adverse effects.

INTRODUCTION

Osteoporosis is a common and often silent disorder causing significant morbidity and mortality and reduced quality of life. It is characterized by low bone density and loss of strength in bone tissue resulting in an increased risk and rate of bone fracture. Osteoporosis is responsible for more than 2 million fractures in the United States annually. Almost 10 million Americans have osteoporosis, and an additional 43 million are classified as having low bone density.[1,2] The cost of care is expected to rise to $25.3 billion by 2025. It is estimated that postmenopausal white women have a 50% lifetime chance of developing an osteoporosis-related fracture, whereas men have a 20% lifetime chance.[1] Common sites of fracture include the spine, hip, and wrist, although almost all sites can be affected.

The fractures associated with osteoporosis have an enormous impact on individual patients, not only causing initial pain, but also chronic pain, loss of mobility, depression, nursing home placement, and death. Patients with vertebral fractures may also experience height loss, kyphosis, and decreased mobility due to limitations in bending and reaching. These patients are also at greater risk of having a future vertebral fracture. Multiple vertebral fractures may lead to restrictive lung disease and altered abdominal anatomy, while patients with hip fractures have added risks associated with surgical intervention to repair the fracture. More than 50% of patients never fully recover or regain preinjury independence. Death is common in the year after a hip fracture.[1]

EPIDEMIOLOGY AND ETIOLOGY

Osteoporosis is the most common skeletal disorder, but only one in three patients with osteoporosis are diagnosed, and only one in seven receives treatment.[2] Osteoporosis can be classified as either primary (no known cause) or secondary (caused by drugs or other diseases). Primary osteoporosis is most often found in postmenopausal women and aging men, but it can occur in other age groups as well.[1,2]

The prevalence of osteoporosis varies by age, gender, and race/ethnicity and increases exponentially after age 50.[3] Most hip fractures occur in postmenopausal white women, who also have the highest incidence of fracture when adjusted for age. The frequency of fracture in African American and Hispanic women trail far behind that of Caucasians, although hip fracture-related mortality may be higher.[4] Although both men and women lose bone as they age, postmenopausal women have accelerated bone loss due to loss of estrogen. Men have some protection from osteoporosis due to their larger initial bone mass and size and lack of accelerated bone loss associated with menopause.[5] Secondary causes of osteoporosis, such as hypogonadism, are found more commonly in men with fragility fractures.[5]

PATHOPHYSIOLOGY

The human skeleton contains both cortical and trabecular bone. Cortical bone comprises approximately 80% of the skeleton, and its density and compactness account for much of bone strength. It is generally found on the surfaces of long and flat bones. Trabecular (or cancellous) bone has a sponge-like appearance and is found along the inner surfaces of long bones and throughout the vertebrae, pelvis, and ribs.

Under normal circumstances, the skeleton undergoes a dynamic process of bone remodeling, responding to stress and injury through continuous replacement and repair. This process is completed by the basic multicellular unit, including both osteoblasts and osteoclasts. Osteoclasts are involved

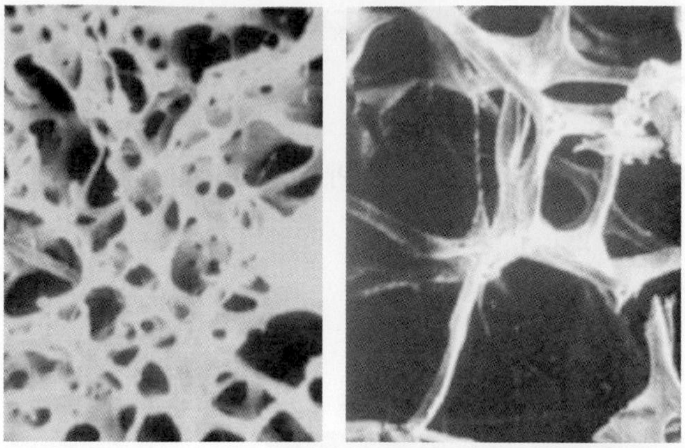

FIGURE 56–1. Normal trabecular bone (left) compared with trabecular bone from a patient with osteoporosis (right). The loss of mass in osteoporosis leaves bones more susceptible to breakage. From Barnett KE, Barman SM, Boitano S. Brooks H. Ganong's Review of Medical Physiology, 24th ed. New York: McGraw-Hill; 2012: Figure 21–11; With permission. http://www.accesspharmacy.com.

with resorption or breakdown of bone and continuously create microscopic cavities in bone tissue. Osteoblasts are involved in bone formation and continuously mineralize new bone in the cavities created by osteoclasts. Until peak bone mass is achieved between the ages of 25 and 35, bone formation exceeds bone resorption for an overall increase in bone mass. Trabecular bone is more susceptible to bone remodeling, and therefore osteoporotic fractures, in part due to its larger surface area. Figure 56–1 illustrates the difference between normal and osteoporotic bone.

In osteoporosis, an imbalance in bone remodeling occurs. Most commonly, osteoclastic activity is enhanced, resulting in overall bone loss. However, a reduction in osteoblastic activity and bone formation also occurs in certain types of osteoporosis. Due to a decrease in endogenous estrogen, bone remodeling accelerates during menopause, and up to 15% of bone is lost during the first 5 years postmenopause. After this initial decline, bone loss continues to occur at a slower rate of up to 1% per year. The resultant bone loss and change in bone quality predispose patients to low-impact or fragility fractures.

CLINICAL PRESENTATION AND DIAGNOSIS

See accompanying text box for the clinical presentation of osteoporosis.

Clinical Presentation of Osteoporosis

General

Many patients with osteoporosis are asymptomatic unless they experience a fragility fracture.

Symptoms of Fragility Fracture

Pain at the site of the fracture or immobility.

Signs

Height loss (greater than 2 cm), spinal kyphosis ("dowager's hump"), fragility fracture especially of the hip or spine.

Table 56–1

Risk Factors for Osteoporosis and Osteoporotic Fractures[1,2]

Risk Factors for Osteoporosis	Risk Factors for Falling and Fractures
Low bone mineral density[a]	Poor health/frailty
Female sex[a]	Impaired gait or balance
Advanced age[a]	Recent falls
Race/ethnicity[a]	Cognitive impairment
History of previous low trauma (fragility) fracture as an adult[a]	Impaired vision
Osteoporotic fracture in a first-degree relative (especially parental hip fracture[a])	Environmental factors (eg, stairs, throw rugs, pets, poor lighting)
Low body weight or body mass index[a]	
Premature menopause (before 45 years old)[b]	
Secondary osteoporosis[b] (especially rheumatoid arthritis[a])	
Past or present systemic oral glucocorticoid therapy[a]	
Current cigarette smoking[a]	
Alcohol intake of three or more drinks per day[a]	
Low calcium intake	
Low physical activity	
Minimal sun exposure	

[a]Major risk factors used in the World Health Organization (WHO) fracture risk model.

[b]Secondary causes included in the FRAX tool question are type 1 diabetes, osteogenesis imperfecta as an adult, longstanding untreated hyperthyroidism, hypogonadism, premature menopause (before 45 years of age), chronic malnutrition, malabsorption, and chronic liver disease.

Adapted from DiPiro JT et al., eds. Pharmacotherapy: A Pathophysiologic Approach. 9th ed. New York: McGraw-Hill; 2014: Table 73–1; With permission.

KEY CONCEPT *The National Osteoporosis Foundation (NOF) recommends evaluating all postmenopausal women and men older than 50 years for osteoporosis risk and need for further diagnostic assessment.* Many risk factors for osteoporosis and osteoporotic fractures are predictors of low bone mineral density (BMD), such as age and ethnicity (Table 56–1). The risk for osteoporosis generally increases as the number of risk factors increases, and the risk of fractures increases as BMD decreases. However, the threshold at which individual patients develop a fracture varies, and other factors, such as fall risk, may play a role in fracture susceptibility. For this reason, fall history and evaluation of risk factors for falling should also be included in the initial evaluation. Because osteoporosis is commonly caused by secondary factors (Table 56–2), medical history, medication history, and laboratory values should be evaluated to determine if further work-up is needed.

Diagnostic Assessment

The diagnostic assessment for osteoporosis may include an assessment of BMD, vertebral imaging, laboratory work-up, and other factors for secondary causes of osteoporosis, and

Table 56–2[1,2]

Medical Conditions and Drugs Associated with Osteoporosis or Low Bone Mass

Medical Conditions	Drugs
Alcoholism	Anticoagulants (heparin, warfarin)
Chronic kidney disease	Anticonvulsants (phenytoin, phenobarbital)
Chronic obstructive pulmonary disease	Aromatase inhibitors (anastrozole, exemestane, letrozole)
Cushing syndrome	Cytotoxic drugs (eg, methotrexate, cisplatin)
Cystic fibrosis	Glucocorticoids (5 mg or more of prednisone daily or equivalent for at least 3 months)
Diabetes mellitus	Gonadotropin-releasing hormone analogs (leuprolide acetate, nafarelin, goserelin)
Eating disorders	Immunosuppressants (eg, tacrolimus)
GI disorders (eg, gastrectomy, malabsorption syndromes)	Lithium
Hematologic disorders (eg, hemophilia)	Medroxyprogesterone acetate
Hyperparathyroidism	Proton pump inhibitors
Hyperthyroidism	Selective serotonin reuptake inhibitors
Hypogonadal states	Thiazolidinediones
Organ transplantation	Thyroid supplements (due to over-replacement)
Skeletal cancer (eg, myeloma)	Total parenteral nutrition
Vitamin D deficiency	

biochemical markers of bone turnover. KEY CONCEPT *Osteoporosis may be diagnosed by low bone density as determined by BMD or established history of low-trauma hip or vertebral fracture in adulthood.*[1]

▶ *Measurement of Bone Mineral Density*

Osteoporosis is characterized by weakened bone tissue, and BMD is the best measure of bone strength, representing approximately 70% of bone strength.[6] Low BMD is associated with an increased risk of fractures. BMD can be measured at various sites throughout the skeletal system and by various methods. Dual-energy x-ray absorptiometry (DXA) can be used to measure central (hip and/or spine) and peripheral (heel, forearm, or hand) sites. Quantitative ultrasound, peripheral quantitative computed tomography, radiographic absorptiometry, and single-energy x-ray absorptiometry are used to measure peripheral sites.

The World Health Organization (WHO) recommends a standardized approach to measuring BMD for diagnosis of osteoporosis using central measurement of BMD by DXA.[2] Preferred sites for central measurement include the total hip, femoral neck, and lumbar spine. Some instruments used for peripheral bone densitometry are portable, allowing bone density to be measured in pharmacies and health-fair screening booths. In addition to accessibility, peripheral measurement of BMD is generally less expensive than central DXA, making it an attractive option for many patients. Peripheral BMD testing is useful in identifying patients who are candidates for central DXA and who are at increased risk of fracture, but it should not be used for diagnosis.

Once the BMD report is available, *T*-scores and *Z*-scores are used to interpret the data. The *T*-score is the number of standard deviations from the mean BMD in healthy, young, white women. Osteoporosis is defined as a *T*-score at least −2.5

Table 56–3

World Health Organization (WHO) Definition of Osteoporosis

Skeletal Disorder	*T*-Score[a]
Normal	−1 or greater
Osteopenia	Less than −1 to −2.5 or greater
Osteoporosis	Less than −2.5

[a]*T*-score is the number of standard deviations above or below the mean bone mineral density in young adults.

standard deviations below the mean BMD in young adults (Table 56–3). **Osteopenia**, or low bone mass that may eventually lead to osteoporosis, is defined as a *T*-score between −2.5 and −1.0. The *Z*-score, defined as the number of standard deviations from the mean BMD of age- and sex-matched controls, is similar to the *T*-score but is corrected for both age and sex of the patient. *Z*-scores may be more clinically relevant in evaluating BMD in premenopausal women, men younger than the age of 50, and patients who may have secondary causes for low BMD.

▶ *Screening and Risk Factor Assessment*

The NOF recommends BMD measurements in the following groups: women age 65 and older, men age 70 and older, perimenopausal women and men age 50 to 69 with risk factors, anyone with a fracture after age 50, and adults with a secondary cause for osteoporosis.[1]

FRAX (see *www.shef.ac.uk/FRAX*) is an additional tool developed by the WHO to evaluate an individual's 10-year probability of developing hip and major osteoporotic fractures based on femoral neck BMD *T*-score, age, and other risk factors.[1] Its intended use is for men and women older than 40 years. The FRAX tool has not been validated for patients with previous or current use of pharmacotherapy to treat osteoporosis. Although the *T*-score is helpful in calculating risk of fracture with FRAX, fracture risk may be calculated without it.

▶ *Vertebral Imaging*

Vertebral fractures cause significant morbidity and mortality among patients with osteoporosis. They are often clinically silent, widespread, frequently recur, and commonly go undiagnosed. For these reasons, vertebral imaging is recommended in high-risk patients: central *T*-score less than −1.0 in women age 70 and older and men age 80 and older; central *T*-score less than −1.5 in women age 65 to 69 or men age 70 to 79; and postmenopausal women and men age 50 and older who have had a fragility fracture in adulthood, height loss of 4 or more centimeters from adulthood, prospective height loss of 2 or more centimeters, or long-term glucocorticoid therapy.[1] Patients may receive vertebral imaging through traditional x-ray or lateral vertebral fracture assessment available on some DXA machines.

▶ *Laboratory Evaluation*

Laboratory assessment has little value in diagnosing osteoporosis but can be beneficial in identifying or excluding secondary causes of bone loss, or predicting patients who may be at risk for more rapid bone loss or fractures. Screening laboratory tests for the most common causes of secondary osteoporosis include complete blood cell count, serum chemistries (electrolytes with

Patient Encounter, Part 1: Patient History

HPI: A frail 71-year-old white man presents to the clinic for follow-up. He reports occasional forgetfulness. His erectile dysfunction, poor libido, and fatigue have improved since starting testosterone replacement therapy. He has no complaints with his current medication regimen for COPD. He takes calcium carbonate (Tums) approximately once a week for heartburn after eating spicy meals. He usually spends his day inside the house watching television from his recliner. He states that milk upsets his stomach, so he usually drinks black coffee or diet soda, occasionally fruit juice.

PMH: COPD, DM type 2, HTN, hyperlipidemia, GERD, hypogonadism, lactose intolerance

FH: Father died at age 76 with Alzheimer disease; mother died at age 92 with history of breast cancer and osteoporotic fracture of the hip; sister alive and well at age 69

SH: Retired construction worker; drinks four beers per day; smoked two packs a day for 40 years, now two cigars daily

Meds: Albuterol inhaler two puffs as needed, metformin 500 mg twice daily; lisinopril 10 mg daily; atorvastatin 40 mg daily, omeprazole 20 mg daily; calcium carbonate (Tums) 500 mg as needed; testosterone cypionate 200 mg IM every 2 weeks; tiotropium 18 mcg daily

Do any symptoms suggest the presence of osteoporosis?

What risk factors for osteoporosis does this patient have as defined by the World Health Organization?

What diseases or medications could contribute to osteoporosis in this patient?

What are the recommended daily intakes for calcium and vitamin D?

How could he incorporate more calcium into his diet?

Table 56–4
Calcium-Rich Foods[a]

1 cup[b] skim milk
1 cup soy milk (calcium-fortified)
1 cup yogurt
1½ oz[c] cheddar cheese
1½ oz jack cheese
1½ oz Swiss cheese
1½ oz part-skim mozzarella
4 tablespoonfuls[d] grated Parmesan cheese
8 oz tofu
1 cup greens (collards, kale)
2 cups broccoli
4 oz almonds
2 cups low-fat cottage cheese
3 oz sardines with bones
5 oz canned salmon
1 cup orange juice (calcium-fortified)

[a]Foods containing approximately 300 mg of elemental calcium.
[b]One cup is equivalent to approximately 240 mL.
[c]One ounce (1 oz) is equivalent to approximately 28 g.
[d]One tablespoon is equivalent to approximately 15 mL.

calcium, phosphorus and liver enzymes), vitamin D, and urinalysis. Biochemical markers of bone turnover such as pyridinoline, deoxypyridinoline, N-telopeptides, and C-telopeptides are not intended for widespread clinical use due to variability and limited clinical data but may be beneficial in some patients to monitor response to therapy, medication adherence, or drug absorption.[2]

TREATMENT

Desired Outcomes

KEY CONCEPT *Treatment goals for osteoporosis include: (a) preventing fractures and their complications; (b) maintaining or increasing BMD; (c) preventing secondary causes of bone loss; and (d) reducing morbidity and mortality associated with osteoporosis.* Strategies to prevent fractures include maximizing peak bone mass, reducing bone loss, and using precautions to prevent falls leading to fragility fractures.

Nonpharmacologic Therapy

▸ *Modification of Risk Factors*

Some osteoporosis risk factors (see Tables 56–1 and 56–2) are nonmodifiable, including family history, age, ethnicity, gender, and concomitant disease states. However, certain risk factors for bone loss may be minimized by early intervention, including smoking, low calcium intake, poor nutrition, inactivity, heavy alcohol use, and vitamin D deficiency. To avoid certain risk factors and maximize peak bone mass, efforts must be directed toward osteoporosis prevention at an early age.

▸ *Nutrition*

A healthy diet is essential to ensure sufficient nutrient intake and appropriate weight maintenance. Dietary calcium intake is important for achieving peak bone mass and maintaining bone density. Good dietary sources of calcium include dairy products, fortified juice, cruciferous vegetables (eg, broccoli, kale), salmon, and sardines (Table 56–4). Dietary intake generally provides 600 to 700 mg/day of calcium for men and women 50 and older. Supplementation to achieve recommended intake not attained by diet alone is important for primary prevention, as well as for those with a diagnosis of osteoporosis.

Adequate dietary intake of vitamin D is essential for calcium absorption. The most common source of vitamin D comes from exposure to sunlight. Ultraviolet rays from the sun promote synthesis of vitamin D_3 (cholecalciferol) in the skin, generally occurring within 15 minutes of direct sunlight exposure to exposed skin without sunscreen. However, during the winter months, patients living in northern latitudes are not able to obtain the type of exposure that results in vitamin D synthesis.[2] It is recommended that individuals receive twice weekly sun exposure to ensure optimal synthesis. Vitamin D may also be found in some dietary sources, including fortified milk, egg yolks, salt-water fish, and liver.

▸ *Exercise*

Exercise can help prevent fragility fractures. Weight-bearing exercise such as walking, jogging, dancing, and climbing stairs can help build and maintain bone strength. Muscle-strengthening or resistance exercises can help improve and maintain strength, agility, and balance, which can reduce falls.[1] It is important to develop and maintain a lifelong routine of weight-bearing and resistance exercise, because the benefits on bone can be lost after cessation of the exercise program.[1]

▶ *Falls Prevention*

Another crucial step in avoiding fragility fractures is prevention of falls. Patients with frailty, poor vision, hearing loss, or those taking medications affecting balance are at higher risk for falling and subsequent fragility fractures.[1,2]

A number of medications have been associated with an increased risk of falling, including drugs affecting mental status such as antipsychotics, benzodiazepines, tricyclic antidepressants, sedative/hypnotics, anticholinergics, and corticosteroids. Some cardiovascular and antihypertensive drugs can also contribute to falls, especially those causing orthostatic hypotension.[1] Efforts to decrease the risk of falling include balance training, muscle strengthening, removal of hazards in the home, installation of fall reduction measures such as handrails, and discontinuation of predisposing medications.[1,2]

Pharmacologic Treatment (Figure 56–2)

KEY CONCEPT *The NOF recommends that all men and women older than 50 years be considered for pharmacologic treatment if they meet any of the following criteria: (a) history of hip or vertebral fracture, (b) T-score −2.5 or less at femoral neck or spine, or (c) osteopenia and at least a 3% 10-year probability of hip fracture or at least a 20% 10-year probability of major osteoporosis-related fracture as determined by FRAX.*[1]

▶ *Calcium and Vitamin D*

KEY CONCEPT *Calcium and vitamin D supplements to meet requirements should be added to all drug therapy regimens for osteoporosis to increase BMD and decrease the risk of hip and vertebral fractures.*

Calcium plays an important role in maximizing peak bone mass and decreasing bone turnover, thereby slowing bone loss. When the calcium supply is insufficient, calcium is taken from bone stores to maintain the serum calcium level. Adequate calcium consumption is essential to prevent this from occurring and may also correct secondary hyperparathyroidism in elderly patients.

The NOF recommends a daily calcium intake of 1000 mg for men between the ages of 50 to 70 and a higher intake of 1200 mg for women older than 51 and men older than 71.[1] When these requirements cannot be achieved by diet alone, appropriate calcium supplementation is recommended. Intakes over 1200 to 1500 mg/day may increase the risk of developing kidney stones,[1] and supplementation greater than 2500 mg/day may lead to hypercalciuria and hypercalcemia. Additionally, excessive calcium supplementation may be associated with an increased risk of cardiovascular events.[7,8]

Calcium supplements are available in a variety of calcium salts and dosage forms. Daily calcium requirements are reported as elemental calcium. However, many product labels list calcium content in the salt form, so the percentage of elemental calcium must be known to calculate the elemental calcium content per tablet. A number of factors, including a single large intake of calcium, can limit calcium absorption, and special consideration must be given to calcium dosing to maximize absorption. Supplement doses should be limited to 500 to 600 mg of elemental calcium per dose, and absorption parameters, elemental calcium content, and adherence should be considered when choosing an appropriate supplement (Table 56–5).

Calcium carbonate should be taken with food to maximize absorption. Elderly patients or patients receiving proton pump inhibitors or H_2-receptor antagonists may have difficulty absorbing calcium supplements due to reduced stomach acidity. Calcium citrate may be better absorbed in these situations because an acid environment is not needed for absorption; it may be taken with or without food.

Common adverse effects of calcium salts include constipation, bloating, cramps, and flatulence. Changing to a different salt form may alleviate symptoms for some patients. Calcium salts may reduce the absorption of iron and some antibiotics, such as tetracycline and fluoroquinolones.

Vitamin D is crucial for calcium absorption and maintenance of bone. The goal is to maintain a serum 25-hydroxyvitamin D level above 30 ng/mL (75 nmol/L).[1] The NOF recommends a daily vitamin D intake of 800 to 1000 IU daily for all adults age 50 and older. However, higher doses may be necessary in some patients to meet this goal.

Vitamin D is available as a single entity, in combination with varying amounts of calcium salts, and in many multivitamin preparations. To avoid hypercalciuria and hypercalcemia, the maximum recommended dose for chronic use in most patients is 4000 IU/day.[9] High-dose ergocalciferol (vitamin D_2) is available by prescription only and is generally reserved for patients with vitamin D deficiency, whereas cholecalciferol (vitamin D_3) is available over the counter.

Patients at risk for vitamin D deficiency include elderly patients with malabsorption syndromes, chronic renal insufficiency, other chronic diseases, and those with limited sun exposure.[1] Elderly patients in particular are at increased risk of deficiency due to decreased exposure to sunlight and subsequent decreased vitamin D synthesis in the skin, decreased GI absorption of vitamin D, and reduction in vitamin D_3 synthesis.

Many adults have low vitamin D levels, and vitamin D deficiency is an important secondary cause of osteoporosis.[2,12] Laboratory determination of 25-hydroxyvitamin D levels should occur prior to the start of therapy to determine whether supplementation is adequate or whether treatment of deficiency is needed. The Endocrine Society Vitamin D Deficiency clinical practice guideline recommends treatment with ergocalciferol 50,000 IU once weekly (or cholecalciferol equivalent of 6000 IU daily) for 8 to 12 weeks.[10] After 25-hydroxyvitamin D levels have risen above 30 ng/mL (75 nmol/L), cholecalciferol doses of 1500 to 2000 IU can be used to maintain 25-hydroxyvitamin D levels between 30 and 60 ng/mL (75 and 150 nmol/L).[2,10]

▶ *Bisphosphonates*

KEY CONCEPT *Bisphosphonates are first-line therapy for osteoporosis in both men and women due to established efficacy in preventing hip and vertebral fractures.* They decrease bone resorption by binding to the bone matrix and inhibiting osteoclast activity. They remain in the bone for several years and are released very slowly, thereby increasing BMD. Alendronate, ibandronate, risedronate, and zoledronic acid carry an FDA-approved indication for osteoporosis. All of these agents are approved for use in men and women, with the exception of ibandronate, which is only approved for use in postmenopausal osteoporosis. Ibandronate is generally considered a second-line bisphosphonate due to lack of documented efficacy in nonvertebral fractures in prospective trials.[2,11] Table 56–6 contains comparative dosing and cost information for the bisphosphonates.

Bisphosphonates can increase BMD by up to 5% to 8% in the lumbar spine and up to 3% to 6% in the hip.[12,13] BMD continues

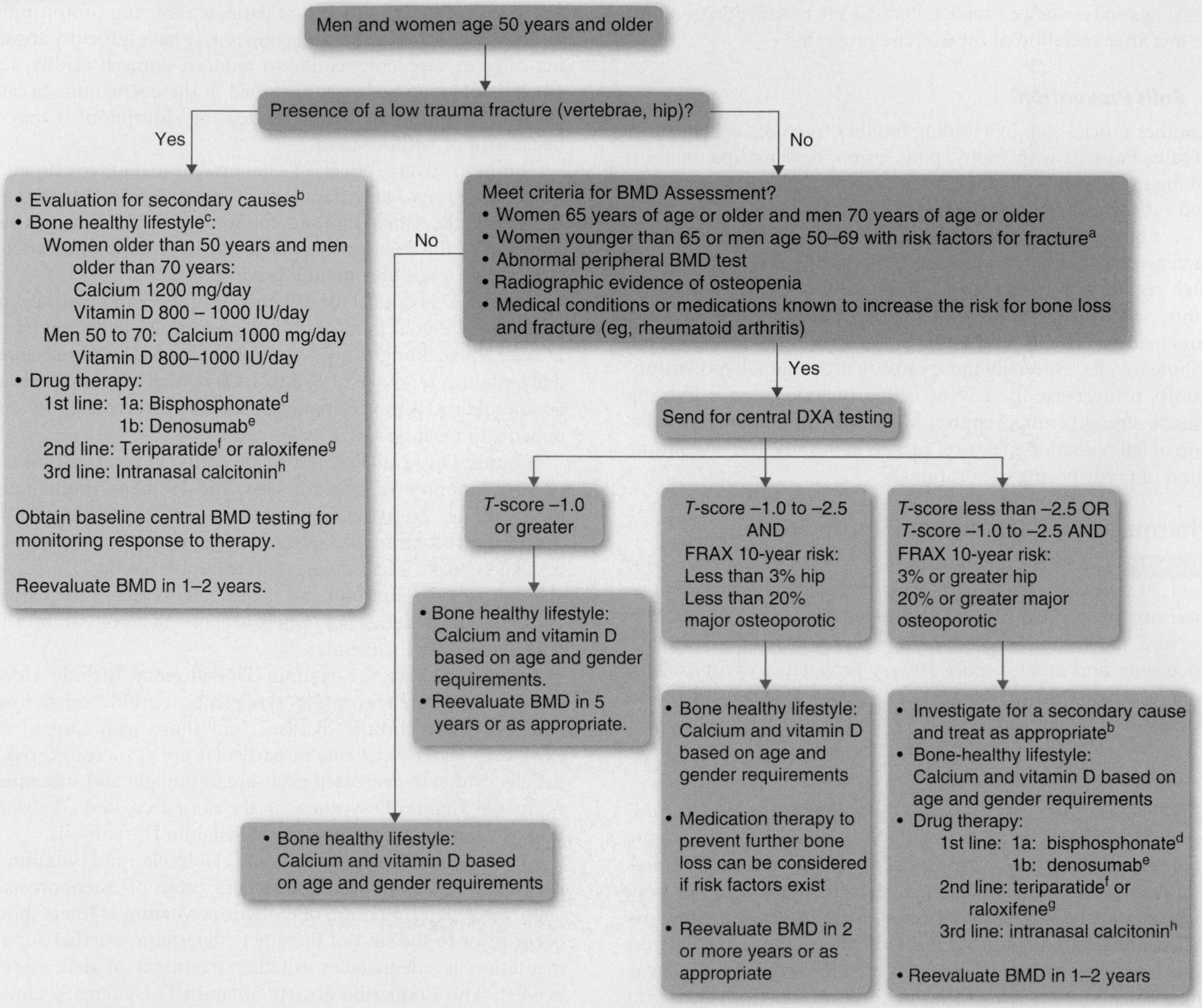

[a]Major risk factors: Current smoker, personal history of fracture as an adult (after age 50 years), history of low-trauma fracture in a first-degree relative, low BMD, low body weight/BMI, excessive alcohol use, chronic glucocorticoid use (3 months or longer).
[b]Secondary causes: Hypogonadism, rheumatoid arthritis, chronic obstructive pulmonary disease, systemic glucocorticoids.
[c]Bone-healthy lifestyle: Smoking cessation, well-balanced diet, weight-bearing/resistance exercise, fall prevention for seniors, and limiting alcohol. Calcium and vitamin D values based on IOM and NOF recommendations for age and gender.
[d]Alendronate, risedronate, and zoledronic acid are first line for men and women. Ibandronate is a second-line bisphosphonate and not FDA approved for use in men. IV bisphosphonates are generally an option if patient cannot tolerate oral bisphosphonates or has significant adherence problems.
[e]Denosumab may be used as a first-line agent per AACE 2010 guidelines.
[f]Teriparatide is FDA approved for use in men and can be considered a first-line option with a *T*- score less than −3.5 or if multiple low trauma factures.
[g]Raloxifene may be a good option for women at high risk for breast cancer.
[h]Calcitonin is not FDA approved for use in men.

Men and women age 50 years and older
Presence of a low trauma fracture (vertebrae, hip)?
Yes
No
• Evaluation for secondary causes[b]
• Bone healthy lifestyle[c]:
Women older than 50 years and men older than 70 years:
Calcium 1200 mg/day
Vitamin D 800 – 1000 IU/day
Men 50 to 70: Calcium 1000 mg/day
Vitamin D 800–1000 IU/day
• Drug therapy:
1st line: 1a: Bisphosphonate[d]
1b: Denosumab[e]
2nd line: Teriparatide[f] or raloxifene[g]
3rd line: Intranasal calcitonin[h]
Obtain baseline central BMD testing for monitoring response to therapy.
Reevaluate BMD in 1–2 years.
Meet criteria for BMD Assessment?
• Women 65 years of age or older and men 70 years of age or older
• Women younger than 65 or men age 50–69 with risk factors for fracture[a]
• Abnormal peripheral BMD test
• Radiographic evidence of osteopenia
• Medical conditions or medications known to increase the risk for bone loss and fracture (eg, rheumatoid arthritis)
No
Yes
Send for central DXA testing
T-score −1.0 or greater
T-score −1.0 to −2.5 AND FRAX 10-year risk: Less than 3% hip Less than 20% major osteoporotic
T-score less than −2.5 OR T-score −1.0 to −2.5 AND FRAX 10-year risk: 3% or greater hip 20% or greater major osteoporotic
• Bone healthy lifestyle: Calcium and vitamin D based on age and gender requirements.
• Reevaluate BMD in 5 years or as appropriate.
• Bone healthy lifestyle: Calcium and vitamin D based on age and gender requirements
• Medication therapy to prevent further bone loss can be considered if risk factors exist
• Reevaluate BMD in 2 or more years or as appropriate
• Investigate for a secondary cause and treat as appropriate[b]
• Bone-healthy lifestyle: Calcium and vitamin D based on age and gender requirements
• Drug therapy:
1st line: 1a: bisphosphonate[d]
1b: denosumab[e]
2nd line: teriparatide[f] or raloxifene[g]
3rd line: intranasal calcitonin[h]
• Reevaluate BMD in 1–2 years
• Bone healthy lifestyle: Calcium and vitamin D based on age and gender requirements

FIGURE 56–2. Algorithm for management of osteoporosis in women and in men aged 50 and older. Adapted from DiPiro JT et al., eds. Pharmacotherapy: A Pathophysiologic Approach, 9th ed. New York: McGraw-Hill; 2014: Figure 73–3; With permission. www.accesspharmacy.com.

to increase with long-term bisphosphonate therapy of 7 to 10 years.[14,15] Although increases in BMD have been reported at other sites, most of the clinically significant increases occur in the hip or spine and are an important marker of treatment effects. Bisphosphonate therapy can also prevent vertebral and nonvertebral fractures, decreasing the vertebral fracture risk by as much as 40% to 50% with oral bisphosphonates and up to 70% with zoledronic acid.[1,16] IV zoledronic acid has also shown a 28% decrease in mortality associated with hip fracture.[17]

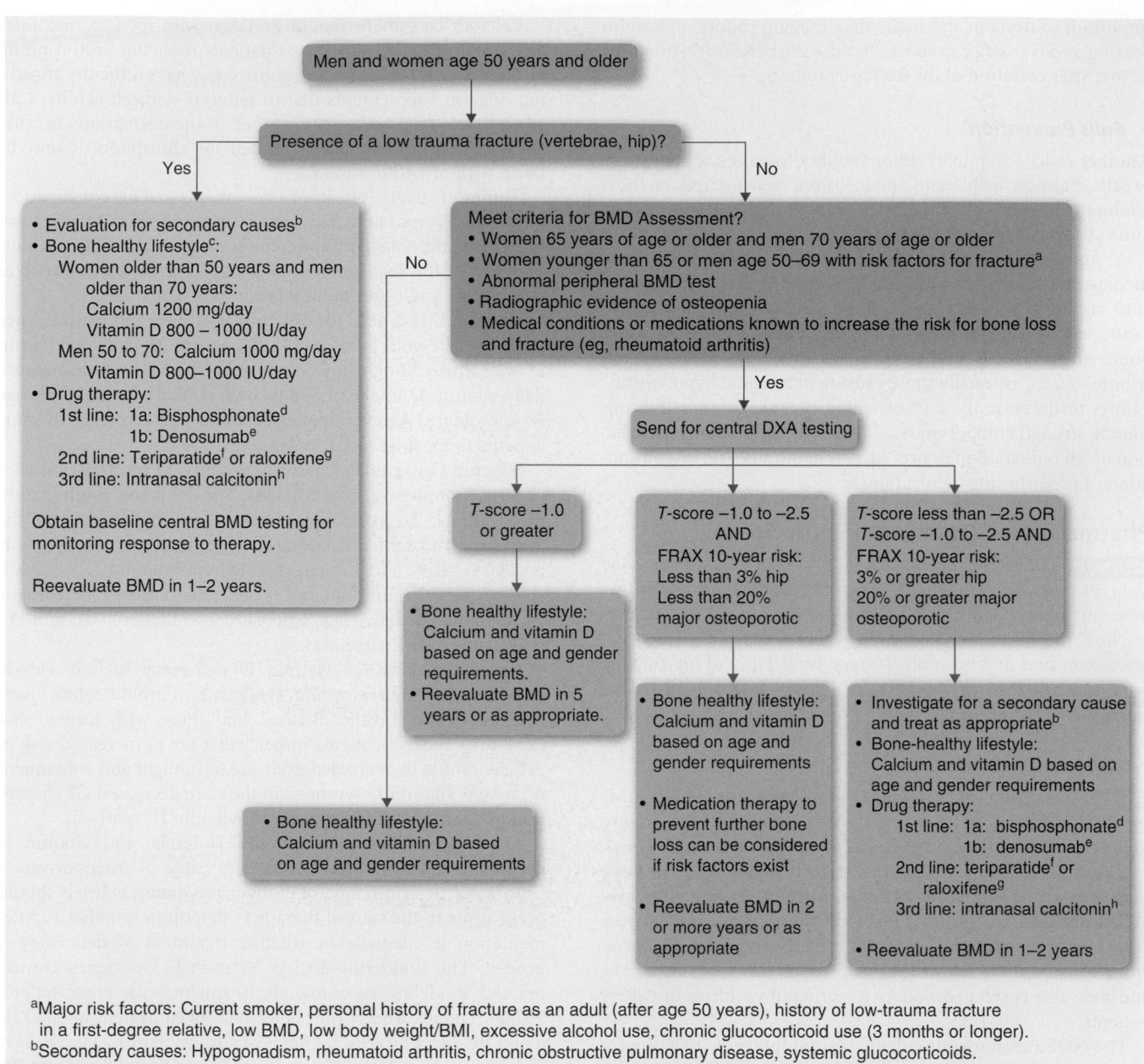

The most notable adverse effects associated with the oral bisphosphonates are GI, ranging from relatively mild nausea, vomiting, and diarrhea to more severe esophageal irritation and

Table 56–5

Calcium and Vitamin D Content of Common Supplements

Product (% Elemental Calcium)	Elemental Calcium per Tablet (mg)	Vitamin D per Tablet (IU)
Calcium Carbonate (40%)		
Tums 500 mg	200	—
Tums E-X 750 mg	300	—
Tums ULTRA 1000 mg	400	—
Os-Cal 500	500	—
Os-Cal 500 + D	500	200
Os-Cal Ultra	600	200
Caltrate 600	600	—
Caltrate 600 + D	600	200
Caltrate 600 + Soy	600	200
One-A-Day Women's Multivitamin	450	400
Rolaids 550 mg	220	—
Viactiv	500	100
Calcium Citrate (24%)		
Citracal	200	—
Citracal 250 mg + D	250	62.5
Citracal + D	315	200
Calcium Phosphate, Tribasic (39%)		
Posture – D	600	125
Calcium Lactate (13%)	85	—
Calcium Gluconate (9%)	60	—

Patient Encounter, Part 2: Physical Examination and Diagnostic Tests

ROS: 4-cm height loss since middle age; (+) back pain

PE:

Gen: Well-developed white man in no acute distress

VS: BP 129/76, P 76, RR 18, T 36.3°C (97.3°F), Wt 64.5 kg (142 lb), Ht 5′11″ (180 cm), BMI 19.8 kg/m^2

Chest: Decreased breath sounds bilaterally, air movement decreased; no crackles or rhonchi

CV: RRR, normal S_1, S_2; no murmurs, rubs, or gallops

Abd: Soft, nontender, nondistended; normal bowel sounds, no hepatosplenomegaly

Ext: No clubbing, cyanosis, or edema

Labs: Na 139 mEq/L (139 mmol/L); K 4.0 mEq/L (4.0 mmol/L); SCr 0.9 mg/dL (80 μmol/L); A1C 6.3% (0.063; 45 mmol/mol hemoglobin); testosterone 408 ng/dL (14.2 nmol/L); 25(OH)D 21 ng/mL (52 nmol/L)

Bone Densitometry by DXA

- BMD of femoral neck: *T*-score = –2.4
- BMD of lumbar spine: *T*-score = –2.1

What additional risk factors and signs of osteoporosis are present in this patient?

Based on the US-adapted WHO algorithm, what is the patient's 10-year probability of a hip fracture and 10-year probability of a major osteoporosis-related fracture?

What are the goals of pharmacologic and nonpharmacologic therapy?

List at least three nonpharmacologic interventions important in his treatment plan.

What factors support pharmacotherapy for osteoporosis in this patient?

What type of supplement(s) would you recommend for this patient to meet his calcium and vitamin D requirements? Why?

esophagitis. Other common adverse reactions include dyspepsia, abdominal pain, nausea, and esophageal reflux. Esophageal ulceration, erosions with bleeding, perforation, stricture, and esophagitis may also occur. Upper GI adverse effects occur in up to 20% of patients and are often related to inappropriate administration. Advanced age, previous upper GI tract disease, and use of nonsteroidal anti-inflammatory drugs also increase the risk for GI adverse events, whereas once-weekly administration of oral bisphosphonates may decrease the risk.

Up to 40% of patients receiving the first dose of IV zoledronic acid may experience acute-phase reactions (flu-like symptoms) that can last for days, such as headache, arthralgia, myalgia, and fever.[1,2,17] Pretreatment with acetaminophen may prevent these symptoms.[2] Patients with moderate to severe renal impairment, severe dehydration, or taking concomitant diuretics or nephrotoxic drugs may be at higher risk of developing acute renal failure with zoledronic acid. Laboratory monitoring, including serum creatinine, alkaline phosphatase, phosphate, magnesium, and calcium, is recommended prior to administration of each zoledronic acid dose.

Long-term administration of bisphosphonates is considered beneficial in patients at high risk for fracture. However, for women who must discontinue bisphosphonate therapy due to intolerance or adverse events, improvements in BMD may be sustained.[15] Although bisphosphonates have demonstrated continued efficacy over time, there are some safety concerns with long-term use. Serious adverse events including **osteonecrosis** of the jaw (ONJ),[18,19] **subtrochanteric** fractures,[18] and nonvertebral atraumatic fractures[19] have been reported. These events may be related to oversuppression of bone turnover causing weakening of bone structure related to inhibition of osteoclastic activity.[20,21] Risk factors for development of ONJ include chemotherapy, radiotherapy, corticosteroids, infection, or preexisting dental disease. Most cases of ONJ occurred in patients receiving high doses of zoledronic acid for cancer-related indications.[18] Patients should complete major dental work prior to initiation of bisphosphonate therapy. The rate of subtrochanteric fractures also increases with more than 5 years of use.[22,23] The NOF recommends reevaluation of therapy after 3 to 5 years of use and to stop treatment in patients who are at moderate risk of fractures.[1] Esophageal cancer has also been reported with long-term therapy, but data are currently inconclusive.[24,25]

Oral bisphosphonates are poorly absorbed (less than 5%). Taking them in the presence of food or calcium supplementation further reduces absorption. After absorption, bisphosphonate uptake to the primary site of action is rapid and sustained. Once attached to bone tissue, bisphosphonates are released very slowly over several years.

Proper drug administration is important for optimal absorption and prevention of adverse effects. Oral bisphosphonates should be taken 30 to 60 minutes prior to the first meal or food in the morning after an overnight fast with 6 to 8 oz

Table 56–6

Prescription Drug Therapy for Osteoporosis

Drug	Product Size	Indication/Usual Dose	Administration
Bisphosphonates			
Alendronate (Fosamax)	5-, 10-, 35-, 70-mg tablets; 70-mg with cholecalciferol 2800 IU; 70-mg with cholecalciferol 5600 IU; 70-mg oral solution	Prevention of PM osteoporosis: 5 mg orally daily or 35 mg orally once weekly Osteoporosis (men and women): 10 mg orally once daily or 70 mg orally once weekly Glucocorticoid-induced osteoporosis: 10 mg once daily Avoid when CrCl < 35 mL/min (0.58 mL/s)	Take after an overnight fast with 6–8 oz (180–240 mL) plain water while sitting or standing upright at least 30 minutes prior to morning meal. Do not lie down for 30 minutes after administration. Do not take with other medications or fluids. Do not chew or suck on the tablet.
Ibandronate (Boniva)	2.5-, 150-mg tablets; 3-mg/3 mL injection	Treatment or prevention of PM osteoporosis: 2.5 mg orally daily or 150 mg orally once monthly; 3 mg IV push over 15–30 seconds every 3 months Avoid when CrCl < 35 mL/min (0.58 mL/s)	Same as alendronate except administer at least 1 hour prior to morning meal and refrain from lying down for 1 hour after administration.
Risedronate (Actonel)	5-, 35-, 75-, 150-mg tablets; 35-mg with 1250-mg calcium carbonate tablets	PM osteoporosis: 5 mg orally daily, 35 mg orally once weekly, 75 mg on 2 consecutive days each month, or 150 mg once monthly Male osteoporosis: 35 mg orally weekly or 150 mg orally monthly Glucocorticoid-induced osteoporosis: 5 mg orally daily Avoid when CrCl < 30 mL/min (0.50 mL/s)	Same as alendronate.
Zoledronic acid (Reclast)	5 mg/100 mL IV infusion	Prevention of PM osteoporosis: 5 mg infused IV over 15 minutes or longer every 24 months Treatment of osteoporosis (men and women), glucocorticoid-induced osteoporosis: 5 mg infused IV over 15 minutes or longer every 12 months Avoid when CrCl < 35 mL/min (0.58 mL/s)	Infuse over at least 15 minutes. May premedicate with acetaminophen.
Monoclonal Antibody			
Denosumab (Prolia)	60 mg/mL SC prefilled syringe	PM or male osteoporosis: 60 mg SC every 6 months	Inject in the upper arm, upper thigh, or abdomen. Keep refrigerated.
Recombinant Human Parathyroid Hormone			
Teriparatide (Forteo)	250 mcg/mL, 2.4-mL prefilled pen	Osteoporosis (men and women), glucocorticoid-induced osteoporosis: 20 mcg SC daily	Inject into thigh or abdominal wall. Keep pen refrigerated.
Estrogen Agonists/Antagonists			
Raloxifene (Evista)	60-mg tablets	PM Osteoporosis: 60 mg daily	May be taken with or without food.
Bazedoxifene/ conjugated estrogens (Duavee)	20 mg/0.45 mg	PM Osteoporosis + menopausal symptoms: one tablet daily	Only for short duration.
Calcitonin			
Calcitonin salmon (Miacalcin)	200 IU/0.9 mL, 3.7-mL nasal spray	PM osteoporosis: Nasal spray: 200 IU daily	Nasal spray: Alternate nostrils on a daily basis.

CrCl, creatinine clearance; PM, postmenopausal; SC, subcutaneously.

(about 180–240 mL) of water (or 2 oz [60 mL] with the oral solution). Administration should be with water only and not combined with other fluids. Patients should remain upright and refrain from lying down for 30 to 60 minutes after administration. The tablets should be swallowed whole without chewing or sucking. Bisphosphonates should not be taken with other medications or dietary supplements. Bisphosphonates are not recommended for use in patients with esophageal abnormalities that may delay transit of the tablet, such as with severe GERD, achalasia, stricture, or Barrett esophagus. They are also not recommended in patients with hypocalcemia or renal insufficiency or failure (creatinine clearance less than 30 to 35 mL/min [0.50–0.58 mL/s]), or in those who are pregnant. For patients who are unable to tolerate or have a contraindication to oral bisphosphonates, IV agents may be used.

▸ *Denosumab*

Denosumab is the first human monoclonal antibody FDA approved for treatment of postmenopausal osteoporosis. It is first-line therapy and should be considered in patients who are unable to tolerate bisphosphonates due to GI contraindications or side effects and for patients with malabsorption or adherence issues.[2] Denosumab reduces nuclear factor-kappa B ligand (RANKL) action, which leads to selective inhibition of osteoclast formation, function, and survival. In contrast to bisphosphonates, the antiresorptive effects of denosumab are reversible.

Denosumab has been shown to increase BMD in the hip and spine by up to 6% and 9%, respectively; and decrease hip, vertebral, and nonvertebral fracture risk by up to 40%, 68%, and 20%, respectively.[26] Patients treated with denosumab had greater increases in hip and spine BMD than patients treated with alendronate, although fracture risk was not reported.[27-29] In a long term, open-label study use of denosumab for 6 years resulted in continued increases in BMD up to 15% in the lumbar spine and up to 7% at the hip; a reduction in fracture rates was sustained compared to denosumab use for 3 years.[30]

Common adverse effects include back pain, arthralgias, fatigue, headache, dermatologic reactions, diarrhea, and nausea. Serious adverse reactions, including hypophosphatemia, hypocalcemia, dyspnea, and skin and other infections, can also occur. Patients should seek medical attention if they experience any symptoms of infection. Denosumab can worsen hypocalcemia in predisposed patients, such as those with severe kidney disease, and preexisting hypocalcemia should be corrected before initiating therapy. Suppression of bone turnover has been associated with denosumab therapy, and ONJ has also been reported.[2]

Denosumab is part of a Risk Evaluation and Mitigation Strategy (REMS) program, in which the manufacturer is required by the FDA to inform patients and health care providers of the risks associated with its use.[31] Denosumab is administered as a subcutaneous injection once every 6 months and should be stored in the refrigerator until administration. Once at room temperature, the vial or prefilled syringe must be used within 14 days. Prescribing information recommends administration of 1000 mg of calcium and at least 400 IU of vitamin D once daily.

▸ *Teriparatide*

Teriparatide, recombinant human parathyroid hormone (1–34), is the first anabolic agent approved by the FDA for treatment of postmenopausal and male osteoporosis. It is generally reserved for patients with very high fracture risk or those in whom other therapies have been ineffective.[2] This agent differs from antiresorptive therapies in that it stimulates osteoblastic activity to form new bone. It is administered as a daily subcutaneous injection. Teriparatide increases BMD in the spine and hip by 9% and 3%, respectively; and reduces fracture risk by 65% and 53% in vertebral and nonvertebral fractures, respectively.[32] Significant reductions in hip fracture have not been demonstrated.

Common adverse effects include nausea, headache, leg cramps, dizziness, injection site discomfort, and hypercalcemia. Orthostatic hypotension may also occur; patients should be seated after the first several doses until drug response is predictable. Teriparatide should not be used in patients with preexisting hypercalcemia. Observations of osteosarcoma in animal studies led to the inclusion of a "black box warning" in the product labeling, but no cases have been reported in humans. Patient-related concerns regarding the use of teriparatide include cost of therapy and need for daily subcutaneous injections. The labeling recommends treatment for a maximum of 2 years because it has not been studied for longer periods.

▸ *Selective Estrogen Receptor Modulators (SERMs)*

Raloxifene is an SERM indicated for prevention and treatment of osteoporosis. It is recommended as alternative therapy after bisphosphonates, denosumab, or teriparatide.[2] It has estrogen-like activity on bones and cholesterol metabolism and estrogen antagonist activity in breast and endometrium. It reduces bone resorption and decreases overall bone turnover.

Raloxifene has been shown to increase BMD in the vertebra (2%–3%) and hip (1%–2%), and reduce vertebral fracture rates by as much as 55%.[33] Significant decreases in nonvertebral fractures have not been demonstrated.[2] Raloxifene has been shown to decrease the incidence of breast cancer in high-risk women. It also decreases total and low-density lipoprotein (LDL) cholesterol, which generated initial enthusiasm for additional cardiovascular benefits. However, mixed results have been seen on cardiovascular disease, stroke, and noncardiovascular mortality.[34,35]

Adverse effects of raloxifene include hot flushes, leg cramps, and increased risk of venous thromboembolism.[34] A previous history of venous thromboembolism is a contraindication to therapy. Hot flushes are very common and may be intolerable in postmenopausal women who are already predisposed to experiencing them. Raloxifene is pregnancy category X and is contraindicated in women who are pregnant or may become pregnant, and in nursing mothers.

Bazedoxifene, a third-generation estrogen agonist/antagonist, has similar effects to raloxifene. At the time of this writing, it was marketed only for short-term use as a combination product with conjugated estrogens (Duavee) for treatment of moderate to severe vasomotor symptoms associated with menopause and for prevention of postmenopausal osteoporosis.[1] A single ingredient product, bazedoxifene acetate (Viviant), was investigational at the time of this writing.

▸ *Calcitonin*

Calcitonin is a naturally occurring mammalian hormone that plays a major role in regulating calcium levels. It inhibits bone resorption by binding to osteoclast receptors. Calcitonin is considered a last-line agent for the treatment of osteoporosis.[2] Calcitonin produces a modest increase in BMD at the spine of 1% to 3% and reduces vertebral fracture risk by up to 30%.[39] However, no benefit has been demonstrated in reducing nonvertebral fractures.[2] Calcitonin was previously thought to provide analgesic effects in women with back pain from vertebral fractures, but recent practice trends favor managing fracture risk and pain separately.

Although salmon calcitonin is approved and available in injectable and intranasal formulations, only the intranasal formulation has documented benefit in clinical trials for management of osteoporosis. Adverse effects associated with the intranasal formulation include rhinitis, nasal irritation, and dryness. Hypersensitivity can develop with either formulation and should be considered before administering to patients with suspected risk.[2]

▸ *Hormone Therapy*

Estrogen, either alone or in combination with a progestin as hormone replacement therapy (HRT), has a long history as an effective treatment of osteoporosis. The Women's Health Initiative (WHI) trial found a 34% reduction in both vertebral and hip fractures and a 23% reduction in other fractures in postmenopausal women receiving conjugated estrogens and medroxyprogesterone.[37] However, significant risks associated with long-term HRT, including breast cancer and venous thromboembolism, have limited its use in osteoporosis.[37,38]

► *Combination and Sequential Therapy*

Interest in combination therapy with two or more osteoporosis drugs is based on the idea that using agents with differing mechanisms would result in greater increases in BMD and reductions in fracture rates. Combination therapies with two antiresorptive agents or an anabolic agent coupled with an antiresorptive agent have shown modest benefit on BMD and markers of bone turnover. Data on fracture reduction are lacking.[1,39,40] Interest in sequential therapy (anabolic agent followed by antiresorptive therapy) stems from the limited duration (2 years) of teriparatide use and the rapid decline in beneficial effects on bone once teriparatide is discontinued.[2] Due to high cost and lack of long-term safety and efficacy data, the AACE does not recommend combination antiresorptive therapy for treating osteoporosis.[2] The NOF prefers sequential therapy over combination therapy but acknowledges that combination antiresorptive and anabolic therapies could be considered for patients with very severe osteoporosis.[1]

► *Investigational Agents*

Several anabolic and antiresorptive therapies are under investigation for treatment of osteoporosis. The most promising antiresorptive therapy may be odanacatib, a selective enzyme inhibitor of cathepsin-K, which prevents enzymatic bone degradation in mature osteoclasts.[41] Anabolic therapies currently under investigation include calcilytic drugs and Wnt pathway modulators.[41-43] Calcilytic drugs increase bone formation by imitating hypocalcemia and cause parathyroid hormone secretion.[42] Wnt signaling pathway modulators promote osteoblastic bone formation. Romosozumab, a monoclonal antisclerostin antibody, binds to sclerostin, a Wnt antagonist, to increase bone formation. These agents are currently in phase 1 and 2 trials.[42,44] Other investigational therapies, strontium ranelate, PTH (1–84), and tibolone, are available outside the United States.[42]

Patient Encounter, Part 3: Development of a Treatment Plan

Considering all of the information presented, develop a treatment plan for this patient. Include the following information:

Recommendations for patient-specific drug therapy including dose and frequency.

Patient education about the chosen regimen, including administration directions.

Monitoring plan for efficacy and adverse effects.

Consideration of alternate therapies if the initial therapy fails or is intolerable.

Treatment of Special Populations

► *Glucocorticoid-Induced Osteoporosis*

Glucocorticoids play a significant role in bone remodeling. Exogenous glucocorticoid administration increases bone resorption, inhibits bone formation, and changes bone quality. Glucocorticoids (eg, prednisone, hydrocortisone, methylprednisolone, and dexamethasone) promote bone resorption through reduced

Patient Care Process

Patient Assessment:

- Assess risk factors for osteoporosis and presence of secondary causes of osteoporosis.
- Assess nonpharmacologic interventions for preventing osteoporotic fractures, including nutrition and weight-bearing and muscle-strengthening exercise regimens. What is the patient's fall risk?
- Determine average calcium intake from diet (see Table 56–4) and supplements (see Table 56–5) and evaluate the patient's sources of vitamin D. Based on age, gender and laboratory values, is the patient receiving appropriate calcium and vitamin D supplementation?
- Test bone densitometry in patients at risk for having low bone mass or bone loss. If *T*-score is between −1.0 and −2.5, use FRAX to estimate fracture risk.

Therapy Evaluation:

- Perform a thorough medication history, including prescription, over-the-counter, and alternative therapies. Does the patient take any calcium and vitamin D supplements?
- If drug therapy is indicated, assess the patient for contraindications.
- If the patient is already receiving pharmacotherapy, assess efficacy, safety, and patient adherence. How long has the patient been on each agent? Was the patient previously trialed with other agents?
- Determine what options are available for the patient. Does the patient have prescription coverage? What agents are recommended on the formulary?

Care Plan Development:

- Select therapy (including agent and dose) likely to be safe and effective for the patient (see Table 56–6).
- Educate the patient on drug therapy selected, including drug name, dose, route and method of administration, common or serious adverse reactions, adherence, and monitoring.
- Educate the patient about nonpharmacologic measures to prevent osteoporotic fractures.
- Discuss therapeutic goals and expectations (eg, changes in individual *T*-scores may not necessarily correlate with benefit in fracture risk reduction).

Follow-Up Evaluation:

- Annually review the need for continued medication. Assess appropriate drug administration, efficacy, adverse effects, and nonpharmacologic measures to prevent fractures.

calcium absorption from the GI tract and increased renal calcium excretion. Bone formation is reduced through inhibition of osteoblasts and decreased estrogen and testosterone production.

Patients receiving long-term glucocorticoids are at increased risk of fracture, which is greater with higher doses and longer-term therapy. Most bone mass is lost during the initial 6 to 12 months of therapy but it continues to decline thereafter.[45] Due to the risk of bone loss and fractures, therapy is recommended for patients receiving long-term supraphysiologic doses of glucocorticoids.[46]

In addition to nonpharmacologic measures, the American College of Rheumatology (ACR) has specific recommendations for preventing and treating patients receiving glucocorticoids.[46] Recommendations for optimal calcium and vitamin D intake are higher and include 1200 to 1500 mg daily of elemental calcium and 800 to 1000 IU daily of vitamin D, or higher as needed to maintain adequate 25(OH)D levels, for all adults receiving glucocorticoids.

KEY CONCEPT *The ACR recommends bisphosphonate therapy with alendronate or risedronate for all patients who are starting treatment with glucocorticoids (prednisone 5 mg or more daily or equivalent) that will continue for 3 months or longer.* Therapy may also be started in patients with lower glucocorticoid doses or shorter duration based on risk factors for fracture. Zoledronic acid and teriparatide may also be considered for moderate- to high-risk patients. Although not FDA approved, denosumab has been studied in this population and may be considered an alternate therapy for patients nonresponsive to or intolerant of other therapies.[45]

OUTCOME EVALUATION

- Evaluate patients for progression of osteoporosis, including signs and symptoms of new fragility fracture (eg, localized pain), loss of height, and physical deformity (eg, kyphosis). Assess patients on an annual basis or more often if new symptoms present
- Monitor for beneficial effects on bone density. The NOF recommends a follow-up DXA scan every 2 years to monitor the effects of therapy
- Assess patients for adverse effects of therapy:
  - Oral bisphosphonates: Dyspepsia, esophageal reflux, esophageal pain, or burning
  - Injectable zoledronic acid: Influenza-type symptoms related to infusion, ONJ (rare)
  - Denosumab: Arthralgias, dermatologic reactions, and hypocalcemia
  - Teriparatide: Nausea, headache, leg cramps, hypercalcemia
  - Raloxifene: Hot flushes, signs, or symptoms of thromboembolic disease (eg, pain, redness, or swelling in one extremity, chest pain, and shortness of breath)
  - Calcitonin salmon: Nasal irritation or burning

Abbreviations Introduced in This Chapter

AACE	American Association of Clinical Endocrinologists
ACR	American College of Rheumatology
BMD	Bone mineral density
BMI	Body mass index
DXA	Dual-energy x-ray absorptiometry
HRT	Hormone replacement therapy
NOF	National Osteoporosis Foundation
ONJ	Osteonecrosis of the jaw
SERM	Selective estrogen receptor modulator
WHI	Women's Health Initiative

REFERENCES

1. National Osteoporosis Foundation [Internet]. Clinician's Guide to Prevention and Treatment of Osteoporosis. Washington, DC, 2014 [cited 2014 Sept 15]. www.nof.org. Accessed Aug. 24, 2015.
2. AACE Osteoporosis Task Force. American Association of Clinical Endocrinologists medical guidelines for clinical practice for the diagnosis and treatment of postmenopausal osteoporosis. Endocr Pract. 2010;16(Suppl 3):1–37.
3. The North American Menopause Society. Management of osteoporosis in postmenopausal women: 2010 position statement of the North American Menopause Society. Menopause. 2010;17:25–54.
4. Cauley JA. Public health impact of osteoporosis. J Gerontol A Biol Sci Med Sci. 2013;68:1243–1251.
5. Khosla S. Update in male osteoporosis. J Clin Endocrinol Metab. 2010;95:3–10.
6. Ammann P, Rizzoli R. Bone strength and its determinants. Osteoporos Int. 2003;14(suppl 3):S13–S18.
7. Xiao Q Murphy RA, Houston DK, Harris TB, et al. Dietary and supplemental calcium intake and cardiovascular disease mortality: The National Institutes of Health-AARP diet and health study. JAMA Intern Med. 2013;173;639–646.
8. Michaelsson K, Melhus H, Warensjo E, et al. Long term calcium intake and rates of all cause and cardiovascular mortality: Community based prospective longitudinal cohort study. BMJ 2013;346:f228. doi: 10.1136/bmj.f228
9. Institute of Medicine [Internet]. Dietary reference intakes for calcium and vitamin D. http://iom.nationalacademies.org/Activities/Nutrition/SummaryDRIs/DRI-Tables.aspx. Accessed Aug. 24, 2015.
10. Holick MF, Binkley NC, Bischoff-Ferrari HA, et al. Evaluation, treatment, and prevention of vitamin D deficiency: An Endocrine Society clinical practice guideline. J Clin Endocrinol Metab. 2011;96:1911–1930.
11. Demas PD, Recker RR, Chesnut CH, et al. Daily and intermittent oral ibandronate normalize bone turnover and provide significant reduction in vertebral fracture risk: Results from the BONE study. Osteoporos Int. 2004;14:792–798.
12. Liberman UA, Weiss SR, Broll J, et al. Effect of oral alendronate on bone mineral density and the incidence of fractures in postmenopausal osteoporosis. N Engl J Med. 1995;333:1437–1443.
13. Brown JP, Kendler DL, McClung MR, et al. The efficacy and tolerability of risedronate once a week for the treatment of postmenopausal osteoporosis. Calcif Tissue Int. 2002;71: 103–111.
14. Boe HG, Hosking D, Devogelaer JP, et al. Ten years' experience with alendronate for osteoporosis in postmenopausal women. N Engl J Med. 2004;350:1189–1199.
15. Mellström DD, Sörensen OH, Goemaere S, et al. Seven years of treatment with risedronate in women with postmenopausal osteoporosis. Calcif Tissue Int. 2004;75:462–468.
16. Boo DM, Delmas PD, Eastell R, et al. Once-yearly zoledronic acid for treatment of postmenopausal osteoporosis. N Engl J Med. 2007;356:1809–1822.
17. Lyles KW, Colón-Emeric CS, Magaziner JS, et al. Zoledronic acid and clinical fractures and mortality after hip fracture. N Engl J Med. 2007;357:1799–1809.
18. Ruggiero SL, Mehrotra B, Rosenberg TJ, Engroff SL. Osteonecrosis of the jaws associated with the use of bisphosphonates: A review of 63 cases. J Oral Maxillofac Surg. 2004;62:527–534.

19. Rizoli R, Akesson K, Bouxsein M, et al. Subtrochanteric fractures after long-term treatment with bisphosphonates: A European Society on Clinical and Economic Aspects of Osteoporosis and Osteoarthritis, and International Osteoporosis Foundation Working Group Report. Osteoporos Int. 2011;22:373–390.
20. Ot SM. Long term safety of bisphosphonates. J Clin Endocrinol Metab. 2005;90:1897–1899.
21. Ovina CV, Zerwekh JE, Rao DS, et al. Severely suppressed bone turnover: A potential complication of alendronate therapy. J Clin Endocrinol Metab. 2005;90:1294–1301.
22. Par-Wyllie YL, Mamdani MM, Juurlink DN, et al. Bisphosphonate use and the risk of subtrochanteric or femoral shaft fractures in older women. JAMA. 2011;305:783–789.
23. FDA [Internet]. FDA Drug Safety Communication: Ongoing safety review of oral bisphosphonates and atypical subtrochanteric femur fractures [cited 2014 Aug 30]. http://www.fda.gov/Drugs/DrugSafety/PostmarketDrugSafetyInformationforPatientsandProviders/ucm203891.htm. Accessed Aug. 24, 2015.
24. Cardwell CR, Abnet CC, Cantwell MM, Murray LJ. Exposure to oral bisphosphonates and risk of esophageal cancer. JAMA 2010;304:657–663.
25. Green J, Czanner G, Reeves G, et al. Oral bisphosphonates and risk of cancer of oesophagus, stomach, and colorectum: Case-control analysis within a UK primary care cohort. BMJ. 2010;341:c4444.
26. Cummings SR, San Martin J, McClung MR, et al. Denosumab for prevention of fractures in postmenopausal women with osteoporosis. N Engl J Med. 2009;361:756–765.
27. Kendler DL, Roux C, Benhamou CL, et al. Effects of denosumab on bone mineral density and bone turnover in postmenopausal women transitioning from alendronate therapy. J Bone Miner Res. 2010;25:72–81.
28. Brown JP, Prince RL, Deal C, et al. Comparison of the effect of denosumab and alendronate on BMD and biochemical markers of bone turnover in postmenopausal women with low bone mass: a randomized, blinded, phase 3 trial. J Bone Miner Res 2009;24:153–161.
29. Lewiecki EM. Treatment of osteoporosis with denosumab. Maturitas 2010;66:182–186.
30. Bone HG, Chapurlat R, Brandi ML, et al. The effect of three or six years of denosumab exposure in women with postmenopausal osteoporosis: Results from the FREEDOM extension. J Clin Endocrinol Metab. 2013;98:4483–4492.
31. Amgen [Internet]. Prolia (denosumab) Risk Evaluation and Mitigation Strategy. http://www.proliahcp.com/risk-evaluation-mitigation-strategy/. Accessed Aug. 24, 2015.
32. Ner RM, Arnaud CD, Zanchetta JR, et al. Effect of parathyroid hormone (1–34) on fractures and bone mineral density in postmenopausal women with osteoporosis. N Engl J Med. 2001;344:1434–1441.
33. Ettinger B, Black DM, Mitlak BH, et al. Reduction of vertebral fracture risk in postmenopausal women with osteoporosis treated with raloxifene: Results from a 3-year randomized clinical trial. JAMA. 1999;282:637–645.
34. Barrett-Connor E, Mosca L, Collins P, et al. For the Raloxifene Use for The Heart (RUTH) Trial Investigators. Effects of raloxifene on cardiovascular events and breast cancer in postmenopausal women. N Engl J Med. 2006;355:125–137.
35. Grady D, Cauley JA, Stock JL, et al. Effect of raloxifene on all-cause mortality. Am J Med. 2010;123:469:e1–e7.
36. Duggan ST, McKeage K. Bazedoxifene: A review of its use in the treatment of postmenopausal osteoporosis. Drugs. 2011;71:2193–2212.
37. Rossouw JE, Anderson GL, Prentice RL, et al. Risks and benefits of estrogen plus progestin in healthy postmenopausal women: Principal results from the Women's Health Initiative randomized controlled trial. JAMA. 2002;288:321–333.
38. Hulley S, Grady D, Bush T, et al. Randomized trial of estrogen plus progestin for secondary prevention of coronary heart disease in postmenopausal women. JAMA. 1998;280:605–613.
39. Leder BZ, Tsai JN, Uihlein AV, et al. Two years of denosumab and teriparatide administration in postmenopausal women with osteoporosis (The DATA Extension Study): A randomized controlled trial. J Clin Endocrinol Metab. 2014;99:1694–1700.
40. Tsai JN, Uihlein AV, Lee H, et al. Teriparatide and denosumab, alone or combined, in women with postmenopausal osteoporosis: The DATA study randomised trial. Lancet. 2013:382:50–56.
41. Eisman JA, Bone HG, Hosking DJ, et al. Odanacatib in the treatment of postmenopausal women with low bone mineral density: Three-year continued therapy and resolution of effect. J Bone Miner Res. 2011;26:242–251.
42. Rachner TD, Khosla S, Hofbauer LC. Osteoporosis: Now and the future. Lancet. 2011;377:1276–1287.
43. Baron R, Hesse E. Update on bone anabolics in osteoporosis treatment: Rationale, current status, and perspectives. J Clin Endocrinol Metab. 2012:97:322–325.
44. McClung MR, Grauer A, Boonen S, et al. Romosozumab in postmenopausal women with low bone mineral density. N Engl J Med. 2014;370:412–420.
45. Weinstein RS. Glucocorticoid-induced bone disease. N Engl J Med. 2011;365:62–70.
46. Grossman JM, Gordon R, Ranganath VK, et al. American College of Rheumatology 2010 recommendations for the prevention and treatment of glucocorticoid induced osteoporosis. Arthritis Care Res (Hoboken). 2010;62:1515–1526.

57 Rheumatoid Arthritis

Susan P. Bruce

LEARNING OBJECTIVES

Upon completion of the chapter, the reader will be able to:

1. Identify risk factors for developing adult rheumatoid arthritis (RA) or juvenile idiopathic arthritis (JIA).
2. Describe the pathophysiology of RA, with emphasis on the specific immunologic components.
3. Discuss the comorbidities associated with RA.
4. Recognize the typical clinical presentation of RA or JIA.
5. Create treatment goals for a patient with RA or JIA.
6. Compare the available pharmacotherapeutic options, selecting the most appropriate regimen for a given patient.
7. Propose a patient education plan that includes nonpharmacologic and pharmacologic treatment measures.
8. Formulate a monitoring plan to evaluate the safety and efficacy of a therapeutic regimen designed for an individual patient with RA or JIA.

INTRODUCTION

Rheumatoid arthritis (RA) is a complex systemic inflammatory condition manifesting initially as symmetric swollen and tender joints of the hands and/or feet. Some patients may experience mild **articular** disease, whereas others may present with aggressive disease and/or extraarticular manifestations. The systemic inflammation of RA leads to joint destruction, disability, and premature death. Juvenile idiopathic arthritis (JIA) is the most common form of arthritis in children.

EPIDEMIOLOGY AND ETIOLOGY

RA has a prevalence of 0.5% to 1%.[1,2] Patients with RA have a 50% increased risk of premature death and a decreased life expectancy of 3 to 10 years compared with individuals without RA.[3] The underlying causes of increased mortality are unclear. RA arises from an immunologic reaction, perhaps in response to a genetic or infectious antigen. Risk factors associated with the development of RA include the following:

- Female gender (3:1 females to males)
- Increasing age (peak onset 35–50 years of age)
- Current tobacco smoking.[4] Tobacco users are more likely to have extraarticular manifestations and to experience treatment nonresponsiveness. This risk is reduced when a patient has remained tobacco-free for at least 10 years.
- Family history of RA. Genetic studies demonstrate a strong correlation between RA and the presence of major histocompatibility complex class II **human leukocyte antigens** (HLA), specifically HLA-DR1 and HLA-DR4.[5,6] HLA is a molecule associated with the presentation of antigens to T lymphocytes.
- Emerging evidence suggests that stress may influence RA onset and disease activity. It appears that individual major stressful life events do not play a significant role. Instead, chronic presence of minor stressors (daily hassles, work and relationship stress, financial pressures) may affect the immune response and RA disease activity.[7]
- The prevalence of JIA is approximately 1 in 1000 children.[8] There are no known risk factors for JIA.

PATHOPHYSIOLOGY

The characteristics of a **synovium** affected by RA are: (a) the presence of a thickened, inflamed membrane lining called **pannus**; (b) development of new blood vessels; and (c) influx of inflammatory cells in the synovial fluid, predominantly T lymphocytes. The pathogenesis of RA is driven by T lymphocytes, but the initial catalyst causing this response is unknown. Understanding specific components of the immune system and their involvement in the pathogenesis of RA will facilitate understanding of current and emerging treatment options for RA. The components of most significance are T lymphocytes, cytokines, B lymphocytes, and kinases.[5,9]

T Lymphocytes

The development and activation of T lymphocytes are important to maintain protection from infection without causing harm to the host.[5] Activation of mature T lymphocytes requires two signals. The first is the presentation of an antigen by antigen-presenting cells to the T-lymphocyte receptor. Second, a ligand-receptor complex (ie, CD80/CD86) on antigen-presenting cells binds to CD28 receptors on T lymphocytes.

Once a cell successfully passes through both stages, the inflammatory cascade is activated.[5] Activation of T lymphocytes: (a) stimulates the release of macrophages or monocytes, which subsequently causes the release of inflammatory cytokines; (b) activates osteoclasts; (c) activates release of matrix metalloproteinases or enzymes responsible for the degradation of connective tissue; and (d) stimulates B lymphocytes and the production of antibodies.[5,9,10]

Cytokines

Cytokines are proteins secreted by cells that serve as intercellular mediators (Table 57–1). An imbalance of proinflammatory and anti-inflammatory cytokines in the synovium leads to inflammation and joint destruction. Some of the proinflammatory cytokines are interleukin 1 (IL-1), tumor necrosis factor-α (TNF-α), IL-6, and IL-17. These proinflammatory cytokines cause activation of other cytokines and adhesion molecules responsible for recruitment of lymphocytes to the site of inflammation. Anti-inflammatory cytokines and mediators (IL-4, IL-10, and IL-1 receptor antagonist) are present in the synovium, although concentrations are not high enough to overcome the effects of the proinflammatory cytokines.[5,9,10]

B Lymphocytes

In addition to serving as antigen-presenting cells to T lymphocytes, B lymphocytes may produce proinflammatory cytokines and antibodies.[6,9] Antibodies of significance in RA are rheumatoid factors (antibodies reactive with the Fc region of IgG) and anticitrullinated protein antibodies (ACPA).[6] Rheumatoid factors are not present in all patients with RA, but their presence is indicative of disease severity, likelihood of extraarticular manifestations, and increased mortality.[11] ACPA are produced early in the course of disease. High levels of ACPA are indicative of aggressive disease and a greater likelihood of poor outcomes. Monitoring ACPA may be useful to predict the severity of disease and match aggressive treatment appropriately.

Kinases

The role of intracellular signaling is an emerging area of interest. Kinases are enzymes involved in communication or signaling activities within and between cells. Activated kinases lead to cell activation and proliferation. Examples include Janus-associated kinases (JAKs) and spleen tyrosine kinase. Research is ongoing to identify therapeutic targets to interrupt signaling and thereby halt the inflammatory process.[12]

Comorbidities Associated with RA

RA reduces a patient's average life expectancy, but RA alone rarely causes death. Instead, specific comorbidities contribute to premature death independent of safety issues surrounding the use of immunomodulating medications. KEY CONCEPT *The comorbidities with the greatest impact on morbidity and mortality associated with RA are: (a) cardiovascular disease, (b) infections, (c) malignancy, and (d) osteoporosis.*

▸ *Cardiovascular Disease*

More than half of all deaths in RA patients are cardiovascular related.[13] Because a patient with RA experiences inflammation and swelling in joints, it is likely that there is inflammation elsewhere, such as in the blood vessels, termed vasculitis. C-reactive protein (CRP), a nonspecific marker of inflammation, is associated with an increased risk of cardiovascular disease; CRP is elevated in patients with RA. Traditional cardiovascular risk factors alone cannot explain the increased cardiovascular mortality in patients with RA. Increasing evidence suggests that the presence of RA is a cardiovascular risk similar to diabetes. Aggressive management of systemic inflammation and traditional cardiovascular risk factors (eg, blood pressure, cholesterol, tobacco use) may reduce cardiovascular mortality in this population.[14]

▸ *Infections*

RA itself leads to changes in cellular immunity and causes a disproportionate increase in infections.[15] Because medications that alter the immune system increase infection risk, it is difficult to distinguish between an increased risk due to RA and the immunosuppressive therapy. Patients and clinicians must pay close attention to signs and symptoms of infection.[15]

Table 57–1

Cytokines Involved in the Pathogenesis of RA[5,9,10]

Cytokine	Source	Activity
Proinflammatory		
TNF-α	Macrophages, monocytes, B lymphocytes, T lymphocytes, fibroblasts	Induces IL-1, IL-6, IL-8, GM-CSF; stimulates fibroblasts to release adhesion molecules
IL-1	Macrophages, monocytes, endothelial cells, B lymphocytes, activated T lymphocytes	Stimulates fibroblasts and chondrocytes to release matrix metalloproteinases
IL-6	T lymphocytes, monocytes, macrophages, synovial fibroblasts	Activates T lymphocytes, induces acute-phase response, stimulates growth and differentiation of hematopoietic precursor cells; stimulates synovial fibroblasts
IL-17	T lymphocytes in synovium	Synergistic effect with IL-1 and TNF leading to increased production of proinflammatory cytokines
Anti-Inflammatory		
IL-4	CD4+ type 2 helper T lymphocytes	Inhibits activation of type 1 helper T lymphocytes, decreases production of IL-1, TNF-α, IL-6, IL-8
IL-10	Monocytes, macrophages, B lymphocytes, T lymphocytes	Inhibits production of IL-1, TNF-α, and proliferation of T lymphocytes

Table 57–2

Comparison of RA and Osteoarthritis

Characteristic	RA	Osteoarthritis
Speed of onset	Rapid (weeks to months)	Slow (years)
Gender prevalence (women: men)	3:1	1:1
Usual age of onset	Juvenile or adult (35–50 years)	Greater than 50 years
Most common joints affected	Small joints of hands (MCPs, PIPs), feet	Hands (DIPs), large weight-bearing joints (hips, knees)
Joint symptoms	Pain, swelling, warmth, stiffness	Pain, bony enlargement
Presence of inflammation	Local and systemic	None or mild, local
Duration of morning joint stiffness	Usually 60 minutes or longer	Usually less than 30 minutes
Joint pattern	Symmetric	Symmetric or asymmetric
ESR	Elevated	Normal
Synovial fluid	Leukocytosis, slightly cloudy	Mild leukocytosis
Systemic manifestations	Yes	No

DIPs, distal interphalangeal joints; ESR, erythrocyte sedimentation rate; MCPs, metacarpophalangeal joints; PIPs, proximal interphalangeal joints.

▸ *Malignancy*

Cancer is the second most common cause of death in RA patients. There is increased risk of developing lymphoproliferative malignancy (eg, lymphoma, leukemia, multiple myeloma), skin, and lung cancer but decreased risk of developing cancer of the breast and digestive tract.[15,16] The relationship between RA and cancer is not clear. To confound the issue, medications for treating RA are undergoing review to determine whether use independently increases cancer risk. Current evidence suggests that the use of biologic medications does not increase the baseline risk associated with disease alone.

▸ *Osteoporosis*

Osteoporosis associated with RA follows a multifaceted pathogenesis, but the primary mechanism likely is mediated by increased osteoclast activity.[15] The cytokines involved in the inflammatory process directly stimulate osteoclast and inhibit osteoblast activity. Additionally, arthritis medications can lead to increased bone loss. Bone mineral density should be evaluated at baseline and routinely using dual-energy x-ray absorptiometry.

CLINICAL PRESENTATION AND DIAGNOSIS

See the box on next page for the clinical presentation of RA.

Diagnosis

Both osteoarthritis and RA are prevalent in the U.S. population, but they differ in presentation (Table 57–2). Because management of the two conditions differs significantly, early evaluation and diagnosis are essential to maximize an individual patient's care.

In 2010, The American College of Rheumatology (ACR) and European League Against Rheumatism (EULAR) released new classification criteria for RA (Table 57–3).[1] The goal was to identify a subset of patients with undifferentiated synovitis who were at high risk for chronic and erosive disease. The criteria are intended to help identify patients earlier in the course of disease. This will allow researchers to determine whether earlier introduction of medications alters the disease process. The criteria were developed as a tool for research purposes, but they are also helpful to guide clinical diagnosis. Patients with at least one joint with definite clinical synovitis that is not explained by another disease should be tested for RA.

Several clinical features of RA are associated with a worse long-term prognosis. The presence of these poor prognostic features should be considered at the time initial treatment decisions are made; more aggressive treatment may be warranted if these features are present. KEY CONCEPT *The most clinically important features associated with poor long-term outcomes include: (a) functional limitation (defined by use of standard measurement scales such as the Health Assessment Questionnaire [HAQ] score),*

Table 57–3

ACR/EULAR 2010 Classification Criteria for Rheumatoid Arthritis[1]

Criteria	Score
Joint involvement	
1 large joint (hips, knees, ankles, elbows, shoulders)	0
2–10 large joints	1
1–3 small joints (MCPS, PIPs, MTPs, wrists)	2
4–10 small joints	3
More than 10 joints (at least one small joint)	5
Serology (need at least one result for classification)	
Negative RF and negative ACPA	0
Low positive RF or low-positive ACPA	2
High-positive RF or high-positive ACPA	3
Acute-phase reactants (need at least one result for classification)	
Normal CRP and normal ESR	0
Abnormal CRP or abnormal ESR	1
Duration of symptoms	
Less than 6 weeks	0
More than 6 weeks	1
TOTAL:	6 or greater indicates definite RA

ACPA, anticitrullinated protein antibodies; ACR, American College of Rheumatology; CRP, C-reactive protein; ESR, erythrocyte sedimentation rate; EULAR, European League Against Rheumatism; MCPs, metacarpophalangeal joints; MTPs, metatarsophalangeal joints; PIPs, proximal interphalangeal joints; RA, rheumatoid arthritis; RF, rheumatoid factor.

Clinical Presentation of RA

General

- About 60% of patients develop symptoms gradually over several weeks to months.
- Patients may present with systemic findings, joint findings, or both.

Symptoms

- Nonspecific systemic symptoms may include fatigue, weakness, anorexia, and diffuse musculoskeletal pain.
- Patients complain of pain in involved joints and prolonged morning joint stiffness.

Signs

- The metacarpophalangeal (MCP), proximal interphalangeal (PIP), metatarsophalangeal (MTP), and wrist joints are involved frequently.
- Joint involvement is usually symmetric.
- There is often limited joint function.
- Signs of joint inflammation are present (tenderness, warmth, swelling, and erythema).
- Low-grade fever may be present.
- Extraarticular manifestations:
  - *Skin:* Subcutaneous nodules
  - *Ocular:* Keratoconjunctivitis sicca, scleritis
  - *Pulmonary:* Interstitial fibrosis, pulmonary nodules, pleuritis, pleural effusions
  - *Vasculitis:* Ischemic ulcers, skin lesions, leukocytoclastic vasculitis
  - *Neurologic:* Peripheral neuropathy, Felty syndrome
  - *Hematologic:* Anemia, thrombocytosis

Laboratory Tests

- Positive rheumatoid factor (the test is negative in up to 30% of patients)
- Elevated ESR (Westergren ESR: greater than 20 mm/hour in men; greater than 30 mm/hour in women)
- Elevated C-reactive protein (CRP) (greater than 0.7 mg/dL or 7 mg/L)
- Complete blood count: Slight elevation in WBC count with a normal differential; slight anemia; thrombocytosis
- Positive anticitrullinated protein antibodies (ACPA)

Other Diagnostic Tests

- *Synovial fluid analysis:* Straw colored, slightly cloudy, WBC 5–25 × 10^3/mm^3 (5–25 × 10^9/L), no bacterial growth if cultured
- *Joint x-rays:* To establish baseline and evaluate joint damage
- *MRI:* May detect erosions earlier in the course of disease than x-rays but is not required for diagnosis

(b) extraarticular disease, (c) positive rheumatoid factor, (d) positive ACPA, and/or (e) bony erosions by radiography.

▶ *Diagnosis of Juvenile Idiopathic Arthritis*

Diagnostic criteria for JIA include: (a) age less than 16 years at disease onset, (b) arthritis in one or more joints for more than 6 weeks, (c) exclusion of other types of arthritis. JIA can be divided into three main types:

1. *Systemic (4%–17% of cases)*: Occurs equally in girls and boys. There are characteristic fever spikes twice daily (greater than 38.3°C or 101°F) and the presence of a pale, pink, transient rash. The peak onset is between ages 1 and 6 years.
2. *Polyarticular (approximately 40% of cases)*: More likely to affect girls than boys (3:1). Arthritis is present in five or more joints. The disorder resembles adult RA more than the other types of JIA.
3. *Oligoarticular (about 50% of cases)*: More likely to affect girls than boys (5:1). Uveitis is more likely to be present. Arthritis is present in four or fewer joints. The peak onset is between ages 1 and 3 years.

TREATMENT

Desired Outcomes

KEY CONCEPT *The goals of treatment in RA are to: (a) reduce or eliminate pain, (b) protect articular structures, (c) control systemic complications, (d) prevent loss of joint function, and (e) improve or maintain quality of life.* The goals for JIA are the same, with the added goals of maintaining normal growth, development, and activity level.[17,18] It is a common misconception that patients with JIA grow out of the disease. Many children with JIA become adults with JIA. Knowing this, it is essential that early, aggressive treatment is initiated to achieve the goals of therapy.

General Approach to Treatment

The clinician must evaluate patient-specific factors and select appropriate treatment to maximize the care of each patient.

Patient Encounter, Part 1

A 68-year-old woman presents to her rheumatologist with complaints of increased joint swelling in her hands and feet over the last 3 months. She is especially disturbed by daily morning joint stiffness that lasts for 90 minutes on average. She is retired but has a small business as a seamstress. She is falling behind on her business projects because of the daily limitations with her hands. She wishes to improve function in her hands as soon as possible before customers start complaining.

What information is suggestive of RA?

What risk factors does she have for RA?

What additional information do you need before creating a treatment plan for this patient?

What other variables in this scenario may inhibit optimal patient care?

Joint damage accumulates over time; therefore, early diagnosis and early aggressive treatment are necessary to reduce disease progression and prevent joint damage. Aggressive treatment is defined as one or more disease-modifying antirheumatic drugs (DMARDs) at effective doses. Delaying treatment will result in more destructive disease that is very difficult to delay or reverse to preserve joint function.

KEY CONCEPT *It is imperative that the initiation of one or more DMARDs occurs in all patients within the first 3 months of diagnosis to reduce joint erosion.* Depending on disease severity and whether poor prognostic features are present, combination therapy may be initiated at the time of diagnosis or after an adequate trial of a DMARD initiated as monotherapy. If a patient has more aggressive disease, a more aggressive treatment plan may be warranted. The following medication classes are prescribed commonly for treatment of RA: (a) nonsteroidal anti-inflammatory drugs (NSAIDs), (b) glucocorticoids, (c) conventional synthetic DMARDs (csDMARDs), (d) biological originator DMARDs (boDMARDs), and (e) targeted synthetic DMARDs (tsDMARDs).

An emerging drug category is biosimilar DMARDs (bsDMARDs). This category will include biological DMARDs that are a copy of the original biologic compound and demonstrate similar efficacy and safety. boDMARDs are currently in development and not yet available for general use. The nomenclature for DMARDs was proposed by an international leader in rheumatology to distinguish the different types of DMARDs.

Figures 57–1 and 57–2 outline the course of treatment for adult RA according to the ACR 2012 Recommendations.[19] The recommendations are based on the disease activity level, presence or absence of poor prognostic features, and duration of disease activity (early vs established). Figure 57–1 applies to patients who have had RA for less than 6 months. csDMARD monotherapy includes hydroxychloroquine, leflunomide, methotrexate, minocycline, or sulfasalazine. Examples of combination therapy for patients with moderate or high disease activity with evidence of poor prognostic features are methotrexate/hydroxychloroquine, methotrexate/sulfasalazine, or methotrexate/sulfasalazine/hydroxychloroquine.

Figure 57–2 outlines the course of treatment for patients with established RA (disease duration 6 months or longer). boDMARDs are usually considered in patients with established RA following inadequate response to csDMARDs. Figure 57–2 establishes a progression for switching from one agent to another in a patient who experiences an inadequate response or adverse event. Because of treatment expense, boDMARDs should be considered only in patients who have no limitations due to cost or insurance coverage. There is no evidence that the benefits of combination boDMARD therapy outweigh the potential risks, especially the increased risk of infections.

Nonpharmacologic Therapy

All patients should receive education about the nonpharmacologic and pharmacologic measures to help manage RA and JIA. Empowered patients take an active role in care by participating in therapy-related decisions. Certain forms of nonpharmacologic therapy benefit all levels of severity, whereas others (ie, surgery) are reserved for severe cases only.

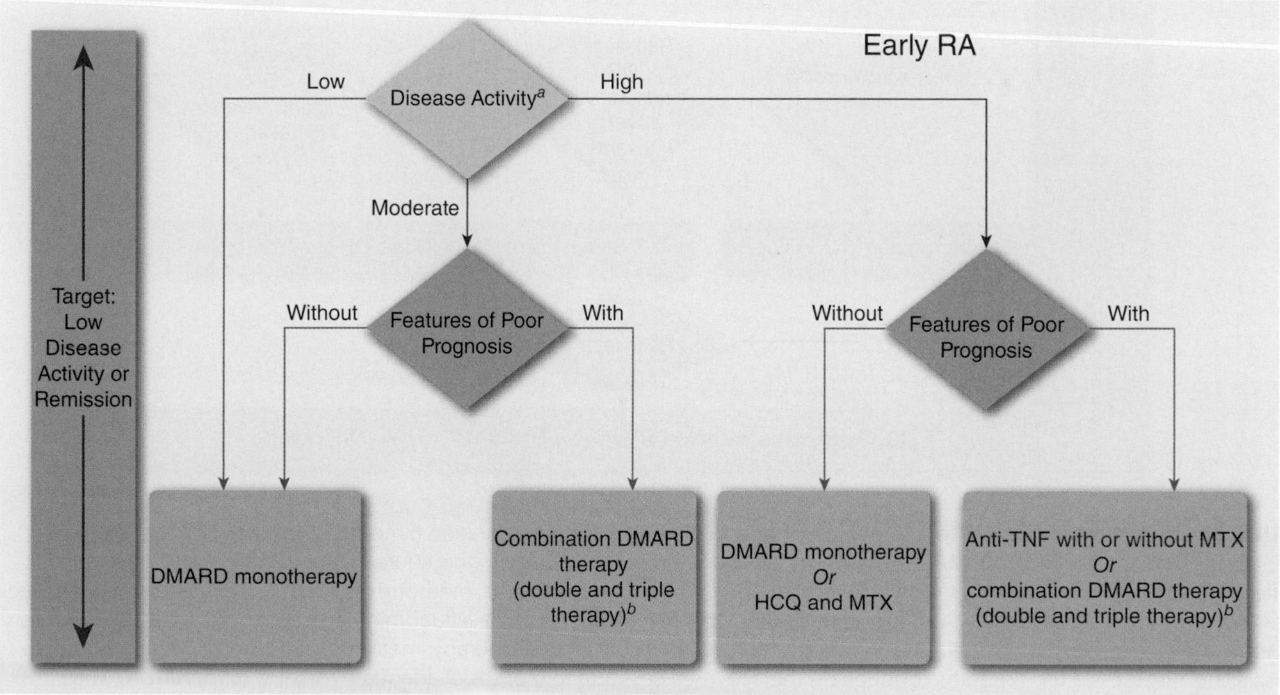

FIGURE 57–1. Recommendations for the treatment of early RA (disease duration < 6 months). DMARD, disease-modifying antirheumatic drug (In this figure, "DMARD" refers to conventional synthetic DMARDs or csDMARDs). [a]See Ref. 19 for definitions of disease activity. [b]Combination DMARD therapy: methotrexate + leflunomide, methotrexate + hydroxychloroquine, methotrexate + sulfasalazine, sulfasalazine + hydroxychloroquine. Triple DMARD therapy: methotrexate + hydroxychloroquine + sulfasalazine. (Reproduced, with permission, from Singh JA, Furst DE, Bharat A, et al. 2012 Update of the 2008 American College of Rheumatology recommendations for the use of disease-modifying antirheumatic drugs and biologic agents in the treatment of rheumatoid arthritis. Arthritis Care Res. 2012;64:625–639.)

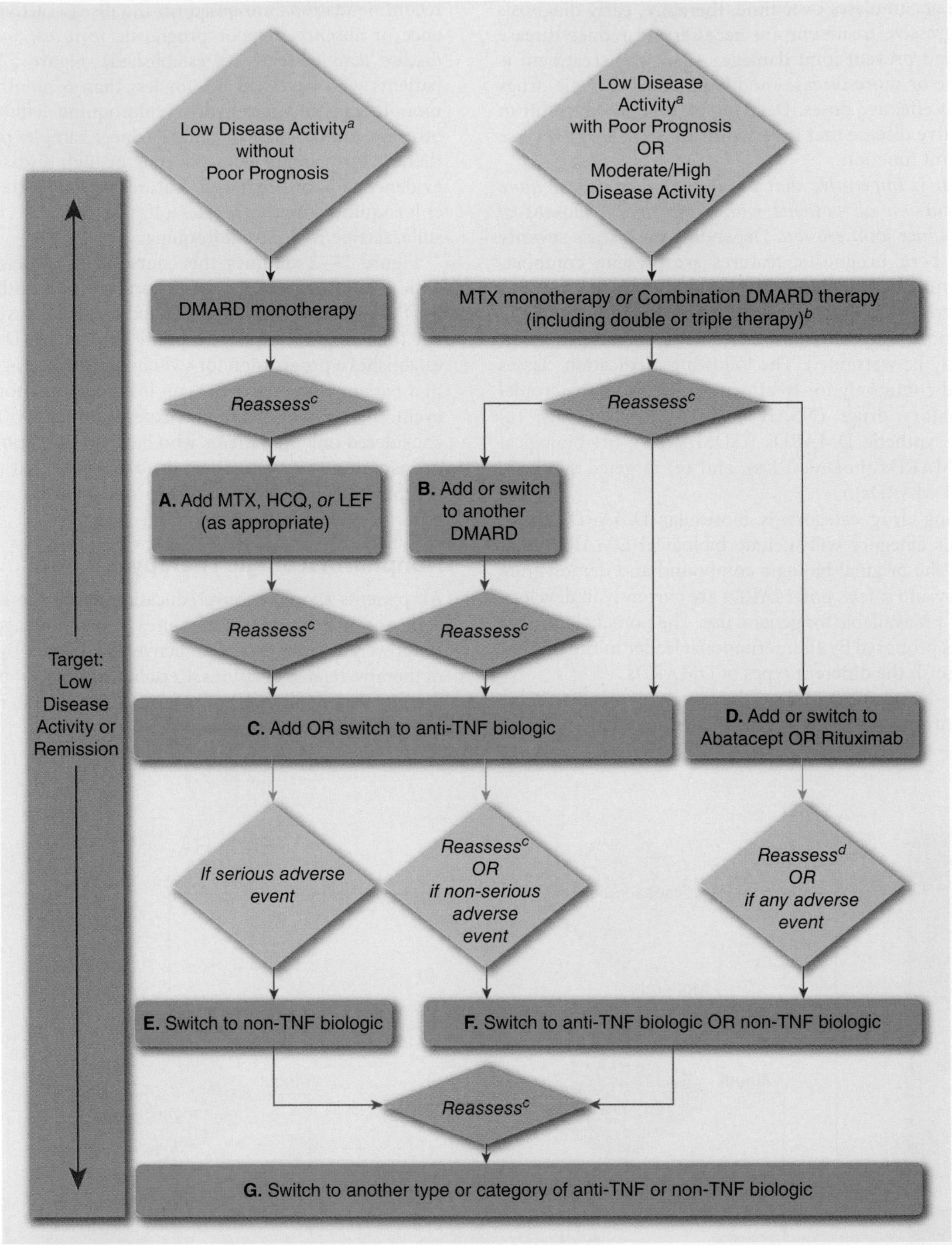

FIGURE 57–2. Recommendations for the treatment of established RA (disease duration 6 month or longer). Biologic, biological originator DMARD or boDMARD; DMARD, disease-modifying antirheumatic drug (In this figure, "DMARD" refers to conventional synthetic DMARDs or csDMARDs); HCQ, hydroxychloroquine; LEF, leflunomide; MTX, methotrexate; TNF, tumor necrosis factor. [a]See Ref. 19 for definitions of disease activity. [b]Combination DMARD therapy: methotrexate + leflunomide, methotrexate + hydroxychloroquine, methotrexate + sulfasalazine, sulfasalazine + hydroxychloroquine. Triple DMARD therapy: methotrexate + hydroxychloroquine + sulfasalazine. [c]Reassess after 3 months of adequate therapy. [d]Reassess after 6 months of adequate therapy. (Reproduced, with permission, from Singh JA, Furst DE, Bharat A, et al. 2012 Update of the 2008 American College of Rheumatology recommendations for the use of disease-modifying antirheumatic drugs and biologic agents in the treatment of rheumatoid arthritis. Arthritis Care Res. 2012;64:625–639.)

Occupational and physical therapy may help patients preserve joint function, extend joint range of motion, and strengthen joints and muscles through strengthening exercises. Patients with joint deformities may benefit from the use of mobility or assistive devices that help to minimize disability and allow continued activities of daily living. When appropriate, patients should also be counseled about stress management (ie, cognitive behavioral therapy, emotional disclosure, tai chi). In situations where the disease has progressed to a severe form with extensive joint erosions, surgery to replace or reconstruct the joint may be necessary.

Pharmacologic Therapy

▶ *Bridge Therapy/Symptomatic Relief*

The current standard of care for RA treatment is to initiate disease-modifying therapy immediately. While this step is critical to control the underlying disease activity, it may take weeks to months for the patient to experience relief. It is acceptable to initiate "bridge therapy" or short-term use of certain medications to provide symptomatic relief until the disease modifying drug reaches its therapeutic effect. The most common classes used for bridge therapy are NSAIDs and glucocorticoids.

NSAIDs These agents provide analgesic and anti-inflammatory benefits for joint pain and swelling. However, they do not prevent joint damage or change the underlying disease. Selecting an NSAID depends on multiple patient-specific factors, including cardiovascular risk, potential for GI-related adverse events, adherence to medication regimens, and insurance coverage or lack thereof. NSAID monotherapy is recommended as initial treatment in children with JIA without prior treatment for a duration of 1 month.[17] Clinicians must carefully evaluate the potential risks of NSAID therapy against the potential benefits.[14] See Chapter 58 for additional discussion of NSAID therapy.

Glucocorticoids In contrast to NSAIDs, low-dose glucocorticoid treatment (equivalent to prednisone 10 mg/day or less) effectively reduces inflammation through inhibition of cytokines and inflammatory mediators and prevents disease progression.[20] However, due to the adverse effect profile, the goal of glucocorticoid use is to keep doses low and use the drugs as infrequently as possible. Patients taking more than 5 mg/day of prednisone or equivalent are at increased risk for clinically significant adverse reactions, especially bone loss leading to osteoporosis. Other glucocorticoid-related adverse reactions include Cushing syndrome, peptic ulcer disease, hypertension, weight gain, infection, mood changes, cataracts, dyslipidemia, and hyperglycemia.[20] A modified-release dosage form of prednisone is available and is intended to improve the benefit-to-risk ratio of glucocorticoid use.

Intraarticular glucocorticoid injections are recommended as initial treatment of JIA for disease affecting four or fewer joints.[17]

▶ *Conventional Synthetic DMARDs (csDMARDs)*

DMARDs are the mainstay of RA treatment because they modify the disease process and prevent or reduce joint damage. In addition to relying on safety and efficacy data, the initial DMARD choice depends on disease severity, patient characteristics (ie, comorbidities, likelihood of adherence), cost, and clinician experience with the medication.[8,19] Methotrexate alone or in combination therapy is the initial treatment of choice for patients with aggressive disease. Agents such as azathioprine, D-penicillamine, gold salts, and anakinra are used rarely today because of concerns about toxicity and reduced efficacy.[19]

Methotrexate KEY CONCEPT *Methotrexate is the csDMARD of choice in RA because of its documented efficacy and safety profile when monitored appropriately.*[1,2] Methotrexate exerts its anti-inflammatory effect through inhibition of dihydrofolate reductase, which causes inhibition of purines and thymidylic acid, and by inhibiting production of certain cytokines.[2] Unless the patient has contraindications to methotrexate, once-weekly doses should be initiated within 3 months of diagnosis and increased steadily until the patient has symptomatic improvement or a maximum dose of 20 mg/wk is reached. If monotherapy does not produce complete resolution of symptoms, methotrexate may be used in combination with other csDMARDs or boDMARDs. Concomitant folic acid is given routinely to reduce the risk of folate-depleting reactions induced by methotrexate therapy (eg, stomatitis, diarrhea, nausea, alopecia, myelosuppression, and elevations in liver function tests).[1]

Methotrexate is recommended as initial treatment for JIA in patients with more than four active joints.[17] There are insufficient published data to assess the risk of serious toxicity in children receiving doses greater than 20 mg/m^2/week. Methotrexate therapy in children should be monitored the same way that is recommended in adults.

Hydroxychloroquine and Sulfasalazine The exact mechanism of action of these drugs is unknown, but both agents are fairly well tolerated. Hydroxychloroquine or sulfasalazine may be initiated on diagnosis of low disease activity. Because of their slow onset of action, each drug must be given at therapeutic doses for at least 6 months before it can be deemed a treatment failure. Hydroxychloroquine and sulfasalazine are relatively inexpensive compared to boDMARDs. If a patient does not respond to methotrexate monotherapy, adding one of these two drugs may provide the benefit necessary to reduce symptoms satisfactorily and ideally induce remission.[2,19]

Hydroxychloroquine is not associated with renal, hepatic, or bone marrow suppression and therefore may be an acceptable treatment option for patients with contraindications to other DMARDs because of their toxicities.

Starting sulfasalazine at low doses and titrating slowly will minimize the nausea and abdominal discomfort caused by the drug. Patients receiving sulfasalazine must undergo routine blood work to monitor for leukopenia.[19] Patients with a sulfa allergy should not receive sulfasalazine.

In patients with JIA, sulfasalazine is recommended only for patients with the enthesitis-related category. Enthesitis-related arthritis is a less common form of JIA that affects boys more than girls and is characterized by lower extremity joint involvement, including heel pain and enthesitis. Hydroxychloroquine is not recommended in JIA patients with active arthritis.[21]

Leflunomide This drug inhibits dihydroorotate dehydrogenase, an enzyme within mitochondria that supplies T lymphocytes with the necessary components to respond to cytokine stimulation.[22] Thus, leflunomide inhibits the T-lymphocyte response to various stimuli and halts the cell cycle. Its efficacy is similar to that of moderate doses of methotrexate or sulfasalazine.[22] Because of its extended half-life, leflunomide therapy begins with a loading dose followed by a maintenance dose. Leflunomide may be used in combination with methotrexate, but the added efficacy comes with a dramatic rise in the risk of hepatotoxicity. If therapy requires abrupt discontinuation (eg, due to toxicity or pregnancy), administering cholestyramine will accelerate leflunomide removal from the body.

Leflunomide is recommended as an alternative to methotrexate in patients with JIA experiencing disease activity in five or more joints.[21] However, leflunomide does not have an FDA-approved indication for this use.

▶ *Biological Originator DMARDs (boDMARDs)*

boDMARDs are indicated in patients who have failed an adequate trial of csDMARD therapy or in combination with csDMARDs in patients with early, aggressive disease. These agents may be added to csDMARD monotherapy (eg, methotrexate) or replace ineffective csDMARD therapy. The decision to select a particular agent generally is based on the prescriber's comfort level with monitoring the safety and efficacy of the medications, severity of disease activity, presence of factors suggestive of poor prognosis, the frequency and route of administration, the patient's comfort level or manual dexterity to self-administer subcutaneous injections, the cost, and the availability of insurance coverage. In general, boDMARDs should be avoided in patients with serious infections, demyelinating disorders (eg, multiple sclerosis), or hepatitis. TNF antagonists should be avoided in patients with heart failure.[19]

Tumor Necrosis Factor Antagonists Etanercept is a recombinant form of human T receptor.[22] Etanercept provides a therapeutic effect by binding to soluble TNF and preventing its binding with TNF receptors. Etanercept is very effective as monotherapy or in combination with other csDMARDs. Etanercept has an FDA-approved indication for treatment of JIA.

Adalimumab is a recombinant human IgG1 monoclonal antibody specific for human TNF.[22] Adalimumab binds to soluble and bound TNF-α. It can be administered in combination with methotrexate or other DMARDs.[2] Adalimumab has an FDA-approved indication for JIA.

Infliximab is a chimeric IgGl monoclonal antibody that binds to soluble and bound TNF-α.[22] Methotrexate typically is given with it to suppress antibody production against the mouse-derived portion of the molecule. Qualified healthcare personnel must be present during the infliximab infusion to respond to infusion-related reactions, if they occur (rash, urticaria, flushing, headache, fever, chills, nausea, tachycardia, dyspnea). These reactions may be treated by: (a) temporarily discontinuing the infusion, (b) slowing the infusion rate, or (c) administering corticosteroids or antihistamines. Patients may be pretreated with corticosteroids or antihistamines if they continue to experience infusion reactions. Infliximab was shown in clinical trials to be effective for treatment of JIA, but it has not yet received FDA approval for this indication.

Golimumab is a human monoclonal antibody that binds to membrane-bound and soluble TNF.[22] Golimumab can be administered in combination with methotrexate in patients with moderate to severe RA. One advantage of this agent over others in the class may be the once-monthly SC dosing or every-other-month IV dosing. Golimumab is not FDA approved for use in JIA.

Certolizumab is a humanized antibody Fab fragment conjugated to polyethylene glycol, which delays its metabolism and elimination.[22] Certolizumab can be administered alone or in combination with methotrexate in patients with moderate to severe RA. Certolizumab is not FDA approved for use in JIA.

Interleukin-1 Receptor Antagonist Anakinra is a recombinant form of human IL-1 receptor antagonist.[22] Anakinra inhibits the activity of IL-1 by binding to it and preventing cell signaling. It is indicated for adults with RA who have failed one or more csDMARDs. It may be used in combination with other csDMARDs in patients not responding to or unable to tolerate csDMARDs or TNF antagonists. Anakinra is not included in the 2012 treatment algorithms due to limited efficacy and infrequent use in RA. Regarding treatment of JIA, anakinra is recommended in the ACR treatment guidelines for patients with systemic arthritis with continued disease activity after a trial with 3 months of methotrexate or leflunomide, a 1-month trial of NSAID monotherapy, or a glucocorticoid injection.[17] Anakinra is not FDA approved for the treatment of JIA.

Costimulation Modulators Abatacept interferes with T-cell signaling, ultimately blocking T-cell activation and leading to anergy, or lack of response to an antigen.[22] Abatacept is indicated as monotherapy or in combination with nonbiologic DMARDs following inadequate response to methotrexate or anti-TNF agents. Abatacept is FDA approved for the treatment of moderate to severe JIA; it is recommended as an option for patients who did not respond to an adequate trial of methotrexate, leflunomide, or anakinra.[17]

Anti-CD20 Monoclonal Antibody Rituximab is a genetically engineered chimeric anti-CD20 monoclonal antibody that causes B-lymphocyte depletion in bone marrow and synovial tissue.[22] The exact role of rituximab in RA is not clearly defined, but it is indicated for patients with moderate to severe active RA and a history of inadequate response to one or more TNF antagonist therapies. Patients with rheumatoid factor positive RA tend to respond more favorably to rituximab than patients with rheumatoid factor negative disease. Rituximab carries a black-box warning of fatal infusion reactions and severe mucocutaneous reactions, even though these events did not occur during the RA clinical trials. The benefits of rituximab must be tempered against the safety concerns reported with use of rituximab in the oncology setting. Rituximab may be used in the treatment of JIA, though its place in therapy is not clear and the medication is not FDA approved for this purpose.[17]

Anti–interleukin-6 Receptor Antibody Interleukin-6 (IL-6) production is increased in patients with RA. High levels are indicative of joint damage and disease activity. In addition, IL-6 plays a significant role in the pathogenesis of anemia associated with RA.[23] Tocilizumab, an anti–IL-6 receptor monoclonal antibody, inhibits the binding of IL-6 to the IL-6 receptor.[23] Studies in patients not responding to methotrexate or TNF antagonists have demonstrated decreased disease activity and improved function and quality of life in patients with RA. In the 2012 recommendations, tocilizumab is considered after inadequate response or adverse event to anti-TNF agents, abatacept, or rituximab.[19] Tocilizumab is FDA approved for the treatment of JIA; it is recommended for patients with inadequate response to glucocorticoid monotherapy, methotrexate, leflunomide, or anakinra.[17]

▶ *Targeted Synthetic DMARDs (tsDMARDs)*

Tofacitinib selectively inhibits Janus kinases, with greatest affinity for JAK3.[24] Tofacitinib is indicated for the treatment of moderate to severe RA as monotherapy or in combination with csDMARDs. Combination administration with boDMARDs is inappropriate due to increased safety concerns. One distinct advantage of tofacitinib over boDMARDs is the oral dosage form. The exact place in therapy of tofacitinib is in the management of RA is not yet known. Presently, it may be initiated if a patient does not have an adequate response to or is otherwise unable to receive csDMARDs or boDMARDs.[24]

▶ *Selecting Disease-Modifying Therapy*

Table 57–4 highlights dosing, safety, monitoring, and patient counseling information for the common DMARDs. Developments in the treatment of RA are tempered by the lack of long-term safety and efficacy data for boDMARDs. In addition, high

Table 57–4

FDA-Approved DMARDs for Treatment of RA

Drug	Dose[a]	Time to Effect (weeks)	ADRs	Dosing in Hepatic Impairment	Dosing in Renal Impairment	Monitoring	Counseling Points
Conventional Synthetic DMARDs (csDMARDs)							
Methotrexate	Adults: 7.5–20 mg orally or IM once weekly Polyarticular-course JIA: Recommended starting dose: 10 mg/m^2 oral, IM, or SC once weekly; usual max dose: 20 mg/m^2 once weekly	4–8	N, D, hepatotoxicity, alopecia, new-onset cough or SOB, MYL	CI	CrCl (mL/min)[b]: 61–80: 75% of dose 51–60: 70% of dose 10–50: 50% of dose Less than 10: Avoid use	CBC, creatinine, LFTs every 4–8 weeks; monitor for signs of infection	Use of folic acid concomitantly Avoid alcohol Use contraception if childbearing potential
Hydroxychloroquine	Adults: 200 mg orally twice daily	8–24	N, D, HA, vision changes, skin pigmentation	Use with caution	No change	Eye examination every 12 months	
Sulfasalazine	Adults: 1000 mg orally two to three times daily Polyarticular-course JIA: Initial: 10 mg/kg/day orally; increase weekly by 10 mg/kg/day; usual dose: 30–50 mg/kg/day orally in two divided doses; max 2 g/day	8–12	N, D, rash, yellow-orange discoloration, photosensitivity, MYL	Avoid use	CrCl (mL/min)[b]: 10–30: Give twice daily Less than 10: Give once daily	CBC every 2–4 weeks for 3 months, then every 3 months	Sunscreen use
Leflunomide (Arava)	Adults: 100 mg orally daily for 3 days; then 20 mg daily	4–12	Hepatotoxicity, D, N, HTN, rash, HA, abdominal pain	Avoid use	Guidelines not available	CBC, creatinine, LFTs every months for 6 months; then every 4–8 weeks Monitor for signs of infection	Avoid alcohol Use contraception if childbearing potential
Biological Originator DMARDs (boDMARDs)							
Etanercept (Enbrel	Adults: 25 mg SC twice weekly or 50 mg SC once weekly Children ages 2–17: 0.8 mg/kg SC once weekly; max 50 mg/wk	1–4	ISR	No change	No change	Monitor for infection	ISR—topical corticosteroids, antipruritics, analgesics, rotate injection sites Screen for tuberculosis
Infliximab (Remicade)	Adults: 3–10 mg/kg by IV infusion at 0, 2, and 6 weeks; then every 8 weeks	1–4	IR (rash, urticaria, flushing, HA, fever, chills, nausea, tachycardia, dyspnea)	No change	No change	Monitor for infection	Screen for tuberculosis
Adalimumab (Humira)	Adults: 40 mg SC every other week Children older than 4 years and weighing 15–29 kg: 20 mg SC every other week Children weighing 30 kg or more: 40 mg SC every other week	1–4	ISR	No change	No change	Monitor for infection	Screen for tuberculosis

(Continued)

Table 57–4

FDA-Approved DMARDs for Treatment of RA (*Continued*)

Drug	Dose[a]	Time to Effect (weeks)	ADRs	Dosing in Hepatic Impairment	Dosing in Renal Impairment	Monitoring	Counseling Points
Golimumab (Simponi)	Adults: 50 mg SC once monthly 2 mg/kg IV infusion at weeks 0, 4, then every 8 weeks	1–4	ISR, IR	No change	No change	Monitor for infection	Screen for tuberculosis
Certolizumab (Cimzia)	Adults: 400 mg SC initially, at 2 weeks, 4 weeks, then every 4 weeks thereafter	1–4	ISR	No change	No change	Monitor for infection	Screen for tuberculosis
Anakinra (Kineret)	Adults: 100 mg SC daily	2–4	HA, N, V, D, ISR	No data available	CrCl < 30 mL/min[b]: consider 100 mg every other day	Monitor for infection	
Abatacept (Orencia)	Adult IV infusion: < 60 kg, 500 mg; 60–100 kg, 750 mg; > 100 kg, 1000 mg IV on days 1, 15 and every 28 days thereafter SC Injection: Weight-based loading dose, then 125 mg SC within 1 day, 125 mg SC once weekly; or 125 mg once weekly in patients unable to receive IV. JIA (> 6 years of age): < 75 kg: 10 mg/kg; 75–100 kg: 750 mg; > 100 kg: 1000 mg IV infusion on days 1, 15, 28 and every 28 days thereafter	2	HA, infection, IR, ISR	No change	No change	Monitor for infection	
Rituximab (Rituxan)	Adults: Two 1000-mg IV infusions separated by 2 weeks; timing of the third dose is based on patient symptoms (no earlier than 16 weeks)	4	IR	No change	No change	Monitor for infection	
Tocilizumab (Actemra)	Adults: 8 mg/kg IV infusion every 4 weeks SC: if > 100 kg, 162 every week; if < 100 kg, 162 every other week JIA (2 years and older): < 30 kg: 12 mg/kg IV infusion every 2 weeks; > 30 kg: 8 mg/kg every 2 weeks		Elevated LFTs, total cholesterol, triglycerides, and high-density lipoprotein; nasopharyngitis, infection	No data available	No data available	Monitor for infection; LFTs	
Targeted Synthetic DMARDs (tsDMARDs)							
Tofacitinib (Xeljanz)	Adults: 5 mg orally twice daily		Infection, headache, HTN, elevated LFTs, D, worsening lipid profile	Mild impairment: no adjustment Moderate: 5 mg once daily Severe: Use not recommended	Mild: no adjustment; Moderate/severe: 5 mg once daily	CBC, Hgb, lipids, LFTs, monitor for infection	

CBC, complete blood count; CI, contraindicated; D, diarrhea; HA, headache; Hgb, hemoglobin; HTN, hypertension; IR, infusion reactions; ISR, injection site reactions; LFTs, liver function tests; MYL, myelosuppression (watch for fever, symptoms of infection, easy bruisability, and bleeding); N, nausea; SC, subcutaneous injection; SOB, shortness of breath.

[a]Geriatric patients should receive the usual adult dose unless renal or hepatic impairment is present. Pediatric doses are provided for drugs that have FDA-approved indications for juvenile idiopathic arthritis (JIA).

[b]To convert to SI units of mL/s, multiply by 0.0167.

Data From Refs. 1, 2,19,22, and 25.

costs can be a deterrent to use. Cost analyses may indicate that the increased expenses associated with these boDMARDs are offset by the costs avoided for treatment of advanced RA.

KEY CONCEPT *The risk of infection in patients treated with boDMARDs must be considered when selecting and monitoring therapy.*[19,26] Influencing the immune response to reduce symptoms of RA may influence the body's response to pathogens. Of particular concern is use of TNF antagonists in patients with a history of tuberculosis exposure. TNF is important in the formation of granulomas that wall off tuberculosis infection. In theory, if TNF is inhibited, patients with latent tuberculosis may have a reactivated infection. Etanercept appears to have the lowest incidence rate of tuberculosis when compared with other TNF antagonists.[22] Patients receiving any boDMARD agent should be screened for tuberculosis and other infections (hepatitis B, hepatitis C). Antituberculosis therapy should be initiated in patients with active or latent tuberculosis.[19] Patients with active tuberculosis should receive the full course of antituberculosis treatment prior to initiating boDMARDs. If there is latent infection, boDMARD therapy may be initiated after at least 1 month of antituberculosis treatment. Patients with untreated hepatitis B should not receive boDMARDs. Etanercept may be a potential treatment option in patients with RA and concomitant hepatitis C.[19] boDMARDs should not be initiated during an acute, serious infection and should be discontinued temporarily during times of infection. boDMARD therapy can be continued during nonserious infections.[27] Concomitant use of two boDMARDs or tsDMARD plus boDMARD is contraindicated due to increased infection risk.

▶ *Fertility, Pregnancy, and Fetal Development*

Women of childbearing potential should be counseled about the impact of antirheumatic drugs on fertility, pregnancy, fetal development, and lactation. Some women may experience a reduction in disease symptoms during pregnancy; however, many agents used to treat RA are known teratogens. In addition, some women may present with signs and symptoms of RA for the first time during the postpartum period. Women desiring motherhood must consult with their physicians to carefully plan for the pregnancy and reduce risks to the developing fetus.[28] Treatment plans selected must also consider the potential effects on breast-feeding babies. Low-dose corticosteroids generally are safe and effective. Certain NSAIDs, hydroxychloroquine, and azathioprine may be considered in severe disease.

Methotrexate use (FDA Pregnancy Category X) is associated with spontaneous abortion, fetal myelosuppression, limb defects, and CNS abnormalities; therefore, pregnancy must be avoided.[28] Methotrexate should be discontinued 3 months prior to attempting conception. Sulfasalazine, on the other hand, may be the drug of choice in women who are pregnant or planning to become pregnant due to its safety profile.[28] There is limited data on safety of boDMARD use in pregnant women. Case reports of pregnancy during boDMARD therapy show no increased risk of fetal toxicity, but long-term data are needed.[28] Based on available data, TNF antagonists are considered safe until the time of conception, and discontinuation during pregnancy is recommended. Rituximab should be discontinued 1 year prior to planned conception. Abatacept should be discontinued 10 weeks prior to planned conception.[28]

Male patients with RA must receive counseling about the effects of certain medications on their fertility and potential harm to the fetus. It is difficult to establish causality between use of a medication by a male and the effect on fertility or fetal development; therefore, a conservative approach must be taken. KEY CONCEPT *Women of childbearing potential and their partners must be counseled to: (a) use proper birth control while undergoing treatment for RA, and (b) involve health care providers in discussions regarding family planning to carefully consider all treatment options.*[28]

Patient Encounter, Part 2: Medical History, Physical Examination, and Laboratory Tests

PMH: Hypertension (20 years), dyslipidemia (20 years), depression (5 years), diabetes (15 years), rheumatoid arthritis (10 years)

FH: Mother died age 70 from MI, also had RA, DM, HTN, dyslipidemia; father died age 82 from lymphoma

SH: Retired but owns a small business. She is a seamstress and relies heavily on her hands for the work of the business. She drinks alcohol occasionally and smokes a half pack of cigarettes daily.

Allergies: aspirin, penicillin

Meds: Lisinopril 10 mg once daily; hydrochlorothiazide 25 mg once daily; simvastatin 40 mg once daily; metformin 500 mg twice daily; paroxetine 20 mg once daily; methotrexate 15 mg orally once weekly; adalimumab 40 mg SC every other week; folic acid 1 mg daily; fish oil 1 g daily

Previous Meds: Etanercept, metoprolol, pravastatin

ROS: (+) Fatigue, (–) N/V/D, HA, SOB, chest pain, cough

PE:

VS: BP 186/92, P 86, RR 22, T 38.0°C (100.4°F); Ht 5′2″ (157 cm), Wt 75 kg (165 lb)

Skin: Warm, dry

HEENT: NC/AT, PERRLA, TMs intact

CV: RRR, normal S1 and S2, no m/r/g

Chest: CTA

Abd: Soft, NT/ND

Neuro: A&O × 3; CN II to XII intact

Ext: Bilateral tender and swollen PIPs and MCPs

Labs: ESR 65 mm/hour, RF (+), HLA-DR4 (+), ACPA (high +)

Synovial fluid analysis: Yellow, cloudy, decreased viscosity

Hand x-rays: Soft-tissue swelling, joint space narrowing, evidence of erosions

Disease Activity Score 28 (DAS-28): 6.63

How would you categorize this patient's disease activity—low, moderate, or high? Why? How does this affect your treatment plan?

What nonpharmacologic and pharmacologic alternatives are appropriate for this patient?

Patient Encounter, Part 3: Creating a Care Plan

Based on the information available, create a care plan for this patient's RA. The plan should include the following:

(a) A statement of the drug-related needs and/or problems

(b) A patient-specific detailed therapeutic plan (including specific medications and associated doses)

(c) Monitoring parameters to assess safety and efficacy

OUTCOME EVALUATION

- Rheumatologists rely on standardized criteria to assess treatment interventions through measurement of disease activity. The ACR uses criteria for improvement based on percentage improvement in tender and swollen joint count and the presence of at least three or more of the following measures: (a) pain, (b) patient global assessment, (c) physician global assessment, (d) self-assessed physical disability, and (e) acute-phase reactants.[29] ACR20, ACR50, and ACR70 are common efficacy endpoints in clinical trials. The number corresponds with the percentage improvement. As drug development continues to evolve, the acceptable criteria for 20% improvement may be too low.
- Common tools to assess disease activity in patients with RA include Patient Activity Scale, Clinical Disease Activity Index, Simplified Disease Activity Index, and Disease Activity in 28 joints (DAS-28).[19] Components involved in the calculation are the number of swollen and tender joints, ESR or CRP, and a subjective measure of the patient's general health. A DAS-28 score of 3.2 or less indicates low disease activity, between 3.2 and 5.1 is considered moderate activity, and 5.1 or more is considered to be high activity. Remission as defined by DAS-28 is a score of less than 2.6.[19]
- Physical disability from RA can be measured through the Stanford Health Assessment Questionnaire (HAQ).[30,31] This patient self-assessment tool was developed to evaluate patient outcomes in five dimensions of chronic conditions: (a) disability, (b) discomfort, (c) drug adverse effects, (d) dollar costs, and (e) death. Clinicians and clinical studies in

Patient Care Process

Patient Assessment:

- Determine whether physical examination findings and patient-reported symptoms are consistent with RA. Evaluate the duration of symptoms and impact on daily living.
- Review the medical history. Does the patient have comorbidities that should also be addressed? Are features of poor prognosis present?
- Review laboratory test results to establish baseline hepatic function, renal function, and blood cell status.

Therapy Evaluation:

- Conduct a medication history and review patient allergies. Are any of the medications causing the noted signs or symptoms?
- If the patient is already receiving pharmacotherapy for RA, assess efficacy, safety and patient adherence.
- Determine whether the patient has prescription coverage. If not, determine if the patient is eligible for prescription assistance programs.

Care Plan Development:

- Educate the patient on nonpharmacologic measures to improve symptoms.
- If the patient is newly diagnosed with RA, make sure s/he receives DMARD therapy immediately to minimize disease progression and joint destruction.
- Select DMARD therapy that is likely to be safe and effective. (see Figures 57–1 and 57–2)
- Ensure that drug doses are optimal (see Table 57–4).
- Screen for tuberculosis if initiation of a boDMARD is under consideration.
- Stress the importance of adherence with medications and laboratory monitoring.
- Evaluate the presence of comorbidities and implement measures to control the increased risk.
    - *Cardiovascular*: Keep doses of NSAIDs and glucocorticoids low; consider initiating folic acid, low-dose aspirin, and/or statin therapy, and encourage smokers to discontinue tobacco use.[13,14] Screen and aggressively treat elevated blood pressure.
    - *Infection*: Inform the patient to wash hands routinely, limit contact with individuals who are ill, and report signs and symptoms of infection immediately (eg, fever, weight loss, and night sweats).
    - *Malignancy*: Have the patient report new signs and symptoms (eg, fever, chills, anorexia, and night sweats) immediately.
    - *Osteoporosis*: Encourage the patient to ingest adequate amounts of calcium and vitamin D; consider initiating medications for osteoporosis if the patient is taking glucocorticoids chronically or has evidence of low bone mineral density.[32]

Follow-Up Evaluation:

- Assess the patient's response to initiation of DMARD therapy after allowing adequate time for the medication to achieve its therapeutic effect.
- Determine whether any adverse reactions to antirheumatic medication are present.
- Monitor laboratory parameters to ensure patient safety and reduce the risk of adverse reactions.
- Longitudinally evaluate the patient's clinical response to therapy and the impact on quality of life and mobility.
- Assess patient understanding of RA and medications they are taking. Provide additional education where appropriate.

rheumatology use the HAQ to assess longitudinal changes that influence the patient's quality of life.[30,31]

- Before starting treatment for RA, assess the subjective and objective evidence of disease. For joint findings, this includes the number of tender and swollen joints, pain, limitations on use, duration of morning stiffness, and presence of joint erosions. Systemic findings may include fatigue and the presence of extraarticular manifestations. Obtain laboratory measurements of CRP and ESR. The impact of the disease on quality of life and functional status is also important.
- At follow-up visits, compare the patient's status to baseline or previous visits using standardized criteria for improvement of disease activity and the influence on quality of life.
- KEY CONCEPT *In addition to designing an individualized therapeutic regimen to control the progression of RA, the clinician must evaluate the presence of comorbidities and implement measures to control the increased risk.*

Abbreviations Introduced in This Chapter

ACPA	Anticitrullinated protein antibodies
ACR	American College of Rheumatology
boDMARD	Biological originator DMARD
bsDMARD	Biosimilar DMARD
COX-2	Cyclooxygenase-2
CRP	C-reactive protein
csDMARD	Conventional synthetic DMARD
DAS	Disease Activity Score
DMARD	Disease-modifying antirheumatic drug
ESR	Erythrocyte sedimentation rate
EULAR	European League against Rheumatism
HAQ	Health Assessment Questionnaire
HLA	Human leukocyte antigen
IL	Interleukin
JIA	Juvenile idiopathic arthritis
MCP	Metacarpophalangeal joint
MTP	Metatarsophalangeal joint
NSAID	Nonsteroidal anti-inflammatory drug
PIP	Proximal interphalangeal joint
RA	Rheumatoid arthritis
TNF	Tumor necrosis factor
tsDMARD	Targeted synthetic DMARD

REFERENCES

1. Aletaha D, Neogi T, Silman A, et al. 2010 Rheumatoid arthritis classification criteria: an American College of Rheumatology/European League against Rheumatism collaborative initiative. Arthritis Rheum. 2010;62:2569–2381.
2. Colmenga I, Ohata B, Menard H. Current understanding of rheumatoid arthritis therapy. Clin Pharmacol Ther. 2012;91:607–620.
3. Myasoedova E, Davis JM, Crowson CS, Gabriel SE. Epidemiology of rheumatoid arthritis: rheumatoid arthritis and mortality. Curr Rheumatol Rep. 2010;12:379–385.
4. Amson Y, Shoenfeld Y, Amital H. Effects of smoking on immunity, inflammation and autoimmunity. J Autoimmun. 2010;34:258–265.
5. Burmester GR, Feist E, Dörner T. Emerging cell and cytokine targets in rheumatoid arthritis. Nat Rev Rheumatol. 2014;10(2):77–88. 2013 doi:10.1038/nrrheum.2013.168.
6. Kotzin BL. The role of B cells in the pathogenesis of rheumatoid arthritis. J Rheumatol. 2005;73(suppl):14–18.
7. McCray C, Agarwal SK. Stress and autoimmunity. Immunol Allergy Clin North Am. 2011;31:1–18.
8. Beukelman T, Patkar NM, Saag KG. 2011 American College of Rheumatology recommendations for the treatment of juvenile idiopathic arthritis: initiation and safety monitoring of therapeutic agents for the treatment of arthritis and systemic features. Arthritis Care Res. 2011;63:465–482.
9. Vital EM, Emery P. The development of targeted therapies in rheumatoid arthritis. J Autoimmun. 2008;31:219–227.
10. Boissier MC. Cell and cytokine imbalances in rheumatoid synovitis. Joint Bone Spine. 2011;78:230–234.
11. Gonzalez A, Icen M, Kremers HM, et al. Mortality trends in rheumatoid arthritis: The role of rheumatoid factor. J Rheumatol. 2008;35:1009–1014.
12. Kelly V, Genovese M. Novel small molecule therapeutics in rheumatoid arthritis. Rheumatology. 2013;52:1155–1162.
13. Pieringer H, Pichler M. Cardiovascular morbidity and mortality in patients with rheumatoid arthritis: vascular alterations and possible clinical implications. QJM. 2011;104:13–26.
14. Gabriel SE, Crowson CS. Risk factors for cardiovascular disease in rheumatoid arthritis. Curr Opin Rheumatol. 2012;24:171–176.
15. Gullick NJ, Scott DL. Co-morbidities in established rheumatoid arthritis. Best Pract Res Clin Rheumatol. 2011;25:469–483.
16. Cush JJ, Dao KH. Malignancy risks with biologic therapies. Rheum Dis Clin North Am. 2012;38:761–770.
17. Ringold S, Weiss PF, Beukelman T, et al. 2013 Update of the 2011 American College of Rheumatology recommendations for the treatment of juvenile idiopathic arthritis: recommendations for the medical therapy of children with systemic juvenile idiopathic arthritis and tuberculosis screening among children receiving biologic medications. Arthritis Rheum. 2013;65:2499–2512.
18. Coulson EJ, Hanson HJ, Foster HE. What does an adult rheumatologist need to know about juvenile idiopathic arthritis? Rheumatology. 2014;53:2155–2166. doi:10.1093/rheumatology/keu257.
19. Singh JA, Furst DE, Bharat A, et al. 2012 Update of the 2008 American College of Rheumatology recommendations for the use of disease-modifying antirheumatic drugs and biologic agents in the treatment of rheumatoid arthritis. Arthritis Care Res. 2012;64:625–639.
20. Caporali R, Toderti M, Sakellariou G, Montecucco C. Glucocorticoids in rheumatoid arthritis. Drugs. 2013;73:31-43.
21. Stoll ML, Cron RQ. Treatment of juvenile idiopathic arthritis: a revolution in care. Pediatr Rheumatol Online J. 2014;12:13.
22. Meier FM, Frerix M, Hermann W, Müller-Ladner U. Current immunotherapy in rheumatoid arthritis. Immunotherapy. 2013;5:955–974.
23. Al-Shakarchi I, Gullick NJ, Scott DL. Current perspectives on tocilizumab for the treatment of rheumatoid arthritis: a review. Patient Prefer Adherence. 2013;7:653–666.
24. Scott LJ. Tofacitinib: a review of its use in adult patients with rheumatoid arthritis. Drugs. 2013;73:857–874.
25. Lexi-Comp Online™, Lexi-Drugs™, Hudson, Ohio: Lexi-Comp Inc.; September 4, 2014.
26. Winthrop KL. Infections and biologic therapy in rheumatoid arthritis: our changing understanding of risk and prevention. Rheum Dis Clin North Am. 2012;38:727–745.
27. Dao KH, Herbert M, Habal N, Cush JJ. Nonserious infections: should there be cause for serious concerns? Rheum Dis Clin North Am. 2012;38:707–725.
28. Parlett R, Roussou E. The treatment of rheumatoid arthritis during pregnancy. Rheumatol Int. 2011;31:445–449.
29. Felson DT, Anderson JJ, Boers M, et al. American College of Rheumatology preliminary definition of improvement in rheumatoid arthritis. Arthritis Rheum. 1995;38:727–735.

30. Bruce B, Fries JF. The Stanford Health Assessment Questionnaire: a review of its history, issues, progress, and documentation. J Rheumatol. 2003;30(1):167–178.
31. Bruce B, Fries JF. The Stanford Health Assessment Questionnaire: dimensions and practical applications. Health Qual Life Outcomes. 2003;1(1):20.
32. Grossman JM, Gordon R, Ranganath VK, et al. American College of Rheumatology 2010 recommendations for the prevention and treatment of glucocorticoid-induced osteoporosis. Arthritis Care Res. 2010;62:1515–1526.

58 Osteoarthritis

Nicholas Carris, Steven M. Smith,
and John G. Gums

LEARNING OBJECTIVES

Upon completion of the chapter, the reader will be able to:

1. Explain the pathophysiologic mechanisms involved in the development of osteoarthritis (OA).
2. Identify risk factors associated with OA.
3. Recognize the clinical presentation of OA.
4. Determine the goals of therapy for individual patients with OA.
5. Formulate a rational nonpharmacologic plan for patients with OA.
6. Recommend a pharmacologic plan for treating OA, taking into consideration patient-specific factors.
7. Develop monitoring parameters to assess effectiveness and adverse effects of pharmacotherapy for OA.
8. Modify an unsuccessful treatment strategy for OA.
9. Deliver effective patient counseling, including lifestyle modifications and drug therapy, to facilitate effective and safe management of OA.

INTRODUCTION

KEY CONCEPT *Osteoarthritis (OA) is the most common form of arthritis and is strongly related to age. Its incidence and cost of care will increase dramatically in the coming years due to a burgeoning senior citizenry.* Weight-bearing joints (eg, hips and knees) are most susceptible, but non–weight-bearing joints, especially the hands, also may be involved. Because of its high prevalence and involvement of joints critical for daily functioning, the disease causes tremendous morbidity and financial burden.[1] OA is the leading cause of chronic mobility disability and the most common reason for total-hip and total-knee replacement.[2]

EPIDEMIOLOGY AND ETIOLOGY

Globally, the age-standardized prevalence of knee and hip OA is at least 3.8% and 0.85%, respectively. High-income countries, which generally have older populations, have a higher prevalence than low-income countries.[3] The National Arthritis Data Workgroup estimates that 27 million Americans have signs and symptoms of OA.[4] Approximately 7% of US adults have daily symptomatic hand OA, whereas 6% and 3% report daily symptoms affecting the knees and hips, respectively.[4] After age 60, 10% to 17% of persons report such symptoms.[4]

The prevalence of OA is greater in women by 1.5- to 2-fold, and they tend to have more generalized disease. Women are also more likely to have inflammation of the proximal and distal interphalangeal joints of the hands, which manifest as **Bouchard nodes** and **Heberden nodes**, respectively. OA of the hip occurs more frequently in men.

The prevalence of OA in whites is similar to that in African Americans, but the latter may experience more severe and disabling disease. Persons of Chinese descent rarely have hip OA; they also are less likely to develop hand OA but more likely to develop knee OA.

PATHOPHYSIOLOGY

OA is characterized by damage to **diarthrodial** joints and joint structures (Figure 58–1). The pathophysiology is multifactorial and typified by progressive destruction of joint cartilage, erratic new bone formation, thickening of **subchondral** bone and the joint capsule, bony remodeling, development of **osteophytes**, variable degrees of mild **synovitis**, and other changes.[5]

The earliest stages of OA are characterized by increasing water content and softening of cartilage in weight-bearing joints. As the disease progresses, **proteoglycan** content of cartilage declines, and eventually, cartilage becomes hypocellular. Protease enzymes proliferate before changes in cartilage, suggesting that catabolic proteinases play an important role in the initiation and progression of OA.

Subchondral bone undergoes metabolic changes, including increased bone turnover, that appear to be precursors to tissue destruction. The normally contiguous bony surface becomes fissured. Persistent use of the joint eventually results in loss of cartilage, permitting bone-to-bone contact that ultimately promotes thickening and **eburnation** of exposed bone. Microfractures may appear in subchondral bone, and **osteonecrosis** may develop beneath the surface especially in individuals with advanced disease.

New bone is formed haphazardly, leading to the formation of osteophytes that extend into the joint capsule and ligament attachments and may encroach on the joint space. Progressive loss of joint cartilage, subchondral damage, narrowing of joint spaces, and changes in the underlying bone and soft tissues may culminate in deformed, painful joints.

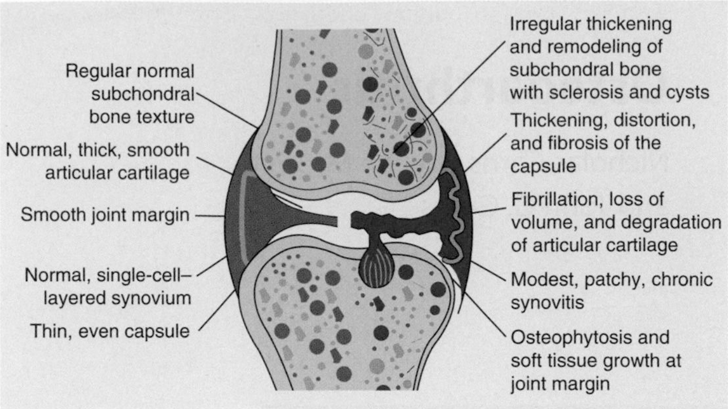

FIGURE 58–1. Characteristics of osteoarthritis in the diarthrodial joint. (From DiPiro JT, Talbert RL, Yee GC, et al., [eds.] Pharmacotherapy: A Pathophysiologic Approach, 8th ed. New York: McGraw-Hill; 2011:1601, Fig. 101–2; With permission.)

Classification

OA can be classified as primary (idiopathic) or secondary. *Primary OA* is the predominant form and occurs in the absence of a known precipitating event. Primary OA may assume a localized, generalized, or erosive pattern. Localized OA is distinguished from generalized disease by the number of sites involved. Erosive disease is characterized by an erosive pattern of bone destruction and marked proliferation of interphalangeal joints of the hands. Secondary OA results from congenital or developmental disorders or inflammatory, metabolic, or endocrine diseases.

Risk Factors

OA develops when systemic factors and biomechanical vulnerabilities combine. Systemic factors include age, gender, genetic predisposition, and nutritional status. Age is the strongest predictor of OA, although advanced age alone is insufficient to cause OA.

Joints exposed to biomechanical factors are at increased risk. Occupational and recreational activities involving repetitive motion or injury can provoke OA, although most daily activities do not produce enough joint trauma to cause OA, even after decades of repeated use. However, daily activities may lead to OA if a joint is susceptible because of previous injury, joint deformity, muscle weakness, or systemic factors. Heavy physical activity is a stronger predictor of subsequent OA than light-to-moderate activities, especially for older individuals, in whom the joint structure is less capable of coping with highly stressful activities.[6] Obesity increases load-bearing stresses on hip and knee joints. The risk of OA increases by 10% for each kilogram of body weight above ideal body weight.[7]

CLINICAL PRESENTATION AND DIAGNOSIS

See the accompanying text box for the clinical presentation of OA. No laboratory tests are specific for diagnosing OA. The erythrocyte sedimentation rate (ESR) and hematologic and chemistry panels are usually unremarkable. Synovial fluid aspirated from an affected joint should be sterile, without crystals, and with a WBC count less than $1.5 \times 10^3/mm^3$ ($1.5 \times 10^9/L$).

Clinical Presentation of OA

General

- Patients usually are more than 50 years old.
- Presentation may range from asymptomatic to severe joint pain and stiffness with functional limitations.
- Joint involvement has an asymmetric local distribution without systemic manifestations.
- In contrast to some other arthritic conditions (eg, rheumatoid arthritis, gout), inflammation usually is absent or mild and localized when present.

Symptoms

- KEY CONCEPT *The most common symptoms are joint pain, reduced range of motion, and brief joint stiffness after periods of inactivity.*
- The cardinal symptoms are use-related joint pain, typically described as deep and aching in character, and stiffness. In advanced cases, pain may be present during rest.
- Weight-bearing joints may be unstable.
- Joint stiffness ("gelling") abates with motion and recurs with rest.
- Joint stiffness generally lasts less than 30 minutes after periods of inactivity, limits the range of joint motion, impairs daily activities, and may be related to weather.

Signs

- One or more joints may be involved, usually in an asymmetric pattern.
- The following sites are most often involved in primary OA:
  - Distal interphalangeal finger joints (Heberden nodes)
  - Proximal interphalangeal finger joints (Bouchard nodes)
  - First carpometacarpal joint
  - Knees, hips, and cervicolumbar spine
  - Metatarsophalangeal joint of the great toe
- Joint examination may reveal local tenderness, bony proliferation, soft tissue swelling, crepitus, muscle atrophy, limited motion with passive/active movement, and effusion.

Radiographic changes are often absent in early OA. As the disease progresses, joint-space narrowing, subchondral bone sclerosis, and osteophytes may be detected. Gross joint deformity and joint effusions may occur in late severe OA.

TREATMENT

Desired Outcomes

KEY CONCEPT *Goals of therapy include: (a) educating the patient and caregivers, (b) relieving pain, (c) maintaining or restoring mobility, (d) minimizing functional impairment and associated adverse outcomes (eg, falls), (e) preserving joint integrity, and (f) improving quality of life.*

General Approach to Treatment

Treatment is individualized considering medical history, physical examination, radiographic findings, distribution and severity of joint involvement, and response to previous treatment. Comorbid diseases, concomitant medications, and allergies are integrated into a holistic treatment approach.

As shown in the treatment algorithm for OA (Figure 58–2), nonpharmacologic treatment is integral to achieving optimal outcomes. Pharmacologic therapy is an adjunctive measure to relieve pain; current treatments do not substantially modify the disease course. Surgical intervention generally is reserved for patients with advanced disease complicated by unremitting pain or severely compromised function.

Nonpharmacologic Therapy

KEY CONCEPT *Nonpharmacologic therapy is the cornerstone of treatment: education, exercise, weight loss, and cognitive behavioral intervention are integral components.*

Educational programs include systematic educational activities designed to improve health behaviors and health status, thereby slowing OA progression. The goal is to increase patient knowledge and self-confidence in adjusting daily activities in the face of evolving symptoms. Effective programs produce positive behavioral changes, decreased pain and disability, and improved functioning. In addition to physical outcomes, psychological outcomes such as depression, self-efficacy, and life satisfaction are positively influenced. Patients can be referred to the Arthritis Foundation (www.arthritis.org) for educational materials and information on support groups.

Lifestyle modification should be encouraged for all patients at risk for and with established OA. Low-impact exercise is advisable for most patients, especially those with knee or hip OA. Aerobic exercise and strength-training programs improve functional capacity in older adults with OA. Stretching and strengthening exercises should target affected and vulnerable joints. Isokinetic and isotonic exercises performed at least three to four times weekly improve physical functioning and decrease disability, pain, and analgesic use.

Obesity's association with both the onset and progression of OA make weight loss a pivotal treatment goal in overweight and obese patients. Women who reduce body weight by 5 kg (11 lb) can cut their risk of developing OA in half. Moreover, symptomatic relief and improved quality of life occur in people with knee OA who lose weight. Weight loss should be pursued through a combination of dietary modification and increased physical activity (see Chapter 102, Overweight and Obesity). The patient's physical capabilities should be considered when implementing an exercise program.

Application of heat or cold to involved joints improves range of motion, reduces pain, and decreases muscle spasms. Applications of heat include warm baths or warm water soaks. Heating pads should be used with caution, especially in the elderly, and patients must be warned of the potential for burns if used inappropriately.

Referral to a physical or occupational therapist may be helpful, particularly in patients with functional disabilities. Physical therapy is tailored to the patient and may include assessment of muscle strength, joint stability, and mobility; use of heat (especially prior to episodes of increased physical activity); structured exercise regimens; and assistive devices such as canes, crutches, and walkers. The occupational therapist ensures optimal joint protection and function, energy conservation, and advice on use of splints and other assistive devices.

Patient Encounter, Part 1

A 67-year-old obese African American man presents to his primary care physician with right knee pain that has significantly worsened over the past several years. He describes the pain as dull and achy, and it is most severe in the morning after awakening until he "loosens up" 10 to 15 minutes later. He believes the morning stiffness is related to a previous knee surgery for his torn meniscus. He also reports feeling "down" because he is no longer able to play golf with his friends due to his knee pain. He is a retired store clerk in a position that required him to be on his feet for long hours in addition to lifting heavy boxes.

What information is suggestive of osteoarthritis (OA)?

What risk factors for OA does this patient have?

What cultural or ethnic factors may contribute to his OA?

What other information will you need to differentiate OA from rheumatoid arthritis (RA)?

What potential comorbidities should be considered in this patient?

What other information will be required before formulating a treatment plan?

Pharmacologic Therapy

Simple analgesics such as acetaminophen and nonsteroidal anti-inflammatory drugs (NSAIDs) are first-line agents for treating OA (Table 58–1).

▶ *Acetaminophen*

Acetaminophen is a centrally acting analgesic that inhibits prostaglandin production in the brain and spinal cord. KEY CONCEPT *Acetaminophen is an effective and inexpensive analgesic with a favorable risk–benefit profile. For treatment of mild-to-moderate pain, acetaminophen should be tried initially at an adequate dose and duration before considering an NSAID.*[8–11] Acetaminophen is generally considered to be as effective as NSAIDs for mild-to-moderate joint pain with a more favorable adverse effect profile.[11]

Acetaminophen should be administered initially on an as-needed basis in daily doses up to 4 g. Single doses should not exceed 1 g. Some patients may require scheduled dosing to achieve adequate pain relief. Periodic assessment of pain control should be performed to maintain the lowest effective dose. A common reason for an inadequate response to acetaminophen is failure

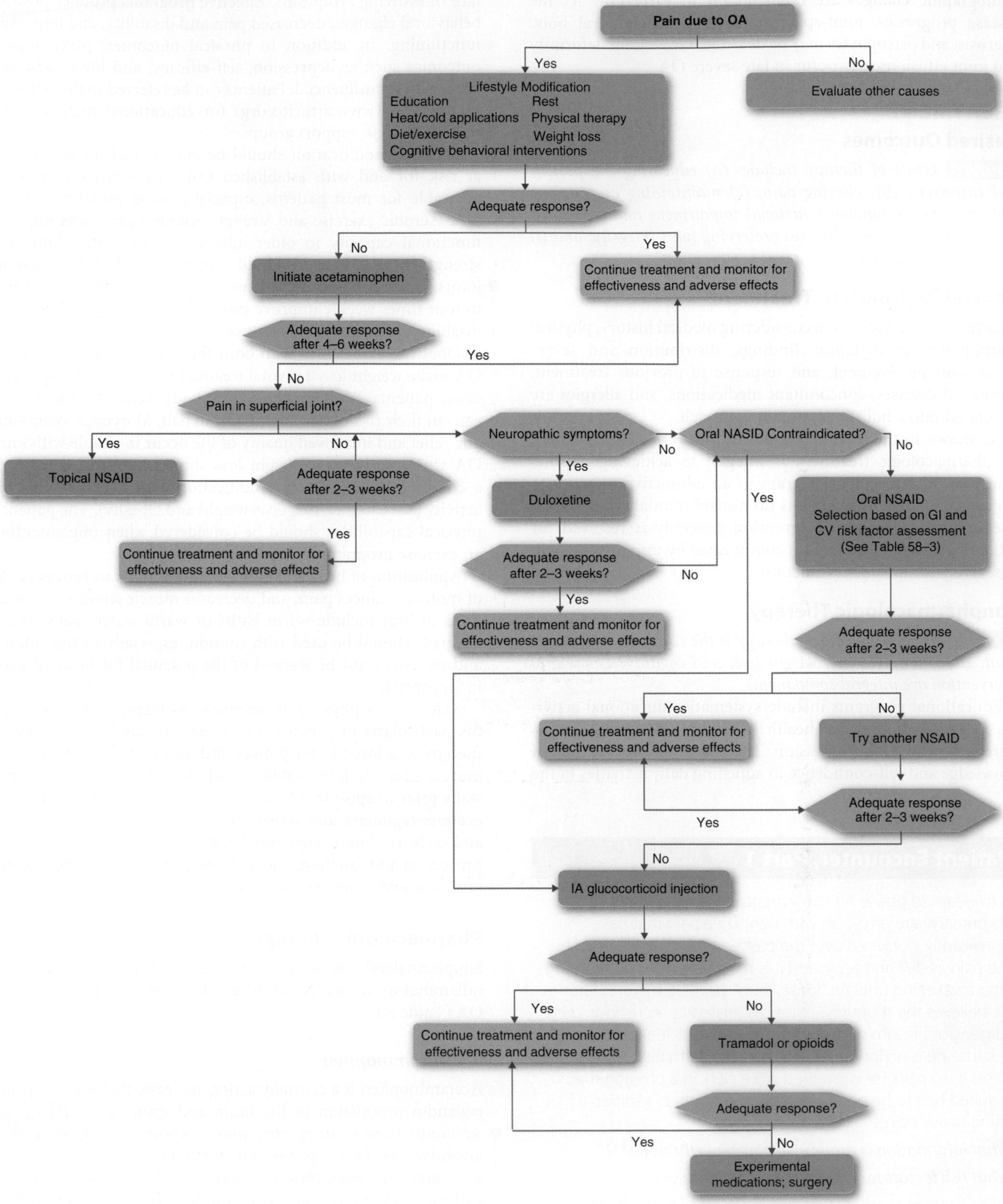

FIGURE 58–2. Treatment of osteoarthritis. (OA, osteoarthritis; CV, cardiovascular; IA, intraarticular; NSAID, nonsteroidal anti-inflammatory drug.)

Table 58–1

Dosing Parameters of Agents Commonly Used to Treat OA

Medication	Dosage and Frequency	Maximum Dosage (mg/day)
Oral Analgesics		
Acetaminophen	325 mg every 4–6 hours or 1 g every 6–8 hours	4000 (consider all products utilized containing acetaminophen)
Tramadol	50–100 mg every 4–6 hours	400 (300 in elderly)
	CrCl < 30 mL/min (0.50 mL/s): 50–100 mg every 12 hours	200
Oxycodone	5–15 mg every 4–6 hours (initial dose for opioid naive)	Dependent on degree of opioid tolerance and patient response
Serotonin-Norepinephrine Reuptake inhibitors		
Duloxetine	30–60 mg once daily	60
Intraarticular Steroid Injection		
Triamcinolone hexacetonide	2–6 mg Smaller joints; 10–20 mg Larger joints	No more often than every 3 months
Methylprednisolone acetate	Small joints 4–10 mg; Medium joints 10–40 mg; Large joins 20–80 mg	No more often than every 3 months
Oral NSAIDs by Chemical Class		
Carboxylic acid (salicylates)		
Aspirin	325–650 mg every 4–6 hours	3600[a]
Salsalate	500–1000 mg two to three times daily	3000[a]
Acetic acid		
Etodolac	300–600 mg twice daily	1200
	400–1000 mg once daily (extended release)	
Diclofenac	50 mg two to three times daily	150
	75 mg twice daily (delayed-release tablets)	
	100 mg once daily (extended-release tablets)	
	35 mg three times daily (submicron particle capsules)	
Indomethacin	25 mg two to three times daily	200
	75 mg one to two times daily (sustained-release)	
Nabumetone	500–1000 mg one to two times daily	2000
Propionic acid		
Ibuprofen	400–800 mg three to four times daily	3200
Naproxen	250–500 mg two times daily	1500
	750–1000 mg once daily (controlled-release)	
	275–550 mg two times daily (naproxen sodium)	1650
Enolic acid		
Meloxicam	7.5–15 mg once daily	15
Piroxicam	20 mg once daily	20
Coxibs		
Celecoxib[c]	100 mg twice daily or 200 mg once daily	200
Topical Analgesics		
Capsaicin 0.025% or 0.075% cream	Apply to affected joint every 6–8 hours	
Diclofenac sodium 1% gel	Upper extremity joints: 2 g four times daily;	8 g[b]
	Lower extremity joints: 4 g four times daily	16 g[b]
Diclofenac sodium 1.5% solution	40 drops per affected knee, four times per day	
Diclofenac sodium 2% solution	40 mg (2 pump actuations) on each painful knee, two times a day	
Dietary Supplements		
Glucosamine sulfate	500 mg three times daily or 1500 mg once daily	
Chondroitin	400–800 mg three times daily with glucosamine	

CrCl, creatinine clearance.

[a]Serum salicylate levels should be monitored for doses greater than 3 g/day.

[b]Total daily dose of diclofenac 1% gel should not exceed 32 g for all affected joints.

[c]Celecoxib is a substrate for CYP2C9, and a 50% reduction in the initial dose should be considered in known or suspected poor metabolizers.

to use a sufficient dose for an adequate duration. A sufficient trial is defined as up to 4 g daily in divided doses for 4 to 6 weeks.

Despite being one of the safest analgesics, acetaminophen can cause significant adverse effects, including hepatic and renal toxicity.[12] Acetaminophen overdose, both intentional and unintentional, is the leading cause of acute liver injury in the United States.[13] Doses greater than 4 g are associated with an increased risk of hepatotoxicity. Total daily doses of 4 g have been associated with significant liver enzyme elevations, but such elevations do not necessarily portend hepatotoxicity.[14] Concomitant use of alcohol may increase the risk of hepatic injury; a maximum acetaminophen dose of 2.5 g daily is recommended in patients who consume more than two to three alcoholic beverages per day. Acetaminophen does not appear to exacerbate stable, chronic liver disease; it can be used with caution and vigilant monitoring of liver function in this population.[12] Prior to developing an acetaminophen regimen, a careful inventory should be taken of all concomitant prescription medications and over-the-counter products to minimize the risk of inadvertent acetaminophen overdose.

Acetaminophen may worsen kidney function and increase blood pressure.[15,16] Nevertheless, acetaminophen remains the preferred oral analgesic for mild-to-moderate pain in patients with hypertension or kidney disease because of the greater risks associated with NSAID use.[17] Monitoring specifically for these adverse effects generally is unnecessary.

▶ *Nonsteroidal Anti-inflammatory Drugs*

Prostaglandins play an important role in the function of several organ systems. These compounds are synthesized via the interaction of two isoforms of the cyclooxygenase enzyme (COX-1 and COX-2) with their substrate, arachidonic acid.

The COX-1 enzyme is expressed constitutively in various body tissues (eg, gastric mucosa, kidney, and platelets). Prostaglandins produced by the actions of the COX-1 enzyme in the gastrointestinal (GI) tract preserve the integrity of the GI mucosa by increasing mucous and bicarbonate secretion, maintaining mucosal blood flow, and decreasing gastric acid secretion. Prostaglandins associated with COX-1 also promote normal platelet activity and function. In the kidney, COX-1–mediated prostaglandins dilate the afferent arteriole, thereby maintaining intraglomerular pressure and glomerular filtration rate when renal blood flow is reduced.

In contrast, the COX-2 enzyme is normally undetectable in most tissues, but its expression can be induced rapidly in the presence of inflammation and local tissue injury. This change leads to the synthesis of prostaglandins involved in pain and inflammation. Consequently, blocking the COX-2 enzyme is thought to result in analgesic and anti-inflammatory effects. All NSAIDs inhibit both the COX-1 and COX-2 enzyme isoforms, but nonselective NSAIDs (eg, ibuprofen, diclofenac, naproxen) are not particularly selective for one isoform over the other, whereas COX-2 inhibitors (ie, celecoxib) preferentially inhibit the COX-2 isoform.

KEY CONCEPT *NSAIDs are a reasonable first-line therapy in patients with moderate-to-severe OA; or, as adjunctive or alternative therapy when acetaminophen fails to provide an acceptable analgesic response.* NSAIDs significantly reduce pain and improve functioning in patients with OA, although individual responses can vary widely. Some clinicians recommend NSAIDs over acetaminophen for the initial treatment of severe pain or when signs and symptoms of inflammation are present. Results from comparative trials of acetaminophen and NSAIDs have been equivocal, but consensus guidelines support the use of NSAIDs as an alternative to acetaminophen if clinical features of peripheral inflammation or severe pain are present.[8–10] Unfortunately, no validated mechanism exists to identify patients who are more likely to respond to NSAIDs than acetaminophen. The route of administration (ie, oral or topical) should be based on affected joint(s), patient preference, ability to administer, and an assessment of risk for adverse effects of systemic NSAIDs.

Topical administration of NSAIDs minimizes systemic exposure while providing pain relief comparable to that of oral NSAIDs, but topical NSAIDs are only appropriate for patients with OA of superficial joints, including hands, wrists, elbows, knees, ankles, and feet. Currently, the only commercially available topical NSAID in the United States is diclofenac, which comes in a variety of preparations, including a solution, gel, and topical patch. These products all decrease pain and improve joint function with no demonstrated superiority for any one product over others.[18–21] Systemic absorption of topical diclofenac is significantly less than that of oral diclofenac. Thus, GI, cardiovascular, and renal adverse effects are rare and similar in incidence to placebo with proper administration. The most common adverse effects include application site dermatitis, pruritus, and phototoxicity.

For patients with OA that affects deeper joints (eg, hip), or who have not achieved an adequate response to topical NSAIDs, an oral NSAID should be considered. KEY CONCEPT *At equipotent doses, the analgesic and anti-inflammatory activity of all oral NSAIDs, including COX-2–selective inhibitors, are similar.* The selection of a specific oral NSAID should be based on patient preference, previous response, tolerability, dosing frequency, cost, and considering underlying GI and cardiovascular risk. Some patients respond to one NSAID better than to another. If an insufficient response is achieved with one NSAID, another agent should be tried. Pain relief occurs rapidly (within hours) with these agents, but anti-inflammatory benefits are not realized until after 2 to 3 weeks of continuous therapy. This period is the minimal duration that should be considered an adequate NSAID trial.

KEY CONCEPT *All NSAIDs are associated with adverse GI, renal, hepatic, cardiovascular, CNS, and blood pressure effects, particularly in the elderly.* Inhibition of the COX-1 enzyme is thought to be responsible primarily for the adverse effects on the gastric mucosa, kidney, and platelets. Direct irritant effects also may contribute to adverse GI events. Minor GI complaints, including nausea, dyspepsia, anorexia, abdominal pain, flatulence, and diarrhea, are reported by 10% to 60% of patients treated with nonselective NSAIDs. Asymptomatic gastric and duodenal mucosal ulceration can be detected in 15% to 45% of patients.[22] Perforation, gastric outlet obstruction, and GI bleeding are the most severe complications and occur in 1.5% to 4% of patients annually.[22]

KEY CONCEPT *COX-2 inhibitors should be reserved for patients at high risk for GI complications and low risk for cardiovascular events* (Table 58–2).[23] Several risk factors predict a greater likelihood of GI complications in NSAID-treated patients (see Chapter 18, Peptic Ulcer Disease). Detecting high-risk patients based on symptoms alone is impractical because the presence of symptoms and actual gastroduodenal damage are poorly correlated. For patients at particularly high GI risk (eg, previous history of NSAID-induced GI bleed), a selective COX-2 inhibitor combined with a proton pump inhibitor reduces risk for GI bleeds compared to a selective COX-2 inhibitor alone, which in turn has lower risk for GI bleeds compared to a nonselective NSAID combined with a proton pump inhibitor.[24–26]

Table 58–2

Treatment Options Based on Cardiovascular and Gastrointestinal Risk

	High CV Risk[a]	Low CV Risk
High GI risk[b]	NS-NSAID[c] *plus* gastroprotection[d]	COX-2[e] *or* NS-NSAID + gastroprotection[d]
Low GI risk	NS-NSAID[c]	NS-NSAID

COX-2, selective cyclooxygenase-2 inhibitor; CV, cardiovascular; NS-NSAID, nonselective nonsteroidal anti-inflammatory drug.

[a]Low-dose aspirin indicated for prevention of cardiovascular event.

[b]History of complicated ulcer or > 2 of the following: Age > 65 years, high dose NSAID, prior uncomplicated ulcer, and current use of aspirin, corticosteroids, or anticoagulants.

[c]Naproxen may be considered initially due to potentially lower CV risk compared with other NS-NSAIDs.

[d]Gastroprotection with either a proton pump inhibitor (preferred) or misoprostol.

[e]A COX-2 inhibitor + gastroprotection can be recommended for patients at very high GI risk (eg, previous upper GI bleed attributable to NS-NSAID therapy).

Although selective COX-2 inhibitors reduce GI events, these agents have been associated with increased risk of cardiovascular events relative to many nonselective NSAIDs.[27–29] The pharmacologic basis for this finding is not fully understood, but multiple factors may be involved, including the degree of COX-2 selectivity, dosage and dosing schedule, and potency of agents.[27] Other mechanisms for increasing cardiovascular risk have been proposed for individual agents.[30] Large scale meta-analyses suggest that COX-2 inhibitors (including celecoxib) and, to a lesser extent, diclofenac and ibuprofen, have the strongest association with major vascular events (eg, stroke, myocardial infarction).[31,32]

In patients at risk for GI events and cardiovascular disease and requiring oral NSAID therapy, a nonselective NSAID plus a proton pump inhibitor is a reasonable option. Naproxen appears to have the lowest incremental cardiovascular risk of the nonselective NSAIDs and should generally be considered first in such patients.[32] Concomitant use of low-dose aspirin mitigates some of the increased cardiovascular risk of selective COX-2 inhibitors but also obliterates the GI safety of COX-2 selectivity.[33–35] Patients treated with a selective COX-2 inhibitor plus aspirin experience GI complications at a rate commensurate with that of patients given a nonselective NSAID. Use of NSAIDs that have more relative COX-2 inhibition but are not selective COX-2 inhibitors (eg, meloxicam) to avoid cardiovascular concerns with selective COX-2 inhibitors may not be justified because neither GI nor cardiovascular safety is optimized.[36]

All NSAIDs can cause renal insufficiency when administered to patients whose renal function depends on prostaglandins. Patients with chronic renal insufficiency or left ventricular dysfunction, the elderly, and those receiving diuretics or drugs that interfere with the renin–angiotensin system are particularly susceptible. These effects may result in decreased glomerular filtration, hyperkalemia, and sodium and water retention. Therefore, both nonselective NSAIDs and selective COX-2 inhibitors should be used with caution in patients with hypertension, heart failure, or chronic renal insufficiency. NSAIDs rarely cause **tubulointerstitial** nephropathy and renal papillary necrosis.

Caution is warranted in pregnant women and women of childbearing potential because the risk of bleeding may be increased if the fetus is subjected to the antiplatelet activity of NSAIDs. Most NSAIDs are Category C before 30 weeks of gestation. After that, all NSAIDs should be avoided because they may promote premature closure of the ductus arteriosus in the fetus.

Nonselective NSAIDs and selective COX-2 inhibitors are prone to drug interactions due to high protein binding, detrimental renal effects, and antiplatelet activity. Interactions are encountered frequently with aspirin, warfarin, oral hypoglycemics, antihypertensives (ie, angiotensin-converting enzyme [ACE] inhibitors, angiotensin receptor blockers [ARBs], β-blockers, diuretics), and lithium. When potential interactions are present, vigilant monitoring is warranted for therapeutic efficacy (eg, NSAIDs blunt the antihypertensive efficacy of diuretics) and adverse effects (eg, NSAIDs increase the risk of bleeding in anticoagulated patients).

▶ Tramadol

Use of opioid analgesics may be warranted when pain is unresponsive to other pharmacologic agents or when such agents are contraindicated. Tramadol is an oral, centrally acting synthetic opioid analgesic that also weakly inhibits the reuptake of serotonin and norepinephrine. Tramadol effectively treats moderate pain but is devoid of anti-inflammatory activity. Tramadol is scheduled as a controlled substance (C-IV) in the United States due to its comparatively low abuse potential.

Tramadol is a reasonable option for patients with contraindications to NSAIDs or in those who have failed to respond to other oral therapies. The addition of tramadol to NSAIDs or acetaminophen may augment the analgesic effects of a failing regimen, thereby securing sufficient pain relief in some patients.[37] Moreover, concomitant tramadol may permit the use of lower NSAID doses. However, the increased risk for side effects associated with tramadol may offset the benefits.[37]

Dizziness, vertigo, nausea, vomiting, constipation, and lethargy are all relatively common adverse events. These effects are more pronounced for several days after initiation and following upward dose titration. Seizures have been reported rarely; the risk is dose-related and appears to increase with concomitant use of antidepressants, such as tricyclic antidepressants or selective serotonin reuptake inhibitors. Tramadol should be avoided in patients receiving monoamine oxidase (MAO) inhibitors due to the potential for serotonin syndrome.

▶ Other Opioid Analgesics

Opioids decrease pain, improve sleep patterns, and increase functioning in patients with OA who are unresponsive to nonpharmacologic therapy and nonopioid analgesics. Evidence suggests that patients can achieve satisfactory analgesia by using nonescalating doses of opioids with minimal risk of addiction.[38] However, clinically significant improvement in pain that is nonresponsive to NSAIDs has only been demonstrated with stronger opioids. Oxycodone is the most extensively studied of the opioids recommended for OA. However, other agents such as morphine, hydromorphone, methadone, and transdermal fentanyl are also effective.[39]

Opioid analgesics should be reserved for patients who experience pain severe enough to require opioid treatment for which alternative treatment options are inadequate. Opioids also may be appropriate in patients with severe OA and conditions that preclude the use of NSAIDs, such as renal failure, heart failure, or anticoagulation.

Opioids should be initiated at low doses in combination with acetaminophen or an NSAID when possible. Combining opioids with other analgesics reduces the opioid requirement, thereby minimizing adverse events. However, use of combination opioid products containing acetaminophen should be accompanied by clear instructions to limit additional over-the-counter acetaminophen use. Conservative initial doses of opioids are warranted, with the dose titrated to the lowest dose achieving an adequate response while minimizing adverse effects. Even with these conservative strategies, adverse effects are common. In clinical trials, more than 80% of opioid-treated patients experienced at least one adverse event, compared with approximately 50% of placebo-treated patients.[39] Common or serious adverse effects include nausea, constipation, sedation, and respiratory depression (see Chapter 34, Pain Management).

If opioid therapy is considered, there should be an initial comprehensive medical history and physical examination, documentation that nonopioid therapy has failed, clearly defined treatment goals, an understanding between the provider and the patient of the true benefits and risks of long-term opioids, use of a single provider and pharmacy whenever possible, and comprehensive follow-up.

▸ Duloxetine

Duloxetine, a serotonin/norepinephrine reuptake inhibitor (SNRI), is effective as adjunctive therapy for knee OA in patients achieving a suboptimal response to acetaminophen or oral NSAIDs alone.[40] Benefits typically are observed only after several weeks of therapy with moderate doses (ie, 60 mg/day); larger doses do not provide additional benefit.[41] Duloxetine may be the preferred adjunctive treatment in patients experiencing concurrent neuropathic and musculoskeletal pain. The most common adverse events are nausea, dry mouth, somnolence, constipation, decreased appetite, and hyperhidrosis.[41] Concomitant use with tramadol should be done cautiously owing to an increased risk of serotonin syndrome.

▸ Intraarticular Therapy

Intraarticular therapies represent an alternative to oral agents for treatment of joint pain. This modality is usually reserved for patients unresponsive to other treatments because of the relative invasiveness of intraarticular injections compared with oral and topical drugs, the small risk of infection, and the cost of the procedure.

Corticosteroids Use of systemic corticosteroids is discouraged in patients with OA. KEY CONCEPT *However, in a subset of patients with an inflammatory component or knee effusion, intraarticular corticosteroids can be useful as monotherapy or as an adjunct to analgesics.*[42] Corticosteroids with reduced solubility, such as methylprednisolone and triamcinolone, are usually preferred. The affected joint can be aspirated and subsequently injected with the corticosteroid. The aspirate should be examined for the presence of crystal formation and infection. Pain relief begins within days after the injection but may wane beyond 3 weeks. Injections should be done as infrequently as possible to avoid joint damage. Specifically, a single joint should not be injected more than three to five times per year to reduce the risk of corticosteroid-induced cartilage and joint damage. Given that the recommended dosing interval greatly exceeds the typical duration of action, these agents are rarely effective as monotherapy for chronic treatment of OA.

The crystalline nature of corticosteroid suspensions can provoke a postinjection flare in some patients. The ensuing flare mimics the flare of arthritis and inflammation that accompanies infection. Cold compresses and analgesics are recommended to treat symptoms in affected patients.

Hyaluronic Acid The mechanism of action of hyaluronic acid is not fully understood. Healthy cartilage and synovial fluid are replete with hyaluronic acid, a viscous substance believed to facilitate lubrication and shock absorbency under varying conditions of load bearing. Patients with OA demonstrate an absolute and functional decline in hyaluronic acid; thus, exogenous administration is referred to as viscosupplementation.

Improvement in pain and joint function following intraarticular hyaluronic acid injections has been evaluated frequently in clinical trials, most of which were of low quality. Evidence is conflicting, but these agents appear to promote only modest improvements in pain and joint function. Consequently, hyaluronic acid is generally not recommended in current treatment guidelines.[43]

Several formulations of hyaluronic acid are available in the United States for treatment of knee OA. Administration typically consists of weekly injections for 3 to 5 weeks, depending on the specific product. Most injections are well tolerated, although some patients may report local reactions. Rarely, postinjection flares and anaphylaxis have been reported. Intra-articular injection is associated with a low risk of infection (approximately 1 joint in 50,000 injections). Patients should be counseled to minimize activity and stress on the joint for several days after each injection.

▸ Over-the-Counter Agents

Glucosamine and Chondroitin Glucosamine is believed to function as a "chondroprotective" agent, stimulating the cartilage matrix and protecting against oxidative chemical damage. Chondroitin, often administered in conjunction with glucosamine, is thought to inhibit degradative enzymes and serve as a substrate for the production of proteoglycans. The highest quality evidence to date suggests no clinically important difference in efficacy between glucosamine, chondroitin, their combination, or placebo in patients with knee OA.[44] Consequently, these products, used alone or in combination, are generally not recommended.[45]

These agents are loosely regulated in the United States as dietary supplements, product standards are inconsistent, and the constituents are not validated by any regulatory agency. The use of glucosamine (derived from crab, lobster, or shrimp shells) and/or chondroitin (derived from cattle or shark cartilage) may warrant caution in patients with shellfish allergies, but preliminary evidence suggests little drug–allergy interaction.[46] Additionally, glucosamine may alter cellular glucose uptake, thus elevating blood glucose levels in diabetic patients.[47] Because the clinical significance of this is unclear, blood glucose levels in diabetic patients should be monitored closely after glucosamine initiation or dosage adjustments.

Other Topical Agents There are limited data to support the use of salicylate-containing rubefacients (eg, methyl salicylate and trolamine salicylate) or other counterirritants (eg, menthol, camphor, and methyl nicotinate) in OA.[48] See Chapter 60 (Musculoskeletal Disorders) for more information on these products when used for musculoskeletal disorders.

Capsaicin achieves pain relief by depleting substance P from sensory neurons in the spine, thereby decreasing pain transmission. Capsaicin is not effective for acute pain; it may take up to 2 weeks of daily administration to achieve pain relief. Capsaicin may provide the greatest benefit to painful superficial joints (eg, hand OA). The lower concentration (0.025%) is typically better tolerated. Most patients experience a local burning sensation at the site of application. The discomfort usually does not result in discontinuation and often abates within the first week. Patients should be cautioned not to allow capsaicin to come into contact with eyes or mucous membranes and to wash their hands after each application.

Surgery

Surgery generally is reserved for patients who fail to respond to medical therapy and have progressive limitations in activities of daily living (ADL). In joint replacement surgery (arthroplasty), the damaged joint surfaces are replaced with metal or plastic prosthetic devices. Hip and knee joints are most commonly replaced, but arthroplasty may also be performed on shoulders, elbows, fingers, and ankles. Most patients achieve significant pain relief and functional restoration after arthroplasty, and it is a reasonable option in carefully selected refractory patients.

Surgical debridement may be performed arthroscopically. With this procedure, a tiny video camera is inserted into the affected joint through a small incision, and the surgeon removes torn cartilage or other debris from the joint. The long-term benefits of arthroscopic surgery for OA are unclear, and it may be no better than optimized physical and medical therapy.[49]

OUTCOME EVALUATION

- At baseline, quantify pain using a visual analogue scale, assess range of motion of affected joints, and identify activities of daily living that are impaired.
- In patients treated with acetaminophen or oral NSAIDs, assess pain control after 2 to 3 weeks. It may take longer for the full anti-inflammatory effect of NSAIDs to occur.
- Incorporate other measures to track disease progress. Use radiography to assess severity of joint destruction, determine 50-ft (~15 m) walking time and grip strength, and administer the Western Ontario and McMaster Universities Osteoarthritis Index (WOMAC) and the Stanford Health Assessment Questionnaire, where appropriate, to assess activities of daily living.
- Ask patients if they are experiencing side effects or other problems with their medications and respond with more specific questions.
- In patients taking oral NSAIDs, monitor for increases in blood pressure, weight gain, edema, skin rash, and CNS adverse effects such as headaches and drowsiness.
- Evaluate serum creatinine, complete blood count, and serum transaminases at baseline and at every 6 to 12 months in patients treated with oral NSAIDs or acetaminophen.
- Perform stool guaiac in patients taking oral NSAIDs when clinically indicated.
- Monitor for drug interactions, including alcohol, at every visit.

Patient Encounter, Part 3: Creating a Care Plan

Based on the available information, create a care plan for this patient's OA. The plan should include:

(a) A statement of the drug-related needs and/or problems

(b) An individualized, detailed therapeutic plan

(c) A plan for follow-up monitoring to document the patient's response and identify adverse reactions

Patient Encounter, Part 2: Medical History, Physical Examination, and Diagnostic Tests

PMH: Obesity (BMI 30 kg/m^2), HTN for 24 years, dyslipidemia, nonischemic cardiomyopathy, COPD, heat failure with reduced ejection fraction

PSH: Torn meniscus s/p repair on right knee 20 years ago

FH: Father had OA of the hip and knee; mother died of MI at age 68

SH: Retired clerk. Denies alcohol use; denies illicit drug use; smoked two packs of cigarettes per day for 35 years but quit 3 years ago

Allergies: NKDA; shellfish allergy

Meds: Lisinopril 40 mg once daily; metoprolol succinate 200 mg once daily; furosemide 20 mg once daily; spironolactone 25 mg once daily; atorvastatin 20 mg once daily; enteric-coated aspirin 81 mg once daily; tiotropium 18 mcg once daily; albuterol 90 mcg as needed for wheezing/shortness of breath; acetaminophen 500 mg one to two tablets two to four times per day as needed for pain

ROS: (+) SOB on exertion, right knee pain 5 out of 10 with movement

PE:

VS: BP 119/72 mm Hg, Pulse 61 beats/min, RR 16 breaths/min, T 98.6°F (37.0°C)

Skin: Warm, dry, cracked skin on feet bilaterally

HEENT: NC/AT, PERRLA, TMs intact

CV: RRR, normal S_1 and S_2, no m/r/g

Chest: CTA

Abd: Soft, NT/ND

Neuro: A&O × 3; CN II to XII intact

Ext: Bilateral ankle nonpitting edema, slight swelling of soft tissue surrounding right knee with crepitus and slight decrease in range of motion

Labs: ESR 12 mm/hour; basic metabolic panel within normal limits

Knee x-rays: Right knee shows joint space narrowing, minor osteophyte formation, and subchondral bone sclerosis

What clinical parameters are consistent with a diagnosis of OA?

What are the treatment goals for this patient?

What nonpharmacologic options are available to treat this patient?

What pharmacologic options are available to treat this patient?

What factors are important to consider when selecting medications for this patient?

Patient Care Process

Patient Assessment:

- Determine whether the patient's symptoms are consistent with OA. Review the medical history to determine whether other rheumatologic diseases may be involved.
- Assess symptoms to determine whether pain warrants additional attention. Does the pain affect quality of life or interfere with activities of daily living?
- Assess radiographs for diagnosis and disease severity (joint-space narrowing, subchondral bone sclerosis, osteophyte formation, joint deformity, joint effusion).
- Consider obtaining laboratory tests depending on degree of clinical suspicion for inflammatory etiology (eg, ESR, CRP, rheumatoid factor, ANA).

Therapy Evaluation:

- Obtain a thorough history of previous device and drug use, including prescription drugs, over-the-counter drugs, and dietary supplements.
- Assess the effectiveness of any current or previous pharmacotherapy, including dose, frequency, and duration to determine whether an adequate trial was given.

Care Plan Development:

- Formulate a plan for lifestyle modifications and alteration/addition of pharmacotherapy that considers risks, benefits, and patient preference given the patient's medical history, concomitant medications, and previous successful/failed OA therapies.
- Address patient concerns related to OA, its treatment, with special focus on the potential adverse effects of medications.
- Emphasize the value of adherence to medication regimens and lifestyle modifications. Facilitate adherence by implementing medication regimens and lifestyle plans that are simple and consistent with the patient's lifestyle.

Follow-Up Evaluation:

- Schedule follow-up to assess the effectiveness of therapy and associated adverse effects; the specific time frame depends on patient factors and the treatment regimen chosen. If laboratory tests (eg, renal function) are required for monitoring drug therapy, provide the patient with an order for the laboratory tests and instructions to complete them prior to the next appointment.
- Document whether the patient has had improvements in pain, quality-of-life measures, mobility and functioning, ability to perform activities of daily living, and well-being.
- Ascertain new OTC medication use; for patients taking acetaminophen, pay particular attention to OTC sources of acetaminophen.
- Evaluate for the presence of adverse drug reactions, drug hypersensitivity, and potential drug interactions.

Abbreviations Introduced in This Chapter

ACR	American College of Rheumatology
APS	American Pain Society
COX	Cyclooxygenase
NSAID	Nonsteroidal anti-inflammatory drug
OA	Osteoarthritis
WOMAC	Western Ontario and McMaster Universities Osteoarthritis Index

REFERENCES

1. Centers for Disease Control and Prevention. National and state medical expenditures and lost earnings attributable to arthritis and other rheumatic conditions—United States, 2003. MMWR Morb Mortal Wkly Rep. 2007;56(1):4–7.
2. Centers for Disease Control and Prevention. Prevalence and most common causes of disability among adults—United States, 2005. MMWR Morb Mortal Wkly Rep. 2009;58:421–426.
3. Cross M, Smith E, Hoy D, et al. The global burden of hip and knee osteoarthritis: Estimates from the Global Burden of Disease 2010 study. Ann Rheum Dis. 2014;73(7):1323–1330.
4. The National Arthritis Data Workgroup. Estimates of the prevalence of arthritis and other rheumatic conditions in the United States: Part II. Arthritis Rheum. 2008;58:26–35.
5. Dijlsma JWJ, Berenbaum F, Lafeber FPJG. Osteoarthritis: An update with relevance for clinical practice. Lancet. 2011;377:2115–2126.
6. McAlindon TE, Wilson PW, Aliabadi P, et al. Level of physical activity and the risk of radiographic and symptomatic knee osteoarthritis in the elderly: The Framingham Study. Am J Med. 1999;106:151–157.
7. Fife RS. Epidemiology, pathology, and pathogenesis. In: Klippel JH, ed. Primer on Rheumatic Diseases, 11th ed. Atlanta, GA: Arthritis Foundation; 1997:216–217.
8. Zhang W, Moskowitz RW, Nuki G, et al. OARSI recommendations for the management of hip and knee osteoarthritis, Part II: OARSI evidence-based, expert consensus guidelines. Osteoarthr Cartil. 2008;16:137–162.
9. Hochberg MC, Altman RD, April KT, et al. American College of Rheumatology 2012 recommendations for the use of nonpharmacologic and pharmacologic therapies in osteoarthritis of the hand, hip, and knee. Arthritis Care Res. 2012;64:465–474.
10. American Pain Society. Guideline for the management of pain in osteoarthritis, rheumatoid arthritis, and juvenile chronic arthritis. American Pain Society 2002;2:43–74.
11. Towheed TE, Maxwell L, Judd MG, et al. Acetaminophen for osteoarthritis. Cochrane Database Syst Rev. 2006;(1):CD004257.
12. Graham GG, Scott KF, Day RO. Tolerability of paracetamol. Drug Saf. 2005;28:227–240.
13. Larson AM, Polson J, Fontana RJ, et al. Acetaminophen-induced acute liver failure: Results of a United States multicenter prospective study. Hepatology. 2005;42:1364–1372.
14. Watkins PB, Kaplowitz N, Slattery JT, et al. Aminotransferase elevations in healthy adults receiving 4 grams of acetaminophen daily. JAMA. 2006;296:87–93.
15. Fored CM, Ejerblad E, Lindblad P, et al. Acetaminophen, aspirin, and chronic renal failure. N Engl J Med. 2001;345:1801–1808.

16. Curhan GC, Knight EL, Rosner B, et al. Lifetime non-narcotic analgesic use and decline in renal function in women. Arch Intern Med. 2004;164:1519–1524.
17. Forman JP, Stampfer MJ, Curhan GC. Non-narcotic analgesic dose and risk of incident hypertension in U.S. women. Hypertension. 2005;46:500–507.
18. Baraf HS, Gloth FM, Barthel HR, et al. Safety and efficacy of topical diclofenac sodium gel for knee osteoarthritis in elderly and younger patients: Pooled data from three randomized, double-blind, parallel-group, placebo-controlled, multicentre trials. Drugs Aging. 2011;28:27–40.
19. Altman RD, Dreiser RL, Fisher CL. Diclofenac sodium gel in patients with primary hand osteoathritis: A randomized, double-blind, placebo-controlled trial. J Rheumatol. 2009;36(9): 1991–1999.
20. Derry, S, Moore RA, Rabbie R. Topical NSAIDs for chronic musculoskeletal pain in adults. Cochrane Database Syst Rev. 2012;12(9):CD007400.
21. Flector Patch [package insert]. Bristol, TN: King Pharmaceuticals, Inc; 2011. http://www.accessdata.fda.gov/drugsatfda_docs/label/2011/021234s005lbl.pdf. Accessed July 11, 2014.
22. Laine L. Approaches to nonsteroidal anti-inflammatory drug use in the high-risk patient. Gastroenterology. 2001;120:594–606.
23. Lanza FL, Chan FKL, Quigley EMM. Guidelines for prevention of NSAID-related ulcer complications. Am J Gastroenterol. 2009; 104:728–738.
24. Chan FKL, Wong VWS, Suen BY, et al. Combination of a cyclo-oxygenase-2 inhibitor and a proton-pump inhibitor for prevention of recurrent ulcer bleeding in patients at very high risk: A double-blind, randomized trial. Lancet. 2007;369:1621–1626.
25. Rahme E, Barkun AN, Toubouti Y, et al. Do proton-pump inhibitors confer additional gastrointestinal protection in patients given celecoxib? Arthritis Rheum. 2007;57:748–755.
26. Chan FK, Lanas A, Scheiman J, Berger MF, Nguyen H, Goldstein JL. Celecoxib versus omeprazole and diclofenac in patients with osteoarthritis and rheumatoid arthritis (CONDOR): A randomised trial. Lancet. 2010;376:173–179.
27. Solomon SD, Wittes J, Finn PV, et al. Cardiovascular risk of celecoxib in 6 randomized placebo-controlled trials: The cross trial safety analysis. Circulation. 2008;117:2104–2113.
28. McGettigan P, Henry D. Cardiovascular risk and inhibition of cyclooxygenase: A systematic review of the observational studies of selective and nonselective inhibitors of cyclooxygenase 2. JAMA. 2006;296:1633–1644.
29. Bresalier RS, Sandler RS, Quan H, et al. Cardiovascular events associated with rofecoxib in a colorectal adenoma chemoprevention trial. N Engl J Med. 2005;352:1092–1102.
30. Zarraga IG, Schwarz ER. Coxibs and heart disease: What we have learned and what else we need to know. J Am Coll Cardiol. 2007;49:1–14.
31. Bhala N, Emberson J, Merhi A, et al. Vascular and upper gastrointestinal effects of non-steroidal anti-inflammatory drugs: Meta-analyses of individual participant data from randomised trials. Lancet. 2013;382:769–779.
32. Trelle S, Reichenbach S, Wandel S, et al. Cardiovascular safety of non-steroidal anti-inflammatory drugs: Network meta-analysis. BMJ. 2011;342:c7086.
33. Silverstein FE, Faich G, Goldstein JL, et al. Gastrointestinal toxicity with celecoxib vs nonsteroidal anti-inflammatory drugs for osteoarthritis and rheumatoid arthritis: The CLASS study: A randomized controlled trial. Celecoxib Long-term Arthritis Safety Study. JAMA. 2000;284:1247–1255.
34. Bombardier C, Laine L, Reicin A, et al. VIGOR Study Group. Comparison of upper gastrointestinal toxicity of rofecoxib and naproxen in patients with rheumatoid arthritis. N Engl J Med. 2000;343:1520–1528.
35. Schnitzer TJ, Burmester GR, Mysler E, et al. Comparison of lumiracoxib with naproxen and ibuprofen in the Therapeutic Arthritis Research and Gastrointestinal Event Trial (TARGET), reduction in ulcer complications: Randomised controlled trial. Lancet. 2004;364:665–674.
36. Gonzalez ELM, Patrignani P, Tacconelli S, Rodriguez LAG. Variability among nonsteroidal antiinflammatory drugs in risk of upper gastrointestinal bleeding. Arthritis Rheum. 2010;62:1592–1601.
37. Cepeda MS, Camargo F, Zea C, Valencia L. Tramadol for osteoarthritis. Cochrane Database Syst Rev. 2006;3:CD005522.
38. Ballantyne JC, Mao J. Opioid therapy for chronic pain. N Engl J Med. 2003;349:1943–1953.
39. Nüesch E, Rutjes AW, Husni E, et al. Oral or transdermal opioids for osteoarthritis of the knee or hip. Cochrane Database Syst Rev. 2009;4:CD003115.
40. McAlindon TE, Bannuru RR, Sullivan MC, et al. OARSI guidelines for the non-surgical management of knee osteoarthritis. Osteoarthritis Cartliage. 2014;22:363–388.
41. Cymbalta [package insert]. Indianapolis, IN: Eli Lilly and Company; 2012. http://dailymed.nlm.nih.gov/dailymed/lookup.cfm?setid=2f7d4d67-10c1-4bf4-a7f2-c185fbad64ba#s145. Accessed July 15, 2014.
42. Bellamy N, Campbell J, Robinson V, et al. Intraarticular corticosteroid for treatment of osteoarthritis of the knee. Cochrane Database Syst Rev. 2006;(2):CD005328.
43. Nelson AE, Allen KD, Golightly YM, Goode AP, Jordan JM. A systematic review of recommendations and guidelines for the management of osteoarthritis: The Chronic Osteoarthritis Management Initiative of the U.S. Bone and Joint Initiative. Semin Arthritis Rheum. 2014;43:701–712.
44. Clegg DO, Reda DJ, Harris CL, et al. Glucosamine, chondroitin sulfate, and the two in combination for painful knee osteoarthritis. N Engl J Med. 2006;354:795–808.
45. Zhang W, Robertson J, Jones AC, Dieppe PA, Doherty M. The placebo effect and its determinants in osteoarthritis: Meta-analysis of randomised controlled trials. Ann Rheum Dis. 2008;67:1716–1723.
46. Gray HC, Hutcheson PS, Gray RG. Is glucosamine safe in patients with seafood allergy? J Allergy Clin Immunol. 2004;114:459–460.
47. Dostrovsky NR, Towheed TE, Hudson RW, Anastassiades TP. The effect of glucosamine on glucose metabolism in humans: A systematic review of the literature. Osteoarthritis Cartilage. 2011;19:375–380.
48. Mason L, Moore RA, Edwards JE, et al. Systematic review of efficacy of topical rubefacients containing salicylates for the treatment of acute and chronic pain. BMJ. 2004;328:995–998.
49. Kirkley A, Birmingham TB, Litchfield RB, et al. A randomized trial of arthroscopic surgery for osteoarthritis of the knee. N Engl J Med. 2008;359:1097–1107.

59 Gout and Hyperuricemia

Maria Miller Thurston

LEARNING OBJECTIVES

Upon completion of the chapter, the reader will be able to:

1. Explain the pathophysiologic mechanisms underlying gout and hyperuricemia.
2. Recognize major risk factors for developing gout in a given person.
3. Assess the signs and symptoms of an acute gout attack.
4. List the treatment goals for a patient with gout.
5. Develop a pharmacotherapeutic plan for a patient with acute gouty arthritis that includes individualized drug selection and monitoring for efficacy and safety.
6. Identify patients for whom prophylactic urate lowering therapy for gout and hyperuricemia is warranted.
7. Select an appropriate drug to reduce serum uric acid (SUA) levels in patients with gout, and outline a plan for monitoring efficacy and toxicity.
8. Formulate appropriate educational information for a patient on lifestyle modifications to help prevent gouty arthritis attacks.

INTRODUCTION

KEY CONCEPT *Gout is an inflammatory condition of the arthritis-type that results from deposition of uric acid crystals in joint spaces, leading to an inflammatory reaction that causes intense pain, erythema, and joint swelling.* It is associated with hyperuricemia, defined as a serum uric acid (SUA) level of 6.8 mg/dL (404 μmol/L) or greater, but not all patients with hyperuricemia demonstrate symptoms.[1] There are presently three published guidelines that provide clinical recommendations for management of patients with gout.[2–7] This chapter will focus primarily on recommendations of the American College of Rheumatology (ACR).[5–7]

EPIDEMIOLOGY AND ETIOLOGY

Gout is the most common inflammatory arthritis in men, with a male:female incidence of about 4:1; it affects over 3% of US adults.[1,8] The National Health and Nutrition Examination Survey (NHANES) 2007–2008 estimated the prevalence of gout among US adults to be 8.3 million.[9] Furthermore, the annual US incidence is approximately 62 cases per 100,000 persons and rising.[1] The incidence increases with age and is rising in part due to a larger number of patients with risk factors for gout.[10]

PATHOPHYSIOLOGY

Gout is caused by an abnormality in uric acid metabolism. Uric acid is a waste product of the breakdown of purines contained in the DNA of degraded body cells and dietary protein. Uric acid is water soluble and excreted primarily by the kidneys, although some is broken down by colonic bacteria and excreted via the gastrointestinal (GI) tract.[11]

The solubility of uric acid depends on concentration and temperature. At high serum concentrations, lower body temperature causes the precipitation of **monosodium urate** (MSU) crystals. Collections of these crystals (called microtophi) can form in joint spaces in the distal extremities. Larger **tophi** may take 10 years or longer to develop.

Free urate crystals can activate several proinflammatory mediators, including tumor necrosis factor α (TNF-α), interleukin 1 (IL-1), and IL-8. Activation of these mediators signals chemotactic movement of neutrophils into the joint space that ingest MSU crystals via phagocytosis. These neutrophils then are lysed and release proteolytic enzymes that trigger the clinical manifestations of an acute gout attack such as pain and swelling. These inflammatory mechanisms in gout, especially in untreated disease, can lead to cartilage and joint destruction.

The increased SUA involves either the underexcretion of uric acid (80% of patients) or its overproduction. The cause of overproduction or underexcretion of uric acid in most gout patients is unknown; this is referred to as primary gout.[1]

The reference range for SUA is 3.6 to 8.3 mg/dL (214–494 μmol/L). The risk of gout increases as the SUA concentration increases. Approximately 30% of patients with levels greater than 10 mg/dL (595 μmol/L) develop symptoms of gout within 5 years.[12] However, most patients with hyperuricemia are asymptomatic.

Dietary risk factors involve ingestion of animal purines, fructose, and alcohol (especially beer). Patients experiencing frequent attacks and those with poorly controlled advanced disease should be educated to avoid sweetbreads, liver, and kidney meat; high-fructose corn syrup; and alcohol use.[5] Other risk factors for gout include male gender, obesity, hypertension, dyslipidemia, and the metabolic syndrome.[8,11,13,14] Gout also occurs frequently in patients with type 2 diabetes mellitus, chronic kidney disease (CKD), and coronary artery disease; however, causal associations have not been established.[15,16] It is known that uric acid excretion is reduced in patients with CKD, putting them at risk for hyperuricemia.

Uric acid nephrolithiasis can occur in up to 25% of patients with persistently acidic urine and hyperuricemia. In severe cases, uric acid stones can cause nephropathy and renal failure.[17] Tumor lysis syndrome (TLS) involves metabolic complications resulting from extreme hyperuricemia due to rapid tumor cell destruction in patients undergoing chemotherapy for certain types of cancer.

KEY CONCEPT *Some drugs can cause hyperuricemia and precipitate gout, such as thiazide and loop diuretics, niacin, pyrazinamide, calcineurin inhibitors, and, occasionally, aspirin.* In most cases, these drugs block uric acid secretion in the kidney.

The effect of aspirin on uric acid is dose dependent. At very high doses (eg, 4000 mg/day), aspirin blocks uric acid reabsorption by the kidneys, increasing uric acid excretion. Smaller aspirin doses inhibit uric acid excretion and can elevate serum uric acid levels. The very low aspirin doses (75–81 mg/day) used for heart attack or stroke prevention do not substantially alter uric acid levels. For these reasons, aspirin in analgesic doses (325–650 mg several times per day) should be avoided.[2] However, patients with hyperuricemia or gout and cardiovascular risk factors should continue low-dose aspirin for cardiovascular prophylaxis because the cardiovascular benefit outweighs the minimal effect on serum urate.[5]

KEY CONCEPT *Long-term consequences of gout and hyperuricemia include joint destruction, tophi, nephrolithiasis, and nephropathy.*

CLINICAL PRESENTATION AND DIAGNOSIS

Refer to the accompanying box for the clinical presentation of acute gouty arthritis.

Diagnosis

A presumptive diagnosis is often based on presenting symptoms and may be confirmed later with laboratory and other diagnostic tests. Severe joint pain, swelling, tenderness, and erythema that rapidly peak are highly suggestive of, but not specific for, gout. For example, it is essential to distinguish between gout and septic arthritis to provide appropriate treatment. Gout is a reasonably accurate clinical diagnosis in patients with recurrent podagra and hyperuricemia.[3]

The serum uric acid level often is elevated but may be normal during an acute attack. In addition, an elevated SUA alone is not diagnostic for gout. The peripheral WBC count may be only mildly elevated. Other laboratory markers of inflammation (eg, increased erythrocyte sedimentation rate) are often present.

Aspiration of affected joint fluid or a tophus is essential for a definitive diagnosis. Needle-shaped negatively birefringent MSU crystals in the aspirate confirm the diagnosis (Figure 59–1). Joint fluid may also have an elevated white blood cell (WBC) count with neutrophils predominating. If infection is suspected, it is imperative to obtain the appropriate diagnosis and treatment.[3,18]

Radiographs of affected joints may have characteristic cystic changes, punched-out lytic lesions with overhanging bony edges, and soft-tissue calcified masses. These signs may also appear in other arthropathies and are generally not apparent with the first acute gout attack. Therefore, radiographs are often reserved for patients with long-standing disease.[3,4,19]

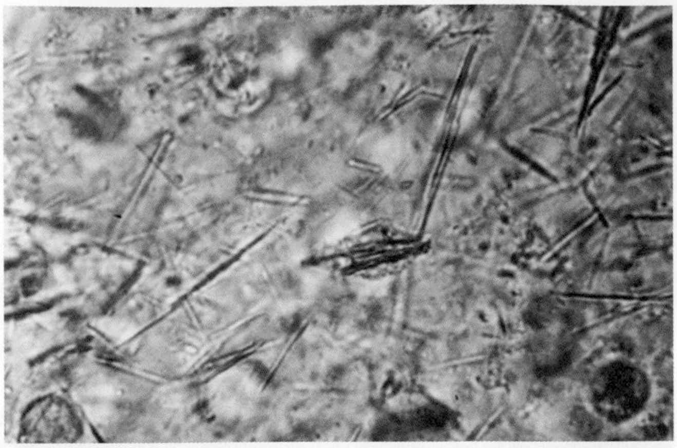

FIGURE 59–1. Synovial fluid containing extracellular and intracellular needle-like, negative birefringent monosodium urate crystals. (From Schumacher H, Chen LX. Chapter 333. Gout and Other Crystal-Associated Arthropathies. In: Longo DL, Fauci AS, Kasper DL, et al., eds. Harrison's Principles of Internal Medicine, 18th ed. New York, NY: McGraw-Hill; 2012. http://accesspharmacy.mhmedical.com/content.aspx?bookid=331&Sectionid=40727136. Accessed August 25, 2014. With permission.)

Although rarely performed, a 24-hour urine collection can be obtained to determine whether the patient is an overproducer or an underexcretor of uric acid. Individuals who excrete more than 800 mg (4.8 mmol) of uric acid in this collection are considered overproducers. Patients with hyperuricemia who excrete less than 600 mg/day (3.6 mmol/day) are classified as underexcretors of uric acid.

Clinical Presentation of Acute Gouty Arthritis

General

- Acute inflammatory monoarthritis.
- Patients are usually in acute distress.

Symptoms

- There is severe pain and swelling in the affected joint(s).
- Symptoms reach maximal intensity within 6 to 12 hours.
- The attack is usually monoarticular; the most common site is the metatarsophalangeal joint.
- In elderly patients, gouty attacks may be atypical with insidious and polyarticular onset, often involving hand or wrist joints.

Signs

- Affected joint(s) are warm, erythematous, and swollen.
- Mild fever may be present.
- Tophi (usually on hands, wrists, elbows, or knees) may be present in chronic, severe disease.

Patient Encounter, Part 1

A 47-year old obese Caucasian man presents to the emergency department with a 16-hour history of rapidly escalating excruciating pain (over 8 hours) in his left big toe unrelated to trauma. On examination, his left great toe is red, swollen, tender, and warm to the touch. During the initial patient interview, he states that this is the second time he has experienced this type of throbbing pain in his toe (last episode occurred 2 months ago and was successfully treated). He rates the pain as 10/10 (10 being the worst pain he has ever experienced). He is an unemployed, single father who did not graduate from high school. He has two young children and is concerned that he will be unable to find work and care for his children if this pain continues to occur frequently.

What information is suggestive of acute gouty arthritis?

What additional information is necessary to differentiate gout from other joint abnormalities?

What additional information do you need before creating a treatment plan for this patient?

What are aspects to consider when providing care for a patient who is unemployed and with limited formal education?

TREATMENT OF ACUTE GOUTY ARTHRITIS

KEY CONCEPT *Treatment of gout involves: (a) acute relief of a gouty arthritis attack with topical application of ice and drug therapy commonly including NSAIDs, colchicine, corticosteroids or a combination thereof, and (b) in some patients, long-term* prophylactic *treatment with urate-lowering therapy (ULT) to prevent subsequent attacks.*

Desired Outcomes

Treatment goals for an acute attack are to: (a) achieve rapid and effective pain relief, (b) maintain joint function, (c) prevent disease complications, (d) avoid treatment-related adverse effects, (e) provide cost-effective therapy, and (f) improve quality of life.[4] Infrequent gouty arthritis is a self-limited disease, and treatment usually focuses on symptomatic relief.

Nonpharmacologic Therapy

Nondrug modalities play an adjunctive role and usually are not effective when used alone. Immobilization of the affected extremity speeds resolution of the attack. Applying ice packs to the joint also decreases pain and swelling, but heat application may be detrimental.[20]

Pharmacologic Therapy

KEY CONCEPT *Nonsteroidal anti-inflammatory drugs (NSAIDs), colchicine, and corticosteroids are considered first-line monotherapy options for acute attacks.[6] Selection depends on number of joints affected, presence/absence of infection, clinician/patient preference, prior response, and patient factors such as comorbidities and renal function* (Figure 59–2). Each drug class has a unique safety and efficacy profile in gout that should be considered carefully before choosing a specific agent (Table 59–1). Generally, the earlier in the course of the arthritic attack these agents are employed (ie, within 24 hours), the better the outcome. Corticotropin (adrenocorticotropic hormone, ACTH) and IL-1 inhibitors are alternatives in select cases.[6] Opioid analgesics have little to no role in acute gout, which results from overwhelming inflammation.[21]

▸ *Nonsteroidal Anti-inflammatory Drugs*

NSAIDs have largely supplanted colchicine as the treatment of choice. These agents are most effective when given within the first 24 hours of the onset of pain. Most studies have shown similar results among agents, and no one NSAID is preferred over another as first-line treatment.[6] Doses at the higher end of the therapeutic range are often needed.[22] NSAIDs are usually continued at full doses until 24 hours after symptoms subside. Clinicians may consider tapering the dose if a patient has multiple comorbidities, including hepatic or renal failure.

Only naproxen, indomethacin, and sulindac are FDA approved for treatment of acute gout. Although indomethacin has been used traditionally, its relative cyclooxygenase-1 (COX-1) selectivity increases its gastropathy risk. Studies comparing indomethacin to other NSAIDs consistency show similar efficacy with higher side effects with indomethacin; thus, other generic NSAIDs may be preferred. The patient's overall clinical status should be evaluated prior to NSAID initiation because adverse effects include gastropathy (primarily peptic ulcers), renal dysfunction, and fluid retention.[23] NSAIDs generally should be avoided in patients at risk for peptic ulcers; those taking anticoagulants; and those with renal insufficiency, uncontrolled hypertension, or heart failure. Gastroprotective agents such as proton pump inhibitors may protect against ulcer development in patients receiving NSAIDs for acute gout.

Cyclooxygenase-2 (COX-2)–selective inhibitors (ie, celecoxib) produce results comparable with those of traditional NSAIDs.[24] However, the need for large COX-2 inhibitor doses, cardiovascular safety concerns, and high cost make the risk-benefit ratio unclear for this disorder.

▸ *Colchicine*

Colchicine has a long history of successful use and was the treatment of choice for many years. It is used less commonly today because of its low therapeutic index and more recently, increased cost. Colchicine is thought to exert its anti-inflammatory effects by interfering with the function of mitotic spindles in neutrophils by binding of tubulin dimers; this inhibits phagocytic activity.[25] Colchicine is not considered to be an analgesic.

About two-thirds of patients with acute gout respond favorably if colchicine is given within the first 24 hours of symptom onset.[26] Presently, colchicine is only indicated if given within 36 hours of attack onset.[6] GI effects (eg, nausea, vomiting, diarrhea, and abdominal pain) are most common and are considered a forerunner of more serious systemic toxicity, including myopathy and bone marrow suppression (usually neutropenia). However, systemic toxicity can occur with oral colchicine without prior GI effects, especially in patients with renal insufficiency.[27,28] In the presence of severe renal impairment (creatinine clearance [CrCl] < 30 mL/min [0.5 mL/s]), dosing should be repeated no more than once every 2 weeks. Dose reductions are required when coadministered with p-glycoprotein or strong CYP3A4 inhibitors (eg, clarithromycin, verapamil, ritonavir, cyclosporine, ranolazine). Because of these problems, colchicine may be reserved for patients who are at risk for NSAID-induced gastropathy or who have failed NSAID therapy.[29]

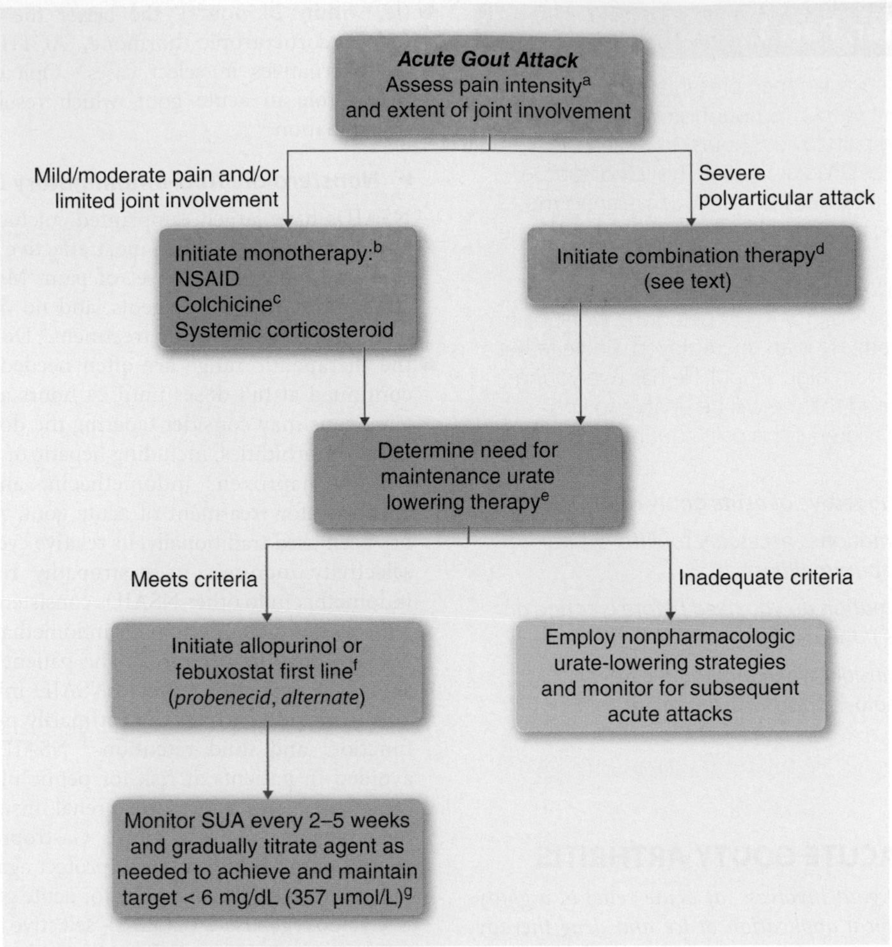

FIGURE 59–2. Treatment algorithm for hyperuricemia in gout. (NSAID, nonsteroidal anti-inflammatory drug; SUA, serum uric acid.) [a]Self-reported pain score using a visual analog scale of 6 or less is considered mild/moderate pain and 7 or more is considered severe pain. [b]May consider switch to alternate monotherapy, add-on combination therapy, or off-label therapy for inadequate response (< 20% improvement in pain score within 24 hours or < 50% at 24 hours or longer). [c]Colchicine recommended only if started within 36 hours of symptom onset. [d]Intraarticular corticosteroids may be used in combination when only one or two large joints are affected. [e]Criteria for ULT initiation include: Recurrent attacks (2 or more per year), evidence of tophus or tophi, chronic kidney disease stage 2 or worse, or past urolithiasis. [f]Initiate concomitant anti-inflammatory prophylaxis and continue for indicated duration. [g]May add on uricosuric therapy if unable to achieve target SUA on maximally dosed xanthine oxidase inhibitor therapy; switch to pegloticase for refractory cases.

Colcrys is the only single-ingredient oral colchicine product FDA approved for treatment of acute gout attacks. For many years prior to its release, generic colchicine products were available without FDA approval. In 2010, the FDA ordered manufacturers to discontinue marketing these unapproved generics. Colcrys is much more expensive than the generic compounds it replaced but has proper labeling and safety data. As part of the approval process, a dosing study showed that one dose initially and a single additional dose after 1 hour was just as effective as and less toxic than continued hourly colchicine dosing.[30] Thus, the approved dosage regimen is 1.2 mg (two 0.6-mg tablets) at the onset of an acute flare, followed by 0.6 mg 1 hour later.[31] The ACR guidelines suggest it can then be continued starting 12 hours later at a dose of 0.6 mg once or twice daily (prophylaxis dosing) until the gout attack is resolved.[6] This is not part of the FDA-approved labeling but is an off-label recommendation based on pharmacokinetic data.[30] Dose adjustment is required for renal insufficiency.

Colchicine should not be used for an acute attack if the patient is currently prescribed colchicine for prophylaxis and was previously treated with colchicine for an acute attack within the last 14 days. Intravenous colchicine (no longer commercially available) should never be used in gout management.[6]

► *Corticosteroids*

It is important to determine the number of joints affected when considering a corticosteroid for first-line therapy. Systemic corticosteroids are a useful option in patients with contraindications to NSAIDs or colchicine (primarily renal impairment) or polyarticular attacks, especially in elderly patients. The ACR recommends initiating oral prednisone or prednisolone at a starting dose of at least 0.5 mg/kg daily for 5 to 10 days, followed by abrupt discontinuation, or full dose therapy for 2 to 5 days with a 7- to 10-day taper to discontinue.[6] Oral methylprednisolone (ie, the 6-day dose pack consisting of a 21-tablet taper of 1 mg tablets, starting with 6 tablets on day 1 [divided into three separate doses] and ending with one tablet on day 6) and naproxen have been shown to be equivalent in treating acute gout attacks.[32]

Table 59–1

Pharmacotherapy Regimens for Acute Gout Treatment

Drug	Usual Dosage Range
NSAIDs[a]	
Etodolac	300–500 mg po two times daily
Fenoprofen	400–600 mg po three to four times daily
Ibuprofen	400–800 mg po three to four times daily
Indomethacin*	50 mg po three times daily initially until pain is tolerable, then quickly taper to discontinue
Ketoprofen	50 mg po four times daily or 75 mg po three times daily
Naproxen*	750 mg po initially, then 250 mg po every 8 hours
Piroxicam	40 mg po once daily for 5–7 days
Sulindac*	150–200 mg po two times daily for 7–10 days
Celecoxib	800 mg po followed by 400 mg po on day 1, then 400 mg po twice daily for 1 week
Oral Colchicine[b] **(Colcrys)**	1.2 mg po at the onset of attack, then 0.6 mg po 1 hour later
Corticosteroids	
Local corticosteroid	
Triamcinolone acetonide	10–40 mg (large joint), 5–20 mg (small joint) for one dose by intraarticular injection
Systemic corticosteroid	
Prednisone (example)	30–60 mg po once daily for 3–5 days, then taper to discontinue by 5 mg decrements over 10–14 days
Triamcinolone acetonide	60 mg by IM injection for one dose[c]
Methylprednisolone	100–150 mg by IM injection once daily for 1–2 days
Corticotropin[d]	40–80 units IM or SC every 24–72 hours
Interleukin-1 Inhibitors[d]	
Anakinra	100 mg SC once daily for 3 days
Canakinumab	150 mg SC for 1 dose

IM, intramuscular; NSAIDs, nonsteroidal anti-inflammatory drugs; po, by mouth; SC, subcutaneous.

[a]NSAIDs that are FDA approved for treatment of gout are indicated with an asterisk.

[b]Dose reduction recommended for renal impairment.

[c]Administration of IM triamcinolone should be followed by oral prednisone or prednisolone.

[d]Not FDA approved for this indication.

Drug regimens derived from various sources.

When only one or two large joints are affected, an **intraarticular** corticosteroid injection can provide rapid relief with a relatively low incidence of side effects, and it may be used in combination with either an NSAID, colchicine, or oral corticosteroid. Joint fluid obtained by **arthrocentesis** should be examined for evidence of joint space infection and crystal identification. If uric acid crystals are present and there is no infection, intraarticular injection can proceed.

Finally, an alternative regimen consisting of a single intramuscular injection of a long-acting corticosteroid such as triamcinolone acetonide, followed by oral prednisone or prednisolone may also be used.[6]

Adverse effects from corticosteroids include fluid retention, hyperglycemia, CNS stimulation, weight gain, GI upset, and increased risk of infection. Patients with diabetes should have blood glucose levels monitored carefully during the corticosteroid course, and caution should be exercised when treating patients with a history of peptic ulcer disease.

▶ *Corticotropin (Adrenocorticotropic Hormone)*

Exogenous administration of intramuscular adrenocorticotropic hormone (ACTH) stimulates production of cortisol and corticosterone by the adrenal cortex. Clinical studies have shown efficacy similar to other agents for acute gout. Although not a first-line option (or FDA approved for this use), the ACR supports its use for patients unable to take medications orally.[6] The product is available in the United States only through specialty pharmacy distribution.

▶ *Interleukin-1 Inhibitors*

Several small clinical trials have demonstrated efficacy of IL-1 inhibitors in inhibiting inflammation associated with acute gout attacks. While their role is unclear and the available products (anakinra and canakinumab) are not FDA approved for this purpose, the ACR guidelines include off-label use as an option for severe acute attacks or for patients refractory to other agents.[6]

▶ *Combination Therapy*

In severe polyarticular attacks, particularly attacks involving multiple large joints, colchicine may be used in combination with an NSAID or oral corticosteroid. Intraarticular corticosteroid injections may be used in combination with any other first-line agent (NSAID, colchicine, oral corticosteroid).[6]

URATE LOWERING THERAPY FOR GOUT PROPHYLAXIS

Gout is an episodic disease, and the number of attacks varies widely from patient to patient. Thus the benefit of long-term prophylaxis against acute gout flares must be weighed against the cost and potential toxicity of therapy that may not be necessary in all patients. KEY CONCEPT *Asymptomatic hyperuricemia generally does not require treatment.*

Nonpharmacologic Therapy

Historically, lifestyle modifications alone have been insufficient for lowering SUA levels in gout patients. Patients should be educated to engage in regular exercise to lose weight if obese, strictly limit or discontinue ethanol consumption, maintain hydration, and manage other comorbidities (eg, hypertension, diabetes). Low-purine diets, including avoiding organ meats, and limiting sardines, shellfish, beef, pork, and lamb are not well tolerated; instead, dietary recommendations should focus on general nutrition principles. Some studies have shown that low-fat dairy products, coffee, and vitamin C may confer a protective effect. Complementary therapies that are considered to be inappropriate for gout due to insufficient evidence of benefit include cherry juice/extract, willow bark extract, ginger, flaxseed, charcoal, strawberries, black current, burdock, sour cream, olive oil, horsetail, pears, and celery root.[6,8] Drugs that may cause or aggravate hyperuricemia should be discontinued if clinically appropriate. Few patients adhere to lifestyle modifications long term, and pharmacologic therapy usually is needed to treat hyperuricemia adequately.[33]

Pharmacologic Therapy

KEY CONCEPT *Patients with recurrent attacks (2 or more per year), evidence of tophus or tophi, CKD stage 2 or worse, or past urolithiasis are candidates for* prophylactic *therapy with allopurinol, febuxostat, probenecid, or pegloticase to lower SUA levels* (see Figure 59–2). Because hyperuricemia is the strongest modifiable risk factor for acute gout, prophylactic therapy commonly involves either decreasing uric acid production or increasing its excretion (Table 59–2). The goal of therapy is to decrease SUA levels significantly, leaving less uric acid available for conversion to MSU crystals.[4]

Ideally, the selection of long-term prophylactic therapy involves determining the cause of hyperuricemia (primarily by analyzing a 24-hour urine collection for uric acid) and tailoring therapy appropriately. If less than 600 mg (3.6 mmol) of uric acid is found in the 24-hour sample, the patient is considered an underexcretor. However, this approach is not used commonly for several reasons. The urine collection is inconvenient for patients and clinicians and does not identify patients who may be both overproducers and underexcretors of uric acid. Also, drugs used to increase uric acid excretion (uricosuric agents) generally are not as well tolerated as drugs that decrease production, and uricosurics increase the risk of uric acid nephrolithiasis.[34]

Because allopurinol (which reduces uric acid production) is effective in both overproducers and underexcretors and is generally well tolerated, many clinicians forego the 24-hour urine collection and treat patients empirically with it. Both allopurinol and febuxostat are xanthine oxidase inhibitors (XOIs) and are considered to be first-line ULT agents. Probenecid, a uricosuric agent, is an alternative first-line option, whereas pegloticase is generally reserved for refractory cases.[5]

KEY CONCEPT *ULT should be continued in patients even during acute flares.*

► Allopurinol

Most patients in the US are treated with allopurinol, which usually is effective if the dosage is titrated appropriately. The drug and its primary active metabolite, oxypurinol, reduce SUA concentrations by inhibiting the enzyme xanthine oxidase, thereby blocking the two-phase oxidation of hypoxanthine and xanthine to uric acid.[4]

Allopurinol is well absorbed, with a short half-life of 2 to 3 hours. The half-life of oxypurinol approaches 24 hours, allowing allopurinol to be dosed once daily. Oxypurinol is cleared primarily by renal mechanisms and can accumulate in patients with reduced kidney function.

Allopurinol may be started during an acute gout attack only if anti-inflammatory treatment is also initiated, because sudden shifts in SUA levels from mobilization of tissue urate stores may precipitate or exacerbate gouty arthritis. Rapid shifts in SUA can change the concentration of MSU crystals in synovial fluid, causing more crystals to precipitate. Thus most clinicians provide anti-inflammatory prophylaxis during initiation of ULT with colchicine (0.6 mg once or twice daily or 0.3 mg daily if severe renal impairment) or a low-dose NSAID (eg, naproxen 250 mg twice daily) with acid-suppressing therapy (eg, omeprazole 20 mg once daily). If a patient is being treated with colchicine for an acute attack, the prophylactic colchicine dose may be administered 12 hours after the last treatment dose. This approach, with colchicine having a stronger evidence grade, is supported by the ACR guidelines. Guidelines recommend that all acute gout patients receive prophylaxis when ULT is started with continuation of therapy for at least 6 months or up to 3 to 6 months after no clinical evidence of gout activity is apparent and the target SUA has been achieved.[6] Patients receiving colchicine for prophylaxis should be screened for drug–drug interactions (via the cytochrome p-450 system) that may increase the risk of colchicine adverse effects. Low-dose prednisone or prednisolone (less than 10 mg/day) is an alternative for patients unable to take colchicine or NSAIDs.

The initial dose of allopurinol is based on the patient's renal function. If renal function is normal, an initial dose no greater than 100 mg daily is recommended. The initial dose should be reduced to 50 mg daily in patients with a CrCl less than 30 mL/min (0.5 mL/s).[5] The relationship between allopurinol dose and its most severe side effects, including allopurinol hypersensitivity syndrome (AHS), is controversial.[35,36] However, the dose can be adjusted upward every 2 to 5 weeks as needed and tolerated, even in patients with renal insufficiency provided that they are monitored and educated appropriately.[5,37] Historically, allopurinol was dosed according to renal function with stringent

Table 59–2

Pharmacotherapy Regimens for Urate Lowering

Drug	Usual Dosage Range
Xanthine Oxidase Inhibitors	
Allopurinol[a]	100 mg po initially, then titrate to achieve SUA level < 6 mg/dL (357 μmol/L); maximum 800 mg po daily
Febuxostat	40 mg po once daily initially, then increase to 80 mg po once daily if SUA does not decline to 6 mg/dL (357 μmol/L) or lower after 2 weeks of treatment
Uricosurics	
Probenecid	250 mg po two times daily for 1 week, then 500 mg po twice daily; may increase by 500 mg every 4 weeks to achieve SUA level < 6 mg/dL (357 μmol/L); maximum 2 g po daily
Other	
Pegloticase	8 mg given as an IV infusion over at least 2 hours once every 2 weeks, optimal duration unknown

po, by mouth; SUA, serum uric acid.

[a]Initiation dose reduction recommended for renal impairment.

Drug regimens derived from various sources.

maximum dosages. The 2012 ACR guidelines recommend titrating the dose to goal SUA regardless of renal function.

SUA levels must be monitored every 2 to 5 weeks during titration, then every 6 months after the target SUA is achieved. The target SUA level is less than 6 mg/dL (357 μmol/L) in all cases and perhaps even less than 5 mg/dL (297 μmol/L) in more severe disease involving tophi. The allopurinol dose should be titrated upward (to a maximum of 800 mg/day) or downward as these levels dictate. The typical dose prescribed is 300 mg/day in patients with normal renal function, but this dose often fails to achieve the target SUA level.[5]

Allopurinol is typically well tolerated; nausea and diarrhea occur uncommonly. A generalized, maculopapular rash occurs in about 2% of patients.[38] Although usually mild, this can progress to severe skin reactions such as Stevens-Johnson syndrome. The most serious side effect is AHS, which may involve severe desquamating skin lesions, high fever (usually greater than 39.0°C [102.2°F]), hepatic dysfunction, leukocytosis with predominant eosinophilia, and renal failure. The risk appears to be highest in the first few months of therapy, and although rare, this severe reaction has a 20% to 25% mortality rate.[5,39,40] Prior to initiating allopurinol, pharmacogenetic screening via human leukocyte antigen (HLA)-B*5801 testing is recommended for patients at an elevated risk for AHS (eg, Koreans with stage 3 or worse CKD and all individuals of Han Chinese and Thai descent). If results are positive, the patient should be provided with an alternative to allopurinol. Patients with a history of AHS should never again receive allopurinol (including desensitization) or oxypurinol (which is available outside the United States). Patients with a mild skin rash who require allopurinol can be desensitized to it using published protocols or be switched to febuxostat.[41,42]

There are several important drug–drug interactions with allopurinol. The effects of both theophylline and warfarin may be potentiated by allopurinol. Azathioprine and 6-mercaptopurine are purines whose metabolism is inhibited by concomitant allopurinol therapy; the dose of these drugs must be reduced by 75% with allopurinol cotherapy. Patients taking allopurinol who receive ampicillin are at increased risk of skin rashes.

► *Febuxostat*

Febuxostat is a nonpurine XOI structurally distinct from allopurinol that is FDA approved for chronic hyperuricemia associated with gout. The initial dose is 40 mg orally once daily. The dose may be increased to 80 mg orally once daily if the SUA does not decrease to 6 mg/dL (357 μmol/L) or less after 2 weeks of treatment. No dosage adjustment is necessary in patients with mild or moderate renal impairment (CrCl 30–89 mL/min [0.5–1.48 mL/s]); however, febuxostat is not recommended in patient with severe renal insufficiency (CrCl < 30 mL/min [0.5 mL/s]).[43,44] Because of its potency and rapid reduction of SUA levels, anti-inflammatory prophylaxis with low-dose colchicine or an NSAID is also recommended during initiation and titration of therapy and for at least 6 months as previously discussed for allopurinol.

Adverse effects of febuxostat include nausea, arthralgias, rash, and transient elevation of hepatic transaminases. Periodic liver function tests are recommended (eg, at baseline, 2 and 4 months after starting therapy, and then periodically thereafter). Due to differences in chemical structure, febuxostat would not be expected to cross-react in patients with a history of allopurinol hypersensitivity syndrome.

Due to cost concerns, febuxostat should generally be reserved for patients who do not tolerate allopurinol and those who

Patient Encounter, Part 2

PMH: Obesity–120 kg (264 lb) and 5′5″ (165 cm) tall, hypertension, dyslipidemia, allergic rhinitis

FH: Father unknown. Mother has coronary artery disease and hypertension. No siblings

SH: He is currently unemployed but previously drove trucks for a local delivery company until losing his job 2 weeks ago. He drinks soda during the day and three to four beers most nights of the week. He denies use of tobacco products or illicit drugs. He admits to a poor diet consisting of many processed and fast foods and likes to snack on candy

Allergies: NKDA

Meds: Hydrochlorothiazide 25 mg once daily (adherent), amlodipine 10 mg once daily (adherent), rosuvastatin 20 mg at bedtime (nonadherent), cimetidine 300 mg at bedtime as needed (self-prescribed), loratadine 10 mg once daily (during allergy season), aspirin 325 mg twice daily as needed (self-prescribed for headaches), colchicine 1.2 mg (two 0.6-mg tablets) for one dose, followed by 0.6 mg 1 hour later and 0.6 mg once daily thereafter until gout attack resolves (completed 10-day course 2 months ago for acute gouty attack)

ROS: (–) Fatigue, (–) N/V/D, HA, SOB, chest pain, cough

PE:

VS: 139/92, P 72, RR 18, T 36.1°C (96.9°F)

Skin: Warm, dry with excessive warmth surrounding left great toe

HEENT: NC/AT, PERRLA, TMs intact

CV: RRR, normal S_1 and S_2, no m/r/g

Chest: CTA

Abd: Soft, NT/ND

Ext: No c/c, trace edema in both ankles

Neuro: A&O × 3, CN II to XII intact

Labs: Serum creatinine 0.9 mg/dL (80 μmol/L), SUA 8.1 mg/dL (482 μmol/L), WBC + diff WNL

Other: 24-hour urine collection, joint aspirate, and x-ray not performed

What risk factors promote gout and hyperuricemia in this patient?

Given this additional information, what is your assessment of the patient's condition?

Identify your gout treatment goals for this patient.

What nonpharmacologic and pharmacologic alternatives are available for this patient's acute gouty attack?

What alternatives are available for urate-lowering therapy for gout prophylaxis in this patient?

Patient Encounter, Part 3

Based on the information available, create a care plan for this patient's gout. The plan should include: (a) a statement of the drug related needs and/or problems, (b) a patient-specific detailed therapeutic plan, and (c) monitoring parameters to assess efficacy and safety.

cannot achieve SUA levels of 6 mg/dL (357 μmol/L) or less despite maximal allopurinol therapy.[1]

▶ *Probenecid*

Probenecid is a uricosuric agent that blocks the tubular reabsorption of uric acid, increasing its excretion. Because of its mechanism of action, probenecid is not recommended for urate overproducers and is contraindicated in patients with a history of urolithiasis or urate nephropathy. Probenecid loses its effectiveness as renal function declines and should be avoided when the CrCl is 50 mL/min (0.83 mL/s) or less.[45] Probenecid is considered an alternate first-line agent if XOI therapy is either not tolerated or contraindicated. It may also be added to XOI therapy that has been titrated to the maximum dose without attainment of the target SUA level.[6]

Although generally well tolerated, probenecid can cause GI side effects such as nausea as well as fever, rash, and rarely, hepatic toxicity. Patients should be instructed to maintain adequate fluid intake and urine output to decrease the risk of uric acid stone formation. Some experts advocate alkalinizing the urine to decrease this risk, but no specific recommendations are provided.

▶ *Other Uricosuric Agents*

Other medications with mild uricosuric effects may be appropriate adjunctive therapy in some patients. Losartan increases both uric acid excretion and urine pH and may be an option in hypertensive patients with gout. Fenofibrate is also uricosuric and may be appropriate in select dyslipidemic patients with gout.[46] Either one of these agents may be combined with a XOI in patients who fail to achieve the target SUA level on maximized therapy.[5]

▶ *Pegloticase*

Gout does not occur in most nonprimate mammals because these species produce the enzyme uricase, which catalyzes oxidation of uric acid into the more soluble compound allantoin, which is readily excreted. Humans lack this enzyme, which allows uric acid to accumulate, leading to gout in some individuals.

Pegloticase is a recombinant form of uricase (also known as urate oxidase) conjugated to polyethylene glycol. It is FDA approved for treatment of chronic gout refractory to other therapies. The approved dose of 8 mg by IV infusion over at least 2 hours every 2 weeks rapidly (within 6 hours) decreased SUA in subjects in published trials.[47] However, pegloticase should be

Patient Care Process

Patient Assessment:

- Assess patient symptoms to determine time of attack onset, joint(s) affected, pain level, and observe physical signs (joint warmth, swelling, and redness).
- Review patient history for contributing lifestyle factors (ie, alcohol use) and comorbidities including CKD that may exacerbate hyperuricemia or help to guide therapy.
- Obtain thorough medication history for prescription and nonprescription drug and dietary supplement use. Determine whether any products such as diuretic therapy may be contributing to hyperuricemia.
- Consider evaluating the SUA level to confirm presence of hyperuricemia.
- If a gout diagnosis has not been confirmed previously, consider aspiration of the affected joint or tophus to identify uric acid crystals.

Therapy Evaluation:

- Discontinue nonessential urate-elevating medications.
- If a patient is currently receiving pharmacotherapy, assess efficacy (ie, frequency and severity of attacks), safety/adverse reactions, adherence, and potential drug interactions.
- Ensure the patient has met criteria for ULT if already prescribed.
- Determine if the patient has prescription insurance and whether recommended agents (eg, colchicine) are included on the formulary.

Care Plan Development: (see Figure 59–2)

- Initiate therapy to treat acute gout attack within 24 hours (see Table 59–1).
- Select therapy based on comorbidities and potential for adverse effects.
- Assess need for continuous ULT (see Table 59–2). Use patient factors such as comorbidities to select an agent.
- Most patients need adjunctive therapy with low-dose colchicine or an NSAID during initiation or titration of ULT to prevent a rebound flare.
- Initiate ULT during an acute attack only in conjunction with effective anti-inflammatory therapy.
- Educate the patient on hyperuricemia/gout, drug therapy, and appropriate lifestyle modifications that may improve symptoms (eg, weight loss, avoidance of ethanol).

Follow-up Evaluation:

- Titrate ULT to achieve the target SUA; monitor the SUA concentration during ULT titration and periodically thereafter.
- Evaluate presence of adverse drug reactions, allergies, and interactions.
- Reinforce adherence with the regimen to prevent future gout attacks and long-term complications.

limited to patients with severe gout with tophi or nephropathy that has not responded to other agents because of significant adverse effects, including gout flares, infusion reactions, anaphylaxis (in up to 5% of patients) that mandates pretreatment with antihistamines and corticosteroids, the inconvenience of IV therapy, and its high cost. Pegloticase is contraindicated in patients with G6PD deficiency due to the risk of hemolysis and methemoglobinemia; therefore, patients should be screened prior to initiation of therapy.

OUTCOME EVALUATION

Acute Gout

- Monitor the patient for pain relief and decreased swelling of the affected joint(s). Both parameters improve significantly within 48 hours of starting therapy.
- Assess the patient's complaints and objective information for adverse effects. For NSAID therapy, be alert for new-onset epigastric pain, dark or tarry stools, blood in vomitus, dizziness or lightheadedness, development of edema, decreased urine output, or shortness of breath. For colchicine, monitor for nausea or vomiting, diarrhea, easy bruising, cold or flu-like symptoms, lightheadedness, muscle weakness, or pain. Advise the patient to inform you of any new medications started or stopped while taking colchicine.
- Monitor patients receiving intraarticular corticosteroid injections for increased swelling or pain at the injection site.
- Assess patients receiving systemic corticosteroids for mental status changes, fluid retention, increased blood glucose, muscle weakness, or development of new infections.

Urate Lowering Therapy

- Monitor the SUA level every 2 to 5 weeks during ULT initiation and titration. Adjust the dose of ULT to achieve a target SUA level of less than 6 mg/dL (357 μmol/L) or optionally less than 5 mg/dL (297 μmol/L) in more severe disease. Then continue measurements every 6 months thereafter.
- Concomitantly initiate anti-inflammatory prophylaxis and continue for the greater of 6 months or 3 to 6 months after achieving target SUA level with no gout signs/symptoms.
- Assess for new gouty arthritis attacks or development of tophi.
- Evaluate patients taking allopurinol for development of rash, nausea, or new fever. These symptoms usually appear within the first 3 months of therapy but can occur anytime.
- Evaluate patients prescribed febuxostat for presence of nausea, arthralgias, rash, and transient elevation of hepatic transaminases.
- Assess patients receiving probenecid for fever, nausea, or skin rash. Reevaluate therapy if a significant decrease in urine output occurs.
- If pegloticase is used, monitor SUA levels before each 2-week IV infusion.
- Evaluate patients on pegloticase for development of gouty flares and infusion reactions, which may include anaphylaxis. The manufacturer recommends giving an antihistamine and perhaps low-dose methylprednisolone before the infusion to minimize reactions.

Abbreviations Introduced in This Chapter

ACR	American College of Rheumatology
ACTH	Adrenocorticotropic hormone
AHS	Allopurinol hypersensitivity syndrome
COX	Cyclooxygenase
G6PD	Glucose-6-phosphate dehydrogenase
HLA	Human leukocyte antigen
IL-1	Interleukin-1
MSU	Monosodium urate
SUA	Serum uric acid
TLS	Tumor lysis syndrome
ULT	Urate lowering therapy
XOI	Xanthine oxidase inhibitor

REFERENCES

1. Neogi T. Clinical practice. Gout. N Engl J Med. 2011;364(5):443–452.
2. Jordan KM, Cameron JS, Snaith M, et al. British Society for Rheumatology and British Health Professionals in Rheumatology guideline for the management of gout. Rheumatol Oxf Engl. 2007;46(8):1372–1374.
3. Zhang W, Doherty M, Pascual E, et al. EULAR evidence based recommendations for gout. Part I: Diagnosis. Report of a task force of the standing committee for international clinical studies including therapeutics (ESCISIT). Ann Rheum Dis. 2006;65(10):1301–1311. doi:10.1136/ard.2006.055251.
4. Zhang W, Doherty M, Bardin T, et al. EULAR evidence based recommendations for gout. Part II: Management. Report of a task force of the EULAR Standing Committee for International Clinical Studies Including Therapeutics (ESCISIT). Ann Rheum Dis. 2006;65(10):1312–1324.
5. Khanna D, Fitzgerald JD, Khanna PP, et al. 2012 American College of Rheumatology guidelines for management of gout. Part 1: Systematic nonpharmacologic and pharmacologic therapeutic approaches to hyperuricemia. Arthritis Care Res. 2012;64(10):1431–1446.
6. Khanna D, Khanna PP, Fitzgerald JD, et al. 2012 American College of Rheumatology guidelines for management of gout. Part 2: Therapy and antiinflammatory prophylaxis of acute gouty arthritis. Arthritis Care Res. 2012;64(10):1447–1461.
7. Nuki G. An appraisal of the 2012 American College of Rheumatology Guidelines for the Management of Gout. Curr Opin Rheumatol. 2014;26(2):152–161. doi:10.1097/BOR.0000000000000034.
8. Roddy E, Choi HK. Epidemiology of gout. Rheum Dis Clin North Am. 2014;40(2):155–175. doi:10.1016/j.rdc.2014.01.001.
9. Zhu Y, Pandya BJ, Choi HK. Prevalence of gout and hyperuricemia in the US general population: The National Health and Nutrition Examination Survey 2007-2008. Arthritis Rheum. 2011;63(10):3136–3141. doi:10.1002/art.30520.
10. Robinson PC, Horsburgh S. Gout: Joints and beyond, epidemiology, clinical features, treatment and co-morbidities. Maturitas. 2014;78(4):245–251. doi:10.1016/j.maturitas.2014.05.001.
11. Cassetta M, Gorevic PD. Crystal arthritis. Gout and pseudogout in the geriatric patient. Geriatrics. 2004;59(9):25–30; quiz 31.
12. Arromdee E, Michet CJ, Crowson CS, et al. Epidemiology of gout: Is the incidence rising? J Rheumatol. 2002;29(11):2403–2406.
13. Johnson RJ, Kang D-H, Feig D, et al. Is there a pathogenetic role for uric acid in hypertension and cardiovascular and renal disease? Hypertension. 2003;41(6):1183–1190. doi:10.1161/01.HYP.0000069700.62727.C5.
14. Cardona F, Tinahones FJ, Collantes E, et al. Contribution of polymorphisms in the apolipoprotein AI-CIII-AIV cluster

to hyperlipidaemia in patients with gout. Ann Rheum Dis. 2005;64(1):85–88. doi:10.1136/ard.2003.019695.
15. Pillinger MH, Goldfarb DS, Keenan RT. Gout and its comorbidities. Bull NYU Hosp Jt Dis. 2010;68(3):199–203.
16. Karis E, Crittenden DB, Pillinger MH. Hyperuricemia, gout, and related comorbidities: Cause and effect on a two-way street. South Med J. 2014;107(4):235–241. doi:10.1097/SMJ.0000000000000082.
17. Shekarriz B, Stoller ML. Uric acid nephrolithiasis: Current concepts and controversies. J Urol. 2002;168(4 Pt 1):1307–1314.
18. Terkeltaub RA. Gout. N Engl J Med. 2003;349(17):1647–1655. doi:10.1056/NEJMcp030733.
19. Schumacher HR. Crystal-induced arthritis: An overview. Am J Med. 1996;100(2A):46S–52S.
20. Schlesinger N, Detry MA, Holland BK, et al. Local ice therapy during bouts of acute gouty arthritis. J Rheumatol. 2002;29(2):331–334.
21. Mandell BF, Edwards NL, Sundy JS, et al. Preventing and treating acute gout attacks across the clinical spectrum: A roundtable discussion. Cleve Clin J Med. 2010;77(Suppl 2):S2–S25. doi:10.3949/ccjm.77.s2.01.
22. Schlesinger N. Management of acute and chronic gouty arthritis: Present state-of-the-art. Drugs. 2004;64(21):2399–2416.
23. Conaghan PG, Day RO. Risks and benefits of drugs used in the management and prevention of gout. Drug Saf Int J Med Toxicol Drug Exp. 1994;11(4):252–258.
24. Schumacher HR, Berger MF, Li-Yu J, et al. Efficacy and tolerability of celecoxib in the treatment of acute gouty arthritis: A randomized controlled trial. J Rheumatol. 2012;39(9):1859–1866. doi:10.3899/jrheum.110916.
25. Smallwood JI, Malawista SE. Colchicine, crystals, and neutrophil tyrosine phosphorylation. J Clin Invest. 1993;92(4):1602–1603. doi:10.1172/JCI116742.
26. Ahern MJ, Reid C, Gordon TP, et al. Does colchicine work? The results of the first controlled study in acute gout. Aust N Z J Med. 1987;17(3):301–304.
27. Wallace SL, Singer JZ, Duncan GJ, et al. Renal function predicts colchicine toxicity: Guidelines for the prophylactic use of colchicine in gout. J Rheumatol. 1991;18(2):264–269.
28. Dixon AJ, Wall GC. Probable colchicine-induced neutropenia not related to intentional overdose. Ann Pharmacother. 2001;35(2):192–195.
29. Terkeltaub R, Zelman D, Scavulli J, et al. Gout Study Group: Update on hyperuricemia and gout. Jt Bone Spine Rev Rhum. 2009;76(4):444–446. doi:10.1016/j.jbspin.2009.05.006.
30. Terkeltaub RA, Furst DE, Bennett K, et al. High versus low dosing of oral colchicine for early acute gout flare: Twenty-four–hour outcome of the first multicenter, randomized, double-blind, placebo-controlled, parallel-group, dose-comparison colchicine study. Arthritis Rheum. 2010;62(4):1060–1068. doi:10.1002/art.27327.
31. Colcrys (colchicine) [product information]. http://dailymed.nlm.nih.gov/dailymed/lookup.cfm?setid=176af20d-d082-47bd-bc56-a21cc1244a33. Accessed August 27, 2014.
32. Janssens HJ, Janssen M, van de Lisdonk EH, et al. Use of oral prednisolone or naproxen for the treatment of gout arthritis: A double-blind, randomised equivalence trial. Lancet. 2008;371(9627):1854–1860. doi:10.1016/S0140-6736(08)60799-0.
33. De Klerk E, van der Heijde D, Landewé R, et al. Patient compliance in rheumatoid arthritis, polymyalgia rheumatica, and gout. J Rheumatol. 2003;30(1):44–54.
34. Pal B, Foxall M, Dysart T, et al. How is gout managed in primary care? A review of current practice and proposed guidelines. Clin Rheumatol. 2000;19(1):21–25.
35. Thurston MM, Phillips BB, Bourg CA. Safety and efficacy of allopurinol in chronic kidney disease. Ann Pharmacother. 2013;47(11):1507–1516. doi:10.1177/1060028013504740.
36. Vazquez-Mellado J, Morales EM, Pacheco-Tena C, Burgos-Vargas R. Relation between adverse events associated with allopurinol and renal function in patients with gout. Ann Rheum Dis. 2001;60(10):981–983.
37. Stamp LK, O'Donnell JL, Zhang M, et al. Using allopurinol above the dose based on creatinine clearance is effective and safe in patients with chronic gout, including those with renal impairment. Arthritis Rheum. 2011;63(2):412–421.
38. Khoo BP, Leow YH. A review of inpatients with adverse drug reactions to allopurinol. Singapore Med J. 2000;41(4):156–160.
39. Zyloprim (allopurinol) [product information]. http://dailymed.nlm.nih.gov/dailymed/lookup.cfm?setid=2298ed2a-e01b-4f7c-9902-7c58a6e06b7a. Accessed August 27, 2014.
40. Zineh I, Mummaneni P, Lyndly J, et al. Allopurinol pharmacogenetics: Assessment of potential clinical usefulness. Pharmacogenomics. 2011;12(12):1741–1749. doi:10.2217/pgs.11.131.
41. Bardin T. Current management of gout in patients unresponsive or allergic to allopurinol. Jt Bone Spine Rev Rhum. 2004;71(6):481–485. doi:10.1016/j.jbspin.2004.07.006.
42. Fam AG, Dunne SM, Iazzetta J, Paton TW. Efficacy and safety of desensitization to allopurinol following cutaneous reactions. Arthritis Rheum. 2001;44(1):231–238. doi:10.1002/1529-0131(200101)44:1<231:AID-ANR30>3.0.CO;2-7.
43. Uloric (febuxostat) [product information]. http://dailymed.nlm.nih.gov/dailymed/lookup.cfm?setid=ae1e0d8a-03fc-419b-9d44-afa68fbd5681. Accessed August 27, 2014.
44. Becker MA, Schumacher HR Jr, Wortmann RL, et al. Febuxostat compared with allopurinol in patients with hyperuricemia and gout. N Engl J Med. 2005;353(23):2450–2461.
45. Benemid (probenecid) [product information]. http://dailymed.nlm.nih.gov/dailymed/lookup.cfm?setid=ab497fd8-00c3-4364-b003-b39d21fbdf38. Accessed August 27, 2014.
46. Takahashi S, Moriwaki Y, Yamamoto T, et al. Effects of combination treatment using anti-hyperuricaemic agents with fenofibrate and/or losartan on uric acid metabolism. Ann Rheum Dis. 2003;62(6):572–575.
47. Sundy JS, Becker MA, Baraf HS, et al. Reduction of plasma urate levels following treatment with multiple doses of pegloticase (polyethylene glycol-conjugated uricase) in patients with treatment-failure gout: Results of a phase II randomized study. Arthritis Rheum. 2008;58(9):2882–2891. doi:10.1002/art.23810.

60 Musculoskeletal Disorders

Jill S. Borchert

LEARNING OBJECTIVES

Upon completion of the chapter, the reader will be able to:

1. Describe the pathophysiologic principles of tissue injury and inflammation.
2. Identify the desired therapeutic outcomes for a patient with musculoskeletal injury or pain.
3. Identify the factors that guide selection of an analgesic or counterirritant for a particular patient.
4. Recommend appropriate nonpharmacologic and pharmacologic therapy for a patient with musculoskeletal injury or pain.
5. Design a patient education plan, including nonpharmacologic therapy and preventative strategies.
6. Develop a monitoring plan to assess treatment of a patient with a musculoskeletal disorder.

INTRODUCTION

The musculoskeletal system consists of muscles, bones, joints, tendons, and ligaments. Disorders related to the musculoskeletal system often are classified by etiology. Acute soft-tissue injuries include strains and sprains of muscles and ligaments.[1] Repeated movements in sports, exercise, work, or activities of daily living can lead to repetitive strain injury, where cumulative damage occurs to the muscles, ligaments, or tendons.[2,3] Although tendonitis and bursitis can arise from acute injury, more commonly these conditions occur as a result of chronic stress.[2,4] Other forms of chronic musculoskeletal pain, such as pain from rheumatoid arthritis (see Chapter 57) or osteoarthritis (see Chapter 58), are discussed elsewhere in this textbook.

EPIDEMIOLOGY AND ETIOLOGY

Musculoskeletal disorders are commonly self-treated, so true estimates of the incidence of both acute and chronic injury are difficult to obtain. In the United States, over 60 million musculoskeletal injuries occur each year, with 60% of episodes treated in ambulatory care offices.[3] These disorders account for a large portion of medical care expenditures and are a leading cause of work absenteeism and disability, resulting in a substantial economic burden from lost productivity and lost wages.

Some musculoskeletal disorders are induced by trauma at the workplace either via a one-time overexertion or through repetition and cumulative trauma.[3] Strains and sprains are the most common workplace injuries, representing over three-fourths of all musculoskeletal injuries. Musculoskeletal injuries are more likely to occur with heavy lifting, exposure to vibration, or working overhead.[5]

In the elderly, musculoskeletal injuries may not be related to work but to daily life. Half of all musculoskeletal injuries occur in the home with falls being the most common cause for those aged 65 and older.[3] In children and adolescents, fractures are more common than muscle and tendon injuries because growth spurts cause bones to weaken while the muscle–tendon unit tightens.[2]

Muscle injuries comprise the majority of sports-related injuries, and roughly half are related to overuse.[6,7] The ankle is the most common site of sports injury.[8] Basketball, which requires rapid acceleration and higher speeds, poses the greatest risk of muscle sprain.[9] Other sports requiring pivoting at higher speeds, such as volleyball and soccer, also pose a high risk of overuse and acute injury, especially to the knee.[7]

Overuse musculoskeletal injury is the phrase used to describe disorders arising from repetitive motion. This injury is common in activities such as running, particularly during periods of increased intensity or duration of training. It also can occur in the workplace with repeated, unvaried motion.[5]

PATHOPHYSIOLOGY

Skeletal muscle consists of muscle fibers linked together by connective tissue. Tendons and ligaments are composed of collagenous fibers that have a restricted capability to stretch. Tendons connect muscle to bone, whereas ligaments connect bone to bone.

Muscle Strains and Sprains

A **sprain** is an overstretching of supporting ligaments that results in a partial or complete tear of the ligament.[1,6,9] Although a **strain** also arises from an overstretching of the muscle–tendon unit, it is marked by damage to the muscle fibers or tendon without tearing of the ligament. The key difference is that a sprain involves damage to ligaments, whereas a strain involves damage primarily to muscle.

Overloading the muscle and connective tissue results in complete or partial tears of the skeletal muscle, tendons, or ligaments.[6,10] This usually occurs when the muscle is activated in an *eccentric contraction*, defined as a contraction in which the muscle is being lengthened.[10] Examples of this type of contraction include putting down a large, heavy laundry basket or lowering oneself from a chin-up bar. Small tears can occur in the muscle because it is lengthening while also trying to contract to support the load. This leads to rupture of blood vessels at the site of the injury, resulting in the formation of a hematoma. Within 24 to 48 hours, an inflammatory response develops. During the inflammatory stage, macrophages remove necrotic fibers.[6,11] The activated neutrophils then release growth factors that will activate myocytes for regeneration. Finally, capillaries grow into the area, and muscle fibers regenerate during the repair and remodeling phases of healing.

Bursitis and Tendonitis

Bursitis is an inflammation of the bursa, the fluid-filled sac near the joint where the tendons and muscles pass over the bone.[4] Overuse of a joint can result in an inflamed bursa. Bursitis causes stiffness and pain because the bursa serves to reduce friction within the joint space.

Tendonitis (or *tendinitis*) refers to inflammation of the tendon that follows incomplete tendon degeneration.[2] Repetitive overuse of a tendon can cause cellular changes in the tissues. Specifically, collagenous tendon tissue is replaced with tissue that lacks the organized collagen arrangement of a normal tendon. In fact, many patients diagnosed with chronic tendonitis may not have inflammation but instead have **tendinosis**, a condition marked by these degenerative changes. As a result of the cellular changes, the tendon progressively loses elasticity and its ability to handle stress or weight. This makes the tendon vulnerable to rupture or inflammation.

Inflammation and Peripheral Pain Sensation

Inflammation is a common pathway in soft-tissue injury of musculoskeletal disorders. Inflammatory processes lead to two outcomes: swelling and pain. Inflammatory processes are considered to be a necessary part of the remodeling process because inflammatory cells remove damaged tissue.[12–14] However, inflammation also contributes to continued pain and swelling that limits range of motion.

The initial injury exposes membrane phospholipids to phospholipase A_2, leading to the formation of arachidonic acid.[12,15] Next, arachidonic acid is transformed by cyclooxygenase (COX) to thromboxanes and prostaglandins (PGs), including prostaglandin E_2 (PGE_2). PGE_2 is the most potent inflammatory mediator; it increases vascular permeability, leading to redness, warmth, and swelling of the affected area. The increased permeability also increases **proteolysis**, or the breakdown of proteins in the damaged tissue.

Neutrophils, lymphocytes, and monocytes are attracted to the area, and monocytes are converted to macrophages, which then stimulate additional PG production.[12] Phagocytic cells release cytokines, including interleukins, interferon, and tumor necrosis factor.

In addition to increasing vascular permeability, PGs also induce pain by sensitizing pain receptors to other substances such as bradykinin. Bradykinin, PGs, leukotrienes, and other inflammatory mediators lower the pain threshold through peripheral pain sensitization. These substances make nerve endings more excitable, and the nerve fibers are more reactive to serotonin, heat, and mechanical stimuli.[16] The increased sensitization in the damaged tissue causes tenderness, soreness, and **hyperalgesia**.[16] The process also facilitates production of additional PGs. In a cyclic fashion, the PGs then sensitize the nerves to bradykinin action.

Without interruption, the neurochemicals ultimately lead to a firing of the unmyelinated or thinly myelinated afferent neurons. This sends messages along the pain pathway in the periphery and communicates the pain message to the CNS. Interruption of this cycle may occur via the effects of anti-inflammatory agents such as aspirin and nonsteroidal anti-inflammatory drugs (NSAIDs).

Nerve receptors, or **nociceptors**, release substance P and other peptides when they are activated.[16] Substance P mediates the production and release of inflammatory mediators and acts as a potent vasodilator. This receptor activation also increases the sensitivity of nociceptors to painful stimuli. Capsaicin relieves pain by stimulating the release of substance P from sensory nerve fibers, ultimately depleting stores of substance P.[17]

CLINICAL PRESENTATION AND DIAGNOSIS

See next page for information on the clinical presentation and diagnosis of musculoskeletal disorders.

TREATMENT

Desired Outcomes

KEY CONCEPT *The two primary goals of treating musculoskeletal disorders are to: (a) relieve pain and (b) maintain functionality.* This is accomplished by decreasing the severity and duration of pain, shortening the recovery period, and preventing acute injury pain from becoming chronic pain. If these goals are achieved, functional limitations are decreased. Ideally, a patient should be able to continue to perform activities of daily living and maintain normal functions in the workplace. Children ideally should be able to maintain usual play activities and sports schedules.

Further goals include a return to usual activity and prevention of future injury. It is also important to minimize the potential for adverse drug events during treatment.

General Approach to Treatment

Treatment of musculoskeletal disorders involves three phases: (a) therapy of an acute injury using the rest, ice, compression, and elevation (RICE) principle; (b) pain relief using oral or topical agents; and (c) lifestyle and behavioral modifications for rehabilitation and to prevent recurrent injury or chronic pain (**Figure 60–1**).

In many cases, musculoskeletal disorders are self-treated with over-the-counter (OTC) oral or topical agents. However, further evaluation may be warranted if acute pain persists longer than

Patient Encounter 1, Part 1

A 28-year-old woman presents with left ankle pain. She stepped on one of her son's toys earlier today after coming down the stairs at home and twisted her ankle. The pain occurs at rest and is worsened with weight bearing on the ankle and with rotation or movement. There is moderate swelling and bruising of the left ankle.

What information is suggestive of a musculoskeletal disorder?

What is your assessment of the patient's ankle pain?

What additional information do you need to formulate a treatment plan?

Clinical Presentation and Diagnosis of Musculoskeletal Disorders

General[2,4,7,13]

- Clinical presentation varies based on etiology of the disorder.
- Repetitive strain or overuse injuries may have a gradual onset.
- Disorders due to acute injury may be associated with other signs of injury such as abrasion.
- Low back pain is often chronic.

Signs and Symptoms of Acute Soft-Tissue Injury (Strains, Sprains)[8,13]

- Discomfort ranging from tenderness to pain may occur at rest or with motion
- Swelling and inflammation of the affected area
- Bruising
- Loss of motion
- Mechanical instability

Signs and Symptoms of Repetitive Strain or Overuse Injury (Tendonitis, Bursitis)[2,4,7]

- Pain and stiffness that occurs either at rest or with motion
- Localized tenderness on palpation
- Mild swelling of the affected area
- Decreased range of motion
- Muscle atrophy

Other Diagnostic Tests and Assessments[8]

- *Radiograph (x-ray)*: Evaluate bony structures to rule out fracture, malalignment, or joint erosion as the primary cause of pain.
- *MRI*: Soft-tissue imaging to evaluate for tendon or ligament tears.
- *Ultrasound*: Superficial soft-tissue imaging to evaluate for tears in tendons or ligaments. Ultrasound does not penetrate bone, so it is of limited usefulness for assessing tendons or ligaments deep within joints.
- *Pain scale*: Patient self-rating on a scale of zero (no pain) to 10 (worst possible pain). Used to assess pain both at rest and with movement. Determined at baseline and to assess response to therapy.

7 to 10 days, symptoms worsen or subside and then return, or there are signs of a more serious condition.[8,18,19] Warning signs of more serious conditions include joint deformity, dislocation, or lack of movement in a joint. Low back pain accompanied by burning, radiating pain, or difficulty urinating requires further evaluation.

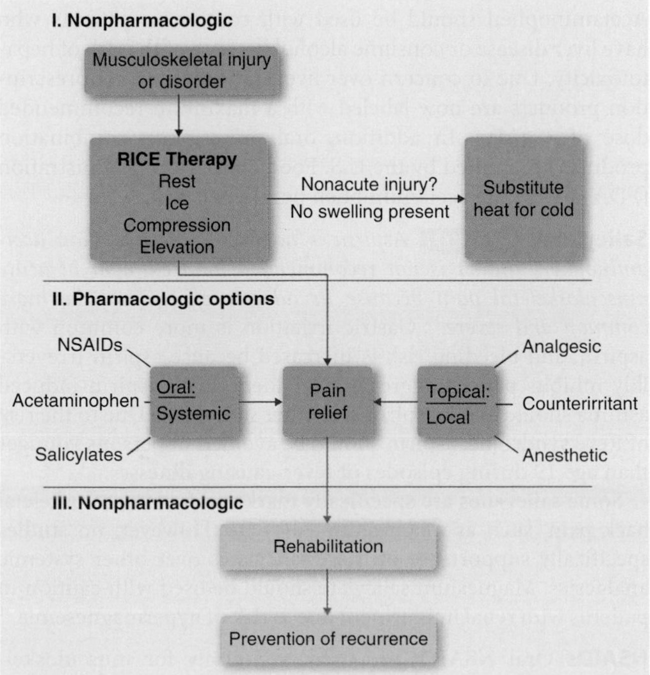

FIGURE 60–1. Treatment plan for musculoskeletal injury or disorder.

In children and adolescents, treatment practices are similar to the approach in adults with a focus on nonpharmacologic therapy and oral analgesics. Children younger than 2 years, elderly persons, and pregnant women also may need special care. Elderly patients may be more prone to systemic effects because of thinning of the skin and increased absorption of topical agents and drug interactions from polypharmacy.

Nonpharmacologic Therapy: RICE

KEY CONCEPT *The cornerstone of nonpharmacologic therapy for acute injury in the first 48 to 72 hours is known by the acronym RICE: rest, ice, compression, and elevation*[6,13,20] (Table 60–1). These four methods initially minimize bleeding from broken blood vessels. Rest eases pressure on the affected area and promotes pain control during the acute inflammatory phase (the first 1–5 days after injury). Cold causes vasoconstriction, assisting in prevention of a large hematoma and providing analgesia by slowing nerve impulses. Immediately after injury, ice also helps to reduce metabolic rate and oxygen demand, thereby reducing tissue damage from hypoxia.[20] Compression, achieved by wrapping the area with an elastic bandage, also reduces the size of the developing hematoma.[6] Preventing hematoma formation is important because a large hematoma can limit mobility and range of motion. Cold and compression also decrease swelling. Elevation decreases blood flow and increases venous return from the affected area.

In addition to minimizing the acute inflammatory response, rest prevents additional injury to the affected area.[6] During acute injury, the ability of muscles and tendons to stretch is limited. Movement in the injured tissue can cause further retraction of the ruptured muscle and increase the size of the gap in the muscle to be healed. Therefore, early activity predisposes a patient to further injury, but prolonged inactivity can lengthen recovery times.

The benefits of ice following injury are well documented, but recommendations for the method of application vary widely.[13,14,20]

Table 60–1

RICE Therapy

Therapy	General Guidelines	Therapeutic Benefit
Rest	Rest the affected area	Analgesia
	Use supports such as slings and crutches as necessary	Anti-inflammatory
	Employ during the acute inflammatory phase, 1–5 days after injury	Prevent further injury
Ice	Cool the affected area by submersion in cool water (13°C [55°F]) or by application of crushed ice in a plastic bag covered with a thin cloth	Analgesia
	Cool the affected area for 15–20 minutes; repeat every 2 hours for the first 48 hours	Anti-inflammatory
Compression	Compress the affected area with an elastic bandage or support	Anti-inflammatory
	Begin wrapping the bandage at the point most distal to the injury (eg, at the toes for an ankle injury); bind firmly but not tightly	Adjunctive analgesia
	If the area distal to the injury (eg, fingers, toes) throbs or turns cold or blue, the bandage is too tight and should be loosened	
Elevation	Elevate the area (especially the extremities) above heart level	Anti-inflammatory

Crushed ice or ice chips should be used because the area will cool more evenly than with large pieces of ice. Patients should not apply ice directly to the affected area or leave it on for longer than the recommended 20 minutes, because extreme cold can cause tissue damage.[13] Similarly, patients should wait at least 1 hour before reapplication of ice to allow the tissue to rewarm. A thin sheet or napkin will protect the skin and also allow for better cold transfer than thicker material such as a towel. Alternatively, soaking the area for 20 minutes in a cool bath (13°C [55°F]) provides effective cooling, provided the area can remain elevated.

For small areas, an ice massage for 5 to 10 minutes can cool the area and add relief.[21] This can be accomplished by freezing water in a paper cup, removing the top part of the cup to expose the ice, and rubbing the exposed ice on the affected area. Any ice application should be stopped if the area becomes white or blue. KEY CONCEPT *Heat should not be applied during the acute injury phase (when edema is present) because it promotes swelling and inflammation.*[14,21] After the acute phase, many patients find that heat decreases pain and eases muscle stiffness. A heating pad, heat wrap, or warm bath can be used as long as no edema is present and no swelling develops after heat is applied. Patients should avoid sleeping with or sitting or lying on heating pads because this can result in burns. Low-level heat, such as that supplied by therapeutic heat wraps (eg, ThermaCare), may provide a safer means of heat application. However, the risk of burns increases with age, and elderly persons should be cautioned about this risk.

Pharmacologic Therapy

KEY CONCEPT *There are two main approaches to pharmacologic intervention for pain relief: oral (systemic) and topical agents.* The choice between systemic or topical options is often guided by patient preference. For example, many topical products have a medicinal odor and require frequent applications. The extent of musculoskeletal pain also guides treatment choice. KEY CONCEPT *Localized pain may be treated effectively with local topical therapy, whereas generalized pain is best treated with systemic agents.* Factors such as alcohol use, liver function, renal function, allergies, age, and comorbid conditions should be considered when choosing among therapeutic options.

► *Oral Analgesics*

Nonopioid analgesics, including acetaminophen, aspirin, and NSAIDs, are used commonly for musculoskeletal disorders. These agents all provide analgesia, but aspirin and NSAIDs also work peripherally by inhibiting the enzyme COX to decrease production of PGE_2, the principal mediator of acute inflammation.[15,16] Although the mechanism of action of acetaminophen is less clear, it appears that acetaminophen acts as a weak inhibitor of PG production via COX-2 inhibition and exerts only a mild anti-inflammatory effect.[22]

Acetaminophen KEY CONCEPT *Acetaminophen is the drug of choice for mild-to-moderate regional musculoskeletal pain without inflammation.*[15,23] Comparative trials between acetaminophen and oral NSAIDs demonstrate equivalent analgesia in some situations, but NSAIDs may be preferred in others. Therefore, if adequate analgesia is not achieved with acetaminophen, switching to an NSAID is a reasonable alternative. Acetaminophen offers the advantage of less GI toxicity than NSAIDs. Although tolerability of acetaminophen is high at therapeutic doses, hepatotoxicity has been reported after overdose and at therapeutic doses, especially in combination with other factors.[15,23] Patients should not exceed 4 g/day of acetaminophen to minimize the risk of liver injury. Acetaminophen should be used with caution in patients who have liver disease or consume alcohol because of the risk of hepatotoxicity. Due to concern over liver injury, many nonprescription products are now labeled with a maximum recommended dose of 3 g/day. In addition, oral prescription combination products are limited by the U.S. Food and Drug Administration (FDA) to 325 mg acetaminophen per dosage unit.

Salicylates KEY CONCEPT *Aspirin is not more effective than acetaminophen, and it is not recommended for treatment of acute musculoskeletal pain because its adverse effects may be more common and severe.*[15] Gastric irritation is more common with aspirin, and bleeding risk is increased because aspirin irreversibly inhibits platelet aggregation. Patients with aspirin-induced asthma should avoid aspirin and other salicylates. Due to the risk of Reye syndrome, aspirin should be avoided in persons younger than age 19 during episodes of fever-causing illnesses.

Some salicylates are specifically marketed for musculoskeletal back pain, such as magnesium salicylate. However, no studies specifically support use of these salicylates over other systemic analgesics. Magnesium salicylate should be used with caution in patients with renal impairment due to risk of hypermagnesemia.[15]

NSAIDs Oral NSAIDs are used commonly for musculoskeletal pain because of their availability without a prescription and anti-inflammatory effects.[15,16] KEY CONCEPT *NSAIDs are a preferred choice over acetaminophen in musculoskeletal disorders in which* *inflammation is the primary problem.*[4,15,23] As a result, NSAIDs are particularly beneficial for chronic overuse injury, in which inflammation is central to the pain and loss of motion. Although NSAIDs may be helpful in relieving pain and inflammation in tendonitis, many tendinopathies are not associated with inflammation. Therefore, use of a simple analgesic such as acetaminophen may relieve pain adequately.[2]

The analgesic effects of NSAIDs are attributed to inhibition of the COX-2 enzyme, whereas the negative GI effects are due to inhibition of COX-1.[15] Patients taking oral anticoagulants, those with a history of peptic ulcer disease, or others at high risk for GI complications may be considered candidates for a COX-2 inhibitor (eg, celecoxib) or a combination of a nonselective NSAID with a gastroprotective agent such as a proton pump inhibitor (see Chapter 58). Combination of any NSAID, including COX-2 inhibitors, with alcohol can increase GI adverse effects. Additionally, all NSAIDs should be used with caution in patients with aspirin-induced asthma.[15]

Both nonselective NSAIDs and COX-2 inhibitors are associated with nephrotoxicity.[23] Furthermore, NSAIDs, including selective COX-2 inhibitors, may increase the risk of myocardial infarction. However, this risk may be higher for the COX-2 inhibitors due to an imbalance in thromboxane A_2 relative to prostacyclin levels creating a prothrombotic environment. A more detailed discussion of the relative risks of nonselective NSAIDs and COX-2 inhibitors and treatment options based on the cardiovascular and GI risk of the individual patient appears elsewhere in this text (see Chapter 58).

Opioids Opioid analgesics can be used for patients not responding adequately to nonopioid analgesics or for moderate-to-severe pain.[4] These agents generally are given alone or in combination with simple analgesics such as acetaminophen. Tolerance and physical dependence are considerations but less of a concern when treating acute pain. When used in equivalent doses, opioids produce similar pain relief and adverse effects such as sedation, nausea, constipation, and respiratory depression (see Chapter 34).

► Topical (External) Analgesics

Topically (or externally) applied drugs that exert a local analgesic, anesthetic, or antipruritic effect by either suppressing cutaneous sensory receptors or by stimulating these receptors in a counterirritant fashion are termed *external analgesics*.[18] These medications are applied directly to the affected area to create high local concentrations of the drug.[17,24] Formulations include gel, cream, lotion, patch, liquid, liniment, or aerosol spray. Negligible systemic concentrations are achieved with intact skin, minimizing systemic adverse effects. Topical application should not be confused with transdermal delivery, in which drug absorption into the bloodstream produces a systemic effect. Musculoskeletal disorders often are treated with topical (but not transdermal) medications.

After application, the topical medication penetrates the skin to the soft tissue and peripheral nerves.[18] At the site, topical analgesics suppress the sensitization of pain receptors, thereby reducing pain and burning. Examples include topical NSAIDs and local anesthetics such as lidocaine. In contrast, *counterirritant* products are external analgesics that stimulate cutaneous sensory receptors, producing a burning, warming, or cooling sensation that masks the underlying pain. In effect, the irritation or inflammation caused by the counterirritant distracts from the underlying pain. Menthol and capsaicin are examples of counterirritants.

Some patients prefer external analgesics to systemic analgesics because the rubbing during application can be comforting.[25] External analgesics are useful adjuvants to nonpharmacologic therapy and systemic analgesic therapy to provide additional relief. These agents are also an option in patients who cannot tolerate systemic analgesics. Because these products are not in pill form and many are available without a prescription, they may be overused or misused. This prompted the FDA to caution consumers that the agents are medicines that may also cause harm.[26] Clinicians should advise patients to read and follow directions on the labels of OTC products.

Topical NSAIDs. In acute soft-tissue injury such as strains and sprains, topical NSAIDs have efficacy that is superior to that of placebo and similar to that of oral NSAIDs.[24,27] Tissue concentrations of topical NSAIDs are high enough to produce anti-inflammatory effects, but systemic concentrations after application remain low.

Diclofenac is the only topical NSAID commercially available in the United States.[27–31] Diclofenac patch (Flector Patch) is indicated specifically for topical treatment of acute pain from minor sprains and strains.[28] The patch is applied to the most painful area twice daily. Diclofenac gel (Voltaren Gel) is indicated for joint pain in the knees and hands secondary to osteoarthritis; it is applied up to four times daily.[29] Diclofenac solution (Pennsaid) is indicated for osteoarthritis of the knee; it is applied to the knee and is available in a solution applied via dropper four times daily or via measured pump two times daily.[27,31] Patient education for topical NSAIDs is outlined in Table 60–2.[27–29,31]

Table 60–2

Patient Education for Topical Diclofenac Products

All Topical Products	Diclofenac Gel	Diclofenac Patch	Diclofenac Solution
Do not apply to damaged or nonintact skin Wash hands after application and/or removal Discontinue use if rash or irritation develops Do not use with oral NSAIDs	Use enclosed dosing card to determine amount for application Avoid bathing or showering for 1 hour after application Avoid sun exposure or tanning beds Do not use with other topical agents (eg, sunscreens, lotions, moisturizers, and insect repellants)	Apply to skin at the most painful area Do not wear during bathing or showering Tape patch in place if it begins to peel off Discard used patches away from children and pets	Apply 40 drops of 1.5% solution (10 drops at a time) four times daily or two pump actuations of 2% solution twice daily to each affected knee Apply directly to knee or first into the hand, then to the knee Rub evenly around front, back, and sides of the knee Do not cover with clothing or apply other topical products until completely dry

Data from Refs. 27–29 and 31.

Table 60–3

Nonprescription Counterirritant External Analgesics

Group and Effect	Agents and Concentration	Example Products (If Applicable)	Comments
Group A			
Rubefacients: Produce redness	Allyl isothiocyanate 0.5%–5%		Mustard derivative; pungent odor; avoid inhalation
	Ammonia water 1%–2.5%		More concentrated solutions are highly caustic; avoid inhalation
	Methyl salicylate 10%–60%	BenGay Ultra Strength[a] Flexall Plus[a] Icy Hot Stick[a]	Caution in aspirin sensitivity May produce systemic concentrations May increase INR with warfarin
Group B			
Produce cooling	Camphor 3%–11% Menthol 1.25%–16%	JointFlex BenGay Patch Icy Hot Patch Mineral Ice	Medicinal odor Sensation of heat follows cooling Mild anesthetic effects at low concentrations
Group C			
Produce vasodilation	Methyl nicotinate 0.25%–1%		May produce systemic vasodilation
Group D			
Irritate without redness	Capsaicin 0.025%–0.25% Capsicum oleoresin 0.025%–0.25%	Capzasin-HP, Zostrix	Must use regularly Burning effect subsides with regular use

INR, international normalized ratio.

[a]Combination products that also contain menthol and/or camphor.

Theoretically, the risk of serious GI adverse events should be less than with oral NSAIDs, but long-term studies evaluating these events are lacking.[24,30] Like oral NSAIDs, topical NSAIDs should be used with caution in patients with a history of GI bleeding or ulcer.[27–29,31] Studies comparing topical NSAIDs with other topical products, including counterirritants, are also needed. Local cutaneous adverse reactions (eg, erythema, rash, pruritus, and irritation) are reported and may be due in part to the vehicle used.[27–29,31]

Local Anesthetics. Nonprescription topical anesthetics such as lidocaine and benzocaine are available in many types of products. Local anesthetics decrease discharges in superficial somatic nerves and cause numbness on the skin surface but do not penetrate deeper structures such as muscle where the pain often lies.[17]

However, local anesthetics are helpful when abrasion accompanies the injury. Application of an OTC antibiotic ointment containing an anesthetic provides soothing relief, promotes healing of abrasions, and prevents soft-tissue infection. Minor abrasions should be cleansed with mild soap and water before application. More severe abrasions may require removal of debris by a clinician followed by irrigation with normal saline.

Counterirritants. Counterirritants are categorized by the FDA into four groups (groups A through D) based on their primary actions (Table 60–3). They produce a feeling of warmth, cooling, or irritation that diverts sensation from the primary source of pain. Because these irritant effects are central to the beneficial actions, counterirritants should not be combined with topical anesthetics or topical analgesics.

Counterirritants are indicated for the temporary relief of minor aches and pains related to muscles and joints.[18] These symptoms may be associated with simple backache, arthritis, strains, sprains, or bruises. Many are available as combination products with ingredients from different counterirritant groups. Active ingredients in marketed products sometimes change; clinicians should be aware of the current ingredients before providing a product recommendation. KEY CONCEPT *Patient education on proper use of counterirritants is essential to therapeutic success* (Table 60–4).[18]

Rubefacients (group A) are counterirritants that produce redness on application. Topical rubefacients containing salicylates (eg, methyl salicylate) are used most commonly. Turpentine oil is no longer judged as either safe or effective but remains in a few products.[18] Clinical trial data evaluating the effect of rubefacients on acute pain from strains, sprains, sports injuries, and chronic musculoskeletal pain are lacking.[32] A systematic review noted that topical salicylates are effective for pain from acute musculoskeletal conditions, but the low quality of the evidence

Table 60–4

Patient Education for Counterirritants

Apply up to three to five times daily to affected area.
Only for external use on the skin; do not ingest.
Do not apply to broken or damaged skin or cover large areas.
Wash hands immediately after application.
Avoid contact with the eyes and mouth.
Do not use with heating pads or other methods of heat application, because burning or blistering can occur.
Do not wrap or bandage the area tightly after application.
Consult a physician if:

- Symptoms worsen
- Symptoms persist for more than 7 days[a]
- Symptoms resolve but then recur

[a]Capsaicin may be used for chronic pain and must be applied consistently for efficacy.

From External analgesics drug products for over-the-counter human use: tentative final monograph. Fed Regist. 1983;48:5851–5869.

led authors to conclude that there are no good data supporting the efficacy of rubefacients.[32]

Methyl salicylate and trolamine salicylate are topical salicylates. Methyl salicylate is considered a counterirritant, but trolamine salicylate is not considered a counterirritant because it does not produce localized irritation after application. Application of both topical salicylates can lead to systemic effects, especially if the product is applied liberally.[33] Repeated application and occlusion with a wrap or bandage also can increase systemic concentrations. Salicylate-containing products should be used with caution in patients in whom systemic salicylates are contraindicated, such as patients with severe asthma or aspirin allergy.[33] Topical salicylates have been reported to increase prothrombin time in patients on warfarin and should be used with caution in patients on oral anticoagulants. Methyl salicylate, including oil of wintergreen, is a common source of pediatric poisonings.[34] Clinicians should advise patients to keep products out of the reach of children.

The FDA advises that there is insufficient evidence to support the effectiveness of trolamine salicylate.[18] However, many patients choose trolamine products because of the lack of medicinal odor.

The group B counterirritants menthol and camphor exert a sensation of cooling through direct action on sensory nerve endings.[33,35] A sensation of warmth follows the cooling effect. The agents also have mild anesthetic activity at low concentrations.[35] In higher concentrations, they act as counterirritants and cause a burning sensation by stimulating cutaneous nociceptors. Menthol and camphor are used often in combination with rubefacients.

Menthol, also known as peppermint oil, is used widely in toothpastes, mouthwashes, gum, lozenges, lip balms, and nasal decongestants. For topical analgesic use, it is available in creams, lotions, ointment, and patches. The patches can be trimmed to fit the affected area.

Menthol and camphor should not be used in children younger than 2 years.[18] Despite limits on the concentration of available products, camphor can be toxic to children even in small amounts, posing a seizure risk.[15] Patients should be advised to keep the products out of the reach of children.

The group C counterirritants methyl nicotinate and histamine dihydrochloride produce vasodilation.[18] Methyl nicotinate produces PG-mediated vasodilation.[36] NSAIDs and aspirin block the production of PGs and decrease methyl nicotinate–induced vasodilation. Application over a large area has been reported to cause systemic symptoms and syncope, possibly due to vasodilation and a decrease in blood pressure.[37] Patients should be educated to apply only scant amounts to the affected area.

The primary counterirritant in group D is capsaicin, a natural substance found in red chili peppers and responsible for the hot, spicy characteristic when used in foods.[15,17,25,38] Capsaicin stimulates the release of substance P from local sensory nerve fibers, depleting substance P stores over time. A period of reduced sensitivity to painful stimuli follows, and transmission of pain impulses to the CNS is reduced.

As with other counterirritants, capsaicin and its derivatives (ie, capsicum and capsicum oleoresin) exert a warming or burning sensation.[15,17] With repeated application, desensitization occurs, and the burning sensation subsides. This typically occurs within the first 1 to 2 weeks. After discontinuation, resensitization occurs gradually and returns completely within a few weeks.

Because of the lag time between initiation and effect, capsaicin is not used for treatment of acute pain from injury. Instead, topical capsaicin is used for chronic pain from musculoskeletal and neuropathic disorders. Capsaicin preparations have been studied for treatment of pain from diabetic neuropathy, osteoarthritis, postherpetic neuralgia, and other disorders.[39] It is often used as an adjuvant to systemic analgesics in these chronic pain conditions.

Although systemic adverse effects to capsaicin are rare, local adverse effects are expected and common.[17,25] Patient education regarding consistent use of capsaicin products is essential to achieving desired outcomes. Product should be applied in a thin layer and rubbed into the skin thoroughly until little remains on the surface.[33] KEY CONCEPT *Patients using capsaicin should be advised to apply it regularly and consistently three to four times daily and that full effect may take 1 to 2 weeks or longer.* Patients should be assured that the burning effects will diminish with repeated application. Adherence to therapy is essential because the burning sensation persists if applications are less frequent than recommended. Because the burning sensation is enhanced with heat, patients should avoid hot showers or baths immediately before or after application. Wearing nitrile gloves during application can decrease the potential for unintended contact with eyes or mucous membranes. Dried product residue has been reported to cause respiratory effects on inhalation, and caution should be used in patients with asthma or other respiratory illnesses.

▶ *Oral Muscle Relaxants*

Where pain is worsened by muscle spasm, oral muscle relaxants serve as a useful adjunct to therapy.[40] Antispasmodic agents are preferred over antispastic agents for musculoskeletal pain. The antispasmodic agents include metaxalone, methocarbamol, carisoprodol, and cyclobenzaprine. Muscle relaxants decrease spasm and stiffness associated with either acute or chronic musculoskeletal disorders. These agents should be used with caution because they all may cause sedation, especially in combination with alcohol or opioid analgesics.

Lifestyle and Behavioral Modifications

After treatment of the acute injury with RICE and pharmacologic therapy, the final phase of therapy is rehabilitation and prevention of future injury. For most injuries, prolonged

Patient Encounter 1, Part 2: Medical History, Physical Examination, and Diagnostic Tests

PMH/PSH: C-section 2 years ago

SH: Smokes two to three cigarettes per week socially; drinks wine with dinner on Fridays

Meds: Women's Multivitamin one tablet by mouth daily, vitamin D 400 IU by mouth daily

Allergies: NKDA

Intolerances: NSAIDS, stomach upset

Preferences: Prefers topical product due to history of adverse effects with oral products

Diagnostic Tests: Radiographs of left ankle show no evidence of fracture

What are your treatment goals and desired outcomes?

What nonpharmacologic and pharmacologic treatments options are available? Are there treatment options that should be avoided? If so, which options and why?

Patient Encounter 1, Part 3: Creating a Care Plan

Based on the information presented, create a care plan to treat this patient's ankle injury. Your plan should include the following:

(a) The goals of therapy and desired outcomes

(b) A patient-specific therapeutic plan, including nonpharmacologic therapy

(c) A plan to monitor the outcome of therapy to determine whether goals of therapy have been met and adverse effects avoided

immobilization can lengthen the recovery time by causing wasting of the healthy muscle fibers.[6,10,14] Rehabilitation starts with the development of range of motion via stretching exercises. The patient should warm the muscle first with light activity or moderate heat. Warmth produces relaxation and increases elasticity. Next, the patient should start general strengthening exercises.[20] Strengthening and stretching exercises should be continued beyond the healing phase to prevent future injury.

After rehabilitation, the patient should be educated about behavior changes to prevent reinjury or the development of chronic pain.[14,20] The warm-up and strengthening routines learned in the rehabilitation phase should be continued. For overuse injury, correction of biomechanical abnormalities with proper footwear and changes in technique may correct misalignments and imbalances. Repetitive trauma can be decreased with proper training (eg, by implementing a gradual increase in mileage in a running plan).[2,7]

Patient Encounter 2

A 14-year-old boy presents with right wrist pain. On questioning, you determine that he spends more than 4 hours a day playing video games and sends text messages often throughout the day. He is right-handed and reports gradual onset of pain over the last few months. When he wakes in the morning he has minimal pain after resting overnight, but the pain intensifies throughout the day. He reports decreased range of motion compared with the left wrist. He has no significant past medical history and his only medication is a daily multivitamin.

Given this information, what is your assessment of the patient's wrist pain? What is the likely etiology of the pain?

What nonpharmacologic and pharmacologic treatment options should be considered?

Based on the information presented, create a care plan for this patient's wrist injury. Your plan should include the following:

(a) The goals of therapy and desired outcomes

(b) A patient-specific therapeutic plan, including nonpharmacologic therapy

(c) A monitoring plan to determine whether goals of therapy have been met and adverse effects avoided

In the workplace, repetitive motion can be decreased through proper ergonomic design and diversification of job tasks.[5] In pain of the back or lower extremity, weight loss in overweight or obese patients can assist in reduction of further inflammation and help to prevent reinjury or repetitive strain injuries.[4]

Patient Care Process

Patient Assessment:

- Assess symptoms. Determine the timing of injury (if applicable), duration, type and degree of pain, and exacerbating factors. Determine if there is interference with usual activities or range of motion.
- Assess exacerbating or alleviating factors. Ask if the patient has tried any nonpharmacologic or pharmacologic treatments.
- Obtain a complete medication history, including prescription and nonprescription drugs and dietary supplement use. Determine whether the patient has used successful or unsuccessful treatments for this condition in the past.
- Gather patient history. Inquire about social history and alcohol use. Ask the patient about drug allergies and chronic health problems such as asthma.
- Assess patient preference for systemic (oral) or local (topical) therapy including acceptability of topical medication with frequent application and/or a medicinal odor.

Therapy Evaluation:

- Based on assessment of symptoms, determine whether empirical care or diagnostic evaluation is appropriate.
- If pain and/or swelling are not controlled, determine if pharmacologic therapy is warranted.

Care Plan Development:

- Select nonpharmacologic and pharmacologic therapy appropriate for the specific patient (see Tables 60–1 and 60–3; see Figure 60–1).
- Educate the patient on nonpharmacologic therapy, including each of the steps in RICE. If swelling is no longer present, consider heat instead of ice (see Table 60–1).
- Educate on proper use of oral or topical agents selected (see Tables 60–2 and 60–4). If a counterirritant is recommended, counsel patients on the irritant effect of the product and recommend washing hands immediately after use and to avoid heating pads. For patients using a capsaicin product, emphasize adherence.

Follow-Up Evaluation:

- If pain is from an acute injury, assess effectiveness within 7 to 10 days. For chronic pain treated with capsaicin, begin to assess pain control in 2 weeks.
- Evaluate for adherence, adverse effects (systemic or local), and drug interactions.

Non–weight-bearing activities, such as swimming or bicycling, can be recommended for initial return to activity.[41]

OUTCOME EVALUATION

- Use a pain scale to monitor treatment interventions to ensure that pain relief is achieved. Ask the patient to rate pain on a scale of zero (no pain) to 10 (worst possible pain) both at rest and with movement. Compare the results with baseline pain assessment to monitor the response to therapy. In pediatric patients, use a visual pain scale with facial expressions depicting various degrees of pain.
- Assess range of motion at baseline and after treatment by comparing movement with the unaffected limb and functionality before the injury. Assess functionality by asking patients if they are able to perform activities of daily living or participate in exercise as desired.
- If pain from acute injury does not decrease greatly within 7 to 10 days, further diagnostic evaluation is warranted.
- For patients using capsaicin products, assess adherence to regular application for therapeutic benefit. Assess chronic pain control in 2 weeks.
- Assess medication adverse effects on a regular basis. When NSAIDs and aspirin are used, ask about GI tolerability, bruising, and bleeding. Inquire about local adverse effects, such as burning, when topical counterirritants are used for treatment.
- Evaluate adherence to preventative rehabilitation measures such as proper footwear, warm-up before activity, strength training, and proper lifting technique.

Abbreviations Introduced in This Chapter

COX	Cyclooxygenase
NSAIDs	Nonsteroidal anti-inflammatory drugs
PG	Prostaglandin

REFERENCES

1. Coleman R, Reiland A. Orthopedic Emergencies. In: Stone CS, Humphries RL, ed. CURRENT Diagnosis & Treatment Emergency Medicine, 7th ed. New York: McGraw-Hill; 2011: 404–441.
2. Rodenberg RE, Bowman E, Ravindran R. Overuse injuries. Prim Care. 2013;40:453–473.
3. Musculoskeletal Injuries. In: United States Bone and Joint Initiative: The Burden of Musculoskeletal Diseases in the United States, 2nd ed. Rosemont, IL: American Academy of Orthopaedic Surgeons; 2011:129–179.
4. Yamada E, Thomas DC. Common musculoskeletal diagnoses of upper and lower extremities in older patients. Mt Sinai J Med. 2011;78:546–557.
5. Centers for Disease Control and Prevention Workplace Health. Work-Related Musculoskeletal Disorders Prevention [Internet]. Center for Disease Control and Prevention; 2013. http://www.cdc.gov/workplacehealthpromotion/evaluation/topics/disorders.html. Accessed June 2, 2014.
6. Järvinen TA, Järvinen TL, Kääriäinen M, et al. Muscle injuries: Optimising recovery. Best Pract Res Clin Rheumatol. 2007;21: 317–331.
7. Paterno MV, Taylor-Haas JA, Myer GD, Hewett TE. Prevention of overuse sports injuries in the young athlete. Orthop Clin North Am. 2013;44:553–564.
8. Boyd AS, Martinez RA, Feden JP. Acute musculoskeletal complaints. In: South-Paul J, Matheny SC, Lewis EL, eds. Current Diagnosis & Treatment in Family Medicine, 3rd ed. New York: McGraw-Hill; 2011:409–424.
9. Tiemstra JD. Update on acute ankle sprains. Am Fam Physician. 2012;85:1170–1176.
10. Howatson G, van Someren KA. The prevention and treatment of exercise-induced muscle damage. Sports Med. 2008;38:483–503.
11. De Carli A, Volpi P, Pelosini I, et al. New therapeutic approaches for management of sport-induced muscle strains. Adv Ther. 2009;26:1072–1083.
12. Widmaier EP, Raff H, Strang KT. Vander's Human Physiology: The Mechanisms of Body Function, 12th ed. New York: McGraw Hill; 2011.
13. Russell JA. Management of acute sport injury. In: Comfort P, Abrahamson E, eds. Sports Rehabilitation and Injury Prevention. Hoboken, NJ: Wiley-Blackwell; 2010:163–184.
14. Prentice WE. Using therapeutic modalities to affect the healing process. In: Prentice WE, Quillen WS, eds. Therapeutic Modalities in Rehabilitation, 4th ed. New York: McGraw-Hill; 2011:19–36.
15. Feucht CL, Patel DR. Analgesics and anti-inflammatory medications in sports: Use and abuse. Pediatr Clin North Am. 2010;57:751–774.
16. Rathmell JP, Fields HL. Pain: Pathophysiology and management. In: Longo D, Fauci A, Kasper D, et al, eds. Harrison's Principles of Internal Medicine, 18th ed. New York: McGraw-Hill; 2011: 93–101.
17. Stanos SP. Topical agents for the management of musculoskeletal pain. J Pain Symptom Manage. 2007;33:342–355.
18. External analgesic drug products for over-the-counter human use: Tentative final monograph. Fed Regist. 1983;48:5851–5869.
19. Last AR, Hulbert K. Chronic low back pain: Evaluation and management. Am Fam Physician. 2009;79:1067–1074.
20. Herrington L, Comfort P. Pathophysiology of skeletal muscle injuries. In: Comfort P, Abrahamson E, eds. Sports Rehabilitation and Injury Prevention, 1st ed. Great Britian: John Wiley & Sons, Ltd.; 2010:67–78.
21. Prentice WE. Cryotherapy and thermotherapy. In: Prentice WE, Quillen WS, eds. Therapeutic Modalities in Rehabilitation, 4th ed. New York: McGraw-Hill; 2011:285–362.
22. Graham GG, Davies MJ, Day RO, et al. The modern pharmacology of paracetamol: Therapeutic actions, mechanism of action, metabolism, toxicity and recent pharmacological findings. Inflammopharmacology. 2013;21:201–232.
23. Hunt RH, Choquette D, Craig BN, et al. Approach to managing musculoskeletal pain: Acetaminophen, cyclooxygenase-2 inhibitors, or traditional NSAIDs? Can Fam Physician. 2007;53: 1177–1184.
24. Haroutiunian S, Drennan DA, Lipman AG. Topical NSAID therapy for musculoskeletal pain. Pain Med. 2010;11:535–549.
25. Jackson KC, Argoff CE. Skeletal muscle relaxants and analgesic balms. In: Bonica's Management of Pain, 4th ed. Baltimore, MD: Lippincott Williams & Wilkins; 2009:1187–1193.
26. FDA Consumer Health Information. Use caution with over-the-counter creams, ointments [Internet]. Food & Drug Administration; 2008 [cited 2014 June 2]. http://www.fda.gov/forconsumers/consumerupdates/ucm049367.htm.
27. Pennsaid (diclofenac sodium topical solution 1.5%) product information. Hazelwood, MO: Mallinckrodt Brand Pharmaceuticals; 2013.
28. Flector Patch (diclofenac epolamine patch 1.3%) product information. Bristol, TN: King Pharmaceuticals; 2011.
29. Voltaren Gel (Diclofenac sodium topical gel 1%) product information. Novartis Consumer Health. Parsippany, NJ; 2009.
30. Zacher J, Altman R, Bellamy N, et al. Topical diclofenac and its role in pain and inflammation: An evidence-based review. Curr Med Res Opin. 2008;24:925–950.

31. Pennsaid (diclofenac sodium topical solution 2%) product information. Hazelwood, MO: Mallinckrodt Brand Pharmaceuticals; 2014.
32. Matthews P, Derry S, Moore RA, McQuay HJ. Topical rubefacients for acute and chronic pain in adults. Cochrane Database Syst Rev. 2009;CD007403.
33. Martindale: The complete drug reference. London: Pharmaceutical Press: Electronic version, Thomson Healthcare, Greenwood Village, CO.
34. Davis JE. Are one or two dangerous? Methyl salicylate exposure in toddlers. J Emerg Med. 2007;32:63–69.
35. Patel T, Ishiuji Y, Yosipovitch G. Menthol: A refreshing look at this ancient compound. J Am Acad Dermatol. 2007;57:873–878.
36. Wilkin JK, Fortner G, Reinhardt LA, et al. Prostaglandins and nicotinate-provoked increase in cutaneous blood flow. Clin Pharmacol Ther. 1985;38:273–277.
37. Fergusson DA. Systemic symptoms associated with a rubefacient. BMJ. 1988;297:1339.
38. McCleane G. Topical analgesic agents. Clin Geriatr Med. 2008;24: 299–312.
39. Stanos SP, Galluzzi KE. Topical therapies in the management of chronic pain. Postgrad Med. 2013;125:25–33.
40. See S, Ginzburg R. Choosing a skeletal muscle relaxant. Am Fam Physician. 2008;78:365–370.
41. Cosca DD, Navazio F. Common problems in endurance athletes. Am Fam Physician. 2007;76:237–244.

61 Glaucoma

Mikael D. Jones

LEARNING OBJECTIVES

Upon completion of the chapter, the reader will be able to:

1. Identify risk factors for the development of primary open-angle glaucoma (POAG) and acute angle-closure glaucoma.
2. Recommend a frequency for glaucoma screening based on patient-specific risk factors.
3. Compare and contrast the pathophysiologic mechanisms responsible for open-angle glaucoma and acute angle-closure glaucoma.
4. Compare and contrast the clinical presentation of chronic open-angle glaucoma and acute angle-closure glaucoma.
5. List the goals of treatment for patients with POAG suspect, POAG, and acute angle-closure glaucoma.
6. Choose the most appropriate therapy based on patient-specific data for open-angle glaucoma, glaucoma suspect, and acute angle-closure glaucoma.
7. Develop a monitoring plan for patients on specific pharmacologic regimens.
8. Counsel patients about glaucoma, drug therapy options, ophthalmic administration techniques, and the importance of adherence to the prescribed regimen.

INTRODUCTION

Glaucoma refers to a spectrum of ophthalmic disorders characterized by neuropathy of the optic nerve and loss of retinal ganglion cells, which typically leads to permanent deterioration of the visual field (peripheral vision) initially and potentially total vision loss (including central vision). It is often, but not always, eye pressure related.[1-3] Table 61–1 describes the general classification of glaucoma. *Glaucoma Suspects* are patients with a higher than average risk of developing glaucoma because of the presence of certain clinical findings, family history, or racial background. Glaucoma suspects can be further classified as open-angle glaucoma suspects or angle-closure glaucoma suspects.

Primary open-angle glaucoma (POAG) and primary angle-closure glaucoma (PACG) represent the most common types of glaucoma and therefore are the focus of this chapter. A common presentation of PACG is acute angle-closure crisis (AACC). AACC is the sudden obstruction of the trabecular meshwork, which leads to rapid increases in IOP resulting in pressure-induced optic neuropathy if untreated.[1-4] KEY CONCEPT *Patients with POAG typically have a slow, insidious loss of vision. This is contrasted by the course of AACC, which can lead to rapid vision loss that develops over hours to days.*

EPIDEMIOLOGY AND ETIOLOGY

It is estimated that almost 65 million people had glaucoma in 2013, making it the second leading cause of blindness after cataracts. By 2040 this number may increase to greater than 110 million people worldwide[5]) In 2010, glaucoma was the second leading cause of blindness worldwide.[6] In North America it is estimated that almost 3 million people are affected by POAG, and by 2040 this number will increase to 4.2 million.[5] The prevalence varies with race and ethnicity, and it is three to five times more prevalent in African Americans than white Americans.[7] The prevalence of POAG increases with age and is rarely seen in patients younger than 40 years.[7,8] The prevalence of POAG suspects is difficult to estimate at this time, but it is estimated that 3.5% to 4.5% of white and Hispanic patients older than 40 years have ocular hypertension.[2]

Approximately 20 million people were estimated to have angle-closure glaucoma in 2013, and this is projected to increase to 32 million people by 2040.[5] The prevalence of angle-closure glaucoma is lower than POAG and varies significantly by race and ethnicity. The prevalence is lower in patients of European ancestry (0.4%) but higher in patients of Asian ancestry (1.2%).[5] PACG is also more prevalent with increasing age and among females.[4]

PATHOPHYSIOLOGY

The pathophysiology of glaucomatous neurodegeneration has not been completely elucidated but appears to be caused by both IOP-dependent and IOP-independent factors. Elevated IOP is clearly associated with damage and eventual death of optic nerves; however, optic neuropathy still occurs in patients without elevated IOP which indicates the presence of independent factors that contribute to ganglion cell death.[9,10] The key to

Table 61–1

Glaucoma Classifications

Classification	Description
Primary glaucoma	Glaucoma that cannot be attributed to a preexisting ocular or systemic disease.
Secondary glaucoma	Glaucoma that can be attributed to preexisting ocular or systemic disease. Examples include pigment dispersion syndrome, neovascular glaucoma, and pseudoexfoliative syndrome.
Open-angle glaucoma	Glaucoma characterized by normal anterior-chamber angles and glaucomatous changes of the optic disc. Can be further classified as primary or secondary.
Angle-closure glaucoma	Glaucoma characterized by the obstruction of the anterior chamber angle resulting in either intermittent or progressive elevated IOP with subsequent damage to the optic nerve. Can be further classified as primary or secondary.

Data from Refs. 3 and 4.

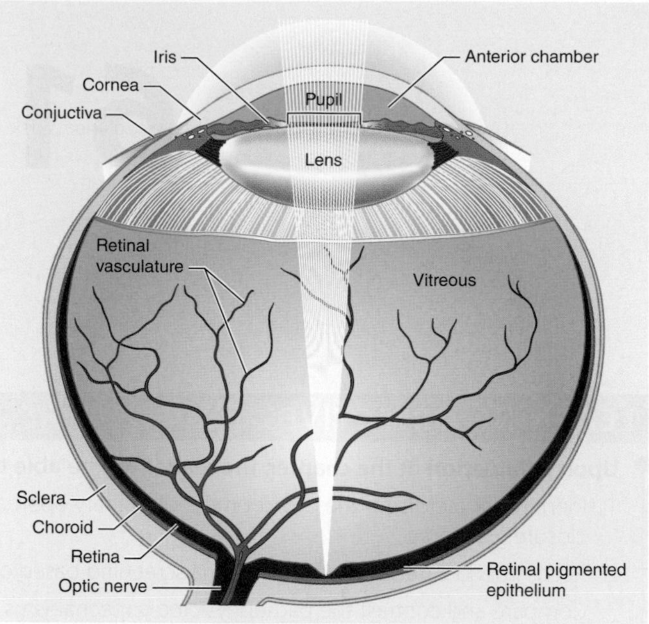

FIGURE 61–1. Anatomy of the eye. (From Lesar Ts, Fiscella Rg, Edward D. Glaucoma. In: Dipiro JT, Talbert RL, Yee GC, et al, eds. Pharmacotherapy: A Pathophysiologic Approach, 9th ed. New York: McGraw-Hill, 2014:1526.)

understanding the pathophysiology and treatment of glaucoma relies on an understanding of aqueous humor dynamics, IOP, and optic nerve anatomy and physiology.

Aqueous Humor and Intraocular Pressure

IOP maintains the curvature of the cornea which is important for the refractive properties of the eye.[11] The distribution of IOP in the general population is 10 to 21 mm Hg (1.3–2.8 kPa) and is slightly skewed toward higher values. However, caution should be used in assigning this as the "normal range" for IOP because some patients may have optic neuropathy in the "normal range" while for other patients optic neuropathy may be absent at higher IOPs. Elevated IOP is generally considered greater than 21 mm Hg (2.8 kPa).[12]

Aqueous humor is an optically neutral fluid that provides oxygen and nutrition to the avascular lens and cornea. IOP is dependent on the balance between aqueous humor production and outflow from the anterior segment. (**Figures 61–1** and **61–2**). The anterior segment of the eye is separated by the iris into the posterior and anterior chambers. The ciliary body, a ring-like structure that surrounds and supports the lens. It also produces aqueous humor through the diffusion and ultrafiltration of plasma. The nonpigmented epithelium of the ciliary body secretes the aqueous humor into the posterior chamber. Aqueous

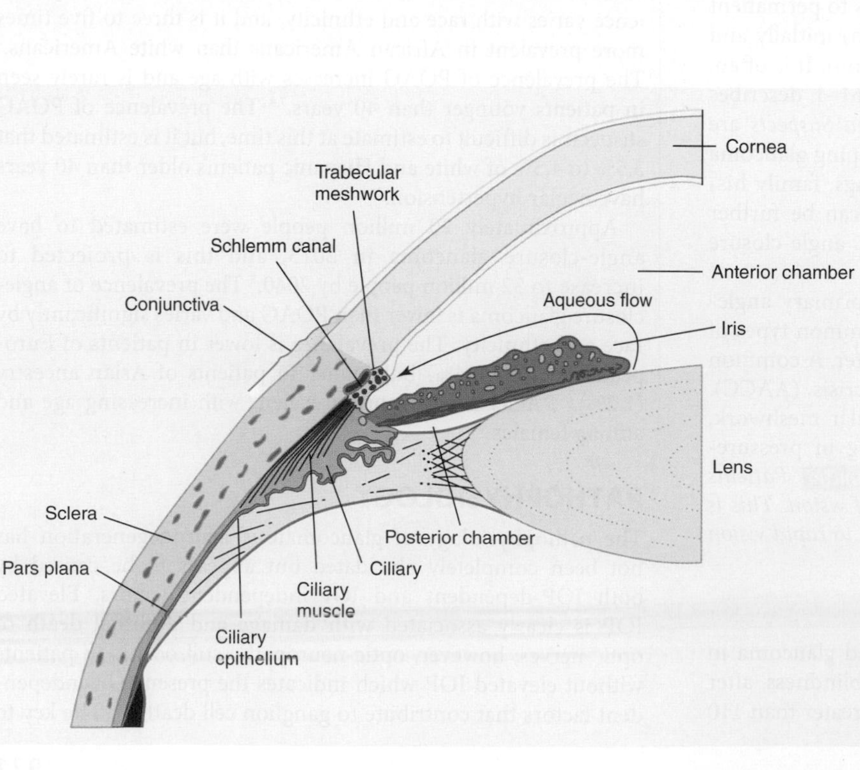

FIGURE 61–2. Anterior chamber of the eye and aqueous humor flow. (From Lesar TS, Fiscella RG, Edward D. Glaucoma. In: DiPiro JT, Talbert RL, Yee GC, et al, eds. Pharmacotherapy: A Pathophysiologic Approach, 9th ed. New York: McGraw-Hill, 2014:1526.)

humor formation can be modified pharmacologically through the α- and β-adrenoceptors, carbonic anhydrase, and sodium and potassium adenosine triphosphatase of the nonpigmented ciliary epithelium.[13,14]

After secretion, the aqueous humor flows from the posterior chamber through the pupil into the anterior chamber. From the anterior chamber, approximately 80% of aqueous humor then exits through the trabecular meshwork while the remaining 20% exits through the uveoscleral pathway.[13,14]

The trabecular meshwork is a lattice of connective tissue that surrounds edge of the anterior chamber located in the inside intersection of the edge of the cornea and the iris insertion. The size of the trabecular meshwork can be altered by the contraction or the relaxation of the ciliary muscle. Stimulation of muscarinic receptors on the ciliary muscle causes contraction, which in turn causes the pores of the trabecular meshwork to open, increasing aqueous humor outflow into Schlemm canal and the episcleral venous system.[13] The contraction can also be decreased by inhibiting Rho Kinases which are involved in the regulation of the contractile tone of the trabecular meshwork tissue.[14]

In the uveoscleral pathway, aqueous humor exits the anterior chamber through the iris root and through spaces in the ciliary muscles, which then drain into the suprachoroidal space. Uveoscleral outflow can be pharmacologically modulated by adrenoceptors, prostanoid receptors, and prostamide receptors.[11,15]

Optic Nerve

In the posterior segment of the eye, retinal ganglion cells are responsible for transmitting visual signaling from the retina to the brain. The axons of the retinal ganglion cells converge at the retinal nerve fiber layer to form the optic nerve. The optic nerve head (also called the optic disc) is the portion of the optic nerve that is visible on funduscopic examination. The optic nerve head is vertically oval and pink to pale yellow with a depression in the center of the optic nerve, called a physiologic cup which is formed as the axons converge and exit the eye as a bundle through the lamina cribrosa. (Figure 61–3). The optic nerve synapses at the lateral geniculate nucleus in the brain.[9,10,16,17]

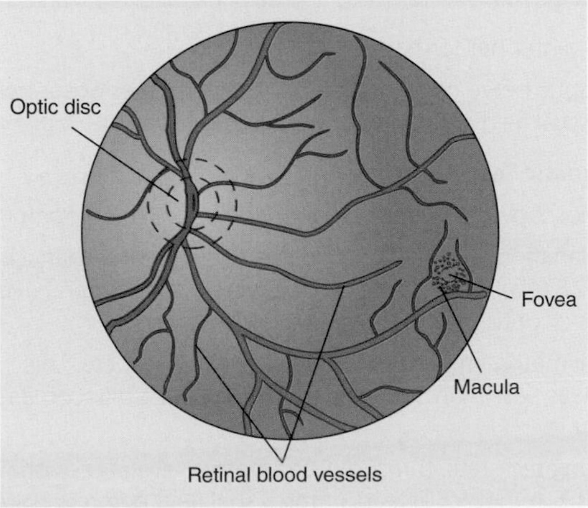

FIGURE 61–3. Normal fundus of the eye and optic disc and cup. (Reprinted with permission from Lesar TS, Fiscella RG, Edward D. Glaucoma. In: DiPiro JT, Talbert RL, Yee GC, et al, eds. Pharmacotherapy: A Pathophysiologic Approach, 9th ed. New York: McGraw-Hill, 2014:1527.)

Pathophysiology of Open-Angle Glaucoma

In patients with POAG, the cause of elevated IOP is not obvious, as obstruction in aqueous humor outflow is not clinically discernible. Possible causes of this increased IOP may be related to an increase in outflow resistance in the trabecular meshwork.[9,10,14,16]

Glaucomatous optic neuropathy may also occur independent of increased IOP. Pressure independent causes of optic neuropathy include abnormal ocular perfusion, oxidative stress, and inflammation.[9,10,12,16]

Regardless of the underlying cause, elevated IOP initiates several detrimental changes to glial cells, the lamina cribrosa, and retinal ganglion cells. The increase in IOP can lead to alterations in retinal blood flow and axonal transport of neurotrophic factors, resulting in cellular stress of the retinal ganglion cells. This stress activates the glial cells in a manner that leads to inappropriate remodeling of the extracellular matrix. Elevated IOP deforms the lamina cribrosa, which places mechanical strain on the retinal ganglion cells. Chronic elevation of IOP ultimately causes the retinal ganglion cells to undergo apoptosis.[9,10,16,18,19]

Current glaucoma therapies fail to target IOP-independent glaucoma pathophysiologic factors. However, IOP reduction may still be beneficial, as the rate of visual field progression is decreased in many patients who exhibit IOP reduction via medical or surgical modalities.[3,9]

Pathophysiology of Angle-Closure Glaucoma

PACG involves a mechanical obstruction of aqueous humor outflow through the trabecular meshwork by the peripheral iris. Two major mechanisms of trabecular meshwork obstruction by the peripheral iris include pupillary block and an abnormality of the iris called *iris plateau*. Pupillary block is the more common mechanism of obstruction and results from a complete or functional apposition of the central iris to the anterior lens and is associated with mid-dilation of the pupil. The trapped aqueous humor in the posterior chamber increases pressure behind the iris, causing the peripheral iris to bow forward and obstruct the trabecular meshwork. Plateau iris refers to an anterior displacement of the peripheral iris caused by anteriorly positioned ciliary

Patient Encounter, Part 1

RJ, a 66-year-old African American woman with a history of COPD and hypertension, presents to your clinic for her yearly checkup. She states that she is concerned about losing her eyesight because her older sister has started losing her vision from glaucoma. She denies any changes in her vision.

Meds: Tiotropium 18 mcg two inhalations of powder contents of a single capsule; albuterol HFA MDI one to two puffs every 4 to 6 hours as needed; amlodipine 10 mg orally once daily; HCTZ 25 mg orally once daily.

Based on the patient's medical and family history, what risk factors does this patient have for glaucoma?

How often would you recommend that this patient receive a comprehensive eye evaluation?

What objective assessments should be gathered in order to fully evaluate her risk factors for glaucoma?

How often would you recommend that this patient receive a comprehensive eye evaluation?

Table 61–2

Recommended Frequency of Comprehensive Adult Medical Eye Evaluation

Age (Years)	With Risk Factors for Glaucoma	No Known Risk Factors for Ocular Disease
65 or above	6–12 months	1–2 years
55–64	1–2 years	1–3 years
40–54	1–3 years	2–4 years

Data from American Academy of Ophthalmology. Preferred Practice Pattern Guidelines Comprehensive Adult Medical Eye Evaluation. San Francisco, CA: American Academy of Ophthalmology, 2010 [cited 2011 Oct 3]. http://www.aao.org/ppp.

processes. In this configuration the peripheral iris bunches as the eye dilates. Both of these mechanisms result in the occlusion of aqueous humor outflow, causing IOP elevation at extreme levels that can lead to vision loss in hours to days.[4,9,20] The degree of iridotrabecular contact (angle closure) can be assessed by visualizing the anatomy of the irido-corneal angle by gonioscopy.

CLINICAL PRESENTATION AND DIAGNOSIS

Risk Factor Evaluation

For POAG, only 4% to 8% of patients may progress to legal blindness. Vision loss does not occur until there has been significant loss of the retinal ganglion cells. It may take 13 to 16 years for a patient to go blind from glaucoma. A patient's quality of life may not be affected until significant visual field loss is present and the patient can no longer perform the activities of daily living.[21] KEY CONCEPT *Practitioners can play an important role in eye care by assessing patients for risk factors and referring to an eye care specialist for appropriate screening and evaluation.* Risk factor evaluation is essential in determining the frequency of comprehensive eye examinations for patients (Table 61–2).

Table 61–3

Risk Factors for Glaucoma

POAG	PACG
Elevated IOP	Advancing age
African or Hispanic descent	Asian or Eskimo ethnicity
Family history of glaucoma	Female sex
Older age	Hyperopia
Thinner CCT	Shallow anterior chamber
Type 2 diabetes	Family history of angle-closure glaucoma
Low ocular perfusion pressures	
Myopia	

CCT, central corneal thickness; IOP, intraocular pressure; PACG, primary angle-closure glaucoma; POAG, primary open-angle glaucoma.
Data from Refs. 3 and 4.

Glaucoma risk factors are also useful in deciding when to start therapy and determining the sequence of pharmacotherapeutic or surgical treatment modalities.[2–4] Table 61–3 lists the major risk factors associated with POAG and PACG.

The development of PACG is associated with several anatomical risk factors that lead to shallow anterior chambers. PACG patients may have a thick, anteriorly displaced lens that results from continued growth of the lens and/or cataractous changes. The anterior chamber depth is typically shallower in many individuals with PACG, which predisposes these eyes to anatomically narrower iridocorneal inlets that are a setup for developing critically narrow angles more susceptible to closure (from an enlarging cataractous lens or other insults).[4,20]

Patients with PACG are characterized by at least 180 degrees of iridotrabecular contact, elevated IOP, and ophthalmic examination characteristic of glaucomatous changes. Recurrent attacks or a prolonged acute attack can lead to the development of peripheral anterior synechia, which partially obstructs the flow of aqueous humor through the trabecular meshwork.[4,20]

Clinical Presentation and Diagnosis of POAG

General

- Adult onset (usually greater than 40 years of age)
- Patients may be unaware that they have glaucoma and may be diagnosed during routine eye evaluation
- POAG is usually bilateral with asymmetric disease progression

Symptoms

- Patients with severe disease progression may report loss of peripheral vision ("tunnel vision") and may describe the presence of paracentral, nasal, and arcuate scotoma (blind spots) in their field of vision

Signs

- Ophthalmoscopic examination may reveal:
  - Optic nerve head (optic disc) cupping
  - Large cup-to-disc ratio
  - Diffuse thinning, focal narrowing, or notching of the optic nerve head rim
  - Splinter hemorrhages
  - Optic nerve head/nerve fiber layer changes occur before visual field changes can be detected

Diagnostic Tests

- Gonioscopy—anterior-chamber angles are to be open
- Applanation tonometry—elevated IOP (greater than 21 mm Hg [2.8 kPa]) may be present. However, patient can have signs of optic neuropathy without elevated IOP
- Pachymetry—measures central corneal thickness. Thin corneas (less than 540 μm) are considered a glaucoma risk factor
- Automated static threshold perimetry—evaluates visual fields. Can detect defects in the visual field before a patient may notice
- Other diagnostic tests—scanning laser polarimetry, confocal scanning laser ophthalmoscopy, and optical coherence tomography

Clinical Presentation and Diagnosis of Acute Angle-Closure Crisis

General

- Medical emergency due to high risk of vision loss
- Unilateral in presentation, but fellow eye is at risk

Symptoms

- Ocular pain
- Red eye
- Blurry vision
- Halos around lights
- Systemic symptoms may develop:
  - Nausea/vomiting
  - Abdominal pain
  - Headache
  - Diaphoresis

Signs

- Cloudy cornea caused by corneal edema
- Conjunctival hyperemia
- Pupil semidilated and fixed to light
- Eye will be harder on palpation through closed eye

Diagnostic Tests

- Gonioscopy—anterior-chamber angles will be closed. Peripheral anterior synechiae may be present
- Applanation tonometry—elevated IOP (greater than 21 mm Hg [2.8 kPa], but when symptoms are present, IOP may be greater than 30 mm Hg [4.0 kPa])
- Slit-lamp biomicroscopy—reveals shallow anterior-chamber depth. Signs of previous attacks include peripheral anterior synechiae, iris atrophy, and pupillary dysfunction

TREATMENT

Primary Open-Angle Glaucoma

▸ Desired Outcomes and Goals

KEY CONCEPT *The goals of therapy are to prevent further loss of visual function; minimize adverse effects of therapy and impact on the patient's vision, general health, and quality of life; maintain IOP at or below a pressure at which further optic nerve damage is unlikely to occur; and educate and involve the patient in the management of their disease.* KEY CONCEPT *Current therapy is directed at altering the flow and production of aqueous humor, which is the major determinant of IOP.*

▸ General Approach

KEY CONCEPT *Because POAG is a chronic, often asymptomatic condition, the decision of when and how to treat patients is difficult, as the treatment modalities are often expensive and have potential adverse effects or complications. Currently lowering IOP is the best method to reduce the risk of visual field loss.*[22,23] *The clinician should evaluate the potential effectiveness, toxicity, and the likelihood of patient adherence for each therapeutic modality. The ideal therapeutic regimen should have maximal effectiveness and patient tolerance to achieve the desired therapeutic response.* The American Academy of Ophthalmology (AAO) publishes Preferred Practice Patterns for POAG and POAG Suspect.[2,3]

Before the selection of a therapeutic modality, the target IOP should be determined for each patient. The target IOP ideally represents an IOP range that will slow the progression of optic neuropathy and not simply obtain an IOP in the range of 10 to 21 mm Hg (1.3–2.8 kPa). Currently, the initial target IOP is an estimate, but it should be modified based on the progression of the disease at each follow-up visit. KEY CONCEPT *The AAO recommends an initial target IOP to be set at least 25% lower than the patient's baseline IOP. The target IOP can be set lower (30%–50% of baseline IOP) for patients who already have severe disease, risk factors for disease progression, or have normal-tension glaucoma (NTG).*[3,24] Risk factors for progression include high IOP, older age, hemorrhage of the optic disc, large cup-to-disc ratio, thinner CCT (central corneal thickness), and established glaucomatous progression (velocity of disease progression is nonlinear).

Initial IOP control can be achieved by medical, laser, surgical, or combination of these therapies. The AAO guidelines[3] do not provide a specific recommendation on which therapeutic modality should be selected first, but patients in the early stages of glaucoma should receive treatment. In general, medical and laser trabeculoplasty are preferred as early treatment options over surgical as surgical interventions are not without potential intraoperative or postoperative complications.[22] The ophthalmologist will individualize therapy based on the risk and benefits for a specific patient. Table 61–4 describes nonpharmacologic treatment modalities for POAG.[3]

Medical treatment is the most commonly selected therapeutic modality. A well-tolerated ocular antihypertensive, at the lowest concentration, should be selected as the initial mediation (Table 61–5). The ocular hypotensive lipids are preferred first-line agents since they are the most effective at lowering at IOP of both peak and trough measurements by at least 25% of baseline

Table 61–4

Select Nonpharmacologic Treatment Options for POAG

Treatment Option	Description
Laser trabeculoplasty	Laser energy aimed at trabecular meshwork Improves aqueous humor outflow
Trabeculectomy	Surgical removal of a portion of the trabecular meshwork Improves aqueous humor outflow Mitomycin C and fluorouracil are used to decrease scarring
Cyclodestructive surgery	Trans-scleral laser reduces rate of aqueous humor production Reserved for patients who have failed other options
Aqueous shunts	Drainage device that redirects the outflow of aqueous humor through a small tube into an outlet chamber placed underneath the conjunctiva

Data from Refs. 3, 4, and 14.

Table 61–5

Pharmacologic Treatment Options for POAG

Drug	Pharmacologic Properties	Common Brand Names	Dose Form	Strength (%)	Usual Dose[a]	Mechanism of Action
β-Adrenergic Blocking Agents						
Betaxolol	Relative β_1-selective	Generic	Solution	0.5	One drop twice a day	All reduce aqueous production of ciliary body
		Betoptic-S	Suspension	0.25	One drop twice a day	
Carteolol	Nonselective, intrinsic sympathomimetic activity	Generic	Solution	1	One drop twice a day	
Levobunolol	Nonselective	Betagan	Solution	0.25, 0.5	One drop twice a day	
Metipranolol	Nonselective	OptiPranolol	Solution	0.3	One drop twice a day	
Timolol	Nonselective	Timoptic, Betimol, Istalol	Solution	0.25, 0.5	One drop every day—one to two times a day	
		Timoptic-XE	Gelling solution	0.25, 0.5	One drop every day[a]	
Nonspecific Adrenergic Agonists						
Dipivefrin	Epinephrine prodrug	Propine	Solution	0.1	One drop twice a day	Increased aqueous humor outflow
α_2-Adrenergic Agonists						
Apraclonidine	Specific α_2-agonists	Iopidine	Solution	0.5, 1	One drop two to three times a day	Both reduce aqueous humor production; brimonidine known to also increase uveoscleral outflow; only brimonidine has primary indication
Brimonidine		Alphagan P	Solution	0.15, 0.1	One drop two to three times a day	
Cholinergic Agonists Direct Acting						
Carbachol	Irreversible	Carboptic, Isopto Carbachol	Solution	1.5, 3	One drop two to three times a day	All increase aqueous humor outflow through trabecular meshwork
Pilocarpine	Irreversible	Isopto Carpine, Pilocar	Solution	0.25, 0.5, 1, 2, 4, 6, 8, 10	One drop two to three times a day	
					One drop four times a day	
		Pilopine HS	Gel	4	Every 24 hours at bedtime	
Cholinesterase Inhibitors						
Echothiophate		Phospholine Iodide	Solution	0.125	Once or twice a day	
Carbonic Anhydrase Inhibitors						
Topical						
Brinzolamide	Carbonic anhydrase type II inhibition	Azopt	Suspension	1	Two to three times a day	All reduce aqueous humor production of ciliary body
Dorzolamide		Trusopt Generic	Solution	2	Two to three times a day	
Systemic						
Acetazolamide		Generic	Tablet	125 mg, 250 mg	125–250 mg two to four times a day	
		Injection	500 mg/vial	250–500 mg		
		Diamox Sequels	Capsule	500 mg	500 mg twice a day	
Methazolamide		Generic	Tablet	25 mg, 50 mg	25–50 mg two to three times a day	

(Continued)

Table 61–5

Pharmacologic Treatment Options for POAG (Continued)

Drug	Pharmacologic Properties	Common Brand Names	Dose Form	Strength (%)	Usual Dose[a]	Mechanism of Action
Prostaglandin Analogs						
Latanoprost	Prostanoid agonist	Xalatan	Solution	0.005	One drop every night	Increases aqueous uveoscleral outflow and to a lesser extent trabecular outflow
Bimatoprost	Prostamide agonist	Lumigan	Solution	0.01, 0.03	One drop every night	
Travoprost	Prostanoid agonist	Travatan Z	Solution	0.004	One drop every night	
Tafluprost	Prostanoid agonist	Zioptan	Preservative free solution	0.0015%	One drop every night	
Combinations						
Timolol—dorzolamide		Cosopt Generic	Solution	Timolol 0.5% dorzolamide 2%	One drop twice daily	
Timolol—brimonidine		Combigan	Solution	Timolol 0.5% brimonide 0.2%	One drop twice daily	
Brinzolamide—brimonidine		Simrinza		Brinzolamide 1% brimonidine 0.2%	One drop three times daily	

Adapted from DiPiro JT, Talbert RL, Yee GC, et al., (eds.) Pharmacotherapy: A Pathophysiologic Approach. 9th ed. New York: McGraw-Hill; 2014.

[a]Use of nasolacrimal occlusion will increase the number of patients successfully treated with longer dosage intervals.

IOP.[25–29] Additionally, these agents lack systemic side effects and are dosed once daily. If monotherapy alone lowers IOP but does not reach target pressure or there is evidence of progression, then combination therapy or switching to another agent is appropriate. The addition of a second agent from another class generally has an additive effect on IOP reduction. The ocular hypotensive lipids, timolol, carbonic anhydrase inhibitors, or brimonidine are reasonable choices for addition as a second agent.[3,9,12] Combination eye-drops reduce the number of drops that need to be administered. Increasing the concentration or dose frequency can also be tried when possible. Adverse effects can be caused by an eye drop's therapeutic agent or inactive excipients, such as preservatives. Benzalkonium chloride is a common eye drop preservative which has been associated with superficial punctate keratitis, corneal erosion, and conjunctival allergy. Intolerances to preservatives can be resolved by changing to a preservative-free eye drop.[30] Figure 61–4 presents an algorithm to select and optimize POAG treatment.

A uniocular trial can be used to assess the safety and effectiveness of a topical medication before initiation in both eyes; however, uniocular drug trials do not always predict the IOP response of the second eye. Ideally, the effectiveness of a medication should be assessed independently using baseline IOP measurements.

▶ *Treatment Considerations for POAG Suspects*

POAG suspects should be considered for topical medication therapy if they are at high risk for developing POAG or have a high IOP in which glaucomatous nerve damage is likely to occur. POAG suspects that develop evidence of glaucomatous damage or visual field defect have developed POAG and should be treated accordingly.[2] The Ocular Hypertension Treatment Study (OHTS) demonstrated that a 20% decrease in IOP can reduce the progression from ocular hypertension to POAG over a 5-year period. The incidence of progression to POAG in the treatment (4.4%) and control (9.5%) groups was small, which underscores the importance of selecting patients at high risk of progressing to POAG.[31] When medical therapy is indicated, a well-tolerated agent should be selected and optimized following the POAG treatment algorithm (see Figure 61–4). The benefit of therapy should be reassessed in patients who may require third- or fourth-line agents to control IOP. Surgical or laser intervention are rarely indicated in the treatment of glaucoma suspects.[2]

Primary Angle-Closure Glaucoma

▶ *Desired Outcomes and Goals*

Therapeutic modalities for PACG are targeted at decreasing IOP. The goals of therapy are to preserve visual function by controlling the elevation in IOP, prevent damage to the optic nerve, and manage or prevent an acute attack of angle closure.[4]

▶ *General Approach*

KEY CONCEPT *Acute angle-closure crisis is a medical emergency and requires urgent laser or surgical intervention.* The treatment of choice for PACG is peripheral laser iridotomy. Laser iridotomy uses laser energy to cut a hole into the iris to alleviate the aqueous humor buildup behind the iris, resulting in reversal of appositional angle closure. Patients currently experiencing an acute angle-closure crisis should receive medical therapy to lower IOP, reduce pain, and reverse corneal edema before the iridotomy. IOP should first be lowered with topical β-blockers, topical α-agonist, prostaglandin $F_{2\alpha}$ analogue, systemic carbonic anhydrase inhibitors, or hyperosmotic agents. Once the IOP has been controlled,

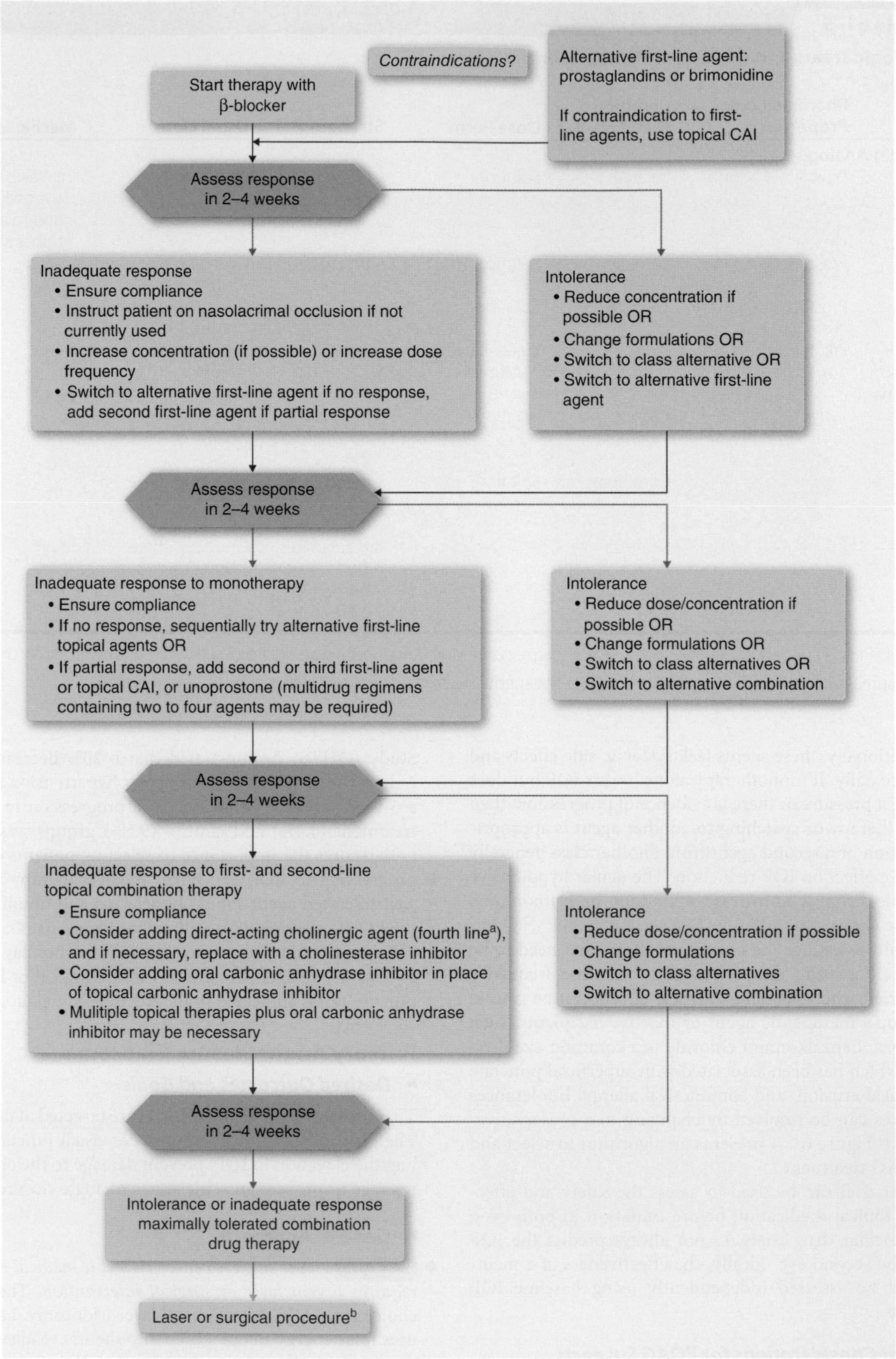

FIGURE 61–4. Algorithm for the pharmacotherapy of open-angle glaucoma. [a]Fourth-line agents not commonly used any longer. [b]Most clinicians believe laser procedures should be performed earlier (eg, after three-drug maximum, poorly adherent patient). CAI, carbonic anhydrase inhibitor. (From Losar TS, Fiscella RG, Edward D. Glaucoma. In: DiPiro JT, Talbert RL, Yee GC, et al, eds. Pharmacotherapy: A Pathophysiologic Approach, 9th ed. New York: McGraw-Hill, 2014:1532.)

miotics (ie, pilocarpine) can be used to break the pupillary block. A topical IOP-lowering agent should be continued to control IOP until laser iridotomy can be performed. Corneal indentation with a cotton-tipped applicator or gonioscopic lens may break pupillary block. If laser iridotomy cannot be performed, then surgical incisional iridectomy is used. Incisional iridectomy is the surgical removal of a small portion of the peripheral iris to allow flow of aqueous humor trapped in the posterior chamber to migrate to the anterior chamber (bypassing the normal flow pattern through the pupil). Topical corticosteroid may be employed to decrease inflammation postoperatively. The fellow eye is at high risk to develop an acute attack and should receive prophylactic iridotomy within a reasonable interval of time. Lens extraction surgery may be another treatment modality as it increases the anterior chamber depth. PACG patients may require chronic medical therapy if the patient has PACG superimposed on preexisting POAG or if synechia formation causes reduced outflow with a continued increase in IOP.[4,9,20]

Pharmacologic Therapy

▸ β-Adrenergic Antagonists

Topical β-adrenergic antagonists (β-blockers) are now considered a second-line agent after the prostaglandin analogues for the treatment of POAG unless contraindications are present.[3,9] Topical β-blockers decrease IOP by reducing the formation of aqueous humor made by the ciliary body, which results in a 20% to 35% reduction in IOP.[28,29,32,33] Timolol, levobunolol, metipranolol, and carteolol are nonselective for β_1- and β_2-adrenergic receptors, whereas betaxolol has β_1-selective properties.[32,33] Betaxolol reduces IOP to a lesser extent than the nonselective β-blockers, but part of its efficacy may be related to a neuroprotective mechanism independent of IOP reduction.[34]

Topical β-blockers are typically administered twice daily. A gel-forming solution of timolol (Timoptic-XE) can be administered once daily. Tachyphylaxis may occur in 20% to 50% of patients on monotherapy with a β-blocker, resulting in the need for a different agent or combination therapy. Patients on concurrent systemic β-blockers may experience less IOP reduction than patients on only topical β-blockers.[32,33]

β-Blockers can cause significant systemic adverse effects through nasolacrimal drainage and subsequent systemic absorption in the mucous membranes in the nasal-pharyngeal cavity. This route bypasses first-pass hepatic metabolism resulting in pharmacologically significant serum drug concentrations.[35] Bronchospasm is the most common pulmonary effect of topical β-blockers. Pulmonary edema, status asthmaticus, and respiratory arrest have been reported with β-blockers as well. Cardiovascular effects include bradycardia, hypotension, and congestive heart failure exacerbation. As with systemic β-blockers, topical β-blockers have also been reported to cause depression and hyperlipidemia and mask symptoms of hypoglycemia. The β_1-selective properties of betaxolol may cause less exacerbation of pulmonary disease. Despite the intrinsic sympathomimetic activity demonstrated by carteolol, this does not translate to a clinically significant decrease in pulmonary or cardiovascular adverse effects. Topical β-blockers are generally contraindicated in patients with asthma, chronic obstructive pulmonary disease (COPD), sinus bradycardia, second- or third-degree heart block, cardiac failure, and hypersensitivity to the product.[30,33,35]

Stinging of the eyes upon instillation is the most common adverse effect. Other local adverse effects include conjunctivitis, keratitis, dry eyes, and uveitis.[30,32]

Patients prescribed topical β-blockers should be counseled on the nasolacrimal occlusion technique to decrease systemic absorption.

▸ Ocular Hypotensive Lipids

The ocular hypotensive lipids in typical ophthalmology practice are considered first-line agents along with β-blockers because of their superior efficacy and safety profiles. Many clinicians may choose to use the ocular hypotensive lipids as first line, especially in patients who have an initial requirement to lower IOP by greater than 25%.[28,29,32,33] All four of the available agents currently have an FDA indication for both POAG and ocular hypertension. Latanoprost and travoprost have dosing aids that help patients administer each medication. Travoprost and tafluprost are available as benzalkonium chloride–free solutions.

Latanoprost, travoprost, tafluprost are analogues of prostaglandin $F_{2\alpha}$ and are agonists of the prostanoid FP receptor, which appears to lower IOP by increasing aqueous humor outflow through the uveoscleral pathway. Bimatoprost is a prostamide analogue and appears to lower IOP by activating prostamide receptors in the uveoscleral pathway and possibly through increasing outflow through the trabecular meshwork. The exact mechanism of how uveoscleral outflow is increased is still unclear, but stimulation of prostanoid FP receptors and prostamide receptors in the ciliary body cause remodeling of the extracellular matrix, making it more permeable to aqueous humor, thus increasing aqueous humor outflow through the ciliary muscles.[32,36,37]

The ocular hypotensive lipids are administered once daily at bedtime and should not be increased to twice daily, as this may decrease effectiveness. The ocular hypotensive lipids can provide a consistent reduction in IOP over a 24-hour period.[33] For patients nonresponsive to latanoprost, switching to bimatoprost may allow some patients to reach their IOP goal, presumably because of the proposed difference in the site of action of each drug.[38,39]

The ocular hypotensive lipids are well tolerated and rarely cause systemic side effects (headache has been reported). Local effects include conjunctival hyperemia, stinging on instillation, increase in iris pigmentation, deepening of the upper eyelid sulcus, hypertrichosis, and darkening of the eyelashes. Increases in iris pigmentation occur most commonly in patients with multicolored irides on long-term prostaglandin analogue therapy. The mechanism of this effect is by its action on melanocytes of the iris, in which the irides become darker because of increased production of melanin in the iris.[30] Increased iris pigmentation appears to be only a cosmetic effect but may affect your product selection, especially when choosing monocular therapy. Conjunctival hyperemia or engorgement of conjunctival blood vessels is a common adverse effect caused by a vasodilatory effect on scleral blood vessels. It is most prominent early in therapy and usually subsides over time. Although generally a benign adverse effect, patients may have a concern if it affects their cosmetic appearance.[30,32]

The ocular hypotensive lipids should be used with caution in patients, since they may worsen anterior uveitis and herpetic keratitis. Cystoid macular edema has been reported during treatment with the ocular hypotensive lipids; therefore, use caution in patients with intraocular inflammation, aphakic patients, pseudophakic patients with a history of intraoperative complications (eg, torn posterior lens capsule), or in patients with risk factors for macular edema.[30]

Patients prescribed ocular hypotensive lipids should be counseled on potential adverse effects and appropriate administration. Patients receiving latanoprost or tafluprost should be instructed to refrigerate unopened medication. Once open latanoprost can stored at room temperature for 6 weeks. Tafluprost single-use containers can be stored at room temperature for up to 28 days.

▶ α_2-Adrenergic Agonists

Brimonidine and apraclonidine are α_2-adrenergic agonists that decrease IOP by reducing aqueous humor production. Brimonidine has a higher selectivity to the α_2-receptor than apraclonidine and has a dual mechanism of action by increasing uveoscleral outflow.[32,33] Apraclonidine is often used for the prevention and treatment of postsurgical IOP elevations and is no longer commonly used for long-term treatment of POAG because of tachyphylaxis and high rate of blepharoconjunctivitis. Brimonidine lowers IOP by 14% to 25%. Peak IOP-lowering effect is similar to that of timolol, but the trough IOP-lowering effect is less than that of timolol.[27,28] Brimonidine may exhibit a neuroprotective effect and has been shown to delay visual field progression compared with timolol but there is insufficient evidence it prevents retinal ganglion cell death.[40]

Brimonidine is typically used as an adjunctive agent in combination with other agents and is usually administered every 8 hours. A 12-hour dosing schedule may be employed when used in combination therapy. Brimonidine-purite 0.1% and 0.15% solution (Alphagan-P) has similar efficacy compared with the brimonidine 0.2% solution, because the purite solution's higher pH allows for more drug to penetrate the cornea.[32,33] Brimonidine cause both local and systemic effects. Local effects include blepharoconjunctivitis, conjunctivitis, and ocular allergy. Systemic effects include headache, dry mouth, and fatigue.[30,32,33]

The frequency of dosing and local adverse effects may lead to nonadherence in some patients. Patients prescribed brimonidine should be counseled on the nasolacrimal occlusion technique to reduce systemic adverse effects and to improve efficacy.[32,33]

▶ Carbonic Anhydrase Inhibitors

Carbonic anhydrase inhibitors decrease aqueous humor production by inhibition of the carbonic anhydrase isoenzyme II located in the ciliary body. In the eye, carbonic anhydrase catalyzes the conversion of H_2O and CO_2 to HCO_3^- and H^+, which is a significant step in aqueous humor production. Carbonic anhydrase inhibitors are available in systemic and topical preparations.[32,33]

Topical Carbonic Anhydrase Inhibitors Dorzolamide and brinzolamide are the only topical carbonic anhydrase inhibitors available on the market. Both medications are administered every 8 hours and are used as adjunctive therapy or as monotherapy for patients who cannot tolerate first-line therapies. Nasolacrimal occlusion may allow for an every-12-hour dosing interval. They lower peak and trough IOP by 17% to 20%.[28,29,32,33]

Local side effects include burning, stinging, itching, foreign body sensation, dry eyes, and conjunctivitis. Brinzolamide may have fewer incidences of these side effects since the drug is in a neutral pH solution. Dorzolamide has been reported to cause irreversible corneal decompensation. Taste abnormalities have been reported with each agent. Both topical carbonic anhydrase inhibitors are sulfonamides and are contraindicated in patients with history of sulfonamide hypersensitivity.[30,32,33]

Systemic Carbonic Anhydrase Inhibitors There are three systemic carbonic anhydrase inhibitors: acetazolamide, dichlorphenamide, and methazolamide. These agents effectively lower IOP by 20% to 30% but are reserved as third-line to fourth-line agents because of their significant adverse effects. They are typically used as bridge therapy from maximal medical therapy to laser or surgical intervention or to control IOP in the perioperative period following a laser or surgical ocular procedure. The systemic carbonic anhydrase inhibitors can also be used to lower IOP in acute angle-closure glaucoma. Acetazolamide has an IV formulation that can be used in patients who are experiencing nausea due to the angle-closure attack. Acetazolamide and methazolamide are the best tolerated of the three agents.[4,32,33]

The systemic carbonic anhydrase inhibitors are associated with significant adverse effects that include paresthesias of the hands and feet, nausea, vomiting, and weight loss. Patients can develop systemic acidosis, hypokalemia, hyponatremia, and nephrolithiasis due to the inhibition of renal carbonic anhydrase. Sulfonamide allergy, renal failure, hepatic insufficiency, COPD, and decreased serum potassium and sodium levels are all contraindications of systemic carbonic anhydrase inhibitor therapy. Blood dyscrasias from bone marrow suppression have been reported and include agranulocytosis, aplastic anemia, neutropenia, and thrombocytopenia.[32,33]

▶ Cholinergic Agents

Cholinergic agents (also called parasympathomimetics or miotics) were the first class of agents to treat glaucoma. The class can be divided into direct-acting and indirect-acting cholinergic agents.

Direct-Acting Cholinergic Agents Pilocarpine directly stimulates the muscarinic (M_3) receptors of the ciliary body, which causes contraction of the ciliary muscle. This results in the widening of spaces in the trabecular meshwork, which causes an increase in aqueous humor outflow and reduces IOP by 20% to 30%.

Pilocarpine requires administration four times daily, since the IOP-lowering effect lasts only 6 hours. Pilocarpine is available in 1%, 2%, and 4% concentrations. Higher concentrations may be needed for patients with dark irides to obtain adequate IOP reduction. A pilocarpine 4% gel is available and allows for once-daily dosing at bedtime.[32] Pilocarpine is considered a fourth-line agent for POAG. In the treatment of PACG, it is important to delay use until IOP has been controlled, because pilocarpine could worsen angle closure by causing anterior displacement of the lens. Once IOP is controlled, pilocarpine can be given to break pupillary block by instilling one drop applied twice in an hour.

Patient Encounter, Part 2

RJ was referred to an ophthalmologist for a comprehensive eye evaluation. The ophthalmology report reveals the patient has an IOP (as assessed by applanation tonometry) of 19 mm Hg (2.5 kPa) in the right eye and 23 mm Hg (3.1 kPa) in the left eye. Gonioscopic examination reveals open anterior angles in both eyes. Ophthalmoscopy reveals cupping of the optic discs in both eyes. Visual field examination reveals a nerve fiber bundle defect consistent with glaucoma in the left eye.

What is your assessment of this patient's glaucoma type?

What pharmacologic and nonpharmacologic treatment modalities are available for this patient?

The adverse effects of pilocarpine are caused by the induction of miosis. The contraction of the ciliary muscle causes the lens to displace forward, which can lead to accommodation spasm and myopia, and can lead to brow ache. Pupillary constriction can also affect night vision. Pilocarpine should be avoided in patients with severe myopia as it increases the risk of developing retinal detachment. Systemic effects may occur at higher concentrations and include nausea, vomiting and diarrhea, and bradycardia.[30]

Carbachol stimulates the same muscarinic receptor as pilocarpine and also inhibits acetylcholinesterase, the enzyme that metabolizes acetylcholine. Carbachol is more potent than pilocarpine, but it causes more accommodation spasm and brow ache and may also cause anterior uveitis. Other reported side effects include corneal clouding, persistent bullous keratopathy, and retinal detachment. Carbachol is rarely used today because of the side-effect profile.[30,32]

Indirect-Acting Cholinergic Agents Echothiophate iodide and demecarium bromide inhibit acetylcholinesterase. Inhibition of this enzyme increases the availability of acetylcholine at the nerve junction, thus increasing the stimulation of the muscarinic (M_3) receptors of the ciliary body. These products are given twice daily and have similar efficacy to pilocarpine in the degree of IOP reduction. The side-effect profile is similar to that of pilocarpine; however, they can deplete systemic cholinesterases and pseudocholinesterases and may cause the formation of cataracts. These agents should be discontinued at least 1 week before general surgical procedures. Succinylcholine and some local anesthetics are metabolized by pseudocholinesterases; therefore, depletion of this enzyme by echothiophate or demecarium may lead to toxic effects. These agents are typically used when other topical agents have failed and are limited to patients who have had their lenses removed or who have artificial lenses.[32]

▶ *Hyperosmotics*

Glycerin, isosorbide, and mannitol are hyperosmotic agents that increase the osmolality of blood. These agents create an osmotic gradient that draws water from the vitreous humor, thus decreasing IOP. The resulting dehydration of the vitreous humor may cause posterior movement of the lens, which then causes the anterior chamber to deepen, thus opening the anterior angle. If the patient is not vomiting, glycerin (1–1.5 g/kg of a 50%) solution and isosorbide (1.5–2 g/kg) can be given orally. Isosorbide is preferred in patients with diabetes because it is not metabolized into glucose. If the patient has nausea or vomiting, mannitol (20%) can be given IV at a dose of 1 to 2 g/kg over 45 minutes. The hyperosmotic agents are rapid acting, reaching peak effect in 30 to 60 minutes. Headache and thirst are common complaints. Patients who are already dehydrated are at risk of developing CNS dehydration, which can lead to coma. These agents should be used with caution in patients with renal or cardiovascular disease, as extracellular water is increased.[33,41]

▶ *Nonselective Adrenergic Agonists*

Epinephrine and its prodrug, dipivefrin, are rarely used for the treatment of glaucoma and are considered last-line agents because of their systemic side-effect profile. Dipivefrin increases the corneal penetration. Once it is absorbed through the cornea, it is enzymatically cleaved to epinephrine. Epinephrine has α- and β-agonist activity and is thought to increase the outflow of aqueous humor through the trabecular meshwork and the uveoscleral pathway. Both products are instilled twice daily and reduce IOP by 15% to 25%. Local adverse effects include mydriasis, conjunctival hyperemia, and ocular irritation. Aphakic patients should not use these medications because they cause a reversible cystoid macular edema. Epinephrine and dipivefrin should not be used in patients with narrow angles since these agents can cause acute angle closure. Systemic side effects include palpitations, increased blood pressure, and arrhythmia, and therefore, these drugs should be used with caution in patients with cardiovascular disease, cerebrovascular disease, and hyperthyroidism. Using the nasolacrimal technique may decrease systemic effects.[32]

SPECIAL CONSIDERATIONS: DRUG-INDUCED GLAUCOMAS

Medications have the potential to cause or exacerbate both POAG and PACG; however, PACG is more likely to be exacerbated by medications than POAG. The use of medications with anticholinergic or sympathomimetic properties can precipitate angle closure. Medications with anticholinergic properties include first-generation antihistamines, tricyclic antidepressants, and antipsychotics. Medications with sympathomimetic properties include phenylephrine and pseudoephedrine. PACG patients who have been treated with laser iridotomy can usually use these agents without causing an exacerbation. Sulfa-based drugs, such as topiramate, acetazolamide, and hydrochlorothiazide, cause swelling of the ciliary body, which causes an anterior displacement of the lens, resulting in a decrease in anterior-chamber depth. Patients with open or closed anterior angles can experience elevated IOP from these drugs. Controlled POAG is rarely exacerbated by anticholinergics and sympathomimetics unless the patient is concomitantly at risk for angle closure. For uncontrolled or untreated POAG, the risk–benefit ratio should be considered before employing these agents. POAG can be exacerbated by any administrated form of corticosteroids. Corticosteroids increase IOP by causing obstruction of the trabecular meshwork with extracellular material. The increase in IOP appears to increase with potency and intraocular penetration. Ophthalmic corticosteroid preparations carry the highest risk of increasing IOP. However, all administrated routes have been shown to raise IOP in some patients. The onset and extent of IOP elevation is dependent on the specific corticosteroid, dose, route, and frequency. Generally corticosteroid-induced IOP elevation typically occurs within a few weeks of beginning steroid therapy. In most cases, the IOP lowers spontaneously to the baseline within a few weeks to months upon stopping the steroid. In rare instances, the IOP remains elevated. Some patients exhibit clinically significant and dangerously high IOP as a result of steroid use.[42]

Patient Encounter, Part 3

The practitioner and RJ agree to start medication therapy. Develop a patient-specific care plan.

Address the patient's (a) drug-related needs, (b) goals of therapy, (c) potential pharmacologic therapies, and (d) plan for follow-up of therapy.

List the monitoring parameters for effectiveness and safety for the chosen therapy.

Explain how you would counsel the patient on the chosen therapy, including the administration of an ophthalmic preparation.

Application of Ophthalmic Solutions or Suspension

1. Clean hands with soap and water.
2. Avoid touching the dropper tip with your fingers or against your eye to maintain sterility of product; shake dropper bottle if product is a suspension.
3. Tilt head back; pull down the lower eye lid with index finger.
4. Hold the dropper bottle with other hand as close as possible without touching the eye. The dropper should be pointing toward the eye with remaining fingers bracing against the face.
5. Gently squeeze the bottle so that one drop is placed into the pocket.
6. Close your eye for 2 to 3 minutes to allow for the maximum corneal penetration of drug.
7. Use a tissue to wipe away any excess liquid.
8. Replace and retighten the cap to the dropper bottle.
9. Wait at least 5 minutes before instilling another ophthalmic drug preparation.
10. Application of some ophthalmic preparations (suspension and gels) may cause blurring of vision.

OUTCOME EVALUATION

Primary Open-Angle Glaucoma

Evaluate patients 2 to 4 weeks after the initiation or alteration of medical therapy. The clinician should elicit the status of ocular health since the last visit, systemic medical history, medication history, and presence of local and ocular adverse effects of medications. IOP measurement, visual acuity assessment, and slit-lamp biomicroscopy at every POAG follow-up visit is necessary. The frequency of visual fields and optic nerve evaluation depends on whether IOP is controlled, the length of time IOP has been controlled, and whether there is progression of the disease. Patients who are at target IOP and have no disease progression should have optic nerve head evaluation and visual field testing every 6 to 12 months. Patients with disease progression and/or who are not at target IOP should receive follow-up evaluation every 1 to 6 months. Assess the patient's ability to use topical eye drops.[3] (See Application of Ophthalmic Solutions or Suspensions textbox.) Finally, evaluate the patient's adherence to their medical regimen. Nonadherence among patients on topical medical therapy ranges from 5% to 80%. Suspect nonadherence in patients who have visual field and optic nerve progression despite a low IOP measurement, as patients may be more adherent to their medical regimen before their visit. Pharmacy refill histories may be useful in assessing adherence but do not confirm that the patient is actually taking the regimen as prescribed.[43] Specific patient factors related to the risk of nonadherence may include health literacy, medication cost, complicated medication regimens, adverse effects, and ethnicity.[44] Using adherence aids, prescribing the least complex regimen, and educating patients about their glaucoma are ways to reduce nonadherence.[45]

KEY CONCEPT *Target IOP should be revised based on the course of the disease and rate of progression.* Adjust therapy if the patient fails to reach his or her target IOP. Patients who have achieved target IOP yet have progressive damage of the optic nerve or who have worsening of their visual fields should have further adjustment of their therapy. Evaluate these patients further for possible reasons of continued disease progression. Consider determining the diurnal pattern of IOP and looking for signs of poor ocular perfusion pressure. Establish a lower target IOP. Adjust therapy in patients who are intolerant, are nonadherent, or develop contraindications to their drug therapy regimen. Consider increasing the target IOP and reducing drug therapy for patients who have stable disease and who have maintained a low IOP; closely follow these patients to assess their response.[3]

Patient Care Process

Patient Assessment:

- Determine whether the patient is experiencing difficulty with vision.
- Review medical and family history. Does the patient have risk factors for glaucoma (Table 61–3)? Review patient's prescription, nonprescription, and natural product use. Does the patient have any causes for drug-induced glaucoma? Does the patient take any medications that interact with any glaucoma medication? Perform/review diagnostic tests (IOP, visual acuity, gonioscopy, visual fields, optic nerve evaluation, etc).

Therapy Evaluation:

- If glaucomatous damage is present or has progressed, determine if medication therapy is indicated.
- If patient is already receiving medication therapy, assess efficacy, safety, and patient adherence. Can the patient appropriately use prescribed ophthalmic preparations? Are there factors contributing to poor adherence? Does the patient report or exhibit signs or symptoms for systemic and ocular adverse drug reactions?

Care Plan Development:

- Select medication therapy that will likely achieve goal IOP with minimal adverse effects.
- Use combination glaucoma eye drops when possible to improve adherence.
- Address patient concerns about glaucoma and its treatment.
- Educate patient on importance of medication adherence. Instruct patient on how to instill eye drops and have them demonstrate their technique.

Follow-Up Evaluation:

- Follow-up in 2 to 4 weeks to reassess patient for progression in glaucomatous damage, achievement of target IOP, adherence, and presence of adverse effects to medication therapy. Review interval medical history. Perform/Review ophthalmic examination findings.

Primary Angle-Closure Glaucoma

Follow-up of acute angle-closure crisis occurs in the postoperative period. Evaluate the patency of the iridotomy and IOP in the postoperative period. Perform gonioscopy and optic nerve head evaluation if not already performed. Stable patients with PACG should be evaluated at least annually, specifically for the presence of peripheral anterior synechia and optic neuropathy. Treat patients according to POAG guidelines if they have underlying POAG or areas of peripheral anterior synechia with the presence of optic neuropathy.[4]

Abbreviations Introduced in This Chapter

AAO	American Academy of Ophthalmology
CCT	Central corneal thickness
IOP	Intraocular pressure
NTG	Normal tension glaucoma
PACG	Primary angle-closure glaucoma
POAG	Primary open-angle glaucoma

REFERENCES

1. Boland MV, Ervin AM, Friedman D, et al. AHRQ Comparative Effectiveness Reviews. Treatment for Glaucoma: Comparative Effectiveness. Rockville (MD): Agency for Healthcare Research and Quality (US); 2012.
2. Panel AAoOG. Primary open-angle glaucoma suspect. Preferred Practice Pattern Guidelines [Internet]. 2010 10/04/2014 [cited 10/04/2014 10/04/2014]. www.aao.org/ppp. Accessed October 4, 2014.
3. Panel AAoOG. Primary open-angle glaucoma. Preferred Practice Pattern Guidelines [Internet]. 2010 10/04/2014 [cited 2014 10/04/2014]. www.aao.org/ppp. Accessed October 4, 2014.
4. Panel AAoOG. Preferred Practice Pattern Guidelines Primary Angle Closure. San Francisco, CA: American Academy of Ophthalmology; 2010 [cited 2014 10/04/2014]. www.aao.org/ppp. Accessed October 4, 2014.
5. Tham YC, Li X, Wong TY, Quigley HA, Aung T, Cheng CY. Global prevalence of glaucoma and projections of glaucoma burden through 2040: A systematic review and meta-analysis. Ophthalmology. 2014;121(11):2081–2090. Epub 2014/07/01. doi: 10.1016/j.ophtha.2014.05.013. PMID: 24974815.
6. Pascolini D, Mariotti SP. Global estimates of visual impairment: 2010. Br J Ophthalmol. 2012;96(5):614–618. Epub 2011/12/03. doi: 10.1136/bjophthalmol-2011-300539. PMID: 22133988.
7. Friedman DS, Wolfs RC, O'Colmain BJ, et al. Prevalence of open-angle glaucoma among adults in the United States. Arch Ophthalmol. 2004;122(4):532–538. Epub 2004/04/14. doi: 10.1001/archopht.122.4.532 [doi] 122/4/532 [pii]. PMID: 15078671.
8. Congdon N, O'Colmain B, Klaver CC, et al. Causes and prevalence of visual impairment among adults in the United States. Arch Ophthalmol. 2004;122(4):477–485. Epub 2004/04/14. doi: 10.1001/archopht.122.4.477. PMID: 15078664.
9. Weinreb RN, Aung T, Medeiros FA. The pathophysiology and treatment of glaucoma: A review. JAMA. 2014;311(18):1901–1911. Epub 2014/05/16. doi: 10.1001/jama.2014.3192. PMID: 24825645.
10. Quigley HA. Glaucoma. Lancet. 2011;377(9774):1367–1377. Epub 2011/04/02. doi: 10.1016/s0140-6736(10)61423-7. PMID: 21453963.
11. Civan MM, Macknight AD. The ins and outs of aqueous humour secretion. Exp Eye Res. 2004;78(3):625–631. PMID: 15106942.
12. King A, Azuara-Blanco A, Tuulonen A. Glaucoma. BMJ. 2013; 346:f3518. Epub 2013/06/13. doi: 10.1136/bmj.f3518. PMID: 23757737.
13. Malihi M, Sit AJ. Aqueous humor dynamics and implications for clinical practice. Int Ophthalmol Clin. 2011;51(3):119–139. Epub 2011/06/03. doi: 10.1097/IIO.0b013e31821e5cea. PMID: 21633243.
14. Wang SK, Chang RT. An emerging treatment option for glaucoma: Rho kinase inhibitors. Clin Ophthalmol (Auckland, NZ). 2014;8:883–890. Epub 2014/05/30. doi: 10.2147/opth.s41000. PMID: 24872673; Central PMCID: PMCPmc4025933.
15. Llobet A, Gasull X, Gual A. Understanding trabecular meshwork physiology: A key to the control of intraocular pressure? News Physiol Sci. 2003;18:205–209. Epub 2003/09/23. PMID: 14500801.
16. Kwon YH, Fingert JH, Kuehn MH, Alward WL. Primary open-angle glaucoma. N Engl J Med. 2009;360(11):1113–1124. Epub 2009/03/13. doi: 360/11/1113 [pii]. 10.1056/NEJMra0804630 [doi]. PMID: 19279343.
17. De Moraes CG. Anatomy of the visual pathways. J Glaucoma. 2013;22 (Suppl 5):S2–S7. Epub 2013/06/14. doi: 10.1097/IJG.0b013e3182934978. PMID: 23733119.
18. Vohra R, Tsai JC, Kolko M. The role of inflammation in the pathogenesis of glaucoma. Surv Ophthalmol. 2013;58(4):311–320. Epub 2013/06/19. doi: 10.1016/j.survophthal.2012.08.010. PMID: 23768921.
19. Ghaffarieh A, Levin LA. Optic nerve disease and axon pathophysiology. Int Rev Neurobiol. 2012;105:1–17. Epub 2012/12/05. doi: 10.1016/b978-0-12-398309-1.00002-0. PMID: 23206593.
20. Patel K, Patel S. Angle-closure glaucoma. Dis Mon. 2014;60(6): 254–262. Epub 2014/06/08. doi: 10.1016/j.disamonth.2014.03.005. PMID: 24906670.
21. Robin AL, Frick KD, Katz J, Budenz D, Tielsch JM. The ocular hypertension treatment study: Intraocular pressure lowering prevents the development of glaucoma, but does that mean we should treat before the onset of disease? Arch Ophthalmol. 2004;122(3):376–378. PMID: 15006854.
22. Boland MV, Ervin AM, Friedman DS, et al. Comparative effectiveness of treatments for open-angle glaucoma: A systematic review for the U.S. Preventive Services Task Force. Ann Intern Med. 2013;158(4):271–279. Epub 2013/02/20. doi: 10.7326/0003-4819-158-4-201302190-00008. PMID: 23420235.
23. Maier PC, Funk J, Schwarzer G, Antes G, Falck-Ytter YT. Treatment of ocular hypertension and open angle glaucoma: Meta-analysis of randomised controlled trials. BMJ. 2005;331(7509):134. Epub 2005/07/05. doi: 10.1136/bmj.38506.594977.E0. PMID: 15994659; Central PMCID: PMCPMC558697.
24. The effectiveness of intraocular pressure reduction in the treatment of normal-tension glaucoma. Collaborative Normal-Tension Glaucoma Study Group. Am J Ophthalmol. 1998;126(4):498–505. PMID: 9780094.
25. Cheng JW, Cai JP, Wei RL. Meta-analysis of medical intervention for normal tension glaucoma. Ophthalmology. 2009;116(7):1243–1249. Epub 2009/05/20. doi: S0161-6420(09)00096-7 [pii]. 10.1016/j.ophtha.2009.01.036 [doi]. PMID: 19450880.
26. Stewart WC, Konstas AG, Kruft B, Mathis HM, Stewart JA. Meta-analysis of 24-h intraocular pressure fluctuation studies and the efficacy of glaucoma medicines. J Ocul Pharmacol Ther. 2010;26(2):175–180. Epub 2010/03/26. doi: 10.1089/jop.2009.0124 [doi]. PMID: 20334538.
27. Stewart WC, Konstas AG, Nelson LA, Kruft B. Meta-analysis of 24-hour intraocular pressure studies evaluating the efficacy of glaucoma medicines. Ophthalmology. 2008;115(7):1117–1122 e1. Epub 2007/12/18. doi: S0161-6420(07)01076-7 [pii]. 10.1016/j.ophtha.2007.10.004 [doi]. PMID: 18082886.

28. van der Valk R, Webers CA, Lumley T, Hendrikse F, Prins MH, Schouten JS. A network meta-analysis combined direct and indirect comparisons between glaucoma drugs to rank effectiveness in lowering intraocular pressure. J Clin Epidemiol. 2009;62(12):1279–1283. Epub 2009/09/01. doi: S0895-4356(09)00176-0 [pii]. 10.1016/j.jclinepi.2008.04.012 [doi]. PMID: 19716679.
29. van der Valk R, Webers CA, Schouten JS, Zeegers MP, Hendrikse F, Prins MH. Intraocular pressure-lowering effects of all commonly used glaucoma drugs: A meta-analysis of randomized clinical trials. Ophthalmology. 2005;112(7):1177–1185. PMID: 15921747.
30. Inoue K. Managing adverse effects of glaucoma medications. Clin Ophthalmol. 2014;8:903–913. Epub 2014/05/30. doi: 10.2147/opth.s44708. PMID: 24872675; Central PMCID: PMCPmc4025938.
31. Kass MA, Heuer DK, Higginbotham EJ, Johnson CA, Keltner JL, Miller JP, et al. The ocular hypertension treatment study: A randomized trial determines that topical ocular hypotensive medication delays or prevents the onset of primary open-angle glaucoma. Arch Ophthalmol. 2002;120(6):701–713; discussion 829-30. Epub 2002/06/07. doi: ecs20045 [pii]. PMID: 12049574.
32. Marquis RE, Whitson JT. Management of glaucoma: Focus on pharmacological therapy. Drugs Aging. 2005;22(1):1–21. Epub 2005/01/25. doi: 2211 [pii]. PMID: 15663346.
33. Sambhara D, Aref AA. Glaucoma management: Relative value and place in therapy of available drug treatments. Therapeutic advances in chronic disease. 2014;5(1):30–43. Epub 2014/01/02. doi: 10.1177/2040622313511286. PMID: 24381726; Central PMCID: PMCPmc3871276.
34. Chidlow G, Wood JP, Casson RJ. Pharmacological neuroprotection for glaucoma. Drugs. 2007;67(5):725-59. Epub 2007/03/28. doi: 6756 [pii]. PMID: 17385943.
35. Vander Zanden JA, Valuck RJ, Bunch CL, Perlman JI, Anderson C, Wortman GI. Systemic adverse effects of ophthalmic beta-blockers. Ann Pharmacother. 2001;35(12):1633–1637. PMID: 11793633.
36. Swymer C, Neville MW. Tafluprost: The first preservative-free prostaglandin to treat open-angle glaucoma and ocular hypertension. Ann Pharmacother. 2012;46(11):1506–1510. Epub 2012/10/25. doi: 10.1345/aph.1R229. PMID: 23092867.
37. Krauss AH, Woodward DF. Update on the mechanism of action of bimatoprost: A review and discussion of new evidence. Surv Ophthalmol. 2004;49 (Suppl 1):S5–S11. PMID: 15016556.
38. Bournias TE, Lee D, Gross R, Mattox C. Ocular hypotensive efficacy of bimatoprost when used as a replacement for latanoprost in the treatment of glaucoma and ocular hypertension. J Ocul Pharmacol Ther. 2003;19(3):193–203. PMID: 12828838.
39. Gandolfi SA, Cimino L. Effect of bimatoprost on patients with primary open-angle glaucoma or ocular hypertension who are nonresponders to latanoprost. Ophthalmology. 2003;110(3):609–614. PMID: 12623831.
40. Sena DF, Lindsley K. Neuroprotection for treatment of glaucoma in adults. Cochrane Database Syst Rev. 2013;2:Cd006539. Epub 2013/03/02. doi: 10.1002/14651858.CD006539.pub3. PMID: 23450569.
41. Hoh ST, Aung T, Chew PT. Medical management of angle closure glaucoma. Semin Ophthalmol. 2002;17(2):79–83. PMID: 15513460.
42. Razeghinejad MR, Myers JS, Katz LJ. Iatrogenic glaucoma secondary to medications. Am J Med. 2011;124(1):20–25. Epub 2010/11/26. doi: 10.1016/j.amjmed.2010.08.011. PMID: 21092926.
43. Olthoff CM, Schouten JS, van de Borne BW, Webers CA. Noncompliance with ocular hypotensive treatment in patients with glaucoma or ocular hypertension an evidence-based review. Ophthalmology. 2005;112(6):953–961. PMID: 15885795.
44. Tsai JC. A comprehensive perspective on patient adherence to topical glaucoma therapy. Ophthalmology. 2009;116(suppl 11):S30–S36. Epub 2009/10/27. doi: S0161-6420(09)00652-6 [pii]. 10.1016/j.ophtha.2009.06.024 [doi]. PMID: 19837258.
45. Gray TA, Orton LC, Henson D, Harper R, Waterman H. Interventions for improving adherence to ocular hypotensive therapy. Cochrane Database Syst Rev. 2009;(2):CD006132. Epub 2009/04/17. doi: 10.1002/14651858.CD006132.pub2 [doi]. PMID: 19370627.

62 Ophthalmic Disorders

Melissa L. Hunter and Michelle L. Hilaire

LEARNING OBJECTIVES

Upon completion of the chapter, the reader will be able to:

1. Differentiate between the various ophthalmic disorders based on patient-specific information.
2. Choose an appropriate treatment regimen for an ophthalmic disorder.
3. Discuss the product differences that direct the selection of ophthalmic medications.
4. Assess when further treatment is required based on patient-specific information.
5. Recommend an ophthalmic monitoring plan given patient-specific information, a diagnosis, and a treatment regimen.
6. Educate patients about ophthalmic disease states and appropriate drug and nondrug therapies.

INTRODUCTION

This chapter provides an overview of common ophthalmic disorders and their treatments. KEY CONCEPT *Many ophthalmic disorders are benign or self-limited, but the clinician must be able to distinguish conditions that lead to serious morbidity, including blindness.* Preserving both visual function and cosmetic appearance is the goal.[1] The clinician must understand when referral is appropriate and the proper time frame for follow-up, based on the patient-specific condition.

OCULAR EMERGENCIES

Etiology and Epidemiology

Ophthalmic problems encompass 3% of all emergency department visits.[2] Corneal abrasions are the most common eye injury in children. Scratches, objects and aggressive eye rubbing may damage the cornea.[3] Healthcare practitioners must know the proper treatment for ocular emergencies and the time frame for follow-up in order to prevent further morbidity (Table 62–1).

CORNEAL ABRASIONS

Treatment

▶ *Desired Outcomes*

- Complete healing of the corneal abrasion with no scarring or vision impairment
- Prevent infection and pain
- Prevent corneal loss or corneal transplant

▶ *General Approach to Treatment*

The five layers of the cornea contain no blood vessels but are nourished by tears, oxygen, and aqueous humor. Minor corneal abrasions heal quickly. Moderate abrasions take 24 to 72 hours to heal. Deep scratches may scar the cornea and require corneal transplant if vision is impaired. Do not use eye patches to treat uncomplicated corneal abrasion.[3]

Corneal Abrasion Prevention[3]

- Wear eye protection during sports
- Wear industrial safety lenses
- Carefully fit and place contact lenses

▶ *Pharmacologic Therapy*

Topical NSAIDs Topical nonsteroidal anti-inflammatory drugs (NSAIDs) decrease pain from corneal abrasion. Available ocular NSAIDs are bromfenac 0.09%, diclofenac 0.1%, ketorolac 0.5%, and nepafenac 0.1%. The usual dose for diclofenac and ketorolac is one drop four times daily; nepafenac is dosed three times daily, and bromfenac is dosed twice daily. Use topical NSAIDs with caution in patients with clotting disorders or those who are on systemic NSAIDs or warfarin therapy. Oral analgesics may be an option for some patients.[3]

Topical Antibiotics Infection slows the healing of a corneal abrasion; therefore, prophylactic antibiotics are often used. Discontinue the use of contact lenses until the abrasion is healed and the antibiotic course complete. KEY CONCEPT *In contact lens wearers, choose an antibiotic that covers* Pseudomonas aeruginosa, like gentamicin ointment or solution or a fluoroquinolone.[3]

Outcome Evaluation

1. Reevaluate patients in 24 hours.
2. If symptoms worsen, recheck for foreign bodies.
3. If not fully healed, evaluate again in 3 to 4 days.
4. Refer to ophthalmologist if[3]:
   - Abrasion greater than 4 mm
   - Contact lens wearers
   - Decreased vision
   - Lack of improvement or worsening symptoms

Table 62–1

Ophthalmic Emergencies: Time to Follow Up by Ophthalmologist

Immediate Consult Required	Within 24 Hours
Foreign body in eye	Acute angle-closure glaucoma
Acute, painless loss of vision	Orbital cellulitis
Acute chemical burn	Blood in the eye (hyphema)
Blunt trauma to eye	Macular edema
	Retinal detachment
	Sudden congestive proptosis (bulging of eye forward)
	Corneal ulcer
	Corneal abrasion

From Ref. 1, Handler JA, Ghezzi KT. General ophthalmologic examination. Emerg Med Clin North Am. 1995;13:521–538.

OTHER OCULAR EMERGENCIES: TREATMENT

Traumatic Injuries

Attempt to remove loose foreign bodies by gentle irrigation with artificial tears or sterile saline. If removal is successful, a topical broad-spectrum antibiotic, such as erythromycin, will prevent infection. If irrigation is unsuccessful, only ophthalmologists should complete mechanical removal of foreign objects. Protect the eye from further injury with a metal eye shield or a paper cup taped over the eye while awaiting the ophthalmologist.[2]

Splash Injuries and Chemical Exposure

Instruct patients by phone to immediately irrigate the eye with water or saline continuously for at least 15 minutes before seeking a clinician. Irrigation dilutes and removes the chemical agent and is the best way to decrease ocular tissue damage. Patients should then seek immediate care from an ophthalmologist or emergency facility.[4]

Clinical Presentation and Diagnosis of Corneal Abrasions[3]

Symptoms

- Photophobia
- Pain with extraocular muscle movement
- Foreign body sensation (or gritty feeling)
- Recent ocular trauma

Signs

- Excessive tearing
- Blepharospasm
- Blurred vision

Diagnostic Test

Use sterile fluorescein dye strips and visualize the cornea under a cobalt-blue filtered light; abrasions appear green; ensure that no foreign body remains in the eye.

Loss of Vision

A variety of disorders may lead to rapid, painless, monocular, or binocular vision loss. These include central retinal artery occlusion, acute narrow-angle glaucoma, trauma, and others.[5] The differential diagnosis is complex and should be undertaken by an emergency department or ophthalmologist.

CONJUNCTIVITIS

Etiology

Conjunctivitis, also known as red eye, is one of the most common ophthalmic complaints seen by clinicians. An inflamed conjunctiva is the most common cause of red eye.[6] Conjunctivitis cases are mostly viral in nature. Use the differential diagnosis algorithm shown in Figure 62–1 to determine the proper treatment or need for referral.

BACTERIAL CONJUNCTIVITIS

Etiology and Pathophysiology

The primary cause of acute bacterial conjunctivitis (ABC) is gram-positive organisms, including *Streptococcus pneumoniae* and *Staphylococcus aureus*, and gram-negative *Haemophilus influenzae*.[6] KEY CONCEPT *Both acute and chronic bacterial conjunctivitis are self-limiting except if caused by* Neisseria.[6] The pathogens are rarely cultured unless the case is unresponsive to treatment.[6] Patients with bacterial conjunctivitis lasting 4 weeks or more should be referred to an ophthalmologist.[7]

Hyperacute bacterial conjunctivitis is associated with gonococcal (*Neisseria gonorrhoeae* or *Neisseria meningitides*) infections in sexually active patients. Prompt workup and treatment is required, as corneal perforation can occur.[6,7]

Treatment

► *Desired Outcomes*

- Complete resolution of the bacterial conjunctivitis
- Prevent adverse consequences of the infection
- Preserve functionality of the eye

► *General Approach to Treatment*

ABC may be treated with broad-spectrum antibiotics. Although the condition is usually self-limiting, antibiotic treatment decreases the spread of disease to others and prevents extraocular infection. Additionally, treatment may help decrease the risk of corneal ulceration or other complications that affect sight. Finally, treatment speeds recovery.[6,7]

► *Pharmacologic Therapy*

The choice of an antibiotic agent for ABC is largely empiric. The initial treatment needs to include *Staphylococcus* coverage, and cost and side-effect profile may be pertinent.[6] In general, ointments are a good dosage form for children. Adults may prefer drops because they do not interfere with vision.

Many broad-spectrum topical antibiotics are approved to treat ABC (Tables 62–2 and 62–3).

- First-line treatments include polymyxin B/trimethoprim solution, polymyxin B with bacitracin ointment, or erythromycin ointment
- The aminoglycosides (tobramycin and gentamicin) are alternatives but have incomplete gram-positive coverage and can cause corneal epithelial toxicity[7]

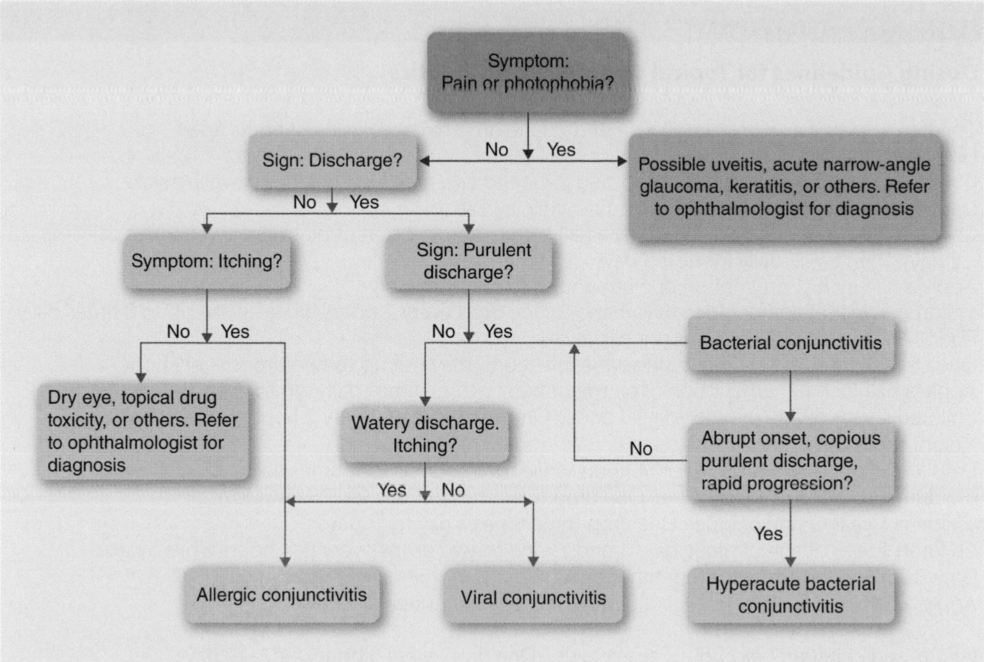

FIGURE 62–1. Differential diagnosis for red eye.

- Sulfacetamide has significant resistance
- If infection recurs or is severe, use a topical fluoroquinolone[6]
- Treat hyperacute bacterial conjunctivitis with a single dose of intramuscular ceftriaxone 1 g in combination with topical antibiotics and refer the patient to an opthalmologist[7]
- If concurrent blepharitis is present, add a lid hygiene regimen to antibiotic treatment[6]

Outcome Evaluation

- Significant improvement of acute bacterial conjunctivitis should be seen within 1 week.[6]

Table 62–2

Adult Bacterial Conjunctivitis Dosing Guidelines for Topical Ophthalmic Antibiotics

Azithromycin 1% solution	Days 1 and 2: One drop twice daily, 8–12 hours apart Days 3–7: 1 drop once daily
Ciprofloxacin 3.5 mg/mL solution	Days 1 and 2: One to two drops every 2 hours while awake Days 3–7: One to two drops every 4 hours while awake
Ciprofloxacin 0.3% ointment	Apply a half inch (~1 cm) ribbon of ointment three times daily for 2 days, then twice daily for next 5 days
Erythromycin 0.5% ointment	Apply a half inch (~1 cm) ribbon of ointment up to six times daily
Gatifloxacin 0.3% solution	Days 1 and 2: One drop every 2 hours while awake up to eight times daily Days 3–7: One drop every 4 hours while awake
Gatifloxacin 0.5% solution	Days 1: One drop every 2 hours while awake up to eight times daily Days 2–7: One drop two to four times per day while awake
Gentamicin 0.3% solution	One to two drops every 4 hours. In severe infections, may use up to two drops every hour
Gentamicin 0.3% ointment	Apply a half inch (~1 cm) ribbon of ointment two to three times daily; up to every 3–4 hours
Levofloxacin 0.5% solution	Days 1 and 2: One to two drops every 2 hours while awake, up to eight times per day Days 3–7: One to two drops every 4 hours while awake, up to four times daily
Moxifloxacin 0.5% solution	One drop two times a day for 7 days (Moxeza) One drop three times a day for 7 days (Vigamox)
Ofloxacin 0.3% solution	Days 1 and 2: One to two drops every 2–4 hours while awake Days 3–7: One to two drops four times daily
Polymyxin B with bacitracin ointment	Apply a half inch (~1 cm) ribbon of ointment every 3–4 hours, or two to three times per day for 7–10 days
Polymyxin B/trimethoprim solution	One drop every 3 hours for 7–10 days
Sulfacetamide 10% ointment	Apply a half inch (~1 cm) ribbon of ointment every 3–4 hours and at bedtime
Sulfacetamide 10% solution	One to two drops every 2–3 hours for 7–10 days
Tobramycin 0.3% ointment	Mild to moderate infections: Apply a half inch (~1 cm) ribbon of ointment two to three times daily; Severe infections: Apply every 3–4 hours
Tobramycin 0.3% solution	Mild to moderate infections: One to two drops every 2–4 hours Severe infections: initially, two drops every hour

From Lacy CF, Armstrong LL, Goldman MP, Lance LL. Drug Information Handbook, 23rd ed. Hudson, OH: Lexi-Comp, Inc., 2014.

Table 62–3

Pediatric Bacterial Conjunctivitis Dosing Guidelines for Topical Ophthalmic Antibiotics

Azithromycin 1% solution	Children 1 year of age or older: Days 1 and 2: One drop twice daily, 8–12 hours apart Days 3–7: One drop once daily
Ciprofloxacin 3.5 mg/mL solution	Children 1 year of age or older, days 1 and 2: One to two drops every 2 hours while awake Days 3–7: One to two drops every 4 hours while awake
Ciprofloxacin 0.3% ointment	Children 2 years of age or older: Apply a half inch (~1 cm) ribbon of ointment three times daily for 2 days, then twice daily for next 5 days
Erythromycin 0.5% ointment	Apply a half inch (1 cm) ribbon of ointment up to six times daily
Gatifloxacin 0.3% solution	Children 1 year of age or older, days 1 and 2: One drop every 2 hours while awake up to 8 times daily Days 3–7: One drop every 4 hours while awake
Gentamicin 0.3% solution	One to two drops every 4 hours. In severe infections, may use up to two drops every hour
Gentamicin 0.3% ointment	Apply a half inch (~1 cm) ribbon of ointment two to three times daily; up to every 3–4 hours
Levofloxacin 0.5% solution	Children 1 year of age or older, days 1 and 2: One to two drops every 2 hours while awake, up to eight times daily Days 3–7: One to two drops every 4 hours while awake, up to four times daily
Moxifloxacin 0.5% solution	Children 4 months of age or older: One drop two times per day for 7 days (Moxeza) Children 1 year of age or older: One drop three times a day for 7 days
Ofloxacin 0.3% solution	Children 1 year of age or older, days 1 and 2: One to two drops every 2–4 hours while awake Days 3–7: One to two drops four times daily
Polymyxin B with bacitracin ointment	Apply a half inch (~1 cm) ribbon of ointment every 3–4 hours for 7–10 days
Polymyxin B/trimethoprim solution	Infants and children 2 months of age or older: One drop every 3 hours for 7–10 days
Sulfacetamide 10% ointment	Apply a half inch (~1 cm) ribbon of ointment every 3–4 hours and at bedtime
Sulfacetamide 10% solution	One to two drops every 2–3 hours for 7–10 days
Tobramycin 0.3% ointment	Infants and children 2 months of age or older: Mild to moderate infections: Apply an approximately half inch (~1 cm) ribbon two to three times daily Severe infections: Apply every 3–4 hours
Tobramycin 0.3% solution	Infants and children 2 months of age or older: Mild to moderate infections: One to two drops every 4 hours Severe infections: initially, two drops every hour

From Lacy CF, Armstrong LL, Goldman MP, Lance LL. Drug Information Handbook, 23rd ed. Hudson, OH: Lexi-Comp, Inc., 2014.

VIRAL CONJUNCTIVITIS

Etiology

Viral conjunctivitis is commonly caused by adenovirus and is often called "pink-eye."[6] Adenovirus is easily spread through swimming pools, camps, and contaminated fingers and medical instruments.[7] Patients often present with an upper respiratory tract infection or recent exposure to viral conjunctivitis.[6] KEY CONCEPT *Viral conjunctivitis is usually self-limiting, resolving within 2 weeks.*[6]

Patient Encounter 1

This morning, a mother brings in her 13-year-old son who has been complaining of irritation, redness, and "goop" coming out of his right eye for the past 13 hours. He woke up terrified this morning because his right eye seemed glued shut. At first, the mother was concerned because his younger sister had "pink-eye" 2 weeks ago. A warm washcloth was used to ease the eye open, and upon examination, the right eye was red and revealed a whitish discharge, whereas the left eye was just red.

What is the probable diagnosis?

Please differentiate between bacterial, hyperacute bacterial, viral, and allergic causes based on physical assessment.

What organisms should be suspected, and what are reasonable treatment regimens?

If the child would have been diagnosed with viral conjunctivitis, what nonpharmacologic measures should be employed to prevent spreading?

Treatment

► *Desired Outcomes*

- Complete resolution of the viral conjunctivitis
- Prevent adverse consequences of the infection
- Avoid spreading infection to other patients

► *Nonpharmacologic Therapy*

KEY CONCEPT *Nonpharmacologic measures are critical to prevent the spread of viral conjunctivitis.* Cold compresses may relieve symptoms.[6,7] Patients should not share towels or other contaminated objects, should avoid close contact with other people, and avoid swimming for 2 weeks.[6,7] Take care in the medical setting to thoroughly decontaminate instruments and wash hands.[6,7]

► *Pharmacologic Therapy*

Patients may obtain further symptomatic relief by using artificial tears and topical decongestants.[6,7] If artificial tear solutions sting, recommend a preservative-free formula.

Topical antivirals are not used to treat adenovirus conjunctivitis. Topical antibiotics are unnecessary and should not be used for a viral infection and to help prevent the development of antibiotic resistance.[7]

Patients with severe subepithelial infiltration may require a topical steroid. However, topical steroids may cause serious ocular complications, increase the period of viral shedding, and may worsen herpetic conjunctivitis, which has similar symptoms as viral conjunctivitis.[7] Only ophthalmologists should prescribe topical steroids.[6]

Outcome Evaluation

Refer patients who do not see improvement within 7 to 10 days to an ophthalmologist to rule out herpetic and other infectious processes.[6,7]

ALLERGIC CONJUNCTIVITIS

Etiology and Clinical Presentation

Ocular allergy is a broad term that includes several diseases with the hallmark symptom of itching, often accompanied by tearing, conjunctival swelling, photophobia, and stringy or sticky mucoid discharge.[8] Allergic conjunctivitis affects up to 40% of patients.[9] Seasonal ocular allergy is the most common type of allergic conjunctivitis. Often, the patient's history is positive for atopic conditions, including allergic rhinitis, asthma, or eczema.[6] Perennial allergic conjunctivitis has similar but less severe symptoms and may not be tied to a specific time of year. Finally, **conjunctivitis medicamentosa** is a drug-induced form of allergic conjunctivitis caused by overuse of topical vasoconstricting agents.[8]

Pathophysiology

The conjunctiva of the eye is often the initial site of contact with an environmental allergen. Mast cell degranulation occurs, and the earliest mediator is histamine, which causes itching, redness, and swelling.[9] Leukotrienes and prostaglandins cause cellular infiltration and increased mucous secretion along with chemosis, resulting in conjunctival vasodilation.

Treatment of ocular allergy is aimed at slowing or stopping these processes. Antihistamines block the histamine receptors, prevent histamine release from the mast cells and stop eosinophil activity.[9] Mast cell stabilizers inhibit the degranulation of mast cells, preventing mediator release. Some topical agents have multiple mechanisms of action, combining antihistaminic, mast cell stabilization, and anti-inflammatory properties (**Tables 62–4, 62–5, and 62–6**).[9]

Patient Encounter 2

AZ is a 17-year-old boy presenting with swollen, teary eyes, and complains of itching. His symptoms seem to be worse in the spring months especially when he's outdoors. He has asthma and smokes (but his parents don't know). He has been using over-the-counter naphazoline for the past 2 weeks that his mother found in their medicine closet.

What information is suggestive of allergic conjunctivitis?

What nonpharmacologic therapies should be recommended for this patient?

What pharmacologic therapies should be recommended for this patient?

How should the patient be monitored?

Table 62–4

Mechanisms of Action of Ocular Allergy Drugs

Drug	Mechanisms
Azelastine	H_1-receptor antagonist
Cromolyn sodium	Mast cell stabilizer
Emedastine	H_1 receptor antagonist
Epinastine	H_1- and H_2-receptor antagonist, mast cell stabilizer
Ketorolac	Inhibitors prostaglandin synthesis
Ketotifen	H_1-receptor antagonist, mast cell stabilizer, eosinophil inhibitor
Lodoxamide	Mast cell stabilizer
Loteprednol	Corticosteroid
Nedocromil	Mast cell stabilizer, eosinophil inhibitor
Olopatadine	H_1-receptor antagonist, mast cell stabilizer
Pemirolast	Mast cell stabilizer

From McEvoy GK, ed. AHFS Drug Information 2014. Bethesda, MD: American Society of Health-System Pharmacists Inc., 2014.

Treatment

▸ *Desired Outcomes*

- Relief of current allergic symptoms
- Prevention of future allergic symptoms
- No adverse effects from treatment

▸ *Nonpharmacologic Therapy*

The primary treatment for ocular allergy is removal and avoidance of the allergen.[6,7] For conjunctivitis medicamentosa, discontinue the offending medication. Apply cold compresses several times daily to reduce redness and itching and to provide symptomatic relief.[8]

▸ *Pharmacologic Therapy*

KEY CONCEPT *Use a step-care approach for the treatment of allergic conjunctivitis.*

- Step 1: Nonmedicated, artificial tears solution. The solution dilutes or removes the allergen, providing relief while lubricating the eye. Solutions are applied two to four times daily as needed. Ointments may be used in the evenings to further moisturize the surface of the eye. Preservative-free formulations may be tried if other products sting or burn.
- Step 2: Topical antihistamine or antihistamine/decongestant combination. The antihistamine/decongestant combination is more effective than either agent alone. Decongestants are vasoconstrictors that reduce redness and seem to have a small synergistic effect with the antihistamine. The only topical decongestant used in combination products is naphazoline. Topical decongestants burn and sting on instillation and commonly cause **mydriasis**, especially in patients with lighter-colored eyes. Topical decongestant use should be limited to less than 10 days to avoid rebound congestion.
- Step 3: A mast cell stabilizer or a multiple-action agent. Use mast cell stabilizers prophylactically throughout the allergy season. Full response may take 4 to 6 weeks.
- Step 4: Short-term topical corticosteroids and immunotherapy.[8,9]

Table 62–5

Pediatric and Adult Dosing and Common Side Effects of Ocular Allergy Drugs

Drug	Dosing	Common Side Effects
Azelastine 0.05%	Children 3 years of age or older and adults: one drop in affected eye(s) twice daily	Ocular stinging, bitter taste, headache
Cromolyn sodium 4%	Children 4 years of age or older and adults: one to two drops in each eye four to six times daily	Ocular stinging
Emedastine 0.05%	Children 3 years of age or older and adults: one drop in affected eye up to four times daily	Ocular stinging, blurred vision, headache
Epinastine 0.05%	Children 3 years of age or older and adults: one drop in each eye twice daily	Ocular burning, ocular itching, cold symptoms
Ketorolac 0.5%	Children 3 years of age or older and adults: one drop four times a day	Ocular stinging, irritation
Ketotifen 0.025%	Children 3 years of age or older and adults: one drop in affected eye(s) twice daily	Red eyes, headache, rhinitis
Lodoxamide 0.1%	Children 2 years of age or older and adults: one to two drops in affected eye(s) four times daily, for up to 3 months	Ocular stinging, discomfort, foreign body sensation
Loteprednol 0.2%	Adults only: one drop in affected eye(s) four times daily	Elevated intraocular pressure, cataracts, secondary ocular infections, systemic side effects possible
Nedocromil 2%	Children 3 years of age or older and adults: one to two drops in each eye twice daily	Headache, ocular stinging, unpleasant taste, nasal congestion
Olopatadine 0.1%; 0.2%	Children 3 years of age or older and adults (0.1%): one drop in affected eye(s) two times daily with minimum 6- to 8-hour interval between doses Children 2 years of age or older: and adults (0.2%): one drop in affected eye(s) once daily	Headache, blurred vision, ocular stinging
Pemirolast 0.1%	Children 3 years of age or older and adults: one to two drops in affected eye(s) four times daily	Headache, cold symptoms

From McEvoy GK, ed. AHFS Drug Information 2014. Bethesda, MD: American Society of Health-System Pharmacists Inc., 2014.

Alomide (lodoxamide tromethamine) solution/drops 0.1%. Fort Worth(TX): Alcon Laboratories, Inc., 2003.

Table 62–6

Risk Factors for Bacterial Keratitis

Exogenous Factors
- Contact lenses
- Loose sutures from ocular surgeries
- Previous corneal surgery
- Previous ocular or eyelid surgery
- Trauma, including foreign bodies, chemical and thermal injuries and local irradiation

Ocular Surface Disease
- Abnormal lid anatomy or function
- Misdirection of eyelashes
- Ocular infection (eg, conjunctivitis, blepharitis)
- Tear film deficiencies

Systemic Conditions
- Atopic dermatitis
- Connective tissue disease
- Debilitating illness (eg, malnourishment or respirator dependence)
- Diabetes mellitus
- Factitious disease (including anesthetic abuse)
- Gonococcal infection
- Immunocompromised
- Stevens-Johnson syndrome
- Substance abuse
- Vitamin A deficiency

Ocular Medications
- Anesthetics
- Antimicrobials
- Contaminated ocular medications
- Glaucoma medications
- Preservatives
- Steroids
- Topical NSAIDs

Corneal Epithelial Abnormalities
- Corneal epithelial edema
- Predisposition to recurrent erosion of the cornea
- Viral keratitis (eg, herpes simplex or zoster keratitis)

Data from Ref. 10, American Academy of Ophthalmology Cornea/External Disease Panel. Preferred Practice Pattern® Guidelines. Bacterial Keratitis [Internet]. San Francisco, CA: American Academy of Ophthalmology, 2013 [cited 2014 Aug 30]. www.aao.org/ppp.

Topical antihistamines are recommended before oral agents in step therapy due to the increased risk of systemic side effects with oral drugs. Topical antihistamines provide faster relief of ocular symptoms. Topical ketorolac tromethamine is approved for ocular itching.[9]

Outcome Evaluation

- Monitor patients for relief of symptoms. Ensure an adequate trial of each agent. Refer severe cases that do not respond to an ophthalmologist.

BACTERIAL KERATITIS

Epidemiology

Thirty thousand cases of microbial keratitis occur annually in the United States.[10] Microbial keratitis encompasses bacterial, fungal, and *Acanthamoeba* keratitis.[10] Only bacterial keratitis, the most common form, is discussed here.

Clinical Presentation and Diagnosis of Bacterial Keratitis[6,10]

General

The rate of progression of signs and symptoms varies depending on the infecting organism. A differential diagnosis for keratitis must include viral, fungal, and nematodal infections in addition to bacterial causes.

Symptoms

- Photophobia
- Rapid onset of ocular pain

Signs

- Red eye
- Conjunctival discharge
- Decreased vision

Laboratory Tests

- Culture if keratitis is severe or sight threatening, chronic, or unresponsive to broad-spectrum antimicrobial therapy.

Pathophysiology

Bacterial keratitis is a broad term for a bacterial infection of the cornea, including corneal ulcers and corneal abscesses. The cornea in a healthy eye has natural resistance to infection, making bacterial keratitis rare. However, many factors may predispose a patient to bacterial infection by compromising the defense mechanisms of the eye (see Table 62–6).[10]

The most common pathogens in bacterial keratitis are *Pseudomonas* (including *Pseudomonas aeruginosa*) and other gram-negative rods, Staphylococci, and Streptococci.[10] If the keratitis is related to the use of contacts, *Pseudomonas* and *Serratia marcescens* are the most common pathogens.[10] KEY CONCEPT *Untreated bacterial keratitis is associated with corneal scarring and potential loss of vision. Corneal perforation may occur, and the patient may lose the eye.*[10] In virulent organisms, this destruction may occur within 24 hours.[10] Central corneal scarring may result in vision loss even after successful eradication of the organism.[10]

Treatment

▶ *Desired Outcomes*[10]

- Resolution of infection and corneal inflammation
- Reduced corneal pain
- Restored corneal integrity with minimal scarring
- Restored visual function

▶ *General Approach to Treatment*

All cases of suspected bacterial keratitis require prompt ophthalmology consultation to prevent permanent vision loss.[6]

▶ *Pharmacologic Therapy*

Dosage Considerations Topical antibiotic drops are preferred. Consider subconjunctival antibiotics if compliance is a concern. Systemic therapy is useful in cases of systemic infection (eg, gonorrhea) or if the sclera is infected. Reserve ointments for minor cases or adjunctive nighttime therapy.[10]

Table 62–7

Pharmacologic Therapies for Bacterial Keratitis

Organism	Drug
Unknown or multiple types of organisms	Cefazolin 50 mg/mL *and* tobramycin/gentamicin 9–14 mg/mL *or* Fluoroquinolones various strengths
Gram-positive cocci	Cefazolin 50 mg/mL *or* Vancomycin[a] 15–50 mg/mL *or* Bacitracin[a] 10,000 international unit *or* Moxifloxacin or gatifloxacin various strengths
Gram-negative rods	Tobramycin 9–14 mg/mL *or* Gentamicin 9–14 mg/mL *or* Ceftazidime 50 mg/mL *or* Fluoroquinolones various strengths
Gram-negative cocci	Ceftriaxone 50 mg/mL *or* Ceftazidime 50 mg/mL *or* Fluoroquinolones various strengths
Nontuberculous mycobacteria	Amikacin 20–40 mg/mL *or* Oral clarithromycin, adults: 500 mg every 12 hours Fluoroquinolones various strengths
Nocardia	Amikacin 20–40 mg/mL *or* Trimethoprim 16 mg/mL *and* sulfamethoxazole 80 mg/mL

Adult Topical Dosing

Severe keratitis: loading dose every 5–15 minutes for the first hour, then every 15 minutes to 1 hour around the clock. Less severe keratitis may use less frequent dosing

[a]Use for resistant *Enterococcus* and *Staphylococcus* species and penicillin allergy. Due to the absence of gram-negative activity, do not use vancomycin or bacitracin for single-agent empiric therapy in bacterial keratitis.

Data from Ref. 10, American Academy of Ophthalmology Cornea/External Disease Panel. Preferred Practice Pattern® Guidelines. Bacterial Keratitis [Internet]. San Francisco, CA: American Academy of Ophthalmology, 2013 [cited 2014 Aug 30]. www.aao.org/ppp.

Drug Choice Start topical broad-spectrum antibiotics empirically. Use a loading dose for severe keratitis (Table 62–7). Single-drug therapy with a fluoroquinolone is as effective as combination therapy. Resistance is seen with some fluoroquinolones, choose moxifloxacin or gatifloxacin in severe keratitis cases.[10] Fortified antibiotic therapy is an option for severe or unresponsive infections but may increase toxicity to the cornea and surrounding tissues. Fortified antibiotics are compounded products that are a higher concentration than the commercially available formulation.[10]

Topical corticosteroids are employed in some cases of bacterial keratitis. The suppression of inflammation may reduce corneal scarring. However, local immunosuppression, increased ocular pressure, and reappearance of the infection are disadvantages to their use. There is no conclusive evidence that they alter clinical outcomes. If the patient is already on topical corticosteroids when the keratitis occurs, discontinue use until the infection is eliminated.[10]

Outcome Evaluation[10]

- Symptomatic improvement is indicative of therapeutic efficacy.
- Adjust treatment based on culture and sensitivity reports.

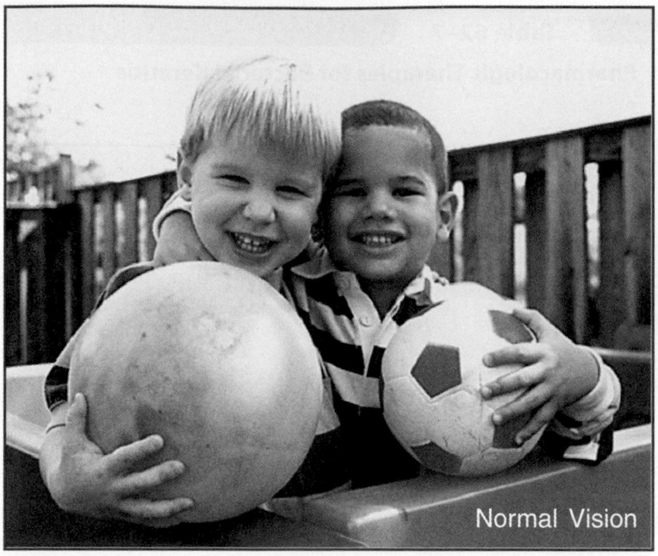

FIGURE 62–2. Normal vision. (From the National Eye Institute, National Institutes of Health Ref. No. EDS01. http://www.nei.nih.gov/photo/)

- Modify the treatment regimen if the patient does not show improvement within 48 hours.
- Gram-negative keratitis will have increased inflammation in the first 24 to 48 hours, even on appropriate therapy.
- Taper therapy based on clinical response.
- Reculture if negative clinical response; discontinue antibiotics 12 to 24 hours before culturing for best results.
- Contact lenses wearers should be educated about the increased risk of infection overnight and continuous wear and the importance of adherence to contact lens hygiene.

MACULAR DEGENERATION

Epidemiology and Etiology

Age-related macular degeneration (AMD) is the primary cause of severe, irreversible vision impairment in developed countries (Figures 62–2 and 62–3). The prevalence increases with age.[11]

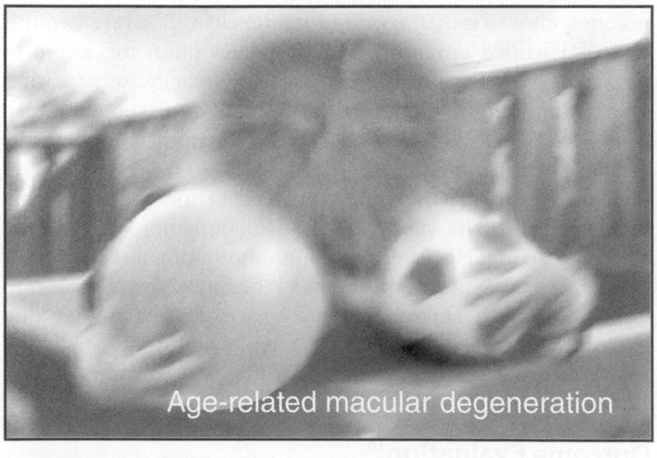

FIGURE 62–3. The scene in Figure 62–2 as it might be viewed by a person with age-related macular degeneration. (From the National Eye Institute, National Institutes of Health Ref. No. EDS05. http://www.nei.nih.gov/photo/)

Table 62–8

Risk Factors for AMD

Definite Risk Factors	Potential Risk Factors
Advancing age	Cardiovascular disease
Light pigmentation (white ethnicity)	Hypertension
Cigarette smoking	Low dietary intake of antioxidant vitamins or zinc
Family history	Increased body mass index
	Higher dietary fat intake

Data from Ref. 11, American Academy of Ophthalmology Retina Panel. Preferred Practice Pattern® Guidelines. Age-Related Macular Degeneration [Internet]. San Francisco, CA: American Academy of Ophthalmology, 2008 [cited 2014 Aug 30]. www.aao.org/ppp.

In the United States, 1.75 million people age 40 or older have advanced AMD, and another 7 million people may have intermediate AMD.[11] It is projected that almost 3 million people will develop AMD by 2020.[12] The causes of AMD are not completely known (Table 62–8).[11]

Pathophysiology

AMD is a deterioration of the macula, the central portion of the retina. The macula facilitates central vision and high-resolution visual acuity because it has the highest concentration of photoreceptors in the retina. The loss of central vision leads to irreversible loss of the ability to drive, read, and perform other fine visual tasks like recognize faces.[13] Peripheral vision is preserved, allowing mobility.[11] AMD is characterized by one or more of the following: drusen formation, retinal pigment abnormalities (eg, hypo- or hyperpigmentation), geographic atrophy, and neovascular maculopathy.[11]

Clinical Presentation and Diagnosis of AMD[12,14]

Symptoms

- Mild blurry central vision
- Difficulty reading
- Trouble with color and contrast
- Painless, progressive, blurring of central vision
- Sudden loss or distortion of vision possible

Signs

- Drusen
- Retinal pigment epithelial mottling

Other Diagnostic Tests

- Amsler grid abnormalities indicate fluid in subretinal space (see Figures 62–4 and 62–5)
- Dilated fundus examination shows drusen and pigmentary abnormalities in the macula
- Rapid sequence fluorescein angiography shows leakage in the neovascular form

Based on clinical presentation, AMD is classified as early, intermediate, or advanced.[11] Early AMD is characterized by small or intermediate drusen and minimal macular pigment abnormalities. These patients generally have normal central vision. Intermediate AMD patients have medium or large drusen in one or both eyes.[11]

Advanced AMD is classified as non-neovascular (also called the atrophic, nonexudative, or dry form) or neovascular (the exudative or wet form).[11,13] In the non-neovascular form, the retina and other layers atrophy.[13] In the neovascular form, new blood vessels appear.[11,13] Generally, vision is already affected when patients progress to advanced AMD; vision loss is seen in both forms.[11] Around 10% to 20% patients with the non-neovascular form will progress to the neovascular form.[14]

Treatment

▶ *Desired Outcomes*

The primary goal of treatment for AMD is to slow the disease progression. This includes slowing the loss of visual acuity and the progression to legal blindness, along with maintaining contrast sensitivity. The secondary goals are maintaining quality of life and minimizing the adverse effects of treatment.[13]

▶ *General Approach to Treatment*

KEY CONCEPT *There is no cure for AMD, and the efficacy of most treatments is low.* Newer drug developments show promise, but no treatment can reverse damage that has already occurred.[14] Early diagnosis is critical. High-risk patients need periodic eye examinations because some patients do not notice any changes, even when neovascularization has occurred.[11]

▶ *Nonpharmacologic Therapy*

Non-neovascular AMD Advise patients to stop smoking, as observational data supports a causal relationship between smoking and AMD.[11]

Drusen ablation by laser has been used however; it is not clear whether the treatment reduces progression to neovascular AMD.[14] Treatments may induce neovascularization and retinal atrophy.[13] Other nonpharmacologic therapies are in trials, but there is insufficient evidence for experts to recommend these procedures at this time.[11]

Neovascular AMD Thermal laser photocoagulation reduces severe visual loss 2 to 5 years after the procedure, but leads to an immediate and permanent reduction in central vision. There is a 50% chance that leakage will recur in the next 2 years after the procedure.[13]

Use of photodynamic therapy in combination with the medication verteporfin has shown success in clinical trials.[15] Verteporfin is reconstituted to achieve the desired dose of 6 mg/m^2 body surface area and diluted with 5% dextrose for injection to a total infusion volume of 30 mL. The drug is given intravenously, and laser light delivery is performed on the patient 15 minutes after the start of the 10-minute infusion with verteporfin. Photodynamic therapy uses nonthermal red light to activate verteporfin, which produces reactive oxygen species that locally damage the neovascular endothelium.[15] Verteporfin treatment reduces the risk of loss of visual acuity and legal blindness over 1 to 2 years. Long-term results are not yet available. Severe photosensitivity for 3 to 5 days after the procedure is common, and some patients experience a severe loss of vision. Eventually, most patients have some visual recovery. This procedure requires multiple treatments over time.[15]

▶ *Pharmacologic Therapy*

There are no approved pharmacologic treatments for non-neovascular AMD.[16] The Age-Related Eye Disease Study showed that a supplement containing ascorbic acid 500 mg, vitamin E 400 IU, β-carotene 15 mg, zinc oxide 80 mg, and cupric oxide 2 mg reduced the rate of clinical progression of all types of AMD by 28% in patients with at least intermediate macular degeneration.[16] No benefit was seen in patients with earlier stages of AMD; however, the duration of the study may have been insufficient to detect this benefit.[16] Currently, experts recommend antioxidant supplementation for intermediate AMD or advanced AMD in one eye.[11] Supplementation is not without risk.[14] For example, β-carotene supplementation in smokers may increase the risk of developing lung cancer.[11,14] At this time, it is not clear from the evidence whether a patient is at a high risk but without symptoms of AMD would benefit from supplementation.[17]

Vascular endothelial growth factor induces **angiogenesis**, increases vascular permeability, and increases inflammation, all of which are thought to contribute to neovascular AMD.[18] Pegaptanib, a vascular endothelial growth factor antagonist, binds to these growth factors in an attempt to suppress neovascularization.[11,18] In clinical studies, patients treated with pegaptanib experienced a slower rate of visual decline than patients treated with a placebo injection.[19] Vision loss continued to occur in patients, and the drug was less effective in the second year of treatment.[18]

Ranibizumab, binds to and inhibits the activity of vascular endothelial growth factor (VEGF) A, a critical protein in angiogenesis.[11] In one clinical study, 95% of patients treated with ranibizumab maintained visual acuity after 12 months compared with 62% of control patients.[11]

Aflibercept, a VEGF-A inhibitor was approved for wet age-related macular degeneration. The dosing of 2 mg every 4 weeks for the first 3 months, followed by 2 mg every 8 weeks thereafter, results in seven injections during the first year of treatment compared with 12 injections with other products.[20] Patients treated with aflibercept or other VEGF-A inhibitors are at risk for arterial thrombotic events. Specifically, stroke, nonfatal heart

Patient Encounter 3, Part 1

JJ, an 82-year-old white man, presents with difficulty seeing license plates on cars while driving. He can still distinguish street signs and other cars, but smaller details seem hazy. He notes that this is only occurring in his left eye, so sometimes he closes that eye and everything is fine.

PMH: Hypertension, osteoporosis, hyperlipidemia, chronic kidney disease, vitamin D Deficiency

FM: Mother died at 70 from cardiovascular disease

Father died at 75 from cancer

SH: Denies drinking, or illicit drugs. Smokes half PPD

Widowed, two adult children

PE: BP 142/82, P 68, R 14, Ht 5′6″ (168 cm), Wt 162 lb (73.5 kg)

Meds: Accupril 10 mg daily; fosamax 70 mg q week (on Fridays); Zocor 20 mg daily; aspirin 81 mg daily; multivitamin daily; vitamin D 2000 IUs daily

Does JJ have any definitive or potential risk factors for age-related macular degeneration?

Patient Encounter 3, Part 2

After meeting with a retinologist, JJ has been diagnosed with early non-neovascular age-related macular degeneration. He has been advised to use a magnifying glass for his left eye instead of closing it while reading. He has been advised to only drive during the day.

What pharmacologic and nonpharmacologic treatment options are available for JJ?

JJ's daughter is very FRUSTRATED that her dad is not on a "medication," as a family friend is being treated for macular degeneration. What information is necessary to relay to JJ's daughter?

What monitoring is appropriate for JJ?

JJ's daughter is concerned that she will develop macular degeneration because she read that it runs in families. What symptoms should JJ's daughter watch for as she gets older?

attack, or vascular deaths were observed were observed in 1.8% of patients in clinical trials.[20]

Outcome Evaluation

Monitor patients for acute and chronic vision changes or loss. The Amsler grid (**Figures 62–4 and 62–5**) and frequent eye examinations may detect changes more quickly. The long-term prognosis for AMD is poor; therefore, it is important to work with patients and families as vision decreases. Monitor patients for inability to drive and remove driving privileges as appropriate.

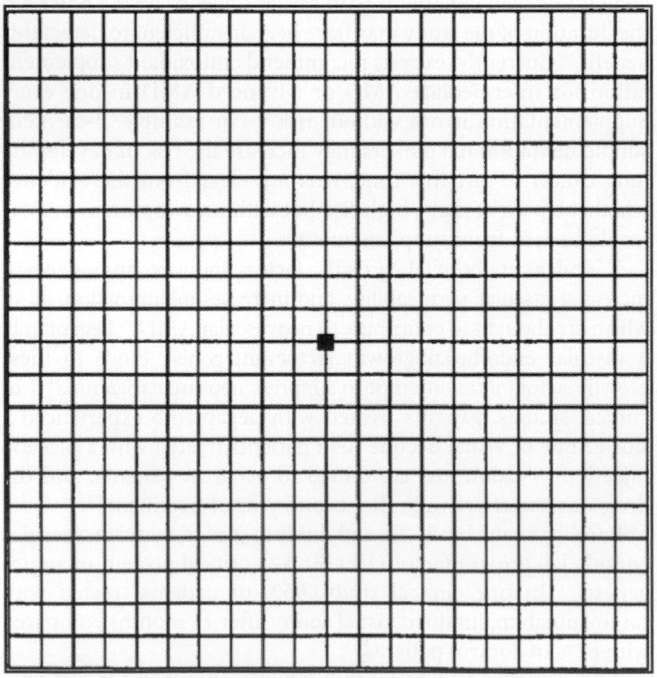

FIGURE 62–4. Amsler grid distortions in the lines of the grid may be caused by subtle changes in central vision due to fluid in the subretinal space. This is the Amsler grid as it appears to someone with normal vision. (From the National Eye Institute, National Institutes of Health Ref. No. EC03. http://www.nei.nih.gov/photo/)

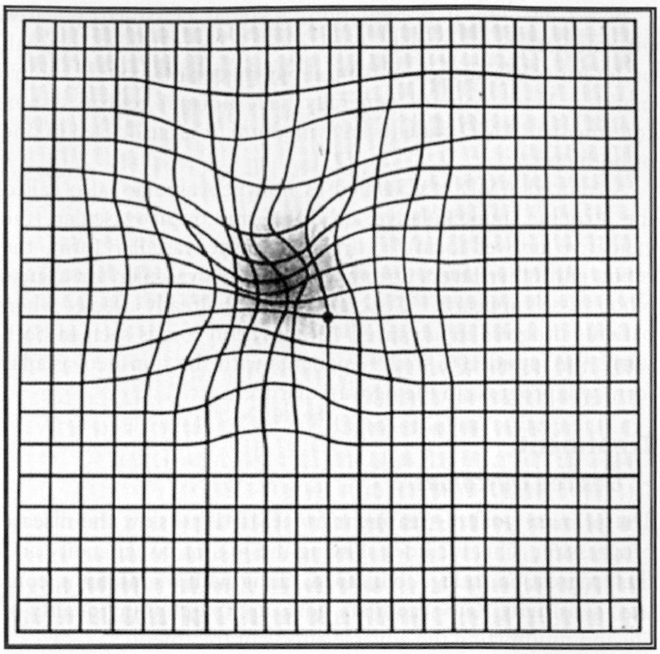

FIGURE 62–5. Amsler grid as it might appear to someone with AMD. (From the National Eye Institute, National Institutes of Health Ref. No. EC04. http://www.nei.nih.gov/photo/)

DRY EYE

Epidemiology and Etiology

Dry eye is a frequent cause of eye irritation. The lack of a single diagnostic test for the condition limits the available epidemiologic data. Reports of the prevalence of dry eye range from 5% to 30%, being more frequent in elderly patients.[21] The risk factors for dry eye are listed in **Table 62–9**. The use of caffeine is associated with a decreased risk of dry eye. Dry eye that is left untreated

Table 62–9

Risk Factors for Dry Eye

Androgen deficiency
Antihistamine use
Connective-tissue disease
Estrogen replacement therapy
Female gender
Hematopoietic stem cell transplantation
Hepatitis C infection
LASIK and refractive excimer laser surgery
Low dietary intake of omega-3 fatty acids
Older age
Radiation therapy
Vitamin A deficiency

Data from Ref. 22, American Academy of Ophthalmology Cornea/External Disease Panel. Preferred Practice Pattern® Guidelines. Dry Eye Syndrome [Internet]. San Francisco, CA: American Academy of Ophthalmology, 2013 [cited 30 Aug 2014]. www.aao.org/ppp.

Clinical Presentation and Diagnosis of Dry Eye[21,22]

General

Many other ocular diseases have similar symptoms. Patients with suggestive symptoms without signs should be placed on a treatment trial. Repeated observations may be required for a clinical diagnosis.

Symptoms

- Dry or foreign body sensation
- Mild itching
- Burning or stinging
- Photophobia
- Ocular irritation or soreness
- Blurry vision
- Contact lens intolerance
- Diurnal fluctuation or symptoms worsening later in the day

Signs

- Redness
- Mucous discharge
- Increased blink frequency
- Tearing

Other Diagnostic Tests

- The tear break-up time test assesses the stability of precorneal tear film. Break-up times of less than 10 seconds are considered abnormal.
- Ocular surface dye staining assesses the ocular surface and will show blotchy areas in the dry eye.
- Schirmer test evaluates aqueous tear production but is not diagnostic. Results of 5 mm or less are considered abnormal.
- Assess corneal sensation if trigeminal nerve dysfunction is suspected.
- Consider an autoimmune disorder if significant dry eyes, other signs and symptoms, or family history are present.

can cause loss of vision, structural damage, an increased risk for infection, and compromised efficacy of ocular surgery.[22]

Pathophysiology

The surface of the eye and the tear-secreting glands work together as an integrated unit that refreshes the tear supply and clears away used tears. Dry eye may be caused by impaired tear secretion and/or increased tear evaporation.[22] It has been suggested that dry eye be called "dysfunctional tear syndrome," as all the predisposing factors cause some disruption of the tear.[21]

Dysfunction may be caused by aging, systemic inflammatory diseases, a decrease in androgen hormones, surgery, ocular surface diseases, systemic diseases, or medications that affect the efferent cholinergic nerves. Dysfunctional tear film may result in an inflammatory response on the ocular surface called **keratoconjunctivitis sicca.**[22]

Table 62–10

Associated Conditions That Cause or Worsen Dry Eye

Ocular Conditions	**Environmental Factors**
Blepharitis	Air travel
Eyelid malposition	Air conditioning or heating
Lagophthalmos	Contact lenses
Meibomian gland dysfunction	Exogenous irritants or allergens
Systemic Diseases	Prolonged use of computer or reading
Amyloidosis	Reduced humidity
Bell palsy	Smoke exposure
Epstein-Barr virus	Wind
Graft-versus-host disease	**Local Trauma**
Hemochromatosis	Injury/scarring
Hepatitis C infection	Orbital surgery
Human immunodeficiency virus infection	Radiation
Lymphoma	**Medications**
Neuromuscular diseases	Anticholinergics
Ocular mucous membrane pemphigoid	Antidepressants
	Antihistamines
Parkinson disease	β-Blockers
Rosacea	Diuretics
Rheumatoid arthritis	Hormone therapy
Sarcoidosis	Systemic retinoids
Scleroderma	Frequent administration of ophthalmic medication
Sjögren syndrome	
Stevens-Johnson syndrome	
Systemic lupus erythematosus	

Data from Ref. 22, American Academy of Ophthalmology Cornea/External Disease Panel. Preferred Practice Pattern® Guidelines. Dry Eye Syndrome [Internet]. San Francisco, CA: American Academy of Ophthalmology, 2013 [cited 30 Aug 2014]. www.aao.org/ppp.

Environmental causes (**Table 62–10**) and an abnormal blink reflex are common causes of increased evaporative loss of tears and worsening of dry eye.[22]

Treatment

▶ *Desired Outcomes*[22]

- Relief of the symptoms of dry eye
- Maintain or improve visual acuity
- Prevention of long-term adverse effects from dry eye

▶ *General Approach to Treatment*

KEY CONCEPT *Dry eye is a chronic condition. Symptoms can be improved with treatment, but unless dry eye is secondary to a disease, it is not usually curable.* Because of this, patient education is critical, and a periodic reassessment of the efficacy of the treatment is appropriate. If the patient is unresponsive to treatment, refer to an ophthalmologist for additional options. If the dry eye is secondary to a systemic disease, the disease should be managed by the appropriate medical specialist.[22]

▶ *Nonpharmacologic Therapy*

Behavioral and environmental modifications may significantly improve dry eye, especially in mild cases. Patients should be counseled to increase their frequency of blinking, use eyelid hygiene and warm compresses, and stop smoking. Reduce air drafts and consider adding a humidifier in low-humidity areas. Schedule regular breaks from computer work or reading. Lower the computer screen to below eye level to decrease lid aperture. Evaluate medication profile and therapeutically substitute medications that do not exacerbate dry eye. Spectacle side shields or goggles may reduce tear evaporation.[21,22]

If pharmacologic and other therapies are not sufficient, punctal occlusion or lateral tarsorrhaphy may be an option.[21,22] Punctal occlusion is the plugging of the punctal drainage sites with collagen or silicone plugs. Lateral tarsorrhaphy sutures portions of the lid margins together to decrease evaporative tear loss.

► *Pharmacologic Therapy*

The mainstay of treatment for dry eye is artificial tears. Artificial tears augment the tear film topically and provide symptom relief. If a patient uses artificial tears more than four times daily, or develops an allergy to ophthalmic preservatives, recommend a preservative-free formulation. Artificial tears are available in gel, ointment, and emulsion forms that provide a longer duration of relief. Ointment use is appropriate at bedtime.[21]

Preliminary data suggest dietary or supplemental intake of omega-3 fatty acids may be beneficial.[6,21,22] Omega-3 fatty acids may block the production of inflammatory cytokines and pro-inflammatory mediators.[21]

Anti-inflammatory agents may be used in conjunction with artificial tears. The only approved agent is cyclosporine emulsion. Cyclosporine emulsion increases tear production in some patients. Fifteen minutes should elapse after instillation of cyclosporine before artificial tears are instilled.[23] Use of topical corticosteroids for short periods (2 weeks) may suppress inflammation and ocular irritation symptoms.[22]

The oral cholinergic agonists pilocarpine and cevimeline are used for patients with Sjögren syndrome (combined dry eye and dry mouth) or severe dry eye. By binding to muscarinic receptors, the cholinergic agonists may increase tear production. Excessive sweating is a common side effect with pilocarpine and may limit its use (Table 62–11).[22]

Outcome Evaluation[22]

- Monitor patient for relief of symptoms and ocular damage.
- Periodically reassess the patient's compliance with therapy and understanding of the disease.
- It may take 6 to 12 weeks before improvement is seen with pilocarpine therapy.[21]

Table 62–11

Pharmacologic Therapies for Dry Eye

Drug	Dosing
Cyclosporine ophthalmic emulsion 0.05%	One drop in each eye twice daily
Loteprednol etabonate suspension 0.5%	One to two drop(s) in affected eye(s) four times daily; short-term use only
Cevimeline capsule	30 mg orally three times daily
Pilocarpine tablet	5 mg orally four times daily

From Ref. 22, American Academy of Ophthalmology Cornea/External Disease Panel. Preferred Practice Pattern® Guidelines. Dry Eye Syndrome [Internet]. San Francisco, CA; American Academy of Ophthalmology, 2013 [cited 30 Aug 2014]. www.aao.org/ppp.

McEvoy GK, ed. AHFS Drug Information 2014. Bethesda, MD: American Society of Health-System Pharmacists Inc., 2014.

Patient Care Process: Patient Counseling

Wash hands before and after instilling medication(s) into the eye

Contact lenses should be removed prior to instilling eye medication, and the patient should wait 10 minutes before reinserting contact lenses

Do not touch the tip of the container with anything

Use of nasolacrimal occlusion decreases systemic absorption up to 60% and may increase ocular bioavailability of the drug. After instilling the eye drop, the patient should close the eye and press a finger gently against the nasolacrimal duct (tear duct) for 2 to 3 minutes[24]

- Cyclosporine therapy may take up to 3 months for full improvement.
- If a patient presents with vision loss, moderate or severe pain, corneal ulceration, or a lack of response to therapy, refer the patient to an ophthalmologist for prompt evaluation.

DRUG-INDUCED OCULAR DISORDERS

Many systemic medications can cause ocular adverse effects. Patients presenting with ocular complaints should have their medication profile evaluated.

Abbreviations Introduced in This Chapter

ABC	Acute bacterial conjunctivitis
AMD	Age-related macular degeneration
NSAID	Nonsteroidal anti-inflammatory drug

REFERENCES

1. Handler JA, Ghezzi KT. General ophthalmologic examination. Emerg Med Clin North Am. 1995;13:521–538.
2. Babineau MR, Sanchez LD. Ophthalmologic procedures in the emergency department. Emerg Med Clin N Am. 2008:26:17–34.
3. Wipperman JL, Dorsch JN. Evaluation and management of corneal abrasions. Am Fam Physician. 2013;87:114-120.
4. Rodrigues Z. Irrigation of the eye after alkaline and acidic burns. Emerg Nurse. 2009;17(8):26–29.
5. Goold L, Durkin S, Crompton J. Sudden loss of vision—History and examination. Aust Fam Physician. 2009;38:764–767.
6. Cronau H, Kankanala RR, Mauger T. Diagnosis and management of red eye in primary care. Am Fam Physician. 2010;81(2): 137–144; patient handout 145.
7. Azari AA, Barney NP. Conjunctivitis: A systematic review of diagnosis and treatment. JAMA. 2013;310:1721–1729.
8. Bielory L. Ocular allergy. Mt Sinai J Med. 2011;78:740–758.
9. O'Brien TP. Allergic conjunctivitis: An update on diagnosis and management. Curr Opin Allergy Clin Immuno. 2013;13:543–549.
10. American Academy of Ophthalmology Cornea/External Disease Panel. Preferred Practice Pattern® Guidelines. Bacterial Keratitis [Internet]. San Francisco, CA: American Academy of Ophthalmology, 2013 [cited 2014 Aug 30]. www.aao.org/ppp.
11. American Academy of Ophthalmology Retina Panel. Preferred Practice Pattern® Guidelines. Age-Related Macular Degeneration [Internet]. San Francisco, CA: American Academy of Ophthalmology, 2008 [cited 2014 Aug 30]. www.aao.org/ppp.

12. Friedman DS, O'Colmain BJ, Munoz B, et al. Prevalence of age-related macular degeneration in the United States. Arch Ophthalmol. 2004;122:564–572.
13. Arnold J, Sarks S. Age related macular degeneration. Clin Evid. 2004;(11):819–834.
14. Comer GM, Ciulla TA, Criswell MH, Tolentino M. Current and future treatment options for nonexudative and exudative age-related macular degeneration. Drugs Aging. 2004;21: 967–992.
15. Visudyne (verteporfin) for injection [package insert]. Menlo Park, CA: Valeant Pharmaceuticals, 2013.
16. Ferris FL, Chew EY, Sperduto R, for the Age-Related Eye Disease Study Group. A randomized, placebo-controlled, clinical trial of high-dose supplementation with vitamins C and E and beta carotene for age-related cataract and vision loss: AREDS report no. 9. Arch Ophthalmol. 2001;119:1439–1452.
17. Mares JA, La Rowe TL, Blodi BA. Doctor, what vitamins should I take for my eyes? Arch Ophthalmol. 2004;122:628–635.
18. Macugen (pegaptanib sodium) injection [package insert]. Palm Beach Gardens, FL: Eyetech, 2011.
19. Gragoudas ES, Adamis AP, Cunningham ET Jr, et al. Pegaptanib for neovascular age-related macular degeneration. N Engl J Med. 2004;351:2805–2816.
20. Eylea (aflibercept) injection [package insert]. Tarrytown, NY: Regeneron Pharmaceuticals, Inc., 2014.
21. Jackson WB. Management of dysfunctional tear syndrome: A Canadian consensus. Can J Ophthalmol. 2009;44:385–394.
22. American Academy of Ophthalmology Cornea/External Disease Panel. Preferred Practice Pattern® Guidelines. Dry Eye Syndrome [Internet]. San Francisco, CA: American Academy of Ophthalmology, 2013 [cited 30 Aug 2014]. www.aao.org/ppp.
23. Restasis (cyclosporine) emulsion [package insert]. Irvine, CA: Allergan, Inc., 2013.
24. Zimmerman TJ, Kooner KS, Kandarakis AS, Ziegler LP. Improving the therapeutic index of topically applied ocular drugs. Arch Ophthalmol. 1984;102:551–553.

63 Allergic Rhinitis

David A. Apgar

LEARNING OBJECTIVES

Upon completion of the chapter, the reader will be able to:

1. Describe the basic pathophysiology of allergic rhinitis (AR).
2. List the four typical symptoms of AR and identify the one that is usually the most troublesome.
3. List at least three reasons for referral to an allergy specialist.
4. Differentiate the categories of pharmacotherapy choices for treatment of AR.
5. Rank the pharmacotherapy choices for efficacy in treating the usual single most troublesome symptom of AR.
6. Describe an approach for treatment of mild AR with over-the-counter (OTC) drugs.
7. Create a therapy plan for treatment of moderate–severe AR.
8. Describe how to monitor patients treated for AR.
9. Identify the differences in approach to the treatment of AR for children, pregnant women, and the elderly compared with the routine approach in adults.

INTRODUCTION

Rhinitis is inflammation of the lining of the nose and contiguous parts of the upper respiratory tract.[1–4] Allergy is only one of numerous causes of rhinitis.[1–5] The most common causes of nonallergic rhinitis are shown in **Table 63–1**.[1–5] Some patients suffer concurrently from both allergic rhinitis (AR) and one or more types of nonallergic rhinitis (NAR). This is sometimes called mixed rhinitis (MR).[1,3] AR will be emphasized in this chapter, but some mention will be made of NAR. Because ocular symptoms frequently occur in association with AR, some sources use the term allergic rhinoconjunctivitis. This acknowledges involvement of the bulbar and palpebral conjunctivae in the allergic process.

KEY CONCEPT *AR is an allergen-induced, immunoglobulin E (IgE)-mediated inflammatory condition of the lining of the nose and upper respiratory tract.*[1,6–9] This pathophysiologic feature differentiates AR from NAR. AR has traditionally been categorized as either seasonal or perennial.[7] Seasonal allergic rhinitis (SAR) is attributed to inhaled allergens (**aeroallergens**) that have a seasonal variation. These allergens are usually encountered outdoors and are most often grass, tree or weed pollens and substances from molds and fungi. Perennial allergic rhinitis (PAR) is attributed to aeroallergens that are present in the patient's environment almost continuously throughout the year and are usually encountered indoors. Common perennial allergens are the house dust mite, indoor molds and fungi, insects (especially cockroaches), and companion animals (pets).[7] Some patients are affected year round, but have seasonal exacerbations. These people are probably allergic to both seasonal and perennial aeroallergens. Other patients have only episodic manifestations. These people are probably allergic to aeroallergens that are only episodically encountered.

Because these traditional categories of seasonal and perennial AR are imperfect and help little with therapeutic management decisions, another system for categorizing AR has been suggested by the international group *Allergic Rhinitis and its Impact on Asthma* (ARIA).[9] This alternative system categorizes the manifestations by a combination of frequency and severity. There are two divisions of frequency: intermittent and persistent. Intermittent frequency is defined as AR manifestations occurring less often than 4 days per week or for fewer than 4 consecutive weeks. Persistent frequency is defined as AR manifestations occurring for 4 or more days per week *and* for 4 or more consecutive weeks. Severity is categorized as either mild or moderate–severe. Mild manifestations are those that do *NOT* cause interference with sleep, daily activities, or work or school performance and that are not "troublesome." Moderate–severe severity includes those patients with manifestations of AR that *DO* cause interference with sleep, impairment of daily activities, problems at work or school, or are "troublesome." The ARIA document uses IAR (for intermittent) and PER (for persistent) for the two frequency categories. It is important to realize that IAR and PER are not synonymous with the classical categories of SAR and PAR, respectively. The ARIA system results in four categories: mild intermittent, mild persistent, moderate–severe intermittent, or moderate–severe persistent. The ARIA approach was updated in 2008 and again in 2010.[9,10] See **Table 63–2** for a summary of these categories of AR.

EPIDEMIOLOGY

AR affects up to 30% of adults and 40% of children in the United States, and there is evidence that the incidence is increasing.[3,5] The total direct and indirect costs of AR in the United States were estimated to be about 11 billion dollars, annually, in 2005.[11]

Table 63–1

Types of Rhinitis

Allergic (see Table 63–2 for details)

Nonallergic

- Vasomotor (also known as perennial nonallergic, idiopathic, and autonomic rhinitis) (triggered by irritants, cold air, exercise/running, or unidentified factors)
- Food/meal related (gustatory)
- Infectious
- NARES (nonallergic rhinitis with eosinophilia syndrome)
- Occupational (caused by protein allergens (IgE-mediated) or by irritants (probably non–IgE-mediated)
- Hormonally related (hypothyroidism, pregnancy, menstrual cycle related, and some drugs [see below])
- Drug-induced
  - Angiotensin-converting enzyme inhibitors (ACEIs)
  - α_1-Blockers (used for treatment of BPH and HT)
  - Phosphodiesterase-5 inhibitors (used for treatment of ED)
  - Aspirin and other NSAIDs (as an isolated side effect of AERD)
  - Oral contraceptives and hormone replacement therapy
  - Miscellaneous agents have been implicated (calcium channel blockers, some diuretics, centrally acting α-2 agonists, risperidone, gabapentin)
- Atrophic rhinitis
- Rhinitis associated with inflammatory or immunologic diseases (eg, granulomatous infections, SLE, Wegener granulomatosis, sarcoidosis, Churg–Strauss syndrome)
- Malignancy

Mixed

- Combination of allergic and nonallergic manifestations

AERD, aspirin-exacerbated respiratory disease; BPH, benign prostatic hyperplasia/hypertrophy; ED, erectile dysfunction; HT, hypertension; NSAIDs, nonsteroidal anti-inflammatory drugs; SLE, systemic lupus erythematosus.

From Refs. 1–5.

Table 63–2

Categories of Allergic Rhinitis

Based on etiologic category

- Seasonal—symptoms present only during specific portions of the year
- Perennial—symptoms present throughout the year
- Episodic—symptoms present only during intermittent exposure to allergen trigger

Based on ARIA 2008 Update

- Mild versus moderate–severe
  - Mild—no interference with sleep, daily activities, work or school function and attendance, and no troublesome symptoms
  - Moderate–severe—presence of any one of the following: abnormal sleep, impairment of daily activities, impairment of work or school function, troublesome symptoms
- Intermittent versus persistent
  - Intermittent—symptoms are present for less than 4 days per week, or for less than 4 consecutive weeks
  - Persistent—symptoms are present for 4 or more days per week and for more than 4 consecutive weeks
  - Any one of the four possibilities of these variables can occur: mild intermittent, mild persistent, moderate–severe intermittent, and moderate–severe persistent

From Refs. 7 and 8.

The major risk factors for AR are a family history of atopy (AR, asthma, eczema, or food allergies); elevated serum IgE levels (especially before the age of 6 years); higher socioeconomic class; positive skin test results; exposure to particulate air pollution; maternal smoking; firstborn status; and emigration into a Western industrialized environment.[5,7,9,11,12]

Certain disorders commonly occur with AR. The most important example is asthma. While different percentages are reported, most patients with asthma have rhinitis symptoms (many of which are AR), and only somewhat fewer with AR have asthma.[5,11] In fact, there is evidence that AR can predispose to the development and/or worsening of asthma.[1,5,12] Other conditions that can occur with AR include allergic conjunctivitis, eczema, sinusitis, sleep disorders, otitis media with effusion, and the oral food allergy syndrome.[5,11,12]

PATHOPHYSIOLOGY[1,5,7–9,12,13]

AR is an IgE-mediated disorder of people who are allergy prone. Initial contact is required to sensitize the patient to subsequent exposures. Patients with an inherited tendency to allergic disorders produce T-helper lymphocyte type 2 (Th-2)-directed responses, including production of specific IgE antibodies, to one or more allergens. Many types of cells, mediators, and intermediate substances (including cytokines) are involved. In response to subsequent exposures to the trigger antigen(s), there is an early-phase and often a late-phase allergic response. This distinction has therapeutic implications.

During the early phase, the trigger allergen becomes bound to IgE that is fixed to mast cells in the nasal mucosa. This occurs within minutes of subsequent exposure to the antigen. Mast cells degranulate and release preformed mediators, the most important of which is histamine. This stimulates more mast cells, as well as macrophages, eosinophils, and basophils to produce more substances, including cysteine leukotrienes and prostaglandin D_2. These mediators bind to receptors in the nose and facilitate many of the manifestations of AR. The resultant vasodilation, mucosal edema, and hypertrophy all contribute to nasal congestion. Clear, watery, and often profuse rhinorrhea is also characteristic in this early phase, a result of mucous secretion and increased vascular permeability. Sneezing and nasal itch are other prominent features of the early phase. Many patients also have ocular symptoms.

The late phase occurs in about 50% of AR sufferers. It can begin as soon as 2 hours after the early phase and usually peaks between 6 and 12 hours. The late phase involves a second release of many of the mediators of the early phase. In addition, the late phase is characterized by an inflammatory component caused by infiltration of several cell types into the nasal mucosa. The most significant manifestation during the late phase is nasal congestion that is often severe and long lasting.

A phenomenon known as the priming response or nasal hyperresponsiveness is also of importance. This means that prolonged and/or repeated allergen exposure makes it easier to stimulate mediator release and symptoms. A vicious cycle results in which smaller doses of allergen can create symptoms (ie, the threshold is lowered). Thus, even when pollen exposure is decreased, symptoms may continue. In some patients, the threshold is lowered to the degree that even irritant substances (eg, formaldehyde, tobacco smoke, perfumes, automobile exhaust, and other environmental pollutants) may cause symptoms, on a nonallergic basis.

Clinical Presentation and Diagnosis of Allergic Rhinitis[1–3,5,6,7–9,11–14]

Typical Symptoms

- Rhinorrhea (usually clear and bilateral; primarily anterior but may be posterior [postnasal drip])
- Sneezing
- Itching (mostly nasal, but also palate, throat, eyes, ears)
- Nasal congestion (not in all patients, but when present, usually the most troublesome symptom)

Other Symptoms

- Ocular manifestations (itch, redness, tearing, chemosis, periorbital edema)
- Sleep disturbances often with fatigue, asthenia, malaise, and irritability
- Presenteeism (impaired performance at work or school)
- Absenteeism from work or school
- Quality of life impairment (including social function)
- Headache, mild facial or ear pain, or fullness
- Cough (especially in those with concurrent asthma)
- Children (especially): snorting, sniffling, clearing the throat, learning or attention problems, poor appetite

Signs (Especially Common in Children)

- Pale, boggy nasal mucosa
- Rubbing the nose upward (allergic salute; may create horizontal crease just above tip of nose)
- Rubbing/scratching of eyes
- Mouth breathing
- Dark circles under the eyes (allergic shiners)
- Dennie-Morgan lines or folds under the eyes

Diagnosis

- Typical symptoms, confirmatory signs, especially in association with exposure to allergen triggers
- Other diagnostic testing usually optional, but may be necessary to rule out nonallergic causes or if immunotherapy is considered (appropriate physical examination, specific IgE antibody testing by either skin testing or in vitro serum testing, other specialized testing)
- Several sources particularly good for differential diagnosis of nonallergic rhinitis.[3,12,14]
- Vasomotor rhinitis—sneezing and itching less common than AR; anosmia more common
- Unilateral symptoms—refer for possible obstruction, anatomic abnormality, tumor, CSF leak
- Atrophic rhinitis—older adults, history of nasal surgery

TREATMENT

Desired Outcomes

KEY CONCEPT *The goals of treatment of AR are to minimize the frequency and severity of symptoms, prevent comorbid disorders and complications, improve the patient's quality of life, improve work attendance and productivity and/or school attendance and performance, and minimize adverse effects of therapy.* Until a cure is established, these are the only realistic goals.

Nonpharmacologic Therapy

KEY CONCEPT *The general approach for treatment of AR is fourfold: avoidance of allergen triggers, pharmacotherapy, immunotherapy, and patient/family education.*[8,12] Immunotherapy could be considered a type of pharmacotherapy. However, even with availability of patient-administered sublingual immunotherapy (SLIT), referral for specific diagnostic testing is required. Therefore, immunotherapy will be discussed separately.

Avoidance of allergen triggers, to the extent they have been identified and to the extent such avoidance is possible, underlies the treatment for all patients with AR (Table 63–3).[7,8]

Immunotherapy is almost always initiated by an allergist or otolaryngologist, after referral for specific allergen testing to determine individualized therapy. Historically, immunotherapy was considered for patients in three categories.[5] The first were those with severe, complicated or worsening rhinitis. This was partly for additional diagnostic testing to rule out nonallergic causes of rhinitis. The second were those patients with AR who did not tolerate or responded poorly to appropriate pharmacotherapy. The third were those patients who had a single, or one major allergen identified, for which there was an immunotherapy product available for treatment. In addition, some patients requested immunotherapy, on the basis of superior and durable effectiveness. Currently, the role of any other health care provider is limited to referral of appropriate candidates. However, this may change in the future with the introduction of several products for sublingual self-administration. As of April, 2014, three products have been approved for administration as sublingual immunotherapy (SLIT). Until that time, only subcutaneous immunotherapy (SCIT) had been available as an approved therapy in the United States.[15–17] The major advantage of SLIT over SCIT is ease of administration. The first dose is given in the prescriber's office, for purposes of safety. Subsequent doses are self-administered by the patient. Questions remain, however, about comparative efficacy and the details of optimal dosage, frequency of administration, and duration of therapy. The current cumulative wisdom is that SCIT is somewhat more effective than SLIT, but that SLIT is somewhat safer and easier to administer than SCIT.[15,18–23]

Education of the patient and the patient's support system is essential.[7] All parties need to understand the potential seriousness of AR (including complications such as asthma) and the chronic, recurrent nature of AR. All should be told about the treatment options, including their relative advantages and disadvantages. Proper understanding and use of current medication in the patient's regimen should be assured. A better educated patient and support system will result in a better relationship with health care providers and hopefully will optimize patient outcomes.

Pharmacologic Therapy

Guideline documents have been published on AR.[7–9,10,14] They provide some of the basis for the summary that follows.

Table 63–3

Allergen Avoidance Measures

Allergen avoidance underlies all other treatments of AR

There are several limitations to allergen avoidance:

- Allergen(s) must be identified.
- Literature support for a clinically significant improvement in symptoms from allergen avoidance is meager.
- Quality of life may be negatively impacted by forced removal of a pet from the household.

Outdoor plant pollen and mold/fungi parts:

- Limit outdoor exposure, especially during high pollen conditions (warm sunny days with wind and low humidity) and during mold/fungi spore release (shortly after rains).
- Wear a face mask during activities that disturb soil and decaying vegetation.
- Keep windows and doors closed.
- Use air conditioning, but maintain clean equipment.

Indoor allergens (house dust mite, mold/fungi, cockroaches, and pets):

- Use air-conditioning, as above.
- Maintain humidity below 50%, and maintain clean equipment.
- Clean frequently to prevent mold growth (dilute bleach with detergent).
- Avoid exposed food and garbage to deter insects.
- Clean kitchen frequently.
- Use roach traps that facilitate their removal.
- Vacuum frequently, and use a high-efficiency particulate air (HEPA) (filter).
- Minimize carpeting, fabric-covered furniture, and fabric wall/window coverings.
- Cover bedding (pillows, mattresses, box springs) with allergen-proof, zippered cases.
- Launder bedding frequently, in hot water (> 130°F or 54°C) to kill mite ova.
- Consider acaricide (eg, benzyl benzoate) treatment of carpets to kill mites and ova.
- Put items that cannot be laundered (eg, soft toys) in a plastic bag and freeze.
- Keep pets out of bedroom and bathe cats weekly, if possible.

Irritants:

- Avoid, as possible, all exposure to smoke, chlorine fumes, formaldehyde fumes, and other substances identified as irritant triggers (eg, perfumes, newspaper ink).

From Refs. 7 and 8.

Patient Encounter 1, Part 1

Evelyn M, a regular customer in your community pharmacy, asks your advice about helping her 8-year-old son, Aaron. He has a diagnosis of "mild" asthma that is primarily exercise induced. His symptoms are usually well controlled by prophylactic use of an albuterol metered-dose inhaler. Both of his parents told the doctor that they do not want Aaron to be treated with "steroids." However, a new issue is that in recent months, he has also had frequent trouble with runny nose, sneezing, and "throat" itching.

What additional information should you get before making any suggestions?

Although guideline documents are highly regarded by many, the patients enrolled in the randomized clinical trials that are a major basis for their conclusions and recommendations are not always representative of patients in a primary practice population.[24] Other sources provide additional information for the treatment of AR.[1,2,5,6,25–27] The recommended approaches begin with allergen avoidance, emphasize patient/family education and pharmacotherapy, and include immunotherapy as an option in selected patients.

KEY CONCEPT *Routine first-line agents for the treatment of AR are intranasal corticosteroids and oral (or possibly intranasal) antihistamines. Secondary agents, each of which may have a first-line role in selected patients, include oral (and rarely intranasal) decongestants, the intranasal mast cell stabilizer cromone (cromolyn), the oral leukotriene receptor antagonist (LTRA) (montelukast), the intranasal antimuscarinic (ipratropium), and intranasal saline irrigation.* In all cases, therapy must be individualized, in cooperation with the patient. Considerations include frequency and severity of specific symptoms, realistic avoidance measures, patient age, patient preferences for route of administration, tolerance of side effects, adherence issues, comorbid disorders, and concurrent therapy. See Table 63–4 for intranasal and oral medications for the treatment of AR.

Table 63–4

Intranasal and Oral Medications for AR

Corticosteroids
Intranasal[a] (budesonide, beclomethasone, ciclesonide, flunisolide, fluticasone furoate, mometasone, OTC: triamcinolone, fluticasone propionate)
Oral (rarely used)

Antihistamines
Intranasal[a] (azelastine, olopatadine)
Oral[b]

- First generation/sedating (cautious use in selected patients) (most OTC depending on strength: diphenhydramine, chlorpheniramine, clemastine, and others)
- Second generation/low- or nonsedating (desloratadine, levocetirizine; OTC: loratadine, cetirizine, fexofenadine)[a]

Combination antihistamine/corticosteroid
Intranasal (azelastine and fluticasone propionate)

Mast cell stabilizer/cromone
Intranasal (OTC: cromolyn)

LTRA
Oral (montelukast)

Antimuscarinic
Intranasal (ipratropium)

Decongestant
Intranasal (short-term use) (tetrahydrozoline; OTC: phenylephrine, naphazoline, oxymetazoline)
Oral[b] (OTC: phenylephrine; BTC[c]: pseudoephedrine)

[a]First-line choices.

[b]Some products combine an antihistamine with a decongestant, sometimes with other ingredients.

[c]Behind the counter (OTC plus other requirements necessary; see the Decongestants section of text).

From Refs. 2,5,7–10,12,25–27, and 29.

Patient Encounter 1, Part 2

Additional history from both Evelyn and Aaron reveals the following information. Aaron does have eye symptoms, including bilateral itching, watering, and redness. He thinks all his nose and eye symptoms are worse in the spring when plants are blooming. Both Evelyn and her husband have "hay fever." Aaron's symptoms have occurred most days of the week for the last 6 to 8 weeks, but he does not think they are "bad or troublesome." He denies unilateral nasal symptoms, significant decreased smell, significant nasal congestion, cough, frequent nighttime awakenings, facial pain, and ear symptoms. Evelyn is not aware of significant changes in Aaron's school performance. The family does not have animal companions (pets). Aaron has not been given any medications for these new nasal symptoms.

You notice bilateral allergic shiners, and Aaron does rub his nose and sniffle frequently during your encounter. You are not able to examine his nasal mucosa or throat.

Explain the reasons for how you would classify Aaron's presumed allergic rhinitis.

What recommendations would you make for initial management of Aaron's presumed AR?

One publication includes an action plan for AR, similar to that used for asthma.[7] The entire article, with a sample Rhinitis Action Plan, is available for universal access on the following website: *http://www.aaaai.org/Aaaai/media/MediaLibrary/PDF%20Documents/Practice%20and%20Parameters/rhinitis2008-diagnosis management.pdf*. Many patients will benefit from having an AR action plan.

▸ First-Line Agents

Corticosteroids Corticosteroids are usually administered by the intranasal route for the treatment of AR. Occasionally, a short course of oral therapy (burst and taper) is necessary. Oral corticosteroids are best applied to overcome severe nasal congestion, particularly that due to rhinitis medicamentosa (see the section on Decongestants). Parenteral administration of corticosteroids for AR is discouraged due to side effects.[5,7,10]

Intranasal corticosteroids (INCSs) provide very good relief for sneezing, itching, and rhinorrhea, and even nasal congestion and ocular symptoms. Nasal congestion is often the most bothersome symptom of AR, and the most difficult to control. This is probably because it results from inflammation that predominates in the late phase of the allergic response. KEY CONCEPT *Intranasal corticosteroids (INCSs) are the most effective therapy for AR, especially for nasal congestion. They are first-line agents for severe manifestations and are also used for those with moderate disease not controlled with oral and/or intranasal antihistamines. Their anti-inflammatory mechanism of action probably contributes to this superiority.*[5,6,12,25,27] The majority of contemporary literature suggests that INCSs are superior to intranasal antihistamines, to oral antihistamines even when combined with a leukotriene antagonist, and to a leukotriene antagonist alone.[5,12,25]

There are currently eight intranasal corticosteroid products available in the United States, including two different salt forms of fluticasone. Most (budesonide, ciclesonide, fluticasone furoate, mometasone, and triamcinolone) are used once daily. However, fluticasone propionate may be given either once or twice daily; beclomethasone is usually given twice daily, and flunisolide is given two or three times daily. There is no good evidence that any single product is superior in efficacy. INCSs are best given regularly, as the onset of action usually takes up to 12 hours and the maximum effects may be delayed up to 14 days.[5,25,27] In some people the onset is within 3 to 4 hours, so these agents may even be used on an as needed basis.[7,28] When nasal congestion is severe, intranasal administration may not be effective due to limited exposure to the nasal mucosa. Short-term use of intranasal decongestants may facilitate better exposure. There have been some recent additions to the marketed ICNSs. Two agents are formulated as HFA metered-dose aerosols: beclomethasone (Qnasl) and ciclesonide (Zetonna).[27] They may be better tolerated. There is a fixed-dose intranasal combination of fluticasone propionate with azelastine (an antihistamine).[26,27] Two OTC products are now available.[29] See Table 63–5 for intranasal corticosteroid products.

The correct technique for administration of intranasal medication is important for optimum efficacy. Consult the individual product labeling for specific instructions. Also see Table 63–6 for general instructions for the optimal administration of intranasal solutions. The technique described maximizes exposure of the drug to the nasal mucosa to optimize efficacy and minimizes both exposure to the nasal septum and loss of medication down the esophagus.

Most patients tolerate intranasal corticosteroids very well. Local side effects include nasal burning, irritation, and dryness, which may occur in 2% to 10% of patients.[5,25,27] Also, 2% to 12% of patients may experience mild epistaxis.[5,25] This may be partly due to administration technique. Perforation of the nasal septum is very rare. This can be minimized by proper administration technique (see Table 63–6), specifically, directing the spray laterally and away from the (medial) nasal septum.[25,27]

The older intranasal corticosteroids (beclomethasone, flunisolide, and budesonide) have significant absorption, whereas, among the newer products, fluticasone and mometasone, have bioavailability of less than 2%.[25] The decreased absorption minimizes systemic side effects. However, there is still some concern for hypothalamic–pituitary–adrenal (HPA) axis suppression (growth suppression), osteoporosis, and ocular effects (glaucoma, cataracts).[5,25,27] There is no confirmation that intranasal corticosteroids *cause* posterior subcapsular cataracts, increased intraocular pressure, or decreased bone density; however, those with risk factors for these conditions should be monitored carefully for their development.[5,25,27] Ultimately, patient preference for a specific intranasal corticosteroid may be determined more by cost, availability, and formulation differences that affect odor and aftertaste.

Antihistamines Antihistamines used for AR treatment are administered by either the oral or the intranasal route. These agents interact with the H_1 (histamine type 1) receptor. They are technically inverse agonists, not competitive antagonists; however, there may be little clinical significance to the difference.[25] These drugs bind H_1 receptors, keeping them in the inactive state. This downregulation of H_1 receptor activity results in a decrease in end organ effects.

Activation of H_1 receptors in the nose, upper airway mucosa, and the eye produce the common manifestations of AR (sneezing, itching, rhinorrhea, nasal congestion, and ocular symptoms). The antihistamines are very effective for the sneezing, itching, and rhinorrhea. There is some improvement of nasal congestion, but less so than for the other symptoms. There is also

Table 63–5

Intranasal Corticosteroids

Generic (Brand) Name	mcg/dose	Usual Adult Dosage (each nostril)	Usual Pediatric Dosage (each nostril)
Beclomethasone dipropionate (Beconase AQ)	42	1–2 sprays twice daily	6 yo or more: 1–2 sprays twice daily
Beclmethasone dipropionate (Qnasl [HFA MDP])	80	2 sprays once daily	12 yo or more: 2 sprays once daily
Budesonide (Rhinocort Aqua)	32	1–4 sprays once daily	6–11 yo or more: 1–2 sprays once daily
Ciclesonide (Omnaris)	50	2 sprays once daily	6 yo or more: 2 sprays once daily (seasonal AR) 12 yo or more: 2 sprays once daily (perennial AR)
Ciclesonide (Zetonna [HFA MDP])	37	1 spray once daily	12 yo or more: 1 spray once daily
Flunisolide	25	2 sprays two or three times daily	6–14 yo or more: 1 spray three times daily or 2 sprays twice daily
Fluticasone furoate (Veramyst)	27.5	2 sprays once daily	2–11 yo or more: 1–2 sprays once daily
Fluticasone propionate (Flonase)[a]	50	1–2 sprays once daily or 1 spray twice daily	4–11 yo or more: 1–2 sprays once daily
Mometasone (Nasonex)	50	2 sprays once daily	2–11 yo or more: 1 spray once daily 12 yo or more: 2 sprays once daily
Triamcinolone acetonide (Nasacort AQ)[a]	55	2 sprays once daily	2–5 yo: 1 spray once daily 6–12 yo: 1–2 sprays once daily

mcg, micrograms; yo, years old; HFA, hydrofluoroalkane (propellant); MDP, metered-dose pump.

Note: All products are FDA Pregnancy category C except budesonide, which is B.

[a]available OTC.

From Refs. 25 and 27.

Table 63–6

Administration Instructions for Intranasal Solution Medications (Not HFA MDP Products)

1. Clear the nose of mucus and debris.
2. Consult product labeling for preadministration instructions (eg, shaking the container, priming the spray pump).
3. Do not tilt head backward. This increases drug lost down the esophagus. This decreases efficacy and increases the potential for systemic absorption and thus systemic side effects.
4. Bend the head forward (flex the chin onto the chest) so that the nose is the lowest portion of the head. This is best for nasal sprays. If possible, lie down with the stomach on a flat surface or kneel down. Then, flex chin onto neck, so that the open nostrils are pointing upward, toward the ceiling. This position may be best for nose drops (more volume than sprays). An alternate position is to lie supine on a flat surface, then bend the neck backward (extend the head), so that the open nostrils point upward toward the ceiling.
5. Use the contralateral hand to insert the spray nozzle or dropper into one nostril (ie, the left hand for right nostril).
6. Use the other hand to occlude the opposite nostril (the one not being medicated).
7. Aim the spray or drops toward the outer (lateral) inside surface of each nostril and away from the nasal septum.
8. Breath in slowly but deeply through the medicated nostril.
9. Repeat this procedure to apply medication to the other nostril.
10. Consult the product labeling for instructions on cleaning the device.
11. See the text for information about preparation and use of saline irrigation.

HFA, hydrofluoroalkane (propellant); MDP, metered-dose pump.

From Refs. 2,6, and 8.

benefit for the ocular symptoms (eg, itching, redness, tearing). Intranasal administration is more effective than oral administration for the nasal congestion, but less effective for the ocular symptoms. The onset of action by oral administration is usually within 1 to 2 hours, and for intranasal administration within 15 minutes.[5,6,12,25,27] Antihistamines probably provide better relief when used continuously during symptomatic periods, but they are also effective used only when needed.

The oral agents are divided into first- and second-generation drugs. The first-generation agents are distributed among six chemical classes, including the more sedating ethanolamine class (eg, diphenhydramine) and the least sedating alkylamine class (eg, chlorpheniramine). Most sources now discourage the routine use of the first-generation agents for AR. This is due to their CNS and antimuscarinic side effects. The CNS effects are primarily sedation and impairment of cognitive function and performance of tasks. Decision making and driving or work performance are impaired even when the patient is unaware of any overt effects.[7,25] There is also evidence of decreased performance at school and impaired learning among pediatric patients.[7,25] The major antimuscarinic effects include blurred vision, dry mouth, urinary retention, and constipation. The only possible advantage of the antimuscarinic properties is an additional effect to decrease rhinorrhea. Another disadvantage of the first-generation antihistamines is that most are administered three to four times daily. Patients who take other sedative substances may have an additive effect from the antihistamine. Those taking any other medications with antimuscarinic properties may experience additive effects from the antihistamine. The elderly are, in general, more sensitive to both types of adverse effects.

Currently available oral second-generation H_1 antihistamines are cetirizine, levocetirizine, loratadine, desloratadine, fexofenadine, and acrivastine. All except acrivastine are available as a single agent, and some are marketed in combination with the decongestant pseudoephedrine. As of August, 2014, cetirizine, loratadine, and fexofenadine are available OTC. The second generation antihistamines have less antimuscarinic activity than the first-generation agents. Based on current literature, no single H_1 antihistamine (first or second generation) is clearly superior in efficacy; however, very few head-to-head comparative studies have been conducted. Individual variation is likely, and patients may need to try more than one product to realize optimal benefit. The oral second-generation antihistamines are effective for the sneezing, itching, and rhinorrhea of AR, but less effective for the nasal congestion. They also improve ocular symptoms. Intranasal antihistamines are somewhat better for nasal congestion.

Fexofenadine has virtually no sedative effects, even at doses higher than recommended. Loratadine and desloratadine are not sedative at recommended doses but can be at higher doses. Cetirizine, levocetirizine, and acrivastine have some sedative effects, even at recommended doses. All the oral second-generation agents require some dosage reduction with impaired renal function, but specific recommendations vary with creatinine clearance.[30,31] Most of the oral second-generation antihistamines can be administered once daily (except for the lower dosage forms of fexofenadine and the acrivastine combination product).

There are only two intranasal antihistamine products available in the US market as of August, 2014. Both azelastine and olopatadine are considered second-generation agents, although they also have anti-inflammatory effects.[25] Both are available only by prescription. The most common side effect of these products is a bitter taste. This is more common with the original formulation of azelastine (Astelin) and less common with olopatadine.[7,25,26] A newer formulation of azelastine (Astepro) has less bitter taste.[26] Also, there is enough systemic absorption to cause sedation in some patients using azelastine (about 10%) and perhaps somewhat fewer on olopatadine.[7,25] See **Table 63–7** for the single-agent second-generation antihistamine products.

KEY CONCEPT *Second-generation antihistamines are first-line agents, and are often effective alone, especially for mild or intermittent AR. They are preferred over first-generation antihistamines because of fewer side effects. Although effective for most symptoms of AR, they are less effective than intranasal corticosteroids for nasal congestion. Intranasal administration is more effective than oral administration for nasal congestion.* Most patients can use oral second-generation products. Others may prefer the intranasal route of administration, but they require a prescription. If nasal congestion is not relieved, addition of a decongestant is reasonable, either alone or as a combination product (see Decongestant section). Perhaps even the combination of an oral with an intranasal antihistamine is reasonable for some patients, depending on their preferences. Other pharmacologic agents can be combined with oral and/or intranasal antihistamines, as necessary for optimal control of symptoms. The new intranasal combination product of azelastine and fluticasone (Dymista) may be appropriate for some patients.

▸ *Adjunctive or Secondary Choice Agents*

Decongestants Decongestant drugs are useful only for nasal congestion.[7–9,25] This results from their α_1-adrenergic agonist

Table 63–7

Single-Agent Second-Generation Antihistamine Products (Oral and Intranasal)

Oral

Generic (Brand) Name	Formulation	Usual Adult Dosage	Usual Pediatric Dosage
Cetirizine[a,b] (Zyrtec, generic)	5, 10 mg tablets/chewable tablets; capsule 5 mg/5 mL syrup	5–10 mg once daily	6–11 mo; 2.5 mg once daily 12–23 mo; 2.5 mg once or twice daily 2–5 yo; 2.5–5 mg once daily or 2.5 mg twice daily
Desloratadine[b] (Clarinex)	5 mg tablets; 2.5-mg/5 mL syrup 2.5, 5 mg orally disintegrating tablets	5 mg once daily	6–11 mo; 1 mg once daily 1–5 yo; 1.25 mg once daily 6–11 yo; 2.5 mg once daily
Fexofenadine[a,b] (Allegra, generic)	30, 60, 180 mg tablets, 6 mg/mL suspension 30 mg orally disintegrating tablets	60 mg twice daily or 180 mg once daily	2–11 yo; 30 mg twice daily
Levocetirizine (Xyzal)	5 mg tablets 2.5 mg/5 mL solution	5 mg once daily	6 mo–5 yo; 1.25 mg once daily 6–11 yo; 2.5 mg once daily
Loratadine[a,b] (Claritin; Alavert, generic)	10 mg tablets and cap; 5 mg/5 mL syrup and susp; 10 mg disintegrating tablets; 5 mg chewable tablet	10 mg once daily	2–5 yo; 5 mg once daily

Intranasal Spray

Generic (Brand) Name	mcg/spray	Usual Adult Dosage (each nostril)	Usual Pediatric Dosage (each nostril)
Azelastine (Astelin, Astepro)	137	1–2 sprays twice daily	5–11 yo; 1 spray twice daily
Olopatadine (Patanase)	665	2 sprays twice daily	6–11 yo: 1 spray twice daily

Note: Acrivastine is available only with pseudoephedrine and so is not included in this table.

mo, months old; yo, years old.

[a]Available OTC

[b]Available in combination with pseudoephedrine (consult labeling for pediatric dosage).

From Refs. 25 and 27.

Patient Encounter 1, Part 3

About 6 months later, Aaron and his mother Evelyn come back to speak with you. Aaron tried using saline irrigations but he did not like the "messiness" it created, so he stopped them. He tried cetirizine but it made him sleepy during the day. Loratadine and fexofenadine just did not seem to work well. His parents still object to trying INCSs, despite your explanation. Montelukast seemed to help the AR symptoms, and even the exercise induced asthma to some extent. However, Aaron's doctor became concerned when Aaron complained of increased sleep disturbance while taking montelukast. The doctor wanted it stopped for what he called "safety" reasons. Ophthalmic ketotifen does help the ocular symptoms, but not the nasal symptoms, which he thinks are actually becoming more frequent and bothersome. They ask your advice.

What suggestions would you offer for control of Aaron's symptoms, now?

activity, which causes vasoconstriction in the nasal mucosa. They provide no benefit for the sneezing, itching, rhinorrhea, or the ocular manifestations. Decongestants can be given alone, either by the oral or by the intranasal route. Also, numerous combination products are available, consisting of a decongestant with an antihistamine (and sometimes other ingredients). There are some special considerations for use of decongestants in pediatric and pregnant patients (see the Special Populations section).

Oral decongestant products are currently limited to pseudoephedrine and phenylephrine.[5,25,27] Pseudoephedrine has been changed from truly OTC to a more controlled "behind the counter" (BTC) status because it is an ingredient in the illicit manufacture of methamphetamine. Some manufacturers changed the ingredients of their products by replacing pseudoephedrine with phenylephrine to maintain shelf presence in the OTC area. However, much controversy surrounds the efficacy of oral phenylephrine. Most contemporary literature suggests that the currently recommended adult dose is minimally effective as a nasal decongestant.[5,25,27]

The side effects of orally administered decongestants most often affect cardiovascular function or the CNS. The side effects are primarily due to sympathetic stimulation and are usually dose related. Some elevation of blood pressure may occur, but in normotensive and well-controlled hypertensive patients, the elevation is usually small. It is not of clinical significance in most situations, especially considering that these drugs are most appropriately used only briefly or intermittently. Insomnia, nervousness, irritability, and anxiety are relatively common CNS side effects. Some patients may have decreased appetite, tremors, headache, and even hallucinations. Men with benign prostatic hyperplasia (BPH) and other patients with disorders causing bladder outlet obstruction may have increased urinary retention due to α_1 stimulation of the urethral sphincter.

The intranasal agents currently available include the OTC products phenylephrine, oxymetazoline, and naphazoline. Intranasal application of decongestants provides rapid and effective relief of nasal congestion. This therapy may provide relief for nasal congestion, even for those patients already on intranasal corticosteroids.[25,27] However, the continuous use of intranasal decongestants often causes a paradoxical rebound phenomenon of persistent nasal congestion, called rhinitis medicamentosa.[5,25,27] Although some patients do not develop rhinitis medicamentosa, even after several weeks of continuous use of intranasal decongestants, the usual recommendation is to use them for no more than 3 consecutive days.[7] Intranasal decongestants can cause local side effects, including stinging, burning, dryness, and even sneezing. These are usually mild and well tolerated. Due to very limited absorption, the intranasal route rarely causes systemic side effects.[5,7] Administration technique should be optimized as described in Table 63–6. Should rhinitis medicamentosa occur, the best management is first to discontinue the decongestant, possibly with a taper to minimize worsening the situation. However, the response to withdrawal is often delayed for days. Therefore, it may be necessary to start intranasal corticosteroids and/or begin a short course of oral corticosteroid.[32]

KEY CONCEPT *The best applications of decongestants in AR are short-term use to overcome severe nasal congestion and to facilitate improved efficacy of other intranasal agents. The intranasal administration of decongestants should usually not exceed 3 consecutive days.* Despite the usual good tolerance of recommended doses of oral decongestants, caution is warranted when they are used in patients with cardiac disease (dysrhythmias, angina pectoris, heart failure), hypertension, cerebrovascular disease, bladder outlet obstruction (including BPH), glaucoma (especially closed angle), hyperthyroidism, and possibly diabetes.[5,25,27] The choice between the two routes of administration is based on several considerations, including cost, convenience, patient preference, speed of onset (within 30 minutes orally, within 5 to 10 minutes intranasally), and side effects.[7,12]

Mast Cell Stabilizer/Cromone[5–7,12,25,27] Cromolyn is the only cromone that is approved in the United States for treatment of AR. It is available as an OTC intranasal product. The mechanism of action in AR is mast cell stabilization. The drug binds to mast cells and prevents release of the mediators of AR that would otherwise result from allergen exposure. The drug is moderately effective, but less so than both intranasal corticosteroids and oral or intranasal antihistamines. It does have effects on both early and late phases of AR. Its effects begin within 4 to 7 days of use but may not be maximal for up to 2 weeks.[7] However, it can be used effectively on an as needed basis for episodic exposures to allergen.[7,27] Cromolyn is very well tolerated. The most common side effects are mild local stinging and/or burning, sneezing, unpleasant taste, and possibly nose bleed. A disadvantage is the frequency of administration. At least initially, it should be used four times daily. Some patients may need only two or three daily doses when used continuously after the first few weeks at four times daily. It is most useful for patients with mild or intermittent symptoms, especially in the pediatric population and in pregnant women.

Leukotriene Receptor Antagonist (LTRA) Leukotrienes are involved in the pathophysiology of AR and in particular contribute to the nasal congestion in the late phase.[1,5,7–9,12,13] There is some difference of opinion about benefits of LTRAs. Most sources indicate good benefit for nasal congestion and rhinorrhea, some benefit for ocular symptoms, but less for nasal itch and sneezing compared to INCSs and antihistamines.[5,6,25,27] Montelukast is the only LTRA approved for treatment of AR. It is marketed as oral granules and as both chewable and regular tablets. The combination of montelukast with an oral antihistamine shows improved efficacy over either agent alone, according to some sources, however, even the combination is probably not better than intranasal corticosteroids.[5,25] The onset of action of montelukast is delayed for a day or more.[7] The drug is usually considered to be very well tolerated. However, there are case reports of neuropsychiatric events, including sleep disturbances, depression and suicidal ideation, as well as headache, GI disturbances, skin rash, and Churg-Strauss syndrome.[12,25,27] It is administered once daily, considered safe (FDA Pregnancy Category B and indicated for children as young as 6 months of age), and particularly well suited to those patients who also have asthma. It may have some benefit in vasomotor (idiopathic, autonomic) rhinitis.[4]

Antimuscarinic Agent[5,7,12,25,27] Ipratropium is currently the only antimuscarinic agent indicated for treatment of AR. Systemic absorption is minimal. It is available by prescription as an intranasal spray. Its use is limited to those patients whose rhinorrhea has not been controlled by other therapy (antihistamines and/or INCSs). There are two strengths available. The 0.03% product is approved for AR in children as young as 6 years of age. This agent may be particularly helpful for patients who have vasomotor (idiopathic, autonomic) rhinitis, or those who may have a mixed etiology.[5,25] Local side effects are usually limited to nasal and oral dryness, throat irritation, and mild epistaxis.[27]

Saline Nasal administration of saline is an alternative for treatment of AR.[5,7,25,33,34] This therapy may benefit any patient with rhinitis, including those with vasomotor rhinitis.[5] Saline may be administered as drops or a spray, but the irrigation mode of administration is popularly known by several terms, including neti pot, nasal wash, nasal douche, nose bidet, and as nasal irrigation. Although less effective than intranasal corticosteroids, it has been shown to improve sneezing and nasal congestion. It can be used either alone or as add-on therapy. The formula provided by the American Academy of Allergy, Asthma and Immunology (AAAAI) should be followed for those making their own saline nasal irrigation solution.[34] Iodized salt is not recommended as it may be irritating. Hypertonic saline seems to have no advantage over 0.9% sodium chloride. Administration can be accomplished while the patient is in the shower or leaning over a sink. The head is bent forward and downward, then tilted to the side opposite the treated nostril. Then, with a bulb syringe or similar device, slowly introduce about 4 oz (118 mL) of the warm saline solution into one nostril. Soon, the solution will run out of the opposite nostril. The position of the head should be adjusted as necessary to avoid the solution running into the ears or down the throat.

Nasal irrigation is one delivery method, although the optimal method (spray, drops, nebulizer, or irrigation) is not known. Optimal frequency of administration is also not known. Nasal irrigation is usually given twice daily, but use of smaller volumes as spray products may be given up to four times daily. Side effects are usually limited to minor local nasal irritation, but nausea has been reported.

Omalizumab[7,25,35] Omalizumab is a monoclonal antibody that binds to IgE. The product is approved for asthma, but not for AR as of August, 2014. It is administered by subcutaneous injection. Dosage is determined by the patient's circulating IgE levels. The cost is high compared with that of other modes of therapy. Investigational use has demonstrated efficacy in AR, although relative efficacy is unknown. Its use is best limited to those with concurrent asthma and AR.

Complementary and Alternative Medicine Therapy Complementary and alternative therapy for AR has been reviewed.[25,36] Consistent evidence for efficacy has not been established, and there are some safety concerns.

► *Special Populations*

Children KEY CONCEPT *Generally speaking, the treatment of AR in children is the same as it is for adults. There are, however, limitations in terms of FDA-approved products for different age groups. Also, depending on the age of the patient, there may be administration issues with some products.* Most children affected by AR are older than 2 years, because usually, several years of antigen exposure is required to establish sensitization.[11] Children who have rhinitis before the age of 2 should be evaluated for other etiologies.[7,25]

There has been concern about use of combination cough and cold products (many contain an antihistamine and a decongestant) in children due to side effects. Most negative outcomes have resulted from inadvertent overdosage, often by giving the same drug from more than one product concurrently. These products are discouraged in children younger than 4 years.[37]

First-generation H_1 antihistamines are discouraged for children as they are for adults, due to the possible detrimental effects on school performance and learning. They may also cause paradoxical CNS stimulation in the very young (< 2 years old).[25] Second-generation (less sedating) H_1 antihistamines (primarily for mild or intermittent symptoms) or intranasal corticosteroids (for moderate–severe or persistent manifestations) are first-line modes of therapy. Antihistamines may need to be used even for more severe and/or persistent symptoms in those children who have difficulty with use of intranasal products. If necessary, these two classes can be combined.

See Table 63–7 for dosages of second-generation antihistamines by age groups for which they are indicated. Special care should be given to avoid administration of the same medication from different (especially combination) products. The side effects of second-generation antihistamines in children are similar to those for adults.

See Table 63–5 for dosages of intranasal corticosteroids by age groups. The consensus of opinion about intranasal corticosteroids and systemic side effects, especially delay in growth, is that most products are safe. Three INCSs, mometasone, fluticasone furoate, and triamcinolone, are FDA approved for children as young as 2 years of age.[25,27]. The local side effects of intranasal corticosteroids are the same in children as for adults.

Other therapy options may be worth consideration for some pediatric patients. Montelukast provides an oral alternative, especially for those who are too young to cooperate with

Patient Encounter 2, Part 1

Mrs. AL presents to your place of work to ask some questions. She is 32 years old, married, with no children. She does not work, but volunteers at several nonprofit organizations. This occupies several hours of her day, 4 days each week. Her husband works full time for a landscaping business. Her only chronic illness is allergic rhinitis that is caused by what her doctor calls "bad pollen allergies." She complains of "attacks" of repeated sneezing; copious watery runny nose; itchy nose and throat; often accompanied by itchy, watery eyes. Her only medications are Dymista (combination azelastine/fluticasone propionate) intranasal spray and oral fexofenadine 180 mg once daily. The dosage of Dymista is supposed to be one spray into each nostril twice daily. However, since starting it about 3 months ago, she has figured out that it makes her sleepy. She often skips the morning dose, especially, if she is volunteering that day.

What additional information do you need to better evaluate Mrs AL's problem?

What preliminary suggestions would you make?

intranasal administration of corticosteroids.[14] It may be used in combination with an oral antihistamine for additional efficacy. Another option for mild or intermittent symptoms is intranasal cromolyn, primarily due to its excellent safety.[25] This OTC product is labeled for use in children 2 years of age and older.[27] Intranasal ipratropium is indicated for patients 6 years of age or older and may benefit unresponsive rhinorrhea.

Pregnant Women[5,38] Women who have AR may suffer an exacerbation of symptoms during pregnancy.[38] However, only minor changes in the routine approach to therapy are necessary as a result of the pregnancy. Nasal saline irrigations are safe, effective, and improve the response to most other modes of therapy. They can be the foundation of AR therapy for pregnant patients.[5,38] Physical exercise increases vasoconstriction of the nasal mucosa, decreasing congestion, and rhinorrhea.[38] External adhesive strips can be used to help keep the nares open, especially during sleep.[38] Second-generation antihistamines are generally considered safe, based on an increasing number of studies and experience.[5,38] The same generalization applies to intranasal corticosteroids. While budesonide is the only product which is FDA pregnancy category B, no evidence exists of fetal harm from either INCSs or inhaled corticosteroids used for asthma.[39] Cromolyn is also FDA Pregnancy Category B and is considered safe.[38] The disadvantages are frequent administration and less efficacy than antihistamines and INCSs. Montelukast is also FDA Pregnancy Category B, but some recommend it primarily in those with concurrent asthma or who have demonstrated a good response prior to pregnancy.[7] Ipratropium is FDA Pregnancy Category B and is useful for troublesome rhinorrhea.[14] Oral decongestants are best avoided, especially in the first trimester. If nasal congestion is severe enough to warrant a decongestant, the intranasal route of administration is preferable, due to decreased systemic exposure.[7,38] Limiting the duration of use to 2 to 3 days is wise.[7,38]

Breast-Feeding Women One source has information about the relative safety of AR medication use in breast-feeding women.[40] Budesonide is probably the safest INCS and loratadine is probably the safest antihistamine. Intranasal cromolyn is also considered safe. Nasal saline irrigation could also be considered as a safe alternative in breast-feeding women.

Elderly AR in elderly patients is treated generally as it is in younger adults. Therefore, first-line agents are primarily INCSs and second-generation oral or possibly intranasal antihistamines.[5,7,25] Older patients may also have a component of atrophy of nasal tissues that can result in more nasal congestion. Most will benefit from regular nasal saline irrigation.[5] The elderly are more sensitive to the sedative and antimuscarinic effects of (especially first-generation) antihistamines and to the cardiovascular and CNS-stimulant effects of decongestants. These drugs should be used cautiously if at all. An increase in cholinergic activity may result in more rhinorrhea. This may respond well to ipratropium.

▶ *Ocular Symptoms*[5,27,41,42]

Several products are available for instillation directly into the eyes for those patients with predominant or unresponsive ocular manifestations. They may be appropriate for occasional moderate–severe flares or episodic AR when other modes of therapy are not optimally effective. The combination (antihistamine and mast cell stabilizing) agents may be the most effective, and they have the advantages of rapid onset of action and (usually) only twice daily administration. Ketotifen is in this category and because it is available OTC, it can be an appropriate initial agent. See Table 63–8 for these products.

Summary of Treatment

Once an agent appropriate for initial therapy is chosen, ongoing management requires repeated checks to ascertain response and freedom from intolerable or adherence limiting side effects. Either "step-up" or "step-down" therapy may be appropriate, depending on individual response. See Table 63–9 for a summary of the approach to treatment of AR. Table 63–10 attempts

Table 63–8

Intraocular Medications

Category	Generic (Brand) Name	Formulation	Frequency	Age
Decongestant/vasoconstrictor	Naphazoline[a] (Naphcon, Privine, others)	0.012% + 0.025%	Four times daily	Adult
Decongestant/vasoconstrictor + antihistamine	Naphazoline + pheniramine[a] (Visine A)	0.025%/0.3%	Four times daily	6 yo or more
Antihistamine	Emedastine (Emadine)	0.05%	Four times daily	3 yo or more
	Alcaftadine (Lastacaft)	0.25%	Once daily	2 yo or more
Mast cell stabilizer	Cromolyn (Generic)	4%	Every 4–6 hours	4 yo or more
	Lodoxamide (Alomide)	0.1%	Four times daily	2 yo or more
	Nedocromil (Alocril)	2%	Twice daily	3 yo or more
	Pemirolast (Alamast)	0.1%	Four times daily	3 yo or more
Antihistamine + mast cell stabilizer	Azelastine (Optivar)	0.05%	Twice daily	3 yo or more
	Epinastine (Elestat)	0.05%	Twice daily	2 yo or more
	Ketotifen[a] (Zaditor, Alaway, Claritin, Zyrtec, generic)	0.025%	Every 8–12 hours	3 yo or more
	Olopatadine (Patanol/Pataday)	0.1%/0.2%	Twice daily/once daily	3 yo or more
	Bepotastine (Bepreve)	1.5%	Twice daily	2 yo or more
NSAIDs	Ketorolac (Acular)	0.5%	Four times daily	3 yo or more
Corticosteroid	Loteprednol (Alrex)	0.2%	Four times daily	Adult

NSAID, nonsteroidal anti-inflammatory drug; yo, years old.

[a]Available OTC.

From Refs. 7,27,40, and 41.

Also, see Chapter 62, Ophthalmic Disorders for more details.

Table 63–9

Routine Approach to Therapy of AR

All patients should practice avoidance of identified allergens

Mild intermittent

First line:

- Oral antihistamine (OTC, initially; preferably second generation)

Adjunctive/secondary (may use more than one; no specific order intended):

- Add nasal saline (eg, as irrigation)
- Consider intranasal cromolyn, especially preexposure for episodic AR
- Consider OTC INCS for refractory symptoms
- Consider intraocular medications, as needed for ocular symptoms (See Table 63–8)
- Consider OTC oral decongestant for nasal congestion
- Consider OTC intranasal decongestant for refractory nasal congestion (not > 3 days)
- Consider prescription therapy for inadequate response (see below)

Possibly consider referral for immunotherapy

Persistent or moderate–severe

First line:

- Intranasal corticosteroid (could try OTC product first)
- Add oral antihistamine for possible additional benefit if necessary

Adjunctive/secondary (may use more than one):

- Add nasal saline (eg, as irrigation)
- Consider intraocular medications, as needed for ocular symptoms (See Table 63–8)
- Consider OTC oral decongestant for nasal congestion
- Consider short-term intranasal decongestant for refractory nasal congestion
- Consider replacement of one first-line agent, if poorly tolerated, with montelukast
- Consider ipratropium for inadequately controlled rhinorrhea
- Consider intranasal antihistamine
- Consider combination intranasal antihistamine with corticosteroid

Consider referral for immunotherapy

Episodic (no order of preference intended)

- Oral antihistamine (OTC, initially; preferably second generation)
- Consider addition of or replacement with intranasal cromolyn (OTC) or intranasal antihistamine or intranasal corticosteroid

Special situations (children, pregnant women, elderly, ocular symptoms)

- See Special Populations section of text

From Refs. 2,5–10,12,14,25,29,33, and 34.

Table 63–10

Relative Efficacy (Semiquantitative) by Classes of Agents for Specific Symptoms of Allergic Rhinitis

Drug Class	Nasal Congestion	Sneezing	Rhinorrhea	Nasal Itch	Ocular Symptoms
Intranasal corticosteroids	6	6	6	5	4
Oral antihistamines[a]	2	4	4	6	4
Intranasal antihistamines	3	4	4	5	0
Oral decongestants[a]	3	0	0	0	0
Intranasal decongestants[a,b]	6	0	0	0	0
Oral leukotriene antagonist	4	1	4	1	4
Intranasal mast cell stabilizer[a]	3	3	3	3	2
Intranasal antimuscarinic	0	0	5	0	0

Note: The information in this table is a composite from numerous sources. There are different opinions about some of the rankings, partly due to inadequate study. Individual variation may create different relative efficacy in some patients. Higher number equals greater activity.

[a]Some products in these classes are available OTC.

[b]Intranasal decongestants are best used for severe, unresponsive nasal congestion, or to facilitate mucosal contact of other intranasal medications, but in either case, should usually be limited to no more than 3 days.

From Refs. 2,5–10,12,14,25,29,33, and 34.

Patient Encounter 2, Part 2

Mrs. AL returns in 2 weeks. She took your advice. She continued the fexofenadine. She replaced Dymista with OTC triamcinolone intranasal spray. And, she tried saline nasal irrigations. Formal allergy skin testing done by her doctor showed that she is allergic to "… just about every tree and flower that blossoms…" in this area! However, she is not allergic to animals, molds, fungi, house dust mite, or cockroaches! Her doctor made some suggestions for allergen avoidance, mostly to stay indoors, keep doors and windows closed, and use an air conditioner. She has noticed some improvement with the new regimen. She does not feel quite as sleepy, having stopped the Dymista. She thinks both the saline irrigations and the triamcinolone help. However, she still has significant symptoms while in her house, during the evening and often during the night.

Additional information gathered at this visit follows.

She is unaware of her family history. They have lived in the same city for more than 15 years. She moved to another part of town when she got married six years ago. Her current home has some plants in the yard, but her husband does all the yard upkeep. Her AR symptoms started as a child, but seem quite a bit worse in the last 5 years or so. She is not exposed to animal dander. She does not think her home is a source of mold or cockroaches. She does have symptoms during the night (while in her bedroom), but she also has symptoms in every other room of the house (see below).

She admits to some nasal congestion and mouth breathing especially at night. Other symptoms include some difficulty sleeping due to "attacks" in the evenings and even during the night. Overall, she considers her symptoms, troublesome. She has AR symptoms virtually every day even with her current regimen. Therefore, she probably has ARIA category moderate-severe persistent AR.

She thinks that her symptoms are worse when she is home and better when she is at the nonprofit organizations where she volunteers at least half a day, 4 days each week.

Before the allergy testing was done, she did not know what specific pollens she was allergic to. She had noticed more frequent and severe symptoms when plants are blooming. Now she knows what she is allergic to (see above). Curiously, however, she has symptoms both indoors and outdoors.

She tried Benadryl several years ago. It made her sleepy and caused dry mouth, so she gave up.

She has an IUD in place. It is called Mirena, which is replaced every 5 years. A new one (her third) was placed about 1 year ago. Since having this IUD, she notices that her menses are a bit lighter, although she is very regular. Her last menses started 7 days ago, and lasted the usual 2 days. She also has fewer problems with cramping. She and her husband have no plans to have children at this time.

Explain the rationale for your plan at this time.

Patient Encounter 2, Part 3

After the second visit with Mrs. AL (Patient encounter 2, part 2), you had an uneasy feeling. Later that evening, you began to wonder about some of the elements in her story. You formulate a theory about the source of her symptoms, and plan to phone Mrs. AL to ask more specific information. If your theory is correct, you may be able to significantly improve her symptom control.

What is the theory about Mrs. AL's symptoms?

Presuming the theory is correct, what specific plan could be suggested?

Patient Encounter 3, Part 1

EM presents to your place of business to ask your advice about his "nose and eye" symptoms. EM is a 50-year-old man, who works as a tax accountant. About 25 years ago, he moved from New England to the Southwest, for employment reasons. The environment was much warmer than he was used to, but like the local people said, it was "…a dry heat!" Within a few months of the move, he began having problems with watery, sometimes profuse runny nose. At that time, the only other symptom he had was a decrease in his sense of smell.

He thought he had allergies to the new plants in the area, but the doctor he saw said that by examination his nose, throat, and ears looked normal. The doc called it "non-allergic rhinitis." He was given a prescription for intranasal flunisolide spray and told to use it three times a day. Over the years, it seemed to work sometimes, but not always. And, he always had problems remembering to use it regularly. He added an OTC oral antihistamine years ago, but it did not help much, and it caused so much sleepiness that he couldn't work. He stopped it, and just continued irregular use of the flunisolide.

More recently, in the last year, he notices even more symptoms, including some sneezing, some nasal itch, and some eye symptoms (redness, wateriness, and itchiness). EM denies all other chronic illnesses and he takes no other medications on a regular basis. He asks your advice for treatment options for his current symptoms.

How would you characterize EM's problem?

What are your recommendations for his therapy?

Patient Encounter 3, Part 2

EM returns 2 weeks later. He took most of your advice. He tried saline irrigations, but found them difficult to do twice every day. He switched from intranasal flunisolide to triamcinolone, which was easier to use and more effective. He tried oral cetirizine, but it seemed to make him tired, so he stopped. The major remaining problems are relatively persistent, and sometimes profuse, watery nasal discharge and itchy eyes.

What additional advice can you suggest?

to rank the relative effectiveness of the classes of agents for treatment of AR by specific symptoms.

OUTCOME EVALUATION

- Confirm the patient's understanding of the disorder (see Clinical Presentation and Diagnosis).
- Confirm the patient's understanding about allergen avoidance measures (see Table 63–3).
- Assess the patient's symptom response, tolerance, and adherence.
- Assess the patient's administration technique with intranasal products.
- Recommend second-generation oral antihistamine therapy for most patients with mild or intermittent symptoms (see Clinical Presentation and Diagnosis and Table 63–9).
- Recommend intranasal corticosteroid therapy for moderate–severe or persistent symptoms (two products are OTC). Suggest additional therapy for those with incomplete control (see Clinical Presentation and Diagnosis and Table 63–9).
- Consider step-up therapy for exacerbations or incomplete response.
- Consider step-down therapy if symptoms are minimal or stable for several months.
- Consider referral to rule out nonallergic causes of rhinitis in nonresponding patients or those with an atypical presentation (see Clinical Presentation and Diagnosis).
- Consider referral for patients who request immunotherapy.
- Consider referral for patients with comorbid conditions, especially asthma.

Patient Care Process

Patient Assessment:

- Determine that the patient probably does not have a nonallergic type of rhinitis (see Table 63–1)
- Determine extent and severity of patient's signs and symptoms of AR. This should be done by combination of History of Present Illness (HPI), Past Medical history (PMHx) and appropriate physical assessment
- Assessment of HPI includes seven elements, using eg, the acronym LOQQSAM (location; onset; quality; quantity; setting; associated symptoms; modifying factors) (see Clinical Presentation and Diagnosis box)
- Appropriate PMHx should include conditions associated with AR and its complications (see Epidemiology section)
- Appropriate physical assessment is usually limited to observation of the patient, and sometimes examination of the nasal mucosa and oropharynx (see Clinical Presentation and Diagnosis box)
- This assessment should be expressed in terms of the frequency and severity of AR, as defined by the ARIA system (see Table 63–2)

Therapy Evaluation:

- Determine the patient's understanding of the nature of AR.
- Determine what modes of therapy the patient has already tried (allergen avoidance, pharmacotherapy, immunotherapy).
- Assess the appropriateness of current therapy, relative to the clinical response.
- If the clinical response is inadequate or suboptimal, determine first, if poor adherence and/or administration technique (ie, with intranasal agents) are involved. See Table 63–6.
- If nonadherence and poor technique do not explain a suboptimal response, consider alternative therapeutic modes. See Table 63–9.
- If specific patient features exist (female who is currently or may become pregnant, woman who is breast-feeding, child, or elderly), see Selected Populations section.

Care Plan Development:

- Advise allergen avoidance to the degree possible. See Table 63–3.
- Educate and counsel about optimal administration technique and adherence.
- Base subsequent, specific recommendations for therapy on symptom pattern (nasal congestion, rhinorrhea, ocular manifestations, concurrent asthma), previous response to therapy and availability (OTC, Rx, referral).

Follow-up Evaluation:

- Follow up weekly at first, especially during worse times or seasons.
- When optimal control is approached, increase duration between follow-up visits (eg, monthly, every 2–3 months, or less frequently).

Abbreviations Introduced in This Chapter

AAAAI	American Academy of Allergy, Asthma, and Immunology
ACEI	Angiotensin-converting enzyme inhibitor
AERD	Aspirin-exacerbated respiratory disease
AR	Allergic rhinitis
ARIA	Allergic Rhinitis and its Impact on Asthma
BPH	Benign prostatic hyperplasia/hypertrophy
BTC	Behind-the-counter
H_1	Histamine type 1 (receptor)
HEPA	High-efficiency particulate air (filter)
HFA	Hydrofluoroalkane ("green" propellant for metered-dose INCSs)
HPA	Hypothalamic–pituitary–adrenal (axis)
HPI	History of Present Illness
HT	(essential or primary) hypertension
IAR	Intermittent allergic rhinitis (ARIA system)
IgE	Immunoglobulin E
INCS(s)	Intranasal corticosteroid(s)
LTRA	Leukotriene receptor antagonist
NARES	Nonallergic rhinitis with eosinophilia (on nasal smear) syndrome
NSAID	Nonsteroidal anti-inflammatory drug
OTC	Over-the-counter
PAR	Perennial allergic rhinitis (AAAAI/ACAAI system)
PDE-5	Phosphodiesterase (isoenzyme)-5
PER	Persistent allergic rhinitis (ARIA system)
PMHx	Past Medical history
QT	Interval between the Q and T waves in an ECG
SAR	Seasonal allergic rhinitis (AAAAI/ACAAI system)

REFERENCES

1. Dion GR, Weitzel EK, McMains KC. Current approaches to diagnosis and management of rhinitis. South Med J. 2013; 106(9):526–531.
2. Simon C. Rhinitis. InnovAiT. 2008;1:412–416.
3. Fletcher RH, Peden D. An overview of rhinitis [Internet]. Waltham, MA: UpToDate, Inc.; 2014 Mar [cited 2014 Aug 5]. http://www.uptodate.com/contents/an-overview-of-rhinitis. Accessed December 6, 2014.
4. Smith H, Glew S. Vasomotor rhinitis. InnovAiT. 2012;5:401–406.
5. Corren J, Baroody FM, Pawankar R. Allergic and nonallergic rhinitis. In: Adkinson Jr NF, Bochner BS, Burks WA, et al. eds. Middleton's Allergy—Principles and Practice. 8th ed. Philadelphia: Saunders-Elsevier; 2014:664–685.
6. Smith H. Hay fever and allergic rhinitis. InnovAiT. 2012;5: 220–225.
7. Wallace DV, Dykewicz MS, Bernstein DI, et al, eds. The diagnosis and management of rhinitis: An updated practice parameter. J Allergy Clin Immunol. 2008;122(2):S1–S84.
8. Scadding GK, Durham SR, Mirakian R, et al. BSACI guidelines for the management of allergic and nonallergic rhinitis. Clin Exp Allergy. 2008;38:19–42.
9. Bousquet J, Khaltaev N, Cruz AA, et al. Allergic rhinitis and its impact on asthma (ARIA) 2008 update. Allergy. 2008;63(Suppl 86): S8–S160.
10. Brożek JL, Bousquet J, Baena-Cagnani CE, et al. Allergic rhinitis and its impact on asthma (ARIA) guideline: 2010 revision. J Allergy Clin Immunol. 2010;126:466–476.
11. de Shazo, RD, Kemp SF. Allergic rhinitis: Clinical manifestations, epidemiology, and diagnosis [Internet]. Waltham, MA: UpToDate, Inc.; 2014 Mar [cited 2014 Aug 5]. http://www.uptodate.com/contents/allergic-rhinitis-clinical-manifestations-epidemiology-and-diagnosis. Accessed December 6, 2014.
12. Greiner AN, Hellings PW, Rotiroti G, et al. Allergic rhinitis. Lancet. 2011;378:2112–2122.
13. de Shazo, RD, Kemp SF. Pathogenesis of allergic rhinitis Internet]. Waltham, MA: UpToDate, Inc.; 2014 Jul [cited 2014 Aug 5]. http://www.uptodate.com/contents/pathogenesis-of-allergic-rhinitis-rhinosinusitis. Accessed December 6, 2014.
14. Angier E, Willington J, Scadding G, et al. Management of allergic and non-allergic rhinitis: A primary care summary of the BSACI guideline. Prim Care Respir J. 2010;19(3):217–222.
15. Creticos PS. Sublingual immunotherapy for allergic rhinitis [Internet]. Waltham, MA: UpToDate, Inc.; 2014 May [cited 2014 Aug 5]. http://www.uptodate.com/contents/sublingual-immunotherapy-for-allergic-rhinitis. Accessed December 6, 2014.
16. Sublingual immunotherapy for allergic rhinitis. Med Lett Drugs Ther. 2014;56(1444):47–48.
17. PL Detail-Document, Oralair, Grastek, and Ragwitek: Sublingual immunotherapy for allergies. Pharmacist's Letter/Prescriber's Letter June, 2014.
18. DeShazo RD, Kemp SF. Overview of immunologic treatments for allergic rhinitis [Internet]. Waltham, MA: UpToDate, Inc.; 2013 Dec [cited 2014 Aug 5]. http://www.uptodate.com/contents/overview-of-immunologic-treatments-for-allergic-rhinitis. Accessed December 6, 2014.
19. Lin SY, Erekosima N, Kim JM, et al. Sublingual immunotherapy for the treatment of allergic rhinoconjunctivitis and asthma—a systematic review. JAMA. 2013;309(12):1278–1288.
20. Kim JM, Lin SY, Suarez-Cuervo C, et al. Allergen-specific immunotherapy for pediatric asthma and rhinoconjunctivitis: A systematic review. Pediatr. 2013;131(6):1–13.
21. Chelladurai Y, Suarez-Cuervo C, Erekosima N, et al. Effectiveness of subcutaneous versus sublingual immunotherapy for the treatment of allergic rhinoconjunctivitis and asthma: A systematic review. J Allergy Clin Immunol Pract. 2013;1(4):361–369.
22. Norman PS. Subcutaneous immunotherapy for allergic disease: Indications and efficacy [Internet]. Waltham, MA: UpToDate, Inc.; 2013 May [cited 2014 Aug 5]. http://www.uptodate.com/contents/subcutaneous-immunotherapy-for-allergic-disease-indications-and-efficacy. Accessed December 6, 2014.
23. Norman PS. Subcutaneous immunotherapy for allergic disease: Therapeutic mechanisms [Internet]. Waltham, MA: UpToDate, Inc.; 2013 May [cited 2014 Aug 5]. http://www.uptodate.com/contents/subcutaneous-immunotherapy-for-allergic-disease-therapeutic-mechanisms. Accessed December 6, 2014.
24. Costa DJ, Amouyal M, Lambert P, et al. How representative are clinical study patients with allergic rhinitis in primary care? J Allergy Clin Immunol. 2011;127(4):920–926.
25. de Shazo, RD, Kemp SF. Pharmacotherapy of allergic rhinitis [Internet]. Waltham, MA: UpToDate, Inc.; 2014 Jun [cited 2014 Aug 5]. http://www.uptodate.com/contents/pharmacotherapy-of-allergic-rhinitis. Accessed December 6, 2014.
26. Azelastine/fluticasone propionate (Dymista) for seasonal allergic rhinitis. Med Lett Drugs Ther. 2012;56(1402):85–87.
27. Drugs for allergic disorders. Treat Guidel Med Lett. 2013; 11(129):43–52.
28. Kirtsreesakul V, Chansaksung P, Ruttanaphol S. Dose-related effect of intranasal corticosteroids on treatment outcome of persistent allergic rhinitis. Otolaryngol Head Neck Surg. 2008; 139(4):565–569.
29. OTC fluticasone nasal spray for allergic rhinitis. Med Lett Drugs Ther. 2015;57(1465):48-49.
30. Aranoff GR, Bennett WM, Berns JS, et al. Drug Prescribing in Renal Failure: Dosing Guidelines for Adults and Children, 5th ed. Philadelphia, PA: American College of Physicians, 2007.
31. Golightly LK, Teitelbaum I, Kiser TH, et al, eds. Renal Pharmacotherapy—Dosage Adjustment of Medications Eliminated by the Kidneys. New York: Springer, 2013.

32. Lockey RF. Rhinitis medicamentosa and the stuffy nose. J Allergy Clin Immunol. 2006;118:1017–1018.

33. Rabago D, Zgierska A. Saline nasal irrigation for upper respiratory conditions. Am Fam Physician. 2009;80(10):1117–1119, 1121–1121.

34. American Academy of Allergy Asthma & Immunology. Saline sinus rinse recipe [Internet]. [cited 2014 Aug 21]. http://www.aaaai.org/conditions-and-treatments/Treatments/Saline-Sinus-Rinse-Recipe.aspx. Accessed December 6, 2014.

35. Tsabouri S, Tseretopoulou X, Priftis K, Ntzani EE. Omalizumab for the treatment of inadequately controlled allergic rhinitis: A systematic review and meta-analysis of randomized clinical trials. J Allergy Clin Immunol Pract. 2014;2:332–340.

36. Bielory L. Complementary and alternative therapies for allergic rhinitis and conjunctivitis [Internet]. Waltham, MA: UpToDate, Inc.; 2013 Sep [cited 2014 Aug 22]. http://www.uptodate.com/contents/complementary-and-alternative-therapies-for-allergic-rhinitis-and-conjunctivitis. Accessed December 6, 2014.

37. U.S. Department of Health & Human Services. U.S. Food and Drug Administration. Drugs. Resources for You. Special Features. An important FDA reminder to parents: Do not give infants cough and cold products designed for older children [updated 2011 Aug 3; cited 2014 Aug 22]. http://www.fda.gov/Drugs/ResourcesforYou/SpecialFeatures/ucm263948.htm. Accessed December 6, 2014.

38. Schatz M. Recognition and management of allergic disease during pregnancy [Internet]. Waltham, MA: UpToDate, Inc.; 2014 Jan [cited 2014 Aug 22]. http://www.uptodate.com/contents/recognition-and-management-of-allergic-disease-during-pregnancy. Accessed December 6, 2014.

39. Rahimi R, Nikfar S, Abdollahi M. Meta-analysis finds use of inhaled corticosteroids during pregnancy safe: A systematic meta-analysis review. Hum Exp Toxicol. 2006;25:447–452.

40. Hale TW. Medications and Mothers' Milk—A Manual of Lactational Pharmacology—2012. 15th ed. Amarillo, TX: Hale Publishing, Inc.; 2012.

41. U.S. Department of Health & Human Services. U.S. Food and Drug Administration. Drugs@FDA. FDA Approved Drug Products. [cited 2012 Feb 6]. http://www.accessdata.fda.gov/scripts/cder/drugsatfda/.Accessed December 6, 2014.

42. Corbett AH, Dana WJ, Fuller MA, et al, eds. Drug Information Handbook 2014-2015, 23rd ed. Hudson, OH: Lexicomp, 2014.

64 Psoriasis

Miriam Ansong, Samson Amos, and Victor Padron

LEARNING OBJECTIVES

Upon completion of this chapter, the reader will be able to:

1. Discuss the etiology and risk factors of psoriasis.
2. Describe the pathophysiology and clinical presentations of psoriasis.
3. Evaluate the assessment strategies of patients with the disease state.
4. Recommend nonpharmacological approaches for the treatment of psoriasis.
5. Develop appropriate treatment and care plan for psoriasis patients.
6. Recommend appropriate monitoring parameters for a patient with psoriasis.
7. Propose patient education and counseling information for patients and caregivers as part of the care plan.

INTRODUCTION

KEY CONCEPT *Psoriasis is a chronic inflammatory condition that exhibits a normal pattern of relapse and remission. There is currently no cure for the disease and treatment is aimed toward management of signs and symptoms associated with the condition.*[1] Remission may last years in some patients, whereas, in others, exacerbations may occur every few months. Things known to exacerbate the condition are stress, seasonal changes, environmental factors, life crises, and certain medications.[2] The severity of the condition ranges from mild and moderate to severely disabling. Depression, alcohol-related problems, cardiovascular diseases, metabolic syndrome, and skin cancers are select comorbidities associated with the severe form of the disease.[1] Thus, management of patients with psoriasis is long term and management modalities may change according to the severity of illness at the time. Treatment should be individualized to meet patient needs. The disease may precipitate emotional distress that requires empathy and a caring attitude.

EPIDEMIOLOGY AND ETIOLOGY

Psoriasis is a chronic common inflammatory skin disorder with a population prevalence of 2% to 3% worldwide. The prevalence is found in Americans and Canadians in a range of 4.6% to 4.7%. African, African American, and Asian populations have an estimated 0.4% to 0.7% prevalence of the disease.[3] Male patients tend to die at least 3.5 years earlier and females 4.5 years earlier than nonpsoriasis patients normalized for differences in mortality by gender.[3] The disease may present at any age, but peaks between age 15 and 30 and again from 50 to 60 years.[3,4] Types of psoriasis manifest as **plaque, flexural (aka inverse or intertriginous), erythrodermic, pustular, guttate, nail,** and **psoriatic arthritis (PsA)**. Eighty to ninety percent of psoriatic patients present with plaque psoriasis. Plaque psoriasis presents with red-pink lesions of varying sizes covered with silvery scales.[2] Up to 42% of patients with psoriasis have been reported to also have PsA.[1,5] PsA is mostly limited to joints, ligaments, and tendons, and manifests in the presence of psoriasis disease. Clinical presentations include pain, stiffness, swelling, and tenderness. PsA progresses from mild symptoms to the destruction of joints affecting quality of life for patients. Some patients may have deforming PsA without cutaneous involvement.[1,5]

Recent research has shown that psoriatic patients have an increased risk of cardiovascular diseases, especially myocardial infarction.[5–7] The risk is increased in patients with both mild and severe psoriasis, with the highest risk in younger patients with severe disease.[7] These findings persist even when corrected for other cardiovascular risk factors.[7–9]

KEY CONCEPT *Even though study results are inconclusive, genetic association has been documented for both psoriasis and psoriatic arthritis.*[2] The histocompatibility complex region of chromosome 6 (HLA-Cw*06) has been suspected in the disease.[2] Even though the linkage to HLA-Cw*06 has long been known, there is further support for this linkage in recent studies.[2,10,11] Studies have also shown that HLA-A2, B8, B17, and B44 are involved.[12] Women exposed to tobacco smoke have a higher risk of psoriasis than their male counterparts with the same exposure. Four life events: divorce, death of a close friend, death of a family member, and change in work environment can increase the risk of developing psoriasis. First-degree relatives with psoriasis is another risk factor, affecting males more than females. Risk is also found to be higher in urban settings versus rural settings. Additional factors exacerbating psoriasis include drugs such as lithium, NSAIDs, antimalarials, β-adrenergic blockers, and withdrawal of corticosteroids.[13] Cytokines such as interleukins and tumor necrosis factor α (TNF-α), T cells, and keratinocytes play significant roles in the inflammatory process that constitutes the disease mechanism.[2]

The emotional and psychological impact of psoriasis may not correlate with the severity of the skin presentation, and it is important to always evaluate the psychosocial effects of psoriasis on the patient.[8,9]

PATHOPHYSIOLOGY

The pathogenesis of psoriasis involves multiple components of the immune system. Cytokines, T cells, and keratinocytes are central to the inflammatory process associated with psoriasis. Additionally, it has been found that when keratinocytes are perturbed, the release of antimicrobial peptide LL-37 takes place. This peptide binds with DNA and RNA. This complex potentially leads to the activation of plasmacytoid and myeloid dendritic cells. These activated dendritic cells secrete interleukin IL-12 and IL-13. The production of these two interleukins eventually results in IL-17 and T helper cell type 1 differentiation.[2] The T cells then release Interleukin IL-17A, IL-17F, IL-22, and IL-23 as mediators which then subsequently activate keratinocytes. This process then generates a complex cascade including proinflammatory cytokines such as TNF-α, interferon (IFN-α and IFN-γ), and interleukin (IL-1β and IL-6). The entire process then leads to alteration of the immune system and chronic inflammation that manifests in the skin causing vascular changes and formation of psoriatic lesions.[2] Keratinocyte proliferation is central to the clinical presentation of psoriasis. Keratinocytes are skin cells producing keratin, which act as a skin barrier.[14] Hyperkeratosis that results from immune derangements causes the characteristic thick, scaly skin lesions seen in patients with psoriasis.[14] The pathologic pathway of psoriatic arthritis is the same, except that the changes that occur as a result of T-cell mediators happen in the synovial fluid within the joints. Osteoclast activation, osteolysis, and bone resorption produces the damage that occurs within the joints.[2]

CLINICAL PRESENTATION AND DIAGNOSIS

KEY CONCEPT *Diagnosis of psoriasis is usually based on recognition of the characteristic plaque lesion and is not based on lab tests.*

"The severity of the disease is classified as mild/limited disease, moderate, or severe disease based on body surface area (BSA) involvement (Table 64–1)." Additionally, classification may be based on assessment tools used such as the Psoriasis Area and Severity Index (PASI) and the Dermatology Life Quality Index (DLQI).[15,16]

TREATMENT

Desired Outcomes and Goals

KEY CONCEPT *Given its manifestations, inflammation, involvement of multiple areas of the affected skin, and the chronic nature of psoriasis, treatment goals must be well targeted. The goals of treatment must be set based on clinical presentations, disease-related comorbidities, treatment-related morbidity, mortality, quality of life, staging of the disease, and recurrent and remission status of the disease at any given point in time.*[5,17,18] It is paramount to know

Patient Encounter, Part 1

AD is a 52-year-old woman who has noticed dark, red, and smooth lesions covering the majority of her upper body. When questioned, the patient says her skin has been relatively clear, until about a month ago. Since then, the lesions have been becoming more uncomfortable, spreading from her back and abdomen to her arms. She is feeling self-conscious about what is happening and does not know what to do.

What type of psoriasis is AD experiencing?

Clinical Presentation and Diagnosis of Plaque Psoriasis

General characteristics

Small, discrete lesions to generalized confluent lesions over a large BSA.

Symptoms

Severe itching.

Signs

- Raised lesion red to violet or silvery in color (commonly known as plaques).
- Sharply demarcated borders lesions, except where confluent.
- Lesions are loosely covered with silvery-white scales, which if lifted off, show small pinpoints of bleeding (Auspitz sign).
- Plaques show on the elbows, knees, scalp, umbilicus, and lumbar areas, and often extend to involve the trunk, arms, legs, face, ears, palms, soles, and nails.
- Nail involvement presents as pitting, discoloration ("oil spots"), crumbling, splinter hemorrhages, growth arrest lines, or tissue buildup around the nails.

Clinical Presentation and Diagnosis of Other Types of Psoriasis

- Flexural psoriasis:
  - Appears in intertriginous area
  - Scaling is minimal
- Guttate psoriasis:
  - Sudden eruption of small, disseminated erythematosquamous papules and plaques
  - Often preceded by a streptococcal infection 2 to 3 weeks prior
- Pustular psoriasis:
  - May be localized or generalized
  - May be an acute emergency requiring systemic therapy. The others are given physical descriptions, but this one is not
- Generalized pustular psoriasis:
  - Disseminated deep-red erythematous areas and pustules
  - May merge to become "lakes of pus"
- Erythrodermic psoriasis: generalized, life-threatening condition
  - Erythema, desquamation, and edema
  - May require life support measures as well as systemic therapy

Table 64–1

Disease Severity Classification[15,16]

Mild or limited disease	Less than or equal to 5% BSA involvement
Moderate disease	PASI greater than or equal to 8 (higher in trials of biologics)
Severe disease	The Rule of Tens: PASI greater than or equal to 10 or DLQI greater than or equal to 10 or BSA greater than or equal to 10% (in some phototherapy trials, BSA greater than or equal to 20% is used as the lower limit

that no cure currently exists for any type of psoriasis disease. However, evidence supports an increase in remission period and reduction in severity of the disease with current treatment options.[17] The goals must therefore include the following:

- Minimizing or eliminating the signs of psoriasis, such as plaques and scales
- Alleviating pruritus and minimizing excoriations
- Reducing flare-up frequency
- Ensuring appropriate management of associated comorbidities such as psoriatic arthritis, cardiovascular disorders, Crohn disease, clinical depression, or itching
- Avoiding or minimizing adverse effects from treatments used
- Providing cost-effective therapy
- Providing guidance or counseling as needed (eg, stress-reduction techniques)
- Maintaining or improving the patient's quality of life
- Ensuring that patients are partners in their own care
- Implementing motivational interviewing skills in all communications with the patient

General Approach to Treatment

Management of the disease must be structured to target the type of psoriasis. Plaque, guttate, flexural, pustular, and erythrodermic are the types that currently manifest clinically in patients, with plaque psoriasis being the most common.[19] General treatment modalities must include location, the extent of BSA involvement, and lifestyle modifications. Additionally, the choice of management approach must take into consideration whether the disease is mild, moderate, or severe.[17]

For PsA, the goal of treatment is to keep the patient pain free, reduce swelling, retard or minimize joint damage and keep the joints functioning.[2,5,8,9] The goals to achieve for patients living with this skin condition are significant improvement of skin appearance and ensuring that unpleasant side effects of drugs are fairly minimized. KEY CONCEPT *Patients are managed with both pharmacologic and nonpharmacologic approaches (Figure 64–1).*[19]

Nonpharmacologic Management

Several effective nonpharmacologic options are available to patients with psoriasis. However, considering the nature of the disease, these treatments may be used as adjunctive treatments to therapeutic agents when appropriate.[16]

KEY CONCEPT *Stress reduction techniques such as psychotherapy, guided imagery, and relaxation techniques have been shown to improve the extent and severity of psoriasis.*[20] *Oatmeal baths in tepid water may help soothe the itching associated with psoriasis.* Nonmedicated moisturizers (occlusive agents, humectants, and/or emollients) help the skin to retain moisture and reduce the scaling of the skin lesions. *Aloe vera* is a common emollient used to help manage skin dryness. These can be applied multiple times during the day to prevent skin dryness. Patients with skin sensitivities should consider the use of fragrance-free products.[21] Harsh soaps, detergents, and other skin irritants must be prohibited as they may worsen the skin condition. Skin cleansing is appropriate; however, it should be done with lipid-free cleansers. Trauma to the skin must always be avoided. Psoriasis can manifest around sites of skin trauma including surgery. The use of sun protection factor (SPF) of 30 or less is recommended to prevent sunburns, as they can induce disease flare-ups. Loose-fitting clothes are desired to help reduce skin irritation.[21]

Pharmacologic Therapy

The pathogenesis of the disease involves a complex mechanism that disturbs the immune system, causes vascular changes, and the development of skin lesions.[2] It is paramount that therapeutic agents that antagonize these processes are well represented in the treatment of psoriasis. KEY CONCEPT *These agents are anti-inflammatory, anticytokines, and biologic therapies. They are classified into topical, phototherapy, conventional systemic therapy, and biologics.*[2,19]

► *Topical Treatment*

"These agents are marked as first-line treatment for mild to moderate psoriasis (Table 64–2 and 64–3)." They are specifically known for their anti-inflammatory, antiproliferative, and anti-immunologic properties. They are classified as corticosteroids, vitamin D analogues, retinoids, calcineurin inhibitors, anthralin, and salicylic acid derivatives. Different dosage forms are available such as creams, lotions, gels, foams, ointments, shampoos, oil solutions, tapes, and sprays. KEY CONCEPT *The choice of specific dosage form or vehicle is dependent on several factors such as the surface area involved, location, thickness of the lesions, and the appearance of the plaques.*[17,19,22] Ointments are recommended for dry and thick lesions to enhance absorption and reduce loss of skin moisture. Creams are indicated for acute, but moist appearing, lesions that do not require ointment-based products. Solutions and gels are recommended for scalp lesions and foams and sprays are usually used for lesions in genital areas.[21,22]

Vehicle selection is an important consideration and may vary from one body part to another. Ointments and tapes provide occlusion, enhancing drug penetration to improve efficacy. Creams and lotions are easier to spread, especially in hairy areas. Gels may have drying and cooling effects, in addition to easy spreadability. Foams may have enhanced drug delivery and/or efficacy compared to lotions or creams that can become cosmetically elegant liquids upon skin contact, providing good patient acceptance. Shampoos incorporating tar distillates or salicylic acid are useful for scalp psoriasis. Pastes, such as Lassar's paste, have an inherent stiffness, minimizing the spread of medication, and are useful for incorporating drugs such as anthralin, which, especially in higher concentrations used in short-contact methods, may cause skin irritation and burning if in contact with normal skin. It is important to remember that changing to a different vehicle may significantly alter drug potency. For example, a tape formulation (highly occlusive) is much more potent than a cream formulation. Ultimately, the optimal vehicle may be the vehicle that the patient is willing to use. Occlusive ointments may be too

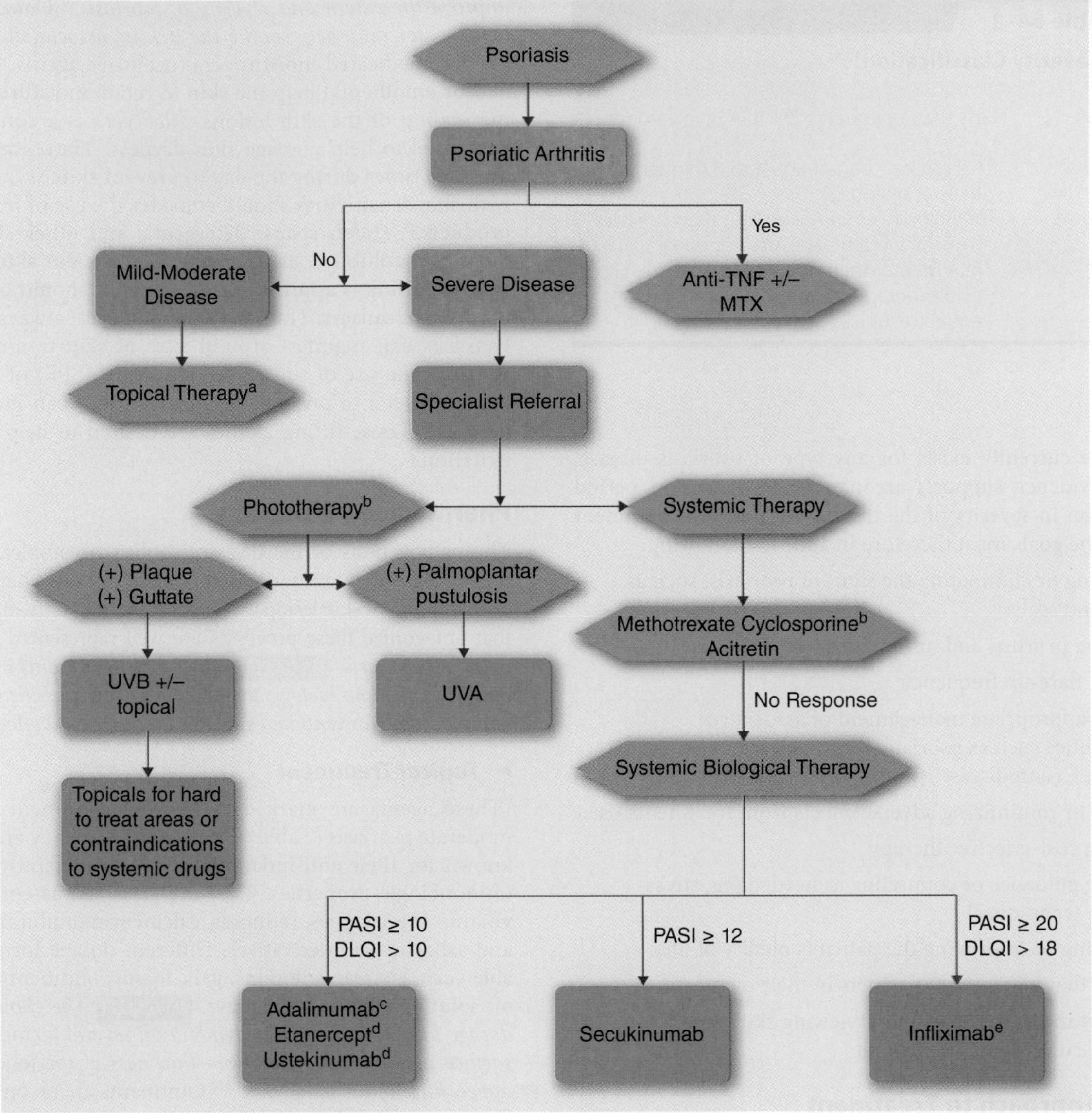

FIGURE 64–1. Treatment algorithm for psoriasis.[5,8,9,21,22,24,27]

[a]Review appointment at 4 weeks for efficacy. [b]Relapse < 50% over 3 months, move to systemic therapy; cyclosporine: no more than 1 year.
[c]Discontinue by 16 weeks if adequate response not met.
[d]Discontinue by 12 weeks if adequate response not met.
[e]Continue treatment beyond 10 weeks if patients shows adequate response.

greasy and cosmetically unappealing, resulting in poor compliance. Sometimes using a cream formulation during the day and an ointment at night may be the best option.[18] Keratolytic agents, such as salicylic acid, are often added to bath oil or shampoos (typically 3%–4%) for scalp psoriasis.[16,21,22] Salicylic acid can also be added to topical corticosteroid preparations to enhance steroid penetration (salicylic acid breaks down keratin).[15,23]

Diagnostic Assessment

Efficacy measurements are guided by three main instruments described as Physicians Global Assessment (PGA) scale, National Psoriasis Foundation-Psoriasis Score (NPF-PS), and PASI with PASI being the most common. Unfortunately, these tools are used predominately in clinical trials and infrequently in clinical practice. The PASI is a scoring instrument that ranges from 0 (absence of disease) to 72 (most severe form of the disease). This tool is commonly used because it takes into consideration severity of the disease and the BSA affected. Effective response to treatment in patients with psoriasis is indicated by a 75% reduction in PASI score.[17]

The National Institute for Health and Care Excellence (NICE) clinical guidelines on psoriasis outline other qualitative measures to be used in assessing the holistic approach to disease management.[1] It emphasizes evaluating the physical, psychological, and social impact of the disease on the patients' quality of life. The impact of psoriasis on the patients' daily living activities should be assessed. Depending on how the patient is coping, advice and support may be needed in the overall treatment plan for

Table 64–2

Topical Medications[2,16,17,23,24]

Actions and Effects	Selected Agents	Criteria	Approach to Therapy	Efficacy Assessment (PGA) Scores	Dosage Form/ Strength	Place in Therapy
Corticosteroids						
Anti-inflammatory Vasoconstriction Immunosuppression Antiproliferative	**Very High Potency** -Bethamethasone -Clobetasol -Diflorasone	Mild to moderate	Monotherapy for acute episode	41%–92% with increase in potency	Ointment Creams Lotions Gel Foams Solutions Shampoo, spray and tape **Available Strengths:** 0.05%–2.5%	First line
	High Potency -Amcinoride -Betamethasone dipropionate and valerate -Desoximetasone		Monotherapy for acute episode			
	Intermediate Potency -Betamethasone -Desoximetasone		Monotherapy for acute episode			
	Low Potency -Alclometasone -Desonide -Hydrocortisone		Monotherapy for acute episode			
Vitamin D Analogues						
Not well-known Vitamin D receptor binding is proposed keratinocytes proliferation is attenuated	Calcipotriene	Mild to moderate	Mono or steroid sparing adjunctive therapy First consideration with steroid when rapid lesion eradication is desired	60%–70%	Cream Scalp solution	First line with or without steroid
	calcitriol			60%–70%	Ointment	
Retinoids						
Not well-known. Modifies gene transcription Decrease inflammation and proliferation due to its retinoid acid receptors binding	Tazarotene	Mild to moderate	Mono or adjunctive therapy with steroid. More effective with high potency steroids	63%	Gel	Second line
Calcineurin Inhibitors						
Decrease lymphokines activity by phosphatase inhibition. Act as immunomudulators	Tacrolimus (Protopic)	Mild to Moderate	Monotherapy for more sensitive areas such as face	65%–70%	**Ointment Strengths:** 0.03% and 0.1%	Third line
	Pimecrolimus (Elidel)	Mild to Moderate	Monotherapy for more sensitive areas of the skin such as face		Cream **Strength:** 1%	

(Continued)

Table 64–2

Topical Medications[2,16,17,23,24] (*Continued*)

OTHER AGENTS						
Moisturizers						
Actions/Effects	**Selected Agents**	**Mild to Moderate**	**Approach to Therapy**	**Partly Indicated**	**Various**	**Not Specified**
Unknown	Nonmedicated moisturizers	Mild to moderate	Commonly used throughout the day	31%	Creams and ointments	
Salicylates						
Acts as a keratolytic agent and reduce lesion scaling to improve absorption of applied medications	Salicylic acid	Mild to moderate	More effective when used as an adjunctive therapy to other topical agents	unknown	Creams Foams Ointments Shampoos **Strengths** 1.8 to 2.5% and 3%	
Anthralin						
Inhibition of T-cell proliferation and migration of neutrophils Keratolytic agent	Anthralin	Mild to moderate	Use infrequently due to irritation	unknown	Creams and shampoos **Strengths** 1%–1.2%	
Coal Tar						
Inhibition of cell proliferation Acts as keratoplastic Agent	Coal tar crude Coal tar combinations (Polytar and Sebutone)	Mild to moderate	Use infrequently due to skin irritation	Unknown	Creams, Gels Shampoo Solutions Lotions Oil **Strengths** 0.5%–3%	

the patient. Efficacy achievement alone may not have the overall desired effect on patients wellbeing.[1,22] Dermatology Quality of Life Scales, Dermatology Life Quality Index (DLQI), Dermatology Specific Quality of Life Instrument, and Skindex-29 are validated instruments that are used to measure these quality outcomes in patients with psoriasis by specialists.[16,22]

Phototherapy for Psoriasis

Phototherapy and photochemotherapy are generally used in the management of moderate to severe disease. Systemic therapies are used for patients with extensive or moderate to severe disease. To minimize drug toxicities or increase efficacy, systemic therapies are sometimes used in conjunction with topical or phototherapy.[15,16]

Phototherapy is traditionally done by using ultraviolet B (UVB) radiation. It can be used as monotherapy or in combination with topical or systemic agents. The UVB disrupts the synthesis of proteins and nucleic acids in skin, which reduces epidermal keratin proliferation. Education should be provided to all patients and include information about the importance of wearing goggles for eye protection. Dosing is administered by the Fitzpatrick skin type, which deals with the skin tones of the patient. Phototherapy may be administered during pregnancy and is considered a first-line therapy.[25]

Photochemotherapy is the administration of phototherapy together with topical or systemic agents.[15,21,25] UVA has a long wavelength, and therapy with UVA is always combined with psoralens (eg, methoxsalen or trioxsalen), which are used as photosensitizers to increase efficacy. The use of psoralens + ultraviolet A (PUVA) for psoriasis causes two types of reaction: (a) an anoxic reaction that affects cellular DNA that inhibits the proliferation of epidermal cells and induces cell death (apoptosis), and (b) an oxygen dependent reaction that gives rise to the formation of free radicals and reactive oxygen that may damage membranes by lipid peroxidation.[26,27]

PUVA (psoralen ultraviolet A therapy) applies to a group of therapies utilizing psoralens to sensitize cells to UVA light.[25] Bath PUVA, topical PUVA, and oral PUVA regimens are available.[15,25] Oral PUVA consists of 8-methoxypsoralen, but in Europe 5-methoxypsoralen is more common. 5-methoxypsoralen is less toxic, but not approved in the United States. Bath PUVA involves soaking in a bath of psoralens (trimethylpsoralen) liquid for 15 minutes prior to UVA treatment and is commonly used in Scandinavian countries for generalized psoriasis to reduce systemic toxicities from psoralens.[19] Topical PUVA uses psoralens directly on the skin, then followed by UVA therapy.[25] Psoralens act much more on cells that are actively dividing than on resting cells. This explains why they are effective only in the active stage of scleroderma and not in the fibrotic stage. Their action on actively dividing or activated immune cells, especially on T cells, explains their action in immune-mediated diseases like psoriasis.

Table 64–3

Topical Medications [2,16,17,23,24]

Drug Class	Dosing and Application	Administration Guidelines	Cautions and Side Effects
Corticosteroid	• Mostly once or twice daily • Every other day or weekends only application may be suitable for chronic conditions • Treatment is recommended for 2–3 weeks • Low and intermediate potency can be used up to 3 months	• Intermediate and low potency agents are indicated for acute and mild lesions and tapering is recommended with the lowest dose when the condition improves • Low potency agents are suitable for lesions in infants due to large body surface area and elderly for the sensitive and thin layer of the skin • High and very high potency agents are indicated for chronic and severe lesions • Palms and soles of the skin require high and very high potency agents to maximize absorption and penetration due to the thickness of the skin	• Skin irritation • Dryness • Withdrawal effects
Vitamin D analogues	Mostly once or twice daily for a maximum of 2 months for effective result	• Recommended to be used with topical steroids to speed up the healing process • Considered less toxic than topical steroids • Combination therapy with steroids has shown to be more effective than the single agent • Onset of action is slow • Avoid calcipotriene use with salicylic acid due to instability of calcipotriene	• Pruritus • Skin irritation on facial area and skin folds • Skin irritation is less with Calcitriol • Skin Rashes • Burning • Changes in systemic vitamin D levels
Retinoids	Preferred as once daily at bedtime	• Best used to achieve better efficacy results with high potent steroids or UVB phototherapy	• Skin irritation • Pruritus • Dryness • Photosensitivity
Calcineurin inhibitors	Mostly once or twice daily depending on the product until effective result is observed	• Comparison data to other agents or in combination is lacking • Use with salicylic acid for 8 weeks showed efficacy improvement in facial lesions	• Skin irritation • Pruritus • Photosensitivity • Risk of malignancy
Other agents **Salicylic acid** **Coal tar** **Anthralin**	As directed	• Decreases the scaling of the skin lesion to allow application of other agents • Infrequent use of Tars and anthralins due to irritation and stain	• Skin irritation • Potential salicylic acid toxicity through nausea and ringing in ears

Patient Encounter, Part 2

Additional relevant information was obtained from the patient, including the following history

FH: Father has psoriasis. Mother passed away 6 months ago from a stroke at the age of 65. Younger sister has Stage I HTN and hyperlipidemia

SH: AD is married with three children: ages 5, 3, and 1. She owns her own landscaping business and tries to join her team in the yards as often as possible. She is an occasional drinker (one to two glasses of wine per week) and admits to smoking when she has "a particularly difficult client"

Meds: Lisinopril 10 mg daily; ibuprofen 400 mg every 8 hours as needed (headaches)

PE:

Gen: She appears very distressed about the lesions

VS: BP 134/87 mm Hg, P 88 beats/min, RR 18 breaths/min, T 37.0°C (98.6°F), Ht 5′ 5″ (165 cm), Wt 175 lb (79.4 kg)

Abd: Soft, NTND; (+) bowel sounds; lesions on abdomen

Exts: Within normal limits; no joint pains; lesions spreading onto arms

Skin: Dark red lesions on abdomen, back, and arms

Labs: All within normal limits, including lipids, renal function tests, and LFTs

What risk factors does she have for psoriasis?

Patient Encounter, Part 3

The diagnosis is that the patient has erythrodermic psoriasis.

Patient expresses to you at this time that she "does not have the best insurance," but she wants something that will take care of her psoriasis.

What nonpharmacologic alternatives are appropriate for this patient?

What pharmacologic agents are appropriate for this patient?

Systemic Therapy

Systemic therapies are usually recommended for moderate to severe psoriasis.[5,15,16,28] These oral agents are classified into immunosuppressants, oral retinoids, T-cell activation inhibitors, cytokine modulators, TNF-α inhibitors, and interleukin 12 and 23 blockers.[1] See Tables 64–4 and 64–5.

Acitretin is an oral retinoid that is likely safer than methotrexate or cyclosporine since potentially serious adverse effects can usually be minimized by appropriate patient selection, careful dosing, and monitoring.[24] Acitretin given concurrently with phototherapy, acitretin +ultraviolet B (ReUVB) or oral retinoid + PUVA (RePUVA), has a synergistic treatment effect. Acitretin monotherapy is usually given for 14 days before instituting UVB or PUVA.[18] The ultraviolet light dose should be reduced by 30% to 50%.[18] ReUVB and RePUVA are well-established treatment regimens for psoriasis.[5,8,9,15,25,28,29]

Acitretin is teratogenic (Pregnancy Category X) and contraindicated in women of childbearing potential. Pregnancy must be avoided during or for 3 years after discontinuation of therapy.[8,9,16,28] Acitretin can transform spontaneously or be converted by ethanol (transesterification) into etretinate, which may take up to 3 years for body clearance.[19] Abstinence from alcoholic beverages should be observed during therapy and for at least 2 months after acitretin is discontinued. Common side effects of acitretin include mucocutaneous dryness and hyperlipidemia.[15,28] Long-term continuous use has caused diffuse idiopathic skeletal hyperostosis (DISH) and periungual pyogenic granulomas.[15,25] Drug interactions include vitamin A (due to the increased risk of hypervitaminosis A), and drugs that interfere with cytochrome P-450 metabolism or have significant plasma albumin binding, which should be used with caution.[25]

Methotrexate is a folic acid antagonist that interferes with purine synthesis and thus inhibits DNA synthesis and cell replication. In addition to the antimitotic effect, it has a specific activity of T-cell suppression and, in low doses, anti-inflammatory and antiproliferative effects.[30] Compared with cyclosporine, methotrexate has a more modest effect but can be used continuously for years, with durable benefits.[15] Folic acid is added to the treatment with methotrexate to reduce gastrointestinal symptoms. It may take up to 4 weeks to see a clinical response after a dose increase.[28] Methotrexate is contraindicated in pregnancy, renal impairment, hepatitis, cirrhosis, alcoholics, unreliable patients, and patients with leukemia or thrombocytopenia.[8,9]

Cyclosporine is an immunosuppressant that specifically inhibits helper T cells and keratinocyte activation and proliferation. Cyclosporine is efficacious in both inducing remission and in maintenance therapy for patients with moderate to severe plaque psoriasis and is also effective in treating pustular, erythrodermic, and nail psoriasis.[15,16,31,32]

Mycophenolate mofetil was found useful in patients with cyclosporine-induced nephrotoxicity as a switch-over agent. Although PASI increased, patients' renal function improved.[33] As adjunctive or monotherapy, there are a few studies in relatively small groups of patients with moderate to severe psoriasis that showed some benefit (at least a 50% reduction in *PASI).*[28,33] For PsA, the systemic drugs used for rheumatoid arthritis are commonly used. This may include NSAIDS, aspirin, but also methotrexate, retinoids, corticosteroids (oral or intrasynovial injection), and cyclooxygenase inhibitors (COX-2s).[8,9]

Patient Encounter, Part 4

The patient was started on methotrexate and has been doing well for 18 months. She reports that her condition was well controlled during this time, but recently, she and her husband have been fighting more frequently and she has noticed the lesions have reappeared. She continued her methotrexate regimen, even after the fighting had stopped and has seen no improvement.

Current Meds: Nonmedicated moisturizer after bathing and ad lib; methotrexate 2.5 mg every 12 hours for a total of three doses per week

What is your main treatment goal for this patient?

What pharmacologic treatments would be appropriate for this patient at this time?

What are the monitoring parameters of your proposed treatment?

Biologic Response Modifiers

Biologic response modifiers (BRMs) are currently recommended for consideration as first-line therapies alongside traditional systemic agents for moderate to severe disease.[15] These are agents employed in the treatment of psoriasis that act by inhibiting various molecular signaling steps of the immunological signaling cascade that are key determinants of the pathogenesis of psoriasis. The following agents are recommended for chronic plaque psoriasis[39]:

1. Inhibitors of TNF, which includes biologic agents such as etanercept, adalimumab, infliximab
2. Inhibitors of interleukin which includes ustekinumab and secukinumab

Their safety profile in comparison with other systemic agents and relatively good acceptability by patients are all positive factors.[13] However, due to a significant cost difference, biologic agents are often reserved for cases in which traditional systemic agents provide inadequate control or for patients with comorbidities such as depression or diabetes (eg, in a patient with PsA or for whom traditional systemic agents may be inappropriate due to potential adverse effects).

Oral apremilast is one of a class of "small molecule" systemic BRMs specifically approved for PsA. It inhibits phosphodiesterase 4 (PDE4) which controls part of the inflammatory actions within cells via cAMP to decrease nitric oxide synthase, TNF-α and interleukin [IL] 23 and increase IL-10. Other BRMs may also be used.

Table 64–4

Systemic Agents[17,39,40]

Drug	Mechanism of Action	Doses and Administration	Dosage Forms	Adverse Effects	Therapeutic Efficacy on PASI 75	Therapeutic Application	Therapeutic Monitoring
Immunosuppressants							
Cyclosporine	An immunosuppressive agent that specifically inhibits helper T cell and keratinocyte activation and proliferation	2.5 mg/kg/day in two divided doses for at least 4 weeks This dose may be subsequently titrated and increased by 0.5 mg/kg/day every 2 weeks until there is control of plaques	Oral and IV solution	Nephrotoxicity, lowering of seizure threshold, tremor, gingival hyperplasia, hypertension, squamous cell carcinoma (cutaneous)	~41%–71%	First-line agent	-LFTs (Baseline and routine) -SCR, BUN -CBC -Uric acid -Blood pressure -Drug Interaction with cytochrome P-450 substrate and inhibitors -pregnancy
Methotrexate	Folic acid antagonist Act by interfering with purine synthesis, thus inhibit DNA synthesis and cell replication	-7.5 to 10 mg weekly -2.5 mg Q12 hours times 3 doses	Oral and injectable	Nausea, vomiting, stomatitis, fatigue, hepatotoxicity, bone marrow suppression, pulmonary fibrosis	24%–60%	First-line agent	-CBC -SCR, BUN -LFTs (baseline and Q 4 weeks) -Pregnancy category X
Oral Retinoids							
Acitretin	Stimulates differentiation and normalizes epidermal cell proliferation	10–50 mg/day	Oral capsule	Myalgia, hair loss, hepatotoxicity, pancreatitis	70%–75%	Second-line agent	Lipids -CBC -SCR, BUN (baseline and every 3 months) -Pregnancy category X

Table 64–5

Biological Therapy[17,34,39-43]

Medication	Mechanism of Action	Dose and Administration	Dosage Forms	Adverse Effects	Therapeutic Effects on PASI	Place in Therapy	Therapeutic Monitoring
Cytokine Modulators-Tumor Necrosis Factors							
Etanercept	Fusion protein that binds to both TNF-α and TNF-β	50 mg SC twice weekly for 12 weeks then 50 mg SC quickly	Subcutaneous solution	Upper respiratory tract infection, nausea, vomiting, headaches Injection site reaction	47%–59% at weeks 12 and 24	Second-line agent	CBC LFTs PPD (tuberculosis)
Adalimumab	Human Monoclonal antibody that targets TNF-α	80 mg SC, first dose then 40 mg SC on week 2, then 40 mg SC Q 2 weeks	Subcutaneous solution	Upper respiratory tract infection, pharyngitis, nausea, dyspepsia, fatigue, headaches Injection site reaction	53%–80% at weeks 12 and 16	First line	CBC LFTs PPD (tuberculosis)
Infliximab	Chimeric monoclonal antibody that targets TNF-α	5 mg/kg IV on weeks 0, 2, 6 and then 5 mg every 8 weeks	Intravenous and subcutaneous solutions	Upper Respiratory Tract Infection, pharyngitis, diarrhea, fatigue, hypersensitivity reaction	76%–82% at weeks 10 and 24	First line	PPD (tuberculosis)
Cytokine Modulators: Interleukin Blockers							
Ustekinumab	Human monoclonal antibody that targets IL12/23 p40	45–90 mg SC on week 0 and 4, then every 12 weeks	Subcutaneous solution	Headache, upper respiratory tract infection pharyngitis, abdominal pain	66%–78% at weeks 12 and 28		None
Secukinumab	Human monoclonal antibody that antagonizes IL17A	300 mg SC at weeks 0, 1, 2, 3, and 4 then 300 mg every 4 weeks	Subcutaneous solution	nasopharyngitis, diarrhea, upper respiratory tract infection	82%–86% at week 12		PPD (tuberculosis), Crohn Disease exacerbations, caution in patients with chronic or recurrent infection

IV, intravenously; SC, subcutaneously.

Table 64–6

Natural Plant Products[35,36,41]

Plant/Product	Plant Taxonomical Family	Evidence	Route of Administration/Dose	Clinical Study Model	References
Aloe vera (AV)	*Liliaceae*	AV improved PASI scores over triamcinolone	Administered topically three times daily for 5 consecutive days per week for 4 weeks	Randomized control trial equivalence design	Choonhakarn et al 2010
Avocado		B12 cream containing avocado oil showed clinical promise in psoriasis	12 weeks study Topical cream	Randomized trial	Stucker et al 2001
Mahonia aquifolium	*Berberidaceae*	Relieva compared to placebo	Topical cream of fruits	Randomized double blind trial	Bernstein et al 2006

▸ *Natural Health Products and Treatments*

Some patients with psoriasis are inclined to use nonmedical and synthetic preparations, such as those containing natural substances. The choice in many cases is motivated by the unwanted side effects and contraindications of conventional medications. These preparations are either used alone or in combination with the medication prescribed by the physician. KEY CONCEPT The following products have clinical evidence in the literature that is inconclusive to support their use in patients with psoriasis. Examples of these products are aloe vera, oil of avocado, and Oregon grape (*Mahonia aqulifolium*).[35–37] Some products have been tested in animal studies but their efficacy has not yet been validated in humans. Examples are capsaicin, chamomile, Indigo, and *naturalis.* A short list of plants and plant products with purported efficacy against psoriasis appears in Table 64–6.

▸ *Investigation Drugs*

KEY CONCEPT *There are several agents including topical, oral and biologic modifiers under investigation at various levels including the combination of topical corticosteroids with vitamin D analogues. Micellar paclitaxel, voclosporin, and pioglitazone are among the oral agents currently being studied.* Biological agents such as IL-11 inhibitor daclizumab, IL-10, protein kinase blocker AEB071, IL-12 and 23 monoclonal antibodies are all in the pipeline under various stages of investigations.[2,17]

OUTCOME EVALUATION

- Monitor for clearance of skin lesions. Depending on the agent(s) used and site of lesions, it may take 2 to 6 weeks or longer to see a response. Complete clearance may not be achieved for all patients.
- Monitor for specific adverse effects and drug interactions, depending on agent(s) used.
- Methotrexate: Monitor CBC and liver function tests at baseline and on a regular basis. Consider liver biopsy prior to treatment and again at a cumulative dose of 1.5 g for high-risk patients.
- Cyclosporine: Monitor serum creatinine, blood urea nitrogen, serum lipids, magnesium, and blood pressure at baseline. Reassess biweekly for at least 12 weeks or until drug levels stabilize then adjust doses accordingly.
- Acitretin: Monitor serum lipids, liver function tests and perform pregnancy testing.
- Topical corticosteroids: Monitor for skin thinning, irritation telangiectasias, and possible hypothalamic–pituitary–adrenal axis suppression.
- Total clearance of skin disease is not impossible during periods of remission; remissions may be days, months, years, and even decades in length with patients being weaned from their medications entirely or have them reduced to a low maintenance dose.

DISCUSSION

Several factors must be taken into consideration in identifying the right therapy for a patient with psoriasis. Some of these factors are the affected area of the disease, cost, availability of medication, and the preferred lifestyle of the patient. Full patient history including allergies must be collected to make therapeutic approach a success. Topical agents are recommended for mild to moderate disease due to the low cost and fewer adverse effects of the products. Low potency corticosteroids are used as first line for mild conditions. If the condition persists, it is recommended to switch to a very high potency steroid in combination with vitamin D analogue or topical retinoids. In general, a patient disease surface area should be less than 5% to qualify for topical therapy. A general recommendation after unsuccessful treatment with topical agents is to add phototherapy. PUVA was found to be more effective that UVB in the treatment of patients with moderate to severe psoriasis.[38] The traditional systemic agents should be the next in line for patients with severe diseases. Clinical trials indicate that immunosuppressants are more effective than oral retinoids. Due to the cost associated with biological agents, they are reserved as a last resort for patients with severe diseases not responding to traditional systemic agents or intolerant to the side effects of these agents. Biologics are known for their fewer adverse effects. The choice of biologic agents depends on the patient's preference. Infliximab and adalimumab are more effective than alefacept or etanercept. A disease affecting more than 5% of the BSA should be the justification for initiating systemic therapy. For patients with liver disease, kidney dysfunction, and skin cancer, it is recommended to avoid methotrexate, cyclosporine, and PUVA treatment, respectively.[17,19,24]

SUMMARY

It should be recognized that psoriasis is a chronic disease with no current cure but requires lifelong management of the disease state. No two cases of psoriasis are identical and treatment modalities must be tailored to the patient with the help of a dermatologist. The disease can severely impact the patients' quality of life by affecting their physical, psychological, and social well-being. The NICE guidelines recommend a holistic approach in assessing all areas of life in caring for patients that live with this disease.

Patient Care Process

Patient Assessment:

- Based on physical exam and review of systems, determine severity of disease.
- Review medical history: What risk factors does the patient have? Does the patient have any comorbid conditions?
- Conduct medication history: Include prescriptions, OTC products, herbal and dietary supplements. Does the patient have any drug allergies? Is this patient experiencing side effects from a medication? What have they tried already?

Therapy Evaluation:

- Is pharmacologic therapy indicated based on current presentation?
- Would patient benefit from nonpharmacologic therapy?
- If patient is already receiving treatment, assess efficacy, safety, and adherence. Are there any significant drug interactions with patients other medications?
- What kind of prescription coverage does the patient have? Determine if recommended agents are included on the institution's formulary.

Care Plan Development:

- Select lifestyle and nonpharmacologic therapy that are likely to be effective and safe.
- Determine if drug doses are optimal. Utilize combination therapy when appropriate to take advantage of synergistic effects and to reduce side effects.
- Address patient concerns about psoriasis.
- Discuss importance of medication adherence and lifestyle modifications to reduce psoriasis.
- Give patients an approximate time frame for improvement.
- Counsel on appropriate application techniques, administration, and potential toxicities of drug therapy.
- Interact with patient's other health care providers to discuss pertinent information about the patient's care.
- Reinforce importance of regular follow-up visits.

Follow-up Evaluation:

- Follow-up at appropriate intervals to assess effectiveness and safety of therapy.
- Review physical exam findings, labs, and other pertinent diagnostic tests.

ACKNOWLEDGMENTS

The authors and editors wish to acknowledge and thank Dr. Rebecca Law, the primary author of this chapter in the 3rd edition of this book. Additionally, the current authors would like to acknowledge the student research assistants that contributed to this chapter, Sarah Anderson, Rebecca Kyper, Heather Rose, and Rebecca Widder from Cedarville University School of Pharmacy.

Abbreviations Introduced in This Chapter

BB-UVB	Broadband ultraviolet B
BRM	Biologic response modifier
BSA	Body surface area
cAMP	Cyclic 3'-5'-adenosine monophosphate
DISH	Diffuse idiopathic skeletal hyperostosis
IF-γ	Interferon-γ
IL-2	Interleukin-2
IL-10	Interleukin-10
IL-12/23	Interleukin-12 and interleukin-23
LFT	Liver function test
NSAIDs	Nonsteroidal anti-inflammatory drugs
PASI	Psoriasis Area and Severity Index
PPD	Purified protein derivative
PUVA	Psoralen ultraviolet A therapy
Q	Every
PsA	Psoriatic arthritis
RePUVA	Oral retinoid + PUVA
ReUVB	Acitretin + ultraviolet B
TNF	Tumor necrosis factor
UVB	Ultraviolet B

REFERENCES

1. Smith CH, Samarasekera EJ. Psoriasis: Guidance on assessment and referral. Clin Med. 2014;14(2):178–182.
2. Papoutsaki M, Costanzo A. Treatment of psoriasis and psoriatic arthritis. Biodrugs. 2013;27(Suppl 1):3–12.
3. Perera GK, Di Meglio P, Nestle FO. Psoriasis. Annu Rev Pathol. 2012;7:385–422.
4. Godic A. New approaches to psoriasis treatment. A review. Acta Dermatovenerol Alp Panonica Adriat. 2004;13(2):50–57.
5. Menter A, Korman NJ, Elmets CA, et al. Guidelines of care for the management of psoriasis and psoriatic arthritis: Section 6. Guidelines of care for the treatment of psoriasis and psoriatic arthritis: Case-based presentations and evidence-based conclusions. J Am Acad Dermatol. 2011;65(1):137–174.
6. Kimball AB, Gladman D, Gelfand JM, et al. National Psoriasis Foundation clinical consensus on psoriasis comorbidities and recommendations for screening. J Am Acad Dermatol. 2008;58 (6):1031–1042.
7. Kremers HM, McEvoy MT, Dann FJ, et al. Heart disease in psoriasis. J Am Acad Dermatol. 2007;57(2):347–354.
8. Menter A. Gottlieb A, Feldman SR, et al. Guidelines of care for the management of psoriasis and psoriatic arthritis: Section 1. Overview of psoriasis and guidelines of care for the treatment of psoriasis with biologics. J Am Acad Dermatol. 2008;58(5):826–850.
9. Gottlieb A, Korman NJ, Gordon KB, et al. Guidelines of care for the management of psoriasis and psoriatic arthritis: Section 2. Psoriatic arthritis: Overview and guidelines of care for treatment with an emphasis on the biologics. J Am Acad Dermatol. 2008;59(5):851–864.

10. Kreuter A, Sommer A, Hyun J, et al. 1% pimecrolimus, 0.005% calcipotriol, and 0.1% betamethasone in the treatment of intertriginous psoriasis: A double-blind randomized controlled study. Arch Dermatol. 2006;142(9):1136–1143.
11. Ashcroft D, Po A, Williams H, et al. Systematic review of comparative efficacy and tolerability of calcipotriol in treating chronic plaque psoriasis. BMJ. 2000;320(7240):963–967.
12. Umapathy S, Pawar A, Mitra R, et al. HLA-A and HLA-B alleles associated in psoriasis patients from Mumbai, Western India. Indian J Dermatol. 2011;56(5):497.
13. Jankovic S, Raznatovic M, Marinkovic J, Jankovic J, Maksimovic N. Risk factors for psoriasis: A case–control study. J Dermatol. 2009;36(6):328–334.
14. Ellis CN, Krueger GG. Treatment of chronic plaque psoriasis by selective targeting of memory effector T lymphocytes. N Engl J Med. 2001;345(4):248–255.
15. Papp K, Gulliver W, Lynde C, Poulin Y, Ashkenas J, Canadian Psoriasis Guidelines Committee. Canadian guidelines for the management of plaque psoriasis: Overview. J Cutan Med Surg. 2011;15(4):210–219.
16. Law RM, Gulliver WP. Chapter 78. Psoriasis. In: DiPiro JT, Talbert RL, Yee GC, Matzke GR, Wells BG, Posey LM, eds. Pharmacotherapy: A Pathophysiologic Approach, 9th ed. New York, NY: McGraw-Hill; 2014.
17. Ballantini K, Flesner J, Pitlick M. Plaque psoriasis: A review of recent guidelines and pharmacologic therapies. Formulary. 2011;46:18–26.
18. Mason A, Mason J,Cork M, Hancock H, Dooley G. Topical treatments for chronic plaque psoriasis: An abridged Cochrane systematic review. J Am Acad Dermatol. 2013;69(5):799–807.
19. Loss LC and Kalb RE. Psoriasis therapy. Dermatol Nurs. 2010:22(5):15–20.
20. Rosenkranz MA, Davidson RJ, MacCoon DG, Sheridan JF, Kalin NH, Lutz A. A comparison of mindfulness-based stress reduction and an active control in modulation of neurogenic inflammation. Brain Behav Immun. 2013;27:174–184.
21. Menter A, Korman NJ, Elmets CA, et al. Guidelines of care for the management of psoriasis and psoriatic arthritis. Section 3. Guidelines of care for the management and treatment of psoriasis with topical therapies. J Am Acad Dermatol. 2009;60(4):643–659.
22. Psoriasis: The assessment and management of psoriasis. NICE 153 clinical guidelines 2012. http://guidance.nice.org.uk/cg153. Updated October 2012. Accessed April 7, 2014.
23. Lexi-Comp Online", Lexi-Drugs Online", Hudson, Ohio: Lexi-Comp, Inc.; 2014; August 15, 2014.
24. Feldman SR, Matheson R, Bruce S, et al. Efficacy and safety of calcipotriene 0.005% foam for the treatment of plaque-type psoriasis: Results of two multicenter, randomized, double-blind, vehicle-controlled phase III clinical trials. Am J Clin Dermatol. 2012;13(4):261–271.
25. Menter A, Korman NJ, Elmets CA, et al. Guidelines of care for the management of psoriasis and psoriatic arthritis: Section 5. Guidelines of care for the treatment of psoriasis with phototherapy and photochemotherapy. J Am Acad Dermatol. 2010;62(1):114–135.
26. Mouli P, Selvakumar T, Kumar S, Parthiban S, Priya R, Deivanayagi M. Photochemotherapy: A review. Internat J Nutrit, Pharmacol, Neurological Dis. 2013;3(3):229–235.
27. Benáková N. Phototherapy of psoriasis in the era of biologics: Still in. Acta Dermatovenerol Croat. 2011;19(3):195–205.
28. Menter A, Korman NJ, Elmets CA, et al. Guidelines of care for the management of psoriasis and psoriatic arthritis: Section 4. Guidelines of care for the management and treatment of psoriasis with traditional systemic agents. J Am Acad Dermatol. 2009;61(3): 451–485.
29. Schon MP, Boehncke WH. Psoriasis. N Engl J Med. 2005;352(18): 1899–1912.
30. Kalb RE, Strober B, Weinstein G, Lebwohl M. Methotrexate and psoriasis: 2009 National Psoriasis Foundation Consensus Conference. J Am Acad Dermatol. 2009;60(5):824–837.
31. Rosmarin DM, Lebwohl M, Elewski BE, et al. Cyclosporine and psoriasis: 2008 National psoriasis Foundation Consensus Conference. J Am Acad Dermatol. 2010;62(5):838–853.
32. Amor KT, Ryan C, Menter A. The use of cyclosporine in dermatology: Part I. J Am Acad Dermatol. 2010;63(6):925–946.
33. Walsh SRA, Shear NH. Psoriasis and the new biologic agents: Interrupting a T-AP dance. CMAJ. 2004;170(13):1933–1941.
34. Panchal MR, Coope H, McKenna DJ, Alexandroff AB. Long-term safety of biologics in the treatment of psoriasis. Psoriasis: Targets and Therapy. 2014;4: 1–9.
35. Stücker M, Memmel U, Hoffmann M, Hartung J, Altmeyer P. Vitamin B12 cream containing avocado oil in the therapy of plaque psoriasis. Dermatology. 2001;203(2):141–147.
36. Choonhakarn C, Busaracome P, Sripanidkulchai B, Sarakarn P. A prospective, randomized clinical trial comparing topical aloe vera with 0.1% triamcinolone acetonide in mild to moderate plaque psoriasis. J Eur Acad Dermatol Venereol. 2010;24(2):168–172.
37. Bernstein S, Donsky H, Gulliver W, Hamilton D, Nobel S, Norman R. Treatment of mild to moderate psoriasis with Relieva, a Mahonia aquifolium extract a double blind placebo controlled study. Am J Ther. 2006;13(2):121–126.
38. Almutawa F, Alnomair N, Wang Y, Hamzavi I, Lim HW. Systematic review of UV-based therapy for psoriasis. Am J Clin Dermatol. 2013;14:87–109.
39. Boca AN, Badalica-Petrescu M, Buzoianu AD. Current therapeutic options in psoriasis. International Journal of Bioflux Society. 2014;6(1):6–10.
40. Nelson AA, Pearce DJ, Fleisher AN, Balkrishhan R, Feldman SR. New treatments for psoriasis. Which biologic is best? J Dermatol Treat. 2006;17(2):96–107.
41. Leonardi CL1, Powers JL, Matheson RT, et al. Etanercept as monotherapy in patients with psoriasis. N Engl J Med. 2003;349(21):2014–2022.
42. Ohtsuki M, Morita A, Abe M, et al. Secukinumab efficacy and safety in Japanese patients with moderate-to-severe plaque psoriasis: Subanalysis from ERASURE, a randomized, placebo-controlled, phase 3 study. J Dermatol. 2014;41(12):1039–1046.
43. Paul C, Lacour JP, Tedremets L, et al. Efficacy, safety and usability of secukinumab administration by autoinjector/pen in psoriasis: A randomized, controlled trial (JUNCTURE). J Eur Acad Dermatol Venereol. 2014.

65 Common Skin Disorders

Laura A. Perry and Lori J. Ernsthausen

LEARNING OBJECTIVES

Upon completion of the chapter, the reader will be able to:

1. Describe the pathophysiology of common skin disorders.
2. Assess the signs and symptoms of common skin disorders in a presenting patient.
3. List the goals of treatment for patients with common skin disorders.
4. Select appropriate nonpharmacologic and pharmacologic treatment regimens for patients presenting with common skin disorders.
5. Identify adverse effects that may result from pharmacologic agents used in the treatment of common skin disorders.
6. Develop a monitoring plan that will assess the safety and efficacy of the overall disease state management of common skin disorders.
7. Create educational information for patients about common skin disorders, including appropriate self-management, available drug treatment options, and anticipated therapeutic responses.

INTRODUCTION

Several thousand skin disorders are currently documented, and many patients seek the assistance of a health care provider when a complication with their skin develops. Others will utilize self-care to effectively treat their symptoms.

This chapter discusses acne vulgaris, contact dermatitis (irritant and allergic), and diaper dermatitis; other common skin and soft tissue infections and superficial fungal infections are discussed in Chapters 73 and 83, respectively. Providing patients with appropriate therapy options, as well as patient education on treatment and prevention, will assist the successful management of many common skin disorders.

ACNE VULGARIS

Acne vulgaris is an inflammatory skin disorder of the pilosebaceous units of the skin. Although most commonly seen on the face, acne can also be present on the chest, back, neck, and shoulders (Figure 65–1).[1] Acne is not just a self-limiting disorder of teenagers. The clinical course of acne can be prolonged or recur, resulting in long-term physical complications such as extensive scarring and psychological distress.[2]

EPIDEMIOLOGY AND ETIOLOGY

With an estimated 40 to 50 million people affected, acne vulgaris is the number one skin disease in the United States.[3] Acne affects approximately 85% of adolescents and adults aged 12 to 25 years, with severity of acne correlating with pubertal maturity.[3,4] Additionally, acne may persist beyond puberty and has been found to affect 64% and 43% of individuals into the 1920s and 1930s, respectively. Acne is more likely to occur in males during adolescence and females during adulthood. Individuals with a positive family history of acne have been shown to develop more severe cases of acne at an earlier age. Prevalence of acne among ethnic groups is similar.[4]

While the link between diet and acne has continued to be controversial, there is evidence to suggest that high glycemic load diets may exacerbate acne.[5,6] Local irritation from occlusive clothing or athletic equipment, oil-based cosmetics or beauty products, prolonged sweating or environments of high humidity, and a variety of medications may also worsen acne.[7]

PATHOPHYSIOLOGY

KEY CONCEPT *The development of acne lesions results from four pathogenic factors: excess sebum production, keratinization, bacterial growth, and inflammation.*[1,2,6]

The pilosebaceous unit of the skin consists of a hair follicle and the surrounding sebaceous glands. An initial acne lesion, called a comedo, forms when there is a blockage in the pilosebaceous unit.

Sebum is released by the sebaceous glands and naturally maintains hair and skin hydration. Increased androgen levels, especially during puberty, can cause an increased size of the sebaceous gland and production of abnormally high levels of sebum within those glands. This excess sebum can result in plugged follicles and acne formation.

Keratinization, the sloughing of epithelial cells in the hair follicle, is also a natural process. In acne, however, *hyper*keratinization occurs and causes increased adhesiveness of the sloughed cells. Accumulation of these cells clogs the hair follicle, blocks the flow of sebum, and forms an acne lesion called an open comedo or "blackhead."

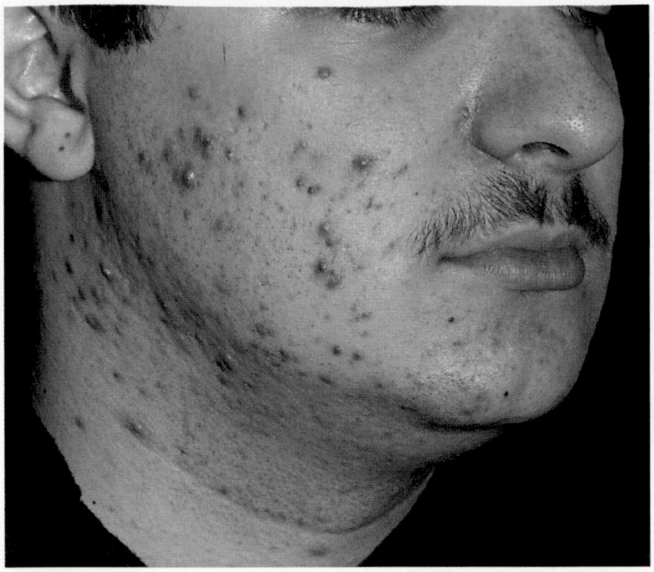

FIGURE 65–1. Twenty-year-old man. In this case of papulopustular acne, some inflammatory papules become nodular and thus represent early stages of nodulocystic acne. (From Wolff K, Johnson RA. Disorders of sebaceous and apocrine glands. Fitzpatrick's Color Atlas & Synopsis of Clinical Dermatology. 6th ed. New York: McGraw-Hill; 2009: 3.)

Propionibacterium acnes (*P. acnes*), an anaerobic organism, is also found in the normal flora of the skin. This bacteria proliferates in the mixture of sebum and keratinocytes and can result in an inflammatory response producing a closed comedo or "whitehead." More severe acne lesions such as pustules, papules, and nodules also form with inflammatory acne and result in significant scarring if treated inadequately.

TREATMENT

Desired Outcomes and Goals

Although traditionally thought of as a self-limiting disorder, acne can have patterns of recurrence. Because acne cannot be cured, proper treatment must involve both short-term and long-term strategies. KEY CONCEPT Goals of therapy are to (1) *Reduce the number and severity of existing lesions,* (2) *Prevent the development of new lesions, and* (3) *Prevent long-term disfigurement and permanent scarring.*[6,10] Acne can cause psychological symptoms of stress, anxiety, frustration, embarrassment, and even depression.[2,6] Evaluating both physical and psychological aspects of acne is imperative.

General Approach to Treatment

KEY CONCEPT *Acne treatment regimens should be based on acne severity and type of acne lesion. Other factors such as response to previous treatment, patient preference, cost and adherence should also be considered.* Topical therapy is considered first line for mild acne with oral therapies added to topical therapy in moderate to severe acne. Optimal management includes induction and maintenance therapy.[2,9] Improvement of symptoms following induction therapy occurs gradually, sometimes taking 6 to 8 weeks for results to be physically apparent.[6] Patients need to be educated on continual treatment compliance during this time and should not get discouraged if acne lesions appear to worsen before getting better. Maintenance therapy should begin after 12 weeks of induction therapy and continues for 3 to 4 months.[6,9]

Nonpharmacologic Therapy

There is significant variance in the clinical benefit of many nonpharmacologic interventions for acne vulgaris. Patients should be counseled to avoid aggressive skin washing and to use a mild, noncomedogenic facial soap twice daily. Furthermore, discourage the use of abrasive cleansers and manipulating or squeezing

Clinical Presentation and Diagnosis of Acne

Acne lesions are most often seen on the face, but can also present on the chest, back, neck, and shoulders and are described as either noninflammatory or inflammatory. Severe inflammatory lesions may lead to scarring and hyperpigmentation.

Noninflammatory Lesions

Open comedo or "blackhead": A plugged follicle of sebum, keratinocytes, and bacteria that protrudes from the surface of the skin and appears black or brown in color. Although dark in color, blackheads do not indicate the presence of dirt, but rather, an accumulation of melanin.

Closed comedo or "whitehead": A plugged follicle of sebum, keratinocytes, and bacteria that remains beneath the surface of the skin. Closed comedos usually appear as small white bumps about 1 to 2 mm in diameter.

Inflammatory Lesions

Papules: Solid, elevated lesion less than 0.5 cm in diameter

Pustules: Vesicles filled with purulent fluid less than 0.5 cm in diameter

Nodules: Lesions greater than 0.5 cm in both width and depth

Cysts: Nodules filled with a fluid or semisolid that can be expressed

Scars

Inflammatory acne can result in permanent scarring that ranges from small depressed pits to large elevated blemishes.

Hyperpigmentation

Inflammatory acne may result in hyperpigmentation of the skin that can last for weeks to months.

Diagnosis

The diagnosis of acne vulgaris is clinical. Lesion cultures may be warranted when treatment regimens fail to rule out other skin infections.

Assessment

No standard acne grading scale has been identified. While several grading scale exist,[2,8,9] most clinicians describe acne as mild (few noninflammatory lesions), moderate (many inflammatory lesions) or severe (numerous severe inflammatory lesions and evidence of scarring).

lesions to minimize scarring. Use of an oil-free, noncomedogenic moisturizer may improve the tolerability of topical drug therapy.[7]

Pharmacologic Therapy

▸ *Topical Agents*

Benzoyl Peroxide Benzoyl peroxide is easy to use and is recommended as an alternative to or in combination with topical retinoids or topical antibiotics in the treatment of acne of all severities.[2,9] Benzoyl peroxide has a comedolytic effect that increases the rate of epithelial cell turnover and helps to unclog blocked pores. It also has antibacterial activity against *P. acnes*, which appears to be the main reason for its effectiveness.[11,12]

Benzoyl peroxide is available with or without a prescription and remains the most commonly purchased over-the-counter topical treatment for acne.[7] Some data suggests that lower strengths offer similar efficacy to higher strengths. Beginning benzoyl peroxide treatment regimen with the lowest strength and titrating to higher effective strengths over several weeks, if needed, will reduce the incidence of localized adverse effects. Newer formulations of benzoyl peroxide are combined with moisturizers to help decrease skin redness and irritation.[11,12]

A typical regimen for benzoyl peroxide is to apply the product to clean, dry skin no more than two times a day. The strength and dosage form selected may vary from patient to patient depending on acne severity and the sensitivity of the patient's skin. Gel preparations are the most potent dosage form. Patients with dry or overly sensitive skin should try a cream, lotion, or facial wash first.[6] If severe irritation or an allergic reaction develops, benzoyl peroxide should be discontinued. Table 65–1 describes available products and adverse effects.

Retinoids Highly effective in the treatment of acne, retinoids stimulate epithelial cell turnover and aid in unclogging blocked pores. Retinoids also exhibit anti-inflammatory properties through the inhibition of neutrophil and monocyte chemotaxis.[11] Due to the ability to target multiple pathogenic features of acne, topical retinoids are recommended as first-line therapy for induction and maintenance regimens in all forms of acne. Although success is seen with monotherapy, using topical retinoids in combination with benzoyl peroxide or topical antibacterial agents is preferred for inflammatory acne lesions.[2,9]

Available topical retinoids include tretinoin, adapalene, and tazarotene. Adapalene is considered the drug of first choice because it has similar efficacy and a lower incidence of adverse effects.[9,13] Newer formulations involving a microsphere gel (Retin-A Micro) or prepolyolprepolymer-2 gel or cream (Avita) gradually release the active ingredient over time and may also cause less initial skin discomfort.[13] Table 65–1 describes available products and adverse effects of topical retinoids.

Topical retinoids should be applied once daily at bedtime, beginning with a low-potency formulation. Increased strengths are then initiated according to treatment results and tolerance. Patients should be advised that a worsening of acne symptoms generally occurs in the first few weeks of therapy, with lesion improvement occurring in 3 to 4 months.[14,15] The use of topical retinoids should be avoided in children younger than 12 years and in pregnant women.[13]

Antibacterials Topical antibacterials directly suppress *P. acnes* and are first-line agents used in combination with benzoyl peroxide, topical retinoids or azelaic acid for the treatment of mild to moderate inflammatory acne. To reduce the likelihood of bacterial resistance, topical antibiotics should never be used as monotherapy or as long-term maintenance therapy.[2,9]

Clindamycin and erythromycin preparations, applied once or twice daily for 3 months, have similar effects and are the most commonly prescribed topical antibacterial agents.[2,9,11] These agents are available in various formulations and combinations with benzoyl peroxide and retinoids. Table 65–1 describes the strengths, formulations, and adverse effects of the available antimicrobial agents.

Azelaic Acid With antibacterial and anti-inflammatory properties, and the ability to stabilize keratinization, azelaic acid is an effective alternative in the treatment of mild to moderate acne in patients who cannot tolerate benzoyl peroxide or topical retinoids.[2,9,15] It can also even out skin tone and may prove effective in patients who are prone to postinflammatory hyperpigmentation resulting from acne.[15,16] Azelaic acid 20% cream should be applied twice daily, with improvement of symptoms seen in 4 weeks.[15]

Dapsone Dapsone gel, a sulfone drug, has antimicrobial and anti-inflammatory properties.[17] Although approved for the treatment of mild to moderate acne, due to the lack of comparative efficacy trials, current guidelines do not comment on the place of dapsone in the treatment of acne.[2,9]

Dapsone 5% (Aczone) is a gritty gel that should be applied in a thin layer to the affected areas twice daily. If no improvement is seen after 12 weeks, treatment should be reevaluated.[18]

Keratolytics Sulfur, resorcinol, and salicylic acid are not as effective as other topical agents, but can be used as second-line therapies in the treatment of mild to moderate acne.[2,7]

Although these agents may cause less skin irritation than benzoyl peroxide or the topical retinoids, several disadvantages exist. Sulfur preparations produce an unpleasant odor when applied to the skin, whereas resorcinol may cause brown scaling. And although rare, the possibility of salicylism exists with continual salicylic acid use.[7,15]

▸ *Oral Agents*

Antibacterials Moderate to severe acne can be effectively treated with oral antibiotics, especially when treatment with topical therapy has failed.[2,9] Because of the ability to decrease *P. acnes* colonization, oral antibiotics can prevent acne lesions from developing. Use of oral antibiotics should be limited to short periods of time, ideally 3 months or less. Assessment of response to oral antibiotics after 6 to 8 weeks of therapy is recommended. As with topical antibiotics, oral antibiotics should never be used as monotherapy or as long-term maintenance therapy. Additionally, the use of topical antibiotics in combination with oral antibiotics is should be avoided.[2]

Tetracycline, doxycycline, and minocycline are the most commonly prescribed oral antibiotics for acne. Erythromycin, azithromycin, and trimethoprim (± sulfamethoxazole) are appropriate second-line agents for use when patients cannot tolerate or have developed resistance to tetracycline or its derivatives. Although effectiveness is similar to the tetracyclines, erythromycin use is often limited due to potential adverse outcomes and increased bacterial resistance.[19] (See Table 65–2 for antibiotic dosing guidelines and adverse effects.)

Isotretinoin Isotretinoin works on the four pathogenic factors that contribute to acne development and can produce acne remission rates of up to several years. Oral isotretinoin is Food and Drug Administration (FDA) approved for patients with severe recalcitrant nodular acne unresponsive to other topical and oral treatment regimens. Although studies are lacking, expert clinicians suggest that oral isotretinoin may be useful in treatment resistant acne of lower severity.[2,9] Contrary to some expert clinicians, the 2012 European Guidelines suggest that oral

Table 65–1

Topical Agents Used in the Treatment of Acne

Drug	Brand	Dosage Form	Adverse Reactions	Comments
Retinoids				
Tretinoin	Atralin Avita	0.05% gel 0.025% cream; 0.025% gel 0.025%, 0.05%, 0.1% cream	Erythema, dryness, scaling, stinging/burning, pruritus, initially may worsen acne	Local adverse reactions most likely occur in first 2 to 4 weeks of use and will usually lessen with continued use.
	Retin-A Retin-A Micro Tretin-X	0.01%, 0.025% gel 0.04%, 0.1% gel 0.038%, 0.075% cream	Possibly teratogenic Photosensitivity	Category C. Use cautiously in pregnancy. Minimize exposure to sun light and sun lamps. Sunscreen use and protective clothing recommended.
Tazarotene	Tazorac Fabior	0.05%, 0.1% cream 0.05%, 0.1% gel 0.1% foam	Erythema, dryness, scaling, stinging/burning, pruritus, initially may worsen acne Teratogenic Photosensitivity	Local adverse reactions most likely occur in first 2 to 4 weeks of use and will usually lessen with continued use. Category X. Use in pregnancy is contraindicated. Minimize exposure to sun light and sun lamps. Sunscreen use and protective clothing recommended.
Adapalene	Differin	0.1% cream 0.1%, 0.3% gel 0.1% lotion	Erythema, dryness, scaling, stinging/burning, pruritus, initially may worsen acne Photosensitivity	Local adverse reactions most likely occur in first 2 to 4 weeks of use and will usually lessen with continued use Less irritation compared to other retinoids. Minimize exposure to sun light and sun lamps. Sunscreen use and protective clothing recommended.
Other topical Agents				
Benzoyl peroxide	1%–10%, Various over the counter and prescription products	Lotion, gel, foam, pads	Excessive drying, peeling, erythema, allergic contact sensitization/ dermatitis Bleaching of hair and colored fabric. Photosensitivity	Local reactions are dose dependent. Gradually increase dose as tolerance develops. Minimize exposure to sun light and sun lamps. Sunscreen use and protective clothing recommended. Pregnancy Category C
Azelaic Acid	Azelex	20% cream	Erythema, skin irritation	Alternative to benzoyl peroxide. Pregnancy Category B
Clindamycin	Cleocin T Clindagel ClindaMax Evoclin BenzaClin Duac	1% solution, lotion, gel 1% gel 1% gel, lotion 1% foam 1%–5% benzoyl peroxide combination gel 1.2%–5% benzoyl peroxide combination gel	Burning, itching, dryness, erythema, peeling Diarrhea, colitis (pseudomembranous colitis)	Rare cases of colitis have been observed with topical use. Discontinue immediately and seek medical attention if diarrhea occurs. Should be combined with topical benzoyl peroxide.
Erythromycin	ERYGEL Ery Benzamycin	2% gel 2% pad 5%–3% benzoyl peroxide combination gel	Burning, peeling, dryness, pruritus, erythema	Should be combined with topical benzoyl peroxide.
Dapsone	Aczone	5% gel	Dryness, erythema, oiliness, and peeling	Does not have a risk of phototoxicity.

Data from (1) Lexicomp [Internet]. Hudson (OH): Wolters Kluwer Health, Inc.1978-2014 [cited 2014 July 25]. http://online.lexi.com/lco/action/home/switch. (2) Facts & Comparisons eAnswers. St. Louis (MO) 2014: Wolters Kluwer health, Inc. 2014 [cited 2014 July 25]. http://online.factsandcomparisons.com/index.aspx

Table 65–2

Oral Agents Used in the Treatment of Acne

Drug	Dosage form (mg)	Dosing Regimen	Adverse Reactions	Comments
Oral Antibiotics				
Tetracycline	250, 500 capsule	250–500 mg twice daily	GI upset, headache, blurry vision, vaginal candidiasis, possible teratogenic risk, tooth discoloration in children Photosensitivity Drug–food interactions	Avoid use in in children < 8 years. Pregnancy Category D. Avoid use in pregnancy. Minimize exposure to sun light and sun lamps. Sunscreen use and protective clothing recommended. Take 1 hour before or 2 hours after dairy products, antacids, vitamins, or iron supplements.
Doxycycline	50, 75, 100 tablets and capsules 200 delayed-release tablet	Immediate release: 50–100 mg once or twice daily Extended release: 200 mg once daily	GI upset, headache, blurry vision, possible teratogenic risk, tooth discoloration in children Photosensitivity Drug–food interactions	Avoid use in in children < 8 years. Pregnancy Category D. Avoid use in pregnancy. Minimize exposure to sun light and sun lamps. Sunscreen use and protective clothing recommended. Take 1 hour before or 2 hours after dairy products, antacids, vitamins, or iron supplements.
Minocycline	50, 75, 100 immediate-release tablets 45, 55, 65, 80, 90, 105, 115, 135 extended-release tablets 50, 75, 100 immediate release capsules	Immediate release: 50–100 mg twice daily. Extended release: 1 mg/kg daily for 12 weeks.	GI upset, headache, blurry vision, lupus-like syndrome, hepatitis, exfoliative dermatitis, possible teratogenic risk, tooth discoloration in children Photosensitivity Drug–food interactions	Avoid use in in children < 8 years. Pregnancy Category D. Avoid use in pregnancy. Minimize exposure to sun light and sun lamps. Sunscreen use and protective clothing recommended. Take 1 hour before or 2 hours after dairy products, antacids, vitamins, or iron supplements.
Erythromycin	250, 500 tablets	250–500 mg twice daily	GI upset, rash, hearing loss, hypersensitivity reactions	Highest incidence of GI intolerance and increasing bacterial resistance. Possible drug interactions: CYP3A4 substrate and P-glycoprotein inhibitor Alternative to tetracyclines. Drug of choice in pregnant women and children < 8 years.
Azithromycin	500 tablet	500 mg per dose 2 to 4 days a week	GI upset, rash, headache, drowsiness	Alternative if other antibiotics cannot be used.
Clindamycin	75, 150, 300 capsules	150–300 mg daily	GI upset, pruritus, rash, vaginitis, pseudomembranous colitis	Alternative if other antibiotics cannot be used. Discontinue immediately and seek medical attention if diarrhea occurs.
Sulfamethoxazole + trimethoprim	400/80, 800/160 tablet	400–800/80–160 mg one to two times daily	GI upset, allergic rash, urticaria, Stevens-Johnson syndrome, possible teratogenicity Photosensitivity	Alternative if other antibiotics cannot be used. Pregnancy Category D. Avoid use in pregnancy. Minimize exposure to sun light and sun lamps. Sunscreen use and protective clothing recommended.
Hormonal Agents				
Oral Contraceptives	Norgestimate/ethinyl estradiol (Ortho Tri-Cyclen) Norethindrone acetate/ethinyl estradiol (Estrostep)	One tablet daily	Nausea, headache, weight gain, breast tenderness, break through bleeding, venous thromboembolism	Not for treatment of acne in men. Use only in females ≥ 15 years of age. Increased risk of venous thromboembolism in women who use tobacco products.

(Continued)

Table 65–2

Oral Agents Used in the Treatment of Acne (*Continued*)

Drug	Dosage form (mg)	Dosing Regimen	Adverse Reactions	Comments
Spironolactone	25, 50, 100	50–200 mg daily	Menstrual irregularities, breast tenderness, nausea, dizziness, headache, transient diuretic effect, hyperkalemia	Not recommended for treatment of acne in men. Monitor serum creatinine and potassium.
Oral Retinoid				
Isotretinoin	10, 20, 30, 40 tablets	0.5–1 mg/kg/day in two divided doses	Cheilitis, dryness of the nose, eyes, and mouth, peeling, pruritus, and drying of the face and skin, alopecia, acne flair up at start of therapy Teratogenicity Depression/suicidality Musculoskeletal pain Increased serum lipids, creatine phosphokinase, and blood glucose Photosensitivity	Nasal sprays, lip moisturizers, and hard candy may help to reduce drying of mucous membranes. Apply oil-free moisturizers to face to relieve drying of skin. Category X. Contraindicated in pregnancy. Monitor patient closely for changes in mood May use nonsteroidal anti-inflammatory drugs to relieve pain Monitor lipid panel, liver function tests, and blood glucose Minimize exposure to sun light and sun lamps. Sunscreen use and protective clothing recommended.

Data from (1) Lexicomp [Internet]. Hudson (OH): Wolters Kluwer Health, Inc.1978-2014 [cited 2014 July 25]. http://online.lexi.com/lco/action/home/switch. (2) Facts & Comparisons eAnswers. St. Louis (MO) 2014: Wolters Kluwer health, Inc. 2014 [cited 2014 July 25]. http://online.factsandcomparisons.com/index.aspx

isotretinoin therapy may be used as first-line therapy in patients with severe nodular acne due to clinical effectiveness, prevention of scarring, and quick improvements in patient quality of life.[9]

Adverse effects with the use of isotretinoin are frequent and generally dose related. Table 65–2 lists common isotretinoin adverse effects and management strategies for those symptoms.

Because isotretinoin is teratogenic and classified as Pregnancy Category X, the FDA mandates an online registry program called iPLEDGE to ensure that females do not become pregnant while taking isotretinoin. Wholesalers, pharmacies, doctors, and patients must be registered in the iPLEDGE computer-based system in order to control the distribution, prescribing, and dispensing of isotretinoin. Two negative pregnancy tests prior to initiating therapy and one negative pregnancy test each month thereafter must be obtained and confirmed in the system before a prescription can be dispensed to female patients of child-bearing potential. These patients must also commit to using two effective forms of birth control 1 month prior, during, and at least 1 month after discontinuation of isotretinoin therapy. Contact the program at their website: https://www.ipledgeprogram.com/ for further details.

Initial dose ranges for treatment are 0.5 to 1 mg/kg daily in two divided doses, with beneficial results generally reported at total daily doses of 120 to 150 mg/day. Treatment with oral isotretinoin should be continued for 6 months, but may be extended for patients with an insufficient response.[2,9,20]

Hormonal Agents Oral contraceptives and antiandrogens (spironolactone and cyproterone acetate) are valuable second-line treatment options for moderate to severe acne in female patients. Hormonal agents primarily work by decreasing androgen production resulting in reduced sebum formation. Because sebum production occurs early in the pathogenesis of acne, it may take up to 3 to 6 months to see the full effect of hormonal agents.[10]

Although many contraceptives are effective, agents containing norgestimate with ethinyl estradiol, norethindrone acetate with ethinyl estradiol, and drospirenone with ethinyl estradiol (Yaz) have been FDA approved for the treatment of acne.[20,21,22] Spironolactone at higher doses is effective for acne through antiandrogenic properties. While not approved for use in the United States, cyproterone acetate combined with an ethinyl estradiol containing oral contraceptive has demonstrated efficacy.[2,9,20] (See Table 65–2 for hormonal agent dosing guidelines and adverse effects.)

Other Agents Although use is infrequent, several other agents are available as second- or third-line treatment options for acne when first-line therapies fail[2,9,20]:

- Corticosteroids
- Chemical peels
- Surgical extraction
- Phototherapy/photodynamic therapy
- Laser treatments

Figure 65–2 shows useful algorithms for the effective treatment of the various stages of acne.

OUTCOME EVALUATION

Depending on severity, complete resolution of acne lesions may take weeks to months. Monitor patients every 4 to 8 weeks during pharmacologic therapy to assess for efficacy.[6,8]

- Decreased number of lesions
- Decreased severity of lesions

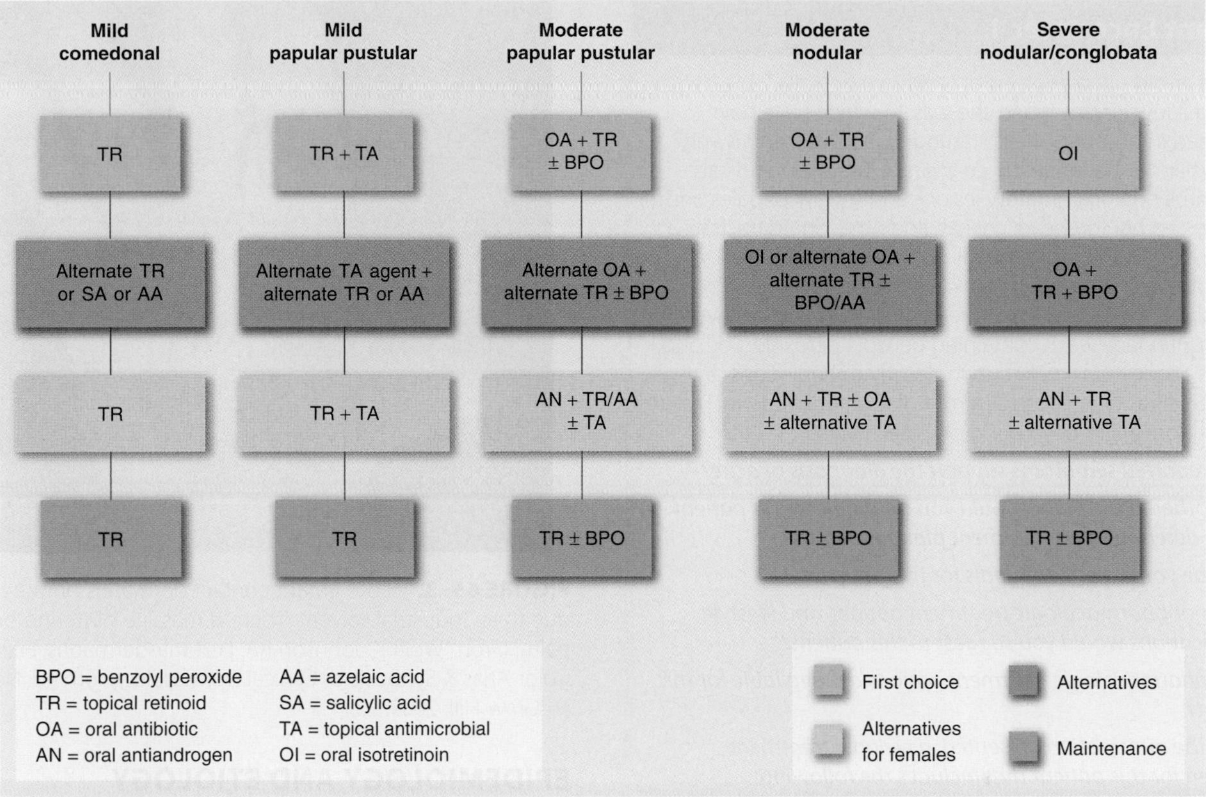

FIGURE 65–2. Algorithms for acne treatment. (From Thiboutot D, Gollnick H, Bettoli V, et. al. New insights into the management of acne: an update from the global alliance to improve outcomes in acne group. J Am Acad Dermatol. 2009;60:S1–S50.

Patient Care Process: Acne

Patient Assessment:

- Assess patient symptoms and acne lesions to determine acne severity: mild, moderate, or severe.
- Determine family history of acne, including severity.
- Evaluate skin care routine, including the use of cosmetics, facial washes, moisturizers, and other possible exacerbating factors.
- Conduct a medication history (nonprescription, prescription, and herbal medications). Identify previous acne treatment regimens.
- Identify any drug allergies.

Therapy Evaluation:

- If the patient is already receiving pharmacotherapy, assess whether active and/or previously tried therapies were effective, safe, and used as directed.
- If the patient is not well controlled, determine appropriate pharmacotherapy options for the patient's acne severity (see Figure 65–2).
- Determine whether the patient has prescription medication coverage to identify possible recommendations included in the plan formulary.

Care Plan Development:

- Select nondrug and drug therapy likely to be effective and safe (see Tables 65–1 and 65–2).
- Address any patient concerns.
- Provide patient education on acne and its management:
  - What is acne and how does it develop?
  - Physical and psychological complications that can result from acne.
  - Proper administration technique. Topical acne therapy should be applied to acne prone areas and existing lesions.
  - Possible side effects of drug therapy.
  - Inform patient of possible initial worsening of acne and/or delay of therapeutic effectiveness of acne drug therapy.
  - Emphasize medication compliance and adherence to lifestyle modifications.

Follow-up Evaluation:

- Follow-up every 1 to 2 months to assess effectiveness and safety of nondrug and drug therapy (see Tables 65–1 and 65–2).
- If acne lesions do not respond after 3 months of drug therapy, consider an alternative acne regimen (see Figure 65–2).
- If the patient experiences resolution of acne symptoms, transition to maintenance drug therapy.

Patient Encounter 1

A 15-year-old girl complains of "embarrassing zits." She began getting a few lesions when she was 14 which have now increased in number. She is starting high school and is very anxious about her appearance. Visual examination reveals numerous noninflammatory lesions and several papules and pustules on her forehead, cheeks, and nose. She is frustrated because she thinks acne means she is not a "clean person" and nothing she has tried has "cured her acne." She admits to washing her face at least three times a day with an over-the-counter face wash containing benzoyl peroxide. She also applies a salicylic acid 2% cream directly to her lesions once a day. She has never seen a dermatologist for her acne. The patient appears to be in good physical health.

What reported symptoms support the diagnosis of acne?

What other information would you obtain from this patient before determining a treatment plan for her?

Describe your treatment goals for this patient.

What nonpharmacologic treatment options and lifestyle modifications would you suggest to this patient?

What pharmacologic treatment options are available for this patient?

Given the information presented, develop a treatment regimen for this patient that includes the following:

(a) A statement of the drug-related needs and/or problem

(b) A patient-specific therapeutic plan

(c) Monitoring parameters to assess efficacy and safety

- Relief of pain/irritation
- Presence of scarring or pigmentation
- Psychological effects

If no improvement is reported after 6 weeks of drug therapy or if symptoms have worsened, patients should be reevaluated and a change to an alternative drug regimen may be necessary (see Figure 65–2).

Educate patients on potential adverse effects of drug therapy (see Tables 65–1 and 65–2). Consider changing therapy if a patient experiences effects that are not tolerated or are a compromise to their health.

CONTACT DERMATITIS

Contact dermatitis is a condition in which exposure to an offending substance produces inflammation, erythema, and pruritus of the skin.[23,24] More specifically, contact dermatitis can be divided into either irritant or allergic forms.[29,30] KEY CONCEPT *Irritant contact dermatitis (ICD) results from first-time exposure to irritating substances such as soaps, plants, cleaning solutions, or solvents. Allergic contact dermatitis (ACD) is a delayed hypersensitivity reaction that occurs after an initial exposure to an allergen results in sensitization. With additional exposure, activation of the immune system results in dermatitis. Allergens that commonly cause ACD include poison ivy, latex, and certain types of metal.*[25,26,27] (Figures 65–3 and 65–4.) Table 65–3 lists agents commonly responsible for irritant and ACD. Although generally occurring on the exposed skin, such as the hands and face, contact dermatitis can appear anywhere on the body.[29]

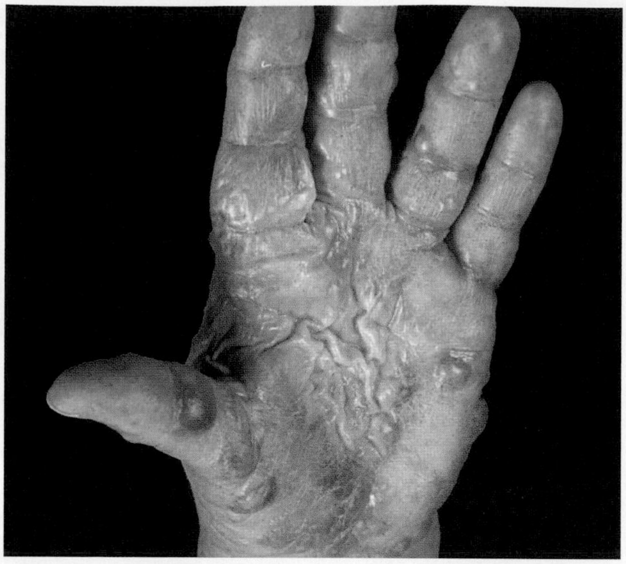

FIGURE 65–3. Acute irritant contact dermatitis on the hand due to an industrial solvent. There is massive blistering on the palm. (From Wolff K, Johnson RA. Eczema/dermatitis. Fitzpatrick's Color Atlas & Synopsis of Clinical Dermatology. 6th ed. New York: McGraw-Hill; 2009: 23.)

EPIDEMIOLOGY AND ETIOLOGY

Contact dermatitis is the most common occupational related skin disease.[28] Although most often seen in adults, contact dermatitis can affect all age groups, with females at slightly greater risk than males due to increased risk of exposure.[26]

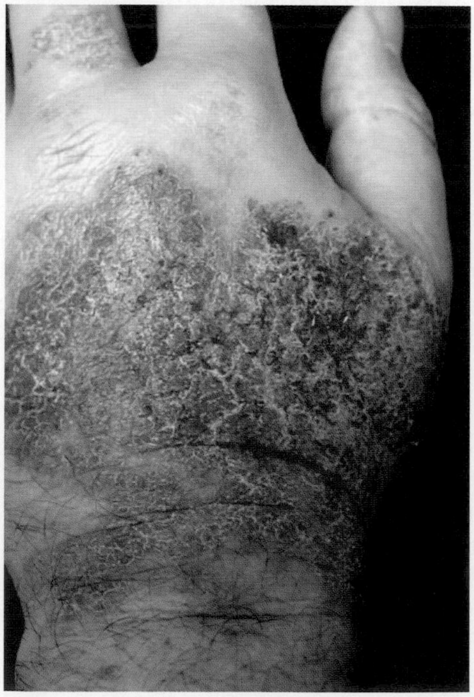

FIGURE 65–4. Allergic contact dermatitis of the hand: chromates. Confluent papules, vesicles, erosions, and crusts on the dorsum of the left hand in a construction worker who was allergic to chromates. (From Wolff K, Johnson RA. Eczema/dermatitis. Fitzpatrick's Color Atlas & Synopsis of Clinical Dermatology. 6th ed. New York: McGraw-Hill; 2009: 27.)

Table 65–3

Common Agents Causing Contact Dermatitis

Irritant Contact Dermatitis
Soaps
Detergents
Cosmetics
Solvents
Acid, mild or strong
Alkali, mild or strong

Allergic Contact Dermatitis
Plant resins, poison ivy, poison oak, sumac
Metals (nickel or gold in jewelry)
Latex and rubber
Cigarette smoke
Local anesthetics (lidocaine, benzocaine)

PATHOPHYSIOLOGY

Irritant contact dermatitis is not the result of an immunologic process, but rather occurs from direct injury to the skin. An irritating agent comes into contact with the skin, damages the protective layers of the epidermis, and can cause erythema, the formation of vesicles and pruritus.[23,29,30] Symptoms occur within minutes to hours of exposure and begin to heal soon after removal of the offending substance.

Clinical Presentation and Diagnosis of Contact Dermatitis

Contact dermatitis is generally confined to the area of contact, but in a highly sensitive person, a widespread or even generalized eruption may occur. Contact dermatitis is divided into two forms—irritant and allergic. Both forms may include, but are not limited to:

- Erythema
- Pruritus
- Vesicles
- Papules
- Crusts
- Burning
- Pain

Irritant Form

The irritant form usually presents within hours of exposure and the rash is often localized. ICD may also result in fissuring and scaling.

Allergic Form

The allergic form can take several days to present and the condition may extend beyond the borders of the region exposed. ACD may cause intense itching and include oozing pustules and skin erosion.

Diagnosis

When the causative agent is known, the diagnosis of contact dermatitis is clinical. Patch testing is done if the allergens are unknown and is usually performed several weeks after the resolution of the original dermatitis.

Allergic contact dermatitis is a type IV hypersensitivity reaction.[25] Upon initial exposure, a substance penetrates the skin, is processed by antigen presenting cells, and subsequently activate allergen-specific T cells. Subsequent exposures to that substance will elicit a response by circulating memory T cells, resulting in an allergic reaction.[23,25,29,30] Symptoms of ACD are similar to those of the irritant type, but may take several hours to several days to develop following reexposure.[23,31]

TREATMENT

Desired Outcomes and Goals

KEY CONCEPT *Identifying the causative substance and eliminating its exposure is the initial treatment goal for contact dermatitis.* Although physical symptoms can develop almost immediately after contact, removal of the offending agent will improve existing symptoms and prevent further complications.[5] Removing the offending agent includes washing the skin and any clothing or objects that may have come into contact with the agent to prevent reexposure. *The second treatment goal is symptom relief.* Since inflammation and pruritus, as well as lesion formation, are likely to result from contact dermatitis, appropriate selection of nonpharmacologic and pharmacologic agents for these symptoms is necessary.

Nonpharmacologic Therapy

In many cases, contact dermatitis may not require medical treatment. Nondrug therapy for contact dermatitis is aimed at relieving pruritus and maintaining skin hydration.[25] Effective agents used for this include the following[23,32]:

- Colloidal oatmeal baths
- Cool or tepid soapless showers
- Cool, moist compresses applied to the area for 20 to 30 minutes as often as needed
- Emollients applied to the area after bathing

Pharmacologic Therapy

► *Astringents*

The drying effect of astringents will decrease oozing from lesions and relieve itching.[23,31] Due to their ability to cause blood vessel constriction, astringents can also decrease inflammation. Aluminum acetate (Burow solution), aluminum sulfate/calcium acetate solution (Domeboro), calamine lotion, colloidal oatmeal baths/soaks, and witch hazel are safe and effective.[23] Aluminum acetate or aluminum sulfate/calcium acetate may be applied as a compress for 30 minutes at least four times daily as needed. Colloidal oatmeal baths or soaks may be applied for 15 to 20 minutes at least twice daily.

Adverse effects reported with these agents are minimal and include drying and tightening of the skin.

► *Topical Steroids*

Erythema, inflammation, pain, and itching caused by ACD can be effectively treated with topically applied corticosteroids. The use of topical corticosteroids for the management of ICD is controversial, as patients with ACD generally respond better to therapy than those with ICD.[31,33] With such a wide range of products and potencies, appropriate steroid selection is based on severity and location of lesions (see Table 65–4 for a list of topical steroids and potencies.) Higher potency preparations are used in areas where

Table 65–4

Potency Rating	Topical Dosage Forms
Class 1: Superpotent	Betamethasone dipropionate 0.05% ointment (Diprolene and Diprosone ointment) Clobetasone propionate 0.05% lotion/spray/shampoo (Clobex lotion/spray/shampoo, OLUX foam) Clobetasone propionate 0.05% cream and ointment (Cormax, Temovate) Diflorasone diacetate 0.05% ointment (Florone, Psorcon) Halobetasol propionate 0.05% cream and ointment (Ultravate) Flurandrenolide tape 4 mcg/cm^2 (Cordran)
Class 2: Potent	Amcinonide 0.1% ointment (Cyclocort ointment) Betamethasone dipropionate 0.05% cream/gel (Diprolene cream, gel, and Diprosone cream) Desoximetasone 0.25% cream (Topicort) Fluocinonide 0.05% cream, gel, ointment (Lidex) Halcinonide 0.1% cream (Halog)
Class 3: Upper mid-strength	Amcinonide 0.1% cream (Cyclocort cream) Betamethasone valerate 0.1% ointment (Betnovate/Valisone ointment) Diflorasone diacetate 0.05% cream (Psorcon cream) Fluticasone propionate 0.005% ointment (Cutivate ointment) Mometasone furoate 0.1% ointment (Elocon ointment) Triamcinolone acetonide 0.5% cream and ointment (Aristocort)
Class 4: Mid-strength	Betamethasone valerate 0.12% foam (Luxiq) Clocortolone pivalate 0.1% cream (Cloderm) Desoximetasone 0.05% cream and gel (Topicort LP) Fluocinolone acetonide 0.025% ointment (Synalar ointment) Fluocinolone acetonide 0.2% cream (Synalar-HP) Hydrocortisone valerate 0.2% ointment (Westcort ointment) Mometasone furoate 0.1% cream (Elocon cream) Triamcinolone acetonide 0.1% ointment (Kenalog)
Class 5: Lower mid-strength	Betamethasone dipropionate 0.05% lotion (Diprosone lotion) Betamethasone valerate 0.1% cream and lotion (Betnovate/Valisone cream & lotion) Desonide 0.05% lotion (DesOwen) Fluocinolone acetonide 0.01% shampoo (Capex shampoo) Fluocinolone acetonide 0.01%, 0.025%, 0.03% cream (Synalar cream) Flurandrenolide 0.05% cream and lotion (Cordran) Fluticasone propionate 0.05% cream and lotion (Cutivate cream and lotion) Hydrocortisone butyrate 0.1% cream (Locoid) Hydrocortisone valerate 0.2% cream (Westcort cream) Prednicarbate 0.1% cream (Dermatop) Triamcinolone acetonide 0.1% cream and lotion (Kenalog cream and lotion)
Class 6: Mild	Alclometasone dipropionate 0.05% cream and ointment (Aclovate) Betamethasone valerate 0.05% cream and ointment Desonide 0.05% cream, ointment, gel (DesOwen, Desonate, Tridesilon) Desonide 0.05% foam (Verdeso) Fluocinonide acetonide 0.01% cream and solution (Synalar) Fluocinonide acetonide 0.01% FS oil (Derma-Smoothe)
Class 7: Least Potent	Hydrocortisone 0.5%, 1%, 2%, 2.5% cream, lotion, spray, and ointment (various brands)

From Law RM, Gulliver WP. Psoriasis. In: Dipiro JT, Talbert RL, Yee GC, et al, eds. Pharmacotherapy: A Pathophysiological Approach. 9th ed. New York: McGraw-Hill; 2014:1583.

penetration is poor, such as the elbows and knees. Lower potency products should be reserved for areas of higher penetration, such as the face, axillae, and groin. Low-potency steroids are also recommended for the treatment of infants and children.[34,35]

Adverse effects from topical steroids are usually related to the potency of the steroid, frequency of application, duration of therapy, and the site of application. Skin atrophy, hypopigmentation, striae, and steroid-induced acne are all possible side effects associated with long-term use.[30] Ointments, because of their occlusive properties, should be avoided on weeping lesions.[23,36]

Topical steroids are typically applied two to four times daily. As improvement begins, maintenance therapy should be limited to the lowest strength steroid that continues to control the condition. Once symptoms are completely resolved, use should be discontinued and should not exceed 1 to 2 weeks.[34]

▸ *Antihistamines*

Whether due to their antihistaminic activity or their sedative side effects, pruritus caused by contact dermatitis can be relieved with the use of sedating oral antihistamines such as diphenhydramine or hydroxyzine. Topical antihistamines are available, but use is limited due to their high-sensitizing potential.[23,34] In addition to sedation, many oral antihistamines can cause hypotension, dizziness, blurred vision, and confusion.

Outcome Evaluation

With adequate treatment, most cases of contact dermatitis should improve within 7 days. Complete resolution of symptoms may take up to 3 weeks.[23] If patients experiences severe symptoms associated with fever or difficulty breathing, they should be instructed to

Patient Care Process: Contact Dermatitis

Patient Assessment:

- Assess symptoms.
- Obtain a thorough patient history. Can the agent/exposure be identified? Has there been prior exposure to that agent? If so, what treatment regimens were used to alleviate symptoms?
- Obtain patient's allergy status.

Therapy Evaluation:

- Determine whether the patient has ICD or ACD.
- Discuss testing needed to suggest or confirm the etiologic agent (patch testing).

Care Plan Development:

- Develop a treatment plan for ICD or ACD. In most cases, nondrug and nonprescription treatment options are most appropriate. If case is severe or if the patient has ACD, the plan may also include prescription therapy.
- Provide patient education on ICD or ACD and treatment:
  - Possible adverse effects of drug therapy
  - Symptoms that warrant physician referral?
  - Importance of treatment compliance.
  - Educate on the recognition of agents that may cause contact dermatitis.

Follow-up Evaluation:

- Symptoms should improve within 2 to 3 days. If no improvement, the patient should be advised to follow-up with the provider.

seek medical attention immediately. Furthermore, patients should return to their health care provider if any of the following occur:

- Rash has not improved (increased in size or spread to other locations) after several days of treatment
- Patient is experiencing adverse effects from the treatment regimen

Patient Encounter 2

A 25-year-old man presents to your pharmacy with complaints of intense itching and shows you a red, raised rash with papules on his arms. The patient tells you several days ago he spent the day clearing brush with his father on his family's property. He states that he was wearing gloves and work boots, but had on a T-shirt and shorts. He suspects he came into contact with poison ivy, because his rash looks similar to the one he had before when he came into contact with poison ivy while camping. The patient indicates that he took a shower several hours after exposure, but hasn't tried anything else to manage his symptoms. From the information he has presented, you conclude that he did likely come in contact with an agent while working that caused an allergic contact dermatitis to develop.

What information supports the possibility of exposure to an allergic agent?

Describe the symptoms that support this diagnosis.

Determine what the patient has tried to relieve her symptoms.

Describe the differences between allergic and irritant contact dermatitis.

What are your treatment goals for this patient?

What nonpharmacologic and pharmacologic treatment options are available for this diagnosis?

Given the information presented, develop a treatment regimen for this patient that includes the following:

(a) A statement of the problem

(b) A patient-specific therapeutic plan

(c) Monitoring parameters to assess efficacy and safety

DIAPER DERMATITIS

EPIDEMIOLOGY AND ETIOLOGY

Diaper dermatitis, more commonly known as diaper rash, is a form of ICD that affects the buttocks, upper thighs, lower abdomen, and genitalia of an estimated 7% to 35% of all infants.[37] Onset of occurrence is usually between 3 weeks and 2 years of age, with the most cases reported between 9 and 12 months of age.[38] The rise in the number of adults who use diapers for incontinence also increases the risk of developing diaper dermatitis.[39]

PATHOPHYSIOLOGY

KEY CONCEPT *Although many factors contribute to diaper rash, it is most likely the result of prolonged contact of the skin with urine and feces in the diaper.* If a diaper is not changed soon after urination or defecation, the protective layer of the skin can break down and make the area more susceptible to irritation and infection.[40] Although most mild cases of diaper rash present as erythema, moderate to severe cases can result in the formation of papules, vesicles, and even ulceration. If these cases are not effectively treated, the likelihood of secondary fungal or bacterial infections developing is greatly increased.[39]

TREATMENT

Desired Outcomes and Goals

KEY CONCEPT *The primary goal in the treatment of diaper rash is prevention and is most often accomplished through frequent diaper changes.* KEY CONCEPT *When a diaper rash is already present, repairing the damaged skin, relieving discomfort, and preventing secondary infections from occurring are important factors to consider when developing an effective treatment regimen.*[40]

Nonpharmacologic Therapy

Most mild cases of diaper rash can be resolved with the use of nonpharmacologic therapies. Keeping the diaper area clean and dry by changing diapers as soon as practically possible (at least every 2 hours or more frequently) is highly effective for treatment and prevention.[39,41] Other nondrug options include[31,39,41]:

Clinical Presentation and Diagnosis of Diaper Dermatitis

Typical Symptoms

- Erythema is the most common symptom presented with a diaper rash. The rash may begin as light to medium pink with poorly defined edges, but may become dark red and raised lesions with distinct edges.
- Rashes generally appear in the folds of the skin around the diaper area, thighs, genitals, and buttocks.
- Other typical symptoms include irritation and pruritus.

Atypical Symptoms

Patients presenting with the following symptoms may indicate the need for more aggressive antibiotic or antifungal therapy and should be referred to a physician for further evaluation:

- Rashes not responding to typical creams and concurrent nonpharmacologic treatment
- Rashes extending beyond the diaper region (upper abdomen, back)
- Formation of papules, bullae, and ulceration
- Excessive oozing
- Presence of genital discharge
- Concurrent fever
- Rashes appearing when diapers have not been used or rashes that fail to improve upon discontinuing diaper usage for extended periods of time (several days or more)
- Bleeding or open skin

Diagnosis

The diagnosis of diaper dermatitis is clinical. The presence of *Candida albicans* can be determined by KOH testing or culture, but is generally not necessary.

- Washing the area with lukewarm water and mild soap and allowing to completely dry before applying a new diaper
- Use water and a cotton cloth or commercial "baby wipes" without coloring, fragrances, or other additives
- Keeping diapers loose and well ventilated
- Avoiding plastic pants over diapers
- Allowing infants to take naps on an open diaper or absorbent pad to promote drying and healing

Pharmacologic Therapy

▶ *Protectants*

Protectants form an occlusive barrier between the skin and moisture from the diaper. Cream and ointment preparations are effective in providing a sufficient barrier in mild, irritant, and noninfected diaper rashes. For more severe cases, a paste is the topical agent of choice. Pastes are thicker and often contain additional ingredients (petrolatum, moisturizers) to decrease discomfort and promote healing.[38] Zinc oxide is one of the most commonly used topical protectants. In addition to forming an effective barrier against moisture, it has astringent and antiseptic properties that provide added symptom relief.[39]

Protectants are generally applied to the affected area after every diaper change and can be discontinued when the rash resolves. Other available protectants that can be used alone or in combination for the safe and effective treatment of diaper rash include white petrolatum, Vitamins A and D, lanolin, and topical cornstarch. Many agents contain a combination of occlusive and protective agents such as Triple Paste and Calmoseptine.

▶ *Topical Steroids*

Because of the increased permeability of their skin, infants are at risk for excessive absorption and toxicity from the use of topical steroids. Although effective in decreasing inflammation and relieving pruritus, steroid use in infants for the treatment of diaper dermatitis should be limited to only low-potency preparations.[42]

A thin layer of hydrocortisone cream (0.25%–1%) applied twice a day for no more than 2 weeks is an appropriate regimen. Use of higher potency steroids or use extending beyond 2 weeks should be at the discretion of a physician only.

▶ *Antifungals*

Diaper rashes lasting longer than 48 to 72 hours are at increased risk for the development of fungal infections. These complications are most frequently caused by *Candida albicans* and will require treatment with a topical antifungal.[38] (Figure 65–5.)

Adverse events with the use of topical antifungals are generally limited to local irritation at the site of application.

Nystatin, clotrimazole, and miconazole creams or ointments applied two to four times daily with diaper changes have all shown to be effective in the treatment of candidal diaper rash.[43] Although some of these products are available over the counter, parents and caregivers should be advised to initiate treatment with antifungal agents only after physician recommendation.

▶ *Antibacterials*

If conventional treatment fails, unresolved diaper rash can also lead to secondary bacterial infections. *Staphylococcus aureus* and

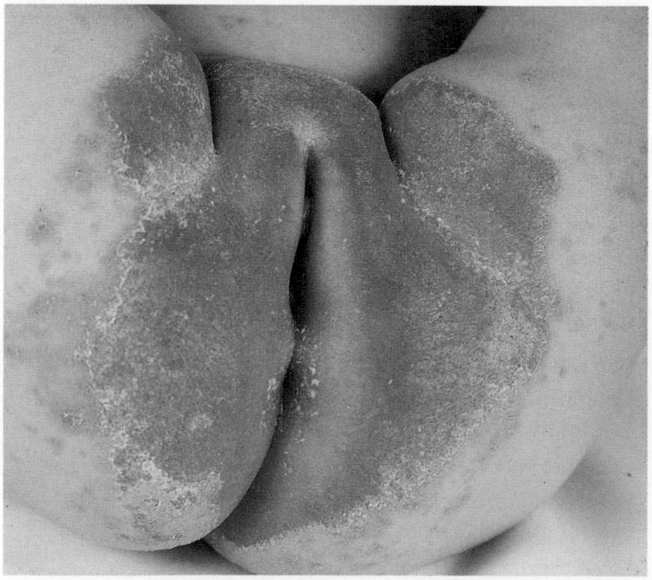

FIGURE 65–5. Candidiasis: diaper dermatitis. Confluent erosions, marginal scaling, and "satellite pustules" in the area covered by a diaper in an infant. (From Wolff K, Johnson RA. Cutaneous fungal infections. Fitzpatrick's Color Atlas & Synopsis of Clinical Dermatology. 5th ed. New York: McGraw-Hill; 2009: 723.)

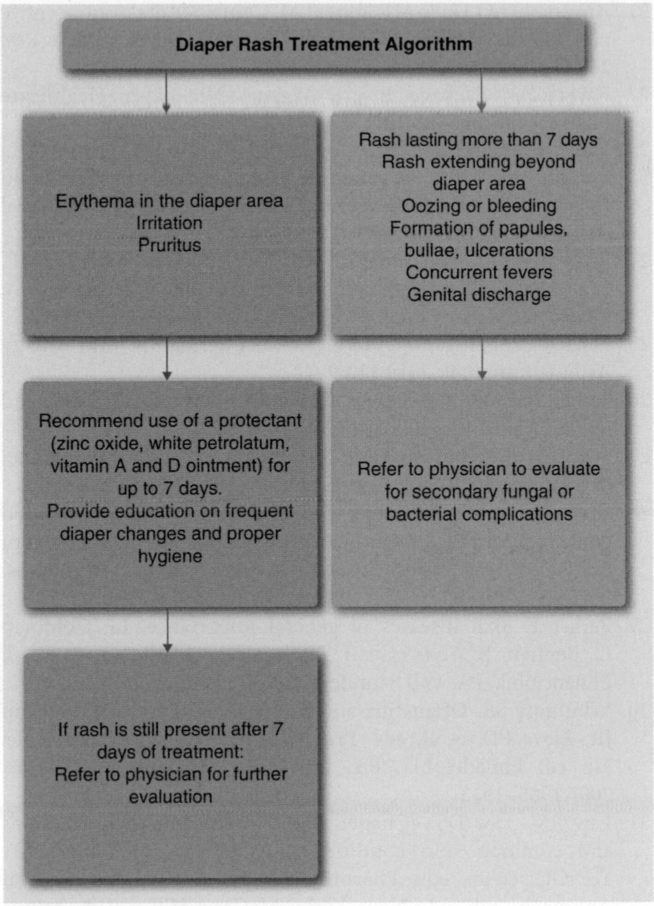

FIGURE 65–6. Diaper dermatitis treatment algorithm.

Streptococcus are the most likely pathogens responsible for these infections and require treatment with systemic antibiotics.[38,40] While topical protectants may be used as an adjunct in treatment, suspected bacterial infections should always be referred to a physician for accurate diagnosis and the selection of an appropriate antibacterial regimen.[39] Figure 65–6 shows a useful algorithm for the effective treatment of diaper dermatitis.

Patient Encounter 3

A woman presents to a community pharmacy inquiring about a product to purchase for her 4-month-old son who recently developed a rash in his diaper area. She says the rash has worsened from light pink to bright red. After further questioning, it is determined that the rash has lasted about 2 to 3 days, seems to be painful for her son when she cleans him with diaper wipes during changing. She has tried using white petrolatum a few times and is now concerned about the rash becoming infected.

What reported symptoms support the diagnosis of diaper rash?

What additional information would aid in your assessment of this patient?

What are your treatment goals for this patient?

What nonpharmacologic and pharmacologic treatment options are available for this diagnosis?

Given the information presented, develop a treatment regimen for this patient that includes the following:

(a) A statement of the problem

(b) A patient-specific therapeutic plan

(c) Monitoring parameters to assess efficacy and safety

OUTCOME EVALUATION

Most diaper rashes can be effectively treated in less than 1 week. If symptoms do not resolve or begin to worsen, advise caregivers to seek medical attention to determine the presence of secondary fungal or bacterial infections. In addition, provide educational information on proper diaper hygiene techniques in order to prevent the development of future diaper rashes.

Patient Care Process: Diaper Dermatitis

Patient Assessment:

- Assess rash symptoms. Determine the level of severity—is there a possibility of a secondary fungal or bacterial infection?
- Identify signs and symptoms that require immediate physician referral.
- Inquire about the patient's history, including similar rashes in the past.
- Obtain patient allergy status.

Therapy Evaluation:

- Determine what treatment options, if any, have been tried and if they were successful.
- Discuss labs that may be necessary if a secondary infection is suspected (cultures, biopsies).

Care Plan Development:

- Discuss available barrier treatment options with the caregiver and develop a treatment plan.
- Include proper usage instructions and potential side effects in patient counseling.
- Educate the caregiver on the importance of frequent diaper changes and proper hygiene.
- Emphasize importance of treatment compliance and use of preventative measures

Follow-Up Evaluation:

- Provide any further patient education about diaper rash etiology, treatment, and prevention.
- Discuss symptoms to report to a physician (blistering, oozing, bleeding, changes in rash, or no improvement in symptoms within 2 to 3 days).

Abbreviations Introduced in This Chapter

ACD Allergic contact dermatitis
ICD Irritant contact dermatitis

REFERENCES

1. McCalmont TH. Diseases of the skin. In: McPhee SJ, Hammer GD. Pathophysiology of diseases: An Introduction to Clinical Medicine. 6th ed. New-York: McGraw-Hill; 2010.
2. Thiboutot D, Gollnick H, Bettoli V, et al. New insights into the management of acne: an update from the global alliance to improve outcomes in acne group. J Am Acad Dermatol. 2009;60:S1–S50.
3. White GM. Recent findings in the epidemiologic evidence, classification, and subtypes of acne vulgaris. J Am Acad Dermatol. 1998;39(2 pt 3):S34–S37.
4. Bhate K, Williams HC. Epidemiology of acne vulgaris. BJD. 2013;168:474–485.
5. Bowe WP, Joshi SS, Shalita AR. Diet and acne. J Am Acad Dermatol. 2010;63:124–141.
6. Sibbald D. Acne Vulgaris. In: Dipiro JT, Talbert RL, Yee GC, et al, eds. Pharmacotherapy: A Pathophysiological Approach. 9th ed. New York: McGraw-Hill; 2014:1555–1578.
7. Foster KT, Coffey CW. Acne. In: Krinsky DL, Berardi RR, Ferreri SP, et al, eds. The Handbook of Nonprescription Drugs. 17th ed. Washington, DC: American Pharmaceutical Association; 2012: 693–705.
8. U.S. Department of Health and Human Services Food and Drug Administration Center for Drug Evaluation and Research (CDER). Guidance for Industry. Acne vulgaris: developing drugs for treatment, 2005.
9. Nast A, Dreno B, Bettoli V, et al. Guidelines for the treatment of acne. J Eur Acad Dermatol Venereol. 2012;26(suppl 1):1–29.
10. DeGrasse ER, Cavanaugh JJ. Acne. In: Alldredge BK, Corelli RL, Ernst ME, et al, eds. Applied therapeutics: the clinical use of drugs. 10th ed. Philadelphia, PA: Lippincott Williams & Wilkins; 2013:944–955.
11. Gamble R, Dunn J, Petersen B, et al. Topical antimicrobial treatment of acne vulgaris: an evidence based review. Am J Clin Demnotol. 2012;13(3):141–162.
12. Fakhouri T, Yentzer BA, Feldman SR. Advancement in benzoyl peroxide-based acne treatment: methods to increase both efficacy and tolerability. J Drugs Dermatol. 2009;8(7):657–661.
13. Thielitz A, Abdel-Naser MB, Fluhr JW, et al. Topical retinoids in acne—an evidence based overview. J Dtsch Dermatol Ges. 2008;6:1023–1031.
14. Thielitz A, Gollnick H. Topical retinoids in acne vulgaris: update on safety and efficacy. Am J Clin Dermatol. 2008;9(6):369–381.
15. Akhavan A, Bershad S. Topical acne drugs: review of clinical properties, systemic exposure, and safety. Am J Clin Dermatol. 2003;4(7):473–492.
16. Kircik, LH. Efficacy and safety of azelaic acid (AzA) gel 15% in the treatment of post-inflammatory hyperpigmentation and acne: a 16-week, baseline-controlled study. J Drugs Dermatol. 2011;10(6):586–590.
17. Stotland M, Shalita AR, Kissling RF. Dapsone 5% gel. A review of its efficacy and safety in the treatment of acne vulgaris. Am J Clin Dermatol. 2008;10(4):221–227.
18. Allergan. Aczone Package Insert. Irvine, CA: Allergan; 2012.
19. Tan HH. Antibacterial therapy for acne: a guide to selection and use of systemic agents. Am J Clin Dermatol. 2003;4(5):307–314.
20. Strauss JS, Krowchuk DP, Leyden JJ, et al. Guidelines of care for acne vulgaris management. J Am Acad Dermatol. 2007;56:651–663.
21. Arowojolu AO, Gallo MF, Lopez LM. Combined oral contraceptive pills for the treatment of acne. Cochrane Database Syst Rev. 2009;7:CD004425.
22. Bayer. Yaz Package Insert. Wayne, NJ: Bayer Healthcare Pharmaceuticals Inc; 2012.
23. Plake KS, Darbishire PL. Contact dermatitis. In: Krinsky DL, Berardi RR, Ferreri SP, et al, eds. Handbook of Nonprescription Drugs. 17th ed. Washington, DC: American Pharmaceutical Association; 2012:645–659.
24. Rustemeyer T. van Hoogstraten IMW, von Blomberg BME, et al. Mechanisms of irritant and allergic contact dermatitis. In: Johansen JD, eds. Contact Dermatitis. 5th ed. 2011:43–90.
25. Fonacier LS, Sher JM. Allergic contact dermatitis. Ann Allergy Asthma Immunol. 2014;113:9–12.
26. Tan C, Rasool S, Johnston GA. Contact dermatitis: allergic and irritant. Clin Dermatol. 2014;32:116–124.
27. Swinnen I, Goossens A. An update on airborne contact dermatitis: 2007–2011. Contact Dermatitis. 2013;68:232–238.
28. Nicholson PJ, Llewellyn D, English JS. Evidence-based guidelines for the prevention, identification and management of occupation contact dermatitis and urticarial. Contact Dermatitis. 2010;63:177–186.
29. Parker F. Skin diseases of general importance. In: Goldman L, Bennett JC, eds. Cecil Textbook of Medicine. 21st ed. Philadelphia, PA: WB Saunders; 2000:2276–2298.
30. Whitmore SE. Dermatitis and psoriasis. In: Barker LB, Burton JR, Zieve PD, et al, eds. Principles of Ambulatory Medicine. 7th ed. Philadelphia, PA: Lippincott Williams & Wilkins; 2007:1905–1913.
31. Law RM, Law DS. eChapter 23. Dermatologic drug reactions and common skin conditions. In: Dipiro JT, Talbert RL, Yee GC, et al., eds. Pharmacotherapy: A Pathophysiological Approach, 9th ed. New York: McGraw-Hill; 2014. http://accesspharmacy.mhmedical.com/content.aspx?bookid=689&Sectionid=48811448. Accessed August 26, 2014.
32. Slodownik D, Lee A, Nixon R. Irritant contact dermatitis: a review. Australasian J Dermatol. 2008;49:1–11.
33. Cohen DE, Heidary N. Treatment of irritant and allergic contact dermatitis. Dermatol Ther. 2004;17:334–340.
34. Law RM, Kwa P. Atopic dermatitis. In: Dipiro JT, Talbert RL, Yee GC, et al, eds. Pharmacotherapy: A Pathophysiological Approach. 9th ed. New York: McGraw-Hill; 2014:1595–1604.
35. Burkhart C, Morrell D, Goldsmith L. Dermatological Pharmacology. In: Brunton LL, Chabner BA, Knollman BC, eds. Goodman & Gillman's: The Pharmacological Basis of Therapeutics. 12th ed. New York: McGraw-Hill; 2011:1803–1832.
36. Lee NP, Arriola ER. Poison ivy, oak, and sumac dermatitis. West J Med. 1999;171:354–355.
37. Ward DB, Fleischer AB, Feldman SR, Krowchuk DP. Characterization of diaper dermatitis in the United States. Arch Pediatr Adolesc Med. 2000;154:943–946.
38. Borkowski S. Diaper rash care and management. Pediatr Nurs. 2004;30(6):467–470.
39. Hagemeir NE. Diaper dermatitis and prickly heat. In: Krinsky DL, Berardi RR, Ferreri SP, et al., eds. Handbook of Nonprescription Drugs. 17th ed. Washington, DC: American Pharmaceutical Association; 2012:661–674.
40. Atherton JD. A review of the pathophysiology, prevention and treatment of irritant diaper dermatitis. Curr Med Res Opin. 2004;20(5):645–649.
41. Nield LS, Kamat D. Prevention, diagnosis, and management of diaper dermatitis. Clin Pediatr. 2007;46(6):480–486.
42. Raimer SS. The safe use of topical corticosteroids in children. Pediatr Ann. 2001;30(4):225–229.
43. Gupta AK, Skinner AR. Management of diaper dermatitis. Int J Dermatol. 2004;43:830–834.

66 Anemia

Robert K. Sylvester

LEARNING OBJECTIVES

Upon completion of the chapter, the reader will be able to:

1. Identify common causes of anemia.
2. Describe common signs and symptoms of anemia.
3. Describe diagnostic evaluation required to determine the etiology of anemia.
4. Recommend a treatment regimen considering the underlying cause and patient-specific variables.
5. Compare and contrast oral and parenteral iron preparations.
6. Explain the optimal use of folic acid and vitamin B_{12} in patients with macrocytic anemia.
7. Evaluate the proper use of epoetin and darbepoetin in patients with anemia caused by cancer chemotherapy or chronic kidney disease.
8. Develop a plan to monitor the outcomes of pharmacotherapy for the treatment of anemia.

INTRODUCTION

KEY CONCEPT *Anemia is a reduction in the concentration of hemoglobin (Hgb) that results in reduced oxygen-carrying capacity of the blood.* Some patients with anemia may be asymptomatic initially, but eventually, the lack of oxygen to tissues results in fatigue, lethargy, shortness of breath, headache, edema, and tachycardia. Common causes include blood loss, decreased red blood cell (RBC) production, and increased RBC destruction. Determination of the underlying cause of anemia is essential for successful management.

EPIDEMIOLOGY AND ETIOLOGY

Anemia is a common diagnosis with a prevalence that varies widely based on age, gender, and race/ethnicity (Table 66–1).[1,2] Patients with specific comorbidities such as cancer and chronic kidney disease (CKD) have significantly higher rates of anemia. The incidence of anemia in cancer patients ranges from 30% to 90%.[3] Contributing factors include the underlying malignancy and myelosuppressive antineoplastic therapy.[4] The prevalence of anemia in patients with CKD ranges from 15% to 20% in patients with CKD stages 1 through 3 and up to 70% in patients with stage 5.[5]

A decrease in erythrocyte production can be multifactorial. Nutritional deficiencies (iron, vitamin B_{12}, and folic acid) are common causes and often easily treatable. Patients with cancer or CKD are at risk for developing anemia caused by dysregulation of iron and erythropoietin (EPO) hemostasis. Patients with chronic immune-related diseases such as rheumatoid arthritis and systemic lupus erythematosus are also at increased risk to develop anemia as a complication of their disease. Anemia related to chronic inflammatory conditions is termed anemia of chronic disease (ACD).[6]

Drug therapy is the mainstay of treatment for anemias caused by reduced RBC production and is the focus of this chapter; anemia due to destruction of erythrocytes will not be discussed.

PATHOPHYSIOLOGY

Erythropoiesis

Erythropoiesis begins with a pluripotent stem cell in the bone marrow undergoing differentiation and ends with the appearance of RBCs in peripheral blood. The production of RBCs is stimulated by EPO, a hormone secreted by the kidney in response to detection of decreased oxygen-carrying capacity of blood. EPO stimulates RBC production by stimulating differentiation of RBC precursors in the bone marrow to become reticulocytes (Figure 66–1). Reticulocytes become erythrocytes after 1 to 2 days in the bloodstream.[7]

Decreased-Production Anemias

▶ Nutritional Deficiencies

Deficiencies in folic acid and vitamin B_{12} may hinder the process of erythrocyte maturation. Folic acid and vitamin B_{12} are required for the formation of DNA. Significant decreases in the amount of either nutrient inhibits DNA synthesis and consequently RBC production.[7,8] Poor diet can contribute to folic acid and vitamin B_{12} deficiencies. Pernicious anemia describes a severe anemia caused by the malabsorption of vitamin B_{12} due to the absence of intrinsic factor, a glycoprotein produced by gastric parietal cells that binds to vitamin B_{12} and facilitates its absorption in the ileum. This condition results in B_{12} deficiency despite adequate dietary B_{12} intake.[9]

Iron is also essential for RBC production. It is required for formation of Hgb. Lack of iron leads to a decrease in Hgb synthesis and decreased RBC production. Normal homeostasis of iron transport and metabolism is depicted in Figure 66–2.[10]

Table 66–1

Prevalence of Anemia[1,2]

Children (1–16 years)	6%–9%
Males (16–69 years)	2%
Males (85+ years)	26%
Females (16–19 years)	16%
Females (20–49 years, nonpregnant)	12%
White, non-Hispanic	10%
Black, non-Hispanic	19%
Mexican American	22%
Females (85+ years)	20.1%

Approximately 1 to 2 mg of iron is absorbed through the duodenum daily, and the same amount is lost via blood loss, desquamation of mucosal cells, or menstruation.

Iron-deficiency anemia (IDA) typically occurs because of inadequate absorption of iron or excessive blood loss. Inadequate absorption may occur in patients who have congenital or acquired intestinal conditions, such as inflammatory bowel disease, celiac disease, or bowel resection. Achlorhydria and diets poor in iron, also may contribute to iron deficiency states. Iron deficiency also may occur following excessive iron loss. Common etiologies include excessive menstruation, ulcers or neoplastic lesions, and excessive bleeding following surgery or trauma.[10]

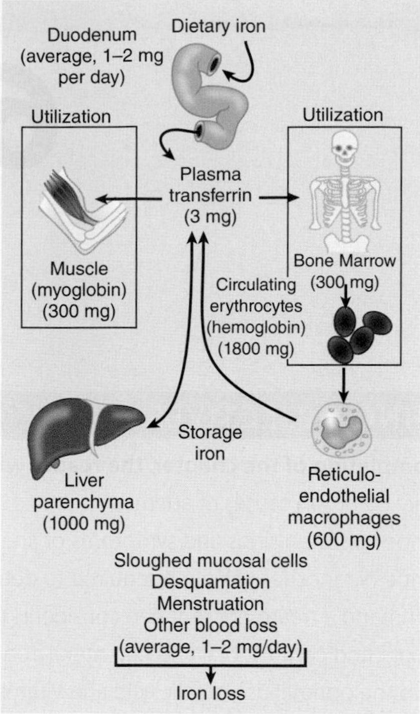

FIGURE 66–2. The distribution of iron use in adults. (From Andrews NC. Disorders of iron metabolism. N Engl J Med. 1999;341:1986–1995.)

► *Dysregulation of Iron Homeostasis and Impaired Marrow Production*

Chronic diseases associated with ACD include infection, autoimmune disease, CKD, and cancer. A major contributing factor for development of ACD is disturbance of iron homeostasis related to activation of the immune system. Hepcidin is an acute-phase protein expressed in response to upregulation of interleukin-6 and exposure to lipopolysaccharide. Increased expression of hepcidin causes decreased iron absorption from the gastrointestinal (GI) tract and inhibition of iron release from macrophages. In addition, immune activation can cause upregulation of cytokines that impair the proliferation and differentiation of erythroid precursors. Decreased production and blunted responsiveness to EPO can also contribute to ACD; this is best documented in patients with CKD. Finally, disruption of erythropoiesis secondary to infiltration of the bone marrow by cancer can lead to anemia.[4–6]

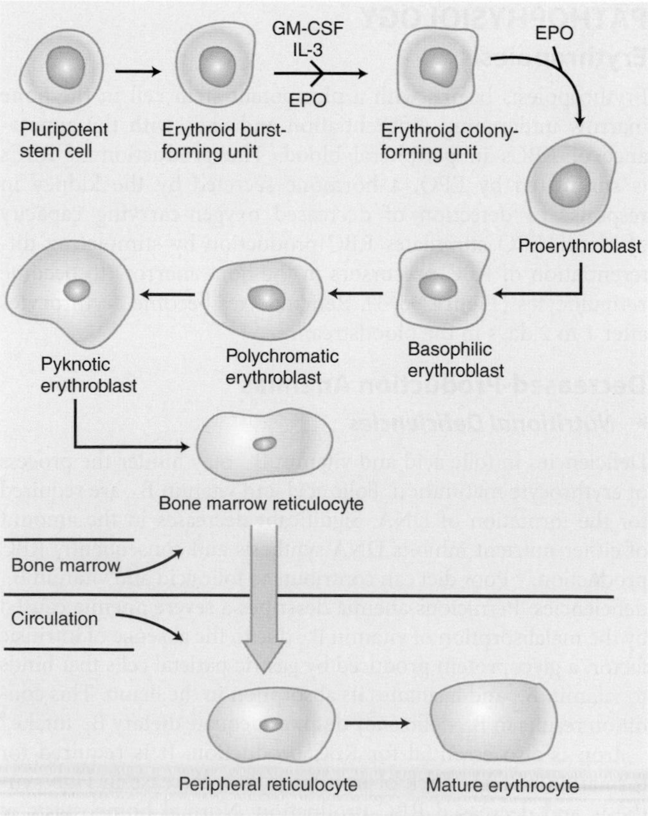

FIGURE 66–1. The process of erythropoiesis.

TREATMENT

Desired Outcomes

KEY CONCEPT *The goal of anemia therapy is to increase Hgb to levels that improve red cell oxygen-carrying capacity, alleviate symptoms, and prevent complications from anemia.* Normal Hgb values are 14.0 to 17.5 g/dL (140–175 g/L or 8.69–10.9 mmol/L) for males and 12.3 to 15.3 g/dL (123–153 g/L or 7.63–9.50 mmol/L) for females. It is important to note that continuation of therapy should be assessed primarily by resolution of clinical symptoms. Patients who experience a resolution in their symptoms (eg, shortness of breath, tachycardia, fatigue, dizziness,) may not require aggressive therapy to maintain their Hgb values within normal limits. Hypoxia and cardiovascular sequelae due to anemia can be avoided if Hgb levels are greater than 7.0 g/dL (70 g/L or 4.34 mmol/L).[11]

General Approach to the Anemic Patient

KEY CONCEPT *The underlying cause of anemia must be determined and used to guide therapy. A complete blood count (CBC) is the laboratory evaluation that provides objective characteristics of RBCs useful in determining etiology and appropriate treatment.*

Clinical Presentation and Diagnosis of Anemia

Signs and Symptoms

Generally, the signs and symptoms of anemia are nonspecific and may include the following:

- Fatigue, lethargy, dizziness
- Shortness of breath
- Headache
- Edema
- Tachycardia

Other findings that may be present in some patients include:

- Dry skin, chapped lips
- Nail brittleness
- Hunger for ice, starch, or clay (termed pica)

Past Medical History

Inquire about the following conditions:

- History of blood loss, such as hemorrhoids, melena, or menorrhagia (IDA)
- Malnourished or recent weight loss (vitamin B_{12} or folate deficiency)
- Alcoholism (folate deficiency)
- Cancer or chronic kidney disease (CKD)
- Chronic autoimmune disorders or infections, such as HIV infection or rheumatoid arthritis (anemia of chronic disease)

Physical Examination

These findings aid the clinician in determining the severity of the anemia:

- Orthostatic hypotension and tachycardia secondary to volume depletion
- Cutaneous changes such as pallor, jaundice, and nail brittleness

Laboratory Evaluation

Table 66–2 describes common tests used to determine the etiology of anemia. A diagnostic and treatment algorithm for anemia is outlined in Figure 66–3.

1. A CBC is a necessary first step in evaluating a patient with anemia. If the Hgb and Hct are less than the normal range, the patient is anemic. Subsequent evaluations of RBC indices and the peripheral smear often are necessary to determine the etiology (and ultimately, the treatment) of the anemia.
2. Evaluating the mean corpuscular volume (MCV) is the next step in an anemia workup. It is classified as microcytic, normocytic, or macrocytic if the MCV is below, within, or above the normal range of 80 to 96 fL/cell, respectively.

Microcytic Anemia and Iron Evaluation

Iron studies (see Table 66–2) should be evaluated in the setting of a low MCV. These include:

- Serum iron
- Serum ferritin—the best indirect determinant of body iron stores. It is commonly decreased in patients with IDA
- Total iron-binding capacity (TIBC)—quantifies the iron-binding capacity of transferrin and is increased in IDA
- Transferrin saturation (serum iron/TIBC)—indicates the amount of transferrin that is bound with iron; it is lower in IDA

Macrocytic Anemia

- Evaluate folic acid and vitamin B_{12} levels in the setting of an elevated MCV
- Further investigation by administering radiolabeled B_{12} (ie, Schilling test) to determine if lack of intrinsic factor

Normocytic Anemia

- Evaluate reticulocytes and CBC
- High reticulocyte counts may indicate RBCs loss via acute blood loss, hemolysis, or splenic sequestration
- Low serum iron with normal to increased ferritin consistent with ACD

Patient Encounter 1, Part 1

A 27-year-old African American woman scheduled a prenatal visit after a positive home pregnancy test. Previous pregnancies and deliveries were uncomplicated; she has healthy children ages 1.5 and 3 years. No other significant past medical history. Earlier this week she states feeling dizzy and short of breath after walking up stairs.

What aspects of this patient's history suggest she may be anemic?

What laboratory assessments are required to make an appropriate diagnosis and therapeutic plan?

How would the requested laboratory parameter(s) aid your decision making?

The mean corpuscular volume and determination of iron, ferritin, folate, and vitamin B_{12} levels are required to correctly diagnose a patient's anemia. Figure 66–3 and Table 66–2 illustrate how laboratory test results determine the correct diagnosis.

Nonpharmacologic Therapy

The primary nonpharmacologic treatment of anemia is transfusion of RBCs. Safety concerns, cost, and the limited availability of this therapy support efforts to establish the "optimum" threshold for administering RBC transfusions. A Cochrane review concluded it is appropriate to use "restrictive transfusion triggers in patients free of serious cardiac disease." The authors concluded a reasonable "trigger for transfusion" for patients without significant cardiovascular disease is 7.0 g/dL (70 g/L or 4.34 mmol/L).[12] The Transfusion Requirements In Critical Care trial reported no significant differences in in-hospital mortality between patients

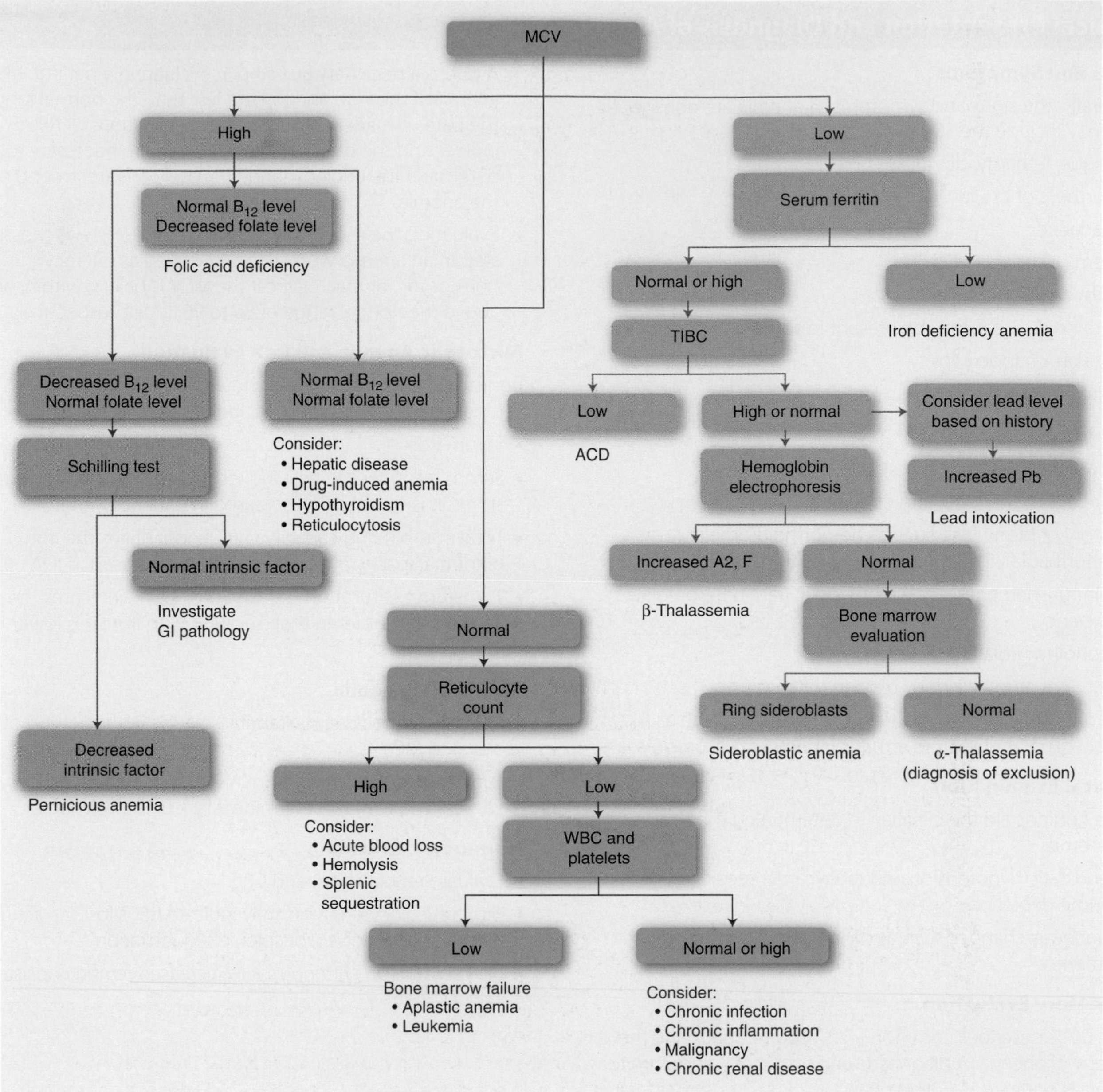

FIGURE 66–3. The anemia evaluation process. ACD, anemia of chronic disease; MCV, mean corpuscular volume; Pb, lead; TIBC, total iron-binding capacity. A2, hemoglobin A2 type; F, hemoglobin F type.

randomly assigned to maintain Hgb levels of 7.0 to 9.0 g/dL (70–90 g/L or 4.34–5.59 mmol/L) and 10.0 to 12.0 g/dL (100–120 g/L or 6.21–7.45 mmol/L).[13] Typically, only patients with acute symptoms (ie, dyspnea, chest pain) and Hgb concentrations in the range of 7.0 to 9.0 g/dL (70–90 g/L or 4.34–5.59 mmol/L) require blood transfusions.

Anemia can be attributed to diets poor in iron, folic acid, or vitamin B_{12}. However, in the United States, nutrient-poor diets rarely cause anemia. Therefore, ingesting a diet that is rich in iron, folic acid, or vitamin B_{12} should be encouraged, but is rarely the sole modality of treatment. Food sources of iron, folic acid, and vitamin B_{12} are listed in Table 66–3.[8]

Pharmacologic Therapy

▶ *Iron-Deficiency Anemia*

KEY CONCEPT *The initial treatment of IDA is oral iron therapy that provides 150 to 200 mg of elemental iron daily.* Many different iron products and salt forms are available. Table 66–4 lists commonly prescribed oral iron products and the amount of elemental iron provided by each.

Iron supplementation resolves anemia by replenishing iron stores to levels necessary for RBC production and maturation. Reticulocytosis should occur in 7 to 10 days, and Hgb values should rise by about 1.0 g/dL (10 g/L or 0.62 mmol/L) per week. Patients should be reassessed if Hgb does not increase by 2.0 g/dL (20 g/L or 1.24 mmol/L) in 3 weeks.[14]

The preferred regimen for oral iron is 50 to 65 mg of elemental iron two to three doses daily on an empty stomach. Administration on an empty stomach (1 hour before or 2 hours after a meal) is preferred for maximal absorption. If patients develop intolerable GI side effects (ie, heartburn, nausea, bloating) after taking iron on an empty stomach, they should be advised to take it with meals. After absorption, iron binds to transferrin in the plasma and is transported to the muscles (for myoglobin), liver

Table 66–2

Pertinent Laboratory Tests in the Evaluation of Anemia

Test Name	Normal Range	Description/Significance
CBC		
Hgb	Males: 14.0–17.5 g/dL (140–175 g/L or 8.69–10.9 mmol/L) Females: 12.3–15.3 g/dL (123–153 g/L or 7.63–9.50 mmol/L)	Amount of Hgb in the blood; signifies oxygen-carrying capacity of the blood and determines whether a patient is anemic
Hct	Males: 40.7%–50.3% (0.407–0.503) Females: 36.1%–44.3% (0.361–0.44.3)	The percent of blood that the erythrocytes encompass; also indicates anemia; the Hgb is measured, and the Hct is calculated
RBC	Males: 4.5–5.9 × 10^6 cells/μL (4.5–5.9 × 10^{12} cells/L) Females: 4.1–5.1 × 10^6 cells/μL (4.1–5.1 × 10^{12} cells/L)	The number of erythrocytes in a volume of blood; also indicates anemia, but seldom used
RBC Indices		
MCV	80–97.6 μm³/cell (80–97.6 fL/cell)	A widely used laboratory value to measure RBC "size"; higher values indicate macrocytosis and lower values indicate microcytosis
MCH	27–33 pg/cell	Amount of Hgb per RBC; may be decreased in IDA
MCHC	32–36 g/dL (320–360 g/L)	Hgb divided by the Hct; also low in IDA
Iron Studies		
Serum iron		
Males	45–160 mcg/dL (8.1–28.6 μmol/L)	Measures amount of iron bound to transferrin; low in IDA
Females	30–160 mcg/dL (5.4–28.6 μmol/L)	
Serum ferritin		
Males	20–250 ng/mL (20–250 mcg/L; 45–562 pmol/L)	Ferritin is the protein–iron complex found in macrophages used for iron storage; low in IDA
Females	10–150 ng/mL (10–150 mcg/L; 22–337 pmol/L)	
TIBC	220–420 mcg/dL (39.4–75.2 μmol/L)	Measures the capacity of transferrin to bind iron; high in IDA
TSAT	15%–50% (0.15–0.50)	TSAT(%) = (serum iron/TIDC) × 100, a saturation of less than 15% (0.15) is common in IDA
Other Tests		
RBC distribution width (RDW)	11.5%–14.5% (0.115–0.145)	A higher value means the presence of many different sizes of RBCs; the MCV is therefore less reliable
Reticulocyte count		
Males	0.5%–1.5% of RBCs (0.005–0.015)	Should be elevated in patients who are responding to treatment
Females	0.5%–2.5% of RBCs (0.005–0.025)	
Folic acid (plasma)	3.1–12.4 ng/mL or mcg/L (7.0–28.1 nmol/L)	Used to determine folic acid deficiency
Folic acid (RBC)	125–600 ng/mL (283–1360 nmol/L)	Used to determine folic acid deficiency
Vitamin B_{12}	180–1000 pg/mL (133–738 pmol/L)	Used to determine vitamin B_{12} deficiency
EPO level	2–25 mIU/mL (2–25 IU/L)	Patients may benefit from EPO therapy if they are anemic and EPO levels are normal or mildly elevated

EPO, erythropoietin; Hct, hematocrit; Hgb, hemoglobin; IDA, iron-deficiency anemia; MCH, mean cell hemoglobin; MCHC, mean cell hemoglobin concentration; MCV, mean cell volume; RDW, RBC distribution width; TIBC, total iron-binding capacity; TSAT, transferrin saturation.

(for storage), or bone marrow (for red cell production). Common toxicities associated with oral iron include abdominal pain, nausea, heartburn, constipation, and dark stools.[14] Potentially clinically significant drug interactions involving iron products include fluoroquinolones, tetracyclines, eltrombopag, and mycophenolate mofetil. Iron decreases the absorption of these drugs. The absorption of iron is influenced by gastric acidity. Limited data support drugs that decrease gastric acidity (antacids, proton pump inhibitors, and H_2-receptor antagonists) may impair the absorption of iron. If concurrent administration cannot be avoided, to minimize this effect oral iron should be administered at least several hours before or after the affected drug.

Table 66–3

Food Sources of Iron, Folic Acid, or Vitamin B_{12}

Nutrient	Food Sources
Iron	Red meat, organ meats, wheat germ, egg yolks, oysters
Folic acid	Green vegetables, liver, yeast, fruits
Vitamin B_{12}	Animal by-products, legumes

Table 66–4

Oral Iron Products and Elemental Iron Content

Salt Form	Brand Name(s)	Elemental Iron Content per Dose Form
Ferrous sulfate	Feosol	65-mg/325-mg tablet 60-mg/300-mg tablet
Ferrous sulfate, anhydrous	N/A	65-mg/200-mg tablet
Ferrous gluconate	Fergon	39-mg/325-mg tablet 37-mg/300-mg tablet
Ferrous fumarate	Feostat	33-mg/100-mg tablet
Polysaccharide–iron complex	Niferex, Ferrex	150-mg/150-mg capsule 50-mg/50-mg tablet

Table 66–5

Parenteral Iron Products

Product (Brand Name)	Max. Approved Dose (mg)[a]	Max. Infusion Rate Undiluted[a]	TDI Possible	Test Dose Required	Black-Box Warning	Absolute Rates LT ADEs/Million[b]
Iron dextran injection (Dexferrum)	100	50 mg/min	Yes	Yes	Yes	11.3
Iron dextran injection (INFed)	100	50 mg/min	Yes	Yes	Yes	3.3
Sodium ferric gluconate complex (Ferrlecit)	125	12.5 mg/min	No	No	No	0.9
Iron sucrose injection (Venofer)	200	40 mg/min	No	No	No	0.6
Ferumoxytol injection (Feraheme)	510	30 mg/sec	No	No	No	NR
Ferric carboxymaltose (Injectafer)	750	100 mg/min	No	No	No	NR

Max, maximum; NR, not reported; TDI, total dose infusion. LT ADEs, Life threatening adverse drug reactions.

[a]From FDA product labeling.

[b]From Auerbach M, Ballard H. Clinical use of intravenous iron: Administration, efficacy and safety. Hematology Am Soc Hematol Educ Program 2010:338–347.

Parenteral iron therapy is indicated when patients cannot tolerate oral formulations, are noncompliant, or fail to respond to oral iron because of malabsorption syndromes. Six parenteral iron formulations are available in the United States.[15-20] Table 66–5 provides details pertinent to the use of these products. The iron dextran products available in the United States differ markedly. As noted Dexferrum (the high-molecular-weight [HMW] product) is associated with a much higher incidence of life-threatening adverse effects, typically anaphylactic-like reactions. This significant difference in safety has resulted in recommendations that the use of HMW iron dextran (ID) be abandoned.[21,22] Although total dose infusion (TDI) is not an approved method of administration in the United States, low-molecular-weight ID is approved for TDI in Europe. TDI administration has been shown to achieve similar patient outcomes while lowering cost. Sodium ferric gluconate complex, iron sucrose, ferumoxytol, and ferric carboxymaltose received FDA labeling for the treatment of patients with anemia and CKD in the last decade.[15-20] Although the occurrence of life-threatening adverse events caused by parenteral iron is extremely low, the absolute rate of life-threatening events is substantially higher for HMW ID.[21,22] Table 66–5 provides details pertinent to the use of these products.

The dose of iron dextran is calculated by the following equation: dose (mL) = 0.0442 (desired Hgb − observed Hgb) × body weight + (0.26 × body weight). The body weight that should be used is lean body weight for adults and children weighing more than 15 kg and actual body weight for children weighing 5 to 15 kg. Hemoglobin should be expressed units of g/dL (hemoglobin expressed in g/L × 0.10, or mmol/L × 1.61).The dose in milligrams can be calculated based on a standard concentration of 50 mg of elemental iron per milliliter.[15] Prescribing information recommends administering iron dextran in 100-mg aliquots daily until the total dose is achieved. However, anecdotal evidence reports that the total calculated dose can be administered safely over 4 to 6 hours in 1 day. Because of the risk of anaphylaxis, a test dose of iron dextran (0.5 mL over at least 30 seconds) must be administered to patients before their first dose of iron dextran. Patients should be monitored for signs of anaphylaxis

Patient Encounter 1, Part 2

Laboratory parameters are ordered, and the following is reported

CBC

- WBC: $6.50 \times 10^3/\mu L$ ($6.50 \times 10^9/L$)
- Hgb: 8.3 g/dL (83 g/L; 5.15 mmol/L)
- Hct: 24.8% (0.248)
- Plt: $210 \times 10^3/\mu L$ ($210 \times 10^9/L$)

Red Blood Cell Indices

- MCV: 103.4 μm^3 (103.4 fL)
- MCH: 28.4 pg/cell
- MCHC: 35.3 g/dL (353 g/L; 21.9 mmol/L)

Others

- RBC count: $3.6 \times 10^6/\mu L$ ($3.6 \times 10^{12}/L$)
- RDW: 22% (0.22)

Iron Studies

- Serum iron: 100 mcg/dL (17.9 μmol/L)
- Serum ferritin: 123 ng/L (123 mcg/L; 276 pmol/L)
- TIBC: 300 mcg/dL (53.7 μmol/L)
- Transferrin saturation: 36% (0.36)

B_{12} and Folate

- Serum folate: 2.3 ng/mL (5.2 nmol/L)
- Serum B_{12}: 496 pg/mL (366 pmol/L)

Is this a macrocytic or microcytic anemia?

Specifically, what is the etiology of the anemia?

Recommend the most appropriate drug regimen (drug, dosage form, and schedule).

Patient Encounter 1, Part 3

The patient is diagnosed with folic acid deficiency anemia and is started on a generic prenatal vitamin containing I mg of folic acid. Follow-up CBC 1 month later reveals Hgb of 10 g/dL (100 g/L or 6.2 mmol/L), previously 8.3 g/dL (83 g/L or 5.15 mmol/L). The patient reports no shortness of breath or dizziness in the past 2 weeks. She also states she occasionally misses doses due to her hectic days.

What hemoglobin level would constitute a therapeutic response in this patient?

How can compliance be improved in this patient?

for at least 1 hour before administering the total dose. Other adverse effects include arthralgias, arrhythmias, hypotension, flushing, and pruritus.[20]

▶ Vitamin B_{12} and Folic Acid Anemia

KEY CONCEPT *Anemia from vitamin B_{12} or folic acid deficiency is treated by replacing the missing nutrient.* Both folic acid and vitamin B_{12} are essential for erythrocyte production and maturation.

Oral and parenteral vitamin B_{12} (cyanocobalamin) replacement therapies are equally effective. Vitamin B_{12} is absorbed completely following parenteral administration, whereas oral vitamin B_{12} is absorbed poorly via the GI tract. Consequently, cyanocobalamin is commonly administered as an intramuscular or subcutaneous injection of 1000 mcg/day for 1 week, followed by 1000 mcg/week for a month or until the Hgb normalizes. Life-long maintenance therapy (1000 mcg/month) is required for patients with pernicious anemia or surgical resection of the terminal ileum. If the etiology was a dietary deficiency or reversible malabsorption syndrome, treatment can be discontinued after the underlying cause is corrected and vitamin B_{12} stores normalized. A common oral dosing regimen is from 1000 to 2000 mcg/day. If parenteral cyanocobalamin is used initially, oral vitamin B_{12} can be useful as maintenance therapy. Typically, resolution of neurologic symptoms, disappearance of megaloblastic RBCs, and increased Hgb levels occur within a week of therapy.

Vitamin B_{12} is well tolerated. Reported adverse effects include injection-site pain, pruritus, and rash. Clinical significance of decreases in protein-bound cyanocobalamin related to proton pump inhibitor therapy has not been established.[23]

The effective dose of folic acid is 1 mg/day by mouth. Absorption of folic acid is rapid and complete. However, patients with malabsorption syndromes may require doses up to 5 mg/day. Resolution of symptoms and reticulocytosis occurs within days of commencing therapy. Typically a patient's Hgb will start to rise after 2 weeks of therapy and normalize after 2 to 4 months of therapy.

Folic acid is well tolerated. Nonspecific adverse effects include allergic reactions, flushing, and rash. A small study evaluating the effect of folic acid doses of 10 mg/day on phenytoin levels reported decreased phenytoin levels in 3 of 4 subjects. However, the occurrence of this interaction at folic acid doses of 1 mg/day has not been reported.[23]

▶ Anemia of Chronic Disease

KEY CONCEPT *Decreased RBC transfusion requirements is an outcome achieved in patients with ACD treated with the erythropoietin stimulating agent (ESAs). However, in 2007, the FDA product labeling for epoetin and darbepoetin were revised to include new data documenting safety concerns.* Subsequently, the Centers for Medicare and Medicaid Services (CMS) implemented more restrictive ESA coverage determination guidelines. In 2010, the FDA implemented a risk evaluation and mitigation strategy (REMS) for ESAs administered to treat patients with cancer who are undergoing chemotherapy. Table 66–6 summarizes the FDA-labeled dosing regimens for patients whose anemia is related to cancer chemotherapy, CKD, or zidovudine treatment.

Anemia Due to Chemotherapy in Patients with Cancer Epoetin, a recombinant human EPO, and darbepoetin, a synthetic EPO analog, bind to the EPO receptors on RBC precursor cells in the bone marrow and result in increased RBC production. Darbepoetin differs from epoetin in that it is a glycosylated protein and exhibits a longer half-life, allowing for a longer dosing interval. Clinical practice guidelines consider epoetin and darbepoetin to be therapeutic equivalents.[4,25] KEY CONCEPT *ESAs should only be used to prevent a transfusion and should not be initiated unless the hemoglobin is less than 10.0 g/dL (100 g/L, 6.21 mmol/L) and chemotherapy is planned for a minimum of two additional months.* ESA-labeled dosing regimens for treatment of patients receiving chemotherapy are summarized in Table 66–6.

Postmarketing outcome data documented that patients administered ESAs experienced increased thrombotic events and

Table 66–6

ESA Products and Usual Doses for Anemia from Cancer/Chemotherapy, CKD, and Zidovudine/HIV Infection[a]

	Epoetin-α (Epogen, Procrit)	Darbepoetin-α (Aranesp)
Cancer/chemotherapy dosing regimens	150 units/kg SC or IV three times per week 40,000 units SC or IV once every week	2.25 mcg/kg SC or IV once every week 500 mcg SC or IV fixed dose every 3 weeks
CKD dosing regimens	50–100 units/kg SC or IV three times per week	0.45 mcg/kg SC or IV once every week[b] 0.75 mcg/kg SC or IV once every 2 weeks[b] 0.45 mcg/kg SC or IV once every 4 weeks[c]
Zidovudine/HIV dosing regimen[d]	100 units/kg IV or SC three times per week	Not recommended

[a]Indications and dosage regimens per FDA product labeling.
[b]for patients on dialysis.
[c]for patients not on dialysis.
[d]FDA labeled indication for Procrit (epoetin-α), not Epogen (epoetin-α) or darbepoetin.

Patient Encounter 2, Part 1

A 55-year-old woman presents to her primary care physician complaining of lack of energy that has gotten more noticeable the last month. She reports she has been unable to keep up her marathon training because of this. She is a vegetarian for the past 30 years. She is a dental hygienist and works part time. Her physical exam was notable for pallor. Past medical history is negative.

What aspects of this patient's history suggest she may be anemic?

What laboratory assessments are required to make an appropriate diagnosis and therapeutic plan?

shorter progression-free and overall survival.[24] ESAs increased on study mortality (combined hazard ratio [cHR] 1.17; 95% confidence interval [CI] 1.06–1.30) and worsened overall survival (cHR 1.06; 95% CI 1.00–1.12). This corresponds to a 17% increased risk of mortality for patients treated with ESAs while on study and a 6% increase overall. Based on these data, the FDA revised ESA product labeling, restricting their administration to patients with chemotherapy-induced anemia without a curative intent. The 2010 update of the American Society of Clinical Oncology/American Society of Hematology clinical practice guideline on the use of ESAs in patients with cancer adopted FDA recommendations for more restrictive use of ESA in patients with cancer.[25]

CMS published more restrictive coverage criteria for ESA treatment of anemia associated with cancer chemotherapy in 2008. Patients should be monitored every 4 weeks. If Hgb has not increased by 1.0 g/dL (10 g/L, 0.62 mmol/L) after 4 weeks and remains less than 10.0 g/dL (100 g/L, 6.21 mmol/L), a one-time dose escalation of 25% is appropriate. If Hgb increases by more than 1.0 g/dL (10 g/L, 0.62 mmol/L), or is more than 10.0 g/dL (100 g/L, 6.21 mmol/L), the ESA should be discontinued. At 8 weeks if Hgb has increased by 1 g/dL (10 g/L, 0.62 mmol/L) but remains less than 10.0 g/dL(100 g/L, 6.21 mmol/L), continued ESA administration is covered. However, if after 8 weeks Hgb fails to increase by 1 g/dL (10 g/L, 0.62 mmol/L), CMS payment of therapy is not covered. CMS covers ESA therapy for up to 8 weeks after completion of chemotherapy for patients achieving respones.[26]

"Functional" iron deficiency exists when total iron stores are normal or increased but disruption of iron homeostasis prevents utilization of the stored iron for erythropoiesis.

"Functional" iron deficiency has been described in patients with ACD. Therefore, it is imperative that patients starting ESA therapy have laboratory studies performed to assess iron stores. If results document a patient has suboptimal iron stores, iron replacement therapy is indicated.

Anemia Due to CKD Anemia is common in patients with CKD. Early treatment of anemia in patients with CKD on dialysis has been associated with slower disease progression and lower risk of death. It is essential to evaluate and treat anemia in patients before they progress to stage 5 CKD (glomerular filtration rate [GFR] of less than 15 mL/min/1.73 m^2 [0.14 mL/s/m^2]).[27]

Patients with CKD typically develop normocytic, normochromic anemia as a result of EPO deficiency. However, a thorough workup of anemia should be performed to rule out other etiologies.[27] Regardless, ESA therapy is effective in treating CKD anemia. The National Kidney Foundation Clinical Practice Recommendations 2007 update recommend a Hgb target range of 11.0 to 12.0 g/dL (110–120 g/L or 6.83–7.45 mmol/L) in dialysis and nondialysis patients.[27] However, in June 2011, the FDA notified health care providers that the target Hgb range in patients with CKD was lowered to 11.0 g/dL (110 g/L or 6.83 mmol/L) in patients on hemodialysis and to 10.0 g/dL (100 g/dL or 6.21 mmol/L) in CKD patients not on hemodialysis.[28] This revision was adopted to decrease the risk of serious adverse

Patient Encounter 2, Part 2

Laboratory results:

CBC

- WBC: 7.7 × 10^3/mm^3 (7.7 × 10^9/L)
- Hgb: 8.7 g/dL (87 g/L; 5.40 mmol/L)
- Hct: 30.8% (0.308)
- Plt: 210 × 10^3/μL (210 × 10^9/L)

Red Blood Cell Indices

- MCV: 71 μm^3 71 fL
- MCH: 23 pg/cell
- MCHC: 28.3 g/dL (283 g/L; 17.6 mmol/L)

Iron Studies

- Serum iron: 27 mcg/dL (4.8 μmol/L)
- Serum ferritin: 6.9 ng/mL (6.9 mcg/L; 16 pmol/L)
- TIBC: 459 mcg/dL (82.2 μmol/L)
- Transferrin saturation: 11% (0.11)

B_{12} and Folate

- Serum B_{12}: 707 pg/mL (522 pmol/L)
- Serum folate: 10 ng/mL (22.7 nmol/L)

Is this a macrocytic or microcytic anemia?

Specifically, what is the etiology of the anemia?

What would be the preferred drug regimen (drug, dosage form, and schedule)?

Patient Encounter 2, Part 3

The patient is diagnosed with iron-deficiency anemia and is started on ferrous sulfate 325 mg orally three times daily to be taken on an empty stomach. Follow-up CBC 1 month later reveals Hgb of 10.5 g/dL (105 g/L; 6.52 mmol/L), previously 8.3 g/dL (83 g/L; 5.15 mmol/L). The patient reports improvement in energy level and has resumed running. However, she often develops heartburn after taking the iron tablets.

What hemoglobin level would constitute a therapeutic response in this patient?

What recommendation would you make regarding the heartburn?

Patient Care Process

Patient Assessment:

- Based on physical exam and review of systems, determine if the patient exhibits signs or symptoms of anemia.
- Review CBC, if anemia present, assess RBC indices to determine if microcytic, normocytic, or macrocytic.
- Determine whether transfusion or pharmacotherapy is indicated.
- Assess iron, folic acid, and vitamin B_{12} studies to determine etiology of anemia.
- When initiating ESAs, assess the patient's iron status.
- Initiate appropriate therapy.

Therapy Evaluation:

- Monitor symptoms such as fatigue, shortness of breath, lethargy, headache, edema, and tachycardia for resolution.

Care Plan Development:

- Discuss importance of medication adherence.

Follow-Up Evaluation:

- Follow up monthly to assess efficacy and tolerance of therapy until resolution of symptoms and Hgb goal achieved.
- Monitor the CBC monthly.
- Monitor side effects of therapy, such as
  - Oral iron: nausea, vomiting, abdominal pain, heartburn, constipation, and dark stools
  - Parenteral iron: anaphylaxis (test dose required for iron dextran and observe for 1 hour after), injection-site pain/irritation, arthralgias, myalgias, flushing, malaise, and fever
  - Folic acid: bad taste and nausea, rash, and allergic reactions
  - Vitamin B_{12}: pain and erythema at injection site
  - ESAs: hypertension (monitor blood pressure), thrombosis (eg, deep vein thrombosis/pulmonary embolism, myocardial infarction, cerebrovascular accident, and transient ischemic attack), arthralgias, and headache

cardiovascular events. ESA-labeled dosing regimens for patients with CKD are summarized in Table 66–6.

Although EPO deficiency is the primary cause of CKD anemia, iron deficiency may also exist. Iron stores in patients with CKD should be maintained so that transferrin saturation is greater than 20% (0.20) and serum ferritin is greater than 100 ng/mL (100 mcg/L or 225 pmol/L). If iron stores are not maintained appropriately, epoetin or darbepoetin will not be effective. Most CKD patients will require iron supplementation.[27]

Anemia Due to Zidovudine in HIV-Infected Patients Early clinical trials evaluating the efficacy of zidovudine in patients with HIV documented that nearly 50% of patients treated with zidovudine develop anemia requiring RBC transfusions. Subsequently, results from numerous clinical trials reported that epoetin resulted in statistically significant decreases in transfusion requirements for patients with serum EPO levels less than 500 mUnits/mL (500 U/L). Currently, epoetin has a labeled indication for the treatment of anemia in patients with EPO levels less than 500 mUnits/mL (500 U/L) and administered zidovudine doses less than 4200 mg/week.[32]

OUTCOME EVALUATION

KEY CONCEPT *Patients should be monitored for Hgb response, symptom resolution, and adverse effects at appropriate intervals, and treatment regimens adjusted accordingly.* The goal of anemia therapy is to correct the underlying etiology of the anemia, normalize the Hgb, and alleviate associated symptoms.

- To ensure response for patients with IDA, monitor CBC with special attention to occurrence of reticulocytosis and iron studies.
- A 1.0-g/dL (10 g/L or 0.62 mmol/L) per week increase in Hgb is desirable in patients with IDA. Reevaluate patients with increases less than 2.0 g/dL (20 g/L or 1.24 mmol/L) in 3 weeks.
- For patients with folic acid deficiency, monitor Hgb periodically and reevaluate patients who fail to normalize Hgb levels after 2 months of therapy.
- For patients with vitamin B_{12} deficiency, monitor for resolution of neurologic symptoms (ie, confusion and paresthesias), if applicable, and Hgb levels weekly until the levels normalize.
- For patients treated with chemotherapy, initiate ESA treatment when Hgb levels are less than 10.0 g/dL (100 g/L or 6.21 mmol/L) and monitor Hgb levels weekly. If Hgb increases exceed 1.0 g/dL (10 g/L or 0.62 mmol/L) or exceed 10.0 g/dL (100 g/L or 6.21 mmol/L), hold therapy until the level drops below 10.0 g/dL (100 g/L or 6.21 mmol/L). Restart the ESA at the lowest dose sufficient to reduce transfusions.
- For patients with CKD on dialysis, initiate ESA treatment when Hgb levels are less than 10.0 g/dL (100 g/L or 6.21 mmol/L) and monitor Hgb levels weekly. If Hgb levels approach or exceed 11.0 g/dL (110 g/L or 6.83 mmol/L), reduce or hold further doses until the level drops below 10.0 g/dL (100 g/L or 6.21 mmol/L). Restart the ESA at the lowest dose sufficient to reduce transfusions.
- For patients with CKD not on dialysis, initiate ESA treatment when Hgb levels are less than 10.0 g/dL (100 g/L or 6.21 mmol/L) and monitor Hgb levels weekly. If Hgb levels exceed 10.0 g/dL (100 g/L or 6.21 mmol/L), reduce or hold further doses until the level drops below 10.0 g/dL (100 g/L or 6.21 mmol/L). Restart the ESA at the lowest dose sufficient to reduce transfusions.

Abbreviations Introduced in This Chapter

CFU-E	Erythroid colony-forming unit
CKD	Chronic kidney disease
EPO	Erythropoietin
ESA	Erythropoietin stimulating agent
GFR	Glomerular filtration rate
GM-CSF	Granulocyte-monocyte colony-stimulating factor
Hct	Hematocrit
Hgb	Hemoglobin

IDA	Iron-deficiency anemia
IL-3	Interleukin 3
MCV	Mean corpuscular volume
MCH	Mean corpuscular hemoglobin
TIBC	Total iron-binding capacity

REFERENCES

1. Centers for Disease Control and Prevention. Iron deficiency—United States, 1999-2000. MMWR Morb Mortal Wkly Rep. 2002; 51:897–899.
2. Guralnik JM, Eisenstaedt RS, Ferrucci L, et al. Prevalence of anemia in persons 65 years and older in the United States: Evidence for a high rate of unexplained anemia. Blood. 2004;104(8):2263–2268.
3. Knight K, Wade S, Balducci L. Prevalence and outcomes of anemia in cancer: A systematic review of the literature. Am J Med. 2004;116(Suppl 7A):S11–S26.
4. National Comprehensive Cancer Network [Internet]. Cancer- and chemotherapy-induced anemia. NCCN Practice Guidelines in Oncology- V.2.2015 [cited 2014 June 30]. http://www.nccn.org/professionals/physician_gls/pdf/anemia.pdf
5. McFarlane SI, Chen SC, Whaley-Connell AT, et al. Prevalence and associations of anemia of CKD: Kidney Early Evaluation Program (KEEP) and National Health and Nutrition Examination Survey (NHANES) 1999-2004. Am J Kidney Dis. 2008:51(Suppl 2): S46–S55.
6. Weiss G, Goodnough LT. Anemia of chronic disease. N Engl J Med. 2005;352(10):1011–1023.
7. Guyton AC, Hall JE. Red blood cells, anemia, and polycythemia. In: Guyton AC, Hall JE, eds. Textbook of Medical Physiology. 11th ed. Philadelphia, PA: WB Saunders; 2006:419–428.
8. Kaushansky K, Kipps TJ. Hemapoietic Agents: Growth factors, minerals, and vitamins. In: Brunton LL, Laza LS, Parker KL, eds. Goodman & Gilman's the Pharmacological Basis of Therapeutics. 11th ed. New York: McGraw-Hill; 2006:1433–1466.
9. Toh BH, van Driel IR, Gleeson PA. Pernicious anemia. N Engl J Med. 1997;337(20):1441–1448.
10. Andrews NC. Disorders of iron metabolism. N Engl J Med. 1999;341(26):1986–1995.
11. Aird William C. Anemia. In: Furie Bruce, Cassileth Peter A, Atkins Michael B, Mayer Robert J, eds. Clinical Hematology and Oncology. Philadelphia, PA: Churchill Livingstone; 2003: 232–240.
12. Carless PA, Henry DA, Carson JL, et al. Transfusion thresholds and other strategies for guiding allogeneic red blood cell transfusion. Cochran Database Syst Rev. 2010;6:CD002042.
13. Hebert PC, Wells G, Blajchman MA, et al. A multicenter, randomized, controlled clinical trial of transfusion requirements in critical care. N Engl J Med. 1999;340:409–417.
14. Alleyne M, Horne MK, Miller JL. Individualized treatment for iron-deficiency anemia in adults. Am J Med. 2008;121:943–948.
15. INFed (iron dextran) prescribing information. Morristown, NJ: Watson Pharma; August 2009.
16. Dexferrum (iron dextran) prescribing information. Shirley, NY: American Regent; August 2008.
17. Ferrlecit (sodium ferric gluconate complex in sucrose injection) prescribing information. Bridgewater, NJ: Sanofi-Aventis; August 2011.
18. Venofer (iron sucrose injection) prescribing information. Shirley, NY: American Regent; January 2014.
19. Feraheme (ferumoxytol injection) prescribing information. Lexington, MA: AMAG Pharmaceuticals; December 2013.
20. Injectafer (ferric carboxymaltose injection) prescribing information. Shirley, NY: American Regent, Inc.; July 2013.
21. Auerbach M, Ballard H. Clinical use of intravenous iron: Administration, efficacy and safety. Hematology Am Soc Hematol Educ Program. 2010;2010:338–347.
22. Chertow GM, Mason PD, Vaage-Nilsen O, et al. Update on adverse drug events associated with parenteral iron. Nephrol Dial Transplant. 2006;21:378–382.
23. Zucchero FJ, Hogan MJ, Sommer CD, eds. Evaluations of Drug Interactions. San Bruno, CA: First DataBank; 2007.
24. Bohlius J, Schmidlin K, Brillant C, et al. Erythropoietin or darbepoetin for patients with cancer—meta-analysis based on individual patient data. Cochrane Database Syst Rev. 2009;8: CD007303.
25. Rizzo JD, Brouwers M, Hurley P, et al. American Society of Clinical Oncology/American Society of Hematology clinical practice guideline update on the use of epoetin and darbeopetin in adult patients with cancer. J Clin Oncol. 2010;28:4996–5010.
26. Centers for Medicare and Medicaid Services [Internet]. Decision memo for erythropoiesis stimulating agents (ESAs) in cancer and related neoplastic conditions [cited 2014 July 22]. https://www.cms.gov/transmittals/downloads/R80NCD.pdf
27. NKF/DOQI Clinical Practice Guideline and Clinical Practice Recommendations for anemia in chronic kidney disease: 2007 update of hemoglobin target. Am J Kid Dis. 2007;50:471–530.
28. FDA [Internet]. FDA Drug Safety Communication: Modified dosing recommendations to improve the safe us of erythropoiesis-stimulating agents (ESAs) in chronic kidney disease [cited 2014 July 22]. http://www.fda.gov/drugs/drugsafety/ucm259639.htm
29. Aranesp (darbepoetin alfa) prescribing information. Thousand Oaks, CA: Amgen; December 2013.
30. Epogen (epoetin alfa) prescribing information. Centocor Ortho Biotech Products, April 2014.
31. Procrit (epoetin alfa) prescribing information. Thousand Oaks, CA: Amgen; December 2013.
32. Henry DH, Beall GN, Benson CA, et al. Recombinant human erythropoietin in the treatment of anemia associated with human immunodeficiency virus (HIV) infection and zidovudine therapy. Overview of four clinical trials. Ann Intern Med. 1992; 117:739–748.

67 Coagulation and Platelet Disorders

Anastasia Rivkin and Sandeep Vansal

LEARNING OBJECTIVES

Upon completion of this chapter, the reader will be able to:

1. Describe the basics of the regulation of hemostasis and thrombosis.
2. Select appropriate nonpharmacological and pharmacological therapy for a patient with hemophilia in a given clinical situation and patient-specific scenario.
3. Calculate an appropriate factor-concentrate dose for a product, given the percentage correction desired based on clinical situation.
4. List possible complications from hemophilia bleeding episodes.
5. Choose an appropriate treatment strategy for patients with factor VIII or IX inhibitors.
6. Devise a treatment plan for a patient with a specific variant of von Willebrand disease.
7. Describe various recessively inherited coagulation disorders (RICDs) and role of specific factor replacement in RICD management.
8. Recommend first-line and a second-line treatment approaches for immune thrombocytopenic purpura.
9. Identify basic clinical features, causes, and management of thrombotic thrombocytopenic purpura.

INTRODUCTION

Components of the Hemostatic System

Following endothelial injury, vessel-wall response involves vasoconstriction, platelet plug formation, coagulation, and **fibrinolysis** regulation. In normal circumstances, platelets circulate in the blood in an inactive form. After injury, platelets undergo activation, which consists of (a) adhesion to the subendothelium, (b) secretion of granules containing chemical mediators (eg, adenosine diphosphate, thromboxane A2, thrombin, etc), and (c) aggregation. Chemical factors released from the injured tissue and platelets stimulate the coagulation cascade and thrombin formation. In turn, thrombin catalyzes the conversion of fibrinogen to fibrin and its subsequent incorporation into the platelet plug.

The coagulation system consists of intrinsic and extrinsic pathways. Both pathways are composed of a series of enzymatic reactions that ultimately produce thrombin, fibrin, and a stable clot. In parallel with the coagulation, the fibrinolytic system is activated locally. Plasminogen is converted to plasmin, which dissolves the fibrin mesh (Figure 67–1).[1]

INHERITED COAGULATION DISORDERS

HEMOPHILIA

Etiology and Epidemiology

Hemophilia A and B are coagulation disorders that result from defects in the genes encoding for plasma coagulation proteins. Hemophilia A (classic hemophilia) is caused by the deficiency of factor VIII, and hemophilia B (Christmas disease) is caused by the deficiency of factor IX. The incidences of hemophilia A and B are estimated at 1 in 5000 and 1 in 30,000 male births, respectively. Both types of hemophilia are evenly distributed across all ethnic and racial groups.[1]

Pathophysiology

The pathophysiology of hemophilia is based on the deficiency of factor VIII or IX resulting in inadequate thrombin generation and an impaired intrinsic-pathway coagulation cascade (see Figure 67–1). Factor VIII and IX genes are located on the X chromosome. Hemophilias are recessive X-linked diseases. Generally, affected males carrying either defective allele on their X chromosome do not transmit the gene to their sons. However, their daughters are obligate carriers. More than 1000 mutations in factor VIII and IX genes have been identified to cause clinical hemophilia.[2]

Consequently, hemophilia is not a result of a single genetic mutation. However, inversion at intron 22 of the factor VIII gene accounts for 40% of severe hemophilia A cases. Owing to the high incidence, this mutation is used for carrier and prenatal testing.[3]

Complications of Hemophilia

The severity of bleeding associated with hemophilia correlates with the degree of factor VIII or factor IX deficiency as measured against the normal plasma standard. Table 67–1 summarizes the age at onset and laboratory and clinical manifestations of hemophilia A and B.[4]

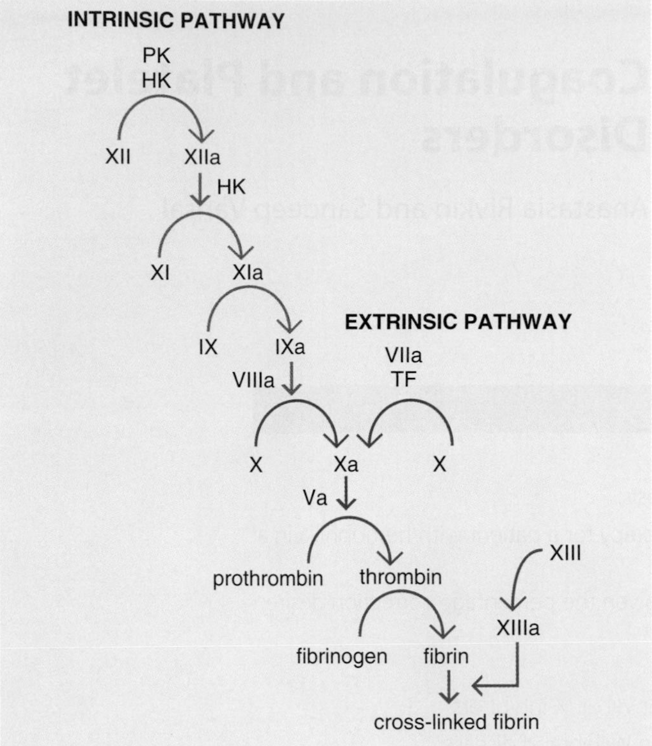

FIGURE 67–1. Cascade model of coagulation demonstrates activation via the intrinsic or extrinsic pathway. This model shows successive activation of coagulation factors proceeding from the top to the bottom where thrombin and fibrin are generated. (PK, prekallikrein; HK, high–molecular weight kininogen; TF, tissue factor.) (From Roberts HR et al. Molecular biology and biochemistry of the coagulation factors and pathways of hemostasis. In: Lichtman MA, Beutler E, Coller BS et al, eds. Williams Hematology, 7th ed. New York: McGraw-Hill, 2006:1665–1694.)

Treatment

▶ *Desired Outcomes*

Currently, there is no cure for hemophilia A or B. The life expectancy of hemophiliacs was only 8 to 11 years in the 1920s and 1930s. With the development of effective treatment strategies, life expectancy is currently about 63 to 75 years, or nearly that of the normal population.[5]

The short-term goals of hemophilia treatment are to:

- Decrease the number of bleeding episodes per year or bleeding frequency
- Normalize or improve clotting factor concentrate levels

The long-term goals of hemophilia treatment are to:

- Maintain clinical joint function
- Normalize orthopedic joint score
- Normalize radiologic joint score
- Maintain quality-of-life measurements

▶ *General Approach to Treatment*

KEY CONCEPT *Intravenous factor replacement with recombinant or plasma-derived products to treat or prevent bleeding is the primary treatment of hemophilia.* Primary prophylaxis is defined as the regular administration of factor concentrates with the intention of preventing joint bleeds.[6] The rationale for primary prophylaxis is that individuals with factor levels of greater than 0.02 IU/mL (20 IU/L) rarely suffer from spontaneous bleeds and arthropathy. Therefore, to maintain a trough level above this might convert "severe" hemophilia to "moderate" disease, with the abolition of joint bleeds and the associated arthropathy.[7]

Although primary prophylaxis is expensive, historical cohorts show progressively better outcomes (joint function and radiologic appearances) with its use. The Medical and Scientific Advisory Council of the National Hemophilia Foundation of the United States recommends primary prophylaxis in patients with

Table 67–1

Laboratory and Clinical Manifestations of Hemophilia

	Severe (< 0.01 IU/mL [10 IU/L])[a]	Moderate (0.01–0.05 IU/mL [10–50 IU/L])	Mild (> 0.05 IU/mL [50 IU/L])
Age at onset	1 year or less	1–2 years	2 years–adult
Neonatal symptoms			
PCB	Usual	Usual	Rare
ICH	Occasional	Uncommon	Rare
Muscle/joint hemorrhage	Spontaneous	Minor trauma	Minor trauma
CNS hemorrhage	High risk	Moderate risk	Rare
Postsurgical hemorrhage (without prophylaxis)	Frank bleeding, severe	Wound bleeding, common	Wound bleeding
Oral hemorrhage following trauma, tooth extraction	Usual	Common	Common

CNS, central nervous system; ICH, intracranial hemorrhage; PCB, postcircumcisional bleeding.

Normal range of factor VIII/IX activity level is 0.5–1.5 IU/mL (500–1500 IU/L). 1 IU/mL (1000 IU/L) corresponds to 100% of the factor found in 1 mL of normal plasma.

Clinical Presentation and Diagnosis of Hemophilias A and B

Hemophilias A and B are clinically indistinguishable.

Symptoms

- Ecchymoses
- Hemarthrosis—bleeding into joint spaces[a] (especially knee, elbow, and ankle)
  - Joint pain, swelling, and erythema
  - Cutaneous warmth
  - Decreased range of motion
- Muscle hemorrhage
  - Swelling
  - Pain with motion of affected muscle
  - Signs of nerve compression
  - Potential life-threatening blood loss, especially with thigh bleeding
- Mouth bleeding with dental extractions or trauma
- Genitourinary bleeding
- Gastrointestinal (GI) bleeding
- Hematuria
- Intracranial hemorrhage (spontaneous or following trauma), with headache, vomiting, change in mental status, and focal neurologic signs
- Excessive bleeding with surgery

Diagnostic Parameters/Laboratory testing

- Family history
- Normal prothrombin time (PT)
- Normal platelet count
- Prolonged activated partial thromboplastin time (aPTT)
- Low factor VIII level (hemophilia A)
- Low factor IX level (hemophilia B)

[a]Hallmark of hemophilia; recurrent inadequately managed hemarthrosis leads to deformity and chronic pain (hemophilic arthropathy).

severe hemophilia A and B (factor VIII or factor IX less than 1%). The optimal duration of prophylactic therapy is unknown.[8,9]

▶ *Nonpharmacologic Therapy*

Supportive Care Rest, ice, compression, elevation (RICE) can be used during the bleeding episode, following with casts, splints, and crutches after the bleeding has been controlled.

Surgery Surgical arthroscopic synovectomy reduces replacement therapy–resistant disease and repetitive hemarthrosis of a single joint. This procedure removes inflamed joint tissue. Patients may have decreased range of motion after the surgery.

Orthotics Joint prostheses do not deal with the deformities directly. Orthotics in hemophilia serve as an important supportive measure before or after surgery.

▶ *Pharmacologic Therapy*

Hemophilia A

DDAVP Primary therapy is based on disease severity and type of hemorrhage.[10] Most patients with mild to moderate disease and a minor bleeding episode can be treated with 1-desamino-8-D-arginine vasopressin (desmopressin acetate [DDAVP]), a synthetic analogue of the antidiuretic hormone, vasopressin. DDAVP causes release of von Willebrand factor (vWF) and factor VIII from endothelial storage sites. DDAVP increases plasma factor VIII levels by threefold to fivefold within 30 minutes. The recommended dose is 0.3 mcg/kg IV (in 50 mL of normal saline infused over 15–30 minutes) or subcutaneously (in < 1.5 mL) or 150 to 300 mcg intranasally via concentrated nasal spray, may repeat after 24 hours. [10] Peak effect with intranasal administration

Patient Encounter 1, Part 1: Hemophilia

A 2-month-old boy without any significant past medical history developed mild bleeding into the joint spaces of the knees and elbows. The baby is irritable and has warm swollen joints. Patient's parents report family history significant for maternal grandfather with hemophilia.

What additional information do you need to create a treatment plan for this patient?

What are this patient's risk factors for hemophilia?

Patient Encounter 1, Part 2: Hemophilia

Meds: None

PE:

- Swollen red joints of elbows and knees bilaterally. Wt 11.1 lb (5.04 kg)

Labs:

- Platelet count: $145 \times 10^3/mm^3$ ($145 \times 10^9/L$) (normal $140–440 \times 10^3/mm^3$ [$140–440 \times 10^9/L$])
- aPTT: 90 seconds (normal 25–40 seconds)
- INR: 1 (normal 0.8–1.2)
- Factor VIII: 5% (normal 50%–150%)
- Ristocetin cofactor activity (vWF:RCo): 150 IU/dL or 1500 IU/L (normal 50–200 IU/dL or 500–2000 IU/L)

Given this additional information, is this patient's presentation consistent with hemophilia? Which type of hemophilia does this patient have?

Identify your treatment goals for this patient.

occurs 60 to 90 minutes after administration, which is somewhat later than with IV administration. Desmopressin infusion may be administered daily for up to 2 to 3 days. Facial flushing, hypertension or hypotension, GI upset, and headache are common side effects of desmopressin. Water retention and hyponatremia may occur; patients should be instructed to limit water intake while taking desmopressin. Serious side effects include seizures related to hyponatremia and myocardial infarction. Due to higher incidence of hyponatremia-related seizures in patients less than 2 years old, use of desmopressin is not recommended in this population. Tachyphylaxis, an attenuated response with repeated administration, may occur after several doses.[11]

According to the manufacturer, use of DDAVP is contraindicated in patients with creatinine clearance less than 50 mL/min (0.83 mL/s); however, it has been used off label in patients with impaired renal function.

Antifibrinolytic Therapy Aminocaproic acid and tranexamic acid are antifibrinolytic agents that reduce plasminogen activity leading to inhibition of clot lysis and clot stabilization. These agents are usually used as adjuncts in dental procedures or in difficult-to-control epistaxis and menorrhagia episodes and have to be administered with appropriate factor concentrates to form a clot.[10]

Factor VIII Replacement Patients with severe hemophilia may receive primary (before the first major bleed) or secondary (after the first major bleed) prophylaxis. All hemophiliacs with a major bleed require factor VIII replacement.[12] The therapy may include recombinant (produced via transfection of mammalian cells with the human factor VIII gene) or plasma-derived (concentrate from pooled plasma) factor VIII (Table 67–2). The choice of product and dose are based on the overall clinical scenario because the efficacy of various preparations does not differ. Newer generation plasma-derived coagulation factor concentrates are considerably safer owing to advancements in viral testing and inactivation technology. Although original recombinant factor VIII concentrates were stabilized with human serum albumin, potentially creating a source for viral contamination, new-generation recombinant factor VIII concentrates are stabilized with sucrose, eliminating the concern for viral transmission.[10]

The severity of hemorrhage and its location are major determinants of percentage correction to target, as well as duration of therapy (Table 67–3). The normal range of factor VIII activity level is 1 IU/mL (1000 IU/L), which corresponds to 100% of the factor found in 1 mL of normal plasma. Minor bleeding may be treated with a goal of 25% to 30% (0.25–0.30 IU/mL [250–300 IU/L]) of normal activity, whereas serious or life-threatening bleeding requires greater than 75% of normal activity. Factor VIII is a large molecule that remains in the intravascular space, and its estimated volume of distribution is approximately 50 mL/kg. Generally, factor VIII levels increase by 2% (0.02 IU/mL

Table 67–2

Factor Concentrates

Brand Name	Product Type	Viral Inactivation or Exclusion Method	Other Contents
Factor VIII Concentrates			
Alphanate	Plasma	Solvent detergent, dry heat	Albumin, heparin, vWF
Advate	Recombinant	None	Trehalose
Bioclate	Recombinant	None	Albumin
Eloctate	Recombinant	None	Sucrose
Helixate FS	Recombinant	Solvent detergent	Sucrose
Hemofil M	Plasma	Solvent detergent, monoclonal antibody	Albumin
Humate-P	Plasma	Pasteurization	Albumin, vWF
Koāte-DVI	Plasma	Solvent detergent, dry heat	Albumin, vWF
Kogenate FS	Recombinant	Solvent detergent, monoclonal antibody	Sucrose
Monoclate P	Plasma	Pasteurization, monoclonal antibody	Albumin
Recombinate	Recombinant	Monoclonal antibody	Albumin
ReFacto	Recombinant B domain deleted	None	Sucrose
Xyntha	Recombinant B domain deleted	Solvent-detergent, nanofiltration	Sucrose
Factor IX Concentrates			
AlphaNine SD	Plasma	Solvent detergent, nanofiltration	Heparin
BeneFIX	Recombinant	None	Sucrose
Mononine	Plasma	Monoclonal antibody, nanofiltration	
Rixubis	Recombinant	None	
Alprolix	Recombinant	None	
APCC			
Feiba VH or NF	Plasma	Vapor heat	II, VIIa, IX, X, factor VIII coagulant antigen
PCC			
Bebulin VH	Plasma	Vapor heat	Heparin, II, IX, X
Profilnine SD	Plasma	Solvent detergent	II, VII, IX, X
Proplex T	Plasma	Dry heat	Heparin, II, VII, IX, X
Other			
NovoSeven RT	Recombinant VII	None	Sucrose
Wilate	Plasma vWF/VIII complex	Solvent detergent and dry heat	Sucrose

APCC, activated prothrombin complex concentrate; PCC, prothrombin complex concentrate; vWF, von Willebrand factor.

Table 67–3

Guidelines for Replacement Dosing with Factor VIII and Factor IX

Type of Hemorrhage	Desired Plasma Factor VIII Level (% of Normal)	Desired Plasma Factor XI Level (% of Normal)	Duration of Therapy (days)
CNS, intracranial, retropharyngeal, retroperitoneal, surgical prophylaxis	80–100	80–100	Factor VIII: every 8–12 hours over 10–14 days Factor IX: every 12 hours over 10–14 days
Mild hemarthrosis, mucosal (eg, epistaxis), superficial hematoma	30	20–30	Factor VIII: every 8–12 hours over 1–2 days Factor IX: every 12–24 hours over 1–2 days

[20 IU/L]) for every 1 unit/kg of factor VIII concentrate infused. To calculate factor VIII replacement dose, the following equation can be used:

$$\text{Dose of factor VIII (units)} = \text{weight (kg)} \times \text{(desired percentage increase)} \times 0.5$$

Thus, to increase factor VIII levels by 50% (eg, from 0 to 50%) in a 70-kg (154-lb) patient, an IV dose of 1750 units is required. The median half-life of factor VIII ranges from 9.4 hours (in 1–6 year olds) to 10.4 hours (in 10–65 year olds).[13,14] Half the initial dose is given every half-life (every 8–12 hours) to maintain the desired factor VIII level. Although intermittent bolus infusions of factor VIII concentrates have been used successfully, continuous-infusion protocols are being instituted successfully in patients requiring prolonged treatment of acute hemorrhage to avoid dangerously low trough levels and decrease the overall cost of therapy. Factor VIII can be administered as a continuous infusion at 2 to 4 units/kg/hour with daily factor level monitoring to ensure appropriate rate of infusion.[15,16]

▸ *Hemophilia B*

Factor IX Replacement Hemophilia B therapy may include recombinant (produced via transfection of mammalian cells with the human factor IX gene) or plasma-derived (concentrate from pooled plasma) factor IX (see Table 67–2). Guidelines for choosing the factor-concentrate formulation for hemophilia B are similar to the guidelines for hemophilia A. However, older generation factor IX concentrates containing other vitamin K–dependent proteins (eg, factors II, VII, and IX), called prothrombin complex concentrates (PCCs), have been associated with thrombogenic side effects. Consequently, these products are not first-line treatment for hemophilia B. Because it is a small protein, the factor IX molecule passes into both the intravascular and the extravascular spaces. Therefore, the volume of distribution of recombinant factor IX is twice that of factor VIII. Consequently, 1 unit of factor IX administered per kilogram of body weight yields a 1% rise in the plasma factor IX level (0.01 IU/mL [10 IU/L]). To calculate the factor IX replacement dose, the following equation can be used:

$$\text{Dose of factor IX (units)} = \text{weight (kg)} \times \text{(desired percentage increase)} \times F$$

Where (F = 1 for human plasma-derived products; F = 1.1 for Rixubis; F = 1.4 for Benefix in adults and 1.2 in children).

Thus, to increase factor IX levels by 50% (eg, from 0% to 50%) in a 70-kg (154-lb) patient, the required dose of factor IX is 4900 units IV (using Benefix). The half-life of factor IX ranges from 16 to 17 hours; therefore, doses are given every 18 to 24 hours. Factor IX fusion protein can be given every 1 to 2 weeks.[17]

Gene therapy for the treatment of hemophilia is currently under investigation. A recent clinical trial has shown long-term therapeutic levels of factor IX in six subjects with severe hemophilia B receiving a single infusion of a factor IX transgene vector.[18,19]

▸ *Treatment of Patients with Factor VIII or IX Inhibitors*

Factor VIII and IX inhibitors are antibodies that develop in approximately 30% and 5% of hemophilia A and hemophilia B patients, respectively, in response to replacement therapy. There is no difference between plasma-derived and recombinant products in their potential for inhibitor development. These antibodies bind to and neutralize the activity of infused factor concentrates. Although the inhibitors do not increase hemorrhage frequency, their existence challenges the treatment of bleeding episodes. Titers of inhibitors are measured and reported in Bethesda units (BU), and this measurement is used to guide therapy (Figure 67–2). Management options for acute bleeding in patients with factor inhibitors include the administration of factor VIII concentrates, PCCs, recombinant factor VIIa (rFVIIa), and porcine factor VIII (currently, recombinant porcine factor VIII is in phase II/III clinical trials in the United States). Immune tolerance induction can be attempted to prevent future bleeding episodes.

Factor VIII concentrates can be used in patients with low inhibitor levels to control acute bleeding episodes. The dose of factor VIII is determined based on clinical response (see Figure 67–2).

PCCs contain the vitamin K–dependent factors II, VII, IX, and X. These agents bypass factor VIII at which the antibody is directed (see Figure 67–2). However, PCCs carry the risk of serious thrombotic complications.

Factor VIIa (rFVIIa) is a bypassing agent designed to generate thrombin only at tissue injury sites, where it binds tissue factor. Due to its local action, rFVIIa is associated with fewer systemic thrombotic events than PCC. rFVIIa is used effectively in surgeries and spontaneous bleeds.[20]

Plasma-derived porcine factor VIII participates in the coagulation cascade in place of human factor VIII. However, due to contamination with parvovirus, it is no longer available. Recombinant porcine factor VIII is currently under review and could serve as a third-line agent (only after factor VIIa and a PCC have failed) owing to the relatively high incidence of cross-reactivity with factor VIII inhibitors.

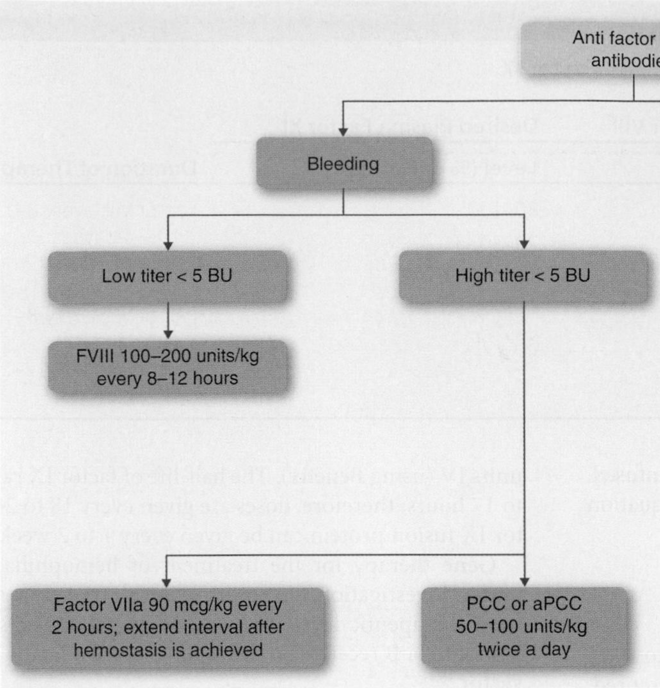

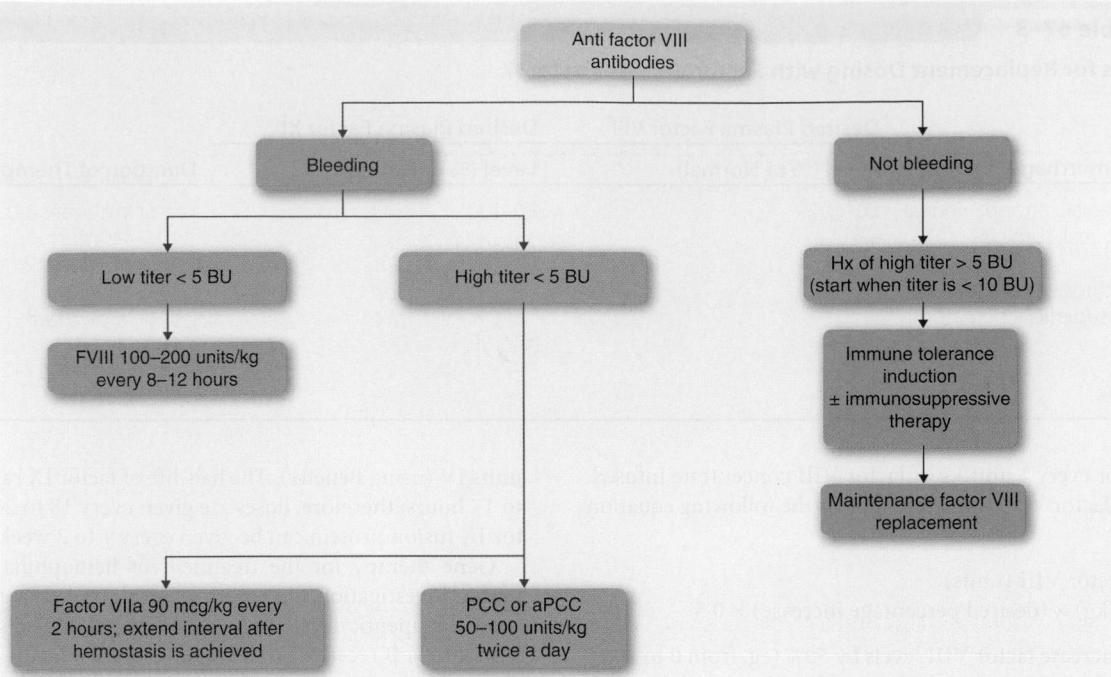

FIGURE 67–2. Treatment algorithm for the management of patients with hemophilia A and factor VIII antibodies. (aPCC, activated prothrombin complex concentrate; BU, Bethesda unit.) (Modified from DiPiro JT, Talbert RL, Yee GC, et al., eds. Pharmacotherapy: A Pathophysiologic Approach. 9th ed. New York: McGraw-Hill; 2014, Figure 81–1.)

Induction of immune tolerance is often performed with the goal of eliminating the inhibitor. Immune tolerance induction is accomplished by the administration of repetitive doses of factor VIII or IX with or without immunosuppressive therapy. It is effective in 70% of patients with hemophilia A and 30% of patients with hemophilia B.

Pain Associated with Hemophilia

Pain commonly occurs in patients with hemophilia. Acute bleeding episodes and long-term joint destruction are common sources of pain. Acetaminophen and opioid analgesics are recommended to control mild to moderate and severe pain, respectively. Nonsteroidal anti-inflammatory drugs and aspirin should be avoided if possible, because these drugs bind to platelets and increase the risk of bleeding episodes. Cyclooxygenase-2 (COX-2) inhibitors can be used with caution.[21]

Outcome Evaluation

The main goal of hemophilia treatment is to prevent bleeding episodes and their long-term complications. Clinicians should evaluate patients for the following:

- Musculoskeletal status, including joint range of motion and radiologic assessment, as indicated.
- Number and type of bleeding episodes to assess adequacy of prophylactic treatment and home therapy.
- Use of clotting-factor concentrates to check for the development of inhibitors, especially in patients with severe disease and poor treatment responders.
- Vaccination against hepatitis A and B is recommended in all hemophiliacs without evidence of immunity.

Patient Encounter 1, Part 3: Hemophilia: Creating a Care Plan

Based on the information presented, create a care plan for this patient with hemophilia.

VON WILLEBRAND DISEASE

Epidemiology and Etiology

von Willebrand disease (vWD) is the most common inherited bleeding disorder caused by a deficiency or dysfunction of vWF. It is classified based on the quantitative deficiency of vWF or qualitative abnormalities of vWF. The disease prevalence is estimated at 30 to 100 cases per million. In contrast to hemophilia, the majority of vWD cases are inherited as an autosomal dominant disorder, ensuing equal frequency in males and females.[22]

Pathophysiology

vWF is a large multimeric glycoprotein with two main functions in **hemostasis**: to aid platelet adhesion to injured blood vessel walls and to carry and stabilize factor VIII in plasma. Table 67–4 represents three main vWD phenotypes, their frequency, and genetic transmission.[23]

Treatment

▶ *Desired Outcomes*

Unlike hemophilia, the bleeding tendency in vWD is less frequent and generally less severe. Consequently, chronic prophylaxis is usually unwarranted. The goal of two mainstay therapeutic options in vWD is:

- To stop spontaneous bleeding as necessary
- To prevent surgical and postpartum bleeding

Table 67–4
Classification of vWD

Phenotype	Mechanism of Disease	Percentage of Cases	Genetic Transmission
Type 1 vWD	Partial (mild to moderate) quantitative deficiency of vWF and factor VIII	70–80	Autosomal dominant
Type 2 vWD	Qualitative abnormalities of vWF	10–30	
2A	Decreased platelet-dependent vWF function owing to lack of larger multimers	10–20	Autosomal dominant (or recessive)
2B	Decreased vWF function due to increased affinity to platelet GP 1b and resultant sequestration or loss	5	Autosomal dominant
2M	Defective platelet-dependent vWF functions not associated with multimer defects	Uncommon	Autosomal dominant (or recessive)
2N	Defective vWF binding to factor VIII	Uncommon	Autosomal recessive
Type 3 vWD	Severe quantitative deficiency of vWF	Rare	Autosomal recessive

▸ *Nonpharmacologic Therapy*

Local measures, including pressure and ice, may be used to control superficial bleeding.

▸ *Pharmacologic Therapy*

Systemic therapy is used to prevent bleeding associated with surgery, childbirth, and dental extractions and to treat bleeding that cannot be controlled with local measures. The two systemic approaches involve using desmopressin, which stimulates the release of endogenous vWF, or administering products that contain vWF. The general approach to the treatment of vWD is depicted in Figure 67–3. In 2008, The National Heart, Lung, and Blood Institute issued comprehensive evidence-based guidelines for the diagnosis and management of vWD.[24]

DDAVP Most patients with type 1 vWD (functionally normal vWF) and a minor bleeding episode can be treated successfully with desmopressin, which induces release of factor VIII and vWF from endothelial cells through interaction with vasopressin V2 receptors. The recommended dose is the same as that used to treat mild factor VIII deficiency (0.3 mcg/kg IV in 50 mL of normal saline infused over 15 to 30 min or 150 to 300 mcg intranasally via concentrated nasal spray, may repeat after 24 hours). This therapy is generally ineffective in type 2A patients, who secrete abnormal vWF. It is recommended in type 2B patients who respond to it. It may increase the risk of postinfusion thrombocytopenia, in which case a concomitant platelet infusion is administered. Type 3 vWD patients who lack releasable stores of vWF do not respond to DDAVP therapy.[25]

The individual responsiveness to desmopressin is consistent, and a test dose administered at the time of diagnosis or prior to therapy is the best predictor of response. Generally, DDAVP is more effective in vWD than in hemophilia patients, with an average twofold to fivefold increase in vWF and factor VIII levels over baseline. In patients with an adequate response, desmopressin is first-line therapy because it allows for once-daily administration (elevates plasma levels for 8 to 10 hours), does not pose a threat in terms of viral transmission, and costs substantially less than the plasma-derived products.

Antifibrinolytic Therapy Fibrinolysis inhibitors and oral contraceptives are used successfully in the management of epistaxis and menorrhagia or as adjuvant treatments.[26] Fibrinolysis inhibitors include aminocaproic acid (25–60 mg/kg orally or IV (or 4–5 g) every 4 to 6 hours, to a maximum dose of 24 g/day) and tranexamic acid (10 mg/kg IV every 8 hours). Oral tranexamic

Clinical Presentation and Diagnosis of vWD

Clinical manifestations vary depending on the subtype. Patients with mild disease may be asymptomatic into adulthood.

Symptoms

- Bruising
- Mucocutaneous bleeding
  - Epistaxis
  - Oral cavity bleeding
  - Menorrhagia
  - GI bleeding
- Joint and deep tissue bleeding
- Postoperative bleeding

Laboratory Testing

- Low or normal von Willebrand factor antigen concentration in plasma (vWF:Ag)
- Low or normal factor VIII coagulation assay (FVIII:C)[a]
- Low ristocetin cofactor activity (vWF:RCo)[b]

[a]Factor VIII coagulation assay measures the ability of vWF to bind and maintain adequate levels of factor VIII.

[b]Ristocetin cofactor activity (vWF:RCo) assay measures the ability of vWF to interact with intact platelets (normal 50–200 IU/dL [500–2000 IU/L]).

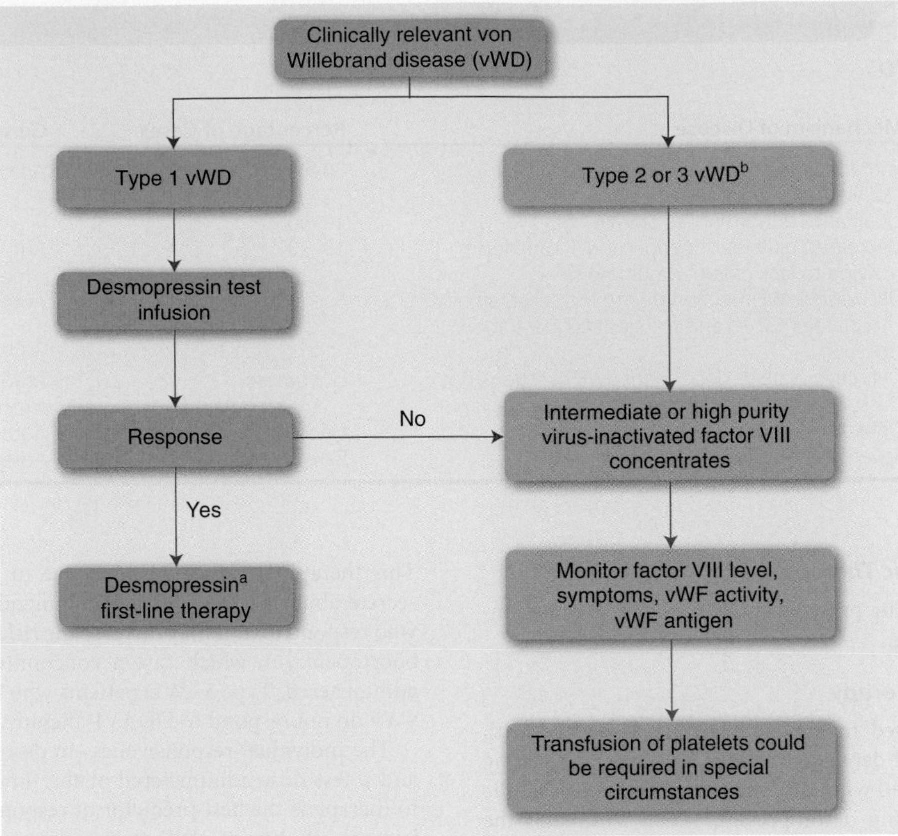

FIGURE 67–3. Guidelines for the treatment of vWD. [a]Use factor VIII concentrate for life-threatening bleeding. [b]Some patients with type 2 or 3 vWD may respond to desmopressin. (From DiPiro JT, Talbert RL, Yee GC, et al., eds. Pharmacotherapy: A Pathophysiologic Approach. 8th ed. New York: McGraw-Hill; 2011:1754, Figure 110–4.)

acid recently received FDA approval for the treatment of cyclic heavy menstrual bleeding; its use is currently not approved for vWD patients. The IV form of tranexamic acid given as swish and swallow or spit every 6 to 8 hours has been used as bleeding prophylaxis in dental surgery. Both aminocaproic acid and tranexamic acid are dose adjusted for patients with renal insufficiency.

Replacement Therapy KEY CONCEPT *Type 1 patients unresponsive to desmopressin, patients with types 2 and 3 vWD, and major surgery patients require replacement therapy with plasma-derived, intermediate- and high-purity virus-inactivated factor VIII concentrates containing vWF.*

Table 67–5 provides typical dosing guidelines and target levels of replacement therapy–concentrates to control various types of hemorrhage. Ultra-high-purity (monoclonal) plasma-derived and recombinant factor VIII concentrates do not contain vWF and should not be used in the treatment of vWD.

Table 67–5

Replacement Therapy in vWD

Condition	Therapy	Recommended Dosage
Major surgery	Maintain vWF:RCo and factor VIII levels at least 100 IU/dL (1000 IU/L) followed by 50 IU/dL (500 IU/L) for 7–14 days To minimize risk of thrombosis: vWF:RCo levels should not exceed 200 IU/dL (2000 IU/L), and factor VIII levels should not exceed 250 IU/dL (2500 IU/L)	40–60 units/kg[a] loading dose, followed by 20–40 units/kg every 12–24 hours DDAVP may be added after a few days
Minor surgery	Prophylaxis: maintain vWF:RCo and factor VIII levels at least 30 IU/dL (300 IU/L) (preferably > 50 IU/dL [> 500 IU/L]) Minor surgery: maintain vWF:RCo and factor VIII levels at least 30 IU/dL (300 IU/L) (preferably > 50 IU/dL [> 500 IU/L]) for 3–5 days	30–60 units/kg loading dose, followed by 20–40 units/kg every 12–48 hours DDAVP may be added after a few days

[a]vWF concentrates are dosed based on vWF:RCo units concentration in the preparation to achieve the desired vWF:RCo levels.

Table 67–6
Clotting Factor Deficiency Characteristics

Factor Deficient	Inheritance Pattern	Estimated Incidence	Laboratory Abnormalities	Severity and Site of Bleeding
II	Autosomal dominant or recessive	Extremely rare	Prolonged PT and aPTT	Mild to moderate umbilical cord, joint, and mucosal tract
V	Autosomal recessive	1:1,000,000	Prolonged PT and aPTT	Mild to moderate mucosal tract
VII	Autosomal recessive	1:500,000	Prolonged PT	Mild to severe mucosal tract and joint
X	Autosomal recessive	1:1,000,000	Prolonged PT and aPTT	Mild to severe umbilical cord, joint, and muscle
XI	Autosomal recessive	4% of Ashkenazi Jews: otherwise rare	Prolonged aPTT	Mild to moderate posttraumatic bleeding
XII	Unknown	Unknown	Prolonged aPTT	No bleeding
XIII	Autosomal recessive	Less than 1:2,000,000	Normal PT and aPTT	Moderate to severe umbilical cord, intracranial, and joint bleeding; recurrent miscarriages, impaired wound healing

aPTT, activated partial thromboplastin time; PT, prothrombin time.

Outcome Evaluation

The main goal of vWF treatment is to prevent bleeding with surgery or dental procedures. Clinicians should evaluate patients every 6 to 12 months for the following:

- Number and type of bleeding episodes to assess the need for prophylactic treatment.
- Ensure adequate levels of vWF and factor VIII prior to minor and major surgical procedures and for the treatment of bleeding.
- Vaccination against hepatitis A and B is recommended in all patients with vWF deficiency with no evidence of immunity.

OTHER CLOTTING FACTOR DEFICIENCIES

Etiology and Epidemiology

Recessively inherited coagulation disorders (RICDs) refer to relatively rare deficiencies in factor II, V, VII, and X to XIII resulting in either decreased clotting factor production or production of a dysfunctional molecule with reduced activity.[27] The clinical severity of bleeding varies and generally is poorly correlated with the factor blood levels. Table 67–6 illustrates these clotting factor deficiencies and some of their characteristics.

Pathophysiology

The RICDs are rare genetic disorders. Mutations in the genes responsible for the respective clotting factors result in impaired functionality or production of the factor.

Treatment

▶ *Desired Outcomes*

Therapeutic options for RICDs improve hemostasis via replacement of deficient blood coagulation factors while minimizing the development of immune tolerance.[28]

Hemostatic levels should be maintained for the following conditions:

- Spontaneous bleeding—until bleeding stops
- Minor surgery—for 2 to 3 days
- Major surgery—until incision site has healed

▶ *Nonpharmacologic Therapy*

Transfusional Therapies KEY CONCEPT *The primary treatment of RICDs is single-donor fresh-frozen plasma (FFP) that contains all coagulation factors.* Disadvantages of FFP treatment include the risk of the patient becoming volume overloaded, especially when repeated infusions are administered to improve and maintain hemostasis; risk of infections; and risk of inhibitor development. PCCs licensed for the treatment of hemophilia B also contain significant levels of vitamin K–dependent factors and may be used off label for treatment of RICD. Table 67–7 lists the recommended RICD treatment schedules in different clinical scenarios.

▶ *Pharmacologic Therapy*

Less severe hemorrhages may be treated successfully with antifibrinolytic amino acids alone or in combination with factor replacement therapy. Tranexamic acid and aminocaproic acid may be administered IV or orally (for doses, see von Willebrand Disease, Pharmacologic Therapy mentioned earlier).

Table 67–7
Treatment of Factor Deficiencies

Factor Deficient	Major Surgery	Spontaneous Bleeding
II	1. PCC: 20–30 units/kg 2. FFP: 15–20 mL/kg	1. FFP: 15–20 mL/kg
V	1. FFP: 15–20 mL/kg	1. FFP: 15–20 mL/kg
VII	1. rFVIIa: 15–30 mcg/kg every 4–6 hours	1. rFVIIa: 15–30 mcg/kg every 4–6 hours
X	1. PCC: 20–30 units/kg 2. FFP: 15–20 mL/kg	1. PCC: 20–30 units/kg 2. FFP: 15–20 mL/kg
XI	1. FFP: 15–20 mL/kg	1. FFP: 15–20 mL/kg
XIII	1. Pasteurized plasma concentrate: 10–20 units/kg 2. FFP: 15–20 mL/kg 3. Cryoprecipitate (1 bag per 10 kg)	1. FFP: 3–5 mL/kg

Numbers indicate lines of therapy. FFP, fresh-frozen plasma; PCC, prothrombin complex concentrates.

Patient Care Process Hemophilias, vWD disease, and RICD

Patient Assessment:

- Obtain a complete medical and family history.
- Evaluate CBC, vital signs, and coagulation studies. If a bleeding disorder is diagnosed, evaluate specific coagulation assays to determine the etiology of the bleeding disorder.

Therapy Evaluation and Care Plan Development:

- Institute nonpharmacological therapy to minimize minor bleeding.
- Depending on the specific diagnosis and disease severity, select appropriate therapy with desmopressin, antifibrinolytic medications, and/or disease-specific factor replacement therapies.
- Recommend prophylactic therapies before major and minor surgical procedures based on bleeding risk assessment.
- Evaluate pain and treat if necessary, selecting medication that do not increase the risk of bleeding.
- Review vaccination history and recommend appropriate vaccinations.

Follow-Up Evaluation:

- If clotting factor replacement is utilized, continuously evaluate its efficacy and test for inhibitors development if loss of efficacy is observed.
- Monitor number/severity of bleeding episodes, joint count/joint destruction, and pain associated with some coagulation/bleeding disorders.

PLATELET DISORDERS

Platelets, in combination with several other factors such as blood vessel wall and coagulation factors, play key role in hemostasis. Normal platelet count is 150–450 × 10^3/mm^3 (150–450 × 10^9/L). Thrombopoietin, a hormone synthesized in the liver, regulates platelet production. Several congenital and iatrogenic disorders may result in low platelet count; among them, drug-induced thrombocytopenia, infection-induced thrombocytopenia, disseminated intravascular coagulation, congenital thrombocytopenia, and idiopathic immune thrombocytopenia. Two types of thrombocytopenic disorders and their treatments are discussed below.

IMMUNE THROMBOCYTOPENIC PURPURA

Etiology and Epidemiology

Immune (or idiopathic) thrombocytopenic purpura (ITP) is one of the most common causes of acquired thrombocytopenia. The estimated incidence is 1.9 to 6.4 cases per 100,000 persons in children and 3.3 cases per 100,000 in adults.[29] ITP is an autoimmune disorder caused by the binding of antibodies (usually immunoglobulin G [IgG]) to platelet surface antigens, resulting in shortened platelet life span. ITP can occur as an isolated condition or secondary to an underlying disorder. Childhood-onset and adult-onset ITP present very differently. Adult-onset ITP is generally chronic (> 6 months) and affects women two to three times more often than men. By contrast, childhood-onset ITP is acute in onset and usually follows an infectious illness, and both sexes are equally affected. Childhood ITP typically resolves on its own within 4 to 6 weeks without major sequelae. In adults presenting with ITP, testing for human immunodeficiency virus (HIV) and hepatitis C virus (HCV) is recommended, because treating these infections may improve ITP course. ITP occurs in 1 to 2 of every 1000 pregnancies. In pregnant women with preexisting ITP, both maternal and fetal complications may occur, requiring separate management.

Pathophysiology

In ITP, IgG autoantibodies bind to platelet-antigen complex and are cleared from the blood via binding to mononuclear phagocytes by macrophage Fcγ receptor, leading to thrombocytopenia. Platelet survival time is significantly shorter in patients with ITP (from minutes to 2–3 days compared with normal 7–10 days). Sequestration in spleen, liver, and bone marrow is partially responsible for decreased platelet survival. Megakaryopoiesis may be reduced due to antibody binding to megakaryocyte precursors in the bone marrow.

Clinical Presentation and Diagnosis of ITP

General

The typical patient is well with the exception of bleeding.

Symptoms

- Petechiae
- Purpura, wet purpura
- Ecchymoses
- Cutaneous bleeding
- Mucosal site bleeding
- Epistaxis
- Gingival bleeding
- Hematuria
- Menorrhagia
- Intracranial hemorrhage (rare)

Diagnostic Criteria

- Platelet count less than 100 × 10^3/mm^3 (100 × 10^9/L)
- Otherwise normal complete blood count with differential
- Normal reticulocyte count
- Normal peripheral blood smear (no hemolysis or blast cells)
- History and physical exam ruling out other possible causes of thrombocytopenia[30]

Other Laboratory Testing

Laboratory testing to rule out other courses of thrombocytopenia, such as HCV, HIV, SLE, Evan syndrome, and others

Patient Encounter 2, Part 1: ITP

A 30-year-old woman with past medical history significant for mild intermittent asthma. Presents with complaints of significant mucosal bleeding from her mouth that was slow to respond to placing ice cubes and swishing cold water. A laboratory analysis reveals platelet count of $8 \times 10^3/mm^3$ ($8 \times 10^9/L$). Her medications at home include albuterol MDI one to two inhalations every 4 hours as needed; she has no known drug allergies.

What information is suggestive of immune thrombocytopenic purpura (ITP)?

What additional information do you need to create a treatment plan for this patient?

Treatment

▶ Desired Outcomes

In children, the main goal of ITP treatment is to maintain the platelet count associated with sufficient hemostasis, while awaiting spontaneous or treatment-induced remission. In adults, the main goal is to maintain platelet count greater than $30 \times 10^3/mm^3$ ($30 \times 10^9/L$), because below this count, the incidence of bleeding in increased.[31]

▶ General Approach to Treatment

KEY CONCEPT *The treatment of ITP is determined by the symptom severity. In some cases, no therapy is needed* (Table 67–8). The initial treatment of children with ITP is controversial because greater than 75% to 80% of cases resolve spontaneously irrespective of pharmacologic intervention. Therapy should be given to children with severe hemorrhage. Therapy may be considered in children meeting one of the following criteria: platelet counts less than $10 \times 10^3/mm^3$ ($10 \times 10^9/L$) and mucocutaneous bleeding; platelet counts less than $30 \times 10^3/mm^3$ ($30 \times 10^9/L$) and moderate systemic or mucosal bleeding; or factors that may increase the risk of bleeding (such as participation in active contact sports increasing risk of head injury).[32] In adults, treatment is indicated when platelet counts are less than $30 \times 10^3/mm^3$ ($30 \times 10^9/L$).[31]

Patient Encounter 2, Part 2: ITP

PE:

Wt 75 kg; vital signs within normal limits. Petechial rash present on lower extremities; bleeding mucous surfaces noted within oral cavity.

Labs:

- Platelet count: $8 \times 10^3/mm^3$ ($8 \times 10^9/L$) (normal 140–440 × $10^3/mm^3$ [140–440 × $10^9/L$])
- aPTT: 35 seconds (normal 25–40 seconds)
- PT: 11 seconds (normal 10–12 seconds)
- Hemoglobin 13 g/dL (130 g/L or 8.07 mmol/L) (normal 13.8–17.2 g/dL or 138–172 g/L or 8.57–10.68 mmol/L)
- HCV antibody negative
- HIV negative

Given this additional information, is this patient's presentation consistent with ITP?

Identify your treatment goals for this patient.

Table 67–8
Guidelines for the Management of Adult ITP

Greater than 30×10^3 platelets/mm^3 ($30 \times 10^9/L$), no bleeding	No treatment
First line	Prednisone (1 mg/kg/day)
Less than 30×10^3 platelets/mm^3 ($30 \times 10^9/L$), bleeding symptoms	Anti-D immune globulin (50–75 mcg/kg/day, × once dose) if corticosteroids contraindicated IVIg (1 g/kg/day × one dose, repeat as necessary) if corticosteroids contraindicated
Second line	Splenectomy
Reserved for patients with bleeding symptoms and platelets < 30×10^3 platelets/mm^3 ($30 \times 10^9/L$) after an adequate trial of first-line agents	Rituximab (375 mg/m^2 once weekly for four doses) Eltrombopag (25–75 mg daily) Romiplostim (1–10 mcg/kg) Immunosuppressants
Hemorrhage	Platelet transfusion IVIg (1 g/kg/day × one dose, repeat as necessary) Methylprednisolone (1 g/day for 3 days)

▶ Nonpharmacologic Therapy

Splenectomy In adults, splenectomy is generally considered after 3 to 6 months if the patient continues to require 10 to 20 mg/day of prednisone to maintain the platelet count greater than $30 \times 10^3/mm^3$ ($30 \times 10^9/L$). Splenectomy may also be considered for urgent treatment of neurologic symptoms or for managing relapse despite an adequate trial of corticosteroids, IV immunoglobulin (IVIg), or anti-Rh(D). Even though individual patient response cannot be predicted, approximately two-thirds of refractory adult patients have a favorable response to splenectomy within several days; however, 30% to 40% will have no response or will experience a relapse sometime after splenectomy.

In children, splenectomy is usually reserved due to the self-limited nature of ITP and fear of infectious complications of splenectomy. Splenectomy is recommended in children with ITP duration greater than 1 year with significant bleeding symptoms and unresponsive or intolerant of pharmacological therapies. Between 70% and 80% of children attain complete remission following splenectomy. Laparoscopic splenectomy is preferable to open splenectomy because it speeds the recovery and shortens the duration of hospitalization. The major drawback of splenectomy is bacterial sepsis, occurring at incidence rates of approximately 1%. Immunization with *Haemophilus influenzae* type b, pneumococcal, and meningococcal vaccines is indicated in all patients 2 weeks prior to splenectomy.[33]

Platelet Transfusions Platelet transfusions are indicated if a patient has severe life-threatening bleeding, such as intracranial hemorrhage. In such situations, platelet transfusions are administered along with IV Immunoglobulin and glucocorticoids (see below).[32]

▸ Pharmacologic Therapy

The general approach to management of ITP in adults is summarized in Table 67–8.

Glucocorticoids Glucocorticoids may decrease splenic sequestration of antibody-coated platelets, diminish antibody generation by the spleen and the bone marrow, and increase platelet output by the bone marrow. In adults, the response rate to oral prednisone (1 mg/kg/day) is 50% to 75%, with patients usually responding within the first 1 to 2 weeks. The duration of therapy depends on the platelet count response; guidelines advocate longer course of prednisone therapy (21 days), followed by a taper. High-dose dexamethasone (40 mg orally or intravenously daily) administered for 4 to 8 days in 14- to 28-day cycles has also been used successfully. In children, oral or parenteral corticosteroids (prednisone, dexamethasone, methylprednisolone) can be used; various dosage regimens have been studied with no specific drug or dosage regimen showing superiority.[31]

IV Immunoglobulin (IVIg) IVIg impairs the clearance of platelets coated with IgG by activating inhibitory receptor FcRγIIb. Roughly 80% of adults will respond to IVIg, but remission usually is not sustained. In adults, use of IVIg (1 g/kg/day given as a single dose, repeated if necessary) is reserved for situations in which rapid increase in platelet count is necessary, such as life-threatening bleeding and very low platelet count, or for patients who have contraindications to glucocorticoids. If treatment is indicated in children, a single dose of IVIg (0.8–1 g/kg) is usually effective. IVIg use is complicated by many serious adverse effects and high cost.

Anti-Rh(D) Anti-Rh(D) can be used only in Rh(D)-positive patients who have not had splenectomy. It is as efficacious as IVIg and is generally less expensive. The indications for use of anti-Rh(D) are identical to those for IVIg. Anti-Rh(D) is a desirable form of treatment in chronic ITP when the goal is to circumvent long-term exposure to corticosteroids. At doses of 50 to 75 mcg/kg/day, anti-Rh(D) may increase the platelet count in about 70% to 80% of children with ITP. Dosage adjustment is recommended based on hemoglobin levels. Response to anti-Rh(D) lasts about 3 to 5 weeks, and substantial numbers of patients treated repetitively with anti-Rh(D) can postpone or avoid splenectomy. Rare fatal intravascular hemolysis has been reported with use of anti-Rh(D); special monitoring for this side effect is recommended.

Immunosuppressants Immunosuppressant therapy is generally utilized for patients who are refractory to or intolerant of all other ITP treatments. Rituximab, an anti-CD20 antibody, at a dose of 375 mg/m^2 once weekly for four doses, can induce long-term response in 21% to 27% of patients.[34] Progressive multifocal leukoencephalopathy has been rarely reported with rituximab use. Rituximab can be considered as a second- or third-line therapy in patients who have experienced treatment failure with corticosteroids, IVIg, or splenectomy. Azathioprine and cyclophosphamide produce response rates of 20% to 40% in adult patients who are treated for 2 to 6 months. Other medications used in ITP include vincristine, vinblastine, cyclosporine, danazol, and mycophenolate mofetil; due to major toxicities and lack of adequate evidence-based recommendations, their use is reserved for refractory ITP.

Thrombopoietic Growth Factors Additional treatment options for ITP include a thrombopoiesis-stimulating protein and a small-molecule thrombopoietin (TPO) receptor agonist. These agents stimulate the bone marrow to make enough platelets to overcome the body's premature destruction of platelets. Romiplostim and eltrombopag are two TPO mimetics that have been approved by the FDA for the treatment of thrombocytopenia in patients with chronic ITP who have had an insufficient response to corticosteroids, immunoglobulins, or splenectomy. Currently, these agents are not FDA approved for use in children; several clinical trials are underway to establish role of these agents in managing childhood ITP.

Romiplostim is a TPO peptide mimetic that binds to and activates the human TPO receptor. As a once weekly subcutaneous injection, romiplostim stimulates megakaryopoiesis, resulting in enhanced platelet production. Initial dose of romiplostim is based on the actual body weight, adjusted weekly by increments of 1 mcg/kg subcutaneously until a maximum of 10 mcg/kg and the patient achieves a platelet count greater than or equal to 50×10^3/mm^3 (50×10^9/L) as necessary to reduce the risk for bleeding. Eltrombopag is a once-daily oral nonpeptide thrombopoietin receptor agonist with a low immunogenic potential that stimulates megakaryocyte proliferation and differentiation.

For most patients, the initial dose of eltrombopag is 50 mg once daily. The daily dose is subsequently adjusted to a maximum dose of 75 mg daily in order to achieve and maintain a platelet count greater than or equal to 50×10^3/mm^3 (50×10^9/L) in order to reduce the risk for bleeding.

Both agents need to be discontinued if platelet counts do not increase after 4 weeks at a maximum dose.

Romiplostim and eltrombopag are effective in increasing platelet counts in patients with ITP and can be used in combination with therapies that inhibit platelet destruction. Although usually well tolerated, a number of rare but serious risks have been reported, including changes in the bone marrow, worsened thrombocytopenia and the risk of bleeding after cessation of the medication, thrombotic/thromboembolic complications (including portal vein thrombosis with eltrombopag), and worsening of blood cancers. Eltrombopag carries a "black box warning" regarding hepatic decompensation in patients with hepatitis C treated with interferon and ribavirin. It is also associated with development of cataracts and has drug–drug interactions with antacids and several minerals (calcium, iron, aluminum, magnesium, selenium, zinc).

Use of TPO-mimetic agents is reserved for refractory ITP due to cost considerations, lack of durability of response after discontinuation, and limited knowledge of long-term side effects.

Outcome Evaluation

- Monitor platelet counts as indicated clinically.
- In adults, the goal of therapy is to maintain platelet count greater than or equal to 30×10^3/mm^3 (30×10^9/L).
- Monitor for signs and symptoms of bleeding.

Patient Encounter 2, Part 3: ITP: Creating a Care Plan

Based on the information presented, create a care plan for this patient. Please include whether pharmacologic therapy is indicated, and if so, please list first-line and alternative therapies.

Patient Care Process ITP

Patient Assessment:

- Conduct physical examination evaluating sites of bleeding. Obtain a complete medical and medication history.
- Evaluate CBC, peripheral blood smear, order tests to rule out other diseases commonly associated with thrombocytopenia.

Therapy Evaluation and Care Plan Development:

- If patient meets clinical criteria for diagnosis of ITP and is a candidate for treatment, evaluation of platelet count, occupational risks of bleeding, and actual bleeding severity dictates initial treatment approach.
- First-line treatment for patients meeting criteria for pharmacotherapy is corticosteroids for up to 21 days. Anti-D or IVIg can be considered if corticosteroids are contraindicated or rapid rise in platelet count is necessary. Alternatives to first-line agents include immunosuppressants and TPO mimetics, which are reserved for patients failing to respond after adequate trial of first-line agents. Surgical splenectomy is reserved for refractory ITP.

Follow-Up Evaluation:

- In adults, monitor regularly to ensure platelet counts stay above $30 \times 10^3/\text{mm}^3$ (30×10^9/L).
- Patients should be instructed to contact their primary health care provider at new signs of bleeding.

THROMBOTIC THROMBOCYTOPENIC PURPURA

Etiology and Epidemiology

Thrombotic thrombocytopenic purpura (TTP) is a severe systemic disorder characterized by thrombi formation within the circulation that results in the platelet consumption and subsequent thrombocytopenia. Acute idiopathic TTP is more common in women and African Americans and most frequently occurs in people between 30 and 40 years of age. The estimated annual incidence of TTP is 4.5 cases per million.[35] Common conditions associated with TTP are summarized in Table 67–9.

Pathophysiology

Endothelial cells normally synthesize vWF in the form of a high-molecular-weight multimer composed of smaller identical monomers. Each monomer is able to bind platelets, and the number of monomers on the vWF multimer is directly proportional to its platelet-binding capacity. Consequently, particularly adherent ultra-large molecules of the vWF (ULvWF) are broken down to smaller size by vWF-cleaving proteases such as ADAMTS13 (a disintegrin and metalloprotease with thrombospondin type 1 repeats) to avoid undesired clot formation. TTP results from genetic or acquired deficiency in the vWF-cleaving protease ADAMTS13 activity. This, in turn, elevates circulating levels of ULvWF, leading to inappropriate platelet agglutination. Thrombocytopenia develops because the rate of aggregated platelet consumption is faster than megakaryocyte bone marrow production. Microangiopathic hemolytic anemia generally follows as a consequence of red blood cell damage by platelet clumps occluding the microcirculation. Occlusive ischemia of the brain or GI tract is common, and renal dysfunction may occur.

Clinical Presentation and Diagnosis of TTP

Typical Pentad of Symptoms (Rare That All Five Are Present)[a]

1. Thrombocytopenia
   - Thrombocytopenic purpura
   - Bleeding
2. Fever
3. Microangiopathic hemolytic anemia
4. Neurologic symptoms
   - Headache, confusion, difficulty speaking, transient paralysis, numbness
5. Renal abnormalities
   - Proteinuria, hematuria, mild renal insufficiency

Laboratory Testing

- Decreased hemoglobin, hematocrit, and platelets
- Peripheral blood smear showing schistocytes
- Decreased serum haptoglobin
- Elevated lactate dehydrogenase (LDH)
- Elevated indirect bilirubin level
- Elevated reticulocyte count
- Normal PT and aPTT
- Elevated urine protein, red blood cells, and/or serum creatinine

[a]TTP diagnosis can be based on the presence of thrombocytopenia and microangiopathic hemolytic anemia in the absence of other possible causes.

In patients suspected to have TTP, the differential diagnosis includes disseminated intravascular coagulation (DIC) and hemolytic uremic syndrome (HUS). Both TTP and HUS can present with thrombotic microangiopathic anemia; however, HUS is usually linked to a diarrheal illness and acute renal failure. Some sources advocate for TTP-HUS spectrum as a single disease since clinical presentation is essentially identical.

Table 67–9

Conditions Associated with TTP

- Infections
- Bacterial, fungal, viral, atypical
- Transplantation
- Solid organ or bone marrow
- Malignancy
- Pregnancy
- Collagen vascular diseases
- Medications
- Antineoplastic agents, ticlopidine, clopidogrel, antibiotics, immunosuppressants, others

Treatment

▶ *Desired Outcomes*

The main goal of TTP treatment is to prevent end-organ damage.

▶ *Nonpharmacologic Therapy*

KEY CONCEPT *The present standard of treatment for TTP is urgent plasma exchange (PEX). If PEX is unavailable, treatment with plasma infusion and glucocorticoids is indicated until PEX is available.*[36]

Plasma Exchange The procedure involves removal of the patient's plasma and its substitution with donor plasma. In this manner, circulating antibody inhibitor of ADAMTS13 is removed and enzyme is replenished. PEX involves placement of two IV lines (cannulae) into two separate veins. Blood removed through one cannula is centrifuged to separate the blood cells from the plasma. The blood cells are mixed subsequently with donor plasma and returned to the patient via the second cannula. The goal is to exchange 1 to 1.5 plasma volumes (40–60 mL/kg). The procedure generally is repeated daily until neurologic symptoms resolve and normal lactate dehydrogenase (LDH) and platelet counts are maintained for several days. After complete remission is achieved, PEX frequency can be reduced to every other day for an additional few days, with subsequent PEX discontinuation and close patient follow-up. When PEX is started immediately upon diagnosis, remission and survival rates at 6 months are approximately 80%. Although generally considered safe, complications from catheter insertion or catheter infection may occur and include hemorrhage, pneumothorax, sepsis, and thrombosis. Allergic reactions to plasma can cause severe hypotension and hypoxia.[37]

Splenectomy Splenectomy is reserved for patients with frequently relapsing disease who are refractory to PEX or immunosuppressive therapy.

▶ *Pharmacologic Therapy*

Glucocorticoids Glucocorticoids can be used for their immunosuppressive effect in combination with PEX; however, they are not as efficacious as monotherapy in TTP. The most commonly used agents are methylprednisolone 250 mg/day IV for or prednisone 1 mg/kg/day orally for the duration of PEX therapy and 1 to 2 weeks after normalized platelet counts are maintained.

Immunosuppressants TTP that fails to respond adequately to PEX can be treated with immunosuppressive agents. Cytotoxic immunosuppressive therapies with the most potential benefit in refractory TTP include cyclosporine and rituximab. Other agents that had been used include vincristine, cyclophosphamide, azathioprine, and IVIg.[36]

Patient Encounter 3, Part 1: TTP

A 35-year-old African American woman presented to her primary care physician complaining of headache, weakness, fever, chills, nausea, vomiting, and vaginal bleeding. She was recently diagnosed with genital herpes and prescribed valacyclovir 1 g twice daily for 10 days, which she's been taking for 9 days now. Otherwise, she suffers from seasonal allergies for which she takes loratadine 10 mg by mouth daily. She is allergic to ibuprofen (rash).

What information is suggestive of TTP?

What additional information do you need to create a treatment plan for this patient?

Patient Encounter 3, Part 2: TTP

PE/ROS:

Wt 55 kg, T 100.8°F (38.2°C), patient appears lethargic and has difficulty concentrating

Labs:

- Platelet count: $9 \times 10^3/mm^3$ ($9 \times 10^9/L$) (normal 140–440 × $10^3/mm^3$ [140–440 × $10^9/L$])
- aPTT: 35 seconds (normal 25–40 seconds)
- PT: 11 seconds (normal 10–12 seconds)
- Haptoglobin 10 mg/dL (100 mg/L) (normal 30–200 mg/dL or 300–2000 mg/L)
- LDH 1900 U/L (31.7 μkat/L) (normal 100–250 U/L, or 1.67–4.17 μkat/L)
- Hemoglobin 9 g/dL (90 g/L; 5.59 mmol/L) (normal 12.1–15.1 g/dL or 121–151 g/L or 7.51–9.37 mmol/L)
- Blood peripheral smear: numerous schistocytes (10–15 per high power field)
- Serum creatinine 1.8 mg/dL (159 μmol/L) (increased from 0.8 mg/dL [71 μmol/L] on record from last year's physical exam) (normal 0.6–1.2 mg/dL [53–106 μmol/L])

Given this additional information, is this patient's presentation consistent with TTP?

What is the likely etiology of this patient's TTP?

Identify your treatment goals for this patient.

Patient Encounter 3, Part 3: TTP: Creating a Care Plan

Based on the information presented, create a care plan for this patient's TTP.

Patient Care Process TTP

Patient Assessment:

- Obtain a complete medical and medication history.
- Evaluate CBC, vital signs, neurologic symptoms, chemistry 7 panel, and urinalysis for presence of thrombocytopenia, fever, anemia, and renal abnormalities. Evaluate neurologic symptoms.

Therapy Evaluation and Care Plan Development:

- If patient meets clinical criteria for diagnosis of TTP, start daily PEX. If ADAMTS13 deficiency is suspected, start glucocorticoids.

Follow-up Evaluation:

- When platelet counts stay above $150 \times 10^3/mm^3$ ($150 \times 10^9/L$) for 2 days, PEX may be discontinued; glucocorticoids may be continued for additional 1 to 2 weeks.
- Follow patients indefinitely with periodic CBC/LDH measurements to screen for possible relapse of TTP.

Outcome Evaluation

Monitor platelet counts, hemoglobin, and LDH.

Abbreviations Introduced in This Chapter

ADAMTS13	A disintegrin and metalloprotease with thrombospondin type 1 repeats (vWF-cleaving metalloprotease)
BU	Bethesda units
DDAVP	1-Desamino-8-D-arginine vasopressin (desmopressin acetate)
DIC	Disseminated intravascular coagulation
FFP	Fresh-frozen plasma
HCV	Hepatitis C virus
ICH	Intracranial hemorrhage
ITP	Immune thrombocytopenic purpura
IVIg	IV immunoglobulin
PCC	Prothrombin complex concentrate
PEX	Plasma exchange
rFVIIa	Recombinant factor VIIa
RICD	Recessively inherited coagulation disorder
TTP	Thrombotic thrombocytopenic purpura
ULvWF	Ultra-large molecules of vWF
vWD	von Willebrand disease
vWF	von Willebrand factor

REFERENCES

1. Soucie JM, Evatt B, and Jackson D. Occurrence of hemophilia in the United States. The Hemophilia Surveillance System Project Investigators. Am J Hematol. 1998;59(4):288–294.
2. Zimmerman B and Valentino LA. Hemophilia: In review. Pediatr Rev. 2013;34(7):289–294; quiz 295.
3. Antonarakis SE, Rossiter JP, Young M, et al. Factor VIII gene inversions in severe hemophilia A: Results of an international consortium study. Blood. 1995;86(6):2206–2212.
4. Bhat R and Cabey W. Evaluation and management of congenital bleeding disorders. Emerg Med Clin North Am. 2014;32(3):673–690.
5. Darby SC, Kan SW, Spooner RJ, et al. Mortality rates, life expectancy, and causes of death in people with hemophilia A or B in the United Kingdom who were not infected with HIV. Blood 2007; 110(3):815–825.
6. Berntorp, E. Prophylactic therapy for haemophilia: Early experience. Haemophilia 2003; 9 Suppl 1:5–9; discussion 9.
7. Blanchette VS, Manco-Johnson M, Santagostino E, et al. Optimizing factor prophylaxis for the haemophilia population: Where do we stand? Haemophilia. 2004;10 Suppl 4:97–104.
8. Manco-Johnson MJ, Abshire TC, Shapiro AD, et al. Prophylaxis versus episodic treatment to prevent joint disease in boys with severe hemophilia. N Engl J Med. 2007;357(6):535–544.
9. MASAC, *Recommendation Concerning Prophylaxis (Regular Administration of Clotting Factor Concentrate to Prevent Bleeding). MASAC Document #179. New York: National Hemophilia Foundation*, 2007.
10. MASAC, *Recommendations Concerning Products Licensed for the Treatment of Hemophilia and Other Bleeding Disorders. MASAC Document # 225. New York: National Hemophilia Foundation*, 2014.
11. Srivastava A. Optimizing clotting factor replacement therapy in hemophilia: A global need. Hematology. 2005;10(Suppl 1): 229–230.
12. MASAC, *Recommendations Concerning the Treatment of Hemophilia and Other Bleeding Disorders. MASAC Document #182. New York: National Hemophilia Foundation*, 2008.
13. Collins PW, Bjorkman S, Fischer K, et al. Factor VIII requirement to maintain a target plasma level in the prophylactic treatment of severe hemophilia A: Influences of variance in pharmacokinetics and treatment regimens. J Thromb Haemost. 2010;8(2):269–275.
14. Collins PW, Blanchette VS, Fischer K, et al. Break-through bleeding in relation to predicted factor VIII levels in patients receiving prophylactic treatment for severe hemophilia A. J Thromb Haemost. 2009;7(3):413–420.
15. Batorova A and Martinowitz U. Continuous infusion of coagulation factors: Current opinion. Curr Opin Hematol. 2006;13(5):308–315.
16. Schulman S. Continuous infusion. Haemophilia. 2003;9(4): 368–375.
17. Powell JS, Pasi KJ, Ragni MV, et al. Phase 3 study of recombinant factor IX Fc fusion protein in hemophilia B. N Engl J Med. 2013;369(24):2313–2323.
18. Nathwani AC, Tuddenham EG, Rangarajan S, et al. Adenovirus-associated virus vector-mediated gene transfer in hemophilia B. N Engl J Med. 2011;365(25):2357–2365.
19. High KA. The gene therapy journey for hemophilia: Are we there yet? Hematology Am Soc Hematol Educ Program. 2012;2012:375–381.
20. Shord SS and Lindley CM. Coagulation products and their uses. Am J Health Syst Pharm. 2000;57(15):1403–1417; quiz 1418-1420.
21. MASAC, *Recommendations on Use of COX-2 Inhibitors in Patients with Bleeding Disorders. MASAC Document #162. New York: National Hemophilia Foundation*, 2005.
22. Rodeghiero F, Castaman G, and Dini E. Epidemiological investigation of the prevalence of von Willebrand's disease. Blood. 1987;69(2):454–459.
23. Werner EJ, Broxson EH, Tucker EL, et al. Prevalence of von Willebrand disease in children: A multiethnic study. J Pediatr. 1993;123(6):893–898.
24. Nichols WL, Hultin MB, James AH, et al. von Willebrand disease (VWD): Evidence-based diagnosis and management guidelines, the National Heart, Lung, and Blood Institute (NHLBI) Expert Panel report (USA). Haemophilia. 2008;14(2):171–232.
25. Mannucci PM. Treatment of von Willebrand's Disease. N Engl J Med. 2004;351(7):683–694.

26. Kouides PA, Byams VR, Philipp CS, et al. Multisite management study of menorrhagia with abnormal laboratory haemostasis: A prospective crossover study of intranasal desmopressin and oral tranexamic acid. Br J Haematol. 2009;145(2):212–220.
27. Mannucci PM, Duga S, and Peyvandi F. Recessively inherited coagulation disorders. Blood. 2004;104(5):1243–1252.
28. Roberts HR and Escobar MA, Other clotting factor deficiencies, in Hoffman P, Benz EJJ, and Shatil SJ, eds. Hematology, Basic Principles and Practice, Philadelphia, PA: Elsevier. 2005:2047–2069.
29. Terrell DR, Beebe LA, Vesely SK, et al. The incidence of immune thrombocytopenic purpura in children and adults: A critical review of published reports. Am J Hematol. 2010;85(3):174–180.
30. Rodeghiero F, Stasi R, Gernsheimer T, et al. Standardization of terminology, definitions and outcome criteria in immune thrombocytopenic purpura of adults and children: Report from an international working group. Blood. 2009;113(11):2386–2393.
31. Neunert C, Lim W, Crowther M, et al. The American Society of Hematology 2011 evidence-based practice guideline for immune thrombocytopenia. Blood. 2011;117(16):4190–4207.
32. Provan D, Stasi R, Newland AC, et al. International consensus report on the investigation and management of primary immune thrombocytopenia. Blood. 2010;115(2):168–186.
33. George JN, Woolf SH, Raskob GE, et al. Idiopathic thrombocytopenic purpura: A practice guideline developed by explicit methods for the American Society of Hematology. Blood. 1996;88(1):3–40.
34. Patel VL, Mahevas M, Lee SY, et al. Outcomes 5 years after response to rituximab therapy in children and adults with immune thrombocytopenia. Blood. 2012;119(25):5989–5995.
35. Terrell DR, Williams LA, Vesely SK, et al. The incidence of thrombotic thrombocytopenic purpura-hemolytic uremic syndrome: All patients, idiopathic patients, and patients with severe ADAMTS-13 deficiency. J Thromb Haemost. 2005;3(7):1432–1436.
36. Scully M, Hunt BJ, Benjamin S, et al. Guidelines on the diagnosis and management of thrombotic thrombocytopenic purpura and other thrombotic microangiopathies. Br J Haematol. 2012;158(3):323–335.
37. Som S, Deford CC, Kaiser ML, et al. Decreasing frequency of plasma exchange complications in patients treated for thrombotic thrombocytopenic purpura-hemolytic uremic syndrome, 1996 to 2011. Transfusion. 2012;52(12):2525-2532; quiz 2524.

68 Sickle Cell Disease

Tracy M. Hagemann and Teresa V. Lewis

LEARNING OBJECTIVES

Upon completion of the chapter, the reader will be able to:

1. Explain the underlying causes of sickle cell disease (SCD) and their relationship to patient signs and symptoms.
2. Identify the typical characteristics of SCD as well as symptoms that indicate complicated disease.
3. Identify the desired therapeutic outcomes for patients with SCD.
4. Recommend appropriate pharmacotherapy and nonpharmacotherapy interventions for patients with SCD.
5. Recognize when chronic maintenance therapy is indicated for a patient with SCD.
6. Describe the components of a monitoring plan to assess effectiveness and adverse effects of pharmacotherapy for SCD.
7. Educate patients about the disease state, appropriate therapy, and drug therapy required for effective treatment and prevention of complications.

INTRODUCTION

KEY CONCEPT *"Sickle cell syndrome" refers to a collection of autosomal recessive genetic disorders that are characterized by the presence of at least one sickle hemoglobin gene (HbS).*[1,2]

Sickle cell disease (SCD) is a chronic illness that is associated with frequent crisis episodes. Acute complications are unpredictable and potentially fatal. Common symptoms include excruciating musculoskeletal pain, life-threatening pneumonia-like illness, cerebrovascular accidents, and splenic and renal dysfunction.[2] As the disease progresses, patients may develop organ damage from the combination of hemolysis and infarction. Because of the complexity and severity of SCD, it is imperative that patients have access to comprehensive care with providers who have a good understanding of the countless clinical presentations and the management options of this disorder.

EPIDEMIOLOGY AND ETIOLOGY

Sickle cell trait (SCT) is the heterozygous form (HbAS) of SCD in which a person inherits one normal adult hemoglobin (*HbA*) gene and one sickle hemoglobin (*HbS*) gene. These individuals are carriers of the SCT and are usually asymptomatic.[2] Symptomatic disease is seen in homozygous and compound heterozygous genotypes of SCD. Sickle cell anemia (SCA) is the homozygous (HbSS) state of SCD.[2] It is the most common and severe form of SCD. SCD affects both males and females equally because it is not a sex-linked disease.

KEY CONCEPT *Around 90,000 to 100,000 Americans have SCD and it occurs in approximately 1 out of every 500 African American births.*[3] *HbSS* (~45%) is the most common genotype, followed by HbSC (~25%), HbSβ^+-thalassemia (~8%), and HbSβ^0-thalassemia (~2%). Other variants account for fewer than 1% of patients.[2,4] For every infant diagnosed with SCD, 50 are identified as carriers.[4]

Having the sickle hemoglobin gene protects heterozygous carriers from succumbing to *Plasmodium falciparum* (malaria) infection.[1] The microorganism cannot parasitize abnormal red blood cells (RBCs) as easily as normal RBCs. Consequently, persons with heterozygous sickle gene (SCT) have a selective advantage in tropical regions where malaria is endemic.

The highest incidence of SCD is seen in those with African heritage, but SCD also affects persons of Indian, Saudi Arabian, Mediterranean, South and Central American, and Caribbean ancestry.[4,5]

Normal HbA is composed of two α-chains and two β-chains (α2β2).[1] A single substitution of the amino acid valine for glutamic acid at position 6 of the β-polypeptide chain is responsible for the production of a defective form of hemoglobin called HbS.[1] Different genetic mutations encode for other hemoglobin variants such as hemoglobin C (HbC).[1] The α-chains of HbS, HbA, and HbC are structurally identical. The chemical differences in the β-chain are responsible for RBC sickling and its associated sequelae.

SCD is the HbSS state of SCD in which individuals inherit the mutant hemoglobin gene (*HbS*) from both parents. The progeny of two carriers will have a 25% probability of having SCD and a 50% risk of being a carrier. β-Thalassemia can be found in conjunction with HbS. Patients with HbSS and HbSβ^0-thalassemia do not have normal β-globulin production and usually have a more severe course than those with HbSC and HbSβ^+-thalassemia.

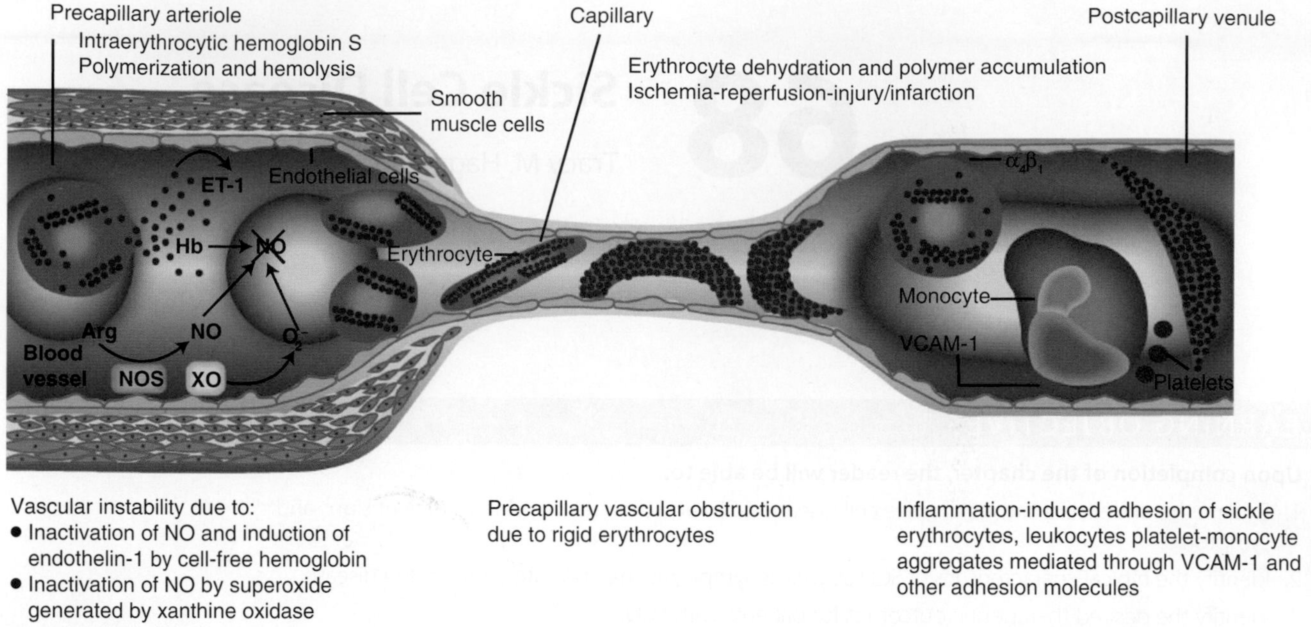

FIGURE 68–1. Pathophysiology of SCD. (Arg, arginine; ET-1, endothelin-1; Hb, hemoglobin; NO, nitric oxide; NOS, nitrous oxide synthase; VCAM-1, vascular cell adhesion molecule 1; XO, xanthine oxidase.) (From Kato GJ, Gladwin MT. Sickle cell disease. In: Hall JB, Schmidt GA, Wood LDH, eds. Principles of Critical Care. 3rd ed. New York: McGraw-Hill; 2005: 1658.)

Impaired circulation, destruction of RBCs, and vascular stasis are three known problems that are primarily responsible for the clinical manifestations of SCD (Figure 68–1).

PATHOPHYSIOLOGY

KEY CONCEPT *SCD involves multiple organ systems, and its clinical manifestations vary greatly between and among genotypes.*

Sickle Hemoglobin Polymerization

The primary event in the molecular pathogenesis of SCD involves polymerization of deoxygenated HbS. HbS carries oxygen normally, and when oxygenated, the solubility of HbS and HbA are the same. Once the oxygen is unloaded to the tissues, HbS solubility decreases. This promotes hydrophobic interactions between the hemoglobin molecules and polymerization, which leads to the distortion of the RBC into the characteristic crescent or sickle shape.[1]

Viscosity of Erythrocytes and Sickle Cell Adhesion

When HbS becomes reoxygenated, the polymers within the RBCs disappear, and the cells eventually return to normal shape. Vasoocclussion is caused by a combination of factors. Repeated assaults on RBCs from sickling and unsickling can lead to cell membrane damage, loss of membrane flexibility, and rearrangement of surface phospholipids. The life span of sickled RBCs is markedly shorter (10–20 days) than that of normal RBCs (100–120 days). As intracellular membrane viscosity of HbS-containing RBCs increases, blood viscosity increases, which further contributes to vasoocclusion.[6] There is also increasing evidence that suggest sickle cells adhere to vascular endothelium.[1,6] The combined effects of decreased RBC deformability, slow transit through microcirculation, and adhesion to vascular endothelium contribute to obstruction of small and sometimes large blood vessels. The resulting local tissue hypoxia can accentuate the pathologic process of SCD.

Protective Hemoglobin Types

Fetal hemoglobin (HbF) binds oxygen more tightly than HbA, and it has a decreased propensity to sickling. HbA2 also possesses this characteristic but to a lesser extent. RBCs that contain HbF sickle less readily than cells without. HbF is composed of two α chains and two β chains; therefore, it is not affected by point mutations on β chains. Irreversibly sickled cells (ISCs) are found to have low HbF concentrations. In some patients, higher HbF may ameliorate the disease.

Other Pathophysiologic Effects

Other factors may be responsible for the pathogenesis of some of the clinical features of SCD. Sickle cells can obstruct blood flow to the spleen leading to functional asplenia. Impaired splenic function can increase the propensity to infection by encapsulated organisms, particularly *Streptococcus pneumoniae*.[1] Additionally,

Clinical Presentation and Diagnosis of SCT

General

- Generally asymptomatic

Symptoms

- Females may have frequent urinary tract infections

Signs

- Microscopic hematuria occurs rarely
- Gross hematuria may occur spontaneously or with heavy-intensity exercise

Laboratory Tests

- Normal Hgb values

Clinical Presentation and Diagnosis of SCD

General

- Identified by neonatal screening before 2 months of age

Symptoms

- Painful vasoocclusive crises are the hallmark of SCD
- Dactylitis (hand–foot syndrome) before age 1 year
- May develop infarction of the spleen, liver, bone marrow, kidney, brain, and lungs
- Gallstones
- Priapism in males
- Slow-healing lower extremity ulcers after trauma or infection
- Weakness, fatigue

Signs

- Chronic hemolytic anemia is common
- Enlargement of spleen and heart
- Scleral icterus

Laboratory Tests

- Hgb 7.0 to 10.0 g/dL (70–100 g/L or 4.34–.21 mmol/L)
- Low HgF and increased reticulocytes, platelets, and white blood cells (WBCs)
- Presence of sickled cells on blood smear
- Neonatal screening: hemoglobin electrophoresis, isoelectric focusing, or DNA analysis

coagulation abnormalities are not uncommon since almost every component of hemostasis is altered in SCD.

TREATMENT

Desired Outcomes

Multidisciplinary, regularly scheduled care is required over the lifetime of the SCD patient, with the goal of reduction of complications and hospitalizations. Comprehensive care should include medical, educational, and psychosocial aspects as well as genetic and medication counseling.

Therapeutic interventions for SCD should be targeted at preventing and/or minimizing the symptoms related to the disease and its complications. The goals of treatment are to reduce or eliminate the patient's symptoms; decrease the frequency of sickle crises, including vasoocclusive pain crises; prevent the development of complications; and maintain or improve the quality of life through decreased hospitalizations and decreased morbidity. Specific therapeutic options may:

- Maintain or increase the hemoglobin level to the patient's baseline
- Increase the HbF concentration
- Decrease the HbS concentration
- Prevent infectious complications
- Prevent or effectively manage pain
- Prevent central nervous system (CNS) damage, including stroke

General Approach to Treatment

Patients should be educated to recognize the signs and symptoms of complications that would require urgent evaluation. Patients and parents of children with SCD should be educated to seek immediate medical care when a fever develops or signs of infection occur. With acute illnesses, prompt evaluation is important, as deterioration may occur rapidly. Fluid status should be monitored to avoid dehydration or overhydration, both of which may worsen complications of SCD. Patients in acute distress should maintain oxygen saturation at 92% (0.92) or at their baseline. Any supplemental oxygen requirements should be evaluated.[4]

Nonpharmacologic Therapy

Patients should avoid smoking and excessive alcohol intake. Patients with SCD should maintain adequate hydration in order to help decrease blood viscosity and should be educated to avoid extreme temperature changes and to dress properly in hot and cold weather. Physical exertion that leads to complications should be avoided.[4] Regular exams, including ophthalmic, dental, renal, pulmonary, and cardiac function, are required to monitor for organ damage. A treatment overview is shown in Table 68–1.

Pharmacologic Therapy

▶ *Health Maintenance*

Immunizations Children with SCD should receive the required immunizations as recommended by the American Academy of Pediatrics and the Advisory Committee on Immunization Practices.[7] Additionally, influenza vaccine should be administered yearly to SCD patients 6 months of age and older, including adult patients. All adult patients with SCD should also receive the vaccine for meningococcal disease as well as a one-time dose of *Haemophilus influenzae* type b vaccine. The quadrivalent meningococcal vaccine should be administered in two doses at least 2 months apart.[8]

Because patients with SCD have impaired splenic function, they are less adequately protected against encapsulated organisms such as *S. pneumoniae, H. influenzae,* and *Salmonella.* KEY CONCEPT *The use of pneumococcal vaccine in SCD patients has dramatically decreased the rates of morbidity and mortality; however, there are still groups of SCD children who continue to have high rates of invasive pneumococcal infections.*[9–11] Infection is the leading cause of death in children with SCD younger than 3 years of age.[11,12] Two pneumococcal vaccines are available. The 13-valent conjugate vaccine (PCV 13: Prevnar) is routinely administered to infants and children and provides good protection against the 13 most common isolates seen in this age range. Administer the first dose of PCV 13 between 6 weeks and 6 months of age, followed by two additional doses at 2-month intervals and a fourth dose at 12 to 15 months of age. The 23-valent polysaccharide vaccine (PPSV 23: Pneumovax 23) is indicated for children older than 2 years and adults. Because PPSV 23 is a polysaccharide vaccine, children younger than 2 years do not respond well. PPV 23 contains the 23 most common isolates of *S. pneumoniae* seen in older children and adults. Because of the different serotypes seen in the two vaccines, it is recommended that SCD children receive both vaccines, with a dose of PPSV 23 administered after the child turns 2 years of age. The dose of PPSV 23 should be separated from the last dose of PCV 13 by at least 2 months. An additional dose of PPSV 23 should be given to children 3 to 5 years of age to ensure antibody response. This second dose should be administered 5 years after the first PPSV 23 dose. All adults with

Table 68–1

Management of SCD

	Options and Comments
Health maintenance	
Infection prophylaxis	• Pneumococcal vaccines (PCV 13 and PPV 23) • Penicillin prophylaxis for children younger than 5 years of age • Annual influenza vaccine
Induction of fetal hemoglobin	• Hydroxyurea is the primary agent • Other agents are butyrates (arginine butyrate and sodium phenylbutyrate), decitabine, clotrimazole, and erythropoietin • Combination HbF inducers have been proposed
Chronic transfusion therapy	• Primary indication: stroke prevention in pediatric patients • May also reduce pain crisis and acute chest syndrome • Goal: maintain HbS less than 30% (0.30)
Future prospects	
Transplantation	• May potentially cure the disease • Most experience is with HLA-matched donors; umbilical cord blood transplantation is being evaluated
Crises and complications	
Fever and infection	• Broad-spectrum antibiotic: cefotaxime or ceftriaxone (clindamycin for cephalosporin allergy); vancomycin for staphylococcal and resistant pneumococcal organisms • Fluids • Acetaminophen or ibuprofen for fever
Stroke	• Exchange transfusion • Initiate chronic transfusion therapy to prevent recurrent strokes
Acute chest syndrome	• Broad-spectrum antibiotics (include Mycoplasma coverage) • Bronchodilator if wheezing or history of reactive airway disease • Fluids • Pain management • Transfusion
Pain crisis	• Hydration • Analgesics

SCD should be vaccinated with both PCV 13 as well as PPSV 23. Adults and children who have not previously received PCV13 or PPSV 23 should receive one dose of PCV 13 followed by a single dose of PPSV 23 at a minimum of 8 weeks later.[8] If an adult or child with SCD has already received at least one dose of PPSV 23, they should additionally received on dose of PCV 13 at least 1 year after the dose of PPSV 23. When both vaccines are indicated in an unvaccinated patient with SCD, PCV 13 should be administered first, followed by a dose of PPSV 23 at least 8 weeks later.[8] A one-time revaccination with PPSV 23 should occur 5 years after the first dose of PPSV 23.[8] Because some children fall behind on their childhood vaccinations, a catch-up schedule is presented in Table 68–2.[7]

Penicillin KEY CONCEPT *Children with SCD should receive prophylactic penicillin until at least the age of 5 years, even if they have been appropriately immunized with PCV 13 against pneumococcal infections.* Penicillin V potassium is typically initiated at age 2 months, with a dose of 125 mg orally twice daily until age 3 years, then 250 mg orally twice daily until 5 years of age. The intramuscular use of benzathine penicillin 600,000 units every 4 weeks from age 6 months to 6 years is also an option for nonadherent patients. Penicillin-allergic patients may receive erythromycin 10 mg/kg twice daily. Penicillin prophylaxis usually is not continued in children older than 6 years, but may be considered in patients with a history of invasive pneumococcal infection or surgical splenectomy.[4,13,14]

Folic Acid Folic acid supplementation with 1 mg daily is generally recommended in adult SCD patients, women considering pregnancy, and any SCD patient with chronic hemolysis.[4] Because of accelerated erythropoiesis, these patients have an increased need for folic acid. There are conflicting studies in the SCD population, especially among infants and children, but if the child has chronic hemolysis, supplementation is recommended.[15]

Fetal Hemoglobin Inducers Fetal hemoglobin (HbF) induction in patients with SCD, especially those with frequent crises, has been shown to decrease RBC sickling and RBC adhesion. A direct relationship between HbF concentrations and the severity of disease has been demonstrated in studies.[2]

Hydroxyurea Hydroxyurea is a ribonucleotide reductase inhibitor that prevents DNA synthesis and traditionally has been

Patient Encounter 1

A 6-year-old girl with SCD is currently taking penicillin V potassium 250 mg orally twice daily, folic acid 0.4 mg orally daily, and acetaminophen/codeine 120/12 mg per 5 mL orally every 6 hours as needed for pain. She fully completed all her routine childhood vaccinations and is up to date. She has not been hospitalized since age 2 when she had an aplastic crisis.

What are the general prophylaxis recommendations for children with SCD?

What interventions do you want to make today to her medication/immunization regimens?

Design an infection prevention plan for this patient.

Table 68–2

Pneumococcal Immunization for Children with SCD[7,9]

	Recommended Schedule
Previously unvaccinated	
Age 2–6 months	PCV 13 (Prevnar): three doses 8 weeks apart; then one dose at 12–15 months
Age 7–11 months	PCV 13 (Prevnar): two doses 8 weeks apart; then one dose at 12–15 months
Age 12–23 months	PCV 13 (Prevnar): two doses 8 weeks apart
Age 24–71 months	PCV 13 (Prevnar): two doses 8 weeks apart PPV 23 (Pneumovax): two doses; first dose at least 8 weeks after last PCV 13 dose; second dose 5 years after the first PPV 23 dose
Age 5 years or older	PCV 13 (Prevnar): one dose PPV 23 (Pneumovax): one dose at least 8 weeks after last PCV 13 dose; second dose 5 years after the first PPV 23 dose
Previously vaccinated	
Age 12–23 months, incomplete PCV 13 series	PCV 13 (Prevnar): two doses 8 weeks apart
Age 24–71 months, any incomplete schedule or completed less than three doses with PCV 13	PCV 13 (Prevnar): two doses 8 weeks apart PPV 23 (Pneumovax): two doses; first dose at least 6–8 weeks after last PCV 13 dose; second dose 5 years after the first PPV 23
Age 24–71 months, any incomplete schedule of three doses or four doses of PCV 13	PCV 13 (Prevnar): one dose at least 8 weeks after the most recent dose PPV 23 (Pneumovax): two doses; first dose at least 6–8 weeks after last PCV 13 dose; second dose 5 years after the first PPV 23
Age 24–71 months, one dose PPV 23 given	PCV 13 (Prevnar): one dose at least 8 weeks after PPV 23 dose PPV 23 (Pneumovax): second dose 5 years after first PPV 23
Age 5–18 years, received one dose PPV 23	PCV 13 (Prevnar): one dose at least 8 weeks after PPV 23 If only received one dose of PPV 23 (Pneumovax): second dose 5 years after the first PPV 23 dose

used in chemotherapy regimens. Studies in the 1990s found that hydroxyurea increases HbF levels as well as increasing the number of HbF-containing reticulocytes and intracellular HbF. Other beneficial effects of hydroxyurea include antioxidant properties, reduction of neutrophils and monocytes, increased intracellular water content leading to increased red cell deformability, decreased red cell adhesion to endothelium, and increased levels of nitric oxide, which is a regulator involved in physiologic disturbances.[16]

KEY CONCEPT *Hydroxyurea reduced the frequency of hospitalizations and the incidences of pain, acute chest syndrome (ACS), and blood transfusions by almost 50% in a landmark trial in adult SCD patients with moderate to severe disease.* Hemoglobin and HbF concentrations increased and hemolysis decreased.[16] A follow-up study demonstrated a 40% reduction in mortality over a 9-year period in patients continuing to receive hydroxyurea.[17] Not all patients responded equally; therefore, hydroxyurea may not be the best option for all patients.

The use of hydroxyurea in children and adolescents with SCD has been investigated, and similar results were reported as in adult trials, with no adverse effects on growth and development.[4,18,19] Hydroxyurea is recommended as an option for children with moderate to severe SCD.[20]

The most common adverse effect of hydroxyurea is myelosuppression. Long-term adverse effects are unknown, but myelodysplasia, acute leukemia, and chronic opportunistic infections have been reported.[16] Hydroxyurea is teratogenic in high doses in animal studies and this is a concern, which should be addressed with patients. Normal pregnancies with no birth defects have been reported in some women receiving hydroxyurea, but close monitoring and weighing risk versus benefit to the patient are vitally important. Hydroxyurea is excreted in breast milk and should be avoided in lactating mothers.[16]

Hydroxyurea should be considered in SCD with frequent vasoocclusive crises, severe symptomatic anemia, repeated history of ACS, or other history of severe vasoocclusive crisis (VOC) complications.[4] The prevention of organ damage or reversal of previous damage has not been shown to occur with chronic use of hydroxyurea.[17] The goals of therapy with hydroxyurea are to decrease the acute complications of SCD, improve quality of life, and reduce the number and severity of pain crises.

Hydroxyurea is available in 200-, 300-, 400-, and 500-mg capsules. Extemporaneous liquid preparations can be prepared for children who cannot swallow capsules. Doses should start at 10 to 15 mg/kg daily in a single oral dose, which can be increased after 8 to 12 weeks if blood counts are stable and there are no side effects. Individualize the dosage based on the patient's response and the toxicity seen. With close monitoring, doses can be increased 5 mg/kg/day up to 35 mg/kg daily.[16] In patients with renal failure, dosing of hydroxyurea will need to be adjusted according to the creatinine clearance, as shown in Table 68–3.

Closely monitor patients for efficacy and toxicity while they are receiving hydroxyurea. Monitor mean corpuscular volume (MCV), since it typically increases as the level of HbF increases. If the MCV does not increase with hydroxyurea use, the marrow may be unable to respond, the dose may not be adequate, or the patient may be nonadherent.[16] However, lack of increase in MCV or in HbF is not an indication to discontinue therapy; the clinical response to therapy may take 3 to 6 months. A 6-month trial on the maximum tolerated dose is required prior to consideration of discontinuation due to treatment failure, whether secondary to lack of adherence or failure to respond to therapy. HbF levels can also be monitored to assess response with a goal of increasing HbF to 15% to 20% (0.15–0.20). Assess blood counts every 2 weeks during dose titration and then every 4 to 6 weeks once the dose is stabilized. Temporary discontinuation of therapy is

Table 68–3

Dosage Adjustments for Renal and Hepatic Dysfunction

Medication	Renal Adjustment	Hepatic Adjustment
Decitabine (Decagon)	For Scr ≥ 2 mg/dl (177 μmol/L): hold therapy until values return to baseline	For serum alanine transaminase (ALT), serum glutamic pyruvic transaminase (SGPT), or total bilirubin values more than two times the upper limit of normal: hold therapy until values return to baseline
Deferoxamine (Desferal)	Cl_{cr} < 10 mL/min (0.17 mL/s): decrease the dose by 50%	
Deferasirox (Exjade) children	Greater than 33% increase in Scr (on two consecutive readings) and above the age-appropriate upper limits of normal: decrease daily dose by 10 mg/kg	Severe or persistent elevations in liver function tests: decrease the daily dose or discontinue therapy
Adults	Greater than 33% increase in Scr above pretreatment values on two consecutive readings: decrease daily dose by 10 mg/kg	Severe or persistent elevations in liver function tests: decrease the daily dose or discontinue therapy
Folic acid	No adjustment necessary	No adjustment necessary
Hydroxyurea	Cl_{cr} < 60 mL/min (1.00 mL/s): Initial dose of 7.5 mg/kg/day Cl_{cr} 10–50 mL/min (0.17–0.83 mL/s): reduce the daily dose by 50% Cl_{cr} < 10 mL/min (0.17 mL/s): administer 20% of the usual dose Hemodialysis: 7.5 mg/kg/day given after dialysis	Monitor patient for bone marrow toxicity

Data from Refs. 21–26.

warranted if hemoglobin level is less than 4.5 g/dL (45 g/L or 2.79 mmol/L), absolute neutrophil count is less than $2 \times 10^3/mm^3$ ($2 \times 10^9/L$), platelets are less than $80 \times 10^3/mm^3$ ($80 \times 10^9/L$), or the reticulocytes are less than $80 \times 10^3/mm^3$ ($80 \times 10^9/L$). Monitor for increases in serum creatinine and transaminases. Once the patient's blood counts have returned to baseline, hydroxyurea may be restarted with a dose that is 2.5 to 5 mg/kg less than the dose associated with the patient's toxicity. Doses may then be increased by 2.5 to 5 mg/kg daily after 12 weeks with no toxicity.

Administer prophylactic folic acid supplementation to SCD patients receiving hydroxyurea, because folate deficiency may be masked by the use of hydroxyurea.

5-Aza-2′-Deoxycytine (Decitabine) For patients who do not respond to hydroxyurea, or cannot tolerate the side effects of hydroyurea, 5-azacytidine and 5-aza-2′-deoxycytidine (decitabine) may be useful. Both induce HbF by inhibiting methylation of DNA, preventing the switch from γ- to β-globin production. Decitabine appears to be safer and more potent than 5-azacytadine.

Patient Encounter 2, Part 1

A 16-year-old African American girl with SCD is admitted to the hospital for progressive neck, shoulder, and back pain that began 2 days ago. The patient denies injury.

PMH: Sickle cell anemia (HbSS); admitted for vasoocclusive crises five times over the past year; acute chest syndrome at age 9, 12, and 14; multiple blood transfusions

PSH: Cholecystectomy, splenectomy

FH: Father with SC trait. Mother with SCD

Allergies: NKDA

SH: Occasional alcohol and marijuana use. Is not sexually active

Home Meds: Hydrocodone/acetaminophen 7.5/500 mg, one tablet every 6 hours as needed for pain; folic acid 1 mg daily by mouth

PE:

VS: T 39.0° C (102.2° F), BP 113/66, P 78, RR 22, O_2 Sat 99% (0.99) on 2 L nasal cannula, Ht 163 cm (5′4″), Wt 62.7 kg (138 lb)

Gen: Awake, alert × 3, in no acute distress, but obviously in pain

HEENT: Normocephalic, atraumatic. PERRLA. No lymphadenopathy

Chest: Normal to inspection and palpation. No rhonchi, rales, or wheezes

CV: RRR, no m/g/r

Abd: Soft, NT/ND

Ext: No clubbing, cyanosis, or edema. Shoulder pain with palpation

Neuro: Cranial nerves II through XII are grossly intact. Nonfocal

Labs: Hgb 7.3 g/dL (73 g/L or 4.53 mmol/L), Hct 23.1% (0.231 fraction), WBC $19 \times 10^3/\mu L$ ($19 \times 10^9/L$), BMP WNL

Chest x-ray was within normal limits.

What is your assessment of this patient's condition?

List treatment goals for this patient.

Devise a detailed therapeutic plan for this patient's hospital management.

Is the patient a candidate for hydroxyurea? Why or why not?

Patient Encounter 2, Part 2

Four months later, the patient is seen on follow-up in the outpatient clinic for management of her SCD. She reports that she has a boyfriend and that they are sexually active.

What are the concerns for using hydroxyurea in this patient? Are there any implications now that she is sexually active?

In a small study in adults refractory to hydroxyurea, decitabine 0.2 mg/kg subcutaneously one to three times weekly was associated with an increase in HbF in all patients. Additionally, RBC adhesion was reduced. Neutropenia was the only significant toxicity reported.[27]

Chronic Transfusion Therapy Chronic transfusion therapy is warranted to prevent serious complications from SCD, including stroke prevention and recurrence. KEY CONCEPT *Especially in children, chronic transfusions have been shown to decrease stroke recurrence from approximately 50% to 10% over 3 years.* Without chronic transfusions, approximately 70% of ischemic stroke patients will have another stroke. Chronic transfusion therapy also may be used to prevent vasoocclusive pain and ACS, as well as prevent progression of organ damage.[4]

The goal of chronic transfusion therapy is to maintain the HbS level at less than 30% (0.30) of total hemoglobin concentration. Transfusions are usually administered every 3 to 4 weeks depending on the HbS concentration. For secondary stroke prevention, current studies have indicated that lifelong transfusion may be required, with increased incidence of recurrence once transfusions are stopped.[4]

The benefits of transfusion should be weighed with the risks. Risks associated with transfusions include alloimmunization (sensitization to the blood received), hyperviscosity, viral transmission, volume overload, iron overload, and transfusion reactions. Although the risk of contracting AIDS has decreased dramatically, hepatitis C remains a concern. All SCD patients should be vaccinated for hepatitis A and B and should be serially monitored for hepatitis C and other infections. Parvovirus occurs in 1 of every 40,000 units of RBCs and can be associated with acute anemia and multiple sickle cell complications.[4] Iron overload is a risk for patients maintained on chronic transfusions for more than 1 year. Counsel patients to avoid excessive dietary iron, and monitor serum ferritin regularly. Chelation therapy with deferoxamine or deferasirox should be considered when the serum ferritin level is greater than 1500 to 2000 ng/mL (1500–2000 mcg/L; 3400–4500 pmol/L). Deferoxamine should be initiated at 20 to 40 mg/kg daily (to a maximum of 1–2 g/day) over 8 to 12 hours subcutaneously and has been associated with growth failure.[4] Monitor children receiving deferoxamine for adequate growth and development on a regular basis. Deferasirox should be initiated at 20 mg/kg daily and is available in a tablet that should be dispersed in water, orange juice, or apple juice and taken orally 30 minutes before food.[28,29] Monitor all chelation patients for auditory and ocular changes on a yearly basis. Exchange transfusions may also be helpful in cases of iron overload.

Sickle cell hemolytic transfusion reaction syndrome is a unique problem in SCD patients. Due to alloimmunization, an acute or delayed transfusion reaction may occur 5 to 20 days posttransfusion. Patients may develop symptoms suggestive of a pain crisis or worsening symptoms if they are already in crisis. A severe anemia after transfusion also may occur due to a rapid decrease in hemoglobin and hematocrit, along with a suppression of erythropoiesis. Further transfusions may worsen the clinical picture due to autoimmune antibodies. Recovery may occur only after ceasing all transfusions and is evidenced by a gradual increase in hemoglobin with reticulocytosis, which indicates the patient is now making their own RBCs.[4]

Allogeneic Hematopoietic Stem Cell Transplant Allogeneic hematopoietic stem-cell transplantation (HSCT) is the only potential cure for SCD. The best candidates are children with SCD who are younger than 16 years of age with severe complications, who have an identical human leukocyte antigen (HLA)-matched donor, usually a sibling. The transplant-related mortality rate is between 5% and 10%, and graft rejection is approximately 10%. Other risks include secondary malignancies, development of seizures or intracranial bleeding, and infection in the immediate posttransplant period.[4,30,31]

Experience with HSCT in adult patients with SCD is still somewhat limited. The use of less intense preparative regimens has made HSCT more available for the older patient with SCD. The best results have been seen in the use of progenitor cells (from bone marrow, cord blood, or peripheral blood stem cells) from matched sibling or related donors. The largest published trial to date in adults undergoing nonmyeloablative transplant involved 30 patients with an 87% rate of disease free survival.[5,31]

▸ *Acute Complications*

Transfusions for Acute Complications Red cell transfusion is indicated in patients with acute exacerbations of baseline anemia; in cases of severe vasoocclusive episodes, including ACS, stroke, and acute multiorgan failure; and in preparation for procedures that will require the use of general anesthesia or ionic contrast products. Transfusions also may be useful in patients with complicated obstetric problems, refractory leg ulcers, refractory and prolonged pain crises, or severe priapism. Hyperviscosity may occur if the hemoglobin level is increased to greater than 10.0 to 11.0 g/dL (100–110 g/L or 6.21–6.83 mmol/L). Volume overload leading to congestive heart failure is more likely to occur if the anemia is corrected too rapidly in patients with severe anemia and should be avoided.[4]

Infection and Fever KEY CONCEPT *Any fever greater than 38.5°C (101.3°F) in a SCD patient should be immediately evaluated, and the patient should have a blood culture drawn and be started on antibiotics that provide empirical coverage for encapsulated organisms.*[4]

Patients who should be hospitalized include the following:

- Infants younger than 1 year of age
- Patients with a previous sepsis or bacteremia episode
- Patients with temperatures in excess of 40°C (104°F)
- Patients with WBC counts greater than $30 \times 10^3/mm^3$ ($30 \times 10^9/L$) or less than $0.5 \times 10^3/mm^3$ ($0.5 \times 10^9/L$) and/or platelets less than $100 \times 10^3/mm^3$ ($100 \times 10^9/L$) with evidence of other acute complications
- Acutely ill-appearing individuals

Broad IV antibiotic coverage for the encapsulated organisms can include ceftriaxone or cefotaxime. For patients with true cephalosporin allergy, clindamycin may be used. If staphylococcal infection is suspected due to previous history or the patient appears acutely ill, vancomycin should be initiated. Macrolide antibiotics, such as erythromycin or azithromycin, may be initiated if mycoplasma pneumonia is suspected. While the patient is receiving broad-spectrum antibiotics, their regular use of penicillin for prophylaxis can be suspended. Fever should be controlled with acetaminophen or ibuprofen. Because of the risk of dehydration during infection with fever, increased fluid may be needed.[1,4]

Bone infarcts or sickling in the periosteum usually is indicated by pain and swelling over an extremity. Osteomyelitis also should also be considered. *Salmonella* species are the most common cause of osteomyelitis in SCD children, followed by *Staphylococcus aureus*.[1] Select an appropriate antibiotic to cover the suspected organisms empirically.

Cerebrovascular Accidents Acute neurologic events, such as stroke, will require hospitalization and close monitoring. Patients should have physical and neurologic examinations every 2 hours.[4] Acute treatment may include exchange transfusion or simple transfusion to maintain hemoglobin at approximately 10.0 g/dL (100 g/L or 6.21 mmol/L) and HbS concentration at less than 30% (0.30). Patients with a history of seizure may need anticonvulsants, and interventions for increased intracranial pressure should be initiated if necessary. Children with history of stroke should be initiated on chronic transfusion therapy.[4]

Early detection of ischemic stroke can be done with the use of transcranial Doppler ultrasonography. In the Stroke Prevention Trial in Sickle Cell Anemia (STOP) study, screening with this method followed by chronic transfusion therapy significantly reduced the incidence of stroke.[32–34] Screening is recommended in all patients older than 2 years.

Acute Chest Syndrome ACS will require hospitalization for appropriate management of symptoms and to avoid complications. Patients should be encouraged to use incentive spirometry at least every 2 hours. Incentive spirometry helps the patient take long, slow breaths to increase lung expansion. Appropriate management of pain is important, but analgesic-induced hypoventilation should be avoided. Patients should maintain appropriate fluid balance because overhydration can lead to pulmonary edema and respiratory distress. Infection with gram-negative, gram-positive, or atypical bacteria is common in ACS, and early use of broad-spectrum antibiotics, including a macrolide, quinolone, or cephalosporin is recommended. Fat emboli, from infarction of the long bones, may lead to ACS. Oxygen therapy should be utilized in any patient presenting with respiratory distress or hypoxia. Oxygen saturations, measured by pulse oximeter, should be maintained at 92% (0.92) or above. Exchanges transfusions are often indicated when there is a rapid progression of ACS symptoms, such as increased needs for supplemental oxygen, increased respiratory distress, or progression of pulmonary infiltrates, and patients who present with wheezing may require inhaled bronchodilators.[4,35,36]

The use of corticosteroids is controversial. Although they may decrease the inflammation and endothelial cell adhesion seen with ACS, their use has also been associated with higher readmission rates for other complications.

Priapism By age 18, approximately 90% of SCD males will have had at least one episode of priapism. Stuttering priapism, where erection episodes last anywhere from a few minutes to less than 2 hours, resolves spontaneously. Erections lasting more than 2 hours should be evaluated promptly. Goals of therapy are to provide pain relief, reduce anxiety, provide detumescence, and preserve testicular function and fertility. Initial treatment should include aggressive hydration and analgesia. Transfusion may or may not be helpful, but should be considered in anemic patients. Avoid the use of ice packs due to the risk of tissue damage.[4]

Both vasoconstrictors and vasodilators have been used in the treatment of priapism. Vasoconstrictors are thought to work by forcing blood out of the cavernosum and into the venous return.

Clinical Presentation and Diagnosis of ACS in SCD

General

- Occurs in 15% to 43% of patients and is responsible for 25% of deaths
- Risk factors include young age, low HbF level, high Hgb and WBCs, winter seasons, reactive airway disease
- Recurrences are up to 80% and can lead to chronic lung disease

Symptoms

- Patients may complain of cough, fever, dyspnea, chest pain

Signs

- Temperature greater than 38.5°C (101.3°F)
- Hypoxia
- New infiltrate on chest x-ray

Laboratory Tests

- CBC with reticulocyte count
- Blood gases
- Oxygen saturation
- Cultures (blood and sputum)

Other

- Closely monitor pulmonary status

Clinical Presentation and Diagnosis of Priapism in SCD

General

- Mean age of initial episode is 12 years of age
- Most males with SCD will have one episode by age 20
- Repeated episodes can lead to fibrosis and impotence

Symptoms

- Patients may complain of painful and unwanted erection lasting anywhere from less than 2 hours (stuttering type) to more than 2 hours (prolonged type)

Signs

- Urinary obstruction

Laboratory Tests

- CBC with reticulocyte count

Other

- Monitor for duration of episode
- Prolonged episodes should be considered medical emergencies

Clinical Presentation and Diagnosis of Acute Aplastic Crisis in SCD

General

- Transient suppression of RBC production in response to bacterial or viral infection
- Most commonly due to infection with parvovirus B19

Symptoms

- Patients may complain of headache, fatigue, dyspnea, pallor, or fever
- Patients may also complain of upper respiratory or GI infection symptoms

Signs

- Temperature greater than 38.5°C (101.3°F) may occur
- Hypoxia
- Tachycardia
- Acute decrease in Hgb with decreased reticulocyte count

Laboratory Tests

- CBC with reticulocyte count
- Chest x-ray
- Parvovirus titers
- Cultures (blood, urine, and throat)

Aspiration of the penile blood followed by intracavernous irrigation with epinephrine (1:1,000,000 solution) has been effective with minimal complications.[37] In severe cases, surgical intervention to place penile shunts has been used, but there is a high failure rate, and the risk of complications, from skin sloughing to fistulas, limits its use.

Pseudoephedrine dosed at 30 to 60 mg daily taken at bedtime has been used to prevent or decrease the number of episodes of priapism.[4] Terbutaline 5 mg has been used orally to prevent priapism, with mixed results.[37,38] Leuprolide, a gonadotropin-releasing hormone, also has been used for this indication. Hydroxyurea may be helpful in some patients.[37,39] The use of antiandrogens is under investigation.[4]

► *Treatment of Acute Complications*

Aplastic Crisis Most patients in aplastic crisis will recover spontaneously and therefore treatment is supportive. If anemia is severe or symptomatic, transfusion may be indicated. Infection with human parvovirus B19 is the most common cause of aplastic crisis. Isolate infected patients because parvovirus is highly contagious. Pregnant individuals should avoid contact with infected patients because midtrimester infection with parvovirus may cause hydrops fetalis and still birth.[1,4]

Sequestration Crisis RBC sequestration in the spleen in young children may lead to a rapid drop in hematocrit, resulting in hypovolemia, shock, and death. Treatment is RBC transfusion to correct the hypovolemia, as well as broad-spectrum antibiotics, because infections may precipitate the crisis.[1,4]

Clinical Presentation and Diagnosis of Sequestration Crisis in SCD

General

- Acute exacerbation of anemia due to sequestration of large blood volume by the spleen
- More common in patients with functioning spleens
- Onset often associated with viral or bacterial infections
- Recurrence is common and can be fatal

Symptoms

- Sudden onset of fatigue, dyspnea, and distended abdomen
- Patients may present with vomiting and abdominal pain

Signs

- Rapid decrease in Hgb and Hct with elevated reticulocyte count
- Splenomegaly
- May exhibit hypotension and shock

Evaluation

- Vital signs
- Spleen size changes
- Oxygen saturations
- CBC with reticulocyte count
- Cultures (blood, urine, throat)

Clinical Presentation and Diagnosis of Vasoocclusive Crisis in SCD

General

- Most often involves the bones, liver, spleen, brain, lungs, and penis
- Precipitating factors include infection, extreme weather conditions, dehydration, and stresses
- Recurrent acute crises result in bone, joint, and organ damage and chronic pain

Symptoms

- Patients may complain of deep throbbing pain, local tenderness

Signs

- Erythema and swelling of painful area
- Dactylitis in young infants
- Temperature greater than 38.5°C (101.3°F)
- Leukocytosis

Laboratory tests

- CBC with reticulocyte count
- Urinalysis
- Abdominal studies (if symptoms exist)
- Cultures (blood and urine)
- Liver function tests and bilirubin
- Chest x-ray

Table 68–4

Management of Acute Pain of SCD

Principles

Treat underlying precipitating factors.

- Avoid delays in analgesia administration.
- Use pain scale to assess severity.
- Choice of initial analgesic should be based on previous pain crisis pattern, history of response, current status, and other medical conditions.
- Schedule pain medication; avoid as-needed dosing.
- Provide rescue dose for breakthrough pain.
- If adequate pain relief can be achieved with one or two doses of morphine, consider outpatient management with a weak opioid; otherwise hospitalization is needed for parenteral analgesics.
- Frequently assess to evaluate pain severity and side effects; titrate dose as needed.
- Treating adverse effects of opioids is part of pain management.
- Consider nonpharmacologic intervention.
- Transition to oral analgesics as the patient improves; choose an oral agent based on previous history, anticipated duration, and ability to swallow tablets; if sustained-release products are used, a fast-release product is also needed for breakthrough pain.

Analgesic Regimens

Mild to moderate pain:

Acetaminophen with codeine:

- Dose based on codeine—children: 1 mg/kg per dose every 6 hours; adults: 30–60 mg/dose

Hydrocodone + acetaminophen:

- Dose based on hydrocodone—children: 0.2 mg/kg per dose every 6 hours; adults: 5–10 mg/dose

Anti-inflammatory agents:

- Use with caution in patients with renal failure (dehydration) and bleeding
- Ibuprofen (oral): children: 10 mg/kg every 6–8 hours; adults: 200–400 mg/dose
- Naproxen: 5 mg/kg every 12 hours; adults: 250–500 mg/dose
- Ibuprofen + hydrocodone: Each tablet contains 200 mg ibuprofen and 7.5 mg hydrocodone per tablet; only for older children who can swallow tablets

Moderate to severe pain:

Morphine—children: 0.1–0.15 mg/kg per dose every 3–4 hours; adults: 5–10 mg/dose

- Continuous infusion: 0.04–0.05 mg/kg/hour; titrate to effect

Hydromorphone—children: 0.015 mg/kg per dose every 3–4 hours; adults: 1.5–2 mg/dose

- Continuous infusion: 0.004 mg/kg/hour; titrate to effect

IV anti-inflammatory agents:

- Ketorolac: 0.5 mg/kg up to 30 mg/dose every 6 hours

Patient-controlled analgesics:

- Morphine: 0.01–0.03 mg/kg/hour basal; demand 0.01–0.03 mg/kg every 6–10 minutes; 4 hours lockout 0.04–0.06 mg/kg
- Hydromorphone: 0.003–0.005 mg/kg/hour basal; demand 0.003–0.05 mg/kg every 6–10 minutes; 4 hours lock out 0.4–0.6 mg/kg

Recurrent episodes are common and can be managed with chronic transfusion and splenectomy. Observation is used commonly in adults because their episodes are milder. Splenectomy is usually delayed until after 2 years of age to lessen the risk of postsplenectomy septicemia. Patients with chronic hypersplenism should be considered for splenectomy.[4,40]

Vasoocclusive Pain Crisis The mainstay of treatment for vasoocclusive crisis includes hydration and analgesia (Table 68–4). Pain may involve the extremities, back, chest, and abdomen. KEY CONCEPT *Patients with mild pain crisis may be treated as outpatients with rest, warm compresses to the affected (painful) area, increased fluid intake, and oral analgesia.* Patients with moderate to severe crises should be hospitalized. Infection should be ruled out because it may trigger a pain crisis, and any patient presenting with fever or critical illness should be started on empirical broad-spectrum antibiotics. Patients who are anemic should be transfused to their baseline. IV or oral fluids at 1.5 times maintenance is recommended. Close monitoring of the patient's fluid status is important to avoid overhydration, which can lead to ACS, volume overload, or heart failure.[4]

Aggressive pain management is required in patients presenting in pain crisis. Assess pain on a regular basis (every 2 to 4 hours), and individualize management to the patient. The use of pain scales may help with quantifying the pain rating. Obtain a good medication history of what has worked well for the patient in the past. Use acetaminophen or a nonsteroidal anti-inflammatory drug (NSAID) for treatment of mild to moderate pain. Patients with bone or joint pain who require IV medications may be helped by the use of ketorolac, an injectable NSAID. Because of the concern for side effects, including GI bleeding, ketorolac should be used only for a maximum of 5 consecutive days. Monitor for the total amount of acetaminophen given daily, because many products contain acetaminophen. Maximum daily dose of acetaminophen for adults is 4 g/day, and for children, five doses over a 24-hour period.[41] Add an opioid if pain persists or if pain is moderate to severe in nature. Combining an opioid with an NSAID can enhance the analgesic effects without increasing adverse effects.[42–45]

Severe pain should be treated with an opioid such as morphine, hydromorphone, methadone, or fentanyl. Moderate pain can be effectively treated in most cases with a weak opioid such as codeine or hydrocodone, usually in combination with acetaminophen. Meperidine should be avoided because of its relatively short analgesic effect and its toxic metabolite, normeperidine. Normeperidine may accumulate with repeated dosing and can lead to CNS side effects including seizures.

IV opioids are recommended for use in treatment of severe pain because of their rapid onset of action and ease in titration. Intramuscular injection should be avoided. Analgesia should be individualized and titrated to effect, either by scheduled doses or continuous infusion. The use of continuous infusion will avoid the fluctuations in blood levels between doses that are seen with bolus dosing. As-needed dosing of analgesia is only appropriate for breakthrough pain or uncontrolled pain. Patient-controlled analgesia (PCA) is commonly used and allows the patient to have control over his or her analgesic breakthrough dosing. As the pain crisis resolves, the pain medications can be tapered. Physical therapy and relaxation therapy can be helpful adjuvants to analgesia.[42–45]

Tolerance to opioids is seen when patients have had continuous long-term use of the medications and can be managed during acute crises by using a different potent opioid or using a larger dose of the same medication. Adverse effects associated with the use of opioids include respiratory depression, itching, nausea and vomiting, constipation, and drowsiness. Patients on continuous infusions of opioids should be on continuous pulse oximeter to assess oxygen saturations. Monitor the patient for oxygen saturations less than 92% (0.92). Oxygen should be administered as needed to keep the saturations above 92% (0.92). Itching can be managed with an antihistamine such as diphenhydramine. Nausea and vomiting can be treated and managed with the administration of antiemetics such as promethazine or the 5HT3 antagonists, but the use of promethazine is contraindicated in children younger than 2 years of age. Assess stool frequency in all patients on a continuous opioid, and start stool softeners or laxatives as needed. Excessive sedation is difficult to control, and the concurrent use of an opioid with diphenhydramine or other sedative medications can exacerbate the drowsiness, leading to hypoxemia. A continuous very low dose of naloxone, an opioid antagonist, has been used successfully when the adverse effects such as itching are unbearable.[46]

OUTCOME EVALUATION

SCD treatment and prevention are considered successful when complications are minimized. The major outcome parameters are a decrease in morbidity and mortality, measured by the number of hospitalizations, and the extent of end-organ damage seen over time. Today, with longer survival for SCD, chronic manifestations of the disease contribute to the morbidity later in life (Table 68–5). Thirty years ago, complications from SCD contributed to high mortality. It was estimated that approximately 50% of patients with SCD did not survive to reach adulthood.[1] Since that time, data suggest improvement in mortality rates for patients with SCD. The survival age for individuals with HbSS has increased to at least the fifth decade of life. Recent reports suggest 85% survival by 18 years of age.[4] SCD is a chronic disease and cannot be cured, except in some patients with transplant.

Starting with birth, SCD patients should have regularly scheduled health assessments and interventions when necessary. Obtain a urine analysis, complete blood count, liver function tests, ferritin or serum iron level and total iron-binding capacity, blood urea nitrogen (BUN), and creatinine on at least a yearly basis and more often for children younger than 5 years of age to monitor for complications. All SCD patients should have regular screening of their hearing and vision.

All patients and parents of children with SCD should have a plan for what to do in the event of symptoms of infection or pain. Obtain a medication history when patients are admitted to the hospital. Assess adherence with prophylactic penicillin and childhood immunization schedules in all pediatric SCD patients.

Table 68–5

Chronic Complications of SCD

System	Complications
Auditory	Sensorineural hearing loss due to sickling in cochlear vasculature with hair cell damage
Cardiovascular	Cardiomegaly, myocardial ischemia, murmurs, and abnormal ECG; patients with SCD have lower BP than the normal population; normal BP values for SCD should be used for diagnosis of hypertension ("relative" hypertension); heart failure usually is related to fluid overload
Dermatologic	Painful leg ulcers; failure to heal occurs in 50% of patients; recurrences are common
Genitourinary	Renal papillary necrosis, hematuria, hyposthenuria, proteinuria, nephrotic syndrome, tubular dysfunction, chronic renal failure, impotence
Growth and development	Delay in growth (weight and height) and sexual development; decreased fertility; increased complications during pregnancy; depression may be more prevalent than in general population, especially in patients with unstable disease
Hepatic and biliary	Cholelithiasis, biliary sludge, acute and chronic cholecystitis, and cholestasis (can be progressive and life-threatening)
Neurologic	"Silent" brain lesions on MRI are associated with poor cognitive and fine motor functions; pseudotumor cerebri (rare)
Ocular	Retinal or vitreous hemorrhage, retinal detachment, transient or permanent visual loss; central retinal vein occlusion
Pulmonary	Pulmonary fibrosis, pulmonary hypertension, cor pulmonale
Renal	Hematuria, hyposthenuria (inability to concentrate urine maximally), tubular dysfunction, enuresis during early childhood, acute renal failure can also occur
Skeletal	Aseptic necrosis of ball-and-socket joints (shoulder and hip); prostheses may be needed due to permanent damage; bone marrow hyperplasia resulting in growth disturbances of maxilla and vertebrae
Spleen	Asplenia (autosplenectomy or surgical splenectomy)

Patient Care Process

Patient Assessment:

- Based on physical exam and review of systems, determine whether the patient is experiencing any signs or symptoms of an acute or chronic SCD complication (see Tables 68–1 and 68–5)
- Review the patient's medical history. Does the patient have a history of previous complications from SCD that would necessitate chronic medication therapy? When was the patient last hospitalized for SCD complications?
- Conduct a medication history including prescriptions, OTC medications, and dietary supplements. Does the patient take any medications routinely for SCD? Does the patient take any analgesics as needed for pain? Does the patient have any medication allergies? Is the patient experiencing any side effects from their current medication therapy? Is the patient adherent with their chronic medication therapy?
- Review available laboratory tests.
- Is the patient up to date on their immunizations? Have they received their annual influenza vaccine?

Therapy Evaluation:

- Which analgesics have been helpful to the patient in the past? Is the patient taking appropriate doses of their pain medication to achieve the desired analgesic effect? If not, why?
- If the patient is having an acute complication of SCD, arrange for referral and/or admission to the hospital.
- If the patient is receiving hydroxyurea, review appropriate laboratory tests. Assess efficacy, safety, and patient adherence.
- If the patient is receiving chelation therapy, review appropriate laboratory tests. Assess efficacy, safety, and patient adherence.
- Determine if the patient has prescription coverage or whether recommended agents are included on the institution's formulary.

Care Plan Development:

- Select lifestyle modifications that are likely to be effective and safe for the patient.
- Determine whether drug doses are optimal.
- Arrange for vaccination if the patient is not up to date with recommendations.
- Address any patient concerns about SCD and its management.
- Discuss the importance of medication adherence and lifestyle modifications to reduce complications of SCD.

Follow-Up Evaluation:

- Follow-up at monthly intervals or more frequently to assess effectiveness and safety of therapy, to avoid complications from SCD and improve quality of life for the patient.
- Review medication history and physical exam findings, laboratory tests and results of other diagnostic tests.
- Assess for adverse effects from medications that the patient is taking.
- Stress the importance of adherence with the therapeutic regimen, including lifestyle modifications. Adjust therapeutic regimens as needed based on patient response and adverse effects.

Abbreviations Introduced in This Chapter

ACS	Acute chest syndrome
CNS	Central nervous system
HbA	Normal adult hemoglobin
HbAS	One normal and one sickle hemoglobin gene
HbC	Hemoglobin C
HbF	Fetal hemoglobin
HbS	Sickle hemoglobin
HbSβ^0-thalassemia	One sickle hemoglobin and one β^0-thalassemia gene
HbSβ^+-thalassemia	One sickle hemoglobin and one β^+-thalassemia gene
HbSC	One sickle hemoglobin and one hemoglobin C gene
HbSS	Homozygous sickle hemoglobin
Hgb	Hemoglobin
HLA	Human leukocyte antigen
HSCT	Hematopoietic stem cell transplantation
ISC	Irreversibly sickled cell
MCHC	Mean corpuscular hemoglobin concentration
MCV	Mean corpuscular volume
NSAID	Nonsteroidal anti-inflammatory drug
PCA	Patient-controlled analgesia
PCV 13	13-Valent pneumococcal conjugate vaccine
PPV 23	23-Valent pneumococcal polysaccharide vaccine
SCA	Sickle cell anemia
SCD	Sickle cell disease
SCT	Sickle cell trait
STOP	Stroke Prevention Trial in Sickle Cell Anemia
VOC	Vasoocclusive crisis
WBC	White blood cell

REFERENCES

1. Stuart MJ, Nagel RL. Sickle-cell disease. Lancet. 2004;364 (9442):1343–1360. Review.
2. Ashley-Koch A, Yang Q, Olney RS. Sickle hemoglobin (HbS) allele and sickle cell disease: A huge review. Am J Epidemiol. 2000;151:839–844.
3. Centers for Disease Control and Prevention [Internet]. Sickle Cell Disease. [cited 2015 Sept 22]. www.cdc.gov/ncbddd/sicklecell/data.htm
4. Yawn BP, Buchanan GR, Afenyi-Annan AN, et al. Management of sickle cell disease: Summary of the 2014 evidence-based report by expert panel members. JAMA. 2014;312(10): 1033–1058.

5. World Health Organization [Internet]. The Health of the People: What Works. Chapter 4: Disease Threats. [cited 2015 Sept 22]. http://www.who.int/bulletin/africanhealth2014/disease_threats/en/.
6. Rees DC, Williams TN, Gladwin MT. Sickle-cell disease. Lancet. 2010;376:2018–2031.
7. American Academy of Pediatrics Policy Statement. Recommended Childhood and Adolescent Immunization Schedule—United States, 2014. Pediatrics. 2014;133;357–363.
8. Centers for Disease Control and Prevention [Internet]. Recommended Adult Immunization Schedule—United States 2014. [cited 2015 Sept 22] http://www.cdc.gov/vaccines/schedules/downloads/adult/adult-schedule.pdf
9. Nuorti JP, Whitney CG. Prevention of pneumococcal disease among infants and children—use of 13-valent pneumococcal conjugate vaccine and 23-valent pneumococcal polysaccharide vaccine—recommendations of the Advisory Committee on Immunization Practices (ACIP). MMWR Recomm Rep. 2010;59:1–18.
10. Adamkiewicz TV, Silk BJ, Howgate J, et al. Effectiveness of the 7-valent pneumococcal conjugate vaccine in children with sickle cell disease in the first decade of life. Pediatrics. 2008;121:562–569.
11. Battersby AJ, Knox-Macaulay HHM, Carrol ED. Susceptibility to invasive bacterial infections in children with sickle cell disease. Pediatr Blood Cancer. 2010;55:401–406.
12. Quinn CT, Lee NJ, Shull EP, Ahmad N, Rogers ZR, Buchanan GR. Prediction of adverse outcomes in children with sickle cell anemia: A study of the Dallas Newborn Cohort. Blood. 2008;111:544–548.
13. Falletta JM, Woods RM, Verter JI, et al. Discontinuing penicillin prophylaxis in children with sickle cell anemia. J Pediatr. 1995;127:685–690.
14. Hirst C, Owusu-Ofori S. Cochrane Review: Prophylactic antibiotics for preventing pneumococcal infections in children with sickle cell disease. Evidence-Based Child Health 2007;2:993–1009.
15. Kennedy TS, Fung EB, Kawchak DA, et al. Red blood cell folate and serum B12 status in children with sickle cell disease. J Pediatr Hematol Oncol. 2001;23:165–169.
16. Brawley OW, Cornelius LJ, Edwards LR, et al. National Institutes of Health consensus development conference statement: Hydroxyurea treatment for sickle cell disease. Ann Intern Med. 2008;148:932–938.
17. Steinberg MH, Bartin F, Castro O, et al. Effect of hydroxyurea on mortality and morbidity in adult sickle cell anemia. Risks and benefits up to 9 years of treatment. JAMA. 2003;289:1645–1651.
18. Kinney TR, Helms RW, O'Branski EE, Ohene-Frempong K, et al. Safety of hydroxyurea in children with sickle cell anemia: Results of the HUG-KIDS study, a phase I/II trial. Pediatric Hydroxyurea Group. Blood. 1999;94(5):1550–1554.
19. Strouse JJ, Lanzkron S, Beach MC, et al. Hydroxyurea for sickle cell disease: A systematic review for efficacy and toxicity in children. Pediatrics. 2008;122:1332–1342.
20. Hankins JS, Ware RE, Rogers ZR, et al. Long-term hydroxyurea therapy for infants with sickle cell anemia: The HUSOFT extension study. Blood. 2005;106:2269–2275.
21. Lexi-Comp. Hydroxyurea monograph. Lexi-Comp Online,™ Pediatric Lexi-Drugs Online.™ Hudson, OH: Lexi-Comp; August 30, 2014.
22. Lexi-Comp. Deferoxamine monograph. Lexi-Comp Online,™ Pediatric Lexi-Drugs Online.™ Hudson, OH: Lexi-Comp; August 30, 2014.
23. Lexi-Comp. Deferasirox monograph. Lexi-Comp Online,™ Pediatric Lexi-Drugs Online.™ Hudson, OH: Lexi-Comp; August 30, 2014.
24. Lexi-Comp. Decitabine monograph. Lexi-Comp Online,™ Lexi-Drugs Online,™ Hudson, OH: Lexi-Comp, August 30, 2014.
25. Lexi-Comp. Folic acid monograph. Lexi-Comp Online,™ Lexi-Drugs Online,™ Hudson, OH: Lexi-Comp; August 30, 2014.
26. Aronoff GR, Bennett WM, Berns JS, et al., eds. Drug Prescribing in Renal Failure. 5th ed. Philadelphia, PA: American College of Physicians; 2007.
27. Hankins J, Aygun B. Pharmacotherapy in sickle-cell disease—state of the art and future prospects. Br J Haematol. 2009;145:296–308.
28. Porter J, Vinchinsky E, Rose C, et al. A phase II study with ICL670 (Exjade), a once-daily oral iron chelator, in patients with various transfusion dependent anemias and iron overload (abstract). Blood. 2004;104:3193.
29. Brittenham GM. Iron-chelating therapy for transfusional iron overload. N Engl J Med. 2011;364:146–156.
30. Bolanos-Meade J, Brodsky RA. Blood and marrow transplantation for sickle cell disease: Overcoming barriers to success Curr Opin Oncol. 2009;21:158–161.
31. Hsieh MM, Fitzhugh CD, Weitzel P, et al. Nonmyeloablative HLA-matched sibling allogeneic hematopoietic stem cell transplantation for severe sickle phenotype. JAMA. 2014;312(1):48–56.
32. Adams RJ, Brambilla DJ, Granger S, et al. Stroke and conversion to high risk in children screened with transcranial Doppler ultrasound during the STOP study. Blood. 2004;103:3689–3694.
33. Lee MT, Piomelli S, Granger S, et al. Stroke Prevention Trial in Sickle Cell Anemia (STOP): Extended follow-up and final results. Blood. 2006;108:847–852.
34. Kwiatkowski JL, Granger S, Brambilla DJ, Brown RC, Miller ST, Adams RJ. Elevated blood flow velocity in the anterior cerebral artery and stroke risk in sickle cell disease; extended analysis from the STOP trial. Br J Haematol. 2006;134:333–339.
35. Caboot JB, Allen JL. Pulmonary complications of sickle cell disease in children. Curr Opin Pediatr. 2008;20:279–287.
36. Johnson CS. The acute chest syndrome. Hematol Oncol Clin North Am. 2005;198:857–879.
37. Maples BL, Hagemann TM. Treatment of priapism in pediatric patients with sickle cell disease. Am J Health Syst Pharm. 2004;61:355–363.
38. Fuh BR, Perkin RM. Sickle cell disease emergencies in children. Ped Emer Med Report. 2009;14:145–155.
39. Saad STO, Lajolo C, Gilli S, et al. Follow-up of sickle cell disease patients with priapism treated by hydroxyurea. Am J Hematol. 2004;77:45–49.
40. Owusu-Ofori S, Riddington C. Splenectomy versus conservative management for acute sequestration crises in people with sickle cell disease. Cochrane Database Syst Rev. 2002;(4):CD003425.
41. Changes for acetaminophen-containing prescription products. Pharm Lett Prescribe Lett 2011;27(2):270203.
42. Field JJ, Knight-Perry JE, Debaun MR. Acute pain in children and adults with sickle cell disease: Management in the absence of evidence-based guidelines. Curr Opin Hematol. 2009;16:173–178.
43. Jerrell JM, Tripathi A, Stallworth JR. Pain management in children and adolescents with sickle cell disease. Am J Hematol. 2011;86:82–84.
44. Frei-Jones MJ, Baxter AL, Rogers ZR, Buchanan GR. Vaso-occlusive episodes in older children with sickle cell disease: Emergency department management and pain assessment. J Pediatr. 2008;152:281–285.
45. Mousa SA, Al Momen A, Al Sayegh F, et al. Management of painful vaso-occlusive crisis of sickle-cell anemia: Consensus opinion. Clin Appl Thromb Hemost. 2010;16:365–376.
46. Miller JM, Hagemann TM. Use of pure opioid antagonists for management of opioid-induced pruritus. Am J Health-Syst Pharm. 2011;68:1419–1425.

69 Antimicrobial Regimen Selection

Catherine M. Oliphant

LEARNING OBJECTIVES

Upon completion of the chapter, the reader will be able to:

1. Recognize that antimicrobial resistance is an inevitable consequence of antimicrobial therapy.
2. Describe how antimicrobials differ from other drug classes in terms of their effects on individual patients as well as on society as a whole.
3. Identify two guiding principles to consider when treating patients with antimicrobials, and apply these principles in patient care.
4. Differentiate between microbial colonization and infection based on patient history, physical examination, and laboratory and culture results.
5. Evaluate and apply at least six major drug-specific considerations when selecting antimicrobial therapy.
6. Evaluate and apply at least seven major patient-specific considerations when selecting antimicrobial therapy.
7. Select empirical antimicrobial therapy based on spectrum-of-activity considerations that provide a measured response proportional to the severity of illness. Provide a rationale for why a measured response in antimicrobial selection is appropriate.
8. Identify and apply five major principles of patient education and monitoring response to antimicrobial therapy.
9. Identify two common causes of patients failing to improve while on antimicrobials, and recognize other less common but potential reasons for antimicrobial failure.

INTRODUCTION

Since 1980, infectious disease–related mortality in the United States has increased, in part owing to increases in antimicrobial resistance. The discovery of virtually every new class of antimicrobials has occurred in response to the development of bacterial resistance and loss of clinical effectiveness of existing antimicrobials. KEY CONCEPT *An inevitable consequence of exposing microbes to antimicrobials is that some organisms will develop resistance to the antimicrobial.* Today, there are many antimicrobial classes and antimicrobials available for clinical use. However, in many cases, differences in mechanisms of action between antimicrobials are minor, and the microbiologic properties of the agents are similar. KEY CONCEPT *Antimicrobials are different from other classes of pharmaceuticals because they exert their action on bacteria infecting the host as opposed to acting directly on the host.* Because antimicrobial use in one patient affects not only that patient but also other patients if they become infected with resistant bacteria, correct selection, use, and monitoring of clinical response are paramount.

KEY CONCEPT *There are two guiding principles to consider when treating patients with antimicrobials: (a) make the correct diagnosis and (b) do no harm!* Patients with infections frequently present with signs and symptoms that are nonspecific and may be confused with other noninfectious disease. Not only is it important to determine whether a disease process is of infectious origin, but it is also important to determine the specific causative pathogen of the infection. Antimicrobials vary in their **spectrum of activity**, the ability to inhibit or kill different species of bacteria. Antimicrobials that kill many different species of bacteria are called *broad-spectrum antimicrobials*, whereas antimicrobials that kill only a few species of bacteria are called *narrow-spectrum antimicrobials*. One might argue that treating everybody with broad spectrum antimicrobials will increase the likelihood that a patient will get better even without knowing the bacteria causing infection. However, counter to this argument is the principle of "Do no harm!" Broad antimicrobial coverage does increase the likelihood of empirically killing a causative pathogen; unfortunately, the development of secondary infections can be caused by selection of antimicrobial-resistant nontargeted pathogens. In addition, adverse events are thought to complicate up to 10% of all antimicrobial therapy, and for select agents, the adverse-event rates are similar to high-risk medications such as warfarin, digoxin, or insulin.[1] Therefore, the overall goal of antimicrobial therapy should be to cure the patient's infection; limit harm by minimizing patient risk for adverse effects, including secondary infections; and limit societal risk from antimicrobial-resistant bacteria.

EPIDEMIOLOGY AND ETIOLOGY

Infectious disease–related illnesses, particularly respiratory tract infections, are among the most common reasons patients seek medical care.[2] Antimicrobial prescribing has been associated with inappropriate use of antimicrobial agents. During the late 1990s/early 2000s, many organizations initiated campaigns to promote appropriate antimicrobial use. Recent trends in prescribing suggest a modest reduction in antimicrobial use for these infections, suggesting an increased recognition of the negative consequences of antimicrobial use.[3,4] Up to one-half of all patients receive at least one antimicrobial during hospitalization. In 2011, the number of health care–associated infections in acute care hospitals in the United States was estimated at 721,800, with approximately 75,000 deaths.[5] In 2014, the CDC reported that there were reductions in central line–associated bloodstream infections (44% reduction between 2008 and 2012) and surgical site infections (20% reduction between 2008 and 2012) as well as a slight reduction in hospital-onset MRSA bloodstream infection (4% reduction from 2011 to 2012).[6] Nosocomial infections tend be associated with antimicrobial-resistant strains of bacteria. However, there has been a shift in the etiology of some community-acquired infections. Increasingly, infections caused by antimicrobial-resistant pathogens, traditionally nosocomial in origin, are being identified in ambulatory care settings. Reasons for this change include an aging populace, improvement in the management of chronic comorbid conditions including immunosuppressive conditions, and increases in outpatient management of more debilitated patients. The majority of infections caused by antimicrobial-resistant pathogens in the ambulatory care setting occur in patients who have had recent exposure to the health care system. The converging bacterial etiologies and increasing resistance in all health care environments emphasize the need to "make the diagnosis."

PATHOPHYSIOLOGY

Normal Flora and Endogenous Infection

Many areas of the human body are colonized with bacteria—this is known as **normal flora**. Infections often arise from one's own normal flora (called an *endogenous infection*). Endogenous infection may occur when there are alterations in the normal flora (eg, recent antimicrobial use may allow for overgrowth of other normal flora) or disruption of host defenses (eg, a break or entry in the skin). Knowing what organisms reside where can help guide empirical antimicrobial therapy (Figure 69–1). In addition, it is beneficial to know what anatomic sites are normally sterile. These include the cerebrospinal fluid, blood, and urine.

Determining Colonization versus Infection

Infection refers to the presence of bacteria that are causing disease (eg, the organisms are found in normally sterile anatomic sites or in nonsterile sites with signs/symptoms of infection). *Colonization* refers to the presence of bacteria that are not causing disease. KEY CONCEPT *Only bacteria that cause disease should be targeted with antimicrobial therapy, and non–disease-producing colonizing flora should be left intact.* It is important to differentiate infection from colonization because antimicrobial therapy targeting colonization is inappropriate and may lead to the development of resistant bacteria.

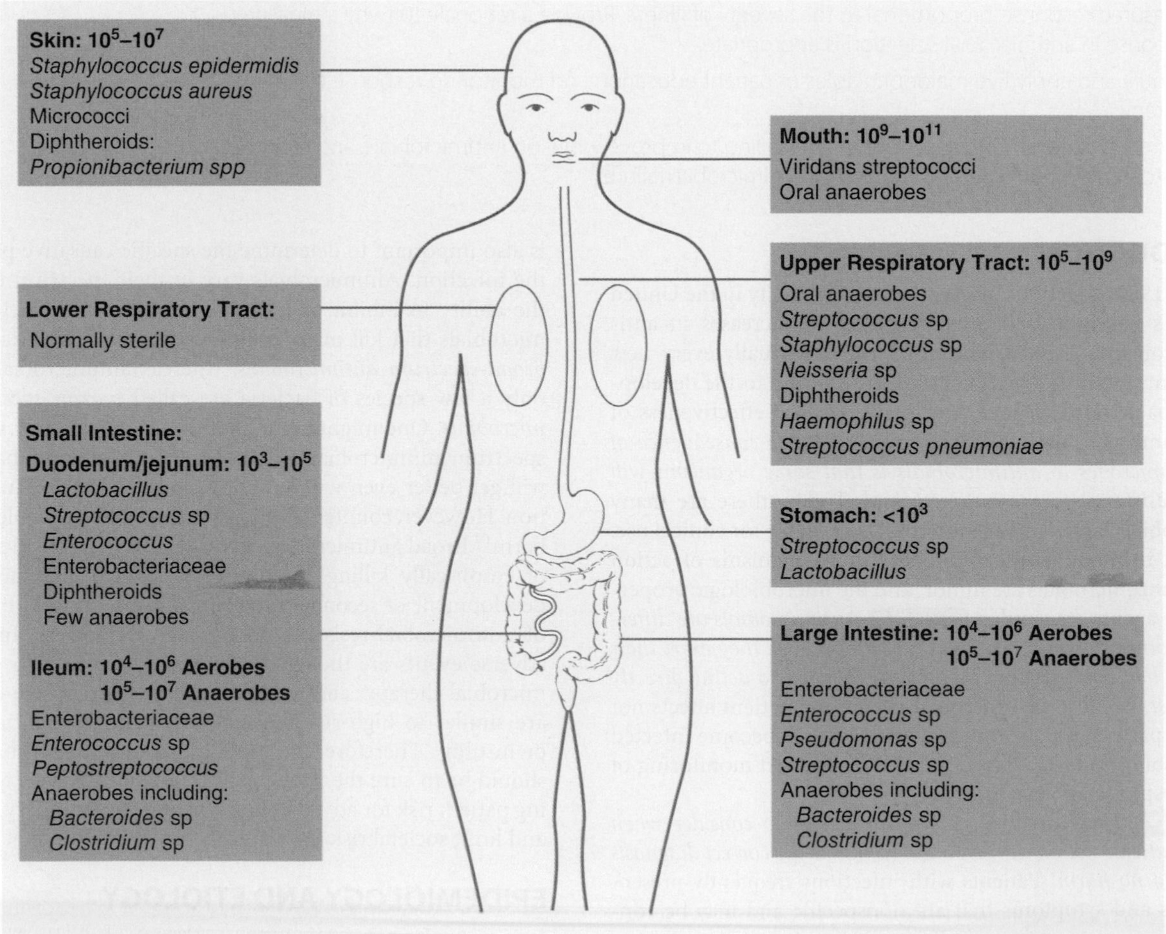

FIGURE 69–1. Normal flora and concentrations of bacteria (organisms per milliliter).

Exogenously Acquired Bacterial Infections

Infections acquired from an external source are referred to as *exogenous infections*. These infections may occur as a result of human-to-human transmission, contact with exogenous bacterial populations in the environment, and animal contact. Resistant pathogens such as methicillin-resistant *Staphylococcus aureus* (MRSA) and vancomycin-resistant *Enterococcus* spp (VRE) may colonize hospitalized patients or patients who access the health care system frequently. It is important to know which patients have acquired these organisms because patients generally become colonized prior to developing infection, and colonized patients should be placed in isolation to minimize transmission.

Contrasting Bacterial Virulence and Resistance

Virulence refers to the pathogenicity or disease severity produced by an organism. Bacteria may produce toxins or possess characteristics that contribute to their pathogenicity. Some virulence factors allow the organism to avoid the immune response of the host and cause significant disease. Virulence and resistance are different microbial characteristics. For example, *Streptococcus pyogenes*, a common cause of skin infections, produces toxins that can cause severe disease, yet it is very susceptible to penicillin. *Enterococcus faecium* is a highly resistant organism but is frequently a colonizing flora that causes disease primarily in the immunocompromised.

CLINICAL PRESENTATION AND DIAGNOSIS

Physical Examination

Findings on physical examination, along with the clinical presentation, can help identify the anatomic location of the infection. Once the anatomic site is identified, the most probable pathogens associated with disease can be determined based on likely endogenous or exogenous flora.

Fever often accompanies infection and is defined as a rise in body temperature above the normal 37°C (98.6°F). Oral and axillary temperatures may underestimate core temperature by at least 0.6°C (1°F), whereas rectal temperatures best approximate core temperatures. Fever is a host response to bacterial toxins. However, bacterial infections are not the sole cause of fever. Fever also may be caused by other infections (eg, fungal or viral), medications (eg, penicillins, cephalosporins, salicylates, and phenytoin), trauma, or other medical conditions (eg, autoimmune disease, malignancy, pulmonary embolism, and hyperthyroidism). Some patients with infections may present with hypothermia (eg, patients with overwhelming infection). Elderly patients may be afebrile, as may those with localized infections (eg, urinary tract infection).[7] For others, fever may be the only indication of infection. Neutropenic patients may not have the ability to mount normal immune responses to infection (eg, infiltrate on chest x-ray, pyuria on urinalysis, or erythema or induration around catheter site), and the only finding may be fever.

Imaging Studies

Imaging studies also may help to identify anatomic localization of the infection. These studies usually are performed in conjunction with other tests to establish or rule out the presence of an infection. Radiographs are performed commonly to establish the diagnosis of pneumonia, as well as to determine the severity of disease. Computed tomography (CT) scans are a type of x-ray that produces a three-dimensional image of the combination of soft tissue, bone, and blood vessels. In contrast, magnetic resonance imaging (MRI) uses electromagnetic radio waves to

Clinical Presentation

- Review of symptoms consistent with an infectious etiology.
- Signs and symptoms may be nonspecific (eg, fever) or specific.
- Specific signs and symptoms are beyond the scope of this chapter (see disease state–specific chapters for these findings).

Patient History

- History of present illness
- Comorbidities
- Current medications
- Allergies
- Previous antibiotic exposure (may provide clues regarding colonization or infection with new specific pathogens or pathogens that may be resistant to certain antimicrobials)
- Previous hospitalization or health care utilization (also a key determinant in selecting therapy because the patient may be at risk for specific pathogens and/or resistant pathogens)
- Travel history
- Social history
- Pet/animal exposure
- Occupational exposure
- Environmental exposure

Physical Findings

- Findings consistent with an infectious etiology
- Vital signs
- Body system abnormalities (eg, rales, altered mental status, localized inflammation, erythema, warmth, edema, pain, and pus)

Diagnostic Imaging

- Radiographs (x-rays)
- CT scans
- MRI
- Labeled leukocyte scans

Nonmicrobiologic Laboratory Studies

- White blood cell count (WBC) with differential
- Erythrocyte sedimentation rate (ESR)
- C-reactive protein
- Procalcitonin

Microbiologic Studies

- Gram stain
- Culture and susceptibility testing

produce two- or three-dimensional images of soft tissue and blood vessels with less detail of bony structures.

Nonmicrobiologic Laboratory Studies

Nonmicrobiological laboratory tests include the white blood cell count (WBC) and differential, erythrocyte sedimentation rate (ESR), C-reactive protein (CRP) and procalcitonin levels. In most cases, the WBC count is elevated in response to infection, but it may be decreased owing to overwhelming or long-standing infection. The differential is the percentage of each type of WBC (Table 69–1). In response to physiologic stress, neutrophils leave the bloodstream and enter the tissue to "fight" against the offending pathogens (ie, leukocytosis). It is important to recognize that leukocytosis is nonspecific for infection and may temporarily occur in response to noninfectious conditions such as acute myocardial infarction. During an infection, immature neutrophils (eg, bands) are released at an increased rate to help fight infection, leading to what is known as a "bandemia" or "left shift". Therefore, a WBC count differential is key to determining whether an infection is present. Some patients may present with a normal total WBC with a left shift (eg, the elderly). ESR and CRP are nonspecific markers of inflammation that increase as a result of the acute-phase reactant response, which is a response to inflammatory stimuli such as infection or tissue injury. These tests may be used as markers of infectious disease response because they are elevated when the disease is acutely active and usually fall in response to successful treatment. Clinicians may use these tests to monitor a patient's response to therapy in osteomyelitis and infective endocarditis. These tests should not be used to diagnose infection because they may be elevated in noninfectious inflammatory conditions. In contrast, procalcitonin, a prohormone of calcitonin, is rapidly produced in response to bacterial infection. Procalcitonin serum levels in conjunction with clinical findings are increasingly being utilized to assess both the need to initiate antibiotic therapy as well as determine when antibiotic therapy may be safely discontinued.[8,9]

Table 69–1

WBC and Differential

Type of Cell	Normal Value % (or Fraction)	Function	Abnormalities
Neutrophil	Segs 40–60 (0.40–0.60) Bands 3–5 (0.03–0.05)	Phagocytic	Leukocytosis • Bacterial infections • Fungal infections • Physiologic stress • Tissue injury (eg, myocardial Infarction) • Medications (eg, corticosteroids) Leukopenia • Long-standing infection • Cancer • Medications (eg, chemotherapy)
Lymphocyte	20–40 (0.20–0.40)	T cells (cell-mediated immunity) B cells (humoral antibody response)	Lymphocytosis • Viral infections (eg, mononucleosis) • Tuberculosis • Fungal infections Lymphopenia • HIV
Monocyte	2–8 (0.02–0.08)	Phagocytic precursor to macrophage	Monocytosis • Tuberculosis • Protozoal infections • Leukemia
Eosinophil	1–4 (0.01–0.04)	Antigen-antibody reactions	Eosinophilia • Hypersensitivity reactions, including medications • Parasitic infections
Basophil	< 1 (0.01)		Hypersensitivity reactions

Microbiologic Studies

Microbiologic studies that allow for direct examination of a specimen (eg, sputum, blood, or urine) may aid in a presumptive diagnosis and give an indication of the characteristics of the infecting organism. Generally, microbial cultures are obtained with a Gram stain of the cultured material.

Patient Encounter 1

HPI: A 72 year old woman with a history of hypertension, diabetes, hyperlipidemia, chronic back pain, osteoarthritis, and a history of frequent urinary tract infections who began feeling poorly 48 hours prior to presenting to the emergency room. She reports extreme fatigue, chills, fever (100.6°F [38.1°C]), nausea, and headache. Her daughter, who is accompanying the patient to the emergency room, notes increasing confusion over the same time period. She has recently been treated for recurrent urinary tract infections 2 and 5 weeks ago with Bactrim DS and levofloxacin.

PMH: Hypertension, diabetes, hyperlipidemia, chronic back pain, osteoarthritis, and frequent urinary tract infections (5–10 per year) with the most recent being treated 2 and 5 weeks ago with Bactrim DS and levofloxacin, respectively

FH: Father died of colon cancer at age 72. Mother died of congestive heart failure at age 83

SH: Lives at home. Has 2 daughters and 1 son

Allergies: NKDA

Meds: Lisinopril 10 mg daily; hydrochlorothiazide 25 mg daily; metoprolol XL 50 mg daily; atorvastatin 20 mg daily; metformin 1000 mg twice daily; glipizide 5 mg twice daily; pregabalin 150 mg daily; oxycodone 5 mg three times; aspirin 81 mg daily; alendronate 70 mg weekly; calcium carbonate 500 mg twice daily; multivitamin 1 daily; cranberry supplement 300 mg daily

What information in the history supports an infectious etiology?

Is this patient at risk for resistant pathogens? Why?

A Gram stain of collected specimens can give rapid information that can be applied immediately to patient care. A Gram stain is performed to identify whether bacteria are present and to determine morphologic characteristics of bacteria (eg, gram-positive or gram-negative and shape—cocci, bacilli). Certain specimens do not stain well or at all and must be identified by alternative staining techniques (*Mycoplasma* spp., *Legionella* spp., *Mycobacterium* spp.). Figure 69–2 identifies bacterial pathogens classified by Gram stain and morphologic characteristics. The presence of WBCs on a Gram stain indicates inflammation and suggests that the identified bacteria are pathogenic. The Gram stain may be useful in evaluating a sputum specimen's adequacy (eg, the presence of epithelial cells on sputum Gram stain suggests that the specimen is either poorly collected or contaminated). A poor specimen can give misleading information regarding the underlying pathogen and may result in inappropriate antimicrobial use.

Culture and susceptibility testing provides additional information to the clinician to select appropriate therapy. Specimens are placed in or on culture media that provide proper growth

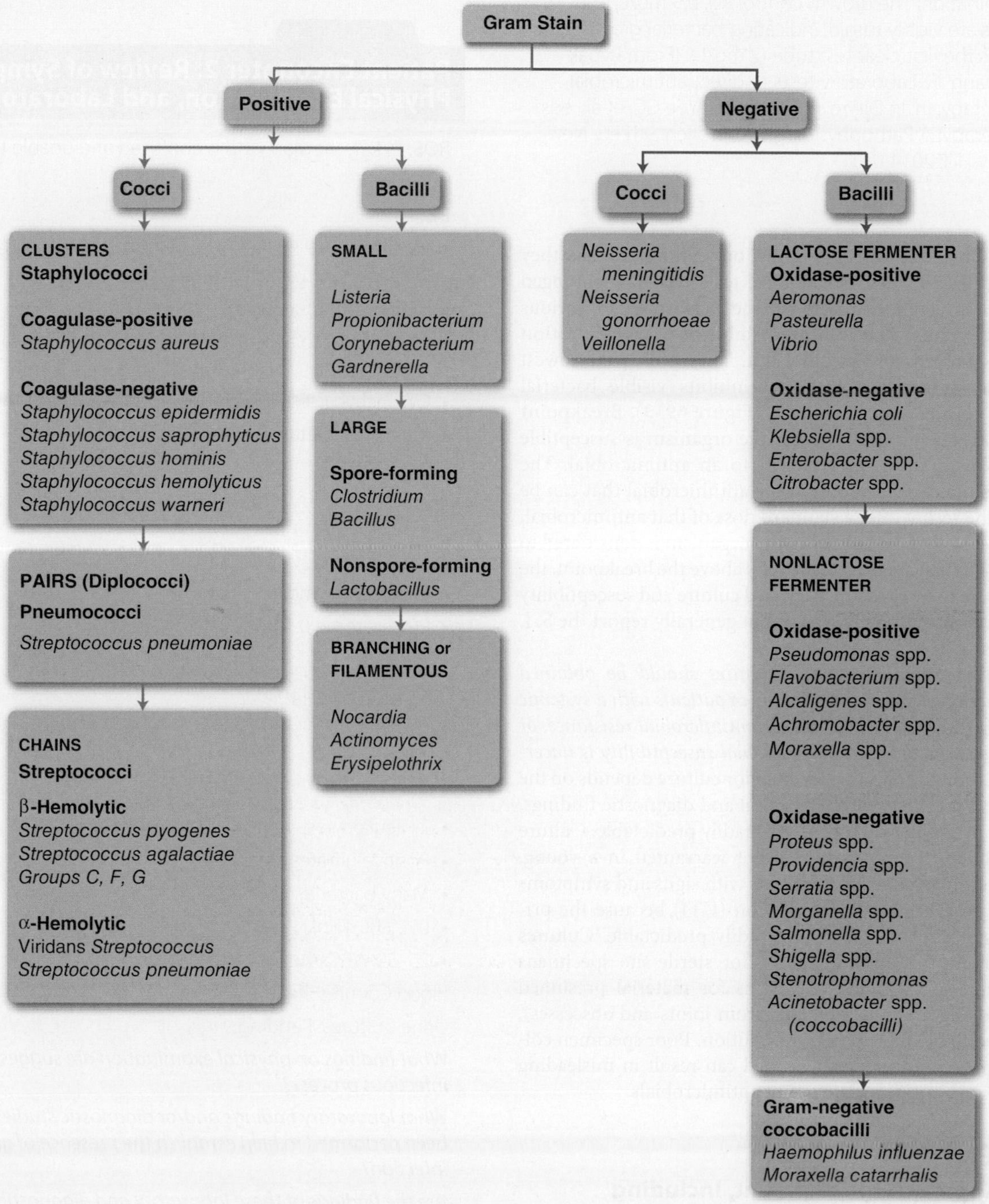

FIGURE 69–2. Important bacterial pathogens classified according to Gram stain and morphologic characteristics. (From Rybak MJ, Aeschlimann JR. Laboratory tests to direct antimicrobial pharmacotherapy. In: In DiPiro JT, Talbert RL, Yee GC, et al., eds. Pharmacotherapy: A Pathophysiologic Approach. 9th ed. New York: McGraw-Hill; 2014.)

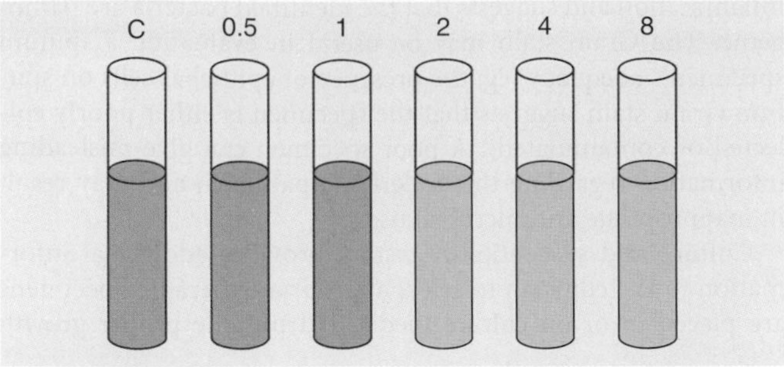

FIGURE 69–3. Macrotube minimal inhibitory concentration (MIC) determination. The growth control (C), 0.5 mg/L, and 1 mg/L tubes are visibly turgid, indicating bacterial growth. The MIC is read as the first clear test tube (2 mg/L). (From Rybak MJ, Aeschlimann JR. Laboratory tests to direct antimicrobial pharmacotherapy. In: In DiPiro JT, Talbert RL, Yee GC, et al., eds. Pharmacotherapy: A Pathophysiologic Approach. 9th ed. New York: McGraw-Hill; 2014.)

conditions. Once the bacteria grow on culture media, they can be identified through biochemical tests. When a pathogen is identified, susceptibility tests can be performed to various antimicrobial agents. The **minimum inhibitory concentration (MIC)** is a standard susceptibility test. The MIC is the lowest concentration of antimicrobial that inhibits visible bacterial growth after approximately 24 hours (Figure 69–3). **Breakpoint** and MIC values determine whether the organism is susceptible (S), intermediate (I), or resistant (R) to an antimicrobial. The breakpoint is the concentration of the antimicrobial that can be achieved in the serum after a standard dose of that antimicrobial. If the MIC is below the breakpoint, the organism is considered to be susceptible to that agent. If the MIC is above the breakpoint, the organism is said to be resistant. Reported culture and susceptibility results may not provide MIC values but generally report the S, I, and R results.

KEY CONCEPT *In general, bacterial cultures should be obtained prior to initiating antimicrobial therapy in patients with a systemic inflammatory response, risk factors for antimicrobial resistance, or infections where diagnosis or antimicrobial susceptibility is uncertain.* The decision to collect a specimen for culture depends on the sensitivity and specificity of the physical and diagnostic findings, and whether or not the pathogens are readily predictable. Culture and susceptibility testing usually is not warranted in a young, otherwise healthy woman who presents with signs and symptoms consistent with a urinary tract infection (UTI) because the primary pathogen, *Escherichia coli*, is readily predictable. Cultures and susceptibility testing are routine for sterile-site specimens (eg, blood and spinal fluid), as well as for material presumed to be infected (eg, material obtained from joints and abscesses). Cultures need to be interpreted with caution. Poor specimen collection technique and processing speed can result in misleading information and inappropriate use of antimicrobials.

TREATMENT

General Approach to Treatment, Including Nonantimicrobial Treatment

While selection of antimicrobial therapy may be a major consideration in treating infectious diseases, it may not be the only therapeutic intervention. Other important therapies may include adequate hydration, ventilatory support, and supportive medications. In addition, antimicrobials are unlikely to be effective if the source that leads to the infection is not controlled. **Source control** refers to this process and may involve removal of prosthetic materials such as catheters and infected tissue or drainage of an abscess. Source control considerations should be a fundamental component of any infectious diseases treatment. It is also important to recognize that there may be many different antimicrobial regimens that may cure the patient. While the following therapy sections provide factors to consider when selecting antimicrobial regimens, excellent and more in-depth

Patient Encounter 2: Review of Symptoms, Physical Examination, and Laboratory Data

ROS: Elderly woman who is confused and unable to answer questions.

PE:

- **VS:** BP 89/55 P 92, RR 20, T 38.7°C (101.7° F), O_2 sat 94% (0.94) on room air, Ht 5′3″ (160 cm), Wt 68 kg
- **HEENT:** Dry mucous membranes
- **Chest:** Clear to auscultation without wheezes, rales or rhonchi
- **CV:** Tachycardic with irregularly irregular rhythm
- **Musculoskeletal:** CVA tenderness

Labs:

- WBC 16.5 × 10^3/mm^3 (16.5 × 10^9/L), segs 82% (0.82), bands 11% (0.11), lymphs 7% (0.07)
- SCr 1.8 mg/dL (159 μmol/L)
- Glucose 242 mg/dL (13.4 mmol/L)
- Procalcitonin 0.5 μg/L
- Urinalysis:

Specific gravity 1.015

- pH 6.0
- 1+ protein
- 2+ blood
- 2+ leukocytes
- Positive nitrates
- Many bacteria
- 0–2 RBCs/hpf
- 25–50 WBCs/hpf

Blood Cultures: Pending

Urine Cultures: Pending

What findings on physical examination are suggestive of an infectious process?

What laboratory findings and/or diagnostic studies have been performed to help establish the presence of an infection?

Are the findings of these laboratory and diagnostic studies suggestive of an infection?

What is your working diagnosis based on this patient encounter?

Table 69–2

Considerations for Selecting Antimicrobial Regimens

Drug Specific	Patient Specific
Spectrum of activity and effects on nontargeted flora	Anatomic location of infection
Dosing	Antimicrobial history
Pharmacokinetic properties	Drug allergy history
Pharmacodynamic properties	Renal and hepatic function
Adverse-effect potential	Concomitant medications
Drug-interaction potential	Pregnancy or lactation
Cost	Compliance potential

resources for selecting antimicrobial regimens for a variety of infectious diseases are the *Infectious Diseases Society of America Guidelines*.[10]

Antimicrobial Considerations in Selecting Therapy

KEY CONCEPT *Drug-specific considerations in antimicrobial selection include spectrum of activity, effects on nontargeted microbial flora, appropriate dose, pharmacokinetic and pharmacodynamic properties, adverse-effect and drug-interaction profile, and cost* (Table 69–2).

▶ *Spectrum of Activity and Effects on Nontargeted Flora*

Most initial antimicrobial therapy is empirical because cultures have not had sufficient time for identification of a pathogen. KEY CONCEPT *Empirical therapy should be based on patient- and antimicrobial-specific factors such as the anatomic location of the infection, the likely pathogens associated with the presentation, the potential for adverse effects in a given patient, and the antimicrobial spectrum of activity.* Prompt initiation of appropriate therapy is paramount in hospitalized patients who are critically ill. Patients who receive appropriate initial antimicrobial therapy survive at twice the rate of patients who receive inadequate therapy.[11] Empirical selection of antimicrobial spectrum of activity should be related to the severity of the illness. Generally, acutely ill patients require broader-spectrum antimicrobial coverage, whereas less ill patients may be managed initially with narrow-spectrum therapy. While a detailed description of antimicrobial pathogen-specific spectrum of activity is beyond the scope of this chapter, this information can be obtained readily from a number of sources.[12,13]

Collateral damage is defined as the development of resistance occurring in a patient's nontargeted flora that can cause secondary infections. *Clostridium difficile* infection (CDI) is an example of a disease that occurs secondary to collateral damage. Antibiotics can increase the risk of CDI by suppressing normal intestinal flora, resulting in overgrowth of the nonsusceptible *C. difficile* bacteria. In addition, CDI is associated with the prior use of broad-spectrum antibiotics; particularly fluoroquinolones.[14] If several different antimicrobials possess activity against a targeted pathogen, the antimicrobial that is least likely to be associated with collateral damage may be preferred.

▶ *Single versus Combination Therapy*

A common debate involves the need for coverage with two antimicrobials for serious infections. Proponents state that double coverage may be synergistic, prevent the emergence of resistance, and improve outcome. However, there are few clinical examples in the literature to support these assertions. Examples where double coverage is considered superior are limited to infections associated with large bacterial loads and in species that are known to readily develop resistance such as active tuberculosis or enterococcal endocarditis.[15,16] A study of patients with *Pseudomonas aeruginosa* infections, an intrinsically resistant organism, demonstrated that empirical double coverage with two antipseudomonal antimicrobials improved survival.[17] Combination therapy increased the likelihood of appropriate empirical coverage; however, once organism susceptibilities were known, there was no difference in outcome between double coverage and monotherapy. Double antimicrobial coverage with two agents of similar spectra of activity may be beneficial for selected infections associated with high bacterial loads or for initial empirical coverage of critically ill patients in whom antimicrobial-resistant organisms are suspected. Monotherapy usually is satisfactory once antimicrobial susceptibilities are established.

▶ *Antimicrobial Dose*

Clinicians should be aware that antimicrobial dosage regimens may be different depending on the infectious process. For example, ciprofloxacin, a fluoroquinolone, has various dosage regimens based on site of infection. The dosing for uncomplicated UTIs is 250 mg twice daily for 3 days. For complicated UTIs, the dose is 500 mg twice daily for 7 to 14 days. Severe complicated pneumonia requires a dosage regimen of 750 mg twice daily for 7 to 14 days. Clinicians are encouraged to use dosing regimens designed for treatment of the diagnosed infection because they have demonstrated proven efficacy and are most likely to minimize harm.

▶ *Pharmacokinetic Properties*

Pharmacokinetic properties of an antimicrobial may be important in antimicrobial regimens. Pharmacokinetics refers to a mathematical method of describing a patient's drug exposure in vivo in terms of absorption, distribution, metabolism, and elimination. Bioavailability refers to the amount of antimicrobial that is absorbed orally relative to an equivalent IV dose administered. Drug-related factors that may affect oral bioavailability include the formulation of the antimicrobial, dosage form, and stability of the drug in the gastrointestinal (GI) tract. Patients with systemic signs of infection such as hypotension should receive intravenous antimicrobials to ensure drug delivery as absorption is affected by GI blood flow. In cases where patients have a functioning GI tract and are not hypotensive, antimicrobials with almost complete bioavailability (greater than 80%) such as the fluoroquinolones, fluconazole, and linezolid may be given orally. With antimicrobials with modest bioavailability (eg, many β-lactams), the decision to choose an oral product will depend more on the severity of the illness and the anatomic location of the infection. In sequestered infections, where higher systemic concentrations of antimicrobial may be necessary to reach the infected source (eg, meningitis) or for antimicrobials with poor bioavailability, IV formulations should be used.

Some antimicrobials may be bound to proteins in serum. Only unbound drug is biologically active and distributes freely between tissues. Protein binding is clinically relevant in highly protein-bound antimicrobials (greater than 50%) as the agents may not be able to penetrate sequestered compartments, such as cerebral spinal fluid, resulting in insufficient concentrations to inhibit bacteria. In addition, some drugs may not achieve sufficient concentrations in specific compartments based on distribution characteristics. For example, *Legionella pneumophila*, an organism that causes severe pneumonia, is known to survive and reside inside pulmonary macrophages. Treatment with an antibiotic that inhibits bacterial cell wall synthesis, such as a cephalosporin, will be ineffective because it only distributes into extracellular host tissues. However, macrolide or fluoroquinolone antimicrobials, which concentrate in human pulmonary macrophages, are highly effective against this organism.

Many antimicrobials undergo some degree of metabolism once ingested. Metabolism may occur via hepatic, renal, or nonorgan-specific enzymatic processes. The route of elimination of the metabolic pathway may be exploited for infections associated with tissues related to the metabolic pathways. For example, many fluoroquinolone antimicrobials are partially metabolized and undergo renal elimination. Urinary concentrations of active drug are many times those achieved in the systemic circulation, making several of these agents good choices for complicated urinary tract infections.

▶ *Pharmacodynamic Properties*

Pharmacodynamics describes the relationship between drug exposure and pharmacologic effect of antibacterial activity or human toxicology. Antimicrobials are categorized based on their concentration-related effects on bacteria. Concentration-dependent pharmacodynamic activity occurs where higher drug concentrations are associated with greater rates and extents of bacterial killing. Concentration-dependent antimicrobial activity is maximized when peak antimicrobial concentrations are high. In contrast, concentration-independent (or time-dependent) activity refers to a minimal increase in the rate or extent of bacterial killing with an increase in antimicrobial dose. Concentration-independent antimicrobial activity is maximized when these antimicrobials are dosed to maintain blood and/or tissue concentrations above the MIC in a time-dependent manner. Fluoroquinolones, aminoglycosides, and metronidazole are examples of antimicrobials that exhibit concentration-dependent activity, whereas β-lactam and glycopeptide antimicrobials exhibit concentration-independent activity. Pharmacodynamic properties have been optimized to develop new dosing strategies for older antimicrobials. Examples include single-daily-dose aminoglycoside or β-lactam therapy administered by continuous or extended infusion. The product labeling for many new antimicrobials takes pharmacodynamic properties into account.

Antimicrobials also can be classified as possessing bactericidal or bacteriostatic activity in vitro. Bactericidal antibiotics generally kill at least 99.9% of a bacterial population, whereas bacteriostatic antibiotics possess antimicrobial activity but reduce bacterial load by less than 3 logs (99.9%). Clinically, bactericidal antibiotics may be necessary to achieve success in infections such as endocarditis or meningitis. A full discussion of the application of antimicrobial pharmacodynamics is beyond the scope of this chapter, but excellent sources of information are available.[18]

▶ *Adverse-Effect and Drug-Interaction Properties*

A major concern when selecting antimicrobial regimens should be the propensity for the regimen to cause adverse effects and the potential for drug interactions. In general, if several different antimicrobial options are available, antimicrobials with a low propensity to cause adverse events should be selected, particularly for patients with risk factors for a particular complication. Risk factors for adverse events may include the coadministration of other drugs that are associated with a similar type of adverse event. For example, coadministration of the known nephrotoxin gentamicin with vancomycin increases the risk for nephrotoxicity compared with administration of either drug alone.[19] Other drug interactions may predispose the patient to dose-related toxicity through inhibition of drug metabolism. For example, erythromycin has the potential to prolong cardiac QT intervals in a dose-dependent manner, potentially increasing the risk for sudden cardiac death.[20]

▶ *Antimicrobial Cost*

A final consideration in selecting antimicrobial therapy relates to cost. The least expensive antimicrobial is not necessarily the most cost-effective antimicrobial. Antimicrobial costs constitute a relatively small portion of the overall cost of care. Careful consideration of antimicrobial microbiologic, pharmacologic, and patient-related factors such as compliance and a variety of clinical outcomes is necessary to establish the cost versus benefit of an antimicrobial in a given patient. If there is no difference or a small difference in these factors, the least costly antimicrobial may be the best choice.

Patient Considerations in Antimicrobial Selection

KEY CONCEPT *Key patient-specific considerations in antimicrobial selection include recent previous antimicrobial exposures, identification of the anatomic location of infection through physical examination and diagnostic imaging, history of drug allergies, pregnancy or breast-feeding status, organ dysfunction that may affect drug clearance, immunosuppression, compliance, and the severity of illness (see Table 69–2).*

▶ *Host Factors*

Host factors can help to ensure selection of the most appropriate antimicrobial agent. Age is an important factor in antimicrobial selection. Populations with diminished renal function include neonates and the elderly. Hepatic function in the neonate is not fully developed, and drugs that are metabolized or eliminated by this route may produce adverse effects. For example, sulfonamides and ceftriaxone may compete with bilirubin for binding sites and may result in hyperbilirubinemia and kernicterus. Gastric acidity also depends on age; the elderly and children younger than 3 years tend to be achlorhydric. Drugs that need an acidic environment (eg, ketoconazole) are not well absorbed, and those whose absorption is enhanced in an alkaline environment will have increased concentrations (eg, penicillin G).

Disruption of host defenses due to IV or indwelling Foley catheters, burns, trauma, surgery, and increased gastric pH may place patients at higher risk for infection. Breaks in skin integrity provide a route for infection because the natural barrier of the skin is disrupted. Increased gastric pH can allow for bacterial overgrowth and has been associated with an increased risk of pneumonia.[21]

Recognizing the presumed site of infection and most common pathogens associated with the infectious source should guide antimicrobial choice, dose, and route of administration. For example, community-acquired pneumonia is caused most commonly by *Streptococcus pneumoniae*, *E. coli* is the primary cause of uncomplicated UTIs, and staphylococci and streptococci are implicated most frequently in skin and skin-structure infections (eg, cellulitis).

Patient Encounter 3: Empirical Selection of Antibiotics

Based on the information presented, select an empirical antimicrobial regimen for this patient. Your plan should include:

(a) A tentative infectious diagnosis or source, including likely pathogens or resistant organisms

(b) A specific antimicrobial(s) regimen, including drug(s), dose, and route of administration

(c) Description of any ancillary treatments

(d) A rationale for your empirical antimicrobial selection based on drug- and patient-specific considerations

Patients with a history of recent antimicrobial use may have altered normal flora or harbor resistant organisms. If a patient develops a new infection while on therapy, fails therapy, or has received antimicrobials recently, it is prudent to prescribe a different class of antimicrobial because resistance to the current treatment is likely. Previous hospitalization or health care utilization (eg, residing in a nursing home, hemodialysis, and outpatient antimicrobial therapy) are risk factors for the acquisition of nosocomial pathogens, which are often resistant organisms.

Antimicrobial allergies are some of the most common drug-related allergies reported and have significant potential to cause adverse events. In particular, penicillin-related allergy is common and can be problematic because there is an approximately 4% cross-reactivity with cephalosporins as well as carbapenems.[22,23] A patient's medical history should be reviewed to determine the offending β-lactam and nature of the allergic reaction. In some cases, patients with mild or nonimmunologic reactions to penicillins may receive a β-lactam antimicrobial with low cross-reactive potential (such as cephalosporins). However, patients with a history of findings consistent with IgE-mediated reactions such as anaphylaxis, urticaria, or bronchospasm should not be administered any type of β-lactam antimicrobial, including cephalosporins, unless there are no other alternatives, and even then they should be administered with caution. Administration of potentially cross-reactive agents in this situation should occur under close observation in a health care setting prepared to treat serious reactions, and some patients may need to undergo desensitization. If the specific medical history relating to a reported allergy cannot be obtained, the patient should be assumed to have had an IgE-mediated reaction and should be managed in a similar manner. Monobactams (ie, aztreonam) may be administered to patients with IgE-mediated allergic reactions to penicillin.

Renal and/or hepatic function should be considered prior to initiation of antimicrobial therapy. Most antimicrobials undergo renal elimination and dosing adjustments are frequently necessary and recommendations for adjustment are available in the literature.[24] In contrast, dosing adjustments for antimicrobials that undergo nonrenal elimination are less well documented. Failure to adjust the antimicrobial dose or interval may result in drug accumulation and adverse effects.

Concomitant administration of other medications may influence the selection of the antimicrobial, dose, and monitoring. Medications that commonly interact with antibiotics include, but are not limited to, warfarin, rifampin, phenytoin, digoxin, theophylline, multivalent cations (eg, calcium, magnesium, and zinc), and sucralfate. Drug interactions between antimicrobials and other medications may occur via the cytochrome P-450 system, protein-binding displacement, and alteration of vitamin K–producing bacteria. Interactions may result in increased concentrations of one or both agents, increasing the risk of adverse effects or additive toxicity. A key consideration in selecting antimicrobial regimens starts with obtaining a good patient medical and drug history, recognizing drug-specific adverse-event characteristics, and anticipating potential problems proactively. If it is necessary to use an antimicrobial with a relatively high frequency of adverse effects, informing patients of the risks and benefits of therapy, as well as what to do if an adverse effect occurs, may improve patient compliance and safety.

Antimicrobial agents must be used with caution in pregnant and nursing women. Some agents pose potential threats to the fetus or infant (eg, quinolones, tetracyclines, and sulfonamides). For some agents, avoidance during a specific trimester of pregnancy is warranted (eg, the first trimester with trimethoprim/sulfamethoxazole). Pharmacokinetic variables also are altered during pregnancy. Both the clearance and volume of distribution are increased during pregnancy. As a result, increased dosages and/or more frequent administration of certain drugs may be required to achieve adequate concentrations. This information can be obtained from a number of sources.[25,26]

Adherence is essential to ensure efficacy. Patients may stop taking their antibiotics once the symptoms subside and save them for a "future" infection. If the patient does not complete the course of therapy, the infection may not be eradicated, and resistance may emerge. Self-medication of saved antibiotics may be harmful, leading to overtreatment, which may further contribute to antibiotic resistance. Poor adherence may be due to adverse effects, tolerability, cost, and lack of patient education.

OUTCOME EVALUATION

Figure 69–4 provides an overview of patient- and antimicrobial agent–specific factors to consider when selecting an antimicrobial regimen. It further delineates monitoring of therapy and actions to take depending on the response to therapy. Duration of therapy depends on patient response and type of infection being treated.

After selection and initiation of an antimicrobial regimen, there are additional patient care and monitoring considerations that should be addressed to improve the likelihood of a successful outcome. KEY CONCEPT *Patient education, de-escalation of antimicrobial therapy based on culture results, monitoring for clinical response and adverse effects, and appropriate duration of therapy are important.*

Modifying Empirical Therapy Based on Cultures and Clinical Response

If a successful clinical response occurs and culture results are available, therapy should be de-escalated. Antibiotic de-escalation generally refers to the discontinuation of antibiotics that are providing a spectrum of activity greater than necessary to treat the infection, discontinuation of duplicative spectrum antibiotics, or switching to a narrower spectrum antibiotic once a patient is clinically stable. De-escalation of empirical therapy

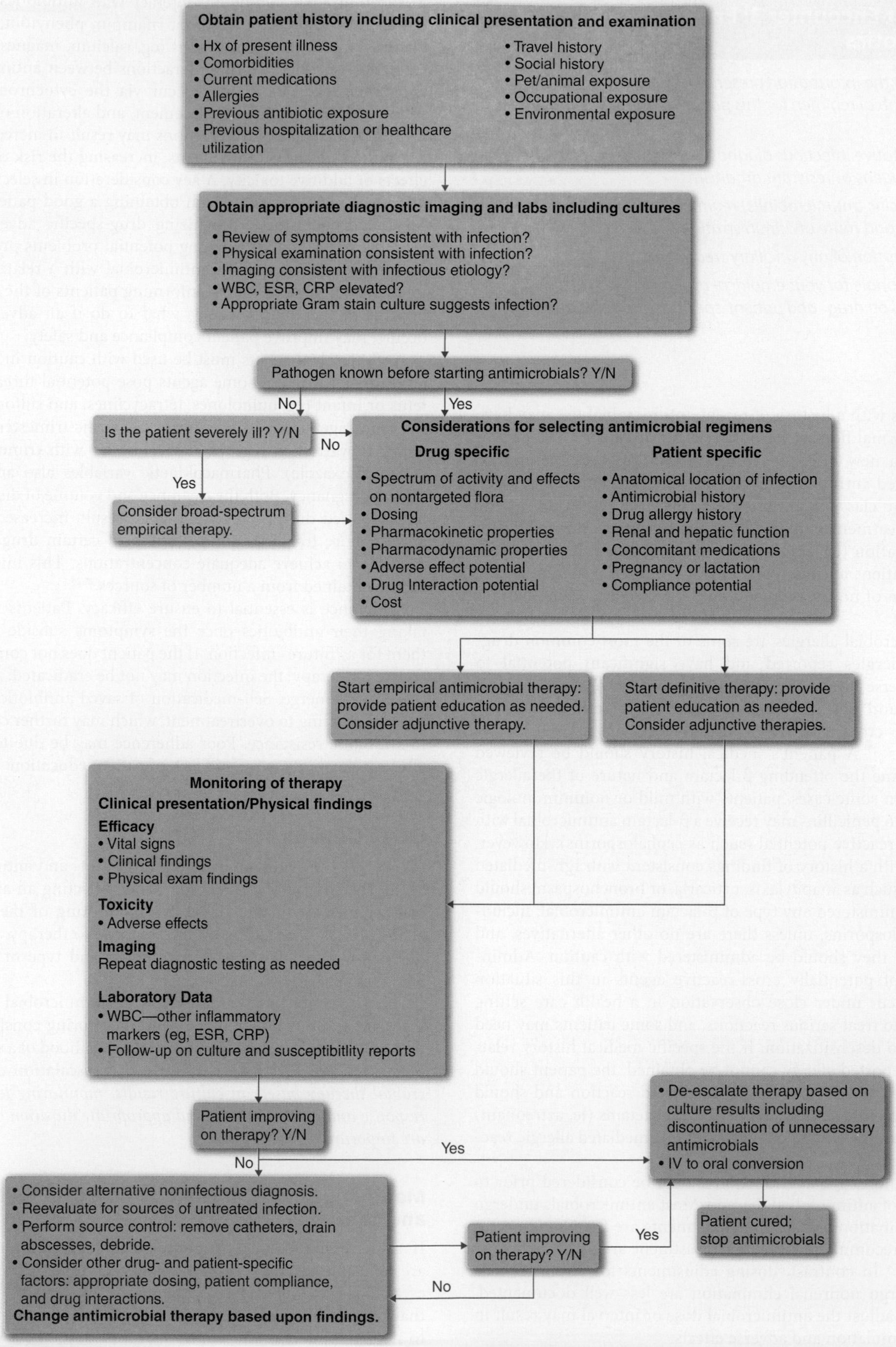

FIGURE 69–4. Approach to selection of antimicrobial therapy.

may also include discontinuing antibiotics based on clinical criteria and negative culture results, such as the absence of antibiotic-resistant pathogens.[27] The purpose of de-escalation therapy is to minimize the likelihood of secondary infections owing to antimicrobial-resistant organisms. In cases in which a specific organism is recovered that has a known preferred antimicrobial treatment of choice, therapy might be changed to that specific agent. For example, antistaphylococcal penicillins are considered to be the agents of choice for methicillin-susceptible *S. aureus* owing to their bactericidal activity and narrow-spectrum activity and may be preferable to other antibiotic regimens. In other cases, empirical coverage might be discontinued if a specific suspected pathogen is excluded by culture or an alternative, noninfectious diagnosis is established. In addition, IV antimicrobials frequently are more expensive than oral therapy. Therefore, it is usually desirable to convert therapy to oral antimicrobials with a comparable antimicrobial spectrum or specific pathogen sensitivity as soon as the patient improves clinically.[28]

Failure of Antimicrobial Therapy

While many infections respond readily to antimicrobials, some infections do not. A common question when a patient fails to improve relates to whether the antimicrobial therapy has failed. Changing antimicrobials generally is one of the easiest interventions relative to other options. However, it is important to remember that antimicrobial therapy comprises only a portion of the overall disease treatment, and there may be many factors that contribute to a lack of improvement. KEY CONCEPT *In general, inadequate diagnosis resulting in poor initial antimicrobial or other nonantibiotic drug selection, poor source control, or the development of a new infection with a resistant organism are relatively common causes of antimicrobial failure.* An infection-related diagnosis may be difficult to establish and generally has two components: (a) differentiating infection from noninfectious disease and (b) providing adequate empirical spectrum of activity if the cause is infectious. Failure of improvement in a patient's condition should warrant broadening the differential diagnosis to include noninfectious causes, as well as considering other potential infectious sources and/or pathogenic organisms. Another common cause of failure is poor source control. A diagnostic search for unknown sources of infection and removal of indwelling devices in the infected environment or surgical drainage of abscesses should be undertaken if the patient's condition is not improving. Less common causes of therapeutic failure include the development of secondary infections. In this case, the patient generally improves, but then develops a new infection caused by an antimicrobial-resistant pathogen and relapses. The emergence of resistance to a targeted pathogen while on antimicrobial therapy can be associated with clinical failure but usually is limited to tuberculosis, pseudomonads, or other gram-negative enterics. Drug- and patient-specific factors such as appropriate dosing, patient compliance, and drug interactions can be associated with therapeutic failure and also should be considered. A common assumption is that the correct diagnosis was made, but the patient was not treated long enough with antimicrobials. There are certain types of infections (eg, endocarditis or osteomyelitis) where the standard of care is to treat for prolonged periods of time (ie, weeks or months). However, the optimal duration of therapy for many infectious diseases is somewhat subjective. Studies of several infectious processes have suggested that shorter durations of therapy can result in similar clinical outcomes as longer durations of therapy, frequently with fewer complications or secondary infections.[29–31] In this period of extensive antimicrobial resistance, clinicians should keep abreast of changing recommendations emphasizing shorter durations of therapy.

Patient Encounter 4: Patient Care and Monitoring

Update: The patient was admitted to the hospital with a presumptive diagnosis of pyelonephritis, sepsis, and acute kidney injury. She received IV hydration with normal saline, 4 L oxygen, and empirical antibiotic therapy with piperacillin/tazobactam.

After 48 hours of therapy, the following parameters are obtained:

PE:

- VS: BP 130/70, P 70, RR 22, T 37.2°C (98.9°F), O_2 sat 94% (0.94) on room air

Labs:

- WBC $9.2 \times 10^3/mm^3$ ($9.2 \times 10^9/L$)
- WBC differential 85% (0.85) segs, 10% (0.10) lymphs, 5% (0.05) monos
- SCr 1.1 mg/dL (97 μmol/L)
- Glucose 126 mg/dL (7.0 mmol/L)
- Blood cultures × 2: *Escherichia coli (confirmed as an extended spectrum beta lactamase [ESBL] enzyme producer)*
- Urine culture: *Escherichia coli (confirmed as an extended spectrum beta lactamase [ESBL] enzyme producer)*

Susceptibility Report:

Cefazolin resistant (MIC greater than 16 mg/L)
Cefepime resistant (MIC greater than 16 mg/L)
Ceftriaxone resistant (MIC greater than 32 mg/L)
Piperacillin/tazo susceptible (MIC less than equal to 16 mg/L)
Meropenem susceptible (MIC less than equal to 1 mg/L)
Gentamicin susceptible (MIC less than equal to 4 mg/L)
Tobramycin resistant (MIC greater than 8 mg/L)
Nitrofurantoin susceptible (MIC less than equal to 32 mg/L)
Ciprofloxacin resistant (MIC greater than 4 mg/L)
Levofloxacin resistant (MIC greater than 4 mg/L)
Trimethoprim/sulfamethoxazole resistant (MIC greater than 2/38)

What information suggests improvement in the patient's condition?

Do any of the antimicrobial doses need to be adjusted for changes in organ function?

Should antimicrobial therapy be modified based on the culture results?

Can the antimicrobial therapy be converted from IV to oral therapy?

Patient Care Process

Patient Assessment:

- Based on patient presentation, physical examination, and review of systems, determine whether the patient is experiencing signs or symptoms that are consistent with an infection.
- Review the medical history. Does the patient have risk factors for infection? Does the patient have risk factors for resistant pathogens?
- Conduct a medication history. Has the patient received recent antimicrobial therapy?
- Review available laboratory tests. Do laboratory findings suggest infection?

Therapy Evaluation:

- Determine whether antimicrobial therapy is indicated.
- Do no harm.
- Determine whether the patient has prescription coverage or whether recommended agents are included on institution's formulary.

Care Plan Development:

- Select appropriate antimicrobial therapy based on presumed site of infection, likely pathogens, supporting laboratory data, previous antimicrobial therapy (if applicable), patient's renal/hepatic function, and other pertinent patient factors (eg, age, concomitant disease states, concomitant medications, pregnant/lactating).
- For further guidance on appropriate antimicrobial therapy selection, refer to The Infectious Diseases Society of America practice guidelines (www.idsociety.org).
- Determine whether antimicrobial therapy doses are optimal.
- Address patient concerns about antimicrobial therapy and management of the infection.
- Discuss importance of medication adherence.

Follow-Up Evaluation:

- Follow up daily (if in-patient or at appropriate intervals if outpatient) to assess efficacy and toxicity of therapy until resolution of infection.
- Review medical history, clinical and physical examination findings, laboratory tests (including culture and susceptibility data), and results of other diagnostic tests to evaluate response to therapy.
- Follow up on culture and susceptibility reports with subsequent de-escalation of therapy, if possible.
- Reculture of specimens is not performed routinely except in few cases (eg, endocarditis) or where a secondary infection is suspected because data may be misleading and lead to the addition of broader or more powerful antimicrobials.

Abbreviations Introduced in This Chapter

CDC	Centers for Disease Control and Prevention
CRP	C-reactive protein
ESR	Erythrocyte sedimentation rate
HPI	History of present illness
MIC	Minimum inhibitory concentration
MRSA	Methicillin-resistant *Staphylococcus aureus*
PMH	Past medical history
UTI	Urinary tract infection
VRE	Vancomycin-resistant *Enterococcus*
WBC	White blood cell count

REFERENCES

1. Shehab N, Patel PR, Srinivasan A, Budnitz DS. Emergency department visits for antibiotic-associated adverse events. Clin Infect Dis. 2008;47:735–743.
2. Chow AC, Benninger MS, Brook I, et al. IDSA clinical practice guideline for acute bacterial rhinosinusitis in children and adults. Clin Infect Dis. 2012;54(8):e72–e112.
3. Centers for Disease Control and Prevention. Get Smart Campaign. www.cdc.gov/getsmart.
4. Vanderweil SG, Pelletier AJ, Hamedani AG, Gonzales R, Metlay JP, Camargo CA Jr. Declining antibiotic prescriptions for upper respiratory infections, 1993–2004. Acad Emerg Med. 2007;14:366–369.
5. Magill SS, Edwards JR, Bamberg W, et al. Multistate Point-Prevalence Survey of Health Care–Associated Infections. N Engl J Med. 2014;370:1198–1208.
6. Centers for Disease Control. National and State Healthcare Associated infection progress report. Published March 2014. http://www.cdc.gov/HAI/pdfs/progress-report/hai-progress-report.pdf
7. Mackowiak PA. Temperature regulation and the pathogenesis of fever. In: Mandell GL, Bennett JE, Dolin R, eds. Principles and Practice of Infectious Diseases. 7th ed. Philadelphia, PA: Elsevier Churchill-Livingstone; 2009:Chap 50.
8. Simon L, Gauvin F, Amre DK, Saint-Louis P, Lacroix J. Serum calcitonin and C-reactive protein levels as markers of bacterial infection: A systematic review and meta-analysis. Clin Infect Dis. 2004;39:206–217.
9. Agarwal R, Schwartz DN. Procalcitonin to guide duration of antimicrobial therapy in intensive care units: A systematic review. Clin Infect Dis. 2011;53(4):379–387.
10. Infectious Diseases Society of America. Practice Guidelines from the Infectious Diseases Society of America [online]. http://www.idsociety.org/Guidelines_Patient_Care/. Accessed September 1, 2015.
11. Kollef MH, Sherman G, Ward S, Fraser VJ. Inadequate antimicrobial treatment of infections: A risk factor for hospital mortality among critically ill patients. Chest. 1999;115:462–474.
12. Antimicrobial spectra. In: Gilbert DN, Chambers HF, Eliopoulos GM, Saag MS, eds. The Sanford Guide to Antimicrobial Therapy 2014. 44th ed. Sperryville, VA: Antimicrobial Inc; 2014.
13. Bartlett JB, ed. The John Hopkins POC-IT Antibiotic Guide. [Cited 2014 Aug 28]. http://www.hopkinsguides.com/hopkins/ub/index/Johns_Hopkins_ABX_Guide/Antibiotics. Accessed August 28, 2014.
14. Cohen SH, Gerding DN, Johnson S, et al. Clinical Practice Guidelines for Clostridium difficile Infection in Adults: 2010 Update by the Society for Healthcare Epidemiology of America (SHEA) and the Infectious Diseases Society of America (IDSA). Infect Control Hosp Epidemiol. 2010;31(5):431–455.

15. Namdar R, Lauzardo M, Peloquin CA,. Tuberculosis. In: DiPiro JT, Talbert RL, Yee GC, et al., eds. Pharmacotherapy: A Pathophysiological Approach. 9th ed. New York: McGraw-Hill; 2014:1787–1806.
16. Baddour LM, Wilson WR, Bayer AS, et al. Infective endocarditis: Diagnosis, antimicrobial therapy, and management of complications: A statement for healthcare professionals from the Committee on Rheumatic Fever, Endocarditis, and Kawasaki Disease, Council on Cardiovascular Disease in the Young, and the Councils on Clinical Cardiology, Stroke, and Cardiovascular Surgery and Anesthesia, American Heart Association: Endorsed by the Infectious Diseases Society of America. Circulation. 2005;111:394–434.
17. Chamot E, Boffi E, Amari E, et al. Effectiveness of combination antimicrobial therapy for Pseudomonas aeruginosa bacteremia. Antimicrob Agents Chemother. 2003;47:2756–2764.
18. Craig WA. Pharmacodynamics of antimicrobials: General concepts and applications. In: Nightingale CH, Ambrose PG, Drusano GL, eds. Antimicrobial Pharmacodynamics in Theory and Clinical Practice. 2nd ed. New York: Informa Healthcare; 2007:1–19.
19. Rybak M, Lomaestro B, Rotschafer JC et al. Therapeutic monitoring of vancomycin in adult patients: A consensus review of the American Society of Health-System Pharmacists, the Infectious Diseases Society of America, and the Society of Infectious Diseases Pharmacists. Am J Health-Syst Pharm. 2009;66:82–98.
20. Ray WA, Murray KT, Meredith S, et al. Oral erythromycin and the risk of sudden death from cardiac causes. N Engl J Med. 2004;351:1089–1096.
21. Laheij RJ, Sturkenboom MC, Hassing R, et al. Risk of community-acquired pneumonia and use of gastric acid-suppressing drugs. JAMA. 2004;292:1955–1960.
22. Gruchalla RS, Pirmohamed M. Clinical practice. Antibiotic allergy. N Engl J Med. 2006;354:601–609.
23. Weiss ME, Adkinson NF. β-lactam allergy. In: Mandell GL, Bennett JE, Dolin R, eds. Principles and Practice of Infectious Diseases. 7th ed. Philadelphia, PA: Churchill Livingstone; 2009;347–354.
24. Mohammad RA, Matzke GR. Drug therapy individualization for patients with chronic kidney disease. In: DiPiro JT, Talbert RL, Yee GC, et al., eds. Pharmacotherapy: A Pathophysiological Approach. 9th ed. New York: McGraw-Hill; 2014:729–744.
25. Briggs GG, Freeman RK, Yaffe SJ. Drugs in Pregnancy and Lactation. 9th ed. Philadelphia, PA: Lippincott Williams & Wilkins; 2011. 5 ed. Amarillo, TX: Hale Publishing; 2012.
27. Dellit TH, Owens RC, McGowan JE, et al. Infectious Diseases Society of America and the Society for Healthcare Epidemiology of America Guidelines for Developing an Institutional Program to Enhance Antimicrobial Stewardship. Clin Infect Dis. 2007;44(2):159–177.
28. Athanassa Z, Makris G, Dimopoulos G, Falagas ME. Early switch to oral treatment in patients with moderate to severe community-acquired pneumonia: A meta-analysis. Drugs. 2008;68:2469–2481.
29. Mandell LA, Wunderink RG, Anzueo A, et al. Infectious Diseases Society of American/American Thoracic Society consensus guideline on the management of community-acquired pneumonia in adults. Clin Infect Dis. 2007;44(Suppl 2): S27–S72.
30. American Thoracic Society, Infectious Diseases Society of America. Guidelines for the management of adults with hospital-acquired, ventilator-associated, and healthcare-associated pneumonia. Am J Respir Crit Care Med. 2005;171: 388–416.
31. Kollef MH, Napolitano LM, Solomkin JS, et al. Healthcare-associated infection (HAI): A critical appraisal of the emerging threat-proceedings of the HAI Summit. Clin Infect Dis. 2008;2(Suppl 47):S55–S99.

70 Central Nervous System Infections

P. Brandon Bookstaver and April Miller Quidley

LEARNING OBJECTIVES

Upon completion of the chapter, the reader will be able to:

1. Discuss the pathophysiology of CNS infections and the impact on antimicrobial treatment regimens (including antimicrobial dosing and CNS penetration).
2. Describe the signs, symptoms, and clinical presentation of CNS infections.
3. List the most common pathogens causing CNS infections and identify risk factors for infection with each pathogen.
4. State the goals of therapy for CNS infections.
5. Design appropriate empirical antimicrobial regimens for patients suspected of having CNS infections caused by each of the following pathogens (taking age, vaccine history, and other patient-specific information into account), and analyze the impact of antimicrobial resistance on both empirical and definitive therapy: *Neisseria meningitidis* meningitis, *Haemophilus influenzae* meningitis, *Listeria monocytogenes* meningitis, group B *Streptococcus* meningitis, gram-negative bacillary meningitis, postneurosurgical infection, CNS shunt infection, herpes simplex encephalitis.
6. Modify empirical antimicrobial regimens based on laboratory data and other diagnostic criteria.
7. Discuss the management of close contacts of patients diagnosed with CNS infections.
8. Identify candidates for vaccines and other prophylactic therapies to prevent CNS infections.
9. Describe the role of adjunctive agents (eg, dexamethasone) in the management of CNS infections.
10. Formulate a monitoring plan to assess efficacy and adverse effects of therapy for CNS infections.

INTRODUCTION

The term *CNS infections* describes a variety of infections involving the brain and spinal cord and associated tissues, fluids, and membranes, including meningitis, encephalitis, brain abscess, cerebrospinal fluid shunt infections, and postoperative infections. KEY CONCEPT *CNS infections, such as meningitis, are considered neurologic emergencies that require prompt recognition, diagnosis, and management to prevent death and residual neurologic deficits.* Improperly treated, CNS infections are associated with high rates of morbidity and mortality. Despite advances in care, the overall mortality of bacterial meningitis in the United States remains at approximately 15%, and at least 10% to 30% of survivors are afflicted with neurologic impairment, including hearing loss, **hemiparesis**, and learning disabilities.[1–3] Antimicrobial therapy and preventive vaccines have revolutionized management and improved outcomes of bacterial meningitis and other CNS infections dramatically.

EPIDEMIOLOGY AND ETIOLOGY

CNS infections are uncommon, with an incidence 1.38 cases per 100,000 in 2006 and 2007.[3] However, the severity of these infections demands prompt medical intervention and treatment. CNS infections can be caused by bacteria, fungi, mycobacteria, viruses, parasites, and spirochetes.

Bacterial meningitis is the most common cause of CNS infections. While vaccination has reduced the incidence of disease by many common pathogens as of 2010, *Streptococcus pneumoniae* (pneumococcus) was the most common pathogen for bacterial meningitis (0.306 cases per 100,000), followed by *Neisseria meningitidis* (meningococcus, 0.123 cases per 100,000).[4] *Haemophilus influenza was a top causative pathogen; however, its incidence has declined to 0.058 cases per 100,000*). Staphylococcal species and gram-negative bacteria account for 0.114 and 0.127 cases per 100,000 persons, respectively in the United States.[4] Group B *Streptococcus and Listeria monocytogenes* remain important causes, but current data on their incidence are lacking.[3] Vaccines directed against bacteria causing meningitis and related infections (eg, pneumonia and ear infections) have reduced the risk of infections due to *S. pneumoniae*, *N. meningitidis*, and *H. influenzae* type b (Hib) dramatically.[3,4] Prior to the availability of Hib conjugate vaccines, Hib meningitis or other invasive disease was documented in one in 200 children by the age of 5 years and due to widespread use, its incidence has decreased such that it is no longer a leading pathogen.[4] Historically, a 7-valent conjugate pneumococcal vaccine (PCV7) was administered, but despite use of the PCV7, *S. pneumoniae* remained the most common pathogen for pediatric bacterial meningitis. In 2010, a 13-valent conjugate pneumococcal vaccine was licensed for use in the United States; however, its impact on the epidemiology of disease in the United States is still unknown. In France the 13-valent vaccine reduced the incidence of pneumococcal meningitis by 27.4%.[5]

Encephalitis may result from viral, bacterial, parasitic, or other noninfectious causes. Herpes simplex virus (HSV) is the most common cause of encephalitis in the United States, accounting for 10% of all cases.[10] The annual incidence of viral encephalitis is 3.5 to 7.4 infections per 100,000 persons.[6] Other pathogens including common bacterial meningitis causes, *Ricksettsia* species, enteroviruses, arboviruses, varicella-zoster virus, rotavirus, coronavirus, influenza viruses A and B, West Nile virus, and Epstein-Barr virus may be associated with a meningoencephalopathic presentation.[7] Approximately 20,000 hospitalizations each year are secondary to encephalitis, accounting for $650 million in health care costs.[8] Over the past 10 to 20 years, mortality secondary to encephalitis has remained constant, correlating well with the increased number of people living with human immunodeficiency virus (HIV) and acquired immune deficiency syndrome (AIDS).

Neurosurgical procedures may place patients at risk for meningitis due to bacteria acquired at the time of surgery or in the postoperative period, including *Staphylococcus aureus*, coagulase-negative staphylococci, and gram-negative bacilli. In addition to bacteria, other pathogens may cause meningitis in at-risk patients. Immunocompromised patients, such as solid-organ transplant patients and patients living with HIV infection, are at risk for fungal meningitis with *Cryptococcus neoformans* and encephalitis secondary to *Toxoplasma gondii* and JC virus. Tuberculosis can spread from pulmonary sites to cause clinical disease in the CNS. Life-threatening viral encephalitis and meningitis can occur in otherwise healthy, young individuals, as well as in patients immunocompromised by age or other factors. Risk factors for CNS infections can be classified as follows:

- *Environmental*: Recent exposures (eg, close contact with meningitis or respiratory tract infection, contaminated foods), active or passive exposure to cigarette smoke, close living conditions
- *Recent infection in the patient:* Respiratory infection, otitis media, sinusitis, mastoiditis
- *Immunosuppression:* Anatomic or functional asplenia, sickle cell disease, alcoholism, cirrhosis, immunoglobulin or complement deficiency, cancer, HIV/AIDS, uncontrolled diabetes mellitus, debilitated state of health
- *Surgery, trauma:* Neurosurgery, head trauma, CSF shunt, cochlear implant
- Noninfectious causes of meningitis include malignancy, medications (eg, sulfonamides, nonsteroidal anti-inflammatory drugs [NSAIDs], IV immunoglobulin), autoimmune disease (eg, lupus), and trauma.[6,7]
- The most common pathogens causing bacterial meningitis, by age group and other risk factors, are found in Table 70–1.

Table 70–1

Most Likely Pathogens and Recommended Empirical Therapy, by Risk Factor, for Bacterial Meningitis[15,25]

Predisposing Factor	Most Likely Pathogens	Recommended Empirical Antibiotic Therapy
Age		
Less than 3 months	Group B *Streptococcus* *Escherichia coli* *Klebsiella pneumoniae* *Listeria monocytogenes*	Ampicillin *plus* cefotaxime *or* aminoglycoside
3 months to less than 18 years	*Streptococcus pneumoniae* *Neisseria meningitidis*	Cefotaxime *or* ceftriaxone *plus* vancomycin
18 years to less than 60 years	*S. pneumoniae* *N. meningitidis*	Cefotaxime *or* ceftriaxone *plus* vancomycin
60 years *or* older	*S. pneumoniae* Gram-negative bacilli *L. monocytogenes*	Cefotaxime *or* ceftriaxone *plus* vancomycin *plus* ampicillin
Immunocompromised	*S. pneumoniae* *N. meningitidis* *L. monocytogenes* Gram-negative bacilli (including *Pseudomonas aeruginosa*)	Cefotaxime *or* ceftriaxone *plus* vancomycin *plus* ampicillin (consider double antibiotic coverage against *Pseudomonas* spp. if suspected)
Surgery, Trauma		
Postneurosurgical infection	*S. aureus* (including MRSA) Coagulase-negative *Staphylococcus* (including MRSE) Gram-negative bacilli (including *P. aeruginosa*)	Vancomycin *or* linezolid *plus* cefepime or ceftazidime *or* meropenem (consider empiric use of two active antibiotics against *Pseudomonas* spp. if suspected)
Penetrating head trauma	*S. aureus* (including MRSA) coagulase-negative *Staphylococcus* Gram-negative bacilli (including *P. aeruginosa*)	Vancomycin *or* linezolid *plus* cefepime or ceftazidime *or* meropenem (consider empiric use of two active antibiotics against *Pseudomonas* spp. if suspected)
CSF shunt	Coagulase-negative *Staphylococcus (including MRSE)* *S. aureus (including MRSA)* Gram negative bacilli *(including P. aeruginosa)*	Vancomycin *or* linezolid *plus* cefepime or ceftazidime or meropenem (consider empiric use of two active antibiotics against *Pseudomonas* spp. if suspected)

MRSA, methicillin-resistant *Staphylococcus aureus*; MRSE, methicillin-resistant *Staphylococcus epidermidis*.

Patient Encounter 1, Part 1

NB is a 57-year-old woman resident of an elderly singles living facility. She maintains her activities of daily living on her own. NB participates in group activities with coresidents on a weekly basis, with the most recent being a knitting party a week ago. She now presents to the emergency department with a 2-day history of headache, fever, and photophobia. Physical findings and laboratory values include temperature of 38.3°C (101°F) and WBC of $13.4 \times 10^3/mm^3$ ($13.4 \times 10^9/L$), with 70% (0.70) polymorphonuclear cells. Examination reveals nuchal rigidity; remainder is benign for additional findings. NB also reports occasional nausea. She has a significant history for osteoporosis for which she takes alendronate and calcium with vitamin D. She receives the influenza vaccine yearly.

What signs and symptoms consistent with meningitis are present in NB?

What causative pathogens should be suspected in NB?

What empiric antimicrobials should be started?

PATHOPHYSIOLOGY

Meningitis is an inflammation of the membranes of the brain and spinal cord (**meninges**) and the CSF in contact with these membranes, whereas encephalitis is an inflammation of the brain tissue. CSF produced in the brain ventricles flows through the subarachnoid space and downward through the spinal cord, insulating and protecting delicate CNS tissue.

To initiate a CNS infection, pathogens must gain entry into the CNS by **contiguous** spread, **hematogenous** seeding, direct inoculation, or reactivation of latent infection. Contiguous spread occurs when infections in adjacent structures (eg, sinus cavities or the middle ear) invade directly through the blood–brain barrier. Hematogenous seeding occurs when a remote infection causes bacteremia that seeds the CSF, such as pneumococcal pneumonia. Reactivation of latent infection results from dormant viral, fungal, or mycobacterial pathogens in the spine, brain, or nerve tracts. Direct inoculation of bacteria into the CNS is the result of trauma, congenital malformations, or complications of neurosurgery.

Once through the blood–brain barrier, pathogens replicate due to limited host defenses in the CNS. Figure 70–1 depicts the pathophysiologic changes associated with meningitis. Neurologic tissue damage is the result of the host's immune reaction to bacterial cellular components, which trigger **cytokine** production, particularly tumor necrosis factor alpha (TNF-α) and interleukin 1 (IL-1), and other inflammatory mediators.[9] Bacteriolysis resulting from antibiotic therapy further contributes to the inflammatory process. Cytokines increase permeability of the blood–brain barrier, allowing influx of neutrophils and other host defense cells that contribute to the development of cerebral edema and increased intracranial pressure characteristic of meningitis.[10] The increase in intracranial pressure is responsible for the hallmark clinical signs and symptoms of meningitis: headache, neck stiffness, altered mental status, photophobia, and seizures. Untreated, these pathophysiologic changes may result in cerebral ischemia and death.

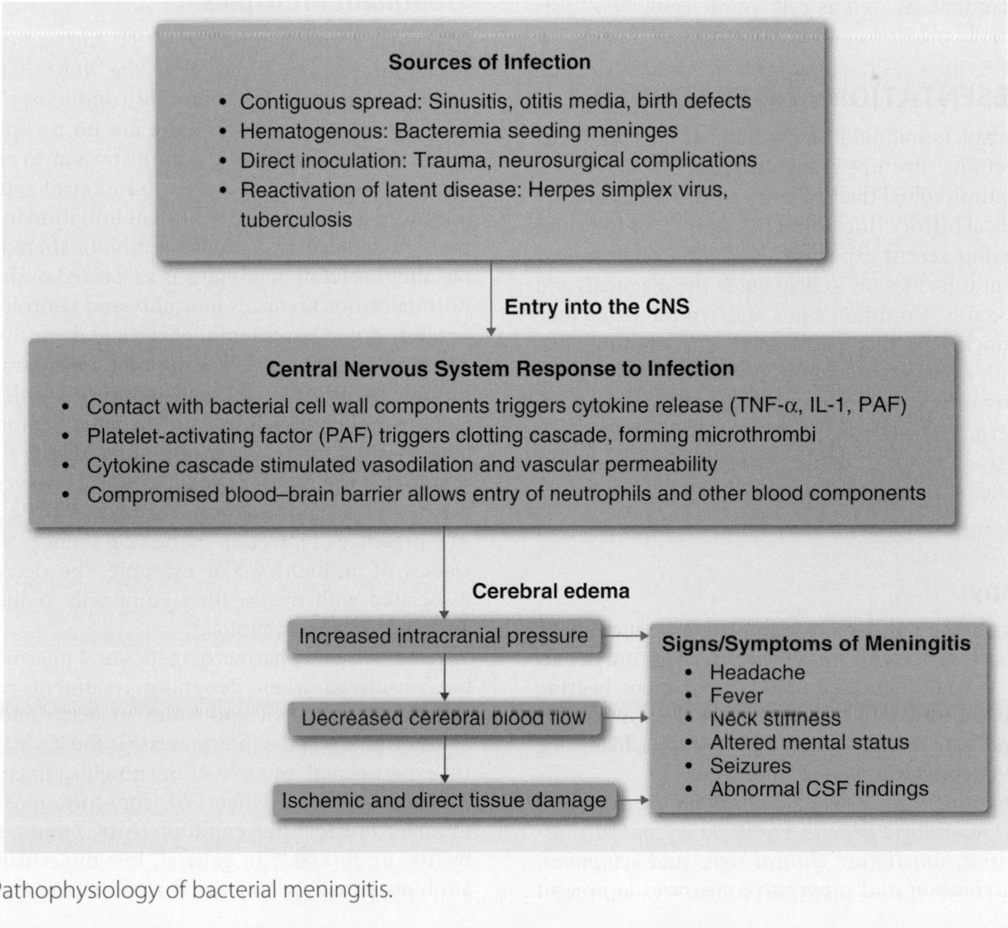

FIGURE 70–1. Pathophysiology of bacterial meningitis.

Table 70–2

CNS Response to Infection (CSF Findings)

	Normal CSF	Bacterial Infection	Viral Infection	Fungal Infection	Tuberculosis
WBC (× 10^3/mm^3 *or* × 10^9/L)	< 0.005	1.0–greater than 5.0	0.1–1	0.1–0.4	50–500
WBC differential (% or fraction in brackets, predominant cell type)	> 85% (0.85) monocytes	At least 80% (0.80) PMNs	50% (0.50) lymphocytes (PMN early)	> 50% (0.50) lymphocytes	> 80% (0.80) lymphocytes (PMNs early)
Protein (mg/dL, mg/L)	20–45 (200–450)	> 100 (> 1000)	50–100 (500–1000)	100–200 (1000–2000)	40–150 (400–1500)
Glucose (mg/dL, mmol/L)	45–80 (2.5–4.4)	5–40 (0.3–2.2)	30–70 (1. 7–3. 9)	< 30–70 (< 1. 7–3. 9)	< 30–70 (< 1. 7–3. 9)
CSF: serum glucose ratio	At least 0.6 serum glucose	< 0.4 serum glucose	At least 0.6 serum glucose	< 0.4 serum glucose	< 0.4 serum glucose
CSF stain	Negative	Positive Gram stain (60%–90%)	Negative	Positive India ink stain (Cryptococcus)	Positive acid-fast bacilli stain
Opening pressure	< 20 mm Hg	> 20 mm Hg	< 20 mm Hg	> 20 mm Hg	> 20 mm Hg

CSF, cerebrospinal fluid; PMNs, polymorphonuclear neutrophils.

Data from Refs. 5, 11, 20, and 33.

The CNS response to infection is cellular and chemical changes in the CSF. KEY CONCEPT *Ideally, LP to obtain CSF for direct examination and laboratory analysis, as well as blood cultures and other relevant cultures, should be obtained before initiation of antimicrobial therapy. However, initiation of antimicrobial therapy should not be delayed if a pretreatment LP cannot be performed.*

Normal CSF has a characteristic composition in terms of protein and glucose content, as well as cell count. Table 70–2 lists CSF findings normally observed and in the setting of meningitis.

CLINICAL PRESENTATION AND DIAGNOSIS

A high index of suspicion should be maintained for patients at risk for CNS infections. Prompt recognition and diagnosis are essential so that antimicrobial therapy can be initiated as quickly as possible. A medical history (including risk factors for infection and history of possible recent exposures) and physical examination yield important information to help guide the diagnosis and treatment of meningitis. Common signs and symptoms include fever, headache, nuchal rigidity (stiff neck), and photophobia. Infants present with nonspecific signs and symptoms, including excessive irritability or crying, vomiting or diarrhea, tachypnea, altered sleep pattern, and poor eating. Depending on involved pathogens and disease severity, patients may also present with altered mental status, stupor, and seizures.

TREATMENT

Goals of Therapy

Prior to antibiotic therapy and vaccination bacterial meningitis was almost universally fatal, with survivors suffering from debilitating residual neurologic deficits, such as permanent hearing loss.[1,2] Although significant improvements have been made, the fatality rate of meningitis remains above 15% in adults, likely due to its occurrence in debilitated patient populations.[2]

KEY CONCEPT *The treatment goals for CNS infections are to prevent death and residual neurologic deficits, eradicate or control causative micro-organisms, ameliorate clinical signs and symptoms, and implement vaccination and suppressive measures to prevent future infections.* Surgical debridement should be employed, if appropriate (as in postneurosurgical infections and brain abscess). Supportive care, consisting of hydration, electrolyte replacement, antipyretics, antiemetics, analgesics, antiepileptic drugs, and wound care (for surgical wounds), is an important adjunct to antimicrobial therapy, particularly early in the treatment course.

Treatment Principles

KEY CONCEPT *Prompt initiation of IV high-dose bactericidal antimicrobial therapy directed at the most likely pathogen(s) is essential due to the high morbidity and mortality associated with CNS infections.* Although there are no prospective studies that relate timing of antibiotic administration to clinical outcome in bacterial meningitis, a longer duration of symptoms and more advanced disease before treatment initiation increase the risk of a poor outcome.[2,11] Initiation of antibiotic therapy as soon as possible after bacterial meningitis is suspected or proven (even before hospitalization) reduces mortality and neurologic sequelae.[11–13]

High-dose parenteral bactericidal antibiotic therapy is required to achieve CSF antibiotic concentrations adequate to rapidly sterilize the CSF and reduce the risk of complications. Data from animal studies and patients demonstrate better outcomes when bactericidal antibiotic therapy (vs bacteriostatic therapy) is used to sterilize the CSF.[14] However, successful treatment of meningitis has been reported with bacteriostatic agents. The presence of infection in the CSF reduces the activity of some classes of antibiotics. For example, the decreased pH of CSF associated with meningitis significantly reduces the activity of aminoglycoside antibiotics.[15]

Antimicrobial pharmacokinetics and pharmacodynamics must be considered when designing treatment regimens for CNS infections. Ability of antibiotics to reach and achieve effective concentrations at the infection site is the key to treatment success. In experimental models of meningitis, maximum bactericidal activity is achieved when CSF concentrations exceed the minimum bactericidal concentration (MBC) of the infecting pathogen by 10- to 30-fold.[16] In general, low-molecular-weight lipophilic antibiotics that are unionized at physiologic pH and not highly

Clinical Presentation and Diagnosis of CNS Infections

General

- Evaluate patient risk factors and recent exposures
- Evaluate other possible causes: space-occupying lesion (which may *or* may not be malignant), drug-induced CNS pathology autoimmune disease, and trauma[12,13]

Signs and Symptoms[2]

- 95% of patients with bacterial meningitis have two of the following: headache, fever, neck stiffness, and altered mental status
- Headache (87%)
- Nuchal rigidity (stiff neck) (83%)
- Fever (77%)
- Nausea (74%)
- Altered mental status (ie, confusion, lethargy, and obtundation) (69%)
- Focal neurologic defects (including positive Brudzinski sign and Kernig sign) (33%)
- Seizures
- Malaise, restlessness
- Photophobia
- Skin lesions (diffuse petechial rash observed in 50% of patients with meningococcal meningitis)
- Signs and symptoms in neonates, infants, and young children: nonspecific findings, such as altered feeding and sleep patterns, vomiting, irritability, lethargy, bulging fontanel, seizures, respiratory distress, and petechial/purpuric rash[17]
- Predictors of an unfavorable outcome: seizures, focal neurologic findings, altered mental status, papilledema, hypotension, septic shock, and pneumococcal meningitis[4]

Laboratory Tests[5,18,44]

- CSF examination via lumbar puncture (LP, spinal tap); contraindicated in patients with cardiorespiratory compromise, increased intracranial pressure and papilledema, focal neurologic signs, seizures, bleeding disorders, abnormal level of consciousness, and possible brain herniation (a CT scan should be performed before LP if there is a question of a CNS mass to avoid potential for brain herniation) (see Table 70–2 for specific CSF findings)
- Elevated opening pressure (may be decreased in neonates, infants, and children)
- Cloudy CSF
- Decreased glucose
- Elevated protein
- Elevated WBC (differential provides clues to offending pathogen)
- Gram stain (adequate for diagnosis in 60%–90% of patients with bacterial meningitis)
- Culture and sensitivity (positive in 70%–85% without prior antibiotic therapy, positive in less than 20% who have had prior therapy)
- If CSF Gram stain and/or culture is negative, rapid diagnostic tests (such as latex agglutination) may be useful; these tests are positive even if bacteria are dead
- Polymerase chain reaction (PCR; DNA amplification of the most common bacterial meningitis pathogens) may be useful to help exclude bacterial meningitis
- Elevated CSF lactate and C-reactive protein
- Blood cultures (at least two cultures, one "set"; positive in 66%)
- Scraping of skin lesions (eg, rash) for direct microscopic examination and culture
- Other cultures should be obtained as clinically indicated (eg, sputum)
- WBC with differential
- Fungal meningitis: CSF culture, CSF and serum cryptococcal antigen titers, microscopic examination of CSF specimens
- Tuberculous meningitis: CSF culture, PCR evaluation (preferred), and acid-fast stain

Patient Encounter 1, Part 2

The 67-year-old patient with signs and symptoms of meningitis underwent lumbar puncture. Initial results from CSF studies are WBC $1.8 \times 10^3/mm^3$ ($1.8 \times 10^9/L$) with 82% (0.82) PMNs and 41% (0.41) monocytes, protein 176 mg/dL (1,760 mg/L), glucose 18 mg/dL (1.0 mmol/L). Gram stain shows gram-negative diplococci. Vital signs remain stable in the ED. First doses of antimicrobial therapy are initiated in the ED, and NB is admitted to a medicine ward for continued treatment and confirmation of final diagnosis. Culture results confirm *Neisseria meningitidis* infection. Antimicrobials are streamlined and continued for the full duration.

What clues in the CSF results are suggestive of bacterial meningitis?

Would adjunctive steroids offer additional benefit in this patient?

How can her antibiotic regimen be streamlined at this time?

Patient Encounter 1, Part 3

NB has clinically improved on hospital day 3 and would like to be discharged home to continue therapy, but would prefer oral therapy if available. As her friends at the home learn of her illness, they are concerned about the possibility of getting sick and begin to follow up with the on-call physician at the group home. They wonder about medications and vaccinations to prevent the disease.

How long should therapy be continued in NB?

What oral options are viable options for continuation as an outpatient in this case?

Who should receive antimicrobial prophylaxis for Neisseria?

protein bound penetrate best into CSF and other body tissues and fluids.[15,17] In addition to drug characteristics, integrity of the blood–brain barrier determines antibiotic penetration into CSF. The CSF penetration of most, but not all, antibiotics is enhanced by the presence of infection and inflammation. Sulfonamides, trimethoprim, chloramphenicol, rifampin, and most antitubercular drugs achieve therapeutic CSF levels even without meningeal inflammation.[7] Most β-lactams and related antibiotics (ie, carbapenems and monobactams), vancomycin, quinolones, acyclovir, linezolid, daptomycin, and colistin achieve therapeutic CSF levels in the presence of meningeal inflammation.[7] Aminoglycosides, first-generation cephalosporins, second-generation cephalosporins (except cefuroxime), clindamycin, and amphotericin do not achieve therapeutic CSF levels, even with inflammation, but clindamycin does achieve therapeutic brain tissue levels.[7]

An adequate duration of therapy is required to treat meningitis successfully (Table 70–3). KEY CONCEPT *Parenteral (IV) therapy is administered for the full course of therapy for CNS infections to ensure adequate CSF penetration throughout the course of treatment.* Antibiotic treatment (and dexamethasone, if used as a treatment adjunct) reduces the inflammation associated with meningitis, which, in turn, reduces the penetration of some antibiotics into the CSF, and parenteral therapy must be used throughout the entire treatment course to ensure adequate concentrations. Carefully selected patients who have close medical monitoring and follow-up may be able to receive a portion of their parenteral meningitis treatment on an outpatient basis.[11,18] A management algorithm for adults with suspected bacterial meningitis, as recommended by the Infectious Diseases Society of America (IDSA), is summarized in Figure 70–2.

Empirical Antimicrobial Therapy

After diagnosis, prompt and aggressive antimicrobial therapy with an appropriate empirical treatment is of the utmost importance in patients with suspected CNS infections. In most patients, a diagnostic LP will be performed before beginning antibiotics, but this never should delay initiation of antimicrobials. Antibiotic pretreatment may alter the CSF profile and complicate interpretation. KEY CONCEPT *Empirical therapy should be directed at the most likely pathogen(s) for a specific patient, taking into account age, risk factors for infection (including underlying disease and immune dysfunction, vaccine history, and recent exposures), CSF Gram stain results, CSF antibiotic penetration, and local antimicrobial resistance patterns.* Results of the CSF Gram stain may be used to help narrow empirical therapy for bacterial meningitis. In the absence of a positive Gram stain, empirical therapy should be continued for at least 48 to 72 hours, when meningitis may, in most cases, be ruled out by CSF findings inconsistent with bacterial meningitis, negative CSF culture, and negative polymerase chain reaction (PCR) evaluations. A repeat LP may be useful in the absence of other findings. Table 70–1 outlines recommendations for empirical antibiotic therapy for bacterial meningitis by most likely pathogen(s) and patient risk factors.

Impact of Antimicrobial Resistance on Treatment Regimens for Meningitis

Development of resistance to β-lactam antibiotics, including penicillins and cephalosporins, has significantly impacted the management of bacterial meningitis with one-fifth of CSF isolates resistant to penicillin and 3.5% of isolates resistant to cephalosporins.[19] The Clinical and Laboratory Standards Institute (CLSI) has set a lower ceftriaxone susceptibility breakpoint for pneumococcal CSF isolates (1 mg/L) than for isolates from non-CNS sites (2 mg/L). Empirical treatment regimens now include the combination of a third-generation cephalosporin plus vancomycin. Recognition of relative and high-level resistance to *N. meningitidis* in the laboratory, as well as in clinical treatment failures, has led to greater use of third-generation cephalosporins for empirical therapy of meningococcal meningitis.[3,11] Treatment of suspected or proven β-lactamase-mediated Hib meningitis also requires a third-generation cephalosporin. Increasing rates of methicillin-resistant *S. aureus* (about one-third of staphylococcal CSF isolates) and coagulase-negative staphylococci require the use of vancomycin for empirical therapy when these pathogens are suspected.[11,18]

The emergence and continued rise of multidrug-resistant strains of gram-negative organisms such as *Pseudomonas aeruginosa*, *Acinetobacter* species, AmpC, and extended-spectrum β-lactamase (ESBL) producing strains of Enterobacteriaceae have become a recognized threat nationally, and broad-spectrum therapy taking into account local resistance patterns should be used.

Pathogen-Directed Antimicrobial Therapy

KEY CONCEPT *Empirical antimicrobial therapy should be modified on the basis of laboratory data and clinical response.* If cultures, CSF Gram stain, or antigen/antibody testing indicate a specific pathogen, therapy should be adjusted quickly as needed to ensure adequate coverage for the offending pathogen(s). Table 70–3 outlines recommended definitive pathogen-directed treatment regimens, recommended treatment duration, and key adverse effects that should be monitored during antibiotic therapy for meningitis. Table 70–4 provides pediatric doses of selected agents used in bacterial meningitis treatment.

► *Neisseria Meningitidis Meningitis*

N. meningitidis CNS infections most commonly occur in children and young adults. From 11% to 19% of survivors of meningococcal meningitis experience long-term sequelae, including hearing loss, limb loss, and neurologic deficits.[20] Nearly all meningococcal disease is caused by five serogroups: A, B, C, Y, and W-135. In the United States, serotypes B, C, and Y each are responsible for approximately 30% of cases.[3,4]

Meningococcal meningitis is observed most commonly in individuals living in close quarters (eg, college students, military personnel). Infants younger than 1 year are at highest risk, possibly because pneumococcal vaccination reduces bactericidal antibodies.[21] However, nearly 60% of cases occur in patients over 11 years of age.[20,22] *N. meningitidis* colonizes the nasopharynx and usually is transmitted via inhaled respiratory droplets from patients or asymptomatic carriers. A subclinical bacteremia typically ensues, seeding the meninges. Meningococcal disease is often (approximately 50%) associated with a diffuse petechial rash, and patients may experience behavioral changes. Patients may develop fulminant meningococcal sepsis, characterized by shock, disseminated intravascular coagulation, and multiorgan failure.[23] Meningococcal sepsis has a poor prognosis and carries a mortality rate of up to 80%, whereas the mortality rate with meningococcal meningitis alone is 13%.[23,24] Patients with suspected meningococcal infection should be kept on respiratory isolation for the first 24 hours of treatment.[20]

Increasing penicillin resistance requires that third-generation cephalosporins now be used for empirical treatment until in vitro susceptibilities are known.[11,15] Patients with a history of type I penicillin allergy or cephalosporin allergy may be treated with vancomycin. Treatment should be continued for 7 days, after which no further treatment is necessary.

Table 70–3

Pathogen-Based Definitive Treatment for CNS Infections[14,55]

Pathogen	Recommended and Alternative Antimicrobial Therapy (Adult Doses)	Adverse Effects/Safety Monitoring	Renal and Hepatic Dose Adjustment	Duration (Days)
Neisseria meningitidis[a]	*Standard Therapy*			
Penicillin MIC 0.1 mg/L	Penicillin G 4 million units IV every 4 hours or	Hypersensitivity (rash, anaphylaxis), diarrhea	*Renal*: CrCl < 50 mL/min (0.83 mL/s): 3 million units IV every 4 hours; CrCl < 10 mL/min (0.17 mL/s): 2 million units IV every 4 hours *Hepatic*: No dose adjustment	7
	Ampicillin 2 g IV every 4 hours	Hypersensitivity (rash, anaphylaxis), diarrhea	*Renal*: CrCl < 50 mL/min (0.83 mL/s): 2 g IV every 8 hours; CrCl < 30 mL/min (0.50 mL/s): 2 g IV every 12 hours; CrCl < 10 mL/min (0.17 mL/s): 2 g IV every 24 hours *Hepatic*: No dose adjustment	
	Alternative Therapies Ceftriaxone 2 g IV every 12 hours or	LFT elevation, cholecystitis	*Renal*: No dose adjustment *Hepatic*: Caution in severe hepatic impairment	
	Cefotaxime 2 g IV every 4 hours	Pseudocholelithiasis	*Renal*: CrCl < 80 mL/min (1.34 mL/s): 2 g IV every 6–8 hours; CrCl < 50 mL/min (0.83 mL/s): 2 g IV every 8–12 hours; CrCl < 30 mL/min (0.50 mL/s): 2 g IV every 12 hours; CrCl < 10 mL/min (0.17 mL/s): 2 g IV every 24 hours *Hepatic:* No dose adjustment	
Penicillin MIC 0.1–1 mg/L	*Standard Therapy* Ceftriaxone *or* cefotaxime *Alternative Therapies*			
	Moxifloxacin 400 mg IV every 24 hours *or*	Nausea/vomiting/diarrhea, dizziness, headache, QT prolongation	*Renal*: No dose adjustment *Hepatic*: Caution in severe hepatic impairment	
	Meropenem 2 g IV every 8 hours *or*	Rash, hypersensitivity, diarrhea, decreased seizure threshold	*Renal*: CrCl < 50 mL/min (0.83 mL/s): 2 g IV every 12 hours; CrCl < 30 mL/min (0.50 mL/s): 500 mg to 1 g IV every 12 hours; CrCl < 10 mL/min (0.17 mL/s): 500 mg to 1 g IV every 24 hours *Hepatic*: No dose adjustment	
	Chloramphenicol 1–1.5 g IV every 6 hours	Rash, diarrhea, seizures, anemia, gray baby syndrome, hypersensitivity, neurotoxicity (last choice due to toxicities)	*Renal*: No dose adjustment *Hepatic*: Reduce dose in moderate to severe impairment; consider serum drug monitoring	
Streptococcus pneumoniae				
Penicillin MIC 0.1 mg/L	*Standard Therapy* Penicillin G *or* ampicillin *Alternative Therapies* Ceftriaxone *or* cefotaxime *or* chloramphenicol			10–14
Penicillin MIC 0.1–1 mg/L (ceftriaxone/cefotaxime-sensitive strains)	*Standard Therapy* Ceftriaxone *or* cefotaxime			

(*Continued*)

Table 70–3

Pathogen-Based Definitive Treatment for CNS Infections[14,55] (Continued)

Pathogen	Recommended and Alternative Antimicrobial Therapy (Adult Doses)	Adverse Effects/Safety Monitoring	Renal and Hepatic Dose Adjustment	Duration (Days)
	Alternative Therapies Cefepime 2 g IV every 8 hours *or* meropenem	Hypersensitivity (rash, anaphylaxis), decreased seizure threshold	*Renal:* CrCl < 50 mL/min (0.83 mL/s): 2 g IV every 12–24 hours; CrCl < 30 mL/min (0.50 mL/s): 1–2 g IV every 24 hours *Hepatic*: No dose adjustment	
Penicillin MIC 2 mg/L *or* greater	*Standard Therapy* Vancomycin 15 mg/kg IV every 8–12 hours (with dosing based on serum concentrations) plus ceftriaxone *or* cefotaxime	Vancomycin: rash, red man's syndrome (if infused too quickly) nephrotoxicity, thrombocytopenia	*Renal:* CrCl < 50 mL/min (0.83 mL/s): dosing every 24 hours; CrCl < 20 mL/min (0.33 mL/s): dosing based on serum concentrations; all dose adjustments should be made based on serum concentrations *Hepatic:* No dose adjustment	
	Alternative Therapies Moxifloxacin			
Cefotaxime/ ceftriaxone MIC at least 1 mg/L	*Standard Therapy* Vancomycin *plus* ceftriaxone *or* cefotaxime *Alternative Therapies* Moxifloxacin			
H. influenzae β-Lactamase-negative	*Standard Therapy* Ampicillin *Alternative Therapies* Ceftriaxone *or* cefotaxime *or* cefepime *or* moxifloxacin *or* chloramphenicol			7
β-Lactamase-positive	*Standard Therapy* Ceftriaxone *or* cefotaxime *Alternative Therapies* Cefepime *or* moxifloxacin *or* chloramphenicol			
Listeria monocytogenes	*Standard Therapy* Ampicillin *or* penicillin G *plus* gentamicin (5 mg/kg/day, dosing based on serum concentrations)	Gentamicin: nephrotoxicity, ototoxicity	*Renal:* CrCl < 60 mL/min (1.00 mL/s): Use of traditional pharmacokinetic dosing; dose adjustments per serum concentrations *Hepatic:* No dose adjustment	21
	Alternative Therapies Trimethoprim-sulfamethoxazole (10–20 mg/kg trimethoprim) IV per day in divided doses every 6–8 hours *or* meropenem	Trimethoprim-sulfamethoxazole: rash, SJS, bone marrow suppression, hepatotoxicity, elevated serum creatinine, hyperkalemia	*Renal*: CrCl < 50 mL/min (0.83 mL/s): 10–15 mg/kg trimethoprim IV per day divided every 8 hours; CrCl < 10 mL/min (0.17 mL/s): 7–10 mg/kg trimethoprim IV per day divided every 8–12 hours *Hepatic:* No dose adjustment	
Streptococcus agalactiae (group B. *Streptococcus*)	*Standard Therapy* Ampicillin *or* penicillin G *Alternative Therapies* Ceftriaxone *or* cefotaxime			14–21
Enterobacteriaceae	*Standard Therapy* Ceftriaxone *or* cefotaxime *Alternative Therapies*			

(Continued)

Table 70–3

Pathogen-Based Definitive Treatment for CNS Infections[14,55] (Continued)

Pathogen	Recommended and Alternative Antimicrobial Therapy (Adult Doses)	Adverse Effects/Safety Monitoring	Renal and Hepatic Dose Adjustment	Duration (Days)
	Aztreonam 2 g IV every 6–8 hours	Phlebitis, fever, rash, headache, confusion, seizures	*Renal*: CrCl < 50 mL/min (0.83 mL/s): 2 g IV every 8 hours; CrCl < 30 mL/min (0.50 mL/s): 2 g IV every 12 hours; CrCl < 10 mL/min (0.17 mL/s): 1 g IV every 12 hours *Hepatic:* No dose adjustment	
	Moxifloxacin *or* meropenem *or* trimethoprim-sulfamethoxazole *or* ampicillin			
Pseudomonas aeruginosa	*Standard Therapy* Cefepime *or* ceftazidime 2 g IV every 8 hours *or* meropenem (addition of aminoglycoside should be considered)	Hypersensitivity, rash, anemia, neutropenia, eosinophilia, LFT elevation	*Renal*: CrCl < 50 mL/min (0.83 mL/s): 1–2 g IV every 12 hours; CrCl < 30 mL/min (0.50 mL/s): 1–2 g IV every 24 hours; CrCl < 10 mL/min (0.17 mL/s): 1 g IV every 24 hours *Hepatic*: No dose adjustment	
	Alternative Therapies Aztreonam *or* ciprofloxacin 400 mg IV every 8–12 hours (addition of aminoglycoside should be considered)	Nausea/vomiting/diarrhea, dizziness, headache, rash, confusion, seizures	Ciprofloxacin: *Renal*: CrCl < 30 mL/min (0.50 mL/s): 400 mg IV every 24 hours *or* 200 mg IV every 12 hours *Hepatic*: No dose adjustment	
Staphylococcus aureus	*Standard Therapy*			
Methicillin susceptible	Nafcillin *or* oxacillin 1.5–3 g every 4 hours	Rash, nausea/vomiting/diarrhea, acute interstitial nephritis	*Renal*: No dose adjustment *Hepatic*: No dose adjustment (combined renal and hepatic impairment may require dose adjustment)	
	Alternative Therapies Vancomycin *or* meropenem	Rifampin: hepatotoxicity, red-orange discoloration of body fluids, skin rash, hepatic enzyme induction		
Methicillin-resistant	*Standard Therapy* Vancomycin *plus* rifampin 600 mg po *or* IV daily if shunt involved		*Renal*: No dose adjustment *Hepatic*: Caution in moderate/severe hepatic impairment	
	Alternative Therapies Linezolid 600 mg IV every 12 hours *or* trimethoprim-sulfamethoxazole	Linezolid: blood dyscrasias, myalgias, arthralgias, neuropathy	*Renal*: No dose adjustment *Hepatic*: No dose adjustment	
Staphylococcus epidermidis	*Standard Therapy* Vancomycin *plus* rifampin 600 mg po *or* IV daily if shunt involved *Alternative Therapies* Linezolid			
Herpes simplex virus	*Standard Therapy* Acyclovir 10 mg/kg IV every 8 hours (adults); 20 mg/kg IV every 8 hours (neonates)	Nephrotoxicity, crystalluria, nausea/vomiting, neurotoxicity, phlebitis	*Renal*: CrCl < 50 mL/min (0.83 mL/s): 10 mg/kg IV every 12 hours; CrCl < 30 mL/min (0.50 mL/s): 10 mg/kg IV every 24 hours; CrCl < 10 mL/min (0.17 mL/s): 5 mg/kg IV every 24 hours *Hepatic*: No dose adjustment	

(*Continued*)

Table 70–3

Pathogen-Based Definitive Treatment for CNS Infections[14,55] (Continued)

Pathogen	Recommended and Alternative Antimicrobial Therapy (Adult Doses)	Adverse Effects/Safety Monitoring	Renal and Hepatic Dose Adjustment	Duration (Days)
	Alternative Therapy Foscarnet 120–200 mg/kg IV per day in divided doses every 8–12 hours	Nephrotoxicity, electrolyte imbalances, nausea/vomiting, headache, penile ulceration, thrombophlebitis, seizures	*Renal*: CrCl: 1.0–1.4 mL/min/kg (0.017–0.023 mL/s/kg): 70 mg/kg IV every 12 hours; CrCl: 0.8–1.0 mL/min/kg (0.013–0.017 mL/s/kg): 50 mg/kg IV every 12 hours; CrCl: 0.6–0.8 mL/min/kg (0.010–0.013 mL/s/kg): 80 mg/kg IV every 24 hours; CrCl: 0.5–0.6 mL/min/kg (0.008–0.010 mL/s/kg): 60 mg/kg IV every 24 hours; CrCl: 0.4–0.5 mL/min/kg (0.007–0.008 mL/s/kg): 50 mg/kg IV every 24 hours; CrCl < 0.4 mL/min/kg (0.007 mL/s/kg) *or* < 20 mL/min (0.33 mL/s) not recommended *Hepatic*: No dose adjustment	
Cryptococcus neoformans	Amphotericin B 0.7mg/kg IV daily *plus* flucytosine 100–150 mg/kg/day in divided doses every 6 hours (induction) Fluconazole 400–800 mg (maintenance) Fluconazole 200 mg (secondary prophylaxis)	Amphotericin: nephrotoxicity, electrolyte imbalances Flucytosine: bone marrow suppression, rash Fluconazole: transaminitis; QTc prolongation	*Renal*: Caution in severe renal dysfunction; consider alternative dosing strategy or change to lipid formulation *Hepatic*: No dose adjustment Flucytosine: *Renal*: CrCl 25–50 mL/min (0.42–0.83 mL/s): every 12 hours; CrCl 10–25 mL/min (0.17–0.42 mL/s) every 24 hours; CrCl < 10 mL/min (0.17 mL/s) 12.5 mg/kg every 24 hours *Hepatic*: No dose adjustment Fluconazole: *Renal*: CrCl < 50 mL/min (0.83 mL/s) decrease dose by 50% *Hepatic*: Consider 50% reduction in mild-moderate hepatic insufficiency; risk-benefit in severe hepatic dysfunction	
Toxoplasmosis gondii	Pyrimethamine 200 mg po x 1, then 50 mg (< 60 kg) to 75 mg (≥ 60 kg) daily *plus* sulfadiazine 1000 mg (< 60 kg) to 1500 mg (≥ 60 kg) po every 6 hours plus leucovorin 10–25 mg po daily	Pyrimethamine: bone marrow suppression, high-risk for anemia Sulfadiazine: nephrotoxicity, bone marrow suppression, rash, SJS	*Renal*: No dose adjustment *Hepatic*: No dose adjustment *Renal*: CrCL 25–50 mL/min (0.42–0.83 mL/s): every 12 hours; CrCl 10–25 mL/min (0.17–0.42 mL/s) every 24 hours; CrCl less than 10ml/min (< 0.17 mL/s) caution use due to high risk of crystalluria *Hepatic*: No dose adjustment	

LFTs, liver function tests; MIC, minimum inhibitory concentration; SJS, Stevens-Johnson Syndrome.

[a]Empiric therapy with a third-generation cephalosporin should be used until in vitro susceptibility data are known.

Prevention of meningococcal disease by vaccination is a key to reducing the incidence of meningococcal meningitis. Routine vaccination should be administered between ages 11 and 21 years (preferably as soon as possible), with quadrivalent vaccine that provides protection against serogroups A, C, Y, and W.[20] In addition, individuals aged 2 through 54 years who are immunocompromised (including those with complement deficiencies, who have HIV, or who have asplenia) or those with recent disease exposure during community outbreaks should receive the quadrivalent vaccine.[20] Additionally, children less than 2 years may also need quadrivalent vaccine, depending on risk factors. The quadrivalent conjugate meningococcal vaccine protects against four of the five serotypes causing invasive disease (A, C, Y, and W-135). Meningococcal vaccines do not protect against serotype B, which causes more than 50% of the cases of meningococcal meningitis in children younger than 2 years.[20]

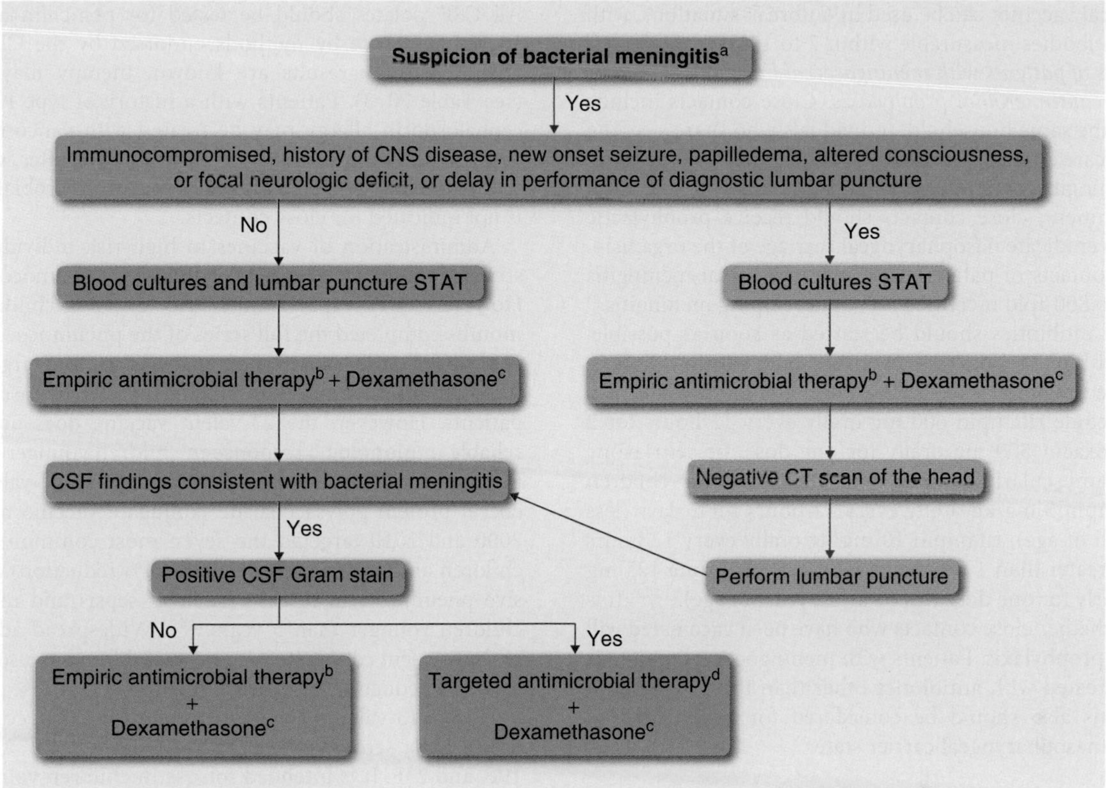

FIGURE 70–2. Management algorithm for adults with suspected bacterial meningitis. [a]Management algorithm is similar for infants and children with suspected bacterial meningitis. [b]See Table 70–1 for empirical treatment recommendations. [c]See text for specific recommendations for use of adjunctive dexamethasone in adults with bacterial meningitis. [d]See Table 70–3 for pathogen-based definitive treatment recommendations. (Adapted, with permission, from Moris G, Garcia-Monco JC. The challenge of drug-induced aseptic meningitis. Arch Intern Med. 1999;159:1185–1194.)

Table 70–4

Pediatric Doses of Selected Agents Used in Bacterial Meningitis Treatment

	Neonates, 0–7 Days	Neonates, 8–28 Days	Infants and Children
Ampicillin	150 mg/kg IV per day in divided doses every 8 hours	200 mg/kg IV per day in divided doses every 6–8 hours	300 mg/kg IV per day in divided doses every 8 hours
Cefepime	—	—	150 mg/kg/day in divided doses every 8 hours
Cefotaxime	100–150 mg/kg IV per day in divided doses every 8–12 hours	150–200 mg/kg IV per day in divided doses every 6–8 hours	225–300 mg/kg/day in divided doses every 6–8 hours
Ceftriaxone	—	—	80–100 mg/kg IV per day in divided doses every 12 hours
Gentamicin	5 mg/kg IV per day in divided doses every 12 hours (with dosing based on serum levels)	7.5 mg/kg IV per day in divided doses every 8 hours (with dosing based on serum levels	7.5 mg/kg IV per day in divided doses every 8 hours based on serum levels)
Meropenem	—	—	120 mg/kg IV per day in divided doses every 8 hours
Nafcillin/ oxacillin	75 mg/kg IV per day in divided doses every 8–12 hours	Nafcillin: 100–150 mg/kg IV per day in divided doses every 6–8 hours; Oxacillin: 150–200 mg/kg IV per day in divided doses every 6–8 hours	200 mg/kg IV per day in divided doses every 6 hours max, 2 g pediatrics > 3 months of age
Penicillin G	0.15 million units/kg IV per day in divided doses 8–12 hours	0.2 million units/kg IV per day in divided doses every 6–8 hours	0.3 million units/kg IV per day in divided doses every 4–6 hours
Vancomycin	20–30 mg/kg IV per day in divided doses every 8–12 hours	30–45 mg/kg IV per day in divided doses every 6–8 hours	60 mg/kg IV per day in divided doses every 6 hours

LFTs, liver function tests; MIC, minimum inhibitory concentration.

Adapted, with permission, from Scheld WM, Koedel U, Nathan B, Pfister HW. Pathophysiology of bacterial meningitis: mechanism(s) of neuronal injury. J Infect Dis. 2002;186(Suppl 2):S225–S233.

Meningococcal vaccines can be used in outbreak situations, with protective antibodies measurable within 7 to 10 days. KEY CONCEPT *Close contacts of patients with meningococcal infections should be evaluated for antimicrobial prophylaxis.* Close contacts include members of the same household, individuals who share sleeping quarters, daycare contacts, and individuals exposed to oral secretions of meningitis patients. After consultation with the local health department, close contacts should receive prophylactic antibiotics to eradicate nasopharyngeal carriage of the organism. Household contacts of patients with meningococcal meningitis have a 400- to 800-fold increased risk of developing meningitis.[23] Prophylactic antibiotics should be started as soon as possible, preferably within 24 hours of exposure and within 14 days. Recommended regimens, all of which are 90% to 95% effective, for adults include rifampin 600 mg orally every 12 hours for 2 days, ciprofloxacin 500 mg orally for one dose, or ceftriaxone 250 mg intramuscularly for one dose. Regimens for children include rifampin 5 mg/kg orally every 12 hours for 2 days (less than 1 month of age), rifampin 10 mg/kg orally every 12 hours for 2 days (greater than 1 month of age), or ceftriaxone 125 mg intramuscularly for one dose (less than 12 years of age).[11,20,23] It is not known whether close contacts who have been vaccinated will benefit from prophylaxis. Patients with meningococcal meningitis who are treated with antibiotics other than third-generation cephalosporins also should be considered for prophylaxis to eradicate the nasopharyngeal carrier state.[22]

▶ *Streptococcus Pneumoniae Meningitis*

S. pneumoniae is the most common cause of meningitis in adults and in children younger than 2 years of age. Pneumococcus is associated with the highest mortality observed with bacterial meningitis in adults (14%–18%), and coma and seizures are more common in pneumococcal meningitis.[1-3] Patients at high risk for pneumococcal meningitis include the elderly, alcoholics, splenectomized patients, patients with sickle cell disease, and patients with cochlear implants. At least 50% of pneumococcal meningitis cases are due to a primary infection of the ears, sinuses, or lungs.

Due to increases in pneumococcal resistance to high-dose penicillin G, the preferred empirical treatment now includes a third-generation cephalosporin in combination with vancomycin.[11]

Patient Encounter 2, Part 1

BB is a 4-year-old boy who is brought to the ED with a 3-day history of fever and irritability. In the past 24 hours, he has become more lethargic, sleeping for 18 hours, and is difficult to arouse. Vital signs and laboratory values include a rectal temperature of 39.4°C (103°F), respirations 40 per minute, heart rate 145 beats/min, and peripheral WBC of $15.9 \times 10^3/mm^3$ ($15.9 \times 10^9/L$), with 68% (0.68) PMNs. Physical examination reveals that the patient is more comfortable when lying flat and has some nuchal rigidity. BB also has a 9-year-old brother with autism and therefore he has not received any routine vaccinations.

What signs and symptoms consistent with meningitis are present in BB?

What clues to causative pathogen are present in BB?

What empiric antimicrobial regimen should be started?

All CSF isolates should be tested for penicillin and cephalosporin resistance by methods endorsed by the CLSI. Once in vitro sensitivity results are known, therapy may be tailored (see Table 70–3). Patients with a history of type I penicillin or cephalosporin allergy may be treated with vancomycin. Treatment should be continued for 10 to 14 days, after which no further maintenance therapy is required. Antimicrobial prophylaxis is not indicated for close contacts.

Administration of vaccines to high-risk individuals is a key strategy to reduce the risk of invasive pneumococcal disease. However, 2013 reports note only 82% of children aged 35 months completed the full series of the pneumococcal conjugate vaccine.[25] The 23-valent pneumococcal vaccine targets serotypes that account for more than 90% of invasive disease in high-risk patients. However, the 23-valent vaccine does not produce a reliable immunologic response in children younger than 2 years, nor does it reduce pneumococcal carriage. The 7-valent pneumococcal protein-polysaccharide conjugate vaccine used between 2000 and 2010 targeted the seven most common serotypes in children and provided protection (94% reduction) against invasive pneumococcal disease (such as sepsis and meningitis) in children younger than 5 years.[4,26,27] Widespread administration of the 7-valent conjugate vaccine to children has also contributed to a 28% reduction in invasive pneumococcal disease in adults.[4] PCV13, a 13-valent vaccine introduced in 2010, confers protection against serotypes 1, 3, 4, 5, 6A, 6B, 7F, 9V, 14, 18C, 19A, 19F, and 23F. It is intended for use in children younger than 18 years in the same schedule as the 7-valent conjugate vaccine.[27] PCV13 is specifically recommended for immunocompromised children aged 6 to 18 years.[28] Immunization schedules provided by CDC are updated at least annually and should be consulted for additional details.

▶ *Haemophilus Influenzae Meningitis*

Prior to the introduction of the Hib conjugate vaccine, *H. influenzae* type b was the most common cause of bacterial meningitis in the United States.[3,4] Routine inoculation of pediatric patients against Hib has significantly reduced the incidence of Hib meningitis between 1998 and 2007.[3,4] The Hib vaccine is also recommended for patients undergoing splenectomy. Hib meningeal disease is often associated with a parameningeal focus such as a sinus or middle ear infection. Due to β-lactamase–mediated resistance, the empirical treatment of choice is third-generation cephalosporins (eg, ceftriaxone and cefotaxime). Treatment should be continued for 7 days, after which no further maintenance therapy is required.

KEY CONCEPT *Close contacts of patients with H. influenzae type B meningitis should be evaluated for antimicrobial prophylaxis.* The risk of Hib meningitis in close contacts may be up to 200- to 1000-fold higher than in the general population.[7] Invasive Hib disease, including meningitis, should be reported to the local health department and the CDC. Prophylaxis to eliminate nasal and oropharyngeal carriage of Hib in exposed individuals should be initiated after consultation with local health officials. Rifampin (600 mg/day for adults; 20 mg/kg/day for children, maximum of 600 mg/day) is administered for 4 days.[11,16] Rifampin prophylaxis is not necessary for individuals who have received the full Hib vaccine series. Exposed, unvaccinated children between 12 and 48 months of age should receive one dose of vaccine, and unvaccinated children 2 to 11 months of age should receive three doses of vaccine, as well as rifampin prophylaxis.[11,16] According to the CDC, up to 18% of children at 35 months have not completed the HiB vaccine series.[25]

Patient Encounter 2, Part 2

BB underwent lumbar puncture. Initial results from CSF studies are WBC 1.76×10^3/mm^3 (1.76×10^9/L) with 79% (0.79) PMNs, protein 265 mg/dL (2650 mg/L), glucose 30 mg/dL (1.7 mmol/l), with a concurrent serum glucose of 110 mg/dL (6.1 mmol/L). Gram stain shows gram-negative rods and culture results identify *H. influenzae* infection. The patient is admitted to an acute care unit and remains clinically stable.

What complications is BB at risk for acutely? What potential long-term complications may result?

How can his antibiotic regimen be streamlined at this time?

How long should the antibiotics be continued?

▸ *Listeria monocytogenes* Meningitis

L. monocytogenes is an intracellular gram-positive bacillus that contaminates foods, such as soft cheese, unpasteurized milk, raw meats and fish, processed meats, and raw vegetables. Bacteria from contaminated foods colonize the GI tract, pass into the bloodstream, and overcome natural cellular immune responses to cause infection. *L. monocytogenes* meningitis, usually observed in patients at extremes of age and in immunocompromised patients with depressed cellular immunity (including patients with leukemia, solid-organ transplants, and HIV/AIDS) has an overall mortality rate of up to 30%.[29,30]

Only a limited number of antibiotics show bactericidal activity against *Listeria*. The combination of high-dose ampicillin or penicillin G and an aminoglycoside is synergistic and bactericidal against *Listeria*. A total treatment course of at least 3 weeks is required. Because of concerns about the risk of nephrotoxicity with an extended treatment course of aminoglycosides, patients are treated with combination therapy for 10 days and may finish out the remainder of their treatment with ampicillin or penicillin alone.[30] In penicillin-allergic patients, trimethoprim-sulfamethoxazole is the agent of choice due to documented in vitro bactericidal activity against *Listeria*, as well as good CNS penetration. Vancomycin and cephalosporins are not effective treatments for *Listeria* meningitis. Prophylaxis is not needed for close contacts, nor is suppressive therapy indicated. Patients with severe depression of cell-mediated immunity should be advised to avoid foods that may be contaminated with *Listeria*.

▸ Group B Streptococcus Meningitis

Infection with group B *Streptococcus* (eg, *S. agalactiae*) is the most common cause of neonatal sepsis and meningitis. Around 15% to 35% of pregnant women are a carrier of group B *Streptococcus* in the vagina or rectum. Group B streptococci can be acquired during childbirth after exposure to infected secretions from the mother's birth canal or rectum. Neonates born to women who are carriers are at very high risk (1 of every 100–200 babies) of developing invasive group B streptococcal disease.[31] Neonatal meningitis is associated with significant morbidity and mortality. Synergistic treatment with penicillin or ampicillin, plus gentamicin, for 14 to 21 days is recommended for group B streptococcal meningitis.[11]

To reduce the risk of clinical group B streptococcal disease in neonates, pregnant women should be screened at 35 to 37 weeks' gestation to determine whether they are carriers of group B streptococci.[31] Intrapartum antibiotics (eg, penicillin or ampicillin) are recommended for pregnant women with the following characteristics: group B streptococcal carrier state detected at screening, history of group B streptococcal bacteriuria at any time during pregnancy, and history of delivery of infant with invasive group B streptococcal disease.[31]

▸ Gram-Negative Bacillary Meningitis

Meningitis caused by enteric gram-negative bacilli is an important cause of morbidity and mortality in populations at risk, including those with diabetes, malignancy, cirrhosis, immunosuppression, advanced age, parameningeal infection, and/or a defect allowing communication from skin to CNS (eg, neurosurgery, congenital defects, cranial trauma).[7]

The optimal treatment for gram-negative bacillary meningitis is not well defined. The introduction of extended-spectrum cephalosporins has improved patient outcomes significantly. Although the third-generation cephalosporins ceftriaxone and cefotaxime provide good coverage for most Enterobacteriaceae, these antibiotics are not active against *P. aeruginosa*. Ceftazidime, cefepime, and carbapenems are effective in pseudomonal meningitis.[15,17] Addition of an aminoglycoside may improve treatment results; however, CNS penetration of aminoglycosides is extremely poor, even in the setting of inflamed meninges. Intrathecal or intraventricular administration of aminoglycosides may be useful, but intraventricular antibiotics have been associated with increased mortality in neonates.[15,32] Intrathecal therapy is accomplished by administering the antibiotic into the CSF via LP, whereas intraventricular therapy is usually administered into a reservoir implanted in the ventricles of the brain.

Initial therapy of suspected or documented pseudomonal meningitis should include an antipsuedomonal β-lactam (eg, cefepime, meropenem) plus an aminoglycoside (eg tobramycin, amikacin). Although the carbapenem imipenem-cilastatin has similar activity to these β-lactams, its use is not recommended in meningitis because of the risk of seizures. Aztreonam, high-dose ciprofloxacin, and colistin are alternative treatments for pseudomonal meningitis, although local susceptibility rates should be considered before initiating alternative therapy. Local therapy (ie, intrathecal or intraventricular therapy) may be indicated in patients with multidrug-resistant gram-negative bacillary meningitis or in patients who fail to improve on IV antibiotics alone. In cases of multidrug-resistant pathogens, alternative pharmacodynamic dosing strategies such as continuous or extended infusion of β-lactam antimicrobials may be considered to optimize target attainment (time greater than minimum inhibitory concentration). Given the differences in local hospital resistance patterns, administration of pathogen-directed treatment is very important after microbiology results become available. Therapy for gram-negative bacillary meningitis should be continued for at least 21 days.

▸ Postoperative Infections in the Neurosurgical Patient and Shunt Infections

Patients who undergo neurosurgical procedures or have invasive or implanted foreign devices (eg, CSF shunts, intraspinal pumps or catheters, epidural catheters) are at risk for CNS infections. Key pathogens in postneurosurgical infections include coagulase-negative staphylococci, *S. aureus*, streptococci, propionibacteria, and gram-negative bacilli, including *P. aeruginosa*. Clinical signs and symptoms may be similar to those of other CNS infections, and there also may be evidence of malfunction of implanted hardware or visible signs of a postoperative wound infection.

Empirical therapy for postoperative infections in neurosurgical patients (including patients with CSF shunts) should include vancomycin in combination with either cefepime, ceftazidime, or meropenem. Linezolid reaches adequate CSF concentrations and resolves cases of meningitis refractory to vancomycin.[30,33] However, data with linezolid are limited. The addition of rifampin may be considered for treatment of shunt infections. Removal of infected devices is desirable; aggressive antibiotic therapy (including high-dose IV antibiotic therapy plus intraventricular vancomycin and/or tobramycin) may be effective for patients in whom hardware removal is not possible.[34] If methicillin-resistant *S. aureus* is identified as the causative organism, daptomycin may be considered an alternative therapy.[35]

The use of prophylactic antibiotics against meningitis postcraniotomy remains controversial.[36,37] One meta-analysis suggests that prophylaxis reduces rates of postoperative meningitis by nearly one-half.[36] Breakthrough meningitis that does occur may be a result of drug-resistant pathogens.[37]

Brain abscesses are localized collections of pus within the cranium. These infections are difficult to treat due to the presence of walled-off infections in the brain tissue reducing antibiotic penetration. In addition to appropriate antimicrobial therapy (a discussion of which is beyond the scope of this chapter), surgical debridement is often required as an adjunctive measure. Surgical debridement may also be required in the management of neurosurgical postoperative infections.

▶ *Viral Encephalitis and Meningitis*

Viral encephalitis and meningitis may mimic bacterial meningitis on clinical presentation but often can be differentiated by CSF findings (see Table 70–2). The most common viral pathogens are enteroviruses, which cause approximately 85% of cases of viral CNS infections.[7] Other viruses that may cause CNS infections include arboviruses, HSV, cytomegalovirus, varicella-zoster virus, rotavirus, coronavirus, influenza viruses A and B, West Nile virus, and Epstein-Barr virus. Viral CNS infections are acquired through hematogenous or neuronal spread.[7] Most cases of enteroviral meningitis or encephalitis are self-limiting with supportive treatment.[38] However, arbovirus, West Nile virus, and Eastern equine virus infections are associated with a less favorable prognosis.

In contrast to other viral encephalitides, HSV type 1 and 2 encephalitis are treatable. Although rare (one case per 250,000 population per year in the United States), HSV encephalitis is a serious, life-threatening infection.[39] More than 90% of HSV encephalitis in adults is due to HSV type 1, whereas HSV type 2 predominates in neonatal HSV encephalitis (greater than 70%).[40] HSV encephalitis is the result of reactivation of a latent infection (two-thirds of cases) or a severe case of primary infection (one-third). Without effective treatment, the mortality rate may be as high as 85%, and survivors often have significant residual neurologic deficits. In accordance with 2008 IDSA guidelines, high-dose IV acyclovir is the drug of choice, given for 2 to 3 weeks at a dose of 10 mg/kg IV every 8 hours in adults, based on ideal body weight, and for 3 weeks at a dose of 20 mg/kg IV every 8 hours in neonates.[41] Patients receiving acyclovir should maintain adequate hydration (consider continuous IV hydration) to help prevent acute kidney injury secondary to crystal nephropathy.[41] Foscarnet 120 to 200 mg/kg/day divided every 8 to 12 hours for 2 to 3 weeks is the treatment of choice for acyclovir-resistant HSV.[41]

▶ *Opportunistic CNS Infections*

Cerebral Toxoplasmosis Across the globe, cerebral toxoplasmosis represents the most common focal brain infection in HIV-infected patients. Infection rates in the United States vary but are reported to be approximately 15% among patients with AIDS.[42] The majority of cases occur in patients with $CD4^+$ cell counts less than 100 cells/mm^3 (100 × 10^6/L). Potent antiretroviral therapy and primary prophylaxis (first-line option is sulfamethoxazole-trimethoprim) in IgG-positive patients has greatly reduced the disease burden.[43] First-line therapy in toxoplasmosis encephalitis is pyrimethamine plus sulfadiazine, given concomitantly with leucovorin to prevent severe hematologic adverse effects secondary to pyrimethamine (see tables for dosing).[43] Clindamycin may be substituted for sulfadiazine in cases of contraindications to sulfa-based therapy. Sulfamethoxazole-trimethoprim may also be an option, specifically in patients unable to take oral therapy. Adjunctive corticosteroids and anticonvulsant therapy should be considered to reduce sequelae from the inflammatory process and control active seizures, respectively.[43]

Cryptococcal Meningitis CNS disease secondary to *Cryptococcus neoformans* is primarily observed in severely immunocompromised hosts, such as those with HIV infection. Potent antiretroviral therapy has significantly reduced the disease burden from preantiretroviral therapy rates of 5% to 8% in developed countries. The majority of disease occurs in patients with $CD4^+$ cell counts less than 50 cells/mm^3 (50 × 10^6/L). First-line therapy is considered amphotericin B deoxycholate 0.7 mg/kg IV daily plus flucytosine 100 mg/kg/day orally in four divided doses for a minimum of 2 weeks.[43] Therapeutic drug monitoring may be considered for flucytosine to help reduce the risk of adverse effects. Development of renal dysfunction as a result of disease and/or drug toxicity should be closely monitored and may prompt dose reduction or possible switch to alternative lipid formulations of amphotericin, which may be less nephrotoxic. High-dose fluconazole is considered an alternative first-line therapy, especially in resource-limited areas. Secondary prophylaxis with fluconazole for an indefinite period is recommended following the completion of at least 2 weeks of induction therapy and 8 weeks of maintenance therapy with fluconazole.[43]

▶ *Adjunctive Dexamethasone Therapy*

The adjunctive agent dexamethasone improves outcomes in selected patient populations with bacterial meningitis. Dexamethasone inhibits the release of proinflammatory cytokines and limits the CNS inflammatory response stimulated by infection and antibiotic therapy.

Clinical benefit in reducing neurologic deficits (primarily by reducing hearing loss) has been observed in infants and children, if dexamethasone is initiated prior to antibiotic therapy.[1,44] The American Academy of Pediatrics recommends dexamethasone (0.15 mg/kg IV every 6 hours for 2 to 4 days) for infants and children at least 6 weeks of age with Hib meningitis and consideration of dexamethasone in pneumococcal meningitis.[11,45] In contrast to this recommendation, a large multicenter cohort study failed to show any mortality benefit of adjunctive dexamethasone therapy regardless of age or responsible pathogen (*S. pneumoniae* or *N. meningitidis*).[46] Dexamethasone should be initiated 10 to 20 minutes before or no later than the time of initiation of antibiotic therapy; it is not recommended for infants and children who have already received antibiotic therapy because it is unlikely to improve treatment outcome in these patients. There are insufficient data to make a recommendation regarding the use of adjunctive dexamethasone therapy in neonatal meningitis.

In adults, a significant benefit was observed with dexamethasone in reducing meningitis complications, including death, particularly in patients with pneumococcal meningitis.[47] The IDSA recommends dexamethasone 0.15 mg/kg IV every 6 hours for 2 to 4 days (with the first dose administered 10 to 20 minutes before or with the first dose of antibiotics) in adults with suspected or proven pneumococcal meningitis.[11] Dexamethasone is not recommended for adults who have already received antibiotic therapy. Some clinicians would administer dexamethasone to all adults with meningitis pending results of laboratory tests. Benefit of dexamethasone in bacterial meningitis in a HIV-positive population has not been clearly established.[48]

There is controversy regarding the administration of dexamethasone to patients requiring vancomycin for pneumococcal meningitis. Animal models indicate that concurrent steroid use reduces vancomycin penetration into the CSF by 42% to 77% and delays CSF sterilization.[15] A prospective evaluation in patients with pneumococcal meningitis receiving vancomycin and adjunctive dexamethasone demonstrated that adequate concentrations of vancomycin (nearly 30% of serum concentrations) were achievable in the CSF, provided appropriate vancomycin dosage was utilized.[49] Treatment failures have been reported in adults with resistant pneumococcal meningitis who were treated with dexamethasone, but the risk–benefit of using dexamethasone in these patients cannot be defined at this time. Animal models indicate a benefit of adding rifampin in patients with resistant pneumococcal meningitis whenever dexamethasone is used.[15,17]

OUTCOME EVALUATION

Monitor patients with CNS infections continuously throughout their treatment course to evaluate their progress toward achieving treatment goals, including relief of symptoms, eradication of infection, and reduction of inflammation to prevent death and the development of neurologic deficits. These treatment goals are best achieved by appropriate parenteral antimicrobial therapy, including empirical therapy to cover the most likely pathogens, followed by directed therapy after culture and sensitivity results are known. KEY CONCEPT *Components of a monitoring plan to assess efficacy and safety of antimicrobial therapy of CNS infections include clinical signs and symptoms and laboratory data (eg, CSF findings, culture, sensitivity data).*

Patient Encounter 2, Part 3

As noted, BB had not received any vaccinations since birth. The parents are concerned and inquire about the need for antibiotic prophylaxis for the family and now are considering vaccination for BB.

Who should receive antimicrobial prophylaxis for H. influenzae?

Who should receive vaccination against Hib disease?

How is vaccination important in the prevention of Hib disease, especially for BB?

Patient Care Process

Patient Assessment:

- Assess patient allergies, including severity of reactions
- Determine if patient has received recent antibiotics that may influence LP results or treatment decisions
- Determine from a medication history if any medicines may be associated with drug-induced aseptic meningitis

Therapy Evaluation:

- Assess LP results, results of antigenic testing, and culture and susceptibility for additional data to help streamline therapy
- Monitor patient for any antimicrobial-related adverse events. Provide recommendations for necessary prophylaxis based on causative pathogen and exposure history

Care Plan Development:

- Based on patient-specific factors and local susceptibility patterns, determine appropriate empirical antimicrobial treatment plan
- Collaborate with treatment team to ensure timely administration of antibiotic in relation to performing LP and obtaining blood cultures
- Collaborate with treatment team to determine appropriate administration of adjunctive corticosteroid therapy

Follow-up Evaluation:

- Determine appropriate length of therapy for diagnosed CNS infection
- Provide recommendations for outpatient parenteral therapy as needed upon discharge from acute care facility

During the patient's treatment course, monitor clinical signs and symptoms at least three times daily. Trends are more important than one-time assessments. Expect fever, headache, nausea and vomiting, and malaise to begin to improve within 24 to 48 hours of initiation of antimicrobial therapy and supportive care. Evaluate the patient for resolution of neurologic signs and symptoms, such as altered mental status and nuchal rigidity, as the infection is eradicated and inflammation is reduced within the CNS. Expect improvement and subsequent resolution of signs and symptoms as the treatment course continues. At the time of hospital discharge, arrange outpatient follow-up for several weeks to months depending on the causative pathogen, clinical treatment course, and patient's underlying comorbidities.

Monitoring of laboratory tests is important in patients receiving treatment for CNS infections. Monitor CSF and blood cultures so that antimicrobial therapy can be tailored to the etiologic organisms. Follow-up cultures may be obtained to prove eradication of the organism(s) or treatment failure. Although repeat LP generally is not performed, consider repeat LP for patients who do not respond clinically after 48 hours of appropriate antimicrobial therapy, especially those with resistant pneumococcus who receive dexamethasone.[11] Other candidates for repeat LP include those with infection with gram-negative bacilli, prolonged fever, and recurrent meningitis. Repeat the

LP in neonates to determine the duration of therapy. Repeat LP also may be performed to relieve elevated intracranial pressure. Expect repeat blood cultures to become negative quickly during therapy and the serum WBC count to improve and normalize with appropriate antimicrobial therapy.

Evaluate antimicrobial dosing regimens to ensure efficacy of the treatment regimen. Trough vancomycin concentrations of 15 to 20 mg/L (10–14 μmol/L) are recommended for the treatment of CNS infections.[44] Monitor patients for drug adverse effects, drug allergies, and drug interactions. The specific safety monitoring plan will depend on the antibiotic(s) used (Table 70–3). Pay close attention to concomitant medications in patients on rifampin for treatment or prophylaxis. Rifampin is a potent inducer of hepatic metabolism and may reduce the efficacy of other drugs metabolized by the cytochrome P-450 enzyme pathway.

Abbreviations Introduced in This Chapter

CDC	Centers for Disease Control and Prevention
CLSI	Clinical and Laboratory Standards Institute
CNS	Central nervous system
CSF	Cerebrospinal fluid
DIC	Disseminated intravascular coagulation
ESBL	Extended spectrum beta-lactamase
GBS	Group B *Streptococcus*
Hib	*Haemophilus influenzae* type B
HSV	Herpes simplex virus
IDSA	Infectious Diseases Society of America
IL-1	Interleukin 1
LP	Lumbar puncture
MBC	Minimum bactericidal concentration
MIC	Minimum inhibitory concentration
MRSA	Methicillin-resistant *Staphylococcus aureus*
MRSE	Methicillin-resistant *Staphylococcus epidermidis*
NSAIDs	Nonsteroidal anti-inflammatory drugs
PCR	Polymerase chain reaction
PMN	Polymorphonuclear cell
SJS	Stevens-Johnson Syndrome
TNF-α	Tumor necrosis factor-alpha

REFERENCES

1. van de Beek D, de Gans J, McIntyre P, Prasad K. Corticosteroids for acute bacterial meningitis. Cochrane Database Syst Rev. 2003;3:CD004405.
2. van de Beek D, de Gans J, Spanjaard L, et al. Clinical features and prognostic factors in adults with bacterial meningitis. N Engl J Med. 2004;351(18):1849–1859.
3. Thigpen MC, Whitney CG, Messonnier NE, et al. Bacterial meningitis in the United States, 1998-2007. N Engl J Med. 2011;364(21):2016–2025.
4. Castelblanco RL, Lee M, Hasbun R. Epidemiology of bacterial meningitis in the USA from 1997 to 2010: A population-based observational study. Lancet Infect Dis. 2014;14(9):813–819.
5. Levy C, Varon E, Picard C, Bechet S, Martinot A, Bonacorsi S, Cohen R. Trends of Pneumococcal meningitis in children after introduction of the 13-valent pneumococcal conjugate vaccine in France. Ped Infect Dis. 2014 Jul 16 (E-pub ahead of print).
6. Sejvar JJ. The evolving epidemiology of viral encephalitis. Curr Opin Neurol. 2006;19:350–357.
7. Mitropoulous IF, Hermsen ED, Schafer JA, Rotschafer JC. Central nervous system infections. In: DiPiro JT, Talbert RL, Yee GC, et al., eds. Pharmacotherapy: A Pathophysiologic Approach. 7th ed. New York City: McGraw-Hill; 2008:1743–1760.
8. Khetsuriani N, Holman RC, Anderson LJ. Burden of encephalitis-associated hospitalizations in the United States, 1988–1997. Clin Infect Dis. 2002;35:175–182.
9. Scheld WM, Koedel U, Nathan B, Pfister HW. Pathophysiology of bacterial meningitis: mechanism(s) of neuronal injury. J Infect Dis. 2002;186(Suppl 2):S225–S233.
10. Kim KS. Pathogenesis of bacterial meningitis: From bacteraemia to neuronal injury. Nat Rev Neurosci. 2003;4:376–385.
11. Tunkel AR, Hartman BJ, Kaplan SL, et al. Practice guidelines for the management of bacterial meningitis. Clin Infect Dis. 2004;39:1267–1284.
12. Lu CH, Huang CR, Chang, WN, et al. Community-acquired bacterial meningitis in adults: the epidemiology, timing of appropriate antimicrobial therapy, and prognostic factors. Clin Neurol Neurosurg. 2002;104:352–358.
13. van de Beek D, de Gans J, Tunkel AR, Wijdicks EFM. Community-acquired bacterial meningitis in adults. N Engl J Med. 2006;354:44–53.
14. Pankey GA, Sabath LR. Clinical relevance of bacterio-static versus bactericidal mechanisms of action in the treatment of gram-positive bacterial infections. Clin Infect Dis. 2004;38:864–870.
15. Sinner SW, Tunkel AR. Antimicrobial agents in the treatment of bacterial meningitis. Infect Dis Clin N Am. 2004;18:581–602.
16. Bashir HE, Laundy M, Booy R. Diagnosis and treatment of bacterial meningitis. Arch Dis Child. 2003;88:615–620.
17. Quagliarello VJ, Scheld WM. Treatment of bacterial meningitis. N Engl J Med. 1997;336(10):708–716.
18. Tice AD, Strait K, Ramey R, et al. Outpatient parenteral antimicrobial therapy for central nervous system infections. Clin Infect Dis. 1999;29:1394–1399.
19. Jones ME, Draghi DC, Karlowsky JA, Sahm DF, Bradley JS. Prevalence of antimicrobial resistance in bacteria isolated from central nervous system specimens as reported by U.S. hospital laboratories from 2000 to 2002 Ann Clin Microb. 2004;3:3 (online journal published March 25, 2004).
20. Centers for Disease Control and Prevention. Prevention and control of Meningococcal Disease: Recommendations of the Advisory Committee on Immunization Practices. MMWR. 2013;62(No. RR#2):1–27.
21. Kim KS. Acute Bacterial Meningitis in Infants and Children. Lancet Infect Dis. 2010;10(1):32–42.
22. Campos-Outcalt D. Meningococcal vaccine: New product, new recommendations. J Fam Pract. 2005;54(4):324–326.
23. Rosenstein NE, Perkins BA, Stephens DS, Popovic T, Hughes JM. Meningococcal disease. N Engl J Med. 2001;344(18):1378–1388.
24. Nudelman Y, Tunkel AR. Bacterial meningitis epidemiology, pathogenesis, and management update. Drugs. 2009;69(18):2577–2596.
25. Centers for Disease Control and Prevention. National, state and selected local area vaccination coverage among children aged 19–35 months—United States, 2013. MMWR. 2014;63(No. RR#34):741–748.
26. Centers for Disease Control and Prevention. Direct and indirect effects of routine vaccination of children with 7-valent pneumococcal conjugate vaccine on incidence of invasive pneumococcal disease—United States, 1998–2003. MMWR. 2005;54(36):893–897.
27. Advisory Committee on Immunization Practices (ACIP). Prevention of pneumococcal disease among infants and children—use of 13-valent pneumococcal conjugate vaccine and 23-valent pneumococcal polysaccharide vaccine. MMWR. 2011;59:RR-11.
28. Centers for Disease Control and Prevention. Use of 13-Valent Pneumococcal Conjugate Vaccine and 23-Valent Pneumococcal

polysaccharide vaccine among children aged 6-18 years with immunocompromising conditions: Recommendations of the Advisory Committee on Immunization Practices (ACIP). MMWR. 2013;62 (RR# 25);521–524.

29. Mylonakis D, Hohmann EL, Calderwood SB. Central nervous system infection with Listeria monocytogenes: 33 years' experience at a general hospital and review of 776 episodes from the literature. Medicine. 1998;77(5):313–336.
30. Hof H. An update on the medical management of Listeriosis. Expert Opin Pharmacother. 2004;5(8):1727–1735.
31. Department of Health and Human Services/CDC. Prevention of perinatal group B streptococcal disease. MMWR. 2010;59: RR-10.
32. Shah S, Ohlsson A, Shah V. Intraventricular antibiotics for bacterial meningitis in neonates. Cochrane Database Syst Rev. 2004;4:CD004496.
33. Villani P, Regazzi MB, Marubbi F, et al. Cerebrospinal fluid linezolid concentrations in postneurosurgical central nervous system infections. Antimicrob Agents Chemother. 2002;46(3):936–937.
34. Anderson EJ, Yogev R. A rational approach to the management of ventricular shunt infections. Pediatr Infect Dis J. 2005;24:557–558.
35. Lee DH, Palermo B, Chowdhury M. Successful treatment of methicillin-resistant *Staphylococcus aureus* meningitis with daptomycin. Clin Infect Dis. 2008;47:588–589.
36. Barker FG. Efficacy of prophylactic antibiotics against meningitis after craniotomy: A meta-analysis. Neurosurgery. 2007;60:887–894.
37. Korinek AM, Golmard JL, Elcheick A, et al. Risk factors for neurosurgical site infections after craniotomy: A critical reappraisal of antibiotic prophylaxis on 4,578 patients. Br J Neurosurg. 2005;19: 155–162.
38. Sawyer MH. Enterovirus infections: Diagnosis and treatment. Pediatr Infect Dis J. 1999;18(12):1033–1040.
39. Tyler KL. Herpes simplex virus infections of the central nervous system: Encephalitis and meningitis, including Mollaret's. Herpes. 2004;11(Suppl 2):57A–64A.
40. Kimberlin D. Herpes simplex virus, meningitis and encephalitis in neonates. Herpes. 2004;11(Suppl 2):65A–76A.
41. Tunkel AR, Glaser CA, Bloch KC, et al. The management of encephalitis: Clinical practice guidelines by the Infectious Diseases Society of America. Clin Infect Dis. 2008;47:303–327.
42. Pereira-Chioccola VL, Vidal JE, Su C. Toxoplasma gondii infection and cerebral toxoplasmosis in HIV-infected patients. Future Microbiol. 2009;4(10):1363–1379.
43. Panel on Opportunistic Infections in HIV-Infected Adults and Adolescents. Guidelines for the prevention and treatment of opportunistic infections in HIV-infected adults and adolescents: Recommendations from the Centers for Disease Control and Prevention, the National Institutes of Health, and the HIV Medicine Association of the Infectious Diseases Society of America. http://aidsinfo.nih.gov/contentfiles/lvguidelines/adult_oi.pdf. Accessed August 21, 2014.
44. Moris G, Garcia-Monco JC. The challenge of drug-induced aseptic meningitis. Arch Intern Med. 1999;159(11):1185–1194.
45. American Academy of Pediatrics. Pneumococcal infections. In: Pickering, LK, ed. Red Book: 2003 Report of the Committee on Infectious Diseases. 26th ed. Elk Grove Village, IL: American Academy of Pediatrics; 2003:490–500.
46. Mongelluzzo J, Mohamad Z, Ten Have TR, Shah SS. Corticosteroids and mortality in children with bacterial meningitis. JAMA. 2008;299(17):2048–2055.
47. de Gans J, van de Beek D, for the European Dexamethasone in Adulthood Bacterial Meningitis Study Investigators. N Engl J Med. 2002;347(20):1549–1556.
48. Scarborough M, Gordon SB, Whitty CJM, et al. Corticosteroids for bacterial meningitis in adults in Sub-Saharan Africa. N Engl J Med. 2007;357:2441–2450.
49. Ricard JD, Wolff M, Lacherade JC, et al. Levels of vancomycin in cerebrospinal fluid of adult patients receiving adjunctive corticosteroids to treat pneumococcal meningitis: A prospective multicenter observational study. Clin Infect Dis. 2007;44:250–255.

71 Lower Respiratory Tract Infections

Diane M. Cappelletty

LEARNING OBJECTIVES

Upon completion of the chapter, the reader will be able to:

1. List the common pathogens that cause community-acquired pneumonia (CAP), aspiration pneumonia, ventilator-associated pneumonia (VAP; early versus late onset), and health care–associated pneumonia.
2. Explain the host defenses that protect against infection.
3. Explain the pathophysiology of pneumonia.
4. List the signs and symptoms associated with CAP and VAP.
5. Identify patient and organism factors required to guide the selection of a specific antimicrobial regimen for an individual patient.
6. Design an appropriate empirical antimicrobial regimen based on patient-specific data for an individual with CAP, aspiration pneumonia, and VAP or health care–associated pneumonia (early vs late onset).
7. Design an appropriate antimicrobial regimen based on both patient- and organism-specific data.
8. Develop a monitoring plan based on patient-specific information for a patient with CAP and health care–associated pneumonia or VAP.
9. Formulate appropriate educational information to be provided to a patient with pneumonia.

INTRODUCTION

Pneumonia is inflammation of the lung with consolidation. The cause of the inflammation is infection, which can be caused by a wide range of organisms. KEY CONCEPT *There are five classifications of pneumonia: community-acquired, aspiration, hospital-acquired, ventilator-associated, and health care-associated.* Patients who develop pneumonia in the outpatient setting and have not been in any health care facilities, which include wound care and hemodialysis clinics, have community-acquired pneumonia (CAP). Pneumonia can be caused by aspiration of either oropharyngeal or gastrointestinal contents. Hospital-acquired pneumonia (HAP) is defined as pneumonia that occurs 48 hours or more after admission.[1,2] Ventilator-associated pneumonia (VAP) requires endotracheal intubation for at least 48 to 72 hours before the onset of pneumonia.[2] Health care–associated pneumonia (HCAP), which is defined as pneumonia occurring in any patient hospitalized for at least 2 days within 90 days of the onset of the infection; residing in a nursing home or long-term care facility; received IV antibiotic therapy, wound care, or chemotherapy within the last 30 days prior to the onset of the infection, or having attended a hemodialysis clinic.[2,3]

EPIDEMIOLOGY AND ETIOLOGY

Etiology and Mortality Rates

KEY CONCEPT *The etiology of bacterial pneumonia varies in accordance with the type of pneumonia.* Table 71–1 lists the more common pathogens associated with the various types or classifications of pneumonia. *Streptococcus pneumoniae* colonizes the nasopharyngeal flora in up to 50% of healthy adults and may colonize the lower airways in individuals with chronic bronchitis.[4,5] It possesses many virulence factors, enhancing its ability to cause infection in the respiratory tract. KEY CONCEPT Therefore, *it is not surprising that S. pneumoniae is the predominant bacterial pathogen associated with CAP.* The second most common pathogen is one of the atypical organisms, *Mycoplasma pneumoniae*. Nontypeable *Haemophilus influenzae* intermittently colonizes about 80% of the population, and the incidence of permanent colonization increases in chronic obstructive pulmonary disease (COPD) patients and those with cystic fibrosis. Therefore, the likelihood of nontypeable *H. influenzae* causing pneumonia increases in COPD patients. *Moraxella catarrhalis* is a more common cause of pneumonia in the very young and the very old. *Chlamydophila pneumoniae* and *Legionella pneumophila* are less frequent causes than the other bacterial and atypical organisms. Community-acquired methicillin-resistant *Staphylococcus aureus* (CA-MRSA) is associated with necrotizing and severe pneumonia in healthy children and young adults. Less than 2% of all CA-MRSA infections are pneumonia (most are skin and soft tissue); however, the number of reports of pneumonia are increasing.[6]

Viruses are a common cause of CAP in children (about 65%) and in adults ranges from 12% to 29%.[7–9] Mixed infections of viruses and bacteria have been increasingly identified in 11% to 56% of cases.[8–10] Viruses most often associated with pneumonia in adults include influenza A and B and rhinoviruses, but can be caused by adenoviruses, enteroviruses, cytomegalovirus,

Table 71–1

Common Pathogens by Type of Pneumonia

Type of Pneumonia	Common Pathogens
Community	Aerobic bacteria: *S. pneumoniae, H. influenzae, M. catarrhalis* Atypical: *M. pneumoniae, C. pneumoniae, L. pneumophila*, respiratory viruses (rhinoviruses and influenza most common)
Aspiration	Oral contents: Anaerobes, *Viridans* streptococci GI contents with pH increase Enteric gram-negative bacilli
Hospital	(Early onset, no risk factors for resistant pathogens)
Ventilator health care	*S. pneumoniae*, MSSA, *E. coli, K. pneumoniae*, (*M. pneumoniae, C. pneumoniae* are rare)
Hospital	(Late onset and/or risk factors for resistant pathogens)
Ventilator health care	MRSA, extended-spectrum β-lactamase-producing *K. pneumoniae, P. aeruginosa, Acinetobacter* spp.

MRSA, methicillin-resistant *Staphylococcus aureus*; MSSA, methicillin-susceptible *S. aureus.*

varicella-zoster virus, herpes simplex virus, and others. In children, viral pneumonia is more commonly caused by respiratory syncytial virus, influenza A, and parainfluenza, and less commonly those listed previously for adults. Influenza is associated with seasonal local outbreaks (epidemics) and global outbreaks (pandemics). Influenza viruses are characterized and named for the hemagglutinin (H) and neuraminidase (N) proteins on the surface of the viruses. There are 16 hemagglutinin and 9 neuraminidase subtypes of influenza A, and H1–3 and N1 and 2 are the principal antigenic types found in humans.[11]

Mortality associated with CAP is dependent on the severity of the illness and the age of the patient. In elderly patients admitted to the hospital with severe pneumonia, the mortality rate is up to 40%.[12–15] In the outpatient setting (mild to moderate disease), the mortality rate is less than 5%.[16] Mortality among case reports of CA-MRSA necrotizing pneumonia is 42%.[6] Pneumonia owing to aspiration of oral contents is caused by a variety of anaerobes (*Bacteroides* spp., *Fusobacterium* spp., *Prevotella* spp., and anaerobic gram-positive cocci) as well as *Streptococcus spp. Moraxella catarrhalis,* and *Eikenella corrodens* may be involved but much less frequently.[17,18] When gastric contents are aspirated, enteric gram-negative bacilli and *Staphylococcus aureus* are more commonly the pathogens.[18]

HAP, VAP, and HCAP may be caused by a wide spectrum of organisms. HCAP, early onset HAP and VAP are commonly caused by enteric gram-negative bacilli in addition to the bacteria listed previously for CAP. Late-onset HAP and VAP are more likely to be caused by more resistant enteric gram-negative bacilli, *Pseudomonas aeruginosa, Acinetobacter* spp., or *S. aureus.* Rarely are viruses or fungi a cause of HAP, VAP, or HCAP. The number of infections caused by multidrug-resistant (MDR) bacteria is increasing significantly in hospitalized patients.[3,15,19–21]

PATHOPHYSIOLOGY

Local Host Defenses

Local host defenses of both the upper and lower respiratory tract along with the anatomy of the airways are important in preventing infection. Upper respiratory defenses include the mucociliary apparatus of the nasopharynx, nasal hair, normal bacterial flora, IgA, and complement. Local host defenses of the lower respiratory tract include cough, mucociliary apparatus of the trachea and bronchi, antibodies (IgA, IgM, and IgG), complement, and alveolar macrophages. Mucous lines the cells of the respiratory tract, forming a protective barrier for the cells. This minimizes the ability of organisms to attach to the cells and initiate the infectious process. The squamous epithelial cells of the upper respiratory tract are not ciliated, but those of the columnar epithelial cells of the lower tract are. The cilia beat in a uniform fashion, moving particles up and out of the lower respiratory tract.

Particles greater than 10 microns (μm) are efficiently trapped by mechanisms of the upper airway and are removed from the nasopharynx either by swallowing or by expulsion. The mucociliary apparatus of the trachea and bronchi along with the sharp angles of the bronchi often are effective at trapping and eliminating particles that are 2 to 10 μm in size. Particles in the range of 0.5 to 1 μm may consistently reach the alveolar sacs of the lung. Microorganisms fall within this size range, and if they reach the alveolar sacs, then infection may result if alveolar macrophages and other defenses cannot contain the organisms.

Aspiration

Aspiration of the oropharyngeal or gastric contents may lead to aspiration pneumonia or chemical (acid) pneumonitis. Risk factors for aspiration include dysphagia, change in oropharyngeal colonization, gastroesophageal reflux (GER), and decreased host defenses.

Dysphagia can be caused by stroke or other neurologic disorders, seizures, alcoholism, and aging.[17] Oropharyngeal colonization may be altered by oral/dental disease, poor oral hygiene, tube feedings, or medications. This could result in a higher number

Patient Encounter 1

A 65-year-old man, who only speaks Spanish, presents to your ED complaining of difficulty breathing and shortness of breath. He is accompanied by his daughter and she serves as his translator. His physical examination reveals that he is alert and oriented ×3, has decreased breath sounds on the left side compared with the right, and has rales and crackles in the left lower lobe. His temperature is 38.3°C (100.9°F), respiratory rate is 16 breaths/min, and blood pressure is 120/80 mm Hg. She indicates he is a bit confused and this is not normal for him.

What are his signs and symptoms of pneumonia?

What are the top two bacterial organisms that could be causing the pneumonia?

What are the top two atypical organisms and top two viruses that could be causing the pneumonia?

What are the advantages and disadvantages of having a family member serve as an interpreter for the patient?

of anaerobic organisms in the oral cavity or colonization with enteric gram-negative bacilli.[17] Acid suppression is an important factor in the treatment of GER disease, which may allow enteric gram-negative bacilli to colonize the gastric contents. Finally, impaired mucous production or cilia function, decreased immunoglobulin in secretions, and altered cough reflex may increase the likelihood of infection following an aspiration. The infection can result in a necrotizing pneumonia or lung abscess.

HAP, VAP, HCAP

Risk factors for the development of HAP fall into four general categories: intubation and mechanical ventilation, aspiration, oropharyngeal colonization, and hyperglycemia.

Intubation and mechanical ventilation increase the risk of HAP/VAP 6- to 21-fold.[2,22] VAP may also be related to colonization of the ventilator circuit.[22] Risk of aspiration is increased in these patients due to the supine positioning of the patient, the presence of the endotracheal tube preventing the closure of the epiglottis over the glottis, enteral feedings, GER, and medications.[22] Oropharyngeal colonization is affected by the use of antibiotics, oral antiseptics, and poor infection control measures, which may decrease normal commensal flora and allow pathogenic organisms to colonize the oral cavity. Hyperglycemia may directly or indirectly promote infection; two proposed mechanisms are inhibiting phagocytosis and providing additional nutrients for bacteria.

Once breakdown of the local host defenses occurs and organisms invade the lung tissue, an inflammatory response is generated either by the organisms causing tissue damage or by the immune response to the presence of the organisms. This inflammatory response either can remain localized in the infected tissue or can become systemic. The role of the alveolar macrophages is twofold. First, to engulf the organisms and to contain the infection, and second, to process the antigens for presentation in order to generate a specific immune response by either the cell-mediated or humoral system, or both. The macrophages release cytokines in the area of the infection, which result in increased mucous production, constricting the local vasculature, and lymphatic vessels and attraction of other immune cells to the site. The increase in mucus is associated with symptoms such as cough and sputum production. If tumor necrosis factor alpha (TNF-α) and interleukins-1 and -6 are released systemically, then the symptoms become more severe and include hypotension, organ dysfunction, and/or a septic or septic-shock clinical presentation.

Patient Encounter 2

A 68-year-old woman was admitted to the hospital secondary to a motor vehicle accident. One day after admission she developed respiratory failure and was intubated. She has remained intubated and on day 9 the chest x-ray revealed bilateral lower lobe infiltrates. She is sedated but does respond to commands. Her temperature is 38.9°C (102°F), her blood pressure is 110/75 mm Hg, and her WBC is $20.4 \times 10^3/mm^3$ ($20.4 \times 10^9/L$) with a cell differential of 75% (0.75) neutrophils, 7% (0.07) bands, 15% (0.15) lymphocytes, and 3% (0.03) monocytes.

What are her signs and symptoms of pneumonia?

What are the top three bacterial organisms that could be causing the pneumonia?

CLINICAL PRESENTATION AND DIAGNOSIS

Several scoring systems are available for assessing the severity of the pneumonia: the Pneumonia Severity Index (PSI); confusion, uremia, respiratory rate, blood pressure (CURB); CURB-65 (for those greater than equal to 65 years of age), and systolic BP, oxygenation, age, and respiratory rate (SOAR).[12,15,23] PSI or CURB-65 scores less than or equal to 70 and less than 2 respectively, correlate with mild disease that should be treated in the outpatient setting. These models are used by physicians to help determine the severity of illness, prognosis (mortality risk), and the need for hospitalization and then to help guide in the selection of antimicrobial therapy, along with the use of published guidelines.[12,15,16]

TREATMENT

KEY CONCEPT *The goal of antibiotic therapy is to eliminate the patient's symptoms, minimize or prevent complications, and decrease mortality.* Potential complications secondary to pneumonia include further decline in pulmonary function in patients with underlying pulmonary disease, prolonged mechanical ventilation, bacteremia/sepsis/septic shock, and death. Use of an antimicrobial agent with the narrowest spectrum of activity that covers the suspected pathogen(s) without having activity against organisms not involved in the infection is preferred to minimize the development of resistance.

General Approach to Treatment

Designing a therapeutic regimen for any patient with any type of pneumonia begins with three general categories of consideration:

1. Patient-specific factors that will impact therapy.
2. The top two to three organisms likely causing the infection and resistance issues associated with each organism.
3. The antimicrobials that will cover these organisms. The spectrum should not be too broad or narrow; they should penetrate into the site of infection and be the most cost effective.

Patient factors that need to be considered include age, renal function, drug allergies and/or drug intolerances, immune status (diabetes, neutropenia, or immunocompromised host), cardiopulmonary disease, pregnancy, medical insurance and prescription coverage, exposure to resistant organisms, and prior antibiotic exposure(s).

- The most common pathogens vary with the type of pneumonia, and they are listed in Table 71–1. *M. pneumoniae* lack a cell wall; therefore, β-lactam drugs have no activity against this organism. The atypical organisms have not changed in recent years with respect to antibiotic resistance. β-Lactamase production in *H. influenzae* has remained relatively steady over the last 5 to 10 years, and the rate is approximately 25%.[24] *S. pneumoniae* has developed resistance mechanisms against many classes of antimicrobials, and the mechanisms include the following:
- Alteration of the penicillin-binding proteins (PBPs), inactivating β-lactams
- Efflux or methylation of the ribosome-inactivating macrolides

Clinical Presentation of CAP or Aspiration Pneumonia

General

Patients may experience nonrespiratory symptoms in addition to respiratory symptoms. With increasing age, both respiratory and nonrespiratory symptoms decrease in frequency.

KEY CONCEPT ***Symptoms***

- Respiratory—cough (productive or nonproductive), shortness of breath, and difficulty breathing
- Nonrespiratory—fever, fatigue, sweats, headache, myalgias, mental status changes

KEY CONCEPT ***Signs***

- Temperature may increase or decrease from baseline, but most often it is elevated. The temperature may be sustained or intermittent.
- Respiratory rate is often increased. Cyanosis, increased respiratory rate, and use of accessory muscles of respiration are suggestive of severe respiratory compromise.
- Breath sounds may be diminished. Rales or rhonchi may be heard.
- Confusion, lethargy, and disorientation are relatively common in elderly patients.

Diagnostic Tests

- Chest x-ray should reveal single or multiple infiltrates.
- Oxygen saturation should be more than 90% (0.90), as determined by pulse oximetry.
- Arterial blood gases are beneficial primarily in patients with severe pneumonia.

Laboratory Tests

- The WBC may or may not be elevated. In elderly patients, a drop in WBCs also can be a sign of infection. The differential should show a predominance of neutrophils if a bacterial infection is present. The presence of bands also could be an indicator of bacterial infection. Elevated lymphocytes are an indication of viral infection.
- Blood urea nitrogen (BUN) and serum creatinine are needed to dose antibiotics appropriately and to minimize or prevent drug toxicity (especially in the elderly patient).

Microbiology Tests

- Sputum Gram stain should demonstrate the presence of WBCs and the absence of squamous epithelial cells. It may or may not show a predominance of one type of organism.
- Sputum culture and susceptibility are not obtained in the outpatient setting. The value of culturing is debated owing to the rapidity in which *S. pneumoniae* dies in transport media and the inability to reliably or routinely culture atypical organisms.
- Bronchoscopy may be performed to improve the ability to diagnose pneumonia. Tracheal secretions often are better specimens than sputum owing to the lack of oral contamination.
- Serology (IgM and IgG) is useful in determining the presence of atypical organisms such as *Mycoplasma* and *Chlamydia*.
- Urinary Legionella antigen is used to diagnose *L. pneumophila*.
- Polymerase chain reaction (PCR) is being used more frequently to detect the DNA of respiratory pathogens.
- Blood cultures should be obtained in all patients admitted to the ICU with pneumonia. Positive blood cultures are present in about 1% to 20% of patients with CAP.

Clinical Presentation of Severe CAP or Aspiration Pneumonia

General

In approximately 10% of patients, CAP will be severe enough to require intensive care or mechanical ventilation.

KEY CONCEPT ***Symptoms***

- Respiratory—cough (productive or nonproductive), shortness of breath, difficulty breathing
- Nonrespiratory—fever, fatigue, sweats, headache, myalgias, mental status changes

Signs

- Temperature may increase or decrease from baseline, but most often it is elevated. The temperature may be sustained or intermittent.
- Respiratory rate greater than 30 breaths/min. Cyanosis and use of accessory muscles of respiration along with the increased respiratory rate are suggestive of severe respiratory compromise.
- Hypotension (systolic blood pressure less than 90 mm Hg or diastolic blood pressure less than 60 mm Hg).
- Requirement for vasopressors.
- Breath sounds may be diminished. Rales or rhonchi may be heard.
- Urine output less than 20 mL/hour or less than 80 mL over 4 hours.
- Confusion, lethargy, and disorientation are relatively common in elderly patients.

Diagnostic Tests

As stated in the clinical presentation of community-acquired or aspiration pneumonia.

Laboratory Tests

As stated in the clinical presentation of community-acquired or aspiration pneumonia.

Microbiology Tests

As stated in the clinical presentation of community acquired or aspiration pneumonia.

Diagnosis of VAP

Clinical Strategy

- Chest x-ray should reveal a new infiltrate *plus* two of the following:
  - Temperature greater than 38.0°C (100.4°F)
  - Leukocytosis or leukopenia
  - Purulent secretions
  - Semiquantitative cultures are obtained to identify the pathogen(s)
- Tracheal aspirates grow more organisms than invasive quantitative cultures and often result in overuse of antibiotics
- The major limitation of the clinical strategy is the consistent overprescribing of antibiotics

Bacteriologic Strategy

- Uses quantitative culture of endotracheal aspirates, bronchoalveolar lavage (BAL), or protected specimen brush (PSB)
- Greater than or equal to 10^6 cfu/mL (10^9cfu/L) for endotracheal aspirates
- Greater than or equal to 10^4 to 10^5 cfu/mL (10^7–10^8cfu/L) for BAL
- Greater than or equal to 10^3 cfu/mL (10^6cfu/L) for PSB
- The advantage of this method is that it separates colonization from infection better than culturing tracheal aspirates
- The limitation is the potential misinterpretation of negative culture results. These samples should be obtained prior to antibiotics being started

Recommended Diagnostic Strategy

- Combination of the preceding two methods:
  - Obtain either a quantitative or semiquantitative culture of a lower respiratory sample. Initiate empirical broad-spectrum antibiotic therapy
  - Days 2 and 3: Check culture results, and assess clinical response to therapy: temperature, WBCs, chest x-ray, oxygenation, purulent sputum, hemodynamic changes, and organ function
- Assess clinical improvement at 48 to 72 hours:
  - Improvement and culture negative—stop antibiotics
  - Improvement and culture positive—narrow antibiotic therapy
  - No improvement and culture negative—consider other pathogens, complications, or other diagnosis
  - No improvement and culture positive—change antibiotic therapy and consider other pathogens, complications, or other diagnosis

Patient Encounter 3, Part 1: Medical History, Physical Examination, and Diagnostic Tests

A 65-year-old man presents to your ED complaining of difficulty breathing and shortness of breath.

PMH: Hypertension for 8 years, COPD for 5 years, currently controlled

FH: Father died of lung cancer at the age of 68 years; mother died of natural causes

SH: Denies alcohol use, smokes 1 pack per day for 15 years. Lives alone and has 2 children. He is 5′8″ (173 cm) and weighs 140 lb (63.6 kg)

Allergies: NKDA

Meds: Hydrochlorothiazide 25 mg orally once daily; fluticasone propionate/salmeterol 250/50 mcg one inhalation twice daily; albuterol inhaler 1 to 2 inhalations every 4 hours as needed for shortness of breath

ROS: (+) difficulty breathing and shortness of breath; (–) chest pain, N/V/D, change in appetite

PE:

VS: BP 120/80, P 82, RR 22, T 38.6°C (101.5°F)

CV: RRR, normal S_1, S_2; no murmurs, rubs, or gallops

Lungs: Decreased breath sounds on the left side compared with the right with rales and crackles in the left lower lobe

Abd: Soft, nontender, nondistended; (+) bowel sounds, no hepatosplenomegaly, heme (–) stool

Neuro: Oriented to name and place, confused

Diagnostic Tests: Chest x-ray: left lower lobe infiltrates; oxygen saturation 84% (0.84) on room air

Labs: WBCs 14.2×10^3/mm^3 (14.2×10^9/L) with a cell differential of 70% (0.70) neutrophils, 2% (0.02) bands, 20% (0.20) lymphocytes, and 8% (0.08) monocytes; BUN 9 mg/dL (3.2 mmol/L), SCr 0.9 mg/dL (80 μmol/L), glucose 90 mg/dL (5.0 mmol/L); sputum Gram stain: moderate gram-positive cocci, few gram-negative bacilli, many WBCs; sputum culture is pending

Given this additional information, what is your assessment of the patient's condition?

Identify your treatment goals for the patient.

What organisms should you include in your list of potential pathogens?

What pharmacologic agents are available for treating this patient?

- Ribosome protection (tetM gene) inactivating tetracyclines
- Alteration of DNA gyrase or topoisomerase IV inactivating fluoroquinolones

S. pneumoniae resistance to commonly prescribed antimicrobials such as the penicillins and macrolides/azalides dramatically increased in the late 1980s through the mid- to late 1990s and has remained relatively flat in the 2000s. Resistance information collected nationally along with susceptibility testing for a new antimicrobials, demonstrates that average national rates of resistance to penicillin and macrolides were approximately 13% and 38%, respectively.[25,26] Resistance to trimethoprim/sulfamethoxazole is approximately 25%, and fluoroquinolone resistance remains less than 0.5%.[26]

For HCAP, HAP, and VAP, the risk of infection from an MDR pathogen is relatively high. The number and type of organisms that are MDR vary from hospital to hospital, making it more difficult to generate guidelines for treatment. Therefore, the treatment recommendations may be too broad or too narrow for any given institution. Treating patients with HCAP, HAP, or VAP is more complex than treating patients with CAP. There are many factors to consider, and one of those relates to the timing of infection to the most likely pathogens. Early-onset infection is less likely to be caused by MDR pathogens than late-onset infection. In early-onset infection, community pathogens such as pneumococcus, *Legionella*, and *Mycoplasma* need to be considered as well as some of the hospital pathogens. Patients developing late-onset pneumonia are at increased risk for resistant pathogens or MDR pathogens such as MRSA, enteric gram-negative bacilli, *Pseudomonas*, and *Acinetobacter*. Risk factors for developing infection caused by a resistant pathogen are as follows:

- Antimicrobial therapy in preceding 90 days
- Current hospitalization of at least 5 days
- High occurrence of antibiotic resistance in the community or in the specific hospital unit
- Immunosuppressive disease and/or therapy
- Presence of risk factors for HCAP:
  - Hospitalization for 2 days or more in the preceding 90 days
  - Residence in a nursing home or extended-care facility
  - Home infusion therapy (including antibiotics)
  - Peritoneal or hemodialysis within 30 days
  - Home wound care
  - Close contact family member with MDR pathogen

Once these issues are addressed, antimicrobial therapy can be selected and initiated. The patient- and drug-related categories are common to all types of pneumonia, but the organisms vary with the type of pneumonia. Guidelines have been generated by experts in the field for all types of pneumonia. These guidelines were generated to provide practitioners with evidence-based therapeutic options for the management of patients with pneumonia. The evidence-based guidelines generated by the American Thoracic Society and Infectious Diseases Society of America were derived from VAP and applied to HCAP and HAP.

Pharmacologic Therapy for CAP

KEY CONCEPT *Treatment of CAP is predominantly empiric, that is, treatment is started without knowing the causative pathogen.* The most recent guidelines are the result of a collaboration between the Infectious Diseases Society of America and the American Thoracic Society.[27] The approach to patient care is based on the classification of patients into two broad categories, outpatient and inpatient, and then further dividing the groups by comorbid conditions and location in the hospital, respectively. These guidelines use patient-specific data along with predominant pathogen information to design appropriate empirical antimicrobial regimens. Table 71–2 summarizes these therapeutic options.

▶ *Adult Outpatient Previously Healthy*

First-line therapeutic options for treating previously healthy adults include use of a macrolide (erythromycin, clarithromycin)

Patient Encounter 3, Part 2: Medical History, Physical Examination, and Diagnostic Tests

A 68-year-old woman was admitted to the hospital secondary to a motor vehicle accident. One day after admission she developed respiratory failure and was intubated. She has remained intubated and on day 9 the chest x-ray revealed bilateral lower lobe infiltrates. She is sedated but does respond to commands.

PMH: Hypertension for 15 years, currently controlled

FH: Father and mother deceased from natural causes. Both had hypertension, mother had hypothyroidism

SH: Denies tobacco, social alcohol one to two glasses of wine per week. She lives with her husband; retired teacher. She is 5′6″ in (168 cm) and weighs 68.2 kg (150 lb)

Allergies: Penicillin—hives

Meds: Losartan 50 mg orally once daily

PE:

VS: BP 100/70, P 78, T 38.7°C (101.6°F)

CV: RRR, normal S_1, S_2; no murmurs, rubs, or gallops

Abd: Soft, nontender, nondistended; (+) bowel sounds, no hepatosplenomegaly

Diagnostic Tests: Chest x-ray: bilateral lower lobe infiltrates; oxygen saturation 98% (0.98) on ventilator

Labs: WBC is $20.4 \times 10^3/mm^3$ ($20.4 \times 10^9/L$) with a cell differential of 75% (0.75) neutrophils, 7% (0.07) bands, 15% (0.15) lymphocytes, and 3% (0.03) monocytes; BUN 10 mg/dL (3.6 mmol/L), SCr 0.9 mg/dL (80 μmol/L); BAL Gram stain: many gram-negative bacilli, moderate gram-positive cocci in clusters, many WBCs; culture is pending

Given this additional information, what is your assessment of the patient's condition?

Identify your treatment goals for the patient.

What organisms should you include in your list of potential pathogens?

What pharmacologic agents are available for treating this patient?

Table 71–2

Summary of CAP Treatment

Adult outpatient otherwise healthy Empirical coverage against *S. pneumoniae, M. pneumoniae, C. pneumoniae,* and *H. influenzae*	*Monotherapy* Azithromycin, clarithromycin, erythromycin, doxycycline
Adult outpatient comorbidities Empirical coverage against *S. pneumoniae, M. pneumoniae, C. pneumoniae,* and *H. influenzae*	*Combination therapy* High-dose amoxicillin, or high-dose amoxicillin-clavulanate (alternatives are cefpodoxime, or cefuroxime, or ceftriaxone) *plus* azithromycin, or clarithromycin or, doxycycline *Monotherapy* Gemifloxacin, levofloxacin, moxifloxacin
Adult inpatient (non-ICU) Empirical coverage against *S. pneumoniae, H. influenzae, M. pneumoniae,* and *C. pneumoniae*	*Combination therapy* Cefotaxime, or ceftriaxone, or ampicillin-sulbactam, or ertapenem *plus* azithromycin, or clarithromycin, or doxycycline *Monotherapy* Gemifloxacin, levofloxacin, moxifloxacin
Adult inpatient ICU (no Pseudomonas*)* Empirical coverage against *S. pneumoniae, L. pneumophila, H. influenzae,* enteric GNB, and *S. aureus*	*Combination therapy* Cefotaxime or ceftriaxone *plus* azithromycin, or levofloxacin, or moxifloxacin
Adult inpatient ICU (Pseudomonas is a concern) Empirical coverage against *P. aeruginosa, S. pneumoniae, L. pneumophila, H. influenzae,* enteric GNB, and *S. aureus*	*Combination therapy* Cefepime, or ceftazidime, or piperacillin-tazobactam, or imipenem, or meropenem *plus* or ciprofloxacin or levofloxacin or an aminoglycoside If an aminoglycoside is chosen, then add azithromycin or levofloxacin or moxifloxacin
Adult inpatient non-ICU or ICU (MRSA is a concern) Empirical coverage against *S. pneumoniae, L. pneumophila, H. influenzae,* enteric GNB, and *S. aureus (Pseudomonas* if ICU)	Add vancomycin or linezolid to the regimens listed above
Pediatric outpatient Empirical coverage against *S. pneumoniae, M. pneumoniae,* and *C. pneumoniae*	*Monotherapy* High-dose amoxicillin, or high-dose amoxicillin-clavulanate, or intramuscular ceftriaxone, or azithromycin, or clarithromycin
Pediatric inpatient (non-ICU) Empirical coverage against *S. pneumoniae*	*Monotherapy* Fully immunized child—ampicillin or penicillin G Partially immunized child—ceftriaxone or cefotaxime
Empirical coverage against *S. pneumoniae, H. influenzae, M. pneumoniae,* and *C. pneumoniae*	*Combination therapy* IV cefuroxime, or cefotaxime, or ceftriaxone, or ampicillin-sulbactam plus azithromycin, or clarithromycin
Pediatric inpatient ICU Empirical coverage against *S. pneumoniae, L. pneumophila, H. influenzae,* enteric GNB, and *S. aureus*	*Combination therapy* Cefotaxime, or ceftriaxone plus azithromycin, or clarithromycin

CA-MRSA, community-acquired methicillin-resistant *Staphylococcus aureus;* GNB, gram-negative bacteria; ICU, intensive care unit.

or an azalide (azithromycin) or doxycycline.[27] If a patient has failed therapy with a macrolide, azalide, or doxycycline, one has to consider why the patient failed. The most common reasons are either medication adherence issues or the presence of resistant organisms. If a resistant organism is suspected, then use of one of the respiratory fluoroquinolones active against *S. pneumoniae* (gemifloxacin, levofloxacin, or moxifloxacin) is warranted.

▸ *Adult Outpatient with Comorbid Conditions*

The comorbid conditions that can impact therapy and outcomes in patients with CAP include diabetes mellitus, COPD, chronic heart, liver, or renal disease, alcoholism, malignancy, asplenia, and immunosuppressive condition or use of immunosuppressive drugs.[27] If the patient did not receive antibiotics in the last 3 months, then either a respiratory fluoroquinolone alone or a combination of an oral β-lactam agent plus a macrolide or azalide is recommended. If the patient received an antibiotic in the last 3 months, the recommendation is to use an agent from a different class. Doxycycline is an acceptable alternative to a macrolide or azalide.

The preferred β-lactam antimicrobial agents are high-dose (3 g daily) amoxicillin or high-dose (4 g daily) amoxicillin-clavulanate. Alternative β-lactams are second- and third-generation cephalosporins such as cefuroxime, cefpodoxime, or ceftriaxone.

▸ *Adult Inpatient Not in the ICU*

For patients admitted to the hospital with CAP, the severity of illness is generally increased (caused either by the organism itself

Patient Encounter 4, Part 1: Creating a Care Plan

Based on the information presented, create a care plan for this patient's pneumonia. Your plan should include:

(a) A statement of drug-related needs and/or problems

(b) A patient-specific detailed therapeutic plan

(c) Monitoring parameters to assess efficacy and safety

or underlying comorbidities in the patient), and the pathogens are essentially the same as in the outpatient setting. Recommendations are to use either a respiratory fluoroquinolone alone or a combination of an IV β-lactam antimicrobial agent plus an advanced macrolide/azalide (clarithromycin/azithromycin) or doxycycline. The recommended β-lactams include cefotaxime, ceftriaxone, ampicillin-sulbactam, or ertapenem.[27] The first antibiotic dose should be administered within the first 24 hours of admission. Conversion to oral therapy should occur when the patient is hemodynamically stable, improving clinically, and able to take oral medications, which often is within 48 to 72 hours for most patients. Discharge from the hospital should be as soon as the patient is stable and without other medical complications. The need to observe the patient in the hospital on their oral antibiotic is not necessary.[27]

► *Adult Inpatient in the ICU*

Patients admitted to the ICU have severe pneumonia, and the likely etiology includes *S. pneumoniae* and *H. influenzae* as in the other categories; however, the incidence of *L. pneumophila* increases in this setting and should be considered a potential pathogen. In addition, enteric gram-negative bacilli and *S. aureus* are more frequently the cause of the pneumonia in these patients. The recommendations are to treat with an IV β-lactam plus either azithromycin or a respiratory fluoroquinolone. These combination therapies minimize the risk of treatment failure due to a resistant pathogen as well as provide broad coverage.[27] The β-lactams are the same as for inpatient non-ICU treatment. If the patient is allergic to β-lactams, then aztreonam plus a respiratory fluoroquinolone are preferred.

If *P. aeruginosa* is suspected, then the antimicrobial treatment must be broadened to cover *Pseudomonas* as well as the organisms listed previously. Owing to the high resistance rates observed with *Pseudomonas*, the recommended regimens empirically double cover the *Pseudomonas* to ensure at least one of the antibiotics is active against it. The regimens include the use of an antipneumococcal, antipseudomonal β-lactam (cefepime, ceftazidime, piperacillin/tazobactam, imipenem, or meropenem), plus either ciprofloxacin or levofloxacin or an aminoglycoside. If the aminoglycoside is chosen, then either IV azithromycin or a respiratory fluoroquinolone should be added to cover *S. pneumoniae* and the atypical bacterial organisms.[27]

If CA-MRSA is suspected in the patient, then the addition of vancomycin or linezolid to the preceding regimen should be considered. Daptomycin cannot be used because surfactant in the lung inactivates the drug, thus rendering it ineffective for pneumonia. CA-MRSA can cause a necrotizing pneumonia, and the cause is believed to be due to its many virulence factors, including the Panton-Valentine leukocidin toxin.[6] In these patients the use of an agent that decreases toxin production may be beneficial. Linezolid decreases toxin production; the other recommended agents to decrease toxin production and added to vancomycin therapy are clindamycin or a respiratory fluoroquinolone.[27]

► *Influenza*

Influenza viruses A and B can cause pneumonia in pediatric and adult patients. Amantadine and rimantadine are available oral agents with activity against influenza virus type A. If started within 48 hours of the onset of the first symptoms, they reduce the duration of the illness by about 1.3 days. Oseltamivir and zanamivir are oral agents active against both type A and B influenza that reduce the duration of the illness by about 1.3 days if initiated within 40 to 48 hours of the first symptoms.[28] For active infection beyond the first 48 hours, none of these agents are effective in treating infection, and supportive care is the best treatment for these patients.

> **Patient Encounter 4, Part 2: Creating a Care Plan**
>
> *Based on the information presented, create a care plan for this patient's pneumonia. Your plan should include:*
>
> *(a) A statement of drug-related needs and/or problems*
>
> *(b) A patient-specific detailed therapeutic plan*
>
> *(c) Monitoring parameters to assess efficacy and safety*

► *Aspiration*

Anaerobes and *Streptococcus* spp. are the primary pathogens if a patient aspirates their oral contents and develops pneumonia. Antibiotics active against these organisms include penicillin G, ampicillin/sulbactam, and clindamycin. If the patient aspirates oral and gastric contents, then anaerobes and gram-negative bacilli are the primary pathogens. The preferred treatment regimen is a β-lactam/β-lactamase inhibitor combination (ampicillin/sulbactam, amoxicillin/clavulanate, piperacillin/tazobactam, or ticarcillin/clavulanate).[27]

► *Pediatric Outpatient*

Guidelines have been published for treating CAP in children. The most predominant pathogens in preschool children in the outpatient setting are viruses, and often supportive therapy (maintaining hydration, antipyretics) is all that is needed.[29] For appropriately immunized infants, children, and adolescents with mild-to-moderate pneumonia in an area lacking high-level penicillin-resistant pneumococcus, high-dose amoxicillin is the recommended first-line therapy. If atypical organisms are considered likely, then a macrolide is recommended. If moderate to severe CAP is diagnosed and it is during influenza season, then treatment with oseltamivir, zanamivir (Relenza), amantadine, or rimantadine is recommended.[29] Fluoroquinolones and tetracyclines should not be used in children younger than 5 years. Dosing of antibiotics for pediatric patients is presented in Table 71–3.

► *Pediatric Inpatient*

If the infant or child is fully immunized, then the guidelines recommend the use of IV penicillin G or ampicillin. Alternative β-lactams include IV cefotaxime or ceftriaxone. If the infant or child is not fully immunized, then the third-generation cephalosporins (cefotaxime or ceftriaxone) should be administered.[29] If atypical organisms are suspected, add azithromycin to the β-lactam. If community-acquired MRSA is suspected, then vancomycin or clindamycin should be added to the regimen.[29]

Pharmacologic Therapy for HCAP/HAP/VAP

Nosocomial pneumonia has since been replaced by the terms *health care–associated pneumonia*, *hospital-associated pneumonia*, and *ventilator-associated pneumonia*. KEY CONCEPT *Empirical selection of antimicrobial therapy for ventilator-, health care–, and hospital-associated pneumonia is broad spectrum; however, once culture and susceptibility information are available, the therapy should be narrowed (de-escalation) to cover the identified*

Table 71–3

CAP Antimicrobial Dosing in Pediatric Patients

	Body Weight < 2000 g		Body Weight > 2000 g		
Drug (Route)	**0–7 Days Old**	**7–28 Days Old**	**0–7 Days Old**	**7–28 Days Old**	**> 28 Days Old**
Amoxicillin (po)				15 mg/kg every 12 hours	17 mg/kg every 8 hours
Amoxicillin-clavulanate (po)			15 mg/kg every 12 hours	15 mg/kg every 12 hours	45 mg/kg every 12 hours
Cefotaxime (IV)	50 mg/kg every 12 hours	50 mg/kg every 8 hours	50 mg/kg every 12 hours	50 mg/kg every 8 hours	50 mg/kg every 8 hours
Ceftriaxone (IM/IV)	25 mg/kg every 24 hours	50 mg/kg every 24 hours	25 mg/kg every 24 hours	50 mg/kg every 24 hours	50 mg/kg every 24 hours
Cefuroxime (po)					15 mg/kg every 12 hours
Azithromycin (po/IV)	5 mg/kg every 24 hours	10 mg/kg every 24 hours	5 mg/kg every 24 hours	10 mg/kg every 24 hours	10 mg/kg every 24 hours
Clarithromycin (po)					7.5 mg/kg every 12 hours

pathogen(s). Two factors important to the empirical selection of antibiotics for these types of pneumonia are onset time after admission and risk factors for MDR organisms. If it is early onset (less than equal to 5 days since admission), and there are no risk factors for MDR organisms, then the most frequent pathogens include *S. pneumoniae, H. influenzae*, methicillin-susceptible *Staphylococcus aureus* (MSSA), and enteric gram-negative bacilli. Recommendations for therapy include third-generation cephalosporins such as ceftriaxone or cefotaxime; a respiratory fluoroquinolone such as gemifloxacin, levofloxacin, or moxifloxacin; ampicillin/sulbactam; or ertapenem.[7] If it is late onset pneumonia and/or there are risk factors for MDR organisms, then the pathogen list includes *P. aeruginosa*, extended-spectrum β-lactamase–producing *K. pneumoniae, Acinetobacter* spp., and MRSA. Empirical antibiotic selection must cover *P. aeruginosa*, which often then covers the other gram-negative pathogens. Available antibiotics include cefepime, ceftazidime, imipenem, meropenem, piperacillin/tazobactam, ticarcillin/clavulanate, levofloxacin, ciprofloxacin, gentamicin, tobramycin, and amikacin. Empirical therapy for late-onset pneumonia (listed in Table 71–4) could include any of the β-lactams, carbapenems, or fluoroquinolones alone or in combination with one of the aminoglycosides. If MRSA is suspected, then either vancomycin or linezolid should be added to the regimen. Recommendations for vancomycin trough concentrations of 15 to 20 mcg/mL (15–20 mg/L; 10–14 μmol/L) were based on expert opinion, not evidence from clinical trials.[2]

Currently there is debate over whether or not double coverage for *Pseudomonas* is required. In vitro studies have shown that aminoglycosides exhibit synergistic killing against gram-negative bacilli when combined with β-lactams. Dosing of the aminoglycosides is dependent on the patient's renal function. A high-dose once-daily regimen (eg, 4–7 mg/kg gentamicin or tobramycin or 15–20 mg/kg amikacin) can be utilized in patients with good renal function. Most of the studies enrolled patients with estimated creatinine clearances of at least 70 mL/min (1.17 mL/s). Meta-analyses have shown high-dose once-daily regimens to be as efficacious as and less toxic than divided daily dosing.[30–34] Divided daily dosing (eg, 1 to 2 mg/kg gentamicin or tobramycin or 7.5 mg/kg amikacin) has been utilized since the 1970s, and the dosing interval is based on the patient's renal function to achieve a trough concentration of less than 2 mcg/mL (2 mg/L; 4 μmol/L) for gentamicin and tobramycin and less than 5 mcg/mL (5 mg/L; 9 μmol/L) for amikacin.

In addition to obtaining a synergistic effect, another reason for double coverage when treating VAP, HAP, or HCAP is to broaden the coverage empirically to increase the likelihood of covering the majority of resistant pathogens. VAP is the most studied of these types of pneumonias and is often the most severe. There is an increase in mortality when inadequate therapy is initiated for VAP. Crude mortality ranges are quite large (35%–92%) compared with estimates of attributable mortality (approximately 9%); however, attributable mortality studies are limited by the large sample size needed to accurately measure this outcome.[35–37]

KEY CONCEPT *Once a pathogen or pathogens have been identified, therapy should be narrowed (de-escalated) to cover only those*

Table 71–4

Empirical Therapy for Late-Onset HAP, HCAP, or VAP in Adults

Antibiotic (Route)	Dosage[a]
Cefepime (IV)	2 g every 8–12 hour
Ceftazidime (IV)	2 g every 8 hour
Imipenem (IV)	500 mg every 6 hour
Meropenem (IV)	1 g every 8 hour
Piperacillin-tazobactam (IV)	4.5 g every 6 hour
Ticarcillin-clavulanate (IV)	
Levofloxacin (IV/po)	750 mg every 24 hour
Ciprofloxacin (IV)	400 mg every 8 hour
Ciprofloxacin (po)	500 mg every 8 hour
Gentamicin or Tobramcyin[b] (IV)	5–7 mg/kg every 24 hour
Amikacin[b] (IV)	20 mg/kg every 24 hour
Vancomycin (IV)	15–20 mg/kg every 12 hour
Linezolid (IV/po)	600 mg every 12 hour

[a]Dosages are based on normal renal and hepatic function and should be adjusted as appropriate for each patient.

[b]Trough concentrations ideally should be nondetectable; less than 1 mcg/mL for gentamicin and tobramycin (1 mg/L; 2 μmol/L) and less than 4 to 5 mcg/mL (4–5 mg/L; 7–9 μmol/L) for amikacin.

pathogens. Use of broad-spectrum antibiotics for prolonged durations increases the risk of colonization with MDR pathogens.

Duration of Antimicrobial Therapy

KEY CONCEPT *The duration of therapy for pneumonia should be kept as short as possible* and depends on several factors: type of pneumonia, inpatient or outpatient status, patient comorbidities, bacteremia/sepsis, and the antibiotic chosen. If the duration of therapy is too prolonged, then it can have a negative impact on the patient's normal flora in the respiratory and gastrointestinal tracts, vaginal tract of women, and on the skin. This can result in colonization with resistant pathogens, *Clostridium difficile* colitis, or overgrowth of yeast. In addition, the longer antibiotics are administered, the greater the chance for toxicity from the agent, as well as an increase in cost.

For treating adult outpatient CAP, two antibiotics are approved for a 5-day duration of therapy, levofloxacin (the 750-mg dose) and azithromycin. The recommended duration of therapy for all other therapies is 7 to 10 days. For treatment of CAP in adult patients admitted to the hospital, the duration is dependent on whether or not blood cultures were positive. In the absence of positive blood cultures, the duration of therapy is 7 to 10 days. If blood cultures were positive, the duration of therapy should be 2 weeks from the day blood cultures first became negative. The duration of therapy in pediatric patients is 10 days for uncomplicated CAP, with the exception of azithromycin, which is approved for 5 days.[29]

The duration of therapy cited in the literature for HCAP, HAP, or VAP ranges from 10 to 21 days. Efforts should be made to shorten the duration of therapy from the traditional 14 to 21 days to periods as short as 7 days, provided that the etiologic pathogen is not *P. aeruginosa* and that the patient has a good clinical response with resolution of clinical features of infection. Shortening the duration of therapy is beneficial because of the colonization, toxicity, and cost issues. Several studies evaluated mortality, clinical success, recurrence, or the development of resistance with shorter courses of therapy for VAP and found no differences when compared with longer courses of therapy.[36,38] The Clinical Pulmonary Infection Score (CPIS) has been used to determine when to end therapy for VAP. Using CPIS, patients who survived VAP and were treated with adequate therapy clinically improved within 3 to 5 days.[39] This study was instrumental in recommending a shortened duration of therapy of 6 days.

OUTCOME EVALUATION

For CAP, outcomes include preventing hospitalization, shortening the duration of hospitalization, and minimizing mortality. Improvement of symptoms should occur within 24 to 72 hours after initiation of therapy for most patients with CAP. Response to therapy could be slowed in patients with underlying pulmonary disease such as moderate to severe asthma, COPD, or emphysema. In patients not responding to therapy consider patient comorbid conditions, other infectious and noninfectious reasons, and a drug-resistant pathogen must be considered. Noninfectious reasons to consider include pulmonary embolus, congestive heart failure, carcinoma, lymphoma, intrapulmonary hemorrhage, and certain inflammatory lung diseases.

Outcome parameters for VAP, HAP, and HCAP are similar to those with CAP. Clinical improvement should occur within 48 to 72 hours of the start of therapy. If a patient is not responding to therapy, then, again, consider infectious and noninfectious reasons. Infectious explanations are the same as for CAP stated above, but noninfectious are not. They include atelectasis, acute respiratory distress syndrome (ARDS), pulmonary embolism or hemorrhage, cancer, empyema, or lung abscess.

PREVENTION

KEY CONCEPT *Prevention of both pneumococcal and influenza pneumonia by use of vaccination is a national goal.* Vaccination is used to prevent or minimize the severity of pneumonia caused by *S. pneumoniae* or the influenza virus.

The influenza vaccine is available in two forms, injectable and nasal inhalation. There are two forms of the injectable inactivated vaccine (containing killed virus). The regular influenza vaccine is approved for use in people older than 6 months of age, including healthy people and people with chronic medical conditions. Fluzone intradermal vaccine is indicated for adults 18 through 64 years of age against influenza disease caused by virus subtypes A and type B. The high-dose influenza vaccine

Patient Care Process

KEY CONCEPT *Monitoring response to therapy is essential for determining efficacy, identifying adverse reactions, and determining the duration of therapy.*

Patient Assessment:

- Symptoms and status (ie, inpatient, outpatient, or intubated) to determine the type of pneumonia.
- Comorbid conditions of asthma, COPD, or emphysema, smoking history.
- Chest x-ray, pulse oximetry.
- Allergies and drug intolerances, noting the severity of the reaction.

Therapy Evaluation:

- What are the top two to three organisms associated with the type of pneumonia the patient has?
- Select an appropriate empirical antibiotic regimen for the patient and type of pneumonia, ensuring that the doses are correct for renal function (see Tables 71–2 and 71–3).

Care Plan:

- Assess the effectiveness of the antibiotic therapy after 24 to 72 hours looking for improvement in signs and symptoms.
- If the patient is not improving, then reevaluate the diagnosis and pathogen list, and make appropriate changes to therapy.
- Assess the patient for conversion from IV to oral therapy.
- Assess the patient for the presence of adverse drug reactions, drug allergies, and drug interactions.

Follow-up Evaluation:

- If the patient responds to therapy within the first 72 hours consider a short course of therapy.

is recommended for those 65 years of age and older. The nasal-spray influenza vaccine is made with live, weakened influenza viruses that do not cause the influenza (live attenuated influenza vaccine). This formulation is approved for use in healthy people 2 to 49 years of age who are not pregnant. The ability of influenza vaccine to protect a person depends on two key factors: the age and health status of the person getting the vaccine, and the similarity or "match" between the virus strains in the vaccine and those in circulation. Protective antibodies are detected approximately 2 weeks after vaccination. In February 2010, the Centers for Disease Control and Prevention (CDC) adopted a universal influenza vaccination policy, thus recommending all persons 6 months of age and older to be vaccinated annually. The CDC indentified high risk groups in whom vaccination is especially important[40]:

1. Pregnant women
2. Children younger than 5, but especially children younger than 2 years old
3. People 50 years of age and older
4. People of any age with certain chronic medical conditions
5. People who live in nursing homes and other long-term care facilities
6. People who live with or care for those at high risk for complications from flu, including:
    - Health care workers
    - Household contacts of persons at high risk for complications from the flu
    - Household contacts and out-of-home caregivers of children less than 6 months (these children are too young to be vaccinated)

The 13-valent conjugated pneumococcal vaccine (PCV13) is recommended for children younger than 5 years (6 years if chronic health conditions are present) and the 23-purified-capsular polysaccharide antigen vaccine (PPSV23) for children 5 years of age and older and adults. The serotypes in the PCV13 are the most common disease-causing strains of pneumococcus.[41,42] The minimum age to receive the PCV is 6 weeks, and the recommended age range is between 12 and 15 months. A reliable immunologic response to the PCV13 has been demonstrated, along with a favorable safety profile.[42,43] The PCV13 is also recommended for adults aged 19 years or older with immunocompromising conditions, functional or anatomic asplenia, cerebrospinal fluid (CSF) leaks, or cochlear implants in addition to receiving the PPSV23 vaccine.[40] The 23 capsular types in the PPSV23 represent at least 85% to 90% of the serotypes that cause invasive pneumococcal infections among children and adults in the United States. Ten years after vaccination, a sample of elderly individuals demonstrated significant quantity of protective antibodies.[44] Those who should receive the polysaccharide vaccine include the following[40]:

1. *All adults 65 years or older should receive one dose.*
2. *Anyone older than 6 years who has a long-term health* problem such as heart disease, lung disease, sickle cell disease, diabetes, alcoholism, cirrhosis, and leakage of cerebrospinal fluid.
3. *Anyone older than 6 years who has a disease or condition* or *is taking any drug that lowers the body's resistance to infection*, such as Hodgkin disease, lymphoma, leukemia, kidney failure, multiple myeloma, nephrotic syndrome, HIV infection or AIDS, damaged spleen or no spleen, organ transplant, long-term steroids, certain cancer drugs, or radiation therapy.

For patients who meet the qualifications, discuss the value of vaccination against *S. pneumoniae* and/or influenza.

Abbreviations Introduced in This Chapter

ARDS	Acute respiratory distress syndrome
ATS	American Thoracic Society
BUN	Blood urea nitrogen
CA-MRSA	Community-acquired methicillin-resistant *Staphylococcus aureus*
CAP	Community-acquired pneumonia
CDC	Center for Disease Control and Prevention
COPD	Chronic obstructive pulmonary disease
CPIS	Clinical Pulmonary Infection Score
DFA	Direct fluorescence antigen
GER(D)	Gastroesophageal reflux (disease)
H	Hemagglutinin
HAP	Hospital-acquired pneumonia
HCAP	Health care–associated pneumonia
IDDM	Insulin-dependent diabetes mellitus
IDSA	Infectious Diseases Society of America
MDR	Multidrug resistant
MRSA	Methicillin-resistant *Staphylococcus aureus*
MSSA	Methicillin-susceptible *Staphylococcus aureus*
N	Neuraminidase
Pao_2/Fio_2	Arterial oxygen pressure/fraction of inspired oxygen
PBP	Penicillin-binding protein
PCR	Polymerase chain reaction
PCV13	Pneumococcal 13-valent conjugated vaccine
PPSV23	Purified-capsular polysaccharide 23 antigen vaccine
TNF-α	Tumor necrosis factor alpha
VAP	Ventilator-associated pneumonia

REFERENCES

1. Masterton R. The place of guidelines in hospital-acquired pneumonia. J Hosp Infect. 2007;66(2):116–122.
2. Niederman MS, Craven DE. Guidelines for the management of adults with hospital-acquired, ventilator-associated, and healthcare-associated pneumonia. Am J Resp Crit Care. Med 2005;171(4):388–416.
3. Polverino E, Dambrava P, Cill, et al. Nursing home-acquired pneumonia: A 10 year single-centre experience. Thorax. 2010;65(4):354.
4. Lees AW, McNaught W. Bacteriology of lower-respiratory-tract secretions, sputum, and upper-respiratory-tract secretions in "normals" and chronic bronchitics. Lancet. 1959;2:1112–1115.
5. Hendley JO, Sande MA, Stewart PM, Gwaltney JMJ. Spread of *Streptococcus pneumoniae* in families. I. Carriage rates and distribution of types. J Inect Dis. 1975;132(1):55–61.
6. Wallin TR, Hern HG, Frazee BW. Community-associated methicillin-resistant *Staphylococcus aureus*. Emerg Med Clin North Am. 2008;26(2): 431–455, ix.
7. Howard LS, Sillis M, Pasteur MC, Kamath AV, Harrison BDW. Microbiological profile of community-acquired pneumonia in adults over the last 20 years. J Infect. 2005;50(2):107–113.
8. Jennings LC, Anderson TP, Beynon KA, et al. Incidence and characteristics of viral community-acquired pneumonia. Thorax. 2008;63:42–48.

9. Van Gageldonk-Lafeber AB, Wever PC, van der Lubben IM, et al. The aetiology of community-acquired pneumonia and implications for patient management. J Med. 2013;71(7):418–425.
10. Templeton KE, Scheltinga SA, va den Eeden WCJFM, et al. Improved diagnosis of the etiology of community-acquired pneumonia with real-time polymerase chain reaction. Clin Infect Dis. 2005;41:345–351.
11. Petric M, Comanor L, Petti C. Role of the laboratory in diagnosis of influenza during seasonal epidemics and potential pandemics. J Infect Dis. 2006;194(Suppl)2:S98.
12. Barlow GD, Lamping DL, Davey PG, Nathwani D. Evaluation of outcomes in community-acquired pneumonia: A guide for patients, physicians, and policy-makers. Lancet Infect Dis. 2003;3(8):476–488.
13. Lim WS, van der Eerden MM, Laing R, et al. Defining community acquired pneumonia severity on presentation to hospital: An international derivation and validation study. Thorax. 2003;58(5):377–382.
14. Ewig S, de Roux A, Bauer T, et al. Validation of predictive rules and indices of severity for community acquired pneumonia. Thorax. 2004; 59(5):421–427.
15. Myint PK, Kamath AV, Vowler SL, Maisey DN, Harrison BDW. Severity assessment criteria recommended by the British Thoracic Society (BTS) for community-acquired pneumonia (CAP) and older patients. Should SOAR (systolic blood pressure, oxygenation, age and respiratory rate) criteria be used in older people? A compilation study of two prospective cohorts. Age Ageing. 2006;35(3):286–291.
16. Aujesky D, Auble TE, Yealy DM, et al. Prospective comparison of three validated prediction rules for prognosis in community-acquired pneumonia. Am J Med. 2005;118(4):384–392.
17. Kikawada M, Iwamoto T, Takasaki M. Aspiration and infection in the elderly: Epidemiology, diagnosis and management. Drugs Aging. 2005;22(2):115–130.
18. Allewelt M, Schuler P, Bolcskei PL, Mauch H, Lode H. Ampicillin + sulbactam vs clindamycin +/– cephalosporin for the treatment of aspiration pneumonia and primary lung abscess. Clin Microbiol Infect. 2004;10(2):163–170.
19. Wunderink RG. Nosocomial pneumonia, including ventilator-associated pneumonia. Proc Am Thorac Soc. 2005;2(5):440–444.
20. Edwards JR, Peterson KD, Andrus ML, et al. National Healthcare Safety Network (NHSN) Report, data summary for 2006, issued June 2007. Am J Infect Control. 2007;35(5):290–301.
21. Hidron A, Edwards J, Patel J, et al. NHSN annual update: Antimicrobial-resistant pathogens associated with healthcare-associated infections: Annual summary of data reported to the National Healthcare Safety Network at the Centers for Disease Control and Prevention, 2006-2007. Infect Control Hosp Epidemiol. 2008;29(11):996.
22. Coffin SE, Klompas M, Classen D, et al. Strategies to prevent ventilator-associated pneumonia in acute care hospitals. Infect Control Hosp Epidemiol. 2008;29:S31–S40.
23. Levy ML, Le Jeune I, Woodhead MA, Macfarlaned JT, Lim WS, on behalf of the British Thoracic Society Community Acquired Pneumonia in Adults Guideline G. Primary care summary of the British Thoracic Society Guidelines for the management of community acquired pneumonia in adults: 2009 update. Primary Care Resp J. 2010;19(1):21–27.
24. Darabi A, Hocquet D, Dowzicky MJ. Antimicrobial activity against Streptococcus pneumoniae and Haemophilus influenzae collected globally between 2004 and 2008 as part of the Tigecycline Evaluation and Surveillance Trial. Diagnost Microbiol Infect Dis. 2010;67(1):78–86.
25. Ortho-McNeil Pharmaceutical. TRUST Surveillance Database, 1999-2007. Raritan, NJ: Ortho-McNeil Pharmaceutical.
26. Jones R, Farrell D, Mendes R, Sader H. Comparative ceftaroline activity tested against pathogens associated with community-acquired pneumonia: Results from an international surveillance study. J Antimicrobiol Chemother. 2011;66(Suppl 3):iii69.
27. Mandell LA, Wunderink RG, Anzueto A, et al. Infectious Diseases Society of America/American Thoracic Society consensus guidelines on the management of community-acquired pneumonia in adults. Clin Infect Dis. 2007;44(Suppl 2): S27–S72.
28. Clark N, Lynch J. Influenza: Epidemiology, clinical features, therapy, and prevention. Semin Resp Crit Care Med. 2011;32(4):373.
29. Bradley J, Byington C, Shah S, et al. The management of community-acquired pneumonia in infants and children older than 3 months of age: Clinical practice guidelines by the pediatric infectious diseases society and the infectious diseases society of america. Clin Infect Dis. 2011;53(7):e25.
30. Contopoulos-Ioannidis DG, Giotis ND, Baliatsa DV, Ioannidis JPA. Extended-interval aminoglycoside administration for children: A meta-analysis. Pediatrics. 2004;114(1):e111–e118.
31. Ferriols-Lisart R, Alos-Alminana M. Effectiveness and safety of once-daily aminoglycosides: A meta-analysis. Am J Health-Sys Pharm. 1996;53(10):1141–1150.
32. Hatala R, Dinh T, Cook DJ. Once-daily aminoglycoside dosing in immunocompetent adults: A meta-analysis. Ann Intern Med. 1996;124(8):717–725.
33. Munckhof WJ, Grayson ML, Turnidge JD. A meta-analysis of studies on the safety and efficacy of aminoglycosides given either once daily or as divided doses. J Antimicrob Chemother. 1996;37(4):645–663.
34. Nestaas E, Bangstad HJ, Sandvik L, Wathne KO. Aminoglycoside extended interval dosing in neonates is safe and effective: A meta-analysis. Arch Dis Child. 2005;90(4):F294–F300.
35. Melsen WG, Rovers MM, Koeman M, Bonten MJM. Estimating the attributable mortality of ventilator-associated pneumonia from randomized prevention studies. Crit Care Med. 2011;39:2736–2742.
36. Chastre J, Wolff M, Fagon J, et al. Comparison of 8 vs 15 days of antibiotic therapy for ventilator-associated pneumonia in adults: A randomized trial. JAMA. 2003;290(19):2588.
37. Klompas M, Khan Y, Kleinman K, et al. Multicenter evaluation of a novel surveillance paradigm for complications of mechanical ventilation. PLoS ONE. 2011;6(3):e18062.
38. Pugh RJ, Cooke RPD, Dempsey G. Short course antibiotic therapy for Gram-negative hospital-acquired pneumonia in the critically ill. J Hosp Infect. 2010;74(4):337–343.
39. Luna CM, Blanzaco D, Niederman MS, et al. Resolution of ventilator-associated pneumonia: Prospective evaluation of the clinical pulmonary infection score as an early clinical predictor of outcome. Crit Care Med. 2003;31(3):676–682.
40. Center for Disease Control and Prevention. Seasonal Influenza [cited 2014 Aug 26]. www.cdc.gov/flu.
41. Greenberg D. The shifting dynamics of pneumococcal invasive disease after the introduction of the pneumococcal 7-valent conjugated vaccine: Toward the new pneumococcal conjugated vaccines. Clin Infect Dis. 2009;49(2):213.
42. Paradiso PR. Advances in pneumococcal disease prevention: 13-valent pneumococcal conjugate vaccine for infants and children. Clin Infect Dis. 2011;52(10):1241–1247.
43. Nunes M, Madhi S. Review on the immunogenicity and safety of PCV-13 in infants and toddlers. Exp Rev Vac. 2011;10(7):951.
44. Musher D, Manoff S, McFetridge R, et al. Antibody persistence 10 years after 1st and 2nd doses of 23-valent pneumococcal polysaccharide vaccine, and immunogenicity and safety of 2nd and 3rd doses in older adults. Hum Vaccin. 2011;7(9):919-926.

72 Upper Respiratory Tract Infections

Heather L. Girand

LEARNING OBJECTIVES

Upon completion of the chapter, the reader will be able to:

1. List common bacteria that cause acute otitis media (AOM), acute bacterial rhinosinusitis (ABRS), and acute pharyngitis.
2. Explain the pathophysiology of and risk factors for AOM, bacterial rhinosinusitis, and streptococcal pharyngitis.
3. Identify clinical signs and symptoms associated with AOM, bacterial rhinosinusitis, streptococcal pharyngitis, and the common cold.
4. List treatment goals for AOM, bacterial rhinosinusitis, streptococcal pharyngitis, and the common cold.
5. Develop a treatment plan for a patient with an upper respiratory tract infection (URI) based on patient-specific information.
6. Create a monitoring plan for a patient being treated for a URI using patient-specific information and prescribed therapy.
7. Educate patients about URIs and proper antibiotic use.

INTRODUCTION

Upper respiratory tract infection (URI) is a comprehensive term for upper airway infections, including otitis media, sinusitis, pharyngitis, laryngitis, and the common cold. Over 1 billion URIs occur annually in the United States, triggering millions of ambulatory care visits and antibiotic prescriptions each year.[1] KEY CONCEPT *Most URIs are caused by viruses, have nonspecific symptoms, and resolve spontaneously.*[2] Antibiotics are not effective for viral URIs, and their excessive use has contributed to resistance, which has prompted development of clinical guidelines to reduce inappropriate prescribing. This chapter focuses on **acute otitis media** (AOM), sinusitis, and pharyngitis which are frequently caused by bacteria. Proper management of the common cold is also reviewed.

OTITIS MEDIA

Otitis media, or middle ear inflammation, is the most common childhood illness treated with antibiotics. It usually results from a nasopharyngeal viral infection and can be subclassified as AOM or **otitis media with effusion** (OME). AOM is a rapid, symptomatic infection with effusion, or fluid, in the middle ear. OME is not an acute illness but is characterized by middle ear effusion. Antibiotics are only useful for the treatment of AOM.

EPIDEMIOLOGY AND ETIOLOGY

AOM occurs in all ages but is most common between 6 months and 2 years of age. By 3 years of age, more than 80% of children have at least one episode, and up to 65% have recurrent infections by 5 years of age.[3,4] Many risk factors (Table 72–1) predispose children to otitis media.[4,5] While the use of antibiotics for otitis media has declined since the mid-1990s, the proportion of health care visits resulting in antibiotic prescriptions remains close to 60%.[6–8]

Although AOM occurs frequently with viral URIs, bacteria are isolated from middle ear fluid in up to 90% of children with AOM.[9] Historically, *Streptococcus pneumoniae* was the most common organism, responsible for up to half of bacterial cases.[9,10] *Haemophilus influenzae* and *Moraxella catarrhalis* caused up to 30% and 20% of cases, respectively. Routine childhood pneumococcal vaccination has altered the microbiology such that the prevalence of *H. influenzae* and *S. pneumoniae* is now nearly equal.[9–11] Viruses are isolated from middle ear fluid with or without concomitant bacteria in up to half of cases.[5,12] Lack of improvement with antibiotics is usually a result of viral infection and subsequent inflammation rather than antibiotic resistance.

KEY CONCEPT *Antibiotic resistance heavily influences the treatment options for AOM.* Penicillin-resistant *S. pneumoniae* (PRSP) exhibit intermediate resistance (minimum inhibitory concentrations between 0.12 and 1.0 mcg/mL [0.12 and 1.0 mg/L]) or high-level resistance (minimum inhibitory concentration of 2.0 mcg/mL [2.0 mg/L] and higher). Altered penicillin-binding proteins cause resistance in approximately 44% of pneumococci, where one-third are highly penicillin-resistant.[13] Amoxicillin resistance is less common, occurring in approximately 19% of pneumococci.[13] PRSP are frequently resistant to other drug classes, including sulfonamides, macrolides, and clindamycin, but are usually susceptible to levofloxacin. Treatment should be aimed at *S. pneumoniae* because pneumococcal AOM is unlikely to

Table 72–1

Risk Factors for Otitis Media[4,8]

Allergies	Native American or Inuit ethnicity
Anatomic defects such as cleft palate	Pacifier use
Daycare attendance	Positive family history/genetic predisposition
Gastroesophageal reflux	Siblings
Immunodeficiency	Tobacco smoke exposure
Lack of breast-feeding	Viral respiratory tract infection/winter season
Low socioeconomic status	Young age at first diagnosis
Male sex	

resolve spontaneously and commonly results in recurrent infections.[5,9] β-Lactamase production occurs in nearly 30% and 90% of *H. influenzae* and *M. catarrhalis*, respectively.[14] Although infections caused by these organisms are more likely to resolve without treatment, they should be considered when failure occurs.

PATHOPHYSIOLOGY

AOM is caused by an interplay of factors. Viral URIs impair eustachian tube function and cause mucosal inflammation, impairing mucociliary clearance and promoting bacterial proliferation and infection. Children are predisposed because they have shorter, more flaccid, and more horizontal eustachian tubes than adults, which are less functional for middle ear drainage and protection. Clinical manifestations of AOM result from host immune response and cellular damage from inflammatory mediators released by bacteria.

Viscous effusions caused by allergy or irritant exposure contribute to impaired mucociliary clearance and AOM in susceptible individuals. Effusions can persist for up to 6 months after an episode of AOM. Atopic children experience chronic OME that may require tympanostomy tube placement to reduce complications such as hearing and speech impairment and recurrent AOM.

TREATMENT

The goals of treatment are to alleviate ear pain and fever, if present; eradicate infection; prevent complications; and avoid unnecessary antibiotic use.

Patient Encounter 1, Part 1

A 13-month-old boy presents to the pediatric clinic with 2 days of fever (maximum temperature of 39.3°C [102.7°F]), rhinorrhea, and fussiness. His mother reports that he was rubbing his left ear throughout the day yesterday. She states that he is irritable and he was crying intermittently throughout the night last night. He has not eaten much today. He attends daycare 3 days a week and has a 5-year-old sister who recently had a cold.

What information is suggestive of acute otitis media (AOM)?

What risk factors does this child have for AOM?

Is there any additional information you need to know before recommending a treatment plan?

General Approach to Treatment

KEY CONCEPT *The majority of uncomplicated cases resolve spontaneously.* Untreated AOM improves in over 80% of children between days 2 and 7 of illness without increasing complications.[15] Antibiotics improve otalgia in only 5% of children between days 2 and 7 of therapy while *increasing* the risk of adverse events by 7%.[15] Antibiotics significantly improve recovery in children younger than 2 years with bilateral AOM and in those with AOM and otorrhea.[15] Children younger than 2 years have a higher incidence of PRSP infections, and children between 6 months and 3 years have higher clinical and bacteriologic failure rates and complications without initial antibiotic treatment as compared with older children.[9,16] Patients with severe AOM have lower spontaneous recovery rates than those with less severe disease, particularly in children less than 2 years.[9,17] KEY CONCEPT *Therefore, antibiotics should be reserved for patients most likely to benefit, which is dependent on proper diagnosis, patient age, and illness severity.* Current guidelines stratify patients using these criteria in order to identify those most likely to benefit from antibiotics.[9]

Nonpharmacologic Therapy

Watchful waiting and "safety-net" antibiotic prescriptions (prescription given to the patient but only filled if symptoms persist or worsen within 48–72 hours after diagnosis) are approaches used to attenuate microbial resistance and avoid unnecessary antibiotic adverse events and costs. Initial observation and use of delayed prescriptions in older children and those with less severe disease can reduce antibiotic use by 67% without increasing complications.[15,18] These approaches should only be considered in otherwise healthy children (Figure 72–1) as a joint decision between the clinician and the parent/caregiver and only if close follow-up and good communication exist.[3,9,18]

Children with recurrent AOM or chronic OME with impaired hearing or speech may benefit from surgery (tympanostomy tube placement with or without adenoidectomy).

Pharmacologic Therapy

▶ *Antibiotic Therapy*

When antibiotics are necessary, clinicians must consider drug factors (eg, antimicrobial spectrum, likelihood of response, middle ear fluid penetration, side effects, drug interactions, cost) and patient factors (eg, risk factors for resistance, allergies, regimen complexity, medication palatability, and presence of other medical conditions). Studies in uncomplicated AOM have not revealed significant differences between antibiotics in clinical response rates, but most were confounded by spontaneous resolution in children likely to have had viral URIs. Bacteriologic response varies among antibiotics and does not always correlate well with clinical response but is considered important when selecting therapy.[5,9]

The American Academy of Pediatrics (AAP) developed clinical guidelines for healthy children between 6 months and 12 years of age with uncomplicated AOM (Figure 72–2).[9] KEY CONCEPT *Amoxicillin is the drug of choice in most patients because of its proven effectiveness, high middle ear concentrations, excellent safety profile, low cost, good-tasting suspension, and relatively narrow spectrum* (Table 72–2). High-dose amoxicillin (80–90 mg/kg/day) is preferred over conventional doses (40–45 mg/kg/day) because higher middle ear fluid concentrations can overcome pneumococcal penicillin resistance without substantially increasing adverse effects.[19] KEY CONCEPT *High dose amoxicillin-clavulanate is preferred for children who received amoxicillin in the previous*

Clinical Presentation and Diagnosis of AOM

Patients with AOM usually have cold symptoms, including rhinorrhea, cough, or nasal congestion, before or at diagnosis.

Symptoms

- Young children: ear tugging or rubbing, irritable, poor sleeping and eating
- Older patients: ear pain, ear fullness, hearing impairment

Signs[5,9]

- Fever: present in fewer than 25% of patients; often in younger children
- Middle ear effusion
- Otorrhea with tympanic membrane perforation
- Bulging tympanic membrane
- Limited or absent mobility of tympanic membrane
- Distinct erythema of tympanic membrane
- Opaque tympanic membrane that obscures middle ear visibility

Laboratory Tests

- Gram stain, culture, and sensitivities of ear fluid if draining spontaneously or obtained via tympanocentesis (not performed routinely in practice)

Complications

- Infectious: mastoiditis, meningitis, osteomyelitis, intracranial abscess
- Structural: perforated eardrum, cholesteatoma
- Hearing and/or speech impairment

Diagnosis[9]

AOM should be diagnosed if any of the following are met:

- Moderate to severe bulging of tympanic membrane (usually with impaired mobility as assessed by pneumatic otoscopy)
- Mild bulging of tympanic membrane *and* recent onset (less than 48 hours) of otalgia (or ear rubbing/tugging in nonverbal child) or intense erythema of tympanic membrane
- New onset otorrhea not caused by acute otitis externa

Severe AOM: Moderate to severe otalgia or otalgia for at least 48 hours *or* temperature of 39.0°C (102.2°F) or greater

30 days, have concurrent purulent conjunctivitis, have a history of recurrent AOM unresponsive to amoxicillin, and when coverage for β-lactamase-producing organisms is desired. Patients with penicillin allergies require alternative therapy (see Figure 72–2). There is limited cross-reactivity between penicillins and newer cephalosporins which supports AAP recommendations to use cephalosporins in penicillin-allergic patients because they are more effective than alternatives.[9,20] Trimethoprim-sulfamethoxazole and macrolides have limited efficacy against *S. pneumoniae* and *H. influenzae*, making them less desirable for most

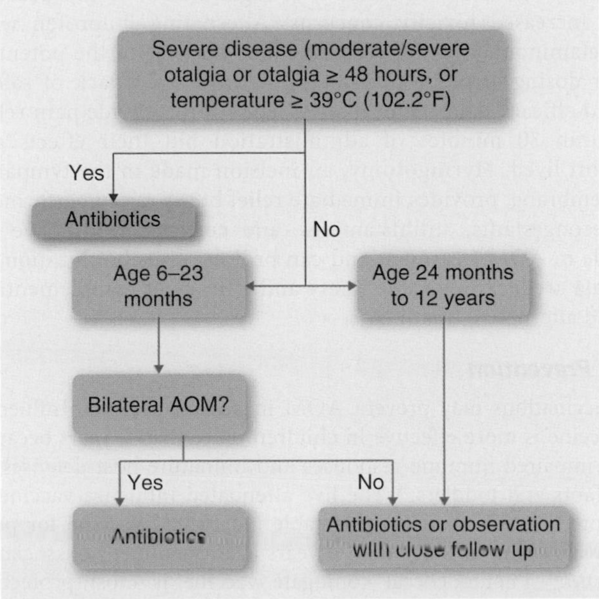

FIGURE 72–1. Treatment algorithm for initial antibiotics or observation in children 6 months to 12 years of age with uncomplicated AOM. (Data from Lieberthal AS, Carroll AE, Chonmaitree T, et al. The diagnosis and management of acute otitis media. Pediatrics. 2013;131(3):e964–e999.)

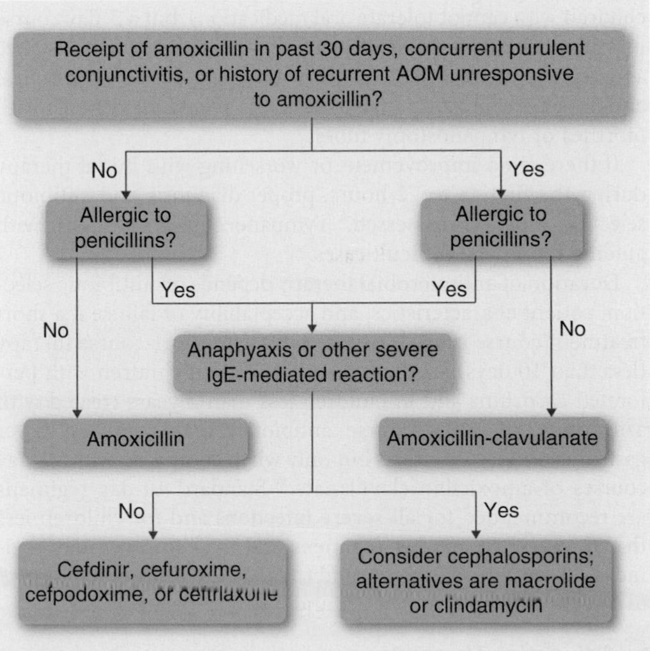

FIGURE 72–2. Treatment algorithm for uncomplicated AOM in children 6 months to 12 years of age. (Data from Lieberthal AS, Carroll AE, Chonmaitree T, et al. The diagnosis and management of acute otitis media. Pediatrics 2013;131(3):e964–e999.)

Table 72–2

Antibiotics[a] for the Treatment of Acute Otitis Media

Drug	Usual Dose and Schedule	Common Adverse Effects	Relative Cost[b]	Comments
Amoxicillin	80–90 mg/kg/day in two doses (adult: 875 mg twice daily)	Nausea, vomiting, diarrhea, rash	$	Drug of choice for AOM; experts recommend high dose to overcome penicillin resistance
Amoxicillin-clavulanate	90 mg/kg/day in two doses (adult: 875 mg twice daily)	Nausea, vomiting, diarrhea, rash, diaper rash	$$$–$$$$	More diarrhea than amoxicillin; amoxicillin:clavulanate ratio of 14:1 preferred because of lower daily clavulanate component
Cefuroxime axetil	30 mg/kg/day in two doses (max 1 g/day with suspension; adult: 250 mg twice daily)	Nausea, vomiting, diarrhea, rash, diaper rash	$$–$$$	Suspension gritty and bitter tasting; not interchangeable with tablets (less bioavailable)
Cefdinir	14 mg/kg/day in one to two doses (adult: 300 mg twice daily or 600 mg once daily)	Diarrhea, rash, vomiting, diaper rash, yeast infections	$$$–$$$$	Preferred oral cephalosporin (good taste); separate from Fe supplements by 3 hours
Cefpodoxime proxetil	10 mg/kg/day in two doses (adult: 200 mg twice daily)	Diarrhea, diaper rash, vomiting, rash, yeast infections	$$$–$$$$	Suspension is bitter tasting
Ceftriaxone	50 mg/kg IM or IV for 1 or 3 days (max 1 g/dose)	Injection site pain, swelling, or erythema, diarrhea, rash	$$$–$$$$	3-day regimen preferred for PRSP
Clindamycin	30–40 mg/kg/day in three doses (adult: 300–450 mg 3 times daily)	Nausea, diarrhea, *C. difficile* colitis, anorexia	$$	Oral liquid poor tasting; only for pneumococcal infection

[a]Other FDA-approved antibiotics for AOM not recommended in AAP guidelines: azithromycin, cefaclor, cefixime, cefprozil, ceftibuten, cephalexin, clarithromycin, erythromycin-sulfisoxazole, and trimethoprim-sulfamethoxazole.

[b]Approximate cost per course: $ (under $25), $$ ($25–$50), $$$ ($50–$100), $$$$ (over $100).

AOM, acute otitis media; Fe, iron; IM, intramuscular; IV, intravenous, PRSP, penicillin-resistant *S. pneumoniae*.

Data from Lieberthal AS, Carroll AE, Chonmaitree T, et al. The diagnosis and management of acute otitis media. Pediatrics 2013;131(3):e964-e999.

patients.[9,13,14] Single-dose intramuscular ceftriaxone is effective for children who cannot tolerate oral medications, but a 3-day course may be preferred because of increasing pneumococcal resistance and reports of treatment failure with single doses.[21] Ototopical antibiotics are an alternative to systemic agents for patients with otorrhea or tympanostomy tubes.[22]

If there is no improvement or worsening with initial therapy during the first 48 to 72 hours, proper diagnosis and antibiotic selection must be reassessed.[9] Tympanocentesis can assist with guiding therapy in difficult cases.

Duration of antimicrobial therapy depends on antibiotic selection, patient characteristics, and acceptability of failure if a short treatment course is used. Failure rates with short-course therapy (less than 10 days) are significantly higher in children with perforated eardrums and in children less than 2 years treated with azithromycin.[23] Short-course antibiotics may result in fewer gastrointestinal side effects but only when compared with 10-day courses of amoxicillin-clavulanate.[23] Standard 10-day regimens are recommended for all severe infections and for children less than 2 years.[9] Seven-day regimens and five- to seven-day regimens can be considered for mild to moderate AOM in children 2 to 5 years and children 6 years and older, respectively.[9]

▸ *Adjunctive Therapy*

Pain is a central feature of AOM but it is often overlooked. Analgesics provide relief within 24 hours and should be used regardless of antibiotic therapy.[9] Acetaminophen and ibuprofen are commonly used for mild to moderate pain. Ibuprofen provides longer relief than acetaminophen but should be avoided in children younger than 6 months because of increased toxicity concerns. Alternating ibuprofen with acetaminophen is not recommended because of the potential for dosing error in ambulatory settings and a lack of safety and efficacy data. Topical anesthetic drops provide pain relief within 30 minutes of administration but their effects are short lived. **Myringotomy**, an incision made in the tympanic membrane, provides immediate relief but is rarely performed. Decongestants, antihistamines, and corticosteroids have no role in AOM treatment and can prolong effusion duration.[9,24] Data are lacking on the safety and efficacy of complementary and alternative treatments.

▸ *Prevention*

Vaccinations may prevent AOM in certain patients. Influenza vaccine is more effective in children older than 2 years because of impaired immune responses and immature host defenses in infants and toddlers.[25] The live attenuated influenza vaccine is more effective than the injectable inactivated vaccine for protecting children older than 2 years against influenza-associated AOM.[26] Pneumococcal conjugate vaccine is most protective against infection from pneumococcal serotypes contained in the vaccine and in infants at low-risk for AOM.[27] Antibiotic prophylaxis is not recommended because of antibiotic resistance trends. Exclusive breast-feeding for the first 6 months of life and avoidance of tobacco smoke are advised, but the effects of these interventions remain unproven.

Patient Encounter 1, Part 2

On further questioning, his mother states that he is "allergic" to trimethoprim/sulfamethoxazole. He was treated for a urinary tract infection 7 months ago and experienced diarrhea while taking this antibiotic. He has not received antibiotics since that time, and this is his first ear infection.

Immunizations: up-to-date

Meds: Acetaminophen drops 120 mg orally every 4 to 6 hours as needed for fever

ROS: (+) rhinorrhea and fever, (–) vomiting, diarrhea, or cough

PE:

Gen: Irritable child but consolable

VS: BP 100/64 mm Hg, P 130 beats/min, RR 22 breaths/min, T 39.1°C (102.4°F)

HEENT: Erythema and severe bulging of the left tympanic membrane with the presence of middle ear fluid; the right tympanic membrane is obscured with cerumen.

Identify your treatment goals for this child.

Given this information, what nonpharmacologic and pharmacologic therapy do you recommend?

Patient Care Process for Acute Otitis Media

Patient Assessment:

- Based on patient history, review of systems, and physical examination (including pneumatic otoscopy findings), determine if the patient has AOM and if it is severe.
- Perform a medical review and conduct a medication history (including prescription and nonprescription medications and natural products). Does the patient have any medication allergies or adverse reactions? Is the patient up-to-date on immunizations?

Therapy Evaluation:

- If the patient is receiving pharmacotherapy, assess efficacy, safety, and adherence.
- Determine if antibiotic therapy is indicated or if observation can be employed (see Figure 72–1).
- Determine whether the patient has prescription coverage and if the desired antibiotic is covered by their insurance.

Care Plan Development:

- If appropriate, select analgesic therapy that will provide optimal pain relief.
- If appropriate, select antibiotic therapy that is likely to be effective and safe (see Figure 72–2).
- Select an optimal antibiotic dose (see Table 72–2) and an appropriate duration of treatment based on patient age and illness severity.
- Discuss potential adverse effects and how to manage them.
- Discuss importance of medication adherence to treat infection and pain.
- Determine the need for influenza and pneumococcal vaccinations to reduce risk for future infection.

Follow-up Evaluation:

- Reevaluate patient within 48 to 72 hours if symptoms persist or worsen.
- Monitor for middle ear effusion resolution at an appropriate interval based on age and presence of conditions that interfere with recognition of hearing impairment.

OUTCOME EVALUATION

Improvement of signs and symptoms (ie, pain, fever, and tympanic membrane inflammation) should be evident by 72 hours of proper therapy. Children can appear clinically worse during the first 24 hours but often stabilize during the second day. If symptoms persist or worsen, reevaluate the patient for the proper diagnosis and treatment. Counsel patients and caregivers regarding common antibiotic adverse effects such as rash, diarrhea, and vomiting that may prompt additional medical attention.

Presence of middle ear effusion in the absence of symptoms is not an indicator of treatment failure. Evaluate hearing in children who are otherwise healthy and have persistent effusion lasting 3 months in duration. Preschool-aged and younger children or those at risk for developmental difficulties may need reexamination earlier because speech and hearing impairment is more difficult to assess in these populations.

SINUSITIS

Sinusitis, or paranasal sinus inflammation, is often described as **rhinosinusitis** because it involves contiguous nasal mucosa and occurs in nearly all viral URIs. Acute rhinosinusitis is characterized by symptoms that persist for up to 4 weeks, whereas chronic rhinosinusitis lasts for more than 12 weeks. Acute bacterial rhinosinusitis (ABRS) refers to an acute bacterial sinus infection that occurs independently of or is superimposed on chronic sinusitis. This section will focus on ABRS.

EPIDEMIOLOGY AND ETIOLOGY

Rhinosinusitis affects about 1 billion people annually in the United States.[1] It is caused mainly by respiratory viruses but can also be triggered by allergies or environmental irritants. Viral rhinosinusitis is complicated by secondary bacterial infection in 0.2% to 2% of adults and 5% to 13% of children.[1,28] URIs of less than 7 days' duration are usually viral, whereas more prolonged or severe symptoms are often caused by bacteria. Risk factors for ABRS include prior viral URI, allergic rhinitis, and anatomic defects (Table 72–3).[29,30]

Bacteria that cause sinusitis are similar to those in AOM. *S. pneumoniae* and *H. influenzae* cause more than half of ABRS cases, with an additional 8% to 16% of cases caused by *M. catarrhalis*.[29,30] Similar to AOM, an increased prevalence of *H. influenzae* has been reported in ABRS, and certain factors predict the presence of drug-resistant pathogens.[1,30]

PATHOPHYSIOLOGY

Rhinosinusitis is caused by mucosal inflammation and mucociliary dysfunction from viral infection or allergy. Increased mucous production and reduced clearance lead to blockage of the sinus

Table 72–3
Risk Factors for Acute Bacterial Rhinosinusitis[29,30,31]

Allergic or nonallergic rhinitis	Intranasal medications or illicit drugs
Anatomic defects (eg, septal deviation)	Mechanical ventilation
Aspirin allergy, nasal polyps, and asthma	Nasogastric tubes
Cystic fibrosis or ciliary dyskinesia	Swimming or diving
Dental infections or procedures	Tobacco smoke exposure
Female sex	Traumatic head injury
Gastroesophageal reflux	Viral respiratory tract infection or winter season
Immunodeficiency	

ostia. This environment is ideal for bacterial growth and promotes a cycle of local inflammation and mucosal injury characterized by increased concentrations of interleukins, histamine, and tumor necrosis factor.[31] Damage to the host defense system perpetuates bacterial overgrowth and persistence of infection.

TREATMENT

The goals of treatment are to relieve symptoms, promote sinus drainage, use antibiotics when appropriate that minimize resistance, and prevent development of chronic disease or complications.

General Approach to Treatment

Initial management focuses on symptom relief. Clinicians often inappropriately prescribe antibiotics for rhinosinusitis, which usually is viral and self-limited. Studies in adults with clinically diagnosed nonsevere sinusitis report cure rates of nearly 50% by day 10 with no differences between antibiotics and placebo but significantly more adverse events with antibiotics.[33] Studies in children with persistent nasal discharge for at least 10 days report modest benefits with antibiotic therapy.[34] KEY CONCEPT *Antibiotics should be prescribed only when ABRS is most likely: persistent symptoms for greater than 10 days with no improvement; sudden worsening of symptoms within 5 to 10 days of initial improvement; and severe symptoms for 3 to 4 days at illness onset.*[28,30,32] In patients with mild persistent illness for at least 10 days, observation for another 3 days can be employed if there is adequate follow-up.[28,30]

Nonpharmacologic Therapy

Humidifiers and saline nasal sprays or drops moisturize the nasal canal, impair crusting of secretions, and promote ciliary function. Although many patients report benefit from such therapies, there are no controlled studies that support their efficacy. Nasal irrigation with isotonic or hypertonic saline may reduce medication use and improve symptoms, especially in patients with recurrent or chronic sinusitis.[28,35]

Pharmacologic Therapy

▶ *Adjunctive Therapy*

Medications that target symptoms are commonly used in rhinosinusitis despite a lack of evidence demonstrating their efficacy. Analgesics/antipyretics should be used to treat facial pain and fever. Oral decongestants relieve congestion but should be avoided in children younger than 4 years and patients with ischemic heart disease or uncontrolled hypertension. Intranasal decongestants can be used for severe congestion in patients 6 years of age or older, but use should be limited to 3 days to avoid rebound nasal congestion. Avoid antihistamines because they thicken mucus and impair clearance, but they may be useful in patients with allergic rhinitis or chronic sinusitis. Similarly, intranasal corticosteroids usually are reserved for patients with allergies or chronic sinusitis, but they may be beneficial as monotherapy or with antibiotics in ABRS.[28,36]

▶ *Antibiotic Therapy*

No randomized, double-blind, placebo-controlled antibiotic studies have used pre- and posttreatment sinus aspirate cultures as an outcome measure. In some studies, antibiotics resulted in

Clinical Presentation and Diagnosis of Acute Bacterial Rhinosinusitis

KEY CONCEPT *It is important to differentiate between viral sinusitis and ABRS to avoid inappropriate antibiotic use.*

Signs and Symptoms[28,30,31]

- *Adults:* Nasal congestion or obstruction, purulent nasal or postnasal discharge, facial pain or pressure (especially unilateral), diminished sense of smell, fever, cough, maxillary tooth pain, fatigue, ear fullness or pain
- *Children:* Persistent nasal or postnasal drainage, nasal congestion, mouth breathing, persistent cough (particularly at night) or throat clearing, fever, pharyngitis, ear discomfort, halitosis, morning periorbital edema or facial swelling, fatigue, facial or tooth pain

Complications

Orbital cellulitis or abscess, periorbital cellulitis, meningitis, cavernous sinus thrombosis, ethmoid or frontal sinus erosion, chronic sinusitis, and exacerbation of asthma or bronchitis

Diagnosis[28,30,32]

- *Clinical diagnosis:* Most common method; signs and symptoms that persist for more than 10 days with no improvement *or* that worsen after initial improvement, *or* severe symptoms (fever greater than or equal to 39.0°C [102.2°F] and purulent nasal discharge) for at least 3 to 4 days at illness onset. Respiratory secretion color is unreliable for diagnosis because neutrophil presence causes color and is found in viral sinusitis.[32]
- *Radiographic studies:* Useful for assessing presence of complications
- *Paranasal sinus puncture:* "Gold standard"; not routine but can be useful in complicated or chronic cases
- *Laboratory studies/nasopharyngeal cultures:* not recommended

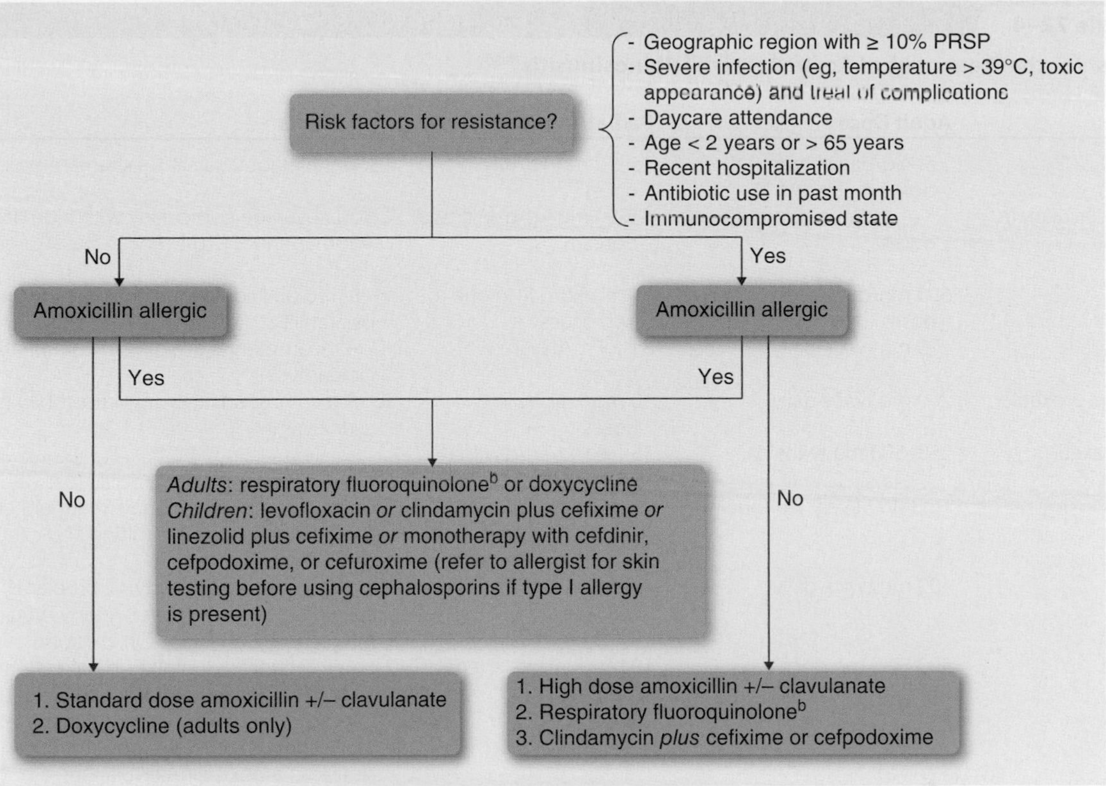

FIGURE 72–3. Treatment algorithm[a] for ABRS. [a]Antibiotics are listed in order of preference based on predicted clinical and bacteriologic efficacy rates, clinical studies, safety, and tolerability. Doses can be found in Table 72–4. [b]Respiratory fluoroquinolone = levofloxacin, moxifloxacin.[28,30]

faster symptom resolution with lower failure rates compared with no treatment, particularly with more severe infection.[28,30,32] Because diagnosis is usually based on clinical presentation, clinicians must differentiate ABRS from viral rhinosinusitis in order to minimize inappropriate antibiotic use. Empiric antibiotic selection is usually used and should target commonly infecting bacteria. KEY CONCEPT *Treatment guidelines outline antibiotic choices that are likely to result in favorable clinical and bacteriologic outcomes based on causative pathogens and nationwide resistance patterns (Figure 72–3).*[28,30] Severe disease should be treated in conjunction with specialists such as otolaryngologists or infectious disease physicians.

Antibiotics (Table 72–4) should target *S. pneumoniae* and *H. influenzae*, but consideration must also be given to other bacteria and local resistance patterns. KEY CONCEPT *Standard dose amoxicillin or amoxicillin-clavulanate is recommended for most patients.*[28,30] Amoxicillin is effective for most infections and is less expensive and better tolerated than amoxicillin-clavulanate, which provides expanded coverage against β-lactamase–producers. High-dose amoxicillin or amoxicillin-clavulanate is recommended for patients who are at risk for infection from resistant bacteria, such as those who attend daycare, and when PRSP and other resistant bacteria are frequent in a community (see Figure 72–3). Patients with penicillin allergies can be treated with an appropriate cephalosporin, doxycycline, or a respiratory fluoroquinolone depending on age and allergy severity. Cephalosporin monotherapy is less desirable because of increased pneumococcal resistance, so combination therapy may be required to optimize coverage for PRSP and β-lactamase producers.[28] Macrolides and trimethoprim-sulfamethoxazole are not recommended because of high pneumococcal and *H. influenzae* resistance. For uncomplicated infections, treatment duration ranges from 5 to 10 days in adults and 10 to 14 days in children.[28,30] While short-course therapy with some fluoroquinolones and β-lactams are as effective as longer courses in adults with uncomplicated acute maxillary sinusitis, data are lacking to support shorter courses in more severe infections or in children.[37]

Failure to improve within 3 to 5 days of therapy or worsening at any time requires reevaluation to confirm the diagnosis, consider changing antibiotics, and examine for complications.[28,30]

OUTCOME EVALUATION

Clinical improvement (eg, defervescence, reduced nasal congestion and discharge, improvements in pain or facial pressure) should be evident within 5 days of therapy. Monitor for common adverse effects and refer to a specialist if clinical response is not obtained with first- or second-line therapy. Referral is also important for severe, recurrent, or chronic infection. Surgery may be indicated in complicated cases.

PHARYNGITIS

Pharyngitis is an inflammation of the throat often caused by infection. Acute pharyngitis is responsible for 1% to 2% of physician visits in adults and 6% to 8% of pediatric visits, but it is generally self-limited.[38,39] Antibiotics are frequently prescribed because it can be difficult to clinically distinguish between viral and bacterial infection and the fear of untreated streptococcal illness.

Table 72–4

Antibiotics[a] for the Treatment of Acute Bacterial Rhinosinusitis[28,30]

Drug	Adult Dose	Pediatric Dose[b]	Comments
Amoxicillin	1.5–4 g/day in two to three doses	45–90 mg/kg/day in two doses	Lacks coverage against β-lactamase producers
Amoxicillin-clavulanate	1.5–4 g/day in two to three doses	45–90 mg/kg/day in two doses	Broad coverage particularly with high doses; Augmentin XR (2 g every 12 hour) targeted toward PRSP
Cefdinir	600 mg/day in one to two doses	14 mg/kg/day in one to two doses	Preferred oral liquid cephalosporin owing to good palatability
Cefixime	200 mg twice daily	8 mg/kg/day in two doses	IDSA recommends use only in combination with clindamycin
Cefpodoxime proxetil	200 mg twice daily	10 mg/kg/day in two doses	IDSA recommends use only in combination with clindamycin
Cefuroxime axetil	250–500 mg twice daily	15–30 mg/kg/day in two doses	
Ceftriaxone	1 g IM/IV every 24 hours	50 mg/kg IM/IV every 24 hours	Experts recommend a 5-day treatment course; useful for patients who are vomiting and cannot tolerate oral therapy
Doxycycline	100 mg twice daily	Avoid in children < 8 years	Can cause photosensitivity, GI problems, tooth staining in young children; many drug–drug interactions (antacids, iron, calcium)
Levofloxacin	500–750 mg once daily (750 mg × 5 days)	10 mg/kg/dose every 12–24 hours	Common fluoroquinolone side effects are nausea, vaginitis, diarrhea, dizziness; many drug–drug interactions (antacids, iron, calcium); tendon rupture, photosensitivity, QT prolongation possible; cost similar to amoxicillin/clavulanate
Moxifloxacin	400 mg once daily	Not available	
Clindamycin	300–450 mg three times daily	30–40 mg/kg/day in three doses	No gram-negative coverage; use only in combination with cephalosporin
Linezolid	600 mg twice daily	10 mg/kg/dose every 8–12 hours	No gram-negative coverage; use only in combination as an alternative to clindamycin

[a]Refer to Table 72–2 for more information on antibiotics. Other FDA-approved antibiotics for ABRS not included in the Infectious Diseases Society of America or American Academy of Pediatrics guidelines: azithromycin, cefaclor, cefprozil, clarithromycin, ciprofloxacin, erythromycin, and trimethoprim-sulfamethoxazole.

[b]Maximum dose not to exceed adult dose.

ABRS, acute bacterial rhinosinusitis; IDSA, Infectious Diseases Society of America; PRSP, penicillin-resistant *S. pneumoniae*; IM, intramuscular.

EPIDEMIOLOGY AND ETIOLOGY

Pharyngitis is a common manifestation of viral URIs. *Streptococcus pyogenes* (Group A streptococci) is the most common bacterial cause, responsible for 20% to 30% of cases in children and 5% to 15% of adult infections.[40,41] It is most common in late winter and early spring and spreads easily through direct contact with contaminated secretions. Clusters of infection are common within families, classrooms, and other crowded settings.

PATHOPHYSIOLOGY

Group A streptococci colonize the pharynx in up to 20% of children and is a risk factor for developing pharyngitis if there is disruption in mucosal integrity.[40] Symptoms of streptococcal pharyngitis usually are self-limited and resolve within a few days of onset *without* antibiotic treatment.[40] Historically, untreated or inappropriately treated infection caused acute rheumatic fever, heart valve damage, and other infectious complications. Delayed antibiotic therapy given up to 9 days after symptom onset can prevent these sequelae, so KEY CONCEPT *proper diagnosis is important to minimize unnecessary antibiotic use for viral pharyngitis and prevent complications of untreated streptococcal infection.*[39–41]

TREATMENT

KEY CONCEPT *The goals of therapy for streptococcal pharyngitis are to shorten the disease course, reduce spread, and prevent complications, including peritonsillar or retropharyngeal abscesses, cervical lymphadenitis, and rheumatic fever.* Immune-mediated, nonsuppurative complications such as **glomerulonephritis** and reactive arthritis are not impacted by antibiotics.[38]

Pharmacologic Therapy

Pain is a key feature of pharyngitis. Oral analgesics provide pain relief and can allow patients to maintain normal eating and drinking habits. KEY CONCEPT *Antibiotics should be used only in cases of laboratory-confirmed streptococcal pharyngitis with associated clinical symptoms* (Figure 72–4).[38,40,41] Effective therapy (Table 72–5) reduces the infectious period from approximately 10 days to 24 hours and shortens symptom duration by 1 to 2 days.[2,38,40] KEY CONCEPT *Penicillin is the drug of choice because of its narrow spectrum, documented safety and efficacy in nasopharyngeal streptococcal eradication, and low cost.*[40,41] Amoxicillin is an alternative agent, particularly for children because of its improved taste and its enhanced adherence with once-daily dosing.[40,41]

Patient Encounter 2

A 45-year-old man presents to his primary care physician with purulent postnasal discharge, nasal congestion, headache, and fatigue. He reports that his symptoms began 6 days ago and have worsened over the past 2 days. He states that his "head hurts" when he bends forward and he noticed that his upper molars ache when he eats or brushes his teeth. He tried acetaminophen and phenylephrine but received no relief. He has sinus infections every few years. His last course of antibiotics was 8 months ago when he received penicillin for streptococcal pharyngitis. He has two daughters (9 years and 13 years of age).

Immunizations: Up-to-date; he has not received his influenza vaccine this season

Allergies: Grass and tree pollens; ragweed

Meds: Fexofenadine 60 mg orally twice daily during allergy season; intranasal fluticasone one spray each nostril twice daily; acetaminophen 500 mg orally as needed; phenylephrine 10 mg orally every 4 hours as needed

PE:

Gen: Tired-appearing, moderate distress, appears uncomfortable

VS: BP 132/74 mm Hg, P 88 beats/min, RR 14 breaths/min, T 38.2°C (100.8°F), Wt 95.5 kg (210 lb)

HEENT: Thick, purulent brown postnasal discharge; nasal mucosal edema; right maxillary facial pain and right upper molar hypersensitivity upon tapping; no oral lesions; erythematous pharynx with mild tonsillar hypertrophy

What information is suggestive of acute bacterial rhinosinusitis (ABRS)?

What risk factors are present?

What other diagnostic studies, if any, should be performed?

What are the treatment goals for this patient?

Create a care plan for this patient that includes nonpharmacologic and pharmacologic therapies and a monitoring plan.

Patient Care Process for Acute Bacterial Rhinosinusitis

Patient Assessment:

- Based on patient history, review of systems, and physical examination, determine if the patient has ABRS and its severity.
- Perform a medical review and conduct a medication history (including prescription and nonprescription medications and natural products). Does the patient have any medication allergies or adverse reactions? Is the patient up-to-date on immunizations?

Therapy Evaluation:

- If the patient is receiving pharmacotherapy, assess efficacy, safety, and patient adherence.
- Determine if antibiotic therapy is indicated or if observation can be used.
- Determine whether the patient has prescription coverage and if the desired antibiotic is covered by their insurance.

Care Plan Development:

- Select analgesic therapy that will provide optimal pain relief and appropriate adjunctive therapies to relieve symptoms.
- If appropriate, select antibiotic therapy that is likely to be effective and safe (see Figure 72–3).
- Select an optimal antibiotic dose (see Table 72–4) and an appropriate duration of treatment based on patient age and severity of illness.
- Discuss potential adverse effects and how to manage them.
- Discuss importance of medication adherence to treat infection and clinical symptoms.

Follow-up Evaluation:

- Reevaluate patient if symptoms persist beyond 5 days or worsen at any time.
- If recurrent infections or chronic sinusitis develop, refer to a specialist.

Cephalosporins may be more effective than penicillin for relapse prevention and nasopharyngeal eradication, particularly in asymptomatic carriers.[41,42] Usual duration of therapy is 10 days, but 5-day courses of some cephalosporins are as effective for streptococcal eradication as 10 days of penicillin.[43]

Resistance plays a smaller role in pharyngitis treatment compared with other URIs. KEY CONCEPT *Penicillin resistance has not been documented in group A streptococci, but resistance and clinical failures occur more frequently with tetracyclines, trimethoprim-sulfamethoxazole, and to a lesser degree macrolides.* Patients with penicillin allergies should be treated with a first-generation cephalosporin (if non–type I allergy), a macrolide/azalide, or clindamycin.[40,41] Recurrent infections or treatment failures can be retreated with the same initial antibiotic or treated with amoxicillin-clavulanate, a first-generation cephalosporin, clindamycin, or penicillin G benzathine.[40,41]

OUTCOME EVALUATION

Antibiotics relieve symptoms of streptococcal pharyngitis within 3 to 5 days, and patients can return to work or school if improved after the first 24 hours of therapy. Lack of improvement or worsening after 72 hours of therapy requires reevaluation. Follow-up throat cultures are not recommended unless symptoms persist or recur. Recurrent symptoms following an appropriate treatment course should prompt reevaluation for possible retreatment.

COMMON COLD

The common cold is a viral URI associated with significant health care resource utilization, including physician office and emergency department visits and nearly universal use of cough and cold medication for treatment or prevention.[44,45] Clinicians

Clinical Presentation and Diagnosis of Streptococcal Pharyngitis

Children between 5 and 15 years have the highest incidence of streptococcal pharyngitis.

Signs and Symptoms of Streptococcal Pharyngitis[40,41]

- Sudden sore throat with severe pain while swallowing
- Fever
- Headache, abdominal pain, nausea, or vomiting (especially children)
- Tonsillopharyngeal erythema with or without exudates
- Tender, anterior cervical lymphadenitis
- Swollen red uvula
- Halitosis
- Soft palate petechiae
- Scarlatiniform rash
- Absence of conjunctivitis, hoarseness, cough, rhinorrhea, discrete ulcerations, and diarrhea (suggestive of viral etiology)

Diagnosis[38,40,41]

- Rapid antigen detection test (RADT): 70% to 90% sensitivity; results available within minutes.
- Throat culture: "gold standard"; results available within 24 to 48 hours. Should be performed after all negative RADTs in children and adolescents, and adults with significant pediatric contact. Also recommended in outbreaks and to monitor for resistance.
- Tests should be performed *only* when there is clinical suspicion for streptococcal pharyngitis. Pharyngeal carriage occurs in up to 20% of healthy children.

must be aware of evidence regarding the use of cough and cold products in order to make appropriate recommendations for this commonly encountered condition.

EPIDEMIOLOGY AND ETIOLOGY

Many viruses cause the common cold, including rhinoviruses (most common), coronaviruses, parainfluenza viruses, respiratory syncytial virus, and adenoviruses. Infection rates increase during the fall through spring seasons and are highest in the winter months. Adults experience 2 to 4 colds each year, whereas children have 6 to 10 colds per year.[46] Colds usually resolve over 10 to 14 days but can be complicated by bacterial superinfections, including AOM and ABRS. Factors associated with an increased incidence of colds are young age, contact with school-age children, crowded conditions and poorly ventilated areas, and cigarette smoking. Children are more likely than adults to transmit viruses because of poorer hand hygiene, closer casual contacts, and sharing of toys.[45] Viral antigenic drifts and host immune system evasion contribute to the persistence of URIs in the community.

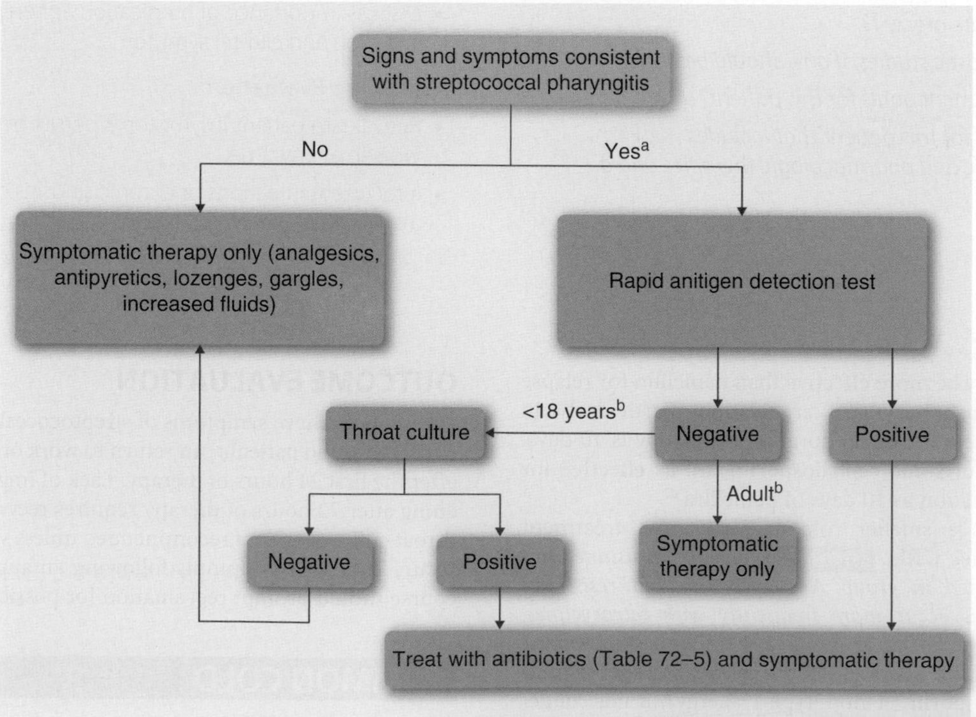

FIGURE 72–4. Treatment algorithm for management of pharyngitis in children and adults. [a]Rapid antigen detection tests (RADTs) are preferred if the test sensitivity exceeds 80%. [b]It is the clinician's discretion to perform a throat culture in adults who have a negative RADT.[40,41]

Table 72–5

Antibiotics[a] for the Treatment of Streptococcal Pharyngitis[40,41]

Drug	Adult Dose	Pediatric Dose	Duration	Comments
Penicillin V	500 mg two to three times daily	250 mg two to three times daily (if ≤ 27 kg), 500 mg two to three times daily (if > 27 kg)	10 days	Drug of choice but increasing reports of treatment failures
Penicillin G benzathine	1.2 million units	600,000 units (if ≤ 27 kg); 1.2 million units (if > 27 kg)	1 IM dose	Useful for patients with poor adherence or emesis; painful injection but pain can be reduced if warmed to room temperature prior to administration
Amoxicillin	775 mg to 1 g once daily (Moxatag 775 mg is a time-released formulation given once daily for patients 12 years of age and older)	50 mg/kg once daily; max 1 g	10 days	Preferred drug for young children because of improved palatability and once daily dosing
Cephalexin	500 mg twice daily	25–50 mg/kg/day in two doses	10 days	Recommended in non–type I penicillin allergy
Cefadroxil	1 g once daily	30 mg/kg once daily	10 days	Recommended in non–type I penicillin allergy
Cefuroxime axetil	250 mg twice daily	20 mg/kg/day in two doses	10 days	
Cefdinir	300 mg twice daily or 600 mg once daily	14 mg/kg/day in one to two doses	5–10 days	Broad spectrum; expensive
Azithromycin	500 mg once daily	12 mg/kg once daily	5 days	Recommended in immediate-type penicillin hypersensitivity; increasing resistance
Clindamycin	300 mg 3 times daily	20 mg/kg/day in three doses	10 days	Recommended in immediate-type penicillin hypersensitivity; useful for recurrent infections

[a]Other FDA-approved agents include amoxicillin-clavulanate, cefixime, cefaclor, cefprozil, cefpodoxime, erythromycin, clarithromycin, and others.

IM, intramuscular.

PATHOPHYSIOLOGY

Viruses enter the respiratory tract mucosa via inhalation of aerosols or infected droplets or direct contact with contaminated secretions. After cell entry, viral replication and shedding occur for several days to weeks. Symptoms arise from epithelial cell damage, inflammation, vasodilation, local tissue edema, increased mucous production, and impaired mucociliary clearance. Tracheobronchial inflammation and irritation induce cough via afferent nerve impulse transmission to the medulla.[45] Antibody production halts viral replication and inflammation as symptoms diminish.

TREATMENT

The treatment goal is to minimize discomfort from symptoms to allow patients to function as normally as possible. Preventative measures are also important to limit the spread of infection.

Antibiotics are not effective, but they are often prescribed to patients with viral URIs and purulent secretions, which have contributed to increased resistance.[2] Treatment should focus on symptom relief.

Supportive measures include air humidification, intranasal saline drops or sprays with or without bulb suctioning, increased fluid intake, throat lozenges or saline gargles, and rest. Nasal strips may relieve congestion by lifting the nares and opening the anterior nasal passages. These nondrug measures are particularly important for children younger than 6 years and pregnant women, for whom medication safety is a significant concern. Although studies proving their benefits are lacking, these nondrug treatments are safe.

Nonprescription cough and cold preparations are used frequently despite a lack of evidence to support their safety and efficacy. Reports of serious adverse events and deaths led to efforts to eliminate use of these medications in young children.[47] Manufacturers have removed product labeling for all children younger than 4 years. Hundreds of products are available to manage cold symptoms. KEY CONCEPT *Choice of therapy is influenced by patient age, presence of comorbid conditions, and balance of effectiveness and safety.* Single-ingredient agents are preferred to target only symptoms that are present and to minimize toxicity that can result from confusion and lack of knowledge about active ingredients in multiple ingredient formulations. Cautious use of nonprescription products is warranted in certain patient populations: pregnant or lactating women, elderly, and patients with cardiovascular disease, diabetes, or glaucoma. Table 72–6 summarizes some of the available agents used for cold symptoms. Antipyretics and analgesics can be used for fever, pain, and discomfort. Local anesthetics (eg, benzocaine, dyclonine) relieve throat pain and are available in lozenges and sprays. Decongestants cause vasoconstriction that can improve congestion, but use of intranasal products should be limited to 3 days to avoid rebound congestion.[44,49]

Patient Care Process for Streptococcal Pharyngitis

Patient Assessment:

- Based on patient history, review of systems, and physical examination, determine if streptococcal pharyngitis is likely. If so, perform a rapid antigen detection test and/or follow-up throat culture to confirm the diagnosis.
- Perform a medical review and conduct a medication history (including prescription and nonprescription medications and natural products). Does the patient have any medication allergies or adverse reactions?

Therapy Evaluation:

- If the patient is receiving pharmacotherapy, assess efficacy, safety, and patient adherence.
- Determine if antibiotic therapy is indicated (see Figure 72–4).
- Determine whether the patient has prescription coverage and if the desired antibiotic is covered by their insurance.

Care Plan Development:

- If appropriate, select analgesic therapy that will provide optimal pain relief.
- If appropriate, select antibiotic therapy that is likely to be effective and safe (Table 72–5). Select an optimal dose and appropriate duration of treatment.
- Discuss potential adverse effects and how to manage them.
- Discuss importance of medication adherence to treat infection, minimize spread, and reduce chances of recurrence.
- Discuss the need to avoid close contact with others for 24 hours to minimize spread.

Follow-up Evaluation:

- Reevaluate patient if symptoms persist after 72 hours or worsen.
- Reevaluate patient if infection recurs after completion of therapy.

Patient Encounter 3

A 7-year-old girl presents to the pediatrician with a sore throat and fever of 39.1°C (102.4°F) for the past 12 hours. She has pain while swallowing, so she is unable to eat or drink as much as usual. She also complains of a "belly ache." She has no other symptoms and takes no medications. She is allergic to amoxicillin (rash). Her mother reports that two children in her daughter's class had "strep throat" recently. Physical examination reveals halitosis, pharyngeal and tonsillar erythema with exudates, and cervical lymphadenopathy.

Does this child have streptococcal pharyngitis?

Is antibiotic therapy indicated? If so, what agent should be initiated and for how long?

What education should be provided to her mother regarding treatment?

Clinical Presentation and Diagnosis of the Common Cold

Symptoms begin 24 to 72 hours after infectious contact. They peak at day 3 to 4, begin to wane by day 7, and resolve by day 10 to 14.

Signs and Symptoms[44,45]

- *Onset:* Malaise, fatigue, headache, pharyngitis, low-grade fever (can be higher in infants and children)
- *Secondary:* Nasal and/or postnasal drainage (often clear at onset, but can become thick and purulent); congestion; cough and/or throat clearing; sneezing; conjunctivitis; irritability; impaired smell or taste

Complications

- AOM, ABRS, chronic bronchitis, bronchiolitis (in infants and children less than 2 years), pneumonia, asthma exacerbation

Diagnosis

- *Clinical diagnosis:* Most common method; based on history, presence of symptoms, and physical examination
- *Radiographic studies:* Useful for assessing complications such as pneumonia
- *Laboratory studies:* Rapid viral antigen tests and nasopharyngeal cultures helpful for epidemiology and diagnosis in acutely ill young infants

Patient Encounter 4

A 20-year-old woman presents to the university health center clinic with a "sinus infection." Three days ago, she developed a sore throat and a "runny nose." Today, her nasal discharge is thicker and yellow in color, she is congested, and she has a headache. She took acetaminophen 500 mg this morning, which provided some relief. She has exercise-induced asthma. She attends college and lives in an apartment with two friends who also have similar symptoms.

Immunizations: Up-to-date; needs influenza vaccine this season

Meds: Ortho Tri-Cyclen orally daily, albuterol inhaler as needed before exercise

Allergies: Cephalexin (rash)

PE:

Gen: No apparent distress

VS: BP 118/66 mm Hg, P 66 beats/min, RR 16 breaths/min, T 37.3°C (99.2°F), Wt 54.5 kg (120 lb)

HEENT: Conjunctiva clear; no photophobia; yellow nasal discharge with swollen nasal mucosa; erythematous pharynx; no facial pain upon palpation; tympanic membranes normal appearing

Lungs: Clear to auscultation; no crackles

What signs and symptoms are suggestive of the common cold? Which are suggestive of ABRS?

What diagnostic studies should be performed?

Create a care plan that includes nonpharmacologic and pharmacologic therapies and a monitoring plan. Include preventative measures in your plan.

Table 72–6

Select Nonprescription Medications for the Common Cold for Patients 6 Years of Age and Older[44,47,48]

Class/Drug	Adult Dose[a]	Pediatric Dose[b]	Comments
Analgesics/Antipyretics			
Acetaminophen[c,d]	325–1000 mg every 4–6 hours (max 4 g/day)	10–15 mg/kg/dose every 4–6 hours (max 5 doses/day)	Use with caution in preexisting liver disease
Ibuprofen[e]	200–400 mg every 6–8 hours (max 1200 mg/day)	5–10 mg/kg/dose every 6–8 hours (max 4 doses/day)	Use with caution in cardiovascular disease; avoid use in elderly, renal impairment, and heart failure; avoid in third trimester of pregnancy
Decongestants			
Intranasal:			
Oxymetazoline 0.05%[d]	Two to three sprays every 12 hours (max 2 doses/24 hours)	One to two sprays every 12 hours (max 2 doses/24 hours)	Limit use of intranasal decongestants to 3–5 days to minimize risk of rebound congestion; use with caution in patients with cardiovascular disease
Phenylephrine 0.25%, 0.5%, 1%	Two to three sprays no more than every 4 hours	Two to three sprays no more than every 4 hours (0.25% only)	
Systemic:			
Pseudoephedrine	60 mg every 4–6 hours (max 240 mg/day)	30 mg every 4–6 hours (max 120 mg/day)	Avoid use in patients with cardiovascular disease; children and elderly have increased risk of adverse effects (cardiovascular or CNS stimulation); use with caution in patients with diabetes, hyperthyroidism, prostatic hypertrophy; avoid in first trimester of pregnancy
Phenylephrine	10 mg every 4 hours (max 60 mg/day)	5 mg every 4 hours (max 30 mg/day)	
Cough Suppressants			
Dextromethorphan[d]	10–20 mg every 4 hours or 30 mg every 6–8 hours or 60 mg every 12 hours (max 120 mg/day)	5–10 mg every 4 hours or 15 mg every 6–8 hours or 30 mg every 12 hours (max 60 mg/day)	Increased adverse effects in children and poor metabolizers (5%–10% of white patients); can cause dysphoria and serotonin syndrome; use caution in those taking psychotropic medications
Expectorants			
Guaifenesin	200–400 mg every 4 hours or 600–1200 mg every 12 hours (max 2.4 g/day)	100 200 mg every 4 hours (max 1.2 g/day)	May cause nausea and abdominal pain, particularly in higher doses
Anticholinergics			
Intranasal ipratropium 0.06%[d]	Two sprays three to four times/day	Two sprays three times/day	Used for rhinorrhea only; does not improve congestion, postnasal drip, or sneezing

[a]Also for children older than 12 years.

[b]For children 6 to 12 years of age.

[c]Preferred antipyretic/analgesic for children; can be used in newborns.

[d]Safe to use in pregnancy.

[e]Can be used in children older than 6 months of age.

Antihistamines should be avoided: first-generation agents may dry secretions through their anticholinergic effects, but they impair mucociliary clearance of thick mucus, which can worsen congestion, and there is not a clear benefit for cough or cold symptoms when these agents are used alone.[44,49] Cough suppressant use is not supported by strong evidence showing benefit. They can cause significant neurologic adverse effects and have been linked to abuse by teens for their euphoric effects in high doses.[44–46,49] Guaifenesin, an expectorant, may reduce sputum thickness in adults, but it has been poorly studied in children.[49] High-dose vitamin C (greater than 200 mg/day) supplementation does not significantly impact cold severity or duration, but it may be useful for prevention in patients exposed to severe physical exercise or cold stress.[49] Echinacea has limited benefit for treatment in adults, and its use is discouraged for prevention and in all children because of adverse effects.[50] Zinc lozenges are not consistently effective, and concerns exist regarding the loss of smell with intranasal preparations, so they should be avoided.

PREVENTION

Prevention of the common cold is best achieved by minimizing contact with infected people and secretions. Frequent hand-washing with soap and water or use of alcohol-based products is vital. Coughing and sneezing into the arm sleeve should be taught rather than using tissues or covering the mouth and nose with hands. Other methods that are advocated for preventing the spread include smoking cessation, maintenance of a healthy lifestyle through diet and exercise, and minimizing stress.

Patient Care Process for Common Cold

Patient Assessment:

- Based on patient history, review of systems, and physical examination, determine if the presentation is consistent with the common cold.
- Perform a medical review and conduct a medication history (including prescription and nonprescription medications and natural products). Does the patient have any medication allergies or adverse reactions? Is the patient up-to-date on immunizations?

Therapy Evaluation:

- If the patient is receiving pharmacotherapy, assess efficacy, safety, and patient adherence.
- Determine if pharmacologic therapy is indicated or if nonpharmacologic measures alone can be employed.

Care Plan Development:

- Select nonpharmacologic and/or nonprescription therapies that will provide optimal relief of symptoms and that are safe for the patient.
- Discuss importance of medication adherence to provide symptom relief and minimize adverse effects.
- Discuss preventative measures for minimizing spread and future illnesses.

Follow-up Evaluation:

- Reevaluate patient if symptoms persist beyond 10 to 14 days or worsen at any time.

OUTCOME EVALUATION

Most colds resolve within 7 to 10 days. Monitor patients for persistent symptoms lasting longer than 10 to 14 days, worsening symptoms, and complications such as wheezing, difficulty breathing, significant facial or ear pain, and high fevers. If complications are suspected, refer to a clinician for evaluation.

Abbreviations Introduced in This Chapter

ABRS	Acute bacterial rhinosinusitis
AOM	Acute otitis media
OME	Otitis media with effusion
PRSP	Penicillin-resistant *S. pneumoniae*
RADT	Rapid antigen detection test
URI	Upper respiratory tract infection

REFERENCES

1. Anon JB. Upper respiratory infections. Am J Med. 2010; 123:S16–S25.
2. Hersh AL, Jackson MA, Hicks LA; American Academy of Pediatrics Committee on Infectious Diseases. Principles of judicious antibiotic prescribing for upper respiratory tract infections in pediatrics. Pediatrics. 2013;132:1146–1154.
3. Vergison A, Dagan R, Arguedas A, et al. Otitis media and its consequences: Beyond the earache. Lancet Infect Dis. 2010;10:195–220.
4. Rovers MM. The burden of otitis media. Vaccine. 2008;26 Suppl 7:G2–G4.
5. Corbeel L. What is new in otitis media? Eur J Pediatr. 2007;166:511–519.
6. Grijalva CG, Nuorti JP, Griffin MR. Antibiotic prescription rates for acute respiratory tract infections in US ambulatory settings. JAMA. 2009;302:758–766.
7. Hersh AL, Shapiro DJ, Pavia AT, Shah SS. Antibiotic prescribing in ambulatory pediatrics in the United States. Pediatrics. 2011;128:1053–1061.
8. McGrath LJ, Becker-Dreps S, Pate V, Brookhart MA. Trends in antibiotic treatment of acute otitis media and treatment failure in children, 2000-2011. PLoS One. 2013;8:e81210.
9. Lieberthal AS, Carroll AE, Chonmaitree T, et al. The diagnosis and management of acute otitis media. Pediatrics. 2013;131:e964–e999.
10. Coker TR, Chan LS, Newberry SJ, et al. Diagnosis, microbial epidemiology, and antibiotic treatment of acute otitis media in children: A systematic review. JAMA. 2010;304:2161–2169.
11. Jokinen J, Palmu AA, Kilpi T. Acute otitis media replacement and recurrence in the Finnish otitis media vaccine trial. Clin Infect Dis. 2012;55:1673–1676.
12. Bulut Y, Güven M, Otlu B, et al. Acute otitis media and respiratory viruses. Eur J Pediatr. 2007;166:223–228.
13. Jones RN, Sader HS, Mendes RE, Flamm RK. Update on antimicrobial susceptibility trends among *Streptococcus pneumoniae* in the United States: Report of ceftaroline activity from the SENTRY Antimicrobial Surveillance Program (1998-2011). Diagn Microbiol Infect Dis. 2013;75:107–109.
14. Critchley IA, Brown SD, Traczewski MM. National and regional assessment of antimicrobial resistance among community-acquired respiratory tract pathogens identified in a 2005-2006 U.S. Faropenem surveillance study. Antimicrob Agents Chemother. 2007;51:4382–4389.
15. Venekamp RP, Sanders S, Glasziou PP, et al. Antibiotics for acute otitis media in children. Cochrane Database Syst Rev. 2013;1:CD000219.
16. Tähtinen PA, Laine MK, Huovinen P, et al. A placebo-controlled trial of antimicrobial treatment for acute otitis media. N Engl J Med. 2011;364:116–126.
17. Hoberman A, Paradise JL, Rockette HE, et al. Treatment of acute otitis media in children under 2 years of age. N Engl J Med. 2011;364:105–115.
18. Spiro DM, Arnold DH. The concept and practice of a wait-and-see approach to acute otitis media. Curr Opin Pediatr. 2008;20:72–78.
19. Piglansky L, Leibovitz E, Raiz S, et al. Bacteriologic and clinical efficacy of high dose amoxicillin for therapy of acute otitis media in children. Pediatr Infect Dis J. 2003;22:405–413.
20. Pichichero ME. Use of selected cephalosporins in penicillin-allergic patients: A paradigm shift. Diagn Microbiol Infect Dis. 2007;57(suppl 3):13S–18S.

21. Leibovitz E, Piglansky L, Raiz S, et al. Bacteriologic and clinical efficacy of one day vs. three day intramuscular ceftriaxone for treatment of nonresponsive acute otitis media in children. Pediatr Infect Dis J. 2000;19:1040–1045.
22. Schmelzle J, Birtwhistle RV, Tan AK. Acute otitis media in children with tympanostomy tubes. Can Fam Physician. 2008;54:1123–1127.
23. Kozyrskyj AL, Klassen TP, Moffatt M, Harvey K. Short-course antibiotics for acute otitis media. Cochrane Database Syst Rev. 2010;CD001095.
24. Coleman C, Moore M. Decongestants and antihistamines for acute otitis media in children. Cochrane Database Syst Rev. 2008;CD001727.
25. Jenson HB, Baltimore RS. Impact of influenza and pneumococcal vaccines on otitis media. Curr Opin Pediatr. 2004;16:58–60.
26. Block SL, Heikkinen T, Toback SL, Zheng W, Ambrose CS. The efficacy of live attenuated influenza vaccine against influenza-associated acute otitis media in children. Pediatr Infect Dis J. 2011;30:203–207.
27. Fortanier AC, Venekamp RP, Boonacker CW, et al. Pneumococcal conjugate vaccines for preventing otitis media. Cochrane Database Syst Rev. 2014;4:CD001480.
28. Chow AW, Benninger MS, Brook I, et al. IDSA clinical practice guideline for acute bacterial rhinosinusitis in children and adults. Clin Infect Dis. 2012;54:e72–e112.
29. Duse M, Caminiti S, Zicari AM. Rhinosinusitis: Prevention strategies. Pediatr Allergy Immunol. 2007;18 Suppl 18:71–74.
30. Wald ER, Applegate KE, Bordley C, et al. Clinical practice guideline for the diagnosis and management of acute bacterial sinusitis in children aged 1 to 18 years. Pediatrics. 2013;132:e262–e280.
31. Eloy P, Poirrier AL, De Dorlodot C, et al. Actual concepts in rhinosinusitis: A review of clinical presentations, inflammatory pathways, cytokine profiles, remodeling, and management. Curr Allergy Asthma Rep. 2011;11:146–162.
32. Rosenfeld RM, Andes D, Bhattacharyya N, et al. Clinical practice guideline: Adult sinusitis. Otolaryngol Head Neck Surg. 2007;137:S1–S31.
33. Lemiengre MB, van Driel ML, Merenstein D, et al. Antibiotics for clinically diagnosed acute rhinosinusitis in adults. Cochrane Database Syst Rev. 2012;10:CD006089.
34. Smith MJ. Evidence for the diagnosis and treatment of acute uncomplicated sinusitis in children: A systematic review. Pediatrics. 2013;132:e284–e296.
35. Achilles N, Mösges R. Nasal saline irrigations for the symptoms of acute and chronic rhinosinusitis. Curr Allergy Asthma Rep. 2013;13:229–235.
36. Zalmanovici Trestioreanu A, Yaphe J. Intranasal steroids for acute sinusitis. Cochrane Database Syst Rev. 2013;12:CD005149.
37. Falagas ME, Karageorgopoulos DE, Grammatikos AP, Matthaiou DK. Effectiveness and safety of short vs. long duration of antibiotic therapy for acute bacterial sinusitis: A meta-analysis of randomized trials. Br J Clin Pharmacol. 2009;67:161–171.
38. Cooper RJ, Hoffman JR, Bartlett JG, et al. Principles of appropriate antibiotic use for acute pharyngitis in adults: background. Ann Intern Med. 2001;134:509–517.
39. Linder JA, Bates DW, Lee GM, Finkelstein JA. Antibiotic treatment of children with sore throat. JAMA. 2005;294:2315–2322.
40. Shulman ST, Bisno AL, Clegg HW, et al. Clinical practice guideline for the diagnosis and management of group A streptococcal pharyngitis: 2012 update by the Infectious Diseases Society of America. Clin Infect Dis. 2012;55:e86–e102.
41. Gerber MA, Baltimore RS, Eaton CB, et al. Prevention of rheumatic fever and diagnosis and treatment of acute streptococcal pharyngitis. A scientific statement from the American Heart Association Rheumatic Fever, Endocarditis, and Kawasaki Disease Committee of the Council on Cardiovascular Disease in the Young, the Interdisciplinary Council on Functional Genomics and Translational Biology, and the Interdisciplinary Council on Quality of Care and Outcomes Research: endorsed by the American Academy of Pediatrics. Circulation. 2009;119:1541–1551.
42. van Driel ML, De Sutter AI, Keber N, Habraken H, et al. Different antibiotic treatments for group A streptococcal pharyngitis. Cochrane Database Syst Rev. 2013;4:CD004406.
43. Casey JR, Pichichero ME. Metaanalysis of short course antibiotic treatment for group a streptococcal tonsillopharyngitis. Pediatr Infect Dis J. 2005;24:909–917.
44. Fashner J, Ericson K, Werner S. Treatment of the common cold in children and adults. Am Fam Physician. 2012;86:153–159.
45. Kelley LK, Allen PJ. Managing acute cough in children: Evidence-based guidelines. Pediatr Nurs. 2007;33:515–524.
46. Pratter MR. Cough and the common cold. ACCP evidence-based clinical practice guidelines. Chest. 2006;129:S72–S74.
47. Yang M, So TY. Revisiting the safety of over-the-counter cough and cold medications in the pediatric population. Clin Pediatr (Phila). 2014;53:326–330.
48. Erebara A, Bozzo P, Einarson A, Koren G. Treating the common cold during pregnancy. Can Fam Physician. 2008;54:687–689.
49. Arroll B. Non-antibiotic treatments for upper-respiratory tract infections (common cold). Respir Med. 2005;99:1477–1484.
50. Karsch-Völk M, Barrett B, Kiefer D, et al. Echinacea for preventing and treating the common cold. Cochrane Database Syst Rev. 2014;2:CD000530.

73 Skin and Soft Tissue Infections

Jaime R. Hornecker

LEARNING OBJECTIVES

Upon completion of the chapter, the reader will be able to:

1. Discuss characteristics of the skin that render it resistant to infection.
2. Describe the epidemiology, etiology, pathogenesis, clinical manifestations, diagnostic criteria, and complications associated with skin and soft tissue infections (SSTIs).
3. Identify the desired therapeutic outcomes for patients with SSTIs.
4. Recommend appropriate empirical and definitive antimicrobial regimens when given a diagnosis, patient history, physical examination, and laboratory findings.
5. Monitor chosen antimicrobial therapy for safety and efficacy.

INTRODUCTION

Skin and soft tissue infections (SSTIs) are frequently encountered in both acute and ambulatory care settings. They can range in severity from mild, superficial, and self-limiting, to life-threatening deep tissue infections that require intensive care, surgical intervention, and IV broad-spectrum antibiotics. Gram-positive pathogens, primarily *Staphylococcus aureus* and *Streptococcus* species, are the most common causative bacteria.[1–4] Polymicrobial infections are more likely in complicated infections involving deeper layers of the skin, fascia, or muscle in persons with immune suppression, diabetes, and vascular insufficiency, and in postsurgical patients.[1,4]

The role of methicillin-resistant *S. aureus* (MRSA), particularly community-acquired methicillin-resistant *S. aureus* (CA-MRSA), in SSTI is of increasing importance. In many US cities, MRSA is the most frequently isolated pathogen from patients presenting to emergency departments with SSTI, and antimicrobial prescribing has largely shifted to empiric use of MRSA-active agents.[2,5] MRSA infections were historically associated with exposures to health care settings and more defined populations such as injection drug users or athletes; however, the prevalence of MRSA in the community and its rise in otherwise healthy individuals means that historical high-risk groups have little clinical relevance in most areas. In areas with high rates of CA-MRSA, and in those with recurrent infections or infections that persist despite appropriate antimicrobial therapy, empiric therapy including antibiotics active against this pathogen must be considered.[1,6] This chapter covers the epidemiology, pathogenesis, clinical manifestations, and pharmacologic management of the more common and severe bacterial SSTIs.

Intact skin generally is resistant to infection. In addition to providing a mechanical barrier, its relative dryness, slightly acidic pH, colonizing bacteria, frequent desquamation, and production of various antimicrobial defense chemicals, including sweat (which contains IgG and IgA), prevent invasion by various microorganisms.[7] Conditions that predispose a patient to SSTIs include: (a) high bacterial load (greater than 10^5 microorganisms); (b) excessive skin moisture; (c) decreased skin perfusion; (d) availability of bacterial nutrients; and (e) damage to the corneal layer of the skin.[8]

IMPETIGO

EPIDEMIOLOGY AND ETIOLOGY

KEY CONCEPT *Impetigo is a common skin infection worldwide that can occur in any age group, but most frequently affects children between 2 and 5 years.*[9] β-Hemolytic streptococci and *S. aureus* are the most common causative pathogens.[4] Impetigo is a superficial infection and spreads easily, especially in settings of poor hygiene and crowding, and particularly during the summer months. The offending microorganisms colonize the skin surface and invade through abrasions, insect bites, or other small traumas. The scabby, crusty eruption of impetigo ensues. These lesions may occur anywhere on the body, but are most common on the face and extremities.[10]

CLINICAL PRESENTATION AND DIAGNOSIS

Impetigo lesions are numerous, well localized, and **erythematous**. KEY CONCEPT *They begin as small, thin-walled blisters that can quickly evolve into ruptured lesions, with the dried discharge forming a honey-colored crust reminiscent of cornflakes.*[4] *S. aureus* and β-hemolytic Strep is most often implicated in impetigo.[4] The lesions of impetigo are rarely painful, but are **pruritic**. Scratching the lesions can spread the infection to other areas of the body. Scarring is rarely problematic, unless ulceration occurs, as in ecthyma.[4]

In order to avoid further spread and complications, antibiotic therapy is usually indicated. Sequelae of impetigo are uncommon, but rarely, glomerulonephritis secondary to group A

Streptococcus (GAS) may occur.[4] Development of impetigo into more serious infections such as cellulitis or sepsis is another rare, but serious consequence.

TREATMENT

The primary goals of therapy for impetigo include preventing the spread of infection within the patient and to others, resolution of infection, and preventing recurrence. Secondarily, relief of symptoms associated with impetigo, such as itching, and improving cosmetic appearance are also important. Prevention of the rare, but serious complications of impetigo is an alternative goal.[11]

Nonpharmacologic Treatment

Because impetigo is rarely painful, there is often a delay in seeking medical attention. Lesions may improve with time and increased hygiene, and soaking and cleansing the lesions with mild soap and water and the use of skin emollients to dry skin areas may reduce spread.[11]

Pharmacologic Treatment

Antibiotic therapy is recommended to achieve the desired outcomes of preventing the spread of infection and complications. Although GAS historically has been the primary causative organism and penicillin is recommended when cultures yield streptococci alone, KEY CONCEPT *the incidence of* S. aureus *impetigo is common, and oral penicillinase-stable penicillins* (such as dicloxacillin) *or first-generation cephalosporins* (such as cephalexin) *are preferred.* Clindamycin, sulfamethoxazole-trimethoprim, or doxycycline is preferred when MRSA is suspected, or as alternative choices when penicillin allergy is a concern; however, tetracyclines should be avoided in children younger than 8 years. KEY CONCEPT *Topical mupirocin or retapamulin twice daily for 5 days may be used alone in mild cases with few lesions or in individual outbreaks.*[4,6]

FOLLICULITIS, FURUNCLES, AND CARBUNCLES

See Table 73-1 for summary.

CELLULITIS AND ERYSIPELAS

EPIDEMIOLOGY AND ETIOLOGY

Cellulitis and erysipelas are bacterial infections involving the skin. KEY CONCEPT *Cellulitis is an infection of the dermis and subcutaneous tissue, whereas erysipelas is a more superficial infection of the upper dermis and superficial lymphatics. Although both can occur on any part of the body, many infections involve the leg.*[13,14] These infections develop after a break in skin integrity, resulting from trauma, surgery, ulceration, burns, tinea infection, or other skin disorder. However, they may occur after an inapparent break in the skin, and the skin may appear previously intact. In rare cases, cellulitis develops from bloodborne or contiguous spread of pathogens.[4,14]

Etiologic microorganisms vary according to the area involved, host factors, and exposures. KEY CONCEPT *The predominant pathogens associated with cellulitis are streptococci, mainly group A, and less frequently* S. aureus, *including methicillin-resistant strains. Persons who are immunocompromised have diabetes or vascular insufficiency, or use injection drugs, are at risk for polymicrobial cellulitis.*[4]

CLINICAL PRESENTATION AND DIAGNOSIS

The manifestations of and diagnostic criteria for erysipelas and cellulitis are presented in Table 73–2.

With early diagnosis and appropriate therapy, the prognoses for cellulitis and erysipelas are excellent. Severe or repeated episodes can cause lymphedema. Rare complications include the spread of infection to deeper skin and soft tissue layers, bacteremia, and sepsis.[4] Although rates of bacteremia were traditionally low, prevalence may be increasing and associated with increased length of hospitalization and costs, and higher readmission rates.[15]

Recurrent cellulitis can be problematic. Annual recurrence rates, especially for cellulitis of the leg, can be as high as 20%. Vascular and lymphatic insufficiencies increase the risk of recurrences; obesity, tobacco use, history of cancer, and homelessness also increase risk.[4]

TREATMENT

The goals of therapy for cellulitis and erysipelas are rapid and successful eradication of the infection and prevention of related complications.

Nonpharmacologic Treatment

Nonpharmacologic treatment includes elevating the involved limb to decrease swelling. Sterile saline dressings may be placed on any open lesions to cleanse them of purulent materials. Surgical débridement may be indicated for severe infection and to rule out any necrotizing process. Drainage of abscesses is imperative to achieving clinical cure and may be the only treatment necessary if the abscess is small (less than 5 cm) with limited cellulitis.[4,14]

Pharmacologic Treatment

Most patients with erysipelas or cellulitis are effectively treated with outpatient therapy. Hospitalization and treatment with IV antibiotics is recommended in the presence of systemic inflammatory response syndrome (SIRS) (eg, temperature greater than 38°C or less than 36°C, tachypnea greater than 24 breaths/min, tachycardia greater than 90 beats/min, or white blood cell count greater than $12 \times 10^3/mm^3$ [$12 \times 10^9/L$] or less than $400/mm^3$ [$0.4 \times 10^9/L$]), altered mental status, or hemodynamic instability. Outpatient treatment should also be avoided when deep or necrotizing infection is present, in severe immunocompromise, or when outpatient treatment is failing or adherence to therapy is poor.[4]

Antibiotic choices for typical cases of cellulitis should have activity against streptococci, and include penicillin, amoxicillin, amoxicillin-clavulanate, dicloxacillin, cephalexin, or clindamycin. In uncomplicated cases, a 5-day course is as effective as a 10-day course.[4] Monotherapy with a β-lactam is appropriate in uncomplicated cases[16]; however, when purulent drainage, abscess, or ulcer is present, or in cases of penetrating trauma, particularly IV drug use, coverage for MRSA should be initiated.

Vancomycin continues to be the drug of choice for severe cellulitis due to MRSA because of its efficacy, safety, and low cost. Daptomycin, linezolid, telavancin, or ceftaroline are also acceptable and should be considered over vancomycin when the isolated organism has a minimum inhibitory concentration (MIC) of greater than 2 mcg/mL (greater than 2 mg/L) (eg, vancomycin-intermediate *S. aureus* [VISA] or vancomycin-resistant *S. aureus* [VRSA]).[6] Tigecycline is an alternative; however, due to its broad spectrum of activity, it is best reserved for patients with intolerances to the aforementioned drugs or in those with polymicrobial infections. Several new agents for SSTI, including tedizolid,

Table 73–1
Folliculitis, Furuncles, and Carbuncles

	Folliculitis	Furuncles	Carbuncles
Epidemiology/ etiology	KEY CONCEPT *Folliculitis is a superficial inflammatory reaction involving the hair follicle. The most familiar form of folliculitis is acne.* It can be infectious, caused by microorganisms such as *S. aureus, Pseudomonas, and Candida.* Folliculitis can also be chemically induced.	Also known as boils, furuncles might be described as a deep form of folliculitis. A furuncle is a bacterial infection that has spread into the subcutaneous skin layers but still only involves individual follicles. Furuncles occur primarily in young men. Diabetes and obesity are other predisposing factors. Staphylococci are the most common cause.	Carbuncles share all the characteristics of furuncles. However, a carbuncle is larger and involves several adjacent follicles and may extend into the subcutaneous fat. Carbuncles are more likely to occur in patients with diabetes and tend to form on the back of the neck.
Presentation and diagnosis	Folliculitis presents as small, pruritic, erythematous papules. Location of the lesions and a good patient history are often all that are required in the diagnosis of folliculitis. Although Gram stain and culture of the papules may be considered to help determine the causative agent, they are not generally required as folliculitis typically resolves spontaneously.	Furuncles most commonly develop on the face, neck, axilla, and buttock. A furuncle typically starts as a small, red, tender nodule. Within a few days, the nodule becomes painful and pustular. Typically, a furuncle will spontaneously discharge pus, heal, and leave a small scar.	Carbuncles are similar to furuncles; only they are larger and exquisitely painful.
Desired outcomes	The goals of therapy for folliculitis, furuncles, and carbuncles are resolution of infection with no or minimal scarring. A secondary goal of therapy for larger furuncles and all carbuncles is to minimize the risk of endocarditis or osteomyelitis by reducing bloodstream invasion.		
Nonpharmacologic treatment	KEY CONCEPT *Warm compresses are generally sufficient.*	*Moist heat is indicated to facilitate drainage. Large furuncles require incision and drainage.*	*Incision and drainage are indicated.*
Pharmacologic treatment	KEY CONCEPT *Often resolves spontaneously. A topical antibiotic or antifungal may be used to control the spread of infection but generally is unnecessary.* For staphylococcal or streptococcal folliculitis, antibiotic ointments such as mupirocin might be administered. Antifungal shampoo can be used for dermatophytes.	*Carbuncles and furuncles that are purulent with signs of infection (ie, fever) should be treated systemically with an antibiotic that will cover S. aureus, such as dicloxacillin or cephalexin. Trimethoprim-sulfamethoxazole or doxycycline is preferred if CA-MRSA is suspected or if the patient has a severe allergy to penicillin.* Treatment should continue until acute inflammation has resolved, usually a 5- to 10-day course. Immunocompromised patients and severe infections or abscesses in patients who fail incision and drainage plus oral antibiotics should be treated empirically with vancomycin, daptomycin, linezolid, televancin, or ceftaroline. Prevention for recurrent episodes may be warranted, including adequate skin hygiene with the use of soap and water, and handwashing after contact with lesions. Proper care of clothing and dressings is also recommended to prevent autoinoculation.	

Data from Refs. 4, 10, and 12.

Patient Encounter 1, Part 1: Cellulitis

A 57-year-old man presents to the ambulatory care clinic with a 3-day history of progressively worsening pain and swelling of his left lower extremity. Upon examination, you notice that in addition to the patient's complaints, the area is visibly erythematous. Poorly defined areas of redness and streaking extend from just below the knee up toward his hip. A small, nonpurulent scabbed area is present over the kneecap. He reports running a low-grade fever and some feelings of fatigue, but otherwise feels fine. When questioned, he indicates that he recently fell from a ladder while working on the gutters of his home and landed primarily on his left side. His vitals at the clinic reveal a temperature of 38.8°C, pulse 90 beats/min, blood pressure 128/89 mm Hg, and respiratory rate 18 breaths/min. The physician diagnoses the patient with cellulitis.

What subjective and objective clinical manifestations are suggestive of cellulitis?

What additional information do you need before developing a therapeutic plan for this patient?

Table 73–2

Presentation of Erysipelas and Cellulitis

Symptoms

- The infected area is described as painful or tender. In the case of erysipelas, the patient may complain of "burning pain" at the lesion site. CA-MRSA infections often start as a localized skin lesion and may be described by the patient as looking like a "spider bite."

Signs

- Both erysipelas and cellulitis are manifested by rapidly spreading areas of redness, edema, warmth, and tenderness. Lymphangitis and regional lymphadenopathy may be observed.
- The affected area may have an "orange peel" appearance due to superficial skin edema causing skin dimpling around the hair follicles.
- Low-grade fever, flu-like illness, and other systemic symptoms may occur prior to development of the lesion.

Laboratory Tests

- Leukocytosis may be present.
- Cultures and sensitivities:
  - Blood cultures should be obtained for complicated or severe cases, although their yield is often low as bacteremia is an infrequent, but growing, occurrence; facial cellulitis may increase risk. Cultures aspirated from the lesion have a low organism isolation rate, but also may be considered.
  - Abscess drainage and débrided tissue, if obtainable, should be cultured and will frequently yield the causative organism(s).

Imaging Studies

- Imaging studies may identify abscess formation, gas in the soft tissues, or osteomyelitis.

Data from Stevens DL, Bisno AL, Chambers HF, et al. Practice guidelines for the diagnosis and management of skin and soft tissue infections. Clin Infect Dis 2014;41:1373–1406.

dalbavancin and oritavancin, may have advantages over traditional therapy in terms of duration of activity and administration.[17,18] For less severe, uncomplicated infections, many CA-MRSA strains can be treated with clindamycin (isolates resistant to erythromycin should be evaluated with a D-test), doxycycline, or trimethoprim-sulfamethoxazole.[4,6] Trimethoprim-sulfamethoxazole and doxycycline should be empirically combined with a β-lactam if GAS is also a suspected causative organism, since the activity of these agents against β-hemolytic streptococci is unknown.[4]

KEY CONCEPT *In addition to coverage for staphylococcal and streptococcal cellulitis, patients with severe infections should receive treatment for gram-negative bacilli such as Escherichia coli and Pseudomonas aeruginosa, with or without anaerobic coverage. Empirical broad-spectrum antimicrobial coverage, including coverage for resistant organisms such as health care-associated MRSA (HA-MRSA) and P. aeruginosa, is appropriate for severe cellulitis and/or severe systemic illness.* Vancomycin plus piperacillin/tazobactam is recommended in these cases. Therapy continuation is recommended in polymicrobial infections, whereas more defined therapy is recommended when a causative pathogen is isolated.[4]

Table 73–3 lists some recommended antibiotic regimens for the treatment of cellulitis. Because antimicrobial susceptibilities vary considerably between geographic locations, clinicians should select empirical treatment based on the antibiograms at their respective institutions. To decrease the spread of resistance, antibiotic therapy should be narrowed based on culture and sensitivity results whenever possible. The duration of therapy for uncomplicated cellulitis typically ranges from 5 to 10 days. For complicated cellulitis, therapy with IV antibiotics is generally initiated, and a switch to oral therapy can be made once the patient is afebrile and skin findings begin to resolve. Typically, this is done after 3 to 5 days. The complete duration of therapy can range from 10 to 14 days and longer in cases in which abscess, tissue necrosis, underlying skin wounds, or delayed response to therapy are involved.[4,14]

Patient Encounter 1, Part 2: Cellulitis: Medical History, Physical Examination, and Diagnostic Tests

PMH: Hypertension, dyslipidemia, GERD.

FH: Father (age 79) and mother (age 77) are both alive. Father has hypertension and CAD; mother is otherwise healthy. One brother, age 54, also has hypertension.

SH: Denies alcohol or illicit drug use. Married, with two sons who attend the local community college. Works full-time in construction.

Meds: Lisinopril 20 mg daily; simvastatin 20 mg daily; omeprazole 20 mg daily as needed.

Allergies: No known drug allergies.

ROS: (+) pain, edema, and erythema in the left lower extremity; (-) headache, chest pain, shortness of breath, cough, nausea, vomiting, diarrhea, and weight loss.

PE:

Gen: Patient is in no acute distress. Wt 88.2 kg (194 lb); Ht 5'11" (180 cm).

Chest: Lungs bilaterally clear to auscultation.

CV: Regular rate, rhythm. No murmurs/rubs/gallops.

Ext: Left lower extremity with erythema and edema from the knee to just below the hip. Warm to the touch. RLE within normal limits.

Labs: WBC 15.8 × 10^3/mm^3 (15.8 × 10^9/L), serum creatinine 0.8 mg/dL (71 μmol/L).

What are the most likely causative organisms in this case of cellulitis?

What are the goals of therapy for this patient?

What nonpharmacologic interventions would you recommend for him?

What antimicrobial therapy would you recommend? Include drug, dosage, route, interval, and duration of therapy.

How would you monitor your selected regimen for safety and efficacy?

How would your initial choice of an antimicrobial agent change if this patient was at high risk for MRSA?

Table 73–3

Empirical Antimicrobial Therapy for Cellulitis

Host Factors	Probable Etiologic Bacteria	Mild Infection or Step-Down Therapy[a] (Oral Antibiotic Therapy)	Moderate–Severe Infection[a] (IV Antibiotic Therapy)
Previously healthy	MSSA GAS CA-MRSA	Dicloxacillin 500 mg every 6 hours Cephalexin 500 mg every 6 hours Clindamycin 300–600 mg every 6–8 hours CA-MRSA suspected or allergy to PCNs: Clindamycin[b] 300–600 mg every 6–8 hours Trimethoprim-sulfamethoxazole DS[c] one to two tablets every 12 hours Doxycycline[c] 100 mg every 12 hours	Nafcillin 1–2 g every 4 hours Cefazolin 1–2 g every 8 hours Clindamycin 600–900 mg every 8 hours CA-MRSA suspected or allergy to PCNs: Vancomycin 15–20 mg/kg every 8–12 hours (individualize dose to achieve a trough of 15–20 mcg/mL [15–20 mg/L; 10.4–13.8 μmol/L]) Linezolid 600 mg every 12 hours Daptomycin 4 mg/kg every 24 hours Telavancin 10 mg/kg every 24 hours Ceftaroline[f] 600 mg every 12 hours
Immunocompromise, diabetes mellitus, vascular insufficiency, pressure ulcer infection, or other polymicrobial infection suspected	MSSA HA-MRSA CA-MRSA Enterobacteriaceae *P. aeruginosa* Anaerobes	Amoxicillin-clavulanate[d] 875 mg every 12 hours Levofloxacin[e] 750 mg every 24 hours + clindamycin 300–600 mg every 6 hours Moxifloxacin[d] 400 mg every 24 hours	Vancomycin, daptomycin, linezolid, or telavancin[g] In combination with one of the following choices: Piperacillin-tazobactam[e] 3.375 g every 6 hours Ampicillin-sulbactam 3 g every 6 hours Imipenem-cilastatin[e] 500 mg every 6 hours Ertapenem 1 g every 24 hours Meropenem 500 mg every 8 hours Cefepime[e] 2 g every 12 hours ± metronidazole 500 mg every 8 hours Ceftazidime[e] 2 g every 8 hours + clindamycin 600–900 mg every 8 hours OR Ceftaroline 600 mg every 12 hours + clindamycin 600–900 mg every 8 hours or metronidazole 500 mg every 8 hours OR Tigecycline 100 mg load, then 50 mg every 12 hours

[a]Doses given are for adults with normal renal function. IV therapy can be switched to oral therapy (as for mild infection) when the patient is afebrile and signs of infection are resolving.

[b]CA-MRSA isolates resistant to erythromycin should be evaluated for inducible clindamycin resistance via a D-test.

[c]Limited clinical data exist for the treatment of MRSA infections. Poor activity against GAS; consider using in combination with clindamycin or cephalexin if empirical coverage for GAS is desired.

[d]If CA-MRSA suspected, clindamycin, trimethoprim-sulfamethoxazole, or doxycycline must be added to this regimen.

[e]*P. aeruginosa* generally is susceptible to this agent.

[f]Use caution in patients with known hypersensitivity to β-lactam antibiotics.

[g]MRSA coverage indicated for patients with severe cellulitis or systemic illness, who have risk factors for HA-MRSA or CA-MRSA infection, or reside in areas with high CA-MRSA prevalence. Otherwise, the broad-spectrum regimens listed below, without MRSA coverage, are appropriate.

Data from Refs. 4, 10 and 14.

Recurrent cellulitis can be problematic, especially in the lower extremities. Reducing risk factors may help with preventing recurrences.[4] Low-dose antibiotic prophylaxis with penicillin may reduce recurrences, but the benefit subsides when therapy is discontinued.[4,13]

NECROTIZING FASCIITIS

EPIDEMIOLOGY AND ETIOLOGY

Necrotizing fasciitis (NF) is an uncommon, rapidly progressive, life-threatening infection that causes necrosis of the subcutaneous tissue and fascia. When due to GAS infection, its associated mortality rate approaches 25%.[19] NF can affect any age group.

Patient Encounter 1, Part 3: Cellulitis: Clinical Course

Three days later, the patient returns to the clinic with moderate improvement of his cellulitis, but with a new presentation of a maculopapular skin rash. It is presumed that he has developed an allergy to penicillin.

What would you suggest for modification of his antimicrobial regimen?

How would you monitor his new regimen for safety and efficacy?

How would your choice of an agent change if this patient's cellulitis was severe enough to warrant hospitalization?

Although the risk of NF is higher in injection drug users and in patients with diabetes or vascular insufficiency, healthy hosts can become infected as well.[4]

NF typically erupts after an initial trauma, which can range from a small abrasion to a deep penetrating wound. The infection begins in the fascia, where bacteria replicate and release toxins that facilitate their spread.[4]

NF may be monomicrobial, most often involving *S. pyogenes, S. aureus, Vibrio vulnificus, Aeromonas hydrophilia*, and anaerobic streptococci (*Peptostreptococcus*). Polymicrobial NF develops in the following clinical settings: after surgery or deep penetrating wounds involving the bowel; from decubitous ulcer, perianal, or vulvovaginal infection; or from the injection site in an IV drug user.[4]

CLINICAL PRESENTATION AND DIAGNOSIS

Patient outcomes rely on the clinician's ability to recognize NF early in the course of disease. This is often difficult because early disease tends to be indistinguishable from cellulitis. The clinical presentation of NF is presented in Table 73–4.

NF is perhaps the most devastating SSTI. Left untreated, it can invade the muscles and circulation, resulting in myonecrosis and septic shock, respectively. Half of the cases caused by GAS are accompanied by GAS toxic shock–like syndrome. The syndrome is endotoxin mediated, manifested by hypotension and multiorgan dysfunction, and highly lethal.[20] Amputation is common in patients with extremity infections. Once the patient recovers from acute NF, he or she often requires skin and/or muscle grafting and consequent physical rehabilitation depending on the amount and types of tissues removed during surgical intervention and the duration of hospital stay.[21]

Table 73–4

Presentation of Necrotizing Fasciitis

Symptoms

- Early: Severe pain that is disproportionate to clinical signs and extends beyond the margins of the infected area.
- Late: Area may become numb secondary to muscle and nerve involvement.

Signs

- Early: Skin is erythematous, edematous, and warm; the clinical presentation is similar to that of cellulitis.
- Intermediate (within 24–48 hours): Blisters and bullae indicate severe skin and tissue ischemia.
- Late: The skin becomes violaceous and progressively gangrenous, and subcutaneous tissues have wooden-hard induration; hemorrhagic bullae may be present. Systemic signs may include fever, tachycardia, hypotension, and shock.

Laboratory Tests

- White blood count, serum creatinine, and C-reactive protein may be elevated.
- Deep tissue specimens obtained during surgical irrigation and débridement should be sent for Gram stain, culture, and sensitivity.

Imaging Studies

- MRI and CT scans may reveal fluid and gas along fascial planes.
- Typically, imaging studies are avoided when making a diagnosis because they may delay surgical intervention and increase mortality.

NF, Necrotizing fasciitis.

Data from Refs. 4 and 20.

TREATMENT

The goals of therapy for NF include eradication of infection and reduction of related morbidity and mortality.

Nonpharmacologic Treatment

KEY CONCEPT After resuscitation and hemodynamic stabilization, *prompt surgical intervention is key in the treatment of NF. Delayed operative débridement increases mortality, and most patients should return to the operating room frequently until debridement is no longer indicated.*[4,22]

Pharmacologic Treatment

As an adjunct to surgery, high-dose, broad-spectrum IV antibiotic therapy should be initiated immediately in patients with NF until the patient has improved clinically and is afebrile for 48 to 72 hours, and no further need for debridement exists. Piperacillin-tazobactam, a carbapenem, or ceftriaxone or a fluoroquinolone plus metronidazole is appropriate for empiric therapy. These agents should be used in combination with vancomycin, daptomycin, or linezolid until MRSA infection is ruled out.[4] The protein synthesis inhibitors clindamycin or linezolid are often utilized to decrease bacterial toxin production, thereby limiting tissue damage. This is particularly beneficial in streptococcal or clostridial infection.[20]

IV immunoglobulin (IVIG) dosed at 2 g/kg may also be a useful adjunctive treatment in patients with GAS NF who present with shock. Anecdotal evidence and data from small studies strongly support its use in improving 30-day survival and reducing mortality, although additional evidence is needed for a definitive recommendation.[4]

DIABETIC FOOT INFECTIONS

EPIDEMIOLOGY AND ETIOLOGY

Foot ulcers and related infections are among the most common, severe, and costly complications of diabetes mellitus. For the approximately 25 million patients with diabetes in the United States, the lifetime risk of developing at least one foot ulcer is estimated at 25%.[22] In addition to significant morbidity, the health care costs associated with treating infected foot ulcers are enormous.

Infected diabetic foot ulcers typically contain a multitude of microorganisms. KEY CONCEPT *Aerobic gram-positive cocci, such as* S. aureus *and β-hemolytic streptococci, are the predominant pathogens in acutely infected diabetic foot ulcers. However, severe, or more extensive chronically infected wounds are subject to polymicrobial infection.* The clinician should suspect the involvement of gram-negative (such as *P. aeruginosa*) and possibly low-virulence pathogens (including enterococci and *S. epidermidis*) in polymicrobial infections. Foul-smelling, necrotic, or gangrenous wounds are also commonly infected with anaerobic bacteria. Patients recently hospitalized or treated with broad-spectrum antibiotics, or those with a previous history of MRSA infection are at risk for MRSA as a causative agent.[23]

Patient Encounter 2, Part 1: Diabetic Foot Infection

A 66-year-old man with type 2 diabetes mellitus presents to the emergency department with complaints of soreness and swelling of his right foot, accompanied by difficulty walking. Upon examination, you see a purulent lesion on the plantar aspect of his right great toe approximately 3 cm (1.2 in) in diameter. His foot is erythematous, warm, and foul-smelling, and cellulitis and lymphangitic streaking extend beyond his ankle. The patient indicates that his doctor told him at his last visit 8 months ago that his feet had some areas of redness that should be watched, especially with his history of a prior amputation, but because of ongoing chronic back pain and diabetic neuropathy, the patient admits to poor foot hygiene at home. The patient is afebrile, and other vital signs are within normal limits.

What signs and symptoms present in this patient are indicative of a diabetic foot infection?

Based on presentation, classify this patient's diabetic foot infection using the PEDIS grading scale.

What additional information do you need before developing a therapeutic plan for this patient?

PATHOPHYSIOLOGY

KEY CONCEPT *The pathogenesis of diabetic foot infection stems from two key factors:* peripheral *neuropathy and ischemia from peripheral vascular disease.*[22] Neuropathy, the most prominent risk factor for diabetic foot ulcers, develops when continuously high blood glucose levels damage motor, autonomic, and sensory nerves. Damage to motor neurons that supply the small intrinsic muscles of the foot causes deformation, resulting in altered muscular balance, abnormal areas of pressure on tissues and bone, and repetitive injuries. Damage to autonomic neurons results in the shunting of blood through direct arteriole-venous communications, thereby decreasing capillary flow. The secretion of sweat and oil is also diminished, producing dry, cracked skin that is more prone to infection. Finally, damage to sensory neurons produces a loss of protective sensation so that the patient becomes unaware of injury or ulceration.[22]

Dysfunction of the endothelial cells and abnormalities of the smooth muscles of the peripheral vessels is also the result of high blood glucose concentrations. Vasoconstriction can occur due to decreased levels of endothelium-derived vasodilators, as well as in the presence of other risk factors, including hypertension, dyslipidemia, and smoking. Together, ischemia and skin breakdown can occur as a cumulative result.[22]

Finally, persons with diabetes have altered immune function that predisposes them to infection. Leukocyte function, and cell-mediated and humoral immunity are compromised in poorly controlled disease.[23] Achieving and maintaining controlled blood glucose levels should be a component of the prevention and management of diabetic foot infections.

CLINICAL PRESENTATION AND DIAGNOSIS

Not all diabetic foot ulcers are infected. However, infection is often difficult to detect when perfusion and the inflammatory response are limited in the patient with diabetes. The common signs and symptoms (ie, pain, erythema, and edema) of infection

Patient Encounter 2, Part 2: Diabetic Foot Infection: Medical History, Physical Examination, and Diagnostic Tests

PMH: Type 2 diabetes mellitus for 21 years, hypertension, hypertriglyceridemia, peripheral neuropathy, and chronic back pain. Left second toe amputation secondary to diabetic foot infection.

FH: Father died of an MI at age 69; mother (age 87) is living with Alzheimer dementia, type 2 diabetes mellitus. One sister alive with type 2 diabetes mellitus.

SH: Married, three grown children. Retired truck driver. Denies alcohol and tobacco use.

Meds: Lantus 35 units at bedtime; Humalog 12 units with meals; losartan 100 mg daily; hydrochlorothiazide 25 mg daily; gemfibrozil 600 mg twice daily; gabapentin 600 mg three times daily; hydrocodone/acetaminophen 5/500 mg every 6 hours as needed; aspirin 81 mg daily.

Allergies: Sulfa (rash), lisinopril (cough).

ROS. (+) right foot findings per HPI; (–) headache, chest pain, shortness of breath, cough, nausea, vomiting, diarrhea, and weight loss.

PE:

Gen: Patient is in no acute distress. Wt 107.7 kg (237 lb); Ht 5′9″ (175 cm).

Chest: CTAB.

CV: RRR. No murmurs/rubs/gallops.

Ext: 3-cm purulent, erythematous lesion present on the plantar aspect of the right great toe. 1+ edema in the right foot; diminished sensation bilaterally. Lymphangitic streaking present; wound probe 1.5 cm deep.

Labs: Most recent laboratory test results were drawn at last visit 8 months ago: BUN 14 mg/dL (5.0 mmol/L), SCr 1.2 mg/dL (106 μmol/L), Glu 154 mg/dL (8.5 mmol/L), A1C 8.8% (0.088; 73 mmol/mol hemoglobin).

The patient is diagnosed with a diabetic foot infection and is admitted to the local hospital.

Explain the role of neuropathy, ischemia, and immunopathy in the development of this patient's diabetic foot infection.

What are the best preventative strategies for diabetic foot infections and complications such as lower extremity amputation?

Antimicrobial therapy for this patient's infection should provide coverage for which microorganisms?

What antimicrobial therapy would you recommend? Include drug, dosage, route, interval, and duration of therapy.

How would you monitor your selected regimen for safety and efficacy?

Table 73–5

Clinical Classification of a Diabetic Foot Infection

Infection Severity	PEDIS Grade	Clinical Manifestations of Infection
Uninfected	1	Wound lacking purulence or any manifestations of inflammation
Mild	2	Presence of at least two manifestations of inflammation (purulence or erythema, pain, tenderness, warmth, or induration), but any cellulitis/erythema extends no more than 2 cm around the ulcer, and infection is limited to the skin or superficial subcutaneous tissues; no other local complications or systemic illness
Moderate	3	Infection (as above) in a patient who is systemically well and metabolically stable but who has at least one of the following characteristics: cellulitis extending > 2 cm, lymphangitic streaking, spread beneath the superficial fascia, deep tissue abscess, gangrene, and involvement of muscle, tendon, joint, or bone
Severe	4	Infection in a patient with systemic toxicity or metabolic instability (eg, fever, chills, tachycardia, hypotension, confusion, vomiting, leukocytosis, acidosis, severe hyperglycemia, or azotemia)

From Lipsky BA, Berendt AR, Cornia PB, et al., 2012 Infectious Diseases Society of America clinical practice guideline for the diagnosis and treatment of diabetic foot infections. Clin Infect Dis 2012;54(12)132–173.

may be absent.[24] Still, the diagnosis of diabetic foot infection depends mostly on clinical evaluation.

Purulent drainage from the ulcer is indicative of infection. When pus and inflammatory symptoms are not present, the clinician must be astute to more subtle findings. These include delayed healing, increase in lesion size, prolonged exudate production, malodor, and tissue friability. Abnormal granulation tissue also may be present, as evidenced by color change (from bright red to dark red, brown, or gray) and increased bleeding. The ability to probe the ulcer to the underlying bone is highly indicative of osteomyelitis.[24]

Diabetic foot infections are classified into four categories based on clinical presentation using the PEDIS scale (perfusion, extent/size, depth/tissue loss, infection, sensation). Grade 1 signifies no infection; grade 2, involvement of skin and subcutaneous tissue only; grade 3, extensive cellulitis or deeper infection; and grade 4, presence of systemic inflammatory response syndrome.[23] Table 73–5 provides detailed information regarding these grades.

Imaging studies, such as x-ray and magnetic resonance imaging (MRI), can identify osteomyelitis. Blood cultures should be obtained from all patients with signs and symptoms of systemic illness. Deep tissue cultures may help to direct therapy. Bone also may be sent for culture in cases of osteomyelitis. Superficial cultures of ulcers are unreliable and should be avoided.[23]

Spreading soft tissue infection and osteomyelitis are often the first complications that develop from diabetic foot infection. Some patients develop bacteremia and sepsis.

Patient Encounter 2, Part 3: Diabetic Foot Infection: Clinical Course

The patient received the empiric therapy you recommended for his diabetic foot infection. Two days later, deep wound cultures were reported positive for *P. aeruginosa*. Blood cultures revealed no growth. The patient remained hospitalized for an additional week, during which time his cellulitis improved on directed antimicrobial therapy. He was discharged to complete his antibiotic therapy and to follow up as an outpatient in 1 week.

What modifications would you make to this patient's antimicrobial regimen knowing that the causative agent is P. aeruginosa?

What individualized foot care strategies can you suggest to this patient to prevent further infections?

The most feared complication of infected diabetic foot ulcers is lower extremity amputation. More than 80% of all nontraumatic lower extremity amputations performed each year in the United States are linked to diabetic foot infections, about half of which could be potentially avoided.[22]

TREATMENT

The goals of therapy for diabetic foot infection are eradication of the infection and avoidance of soft tissue loss and amputation.

Prevention

Comprehensive foot care programs and the utilization of multidisciplinary care teams can improve outcomes and decrease amputation rates.[23] Periodic foot examinations with monofilament testing and patient education regarding proper foot care, optimal glycemic control, and smoking cessation are key preventative strategies.

Nonpharmacologic Treatment

The nonpharmacologic treatment of diabetic foot ulcers may include débridement of necrotic or nonviable tissue, wound dressings, vascular or orthopedic surgery, and off-loading pressure from the wound.[23]

Pharmacologic Treatment

The severity of a patient's infection, based on the PEDIS scale, can help guide the selection of empirical antimicrobial therapy. Although most patients with grade 2 diabetic foot infections can be treated as outpatients with oral antimicrobial agents, all grade 4 and many grade 3 infections require hospitalization, stabilization of the patient, and broad-spectrum IV antibiotic therapy.[23]

Multiple antibiotic options exist for the treatment of diabetic wound infections. Table 73–6 provides both general treatment strategies and specific, although not all-inclusive, antibiotic recommendations. The duration of therapy correlates with infection severity. Antibiotics should be continued until the infection has resolved, but not necessarily until the ulcer has healed. Milder infections generally require 7 to 14 days of therapy, whereas more severe infections may necessitate longer treatment durations. Patients with osteomyelitis may require days to weeks of

Table 73–6

Empirical Pharmacologic Treatment of Diabetic Foot Infection

Infection Severity	PEDIS Grade	General Approach to Empirical Pharmacologic Treatment	Examples of Appropriate Empirical Antibiotics[a]
Uninfected	1	None. Avoid treating uninfected diabetic foot ulcers.	Not applicable
Mild	2	Oral, narrow-spectrum antibiotic therapy with activity against *S. aureus* and streptococcal species. Include coverage for MRSA according to patient history and resistance patterns in the area.	MRSA not suspected: cephalexin, dicloxacillin, clindamycin, amoxicillin-clavulanate MRSA suspected: clindamycin[b], trimethoprim-sulfamethoxazole[c], or doxycycline[c]
Moderate	3	Difficult to define a general approach. In many patients, highly bioavailable oral therapy is appropriate. IV therapy should be initiated in patients with more extensive or chronic infections, or those with abscess, deep tissue or bone involvement, or gangrene.	Oral options for grade 3 infections: amoxicillin-clavulanate, levofloxacin[d] + clindamycin, or moxifloxacin MRSA suspected: clindamycin[b], trimethoprim-sulfamethoxazole[c] or doxycycline[c]
Severe	4	Parenteral, broad-spectrum antibiotic therapy should be initiated. Ideally, drugs with activity against gram-positive, gram-negative, and anaerobic bacteria (especially if wound is malodorous) should be selected. Include coverage for MRSA.	IV options for grade 3–4 infection: MRSA not suspected: ampicillin-sulbactam, ertapenem, imipenem-cilastatin[d], moxifloxacin, levofloxacin[d] + clindamycin MRSA suspected: vancomycin, daptomycin, or linezolid *P. aeruginosa:* piperacillin-tazobactam

[a]Please refer to Table 73–3 for dosing in adults with normal renal function.

[b]CA-MRSA isolates resistant to erythromycin should be evaluated for inducible clindamycin resistance via a D-test.

[c]Poor activity against GAS; consider using in combination with clindamycin or cephalexin if empirical coverage for GAS is desired.

[d]*P. aeruginosa* generally is susceptible to this agent.

From Williams DT, Hilton JR, Harding KG. Diagnosing foot infection in diabetes. Clin Infect Dis 2004;39(2):S83–S86.

antibiotic therapy depending on whether infected and necrotic bone is surgically debrided.[23]

INFECTED PRESSURE SORES

EPIDEMIOLOGY AND ETIOLOGY

Pressures sores, also known as *decubitus ulcers* or *bedsores*, affect approximately 3 million adults, with an annual prevalence in the United States of about 12.5%. Patients of advanced age and those with spinal cord or orthopedic injuries are at highest risk.[25]

A pressure sore is a chronic wound that results from continuous pressure on the tissue overlying a bony prominence. This pressure impedes blood flow to the dermis and subcutaneous fat, resulting in tissue damage and necrosis.[26] Pressure sore infections develop from breaks in skin integrity and contamination from dirty areas of close proximity, and are often polymicrobial.[27]

CLINICAL PRESENTATION AND DIAGNOSIS

Approximately two-thirds of all pressure sores occur on the sacrum and heels.[27] Pressure sores are classified according to the extent of tissue destruction.[28] The most commonly used system for staging of pressure sores is presented in Table 73–7.

Bacterial colonization of pressure sores is common. Because infection impairs wound healing and may require systemic antimicrobial therapy, the clinician must be able to distinguish it from colonization. Table 73–8 describes the clinical presentation of infected pressure sores.

Most complications are infectious. The most common is osteomyelitis; less frequently, NF, clostridial myonecrosis, and sepsis can occur.

TREATMENT

The goals of therapy for infected pressure sores include resolution of infection, promotion of wound healing, and establishment of effective infection control.[30]

Prevention

KEY CONCEPT *Prevention is the most humane and cost-effective component for the management of pressure sores.* Key prevention strategies include monitoring of high-risk patients, reducing skin exposure to pressure and moisture, and promoting good nutritional status.

Careful monitoring and preventative care of high-risk patients can begin once these patients are identified. Intrinsic or host-related risk factors for the development of pressure sores include age more than 75 years, limited mobility, loss of sensation, unconsciousness or altered sense of awareness, and malnutrition. Extrinsic or environmental risk factors include pressure, **friction**, **shear stress**, and moisture.[31]

Turning and repositioning the patient at least every 2 hours can reduce skin pressure and prevent pressure sores. However, because this level of care is difficult to achieve in most hospital and nursing home environments, multitudes of pressure-reducing mattresses have been manufactured. Although these can help to decrease pressure on susceptible areas, they do not negate the need for position changes.[31]

Maintaining a clean, dry environment can prevent skin **maceration** and subsequent tissue damage. This can be accomplished with

Table 73–7

Staging of Pressure Ulcers

Suspected Deep Tissue Injury

- Intact skin with localized area of purple or maroon discoloration or presence of a blood-filled blister.
- The area may be preceded by tissue that is painful, firm, mushy, boggy, and warmer or cooler as compared with adjacent tissue.

Stage I

- Intact skin with localized area of nonblanchable redness, usually over a bony prominence.
- May be difficult to detect in darkly pigmented skin; its color may differ from the surrounding area.

Stage II

- Partial-thickness loss of dermis presenting as a shallow open ulcer with a red-pink wound bed or an intact or ruptured serum-filled blister.
- This stage should not be used to describe skin tears, tape burns, perineal dermatitis, maceration, or excoriation.

Stage III

- Full-thickness tissue loss. Subcutaneous fat may be visible, but bone, tendon, or muscle is not exposed. Slough may be present but does not obscure the depth of tissue loss. May include undermining and tunneling.

Stage IV

- Full-thickness tissue loss with exposed bone, tendon, or muscle. Slough or eschar may be present on some parts of the wound bed. Often include undermining and tunneling.

Unstageable

- Full-thickness tissue loss in which the base of the ulcer is covered by slough (yellow, tan, gray, green, or brown) and/or eschar (tan, brown, or black) in the wound bed.
- Until enough slough and/or eschar is removed to expose the base of the wound, the true depth, and therefore stage, cannot be determined. Stable (dry, adherent, intact without erythema or fluctuance) eschar on the heels serves as "the body's natural (biological) cover" and should not be removed.

From National Pressure Ulcer Advisory Panel. Updated staging system [online]. 2007. [cited 2014 September 1]. Available from: http://www.npuap.org/resources/educational-and-clinical-resources/npuap-pressure-ulcer-stagescategories/

frequent changes of bed sheets and clothing, thorough drying of skin after bathing, and prompt disposal of incontinent stool or urine.

Malnutrition is a significant but reversible risk factor. High-protein diets improve wound healing in patients with pressure sores.[31]

Nonpharmacologic Treatment

Pressure relief, adequate nutrition (high-protein diet), and surgical débridement or abscess drainage are the mainstays of nonpharmacologic treatment.[30]

Pharmacologic Treatment

Systemic antibiotics are indicated for serious pressure ulcer infections, including those associated with spreading cellulitis, osteomyelitis, or bacteremia.[30] Pressure ulcer infections are generally polymicrobial; thus, antimicrobial agents with a broad spectrum of activity should be initiated and narrowed according to the results of cultures obtained surgically. The duration of treatment is generally 10 to 14 days, unless osteomyelitis is present.[30]

Table 73–8

Presentation of Infected Pressure Sores

Symptoms

- Because many high-risk patients lack sensation, pain may not be a primary symptom.

Signs

- Infection generally is diagnosed when erythema and edema of the surrounding skin, purulent drainage, malodor, or delayed wound healing are present.

Patients with bacteremia often develop fever, chills, confusion, and/or hypotension.

Laboratory Tests

- Deep tissue cultures may help to direct therapy. Bone also may be sent for culture in cases of osteomyelitis. Superficial cultures are unreliable and should be avoided.

Imaging Studies

- Imaging studies, such as CT, MRI, or bone scan, can be used to detect osteomyelitis and to determine the depth and extent of tissue destruction.

From Refs. 29 and 30.

Mild superficial infections, such as those that present clinically with delayed wound healing or minimal cellulitis, may be treated with topical antimicrobial agents such as silver sulfadiazine 1% cream or combination antibiotic ointments.[26] Systemic options for more extensive cellulitis are available in Table 73–3.

INFECTED BITE WOUNDS

EPIDEMIOLOGY AND ETIOLOGY

Many Americans will be bitten by an animal at least once during their lifetimes. Although most of these injuries are minor, some will require medical treatment.

Dogs cause most animal bites, typically open lacerations, of which approximately 20% become infected. Cat bites are the second most common animal bite, most often puncture wounds involving the hand. Because cat bites are deep and penetrating, up to 80% may become infected.[32]

Human bites are the third most common and the most serious. Before the availability of antibiotics, up to 20% resulted in amputation. Currently, human bite–associated amputation rates remain at 5%, secondary to vascular compromise and infectious complications.[33]

There are two types of human bite injuries. Occlusal injuries are inflicted by actual biting, whereas clenched-fist injuries are sustained when a person's closed fist hits another's teeth. Of the two, clenched-fist injuries typically are more prone to infectious complications.[32,33]

KEY CONCEPT *Bite wound infections generally are polymicrobial.*[4] Both the normal flora of the biter's mouth and that of the bite recipient's skin can be implicated. The bacteriology of the cat and dog mouth is quite similar. *Pasteurella multocida*, a gram-negative aerobe, is one of the predominant pathogens. Viridans streptococci are the most frequently cultured bacteria from human bite wounds, although empiric treatment should also provide coverage for *Eikenella corrodens*.[4,33] Table 73–9 provides a comprehensive list of cat-, dog-, and human bite-wound pathogens.

Table 73–9

Etiology and Presentation of Infected Bite Wounds

Bacterial Pathogens

- *Dog and cat: Pasteurella multocida*, staphylococci, streptococci *Moraxella* spp., *Eikenella corrodens, Capnocytophaga canimorsus, Actinomyces, Fusobacterium, Prevotella*, and *Porphyromonas* spp.
- *Human:* Viridans streptococci, *S. aureus, E. corrodens, Haemophilus influenzae*, and β-lactamase–producing anaerobic bacteria.

Signs and Symptoms

- The onset of infectious symptomatology is typically 12–24 hours after the bite.
- Pain at the wound site is common.
- Erythema, edema, and purulent or malodorous drainage at the wound site are manifestations of infected wounds. The patient may be febrile.
- Limited range of motion may be present, especially if the hand is bitten.

Laboratory Tests

- Leukocytosis may be present.
- The clinician should obtain anaerobic and aerobic wound cultures only if the wound appears clinically infected.

Imaging Studies

- Radiographs should be obtained if the bite is on the hand, could have damaged bone or joints, or if an embedded object or tooth fragment is suspected.

Data from Refs. 4 and 33.

CLINICAL PRESENTATION AND DIAGNOSIS

The clinical presentation of infected bite wounds is presented in Table 73–9.

Complications of infected bite wounds include **lymphangitis**, abscess, septic arthritis, tenosynovitis, and osteomyelitis. Bites to the hand are particularly complication-prone.[33]

TREATMENT

The goals of therapy for an infected bite wound are rapid and successful eradication of infection and prevention of related complications.

Nonpharmacologic Treatment

Thorough irrigation with normal saline is the first step in the care of an infected bite wound. The wound should be elevated and immobilized. Surgical closure may be advocated, especially for facial wounds. Wounds that are infected, at higher risk for infection, or older than 24 hours should be left open because premature closure can lead to disastrous infectious complications.[33]

Pharmacologic Treatment

Most bite wounds require antibiotic therapy only when clinical infection is present. *However, prophylactic therapy is recommended for wounds at higher risk for infection and bites requiring surgical repair.*[33] Bites to the hand and human bites may benefit the most from prophylaxis.[32]

The most effective agent for the treatment (and prophylaxis) of human and animal bite-wound infections is amoxicillin-clavulanate. Alternatives include second-generation cephalosporins, such as cefuroxime, plus coverage for anaerobes, such as clindamycin or metronidazole. Moxifloxacin, doxycycline, or a carbapenem may also be used. The durations of prophylaxis and treatment are generally 3 to 5 days.[4]

If the wound is associated with significant cellulitis and edema, systemic signs of infection, or possible joint or bone involvement, hospitalization and IV antibiotics (typically ampicillin-sulbactam 3 g IV every 6 hours) should be initiated. Bone and joint infections will require longer durations of therapy of up to 6 weeks.[4,33]

OUTCOME EVALUATION

Education of the patient, caregivers, and household members is important to limit further spread of infection and is a key component in SSTI case management. **Table 73–10** lists several key prevention messages for patients with SSTIs.

Patients receiving antibiotic therapy for SSTIs require monitoring for efficacy and safety. Efficacy typically is manifested by reductions in temperature, white blood cell count, erythema, edema, and pain. Initially, signs and symptoms of infection may worsen owing to toxin release from certain organisms (ie, GAS); however, they should begin to resolve within 48 to 72 hours of treatment initiation. If no response or worsening infection is noted after the first 3 days of antibiotics, reevaluate the patient.[4] Lack of response may be due to a noninfectious or nonbacterial diagnosis, a pathogen not covered by or resistant to current antibiotic therapy, poor patient adherence, drug or disease interactions causing decreased antibiotic absorption or increased clearance, immunodeficiency, or the need for surgical intervention. To ensure the safety of the regimen, dose antibiotics according to renal and hepatic function as appropriate, and monitor for or minimize adverse drug reactions, allergic reactions, and drug interactions.

Table 73–10

Prevention Education for Patients with SSTIs

1. Draining wounds should be covered with clean, dry bandages.
2. Hands should be cleaned regularly with soap and water (or with alcohol-based hand gel if not visibly soiled) and immediately after touching infected skin or any item directly contacting a draining wound.
3. General hygiene should be maintained with regular bathing.
4. Items that may become contaminated with wound drainage or that directly touch the skin should not be shared.
5. Wash and dry thoroughly any clothing that has come in contact with wound drainage after each use.
6. If the wound is unable to be covered with a clean, dry bandage at all times, avoid activities with skin-to-skin contact until the wound is healed.
7. Equipment and environmental surfaces with bare skin contact should be cleaned with *S. aureus*–active detergents or disinfectants.

From Gorwitz RF, Jernigan DB, Powers JH, et al. Strategies for clinical management of MRSA in the community: Summary of an experts' meeting convened by the Centers for Disease Control and Prevention [online]. 2006. [cited 2011 Oct 10]. http://www.cdc.gov/ncidod/dhqp/ar_mrsa_ca.html.50

Patient Care Process

Patient Assessment:

- Based on physical examination and review of systems, determine whether the patient is experiencing signs or symptoms of an SSTI and if so, its severity.
- Review the medical history. Does the patient have any risk factors or chronic conditions that lend to the diagnosis of an SSTI or a particular causative pathogen?
- Conduct a medication history (including prescriptions, OTC medications, and dietary supplements). Does the patient have any drug allergies? Is the patient experiencing side effects from therapy?
- Review available laboratory tests, especially white blood cell counts and renal function.

Therapy Evaluation:

- Determine whether oral or IV therapy is indicated based on severity of infection.
- If the patient is already receiving pharmacotherapy, assess efficacy, safety, and patient adherence. Are there any significant drug interactions?
- Determine whether the patient has prescription coverage or whether recommended agents are included on the institution's formulary.

Care Plan Development:

- Select an empirical antibiotic agent based on patient assessment that is likely to be effective and safe.
- Determine whether drug doses, dosing frequency, and duration of therapy are optimal.
- Address any patient concerns about SSTIs and their management.
- In pediatric patients especially, consider method and ease of administration, and palatability and tolerability of oral formulations.

Follow-Up Evaluation:

- Ensure that antimicrobial therapy is effective by monitoring for resolution of local and systemic signs and symptoms of infection.
- Monitor for laboratory evidence of infection resolution.
- Narrow antibiotic coverage when possible with the use of culture and sensitivity data.
- Determine whether patient is experiencing any adverse reactions or drug interactions.

Abbreviations Introduced in This Chapter

CA-MRSA	Community-acquired methicillin-resistant *S. aureus*
GAS	Group A *Streptococcus* (also known as *Streptococcus pyogenes*, one of the β-hemolytic streptococci)
GERD	Gastroesophageal reflux disease
HA-MRSA	Health care-associated methicillin-resistant *S. aureus*
IVIG	Intravenous immunoglobulin
MIC	Minimum inhibitory concentration
MRI	Magnetic resonance imaging
MRSA	Methicillin-resistant *S. aureus*
MSSA	Methicillin-sensitive *S. aureus*
NF	Necrotizing fasciitis
SIRS	Systemic inflammatory response syndrome
SSTI	Skin and soft tissue infection
VISA	Vancomycin-intermediate *S. aureus*
VRE	Vancomycin-resistant enterococci
VRSA	Vancomycin-resistant *S. aureus*

REFERENCES

1. Amin AN, Cerceo EA, Deitelzweig ST, et al. Hospitalist perspective on the treatment of skin and soft tissue infections. May Clin Proc. 2014;1–16.
2. Moran GJ, Abrahamian FM, LoVecchio F, et al. Acute bacterial skin infections: Developments since the 2005 Infectious Diseases Society of America (IDSA) guidelines. J Emer Med 2013;44(6):e397–e412.
3. Pallin DJ, Espinola JA, Leung DY, et al. Epidemiology of dermatitis and skin infections in United States physicians offices, 1993-2005. Clin Infect Dis 2009;49:901–907.
4. Stevens DL, Bisno AL, Chambers HF, et al. Practice guidelines for the diagnosis and management of skin and soft tissue infections. Clin Infect Dis 2014;41:1373–1406.
5. Moran GJ, Krishnadasan A, Gorwitz RJ, et al. Methicillin-resistant *S. aureus* infection among patients in the emergency department. N Engl J Med 2006;355(7):666–674.
6. Liu C, Bayer A, Cosgrove SE, et al. Clinical practice guidelines by the Infectious Disease Society of America for the treatment of methicillin-resistant *Staphylococcus aureus* infections in adults and children. Clin Infect Dis 2011;52:1–38.
7. Dieffenbach CW, Tramont EC, Plaeger SF. Innate (general or nonspecific) host defense mechanisms. In: Mandell GL, Bennett JE, Dolin R, eds. Principles and Practice of Infectious Diseases. 7th ed. Philadelphia, PA: Elsevier; 2010:37–47.
8. Yagupski P. Bacteriologic aspects of skin and soft tissue infections. Pediatr Ann 1993;22:217–224.
9. Stevens DL, Bisno AL, Chambers HF, et al. Practice guidelines for the diagnosis and management of skin and soft tissue infections. Clin Infect Dis 2005;41:1373–1406.
10. Pasternack MS, Swartz MN. Cellulitis, necrotizing fasciitis, and subcutaneous tissue infections. In: Mandell GL, Bennett JE, Dolin R, eds. Principles and Practice of Infectious Diseases. 7th ed. Philadelphia, PA: Elsevier; 2010:1289–1312.
11. Cole C, Gazewood J. Diagnosis and treatment of impetigo. Am Fam Physician 2007;75:859–864, 868.
12. Luelmo-Aguilar J, Santandreu MS. Folliculitis: Recognition and management. Am J Clin Dermatol 2004;5(5):301–310.
13. Thomas KS, Crook AM, Nunn AJ, et al. Penicillin to prevent recurrent leg cellulitis. N Engl J Med 2013;368;(18):1695–1703.
14. Swartz MN. Clinical practice. Cellulitis. N Engl J Med 2004;350(9):904–912.
15. Micek ST, Hoban AP, Pham V, Doherty JA, Kollef MH. Institutional perspective on the impact of positive blood cultures on the economic and clinical outcomes of patients with

complicated skin and skin structure infections: Focus on gram-positive infections. Clin Ther 2011;33:1759–1768.

16. Pallin DJ, Binder WD, Allen MB, et al. Clinical trial: Comparative effectiveness of cephalexin plus trimethoprim-sulfamethoxazole versus cephalexin alone for treatment of uncomplicated cellulitis: A randomized controlled trial. Clin Infect Dis 2013;56:1754–1762.
17. Corey GR, Kabler H, Mehra P, et al. Single-dose oritavancin in the treatment of acute bacterial skin infections. N Engl J Med 2014;370:2180–2190.
18. Boucher HW, Wilcox M, Talbot GH, et al. Once-weekly dalbavancin versus daily conventional therapy for skin infection. N Engl J Med 2014;370:2169–2179.
19. Group A Streptococcal (GAS) Disease [online]. Department of Health and Human Services. Centers for Disease Control and Prevention. May 1, 2014. [cited 2014 Sept 1]. http://www.cdc.gov/groupastrep/clinicians.html
20. Anaya DA, Dellinger EP. Necrotizing soft-tissue infection: Diagnosis and management. Clin Infect Dis 2007;44:705–710.
21. Hakkarainen TW, Burkette Ikebata N, Bulger E, et al. Necrotizing soft tissue infections: Review and current concepts in treatment, systems of care, and outcomes. Curr Prob Surg 2014;51:344–362.
22. Clayton W, Elasy TA. A review of the pathophysiology, classification, and treatment of foot ulcers in diabetic patients. Clin Diabetes 2009;27:52–58.
23. Lipsky BA, Berendt AR, Cornia PB, et al. 2012 Infectious Diseases Society of America clinical practice guideline for the diagnosis and treatment of diabetic foot infections. Clin Infect Dis 2012;54(12):132–173.
24. Williams DT, Hilton JR, Harding KG. Diagnosing foot infection in diabetes. Clin Infect Dis 2004;39(2):S83–S86.
25. Agency for Healthcare Research and Quality. Pressure Ulcer Risk Assessment and prevention: A comparative effectiveness review. Published online January 10, 2012 at http://www.effectivehealthcare.ahrq.gov. Accessed September 1, 2014.
26. National Pressure Ulcer Advisory Panel, European Pressure Ulcer Advisory Panel, and Pan Pacific Pressure Injury Alliance. Prevention and treatment of pressure ulcers: Quick reference guide. 2014. Emily Haesler (Ed.). Cambridge Media: Osborne Park, Western Australia; 2014.
27. Smith DM, Snow DE, Rees E, et al. Evaluation of the bacterial diversity of pressure ulcers using bTEFAP pyrosequencing. BMC Medical Genomics 2010;3:41.
28. National Pressure Ulcer Advisory Panel. Updated staging system [online]. 2007. [cited 2014 September 1]. Available from: http://www.npuap.org/resources/educational-and-clinical-resources/npuap-pressure-ulcer-stagescategories/
29. Livesley NJ, Chow AW. Pressure ulcers in elderly individuals. Clin Infect Dis 2002;35:1390–1396.
30. Cannon BC, Cannon JP. Management of pressure ulcers. Am J Health Syst Pharm 2004;61:1895–1907.
31. Thomas DR. Prevention and treatment of pressure ulcers: What works? What doesn't? Cleve Clin J Med 2001;68(8):704–707.
32. Singer AJ, Dagum AB. Current management of acute cutaneous wounds. N Engl J Med 2008;359:1037–1046.
33. Bower MG. Managing dog, cat, and human bite wounds. Nurs Pract 2001;26(4):36–38, 41, 42, 45.

74 Infective Endocarditis

Ronda L. Akins and Katie E. Barber

LEARNING OBJECTIVES

Upon completion of the chapter, the reader will be able to:

1. Differentiate the causes and development of infective endocarditis (IE).
2. Identify the clinical presentation and laboratory evaluation for IE.
3. Assess diagnostic criteria used to evaluate a patient suspected of having IE.
4. Describe the most likely causative pathogens of IE, particularly in specific patient populations.
5. Develop appropriate pharmacologic treatment recommendations for patients with IE.
6. Define appropriate patient populations requiring prophylactic treatment, and differentiate appropriate drug regimens.
7. Devise a monitoring plan for patients with IE to determine treatment efficacy and discern any adverse effects.

INTRODUCTION

Infective endocarditis (IE) is a serious infection affecting the lining and valves of the heart. Although this disease is mostly associated with infection of the heart valves, septal defects may become involved in some cases. Infections also occur in patients with prosthetic or mechanical devices or who are intravenous drug users (IVDUs). Bacteria are the primary cause of IE; however, fungi and atypical organisms may also be responsible pathogens.

Typically IE is classified into two categories: acute or subacute. Differences between the two categories are based on the progression and severity of the disease. Acute disease is more aggressive, characterized by high fevers, leukocytosis, and systemic toxicity, with death occurring within a few days to weeks. This type of IE is often caused by more virulent organisms, particularly *Staphylococcus aureus*. Subacute disease is typically caused by less virulent organisms, such as viridans group streptococci, producing a slower and more subtle presentation. It is characterized by weakness, fatigue, low-grade fever, night sweats, weight loss, and other nonspecific symptoms, with death occurring in several months.

Successful management of patients with IE is based on proper diagnosis, treatment with appropriate therapy, and monitoring for complications, adverse events, or development of resistance. The treatment and management of IE are best determined through identification of the causative organism. IE has varied clinical presentations; therefore, patients with this infection may be found in any medical subspecialty (ie, medicine, surgery, critical care, etc).

EPIDEMIOLOGY AND ETIOLOGY

Despite IE being a fairly uncommon infection, in the United States, there are about 10,000 to 20,000 new cases annually, accounting for an incidence of approximately five to seven cases per 100,000 persons-years.[1] Although the exact number of cases is often difficult to determine, owing to the diagnostic criteria and reporting methods for this disease, it continues to rise. IE is now considered the fourth leading cause of serious infectious diseases syndromes following sepsis secondary to urinary tract infection, pneumonia, and intraabdominal sepsis.[2] Although IE occurs at any age, more than 50% of cases occur in patients older than 50 years.[1] IE in children continues to be uncommon and is mainly associated with underlying structural defects, surgical repair of the defects, or nosocomial catheter-related bacteremia.[1] With the increased use of mechanical valves, prosthetic-valve endocarditis (PVE) now accounts for approximately 10% to 30%.[3] Patients who are IVDUs are also at an increased risk for IE, with 150 to 2000 cases per 100,000 persons per year, most being younger adults.[4] Additionally, others at high risk for IE include patients with any congenital or structural cardiac defects, including valvular disease, long-term hemodialysis, diabetes mellitus; poor oral hygiene, major dental treatment, previous endocarditis, hypertrophic cardiomyopathy, and mitral valve prolapse with regurgitation.[5–7]

Although almost any type of microorganism is capable of causing IE, the majority of cases are caused by gram-positive organisms. These consist primarily of streptococci, staphylococci, and enterococci. Consideration of gram-negative, fungal, and other atypical organisms must be taken into account, particularly in certain patient populations. In Table 74–1, approximate percentages are given for each organism based on the type of IE, including native valve (community-acquired vs health care–associated), prosthetic valve (grouped by months post-surgery), and IVDUs.

Table 74–1

Etiologic Organisms of Infective Endocarditis

	Percent of Cases					
	Native-Valve IE		**PVE (Indicated in Months After Valve Surgery)**		**IVDU (Right- and Left-Sided)**	
	Community-Acquired	**Health Care-Associated**	**< 2**	**2–12**	**> 12**	**Total**
Streptococci[a]	40	9	1	9	31	12
Pneumococci	2	—	—	—	—	—
Enterococci	9	13	8	12	11	9
Staphylococcus aureus	28	53[b]	22	12	18	57
CNS	5	12	33	32	11	—
HACEK group	3	—	—	—	6	—
Gram-negative bacilli	1	2	13	3	6	7
Fungi (*Candida* spp.)	< 1	2	8	12	1	4
Polymicrobial/ miscellaneous	3	4	3	6	5	7
Diphtheroids	—	< 1	6	—	3	0.1
Culture-negative	9	5	5	6	8	3

CNS, coagulase-negative staphylococci; HACEK, *Haemophilus* spp. (primarily *H. paraphrophilus, H. parainfluenzae*, and *H. aphrophilus*), *Aggregatibacter actinomycetemcomitans, Cardiobacterium hominis, Eikenella corrodens*, and *Kingella kingae*.

[a]Includes viridans group streptococci; *S. bovis*; other nongroup A, groupable streptococci; and nutritionally variant streptococci.

[b]Methicillin resistance is common among these *S. aureus* strains.

Modified from Karchmer AW. Infective endocarditis. In: Fauci AS, Braunwald E, Kasper DL, Hauser SL, Longo DL, Jameson JL, Loscalzo J, eds. Harrison's Principles of Internal Medicine. 18th ed. New York: McGraw Hill; 2012: Chap. 124.

Patient Encounter, Part 1

A 62-year-old woman with a history of end-stage renal disease (ESRD) on hemodialysis presents to the emergency department with complaints of weakness, fever, and chills. Her current weight is 105 kg (231 lb). On interviewing the patient, you determine she has had type 2 diabetes for 25 years and has been receiving dialysis Monday, Wednesday, and Friday for the past 6 months. She denies any use of alcohol, illicit drugs, or tobacco.

What information would make you suspect IE?

Does she have any risk factors for IE?

What additional information would you like to know before deciding on an empirical treatment for this patient?

PATHOPHYSIOLOGY

KEY CONCEPT *For IE to develop, the occurrence of several factors is required. Typically, there must be an alteration of the endothelial surfaces of the heart valves to allow for organism attachment and colonization.* These alterations may be produced by an inflammatory process such as rheumatic heart disease or by injury from turbulent blood flow. Platelets and fibrin are then capable of depositing on the damaged valves, forming a nonbacterial thrombotic endocarditis (NBTE). At this point, bacteria, through hematogenous spread (ie, bacteremia), adhere to and colonize the **nidus**, forming a vegetation. Further deposits of platelets and fibrin cover the bacteria, providing a protective coating that allows for development of a suitable environment for continued organism and vegetation progression, often producing an organism density of 10^9 to 10^{10} **colony-forming units** (CFU) per gram.

Acquisition of PVE differs in early stages, where direct inoculation may occur during surgery rather than through hematogenous seeding. In addition, causative organisms in early PVE are typically nosocomial, with increased likelihood of being drug resistant.[7,8] The prosthetic valve also has a greater propensity for organism colonization than native valves.[8] However, in late PVE, the process of colonization and vegetation formation is similar to that of native-valve IE, as described earlier.[7,8]

Typically, vegetations are located on the line along valve closure on the atrial surface of the atrioventricular valves (tricuspid and mitral) or on the ventricular surface of the semilunar valves (pulmonary and aortic). The vegetations can vary significantly in size, ranging from millimeters to several centimeters and may be single or multiple masses. Often, destruction of underlying tissue occurs and may cause perforation of the valve leaflet or rupture of the chordae tendineae, interventricular septum, or papillary muscle. Valve ring abscesses may occur, resulting in fistulas penetrating into the myocardium or pericardial sac, particularly with staphylococcal endocarditis.

Embolic events are also common. Embolization occurs as portions of the friable vegetation break loose and enter the bloodstream. These infected pieces are called *septic emboli*. Pulmonary abscesses are commonly formed as a result of septic emboli from right-sided IE (tricuspid and pulmonary valves). However, left-sided IE (mitral and aortic valves) is more likely to have an embolus travel to any organ, especially kidneys, spleen, and brain. Along with emboli, immune complex deposition may occur in organ systems, causing extracardiac manifestations of the disease. This commonly occurs in the kidneys, producing abscesses, infarction, or glomerulonephritis. Immune complexes or emboli may also produce skin manifestations of the disease, as seen with petechiae, Osler nodes, and Janeway lesions, or within the eye (eg, Roth spots).

CLINICAL PRESENTATION AND DIAGNOSIS

The clinical presentation for IE is quite variable and often nonspecific. KEY CONCEPT *A fever is the most frequent and persistent symptom in patients but may be blunted with previous antibiotic use, congestive heart failure, chronic liver or renal failure, or infection caused by a less virulent organism (ie, subacute disease).*[1,3,4] Other signs and symptoms that may also occur are listed below, with some discussed in further detail.

Heart murmurs are heard frequently on auscultation (greater than 85% of cases), but a new murmur or change in murmurs is only found in 3% to 5% or 5% to 10%, respectively.[1] Additionally, more than 90% of patients who have a new murmur will develop congestive heart failure, which is a major cause of morbidity and mortality. Splenomegaly and mycotic aneurysms are also noted in many cases of IE.

This disease is also characterized by the following peripheral manifestations. Some of these clinical findings are found in up to one-half of adult patients with IE, although recently the prevalence has been decreasing and is rarely seen in children.[1,3]

- **Skin:** *Petechiae* are very small (usually less than 3 mm), pinpoint, flat red spots beneath the skin surface caused by microhemorrhaging. They occur in 20% to 40% of patients with chronic IE and are often found on the buccal mucosa, conjunctivae (Figure 74–1A), and extremities.[1] *Splinter hemorrhages* appear as small dark streaks beneath the fingernails or toenails and occur most commonly proximally with IE, typically as a result of local vasculitis or microemboli in about 20% of patients (Figure 74–1B). *Osler nodes* are small (usually 2–15 mm), painful, tender subcutaneous nodules located on the pads of the fingers and toes (Figure 74–1D) caused primarily by either septic emboli or vasculitis. These nodes are rare in acute disease but are also nonspecific for IE despite occurring in 10% to 25% of all patients.[1] *Janeway lesions* are small, painless, hemorrhagic macular plaques on the palms of the hands or soles of the feet due to septic emboli (in ~5% of patients) and more commonly associated with acute *S. aureus* IE (Figure 74–1E).
- **Extremities:** *Clubbing* of the finger tips typically occurs in long-standing illness and is present in approximately 10% to 20% of patients (Figure 74–1C).[1]
- **Eye:** *Roth spots* occur rarely (less than 5% of IE cases) and are oval-shaped retinal hemorrhages with a pale center near the optic disc (Figure 74–1F).

Laboratory Studies

KEY CONCEPT *Blood cultures are the essential laboratory test for the diagnosis and treatment of IE. Typically, patients with IE have a low-grade consistent bacteremia, with approximately 80% of cases having less than 100 CFU/mL (100,000 CFU/L) in the bloodstream.*[1] *Blood culture results are critical for determining the most appropriate therapy.* Three blood culture sets should be drawn within the initial 24 hours to determine the etiologic agent. Approximately 90% of the first two cultures will yield a positive result. If a positive blood culture is not obtained from a patient with suspected IE, the microbiology laboratory should be notified to monitor cultures for growth of fastidious organisms (eg, HACEK) for up to 1 month.

KEY CONCEPT *Another important tool aiding in the diagnosis of IE is the echocardiogram. This imaging tool is used to visualize vegetations. Two methods of the echocardiogram are used: the transthoracic echocardiogram (TTE) and the transesophageal*

Clinical Presentation and Diagnosis of IE KEY CONCEPT

General

Patients typically present with nonspecific and variable signs or symptoms.

Symptoms

Complaints from patients may include:

- Fever
- Chills
- Night sweats
- Weakness
- Dyspnea
- Weight loss
- Myalgia or arthralgias

Signs

- Fever is the most common sign of IE
- New or changing heart murmur
- Embolic phenomena (emboli affect the kidneys, spleen, brain, lung, or extremities)
- Skin manifestations (eg, petechiae, splinter hemorrhages, Osler nodes, Janeway lesions)
- Splenomegaly
- Clubbing of extremities

Laboratory Tests

- Blood cultures are the most important laboratory assessment for persistent bacteremia, which occurs commonly in IE. A minimum of three blood culture sets should be collected during the initial 24 hours
- Hematologic tests for anemia (normochromic, normocytic)
- WBC count may be elevated in acute disease but could be normal in subacute IE
- Nonspecific findings such as thrombocytopenia, elevated erythrocyte sedimentation rate or C-reactive protein, and abnormal urinalysis (ie, proteinuria or microscopic hematuria)

Other Diagnostic Tests

An echocardiogram (TTE or TEE) should be performed on any patient with suspected IE to detect the presence of vegetations.

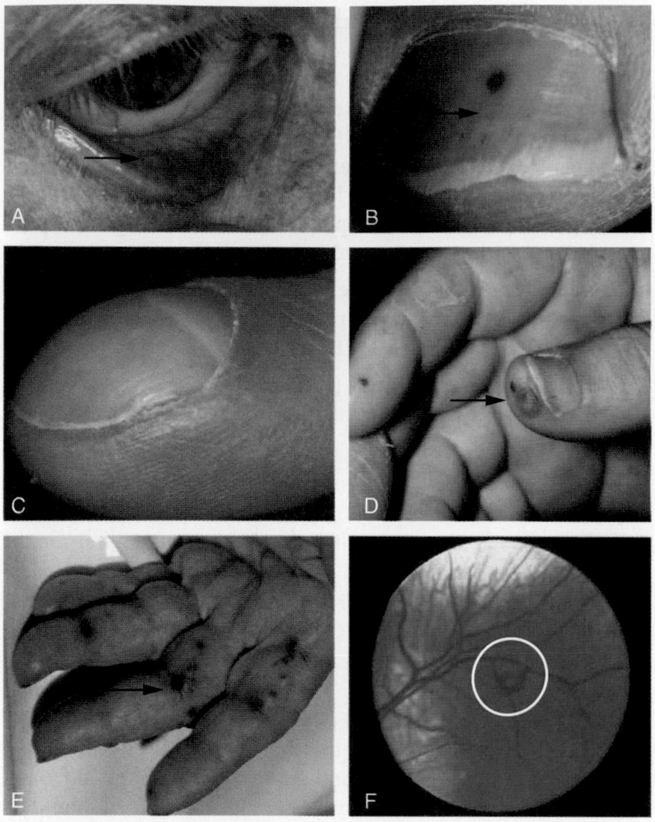

FIGURE 74–1. **(A)** Conjunctival petechiae. (From Wolff K, Johnson R, Saavedra AP. In: Fitzpatrick's Color Atlas & Synopsis of Clinical Dermatology. 7th ed. New York: McGraw Hill. Copyright 2013.) **(B)** Splinter hemorrhage. (From Knoop KJ, Stack LB, Storrow AB, Thurman AB. In: Atlas of Emergency Medicine. 3rd ed. New York: McGraw Hill. Copyright 2010.) **(C)** Clubbing of finger. (From Tosti A, Piraccini BM. In: Fitzpatrick's Dermatology in General Medicine. 7th ed. New York: McGraw Hill. Copyright 2007.) **(D)** Osler nodes. (From Knoop KJ, Stack LB, Storrow AB, Thurman AB. In: Atlas of Emergency Medicine. 3rd ed. New York: McGraw Hill. Copyright 2010.) **(E)** Janeway lesions. (From Wolff K, Johnson R, Saavedra AP. In: Fitzpatrick's Color Atlas & Synopsis of Clinical Dermatology. 7th ed. New York: McGraw Hill. Copyright 2013.) **(F)** Roth spots. (From Effron D, Forcier BC, Wyszynski RE. In: Atlas of Emergency Medicine. 3rd ed. New York: McGraw Hill. Copyright 2010.)

echocardiogram (TEE). The TTE has been used since the 1970s; however, it is less sensitive (45%–65%) than the TEE (85%–95%).[3] Despite the TEE being more sensitive, use of the TTE for patients with suspected native-valve IE is usually sufficient.[9,10] The TEE may be used as a secondary test for patients whose TTE was negative when a high clinical suspicion of IE exists. On the other hand, a TEE is often preferred in patients who have complicated disease, including left-sided IE, prosthetic valves, or perivalvular extension of the vegetation.[2,10,11] Echocardiograms may also be employed to assess the need for surgical intervention or to determine the possible source of emboli.[10]

Additional nonspecific tests for IE may be performed. These include hematologic parameters to determine whether the patient is anemic, which occurs in the majority of patients. The white blood cells (WBCs) may be elevated, particularly in acute disease. However, in a subacute infection, WBCs may be normal. An erythrocyte sedimentation rate (ESR) may also be obtained to determine the presence of inflammation, although this test is highly nonspecific and almost always elevated in IE.

Diagnostic Criteria

A definitive diagnosis of IE would consist of a biopsy or culture directly from pathologic specimens from the endocardium. However, this would be a highly invasive test. Therefore, diagnosis of IE relies on clinical presentation as well as laboratory and echocardiographic results. To guide the clinical diagnosis of IE, major and minor criteria have been established (Table 74–2A).[12] Depending on the number of major or minor criteria a patient demonstrates, leads to a classification of definite, possible, or rejected diagnosis of IE (Table 74–2B).

Causative Organisms

Gram-positive bacteria are the most common causative organisms to produce IE. Streptococci and staphylococci species account for the majority of cases at more than 80%.[1,7] Viridans group streptococci have been considered the primary pathogens in IE. However, staphylococci have been increasing in prevalence and are now the dominant causative organisms in some reports (see Table 74–1).[12,13] Other gram-positive, gram-negative, atypical, and fungal organisms are less common but still must be considered in certain patient populations.

▶ *Streptococci*

Streptococci causing IE are typically a group of species called viridans group streptococci. The most common of this group are *Streptococcus salivarius, Streptococcus mutans, Streptococcus mitis*, and *Streptococcus sanguis*. This group of bacteria, considered normal flora in the human mouth, is α-hemolytic, with most clinical microbiology laboratories not differentiating to the exact species. These organisms may cause bacteremia after dental procedures, which can lead to the development of IE in at-risk patients. Viridans group streptococci are also the predominant pathogen of IE associated with mitral valve prolapse, native valves and in children.[14] Another streptococcal species commonly associated with IE is *Streptococcus bovis*, classified as group D streptococci and is frequently found in the GI tract. However, owing to the similarities of these streptococci, including microbiologic susceptibility, treatment is similar regardless of species.

IE caused by these streptococci typically have a subacute clinical course. The current cure rate is often greater than 90% unless complications arise, which do occur in more than 30% of patients.[14,15] The majority of viridans group streptococci remain very susceptible to penicillin, with most strains having a *minimum inhibitory concentration* (MIC) of less than 0.125 mcg/mL (0.125 mg/L).[16] However, isolation of organisms with decreased susceptibilities is increasing. Therefore, antibiotic susceptibilities need to be assessed in order to determine the most appropriate treatment regimen.

▶ *Staphylococci*

Staphylococcal endocarditis continues to increase in prevalence, causing 30% or more of all cases of IE, with the majority (80%–90%) being due to *S. aureus* (coagulase-positive staphylococci).[17,18] This increase in staphylococci has been primarily attributed to expanded use of venous catheters, more frequent valve replacement, and increased IVDU.[17] Coagulase-negative

Table 74–2

Modified Duke Criteria for IE

2A. Definitions of Modified Duke Criteria

Major Criteria

Blood culture positive for IE:

Typical microorganisms consistent with IE from two separate blood cultures:

Viridans streptococci, *S. bovis*, HACEK group, *S. aureus*, or community-acquired enterococci in the absence of a primary focus, or

Microorganisms consistent with IE from persistently positive blood cultures, defined as follows:

At least two positive cultures of blood samples drawn greater than 12 hours apart, or

All of three or a majority of four separate cultures of blood (with first and last sample drawn at least 1 hour apart)

Single positive blood culture for *C. burnetii* or antiphase I IgG antibody titer greater than 1:800

Evidence of endocardial involvement:

Echocardiogram positive for IE (TEE recommended in patients with prosthetic valves, rated at least "possible IE" by clinical criteria, or complicated IE [paravalvular abscess] TTE as first test in other patients), defined as follows:

Oscillating intracardiac mass on valve or supporting structures, in the path of regurgitant, or on implanted material in the absence of an alternative anatomic explanation, or

Abscess, or

New partial dehiscence of prosthetic valve

New valvular regurgitation (worsening or changing of preexisting murmur not sufficient)

Minor Criteria

Predisposition: predisposing heart condition or injection drug use

Fever: temperature greater than 38°C (100.4°F)

Vascular phenomena: major arterial emboli, septic pulmonary infarcts, mycotic aneurysm, intracranial hemorrhage, conjunctival hemorrhages, and Janeway lesions

Immunologic phenomena: glomerulonephritis, Osler nodes, Roth spots, and rheumatoid factor

Microbiologic evidence: positive blood culture but does not meet a major criterion as noted above[a] or serologic evidence of active infection with organism consistent with IE

2B. Modified Duke Criteria for the Diagnosis of IE

Definite IE

Pathologic criteria:

(1) Microorganisms demonstrated by culture or histologic examination of a vegetation that has embolized, or an intracardiac abscess specimen, or

(2) Pathologic lesions; vegetation or intracardiac abscess confirmed by histologic examination showing active endocarditis

Clinical criteria[b]:

(1) Two major criteria, or

(2) One major criterion and three minor criteria, or

(3) Five minor criteria

Possible IE

(1) One major criterion and one minor criterion, or

(2) Three minor criteria

Rejected

(1) Firm alternate diagnosis explaining evidence of IE, or

(2) Resolution of IE syndrome with antibiotic therapy for less than or equal to 4 days, or

(3) No pathologic evidence of IE at surgery or autopsy, with antibiotic therapy for less than or equal to 4 days, or

(4) Does not meet criteria for possible IE, as above

TEE, transesophageal echocardiography; TTE, transthoracic echocardiography.

[a]Excludes single positive cultures for CNS and organisms that do not cause endocarditis.

[b]See above for definitions of major and minor criteria.

From Li JS, Sexton DJ, Mick N, et al. Proposed modifications to the Duke criteria for the diagnosis of infective endocarditis. Clin Infect Dis 2000;30:633–638; by permission of Oxford University Press, 2000 by the Infectious Diseases Society of America.

staphylococci (CNS) also cause IE; however, these organisms typically infect prosthetic valves or indwelling catheters.[19]

Patients with *S. aureus* bacteremia are at an increased risk of developing IE. *S. aureus* may infect "normal" heart valves (no prior detected valvular disease) in one-third of cases.[1,17] Therefore, it is imperative to assess these patients adequately for the presence of vegetations. Any heart valve may be affected; however, when the mitral or aortic valve is involved, it often results in extensive systemic infection with a mortality rate of approximately 20% to 65%.[1,17] When treating *S. aureus* IE, one must consider whether the isolate displays methicillin-resistance, the location of infection (right or left side), presence of prosthetic valves, and history of IVDU. Despite significant resistance to penicillinase-resistant penicillins (eg, methicillin and nafcillin), most isolates remain susceptible to vancomycin. However, there is an increasing incidence of *S. aureus* with an elevated MIC of 2 mcg/mL (2 mg/L) which may require use of an alternative agent such as daptomycin.[20] Additionally, strains that are intermediately-resistant or fully resistant to vancomycin have been reported.[21–23] Fortunately, these strains are not widespread enough to affect empirical antibiotic selection. Susceptibility reports along with clinical response should be assessed to ensure appropriate antimicrobial coverage.

Over the past decade, there has been an increasing emergence of community-acquired methicillin-resistant *S. aureus* (CA-MRSA) that differs from healthcare-associated MRSA. This organism tends to be less resistant to many antibiotics, with sensitivity to clindamycin, trimethoprim-sulfamethoxazole, and minocycline, as well as vancomycin, linezolid, and daptomycin. In addition, this organism has a virulence gene (Panton-Valentine-leukocidin), which produces a toxin that causes necrosis. To date, this organism primarily causes skin/skin-structure infections or pneumonias (see Chapter 73: Skin and Soft Tissue Infections). There have been a limited number of cases of IE caused by CA-MRSA.[24] If CA-MRSA is suspected, treatment with vancomycin with or without gentamicin and/or rifampin remains standard of care.

The predominant coagulase-negative organism causing IE has been *S. epidermidis*. However, in the past few years there has been an increase in isolation of another coagulase-negative species, *S. lugdunensis*.[25,26] Typically, coagulase-negative staphylococcal IE has a subacute course with numerous complications. Treatment (with or without surgical intervention) is usually successful. On the other hand, *S. lugdunensis* produces a more virulent infection and, despite similar antibiotic susceptibilities, has a much higher mortality rate.[25,26]

► Enterococci

Enterococci are normal flora of the human GI tract and sometimes found in the anterior urethra. Affected patients are typically older males who have undergone genitourinary manipulations or younger females who have had obstetric procedures. Although enterococci are a less common cause of IE, there are two predominant species: *Enterococcus faecium* and *Enterococcus faecalis*. *E. faecalis* is the most common and more susceptible of the strains. However, enterococci overall are more intrinsically resistant, with enterococcal IE representing one of the most problematic gram-positive infections to treat and cure. Frequently, enterococci display resistance to multiple antibiotics, including penicillins, vancomycin, aminoglycosides, as well as being described in some of the newer agents (eg, linezolid, quinupristin/dalfopristin, or daptomycin).[27]

► Gram-Negative Organisms

Gram-negative IE is much less common (~2%) but is typically much more difficult to treat than gram-positive infections.[1,28] Fastidious organisms, such as the HACEK group, tend to be seen most commonly, causing approximately 3% of all IE.[4,29,30] This group consists of *Haemophilus* spp. (primarily *H. paraphrophilus, H. parainfluenzae*, and *H. aphrophilus*), *Aggregatibacter actinomycetemcomitans, Cardiobacterium hominis, Eikenella corrodens*, and *Kingella kingae*. The clinical presentation of IE by these organisms is subacute, with approximately 50% of patients developing complications. These complications are primarily due to the presence of large, friable vegetations and numerous emboli along with development of acute congestive heart failure often requiring valve replacement.[30,31] It is important to allow cultures sufficient incubation time (often 2–3 weeks) in order to isolate these organisms. Despite prolonged incubation, these organisms may not be isolated on culture and thus present as culture-negative IE.

Other gram-negative organisms, such as *Pseudomonas* spp., cause IE, especially in IVDUs and patients with prosthetic valves. Additionally, IE may be caused by *Salmonella* spp., *Escherichia coli, Citrobacter* spp., *Klebsiella* spp., *Enterobacter* spp., *Serratia marcescens, Proteus* spp., and *Providencia* spp.[1,28]

Historically, gram-negative IE typically had a poor prognosis with high mortality rates. However, as nondrug therapy advances to include cardiac surgery in more than half of patients, in-hospital mortality has improved to 24%.[1,28] Treatment usually consists of high-dose combination antimicrobial therapy, with valve replacement often necessary in many patients.

► Culture Negative

Negative blood cultures are reported in approximately 5% of confirmed IE cases, often delaying diagnosis and treatment.[1,4,32] Cultures that do not grow bacteria may be the result of previous antibiotic use, subacute right-sided disease, slow growth of fastidious organisms, nonbacterial endocarditis (eg, fungal or intracellular parasitic infections), noninfective endocarditis, or improper collection of blood cultures. If nonbacterial or fastidious organisms are suspected, additional testing is essential. The choice of treatment regimen depends on patient history and risk factors.

► Other Organisms

Numerous bacteria, including gram-positive bacilli, unusual gram-negative bacteria, atypical bacteria, and anaerobes, as well as spirochetes, may be a rare cause IE.[29] Some of the more common organisms include *Legionella, Coxiella burnetii* (Q fever), and *Brucella*. These rare organisms occur primarily in at-risk patients such as those with prosthetic valves or IVDUs. A comprehensive discussion of these organisms is not feasible for this chapter; for further information, other references sources (particularly references 1–5) should be examined. Treatment of these organisms is difficult, and cure rates are low. Therefore, consulting an infectious diseases specialist is warranted.

► Fungi

Fungal endocarditis is quite uncommon but has significant mortality, typically affecting patients who have had cardiovascular surgery, received total parenteral nutrition (TPN) or prolonged course of broad-spectrum antibiotics, have long-term catheter placement, immunocompromised, or IVDUs.[3,33] Survival rates remain poor, at approximately 15%, but improvements (survival rates ~30%) have been reported owing to advances in diagnosis and treatment.[33] Poor prognosis has been attributed to large vegetations, propensity for organism invasion into the myocardium, extensive septic emboli, poor antifungal penetration into vegetations, and low toxic-to-therapeutic ratio and lack of cidal activity of certain antifungals.[30,33] The two most commonly associated organisms are *Candida* spp. and *Aspergillus* spp. Lack of clinical studies makes treatment decisions difficult. Typically, combination and/or high-dose therapy in conjunction with surgery is required.

TREATMENT

Therapeutic Considerations

Treatment of IE often is complicated and difficult. Numerous factors involving vegetations influence the effectiveness of antimicrobial agents. Vegetations consist of a fibrin matrix (as discussed earlier) that provides an environment where organisms are relatively free to replicate unimpeded, allowing the microbial density to reach very high concentrations (10^9–10^{10} CFU/g). Once organism density has reached this level, the organisms are virtually in a static growth phase. These factors hinder host defenses, as well as the ability of antimicrobials to produce sufficient kill. This is often seen with β-lactams and glycopeptides as their effectiveness can be significantly affected by bacterial inoculum and stationary growth phase.

KEY CONCEPT *Selection of an appropriate antimicrobial agent must combine characteristics such as the ability to penetrate into the vegetation, the ability to achieve adequate drug concentrations, and the ability to be minimally affected by high bacterial inoculum in order to achieve adequate kill rates.*

KEY CONCEPT *To accomplish this, antimicrobials typically have to be given parenterally at high doses, with an extended treatment course of 4 to 6 weeks (in most cases).* Other desirable drug characteristics include bactericidal and synergistic activity.

Empirical Therapy

KEY CONCEPT *The overall goal of therapy is to eradicate the infection and minimize/prevent any complications.* Patients with suspected IE should be evaluated for risk factors that may provide some indication of the most likely causative organism. If no risk factors can be determined, empirical therapy should primarily cover gram-positive organisms. Generally, if streptococci are suspected, empirical treatment should consist of penicillin plus gentamicin. However, if staphylococci or enterococci are suspected, empirical treatment should consist of vancomycin plus gentamicin. It is important to monitor the patient's response to therapy closely until cultures and susceptibilities are determined to ensure adequate treatment.

Specific Therapy

The American Heart Association (AHA) has published guidelines for the management of IE, including specific treatment recommendations.[5] A summary of these treatments for the most common organisms (streptococci, staphylococci, and enterococci) is provided in Tables 74–3 through 74–6. However, for more detailed information, refer to the complete guidelines.[5]

▶ *Streptococci*

Most isolates are highly susceptible to penicillin; therefore, penicillin G remains the regimen of choice. However, ceftriaxone may be used as an alternative agent if the patient is allergic or penicillin resistance is suspected. Typically, length of treatment is 4 weeks and remains the most common duration. However, a shorter course (ie, 2 weeks) may be employed for a patient with uncomplicated IE due to highly penicillin-susceptible strains with no extracardiac infection or whose creatinine clearance is greater than 20 mL/min (0.33 mL/s). If the shorter length of therapy is chosen, gentamicin should be added to the previous regimens for the entire course (ie, 2 weeks). Recommended therapies for highly penicillin-susceptible viridans streptococci are summarized in Table 74–3.

When penicillin MICs for viridans group streptococci are greater than 0.12 mcg/mL [0.12 mg/L] but less than or equal to 0.5 mcg/mL [0.5 mg/L], antimicrobial doses should be increased with 4 weeks therapy suggested. In addition, combination therapy with gentamicin is recommended during the first 2 weeks. In patients who are allergic or intolerant to β-lactams, vancomycin is an alternative treatment option. In patients with resistant strains of viridans group streptococci (MIC greater than 0.5 mcg/mL [0.5 mg/L]), treatment should include antimicrobial agents for enterococcal IE (precise agents determined by the susceptibility report).

Patients with PVE caused by penicillin-susceptible strains of viridans streptococci require treatment for 6 weeks with penicillin G or ceftriaxone with or without gentamicin during the initial 2 weeks of therapy. However, if the organism demonstrates less susceptibility to penicillin (MIC greater than > 0.12 mcg/mL [0.12 mg/L]), combination therapy with penicillin G or ceftriaxone plus gentamicin should be given for the entire 6 weeks. Vancomycin remains the primary alternative for β-lactam (eg, penicillins, cephalosporins) allergic patients.

Patient Encounter, Part 2: Medical History, Physical Examination, and Diagnostic Tests

PMH: ESRD on hemodialysis (MWF), type 2 diabetes

FH: Mother had a history of hypertension and died at the age of 70 from a stroke; father's history is unknown

SH: She began dialysis 6 months ago. She denied alcohol, illicit drug, and tobacco usage

Meds: Novolog (insulin aspart) 90 units/24 hour basal rate with 20 units bolus prior to each meal via an insulin pump; sevelamer 800 mg three times daily; epogen 10,000 units post-HD

Allergies: No known allergies

ROS: Fatigue, decreased appetite

PE:

VS: BP 105/65 mm Hg, P 115 beats/min, RR 22 breaths/min, T 39.5°C

Cardiovascular: Tachycardia, positive new murmur

Abd: Normal weight, soft, nontender, nondistended; (–) bowel sounds

Labs: Within normal limits, except WBC = $18.6 \times 10^3/\mu L$ ($18.6 \times 10^9/L$), SCr = 4.2mg/dL (371 μmol/L)

Given this additional information, what is your assessment of the patient's condition?

Identify your empirical treatment recommendations for this patient.

What other information would be beneficial to obtain?

Table 74–3

Therapy of Native-Valve Endocarditis Caused by Highly Penicillin-Susceptible Viridans Group Streptococci and *S. bovis*

Regimen	Dosage[a] and Route	Duration (weeks)	Strength of Recommendation[b]	Comments
Aqueous crystalline penicillin G sodium *OR*	12–18 million units/24 hour (IV either continuously or in four or six equally divided doses	4	IA	Preferred in most patients 65 years of age or older or patients with impairment of eighth cranial nerve function or renal function
Ceftriaxone sodium	2 g/24 hour IV/IM in one dose *Pediatric dose*[c]: penicillin 200,000 units/kg/24 hour IV in four to six equally divided doses; ceftriaxone 100 mg/kg/24 hour IV/IM in one dose	4	IA	
Aqueous crystalline penicillin G sodium *OR*	12–18 million units/24 hour IV either continuously or in six equally divided doses	2	IB	2-week regimen not intended for patients with cardiac or extracardiac abscess or for those with creatinine clearance of < 20 mL/min (0.33 mL/s), impaired eighth cranial nerve function, or *Abiotrophia, Granulicatella, or Gemella* spp. infection; gentamicin dosage should be adjusted to achieve peak serum concentration of 3–4 mcg/mL (3–4 mg/L; 6.3–8.4 μmol/L) and trough serum concentration of < 1 mcg/mL (1 mg/L; 2.1 μmol/L) when three divided doses are used; nomogram used for single daily dosing[e]
Ceftriaxone plus gentamicin sulfate[d]	2 g/24 hour IV/IM in one dose 3 mg/kg/24 hour IV/IM in one dose *Pediatric dose*: penicillin 200,000 units/kg/24 hour IV in four to six equally divided doses; ceftriaxone 100 mg/kg/24 hour IV/IM in one dose; gentamicin 3 mg/kg/24 hour IV/IM in one dose or three equally divided doses[f]			
Vancomycin hydrochloride[g]	30 mg/kg/24 hour IV in two equally divided doses not to exceed 2 g/24 hour unless concentrations in serum are inappropriately low *Pediatric dose*: 40 mg/kg/24 hour IV in two to three equally divided doses MIC ≤ 0.12 mcg/mL (0.12 mg/L)	4	IB	Vancomycin therapy recommended only for patients unable to tolerate penicillin or ceftriaxone; vancomycin dosage should be adjusted to obtain peak (1 hour after infusion completed) serum concentration of 30–35 mcg/mL (30–35 mg/L; 21–24 μmol/L) and a trough concentration range of 10–15 mcg/mL (10–15 mg/L; 6.9–10.4 μmol/L)

IM, intramuscularly; MIC, minimum inhibitory concentration.

[a]Dosage recommended are for patients with normal renal function.

[b]IA, condition with evidence and/or general agreement that a procedure or treatment is useful and effective, based on data from multiple randomized clinical trials; IB, condition with evidence and/or general agreement that a procedure or treatment is useful and effective based on data from a single randomized trial or nonrandomized studies.

[c]Pediatric dose should not exceed that of a normal adult.

[d]Other potentially nephrotoxic drugs (eg, nonsteroidal anti-inflammatory drugs) should be used with caution in patients receiving gentamicin therapy.

[e]See Nicolau DP, Freeman CD, Belliveau PB, et al. Experience with a once-daily aminoglycoside program administered to 2184 adult patients. Antimicrob Agents Chemother 1995;39:650–655.

[f]Data for once-daily dosing of aminoglycosides for children exist, but no data for treatment of IE exist.

[g]Vancomycin dosages should be infused during course of at least 1 hour to reduce risk of histamine-release "red man" syndrome.

Reprinted with permission. Baddour LM, Wilson WR, Bayer AS, et al. American Heart Association Scientific Statement. Infective endocarditis: Diagnosis, antimicrobial therapy, and management of complications. Circulation 2005;111:e394–e433. ©2005, American Heart Association, Inc.

Table 74–4

Therapy for Endocarditis Caused by Staphylococci in the Absence of Prosthetic Materials

Regimen	Dosage[a] and Route	Duration (weeks)	Strength of Recommendation[b]	Comments
Oxacillin-Susceptible Strains				
Nafcillin or oxacillin[c]	12 g/24 hour IV in four to six equally divided doses	6	IA	For complicated right-sided IE and for left-sided IE, 6-week treatment; for uncomplicated right-sided IE, 2-week treatment
With optional addition of gentamicin sulfate[d]	3 mg/kg/24 hour IV/IM in two or three equally divided doses *Pediatric dose*[e]: nafcillin or oxacillin 200 mg/kg/24 hour IV in four to six equally divided doses; gentamicin 3 mg/kg/24 hour IV/IM in three equally divided doses	3–5 days		Clinical benefit of aminoglycosides has not been established
For penicillin-allergic (nonanaphylactoid type) allergy: cefazolin	6 g/24 hour IV in three equally divided doses	6	IB	Consider skin testing for oxacillin-susceptible staphylococci and questionable history of immediate-type hypersensitivity to penicillin; cephalosporins should be avoided in patients with anaphylactoid-type hypersensitivity to β-lactams; vancomycin should be used in these cases[e]
With optional addition of gentamicin sulfate	3 mg/kg/24 hour IV/IM in two or three equally divided doses *Pediatric dose*: cefazolin 100 mg/kg/24 hour IV in three equally divided doses; gentamicin 3 mg/kg/24 hour IV/IM in three equally divided doses	3–5 days		Clinical benefit of aminoglycosides has not been established
Oxacillin-Resistant Strains				
Vancomycin hydrochloride[f]	30 mg/kg/24 hour IV in two equally divided doses *Pediatric dose*: 40 mg/kg/24 hour IV in two to three equally divided doses	6	IB	Adjust vancomycin dosage to achieve 1 hour (peak) serum concentration of 30–45 mcg/mL (30–45 mg/L; 21–31 μmol/L) and trough concentration of 10–15 mcg/mL (10–15 mg/L; 6.9–10.4 μmol/L) (see text for vancomycin alternatives)

IM, intramuscular.

[a]Dosages recommended are for patients with normal renal function.

[b]IA, condition with evidence and/or general agreement that a procedure or treatment is useful and effective, based on data from multiple randomized clinical trails; IB, condition with evidence and/or general agreement that a procedure or treatment is useful and effective based on data from a single randomized trial or nonrandomized studies.

[c]Penicillin G 24 million units/24 hour IV in four to six equally divided doses may be used in place of nafcillin or oxacillin if strain is penicillin-susceptible (MIC less than or equal to 0.1 mcg/mL [0.1 mg/L]) and does not produce β-lactamase.

[d]Gentamicin should be administered in close temporal proximity to vancomycin, nafcillin, or oxacillin dosing.

[e]Pediatric dose should not exceed that of a normal adult.

[f]For specific dosing adjustment and issues concerning vancomycin, see Table 74–3 footnotes.

Reprinted with permission. Baddour LM, Wilson WR, Bayer AS, et al. American Heart Association Scientific Statement. Infective endocarditis: diagnosis, antimicrobial therapy, and management of complications. Circulation 2005;111:e394–e433. ©2005, American Heart Association, Inc.

Table 74–5

Therapy for PVE Caused by Staphylococci

Regimen	Dosage[a] and Route	Duration (weeks)	Strength of Recommendation[b]	Comments
Oxacillin-Susceptible Strains				
Nafcillin or oxacillin *plus*	12 g/24 hour IV in four to six equally divided doses	6 weeks or longer	IB	Penicillin G 24 million units/24 hour IV in four to six equally divided doses may be used in place of nafcillin or oxacillin if strain is penicillin-susceptible (MIC ≤ 0.1 mcg/mL [0.1 mg/L]) and does not produce β-lactamase; vancomycin should be used in patients with immediate-type hypersensitivity reactions to β-lactam antibiotics (see Table 74–3 for dosing guidelines); cefazolin may be substituted for nafcillin or oxacillin in patients with nonimmediate-type hypersensitivity reactions to penicillins
Rifampin *plus*	900 mg/24 hour IV/orally in three equally divided doses	6 weeks or longer		
Gentamicin sulfate[c]	3 mg/kg/24 hour IV/IM in two or three equally divided doses	2		
	Pediatric dose[d]: nafcillin or oxacillin 200 mg/kg/24 hour IV in four to six equally divided doses; rifampin 20 mg/kg/24 hour IV/oral doses; in three equally divided doses; gentamicin 3 mg/kg/24 hour in three equally divided doses			
Oxacillin-Resistant Strains				
Vancomycin hydrochloride *plus*	30 mg/kg/24 hour IV in two equally divided doses	6 weeks or longer	IB	Adjust vancomycin to achieve 1 hour (peak) serum concentration of 30–45 mcg/mL (30–45 mg/L; 21–31 µmol/L) and trough concentration of 10–15 mcg/mL (10–15 mg/L; 6.9–10.4 µmol/L)
Rifampin *plus*	900 mg/24 hour IV/oral in three equally divided doses	6 weeks or longer		
Gentamicin sulfate	3 mg/kg/24 hour IV/IM in two or three equally divided doses	2		
	Pediatric dose: vancomycin 40 mg/kg/24 hour IV in two or three equally divided doses; rifampin 20 mg/kg/24 hour IV/oral in three equally divided doses (up to adult dose); gentamicin 3 mg/kg/24 hour IV/IM in three equally divided doses			

[a]Dosages recommended are for patients with normal renal function.

[b]IB, condition with evidence and/or general agreement that a procedure or treatment is useful and effective, based on data from a single randomized trial or nonrandomized studies.

[c]Gentamicin should be administered in close proximity to vancomycin, nafcillin, or oxacillin dosing.

[d]Pediatric dose should not exceed that of a normal adult.

Reprinted with permission from Baddour LM, Wilson WR, Bayer AS, et al. American Heart Association Scientific Statement. Infective endocarditis: Diagnosis, antimicrobial therapy, and management of complications. Circulation 2005;111:e394–e433. ©2005, American Heart Association, Inc.

▸ *Staphylococci*

It is important to determine (a) whether the isolate is methicillin-susceptible versus methicillin-resistant and (b) whether the patient has a native versus prosthetic valve. For patients with no prosthetic material, methicillin-susceptible staphylococcal treatment should consist of a penicillinase-resistant penicillin (eg, nafcillin or oxacillin) or cefazolin with or without gentamicin, and for methicillin-resistant strains, therapy should consist of vancomycin (see Table 74–4). Combination therapy with aminoglycosides, when used in these patients, typically is given only during the first 3 to 5 days of therapy to decrease bacterial burden. In the absence of prosthetic material, some treatment guidelines do not recommend combination therapy against MRSA. However, many clinicians may combine either gentamicin or rifampin with vancomycin if the patient is unresponsive to monotherapy.

Increasing resistance of staphylococci necessitates the expanded use of alternative therapies. Daptomycin demonstrated similar efficacy when compared with standard therapy (ie, penicillinase-resistant penicillin for methicillin-sensitive *S. aureus* [MSSA] or vancomycin for MRSA) in patients with staphylococcal IE and is FDA approved for the treatment of right-sided IE or bacteremia caused by *S. aureus*.[34] Recommended daptomycin dosing for these indications is 6 mg/kg/day (unless renal adjustments are necessary); although dosages of 8 to 10 mg/kg/day have been suggested in IE.[20,34] Daptomycin was shown to be safe and well tolerated.[34,35] Additionally, other antibiotics, such as ceftaroline, linezolid, quinupristin/dalfopristin, telavancin, or tigecycline alone or in combination, have been used in patients who were unresponsive to standard therapy, although they have had variable response rates.[36–39] These therapies often are reserved for patients who have been unresponsive to traditional therapy (eg, β-lactams or vancomycin) or for organisms that remain susceptible to these agents when resistant to traditional therapy.

Table 74–6

Therapy for Native-Valve or Prosthetic-Valve Enterococcal Endocarditis Caused by Strains Susceptible to Penicillin, Gentamicin, and Vancomycin

Regimen	Dosage[a] and Route	Duration (weeks)	Strength of Recommendation[b]	Comments
Ampicillin sodium *OR*	12 g/24 hour IV in six divided doses	4–6	IA	Native valve: 4-week therapy recommended for patients with symptoms of illness ≤ 3 months; 6-week therapy recommended for patients with symptoms > 3 months
Aqueous crystalline penicillin G sodium *plus* gentamicin sulfate[c]	18–30 million units/24 hour IV either continuously or in six equally divided doses	4–6	IA	Prosthetic valve or other prosthetic cardiac material: minimum of 6 weeks of therapy recommended
	3 mg/kg/24 hour IV/IM in three equally divided doses *Pediatric dose*[d]: ampicillin 300 mg/kg/24 hour IV in four to six equally divided doses; penicillin 300,000 units/kg/24 hour IV in four to six equally divided doses; gentamicin 3 mg/kg/24 hour IV/IM in three equally divided doses	4–6		
Vancomycin hydrochloride[e]	30 mg/kg/24 hour IV in two equally divided doses	6	IB	Vancomycin therapy recommended only for patients unable to tolerate penicillin or ampicillin
plus gentamicin sulfate	3 mg/kg/24 hour IV/IM in three equally divided doses *Pediatric dose:* vancomycin 40 mg/kg/24 hour IV in two or three equally divided doses; gentamicin 3 mg/kg/24 hour IV/IM in three equally divided doses	6		6 weeks of vancomycin therapy recommended because of decreased activity against enterococci

[a]Dosages recommended are for patients with normal renal function.

[b]IA, condition with evidence and/or general agreement that a procedure or treatment is useful and effective, based on data from multiple randomized clinical trials; IB, condition with evidence and/or general agreement that a procedure or treatment is useful and effective, based on data from a single randomized trial or nonrandomized studies.

[c]Dosage of gentamicin should be adjusted to achieve peak serum concentration of 3 to 4 mcg/mL (3–4 mg/L; 6.3–8.4 μmol/L) and a trough concentration of less than 1 mcg/mL (1 mg/L; 2.1 μmol/L). Patients with a creatinine clearance of less than 50 mL/min (0.83 mL/s) should be treated in consultation with an infectious diseases specialist.

[d]Pediatric dose should not exceed that of a normal adult.

[e]See Table 74–3 for appropriate dosage of vancomycin.

Reprinted with permission from Baddour LM, Wilson WR, Bayer AS, et al. American Heart Association Scientific Statement. Infective endocarditis: Diagnosis, antimicrobial therapy, and management of complications. Circulation 2005;111:e394–e433. ©2005, American Heart Association, Inc.

For staphylococcal PVE, treatment length increases significantly, typically requiring a minimum of 6 weeks (see Table 74–5). For MSSA, a penicillinase-resistant penicillin should still be used, as well as vancomycin for MRSA. However, with either regimen, addition of gentamicin for first 2 weeks and rifampin for the entire length of treatment is recommended. Infectious Diseases consultation is recommended for all patients with *S. aureus* IE, irrespective of methicillin-susceptibility, due to an observed reduction in mortality in this patient population.

▸ *Enterococci*

For enterococci, it is imperative to determine species and antibiotic susceptibilities. If the organism is susceptible to penicillin and vancomycin, treatment may consist of high-dose penicillin G, ampicillin, or vancomycin plus an aminoglycoside (gentamicin [see Table 74–6] or streptomycin for gentamicin-resistant strains). Treatment length is usually 4 to 6 weeks, with the aminoglycoside used over the entire course. As resistance develops to penicillin, ampicillin and vancomycin remain treatment options. If the isolate becomes resistant to ampicillin, vancomycin is considered the treatment of choice.

If the isolate is determined to be vancomycin-resistant, it is crucial to know the exact species because some treatment options, such as quinupristin/dalfopristin, are not active against *E. faecalis*. Treatment options for vancomycin-resistant enterococci (VRE) have not been well established. Currently,

Patient Encounter, Part 3: Additional Laboratory and Diagnostic Tests

Blood Cultures: All cultures are positive for gram-positive cocci in clusters, coagulase positive; *S. aureus*.

Labs: Within normal limits, excluding WBC and SCr.

Echo: 0.7 × 1.2 cm vegetation on the mitral valve.

Given this additional information, are there any changes in your assessment of the patient?

How would you tailor your treatment based on these new data?

What would be your treatment goals, including length of treatment?

What other information would be beneficial to have?

recommendations for treating vancomycin-resistant *E. faecium* include linezolid or quinupristin/dalfopristin for a minimum of 8 weeks. However, newer agents, such as daptomycin, provide another option for treatment for either enterococci species (*E. faecium* and *E. faecalis*). The guidelines also suggest the use of imipenem/cilastatin plus ampicillin or ceftriaxone plus ampicillin for the treatment of *E. faecalis*, with a minimum of 8 weeks of therapy; although these regimens are not commonly used. Even with newer agents, combination therapy is often warranted; therefore, consultation with an infectious diseases specialist is recommended if VRE is identified.

▶ *Gram-Negative Organisms*

Identification of the exact pathogen is crucial in gram-negative IE as treatment decisions depend on which organism is isolated. Therapy is usually targeted to the most susceptible antibiotics. Combination therapy (usually the addition of an aminoglycoside) is commonly used. For example, *Pseudomonas* spp. are treated with an antipseudomonal β-lactam (eg, piperacillin/tazobactam, cefepime, imipenem/cilastatin) plus high-dose aminoglycoside (typically tobramycin 8 mg/kg/day). However, exact dosing of antibiotics depends on the organism isolated. Length of treatment is usually a minimum of 6 weeks.

Patient Encounter, Part 4: Additional Laboratory

Susceptibility Report: *S. aureus*

Drug	MIC (mg/L)
Oxacillin	0.25
Vancomycin	2
Clindamycin	less than or equal to 0.5
Trimethoprim-sulfamethoxazole	less than or equal to 0.5/9.5
Daptomycin	0.125

Given this additional information, are there any changes in your assessment of the patient?

Do you need to adjust your treatment regimen based on these data?

Would your treatment goals, particularly length of treatment, change?

▶ *HACEK Group*

The HACEK group bacteria are difficult to isolate, often taking weeks for identification. If one of these organisms is suspected, it is important to initiate appropriate empirical treatment. The preferred regimen is ceftriaxone (or another third- or fourth-generation cephalosporin), followed by ampicillin-sulbactam. However, for patients who are intolerant of these treatments, ciprofloxacin may be used. The length of treatment typically is 4 weeks for these organisms.

▶ *Culture-Negative*

Treatment for culture-negative IE presents a significant dilemma. Therapeutic regimens are guided by isolated organisms. When cultures fail to identify a specific organism, decisions regarding treatment should cover the most common causative pathogens. If the patient is unresponsive to this initial treatment, additional coverage for less common organisms becomes warranted. An infectious diseases specialist should be consulted for managing culture-negative IE.

▶ *Fungi*

Treatment of fungal IE is exceptionally difficult. There is a significant lack of evidence to identify the most appropriate therapy. Currently, amphotericin B is the most common treatment. However, valve replacement surgery is often considered a necessary adjunctive therapy. Intravenous antifungal therapy requires high doses for a minimum of 8 weeks of treatment. Oral azoles (eg, fluconazole) are used as long-term suppressive therapy to prevent relapse. Newer antifungals may be effective options, including the echinocandins (eg, caspofungin) and voriconazole, depending on the organism and susceptibilities.[33]

Surgery

Surgical intervention has become an integral therapy in combination with pharmacologic management of IE. Valve replacement is the predominant intervention, and is used in almost one-half of all cases of IE.[1] Surgery may be indicated if the patient has unresolved infection, ineffective antimicrobial therapy, more than one episode of serious emboli, refractory congestive heart failure, significant valvular dysfunction, mycotic aneurysm requiring resection, local complications (perivalvular or myocardial abscesses), or prosthetic-valve infection associated with a pathogen demonstrating higher antimicrobial resistance.[40,41] Often a patient's hemodynamic status (ie, blood pressure, heart rate, pulmonary artery pressure, etc) is used to determine when surgical intervention is warranted.[1] Despite appropriate medical management and cure, a significant number of people who develop native-valve endocarditis require valve replacement surgery. Involvement of the aorta or development of IE complications is considered an indication for surgery in the majority of patients with PVE.[42,43]

Antimicrobial Dosing Considerations

The majority of antibiotic and antifungal agents used for the treatment of IE require dosing modifications based on renal or hepatic function. However, the most closely monitored are vancomycin and aminoglycosides. This is due in part because (a) serum levels are normally monitored to guide therapy, and (b) there is an increased likelihood of developing toxicities (ie, nephrotoxicity, ototoxicity) if the level is too high or adverse outcomes (ie, clinical failure or resistance development) if level is too low. General dosing considerations are included in Table 74–7 for

Table 74–7

Dosage Considerations for Standard Antibiotics for Treatment of IE[a]

Drug	Renal Adjustments	Hepatic Adjustments	Comments
Penicillin G	Required	None	Extension of dosing interval primarily used for adjustment
Ampicillin	Required	None	Seizures most common AE if dosing not adjusted
Nafcillin	None	Severe (see comment)	Adjustments necessary ONLY in patients with severe hepatic AND renal impairment
Oxacillin	Severe (see comment)	None	Adjustments for CrCl < 10 mL/min (0.17 mL/s) to lower range of normal dose
Cefazolin	Required	None	Dose and/or dosing interval require adjustment. Based on patient's CrCl
Ceftriaxone	Severe (see comment)	None	Do not exceed 2 g/day if patient has BOTH severe renal AND hepatic impairment
Vancomycin	Required	None	Monitor therapeutic levels to guide dosage adjustments (see treatment guidelines for target ranges)
Gentamicin	Required	None	Used for synergy only with gram-positives. Therapeutic levels vary for gram-negative organisms Monitor therapeutic levels to guide dosage adjustments Synergy target levels: peak 3–4 mcg/mL (3–4 mg/L; 6.3–8.4 μmol/L) and trough < 1 mcg/mL (1 mg/L; 2.1 μmol/L)
Rifampin	None	Required	Adjustment based on hepatic dysfunction
Newer and Salvage Drugs			
Ceftaroline	Required	None	Adjustments in dose (33%–67% reduction) are based on patient's CrCl. Suggested dosages in off-label use for IE are higher than standard dosing (ie, 600 mg every 8 hours)
Daptomycin	Required	None	Adjustment in dosing interval CrCl < 30 mL/min (0.50 mL/s) CPK should be monitored prior to and during therapy
Linezolid	None	None	Metabolites may accumulate in severe renal impairment Monitor for hematologic AE Use in severe hepatic impairment not established
Quinupristin/dalfopristin	None	Possibly	Adjustments suggested based on pharmacokinetic data. However, no specific recommendations are described
Telavancin	Required	None	Decrease daily dose by 25% if CrCl 30–50 mL/min (0.50–0.83 mL/s) or if CrCl < 30 mL/min (0.50 mL/s)—extend interval to every 48 hours
Tigecycline	None	Severe (see comment)	In severe hepatic impairment (Child-Pugh class C)—decrease maintenance dose 50%
Streptomycin	Required	None	Used for synergy only with gram-positives. Therapeutic levels vary for gram-negative organisms Monitor therapeutic levels to guide dosage adjustments Synergy target levels: peak 20–35 mcg/mL (20–35 mg/L; 34–60 μmol/L) and trough < 10 mcg/mL (10 mg/L; 17 μmol/L)

AE, adverse event; CPK, creatinine phosphokinase; CrCl, creatinine clearance.

[a]Gram-negative bacteria, fungal, or atypical treatments are not listed. It is suggested that an Infectious Diseases Consult be obtained if a patient has IE caused by one of these organisms due to the complexity and difficulty in managing these patients.

the most commonly used drugs for treating IE. However, specific dosing adjustments for individual patients should be determined by referring to an appropriate drug dosing reference.

Prophylaxis

KEY CONCEPT *Certain conditions have been associated more commonly with IE due to preexisting cardiac disease in the presence of a transient bacteremia. In an effort to prevent the development of IE, prophylactic treatment is generally considered appropriate for these at-risk patients.* Although there are no well-controlled clinical studies of these recommendations, it is thought that if antibiotics are given just prior to a procedure, the number of bacteria may be decreased in the bloodstream and prevent the bacteria from adhering to the valves.

Cardiac conditions in which prophylaxis is reasonable include presence of prosthetic valves or material, prior IE, congenital cardiac disease (specific forms only), and cardiac transplant patients with cardiac valvulopathy (Table 74–8).[6] Although many patients have other cardiac dysfunction, only patients with these conditions are considered to be at a high risk of developing IE. No prophylaxis is advised in other patients.

Transient bacteremia may occur due to many types of dental and surgical procedures. However, the AHA guidelines significantly limit the types of procedures where prophylaxis is appropriate. Only dental procedures involving manipulation of gingival tissue or periapical region of teeth or perforation of the oral mucosa are considered to increase the likelihood that high-risk patients will develop IE.[6] Viridans group streptococci are the primary bacteria targeted for prophylaxis in this circumstance. On the other hand, prophylaxis for GI or genitourinary surgeries primarily targets enterococci.

The AHA guidelines include suggested antibiotic regimens for dental procedures for which prophylaxis is warranted.[6] Recommended regimens for dental procedures are listed in Table 74–9.

Table 74–8

Cardiac Conditions Associated with the Highest Risk of Adverse Outcome from Endocarditis for Which Prophylaxis with Dental Procedures Is Reasonable[a]

Prosthetic cardiac valve or prosthetic material used for cardiac-valve repair
Previous IE
Congenital heart disease[b]
Unrepaired cyanotic congenital heart disease, including palliative shunts and conduits
Completely repaired congenital heart defect with prosthetic material or device, whether placed by surgery or by catheter intervention, during the first 6 months after the procedure[c]
Repaired congenital heart disease with residual defects at the site or adjacent to the site of a prosthetic patch or prosthetic device (which inhibit endothelialization)
Cardiac transplantation recipients who develop cardiac valvulopathy

[a]*All dental procedures* that involve manipulation of gingival tissue or the periapical region of teeth or perforation of the oral mucosa is reasonable to give prophylaxis in the patient conditions listed above.

[b]Except for the conditions listed above, antibiotic prophylaxis is no longer recommended for any other form of CHD.

[c]Prophylaxis is reasonable because endothelialization of prosthetic material occurs within 6 months after the procedure.

Reprinted with permission from Wilson W, Taubert KA, Gewitz M, et al. Prevention of infective endocarditis: Guidelines from the American Heart Association. Circulation 2007;116:1736–1754. ©2007, American Heart Association, Inc.

These guidelines recommend a single oral or intramuscular/intravenous dose initiated shortly before the procedure. The regimen for dental procedures consists primarily of a penicillin as first choice, with a cephalosporin for penicillin-allergic patients who have not had an anaphylactic reaction and clindamycin or a macrolide for penicillin-allergic patients. A second prophylactic dose is not recommended. However, if an infection develops at the procedure site, additional antibiotics (ie, a therapeutic course) may be required.

Patient Encounter, Part 5: Create a Care Plan

Based on this patient's information, create a care plan for the management of her IE. Be sure to include:

(a) A statement regarding treatment requirements and/or possible problems

(b) Goals of therapy

(c) A patient-specific plan, including preventive plans

(d) A follow-up plan to assess whether the goals have been met and to determine whether the patient experienced any adverse effects

OUTCOME EVALUATION

KEY CONCEPT *Monitoring for successful therapy is critical for this serious infection to prevent complications, prevent development of resistance, and decrease mortality.* Routine assessment of clinical signs and symptoms, as well as laboratory tests (ie, repeat blood cultures), microbiologic testing, and serum drug concentrations (if appropriate), must be performed.

Resolution of signs and symptoms typically occurs within a few days to a week in most cases. Monitor the patient daily for febrile episodes, as well as other vital signs, with expected normal values within 2 to 3 days of initiating antimicrobial therapy.[4] Persistent signs or symptoms could be indicative of inadequate treatment or development of resistance.

Blood cultures are the primary laboratory evaluation to assess response to therapy. Typically, with appropriate treatment, they should become negative within 3 to 7 days. Perform additional blood cultures if the patient appears unresponsive to current therapy or upon treatment completion to confirm eradication of infection. Evaluate all susceptibility reports to assess for appropriateness of antimicrobial therapy.

Table 74–9

Prophylactic Regimens for Dental Procedure

		Regimen: Single Dose 30–60 Minutes Before Procedure	
Situation	**Agent**	**Adults**	**Children**
Oral	Amoxicillin	2 g	50 mg/kg
Unable to take oral medications	Ampicillin or Cefazolin or Ceftriaxone	2 g IM or IV	50 mg/kg IM or IV
Allergic to penicillins or ampicillin—oral	Cephalexin[a,b] or Clindamycin or Azithromycin or Clarithromycin	2 g 600 mg 500 mg	50 mg/kg 20 mg/kg 15 mg/kg
Allergic to penicillins or ampicillin and unable to take oral medications	Cefazolin or Ceftriaxone[b] or Clindamycin	1g IM or IV 600 mg IM or IV	50 mg/kg IM or IV 20 mg/kg IM or IV

IM, intramuscular.

[a]Or other first- or second-generation oral cephalosporin in equivalent adult or pediatric dosage.

[b]Cephalosporins should not be used in an individual with a history of anaphylaxis, angioedema, or urticaria with penicillins or ampicillin.

Reprinted with permission from Wilson W, Taubert KA, Gewitz M, et al. Prevention of infective endocarditis: Guidelines from the American Heart Association. Circulation 2007;116:1736–1754. © 2007, American Heart Association, Inc.

Patient Care Process

Patient Assessment:

- Review patient history (social, medical, and surgical), physical exam, laboratory tests (especially blood cultures) and diagnostic imaging (particularly echocardiogram results), assess whether patient has clinical features of IE utilizing modified Duke criteria (see Table 74–2).
- Review patient past medical and medication history. Does patient have any allergies which could limit antimicrobial therapy? Does patient have any risk factors for resistant-pathogens (prior use of broad-spectrum antibiotics, multiple hospital admissions, hemodialysis patient, etc)?
- Conduct a personal history to identify possible causes of IE.

Therapy Evaluation:

- Once blood culture identification/susceptibility reported, determine if patient is on appropriate antimicrobial therapy.
- If bacteremia not cleared after repeat blood cultures, reassess appropriateness of antimicrobial(s) including new cultures/susceptibility and drug dosage and/or frequency.
- Monitor subsequent blood cultures for growth. Determine end of therapy based on first negative blood culture.
- Monitor vital signs/symptoms for return to baseline. If continued to be abnormal, reassessment of therapy/other diagnostic testing is necessary.
- Is patient experiencing any adverse effects from their antimicrobial(s)? Are there any potential drug–drug interactions from this medication?
- Determine whether recommended agent is on institution's formulary. If not, is there a formulary alternative? If no alternative, is there anything specific to institution to utilize nonformulary agent?
- Determine whether patient has prescription coverage. Is patient able to afford medication if completing therapy as an outpatient?

Care Plan Development:

- Determine whether drug doses are optimal. Change therapy if pathogen not susceptible to current antimicrobial(s) or if patient not improving on current therapy.
- Address any patient concerns about IE and its management.
- Discuss importance of lifestyle modifications if applicable.

Follow-Up Evaluation:

- Follow-up with blood cultures and physical exam. Review medical history and any other pertinent laboratory tests and results of other diagnostic tests.
- Discuss with patient preventative antibiotics prior to future invasive dental procedures.

Additionally, counsel patients at risk on the necessity of prophylactic antibiotics prior to major dental treatments in order to prevent recurrent infections. This is critical in patients with risk factors that predispose them to developing IE, such as prosthetic heart valves, other valvular defects, or previous IE.

Develop a follow-up plan to determine whether the patient has achieved a cure, which includes a clinical evaluation of signs/symptoms, repeat blood cultures, and possibly a repeat echocardiogram. The patient should also be assessed for any adverse events. This should be performed usually within a few weeks after the completion of therapy.

Abbreviations Introduced in This Chapter

AHA	American Heart Association
CFU	Colony-forming units
CNS	Coagulase-negative staphylococci
ESR	Erythrocyte sedimentation rate
HACEK	Group of bacteria consisting of *Haemophilus* spp., *Aggregatibacter actinomycetemcomitans, Cardiobacterium hominis, Eikenella corrodens*, and *Kingella kingae*
IE	Infective endocarditis
IVDUs	Intravenous drug users
MIC	Minimum inhibitory concentration
MRSA	Methicillin-resistant *S. aureus*
MSSA	Methicillin-sensitive *S. aureus*
NBTE	Nonbacterial thrombotic endocarditis
PVE	Prosthetic-valve endocarditis
TEE	Transesophageal echocardiogram
TTE	Transthoracic echocardiogram
VRE	Vancomycin-resistant enterococci

REFERENCES

1. Fowler VG Jr, Scheld WM, Bayer AS. Endocarditis and intravascular infections. In: Mandell GL, Bennett JE, Dolin R, eds. Principles and Practice of Infectious Diseases. 7th ed. Philadelphia, PA: Elsevier; 2009:1067–1111.
2. Bayer AS, Bolger AF, Taubert KA, et al. Diagnosis and management of infective endocarditis and its complications. Circulation. 1998;98:2936–2948.
3. Karchmer AW. Infective endocarditis. In: Bonow: Braunwald E, ed. Heart Disease: A Textbook of Cardiovascular Medicine. 9th ed. Philadelphia, PA: Saunders; 2012:1540–1560.
4. Mylonakis E, Calderwood SB. Infective endocarditis in adults. N Engl J Med. 2001;345:1318–1320.
5. Baddour LM, Wilson WR, Bayer AS, et al. American Heart Association Scientific Statement. Infective endocarditis: Diagnosis, antimicrobial therapy, and management of complications. Circulation. 2005;111:e394–e433.
6. Wilson W, Taubert KA, Gewitz M, et al. Prevention of infective endocarditis: Guidelines from the American Heart Association. Circulation. 2007;116:1736–1754.
7. Que Y, Moreillon P. Infective endocarditis. Nat Rev Cardiol. 2011;8:322–336.
8. Knoll BM, Baddour LM, Wilson WR. Prosthetic valve endocarditis. In: Mandell GL, Bennett JE, Dolin R, eds. Principles and Practice of Infectious Diseases. 7th ed. Philadelphia, PA: Elsevier; 2009:1113–1126.
9. Cecchi E, Imazio M, Trinchero R. Infective endocarditis: Diagnostic issues and practical clinical approach based on echocardiography. J Cardiovasc Med. 2008;9:414–418.
10. Mestres CA, Fita G, Azqueta M, Miro JM. Role of echocardiogram in decision making for surgery in endocarditis. Curr Infect Dis Rep. 2010;12:321–328.

11. Habib G, Badano L, Tribouilloy C, Vilacosta I, Zamorano JL. Recommendations for the practice of echocardiography in infective endocarditis. Eur J Echocardiogr. 2010;11:202–219.
12. Li JS, Sexton DJ, Mick N, et al. Proposed modifications to the Duke criteria for the diagnosis of infective endocarditis. Clin Infect Dis. 2000;30:633–638.
13. Murdoch DR, Corey GR, Hoen B, et al. Clinical presentation, etiology, and outcome of infective endocarditis in the 21st century. Arch Intern Med. 2009;169:463–473.
14. Ferrieri P, Gewitz MH, Gerber MA, et al. Unique features of infective endocarditis in childhood. Circulation. 2002;105: 2115–2127.
15. Knoll B, Tleyjeh IM, Steckelberg JM, et al. Infective endocarditis due to penicillin-resistant viridans group streptococci. Clin Infect Dis. 2007;44:1585–1592.
16. Upton A, Drinkovic D, Pottumarthy S, et al. Culture results of heart valves resected because of streptococcal endocarditis: Insights into duration of treatment to achieve valve sterilization. J Antimicrob Chemother. 2005;55:234–239.
17. Murray RJ. Staphylococcus aureus infective endocarditis: Diagnosis and management guidelines. Intern Med J. 2005;35:S25–S44.
18. Bor DH, Woolhandler S, Nardin R, et al. Infective endocarditis in the U.S., 1998-2009: A nationwide study. PLoS One. 2013; 8(3):e60033.
19. Lopez J, Revilla A, Vilacosta I, et al. Definition, clinical profile, microbiological spectrum, and prognostic factors of early-onset prosthetic valve endocarditis. Eur Heart J. 2007;28:760–765.
20. Liu C, Bayer A, Cosgrove SE, et. al. Clinical practice guidelines by the Infectious Diseases Society of America for the treatment of methicillin-resistant *Staphylococcus aureus* infections in adults and children: executive summary. Clin Infect Dis. 2011;52: 285–292.
21. Huang YT, Hsiao CH, Liao CH, Lee CW, Hsueh PR. Bacteremia and infective endocarditis caused by a non-daptomycin-susceptible, vancomycin-intermediate, and methicillin-resistant *Staphylococcus aureus* strain in Taiwan. J Clin Microbiol. 2008;46:1132–1136.
22. Bae IG, Federspiel JJ, Miro JM, et al. Heterogeneous vancomycin-intermediate susceptibility phenotype in bloodstream methicillin-resistant *Staphylococcus aureus* isolates from an international cohort of patients with infective endocarditis: Prevalence, genotype, and clinical significance. J Infect Dis. 2009;200:1355–1366.
23. Woods CW, Cheng AC, Fowler VG Jr, et al. Endocarditis caused by Staphylococcus aureus with reduced susceptibility to vancomycin. Clin Infect Dis. 2004;38:1188–1191.
24. Millar BC, Prendergast BD, Moore JE. Community-associated MRSA (CA-MRSA): An emerging pathogen in infective endocarditis. J Antimicrob Chemother. 2008;61:1–7.
25. Sabe MA, Shrestha NK, Gordon S, Menon V. Staphylococcus lugdunensis: A rare but destructive cause of coagulase-negative staphylococcus infective endocarditis. Eur Heart J Acute Cardiovasc Care. 2014;3:275–280.
26. Frank KL, Luiz del Pozo J, Patel R. From clinical microbiology to infection pathogenesis: How daring to be different works for Staphylococcus lugdunensis. Clin Microbiol Rev. 2008;21:111–133.
27. Linden PK. Optimizing therapy for vancomycin-resistant enterococci (VRE). Semin Respir Crit Care Med. 2007;28:632–645.
28. Morpeth S, Murdoch D, Cabell CH, et al. Non-HACEK gram-negative bacillus endocarditis. Ann Intern Med. 2007;147:829–835.
29. Brouqui P, Raoult D. Endocarditis due to rare and fastidious bacteria. Clin Microbiol Rev. 2001;14:177–207.
30. Durante-Mangoni E, Tripodi MF, Albisinni R, Utili R. Management of Gram-negative and fungal endocarditis. Int J Antimicrob Agents. 2010;36S:s40–s45.
31. Raza SS, Sultan OW, Sohail MR. Gram-negative bacterial endocarditis in adults: State-of-the-heart. Expert Rev Anti Infect Ther. 2010;8:879–885.
32. Katsouli A, Massad MG. Current issues in the diagnosis and management of blood culture-negative infective and non-infective endocarditis. Ann Thorac Surg. 2013;95:1467–1474.
33. Tacke D, Koehler P, Cornely OA. Fungal endocarditis. Curr Opin Infect Dis. 2013;26:501–507.
34. Fowler V, Boucher HW, Corey GR, et al. Daptomycin versus standard therapy for bacteremia and infective endocarditis caused by Staphylococcus aureus. N Engl J Med. 2006;355:653–665.
35. Kaya S, Yilmaz G, Kalkan A, Ertunc B, Koksal I. Treatment of Gram-positive left-sided infective endocarditis with daptomycin. J Infect Chemother. 2013;19:698–702.
36. Tascini C, Bongiorni MG, Doria R, et al. Linezolid for endocarditis: A case series of 14 patients. J Antimicrob Chemother. 2011;66:679–682.
37. Ho TT, Cadena J, Childs LM, et al. Methicillin-resistant *Staphylococcus aureus* bacteraemia and endocarditis treated with ceftaroline salvage therapy. J Antimicrob Chemother. 2012;67:1267–1270.
38. Drees M, Boucher H. New agents for *Staphylococcus aureus* endocarditis. Curr Opin Infect Dis. 2006;19:544–550.
39. Marcos LA, Camins BC. Successful treatment of vancomycin-intermediate *Staphylococcus aureus* pacemaker lead infective endocarditis with telavancin. Antimicrob Agents Chemother. 2010;54:5376–5378.
40. Sohail MR, Martin KR, Wilson WR, et al. Medical versus surgical management of Staphylococcus aureus prosthetic valve endocarditis. Am J Med. 2006;119:147–154.
41. Rivas P, Alonso J, Moya J, et al. The impact of hospital-acquired infections on the microbial etiology and prognosis of late-onset prosthetic valve endocarditis. Chest. 2005;128:764–771.
42. Head SJ, Mokhles MM, Osnabrugge RLJ, et al. Surgery in current therapy for infective endocarditis. Vascular Health and Risk Management 2011;7:255–263.
43. Leontyev S, Borger MA, Modi P, et al. Surgical management of aortic root abscess: A 13 year experience in 172 patients with 100% follow-up. J Thorac Cardiovasc Surg. 2012;143:332–337.

75 Tuberculosis

Rocsanna Namdar, Michael Lauzardo, and Charles Peloquin

LEARNING OBJECTIVES

Upon completion of the chapter, the reader will be able to:

1. Compare the risk for active tuberculosis (TB) disease among patients based on their age, immune status, place of birth, and time since exposure to an active case.
2. Design an appropriate therapeutic plan for a patient with active TB disease.
3. Distinguish among the diagnostic tests used for patients potentially infected with TB.
4. Assess the effectiveness of therapy in TB patients.
5. Describe the common and important adverse drug effects caused by TB drugs.
6. Select patients for whom therapeutic drug monitoring (TDM) may be valuable and identify the necessary laboratory monitoring parameters for patients on antituberculosis medications.
7. Design appropriate antimicrobial regimens for the treatment of latent TB infection.

INTRODUCTION

Tuberculosis (TB) remains one of the leading infectious causes of death worldwide. In 2012, about 8.6 million people developed TB and 1.3 million people died from the disease.[1] Most deaths are preventable if access to health care for diagnosis and correct treatment are provided.

EPIDEMIOLOGY AND ETIOLOGY

KEY CONCEPT *Roughly one-third of the world's population is infected and drug resistance is increasing in many areas.*[1] *The majority of cases worldwide are found in South-East Asia and Africa. In the United States, about 13 million people have latent TB infection (LTBI), evidenced by a positive skin test (***purified protein derivative** *[PPD]) but no signs or symptoms of disease.* The PPD is the antigen derived from *Mycobacterium tuberculosis* used to determine the presence of an immune response in patients with previous exposure. Patients testing positive have roughly a 1 in 10 chance of active disease during their lives, with the greatest risk in the first 2 years after infection. In 2013, 9588 new TB cases were reported in the United States; a 4.2% decline from 2012.[2]

The most recent data from the Centers for Disease Control and Prevention (CDC) indicate that TB deaths in the United States have increased slightly to 7.6%, from 529 deaths in 2009 to 569 deaths in 2010.[3] (For details, visit the CDC website at www.cdc.gov/nchstp/tb.)

Risk Factors for Infection

▶ *Location and Place of Birth*

California, New York, Florida, and Texas accounted for approximately 50% of all TB cases in 2013.[2] These higher numbers may reflect the high immigration rates into these states.[2] Mexico, the Philippines, Vietnam, India, and China account for the largest numbers of these immigrants.[2] TB is most prevalent in large urban areas and is exacerbated by crowded living conditions.[2] Those in close contact with patients with active pulmonary TB are most likely to become infected.[2,3]

▶ *Race, Ethnicity, Age, and Gender*

In 2012, Asians accounted for 30% of new TB cases, followed by Hispanics (28%) and African Americans (22%), whereas non-Hispanic whites accounted for 16% of new TB cases in the United States.[3] TB is most common among people 25 to 44 years of age, and those 45 to 64 years of age.[3]

Risk Factors for Disease

Once infected, a person's lifetime risk of active TB is about 10%, with about half this risk during the first 2 years.[2–4] *Young children, the elderly, and immunocompromised patients have greater risks.* KEY CONCEPT *HIV is the most important risk factor for active TB because the immune deficit prevents patients from containing the initial infection.*[1–4] *HIV-infected patients with M. tuberculosis infection are roughly 100 times more likely to develop active TB than normal hosts.*[1,3,4]

TB is caused by *M. tuberculosis*, a rod-shaped thin aerobic bacterium. It presents either as LTBI or as progressive active disease.[4] The latter typically causes progressive destruction of the lungs, leading to death in most patients who do not receive treatment. *M. tuberculosis* are acid-fast bacilli (AFB). Acid-fast organisms are characterized by wax-like nearly impermeable cells walls which often do not stain with Gram stain and cannot be decolorized by acid alcohol. The cell wall contains a high amount of mycolic acids, long-chain fatty acids, and cell wall lipids which make the wall difficult to attack with conventional antibiotics. The acid-fast stain is a differential stain used to identify acid-fast organisms.

Culture and Susceptibility Testing

KEY CONCEPT *Microscopic examination of infected material ("sputum smear" of material on a glass slide) is the most rapid and readily available test to detect AFB in clinical specimens.* Three sputum specimens should be collected in patients suspected of pulmonary TB to increase the likelihood of finding AFB. *The sensitivity of the sputum smear is only about 40%, so culture based TB diagnosis is the current gold standard.*[5] Unfortunately, culture is much slower due to the roughly 20-hour doubling time of the bacilli. Furthermore, microscopic examination for AFB through sputum smear alone cannot determine which of over 100 mycobacterial species is present. Depending on the presence of epidemiological risk factors, the usual practice is to isolate the patient and treat empirically until presence of *M. tuberculosis* is confirmed by genetic probe or positive culture.

Antimicrobial susceptibility testing is essential for directing proper treatment. The most common method utilizing solid growth media, known as the *proportion method,* takes 3 to 8 weeks to produce results. Growth in liquid media is faster and can detect live mycobacteria in about 2 weeks.[5,6] Rapid-identification tests include nucleic acid amplification tests utilizing the polymerase chain reaction (PCR).[7–9] Three nucleic acid amplification tests have been approved for use in the United States to detect *M. tuberculosis* in respiratory secretions. These tests are highly sensitive and specific for smear positive patients and somewhat less sensitive in smear negative patients, but only need as few as 1 to 10 organisms/mL (10^3–10^4/L) to give a positive result.[7–9] The Cepheid MTB/RIF Assay performed on the Xpert System is a qualitative test designed for rapid detection of *M. tuberculosis* and rifampin resistance.[10] New tests looking for specific mutations such as the katG gene associated with isoniazid resistance may facilitate rapid drug therapy decisions in the future. Nitrate reductase assays and porous ceramic support systems are among other rapid drug susceptibility testing techniques currently being investigated.[11] DNA fingerprinting is performed to assist surveillance programs and contact investigations. Various techniques are employed including **restriction fragment length polymorphism** (RFLP) analysis, spoligotyping, and mycobacterial interspersed repeat units. These techniques exploit conserved fragments in the TB genome that change gradually over time and allow investigators to determine if strains are related to one another. Strains that are related to one another are referred to as clusters. Clusters generally indicate recent transmission and are then targeted for interventions by TB programs.[12]

PATHOPHYSIOLOGY

Primary Infection

KEY CONCEPT *M. tuberculosis* is transmitted from person to person by coughing or any other aerosol producing activities.[4,13] This produces small particles known as *droplet nuclei* that float in the air for long periods of time. Primary infection usually results from inhaling droplet nuclei that contain *M. tuberculosis.*[4,13] The progression to clinical disease depends on three factors: (1) the number of *M. tuberculosis* organisms inhaled (infecting dose), (2) the virulence of these organisms, and (3) the host's cell-mediated immune response.[4,13,14] If pulmonary macrophages inhibit or kill the bacilli, the infection is aborted.[13] If not, *M. tuberculosis* eventually spreads throughout the body through the bloodstream.[4,13] *M. tuberculosis* most commonly infects the posterior apical region of the lungs, where conditions are most favorable for its survival.

T lymphocytes become activated over the course of 3 to 4 weeks, producing interferon-γ (IFN-γ) and other cytokines. These stimulate microbicidal macrophages to surround the tuberculous foci and form **granulomas** to prevent further extension.[13] A granuloma is a nodular aggregation of mononuclear inflammatory cells formed when the immune system attempts to wall off foreign substances. At this point, the infection is largely under control, and bacillary replication falls off dramatically. Any remaining mycobacteria are believed to reside primarily within granulomas or within macrophages that have avoided detection and lysis. Over 1 to 3 months, tissue hypersensitivity occurs, resulting in a positive tuberculin skin test.[4,13] Approximately 95% of individuals with an intact immune system will enter into this latent phase. KEY CONCEPT *Progressive primary disease occurs in roughly 5% of patients, especially children, the elderly, and immunocompromised patients.*[15] *This presents as a progressive pneumonia and frequently spreads, leading to meningitis and other severe forms of TB, often before patients develop positive skin tests or interferon-γ release assays.*[15]

Reactivation Disease

About 10% of infected patients develop reactivation TB, with half occurring in the first 2 years after infection.[4,8] Reactivation TB results when a previously "dormant" focus is reactivated and causes disease. Progression involves the development of caseating granulomas as a result of a vigorous immune response. Liquefaction leads to local spread and a pulmonary cavity results. This provides a portal to the airways and subsequently ambient

Patient Encounter, Part 1

HPI: AF is a 43-year-old man who presents to the medical clinic complaining of a 2-month history of a persistent cough that has become productive over the past 3 weeks. He also complains of fever, malaise and a 6-kg (13-lb) weight loss over the past 2 months.

PMH: Type 2 diabetes mellitus (NIDDM)—not well controlled; hypertension (HTN) × 5 years—not controlled, rheumatoid arthritis

FH: Mother and father died in an MVA 10 years ago; one brother, age 50, lives with the patient; one sister, age 53, is alive and currently undergoing chemotherapy treatment for breast cancer

SH: Born and raised in Mexico city until the age of 19 when he moved to Los Angeles, California. Single, one daughter. He reports IV drug use but last use was 5 years ago. He had a 20-year history of alcohol abuse but has been sober for 5 years. He owns his own import/export business and travels internationally to Mexico and parts of South America

Meds: Lisinopril 20 mg daily; amlodipine 5 mg daily; metformin 500 mg twice daily, adalimumab 40 mg every other week. Patient reports that he tries to be compliant with his therapies and takes them regularly except when he is unable to get his refills; over the past 2 months, he has only gone 3 to 4 days without medication

What information is suggestive of TB?

What factors place this patient at increased risk for acquiring TB?

air that enhances person-to-person spread. Bacterial counts in the cavities can be as high as 10^8/mL (10^{11}/L) of cavitary fluid.[4,13] Prior to the chemotherapy era, pulmonary TB usually was associated with hypoxia, respiratory acidosis, and eventually death related to asphyxia; a fate that remains all too common in poor countries where patients do not have access to effective therapy.

Extrapulmonary and Miliary Tuberculosis

Caseating granulomas, regardless of location, can spread tubercle bacilli, and cause symptoms.[4] Because of muted or altered symptoms, the diagnosis of TB is difficult and often delayed in immunocompromised hosts.[4,13] HIV-infected patients may present with only extrapulmonary TB, which is uncommon in HIV-negative persons. A widely disseminated form of the disease called *miliary TB* can occur, particularly in children and immunocompromised hosts. It can be rapidly fatal and immediate treatment is required.[13]

Influence of HIV Infection on Pathogenesis

HIV infection is the most important risk factor for active TB.[13] As $CD4^+$ lymphocytes multiply in response to the mycobacterial infection, HIV multiplies within these cells and selectively destroys them, gradually eliminating the TB-fighting lymphocytes.[16,17] HIV-positive patients often have negative skin tests and fail to produce cavitary lesions, and fever may be absent. Cavitary lesions are present in a wide variety of pathological processes involving the lung and are observed radiographically as gas or fluid filled areas of the lung in the center of a nodule. Approximately 5% of HIV-infected patients with pulmonary TB who are not being treated effectively with antiretroviral medications will have positive results on acid-fast staining, yet have a normal chest radiograph. Patients coinfected with HIV and TB have a substantially higher risk of early mortality compared with HIV-negative patients with TB.[17]

CLINICAL PRESENTATION AND DIAGNOSIS

Fever, night sweats, weight loss, fatigue, and a productive cough are the classic symptoms of TB.[4,13,14] Onset may be gradual, and the diagnosis is easily missed if the symptoms are muted.[4,13,14] Progressive pulmonary disease leads to cavitary lesions visible on x-ray. Physical examination is nonspecific but may be consistent with pneumonia. Dullness to chest percussion, rales, and increased vocal fremitus may be observed on examination. Laboratory data often are uninformative, but a modest increase in the white blood cell (WBC) count with a lymphocytic predominance can be seen. Frequently however, the physical exam is largely unremarkable.

Atypical presentations are common in patients coinfected with HIV.[4,13,17] Symptoms for these patients range from classic pulmonary to muted and nonspecific. Extrapulmonary TB typically presents either as a slowly progressive decline in the effected organ's function or commonly as a mass lesion. Lymphadenopathy is relatively common.[13,14] Abnormal behavior, headaches, or convulsions suggest tuberculous meningitis, although other acute central nervous system (CNS) infections must be excluded.[4,14]

The Elderly

Positive skin tests, fevers, night sweats, sputum production, or hemoptysis may be absent, making TB hard to distinguish from other bacterial or viral infections or chronic lung diseases.[4,18,19] In contrast, mental status changes are twice as common in the elderly, and CNS disease must be considered when TB is entertained. Mortality is six times higher in the elderly, in part owing to delays in diagnosis.[4,18,19]

Children

TB in children may present as atypical bacterial pneumonia, and often involves the lower and middle lobes.[4,14,19] Extrapulmonary TB is more common in children. The Bacille Calmette-Guérin (BCG) is a vaccine made from strains of tubercle bacilii and is used to produce immunity against human TB. It is administered in countries where TB remains common appears to stimulate children's immune systems to ward off the most serious forms of the disease. In fact, BCG is most effective in reducing infant mortality from TB meningitis and miliary disease. BCG does not block infection, and these same children often experience reactivation TB as young adults.

Skin Testing

TB skin testing with PPD (commercially available as Tubersol or Aplisol) is one of the oldest diagnostic tests still in clinical use.[4,14,16] Also known as the tuberculin skin test, the product is injected into the skin (not subcutaneously) with a fine (27-gauge) needle, a technique referred to as the Mantoux method, and produces a small, raised, blanched wheal to be read by an experienced professional in 48 to 72 hours. The chance of a false-negative result is increased when the patient is immunosuppressed. The CDC does not recommend the routine use of anergy panels to determine if a patient's T-cell immune system reacts to common antigens.[16,20]

Criteria for interpretation are listed in Table 75–1.[14]

The "booster effect" occurs in patients who do not respond to an initial skin test but show a positive reaction if retested 1 to 3 weeks later.[14,20] In order to reduce the likelihood that a boosted reaction is misinterpreted as a new infection, the two-step method is recommended at the time of initial testing for individuals such as health care workers or nursing home residents who may be tested periodically. If the first PPD skin test is negative, repeat the test in 1 to 3 weeks. If the second test is positive, it is most likely a boosted reaction, and the person should be classified as previously infected.

Newer Diagnostic Tests

Newer technology has led to the development of blood tests or interferon-γ release assays (IGRAs) that may replace the PPD test.[20] These methods measure the release of interferon-γ in blood in response to TB antigens. The sensitivity of IGRAs ranges from 80% to 90%, and specificity of 95% for diagnosis of latent TB. The IGRAs do not cause the booster phenomenon and are unaffected by BCG, or infection by most nontuberculosis mycobacteria. Results of the IGRAs are available in less than 24 hours, versus the 3 days required for the traditional PPD skin test. Data are limited for use of IGRAs in children younger than 5 years of age, persons recently exposed to TB, health care workers, and immunodeficient patients.[20] **KEY CONCEPT** *The CDC has endorsed the use of IGRA tests in all circumstances where the PPD is used.* IGRAs are approved for the diagnosis of LTBI in HIV-infected patients, but sensitivity is diminished.[20] *IGRAs are preferred for testing patients who have received BCG and in patients who have poor rates of return for PPD skin test reading.* Testing with both PPD and IGRA generally is not recommended, but may be useful in certain situations (eg, if the initial PPD test is negative and the risk for infection, clinical suspicion, or the

Table 75–1

Criteria for Tuberculin Positivity, by Risk Group

Reaction ≥ 5 mm of Induration	Reaction ≥ 10 mm of Induration	Reaction ≥ 15 mm of Induration
HIV-infected persons	Recent immigrants (ie, within the last 5 years) from high-prevalence countries	Persons with no risk factors for TB
A recent contact of a person with TB disease	Injection drug users	
Fibrotic changes on chest radiograph consistent with prior TB	Residents and employees[a] of the following high-risk congregate settings: prisons and jails, nursing homes and other long-term facilities for the elderly, hospitals and other health care facilities, residential facilities for patients with AIDS, and homeless shelters	
Patients with organ transplants and other immunosuppressed patients (receiving the equivalent of 15 mg/day or more of prednisone for 1 month or longer, taking TNF-α antagonists)[b]	Mycobacteriology laboratory personnel, persons with the following clinical conditions that place them at high risk: silicosis, diabetes mellitus, chronic renal failure, some hematologic disorders, other specific malignancies, gastrectomy, and jejunoileal bypass	
	Children younger than 4 years of age or infants, children, and adolescents exposed to adults at high risk	

[a]For persons who are otherwise at low risk and are tested at the start of employment, a reaction of 15 mm or more of induration is considered positive.

[b]Risk of TB in patients treated with corticosteroids increases with higher dose and longer duration.

risk for poor outcome is high; or if the initial PPD test is positive and additional evidence of infection is required; or the patient has a low risk of infection or progression).[20,21] IGRAs, and for that matter the PPD, should not be used to rule in or rule out the diagnosis of active TB disease.[21]

TREATMENT

General Approaches to Treatment

The primary treatment approach is the use of antimicrobials active against *M. tuberculosis*. Monotherapy can be used only for patients with LTBI, as evidenced by a positive skin test or positive IGRA in the absence of signs or symptoms of disease. Once active disease is present, typically *three or four drugs* must be used simultaneously from the outset of treatment.[4,13,20,16] The shortest duration of treatment is 4 months in the unusual case of smear and culture negative clinical cases of pulmonary TB, and up to 2 years of treatment may be necessary for advanced cases of Multidrug-resistant tuberculosis (MDR-TB).[20,22] **Directly observed treatment** (DOT) is a method used to ensure adherence in which patients are directly observed by a health care worker while taking their antituberculosis medication.[23] This also is a cost-effective way to ensure completion of treatment.

Desired Outcomes

Steps should be taken to (a) prevent the spread of TB (respiratory isolation); (b) find where TB has already spread (contact investigation); and (c) return the patient to a state of normal weight and well-being. Items (a) and (b) are performed by public health departments. Clinicians involved in the treatment of TB should verify that the local health department has been notified of all new cases of TB. In rare instances, surgery may be needed.[16]

Pharmacologic Therapy

▸ Treating LTBI

KEY CONCEPT *Isoniazid is used for treating LTBI. Typically, isoniazid 300 mg daily (5–10 mg/kg of body weight) is given alone for 9 months. Lower doses usually are less effective.*[16] *In some instances, a 6 month duration of treatment with isoniazid alone is an acceptable alternative. Pyridoxine (25–50 mg/day in adults) can reduce the risk of peripheral neuropathy.*[16,24] Treatment of LTBI reduces a person's lifetime risk of active TB from about 10% to about 1%.[16,24] Rifampin 600 mg daily for 4 months can be used when isoniazid resistance is suspected or when the patient cannot tolerate isoniazid.[16,24] Rifabutin 300 mg daily might be substituted for rifampin in patients at high risk of drug interactions.[25] The combination of pyrazinamide and rifampin is no longer recommended.[25,26] Once-weekly doses of isoniazid 900 mg and rifapentine 900 mg given as DOT for 3 months are as effective as 9 months of self-administered isoniazid 300 mg daily.[27] When resistance to isoniazid and rifampin is suspected, there is no regimen proven to be effective (Table 75–2).[24] Note that patients with LTBI are not infectious and there is no isolate on which to perform susceptibility testing. Susceptibility patterns must be inferred based on the most likely source of infection.

▸ Treating Active Disease

In the United States, TB patients can receive free treatment through the local health department. Treating active TB disease requires combination chemotherapy. KEY CONCEPT *Generally, four drugs are started. In particular, isoniazid and rifampin should be included because they are the best drugs available for preventing drug resistance.*[16,24] *Drug susceptibility testing should be done on the initial isolate for all patients.*[16,24] Susceptibility testing is repeated if the patient remains culture-positive 8 weeks or more into therapy.[22]

The standard TB treatment regimen for susceptible TB is isoniazid, rifampin, pyrazinamide, and ethambutol for 2 months, followed by isoniazid and rifampin for 4 months, for a total of 6 months of treatment.[16,24] *Extending treatment to 9 months of isoniazid and rifampin treatment is recommended for patients at greater risk of failure and relapse, including those with cavitary lesions on initial chest radiograph and positive cultures at the completion of the initial 2-month phase of treatment, as well as for patients treated initially without pyrazinamide. Ideally, treatment should be continued for at least 6 months from the time*

Patient Encounter, Part 2

VS: BP 142/82, P 90 beats/min, RR 18 breaths/min, T 38°C (100.4°F), O_2 sat 82% (0.82) on room air, Wt 51 kg (112 lb), Ht 5′8″ (173 cm)

HEENT: PERRLA; EOMI

Neck: Supple; no lymphadenopathy, bruits, or JVD; no thyromegaly

Chest: Diffuse rhonchi, decreased breath sounds on left

CV: RRR; no murmurs, rubs, gallops

Abd: (+) BS; nontender, nondistended

Neuro: A&O × 3

Laboratory Values (US Units)

Lab	Normal	Lab	Normal
Na 139 mEq/L	135–145 mEq/L	Hgb 13.5 g/dL	13.5–17.5 g/dL
K 3.9 mEq/L	3.5–5 mEq/L	Hct 40%	40%–54%
Cl 98 mEq/L	95–105 mEq/L	RBC 4.6 × 10^6 mm^3	4.6–6.0 × 10^6 mm^3
CO_2 38 mEq/L	22–30 mEq/L	WBC 4.0 × 10^3 mm^3	4.0–10 × 10^3 mm^3
BUN 20 mg/dL	5–25 mg/dL	PMN 51%	50%–65%
SCr 1.0 mg/dL	0.8–1.3 mg/dL	Lymph 25%	25%–35%
Gluc 150 mg/dL	< 140 mg/dL	Mono 2%	2%–6%
AST 36 IU/L	5–40 IU/L		
ALT 28 IU/L	5–35 IU/L		
Tbili 1 mg/dL	0.1–1.2 mg/dL		
PT 10 seconds	10–12 seconds		

Laboratory Values (SI Units)

Lab	Normal	Lab	Normal
Na 139 mmol/L	135–145 mmol/L	Hgb 135 g/L or 8.38 mmol/L	135–175 g/L or 8.38–10.86 mmol/L
K 3.9 mmol/L	3.5–5 mmol/L	Hct 0.40 vol fraction	0.40–0.54 vol fraction
Cl 98 mmol/L	95–105 mmol/L	RBC 4.6 × 10^{12}/L	4.6–6.0 × 10^{12}/L
CO_2 38 mmol/L	22–30 mmol/L	WBC 4.0 × 10^9/L	4.0–10.0 × 10^9/L
BUN 7.1 mmol/L	1.8–8.9 mmol/L	PMN 0.51	0.50–0.65
SCr 88 μmol/L	71–115 μmol/L	Lymph 0.25	0.25–0.35
Gluc 8.3 mmol/L	< 7.8 mmol/L	Mono 0.02	0.02–0.06
AST 0.60 μkat/L	0.08–0.67 μkat/L		
ALT 0.47 μkat/L	0.08–0.58 μkat/L		
Tbili 17.1 μmol/L	1.7–20.5 μmol/L		
PT 10 seconds	10–12 seconds		

CXR: Bilateral upper lobe infiltrates with cavitary lesions on left; small left pneumothorax

Clinical Course: The patient was admitted and placed on respiratory isolation. Three separate sputum AFB stain specimens were reported to contain 3+ AFB. IFN-γ was sent and a PPD tuberculin skin test was placed. Sputum samples were sent for AFB, fungi, and bacterial cultures and sensitivities. After 48 hours, the PPD skin test was read as a 7-mm area of induration

Assessment: Active pulmonary TB; pneumothorax; hypertension; type 2 diabetes mellitus; rheumatoid arthritis

Which signs, symptoms, and other findings are consistent with active TB infection?

that patients convert to a negative culture.[16,24] When the patients' sputum smears convert to negative, the risk of infecting others is greatly reduced, but it is not zero.[10,24] Such patients can be removed from respiratory isolation if they are responding clinically. The decision to discontinue isolation should be done by medical providers experienced in TB control. Table 75–3 shows the recommended treatment regimens. When intermittent therapy is used, DOT is essential. Doses missed during an intermittent TB regimen decrease the efficacy of the regimen and increase the relapse rate.

Adjustments to the regimen should be based upon susceptibility data.[8,24] Drug resistance should be suspected in patients who have been treated previously for TB. If adjustments are needed, two or more drugs with in vitro activity against the patient's isolate and that were not used previously should be added to the regimen.[8,24] When isoniazid and rifampin cannot be used, either because of drug resistance or intolerance, treatment durations typically become 2 years or more, regardless of immune status.[8,24,30] TB specialists should be consulted regarding cases of drug-resistant TB, or whenever treatment is uncertain.[8,24] Therapeutic drug monitoring (TDM) can direct dosing for such patients. One of the proven reasons for treatment failure is malabsorption of orally administered drugs.[24,28,29] KEY CONCEPT *Due to the risk of further drug resistance, it is critical to avoid adding only a single drug to a failing regimen.*[8,24]

Table 75–2

Recommended Drug Regimens for Treatment of LTBI in Adults

Drug	Interval and Duration	Comments	Rating[a] HIV–	Evidence HIV+
Isoniazid	Daily for 9 months[c,d]	In HIV-infected patients, isoniazid may be administered concurrently with nucleoside reverse transcriptase inhibitors (NRTIs), protease inhibitors, or non-NRTIs (NNRTIs) Preferred regimen in children 2–11 years	A (II)	A (II)
	Twice weekly for 9 months[c,d]	Directly observed treatment (DOT) must be used with twice-weekly dosing	B (II)	B (II)
Isoniazid and Rifapentine	Once weekly	Equal alternative to 9 months of daily isoniazid for otherwise healthy patients age > 12 years DOT is recommended Not recommended for children < 2 years HIV-infected patients taking antiretroviral therapy, presumed resistance, pregnant women or women expecting to become pregnant during the treatment period	B(I)	B(I)
Isoniazid	Daily for 6 months[d]	Not indicated for HIV-infected persons, those with fibrotic lesions on chest radiographs, or children	B (I)	C (I)
	Twice weekly for 6 months[d]	DOT must be used with twice-weekly dosing	B (II)	C (I)
Rifampin	Daily for 4 months	For persons who are contacts of patients with isoniazid-resistant rifampin-susceptible TB In HIV-infected patients, protease inhibitors or NNRTIs generally should not be administered concurrently with rifampin; rifabutin can be used as an alternative for patients treated with indinavir, nelfinavir, amprenavir, ritonavir, or efavirenz, and possibly with nevirapine or soft-gel saquinavir[e]	B (II)	B (III)

[a]Strength of recommendation: A = preferred; B = acceptable alternative; C = offer when A and B cannot be given.

[b]Quality of evidence: I = randomized clinical trial data; II = data from clinical trials that are not randomized or were conducted in other populations; III = expert opinion.

[c]Recommended regimen for children younger than 18 years.

[d]Recommended regimens for pregnant women. Pyrazinamide should be avoided during the first trimester.

[e]Rifabutin should not be used with hard-gel saquinavir or delavirdine. When used with other protease inhibitors or NNRTIs, dose adjustment of rifabutin may be required.

Special Populations

Treatment for extrapulmonary TB is the same as for pulmonary disease. Patients with CNS TB usually are treated for 12 months.[8,24] Isoniazid and pyrazinamide cross the blood–brain barrier well, but rifampin, ethambutol, and streptomycin can penetrate inflamed meninges. TB osteomyelitis typically is treated for 9 months, occasionally with surgical débridement.[8,24] TB of the soft tissues can be treated with conventional regimens.[8,24] Patients with diabetes mellitus have been shown to have low 2-hour peak serum concentrations of antimicrobials. TDM can be considered to optimize treatment response.[30] TB in children may be treated with regimens similar to those used in adults, although some physicians extend treatment to 9 months.[8,14,15,16,24] Pediatric doses of isoniazid and rifampin on a milligram per kilogram basis are higher than those used in adults (Table 75–4).[24]

Pregnant women receive the usual treatment of isoniazid, rifampin, and ethambutol for 9 months.[24] Pyrazinamide has not been studied in large numbers of pregnant women, but anecdotal data suggest that it may be safe.[24,31] The clinician should always determine risk versus benefit and determine if a drug is safe to administer in pregnancy.

▶ *Human Immunodeficiency Virus*

HIV-infected adults may receive a 6-month regimen of phase of isoniazid, a rifamycin, pyrazinamide, and ethambutol for the first 2 months followed by isoniazid and a rifamycin for 4 months.[8,24,32] *Some clinicians recommend extending treatment to 9 months. Rifabutin is used to reduce drug interactions with protease inhibitors and some non-nucleoside reverse transcriptase inhibitors.* Integrated antiretroviral therapy (ART) is superior to sequential ART in the treatment of naïve HIV seropositive patients with TB.[33] The optimal timing of integrated HIV and TB therapy is influenced by the patient's immune status.[33] It is recommended to start integrated ART therapy 2 to 12 weeks after initiating anti-TB therapy.[31] TB-HIV experts should manage such patients. Highly intermittent regimens (twice or once weekly) are not recommended for HIV-positive TB patients.[24,32] Some patients with AIDS malabsorb their oral medications, and drug interactions are common, so TDM can be useful.[24,28,29]

Table 75–3

Drug Regimens for Culture-Positive Pulmonary Tuberculosis Caused by Drug-Susceptible Organisms

Initial Phase			Continuation Phase		
Regimen	**Drugs**	**Interval and Doses[a] (Minimal Duration)**	**Drugs**	**Interval and Doses[a,b] (Minimal Duration)**	**Range of total doses (minimum duration)**
1	Isoniazid Rifampin Pyrazinamide Ethambutol	7 days per week for 56 doses (8 weeks) or 5 doses per week for 40 doses (8 weeks)[c]	Isoniazid/Rifampin Isoniazid/Rifampin Isoniazid/Rifapentine	7 days per week for 126 doses (18 weeks) or 5 days per week for 90 doses (18 weeks)[c] Twice weekly for 36 doses (18 weeks)[d] Once weekly for 18 doses (18 weeks)[e]	182–130 (26 weeks) 92–76 (26 weeks)[d] 74–58 (26 weeks)
2	Isoniazid Rifampin Pyrazinamide Ethambutol	7 days per week for 14 doses (2 weeks)[c], *then* twice weekly for 12 doses (6 weeks) or 5 days per week for 10 doses (2 weeks), *then* twice weekly for 12 doses (6 weeks)	Isoniazid/Rifampin Isoniazid/Rifapentine	Twice weekly for 36 doses (18 weeks)[d] Once weekly for 18 doses (18 weeks)[e]	62–58 (26 weeks) 44–40 (26 weeks)
3	Isoniazid Rifampin Pyrazinamide Ethambutol	three times weekly for 24 doses (8 weeks)	Isoniazid/Rifampin	Three times weekly for 54 doses (18 weeks)	78 (26 weeks)
4	Isoniazid Rifampin Ethambutol	7 days per week for 56 doses (8 weeks) or 5 days per week for 40 doses (8 weeks)[c]	Isoniazid/Rifampin	7 days per week for 217 doses (31 weeks) or 5 days per week for 155 doses (31 weeks)[c]	273–195 (39 weeks)
			Isoniazid/Rifampin	Twice weekly for 62 doses (31 weeks)	118–102 (39 weeks)

[a]When DOT is used, drugs may be given 5 days per week and the necessary umber of doses adjusted accordingly. Although there are no studies that compare five with seven daily doses. Extensive experience indicates this would be an effective practice.

[b]Patients with cavitation on initial chest radiograph and positive cultures at completion of 2 months of therapy should receive 7-month continuation phase

[c]Five days a week administration is always given by DOT.

[d]Not recommended for HIV infected patients with CD4 counts < 100 cells/μl (100 × 10^6/L).

[e]Once weekly options with rifapentine should be used only in HIV negative patients who have negative sputum smears at the time of completion of 2 months of therapy and who do not have cavitation on initial chest radiograph. For patients started on this regimen and found to have a positive culture form the 2-month specimen, treatment should be extended an extra 3 months. Centers for Disease Control and Prevention. Treatment of Tuberculosis, American Thoracic Society, CDC, and Infectious Diseases Society of America. MMWR 2003;52(No. RR-11):[inclusive page numbers].

For complete recommendations on management of TB and HIV visit the CDC website: www.cdc.gov/tb/publications/guidelines/HIV_AIDS.htm.

▶ *Multidrug-Resistant TB*

If drug-resistant TB is suspected, the empiric regimen should be modified based on patterns of suspected resistance. Once susceptibilities are confirmed, regimens can be modified appropriately. Patients with MDR-TB are at high risk of failure and should be treated by specialists or centers with experience treating drug resistant TB.

▶ *Renal Failure*

Isoniazid and rifampin usually do not require dose modification in renal failure.[27,34] Pyrazinamide and ethambutol typically are reduced to three times weekly to avoid accumulation of the parent drug (ethambutol) or metabolites (pyrazinamide).[28,29] Renally cleared TB drugs include the aminoglycosides, ethambutol, cycloserine, and levofloxacin.[28,29] With renal impairment, dosing intervals need to be extended for these drugs. TB drugs should be administered after hemodialysis; three times weekly regimens may be more convenient. Serum concentration monitoring should be performed for cycloserine and ethambutol to avoid dose-related toxicities in renal failure patients.[29,34,35]

Patient Encounter, Part 3

Based on the information provided, what are the goals of therapy for this patient?

Select and recommend a therapeutic plan for treatment of this patient's TB infection. What drugs, dose, schedule, and duration of therapy are best for this patient?

Who else should be tested? How should any contacts infected by this patient be evaluated and treated?

Table 75–4

Antituberculosis Drugs for Adults and Children

Drug	Daily Doses[a,b,c]	Adverse Effects	Monitoring
Isoniazid	*Adults*: 5 mg/kg (300 mg) *Children*: 10–15 mg/kg (300 mg)	Asymptomatic elevation of aminotransferases, clinical hepatitis, fatal hepatitis, peripheral neurotoxicity, CNS system effects, lupus-like syndrome, hypersensitivity, monoamine poisoning, diarrhea	LFT monthly in patients who have preexisting liver disease or who develop abnormal liver function that does not require discontinuation of drug Dosage adjustments may be necessary in patients receiving anticonvulsants or warfarin
Rifampin[d]	*Adults*: 10 mg/kg (600 mg) *Children*: 10–20 mg/kg (600 mg)	Cutaneous reactions, GI reactions (nausea, anorexia, abdominal pain), flu-like syndrome, hepatotoxicity, severe immunologic reactions, orange discoloration of bodily fluids (sputum, urine, sweat, tears), drug interactions owing to induction of hepatic microsomal enzymes	Rifampin causes many drug interactions. For a complete list of drug interactions and effects, refer to CDC website: www.cdc.gov/nchstp/tb/tb
Rifabutin[d]	*Adults*: 5 mg/kg (300 mg) *Children*: Appropriate dosing unknown	Hematologic toxicity, uveitis, GI symptoms, polyarthralgias, hepatotoxicity, pseudojaundice (skin discoloration with normal bilirubin), rash, flu-like syndrome, orange discoloration of bodily fluids (sputum, urine, sweat, tears)	Drug interactions are less problematic than rifampin
Rifapentine[d]	*Adults*: 10 mg/kg (continuation phase) (600 mg) dosed weekly *Children*: The drug is not approved for use in children	Similar to those associated with rifampin	Drug interactions are being investigated and are likely similar to rifampin
Pyrazinamide	*Adults*: Based on IBW: 40–55 kg: 1000 mg; 56–75 kg: 1500 mg; 76–90 kg: 2000 mg *Children*: 15–30 mg/kg	Hepatotoxicity, GI symptoms (nausea, vomiting), nongouty polyarthralgia, asymptomatic hyperuricemia, acute gouty arthritis, transient morbilliform rash, dermatitis	Serum uric acid can serve as a surrogate marker for compliance LFTs in patients with underlying liver disease
Ethambutol[e]	*Adults*: Based on IBW: 40–55 kg: 800 mg; 56–75 kg: 1200 mg; 76–90 kg: 1600 mg *Children*[c]: 15–20 mg/kg daily	Retrobulbar neuritis, peripheral neuritis, cutaneous reactions	Baseline visual acuity testing and testing of color discrimination Monthly testing of visual acuity and color discrimination in patients taking > 15–20 mg/kg, renal insufficiency, or receiving the drug for > 2 months
Cycloserine[f]	*Adults*: 10–15 mg/kg/day, usually 500–750 mg/day in two doses *Children*: 10–15 mg/kg/day	CNS effects	Monthly assessments of neuropsychiatric status Serum concentration may be necessary until appropriate dose is established
Ethionamide[g]	*Adults*: 15–20 mg/kg/day, usually 500–750 mg/day in a single daily dose or two divided doses *Children*: 15–20 mg/kg/day	GI effects, hepatotoxicity, neurotoxicity, endocrine effects	Baseline LFTs Monthly LFTs if underlying liver disease is present TSH at baseline and monthly intervals
Streptomycin	*Adults*[h] *Children*: 20–40 mg/kg/day	Ototoxicity, neurotoxicity, nephrotoxicity	Baseline audiogram, vestibular testing, Romberg testing and SCr Monthly assessments of renal function and auditory or vestibular symptoms
Amikacin/ kanamycin	*Adults*[h] *Children*: 15–30 mg/kg/day IV or intramuscular as a single daily dose	Ototoxicity, nephrotoxicity	Baseline audiogram, vestibular testing, Romberg testing and SCr Monthly assessments of renal function and auditory or vestibular symptoms
Capreomycin	*Adults*[h] *Children*: 15–30 mg/kg/day as a single daily dose	Nephrotoxicity, ototoxicity	Baseline audiogram, vestibular testing, Romberg testing and SCr Monthly assessments of renal function and auditory or vestibular symptoms Baseline and monthly serum K^+ and Mg^{2+}

(Continued)

Table 75–4

Antituberculosis Drugs for Adults and Children (*Continued*)

Drug	Daily Doses[a,b,c]	Adverse Effects	Monitoring
p-Aminosalicylic acid (PAS)	*Adults*: 8–12 g/day in two or three doses *Children*: 200–300 mg/kg/day in two to four divided doses	Hepatotoxicity, GI distress, malabsorption syndrome, hypothyroidism, coagulopathy	Baseline LFTs and TSH TSH every 3 months
Levofloxacin	Adults: 500–1000 mg daily *Children*[i]: Not recommended	GI disturbance, neurologic effects	No specific monitoring recommended
Moxifloxacin	*Adults*: 400 mg daily *Children*[j]: Not recommended		
Bedaquiline	*Adults:* Weeks 1–2: 400 mg daily Weeks 3–24: 200 mg three times weekly *Children:* Not recommended	GI disturbances, dizziness, headache, rash, arthralgia	Serum K, Ca, Mg ECG at baseline, weeks 2, 12, 24 Weekly ECG for persons taking other QTc prolonging drugs, history of arrhythmias, hypothyroidism, uncompensated heart failure, or have serum K, Ca or Mg below normal limits

[a]Dose per weight is based on ideal body weight. Children weighing more than 40 kg should be dosed as adults.

[b]For purposes of this document adult dosing begins at age 15 years.

[c]The authors of this chapter do not agree with the use of maximum doses, since this arbitrarily caps doses for patients who otherwise might need larger doses. These maximum doses were not based on prospective studies in large or overweight individuals, and do not consider patients with documented malabsorption of their medications. Clinical judgment should be used in such circumstances.

[d]Higher doses of rifampin and rifapentine are being studied. Rifabutin dose may need to be adjusted when there is concomitant use of protease inhibitors or nonnucleoside reverse transcriptase inhibitors.

[e]The drug can likely be used safely in older children but should be used with caution in children less than 5 years of age, in whom visual acuity cannot be monitored. In younger children, ethambutol at the dose of 15 mg/kg/day can be used if there is suspected or proven resistance to isoniazid or rifampin.

[f]It should be noted that, although this is the dose recommended generally, most clinicians with experience using cycloserine indicate that it is unusual for patients to be able to tolerate this amount. Serum concentration measurements are often useful in determining the optimal dose for a given patient.

[g]The single daily dose can be given at bedtime or with the main meal.

[h]Dose: 15 mg/kg/day (1 g), and 10 mg/kg in persons older than 59 years of age (750 mg). Usual dose: 750–1000 mg administered intramuscularly or intravenously, given as a single dose 5–7 days/week and reduced to two or three times per week after the first 2 to 4 months or after culture conversion, depending on the efficacy of the other drugs in the regimen.

[i]The long-term (more than several weeks) use of levofloxacin in children and adolescents has not been approved because of concerns about effects on bone and cartilage growth. However, most experts agree that the drug should be considered for children with tuberculosis caused by organisms resistant to both isoniazid and rifampin. The optimal dose is not known.

[j]The long-term (more than several weeks) use of moxifloxacin in children and adolescents has not been approved because of concerns about effects on bone and cartilage growth. The optimal dose is not known.

Data from Centers for Disease Control and Prevention. Treatment of tuberculosis. MMWR 2003;52 (RR-11).

▶ *Hepatic Failure*

Hepatically cleared TB drugs include isoniazid, rifampin, pyrazinamide, ethionamide, and *p*-aminosalicylic acid.[22] Ciprofloxacin and moxifloxacin are about 50% cleared by the liver. Isoniazid, rifampin, pyrazinamide, and to a lesser degree ethionamide, *p*-aminosalicylic acid, and rarely ethambutol may cause hepatotoxicity.[26,28,] These patients require close monitoring, and serum concentration monitoring may be the most accurate way to dose them.[29]

TB Drugs

Detailed information regarding TB drugs can be accessed at the following references.[22,24,28,29] A summary is provided in Table 75–4.[23] Isoniazid, rifampin, and pyrazinamide are the key drugs. Other drugs are used in selected circumstances. Quinolones eventually may be used as first-line drugs, but currently are not.[36,37] In 2012, the Food and Drug Administration approved bedaquiline for the treatment of MDR-TB.[38] It should be used with three or more drugs that are active against the patient's isolate. Bedaquiline carries a black-box warning due to prolongation of QTc interval. Baseline and follow-up electrocardiograms are recommended. Other new therapies include investigational vaccines, and investigational drugs such as PA-824, OPC-67683, and SQ109, which are in clinical trials.[39]

OUTCOME EVALUATION

● *Effectiveness of TB therapy is determined by AFB smears and cultures. Send sputum samples for AFB staining and microscopic examination (sputum smears) every 1 to 2 weeks until two consecutive smears are negative. This provides early evidence of a response to treatment.*[24] *Once on maintenance therapy,* sputum cultures *can be performed monthly until two consecutive cultures are negative, which generally occurs over 2 to 3 months. If sputum cultures continue to be positive after 2 months, repeat drug susceptibility testing and check serum concentrations of the drugs.*

KEY CONCEPT *The most serious problem with TB therapy is patient nonadherence.*[24,40] *There is no reliable way to identify such patients a priori, therefore DOT should be used.*[8,24,40] DOT also provides increased opportunities to observe the patient for any apparent toxicities, thus improving overall care.[40]

Check serum chemistries, including blood urea nitrogen (BUN), creatinine, aspartate transaminase (AST), and alanine transaminase (ALT) and a complete blood count with platelets at baseline and periodically thereafter depending on the presence of other factors that may increase the likelihood of toxicity (eg, advanced age, alcohol abuse, pregnancy).[24] Suspect hepatotoxicity in patients whose transaminases exceed five times the upper limit of normal (ULN) or whose total bilirubin exceeds 3 mg/dL (51 μmol/L), and in patients with symptoms such as nausea, vomiting, and jaundice with liver enzyme elevations of more than three times ULN. At this point, discontinue the offending agents. Typically, all TB drugs are stopped, followed by the sequential reintroduction of the drugs, along with frequent testing of liver enzymes. This usually is successful in identifying the offending agent; other agents may be continued (see Table 75–4).[24]

Therapeutic Drug Monitoring

TDM is the use of serum drug concentrations to optimize therapy.[24,28,29] Patients with uncomplicated, drug-susceptible TB generally do well. Pharmacokinetic variability of anti-TB drugs can contribute to poor outcomes despite adherence. TDM can be used to shorten the time to response and to treatment completion. The evidence to support the use of TDM in the treatment of TB is growing.[29] *TDM can assist in patients failing appropriate DOT (no clinical improvement after 2 to 4 weeks or smear-positive after 4 to 6 weeks). Patients with AIDS, diabetes, and various GI disorders often fail to absorb these drugs properly and also are candidates for TDM. Drug levels in patients with hepatic or renal disease should be monitored, given their potential for toxicities. In the treatment of MDR-TB, TDM may be particularly useful.*[22] *Finally, TDM of the TB and HIV drugs is perhaps the most logical way to untangle the complex drug interactions that take place.*

For a complete list of drug interactions, visit the CDC website: www.cdc.gov/tb/publications/guidelines/TB_HIV_DRUGS/default.htm.[41] In particular, interactions between the rifamycins (eg, rifampin, rifapentine, rifabutin) and the HIV protease inhibitors and non-nucleoside reverse transcriptase inhibitors are common and require dose and frequency modifications in many cases. Because these are constantly being updated, the preceding link is an excellent way to keep current.

Patient Encounter, Part 4

Based on the information provided, which clinical and laboratory parameters should be monitored in this patient to determine efficacy and avoid toxicity?

Is this patient a candidate for therapeutic drug monitoring? Why or why not?

Patient Care Process

- Rapidly identify a new TB case.
- Assess the patient's risk factors and signs and symptoms to determine whether the patient might be infected with TB.
- Isolate the patient with active disease to prevent the spread of the disease.
- Collect appropriate samples for smears and cultures.

Therapy Evaluation:

- Obtain a thorough medication history.
- Select and recommend appropriate antituberculosis treatment. Consider HIV status, type of TB infection, renal function, liver function, etc.

Care Plan Development:

- Ensure adherence to the treatment regimen by the patient.
- Obtain AFB stains to evaluate the effectiveness of treatment.
- Consider TDM if no clinical improvement.

Follow-up Evaluation:

- Continue treatment for at least 6 months from the time that the patient converts to a negative culture.
- Identify the index case that infected the patient, identify of all persons infected by both the index case and the new case of TB, and the complete of appropriate treatments for those individuals.

Abbreviations Introduced in This Chapter

AFB	Acid-fast bacillus
AIDS	Acquired immunodeficiency syndrome
ALT	Alanine transaminase
ART	antiretroviral therapy
AST	Aspartate transaminase
BCG	Bacille Calmette-Guérin
CDC	Centers for Disease Control and Prevention
CNS	Central nervous system
DOT	Directly observed therapy
HIV	Human immunodeficiency virus
HTN	Hypertension
IGRA	Interferon-γ release assay
INF	Interferon
LTBI	Latent tuberculosis infection
MDR-TB	Multidrug-resistant tuberculosis
MGIT	Mycobacterial growth indicator tube
NIDDM	Noninsulin-dependent diabetes mellitus
PCR	Polymerase chain reaction
PPD	Purified protein derivative
RFLP	Restriction fragment length polymorphism
TB	Tuberculosis
TDM	Therapeutic drug monitoring
ULN	Upper limit of normal
WBC	White blood cell

REFERENCES

1. World Health Organization Report on the Global Tuberculosis 2013 [online]. [cited 2013 Sept 25]. http://www.who.int/tb/publications/global_report/en/. Accessed September 2013.
2. Centers for Disease Control and Prevention. Trends in tuberculosis - United States, 2013. MMWR Morb Mortal Wkly Rep. 2014;63:229–233.
3. Centers for Disease Control and Prevention. Reported tuberculosis in the United States, 2012. Atlanta, GA: U.S. Department of Health and Human Services. MMWR Morb Mortal Wkly Rep. 2013;62(11):201–205.
4. Fitzgerald DW, Sterling TR, Haas DW. Mycobacterium tuberculosis. In: Mandell GL, Bennett JE, Dolin R, eds. Principles and Practice of Infectious Diseases. 7th ed. New York: Churchill Livingstone; 2009:3129–3165.
5. Heifets L. Mycobacteriology laboratory. Clin Chest Med. 1997;18:35–53.
6. Heifets LB. Drug susceptibility tests in the management of chemotherapy of tuberculosis. In: Heifets LB, ed. Drug Susceptibility in the Chemotherapy of Mycobacterial Infections. Boca Raton, FL: CRC Press; 1991:89–122.
7. Issa R, Mohd Hassan NA, Abdul H, et al. Detection and discrimination of Mycobacterium tuberculosis complex. Diagn Microbiol Infect Dis. 2012;72:62–67.
8. Kiraz N, Sglik I, Kiremitci A, et al. Evaluation of the genotype mycobacteria direct assay for direct detection of the Mycobacterium tuberculosis complex obtained from sputum samples. J Med Microbiol. 2010;59:930–934.
9. Hillemann D, Weizenegger M, Kubica T, et al. Use of the genotype MTBDR assay for rapid detection of rifampin and isoniazid resistance in Mycobacterium tuberculosis complex isolates. J Clin Microbiol. 2005;43:3699–3703.
10. Marlowe EM, Novack-Weekley SM, Cumpio J, et al. Evaluation of the Cepheid Xpert MTB/RIF assay for direct detection of Mycobacterium tuberculosis complex in respiratory specimens. J Clin Microbiol. 2011;49:1621–1623.
11. Martin A, Panaiotov S, Portaels F, et al. The nitrate reductase assay for the rapid detection of isoniazid and rifampicin resistance in Mycobacterium tuberculosis: A systematic review and meta-analysis. J Antimicrob Chemother. 2008;62(1):56–64.
12. Guide to the application of genotyping to tuberculosis prevention and control. CDC; 2004 [cited 2014 Sept 25]. http://www.cdc.gov/tb/programs/genotyping/manual.htm
13. Woolwine SC, Bishai WR. Pathogenesis of tuberculosis from a cellular and molecular perspective. In: Reichman LB, Hershfield ES. Tuberculosis. A Comprehensive International Approach. 3rd ed. New York: Marcel Dekker; 2006:101–17.
14. American Thoracic Society/Centers for Disease Control and Prevention. Diagnostic standards and classification of tuberculosis in adults and children. Am J Respir Crit Care Med. 2000;161:1376–1395.
15. Cruz AT, Starke JR. Clinical manifestations of tuberculosis in children. Paediatr Respir Rev. 2007;8:107–117.
16. American Thoracic Society/Centers for Disease Control and Prevention. Targeted tuberculin skin testing and treatment of latent tuberculosis infection. Am J Respir Crit Care Med. 2000;161:S221–S247.
17. Kwan CK, Ernst JD. HIV and tuberculosis: A deadly human syndemic. Clin Microbiol Rev. 2011;24:351–376.
18. Zevallos M, Justman JE. Tuberculosis in elderly. Clin Geriatr Med. 2003;19:121–138.
19. Umeki S. Comparison of younger and elderly patients with pulmonary tuberculosis. Respiration. 1989;55:75–83.
20. Centers for Disease Control and Prevention. Guidelines for using Interferon Gamma Release Assays to detect Mycobacterium tuberculosis infection - United States, 2010. MMWR Recomm Rep. 2010;59(RR-5):1–25.
21. Nienhaus A, Schablon A, Diel R. Interferon-gamma release assay for the diagnosis of latent TB infection analysis of discordant results, when compared to the tuberculin skin test. PLoS One. 2008;3(7):e2665.
22. Peloquin CA. Antituberculosis drugs: Pharmacokinetics. In: Heifets LB, ed. Drug Susceptibility in the Chemotherapy of Mycobacterial Infections. Boca Raton, FL: CRC Press; 1991:59–88.
23. Fujiwara PI, Larkin C, Frieden TR. Directly observed therapy in New York City. Clin Chest Med. 1997;18:135–148.
24. American Thoracic Society/Centers for Disease Control/Infectious Disease Society of America. Treatment of tuberculosis. Am J Respir Crit Care Med. 2003;167:603–662.
25. Volmink J, Garner P. Directly observed therapy for treating tuberculosis. Cochrane Database Syst Rev. 2007;17:CD003343.
26. Centers for Disease Control and Prevention. Update: Fatal and severe liver injuries associated with rifampin and pyrazinamide for latent tuberculosis infection, and revisions in the American Thoracic Society/CDC recommendations—United States, 2001. MMWR Morb Mortal Wkly Rep. 2001;50(34):733–735.
27. Centers for Disease Control and Prevention. Recommendations for use of an isoniazid-rifapentine regimen with observation to treat latent Mycobacterium tuberculosis. MMWR Morb Mortal Wkly Rep. 2011;60(48);1650–1653.
28. Peloquin CA. Pharmacological issues in the treatment of tuberculosis. Ann N Y Acad Sci. 2001;953:157–164.
29. Peloquin CA. Therapeutic drug monitoring in the treatment of tuberculosis. Drugs. 2014;74:839–854.
30. Heysell SK, Moore JL, Staley D, et al. Early Therapeutic Drug Monitoring for Isoniazid and Rifampin among Diabetics with Newly Diagnosed Tuberculosis in Virginia, USA. Tuberc Res Treat. 2013;2013:1–6.
31. Mnyani CN, McIntyre JA. Tuberculosis in pregnancy. BJOG: An International J Obstet Gynaecol 2010;118:226–231.
32. Centers for Disease Control and Prevention. Guidelines for prevention and treatment of opportunistic infections in HIV-infected adults and adolescents: Recommendations from CDC, the National Institutes of Health, and the HIV Medicine Association of the Infectious Diseases Society of America. MMWR Recomm Rep. 2009;58:1–207.
33. Abdool Karim SS, Naidoo K, Padayatchi N, et al. Timing of initiation of antiretroviral drugs during tuberculosis therapy. N Engl J Med. 2010; 362;697–706.
34. Malone RS, Fish DN, Spiegel DM, et al. The effect of hemodialysis on isoniazid, rifampin, pyrazinamide, and ethambutol. Am J Respir Crit Care Med. 1999;159:1580–1584.
35. Malone RS, Fish DN, Spiegel DM, et al. The effect of hemodialysis on cycloserine, ethionamide, paraminosalicylate acid, and clofazamine. Chest. 1999; 116:984–990.
36. Burman WJ. Moxifloxacin versus ethambutol in the first 2 months of treatment for pulmonary tuberculosis. Am J Respir Crit Care Med. 2006;174:331–338.
37. Conde MB, Efron A, Loredo C, et al. Moxifloxacin versus ethambutol in the initial treatment of tuberculosis: A double-blind, randomized, controlled phase II trial. Lancet. 2009;373:1183–1189.
38. Diacon AH, Pym A, Grobusch MP, et al. Multidrug-resistant tuberculosis and culture conversion with bedaquiline. N Engl J Med. 2014; 371:723–732.
39. Zhang Y. Advances in the treatment of tuberculosis. Clin Pharmacol Ther. 2007;82:595–600.
40. Volmink J, Garner P. Directly observed therapy for treating tuberculosis. Cochrane Database Syst Rev. 2009;4:CD0003343.
41. Centers for Disease Control and Prevention. Drug Interactions in the Treatment of HIV-Related Tuberculosis [online]. [cited 2014 Sept 29]. www.cdc.gov/tb/publications/guidelines/TB_HIV_Drugs/default.htm. Accessed Sept 2014.

76 Gastrointestinal Infections

Bradley W. Shinn and Sharon Ternullo

LEARNING OBJECTIVES

Upon completion of the chapter, the reader will be able to:

1. Describe the epidemiology and clinical presentation of commonly encountered gastrointestinal (GI) infections.
2. Summarize common risk factors associated with the development of a GI infection.
3. Given a patient with a GI infection, develop an individualized treatment plan.
4. Outline the impact of widespread antimicrobial resistance on current treatment recommendations for GI infections.
5. Discuss the effect of host immunosuppression on the risk of disease complications and treatment strategies associated with GI infections.
6. Educate patients on appropriate prevention measures of GI infections.
7. Describe the role of antimicrobial prophylaxis and/or vaccination for GI infections.

INTRODUCTION

One of the primary concerns related to gastrointestinal (GI) infection, regardless of the cause, is dehydration, which is the second leading cause of worldwide morbidity and mortality.[1] Dehydration is especially problematic for children younger than age 5; however, the highest rate of death in the United States occurs among the elderly.[1] KEY CONCEPT *Rehydration is the foundation of therapy for GI infections, and oral rehydration therapy (ORT) is usually preferred* (Table 76–1).[2] Single-dose oral ondansetron should be considered the first-line antiemetic in children who are dehydrated with significant vomiting.[3] In nonimmunocompromised hospitalized pediatric patients, *Lactobacillus* supplementation may reduce the length of hospitalization.[4]

In the United States, each year 31 major pathogens cause about 9 million episodes of foodborne illness, almost 56,000 hospitalizations, and 1350 deaths. Most illnesses are caused by norovirus, nontyphoidal *Salmonella* (NTS), *Clostridium perfringens*, and *Campylobacter*.[5] KEY CONCEPT *The indiscriminate use of proton-pump inhibitor (PPI) therapy leads to GI-tract bacterial colonization and increased susceptibility to enteric bacterial infections.*[6]

BACTERIAL INFECTIONS

SHIGELLOSIS

Epidemiology

Shigella causes bacillary dysentery, which refers to diarrheal stool containing pus and blood. Worldwide, there are an estimated 165 million annual cases of shigellosis, with 1 million associated deaths, and approximately 450,000 infections each year in the United States, which results in more than 6000 hospitalizations.[7] Shigellosis usually affects children 6 months to 10 years of age. In the United States, shigellosis is a serious problem in daycare centers and in areas with crowded living conditions or poor sanitation. Most cases of shigellosis are transmitted through the fecal–oral route. Activities that may lead to shigellosis include handling toddlers' diapers, ingesting pool water, or consuming vegetables from a sewage-contaminated field. *Shigella* transmission from contaminated food and water, although less common, is associated with large outbreaks.

Pathogenesis

Shigella organisms are nonmotile, nonlactose-fermenting, gram-negative rods and are members of the Enterobacteriaceae family. *S. sonnei* (serogroup D) is responsible for most shigellosis cases in the United States. Infection with Shigella occurs after ingestion of as few as 10 to 100 organisms, which may explain the ease of person-to-person spread. Symptoms develop in about 3 days (range, 1–7) after contracting the bacteria.[8]

Shigella strains invade intestinal epithelial cells, with subsequent multiplication, inflammation, and destruction. This organism only rarely invades the bloodstream; but, bacteremia can occur in malnourished children and immunocompromised patients and is associated with a mortality rate as high as 20%.[9]

Treatment and Monitoring

Although infection with *Shigella* is generally self-limited and responds to supportive care, antibiotic therapy is indicated because it shortens the duration of illness and reduces the risk of transmission.[10] Several antimicrobial agents are available for the treatment of shigellosis, although options are increasingly limited due to globally emerging drug resistance. If antimicrobial susceptibility results are not available, the recommended

Table 76–1

Clinical Assessment of Degree of Dehydration in Children Based on Percentage of Body Weight Loss

Variable	Mild (3%–5%)	Moderate (6%–9%)	Severe (10% or More)
Blood pressure	Normal	Normal	Normal to reduced
Quality of pulses	Normal	Normal to slightly decreased	Moderately decreased
Heart rate	Normal	Increased	Increased (bradycardia in severe cases)
Skin turgor	Normal	Decreased	Decreased
Fontanelle	Normal	Sunken	Sunken
Mucous membranes	Slightly dry	Dry	Dry
Eyes	Normal	Sunken orbits/decreased tears	Deeply sunken orbits/decreased tears
Extremities	Warm, normal capillary refill	Delayed capillary refill	Cool, mottled
Mental status	Normal	Normal to listless	Normal to lethargic to comatose
Urine output	Slightly decreased	< 1 mL/kg/hour	< 1 mL/kg/hour
Thirst	Slightly increased	Moderately increased	Very thirsty
Fluid replacement	ORT 50 mL/kg over 2–4 hours	ORT 100 mL/kg over 2–4 hours	Lactated Ringer 40 mL/kg in 15–30 minutes, then 20–40 mL/kg if skin turgor, alertness, and pulse have not returned to normal *or* Lactated Ringer or normal saline 20 mL/kg, repeat if necessary, and then replace water and electrolyte deficits over 1–2 days, followed by ORT 100 mL/kg over 4 hours

From Martin S, Jung R. Gastrointestinal infections and enterotoxigenic poisonings. In: DiPiro JT, Talbert RL, Yee GC, et al, eds. Pharmacotherapy: A Pathophysiologic Approach. 9th ed. New York: McGraw-Hill; 2014:1951–1967.

first-line drugs are ciprofloxacin or levofloxacin. Alternative agents include azithromycin and ceftriaxone.[11] However, the choice of antibiotic should also be influenced by periodically updated local antimicrobial susceptibility patterns. Treatment should be continued for a total of 5 days. Antimotility agents are not recommended because they can worsen dysentery and may be related to the development of toxic megacolon. No vaccines are available for the prevention of shigellosis.

SALMONELLOSIS

Epidemiology

Salmonella are gram-negative facultative rods that cause a wide variety of disease manifestations. *Salmonella typhi* and *Salmonella paratyphi* cause typhoid (or enteric) fever. Although typhoid fever is now a rare disease in the United States with approximately 300 clinical cases reported per year, these infections cause an estimated 20 million cases and 200,000 deaths annually worldwide.[12] Nontyphoidal *Salmonella* (NTS) are important causes of reportable food-borne infection. There are an estimated 1.4 million cases of NTS illness annually in the United States, and almost 94 million worldwide.[13] The highest incidence is in those younger than 1 year of age and older than 65 years of age or in those with HIV/AIDS. Exotic pets, especially reptiles, are an increasing source of human salmonellosis. NTS strains may also result in bacteremia and focal disease, such as endovascular infections, osteomyelitis, meningitis, and septic arthritis. Antimicrobial-resistant strains are associated with excess bloodstream infections and hospitalizations.[14] Recurrent *Salmonella* bacteremia is an AIDS-defining illness.

Risk factors for salmonellosis include extremes of age; alteration of endogenous GI flora due to antimicrobial therapy, surgery, or acid-suppressive therapy[5]; diabetes; malignancy; rheumatologic disorders; HIV infection; and therapeutic immunosuppression.

Clinical Presentation and Diagnosis of Shigellosis

- Biphasic illness
  - Early—high fever, watery diarrhea without blood
  - Later—after approximately 48 hours, colitis develops with urgency, **tenesmus**, and dysentery
  - Low-grade fever
  - More frequent small-volume stools ("fractional stools")
  - Vomiting (35%)
- Complications of shigellosis
  - **Proctitis** or rectal prolapse—more common in infants and young children
  - Intestinal obstruction
  - Colonic perforation
  - Bacteremia—more common in children
  - Metabolic disturbances
  - Neurologic disease—most commonly seizures (approximately 10% of patients)
  - Hemolytic-uremic syndrome (HUS)
- Microscopic examination of stool is extremely useful and reveals multiple polymorphonuclear leukocytes and red blood cells (RBCs). Diagnosis is usually confirmed by stool culture

Patient Encounter 1

A 3-year-old child who attends daycare four days each week complains that his "stomach hurts" and that he does not want to eat anything. His mother notes that his stools are loose and that the child has a low-grade fever. The next day, his mother notices blood and some pus in his stools.

By what method did this child most likely acquire this infection?

What is the most likely microorganism to be causing this infection?

What antibiotic (if any) should be recommended to treat this child's infection?

Proper food handling and storage can help prevent *Salmonella* gastroenteritis. Effective handwashing is important, especially when handling eggs and poultry.

Treatment and Monitoring

▶ *Gastroenteritis*

Salmonella gastroenteritis is usually self-limited, and antibiotics have no proven value. Patients respond well to ORT. Symptoms typically diminish in 3 to 7 days without sequelae. Antibiotic use may result in a higher rate of chronic carriage and relapse. Antimicrobial use should be limited to preemptive therapy among patients at higher risk for extraintestinal spread or invasive disease (Table 76–2). Antimotility agents should not be used.

▶ *Enteric Fever*

The current drug of choice for typhoid fever in adults is a fluoroquinolone, such as ciprofloxacin. Azithromycin or ceftriaxone are preferred in children. The recommended adult dose of ciprofloxacin for uncomplicated typhoid fever is 500 mg orally twice daily for 5 to 7 days; however, decreased susceptibility to ciprofloxacin is a significant problem in many parts of the world. In the United States, *S. typhi* with decreased ciprofloxacin susceptibility is associated with travel to the Indian subcontinent.[12] If ciprofloxacin resistance is present, ceftriaxone may be used; however, this agent may be less suitable in some low- and middle-income countries due to cost and route of administration. Azithromycin is an effective alternative for uncomplicated typhoid fever.[15]

Table 76–2

Antimicrobial Indications for Nontyphoidal Salmonellosis (NTS)

Age 3 months or less or 65 years or more
Fever and systemic toxicity
HIV/AIDS
Other immunodeficiency (eg, steroid use, organ transplantation)
Uremia or hemodialysis or renal transplant
Malignancy
Sickle cell anemia or hemoglobinopathy
Inflammatory bowel disease
Aortic aneurysm, prosthetic heart valve, vascular or orthopedic prosthesis

Clinical Presentation and Diagnosis of Salmonellosis

Gastroenteritis

- Onset 8 to 48 hours after ingestion of contaminated food.
- Fever, diarrhea, and cramping.
- Stools are loose, of moderate volume, and without blood.
- Headache, myalgias, and other systemic symptoms can occur.
- Certain underlying conditions (eg, AIDS, inflammatory bowel disease, and prior gastric surgery) predispose the patient to more severe disease.

Enteric Fever

- Febrile illness 5 to 21 days after ingestion of contaminated food or water, which may be persistent and high-grade. A relative bradycardia may be noted at the fever peak.
- Chills, diaphoresis, headache, anorexia, cough, weakness, sore throat, dizziness, muscle pain, and diarrhea may be present before onset of fever.
- Rose spots, a coated tongue, and/or hepatosplenomegaly may be noted.
- Intestinal hemorrhage or perforation, leukopenia, anemia, and subclinical disseminated intravascular coagulopathy may occur.
- Culture of stool, blood, or bone marrow for *Salmonella* species is helpful.

Two typhoid vaccines are available for use in the United States. Immunization is recommended for travelers going to endemic areas such as Latin America, Asia, and Africa; household contacts of a chronic carrier; and laboratory personnel who frequently work with *S. typhi*.

▶ *Bacteremia and Focal Infections*

Treatment of *Salmonella* bacteremia should be initiated with either a fluoroquinolone (eg, levofloxacin, ciprofloxacin) or a third-generation cephalosporin (eg, ceftriaxone).[11] Given increasing antimicrobial resistance, life-threatening infections should be treated with both agents until susceptibilities are available.[13] If there is no evidence of an endovascular infection, therapy for bacteremia should continue for 10 to 14 days. For patients with suspected meningitis, high-dose ceftriaxone is preferred because of its optimal penetration of the blood–brain barrier. Osteomyelitis and joint infections, often associated with sickle-cell anemia, are difficult to eradicate and require longer durations of antimicrobial therapy (at least 4–6 weeks), as do patients who are infected with HIV.[13]

▶ *Chronic Carrier State*

A chronic carrier state, defined as positive stool or urine cultures for more than 12 months, develops in 1% to 4% of adults with typhoid fever. Effective agents for eradication of chronic carriage include amoxicillin (3 g orally divided three times a day in adults for 3 months), trimethoprim-sulfamethoxazole (one double-strength tablet orally twice a day for 3 months), or ciprofloxacin (750 mg orally twice daily for 4 weeks). Surgery in combination with antibiotic therapy is indicated in patients with biliary tract abnormalities.

CAMPYLOBACTERIOSIS

Epidemiology

Campylobacter jejuni is the most commonly identified cause of bacterial diarrhea worldwide. In the United States, this organism accounts for an estimated 1.4 million infections, 13,000 hospitalizations, and 100 deaths annually.[16] Risk factors for *Campylobacter* infection include consumption of contaminated foods of animal origin, especially undercooked poultry or other foods that are cross-contaminated by raw poultry meat during food preparation; unpasteurized milk; contaminated water; foreign travel; contact with farm animals and pets; and the use of antimicrobial therapy.[17] People should be instructed to wash their hands after contact with raw meats and animals.

In developed countries, there are two distinct age peaks for Campylobacter infection: younger than 1 year of age and 15 to 44 years of age, with a mild male predominance. In developing countries, *Campylobacter* diarrhea is primarily a pediatric disease.

Pathophysiology

Campylobacter spp. are gram-negative bacilli that have a curved or spiral shape. *Campylobacter* are sensitive to stomach acidity; as a result, diseases or medications that buffer gastric acidity may increase the risk of infection. The infectious inoculum for *C. jejuni* is low, similar to that for *Salmonella* spp. After an incubation period, infection is established in the jejunum, ileum, colon, and rectum.

Treatment

Effective fluid and electrolyte replacement is the cornerstone of therapy for patients with *Campylobacter* infection. In most cases, this can be accomplished with the use of oral glucose–electrolyte solutions. Antibiotic therapy should be considered in patients with high fevers, bloody stools, symptoms lasting longer than 1 week, pregnancy, infection with HIV, and other immunocompromising conditions.

Macrolides are the recommended first-line drug class for the treatment of *Campylobacter* infections.[11] A fluoroquinolone or a tetracycline are alternatives; however, the widespread use of these agents in food animals has resulted in fluoroquinolone-resistant *Campylobacter* strains worldwide.[17] *Campylobacter fetus* is the most commonly identified species in patients with bacteremia, which primarily occurs in patients who are elderly or immunocompromised. In addition, focal infections such as cellulitis, vascular infections, meningitis, and abscesses may be present. *C. fetus* has a predilection for the vascular endothelium and implanted medical devices.[18] For these serious infections, treatment with a third-generation cephalosporin, gentamicin, ampicillin, or a carbapenem is recommended.[11] Antimotility agents should be avoided because they may prolong the duration of symptoms and have been associated with worse outcomes. Postinfectious complications associated with *Campylobacter* infection include reactive arthritis (1%) and Guillain-Barré syndrome (0.1%).

Clinical Presentation and Diagnosis of Campylobacteriosis

- Incubation period of 1 to 7 days.
- A brief prodrome of fever, headache, and myalgias is followed by crampy abdominal pain, a high fever, and several bowel movements per day, which may be watery or bloody.
- The abdominal pain and tenderness may be localized, and pain in the right lower quadrant may mimic acute appendicitis. Abdominal pain is more prevalent in *Campylobacter* infection than in either *Shigella* or *Salmonella* infections.
- Tenesmus occurs in approximately 25% of patients.
- Fecal leukocytes and red blood cells (RBCs) are detected in the stools of 75% of infected individuals. Diagnosis of *Campylobacter* is established by stool culture.

Patient Encounter 2

A 55-year-old man with a 20-year history of HIV infection has recently purchased a pet snake. About two months after getting the snake, he presents to his local emergency center with a 3-day history of nausea, several episodes of vomiting, abdominal pain, and nonbloody diarrhea. He also complains of episodes of chills and nightsweats over the past two days. Upon further questioning, it is noted that he recently lost his health insurance coverage and he has been unable to refill his HIV medications the past two months. STAT blood cultures are positive for nontyphoidal *Salmonella* (NTS).

What risk factors does this patient have for a disseminated Salmonella infection?

What treatment do you recommend? Are there any special considerations due to this patient's HIV infection?

ENTEROHEMORRHAGIC *ESCHERICHIA COLI*

Epidemiology

KEY CONCEPT *Blood in the stool indicates the possibility of inflammatory mucosal disease of the colon such as enterohemorrhagic Escherchia coli (EHEC), a pathogenic subgroup of shiga toxin-producing organisms and an important cause of bloody diarrhea in the United States.* Acute hemorrhagic colitis has been primarily associated with the O157:H7 serotype. This serotype has been responsible for large outbreaks of infection, has higher rates of complications, and appears to be more pathogenic than non-EHEC STEC strains. The spectrum of disease associated with *E. coli* O157:H7 includes bloody diarrhea, which is seen in up to 95% of patients; nonbloody diarrhea; hemolytic-uremic syndrome (HUS); and thrombotic thrombocytopenic purpura (TTP). The incidence of HUS has declined in recent years and NSAIDs are increasingly recognized as an important contributor to acute kidney injury in children, especially if volume depleted.[19]

Approximately 70,000 cases of EHEC illness occur every year in the United States and lead to more than 2000 hospitalizations. The highest incidence is in patients aged 5 to 9 years and 50 to 59 years. Both young and old patients are at risk to develop postinfectious complications, TTP, and HUS.[20] Outbreaks of diarrhea due to *E. coli* O157:H7 and other STECs have occurred following ingestion of contaminated beef, unpasteurized milk, vegetables (eg, alfalfa sprouts, coleslaw, and lettuce), and apple juice. The most important reservoir for *E. coli* O157:H7 is the GI tract of cattle. Person-to-person transmission also occurs,

Clinical Presentation and Diagnosis of EHEC

- Incubation period of 3 to 5 days
- Bloody stools
- Leukocytosis is often present; fever is frequently absent
- Abdominal tenderness
- HUS in 2% to 10% of patients (especially children 1 to 5 years of age and the elderly in nursing homes); develops on average 1 week after the onset of diarrhea.
- EHEC belonging to serotype 0157:H7 characteristically do not ferment sorbitol, whereas more than 70% of intestinal floral *E. coli* do. To properly screen EHEC strains in cases of diarrhea, stool should be placed on special sorbitol-MacConkey agar. In addition, stool should be tested directly for the presence of Stx I and II by enzyme immunoassay (EIA).

Patient Encounter 3

A very pleasant 73-year-old white woman with a 48-hour history of hematochezia presents to the ED. She denies any recent travel, exotic foods, raw foods, or sick contacts. She does note that she ate cold-cut sandwiches at a fundraiser approximately 3 days before her symptoms started. She also noticed that she has three friends who developed bloody diarrhea who also ate at this same fundraiser. She denies any fevers, shakes, chills, cough, sore throat, shortness of breath, chest pain, nausea or vomiting, dysuria, hematuria, edema, or night sweats. On her initial presentation, she had a CT that showed pan-colitis and terminal ileitis. She was started on antibiotic therapy including ciprofloxacin and metronidazole. Fecal leukocytes were negative. A stool culture was sent and was positive for Stx. The final culture result was positive for *Escherichia coli* O157:H7.

What would be your antibiotic recommendation for this patient?

Two days later, she develops acute kidney injury and thrombocytopenia.

What is the most likely diagnosis?

and swimming in infant pools or contaminated lakes or drinking municipal water are additional risk factors. The incidence of diagnosed *E. coli* O157:H7 infections in the United States are greater among rural populations and usually occur in summer and autumn months.

Pathophysiology

The infectious inoculum of EHEC is very low, between 1 and 100 colony-forming units (CFUs). The major virulence factor for EHEC is the production of two Shiga-like cytotoxins (Shiga toxin [Stx] I and II), which are responsible for vascular damage and systemic effects such as HUS. Adhesion mediates initial attachment of EHEC to intestinal epithelial cells. Following attachment, these organisms produce lesions on individual intestinal epithelial cells in the small or large intestine resulting in diarrhea.

Treatment

The only recommended treatment of EHEC infection is supportive, including fluid and electrolyte replacement, usually in the form of ORT. Most illnesses resolve in 5 to 7 days. Patients should be monitored for the development of HUS. Antibiotics are currently contraindicated because they can induce the expression and release of toxin. Antimotility agents should be avoided because they delay clearance of the pathogen and toxin, which increases the risk of systemic complications. The use of narcotics and nonsteroidal anti-inflammatory drugs (NSAIDs) should also be avoided in acutely infected patients.[21]

Prevention of EHEC infection is especially important because no therapeutic interventions are available to lessen the risk of the development of HUS.[20] Hamburgers should be cooked thoroughly until the temperature of the thickest part of the patty is 72°C. All surfaces and utensils that contact raw meat should be washed thoroughly before reuse. Fruits and vegetables should be washed thoroughly, especially those that will not be cooked. Handwashing is also very important and should include the supervision of handwashing by children in daycare centers.

CHOLERA

Epidemiology

Cholera is an intestinal infection that is caused by the bacterium *Vibrio cholerae* that leads to a massive loss of fluid through the GI tract and often results in life-threatening dehydration and shock. The biotypes of *V. cholerae* responsible for pandemics are serogroup O1 (El Tor) and serogroup O139. Worldwide this infection affects 3 to 5 million people and causes more than 100,000 deaths per year. Cholera can be transmitted by water or by food tainted with contaminated water, particularly undercooked seafood.[22] Research on cholera has led to the refinement of general rehydration therapy, including the proper use of IV and oral rehydration solutions.

Pathophysiology

V. cholerae is a gram-negative bacillus. Vibrios pass through the stomach to colonize the upper small intestine. They possess filamentous protein extensions that attach to receptors on the intestinal mucosa, and their motility assists with penetration of the mucus layer. The cholera enterotoxin consists of two subunits, one of which (subunit A) is transported into the cells and causes an increase in cyclic adenosine monophosphate (cAMP), which leads to the secretion of fluid into the small intestine. This large volume of GI fluid results in the watery diarrhea that is characteristic of cholera. The stools consist of an electrolyte-rich isotonic fluid that is highly infectious.[22]

Treatment

The cornerstone of cholera treatment is fluid replacement. Without treatment, the case-fatality rate for severe cholera is approximately 50%. For cholera, rice-based ORT is better than glucose-based ORT because it reduces the number of stools.[23] Antibiotic prophylaxis is not warranted. The current WHO treatment protocol recommends antibiotics for only "severe" symptoms; however, this is controversial and some expert groups argue that antibiotics should be used more liberally in significant outbreaks.[24] With effective antibiotic therapy, the illness is shortened by about 50%, and the duration of excretion of *V. cholerae* in the stool is shortened to 1 or 2 days.[25] A tetracycline (eg, doxycycline) is recommended as first-line therapy; however, some

Clinical Presentation and Diagnosis of Cholera

- Incubation period of 18 hours to 5 days
- Abrupt, painless onset of watery diarrhea and vomiting. The diarrheal fluid is usually clear and may be as much as 10 to 20 liters per day
- Large volumes of rice-water stools, which may have fishy odor
- Dehydration is often severe and puts patients at risk for death within hours of disease onset. Symptoms of severe dehydration include low blood pressure, poor skin turgor, sunken eyes, and rapid pulse
- Severe muscle cramps in extremities are due to electrolyte imbalances caused by fluid loss. These cramps should resolve with treatment
- Metabolic acidosis

strains are resistant. Other therapeutic options include a fluoroquinolone, trimethoprim-sulfamethoxazole, and azithromycin,[11] which is increasingly utilized in areas where multidrug-resistant strains are prevalent.[26]

Primary preventive strategies include ensuring a safe water supply and safe food preparation, improving sanitation, and patient education. Safe and effective oral vaccines for cholera are available; however, cholera vaccination is not recommended by the Centers for Disease Control and Prevention (CDC) for most people traveling from the United States to endemic areas. The WHO recommends immunization of high-risk groups, such as children and patients infected with HIV, in countries where the disease is endemic.[24]

TRAVELER DIARRHEA

Epidemiology

Traveler diarrhea (TD) commonly occurs when visitors from developed countries travel to developing countries. More than 50 million people are at risk for TD each year.[27] These infections arise following the consumption of food or water contaminated with bacteria, viruses, or parasites. KEY CONCEPT *Bacteria such as* Shigella, Salmonella, Campylobacter, *and enterotoxigenic E. coli (ETEC) are responsible for 60% to 85% of TD cases.*[27] *Noroviruses are increasingly recognized as a significant cause of TD as well.*[28] Most of these illnesses occur during the first 2 weeks of travel and last about 4 days without therapy.[29] Protozoans are an uncommon cause but should be suspected if diarrhea lasts for more than 2 weeks.

Food and water contaminated with fecal matter are the main sources of pathogens that lead to TD. Particularly problematic foods and beverages include salads, unpeeled fruits, raw or poorly cooked meats and seafood, unpasteurized dairy products, and tap water (including ice).[29] Food from street vendors and buffet-style meals are particularly risky. The consumption of more than five alcoholic drinks per day is a risk factor for TD, especially in males.[30] Providing effective education about the types of foods and activities to avoid during travel may decrease the number of cases of TD.

Clinical Presentation and Diagnosis of Traveler Diarrhea

- Frequent, loose stools
- Nausea and vomiting
- Abdominal pain
- Fecal urgency
- Dysentery
- Signs and symptoms related to specific causative pathogen

Pathophysiology

Enterotoxigenic *E. coli*, which is responsible for up to 70% of TD cases in Mexico, produces both heat-labile enterotoxins (LT) and heat-stable enterotoxins (ST). Both toxins demonstrate cellular mechanisms similar to those of cholera toxins and lead to a great increase in both fluid and electrolyte secretion. These *E. coli* strains are not invasive, as are the Shiga-toxin–producing EHEC strains. These organisms lead to a profuse, watery diarrhea without blood, leukocytes, or abdominal cramping.

Treatment

The goal of treatment is to maintain hydration and functional status and to prevent disruption of travel plans. For travelers with mild cases of diarrhea, oral rehydration salts can prevent and treat dehydration and may be particularly important for children and the elderly.[31] Loperamide (to a maximum dose of 16 mg/day) may be used for milder diarrhea; however, this agent is not recommended if bloody diarrhea or fever is present. Antibiotics are effective at reducing the duration of illness to 1 or 2 days. Providing the traveler with a means for empiric self-treatment is an effective method of treating this illness without promoting the inappropriate use of antibiotics. Therapy should be initiated after the first episode of diarrhea that is uncomfortable or interferes with activities.[32] In general, levofloxacin or ciprofloxacin are recommended as first-line agents for travel to most parts of the world.[29,31] Azithromycin is an alternative and is preferred in areas where quinolone-resistant *Campylobacter* is prevalent (eg, Thailand, India).[29] Azithromycin can also be used in pregnant women and children (10 mg/kg/day orally for 3 days).[31] Rifaximin, a nonabsorbed oral antibiotic, is approved for treatment of TD caused by ETEC in persons at least 12 years old and has been used off-label in younger children at a dose of 20 to 40 mg/kg/day for 4 days. This agent may be a good choice for persons traveling to destinations where ETEC is the predominant pathogen, such as Mexico. Many clinicians will recommend the use of loperamide in dysentery if it is combined with an antibiotic.[29]

KEY CONCEPT *The education of travelers about high-risk food and beverages is an important component in the prevention of TD.* Slogans such as "peel it, boil it, cook it, or forget it" can help to remind travelers of the foods that may be contaminated. However, many travelers find it difficult to follow dietary recommendations. In a study of American travelers, almost 50% developed diarrhea despite receiving advice on preventive dietary measures.[33] Antibiotic prophylaxis is not recommended by the CDC because it can lead to drug-resistant organisms and may give travelers a false sense of security.[29] However, some health care professionals do prescribe prophylactic antibiotics for those who are at high risk of developing TD (eg, immunocompromised persons, patients with impaired gastric acid production) or for those who cannot risk temporary incapacitation (eg, athletes, diplomats, business people). A fluoroquinolone antibiotic, such as levofloxacin or ciprofloxacin, is usually used first line for this purpose at a dose of one tablet daily during travel and for 2 days following return.[31] Although not approved for prophylaxis, rifaximin may be an option for travelers to Mexico because it is not absorbed and should be less likely to select out resistant organisms than are the fluoroquinolones. Bismuth subsalicylate (Pepto-Bismol; 525 mg orally four times daily for up to 3 weeks) provides a rate of protection of about 60% against TD.[29] However, this agent should not be used in persons taking anticoagulants or other salicylates. Probiotics colonize the GI tract and may prevent pathogenic organisms from causing infections. These agents may provide protection rates as high as 50%, but additional studies are needed, and these products suffer from lack of standardization. No effective vaccines are available for TD.

CLOSTRIDIUM DIFFICILE INFECTION

Epidemiology

C. difficile is the primary cause of hospital-acquired infectious diarrhea in hospitalized patients, including children. Both the incidence and severity of *C. difficile* infection (CDI) have been increasing in the United States.[34] The number of *C. difficile* cases that were reported in 2005 (84 per 100,000) was nearly three times higher than the 1996 rate.[35] There has also been a significant increase in severe cases, colectomies, and death related to CDI.[36] A more virulent, epidemic strain (NAP1/B1/027) was initially identified in the 1980s and is now commonly associated with outbreaks. These strains are associated with an increased production of toxins A and B, which are the primary virulence determinants for *C. difficile*.[35] An increasing proportion of CDI patients have a community acquired infection. These patients are often younger, lack traditional risk factors, and generally have less severe disease compared with those with hospital-acquired infections.[34] A primary risk factor for these community-acquired infections appears to be therapeutic gastric acid suppression.[37] Common risk factors for hospital-acquired CDI include increasing age, severe underlying illness, intensive care unit admission, gastric acid suppression,[38] and exposure to antimicrobials, especially broad-spectrum, multiple-drug regimens.[39] KEY CONCEPT *Nosocomial Clostridium difficile-associated diarrhea (CDAD) is almost always associated with antimicrobial use; therefore, unnecessary and inappropriate antibiotic therapy should be avoided. Clindamycin, cephalosporins, and penicillins are the antibiotics most commonly associated with CDAD, but almost all antibiotics except aminoglycosides have been implicated.*[40] Fluoroquinolones are also strongly associated with CDAD, especially in community-acquired infections.[41]

Pathophysiology

C. difficile, a gram-positive, spore-forming anaerobe, is spread by the fecal–oral route, and patient-to-patient spread is an important mode of transmission within the hospital. The organism is ingested either as the vegetative form or spores, which can survive for long periods in the environment and can traverse the acidic stomach. In the small intestine, spores germinate into the vegetative form. Once the GI tract is colonized with spores, disruption of the gut flora, which occurs with antibiotic therapy, allows *C. difficile* to proliferate. Toxin production is essential for the disease to occur and is responsible for the inflammation, fluid and mucus secretion, and mucosal damage that lead to diarrhea or colitis.

Treatment

Patients who develop CDI while receiving an antibiotic should have the antibiotic discontinued, if possible. If antimicrobial therapy must continue, an attempt should be made to switch the patient to an agent with a lower risk of CDI.[42] The use of concurrent antibiotics during CDI therapy, or soon thereafter, lowers the chances of a clinical cure. Clinical practice guidelines recommend that initial antimicrobial therapy should be based on the severity of illness.[43]

Metronidazole (500 mg orally three times daily for 7–14 days; or, 30 mg/kg/day divided into four daily doses for children) is the recommended first-line drug for initial treatment of mild-to-moderate CDI. Oral vancomycin (125 mg four times daily for 7 to 14 days; or, 40 to 50 mg/kg/day divided into four daily doses for children) is the recommended first-line drug therapy for initial treatment of severe CDI,[43] which is usually defined as a serum creatinine increase to more than 1.5 times baseline or a white blood cell count greater than 15,000 cells/mm^3(15 × 10^9/L). Other risk factors for severe disease include age more than 65 years, hypoalbuminemia, immunosuppression, and severe underlying disease.[39] For the treatment of severe, complicated CDI (refractory hypotension, ileus, and/or toxic megacolon), a higher dose of vancomycin (500 mg orally four times daily) may be combined with IV metronidazole (500 mg every 8 hours). Vancomycin may be given as a retention enema (500 mg in 100 mL of normal saline every 6 hours) if a complete ileus is present.[43] The use of antimotility agents should be avoided because they may precipitate toxic megacolon. Surgical intervention may be lifesaving, particularly in cases complicated by toxic megacolon or colonic perforation. Antimicrobial stewardship programs can decrease the incidence of CDIs and better assure appropriate initial therapy.[44]

The cost of oral vancomycin capsules (~$1,000 for a 10-day course) is much higher than metronidazole; however, vancomycin for IV use can be prepared for oral use at a much lower cost.[39] The FDA has also approved fidaxomicin, an oral macrolide antibiotic, for the treatment of CDI in patients who are at least 18 years old. This drug is minimally absorbed and has no activity against organisms other than clostridia, which allows for preservation of normal gut flora. The recommended dose of fidaxomicin is 200 mg orally twice daily for 10 days. In clinical trials, fidaxomicin resulted in clinical cure rates that were similar to those achieved with oral vancomycin, but there were significantly fewer recurrences in those treated with fidaxomicin. However, recurrence rates were similar among patients infected with the more virulent NAP1/B1/027 strain.[45] Fidaxomicin is expensive (~$3000 for a 10-day course) and its place in therapy has not been clearly established.

The recurrence rate after an initial episode of CDI is approximately 20% to 25%, with the highest risk within the first 2 weeks.[39] This rate is independent of which agent is used initially. Treatment of the first recurrence of CDI is usually treated with the same regimen used for the initial episode; however, this choice should also depend on the clinical condition of the patient, as recommended for the initial therapy choice.[43] Metronidazole should not be used beyond the first recurrence or for long-term chronic treatment due to the risk of neurotoxicity. The treatment of second or later recurrences of CDI should be undertaken with vancomycin using a tapered and/or pulse regimen.[35,43] Fidaxomicin may be superior to vancomycin at preventing CDAD recurrences secondary to non-NAP1/B1/027 strains. Rifaximin, administered directly following a course of metronidazole or vancomycin, may be an option for the prevention of recurrent

Clinical Presentation and Diagnosis of CDAD

- Symptoms can start as early as the first day of antimicrobial therapy or several weeks after antibiotic therapy is completed.
- Asymptomatic carriage.
- Diarrhea:
  - Acute watery diarrhea with lower abdominal pain, low-grade fever, and mild or absent leukocytosis.
  - Mild, with only three or four loose watery stools per day.
  - *C. difficile* toxins are present in stool, but sigmoidoscopic examination is normal.
- Colitis:
  - Profuse, watery diarrhea with 5 to 15 bowel movements per day, abdominal pain, abdominal distention, nausea, and anorexia.
  - Left or right lower quadrant abdominal pain and cramps that are relieved by passage of diarrhea.
  - Dehydration and low-grade fever.
  - Sigmoidoscopic examination may reveal a nonspecific diffuse or patchy erythematous colitis with or without pseudomembranes.
- Toxic megacolon: Suggested by acute dilation of the colon to a diameter greater than 6 cm, associated systemic toxicity, and the absence of mechanical obstruction. It carries a high mortality rate.
- Fulminant colitis: Acute abdomen and systemic symptoms such as fever, tachycardia, dehydration, and hypotension. Some patients have marked leukocytosis (up to 40×10^3 white blood cells/mm^3 [40×10^9/L]). Diarrhea is usually prominent but may not occur in patients with paralytic ileus and toxic megacolon.
- Recurrent disease:
  - Risk factors include increased age, recent abdominal surgery, increased number of *C. difficile* diarrheal episodes, and leukocytosis.
  - 20% to 25% of patients develop a second episode of CDAD within 2 months of the initial diagnosis.
- In most cases, *C. difficile* toxin testing of a single unformed stool specimen effectively establishes the diagnosis. Stool culture is the most sensitive test, but it is not clinically practical due to slow turnaround time. Enzyme immunoassay (EIA) testing for toxin A and B is used in most labs. This test is rapid, but less sensitive, and repeat testing may be necessary if the initial test is negative. Newer tests, such as EIA detection of glutamate dehydrogenase or use of polymerase chain reaction technology, may ultimately improve diagnostic testing for CDI.
- Leukocytosis, hypoalbuminemia, and fecal leukocytes are nonspecific but suggestive of *C. difficile* infection.
- In selected patients, sigmoidoscopy, colonoscopy, or abdominal CT scan can provide useful diagnostic information.

episodes of CDI in some patients. Fecal microbiota transplantation (FMT) has a reported efficacy of about 90% in preventing recurrent CDI, and this therapy is emerging as a first-line option for patients with multiple recurrent episodes of CDI.[46]

Strict infection control measures, including contact precautions, should be instituted for all patients with CDAD. Environmental cleaning with chlorine-containing agents should be used to eliminate *C. difficile* spores. Because alcohol is ineffective in killing spores, it is essential that health care workers wash their hands with soap and water rather than using alcohol-based hand sanitizers. Meticulous handwashing is the single most important strategy to decrease the patient-to-patient transmission of *C. difficile*. The administration of currently available probiotic agents is not recommended to prevent primary CDI or to treat recurrences.[43]

Patient Encounter 4

A 58-year-old man presents to his local medical clinic complaining of new-onset diarrhea, which he describes as watery and "constant." He also states that he has some lower abdominal pain. Upon physical examination, the patient is noted to have a low-grade fever and initial lab studies show a mild leukocytosis. Upon further review of this patient's electronic medical record, you note that he was hospitalized about two months earlier for an acute small bowel obstruction which required surgery. Following surgery, he developed a ventilator-associated pneumonia and was treated with broad-spectrum antibiotics for ten days. Shortly after finishing this course of antibiotics, he was diagnosed with a moderately severe *C. difficile* infection (CDI) and completed a 10 day course of oral metronidazole (500 mg). About one month ago, he was diagnosed with recurrent CDI that was described as "mild." At that time he completed a second 10-day course of oral metronidazole. About 2 weeks before this presentation, this patient was treated with a 10-day course of oral levofloxacin for an episode of acute bacterial rhinosinusitis. He now presents with what is presumed to be a third episode of CDI. His current outpatient medications include lisinopril, carvedilol, citalopram, esomeprazole, albuterol (prn), and ibuprofen (prn).

What was the primary risk factor that led to this patient's initial episode of CDI?

What risk factors are present for this patient's recurrent infections?

What drug and/or nondrug therapies could be considered for this patient's third C. difficile infection?

CRYPTOSPORIDIOSIS

Epidemiology

Cryptosporidiosis has been recognized as a human disease since the 1970s, with increasing importance in the 1980s and 1990s because of its relationship with HIV/AIDS. *Cryptosporidium* accounts for 2.2% and 6.1% of diarrhea cases in immunocompetent people in developed and developing countries, respectively.[47] In the United States, the number of reported cases of cryptosporidiosis increased from 6479 in 2006 to 10,500 in 2008. This increase was partially attributed to multiple large recreational water outbreaks and likely reflects increased use of communal swimming venues (eg, lakes, swimming pools, and water parks) by young children.[48]

Cryptosporidiosis is spread person-to-person, usually via the fecal–oral route; by animals, particularly cattle and sheep; and through the environment, especially water.

Pathophysiology

Cryptosporidium is an intracellular protozoan parasite that is capable of completing its entire life cycle within one host. Humans become infected upon ingestion of the oocysts, and autoinfection and persistent infections are possible owing to repeated life cycles within the GI tract. As few as 10 to 100 oocysts can cause infection.[47]

Treatment

In general, immunocompetent persons and those with asymptomatic infection do not require antimicrobial therapy. In patients with HIV/AIDS, the optimal therapy is restoration of immune function through the use of antiretroviral therapy (ART). In persons in whom antimicrobial therapy is deemed necessary or in HIV/AIDS patients in whom ART is ineffective, a combination of an antimicrobial and an antidiarrheal agent is recommended.[47]

Nitazoxanide is the only FDA-approved agent for the treatment of cryptosporidiosis in adults and children 1 year and older. This agent has demonstrated efficacy in cryptosporidiosis in immunocompetent persons, malnourished children, and HIV/AIDS patients. Patients who are infected with both HIV and *Cryptosporidium* usually require longer therapy durations and higher doses than immunocompetent patients. Alternative agents include paromomycin, azithromycin, and clarithromycin.

Prevention of cryptosporidiosis can prove difficult because the oocysts are resilient to many disinfectants and antiseptics, including ammonia, alcohol, and chlorine. Routine screening of drinking water should be considered for water treatment plants, and severely immunocompromised individuals should be advised to avoid water in lakes and streams and contact with young animals.[47]

Clinical Presentation and Diagnosis of Cryptosporidiosis

General

- 7- to 10-day incubation period.
- Profuse, watery diarrhea with mucus but not blood or leukocytes that lasts for approximately 2 weeks.
- Nausea, vomiting, fever, and abdominal cramps may accompany the diarrhea.
- Simplest method of diagnosis is detection of oocysts by modified acid-fast staining of a stool specimen. Standard ova and parasite test does not include *Cryptosporidium*.

Immunocompetent

- May manifest as asymptomatic disease, acute diarrhea, or persistent diarrhea lasting for several weeks.
- Usually self-limiting.

Immunocompromised

- May manifest as asymptomatic disease, chronic diarrhea lasting at least 2 months, or fulminant infection with at least 2 L of watery stool per day.
- In HIV-infected individuals, asymptomatic disease is more common in those with a $CD4^+$ cell count greater than 200 cells/mm^3 (200×10^6/L), and fulminant infection is more common in those with a $CD4^+$ cell count of less than 50 cells/mm^3 (50×10^6/L).

VIRAL GASTROENTERITIS

KEY CONCEPT *Viruses are the most common cause of diarrheal illness in the world and, in the United States, account for 450,000 illnesses and 160,000 hospitalizations for adults and children, respectively, and more than 4000 deaths.* Many viruses may cause gastroenteritis, including rotaviruses, noroviruses, astroviruses, enteric adenoviruses, and coronaviruses (Table 76–3). This chapter focuses on rotaviruses.

Table 76–3

Agents Responsible for Acute Viral Gastroenteritis and Diarrhea

Virus	Peak Age	Peak Time	Duration	Transmission	Symptoms
Rotavirus	6 months–2 years	Winter	3–8 days	Fecal–oral, water, food	Diarrhea, vomiting, fever, abdominal pain
Enteric adenovirus	< 2 years	Year-round	7–9 days	Fecal–oral	Diarrhea, respiratory symptoms, vomiting, fever
Astrovirus	< 7 years	Winter	1–4 days	Fecal–oral, water, shellfish	Vomiting, diarrhea, fever, abdominal pain
Noroviruses	> 5 years	Variable	12–24 hours	Fecal–oral, food, aerosol	Nausea, vomiting, diarrhea, abdominal cramps, headache, fever, chills, myalgia

Modified from Martin S, Jung R. Gastrointestinal infections and enterotoxigenic poisonings. In: DiPiro JT, Talbert RL, Yee GC, et al., eds. Pharmacotherapy: A Pathophysiologic Approach. 8th ed. New York: McGraw-Hill; 2011:1951–1967.

Clinical Presentation and Diagnosis of Rotavirus Infection

- Incubation period of 2 days.
- 2- to 3-day **prodrome** of fever and vomiting.
- Profuse diarrhea without blood or leukocytes (up to 10 to 20 stools per day).
- Severe dehydration.
- Anorexia.
- Fever may be present.
- Presentation in adults may vary from asymptomatic to nonspecific symptoms of headache, malaise, and chills to severe diarrhea, nausea, and vomiting.
- Diagnosis can be made by polymerase chain reaction (PCR) of the stool.

Patient Encounter 5

A 28-year-old woman who has an occasional prescription filled in your community pharmacy, now comes in to ask if she needs to get a flu shot. Since you know she has a 4-month-old child, you ask if her child has started the vaccine series for rotavirus. The mother tells you that she doesn't believe in giving her child a lot of vaccines because she is concerned that there are a lot of potential long-term effects from vaccines that we don't know about.

What scientific findings could you discuss with this mother to persuade her to get all recommended vaccinations for her child, especially the rotavirus vaccine?

ROTAVIRUS

Rotavirus causes between 600,000 and 875,000 deaths each year, with the highest rates in the very young and in developing countries. Rotavirus is the leading cause of childhood gastroenteritis and death worldwide. Most infections occur in children between 6 months and 2 years of age, typically during the winter season, but adults may be infected as well. Worldwide, rotavirus causes more than 2 million hospitalizations and 600,000 deaths per year in children younger than 5 years of age and approximately 60,000 hospitalizations in the United States each year. Almost all children will experience at least one episode of rotavirus infection before 5 years of age. Person-to-person transmission occurs through the fecal–oral route.

The mechanism of diarrhea has not been clearly elucidated, but theories include a reduction in the absorptive surface along with impaired absorption owing to cellular damage, enterotoxigenic effects of a rotavirus protein, and stimulation of the enteric nervous system.

The cornerstone of rotavirus treatment is supportive care and rehydration with ORT or IV fluids. Antimotility and antisecretory agents should not be used owing to their potential side effects in children and the self-limited nature of the disease. KEY CONCEPT Two oral rotavirus vaccine products are currently approved by the FDA and, since their introduction, these vaccines have reduced diarrhea-related health care use in children by as much as 94% and has conferred protection on unvaccinated children (herd immunity). This reduction in health care usage has saved an estimated $1 billion over a 4-year period.[49,50] The CDC Advisory Committee on Immunization Practices recommends vaccination at 2, 4, and 6 months.

FOOD POISONING

Each year in the United States, approximately 76 million food-borne illnesses occur, leading to 325,000 hospitalizations and more than 5000 deaths. Many bacterial and viral pathogens that have been discussed previously in this chapter (eg, *Salmonella, Shigella, Campylobacter, E. coli,* and noroviruses) can cause food poisoning. Other bacteria that can cause food-borne illness include *Staphylococcus aureus, C. perfringens, Clostridium botulinum,* and *Bacillus cereus* (Table 76–4). Food poisoning should be suspected if at least two individuals present with similar symptoms after the ingestion of a common food in the prior 72 hours.

Table 76–4

Food Poisonings

Organism	Onset (Hours)	Associated Foods	Duration	Symptoms	Treatment
Staphylococcus aureus	1–6	Salad, pastries, ham, poultry	12 hours	Nausea, vomiting	Supportive
Bacillus cereus—emetic	0.5–6	Rice, noodles, pasta, pastries	24 hours	Vomiting	Supportive
Bacillus cereus—diarrheal	8–16	Meats, vegetables, soups, sauces, milk products	24 hours	Diarrhea, abdominal pain	Supportive
Clostridium perfringens (type A)	8–12	Meats, poultry	24 hours	Nausea; abdominal cramps; profuse, watery diarrhea	Supportive
Clostridium botulinum	18–24	Canned fruits, vegetables, meats, honey, salsa, relish	Weeks	Acute GI symptoms followed by symmetric, descending, flaccid paralysis; death is possible	Supportive (including mechanical ventilation); trivalent antitoxin

Patient Care Process

Patient Assessment:

- Based on physical examination, review of systems, and laboratory findings, determine the degree of fluid and electrolyte depletion and estimate current renal function.
- Review the medical history with particular attention to risk factors or medical conditions associated with more severe infection outcomes, such as immunosuppression.
- Conduct a medication history focusing on holding drugs that may worsen the current fluid status or renal function, immunosuppressive therapies, and antibiotic allergies.

Therapy Evaluation:

- Review all available tests to determine the etiology and antimicrobial susceptibilities of the suspected pathogen.
- Based on suspected pathogen, patient age, assessment of immune status, and other risk factors for severe complications, determine if antibiotic therapy is indicated.

Care Plan Development:

- Determine that appropriate fluids and other supportive measures have been initiated.
- If indicated, select an antibiotic that is appropriate for the pathogen, not unnecessarily broad in its coverage, and is cost-effective for the patient and the health care system.

Follow-Up Evaluation:

- Determine that signs of fluid depletion and electrolyte imbalances have been corrected. If acute renal dysfunction was initially present, assess for clinical improvement and reassess medication doses.
- Assess for increase in stool consistency and decrease in stool frequency.
- Assure that all indicated chronic medications that were initially held have been restarted, as appropriate.
- Provide patient counseling on measures to avoid gastrointestinal pathogens and vaccinations, as appropriate.

Abbreviations Introduced in This Chapter

ART	Antiretroviral therapy
CDAD	*Clostridium difficile*–associated diarrhea
CDC	Centers for Disease Control and Prevention
CDI	*Clostridium difficile* infection
CFUs	Colony-forming units
EHEC	Enterohemorrhagic *Escherichia coli*
ETEC	Enterotoxigenic *Escherichia coli*
FMT	Fecal microbiota transplant
HUS	Hemolytic-uremic syndrome
ORT	Oral rehydration therapy
LT	Heat-labile enterotoxin
MIC	Minimum inhibitory concentration
NSAID	Nonsteroidal anti-inflammatory drug
NTS	Nontyphoidal *Salmonella*
PPI	Proton-pump inhibitor
ST	Heat-stable enterotoxin
STEC	Shiga toxin-producing *E. coli*
TD	Traveler diarrhea
TTP	Thrombotic thrombocytopenic purpura
WHO	World Health Organization

REFERENCES

1. Martin S, Jung R. Gastrointestinal infections and enterotoxigenic poisonings. In: DiPiro JT, Talbert RL, Yee GC, et al, eds. Pharmacotherapy: A Pathophysiologic Approach. 9th ed. New York: McGraw-Hill; 2014:1807–1820.
2. Hartling L, Bellemare S, Wiebe N, et al. Oral versus intravenous rehydration for treating dehydration due to gastronenteritis in children. Cochrane Database Syst Rev. 2006:CD004390.
3. Freedman SB, Ali S, Oleszczuk M, et al. Treatment of acute gastronenteritis in children: An overview of systematic reviews of interventions commonly used in developed countries. Evid Based Child Health. 2013;8:1123–1137.
4. Salari P, Nikfar S, Abdollahi M. A meta-analysis and systematic review on the effect of probiotics in acute diarrhea. Inflamm Allergy Drug Targets. 2012;11:3–14.
5. Scallan E, Hoekstra RM, Angulo FJ, et al. Foodborne illness acquired in the United States—major pathogens. Emerg Infect Dis. 2011;17:7–15.
6. Bavishi C, Dupont HL. Systematic review: The use of proton pump inhibitors and increased susceptibility to enteric infection. Aliment Pharmacol Ther. 2011;34:1269–1281.
7. Kotloff KL, Winickoff JP, Ivanoff B, et al. Global burden of *Shigella* infections: Implications for vaccine development and implementation of control strategies. Bull World Health Organ. 1999;77:651–666.
8. Dupont HL. *Shigella* species (bacillary dysentery). In: Mandell GL, Bennett JE, Dolin R, eds. Principles and Practice of Infectious Diseases. 7th ed. Philadelphia, PA: Elsevier Churchill Livingstone; 2009, Chap. 224.
9. Moralez EI, Lofland D. Shigellosis with resultant septic shock and renal failure. Clin Lab Sci Summer. 2011;24(3):147–152.
10. Christopher PRH, David KV, John SM, Sankarapandian V. Antibiotic therapy for Shigella dysentery. Cochrane Database Syst Rev. 2010:CD006784.
11. The choice of antibacterial drugs. Treat Guidel Med Lett. 2013; 11:65–74.
12. Lynch MF, Blanton EM, Bulens S, et al. Typhoid fever in the United States, 1999-2006. JAMA. 2009;302:859–865.
13. Hohmann EL. Nontyphoidal salmonellosis. Clin Infect Dis. 2001;32:263–269.
14. Crump JA, Medalla FM, Joyce KW, et al. Antimicrobial resistance among invasive nontyphoidal *Salmonella enterica* isolates in the United States: National Antimicrobial Resistance Monitoring System, 1996 to 2007. Antimicrob Agents Chemother. 2011;55: 1148–1154.
15. Crump JA, Mintz ED. Global trends in typhoid and paratyphoid fever. Clin Infect Dis. 2010;50:241–246.
16. Nelson JM, Chiller TM, Powers JH, Angulo FJ. Fluoroquinolone-resistant *Campylobacter* species and the withdrawal of

fluoroquinolones from use in poultry: A public health success story. Clin Infect Dis. 2007;44:977–980.

17. Luangtongkum T, Jeon B, Han J, et al. Antibiotic resistance in *Campylobacter*: Emergence, transmission, and persistence. Future Microbiol. 2009;4:189–200.
18. Pacanowski J, Lalande V, Lacombe K, et al. *Campylobacter* bacteremia: Clinical features and factors associated with fatal outcome. Clin Infect Dis. 2008;47:790–796.
19. Chandramobhan G, Anand SK. Acute kidney injury. In: Berkowitz C ed. Berkowitz's Pediatrics. 4th Ed. Elk Grove, IA: American Academy of Pediatrics; 2012.
20. Pennington H. *Escherichia coli* O157. Lancet. 2010;376:1428–1435.
21. Tarr PI, Gordon CA, Chandler WL. Shiga-toxin-producing *Escherichia coli* and hemolytic uremic syndrome. Lancet. 2005;365:1073–1086.
22. Sack DA, Sack RB, Nair GB, Siddique AK. Cholera. Lancet. 2004;363:223–233.
23. Zaman K, Yunus M, Rahman A, et al. Efficacy of a packaged rice oral rehydration solution among children with cholera and cholera-like illness. ActaPaediatr. 2001;90:505–510.
24. Sack DA, Sack RB, Chaignat CL. Getting serious about cholera. N Engl J Med. 2006;355:649–651.
25. Nelson EJ, Nelson DS, Salam MA, Sack DA. Antibiotics for both moderate and severe cholera. N Engl J Med. 2011;364:5–7.
26. Saha D, Karim MM, Khan WA, et al. Single-dose azithromycin for the treatment of cholera in adults. N Engl J Med. 2006;354:2452–2462.
27. Okhuysen PC. Current concepts in travelers' diarrhea: Epidemiology, antimicrobial resistance and treatment. Curr Opin Infect Dis. 2005;18:522–526.
28. Chapin AR, Carpenter CM, Dudley WC, et al. Prevalence of norovirus among visitors from the United States to Mexico and Guatemala who experience traveler's diarrhea. J Clin Microbiol. 2005;43:1112–1117.
29. Yates J. Traveler's diarrhea. Am Fam Physician. 2005;71:2095–2100.
30. Huang DB, Sanchez AP, Triana E, et al. United States male students who heavily consume alcohol in Mexico are at greater risk of travelers' diarrhea than their female counterparts. J Travel Med. 2004;11:143–145.
31. Centers for Disease Control (U.S.). Advice for travelers. Treat Guidel Med Lett. 2009;7:83–94.
32. Ericsson CD. Travelers' diarrhea: Epidemiology, prevention, and self-treatment. Infect Dis Clin North Am. 1998;12:285–303.
33. Hill DR. Occurrence and self-treatment of diarrhea in a large cohort of Americans traveling to developing countries. Am J Trop Med Hyg. 2000;62:585–589.
34. Khanna S, Pardi DS, Aronson SL. The epidemiology of community-acquired *Clostridium difficile* infection: A population-based study. Am J Gastroenterol. 2012;107:89–95.
35. Kelly CP, LaMont JT. *Clostridium difficile*—more difficult than ever. N Engl J Med. 2008;359:1932–1940.
36. Oake N, Taljaard M, van Walraven C, et al. The effect of hospital-acquired *Clostridium difficile* infection on in-hospital mortality. Arch Intern Med. 2010;170:1804–1810.
37. Dial S, Delaney JA, Barkun AN, Suissa S. Use of gastric acid-suppressive agents and the risk of community-acquired *Clostridium difficile*-associated disease. JAMA. 2005;294: 2989–2995.
38. King RN, Lager SL. Incidence of *Clostridium difficile* infections in patients receiving antimicrobial and acid-suppression therapy. Pharmacotherapy. 2011;31:642–648.
39. Treatment of *Clostridium difficile* infection. Med Lett Drugs Ther. 2011;53:14–16.
40. Wistrom J, Norrby SR, Myhre EB, et al. Frequency of antibiotic-associated diarrhoea in 2462 antibiotic-treated hospitalized patients: A prospective study. J Antimicrob Chemother. 2001; 47:43–50.
41. Deshpande A, Pasupuleti V, Thota P, et al. Community-associated *Clostridium difficile* infection and antibiotics: A meta-analysis. J Antimicrob Chemother. 2013;68:1951–1961.
42. Gerding DN, Muto CA, Owens RC Jr. Treatment of *Clostridium difficile* infection. Clin Infect Dis. 2008;46(Suppl 1):S32–S42.
43. Cohen SH, Gerding DN, Johnson S, et al. Clinical practice guidelines for *Clostridium difficile* infection in adults: 2010 update by the Society for Healthcare Epidemiology of America (SHEA) and the Infectious Diseases Society of America (IDSA). Infect Control Hosp Epidemiol. 2010;31:431–455.
44. Le F, Arora V, Shah DN, et al. A real-world evaluation of oral vancomycin for severe *Clostridium difficile* infection: Implications for antibiotic stewardship programs. Pharmacotherapy. 2012;32: 129–134.
45. Louie TJ, Miller MA, Mullane KM, et al. Fidaxomicin versus vancomycin for *Clostridium difficile* infection. N Engl J Med. 2011;364:422–431.
46. van Nood E, Vrieze A, Nieuwdorp M, et al. Duodenal infusion of donor feces for recurrent *Clostridium difficile*. N Engl J Med 2013;368:407–415.
47. Chen XM, Keithly JS, Paya CV, LaRusso NF. Cryptosporidiosis. N Engl J Med. 2002;346:1723–1731.
48. Yoder JS, Harral C, Beach MJ. Cryptosporidiosis surveillance—United States, 2006-2008. MMWR Surveill Summ. 2010;59:1–14.
49. Panozzo CA, Becker-Dreps S, Pate V, et al. Direct, indirect, total, and overall effectiveness of the rotavirus vaccines for the prevention of gastroenteritis hospitalizations in privately insured US children, 2007–2010. Am J Epidemiol. 2014;179:895–909.
50. Leshem E, Moritz RE, Curns AT, et al. Rotavirus vaccines and health care utilization for diarrhea in the United States (2007–2011). Pediatrics. 2014;134:15–23.

77 Intra-Abdominal Infections

Joseph E. Mazur and Joseph T. DiPiro

LEARNING OBJECTIVES

Upon completion of the chapter, the reader will be able to:

1. Define and differentiate between primary and secondary intra-abdominal infections (IAIs).
2. Describe the microbiology typically seen with primary and secondary IAIs.
3. Describe the clinical presentation typically seen with primary and secondary IAIs.
4. Describe the role of culture and susceptibility information for diagnosis and treatment of IAIs.
5. Recommend the most appropriate drug and nondrug measures to treat IAIs.
6. Recommend an appropriate antimicrobial regimen for treatment of a primary and a secondary IAIs.
7. Describe the patient-assessment process during the treatment of IAIs.

INTRODUCTION

Intra-abdominal infections (IAIs) are those contained within the peritoneal cavity or retroperitoneal space. The peritoneal cavity extends from the undersurface of the diaphragm to the floor of the pelvis and contains the stomach, small bowel, large bowel, liver, gallbladder, and spleen. The duodenum, pancreas, kidneys, adrenal glands, great vessels (aorta and vena cava), and most mesenteric vascular structures reside in the retroperitoneum. IAIs may be generalized or localized. They may be contained within visceral structures, such as the liver, gallbladder, spleen, pancreas, kidney, or female reproductive organs. Two general types of IAI are discussed throughout this chapter: **peritonitis** and **abscess**. (*Peritonitis* is defined as the acute inflammatory response of the peritoneal lining to microorganisms, chemicals, irradiation, or foreign-body injury.)

An *abscess* is a purulent collection of fluid separated from surrounding tissue by a wall consisting of inflammatory cells and adjacent organs. It usually contains necrotic debris, bacteria, and inflammatory cells. Peritonitis and abscess differ considerably in presentation and approach to treatment.

EPIDEMIOLOGY AND ETIOLOGY

Peritonitis may be classified as primary, secondary, or tertiary. Primary peritonitis, also called *spontaneous bacterial peritonitis*, is an infection of the peritoneal cavity without an evident source of bacteria from the abdomen.[1,2] In secondary peritonitis, a focal disease process is evident within the abdomen. Secondary peritonitis may involve perforation of the gastrointestinal (GI) tract (possibly because of ulceration, ischemia, or obstruction), postoperative peritonitis, or posttraumatic peritonitis (eg, blunt or penetrating trauma). Tertiary peritonitis occurs in critically ill patients, and it is an infection that persists or recurs at least 48 hours after apparently adequate management of primary or secondary peritonitis.

KEY CONCEPT Most IAIs are secondary infections that are caused by a defect in the GI tract that must be treated by surgical drainage, resection, and/or repair. *Primary peritonitis develops in 10% to 30% of hospitalized patients with alcoholic cirrhosis.*[3] Patients undergoing continuous ambulatory peritoneal dialysis (CAPD) average one episode of peritonitis every 2 years.[4] Secondary peritonitis may be caused by perforation of a peptic ulcer; traumatic perforation of the stomach, small or large bowel, uterus, or urinary bladder; appendicitis; pancreatitis; diverticulitis; bowel infarction; inflammatory bowel disease; cholecystitis; operative contamination of the peritoneum; or diseases of the female genital tract such as septic abortion, postoperative uterine infection, endometritis, or salpingitis. Appendicitis is one of the most common causes of IAI. In 2010, approximately 305,000 appendectomies were performed in the United States for suspected appendicitis.[5]

Primary peritonitis in adults occurs most commonly in association with alcoholic cirrhosis, especially in the end stage, or with ascites caused by postnecrotic cirrhosis, chronic active hepatitis, acute viral hepatitis, congestive heart failure, malignancy, systemic lupus erythematosus, and nephrotic syndrome. It also may result from the use of a peritoneal catheter for dialysis with renal failure or central nervous system ventriculoperitoneal shunting for hydrocephalus. Abscesses are the result of chronic inflammation and may occur without preceding generalized peritonitis. They may be located within the peritoneal cavity or in a visceral organ and may vary in size, taking a few weeks to years to form.

PATHOPHYSIOLOGY

IAI results from bacterial entry into the peritoneal or retroperitoneal spaces or from bacterial collections within intra-abdominal organs. In primary peritonitis, bacteria may enter the abdomen via the bloodstream or the lymphatic system by transmigration through the bowel wall, through an indwelling peritoneal dialysis (PD)

Patient Encounter 1, Part 1

A 32-year-old woman with a history of sickle cell disease presents to the surgery clinic with chief complaints of abdominal pain. She had an appendectomy 4 weeks ago and had an uneventful course. Her current medications are oxycodone 10 mg orally every 12 hours, zolpidem 5 mg orally at bedtime, and two herbals (ginseng and ginko biloba). On the previous hospital course, she was treated with a 2-day course of fluconazole.

PMH: Sickle cell disease and early onset ESRD for the last 7 years

Meds: Oxycodone 10 mg orally every 12 hours, zolpidem 5 mg orally every 12 hours, plus herbals

SOC: Single, no alcohol, smoking, or illicit drugs

PE:

Tender, hard, distended abdomen, negative bowel sounds. Rest of the physical exam is noncontributory

VS: T 100°F (37.8°C), BP 75/35 mm Hg, P 136 beats/min, RR 22 breaths/min, Wt 115 lb (52.3 kg), Ht 5′5″ (165 cm)

Labs: Hct 15.0% (0.150), Hgb 5.1 g/dL (51 g/L; 3.17 mmol/L), WBC 20×10^3/mm^3 (20×10^9/L), serum creatinine 3.2 mg/dL (283 μmol/L), BUN 30 mg/dL (10.7 mmol/L), Na 140 mEq/L (140 mmol/L), K 4.9 mEq/L (4.9 mmol/L), Cl 95 mEq/L (95 mmol/L), CO_2 20 mEq/L (20 mmol/L), total bilirubin 1.8 mg/dL (30.8 μmol/L), aPTT 32.0 seconds

Comment on the diagnostic approach which should be taken in this patient in order to determine a diagnosis.

What are the top two diagnoses that could be made for this patient?

Based on your assessment of her medication history, are there any of her medications or herbals that could be potentiating her clinical condition?

What pharmacotherapeutic treatments should the pharmacy clinician focus on?

catheter, or via the fallopian tubes in females. Hematogenous bacterial spread (through the bloodstream) occurs more frequently with tuberculosis peritonitis or peritonitis associated with cirrhotic ascites. When peritonitis results from PD, skin-surface flora are introduced via the peritoneal catheter. In secondary peritonitis, bacteria most often enter the peritoneum or retroperitoneum as a result of perforation of the GI or female genital tracts caused by diseases or traumatic injuries.

If bacteria that enter the abdomen are not contained by cellular and humoral defense mechanisms, bacterial dissemination occurs throughout the peritoneal cavity, resulting in peritonitis. This is more likely to occur in the presence of a foreign body, hematoma, necrotic tissue, large bacterial inoculum, continuing bacterial contamination, and contamination involving a mixture of synergistic organisms.

The fluid and protein shift into the abdomen (called *third spacing*) may be so dramatic that circulating blood volume is decreased, which causes decreased cardiac output and hypovolemic shock. Accompanying fever, vomiting, or diarrhea may worsen the fluid imbalance. A reflex sympathetic response, manifested by sweating, tachycardia, and vasoconstriction, may be evident. With an inflamed peritoneum, bacteria and endotoxins are absorbed easily into the bloodstream (**translocation**), and this may result in septic shock.[1] Other foreign substances present in the peritoneal cavity potentiate peritonitis, notably feces, dead tissues, barium, mucus, bile, and blood.

Many of the manifestations of IAIs, particularly peritonitis, result from cytokine activity. Inflammatory cytokines are produced by macrophages and neutrophils in response to bacteria and bacterial products or to tissue injury, resulting from the

Patient Encounter 2, Part 1

A 65-year-old man with a recent history of gastric cancer (diagnosed 1 year back) presents to the emergency room with a 3-day history of fevers and night sweats. He has just completed an 8-week course of chemotherapy that ended 1 week ago. His surgical history comprises a subtotal gastrectomy done at the onset of his diagnosis. His lab values are as follows:

PE:

The patient is tender to palpation and winces in pain

VS: T 101°F (38.3°C), BP 110/75 mm Hg, P 99 beats/min, RR 12 breaths/min, Wt 250 lb (dry weight on admission [114 kg]), Ht 6′2″ (188 cm)

Labs: Na 142 mEq/L (142 mmol/L), K 4.5 mEq/L (4.5 mmol/L), Cl 95 mEq/L (95 mmol/L), CO_2 22 mEq/L (22 mmol/L), glucose 250 mg/dL (13.9 mmol/L), BUN 42 mg/dL (15.0 mmol/L), serum creatinine 1 mg/dL (88 μmol/L), total bilirubin 1.2 mg/dL (20.5 μmol/L), lactate 4.0 mg/dL (0.44 mmol/L), Hct 30% (0.30), Hgb 10 g/dL (100 g/L; 6.21 mmol/L), WBC 1.5×10^3/mm^3 (1.5×10^9/L) with an absolute neutrophil count (ANC) of 1050/mm^3 (1.050×10^9/L).

The patient's blood pressure is dropping, and the patient is still hypotensive.

What test(s) should be done to ascertain the cause of his continued fevers and night sweats?

Comment on the monitoring parameters that should be displayed in assisting this patient through the next 24 to 48 hours?

What pharmacological treatment should be used for this patient focusing on empiric antibiotics, doses, and addressing any toxicity that may result?

List the most likely resistance patterns than can result from overuse of antimicrobials for intra-abdominal processes.

surgical incision.[1] The outer membrane components of gram-negative and gram-positive organisms contribute to the cascade of proinflammatory cytokines, ultimately leading to end-organ dysfunction (lungs, heart, kidneys) and septic shock.[6] Peritonitis may result in death because of the effects on major organ systems.

An abscess occurs if peritoneal contamination is localized but bacterial elimination is incomplete. The location of the abscess often is related to the site of primary disease. For example, abscesses resulting from appendicitis tend to appear in the right lower quadrant or the pelvis; those resulting from diverticulitis tend to appear in the left lower quadrant or pelvis. A mature abscess may have a fibrinous capsule that isolates bacteria and the liquid core from antimicrobials and immunologic defenses.

Microbiology of Intra-Abdominal Infection

KEY CONCEPT *Primary bacterial peritonitis is often caused by a single organism.* In children, the pathogen is usually *Streptococcus pneumoniae* or a group A *Streptococcus*, *Escherichia coli*, *S. pneumoniae*, or *Bacteroides* species.[4,7] When peritonitis occurs in association with cirrhotic ascites, *E. coli* and *Klebsiella* are isolated most frequently.[8] Other potential pathogens are *Haemophilus pneumoniae*, *Klebsiella*, *Pseudomonas*, anaerobes, and *S. pneumoniae*.[9] Occasionally, primary peritonitis may be caused by *Mycobacterium tuberculosis*. Peritonitis in patients undergoing PD is caused most often by common skin organisms ranging from *S. aureus* to *S. epidermidis*, to *Pseudomonas aeruginosa*.[10] Occasionally, aerobic gram-negative bacilli may cause infections, particularly in patients undergoing dialysis during hospitalization.

KEY CONCEPT *Because of the diverse bacteria present in the GI tract, secondary IAIs are often polymicrobial.*[2,11]

Bacterial Synergism and Other Factors

A combination of aerobic and anaerobic organisms appears to increase the severity of infection (**synergism**). Facultative bacteria (eg, *E. coli*) may provide an environment conducive to the growth of anaerobic bacteria.[2] Although many bacteria isolated in mixed infections are nonpathogenic by themselves, their presence may be essential for the pathogenicity of the bacterial mixture.[3]

Complicating the clinical picture for treatment are polymicrobial IAIs with certain bacterial species being isolated such as enterococci or *P. aeruginosa*. Depending on the patients' immune system (immunocompromised host), targeting these organisms may be necessary to avoid treatment failure or mortality.[12]

CLINICAL PRESENTATION AND DIAGNOSIS

IAIs have a wide spectrum of clinical features. Peritonitis usually is easily recognized, but intra-abdominal abscess often may continue unrecognized for long periods of time. Patients with primary and secondary peritonitis present quite differently.

TREATMENT

The primary goals of treatment are correction of the intra-abdominal disease processes or injuries that have caused infection and drainage of collections (**source control**) of purulent material (abscess). A secondary objective is to resolve the infection without major organ system complications (eg, pulmonary, hepatic, cardiovascular, or renal failure) or adverse drug effects. Ideally, the patient should be discharged from the hospital with full function for self-care and routine daily activities.

General Approach to Treatment

The treatment of IAI most often requires the coordinated use of three major modalities: (a) prompt drainage; (b) support of vital functions; and (c) appropriate antimicrobial therapy to treat infection not eradicated by surgery.[13] Antimicrobials are an important adjunct to drainage procedures in the treatment of secondary IAIs; however, the use of antimicrobial agents without surgical intervention usually is inadequate. For most cases of primary peritonitis, drainage procedures may not be required, and antimicrobial agents become the mainstay of therapy.

KEY CONCEPT *In the early phase of serious IAIs, attention should be given to preserving major organ system function.* With generalized peritonitis, large volumes of IV fluids are required to maintain intravascular volume, to improve cardiovascular function, and to ensure adequate tissue perfusion and oxygenation. Adequate urine output should be maintained to ensure appropriate fluid resuscitation and to preserve renal function. A common cause of early death is hypovolemic shock caused by inadequate intravascular volume expansion and tissue perfusion.

An additional important component of therapy is nutrition. IAIs often involve the GI tract directly or disrupt its function

Clinical Presentation of Primary Peritonitis

General

Patients may not be in acute distress, particularly with peritoneal dialysis.

Symptoms

Patient may complain of nausea, vomiting (sometimes with diarrhea), and abdominal tenderness.

Signs

- Temperature may be only mildly elevated or not elevated in patients undergoing peritoneal dialysis.
- Bowel sounds are hypoactive.
- Cirrhotic patients may have worsening encephalopathy.
- There may be cloudy dialysate fluid with peritoneal dialysis.

Laboratory Tests

- The WBC may be only mildly elevated.
- Ascitic fluid usually contains more than $0.3 \times 10^3/mm^3$ ($0.3 \times 10^9/L$) leukocytes, and bacteria may be evident on Gram stain of a centrifuged specimen.

Other Diagnostic Tests

Culture of peritoneal dialysate or ascitic fluid should be positive.

Clinical Presentation of Secondary Peritonitis

General

Patients may be in acute distress.

Symptoms

- Patients may complain of nausea, vomiting, and generalized abdominal pain.
- Patients may demonstrate abdominal guarding and a "boardlike abdomen."

Signs

- Tachypnea and tachycardia are present.
- Temperature is normal initially, then may increase to 100°F to 102°F (37.8°C–38.9°C) within the first few hours, and may continue to rise for the next several hours.
- Hypotension and shock may develop if intravascular volume is not restored.
- Decreased urine output may develop owing to dehydration.
- Bowel sounds are faint initially and eventually cease.

Laboratory Tests

- The WBC is high (WBCs 15–20 × 10^3/mm^3 [15–20 × 10^9/L]), with neutrophils predominating and an elevated percentage of immature neutrophils (bands).
- The hematocrit and blood urea nitrogen increase because of dehydration.
- Hyperventilation and vomiting result in early alkalosis, which changes to acidosis and lactic academia to reduced intravascular volume and diminished tissue perfusion.

Other Diagnostic Tests

Abdominal radiographs may be useful because free air in the abdomen (indicating intestinal perforation) or distension of the small or large bowel is often evident.

(paralytic ileus). The return of GI motility may take days, weeks, and occasionally, months. In the interim, enteral or parenteral nutrition as indicated facilitates improved immune function and wound healing to ensure recovery.

Nonpharmacologic Therapy

▶ *Drainage Procedures*

Primary peritonitis is treated with antimicrobials and rarely requires drainage. Secondary peritonitis requires surgical removal of the inflamed or gangrenous tissue to prevent further bacterial contamination. If the surgical procedure is suboptimal, attempts are made to provide drainage of the infected or gangrenous structures.

The drainage of purulent material is the critical component of management of an intra-abdominal abscess. This may be performed surgically or with percutaneous image-guided techniques.[14] Without adequate drainage of the abscess, antimicrobial therapy and fluid resuscitation can be expected to fail. The most valuable microbiologic information may be obtained at the time of percutaneous or operative abscess drainage.

▶ *Fluid Therapy*

In patients with peritonitis, hypovolemia is often accompanied by acidosis, and large volumes of an intravenous solution such as lactated Ringer may be required initially to restore intravascular volume. Maintenance fluids should be instituted (after intravascular volume is restored) with 0.9% sodium chloride and potassium chloride (20 mEq/L [20 mmol/L]) or 5% dextrose and 0.45% sodium chloride with potassium chloride (20 mEq/L [20 mmol/L]). The administration rate should be based on estimated daily fluid loss through urine and nasogastric suction, including 0.5 to 1.0 L for insensible fluid loss. Aggressive fluid therapy often must be continued in the postoperative period because fluid will continue to sequester in the peritoneal cavity, bowel wall, and lumen.

Pharmacologic Therapy

▶ *Antimicrobial Therapy*

The goals of antimicrobial therapy are as follows:

- To control bacteremia and prevent the establishment of metastatic foci of infection

Patient Encounter 1, Part 2: Physical Examination and Diagnostic Tests

PE:

The patient is becoming more encephalopathic and somnolent, and she is still having a lot of pain (7/10 pain scale) the attending physician decides to perform an invasive test.

Ascitic fluid analysis is reported as following: hazy yellow color with 2125 cu/mm^3 (2.125 × 10^9/L) WBC, (38% [0.38] neutrophils, 5% [0.05] lymphocytes, 57% [0.57] macrophages). Urinalysis is not significant because the patient is oliguric and almost anuric. Other physical exam findings are nonsignificant.

VS: As noted previously

Labs: As noted previously

Serum: As noted previously

KUB: Negative findings

DPL (diagnostic peritoneal lavage): 2125 cu/mm^3 (2.125 × 10^9/L)

Microbiological cultures: 2/2 bottles from the blood positive for gram-positive pairs in chains and gram-negative bacilli cultured the small amount of urine collected.

Discuss the most appropriate pharmacologic course of treatment, outlining medications, dosing, and monitoring parameters.

List the goals of treatment and follow-up plan that should be developed by the clinician to ensure positive patient outcomes.

Patient Encounter 2, Part 2

The patient's clinical status grows worse over the next couple of hours despite the efforts of the team. He is now placed on vasopressor therapy combined with fluid, antibiotics are begun emergently, and steroids are also begun. His urine output is less than 15 mL/hour and the patient is still mechanically ventilated.

What are your next steps in terms of a care plan as well as monitoring parameters for this patient?

What is the overall goal of treatment in patients with intra-abdominal infections?

How do the pharmacologic versus nonpharmacologic goals compare in this patient?

- To reduce suppurative complications after bacterial contamination
- To prevent local spread of existing infection

After suppuration has occurred (eg, an abscess has formed), a cure by antibiotic therapy alone is difficult to achieve; antimicrobials may serve to improve the results with surgery.

KEY CONCEPT *An empirical antimicrobial regimen should be started as soon as the presence of IAI is suspected and before identification of the infecting organisms is complete.* Therapy must be initiated based on the likely pathogens, which vary depending on the site of IAI and the underlying disease process. Cultures of secondary IAI sites generally are not useful for directing antimicrobial therapy. Table 77–1 lists the likely pathogens against which antimicrobial agents should be directed.

Table 77–1

Likely Intraabdominal Pathogens

Type of Infection	Aerobes	Anaerobes
Primary (Spontaneous) Bacterial Peritonitis		
Children	Group A *Streptococcus*, *E. coli*, pneumococci	—
Cirrhosis	*E. coli*, *Klebsiella*, pneumococci (many others)	—
Peritoneal dialysis	*Staphylococcus*, *Streptococcus*, *E. coli*, *Klebsiella*, *Pseudomonas*	—
Secondary Bacterial Peritonitis		
Gastroduodenal	*Streptococcus*, *E. coli*	—
Biliary tract	*E. coli*, *Klebsiella*, enterococci	*Clostridium* or *Bacteroides* (infrequent)
Small or large bowel	*E. coli*, *Klebsiella*, *Proteus*	*B. fragilis* and other *Bacteroides*, *Clostridium*
Appendicitis	*E. coli*, *Pseudomonas*	*Bacteroides*
Abscesses	*E. coli*, *Klebsiella*, *Streptococcus*, enterococci	*B. fragilis* and other *Bacteroides*, *Clostridium*, anaerobic cocci
Liver	*E. coli*, *Klebsiella*, *Streptococcus*, enterococci, *Staphylococcus*, amoeba	*Bacteroides* (infrequent)
Spleen	*Staphylococcus*, *Streptococcus*, *E. coli*, *Salmonella*	

▶ *Antimicrobial Experience*

Important findings from the last 25 years of clinical trials regarding selection of antimicrobials for IAIs are as follows:

- Antimicrobial regimens for secondary IAIs should cover a broad spectrum of aerobic and anaerobic bacteria from the GI tract. Worrisome is the development of hospital-acquired IAIs with bacteria such as *P. aeruginosa*, *Acinetobacter* spp., *Proteus* spp., B-lactamase producing bacteria, methicillin-resistant *S. aureus* (MRSA), *Enterobacteriaceae*, *Candida* spp., and Enterococci that make the clinical management of these patients challenging.
- Single-agent regimens (such as antianaerobic cephalosporins, extended-spectrum penicillins with β-lactamase inhibitors, or carbapenems) are as effective as combinations of aminoglycosides or fluoroquinolones with antianaerobic agents. This is also true for antimicrobial treatment of acute bacterial contamination from penetrating abdominal trauma.
- Newer agents such as tigecycline and ertapenem may offer some theoretical advantages in the treatment of IAIs, but have some limitations. Tigecycline has a broad spectrum of activity against both aerobic and anaerobic gram negative rods, but lacks sufficient anti-*Pseudomonal* activity. Ertapenem is an example of a carbapenem that has a favorable pharmacokinetic profile (once daily dosing) and, like the other agents, lacks MRSA activity.
- Clindamycin and metronidazole appear to be equivalent in efficacy when combined with agents effective against aerobic gram-negative bacilli (eg, gentamicin or aztreonam).
- For most patients, antimicrobial treatment can be completed orally with moxifloxacin, ciprofloxacin and metronidazole, levofloxacin plus metronidazole, or amoxicillin–clavulanate or the combination of ciprofloxacin and metronidazole.
- Four to 7 days of antimicrobial treatment are sufficient for most IAIs of mild to moderate severity.

IAI presents in many different ways and with a wide spectrum of severity. The antibiotic regimen employed and duration of treatment depends on the specific clinical circumstances (ie, the nature of the underlying disease process and the condition of the patient).

Recommendations

KEY CONCEPT *For most IAIs, the antimicrobial regimen should be effective against both aerobic and anaerobic bacteria.*[15] Although it is impossible to provide antimicrobial activity against every possible pathogen, agents with activity against enteric gram-negative bacilli, such as *E. coli* and *Klebsiella*, and anaerobes, such as *B. fragilis* and *Clostridia* spp., should be administered.

Table 77–2 presents the recommended agents for treatment of community-acquired and complicated IAIs from the Infectious Diseases Society of America and the Surgical Infection Society.[15] These recommendations were formulated using an

Table 77–2

Recommended Agents for the Treatment of Community-Acquired Complicated Intraabdominal Infections in Adults

Agents Recommended for Mild-to-Moderate Infections	Agents Recommended for High Risk or High Severity Infections
Single Agent	
Cefoxitin[a]	Piperacillin–tazobactam
Ticarcillin–clavulanate	
Moxifloxacin[b]	Imipenem–cilastatin,[c]
Ertapenem[c]	Meropenem,[c] doripenem[c]
Combination Regimens	
Cefazolin,[a] cefuroxime,[a] ceftriaxone, cefotaxime each in combination with metronidazole	Cefepime or ceftazidime each in combination with metronidazole
Ciprofloxacin[b] or levofloxacin[b] each in combination with metronidazole	Ciprofloxacin[b] or levofloxacin[b] each in combination with metronidazole

[a]Empiric first- and second-generation cephalosporin use should be avoided unless local antibiograms show > 80% to 90% susceptibility of *E. coli* to these agents.

[b]Use of quinolones may be associated with treatment failure due to increasing resistance of enteric pathogens including *E. coli*. Empiric quinolone use should be avoided unless local antibiograms show > 80% to 90% susceptibility of *E. coli* to quinolones.

[c]Carbapenems should typically be reserved for settings where there is a high risk of resistance to other agents.

Data from Pharmacotherapy: A Pathophysiologic Approach, 9th edition Adapted from Solomkin et al.

evidence-based approach. Most community-acquired infections are "mild to moderate," whereas health care-associated infections tend to be more severe and difficult to treat. Table 77–3 presents guidelines for treatment and alternative regimens for specific situations. These are general guidelines; there are many factors that cannot be incorporated into such a table.

When used for IAI, aminoglycosides should be combined with agents that are effective against the majority of *B. fragilis*; however, their side-effect profile may prohibit use secondary to nephrotoxicity. Clindamycin or metronidazole is the agent of first choice, but others, such as antianaerobic cephalosporins (eg, cefoxitin, cefotetan, or ceftizoxime), piperacillin, mezlocillin, and combinations of extended-spectrum penicillins with β-lactamase inhibitors would be suitable alternative. Preemptive antifungal therapy should maybe be indicated with either an azole antifungal (fluconazole) or an echinocandin (caspofungin) in patients who are immunocompromised or postsurgical with recurrent infection.

In immunocompromised patients or patients with valvular heart disease or a prosthetic heart valve, there is justification to provide specific antimicrobial activity against enterococci. Ampicillin or other penicillins that are active against enterococci (eg, penicillin, piperacillin, and mezlocillin) should be used in patients at high-risk, patients with persistent or recurrent IAI, or patients who are immunosuppressed, such as after organ transplantation. Ampicillin remains the drug of choice for this indication because it is most active in vitro against enterococci and is relatively inexpensive. Vancomycin is active against most enterococci; however, resistance is increasing, and this agent should be reserved for established infections when first-line therapies cannot be used.

Intraperitoneal (IP) administration of antibiotics is preferred over IV therapy in the treatment of peritonitis that occurs in patients undergoing CAPD.[16] The International Society of Peritoneal Dialysis guidelines for the diagnosis and pharmacotherapy of PD-associated infections provide dosing recommendations for intermittent and continuous therapy based on the modality of dialysis (CAPD or automated PD [APD]) and the extent of the patient's residual renal function.[10]

KEY CONCEPT *Antimicrobial agents effective against both gram-positive and gram-negative organisms should be used for initial IP empirical therapy for peritonitis in PD patients.* The most important factors to take into consideration for initial antimicrobial selection are the dialysis center's and the patient's history of infecting organisms and their sensitivities. The use of cefazolin (loading dose [LD] 500 mg/L, maintenance dose [MD] 125 mg/L) plus ceftazidime (LD 500 mg/L, MD 125 mg/L) or cefepime (LD 500 mg/L, MD 125 mg/L) or an aminoglycoside (gentamicin-tobramycin LD 8 mg/L, MD 4 mg/L) is suitable for initial empirical therapy; if patients are allergic to cephalosporin antibiotics, vancomycin (LD 1000 mg/L, MD 25 mg/L) or an aminoglycoside should be substituted. Aztreonam is an alternative to ceftazidime or cefepime in this patient population. Another option is monotherapy with imipenem-cilastin (LD 750 mg/L, MD 50 mg/L) or cefepime. Antimicrobial doses should be increased empirically by 25% in patients with residual renal function (greater than 100 mL/day urine output).[10] Antimicrobial therapy should be continued for at least 1 week after the dialysate fluid is clear and for a total of at least 14 days. The reader is referred to these guidelines for additional information.[10]

After acute bacterial contamination, such as with abdominal trauma where GI contents spill into the peritoneum, combination antimicrobial regimens are not required. If the patient is seen soon after injury (within 2 hours) and surgical measures are instituted promptly, antianaerobic cephalosporins (eg, cefoxitin or cefotetan) or extended-spectrum penicillins are effective in preventing most infectious complications. Antimicrobials should be administered as soon as possible after injury.[17]

For appendicitis, the antimicrobial regimen used should depend on the appearance of the appendix at the time of operation, which may be normal, inflamed, gangrenous, or perforated. Because the condition of the appendix is unknown preoperatively, it is advisable to begin antimicrobial agents before the appendectomy is performed. Reasonable regimens would be antianaerobic cephalosporins or, if the patient is seriously ill, a carbapenem or β-lactam–β-lactamase-inhibitor combination. If, at operation, the appendix were normal or inflamed, postoperative antimicrobials would not be required. If the appendix is gangrenous or perforated, a treatment course of 5 to 7 days with the agents listed in Table 77–2 is appropriate.

KEY CONCEPT *Acute intra-abdominal contamination, such as after a traumatic injury, may be treated with a short course (24 hours) of antimicrobials.*[17] *For established infections (ie, peritonitis or intra-abdominal abscess), an antimicrobial course limited to 4 to 7 days is justified.* Under certain conditions, therapy for longer than 7 days would be justified, for example, if the patient remains febrile or is in poor general condition, when relatively resistant bacteria are isolated, or when a focus of infection in the abdomen still may be present. For some abscesses, such as pyogenic liver abscess, antimicrobials may be required for a month or longer.

Table 77–3

Guidelines for Empiric Antimicrobial Agents for Intraabdominal Infections [39,49]

	Primary Agents	Alternatives
Primary (Spontaneous) Bacterial Peritonitis		
Cirrhosis	Ceftriaxone, cefotaxime	1. Piperacillin–tazobactam, carbapenems 2. Aztreonam combined with an agent active against *Streptococcus* spp. (e.g., vancomycin) or quinolones with significant *Streptococcus* spp. activity (levofloxacin, moxifloxacin)
Peritoneal dialysis	Initial empiric regimens should be active against both gram-positive (including *S. aureus*) and gram-negative pathogens: Gram-positive agent (first-generation cephalosporin or vancomycin) plus a gram-negative agent (third-generation cephalosporin or aminoglycoside)	1. Cefepime or carbapenems may be used alone 2. Aztreonam or an aminoglycoside may be used in place of ceftazidime or cefepime as long as combined with a gram-positive agent 3. Quinolones may be used in place of gram-negative agents if local susceptibilities allow
	1. *Staphylococcus* spp.:oxacillin/nafcillin or first-generation cephalosporin	1. Vancomycin should be used if concern for methicillin-resistant *Staphylococcus* spp. 2. Add rifampin for 5–7 days with vancomycin for methicillin-resistant *Staphylococcus aureus*
	2. *Streptococcus* or *Enterococcus*: ampicillin	1. An aminoglycoside may be added for *Enterococcus* spp. 2. Linezolid, daptomycin, or quinupristin/dalfopristin should be used to treat vancomycin-resistant *Enterococcus* spp. not susceptible to ampicillin
	3. Aerobic gram-negative bacilli: ceftazidime or cefepime	1. The regimen should be based on in vitro sensitivity tests
	4. *Pseudomonas aeruginosa*: two agents with differing mechanisms of action, such as an oral quinolone plus ceftazidime, cefepime, tobramycin, or piperacillin	
Secondary Bacterial Peritonitis		
Perforated peptic ulcer	First-generation cephalosporins	1. Ceftriaxone, cefotaxime, or antianaerobic cephalosporins[a]
Other	Third- or fourth-generation cephalosporin with metronidazole, piperacillin–tazobactam or ticarcillin–clavulanate, carbapenem	1. Ciprofloxacin[b] or levofloxacin[b] each with metronidazole or *moxifloxacin*[b] alone 2. Aztreonam with vancomycin and metronidazole 3. Antianaerobic cephalosporins[a]
Abscess		
General	Third- or fourth-generation cephalosporin with metronidazole, piperacillin–tazobactam, or ticarcillin–clavulanate	1. Imipenem–cilastatin, meropenem, doripenem, or ertapenem 2. Ciprofloxacin[b] or levofloxacin[b] each with metronidazole or moxifloxacin alone
Liver	As above	Use metronidazole if amoebic liver abscess is suspected
Spleen	Ceftriaxone or cefotaxime	Moxifloxacin[b] or levofloxacin[b]
Other Intraabdominal Infections		
Appendicitis	Same management as for community-acquired complicated intraabdominal infections as listed in Table 92-6[39]	
Community-Acquired Acute Cholecystitis	Ceftriaxone or cefotaxime	Severe infection, piperacillin/tazobactam, antipseuodomonal carbapenem, aztreonam with metronidazole
Cholangitis	Ceftriaxone or cefotaxime each with or without metronidazole	Vancomycin with aztreonam with or without metronidazole
Acute Contamination from Abdominal Trauma	Antianaerobic cephalosporins[a] or metronidazole with either ceftriaxone or cefotaxime	1. Piperacillin/tazobactam or a carbapenem 2. Ciprofloxacin[b] or levofloxacin[b] each with metronidazole or moxifloxacin alone

[a]Cefoxitin or ceftizoxime; these agents should be avoided empirically unless local antibiograms show > 80% to 90% susceptibility of *E. coli* to these agents.

[b]Use of quinolones may be associated with treatment failure due to increasing resistance of enteric pathogens including *E. coli*. Empiric quinolone use should be avoided unless local antibiograms show > 80% to 90% susceptibility of *E. coli* to quinolones.

OUTCOME EVALUATION

Whether diagnosed with primary or secondary peritonitis, monitor the patient for relief of symptoms. Once antimicrobials are initiated and the other important therapies described earlier are used, most patients should show improvement within 2 to 3 days.

Successful antimicrobial therapy with resolution of infection will result in decreased pain, manifested as resolution of abdominal guarding and decreased use of pain medications over time. The patient should not appear in distress, with the exception of recognized discomfort and pain from incisions, drains, and a nasogastric tube.

Monitor vital signs and WBC count with differential; each should normalize as the infection resolves. At 24 to 48 hours, aerobic bacterial culture results should be available. If a suspected pathogen is not sensitive to the antimicrobial agents being given, the regimen should be changed if the patient has not shown sufficient improvement. If the isolated pathogen is extremely sensitive to one antimicrobial and the patient is progressing well, concurrent antimicrobial therapy often may be discontinued.

With anaerobic culturing techniques and the slow growth of these organisms, anaerobes often are not identified until 4 to 7 days after culture, and sensitivity information is difficult to obtain. For this reason, anaerobic culture information generally is not helpful for selection of the antianaerobic component of the antimicrobial regimen.

Once the patient's temperature is normal for 48 to 72 hours and the patient is eating, consider changing the IV antibiotic to an oral regimen for the duration of antibiotic treatment. Monitor the serum creatinine level to evaluate for renal complications as well as potential drug toxicity, especially if an aminoglycoside is a component of the antibiotic regimen. Bowel sounds should return to normal. Evaluate the patient daily for development of rash or other drug-related adverse effects.

For patients with primary peritonitis, if peritoneal dialysate cultures were positive initially, repeat cultures should be negative. For patients with secondary peritonitis, monitor the amount of fluid draining if a drain was placed. The volume of drainage should lessen as the infection resolves. Repeat abdominal radiographs should return to normal.

If symptoms do not improve, the patient should be evaluated for persistent infection. There are many reasons for poor patient outcome with IAI; improper antimicrobial selection is only one. The patient may be immunocompromised, which decreases the likelihood of successful outcome with any regimen. It is impossible for antimicrobials to compensate for a nonfunctioning immune system. There may be surgical reasons for poor patient outcome. Failure to identify all intra-abdominal foci of infection or leaks from a GI anastomosis may cause continued IAI. Even when IAI is controlled, accompanying organ system failure, most often renal or respiratory, may lead to patient demise.

KEY CONCEPT *Health care-associated infections are becoming more common for IAIs secondary to acute care hospital admissions or admissions from chronic care settings. The major pathogens include more resistant gram-negative flora,* Candida *infections causing peritonitis, and Enterococcal species.*

The outcome from IAI is not determined solely by what transpires in the abdomen. Unsatisfactory outcomes in patients with IAIs may result from complications that arise in other organ systems. Infectious complications commonly associated with mortality after IAI are urinary tract infections and pneumonia.[18] Reasons for antimicrobial failure may not always be apparent. Even when antimicrobial susceptibility tests indicate that an organism is susceptible in vitro to the antimicrobial agent, therapeutic failures may occur. Possibly there is poor penetration of the antimicrobial agent into the focus of infection, or bacterial resistance may develop after initiation of antimicrobial therapy. Also, it is possible that an antimicrobial regimen may encourage the development of infection by organisms not susceptible to the regimen being used. Superinfection in patients being treated for IAI can be caused by *Candida*; however, Enterococci or opportunistic gram-negative bacilli such as *Pseudomonas* and *Serratia* may be involved.

Treatment regimens for IAI can be judged as successful if the patient recovers from the infection without recurrent peritonitis or intra-abdominal abscess and without the need for additional antimicrobials. A regimen can be considered unsuccessful if a significant adverse drug reaction occurs, reoperation or percutaneous drainage is necessary, or patient improvement is delayed beyond 1 or 2 weeks.

Patient Care Process

Patient Assessment:

- You should do a thorough patient medication history at the time of admission to document all recent medication use, including nonprescription medications and use of complementary or alternative medicines. You should also document any drug allergies or intolerances for your patient you are working up.

Therapeutic Evaluation:

- Be cognizant for the initial antimicrobial regimen conforming to standard guidelines (unless an appropriate justification for an alternative regimen is evident). See Table 77–3.

Care Plan Development:

- You need to review the dosages of all medications to be sure that they are appropriate for age, weight, and major organ function.
- You should also verify that the drugs selected are not contraindicated in the patient with allergies or other intolerances.
- You should select antimicrobials that are appropriate based on the susceptibility information, while reviewing the results of the obtained both preoperatively or during the surgical procedure.
- On the fifth day of antimicrobial treatment or when GI function returns, determine whether parenteral antimicrobial agents can be switched to oral agents to complete therapy.
- Assess nutritional needs and recommend appropriate supplementation. When the patient is tolerating an oral diet, determine whether any parenteral medications can be switched to the oral route.

Follow-Up Evaluation:

- You should monitor the patient for the development of potential complications of treatment such as delayed hypersensitivity reactions, antibiotic-induced diarrhea, pseudomembranous colitis, or fungal superinfections (manifested as oral thrush).
- You should also provide information to the patient concerning the medications administered in the hospital as well as any new medications prescribed for use at home.
- You should also advise the patient to contact his or her doctor or pharmacist if he or she experiences any adverse effects from medications.

Abbreviations Introduced in This Chapter

ANC	Absolute neutrophil count
APD	Automated peritoneal dialysis
CAPD	Continuous ambulatory peritoneal dialysis
DPL	Diagnostic peritoneal lavage
IAIs	Intra-abdominal infections
IP	Intraperitoneal
LD	Loading dose
MD	Maintenance dose
MRSA	Methicillin-resistant *S. aureus*
PD	Peritoneal dialysis

REFERENCES

1. Ordonez CA, Puyana JC. Management of peritonitis in the critically ill patient. Surg Clin North Am. 2006;86:1323–1349.
2. Marshall JC. Intra-abdominal infections. Microbes Infect. 2004;6:1015–1025.
3. Mowat C, Stanley AJ. Spontaneous bacterial peritonitis—Diagnosis, treatment, and prevention. Aliment Pharmacol Therap. 2001;15:1851–1859.
4. Vas S, Oreopoulos DG. Infections in patients undergoing peritoneal dialysis. Infect Dis Clin North Am. 2001;15:743–774.
5. CDC/NCHS National Hospital Discharge Survey./ftp://ftp.cdc.gov/pub/Health_Statistics/NCGS/Dataset_Documentation/NHDS/NHDS_2010_Documentation.pdf
6. Sartelli M, Viale P, Catena F et al. WSES guidelines for management of intra-abdominal infections. World J Emerg Surg. 2013;8:1–29.
7. Thompson AE, Marshall JC, Opal SM. Intraabdominal infections in infants and children: Descriptions and definitions. Pediatr Crit Care Med. 2005;6:S30–S35.
8. Căruntu FA, Benea L. Spontaneous bacterial peritonitis: Pathogenesis, diagnosis, treatment. J Gastroint Liver Dis. 2006;15:51–56.
9. Johnson DH, Cuhna BA. Infections in cirrhosis. Infect Dis Clin North Am. 2001;15:363–371.
10. Li PK, Szeto CC, Piraino B, et al. Peritoneal dialysis-related infections: 2010 update. Perit Dial Int. 2010;30:393–423.
11. Brook I. Microbiology and management of abdominal infections. Dig Dis Sci. 2008;53:2585–2591.
12. Ball CG, Hansen G, Harding G, et al. Canadian practice guidelines for surgical intra-abdominal infections. Can J Infect Dis Med Microbiol. 2010;21:11–37.
13. Gauzit R, Pean Y, Barth X, etal. Epidemiology, management, and prognosis of secondary non-postoperative peritonitis: A French prospective observational multicenter study. Surg Infect. 2009;10(2):119–127.
14. Jaffe TA, Nelson RC, Delong DM, Paulson EK. Practice patterns in percutaneous image-guided intraabdominal abscess drainage: Survey of academic and private practice centers. Radiology. 2004;233:750–756.
15. Solomkin JS, Mazuski JE, Bradley JS, et al. Diagnosis and management of complicated intra-abdominal infection in adults and children: Guidelines by the Surgical Infection Society and the Infectious Diseases Society of America. Clin Infect Dis. 2010;50:133–164.
16. Wiggins KJ, Craig JC, Johnson DW, Strippoli GF. Treatment for peritoneal dialysis-associated peritonitis. Cochrane Database Syst Rev. 2008;(1):CD005284.
17. Bozorgzadeh A, Pizzi WF, Barie PS, et al. The duration of antibiotic administration in penetrating abdominal trauma. Am J Surg. 1999;172:125–135.
18. Merlino JI, Yowler CJ, Malangoni MA. Nosocomial infections adversely affect the outcomes of patients with serious intraabdominal infections. Surg Infect (Larchmt). 2004;5:21–27.

78 Parasitic Diseases

J. V. Anandan

LEARNING OBJECTIVES

Upon completion of the chapter, the reader will be able to:

1. Identify the primary reasons why some parasitic diseases may be more prevalent in the US population.
2. Describe the treatment algorithm for giardiasis and amebiasis.
3. List one effective therapy for nematodes and select the drugs of choice for strongyloidiasis and tapeworms.
4. List three major reasons why travelers are infected with malaria.
5. Describe the presenting signs and symptoms of malaria.
6. List some specific toxicities of mefloquine.
7. Identify the monitoring parameters for quinidine gluconate in severe malaria.
8. Define the major complications of falciparum malaria.
9. Discuss the cardiovascular complications of chronic South American trypanosomiasis.
10. Describe the steps to take to eradicate lice infestation and scabies.

INTRODUCTION

The increased desire of large segments of the US population to travel to Asia, Africa, and other parts of the world can expose them to parasitic infections that are endemic in those areas. The influx of refugees and new immigrant populations from Asia and other parts of the world have brought new parasitic infections to our shores. Migrant farm workers, the large and growing Central and South American immigrant population, and the presence of immunosuppressed populations (eg, those with the AIDS and transplant patients) represent significant sources of parasitic infections in the United States.[1–5]

Terms that are frequently used when discussing parasitic diseases are as follows.[6] *Symbiosis* means "living together," when two species are dependent on each other for food and protection. The term *commensalism*, implies a mutual association in which both organisms may benefit, or at least one benefits but does no harm to the other. In contrast, *parasitism*, although resembling symbiosis in that it is also an intimate relationship between two species does not represent a mutually beneficial association. One species (the host) does not benefit from the relationship, and in fact the relationship may be detrimental to its survival.

Parasites have made metabolic and other defensive adaptations over time to increase their ability to survive host defenses and have allowed them to utilize the host's biochemical systems to synthesize necessary cellular components. Beef and pork tapeworms (cestodes) possess highly developed reproductive systems that allow them to transfer easily to new hosts. Because of the lack of digestive systems, cestodes are completely host-dependent for all nutrients. Cestodes (tapeworms) (*Taenia saginata* and *Taenia solium*) use specialized suckers that enable them to obtain blood and vital nutrients from their host. *Entamoeba histolytica*, once it has gained access to the human colon or large intestine is able to invade and utilize its specialized proteolytic enzyme to erode the GI mucosa. *E. histolytica* is also able to survive in adverse conditions by walling itself off and forming cysts; this protects the parasite from environmental conditions until it is ready to infect the next host.

Although acquired immunity to some parasitic diseases may lower the level of infection, absolute immunity as seen in bacterial and viral infections is seldom seen in parasitic diseases. Since parasitic infections produce a wide variety of antigens because of the many life cycle phases, it is more difficult to identify a constant antigenic protein against which specific antibodies are protective. However, malaria remains a likely candidate for a vaccine and there are ongoing studies to develop one.

For more detailed discussions of the world of parasites, clinicians and students are directed to some excellent resources on parasites and parasitic diseases.[5,6] Discussion in this chapter includes parasitic diseases more likely seen in the United States and includes GI parasites (primarily giardiasis and amebiasis), protozoan infections (malaria and South American trypanosomiasis), some common helminthic diseases (specifically those caused by nematodes and cestodes), and ectoparasites (lice and scabies).

GIARDIASIS

Epidemiology and Etiology

Giardia lamblia (*G. intestinalis* or *G. duodenalis*), is the most common intestinal parasite responsible for diarrheal syndromes throughout the world and is the most frequently identified

Patient Encounter 1: Giardiasis

LA is a 29-year-old recently returned US resident who had traveled to Texcoco in Mexico to visit a friend he had met at a meeting in Mexico city. Although the majority of his meals were in his friend's house, the night before returning home he had a meal at a local restaurant. Three days after his return from Texcoco he developed severe nausea, diarrhea, alternating with constipation. When he is seen at the travel clinic at a local hospital, he reports nausea and crampy, watery diarrhea with foul-smelling stools for four days. LA also reported that his stool was "light-colored."

Are his symptoms characteristic of parasitic-associated diarrhea?

How would you differentiate giardiasis from an Escherichia coli–induced diarrhea?

intestinal parasites in the United States, with a prevalence rate of 5% to 15% in some areas. *G. lamblia* has been identified as the first enteric pathogen in children in developing countries, with prevalence rates between 15% and 30%.[7,8]

There are two stages in the life cycle of *G. lamblia*: the trophozoite and the cyst. *G. lamblia* is found in the small intestine, the gallbladder, and in biliary drainage.[7,8] The distribution of giardiasis is worldwide, with children being more susceptible than adults.

Pathophysiology

Giardiasis is caused by ingestion of *G. lamblia* cysts in fecally contaminated water or food.[7,8] The protozoan excysts in the low gastric pH to release the trophozoite. Colonization and multiplication of the trophozoite lead to mucosal invasion, localized edema, and flattening of the villi, resulting in malabsorption states in the host. Achlorhydria, hypogammaglobulinemia, or deficiency in secretory immunoglobulin A (IgA) predispose to giardiasis.[7] Individuals with HIV infection and AIDS may have higher carriage rates than the general population. Some patients may develop lactose intolerance after chronic giardiasis.

Pharmacologic Therapy

KEY CONCEPT *All symptomatic adults and children over the age of 8 years with giardiasis should be treated with metronidazole 250 mg three times daily for 7 days, or tinidazole 2 g as a single dose, or nitazoxanide (Alina) 500 mg twice daily for 3 days.*[9] The pediatric dose of metronidazole is 15 mg/kg/day three times daily for 7 days. Alternative drugs include furazolidone 100 mg four times daily or paromomycin 25 to 35 mg/kg/day in divided doses daily for 7 days. Paromomycin may be used in pregnancy instead of metronidazole. Pediatric patients can also be treated with suspensions of furazolidone 6 mg/kg/day in four divided doses for 7 days.

Quinacrine 100 mg three times in adults or 5 mg/kg/day in pediatric patients for 5 to 7 days, is available from a specialized pharmacy (eg, Panorama Compounding Pharmacy).[9]

Outcome Evaluation

Patients with symptomatic giardiasis and positive stool samples or positive enzyme-linked immunosorbent assay (ELISA) tests should be treated with metronidazole for 7 days. Patients who

Clinical Presentation and Diagnosis of Giardiasis

Acute Onset

- Diarrhea, cramp-like abdominal pain, bloating, and flatulence
- Malaise, anorexia, nausea, and belching

Chronic Symptoms

- Diarrhea: Foul-smelling, copious, light-colored, and greasy stools
- Weight loss, steatorrhea, and vitamin B_{12} and fat-soluble vitamin deficiencies
- Constipation alternating with diarrhea

Diagnosis

- Diagnosis is made by examination of fresh stool or a preserved specimen during acute diarrheal phase
- Fresh stool may show trophozoites, whereas preserved specimens yield cysts. (*Note:* stool for ova may show the presence of other parasites [eg, *Cryptosporidium parvum, E. histolytica*, or *E. hartmanni*]; multiple stool samples may be needed.)
- Stool examination for ova and parasites is the major means of diagnosis, and other diagnostic tests include enzyme-linked immunosorbent assay (ELISA), which is considered to be between 85% and 98% sensitive and almost 100% specific (ProSpec T, Giardia Microplate Assay, Remel, Lenexa, KS.)

Patient Care Process: Giardiasis

Patient Assessment:

- Evaluate patient medical history, recent travel, signs, and symptoms.
- Conduct a medication history, review laboratory findings and consider if stool for O/P and other tests may be necessary for diagnosis of giardiasis.

Therapy Evaluation:

- Based on symptoms and laboratory findings, consider the appropriate pharmacotherapy for the patient.
- Discuss expected side effects, any drug interactions and availability of the prescribed medication in the community or hospital.

Care Plan Development:

- Consider any dietary or other considerations for giardiasis—fluids and replacements for deficiencies if warranted.
- Address patient concerns about the infection and the therapy.

Follow-Up Evaluation:

- Decide when patient should come back for follow-up.
- Inform patient for repeat stool for O/P and the need for reevaluation at the end of therapy.

fail initial therapy with metronidazole should receive a second course of therapy. Pregnant patients can receive paromomycin 25 to 35 mg/kg/day in divided doses for 7 days. Giardiasis can be prevented by good hygiene and by using caution in food and drink consumption.

AMEBIASIS

Epidemiology and Etiology

Amebiasis remains one of the most important parasitic diseases because of its worldwide distribution and serious GI manifestations. The major causative agent in amebiasis is *E. histolytica*, which invades the colon and must be differentiated from *Entamoeba dispar*, which is associated with an asymptomatic carrier state and is considered nonpathogenic.[10,11] Invasive amebiasis is almost exclusively the result of ingesting *E. histolytica* cysts found in fecally contaminated food or water. Approximately 50 million cases of invasive disease result each year worldwide, leading to an excess of 100,000 deaths. In the general population, the highest incidence is found in institutionalized mentally retarded patients, sexually active homosexuals, AIDS patients, the Native American population, and new immigrants from endemic areas (eg, Mexico, South and Southeast Asia, West and South Africa, and portions of Central and South America).[10,11]

Pathophysiology

E. histolytica invades mucosal cells of colonic epithelium, producing the classic flask-shaped ulcer in the submucosa. The trophozoite toxin has a cytocidal effect on cells. If the trophozoite gets into the portal circulation, it will be carried to the liver, where it produces abscess and periportal fibrosis. Liver abscesses are more common in men than women and are rarely seen in children.[11,12] Amebic ulcerations can affect the perineum and genitalia, and abscesses may occur in the lung and brain.

Erosion of liver abscesses can result in peritonitis. Liver abscesses that are located in the right lobe can spread to the lungs and pleura. Pericardial infection, although rare, may be associated with extension of the amebic abscesses from the liver.[11,12]

Patient Encounter 2: Amebiasis

DR is a 32-year-old computer programmer who, on returning from visiting Angkor Wat in Siem Reap, Cambodia, is seen in the emergency department at Detroit Receiving Hospital with complaints of a 3-day history of severe diarrhea, cramps, and postprandial abdominal pain. The abdominal pain is over the right lower quadrant and associated with nausea and flatulence. DR indicates that he had some diarrhea the night after he had visited a local restaurant in Siem Reap. The diarrhea subsided after treatment from a local physician. However, 5 days later after his return to the States, his symptoms came back.

What specific findings in this patient suggest that he may have giardiasis, amebiasis or an E. coli-associated diarrhea?

What specific laboratory or diagnostic test will confirm a diagnosis of amebiasis?

Describe some of the complications associated with amebiasis.

Clinical Presentation and Diagnosis of Amebiasis

Review of the patient's history should include the following: recent travel, type of foods ingested (eg, salads or unpeeled fruit), the nature of water and fluid consumed, and description of any symptoms of friends or relatives who ate the same food

Intestinal Disease

- Vague abdominal discomfort
- Symptoms may range from malaise to severe abdominal cramps, flatulence, and nonbloody or bloody diarrhea (heme-positive in 100% of cases) with mucus
- May have low-grade fever, but this may be absent in many patients
- Eosinophilia is usually absent, although mild leukocytosis is not unusual

Note: Fecal screening may show other intestinal parasites, including *Cryptosporidium* spp., *Balantidium coli, Dientamoeba fragilis, Isospora belli, G. lamblia,* or *Blastocystis hominis.*

Amebic Liver Abscess

- May present with high fever with significant leukocytosis with **left shift**, anemia, elevated alanine aminotransferase, and dull abdominal pain on palpation
- *Physical findings:* Right upper quadrant pain, hepatomegaly, and liver tenderness, with referred pain to the left or right shoulder (*Note*: Erosion of liver abscesses may present as peritonitis.)

KEY CONCEPT Diagnosis

- *Intestinal amebiasis is diagnosed by demonstrating E. histolytica cysts or trophozoites (may contain ingested erythrocytes) in fresh stool or from a specimen obtained by sigmoidoscopy*
- *Microscopy may not differentiate between the pathogenic E. histolytica and the nonpathogenic (commensal) E. dispar or E. moshkovskii in stools*
- *Sensitive techniques are available to detect E. histolytica in stool: antigen detection, antibody test (ELISA) and polymerase chain reaction (PCR)*
- **Endoscopy** with scrapings or biopsy and stained slides (iron hematoxylin or trichrome) may provide more definitive diagnosis of amebiasis
- Diagnosis for liver abscess includes serology and liver scans (using isotopes by ultrasound or computed tomography [CT]) or MRI; however, none of these are specific for liver abcess. In rare instances, needle aspiration of hepatic abscess may be attempted using ultrasound guidance

Pharmacologic Therapy

Metronidazole (Flagyl), dehydroemetine, and chloroquine (Aralen) are tissue-acting agents, and iodoquinol (Yodoxin), diloxanide furoate (Furamide), and paromomycin (Humatin) are well absorbed that the amounts of the drug remaining in the bowel may be insufficient to have luminal or local effects. A agent active in the GI lumen, on the other hand, may not attain effective enough levels in the tissue to be efficacious. Asymptomatic cyst passers (identified by stool examinations, and who may develop invasive disease) and patients with mild intestinal amebiasis should receive a luminal agent: paromomycin 25 to 35 mg/kg/day three times daily for 7 days, or iodoquinol 650 mg three times daily for 20 days. These regimens have cure rates of between 84% and 96%. The pediatric dose of paromomycin is the same as that used in adults, whereas the pediatric dose of iodoquinol is 30 to 40 mg/kg (maximum: 2 g) per day in three doses for 20 days, and the pediatric dose of diloxanide furoate is 20 mg/kg/day in three doses for 10 days. Paromomycin is the preferred agent in pregnant patients.[9,11]

Patients with severe intestinal disease or liver abscess should receive metronidazole 750 mg three times daily for 10 days, followed by the luminal agents indicated previously. The pediatric dose of metronidazole is 50 mg/kg/day in divided doses, which should be followed by a luminal agent.[11–14] An alternative regimen of metronidazole is 2.4 g/day for 2 days in combination with the luminal agent.[9,11,12] Tinidazole administered in a dose of 2 g daily for 3 days (pediatric dose: 50 mg/kg for 3 days; can be crushed and added to cherry syrup) is an alternative to metronidazole.[9] If there is no prompt response to metronidazole or aspiration of the abscess, an antibiotic regimen should be added. Patients who cannot tolerate oral doses of metronidazole should receive an IV dose of metronidazole.[11,12]

Outcome Evaluation

Follow-up in patients with amebiasis should include repeat stool examinations, serology, colonoscopy (in colitis), or CT scan a month after the end of therapy. Serial liver scans have demonstrated healing of liver abscesses over 4 to 8 months after adequate therapy.[12,14]

Patient Care Process: Amebiasis

Patient Assessment:

- Based on physical exam, review of systems and travel history, determine if these findings are consistent with giardiasis or amebiasis.
- Address what specific diagnostic tests would be required to make a definitive diagnosis for amebiasis.
- Conduct a medication history and check for allergies.

Therapy Evaluation:

- Determine, based on the results of the diagnostic tests, whether this is amebic colitis or colitis with liver abscess.
- Verify whether the drug or drugs you intend to use is on the hospital formulary or readily available at a local pharmacy.

Care Plan Development:

- Select pharmacotherapy and appropriate regimen and check for any potential drug interactions.
- Address any patient concerns and discuss the need for medication adherence and dietary restrictions.

Follow-Up Evaluation:

- Follow-up in 10 days and repeat tests to evaluate therapy.
- Monitor for efficacy and toxicity.

HELMINTHIC DISEASES

Helminthic infections include three groups of organisms: roundworms or nematodes, flukes (trematodes), and tapeworms (cestodes). Brief descriptions of some of the helminthic infections most commonly seen in North America and their treatments are provided here. Although helminthic infections may not produce clinical manifestations, they can cause significant pathology. One factor that determines the pathogenicity of helminthic infections is their population density; a high-density population ("worm burden") results in predictable disease presentation. In the United States, these infections are reported most frequently in recent immigrants from Southeast Asia, the Caribbean, Mexico, and Central America.[1,15–17] Populations at risk include institutionalized patients (both young and elderly), preschool children in daycare centers, residents of Native American reservations, and homosexuals.[15,16] Certain conditions and drugs (anesthesia and corticosteroids) can cause atypical localization of worms. Immunocompromised hosts can be overwhelmed by some helminthic infections, such as *Strongyloides stercoralis*.

Nematodes

▸ *Hookworm Disease*

Hookworm infection is caused by *Ancylostoma duodenale* or *Necator americanus*. *N. americanus* is found in the southeastern United States.[15–17] Infective larvae enter the host in contaminated food or water or penetrate the skin and migrate to the small intestine. The adult worm attaches to GI mucosa and causes injury by lytic destruction of the tissue. Over a period of time, the adult worm can cause anemia and hypoproteinemia in the host.[18–20]

▸ *Treatment*

KEY CONCEPT *The drug of choice is mebendazole (Vermox), which is also active against ascariasis, enterobiasis, trichuriasis, and hookworm.*[9,21] The adult and pediatric (age greater than 2 years) oral dose of mebendazole for hookworm is 100 mg twice daily for 3 days. An alternative agent that can be used in both pediatric and adult patients is albendazole (Zentel), 400 mg as a single oral dose. Diagnosis is by detection of eggs or larvae in stool. Stool examination for eggs and the larvae should be repeated in 2 weeks and the patient retreated if necessary.

Ascariasis

The causative agent in ascariasis is the giant roundworm *Ascaris lumbricoides,* which is found worldwide and is responsible for about 4 million infections in the United States (it primarily affects residents of the Appalachian mountain range and the Gulf Coast states).[15–17] Migration of the worm into the lungs usually produces pneumonitis, fever, cough, eosinophilia, and pulmonary infiltrates. *Ascaris* infection can also cause abdominal discomfort, intestinal obstruction, and appendicitis. Diagnosis is made by detection of the characteristic eggs in the stool or passed worms.

▸ *Treatment*

In both adults and pediatric patients older than 2 years of age, mebendazole 100 mg orally twice daily for 3 days is the treatment to use. An alternative agent is pyrantel pamoate (Antiminth).[9] The stool should be checked within 2 weeks and the patient retreated when warranted.

Enterobiasis

Enterobiasis, or pinworm infection, is caused by *Enterobius vermicularis*. It is the most widely distributed helminthic infection in the world.[15–17] There are approximately 42 million cases in the United States, primarily affecting children. The most common manifestation of the infection is cutaneous irritation in the perianal region, resulting from the migrating female or the presence of eggs. The intense pruritus may lead to dermatitis and secondary bacterial infections. Diagnosis is made by the use of a perianal swab and cellophane tape sampling, which will aid in egg identification.

▸ *Treatment*

The three agents that are administered for enterobiasis include pyrantel pamoate, mebendazole, and albendazole.[9] The oral dose of pyrantel pamoate is 11 mg/kg (maximum: 1 g) as a single dose that can be repeated in 2 weeks. The oral dose of mebendazole for both adults and children older than 2 years of age is 100 mg as a single dose. This may be repeated in 2 weeks.[9] Following treatment, to eradicate the eggs, all bedding and underclothing should be sterilized by steaming or washing in the hot cycle of the washing machine.

Strongyloidiasis

Strongyloidiasis is caused by *Strongyloides stercoralis,* which has a worldwide distribution and is predominantly prevalent in South America (Brazil and Columbia) and in Southeast Asia.[33–38] Strongyloidiasis is primarily seen among institutionalized populations (those in mental hospitals and children's hospitals) and immunocompromised individuals (those with HIV infection, AIDS, and patients with hematologic malignancies).[22–24] The worm is usually found in the upper intestine, where the eggs are deposited and hatch to form the rhabditiform larvae. The rhabditiform larva (male and female) migrate to the bowel where they may be excreted in the feces. If excreted in the feces, the larva can evolve into either one of two forms after copulation: a free-living noninfectious rhabditiform larvae, or an infectious filariform larvae. The filariform larva can penetrate host skin and migrate to the lungs and produce progeny, a process called **autoinfection**. This can result in hyperinfection (ie, an increased number of larva in the intestine, lungs, and other internal organs), especially in an immunocompromised host.

Patients with acute infection may develop a localized pruritic rash, but heavy infestations can produce eosinophilia (10%–15% eosinophils [0.10–0.15]), diarrhea, abdominal pain, and intestinal obstruction. Administration of corticosteroids or other immunosuppressive drugs to an infected individual can result in hyperinfections and disseminated strongyloidiasis.[23,24] Diagnosis of strongyloidiasis is made by identification of the rhabditiform larva in stool, sputum, or duodenal fluid, or from small bowel biopsy specimens. Even though antigen testing (ELISA essay) remains the most sensitive method, stool examinations and other body fluids should also be utilized in the diagnosis.[22,24]

▸ *Treatment*

KEY CONCEPT *The drug of choice for strongyloidiasis is oral ivermectin 200 mcg/kg/day for 2 days, whereas albendazole 400 mg twice daily is given for 7 days as an alternative.*[9] With hyperinfection or disseminated strongyloidiasis, immunosuppressive drugs should be discontinued and treatment should be initiated with ivermectin 200 mcg/kg/day until all symptoms are resolved. Patients should be tested periodically to ensure the elimination of the larva. Individuals from an endemic area who are candidates for organ transplantation must be screened for *S. stercoralis*.[24]

Cestodiasis

Cestodiasis (tapeworm infection) is caused by species of the phylum Platyhelminthes (flatworms) and include, among others, the pork tapeworm (*Taenia solium*) and the beef tapeworm (*T. saginata*).[6,25] The tapeworm attaches itself to the mucosal wall of the upper jejunum by the scolex (mouth parts) and by two to four cup-shaped suckers and a structure called a rostellum, which may have hooks in some species. Since the parasite lacks a digestive system, it obtains all nutrients directly from the host. The scolex, proglottids (segments), and eggs are specific for each species and used for identification of tapeworms. Tapeworm infections are caused by ingestion of poorly cooked meat that contains the larva or cysticerci. Cysticerci, when released from the contaminated meat by host digestive juices, mature in the host jejunum. Cystericercosis is a systemic disease caused by the larva of *T. solium* (oncosphere or hexacanth) and is usually acquired by ingestion of eggs in contaminated food or by autoinfection.[6,25] The larvae can penetrate the bowel and migrate through the bloodstream to infect different organs, including the central nervous system (CNS) (neurocysticercosis). Diagnosis of both *T. saginata* and *T. solium* is accomplished by recovery of the gravid proglottids and the scolex in the stool. Newer diagnostic tools for neurocysticercosis include serum and cerebrospinal antigen and antibody testing.[25]

▸ *Treatment*

KEY CONCEPT *Tapeworm infections (T. saginata and T. solium) are treated with praziquantel 5 to 10 mg/kg as a single dose (use the same dose for adults and pediatric patients).*[9] The treatment for cysticercosis and neurocysticercosis may include surgery, anticonvulsants (neurocysticercosis can cause seizures), and anthelmintic therapy. The anthelmintic therapy of choice is albendazole 400 mg twice daily for 5 to 30 days.[25–29] The pediatric dose of albendazole is 15 mg/kg (maximum: 800 mg) in two divided doses for 8 to 30 days. The doses for both adults and pediatric subjects can be repeated if necessary. Praziquantel is an alternative therapy.[9]

Outcome Evaluation

Morbidity and disease due to helminthic infections is related to the intensity of infection. The major adverse effects of helminthic infections are malnutrition, fatigue, and diminished work capacity. Unlike other helminthic infections, strongyloidiasis can cause autoinfection, and in the presence of immunosuppression, it can cause CNS and disseminated infections, which have high mortality.[23,24]

The most serious complication of cysticercosis is neurocysticercosis that can cause strokes and seizures.[26,27] Treatment of neurocysticercosis with anthelmintic treatment remains controversial.

MALARIA

Malaria is one of the most devastating parasitic diseases, affecting a population in excess of 500 million and causing in excess of 660,000 deaths a year worldwide.[2,3] In the year 2000, approximately 27 million US travelers visited countries where malaria is endemic. In 2011, the Centers for Disease Control and Prevention indicated that there were 1925 cases of malaria, an increase of 14% over 2010 and the highest number reported since 1971.[3] There were five fatalities, three due to *Plasmodium falciparum*

Patient Encounter 3, Part 1: Malaria

AR is a 52-year-old West African man who had returned recently from Cameroon. He was well since returning from Cameroon until 2 days ago, when he developed a temperature as high as 39.0°C (102.2°F), with anorexia, headache, chills, sweats, myalgias, and abdominal pain. AR comes to the emergency department with high fever (greater than 39.8°C [greater than 103.6°F]), headache, abdominal pain, nausea, stiffness of the neck, and back pain. AR indicates that he took some antimalarials but missed some days and is not able to name the exact medication or doses taken.

What are the symptoms in this patient that are consistent with malaria?

Why is this patient at risk for malaria?

Are there any additional information you like to have, to be able to develop a pharmacotherapy plan for this patient?

and one due P. vivax (the malaria species in one case was not reported).[3] KEY CONCEPT *The primary reasons for morbidity and death in malaria are failure to take recommended chemoprophylaxis, inappropriate chemoprophylaxis, delay in seeking medical care or in initiating therapy promptly, and misdiagnosis.*[3] Evaluation of a patient should include specific travel history, details of chemoprophylaxis, and physical findings (eg, splenomegaly).

Malaria is transmitted by the bites of the *Anopheles* mosquitoes, which introduce into the bloodstream one of five species of sporozoites of the plasmodia (*Plasmodium falciparum, P. ovale, P. vivax, P. malariae, and P.knowlesi*).[30–33] Initial symptoms of malaria are nonspecific and may resemble influenza and include chills, headache, fatigue, muscle pain, rigors, and nausea. The onset of the symptoms is between 1 and 3 weeks following exposure. Fever may appear 2 to 3 days after initial symptoms and may follow a pattern and occur every 2 or 3 days (*P. vivax, P. ovale,* and *P. malariae*). Fever with *P. falciparum* can be erratic and may not follow specific patterns. It is not unusual for patients to have concomitant infections with *P. vivax* and *P. falciparum*. Falciparum malaria (or *P. knowlesi*) must always be regarded as a life-threatening medical emergency.

Epidemiology and Etiology

The distribution of the various species of malaria is not well defined, but *P. vivax* is reported to be prevalent in the Indian subcontinent, Central America, North Africa, and the Middle East, whereas *P. falciparum* is predominantly in Africa (including sub-Saharan Africa), both East and West Africa, Haiti, the Dominican Republic, the Amazon region of South America, Southeast Asia, and New Guinea.[3,30,31] Most *P. ovale* infections occur in Africa, whereas the distribution of *P. malariae* is worldwide.[3,30] Most infections in the United States are reported in American travelers, recent immigrants, or immigrants who have visited friends and family in an endemic area.[3,30] Placental transmission and blood transfusions are also sources of malaria.

Pathophysiology

Within minutes after the bite of the *Anopheles* mosquito, the sporozoites invade hepatocytes and begin an asexual phase called schizonts (exoerythrocytic stage or schizogony). The patient may be asymptomatic during this period. After a lapse of between 5 and 15 days (depending on the species), schizonts rupture to release daughter cells (merozoites) into the blood, which then invade erythrocytes. In erythrocytes, the merozoites undergo a number of sequential forms: a ring form, trophozoite, schizont, and merozoite, which then invade new erythrocytes. This asexual phase is about 48 hours for *P. falciparum, P. vivax,* and *P. ovale,* and 72 hours for *P. malariae*. Subsequently, the merozoites develop into gametocytes and undergo a sexual phase (sporogony) in the *Anopheles* mosquito. In the mosquito, the gametocytes undergo a number of stages: zygote, ookinete, and oocyst, and finally transform into sporozoites in the salivary glands, where it is again able to infect the next host. Unlike *P. falciparum* and *P. malariae*, which only remain in the liver for about 3 weeks before invading erythrocytes, *P. ovale* and *P. vivax* can remain in the liver for extended periods in a latent stage (as hypnozoites); this can result in the recurrence of the infection after weeks or months. Primaquine therapy is necessary to eradicate this stage of the infection.[9]

Clinical Presentation and Diagnosis

The clinical presentation of malaria can be quite variable. Normally, the appearance of a prodrome with headache, abdominal pain, fatigue, fever, and chills, which coincides with the erythrocytic phase of malaria, occurs frequently between 10 and 21 days after being exposed.[3,30,31] This phase causes extensive hemolysis, which results in anemia and splenomegaly. The most serious complications are caused by *P. falciparum* infections. Infants and children younger than 5 years and nonimmune pregnant women are at high risk for severe complications with falciparum infections.[30,31,34] The complications associated with falciparum malaria are related to two unique features of *P. falciparum*: (a) its ability to produce high parasitism (up to 80%) of red cells of all ages; and (b) the propensity to be sequestered in post-capillary venules of critical organs such as brain, liver, heart, lungs, and kidneys.[30,34] It has been postulated that tissue hypoxia from anemia, together with *P. falciparum*–parasitized red blood cell adherence to endothelial cells in capillaries, contributes to severe ischemia and metabolic derangements.[34] *P. malariae* is implicated in immune-mediated glomerulonephritis and nephrotic syndrome.[35]

Clinical Presentation and Diagnosis

Innovations for detecting malaria include DNA or RNA probes by PCR and monoclonal antibody testing.[3,30] These, however, are not widely available for clinical use. A *P. falciparum*–specific monoclonal antibody test, histidine-rich protein 2 (HRP-2), is fairly sensitive for *P. falciparum* and is recommended by the World Health Organization as an alternative for microscopic test (the "gold standard"). However, the rapid malaria diagnostic tests (MRDTs) are restricted from wide use by cost, regulatory standards, operative expertise, and availability.[2,3,30]

Treatment

The primary goal in the management of malaria is the rapid identification of the *Plasmodium* species by blood smears (both thick and thin smears repeated every 12 hours for 3 days). Antimalarial therapy should be initiated promptly to eradicate the infection within 48 to 72 hours and avoid complications such as hypoglycemia, pulmonary edema, and renal failure.[3,31,34,36]

Pharmacologic Therapy

In an uncomplicated attack of malaria (for all plasmodia except chloroquine-resistant *P. falciparum and P. vivax*), the

Patient Encounter 3, Part 2: Falciparum Malaria

TW presents with fever, nausea, headache, myalgias, chills, and body aches including back pain.

PMH: Otherwise healthy 52-year-old man

FH: Father died of colon cancer at age 62 years; mother, who is 82-year-old, has osteoarthritis and lives with an unmarried daughter

SH: Works for an office supply company; infrequently drinks a beer

Meds: Amlodipine 10 mg; furosemide 40 mg

ROS: In addition to the complaints noted previously, he complains of severe nausea and fatigue

PE:

Gen: Patient is slightly agitated and febrile

VS: BP 170/98 mm Hg; P 120 beats/min, RR 36 breaths/min, T 40.1°C (104.2°F)

Skin: Warm and dry to touch

HEENT: Slightly dry oral mucosa

ABD: Splenomegaly

Rest of the systems were WNL

Labs: Sodium 148 mEq/L (148 mmol/L), hemoglobin 10.2 g/dL (102 g/L or 6.33 mmol/L), potassium 4.1 mEq/L (4.1 mmol/L), hematocrit 31% (0.31), chloride 96 mEq/L (96 mmol/L), WBC $14.8 \times 10^3/mm^3$ ($14.8 \times 10^9/L$), BUN 28 mg/dL (10.0 mmol/L), total bilirubin 1.8 mg/dL (30.8 μmol/L), Scr 1.4 mg/dL (124 μmol/L), platelets $110 \times 10^3/mm^3$ ($110 \times 10^9/L$), glucose 77 mg/dL (4.3 mmol/L), aspartate aminotransferase 87 U/L (1.45 μkat/L), albumin 3.2 g/dL (32 g/L), alanine aminotransferase 94 U/L (1.57 μkat/L), blood smear (Giemsa stain): *P. falciparum*.

As a result of above findings, what is your approach in the management of TW?

Describe the specific steps one need to take to ensure a good outcome and minimize the associated complications with P. falciparum infection.

recommended oral regimen is chloroquine 600 mg (base) initially, followed by 300 mg (base) 6 hours later, and then 300 mg (base) daily for 2 days.[9,36] KEY CONCEPT *In severe illness or falciparum malaria, patients should be admitted to an acute care unit, and quinidine gluconate 10 mg salt/kg as a loading dose (maximum 600 mg) in 250 mL normal saline should be administered IV slowly over 1 to 2 hours. This should be followed by continuous infusion of 0.02 mg/kg/min of quinidine for at least 24 hours until oral therapy can be started. In patients who have received either quinine or mefloquine, the loading dose of quinidine should be omitted. Oral quinine salt (650 mg every 8 hours) plus doxycycline 100 mg twice daily should follow the IV dose of quinidine to complete 7 days of therapy.*[9,36] The pediatric dose of IV quinidine gluconate is the same as the dose for adults. The pediatric dose of oral quinine is 25 mg/kg/day in three divided doses, whereas the dose of doxycycline (children greater than 8 years) is 4 mg/kg in two divided doses for 7 days. An alternative to doxycycline is clindamycin 900 mg (20 mg/kg/day) three times daily for 3 days. The pediatric dose of clindamycin is the same as in adults. *(In patients who cannot tolerate quinidine or if quinidine is not readily available, IV artesunate 2.4 mg/kg/dose for 3 days, at 0, 12, 24, 48, and 72 hours may be used, followed by oral therapy. Artesunate is available from the Centers for Disease Control and Prevention [CDC] under an investigational new drug application. The pediatric dose of artesunate is same as in adults. Oral therapy may include atovaquone/proguanil, doxycycline, mefloquine or clindamycin.)*[9,36]

Clinical Presentation and Diagnosis of Malaria

Initial Presentation

Include a careful travel history of patient and physical findings (eg, splenomegaly) and details of antimalarial chemoprophylaxis, when obtainable

Erythrocytic Phase

1. Prodrome: Headache, anorexia, malaise, fatigue, and myalgia
2. Nonspecific complaints include abdominal pain, diarrhea, chest pain, and arthralgia
3. Paroxysm: High fever, chills, and rigor
4. Cold phase: Severe pallor, cyanosis of the lips and nail beds
5. Hot phase: Fever between 40.5°C (104.9°F) and 41.0°C (105.8°F) (seen more frequently with *P. falciparum*)
6. Sweating phase: Follows the hot phase by 2 to 6 hours
7. When fever resolves, it is followed by marked fatigue and drowsiness, warm dry skin, tachycardia, cough, headache, nausea, vomiting, abdominal pain, diarrhea and delirium, anemia, and splenomegaly

KEY CONCEPT *P. falciparum malaria is a life-threatening emergency. Complications include hypoglycemia, acute renal failure, pulmonary edema, severe anemia (high parasitism), thrombocytopenia, heart failure, cerebral congestion, seizures, coma, and adult respiratory distress syndrome*

Diagnostic Procedures for Malaria

1. To ensure a positive diagnosis, blood smears (both thick and thin films) should be obtained every 12 to 24 hours for 3 consecutive days
2. The presence of parasites in the blood 3 to 5 days after initiation of therapy suggests resistance to the drug regimen

In *P. falciparum, P. vivax, P. ovale*, or *P. malariae* (chloroquine-resistant) infections, a dose of 750 mg of mefloquine followed by 500 mg 12 hours later is recommended.[9,36] The pediatric dose of mefloquine is 15 mg/kg (less than 45 kg) followed by 10 mg/kg 8 to 12 hours later. Mefloquine is associated with sinus bradycardia, confusion, hallucinations, and psychosis and should be avoided in patients with a history of epilepsy, cardiovascular problems or depression. IV quinidine gluconate followed by quinine plus doxycycline or clindamycin should be administered for severe illness as indicated previously. The IV quinidine regimen requires close monitoring of the ECG (QT-segment) and other vital signs (hypotension and hypoglycemia). An alternative oral treatment for *P. falciparum* infections in adults, especially those with history of seizures, psychiatric disorders, or cardiovascular problems, is the combination of atovaquone 250 mg and proguanil 100 mg (Malarone) (two tablets twice daily for 3 days).[12] The pediatric dose of Malarone is as follows: it is not indicted for children less than 5 kg; 9 to 10 kg: three pediatric tablets per day for 3 days; 11 to 20 kg: one adult tablet per day for 3 days; 21 to 30 kg: two adult tablets per day for 3 days; 31 to 40 kg: three adult tablets per day for 3 days; greater than 40 kg: two adults tablets twice daily for 3 days. KEY CONCEPT *Since falciparum malaria is associated with serious complications, including pulmonary edema, hypoglycemia, jaundice, renal failure, confusion, delirium, seizures, coma, and death, careful monitoring of fluid status and hemodynamic parameters is mandatory.* Exchange transfusion that may be required in patients with *P. falciparum* malaria in whom parasitemia may be between 5% and 15% remains a controversial modality.[3,36] Either peritoneal or hemodialysis may be indicated in renal failure.

Outcome Evaluation

Acute *P. falciparum* malaria resistant to chloroquine should be treated with IV quinidine and the loading dose of quinidine should be omitted in patients who have received quinine or mefloquine. Hypoglycemia, that is associated with both *P. falciparum* and quinidine administration, should be checked every 6 hours and when necessary, corrected with dextrose (5%–10%) infusions. Quinidine infusions should be slowed or stopped if the QT interval is greater than 0.6 second, the increase in the QRS complex is greater than 25%, or hypotension unresponsive to fluid challenge results. Quinidine levels should be maintained at 3 to 7 mg/dL (9.2–21.6 μmol/L). If quinidine is not readily available, artesunate (investigational protocol) should be obtained from the Centers for Disease Control and Prevention (www.cdc.gov/malaria/features/artesunate_now available.htm).[9,36]

When advising potential travelers on prophylaxis for malaria, be aware of the incidence of chloroquine-resistant *P. falciparum* malaria and the countries where it is prevalent.[36,37] In patients who have *P. vivax* or *P. ovale* malaria (note that some patients can have *P. falciparum* and one of these species), following the treatment of the acute phase of malaria and screening for glucose-6-phosphate dehydrogenase deficiency, patients should receive a regimen of primaquine for 14 days to ensure eradication of the hypnozoite stage of *P. vivax* or *P. ovale*.[9,36] For detailed recommendations for prevention of malaria, go to www.cdc.gov/travel/. *Vaccines for malaria are under investigation.*[37]

AMERICAN TRYPANOSOMIASIS

Etiology

Two distinct forms of the genus *Trypanosoma* occur in humans. One is associated with African trypanosomiasis (sleeping sickness) and the other with American trypanosomiasis (Chagas disease). *Trypanosoma brucei gambiense* and *Trypanosoma brucei rhodesiense* are the causative organisms for the East African and West African trypanosomiasis, respectively. *T. brucei rhodesiense* causes the acute disease and is the more virulent of the two species. Both East and West African trypanosomiasis are transmitted by various species of tsetse fly belonging to the genus *Glossina*. Further discussion of this subject will focus on American trypanosomiasis.

Trypanosoma cruzi is the agent that causes American trypanosomiasis. American trypanosomiasis is transmitted by a number of species of reduviid bugs *(Triatoma infestans* and *Rhodium prolixus)* that live in wall cracks of houses in rural areas of North, Central, and South America.[38–41] The reduviid bug is infected by sucking blood from animals (eg, opossums, dogs, and cats) or humans infected with circulating trypomastigotes. American trypanosomiasis is endemic in all Latin American countries and can be transmitted congenitally, by blood transfusion, and by organ transplantation.[42]

▸ *Pharmacologic Therapy*

The drugs used for *T. cruzi* include nifurtimox (Lampit) and benznidazole (Rochagan). Oral nifurtimox is available from

Patient Care Process: Malaria

Patient Assessment:

- Based on the physical exam and review of systems, determine whether patient has acute malaria.
- Review all laboratory tests and take note of blood work that identifies the species of plasmodia reported.
- Conduct a medication history and identify any allergies.

Therapy Evaluation:

- Determine, based on patient presentation and previous therapy, if acute malaria is chloroquine sensitive or chloroquine-resistant.
- Assess the efficacy of present therapy and patient adherence.
- Recheck blood smears and parasite load.

Care Plan Development:

- Determine what modification in therapy is warranted.
- Review new regimen, consider whether a combination therapy is needed and check for any drug interactions.
- Check the CDC Malaria Website for recommended therapy.

Follow-Up Evaluation:

- Monitor patient for efficacy and toxicity.
- Review physical exam findings, lab tests, and diagnostic tests.

Clinical Presentation and Diagnosis of Trypanosomiasis

Acute

- Unilateral orbital edema (Romana sign)
- Granuloma (chagoma)
- Fever, hepatosplenomegaly, and lymphadenopathy

KEY CONCEPT Chronic

- *Cardiac: cardiomyopathy and heart failure*
- *ECG: first-degree heart block, right bundle-branch block, and arrhythmias*
- *GI: enlargement of the esophagus and colon ("mega" syndrome)*
- *CNS: meningoencephalitis, strokes, seizures, and focal paralysis*

Diagnosis

Positive history of exposure and use of serology: indirect hemagglutination test, ELISA (Chagas EIA, Abbott Labs, Abbott Park, IL), and complement fixation (CF) test. (*Note:* CF may produce false-positive reactions in those exposed to leishmaniasis, syphilis, and malaria. PCR may be more definitive for diagnosis.)

the CDC, whereas benznidazole is only available in Brazil.[9,42–44] The adult dose of nifurtimox is 8 to 10 mg/kg/day in divided doses for 120 days. Since children seem to tolerate the dose better than adults, the pediatric dose of nifurtimox for 1- to 10-year-old children is 15 to 20 mg/kg/day, and for 11- to 16-year-old children is 12.5 to 15 mg/kg/day in divided doses.[9] Symptomatic treatment for heart failure associated with Chagas disease should be initiated. The GI complications may require surgical revisions and reconstruction.

Outcome Evaluation

Treatment of the acute phase of the disease (ie, fever, malaise, edema of the face, and hepatosplenomegaly) is nifurtimox. The congestive heart failure associated with cardiomyopathy of Chagas disease is treated the same way as cardiomyopathy from other causes.[38,39]

ECTOPARASITES

A parasite that lives outside the body of the host is called an ectoparasite. Approximately 6 to 12 million subjects become infested with pediculosis (lice infestation) yearly in the United States. Pediculosis is usually associated with poor hygiene, and infections are passed from person to person through social and sexual contact.

Lice

The two species that belong to this group include *Pediculus humanus capitis* (head louse) and *Pediculus humanus corporis* (body louse).[45–47] The eggs (or nits) remain firmly attached to the hair, and in about 10 days the lice hatch to form nymphs, which mature in 2 weeks. The lice become attached to the base of the hair follicle and feed on the blood of the host.[10] Pubic or crab lice is found on the hairs around the genitals but may occur in other parts of the body (eg, eyelashes or axillae). Hypersensitivity to the secretions from lice can produce macular swellings and lead to secondary bacterial infections.

▸ *Treatment*

KEY CONCEPT *The agent of choice for all three infections (body, head, and crab lice) is 1% permethrin (Nix).*[9,45–47] Permethrin has both pediculicidal and ovicidal activity against *P. humanus capitis*. The cure rate is reported to be between 90% and 97%. A cream rinse of permethrin 1% (Nix-Crème Rinse) is also available. Individuals with a history of hypersensitivity to ragweed or chrysanthemum may react to permethrin and should avoid this preparation. An alternative agent is oral ivermectin 100 mcg/kg for 3 days (days 1, 2, and 10). Permethrin can cause itching, burning, stinging, and tingling with application. Permethrin 1% should be applied to the dry scalp after shampooing and be left on the scalp for 10 minutes. The application may need to be repeated. Because of the reports of resistance to permethrin, an alternative agent is 0.5% malathion (Ovide), which has to be left on the scalp for 90 minutes and has also been found to be effective. Two applications of malathion, 7 days apart, may be necessary to eradicate the infection.[9] An alternative for head lice is Spinosad 0.9% Creme which became available for patients who may not tolerate permethrin.[47] Benzyl alcohol 5% (Ulesfia) is a recently available lice therapy for subjects over 6 months. For the relief of pruritus, calamine lotion with 0.1% menthol or an equivalent agent may be used. *All individuals, including immediate family members and sexual*

Patient Care Process: Trypanosomiasis (Chagas Disease)

Patient Assessment:

- Review medical history and laboratory tests including serology to establish the diagnosis for *T. cruzi*.
- Identify common complications associated with *T. cruzi*.

Therapy Evaluation:

- Determine if patient needs to be treated for primary disease and any secondary complications.
- Assess efficacy, safety, and potential drug interactions.

Care Plan Development:

- Determine the doses and regimen for pharmacotherapy.
- Address patient concerns and discuss the importance of adherence.

Follow-Up Evaluation:

- Review medical history, physical exam findings, and lab tests monthly.
- Determine, after assessing efficacy and toxicities of pharmacotherapy, if changes in regimen are necessary.

partners of the primary host, should be treated. All bedding and clothes should be sterilized as previously indicated for enterobiasis.

SCABIES

KEY CONCEPT *Scabies is caused by the itch mite Sarcoptes scabiei hominis, which affects both humans and animals. Infection usually affects the interdigital and popliteal folds, axillary folds, the umbilicus, and the scrotum.* The infection causes severe itching and excoriations in the interdigital web spaces, buttocks, groin, and scalp.[48–50] *Diagnosis is made by identifying the mite from skin scrapings on a wet mount.*

Treatment

KEY CONCEPT *The agent of choice for scabies is permethrin 5% (Elimite) cream.*[9] Alternative agents in subjects who cannot use permethrin are crotamiton 10% (Eurax) and oral ivermectin (Stromectol) 200 mcg/kg as a single dose. To initiate the treatment with permethrin, the skin should be scrubbed in a warm soapy bath to remove the scabs. The permethrin lotion should then be applied to the whole body, avoiding the face, mucous membranes, and eyes, and left on for 8 to 14 hours. A single application eradicates 97% of scabies. However, in subjects with poor response, permethrin application can be combined with oral ivermectin therapy.[48–50] All close contacts should be treated appropriately. The pruritus associated with scabies may persist for 2 to 4 weeks because of the remnants of mite parts in the skin.

Outcome Evaluation

Infections due to arthropods can be controlled by preventing their access to the host. Improving living conditions and avoiding sharing common personal items like hats and hair brushes may minimize these infections due to arthropods. Permethrin (1%–5%) is an effective agent for all these infections.

Abbreviations Introduced in This Chapter

CDC	Centers for Disease Control and Prevention
CF	Complement fixation
ELISA	Enzyme-linked immunosorbent assay
IgA	Immunoglobulin A
PCR	Polymerase chain reaction

REFERENCES

1. Goswami ND, Shah JS, Corey GR, Stout JE. Short report: Persistent eosinophilia and *Strongyloides* infection in Montagnard refugees after presumptive albendazole therapy. Am J Trop Med Hyg. 2009;81:302–304.
2. Garcia LS. Malaria. Clin Lab Med. 2010;30:93–129.
3. Cullen KA, Arguin PM. Malaria Surveillance – United States, 2011; MMWR Surveill Summ. 2013;62:1–17.
4. Russ AGP, Olds GR, Cripps AW, Farrar JJ, McManus DP. Enteropathogens and chronic illness in returning travelers. N Engl J Med. 2013;368:1817–1825.
5. Munoz P, Valerio M, Puga D, Bouza E. Parasitic infections in solid organ transplant recipients. Infect Dis Clin N Amer. 2010;24:461–495.
6. John DT, Petri WA Jr. Markell and Voge's Medical Parasitology. 9th ed. Philadelphia, PA: Saunders; 2006.
7. Hill DR, Nash TE. Giardia lamblia. In: Mandell GL, Bennett JE, Dolin R, eds. Principles and Practice of Infectious Diseases. 7th ed. New York: Elsevier Churchill-Livingstone; 2010:3527–3534.
8. Yoder JS, Harral C, Bach MJ. Giardiasis Surveillance – United States, 2006–2008. MMWR Suveill Summ. 2010;59:15–24.
9. Drugs for parasitic infections. In: Handbook of Antimicrobial Therapy. 18th ed. New Rochelle, NY: Medical Letter; 2008:225–280.
10. Wright SG. Protozoan infections of the gastrointestinal tract. Infect Dis Clin N Amer. 2012;26:323–339.
11. Farthing MJG. Intestinal protozoa. *Entamoeba histolytica*. In: Manson's Tropical Diseases. 22nd ed. London: WB Saunders; 2009:1375–1386.
12. Petri WA Jr, Haque R. Entamoeba species, including amebiasis. In: Mandell GL, Bennett JA, Dolin R, eds. Principles and Practice of Infectious Diseases. 7th ed. New York: Elsevier Churchill-Livingstone; 2010:3411–3425.
13. Rao S, Solaymani-Mohammadi S, Petri WA Jr, Parker SK. Hepatic amebiasis: A reminder of the complications. Curr Opin Pediat. 2009;21:145–149.
14. Athie-Gutierrez C, Rodea-Rosas H, Guizar-Bermudez C, Alcantara A, MontalvoJave E. Evolution of surgical treatment of amebiasis-associated colon perforation. J Gastrointest Surg. 2010;14:82–87.
15. Maguire JH. Intestinal nematodes (roundworms). In: Mandell GL, Bennett JE, Dolin R, eds. Principles and Practice of Infectious Diseases. 7th ed. New York: Elsevier Churchill-Livingstone; 2010:3577–3586.
16. Starr MC, Montgomery SP. Soil-transmitted helminthiasis in the United States: A systematic review – 1940–2010. Am J Trop Med Hyg. 2011;85:680–684.
17. Knopp S, Steinmann P, Keiser J, Utzinger J. Nematode infection: Soil-transmitted helminthes and Trichnella. Infect Dis Clin N Amer. 2012;26:341–358.
18. Pasricha S-R, Caruana SR, Phu TQ, et al. Anemia, iron deficiency, meat consumption, and hookworm infection in women of reproductive age in Northwest Vietnam. Am J Trop Med Hyg. 2008;78:375–381.
19. Jardin-Botelho A, Raff S, Hoffman HJ, et al. Hookworm, *Ascaris lumbricoides* infection and polyparasitism associated with poor cognitive performance in Brazilian schoolchildren. Trop Med Int Health. 2008;13:994–1004.
20. Shah JJ, Maloney SA, Liu Y, et al. Evaluation of the impact of overseas pre-departure treatment for infection with intestinal parasites among Montagnard refugees migrating from Cambodia to North Carolina. Am J Trop Med Hyg. 2008;78:754–759.
21. Keiser J, Utzinger J. Efficacy of current drugs against soil-transmitted helminth infections. Systematic review and meta-analysis. JAMA. 2008;299:1937–1948.
22. Krolewiecki AJ, Lammie P, Jacobson J, et al. A public health response against Strongyloides stercoralis: Time to look at soil-transmitted helminthiasis in full. PLoS Negl Trop Dis. 2013;7:e2165 (1–7).
23. Buonfrate D, Requena-Mendez A, Angheben A, et al. Severe strongyloidiasis: A systematic review of case reports. BMC Infect Dis. 2013;13:78 (1–10).
24. Marcos LA, Terashima A, Canales M, Gotuzzo E. Update on strongyloidiasis in the immunocompromised host. Curr Infect Rep. 2011;13:35–46.
25. King CH, Fairley JK. Cestodes (tapeworms). In: Mandell GL, Dolin R, Bennett JE, eds. Principles and Practice of Infectious Diseases. 7th ed. New York: Elsevier Churchill-Livingstone; 2010:3607–3616.
26. Serpa JA, Graviss EA, Kass JS, White AC Jr. Neurocysticercosis in Houston, Texas. An Update. Medicine 2011;90:81–86.
27. Del Brutto OH. Neurocysticercosis. Cont Lifelong Learn Neurol. 2012;18:1392–1416.
28. Baird RA, Wiebe S, Zunt JR, Halperin JJ, Gronseth G, Roos KL. Evidence-based guideline: Treatment of parenchymal neurocysticercosis. Neurology. 2013;80:1424–1429.

29. Del Brutto OH. Neurocysticercosis: New thoughts on controversial issues. Curr Opin Neurol. 2013;26:289–294.
30. Fairhurst RM, Wellems TE. Plasmodium species (malaria). In: Mandell GL, Dolin R, Bennett JE, eds. Principles and Practice of Infectious Diseases. 7th ed. New York: Elsevier Churchill-Livingstone; 2010:3437–3462.
31. White NJ. Malaria. In: Cook GC, Zumla A, eds. Manson's Tropical Diseases. 22nd ed. London: WB Saunders; 2009:1201–1300.
32. Scuracchio P, Viera SD, Dourado DA, et al. Transfusion-transmitted malaria: A case report of asymptomatic donor harboring *Plasmodium malariae*. Rev Inst Med Trop Sao Paulo. 2011; 53:55–59.
33. Kantle A, Jokiranta TS. Review of cases with the emerging fifth human malaria parasite, Plasmodium knowlesi. Clin Infect Dis. 2011;52:1356–1362.
34. Marks M, Gupta-Wright A, Doherty JF, Singer M, Walker D. Managing malaria in the intensive care unit. Br J Anesth. 2014;113(6):910–921 (doi:10.1093/bja/aeu157).
35. Badiane AS, Diongue K, Diallo S, et al. Acute kidney injury associated with Plasmodium malariae infection. Malaria J. 2014;13:226 (1–5).
36. CDC Guidelines for treatment of Malaria in the United States. http://www.cdc.gov/malaria.resources/pdf/treatmenttable.pdf 2013
37. Hill AVS. Vaccines against malaria. Phil Trans R Soc Lond B Biol Sci. 2011;366:2806–2814.
38. Kirchhoff LV. Trypanosoma species (American trypanosomiasis, Chagas' disease): Biology of trypanosomes. In: Mandell GL, Bennett JE, Dolin R, eds. Principles and Practice of Infectious Diseases. 7th ed. New York: Elsevier Churchill-Livingstone; 2010:3481–3488.
39. Rassi Jr A, Rassi A, Marcondes de Rezende J. American Trypanosomiasis (Chagas Disease). Infect Dis Clin N Amer. 2012;26:275–291.
40. Carter YL, Juliano JJ, Montgomery SP, Ovarnstrom Y. Acute Chagas disease in a returning traveler. Am J Trop Med Hyg. 2012;87:1038–1040.
41. Fox MC, Lakdawala N, Miller AL, Loscalzo J. A patient with syncope. N Engl J Med. 2013;369:966–972.
42. Kransdorf EP, Czer LSC, Luthringer DJ, et al. Heart transplantation for Chagas cardiomyopathy in the United States. Am J Transpl. 2013;20:1–7.
43. Molina I, Prat JG, Salvador F, et al. Randomized trial of posaconazole and benznidazole for chronic Chagas's disease. N Engl J Med. 2014;370:1899–1908.
44. Moore TA. Agents used to treat Parasitic Infections. In: Longo DL, Kasper DL, Fauci AS, et al., eds. Harrison's Principles of Internal Medicine. 18th ed. New York: McGraw-Hill; 2012:1675–1682.
45. Diaz SH. Lice (pediculosis). In: Mandell GL, Bennett JR, Dolin R, eds. Principles and Practice of Infectious Diseases. 7th ed. New York: Elsevier Churchill-Livingstone; 2010:3629–3632.
46. Chosidow O, Giraudeau B, Cottrell J, et al. Oral ivermectin versus malathion lotion for difficult-to-treat head lice. N Engl J Med. 2010;362:896–905.
47. Villegas SC, Breitzka RL. Head Lice and the use of Spinosad. Clin Therap. 2012;34:14–23.
48. Shimose L, Muinoz-Price LS. Diagnosis, Prevention, and Treatment of Scabies. Curr Infect Dis Rep. 2013;15:426–431.
49. Currie BJ, McCarthy JS. Permethrin and ivermectin for scabies. N Engl J Med. 2010;362:717–725.
50. Panuganti B, Tarbox M. Evaluation and management of pruritus and scabies in the elderly population. Clin Geriatr Med. 2013;29: 479–499.

79 Urinary Tract Infections

Warren E. Rose

LEARNING OBJECTIVES

Upon completion of the chapter, the reader will be able to:

1. Determine the diagnostic criteria for significant bacteriuria.
2. Interpret the signs and symptoms of urinary tract infections (UTIs) and differentiate those of upper versus lower urinary tract disease.
3. Identify the organism responsible for the majority of uncomplicated UTIs.
4. Assess the laboratory tests that help in diagnosing patients with UTI.
5. Recommend appropriate drug, dose, and duration for uncomplicated and complicated UTI prophylaxis and empiric treatment.
6. Evaluate and select therapy for uncomplicated and complicated UTIs based on specific urine culture results and patient characteristics.
7. Formulate appropriate monitoring and education information for patients with UTIs.

INTRODUCTION

Urinary tract infections (UTIs) are comprised of a diverse array of syndromes depending on the location of the infection within the urinary tract.[1–3] UTIs are one of the most common infectious diseases accounting for approximately 10.5 million annual ambulatory patient visits.[4] In hospitalized patients, UTIs are also common and are reported in 3.7% of catheterized and 0.9% of non-catheterized patients.[5] A UTI is defined by microorganism(s) in the urinary tract, which does not represent contamination.

EPIDEMIOLOGY AND ETIOLOGY

The prevalence and type of UTIs generally vary by age and gender.[7,8] Premature infants have a higher rate than full-term infants, and neonatal boys are five to eight times more likely to have UTIs than neonatal girls. In young children 1 to 5 years of age, significant **bacteriuria** occurs more in girls than boys, 4.5% compared with 0.5%, respectively.[9] Once adulthood is reached, bacteriuria increases in young, nonpregnant women (range, 1%–3%), yet remains low in men (up to 0.1%).[10] Symptomatic UTI affects 30% of women between 20 and 40 years of age, which represents a prevalence that is 30 times greater than that of men in the same age group. The lifetime risk of UTIs in women is as high as 50% based on symptomatic reporting.[11]

The etiology of UTIs has remained relatively unchanged over the past several decades. **KEY CONCEPT** *UTIs are either uncomplicated or complicated.* There is a lack of consensus regarding the definition of what makes a UTI complicated (specifically in postmenopausal women or patients with diabetes mellitus), but in general, a complicated UTI refers to a structural or functional abnormality of the urinary tract.[1] Patients with complicated UTIs are typically given longer treatment durations than those patients with uncomplicated infections. Those with complicated UTIs by definition are also prone to more frequent infections. It is important to note that an upper UTI does not necessarily imply complicated UTI, nor does lower UTI imply uncomplicated UTI.

PATHOPHYSIOLOGY

There are three potential ways for bacteria to enter into the urinary tract and cause infection: the ascending, hematogenous, and lymphatic pathways.

Ascending Pathway

The ascending pathway is involved when bacteria colonizing the urethra subsequently travel upwards, or ascend, the urethra to the bladder and cause **cystitis** (**Figure 79–1**). Women have a shorter urethra than men, and colonization of the female urethra is likely due to its proximity to the perirectal area.[12–14] Once in the bladder, bacteria are not limited to causing cystitis. These bacteria may continue to ascend the urinary tract via the ureters and cause more complicated infections, such as **pyelonephritis**.

Hematogenous Pathway

The hematogenous route is involved through the seeding of the urinary tract with pathogens carried by the blood supply. These pathogens represent an infection at some other primary site in the body. *Staphylococcus aureus* **bacteremia** can cause renal abscesses via the hematogenous route,[15] and pyelonephritis can be experimentally produced in rabbits by intravenous (IV) injection of *Salmonella* spp., *Mycobacterium tuberculosis*, or even yeast (*Candida* spp.).[16] *E. coli* and *P. aeruginosa* are less likely to seed the kidneys via hematogenous spread.[16]

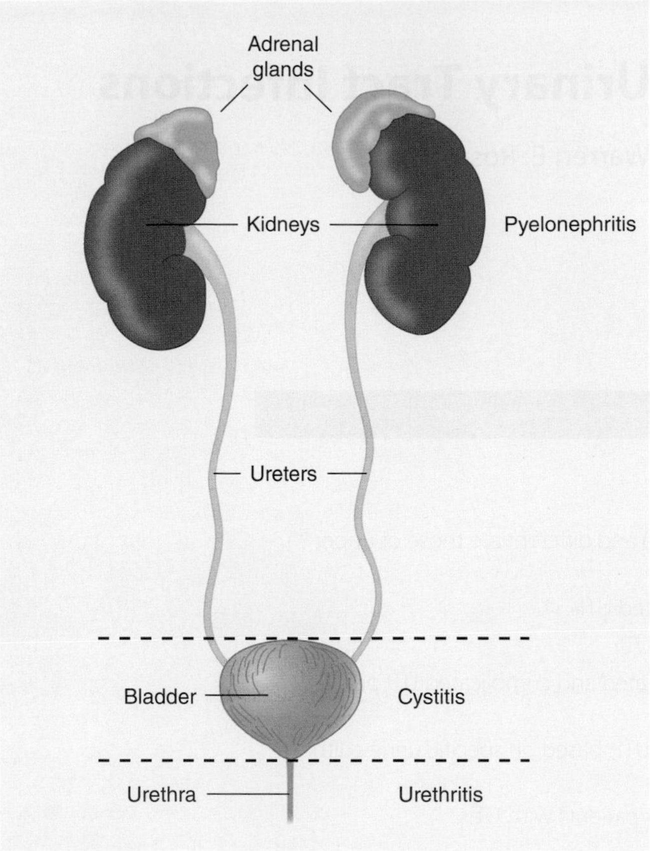

FIGURE 79–1. Anatomy and associated infection of the urinary tract. (From Sprandel KA, Lesch CA, Rodvold KA. Lower urinary tract infection. IN: Schwinghammer TL (ed). 6th ed. New York: McGraw-Hill; 2005; 315; with permission.)

Host Defense Mechanisms

Urine possesses characteristics that are not ideal for bacterial metabolism and growth such as low pH, high urea concentration, and high osmolality. Bacteria in the bladder can stimulate an urge to urinate and increase bacterial voiding. In men, prostatic fluid secretions in can inhibit bacterial growth, whereas normal vaginal flora in women such as *Lactobacillus* spp. can secrete lactic acid that further lowers the pH of the enviroment.[17–19]

Innate host response and adaptive immunity are a primary defense against bacterial infections including UTIs.[20] Several other secreted host factors specifically inhibit bacterial virulence factors. Virulence factors are mechanisms that bacteria utilize to cause infection and/or ensure their survival. Glycosaminoglycan is compound produced by the bladder that coats the epithelial cells. This separates the bladder from the urine by forming a protective layer against bacterial adhesion.[21] Tamm-Horsfall protein is also secreted into the urine and prevents *E. coli* from binding to receptors present on the surface of the bladder.

Risk Factors

There are several risk factors for development of UTIs.[10] Common risk factors for UTIs in women include sexual intercourse, use of a cervical diaphragm, use of spermicidal jellies, diabetes, and pregnancy.[22–24] In men, the risks are increased in uncircumcised males and older age men with prostatic hyperplasia. Common risk factors for both men and women include urologic instrumentation, urethral catheterization, renal transplantation, neurogenic bladder, and urinary tract obstruction.[25,26]

Table 79–1

Diagnostic Criteria for Significant Bacteriuria

- Greater than or equal to 10^2 CFU coliforms/mL (10^5 CFU/L) or greater than or equal to 10^5 CFU noncoliforms/mL (10^8 CFU/L) in a symptomatic female
- Greater than or equal to 10^3 CFU organisms/mL (10^6 CFU/L) in a symptomatic male
- Greater than or equal to 10^5 CFU same organisms/mL (10^8 CFU/L) in asymptomatic individuals on two consecutive specimens
- Any growth of bacteria on suprapubic catheterization in a symptomatic patient
- Greater than or equal to 10^2 CFU organisms/mL (10^5 CFU/L) in a catheterized patient

CLINICAL PRESENTATION AND DIAGNOSIS

Bacteriuria, or bacteria in the urine, does not always represent infection. For this reason, quantitative diagnostic criteria have been created (Table 79–1) to identify the amount of bacteria in

Clinical Presentation and Diagnosis of UTIs

General

- Most women present with hematuria; however, this is not a presentation restricted only to UTIs.
- Elderly patients frequently will not present with common signs and symptoms of UTI, but may present with altered mental status.
- More than 95% of uncomplicated UTIs are caused by a single organism.
- Patients may present with urosepsis.

KEY CONCEPT *Signs and Symptoms of Lower UTI*

- *Dysuria, gross hematuria, suprapubic heaviness, nocturia, increased urinary frequency and urgency*

KEY CONCEPT *Signs and Symptoms of Upper UTI*

- *Fever, nausea, vomiting, malaise, and often severe flank pain*

Laboratory Tests

Urinalysis should show:

- **Pyuria** typically greater than 10 white blood cells/mm^3 urine (10×10^6/L)
- Bacteriuria, usually greater than 10^5 CFU organisms/mL (10^8 CFU/L)
- Nitrites present
- Leukocyte esterase present

Other Diagnostic Tests

- Bacterial urine culture
- Presence of costovertebral tenderness (upper UTI only)

Patient Encounter, Part 1

AC is a 30-year-old woman who presents to an acute care clinic with complaints of a 3-day history of dysuria and urgency. She has had three prior UTI episodes in the last 6 months each treated with oral trimethoprim/sulfamethoxazole 800/160 mg daily for 3 days. Her last antibiotic course finished 6 days ago. She denies vomiting, fever, nausea, or flank pain. Urine culture information is not available from previous UTI episodes.

What signs and symptoms are suggestive of a lower urinary tract infection (UTI)?

Would you classify this patient as noncomplicated or complicated UTI?

How does this change your treatment approach?

What additional patient information is required before creating an appropriate treatment plan for this patient?

the urine that most likely represents true infection. Clinically this is referred to as significant bacteriuria.[6] UTIs are classified as lower tract or upper tract disease. Lower tract urinary infections are usually less severe and are treated in the outpatient setting. Cystitis, a common lower tract syndrome, involves inflammation of the bladder and is associated with symptoms of dysuria, nocturia, gross hematuria, and occasional suprapubic tenderness. Upper tract disease such as pyelonephritis is generally more severe infection, and patients more often present with symptoms of systemic response such as fever, chills, and elevated white blood cell count. Patients with upper tract infection are more likely to be admitted to the hospital for treatment.

TREATMENT

KEY CONCEPT *The goals of treatment are to eradicate the causative pathogen, prevent or treat consequences of infection, administer targeted antimicrobial therapy for the identified or most likely pathogen, minimize unnecessary exposure to noncausative organisms, and prevent, if possible, recurrence of infection.* Therapy is directed at microbiologic eradication of the offending organism through antibiotics with a defined duration of treatment based on the UTI classification.

Antimicrobial therapy is the cornerstone of treatment in symptomatic UTIs. The selected antimicrobial should ideally be well tolerated, lend itself to patient compliance (low total number of doses), have adequate concentrations at the site of the infection in the urinary tract, have good oral bioavailability, and be narrow in antimicrobial spectrum to limit collateral damage and resistance development in human flora not affiliated with the infection.[1]

Nonpharmacologic Therapy

Several nonpharmacologic therapies have been proposed for prevention of UTIs. The intake of large volumes of cranberry juice has been associated with a decrease in the number of UTIs over a year period in patients with recurrent UTIs in small randomized controlled trials. The efficacy is uncertain in the general population and with smaller intake volumes.[27–29] Probiotics such as *Lactobacillus* spp. lower urinary pH and may reduce the growth of pathogenic bacteria[18,19], and the agents have demonstrated promise in preventing recurrent UTIs in women.[30] Topical estrogen replacement therapy significantly decreases the incidence of UTIs in postmenopausal women as compared with placebo.[31] Methenamine hippurate and methenamine mandelate are hydrolyzed in acidic urine to the antimicrobial formaldehyde and are effective in preventing UTIs in patient without renal tract abnormalities.[32] Patient education of common risk factors is important.

Pharmacologic Therapy

Table 79–2 reviews oral and IV antibiotics frequently used to treat UTIs with comments on their use, and Table 79–3 reviews frequency, duration, and doses of oral antibiotics used commonly for outpatient treatment of UTIs.

▸ *Uncomplicated UTIs*

Cystitis Uncomplicated cystitis is frequently managed in the outpatient setting and occurs mostly in women of childbearing age.[1]

Table 79–2

Commonly Used Antimicrobial Agents for the Treatment of UTIs

Agent	Comments
Oral Therapy	
Penicillins	
Amoxicillin Amoxicillin-clavulanic acid	Increasing *E. coli* resistance has limited amoxicillin use in acute cystitis despite broad-spectrum activity. Amoxicillin-clavulanic acid is empirically preferred due to resistance. Ampicillin is the drug of choice for enterococci-sensitive to penicillin, but oral bioavailability is approximately 50%.
Pivmecillinam	Pivmecillinam is a prodrug of mecillinam and is recommended for treatment of acute cystitis. It should be avoided in patients with suspected pyelonephritis. Neither pivmecillinam nor mecillinam are currently approved for use by the US FDA.
Cephalosporins	
Cefaclor Cefadroxil Cefixime Cefpodoxime Cefuroxime Cephalexin Cephradine	There are no major advantages of these agents over other oral agents in the treatment of UTIs, and they may have inferior efficacy as compared with other oral agents such as fluoroquinolones. They may be useful in cases of resistance to amoxicillin and trimethoprim-sulfamethoxazole, but concern exists for use as a first-line agent for uncomplicated cystitis therapy due to potential selection of cephalosporin resistant organisms (collateral damage). These agents are not active against enterococci. Susceptibility of cephalexin cannot be accurately predicted based on cefazolin susceptibility testing.

(Continued)

Table 79–2

Commonly Used Antimicrobial Agents for the Treatment of UTIs (*Continued*)

Agent	Comments
Tetracyclines	
Doxycycline Minocycline Tetracycline	These agents have been effective for initial episodes of UTI; however, resistance can develop rapidly. Avoid during pregnancy.
Fluoroquinolones	
Ciprofloxacin Levofloxacin Norfloxacin Ofloxacin	The newer quinolones have a greater spectrum of activity; rates of resistance are increasing. Concern for use as a first-line agent for uncomplicated UTI therapy exists due to potential selection of multidrug resistant organisms (collateral damage). These agents are often effective for pyelonephritis. Avoid in pregnancy and children. Moxifloxacin is not listed due to limited urinary excretion.
Miscellaneous	
Trimethoprim-sulfamethoxazole	This combination is highly effective against most aerobic enteric bacteria except *P. aeruginosa*. High urinary tract tissue levels and urine levels are achieved, which may be important in complicated UTI treatment. Also effective as prophylaxis for recurrent infections. Generally well tolerated and low cost but increasing resistance rates above 20% in certain regions has limited empiric use. Its use may be precluded in patients with sulfa allergies.
Nitrofurantoin	This agent is effective in treatment and prophylaxis in patients with uncomplicated or recurrent lower tract UTIs. Should not be used in patients with low estimated CrCl (< 40–60 mL/min [0.67–1.00 mL/s]) due to limited urine concentrations and potential increased risk of neuropathy.
Azithromycin	Commonly used for sexually transmitted diseases (ie, chlamydia infections) rather than for UTIs.
Fosfomycin	Single-dose therapy for uncomplicated cystitis. Has been recommended for empiric therapy since resistance rates are low but may have inferior efficacy when compared with short courses of other oral antibiotic agents.
Parenteral Therapy	
Aminoglycosides	
Amikacin Gentamicin Tobramycin	Gentamicin and tobramycin are generally equally effective, whereas tobramycin has slightly better coverage of certain *Pseudomonas* spp. Amikacin generally is reserved for multidrug-resistant bacteria. Typically used as a short course of therapy followed by a switch to an oral agent. Concern for neurotoxicity and ototoxicity generally limit use, especially in patients with impaired renal function.
Penicillins	
Ampicillin Ampicillin-sulbactam Piperacillin Piperacillin-tazobactam	These agents are generally effective for susceptible bacteria. The extended-spectrum penicillins are active against certain strains of *Pseudomonas* spp. They are very useful in renally impaired patients since urine concentration can remain adequate or when an aminoglycoside is avoided. Empiric use of ampicillin with an aminoglycoside is recommended only in patients with suspected infection due to *Enterococcus* spp.
Cephalosporins	
First-, second-, third-, and fourth-generation	Second- and third-generation cephalosporins have a broad spectrum of activity against gram-negative bacteria, but are not active against enterococci. Only ceftazidime and cefepime have activity against certain strains of *Pseudomonas* spp. They are useful for nosocomial infections and urosepsis due to susceptible pathogens. A single ceftriaxone dose could be used in lieu of an IV fluoroquinolone for acute uncomplicated pyelonephritis.
Carbapenems	
Doripenem Ertapenem Imipenem-cilastatin Meropenem	These agents have broad-spectrum activity, including gram-positive, gram-negative, and anaerobic bacteria. Ertapenem is not active against *Pseudomonas* spp. All may be associated with *Candida* spp. superinfections. Rarely used for UTIs.
Fluoroquinolones	
Ciprofloxacin Levofloxacin	These agents have broad-spectrum activity against both gram-negative and gram-positive bacteria. They provide high urine and tissue concentrations and are actively secreted in reduced renal function. Switch to oral therapy when possible due to excellent bioavailability.
Monobactam	
Aztreonam	Only active against gram-negative bacteria, including some strains of *P. aeruginosa*. Generally useful for nosocomial infections when aminoglycosides are to be avoided and in patients with type 1/immediate hypersensitivity to penicillins.
Glycopeptide	
Vancomycin	May be considered in combination for empiric therapy based on patient risk factors for multidrug-resistant organisms and gram-positive cocci shown in urinalysis.

KEY CONCEPT *E. coli represent the vast majority of causal organisms in this setting, but Staphylococcus saprophyticus, Klebsiella pneumoniae, Proteus mirabilis, Enterococcus spp. are also known pathogens.*[33–36] Treatment in the outpatient setting is frequently relegated to a urinalysis and empiric therapy without a urine culture.[1,37,38] Patients are subsequently monitored for resolution of signs and symptoms. KEY CONCEPT *Uncomplicated UTIs may be managed with a short-course antimicrobial therapy with one-dose, 3-day, or 5-day regimens depending on the clinical factors involved.*

Table 79–3

Overview of Outpatient, Oral Antimicrobial Therapy for Lower and Upper Tract UTIs

Indications	Antibiotic	Adult Dose[a]	Frequency	Duration
Lower Tract UTIs				
Uncomplicated	Nitrofurantoin macrocrystals	100 mg	Every 12 hours	5–7 days
	Nitrofurantoin monohydrate	100 mg	Every 12 hours	5–7 days
Alternative options:	Trimethoprim-sulfamethoxazole	One DS[b] tablet	Every 12 hours	3 days
	Trimethoprim	100 mg	Every 12 hours	3 days
	Fosfomycin	3000 mg	Single dose	1 day
	Pivmecillinam[c]	400 mg	Every 12 hours	3–7 days
	Ciprofloxacin	250 mg	Every 12 hours	3 days
	Levofloxacin	250 mg	Every 24 hours	3 days
	Ofloxacin	200 mg	Every 12 hours	3 days
	Amoxicillin-clavulanic acid	500 mg	Every 8 hours	3 days
	Cefdinir	100 mg	Every 12 hours	7 days
	Cefaclor	250–500 mg	Every 8 hours	7 days
	Cefpodoxime-proxetil	100 mg	Every 12 hours	7 days
Complicated	Trimethoprim-sulfamethoxazole	One DS[b] tablet	Every 12 hours	7–10 days
	Trimethoprim	100 mg	Every 12 hours	7–10 days
	Ciprofloxacin	500 mg	Every 12 hours	7–10 days
	Norfloxacin	400 mg	Every 12 hours	7–10 days
	Levofloxacin	250 mg	Every 24 hours	7–10 days
	Amoxicillin-clavulanic acid	500 mg	Every 8 hours	7–10 days
Recurrent infections—continuous prophylaxis	Trimethoprim-sulfamethoxazole	½ SS[d] tablet	Every 24 hours	6 months
	Trimethoprim	100 mg	Every 24 hours	6 months
	Ciprofloxacin	125 mg	Every 24 hours	6 months
	Nitrofurantoin	50 *or* 100 mg	Every 24 hours	6 months
	Cefaclor	250 mg	Every 24 hours	6 months
	Cephalexin	125 mg	Every 24 hours	6 months
Upper Tract UTIs				
Uncomplicated Acute pyelonephritis[e]	Ciprofloxacin	500 mg	Every 12 hours	7 days
	Ciprofloxacin (extended release)	1000 mg	Every 24 hours	7 days
	Levofloxacin (extended release)	750 mg	Every 24 hours	5 days
	Trimethoprim-sulfamethoxazole	One DS[b] tablet	Every 12 hours	14 days

[a]Majority of listed antimicrobial agents require dosage adjustment in patients with significant renal dysfunction.
[b]DS, double strength (160 mg trimethoprim/800 mg sulfamethoxazole).
[c]Not approved for use by the US FDA as of November 2011.
[d]SS, single strength (80 mg trimethoprim/400 mg sulfamethoxazole).
[e]Doses listed for acute pyelonephritis are for oral regimens.

For acute uncomplicated UTIs, it is reasonable to pursue oral empiric therapy with one dose (3000 mg) of fosfomycin, a 3-day course of trimethoprim-sulfamethoxazole (one double-strength tablet twice daily), or a 5-day course of nitrofurantoin (100 mg twice daily) depending on the patient's characteristics and risk factors.[1] For treatment of multidrug resistant organisms, multiple doses of fosfomycin (given every other day) have been used.[39] The antibiotic selection for empiric therapy partly depends on known resistance rates in the geographic region, particularly *E. coli* resistance to trimethoprim-sulfamethoxazole.[33,40] Empiric therapy with trimethoprim-sulfamethoxazole should be considered only if the local resistance rates in *E. coli* is less than 20%, due to poor UTI treatment responses with trimethoprim-sulfamethoxazole when resistance rates are above this threshold.[1,40] Although fluoroquinolone antibiotics and certain β-lactam agents can be highly active and efficacious against *E. coli*, these agents should be considered alternative agents in uncomplicated UTIs due to their broad-spectrum activity and risk of resistance development in bacteria unaffiliated with the infection.[1]

▶ *Complicated UTIs*

KEY CONCEPT *Complicated UTIs including acute pyelonephritis should be treated for at least 7 days and sometimes 2 weeks or longer.*

▶ *Acute Pyelonephritis*

Patients who present with pyelonephritis usually have high-grade fever (greater than 38.3°C [100.9°F]) and severe flank pain. Select patients with pyelonephritis may be treated in the outpatient setting; however, patients with infection-related vomiting, decreased food intake, and dehydration may need to be treated in the hospital. These patients will often receive IV antibiotics initially before being switched to oral therapy depending on susceptibility testing.

Patients with pyelonephritis are traditionally given 14 days of therapy. Shorter course fluoroquinolone therapy for 7 days has been successful in women with acute pyelonephritis[41], but further studies are needed for validation.[1] Gram stain and culture are important in ensuring that appropriate antimicrobial coverage is selected. Women who present with mild cases of pyelonephritis

Patient Encounter, Part 2 of Patient AC: Medical History, Physical Exam, and Diagnostic Tests

PMH: Obesity (body mass index 32); history of UTI with three episodes in last 6 months

FH: Mother living with hypertension; father living with chronic obstructive pulmonary disease, hypertension, and dyslipidemia

SH: Unmarried, sexually active with two partners in last 6 months, occupation: store clerk

Allergies: None

Meds: Norethindrone 0.5 mg/ethinyl estradiol daily

ROS: (+) dysuria, urinary frequency; (–) fever, nausea, vomiting, flank pain

VS: BP 125/77 mm Hg, P 70 beats/min, RR 16 breaths/min, T 37.0°C

CV: RRR, normal S1, S2; normal findings

Abd: Soft, nontender, nondistended; (+) bowel sounds, no hepatosplenomegaly, heme (–) stool

Lab: Within normal limits including blood glucose; (–) pregnancy test

Urinalysis: Greater than 200 white blood cells/mm^3 (200 × 10^6/L); urine nitrates positive; leukocyte esterase positive

Urine Gram Stain: Gram-negative rods, more than 10^5 CFU/mL (10^8 CFU/L)

Given this additional information, what is your assessment of the patient's condition?

Identify your treatment goals for the patient.

What nonpharmacologic and pharmacologic alternatives are available for the patient?

What duration of antibiotic therapy is appropriate for this patient?

(defined as low-grade fever and a normal to slightly elevated peripheral white blood count, without nausea or vomiting) may be treated as outpatients. Outpatient antibiotic therapy with trimethoprim-sulfamethoxazole, fluoroquinolones, or even β-lactam/β-lactamase inhibitor, such as amoxicillin-clavulanic acid is recommended.[1] In cases where an initial, one-time IV antibiotic is used as supplemental therapy, a single ceftriaxone dose or single high-dose aminoglycoside therapy could be used in lieu of an IV fluoroquinolone. This practice is a recommended addition to therapy if local prevalence of fluoroquinolone resistance exceeds 10%.[1] Those patients who exhibit more severe signs and symptoms will need to be admitted to an acute care setting for appropriate treatment. The same holds true for antibiotic selection in these patients. Hospitalized patients, suspected of having bacteremia or urosepsis, typically receive IV therapy such as a fluoroquinolone or a β-lactam plus an aminoglycoside.[1,42] When selecting fluoroquinolone antibiotics, ciprofloxacin may be ideal due to its relatively narrow spectrum of activity directed against gram-negative organisms.[1]

Special Populations

▸ Pregnant Women

Changes to the urinary tract in pregnant women predispose them to an increased incidence of bacteriuria and subsequent UTIs that may follow. These changes include alterations in amino acid and other nutrient concentrations in the urine along with physiologic changes such as reduced bladder tone and dilation of the renal pelvis and ureters.[43,44]

An association exists between maternal UTI during pregnancy and fetal death, labor complications, mental retardation, and developmental delay.[45,46] Therefore, screening for UTI during pregnancy is necessary.[22,47] In pregnant patients with significant bacteriuria, whether symptomatic or asymptomatic, treatment is recommended to avoid these complications. In the majority of patients, a sulfonamide (with the exception of use during the third trimester due to concerns for kernicterus), amoxicillin-clavulanic acid, cephalexin, or nitrofurantoin are effective treatment options. Tetracyclines and fluoroquinolones should be avoided due to risk of teratogenicity and ability to inhibit cartilage and bone development, respectively. Follow-up usually consists of a urine culture 1 to 2 weeks after completion of therapy and then subsequent monthly urine cultures until birth.

▸ Catheterized Patients

An indwelling catheter is commonly used in various health care settings and is associated with UTIs.[25,48] Bacteria may be introduced into the bladder via the catheter by colonization and direct introduction during catheterization. UTIs as a result of an indwelling catheter are common and occur at a rate of 3% to 8% per day of catheter presence.[48]

The approach to management of a patient with bacteriuria and an indwelling urinary catheter follows two paths.[48] KEY CONCEPT *The first, in asymptomatic patients with catheterization, is to hold antibiotics and remove the catheter if possible. The second, in symptomatic patients with catheterization, is to initiate antibiotic therapy and remove the catheter if possible.* In both of the above situations, if discontinuation of the catheter is not possible, the patient should be recatheterized with a new urinary catheter if the previous catheter is greater than 2 weeks old.[48]

▸ UTIs in Men

KEY CONCEPT *Although UTIs in men are not always complicated by definition, due to the relative infrequency of UTIs in men compared*

Patient Encounter, Part 3: Creating a Care Plan for AC

Based on the information presented, create a care plan for this patient's UTI. Your plan should include:

(a) A statement of the drug-related needs and/or problems

(b) A patient-specific detailed therapeutic plan

(c) Monitoring parameters to assess efficacy and safety

Table 79–4

Monitoring Parameters for Select Antibiotics Used in the Treatment of UTIs

Drug Class or Drug	What to Monitor	Frequency	Endpoint
Aminoglycosides	SCr, urine output	Every 24 hours	Prevention of nephrotoxicity manifested by a rise in SCr
	Aminoglycoside serum concentrations	Depends on duration of therapy. At least once weekly; more frequently if evidence of changing renal function	Trough serum concentrations < 2 mg/L (< 4.2 μmol/L for gentamicin and < 4.3 μmol/L for tobramycin) or < 8 mg/L (13.7 μmol/L) for amikacin,[a] to decrease risk of nephrotoxicity and ototoxicity
Nitrofurantoin	SCr	Only if renal function changing or unstable	Nitrofurantoin metabolites may accumulate in renal insufficiency and lead to neuropathy; avoid if CrCl < 40 mL/min (0.67 mL/s)
	Liver profile	Periodic monitoring	Prevention of cholestasis
Aminoglycosides Nitrofurantoin Tetracyclines Sulfonamides	SCr	Only if renal function changing or unstable	Decreases in glomerular filtrate rate can significantly decrease the urine concentration of these agents

[a]Streptomycin concentrations are different than those listed here; because streptomycin is not used to treat UTIs, monitoring for this agent is not included.

with women, an abnormality (structural or functional) should be suspected and therefore treated as a probable complicated infection until proven otherwise.[49] For this reason, men should not be treated with a single dose or short course of therapy if diagnosed with a UTI. Typically, these patients will receive 2 weeks of therapy and in situations of failure may be treated up to 6 weeks, particularly if a prostatic source of infection is suspected.

Outcome Evaluation

- Monitor the patient for resolution of symptoms with the goal of 48 to 72 hours to resolution after start of antimicrobial therapy
- If possible, follow-up on susceptibilities of the infecting organism detected by the urine culture
- Repeat urine culture is necessary only if symptoms do not acutely abate or reinfection or recurrence occurs. Resistance rates to *E. coli* are increasing to antibiotics commonly prescribed for UTI, and certain isolates are multidrug resistant.[50]
- Depending on the chosen antibiotic therapy, evaluate the patient based on drug therapy monitoring parameters including those presented in Table 79–4 to optimize therapy and decrease incidence of adverse events.

Patient Care Process

Patient Assessment:

- Based on physical exam, review of systems, and urinalysis, determine whether the patient is experiencing signs and symptoms of UTI.
- Assess patient medication history and risk factors for drug the potential of an antibiotic resistant infection.
- Assess patient renal function and other laboratory tests for antibiotic dosing and systemic complications.
- Identify potential sources of infection such as urinary catheters.

Therapy Evaluation:

- Based on urinalysis and Gram stain (if available), determine whether the empiric antibiotic selection is appropriate.
- Based on culture and susceptibility data (if available), determine whether any changes should be made from your initial empiric antimicrobial selection (ie, resistance to the regimen initially selected).
- Evaluate the patient's symptoms to determine response to the antimicrobial regimen you have chosen.
- Evaluate the patient for the presence of adverse drug reactions, drug allergies, and potential drug interactions.

Care Plan Development:

- Determine the optimal antibiotic dose and duration of therapy based on the patient and infection type (complicated vs uncomplicated).
- Determine whether the patient may benefit from prophylactic therapy (ie, recurrent UTIs secondary to chronic urinary catheterization due to paraplegia).
- Recommend lifestyle modifications as needed to minimize UTI recurrence.
- Discuss the importance of medication adherence throughout the entire recommended treatment duration.

Follow-Up Evaluation:

- Stress the importance of complying with the prescribed antimicrobial regimen and to follow up with the health care provider if signs and symptoms recur.

Abbreviations Introduced in This Chapter

CFU	Colony-forming units
CrCl	Creatinine clearance
IV	Intravenous
SCr	Serum creatinine
UTI	Urinary tract infection

REFERENCES

1. Gupta K, Hooton TM, Naber KG, et al. International clinical practice guidelines for the treatment of acute uncomplicated cystitis and pyelonephritis in women: A 2010 update by the Infectious Diseases Society of America and the European Society of Microbiology and Infectious Diseases. Clin Infect Dis. 2011;52:e103–e120.
2. Nicolle LE, Bradley S, Colgan R, et al. Infectious Diseases Society of America guidelines for the diagnosis and treatment of asymptomatic bacteriuria in adults. Clin Infect Dis. 2005;40:643–654.
3. Fihn SD. Clinical practice. Acute uncomplicated urinary tract infection in women. N Engl J Med. 2003;349:259–266.
4. Foxman B. Urinary tract infection syndromes: Occurrence, recurrence, bacteriology, risk factors, and disease burden. Infect Dis Clin North Am. 2014;28:1–13.
5. Uckay, I, Sax H, Gayet-Ageron, et al. High proportion of healthcare associated urinary tract infection in the absence of prior exposure to urinary catheter: A cross sectional study. Antimicrob Resist Infect Control. 2013;2:5.
6. Bent S, Nallamothu BK, Simel DL, et al. Does this woman have an acute, uncomplicated urinary tract infection? JAMA. 2002;287:2701–2710.
7. American Academy of Pediatrics, Subcommittee on Urinary Tract Infection, Steering Committee on Quality Improvement Management. Urinary tract infection: Clinical practice guideline for the diagnosis and management of the initial UTI in febrile infants and children 2 to 24 months. Pediatrics. 2011;128:595–610.
8. Alper BS, Curry SH. Urinary tract infection in children. Am Fam Physician. 2005;72:2483–2488.
9. Smellie JM, Prescod NP, Shaw PJ, et al. Childhood reflux and urinary infection: A follow-up of 10–41 years in 225 adults. Pediatr Nephrol. 1998;12:727–736.
10. Ronald AR, Pattullo AL. The natural history of urinary tract infection in adults. Med Clin North Am. 1991;75:299–312.
11. Foxman B. Epidemiology of urinary tract infections: Incidence, morbidity, and economic costs. Am J Med. 2002;113:5S–13S.
12. Hooten TM, Hillier S, Johnson C, et al. *Escherichia coli* bacteriuria and contraceptive method. JAMA. 1991;265:64–69.
13. Stamatiou C, Bovis C, Panaguopoulos P, et al. Sex-induced cystitis—patient burden and other epidemiological features. Clin Exp Obstet Gynecol. 2005;32:180–182.
14. Bran JL, Levison ME, Kaye D. Entrance of bacteria into the female urinary bladder. N Engl J Med. 1972;286:626–629.
15. Freedman LR. Experimental pyelonephritis. VI. Observation on susceptibility of the rabbit kidney to infection by a virulent strain of *Staphylococcus aureus*. Yale J Biol Med. 1960;32:272–279.
16. Gorrill RH, DeNavasquez SJ. Experimental pyelonephritis in the mouse produced by *Escherichia coli*, *Pseudomonas aeruginosa*, and *Proteus mirabilis*. J Pathol Bacteriol. 1964;87:79–87.
17. Stamey TA, Fair WR, Timothy MM, et al. Antibacterial nature of prostatic fluid. Nature. 1968;218:444–447.
18. Kwok L, Staphleton AE, Stamm WE, et al. Adherence of *Lactobacillus crispatus* to vaginal epithelial cells from women with or without a history of recurrent urinary tract infection. J Urol. 2006;176;2050–2054.
19. Gupta K, Stapleton AE, Hooton TM, et al. Inverse association of H_2O_2-producing lactobacilli and vaginal *Escherichia coli* colonization in women with recurrent urinary tract infections. J Infect Dis. 1998;178:446–450.
20. Medzhitov R. Toll-like receptors and innate immunity Nat Rev Immunol. 2001;1:135–45.
21. Parsons CL, Schrom SH, Hanno PM, Mulholland SG. Bladder surface mucin. Examination of possible mechanisms for its antibacterial effect. Invest Urol. 1978;6:196–200.
22. U.S. Preventive Services Task Force. Screening for asymptomatic bacteriuria in adults: U.S. Preventive Services Task Force reaffirmation recommendation statement. Ann Intern Med. 2008; 149:43–47.
23. Nicolle LE. Urinary tract infection in diabetes. Curr Opin Infect Dis. 2005;18:49–53.
24. Harding GK, Zhanel GG, Nicolle LE, et al. Antimicrobial treatment in diabetic women with asymptomatic bacteriuria. N Engl J Med. 2002;347:1576–1583.
25. Niël-Weise BS, van den Broek PJ. Urinary catheter policies for long-term bladder drainage. Cochrane Database Syst Rev. 2005;1:CD004201.
26. Sobel JD, Kaye D. Urinary tract infection. In: Mandell GL, Bennett JE, Dolin R, eds. Principles and Practice of Infectious Diseases. 8th ed. Philadelphia, PA: Elsevier; 2014:74.
27. Jepson RG, Craig JC. Cranberries for preventing urinary tract infection. Cochrane Database Syst Rev. 2008;1:CD001321.
28. Salo J, Uhari M, Helminen M, et al. Cranberry juice for the prevention of recurrences of urinary tract infections in children: A randomized placebo-controlled trail. Clin Infect Dis. 2012;54:340–346.
29. Barbosa-Cesnik C, Brown MB, Buxton M, et al. Cranberry juice fails to prevent recurrent urinary tract infection: Results from a randomized placebo-controlled trail. Clin Infect Dis. 2011;52:23–30.
30. Grin PM, Kowalewska PM, Alhazzan W, Fox-Robichaud AE. Lactobacillus for preventing recurrent urinary tract infections in women: Meta-analysis. Can J Urol. 2013 Feb;20(1):6607–6614.
31. Raz R, Stamm WE. A controlled trial of intravaginal estriol in post-menopausal women with recurrent urinary tract infections. N Engl J Med. 1993;329:753–756.
32. Lee BS, Bhuta T, Simpson JM, Craig JC. Methenamine hippurate for preventing urinary tract infections. Cochrane Database Syst Rev. 2012;10:CD003265.
33. Zhanel GG, Hisanaga TL, Laing NM, et al. Antibiotic resistance in *Escherichia coli* outpatient urinary isolates: Final results from the North American Urinary Tract Infection Collaborative Alliance (NAUTICA). Int J Antimicrob Agents. 2006;27:468–475.
34. Stamm WE, Hooton TM. Management of urinary tract infections in adults. N Engl J Med. 1993;329:1328–1334.
35. Ronald A. The etiology of urinary tract infection: Traditional and emerging pathogens. Am J Med. 2002;113:S14–S19.
36. Raz R, Colodner R, Kunin CM. Who are you—*Staphylococcus saprophyticus*? Clin Infect Dis. 2005;40:896–898.
37. Carson C, Naber KG. Role of fluoroquinolones in the treatment of serious bacterial urinary tract infections. Drugs. 2004;64:1359–1373.
38. Miller LG, Tang AW. Treatment of uncomplicated urinary tract infections in an era of increasing antimicrobial resistance. Mayo Clin Proc. 2004;79:1048–1054.
39. Reffert JL1, Smith WJ. Fosfomycin for the treatment of resistant gram-negative bacterial infections. Insights from the Society of Infectious Diseases Pharmacists. Pharmacotherapy. 2014;34:845–857.

40. Gupta K, Sahm DF, Mayfield D, et al. Antimicrobial resistance among uropathogens that cause community-acquired urinary tract infections in women: A nationwide analysis. Clin Infect Dis. 2001;33:89–94.
41. Sandberg T, Skoog G, Hermansson AB, et al. Ciprofloxacin for 7 days versus 14 days in women with acute pyelonephritis: A randomised, open-label and double-blind, placebo-controlled, non-inferiority trial. Lancet. 2012;380:484–490.
42. Rubenstein JN, Schaeffer AJ. Managing complicated urinary tract infections: The urologic view. Infect Dis Clin North Am. 2003;17:333–351.
43. Ovalle A, Levancini M. Urinary tract infections in pregnancy. Curr Opin Urol. 2001;11:55–59.
44. Christensen B. Which antibiotics are appropriate for treating bacteriuria in pregnancy? J Antimicrob Chemother. 2000;46: 29–34.
45. McDermott S, Daguise V, Mann H, et al. Perinatal risk for mortality and mental retardation associated with maternal urinary tract infections. J Fam Pract. 2001;50:433–437.
46. Sheiner E, Mazor-Drey E, Levy A. Asymptomatic bacteriuria during pregnancy. J Matern Fetal Neonatal Med. 2009 May;22(5): 423–427.
47. Nicolle LE, Bradley S, Colgan R, et al. Infectious Diseases Society of America guidelines for the diagnosis and treatment of asymptomatic bacteriuria in adults. Clin Infect Dis. 2005;40: 643–654.
48. Hooton TM, Bradley SF, Cardenas DD, et al. Diagnosis, prevention, and treatment of catheter-associated urinary tract infection in adults: 2009 International Clinical Practice Guidelines from the Infectious Diseases Society of America. Clin Infect Dis. 2010;50:625–663.
49. Naber KG, Bergman B, Bishop MC, et al. EAU guidelines for management of urinary and male genital tract infections. Urinary Tract Infection Working Group of the Health Care Office of the European Associated of Urology. Eur Urol. 2001;40:576–588.
50. Johnson JR, Johnston B, Clabots C, et al. *Escherichia coli* sequence type ST131 as the major cause of serious multidrug-resistant *E. coli* in the United States. Clin Infect Dis. 2010;51:286–294.

80 Sexually Transmitted Infections

Marlon S. Honeywell and Evans Branch III

LEARNING OBJECTIVES

Upon completion of the chapter, the reader will be able to:

1. Analyze the behavioral considerations and assess the importance of contraception with regard to the contributing factors of sexually transmitted infections (STIs).
2. Apply the "expedited partner treatment" method when recommending treatment for STIs.
3. Identify the patient populations that are typically affected by specific STIs.
4. Identify causative organisms for STIs.
5. Devise a list of the clinical signs and symptoms corresponding to each type of STI and classify patients based on recommended criteria.
6. Select appropriate diagnostic procedures for STIs.
7. Identify STI treatment regimens and recommend therapy when appropriate.
8. Design a patient care plan based on the monitoring parameters.

INTRODUCTION

Though we have made progress in medicine, age-old problems of infectious disease continue to plague us.[1] Even with the discovery of newly improved antibiotics, sexually transmitted infections (STIs) have not been eradicated. Many have reemerged secondary to modern social trends of sexual activity, and some as a result of the HIV epidemic, socioeconomic concerns, and the global lack of preventive education. KEY CONCEPT *Optimal detection and treatment of sexually transmitted diseases depends on counseling by a patient-friendly and knowledgeable clinician who can establish open communication with the patient.*

The correlation between risky sexual behavior and STIs is well documented.[2] Inconsistent and incorrect condom use increases the incidence of new STIs. KEY CONCEPT However, counseling patients on the consistent use of condoms, spermicides, or diaphragms is an important component in reducing the overall incidence of STIs.[3] Health care providers who manage persons at risk for STIs should counsel women concerning the option for emergency contraception, if indicated, and provide it in a timely fashion if desired by the woman or the couple. Plan B (two 750 mcg levonorgestrol) is approved in the United States for the prevention of unintended pregnancy.[4]

In addition to the increasing number of adolescents engaging in unsafe sexual practices is a high incidence of men who have sex with men (MSM) and women who have sex with women (WSW). Many MSM do not disclose their HIV status. This "don't ask, don't tell" practice has been linked to an upsurge in newly diagnosed HIV infections and STIs among previously noninfected people.[5] Although limited data are available with regard to STIs in WSW, risk of transmission probably varies by the specific STI and sexual techniques. Sharing penetrative items or employing practices involving digital vaginal or digital anal contact most likely represent common modes of transmission. This possibility is supported by reports of metronidazole-resistant trichomoniasis and genotype-specific HIV transmitted sexually between women who reported such behaviors and an increased prevalence of bacterial vaginosis (BV) among monogamous WSW.[6]

Sexual abuse in adolescents and children is becoming prevalent in the United States. Any child or adolescent with a STI should be evaluated for sexual abuse.[7] In cases of abusive contact, commonly found infections include *Neisseria gonorrhoeae* or *Chlamydia trachomatis*. Abusive cases should be reported to Child Protective Services.

Defined as a person who engages in the exchanging of spouses for sexual activities, the emergence of "swingers" as a new category of at-risk patients has been seen in STI clinics throughout the world. In fact, in one Canadian clinic, swingers composed 40.8% of patients that rarely accessed STI health services.[8] To this end, although little data exists, swingers now represent a group with risky behaviors that must be identified and treated, when necessary.

KEY CONCEPT *Optimally, both sex partners should be treated simultaneously for a STI; however, this is difficult to accomplish. Clinics and health departments often proactively attempt dual treatment by providing a prescription for the partner to the index patient (the patient who is evaluated by a clinician), a practice commonly known as patient-delivered partner therapy. Medications or prescriptions should be accompanied by treatment instructions and appropriate warnings.* Counseling regarding the appropriate use of condoms, cervical diaphragms, spermicides, and emergency contraception is also important to mitigate the occurrence of reinfection.

Accurate reporting of STIs is imperative to the evaluation of trends in sexual behaviors; reporting may be provider- or laboratory-based. State and local health departments may assist with the mechanism by which STIs are reported and cases must be conveyed in accordance with statutory requirements. Confidentiality should always be exercised in such cases.[9,10]

GONORRHEA

Gonorrhea is a curable STI caused by the gram-negative diplococcus *Neisseria gonorrhoeae*. Gonorrhea may be the second most commonly reported bacterial STI. Proper therapeutic management with antimicrobial agents is essential to eradicate this infection and prevent the development of associated sequelae such as a urethritis, cervicitis, or dysuria.

In the United States, the highest rate of gonococcal infection is seen within the 15- to 24-year-old age groups for both sexes; although more cases are reported in men. Approximately 700,000 new cases occur annually in the United States.[9,10] Factors associated with an increased risk of infection include ethnicity, low socioeconomic status, illicit drug use, and age. Targeted screening of young women, less than 25 years of age, who are at an increased risk has been correlated to gonorrhea control in the United States.[9] In fact, the risk of a cervical infection after a single episode of vaginal intercourse is approximately 50% and increases with multiple exposures. Furthermore, rates of reinfection are significantly higher among ethnic minorities.

PATHOPHYSIOLOGY

Attachment to mucosal epithelium, mediated in part by pili and opa (outer membrane opacity proteins), is followed by penetration of *N. gonorrhoeae* through epithelial cells to the submucosal tissue within 24 to 48 hours. A vigorous response by neutrophils begins with sloughing of the epithelium, development of submucosal microabscesses, and exudation of pus. Stained smears usually reveal large numbers of gonococci within a few neutrophils, whereas most cells contain no organisms.[11]

DIAGNOSIS

Several laboratory tests are available to aid in the diagnosis of gonorrhea and include Gram-stained smears, endocervical or vaginal specimens, culture, or the DNA hybridization probe. A Gram stain of a male urethral specimen that demonstrates polymorphonuclear leukocytes with intracellular gram-negative

Clinical Presentation of Gonorrhea[9,10]

General

- Purulent discharge

Signs

- Painful or swollen testicles
- Tubal scarring

Symptoms

Men:

- May be asymptomatic, though acute urethritis is the predominant manifestation
- Urethral discharge and dysuria, usually without urinary frequency or urgency
- When compared with nongonococcal urethritis, the discharge in gonococcal urethritis is generally more profuse and purulent
- Pain during urination

Women:

- Cervicitis, urethritis, increased vaginal discharge, dysuria, and intermenstrual bleeding
- Pain during urination
- Abdominal pain

Patient Encounter 1, Part 1

BJ is a 52-year-old man who visits a clinic complaining of profuse urethral discharge and swollen testicles for the past several days. The patient admits to having sexual intercourse with his wife and with another woman without barrier contraception (condoms). He also admits to having sexual intercourse with the other woman for more than 6 months.

What information is suggestive of gonorrhea?

What potential risk factors for STIs are present?

What other diagnostic tests should be ordered?

Patient Encounter 1, Part 2

PMH: Hypertension, diabetes, hyperlipidemia; no prior history of STIs; no drug allergies noted

Meds: Amlodipine 10 mg by mouth daily; furosemide 40 mg by mouth daily; metformin 500 mg by mouth three times daily; glipizide XL 5 mg by mouth daily; simvistatin 40 mg by mouth at bedtime

FH: Mother has diabetes and hypertension. Father is deceased

SH: Admits to having unprotected sex with wife and another woman. Does not smoke; drinks alcohol occasionally

ROS: C/o urethral discharge and swollen testicles

PE:

VS: BP 145/88 mm Hg, post prandial glucose 132 mg/dL (7.3 mmol/L), total cholesterol 188 mg/dL (4.86 mmol/L), P 70 beats/min, T 37.0°C (98.6°F)

Lab: Urethral discharge swab revealed *N. gonorrhoeae*; rapid plasma reagin (RPR) test was positive

Given this additional information, what is your assessment of the patient's condition?

What consideration should be given to other STIs?

Identify your treatment goals for this patient.

What pharmacologic alternatives are available for this patient?

diplococci may be considered diagnostic in symptomatic men. A gram-negative stain should not be considered sufficient for ruling out infection in asymptomatic men.[9] Additionally, Gram stain of endocervical, pharyngeal, or rectal specimens are also insufficient to detect infections. All patients who test positive for gonorrhea should be tested for other STIs, including chlamydia, syphilis, and HIV.

TREATMENT

The desired outcome is complete eradication of *N. gonorrhoeae* and avoidance of sequelae.

Pharmacologic Therapy[4,9,12,13]

KEY CONCEPT *Patients infected with gonorrhea often are coinfected with C. trachomatis and should receive therapy to eradicate both organisms concurrently.* To mitigate the probability of resistance, the combination of doxycycline and azithromycin have been prescribed.[9] Cephalosporins are now a secondary treatment option; if used, dual treatment may increase efficacy for pharyngeal infections. However, treatment failures involving cephalosporins have been noted in Hawaii and Asian countries. As such, clinicians should determine whether sexual activity may have occurred in these countries before recommending antibiotic therapy. Fluoroquinolones should not be prescribed for infections in MSM, in those with a history of recent foreign travel or partners' travel, or for infections acquired in California, Hawaii, and in Asian countries or for infections in other areas with increased gonococcal resistance.[14]

Gonoccocal resistance to some cephalosporins has emerged.[15] The recommended first-line treatment for gonorrhea in most countries is third generation cephalosporins, and in some cases, spectinomycin, doxycycline, and azithromycin.[16] The mechanism of resistance appears to be associated with a mosaic penicillin-binding protein in addition to other chromosomal mutations previously found to confer resistance to β-lactam antimicrobials. To mitigate the prevalence of cephalosporin resistance, strong antimicrobial management programs, expanding surveillance networks and procedures, and STI control and prevention is warranted.

Oral hormonal contraception has been evaluated to determine if it deters the acquisition of gonnococal infections in women. Though transmission of *N. gonorrhea* is poorly understood, one study suggested that oral hormonal contraception may lessen the probability of infection.[17] More studies are required to support this theory as a viable option for prevention.

Treatment of gonorrhea may vary according to clinical presentation and is indicated as follows[9]:

Uncomplicated Gonococcal Infection of the Cervix, Urethra, and Rectum*: Ceftriaxone 250 mg intramuscularly *or* cefixime 400 mg orally *or* single-dose injectable cephalosporin regimens *plus* azithromycin 1 g orally *or* doxycycline 100 mg orally twice daily for 7 days. Several alternative agents possess notable activity; however, they should not be used if pharyngeal infection is suspected. Alternatives include cefpodoxime 400 mg orally or cefuroxime axetil 1 g orally or azithromycin 2 g. Though unavailable in the United States, spectinomycin has also been prescribed.

MSM or Heterosexuals with a History of Recent Travel* Ceftriaxone 250 mg intramuscularly *or* cefixime 400 mg orally *plus* treatment for chlamydial infection if it has not been ruled out.

Uncomplicated Gonococcal Infection of the Pharnyx, Cervix, Urethra, or Rectum Ceftriaxone 250 mg intramuscularly plus azithromycin 1 g orally or doxycycline 100 mg orally twice daily for 7 days.

Coverage for Coinfection with *C. trachomatis* Azithromycin 1 g orally as a single dose *or* doxycycline 100 mg orally twice daily for 7 days. Since most gonococcal infections in the United States are susceptible to azithromycin and doxycycline, routine cotreatment might hinder the development of resistance.

Treatment of Gonorrhea in Special Situations

Uncomplicated infections of the cervix, urethra, and rectum can be treated with one of the following regimens in adults:

► ***Recommendations During Pregnancy***

- Pregnant women should be treated with a recommended or alternative cephalosporin. For women who cannot tolerate a cephalosporin, azithromycin 2 g orally may be prescribed. For treatment of presumptive or diagnosed *C. trachomatis*, azithromycin or amoxicillin is recommended.
- Doxycycline and fluoroquinolones are contraindicated.

Recommendations for Disseminated Gonococcal Infection (Regimens Should Be Continued for 24 to 48 Hours) Ceftriaxone 1 g intramuscularly or IV every 24 hours *or* cefotaxime 1 g IV every 8 hours *or* ceftizoxime 1 g IV every 8 hours. Continue regimens for 24 to 48 hours after improvement is noted. Once improvement begins, therapy should be converted to Cefixime 400 mg orally twice daily for at least one week.

Uncomplicated Infections of the Cervix, Urethra, and Rectum in Children Less Than 45 kg Ceftriaxone 250 mg intramuscularly as a single dose *or* spectinomycin 40 mg/kg intramuscularly as a single dose (not to exceed 2 g).

Gonococcal Conjunctivitis Ceftriaxone 1 g intramuscularly once for adults has demonstrated excellent response rates. Lavage of the infected eye(s) once with saline solution should also be considered. Patients treated for gonococcal conjunctivitis should also be treated prophylactically for *C. trachomatis* infection.

Patient Encounter 1, Part 3

Unprotected sex is a major risk factor for contracting STIs. Although the purulent discharge is consistent with gonorrhea infection, a positive urethral swab coupled with an incubation period consistent with gonorrhea confirms the diagnosis. A serologic test for HIV should be performed. Although gonorrhea has been confirmed in this patient, infection with *C. trachomatis* occurs commonly in this setting. The expedited partner treatment approach should be employed and treatment should effectively cover gonorrhea and chlamydia.

If this patient has an allergy to penicillin, how would the therapeutic management of the identified problems change?

*Regimens are given for one dose only.

Ophthalmic Neonatorum or Prophylactic Treatment for Infants Whose Mothers Have Gonococcal Infection Ceftriaxone 25 to 50 mg/kg IV or intramuscularly in a single dose, not to exceed 125 mg.

Gonococcal Scalp Access in Newborns Ceftriaxone 25 to 50 mg/kg/day IV or intramuscularly in a single daily dose for 7 days or cefotaxime 25 mg/kg IV or intramuscularly every 12 hours for 7 days may be used. If meningitis is noted, treatment duration of both medications should be extended for a total of 10 to 14 days.

Ophthalmic Neonatorum Prophylaxis Erythromycin (0.5%) ophthalmic ointment in a single application to the eyes *or* ceftriaxone 25 to 50 mg/kg IV or intramuscularly, not to exceed 125 mg in a single dose.

Outcome Evaluation

- Order diagnostic test for gonorrhea. If positive, recommend antibiotics that cover gonorrhea and chlamydia.
- Subsequent to treatment, expect the eradication of organisms responsible for gonorrhea and chlamydia.
- Monitoring is generally not required.

CHLAMYDIA

Epidemiology

Infection with *C. trachomatis* has increased dramatically in recent years. This bacterium is the most common cause of nongonococcal urethritis, accounting for as many as 40% of cases. Worldwide, this intracellular, gram-negative bacterium produces around 92 million new genital infections. The prevalence is highest in individuals less than or equal to 25 years. Associated sequelae include pelvic inflammatory disease (PID), ectopic pregnancy, and infertility.

PATHOPHYSIOLOGY

C. trachomatis possesses characteristics resembling both bacteria and viruses. Its major membrane is comparable to that of gram-negative bacteria, although it lacks a peptidoglycan cell wall and requires cellular components from the host for replication. Chlamydia transmission risk is thought to be less than that of gonorrhea.

CLINICAL PRESENTATION AND DIAGNOSIS

Common tests used to diagnose *C. trachomatis* include culture, enzyme immunoassay, DNA hybridization probe, or the direct fluorescent monoclonal antibody test. Diagnosis has been confirmed in women through urine or swab specimen collected from the endocervix and in men using a urethral swab or urine specimen. Most women are asymptomatic; therefore, an annual screening or physical is necessary, as early detection may reduce rates of transmission.

TREATMENT[9,18]

Uncomplicated Urethral, Endocervical, or Rectal Infection in Adults

The recommended adult regimen is azithromycin 1 g orally in a single dose *or* doxycycline 100 mg orally twice daily for 7 days. An alternate regimen *is* erythromycin ethylsuccinate 800 mg orally four times daily for 7 days *or* erythromycin base 500 mg orally four times daily for 7 days *or* levofloxacin 500 mg orally once daily for 7 days *or* ofloxacin 300mg orally twice daily for 7 days.

The recommended regimen for pregnant patients is azithromycin 1 g orally in a single dose *or* amoxicillin 1 g orally in a single dose *or* amoxicillin 500 mg orally three times daily for 7 days.

Alternate regimens include erythromycin base 500 mg orally four times daily for 7 days *or* 250 mg orally four times daily for 14 days *or* erythromycin ethylsuccinate 800 mg orally four times daily for 7 days *or* 400 mg orally four times daily for 14 days.

C. trachomatis Infection in Infants

Treatment of ophthalmia neonatorum or infant pneumonia should be with erythromycin base or ethylsuccinate 50 mg/kg/day orally divided into four doses daily for 14 days. An association between oral erythromycin and infantile hypertrophic pyloric stenosis (IHPS) has been reported in infants aged less than 6 weeks

Patient Care Process

Patient Assessment:

- Review the patient's medical history and determine whether the patient's symptoms are consistent with gonorrhea.
- Order a culture to identify whether *N. gonorrhea* is present.

Therapy Evaluation:

- Recommend therapy consistent with the treatment of gonorrhea and chlamydia.
- Ensure that the patient and partner receive adequate treatment for both organisms.

Care Plan Development:

- Counsel the patient on effective methods of contraception and on the possibility of side effects or of an allergy to the drug.

Clinical Presentation of Chlamydia[9,10,13]

General

- Asymptomatic

Signs

- Beefy red cervix that bleeds easily (women)

Symptoms

- When present, the urethral discharge is watery and less purulent than that seen with acute gonococcal urethritis. Complications resulting from lack of treatment or inadequate treatment include: epididymitis (in males), and PID including associated complications in women.

Other Diagnostic Tests

- Culture is usually positive for both chlamydia and gonorrhea.

Patient Care Process

Patient Assessment:

- Review the patient's medical history and determine whether the patient's symptoms are consistent with chlamydia.
- Order a culture to identify whether *C. trachomatis* is present.

Therapy Evaluation:

- Recommend therapy consistent with the treatment of gonorrhea and chlamydia.
- Ensure that the patient and partner receive adequate treatment for both organisms.

Care Plan Development:

- Counsel the patient on effective methods of contraception and on the possibility of side effects or of an allergy to the drug.

who were treated with this drug. Infants treated with erythromycin should be monitored for signs and symptoms of IHPS.

▸ ***Infant Pneumonia Caused by C. Trachomatis***

Erythromycin base or ethylsuccinate 50 mg/kg/day orally divided into four doses daily for 14 days.

Outcome Evaluation

- Order diagnostic test for chlamydia. If positive, recommend antibiotics that cover gonorrhea and chlamydia.
- Subsequent to treatment, expect the eradication of organisms responsible for gonorrhea and chlamydia.
- Monitoring is generally not required.

SYPHILIS

Syphilis, attributed to the spirochete *Treponema pallidum*, can have numerous and complex manifestations. Clinician familiarity, stage-specific diagnosis, and effective treatment are vital. Missed or inappropriately treated syphilis may result in cardiovascular complications, neurologic disease, or congenital syphilis.

EPIDEMIOLOGY AND ETIOLOGY

Since the 1940s, the incidence of syphilis declined drastically following the introduction of penicillin, but rose when HIV arrived from obscurity in the 1980s. In 2009, rates of primary and secondary syphilis increased for the tenth consecutive year, reaching the highest rate reported since 1995. Although increases have occurred mostly among men, in 2013, the rate of reported primary and secondary syphilis in the United States was 5.3 cases per 100,000 population. Additionally, from 2005 to 2013, the number of primary and secondary cases nearly doubled. The primary and secondary syphilis rate among black men was 5.2 times that among white men; the rate among black women was 13.3 times that among white women, emphasizing the need for enhanced preventive measures among blacks and MSM. The disparity among men and women has been observed across racial and ethnic groups and is highest in the South and among non-Hispanic blacks.[19]

PATHOPHYSIOLOGY

T. pallidum rapidly penetrates intact mucous membranes or microscopic dermal abrasions, and within a few hours, enters the lymphatics and blood to produce systemic illness. During the secondary stage, examinations commonly demonstrate abnormal findings in the cerebrospinal fluid (CSF). As the infection progresses, the parenchyma of the brain and spinal cord may subsequently be damaged.

Diagnosis and Clinical Presentation

▸ ***Stages of Syphilis***

Primary Syphilis Usually manifests as a solitary, painless chancre. Primary syphilis develops at the site of infection approximately 3 weeks after exposure to *T. pallidum*; the chancre is highly infectious.[9,20]

Secondary Syphilis Without appropriate treatment, primary syphilis will advance to secondary syphilis, a stage usually apparent from its clinical symptomatology. Symptoms include fatigue, diffuse rash, fever, lymphadenopathy, and genital or perineal condyloma latum. Additionally, the skin is most often affected and a rash may present as macular, macropapular, or pustular lesions or may involve skin surfaces including the palms of the hands and soles of the feet.

Latent Syphilis

Early Latent Usually occurs during the first year after infection and may be established in patients who have seroconverted, who had symptoms of primary or secondary syphilis, or who had sex with a partner with primary, secondary, or latent syphilis

Late Latent Patients should be considered to have late latent syphilis if the aforementioned criteria (early latent) are not met. In both stages, patients are usually asymptomatic and the lesions noted in the primary and secondary phase usually resolve; however, individuals are still seropositive for *T. pallidum*.

Tertiary Syphilis Develops years after the initial infection and may involve any organ in the body.

Congenital Syphilis

Congenital syphilis is a condition in which the fetus is infected with *T. pallidum* as a result of the hematogenous spread from an infected mother, although transmission may also occur from direct contact with the infectious genitalia of the mother. Since the primary stage of syphilis is characterized by spirochetemia, infectious rates of the fetus are nearly 100% if the mother has primary syphilis.[20,21]

Diagnostic procedures include dark-field microscopy, nontreponemal exams[9,20] (ie, the Venereal Disease Laboratory [VDRL] and the rapid plasma reagin [RPR] test), and treponemal exams (ie, enzyme immunoassay, the *T. pallidum* hemagglutination test, the fluorescent treponemal antibody test, and the enzyme-linked immunosorbent assay).

TREATMENT

After confirming the diagnosis of syphilis, the desired outcome is a fourfold decrease in quantitative nontreponemal titers over a 6-month period and within 12 to 24 months after treatment of

Patient Encounter 2

RM is a HIV-positive male who complains of first observing the appearance of a "sore" on his penis. He admits to disregarding the lesion; however, he is now experiencing fatigue, diffuse rash, fever, and perineal condyloma latum. He reports having unprotected sexual intercourse with two male partners. He denies pain or itching at the original site of the lesion, dysuria, or frequent urination. Additionally, there appears to be no vesicles in the genital area.

What information is suggestive of syphilis?

What stage of syphilis is present?

What potential risk factors for STIs are present?

How should the diagnosis of syphilis be confirmed in this patient?

If the diagnosis of syphilis is confirmed, what therapeutic options exist for this patient?

latent or late syphilis. An algorithm for the treatment of syphilis is shown in Figure 80–1.

With regard to neurosyphilis, a reduction in neurologic manifestations is desired, which may include seizures, paresis, meningitis, stroke, hyperreflexia, visual disturbances, hearing loss, neuropathy, or loss of bowel and bladder function. In late neurosyphilis, vascular lesions (meningovascular neurosyphilis) may also be observed; thus, a reduction in the number of observed lesions is warranted. A diminution in CSF WBC (less than $10 \times 10^3/mm^3$ [$10 \times 10^9/L$]) or protein levels (0.05 g/dL [0.5 g/L]) is also preferred.

Pharmacologic Therapy

KEY CONCEPT *Parenterally administered penicillin is recommended for all stages of syphilis* (*Table 80–1*). Although penicillin is the drug of choice, combinations of benzathine penicillin with procaine penicillin or oral penicillin preparations are not considered appropriate treatment regimens. Several reports demonstrated the misuse of the benzathine–procaine combination (Bicillin C-R) instead of the standard benzathine penicillin (Bicillin L-A) for treatment of syphilis.[20,22] Clinicians and purchasing agents should be aware of the similarities in product names to avoid errors in the prescribing and administration of these agents. Pertinent information germane to benzathine penicillin G is found in Table 80–1.

Alternative agents may be used in allergic individuals and include doxycycline, minocycline, tetracycline, or erythromycin base or stearate. Some patients (such as young children or pregnant women) may not respond favorably to alternative modalities or should not receive tetracyclines. Therefore, in patients who must be administered penicillin (ie, patients who are pregnant or have central nervous system [CNS] involvement) or are allergic, desensitization should be performed before the drug is initiated.

Patients may experience fever, chills, tachycardia, and tachypnea, a condition commonly known as the Jarisch-Herxheimer reaction, an acute febrile reaction accompanied by headache, myalgia, fever, and other symptoms within the first 24 hours after the initiation of therapy. This reaction is postulated to occur secondary to spirochete lysis and proinflammatory cytokine cascades. Treatment is supportive and may include antipyretic and anti-inflammatory agents, as well as fluid resuscitation and bed rest.

▶ *Primary Syphilis*

Drug of Choice

Adults Benzathine penicillin, 2.4 million units intramuscularly as a single dose. Additional doses of benzathine penicillin or other antibiotics do not enhance efficacy, regardless of HIV status.[9]

Children Benzathine penicillin 50,000 units/kg intramuscularly, up to the adult dose of 2.4 million units in a single dose. Infants less than 1 month of age diagnosed with syphilis should have a CSF test to determine if asymptomatic neurosyphilis is present. Patient records should be reviewed to decipher whether syphilis is congenital or acquired.

Alternatives Oral doxycycline 100 mg twice daily for 2 weeks *or* tetracycline 500 mg by mouth four times daily for 2 weeks. Limited literature also supports the use of ceftriaxone 1 g intramuscularly or IV once daily for 10 days *or* oral azithromycin as a single 2 g dose.[9,21]

▶ *Secondary and Early Latent Syphilis*

Treatment modalities administered in primary syphilis are also effective in secondary syphilis and early latent syphilis (less than 1 year duration).

Children with early latent syphilis should receive benzathine pencillin G 50,000 units/kg intramuscularly, up to the adult dose of 2.4 million units in a single dose.

▶ *Late Latent Syphilis*

Benzathine penicillin, 7.2 million units total, administered as three doses of 2.4 million units intramuscularly each at 1-week intervals.

Children with late latent syphilis should be treated with benzathine penicillin G 50,000 units/kg intramuscularly, up to the adult dose of 2.4 million units, administered as three doses at 1-week intervals (total 150,000 units/kg up to the adult dose of 7.2 million units)

▶ *Tertiary Syphilis*

Drug of Choice Benzathine penicillin 2.4 million units administered intramuscularly once weekly for 3 weeks. A total of 7.2 million units should be administered.

Alternatives In nonpregnant patients with a penicillin allergy, alternative regimens include doxycycline 100 mg orally two times daily for 4 weeks *or* tetracycline 500 mg orally four times daily for 4 weeks.

▶ *Gummatous and Cardiovascular Syphilis*

As long as no evidence of CNS involvement exists, antibiotic therapy for gummatous and cardiovascular syphilis is identical to that for tertiary syphilis.

▶ *Neurosyphilis*

As an effective treatment for neurosyphilis, the Centers for Disease Control and Prevention (CDC) endorse two regimens of penicillin. Alternatively, ceftriaxone may also be prescribed.[25]

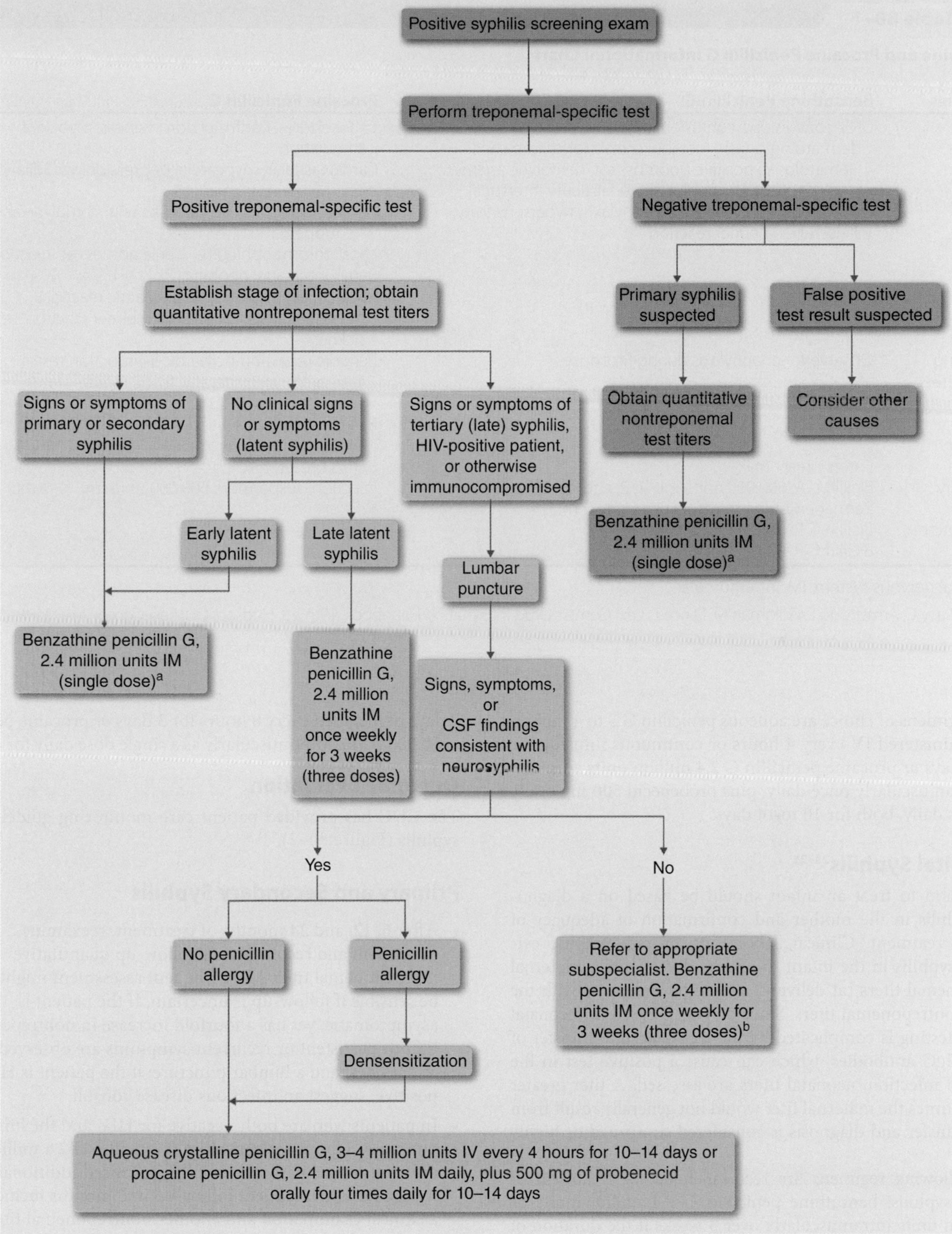

FIGURE 80–1. Treatment of syphilis. (CSF, cerebrospinal fluid; IM, intramuscularly.) (From Brown D, Frank J. Diagnosis and management of syphilis. Am Fam Physician. 2003;68(2):283–290.) [a]Alternative treatments for nonpregnant penicillin-allergic patients: doxycycline 100 mg orally twice daily for 2 weeks, or tetracycline 500 mg four times daily for 2 weeks; limited data support ceftriaxone 1 g once daily IM or IV for 8 to 10 days; or azithromycin, 2 g orally (single dose). [b]Alternative treatments for nonpregnant penicillin-allergic patients: doxycycline, 100 mg orally twice daily for 4 weeks, or tetracycline 500 mg orally four times daily for 4 weeks.

Table 80–1

Benzathine and Procaine Penicillin G Informational Chart

Categories	Benzathine Penicillin G	Procaine Penicillin G
Potential adverse reactions	CNS: convulsions, confusion, drowsiness, myoclonus, fever; dermatologic: rash; metabolic: electrolyte imbalance; Hematologic: positive Coombs test, hemolytic anemia; local: pain, thrombophlebitis; renal: acute interstitial nephritis; miscellaneous: anaphylaxis, hypersensitivity, Jarisch-Herxheimer reaction	CNS: seizures, confusion, drowsiness, myoclonus, CNS stimulation Cardiovascular: myocardial depression, vasodilation, conduction disturbances Hematologic: positive Coombs test, hemolytic anemia, neutropenia Local: thrombophlebitis, sterile abscess at injection site Renal: interstitial nephritis Miscellaneous: pseudoanaphylactic reactions, hypersensitivity, Jarisch-Herxheimer reaction, serum sickness
Monitoring parameters	Observe for anaphylaxis during first dose	Periodic renal and hematologic function tests with prolonged therapy; fever, mental status, WBC
Pregnancy category	B	B
Lactation	Enters breast milk	Enters breast milk
Availability	Bicillin L-A: 600,000 units/mL (1, 2, and 4 mL); Permapen Isoject: 600,000 units/mL (2 mL)	Injection, suspension: 600,000 units/mL (1, 2 mL)
Combination	Bicillin C-R: (1, 2, 4 mL) Bicillin C-R: 900/300: (2 mL)	Same

CNS, central nervous system; IM, intramuscular.

Data from Lacy C, Armstrong L, Goldman M, Lance L. Lexi-Comp's Drug Information Handbook, 19th ed. Hudson, OH: Lexi-Comp; 2010:1128–1132.

The regimens of choice are aqueous penicillin G 3 to 4 million units administered IV every 4 hours or continuous infusion for 10 to 14 days *or* procaine penicillin G 2.4 million units administered intramuscularly once daily, plus probenecid 500 mg orally four times daily, both for 10 to 14 days.

Congenital Syphilis[23-25]

The decision to treat an infant should be based on a diagnosis of syphilis in the mother and confirmation of adequacy of maternal treatment. Clinical, laboratory, or radiographic evidence of syphilis in the infant should be documented. Maternal nontreponemal titers (at delivery) should be compared with the infant's nontreponemal titers. Since diagnosis based on neonatal serologic testing is complicated by the transplacental transfer of maternal IgG antibodies, which can cause a positive test in the absence of infection, neonatal titers are assessed. A titer greater than four times the maternal titer would not generally result from passive transfer and diagnosis is considered confirmed or highly probable.

The following regimens are recommended for treatment of maternal syphilis: benzathine penicillin G 2.4 million units or 7.2 million units intramuscularly over 3 weeks if the duration of syphilis has been at least a year. An alternative regimen is procaine penicillin 0.6 to 0.9 million units intramuscularly for 10 to 14 days, or ceftriaxone 1 g daily intramuscularly or IV for 8 to 10 days.

In women who experience uterine cramping, pelvic pain, or fever, administer acetaminophen to combat these symptoms. Additionally, the patient should be well hydrated and rested.

Treatment of asymptomatic neonates is with 50,000 units/kg of benzathine penicillin G in a single intramuscular dose. Symptomatic neonates should receive 50,000 units/kg of aqueous crystalline penicillin G every 12 hours intramuscularly for the first 7 days of life, then every 8 hours for 3 days *or* procaine penicillin G 50,000 IU/kg intramuscularly as a single dose daily for 10 days.

Outcome Evaluation

The CDC has provided patient care monitoring guidelines for syphilis (Figure 80–2).[9,11,20]

Primary and Secondary Syphilis

- After 6, 12, and 24 months of treatment, reexamine the patient and recommend a follow-up quantitative nontreponemal titer. More frequent assessment might be sensible if follow-up is uncertain. If the patient is asymptomatic, yet has a fourfold increase in nontreponemal titer or persistent or recurrent symptoms are observed, order an HIV test and a lumbar puncture; if the patient is HIV-positive, suggest an infectious disease consult.
- In patients who are both negative for HIV and the lumbar puncture, administer benzathine penicillin G 2.4 million units intramuscularly once weekly for three additional weeks. Perform a patient follow-up in 6 months including a clinical examination and another nontreponemal titer. In HIV-negative patients with lumbar puncture findings compatible with neurosyphilis, treat the patient accordingly for neurosyphilis.
- Six months after the original diagnosis, institute a standard clinical follow-up exam in patients who show no symptomatology and a fourfold decrease in nontreponemal titers. By testing and observing the patient for signs of remission, you may be able to initiate proper treatment or recommend a consult in a timely fashion, thereby decreasing the propensity of the patient's condition to advance to a higher stage.

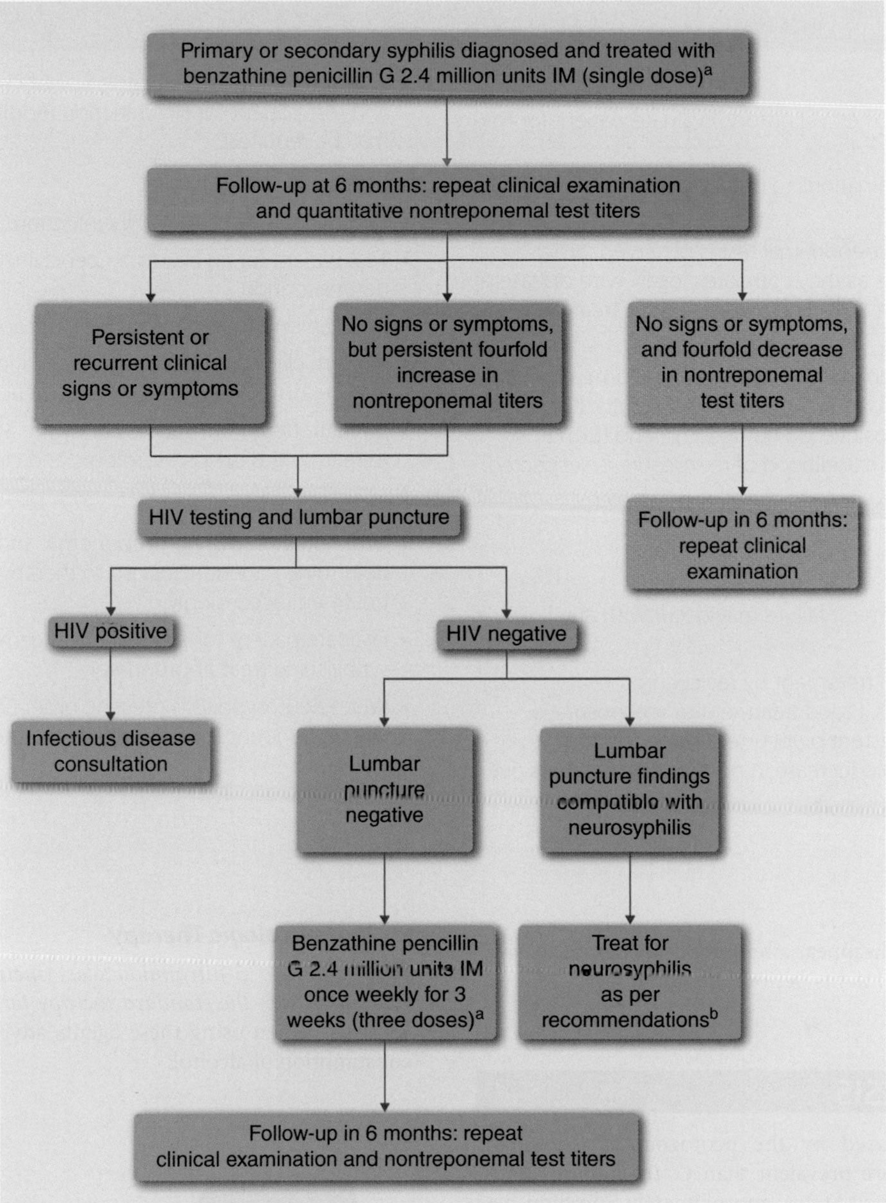

FIGURE 80–2. Patient care monitoring for syphilis. (From Brown D, Frank J. Diagnosis and management of syphilis. Am Fam Physician. 2003;68(2):283–290.) ([a]See text for alternative treatment recommendations for nonpregnant penicillin-allergic patients. [b]See text for treatment recommendations for neurosyphilis.)

- If serologic titers do not decline despite a negative CSF examination and a repeated course of therapy, it is unclear whether additional therapy or CSF examinations are needed; additional testing or repeated therapy is not generally recommended.

Early and Late Latent Syphilis

- Order nontreponemal titers 6, 12, and 24 months after instituting treatment for early or late latent syphilis. Neurosyphilis should be strongly considered in patients who show a fourfold increase in titers, patients who have an initially high titer (1:32 or greater) that fails to decline at least fourfold within 12 to 24 months of therapy, HIV-infected patients, and patients who develop signs or symptoms associated with neurosyphilis.

Neurosyphilis

- Follow-up is dependent on the CSF findings. If pleocytosis is present, reexamine the CSF every 6 months until the WBC count normalizes. Consider recommending a second course of treatment if the CSF white count does not decline after 6 months or completely normalize after 2 years.[4,9,20] Failure to normalize may require retreatment; most treatment failures occur in immunocompromised patients.

Congenital Syphilis

- Observe the patient for changes in clinical features; hepatomegaly, jaundice, and bone changes will usually resolve in 3 months.
- Monitor elevated serologic markers (nontreponemal tests) for reduction in titer levels. Given effective treatment, clinical

Patient Care Process

Patient Assessment:

- Review the patient's medical history. Evaluate patient for HIV infection.
- Order darkfield examinations to detect *T. pallidum* in lesion exudate or tissue.
- If positive, a positive treponemal test is observed, order nontreponemal titers as they correlate closely with disease activity. Titers generally decline subsequent to treatment initation.
- If a negative treponemal test is observed, perform a different treponemal test to confirm initial results. If second treponemal test is positive, do not recommend further management unless a likelihood of reexposure is suspected.
- Offer treatment to those without prior exposure to *T. pallidum*.

Therapy Evaluation:

- Recognize that treatment failure may occur with any regimen.
- Evaluate response to treatment by reviewing the nontreponemal titers. Failed treatment or reexposure is consistent with persistent or recurrent signs and symptoms or a sustained fourfold increase in nontreponemal titers over a 6- to 12-month period.
- If treatment failure is observed, analyze CSF for neurosyphilis and test patient for HIV infection. Additional serologic tests may be required.

Care Plan Development:

- Test patient for possible HIV infection.
- Test patient for an allergy to pencillin. If allergic, recommend desensitization.
- Recommend treatment for the appropriate stage of syphilis.
- Perform clinical and serologic evaluation at 6 and 12 months after treatment to assess for treatment success of failure.
- Evaluate treatment success or failure and the necessity of retreatment based on serologic and clinical exams.

Follow-Up Evaluation:

- Order quantitative nontreponemal and CSF tests to determine patient response to therapy. Adjust doses and treatment accordingly.
- Evaluate patient for signs of advancement in stages of syphilis and treat appropriately.
- When neurosyphilis is present, order CSF exams and leukocyte count to evaluate effectiveness of treatment.

features will usually disappear after 6 months. On this basis, evaluate seropositive infants periodically for at least 6 months.[24]

TRICHOMONIASIS

Trichomoniasis is caused by the protozoan *Trichomonas vaginalis* and is far more prevalent than *C. trachomatis* or *N. gonorrhoeae*. In the United States, approximately 5 million new cases appear annually, compared with 3 million chlamydial and 650,000 gonococcal cases annually.[26]

PATHOPHYSIOLOGY

T. vaginalis, a protozoa, may be isolated from the vagina, urethra, and Bartholin or Skene glands. After attachment to the host cells, it ignites an inflammatory response exhibited as a discharge containing elevated levels of polymorphonuclear leukocytes. The pathogen causes direct damage to the epithelium, leading to microulcerations.

Clinical Presentation and Diagnosis

Diagnosis is usually performed with a wet mount or Papanicolaou smear. In women, symptoms are characterized by diffuse, malodorous, yellow-green vaginal discharge with vulvar irritation. Some women may be asymptomatic.

Treatment

The desired outcome is the complete eradication of *T. vaginalis* in both partners and elimination of the signs and symptoms observed.

▶ *Pharmacologic Therapy*

KEY CONCEPT *The 5-nitroimidazoles (metronidazole and tinidazole) have been the standard therapy for trichomoniasis for over 45 years.* When using these agents advise patients to avoid the consumption of alcohol.

Clinical Presentation of Trichomoniasis[9,26]

General

- Asymptomatic

Signs

- Strawberry cervix (women)
- Colpitis macularis (women)
- Prostatitis or epididymitis (men)

Symptoms

- Vaginal/vulvar erythema
- Excessive yellow-green discharge
- Vulvar itching
- Vaginal odor
- Urethral discharge or irritation
- Dysuria
- Vaginal pH greater than 4.5

Patient Care Process

Patient Assessment:

- Review the patient's medical history and determine whether the patient's symptoms are consistent with trichomoniasis.
- Order a Papanicolaou smear to identify whether *T. vaginalis* is present.

Therapy Evaluation:

- Recommend therapy consistent with the treatment of trichomoniasis.
- Ensure that the patient and partner receive adequate treatment.

Care Plan Development:

- Counsel the patient on effective methods of contraception and on the possibility of side effects or of an allergy to the drug.

Metronidazole Metronidazole may be administered orally as a single 2 g dose or 500 mg twice daily for 7 days.[9,26] Pregnant women should be prescribed the single dose of metronidazole. Cure rates are greater than 90% when metronidazole is administered as either a single 2 g dose or a 7-day regimen. Possible adverse effects include an unpleasant metallic taste, reversible neutropenia, urticaria, rash, flushing, dry mouth, darkened urine, and a disulfiram-like reaction.

Tinidazole Tinidazole, a second-generation nitroimidazole with protozoal and anaerobic activity.[27] As a single 2 g dose, tinidazole has an efficacy equivalent to a 2 g dose of metronidazole. Tindazole also has a longer half-life than metronidazole, 14 and 7 hours, respectively, and penetrates into male reproductive tissue better than metronidazole.

Tinidazole is effective for metronidazole-resistant trichomoniasis.[26,27] Possible side effects include an unpleasant metallic taste, dizziness, loss of coordination, seizures, severe diarrhea, darkened urine, nausea, vomiting, and a swollen or discolored tongue.

Outcome Evaluation

- Order diagnostic test for trichomoniasis. If positive, recommend antibiotics that cover *T. vaginalis*.
- Subsequent to treatment, expect the eradication of the protozoa.
- Monitoring is generally not required.

GENITAL WARTS

Genital warts, caused by the human papillomavirus (HPV), usually appear in the genital area as very contagious, small bumps. Responsible for various visible, keratotic, and nonkeratotic manifestations, HPV has more than 120 noted strains, some of which have been linked to squamous cell carcinoma.[28] More than 40 strains have been linked to the genital area.[9]

EPIDEMIOLOGY AND ETIOLOGY

Genital warts are caused by several strains of HPV and are spread by skin-to-skin contact during sexual activity.[29] Affecting over 20 million Americans, HPV is the most common newly diagnosed STI in the United States, with prevalence just about 15.2%. Approximately 6.2 million new HPV infections occur every year in the United States.[30] Condoms offer incomplete (grade B, level II [fair research-based evidence to support the recommendation]) protection against HPV.[29]

The frequency of cervicovaginal HPV infection among sexually active women has been observed at 43%, with the greatest incidence noticed in men with three or more sex partners and women whose most recent regular sexual partner had two or more lifetime partners. Most people with HPV do not develop symptoms. At least half of sexually active persons will become infected at least once in their lifetime. In 90% of the cases, the body immune system clears HPV naturally within 2 years. Routine testing for HPV infection is not recommended. HPV types 16 and 18 cause 99.7% of all cervical cancer while HPV types 6 and 11 are responsible for about 90% of genital warts.[31]

PATHOPHYSIOLOGY

HPV replicates in terminally differentiated squamous cells in the intermediate layers of the genital mucosa. Hence, these effects of the viral early region genes on DNA synthesis are critical for viral survival. Genital warts are the clinical manifestation of active viral replication and virion production at the infection site.

Clinical Presentation and Diagnosis

- A definitive diagnosis of HPV is based on DNA or RNA or capsid protein detection.
- Diagnosis is generally made from the clinical presentation and may be classified into several categories: classic condyloma acuminata, which are pointed or cauliform; keratotic warts with a thick, horny surface resembling common skin warts; and flat warts, frequently observed on the surface.
- Tissue biopsy or viral typing is only indicated if the diagnosis is uncertain and is not recommended for patients with routine or typical lesions.
- Since HPV is highly associated with cervical cancer and has more than 20 different cancer-associated HPV types, patients who are diagnosed with HPV should be tested for cervical cancer.

Clinical Presentation of Genital Warts[9,30,31]

General

- Appear as rough, thick, cauliflower-like lesions

Signs

- Black dots within warts
- Disrupted surface

Symptoms

- Anogenital pruritus
- Burning
- Vaginal discharge or bleeding
- Although rare, dyspareunia may occur with vulvovaginal condyloma

Table 80–2

Comparison of Adverse Effects Seen With Treatments for Genital Warts

Treatment	Adverse Effects
Podofilox	Burning at site of application, pain, inflammation
Imiquimod	Erythema, irritation, ulceration, pain, burning, edema, pigmentary changes
Sinecatechins	Burning at site of application, erythema, pruritus, edema
Podophyllin resin	Local irritation, erythema, burning, soreness at application site; possibly oncogenic
Bichloroacetic and trichloroacetic acid	Local irritation and pain, minimal systemic effects
Cryotherapy	Pain or blisters at application site
Surgical excision	Pain, bleeding, scarring; possible burning or allergic reaction to local anesthetic
Vaporization	Pain, bleeding, scarring; risk of HPV spreading via smoke plumes
Intralesional interferon	Burning, itching, irritation at injection site, systemic myalgia, headache, fever, chills, leukopenia, elevated liver enzymes, and thrombocytopenia

HPV, human papillomavirus.

Data from Refs. 9, 28, and 31.

Treatment

Approximately 40% to 60% of untreated warts will spontaneously resolve in 9 to 12 months if left untreated.[29] Treatment of benign, symptomatic genital warts is aimed at alleviation of physical symptoms and cosmetic improvement. Removal of visible warts and reduction of infectivity are the goals of treatment.

A comparison of adverse effects related to treatment options may be found in Table 80–2.[32]

▶ *Patient-Applied Treatment*

Podofilox Available as a 0.5% gel or solution containing purified extract of the most active compound of podophyllin, podofilox arrests the formation of the mitotic spindle, prevents cell division, and may also induce damage in blood vessels within the warts. The surface area treated must not exceed 10 cm^2, and a maximum of 0.5 mL should be used on a daily basis.

Apply podofilox twice daily for 3 consecutive days followed by 4 consecutive days without treatment. This cycle may be repeated until there are no visible warts or for a maximum of 4 weeks. Side effects are generally local and may include erythema, swelling, and erosions. Podofilox is not recommended for use in the vagina, anus, or during pregnancy.

Imiquimod Imiquimod is a cell-mediated immune-response modifier, available as a topical 5% cream in single-dose application packets. There are two recommended dosage regimens:

a. Apply at bedtime, three times a week for up to 16 weeks.
b. Apply every other day for three applications.

The treatment area should be washed with soap and water 6 to 10 hours after application. Mild to moderate erythema has been noted with imiquimod use; however, this generally suggests that the drug is reaching a therapeutic range and may be clearing the lesion.[33,34]

Sinecatechins A green tea extract with an active product (catechins), is available as a 15% ointment. Apply a thin layer (0.5 cm) using a finger to each wart, three times a day until complete clearance of warts. Do not wash off after use and all sexual contact should be avoided while ointment is on the skin. This product should not be continued for longer than 16 weeks.[9]

▶ *Physician-Applied Treatments*

Podophyllin Resin A 10% to 25% solution of podophyllin resin has been the standard in-office treatment for genital warts. Because podophyllin is neurotoxic and easily systemically absorbed, only a small amount (no more than 0.5 mL) should be applied, avoiding normal tissue. Application should be limited to less than 0.5 mL of podophyllin on an area of less than 10 cm^2 of warts per session and no open lesions or wounds should exist in the area to which treatment is administered. The affected area will likely become erythematous and painful within 48 hours of application.[34]

Topical podophyllin is applied once weekly and the area should be allowed to dry. Immediately following treatment, the dried drug should be removed using alcohol or soap and water. It is contraindicated in pregnant patients.

Bichloroacetic (BCA) and Trichloroacetic (TCA) Acids These products are available in 80% to 90% concentrations and are not systemically absorbed. The products are effective when used to treat a few, small, moist lesions. Apply once a week until wart is resolved. They may be applied to both keratinized epithelial and mucosal surfaces and may be used in pregnancy.

A noted reaction to these medications is transient burning; contact with surrounding epithelium may prove to be painful, producing significant local erythema and swelling. To avoid these effects, place petroleum jelly around the external lesion, including unaffected skin, and carefully apply the agent with a small applicator. If an excess amount of acid is used, talc or sodium bicarbonate (baking soda) may be administered to neutralize unreacted acid.

Other Treatments Other treatments may include fluorouracil/epinephrine/bovine collagen gel, an intralesional injection that has been proven effective in clinical trials for refractory patients or an intralesional injection of interferon.[31]

▶ *Ablative Therapy*

Several ablative options have been employed in the treatment of genital warts and include cryotherapy, surgical removal, and vaporization.

▶ *Special Therapeutic Issues* [32–35]

Large Warts Treat warts greater than 10 mm in diameter with surgical excision. Use imiquimod for three to four treatment cycles to reduce the number of warts and improve surgical outcomes. Fifty percent reduction in wart size after four treatment cycles warrants continued use of imiquimod until warts clear or eight cycles have been completed; less than 50% reduction warrants surgical excision or other ablative therapy.

Subclinical Warts Subclinical warts may be identified through colonoscopy, biopsy, acetic acid application, or laboratory serology. However, early treatment has not been linked to a favorable effect during the course of therapy in the index patient or the partner with regard to reduction of the transmission rate.

Pregnancy Agents contraindicated in pregnancy include podofilox, sinecatechins, fluorouracil, and podophyllin. Imiquimod is not approved for use in pregnancy, although it has been

Patient Care Process

Patient Assessment:

- Physical examination should be done.
- Order a pregnancy test.
- Review symptoms.
- Verify sexual history.
- Determine if lesions are a first episode or reoccurrence.
- Review all medical conditions and medications.

Therapy Evaluation:

- Discuss the treatment options with the patient including observation without active treatment.
- Determine the choice of therapy based on the size, site, and morphology of the lesion.
- Include patient preference, treatment cost, adverse effects, and convenience before making a decision.

Care Plan Development:

- Emphasize to the patient that sexually active people can lower the chance of getting HPV by limiting the number of partners.
- Order oral contraception for fertile women.
- Start patient treatment and continue for the recommended duration.
- Switch to an alternate therapy if there has been no response after two to three treatment cycles.

Follow-up Evaluation:

- Follow-up every 2 to 3 months for a reduction in lesions or disease remission.
- Monitor patient compliance, disease remission, and benign or cancerous tumors.

considered after signed consent has been obtained. Bichloroacetic and trichloroacetic acids have been used without problems. Ablative therapy is also a viable option.

Outcome Evaluation

- Monitor the patient for any visible warts and relief of symptoms.
- Apply powder with talc, baking soda, or liquid soap to remove unreacted trichloracetic or bichloroacetic acid.
- Dry area before contact with normal mucosa after application of podophyllin.
- Repeat TCA, BCA, podophyllin treatment weekly if necessary.
- Administer a different agent if warts persist after one type of therapy.
- Refer all recalcitrant patients to local STI clinic, gynecologists, dermatologists, or urologists.

Vaccinations

Several HPV genotypes have been linked to the development of cervical cancer. Gardasil, developed to protect against HPV genotypes 6, 11, 16, and 18, was the first vaccine employed to prevent cervical cancer, precancerous genital lesions, and genital warts due to HPV. Cervarix vaccine prevents cervical cancer and precancers caused by HPV types 16 and 18. The CDC recommends the HPV vaccine for all 11- and 12-year-old females and males. Vaccination is also recommended for females aged 13 through 26 years and males 13 to 21 years old who have not been previously vaccinated or who have not completed the full series of shots.[36] The quadrivalent vaccine Gardasil is FDA-approved for females and males 9 to 26 years old.[37]

Both inactivated vaccines are given in a series of three injections over a 6-month period. The second and third doses should be given at 2 and 6 months (respectively) after the first dose. HPV vaccine may be given at the same time as other vaccines. Vaccines are efficacious in preventing genital warts; however, they will not clear those that are already present.

GENITAL HERPES

Genital herpes (GH) is caused by herpes simplex virus (HSV) types 1 and 2. HSV is a chronic, lifelong viral infection, for which there is no cure. Once latency is established, neither competent host immunity nor therapeutic agents can eradicate the virus.[9] Currently, there is no vaccine available for HSV, and it seems that the development of one is unlikely in the near future.

EPIDEMIOLOGY AND ETIOLOGY

Approximately 50 million Americans have GH. HSV-2 is the most common cause of recurrent genital herpes. Roughly 1 in 6 people in the United States (16.2%) aged 14–49 is infected with HSV-2. Prevalence of HSV-2 infection has grown by approximately slightly since the late 1970s (16.4%–17.2%), and currently over 500,000 new cases of HSV-2 occur annually.

PATHOPHYSIOLOGY

Nearly all HSV-2 infections are sexually acquired. Since HSV is only found in humans, infection may only be transmitted from infectious secretions onto mucosal surfaces (ie, cervix or urethra) or direct contact with an active lesion (abraded skin). The virus may survive for a limited amount of time on environmental surfaces. Most sexual transmission occurs while the source case is asymptomatic. Most patients with asymptomatic or unrecognized genital HSV infections will still shed virus intermittently in the genital tract. Patients will have small, painful blisters that are filled with fluid. The first outbreak takes 2 to 4 weeks to heal, with later attacks being less severe. Because there is no cure for this illness, treatment will only help reduce the signs, symptoms, and number of attacks.

Clinical Presentation and Diagnosis

Ulcerative or multiple vesicular lesions are absent in many infected persons. Laboratory confirmation is vital to effective treatment of HSV, especially in individuals in whom a clinical diagnosis cannot be obtained. There are several methods by which a definitive diagnosis may be acquired, and these include virologic typing, serologic diagnosis, rapid point-of-care antigen detection, enzyme-linked immunosorbent assay (ELISA), immunoblot, and DNA polymerase chain reaction.[38] Glycoprotein G-based assays may also be used to aid in the diagnosis of HSV.

Treatment

The desired outcome is to curtail the number of episodic prodromes and to minimize any side effects experienced due to the

Clinical Presentation of Genital Herpes[9,38,39]

General

- Asymptomatic

Classic Sign

- A cluster of painful vesicles on an erythematous base

Symptoms

- Itching
- Burning
- Tingling
- Groin lump
- Dysuria
- Dyspareunia
- Increased urinary frequency

Other Symptoms

- Ulcerative lesions, fissures, cervicitis

antivirals. Counseling of infected persons and their partners is vital to the management of HSV.

► *First Episode*

The first episode is a systemic illness associated with the vesicular lesions, may last up to 21 days, usually has an uncomplicated course of infection, and in severe cases may require hospitalization. Several agents are effective during this period (Table 80–3).[39–41] At the cited dosages, these agents have had excellent outcomes with regard to lesion healing time, viral shedding, and loss of pain. Common adverse effects are nausea, headache, and diarrhea. It is important to note that the first episode does not necessarily indicate recent infection and the genital symptoms may develop several years after the infection was acquired. Condom use in new or uninfected partners particularly in the 12 months after the first attack is recommended.

► *Episodic Therapy*

In a patient with a previous diagnosis of genital herpes, the appearance of new vesicular lesions is synonymous with HSV reactivation. For most patients, genital herpes recurrence is self-limiting and short-lived, lasting approximately 6 to 7 days.

► *Suppressive Therapy*

Suppressive therapy is effective for controlling all symptoms related to the disease and may impact troublesome complications of infection. Before beginning suppressive therapy, discuss patient expectations. Encourage patients to record any breakthrough episodes, as this may require treatment reevaluation and adjustment.

► *Preventive Therapy*

Valacyclovir 500 mg orally once daily has been used to prevent the sexual transmission of HSV to an uninfected partner. In addition to pharmacologic therapy, counsel patients regarding safe sex practices.

► *Drug Resistance*

All acyclovir resistant strains are resistant to valacyclovir and the majority are resistant to famciclovir. Foscarnet, cidofovir, and trifuridine have been administered in acyclovir-resistant patients.[42] These agents are usually reserved for use after other medications have failed because of their associated toxicities.

► *Pregnancy*

Women who are pregnant may transmit the virus to the neonate during delivery. There are two management strategies: caesarean section and antiviral therapy. Acyclovir 200 to 400 mg every 8 hours has been administered from 38 weeks' gestation until delivery. Acyclovir, famciclovir, and valcyclovir are all classified as category B (no evidence of risk in humans) for use during pregnancy. Suppressive treatment includes the use of acyclovir or valacyclovir from week 36 until delivery. The goal of therapy is to reduce the number of lesions and asymptomatic shedding at delivery.

► *Neonates*

The risk for transmission from an infected mother to a neonate is high among women who acquired GH near time of delivery. HSV infections should be considered in all neonates who present with nonspecific symptoms such as fever, poor feeding, lethargy, or seizures in the first month of life. Infants suspected to have or who are diagnosed with an HSV infection should be treated parenterally. Acyclovir 20 mg/kg/day in three divided doses IV for 21 days for disseminated and CNS disease or 14 days for disease limited to skin, eyes, and mucous membranes.

Outcome Evaluation

- Monitor for systemic symptom improvement and a decrease in viral shedding in initial HSV treatment.
- Take lukewarm baths three to four times a day to ease itching and pain. Pat dry infected areas.
- Wear loose-fitting underwear to help the sore dry.
- Avoid sexual contact until treatment is finished.
- Consider stopping suppressive therapy after 1 year to assess recurrence rate.
- Compound topical 1% cidofovir gel in acyclovir-resistant strains where IV foscarnet is not preferred.

PELVIC INFLAMMATORY DISEASE

Pelvic inflammatory disease (PID) usually affects young, sexually active, reproductive-age women. PID includes a spectrum of inflammatory disorders of the upper female genital tract. In the majority of cases, the pathogens responsible are *C. trachomatis* and *N. gonorrhoeae*; although anaerobes, enteric gram-negative rods, and cytomegalovirus have also been implicated in the pathogenesis.[43] PID has been correlated with ectopic pregnancy, infertility, tubo-ovarian abscess, and chronic pelvic pain.[44]

Epidemiology and Etiology

PID is most common in women younger than 25 years of age, who have more than one sex partner. More than 750,000 women are affected by PID each year in the United States. The highest rates of PID occur in teenagers and first time mothers. Up to 10% to 15% of these women may become infertile as a result of PID. The CDC estimates that more than 1 million women experience

Table 80–3

Comparison of Antiviral Agents Used for Herpes Simplex Infection

Agent	Dose	Side Effects
First Episode		
Acyclovir	*200 mg orally five times a day × 7–10 days* ***Or*** 400 mg orally three times daily × 7–10 days	Headache, confusion, nausea, vomiting, thrombocytopenia, renal insufficiency, rash, pruritus, fever, arthralgias, myalgia, thrombotic thrombocytopenic purpura, hallucinations, somnolence, depression
Valacyclovir	*1 g orally two times daily × 7–10 days*	Refer to acyclovir
Famciclovir	250 mg orally three times daily × 7–10 days	Refer to acyclovir
Episodic		
Acyclovir	*200 mg orally five times daily × 5 days* ***Or*** 400 mg orally every 8 hours × 5 days ***Or*** 800 mg orally two times daily × 5 days ***Or*** 800 mg orally three times daily × 2 days	Refer to acyclovir (WHO)
Valacyclovir	*500 mg orally two times daily × 3 days* ***Or*** 1 g orally once daily × 5 days	Refer to acyclovir
Famciclovir	125 mg orally two times daily × 5 days ***Or*** 1000 mg orally twice daily × 1 day	Refer to acyclovir
Suppressive		
Acyclovir	400 mg orally two times daily continuously ***Or***	Refer to acyclovir
Valacyclovir	500 mg orally once daily continuously ***Or***	Refer to acyclovir
Valacyclovir	1000 mg orally once daily continuously ***Or***	Refer to acyclovir
Famciclovir	250 mg orally two times daily continuously	Refer to acyclovir
Reserved Agents		
Foscarnet	40 mg/kg IV every 8 hours until clinical resolution is attained	Renal insufficiency, metabolic disturbances, hypophosphatemia
Cidofovir	1% topical agent (gel) used daily on a compassionate basis for acyclovir-resistant herpes lesions for 5 days	Application site reactions, lesion recrudescence
Imiquimod	Topical alternative used daily on a compassionate basis for acyclovir-resistant herpes lesions for 5 days	Application site reactions, lesion recrudescence

Italicized data indicate recommended dosages.

Data from Refs. 9 and 33.

Patient Encounter 3

LS is a 27-year-old female model who decides to visit her gynecologist because of a 1-month history of vaginal burning, vaginal bleeding, and rough thick lesions around her perianal area. Currently, LS is not in a monogamous relationship. Upon questioning, LS stated she was treated twice before for STIs in the past decade. Her last sexual encounter was 2 weeks ago and stated they did not utilize protection.

What information is suggestive of genital herpes?

What potential risk factors for STIs are present?

What additional information is required to initiate a treatment plan? What is your opinion about the use of the Gardasil vaccine in this patient?

Patient Encounter 4

BC is the father of patient 1 (LS) only child. BC is a 33-year-old former NBA player that was forced to retire 4 years ago due to a long history of substance abuse. BC has three other children from two different women. BC became mentally and emotionally stress after hearing of LS's diagnosis. BC has experienced symptoms of painful urination, enlarged lymph nodes, and small blisters in his genital area 3 days ago. BC was initially informed of his HSV-2 status during his rookie year in the NBA.

Given this information, what is your assessment of the patient?

Identify the treatment goals for this patient?

BC subsequently states that acyclovir did not work during his last episode. What are his options?

Patient Care Process

Patient Assessment:

- Based on physical exam, ask a series of questions: Do you have sores in the genital area or anywhere else on your body? Do the sores come and go? Do you have frequent urination or burning/stinging with urination? If discharge is present, does it smell or have color? Do you use condoms or birth control? Have you or your partner ever been treated for a STI in the past? Is this your first outbreak?
- Review all medical conditions and medications including dosing.
- Review available laboratory test if available of definitive diagnosis.

Therapy Evaluation:

- Base treatment on likelihood of patient compliance, whether it is first or a recurrent episode, host immunity, and pregnancy.
- Remind patient that response has been linked to the time it takes to initiate treatment with acyclovir, or its analogues, after symptom onset.

Care Plan Development:

- Immediately initiate therapy (within one day of onset) in episodic treatment of systematic recurrent lesions for patient to experience benefit from agent.
- Emphasize that sexually active people can lower their chances of spreading HSV by using condoms.
- Evaluate and educate all sex partners of infected persons.

Follow-up Evaluation:

- Reevaluate the patient's psychosocial and psychosexual status.
- Order tests to detect malignant changes of the female genital tract.
- Order yearly testing for HIV status.
- Review side effects of drugs with the patient.
- Frequently reassess all recurrent episodes and therapy adjustments.

an episode of PID every year. The disease leads to approximately 2.5 million office visits annually. Since many cases of PID go unrecognized and some episodes are asymptomatic, the potential for damage to the reproductive health of women has increased. There is an increased risk for women with past STIs and with partners who have more than one partner.

PATHOPHYSIOLOGY

PID is an infection that occurs when bacteria move upward from a woman's vagina into her reproductive organs. Normally, the cervix prevents bacteria from entering the vagina and spreading to the reproductive organs. However, when the cervix is exposed to STI's such as chlamydia and gonorrhea, the bacteria is disseminated to the female internal organs. Chlamydia may produce a heat-shock protein that causes tissue damage through a delayed hypersensitivity reaction. *C. trachomatis* may also possess DNA evidence of toxin-like genes that code for high-molecular-weight proteins with structures similar to *Clostridium difficile* cytotoxins, enabling inhibition of immune activation. This may explain the observation of a chronic *C. trachomatis* infection in subclinical PID.

Clinical Presentation and Diagnosis[43,46]

Because many women with PID have subtle or mild symptoms, delays in diagnosis and treatment probably led to inflammatory sequelae in the upper reproductive tract. To be diagnosed with PID, patients must have uterine tenderness, cervical motion tenderness, painful urination, lower abdominal pain, painful intercourse, and adnexal tenderness with no other cause of these signs. Additional criteria include:

- Oral temperature greater than 38.3°C (101°F)
- Abnormal cervical or vaginal discharge or that has an unusual color (green or yellow)
- WBC presence on saline microscopy of vaginal secretions
- Elevated erythrocyte sedimentation rate
- Elevated C-reactive protein
- Laboratory documentation of cervical infection with *N. gonorrhoeae or C. trachomatis*

Treatment

The removal of causative bacteria and reduction of any related sequelae are the desired goals of treatment. Resolution of infection (ie, *N. gonorrhoeae, C. trachomatis, Streptococcus* spp., and gram-negative facultative bacteria) and mitigation of sequelae should be the main goal of pharmacologic therapy. Treatment regimens for PID must provide empiric, broad-spectrum coverage of likely pathogens. CDC-approved treatment regimens are shown in Table 80–4.[9,43]

Though outpatient management remains contentious, many feel that outpatient management should be limited to individuals who: remain afebrile, have a WBC counts less than $11 \times 10^3/mm^3$ ($11 \times 10^9/L$), have minimal evidence of peritonitis, have active bowel sounds, and can tolerate oral nourishment. Nonetheless, outpatient therapy with a parenteral cephalosporin followed by doxycycline and metronidazole is recommended.

OUTCOME EVALUATION

- Reevaluate any patient who does not respond significantly within 72 hours of parenteral/oral treatment.
- Initiate parenteral therapy (inpatient or outpatient) for patients that do not respond to oral treatment.
- Continue parenteral therapy for 14 days; however, it may be stopped 24 hours after clinical improvement and doxycycline continued to complete 14 days of therapy.
- Hospitalization and reassessment of the antimicrobial regimen and diagnostics are recommended in women without clinical improvement.
- Repeat testing of all women who have been diagnosed with chlamydia or gonorrhea is recommended 3 to 6 months after treatment, regardless of whether their sex partners were treated.
- Inform the patient that an alteration in sexual behavior should be the first concern, as promiscuous sexual activity augments the probability of infection.

Table 80–4

Treatment Regimens for Pelvic Inflammatory Disease

Parenteral Option A

Cefotetan 2 g IV every 12 hours

Or

Cefoxitin 2 g IV every 6 hours plus doxycycline 100 mg orally or IV every 12 hours

Parenteral Option B

Clindamycin 900 mg IV every 8 hours plus gentamicin, loading dose IV or IM (2 mg/kg) followed by maintenance dose (1.5 mg/kg) every 8 hours. A single daily dose of gentamicin (3–5mg/kg) may be used

Alternative Parenteral treatment

Ampicillin-sulbactam 3 g IV every 6 hours plus doxycycline 100 mg orally or IV every 12 hours

Oral

Ceftriaxone 250 mg intramuscular single dose plus doxycycline 100 mg orally twice daily for 14 days with or without metronidazole 500 mg orally twice daily for 14 days

Or

Cefoxitin 2 g intramuscular single dose and probenecid 1 g single dose, plus doxycycline 100 mg orally twice daily for 14 days with or without metronidazole 500 mg orally twice daily for 14 days

Or

Third-generation cephalosporin (ceftizoxime or cefotaxime) plus doxycycline 100 mg orally twice daily for 14 days with or without metronidazole 500 mg orally twice daily for 14 days

Data from Refs. 9, 45, and 46

Abstinence is the best course of action, especially in patients with herpes during lesional episodes. However, compliance in some may be minimal, in which case, appropriate condom use should always be recommended. To alleviate any possible misconceptions about condom application, either demonstrate how to apply a condom or ask the patient to demonstrate. During

Clinical Presentation of Pelvic Inflammatory Disease[9,46]

General

- Signs and symptoms may vary from mild to severe

Signs

- Vague

Symptoms

- Lower abdominal or pelvic pain
- Malodorous vaginal discharge
- Abnormal uterine bleeding
- Dyspareunia
- Dysuria
- Nausea and/or vomiting
- Fever

Patient Care Process

Patient Assessment:

- Based on a physical exam that includes a pelvic exam, determine if the patient is experiencing and pain in the lower belly or back, vagina discharge with or without color, painful sex, fever, or burning during urination.
- Test for pregnancy, complete blood count, gonorrhea, chlamydia, and bacterial vaginosis.

Therapy Evaluation:

- Optimal management of PID should be individualized based on clinical setting and patient characteristics.
- For some patients, hospitalizations, IV antibiotics, and surgical treatment of complications may be needed.

Care Plan Development:

- If no clinical improvement has occurred within 3 days after parenteral or outpatient oral therapy, perform further assessment.
- Educate the patient about the goals of monitoring patients with PID are related to reducing long-term complications.
- Examine the male sex partners of women with PID if the patient's onset of symptoms occurred within the previous 60 days. Remind women that numerous sex partners increase the risk of developing PID.

Follow-up Evaluation:

- Advise a combination of prevention efforts.
- The primary approach should be prevention and education of at-risk women.
- Secondary prevention includes screening by conducting a pelvic exam during a routine check-up.
- Verify substantial clinical improvement within 72 hours after initiation of therapy.

Patient Encounter 5

PMH: History of chlamydia 2 years ago. Allergy to clindamycin

FH: Noncontributory

SH: 18-year-old college freshman and current girlfriend of BC. Admits that she has a secretive sexual relationship with the starting football quarterback

ROS: Unpleasant vaginal odor, painful sex, and pain in her lower abdomen

PE:

VS: BP 135/85, Ht 5′4″ (163 cm), Wt 117 lb (53.2 kg) T 97.8°F (36.6°C)

In the past, the patient utilized condoms frequently; but states they cause her to have yeast infections and has since discontinued their use.

What consideration should be given to other STIs?

What oral treatment options are available for this patient?

What non-pharmacologic therapy should be recommended for this patient?

the demonstration, explicitly educate the patient with regard to application, storage, and the use of lubricants.[46]

Abbreviations Used in This Chapter

CSF	Cerebrospinal fluid
ELISA	Enzyme-linked immunosorbent assay
GH	Genital herpes
HPV	Human papillomavirus
HSV	Herpes simplex virus
MSM	Men who have sex with men
PID	Pelvic inflammatory disease
RPR	Rapid plasma reagent
STI	Sexually transmitted infection
WSW	Women who have sex with women

REFERENCES

1. Birley H, Duerden B, Hart CA, et al. Sexually transmitted diseases: Microbiology and management. J Med Microbiol. 2002;51:793–807.
2. Aral SO. Sexually risky behaviour and infection: Epidemiological considerations. Sex Transm Infect. 2004;80(Suppl 2):ii8–ii12.
3. Kann L, Kinchen S, Shanklin SL, et al. Youth risk behavior survelliance—United States in 2013. MMWR Surveill Summ. 2014 Jun 13; 63 Suppl 4:1–168.
4. Gemzell-Danielsson K, Berger C, Lalitkumar PG. Emergency Contraception-Mechanism of Action. *Contraception.* 87. 2013. 300–308.
5. Glick S, Golden M. Early male partnership patterns, social support, and sexual risk behavior among young men who have sex with men. AIDS Behav. 2014 Aug;18(8):1466–1475.
6. Fethers K, Marks C, Mindel A, et al. Sexually transmitted infections and risk behaviors in women who have sex with women. Sex Transmit Infect. 2000;76:345–349.
7. Bechtel K. Sexual abuse and sexually transmitted infections in children and adolescents. Curr Opin Pediatr. 2010;22:94–99.
8. O'Byrne P, Watts JA. Exploring sexual networks: A pilot study of swingers' sexual behaviour and health-care-seeking practices. Can J Nurs Res. 2011;43(1):80–97.
9. Sexually transmitted diseases. MMWR Treatment Guidelines. 2010. www.cdc.gov/mmwr. Accessed June 24, 2014.
10. Kodner C. Sexually transmitted infections in men. *Primary Care.* 2003; 30(1):173–191.
11. Mandell, Douglas, and Bennett's Principles and Practice of Infectious Disease. *JAMA.* 2010;304(18):2067-2071.
12. Barbee L, Dombrowski J. Control of Neisseria gonorrhoeae in an era of evolving antimicrobial resistance. Infect Dis Clin North Am. 2013;27(4):723–737.
13. Center for Disease Control and Prevention. Recommendations for the laboratory-based detection of *Chlamydia* and *Neisseria gonorrhoeae*—2014. MMWR Recomm Rep. 2014 Mar 14;63 (RR-02):1–19.
14. Kirkcaldy RD, Kidd S, Weinstock HS, Papp JR, Bolan GA. Trends in antimicrobial resistance in *Neisseria gonorrhoeae* in the USA: the Gonococcal Isolate Surveillance Project (GISP), January 2006–June 2012. Sex Transm Infect. 2013;89 Suppl 4:iv5–iv10.
15. Barbee L. Preparing for an era of untreatable gonorrhea. Curr Opin Infect Dis. 2014;27(3):282–287.
16. Bala M and Sood S. Cephalosporin resistance in Neisseria gonorrhoeae. J Glob Infect Dis. 2010;2(3):284–296.
17. Gursahaney PR, Meyn LA, Hiller SL, Sweet RL, Wiesenfeld HC. Combined hormonal contraception may be protective against Neisseria gonorrhoeae infection. Sex Transm Dis. 2010; 37 (6): 356–360.
18. Young F. Sexually transmitted infections. Genital chlamydia: Practical management in primary care. J Fam Health Care. 2005;15:19–21.
19. Summary of Notifiable Diseases in the United States 2014. Morbidity and Mortality Weekly Report. MMWR (http://www.cdc.gov/mmwr/preview/mmwrhtml/mm6318a4.htm?s_cid=mm6318a4_w). Accessed July 2, 2014.
20. Pastuszczak M, Wojas-Pelc A. Current standards for diagnosis and treatment of syphilis: selection of some practical issues, based on the European (IUSTI) and U.S. (CDC) guidelines. Postepy Dermatol Alergol. 2013;30(4):203–210.
21. Cohen SE, Klausner JD, Engelman J, Philip S. Syphilis in the modern ear: an update for physicians. Infect Dis Clin North Am. 2013;27(4):705–722.
23. Gupta R, Vora RV. Congenital syphilis, still a reality. Indian J Sex Transm Dis. 2013;34(1): 50–52.
24. Peeling RW, Ye H. Diagnostic tools for preventing and managing maternal and congenital syphilis: An overview. Bull World Health Organ. 2004;82(6):439–446.
25. Berman SM. Maternal syphilis: Pathophysiology and treatment. Bull World Health Organ. 2004;82(6):433–438.
26. Seña A, Bachmann LH, Hobbs MM. Persistent and recurrent *Trichomonas vaginalis* infections: Epidemiology, treatment, and management considerations. Expert Rev Anti Infect Ther. 2014;12(6):673–685.
27. Tinidazole (Tindamax)—a new option for treatment of bacterial vaginosis. Med Lett Drugs Ther. 2007;49(1269):73–74.
28. Kodner CM, Nasraty S. Management of genital warts. Am Fam Physician. 2004;70:2335–2342.
29. Lopaschuk CC. New approach to managing genital warts. Can Fam Physician. 2013;59(7): 731–736.
30. Ault K. Epidemiology and natural history of human papillomavirus infections in the female genital tract. Infect Dis Obstet Gynecol. 2006:1-5;Article ID: 40470.
31. Smith GD, Travis L. Getting to know human papillomavirus (HPV) and the HPV vaccines. J Am Osteopath Assoc. 2011;111 (3 suppl 2):S29–S34.
32. Gunter J. Genital and perianal warts: new treatment opportunities for human papillomavirus infection. Am J Obstet Gynecol. 2003;189:S3–S11.
33. Bowden FJ, Tabrizi SN, Garland SM, Fairley CK. Sexually transmitted infections: New diagnostic approaches and treatments. Med J Aust. 2002;176:551–557.
34. World Health Organization. (2003). Guidelines for the management of sexually transmitted infections. http://www.who.int/HIV/pub/sti/en/STIGuidelines2003.pdf.
35. Woodward C, Fisher MA. Drug treatment of common STDs: Part II. Vaginal infections, pelvic inflammatory disease and genital warts. Am Fam Physician. 1999;60:1716–1722.
36. Gardasil. http://www.cdc.gov/vaccines/vpd-vac/hpv/vac-faqs.html. Accessed August 1, 2014.
37. Genital Warts. Women's Health 2013 (May 9). Accessed August 9, 2014.
38. Patel R. Progress in meeting today's demands in genital herpes: an overview of current management. J Infect Dis. 2002;186(Suppl 1):S47–S56.
39. Alexander L, Naisbett B. Patient and physician partnerships in managing genital herpes. J Infect Dis. 2002;186(Suppl 1):S57–S65.
40. Lacy C, Armstrong L, Goldman M, Lance L. Lexi-Comp's Drug Information Handbook, 19th ed. 2013:1128–1132.

41. Kimberlin DW, Rouse DJ. Clinical Practice. Genital herpes. N Eng J Med. 2004;350:1970–1977.
42. Wald A. New therapies and prevention strategies for genital herpes. Clin Infect Dis. 1999;28(Suppl 1):S4–S13.
43. Miller KE, Ruiz DE, Graves JC. Update on the prevention and treatment of sexually transmitted diseases. Am Fam Physician. 2003;67(9):1915–1922.
44. Epperly AT, Viera AJ. Pelvic inflammatory disease. Clin Fam Pract. 2005;7:67–78.
45. Beigi RH, Wiesenfeld HC. Pelvic inflammatory disease: New diagnostic criteria and treatment. Obstet Gynecol Clin North Am. 2003(Dec);30(4):777–793.
46. FDA. Condoms and Sexually Transmitted diseases. http://www.fda.gov/oashi/aids/condom.html. Accessed August 24, 2011.

81 Osteomyelitis

Melinda M. Neuhauser and Susan L. Pendland

LEARNING OBJECTIVES

Upon completion of the chapter, the reader will be able to:

1. List common risk factors for osteomyelitis.
2. Discuss the pathophysiology of osteomyelitis.
3. Compare and contrast the classic signs and symptoms of acute and chronic osteomyelitis.
4. Evaluate microbiology culture data and other laboratory tests and imaging studies utilized for diagnosis of osteomyelitis.
5. List the most common pathogens isolated in acute and chronic osteomyelitis.
6. Develop a treatment plan for osteomyelitis.
7. Recommend parameters to monitor antimicrobial therapy for effectiveness and toxicity.
8. Educate patients regarding disease state and drug therapy.

INTRODUCTION

KEY CONCEPT *Osteomyelitis is an infection of the bone that can be an acute or chronic process.* The inflammatory response associated with acute osteomyelitis can lead to bone necrosis and subsequently chronic infections.[1] Bacterial pathogens, particularly *Staphylococcus aureus*, are the most common microorganisms implicated in these infections.[1–8] Diagnosis and treatment are often difficult due to the heterogeneous nature of osteomyelitis.[1,2] Medical management is the mainstay of treatment for acute infections; however, surgical intervention is necessary for chronic infections that involve bone necrosis.[1,2] Outcomes may vary based on patient-specific risk factors, duration of disease, and site of infection.[1,2]

KEY CONCEPT *Osteomyelitis is most often classified by duration of disease and route of infection.*[1,2,9] Historically, osteomyelitis has been classified as acute or chronic based on duration of disease.[1,2,9] However, there are no established definitions for acute and chronic infections.[1,9,10] Acute infection has been defined as first episode or recent onset of symptoms (within 2 weeks).[2,9–11] Chronic osteomyelitis is generally defined as relapse of the disease or symptoms persisting beyond 2 months.[2,9] Because there is no abrupt demarcation, but rather a gradual shift from acute to chronic infection, others describe chronic osteomyelitis as the presence of necrotic bone.[1,2,10,11]

In the Waldvogel classification scheme, the route of infection is categorized as either hematogenous or contiguous.[9] Osteomyelitis secondary to a contiguous focus is further subdivided into infections with or without vascular insufficiency. Typical bone involvement in osteomyelitis depends on the route of infection.

- Hematogenous: long bones (femur, tibia) in children and vertebra in the elderly[2–5,10]
- Contiguous with vascular insufficiency: lower extremities[2,11,12]
- Contiguous without vascular insufficiency: bones affected by trauma, surgery, or adjacent to soft-tissue infection[1,5]

A single pathogen is most often isolated in hematogenous osteomyelitis, whereas multiple organisms are often isolated in contiguous osteomyelitis.[7,10,11,13]

EPIDEMIOLOGY AND ETIOLOGY

Hematogenous osteomyelitis is the most common type of osteomyelitis in children while osteomyelitis due to contiguous spread is most common in adults.[1–4,6] Hematogenous osteomyelitis is reported in older adults and IV drug users, with the spine (vertebral osteomyelitis) being the most common site of infection.[1,2,5]

KEY CONCEPT *S. aureus is the predominant pathogen seen in all types of osteomyelitis, with methicillin-resistant S. aureus (MRSA) being increasingly reported.*[1–4,6,10] However, the spectrum of potential causative pathogens varies with patient-specific risk factors including the following:

- Patients with uncontrolled diabetes and/or peripheral vascular disease have poor wound healing and often present with nonhealing skin ulcers. These wounds are typically colonized with a mixture of aerobic and anaerobic microorganisms, which can lead to polymicrobial osteomyelitis.[1,11,13,14] Common aerobic pathogens in this setting may include MRSA, Enterobacteriaceae, and *Pseudomonas aeruginosa*.[11,14] Therefore, if a wound is deep or extensive, these patients should be evaluated for underlying osteomyelitis.[11,14]
- Sickle cell patients (*Salmonella* spp)[1,2,7]

- Individuals with prosthetic implants (coagulase-negative staphylococci)[7]
- Neonates (*E. coli* or group B streptococci)[2]
- Patients with pressure sores (polymicrobial)[2,7]

PATHOPHYSIOLOGY

Both microbial and host factors are important determinants in the development of osteomyelitis.[1] Healthy bone tissue is normally resistant to infection but may become susceptible under certain conditions.[1,2] Bone can become infected: (a) via the presence of bacteria in the bloodstream, (b) by direct inoculation from trauma or surgery, and (c) by spread from an adjacent site (eg, soft-tissue infection).[1] The latter is particularly problematic in patients with foreign body implants (eg, hip replacement) and chronic skin ulcers.[1,11]

Staphylococcus species possess bacterial adhesins, which promote their attachment to tissues and foreign devices.[1] Microbial adherence to bone elicits an inflammatory response.[1] The subsequent release of leukocytes and cytokines leads to edema and ischemia. In some cases, these processes can lead to bone necrosis.[1] Pieces of dead bone may become separated, forming sequestra.[1] These areas typically cannot be penetrated by antimicrobials and phagocytic cells and thus require surgical intervention to eradicate the bacterial nidus.[1,11]

CLINICAL PRESENTATION AND DIAGNOSIS

General

The clinical presentations of osteomyelitis may vary depending on route and duration of infection, as well as patient-specific factors such as infection site, age, and comorbidities.[1–4,7,11,14]

KEY CONCEPT *The gold standard for diagnosis of osteomyelitis is a bone biopsy with isolation of microorganism(s) from culture and the presence of inflammatory cells and osteonecrosis on histologic exam.*[1,2,11–14] *Due to the invasive nature of the bone biopsy, the diagnosis of osteomyelitis is often based on clinical findings, laboratory tests, and imaging studies rather than bone biopsy.*[1,12,13]

KEY CONCEPT *Typical signs and symptoms of osteomyelitis include local pain and tenderness over the affected bone, as well as inflammation, erythema, edema, and decreased range of motion.*[1,3,4,6,9] *Patients with acute hematogenous osteomyelitis may also present with fever, chills, and malaise.*[1,3,4,9] A cardinal sign of chronic osteomyelitis is the formation of sinus tracts (a channel from the infected site to the skin) with purulent drainage.[1]

Laboratory Tests

No single noninvasive laboratory test is currently available for the diagnosis of osteomyelitis.[1] Despite low specificity, several tests are commonly used to aid in the diagnosis and to monitor response to therapy.

Nonspecific inflammatory markers for infection include:[1,2,4–6]

- White blood cell count (WBC)
- Erythrocyte sedimentation rate (ESR)
- C-reactive protein (CRP)
- Procalcitonin

WBC, ESR, and CRP are often elevated, but may also be within normal limits. An elevated WBC is mostly seen in patients with acute osteomyelitis.[1,2,6,9] CRP rises faster than ESR during early stages of infection and also returns to normal levels more quickly than ESR. This makes CRP a more useful tool for both diagnosis and monitoring of therapeutic response.[4–6] Similar to CRP, procalcitonin may be useful for both diagnosis and monitoring of therapeutic response; however, it is often more expensive and may not be as readily available.[4]

Microbiologic Evaluation

Isolation of causative pathogen from bone biopsy samples is essential for targeted antimicrobial therapy.[1–3,5,7,11,12] If bone biopsy is not done, quality specimens (eg, two consecutive samples with bone contact [deep samples] in patients with contiguous osteomyelitis[12,15] or blood cultures in patients with acute hematogenous osteomyelitis[1,3,5] may assist in pathogen identification. Superficial swabs often represent colonization rather than infecting organism(s).[1,7,12,14]

Imaging Studies

- Imaging tests are used to assist in the diagnosis of osteomyelitis.[1,3,12,14,16,17]
- Plain film radiographs (x-rays) are the initial imaging study of choice for skeletal infections.[1,5,6,12,16] Although changes in soft tissue may appear within 3 days of infection, bone lesions may not be visible for 10 to 21 days.[1,4,6,11,12,16] Advantages of radiographs are accessibility, cost, low radiation exposure, and they are readily repeatable.[5,16] A disadvantages is the inability to detect early bone infections.[1,3,4,6,11,16]
- Magnetic resonance imaging (MRI) is considered the best overall imaging modality for the diagnosis of osteomyelitis.[1,3,4,11,13,14,16,17] Advantages include early detection (ie, 3–5 days after onset of infection), no radiation exposure, and high resolution.[1,6,16,17] Disadvantages include expense, inconvenience to patients (long examination time), movement artifacts, and the limitations to scanning patients with pacemakers and other implantable metal devices.[3,17]
- Computed tomography (CT) scans have high resolution and reproducibility.[17] CT scans have reduced sensitivity compared to MRI and should not be routinely used to diagnose osteomyelitis.[1,5,16] Advantages are that it is useful for the identification of sequestra, and it is less expensive than MRI.[3,16,17] Disadvantages are the exposure of the patient to radiation and inability to use contrast medium to enhance images in patients with impaired renal function or previous allergic reactions.[3,4,17]
- Radionuclide imaging is also used for the early diagnosis of bone infections.[16] The most widely used nuclear medicine test is the three-phase bone scan.[16,17] An advantage is early detection within 24 to 48 hours after onset of symptoms.[5,6,16] Disadvantages include low specificity (increased risk of false positives) in patients with recent trauma, surgery, orthopedic prosthesis, diabetes, and ischemia, and high radiation dose required.[1,16] Using a labeled WBC scan in combination with the three-phase bone scan can increase sensitivity and specificity.[14,16]

TREATMENT

KEY CONCEPT *The treatment goals for osteomyelitis are to eradicate the infection and prevent recurrence.*[6–8,14,18] In comparison to acute hematogenous osteomyelitis, chronic osteomyelitis is associated with higher failure rates, largely due to the presence of necrotic bone.[1,8,14,19] These patients typically require surgical intervention to remove the necrotic bone and tissue, and if applicable, to

Patient Encounter, Part 1

A 42-year-old man limps into the emergency department complaining of pain and swelling in his left lower leg. He states that he also has a fever and feels tired. After questioning him, you discover that he was recently discharged from the hospital following surgery for an open fracture of his left tibia. He had undergone debridement and irrigation, followed by internal fixation and treatment with IV cefazolin. He was discharged home on oral cephalexin. On physical examination, the area above the fracture is red and swollen (erythematous and inflamed).

What information is suggestive of osteomyelitis?

What risk factors, if any, does he have for osteomyelitis?

replace infected hardware.[7] Comorbidities such as vascular insufficiency can further contribute to the poor outcomes seen with chronic osteomyelitis.[1,7] Due to the high failure rates, treatment in this patient population may require prolonged therapy, with the primary goal of preventing amputation of infected areas.[1,11,14]

General Approach to Treatment

KEY CONCEPT *Antimicrobial therapy alone is the mainstay of treatment for acute osteomyelitis.*[3–5,7] *In comparison, treatment for chronic osteomyelitis typically requires a combination of antimicrobial therapy and surgical intervention.*[7,11,14] If the patient is not a candidate for surgical intervention, prolonged antimicrobial therapy is generally necessary.[11–14]

▸ Nonpharmacologic Therapy

In addition to medical and surgical management, nonpharmacologic interventions for health promotion such as smoking cessation, weight-control and good nutrition should be communicated to the patient. Additionally, a diabetic patient should be counseled regarding the necessity of controlled blood glucose, routine care and self-examination of lower extremities, and aggressive wound care.[14] Patients with chronic immobility should be counseled on skin care and techniques to prevent the development of pressure ulcers.[7]

▸ Pharmacologic Therapy

KEY CONCEPT *Empiric antimicrobial therapy should target likely causative pathogen(s) based on patient-specific risk factors and route of infection.*[6] Empiric antimicrobial coverage against *S. aureus* should be considered for all classifications of osteomyelitis.[2,6] With MRSA increasingly being reported in the hospital and community settings, the use of anti-MRSA antimicrobials (eg, vancomycin) should be considered as first-line therapy for empiric coverage of suspected staphylococcal osteomyelitis.[1,2,6,7,20,21] In addition to anti-MRSA coverage, patients with contiguous osteomyelitis with vascular insufficiency (eg, diabetic) should also receive empiric antimicrobial therapy to cover Enterobacteriaceae, *P. aeruginosa*, and anaerobes.[11,14] Specific recommendations may vary based on factors such as patient allergies, potential for harboring a resistant organism, institution formulary, and cost considerations.[2,3,11]

Antimicrobial therapy should be modified based on culture and sensitivity data of appropriately collected specimens (Table 81–1).[4,6,11,14] If MRSA is isolated, vancomycin is considered first-line therapy unless the minimum inhibitory concentration is greater than 2 mcg/mL (2 mg/L).[10,22,23] Alternate agents include daptomycin, linezolid, clindamycin, and trimethoprim-sulfamethoxazole in combination with oral rifampin.[22] Other anti-MRSA agents (tigecycline, telavancin, ceftaroline, dalbavancin, tedizolid, oritavancin) lack clinical data to support their routine use in osteomyelitis.[10,24] Clindamycin is commonly used in pediatric patients.[3,4,8,22] However, microbiology laboratories must screen with a disk diffusion test (D-test) for inducible resistance via the macrolide-lincosamide-streptogramin gene, as clindamycin failures have been associated with infections caused by isolates that are D-test positive.[3,25] If methicillin-sensitive *S. aureus* is isolated and the patient has no β-lactam allergy, therapy should be changed to nafcillin/oxacillin or cefazolin.[1,2,5–7]

Treatment is initiated with IV antimicrobials in the inpatient or outpatient setting to optimize drug concentrations in bone.[1,6,7,14] Following initial IV therapy, a switch to oral antibiotics may be considered in patients with good clinical response, strict adherence, and outpatient follow-up.[3,4,6,8,11,14,22] Oral agents should possess such characteristics as high bioavailability, good bone penetration, and long half-life (ie, extended dosing interval).[1,3,5–7,10,11,19,22] Antimicrobials commonly used as oral therapy for osteomyelitis include fluoroquinolones, clindamycin, linezolid, and trimethoprim-sulfamethoxazole.[1,6,7,19,22] Additionally, oral rifampin may be used in combination with another antibiotic in patients with foreign devices or MRSA osteomyelitis.[1,7,11,19,22] For chronic osteomyelitis, some clinicians recommend placement of antibiotic impregnated beads or cement.[3,7,11,14] This enables antibiotics such as aminoglycosides and vancomycin to be delivered in high concentrations at the site of infection.[3,7]

KEY CONCEPT *The duration of treatment is typically 4 to 6 weeks for acute and chronic osteomyelitis.*[1–5,8,14,22] Shorter regimens (3 weeks) are often recommended for uncomplicated acute hematogenous infections due to *S. aureus* in children greater than 3 months of age.[4,6,8] *Infectious Diseases Society of America (IDSA) MRSA guidelines recommend a minimum of 8 weeks for treatment of MRSA osteomyelitis in adults.*[22] Prolonged therapy (greater than 3 months) may be necessary for certain populations such as patients with vascular insufficiency or patients with recalcitrant infections that do not respond to 4 to 6 weeks of therapy.[1,5,11,14,22]

Patient Encounter, Part 2

The medical team suspected osteomyelitis and ordered laboratory tests and imaging studies and consulted orthopedic surgery service.

How would you classify the infection in this patient?

What laboratory test(s) should be ordered for this patient?

What imaging study(s) should be ordered for this patient?

OUTCOME EVALUATION

Therapeutic success is measured by the extent to which the care plan (a) resolves signs and symptoms, (b) eradicates the microorganism(s), (c) prevents relapses, and (d) prevents complications such as amputation.[8,11,14] Patients should be evaluated for resolution of clinical signs and symptoms and normalization of laboratory tests (WBC, CRP, ESR, procalcitonin, and cultures).[3–6,8,10,14] Improvement in clinical manifestations may be

Table 81–1

Pathogen-Targeted Antimicrobial Therapy and Dosing Recommendations in Adults and Pediatrics

Microorganism	Antimicrobial Agent	Adult Dose	Pediatric Dose[a]
S. aureus			
MRSA	Vancomycin[b]	15–20 mg/kg IV every 8–12 hours	15 mg/kg IV every 6 hours
	Daptomycin[b]	6 mg/kg IV every 24 hours	6–10 mg/kg IV every 24 hours
	Linezolid	600 mg IV/oral every 12 hours	10 mg/kg IV/oral every 8 hours (< 12 years old)
	Clindamycin[c]	600 mg IV/oral every 8 hours	10–13 mg/kg/dose IV/oral every 6–8 hours
	Trimethoprim-sulfamethoxazole[b] (+ rifampin[c] 600 mg oral daily)	3.5–4.0 mg/kg of trimethoprim component IV/oral every 8–12 hours (trimethoprim-sulfamethoxazole single strength tablet is 80 mg/400 mg; double strength tablet is 160 mg/800 mg)	—
MSSA	Nafcillin[d]/oxacillin[b]	1–2 g IV every 4–6 hours	100–200 mg/kg/day IV in divided doses every 4–6 hours
	Cefazolin[b]	1–2 g IV every 6–8 hours	50–100 mg/kg/day IV in divided doses every 6–8 hours
***Enterococcus* spp.**			
Ampicillin-sensitive	Ampicillin[b]	2 g IV every 4–6 hours	100–400 mg/kg/day IV in divided doses every 6 hours
Ampicillin-resistant	Vancomycin[b]	15–20 mg/kg IV every 8–12 hours	15 mg/kg IV every 6 hours
Vancomycin-resistant	Daptomycin[b]	4–6 mg/kg IV every 24 hours	—
	Linezolid	600 mg IV/oral every 12 hours	10 mg/kg IV/oral every 8 hours (< 12 years old)
***Streptococcus* spp.**	Penicillin G[b]	2–4 million units IV every 4–6 hours	250,000–400,000 units/kg/day IV in divided doses every 4–6 hours
P. aeruginosa			
	Doripenem[b]	500 mg IV every 8 hours	—
	Imipenem/cilastatin[b]	500 mg IV every 6 hours	25 mg/kg IV every 6 hours
	Meropenem[b]	1 g IV every 8 hours	10–20 mg/kg IV every 8 hours
	Ceftazidime[b]	2 g IV every 8 hours	50 mg/kg IV every 8 hours
	Cefepime[b]	2 g IV every 12 hours	50 mg/kg IV every 8–12 hours
	Piperacillin/tazobactam[b]	4.5 g IV every 6 hours	100 mg/kg IV piperacillin component every 8 hours
	Ciprofloxacin[b,e]	400 mg IV every 8–12 hours; 750 mg oral every 12 hours	—
	Levofloxacin[b,e]	750 mg IV/oral every 24 hours	—
Enterobacteriaceae (in addition to antipseudomonal agents listed above)	Ceftriaxone[d]	1–2 g IV every 24 hours	50–100 mg/kg/day IV in divided doses every 12–24 hours
	Cefotaxime[b,d]	1–2 g IV every 8 hours	50–200 mg/kg/day IV in divided doses every 6–8 hours
	Ertapenem[b]	1 g IV every 24 hours	—
	Moxifloxacin[c,e]	400 mg IV/oral every 24 hours	—
Anaerobes[f]	Clindamycin[c]	600–900 mg IV every 8 hours; 300–450 mg oral every 6–8 hours	25–40 mg/kg/day IV in divided doses every 6–8 hours
	Metronidazole[b,c]	500 mg IV/oral every 6–8 hours	30 mg/kg/day IV/oral in divided doses every 6–8 hours

[a]Refer to specialized pediatric reference for maximum neonatal and pediatric dosing recommendations.

[b]Dosage adjustment necessary in renal dysfunction.

[c]Dosage adjustment necessary in severe hepatic dysfunction.

[d]Dosage adjustment necessary in patients with concomitant renal and hepatic dysfunction.

[e]Fluoroquinolones: Not approved by the US FDA for use in children except for anthrax (ciprofloxacin, levofloxacin) and complicated UTI and pyelonephritis (ciprofloxacin).

[f]May consider β-lactam/β-lactamase inhibitor or carbapenem for broad-spectrum activity including anaerobes.

Data from Refs. 1, 3, 4, 7, 8, 10, 11, 19, 20, and 22–26.

seen within 2 to 4 days of initiation of IV antimicrobial therapy in patients acute osteomyelitis.[4,8] A reduction in CRP should be seen within 1 week of therapy and should be monitored weekly throughout therapy for a continued downward trend.[3,4,6] ESR can also be monitored weekly, although normalization will be slower than for CRP.[3,6] Patients should also be monitored for antimicrobial tolerability and toxicity[2] (Table 81–2). If poor response is noted, the following should be evaluated: (a) patient adherence, (b) significant drug–drug or drug–food interactions, (c) appropriate dosage to achieve therapeutic concentrations, (d) development of antimicrobial resistance necessitating a change in the treatment regimen, (e) need for additional imaging studies, and (f) diagnostic reevaluation.[8,14] Treatment is considered successful if all clinical signs and symptoms are resolved and all laboratory tests have returned to normal

Table 81–2

Monitoring Considerations for Select Antistaphylococcal Agents

Antimicrobial	Monitoring Considerations
Daptomycin	Muscle pain or weakness particularly of the distal extremities; monitor CPK weekly with more frequent monitoring in patients with renal insufficiency or receiving (or recent discontinuation) of HMG-CoA reductase inhibitors; Consider temporarily discontinuing HMG-CoA reductase inhibitors while patient receiving daptomycin.
	Peripheral neuropathy: Monitor for neuropathy
	Decreased efficacy was observed in patients with moderate baseline renal impairment.
Linezolid	Myelosuppression: Monitor CBC once weekly
	MAO inhibitors; evaluate for potential drug–drug interactions. Linezolid should not be used concomitantly or within 2 weeks of medications that inhibit monoamine oxidases A or B.
	Serotonin syndrome; evaluate for potential drug–drug and drug-food interactions. Patients taking serotonergic antidepressants should receive linezolid only if no other therapies are available. Discontinue serotonergic antidepressants and monitor patients for signs and symptoms of both serotonin syndrome and antidepressant discontinuation.
	Peripheral and/or optic neuropathy has been reported with long-term therapy; perform routine neurologic and ophthalmic evaluations in these patients.
	Elevation of blood pressure in certain patients (eg, uncontrolled hypertension): monitor blood pressure.
	Hypoglycemia in patients with diabetes mellitus receiving insulin or oral hypoglycemic agents: monitor glucose.
Vancomycin	Targeted steady state trough is 15–20 mcg/mL (15–20 mg/L; 10–14 μmol/L) for serious infections such as osteomyelitis.
	Renal dysfunction: monitor weekly renal function (BUN/SCr) and troughs in stable patients; more often in nonstable patients.
	Potential for additive renal toxicity if being coadministered with a nephrotoxic agent (eg, aminoglycoside).

BUN, blood urea nitrogen; CBC, complete blood count; CPK, creatine phosphokinase; MAO, monoamine oxidase; SCr, serum creatinine.

Data from Refs. 1, 7, 11, 20, and 22–26.

Patient Encounter, Part 3: The Medical History, Physical Exam, and Diagnostic Tests

PMH: Type 2 diabetes mellitus, dyslipidemia, depression

SH: Tobacco smoker (one pack per day for 10 years), two to three cans of beer daily. Employed as mechanic

Allergies: NKDA

Meds: Cephalexin 500 mg orally four times a day; rosuvastatin 20 mg orally at bedtime; metformin 500 mg orally twice daily; fluoxetine 20 mg orally daily

PE:

Gen: Moderate distress with pain and tenderness in lower left leg; limps

Skin: Erythema and inflammation

VS: BP 120/70 mm Hg, P 85 beats/min, RR 20 breaths/min, T 38.4°C (101.2°F), Ht 5′ 7″ (170 cm), Wt 73 kg (161 lb)

Labs: WBC 16.4 × 10³/mm³ (16.4 × 10⁹/L), hemoglobin 13.0 g/dL (130g/L; 8.07 mmol/L), hematocrit 37.0% (0.37), platelets 220 × 10³/uL (220 × 10⁹/L), BUN 23 mg/dL (8.2 mmol/L), serum creatinine (Scr) 1.3 mg/dL (115 μmol/L), total bilirubin 1.1 mg/dL (18.8 μmol/L), alkaline phosphatase 82 U/L (1.37 μkat/L), AST 28U/L (0.47μkat/L), ALT 13 U/L (0.22 μkat/L), albumin 3.7g/dL (37 g/L), fasting blood glucose 180 mg/dL (10.0 mmol/L), ESR 110 mm/h, CRP 14 mg/dL (140 mg/L)

Microbiology: Culture from bone aspirate grew *S. aureus* (sensitive to daptomycin, linezolid, rifampin, trimethoprim-sulfamethoxazole, and vancomycin but resistant to clindamycin, erythromycin, and oxacillin)

Based on the information presented, create a care plan for this patient's osteomyelitis. Your plan should include:

(a) Goals of therapy

(b) Patient-specific detailed therapeutic plan

(c) Nonpharmacologic interventions

(d) Follow-up plan to determine whether outcomes have been achieved

Patient Encounter, Part 4

The patient received 2 weeks of IV antimicrobial therapy following debridement. The patient has shown clinical and laboratory improvement. The multidisciplinary medical team plans to complete therapy with an oral antibiotic.

What oral antimicrobial therapy would you recommend for this patient?

Evaluate the patient's medication profile for drug–drug interactions.

Counsel the patient regarding this drug therapy.

Patient Care Process

Patient Assessment:

- Review the medical history to assess risk factors for osteomyelitis.
- Based on physical exam and review of systems, determine whether the patient is experiencing signs or symptoms of osteomyelitis.
- Review available imaging studies and laboratory tests, especially WBC, ESR, and CRP.
- Obtain a thorough history of prescription, nonprescription, and natural drug product use.

Therapy Evaluation:

- Determine the appropriateness of current antibiotic therapy based upon patient-specific factors and microbiology data (if available).

Care Plan Development:

- Determine whether the antibiotic dosage regimen is optimal based upon patient-specific factors and site of infection.
- Provide patient education with regard to disease state and drug therapy. Stress the importance of adherence to the therapeutic regimen.

Follow-Up Evaluation:

- Patients should be monitored for clinical and laboratory response, development of adverse drug reactions, and potential drug–drug interactions. Patients should also be closely monitored for adherence in the outpatient setting.

following 4 to 8 weeks of appropriate treatment. Due to high rates of relapse, patients should have medical follow-up for at least 1 year following resolution of symptoms.[4] Patients should be evaluated at predefined follow-up intervals (3- to 6- to 12-months) for any clinical manifestations of recurring infection and continued normalization of laboratory tests.[8,11] Follow-up imaging studies at 1 to 2 years may be useful in some patients to confirm therapeutic success.

Disclaimer

The views expressed in this chapter are those of the authors and do not necessarily reflect the position or policy of the Department of Veterans Affairs or the US government.

Abbreviations Introduced in This Chapter

ALT	Alanine aminotransferase
AST	Aspartate aminotransferase
BUN	Blood urea nitrogen
CBC	Complete blood count
CRP	C-reactive protein
CPK	Creatine phosphokinase
CT	Computed tomography
CYP	Cytochrome P-450 isoenzyme
ESR	Erythrocyte sedimentation rate
IV	Intravenous
LFT	Liver function test
MAO	Monoamine oxidase
MRI	Magnetic resonance imaging
MRSA	Methicillin-resistant *Staphylococcus aureus*
MSSA	Methicillin-sensitive *Staphylococcus aureus*
Scr	Serum creatinine
UTI	Urinary tract infection
WBC	White blood cell

REFERENCES

1. Chihara S, Segreti J. Osteomyelitis. Dis Mon. 2010;56:6–31.
2. Howell WR, Goulston C. Osteomyelitis: An update for hospitalists. Hosp Pract (Minneap). 2011;39(1):153–160.
3. Harik NS, Smeltzer MS. Management of acute hematogenous osteomyelitis in children. Expert Rev Anti infect Ther. 2010;8(2):175–181.
4. Peltola H, Pääkkönen M. Acute Osteomyelitis in Children. N Engl J Med. 2014;370:352–360.
5. Zimmerli W. Vertebral osteomyelitis. N Engl J Med. 2010;362: 1022–1029.
6. Conrad DA. Acute hematogenous osteomyelitis. Pediatr Rev. 2010;31:464–471.
7. Rao N, Ziran BH, Lipsky BA. Treating osteomyelitis: antibiotics and surgery. Plast Reconstr Surg. 2011;127(Suppl 1):S177–S187.
8. Howard-Jones AR, Isaacs D. Systemic review of duration and choice of systemic antibiotic therapy for acute haemetagenous bacterial osteomyelitis in children. J Pediatr Child Health. 2013:49:760–768.
9. Waldvogel FA, Medoff G, Swartz MN. Osteomyelitis: A review of clinical features, therapeutic considerations and unusual aspects. N Engl J Med. 1970;282:198–206.
10. Senneville E, Nguyen S. Current pharmacotherapy options for osteomyelitis: Convergences, divergences, and lessons to be drawn. Expert Opin Pharmacother. 2013;14:723–734.
11. Peters EJ, Lipsky BA. Diagnosis and management of infection in the diabetic foot. Med Clin N Am. 2013;97:911–946.
12. Game FL. Osteomyelitis in the diabetic foot. Diagnosis and Management. Med Clin N Am. 2013;97:947–956.
13. Game F. Management of osteomyelitis of the foot in diabetes mellitus; Nat Rev Endocrinol. 2010;6:43–47.
14. Lipsky BA, Berendt AR, Cornia PB, et al. 2012 Infectious Diseases Society of America clinical practice guideline for the diagnosis and treatment of diabetic foot infections. Clin Infect Dis. 2012;54;132–173.
15. Bernard L, Assal M, Garzoni C, Uckay L. Predicting the pathogen of diabetic toe osteomyelitis by two consecutive ulcer cultures with bone contact. Eur J Clin Microbiol Infect Dis. 2011;30:279–281.
16. Hankin D, Bowling FL, Metcalfe SA, et al. Critically evaluating the role of diagnostic imaging in osteomyelitis. Foot Ankle Spec. 2011;4(2):100–105.
17. Gotthardt M, Bleeker-Rovers CP, Boerman OC, Oyen WJG. Imaging of inflammation by PET, conventional scintigraphy, and other imaging techniques. J Nucl Med. 2010;51:1937–1949.
18. Conterno LO, Turchi MD. Antibiotics for treating chronic osteomyelitis in adults. Cochrane Database Syst Rev. 2013;9: CD004439.
19. Spellberg B, Lipsky BA. Systemic antibiotic therapy for chronic osteomyelitis in adults. Clin Infect Dis. 2012:54:393–407.
20. Boucher H, Miller LG, Razonable RR. Serious infections caused by methicillin-resistant *Staphylococcus aureus*. Clin Infect Dis. 2010;51(Suppl 2):S183–S197.

21. Bhavan KP, Marschall J, Olsen MA, et al. The epidemiology of hematogenous vertebral osteomyelitis: A cohort study in a tertiary care hospital. BMC Infect Dis. 2010;10:158.
22. Liu C, Bayer A, Cosgrove SE, et al. Clinical practice guidelines by the Infectious Diseases Society of America for the treatment of methicillin-resistant *Staphylococcus aureus* infections in adults and children. Clin Infect Dis. 2011;52:1–38.
23. Rybak M, Lomaestro B, Rotschafer JC, et al. Therapeutic monitoring of vancomycin in adult patients: a consensus review of the American Society of Health-System Pharmacists, the Infectious Diseases Society of America, and the Society of Infectious Diseases Pharmacists. Am J Health Syst Pharm. 2009;66:82–98.
24. Moenster RP, Linneman TW, Call WB, et al. The potential role of newer gram-positive antibiotics in the setting of osteomyelitis of adults. J Clin Pharm Ther. 2013;38:89–96.
25. Eleftheriadou I, Tentolouris N, Argiana V, et al. Methicillin-resistant *Staphylococcus aureus* in diabetic foot infections. Drugs. 2010;70(14):1785–1797.
26. Lexi-Drugs Online. [cited 2014 Sept 1]. www.crlonline.com. Accessed September 1, 2014.

82 Sepsis and Septic Shock

Trisha N. Branan, Christopher M. Bland, and S. Scott Sutton

LEARNING OBJECTIVES

Upon completion of the chapter, the reader will be able to:

1. Compare and contrast the definitions of syndromes related to sepsis.
2. Identify the pathogens associated with sepsis.
3. Discuss the pathophysiology of sepsis as it relates to pro- and anti-inflammatory mediators.
4. Identify patient symptoms as early or late sepsis and evaluate diagnostic and laboratory tests for patient treatment and monitoring.
5. Assess complications of sepsis and discuss their impact on patient outcomes.
6. Design desired treatment outcomes for septic patients.
7. Formulate a treatment and monitoring plan (pharmacologic and nonpharmacologic) for septic patients.
8. Evaluate patient response and devise alternative treatment regimens for nonresponding septic patients.

INTRODUCTION

KEY CONCEPT *Sepsis occurs across a continuum of physiologic stages in response to infection which manifests as systemic inflammation, coagulation, and tissue hypoperfusion, potentially leading to organ dysfunction known as severe sepsis.*[1] The American College of Chest Physicians and the Society of Critical Care Medicine have defined the nomenclature to standardize sepsis terminology. (Table 82–1).[2,3] Physiologic parameters categorize patients as having systemic inflammatory response syndrome (SIRS), sepsis, severe sepsis, or septic shock.[2]

EPIDEMIOLOGY AND ETIOLOGY

Sepsis is the leading cause of morbidity and mortality for critically ill patients and the tenth leading cause of death overall.[4,5] Mortality rates remain high for patients with severe sepsis and septic shock with septic shock and multiorgan failure as the most common causes of death.[1] There are approximately 750,000 cases of sepsis diagnosed every year in the United States which continues to increase.[1]

Risk factors for sepsis include increased age, cancer, immunodeficiency, chronic organ failure, genetic factors (male gender and nonwhite ethnic origin in North America), and bacteremia.[5–9] Pulmonary infections cause approximately half of all cases, followed by intra-abdominal and genitourinary infections.[2] In approximately one-third of cases of sepsis a pathogen is not identified making de-escalation from broad spectrum to a more narrowed antimicrobial regimen difficult.[2]

KEY CONCEPT *Gram-positive and gram-negative bacteria, fungal species, and viruses may cause sepsis* (Table 82–2). Gram-positive infections account for 30% to 50% of sepsis and septic shock cases.[5–7] The percentages of gram-negative, polymicrobial, and viral sepsis cases are 25%, 25%, and 4%, respectively.[5–7,10] A multinational study of 14,000 critically ill patients showed an increase in gram-negative bacterial causes of sepsis compared to gram-positive bacterial and fungal causes.[2] Multidrug-resistant (MDR) bacteria are responsible for approximately 25% of sepsis cases, are difficult to treat, and increase mortality.[6,7] The rate of fungal infections has significantly increased with *Candida albicans* as the most common fungal species identified; however, non-albicans species (*C. glabrata, C. krusei,* and *C. tropicalis*) have increased from 24% to 46%.[5,10,11] Other fungi identified as causes of sepsis include species of *Cryptococcus, Coccidioides, Fusarium,* and *Aspergillus.*

PATHOPHYSIOLOGY

The development of sepsis is complex and multifactorial. The normal host response to infection is designed to localize and control bacterial invasion and initiate repair of injured tissue through phagocytic cells and inflammatory mediators.[4] KEY CONCEPT *Sepsis results when the interplay between the host's immune, inflammatory, and coagulant responses becomes exaggerated extending to normal tissue distant from the initial tissue site.*

Pro- and Anti-inflammatory Mediators

The key factor in the development of sepsis is inflammation, which is intended to be a local and contained response to infection or injury. Infection or injury is controlled through proinflammatory and anti inflammatory mediators. Proinflammatory mediators facilitate clearance of the injuring stimulus, promote resolution of injury, and are involved in processing of damaged tissue.[4,14–17] To control the intensity and duration of the inflammatory response, anti-inflammatory mediators are released that act to regulate proinflammatory mediators.[16,17] The balance between pro- and anti-inflammatory mediators localizes

Table 82–1

Diagnostic Criteria for Sepsis, Severe Sepsis, and Septic Shock

Sepsis (documented or suspected infection plus ≥ 1 of the following)
General variables
- Hyperthermia (core temperature > 38.3°C)
- Hypothermia (core temperature < 36°C)
- Tachycardia (heart rate > 90 beats/min)
- Tachypnea
- Altered mental status
- Substantial edema or positive fluid balance (> 20 mL/kg of body weight over 24 hours)
- Hyperglycemia (plasma glucose > 120 mg/dL [6.7 mmol/L]) in absence of diabetes

Inflammatory variables
- Leukocytosis (white blood cell count > 12,000/mm^3 [12 × 10^9/L])
- Leukopenia (white blood cell count < 4000/mm^3 [4 × 10^9/L])
- Normal white blood cell count with > 10% (0.10) immature forms (bands)
- Elevated plasma C-reactive protein
- Elevated plasma procalcitonin

Hemodynamic variables
- Arterial hypotension (systolic pressure < 90 mm Hg; mean arterial pressure < 70 mm Hg (9.3 kPa); or decrease in systolic pressure of > 40 mm Hg)
- Organ dysfunction variables
- Arterial hypoxemia (Pao_2/Fio_2 < 300 mm Hg [39.9 kPa])
- Acute oliguria (urine output < 0.5 mL/kg/hour or 45 mL/hour for at least 2 hours)
- Increase in serum creatinine level of > 0.5 mg/dL (> 44 μmol/L)
- Coagulation abnormalities (INR > 1.5; or aPTT > 60 seconds)
- Paralytic ileus (absence of bowel sounds)
- Thrombocytopenia (platelet count < 100,000/mm^3 [100 × 10^9/L])
- Hyperbilirubinemia (plasma total bilirubin > 4 mg/dL [68.4 μmol/L])

Tissue-perfusion variables
- Hyperlactatemia (lactate > 1 mmol/L)
- Decreased capillary refill or mottling

Severe sepsis (sepsis plus organ dysfunction)
Septic shock (sepsis plus either hypotension [refractory to fluid resuscitation] or hyperlactatemia)

Pao_2, partial pressure of oxygen; Fio_2, fraction of inspired oxygen.
Adapted from Dellinger RP, Levy MM, Rhodes A, et al. Surviving sepsis campaign: International guidelines for management of severe sepsis and septic shock: 2012. Crit Care Med. 2013;41:580–637.

infection/injury of host tissue.[14–17] However, systemic responses ensue when equilibrium in the inflammatory process is lost.

The inflammatory process in sepsis is linked to the coagulation system. Proinflammatory mediators may have procoagulant and antifibrinolytic effects, whereas anti-inflammatory mediators may have fibrinolytic effects. A key factor in the inflammation of sepsis is activated protein C, which enhances fibrinolysis and inhibits inflammation. Protein C levels are decreased in many septic patients.

CLINICAL PRESENTATION AND DIAGNOSIS

The clinical presentation of sepsis varies, and the rate of development of clinical manifestations may differ from patient to patient.

Table 82–2

Pathogens in Sepsis

Organism	Frequency (%)
Gram-positive bacteria	30–50
Methicillin-susceptible *Staphylococcus aureus*	14–24
Methicillin-resistant *Staphylococcus aureus*	5–11
Other *Staphylococcus* species	1–3
Streptococcus pneumoniae	9–12
Other *Streptococcus* species	6–11
Enterococcus species	3–13
Anaerobes	1–2
Other gram-positive bacteria	1–5
Gram-negative bacteria	25–30
Escherichia coli	9–27
Pseudomonas aeruginosa	8–15
Klebsiella pneumoniae	2–7
Enterobacter species	6–16
Haemophilus influenzae	2–10
Anaerobes	3–7
Other gram-negative bacteria	3–12
Fungi	
Candida albicans	1–3
Other *Candida* species	1–2
Parasites	1–3
Viruses	2–4

Data from Refs. 5, 6, 12, and 13.

A physical examination should be performed rapidly and efficiently when sepsis is suspected, with efforts directed toward uncovering the most likely cause of sepsis. The patient may not provide any medical history; therefore, historical data may be obtained from medical records and/or family. The patient's medical condition, recent illnesses, infections, or activities may provide valuable information about the cause of sepsis.

Diagnostic and Laboratory Tests

Microbiologic cultures should be obtained before antimicrobial therapy is initiated as long as this does not significantly delay

Physical Examination Results in Sepsis

HEENT: Scleral icterus, dry mucous membranes, pinpoint pupils, dilated and fixed pupils, nystagmus

Neck: Jugular venous distention, carotid bruits

Lungs: Crackles (rales), consolidation, egophony, absent breath sounds

CV: Irregular rhythm, S_3 gallop, murmurs

Abd: Tense, distended, tender, rebound, guarding, hepatosplenomegaly

Rectal: Decreased tone, bright red blood

Exts: Swollen calf, disparity of blood pressure between upper extremities

Neurologic: Agitation, confusion, delirium, obtundation, coma

Skin: Cold, clammy, or warm; hyperemic skin; rashes

Clinical Presentation and Diagnosis of Sepsis

The signs and symptoms of septic patients are referred to as early and late sepsis.

Signs and Symptoms

The initial clinical signs and symptoms represent early sepsis, and they include fever, chills, and change in mental status. Other signs and symptoms include:

- Tachycardia
- Tachypnea
- Nausea and vomiting
- Hyperglycemia
- Myalgias
- Lethargy and malaise
- Proteinuria
- Leukocytosis
- Hypoxia
- Hyperbilirubinemia

Septic patients may have an elevated, low, or normal temperature. The absence of fever is common in neonates and elderly patients. Hypothermia is associated with a poor prognosis. Hyperventilation may occur before fever and chills and may lead to respiratory alkalosis. Disorientation and confusion may develop early in septic patients, particularly in the elderly and patients with preexisting neurologic impairment. Disorientation and confusion may be related to the infection or due to sepsis signs and symptoms (eg, hypoxia).

Late sepsis represents a slow process that develops over several hours of hypoperfusion. Signs and symptoms of late sepsis include:

- Lactic acidosis
- Oliguria
- Leukopenia
- Thrombocytopenia
- Myocardial depression
- Pulmonary edema
- Hypotension
- Hypoglycemia
- Gastrointestinal hemorrhage

Oliguria often follows hypotension because of decreased renal perfusion. Metabolic acidosis ensues because of diminished clearance of lactate by the kidneys and liver.

the start of therapy. However, cultures take 6 to 48 hours for results to be completed and often are negative (no growth of bacterial organisms). Negative cultures do not rule out the presence of infection. Administering antimicrobials before obtaining cultures may lead to a false-negative culture. Rapid diagnostics of blood cultures allows for identification of specific pathogens within as little as 20 minutes to 3 hours after initial growth is identified. However not all health care systems have this technology available.

At least two sets of blood cultures should be obtained to rule out contamination with at least one set drawn percutaneously and one set drawn through each vascular access device present for greater than 48 hours.

Cultures of urine (with urinalysis), respiratory secretions, cerebrospinal fluid, and wounds should be obtained if the clinical presentation suggests infection of these specific fluids, tissues, or organs. Laboratory tests should be performed to evaluate infection or complications of sepsis, including complete blood count (CBC) with differential, coagulation parameters, comprehensive metabolic panel (CMP), serum lactate concentration, arterial blood gas (ABG), and appropriate diagnostic radiographic imaging studies.

The use of biomarkers of sepsis has been controversial. Measurement of endotoxin, procalcitonin, or other markers in blood or serum is not routinely recommended. Concentrations of procalcitonin in serum are usually increased in sepsis, but fail to differentiate between infection and inflammation. However, procalcitonin has a high negative predictive value and may allow for the discontinuation of antibiotics.

Complications of Sepsis

KEY CONCEPT *Recognition and treatment of sepsis complications, particularly organ failure, is essential to improve outcomes. The cumulative burden of sepsis complications is the leading factor of mortality. The risk of death increases 20% with failure of each additional organ. Severe sepsis averages two failed organs, with a mortality rate of 40%.* The most common complications are respiratory and cardiovascular compromise, usually seen as acute respiratory distress syndrome (ARDS), hemodynamic compromise, and elevated serum lactate levels. Other complications include altered mentation, acute kidney injury (AKI) which may require renal replacement therapy, paralytic ileus, disseminated intravascular coagulation (DIC), and adrenal insufficiency.[2]

TREATMENT AND OUTCOME EVALUATION

Desired Outcomes

KEY CONCEPT *The primary treatment goal of sepsis is to prevent morbidity and mortality through rapid recognition and intervention.* Treatment is aimed at early implementation of therapies, such as fluid

Patient Encounter, Part 1

A 35-year-old woman with history of asthma presents to the emergency department with complaints of several days of high fevers, chills, cough, and increased purulent sputum production. The patient appears to be in severe respiratory distress and is becoming increasingly lethargic.

What information is suggestive of infection and/or sepsis?

What information do we need in order to confirm or diagnose sepsis in this patient?

resuscitation and antimicrobials, reducing or eliminating organ dysfunction, eliminating the source of infection, avoiding adverse reactions of treatment, and providing cost-effective therapy.[18–24]

General Approach to Treatment

Similar to the emphasis placed on the expedited treatment of patients with acute myocardial infarction and cerebrovascular accidents, quick, quantitative intervention with appropriate therapies to achieve specific, measurable endpoints once a diagnosis of sepsis has been made is crucial to decrease morbidity and mortality.[18,20]

Pertinent approaches in the management of septic patients are as follows (Figure 82–1)[24]:

1. Prompt recognition of the septic patient and early implementation of therapies.
2. Fluid therapy, using crystalloids initially, to achieve quantitative therapeutic endpoints.
3. Early administration of broad-spectrum antimicrobial therapy.
4. Vasopressor therapy, using norepinephrine initially, to maintain hemodynamic stability (on average a mean arterial pressure of 65 mm Hg [8.6 kPa]) in patients with septic shock refractory to fluid resuscitation.
5. Intravenous (IV) hydrocortisone may be considered for patients who remain hemodynamically unstable despite adequate fluid resuscitation and vasopressor support.
6. Glycemic control via infusion of regular insulin to maintain glucose levels between 140 and 180 mg/dL (7.8 and 10.0 mmol/L).

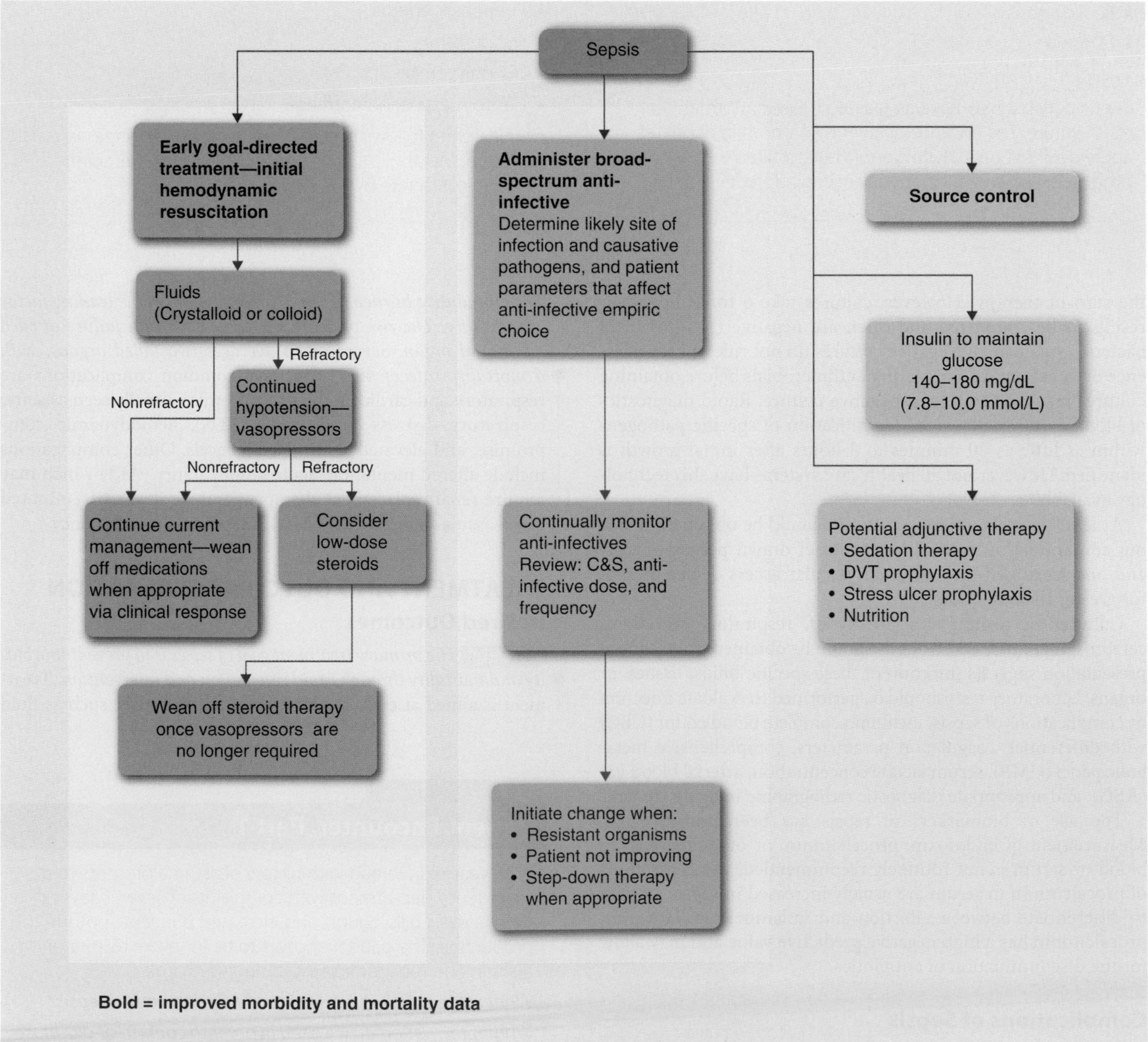

FIGURE 82–1. Therapeutic approach to sepsis. (C&S, culture and sensitivity.)

7. Adjunctive therapies: blood product administration, sedation, analgesia, neuromuscular blockade, renal replacement therapy, deep vein thrombosis (DVT) prophylaxis, stress ulcer prophylaxis, and nutrition.

Treatment for sepsis focuses on infection, inflammation, hypoperfusion, and widespread tissue injury. Septic patients may require multiple simultaneous treatment regimens to achieve desired outcomes of decreased morbidity and mortality.

Initial Resuscitation

A landmark study of early goal directed therapy (EGDT) using a standardized protocol that required the use of a special catheter for central venous oxygen saturation monitoring decreased 28-day mortality in septic patients by approximately 16%.[23] Three subsequent randomized controlled studies comparing EGDT to groups of patients receiving contemporary care (with or without the use of protocols) found no differences in mortality.[25–27] These results may demonstrate that continued focus on early recognition and treatment of these patients may play a more important role than protocol-based therapy. Specifically the placement of central venous catheters for mixed venous oxygen saturation monitoring as well as administration of inotrope therapy and blood transfusions did not improve outcomes compared to standard care. The most current treatment goals of sepsis-induced hypoperfusion (hypotension or blood lactate level greater than or equal to 4 mEq/L [4 mmol/L]) during the first 6 hours include[20,23,24,28]:

- Central venous pressure (CVP) 8 to 12 mm Hg (1.1–1.6 kPa)
- Mean arterial pressure (MAP) greater than or equal to 65 mm Hg (8.6 kPa)
- Urine output greater than or equal to 0.5 mL/kg/h

Emerging noninvasive techniques, such as the use of cardiac ultrasound, have recently shown reliability in assessing intravascular volume status through measuring inferior vena cava diameter changes and collapsibility.[29,30] Resuscitation should also target the normalization of blood lactate levels in patients with an initially elevated blood lactate as a marker of improved tissue perfusion.[20]

Fluid Therapy

Crystalloid fluids (such as 0.9% sodium chloride or lactated Ringer solutions) or colloids (albumin products) are used for resuscitation, and clinical studies comparing the fluids have found them to be equivalent.[28,31,32] Crystalloids require more fluid volume, which may lead to more edema (utilize caution in patients at risk for fluid overload, eg, congestive heart failure and ARDS); however, albumin is significantly more expensive. Hydroxyethyl starches (HES), another type of colloid, should not be used due to studies demonstrating increased morbidity and mortality rates.[33,34] A large, multicenter, randomized controlled trial comparing HES to Ringer acetate in patients with severe sepsis showed an increased 90-day mortality rate and a higher need for renal replacement therapy in patients administered HES for fluid resuscitation.[33] For these reasons, crystalloids are preferred versus colloids for initial resuscitation, except in cases where large amounts of crystalloids are needed and hypervolemia may be harmful to the patient.[20]

Administer an initial fluid challenge in patients with suspected sepsis-induced tissue hypoperfusion and hypovolemia with 30 mL/kg of crystalloid fluid. Most patients require aggressive fluid resuscitation during the first 24 hours because of persistent venodilation and capillary leak.[20,24]

Anti-infective Therapy

KEY CONCEPT *Appropriate empiric antimicrobial therapy decreases 28-day mortality compared with inappropriate empiric therapy (24% vs 39%).*[18,19,35] Additionally, appropriate therapy administered within 1 hour of sepsis recognition also decreases complications and mortality.[18,19,35] Empiric antimicrobial therapy should include multiple agents for most cases, depending on the likely site of infection and causative pathogens. Anti-infective clinical trials in sepsis and septic shock patients are scarce and have not demonstrated differences among agents; therefore, factors that determine selection are:

- Site of infection
- Causative pathogens
- Community- or nosocomial-acquired infection
- Immune status of patient
- Antibiotic susceptibility and resistance profile for the institution and local community. Clinicians should be cognizant of growing prevalence of bacterial resistance in community and health care settings.

Patient Encounter, Part 2: Medical History, Physical Exam, and Diagnostic Tests

PMH: Asthma diagnosed at 3 years of age

FH: Father had stroke at age 62; mother has history of hypertension and diabetes mellitus

SH: Teacher; nonsmoker; rare alcohol intake

Allergies: NKDA

Meds: Fluticasone/Salmeterol 250/50 mg one puff twice daily; albuterol 90 mcg inhaler two puffs every 4 hours as needed for shortness of breath

ROS: Unable to obtain; patient has become more confused

PE:

Within normal limits except as noted below

VS: BP 79/44 mm Hg, P 124 beats/min, RR 29 breaths/min, T 39.3°C (102.7°F)

Lungs: Decreased breath sounds, bilateral crackles

Labs: Serum creatinine 2.7 mg/dL (239 μmol/L); glucose 298 mg/dL (16.5 mmol/L); white blood cells: leukocytosis (15,000/mm^3 [15 × 10^9/L]) with left shift.; lactic acid 5.1 mEq/L (5.1 mmol/L)

Cultures: Blood, urine, and respiratory cultures pending

Radiology: Bilateral pulmonary infiltrates seen on chest x-ray

According to the patient's parameters, what does she have (ie, systemic inflammatory response syndrome, sepsis, or septic shock)?

Identify treatment goals.

Formulate an initial plan for therapy.

- Patient history (underlying disease, previous cultures or infections including any recent antibiotic therapy, and drug allergy/intolerance)
- Adverse reactions
- Cost

Anti-infective regimens should be broad-spectrum since delays in appropriate therapy result in increased mortality.

Monitoring and Treatment Strategies to Maximize Efficacy and Minimize Toxicity for Antimicrobials

- Administer broad-spectrum antimicrobials for initial therapy, as early as possible and within first hour of recognition of sepsis.
- Appropriate cultures should be obtained before initiating antibiotic therapy, but should not prevent prompt administration.
- Administer antibiotics that concentrate at the site of infection.
- Monitor patient parameters to ensure adequate dosing.
- Abnormal renal and hepatic function will increase drug concentration and predispose the patient to toxicity.
  - Ensure antibiotic dosing is changed to normal doses once renal dysfunction has resolved to limit the development of treatment failure, antimicrobial resistance, or both.
- Septic patients may have increased volume of distribution due to initial large volume resuscitation.
- Reevaluate the initial dosing regimen daily to optimize activity, prevent development of resistance, reduce toxicity, and decrease costs.
- Initiate step-down therapy based on microbiologic cultures to: prevent resistance, reduce toxicity, and cost.
- Monotherapy is equivalent to combination therapy once a causative pathogen has been identified in the vast majority of cases. Empiric therapy should include combination regimens to ensure appropriate coverage of causative organisms.

Duration of Anti-Infective Therapy

Average duration of antimicrobial therapy for septic patients is 7 to 10 days. However, durations vary depending on the site of infection and response to therapy. Step-down therapy from IV to oral antimicrobials is recommended in most patients whom are hemodynamically stable, afebrile for 48 to 72 hours, have a normalized WBC, and able to take oral medications.

Source Control

Evaluate septic patients for the presence of a localized infection amenable to source control measures. Common source control measures include drainage and debridement, device removal, and prevention.[20–22] Implementation of source control methods should be instituted as soon as possible following initial fluid resuscitation. The selection of optimal source control methods must weigh benefits and risks of the intervention. Source control measures may cause complications (bleeding, fistulas, and organ injury); therefore, the method with the least risk should be employed.[20]

Patient Encounter, Part 3

Treatment and Outcome Evaluation

The patient remains hypotensive despite previous intervention. Continued hypoxia has led to mechanical ventilation. The patient's serum creatinine has risen to 6.8 mg/dL (601 μmol/L) and she has minimal urine output.

What additional therapies will you consider adding to this patient?

HEMODYNAMIC SUPPORT

Vasopressors and Inotropic Therapy

KEY CONCEPT *When fluid resuscitation does not provide adequate arterial pressure and organ perfusion, vasopressors and/or inotropic agents should be initiated.* Vasopressors are recommended in patients with a systolic blood pressure less than 90 mm Hg or MAP lower than 60 to 65 mm Hg (8.0–8.6 kPa), after failed treatment with crystalloids.[20,23,24] Vasopressors and inotropes are effective in treating life-threatening hypotension and improving cardiac index, but complications such as tachycardia and myocardial ischemia require slow titration of the adrenergic agents to restore MAP without impairing stroke volume. Vasopressor therapy may also be required transiently to sustain life and maintain perfusion in the face of life-threatening hypotension, even when fluid resuscitation is in progress and hypovolemia has not yet been corrected. Agents commonly considered for vasopressor or inotropic support include norepinephrine, epinephrine, dopamine, phenylephrine, vasopressin, and dobutamine. Norepinephrine is the first-line vasopressor to correct hypotension in septic shock.[20]

Norepinephrine is a potent α-adrenergic agent with less pronounced β-adrenergic activity. Doses of 0.01 to 3 mcg/kg/min can reliably increase blood pressure through vasoconstriction with small changes in heart rate or cardiac index. Norepinephrine is a more potent agent than dopamine in refractory septic shock.[20,23,24] Norepinephrine induces less arrhythmias compared with dopamine.[36]

Dopamine is an α- and β-adrenergic agent with dopaminergic activity. Low doses of dopamine (1–5 mcg/kg/min) maintain renal perfusion; higher doses (greater than 5 mcg/kg/min) exhibit α- and β-adrenergic activity and are frequently utilized to support blood pressure and to improve cardiac function, mainly through increasing stroke volume and heart rate. Because of the effects on heart rate, dopamine causes more tachycardia and thus increases potential for arrhythmias versus norepinephrine. Based on these data, dopamine should not be used routinely in the management of septic shock.[20,36] Low doses of dopamine should not be used for renal protection as part of the treatment of severe sepsis.[20,23,24]

Epinephrine is a nonspecific α- and β-adrenergic agonist that can increase cardiac index and produce significant peripheral vasoconstriction. Some human and animal studies suggest it can also increase lactate levels and impair blood flow to the splanchnic system; however, studies comparing norepinephrine to epinephrine show no difference in mortality rates. Epinephrine should be considered the first alternative to norepinephrine in patients with persistent hypotension.[20,23,24]

Phenylephrine is a fast-acting, short-acting pure α_1-agonist. Phenylephrine is the least likely vasopressor to cause tachycardia, but may decrease stroke volume. Phenylephrine should be reserved for use in patients with high cardiac output in whom tachycardia or ischemia limits the use of other vasopressors or as salvage therapy.[20,23,24]

Vasopressin levels are increased during hypotension to maintain blood pressure by vasoconstriction. However, there is a vasopressin deficiency in septic shock. Low, fixed doses of vasopressin increase MAP, leading to the discontinuation of vasopressors. However, routine use of vasopressin with norepinephrine is not recommended because of no difference in mortality compared with norepinephrine monotherapy.[37] Vasopressin is a direct vasoconstrictor without inotropic or chronotropic effects and may result in decreased cardiac output and hepatosplanchnic flow. Vasopressin use may be considered in patients with refractory shock despite adequate fluid resuscitation and high-dose vasopressors.[20,23,24]

Dobutamine is recommended as the first-line inotropic agent. Dobutamine is a β-adrenergic inotropic agent that can be utilized for improvement of cardiac output and oxygen delivery. Doses of 2 to 20 mcg/kg/min increase cardiac index; however, heart rate increases significantly. Dobutamine should be considered in septic patients with adequate filling pressure and blood pressure, but low cardiac index. If used in hypotensive patients, dobutamine should be combined with vasopressor therapy.[20,23,24]

Corticosteroids

Stress-induced adrenal insufficiency complicates 9% to 24% of septic patients and is associated with increased mortality. The role of steroid use in septic shock remains unclear. Previous studies have demonstrated a mortality benefit or quicker reversal of shock in patients with sepsis-induced adrenal insufficiency treated with hydrocortisone.[38] However, a large, multicenter, randomized controlled trial (CORTICUS) showed no difference in mortality rates in septic shock patients treated with hydrocortisone.[39] KEY CONCEPT *For these reasons, the use of IV hydrocortisone at a dose of 200 mg/day should be reserved for patients who remain hemodynamically unstable despite fluid and vasopressor therapy.*[20] Patients should be weaned from steroid therapy when vasopressors are no longer required.

Glucose Control

The optimal blood glucose range in septic patients is unknown. Tight glycemic control (80–110 mg/dL [4.4–6.1 mmol/L]) improved survival in postoperative surgical patients, but did not show a benefit in medical critically ill patients.[40,41] More recent studies, including the large NICE-SUGAR trial, do not demonstrate a mortality benefit in favor of tight glycemic control, but actually a higher incidence of severe hypoglycemia and increased mortality rates.[42] KEY CONCEPT *Following initial stabilization of septic patients, current guidelines recommend initiating insulin therapy when two consecutive blood glucose measurements are greater than 180 mg/dL (10.0 mmol/L) and then maintaining a blood glucose range of 140 to 180 mg/dL (7.8–10.0 mmol/L).* Blood glucose levels should be monitored frequently, every 1 to 2 hours, until glucose values and insulin infusion rates are stable, then every 4 hours thereafter.[20]

Patient Encounter, Part 4

Three days later, the patient's blood pressure begins to respond to therapy with a MAP remaining greater than 65 mm Hg (8.6 kPa) on minimal vasopressor support.

What changes to the patient's medication regimen do you recommend?

Adjunctive Therapies

▶ Blood Product Administration

There are no trials showing the optimal hemoglobin concentration in patients with severe sepsis. However, based on other studies which included subgroups of septic patients, with the exception of myocardial ischemia, severe hypoxemia, acute hemorrhage, or ischemic coronary artery disease, it is recommended to target a hemoglobin concentration of 7 to 9 g/dL (70–90 g/L; 4.34–5.59 mmol/L) and red blood cell transfusion should occur when the hemoglobin concentration is less than 7 g/dL (70 g/L; 4.34 mmol/L).[20,43] Erythropoietin stimulating agents, fresh frozen plasma, and antithrombin should not be administered, unless other compelling indications exist, to treat sepsis-induced abnormalities.[20]

▶ Sedation, Analgesia, and Neuromuscular Blockade

It is common for severe sepsis patients to require mechanical ventilation during their course of therapy. These patients may require analgesic or sedative agents to facilitate mechanical ventilation. Historically, concerns for patient safety and posttraumatic stress disorder emphasized the need for sedation in these patients. However, there continue to be ample data indicating that, while sedation is necessary, limiting exposure to certain sedative medications may improve morbidity and mortality rates. When sedation is needed, a standardized protocol targeting specific endpoints should be utilized.[20,44]

Neuromuscular blockade usually is reserved for patients in whom sedation alone does not improve the effectiveness of mechanical ventilation. Neuromuscular blockers may lead to prolonged skeletal muscle weakness and should be avoided if possible especially if receiving concomitant corticosteroid therapy which can increase the risk of critical illness polyneuropathy. Patients requiring neuromuscular blockade should be monitored, and intermittent bolus doses or continuous infusion should be utilized. Monitor depth of neuromuscular blockade with either train-of-four stimulation or other forms of clinical assessment when using continuous infusion. Patients with early, sepsis-induced ARDS with a Pao_2/Fio_2 less than 150 mm Hg (20.0 kPa), may benefit from a short course of a neuromuscular blocking agent to not exceed 48 hours.[20]

Renal Replacement Therapy

Patients who develop acute kidney injury as a manifestation of severe sepsis may require some type of renal replacement therapy. There are no data currently that suggest superiority for either continuous or intermittent modalities of hemodialysis as both have demonstrated similar mortality rates. In patients who are hemodynamically unstable, continuous renal replacement therapy may be more beneficial due to less overall hypotension during therapy.

Deep Vein Thrombosis Prophylaxis

Combination pharmacologic and mechanical prophylaxis against venous thromboembolism is recommended for septic patients when possible. Low-dose unfractionated heparin, low-molecular-weight heparin (eg, enoxaparin or dalteparin), or pentasaccharide therapy (eg, fondaparinux) may be utilized. Graduated compression stockings or an intermittent compression device is recommended for patients with a contraindication to heparin products (thrombocytopenia, severe coagulopathy, active bleeding, or recent intracerebral hemorrhage).[20]

Patient Care Process

Patient Assessment:

- Based on physical exam and review of systems, determine whether the patient meets criteria for suspected sepsis.
- Review available diagnostic and laboratory data, especially CBC with differential, CMP, lactic acid, and patient specific factors including previous antimicrobial history and microbiologic cultures.
- Measure vital signs, including temperature, heart rate, respiratory rate, and blood pressure.

Therapy Evaluation:

- Institute early intervention initially with crystalloid fluids. Understand which parameters indicate effective/ineffective therapy. Recommend additional resuscitation therapy if the patient remains hypotensive.
- Initiate appropriate, broad-spectrum antimicrobials that cover the most likely pathogens within the first hour of diagnosis.
- Evaluate the source of infection and make recommendations to remove potential sources.
- If patient remains hemodynamically unstable despite fluid administration, start vasopressor therapy and/or corticosteroids with potential inotropic therapy if required.

Care Plan Development:

- Formulate appropriate dosing regimens of medications involved in therapy and revise as needed.
- Patient parameters may change frequently, thus requiring modifications of therapy. This may include the addition or deletion of adjunctive medications, such as antimicrobial agents, analgesics, sedatives, neuromuscular blockers, insulin, blood products, and renal replacement therapy.

Follow-Up Evaluation:

- Continually monitor patient parameters to ensure optimal therapy to minimize morbidity and mortality.

Stress Ulcer Prophylaxis

Patients with severe sepsis are at increased risk for developing a stress ulcer bleeding event. Stress ulcer prophylaxis using either a histamine-receptor antagonist (H-2 blocker) or proton pump inhibitor (PPI) is recommended in septic patients. Patients at greatest risk for stress ulcers include those who are coagulopathic, mechanically ventilated (greater than 48 hours), or hypotensive. Histamine-2 receptor antagonists (eg, ranitidine) are more efficacious than sucralfate. There is ongoing debate to determine if PPIs (eg, omeprazole) are more efficacious than H-2 blockers with low-quality data showing conflicting outcomes.[20,45] Both, however, demonstrate equivalence in the ability to increase gastric pH.[20] The benefit of prophylaxis must be weighed against the potential effect of increased stomach pH and development of infectious complications, such as hospital-acquired pneumonia and/or *Clostridium difficile* infection.

Nutrition

Meeting the nutritional needs of septic patients can be challenging, especially in patients who are hemodynamically unstable. When possible, early initiation of enteral nutrition should be considered to maintain gut mucosa and potentially decrease the risk of bacterial translocation leading to infection. Patients who are hemodynamically unstable may not tolerate enteral nutrition and are at risk for gut ischemia. Parenteral nutrition alone or in conjunction with enteral nutrition should not be initiated in the first 7 days as this has not been shown to improve outcomes.[20]

Prognosis

There are various factors that influence outcome. Gram-negative bacteria are more likely to produce septic shock than gram-positive bacteria (50% vs 25%) and have a higher mortality rate than other pathogens. This may be related to the severity of the underlying condition. Patients with rapidly fatal conditions, such as leukemia, aplastic anemia, and burns, have a worse prognosis than patients with nonfatal underlying conditions, such as diabetes mellitus or chronic renal insufficiency. Other factors that worsen the prognosis of septic patients include advanced age, malnutrition, resistant bacteria, utilization of medical devices, and immunosuppression. Data for long-term mortality are lacking (it is estimated that the mortality for sepsis survivors within the first year is 20%).[12] Patients may have prolonged physical disability related to muscle weakness and posttraumatic stress.

Abbreviations Introduced in This Chapter

ABG	Arterial blood gas
AKI	Acute kidney injury
ARDS	Acute respiratory distress syndrome
CBC	Complete blood count
CMP	Comprehensive metabolic panel
CVP	Central venous pressure
DIC	Disseminated intravascular coagulation
DVT	Deep vein thrombosis
Fio_2	Fraction of inspired oxygen
HES	Hydroxyethyl starch
IV	Intravenous
MAP	Mean arterial pressure
MDR	Multidrug resistant
Pao_2	Partial pressure of oxygen
SIRS	Systemic inflammatory response syndrome

REFERENCES

1. Russell JA. Management of sepsis. N Engl J Med. 2006;355:1699–1713.
2. Angus D, van der Poll T. Severe sepsis and septic shock. N Engl J Med. 2013;369:840–851.
3. Levy M, Fink M, Marshall J, et al. 2001 SCCM/ESICM/ACCP/ATS/SIS International Sepsis Defintions Conference. Crit Care Med. 2003;31:1250–1256.
4. Hotchkiss RS, Karl IE. The pathophysiology and treatment of sepsis. N Engl J Med. 2003;348:138–150.

5. Martin GS, Mannino DM, Eaton S, Moss M. The epidemiology of sepsis in the United States from 1979 through 2000. N Engl J Med. 2003;348:1546–1554.
6. Hoste E, Lameire NH, Vanholder RC, et al. Acute renal failure in patients with sepsis in a surgical ICU: Predictive factors, incidence, comorbidity, and outcome. J Am Soc Nephrol. 2003; 14:1022–1030.
7. Poutsiaka DD, Davidson LE, Kahn KL, et al. Risk factors for death after sepsis in patients immunosuppressed before the onset of sepsis. Scand J Infect Dis. 2009;41(6–7):469–479.
8. Wafaisade A, Lefering R, Bouillon B, et al. Epidemiology and risk factors of sepsis after multiple trauma: An analysis of 29,829 patients from the trauma registry of the German society for trauma surgery. Crit Care Med. 2011;39(4):621–628.
9. Lin MT, Albertson TE. Genomic polymorphisms in sepsis. Crit Care Med. 2004;32:569–579
10. Bodey GP, Mardani M, Hanna HA, et al. The epidemiology of Candida glabrata and Candida albicans fungemia in immunocompromised patients with cancer. Am J Med. 2002;112: 380–385.
11. Costa SF, Marino I, Araujo EA, et al. Nosocomial fungemia: A 2-year prospective study. J Hosp Infect. 2000:45:69–72.
12. Cartin-Ceba R, Kojicic M, Li G, et al. Epidemiology of critical care syndromes, organ failures, and life-support interventions in a suburban US community. Chest. 2011;140(6):1447–1455.
13. Angus DC, Linde-Zwirble WT, Lidicker J, et al. Epidemiology of severe sepsis in the United States: Analysis of incidence, outcome, and associated costs of care. Crit Care Med. 2001;29:1303–1310.
14. Marie C, Muret J, Fitting C, et al. Interleukin-1 receptor antagonist production during infectious and noninfectious systemic inflammatory response syndrome. Crit Care Med. 2000;28:2277–2282.
15. Opal SM, Girard TD, Ely EW. The immunopathogenesis of sepsis in elderly patients. Clin Infect Dis. 2005;41:S504–S512.
16. Kim PK, Deutschman CS. Inflammatory responses and mediators. Surg Clin North Am. 2000;80:885–894.
17. van der Poll T, van Deventer SJH. Cytokines and anticytokines in the pathogenesis of sepsis. Infect Dis Clin North Am. 1999;13: 413–426.
18. Harbarth S, Garbino J, Pugin J, et al. Inappropriate initial antimicrobial therapy and its effects on survival in a clinical trial of immunomodulating therapy for severe sepsis. Am J Med. 2003;115:529–535.
19. Garnacho-Montero J, Garcia-Garmendia JL, Barrero-Almodovar A, et al. Impact of adequate empirical antibiotic therapy on the outcome of patients admitted to the intensive care unit with sepsis. Crit Care Med. 2003;31:2742–2751.
20. Dellinger RP, Levy MM, Rhodes A, et al. Surviving sepsis campaign: International guidelines for management of severe sepsis and septic shock: 2012. Crit Care Med 2013;41:580–637.
21. Jimenez MF, Marshall JC. Source control in the management of sepsis. Intensive Care Med. 2001;27:S49–S62.
22. O'Grady NP, Alexander M, Dellinger EP, et al. Guidelines for the prevention of intravascular catheter-related infections. Centers for Disease Control and Prevention. MMWR 2002;51:1–29.
23. Rivers E, Nguyen B, Havstad S, et al; Early Goal-directed Therapy Collaborative Group. Early goal-directed therapy in the treatment of severe sepsis and septic shock. N Engl J Med. 2001;345:1368–1377.
24. Hollenberg SM, Ahrens TS, Annane D, et al. Practice parameters for hemodynamic support of sepsis in adult patients: 2004 update. Crit Care Med. 2004;32:1928–1948.
25. Yealy D, Kellum J, Huang D, et al; The ProCESS Investigators. A randomized trial of protocol-based care for early septic shock. N Engl J Med. 2014;370:1683–1693.
26. Peake S, Delaney A, Bailey M, et al. Goal-directed resuscitation for patients with early septic shock. N Engl J Med. 2014;371: 1496–1506.
27. Mouncey P, Osborn T, Power S, et al. Trial of early, goal-directed resuscitation for septic shock. N Engl J Med. 2015;372:1301–1311.
28. Finfer S, Bellomo R, Boyce N, et al. A comparison of albumin and saline for fluid resuscitation in the intensive care unit. N Engl J Med. 2004;350:2247–2256.
29. Ferrada P, Anand R, Whelan J, et al. Qualitative assessment of the inferior vena cava: Useful tool for the evaluation of fluid status in critically ill patients. Am Surg. 2012;78:468–470.
30. Schefold J, Storm C, Bercker S, et al. Inferior vena cava diameter correlates with invasive hemodynamic measures in mechanically ventilated intensive care unit patients with sepsis. J Emerg Med. 2010;38:632–637.
31. Caironi P, Tognoni G, Masson S, et al. Albumin replacement in patients with severe sepsis or septic shock. N Engl J Med. 2014; 370:1412–1421.
32. Patel A, Laffan M, Waheed U, et al. Randomised trials of human albumin for adults with sepsis: Systematic review and meta-analysis with trail sequential analysis of all-cause mortality. BMJ. 2014;349:g4561.
33. Perner A, Haase N, Guttormsen AB, et al; 6S Trial Group. Scandinavian Critical Care Trials Group: Hydroxyethyl starch 130/0.42 versus Ringer's acetate in severe sepsis. N Engl J Med. 2012;367:124–134.
34. Myburgh JA, Finfer S, Bellomo R, et al; CHEST Investigators. Australian and New Zealand Intensive Care Society Clinical Trials Group: Hydroxyethyl starch or saline for fluid resuscitation in intensive care. N Engl J Med. 2012;367:1901–1911.
35. MacArthur RD, Miller M, Albertson T, et al. Adequacy of early empiric antibiotic treatment and survival in severe sepsis: Experience from the MONARCS trial. Clin Infect Dis. 2004; 38:284–288.
36. De Backer D, Biston P, Devriendt J, et al. Comparison of dopamine and norepinephrine in the treatment of shock. N Engl J Med. 2010;362:779–789.
37. Russell JA, Walley KR, Singer J, et al. Vasopressin versus norepinephrine infusion in patients with septic shock. N Engl J Med. 2008;358:877–887.
38. Annane D, Sebille V, Charpentier C, et al. Effect of treatment with low doses of hydrocortisone and fludrocortisone on mortality in patients with septic shock. JAMA. 2002;288:862–871.
39. Sprung CL, Annane D, Keh D, et al. Hydrocortisone therapy for patients with septic shock. N Engl J Med. 2008;358:111–124.
40. Van den Berghe G, Wilmer A, Hermans G, et al. Intensive insulin therapy in the medical ICU. N Engl J Med. 2006;354:449–461.
41. van den Berghe G, Wouters P, Weekers F, et al. Intensive insulin therapy in the critically ill patient. N Engl J Med. 2001; 345:1359–1367.
42. Finfer S, Chittock D, Yu-Shuo S, et al; The NICE-SUGAR Study Investigators. Intensive versus conventional glucose control in critically ill patients. N Engl J Med. 2009;360:1283–1297.
43. Hebert PC, Wells G, Blajchman MA, et al; Transfusion Requirements in Critical Care Investigators. A multicenter, randomized, controlled clinical trial or transfusion requirements in critical care. N Engl J Med. 1999;340:409–417.
44. Barr J, Fraser G, Puntillo K, et al. Clinical practice guidelines for the management of pain, agitation, and delirium in adult patients in the intensive care unit. Crit Care Med. 2013;41:263–306.
45. MacLaren R, Reynolds P, Allen R. Histamine-2 receptor antagonists vs proton pump inhibitors on gastrointestinal tract hemorrhage and infectious complications in the intensive care unit. JAMA. 2014;174:564–574.

83 Superficial Fungal Infections

Lauren S. Schlesselman

LEARNING OBJECTIVES

Upon completion of the chapter, the reader will be able to:

1. Explain the underlying pathophysiology of vulvovaginal candidiasis, oropharyngeal candidiasis, esophageal candidiasis, and fungal skin infections.
2. Identify symptoms of vulvovaginal candidiasis, oropharyngeal candidiasis, esophageal candidiasis, and fungal skin infections.
3. Identify the desired therapeutic outcomes for patients with uncomplicated and complicated vulvovaginal candidiasis, oropharyngeal candidiasis, esophageal candidiasis, and fungal skin infections.
4. Recommend appropriate lifestyle modifications and pharmacotherapy interventions for patients with vulvovaginal candidiasis, oropharyngeal candidiasis, esophageal candidiasis, and fungal skin infections.
5. Recognize when long-term suppressive therapy is indicated for a patient with vulvovaginal candidiasis.
6. Recognize when topical versus oral treatment is indicated for a patient with oropharyngeal candidiasis, esophageal candidiasis, vulvovaginal candidiasis, and fungal skin infections.
7. Educate patients about the disease state, appropriate lifestyle modifications, and medication therapy required for effective treatment of vulvovaginal candidiasis, oropharyngeal candidiasis, esophageal candidiasis, and fungal skin infections.

INTRODUCTION

Superficial fungal infections, also referred to as mycoses, are common and treatable conditions seen in everyday practice. Treatment largely depends on the use of azole and allylamine antifungal agents, either topically or orally, depending on the site, severity, and immune status of the patient.

VULVOVAGINAL CANDIDIASIS

Vulvovaginal candidiasis (VVC), whether symptomatic or asymptomatic, refers to infections in women whose vaginal cultures are positive for *Candida* species.

EPIDEMIOLOGY AND ETIOLOGY

Vulvovaginal candidiasis, also known as moniliasis, is a common form of vaginitis, accounting for 20% to 25% of vaginitis cases. Although VVC is uncommon prior to menarche, an estimated 75% of women will have at least one occurrence of VVC.[1]

According to the treatment guidelines of the Centers for Disease Control and Prevention (CDC),[1] VVC can be classified as uncomplicated or complicated. Uncomplicated infections occur sporadically, cause mild to moderate symptoms, and occur in nonimmunocompromised women. Uncomplicated infections, most often caused by *Candida albicans*, often have no identifiable precipitating cause. Complicated infections, including recurrent, severe infections, and those in women with uncontrolled diabetes, debilitation, or immunosuppression, may be caused by nonalbicans or azole-resistant fungal organisms. Recurrent VVC, defined as four or more infections per year, occurs in less than 5% of women, is distinguishable from a persistent infection by the presence of a symptom-free interval between infections.[1]

KEY CONCEPT *Candida albicans is the primary pathogen responsible for VVC, accounting for 66% of cases.*[2] Other cases are caused by nonalbicans species, including *Candida glabrata, Candida tropicalis, Candida krusei*, and *Candida parapsilosis*.[2]

PATHOPHYSIOLOGY

The normal vaginal environment protects women against vaginal infections. Under the influence of estrogen, vaginal epithelium cornifies to reduce the risk of infection. Vaginal discharge, composed of exfoliated cells, cervical mucus, and colonized bacteria, cleans the vagina. The normal pH of vaginal secretions, near 4.0, is toxic to many pathogens and is maintained by *Lactobacillus acidophilus*, diphtheroids, and *Staphylococcus epidermidis*. Alterations in the vaginal environment, including pH changes, allow for overgrowth of organisms that are normally suppressed, increasing the risk of vulvovaginitis.

RISK FACTORS

KEY CONCEPT *Although no risk factors are consistently associated with conversion to symptomatic infection, a variety of factors may increase the risk of developing symptomatic VVC in certain women* (Table 83–1).

Clinical Presentation and Diagnosis of VVC

Patients with VVC may present with vulvar and/or vaginal symptoms. Symptoms often develop the week before menses and resolve with the onset of menses.

Symptoms

- Vaginal itching
- Vaginal soreness
- Vaginal burning
- Irritation
- External dysuria
- Dyspareunia

Signs

- Nonodorous vaginal discharge (may vary from watery to curd-like)
- Yellow or yellowish green discharge
- Erythema and edema of the labia and vulva
- Fissures
- Pustulopapular lesions
- Normal cervix

Diagnostic Testing

- Microscopic investigation for the presence of blastospores or pseudohyphae; saline wet mount has a sensitivity of 40% to 50%, whereas a potassium hydroxide (KOH) preparation has a sensitivity of 50% to 70%.[7] *Asymptomatic vaginal colonization of* Candida albicans *is not diagnostic of VVC since 10% to 20% of women are asymptomatic carriers of* Candida *species. Asymptomatic vaginal colonization does not require treatment; therefore, the presence alone of* Candida *should not determine care.*
- Vaginal pH less than or equal to 4.5; pH should remain normal in cases of fungal infection, whereas an elevated pH suggests bacterial infection.
- *Candida* cultures should be obtained only if signs and microscopy are inconclusive or in cases of recurrent VVC.

Table 83–1

Possible Risk Factors Associated with VVC

Risk Factor	Proposed Mechanism
Broad-spectrum antibiotic use	Altered vaginal flora allowing overgrowth of *Candida* organisms; risk increases with duration of antibiotic use
Systemic corticosteroid or immunosuppressant use	Reduced vaginal protection by immunoglobulins
Sexual activity	VVC is often associated with the onset of sexual activity; partners may have penile or oral colonization; use of vaginal irritants or devices, including diaphragms and intrauterine systems, can irritate vaginal mucosa
Tight-fitting and nonabsorbent clothing	Promotes warm, moist environment for fungus growth
Elevated estrogen levels, hormonal contraceptives, and pregnancy	Estrogen enhances *Candida* adherence to vaginal epithelial cells and yeast-mycelial transformation; this is supported by the fact that infection rates are lower before menarche and after menopause (except in women taking hormone replacement therapy), whereas rates are higher during pregnancy
Vaginal pH	Changes in glycogen and lactic acid levels
Gastrointestinal reservoir of *Candida* organisms	Transfer of organism from rectum to vagina; irritation of the vulvovaginal area during sexual intercourse may enhance invasion of organisms
Diabetes	Enhanced binding of *Candida* to epithelial cells due to hyperglycemia; asymptomatic colonization is more common in patients with diabetes; elevated sugar levels may cause conversion to symptomatic infection

TREATMENT

The goals of treatment of VVC are as follows:

- Relief of symptoms
- Eradication of infection
- Reestablishment of normal vaginal flora
- Prevention of recurrent infections in complicated infections

Nonpharmacologic Treatments

In combination with pharmacologic treatment, the practitioner should recommend basic nonpharmacologic approaches to treatment and prevention of VVC:

- Keep the genital area clean and dry
- Avoid prolonged use of hot tubs
- Avoid constrictive clothing
- Avoid vaginal douching

Patient Encounter 1

A teenaged girl and her mother present to your clinic. The mother reports that her daughter has been complaining of itching in her vaginal area and a white discharge. After questioning the daughter, you determine that she has vaginal burning, soreness, and itching, accompanied by a curd-like discharge. She has never had a vaginal infection before. Upon further questions, you determine that the girl is a lifeguard and on the high school swim team, along with a long-distance runner. Despite the daughter's denial of sexual activity, the mother is concerned that her daughter has contracted a sexually transmitted disease "from the water in the pool." On examination, she has erythema of the labia and a nonodorous discharge.

What information is suggestive of VVC?

What additional information do you need to know before creating a treatment plan for this patient?

- Wear underwear made of breathable materials, such as cotton
- Avoid soaps and perfumes in the genital area
- Although study results are conflicting, possibly due to the strain or concentration studied, the daily consumption of active *Lactobacillus* may reduce recurrence. Newer studies have found ingestion of *Lactobacillus rhamnosus* and *Lactobacillus reuteri* suppressed metabolic activity and killed *C. albicans*,[3] whereas older studies found no difference in infection rates in women who ingested yogurt.[4]

Pharmacologic Treatment of Uncomplicated VVC

For most cases of uncomplicated VVC, the CDC guidelines recommend a short course of therapy (1–3 days) with an oral or vaginal antifungal agent, either prescription or nonprescription.[1] Nonprescription azole antifungal products are available as 1-night, 3-night, and 7-night regimens in a variety of formulations, including cream, suppository, and vaginal tablets (Table 83–2). Oral fluconazole offers the option of treatment with one dose administered without regard to time of day. Some practitioners opt to retreat with a second dose of fluconazole 3 days later. Due to the risk of severe hepatotoxicity, the use of oral ketoconazole should be reserved for severe fungal infections resistant to other antifungal options.

Inability to resolve an infection may indicate a mixed infection, infection owing to a nonalbicans strain, an infection that is not fungal, or indicative of serious underlying conditions, such as diabetes or human immunodeficiency virus (HIV) infection. For these reasons, if infection does not resolve with a single antifungal course or if symptoms return within 2 months, practitioners should check cultures and further evaluate the patient's health status.

KEY CONCEPT *Due to the numerous treatment options available, a variety of factors can influence product selection, with patient preference playing a significant role.* To improve adherence with therapy, the practitioner should discuss with the patient what options are available and what her preferences are.

Adherence rates are greater with oral treatment than with vaginal therapy, possibly due to ease of administration, short duration, and administration flexibility. Vaginal creams provide rapid relief of itching and burning, while symptom resolution may take 1 to 2 days with oral treatment. The practitioner may wish to recommend applying a vaginal cream externally to reduce itching and burning when using an oral agent, although this increases the cost of therapy. Most OTC products cost $10 to $20 per course of therapy. The cost of prescription products can vary based on insurance coverage. If the patient does not have prescription coverage, nonprescription products may prove less expensive than even one or two fluconazole tablets.

▸ Risk of Adverse Effects and Interactions

Systemic adverse effects associated with vaginally administered azoles are less frequent than with oral products. With topical products, local discomfort such as burning, itching, stinging, and redness may occur, particularly with the first application. In contrast, common adverse effects associated with fluconazole include headache, diarrhea, nausea, dizziness, abdominal pain, and taste alterations. Around 15% of patients experience gastrointestinal side effects with orally administered fluconazole.[5]

Oral azoles are associated with significant drug interactions, particularly due to potent inhibition of cytochrome P-450 (CYP) 2C9 and moderate inhibition of CYP 3A4. For patients receiving only a few doses, these interactions do not pose a significant risk but may pose a risk with long-term suppressive therapy for recurrent infections.

TREATMENT OF RECURRENT VVC

The goal of treating recurrent VVC is control of the infection, rather than cure. First, any acute episodes are treated, followed by maintenance therapy. Although acute episodes of recurrent VVC will respond to azole therapy, some patients may require prolonged therapy to achieve remission. To achieve remission, 14 days of topical azole therapy or a second dose of oral fluconazole 150 mg repeated 3 days after the first dose can be used. The practitioner should consider that nonalbicans infections are more common in recurrent VVC; therefore, fluconazole and itraconazole resistance may make these agents less effective.

KEY CONCEPT *After achieving remission, recurrent VVC requires long-term suppressive therapy for 6 months* (Table 83–3). Per CDC

Table 83–2

Treatment Options for Uncomplicated VVC

1-Day Therapies
- Butoconazole 2% sustained-release cream, 5 g intravaginally as a single application
- Fluconazole 150 mg, one tablet orally as a single dose
- Tioconazole 6.5% ointment, 5 g intravaginally as a single application

3-Day Therapies
- Butoconazole 2% cream, 5 g intravaginally for 3 nights
- Clotrimazole 100-mg vaginal tablet, two tablets for 3 nights
- Miconazole 200-mg vaginal suppository, one suppository for 3 nights
- Terconazole 0.8% cream, 5 g intravaginally for 3 nights
- Terconazole 00 mg vaginal suppository, one suppository for 3 nights

7- to 14-Day Therapies
- Boric acid 600-mg vaginal suppository, one suppository intravaginally twice daily for 14 days
- Clotrimazole 1% cream, 5 g intravaginally for 7–14 nights
- Clotrimazole 100-mg vaginal tablet, one tablet for 7 nights
- Miconazole 2% cream, 5 g intravaginally for 7 nights
- Miconazole 100-mg vaginal suppository, one suppository for 7 nights
- Nystatin 100,000-unit vaginal tablet, one tablet for 14 nights
- Terconazole 0.4% cream, 5 g intravaginally for 7 nights

Table 83–3

Treatment Options for Maintenance Therapy

Daily
- Boric acid 600 mg in gelatin capsule vaginally daily during menses (5 days)
- Itraconazole 100 mg orally once daily
- Ketoconazole 100 mg orally once daily

Weekly
- Clotrimazole 500 mg vaginal suppository once weekly
- Fluconazole 100 or 150 mg orally once weekly
- Terconazole 0.8% cream 5 g vaginally once weekly

Monthly
- Fluconazole 150 mg orally once monthly
- Itraconazole 400 mg orally once monthly

guidelines, oral fluconazole 100-, 150-, or 200-mg weekly for 6 months is first-line treatment.[1] Cessation of suppressive therapy is associated with resurgence of symptomatic infection in 30% to 50% of women.[1]

TREATMENT OF NONALBICANS INFECTIONS

Treatment response rates are lower for nonalbicans infections. Although an optimal regimen is unknown, use of nonfluconazole azole therapy for 7 to 14 days is recommended.[1] For second-line therapy, boric acid 600 mg in a gelatin capsule administered vaginally daily for 2 weeks is recommended.[1] This regimen provides mycologic cure rates of 40% to 100%,[6] although local irritation often limits its use. Oral itraconazole 200-mg twice daily one day per month for 6 months is also effective.[7] Topical 4% flucytosine is also effective, but use should be limited due to the potential for resistance.

VVC DURING PREGNANCY

During pregnancy, VVC may prove difficult to treat due to elevated estrogen levels, lower response rates, and frequent recurrences, accompanied by concern for the fetus. Vaginal antifungals remain the preferred treatment during pregnancy, although therapy should continue for 1 to 2 weeks to ensure effectiveness.[8] Most topical antifungals are classified as risk category C, whereas clotrimazole is classified as risk category B. Fluconazole's risk category classification for the single 150-mg dose is risk category C but category D for all other doses due to case studies of congenital limb deformities with doses of 400 to 800 mg daily during the first trimester.[9]

CULTURAL AWARENESS DURING TREATMENT OF VVC

As with all gynecologic issues, the practitioner is faced with cultural perceptions of female genitalia. In particular, practitioners are treating an increased number of patients who have undergone female genital mutilation. Female genital mutilation, formerly known as female circumcision, describes the intentional alteration or injury of female genitalia. More than 100 million women and girls, particularly in Africa and the Middle East, have undergone such procedures for cultural and religious reasons.[10] Some authorities suggest using the term "genital cutting" when dealing with patients to avoid appearing judgmental.[11] Women who have undergone this procedure suffer acute and chronic complications. Patients with female genital mutilation may suffer from recurrent VVC due to inadequate drainage of vaginal fluids. Regardless of the practitioner's opinion on female genital mutilation, the practitioner must be sensitive to the patient's feeling and cultural values.

OUTCOME EVALUATION

Whether using a topical or an oral agent, patients should notice relief of itching and discomfort within 1 to 2 days. The volume of discharge should also begin to decrease within a few days. The entire course of therapy should be continued even if symptoms have resolved. If the condition recurs within 4 weeks or more than four times per year, the patient should be further evaluated for possible non-*Candida* infections, resistant organism, or other complicating factors, along with assessment of need for long-term suppressive therapy.

Patient Care Process for VVC

Patient Assessment:

- Assess the patient's symptoms to determine whether self-treatment with OTC antifungal therapy is appropriate. OTC preparations should only be recommended for patients who have previously been diagnosed with VVC.
- Review any available diagnostic data, including cultures and KOH preps.
- Obtain a thorough history of prescription, nonprescription, and natural drug product use. Is the patient taking any medications, such as steroids, antibiotics, or immunosuppressants, that may contribute to VVC? Is the patient taking any medications that may interfere with treatment? Any allergies?

Therapy Evaluation:

- Determine whether self-treatment with OTC antifungal therapy is appropriate.
- If the patient has had VVC previously, determine what treatments were helpful to the patient in the past.
- Determine whether long-term maintenance therapy is necessary.
- Evaluate the patient for the potential for adverse drug reactions, drug allergies, and drug interactions.
- Determine whether patient has prescription coverage.

Care Plan Development:

- Stress the importance of adherence with the antifungal regimen, including lifestyle modifications.
- Educate the patient on lifestyle modifications that may prevent recurrence, including wearing loose clothing, increased consumption of yogurt containing live cultures, and wearing cotton underwear.
- Provide patient education pertaining to vulvovaginal candidiasis and antifungal therapy, including causes, medication administration, adverse effects of vaginal agents on latex condoms, and potential adverse effects.
- Discuss warning signs to report to a practitioner such as recurrent or difficult-to-cure infections or infections with malodorous discharge.

Follow-Up Evaluation:

- Follow-up only necessary of treatment failure or recurrence.

OROPHARYNGEAL AND ESOPHAGEAL CANDIDIASIS

Oropharyngeal candidiasis (OPC) is a common fungal infection, often associated with immune suppression. If left untreated, it will progress to more serious oral disease, such as esophageal candidiasis.

EPIDEMIOLOGY AND ETIOLOGY

KEY CONCEPT *The occurrence of oropharyngeal and esophageal candidiasis is an indicator of immune suppression, often developing in infants, the elderly, and the immunocompromised.* One-third to one-half of geriatric inpatients develop oropharyngeal candidiasis. Denture stomatitis is present in approximately 40% of denture wearers,[12] more commonly in women than men. Oral candidiasis is the most commonly reported adverse drug event reported by patients receiving inhaled corticosteroids,[13] with the prevalence of esophageal candidiasis reaching 37% among patients treated with inhaled corticosteroids.[14] The incidence of esophageal candidiasis is highest among patients receiving high doses of corticosteroids or with diabetes.

The prevalence of HIV infection plays a significant role in the incidence of oropharyngeal and esophageal candidiasis. In the 1980s, the incidence of oropharyngeal candidiasis increased fivefold, in association with the spread of HIV infections.[15] Although HIV infection remains a risk factor for candidiasis, the introduction of highly active antiretroviral therapy precipitated a decline in the incidence of oral candidiasis to 45.9% to 79.1%, varying by geographic location, race, and therapy.[16]

Oropharyngeal candidiasis remains the most common opportunistic infection in patients with HIV. For the majority of patients, it is the first manifestation of HIV infection.[28] The incidence of oropharyngeal infection increases with decreasing $CD4^+$ lymphocyte counts, with an incidence of 59% in patients with a $CD4^+$ count less than 350 cells/mm^3 (350×10^6/L).[17]

Although esophageal candidiasis represents the first manifestation of HIV infection in less than 10% of cases, it is the most common acquired immunodeficiency syndrome (AIDS)-defining disease.[18] The CDC classifies esophageal candidiasis as a Stage 3-defining opportunistic infection in HIV.[19] As with oropharyngeal candidiasis, the incidence of esophageal candidiasis increases with decreasing $CD4^+$ counts, therefore is a measure of declining $CD4^+$ count or treatment failure.

Candida albicans accounts for 80% of cases of OPC and esophageal candidiasis. Over the last 20 years, an increasing incidence of *C. albicans* resistance has been accompanied by an increased incidence of nonalbicans species infections, including *Candida glabrata, Candida tropicalis, Candida krusei*, and *Candida parapsilosis*. In patients with cancer and HIV, the prevalence of *Candida glabrata* infections or mixed *Candida albicans* and *Candida glabrata* infection has been increasing.[20] Such infections tend to be more severe and require larger doses of antifungal agents for treatment.

PATHOPHYSIOLOGY

Similar to VVC, the development of OPC occurs when the normal environment is altered. *Candida* organisms frequently colonize the oropharynx and mucous membranes. These organisms do not become pathogenic until the environmental balance is disturbed. This occurs in the setting of broad-spectrum antibiotic use, tissue damage (due to chemotherapy, catheter tubing, trauma, or smoking), hyposalivation, or immune deficiency.

RISK FACTORS

Risk factors for OPC can be found in Table 83–4.

Table 83–4

Risk Factors for Oropharyngeal and Esophageal Candidiasis

Factor	Proposed Mechanism
Extremes of age	Immature immunity in infants and reduced immunity in the elderly
Impaired mucosal integrity	Breaks in the protective barrier allows fungal invasion; often due to radiation, surgery, or mucositis
Dentures	Adherence of fungus to dentures, along with reduced salivary flow under dentures; ill-fitting dentures may impair mucosal integrity
Xerostomia	Reduced cleansing and defense factors of saliva
Use of antibiotics	Altered flora of mucosa allowing fungal overgrowth
Use of steroids	Suppression of immunity
Use of immunosuppressants	Suppression of immunity
HIV infection	Decreased CD4 T lymphocytes
Diabetes mellitus	Elevated glucose levels and defense factors in saliva
Nutritional deficiencies	Altered defense mechanisms, impaired mucosal integrity, or enhanced pathogenic potential of fungus

CLINICAL PRESENTATION AND DIAGNOSIS

See text boxes for clinical presentation and diagnosis of OPC and esophageal candidiasis.

TREATMENT

Along with selecting an effective treatment, selection of an appropriate antifungal agent requires consideration of location and severity of infection, medication adherence, potential drug interactions, concomitant medical conditions, and presence of sucrose or dextrose. Topical agents require frequent dosing and prolonged contact time with oral mucosa. Rough surfaces of tablets and troches may irritate sensitive mucosa. Patients with xerostomia may have inadequate saliva to dissolve troches. Topical agents containing sucrose or dextrose may increase the risk of caries or cause elevated blood sugar in patients with diabetes. Along with being expensive, oral azoles exhibit an increased risk of toxicity and drug interactions due to inhibition of CYP-450.

Because oropharyngeal and esophageal candidiasis are signs of immunocompromise, the immune status of the patient should be considered in the therapeutic care plan. For HIV-infected patients, this should also include an evaluation of the patient's antiretroviral therapy because fungal infections may represent immune status deterioration.

KEY CONCEPT *For low-risk patients, topical agents are first-line therapy for oropharyngeal candidiasis, although systemic agents may be used for severe or unresponsive cases.* Infectious Disease Society of America (ISDA) guidelines recommend nystatin suspension four times per day or clotrimazole troches 10 mg five times per day for mild infections.[21] Once-daily oral fluconazole is reserved for moderate-to-severe cases.[21] Two weeks of oral itraconazole 200-mg or posaconazole 400-mg daily, voriconazole 200-mg twice daily, or amphotericin-B suspension are alternatives, typically reserved for refractory cases.

For non–HIV-infected patients who have suppressed immune systems, the practitioner must consider the patient's risk of dissemination. Patients with cell-mediated immune deficiency but near-normal granulocyte function, such as patients with diabetes, solid organ transplant, or solid tumors, are at low risk for dis semination. The risk of dissemination is higher in patients who develop neutropenia, including patients with leukemia or bone

Clinical Presentation and Diagnosis of Oropharyngeal Candidiasis

OPC is often a presumptive diagnosis based on signs and symptoms, along with the resolution of them after treatment with antifungal agents.

Symptoms

- Sore, painful mouth and tongue
- Burning tongue
- Dysphagia
- Metallic taste

Signs

Signs vary depending on the type of oropharyngeal candidiasis.

- Diffuse erythema on the surface of buccal mucosa, throat, tongue, and gums
- White patches on tongue, gums, or buccal mucosa; removal of patches reveals erythematous and bloody tissue; ability to remove patches distinguishes OPC from oral hairy leukoplakia
- Angular cheilitis presents with small cracking lesions, erythema, and soreness at the corners of the mouth; associated with vitamin and iron deficiency
- Denture stomatitis presents with flat, red lesions on mucosa beneath dentures; signs of chronic erythema and edema on mucosa
- Hyperplastic OPC presents with discrete, transparent raised lesions on the inner mucosa of the cheek; typically found in men who smoke
- Pseudomembranous OPC presents with yellow-white plaques that may be small and discrete or confluent; most common form found in HIV patients

Diagnostic Testing

Diagnosis is primarily based on identification of characteristic lesions. Although rarely necessary, diagnostic testing is possible if a definitive diagnosis is required.

- Cytology, although presence of *Candida* is not diagnostic because colonization is common
- Culture to identify species of yeast or presence of resistance
- Biopsy

marrow transplant. These patients should be treated aggressively to prevent invasive fungal infection.

For the treatment of OPC in HIV-infected individuals, initial episodes can be adequately controlled with topical agents, such as clotrimazole troches, so long as symptoms are not severe and no esophageal involvement is suspected. Topical clotrimazole appears to be the most effective topical antifungal, exhibiting clinical responses equivalent to oral fluconazole and itraconazole solution, but mycological cure rates are lower and relapse rates higher with clotrimazole.[18]

KEY CONCEPT *Representing a severe extension of oropharyngeal candidiasis, esophageal candidiasis requires systemic antifungal therapy.* The significant morbidity associated with esophageal candidiasis warrants aggressive treatment.

The ISDA recommends 2 to 3 weeks of fluconazole 200 to 400 mg for esophageal candidiasis, with an echinocandin or amphotericin-B as alternatives in patients unable to tolerate oral therapy, or with resistant or refractory disease.[21] Itraconazole 200-mg daily, posaconazole 400-mg twice daily, or voriconazole 200-mg twice daily are considered second-line therapy. If immunocompromised patients experience frequent or severe recurrences, particularly of esophageal candidiasis, chronic maintenance therapy with fluconazole 100 to 200 mg daily should be considered.

Clinical Presentation and Diagnosis of Esophageal Candidiasis

Symptoms

- Fever
- Odynophagia
- Dysphagia
- Retrosternal pain

Signs

- Fever
- Hyperemic or edematous white plaques
- Ulceration of esophagus
- Increased mucosal friability
- Narrowing of lumen

Diagnostic Testing

Unlike OPC, diagnosis of esophageal candidiasis is not based solely on clinical presentation, instead requiring endoscopic visualization of lesions and culture confirmation. Due to the invasive nature of these procedures, most practitioners opt to treat the infection presumptively, reserving endoscopic evaluation for patients who fail therapy.

- Cytology and culture to identify species of yeast or presence of resistance
- Barium esophagogram
- Endoscopy revealing whitish plaques with progression to superficial ulceration of the esophageal mucosa
- Mucosal biopsy

Patient Encounter 2

A 29-year-old man presents to your clinic stating that he noticed "this funny white stuff" in his mouth, along with "burning and soreness in my mouth." He also mentions that he has a metallic taste in his mouth.

On initial examination, he has white patches on his tongue, gums, and buccal mucosa. These patches are easily removed, revealing erythematous tissue underneath.

His medical record shows that he recently completed a course of azithromycin and steroids for pneumonia.

What additional information do you need to know before creating a treatment plan for this patient?

What underlying medical conditions might make him susceptible to fungal infections?

How is the treatment care plan altered if the patient has a history of frequent and severe OPC? If the patient is HIV-positive? If the patient is neutropenic?

OUTCOME EVALUATION

- Patients should notice symptomatic relief within 2 to 3 days of initiating therapy. Complete resolution typically occurs within 7 to 10 days. The entire course of therapy should be continued even if symptoms have resolved. If the condition does not resolve or worsens, the patient should be referred to a specialist for aggressive therapy.
- Short courses of oral azoles are associated with gastrointestinal upset, whereas courses lasting longer than 7 to 10 days are associated with increased risk of hepatotoxicity and CYP-450 drug interactions. In patients receiving prolonged therapy lasting more than 3 weeks, periodic monitoring of liver function tests should be considered.
- Immunocompetent patients generally do not require reassessment after treatment. Patients with neutropenia exhibit an increased risk of dissemination of infection and therefore should be monitored for signs of systemic fungal infection. Due to an increased risk of recurrence, HIV-positive patients should routinely be evaluated for recurrence at each visit.

MYCOTIC INFECTIONS OF THE SKIN, HAIR, AND NAILS

Tinea infections are superficial fungal infections in which the pathogen remains within the keratinous layers of the skin or nails (Table 83–5). Typically these infections are named for the affected body part, such as tinea pedis (feet), tinea cruris (groin), and tinea corporis (body). Tinea infections are commonly referred to as ringworm due to the characteristic circular lesions. In actuality, tinea lesions can vary from rings to scales and single or multiple lesions.

EPIDEMIOLOGY AND ETIOLOGY

Tinea infections are second only to acne in frequency of reported skin disease. The common tinea infections are tinea pedis, tinea corporis, and tinea cruris. Tinea pedis, the most prevalent cutaneous fungal infection, afflicts more than 25 million people annually in the United States.

Patient Care Process of Oropharyngeal Candidiasis

Patient Assessment:

- Assess the patient's symptoms to determine whether symptoms are consistent with oropharyngeal or esophageal candidiasis.
- Review any available diagnostic data, including cultures.
- Evaluate for risk factor, such as immunocompromise.
- Review the medical history. Does the patient have compelling indications or contraindications for specific antifungal treatment?
- Review available laboratory tests, especially liver function.
- Obtain a thorough history of prescription, nonprescription, and natural drug product use. Is the patient taking any medications that may contribute to candidiasis? Is the patient taking any medications that may interfere with treatment?
- Determine if the patient has any allergies.

Therapy Evaluation:

- If the patient has had oropharyngeal or esophageal candidiasis previously, determine what treatments were helpful to the patient in the past.
- If the patient has had oropharyngeal or esophageal candidiasis previously, determine whether the patient has risk factors for recurrent infection.
- Determine whether long-term suppressive therapy is necessary.
- Evaluate the patient for the potential of adverse drug reactions, drug allergies, or drug interactions.

Care Plan Development:

- Stress the importance of adherence with the antifungal regimen until complete.
- Provide patient education pertaining to oropharyngeal or esophageal candidiasis and antifungal therapy, including causes, risk factors, medication administration, potential adverse effects, potential medication interactions.
- Discuss warning signs to report, include recurrence or worsening symptoms.

Follow-Up Evaluation:

- Follow-up if symptoms do not resolve within 7 days or if symptoms worsen.
- Follow-up on any identifiable precipitating cause, such as immunocompromise.

Table 83–5

Signs, Symptoms, and Risk Factors of Superficial Fungal Infections

Infection	Symptoms, Signs, and Risk Factors
Tinea pedis	• Involves plantar surface and interdigital spaces of foot • Interdigital infections produce itching; presents as fissures, scaling, or macerated skin; can occur between any toes but most often between fourth and fifth toes; may cause foul smell due to superinfection with *Pseudomonas* or diphtheroids • Hyperkeratotic infections present with slivery white scales on a thickened, red base; usually covers entire foot; occasionally may also affect hand • Vesiculobullous tinea pedis presents as pustules or vesicles on soles of feet; associated with maceration, itching, and thickening of sole; may cause lymphangitis and cellulitis; most common during summer months • Ulcerative tinea pedis presents as macerated, denuded, and weeping ulcers on soles; may produce extreme pain and erosion of interdigital spaces; typically complicated by opportunistic gram-negative infections • Risk factors include occlusive footwear, foot trauma, and use of public showers
Tinea manuum	• Infection of the interdigital and palmar surfaces • Presents as white scales in palmar folds; may also develop scales on remainder of palm; may present as singular plaque • More commonly affecting only one hand • Presents with hyperkeratotic skin
Tinea cruris	• Presents with follicular papules and pustules on the medial thigh and inguinal folds • Ringed lesions may extend from inguinal fold over adjacent inner thigh • Lesions usually spare the penis and scrotum, in contrast to candidiasis • Frequency increases during summer • Primarily develops in young men • Risk factors include tight-fitting clothing, excessive sweating, poor hygiene, increased humidity and temperatures • Commonly referred to as "jock itch"
Tinea corporis	• Presents with circular, scaly patch with enlarged border • Lesions may have red papules or plaque in center that clears, leaving hypopigmentation or hyperpigmentation • Itching may be present • Commonly referred to as ringworm of the body • Risk factors include animal to human contact
Tinea versicolor	• Characterized by skin depigmentation but can present as hyperpigmentation, particularly in dark-skinned patients • Typically occurs in areas with sebaceous glands, including neck, trunk, and arms • Depigmentation may persist for years • Primarily develops in young and middle-aged adults • Risk factors include application of oil, greasy skin, high ambient temperature, high relative humidity, tight-fitting clothing, immunodeficiency, malnutrition, hereditary predisposition
Tinea barbae	• Infection of beard area
Tinea capitis	• Infection of the head and scalp • May be asymptomatic initially, then progresses to inflammatory alopecia • "Black dot" alopecia may develop due to breakage of hair at the root • May form kerions (nodular swellings) • Scaling or favus may develop on scalp • Cervical lymphadenopathy is common • Primarily found in infants, children, and young adolescents, often in African American and Hispanic populations • Can be spread from person to person or animal to person
Onychomycosis (tinea unguium)	• Infection of nail plate and bed • Nail becomes opaque, thick, rough, yellow or brownish, and friable; nail may separate from bed • Toenails affected more frequently than fingernails • Prevalence increases with advanced age

Fungal skin infections are primarily caused by **dermatophytes** such as *Trichophyton*, *Microsporum*, and *Epidermophyton*. *Trichophyton rubrum* accounts for more than 75% of all cases in the United States.[22] To a lesser extent, *Candida* and other fungal species cause skin infections. With tinea infections, the causative dermatophyte typically invades the stratum corneum without penetration into the living tissues, leading to a localized infection.

PATHOPHYSIOLOGY

The primary mode of transmission of tinea infections is direct contact with other persons or surface reservoirs. Upon contact, the dermatophytes attach to the keratinized cells, leading to thickening of the cells. Although infection remains localized, bacterial superinfections may develop.

The pathophysiology of onychomycosis depends on the clinical type. With the most common form of onychomycosis, distal

Clinical Presentation and Diagnosis of Mycotic Infections

Symptoms and Signs

(see Table 83–5)

Diagnostic Testing

- KOH prep
- Wood's ultraviolet lamp
- Microscopic examination
- Fungal cultures
- Periodic acid-Schiff (PAS) staining of nail

Treatment of Skin and Hair Infections

The goals of treatment include the following:

- Providing symptomatic relief
- Resolution of infection
- Preventing spread of infection

lateral subungual, the fungus spreads from the plantar skin. The fungus invades the underside of the nail through the distal lateral nail bed, leading to inflammation of the area. In cases of white superficial onychomycosis, the fungus invades the surface of the nail plate directly. With white superficial onychomycosis, the nail bed and hyponychium are infected secondarily. Proximal subungual onychomycosis infections begin in the cuticle and the proximal nail fold, then penetrate the dorsum of the nail plate.

RISK FACTORS

- Prolonged exposure to sweaty clothing
- Excessive skin folds
- Sedentary lifestyle
- Warm, humid climate
- Use of public pools
- Walking barefoot in public areas
- Skin trauma
- Poor nutrition
- Diabetes mellitus
- Immunocompromise
- Impaired circulation

TREATMENT

Nonpharmacologic Therapy

- Because fungi thrive in warm, moist environments, the practitioner should encourage patients to wear loose-fitting clothing and socks, preferably garments made of cotton or other fabrics that wick moisture away from the body. Avoid clothing made with synthetic fibers or wool.
- Sweaty or wet clothing should be removed as soon as possible.
- Clean the infected area daily with soap and water.
- The infected area should be dried completely prior to dressing, paying particular attention to skin folds.

Patient Encounter 3

A middle-aged man presents to the clinic complaining of painful red areas on his feet, particularly between his toes. He said this has been going on for a few weeks and he thought it might be athlete's foot so he sprayed antifungal powder inside his running shoes, rather than on his feet "since my feet are in those shoes for hours each day when I run anyway." When that did not work, the raw skin became so painful that he had to stop training for his next ultra-marathon.

What information is suggestive of tinea pedis?

What risk factors are present for tinea pedis?

What nonpharmacologic approaches can be recommended to prevent recurrence?

- To allow circulation of air, the infected area should not be bandaged.
- For foot infections, cotton socks are recommended, although these should be changed two to three times a day to reduce moisture.
- To prevent spread, towels, clothing, and footwear should not be shared with other persons.
- Wear protective footwear in public showers and pool areas.

Pharmacologic Therapy of Tinea Infections

KEY CONCEPT *Since dermatophyte hyphae seldom penetrate into the living layers of the skin, instead remaining in the stratum corneum, most infections can be treated with topical antifungals. Infections covering large areas of the body, infections involving nails or hair, chronic infections, or infections not responding to topical therapy may require systemic therapy.* Treatment is typically initiated based on symptoms, rather than on microscopic evaluation. For infections accompanied by inflammation, combination therapy with a topical steroid can be considered (Tables 83–6, 83–7, **and** 83–8).

Typically, tinea pedis requires treatment one to two times daily for 4 weeks, whereas tinea corporis and tinea cruris require topical treatment one to two times daily for 2 weeks. When applying treatment, the medication should be applied at least 1 in beyond the affected area. Treatment of infection should continue at least 1 week after resolution of symptoms. Many practitioners opt to initiate therapy with nonprescription clotrimazole, tolnaftate, miconazole, or terbinafine, reserving prescription topical agents, such as naftifine, ciclopirox, and butenafine, for second-line therapy or refractory cases and systemic therapy for refractory cases.

When recommending topical therapy, the selection of vehicle is based on the type of lesion and location of the infection. Solutions and lotions are recommended for hairy areas and oozing lesions, whereas creams and ointments should be avoided in these areas. Creams are better for moderately scaling and nonoozing lesions. For hyperkeratotic lesions, ointments can be considered. The selected formulation should be applied to the affected area after it is cleaned and dried. The medication should be rubbed into the infected area for improved penetration. Because most patients do not rub in sprays and powders, penetration of the epidermis is minimal, making them less effective than other formulations. Sprays and powders should

Table 83–6

Available Topical Antifungal Agents

Medication	Rx/OTC	Cream/Ointment	Gel	Lotion	Spray/Solution	Powder
Butenafine	OTC	X				
Ciclopirox	Rx	X		x	Lacquer and shampoo	
Clotrimazole	OTC	X		x	X	x
Econazole	Rx	x				
Efinaconazole	Rx				X	
Haloprogin	Rx	x			X	
Ketoconazole	Rx/OTC	x			Shampoo	
Miconazole	OTC	x		x	X	x
Naftifine	Rx	x	x			
Nystatin	Rx	x		x		x
Oxiconazole	Rx	x		x		
Sertaconazole	Rx	x				
Sulconazole	Rx	x				
Tavaborole	Rx				X	
Terbinafine	OTC	x	x		X	
Tolnaftate	OTC	x		x	X	

be considered as adjuvant therapy with a cream or lotion or as prophylactic therapy to prevent recurrence.[7]

Due to the severity of infection and inflammation, tinea capitis does not adequately respond to topical agents; therefore, oral agents for 6 to 8 weeks are recommended. Griseofulvin has long been considered the treatment of choice due to its ability to achieve high levels within the stratum corneum. Itraconazole has also demonstrated effectiveness. Due to its lipophilicity, itraconazole achieves high dermal concentrations that are maintained for 4 weeks after discontinuation of therapy.

Treatment of Onychomycosis

For onychomycosis, a chronic infection that rarely remits spontaneously, adequate treatment is essential to prevent spread to other sites, secondary bacterial infections, cellulitis, or gangrene. KEY CONCEPT *Due to the chronic nature and impenetrability of nails, topical agents have low efficacy rates for treating onychomycosis.* Oral agents that can penetrate the nail matrix and nail base, such as itraconazole and terbinafine, are more effective than ciclopirox lacquer, efinaconazole solution, or tavaborole solution. Itraconazole (200 mg twice daily for 1 week per month or 200 mg daily for 12 weeks) and terbinafine (250 mg daily for 12 weeks) demonstrate mycological cure rates of 71% and 77%, respectively, whereas the cure rate range from 29% to 36% for ciclopirox, approximately 55% for efinaconazole, and 35% for tavaborole.[23] For patients with liver disease or who are unable to use oral agents, ciclopirox lacquer, efinaconazole solution, and tavaborole solution remain reasonable alternatives, despite requiring 48 weeks of therapy. Due to low efficacy, griseofulvin should only be considered as second-line therapy with therapy continued for 4 months for fingernail infections or 6 months for toenail infections.

The FDA has released warnings pertaining to itraconazole and terbinafine as there is a small but real risk of developing congestive heart failure with itraconazole therapy due to its negative inotropic effects. Itraconazole should not be administered to patients with ventricular dysfunction such as congestive heart failure. The FDA also released warnings that itraconazole and terbinafine are associated with serious hepatic toxicity, including liver failure and death. Liver failure associated with these medications has occurred in patients with no preexisting living disease or serious underlying medical conditions. Treatment with itraconazole or terbinafine for prolonged periods requires laboratory monitoring of liver function tests before initiation of therapy and at monthly intervals.

Table 83–7

Dosing of Topical Agents for Tinea Infections and Onychomycosis

Agents	Topical Dosing Frequency
Butenafine	Once daily
Ciclopirox	Twice daily; at bedtime (lacquer)
Clotrimazole	Twice daily
Econazole	Once daily
Efinaconazole	Once daily (nail solution)
Haloprogin	Twice daily
Ketoconazole	Once daily
Miconazole	Twice daily
Naftifine	Once daily (cream); twice daily (gel)
Oxiconazole	Twice daily
Sertaconazole	Twice daily
Sulconazole	Twice daily
Tavaborole	Once daily (nail solution)
Terbinafine	Twice daily
Tolnaftate	Two to three times daily

Table 83–8

Dosing of Systemic Therapy for Tinea Infections

Medication	Adult Dosing	Pediatric Dosing
Fluconazole	150 mg/week	6 mg/kg/week
Griseofulvin	0.5–1 g/day	10–20 mg/kg/day
Itraconazole	200 mg twice daily	Not studied
Ketoconazole	200–400 mg/day	3.3–6.6 mg/kg/day
Terbinafine	250 mg/day	< 25 kg: 125 mg/day; 25–35 kg: 187.5 mg/day; > 35 mg: 250 mg/day

Patient Care Process for Mycotic Infections

Patient Assessment:

- Assess the patient's symptoms to determine whether self-treatment with OTC antifungal therapy is appropriate. Exclusions for self-treatment include infection of nails or hair, unsuccessful initial treatment, worsening condition, signs of secondary bacterial or systemic infection, large infected areas, or chronic medical conditions such as diabetes, immunosuppression, or impaired circulation.
- Review any available diagnostic data, including cultures and KOH preps.
- Obtain a thorough history of prescription, nonprescription, and natural drug product use. Any allergies?

Therapy Evaluation:

- If the patient has had a mycotic infection previously, determine what treatments were helpful to the patient in the past.
- Determine whether long-term prophylactic therapy is necessary to prevent recurrence.
- Determine whether the patient has prescription coverage.

Care Plan Development:

- Evaluate the patient for the potential for adverse drug reactions, drug allergies, and drug interactions.
- Educate the patient on lifestyle modifications that will prevent recurrence, including keeping the area dry, wearing shower shoes, washing clothing in hot water, using drying powders, avoiding sharing towels or clothing, and wearing loose-fitting clothing.
- Provide the patient education pertaining to mycotic infections and antifungal therapy, including causes, medication application or administration, length of therapy, how to avoid spread of infection or recurrence, and potential adverse effects.
- Discuss dietary modifications that are necessary with oral agents.
- Discuss medications that may interact with antifungal therapy, particularly with oral agents used for nail infections.
- Discuss warning signs to report such as recurrent or difficult-to-cure infections, infections with malodorous discharge or bleeding.
- Stress the importance of adherence with the antifungal regimen.

Follow-Up Evaluation:

- Follow-up if unresolved or worsens with treatment.

Cultural Awareness When Treating Mycotic Infections

Awareness of cultural beliefs related to feet and hands is essential when treating patients with fungal infections. In Arab countries, showing the bottom of the foot is a grave insult. The foot is considered the dirtiest part of the body. As such, patients from these countries may be hesitant to show their feet to the practitioner. In other countries, the open palm "high five" gesture is considered insulting. When treating patients with infections on the hand, the practitioner should refrain from making this gesture while discussing the patient's hand infection.

OUTCOME EVALUATION

For infections of the skin, patients should notice relief of symptoms, including pruritus, scales, and inflammation, within 1 to 2 weeks. Therapy should be continued at least 1 week after complete resolution of symptoms. If the condition worsens on topical therapy, the patient should be treated with oral therapy.

For onychomycosis, relief of symptoms is slow. The infected nail will need months to grow out. The practitioner should advise the patient not to become frustrated by the slow resolution. Despite the slow progress, the antifungal agent is curing the infection. The practitioner should also advise the patient that even after the infection is cured, the nail may not look "normal."

Abbreviations Introduced in This Chapter

AIDS	Acquired immunodeficiency syndrome
CDC	Centers for Disease Control and Prevention
HIV	Human immunodeficiency virus
KOH	Potassium hydroxide
OPC	Oropharyngeal candidiasis
OTC	Over the counter
PAS	Periodic acid-Schiff test
VVC	Vulvovaginal candidiasis

REFERENCES

1. Center for Disease Control and Prevention. Diseases characterized by vaginal discharge. In: Sexually transmitted diseases treatment guidelines, 2010. MMWR Recomm Rep 2010;59(RR-12):56–63.
2. Vijaya D, Dhanalakshmi A, Kulkarni. Changing trends of vulvovaginal candidiasis. J Lab Physicians 2014;6(1):28-30.
3. Kohler GA, Asseja S, Reid G. Probiotic interference of Lactobacillus rhamnosus GR-1 and Lactobacillus reuteri RC-14 with the opportunistic fungal pathogen Candida albicans. Infect Dis Ob Gyn 2012; Article ID 636474.
4. Pirotta M, Chondros, P, Grover S, et al. Effect of lactobacillus in preventing post-antibiotic vulvovaginal candidiasis: A randomized controlled trial. BMJ 2004;329:548.
5. Pfizer, Incorporated. Diflucan® package insert. New York, NY: Pfizer, Incorporated; 2014.
6. Iavazzo C, Gkegkes ID, Zarkada IM, Falagas ME. Boric acid for recurrent vulvovaginal candidiasis: The clinical evidence. J Women's Hlth 2011;20(8):1245–1255.
7. Davis JD, Harper AL. Treatment of recurrent vulvovaginal candidiasis. Am Fam Physician 2011;83(12):1482–1484.
8. British association for sexual health and HIV. National guideline on the management of vulvovaginal candidiasis. British association for sexual health and HIV [online]. [cited 2014 Aug 10]. Available from: www.bashh.org/documents/50/50.pdf
9. Pursley TJ, Blomquist IK, Abraham J, et al. Fluconazole-induced congenital anomalies in three infants. Clin Infect Dis 1996;22: 336–340.

10. World Health Organization Website. Female genital mutilation [online]. [cited 2014 Aug 10]. Available from: http://www.who.int/mediacentre/factsheets/fs241/en/
11. Braddy CM, Files JA. Female genital mutilation: Cultural awareness and clinical considerations. J Midwifery Womens Health 2007;52: 159–163.
12. Kossioni A. The prevalence of denture stomatitis and its predisposing conditions in an older Greek population. Gerodontology 2011; 28:85–90.
13. Aun MV, Ribeiro MR, Garcia CLC, Agondi RC, Kalil J, Giavina-Bianchi P. Esophageal candidiasis – an adverse effect of inhaled corticosteroids therapy. J Asthma 2009;46:399–401.
14. Kanda N, Yasuba H, Takahashi T, et al. Prevalence of esophageal candidiasis among patients treated with inhaled fluticasone propionate. Am J Gastroenterol 2003;98:2146–2148.
15. Fotos PG, Lilly JP. Clinical management of oral and perioral candidosis. Dermatol Clin 1996;14:273–280.
16. Gaitan-Cepeda LA, Sanchez-Vargas O, Castillo N. Prevalence of oral candidiasis in HIV/AIDS children in highly active antiretroviral therapy-era. A literature analysis. Int J STD AIDS 2014 Aug 25: pii 0956462414548906 [Epub ahead of print].
17. Petruzzi MNMR, Cherubini K, Salum FG, Zancanaro de Figueiredo MA. Risk factors of HIV-related oral lesions in adults. Rev Saude Publica 2013;47(1):52–59.
18. Buchacz K, Baker RK, Palella FJ, et al. AIDS-defining opportunistic illnesses in US patients, 1994-2007: A cohort study. AIDS 2010;24:1549–1559.
19. Center for Disease Control and Prevention. Revised surveillance case definition for HIV infection. MMWR 2014;63(RR-03):1–10
20. Redding SW. Dahiya MC, Kirkpatrick WM, Coco BJ, et al. Candida glabrata is an emergeing cause of oropharyngeal candidiasis in patients receiving radiation for head and neck cancer. Oral Surg Oral Med Oral Pathol Oral Radiol Endo 2004; 97:47–52.
21. Pappas PG, Kauffman CA, Andes D, Benjamin DK, Calandra TF, et al. Clinical practice guidelines for the management of candidiasis: 2009 update by the Infectious Diseases Society of America. Clin Infect Dis 2009;48:503–535.
22. Kemna ME, Elewski BE. A U.S. epidemiologic survey of superficial fungal diseases. J Am Acad Dermatol 1996;35:539–542.
23. Del Rosso JQ. The role of topical antifungal therapy for onychomycosis and the emergency of new agents. J Clin Aesthetic Derm 2014;7(7):10–18.

84 Invasive Fungal Infections

Russell E. Lewis and P. David Rogers

LEARNING OBJECTIVES

Upon completion of the chapter, the reader will be able to:

1. Differentiate epidemiologic differences and host risk factors for acquisition of primary and opportunistic invasive fungal pathogens.
2. Recommend appropriate empiric or targeted antifungal therapy for the treatment of invasive fungal infections.
3. Describe the components of a monitoring plan to assess effectiveness and adverse effects of pharmacotherapy for invasive fungal infections.
4. Evaluate the role of antifungal prophylaxis in the prevention of opportunistic fungal pathogens.

INTRODUCTION

Invasive fungal infection or invasive mycoses are general terms for diseases caused by invasion of living tissue by fungi. In contrast to superficial mycoses (see Chapter 83), invasive fungal infections are much less common, but are of greater medical concern because of their disproportionately higher severity and mortality. Approximately 1.5 million people die each year from the 10 most common invasive fungal infections, which is higher than World Health Organization mortality estimates for tuberculosis (1.4 million) or malaria (1.2 million).[1] However, these numbers probably underestimate the actual mortality burden of invasive fungal disease considering that the four most common infections (cryptococcosis, invasive candidiasis, invasive aspergillosis, and *Pneumocystis jiroveci* pneumonia) are often underdiagnosed and not reportable diseases to public health agencies (Table 84–1).

Invasive fungal infections are broadly categorized as either primary or opportunistic mycoses. Primary invasive fungal infections develop following exposure to fungal spores or conidia in the soil that, when disturbed, can become aerosolized and inhaled leading to infection, even in an immunocompetent patient exposed to a sufficient inoculum. Because these fungi are in specific soil types in select geographic areas, they are also referred to as endemic fungi. In the United States, three Genera (*Histoplasma capsulatum, Blastomyces dermatitidis*, and *Coccidioides immitis/Coccidioides posadasii*) account for most of these infections (see Table 84–1).

In contrast, opportunistic fungal infections are most frequently encountered in setting of compromised host immune defenses, and are caused by a wider spectrum of less virulent fungal species that rarely cause infection in healthy patients (see Table 84–1). Hence, the spectrum, severity, and outcome of opportunistic fungal infections are strongly influenced by the degree, type, and severity of host immunosuppression. As a general rule, opportunistic fungal infections are difficult to diagnose, but often fatal if not diagnosed early and treated aggressively.

Occasionally, opportunistic fungal pathogens may be associated with outbreaks of invasive disease in otherwise nonimmunocompromised patients, especially if they are inadvertently inoculated into patients from contaminated drug solutions or medical devices. For example, in 2012 an outbreak of fungal meningitis and articular infections (n=751 cases) in 20 states was eventually traced by the Centers for Disease Control and state health departments to contaminated preservative-free methylprednisolone solution used for epidural and articular injections in patients with chronic back or joint pain. The dematiaceous mold eventually linked to the fungal meningitis cases, *Exserohilum rostratum*, had rarely been described as a human pathogen prior to the outbreak.[2]

EPIDEMIOLOGY AND ETIOLOGY

Endemic mycoses are capable of infecting otherwise healthy individuals. In immunocompromised patients, endemic fungal infections present with a more fulminant course (in the case of primary infections, or reactivate to cause life-threatening infection). Because initial symptoms of an endemic fungal infection are nonspecific and produce symptoms indistinguishable from other slowly progressing infections (eg, tuberculosis), a careful patient history concerning travel and activities that may have resulted in exposure to endemic fungi is essential for early diagnosis.

Two of the most common endemic fungal infections (histoplasmosis and North American blastomycosis) are found in overlapping regions in the eastern and central river basins of the United States (Figure 84–1).[3,4] *H. capsulatum* var. *capsulatum*, the causative fungus of histoplasmosis, grows heavily in soil contaminated with bird or bat excreta, which serve to enhance sporulation of the fungus. Infections have been associated with activities that disturb soil contaminated with this excreta, including cave exploration (spelunking), working in or demolishing chicken coops or older buildings, or cleaning working in

Table 84–1

Invasive Mycoses

Primary (Endemic) Invasive Fungi
Histoplasma capsulatum[a]
Coccidioides immitis/Coccidioides posadasii[a]
Blastomyces dermatitidis[a]
Opportunistic Invasive Fungi
Yeast
Candida species (*C. albicans, C. glabrata, C. parapsilosis, C. tropicalis, C. krusei,* and others)[a]
Cryptococcus neoformans[a]
Trichosporon spp. and others
Mold
Hyalohyphomycoses (nondematiaceous)
Aspergillus fumigatus, Aspergillus terreus, Aspergillus flavus, and other species[a]
Fusarium solani and *Fusarium oxysporum*
Mucorales (formally *zygomycosis*) (*Mucor, Absidia, Rhizopus, Cunninghamella,* and *Rhizomucor*)
Penicillium species
Phaeohyphomycoses (dematiaceous)
Pseudallescheria boydii (*Scedosporium* spp.)
Bipolaris
Alternaria
Exserohilum rostratum
Other
Pneumocystis jiroveci (formerly *P. carinii*)[a]

[a]Most common.

campsites in heavily wooded areas. For blastomycosis, decaying organic matter, warm humid conditions, and proximity to water or frequent rainfall support growth of this fungus. Outbreaks of blastomycosis have been most frequently associated with occupational or recreational activities around the major waterways such as the Great Lakes region, where soil concentrations of *B. dermatitidis* are elevated.[4]

Coccidioidomycosis differs from histoplasmosis and blastomycosis, as the fungus is associated with arid to semiarid climates, hot summers, low altitude, alkaline soil, and sparse flora. Hence the fungus is found in the southwestern regions of the United States stretching from western Texas to southern California (see Figure 84–1).[5] Epidemics of coccidioidomycosis have been reported in California following dust storms and earthquakes, including cycles of intense drought and rain, which favor the growth of the fungus and enhance dispersion of its specialized spore forms, called arthroconidia.

PATHOPHYSIOLOGY

Endemic fungi share several key biologic and ecologic characteristics that contribute to their pathogenicity in humans. All endemic fungi exhibit temperature-dependent dimorphism, meaning they can propagate as either yeast (single cells that reproduce by budding into daughter cells) or molds (multicellular filamentous fungi that reproduce through production of conidia or spores). At environmental temperatures (25–30°C [77–86°F]), *H. capsulatum*, *B. dermatitidis*, and *C. immitis* grow in the mold form, producing 2- to 10-μm round- to oval-shaped (*Histoplasma* and *Blastomyces*) or barrel-shaped conidia (*Coccidioides*) that are dispersed throughout the environment and in air currents. At physiologic temperatures, the conidia germinate into yeast (*Histoplasma* and *Blastomyces*) or in specialized cell forms called spherules (*Coccidioides*) that are resistant to killing by alveolar macrophages and neutrophils in the host lung.

Control of infection by the host requires the development of antigen-specific T-lymphocyte response that enhances macrophage fungicidal activity and formation of a granuloma to contain the

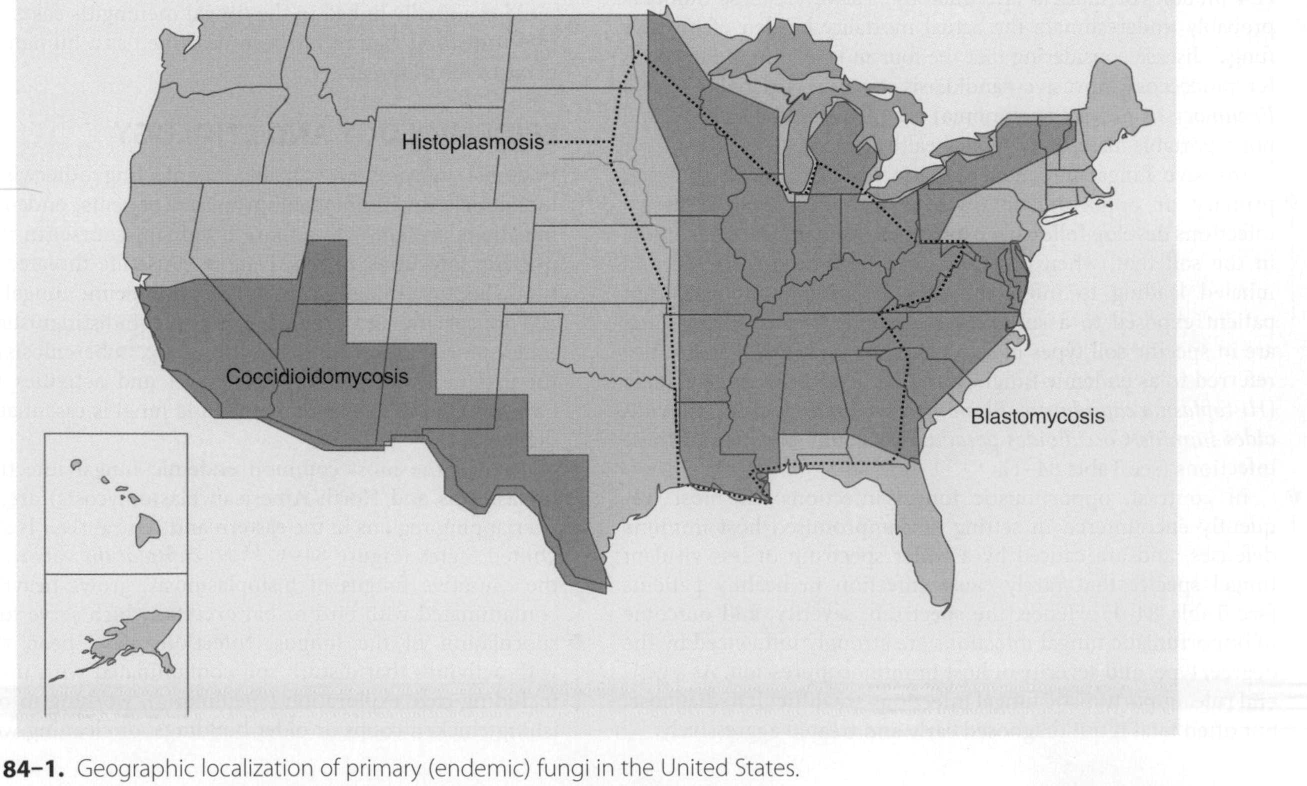

FIGURE 84–1. Geographic localization of primary (endemic) fungi in the United States.

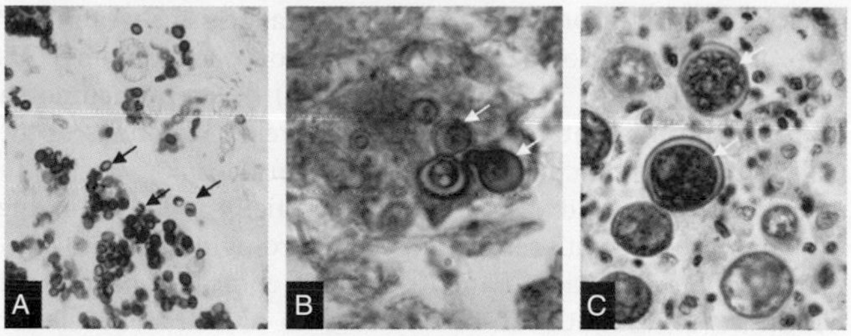

FIGURE 84–2. Histopathology of endemic mycoses in tissue. (A) Histoplasmosis (yeast). (B) Blastomycoses (broad-based budding yeast). (C) Coccidioidomycoses (spherules with endospores).

fungus.[6] Not surprisingly, patients with T-cell–mediated immune deficiency (eg, AIDS patients and transplant recipients) or suppressed cellular immunity due to drug therapy (eg, chemotherapy, high-dose corticosteroids, or tumor necrosis-α blockers such as infliximab) are especially prone to severe reactivation of fungal disease.

The most common route of infection for endemic fungi is the respiratory tract, where conidia aerosolized from contaminated soil are inhaled into the lung. Once in the lung, conidia are phagocytosed but not destroyed by macrophages and neutrophils in the alveoli and bronchioles. Within 2 to 3 days, conidia germinate into facultative yeast resistant to phagocytosis and killing by macrophages and neutrophils (**Figure 84–2A and B**). For *C. immitis*, germination of the arthroconidia results in the formation of a sac-like structure called a spherule filled with endospores (**Figure 84–2C**). Spherules then rupture to release large numbers of endospores, which are the propagating form of the infection. Control of infection in the lungs is typically accomplished through formation of granulomas that contain the infection. However, in patients exposed to an overwhelming inoculum, or lower inocula in the setting of suppressed T-cell–mediated immunity, dissemination outside the lung to the skin and oral mucosa, adrenal glands, bone, spleen, thyroid, GI tract, heart, and central nervous system (CNS) is possible and uniformly fatal if left untreated.

CLINICAL PRESENTATION AND DIAGNOSIS

Histoplasmosis and coccidioidomycosis are frequently asymptomatic infections in immunocompetent patients or present as a self-limiting, influenza-like or mild lower-respiratory tract illness 1 to 3 weeks after inhalation of conidia. The clinical presentation of blastomycosis can range from asymptomatic infection, to acute or chronic pneumonia that develops 30 to 40 days after exposure, to full-blown disseminated disease.

More severe endemic fungal disease presents as persistent pneumonia despite antibiotic therapy that is accompanied by fever, chills, cough, arthralgia, night sweats, and weight loss that may be indistinguishable from other chronic infections such as pulmonary tuberculosis. KEY CONCEPT *The diagnosis of endemic fungal infection is often prompted by a patient history of prolonged infectious symptoms, travel or residence in an endemic area, and/or participation in activities that result in exposures to soil contaminated by endemic fungi.*

Radiographs

- Chest radiographs often reveal either diffuse or nodular infiltrates in the lung, accompanied by enlargement of the hilar and/or mediastinal lymph nodes.
- Fulminant pneumonia may be seen with high inoculum exposures, resulting in diffuse lung infiltrates that precede to acute respiratory distress syndrome (ARDS) and respiratory failure.

Signs and Symptoms

- Rheumatologic symptoms such as severe arthritis, pericarditis, and erythema nodosum may be seen in 10% to 30% of patients with endemic fungi.[3–5]
- Dissemination outside the lung is common in patients with suppressed cellular immunity and frequently produces signs of progressing infection.
- Ulcerative oral and cutaneous lesions may also arise with any endemic fungal infections.
- Verrucose (wart-like) skin lesions on sun-exposed areas on the face are particularly suggestive of progressing blastomycosis and are frequently mistaken for cutaneous malignancy.[4]
- Dissemination of the fungi to bone marrow may result in anemia or thrombocytopenia.
- Hepatomegaly, splenomegaly, and adrenal insufficiency can also occur with dissemination of the endemic fungi to these internal organs.
- Seizures, meningeal signs, and hydrocephalus are common findings with dissemination of the infection to the CNS and portend an especially poor prognosis in the setting of disseminated coccidioidomycosis.

Definitive diagnosis of an endemic fungal infection requires growth of the fungus from body fluids or tissue, or evidence of cellular or tissue invasion in clinical samples by histopathology. However, cultures may only be positive in the setting of high inoculum exposures, pneumonia, or disseminated disease.[7] Serologic testing is helpful in the diagnosis and management of patients with histoplasmosis or coccidioidomycosis, but lacks specificity for diagnosis of *B. dermatitidis*.[4] In general, a fourfold rise in antibody or complement fixation titers of *Histoplasma* or *Coccidioides* or any titer greater than 1:16 suggests active infection. However, many clinicians still consider titers as low as 1:8 as evidence of active disease because undetectable titers may

Patient Encounter 1, Part 1: Endemic Fungal Infection

A 54-year-old African American woman from Phoenix Arizona with a history of steroid-refractory Crohn disease presents with a 3-week history of cough, fever, night sweats, and 7-kg weight loss. Approximately 6 weeks before this presentation, she was treated with infliximab and a 7-day course of amoxicillin-clavulanate. The patient complains of fatigue but is afebrile (37°C), with a normal resting respiratory rate. Laboratory studies revealed anemia (hemoglobin less than 8.7 g/dL [87 g/L or 5.40 mmol/L]). A chest x-ray taken 1-week ago is reported as normal.

What information is suggestive that this patient may have an endemic fungal infection?

What is the most likely endemic fungal pathogen based on this patient's area of residence?

be present in one-third of all active infections.[5] Enzyme-linked immunosorbent assays (ELISAs) have been developed for direct detection of *Histoplasma* antigens in serum and urine. Serial antigen testing can also provide a means for assessing response of histoplasmosis to antifungal therapy and detection of relapsing disease.[3]

TREATMENT

KEY CONCEPT *The approach to antifungal therapy in patients with endemic fungal infections is determined by the severity of clinical presentation, the patient's underlying immunosuppression, and potential toxicities and drug interactions associated with antifungal treatment.* Immunocompetent patients with mild disease following exposure to *H. capsulatum* or *C. immitis* often experience a benign course of infection that does not require antifungal therapy. Persons of Filipino or African descent have a higher risk for dissemination with *C. immitis*, and this may also be taken into consideration for more aggressive treatment.[5] Approximately 9% of patients exposed to coccidioidomycosis (defined by positive IgM or IgG serology) develop pneumonia requiring hospitalization, and 1% may develop infections of the CNS, which are difficult to treat if not incurable.[5]

Patients with mild disease may be initially followed in the outpatient setting with serial antigen or serologic studies to confirm resolving infection. Patients without clinical improvement within the first month can be treated with oral itraconazole for 6 to 12 weeks (Table 84–2).[3,5] Broader-spectrum triazoles such as voriconazole and posaconazole, and in the future possibly isavuconazole, appear to have clinically-useful activity against endemic fungi; but have limited data to recommend their routine first-line use. Fluconazole (400–800 mg/day) is somewhat less effective than itraconazole (higher relapse rates), but has fewer GI adverse effects and drug interactions versus itraconazole. Echinocandins and flucytosine are not clinically useful agents for the treatment of endemic mycoses.

Table 84–2

Common Treatment Regimens for Endemic Fungal Infections

Mycosis	Recommended Treatment Regimens	Comments
Histoplasmosis		
Mild to moderate	Observation or itraconazole 200 mg three times daily for 3 days, then two times daily for 6–12 weeks.	Fluconazole has a higher rate of relapse than itraconazole but is better tolerated by many patients than itraconazole. Echinocandins are not clinically effective against endemic mycoses. Lipid formulations better tolerated than conventional formulations, especially for CNS disease.
	Fluconazole 12 mg/kg/day PO for 6–12 weeks adjusted for renal function.[a]	Patients initially treated with amphotericin B–based regimens are transitioned to itraconazole or fluconazole once they are clinically stable. Corticosteroid therapy should be considered in hypoxic patients with acute pulmonary infection. Itraconazole is less effective for CNS infections.
Severe including CNS disease or immunocompromised host	Amphotericin B 0.7 mg/kg/day IV or liposomal. Amphotericin B 3–5 mg/kg/day for 12 weeks or until clinically stable.	
Blastomycosis		
Mild to moderate	Itraconazole 200 mg three times daily for 3 days, then two times daily for 6–12 months.	Relapses are common in immunocompromised host.
Severe including CNS disease or immunocompromised host	Amphotericin B 0.7 mg/kg/day IV until patient is clinically stable, then Itraconazole (non-CNS) or fluconazole 12 mg/kg/day orally adjusted for renal function.[a]	
Coccidioidomycosis		
Mild to moderate	Observation or itraconazole 200 mg three times daily for 3 days, then two times daily for 3–6 months. OR Fluconazole 6–12 mg/kg/day PO daily adjusted for renal function[a] for 3–6 months.	Itraconazole demonstrated trend toward superiority over fluconazole in a randomized controlled trial for progressive, nonmeningeal coccidioidomycosis; however, fluconazole is better tolerated than itraconazole.
Diffuse pneumonia or disseminated infection	Amphotericin B 1–1.5 mg/kg/day with dose and frequency decreased as improvement occurs. Patient then transitioned to triazole therapy. OR Lipid Amphotericin B formulations 3–5 mg/kg/day. Patient then transitioned to triazole therapy.	Fluconazole 800–1000 mg/day adjusted for renal function[a] is often recommended after initial AMB therapy for meningitis.

CNS, central nervous system; IV, intravenous; PO, oral.

[a]CrCl more than 50–90 mL/min (0.83–1.50 mL/s), 100% of dose; CrCl 10–50 mL/min (0.17–0.83 mL/s), 50% of dose; CrCl less than 10 mL/min (0.17 mL/s) 50%.

Patients with progressive symptoms for longer than 2 weeks, greater than 10% weight loss, extensive pneumonia, or serologic titers greater than 1:8 of histoplasmosis or coccidioidomycosis are candidates for immediate antifungal therapy. Any patient with underlying immunosuppression should also receive immediate antifungal therapy. The following signs and symptoms are considered to be indicators of severe disease that require hospitalization and initial treatment with systemic amphotericin B (see Table 84–2).[3–5]

- Hypoxia indicated by a partial pressure of oxygen less than 80 mm Hg (10.6 kPa)
- Hypotension (systolic blood pressure less than 90 mm Hg)
- Impaired mental status
- Anemia (hemoglobin less than 10 g/dL [100 g/L or 6.2 mmol/L])
- Leukopenia (less than $1 \times 10^3/mm^3$ [$1 \times 10^9/L$])
- Elevated hepatic transaminases (greater than five times upper limit of normal) or bilirubin (greater than 2.5 times upper limit of normal)
- Coagulopathy
- Evidence of dissemination, including cutaneous manifestations
- Meningitis

All patients with blastomycosis require antifungal treatment, even though patients with mild disease can be managed as outpatients with oral itraconazole.[4] Patients with evidence of severe pulmonary disease or dissemination require initial treatment in the hospital with amphotericin B–based regimens until they are clinically stable, whereupon they can complete a 6- to 12-month treatment course as outpatients with oral triazoles.[4] Methylprednisolone (0.5–1 mg/kg daily IV) may be administered during the first 1 to 2 weeks of antifungal therapy if the patient develops respiratory complications, including hypoxemia or significant respiratory distress.

OUTCOME EVALUATION

Response to antifungal therapy may be slow in patients with a prolonged history of infection or severe manifestations. However, gradual improvements in symptoms and reduction in fever are indicators of response to treatment. For histoplasmosis and coccidioidomycosis, decreasing antigen titers or serology are indicative of response to antifungal therapy.[3,5]

Antifungals used for the treatment of endemic mycoses can be associated with clinically significant drug interactions and toxicities, especially with the prolonged treatment courses that are often required for endemic mycoses. Itraconazole is available as a capsule formulation and as a cyclodextrin-solubilized solution. The liquid formulation of itraconazole has several advantages over the capsule: It has a better oral bioavailability and does not require the low gastric pH that is required for dissolution and absorption of the capsule. However, the oral solution is somewhat dilute, has an unpalatable aftertaste (an issue when taking months of therapy), and has a much higher rate of GI intolerance. Therefore, the capsule formulation is often preferred provided patients are not on acid-suppression therapy (ie, proton pump inhibitors, histamine antagonists, or antacids).

Posaconazole is formulated as a micronized suspension that is best absorbed when taken with high-fat meals and when taken in divided doses up to 800 mg/day. A delayed-release tablet formulation with improved bioavailability and fewer gastric pH-associated drug interactions has been introduced, and is probably the preferred oral treatment formulation in most patients unless the patient cannot swallow the tablet.[8] Absorption of voriconazole is not affected by gastric pH, but is generally administered 1 hour prior to or 2 hours after eating.

Drug interactions are an important concern in patients taking long-term triazole therapy. Itraconazole and voriconazole are substrates of the cytochrome P450 (CYP) 3A4 enzyme.[9] Coadministration of itraconazole, voriconazole, and to lesser extent fluconazole and posaconazole, with inducers of this CYP 3A4 (eg, rifampin, phenytoin, and phenobarbital) increases drug clearance resulting in ineffective plasma and tissue concentrations of the drug.[9] In general, coadministration of the broader spectrum triazoles (itraconazole, voriconazole, posaconazole) with these inducers must be avoided. Itraconazole, voriconazole, and posaconazole are also potent inhibitors of CYP 3A4, which predisposes these agents to a large number (estimated greater than 2000) of clinically significant pharmacokinetic drug–drug interactions.[9]

Posaconazole is also a substrate and inhibitor of P-glycoprotein, although the impact of this pathway on drug absorption or distribution into some anatomically protected sites such as the CNS is unknown.[10] Consequently, all patients should have their medication profile carefully reviewed prior to initiating and stopping triazole antifungals, preferably with the aid of a computerized drug-interactions database. Even in the absence of drug interactions, serum drug levels of the broader spectrum triazoles (itraconazole, voriconazole, posaconazole) are often unpredictable.[11] Serum drug concentration monitoring has been recommended in patients receiving triazole antifungals for documented infections, or when inadequate serum concentrations are suspected because of altered absorption, drug interactions. Suspected toxicities, especially CNS toxicity during voriconazole therapy, may also be indicative of excessive drug levels that can be detected by therapeutic drug monitoring (Table 84–3).

All azole antifungals carry the potential for rash, photosensitivity, and hepatotoxicity. In general, hepatotoxicity is mild and reversible, presenting as asymptomatic increases in liver transaminases, and less frequently increases in total bilirubin. Fulminant hepatic failure is less common and typically mediated by immunologic mechanisms. Therefore, serial monitoring of liver function is recommended in all patients receiving triazole antifungals. Long-term therapy with itraconazole has also been associated with reversible adrenal suppression and cardiomyopathy due to negative inotropic effects of the drug. Long-term therapy with voriconazole can be associated with severe phototoxic reactions and cutaneous erythema in sun-exposed skin, which may not be preventable with sunscreen alone. These reactions have been linked to development of squamous cell carcinoma or melanoma.[12] Patients should be instructed to avoid sun exposure while on voriconazole therapy and have frequent

Patient Encounter 1, Part 2: Endemic Fungal Infection

Patient management

The patient's serum titer for coccidiodiodomycosis returns as greater than 1:8. Based on the information presented, select an appropriate treatment plan for the patient's infection.

Should the patient receive antifungal therapy at this time? What factors need to be considered?

Table 84–3

Recommendations for Antifungal Therapeutic Drug Monitoring

Drug	Indication for Monitoring	Time of First Measurement	Target Conc. for Efficacy (mcg/mL or mg/L)	Target Conc. for Safety (mcg/mL or mg/L)
Flucytosine	Routine during first week of therapy, renal insufficiency, or poor clinical response	3–5 days	Peak > 20 (155 μmol/L)	Peak < 50 (387 μmol/L) to reduce risk of marrow toxicity
Itraconazole	Routine during first week of therapy, GI dysfunction, suspected drug interactions	4–7 days	Prophylaxis > 0.5 (0.7 μmol/L); therapy trough > 1–2 (1.4–2.8 μmol/L)	Some evidence to suggest trough greater than 4 (5.7 μmol/L) increased cardiac toxicity
Voriconazole	Lacking response, GI dysfunction, suspected drug interactions, pediatrics,[a] IV to oral switch, unexplained neurological changes	4–7 days	Prophylaxis trough > 0.5 (1.4 μmol/L); therapy trough 1–2 (2.9–5.7 μmol/L)	Trough < 6 (17.2 μmol/L) to reduce risk of CNS toxicities
Posaconazole	Lacking response, GI dysfunction, potent acid suppression therapy (ie, proton pump inhibitor) therapy, suspected drug interactions	4–7 days	Prophylaxis trough greater than 0.5 (0.7 μmol/L); therapy trough 0.5–1.5 (0.7–2.1 μmol/L)	Not established Delayed-release tablet formulation preferred for most patients because fewer pH drug interactions and improved bioavailibility

[a]Pediatric patients display accelerated linear clearance of voriconazole. Therefore, higher daily voriconazole dosing (7 mg/kg every 12 hours) without a loading dose are recommended to achieve similar exposures to adults. Some children may require doses as high as 12 mg/kg every 12 hours to achieve similar serum drug exposures to adults. Therefore, therapeutic drug monitoring is recommended.

skin examinations by a dermatologist. Long-term voriconazole therapy may also predispose patients to periostitis (fluoride toxicity) that presents with nonspecific joint, shoulder and limb pain that can be diagnosed radiographically and with serum fluoride levels.[13] Alopecia, chapped lips and brittle nails, and cognitive difficulties have also been reported with longer-term voriconazole therapy, especially at higher doses.[14] Peripheral neuropathy may develop in 3% to 17% of patients on long-term triazole therapy, and is most frequently reported with itraconazole and voriconazole.[15]

Amphotericin B remains the mainstay of treatment of patients with severe endemic fungal infections. The conventional deoxycholate formulation of the drug can be associated with substantial infusion-related adverse effects (eg, chills, fever, nausea, rigors, and in rare cases hypotension, flushing, respiratory difficulty, and arrhythmias). As-needed premedication with low doses of hydrocortisone, acetaminophen, nonsteroidal anti-inflammatory agents, and meperidine are used to reduce acute infusion-related reactions. Venous irritation associated with the drug can also lead to thrombophlebitis; hence, central venous catheters are the preferred route of administration in patients receiving more than a week of therapy.

The most severe adverse effect associated with amphotericin B therapy is nephrotoxicity, which occurs through the renal vascular effects of the drug (constriction of the afferent arterioles in the kidney tubule) and direct toxicity to the kidney tubular membrane.[11] Generally, nephrotoxicity with amphotericin B is reversible provided the drug is stopped. However, treatment interruptions can be problematic in patients with severe infections. Precipitous decreases in glomerular filtration may occur in patients with marked dehydration or during aggressive diuresis. Infusion of normal saline before and after amphotericin B, a practice known as "sodium loading," can blunt precipitous decreases in renal perfusion pressure and slow the rate of decline in the glomerular filtration rate but may not be tolerated in patients with poor cardiac function. Administration of amphotericin B by continuous infusion reduces the nephrotoxicity of the drug but is generally not advocated because of unproven efficacy. Toxicity can be delayed by avoiding the use of other drugs with known tubular toxicity such as aminoglycosides, cyclosporine, cisplatin, or foscarnet. Generally, tubular toxicity manifests in patients with severe wasting of potassium and magnesium in the urine. Therefore, patient electrolytes must be carefully monitored and potassium and magnesium supplementation is always necessary. Hypokalemia and hypomagnesaemia frequently precede decreases in glomerular filtration (increased serum creatinine), especially in patients who are adequately hydrated.[16] Continued tubular damage eventually results in decreases in renal blood flow and glomerular filtration through tubuloglomerular feedback mechanisms that further constrict the afferent arteriole.

During the 1990s, amphotericin B was reformulated into three different lipid-based formulations (Abelcet, AmBisome, and Amphotec) that have reduced rates of nephrotoxicity compared with the conventional deoxycholate formulation (Fungizone). Two of the formulations (Abelcet and AmBisome) have lower rates of infusion-related reactions. Although these lipid formulations are generally considered to be as effective as conventional amphotericin B deoxycholate, they are not dosed equivalently to the standard formulation (see Table 84–2).

PROPHYLAXIS

Primary prophylaxis, before development of infection, is generally not recommended for endemic fungi, but may be considered in specific situations, including the following:

1. Patients with HIV infection with $CD4^+$ cell counts less than 150 cells/mm³ (150×10^6/L) (histoplasmosis) or less than 250 cells/mm³ (250×10^6/L)(coccidioidomycosis) living in regions with high endemic case rates (more than 10 cases per 100 patient-years), or in any patient with positive IgM or IgG antibodies. The recommended regimen is itraconazole 200 mg daily.

2. Secondary prophylaxis or suppressive therapy with itraconazole 200 mg daily is recommended to prevent recurrence of blastomycosis in immunosuppressed patients if immunosuppression cannot be reversed.[4]
3. In patients with prior CNS disease, fluconazole or voriconazole are preferred over itraconazole and posaconazole due to the lower penetration of itraconazole and posaconazole into the CNS.[5]

OPPORTUNISTIC MYCOSES

KEY CONCEPT *Commensal or environmental fungi that are typically harmless can become invasive mycoses when the host immune defenses are impaired. Host immune suppression and risk for opportunistic mycoses can be broadly classified into three categories:*

1. *Quantitative or qualitative deficits in neutrophil function*
2. *Deficits in cell-mediated immunity*
3. *Disruption of the integument and/or microbiologic barriers*

Quantitative defects in neutrophils (neutropenia) resulting from neoplastic diseases, cytotoxic chemotherapy, marrow transplantation, or bone marrow aplasia are among the most common risk factors for opportunistic mycoses. Qualitative defects may be seen in certain disease states (eg, advanced diabetes mellitus and chronic granulomatous disease) or with high-dose corticosteroid therapy. Deficits in T-cell–mediated immunity associated with HIV infection, high-dose corticosteroid therapy, calcineurin inhibitors or other immunosuppressive drugs, chemotherapy, transplantation, bone marrow failure, and other immunodeficiencies have become increasingly prevalent with the prolonged survival of transplant patients or other chronically-immunosuppressed populations.

Immune deficits arising from disruption of the integument or GI/genitourinary barriers can also predispose patients to fungal infections. The most common types of barrier disruptions include surgery or infections/perforation of the abdominal viscus, use of central venous and urinary catheters, parenteral nutrition, and mucositis associated with cytotoxic chemotherapy and antibiotic therapy. Broad-spectrum antibacterial therapy disrupts the protective microbiologic flora of the gut, which allows overgrowth of *Candida* species that can translocate to the bloodstream and invade internal organs..

All of the opportunistic mycoses are difficult to diagnose and often must be treated empirically before diagnosis is proven. Deciding when to initiate antifungal therapy and what opportunistic pathogens to cover is a decision governed largely by the *cumulative* immune deficits of the host, local epidemiology and experience, or clinical or diagnostic clues suggestive of incipient infection.

INVASIVE CANDIDIASIS

EPIDEMIOLOGY AND ETIOLOGY

Candida species are the most common opportunistic fungal pathogens encountered in hospitals, ranking as the third to fourth most common cause of nosocomial bloodstream infections in the United States.[17] The incidence of nosocomial candidiasis has increased steadily since the early 1980s, with the widespread use of central venous catheters, broad-spectrum antimicrobials, and other advancements in the supportive care of critically ill patients. In the 1980s, *C. albicans* accounted for more than 80% of all bloodstream yeast isolates cultured from patients. By the late 2000s, this relative frequency of *C. albicans* had decreased to less 50% in national surveys of bloodstream infections with increasing proportion of infections caused by non-*albicans* species.[17,18] Because of the inherent resistance (eg, *C. krusei*) or diminished susceptibility (eg, *C. glabrata*) of many the non-*albicans* species, the introduction of fluconazole in the early 1990s is often cited as the key element driving the shift in the microbiology of invasive candidiasis. Nevertheless, other factors, including central venous catheters, higher intensity of cytotoxic/mucotoxic chemotherapy, and broad-spectrum antibiotic therapy have also contributed to this trend. KEY CONCEPT *Familiarity with the local epidemiology and frequency of non-albicans Candida species in the institution or intensive care unit (ICU) is essential before selecting empiric antifungal therapy for invasive candidiasis, as fluconazole is not recommended for the treatment of C. glabrata and C. krusei infections, and echinocandin-resistance among* C. glabrata *is increasing in some centers.*

CLINICAL PRESENTATION AND DIAGNOSIS

Invasive candidiasis encompasses several infectious syndromes broadly categorized as candidemia or deep-seated infections (infections of tissue sites beneath mucosal surfaces).[19] Approximately one-third of all patients with invasive candidiasis fall within three groups at the time of diagnosis: (1) patients with uncomplicated candidemia in the absence of deep-seated candidiasis; most frequently arising from an infected catheter; (2) candidemia associated with deep-seated candidiasis, most frequently arising from the gastrointestinal tract or secondary seeding from a separate infection site; and (3) deep-seated candidiasis without candidemia.[20]

Focal deep-seated invasive candidiasis can involve virtually any organ, even following apparently uncomplicated catheter-related bloodstream infections. The most common sites of infection are the kidney, eye, and bone. *Candida* in the urine can be an indication of renal candidiasis or an obstructing fungus ball; however, it must be distinguished from more benign colonization of the urinary tract, especially in patients with chronic indwelling urinary catheters.[21] Similarly, *Candida* species isolated for respiratory samples (sputum, bronchoalveolar lavage) are indicative of colonization, and almost never reflect true pneumonia, which is an uncommon clinical entity. All patients with candidemia should undergo an eye examination to rule out *Candida* endophthalmitis, which can be sight threatening if not recognized early and may require direct installation of antifungal therapy for adequate treatment.[21]

Invasive candidiasis is most frequently diagnosed by blood culture, which probably identifies the majority of patients with candidemia alone, fewer patients with mixed of deep-seated disease and intermittent candidemia, and virtually no patients who have infection limited to deep tissues at the time of culture.[20] As a result, half of all episodes of invasive candidiasis are not detected by blood cultures alone. Therefore, a negative blood culture cannot rule out the possibility of invasive candidiasis, especially in patients with multiple underlying risk factors for the infection. The development of new diagnostic tools that do not exclusively rely on microbiological isolation of *Candida* has become a major research focus for improving diagnosis of the infection, especially deep-seated disease.[20]

Novel serodiagnostic tests have been developed for the detection *Candida* cell wall antigens, or nucleic acids of *Candida* species, in the hope of improving the detection of invasive disease missed by blood cultures. Currently, the most frequently used test is the Fungitell (1→3)-β-D-glucan test, Associates of Cape Cod Inc.). False-positive results may occur, however, in patients with gram-negative bacteremia, certain gauze dressing or dialysis membranes, or patients heavily colonized with *Candida* species.

Laboratory identification of *Candida* in clinical samples must be performed to the species level whenever possible, as *Candida* species differ considerably in their susceptibility to antifungal agents.[21] Rapid discrimination of *C. albicans* from common non-albicans *Candida* species can be accomplished by the germ-tube test, which presumptively identifies *C. albicans* by the early formation (less than 4 hours) of a hyphae-like structure when the yeast is incubated in serum at 37°C (98.6°F). Definitive species identification, however, may require an additional 48 to 72 hours after the organism is isolated on agar, but can be accelerated with fluorescent in situ hybridization (FISH) of *Candida* species-specific DNA sequences. Matrix-assisted laser desorption/ionization time of flight (MALDI-TOF) and magnetic-resonance based technologies have shown some promise in the early identification of *Candida* species in whole blood specimens in as little as 3 hours, which could shorten the time to earlier diagnosis.

C. albicans remains the most common cause of invasive candidiasis and is the most virulent of *Candida* species, but is the most susceptible to commonly used antifungals including fluconazole.[17,21]Like *C. albicans*, *C. tropicalis* is a relatively virulent species associated with the highest mortality rates,[17,22] but has similar susceptibility profiles as *C. albicans*. *C. parapsilosis* is a less virulent species seen frequently in neonates and in adults with central venous catheters. However, many *C. parapsilosis* isolates form thick biofilms on prosthetic materials and catheters that make the organism difficult to eradicate.[17] *C. parapsilosis* is generally susceptible to most antifungals, including fluconazole, although mean inhibitory concentrations (MICs) for echinocandins are higher than for other *Candida* species. *C. krusei* is considered to be uniformly resistant to fluconazole, although most isolates retain susceptibility to voriconazole and posaconazole.

Patient Encounter 2, Part 1: Invasive Candidiasis

A 44-year-old man recovering in the surgical ICU following a ruptured appendix and diffuse peritonitis develops fever while receiving broad-spectrum antibacterial therapy (meropenem 1 g every 8 hours and linezolid 600 mg every 12 hours). The patient has a central venous catheter and a Foley catheter. Blood cultures are negative at the time, but the patient has yeast growing in the sputum and urine. A serum (1→3)-β-D-glucan test is positive at 80 pg/mL (80 ng/L). Laboratory studies reveal a white blood cell count of 11,500 cells/mm^3 (11.5 × 10^9/L).

What are this patient's risk factors for developing an invasive fungal infection?

What evidence suggests this patient has an invasive fungal infection despite negative blood cultures?

If antifungal therapy is empirically started in this patient, what information should be considered?

C. glabrata has become a common cause of breakthrough infection on fluconazole prophylaxis, and increasingly during treatment with echinocandins. Although *C. glabrata* is generally less virulent than other *C. albicans*, infections with this organism are typically seen in older patients with poor performance status, and therefore mortality remains high. The marginal susceptibility of *C. glabrata* to fluconazole and increasing echinocandin resistance fueled a growing clinical need for susceptibility testing of this species, as some isolates may demonstrate resistance to multiple antifungal classes.[23,24] Generally, fluconazole-resistant strains of *C. glabrata* should be assumed to be cross-resistant to other triazoles.

TREATMENT

Six antifungals (amphotericin B, fluconazole, voriconazole, caspofungin, micafungin, and anidulafungin) have been studied as monotherapy in prospective, randomized comparative clinical trials for the treatment of invasive candidiasis. In a patient-level meta-reanalysis of these trials, increasing patient age, increasing APACHE II score, use of immunosuppressive therapy, and infection with *Candida tropicalis* were independent risk factors for patient mortality.[25] On the other hand, removal of central venous catheters in patients with candidemia and treatment with an echinocandin were variables associated with reduced patient mortality. Based on these findings and treatment guidelines endorsed by the Infectious Diseases Society of America,[21] echinocandins are recommended as the preferred initial treatment for invasive bloodstream candidiasis, even less "critically-ill" patients.[26] Timely initiation of antifungal therapy for invasive candidiasis is critical, as any delay in the initiation of antifungal therapy once a patient has a positive blood culture increases the potential for metastatic seeding of organs and mortality. Clinically stable patients can be transitioned to oral fluconazole or other triazoles once the infecting isolate has been identified and susceptibility is known.[27]

The efficacy of echinocandins for deep-tissue candidiasis is less well established compared to bloodstream infections, and higher failure rates have been reported for infections located in anatomical sites where echinocandin penetration is limited (ie, meninges, endophthalmitis, urine).[10] For other forms of deep tissue candidiasis, triazoles or lipid amphotericin B formulation may be preferable as initial therapy until diagnosis and culture results are available, depending on the suspected organs involved and the clinical severity of illness.[21] Frequently patients are transitioned to oral triazole therapy once stable because of the long-treatment courses that are often required (4–6 weeks minimum) for deep-seated infections.

Another important caveat for empiric use of echinocandins is that cryptococcosis, endemic fungi, or other rare yeast (eg, *Trichosporon* species) occasionally produce fungemia in lymphopenic patients that may initially be mistakenly assumed to be *Candida*. Therefore, initial treatment with a lipid amphotericin B formulation may be judicious in profoundly lymphopenic patients (i.e., CD4$^+$ less than 250/mm^3 [250 × 10^6/L]) with yeast in blood cultures until fungal identification is confirmed, as echinocandins have poor activity against non-*Candida* yeast.

Echinocandins (ie, caspofungin, micafungin, or anidulafungin); voriconazole; or lipid amphotericin B formulation are often administered as empiric treatment for *Candida* spp in patients with prolonged neutropenia (ie, absolute neutrophil count less than 500 PMN/mm^3 [500 × 10^6/L] for greater than 7 days) with fever.[21,28] Fluconazole may be an acceptable option

Table 84–4

Therapeutic Approach to Opportunistic Invasive Fungal Infections

Mycoses	Recommended Treatment Regimens	Comments
Candidiasis		
Catheter-related and acute hematogenous	Fluconazole 12 mg/kg loading dose, then 6–12 mg/kg/day IV every 24 hours adjusted for renal function[a] OR Echinocandin[b] OR Voriconazole 6 mg/kg every 12 hours IV for 1 day, then 3 mg/kg every 12 hours IV *Second line:* Lipid amphotericin B formulation 3–5 mg/kg /day[c] OR Amphotericin B 0.7 mg/kg/day IV OR Amphotericin B + fluconazole	Treat for 14 days after the last positive blood culture and resolution of signs and symptoms; catheter should be removed whenever possible Patients can be switched to oral fluconazole when clinically stable if isolate is susceptible Echinocandins and amphotericin B are preferred agents for fluconazole-resistant species. Voriconazole appears to be effective against fluconazole-resistant *C. krusei*
Empirical therapy in neutropenic patient	Fluconazole 6–12 mg/kg/day (low risk) adjusted for renal function[a] OR Liposomal amphotericin B 3 mg/kg every 24 hours OR Echinocandin OR Amphotericin B 0.7 mg/kg every 24 hours	Antifungals with coverage of *Aspergillus* should be used in higher risk patients or prolonged neutropenia (ie, longer than 2 weeks)
Urinary candidiasis	Fluconazole 200 mg IV or orally for 7–14 days OR Amphotericin B 0.3 mg/kg/day IV for 1–7 days	Asymptomatic candiduria does not require therapy
Cryptococcosis		
Pulmonary-Isolated	Fluconazole 6 mg/kg/day IV or PO for 6–12 months adjusted for renal function[a]	
Severe Pulmonary Infection and Meningitis	*Induction:* Amphotericin B 1 mg/kg/day + flucytosine 100 mg/kg/day orally divided every 6 hours for 2 weeks adjusted for renal function[c] *Consolidation:* Fluconazole 6–12 mg/kg/day for 10 weeks adjusted for renal function[a] *Second line:* Fluconazole + flucytosine for 2 weeks, then fluconazole for 10 weeks adjusted for renal function[a,c] OR Amphotericin + fluconazole for 2 weeks, then fluconazole for 10 weeks adjusted for renal function[a] OR Liposomal amphotericin B 5 mg/kg/day for 2 weeks, then fluconazole for 10 weeks adjusted for renal function[a]	Therapeutic drug monitoring is required for safe use of flucytosine, see Table 84–3 Echinocandins have no activity against cryptococci Use of flucytosine-amphotericin B combination therapy was associated with faster CSF sterilization and improved survival. Similar benefits were not observed with combination fluconazole-amphotericin B regimens

(Continued)

Table 84–4

Therapeutic Approach to Opportunistic Invasive Fungal Infections (*Continued*)

Mycoses	Recommended Treatment Regimens	Comments
Aspergillosis	Voriconazole 6 mg/kg IV every 12 hours × 2 doses, then 4 mg/kg IV every 12 hours Voriconazole 4 mg/kg oral every 12 hours OR Lipid formulations of amphotericin B OR Echinocandin[b] OR Posaconazole 300 mg every 12 hours IV day 1, then 300 mg IV daily Posaconazole delayed-release tablet 300 mg twice daily, day 1, then 300 mg daily Posaconazole suspension 200 mg by mouth four times daily for 14 days, then 400 mg PO twice daily OR Combination therapy	Voriconazole can be administered as oral therapy in patients taking oral medications. However, patients with suspected aspergillosis should initially be stated on IV therapy Therapeutic drug monitoring should be considered in patients receiving voriconazole or posaconazole suspension, see Table 84–3 Combination therapy with triazole and echinocandin associated with improved survival in patients with galactomannan-diagnosed infection *A. terreus* and *A. flavus* should be considered resistant to amphotericin B Tablet formulation of posaconazole is preferred for most patients because of improved bioavailability and fewer drug interactions

[a]Fluconazole renal dosing adjustments: CrCl greater than 50–90 mL/min (0.83–1.50 mL/s), 100% of dose; CrCl 10–50 mL/min (0.17–0.83 mL/s), 50% of dose; CrCl less than 10 mL/min (0.17 mL/s) 50%.

[b]Anidulafungin 200 mg loading dose day 1, then 100 mg daily, caspofungin 70 mg loading dose day 1, then 50 mg daily; or micafungin 100 mg daily.

[c]Flucytosine renal dosing adjustments: CrCl greater than 50–90 mL/min (0.83–1.50 mL/s), 25 mg/kg every 12 hours; CrCl 10–50 mL/min (0.17–0.83 mL/s), 25 mg/kg every 12–24 hours; CrCl less than 10 mL/min (0.17 mL/s) 25 mg/kg every 24 hours. Therapeutic drug monitoring is required for safe use of flucytosine (see Table 84–3).

in patients expected to have short duration of neutropenia (less than 2 weeks) not receiving systemic antifungal prophylaxis with a triazole. Lipid amphotericin B formulations, an echinocandin, or voriconazole are preferred if the patient has or is expected to have prolonged neutropenia (ie, greater than 2 weeks) because of the increased risk for mold infections. If patients are receiving fluconazole prophylaxis, breakthrough infections with *C. glabrata,* and less frequently *C. krusei*, are possible and should be initially treatable with an echinocandin or amphotericin B.

Urinary candidiasis is a term for an ill-defined group of syndromes that can range from benign colonization (candiduria) in the bladder to invasive disease of the renal parenchyma. Asymptomatic candiduria in nonneutropenic patients does not require antifungal therapy, as transient clearance of *Candida* from the urine of asymptomatic patients has no demonstrable clinical benefit.[21] Patients should receive 7 to 14 days of antifungal therapy for urinary candidiasis if they are (a) symptomatic, (b) have clinical or laboratory evidence of infection, (c) are neutropenic, (d) are low-birth-weight infants; (e) will undergo urologic manipulations, or (f) have renal allografts. Removal of urinary tract instruments, including Foley catheters and stents, is essential to prevent relapse. The preferred therapy is fluconazole 200 mg daily, although IV amphotericin B deoxycholate 0.3 to 1 mg/kg/day is also effective. Other antifungal agents (with the exception of flucytosine) do not achieve appreciable concentrations in the urine and therefore should not be considered first-line treatments for urinary candidiasis.[10] Irrigation with amphotericin B is not effective for infections above the bladder and should not be used in higher risk patients with the exception of its use as a diagnostic tool for confirming a localized infection of the bladder. *Candida* infections of the renal parenchyma secondary to metastatic seeding from the bloodstream are treated in a similar fashion to candidemia.

Mucocutaneous candidiasis is not invasive and can be treated with topical azoles (clotrimazole troches), oral azoles (fluconazole, ketoconazole, or itraconazole), or oral polyenes (such as nystatin or oral amphotericin B). Orally administered and absorbed azoles (ketoconazole, fluconazole, or itraconazole solution), amphotericin B suspension, IV echinocandins, or IV amphotericin B are recommended for refractory or recurrent infections.[17]

Although more severe than mucocutaneous candidiasis, esophageal candidiasis typically does not evolve into a life-threatening infection unless the esophagus is ruptured. However, topical

Patient Encounter 2, Part 2: Invasive Candidiasis

The patient was started on fluconazole 400 mg/day, but 4 days later has persistent fever and develops hypotension and decreased urine output. Blood cultures are now growing a germ tube–negative yeast. Laboratory studies revealed a white blood cell count of 14,200/mm^3 (14.2 × 10^9/L), aspartate aminotransferase 68 IU/L (1.13 μkat/L), alanine aminotransferase 75 IU/L (1.25 μkat/L), alkaline phosphatase 168 IU/L (2.80 μkat/L), and normal bilirubin. Serum creatinine has increased from 1.2 to 1.8 mg/dL (106–159 μmol/L) over the last 3 days.

What factors suggest empiric antifungal therapy should be changed in this patient?

What other procedures should be recommended in this patient to improve management and response to antifungal therapy?

therapy is ineffective. Triazole antifungals (fluconazole, itraconazole solution, or voriconazole), echinocandins, or IV amphotericin B (in cases of unresponsive infections) are effective treatment options. Parenteral therapy should be used in patients who are unable to take oral medications.[17]

OUTCOME EVALUATION

Response to antifungal therapy in invasive candidiasis is often more rapid than for endemic fungal infections. Resolution of fever and sterilization of blood cultures are indications of response to antifungal therapy with the caveat that the growth of *Candida* from blood cultures is often delayed by 48 to 72 hours. Adverse effects associated with antifungal therapy are similar in these patients as described earlier, except some toxicities may be more pronounced in critically ill patients with invasive candidiasis. Nephrotoxicity and electrolyte disturbances with amphotericin B can be especially problematic and may not be avoidable even with lipid amphotericin B formulations. Therefore, current treatment guidelines favor less-toxic treatment options, such as the echinocandins, especially in higher-risk patients. Decisions to use one class of antifungal agents over the other are principally driven by concerns of non-*albicans* species, patient tolerability, or history of prior fluconazole exposure (risk factor for non-*albicans* species.) and local susceptibility patterns; especially institutional rates of fluconazole (triazole) and echinocandin-resistance.

PROPHYLAXIS

Fluconazole (400 mg/day) has been studied as a prophylactic regimen to prevent invasive candidiasis in patients with prolonged (greater than 2 weeks) neutropenia.[21] Placebo-controlled, prospective randomized trials performed in the 1990s demonstrated that fluconazole was effective in reducing the frequency, morbidity, and, in some trials, mortality due to invasive candidiasis in neutropenic patients if administered until marrow recovery. However, the major limitation with fluconazole is its lack of mold coverage needed for high-risk patients with prolonged (ie, greater than 3 weeks) neutropenia.[28] Itraconazole, voriconazole, posaconazole, and the echinocandin micafungin have demonstrated a benefit in reducing the incidence of invasive candidiasis when used for prophylaxis in hematopoietic cell transplant recipients until engraftment; however, all of the drugs have limitations with respect to prolonged administration in high-risk patients. Therefore, the approach toward antifungal prophylaxis is highly institution-specific depending on the patient population, epidemiology of invasive fungal infections, and options for outpatient IV drug therapy.

Use of antifungal prophylaxis for invasive candidiasis in non-neutropenic patients remains an area of controversy. Fluconazole prophylaxis can reduce the incidence but not necessarily mortality associated with invasive candidiasis in select high-risk transplant populations (eg, liver, pancreatic, or small-bowel transplantation) or subsets of ICU patients at high risk for infection (ie, neonatal intensive care).[21] However, prophylaxis can result in excessive antifungal use in lower-risk patients; therefore, many experts have advocated preemptive (ie, starting therapy based on biomarkers of infection such as serum β-glucan) or empirical (symptoms of infection) treatment approaches in this population in lieu of prophylaxis.

Nevertheless, a multi-institutional prospective randomized trial of administering empirical fluconazole (800 mg/day versus placebo) in ICU patients with persistent fever, did not demonstrate significant benefits in reducing the incidence or mortality associated with invasive candidiasis.[29] Similarly, a recent multi-institutional study that focused on ICU patients identified as "high risk" for invasive candidiasis using a validated clinical risk prediction score failed to demonstrate significant reductions in the incidence or mortality of invasive candidiasis with caspofungin prophylaxis.[30] However, patients who were treated with an echinocandin after developing a positive serum β-glucan appeared to have lower rates of progression to documented invasive candidiasis. Therefore, many questions persist regarding the optimal approach for preventing or preemptive treating invasive candidiasis in non-neutropenic ICU patients.

CRYPTOCOCCOSIS

EPIDEMIOLOGY

Cryptococcus neoformans is an encapsulated yeast that can infect apparently normal hosts but is more frequently associated with severe infections in immunocompromised patients. *C. neoformans* is divided into two varieties based on serotype: *C. neoformans* var. *neoformans* (serotypes a and d) that is associated with infections in immunocompromised patients, and *C. neoformans* var. *gattii* (serotypes b and c) that is associated with infections in healthy hosts. *C. neoformans* var. *gattii* is found predominantly in tropical and subtropical climates with eucalyptus trees, and has been linked to infectious outbreaks around Vancouver Island and the US Pacific Northwest. *C. neoformans* var. *neoformans* is found worldwide and is associated with pigeon droppings and other avian excreta. Before the AIDS pandemic, cryptococcosis was a relatively uncommon disease, but became a leading cause of meningitis among HIV-infected patients. Although the incidence of this infection has declined in developed countries with the widespread use of highly active antiretroviral therapy (HAART), *C. neoformans* remains an important pathogen in the developing regions with high rates of AIDS and also in immunocompromised patients, including transplant and cancer patients who may present with initially indolent pulmonary forms of the infection.

CLINICAL PRESENTATION AND DIAGNOSIS

C. neoformans is acquired primarily through inhalation of the desiccated yeast particles found in the environment. Inhaled cells reach distal alveolar spaces where they gradually rehydrate and form their characteristic polysaccharide capsules that enable resistance to phagocytosis. Defects in cellular immunity allow reconstitution of the protective capsule and multiplication of yeast in the lungs. Although alveolar macrophages phagocytose the yeast, containment and killing require a coordinated response between innate and adaptive humoral (complement and anti-cryptococcal antibodies) and T-cell–mediated host responses.[6] Deficiencies in cell-mediated immunity allow the yeast to survive as a facultative intracellular pathogen in macrophages as they migrate from the lung to draining lymph nodes, leading to dissemination via the bloodstream to the meninges.

Unlike most opportunistic fungi, true virulence factors have been identified for *C. neoformans*. The capsules, including the soluble polysaccharides released from the yeast cells during infection, impair phagocytosis and binding of anticryptococcal antibodies. Primary cryptococcal infection begins in the lung, presenting as a mildly symptomatic or asymptomatic infection that resolves spontaneously or undergoes encapsulation in non-calcified lung nodules. It is common for these isolated nodules to be detected on chest x-rays during routine workup. Diagnosis of primary cryptococcosis is only made if the nodule is aspirated or removed because of concerns of primary lung cancer.

In the immunocompromised host, infection of the lung may present with more diffuse, bilateral, and interstitial disease that mimics the presentation of *P. jiroveci (carinii)* pneumonia (PCP). Dissemination to other organs, particularly the CNS, eye, and possibly the skin, is more likely to occur in patients with severe deficits in cell-mediated immunity. Fever, cough, dyspnea, and pleural pain are common at presentation, with accompanying hypoxemia that can rapidly evolve to acute respiratory failure. Because the features of diffuse pulmonary cryptococcosis overlap with other opportunistic pathogens, early diagnosis requires bronchoalveolar lavage or transbronchial biopsy, which can effectively diagnose 80% to 100% of cases.[31] The clinical course of diffuse cryptococcal pneumonia can be as severe as PCP, with mortality rates approaching 100% in untreated patients by 48 hours.

C. neoformans readily disseminates from the lung to the CNS, specifically the leptomeninges, and occasionally the parenchyma of the brain. The clinical characteristics of cryptococcal meningitis differ somewhat, however, between patients with and without underlying AIDS. In patients without AIDS, disease presentation is more insidious, and symptoms such as dizziness, irritability, decreased comprehension, and unstable gait may present many weeks to months before the diagnosis is established.[31] Patients with AIDS generally present much later in the course of disease with severe meningoencephalitis.[31] The most common signs and symptoms on presentation are fever, headache, **meningismus**, photophobia, mental status changes, and seizures. CT or more sensitive MRI may reveal cerebral edema, multiple areas of enhanced nodules, or a single mass lesion (cryptococcoma). Examination of the cerebrospinal fluid (CSF) often reveals increased opening pressure upon lumbar puncture, but glucose, protein, and leukocyte levels can be normal.[31]

LABORATORY DIAGNOSIS

Clinical diagnosis is confirmed by cultures from the blood, CSF, or other clinically relevant fluids or tissue. *C. neoformans* can be directly visualized in the CSF when stained with India Ink, which is excluded by the yeast capsule (**Figure 84-3B**). However, infection is most frequently diagnosed (Figure 84–3B), by detection of cryptococcal antigen in either serum or CSF, which has high sensitivity and specificity (greater than 95%) and correlated with fungal burden.[31] A positive serum antigen test of greater than 1:4 strongly suggests cryptococcal infection, and greater than or equal to 1:8 is indicative of active disease. Antigen titers in serum are positive in 99% of patients with cryptococcal meningitis and typically exceed titers of 1:2048 in patients with AIDS.[31] However, the time course of cryptococcal antigen elimination is unknown, and a positive test result can persist for many years. Changes in the CSF cryptococcal antigen titers have limited value in the monitoring of drug therapy for cryptococcal meningitis, although it is expected that a decrease should be seen after 2 or more weeks of antifungal therapy.[31]

TREATMENT

Cryptococcal meningitis is fatal if left untreated. Because pneumonia frequently precedes dissemination of disease and subsequent meningitis, all patients with culture-, histopathology-, or serology-proven disease should receive antifungal therapy. In patients with isolated pulmonary cryptococcosis, fluconazole is generally considered to be the therapy of choice (see Table 84–2).[31] Alternatively, itraconazole, voriconazole, or combination therapy (fluconazole plus flucytosine) has also been used with some success, but these regimens are generally considered inferior to amphotericin B and are recommended only for persons unable to tolerate or unresponsive to standard treatment. Echinocandins do not have activity against *C. neoformans*.

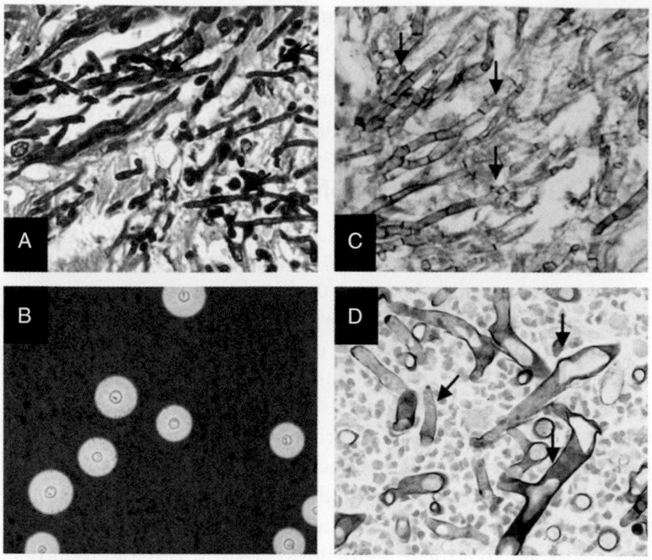

FIGURE 84–3. Opportunistic mycoses in clinical samples. **(A)** Candidiasis (tissue). **(B)** Cryptococcosis (India ink stain of CSF). **(C)** Aspergillosis (tissue). **(D)** Mucormycosis (tissue).

Disseminated or CNS cryptococcosis requires a more aggressive treatment approach. Pretreatment predictors of poor outcome with antifungal therapy include the following:

- Progressive underlying disease or immune dysfunction
- Abnormal mental status at the time of presentation
- Increased opening pressure on lumbar puncture (greater than 260 mm H_2O [2.55 kPa])
- High fungal burden as reflected by a CSF antigen titer (in AIDS patients) of greater than 1:2048

Clinical trials performed by the National Institute of Allergy and Infectious Diseases (NIAID) Mycoses Study Group defined the standard treatment regimen for cryptococcal meningitis consisting of 2 weeks of induction antifungal therapy with combination amphotericin B (0.7 mg/kg/day) plus flucytosine (100 mg/kg/day) for cryptococcal meningitis, followed by consolidation therapy with fluconazole (400 mg daily) for 8 weeks (see Table 84–2).[31] However, other combinations of either fluconazole plus flucytosine, or fluconazole plus amphotericin B were sometimes recommended due difficulties in obtaining flucytosine (especially in developing countries) and toxicity (see Table 84–2).

KEY CONCEPT *In a landmark study addressing which combination is best for cryptococcal meningitis, there were significantly fewer deaths in patients receiving amphotericin B plus flucytosine versus patients receiving amphotericin B alone or a combination of amphotericin B plus fluconazole.*[32] Notably, the amphotericin B–flucytosine combination was associated with more rapid clearance of yeast from the CSF versus other regimens.

PROPHYLAXIS

Fluconazole (200 mg/day) is recommended as maintenance therapy for life in patients with persistent underlying immune dysfunction to prevent recurrent cryptococcal meningitis.[31] Available data suggest it is safe to discontinue maintenance therapy in AIDS patients who have had a sustained immunologic response on effective antiretroviral therapy (ie, $CD4^+$ count greater than 100 cells/microliter (100×10^6/L) with undetectable or very low viral RNA) if they have received at least 12 months of antifungal therapy.[31] Occasionally, initiation of HAART can result in the reactivation of a subclinical, immunologic manifestation of cryptococcal infection (or other opportunistic infections). Manifestations of this *immune reconstitution inflammatory syndrome* (IRIS) may include exacerbations of meningitis or necrotizing pneumonia. Antifungal therapy plus a nonsteroidal anti-inflammatory agent or prednisone has been used successfully in patients with cryptococcal-associated immune reconstitution syndrome.[33] However, the optimal management of this recently defined clinical entity remains unknown.

INVASIVE ASPERGILLOSIS

EPIDEMIOLOGY

Invasive molds, particularly *Aspergillus* species, are a common complication of intensive cancer chemotherapy required for hematologic malignancies, and prolonged immunosuppression following hematopoietic and solid organ transplantation. Four species are commonly associated with invasive infection: *Aspergillus fumigatus*, *Aspergillus flavus*, *Aspergillus terreus*, and *Aspergillus niger*. Of these four species, *A. fumigatus* accounts for most of human infections. However, identification of *Aspergillus* mold in culture to the species level is still essential because the incidence of amphotericin B–resistant *Aspergillus terreus* and *Aspergillus flavus* have increased in some centers over the last 10 years. Additionally, less common mold infections such as fusariosis and mucormycosis often present with similar clinical features aspergillosis, but require different treatment approaches due to their inherent resistance to many antifungal agents. Early and accurate diagnosis of invasive aspergillosis (IA) improves the outcome of infection, reducing mortality rates by 30% to 50% with the timely administration of effective antifungal therapy.[34]

CLINICAL PRESENTATION AND DIAGNOSIS

The pathogenesis of IA is defined largely by the underlying immune dysfunction of the host. The most common route of acquisition for *Aspergillus* is through the respiratory tract. Conidia dispersed in air currents are continuously inhaled through the sinuses and mouth and penetrate down to distal alveolar spaces (see **Figure 84–4**). Most conidia are rapidly phagocytosed and removed by resident macrophages and neutrophils in the upper and lower respiratory tract.[6] However, macrophage function may be suppressed following transplantation, cytotoxic chemotherapy, or in patients who have received high-dose corticosteroid therapy. Conidia that escaped phagocytosis begin to germinate into hyphal forms that invade blood vessels or contiguous tissues or bone (in sinuses), resulting in hemorrhage and/or infarction and coagulative necrosis. Once in the bloodstream, viable hyphal fragments can break off and disseminate to distal organs including the brain. Control of the infection at this stage requires development of an adaptive TH1 or TH17 response to enhance the fungicidal activity of professional effector cells (ie, neutrophils) against hyphal elements.[6]

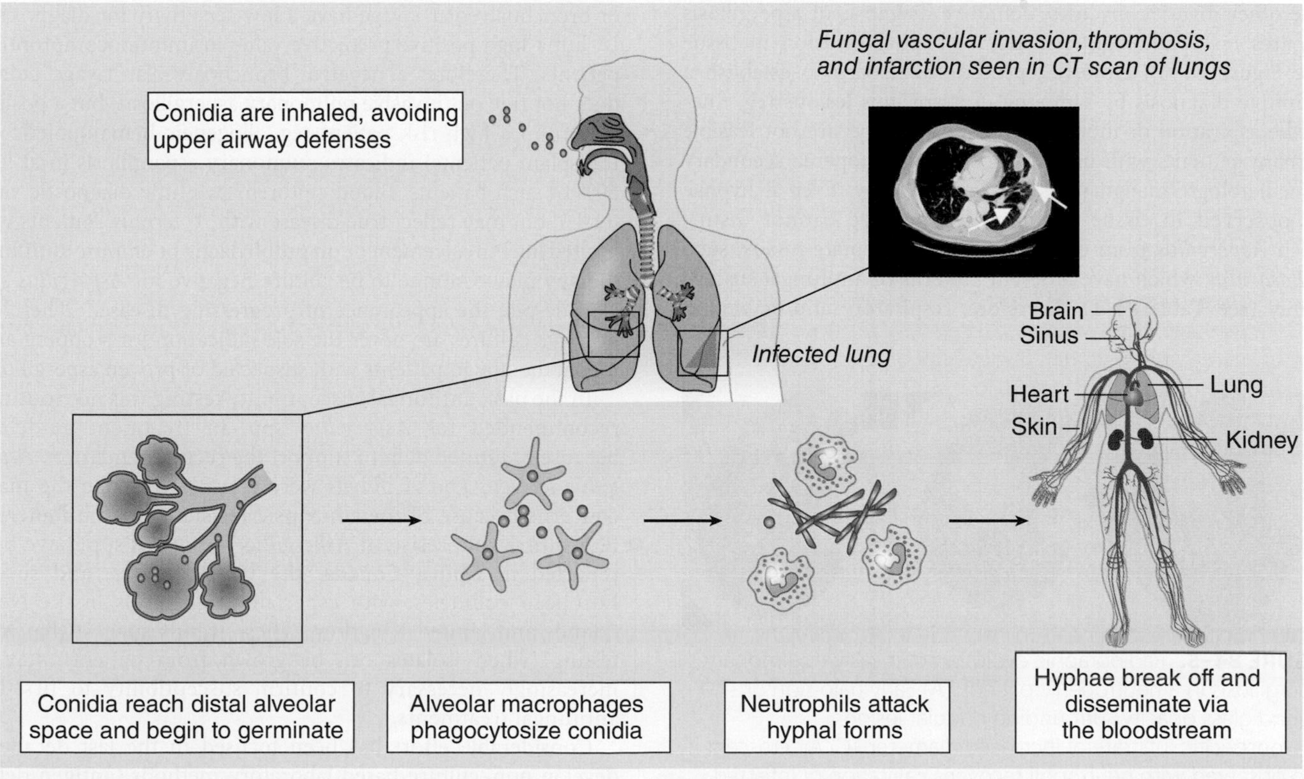
Conidia are inhaled, avoiding upper airway defenses
Fungal vascular invasion, thrombosis, and infarction seen in CT scan of lungs
Infected lung
Brain
Sinus
Heart
Skin
Lung
Kidney
Conidia reach distal alveolar space and begin to germinate
Alveolar macrophages phagocytosize conidia
Neutrophils attack hyphal forms
Hyphae break off and disseminate via the bloodstream

FIGURE 84–4. Pathogenesis of invasive aspergillosis (IA).

Patients with dysregulated, suppressed T-cell–mediated immunity or prolonged neutropenia are unable to control fungal growth and are at high risk for dissemination of the infection. Without early diagnosis and antifungal therapy, IA in persistently immunosuppressed patients is uniformly fatal.

Signs and symptoms of IA are predictably muted in the immunocompromised host. Fever is common but nonspecific for infection and may be accompanied by pleuritic chest pain, cough, hemoptysis, and/or friction rub.[34] Neurologic signs, including seizures, hemiparesis, and stupor, may be present in patients with dissemination to the brain. Cutaneous plaques or papules characterized by a central necrotic ulcer or eschar occur in up to 10% of patients with disseminated disease; however, concomitant blood cultures are often negative. Chest radiographs cannot detect early forms of disease and may remain negative in up to 10% of patients within 1 week of death. Nodular lesions detected by high-resolution computed tomography (HRCT) scans, along with fever, are often the first indication of invasive pulmonary aspergillosis in severely immunocompromised patients. Typically these radiographs reveal wedge-shaped or nodular lesions, surrounded by intermediate attenuation called the "halo sign" (Figure 84–5). These early lesions on CT scans represent hemorrhage and edema surrounding an infarcted blood vessel. Despite "effective" antifungal therapy, lesions on CT scan may continue to increase in size in neutropenic patients until neutrophil counts recover, at which time they begin to cavitate, forming the "air-crescent sign" on chest radiographs, indicative of resolving infection. KEY CONCEPT *Immunocompromised patients on fluconazole with progressive sinus or pulmonary disease by radiography should be considered to have a possible mold infection and receive empiric antifungal therapy directed (at minimum) against Aspergillus species.*[40]

LABORATORY DIAGNOSIS

Like other invasive mycoses, definitive diagnosis of aspergillosis requires histopathologic evidence of hyphal invasion in tissue (see Figure 84–3). However, procedures needed to establish a definitive diagnosis by sampling of suspicious lesions (eg, fine-needle aspiration or thoracoscopic lung biopsy) are not feasible in many patients with underlying thrombocytopenia secondary to hematologic malignancies or chemotherapy. Even if hyphae are observed in tissue, histopathology alone cannot distinguish *Aspergillus* from other angioinvasive septate molds, such as *Fusarium*, which have different patterns of antifungal susceptibility (see Table 84–1). Therefore, respiratory and/or wound cultures (if cutaneous or sinus/hard palate lesions are present) are important factors in the modification of empiric antifungal therapy.

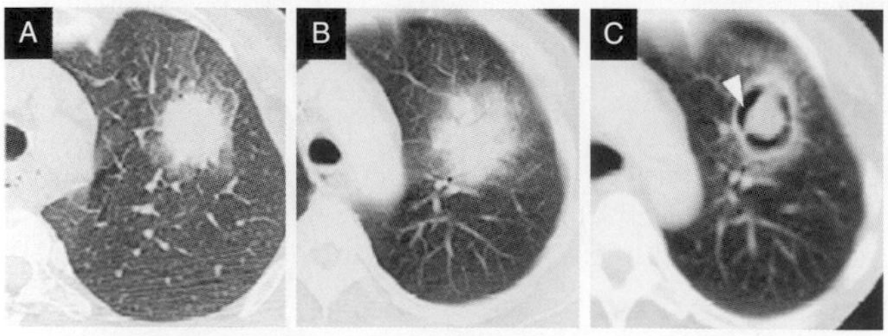

FIGURE 84–5. Radiographic evolution of invasive pulmonary aspergillosis in a neutropenic patient. (**A**) Early halo sign of ground glass opacity surrounding nodular lesions. (**B**) Nonspecific infiltrate of increased diameter. (**C**) Air crescent sign observed with neutrophil recovery, cavitation of infected lung in walled off cavity with air (arrow).

Patient Encounter 3: Invasive Mold Infection

A 52-year-old man with acute myeloid leukemia who received a matched-allogeneic donor hematopoietic stem-cell transplantation presents to the clinic 70 days after transplant with complaints of fever. On laboratory examination, he is noted to have an alanine aminotransferase of 119 IU/L (1.98 μkat/L), aspartate aminotransferase 107 IU/L (1.78 μkat/L), and total bilirubin of 1.8 mg/dL (31 μmol/L). The patient has an absolute neutrophil count of 970 (970×10^6/L). His current medications include tacrolimus 5 mg twice daily (most recent level: 9 ng/mL [9 mcg/L; 11 nmol/L]), prednisone 10 mg daily, levofloxacin 500 mg daily, fluconazole 200 mg/day, valacyclovir 500 mg twice daily. A CT scan of the chest reveals a single dense pleural-based lung nodule in the left lung. A serum galactomannan test is reported to be negative (index 0.4, positive when greater than 0.5). The primary service wishes to start voriconazole.

What are the patient's risk factors and signs that suggest he has an invasive fungal infection?

What problems need to be anticipated in this patient if voriconazole is started?

If the patient's infection appears to resolve and he continues to take voriconazole for months while tapering immunosuppression, what are some of the toxicities potentially associated with prolonged voriconazole therapy?

Respiratory cultures, including sputum, bronchial washings, or bronchoalveolar lavage have a low sensitivity for diagnosis of IA but a high positive predictive value in immunocompromised patients. Therefore, a negative bronchoalveolar lavage culture does not rule out invasive pulmonary aspergillosis, but a positive culture in a high-risk patient (eg, allogeneic hematopoietic cell transplant patients) indicates pulmonary aspergillosis in at least 60% of such patients. Blood cultures have little diagnostic value for IA, but may reflect true disease with *A. terreus*. Patients with limited lung involvement or on prophylactic or empiric antifungal therapy may continue to be culture-negative for *Aspergillus* species, despite the appearance of progressing disease.[34] Therefore, negative cultures are never the sole indication for stopping antifungal therapy in patients with suspected or proven aspergillosis.

In the past, antifungal susceptibility testing was not routinely recommended for *Aspergillus* spp. in treatment guidelines because of limited data to support the recommendation. *Aspergillus terrreus* and *A. flavus* were considered to be the major concerns because of their intrinsic resistance to amphotericin B. Multitriazole-resistant *Aspergillus fumigatus* spp. have been reported in China, Canada, the United States, and several European countries, with especially high levels in the Netherlands and United Kingdom. These trends suggest that MIC testing (when isolates can be grown from patient) may be increasingly necessary to confirm susceptibility to first-line antifungal treatments.

Considerable effort has been focused in the last decade to develop non–culture-based laboratory methods (antigen detection, polymerase chain reaction [PCR], and antigen detection) for the diagnosis of IA. The hope is that these surrogate tests could detect early evidence of *Aspergillus* infection before significant target organ damage eventually detected by CT scans occurs. Currently, most centers use an ELISA-based assay for the detection of a polysaccharide component of the *Aspergillus* cell wall called galactomannan. Although several large prospective studies have found that the sensitivity and specificity of the assay exceeded 90% in neutropenic patients with hematologic malignancies, the median time span between galactomannan detection and clinical signs and symptoms of IA averages less than 6 days. The sensitivity of the galactomannan may be enhanced if the test is performed on bronchial lavage fluid. Other factors such as patient immune status (neutropenia vs graft-versus-host disease), antibacterial therapy, antifungal prophylaxis, and diet may affect the sensitivity and specificity of the galactomannan test.[34] For example, false-positive results have been reported to be higher in the pediatric population, patients receiving piperacillin-tazobactam for neutropenic fever, and following the ingestion of certain cereals, pastas, nutritional supplements, or soy sauce. Accumulating clinical data suggest that rising galactomannan levels are a harbinger of breakthrough infection, and declining galactomannan concentrations are an early indicator of response to treatment. However, antifungal therapy is rarely stopped in patients once the serum galactomannan becomes negative, especially in persistently immunosuppressed patients. Hence, the galactomannan test and other non-culture-based strategies, such as serum β-glucan, which can also be detected during *Aspergillus* infection, serve as complementary methods to confirm results from microbiologic, histopathologic, and radiographic investigations directed toward diagnosing IA.

TREATMENT

Four comparative randomized controlled clinical trials have evaluated antifungal therapies for the treatment of diagnosis-proven IA. Voriconazole is considered by many experts and consensus treatment guidelines to be the preferred antifungal for IA (see Table 84–2).[34] However, patients who are intolerant to voriconazole, have ongoing hepatotoxicity issues, or have received voriconazole prophylaxis in the recent past may initially be treated with a liposomal amphotericin B formulation. Lipid amphotericin B formulations are recommended over other antifungal classes because of their better coverage of Mucorales molds, which are intrinsically resistant to voriconazole, but often present as a breakthrough infection indistinguishable from IA. Once the infection has stabilized and diagnosis is clarified, patients can be transitioned back to an intravenous or oral triazole for the completion of their therapy.

Isavuconazole is a newer triazole unique from other agents because it is administered as a prodrug, isavuconazonium, which is rapidly cleaved in vivo to the active drug (isavuconazole) and an inactive prodrug cleavage product (BAL8728). In a phase 3 trial, patients with proven or probable aspergillosis treated with isavuconazole achieved similar clinical response rates as a standard voriconazole regimen, but with significantly fewer hepatic, skin, and visual adverse effects.[35] Therefore, isavuconazole appears to be a promising alternative to voriconazole for the treatment of IA.

Echinocandins are clinically active against *Aspergillus* spp. and have demonstrated efficacy in the treatment of probable or proven aspergillosis. However, their lack of fungicidal activity and possibly lower response rates reported with monotherapy regimens in noncomparative studies[36] makes them less appealing as a frontline treatment regimen for documented infections, despite their excellent safety profile.

Multiple studies in vitro and in animal models, as well small clinical studies have suggested that administration of an echinocandin with a triazole such as voriconazole may be synergistic and improve survival in IA over monotherapy, but prospective clinical studies, until recently, have been lacking. A multicenter, randomized clinical trial comparing voriconazole-anidulafungin combination therapy to to voriconazole monotherapy for proven or probable aspergillosis reported a trend in improved 6-week survival for patients randomized to combination therapy, that was significant among a post-hoc analyzed group of patients whose disease was diagnosed with galactomannan antigen but not culture (reflecting patients with earlier-diagnosed disease).[37] Nevertheless, the failure of the study to meet its primary endpoint objective raises lingering questions about the efficacy of combination therapy, and many clinicians reserve the use of combination regimens for patients with extensive disease (ie, multifocal or bilateral pneumonia, disseminated infection) or in cases of suspected breakthrough infection.

PROPHYLAXIS

Although published guidelines for preventing opportunistic infections in hematopoietic cell transplant recipients do not provide concrete recommendations for antifungal prophylaxis against *Aspergillus*, prophylaxis should be considered in certain high-risk subgroups with rates of IA exceeding 10%. These groups include (a) patients with prolonged pre-engraftment periods (eg, cord-blood transplant recipients), (b) patients with a history of IA prior to transplantation, (c) patients receiving transplants with a high risk of graft-versus-host disease (eg, haploidentical allogeneic transplant) or infection (eg, T-cell–depleted transplant), any patient with graft-versus-host disease on high-dose corticosteroid therapy (greater than 1 mg/kg prednisone equivalent) with or without antithymocyte globulin or tumor necrosis factor blockade (ie, infliximab), and (d) any transplant recipient with active cytomegalovirus disease, which is associated with an increased risk of subsequent mold infections due to the immunosuppressive effects of the virus. Posaconazole was shown in two prospective randomized trials to reduce *Aspergillus*-associated death in patients with acute high-risk leukemia and reduce mold infections in patients with graft-versus-host disease following hematopoietic stem cell transplantation. Similar data are available for voriconazole, for HSCT[38,39] but less benefit was observed versus standard fluconazole prophylaxis plus intensive galactomannan monitoring in the hematopoietic stem cell transplant patients. Prophylactic approaches, however, are often individualized to institution and patient-specific risk factors.

OUTCOME EVALUATION

Response to antifungal therapy in invasive molds is slow and difficult to judge by clinical signs alone. Resolution of fever and eventual clearing of CT scans (in the case of lung infections) are indications of response to antifungal therapy. Toxicity associated with antifungal therapy is similar in these patients as in those described earlier. Patients who develop breakthrough infections on voriconazole should also undergo a careful clinical workup for other invasive mold pathogens such as mucormycosis (see Table 84–1), which are not susceptible to voriconazole. In most cases, antifungal therapy may be continued until immunosuppression has resolved.

Abbreviations Introduced in This Chapter

AIDS	Acquired immunodeficiency syndrome
ARDS	Acute respiratory distress syndrome
CNS	Central nervous system
CrCl	Estimated creatinine clearance
CSF	Cerebrospinal fluid
CT	Computed tomography
CYP	Cytochrome P-450 isoenzyme
ELISA	Enzyme-linked immunosorbent assay
FISH	Fluorescent in situ hybridization
HAART	Highly active antiretroviral therapy
HRCT	High-resolution computed tomography
IA	Invasive aspergillosis
ICU	Intensive care unit
IRIS	Immune reconstitution inflammatory syndrome
IV	Intravenous
MALDI-TOF	Matrix-assisted laser desorption/ionization time of flight
NIAID	National Institute of Allergy and Infectious Diseases
PCP	*Pneumocystis jiroveci (carinii)* pneumonia
PCR	Polymerase chain reaction
PMN	Polymorphonuclear cell

REFERENCES

1. Brown GD, Denning DW, Gow NAR, Levitz SM, Netea MG, White TC. Hidden killers: Human fungal infections. Sci Transl Med. 2012;4(165):165rv13.
2. Kainer MA, Reagan DR, Nguyen DB, et al. Fungal infections associated with contaminated methylprednisolone in Tennessee. N Engl J Med. 2012;367(23):2194–2203.
3. Wheat LJ, Freifeld AG, Kleiman MB, et al. Clinical practice guidelines for the management of patients with histoplasmosis: 2007 update by the Infectious Diseases Society of America. Clin Infect Dis. 2007;45(7):807–825.
4. Chapman SW, Dismukes WE, Proia LA, et al. Clinical practice guidelines for the management of blastomycosis: 2008 update by the Infectious Diseases Society of America. Clin Infect Dis. 2008;46(12):1801–1812.
5. Galgiani JN, Ampel NM, Blair JE, et al. Coccidioidomycosis. Clin Infect Dis. 2005 Nov 1;41(9):1217–1223.
6. Romani L. Immunity to fungal infections. Nat Rev Immunol. 2011;11(4):275–288.
7. Lortholary O, Denning DW, Dupont B. Endemic mycoses: A treatment update. J Antimicrob Chemother. 1999;43(3):321–331.
8. Duarte RF, López-Jiménez J, Cornely OA, et al. Phase 1b study of new posaconazole tablet for the prevention of invasive fungal infections in high-risk patients with neutropenia. Antimicrob Agents Chemother. 2014;58(10):5758–5765.
9. Brüggemann RJM, Alffenaar J-WC, Blijlevens NMA, et al. Clinical relevance of the pharmacokinetic interactions of azole antifungal drugs with other coadministered agents. Clin Infect Dis. 2009;48(10):1441–1458.
10. Felton T, Troke PF, Hope WW. Tissue penetration of antifungal agents. Clin Microbiol Rev. 2014;27(1):68–88.
11. Ashley ESD, Lewis R, Lewis JS, Martin C, Andes D. Pharmacology of systemic antifungal agents. Clin Infect Dis. 2006;43(Supplement 1):S28–S39.
12. Epaulard O, Villier C, Ravaud P, et al. A multistep voriconazole-related phototoxic pathway may lead to skin carcinoma: Results from a French nationwide study. Clin Infect Dis. 2013;57(12):e182–e188.
13. Wermers RA, Cooper K, Razonable RR, et al. Fluoride excess and periostitis in transplant patients receiving long-term voriconazole therapy. Clin Infect Dis. 2011;52(5):604–611.
14. Malani AN, Kerr L, Obear J, Singal B, Kauffman CA. Alopecia and nail changes associated with voriconazole therapy. Clin Infect Dis. 2014; Aug;59(3):e61–e65.
15. Baxter CG, Marshall A, Roberts M, Felton TW, Denning DW. Peripheral neuropathy in patients on long-term triazole antifungal therapy. J Antimicrob Chemother. 2011;66(9):2136–2139.
16. Groll AH, Piscitelli SC, Walsh TJ. Clinical pharmacology of systemic antifungal agents: a comprehensive review of agents in clinical use, current investigational compounds, and putative targets for antifungal drug development. Adv Pharmacol. 1998; 44:343–500.
17. Pfaller MA, Diekema DJ. Epidemiology of invasive candidiasis: A persistent public health problem. Clin Microbiol Rev. 2007; 20(1):133–163.
18. Wisplinghoff H, Seifert H, Wenzel RP, Edmond MB. Current trends in the epidemiology of nosocomial bloodstream infections in patients with hematological malignancies and solid neoplasms in hospitals in the United States. Clin Infect Dis. 2003;36(9):1103–1110.
19. Clancy CJ, Nguyen MH. Systemic candidiasis: Candidemia and deep-organ infections. In: Calderone RA, Clancy CJ, editors. Candida and Candidiasis, 2nd ed. American Society of Microbiology; 2012. pp. 429–441.
20. Clancy CJ, Nguyen MH. Finding the "Missing 50%" of invasive candidiasis: How nonculture diagnostics will improve understanding of disease spectrum and transform patient care. Clin Infect Dis. 2013;56(9):1284–1292.
21. Pappas PG, Kauffman CA, Andes D, et al. Clinical practice guidelines for the management candidiasis: 2009 update by the Infectious Diseases Society of America. Clin Infect Dis. 2009; 48(5):503–535.
22. Pfaller MA, Andes DR, Diekema DJ, et al. Epidemiology and outcomes of invasive candidiasis due to non-albicans species of candida in 2,496 patients: Data from the prospective antifungal therapy (PATH) registry 2004–2008. PLoS One. 2014; 9(7):e101510.
23. Alexander BD, Johnson MD, Pfeiffer CD, et al. Increasing echinocandin resistance in Candida glabrata: Clinical failure correlates with presence of FKS mutations and elevated minimum inhibitory concentrations. Clin Infect Dis. 2013;56(12): 1724–1732.
24. Beyda ND, John J, Kilic A, Alam MJ, Lasco TM, Garey KW. FKS mutant Candida glabrata: Risk factors and outcomes in patients with candidemia. Clin Infect Dis. 2014 Sep 15;59(6):819–825.
25. Andes DR, Safdar N, Baddley JW, et al. Impact of treatment strategy on outcomes in patients with candidemia and other forms of invasive candidiasis: A patient-level quantitative review of randomized trials. Clin Infect Dis. 2012;54(8):1110–1122.
26. Clancy CJ, Nguyen MH. The end of an era in defining the optimal treatment of invasive candidiasis. Clin Infect Dis. 2012; 54(8):1123–1125.
27. Vazquez J, Reboli AC, Pappas PG, et al. Evaluation of an early step-down strategy from intravenous anidulafungin to oral azole therapy for the treatment of candidemia and other forms of invasive candidiasis: results from an open-label trial. BMC Infect Dis. 2014;14:97.
28. Freifeld AG, Bow EJ, Sepkowitz KA, et al. Clinical practice guideline for the use of antimicrobial agents in neutropenic patients with cancer: 2010 update by the infectious diseases society of america. Clin Infect Dis. 2011;52(4):e56–e93.
29. Schuster MG, Edwards JE, Sobel JD. Empirical fluconazole versus placebo for intensive care unit patients: A randomized Trial. Ann Intern Med. 2008;149:83–90.

30. Ostrosky-Zeichner L, Shoham S. Msg-01: A randomized, double-blind, placebo-controlled trial of caspofungin prophylaxis followed by preemptive therapy for invasive candidiasis in high-risk adults in the critical care setting. Clin Infect Dis. 2014;58(9):1219–1226.
31. Perfect JR, Dismukes WE, Dromer F, et al. Clinical practice guidelines for the management of cryptococcal disease: 2010 update by the Infectious Diseases Society of America. Clin Infect Dis. 2010;50(3):291–322.
32. Day JN, Chau TTH, Wolbers M, et al. Combination antifungal therapy for cryptococcal meningitis. N Engl J Med. 2013; 368(14):1291–1302.
33. Singh N, Perfect JR. Immune reconstitution syndrome associated with opportunistic mycoses. Lancet Infect Dis. 2007;7(6): 395–401.
34. Walsh TJ, Anaissie EJ, Denning DW, et al. Treatment of aspergillosis: clinical practice guidelines of the Infectious Diseases Society of America. Clin Infect Dis. 2008;46(3):327–360.
35. Maertens J, Patterson T, Rahav G, et al. A phase 3 randomized, double-blind trial evaluating isavuconazole versus voriconazole for the primary treatment of invasive fungal infections caused by *Aspergillus* spp. and other filamentous fungi. ECCMID 2014, Barcelona Spain, Oral presentation O230a.
36. Viscoli C, Herbrecht R, Akan H, Baila L, et al. An EORTC Phase II study of caspofungin as first-line therapy of invasive aspergillosis in haematological patients. J Antimicrob Chemother. 2009;64(6):1274–1281.
37. Marr K, Schlamm H, Rottinghaus S, Jagannatha S et al. A randomised, double-blind study of combination antifungal therapy with voriconazole and anidulafungin versus voriconazole monotherapy for primary treatment of invasive aspergillosis. ECCMID 2012, London, England. Abstract LB2812.
38. Cornely OA, Maertens J, Winston DJ, et al. Posaconazole vs. fluconazole or itraconazole prophylaxis in patients with neutropenia. N Engl J Med. 2007;356(4):348–359.
39. Ullmann AJ, Lipton JH, Vesole DH, et al. Posaconazole or fluconazole for prophylaxis in severe graft-versus-host disease. N Engl J Med. 2007;356(4):335–347.

85 Antimicrobial Prophylaxis in Surgery

Mary A. Ullman and John C. Rotschafer

LEARNING OBJECTIVES

Upon completion of the chapter, the reader will be able to:

1. Describe the impact of surgical site infections (SSIs) on patient outcomes and health care costs.
2. Name and differentiate the four different types of wound classifications.
3. Recognize at least three risk factors for postoperative SSIs.
4. Identify likely pathogens associated with different surgical operations.
5. Compare and contrast antimicrobials used for surgical prophylaxis and identify potential advantage and disadvantages for each antimicrobial.
6. Discuss the importance of β-lactam allergy screening and how this could impact resistance and health care costs.
7. Identify nonantimicrobial methods that can reduce the risk of postoperative infection.
8. Discuss the importance of antimicrobial timing, duration, and redosing in relation to antimicrobial prophylaxis in surgery.
9. Recommend appropriate prophylactic antimicrobial(s) given a surgical operation.

INTRODUCTION

KEY CONCEPT *Surgical site infections (SSIs) are a significant cause of morbidity and mortality.* Approximately 2% to 5% of patients undergoing clean extra-abdominal operations and 20% undergoing intra-abdominal operations will develop an SSI.[1] SSIs have become the second most common cause of nosocomial infection, and these data are likely underestimated due to a large number of surgical procedures being performed on an outpatient basis.[1,2]

SSIs negatively affect patient outcomes and increase health care costs. Patients who develop SSIs are five times more likely to be readmitted to the hospital and have twice the mortality of patients who do not develop an SSI.[1] A patient with an SSI is also 60% more likely to be admitted to an ICU.[1] SSIs lengthen hospital stays and increase costs.[1,3,4] Deep SSIs, involving organs or spaces, result in longer durations of hospital stay and higher costs compared with incisional SSIs.[5] Additionally, since 2008, Medicare and Medicaid Services no longer reimburses hospitals for any cost incurred from treating certain hospital-acquired infections, including SSIs.[6]

SSIs are defined and reported according to Centers for Disease Control and Prevention (CDC) criteria.[5] SSIs are classified as either incisional or organ/space. Incisional SSIs are further divided into superficial incisional SSI (skin or subcutaneous tissue) and deep incisional SSI (deeper soft tissues of the incision). Organ/space SSIs involve any anatomic site other than the incised areas (eg, meningitis after brain tumor removal). An infection is considered an SSI if any of the above criteria is met and the infection occurs within 30 days of the operation. If a prosthetic is implanted during the operation, the timeline extends out to 1 year.

EPIDEMIOLOGY AND ETIOLOGY

Risk factors for SSIs can be divided into two categories: patient and operative characteristics.[5,7,8] Patient risk factors for SSI include age, comorbid disease states (especially chronic lung disease and diabetes), malnutrition, immunosuppression, nicotine or steroid use, and colonization of the nares with *Staphylococcus aureus*. Modifying risk factors prior to planned operations may decrease the threat of SSI.

Operative characteristics are based on the actions of both the patient and the operating staff. Shaving of the surgical site prior to operating can produce microscopic lacerations and increase the chance of SSI and is, therefore, not accepted as a method of hair removal.[5] Maintaining aseptic technique and proper sterilization of medical equipment is effective in preventing SSI. Surgical staff should wash their hands thoroughly. In clean operations, most bacterial inoculums introduced postoperatively are generally small. However, subsequent patient contact between contaminated areas (such as the nares or rectum) and the surgical site can lead to SSI. Finally, the appropriate use of antimicrobial prophylaxis can have a significant impact on decreasing SSIs.

PATHOPHYSIOLOGY

Prophylaxis Versus Treatment

Properly identifying the site of an infection is important when using antimicrobial prophylaxis in surgery. Antimicrobial prophylaxis begins with the premise that no infection exists but that during the operation there can be a low-level inoculum of bacteria introduced into the body. However, if sufficient antimicrobial concentrations are present, bacteria can be controlled without infection developing. This is the case when surgery is done under controlled conditions, there are no major breaks in sterile technique or spillage of GI contents, and perforation or damage to the surgical site is absent. An example would be an elective hysterectomy done with optimal surgical technique.

If an infection is already present, or presumed to be present, then antimicrobial use is for treatment, not prophylaxis, and the goal is to resolve the infection. This is the case when there is spillage of GI contents, gross damage or perforation is already present, or the tissue being operated on is actively infected (pus is present and cultures are positive). An example would be a patient undergoing surgery for a ruptured appendix with diffuse peritonitis.

KEY CONCEPT *The distinction between prophylaxis and treatment influences the choice of antimicrobial and duration of therapy.* Appropriate antimicrobial selection, dosing, and duration of therapy differ significantly between these two situations. A regimen for antimicrobial prophylaxis ideally involves one agent and lasts less than 24 hours. Treatment regimens can involve multiple antimicrobials with durations lasting weeks to months depending on desired antimicrobial coverage and the surgical site.

Types of Surgical Operations

KEY CONCEPT *Surgical operations are classified at the time of operation as clean, clean-contaminated, contaminated, or dirty.* Antimicrobial prophylaxis is appropriate for clean, clean-contaminated, and contaminated operations. Dirty operations take place in situations of existing infection and antimicrobials are used for treatment, not prophylaxis (Table 85–1).

Microbiology

KEY CONCEPT *Appropriate prophylactic antimicrobial selection relies on anticipating which organisms will be encountered during the operation.* SSIs associated with extra-abdominal operations are the result of skin flora organisms in nearly all cases. These organisms include gram-positive cocci, with *S. aureus* and *Staphylococcus epidermidis* being among the most frequently isolated SSI pathogens[5,6,9] (Table 85–2). *Streptococcus* spp. may also be implicated.

Intra-abdominal operations involve a diverse flora with the potential for polymicrobial SSIs. *Escherichia coli* make up a large portion of bowel flora and are frequently isolated as pathogens.[5,6] Other enteric gram-negative bacteria, as well as anaerobes (especially *Bacteroides* spp.), may be encountered during intra-abdominal operations.

Candida albicans continues to be an increasing cause of SSIs.[6] Increased use of broad-spectrum antimicrobials and

Table 85–2

Major Pathogens in Surgical Wound Infections[9]

Pathogen	Percentage of Infections
Staphylococcus aureus	30.4
Coagulase-negative Staphylococci	11.7
Escherichia coli	9.4
Enterococcus faecalis	5.9
Pseudomonas aeruginosa	5.5
Streptococcus spp.	4.9
Enterobacter spp.	4
Klebsiella (pneumonia/oxytoca)	4
Enterococcus spp.	3.2
Proteus spp.	3.2
Enterococcus faecium	2.5
Serratia spp.	1.8
Candida albicans	1.3
Acinetobacter baumannii	0.5

Table 85–1

National Red Cross Wound Classification, Risk of SSI, and Antimicrobial Indication

Classification	Description	SSI Risk	Antimicrobial Prophylaxis
Clean	No acute inflammation or transection of GI, oropharyngeal, GU, biliary, or respiratory tracts; elective case, no technique break	Low	Indicated
Clean-contaminated	Controlled opening of aforementioned tracts with minimal spillage or minor technique break; clean procedures performed emergently or with major technique breaks	Medium	Indicated
Contaminated	Acute, nonpurulent inflammation present; major spillage or technique break during clean-contaminated procedures	High	Indicated
Dirty	Obvious preexisting infection present (abscess, pus, or necrotic tissue present)	—	Not indicated; antimicrobials used for treatment

GU, genitourinary.
Data from Refs. 7 and 11.

rising prevalence of immunocompromised and human immunodeficiency virus-infected individuals are factors in fungal SSIs. Despite this increase, antifungal prophylaxis for surgery is not currently recommended.

Choosing an Antibiotic

Ideal criteria for an antimicrobial in surgical prophylaxis include the following:

- Spectrum that covers expected pathogens
- Inexpensive
- Parenteral
- Easy to use
- Minimal adverse-event potential
- Longer half-life to minimize need for redosing during procedure

Operations can be separated into two basic categories: extra-abdominal and intra-abdominal. SSIs resulting from extra-abdominal operations are frequently caused by gram-positive aerobes. Thus an antimicrobial with strong gram-positive coverage is useful. Cefazolin provides a benign adverse-event profile, simple dosing, and low cost, making cefazolin the mainstay for surgical prophylaxis of extra-abdominal procedures. For patients with a β-lactam allergy, clindamycin or vancomycin can be used as an alternative.

Intra-abdominal operations necessitate broad-spectrum coverage of gram-negative organisms and anaerobes. Antianaerobic cephalosporins, cefoxitin and cefotetan, are widely used. Fluoroquinolones or aminoglycosides, paired with clindamycin or metronidazole, should provide adequate coverage for intra-abdominal operations; these regimens are recommended as appropriate regimens for use in patients with β-lactam allergies.

Guidelines do not recommend routine use of vancomycin for surgical procedures.[10,11] Vancomycin should be considered when a cluster of methicillin-resistant *S. aureus* (MRSA) or coagulase-negative staphylococci have been identified. Additionally, vancomycin is appropriate to use in patients with known MRSA colonization or at high risk for MRSA colonization. However, vancomycin use in institutions where MRSA rates are "high" may not translate into a lower incidence of SSI. The incidence of SSI for patients on cefazolin or vancomycin did not differ despite a high MRSA rate at the study institution.[12] However, patients who received cefazolin were more likely to develop an SSI due to MRSA.[11] The increasing prevalence of community-associated methicillin-resistant *S. aureus* (CA-MRSA) in patients admitted to the hospital creates an added concern, although this pathogen is often sensitive to clindamycin. Responsibility for determining appropriate use of vancomycin falls on each institution and interpretation of institutional resistance data.

Newer antimicrobials may be alternative agents for surgical prophylaxis, especially as drug shortages limit availability of routinely used antimicrobials. Ertapenem was superior to standard cefotetan in the prevention of SSIs after elective colorectal surgery.[13] However, the ertapenem treatment group had a larger proportion of *Clostridium difficile* infections than those in the cefotetan treatment group. Ertapenem has been included as an approved antimicrobial for colon surgery.[10] At this time, it is not considered appropriate to routinely use newer antimicrobials for surgical prophylaxis; overuse of these antimicrobials may contribute to **collateral damage** and the development of bacterial resistance.

β-Lactam Allergy

Allergy to β-lactam antimicrobials such as penicillin is one of the most common reported drug allergies. Concerns over cross-reactivity between antimicrobials may limit the use of β-lactams for surgical prophylaxis. KEY CONCEPT *A thorough drug allergy history should be taken to discern true allergy (eg, anaphylaxis) from medication intolerance (eg, upset stomach).* Allergy testing may be helpful in confirming penicillin allergy and could spare vancomycin. However, practitioners should be aware that penicillin allergy testing may be difficult to perform due to the removal of a major component (penicilloyl-polylysine) of the testing from the commercial market.[14] If a practitioner desires to perform allergy testing, the individual reagents required for penicillin allergy testing must be prepared at the health care facility, on a case-by-case basis. Cross-allergenicity between penicillins and cephalosporins is low. The increased risk of cephalosporin allergy in patients with a history of penicillin allergy may be as low as 0.4% for first-generation cephalosporins and nearly zero for second- and third-generation agents.[14] Other studies also found the risk of cross-reactivity to be very low.[16] However, in the case of severe penicillin allergy (anaphylaxis), cephalosporins should be avoided.

Alternative Methods to Decrease SSI

Several nonantimicrobial methods have been studied for reducing the risk of SSI.[18–34] Supplemental warming of patients (36.7°C [98.0°F]) during the intraoperative period reduced infection rates compared with control patients (34.7°C [94.5°F]).[19] Intensive glucose control (maintaining blood glucose to 80–110 mg/dL [4.4–6.1 mmol/L]) versus conventional control (blood glucose < 220 mg/dL [12.2 mmol/L]) reduced operative site infections and improved outcomes in cardiac patients who received intensive insulin control in the ICU after surgery.[20] Also, patients randomized to 80% (0.80) inspired oxygen had lower SSI rates compared with patients on 30% (0.30) oxygen after colorectal resection.[21] Despite these findings, there are insufficient data to make definitive recommendations on the use of these approaches.

Alternative topical routes of antimicrobial prophylaxis such as antimicrobial-impregnated bone cement, implantable antimicrobial collage sponges, antimicrobial irrigations, and topical administration of antimicrobial powders have not been well studied. Studies demonstrating an advantage often lack rigorous design and only show superiority when compared to placebo.[10,20–21] Irrigation with detergent solutions, rather than antimicrobials, appears to provide the same results but with less wound-healing problems encountered with antimicrobial irrigation.[25] Confounding this issue is the lack of standards for topical administration routes. An array of drugs, from aminoglycosides to macrolides, is used in these preparations. Some bone cements are produced commercially, whereas others are made in the operating room. The long-term durability of impregnated cements is also unknown, as the addition of antimicrobials may reduce the tensile strength of bone cement. Irrigation solutions may be compounded in the surgical suites and result in variable concentrations. High concentrations can results in local irritation, systemic absorption, and toxicity. Alternatively, low concentrations can contribute to the development of resistant organisms may occur. Further study is required before topical administration is recommended for use in surgical prophylaxis.

With the increase of CA-MRSA, increased importance has been placed on screening for *S. aureus*, especially MRSA and **decolonization**. Surgical patients with nasal colonization of

S. aureus have a higher risk of an SSI due to *S. aureus*, and decolonization leads to a lower incidence of SSIs.[25–27] Guidelines endorse the use of mupirocin for *S. aureus* decolonization, especially in cardiac and orthopedic surgery. The most studied approach to eradication of methicillin-sensitive *S. aureus* (MSSA) and/or MRSA has been mupirocin applied to the anterior nares for 5 days prior to surgery.[10,30] Additionally, skin decolonization with 4% chlorhexidine for 5 days prior to surgery has also been recommended. Although decolonization of the anterior nares is the most common and most studied, some controversy exists because patients may be colonized elsewhere (rectum, throat, vagina, etc) and often do not receive complete decolonization.[30] Furthermore, decolonization usually does not lead to lifelong eradication. Other drugs, both topical and systemic, have been studied for decolonization/eradication of MRSA, but a review of randomized controlled trials for the eradication of MRSA found insufficient evidence for the use of any agent for eradication of MRSA.[31] A significantly lower incidence of infections was demonstrated in surgical patients who were nasal colonized with *S. aureus* and completed a 5-day treatment of intranasal mupirocin twice daily and chlorhexidine wash daily. Although no MRSA infections were noted in the patients included in this study, the authors suggest that this treatment strategy would be beneficial in MRSA-colonized patients as long as those strains were susceptible to mupirocin. Although MRSA screening has gained more acceptance, less than 10% of centers screen for mupirocin and/or chlorhexidine resistance.[10,33] Mupirocin resistance rates have varied from 1.9% to 5.6% of *S. aureus* isolates.[34] Further studies are needed to elucidate this area of surgical prophylaxis, including cost-effectiveness.

Principles of Antimicrobial Prophylaxis

▶ *Route of Administration*

IV antimicrobial administration is the most common delivery method for surgical prophylaxis. IV administration ensures complete bioavailability while minimizing the impact of patient-specific variables. Oral administration is also used in some bowel operations. Nonabsorbable compounds such as erythromycin base and neomycin are given during the 24 hours prior to surgery to reduce microbial concentrations in the bowel. Note that oral agents are used adjunctively and do not replace IV agents.

▶ *Timing of First Dose*

KEY CONCEPT *For prevention of SSIs, correct timing of antimicrobial administration is imperative so as to allow the persistence of therapeutic concentrations in the blood and wound tissues during the entire course of the operation.* The National Surgical Infection Prevention Project recommends infusing antimicrobials for surgical prophylaxis within 60 minutes of the first incision. Exceptions to this rule are fluoroquinolones and vancomycin, which can be infused 120 minutes prior to avoid infusion-related reactions.[1] No consensus has been reached on whether the infusion should be complete prior to the first incision. However, if a proximal tourniquet is used, antimicrobial administration should be complete prior to inflation.

Administration of the intravenous antimicrobial should begin as close to the first incision as possible. This is important for antimicrobials with short half-lives so that therapeutic concentrations are maintained during the operation and reduce the need for redosing. Beginning the antimicrobial infusion after the first incision is of little value in preventing SSI. Administration of the antimicrobial after the first incision had SSI rates similar to patients who did not receive prophylaxis.[35]

▶ *Dosing and Redosing*

KEY CONCEPT *The goal of antimicrobial dosing for surgical prophylaxis is to optimize the pharmacodynamic parameter of the selected agent against the suspected organism for the duration of the operation.* Dosing recommendations can vary between institutions and guidelines. Clinical judgment should be exercised regarding dose modifications for renal function, age, and especially weight. Obese patients often require higher antimicrobial doses than do nonobese patients. The newest guidelines recommended higher doses of cefazolin based on population pharmacokinetic/pharmacodynamics data: 2 g for all patients less than 120 kg; 3g for patients more than or equal to 120 kg.[10] Clindamycin should be given as a 900-mg preoperative intravenous dose[10].

If an operation exceeds two half-lives of the selected antimicrobial, then another dose should be administered.[1,10] Repeat dosing reduces rates of SSI. For example, cefazolin has a half-life of about 2 hours, thus another dose should be given if the operation exceeds 4 hours. The clinician should have extra doses of antimicrobial ready in case an operation lasts longer than planned.

▶ *Duration*

The National Surgical Infection Prevention Project and published evidence suggest that the continuation of antimicrobial prophylaxis beyond wound closure is unnecessary.[1,10] KEY CONCEPT *The duration of antimicrobial prophylaxis should not exceed 24 hours (48 hours for cardiac surgery); additional doses of antimicrobial past this time point do not demonstrate added benefits.* Antimicrobial prophylaxis does not need to be continued until all drains and catheters have been removed. Longer durations of antimicrobial prophylaxis are advocated by some guidelines and will be discussed later.

PROPHYLAXIS REGIMENS

Antimicrobial Prophylaxis in Specific Surgical Procedures

▶ *Gynecologic and Obstetric*

- Possible pathogens: enteric gram-negative bacilli, anaerobes, group B streptococci, enterococci
- Prophylaxis for hysterectomy: cefazolin, cefotetan, cefoxitin, ampicillin-sulbactam
  - Alternatives for β-lactam allergy: clindamycin or vancomycin combined with aminoglycoside, aztreonam, or fluoroquinolone; metronidazole combined with aminoglycoside or fluoroquinolone
- Prophylaxis for Cesarean section: cefazolin
  - Alternatives for β-lactam allergy: clindamycin and aminoglycoside

Cesarean sections are stratified into low- and high-risk groups. Patients who undergo emergency operations or have cesarean sections after the rupture of membranes and/or onset of labor are considered high risk. Prophylactic antimicrobials are most beneficial for high-risk patients but are used in both groups. Antimicrobials should not be administered until after the first incision and the umbilical cord has been clamped. This practice prevents potentially harmful antimicrobial concentrations from reaching the newborn.

Table 85–3

Recommended Regimens for Antimicrobial Prophylaxis of Specific Surgical Procedures[a]

Type of Operation	Recommended Prophylaxis Regimen *(Duration is for a total of 24 hours unless specified)*	Alternative Regimen for β-Lactam Allergy *(Duration is for a total of 24 hours unless specified)*
Vascular	Cefazolin 2–3 g[b] IV every 8 hours	Clindamycin 900 mg IV every 6–8 hours *or* vancomycin 15 mg/kg every 8–12 hours
Neurosurgery	Cefazolin 2–3 g[b] IV every 8 hours	Clindamycin 900 mg IV every 6–8 hours *or* vancomycin 15 mg/kg IV every 8–12 hours
Head and neck (clean with prosthesis placement excluding tympanostomy tubes)	Cefazolin 2–3 g[b] IV every 8 hours *or* cefuroxime 1.5 g every 8 hours	Clindamycin 900 mg IV every 6–8 hours
Head and neck (clean-contaminated)	(Cefuroxime 1.5 g every 8 hours and metronidazole 500 mg every 8 hours) *or* amipicillin-sulbactam 3 g every 6 hours	Clindamycin 900 mg IV every 6–8 hours
Urologic (clean)	Cefazolin 2–3 g[b] IV × 1	Clindamycin 900 mg IV × 1 *or* vancomycin 15 mg/kg × 1
Urologic (lower tract instrumentation with risk factors for infection, transrectal prostate biopsy)	Ciprofloxacin 400 mg IV × 1 *or* levofloxacin 500 mg IV × 1 *or* trimethoprim-sulfamethoxazole *or* cefazolin 2–3 g[b] × 1	Gentamicin 5 mg/kg × 1 with or without clindamycin 900 mg × 1
Cesarean section	Cefazolin 2–3 g[b] IV × 1	See hysterectomy
Hysterectomy	Cefazolin 2–3 g[b] IV × 1 *or* cefotetan 2 g × 1 *or* cefoxitin 2 g × 1 *or* ampicillin-sulbactam 3 g × 1	(Clindamycin 900 mg × 1 or vancomycin 15 mg/kg × 1) and (gentamicin 5 mg/kg × 1 or aztreonam 2 g *or* ciprofloxacin 400 mg *or* levofloxacin 500 mg)
Gastroduodenal (high-risk only: obstruction, acid suppression, morbid obesity, hemorrhage, malignancy)	Cefazolin 2–3 g[b] IV × 1	(Clindamycin 900 mg × 1 *or* vancomycin 15 mg/kg × 1) and (gentamicin 5 mg/kg × 1 *or* aztreonam 2 g *or* ciprofloxacin 400 mg *or* levofloxacin 500 mg)
Biliary tract (open procedure or high-risk laprascopic only: age > 70 years, acute cholecystitis, obstructive jaundice, duct stones, nonfunctioning gallbladder)	Cefazolin 2–3 g[b] IV × 1 *or* cefotetan 2 g × 1 *or* cefoxitin 2 g × 1 *or* ceftriaxone 2 g × 1 *or* ampicillin-sulbactam 3 g × 1	[(Clindamycin 900 mg × 1 *or* vancomycin 15 mg/kg × 1] and gentamicin 5 mg/kg × 1 *or* aztreonam 2 g *or* ciprofloxacin 400 mg *or* levofloxacin 500 mg)] or ([metronidazole 500 mg × 1 AND [gentamicin 5 mg/kg × 1 *or* ciprofloxacin 400 mg *or* levofloxacin 500 mg])
Colorectal	[c]Oral: neomycin 1 g plus erythromycin base 1 g (give 19, 18, and 9 hours prior to procedure)	
	IV: (Cefazolin 2–3 g[b] × 1 and metronidazole 500 mg × 1) *or* cefoxitin 2 g × 1 *or* cefotetan 2 g × 1 *or* ampicillin-sulbactam 3 g × 1 *or* (ceftriaxone 2 g × 1 AND metronidazole 500 mg × 1) *or* ertapenem 1 g × 1	See biliary tract
Appendectomy	Cefoxitin 2 g IV × 1; cefotetan 2 g IV × 1; cefazolin 2–3g[b] × 1 and metronidazole 500 mg × 1	Metronidazole 0.5–1 g IV *plus* gentamicin 1.5 mg/kg IV × 1
Orthopedic	Cefazolin 2–3 g[b] IV every 8 hours	Vancomycin 15 mg/kg every 8–12 hours *or* clindamycin 900 mg every 6–8 hours
Cardiothoracic	Cefazolin 2–3 g[b] IV every 8 hours for a total of 48 hours *or* cefuroxime 1.5 g IV every 12 hours for a total of 48 hours	Vancomycin 15 mg/kg every 8–12 hours for a total of 48 hours *or* clindamycin 900 mg every 6–8 hours for a total of 48 hours

[a]Dosing recommendations are based on common clinical doses for adult patients with normal renal function; dosing for individual patients and institutions may vary.
[b]3 g dose for weight more than or equal to 120 kg.
[c]Oral regimens should be used in conjunction with IV prophylaxis.

Data from Refs. 10, 11, and 15.

► Orthopedic Surgery

- Possible pathogens: gram-positive cocci, mostly staphylococci
- Prophylaxis for total joint arthroplasty (hip or knee): cefazolin
  - Alternatives for β-lactam allergy: clindamycin, vancomycin

Antimicrobial-impregnated bone cement can be useful in lowering infection rates in orthopedic surgery but has not been approved for prophylaxis.

► Cardiothoracic and Vascular Surgery

- Possible pathogens: gram-positive cocci, mostly staphylococci
- Prophylaxis for cardiac surgeries: cefazolin, cefuroxime
- Prophylaxis for noncardiac thoracic surgeries: cefazolin, ampicillin-sulbactam
- Prophylaxis for vascular surgeries: cefazolin
- For all cardiothoracic and vascular surgeries alternatives for β-lactam allergy: clindamycin, vancomycin

Debate exists on the duration of antimicrobial prophylaxis for cardiothoracic operations. SSIs are rare after cardiothoracic operations, but the potentially devastating consequences lead some clinicians to support longer periods of prophylaxis. The National Surgical Infection Prevention Project cites data that extending prophylaxis beyond 24 hours does not decrease SSI rates and may increase bacterial resistance.[1,10] However, the Society of Thoracic Surgeons issued practice guidelines in 2006 to extend the duration of antimicrobials to 48 hours following cardiac surgeries.[37] Duration of therapy should be based on patient factors and risk of development of an SSI.

► Colorectal Surgery

- Possible pathogens: gram-positive, gram-negative, and anaerobic organisms

Patient Encounter Part 1

RP is a 61-year-old woman with a history of rectal bleeding and recent diagnosis of sigmoid colon cancer. She presents today for a colon resection (colorectal surgery). She has a history of nausea with cephalexin. You have been asked for recommendation for surgical prophylaxis.

VS: BP 127/83 mm Hg, HR 63 beats/min, RR 21 breaths/min, T 98.6°F (37.0°C), Ht 62′ (157 cm), Wt 186 lb (84.5 kg)

Labs: WBC 7 × 10³ mm³ (7 × 10⁹/L), serum creatinine 0.7 mg/dL (62 μmol/L), glucose 95 mg/dL (5.3 mmol/L)

What organisms are likely to be encountered for this operation and why?

What agents need to be avoided considering this patient's previous reaction with cephalosporins?

What drug would you choose for this operation and why?

The surgeon agrees with your decision and wants to begin infusing the antimicrobial 3 hours prior to the first incision. Comment on this.

What other interventions besides antimicrobial use could prove useful in lowering RP's risk of SSI?

Patient Encounter Part 2

RP is transferred to the oncology ward after completion of her surgery. In the procedure notes, the surgeon notes that part of the small bowel was nicked and possible intra-abdominal contamination may have occurred.

Does this patient still require surgical site prophylaxis?

The surgeon asks for your opinion for which antimicrobial the patient should receive. Which antimicrobial do you recommend?

How long should this patient remain on antimicrobials?

- Parenteral prophylaxis: cefazolin and metronidazole; cefoxitin; cefotetan; ampicillin-sulbactam; ceftriaxone and metronidazole; ertapenem
  - Alternatives for β-lactam allergy: clindamycin combined with aminoglycoside, aztreonam, or fluoroquinolone; metronidazole combined with aminoglycoside or fluoroquinolone

Oral routes for prophylaxis include the combination of neomycin with either erythromycin or metronidazole and are administered at 19, 18, and 9 hours prior to surgery. These oral routes should be given with mechanical bowel preparation. For most patients, this oral regimen should be combined with a parenteral regimen.

Appendectomy is one of the most common intra-abdominal operations. Antimicrobial prophylaxis used for appendectomy is similar to that used for colorectal regimens. In the case of ruptured appendix, antimicrobials are used for treatment, not prophylaxis.

OUTCOME EVALUATION

The clinician should consistently follow up postoperative patients and screen for any sign of SSI. KEY CONCEPT *According to CDC criteria, SSIs may appear up to 30 days after an operation and up to 1 year if a prosthesis is implanted.*[5] This period often extends beyond hospitalization, so educate patients on warning signs of SSI and be encouraged to contact a clinician immediately if necessary. The presence of fever or leukocytosis in the immediate postoperative

Patient Encounter Part 3

RP was treated appropriately for her surgical complications based on your recommendations following her surgery. She presents to a 3-week follow-up appointment to the surgical clinic. She notes that her wound site has been increasing in redness over the past 1 to 2 days, accompanied by a slight discharge that started this morning prior to the clinic visit.

VS: BP 104/78 mm Hg, P 82 beats/min, RR 21 breaths/min, T 101.7°F (38.7°C)

Labs: WBC 19 × 10³/mm³ (19 × 10⁹/L) serum creatinine 1.4 mg/dL (124 μmol/L)

Based on the available data, does RP have an SSI?

What further steps should be taken in regard to this possible SSI?

Patient Care Process

Patient Assessment:
- Conduct thorough medication history.
- Obtain serum creatinine and weight.
- Document allergies and the type of reaction.

Therapy Evaluation:
- Consider penicillin allergy testing in patients with unclear documentation of penicillin allergy.
- Document type of operation patient is to receive.
- Start antimicrobials within 1 hour of surgical incision (2 hours for vancomycin, fluoroquinolones).

Care Plan Development:
- Monitor patient for signs of allergic reaction.
- Document any major breaks in surgical technique and adjust length of antimicrobial therapy if surgical classification changes.

Follow-Up Evaluation:
- Monitor for signs and symptoms of postoperative infection (30 days postoperation, up to 1 year if prosthesis involved).
- Draw cultures to further guide therapy if SSI suspected.

period does not constitute SSI and should resolve with proper patient care. Distal infections, such as pneumonia, are not considered SSIs even if these infections occur in the 30-day period. Check the appearance of the surgical site regularly and document any changes (eg, erythema, drainage, or pus). The presence of pus or other signs suggestive of SSI must be treated accordingly. Any wound requiring incision and drainage is considered an SSI regardless of appearance. Collect prompt cultures and initiate appropriate antimicrobial therapy to reduce any chance of morbidity and mortality.

Abbreviations Introduced in This Chapter

ASHP	American Society of Health-System Pharmacists
CA-MRSA	Community-associated methicillin-resistant *Staphylococcus aureus*
MIC	Minimum inhibitory concentration
MRSA	Methicillin-resistant *Staphylococcus aureus*
MSSA	Methicillin-sensitive *Staphylococcus aureus*
NNIS	National Nosocomial Infections Surveillance System
SSI	Surgical site infection

REFERENCES

1. Bratzler DW, Houck PM; Surgical Infection Prevention Guideline Writers Workgroup. Antimicrobial prophylaxis for surgery: An advisory statement from the National Surgical Infection Prevention Project. Am J Surg. 2005;189:395–404.
2. Barie PS, Eachempati SR. Surgical site infections. Surg Clin North Am. 2005;85:1115–1135.
3. Kirkland KB, Briggs JP, Trivette SL, et al. The impact of surgical site infections in the 1990s: Attributable mortality, excess length of hospitalization, and extra costs. Infect Control Hosp Epidemiol. 1999;20:725–730.
4. Hollenbeak CS, Murphy D, Dunagan WC, et al. Nonrandom selection and the attributable cost of surgical-site infections. Infect Control Hosp Epidemiol. 2002;23:174–176.
5. Mangram AJ, Horan TC, Pearson ML, et al. Guideline for prevention of surgical site infection, 1999. Infect Control Hosp Epidemiol. 1999;20:247–266.
6. Department of Health and Human Services: Centers for Medicare & Medicaid Services. Medicare Program; Changes to the Hospital Inpatient Prospective Payment Systems and Fiscal Year 2008; Final Rule. Federal Register 2007;72:47200–47206.
7. Dionigi R, Rovera F, Dionigi G, et al. Risk factors in surgery. J Chemother. 2001;13:6–11.
8. Pessaux P, Atallah D, Lermite E, et al. Risk factors for prediction of surgical site infections in "clean surgery." Am J Infect Control. 2005;33:292–298.
9. Sievert DM, Ricks P, Edwards JR, et al. Antimicrobial-resistant pathogens associated with healthcare-associated infections: Summary of data reported to the National Healthcare Safety Network at the Centers for Disease Control and Preventions. Infect Control Hosp Epidemiol. 2013;34:1–14.
10. Bratzler DW, Dellinger EP, Olsen KM, et al. Clinical Practice Guidelines for Antmicrobial Prophylaxis in Surgery. Am J Health System Pharm. 2013;70:195–283.
11. Devlin JW, Kanji S, Janning SW, et al. Antimicrobial prophylaxis in surgery. In: DiPiro JT, Talbert RL, Yee GC, et al. Pharmacotherapy: A Pathophysiologic Approach. 5th ed. New York: McGraw-Hill; 2002:2111–2122.
12. Finkelstein R, Rabino G, Mashiah T, et al. Vancomycin versus cefazolin prophylaxis for cardiac surgery in the setting of a high prevalence of methicillin-resistant staphylococcal infections. J Thorac Cardiovasc Surg. 2002;123:326–332.
13. Itanu KMF, Wilson SE, Awad SS, et al. Ertapenem versus cefotetan prophylaxis in elective colorectal surgery. N Engl J Med. 2006;355:2640–2651.
14. Schafer JA, Mateo N, Parlier GL, Rotschater JC. Penicillin allergy skin testing: What do we do know? Pharmacotherapy. 2007;27: 542–545.
15. Pichichero ME. A review of evidence supporting the American Academy of Pediatrics recommendation for prescribing cephalosporin antibiotics for penicillin-allergic patients. Pediatrics. 2005;115:1048–1057.
16. Apter AJ, Kinman JL, Bilker WB, et al. Is there cross-reactivity between penicillins and cephalosporins? Am J Med. 2006;119: 354.e11–e20.
17. Weed HG. Antimicrobial prophylaxis in the surgical patient. Med Clin North Am. 2003;87:59–75.
18. Anderson DJ, Kaye KS, Classen D, et al. Strategies to prevent surgical site infections in acute care hospitals. Infect Control Hosp Epidemiol. 2018;29:S51–S61.
19. Kurz A, Sessler D, Lenhardt R. Perioperative normothermia to reduce the incidence of surgical-wound infection and shorten hospitalization. Study of Wound Infection and Temperature Group. N Engl J Med. 1996;334:1209–1215.
20. Ingels C, Debaveye Y, Milants I, et al. Strict blood glucose control with insulin during intensive care after cardiac surgery: Impact on 4-years survival, dependency on medical care, and quality of life. Eur Heart J. 2006;27(22):2716–2724.
21. Greif R, Akca O, Horn E, et al; Outcomes Research Group. Supplemental perioperative oxygen to reduce the incidence of surgical-wound infection. N Engl J Med. 2000;342:161–167.

22. Chiu FY, Chen CM, Lin CF, et al. Cefuroxime-impregnated cement in primary total knee arthroplasty. J Bone Joint Surg. 2002;84:759–762.
23. Joseph TN, Chen AL, Di Cesare PE. Use of antibiotic-impregnated cement in total joint arthroplasty. J Am Acad Orthop Surg. 2003; 11:38–47.
24. Fletcher N, Sofianos D, Berkes MB, Obremskey WT. Prevention of perioperative infection. J Bone Joint Surg Am. 2007;89: 1605–1618.
25. Wilcox MH, Hall J, Pike H, et al. Use of perioperative mupirocin to prevent methicillin-resistant *Staphylococcus aureus* (MRSA) orthopaedic surgical site infections. J Hosp Infect. 2003;54: 196–201.
26. Perl TM, Cullen JJ, Wenzel RP, et al. Intranasal mupirocin to prevent postoperative *Staphylococcus aureus* infections. N Engl J Med. 2002;346:1871–1877.
27. Munoz P, Hortal J, Giannella M, et al. Nasal carriage of *S. aureus* increases the risk of surgical site infection after major heart surgery. J Hosp Infect. 2008;68:25–31.
28. Coia JE, Duckworth GJ, Edwards DI, et al. Guidelines for the control and prevention of meticillin-resistant *Staphylococcus aureus* (MRSA) in healthcare facilities. J Hosp Infect. 2006;63: S1–S44.
29. Harbath S, Fankhauser C, Schrenzel J, et al. Universal screening for methicillin-resistant *Staphylococcus aureus* at hospital admission and noscomial infection in surgical patients. JAMA. 2008;299: 1149–1157.
30. Loveday HP, Pellowe CM, Jones SRLJ, Pratt RJ. A systematic review of the evidence for interventions for the prevention and control of meticillin-resistant *Staphylococcus aureus* (1996–2004): Report to the Joint MRSA Working Party (Subgroup A). J Hosp Infect. 2006;63:S45–S70.
31. Loeb M, Main C, Walker-Dilks C, Eady A. Antimicrobial drugs for treating methicillin-resistant *Staphylococcus aureus* colonization. Cochrane Database Syst Rev. 2003;CD003340.
32. Bode LGM, Kluytmans JAJW, Wertheim HFL, et al. Preventing surgical-site infections in nasal carriers of *Staphylococcus aureus*. N Engl J Med. 2010;362:9–17.
33. Diekema D, Johannsson B, Herwaldt, et al. Current practice in *Staphylococcus aureus* screening and decolonization. Infect Control Hosp Epidemiol. 2011;32:1042–1044.
34. Deshpande LM, Fix AM, Pfaller MA, et al. Emerging elevated mupirocin resistance rates among staphylococcal isolates in the SENTRY Antimicrobial Surveillance Program (2000): correlations of results from disk diffusion, Etest, and reference dilution methods. Diagn Microbiol Infect Dis. 2002;42:283–290.
35. Stone HH, Hooper CA, Kolb LD, et al. Antibiotic prophylaxis in gastric, biliary and colonic surgery. Ann Surg. 1976;184:443–452.
36. Forse RA, Karam B, MacLean LD, et al. Antibiotic prophylaxis for surgery in morbidly obese patients. Surgery. 1989;106:750–756.
37. Edwards FH, Engelman RM, Houck P, et al. The Soceity of Thoracic Surgeons practice guideline series: Antibiotic prophylaxis in cardiac surgery, part I: Duration. Ann Thorac Surg. 2006;81: 397–404.

86 Vaccines and Toxoids

Marianne Billeter

LEARNING OBJECTIVES

Upon completion of the chapter, the reader will be able to:

1. Define vaccination and immunization.
2. Recommend an immunization schedule for a child, including immunocompromised children.
3. Recommend an immunization schedule for an adult based on comorbid conditions and lifestyle choices.
4. Evaluate an adverse reaction and its probable association with a vaccine.

INTRODUCTION

The development and widespread use of vaccines is one of the greatest public health achievements of the 20th century. Other than safe drinking water, no other modality has had a greater impact on reducing mortality from infectious diseases.[1] The first accounts of deliberate inoculation to prevent disease date back as far as the 10th century. However, it wasn't until 1798 that Edward Jenner published his work on inoculation of natural cowpox as a means to prevent infection with smallpox that documented the first scientific attempt to prevent infection by inoculation. Since 1900, the widespread use of vaccines has resulted in the eradication of smallpox worldwide and wild-type poliovirus from the Western hemisphere. There have also been dramatic declines in the incidence of diphtheria, pertussis, tetanus, measles, mumps, rubella, and *Haemophilus influenzae* type b infections. In the United States, there are immunization recommendations against 17-vaccine preventable diseases affecting all age groups.

KEY CONCEPT *Vaccines have traditionally been preparations of killed or attenuated microorganisms that provide active immunity against a variety of viral and bacterial infections.* Most vaccines are designed to prevent acute infections that can be rapidly controlled and cleared by the immune system. Successful immunization involves activation of antigen-presenting cells with processing of the antigen by lysosomal or cytoplasmic pathways. T and B lymphocytes will be activated to replicate and differentiate to form large pools of memory cells for protection against subsequent exposure to the antigen.[2]

Vaccines against viral infections may be **attenuated** live viruses or inactivated viral particles. Attenuation may be accomplished by several methods to decrease the viruses' virulence while retaining their **immunogenicity**. Bacterial vaccines utilize antigenic particles of the outer membrane to elicit an immune response. KEY CONCEPT *Outer membrane polysaccharides are poorly immunogenic in children younger than 2 years* unless conjugated with a carrier protein. Also, bacterial toxins may undergo chemical treatment to render them nontoxic to form **toxoids** against infectious agents.

Often the terms *vaccination* and *immunization* are used interchangeably even though they are distinct concepts. Vaccination refers to the act of administering a vaccine, whereas immunization refers to the development of immunity to a pathogen. The delivery of a vaccine does not imply that the individual mounted an adequate immune response to the vaccine to elicit protection. However, immunization implies that the act of vaccination resulted in the development of protective immunity.

Herd immunity refers to high levels of immunization in one population, resulting in protection of another unvaccinated population. For example, concentrated vaccination of children with the pneumococcal conjugate vaccine resulted in decreased invasive *Streptococcus pneumoniae* infection not only in the vaccinated children, but also in elderly persons within the same community.

Cocoon immunization is a strategy used to immunize all persons surrounding another high-risk individual, such as vaccinating parents, siblings, and grandparents of a new infant who is too young to be vaccinated. This strategy is used to protect individuals who are not able to be vaccinated themselves.

THE ROUTINE VACCINES

Diphtheria, Tetanus, and Pertussis Vaccines

Diphtheria is a contagious bacterial respiratory infection characterized by membranous pharyngitis. The impact of diphtheria is not from the causative bacteria, *Corynebacterium diphtheriae*, but rather from complications attributed to its exotoxin, such as **myocarditis** and peripheral **neuritis**. Diphtheria is rarely reported in the United States since the introduction of vaccination with diphtheria toxoid; however, diphtheria continues to be a major problem in developing countries.

The tetanus vaccine differs from others in that it does not protect against a contagious disease such as diphtheria, but rather against an environmental pathogen. *Clostridium tetani* is widely found in the environment, especially in dirt and soils. Tetanus is rarely seen in developed countries.

Pertussis is a highly contagious respiratory tract infection caused by the bacteria *Bordetella pertussis*. Pertussis is characterized by a protracted severe cough with or without posttussive vomiting, whoop, difficulty breathing, difficulty sleeping, and rib fractures. It is often referred to as "whooping cough" or the 100-day cough.

▶ Use of Diphtheria, Tetanus, and Acellular Pertussis Vaccine

Diphtheria and tetanus toxoids and acellular pertussis vaccine should be administered in a five-shot series to all children beginning at 2 months of age. The shots are given at 2, 4, 6, and 15 to 18 months, and 4 to 6 years. Immunity to diphtheria, tetanus, and pertussis is achieved after the third vaccination.

▶ Use of Tetanus and Diphtheria Toxiod Vaccine

Immunity to tetanus and diphtheria wane with increasing age necessitating the need for booster doses every 10 years. The preferred agent to use in adults is tetanus and diphtheria toxoid in order to also give a booster for diphtheria. Tetanus immunization status should be assessed in the management of moderate and severe wounds or contaminated wounds in individuals seeking medical care. A tetanus booster should be administered if necessary.

▶ Use of Tetanus Toxiod, Reduced Diphtheria, and Acellular Pertussis Vaccine

Pertussis continues to be reported in adolescents and adults of all ages indicating a waning immunity following primary immunization. Additionally, adults with pertussis may infect young infants who have not received the first three doses of primary vaccination resulting in hospitalizations and death. A tetanus toxoid, reduced diphtheria toxoid, and acellular pertussis vaccine is recommended for use in adolescents and adults.

Tetanus toxoid, reduced diphtheria toxoid, and acellular pertussis vaccine should be administered to adolescents 11 through 18 years as a single booster. Ideally it should be given at 11 to 12 years of age. Tetanus toxoid, reduced diphtheria toxoid, and acellular pertussis vaccine is also recommended for adults 19 years and older as a single booster dose in individuals who have not already received it. This may be given as a routine vaccination or for wound management.[3]

Tetanus toxoid, reduced diphtheria toxoid, and acellular pertussis vaccine is also used as part of cocoon immunization strategy to protect young infants. The vaccine should be administered to pregnant women during the third trimester (27–36 weeks preferred) of each pregnancy in order for transfer of maternal antibodies to the newborn infant. Additionally, individuals with close contact to infants less than 12 months of age, such as fathers, grandparents, health care workers, and child care workers, should also be vaccinated. Tetanus toxoid, reduced diphtheria toxoid, and acellular pertussis vaccine may be given at any interval following a tetanus vaccine.[4]

Haemophilus Influenzae Type b Vaccine

H. influenzae is a bacterial respiratory pathogen that causes a wide spectrum of disease ranging from upper respiratory infections to bacterial meningitis. *H. influenzae* type b was the leading cause of invasive disease in children younger than 5 years. Approximately two-thirds of the cases were meningitis that resulted in a high degree of hearing loss among survivors.[5] Since the introduction of the vaccine, invasive disease due to *H. influenzae* type b has been nearly eliminated.

The *H. influenzae* type b vaccine is a protein conjugate that illicits T-lymphocyte-dependent immunity. The T-dependent antigens induce an enhanced immune response in younger children including infants. *H. influenzae* type b conjugate vaccine is a recommended routine childhood vaccination beginning at 2 months of age. There are currently three licensed monovalent *H. influenzae* type b conjugate vaccines and three combination vaccines containing *H. influenzae* type b conjugate. Each vaccine has a different dosing schedule and age range for use. Vaccine providers need to be aware of the brand being used and related dosing schedule. The immune response to *H. influenzae* type b is similar among the different vaccines. The different brands are interchangeable without affecting the primary immune response or booster response.[5]

A booster dose of *H. influenzae* type b vaccine is also recommended in adolescents and adults at high risk for becoming infected with *H. influenzae*. The currently available vaccines are labeled for pediatric use, but can be used in adults when vaccination is indicated.

H. influenzae type b and influenza vaccines have the potential for confusion and medication errors because of the similarity of the names. Care should be taken when ordering, dispensing, and administering these vaccines.

Hepatitis A Vaccine

Hepatitis A virus continues to be a frequent cause of illness despite the availability of a highly effective vaccine. Frequently, children younger than 6 years are asymptomatic with primary infection and play a pivotal role in spreading disease to adults. The economic burden of hepatitis A is greater than $300 million annually in combined direct and indirect costs. Widespread use of the Hepatitis A vaccine significantly decreases the disease burden caused by hepatitis A infection.[6]

Hepatitis A vaccine was licensed in the United States in 1995. It is an inactivated whole virus vaccine that is administered in a two-dose series. More than 94% of children, adolescents, and adults will have protective antibodies 1 month after receiving the first dose and 100% following the second dose. The hepatitis A vaccine is recommended for all children following the first birthday, with the second dose administered 6 months later. Adults who are at high risk for hepatitis A should receive two doses at least 6 months apart. High-risk adults include persons with clotting disorders or chronic liver disease, men who have sex with men, illicit drug users, and international travelers going to areas with high to intermediate endemicity of hepatitis A, persons with anticipated close contact with an international adoptee, or any other person who wishes to become immune.[6]

Hepatitis B Vaccine

Hepatitis B virus is transmitted following exposure to infected blood and body fluids. Individuals with chronic hepatitis B infection are at risk for cirrhosis, liver cancer, liver failure and death. Vaccination with hepatitis B vaccine is the most effective way to prevent hepatitis B infection.[7]

Hepatitis B vaccine is manufactured using recombinant DNA technology to express hepatitis B surface antigen (HBsAg) in yeast. Hepatitis B vaccine is available as a single component or in combination vaccines.

Hepatitis B vaccine is recommended for routine use in infants and children in a three-dose series. The first dose should be given prior to discharge following birth. The remaining two doses should be administered with other routine infant vaccinations during the first 6 months of life. The dosing schedule will depend on the use of single component or combination vaccines. Adolescents should receive the three-dose series if not previously vaccinated.[7]

Hepatitis B vaccine is recommended for adults at high risk for hepatitis B infection and those requesting protection from hepatitis B. The vaccine is administered in a three-dose series over 4 to 6 months.[8] Frequently, individuals do not follow through with the complete three-dose series and questions arise about restarting the series. Hepatitis B vaccine produces an amnesic response; therefore, the series may be continued at any time in order to complete the three doses.

Following vaccination with hepatitis B vaccine, hepatitis B virus serologic markers will remain negative, with the exception of antibody to hepatitis B surface antigen (anti-HBs), which will be positive indicating immunity. Persons with anti-HBs concentration greater than 10 mIU/mL (10 IU/L) after vaccination will have complete protection against acute and chronic infection.[8] There is no need for booster doses in immunocompetent individuals when anti-HBs concentrations fall below 10 mIU/mL (10 IU/L), since a good memory response will occur following exposure to hepatitis B virus. However, a booster dose may be warranted in immunocompromised individuals.

Human Papillomavirus Vaccine

Human papillomavirus (HPV) is the most common sexually transmitted virus and is associated with a wide range of diseases, including cervical cancer and genital warts. More than 150 HPVs have been identified and classified on their ability to cause malignant disease. HPV 16 and 18 are highly associated with causing cervical cancer, as well as anal, oropharyngeal, penile, vaginal, and vulval cancers. HPV 6 and 11 are associated with 90% of genital warts.

There are two HPV vaccines on the market. The bivalent vaccine is effective against HPV 16 and 18, while the quadravalent vaccine is effective against HPV 6, 11, 16, and 18. These vaccines are unique in that preventing infection by HPV will translate into prevention of cancer. Countries with high uptake of HPV vaccine have started to see declines in HPV infections and related diseases such as genital warts and high-grade cervical disease.[9]

HPV vaccination is recommended for females aged 11 or 12 in a three-dose series. Females aged 13 through 26 years should also be vaccinated if they have not previously received the full three-dose series. There is no preference to administering the bivalent or quadravalent vaccine in females.[10]

The HPV quadravalent vaccine is recommended for routine vaccination in males aged 11 or 12 years. Vaccination is also recommended for males 13 through 21 years who have not received the full three-dose series.[10]

The overall rate of HPV vaccination is low among 13 year olds, with 57% of girls and 34% of boys having initiated the HPV series in 2013. The main reasons cited for not vaccinating teens is related to knowledge gaps among clinicians and parents regarding recommendations for use and safety concerns. With over 68 million doses distributed, the adverse event profile is similar to other vaccines administered to adolescents.[10]

Influenza Vaccine

Influenza is a contagious viral respiratory infection that usually occurs during the winter months in the Northern Hemisphere and all year round in the Southern Hemisphere. All age groups are affected by influenza; however, children have the highest rate of infection. Serious illness and death due to influenza usually occurs in extremes of age, those older than 65 years or younger than 2 years.

Influenza A and B viruses are responsible for causing human disease. Both influenza A and B undergo frequent antigenic drift, creating new influenza variants. Immunity to the surface antigens decreases the likelihood of infection. Unfortunately, antibody to one influenza subgroup does not give complete protection against other influenza subtypes.

The best way to protect against seasonal influenza is through vaccination. The current trivalent influenza vaccine contains two A strains, 1 A(H1N1), 1 A(H3N2), and one B strain. The quadravalent influenza vaccine contains the same components of the trivalent and an additional B strain. Inactivated influenza vaccine is available in both trivalent and quadravalent presentations. The live attenuated vaccine is only quadravalent.[11]

All individuals 6 months of age and older should receive yearly seasonal influenza vaccination. There is no preference for vaccine presentation when multiple types are available within an approved age range, except for the following groups. The live attenuated influenza vaccine should preferentially be administered to healthy children aged 2 through 8 years. Live attenuated influenza vaccine is more effective than inactivated influenza vaccine in this age group. However, in adults inactivated influenza vaccine is more effective than live attenuated influenza vaccine.[12] In person 65 years and older, the high-dose trivalent-inactivated influenza vaccine produced increased immunity and protection against confirmed influenza when compared to regular dose influenza vaccine, and should be used for older adults.[13] The recombinant influenza vaccine is used in persons with severe egg allergy.

Measles, Mumps, and Rubella Vaccine

Measles, mumps, and rubella are acute viral infections that can cause serious disease and complications. Aggressive vaccination programs have made these infections uncommon in the United States. Measles and rubella have been eliminated from the United States. Recent outbreaks have been caused from importation of infected persons from other parts of the world where measles are still circulating. Some outbreaks also occur in communities with high levels of unvaccinated individuals.

Measles, mumps, and rubella vaccine is a live attenuated vaccine. It causes a mild subclinical infection producing long-term immunity. Measles, mumps, and rubella vaccine is recommended for routine vaccination after the first birthday and a second dose administered at 4 through 6 years of age. Measles, mumps, and rubella vaccine is available in combination with varicella vaccine. This vaccine is not recommended for the first dose due to the increased risk of febrile seizures when compared to giving measles, mumps, and rubella and varicella separately at the same visit.[14] Measles, mumps, and rubella vaccine should also be given to adults older than 18 years who are found to be nonimmune.

Measles, mumps, and rubella vaccine should be avoided in immunocompromised persons because of the risk of acquiring measles from the vaccine. However, HIV-infected persons, who are not severely immunocompromised, including those on antiretroviral therapy, can be vaccinated if not immune.[14]

Measles, mumps, and rubella vaccine is a safe vaccine and rarely associated with severe reactions. The most common reaction is fever which usually occurs more than a week after vaccination. Children with a personal or family history of febrile seizures or epilepsy are at increased risk for measles, mumps, and rubella vaccine associated febrile seizures.[14]

Patient Encounter 1

A mother brings her 1-year boy to the pediatrician's office with his first yearly check-up. The child is healthy with no chronic health problems. The mother has researched childhood vaccines on the Internet and is reluctant to have any vaccines administered because of the risks of seizures and autism.

What routine vaccines should the child receive?

How should the mother's concerns regarding autism be addressed?

The mother is concerned about the number of shots, and wants to use combination vaccines. What combinations can be administered?

Meningococcal Vaccines

Neisseria meningitidis is a significant cause of meningitis and bacteremia. Invasive meningococcal disease is associated with a high morbidity and mortality rate. Morbidity in survivors is substantial, with approximately 20% having loss of limb or neurologic sequelae. The highest rates of meningococcal disease are among young children; however, rates have been increasing in adolescents and young adults. Thirteen meningococcal serogroups have been identified; however, five serogroups, A, B, C, Y, and W-135, are responsible for epidemic and endemic disease worldwide. Despite the availability of highly active antibacterial agents against *N. meningitidis*, there has been little impact on decreasing the morbidity and mortality due to invasive meningococcal disease.[15]

The meningococcal vaccine is recommended for routine vaccination of adolescents. The first dose should be administered at 11 to 12 years with a booster dose at age 16 years. Meningococcal vaccine is also recommended for high-risk individuals older than 2 months.[15] There are three quadravalent and a bivalent vaccine available for use. The quadravalent vaccines contain serogroups A, C, Y, and W-135. The bivalent contains serogroups C and Y, and is conjugated to *H. influenzae* type B vaccine. Each vaccine is approved for different age groups. The vaccine provider should be cognizant to use the appropriate vaccine for the age of the patient. The quadravalent conjugated vaccines should preferentially be used. The polysaccharide vaccine should be reserved for high-risk individuals older than 55 years.

Pneumococcal Vaccines

S. pneumoniae is the most common bacterial cause of community-acquired respiratory tract infections. *S. pneumoniae* causes approximately 3000 cases of meningitis, 50,000 cases of bacteremia, 500,000 cases of pneumonia, and more than 1 million cases of otitis media each year. The increasing prevalence of drug-resistant *S. pneumoniae* has highlighted the need to prevent infection through vaccination. Pneumococcal vaccines are highly effective in preventing disease from the common *S. pneumoniae* serotypes that cause human disease.

The 13-valent pneumococcal conjugate vaccine contains the serotypes that most commonly cause disease in children. The 23-valent pneumococcal polysaccharide vaccine contains 23 serotypes that are responsible for causing more than 80% of invasive *S. pneumoniae* infections in adults. The pneumococcal vaccines have demonstrated good immunogenicity and prevention of invasive pneumococcal disease.

The 13-valent pneumococcal vaccine is part of the routine childhood immunization schedule beginning at 2 months of age. Children older than 6 years who are at high risk of invasive pneumococcal disease should receive a single 23-valent pneumococcal polysaccharide vaccine, with a booster dose given in 5 years.[16]

Both the 13-valent pneumococcal conjugate and 23-valent pneumococcal polysaccharide vaccines are recommended for routine use in all adults 65 years of age or older. The 13-valent vaccine should be administered first followed by the 23-valent vaccine 6 to 12 months later. If an individual has already received the 23-valent pneumococcal vaccine, the 13-valent vaccine should be administered at least 12 months after the 23-valent vaccine. Adults 19 through 64 years who are at increased risk for invasive pneumococcal disease are recommended to receive a single vaccination with the 13-valent pneumococcal conjugate vaccine. This is followed in 8 weeks with a 23-valent pneumococcal polysaccharide vaccine, and a booster dose in 5 years.[17]

Revaccination with the 23-valent pneumococcal polysaccharide vaccine is recommended for adults older than 65 years if the first dose was administered when they were younger than 65 years and at least 5 years have passed. A dose of the 13-valent pneumococcal vaccine should be administered prior to receiving the 23-valent vaccine.[17]

Poliovirus Vaccine

Poliomyelitis is a highly contagious disease that is often asymptomatic; however, approximately 1 in every 100 to 1000 cases will develop a rapidly progressive paralytic disease. Polio is caused by poliovirus. Since the introduction of the first poliovirus vaccine, there has been a significant reduction in the number of polio cases. Today, polio caused by wild-type poliovirus has been eradicated from the Western hemisphere with the goal of eradicating it from the world.[18]

The oral poliovirus vaccine has been routinely used in the United States. Unfortunately, the oral poliovirus vaccine has the risk of vaccine-associated paralytic poliomyelitis occurring in approximately 1 case of every 2.4 million doses distributed. The risk with the first dose of oral poliovirus vaccine is 1 case in 750,000 doses.[18]

The last reported case of indigenous wild-type poliovirus in the United States was in 1979; subsequent cases were all vaccine associated. In 1997, a transition period to the inactivated poliovirus vaccine was begun to reduce the risk of vaccine-associated paralytic poliomyelitis. By January 2000, the oral vaccine was no longer recommended for routine use. Currently, the inactivated poliovirus vaccine is recommended for routine use in the United States. It is available as a single component or in combination vaccines. A booster dose should be given after age 4 years, no matter how many doses were given in the infant vaccination series.[19]

Rotavirus Vaccine

Rotavirus is the most common cause of severe diarrheal disease in children younger than 5 years. It is a major cause of diarrhea hospitalizations for dehydration worldwide. Rotavirus G1 is the most prevalent strain found in the United States. However, in any given year, other strains (G2, G3, G4, and G9) may predominate.

There are two rotavirus vaccines available for use. They are a pentavalent human-bovine reassortant vaccine that contains outer capsid proteins for G1, G2, G3, G4, and P1, and a monovalent, G1 vaccine. The exact mechanism by which these vaccines produce an immune response is unknown; however, these live virus vaccines replicate in the small intestine and induce immunity.

The rotavirus vaccine is administered in either a two-dose or a three-dose series that is orally administered. The first dose is given to infants between 6 and 12 weeks of age. The impact of the rotavirus vaccine has been dramatic with a significant decrease in rotavirus hospitalizations and all-cause diarrhea hospitalizations in children younger than 5 years. The vaccine has also offered protection to children too old to receive the vaccine and young adults.[20] The most severe adverse events associated with rotavirus vaccine is **intrussusception**, a telescoping of the intestines on to itself. Post-licensure monitoring has shown a minimal risk of the vaccine with 1 to 5 excess cases of intrussusception per 100,000 vaccinated children.

Varicella Vaccine

Varicella zoster virus is a highly contagious herpes virus. Primary infection with varicella zoster causes chickenpox and was one of the most common childhood diseases in the prevaccine era. Following primary infection, varicella becomes latent in cranial nerve, dorsal routes, and autonomic ganglia where it may reactivate to cause shingles (Zoster) in older adults. Since the introduction of the varicella virus vaccine in 1995, there has been a 90% reduction in varicella infections and hospitalization in all age groups.[21]

The varicella vaccine is a live attenuated vaccine. Children younger than 12 years will have a 97% seroconversion rate following a single vaccination. Adolescents and adults older than 13 years will only have 78% seroconversion after a single inoculation, but will have 99% conversion following a second dose. Therefore, varicella vaccine is recommended to be administered in a two-dose series. The first dose should be administered after 12 months of age and a second dose at 4 years of age. Adolescents and adults without evidence of immunity to varicella zoster should receive two doses of varicella vaccine given 4 to 8 weeks apart. Antibody titers appear to persist for at least 20 years following immunization.

Varicella vaccine is well tolerated with tenderness at the injection site and mild rash the most common adverse events. Rashes due to the vaccine strain typically occur more than 20 days following vaccination. A few cases of secondary transmission to household contacts have been reported.[21]

Zoster Vaccine

Later in life, approximately 15% of the population will develop herpes zoster (shingles). Zoster is the reactivation of latent varicella zoster virus in the sensory ganglia. Zoster most frequently occurs in the elderly and immunocompromised individuals who have decreased circulating antibodies to varicella zoster virus.

Zoster vaccine is a more concentrated form of the varicella vaccine. It is FDA approved for use in individuals 50 years and older. However, ACIP recommends its use in individuals 60 years and older even with a previous episode of shingles.[22] Use of the zoster vaccine has shown a reduction in the incidence of zoster and postherpetic neuralgia.

> **Patient Encounter 2**
>
> A 65-year-old patient presents to the pharmacy to pick-up his prescription for blood pressure medication. The pharmacist asks the patient if he would like to receive his vaccines, and the patient accepts.
>
> ***What vaccines should the patient receive?***
>
> ***What warnings should be given to the patient?***

VACCINE ADMINISTRATION SCHEDULES

Most vaccines are administered in two- to four-shot series in order to elicit the best protection. Childhood and adult immunization schedules are revised frequently and published annually by the CDC Advisory Committee on Immunization Practices (ACIP). Current immunization schedules can be found at www.cdc.gov/vaccines/. Recommendations will be published throughout the year in the *Morbidity and Mortality Weekly Report* (*MMWR*) as new vaccines are licensed or new information necessitates a change in previous recommendations.[23] See Table 86-1 for vaccine dosing.

The childhood immunization schedule is complex and requires a large number of injections. In small infants, the number of injections can be intolerable to the infant, parent, and health care provider. Limiting the number of injections at each visit can lead to missed vaccinations and increased expense for return visits. KEY CONCEPT *Use of combination vaccines decreases the number of injections and increases the likelihood that the immunization schedule will be completed.* Using combination vaccine does not adversely affect the immunity or increase adverse effects. Vaccine administration should not be delayed for mild to moderate respiratory tract illnesses or fevers.[23]

VACCINE SAFETY

Vaccination is one of the most powerful tools used to prevent disease. As with all drugs, most vaccines have been reported to cause adverse reactions. The reactions are either acute or are related to the risk of developing another disease. Health care professionals should discuss the risks versus benefits of vaccines with individuals or caregivers prior to vaccination. Vaccine information sheets (VIS) provide written information about each vaccine and are required to be given individuals prior to vaccination.[23]

Vaccine safety is monitored by the FDA and CDC through a passive reporting system that allows anyone, health professionals or lay public, to report any event through the Vaccine Adverse Event Reporting System (VAERS). KEY CONCEPT *Health care professionals are mandated to report certain events through VAERS.* Additionally, any serious, life-threatening or unusual reactions should also be reported.

The VAERS database is continually monitored to determine whether the prevalence of reactions is changing and to identify previously unreported reactions to a particular vaccine. Large epidemiologic safety studies are conducted through the Vaccine Safety Datalink; a partnership between the CDC and 9 large health care organizations.

Pain at the injection site is one of the most commonly reported adverse effects of vaccination. The reaction is usually mild, with complaints of pain and tenderness at the injection site that may or may not be accompanied by erythema. Local reactions tend to be more frequent with repeated doses or booster doses of vaccine.[23] Tetanus-containing vaccines are well known for causing localized reactions.

Fever is the most frequently reported adverse effect in children. Elevated temperature is usually self-limiting and resolves in a few days. Rarely febrile seizures may occur following vaccination with measles, mumps, and rubella vaccine.

Reports of syncope following vaccination have been increasing since the approval of human papillomavirus and tetanus toxoid, reduced diphtheria toxoid, and acellular pertussis vaccines. Syncope most commonly occurs in adolescent girls and young adults. Health care professionals should implement measures to mitigate secondary injuries when vaccinating this age group.[23]

Table 86–1

Vaccine Dosing

Vaccine	Common Abbreviation	Dose	Route	Cautions and Adverse Effects
Diphtheria and tetanus toxoid	DT	0.5 mL	Intramuscular	History of arthus-type hypersensitivity reaction
Diphtheria, tetanus, acellular pertussis	DTaP	0.5 mL	Intramuscular	Systemic neurologic reaction from previous vaccine History of arthus-type hypersensitivity reaction Temperature greater than 40.6°C (105°F)
Haemophilus influenzae type b	HIB	0.5 mL	Intramuscular	
Hepatitis A	HepA	C: 0.5 mL A: 1 mL	Intramuscular	Pregnant women
Hepatitis B	HepB	C: 0.5 mL A: 1 mL	Intramuscular	
Human papillomavirus	HPV (HPV2, HPV4)	0.5 mL	Intramuscular	Pregnant women
Inactivated influenza	IIV3, IIV4	0.5 mL 0.1 mL	Intramuscular Intradermal	Severe egg allergy History of Guillain-Barré syndrome
Live attenuated influenza	LAIV	0.2 mL	Intranasal	Severe egg allergy Asthma Chronic health problems Immunocompromised host Pregnant women History of Guillain-Barré syndrome
Measles, mumps, rubella	MMR	0.5 mL	Subcutaneous	Pregnant women Immunocompromised host
Meningococcal polysaccharide	MPSV4	0.5 mL	Subcutaneous	
Meningococcal conjugate	MCV4	0.5 mL	Intramuscular	
Pneumococcal 13-valent conjugate	PCV13	0.5 mL	Intramuscular	
Pneumococcal polysaccharide	PPV23	0.5 mL	Intramuscular route preferred; subcutaneous	Children < 2 years
Poliovirus, inactivated	IPV	0.5 mL	Intramuscular, subcutaneous	
Rotavirus vaccine	RV (RV1, RV5)	1 or 2 mL	Oral	Immunocompromised host
Tetanus and diphtheria toxoid	Td	0.5 mL	Intramuscular	History of arthus-type hypersensitivity reaction
Tetanus, reduced diphtheria, acellular pertussis	Tdap	0.5 mL	Intramuscular	Systemic neurologic reaction from previous vaccine History of arthus-type hypersensitivity reaction
Varicella	VAR	0.5 mL	Subcutaneous	Pregnant women Immunocompromised host
Zoster	ZOS	0.65 mL	Subcutaneous	Immunocompromised host

A, adult; C, children.

Autism

Thimerosal is a preservative used in vaccines that has been purported to cause autism in children. The assumption is that thimerosal, also known as ethyl mercury, causes similar effects as methyl mercury, which has neurotoxic and nephrotoxic effects at high doses. Numerous epidemiologic studies have not shown a higher rate of autism among children receiving thimerosal-containing vaccines when compared with the normal background rate of autism. Additionally, the mercury exposure with vaccination is much lower than through many other environmental exposures.[24]

Guillain-Barré Syndrome

Guillain-Barré syndrome is a transient neurologic disorder causing flaccid paralysis. It is thought to be caused from the development of autoimmune antibodies that cause damage to the peripheral nerves. Guillain-Barré syndrome has been temporally associated with several bacterial and viral infections as well as vaccinations.

The association with vaccination and Guillain-Barré syndrome was first recognized with the Swine flu vaccine of 1976. Since that time a clear association of influenza vaccination and Guillain-Barré syndrome has not been clearly established. Caution is still recommended with influenza vaccines since the influenza strains contained in the vaccine has the potential to change each year.[25]

Several large epidemiologic studies have sought to establish a temporal association of Guillain-Barré syndrome and other routine vaccines. The evidence is inconclusive in determining a cause-and-effect relationship. Overall the risk of Guillain-Barré syndrome following vaccination is minimal with 1 to 2 cases per 100,000 vaccines administered. The benefits of vaccination far outweigh the risk of Guillain-Barré syndrome.[25]

Patient Encounter 3

A 12-year-old girl is being seen at a school-based clinic with complaints of a common cold. The girl has significant nasal congestion, but no fever. The health provider takes the opportunity to review her vaccination records and finds she is due for her routine adolescent vaccines.

Should this patient wait 2 weeks before being vaccinated?

What vaccines should this patient receive?

What precautions should be taken with this patient when administering vaccines?

SPECIAL POPULATIONS

Immunocompromised Host

The number of immunocompromised persons is continually increasing as advances are made in medicine. The life expectancy for persons with cancer, HIV infection, and solid organ or bone marrow transplantation is increasing. Vaccination provides one tool to prevent infection in the immunocompromised host. However, the individual's immunosuppressed state will alter the response to the vaccine. In general, all vaccinations should be updated prior to the person becoming immunosuppressed. KEY CONCEPT *Once a person becomes significantly immunosuppressed, live virus vaccines should be avoided.*

Infants, children, and adults with HIV should receive all routine vaccinations according to the recommended immunization schedule as long as T-lymphocyte CD4 count is more than 200 cells/mm^3 (200×10^6/L). Live vaccines should be used with caution when T-lymphocyte CD4 counts are less than 200 cells/mm^3 (200×10^6/L). All HIV-infected persons should receive yearly inactivated influenza vaccination.[26]

Following hematopoietic stem-cell transplantation, the patient will need most routine vaccines to be administered 6 to 12 months following transplantation. Diphtheria, tetanus, acellular pertussis, *H. influenzae* type b, hepatitis B, meningococcal, pneumococcal, and inactivated poliovirus should be given. Inactivated influenza vaccine is given yearly, starting 6 months after transplant. Measles, mumps, and rubella can be given 2 years after transplant and varicella and zoster vaccines are contraindicated.[26]

Solid organ transplant recipients have a blunted immune response to vaccines because the immunosuppressive regimens used to prevent organ rejection inhibit both T- and B-cell proliferation. Prior to transplant, children should complete primary immunization schedules if possible. Otherwise primary immunization schedule with inactivated vaccines may continue 2 months following transplantation. Adults should have all vaccinations updated prior to transplantation. Yearly seasonal inactivated influenza vaccination may be given 6 months following transplantation.[26]

Household contacts of immunocompromised persons should have all routine vaccines as scheduled, including yearly influenza vaccination. Children in the household may receive live virus vaccines without special precautions; however, if a rash develops following varicella vaccination, contact should be avoided with the immunocompromised host until the rash resolves.

Pregnancy

Vaccination during pregnancy has the ability to protect not only the mother but also the newborn infant. A fully immunized mother is less likely to infect their infant with critical diseases such as influenza, tetanus, and pertussis. Mothers who are vaccinated in the second half of the pregnancy will have maternal transfer of antibodies through the placenta giving protection to the newborn infant. Pregnant women should be vaccinated with inactivated influenza and tetanus toxoid, reduced diphtheria toxoid, and acellular pertussis vaccines during each pregnancy. Ideally the vaccines should be administered after 20-week gestation, but can be administered at any time during the pregnancy.[27]

Live virus vaccines should be avoided during pregnancy due to the theoretical concern of the virus being transported across the placenta and infecting the fetus. Women found to be nonimmune to rubella or varicella may be vaccinated soon after delivery, but not during the pregnancy. The live attenuated influenza vaccine should also be avoided.[27]

Health Care Professionals

Health care professionals are in a unique position to protect them selves and their patients by receiving immunizations against vaccine preventable diseases. Health care professionals should have documented immunity to measles, mumps, rubella, and varicella. The vaccine series should be administered if found nonimmune. Health care professionals with direct patient contact should also receive the Hepatitis B vaccine series and have proven immunity following the series. As concerns regarding the rise of pertussis among adults, it is now recommended that all health care professionals receive at least one dose of tetanus, reduced diphtheria, and acellular pertussis vaccine to protect against pertussis. This dose may be administered at any interval following a tetanus booster.[28]

The Centers for Diseases Control recommends all health care professionals receive yearly influenza vaccination; there is no preference to the type of influenza vaccine that is given. Many health care facilities are now mandating that employees receive yearly influenza vaccination or wear masks during influenza season.[28]

OUTCOME MEASURES

KEY CONCEPT *Vaccines are a cost-effective means for disease prevention.* From a societal perspective, for every dollar spent on routine childhood vaccines, there will be a $10 savings in direct and indirect costs.[29] The rates of vaccination for young children are 90% or more for most recommended vaccines. This has been attributed to the requirements for proof of vaccination by States for enrollment into daycare centers and school. For vaccines not required by schools, the rate of vaccination is lower.

Adolescents present a unique challenge for vaccinating because they do not have as many encounters with health care professionals as young children do. However, the constantly changing immunization schedules makes this population vulnerable to missing newly approved vaccines and catch-up doses of vaccines that were not recommended when they were younger. Every encounter with a health care establishment should be viewed as an opportunity to evaluate and vaccinate if necessary. Adolescents may also have incomplete medical records due to changes in health care providers. Therefore, it is important for health professionals to regularly utilize universal State immunization databases that document pediatric and adult vaccinations. This eliminates the problems of lost immunization records if a child changes health care providers.[23]

The vaccination rate in adults is much lower than that in children. Only 50% to 60% of adults who meet criteria have received pneumococcal vaccination, and less than 40% have received seasonal influenza vaccine. Comprehensive initiatives need to be implemented to increase the adult vaccination rate.

Some proven concepts are providing reminders to patients that vaccines are due and implementation of standing orders for vaccines. This latter concept allows nurses and pharmacists to screen patients to determine whether pneumococcal, influenza, or other vaccines are needed and to vaccinate without a direct physician's order.

Abbreviations Introduced in This Chapter

ACIP	Advisory Committee on Immunization Practices
anti-HBs	Antibody to hepatitis B surface antigen
CDC	Centers for Disease Control and Prevention
HBsAg	Hepatitis B surface antigen
VAERS	Vaccine Adverse Event Reporting System
VIS	Vaccine information sheets

REFERENCES

1. Centers for Disease Control and Prevention. Achievements in public health 1900-1999. Control of infectious diseases. MMWR. 1999;48:621–629.
2. MacKay IR, Rosen FS. Vaccines and vaccination. N Engl J Med. 2001;345:1042–1053.
3. Centers for Disease Control and Prevention. Updated recommendations for use of tetanus toxoid, reduced diphtheria toxoid, and acellular pertussis (Tdap) vaccine in adults aged 65 years and older—Advisory Committee on Immunization Practices (ACIP), 2012. MMWR. 2012;61:468–470.
4. Centers for Disease Control and Prevention. Updated recommendations for use of tetanus toxoid, reduced diphtheria toxoid, and acellular pertussis vaccine (Tdap) in pregnant women—Advisory Committee on Immunization Practices (ACIP), 2012. MMWR. 2013;62:131–135.
5. Briere EC, Rubin L, Moro PL, Cohn A, Clark T, Messonnier N. Prevention and control of Haemophilus influenzae type b disease. Recommendations of the Advisory Committee on Immunization Practices (ACIP). MMWR. 2014;63 (No. RR-1):1–20.
6. Centers for Disease Control and Prevention. Prevention of Hepatitis A through active or passive immunization: Recommendations of the Advisory Committee on Immunization Practices (ACIP). MMWR. 2006;55(No. RR-7):1–23.
7. Centers for Disease Control and Prevention. A comprehensive immunization strategy to eliminate transmission of hepatitis B virus infection in the United States: Recommendations of the Advisory Committee on Immunization Practices (ACIP); Part 1: immunization of infants, children, and adolescents. MMWR. 2005;54(No. RR-16):1–23.
8. Centers for Disease Control and Prevention. A comprehensive immunization strategy to eliminate transmission of hepatitis B virus infection in the United States: Recommendations of the Advisory Committee on Immunization Practices (ACIP); Part 2: Immunization of adults. MMWR. 2006;55(No. RR-16):1–33.
9. Brotherton JML. Human papillomavirus vaccination: Where are we now? J Paediatr Child Health. 50(12):959–965.2014;10.1111/jpc.12627. Epub 2014 Jun 9.
10. Markowitz LE, Dunne EF, Saraiya M, et al. Human papillomavirus vaccination. Recommendations of Advisory Committee on Immunization Practices (ACIP). MMWR. 2014;63 (RR-No. 5):1–29.
11. Centers for Disease Control and Prevention. Prevention and control of seasonal influenza with vaccines. Recommendations of the Advisory Committee on Immunization Practices—United States, 2013-2014. MMWR. 2013;62(No. RR-7):1–42.
12. Grohskopf LA, Olsen SJ, Sokolow LZ, et al. Prevention and control of seasonal influenza with vaccines: Recommendations of the Advisory Committee on Immunization Practices (ACIP)—United States, 2014-2015 influenza season. MMWR. 2014;63:691–697.
13. DiazGranados CA, Dunning AJ, Kimmel M, et al. Efficacy of high-dose versus standard-dose influenza in older adults. N Engl J Med. 2014;371:635–645.
14. Centers for Disease Control and Prevention. Prevention of measles, rubella, congenital rubella syndrome, and mumps, 2013. Summary recommendations of the Advisory Committee on Immunization Practices (ACIP). MMWR. 2013;62 (No. RR-4):1–34.
15. Centers for Disease Control and Prevention. Prevention and control of meningococcal disease. Recommendations of the Advisory Committee on Immunization Practices (ACIP). MMWR. 2013; 62(RR-2):1–22.
16. Centers for Disease Control and Prevention. Use of 13-valent pneumococcal vaccine and 23-valent pneumococcal polysaccharide vaccine among children aged 6-18 years with immunocompromising conditions: Recommendations of the Advisory Committee on Immunization Practices (ACIP). MMWR. 2013;62:521–524.
17. Tomczyk S, Bennett NM, Stoecker C, et al. Use of 13-valent pneumococcal conjugate vaccine and 23-valent pneumococcal polysaccharide vaccine among adults ≥ 65 years: Recommendations of the Advisory Committee on Immunization Practices (ACIP). MMWR. 2014;63:822–825.
18. Centers for Disease Control and Prevention. Poliomyletis prevention in the United States: Updated recommendations of the Advisory Committee on Immunization Practices (ACIP). MMWR. 2000; 49(RR-5):1–22.
19. Centers for Disease Control and Prevention. Updated recommendations of the Advisory Committee on Immunization Practices (ACIP) regarding routine poliovirus vaccination. MMWR. 2009; 58:829–830.
20. Tate JE, Parashar UD. Rotavirus vaccines in routine use. Clin Infect Dis. 2014 Nov 1;59(9):1291-1301. 2014: Jul 21 [Epub ahead of print].
21. Baxter R, Tran TN, Ray P, et al. Impact of vaccination on the epidemiology of varicella: 1995-2009. Pediatrics. 2014; 134:24–30.
22. Hales CM, Harpaz R, Ortega-Sanchez I, Bialek S. Update on recommendations for use of Herpes zoster vaccine. MMWR. 2014;63:729–731.
23. Centers for Disease Control and Prevention. General recommendations on immunization. Recommendations of the Advisory Committee on Immunization Practices(ACIP). MMWR. 2011; 60(No. RR-2):1–58.
24. Maglione MA, Das L, Raaen L, et al. Safety of vaccines used for routine immunization of US children: A systematic review. Pediatrics. 2014;134:325–337.
25. Haber P, Sejvar J, Mikaeloff Y, DeStefano F. Vaccines and Guillain-Barré syndrome. Drug Saf. 2009; 32:309–323.
26. Rubin LG, Levin MJ, Ljungman P, et al. 2013 IDSA clinical practice guideline for vaccination of the immunocompromised host. Clin Infect Dis. 2014:58:e44–e100.
27. Rasmussen SA, Watson AK, Kennedy ED, Broder KR, Jamieson DJ. Vaccines and pregnancy: Past, present, and future. Semin Fetal Neonatal Med. 2014:19:161–169.
28. Kaltsas A, Sepkowitz K. Vaccinations for healthcare personnel: Update on influenza, hepatitis B, and pertussis. Curr Opin Infect Dis. 2013:26;366–377.
29. Zhou F, Shefer A, Wenger J, et al. Economic evaluation of the routine childhood immunization program in the United States, 2009. Pediatrics. 2014;133:577–585.

87 Human Immunodeficiency Virus Infection

Emily L. Heil, Christine Trezza, and
Amanda H. Corbett

LEARNING OBJECTIVES

Upon completion of the chapter, the reader will be able to:

1. Explain the routes of transmission for HIV and its natural disease progression.
2. Identify typical and atypical signs and symptoms of acute and chronic HIV infection.
3. Identify the desired therapeutic outcomes for patients with HIV infection.
4. Recommend appropriate first-line pharmacotherapy interventions for patients with HIV infection.
5. Recommend appropriate second-line pharmacotherapy interventions for patients with HIV infection.
6. Describe the components of a monitoring plan to assess effectiveness and adverse effects of pharmacotherapy for HIV infection.
7. Educate patients about the disease state, appropriate lifestyle modifications, and drug therapy required for effective treatment.

INTRODUCTION

Human immunodeficiency virus type is the major cause of AIDS. HIV primarily targets $CD4^+$ lymphocytes, which are critical to proper immune system function. If left untreated, patients experience a prolonged asymptomatic period followed by rapid, progressive immunodeficiency. Therefore, most complications experienced by patients with AIDS involve opportunistic infections and cancers. AIDS occurs when a patient with HIV has a CD4 cell count below 200 cells/mm³ (200×10^6/L), a CD4 cell percentage of total lymphocytes less than 14% (0.14), or one of the Centers for Disease Control (CDC) AIDS defining conditions.[1]

EPIDEMIOLOGY AND ETIOLOGY

HIV is primarily transmitted by sexual contact, by contact with blood or blood products, and from mother to child during gestation, delivery, or breast-feeding. Although the global incidence of HIV has fallen 33% since 2001, HIV prevalence has increased, largely due to life-extending antiretroviral therapy. Combination antiretroviral therapy (cART) has increased both the length and quality of life for HIV-infected patients, however, to date, there are no treatments that eradicate HIV from the body.[2]

As of 2012, approximately 35.3 million people are infected with HIV worldwide. Approximately 70% of these cases are in Sub-Saharan Africa, with a prevalence of approximately 5%. Central Asia, Eastern Europe, North Africa, and the Middle East are also seeing rapidly rising infection rates.[2]

In 2012 alone, approximately 1.6 million people worldwide died from AIDS and 2.3 million people were newly infected with HIV. Most of these infections were acquired through heterosexual transmission. As of December 2012, women accounted for 45.6% of all people living with HIV worldwide. Young adults, aged 15 to 24 years, accounted for approximately 39% of new HIV infections worldwide.[2]

In the United States, at the end of 2011, an estimated 1.2 million persons (aged 13 years or older) were living with HIV/AIDS. Approximately 14% of these are undiagnosed and unaware of their HIV infection and could be unknowingly transmitting the virus to others.[3]

In 2010, HIV/AIDS rates for African American men were six times those for white men and twice that for Hispanic males, representing 44% and 21% of cases, respectively. Although HIV/AIDS rates in African American women dropped by 21% in 2010, incidence in this population is 20 times the rate for white females and five times the rate for Hispanic females.[3]

Risk factors for HIV/AIDS infection include men who have sex with men (MSM), history of or current IV drug use (needle or equipment sharing), unprotected sexual intercourse with high-risk individuals, the presence of other sexually transmitted infections (eg, *Chlamydia trachomatis* or *Neisseria gonorrhoeae*), persons with coagulation/hemophilia disorders, and previous blood product recipients.

PATHOPHYSIOLOGY

HIV-1 is a retrovirus and member of the genus *Lentivirus*. There are two molecularly and serologically distinct but related types of HIV: HIV-1 and HIV-2. These viruses have a prolonged latency period. HIV-2 is a less common cause of the epidemic and is found primarily in West Africa. HIV-1 is categorized by phylogenetic lineages into three groups (M [main or major], N [new], and O [outlier]). HIV-1 group M can be further categorized into nine subtypes: A through D, F through H, and J and K. HIV-1 subtype B is primarily responsible for the North American and Western European epidemic.

HIV infection occurs through three primary modes of transmission: sexual, parenteral, and perinatal. The most common method for transmission is receptive anal and vaginal intercourse, with the probability of transmission highest, 138 infections per 10,000 exposures, with receptive anal intercourse.[4] The probability of transmission increases when the infected partner has a high level of viral replication (which occurs at the beginning of infection or late in disease) or when the uninfected partner has ulcerative disease or compromised mucosal surfaces or (in the case of men) has not been circumcised.

Parenteral transmission of HIV primarily occurs through injection drug use by sharing contaminated needles or injection-related supplies. Less than 1% of all cases of HIV infection occur as a result of transfusions of contaminated blood or blood products, or infected transplant organs.[3] Health care workers have a 0.3% estimated risk of acquiring HIV infection through percutaneous needlestick injury.

Perinatal infection (also known as vertical transmission or mother-to-child transmission [MTCT]) can occur during gestation, at or near delivery, and during breast-feeding. In the absence of specific intervention including medications, the risk of MTCT up to and including delivery is approximately 25%, whereas the risk of transmission during breast-feeding is approximately 15% to 20% within the first 6 months of life.[5] Because a high rate of HIV replication in the blood is a significant risk factor for transmission of HIV, it is important to treat women for their HIV infection during pregnancy. After delivery, mothers are strongly recommended not to breast-feed if safe alternatives are available.

Understanding the life cycle of the virus is important to know how antiretroviral drugs are combined for optimal therapy (Figure 87–1). Once HIV enters the body, an outer glycoprotein called gp120 binds to CD4 receptors found on the surface of dendritic cells, T lymphocytes, monocytes, and macrophages. This allows further binding to other chemokine receptors on the cell surface called CCR5 and/or CXCR4. Greater than 95% of newly infected patients have viruses that preferentially use CCR5 to enter the cell, and most patients with advanced disease have viruses that preferentially use CXCR4 to enter the cell.

After the virus has attached to CD4 and chemokine receptors, another viral glycoprotein (gp41) assists with viral fusion to the cell and internalization of the viral contents. The viral contents include single-stranded RNA, an RNA-dependent DNA polymerase (also known as reverse transcriptase), and other enzymes. Using the single-stranded viral RNA as a template, reverse transcriptase synthesizes a complementary strand of DNA. The single-stranded viral RNA is removed from the newly formed DNA strand by ribonuclease H, and reverse transcriptase completes the synthesis of double-stranded DNA. The viral reverse transcriptase enzyme is highly error-prone, and many mutations occur in the conversion of RNA to DNA. This inefficient reverse transcription activity is responsible for HIV's ability to rapidly mutate and develop drug resistance.

A chronic infection is established when the double-stranded DNA migrates to the host cell nucleus and is integrated into the host cell chromosome by an HIV enzyme called integrase. Once the cell becomes activated by antigens or cytokines, HIV replication starts: Host DNA polymerase transcribes viral DNA into messenger RNA, and messenger RNA is translated into viral

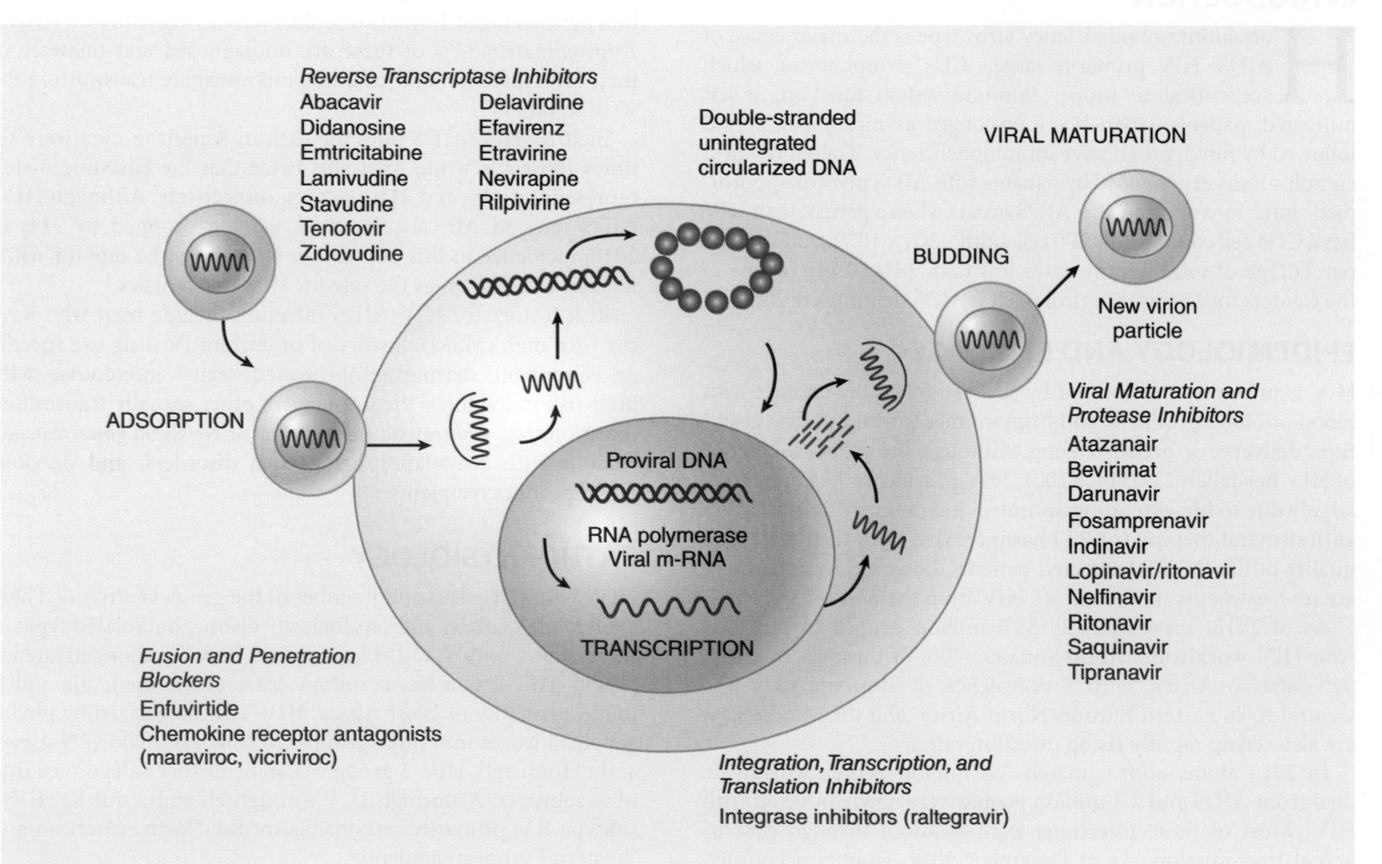

FIGURE 87–1. Life cycle of HIV and targets for antiretroviral drugs. (From Fletcher CV, Kakuda TN. Human immunodeficiency virus infection. In: DiPiro JT, Talbert RL, Yee GC, et al, eds. Pharmacotherapy: A Pathophysiologic Approach. 9th ed. New York: McGraw-Hill; 2005: 2258; With permission.)

proteins. These proteins assemble beneath the bilayer of the host cell, a nucleocapsid forms containing these proteins, and the virus buds from the cell. After budding, the virus matures when an HIV protease enzyme cleaves large polypeptides into smaller functional proteins. Without this process, the virus is unable to infect other cells.

During the early stages of infection, approximately 10 billion virions can be produced each day. Most of the cells containing these viruses will be lysed as a result of budding virions, cytotoxic T-lymphocytes, or undergoing apoptosis. However, HIV will be protected within some cells (macrophages, T cells in lymph nodes), which can stay dormant for years.

The initial immune response against HIV is relatively effective, but it is unable to completely clear the infection, and the patient enters a latent, asymptomatic, or mildly symptomatic stage lasting 5 to 15 years. During this time, a high rate of viral replication can be seen in the lymph nodes. Eventually immune deficiency occurs when the body is no longer able to replenish helper T cells at a rate equal to that at which HIV is destroying them.

KEY CONCEPT *The goal of therapy is to maximally and durably suppress HIV replication to restore and preserve immune system function and minimize morbidity and mortality.* Because HIV replication has been found in all areas of the body, it is important to use potent combination drug therapy that can achieve adequate concentrations in all tissues, including protected sites such as the brain and genital tract.

CLINICAL PRESENTATION AND DIAGNOSIS

Patients who are acutely infected with HIV may be asymptomatic or present with signs and symptoms associated with any viral infection, such as fever, myalgias, lymphadenopathy, pharyngitis, or rash. Taken together, these are the "acute retroviral syndrome," and 40% to 90% of acutely infected individuals will have symptoms.[8] Providers should consider the possibility of HIV infection in any patient with these findings and inquire about recent high-risk sexual encounters or other modes of high-risk exposures. In the United States, 1 in 6 HIV-infected individuals are not aware of their status, thus identifying acutely infected patients and providing referral into HIV care is critical for preventing HIV transmission.[3] In acute infection, HIV RNA concentrations in blood and the genital tract are very high, increasing the risk of transmission to others.[6] Increased infectiousness coupled with undiagnosed HIV infection in these patients may account for a substantial proportion of sexual HIV transmission.

If patients are not identified during acute infection, they may later present with nonspecific symptoms such as myalgias, fatigue, weight loss, thrush, or symptoms associated with opportunistic infections. The U.S. CDC recommends that patients aged 13 to 64 years in all health care settings undergo opt-out HIV testing, meaning that a separate consent form for testing is not needed after the patient has been informed that testing will be performed. For those patients in the high-risk groups mentioned above, HIV testing should be performed on an annual basis, and pregnant women should be tested with each pregnancy.[7]

Diagnosis of HIV is made either by a positive HIV enzyme-linked immunosorbent assay (ELISA) or rapid test (these tests may be positive as soon as 3–6 weeks after infection) and then confirmed by a positive test, usually the HIV western blot (WB) (Table 87–1). At-home HIV-1 test kits (Home Access Systems, OraQuick), allows patients to self-collect blood or oral swab samples, and obtain confidential results in the privacy of their home. Positive results require confirmation by WB.

If the WB is the gold standard confirmatory test and is commonly used. The WB is considered reactive if two of the three major bands (p24, gp41, and/or gp120/160) change color. The test is nonreactive if no viral bands are visible. If the test is indeterminate (one band visible), patients are retested in 2 to

Table 87–1
HIV Diagnostic Tests

Test	Minimum Time to Detection after Exposure	Sample(s) Tested	Comments
Initial Screening Tests			
ELISA	3–6 weeks	Plasma	If nonreactive, no further testing is required, unless acute infection suspected
HIV RNA assay	Up to 14 days	Plasma	Obtain if recent high-risk exposure; if initially negative, repeat at months 1, 3, and 6
Rapid tests (currently FDA-approved products):	Detects HIV antibodies within minutes of sample application		
OraQuick ADVANCE	3–6 weeks	Oral fluid	Detects HIV-1 and HIV-2
SURE CHECK HIV 1/2	3–6 weeks	Whole blood, plasma, or serum	Detects HIV-1 and HIV-2
Multispot HIV-1/HIV-2 Rapid Test	3–6 weeks	Plasma or serum	Detects HIV-1 and HIV-2
Reveal Rapid HIV-1 Antibody Test	3–6 weeks	Plasma or serum	Detects HIV-1
Uni-Gold Recombigen HIV Test	3–6 weeks	Whole blood, plasma, or serum	Detects HIV-1
INSTI™ HIV-1/HIV-2 Rapid Antibody Kit	3–6 weeks	Plasma or whole blood	Detects HIV-1 and HIV-2
Confirmatory Tests			
Western blot (WB)	3–6 weeks	Plasma	Gold standard confirmatory test
Indirect immunofluorescence assay (IFA)	3–6 weeks	Plasma	Simple to perform, but requires expertise to interpret results

ELISA, enzyme-linked immunosorbent assay.

Clinical Presentation and Diagnosis of HIV

Patients with acute HIV infection may display symptoms described as acute retroviral syndrome. Patients with chronic HIV infection may present with these same nonspecific symptoms and/or opportunistic infections.

Acute Retroviral Syndrome

The majority of patients may present with fever, lymphadenopathy, pharyngitis, and/or rash. Other symptoms include the following:

- Myalgia or arthralgia
- Diarrhea
- Headache
- Nausea and vomiting
- Hepatosplenomegaly
- Weight loss
- Thrush
- Neurologic symptoms (meningoencephalitis, aseptic meningitis, peripheral neuropathy, facial palsy, or cognitive impairment or psychosis)

Opportunistic Infections

Depending on the severity of immunosuppression (the CD4+ count), patients may present with the following opportunistic infections (grouped by CD4+ count):

- *Any CD4+ count*
  - *Mycobacterium tuberculosis* disease
  - Bacterial pneumonia (commonly *Streptococcus pneumoniae, Haemophilus influenzae, Pseudomonas aeruginosa*, and *Staphylococcus aureus*)
  - Herpes simplex virus disease
  - Varicella zoster virus disease
  - Bacterial enteric disease (most commonly *Salmonella, Campylobacter*, and *Shigella*)
  - Syphilis
  - Bartonellosis
- *Less than 200 cells/mm³ (200 × 10⁶/L)*
  - Coccidioidomycosis
  - *Pneumocystis jiroveci* (formerly *carinii*) pneumonia (PCP or PJP)
  - Oropharyngeal and esophageal candidiasis
  - Kaposi sarcoma or human herpesvirus-8 disease
- *Less than 150 cells/mm³ (150 × 10⁶/L)*
  - Disseminated histoplasmosis
- *Less than 100 cells/mm³ (100 × 10⁶/L)*
  - *Toxoplasma gondii* encephalitis
  - Cryptosporidiosis
  - Microsporidiosis
- *Less than 50 cells/mm³ (50 × 10⁶/L)*
  - Disseminated *Mycobacterium avium* complex disease
  - Cytomegalovirus disease (CMV)
  - Cryptococcosis, aspergillosis

3 months. This is most likely if a recent (ie, less than 3–6 weeks) infection has occurred, and HIV antibodies have not yet been fully formed. In this case, a plasma HIV RNA concentration (reverse transcriptase polymerase chain reaction [RT-PCR]) should be evaluated. Patients with acute infection will generally have HIV RNA concentrations greater than 10^6 copies/mL (10^9 copies/L). KEY CONCEPT *HIV treatment response and disease progression is determined by following: (a) the CD4+ lymphocyte count (CD4+ count) and percentage and (b) HIV RNA (viral load).* The CD4+ percentage is followed because the absolute count may fluctuate and does not necessarily indicate a change in the patient's condition.

TREATMENT

KEY CONCEPT *The goals of treatment are to maximally and durably suppress viral replication, avoid the development of drug resistance, restore and preserve immune function, prevent opportunistic infections, minimize drug adverse effects, and prevent disease transmission.* Elimination or cure of HIV is not possible with currently available therapies. Instead, maximal suppression of viral replication (defined as HIV RNA concentrations undetectable by the most sensitive assay available) is desired. After the initiation of antiretroviral therapy, a rapid decline to undetectable HIV RNA in 16 to 24 weeks is a predictor of improved clinical outcomes.[8]

KEY CONCEPT *Degree of immune function preservation is also correlated with decreased viral replication and is measured by CD4+ T-cell counts. CD4+ measures are the best predictor of progression to AIDS and help clinicians determine when to initiate treatment.* At CD4+ T-cell counts of 200 cells/mm³ (200 × 10^6/L) and lower, patients require drug prophylaxis for opportunistic infections. Table 87–2 details the monitoring points of HIV treatment for HIV RNA and CD4+ T-cell counts. In addition to these parameters, basic blood chemistry tests, liver function tests, complete blood counts, and lipid profiles should be monitored every 3 to 6 months in patients receiving antiretroviral therapy.[8]

Six classes of drugs are available to treat HIV infection: nucleoside (NRTI)/nucleotide (NtRTI) reverse transcriptase inhibitor, protease inhibitor (PI), nonnucleoside reverse transcriptase inhibitor (NNRTI), fusion inhibitors, CCR5 inhibitors, and integrase strand transfer inhibitors (INSTI). KEY CONCEPT *Currently, combination antiretroviral drug therapy with three or more active drugs is the standard of care, which increases the durability of viral suppression and decreases the potential for the development of resistance. Two nucleoside (nucleotide) reverse transcriptase inhibitors AND an NNRTI OR a ritonavir-boosted PI OR an INSTI are the mainstay regimens of combination therapy in initial treatment.* Combination regimens decrease HIV RNA to less than 50 copies/mL (50 × 10^3 copies/L) in 80% to 90% of patients in clinical trials.[8] Therefore, monotherapy with any agent or the use of NRTIs without another drug class are not recommended

Table 87–2

Monitoring End Points for CD4+ T-Cell Counts and HIV RNA

CD4+ T Cell Counts			HIV RNA Concentration		
When to Monitor?	**Why?**	**Goal**	**When to Monitor?**	**Why?**	**Goal**
Initial diagnosis	Assess immune function	Start therapy in appropriate patients	Initial diagnosis/ evaluation	Establish baseline	Start ART in appropriate patients
	Assess need for OI chemoprophylaxis	Start prophylaxis when counts < 200 cells/mm^3 (200 × 10^6/L)	2–8 weeks after starting or changing ART[a]	Early assessment of regimen efficacy	Undetectable concentrations
Every 3–6 months	Receiving ART: monitor success of treatment[b]	Average increase of 100–150 cells/ mm^3/year (100 × 10^6–150 × 10^6/L/year)	Every 3–6 months	Receiving ART: assess success and durability of virologic suppression and adherence with current regimen	Steadily decreasing and/or consistently undetectable concentrations
	Not receiving ART: assess urgency to begin therapy	Start ART in appropriate patients	Optional[c]	Not receiving ART: monitor changes in viral load	Start therapy in appropriate patients
	Assess need for OI chemoprophylaxis	Start prophylaxis when counts < 200 cells/ mm^3 (200 × 10^6/L)			

ART, antiretroviral therapy; OI, opportunistic infection.

[a]If viral load is detectable, repeat every 4 to 8 weeks until less than 200 copies/mL (200 × 10^3/L), then resume every 3- to 6-month schedule.

[b]In clinically stable patients with viral loads less than 50 copies/mL (50 × 10^3/L) for more than 2 years, monitoring can be extended to every 6 to 12 months.

[c]For patients who choose to delay therapy, repeat viral load testing while not on therapy is optional. HIV RNA concentration should be determined prior to initiating therapy.

Adapted from Panel on Antiretroviral Guidelines for Adults and Adolescents. Guidelines for the use of antiretroviral agents in HIV-1-infected adults and adolescents [online]. Department of Health and Human Services. May 1, 2014;1–166. [cited 2014 June 1]. http://www.aidsinfo.nih .gov/ContentFiles/AdultandAdolescentGL.pdf

Patient Encounter 1, Part 1: Treatment Initiation

A 32-year-old white man presents to the clinic requesting to be tested for HIV. He reports having unprotected receptive anal intercourse with multiple male partners in the past year. Last week, he presented to the urgent care clinic with complaints of fever, malaise, and pharyngitis. He was prescribed azithromycin for a presumed bacterial infection.

PMH: Seizure disorder, Allergic rhinitis, obesity

FH: Mother—HTN, CAD; father—Type II DM, dyslipidemia, prostate cancer

SH: Financial advisor; reports multiple sexual partners in the past 12 months with condom use about 50% of the time. He denies illicit drugs, but drinks about 10 alcoholic drinks weekly

Meds: Carbamazepine 200 mg by mouth twice daily; azithromycin 500 mg by mouth on day 1, 250 mg by mouth days 2 to 5 (completed 2 days ago); fexofenadine by mouth once daily; multivitamin by mouth once daily

All: Penicillin (anaphylaxis)

ROS: Negative for weight loss, decreased appetite, shortness of breath, and cough, chest pain, nausea, vomiting, diarrhea

PE:

Within normal limits

VS: BP 124/84 mm Hg, P 73 beats/min, RR 18 breaths/min, T 39.3°C

HEENT: Within normal limits

CV: RRR, normal S1, S2; no murmurs, rubs, gallops

Abd: Soft, nontender, nondistended; (+) bowel sounds, no hepatosplenomegaly

Rectal: Deferred

Labs: Sodium 135 mEq/L (135 mmol/L), potassium 3.6 mEq/L (3.6 mmol/L), chloride 100 mEq/L (100 mmol/L), bicarbonate 24 mEq/L (24 mmol/L), blood urea nitrogen 14 mg/dL (5 mmol/L), creatinine 1.0 mg/dL (88 μmol/L), WBC 5.2 × 10^3/mm^3 (5.2 × 10^9/L), hemoglobin 11.5 g/dL (115 g/L or 7.14 mmol/L), hematocrit 34.1% (0.341), platelets 151 × 10^3/mm^3 (151 × 10^9/L), neutrophils 58% (0.58), bands 9% (0.09), lymphocytes 32% (0.32), monocytes 1% (0.01), eosinophils 0% (0.00), basophils 0% (0.00)

What information is suggestive of HIV?

What is the likely time frame of this patient's HIV infection?

What are the risk factors present for having HIV?

How can the diagnosis of HIV be made in this patient?

What additional laboratory measurements would be useful?

treatment options. Fusion inhibitors are only FDA approved for use in treatment experienced patients with drug resistance to NRTIs, NNRTIs, and/or PIs. Figure 87–1 details the mechanisms of action of the drug classes within the life cycle of HIV.

Nonpharmacologic Interventions

KEY CONCEPT *Patient adherence is a key component in treatment success.* Drug therapy is required for a lifetime, as the virus begins to replicate at high levels when medications are stopped. HIV combination therapy used in the past was exceedingly complicated for patients, with multiple daily doses, varying food restrictions, and large pill burdens. Advances in delivery and formulations now make possible once- or twice-daily dosing with fewer pills per day. Currently, two combination tablets providing one pill, once daily NNRTI-containing regimens are available: tenofovir + emtricitabine + efavirenz (Atripla) and tenofovir + emtricitabine + rilpivirine (Complera). Additionally, two fixed dose INSTI-containing combination tablets are available: elvitegravir + cobicistat + tenofovir + emtricitabine (Stribild) and dolutegravir + abacavir + lamivudine (Triumeq), both once daily regimens. The use of low-dose ritonavir or cobicistat to enhance the concentrations of other PIs or elvitegravir, respectively (known as pharmacokinetic enhancement, or "boosting" agents) allows for significantly fewer daily doses and lower pill burdens. Cobicistat, unlike ritonavir, does not exert antiviral activity. Atazanavir or darunavir with ritonavir boosting are potent, once-daily PI options; once-daily lopinavir/ritonavir may be used in selected treatment-naïve patients. These advances, however, do not replace the need for patient counseling by a trained pharmacist and a multidisciplinary approach to promoting adherence.

All patients should be counselled initially and repeatedly on ways to prevent viral transmission. Preventing the spread of resistant virus is particularly important. Patients receiving antiretroviral therapy can still transmit virus to sexual partners and to those with whom they share needles or other drug equipment. Where both partners are HIV-positive, safe sex and needle practices reduce the risk of superinfection with differing strains of HIV and the transmission of other sexually transmitted diseases. General guidelines for preventing viral transmission include using condoms with a water-based lubricant for vaginal or anal intercourse, using condoms without lubricant or dental dams for oral sex, and not sharing equipment used to prepare, inject, or inhale drugs. Treating other sexually transmitted infections (STIs), particularly genital herpes, in HIV-infected patients may help to prevent HIV transmission. The presence of STIs increases genital tract HIV viral load and, correspondingly, the risk of HIV transmission to sexual partners.

KEY CONCEPT *Nutrition and dietary counseling should also be included in the care of the HIV patient, as poor nutrition leads to poorer outcomes and complicates treatment.* Antiretroviral therapy itself introduces a host of nutritional issues, including drug–food interactions, GI adverse effects that may affect appetite and limit dietary intake, lipid abnormalities, and fat redistribution. The American Dietetics Association currently recommends assessing HIV-infected patients for their level of nutritional risk and involving a registered dietician as part of the clinical team for optimal nutrition care.[9]

Pharmacologic Therapy for Antiretroviral-Naïve Patients

Two expert panels publish guidelines for the treatment of HIV-infected individuals. Although the recommendations are quite similar, slight differences do exist between the Department of Health and Human Services (DHHS) Guidelines[8] and the International AIDS Society–USA (IAS-USA) Panel Recommendations.[10] The DHHS Guidelines are updated frequently, and current and archived versions are available online at www.aidsinfo.nih.gov. Due to the intense research and constant modifications to therapeutic approaches in the treatment of HIV, the majority of the treatment algorithms and recommendations presented herein follow the most up-to-date information found in the May 2014 DHHS recommendations.

KEY CONCEPT *The decision of when to begin antiretroviral therapy is complex. Initiating highly active antiretroviral therapy should be considered in all HIV-infected individuals willing to adhere to lifelong therapy. The strength of this recommendation is based on the* $CD4^+$ *T-cell count and other comorbid conditions.* Other factors to consider include the patient's viral load, decline in $CD4^+$ counts over time, hepatitis C status, risk for cardiovascular disease, risk of transmission to sex partners, willingness to begin therapy and maintain medication adherence, and the risk versus benefit of treating an asymptomatic patient. The DHHS guidelines recommend initiating antiretroviral therapy in all HIV-infected individuals to reduce the risk of disease progression. The strength and evidence to support this recommendation depends on pretreatment $CD4^+$ T lymphocyte count. The clinical evidence is strongest for beginning treatment at $CD4^+$ counts less than 350 cells/mm^3 (350×10^6/L), but more recent evidence from long-term studies and the availability of potent drugs with improved tolerability support earlier treatment at higher $CD4^+$ counts. Once the decision is made to initiate treatment, the regimen is selected based on patient-specific factors. KEY CONCEPT *All recommended regimens for initial treatment contain an NNRTI, a ritonavir-boosted PI, or an INSTI in combination with two NRTI (tenofovir + emtricitabine or abacavir + lamivudine).* The recommended agents are shown in Table 87–3.

Table 87–3

Recommended Initial ART Regimen Options for All Patients, Regardless of Pre-ART Viral Load or $CD4^+$ Cell Count[8]

NNRTI-Based Regimens:
Efavirenz + tenofovir + emtricitabine
Efavirenz + abacavir + lamivudine *(Only for patients with pre-ART plasma HIV RNA < 100,000 copies/mL [100 x 10⁶/L] AND HLA-B*5701 negative)*
Rilpivirine + tenofovir + emtricitabine *(Only for patients with pre-ART plasma HIV RNA < 100,000 copies/mL [100 x 10⁶/L] AND CD4+ count > 200 cells/mm³ [200 × 10⁶/L])*

PI-Based Regimens:
Atazanavir/ritonavir + tenofovir + emtricitabine
Atazanavir/ritonavir + abacavir + lamivudine *(Only for patients with pre-ART plasma HIV RNA < 100,000 copies/mL [100 × 10⁶/L] AND HLA-B*5701 negative)*
Darunavir/ritonavir + tenofovir + emtricitabine

INSTI-Based Regimens:
Dolutegravir + abacavir + lamivudine *(Only for patients who are HLA-B*5701 negative)*
Dolutegravir + tenofovir + emtricitabine
Elvitegravir + cobicistat + tenofovir + emtricitabine *(Only for patients with pre-ART CrCL > 70 mL/min [1.17 mL/s])*
Raltegravir + tenofovir + emtricitabine

The decision to choose an NNRTI-, PI-, or INSTI-based regimen as initial therapy is based on many patient- and clinician-specific factors. Drug resistance testing should be performed at diagnosis and again prior to initiating treatment if time has elapsed between diagnosis and treatment (see Pharmacologic Therapy for Antiretroviral-Experienced Patients for further discussion of drug resistance testing). The results of resistance testing may dictate which drug class is preferred; a minimum of 10% to 17% of newly diagnosed patients will have drug-resistant virus.[11] This initial resistance pattern often involves the NNRTIs, but may involve other drug classes. NNRTI-based regimens have low pill burdens and may have decreased incidences of long-term adverse effects (eg, dyslipidemia) in comparison with some PI-based regimens. However, this class also has a low threshold for drug resistance (the K103N mutation causes high level cross-class resistance), and patient adherence is a critical consideration. In pregnant women, or women with the potential to become pregnant, a PI-based regimen is preferred due to the potential teratogenicity of efavirenz in early pregnancy (Pregnancy Category D). INSTI-based regimens have the advantage of avoiding many complex drug–drug interactions and toxicities seen with NNRTIs and PIs. However, raltegravir must be dosed twice daily, elvitegravir must be coadministered with cobicistat which is associated with many cytochrome (CYP)-450-mediated drug interactions and should not be initiated in patients with a creatinine clearance less than 70 mL/min (1.17 mL/s). Transmitted INSTI resistance is not yet a major clinical concern, but may develop as integrase inhibitors come into wider use. If transmitted INSTI resistance is a concern, integrase resistance testing must be ordered separately from standard HIV genotyping, which only includes the protease and reverse transcriptase genes.

In patients who cannot tolerate the preferred first-line therapies, or have a compelling reason to choose a different agent, the following alternative regimens are recommended.[8]

1. PI based:
   a. Darunavir/ritonavir + abacavir/lamivudine
   b. Lopinavir/ritonavir (dosed once or twice daily) + either tenofovir/emtricitabine OR abacavir/ lamivudine
2. INSTI:
   a. Raltegravir + abacavir/lamivudine

If abacavir is included in a regimen, patients should undergo human leukocyte antigen (HLA)-B*5701 testing prior to initiation to assess the risk of abacavir hypersensitivity. Patients who test positive for the allele are at high risk (approximately 50%–67%) of developing this reaction and should not be given abacavir.[8] An abacavir allergy should also be documented in the patient's medical record to prevent future administration. Those patients with a negative test may receive abacavir, but should still be counseled and monitored for the development of hypersensitivity.

Regimens with demonstrated efficacy but less desirable, including the CCR5 antagonist maraviroc, the NNRTI nevirapine, unboosted atazanavir, and boosted saquinavir are no longer recommended as first-line therapy for treatment-naïve patients. One of these regimens should only be selected if a first-line regimen is intolerable or the patient has a compelling reason to avoid drugs in a first-line regimen. If maraviroc is under consideration, viral tropism testing should be performed to ensure CCR5-tropic virus for optimal efficacy.

Therapies *not recommended* for initial treatment due to poor potency or significant toxicity include triple-NRTI regimens, delavirdine, nevirapine in patients with moderate to high CD4$^+$ T-cell counts, indinavir ± ritonavir, darunavir, saquinavir or fosamprenavir used without ritonavir ("unboosted"), ritonavir used without another PI, nelfinavir, tipranavir/ritonavir, and tenofovir, lamivudine, or emtricitabine with didanosine. Because of limited data in antiretroviral naïve patients, etravirine is not recommended in the DHHS Guidelines at this time.

Drugs that should *not be combined* due to overlapping toxicities include atazanavir plus indinavir (due to enhanced hyperbilirubinemia), two NNRTIs, and didanosine plus stavudine. Emtricitabine and lamivudine should not be combined because of their similar chemical structures, and antagonism can result when stavudine is combined with zidovudine.

Patient Encounter 1, Part 2

After receiving the diagnosis of HIV and assessing his laboratory values and willingness to initiate therapy, the patient from Part 1 and his medical team decide to start antiretrovirals.

What is the guidance for when to start therapy in a treatment-naïve patient?

What are the recommended regimens according to the DHHS Guidelines?

What is the potential for drug interactions with each of the recommended regimens?

Which concomitant medication complicates initiating therapy in this patient and what are possible ways to manage such drug interactions?

What adverse effects does the patient need to be counseled on with each of the recommended regimens?

Pharmacologic Therapy for Antiretroviral-Experienced Patients

KEY CONCEPT *Ongoing viral replication, whether at low levels in the face of adequate drug concentrations or at higher levels due to inconsistent systemic concentrations (or low concentrations in sanctuary sites, eg, male and female genital fluids, cerebrospinal fluid, or lymph nodes), will eventually lead to resistance to the prescribed medications.* To avoid further progression of resistant mutations, a failing regimen should be discontinued as soon as possible. *Virologic failure is defined as the inability to obtain or maintain an HIV RNA less than 200 copies/mL* (200×10^3 copies/L), *whereas incomplete virologic suppression is defined as two consecutive HIV RNA greater than 200 copies/mL* (200×10^3 copies/L) *after 24 weeks of therapy.*[8] Immunologic failure is defined as the failure to achieve and/or maintain an adequate CD4$^+$ count in the setting of virologic suppression. A typical CD4$^+$ count should increase at least 150 cells/mm^3 (150×10^6/L) over the first year of therapy. The goal of therapy for patients with antiretroviral resistance is to reestablish virologic suppression or HIV RNA lower than the limit of detection of the assay (typically less than 40 *copies/mL* [40×10^3 copies/L]).

Treatment considerations for antiretroviral-experienced patients are much more complex than for patients who are naïve to therapy. Prior to changing therapy, the reasons for treatment failure should be identified. A comprehensive review of the patient's severity of disease, antiretroviral treatment history, adherence to therapy, intolerance or toxicity, concomitant drug therapies, comorbidities, and results of current and past HIV resistance testing should be performed. If patients fail therapy due to poor adherence, the underlying reasons must be determined and addressed prior to initiation of new therapy. Reasons for poor adherence include problems with medication access, active substance abuse, depression and/or denial of the disease, and a lack of education on the importance of 100% adherence to therapy. Medication intolerance or toxicity can be remedied with therapy for the adverse event, exchanging the drug causing the toxicity with another in the same class, or changing the entire regimen. Pharmacokinetics or systemic drug exposure can be optimized by ensuring maximal drug absorption (taking the drug with or without food can alter exposure by up to 30%) and avoiding interactions with concomitant prescription or nonprescription medications and dietary supplements. When causes for treatment failure are identified, appropriate strategies for therapy can be determined.

An additional consideration when stopping or changing therapy is a staggered discontinuation of antiretrovirals with different half-lives. For example, in patients taking Atripla (tenofovir, emtricitabine, and efavirenz), tenofovir and emtricitabine should be continued for at least 4 to 7 days after discontinuation of the Atripla combination pill due to the much prolonged half-life of efavirenz as compared with tenofovir and emtricitabine. Without continued dosing of tenofovir and emtricitabine, patients will have prolonged exposure of only efavirenz resulting in efavirenz monotherapy, which has demonstrated antiretroviral resistance. If new antiretroviral therapy is to be initiated immediately, no overlap is necessary; however, it should be noted that efavirenz concentrations will persist for some period of time.[8]

Drug interactions between antiretrovirals and between antiretrovirals and concomitant medications should be evaluated for each patient to avoid under- and/or overexposure of either therapy. KEY CONCEPT *NNRTIs, PIs, certain INSTIs, and maraviroc are metabolized by CYP-450 enzymes. In addition, NNRTIs, PIs, and cobisistat are inhibitors and/or inducers of this enzyme system.* In addition, some of the antiretrovirals are substrates, inhibitors, and/or inducers of transporters such as P-glycoprotein (P-gp) and therefore may lead to drug interactions. Information provided in Table 87–4 describes the drug interaction potential of each antiretroviral. Due to the ever-changing drug interactions with this class of medications, the regularly updated DHHS Guidelines for the Use of Antiretroviral Agents in HIV-1–Infected Adults and Adolescents are a recommended source of specific drug interactions.[8]

The goals of therapy differ for antiretroviral-experienced patients who have limited drug exposure (ie, developing resistance to their first antiretroviral regimen) versus those with extensive exposure (ie, developing resistance to their third or fourth antiretroviral regimen). It is reasonable to expect maximal viral suppression in those with limited drug exposure. However, this may not be feasible for patients with prior exposure to multiple medications. In antiretroviral-experienced patients, a reasonable goal is to simply preserve immune function and prevent clinical progression.

Several issues need to be considered in choosing a salvage regimen for HIV infection. Knowing prior medication exposure can assist in identifying which drugs to avoid. However, direct HIV resistance testing can better identify the resistance and susceptibility patterns of the major viral strains. Because HIV may be susceptible to certain components of the failing antiretroviral regimen, these drugs can be recycled into future regimens. Resistance testing should be used when all patients enter into care, in patients with virologic failure on an antiretroviral regimen, or with suboptimal suppression after initiation of antiretroviral therapy. Testing is generally preferred for antiretroviral naïve patients. For resistance testing to be useful, the patient should have a plasma HIV RNA of at least 1000 copies/mL (1×10^6 copies/L) and should be currently taking their antiretroviral medications (or be within 4 weeks of discontinuing antiretroviral therapy). This viral concentration is necessary to yield reliable amplification of the virus, and the antiretroviral medications are needed because the dominant viral species reverts to wild-type within 4 to 6 weeks after medications are stopped.

Two types of HIV resistance testing are available, an HIV genotype and an HIV phenotype. Genotyping involves detecting mutations by genetically sequencing the virus, whereas phenotyping determines the ability of the virus to replicate in the presence of varying antiretroviral concentrations. Genotyping is more rapid and less costly than phenotyping, but results in a list of mutations that may be more difficult to interpret than phenotyping. An HIV virtual phenotype report may also be obtained when genotypes are ordered.[8] This compares the patient's viral sequence to a database of matched genotypes and drug susceptibilities. Web-based tools are available to assist with interpretation of resistance mutations (eg, Stanford University's HIV Drug Resistance Database; http://hivdb.stanford.edu/index.html). However, expert interpretation of genotype and phenotype reports is recommended.

Management of antiretroviral-experienced patients is complex, and expert opinion is advised before selecting therapy. KEY CONCEPT *As with antiretrovial-naïve patients, three or more active drugs should be prescribed.*[8] Since considerable cross-resistance can occur between medications within an antiretroviral class, simply using drugs to which the patient has not been exposed may be insufficient. Complete cross-resistance occurs within the first generation of NNRTIs, whereas the NRTIs and PIs have variable overlapping resistance patterns. For this reason, HIV resistance assays are important tools for choosing subsequent effective therapies. The use of antiretrovirals with unique mechanisms of action like enfuvirtide (fusion inhibitor) or maraviroc (CCR5 antagonist) may be warranted as salvage therapy.

If patients fail therapy with resistance to only one drug, one or two active agents may be substituted for this drug while retaining the remaining drugs in the regimen. If patients fail therapy with resistance to more than one drug, changing classes of antiretrovirals and/or adding new active drugs is warranted. New NRTIs should be selected from resistance testing. If this is not available, the assumption should be made that resistance has developed to all NRTIs used in the failing regimen. In general, HIV that is resistant solely to lamivudine and/or emtricitabine will be susceptible to other NRTIs. If HIV develops resistance solely to tenofovir, then it may have reduced susceptibility to didanosine and likely abacavir but should remain susceptible to zidovudine, stavudine, lamivudine, and emtricitabine. Cross-resistance occurs between zidovudine and stavudine.[8]

If a patient appears to fail an antiretroviral regimen without detectable HIV resistance, adherence should be investigated, and the adequacy of the plasma HIV RNA concentration in the resistance sample confirmed. Options include continuing the current regimen or starting a new regimen and repeating the resistance test 2 to 4 weeks after adherence is verified. The availability of new potent antiretrovirals has resulted in a decrease in the number of patients with multiclass drug resistance. Although rare, such patients have very limited treatment options, making it impossible to construct a regimen with two to three active agents.

Table 87–4

Summary of Currently Available Antiretroviral Agents

Generic Name [Abbreviation] (Trade Name)	Dosage Forms	Commonly Prescribed Doses	Dose Adjustments	Food Restrictions	Significant Adverse Events	Drug Interaction Potential
Nucleoside (Tide) Reverse Transcriptase Inhibitors						
Abacavir (Ziagen)	300-mg tablet; 20 mg/mL oral solution	300 mg twice daily or 600 mg once daily	None	None (alcohol increases abacavir conc. by 41%)	Potentially fatal hypersensitivity reaction (rash, fever, malaise, nausea, vomiting, shortness of breath, sore throat, loss of appetite)—HLA B*5701 test before treatment	Alcohol dehydrogenase and glucuronyl transferase, 82% renal excretion of metabolites
Didanosine (Videx EC)	125-, 200-, 250-, 400-mg capsules; 10 mg/mL oral Powder for Suspension:	> 60 kg: 400 mg daily < 60 kg: 250 mg daily	CrCl (mL/min[mL/s]): / Greater than 60 kg: / Less than 60 kg: 30–59 [0.50–0.99]: 200 mg / 125 mg 10–29 [0.17–0.49]: 125 mg / 100 mg less than 10 [0.17]: 125 mg / 75 mg	Take 30 minutes prior or 2 hours after meal (conc. decrease 55% with food)	Pancreatitis; peripheral neuropathy; nausea; diarrhea	Renal excretion
Emtricitabine (Emtriva)	200-mg capsule; 10 mg/mL oral solution	200 mg daily; 240 mg (24 mL) oral solution daily	CrCl (mL/min[mL/s]): / Capsule: / Solution: 30–49 [0.50–0.82]: 200 mg every 48 hours / 120 mg every 24 hours 15–29 [0.25–0.49]: 200 mg every 72 hours / 80 mg every 24 hours < 15/HD [0.25/HD]: 200 mg every 96 hours / 60 mg every 24 hours (Dose after dialysis on dialysis days)	None	Minimal	Renal excretion
Lamivudine (Epivir)	150-mg and 300-mg tablets or 10 mg/mL oral solution	150 mg twice daily or 300 mg once daily	CrCl (mL/min[mL/s]): / Dose: 30–49 [0.50–0.82]: 150 mg every day 15–29 [0.25–0.49]: 150 mg, then 100 mg every day 5–14 [0.08–0.24]: 150 mg, then 50 mg every day < 5/HD [0.08/HD]: 50 mg, then 25 mg every day (Dose after dialysis on dialysis days)	None	Minimal	Renal excretion

(Continued)

Table 87–4

Summary of Currently Available Antiretroviral Agents (*Continued*)

Generic Name [Abbreviation] (Trade Name)	Dosage Forms	Commonly Prescribed Doses	Dose Adjustments	Food Restrictions	Significant Adverse Events	Drug Interaction Potential
Stavudine (Zerit)	15-, 20-, 30-, 40-mg capsules or 1 mg/mL for oral solution	> 60 kg: 40 mg twice daily < 60 kg: 30 mg twice daily	**CrCl (mL/min[mL/s]): / Greater than 60 kg: / Less than 60 kg:** 26–50 [0.43–0.83]: 20 mg every 12 hours / 15 mg every 12 hours 10–25/HD [0.17–0.42/HD]: 20 mg every 24 hours / 15 mg every 24 hours	None	Peripheral neuropathy; lipodystrophy; rapidly progressive ascending neuromuscular weakness (rare); pancreatitis; lactic acidosis with hepatic steatosis (higher incidence with stavudine than with other NRTIs); hyperlipidemia	Renal excretion
Tenofovir disoproxil fumarate (Viread)	150, 200, 250-, 300-mg tablet Oral powder for suspension 40 mg per 1g powder	300 mg daily	**CrCl (mL/min[mL/s]): / Dose:** 30–49 [0.50–0.82]: 300 mg every 48 hours 10–29 [0.17–0.49]: 300 mg twice weekly ESRD/HD: 300 mg every 7 days (Dose after dialysis on dialysis days)	Powder taken with food	Asthenia, headache, diarrhea, nausea, vomiting, and flatulence; renal insufficiency	Renal excretion
Zidovudine (Retrovir)	100-mg capsule, 300-mg tablet, 10 mg/mL IV solution, 10 mg/mL oral solution	600 mg daily in two to three divided doses	100 mg 3 times daily or 300 mg once daily in severe renal impairment (CrCl < 15 mL/min [0.25 mL/s]) or HD	None	Bone marrow suppression: macrocytic anemia or neutropenia; GI intolerance, headache, insomnia, asthenia	Glucuronyl transferase and renal
Zidovudine + lamivudine (Combivir)	Zidovudine 300 mg + Lamivudine 150-mg tablet	One tablet twice daily	Do not use with CrCl < 50 mL/min (0.83 mL/s)	None	See adverse events for zidovudine and lamivudine	See zidovudine and lamivudine
Abacavir + lamivudine + zidovudine (Trizivir)	Abacavir 300 mg + lamivudine 150 mg + zidovudine 300-mg tablet	One tablet twice daily	Do not use with CrCl < 50 mL/min (0.83 mL/s)	None	See adverse events for zidovudine, lamivudine, and abacavir	See zidovudine, lamivudine, and abacavir
Abacavir + lamivudine (Epzicom)	Abacavir 600 mg + lamivudine 300-mg tablet	One tablet daily	Do not use with CrCl < 50 mL/min (0.83 mL/s)	None	See adverse events for abacavir and lamivudine	See abacavir and lamivudine
Tenofovir + emtricitabine (Truvada)	Tenofovir 300 mg + emtricitabine 200-mg tablet	One tablet daily	**CrCl (mL/min[mL/s]): / Dose:** 30–49 [0.50–0.82]: One tablet every 48 hours < 30 [0.50]: Not recommended	None	See adverse events for tenofovir and emtricitabine	See tenofvir and emtricitabine

Nonnucleoside Reverse Transcriptase Inhibitors						
Delavirdine (Rescriptor)	100-, 200-mg tablets	400 mg 3 times daily (100-mg tablet can be dispersed in 3 oz or more of water to produce slurry); 200-mg tablet should be administered whole; separate dosing from buffered didanosine or antacids by 1 hour	Use with caution in patients with hepatic impairment	None	Rash; increased LFTs, headaches	Metabolized by cytochrome P-450 (CYP); CYP3A inhibitor; 51% excreted in urine (< 5% unchanged); 44% in feces
Efavirenz (Sustiva)	50-, 200-mg capsules or 600-mg tablet	600 mg daily at or before bedtime	Use with caution in patients with hepatic impairment	Take on an empty stomach high-fat/calorie meals increases C_{max} of capsule 39% and C_{max} of tablet 79%	Rash; CNS symptoms (insomnia, irritability, lethargy, dizziness, vivid dreams) usually resolve in 2 weeks; increased LFTs; false-positive cannabinoid test; teratogenic in monkeys	Metabolized by CYP2B6 and CYP3A (3A mixed inducer/inhibitor); 14–34% excreted in urine (glucuronidated metabolites, < 1% unchanged); 16%–61% in feces
Etravirine (Intelence)	100-, 200-mg tablets	200 mg twice daily following a meal	No dosage adjustment for Child Pugh Class A or B. Has not been evaluated for Class C	Take following a meal. Fasting decreases by 50%	Rash, nausea	Metabolized by CYP3A, 2C9, and 2C19; Induces 3A4 and inhibits 2C9 and 2C19
Nevirapine (Viramune, Viramune XR)	200-mg tablet, 100 and 400mg XR tablet or 50 mg/5 mL oral suspension,	200 mg once daily for 14 days; then 200 mg twice daily, For XR tablet, lead-in with 200 mg once daily of IR tablet followed by 400 mg daily XR tab	Use with caution in patients with hepatic impairment; avoid use with moderate to severe hepatic impairment	No food restrictions	Rash including Stevens-Johnson syndrome; symptomatic hepatitis, including fatal hepatic necrosis	Metabolized by CYP2B6 and CYP3A (3A inducer); 80% excreted in urine (glucuronidated metabolites; less than 5% unchanged); 10% in feces
Rilpivirine (Edurant)	25-mg tablet	25 mg daily	No dosage adjustment for Child Pugh Class A or B. Has not been evaluated for Class C; Use with caution in severe or end-stage renal impairment	Take with a normal- to high-calorie meal Absorption dependent on gastric pH-special considerations needed when coadministered with antacids	Rash; depressive disorders;	Metabolized by CYP3A4

(*Continued*)

Table 87–4

Summary of Currently Available Antiretroviral Agents (*Continued*)

Generic Name [Abbreviation] (Trade Name)	Dosage Forms	Commonly Prescribed Doses	Dose Adjustments	Food Restrictions	Significant Adverse Events	Drug Interaction Potential
Tenofovir + emtricitabine + efavirenz [tenofovir/emtricitabine/efavirenz] (Atripla)	Tenofovir 300 mg Emtricitabine 200 mg Efavirenz 600 mg	One tablet daily	Do not use in patients with CrCl < 50 mL/min (0.83 mL/s)	High-fat/high-caloric meals increase peak plasma concentrations of efavirenz capsules by 39% and efavirenz tablets by 79%; take on empty stomach	See adverse events of tenofovir, emtricitabine, and efavirenz	See tenofovir, emtricitabine, and efavirenz
Tenofovir + emtricitabine – rilpivirine [tenofovir/emtricitabine/rilpivirine] (Complera)	Tenofovir 300 mg Emtricitabine 200 mg Rilpivirine 25mg	One tablet daily	Do not use in patients with CrCl < 50 mL/min (0.83 mL/s)	Take with a meal (preferrably high fat), avoid acid suppression	See adverse events of tenofovir, emtricitabine, and rilpivirine	See tenofovir, emtricitabine, and rilpivirine
Protease Inhibitors						
Atazanavir (Reyataz)	100-, 150-, 200-, 300-mg capsules	Atazanavir 300mg + ritonavir 100mg or atazanavir 400 mg daily If taken with tenofovir use the following: atazanavir 300 mg daily + ritonavir 100 mg daily If taken with efavirenz in treatment of naïve patients only: atazanavir 400 mg daily + ritonavir 100 mg daily (do not use efavirenz in treatment of experienced patients)	Child-Pugh Class — Dose 7–9 — 300 mg daily > 9 — Not recommended; Treatment-naïve patients on hemodialysis: atazanavir 300 mg + ritonavir 100 mg daily; treatment-experienced patients on hemodialysis: Not recommended	Take with food (AUC increases 30%); pH-sensitive dissolution—special considerations needed when coadministered with antacids	Indirect hyperbilirubinemia; prolonged PR interval (asymptomatic first-degree AV block); use with caution in patients with underlying conduction defects or on concomitant medications that can cause PR prolongation; hyperglycemia; fat maldistribution; increased bleeding episodes in patients with hemophilia	CYP3A4 inhibitor and substrate; UGT1A1 inhibitor

Darunavir (Prezista)	75-g, 150-mg, 600-mg, 800-mg tablets, 100 mg/mL oral suspension	Darunavir 600 mg + ritonavir 100 mg twice daily in treatment experienced patients Darunavir 800 mg daily + ritonavir 100 mg daily in treatment naïve patients	Use with caution in patients with hepatic impairment		Should be given with food	Skin rash (has a sulfonamide moiety, Stevens-Johnson and erythema multiforme have been reported); diarrhea, nausea; headache; hyperlipidemia; transaminase elevation; hyperglycemia; fat maldistribution; possible increased bleeding episodes in patients with hemophilia	CYP3A4 inhibitor and substrate
Fosamprenavir (Lexiva)	700-mg tablet; 50 mg/mL oral suspension	ARV-naïve patients: fosamprenavir 1400 mg twice daily, Fosamprenavir 700 mg + ritonavir 100 mg twice daily, or fosamprenavir 1400 mg + ritonavir 200 mg once daily; PI-experienced *patients:* fosamprenavir 700 mg + ritonavir 100 mg twice daily	Child-Pugh Class 5–8 9–12	Dose 700 mg twice daily Not recommended	None	Skin rash; diarrhea, nausea and vomiting; headache; hyperlipidemia; LFT elevation; hyperglycemia; fat maldistribution; increased bleeding episodes in patients with hemophilia	CYP3A4 inhibitor, inducer, and substrate
		Coadministration with efavirenz: fosamprenavir 700 mg + ritonavir 100 mg twice daily or fosamprenavir 1400 mg + ritonavir 300 mg once daily	Ritonavir should not be used in patients with hepatic impairment				

(*Continued*)

Table 87–4

Summary of Currently Available Antiretroviral Agents (*Continued*)

Generic Name [Abbreviation] (Trade Name)	Dosage Forms	Commonly Prescribed Doses	Dose Adjustments	Food Restrictions	Significant Adverse Events	Drug Interaction Potential
Indinavir (Crixivan)	200-, 400-mg capsules	800 mg every 8 hours; indinavir 800 mg + ritonavir 100 twice daily; indinavir 800 mg + ritonavir 200 mg twice daily	Mild to moderate hepatic insufficiency due to cirrhosis: 600 mg every 8 hours	*For unboosted indinavir:* Take 1 hour before or 2 hours after heavy meals, or concomitantly with low-fat meal. No restrictions when used with ritonavir	Nephrolithiasis; GI intolerance, nausea; indirect hyperbilirubinemia; hyperlipidemia; headache, asthenia, blurred vision, dizziness, rash, metallic taste, thrombocytopenia, alopecia, hemolytic anemia; hyperglycemia; fat maldistribution; increased bleeding episodes in patients with hemophilia	CYP3A4 inhibitor (less than ritonavir)
Lopinavir + ritonavir (Kaletra)	Lopinavir 100 mg + ritonavir 25 mg tablet, Lopinavir 200 mg + ritonavir 50-mg tablet, lopinavir 400 mg + ritonavir 100 mg/5 mL oral solution (contains 42% alcohol)	two 200/50 mg tablets or 5 mL twice daily four 200/50 mg tablets once daily; with efavirenz or nevirapine: 3 tablets or 6.5 mL twice daily	Use with caution in patients with hepatic impairment	Take with food (AUC increases 48%–80%)	Nausea, vomiting, diarrhea; asthenia; hyperlipidemia; LFT elevation; hyperglycemia; fat maldistribution; increased bleeding episodes in hemophiliacs	CYP3A4 inhibitor and susbstrate CYP2C9, 2C19, 1A2 inducer
Nelfinavir (Viracept)	250- to 625-mg tablets, 50 mg/g oral powder	1250 mg twice daily or 750 mg three times daily	Use with caution in patients with hepatic impairment	Take with meal or snack	Diarrhea; hyperlipidemia; hyperglycemia; fat maldistribution; increased bleeding in hemophiliacs; LFT elevation	CYP3A4 inhibitor and substrate

Ritonavir (Norvir)	100-mg tablet or capsule, 600 mg/7.5-mL solution	100–200 mg/dose when used as pharmacokinetic enhancer	No dosage adjustment in mild hepatic impairment No data for moderate to severe impairment; use with caution	Take with food to improve tolerability	GI intolerance, nausea, diarrhea; paresthesias; hyperlipidemia; hepatitis; asthenia; taste perversion; hyperglycemia; fat maldistribution; increased bleeding in hemophiliacs	CYP3A4 inhibitor (potent) and substrate; CYP2D6 substrate; mixed dose-dependent induction and inhibition of other phase I and II enzymes
Saquinavir (Invirase)	200-mg capsule, 500-mg tablet	Unboosted saquinavir not recommended *With* ritonavir: (ritonavir 100 mg + saquinavir 1000 mg) twice daily	Use with caution in patients with hepatic impairment	Take within 2 hours of a meal when taken with ritonavir	Nausea, diarrhea; headache; LFT elevation; hyperlipidemia; hyperglycemia; fat maldistribution; increased bleeding in hemophiliacs	CYP3A4 inhibitor and substrate
Tipranavir (Aptivus)	250-mg capsules, oral solution 100 mg/mL	500 mg twice daily with ritonavir 200 mg twice daily	Contraindicated in patients with moderate to severe hepatic insufficiency	Take with food	Hepatotoxicity; skin rash; hyperlipidemia; hyperglycemia; fat maldistribution; possible increased bleeding in hemophiliacs	Tipranavir/ritonavir mixed CYP inhibitor/inducer; Tipranavir is CYP3A4 substrate
Fusion Inhibitors						
Enfuvirtide (Fuzeon)	Injectable, in lyophilized powder Each single-use vial contains 108 mg of enfuvirtide to be reconstituted with 1.1 mL of sterile water for injection for delivery of approximately 90 mg/1 mL	90 mg (1 mL) subcutaneously twice daily	No dosage recommendation	N/A	Local injection site reaction (pain, erythema, induration, nodules and cysts, pruritus, eachymosis) in most patients; increased rate of bacterial pneumonia; less than 1% hypersensitivity reaction (rash, fever, nausea, vomiting, chills, rigors, hypotension, or elevated serum transaminases); do not rechallenge	Catabolism to amino acids, with subsequent recycling in the body pool

(Continued)

Table 87–4

Summary of Currently Available Antiretroviral Agents (*Continued*)

Generic Name [Abbreviation] (Trade Name)	Dosage Forms	Commonly Prescribed Doses	Dose Adjustments	Food Restrictions	Significant Adverse Events	Drug Interaction Potential
Chemokine Receptor Antagonists (CCR5 Antagonists)						
Maraviroc (Selzentry)	150-mg and 300-mg tablets	150 mg twice daily when given with strong CYP3A inhibitors (with or without CYP3A inducers) including PIs (except tipranavir/ritonavir) 300 mg twice daily when given with NRTIs, enfuvirtide, tipranavir/ritonavir, nevirapine and other drugs that are not potent P450 inhibitors 600 mg twice daily when given with CYP3A inducers, including efavirenz, rifampin, etc. (without a CYP3A inhibitor)	Patients with CrCl < 30 mL/min (0.83 mL/s) should receive maraviroc with a CYP3A inhibitor only if benefit outweighs the risk	No food restrictions	Abdominal pain; cough; dizziness; musculoskeletal symptoms; pyrexia; rash; upper RTI; hepatotoxicity; orthostatic hypotension	CYP3A substrate
Integrase Inhibitors						
Dolutegravir (Tivicay)	50-mg tablet	50 mg daily if treatment naïve 50 mg twice daily if coadministered with efavirenz, fosamprenavir, tipranavir/ritonavir, rifampin OR if INSTI-experienced with known or suspected INSTI resistance	Use with caution if CrCl < 30 mL/min (0.83 mL/s) No dosage adjustment for Child Pugh Class A or B Not recommended in Class C/has not been studied	Separate dose from polyvalent cations (eg, Ca, Mg, Al, Fe, Zn)	Insomnia, headache, increased serum creatinine	UGT1A1/3/9 and CYP3A4 (minor) substrate

Elvitegravir + cobicistat + tenofovir + emtricitabine (Stribild)	Elvitegravir 150 mg + cobicistat 150 mg + tenofovir 300 mg + emtricitabine 200-mg tablet	One tablet daily	CrCl < 70 mL/min (1.17 mL/s) at initiation of therapy: Not recommended CrCl < 50 mL/min (0.83 mL/s) during therapy: Continued use is not recommended	Take with food Separate dose from polyvalent cations (eg, Ca, Mg, Al, Fe, Zn)	Nausea; diarrhea; proteinuria; increased serum creatinine	Elvitegravir: UGT1A1/3 and CYP3A substrate Cobicistat: CYP3A inhibitor See tenofovir and emtricitabine
Raltegravir (Isentress)	400-mg tablet, 25 mg and 100 mg chewable tablets, 100 mg packets for oral suspension	400 mg twice daily 800 mg twice daily if coadministered with rifampin	No dosage adjustment	Separate dose from polyvalent cations (eg, Ca, Mg, Al, Fe, Zn)	Nausea; headache; diarrhea; pyrexia; CPK elevation	UGT1A1 substrate (glucuronidation)
Abacavir + lamivudine + Dolutegravir (Triumeq)	Abacavir 600 mg Lamivudine 300 mg Dolutegravir 50 mg	One tablet daily	Do not use if CrCl < 50 mL/min (0.83 mL/s) No dosage adjustment for Child Pugh Class A or B. Not recommended in Class C/has not been studied		See adverse events of abacavir, lamivudine, and dolutegravir	See abacavir, lamivudine, and dolutegravir

ARV, antiretroviral; AUC, area under the time-concentration curve; AV, atrioventricular; C_{max}, maximum concentration; CrCl, creatinine clearance; ESRD, end-stage renal disease; HD, hemodialysis; INSTI, integrase strand transfer inhibitor; LFT, liver function test; NRTI, nucleoside reverse transcriptase inhibitor; UGT, uridine diphosphate-glucuronsyltransferase.

Adapted from the DHHS Guidelines for the Use of Antiretroviral Agents in HIV-1-Infected Adults and Adolescents, May 1, 2014.

For these patients, continuing the current regimen may be beneficial because drug-resistant virus may have a compromised replication capacity. Other strategies may be considered for this type of patient, including pharmacokinetic enhancement with ritonavir, retreatment with prior antiretroviral agents, treatment with multidrug regimens (four or more antiretroviral drugs), and the use of new agents through expanded access programs or clinical trials.

Treatment Considerations in Special Populations

▶ *Acute HIV Infection*

Diagnosis of acute HIV infection is difficult, since many patients are asymptomatic or have nonspecific clinical symptoms similar to other common respiratory infections. If acute HIV infection is suspected, HIV antibody tests and a plasma HIV RNA concentration should be obtained. A clear diagnosis is made when an HIV antibody test is negative and the plasma HIV RNA concentration is detected or p24 antigen is present.

There is limited outcome data for treating acutely infected patients. Treatment of acute infection can decrease the severity of acute disease and decrease the viral set point; this may decrease progression rates and reduce the rate of viral transmission.[5] Limitations include an increased risk of chronic drug-induced toxicities and the development of viral resistance. Resistance testing should be performed prior to initiation of therapy due to an increase in resistance of antiretroviral naïve patients.[8]

▶ *Adolescent and Young Adult Patients*

As a result of similar modes of HIV transmission, adolescents infected after puberty are treated as adults. In this population, dosing of antiretroviral drugs should not be based on age, but on the Tanner stage (which considers external primary and secondary sexual characteristics).[8] Adolescents in early puberty should be dosed according to pediatric guidelines, whereas those in late puberty should be dosed as adults. During growth spurts, adolescents should be monitored closely for drug efficacy and toxicity, since rapid changes in weight can lead to altered drug concentrations. Adherence is of concern in this population due to denial of the disease, misinformation, distrust of health care professionals, low self-esteem, and lack of family and/or social support. Additionally, asymptomatic patients this age find it more difficult to adhere to therapy while feeling well.

▶ *Pediatric Patients*

There are unique considerations in the treatment of HIV-infected children. Specific treatment guidelines exist,[12] but a thorough review is outside the scope of this chapter. Most children acquire HIV infection through perinatal transmission either in utero, intrapartum, or postpartum through breast-feeding, although antiretroviral interventions have dramatically reduced transmission rates.[8] Antiretroviral therapy research is limited in pediatric patients, as some drugs have no dosing recommendations for this population or are not available in a formulation that can be easily administered to children. Additionally, drug exposures can change dramatically during early childhood development due to altered drug-metabolizing enzyme and drug transporter activities.

▶ *Pregnancy and Women of Reproductive Potential*

The goals of antiretroviral therapy for women of reproductive age and pregnant women are the same as for other adult patients. Specific guidelines for HIV-infected pregnant women are available.[13] If a woman is already virally suppressed on an antiretroviral regimen at the time she becomes pregnant, it is recommended that she remain on that regimen unless it contains efavirenz, which is pregnancy category D. However, because the risk of neural tube defects with efavirenz is highest during the first 5 to 6 weeks of pregnancy, and pregnancy is often not detected before 4 to 6 weeks, it is reasonable for women virologically suppressed on an efavirenz-containing regimen to continue that regimen rather than switch regimens and risk viral rebound. If not already on antiretroviral therapy, recommended therapies in pregnancy include zidovudine, lamivudine, lopinavir/ritonavir, atazanavir/ritonavir, and, if greater than 8 weeks of gestation, efavirenz. Nevirapine may be considered an alternative NNRTI for ARV-naive pregnant women if the $CD4^+$ count is less than 250 cells/mm^3 (250×10^6/L). Although data on the use of raltegravir in pregnancy is limited, it may be considered as an alternative agent if first-line therapies are to be avoided. A dual nucleoside reverse transcriptase inhibitor (NRTI) backbone that includes one or more NRTIs with high levels of transplacental passage, if possible, is recommended. Drugs to be avoided include efavirenz (in the first 8 weeks of pregnancy due to potential teratogenicity), the combination of didanosine and stavudine (due to a high incidence of lactic acidosis), and nevirapine in patients with a $CD4^+$ count greater than 250 cells/mm^3 (250×10^6/L) (due to an increased risk of hepatotoxicity). The goal of therapy is to reduce plasma HIV RNA below detectable levels and prevent MTCT of HIV. Limited data are available on antiretroviral pharmacokinetics in pregnancy, and standard doses of antiretroviral drugs are currently recommended, with close HIV RNA and $CD4^+$ monitoring in the third trimester of pregnancy.

Women of reproductive potential prescribed efavirenz should be counseled on its potentially teratogenic effects and the importance of birth control. Additionally, efavirenz, nevirapine, ritonavir, atazanavir/ritonavir, lopinavir/ritonavir, and tipranavir/ritonavir, darunavir/ritonavir, fosamprenavir/ritonavir, and saquinavir/ritonavir decrease the concentrations of different estrogens and/or progestins in oral contraceptives, which could lead to failure.[8] For patients prescribed these drugs, barrier forms of contraception are preferred to prevent pregnancy. Atazanavir may be taken with oral contraceptives with extreme caution, as it can increase or decrease the exposure to estrogen and progesterone, depending on whether it is used in combination with ritonavir. Depo-Provera is likely the safest alternative, as studies have shown no significant interactions between depot medroxyprogesterone acetate and antiretrovirals.[14] Maraviroc, raltegravir, elvitegravir/cobicistat, and dolutegravir have not shown clinically significant effects when used with oral contraceptives and are safe to use in combination.

▶ *Hepatitis B Coinfection*

HIV-infected patients coinfected with hepatitis B virus (HBV) have higher concentrations of DNA and hepatitis B early antigen (HBeAg) and higher rates of HBV-associated liver disease. Indications to initiate therapy for HBV/HIV coinfected patients are the same as in HIV-negative patients and is based on the HBV DNA level, serum ALT, and severity of liver disease. Options include interferon-α 2a or 2b and nucleoside/tide analogs. Nucleoside/tide analogs that treat HBV but not HIV are adefovir and entecavir. Entecavir, however, exhibits minimal antiviral activity against HIV, and should never be administered to coinfected patients who are not concurrently receiving fully suppressive HIV therapy. If given without suppressive antiretrovirals, entecavir can select for M184 resistance, leading to HIV resistance to emtricitabine and lamivudine. Nucleoside/tide analogs that are used to treat HBV and HIV are lamivudine, emtricitabine, and tenofovir. Combinations of tenofovir + emtricitabine or tenofovir + lamivudine should comprise the NRTI backbone of a fully suppressive regimen.[15] When changing HIV therapy in a patient with HBV viral suppression, the lamivudine, emtricitabine, or tenofovir should be continued for treatment of HBV in addition to the new HIV regimen.[8] Abrupt discontinuation of these antiretrovirals may result in significant hepatic injury due to the exacerbation of hepatitis B.

Vaccination against HBV can effectively prevent transmission. Currently in the United States, all infants should get their first HBV vaccination at birth. If there is no record of vaccination, or immunization history is unknown, HIV-infected patients and adults with high-risk sexual behavior or occupational exposure to HBV should be vaccinated.

► *Hepatitis C Coinfection*

All HIV-infected patients should be screened for hepatitis C infection. Patients coinfected with hepatitis C virus (HCV) and HIV have an increased rate of progression to cirrhosis, decompensated liver disease, hepatocellular carcinoma, and death compared with monoinfected HCV alone.[15] All HCV/HIV coinfected patients should be considered for therapy, taking into consideration the HCV genotype, stage of liver disease, as well as patient specific factors that may contraindicate therapy (eg, nonadherence, depression, substance abuse). The goal of HCV treatment is to achieve sustained virologic response (absence of detectable viremia greater than or equal to 3 months after discontinuation of treatment) and to decrease the progression of liver injury and likelihood of end-stage liver disease. Comprehensive treatment guidelines for HIV/HCV-coinfected patients are available and have recently been updated to reflect the rapidly evolving treatment options for HCV.[16] Recommended treatment regimens for HCV consist of pegylated interferon-α 2a or 2b, ribavirin, sofosbuvir, and simeprevir, with the combinations and duration of treatment determined by HCV genotype. Sofosbuvir and simeprevir are novel direct acting antivirals that exhibit potent antiviral activity and minimal toxicity. However, simeprevir, an HCV protease inhibitor, is metabolized primarily by CYP3A4 and is a substrate for the drug transporter P-glycoprotein (P-gp) and organic anion transporting polypeptide 1B1. Due to the potential for significant drug interactions, simeprevir is not recommended for use with HIV protease inhibitors, cobicistat, or the nonnucleoside reverse transcriptase inhibitors efavirenz, nevirapine, and etravirine. Coadministration of ribavirin with didanosine, and stavudine (due to increased risk of pancreatitis and/or lactic acidosis) and ribavirin with zidovudine (due to increased risk of anemia) should also be avoided. The first-generation protease inhibitors, telepravir and boceprevir, are associated with relatively increased toxicities and extensive drug-drug interactions, and are no longer recommended by the guidelines.[16] With many potent direct-acting antivirals in the HCV pipeline, the landscape of HCV treatment is rapidly evolving, with the hope of multiple curative, interferon-free, regimens to come in the near future.

Preexposure Prophylaxis (PrEP)

Multiple large-scale clinical trials in populations at highest risk for acquiring HIV have demonstrated that antiretrovirals, particularly tenofovir + emtricitabine, in combination with effective risk-reduction services (counseling, access to condoms, treatment of STI, etc.), reduce the rate of HIV transmission. Data from these trials has led to the FDA approval of Truvada (fixed-dose combination of tenofovir disoproxil fumarate 300 mg and emtricitabine 200 mg), as preexposure prophylaxis (PrEP) to reduce the risk of HIV-1 in adult homosexual men who have sex with men, heterosexually active men and women, and injection drug users who are at substantial risk of HIV acquisition.[17] The use of daily Truvada as PrEP should be in combination with effective risk-reduction interventions, as well as, very close follow-up and monitoring. Patients must be tested for HIV at baseline, and minimally every 3 months while taking PrEP. Additionally, due to the potential toxicities associated with tenofovir, renal function must be assessed at baseline and at 6-month intervals in patients taking Truvada as PrEP. Patient counseling, stressing the importance of medication adherence, should be routinely provided, as medication adherence has been linked to PrEP efficacy.[17]

Patient Encounter 2

A 29-year-old African American man presents to your clinic requesting medication to prevent the transmission of HIV. He had heard from his HIV-infected partner that the FDA approved a prescription medication for the prevention of HIV and he wanted to learn more about it. He reports engaging in MSM with an HIV-infected partner and uses condoms about 75% of the time.

What additional information do you need to know before creating a treatment plan for this patient?

What laboratory tests do you recommend?

What pharmacologic and nonpharmacologic options are available for this patient to protect himself from acquiring HIV?

What monitoring assessments and follow-up would you recommend?

OUTCOME EVALUATION

KEY CONCEPT *The success of antiretroviral therapy is measured by the degree to which the therapy (a) restores and preserves immunologic function, (b) maximally and durably suppresses HIV RNA, (c) improves quality of life, (d) reduces HIV-related morbidity and*

Patient Encounter 3

A 43-year-old woman presents to your clinic with complaints that she has noticed yellowing of the whites of her eyes. Four months ago, she initiated a regimen consisting of emtricitabine, tenofovir, and atazanavir/ritonavir. She is very upset because colleagues from work have noticed and as a result she would like to switch therapy.

Which medication is responsible for this adverse event?

What laboratory tests do you recommend?

What additional information do you need to know before creating a treatment plan for this patient?

What monitoring assessments and follow-up would you recommend?

Table 87–5

Serious Adverse Effects and Management

Adverse Effects	Drug	Signs and Symptoms	Risk Factors	Prevention/Monitoring	Management
Hepatotoxicity	Nevirapine	**Onset:** Up to 18 weeks postinitiation **Symptoms:** Abrupt onset of flu-like symptoms, abdominal pain, jaundice, fever ± rash	Increased $CD4^+$ count at initiation Female Elevated baseline AST/ALT Any liver disease High nevirapine concentration	2-week dose escalation Avoid starting nevirapine in women with $CD4^+$ > 250 cells/mm^3 (250 × 10^6/L), men with $CD4^+$ > 400 cells/mm^3 (400 × 10^6/L) AST/ALT every 2 weeks for 1st month, monthly for 3 months, then every 3 months	D/C antiretrovirals; D/C all hepatotoxic agents; rule out other causes; do not rechallenge with nevirapine
	Other NNRTIs, PIs, most NRTIs, and MVC	**Onset:** NNRTI—60% within first 12 weeks PI—weeks to months NRTI—months to years **Symptoms:** NNRTI—asymptomatic to nonspecific symptoms, such as anorexia, weight loss, or fatigue PI—generally asymptomatic, some with anorexia, weight loss, jaundice Didanosine NRTI—zidovudine, didanosine, stavudine may cause hepatotoxicity associated with lactic acidosis; lamivudine, emtricitabine, or tenofovir may cause HBV flare when these drugs are withdrawn	HBV or HCV coinfection Alcoholism Concomitant hepatotoxic drugs	Monitor LFTs at least every 3–4 months	Rule out other causes. For symptomatic patients: D/C all antiretrovirals and other potential hepatotoxic agents; after symptoms and LFTs normalize, begin new antiretroviral regimen (without the potential offending agents). For asymptomatic patients: If ALT > 5–10 × ULN, may consider D/C antiretrovirals or continue with close monitoring; after symptoms and LFTs normalize, begin new antiretroviral regimen (without the potential offending agents)
Lactic acidosis/ hepatic steatosis ± pancreatitis	NRTIs (esp. stavudine, didanosine, zidovudine)	**Onset:** Months after initiation **Symptoms:** Nonspecific GI (nausea, anorexia, abdominal pain, vomiting, weight loss, fatigue) Laboratory values: ↑ lactate, ↓ arterial pH, ↓ serum bicarbonate, ↑ AST/ALT, ↑ PT, ↑ T.bili, ↓ serum albumin, ↑ amylase/lipase (with pancreatitis)	Stavudine + didanosine Female sex Obesity Pregnancy Didanosine + hydroxyurea or ribavirin ↑ Duration of NRTI use	None unless symptoms present Consider lactate concentrations in patients with ↓ serum bicarbonate or ↑ anion gap	D/C all antiretrovirals; symptomatic support with fluids; some patients require IV bicarbonate, hemodialysis, parenteral nutrition, or mechanical ventilation; once syndrome resolves, consider using NRTIs with ↓ mitochondrial toxicity (abacavir, tenofovir, lamivudine, or emtricitabine); monitor lactate after restarting NRTIs; some clinicians use NRTI-sparing regimens

Stevens-Johnson syndrome/toxic epidermal necrosis	Nevirapine greater than efavirenz, delavirdine, etravirine; also, amprenavir, abacavir, zidovudine, didanosine, indinavir lopinavir/r, atazanavir, darunavir, rilpivirine, raltegravir	**Onset:** First day–weeks after therapy start **Symptoms:** Skin eruption with mucosal ulcerations; fever, tachycardia, malaise, myalgia, arthralgia; for nevirapine may also have hepatic toxicity	Nevirapine—female, black, Asian, Hispanic	Nevirapine: use 2-week lead in 200 mg daily, then 200 mg twice a day Avoid corticosteroid use during dose escalation—may increase rash incidence Educate patients to report symptoms as soon as they appear	D/C all antiretrovirals as well as any other possible cause; aggressive symptom support; do not rechallenge patient with offending agent; if caused by nevirapine, avoid NNRTI class, if possible
Hypersensitivity reaction (HSR)	Abacavir	**Onset:** Median = 9 days; 90% within first 6 weeks **Symptoms:** Acute onset of symptoms (most frequent to least): high fever, diffuse skin rash, malaise, nausea, headache, myalgia, chills, diarrhea, vomiting, abdominal pain, dyspnea, arthralgia, respiratory symptoms	HLA-B*5701, HLA-DR7, HLA-DQ3 Antiretroviral-naïve patients Higher incidence with 600 mg every day compared with twice a day dosing	HLA-B*5701 screening prior to abacavir if (+), label as abacavir allergic in medical chart Educate patients about signs and symptoms of HSR and the need of prompt report	D/C abacavir and other antiretrovirals; rule out other causes of symptoms, most signs and symptoms resolve 48 hours after abacavir/D/C; do not rechallenge with abacavir after suspected HSR
Lactic acidosis/ rapidly progressive ascending neuromuscular weakness	Stavudine	**Onset:** Months, then striking motor weakness within days–weeks **Symptoms:** Rapidly progressive ascending demyelinating polyneuropathy (similar to Guillain-Barré); respiratory paralysis	Prolonged stavudine use	Early recognition and D/C of offending agent to avoid progression	D/C antiretrovirals; supportive care; recovery may take months, sometimes irreversible; do not rechallenge with offending agent
Bleeding events	Tipranavir/ritonavir: intracranial hemorrhage (ICH); other PIs: ↑ bleeding in hemophiliacs	**Onset:** ICH: median = 525 days on tipranavir/ ritonavir Hemophiliacs: Few weeks **Symptoms:** ↑ Spontaneous bleeding tendency (in joints, muscles, soft tissues, and hematuria)	ICH: CNS lesions, head trauma, recent neurosurgery, coagulopathy, alcohol abuse, or on anticoagulant or antiplatelet agents Hemophiliac patients: PI use	ICH: Avoid tipranavir/ritonavir use in high risk patients Hemophiliacs: Consider using an NNRTI-based regimen; monitor for spontaneous bleeding	ICH: D/C tipranavir/ritonavir; supportive care Hemophiliacs: May require increased use of factor VIII products
Bone marrow suppression	Zidovudine	**Onset:** Few weeks–months **Symptoms:** Fatigue, risk of ↑ bacterial infections due to neutropenia; anemia, neutropenia	Advanced HIV High-dose zidovudine Preexisting anemia or neutropenia Concomitant use of bone marrow suppressants	Avoid in patients at high risk for bone marrow suppression; avoid other suppressing agents; monitor CBC with differential at least every 3 months	Switch to another NRTI; D/C concomitant bone marrow suppressant, if possible; for anemia: Identify and treat other causes; consider erythropoietin treatment or blood transfusion, if indicated; for neutropenia: Identify and treat other causes; consider filgrastim treatment, if indicated

(Continued)

Table 87–5

Serious Adverse Effects and Management (*Continued*)

Adverse Effects	Drug	Signs and Symptoms	Risk Factors	Prevention/Monitoring	Management
Nephrolithiasis/urolithiasis/crystalluria	Indinavir Atazanavir	**Onset:** Any time after initiation of therapy, especially if ↓ fluid intake **Symptoms:** Flank pain and/or abdominal pain, dysuria, frequency; pyuria, hematuria, crystalluria; rarely, ↑ serum creatinine and acute renal failure	History of nephrolithiasis Patients unable to maintain adequate fluid intake High peak indinavir concentration ↑ duration of exposure	Drink at least 1.5–2 L of noncaffeinated fluid per day; ↑ fluid intake at first sign of darkened urine; monitor urinalysis and serum creatinine every 3–6 months	Increased hydration; pain control; may consider switching to alternative agent; stent placement may be required
Nephrotoxicity	Indinavir, tenofovir	**Onset:** Indinavir—months after therapy Tenofovir—weeks to months after therapy **Symptoms:** Indinavir—asymptomatic; rarely develop end-stage renal disease; ↑ serum creatinine, pyuria; hydronephrosis, renal atrophy Tenofovir—asymptomatic to symptoms of nephrogenic diabetes insipidus, Fanconi syndrome; ↑ serum creatinine, proteinuria, hypophosphatemia, glycosuria, hypokalemia, non–anion gap metabolic acidosis	History of renal disease Concomitant use of nephrotoxic drugs	Avoid use of other nephrotoxic drugs; adequate hydration if on indinavir; monitor creatinine, urinalysis, serum potassium and phosphorus in patients at risk	D/C offending agent, generally reversible; supportive care; electrolyte replacement as indicated
Pancreatitis	Didanosine; didanosine + stavudine; didanosine + hydroxyurea or ribavirin; tenofovir	**Onset:** Usually weeks to months **Symptoms:** Postprandial abdominal pain, nausea, vomiting; ↑ serum amylase and lipase	High intracellular and/or serum Didanosine concentrations History of pancreatitis Alcoholism Hypertriglyceridemia Concomitant use of didanosine with stavudine, hydroxyurea, or ribavirin Use of didanosine + tenofovir without Didanosine dose reduction	Didanosine should not be used in patients with history of pancreatitis; avoid concomitant use of didanosine with stavudine, hydroxyurea, or ribavirin; ↓ didanosine dose when used with tenofovir	D/C offending agents; symptomatic management of pancreatitis—bowel rest, IV hydration, pain control, gradual resumption of oral intake

ALT, alanine aminotransferase; AST, aspartate aminotransferase; CBC, complete blood cell count; CPK, creatine phosphokinase; D/C, discontinue; HBV, hepatitis B virus; HCV, hepatitis C virus; LFT, liver function tests; NNRTI, nonnucleoside reverse transcriptase inhibitor; NRTI, nucleoside reverse transcriptase inhibitor; PI, protease inhibitor; PT, prothrombin time; T.bili, total bilirubin; ULN, upper limit of normal.

Table 87–6

Other Adverse Effects and Management

Adverse Effects	Drug	Signs and Symptoms	Risk Factors	Prevention/Monitoring	Management
Potential Long-Term Complications					
Cardiovascular	Potentially all PIs and other antiretrovirals (efavirenz, stavudine—unfavorable lipid effect; abacavir, didanosine—unknown)	**Onset**: months to years after therapy initiation **Symptoms**: premature CVD	Other risk factors for CVD	Consider non–PI-based regimen; lifestyle modification, counseling	Early diagnosis, prevention, and pharmacologic therapy for hyperlipidemia, HTN, insulin-resistance/diabetes mellitus; assess cardiac risk factors; switch to NNRTI- or atazanavir-based regimen; avoid stavudine
Hyperlipidemia	All PIs (except atazanavir); stavudine; efavirenz (to a lesser extent)	**Onset**: weeks to months after therapy initiation **Symptoms**: all PIs except atazanavir—↑ LDL and total cholesterol (TC), ↓↑ HDL; lopinavir/r and ritonavir—disproportionate ↑ TG; stavudine—↑ TG; may also ↑ LDL and TC; efavirenz or nevirapine—↑ HDL, slight ↑ TG	Underlying hyperlipidemia PI: Tipranavir/r greater than lopinavir/r and ritonavir greater than nelfinavir and amprenavir greater than indinavir and saquinavir greater than atazanavir NNRTI: less than PIs; efavirenz greater than nevirapine, etravirine, or rilpivirine NRTI: stavudine greater than zidovudine and tenofovir most common	Use non-PI, non–stavudine-based regimens; use atazanavir-based regimen; monitor fasting lipid profile at baseline, 3–6 months after new regimen, then at least annually	Assess cardiac risk factor; lifestyle modification; switch to antiretrovirals with fewer lipid effects; Consider statin therapy
Insulin resistance/ diabetes mellitus	All PIs	**Onset**: weeks to months after therapy initiation; **Symptoms**: polyuria, polydipsia, polyphagia, fatigue, weakness; exacerbation of hyperglycemia in patients with underlying diabetes	Underlying hyperglycemia, family history of diabetes mellitus	Use PI-sparing regimens; monitor fasting blood glucose 1–3 months after starting new regimen, then at least every 3–6 months	Diet and exercise; consider switching to an NNRTI-based regimen; if need for pharmacologic therapy, consider metformin, sulfonylurea, "glitazones," or insulin, where indicated
Osteoporosis/ Osteonecrosis	All PIs Tenofovir	**Onset**: insidious; **Symptoms:** mild to moderate periarticular pain; 85% of cases involve one or both femoral heads	Diabetes Prior steroid use Advanced age Alcohol use Hyperlipidemia	Risk reduction (limit steroid and alcohol use): for asymptomatic cases with < 15% bony head involvement, monitor with MRI every 3–6 months × 1 year, then every 6 months × 1 year, then annually	Conservative: reduce weight-bearing activity on affected joint; reduce risk factors; analgesics as needed; surgical: core decompression ± bone grafting (early disease); total joint arthroplasty (severe disease)

(Continued)

Table 87–6

Other Adverse Effects and Management (*Continued*)

Adverse Effects	Drug	Signs and Symptoms	Risk Factors	Prevention/Monitoring	Management
Quality-of-Life Complications					
CNS effects	Efavirenz	**Onset**: first few doses; **Symptoms**: one or more of the following: drowsiness, insomnia, abnormal dreams, dizziness, impaired concentration, depression, hallucination; exacerbation of psychiatric disorders; psychosis; suicidal ideation	Preexisting or unstable psychiatric illness Use of other drugs with CNS effects May be more common in African Americans due to genetic predisposition of ↓ clearance	Take no earlier than 2–3 hours before bedtime; take on an empty stomach; counsel patients to avoid operating machinery during first 2–4 weeks of therapy	Symptoms usually diminish or resolve after 2–4 weeks; may consider discontinuing therapy if symptoms persist and significantly impair daily function or exacerbate psychiatric illness
Fat maldistribution	PIs, thymidine analogs (stavudine more common than zidovudine)	**Onset**: gradually, months after therapy initiation; **Symptoms**: lipoatrophy—peripheral fat loss (facial thinning, thinning of extremities and buttocks); lipohypertrophy—increase in abdominal girth, breast size, and dorsocervical fat pad (buffalo hump)	Lipoatrophy—low baseline body mass index	DEXA scan; lipoatrophy: avoid thymidine analogs or switch from zidovudine or stavudine to abacavir or tenofovir	Switching to other agents may slow or stop progression, but may not reverse effects; injectable poly-L-lactic acid for facial lipoatrophy, human growth hormone
GI intolerance	All PIs, zidovudine, didanosine	**Onset**: first few doses; **Symptoms**: nausea, vomiting, abdominal pain; diarrhea commonly seen with nelfinavir, lopinavir/ritonavir, and didanosine-buffered formulations	All patients	Taking with food may reduce symptoms (not for didanosine or unboosted indinavir); may preemptively need antiemetics or antidiarrheals	May spontaneously resolve or become tolerable with time; nausea and vomiting: consider antiemetic prior to dosing; switch to less emetogenic agent; diarrhea: consider antimotility agents, calcium tablets, bulk-forming agents, and/or pancreatic enzymes
Injection site reactions	Enfuvirtide	**Onset**: first new doses; **symptoms**: pain, pruritus, erythema, ecchymosis warmth, nodules, rarely injection site infection	All patients	Educate regarding use of sterile technique, solution at room temperature, rotation of injection sites, avoidance of sites with little subcutaneous fat or existing reactions	Massaging the area vigorously before and after injection may reduce pain; wear loose clothing around injection site areas; take warm shower or bath prior to injection; rarely, warm compact or analgesics may be necessary
Peripheral neuropathy	Didanosine, stavudine	**Onset**: weeks to months after therapy initiation; **Symptoms**: begins with numbness and paresthesias of toes and feet; may progress to painful neuropathy; upper extremities less frequently involved; may be irreversible despite drug discontinuation	Preexisting peripheral neuropathy Combined use of these NRTIs or other drugs which may cause neuropathy Advanced HIV High dose of offending drugs or drugs that may increase didanosine intracellular activities (hydroxyurea, ribavirin)	Avoid using these agents in patients at risk, if possible; avoid combined use of these agents; ask patient at each encounter	Consider D/C offending agent prior to onset of disabling pain; pharmacologic treatment (variable effectiveness): gabapentin, tricyclic antidepressants, lamotrigine, oxcarbamazepine, topiramate, tramadol, narcotic analgesics, capsaicin cream, topical lidocaine

CVD, cardiovascular disease; D/C, discontinue; DEXA, dual-energy x-ray absorptiometry; HTN, hypertension; LDL, low-density lipoprotein; NNRTI, nonnucleoside reverse transcriptase inhibitor; NRTI, nucleoside reverse transcriptase inhibitor; PI, protease inhibitor; TG, triglyceride.

mortality, and (e) prevents opportunistic infections. KEY CONCEPT *The major outcome parameters are CD4⁺ lymphocyte absolute count and percentage and plasma HIV RNA.* Adequate immunologic response in antiretroviral-naïve patients consists of an increase in $CD4^+$ cell count that averages 50 to 150 cells/mm^3 (50×10^6 to 150×10^6/L) (with a faster response in the first 3 months), and a 1-log decrease in HIV RNA by 2 to 8 weeks after starting medications, followed by concentrations less than 50 copies/mL (50×10^3 copies/L) by 12 to 16 weeks (if HIV RNA less than 100,000/mL [100×10^6/L] or by 16 to 24 weeks if HIV RNA greater than 100,000/mL [100×10^6/L]). Upon initiating or changing antiretroviral therapy, HIV RNA should be measured after 2 to 8 weeks and every 4 to 8 weeks until undetectable. Once stable, HIV RNA and $CD4^+$ count are monitored generally every 3 to 6 months. In highly treatment-experienced patients, adequate immunologic response may be only a stable, or slightly increased, $CD4^+$ count and a stable HIV RNA. This may be enough to prevent clinical progression. However, with the new agents and new therapeutic classes of antiretrovirals available for treatment-experienced patients, the goal of treatment should be to reestablish maximal viral suppression to less than 50 HIV RNA copies/mL (50×10^3 copies/L).[8]

There should be a plan for each patient to assess the effectiveness of antiretroviral therapy after initiation. At each clinic visit, patients should be evaluated for the presence of adverse drug reactions, drug allergies, medication adherence, and potential drug interactions. Antiretrovirals have both class-associated and drug-specific adverse effects (see Table 87–4). If the patient experiences any of the serious, life-threatening effects (Table 87–5), the offending agent should be discontinued promptly, and in most cases the patient cannot be rechallenged. Potential long-term complications that may reduce the quality of life are listed in Table 87–6. For drugs with a high likelihood of intolerability (such as nelfinavir-associated diarrhea), patients should be counseled to anticipate these effects and have concomitant prescriptions available for preemptive management (such as an antidiarrheal agent). Patients should have follow-up within the first week after initiating a new drug regimen. If the patient does not tolerate a medication despite all efforts to the contrary, consider changing the drug.[8]

KEY CONCEPT *Treatment of HIV infection is lifelong.* Unplanned short-term treatment interruptions may be necessary due to drug toxicity or illness that precludes administration of oral therapy. If a patient must interrupt therapy due to toxicity, all drugs of the regimen should be stopped at the same time, regardless of half-life. The strategy of scheduling elective treatment interruptions (where patients stop and start antiretroviral therapy based on $CD4^+$ T-cell count criteria) has been evaluated in several clinical trials. Viral rebound occurs quickly after stopping therapy and worsens immune function, causes clinical progression, and may even result in death. If either short-term (less than 7 days) or long-term treatment interruption is needed, drug half-life must be taken into consideration to assure that monotherapy with longer-acting antiretrovirals is avoided as was described previously for tenofovir/emtricitabine/efavirenz combination. For regimens in which all components have similar half-lives, all drugs can be stopped simultaneously. If the regimen contains components with significantly different half-lives (eg, Atripla), stopping all drugs at the same time could result in the drug with the longest half-life (usually NNRTIs) lingering in the body and functioning as monotherapy. The ideal time to stop the NNRTIs (efavirenz, etravirine, or nevirapine) is unknown, as these drugs can continue to be detectable 1 to 3+ weeks in patients. Options include either (a) stopping the NNRTI first and continuing the

The Patient Care Process: Newly Diagnosed

Patient Assessment:

- Confirm HIV infection (see Table 87–1), screen for additional sexually transmitted infections, and assess the risk for opportunistic infections and need for prophylaxis.
- Create a safe and comfortable environment to obtain a thorough medical and medication history (prescription, nonprescription, and natural drug product use). Review and update patient allergies.
- Acquire baseline laboratory data (see Table 87–2) to stage HIV disease and to assist in the selection of ARV drug regimens (genotypic resistance testing, HLA-B*5701).
- Assess patient's readiness for initiating ART.

Therapy Evaluation:

- Evaluate comorbid conditions (eg, mental illness, substance abuse) and social issues (economic stability, lack of social support, insurance coverage) that may impair medication adherence.
- Utilize results of genotype in conjunction with patient specific factors to construct a recommended ART regimen.
- Assess the potential for clinically significant drug–drug, drug–food, drug–disease interactions.

Care Plan Development:

- Provide patient with basic information regarding HIV infection, progression of HIV/prognosis, treatment options, and support services available.
- Inform patient of the benefits of initiating ART, stressing the importance of strict medication adherence.
- Educate patient on regimen-specific administration and the common adverse drug effects (see Table 87–4). Warn patient of the key signs and symptoms of severe toxicity (ie, jaundice and abacavir hypersensitivity reaction).
- Provide risk reduction counseling on effective strategies to prevent HIV transmission and disclosure to sexual and/or needle-sharing partners.

Follow-up Evaluation:

- Assess response to ARV therapy by drawing plasma HIV RNA within 2 to 4 weeks (no later than 8 weeks) after initiation of ART and every 4 to 8 weeks until viral load is suppressed.
- Monitor immune reconstitution by measuring $CD4^+$ count 3 months after initiation of ART.
- Evaluate tolerability of regimen by assessing for adverse events and medication adherence.

other drugs in the regimen for up to 4 weeks or (b) substituting the NNRTI with a PI and continuing the PI with dual NRTIs for up to 4 weeks. In this situation, therapeutic drug monitoring of the long half-life drug can be useful in determining when to stop the NRTI ± PI coverage.[8]

Abbreviations Introduced in This Chapter

AIDS	Acquired immunodeficiency syndrome
ALT	Alanine aminotransferase
ART	Antiretroviral therapy
AST	Aspartate aminotransferase
CPK	Creatine phosphokinase
CVD	Cardiovascular disease
CYP	Cytochrome P-450 isoenzyme
D/C	Discontinue
DEXA	Dual-energy x-ray absorptiometry
DHHS	Department of Health and Human Services
ELISA	Enzyme-linked immunosorbent assay
GERD	Gastroesophageal reflux disease
gp	Glycoprotein
HAART	Highly active antiretroviral therapy
HBeAg	Hepatitis B early antigen
HBV	Hepatitis B virus
HCV	Hepatitis C virus
HDL	High-density lipoprotein
HIV	Human immunodeficiency virus
HLA	Human leukocyte antigen
HSR	Hypersensitivity reaction
HTN	Hypertension
IAS-USA	International AIDS Society–USA
ICH	Intracranial hemorrhage
IFA	Indirect immunofluorescence assay
LDL	Low-density lipoprotein
LFT	Liver function tests
MSM	Men who have sex with men
MTCT	Mother-to-child transmission
NNRTI	Nonnucleoside reverse transcriptase inhibitor
NRTI	Nucleoside reverse transcriptase inhibitor
NtRTI	Nucleotide reverse transcriptase inhibitor
P-gp	P-glycoprotein
PCP	*Pneumocystis jiroveci* (formerly *carinii*) pneumonia
PI	Protease inhibitor
PrEP	Pre-Exposure Prophylaxis
PT	Prothrombin time
RT-PCR	Reverse transcriptase polymerase chain reaction
SIV	Simian immunodeficiency virus
STI	Sexually transmitted infection
T.bili	Total bilirubin
TDF	Tenofovir disoproxil fumarate
TG	Triglyceride
ULN	Upper limit of normal
WB	Western blot

REFERENCES

1. Centers for Disease Control. Revised classification system for HIV infection and expanded surveillance case definition for AIDS among adolescents and adults. 1993 Morbidity and Mortality Weekly Report, 41 (RR-17).
2. World Heath Organization. UNAIDS report on the global AIDS epidemic 2013 [online]. [cited 2014 Jun 1]. http://www.unaids.org/en/resources/campaigns/globalreport2013/globalreport/. Accessed June 1, 2014.
3. Centers for Disease Control and Prevention. HIV surveillance report [online]. [cited 2014 Jun 1]. http://www.cdc.gov/hiv/library/reports/surveillance/index.html
4. Patel P, Borkowf CB, Brooks JT, et al. Estimating per-act HIV transmission risk: A systematic review. AIDS. 2014;28:1509.
5. World Health Organization. HIV transmission through breastfeeding: A review of available evidence 2007 update [online]. [cited 2015 Jan 12]. http://whqlibdoc.who.int/publications/2008/9789241596596_eng.pdf?ua=119
6. Wawer MJ, Gray RH, Sewankambo NK, et al. Rates of HIV-1 transmission per coital act, by stage of HIV-1 infection, in Rakai, Uganda. J Infect Dis. 2005;191:1403–1409.
7. Branson BM, Handsfield HH, Lampe MA, et al. Revised recommendations for HIV testing of adults, adolescents, and pregnant women in health-care settings. MMWR Recomm Rep. 2006;55:1–17.
8. Panel on Antiretroviral Guidelines for Adults and Adolescents. Guidelines for the use of antiretroviral agents in HIV-1-infected adults and adolescents [online]. Department of Health and Human Services. 2014 May 1;1–284. [cited 2014 June 1]. http://www.aidsinfo.nih.gov/ContentFiles/AdultandAdolescentGL.pdf
9. Fields-Gardner C, Campa A; America Dietetics Association. Position of the American Dietetic Association: Nutrition Intervention and Human Immunodeficiency Virus Infection. J Am Diet Assoc. 2010; 110(7):1105–1119.
10. Gunthard HF, Aberg JA, Eron JJ, et al. Antiretroviral treatment of adult HIV infection: 2014 recommendations of the International AIDS Society-USA panel. JAMA. 2014;312(4):410–425.
11. World Health Organization. HIV resistance report, 2012. http://apps.who.int/iris/bitstream/10665/75183/1/9789241503938_eng.pdf
12. Panel on Antiretroviral Therapy and Medical Management in HIV-infected Children. Working guidelines for the use of antiretroviral agents in pediatric HIV infection [online]. February 12, 2014. [cited 2014 June 1]. http://aidsinfo.nih.gov/contentfiles/PediatricGuidelines.pdf
13. Panel on Treatment of HIV-Infected Pregnant Women and Prevention of Perinatal Transmission. Recommendations for use of antiretroviral drugs in pregnant HIV-1-infected women for maternal health *and* interventions to reduce perinatal HIV transmission in the United States [online]. March 28, 2014. [cited 2014 Jun 1]. http://aidsinfo.nih.gov/contentfiles/PerinatalGL.pdf
14. Cohn SE, Watts D, Lertora J, Park JG, Yu S. Depo-medroxyprogesterone in women on antiretroviral thearpy: Effective contraception and lack of clinically significant interactions. Clin Pharmacol Ther. 2007; 81:222–227.
15. Koziel MJ, Peters MG. Viral hepatitis in HIV infection. N Engl J Med. 2007;356:1445–1454.
16. American Association for the Study of Liver Diseases and Infectious Diseases Society of America. Recommendations for Testing, Managing, and Treating Hepatitis C. August 2014 [cited 2014 Sept 6]. www.hcvguidelines.org
17. US Public Health Service. Preexposure prophylaxis for the prevention of HIV infection in the United States, 2014 Clinical Practice Guideline. May 2014 [cited 2014 Sept 6]. www.cdc.gov/hiv/pdf/prepguidelines2014.pdf

88 Cancer Chemotherapy and Treatment

Amy Robbins Williams

LEARNING OBJECTIVES

Upon completion of the chapter, the reader will be able to:

1. Describe the etiology of cancer.
2. Define the tumor, nodes, metastases (TNM) system of cancer staging.
3. Classify each drug used in the treatment of cancer and compare and contrast the mechanisms of action, uses, and adverse effects.
4. Outline actions for all health professionals to prevent medication errors with cancer treatments.
5. Discuss the impact that increased use of oral chemotherapy agents may have on oncology practice.
6. Describe what cancer survivorship means and how this impacts future health care needs of an individual.
7. Describe the role of health professionals in the care of cancer patients.

INTRODUCTION

KEY CONCEPT *The word cancer covers a diverse array of tumor types that affect a significant number of Americans and individuals worldwide and are a major cause of mortality.* The term *cancer* actually refers to more than 100 different diseases. What is common to all cancers is that the cancerous cell is uncontrollably growing and has the potential for invading local tissue and spreading to other parts of the body, a process called **metastases**. Cancer is now the leading cause of death in Americans younger than 85 years.[1] In 2015, it was projected that just over 1.6 million Americans will be diagnosed with cancer, and that an estimated 589,430 Americans will die from the cancer.[2] **Figure 88–1** describes cancers by gender, new cases, and deaths.

Although cancer in children and adolescents is less common when compared to older adults, it is estimated that about 1 in 285 children in America will be diagnosed before age 20. It is the second leading cause of death in children ages 5 to 14.[2]

Once diagnosed, a cancer patient may encounter many different health professionals. All health professionals need to collaborate to ensure safe and appropriate prescribing, preparation, administration, and monitoring of anticancer agents; management of toxicities; resolution of reimbursement issues; and participation in clinical trials.[3]

As a result of advances in research and technology, available cancer treatments have increased dramatically in the last couple of decades. The fields of radiation therapy, surgery, and drug development have made enormous progress over the years; therefore, patients may not only be receiving less toxic treatments but also treatments that have better outcomes than in the past. Supportive care therapies have improved, and patients now may be at less risk for toxicity and have a better **quality of life** than patients in the past. Twenty years ago, most patients received chemotherapy in the hospital because of side effects. Today, most patients are able to receive chemotherapy in the outpatient clinics and/or take oral anticancer agents at home.

Cancer Prevention

Because most cancers are not curable in advanced stages, cancer prevention is an important and active area of research. Both lifestyle modifications and chemoprevention agents may significantly reduce the risk of developing cancer. Although still an active area of investigation, the Food and Drug Administration (FDA) has approved three vaccines that can help prevent cancer. There are two approved vaccines that prevent infection with human papillomavirus, which can cause cancers of the cervix, vulva, vagina, and anus. Another approved vaccine prevents infection with hepatitis B virus, which can cause liver cancer. In addition to vaccines, there are other medications that can be taken orally and have been used for cancer prevention. An example is the selective estrogen receptor modulator (SERM) tamoxifen, which reduces the risk of breast cancer in premenopausal women. Another SERM, raloxifene and the aromatase inhibitor exemestane both have shown a reduction in breast cancer in high-risk postmenopausal women. Because these agents will have adverse effects and possible long-term complications (eg, an increased risk of endometrial cancer with the use of tamoxifen), benefits versus risks needs to be weighed when making a recommendation.

Tobacco

Tobacco smoking increases the risk of developing not only lung cancer but also many other types of cancer, including cancer of the bladder, mouth, pharynx, larynx, and esophagus as well as renal cell cancer. Smoking cessation is associated with a gradual decrease in the risk of cancer, but more than 5 years is needed before a major decline in risk is detected. In addition, most

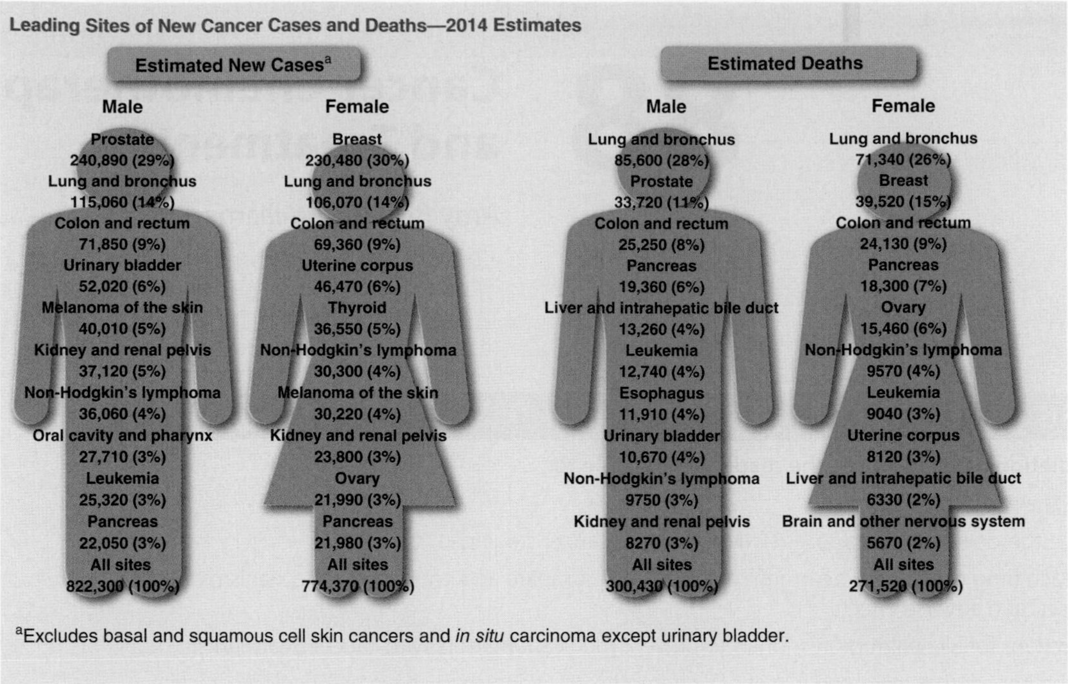

Leading Sites of New Cancer Cases and Deaths—2014 Estimates
Estimated New Cases[a]
Male
Prostate
240,890 (29%)
Lung and bronchus
115,060 (14%)
Colon and rectum
71,850 (9%)
Urinary bladder
52,020 (6%)
Melanoma of the skin
40,010 (5%)
Kidney and renal pelvis
37,120 (5%)
Non-Hodgkin's lymphoma
36,060 (4%)
Oral cavity and pharynx
27,710 (3%)
Leukemia
25,320 (3%)
Pancreas
22,050 (3%)
All sites
822,300 (100%)
Female
Breast
230,480 (30%)
Lung and bronchus
106,070 (14%)
Colon and rectum
69,360 (9%)
Uterine corpus
46,470 (6%)
Thyroid
36,550 (5%)
Non-Hodgkin's lymphoma
30,300 (4%)
Melanoma of the skin
30,220 (4%)
Kidney and renal pelvis
23,800 (3%)
Ovary
21,990 (3%)
Pancreas
21,980 (3%)
All sites
774,370 (100%)
Estimated Deaths
Male
Lung and bronchus
85,600 (28%)
Prostate
33,720 (11%)
Colon and rectum
25,250 (8%)
Pancreas
19,360 (6%)
Liver and intrahepatic bile duct
13,260 (4%)
Leukemia
12,740 (4%)
Esophagus
11,910 (4%)
Urinary bladder
10,670 (4%)
Non-Hodgkin's lymphoma
9750 (3%)
Kidney and renal pelvis
8270 (3%)
All sites
300,430 (100%)
Female
Lung and bronchus
71,340 (26%)
Breast
39,520 (15%)
Colon and rectum
24,130 (9%)
Pancreas
18,300 (7%)
Ovary
15,460 (6%)
Non-Hodgkin's lymphoma
9570 (4%)
Leukemia
9040 (3%)
Uterine corpus
8120 (3%)
Liver and intrahepatic bile duct
6330 (2%)
Brain and other nervous system
5670 (2%)
All sites
271,520 (100%)
[a]Excludes basal and squamous cell skin cancers and *in situ* carcinoma except urinary bladder.

FIGURE 88–1. Cancer Incidences (left) and deaths (right) in the United States for males and females—2014 estimates. Reproduced with permission from American Cancer Society. Cancer facts and figures-2014.

studies have found that passive smoking (ie, secondhand smoke) also increases a person's risk of developing lung cancer.[4]

Ultraviolet Radiation

Ultraviolet light (sunlight or tanning booths and lamps) and increased skin exposure may increase the risk of melanoma and other skin cancers, especially in individuals who have a positive family history, fair skin, light-colored eyes, high degrees of freckling, and a tendency to burn instead of tan. Practitioners can counsel patients on proper sun protection, including minimizing sun exposure, using sunscreens with a sun protection factor (SPF) of 15 or greater on exposed areas, wearing protective clothing and sunglasses, avoiding tanning beds and sun lamps, and the importance of early detection.

CARCINOGENESIS

The exact cause of cancer remains unknown and is probably very diverse given the vast array of diseases called cancer. It is thought that cancer develops from a single cell in which the normal mechanisms for control of growth and proliferation are altered. Current evidence indicates that there are four stages in the cancer development process. The first step, initiation, occurs when a carcinogenic substance encounters a normal cell to produce genetic damage and results in a mutated cell. The environment is altered by carcinogens or other factors to favor the growth of the mutated cell over the normal cell during promotion, the second step. The main difference between initiation and promotion is that promotion is a reversible process. Third, transformation (or conversion) occurs when the mutated cell becomes malignant. Depending on the type of cancer, up to 20 years may elapse between the carcinogenic phases and the development of a clinically detectable tumor. Finally, progression occurs when cell proliferation takes over and the tumor spreads or develops metastases.

There are substances known to have carcinogenic risks, including chemicals, environmental factors, and viruses. Chemicals in the environment, such as aniline and benzene, are associated with the development of bladder cancer and leukemia, respectively. Environmental factors, such as excessive sun exposure, can result in skin cancer, and smoking is widely known as a cause of lung cancer. Viruses, including human papillomavirus (HPV), Epstein-Barr virus, and hepatitis B virus, have been linked to cervical cancers, lymphomas, and liver cancers, respectively. Anticancer agents such as the alkylating agents (eg, melphalan), anthracyclines (eg, doxorubicin), and epipodophyllotoxins (eg, etoposide) can cause secondary malignancies (eg, leukemias) years after therapy has been completed. Additionally, factors such as the patient's age, gender, family history, diet, and chronic irritation or inflammation may be considered to be promoters of carcinogenesis.

Cancer Genetics

Because the human genome has been sequenced and with the great improvements in genetic technology, there is growing knowledge regarding the genetic changes of cancer. There are two major classes of genes involved in carcinogenesis, oncogenes and tumor suppressor genes. Protooncogenes are normal genes that, through some genetic alteration caused by carcinogens, change into oncogenes. Protooncogenes are present in all normal cells and regulate cell function and replication. Genetic damage of the protooncogene may occur through point mutation, chromosomal rearrangement, or an increase in gene function, resulting in the oncogene. The genetic damage may either be inherited from an individual's parents (germline mutations) or by way of carcinogenic agents (eg, smoking). The oncogene produces abnormal or excessive gene product that disrupts normal cell growth and proliferation.[5] As a result, this may cause the cell to have a distinct growth advantage, increasing its likelihood of becoming cancerous. Table 88–1 provides examples of oncogenes by their cellular function and associated cancer.

Tumor suppressor genes inhibit inappropriate cellular growth and proliferation by gene loss or mutation. This results in loss

Table 88–1

Examples of Oncogenes and Tumor Suppressor Genes

Gene	Function	Associated Human Cancer
Oncogenes		
Genes for growth factors or their receptors		
EGFR or Erb-B1	Codes for epidermal growth factor (EGFR) receptor	Glioblastoma, breast, head and neck, and colon cancers
HER-2/neu or Erb-B2	Codes for a growth factor receptor	Breast, salivary gland, prostate, bladder, and ovarian cancers
RET	Codes for a growth factor receptor	Thyroid cancer
Genes for cytoplasmic relays in stimulatory signaling pathways		
K-RAS and N-RAS	Code for guanine nucleotide-proteins with GTPase activity	Lung, ovarian, colon, pancreatic binding cancers Neuroblastoma, acute leukemia
Genes for transcription factors that activate growth-promoting genes		
c-MYC		Leukemia and breast, colon, gastric, and lung cancers
N-MYC		Neuroblastoma, small cell lung cancer, and glioblastoma
Genes for cytoplasmic kinases		
BCR-ABL	Codes for a nonreceptor tyrosine kinase	Chronic myelogenous leukemia
Genes for other molecules		
BCL-2	Codes for a protein that blocks apoptosis	Indolent B-cell lymphomas
BCL-1 or PRAD1	Codes for cyclin D_1, a cell-cycle clock stimulator	Breast, head, and neck cancers
MDM2	Protein antagonist of p53 tumor suppressor protein	Sarcomas
Tumor-Suppressor Genes		
Genes for proteins in the cytoplasm		
APC	Step in a signaling pathway	Colon and gastric cancer
NF-1	Codes for a protein that inhibits the stimulatory Ras protein	Neurofibroma, leukemia, and pheochromocytoma
NF-2	Codes for a protein that inhibits the stimulatory Ras protein	Meningioma, ependymoma, and schwannoma
Genes for proteins in the nucleus		
MTS1	Codes for p16 protein, a cyclin-dependent kinase inhibitor	Involved in a wide range of cancers
RB1	Codes for the pRB protein, a master brake of the cell cycle	Retinoblastoma, osteosarcoma, and bladder, small cell lung, prostate, and breast cancers
p53	Codes for the p53 protein, which can halt cell division and induce apoptosis	Involved in a wide range of cancers
Genes for protein whose cellular location is unclear		
BRCA1	DNA repair, transcriptional regulation	Breast and ovarian cancers
BRCA2	DNA repair	Breast cancer
VHL	Regulator of protein stability	Renal cell cancer
MSH2, MLH1, PMS1, PMS2, MSH6	DNA mismatch repair enzymes	Hereditary nonpolyposis colorectal cancer

From DiPiro JT, Talbert RL, Yee GC, et al. (eds.) Pharmacotherapy: A Pathophysiologic Approach, 8th ed. New York: McGraw-Hill; 2011: Table 135–2.

of control over normal cell growth. The *p53* gene is one of the most common tumor suppressor genes, and mutations of *p53* may occur in up to 50% of all malignancies. This gene stops the cell cycle to enable "repairs" of the cell. If *p53* is inactivated, then the cell allows the mutations to occur. Although mutations of the *p53* gene are found in many tumors, such as breast, colon, and lung cancer, it is also associated with drug resistance of cancer cells. DNA repair genes fix errors in DNA that occur because of environmental factors or errors in replication and can be classified as tumor suppressor genes. Mutations in DNA repair genes have been reported in hereditary nonpolyposis colon cancer and in some breast cancer syndromes.

KEY CONCEPT *Numerous cellular changes occur in the genetic material of the cancer cell so that programmed cell death, or apoptosis, does not occur. Proliferation of cancer cells goes unregulated.* If mutations persist and cells are not repaired or suppressed, cancer may develop. Apoptosis, or programmed cell death, may prevent the mutated cell from becoming cancerous. Loss of *p53* and overexpression of *bcl-2* are two examples of changes within the cell that occur to result in enhanced cell survival. Cellular senescence refers to cell death that occurs after a preset number of cell doublings. Telomeres are DNA segments at the ends of chromosomes that shorten with each replication to the point where senescence is triggered.

Identification of genes involved in cancer may be conducted for various reasons, including cancer screening to determine if an individual is at an increased risk of cancer, to develop new anticancer agents, to aid in diagnosis, and to predict response and/or the toxicity of the agents used in individual patients.

Principles of Tumor Growth

It takes about 10^9 cancer cells to be clinically detectable by palpation or radiography. Figure 88–2 demonstrates the classic Gompertzian kinetics tumor growth cycle. From the diagram, one can see that malignant cell growth occurs many times before a mass may be detected. The number of malignant cells may decrease drastically because of surgery or in decreasing steps by each administration of chemotherapy. One dosing round, or cycle, of

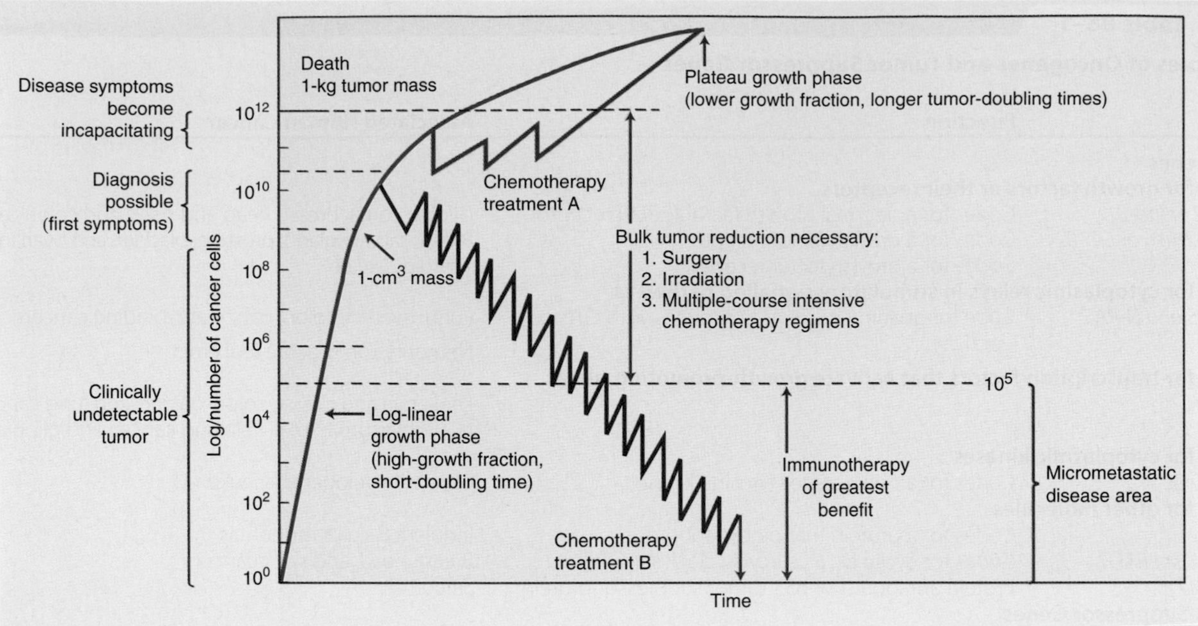

FIGURE 88–2. The Gompertzian growth curve demonstrating symptoms and treatments versus tumor volume.

chemotherapy does not eliminate all malignant cells; therefore, repeated cycles of chemotherapy are administered to eliminate tumor cell burden. The cell kill hypothesis states that a fixed percentage of tumor cells will be killed with each cycle of chemotherapy. According to this hypothesis, the number of tumor cells will never reach zero. This theory assumes that all cancers are equally responsive and that anticancer drug resistance and metastases do not occur, which is not the case.[6]

Metastases

A metastasis is a growth of the same cancer cell found at some distance from the primary tumor site.[7] The metastasis may be large, or it may be just a few cells that may be detected through polymerase chain reaction (PCR); however, the presence of metastasis at staging usually is associated with a poorer prognosis than the patient with no known metastatic disease. As the technology to detect malignant cells evolves, the dilemma exists on how to treat patients based on current guidelines that were not based on cellular detection technology.

Cancers spread usually by two pathways: hematogenous (through the bloodstream) or through the lymphatics (drainage through adjacent lymph nodes). The malignant cells that split from the primary tumor find a suitable environment for growth. It is believed that malignant cells secrete mediators that stimulate the formation of blood vessels for growth and oxygen, the process of angiogenesis. The usual metastatic sites for solid tumors are the brain, bone, lung, and liver.

PATHOPHYSIOLOGY

Tumor Origin

Tumors may arise from the four basic tissue types: epithelial, connective (ie, muscle, bone, and cartilage), lymphoid, or nerve tissue. The suffix *-oma* is added to the name of the cell type if the tumor cells are benign. A *lipoma* is a benign growth that resembles fat tissue.

Precancerous cells have cellular changes that are abnormal but not yet malignant and may be described as *hyperplastic* or *dysplastic*. Hyperplasia occurs when a stimulus is introduced and reverses when the stimulus is removed. Dysplasia is an abnormal change in the size, shape, or organization of cells or tissues.

Malignant cells are divided into categories based on the cells of origin. Carcinomas arise from epithelial cells, whereas sarcomas arise from muscle or connective tissue. Adenocarcinomas arise from glandular tissue. *Carcinoma* in situ refers to cells limited to epithelial origin that have not yet invaded the basement membrane. Malignancies of the bone marrow or lymphoid tissue, such as leukemias or lymphomas, are named differently.

Tumor Characteristics

Tumors are either benign or malignant. Benign tumors often are encapsulated, localized, and indolent; they seldom metastasize; and they rarely recur once removed. Histologically, the cells resemble the cells from which they developed. Malignant tumors are invasive and spread to other locations even if the primary tumor is removed. The cells no longer perform their usual functions, and their cellular architecture changes. This loss of structure and function is called *anaplasia*. Despite improvements in screening procedures, many patients have metastatic disease at the time of diagnosis. Usually, once distant metastases have occurred, the cancer is considered incurable.[8]

DIAGNOSIS OF CANCER

Cancer can present as a number of different signs and symptoms. Unfortunately, many people fear a diagnosis of cancer and may not seek medical attention at the first warning signs when the disease is at its most treatable stage. After the initial visit with the clinician, a variety of tests will be performed, which are somewhat dependent on the initial differential diagnoses. Appropriate laboratory tests, radiologic scans, and tissue samples are necessary. The sample of tissue may be obtained by a biopsy, fine-needle aspiration, or exfoliative cytology. No treatment of cancer should be initiated without a pathologic diagnosis of cancer. During the pathologic workup, genetic analysis may be done. Depending on the type of cancer, the genetic analysis can provide the additional information on prognosis of the malignancy and whether certain therapies may be appropriate.

Once the pathology of cancer is established, then staging of the disease is done before treatment is initiated. KEY CONCEPT *Cancer staging is usually done according to the primary tumor size, extent of lymph node involvement, and the presence or absence of metastases, also referred to as the tumor, nodes, metastases (TNM) system (Table 88–2). The stage of the disease is a compilation of the primary tumor size, the nodal involvement, and metastases and is usually referred to as stages I, II, III, or IV.* Not all cancers can be staged according to this system, but many of the solid tumors are.

Staging of the disease is an important part of determining the prognosis of the cancer. Staging also allows comparison of

Table 88–2

Tumor (T), Node (N), Metastasis (M) Staging for Non–Small Cell Lung Cancer

Primary Tumor		**Description**
T_1		Tumor 3 cm or less diameter, surrounded by lung or visceral pleura, without invasion more proximal than lobar bronchus
	T_{1a}	Tumor 2 cm or less in diameter
	T_{1b}	Tumor greater than 2 cm but 3 cm or less in diameter
T_2		Tumor greater than 3 cm but 7 cm or less, or tumor with any of the following features: –Involves main bronchus, 2 cm or less distal to carina –Invades visceral pleura –Associated with atelectasis or obstructive pneumonitis that extends to the hilar region but does not involve the entire lung
	T_{2a}	Tumor greater than 3 cm but 5 cm or less
	T_{2b}	Tumor greater than 5 cm but 7 cm or less
T_3		Tumor greater than 7 cm or any of the following: –Directly invades any of the following: chestwall, diaphragm, phrenic nerve, mediastinal pleura, parietal pericardium, main bronchus less than 2 cm from carina (without involvement of carina) –Atelectasis or obstructive pneumonitis of the entire lung –Separate tumor nodules in the same lobe
T_4		Tumor of any size that invades the mediastinum, heart, great vessels, trachea, recurrent laryngeal nerve, esophagus, vertebral body, carina, or with separate tumor nodules in a different ipsilateral lobe
Regional lymph nodes (N)		
N_0		No regional lymph node metastases
N_1		Metastasis in ipsilateral peribronchial and/or ipsilateral hilar lymph nodes and intrapulmonary nodes, including involvement by direct extension
N_2		Metastasis in ipsilateral mediastinal and/or subcarinal lymph node(s)
N_3		Metastasis in contralateral mediastinal, contralateral hilar, ipsilateral or contralateral scalene, or supraclavicular lymph node(s)
Distant metastasis (M)		
M_0		No distant metastasis
M_1		Distant metastasis
	M_{1a}	Separate tumor nodule(s) in a contralateral lobe; tumor with pleural nodules or malignant pleural or pericardial effusion
	M_{1b}	Distan metastasis

Stage	**T**	**N**	**M**	**5-Year Survival**
Stage IA:	T_{1a}-T_{1b}	N_0	M_0	73%
Stage IB:	T_{2a}	N_0	M_0	58%
Stage IIA:	T_{1a}, T_{1b}, T_{2a}, T_{2b}	N_1, N_0	M_0, M_0	46%
Stage IIB:	T_{2b}, T_3	N_1, N_0	M_0, M_0	36%
	T_{1a}, T_{1b}, T_{2a}, T_{2b}	N_2	M_0	
Stage IIIA:	T_3	N_1, N_2	M_0	24%
	T_4	N_0, N_1	M_0	
Stage IIIB:	T_4	N_2	M_0	9%
	Any T	N_3	M_0	
Stage IV:	Any T	Any N	M_{1a} or M_{1b}	13%

From DiPiro JT, Talbert RL, Yee GC, et al. (eds.) Pharmacotherapy: A Pathophysiologic Approach. 8th ed. New York: McGraw-Hill; 2011: Table 137–2.

patient groups when examining data from clinical trials; staging reflects the extent of disease. Finally, the clinician uses it as a guide to treatment and may use restaging after treatment to guide further treatment.

Some cancers produce substances (eg, proteins) that are detected by a blood test, that may be useful in following response to therapy or detecting a recurrence; these are referred to as tumor markers. An example of a clinically used tumor marker is the prostate-specific antigen (PSA). The PSA serum level is used to monitor response to treatment. Unfortunately, some tumor markers are nonspecific and may be elevated from nonmalignant causes. In the case of PSA, nonmalignant causes such as prostatitis, trauma, surgery, ejaculation, some medications, benign prostatic hypertrophy, or riding on an exercise bicycle can all cause increased PSA levels.[9] Some tumors may express a marker in some patients and not in others. The full role of tumor markers has not been fully elucidated.

TREATMENT

Desired Outcome

Surgery may be able to remove all macroscopic disease; however, microscopic cells may still be present near the surgical site or may have traveled to other parts of the body. When malignant cells have traveled to other parts of the body and become established there and are able to grow in this new environment, they are called metastatic cancer cells. Thus, for chemotherapy-sensitive diseases, systemic therapies may be administered after surgery to destroy these microscopic malignant cells; this is called adjuvant chemotherapy. The goals of adjuvant chemotherapy are to decrease the recurrence of the cancer and to prolong survival. Chemotherapy may also be given before surgical resection of the tumor; this is referred to as neoadjuvant chemotherapy. Chemotherapy given before surgery should decrease the tumor burden to be removed (which may result in a shorter surgical procedure or less physical disfigurement to the patient) and make the surgery easier to perform because the tumor has shrunk away from vital organs or vessels. Neoadjuvant chemotherapy also gives the clinician an idea of the responsiveness of the tumor to that particular chemotherapy.

Chemotherapy may be given to cure cancers that are curable, or it may be given to help control the symptoms of an incurable cancer, which is referred to as palliative therapy.

Response

The responses to chemotherapy may be referred to as complete response (CR), partial response (PR), stable disease (SD), or disease progression. A cure in oncology implies that the cancer is completely gone, and the patient will have the same life expectancy as a patient without cancer. The Response Evaluation Criteria in Solid Tumors (RECIST) was developed in 2000 and revised in 2009 and is considered to be the standard criteria to evaluate a response to therapy (Table 88–3). The term overall objective response rate refers to the combination of PR and CR. Some cancers, such as leukemia, cannot be measured by size, so biopsy of the bone marrow provides a cellular indication of the absence or presence of disease.[10]

Anticancer treatments can be thought of as being analogous to antiinfectives treatments. Cancer cells may be sensitive to certain chemotherapy agents, but then with repeated exposure, the cells may become resistant to treatment. The resistant cells then may grow and multiply. A number of genetic mutations, including *EGFR*, *KRAS*, and *BRAF*, predict sensitivity to chemotherapy agents that target these mutations. These mutations will be discussed in depth in the following cancer-specific chapters.

Table 88–3

RECIST 1.1 Criteria

Term	Description
Complete response (CR)	Disappearance of all targeted lesions
Partial response (PR)	At least a 30% decrease in the sum of the longest diameter of target lesions from baseline
Progressive disease (PD)	At least a 20% increase in the sum of the longest diameter of target lesions from baseline, including new lesions discovered during treatment
Stable disease (SD)	Neither sufficient shrinkage to qualify for PR nor sufficient increase to qualify for PD

Adapted from Eisenhauer E, Therasse P, Bogaerts J, et al. New response evaluation criteria in solid tumours: Revised RECIST guideline (version 1.1). Eur J Cancer. 2009;45:228–247.

Nonpharmacologic Therapy

The four primary treatment modalities of cancer are surgery, radiation, biotherapy, and pharmacologic therapy. Surgery is useful to gain tissue for diagnosis of cancer and for treatment, especially those cancers with limited disease. Radiation plays a key role not only in the treatment and possible cure of cancer but also in palliative therapy. Together, surgery and radiation therapy may provide local control of symptoms of the disease. However, when cancer is widespread, surgery may play little or no role, but radiation therapy localized to specific areas may palliate symptoms.

Pharmacologic Therapy

Chemotherapy of cancer started in the early 1940s when nitrogen mustard was first administered to patients with lymphoma. Since then, numerous agents have been developed for the treatment of different cancers.

Dosing of Chemotherapy

Chemotherapeutic agents typically have a very narrow therapeutic index. If too much is administered, the patient may suffer from fatal toxicities. If too little is given, the desired effect on cancer cells may not be achieved. Many chemotherapy agents have significant organ toxicities that preclude using steadily increasing doses to treat the cancer. The doses of chemotherapy must be given at a frequency that allows the patient to recover from the toxicity of the chemotherapy; each period of chemotherapy dosing is referred to as a cycle. Each cycle of chemotherapy may have the same dosages; the dosages may be modified based on toxicity; or a chemotherapy regimen may alternate from one set of drugs given during the first, third, and fifth cycles to another set of different drugs given during the second, fourth, and sixth cycles. The dose density of chemotherapy refers to shortening of the period between cycles of chemotherapy. This can accomplish two things: First, the tumor has less time between cycles of chemotherapy to grow, and second, patients receive the total

Clinical Presentation and Diagnosis: Cancer Chemotherapy and Treatment

Signs and Symptoms

The seven warning signs of cancer are:

- Change in bowel or bladder habits
- A sore that does not heal
- Unusual bleeding or discharge
- Thickening or lump in breast or elsewhere
- Indigestion or difficulty in swallowing
- Obvious change in a wart or mole
- Nagging cough or hoarseness

The eight warning signs of cancer in children are:

- Continued, unexplained weight loss
- Headaches with vomiting in the morning
- Increased swelling or persistent pain in bones or joints
- Lump or mass in abdomen, neck, or elsewhere
- Development of a whitish appearance in the pupil of the eye
- Recurrent fevers not caused by infections
- Excessive bruising or bleeding
- Noticeable paleness or prolonged tiredness

Diagnostic Procedures

- Laboratory tests: CBC, lactate dehydrogenase (LDH), renal function, and liver function tests
- Radiologic scans: x-rays, CT scans, MRI, position emission tomography (PET)
- Biopsy of tissue or bone marrow with pathologic evaluation
- Cytogenetics
- Tumor markers

Staging determination of the primary tumor size, extent of lymph node involvement, and the presence or absence of metastases, referred to as the TNM system (see Table 88–2). Most solid tumors are staged according to the TNM classification system. The size of the primary tumor, extent of nodal involvement, and presence of metastases are used to determine the stage. Metastases are cancer cells that have spread to sites distant from the primary tumor site and have started to grow. The most frequently occurring sites of metastases of solid tumors are the brain, bone, liver, and lungs.

number of required cycles in a shorter time period. Administration of dose-dense chemotherapy regimens often requires the use of colony-stimulating factors (eg, filgrastim or granulocyte colony-stimulating factor [G-CSF]) to be administered. These agents shorten the duration and severity of neutropenia. The chemotherapy regimens that are dose dense tend to be adjuvant regimens, and the goal of therapy is cure.

When a chemotherapy regimen is used as palliative therapy (to control symptoms), the dosages of chemotherapy may be decreased based on toxicity or the interval between cycles may be lengthened to maintain quality of life.

Patient and tumor biology also affect how cancer therapy is dosed. Patients with a uridine diphosphate–glucuronosyltransferease 1A1 enzyme (UGT1A1* 28) deficiency can have life-threatening diarrhea and complications from irinotecan related to a decreased ability to metabolize the parent drug. The patient may have a blood test before irinotecan therapy to determine if this genetic mutation is present. In the case of some monoclonal antibodies, flow cytometry results reveal whether the tumor has the receptor where the drug will bind and exert the pharmacologic effect.[11] The therapeutic uses of oncology drugs with valid genomic biomarkers will be discussed briefly in this chapter and in more detail in the following chapters.

Another consideration of chemotherapy administration is the patient. Factors that affect chemotherapy selection and dosing are age, concurrent disease states, and performance status. Performance status can be assessed through either the Eastern Cooperative Oncology Group (ECOG) Scale or the Karnofsky Scale (Table 88–4). Performance status is a very important prognostic factor for many types of cancer. If a patient has renal dysfunction and the chemotherapy is eliminated primarily by the kidney, dosing adjustments will need to be made. If a patient has had a myocardial infarction recently or preexisting heart disease, the clinician will weigh the risks of anthracycline therapy against the benefit of the treatment of the cancer.

Another important consideration for treatment of cancers is reimbursement by third-party payers for compendia off-label use. Off-label use is when a medication is used to treat a cancer that is not an FDA-labeled indication. Because of rapid advancements in oncology, it is estimated that up to 75% of chemotherapy agents are prescribed "off-label." Drugs used according to FDA-approved indications are usually reimbursed. If sufficient supportive literature exists and the use is supported by one of the Medicare-approved compendia (eg, AHFS-DI, Clinical Pharmacology, DRUGDEX, NCCN, others), an insurer should cover the cost of the anticancer treatment that does not have an FDA indication.

During the time of chemotherapy administration, patients will likely experience various toxicities. The National Cancer Institute (NCI) has provided a standardized system for evaluating and grading the toxicity from chemotherapy to provide uniform grading of toxicity and evaluation of new agents and new regimens (Table 88–5).

Combination Chemotherapy

The underlying principles of using combination therapy are to use (1) agents with different pharmacologic actions, (2) agents with different organ toxicities, (3) agents that are active against the tumor and ideally synergistic when used together, and (4) agents that do not result in significant drug interactions (although these can be studied carefully and the interactions addressed). When two or more agents are used together, the risk of development of resistance may be lessened, but toxicity may be increased.

KEY CONCEPT *Traditional chemotherapy agents have some similar side effects, usually manifested on the most rapidly proliferating cells of the body. However, there are unique toxicities of various pharmacologic categories of antineoplastic agents. Anthracyclines (eg, doxorubicin) have the potential to cause cardiac toxicity, which is related to the cumulative dose. Microtubule-targeting agents (eg, vincristine) are associated with various forms of*

Table 88–4

Performance Status Scales

Description: Karnofsky Scale	Karnofsky Scale (%)	Zubrod Scale (ECOG)	Description: ECOG Scale
No complaints; no evidence of disease	100	0	Fully active; able to carry on all predisease activity
Able to carry on normal activity; minor signs or symptoms of disease	90		
Normal activity with effort; some signs or symptoms of disease	80	1	Restricted in strenuous activity but ambulatory and able to carry out work of a light or sedentary nature
Cares for self; unable to carry on normal activity or to do active work	70		
Requires occasional assistance but is able to care for most personal needs	60	2	Out of bed more than 50% of time; ambulatory and capable of self-care but unable to carry out any work activities
Requires considerable assistance and frequent medical care	50		
Disabled; requires special care and assistance	40	3	In bed more than 50% of time; capable of only limited self-care
Severely disabled; hospitalization indicated, although death not imminent	30		
Very sick; hospitalization necessary; requires active supportive treatment	20	4	Bedridden; cannot carry out any self-care; completely disabled
Moribund; fatal processes progressing rapidly	10		
Dead	0		

ECOG, Eastern Cooperative Oncology Group.

Table 88–5

Selected National Cancer Institute Common Toxicity Criteria

Toxicity	Grade 1	Grade 2	Grade 3	Grade 4	Grade 5
General	Mild	Moderate	Severe	Life threatening	Death
Neutropenia	Lowest baseline: 1500/mm^3 (1.5 × 10^9/L)	Less than 1500–1000/mm^3 (1.5–1 × 10^9/L)	Less than 1000–500/mm^3 (1–0.5 × 10^9/L)	Less than 500/mm^3 (0.5 × 10^9/L)	
Thrombocytopenia	Lowest baseline: 75,000/mm^3 (75 × 10^9/L)	Less than 75,000–50,000/mm^3 (75–50 × 10^9/L)	Less than 50,000–25,000/mm^3 (50–25 × 10^9/L)	Less than 25,000 mm^3 (25 × 10^9/L)	Death
Diarrhea	Increase of less than four stools per day over baseline or mild increase in ostomy output	Increase of four to six stools per day over baseline; IV fluids indicated less than 24 hours of moderate increase in ostomy output compared with baseline; not interfering with ADLs	Increase of greater than or equal to seven stools per day over baseline; incontinence; IV fluids greater than or equal to 24 hours; hospitalization; severe increase in ostomy output compared with baseline; interfering with ADLs	Life-threatening consequences (eg, hemodynamic collapse)	Death
Esophagitis	Asymptomatic pathologic, radiographic, or endoscopic findings only	Symptomatic altered eating or swallowing; IV fluids indicated less than 24 hours	Symptomatic and severely altered eating or swallowing; IV fluids, tube feedings, or TPN indicated 24 hours or more	Life-threatening consequences	Death
Nausea	Loss of appetite without alteration in eating habits	Oral intake decreased without significant weight loss, dehydration, or malnutrition; IV fluids indicated less than 24 hours	Inadequate oral caloric or fluid intake; IV fluids, tube feedings, or TPN indicated greater than 24 hours	Life-threatening consequences	Death
Vomiting	One episode in 24 hours	Two to five episodes in 24 hours; IV fluids indicated less than 24 hours	Six episodes or more in 24 hours; IV fluids or TPN indicated greater than or equal to 24 hours	Life-threatening consequences	Death

ADL, activity of daily living; IV, intravenous; TPN, total parenteral nutrition.

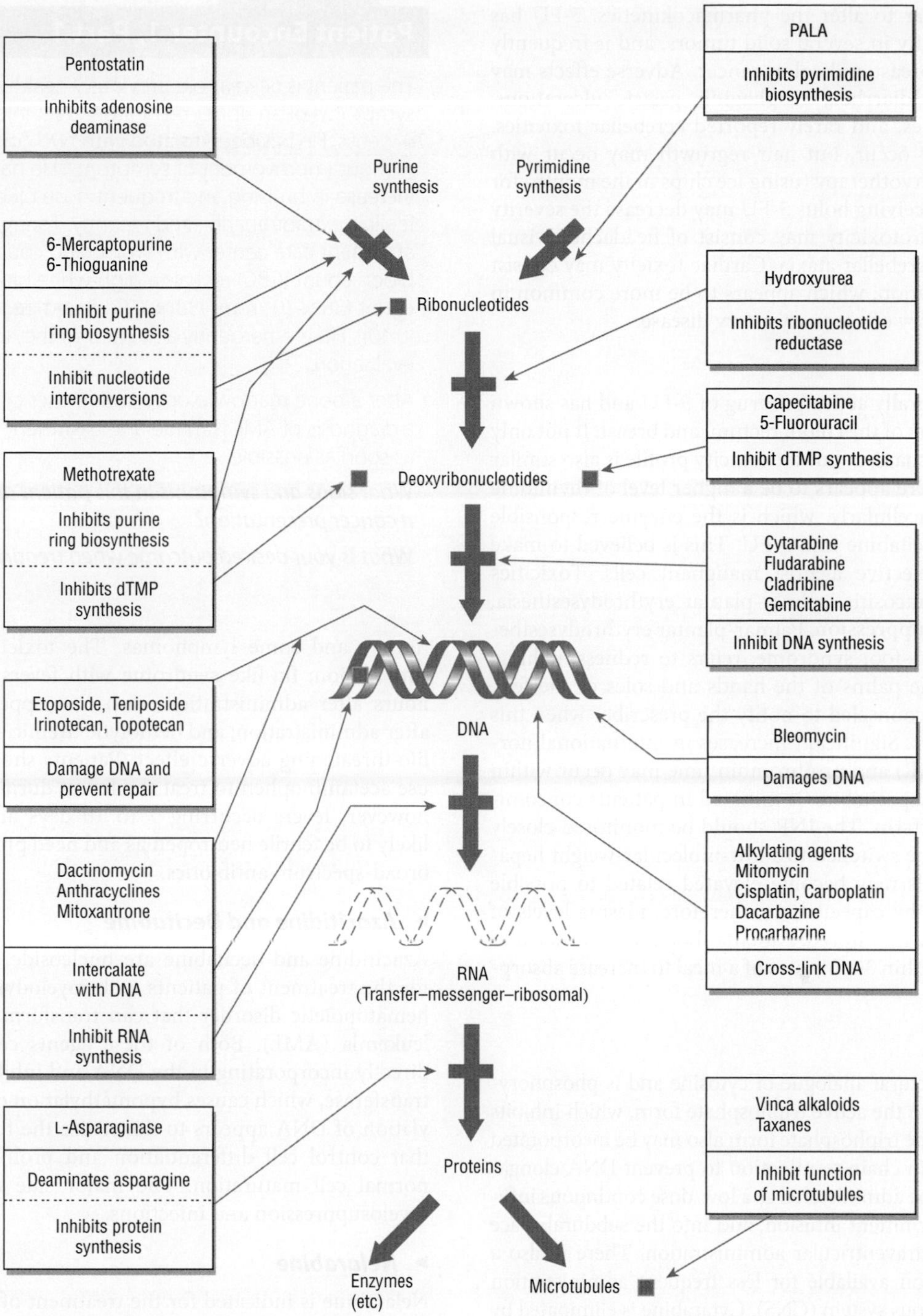

FIGURE 88–3. The mechanisms of action of commonly used antineoplastic agents. Reproduced with permission from Chabner BA. General Principles of Chemotherapy. In: Brunton LL, Chabner BA, Knollman BC (eds). Goodman & Gilman's The Pharmacologic Basis of Therapeutics, 12th ed. New York: McGraw-Hill, 2010.

neurotoxicity. Alkylating agents (eg, melphalan) are associated with secondary malignancies.

Currently, anticancer agents are categorized by the mechanism of action. As depicted in Figure 88–3, different agents work in different parts of the cell.

Antimetabolites: Pyrimidine Analogues

▸ *Fluorouracil*

5-Fluorouracil (5-FU) is a fluorinated analogue of the pyrimidine uracil. Once administered, this prodrug is metabolized by dihydropyrimidine dehydrogenase. 5-FU ultimately is metabolized to fluorodeoxyuridine monophosphate (FdUMP), which interferes with the function of thymidylate synthase (TS), which is required for synthesis of thymidine. The triphosphate metabolite of 5-FU is incorporated into RNA to produce the second cytotoxic effect of 5-FU. Inhibition of thymidylate synthesis occurs with the continuous infusion regimens, whereas the triphosphate form is associated with bolus administration. Patients with a low activity of dihydropyrimidine dehydrogenase appear to be at risk for life-threatening toxicities. Folates increase the stability of FdUMP–TS inhibition, which enhances the activity of the drug in certain cancers. 5-FU is metabolized extensively by the liver, but up to 15% of a dose may be found unchanged in the urine.

Age does not appear to alter the pharmacokinetics. 5-FU has shown clinical activity in several solid tumors, and is frequently used to treat both breast and colon cancer. Adverse effects may include stomatitis, diarrhea, esophagitis, gastric ulcerations, cardiac abnormalities, and rarely reported cerebellar toxicities. Some alopecia may occur, but hair regrowth may occur with subsequent doses. Cryotherapy (using ice chips in the mouth) for 30 minutes while receiving bolus 5-FU may decrease the severity of mucositis.[12] Neurotoxicity may consist of headaches, visual disturbances, and cerebellar ataxia. Cardiac toxicity may consist of ST-segment elevation, which appears to be more common in patients with a history of coronary artery disease.

► *Capecitabine*

Capecitabine is an orally active prodrug of 5-FU and has shown to be active in tumors of the colon, rectum, and breast. It not only shares the same mechanism but the toxicity profile is also similar to that of 5-FU. There appears to be a higher level of thymidine phosphorylase intracellularly, which is the enzyme responsible for converting capecitabine into 5-FU. This is believed to make the agent more selective against malignant cells. Toxicities include diarrhea, mucositis, palmar-plantar erythrodysesthesia, nausea, and myelosuppression. Palmar-plantar erythrodysesthesia, also called hand–foot syndrome, refers to redness, itching, and blistering of the palms of the hands and soles of the feet. Patients should be counseled to notify the prescriber when this adverse effect occurs. Significant increases in international normalization ratio (INR) and prothrombin time may occur within several days when capecitabine is initiated in patients concomitantly receiving warfarin. The INR should be monitored closely or the patient may be switched to a low-molecular-weight heparin. Phenytoin levels may become elevated related to possible CYP2C9 inhibition by capecitabine; therefore, plasma levels of phenytoin should be monitored. Patients should be instructed to take capecitabine within 30 minutes of a meal to increase absorption of the drug.

► *Cytarabine*

Cytarabine is a structural analogue of cytosine and is phosphorylated intracellularly to the active triphosphate form, which inhibits DNA polymerase. The triphosphate form also may be incorporated into DNA to result in chain termination to prevent DNA elongation. The drug may be administered as a low-dose continuous infusion, high-dose intermittent infusion, and into the subdural space via intrathecal or intraventricular administration. There is also a liposomal formulation available for less frequent administration into the central nervous system (CNS). Cytarabine is eliminated by the kidneys with a renal clearance of 90 mL/min (1.5 mL/s). Cytarabine has shown efficacy in the treatment of acute leukemias and some lymphomas. The toxicities of cytarabine in high doses include myelosuppression; cerebellar syndrome (ie, nystagmus, dysarthria, and ataxia); and chemical conjunctivitis, an eye irritation that requires prophylaxis with steroid eye drops. The risk of neurotoxicity is increased with high doses (greater than 1 g/m^2), advanced age, and renal dysfunction. If cerebellar toxicity does occur, the drug needs to be discontinued immediately, and decisions regarding further therapy need to be carefully considered.[13]

► *Gemcitabine*

Gemcitabine is a deoxycytidine analogue that is structurally related to cytarabine. Gemcitabine inhibits DNA polymerase activity and ribonucleotide reductase to result in DNA chain elongation. Gemcitabine has shown activity in several solid tumors and some lymphomas. The toxicities include myelosuppression; flu-like syndrome with fevers during the first 24 hours after administration; rash that appears 48 to 72 hours after administration; and hemolytic uremic syndrome, a rare but life-threatening adverse effect. Patients should be counseled to use acetaminophen to treat the fevers during the first 24 hours; however, fevers occurring 7 to 10 days after gemcitabine are likely to be febrile neutropenias and need prompt treatment with broad-spectrum antibiotics.

> **Patient Encounter 1, Part 1**
>
> The patient is 64-year-old previously healthy man who has had symptoms of an upper respiratory tract infection for about 4 weeks. He has been treated with two courses of antibiotics without improvement of symptoms. He has also noticed an increase in bruising and frequent nose bleeds. He reports feeling extraordinarily tired recently. Today, he presents to an urgent care center with worsening cough. His complete blood count (CBC) reveals a high white blood cell (WBC) count (38 × 10^3/mm^3 [38 × 10^9/L]) and peripheral blasts (40% [0.40]). He is emergently admitted to the hospital for further evaluation.
>
> After a bone marrow biopsy and further cytogenetic testing, a diagnosis of AML is made and treatment is planned to start as soon as possible.
>
> ***What signs and symptoms in this patient are consistent with a cancer presentation?***
>
> ***What is your desired outcome when treating this patient?***

► *Azacitidine and Decitabine*

Azacitidine and decitabine are nucleoside analogues approved for the treatment of patients with myelodysplastic syndrome, a hematopoietic disorder that can transform into acute myeloid leukemia (AML). Both of these agents cause cytotoxicity by directly incorporating in the DNA and inhibiting DNA methyltransferase, which causes hypomethylation of DNA. Hypomethylation of DNA appears to normalize the function of the genes that control cell differentiation and proliferation to promote normal cell maturation. The major side effects reported are myelosuppression and infections.

► *Nelarabine*

Nelarabine is indicated for the treatment of patients with T-cell acute lymphoblastic leukemia and T-cell lymphoblastic lymphoma, whose disease has been already treated with at least two other chemotherapy regimens. Nelarabine is a prodrug that accumulates as the active 5'-triphosphate form in leukemic blasts to result in inhibition of DNA synthesis and cell death. The most common adverse effects are hematologic toxicities, neutropenic fever, headaches, and gastrointestinal toxicities. Severe neurologic toxicities, including mental status change, convulsions, peripheral neuropathies, and effects similar to Guillain–Barré syndrome, have been reported.

Antimetabolites: Purine Analogues

► *Mercaptopurine and Thioguanine*

6-Mercaptopurine (6-MP) and thioguanine are oral purine analogues that are converted to ribonucleotides that inhibit purine synthesis. Mercaptopurine is converted into thiopurine nucleotides, which are catabolized by thiopurine *S*-methyltransferase (TPMT), which is subject to genetic polymorphisms and may cause severe myelosuppression. TPMT status may be assessed before therapy to reduce drug-induced morbidity and the costs of hospitalizations for neutropenic events. Both of these agents are used in the treatment of acute lymphocytic leukemia (ALL) and chronic myeloid leukemia (CML). Because the agents are similar structurally, cross-resistance is observed. Significant side effects include myelosuppression, mild nausea, skin rash, cholestasis, and rarely, veno-occlusive disease. Mercaptopurine is metabolized by xanthine oxidase, an enzyme that is inhibited by allopurinol. This represents a major drug–drug interaction. To avoid toxicities of mercaptopurine when these drugs are used concomitantly, the dose of mercaptopurine must be reduced by 66% to 75%.

▸ *Fludarabine*

Fludarabine is an analogue of the purine adenine. It interferes with DNA polymerase to cause chain termination and inhibits transcription by its incorporation into RNA. Fludarabine is dephosphorylated rapidly and converted to 2-fluoro-Ara-AMP (2-FLAA), which enters the cells and is phosphorylated to 2-fluoro-Ara-ATP, which is cytotoxic. Fludarabine is used in the treatment of chronic lymphocytic leukemia (CLL), some lymphomas, and refractory AML. This drug is given intravenously (IV) usually daily for 5 days every 4 weeks. Significant and prolonged myelosuppression may occur, along with immunosuppression, so patients are susceptible to opportunistic infections. Prophylactic antibiotics and antivirals are recommended until CD4 counts return to normal. Mild nausea and vomiting and diarrhea have been observed. Rarely, interstitial pneumonitis has occurred.

▸ *Cladribine*

Cladribine is a purine nucleoside that is a prodrug. It is activated via phosphorylation to a 5′-triphosphate derivative, which is incorporated into DNA, resulting in inhibition of DNA synthesis and chain termination. It may be administered as a continuous 7-day IV infusion or as a 2-hour infusion daily for 5 days; both regimens deliver the same total dose of drug. The primary indication for cladribine is hairy cell leukemia. Although fairly well tolerated, patients may experience myelosuppression and opportunistic infections. Fever, which is thought to be as a result of cell lysis and endogenous pyrogens being released into the bloodstream, can prompt the clinician to consider initiation of antibiotics. Even though it is likely drug induced, it may be difficult to rule out an infectious cause. Rash occurs in approximately 50% of patients.

▸ *Clofarabine*

Clofarabine was developed based on the structures of fludarabine and cladribine with the hope it would be resistant to deamination by adenosine deaminase. Clofarabine has shown activity in myeloid leukemia and myelodysplastic syndrome.[14] Side effects include bone marrow suppression, severe but transient liver dysfunction in 15% to 25% of patients, skin rashes, and hand–foot syndrome.

▸ *Pentostatin*

Pentostatin is an inhibitor of adenosine deaminase, an enzyme important in purine base metabolism. Pentostatin irreversibly inhibits adenosine deaminase, which blocks DNA synthesis through inhibition of RNA ribonucleotide reductase. Side effects include bone marrow suppression, myalgias, conjunctivitis, and rash.

Antimetabolites: Folate Antagonists

Folates carry one-carbon groups in transfer reactions required for purine and thymidylic acid synthesis. Dihydrofolate reductase is the enzyme responsible for supplying reduced folates intracellularly for thymidylate and purine synthesis.

▸ *Methotrexate*

Methotrexate inhibits dihydrofolate reductase of both malignant and nonmalignant cells. When high doses of methotrexate are given, the "rescue drug" leucovorin, a reduced folate, is administered to bypass the methotrexate inhibition of dihydrofolate reductase of normal cells and is usually initiated 24 hours after methotrexate administration. This is done to prevent potentially fatal myelosuppression and mucositis. For safety purposes, the term folinic acid, another term used for leucovorin, should not be used because of the potential for a medication error in which folic acid might be given instead. Methotrexate concentrations should be monitored to determine when to stop leucovorin administration. Generally, leucovorin administration may be stopped when methotrexate concentrations decrease to 5×10^{-8} M, although this may vary by the chemotherapy regimen. High dosages of methotrexate may cause methotrexate to crystallize out in the kidney, which may result in acute renal failure and decreased methotrexate clearance. Administration of IV hydration with sodium bicarbonate to maintain urinary pH greater than or equal to 7 is necessary to prevent methotrexate-induced renal dysfunction. Methotrexate is eliminated by tubular secretion; therefore, concomitant drugs (eg, probenecid, salicylates, penicillin G, and ketoprofen) that may inhibit or compete for tubular secretion should be avoided. Methotrexate doses must be adjusted for renal dysfunction and close monitoring of methotrexate concentrations is advised. Side effects of methotrexate include myelosuppression, nausea and vomiting, and mucositis. Methotrexate also may be administered via the intrathecal route or via an Ommaya reservoir in very low doses as small as 12 mg, so it is crucial for the clinician to know the correct dose by the correct route in order to avoid substantial toxicity. The methotrexate used for intrathecal and intraventricular injection must be preservative-free to prevent CNS toxicity.

▸ *Pemetrexed*

Pemetrexed inhibits four pathways in thymidine and purine synthesis. Pemetrexed has shown activity in the treatment of mesothelioma and non–small cell lung cancer (NSCLC). Side effects include myelosuppression, rash, diarrhea, and nausea and vomiting. Patients should receive folic acid and cyanocobalamin to reduce bone marrow toxicity and diarrhea. Doses of folic acid of at least 400 mcg/day starting 5 days before treatment and continuing throughout therapy, as well as for 21 days after the last pemetrexed dose, have been used. Cyanocobalamin 1000 mcg is given intramuscularly the week before pemetrexed and then every three cycles thereafter. Dexamethasone 4 mg twice daily the day before, the day of, and the day after pemetrexed administration helps to decrease the incidence and severity of rash.[15]

▸ *Pralatrexate*

Pralatrexate is a folate analogue metabolic inhibitor that is transported into tumor cells via the reduced folate carrier (RFC-1) and competitively inhibits dihydrofolate reductase. It also competitively inhibits polyglutamylation by the enzyme folylpolyglutamyl synthetase, resulting in the depletion of thymidine and other molecules. It is an intravenously administered agent indicated for the treatment of patients with refractory or relapsed peripheral T-cell lymphoma. Pralatrexate was approved based on overall response rates, not survival benefits. Common adverse reactions include mucositis, thrombocytopenia, nausea, and fatigue. In an effort to reduce the treatment-related mucositis and hematologic toxicity associated with pralatrexate, patients should be counseled to take low-dose oral folic acid on a daily basis and vitamin B_{12} intramuscular injections every 8 to 10 weeks.

Microtubule-Targeting Agents

▶ *Vinca Alkaloids (Vincristine, Vinblastine, and Vinorelbine)*

The vinca alkaloids (vincristine, vinblastine, and vinorelbine) are derived from the periwinkle (vinca) plant and cause cytotoxicity by binding to tubulin, disrupting the normal balance between polymerization and depolymerization of microtubules, and inhibiting the assembly of microtubules, which interferes with the formation of the mitotic spindle. As a result, cells are arrested during the metaphase of mitosis. The vinca alkaloids are used in several malignancies, primarily hematologic. Even though these agents have similar structures, the incidence and severity of toxicities vary among the agents. The dose-limiting toxicity of vincristine is neurotoxicity, which can consist of depressed tendon reflexes, paresthesias of the fingers and toes, toxicity to the cranial nerves, or autonomic neuropathy (constipation or ileus, abdominal pain, and/or orthostatic hypotension.) In contrast, the dose-limiting toxicity associated with vinorelbine and vinblastine is myelosuppression. All of the vinca alkaloids are vesicants and can cause tissue damage; therefore, the clinician must take precautions to avoid extravasation injury. Biliary excretion accounts for a significant portion of elimination of vincristine and its metabolites, so doses need to be adjusted for obstructive liver disease.

Vincristine, vinblastine, and vinorelbine have similar sounding names, which is a potential cause of medication errors. As with all chemotherapy prescribing, dispensing, and administration, the clinician must be very careful with sound-alike, look-alike medications. Unfortunately, vincristine has been involved in numerous cases of fatal chemotherapy errors, including inadvertent intrathecal administration. Because the drug is a vesicant, intrathecal administration of the drug can cause widespread tissue damage in the brain and death. An example of a strategy that health systems can use to decrease the likelihood of an error such as this is for the pharmacy to only dispense vincristine in a minibag for IV administration. Many clinicians cap IV vincristine doses at 2 mg to prevent severe neuropathic side effects; however, if the intent of chemotherapy is curative, the vincristine dose may be dosed above the 2-mg cap.[16]

▶ *Taxanes (Paclitaxel, Nanoparticle Albumin-Bound Paclitaxel, Docetaxel, and Cabazitaxel)*

Paclitaxel and docetaxel are taxane plant alkaloids that, similar to the vinca alkaloids, exhibit cytotoxicity during the M phase of the cell cycle by binding to tubulin. Unlike the vinca alkaloids, however, the taxanes do not interfere with tubulin assembly. Rather, the taxanes promote microtubule assembly and inhibit microtubule disassembly. Once the microtubules are polymerized, the taxanes stabilize against depolymerization.

Hepatic metabolism and biliary excretion account for the majority of paclitaxel's elimination. Paclitaxel has demonstrated activity in several solid tumors. Considerable variability exists in paclitaxel dosing, from weekly 1-hour infusions to 24-hour infusions administered every 3 weeks. The diluent for paclitaxel, Cremophor EL, is composed of ethanol and castor oil. Infusions must be prepared and administered in non–polyvinyl chloride–containing bags and tubings, and solutions must be filtered. Patients receive dexamethasone, diphenhydramine, and an H_2 blocker to prevent hypersensitivity reactions caused by Cremophor EL. Patients also may have asymptomatic bradycardia during the infusion. Approximately 3 to 5 days after administration, patients may complain of myalgias and arthralgias that may last several days. Myelosuppression, flushing, neuropathy, ileus, and total-body alopecia are other common side effects. Because paclitaxel is a substrate for CYP 3A4, steady-state concentrations of paclitaxel were 30% lower in patients receiving phenytoin than in patients not receiving phenytoin. Paclitaxel clearance was decreased by 33% when it was administered after cisplatin, so paclitaxel is administered before cisplatin.

A nanoparticle albumin-bound nab-paclitaxel product is also available for the treatment of metastatic breast cancer resistant to conventional chemotherapy or progressing within 6 months of receiving a regimen containing an anthracycline. The nab-paclitaxel formulation uses nanotechnology to combine human albumin with paclitaxel allowing for the delivery of an insoluble drug in the form of nanoparticles. This unique formulation allows for an increased bioavailability and higher intracellular concentrations of the drug. It does not have the serious hypersensitivity reactions encountered with paclitaxel solubilized in Cremophor EL, so premedication with H_1 and H_2 blockers and steroids is not necessary. There is also a significantly lower incidence of severe neutropenia when compared to paclitaxel. The dose is infused over 30 minutes and does not require a special IV bag, tubing, or filter. The dosing of this product is different from that of the original paclitaxel, so practitioners need to be aware of which product is being prescribed. The pharmacokinetics of the albumin-bound paclitaxel displays a higher clearance and larger volume of distribution than paclitaxel. The drug is eliminated primarily via fecal excretion.[17] Bone marrow suppression, neuropathy, ileus, arthralgias, and myalgias still occur.

Docetaxel has activity in the treatment of several solid tumors also. Dexamethasone, 8 mg twice daily for 3 days starting the day before treatment, is used to prevent the fluid-retention syndrome associated with docetaxel and possible hypersensitivity reactions. The fluid-retention syndrome is characterized by edema and weight gain that is unresponsive to diuretic therapy and is associated with cumulative doses greater than 800 mg/m^2. Myelosuppression, alopecia, and neuropathy are other side effects associated with docetaxel treatment.

Cabazitaxel is a newer taxane used in combination with prednisone for the treatment of metastatic hormone-refractory prostate cancer in patients previously treated with a docetaxel-containing treatment regimen. Cabazitaxel has shown to have similar adverse effects as paclitaxel and docetaxel. Premedication with an antihistamine, corticosteroid, and H_2 antagonist to prevent hypersensitivity reactions is required.

▶ *Halichondrins*

Eribulin mesylate is a nontaxane microtubule dynamics inhibitor. It is a synthetic analogue of halichondrin B, which is a product isolated from the sea sponge *Halichondria okadai*. While taxanes inhibit cell division by stabilizing microtubules, eribulin arrests the cell cycle through inhibition of the growth phase of microtubules without interfering with microtubule shortening. The cytotoxicity results from its effects via a tubulin-based antimitotic mechanism, resulting in G_2/M cell-cycle arrest and mitotic blockage. Apoptotic cell death results from prolonged mitotic blockage. Eribulin mesylate is an IV medication that is specifically indicated for the treatment of patients with metastatic breast cancer who have received at least two previous chemotherapy regimens (containing an anthracycline and taxane) for metastatic disease. The most common adverse effects reported are neutropenic fever, anemia, asthenia or fatigue, alopecia, peripheral neuropathy, nausea, and constipation. Eribulin has been reported to cause significant neutropenia and QT interval prolongation. It has vesicant properties. Dosages should be adjusted in renal and hepatic impairment.[18]

▶ *Estramustine*

Estramustine, an oral drug, also inhibits microtubule assembly and has weak estrogenic activity at the estradiol hormone receptors of the cell. This drug is used primarily for the treatment of prostate cancer, but its use is limited by the side effects, which include nausea and vomiting, diarrhea, thromboembolic events, and gynecomastia.

▶ *Ixabepilone*

Ixabepilone, an epothilone analogue, binds to β-tubulin subunits on microtubules, which results in suppression of microtubule dynamics. Ixabepilone is primarily eliminated by the liver by oxidation through the CYP3A4 system. Ixabepilone, in combination with capecitabine or alone if resistant to capecitabine, is indicated for the treatment of metastatic or locally advanced breast cancer after failures of anthracyclines and a taxane. Studies have shown a possible synergy when used in combination with capecitabine. Side effects include hypersensitivity reactions, myelosuppression, and peripheral neuropathy. To minimize the occurrence of hypersensitivity reactions, patients must receive both H_1 and H_2 antagonists before therapy. If a reaction still occurs, corticosteroids should be added to the premedications.

Topoisomerase Inhibitors

Topoisomerase is responsible for relieving the pressure on the DNA structure during unwinding by producing strand breaks. Topoisomerase I produces single-strand breaks, whereas topoisomerase II produces double-strand breaks.

▶ *Epipodophyllotoxins (Etoposide and Teniposide)*

Etoposide and teniposide are semisynthetic podophyllotoxin derivatives that inhibit topoisomerase II, causing multiple DNA double-strand breaks. Etoposide has shown activity in the treatment of several types of lymphoma, testicular and lung cancer, retinoblastoma, and carcinoma of unknown primary. Oral bioavailability is approximately 50%, so oral dosages are approximate two times those of IV doses. Teniposide has shown activity in the treatment of ALL, neuroblastoma, and non-Hodgkin lymphoma. Both of these agents should be slowly administered to prevent hypotension. Side effects of these agents include mucositis, myelosuppression, alopecia, phlebitis, hypersensitivity reactions, and secondary leukemias. Hypersensitivity reactions may be life threatening.

▶ *Camptothecin Derivatives (Irinotecan and Topotecan)*

Irinotecan and topotecan, both camptothecins, inhibit the topoisomerase I enzyme to interfere with DNA synthesis through the active metabolite SN38. Topoisomerase I enzymes stabilize DNA single-strand breaks and inhibit strand resealing. Irinotecan has shown activity in the treatment of cancers of the colon, rectum, cervix, and lung. Irinotecan-induced diarrhea is a serious complication and may be life threatening. One form of diarrhea (acute) can occur during or immediately after the infusion. This is a result of a cholinergic process in which the patient may experience facial flushing, diaphoresis, and abdominal cramping. IV atropine should be administered to treat diarrhea that occurs any time during the first 24 hours of administration. Another form of diarrhea (chronic) can occur several days after administration and can result in severe dehydration. This adverse effect should be treated immediately with loperamide at a dosage of 2 mg every 2 hours or 4 mg every 4 hours until diarrhea has stopped for 12 hours. Other side effects include myelosuppression, fatigue, and alopecia. Individuals homozygous for *UGT1A1* 28* have an increased risk of febrile neutropenia and diarrhea and should be considered for an empiric dose reduction of one level; heterozygotes should receive closer monitoring, including more frequent complete blood counts (CBCs) to detect myelosuppression.

Topotecan has shown clinical activity in the treatment of ovarian and lung cancer, myelodysplastic syndromes, and AML. The IV infusion may be scheduled daily for 5 days or once weekly. Side effects include myelosuppression, mucositis, and diarrhea. Diarrhea is less common than with irinotecan.

Anthracene Derivatives

▶ *Daunorubicin, Doxorubicin, Idarubicin, and Epirubicin*

Anthracyclines (daunorubicin, doxorubicin, idarubicin, and epirubicin) are also referred to as antitumor antibiotics or topoisomerase inhibitors when considering their mechanism of action. All of the anthracyclines contain a four-membered anthracene ring, a chromophore, with an attached sugar portion. Free radicals formed from the anthracyclines combine with oxygen to form superoxide, which can make hydrogen peroxide. These agents are able to insert between base pairs of DNA to cause structural changes in DNA. However, the primary mechanism of cytotoxicity appears to be the inhibition of topoisomerase II. These drugs are widely used in a variety of cancers.

Oxygen-free-radical formation is a cause of cardiac damage and extravasation injury, which is common with these drugs. The anthracyclines can cause cardiac toxicity as manifested by a congestive heart failure or cardiomyopathy symptomatology, alopecia, nausea or vomiting, mucositis, myelosuppression, and urinary discoloration. These drugs are vesicants. Dosage alterations should be made in the presence of biliary dysfunction.[19]

To reduce the risk of cardiotoxicity associated with doxorubicin, the maximum lifetime cumulative dose is 550 mg/m^2. Ventricular ejection fractions should be measured before therapy and periodically if therapy is continued. Therapy should be halted if there is a 10% to 20% decrease from baseline in ejection fraction. Patients at increased risk of cardiotoxicity include patients reaching the upper limit of cumulative lifetime dose; those taking concomitant or previous cardiotoxic drugs, concurrent paclitaxel, or bolus administration; patients with preexisting cardiac disease or mediastinal radiation; and the very young and elderly. Cardioprotectants (eg, dexrazoxane) have been used to decrease risk in some cases. Clinical guidelines exist recommending when cardioprotective agents are warranted.[20]

Liposomal doxorubicin is an **irritant**, not a vesicant, and is dosed differently from doxorubicin, so clinicians need to be very careful when prescribing these two drugs. Liposomal doxorubicin has shown significant activity in the treatment of breast and ovarian cancer along with multiple myeloma and Kaposi sarcoma. Side effects include mucositis, myelosuppression, alopecia, and palmar-plantar erythrodysesthesia. The liposomal doxorubicin may be less cardiotoxic than doxorubicin.

▶ *Mitoxantrone*

This royal blue–colored drug is an anthracenedione that inhibits DNA topoisomerase II. Mitoxantrone has shown clinical activity in the treatment of acute leukemias, breast and prostate cancer, and non-Hodgkin lymphomas. Myelosuppression, mucositis, nausea and vomiting, and cardiac toxicity are side effects of this drug. The total cumulative dose limit is 160 mg/m^2 for patients who have not received prior anthracycline or mediastinal radiation. Patients who have received prior doxorubicin or daunorubicin therapy should not receive a cumulative dose greater than 120 mg/m^2 of mitoxantrone. Patients should be counseled that their urine will turn a blue–green color.[21]

Alkylating Agents

Although still widely used for many malignancies, the alkylating agents are the oldest class of anticancer drugs. The agents cause cytotoxicity via transfer of their alkyl groups to nucleophilic groups of proteins and nucleic acids. The major site of alkylation within DNA is the N7 position of guanine, although alkylation does occur to a lesser degree at other bases. These interactions can either occur on a single strand of DNA (monofunctional agents) or on both strands of DNA through a cross-link (bifunctional agents), which leads to strand breaks. The major toxicities of the alkylating agents are myelosuppression, alopecia, nausea or vomiting, sterility or infertility, and secondary malignancies.

▶ *Nitrogen Mustards (Cyclophosphamide and Ifosfamide)*

Cyclophosphamide and ifosfamide are commonly used bifunctional alkylating agents, therefore, causing cross-linking of DNA. They each share similar adverse effects and spectrum of activity, being used in a variety of solid and hematologic cancers. Cyclophosphamide and ifosfamide are both prodrugs, requiring activation by mixed hepatic oxidase enzymes to get to their active forms, phosphoramide and ifosfamide mustard, respectively. During the activation process, additional byproducts (acrolein and chloroacetaldehyde) are formed. Acrolein has no cytotoxic activity but is responsible for the hemorrhagic cystitis associated with ifosfamide and high-dose cyclophosphamide. Acrolein produces cystitis by directly binding to the bladder wall. Prophylaxis is necessary with aggressive hydration, administration of 2-mercaptoethane sulfonate sodium (MESNA, which binds to and inactivates acrolein in the bladder), frequent voiding, and monitoring in patients receiving ifosfamide and high-dose cyclophosphamide. Patients should be counseled to drink plenty of fluids; void frequently; and report any hematuria, irritation, or flank pain. Dosing regimens of MESNA range from an equal milligram dose to the ifosfamide mixed in the same IV bag to 20% of the dose before ifosfamide and 20% of the dose repeated at 4 and 8 hours after the dose.

Chloroacetaldehyde, a metabolite of ifosfamide, can result in encephalopathy, especially in patients receiving ifosfamide that exhibit risk factors such as renal dysfunction or advanced age. This adverse effect can occur within 48 to 72 hours of administration and is usually reversible.

> **Patient Encounter 1, Part 2**
>
> The decision to treat the patient with a systemic chemotherapy regimen is made. He will be receiving the standard induction regimen of 7 + 3 (idarubicin 12 mg/m^2/day IV every day for 3 days + cytarabine 100 mg/m^2/day continuous IV infusion for 7 days).
>
> ***Before initiating this chemotherapy regimen in the patient, what patient specific issues need to be addressed?***
>
> ***What adverse effects will the patient likely experience with these two chemotherapy drugs?***

> **Patient Encounter 1, Part 3**
>
> The patient goes into complete remission (or a complete response), and now consolidation therapy with high-dose cytarabine (2 g/m^2/dose IV every 12 hours for six doses) will be initiated.
>
> ***What is the mechanism of action of cytarabine?***
>
> ***How do the toxicities of high-dose cytarabine differ from those of conventional (low-dose) cytarabine? What are the risk factors, prophylaxis recommendations, and treatment recommendations for these toxicities?***

▶ *Busulfan*

Busulfan is an alkylating agent that forms DNA–DNA and DNA–protein cross-links to inhibit DNA replication. Oral busulfan is well absorbed, has a terminal half-life of 2 to 2.5 hours, and is eliminated primarily by metabolism. It is also available in an IV formulation, which is useful when using the high doses required in blood and marrow transplantation. Busulfan has shown significant clinical activity in the treatment of AML and CML and has been used as a conditioning regimen prior to stem cell transplant. Side effects include bone marrow suppression; hyperpigmentation of skin creases; and rarely, pulmonary fibrosis. High doses used for bone marrow transplant preparatory regimens result in severe nausea and vomiting, tonic–clonic seizures, and sinusoidal obstruction syndrome. Patients receiving high-dose busulfan should receive anticonvulsant prophylaxis. Toxicities associated with busulfan dosing along with a discussion on adaptive dosing of busulfan can be found in Chapter 98.

▶ *Nitrosoureas (Carmustine and Lomustine)*

Carmustine (BCNU) and lomustine (CCNU) are nitrosoureas that are lipophilic in nature and therefore able to cross the blood–brain barrier. Carmustine, which is reconstituted with ethanol, crosses the blood–brain barrier when given IV. It also comes as a biodegradable wafer formulation that may be implanted to treat residual tumor tissue after surgical resection of brain tumors. Lomustine is available in an oral formulation. Carmustine has shown clinical activity in the treatment of lymphoma, melanoma, and brain tumors. Lomustine has shown clinical activity in the treatment of non-Hodgkin lymphoma and melanoma. Patients should receive only enough lomustine for one cycle at a time to prevent confusion with their drug regimens and the prolonged neutropenia that can occur. Side effects include myelosuppression, severe nausea and vomiting, and pulmonary fibrosis with long-term therapy.

► *Nonclassic Alkylating Agents (Dacarbazine and Temozolomide)*

Although the exact mechanism of action remains unclear, dacarbazine and temozolomide appear to inhibit DNA, RNA, and protein synthesis. Dacarbazine has shown clinical benefit in the treatment of patients with melanoma, Hodgkin lymphoma, and soft tissue sarcomas. Side effects include myelosuppression, severe nausea and vomiting, and a flu-like syndrome that starts about 7 days after treatment and lasts 1 to 3 weeks.

Temozolomide is an orally active agent that is well absorbed and crosses the blood–brain barrier. Temozolomide is converted via pH-dependent hydrolysis to the active metabolite 5-(3-methyltriazeno)-imidazole-4-carboxamide. Temozolomide may be used in the treatment of melanoma, refractory anaplastic astrocytoma, and glioblastoma multiforme. Nausea may be minimized by administering the drug at bedtime. Because patients receiving temozolomide may have confusion secondary to their brain tumors and because dosing can consist of multiple capsule sizes, care must be taken by all providers to simplify regimens to prevent chemotherapy overdose.[22]

► *Procarbazine*

Although the exact mechanism of action of procarbazine is unknown, it does inhibit DNA, RNA, and protein synthesis. Procarbazine is used most often in the treatment of lymphoma. Myelosuppression is the major side effect. Nausea, vomiting, and a flu-like syndrome occur initially with therapy. Patients must be counseled to avoid tyramine-rich foods because procarbazine is a monoamine oxidase inhibitor. Patients should be provided a list of foods and beverages to avoid a hypertensive crisis. A disulfiram-like reaction can occur with the ingestion of alcohol.

► *Bendamustine*

Bendamustine has three chemically active groups: a 2-chlorethyl group, a butyric acid side chain, and a benzimidazole ring. Bendamustine has shown activity in chronic lymphocytic leukemia and non-Hodgkin lymphoma. It is usually given in combination with rituximab as first-line therapy. Side effects include nausea, vomiting, bone marrow suppression, headache and dyspnea.

► *Thiotepa*

Thiotepa is an alkylating agent that reacts with DNA phosphate groups to produce chromosomal cross-linkage. Thiotepa has shown clinical activity in the treatment of breast, bladder, and ovarian cancer, along with carcinomatous meningitis and malignant effusions, and usually is administered IV or as an intravesicular infusion. It also may be used intrathecally. Side effects include myelosuppression, nausea and vomiting, and venous irritation.

Heavy Metal Compounds

Platinum drugs form reactive platinum complexes that bind to cells, so the pharmacokinetics of the individual drug may be of the platinum, both free and bound, rather than of the parent drug.

► *Cisplatin*

Cisplatin forms inter- and intrastrand DNA cross-links to inhibit DNA synthesis. Cisplatin has shown clinical activity in the treatment of numerous tumor types, from head and neck cancers to anal cancer, including many types of lymphoma and carcinoma of unknown primary. Cisplatin is highly emetogenic, even when low doses are given daily for 5 days, and causes delayed nausea and vomiting as well; patients require aggressive antiemetic regimens for both delayed and acute emesis. Significant nephrotoxicity and electrolyte abnormalities can occur if inadequate hydration occurs. Ototoxicity, which manifests as a high-frequency hearing loss, and a glove-and-stocking neuropathy may limit therapy.

► *Carboplatin*

Carboplatin has the same mechanism of action as cisplatin, however, its side effects are similar but less intense than those of cisplatin. Many chemotherapy regimens dose carboplatin based on an area under the curve (AUC), which is also called the Calvert equation. According to the Calvert equation, the dose in milligrams of carboplatin = (CrCl + 25) × AUC desired, where CrCl is expressed in mL/min.[23] Carboplatin has shown clinical activity in the treatment of several solid tumors and lymphoma. Thrombocytopenia, nausea and vomiting, and hypersensitivity reactions are adverse effects.

► *Oxaliplatin*

Oxaliplatin has shown clinical activity in the treatment of colorectal cancer. Oxaliplatin, although similar in action to cisplatin and carboplatin in terms of adverse effects, also, causes a cold-induced neuropathy. Patients should be counseled to avoid cold beverages, to use gloves to remove items from the freezer, and to wear protective clothing in cold climates for the first week after treatment. A glove-and-stocking neuropathy also occurs with long-term dosing. Hypersensitivity reactions and moderate nausea and vomiting are also adverse effects.[24]

mTOR Inhibitors

► *Temsirolimus and Everolimus*

The mammalian target of rapamycin (mTOR) is a downstream mediator in the phosphatidylinositol 3-kinase/Akt signaling pathway that controls translation of proteins that regulate cell growth and proliferation but also angiogenesis and cell survival. The mTOR is an intracellular component that stimulates protein synthesis by phosphorylating translation regulators, and contributes to protein degradation and angiogenesis.

Temsirolimus is approved for the treatment advanced renal cell carcinoma. Temsirolimus and its metabolite sirolimus are substrates of the cytochrome CYP3A4/5 isoenzyme system. The primary side effects of temsirolimus include mucositis, diarrhea, maculopapular rash, nausea, leucopenia, thrombocytopenia, and hyperglycemia.

Everolimus is an oral inhibitor of mTOR that is approved for the treatment of patients with advanced renal cell cancer after failure of treatment with sunitinib or sorafenib and most recently for the treatment of advanced pancreatic neuroendocrine tumors. Drug interactions and adverse reactions are similar to those of temsirolimus.

Miscellaneous Agents

► *Altretamine*

Altretamine, formerly known as hexamethylmelamine, is similar in structure to alkylating agents but is known to have anticancer activity in cancer cells resistant to alkylating agents. Altretamine has shown activity in the treatment of ovarian and lung cancer. This orally administered drug has the dose-limiting side effects of anorexia, nausea, vomiting, diarrhea, and abdominal cramping. Other side effects include neuropathy, agitation, confusion, and depression.

▶ Bleomycin

Bleomycin is a mixture of peptides with drug activity expressed in units, where 1 unit equals to 1 mg. Bleomycin causes DNA strand breakage. Bleomycin has shown clinical activity in the treatment of patients with testicular cancer and malignant effusions, squamous cell carcinomas of the skin, and Kaposi sarcoma. Hypersensitivity reactions and fever may occur, so premedication with acetaminophen may be required. The most serious side effect is the pulmonary toxicity that presents as a pneumonitis with a dry cough, dyspnea, rales, and infiltrates. Pulmonary function studies show decreased carbon monoxide diffusing capacity and restrictive ventilatory changes. "Bleomycin lung" is associated with cumulative dosing greater than 400 units and occurs rarely with a total dose of 150 units. The pulmonary toxicity is potentiated by thoracic radiation and by hyperoxia. Additional side effects include fever with or without chills, mild to moderate alopecia, and nausea and vomiting. Bleomycin has been used to manage malignant plural effusions at doses of 15 to 60 units through installation into the affected area. The drainage tube of the effusion is clamped off for some period of time after administration of bleomycin and then the amount of drainage is monitored to determine efficacy of the treatment.[25]

▶ Hydroxyurea

Hydroxyurea is an oral drug that inhibits ribonucleotide reductase, which converts ribonucleotides into the deoxyribonucleotides used in DNA synthesis and repair. Hydroxyurea has shown clinical activity in the treatment of CML, polycythemia vera, and thrombocytosis. The major side effects are myelosuppression, nausea and vomiting, diarrhea, and constipation. Rash, mucositis, and renal tubular dysfunction occur rarely.

▶ L-Asparaginase

L-Asparaginase is an enzyme that may be produced by *Escherichia coli*. Asparaginase hydrolyzes the reaction of asparagine to aspartic acid and ammonia to deplete lymphoid cells of asparagine, which inhibits protein synthesis. L-Asparaginase has shown clinical activity in the treatment of ALL and childhood AML. Severe allergic reactions may occur when the interval between doses is 7 days or greater, so while a skin test result may be negative, patients should be observed closely after asparaginase administration. Pancreatitis and fibrinogen depletion may also occur during therapy. Repletion of fibrinogen should be done to prevent disseminated intravascular coagulation and fatal bleeding. If the patient suffers an allergic reaction to L-asparaginase, pegaspargase, which is L-asparaginase modified through a linkage with polyethylene glycol, which extends the half-life and allows for lower doses and less frequent administration, may be given. Cost and limited availability are some reasons pegaspargase may not be used first.

▶ Arsenic Trioxide

Arsenic trioxide, which is approved for the treatment of acute promyelocytic leukemia (APL), induces the growth of cancer cells into mature, more normal cells and induces programmed cell death, or apoptosis. Arsenic trioxide causes QT-interval prolongation, so frequent electrocardiograms need to be done before each dose, and other drugs that may prolong the QT interval need to be avoided during therapy. Monitoring of potassium and magnesium should be performed and active replacement undertaken to prevent QT prolongation. Other side effects include dry skin with itching, nausea and vomiting, loss of appetite, and elevations of serum hepatic enzymes. A serious side effect is APL differentiation syndrome, which appears similar to pneumonia but is related to the arsenic therapy.[26]

▶ Mitomycin C

Mitomycin C forms cross-links with DNA to inhibit DNA and RNA synthesis. Mitomycin C has shown clinical activity in the treatment of several solid tumors. Side effects consist of myelosuppression and mucositis, and it is a vesicant.

▶ Tretinoin

Tretinoin, also referred to *ATRA*, which stands for all-trans-retinoic acid, is a retinoic acid that is not cytotoxic but promotes the maturation of early promyelocytic cells and is specific to the t(15;17) cytogenetic marker. The most significant side effect is the APL differentiation syndrome, which may occur anywhere from the first couple of days of therapy until the end of therapy and consists of symptoms of fever, respiratory distress, and hypotension. Chest radiographs are consistent with a pneumonia-like process. The syndrome can be confused easily with pneumonia in a patient with possible neutropenia. The treatment for retinoic acid syndrome is dexamethasone 10 mg IV every 12 hours; the syndrome may resolve within 24 hours of the start of dexamethasone therapy. However, the use of steroids in a febrile neutropenic patient may further compromise the treatment of infection.[27]

▶ Immunomodulatory Agents (Thalidomide, Lenalidomide, and Pomalidomide)

Thalidomide was introduced into the market in Europe on October 1, 1957, as a sedative–hypnotic, and when it was taken by pregnant women, it resulted in severe limb deformities (phocomelia) and its withdrawl from use. Thalidomide is an angiogenesis inhibitor, but the full mechanism of action is still unknown. Possible mechanisms of action include free radical oxidative damage to DNA, inhibiting tumor necrosis factor α production, altering the adhesion of cancer cells, and altering cytokines that affect the growth of cancer cells.[28,29] Thalidomide has shown clinical activity in the treatment of multiple myeloma. Because of thalidomide's potential to cause phocomelia, each patient must be enrolled in the STEPS program and counseled on the risks of thalidomide not only for the patient but also the patient's reproductive partner. Clinicians must be registered to prescribe thalidomide. Common adverse effects include somnolence, constipation, peripheral neuropathy, and deep vein thrombosis (DVT). Recommendations for DVT prophylaxis include standard dose warfarin or low-molecular-weight heparins.

Lenalidomide is approved for the treatment of myelodysplastic syndrome when the 5q deletion is present and multiple myeloma. Because lenalidomide is an analogue of thalidomide, all of the same precautions must be taken to prevent phocomelia. However, lenalidomide has fewer adverse effects than thalidomide. Dosing adjustments are necessary for renal dysfunction. Lenalidomide is used in the treatment of myelodysplastic syndrome and multiple myeloma. Other side effects are neutropenia, thrombocytopenia, deep vein thrombosis (DVT), and pulmonary embolus.

Pomalidomide was approved for the treatment of retractory or progressive multiple myeloma in February 2013. Adverse effects include myelosuppression and infections. The use of the immunomudulatory agents in the treatment of multiple myeloma is discussed thoroughly in Chapter 96.

▶ *Bexarotene*

Bexarotene is a retinoid that selectively activates retinoid X receptors, which affects cellular differentiation and proliferation. Bexarotene is eliminated primarily by the hepatobiliary system. Bexarotene is indicated for the treatment of cutaneous manifestations of cutaneous T-cell lymphoma in patients who are refractory to other therapy. Side effects include hypercholesterolemia, elevations in triglycerides, pancreatitis, hypothyroidism, and leukopenia, headache, and dry skin.

▶ *Proteasome Inhibitors (Bortezomib and Carfilzomib)*

The proteasome is an enzyme complex that exists in all cells and plays an important role in degrading proteins the control the cell cycle. When the proteasome is inhibited, the numerous pathways that are necessary for the growth and survival of cancer cells are disrupted. Bortezomib specifically inhibits the 26S proteasome, which is a large protein complex that degrades ubiquitinated proteins. This pathway plays an essential role in regulating the intracellular concentration of specific proteins, causing the cells to maintain homeostasis. Inhibition of the 26S proteasome prevents this to occur, ultimately causing a disruption in the homeostasis and cell death.

Bortezomib is approved for the treatment of multiple myeloma (MM), mantle cell lymphoma, and in some cases of relapsed/refractory AML. It is administered as an IV injection. The most commonly reported adverse effects are asthenia, gastrointestinal disturbances (nausea, diarrhea, decreased appetite, constipation, vomiting), thrombocytopenia, peripheral neuropathy, anemia, headache, insomnia, and edema. Prophylactic anticoagulation is not routinely required. Reactivation of varicella zoster infection is also common with bortezomib, and antiviral prophylaxis with acyclovir should be considered.

Carfilzomib is a newer second-generation proteasome inhibitor and is used in the treatment of refractory cases of MM.

▶ *Omacetaxine Mepesuccinate*

Omacetaxine mepesuccinate, an alkaloid from *Cephalotaxus harringtonia*, was granted accelerated approval by the FDA in October 2012. The agent reversibly inhibits protein synthesis, causing cell death. It affects both malignant and nonmalignant cells. It is a subcutaneous injection and is indicated for the treatment of CML patients (including those patients with the T315I mutation) showing resistance and/or intolerance to two or more TKIs. The most common nonhematological adverse effects are gastrointestinal disruption, fatigue, and hyperglycemia. Rare but serious adverse reactions include febrile neutropenia, infections, and cerebral hemorrhage.

▶ *Ziv-aflibercept*

Ziv-aflibercept is a recombinant fusion protein that consists of vascular endothelial growth factor (VEGF)-binding portions from the extracellular domains of human VEGF receptors 1 and 2 fused to the Fc portion of the human IgG1 immunoglobulin. It is an intravenously administered and approved for the treatment of metastatic colorectal cancer in combination with FOLFIRI after progression on an oxaliplatin-based regimen. Ziv-aflibercept has black-box warnings, which include hemorrhage, gastrointestinal perforation, and compromised wound healing. Other adverse effects include neutropenia, diarrhea, and a reversible posterior leukoencephalopathy syndrome.

Patient Encounter 2

A 48-year-old man is receiving doxorubicin and ifosfamide for a newly diagnosed osteosarcoma. While receiving chemotherapy, he begins to complain of flank pain and hematuria. His serum creatinine has risen from 0.8 mg/dL to 2.1 mg/dL (71 to 186 μmol/L) in the last 3 days.

What is the likely diagnosis?

What medication should always be included as part of this regimen?

What should patients be counseled to do while receiving ifosfamide therapy?

▶ *HDAC Inhibitors (Vorinostat and Romidepsin)*

Vorinostat is indicated for the treatment of cutaneous T-cell lymphoma in patients with progressive, persistent, or recurrent disease after treatment with two systemic therapies. Romidepsin is approved for the treatment of cutaneous or peripheral T-cell lymphoma in patients who have received at least one systemic therapy. These agents catalyze the removal of acetyl groups from acetylated lysine residues in histones, resulting in the modulation of gene expression. Vorinostat is an orally available agent, and romidepsin is only available in an IV formulation. These drugs are metabolized by CYP3A4, so caution should be exercised with monitoring for drug–drug interactions. Side effects include diarrhea, fatigue, nausea and anorexia, hypercholesterolemia, hypertriglyceridemia, and hyperglycemia. Despite anemia, thrombocytopenia, and neutropenia, patients have developed pulmonary embolism and DVT while on therapy.[30]

Immune Therapies

▶ *Interferons*

The categories of α, β, and γ interferons exist; the α-interferons are used in the treatment of cancer. Interferon enhances the immune system's attack on cancer cells, can decrease new blood vessel formation, and can augment expression of antigen on tumor cell surfaces. Interferon has shown clinical activity in the treatment of melanoma, kidney cancer, Kaposi sarcoma, and CML and CLL. Unfortunately, interferon is not well tolerated by patients because it causes a flu-like syndrome that consists of fevers and chills; depression, malaise, and fatigue are other side effects. Premedication with acetaminophen helps alleviate the flu-like symptoms, which decrease with chronic administration.

▶ *Aldesleukin*

Aldesleukin, which is a human recombinant *interleukin-2 (IL-2)*, is a lymphokine that promotes B- and T-cell proliferation and triggers a cytokine cascade to attack the tumor. Aldesleukin has shown clinical activity in the treatment of kidney cancer and melanoma. Side effects of IL-2 vary by dose and route. IV high-dose IL-2 causes a drug-induced shock-like picture. Patients may develop hypotension despite aggressive IV hydration. Patients develop a red, itchy skin; liver and kidney function tests change; via immune complex formation in the kidneys, fluid and electrolyte imbalances occur; and high fevers occur while receiving scheduled acetaminophen and nonsteroidal anti-inflammatory agents. Severe rigors and chills may require symptom control. All the side effects reverse within 24 hours of stopping the drug. The toxicity profile is much less with subcutaneous administration. However, with subcutaneous administration, nodules form at the injection site and may take months to resolve. Corticosteroids should not be administered to patients while they are receiving aldesleukin unless a life-threatening emergency occurs. Steroids reverse all the symptoms and the antitumor effect even with topical administration. The itching, red skin may be treated with topical creams and antihistamines.

► *Denileukin Diftitox*

Denileukin diftitox is a combination of the active moieties of IL-2 and diphtheria toxin. It binds to high-affinity IL-2 receptors on the cancer cell (and other cells), and the toxin portion of the molecule inhibits protein synthesis to result in cell death. Denileukin diftitox is used for the treatment of persistent or recurrent cutaneous T-cell lymphoma whose cells express the CD25 receptor. Side effects include vascular leak syndrome, fevers or chills, hypersensitivity reactions, hypotension, anorexia, diarrhea, and nausea and vomiting.

► *Peginterferon α-2b*

Sylatron is a covalent conjugate of recombinant α-2b interferon with monomethoxy polyethylene glycol (PEG). The mechanism of cytotoxicity in patients with melanoma is unknown. This agent is specifically indicated for the adjuvant treatment of melanoma with microscopic or gross nodal involvement up to 84 days after definitive surgical resection (including complete lymphadenectomy). Adverse effects include fatigue, increased liver enzymes, pyrexia, headache, anorexia, myalgia, nausea, chills, and pain at the injection site.[31]

► *Sipuleucel-T*

Sipuleucel-T is a novel autologous cellular immunotherapy approved for the treatment of asymptomatic or minimally symptomatic metastatic hormone refractory prostate cancer. Sipuleucel-T is designed to induce an immune response targeted at prostatic acid phosphatase (PAP), which is an antigen expressed in greater than 95% of prostate cancers. Patients receiving sipuleucel-T undergo leukapheresis to collect their own antigen-presenting cells. These cells are then sent to a manufacturing facility and cultured with a recombinant antigen (PAP-GM-CSF, composed of PAP and GM-CSF, an immune cell activator). The cellular product, which is made specifically for each patient, is then delivered to the patient's clinic and infused intravenously into the patient on day 3 or 4. Each course consists of three infusions of activated cells given at 2-week intervals. Adverse effects include chills, fatigue, fever, back pain, nausea, joint pain, and headache.[32]

Monoclonal Antibodies

The cell surface contains molecules, which are referred to as *CD*, which stands for "cluster of differentiation." The antibodies are produced against a specific antigen. When administered, usually by an IV injection, the antibody binds to the antigen, which may trigger the immune system to result in cell death through complement-mediated cellular toxicity, or the antigen–antibody cell complex may be internalized to the cancer cell, which results in cell death. Monoclonal antibodies also may carry radioactivity, sometimes referred to as *hot antibodies*, and are referred to as *radioimmunotherapy*, so the radioactivity is delivered to the cancer cell. Antibodies that contain no radioactivity are referred to as *cold antibodies*.

All monoclonal antibodies end in the suffix *-mab*. The syllable before *-mab* indicates the source of the monoclonal antibody (Table 88–6). When administering an antibody for the first time, one should consider the source. The less humanized an antibody, the greater the chance for the patient to have an allergic-type reaction to the antibody. The more humanized the antibody, the lower the risk of a reaction. The severity of the reactions may range from fever and chills to life-threatening allergic reactions. Premedication with acetaminophen and diphenhydramine is common before the first dose of any antibody. If a severe reaction occurs, the infusion should be stopped and the patient treated with antihistamines, corticosteroids, or other supportive measures.

Table 88–6

Syllable Source Indicators for Monoclonal Antibodies[a]

U	Human
O	Mouse
A	Rat
E	Hamster
I	Primate
Xi	A cross between humanized and animal source

[a]These letters appear before mab, which stands for monoclonal antibody.

From Programme on International Nonproprietary Names (INN) Division of Drug Management and Policies, World Health Organization, Geneva. 1997.

► *Bevacizumab*

Bevacizumab is a humanized monoclonal antibody that binds to vascular endothelial growth factor (VEGF), which prevents it from binding to its receptors, ultimately resulting in inhibition of angiogenesis. Bevacizumab has shown clinical activity in the treatment of colorectal, kidney, lung, breast, and head and neck cancer. Patients may develop hypertension requiring chronic medication during therapy. Impaired wound healing, thromboembolic events, proteinuria, bleeding, and bowel perforation are serious side effects that occur with this drug.

► *Brentuximab*

Brentuximab vedotin is a CD30-directed antibody–drug conjugate (ADC) that consists of the antibody specific for CD30, a microtubule disrupting agent called monomethyl auristatin E (MMAE), and a protease-cleavable linker that covalently attaches MMAE to the antibody. It is reported that the cytotoxic activity is a result of the binding of the ADC to CD30-expressing cells followed by internalization of the ADC–CD30 complex, and then proteolytic cleavage and release of MMAE into the cell. Binding of MMAE to tubulin disrupts the microtubule network, resulting in cell cycle arrest and apoptosis. This IV agent is indicated for Hodgkin lymphoma patients after failure of autologous stem cell transplant (ASCT) or after failure of at least two multidrug regimens in patients who are not eligible for ASCT and for patients with systemic anaplastic large cell lymphoma who have failed at least one systemic chemotherapy regimen. In vitro data suggests that MMAE is a substrate and an inhibitor of CYP3A4/5; therefore, patients need to be monitored for drug–drug interactions. The most common adverse effects are neutropenia, peripheral neuropathy, fatigue, nausea and vomiting, diarrhea, anemia, thrombocytopenia, and upper respiratory infection. Dosing modifications guidelines for peripheral neuropathy can be found in the prescribing information.[33]

▶ *Cetuximab*

Cetuximab is a chimeric antibody that binds to the epidermal growth factor receptor (EGFR) to block its stimulation. Tumors that have *KRAS* mutations do not respond to treatment with cetuximab; therefore, tumors should be tested for *KRAS* mutations before initiating therapy. Cetuximab has shown clinical activity in the treatment of colorectal and head and neck cancers. An acne-like rash may appear on the face and upper torso 1 to 3 weeks after the start of therapy. Other side effects include hypersensitivity reactions, interstitial lung disease, fever, malaise, diarrhea, abdominal pain, and nausea and vomiting.

▶ *Ipilimumab*

Ipilimumab is a recombinant, human monoclonal antibody that binds to the cytotoxic T lymphocytic–associated antigen 4 (CTLA-4), which is a molecule on T cells that causes a suppression of the immune response. CTLA-4 is a negative regulator of T-cell activation. Ipilimumab binds to CTLA-4 and blocks the interaction of CTLA-4 with its ligands. This blockage has been reported to enhance T-cell activation and proliferation. Ipilimumab is approved for patients with unresectable or metastatic melanoma. The antitumor effects appear to be T-cell–mediated immune responses. Ipilimumab administration can result in severe and fatal immune-mediated adverse reactions, including enterocolitis, hepatitis, toxic epidermal necrolysis, neuropathy, and endocrine abnormalities. These symptoms can occur during treatment or weeks to months after discontinuation of the drug. Liver and thyroid function tests should be performed at baseline and before each dose. If this occurs, treatment should be initiated with systemic corticosteroids and the drug should be discontinued permanently. Progressive multifocal leukoencephalopathy has been reported. Additional less serious adverse effects include fatigue, diarrhea, pruritus, rash, and colitis.

▶ *Panitumumab*

Panitumumab binds to the EGFR to prevent receptor autophosphorylation and activation of receptor-associated kinases, which results in inhibition of cell growth and induction of apoptosis. Panitumumab has demonstrated activity against tumors of the colon and rectum. However, panitumumab is not recommended for the treatment of colorectal cancer with *KRAS* mutations in codon 12 or 13. Retrospective subset analyses have not shown a treatment benefit for these mutations. Side effects include dermatitis, pruritus, exfoliative rash, infusion reactions, pulmonary fibrosis, diarrhea, hypomagnesemia, hypocalcemia, and photosensitivity.

▶ *Rituximab*

Rituximab is a monoclonal antibody to the CD20 receptor expressed on the surface of B lymphocytes; the presence of the antibody is determined during flow cytometry of the tumor cells. Cell death results from antibody-dependent cellular cytotoxicity. Rituximab has shown clinical activity in the treatment of B-cell lymphomas that are CD20 positive. Side effects include infusion-related reactions, hypotension, fevers, chills, rash, headache, and mild nausea and vomiting. Premedication with diphenhydramine and acetaminophen is recommended to minimize the first-dose infusion reaction.

▶ *Tositumomab and Ibritumomab Tiuxetan*

Tositumomab, a "hot antibody," is linked to radioactive iodine and binds to the CD20 receptor present on B lymphocytes (see Rituximab). Tositumomab has shown activity in non-Hodgkin lymphoma. Hematologic toxicity occurs several weeks after administration and may persist for months. Because radioactive iodine may have adverse effects on the thyroid, all patients must receive thyroid-blocking agents.

Ibritumomab Tiuxetan, a "hot antibody," is linked to yttrium and binds to the CD20 receptor of B lymphocytes. Similarly, hematologic toxicity may occur several weeks after administration and may take weeks to resolve.

▶ *Ofatumumab and Obinutuzumab*

Ofatumumab and obinutuzumab are two newer monoclonal antibodies that are directed at the CD20 antigen in patients with chronic lymphocytic leukemia that is refractory to fludarabine and alemtuzumab therapy. Obinutuzumab was approved recently for the combination treatment with chlorambucil in patients that have previously untreated CLL. The most common adverse effects include infusion-related reactions, neutropenia, infections, pyrexia, anemia, diarrhea, and nausea. Serious adverse events, including fatal infections, progressive multifocal leukoencephalopathy, and reactivation of hepatitis B, have been reported.

▶ *Alemtuzumab*

Alemtuzumab is an antibody to the CD52 receptor present on B and T lymphocytes. Alemtuzumab has shown clinical activity in the treatment of chronic lymphocytic leukemia. Severe and prolonged (6 months) immunosuppression may result, which necessitates pneumocystis carinii pneumonia (PCP) prophylaxis and antifungal and antiviral prophylaxis to prevent opportunistic infections. Infusion-related reactions typically occur with the first dose and can be severe. Premedication with antihistamines and acetaminophen is recommended. Subcutaneous administration will also alleviate the severity of infusion reactions.

▶ *Ramucirumab*

Ramucirumab is a humanized monoclonal antibody that binds with high affinity to the extracellular domain of vascular endothelial growth factor receptor 2 (VEGFR2, preventing the binding of VEGF-A, VEGF-C, and VEGF-D. This agent was approved in 2014 for the treatment of advanced gastric cancer with disease progression after fluoropyrimidine- or platinum-containing chemotherapy. The most common grade 3 or 4 adverse effects are hypertension, most commonly occurring in patients with preexisting hypertension. There is also a risk of hemorrhage, and the drug should be permanently discontinued in patients experiencing a severe bleeding episode.

▶ *Trastuzumab*

Trastuzumab is a humanized monoclonal antibody directed against human epidermal receptor 2 (HER-2), which is amplified or overexpressed by 15% to 20% of all breast cancers and is associated with aggressive disease and decreased survival. Breast cancer tissue must be tested for the presence of HER-2 because patients who do not express HER-2 do not respond to trastuzumab. It can be used as single agent or in combination with an anthracycline or taxane-based combination chemotherapy. Trastuzumab is also indicated for the treatment of gastric cancer. Severe congestive heart failure may occur with concurrent anthracycline administration. Cardiac toxicity may be seen when the drug is administered months after anthracycline administration, so patients must be counseled on the signs and symptoms of heart failure. A common side effect associated with trastuzumab is a first-dose infusion-related reaction which includes chills. The patient may be given acetaminophen and diphenhydramine and/or the infusion may be slowed. Other side effects which are rare include hypersensitivity reactions and pulmonary reactions.[34] A more detailed discussion of the use of trastuzumab in breast cancer can be found in Chapter 89.

▸ *Trastuzumab-DM1 (T-DM1, Trastuzumab Emtansine)*

Trastuzumab-DM1 or ado-trastuzumab emtansine was approved by the FDA in February 2013. In this compound, trastuzumab is used as a drug vehicle to deliver an anticancer agent known as emtansine (a maytansine derivative). Phase 3 clinical data evaluating the use in progressive HER-2-positive breast cancer patients will be discussed in Chapter 89. The most common serious adverse effect reported in clinical trials was thrombocytopenia. The platelet nadir usually occurred about 7 days after treatment and recovered within a week. Other adverse effects included abnormal liver function tests, fatigue, nausea, headache, and hypokalemia. Cardiac toxicity was not a reason for study withdrawal.

▸ *Pertuzumab*

The FDA approved the new HER-2-targeted pertuzumab in June 2012. When compared to trastuzumab, pertuzumab recognizes different extracellular epitopes, binds uniquely which causes structural changes and therefore interrupts receptor dimerization. These differences were thought to be able to provide greater inhibition of HER-2 when compared to trastuzumab. This has not been proven to be the case, but based on clinical studies is indicated for first-line treatment in combination with trastuzumab and docetaxel for HER-2-positive metastatic breast cancer. Adverse effects seen in clinical trials were diarrhea and a similar incidence of cardiac toxicity as trastuzumab. When used in combination with trastuzumab, it does not appear to increase the incidence of cardiac toxicity.

Tyrosine Kinase Inhibitors

There are more than 100 different types of tyrosine kinases present in the body. Tyrosine kinase inhibitors (TKIs) are also referred to as small-molecule inhibitors. Each of the following drugs was developed to block either several or a specific tyrosine kinase.

▸ *Imatinib*

Imatinib was the first FDA-approved TKI and is considered to be first-generation. Imatinib inhibits phosphorylation during cell proliferation. The drug was designed to block the breakpoint cluster region tyrosine kinase (BCR-ABL) produced by the Philadelphia chromosome associated with CML and ALL. Imatinib also has shown activity against gastrointestinal stromal tumors (GIST) that are positive for c-kit (CD117). Imatinib is usually well tolerated, but common adverse effects include myelosuppression, rash, GI upset, edema, fatigue, arthalgias, myalgias, and headaches. A cumulative cardiotoxicty is a serious but rare adverse effect therefore it is recommended to closely monitor patients with preexisting cardiac conditions. Numerous drug interactions have been reported for imatinib. CYP3A4 inducers, such as rifampicin and St. John's wort, increase the clearance of imatinib.[35,36] Ketoconazole, a CYP3A4 inhibitor, has been shown to decrease imatinib clearance by almost 30%.[37] Imatinib also may increase the exposure of simvastatin, a CYP3A4 substrate.[38] These are various examples of how drug–drug interactions can occur and how important monitoring for these reactions is for the health professionals.

▸ *Advanced-Generation BCR-ABL TKIs*

Advanced generation BCR-ABL TKIs were developed in an effort to overcome the resistance or intolerance to imatinib. These agents are more potent than imatinib and can overcome most BCR-ABL mutations that lead to imatinib resistance. Dasatinib and nilotinib are second-generation TKI that share the same binding site on the BCR-ABL cluster region as imatinib but maintains activity despite imatinib resistance, with higher potency than imatinib. Dasatinib also inhibits SRC kinases, which are tyrosine kinases that mediate cellular differentiation, proliferation, and survival. Dasatinib and nilotinib are used front line in the treatment of CML and in CML with resistance or intolerance to imatinib. Side effects of dasatinib and nilotinib are similar to imatinib and include myelosuppression, nausea and vomiting, headache, fluid retention, and hypocalcemia. Pleural effusions have been reported with dasatinib and imatinib but not with nilotinib. QT prolongation can occur with dasatinib and nilotinib. Abnormalities in indirect bilirubin have been reported with nilotinib.

Nilotinib is a competitive inhibitor of UGT1A1 in vitro, which could increase the concentrations of nilotinib. In a pharmacogenetic analysis, patients with (TA)7/(TA)7 genotype (UGT1A1*28) had a statistically significant increase in bilirubin over other genotypes.[39] Nilotinib should be administered on an empty stomach or 2 hours after a meal.

Bosutinib is indicated for the second-line treatment of CML in cases of resistance or intolerance to prior TKI therapy. With the exception of *T315I*, Bosutinib overcomes most BCR-ABL domain mutations. Gastrointestinal disturbances and rash are common. Bosutinib appears to have a milder side effect profile than other TKIs.

Ponatinib is a third-generation multikinase inhibitor and the only advanced generation TKI that overcomes the *T315I* mutation. Serious adverse effects reported included thrombosis, hepatotoxicity (rare) and death (rare). These are included as black-box warnings. Less serious adverse effects include abdominal pain, dry skin, and rash.

▸ *Ibrutinib and Idelalisib*

Two small molecule inhibitors that target the B-cell receptor pathway have been recently approved. Ibrutinib inhibits Bruton tyrosine kinase and has shown activity in mantle cell lymphoma and CLL. Idelalisib, in combination with rituximab, is approved for relapsed CLL and targets phosphatidylinositol-3-kinase (PI3-K), an essential lipid kinase. Adverse effects associated with these agents are GI disturbances, rash, hematological side effects, fatigue and musculoskeletal pain. Idelalisib has hepatotoxicity, colitis, pneumonitis, and intestinal perforation as black-box warnings.

▸ *Epidermal Growth Factor Receptor Pathway Inibitors (Erlotinib, Afatinib, and Lapatinib)*

Patients with malignancies (eg, non-small cell lung cancer or NSCLC) in which the tumors have mutations in exon 19 and/or 21 in the epidermal growth factor receptor (EGFR) pathway will likely respond to EGFR tyrosine kinase inhibitors such as erlotinib. These agents are believed to inhibit the intracellular phosphorylation of the EGFR. Erlotinib is about 60% absorbed after oral administration. Food increases bioavailability to almost 100%, but this is variable, and experts recommend administering erlotinib on an empty stomach. Erlotinib is eliminated predominately by CYP3A4. Smoking increases the clearance of erlotinib by 24%, which may result in treatment failure.[40] Erlotinib is used in the treatment of NSCLC and cancer of the pancreas. Side effects include interstitial lung disease, rash, diarrhea, anorexia, pruritus, conjunctivitis, and dry skin. Again, significant drug interactions have been documented with CYP3A4 inducers and inhibitors.

Afatinib is an oral, selective EGFR-TKI approved for the treatment of metastatic NSCLC in patients with EGFR exon 19 deletions or exon 21 (L858R) substitution mutations. It is taken on an empty stomach at a dose of 40 mg orally once daily. Adverse effects are similar to those reported with erlotinib.

Lapatinib inhibits the intracellular kinase domains of both EGFR and HER-2 and has been shown to retain activity against breast cancer cells that have become resistant to trastuzumab. Lapatinib is indicated for the treatment of patients with breast cancer whose tumors overexpress HER-2. When used in combination with capecitabine, the adverse effects of lapatinib include decreased left ventricular ejection fraction and QT prolongation, diarrhea, dyspepsia, rash, and hepatotoxicity. When not used as a doublet with capecitabine, the cardiac events and adverse effects were not as common.

▶ *Multikinase Inhibitors (Sorafenib, Sunitinib, Pazopanib)*

Sorafenib is a multikinase inhibitor that inhibits both intracellular and extracellular kinases to decrease renal cell cancer proliferation. Sorafenib is metabolized primarily by the liver by CYP3A4. Sorafenib is used for the treatment of renal cell cancer. The primary side effects of sorafenib include rash, hand–foot skin reaction, diarrhea, pruritus, and elevations in serum lipase.

Sunitinib blocks several tyrosine kinases, including platelet-derived growth factor, VEGF receptor, stem cell factor receptor, fms-like receptor growth factor, colony-stimulating growth factor receptor type 1, and glial cell line–derived neurotrophic factor receptor. The active metabolite of sunitinib blocks these same enzymes with similar potency. Significant side effects include left ventricular dysfunction, hemorrhage, asthenia, hypertension, nausea and vomiting, and diarrhea. Approximately one-third of patients may develop a yellow color of the skin along with dryness and cracking of the skin. Also, hair may become depigmented with doses of 50 mg/day or more; the depigmentation is reversible when therapy is stopped. Clinically significant drug interactions exist with inducers and inhibitors of CYP3A4; ketoconazole has been shown to increase concentrations of sunitinib, whereas rifampin has been shown to decrease concentrations of sunitinib.

Pazopanib is a vascular epidermal growth factor receptor (VEGFR) TKI that acts at VEGFR-1, VEGFR-2, and VEGFR-3. It is specifically indicated for the treatment of patients with advanced renal cell carcinoma. Pazopanib is metabolized through CYP3A4; therefore, drug–drug interactions should be monitored. Pazopanib is an orally administered agent that should be taken on an empty stomach. Common adverse effects include diarrhea, hypertension, hair color change, nausea and vomiting, fatigue, and anorexia. Serious toxicities that have been observed are increased in liver enzymes and bilirubin, including fatal hepatotoxicity, prolonged QT intervals and torsades de pointes, hemorrhagic events, arterial thrombotic events, gastrointestinal perforation, and proteinuria.

▶ *Regorafenib*

Regorafenib is a small molecule inhibitor of multiple membrane-bound and intracellular kinases. It is approved for the treatment of metastatic colorectal cancer in patients who have been previously received fluoropyrimidine-, oxaliplatin-, and irinotecan-based chemotherapy, anti-VEGF therapy, and an anti-EGFR therapy if KRAS wild-type. The proposed mechanism of action is through inhibition of vascular endothelial receptors involved in angiogenesis. It was recently approved for the treatment of gastrointestinal stromal tumor that had been previously treated with imatinib mesylate and sunitinib malate. GI effects, hypertension, mucositis, infection, rash, and fever are commonly occurring adverse effects. Hepatoxicity is listed as a black-box warning; therefore hepatic function should be monitored closely. It is an orally administered agent given for the first 21 days per 28-day cycle and should be taken with a low-fat breakfast.

▶ *Vemurafenib, Trametinib, Dabrafenib*

Vemurafenib is a potent inhibitor of mutated *BRAF* and is indicated for the treatment of unresectable or metastatic melanoma in patients with documented *BRAFV600E* mutation as determined by an FDA-approved test. Vemurafenib produced improved rates of overall and progression-free survival in a phase III trial when compared with dacabarazine. Vemurafenib is not indicated for patients with wild-type *BRAF*. The orally administered vemurafenib is dosed at 960 mg twice daily without regards to meals. Common adverse effects include arthralgia, rash, fatigue, alopecia, keratoacanthoma or squamous cell cancer, photosensitivity, nausea, and diarrhea. Approximately 40% of patients require dosage modifications because of adverse effects.[41]

Trametinib is a reversible inhibitor of mitogen-activated extracellular kinases (MEK)-1 and MEK-2 that is also active against *BRAF V600*-mutated forms of BRAF kinases in melanoma cells. It is indicated as monotherapy and in combination with dabrafenib for unresectable or metastatic malignant melanoma. It is not indicated in patients previously treated with a BRAF inhibitor. Rash, diarrhea, and lymphedema were commonly reported. Cardiomyopathy (defined as heart failure) and bleeding have also been reported.

Dabrafenib is a kinase inhibitor that has activity against BRAF kinases. It is indicated for the treatment of unresectable or metastatic malignant melanoma as monotherapy in patients with *BRAF V600E* mutation or in combination with trametinib in patients with *BRAF V600E* or V600K mutations. Adverse effects associated with this agent include arthralgias, alopecia, headache, palmar-plantar erythrodysesthesia syndrome, elevated liver enzymes, pyrexia, and papilloma.

▶ *Crizotinib and Ceritinib*

Crizotinib is a small-molecule inhibitor of the anaplastic lymphoma kinase gene (ALK) and mesenchymal epithelial transition growth factor (*c-MET*). This orally available agent is approved for the treatment of locally advanced or metastatic NSCLC that is ALK positive (about 2%–7% of NSCLC patients) as detected by an FDA-approved test. Adverse effects reported include mild gastrointestinal symptoms, edema, and visual disturbances, which have been described as trails of light following objects as they move.[42] Ceritinib is newly approved for ALK-positive NSCLC patients who have progressed on or are intolerant to crizotinib. Ceritinib, which has shown to be 20 times more potent than crizotinib in enzymatic assays, primarily targets ALK along with additional targets, including insulin-like growth factor 1 (IFG-1) receptor, insulin receptor (InsR), and ROS1. In comparison with crizotinib, ceritinib does not inhibit the kinase activity of c-MET. GI toxicities and elevated liver function tests were the most common adverse reactions. Visual changes, pulmonary disease, and QT prolongation were also seen in clinical trials.

▸ *Vandetanib*

Vandetanib is an orally available receptor TKI that blocks both the VEGF and EGF receptor kinase. This agent is indicated for the treatment of symptomatic or progressive medullary thyroid cancer in patients with unresectable locally advanced or metastatic disease. Common adverse effects include diarrhea, rash, acne, nausea, hypertension, headache, fatigue, decreased appetite, and abdominal pain.

Hormonal Therapies

A patient's hormonal receptor status (eg, estrogen and progesterone receptor status) can be used clinically as a prognostic indicator and can help predict a response to hormonal therapy. Hormonal or endocrine therapies have shown activity in the treatment of cancers whose growth is affected by gonadal hormonal control. Hormonal treatments either block or decrease the production of endogenous hormones. You will learn more about these treatments and outcomes in chapters 89 and 91, including the breast and prostate cancer chapters.

▸ *Antiandrogens: Bicalutamide, Flutamide, and Nilutamide*

The antiandrogens block androgen receptors to inhibit the action of testosterone and dihydrotestosterone in prostate cancer cells. Unfortunately, prostate cancer cells may become hormone refractory.

Side effects common to these agents are hot flashes, gynecomastia, and decreased libido. Flutamide tends to be associated with more diarrhea and requires three times daily administration, whereas bicalutamide is dosed once daily. Nilutamide may cause interstitial pneumonia and is associated with the visual disturbance of delayed adaptation to darkness.

▸ *Pure Androgen Receptor Antagonist: Enzalutamide*

Enzalutamide is an androgen receptor (AR) antagonist that works by competitively inhibiting androgen binding to androgen receptors and by inhibiting androgen receptor nuclear translocation and coactivator recruitment of the ligand-receptor complex. This agent has shown to competitively inhibit androgen binding to androgen receptors and inhibit androgen receptor nuclear translocation and interaction with DNA. Enzalutamide is indicated for the treatment of metastatic castration-resistant prostate cancer. The oral dosage is 160 mg orally once daily. Adverse effects associated with the agents are musculoskeletal effects, hot flashes, diarrhea, peripheral edema, hypertension, infections, headache, spinal cord compression, and hematuria.

▸ *Luteinizing Hormone–Releasing Hormone Agonists: Goserelin and Leuprolide*

Initially, luteinizing hormone–releasing hormone (LHRH) agonists increase levels of luteinizing hormone and follicle-stimulating hormone, but testosterone and estrogen levels are decreased because of continuous negative-feedback inhibition. Major side effects are testicular atrophy, decreased libido, gynecomastia, and hot flashes. Goserelin is injected as a pellet under the skin, therefore, subcutaneous injection of lidocaine around the injection site before administration helps to decrease the pain associated with goserelin administration. Numerous dosage forms are available for leuprolide with varying strengths and dosing intervals. Antiandrogens may be administered during initial therapy to decrease symptoms of tumor flare (eg, bone pain and urinary tract obstruction).

▸ *Luteinizing Hormone–Releasing Hormone Antagonist: Degarelix*

Degarelix is a gonadotropin-releasing hormone (GnRH) receptor antagonist that works by binding reversibly to the pituitary GnRH receptors, thereby reducing the release of gonadotropins and consequently testosterone. Degarelix is indicated for the treatment of advanced prostate cancer. Adverse events include hot flashes, injection site reactions, and an increase in liver enzymes. An advantage of degarelix over LHRH agonists is the lack of the tumor flare.[43]

▸ *Abiraterone*

Abiraterone is an orally available androgen biosynthesis inhibitor that inhibits 17α-hydroxylase/C17,20-lyase (CYP17), which is expressed in testicular, adrenal, and prostatic tumor tissues. Abiraterone is indicated in combination with prednisone for the treatment of metastatic castration–resistant prostate cancer who has received prior chemotherapy containing docetaxel. Adverse effects include joint swelling, hypokalemia, edema, muscle discomfort, hot flashes, diarrhea, urinary tract infections, nocturia, urinary frequency, dyspepsia, cough, hypertension, and arrhythmia. The patient must be counseled to take the oral medication on an empty stomach because food increases absorption and results in adverse reactions.[44]

▸ *Aromatase Inhibitors*

There are three aromatase inhibitors (AI) currently available, anastrozole, letrozole, and exemestane. Anastrozole and letrozole are selective nonsteroidal aromatase inhibitor that lowers estrogen levels. Anastrozole is a standard adjuvant treatment of postmenopausal women with hormone-positive breast cancer. The length of therapy is usually 5 years; however, evidence exists that suggests a benefit of prolonged treatment in certain situations. Exemestane, a steroidal compound, is an irreversible aromatase inactivator that binds to the aromatase enzyme to block the production of estrogen from androgens. This difference in activity does not appear to translate into improved clinical outcomes when compared to other AI therapies. When compared to tamoxifen, there are less endometrial and uterine cancers, vaginal bleeding, and thrombosis with AI therapy. Common adverse effects associated with the AI therapy include hot flashes and arthralgias. Serious adverse effects include osteoporosis, skeletal-related events, and atherosclerotic cardiovascular disease. The AIs are used exclusively for postmenopausal women. More information on the pharmacology and clinical use of AI therapy can be found in Chapter 89.

▸ *Antiestrogens*

Antiestrogens bind to estrogen receptors and block the effect of estrogen on tissue. There are two classes of antiestrogens: selective estrogen-receptor modulators (SERMs, tamoxifen, raloxifene) and selective estrogen-receptor downregulators (SERDs, Fulvestrant). SERDs were developed in an effort to eliminate the unwanted estrogenic side effects from the SERMs. Tamoxifen is used for the treatment of estrogen receptor (ER) positive premenopausal or postmenopausal metastatic hormone receptor–positive breast cancer, as adjuvant and primary treatment of breast cancer, and in the prevention of breast cancer in high-risk women. It is associated with a significant decrease in disease recurrence and mortality. The agent has a beneficial effect on bone density and the lipid profile. Unwanted side effects include hot flashes, fluid retention, and mood swings. Thrombosis, endometrial and uterine cancer, corneal changes, and cataracts are harmful adverse effects that occur more frequently with this agent. Although uncommon, there is a disease/tumor flare which can occur during the initiation of therapy in metastatic breast cancer patients with bone metastases. Because tamoxifen is a substrate of CYP3A4, decreased tamoxifen levels have occurred with use of St. John's wort and rifampin. Tamoxifen is also a substrate for CYP450 2D6, and evidence suggests that those who are *CYP2D6*4/*4* may have a poorer response and more toxicity with tamoxifen.[45] Routine pharmacogenomics screening of these patients is not currently recommended. Significant drug interactions exist and drug–drug interactions affecting this enzyme should be avoided if possible.

Raloxifene is another SERM and is used for the treatment of osteoporosis in postmenopausal women and is the chemopreventative agent of choice for the prevention of breast cancer in high-risk women. When compared head to head with tamoxifen for breast cancer prevention, it was demonstrated to have equal efficacy with less toxicity. Raloxifene was not studied in premenopausal women; therefore, tamoxifen is still the preventative agent of choice in these women. Hot flashes, arthralgias, and peripheral edema occur frequently with raloxifene, but thrombosis and endometrial cancer is less common than with tamoxifen.

Fulvestrant is used as second-line treatment in hormone receptor–positive metastatic breast cancer, postmenopausal women with disease progression following antiestrogen therapy. Fulvestrant is given as a monthly intramuscular injection, which might be a deterrent to some patients.

Other antiestrogen agents that are used in the treatment of breast cancer include toremifene (SERM) and megestrol acetate. Megestrol acetate can cause fluid retention, hot flashes, vaginal bleeding and spotting, breast tenderness, and thrombosis.

ADMINISTRATION ISSUES

Extravasation

One issue of chemotherapy safety is extravasation. Antineoplastic agents that cause severe tissue damage when they escape from the vasculature are called vesicants. The tissue damage may be severe, with tissue sloughing and loss of mobility, depending on the area of extravasation. Patients need to be educated to notify the nurse immediately if there is any pain on administration. If extravasation of a vesicant occurs, the injection should be stopped and any fluid aspirated out of the injection site. The prevention, risk factors, signs and symptoms, causative agents, and treatment will be discussed thoroughly in Chapter 99.

Hypersensitivity Reactions

Hypersensitivity reactions of cancer treatments is problematic because of cross-reactivity between agents and the desire to continue active therapies against the cancer.[46] For documented immediate hypersensitivity reactions to a particular agent, further administration of the agent may be achieved through extensive premedication with H_1 and H_2 antihistamines and corticosteroids and through use of escalating doses of the offending agent given at doses of one-hundredth, one-tenth, and the balance of the dose (so the total dose administered is equivalent to the normally prescribed dose) administered over a much longer period of time. These treatments must be given in an environment where resuscitation is readily available in case of medical emergency.

Secondary Malignancies

Chemotherapy and radiation therapy treatments may cause cancers later in life; these are referred to as secondary cancers. The most common type of secondary cancer is myelodysplastic syndrome, or AML. The antineoplastic agents most commonly associated with secondary malignancies are alkylating agents, etoposide, teniposide, topoisomerase inhibitors, and anthracyclines. Although the risk for secondary cancers is extremely low, it must outweigh the risk of survival produced by treatment of the primary malignancy. Because secondary malignancies may not occur for several years after treatment, patients with relatively short-term survival owing to the primary malignancy should consider the more immediate benefits of chemotherapy. Radiation therapy rarely may cause solid tumors as secondary cancers decades after treatment. The most common example of radiation therapy–induced secondary malignancy is breast cancer, which rarely occurs after mantle field radiation therapy for Hodgkin disease.

CHEMOTHERAPY SAFETY

One of the first Institute of Medicine reports, the health arm of the National Academy of Sciences, starts out with a patient who died from an overdose of chemotherapy; the patient did not have an immediately life-threatening cancer, so her death was hastened by a medication error. Chemotherapy agents may cause harm to patients, health professionals, and the environment if not handled correctly.

KEY CONCEPT *Because of the risk of severe toxicities associated with many of the chemotherapy agents, safety precautions must be in place to prevent chemotherapy errors or accidental chemotherapy exposures of health professionals or patients.* The Oncology Nursing Society and the American Society of Health-System Pharmacists have information to assist in the safe handling of chemotherapy agents.[16] National, state, and local regulations regarding the safe disposal of chemotherapy agents and the equipment used to administer them need to be followed to protect the environment.

KEY CONCEPT *Each organization should have chemotherapy safety checks built into the prescribing, preparation and administration of chemotherapy.*[16] Dosing based on patient-specific information should be included on every order for chemotherapy, whether it is oral or parenteral. Many chemotherapy regimens are referred to by acronyms (eg, AC, which is doxorubicin cyclophosphamide); these should not be allowed as the only reference to drugs in the prescribing of chemotherapy. Also, abbreviations for the names of chemotherapy agents should be avoided because one abbreviation may stand for two different drug entities. For drugs such as doxorubicin and liposomal doxorubicin, the names should be written out fully, and in this case, the addition of the brand name may help to prevent a mistake.

The measured height and weight, along with the body surface area (BSA), if applicable, should be readily available, along with the dosage in milligrams per meter squared or kilogram, so that the dosage may be checked. If a chemotherapy regimen is a continuous infusion of 800 mg/m^2/day for 4 days, an added safety feature would be to include the total dosage of 3200 mg in order to prevent any ambiguity. In cases where the clinician wants to decrease the dosage based on a laboratory value or side effect, it

Table 88–7

Empiric Dose Modifications in Patients with Renal Dysfunction

Agent	Organ Dysfunction	Dose Modification
Bleomycin	CrCl = 30–60 mL/min (0.50–1.0 mL/s)	25%–50% decrease
	CrCl = 10–30 mL/min (0.17–0.50 mL/s)	25%–50% decrease
	CrCl < 10 mL/min (0.17 mL/s)	50% decrease
Bosutinib	CrCl < 30 ml/min (0.50 mL/s)	Decrease dose to 300 mg daily
Capecitabine	CrCl = 30–50 mL/min (0.50–0.83 mL/s)	25% decrease
	CrCl < 30 mL/min (0.50 mL/s)	Do not use
Carboplatin	Renal insufficiency	Total Dose = AUC × (CrCl [in mL/min] + 25)
Cisplatin	CrCl < 50 mL/min (0.83 mL/s)	Decrease dose by 50%
Crizotinib	CrCl < 30 ml/min (0.50 mL/s)	Use with caution. Decrease dose to 250 mg daily
Cyclophosphamide	Renal failure	Decrease dose 25%
Eribulin	CrCl 30–60 ml/min(0.50–1.00 mL/s)	Decrease dose to 1.1 mg/m^2
	CrCl < 30 ml/min (0.50 mL/s)	Do not use
Etoposide	CrCl: 15–50 mL/min (0.25–0.83 mL/s)	Decrease dose 25%
Fludarabine, hydroxyurea	CrCl < 60 mL/min (1.00 mL/s)	Decrease dose in proportion to CrCl
Ifosfamide	CrCl = 10–50 mL/min (0.17–0.83 mL/s)	Decrease dose 25%
	CrCl = < 10 mL/min (0.17 mL/s)	Decrease dose 50%
Lenalidomide	CrCl < 60 ml/min (1.00 mL/s)	Dose modification varies depending on diagnosis
Methotrexate[a]	80 mL/min (1.33 mL/s)	Full dose
	80 mL/min (1.33 mL/s)	75%
	60 mL/min (1.00 mL/s)	63%
	50 mL/min (0.83 mL/s)	56%
	< 50 mL/min (0.83 mL/s)	Use alternative chemotherapy
Pentostatin	Renal insufficiency	Dose in proportion to CrCl
Pomalidomide	Serum Creatinine ≥ 3.0 mg/dL (265 μmol/L)	Do not use
Streptozocin	Renal Failure	Decrease dose 50%–75%
Topotecan	CrCl 20–39 mL/min (0.33–0.65 mL/s)	Decrease dose 50%
	CrCl < 20 ml/min (0.33 mL/s)	Do not use
Vandetanib	CrCl < 50 ml/min (0.83 mL/s)	Decrease dose 200 mg daily

[a]Monitor levels closely in all patients receiving high-dose therapy (eg, 150 mg/m^2 or greater).

is recommended that the clinician include that information with the order so that everyone understands what the correct dosage is for that patient. Chemotherapy dosages should be checked for route and dose to determine that the dosages prescribed are correct according to the regimen and do not exceed dosing guidelines. Appropriate laboratory values should be checked to verify that dosages are correct for any organ dysfunction present, and drug interactions should be scrutinized closely (Tables 88–7 and 88–8). Health professionals administering chemotherapy should check the dosage calculation for the patient's weight or BSA along with the five Rs of administering medication (ie, right patient, right medication, right dose, and right route, at the right time). If there is any question about the safe dosage or safe administration of a chemotherapy agent, the chemotherapy should not be administered until the question is resolved.

An area of controversy with chemotherapy dosing: What weight should be used for patients who are morbidly obese currently? Based on clinical practice guidelines published by the American Society of Clinical Oncology, it is recommended that clinicians routinely use an obese patient's actual body weight, instead of an ideal body weight or other measurement.

ORAL CHEMOTHERAPY

KEY CONCEPT *Over the past decade, self-administration of oral chemotherapy has increased because of the availability of oral, novel anticancer agents. Although oral chemotherapy has many advantages, such as convenience for the patient, potential increase in quality of life, and decreased treatment-associated costs, it also comes with an increased risk of medication errors, less monitoring of adverse effects and drug, dietary supplements, OTC medication and/or food interactions and accidental exposure to other individuals.* Health professionals have an important role in ensuring safe handling of oral anticancer agents, and should be properly trained and perform competently within guidelines for the storage, handling, and disposal of oral agents. The health professionals are also expected to provide proper training and education on safe handling and proper administration (See Table 88-9) for the patient and caregivers.[47]

CANCER SURVIVORSHIP

KEY CONCEPT *As early detection of cancers and effective therapies have improved over the last several years, the number of cancer survivors has increased. A cancer survivor by definition, according to the National Coalition for Cancer Survivorship, starts at the point of diagnosis. It is estimated that two out of every three people with cancer live at least 5 years after diagnosis.* In 2005, the Institute of Medicine (IOM) released a report, "From Cancer Patient to Cancer Survivor: Lost in Transition," which emphasized that a lack of definitive guidance in this area and identified that increased efforts were needed to raising awareness. In addition to facing a risk of a cancer recurrence, secondary malignancy, and an increased risk of developing other health

Table 88–8

Empiric Dose Modifications for Patients with Hepatic Dysfunction

Abiraterone acetate	Child-Pugh Class B	Decrease dose to 250 mg daily
	Child-Pugh Class C	Do not give
Anthracyclines	Bilirubin 1.2–3.0 mg/dL (20.5–51.3 μmol/L)	Decrease dose 50%
	Bilirubin 3.1–5.0 mg/dL (53.0–85.5 μmol/L)	Decrease dose 75%
	Bilirubin > 5.0 mg/dL (85.5 μmol/L)	Do not give
Axitinib	Child-Pugh Class A	No modification needed
	Child-Pugh Class B	Decrease dose 50%
	Child-Pugh Class C	Has not been studied
Bosutinib	Any baseline hepatic impairment	Decrease dose 200 mg daily
Cabozantinib	Moderate/severe hepatic impairment	Do not give
Carfilzomib	ALT/AST ≥ 3 × ULN and Bilirubin ≥ 2 × ULN	Do not give
Crizotinib	Bilirubin > 1.5 × ULN or AST/ALT > 2.5 × ULN	Use caution
Docetaxel	Bilirubin greater than ULN	Do not give
	AST or ALT > 1.5 ULN and Alk Phos > 2.5 ULN	Do not give
Eribulin	Child-Pugh A	Decrease dose to 1.1 mg/m^2
	Child-Pugh B	Decrease dose to 0.7 mg/m^2
Etoposide	Bilirubin 1.5–3.0 mg/dL (25.7– 51.3 μmol/L)	Decrease dose 50%
	Bilirubin 3.1–5.0 mg/dL (53.0– 85.5 μmol/L)	Do not give
Everolimus	Child-Pugh Class A	Decrease dose to 7.5 mg daily
	Child-Pugh Class B	Decrease dose to 5 mg daily
	Child-Pugh Class C	Decrease dose to 2.5 mg daily
Imatinib	Bilirubin greater than 3 × ULN	Withhold until less than 1.5 ULN
Ixabepilone	As a monotherapy agent if AST or ALT greater than 10 × ULN or bilirubin greater than 3 × ULN	Contraindicated
	In combination with capecitabine AST or ALT greater than 2.5 × ULN or bilirubin greater than 1 × ULN	
Lapatinib	Child–Pugh class C hepatic dysfunction	Dose reduction to 750 mg/day
Paclitaxel	Use with caution in hepatic failure	
Albumin-bound paclitaxel (Abraxane)	Bilirubin > 1.26 × ULN and elevated AST level	Dose modifications recommended (varies by diagnosis)
	Bilirubin > 5 × ULN or SGOT (AST) level > 10 × ULN	Do not give
Pazopanib	Bilirubin > 1.5–3 × ULN	Decrease to 200 mg daily
	Bilirubin > 3 × ULN	Do not give
Pomalidomide	Bilirubin > 2.0 mg/dL (34.2 μmol/L) and AST/ALT greater than 3.0 × ULN	Do not give
Ponatinib	Any baseline hepatic dysfunction (Child-Pugh Class A, B, or C)	Decrease dose 30 mg daily
Thiotepa	Use with caution in hepatic failure	
Vandetanib	Moderate-Severe hepatic impairment	Do not give
Vinblastine, vincristine	Bilirubin 1.5–3.0 mg/dL (25.7–51.3 μmol/L)	Decrease dose 50%
	Bilirubin 3.1–5.0 mg/dL (53.0–85.5 μmol/L)	Do not give
Vinorelbine	Bilirubin 2.1–3.0 mg/dL (35.9–51.3 μmol/L)	Decrease dose 50%
	Bilirubin > 3 mg/dL (51.3 μmol/L)	Decrease dose 75%

ULN, upper limit of normal.

Patient Encounter 3

A 63-year-old woman with a stage IV NSCLC (adenocarcinoma) and a mutation in exon 19 of the EGFR gene presents to the clinic. She will be receiving a new prescription for afatanib 40 mg orally, once daily.

What education and training should be provided to the patient to ensure their understanding of safe handling procedures as well as thorough knowledge of proper administration?

How should the patient be instructed to take this medication, in regards to meals or the time of day?

What adverse reactions would require that a holding treatment or a dose modification be made in therapy?

conditions, cancer survivors often face physical, emotional, financial, and social challenges as a result of the cancer diagnosis and treatment.[48] Agencies such as the American Cancer Society (ACS), National Cancer Institute (NCI), Centers for Disease Control (CDC), and American Society of Clinical Oncology (ASCO) are implementing strategies to meet the needs of these individuals who experience the long-term effects of cancer and its treatment.

OUTCOME EVALUATION

Once a pathologic diagnosis of cancer is made, the patient may be evaluated by a radiation oncologist, a surgical oncologist, and a medical oncologist. Options for treatment are presented that may include surgery, radiation, chemotherapy biotherapy, or some combination of these modalities. The goals of treatment vary by the cancer and the stage of disease. For example, the

Table 88–9

Oral Chemotherapy Administration with Respect to Food

	With Food	Empty Stomach	With or without Food
Abiraterone		X	
Afatinib		X	
Anastrozole			X
Axitinib			X
Bexarotene	X		
Bicalutamide			X
Bosutinib	X		
Cabozantinib		X	
Capecitabine	X		
Ceritinib		X	
Crizotinib			X
Dabrafenib		X	
Dasatinib			X
Enzalutamide			X
Erlotinib		X	
Estramustine			X
Etoposide			X
Everolimus			X
Exemestane	X		
Ibrutinib			X
Idelalisib			X
Imatinib	X		
Lapatinib		X	
Lenalidomide			X
Letrozole			X
Nilotinib		X	
Nilutamide			X
Pazopanib		X	
Pomalidomide		X	
Ponatinib			X
Regorafenib	X(low-fat meal)		
Sorafenib		X	
Sunitinib			X
Tamoxifen			X
Temozolomide		X	
Thalidomide			X
Toremifene			X
Trametinib		X	
Vandetanib			X
Vemurafenib			X
Vismodegib			X
Vorinostat	X		

patient who has metastatic kidney cancer could be presented with several options. They may have a possible cure with high-dose aldesleukin or receive palliative therapy with sorafenib or sunitinib, or the patient may decline any therapy because of fears of significant toxicity that would decrease quality of life. In this case, if the patient's performance status is poor, such as an ECOG performance status 3, then the patient would not be a candidate for aldesleukin therapy because of significant toxicity or even death from treatment. The patient with the poor performance status will receive palliative therapy to control symptoms of the disease to improve the quality of life at the end of life. For the patient with a poor performance status and extensive metastatic disease, no treatment of the cancer may be appropriate, and the patient may be enrolled in a hospice program or provided comfort care.

Patient Care Process

Patient Assessment:

- Based on workup, confirm cancer diagnosis and stage of disease before initiating anticancer treatment.
- Determine treatment goals (ie, cure) considering type of cancer, stage of disease, patient characteristics (eg, age, performance status, etc).
- Review the medical history. Does the patient have any special population precautions (eg, pregnancy, breastfeeding, dialysis, renal/hepatic dysfunction, pharmacogenomic information, etc) or specific concerns that would change your approach with standard of care treatments?
- Ensure that weight and height is accurate and recent. Calculate the BSA (if applicable). Determine if actual, ideal, or adjusted weights are to be used, based on treatment goals and discussion with health care team.
- Check patient laboratory values, physical assessment and any other work-up to ensure that the CBC and organ function studies are normal or within acceptable limits before administering chemotherapy. Does the patient need a measure of ejection fraction or a chest x-ray, for example? Does the patient need a central line (if receiving a vesicant)?
- Conduct a medication history (including prescriptions, OTC medications, herbals and dietary supplements) and nutrition history. Identify any possible drug–drug or drug–food interactions. Does the patient have any allergies or previous treatment with an anticancer agent? For example, has a patient received an anthracycline in the past?

Therapy Evaluation:

- Evaluate the chemotherapy regimen to ensure the correct dose and route of administration.
- If a patient has hematologic, renal or hepatic, or other toxicities, recommend adjustments in chemotherapy and/or doses if necessary.
- Ensure appropriate antiemetic therapy, hydration, and ancillary medications (antihistamines, steroids, folate, anti-infectives, etc) along with any rescue medications (leucovorin, mesna, etc) are ordered for patient.
- Assess the regimen to determine if primary prophylaxis with colony-stimulating factors is needed.

Care Plan Development

- Counsel patient and caregivers on the treatment plan, short- and long-term adverse effects, precautions, supportive care plans.
- Use safe handling and disposal methods.
- For oral chemotherapy, provide specific recommendations to patients and caregivers to ensure their understanding of safe handling procedures as well as thorough knowledge of proper administration of the medication.

Follow-up Evaluation:

- Monitor CT scans or other imaging studies, and categorize patient with a CR, PR, SD, or progressive disease.
- Monitor CBC, renal function, liver function, and other laboratory or diagnostic tests as needed.
- Monitor patient for other known toxicities of the chemotherapy regimen and hold or modify the dose or discontinue the regimen if necessary.
- Ensure that cancer survivorship needs are being met.

Abbreviations Introduced in This Chapter

2-FLAA	2-Fluoro-Ara-AMP
5-FU	Fluorouracil
6-MP	6-Mercaptopurine
6-TG	6-Thioguanine
ADC	Antibody–drug conjugate
AI	Aromatase inhibitor
ALK	Anaplastic lymphoma kinase gene
ALL	Acute lymphocytic leukemia
AML	Acute myeloid leukemia
APL	Acute promyelocytic leukemia
Ara-C	Cytarabine
ASCT	Autologous stem cell transplant
ATRA	All-trans-retinoic acid
AUC	Area under the-curve
c-MET	Mesenchymal epithelial transition growth factor
CD	Cluster of differentiation
CLL	Chronic lymphocytic leukemia
CML	Chronic myeloid leukemia
CTC	Common toxicity criteria
CTLA-4	Cytotoxic T-lymphocytic-associated antigen 4
ECOG	Eastern Cooperative Oncology Group
EGFR	Epidermal growth factor receptor
ER	Estrogen receptor
FdUMP	Fluorodeoxyuridine monophosphate
GIST	Gastrointestinal stromal tumor
GnRH	Gonadotropin-releasing hormone receptor
HER-2	Human epidermal receptor-2
HPV	Human papillomavirus
IL	Interleukin
LHRH	Luteinizing hormone releasing hormone
MEK	Mitogen-activated extracellular kinases
MM	Multiple myeloma
MMAE	Monomethyl auristatin E
mTOR	Mammalian target of rapamycin
NCI	National Cancer Institute
NSCLC	Non–small cell lung cancer
PCR	Polymerase chain reaction
PEG	Polyethylene glycol
PSA	Prostate specific antigen
SERDs	Selective estrogen-receptor downregulators
SERMs	Selective estrogen receptor modulator
TKI	Tyrosine kinase inhibitor
TNM	Tumor, nodes, metastases
TPMT	Thiopurine *S*-methyltransferase
TS	Thymidylate synthase
VEGF	Vascular epidermal growth factor
VEGFR	Vascular epidermal growth factor receptor

REFERENCES

1. Jemal A, Murray T, Ward E, et al. Cancer Statistics, 2005. CA Cancer J Clin. 2005;55(1):10–30.
2. American Cancer Society. *Cancer Facts & Figures 2014*. [Internet]. Atlanta: American Cancer Society; 2014 [cited 2014 Aug 15]. http://www.cancer.org/research/cancerfactsfigures/index. Accessed August 15, 2014.
3. Sessions J, Valgus J, Barbour S, Iacovelli L. Role of Oncology clinical pharmacists in light of the oncology workforce study. J Oncol Pract. 2010;6(5):270–272.
4. Schottenfeld D, Searle JG. The etiology and epidemiology of lung cancer. In: Pass HI, Carbone DP, Johnson DH, Minna JD, Turrisi AT, eds. Lung Cancer: Principles and Practice, 3rd ed. Philadelphia: Lippincott, Williams & Wilkins; 2005:3–24.
5. Blagosklonny MV. Molecular theory of cancer. Cancer Biol Ther. 2005;4(6):621–627.
6. Buick RN. Cellular basis of chemotherapy. In: Dorr RT, Von Hoff DD, eds. Cancer Chemotherapy Handbook, 2nd ed. New York: Elsevier, 1994:3–14.
7. Folkman J. Angiogenesis. Annu Rev Med. 2006;57:1–18.
8. Mountford CE, Doran S, Lean CL, Russell P. Cancer pathology in the year 2000. Biophys Chem. 1997;68(1–3):127.
9. Chang S, Harshman L, Presti J. Impact of common medications on serum total prostate-specific antigen levels: Analysis of the National Health and Nutrition Examination Survey. J Clin Oncol. 2010;28(5):3951–3957.
10. Eisenhauer E, Therasse P, Bogaerts J, et al. New response evaluation criteria in solid tumours: Revised RECIST guideline (version 1.1). Eur J Cancer. 2009;45:228–247.
11. Innocenti F, Schilsky RL, Ramirez J, et al. Dose-finding and pharmacokinetic study to optimize the dosing of irinotecan according to the UGT1A1 genotype of patients with cancer. J Clin Oncol. 2014;32(22):2328–2334.
12. Baydar M, Dikilitas M, Sevinc A, Aydogdu I. Prevention of oral mucositis due to 5-fluorouracil treatment with oral cryotherapy. J Natl Med Assoc. 2005;97(5):1161–1164.
13. Baker J, Royer G, Weiss R. Cytarabine and neurological toxicity. J Clin Oncol. 1991;9(4):679–693.
14. Kantarjian H, Gandhi V, Cortes J, et al. Phase 2 clinical and pharmacologic study of clofarabine in patients with refractory or relapsed acute leukemia. Blood. 2003;1202:2379–2386.
15. Villela LR, Stanford BL, Shah SR. Pemetrexed, a novel antifolate therapeutic alternative for cancer chemotherapy. Pharmacotherapy. 2006;26(5):641–654.
16. American Society of Health-System Pharmacists. ASHP guidelines on preventing medication errors with antineoplastic agents. Am J Health Syst Pharm. 2002;59:1648–1668.
17. Sparreboom A, Scripture CD, Trieu V, et al. Comparative preclinical and clinical pharmacokinetics of a Cremophor-free, nanoparticle albumin-bound paclitaxel (ABI-007) and paclitaxel formulated in Cremophor (Taxol). Clin Cancer Res. 2005;11(11):4136–4143.
18. Cortes J, O'Shaughnessy J, Loesch D, et al. Eribulin monotherapy versus treatment of physician's choice in patients with metastatic breast cancer (EMBRACE): A phase 3 open-label randomised study. Lancet. 2011;377(9769):914–923.
19. Ormrod D, Holm K, Goa K, Spencer C. Epirubicin: A review of its efficacy as adjuvant therapy and in the treatment of metastatic disease in breast cancer. Drugs Aging. 1999;5:389–416.
20. Hensley M, Hagerty K, Kewalramani T, et al. American Society of Clinical Oncology clinical practice guideline update: Use of chemotherapy and radiation therapy protectants. J Clin Oncol. 2009;27(1):127–145.
21. Faulds D, Balfour JA, Chrisp P, Langtry HD. Mitoxantrone: A review of its pharmacodynamic and pharmacokinetic properties, and therapeutic potential in the chemotherapy of cancer. Drugs. 1991;41(3):400–449.
22. Rudek MA, Donehower RC, Statkevich P, et al. Temozolomide in patients with advanced cancer: Phase I and pharmacokinetic study. Pharmacotherapy. 2004;24(1):16–25.
23. Calvert AH, Newell DR, Gumbrell LA, et al. Carboplatin dosage: Prospective evaluation of a simple formula based on renal function. J Clin Oncol. 1989;7(11):1748–1756.
24. Graham MA, Lockwood GF, Greenshade D, et al. Clinical pharmacokinetics of oxaliplatin: A critical review. Clin Cancer Res. 2000;6:1205–1218.
25. Dorr RT. Bleomycin pharmacology: Mechanism of action and resistance, and clinical pharmacokinetics. Semin Oncol. 1992;19(2 suppl 5):3–8.

26. Zhi-Xiang S, Chen, G, Ni J, et al. Use of arsenic trioxide in the treatment of acute promyelocytic leukemia: II. Clinical efficacy and pharmacokinetics in relapsed patients. Blood. 1997; 89(9):3354–3360.
27. Avvisati G, Tallman MS. All-trans retinoic acid in acute promyelocytic leukaemia. Best Pract Res Clin Haematol. 2003;16(3):419–432.
28. Wohl DA, Aweeka FT, Schmitz J, et al. Safety, tolerability, and pharmacokinetic effects of thalidomide in patients infected with human immunodeficiency virus: AIDS clinical trials group 267. J Infect Dis. 2002;185:1359–1363.
29. Chen N, Lau H, Kong L, et al. Pharmacokinetics of lenalidomide in subjects with various degrees of renal impairment and in subjects on hemodialysis. J Clin Pharmacol. 2007;47:1466–1475.
30. Dokmanovic M, Clarke C, Marks P. Histone deacetylase inhibitors: Overview and perspectives. Mol Cancer Res. 2007;5:981–989.
31. Bouwhuis MG, Suciu S, Testori A, et al. Phase III trial comparing adjuvant treatment with pegylated interferon alfa-2b versus observation: Prognostic significance of autoantibodies—EORTC 18991. J Clin Oncol. 2010;28(14):2460–2466.
32. Kantoff P, Higano C, Shore N, et al. Sipuleucel-T immunotherapy for castration-resistant prostate cancer. N Eng J Med. 2010; 363(5):411–422.
33. Adcetris (Brentuximab) package insert. Bothell, WA: Seattle Genetics, 2011.
34. Leyland-Jones B, Gelman K, Ayoub J, et al. Pharmacokinetics, safety, and efficacy of trastuzumab administered every three weeks in combination with paclitaxel. J Clin Oncol. 2003;21: 3965–3971.
35. Bolton AE, Peng B, Hubert M, et al. Effect of rifampicin on the pharmacokinetics of imatinib mesylate in healthy subjects. Cancer Chemother Pharmacol. 2004;53(2):102–106.
36. Frye RF, Fitzgerald SM, Lagattuta TF, et al. Effect of St. John's Wort on imatinib mesylate pharmacokinetics. Clin Pharmacol Ther. 2004;76(4):323–329.
37. Dutreix C, Peng B, Mehring G, et al. Pharmacokinetic interaction between ketoconazole and imatinib mesylate in healthy subjects. Cancer Chemother Pharmacol. 2004;54(4):290–294.
38. O'Brien SG, Meinhardt P, Bond E, et al. Effects of imatinib mesylate on the pharmacokinetics of simvastatin, a cytochrome p450 3A4 substrate, in patients with chronic myeloid leukaemia. Br J Cancer. 2003;89(3):1855–1859.
39. Singer JB, Shou Y, Giles F, et al. UGT1A1 promoter polymorphism increases risk of nilotinib-induced hyperbilirubinemia. Leukemia. 2007;21(11):2311–2315.
40. Hamilton M, Wolf JL, Rusk J, et al. Effects of smoking on the pharmacokinetics of erlotinib. Clin Cancer Res. 2006;12: 2166–2171.
41. Chapman PB, Hauschild A, Robert C, et al. Improved survival with vemurafenib in melanoma with BRAF V600e mutation. N Eng J Med. 2011;264(26):2507–2516.
42. Kwak EL, Bang YJ, Carnidge DR, et al. Anaplastic lymphoma kinase inhibition in non-small cell lung cancer. N Eng J Med. 2010;363(18):1693–1703.
43. Firmagon (Degarelix) package insert. Parsippany, NJ: Ferring Pharmaceuticals, 2009.
44. Bono JS, Logothetis CJ, Molina A, et al. Abiraterone and increased survival in metastatic prostate cancer. N Eng J Med. 2011;364(21):1995–2005.
45. Goetz MP, Knox SK, Suman VJ, et al. The impact of cytochrome P450 2D6 metabolism in women receiving adjuvant tamoxifen. Breast Cancer Res Treat. 2007;101:113–121.
46. Gonzalez ID, Saez RS, Rodilla EM, Yges EL, Toledano FL. Hypersensitivity reactions to chemotherapy drugs. Allerg Immunol Clin. 2000;15:151–181.
47. Goodin S, Griffith N, Chen B, et al. Safe handling of oral chemotherapeutic agents in clinical practice: Reommendations form an international pharmacy panel. J Oncol Pract. 2011;7(1): 7–12.
48. Hewitt M, Greenfield S, Stovall E. From Cancer Patient to Cancer Survivor: Lost in Transition. Washington DC: National Academies Press; 2006.

89 Breast Cancer

Gerald Higa

LEARNING OBJECTIVES

Upon completion of the chapter, the reader will be able to:

1. Explain the relative importance of various risk factors.
2. Summarize the features of the four intrinsic breast cancer subtypes.
3. Articulate some of the reasons for improved patient survival.
4. Recognize signs and symptoms related to early and late stages of the disease.
5. Distinguish between good and poor prognostic factors.
6. Describe the roles of hormone and HER2 receptors.
7. Determine treatment goals for early stage, locally advanced, and metastatic breast cancers.
8. State the rationale for inclusion of adjuvant and neoadjuvant therapies.
9. Discuss the benefits and risks associated with various endocrine therapies.
10. List relevant factors that guide management and treatment of early and metastatic breast cancers.

INTRODUCTION

Two breast cancer trends, the modest decline in new diagnoses and improvement of 5-year survival rates, have continued over the past decade. One factor that could be associated with both the former and latter findings is screening. The link to screening is plausible as detection of more patients with non-invasive (ie, in situ) disease could impact the number of new invasive breast cancer cases, while diagnosis of early-stage disease should translate to improved overall survival.

EPIDEMIOLOGY AND ETIOLOGY

Breast cancer is the most common type of cancer and second only to lung cancer as a cause of cancer death in American women. In 2015, female breast cancer will account for 99% of the projected 235,000 new cases; the median age at diagnosis will be 61 years; and approximately 40,000 deaths will occur as a result of the disease.[1] KEY CONCEPT Even *though the disease occurs more frequently in white women than any other ethnic group, the mortality rate is highest among African Americans.*

Tumor size of most breast cancers at diagnosis is usually small (less than 2 cm); and early-stage disease predominates in all racial and ethnic groups. However, African American women have proportionally more cases of advanced disease compared with white women. It has been suggested that reduced access to proper medical care, including breast cancer screening programs, as well as certain biological factors, contribute to late diagnoses.

KEY CONCEPT *The etiology of breast cancer remains largely unknown though a number of factors have been associated with risk of developing the disease. Evidence also strongly suggests that breast cancer biology involves very complex interactions between sex hormones, genetic factors, environment, and lifestyle.* The intrinsic and extrinsic components associated with the disease are discussed further.

Intrinsic Components

KEY CONCEPT *Aside from gender, the variable most strongly associated with breast cancer is age as disease risk and incidence increase with age.* One of the most frequently quoted breast cancer statistic is the probability that one in eight will develop the disease. However, a more instructive way of explaining the age-related factor is shown in Table 89–1. Although the probability of developing breast cancer increases with age, more than half the risk occurs after 60 years of age.

Both personal and family history can influence the risk of developing breast cancer. For example, a woman who has a history of breast cancer has a fivefold increase in risk of developing contralateral breast cancer. Prior histories of cancers involving the uterus and ovary also appear to be associated with an increased risk of developing breast cancer. Breast tissue with atypical changes appears to be a premalignant lesion. Even though family history is often linked to disease risk, the percentage of familial breast cancer, in reality, is quite low (ie, ~10%). KEY CONCEPT *Nonetheless, clarification of several key elements related to family history includes findings that:*

- A first-degree relative (ie, mother or sister) with breast cancer is associated with a 3-fold increase in risk.
- A first-degree relative diagnosed with breast cancer younger than 45 years is associated with a more than threefold increase in risk.

Table 89–1

Risk of Developing Breast Cancer: SEER Areas, Women, All Races, 2008 to 2010

Age Interval (years)	Probability (%) of Developing Invasive Breast Cancer during the Interval
30–40	0.44 or 1 in 227
40–50	1.45 or 1 in 69
50–60	2.31 or 1 in 43
60–70	3.49 or 1 in 29
From birth to death	12.15 or 1 in 8

SEER, Surveillance, Epidemiology and End Results.

Probability derived by Devcan 6.7.0, June 2013 (http://surveillance.cancer.gov/devcan).

- Multiple first-degree relatives with breast cancer have not been consistently shown to be associated with risk greater than one first-degree relative.
- A second-degree relative with breast cancer is associated with 1.5-fold increase in risk.
- Family members on the paternal side contribute to risk similar to the maternal side.

KEY CONCEPT *A number of endocrine factors have been linked to an increased risk for breast cancer.* Many of the risks relate to the total duration of estrogen exposure. Hence, early menarche (before age 12 years) and late menopause (after age 55 years) are associated with an increased risk of the disease. Support for this association is the finding that bilateral oophorectomy before age 35 years decreases the relative risk of developing breast cancer. Nulliparity and late age at first birth (30 years or older) have been reported to double the lifetime risk of developing breast cancer.

Long-term use of hormone replacement therapy and concurrent use of progestins appear to contribute to breast cancer risk. Use of postmenopausal estrogen replacement therapy in women with a history of breast cancer is generally contraindicated. However, most experts believe that the safety and benefits of low-dose oral contraceptives currently outweigh the potential risks and that changes in the prescribing practice for the use of oral contraceptives are not warranted. Moreover, oral contraceptives are known to reduce the risk of ovarian cancer by about 40% and the risk of endometrial cancer by about 60%.

KEY CONCEPT *In the early 1990s, the BRCA1 gene (locus 17q21) was found to be mutated in a large percentage of hereditary breast and ovarian cancer patients. A second breast cancer gene, called BRCA2, has been mapped to chromosome 13.* Since *BRCA1* and *BRCA2* are tumor suppressor genes, mutations or functional aberrations result in loss of key inhibitory activities of both proteins.[2] Compelling evidence of their critical importance is the observation that women who carry germline mutations of *BRCA1* are at high risk for breast and ovarian cancers (85% and 60% over their lifetimes, respectively). Carriers of the *BRCA2* mutation have similar risks for breast cancer but much lower risks for ovarian cancer. Jewish people of Eastern European descent (Ashkenazi Jews) have an unusually high (2.5%) carrier rate of germline mutations in *BRCA1* and *BRCA2* compared with the rest of the US population. Women with strong family histories of breast cancer are candidates for *BRCA1* and *BRCA2* mutation analysis. If performed, genetic testing should be done under the guidance of a professional genetic counselor.

Extrinsic Components

KEY CONCEPT *Experimental and epidemiologic evidence suggest an association between breast cancer and a diet high in calories, fat, and cooked meats. Obesity in postmenopausal women and distribution of body fat around the abdominal region also appear to increase the risk of breast cancer.* This risk factor may be related, in part, to peripheral conversion of androgens to estrogens in adipose tissue. More dramatic evidence of the negative impact of obesity was presented at the 2014 meeting of American Society of Clinical Oncology (ASCO). In a large-scale analysis investigators reported that among premenopausal women with early-stage, ER positive breast cancer, obesity raised the risk of dying by 34% compared with the other breast cancer patients. Evidence also indicates a modest ingestion-dependent relationship between alcohol and breast cancer. While exercise may have a modest protective effect against breast cancer, neither cigarette smoking nor breast augmentation appears to modify disease risk

Radiation is also associated with an increased risk of breast cancer. Even though the risk appears to be dosage-related, the minimal level of exposure is not well defined. Overt environmental exposure such as that which occurred in survivors of the atomic bomb is associated with an increased risk. However, even radiation exposure during therapeutic management of patients with postpartum mastitis, tuberculosis, and certain hematologic malignancies appears to increase breast cancer risk. Interestingly, this risk appears to be confined to exposure before 40 years of age, which suggests that a "window of initiation" for breast cancer occurs relatively early. On the other hand, it is currently accepted that exposure to radiation doses utilized in diagnostic x-rays, including screening mammography, are not of clinical concern.

Despite what is known to confer risk, the majority of women diagnosed with breast cancer do not have any of the identified factors (other than age). A number of calculators now accessible through the Internet can be used to estimate breast cancer risk. The National Cancer Institute (NCI) has an online version of the Breast Cancer Risk Assessment Tool that is considered to be the most authoritative and accurate (www.cancer.gov/bcrisk-tool). This tool was designed for health professionals to project individualized 5-year and lifetime risks for invasive breast cancer.

Prevention of Breast Cancer

Even though breast cancer is not the most lethal malignancy, disease-related morbidity and mortality is still significant. Current efforts at breast cancer prevention are directed toward the identification and removal of risk factors. Unfortunately, a number of risk factors such as age, family or personal history of the disease or other gynecologic malignancies cannot be modified.

The idea that prevention can be achieved pharmacologically is based on clinical trials of tamoxifen, an antiestrogen used as **adjuvant therapy** for certain women with early breast cancer. These trials demonstrated a reduction of contralateral breast cancer events as well as a survival advantage in this subset of patients who received the drug for 2 to 5 years following mastectomy.[3] Several clinical trials conducted with this antiestrogen provided proof of principle that breast cancer risk reduction could be achieved through chemoprevention.[4,5] A meta-analysis of these trials indicated a consistent (and significant) benefit in reducing the risk of developing estrogen receptor (ER) positive breast cancers in premenopausal and postmenopausal women.

Results of these trials also confirmed the carcinogenic and thrombogenic effects of tamoxifen. Unfortunately, the increased

Patient Encounter, Part 1

A 45-year-old woman who is part owner of a local dry cleaning business comes to clinic. Except for hypertension (controlled with lisinopril + hydrochlorothiazide) and being slightly overweight, she has been in good health. She is happily married with two grown children in college. She has one paternal aunt who died from breast cancer. There is no other breast or gynecologic cancer history in the family. On routine self-examination, she detected a very small lump in her left breast. No other breast changes were noted. Although she had screening mammography nearly a year ago which was officially read as normal, she is still very concerned and makes an appointment to see her personal physician as soon as possible. The following week her doctor also notes the abnormality on clinical examination and orders a mammogram.

Compile a list of considerations integral to screening programs.

Explain why the currently ordered mammogram is not a screening mammogram.

incidence of endometrial cancers and thrombotic events had a negative impact on both patient acceptance and physician willingness to prescribe tamoxifen in this setting. However, studies with another antiestrogen known as raloxifene demonstrated that this agent not only reduced spinal fractures in postmenopausal women, but also decreased the incidence of breast cancer without adversely affecting the endometrium. The latter finding led to a head-to-head clinical study of tamoxifen and raloxifene (STAR), which involved postmenopausal women considered to be at increased risk for developing breast cancer.[6] Although the reduction in the incidence of breast cancer was similar, raloxifene had a superior safety profile with regards to cancer and thromboembolic events. Thus, raloxifene is considered the chemopreventive agent of choice for high-risk postmenopausal women. Because premenopausal women were not included in the STAR trial, tamoxifen is the only agent approved for reducing the risk of breast cancer in young women.

Despite these important findings, the role of tamoxifen in *BRCA* mutation carriers is still not clear. Surgical prophylaxis for these individuals includes bilateral mastectomy or oophorectomy at completion of childbearing. Importantly, the risk of developing breast and ovarian cancer following prophylactic surgery is significantly, but not absolutely, reduced. For those foregoing elective surgical options semiannual mammograms are recommended.

The impressive data of the aromatase inhibitors (AIs) in the adjuvant setting provided the impetus for studying their potential as breast cancer chemopreventive agents. The steroidal AI, exemestane, has been reported to be more effective than placebo in reducing the risk of breast cancer in high risk postmenopausal women.[7] Although exemestane has not been compared directly with either tamoxifen or raloxifene, the superior results of AIs compared to tamoxifen in the adjuvant setting suggest that the AIs could outperform the antiestrogens in reducing breast cancer risk with lower endometrial and thrombotic events.

PATHOPHYSIOLOGY

Histologic evaluation of breast lesions serves to establish a pathologic diagnosis and confirm the presence or absence of other factors believed to influence prognosis. These **prognostic factors** are discussed later.

Invasive Breast Cancer

Breast cancer typically arises in the ducts or lobules of the mammary gland. When tumor cells infiltrate surrounding breast tissue, a diagnosis of invasive breast cancer is made. Even though the vast majority of tumors are adenocarcinomas, this does not imply that breast cancer is one disease. *Substantial progress has been made to further refine the way four intrinsic subtypes of breast cancer are classified. When defined by clinical and pathological features, the classification system also provides a guide to treatment (Table 89–2).*

Noninvasive Carcinoma

The annual breast cancer incidence does not include thousands of cases of carcinomas in situ (ie, noninfiltrating tumors confined to the ducts and lobules). Ductal carcinoma in situ (DCIS) accounts for approximately 85% of all in situ breast cancers;

Table 89–2

Intrinsic Subtypes of Breast Cancer

Subtype	Tumor Features	Treatment Approach	Added Comment
Luminal A	All of the following: ER and PR positive, HER2 negative, and low Ki-67 (proliferation marker)	Endocrine only (usually)	May add chemotherapy if 4 or more positive nodes, grade 3 disease, Oncotype Dx recurrence score higher than 25, or age younger than 35 years
Luminal B (HER2 negative)	ER positive, HER2 negative, and either high Ki-67 or PR negative	Endocrine	Add chemotherapy for most patients
Luminal B (HER2 positive)	ER positive, HER2 positive	Endocrine, HER2 targeted therapy and chemotherapy	
HER2 amplified or overexpressed (nonluminal)	HER2 positive	HER2 targeted and chemotherapy	Opinion differs regarding use of anti-HER2 therapy in tumors
Basal (triple-negative)	ER, PR, and HER2 negative	Chemotherapy only	Less than 5 mm

Adapted with permission from Oxford University Press. The original source for this material Annals of Oncology 2013; 24:2206–2223.

Patient Encounter, Part 2

The repeat mammogram shows a calcified area approximately 2.1 cm in diameter suspicious for cancer. A core biopsy of the lesion is performed and pathology confirms a diagnosis of infiltrating intraductal carcinoma. Tumor samples indicated the absence of ER and PR, but overexpressed HER2 (3+ by IHC). The axillary nodes were negative by clinical examination. **Staging** workup indicated no evidence of distant disease. Surgical options were discussed with the patient. She desired BCS with sentinel node biopsy. Pathologic examination of the sentinel node was positive for tumor.

Explain why the breast cancer is considered early-stage disease.

Classify the intrinsic subtype of this breast cancer.

Describe the treatment goal and management strategy for this patient's breast cancer.

Appraise the patient's overall prognosis.

while lobular carcinoma in situ (LCIS) may not be a true cancer, but rather a high-risk premalignant lesion. The overwhelming majority of cases can be cured by surgery alone. Although there is no proven role for the application of cytotoxic chemotherapy, patients with **hormone receptor-positive** tumors may benefit from the addition of tamoxifen.[8]

CLINICAL PRESENTATION AND DIAGNOSIS

Early Detection

The rationale for early detection of breast cancer is based on the clear relationship between early stage disease at diagnosis and greater probability of long-term survival. Thus, patients with tumors less than 2 cm and negative lymph nodes have a higher likelihood of being cured. KEY CONCEPT *Screening guidelines for early detection of breast cancer have been put forward by the American Cancer Society, the United States Preventive Services Task Force (USPSTF), and the NCI (Table 89–3).* All include recommendations for women at average risk, with some general statements regarding screening for high-risk women as well. Nearly 80% of all breast cancers occur in women 50 years of age or older, and regular use of screening mammography can reduce mortality from breast cancer by 20% to 40% in this age group. Controversy regarding the use of screening mammography is largely confined to women younger than 50 years. After many years of debate, three organizations recommended mammograms in this age group of women every 1 to 2 years except for the USPSTF, which modified its recommendation in 2009.[9]

Clinical Presentation and Diagnosis of Breast Cancer

Common early signs and symptoms include:

Painless lump (90% of cases) that is:

- Solitary
- Unilateral
- Solid
- Hard
- Irregular
- Nontender

Stabbing or aching pain (10% of cases) as the first symptom

Uncommon early signs and symptoms include:

Nipple discharge (3% of women and 20% of men), retraction, or dimpling

- Eczema appearance of the nipple (Paget carcinoma)
- Prominent skin edema, redness, warmth, and induration of the underlying tissue (inflammatory carcinoma)

Metastatic signs and symptoms—tissues most commonly involved with metastases are lymph nodes (other than axillary or internal mammary), skin, bone, liver, lungs, and brain. The following symptoms of metastases will be present in about 10% of patients when they first seek treatment:

- Bone pain
- Difficulty breathing
- Abdominal enlargement
- Jaundice
- Mental status changes

Diagnosis

Unless following up on abnormalities found during screening, the initial workup for women presenting with signs or symptoms (see Clinical Presentation and Diagnosis) suggestive of breast cancer should include a careful history, physical examination of the breast, three-dimensional mammography, and possibly other imaging techniques such as magnetic resonance imaging. Most (80%–85%) breast cancers are visualized on a mammogram as a

Table 89–3

Guidelines for Early Detection of Breast Cancer in Average Risk Individuals

	American Cancer Society	U.S. Preventive Services Task Force	National Cancer Institute
BSE	Age ≥ 20 years: Risk-to-benefit discussion	NR	NR
CBE	Age 20–30 years: Every 3 years Age ≥ 40 years: Every year	Not specifically addressed	All ages: Every year
Mammography	Annual beginning at age 40 years	Age 50–74 years: Every 2 years (with or without CBE)	Age 40–49: Every 1–2 years Age ≥ 50 years: Every 1–2 years

BSE, breast self-examination; CBE, clinical breast examination; NR, not recommended.

Table 89–4

Estimated Stage at Presentation and 5-Year Disease-Free Survival (DFS): Breast Cancer

	Percentage of Total Cases	5-Year DFS[a] (%)
Stage I	40	70–90
Stage II	40	50–70
Stage III	15	20–30
Stage IV	5	0–10[b]

[a] With current conventional local and systemic therapy.

[b]Patients in stage IV are rarely free of disease; however, 10% to 20% of these patients may survive with minimal disease for 5 to 10 years.

mass, a cluster of calcifications, or a combination of both. A breast biopsy is indicated for a mammographic abnormality that suggests malignancy or for a palpable mass on physical examination.

Clinical Staging

Stage is determined by primary tumor size (T), axillary lymph node involvement (N), and presence or absence of distant metastases (M). See Table 88–2 for an example of TMN staging. Aside from carcinoma in situ (stage 0) multiple combinations of T and N are possible within a given stage. Simplistically, stage I disease is represented by tumors less than 2 cm in diameter and usually no lymph node involvement. KEY CONCEPT *Stage I and II disease is referred to as early breast cancer, which carries a relatively good prognosis and correlates with the highest probability of cure (Table 89–4).* Stage III, or locally advanced breast cancer, has poorer disease features, including larger tumor size, positive node involvement, and tumor invasion of the chest wall. Stage IV disease is characterized by the presence of metastases (M_1) to organs or tissue distant from the primary tumor and is often referred to as advanced or metastatic breast cancer.

Prognostic Factors

Prognostic factors are biological or clinical indicators associated with survival independent of therapy. Poor prognostic factors for breast cancer include:

- Age younger than 35 years
- Large tumor size
- High nuclear grade (correlates with tumor growth)
- Lymph node involvement
- Triple-negative disease (ie, absence of ER, PR, and HER2 receptors)
- Overexpression of HER2 alone

EARLY BREAST CANCER

TREATMENT

Desired Outcome

KEY CONCEPT *Most patients presenting with invasive breast cancer today have small tumors with negative lymph nodes (stage I), or a stage II cancer. The goal of therapy for early breast cancer is cure.* While surgery alone may be able to cure approximately one-third to one-half of all patients with early stage breast cancer, certain tumor features warrant addition of systemic therapy.

Patient Encounter, Part 3

Two years after this patient's initial diagnosis, routine follow-up chest x-ray showed two 3-cm nodules in the right upper lobe of the lung. Pulmonary consultants perform a transbronchial lung biopsy of one lung lesion. Pathologic examination reveals recurrent breast cancer. Tumor tissue indicates the same receptor pattern. Imaging of the chest, abdomen, and pelvis is negative for other sites of metastasis.

Formulate a list of clinical factors that should be considered when deciding on therapy.

Conclude what treatment would be appropriate at this time.

Local-Regional Therapy

Surgical procedures have changed drastically over the past 50 years. KEY CONCEPT *Less aggressive surgical options for early invasive breast cancer include total mastectomy and breast conserving surgery (BCS) such as lumpectomy.* The reason for favoring the latter is based on findings that BCS achieves similar survival outcomes as more extensive surgical procedures and is cosmetically superior.[10] Additionally, breast conservation aids in preserving the emotional and psychological well-being of the patient.[11] Only two contraindications to BSC considered absolute (or nearly absolute) include persistence of tumor on surgical margins and inability to perform postsurgery radiation, if indicated.

KEY CONCEPT *Equally important is the issue related to complete axillary lymph node dissection (CALND). Because of the morbidity associated with the procedure, clinical trials were conducted to determine when biopsy of the sentinel lymph nodes was sufficient.* Results of these studies indicated that CALND can be avoided in patients with microscopic disease in the sentinel nodes as well as in patients undergoing BCS with postsurgery radiation to the breast.[12,13]

Except for the elderly and patients with substantial comorbid medical conditions, radiation therapy is an integral adjunct to BCS. However, radiation therapy should also be considered in certain postmastectomy situations, especially in patients with more than three positive nodes or patients with positive sentinel nodes without CALND. What used to entail 4 to 6 weeks of external-beam radiation, newer clinical evidence supports the efficacy of a shorter 3-week course of whole breast irradiation.[14] Complications associated with radiation therapy are usually minor and include erythema of the breast tissue and shrinkage of total breast mass beyond that predicted on the basis of surgical resection alone.

Systemic Adjuvant Therapy

Breast cancer cells can spread by contiguity, lymphatic channels, and blood to distant sites. Tumor cells often metastasize early in cancer growth. Because these deposits cannot be detected with current diagnostic techniques, they are referred to as micrometastases. Systemic adjuvant therapy is treatment that follows definitive local therapy when there is no evidence of disease beyond the axillary nodes but a high likelihood of disease recurrence. Hence, administration of systemic therapy (at a time when the tumor burden is low) should theoretically increase the likelihood of cure and minimize the emergence of drug-resistant tumor cell clones. KEY CONCEPT *Most published results confirm that chemotherapy (in selected patients), hormonal therapy (in patients with hormone receptor–positive disease), anti-HER2 therapy (in tumors with amplification or overexpression of HER2) or appropriate combinations of these therapies improved disease-free survival* (DFS) *and/or overall survival (OS) in patients with early-stage breast cancer (see Table 89–2).*

Among the most influential groups that provide treatment recommendations is the St. Gallen International Expert Consensus panel. Convened every 2 years to review new evidence related to therapies for early breast cancer, the most recent conference was held in 2013.[15] In the 2 years since their previous meeting, additional evidence has emerged to support the various types of systemic therapies (see Table 89–2).

▶ *Adjuvant Chemotherapy*

Cytotoxic drugs that have been used most frequently as adjuvant therapy of breast cancer include cyclophosphamide, anthracyclines, taxanes, methotrexate, and fluorouracil. The most common chemotherapy regimens used in the adjuvant setting are listed in Table 89–5. Dose-limiting and other significant toxicities have been previously described in Chapter 88 and are discussed in Table 89–6.

Chemotherapy is usually initiated within 3 weeks of the surgical procedure. Traditionally, treatment consisted of four to six cycles; and completed in less than 6 months. Dose reduction for standard chemotherapy regimens should be avoided in the absence of severe acute toxicity because of the negative impact on DFS and OS.[16] Even though most patients are able to maintain a reasonable level of functional, emotional, and social well-being during treatment, there are some compelling data indicating that some toxicities can have chronic debilitating effects on quality of life.[17] Various forms of supportive therapy including antiemetics and hematopoietic growth factors for patients receiving systemic adjuvant chemotherapy are discussed in Chapter 99.

As mentioned previously, the usefulness of the intrinsic subtype classification also extends to treatment strategies (see Table 89–2). Since the magnitude of the 10-year survival benefit with cytotoxic agents appears to be only 5% and 10% for patients with negative and positive nodes, respectively, there has been intensive research to identify patients with low-risk disease that could avoid treatment with chemotherapy. One validated multigene assay known as Oncotype DX is used to identify patients with luminal A disease, regardless of nodal involvement, who can be treated with endocrine therapy alone.[18]

KEY CONCEPT *It is generally agreed that patients with luminal B, HER2-positive, and basal-like subtypes should receive*

Table 89–5

Common Chemotherapy Regimens for Breast Cancer

Adjuvant Chemotherapy Regimens

AC
Doxorubicin 60 mg/m^2 IV, day 1
Cyclophosphamide 600 mg/m^2 IV, day 1
Repeat cycles every 21 days for four cycles[a]

FAC[w]
Fluorouracil 500 mg/m^2 IV, days 1 and 4
Doxorubicin 50 mg/m^2 IV continuous infusion over 72 hours[w]
Cyclophosphamide 500 mg/m^2 IV, day 1
Repeat cycles every 21–28 days for six cycles[c]

CAF
Cyclophosphamide 600 mg/m^2 IV, day 1
Doxorubicin 60 mg/m^2 IV bolus, day 1
Fluorouracil 600 mg/m^2 IV, day 1
Repeat cycles every 21–28 days for six cycles[e]

FEC
Fluorouracil 500 mg/m^2 IV, day 1
Epirubicin 100 mg/m^2 IV bolus, day 1
Cyclophosphamide 500 mg/m^2 IV, day 1
Repeat cycle every 21 days for six cycles[g]

CEF
Cyclophosphamide 75 mg/m^2 orally on days 1–14
Epirubicin 60 mg/m^2 IV, days 1 and 8
Fluorouracil 500 mg/m^2 IV, days 1 and 8
Repeat cycles every 28 days for six cycles (requires prophylactic antibiotics or growth factor support)[i,j]

AC → Paclitaxel (CALGB 9344)
Doxorubicin 60 mg/m^2 IV, day 1
Cyclophosphamide 600 mg/m^2 IV, day 1
Repeat cycles every 21 days for four cycles
Paclitaxel 175 mg/m^2 on day 1

TAC (BCIRG 001)
Docetaxel 75 mg/m^2 IV, day 1
Doxorubicin 50 mg/m^2 IV bolus, day 1
Cyclophosphamide 500 mg/m^2 IV, day 1
(doxorubicin should be given first)
Repeat cycles every 21–28 days for six cycles[d]

Paclitaxel→ FAC[f,w]
Paclitaxel 80 mg/m^2/week IV over 1 hour every week for 12 weeks
Followed by:
Fluorouracil 500 mg/m^2 IV, days 1 and 4
Doxorubicin 50 mg/m^2 IV continuous infusion over 72 hours
Cyclophosphamide 500 mg/m^2 IV, day 1
Repeat cycles every 21–28 days for four cycles[n]

CMF
Cyclophosphamide 100 mg/m^2/day orally, days 1–14
Methotrexate 40 mg/m^2 IV, days 1 and 8
Fluorouracil 600 mg/m^2 IV, days 1 and 8
Repeat cycles every 28 days for six cycles[h,j]
or
Cyclophosphamide 600 mg/m^2 IV, day 1
Methotrexate 40 mg/m^2 IV, day 1
Fluorouracil 600 mg/m^2 IV, days 1 and 8
Repeat cycles every 28 days for six cycles[i]

Dose-Dense AC → Paclitaxel
Doxorubicin 60 mg/m^2 IV bolus, day 1
Cyclophosphamide 600 mg/m^2 IV, day 1
Repeat cycles every 14 days for four cycles (must be given with growth factor support)
Followed by:
Paclitaxel 175 mg/m^2 IV over 3 hours
Repeat cycles every 14 days for four cycles (must be given with growth factor support)[k]
Followed by:
Paclitaxel 175 mg/m^2 IV over 3 hours
Repeat cycles every 21 days for four cycles[b]

(*Continued*)

Table 89–5

Common Chemotherapy Regimens for Breast Cancer (*Continued*)

Metastatic Single-Agent Chemotherapy	
Paclitaxel Paclitaxel 175 mg/m² IV over 3 hours Repeat cycles every 21 days *or* Paclitaxel 80 mg/m²/week IV over 1 hour Repeat dose every 7 days[m]	**Vinorelbine** Vinorelbine 30 mg/m² IV, days 1 and 8 Repeat cycles every 21 days or Vinorelbine 25–30 mg/m²/week IV Repeat cycles every 7 days (adjust dose based on absolute neutrophilcount; see product information)[n]

Metastatic Single-Agent Chemotherapy	
Docetaxel Docetaxel 60–100 mg/m² IV over 1 hour Repeat cycles every 21 days[o] *or* Docetaxel 30–35 mg/m²/week IV over 30 minutes Repeat dose every 7 days[p] **Capecitabine** Capecitabine 2000–2500 mg/m²/day orally, divided twice daily for 14 days Repeat cycles every 21 days[q,r] **Docetaxel + Capecitabine** Docetaxel 75 mg/m² IV over 1 hour, day 1 Capecitabine 2000–2500 mg/m²/day orally divided twice daily for 14 days Repeat cycles every 21 days[t] **Epirubicin + Docetaxel[x]** Epirubicin 70–90 mg/m² IV bolus Followed by: Docetaxel 70–90 mg/m² IV over 1 hour Repeat cycles every 21 days[v]	**Gemcitabine** Gemcitabine 600–1000 mg/m²/week IV, days 1, 8, and 15 Repeat cycles every 28 days (may need to hold day-15 dose based on blood counts)[q] **Liposomal Doxorubicin** Liposomal doxorubicin 30–50 mg/m² IV over 90 minutes Repeat cycles every 21–28 days[s] **Doxorubicin + Docetaxel[x]** Doxorubicin 50 mg/m² IV bolus, day 1 Followed by: Docetaxel 75 mg/m² IV over 1 hour, day 1 Repeat cycles every 21 days[u]

[a]From Fisher B, et al. J Clin Oncol 1990;8:1483. [b]From Henderson CI, et al. J Clin Oncol. 2003;21:976. [c]From Buzdar AU, et al. In: Salmon S, ed. Adjuvant Therapy of Cancer, VIII. Philadelphia, Lippincott-Raven, 1997:93–100. [d]From Martin, et al. San Antonio Breast Cancer Symposium 2003;A43. [e]From Wood WC, et al. N Engl J Med. 1994;330:1253. [f]From Martin M, et al. N Engl J Med 2005;325:2302. [g]From Green MC, et al. J Clin Oncol 2005;23:5983. [h]From Bonadonna G, et al. N Engl J Med. 1976;294:405. [i]From Fisher B, et al. N Engl J Med. 1989;32:473. [j]From Levine MN, et al. J Clin Oncol. 1998;16:2651. [k]From Citron, et al. J Clin Oncol. 2003;21;1431. [l]From Taxol (paclitaxel) product information. Bristol-Myers Squibb, April 2003. [m]From Perez EA, et al. Clin Oncol. 2001;19:4216. [n]From Zelek L. Cancer. 2001;92:2267. [o]From Taxotere (docetaxel) product information. Aventis Pharmaceuticals Inc., April 2003. [p]From Hainsworth JD, et al. J Clin Oncol. 1998;16:2164. [q]From Carmichael J, et al. J Clin Oncol. 1995;13:2731. [r]From Michaud, et al. Proc Am Soc Clin Oncol. 2000; A402, and Xeloda product information. [s]From Ranson MR, et al. J Clin Oncol. 1997;15:3185. [t]From O'Shaughnessy, et al. J Clin Oncol. 2002;20:2812. [u]From Nabholtz JM, et al. J Clin Oncol. 2003;21:968. [v]From Levin MN, et al. J Clin Oncol. 1998;16:2651. [w]FAC may also be given with bolus doxorubicin administration, and the fluorouracil dose is then given on days 1 and 8. [x]Paclitaxel may also be given concurrently with doxorubicin or epirubicin as a combination regimen. Pharmacokinetic interactions make these regimens more difficult to give.

IV, intravenous.

chemotherapy (both anthracycline and taxane) with hormonal and/or HER2-targeted therapy if indicated.[19]

▸ *Adjuvant Anti-HER2 Therapy*

HER-2 amplification or overexpression is found in approximately 15% to 20% of all breast cancers. Because of its aggressive features, trastuzumab (plus chemotherapy) is usually indicated in this subset of patients, especially for tumors greater than or equal to 0.5 cm in size. Most experts also agree that HER2-positive tumors appear to derive greater benefit from anthracycline or taxane-based chemotherapy regimens.[20] When used with these agents, trastuzumab is given either following completion of the anthracycline or concurrently with the taxane. Current evidence indicates that the duration of trastuzumab therapy is 12 months.[21]

▸ *Adjuvant Endocrine Therapy*

KEY CONCEPT *Hormone receptors are used clinically as indicators of prognosis, predictors of response to endocrine therapies, and more recently, discriminators of luminal breast cancer subtypes.* Estrogen and progesterone receptors (PR) are cytoplasmic proteins that bind to nuclear DNA and function as transcription factors. Approximately 50% to 70% of patients with primary and metastatic breast cancer have hormone receptor–positive tumors. However, receptor-positivity refers to tumors expressing both ER and PR, as well as either ER or PR alone. Furthermore,

Table 89–6

Toxicities of Common Chemotherapies Used for Breast Cancer

Class	Drug	Dose-Limiting Toxicities	Other Toxicities
Anthracyclines	Doxorubicin, epirubicin	Myelosuppression, cardiomyopathy	Alopecia, nausea, vomiting, stomatitis, ulceration, and necrosis with extravasation, red-colored urine, radiation-recall effect
	Liposomal doxorubicin	Myelosuppression, palmar-plantar erythrodysesthesia (hand–foot syndrome)	Alopecia, infusion reactions, stomatitis, fatigue, nausea, vomiting
Taxanes	Paclitaxel	Neutropenia, peripheral neuropathy, hypersensitivity reactions	Alopecia, fluid retention, myalgia, skin reactions, ulceration, and necrosis with extravasation, bradycardia, stomatitis
	Docetaxel	Myelosuppression, severe fluid retention	Alopecia, fatigue, stomatitis, nausea, vomiting, diarrhea, peripheral neuropathy, nail disorder, skin reactions, hypersensitivity reactions
Antimetabolites	Capecitabine	Diarrhea, palmar-plantar erythrodysesthesia (hand–foot syndrome)	Myelosuppression, stomatitis, nausea, vomiting
	Gemcitabine	Myelosuppression (especially thrombocytopenia)	Flulike syndrome (fever, chills, myalgias, and arthralgias), nausea
	Fluorouracil	Myelosuppression	Stomatitis, diarrhea, alopecia
	Methotrexate	Myelosuppression, stomatitis	Diarrhea, nausea, vomiting, renal toxicity
Vinca alkaloids	Vinorelbine	Neutropenia	Fatigue, nausea, vomiting, ulceration, and necrosis with extravasation
Alkylating agents	Cyclophosphamide	Myelosuppression, hemorrhagic cystitis	Alopecia, stomatitis, amenorrhea, aspermia

"ER positive" tumors traditionally refer to ERα only. Although it is beyond the scope of this discussion, it is noteworthy to mention the existence, and accumulating data regarding the roles of ERβ and the ERα/ERβ heterodimer in breast cancer.[22,23] Tumors with high expression of both ER and PR (ie, luminal A subtype) are associated with favorable prognoses, superior responses to endocrine therapy, and longer disease-free intervals following initial treatment. Hormone receptor–positive tumors are more common in postmenopausal patients. Many experts also believe that the premenopausal breast cancer is biologically more aggressive than breast cancers diagnosed after menopause.

KEY CONCEPT *Hormonal therapies that have been studied in the treatment of early breast cancer include selective estrogen receptor modulators (SERMs, tamoxifen), ovarian suppression (surgical and pharmacologic), and the aromatase inhibitors (AIs).*

Tamoxifen, has been used in the adjuvant setting for nearly four decades. Analysis of long-term data indicates the drug's antagonist (anti-estrogen) effect was associated with a significant reduction in disease recurrence and mortality. This observation, coupled with evidence of the drug's beneficial agonist activity on the lipid profile and bone density supported tamoxifen's role as standard endocrine therapy. However, the agonist properties are also associated with detrimental effects on endometrial tissue and blood coagulation.

In premenopausal women, tamoxifen alone is considered the adjuvant hormonal therapy of choice. Some disagreement exists among experts regarding the utility of combining ovarian function suppression with tamoxifen in women younger than 40 years. Tamoxifen is initiated shortly after surgery or as soon as pathology results are known. However, when chemotherapy is also indicated, tamoxifen is given after all cytotoxic agents have been completed. The rationale for sequential therapy is supported by some data which show a small negative effect on disease-free survival (DFS) when tamoxifen and chemotherapy are given concurrently.

Treatment with adjuvant tamoxifen (20 mg/day) has historically been for 5 years. However, results of a recent clinical trial indicate a survival benefit associated with extending therapy to a total of 10 years.[24] While these data are noteworthy, it should also be noted that the additional 5 years of treatment may not apply to all women. Other issues that make the longer duration of therapy less appealing relate to drug-related toxicities and medication compliance.

Other new evidence of note relates to women who were premenopausal when starting, and postmenopausal at completion, of tamoxifen therapy. In this subset of women, continuation of endocrine therapy with an aromatase inhibitor was associated with a significant improvement in breast cancer-related events, including new primaries in the contralateral breast, disease recurrence, and disease-free survival.[25] So compelling were the results, the clinical trial had to be stopped after a median follow-up of only 2.4 years.

Patient Encounter, Part 4

Four months after beginning treatment for the lung metastasis, repeat imaging indicates a complete response (ie, no radiographic evidence of disease) to therapy. However, the patient now states that she has been having more frequent headaches and some problems with balance. An MRI of the head shows several small ring-enhancing lesions in the cerebellum. Biopsy of one of the lesions indicates brain metastasis.

Explain your choice of therapy in this patient with brain only metastasis.

Patient Encounter, Part 5

Routine mammography in your patient, a 62-year-old grandmother indicates an area on the right breast that appears to be consistent with atypical changes but not highly suspicious for cancer. However, because of her family history (sister with breast cancer), a fine-needle aspirate of the breast tissue was obtained for histologic examination. Molecular markers show great promise as an adjunct to a tissue diagnosis of cancer. On the other hand, we must ensure that these tests are accurate indicators of malignant disease. Pathology used a new molecular test with modest sensitivity (ie, 80%) but very high specificity (ie, 99%) on the tissue sample to further analyze the radiographic abnormality. Although the test was negative, the tissue findings were consistent with atypical hyperplasia.

Summarize what would be appropriate to tell this 62-year-old woman regarding the needle aspirate findings.

Formulate a follow-up plan for this patient.

Finally, the issue regarding the role of pharmacogenomics in tailoring tamoxifen therapy is both persuasive and controversial.[26,27] As such, routine screening for germline variants of CYP2D6 has not been endorsed. Nonetheless, drugs that do inhibit the enzyme should be avoided if possible.

In postmenopausal women, the use of adjuvant AIs has been studied in three different ways: (a) direct comparison with tamoxifen, (b) after 5 years of tamoxifen therapy, and (c) sequentially after 2 to 3 years of tamoxifen.[28] Based on the positive results of several studies, expert panels strongly recommend AIs for postmenopausal women with hormone-dependent breast cancer.[29] Although 5 years of adjuvant AI therapy is considered standard, there is also strong support for continuing hormonal therapy (beyond 5 years) if tamoxifen was used initially, especially in patients with high-risk features such as node-positive disease. Further support of extended endocrine therapy that includes an AI has been noted previously.[25] While these recommendations can be applied to most postmenopausal patients, tamoxifen can still be used first line or as an alternative in those who do not tolerate AI therapy.

AI therapy is associated with several adverse effects, including hypercholesterolemia, atherosclerotic cardiovascular disease, and skeletal-related events. The three available AIs are anastrozole, letrozole, and exemestane (Table 89–7).

LOCALLY ADVANCED BREAST CANCER (STAGE III)

TREATMENT

Desired Outcome

Locally advanced breast cancer is defined by tumors greater than or equal to 5 cm and a high likelihood of nodal involvement in the absence of demonstrable distant metastasis. A wide variety of clinical scenarios can be seen within this group of patients, including tumors that have been neglected for a period of time and inflammatory breast cancer, which is a unique clinical entity. Inflammatory breast cancer has, at times, been misdiagnosed as cellulitis.

Treatment of stage III breast cancer consists of all modalities used in the management of early breast cancer. The goal of therapy is to achieve optimal systemic control of the disease. However, despite treatment, systemic relapse and death are common even when local-regional control is accomplished. One major difference related to the systemic therapies is the use of chemotherapy plus ant-HER2 therapy (if indicated) or hormonal therapy before surgery. This approach, referred to as **neoadjuvant therapy**, can render initially inoperable tumors resectable, even with the possibility of BCS. It is also conceivable that earlier administration of systemic therapy could have therapeutic benefits beyond surgical

Table 89–7

Endocrine Therapies Used for Metastatic Breast Cancer

Class	Drug	Dose	Side Effects
Aromatase inhibitors			
Nonsteroidal	Anastrozole	1 mg/day PO	Hot flashes, arthralgias, myalgias, headaches, diarrhea, mild nausea
	Letrozole	2.5 mg/day PO	
Steroidal	Exemestane	25 mg/day PO	
Antiestrogens			
SERMs	Tamoxifen	20 mg/day PO	Hot flashes, vaginal discharge, mild nausea, thromboembolism, endometrial cancer
	Toremifene	60 mg/day PO	
SERDs	Fulvestrant	250 mg IM every 28 days	Hot flashes, injection site reactions, possibly thromboembolism
LHRH analogues	Goserelin	3.6 mg SC every 28 days	Hot flashes, amenorrhea, menopausal symptoms, injection site reactions
	Leuprolide	7.5 mg IM every 28 days	
	Triptorelin	3.75 mg IM every 28 days	
Progestins	Megestrol acetate	40 mg PO 4 for a day	Weight gain, hot flashes, vaginal bleeding, edema, thromboembolism
	Medroxyprogesterone	400–1000 mg IM every week	
Androgens	Fluoxymesterone	10 mg PO twice a day	Deepening voice, alopecia, hirsutism, facial or truncal acne, fluid retention, menstrual irregularities, cholestatic jaundice

IM, intramuscular; LHRH, luteinizing hormone–releasing hormone; PO, oral; SC, subcutaneous; SERD, selective estrogen receptor downregulator; SERM, selective estrogen receptor modulator.

resection. Other potential advantages include in vivo assessment of treatment response, and an opportunity to evaluate the biologic effects of the systemic therapy. However, nodal status will not be assessable.

Pharmacologic Therapy

For patients with inoperable breast cancer, including inflammatory breast cancer, one of the treatment objectives is to obtain tumor resectability. The guidelines for selection and duration of systemic neoadjuvant chemotherapy are similar to the adjuvant setting. Available data support the use of anthracycline-containing regimens, incorporation of the taxanes, and approaches to improve dose-density or dose-intensity. Neoadjuvant endocrine therapy may be an option for patients who have unresectable, strongly hormone receptor–positive tumors, low risk factors, or are unable to receive chemotherapy because of comorbid medical conditions. When endocrine therapy is used, treatment is continued to maximal response. Even though not an approved indication, several clinical studies have demonstrated the efficacy of neoadjuvant trastuzumab in combination with chemotherapy in patients with HER2-overexpressing tumors. Interestingly, pertuzumab is the only HER2-targeted agent approved in the neoadjuvant setting when used in combination with trastuzumab and docetaxel. Regardless of therapeutic approach, about two-thirds of the tumors can be downstaged.

In terms of local therapy, the extent of surgery will be determined by tumor response to neoadjuvant therapy, patient wishes, and cosmetic results likely to be achieved. To minimize local recurrence, adjuvant radiation therapy should be administered to all patients with locally advanced breast cancer who undergo mastectomy or BCS. Inoperable tumors that are unresponsive to systemic chemotherapy may require radiation for local management; however, these tumors may be ineligible for subsequent surgical resection. This situation is associated with a very poor prognosis though not commonly seen.

METASTATIC BREAST CANCER (STAGE IV)

TREATMENT

Desired Outcome

KEY CONCEPT *The goals of therapy for patients with metastatic breast cancer are maintaining or improving quality of life and prolonging survival, if possible. In order to achieve these goals, an important consideration is selecting therapy with good activity and tolerability.*

General Approach to Treatment

KEY CONCEPT *The choice of therapy for metastatic disease is based on receptor expression status (ie, hormone and HER2) and distant disease sites. In many instances, age and comorbid medical problems will also be considered. While the choice between endocrine and cytotoxic chemotherapy is usually the hormone receptor status of the tumor, sites of metastatic disease may also influence treatment decisions.* For example, in patients with ER positive breast cancer with soft tissue or bone-only metastasis (without impending fracture), endocrine therapy alone is usually warranted. Hormonal therapy can even be considered in patients with asymptomatic visceral involvement. In contrast, chemotherapy is usually the initial treatment option for hormone-dependent breast cancer in patients who present with significant life-threatening metastasis to liver and/or lung. When used, chemotherapy is continued to maximal response. Patient encounters, part 6 and part 7 illustrate these concepts further. Patients with tumors responding initially to endocrine therapies are often treated with chemotherapy when endocrine options are exhausted or symptomatic visceral metastasis develops. Approximately 75% to 80% of tumors positive for both ER and PR respond to initial hormonal therapy; responses decrease to 50% to 60% for ER positive/PR negative tumors. The best predictor of response to second- and, possibly, third-line endocrine therapies is extent and duration of the initial response. Nevertheless, tumor responses are frequently lower and durations shorter with subsequent hormonal therapies.

> **Patient Encounter, Part 6**
>
> The patient missed her next two mammograms and returned to the clinic 30 months later than originally scheduled. Imaging studies performed at this time showed definite changes and an irregular lesion measuring 1.6 × 1.9 cm at its greatest diameters. Core biopsy of the mass lesion was interpreted by pathology as malignant adenocarcinoma of the breast. Further testing indicated an ER-positive/PR-negative, HER2-negative, well-differentiated tumor. Staging indicated several "hot spots" in the femur and pelvis consistent with metastatic disease. There is no tumor involvement of visceral organs, lungs, or brain.
>
> ***Outline the most appropriate way to manage this patient's breast cancer. Appraise the patient's overall prognosis.***

KEY CONCEPT *Endocrine therapy is not indicated for tumors that do not express at least one of the hormone receptors. Patients with receptor negative tumors should be treated with cytotoxic chemotherapy. Objective responses are achieved in 50% to 60% of patients who have not received prior chemotherapy though less than 20% of the responses are complete.* The duration of response to first-line therapy is usually less than 12 months. Although very uncommon, responses to initial treatment can be extremely durable with patients living years without evidence of disease. The response rate to second- and third-line chemotherapy varies from 20% to 40%. Combinations of different hormonal therapies or chemotherapy plus endocrine therapy are not used in the metastatic disease setting because of increased toxicity without added benefit.

In general, the duration of overall survival of patients with advanced breast cancer ranges between 14 and 33 months.

Pharmacologic Systemic Therapy

▶ *Endocrine Therapy*

The operative mode of all endocrine therapies is estrogen deprivation. The pharmacologic goals of treatment include decreasing the levels of circulating estrogen and/or preventing the effects of estrogen on tumor tissue through hormone receptor blockade or downregulating receptor expression. Achievement of these goals is independent of menopausal status. Many available endocrine therapies can accomplish these goals. Combined endocrine therapies also have been studied in an attempt to improve patient outcomes with negative results. As such, patients usually receive sequential endocrine therapies before chemotherapy is considered.

Until the turn of the century, evidence did not support the superiority of one type of endocrine therapy with regards to response or survival. Because of the similarity in efficacy, selection of endocrine therapy was based primarily on their toxicity prolife (see Table 89–7), which favored tamoxifen. The only exception to this choice of therapy occurred in patients who received adjuvant tamoxifen and subsequently developed metastatic disease within 1 year of drug cessation.

Over the past 15 years, accumulating evidence related to the AIs has changed the way postmenopausal women with hormone-dependent metastatic breast cancers are treated. After menopause, estrogens continue to be produced by extragonadal conversion of androstenedione and testosterone to estrone and estradiol. This biosynthetic process, which is dependent on aromatase, occurs in peripheral tissue, including muscle, adipose, and even the breast itself. Therefore, AIs effectively reduce the level of circulating estrogens, as well as estrogens in the target gland. Their toxicity profile has been described in Chapter 88 and Table 89-7. Anastrozole and letrozole are nonsteroidal compounds that competitively inhibit aromatase. Exemestane is a steroidal compound that binds irreversibly (by forming a covalent bond) to aromatase. However, this biochemical distinction does not translate into clinical superiority with exemestane.

The AIs are used as first-line therapy for ER-positive advanced breast cancer in postmenopausal women.[30] Large trials have compared these agents with tamoxifen and have found similar response rates and a longer median time to progression for patients receiving the selective AIs. A consistent observation in these trials was a lower incidence of thromboembolic events, endometrial cancer, and vaginal bleeding in patients treated with an AI. Collectively, these findings led to the recommendation that AI therapy be used as first-line therapy for advanced breast cancer in postmenopausal women. Of note also, several small studies indicate that regardless of which subclass of AI is used initially, approximately 50% of the patients will have further antitumor benefit after switching to the other subclass suggesting that cross-resistance is incomplete. Therefore, postmenopausal patients may receive two AIs as first- and second-line therapies.

The AIs are only used in postmenopausal women. Even though ovarian estrogen production relies on the same enzymatic pathway discussed earlier, premenopausal or perimenopausal women with functioning ovaries are not appropriate candidates for these therapies. The reason is physiologic as evidence indicates that negative endocrine feedback will overcome aromatase inhibition. Early clinical data also suggested that the strategy of combining an AI with ovarian suppression (ie, oophorectomy or LHRH agonists) may be a therapeutic option in premenopausal women. Currently, this option is considered inappropriate unless a strict contraindication to tamoxifen exists.

The use of AIs in men with advanced breast cancer should be avoided. Available data suggest the use of these agents in men increases circulating levels of testosterone, which may negate the therapeutic effects of the drug.

Antiestrogens bind to ERs, preventing receptor-mediated gene transcription, and therefore are used to block the effect of estrogen on the end target. This class of agents is subdivided into two pharmacologic categories, SERMs and SERDs (selective estrogen-receptor downregulators). SERMs like tamoxifen have tissue-specific estrogenic and antiestrogenic activities. The effort to minimize or eliminate the adverse estrogenic effects led to the development of SERDs, which are pure estrogen receptor antagonists. The distinguishing feature of SERDs is their ability to degrade the ligand–ER complex.

Tamoxifen can be used in both premenopausal and postmenopausal women with ER positive, metastatic breast cancer. Toxicities associated with tamoxifen have been previously described. The only additional acute adverse effect, which occurs in about 5% of the patients with bone metastasis is tumor flare or hypercalcemia following initiation of tamoxifen. Generally, this acute reaction is not an indication to discontinue treatment. Conversely, this finding appears to correlate with subsequent response to endocrine therapy.

Fulvestrant is the only SERD approved for clinical use in the United States. The drug is approved as second-line therapy of postmenopausal patients with hormone-dependent advanced breast cancer. Clinical studies conducted in postmenopausal patients with disease progressing on tamoxifen compared fulvestrant against anastrozole. Results of these trials indicated similar efficacy and acceptable tolerability. The side effect observed with fulvestrant only was dermal reactions at the injection site. Even though fulvestrant is a good option for patients who are unable to take an oral medication, some patients may be averse to the drug because it must be given intramuscularly. There is no biological reason why fulvestrant should not produce similar outcomes in premenopausal women; however, safety or efficacy data are lacking.

Estrogen production in premenopausal women can be effectively achieved by surgery, pharmacologic agents, or radiation. Results of two randomized clinical trials evaluating the overall response rate between oophorectomy and tamoxifen were not significantly different. Interestingly, secondary response rates to oophorectomy after tamoxifen treatment were somewhat higher than response rates to tamoxifen after oophorectomy (33% versus 11%). Interpretation of these findings suggests that tamoxifen does not completely antagonize available estrogen, particularly in premenopausal women. Ovarian ablation (surgically or chemically) is still commonly performed in parts of the United States and is considered by some to be the endocrine therapy of choice in premenopausal women with advanced disease. The mortality rate with surgical oophorectomy is less than 3% in appropriately selected patients.

Castration can also be achieved pharmacologically with LHRH agonists. An initial surge in luteinizing hormone (LH) and estrogen production during the first few weeks of treatment can cause a tumor flare reaction similar to tamoxifen. With continued therapy, this strategy induces remission in about one-third of unselected patients. LHRH agonists purportedly downregulates LHRH receptors in the pituitary resulting in decreased LH release and castrate levels of estrogens. Of the three agents available in the United States (ie, leuprolide, goserelin, and triptorelin), only goserelin is approved for the treatment of metastatic breast cancer.

In randomized trials, progestins such as megestrol acetate and medroxyprogesterone acetate have been shown to induce noninferior response rates when compared with tamoxifen. Megestrol acetate is used more frequently in the United States. Despite their efficacy, these agents are generally used after patients have received an AI and/or tamoxifen. The most common side effects are listed in Table 89-7. One side effect, weight gain, occurs in 20% to 50% of patients. Patients experiencing weight gain may have fluid retention, but fluid retention is not responsible for all of the weight gain. In cachectic cancer patients, the weight gain may be desirable, but this is not uniformly true of all patients with metastatic breast cancer.

High-dose estrogens and androgens are rarely used because they are more toxic than other hormonal agents and in some cases less effective. About one-third of patients placed on high-dose estrogens will discontinue the use of these agents because side effects, the most important of which are thromboembolic events, vomiting, and fluid retention.

► *Cytotoxic Chemotherapy*

Except for brain and spine (with impending cord compression), chemotherapy is given as initial treatment of metastasis in patients with hormone receptor–negative tumors. The median time to an objective response is 2 to 3 months, but this period depends largely on the site of measurable disease. For example, time to response is 3 to 6 weeks for disease localized primarily to skin and lymph nodes; 6 to 9 weeks lung lesions; 15 weeks for liver metastasis; and 18 weeks for bone involvement. Once chemotherapy has been initiated, it is usually continued until maximal response, disease progression, or intolerable toxicity.

Unlike endocrine therapy, no clinical characteristic or established test has been shown to predict benefit from chemotherapy. However, a number of factors are associated with likelihood of tumor response, including good performance status, limited number (one or two) of disease sites, treatment naïve status, and previous response to chemotherapy with a long disease-free interval. Tumors that progress while being treated may respond to different agents. Importantly, tumors that do not respond to endocrine therapy are as likely to respond to chemotherapy as tumors treated with cytotoxic agents first. If not used initially, chemotherapy is eventually required in most patients with advanced breast cancer.

Although many chemotherapeutic agents have demonstrated activity in the treatment of breast cancer, the most frequently used agents include all of the agents used in the adjuvant setting plus nab-paclitaxel, capecitabine, gemcitabine, ixabepilone, and vinorelbine. KEY CONCEPT *The most active classes of chemotherapy in metastatic breast cancer are the anthracyclines and the taxanes with response rates as high as 50% to 60% in patients who have not received prior chemotherapy for metastatic disease.* A brief discussion of some chemotherapy-related issues specific to breast cancer extends upon what is described in Chapter 88.

Taxanes

In the metastatic setting the most effective weekly dose of paclitaxel appears to be 80 mg/m²/week with no breaks in therapy. With this approach, the toxicity profile of paclitaxel changes with less myelosuppression and delayed onset of peripheral neuropathy but slightly more fluid retention and skin and nail changes.

A dose-response relationship has been demonstrated with docetaxel. However, at 100 mg/m² every 21 days, the positive impact was limited to ORR. Therefore, asymptomatic patients who may not require a rapid clinical response, dosages in the range of 60 mg/m² to 75 mg/m² are appropriate. While less neuropathy, myalgia, and hypersensitivity reactions are observed with docetaxel (compared to paclitaxel), the incidence of febrile neutropenia, fluid retention, and skin reactions is higher. A weekly schedule of docetaxel, 35 mg/m², six doses of an 8-week cycle is also very active and more tolerable than the 3-weekly schedule.

Nanoparticle albumin-bound (nab)-paclitaxel exhibits some advantages over conventional paclitaxel. Comparatively, treatment with nab-paclitaxel, 260 mg/m², produced significantly better ORRs and median TTP than standard dose paclitaxel, 175 mg/m². Despite the higher dosage, the incidence of severe neutropenia was significantly lower with nab-paclitaxel. Nab-paclitaxel is indicated for patients with metastatic breast cancer resistant to conventional chemotherapy or progressing within 6 months of receiving an adjuvant anthracycline-containing chemotherapy regimen.

Antimetabolites

Capecitabine has activity against tumors progressing on anthracycline-and taxane-containing regimens. Moreover, the drug exhibits somewhat selective activity against cancer cells. This belief is supported by the presence of higher tumor cell levels of thymidine phosphorylase, the enzyme which catalyzes the final step in the conversion of capecitabine to 5-FU. In previously treated patients, capecitabine produced response rates of about 25%, which was impressive compared with other tested chemotherapy agents.

Gemcitabine is another agent that is used frequently in patients with advanced breast cancer. This nucleotide analogue has a unique mechanism of action and a favorable toxicity profile. As a single agent, response rates of nearly 40% have been achieved in the first-line setting. However, ORRs up to 90% have been obtained when gemcitabine was combined with doxorubicin or epirubicin and paclitaxel as first-line treatment. Response rates to gemcitabine monotherapy in the second- and third-line settings are approximately 18% to 26%. When combined with one other agent such as a taxane, vinorelbine, cisplatin, or an anthracycline, results of clinical studies consistently demonstrated higher efficacy than either single agent. In patients who have been exposed to an anthracycline and a taxane, gemcitabine appears to provide similar benefit to capecitabine.

Epothilone

In vitro studies show that the antimicrotubule activity of ixabepilone is similar to the taxanes. The results of a phase 3 clinical trial demonstrated that the combination of ixabepilone plus capecitabine significantly improved PFS by 38% while the ORR was more than twice as high with the combination compared with capecitabine alone (35% vs 14%, respectively).[31] Even in patients with disease intrinsically resistant to previous taxane therapy, response rates were twice as high with the combination. The findings from this study support preclinical data that the antitumor activity between ixabepilone and capecitabine are at least additive and, possibly, synergistic. However, the improved outcomes must be balanced against a much higher incidence of adverse effects involving the bone marrow and peripheral nervous system. Five infection-related deaths occurred with combination therapy. In addition, two-thirds of the patients developed variable grades of sensory neuropathy; 21% of the all patients discontinued treatment because of this adverse effect. Ixabepilone is approved for use in combination with capecitabine for patients with advanced breast cancer resistant to or progressing on previous anthracycline and taxane therapy or for patients

Patient Encounter, Part 7

Unfortunately, this patient's disease progresses after 11 months of treatment. She now complains of right abdominal quadrant pain. Her liver exhibits rebound tenderness. She is nauseated and weak from dehydration. CT of her abdomen indicates multiple lesions in both lobes of the liver, which are consistent with recurrent disease. Liver function tests are two times the upper limit of normal. A month ago, her performance status was 1; now it is 3 and metastasis related.

Propose a plan to manage the patient.

in whom anthracyclines are contraindicated. The use of single-agent ixabepilone is approved for use in patients with disease resistant to capecitabine.

Vinca alkaloid

Although not approved for breast cancer, activity has been observed with vinorelbine therapy in patients with advanced disease. However, some of the more intriguing data are associated with the combination of vinorelbine and trastuzumab. In a small cohort of patients with HER2-positive, metastatic breast cancer, an ORR of 68% was achieved; 38% of patients were progression-free after 1 year. Importantly, none of the antimicrotubule agents appears to be cross-resistant with the anthracyclines.

General Comments

Combination chemotherapy regimens are usually associated with higher response rates than are single-agent therapies, but the higher response rates do not necessarily translate into significant differences in OS. The use of sequential single-agent therapy versus combination chemotherapy regimens has been debated widely for metastatic breast cancer. In fact, current consensus regarding first-line chemotherapy is the use of single agents or combination chemotherapy.[32] In the palliative metastatic setting, the least toxic approach is preferred when efficacy is considered equal. In clinical practice, patients who require a rapid response to chemotherapy (eg, those with symptomatic bulky metastases) often receive combination therapy despite the added toxicity. This decision is complex and should be made on an individual patient basis.

Because many patients receive adjuvant chemotherapy, regimens chosen for first-line use in the metastatic setting often are different from those used in the adjuvant setting with the following caveat. If the patient's cancer recurs more than 1 year after the end of adjuvant chemotherapy, the same agents may have activity in the metastatic disease setting.

▶ *Targeted Biologic Therapy*

All breast cancers are tested for HER2 by immunohistochemistry (IHC) and/or fluorescence in-situ hybridization (FISH). Notably, an IHC score of 2+ (on a 0–3+ scale) for HER2 is associated with little to no benefit with trastuzumab therapy. Moreover, the 2+ IHC score is often negative by the more sensitive and specific FISH technique. As such, targeted anti-HER2 therapies are only indicated for breast cancers that overexpress the receptor at the 3+ level by IHC and/or demonstrate gene amplification by FISH.

Trastuzumab is a humanized monoclonal antibody that recognizes a specific extracellular epitope of HER2. Single-agent treatment with trastuzumab produces responses in approximately 15% to 20% of patients; the clinical benefit rate, which includes CRs, PRs, and stable disease is nearly 40%. Trastuzumab has additive and perhaps synergistic activity with chemotherapeutic agents.[33] Because cardiac toxicity is associated with the antibody, trastuzumab is given after all cycles of the anthracyclines have been completed. A non–anthracycline-containing regimen with excellent activity is the combination of docetaxel and carboplatin with concurrent trastuzumab.[34] Other chemotherapy agents that are being evaluated in combination with trastuzumab include vinorelbine, gemcitabine, capecitabine, and the platinum agents (eg, cisplatin and carboplatin).

Trastuzumab is reasonably well tolerated. The most common adverse effects are first dose infusion-related chills which occur in about 40% of patients. To alleviate the symptoms, acetaminophen and diphenhydramine may be given and/or the infusion rate may be reduced. Rare severe adverse effects including hypersensitivity and/or pulmonary reactions have also been reported. It is important to educate patients regarding the pulmonary reactions because they may occur up to 24 hours after the infusion and can be fatal if not treated promptly. Trastuzumab may increase the incidence of infection, diarrhea, and/or other adverse events when given with chemotherapy. When trastuzumb is given with an anthracycline, the rates of heart failure are unacceptably high; even as a single agent, cardiac events have approached 5%. Fortunately, this toxicity is usually reversible though patients may require pharmacologic management. Some patients have even continued therapy with trastuzumab after their left ventricular ejection fraction has returned to normal. Close monitoring for clinical signs and symptoms of heart failure is important in order to intervene with appropriate cardiac treatments.

Lapatinib is a dual inhibitor of HER2 and the epidermal growth factor receptor (EGFR, HER1). In contrast to the extracellular recognition site of trastuzumab, the specific targets of lapatinib are the receptors' intracellular kinase domain. A pivotal phase 3 clinical trial was conducted to assess the efficacy and safety of lapatinib plus capecitabine versus capecitabine alone in patients with disease progressing on trastuzumab. The trial was terminated early when a preplanned interim analysis indicated a significant reduction in risk of disease progression that favored the combination arm. Of note, the incidence of brain metastasis was significantly lower in the lapatinib-treated group.[35]

The side-effect profile of lapatinib is described in Chapter 88. A few side effects such as diarrhea, dyspepsia, and rash occurred more frequently when lapatinib was combined with capecitabine. Importantly, the lapatinib doublet was not associated with cardiac events resulting in subject withdrawal.

In May 2014, the American Society of Clinical Oncology (ASCO) issued two clinical practice guidelines related to lapatinib for the treatment of advanced, HER2-positive breast cancer. First, depending on hormone receptor status, third-line therapy may include hormonal therapy or chemotherapy with trastuzumab and in some cases with lapatinib or the combination of trastuzumab and lapatinib; and second, in patients with brain metastases systemic therapies with lapatinib and capecitabine is one option that can be considered for patients with a poor prognosis for survival.

A new HER2-targeted agent called pertuzumab received FDA approval in June 2012. Although both pertuzumab and trastuzumab are monoclonal antibodies that inhibit HER2-mediated signaling, a number of differences exist. First, each agent recognizes different extracellular epitopes, a finding that could have important therapeutic ramifications. Second, the unique binding site of pertuzumab induces structural changes that hinder receptor dimerization. Theoretically, by inhibiting HER2 signaling initiated by ligand-activated HER1 or HER3, pertuzumab could provide even greater inhibition of HER2 than trastuzumab. However, this does not appear to be case. In fact, compared to trastuzumab, pertuzumab has exhibited less activity. Based on results of a phase 3 clinical trial, pertuzumab is indicated for use as first-line therapy (in combination with trastuzumab and docetaxel) for HER2-positive metastatic breast cancer.[36] The most frequently reported adverse observed in clinical trials involving pertuzumab was diarrhea; cardiac toxicity was similar to, but does not appear to be increased when used concurrently with, trastuzumab.

One of the most significant limitations of cytotoxic chemotherapy is the lack of tumor specificity. Coupling target selectivity with the observation that trastuzumab's modest antitumor effect was substantially improved by the addition of chemotherapy led to the idea that antibodies could be used to deliver chemotherapy rather specifically to tumor cells. However, the efficacy of antibody-chemotherapy (drug) conjugates (ADCs) has historically been limited by variable expression of the target antigen, defective tumor cell uptake mechanisms, and unreliable linkers used in the conjugation process.

A novel therapeutic compound known as trastuzumab-DM1 (T-DM1, trastuzumab emtansine) has been developed that appears to have resolved all of the above issues. Because HER2 is overexpressed in approximately 20% of breast cancers, trastuzumab was identified as a reasonable vehicle for drug delivery. In order to improve the therapeutic index of the attached chemotherapeutic agent, a maytansine derivative was synthesized. The resulting maytansinoid, emtansine, was configured to have an easily cleavable linker to trastuzumab. The resulting ADC has the potential not only of retaining the antitumor properties of the individual agents but also maintaining a tolerable side-effect profile.

The most significant results were reported in a phase 3 clinical trial which compared T-DM1 against the combination of lapatinib plus capecitabine as second-line therapy for patients with HER2-positive breast cancer progressing on trastuzumab and a taxane.[37] Primary end points were PFS, OS, and tolerability. Compared to the capecitabine/lapatinib arm, T-DM1 significantly reduced the risk of disease progression or death by 35%. Median OS at the second interim analysis crossed the prespecified efficacy stopping boundary. The most common grade more than or equal to 3 toxicity observed in patients receiving T-DM1 arm was thrombocytopenia. Platelet nadirs occurred 7 days after drug administration and recovered within a week. Other frequently occurring side effects included liver function test abnormalities, hypokalemia, fatigue, nausea, and headache. However, none of these adverse events were greater than grade 2. Cardiac toxicity requiring treatment discontinuation was not observed. The results of this study led to FDA approval in February 2013.

Two noteworthy phase 3 clinical trials involving this novel ADC are in progress. The first compares T-DM1 with or without pertuzumab against trastuzuamb plus a taxane as first-line treatment of HER2-positive, progressive or recurrent locally advanced or metastatic breast cancer; the second, T-DM1 versus trastuzumab as adjuvant therapy for patients with HER2 positive primary breast cancer who have residual tumor present pathologically in the breast or axillary lymph nodes following preoperative therapy.

▸ *Bisphosphonates*

For women whose breast cancer has metastasized to bone, bisphosphonates are recommended, in addition to chemotherapy or endocrine therapy, to reduce bone pain and fractures. Pamidronate (90 mg) and zoledronate (4 mg) can be given IV once each month. These bisphosphonates are given in combination with calcium and vitamin D.

Local-Regional Control

▸ *Radiation Therapy*

Radiation is an important modality in the treatment of symptomatic metastatic disease. The most common indication for treatment with radiation therapy is painful bone metastases or other localized sites of disease refractory to systemic therapy. Approximately 90% of patients who are treated for painful bone metastases experience significant pain relief with radiation therapy. Additionally, radiation is an important modality in the palliative treatment of metastatic brain lesions and spinal cord lesions, which respond poorly to systemic therapy, as well as eye or orbit lesions and other sites where significant accumulation of tumor cells occurs. Open or painful skin wounds and/or lymph node metastases confined to the chest wall area may also be treated with radiation therapy for palliation.

Patient Care Process: Breast Cancer

Patient Assessment:

- Detail key aspects of the patient's history related to the breast cancer diagnosis. Describe the circumstances (ie, screening or physical findings) underlying the cancer diagnosis. Determine patient risk factors for the disease.
- Summarize disease stage, prognosis, and treatment goals.

Therapy Evaluation:

- Formulate rational treatment plans for premenopausal and postmenopausal women with early breast cancer in each of the following situations: (1) luminal A; (2) luminal B; (3) HER2 positive; and (4) basal subtype. Determine surgical options, radiation therapy, and systemic therapies as indicated.
- Formulate rational treatment plan for a patient with locally advanced breast cancer (including surgical options, radiation therapy, and systemic therapies as indicated).
- Formulate rational treatment plans for premenopausal and postmenopausal women with metastatic breast cancer in each of the following situations: (1) luminal A; (2) luminal B; (3) HER2 positive; and (4) basal subtype. Determine systemic therapies as indicated.

Care Plan Development:

- Articulate components of the overall management plan with a focus on pharmacologic agents, their relevant side effects especially with regard to probability and timing of occurrence, and appropriate prophylaxis and/or management.
- Propose a plan for the supportive care of the patient.
- Identify and assess key endpoints (especially with regards to quality of life issues) related to pharmacotherapeutic management of the patient.

Follow-Up Evaluation:

- Address adverse events and modify the treatment plan accordingly.
- Reeducate the patient regarding any change(s) to the treatment plan.
- Explain the importance of patient reporting of adverse events and adherence with the prescribed medication regimen.

OUTCOME EVALUATION

Early breast cancer is resected completely with curative intent and adjuvant chemotherapy and/or hormonal therapy with trastuzumab in selected patients are initiated to prevent recurrence. During adjuvant chemotherapy, laboratory values to monitor chemotherapy toxicity are obtained before each cycle of treatment. After completion of adjuvant therapy, patients are monitored every 3 months for the first few years after diagnosis, with intervals between examinations extended as time from diagnosis lengthens. Evaluation includes:

- Physical examination to detect breast cancer recurrence
- Annual mammography
- Symptom-directed workup

Patients with locally advanced breast cancer are often treated with neoadjuvant therapy to make the tumor surgically resectable. However, many believe that neoadjuvant therapy may have benefits that extend beyond downstaging. During neoadjuvant chemotherapy, laboratory values to monitor chemotherapy toxicity are obtained before each cycle and weekly thereafter while on treatment; physical and ultrasound examinations to determine the size of the tumor are performed following a complete course of neoadjuvant therapy. Generally, no further chemotherapy is given after surgery. After complete surgical resection, monitoring proceeds as described for early breast cancer.

Metastatic breast cancer is not curable, and therapy is intended to palliate symptoms and prolong survival. In most cases, hormonal therapy is the mainstay for tumors that are ER positive. While on therapy, patients are monitored monthly for signs of disease progression or metastasis to common sites, such as the bones, brain, or liver. Evaluations include:

- Pain
- Mental status or other neurologic findings
- Laboratory tests
- Liver function tests
- Complete blood count
- Calcium, electrolytes

Abbreviations Introduced in This Chapter

AI	Aromatase inhibitor
DFS	Disease-free survival
ER	Estrogen receptor
HER2	Human epidermal growth factor receptor 2
LHRH	Luteinizing hormone-releasing hormone
ORR	Overall response rate
OS	Overall survival
PFS	Progression-free survival
PR	Progesterone receptor
SERD	Selective estrogen-receptor downregulators
SERM	Selective estrogen receptor modulator
TNM	Tumor, node, metastasis (staging system)
TTP	Time to progression

REFERENCES

1. Siegel RL, Miller KD, Jemal A. Cancer statistics, 2015. CA Cancer J Clin 2015;65:5–29.
2. King MC, Marks JH, Mandell JB. Breast and ovarian cancer risks due to inherited mutations in BRCA1 and BRCA2. Science. 2003;302:643–646.
3. Early Breast Cancer Trialists' Collaborative Group. Effects of chemotherapy and hormonal therapy for early breast cancer on recurrence and 15-year survival: An overview of the randomised trials. Lancet. 2005;365:1687–1717.
4. Fisher B, Costantino JP, Wickerham DL, et al. Tamoxifen for prevention of breast cancer: Report of the National Surgical Adjuvant Breast and Bowel Project P-1 Study. J Natl Cancer Inst. 1998;90:1371–1388.
5. Powles TJ, Ashley S, Tidy A, et al. Twenty-year follow-up of the Royal Marsden randomized double-blinded tamoxifen breast cancer prevention trial. J Natl Cancer Inst. 2007;99:283–290.
6. Vogel VG, Costantino JP, Wickerham DL, et al. The study of tamoxifen and raloxifene (STAR): Report of the National Surgical Adjuvant Breast and Bowel Project P-2 trial. JAMA. 2006;295:2727–2741.
7. Barton MK Exemestane is effective for the chemoprevention of breast cancer. CA Cancer J Clin. 2011;61(6):363–364.
8. Higa GM. Current and evolving therapeutic options in the treatment of early breast cancer. Clin Med Rev Womens Health. 2011; 3:1–21.
9. U.S. Preventive Services Task Force. Screening for breast cancer: U.S. Preventive Services Task Force recommendation statement. Ann Intern Med. 2009;151:716–726.
10. Veronesi U, Cascinelli N, Mariani MD, et al. Twenty-year follow-up of a randomized study comparing breast-conserving surgery with radical mastectomy for early breast cancer. N Engl J Med. 2002;347:1227–1232.
11. Markopoulos C, Tsaroucha AK, Kouskos E, Mantas D, Antonopoulou Z, Karvelis S. Impact of breast cancer surgery on the self-esteem and sexual life of female patients. J Int Med Res. 2009;37:182–188.
12. Galimberti V, Cole BF, Zurrida S et al. Axillary dissection versus no axillary dissection in patients with sentinel-node micrometastases (IBCSG 23-01): A phase 3 randomised controlled trial. Lancet Oncol. 2013;14:297–305.
13. Giuliano AE, Hunt KK, Ballman KV et al. Axillary dissection versus no axillary dissection in women with invasive breast cancer and sentinel node metastasis. JAMA. 2011;305: 569–575.
14. Whelan TJ, Pignol JP, Levine MN et al. Long-term results of hypofractionated radiation therapy for breast cancer. N Eng J Med. 2010;362:513–520.
15. Goldhirsch A, Winer EP, Coates AS, et al. Personalizing the treatment of women with early breast cancer: Highlights of the St Gallen International Expert Consensus on the primary therapy of early breast cancer 2013. Ann Oncol. 2013;24:2206–2223.
16. Bonadonna G, Moliterni A, Zambetti M, et al. 30 years' follow up of randomised studies of adjuvant CMF in operable breast cancer: Cohort study. BMJ. 2005;330:217–222.
17. Azim Jr HA, de Azambuja E, Colozza M, Bines J, Piccart MJ. Long-term toxic effects of adjuvant chemotherapy in breast cancer. Ann Oncol. 2011;22:1939–1947.
18. Goldstein LJ, Gray R, Badve S, et al. Prognostic utility of the 21-gene assay in hormone receptor–positive operable breast cancer compared with classical clinicopathologic features. J Clin Oncol. 2008;26:4063–4071.
19. Cheang MCU, Voduc KD, Tu D, et al. Responsiveness of intrinsic subtypes to adjuvant anthracycline substitution in the NCIC.CTG MA.5 randomized trial. Clin Cancer Res. 2012;18:2402–2412.
20. Dhesy-Thind B, Pritchard KI, Messersmith H, et al. HER2/neu in systemic therapy for women with breast cancer: A systematic review. Breast Cancer Res Treat. 2008;109:209–229.
21. Goldhirsch A, Gelber R, Piccart-Gebhart MJ, et al. 2 years versus 1 year of adjuvant trastuzumab for HER2-positive breast cancer (HERA): An open-label, randomized controlled trial. Lancet. 2013;382:1021–1028.

22. Skliris GP, Leygue E, Curtis-Snell L, Watson PH, Murphy LC. Expression of oestrogen receptor-β in oestrogen receptor-α negative human breast tumours. Br J Cancer. 2006;95:616–626.
23. Papoutsi Z, Zhao C, Putnik M, Gustafsson J-A, Dahlman-Wright K. Binding of estrogen receptor α/β heterodimers to chromatin in MCF-7 cells. J Mol Endocrin. 2009;43:65–72.
24. Davies C, Pan H, Godwin J, et al. Long-term effects of continuing adjuvant tamoxifen to 10 years versus stopping at 5 years after diagnosis of oestrogen receptor-positive breast cancer: ATLAS, a randomised trial. Lancet. 2013;381:805–816.
25. Goss PE, Ingle JN, Martino S, et al. Impact of premenopausal status at breast cancer diagnosis in women entered on the placebo-controlled NCIC CTG MA17 trial of extended adjuvant letrozole. Ann Oncol. 2013;24:355–361.
26. Schroth W, Goetz MP, Hamann U, et al. Association between CYP2D6 polymorphisms and outcomes among women with early stage breast cancer treated with tamoxifen. JAMA. 2009;302: 1429–1436.
27. Dezentjé VO, van Schaik RHN, Vletter-Bogaartz JM, et al. (2013). CYP2D6 genotype in relation to tamoxifen efficacy in a Dutch cohort of the tamoxifen exemestane adjuvant multinational (TEAM) trial. Breast Cancer Res Treat. 2013;140:363–373.
28. Mouridsen H, Giobbie-Hurder A, Goldhirsch A, et al. Letrozole therapy alone or in sequence with tamoxifen in women with breast cancer. N Engl J Med. 2009;361:766–776.
29. Dowsett M, Cuzick J, Ingle J, et al. Meta-analysis of breast cancer outcomes in adjuvant trials of aromatase inhibitors versus tamoxifen. J Clin Oncol. 2010;28:509–518.
30. Lønning PE. The potency and clinical efficacy of aromatase inhibitors across the breast cancer continuum. Ann Oncol. 2011;22:503–514.
31. Thomas ES, Gomez HL, Li RK, et al. Ixabepilone plus capecitabine for metastatic breast cancer progressing after anthracycline and taxane treatment. J Clin Oncol. 2007;25:5210–5217.
32. Partridge AH, Rumble RB, Carey LA, et al. Chemotherapy and targeted therapy for women with human epidermal growth factor receptor 2-negative (or unknown) advanced breast cancer: American Society of Clinical Oncology Clinical Practice Guideline. J Clin Oncol 2014;32:3307–3329.
33. Slamon DJ, Leyland-Jones B, Shak S, et al. Use of chemotherapy plus a monoclonal antibody against HER2 for metastatic breast cancer that overexpresses HER2. N Engl J Med. 2001;344: 783–792.
34. Slamon D, Eiermann W, Robert N, et al. Phase III randomized trial comparing doxorubicin and cyclophosphamide followed by docetaxel (AC->T) with doxorubicin and cyclophosphamide followed by docetaxel and trastuzumab (AC->TH) with docetaxel, carboplatin and trastuzumab (TCH) in Her2neu positive early breast cancer patients: BCIRG 006 Study. Cancer Res. 2010;69:62.
35. Lin NU, Diéras V, Paul D, et al. Multicenter phase II study of lapatinib in patients with brain metastases from HER2-positive breast cancer. Clin Cancer Res. 2009;15:1452–1459.
36. Baselga J, Cortés J, Kim S-B, et al. Pertuzumab plus trastuzumab plus docetaxel for metastatic breast cancer. N Engl J Med. 2012;366: 109–119.
37. Verma S, Miles D, Gianni L, Krop IE, Welslau M, Baselga J, et al. Trastuzumab emtansine for HER2-positive advanced breast cancer. N Engl J Med. 2012;367:1783–1791.

90 Lung Cancer

Val Adams and Justin Balko

LEARNING OBJECTIVES

Upon completion of the chapter, the reader will be able to:

1. Identify major risk factors for the development of lung cancer.
2. Explain the pathologic progression of lung cancer and its relationship with signs and symptoms of the disease.
3. Make appropriate recommendations for screening or preventive measures in high-risk patients.
4. Understand staging of lung cancer patients and how it influences treatment decisions.
5. List the rationale, advantages, disadvantages, and place in therapy for adjuvant and neoadjuvant chemotherapy.
6. Identify the chemotherapeutic or molecularly targeted regimens of choice for limited and extensive small cell lung carcinoma, as well as local, locally advanced, and advanced non–small cell lung carcinoma.
7. Monitor patients for treatment-associated toxicity and recommend appropriate management.
8. Distinguish the treatment goals of palliative care versus those of first-line treatment.

INTRODUCTION

Lung cancer has a major health impact both in the United States and worldwide. Before 1930, lung cancer was a relatively rare disease, but a sharp incline in industrialization and smoking in the early 1900s has bred an epidemic. Lung cancer has a high mortality rate, and although treatment can cure some patients, most therapies only prolong survival for months. Recent advances in lung cancer research provide good reason for optimism but antismoking campaigns still appear to offer the best opportunity to reduce lung cancer incidence and mortality.

EPIDEMIOLOGY AND ETIOLOGY

Incidence and Mortality

Cancers of the lung and bronchus rank first in cancer-related mortality, comprising more than 28% of cancer-related deaths.[1] In 2015, more than 1,500 new cases of lung cancer are expected. A close correlation exists between incidence and mortality of lung cancer, reflecting the reality that approximately 70% of lung cancer patients ultimately die of the disease.

Clinical Risk Factors

▶ Smoking

KEY CONCEPT *The most important risk factor for the development of lung cancer is smoking.* One of the most predictive factors on lung cancer epidemiology is prevalence of cigarette smoking. Because lung cancer is a fatal disease in most cases, both incidence and mortality strongly reflect the smoking prevalence of the population on a 20- to 30-year lag. In other words, decreases in tobacco use now would be expected to affect lung cancer incidence in 2040. With this knowledge, the current expectation is that lung cancer incidence and mortality will decrease steadily until 2020, reflecting decreases in cigarette smoking between 1970 and 1990. Because smoking prevalence has been constant since 1990, lung cancer incidence is expected to plateau.[2] Correlation between smoking and lung cancer continues to drive antismoking and clean indoor air campaigns and should be considered an investment in the future health care of the nation. Furthermore, smoking cessation plays an important role in reducing lung cancer risk on a patient-to-patient basis, and appropriately guiding such therapy is a crucial part of preventing lung cancer in at-risk patients.[3] Both total smoke exposure and current use correlate with the individual's risk of developing malignancy. The risk of lung cancer decreases to near-normal levels 10 to 15 years following successful smoking cessation. Total smoke exposure is reported as pack-years. One pack-year is the equivalent of smoking one pack per day for 1 year. A patient who smokes 40 cigarettes per day (two packs) for 5 years would have a 10 pack-year history (2 packs/day for 5 years).

▶ Other Air-Related Risks

In addition to direct inhalation of cigarette smoke, other environmental factors have been identified as risks for the development of primary lung tumors. Environmental tobacco smoke (ETS) presents a significant occupational hazard for nonsmokers working in environments that have a high smoking population, such as bars or restaurants. Each year approximately 3000 cases of lung cancer in nonsmokers are caused by ETS. In response, the majority of states have enacted clean indoor air acts. Other environmental factors linked to lung cancer include radon, arsenic, nickel, and chloromethyl ethers. Those who live in an urban environment are also at an increased risk for lung cancer owing to exposure to high concentrations of combustion fumes.[4] Asbestos exposure increases the risk of developing a distinct but rare type of lung cancer called **mesothelioma**.

▶ *Nutrition*

Diet and nutrition are suspected to play a role in cancer susceptibility, and many studies have sought to define specific foods or nutrients that influence cancer risk. Because not all heavy smokers develop lung cancer, nutritional factors may explain part of this variation. Epidemiologic studies focusing on diet and nutrition in lung cancer have shown reduced rates of lung cancer in smoking individuals who report higher fruit and vegetable consumption. However, studies attempting to identify specific chemical components of fruits and vegetables that are responsible for this effect have not been successful.[5] KEY CONCEPT *Recommendations to patients who are at risk owing to smoking or other factors or those who are simply interested in reducing their risk of cancer should include an increase in dietary intake of fruits and vegetables.*

Hereditary or Genetic Risk Factors

Although smoking is a key risk factor for lung cancer, the majority of people who smoke never develop lung cancer. Genetic risk factors may predispose certain smokers to lung cancer. After adjustments for age, smoke exposure, occupation, and gender, relatives of a lung cancer patient have approximately a twofold risk of developing lung cancer. The degree of inherited risk inversely correlates with the age of the relative at the time of diagnosis. First-degree relatives of a lung cancer patient diagnosed between the ages of 40 and 59 years have a sixfold relative risk for lung cancer. Familial lung cancer that develops at an early age in nonsmokers fits a Mendelian codominant inheritance model. However, a lung cancer gene has not been identified.

Chemoprevention

Chemoprevention refers to the use of prophylactic medications to prevent the development of cancer. Many studies have been conducted testing potential chemopreventatives, including nonsteroidal anti-inflammatory drugs, retinoids, inhaled glucocorticoids, vitamin E, selenium, and green tea extracts, but none have been successful. A large randomized trial testing the effects of selenium, previously considered a promising chemopreventative agent for lung cancer, was stopped early due to lack of any observable effect at its first interim analysis.[6]

Interestingly, data from a placebo-controlled double blind study demonstrated that selective cyclooxygenase-2 (COX-2) inhibition with celecoxib reduces the proliferation of bronchial epithelial cells, lowers inflammatory markers, and may resolve benign or premalignant lung nodules in former smokers.[7] Existing data suggest that bronchial epithelial cell proliferation may be a surrogate endpoint for chemopreventative lung cancer trials. However, at this time, routine use of celecoxib as a chemopreventative agent is not warranted.

Screening and Early Detection

Overall 5-year survival in lung cancer is only 15%, but those who are diagnosed at a localized stage exhibit a 5-year survival rate of 50%. Currently, more than three quarters of newly diagnosed lung cancers present with locally advanced or metastatic disease, and therefore, very few patients are able to undergo surgical resection.[1] In an attempt to identify tumors when they are localized and have higher cure rates, many studies have evaluated different screening modalities, which have led to screening recommendations.

The landmark trial, the National Lung Screening Trial (NLST) randomized more than 53,000 patients at high risk for lung cancer to three annual low-dose spiral computed tomography (CT) scans or chest x-ray. Chest x-ray has been shown in large trials to be equivalent to no screening and can be considered a placebo control for mortality. In the CT arm 6.9% of patients were diagnosed with lung cancer and 63% were diagnosed with stage Ia or Ib disease with over 90% having surgery with curative intent. Screening by CT reduced lung cancer mortality by 20% and was subsequently approved and recommended for high-risk patients. High-risk patients are defined by the following criteria:

1. Age greater than or equal to 55 years
2. Smoking within the last 15 years
3. A 20 pack-year history plus an additional risk factor or greater than a 30 pack-year history

The challenge with utilizing low-dose CT scans in screening is the high sensitivity, which translates into frequent detection of nonmalignant lesions. In the NLST, the CT screening arm had positive findings in 24.2% of patients with 96.4% of the lesions being benign (false positives). Due to this high false positive rate, screening should be perceived as a two-step process in order to prevent excessive patient workup and anxiety. The plan for a patient (biopsy, PET scan evaluation, or repeat CT scan at 3, 6, or 12 months) with a positive finding on spiral CT is determined by an algorithm that evaluates the number, size, and characteristics of lesions.

The United States Preventative Services Task Force guidelines provide lung cancer screening a grade B recommendation, which means the magnitude of benefit is moderate. The proposed action for grade B recommendations is to offer or provide this service for qualifying patients.

PATHOPHYSIOLOGY

Most lung cancers arise from the epithelium of the airways and are classified as **carcinomas**. There are four major and several rare histologic types of lung cancer. They appear to form through different mutagenic pathways; however, they all appear to transition through a premalignant state. The presence of a transitional state from normal tissue to cancerous tissue is important because the premalignant cells contain damage that is generally thought to be reversible. Researchers are currently trying to develop methods to identify people with premalignant lesions as well as drugs that can reverse the damage.

Continued damage to premalignant cells can lead to cancer. The first appearance of cancer cells that have not yet become invasive is referred to as carcinoma in situ. Patients are rarely diagnosed with this early stage of cancer owing to a lack of symptoms and relatively rapid progression from this state to larger invasive tumors. As the tumor grows, cells may become dislodged from the tumor bulk and enter the hematologic or lymphatic circulatory systems, where they can travel to either local or distant parts of the body. Hematologic spread usually results in metastatic sites in the bones, liver, and central nervous system (CNS). Lymphatic spread is more orderly in nature, with the hilar and mediastinal lymph nodes in the pleural cavity commonly being involved. Once the tumor has spread to multiple

Table 90–1

Lung Tumor Histopathology[32]

Tumor Type	Percent of Tumors	Approximate Cell Doubling Time (days)	Sensitivity to Chemotherapy and Radiotherapy	Relative Risk of Metastasis
Small cell	15–20	30	High	High
Non–small cell				
Adenocarcinoma	35–40	180	Low	Medium
Large cell (giant)	10	100	Low	Low
Squamous (epidermoid)	25–30	180	Low	Low

locations, curative treatment is rare because surgical excision and radiotherapy cannot remove all or nearly all of the cancer cells.

Histologic Classification

Histologic classification of lung cancer involves determining the cellular origin of the tumor. Knowing the histology of the tumor influences treatment decisions as well as prognosis.

There are four major histologic types of lung cancer that are divided into three classes based on response to treatment and prognosis: small cell lung cancer (SCLC), squamous cell non-small cell lung cancer (NSCLC) and non–squamous NSCLC. The four major types of lung cancer are outlined by class in Table 90–1. However, it is important to note that certain other rare malignancies can be seen and many lung cancers may consist of multiple histologic subtypes. Furthermore, a recent phenomenon has been observed where pharmacologic treatments may selectively kill different components of the tumor, resulting in a conversion of the remaining tumor to a different subtype (ie, NSCLC becomes SCLC after treatment). Therefore, repeat biopsies of lung tumors before each line of treatment may become a standard of care, although it is not routinely performed at this time.

Clinical Staging

Once the diagnosis of lung cancer is confirmed through visualization and biopsy, the extent of disease must be determined. NSCLC (squamous and non–squamous subsets) are staged using the American Joint Committee on Cancer (AJCC) tumor, node, and metastasis (TNM) staging system. SCLC is typically staged using the Veterans Administration Lung Cancer Study Group method. Clinical staging serves two primary purposes: predicting prognosis and guiding therapy.

Patient Encounter, Part 1

A 61-year-old woman presents at your clinic complaining of new-onset cough. She has had several upper respiratory infections in the last 2 months, with occasional hemoptysis. She smoked about a pack of cigarettes per day beginning in her early 30s, but quit about 10 years later, and has not smoked since. She lives downtown in the city and has worked at her own restaurant/bar since she bought the establishment 10 years ago.

What risk factors for lung cancer are present?

Calculate this patient's pack-year history.

▸ *Non–Small Cell Lung Cancer*

Clinical staging of NSCLC with the TNM system evaluates the size of the tumor (T), extent of nodal involvement (N), and presence of metastatic sites (M). The combination of these three evaluations determines the stage. Clinical stages and associated survival rates are outlined in Table 90–2. Local disease includes tumors that are confined to a single **hemithorax** and those cancers which have spread to the ipsilateral hilar lymph nodes. Once malignancy invades the mediastinal lymph nodes or contralateral hilar nodes, the disease becomes locally advanced. When signs of cancer are detected outside the pleural cavity, it is classified as advanced disease. Local disease is associated with the highest cure and survival rates, whereas those with advanced disease have a 5-year survival rate of less than 5%.

Mutation (genetic) testing plays a key role in the treatment plan for NSCLC. Tumors bearing mutations or rearrangements of the EGFR or ALK genes have specific treatment options that offer improved response rates over traditional therapies. In non–squamous NSCLC histology, mutational testing should always be performed to further guide therapy.

▸ *Small Cell Lung Cancer*

The most common system for staging SCLC was developed originally by the Veterans Administration Lung Cancer Study Group. This system categorizes SCLC into two classifications, limited and extensive disease.[8]

- Limited disease: evidence of the tumor is confined to a single hemithorax and can be encompassed by a single radiation port
- Extensive disease: any progression beyond limited disease

Table 90–2

Clinical Stage and Prognosis[8]

	Survival Rate (%)	
Clinical Stage	**1 Year**	**5 Year**
Local		
IA	94	67
IB	87	53
IIA	89	40
Locally Advanced		
IIB	73	30
IIIA	58	15
IIIB	37	10
Advanced		
IIIB	37	10
IV	18	< 5

Clinical Presentation and Diagnosis

Pulmonary Symptoms

Symptoms related to the direct effects of the primary tumor often appear first and are the most common. These include the following:

- Cough
- Chest pain
- Shortness of breath
- Dysphagia
- Hemoptysis

Extrapulmonary Symptoms

Once the tumor invades tissues outside the pleural cavity, it can produce a wide array of symptoms, including:

- General bone pain
- Adrenal insufficiency
- Confusion
- Personality changes
- Enlarged lymph nodes
- Weight loss
- Seizures
- Nausea and vomiting
- Focal neurologic symptoms
- Horner syndrome
- Fatigue
- Headache
- Pancoast syndrome
- Subcutaneous skin nodules

Paraneoplastic Syndromes

Symptoms that are not a result of the direct effects of the tumor are termed paraneoplastic syndromes. They may be caused by substances secreted by the tumor or in response to the tumor and often occur in tissues far from the site of malignancy. Paraneoplastic syndromes are numerous and affect a wide variety of systems, including the endocrine, neurologic, skeletal, renal, metabolic, vascular, and hematologic systems.

Diagnosis

Diagnosis requires visualization of one or more lesions as well as biopsy of the lesion to confirm malignancy. Both visualization and sampling can be performed by invasive or noninvasive methods. These methods are summarized in Table 90–3.

CLINICAL PRESENTATION AND DIAGNOSIS

KEY CONCEPT *Signs and symptoms of lung cancer can be classified into three subdivisions: pulmonary, extrapulmonary, and paraneoplastic syndromes. Distinguishing among these classes of symptoms is important because it can aid in determining the severity of the disease, guide treatment options, and affect prognosis.*

TREATMENT

Desired Outcome and General Approach to Patient

The treatment of lung cancer depends on tumor histology, genetic alterations; stage of disease; and patient characteristics such as age, gender, history, and performance status (PS). All these aspects must be assessed before appropriate treatment can

Table 90–3

Diagnostic Tools

	Technique	Description
Visualization	Chest x-ray	The least expensive visualization method in the diagnosis of lung cancer. Readily accessible and does not require systemic administration of contrast dye. However, it often detects lesions that are not cancerous and is not capable of assessing lymph node status.
	CT	More accurate when providing information on size, location, and invasion than chest radiography. It is recommended as part of the standard workup in most cases.
	PET scanning	Uses a substance called 5-FDG to produce a functional image of the lungs. Cells that are actively growing and dividing use greater amounts of glucose and therefore take up more 5-FDG. Focal regions of fluorescence can be visualized in cancerous lesions. PET scanning combined with a CT scan is more accurate than CT scan alone; however, the exact role of PET scanning in staging and monitoring is unclear. The apparent benefit and common role in staging is to evaluate mediastinal disease when it can influence the tumor resectability.
Tumor sampling	Fine-needle aspiration	A method of aspirating cells from the tumor via insertion of a small-bore needle into the lesion and aspirating. Commonly used to evaluate lymph nodes or other poorly accessible sites, it has the advantage of being faster and less invasive than other biopsy methods; however, it does not preserve the architecture of the tumor and may return cells that are undergoing cell death, which negates histologic analysis.
	Bronchoscopy	A fiberoptic camera is inserted through the airways to examine the site of the suspected lesion. Once the lesion is visualized, a tool attached to the camera allows for a tissue biopsy. Newer technologies incorporate fluorescence to differentiate malignant tissue from premalignant lesions.
	Core needle biopsy	A method of obtaining tissue and preserving the tumor architecture. A large-bore needle is inserted into a lesion, where it cuts a core of tissue out that then can be evaluated.
	Thoracentesis	Involves removal of fluid in the pleural cavity via a needle. The fluid then is assayed for presence cancerous cells. This procedure has low sensitivity and depends on the presence of a pleural effusion.
	Sputum cytology	Detects cancerous cells that become dislodged from the airways into the sputum. Sputum cytology is useful because it is not invasive, but it has much lower sensitivity for detecting cancer.

CT, computed tomography; 5-FDG, 5-fluorodeoxyglucose; PET, positron emission tomography.

Patient Encounter, Part 2

Medical History, Physical Examination, and Diagnosis

PMH: GERD (controlled with PPIs), and moderate hypertension (controlled)

FH: Father recently diagnosed with colorectal cancer, but alive, mother living and healthy

Meds: Lisinopril 20 mg daily; lansoprazole 30 mg daily

ROS: (+) Chest pain, shortness of breath, hemoptysis; (–) recent weight loss

PE

VS: BP 125/69, RR 26, P 80, T 99°F (37.2°C)

CV: RRR

Labs: Slightly elevated ionized calcium and LFTs; all others WNL; CXR reveals a solitary nodule in right lower lobe; fine-needle aspiration confirms adenocarcinoma of the lung; further evaluation with CT and PET scans reveal a 3-cm mass, with possible ipsilateral lymph node involvement.

What clinical stage is this patient's disease?

What is the estimated survival time for this stage of NSCLC?

Does this patient have any factors that may negatively or positively influence survival?

be recommended. In the development of a patient care plan, keep in mind the ultimate goals of therapy. Treatment modality based on histology and stage is outlined in Figure 90–1. KEY CONCEPT *In general patients with early stage disease, a definitive cure is the primary goal of treatment, although this end point is not always met. Additional goals of treating lung cancer patients include prolongation of survival and improvement of quality of life through alleviation of symptoms.* The goals of treatment must be considered when selecting a therapeutic plan. Some treatments may prolong survival by a few months but at the expense of

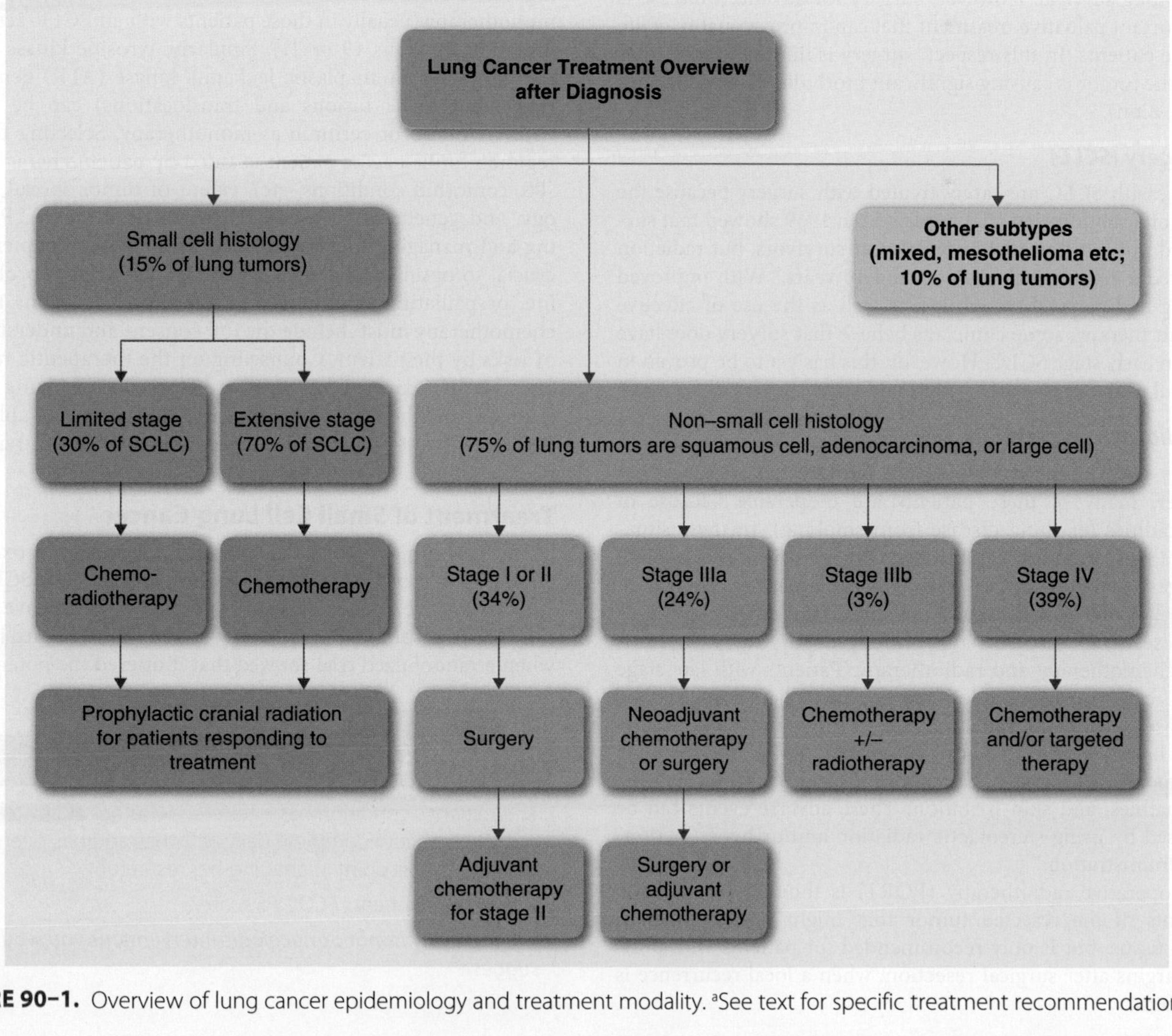

FIGURE 90–1. Overview of lung cancer epidemiology and treatment modality. [a]See text for specific treatment recommendations.

significant decreases in patient quality of life. Treatment decisions must include both the health care team and an informed and well-counseled patient.

▶ *Performance Status*

The performance status (PS) of an individual patient predicts response and likelihood of toxicity to chemotherapy as well as overall survival. The PS evaluation system used most frequently was developed by the Eastern Cooperative Oncology Group (ECOG) (see Chapter 88). KEY CONCEPT *Categorizing patients by their ECOG PS allows for an objective measure of capability to tolerate systemic therapies that may severely compromise the patient's health. Patients with a good PS (0–1) are more likely to tolerate intense therapy. PS 2 may receive chemotherapy, and PS 3 to 4 may receive supportive therapy or treatment with targeted therapies if they have targetable activating mutations.* Patients with localized disease may be treated more aggressively in this scenario because the intent of treatment is curative.

Treatment Modality

▶ *Surgery (NSCLC)*

KEY CONCEPT *Of all treatment modalities, surgical resection of the affected lobe or lung leads to the greatest improvement in survival for patients with early stage and locally advanced NSCLC tumors (clinical stage IA, IB, or IIA).* In patients with advanced disease NSCLC, surgery is not curative and as a general approach does not prolong survival. However, surgery for advanced disease is an important palliative treatment that can improve quality of life in some patients. In this respect, surgery is limited to local sites where the tumor is causing significant morbidity (eg, spinal cord compression).

▶ *Surgery (SCLC)*

Patients with SCLC are rarely treated with surgery because the results of a randomized trial published in 1969 showed that surgery did not result in any 5- or 10-year survivors, but radiation produced a 4% survival rate at 5 and 10 years.[9] With improved imaging and surgical techniques as well as the use of effective adjuvant therapy, some clinicians believe that surgery does have a role in early stage SCLC. However, this has yet to be proven in a clinical trial.

▶ *Radiotherapy (NSCLC)*

Patients with localized NSCLC are best treated with surgery; however, many of these patients are inoperable because of comorbidities (eg, lung disease from smoking). In these situations, radiation therapy can be used with curative intent in place of surgery, and the success rate is approximately 50% that of surgery.[10] Patients with locally advanced (stage IIIB, nonsurgically resectable) disease have prolonged survival with combined chemotherapy and radiotherapy. Patients with late stage NSCLC can receive radiation therapy to palliate symptomatic metastases. Although radiation is less invasive than surgery, it can have marked toxicity on normal tissue, and patients may experience esophagitis, pneumonitis, cardiac abnormalities, myelopathies, and skin irritation. These adverse events can be decreased by using stereotactic radiation and/or hyperfractionated administration.[11]

Postoperative radiotherapy (PORT) is thought to eliminate remnants of the resected tumor that might be deposited in nearby tissue, but is only recommended for patients with positive margins after surgical resection, when a local recurrence is of concern.

▶ *Radiotherapy (SCLC)*

Radiotherapy (concurrent with chemotherapy) is the treatment of choice for limited-stage SCLC. Limited- and extensive-stage SCLC patients who respond to therapy should also receive prophylactic cranial irradiation (PCI), which treats micrometastatic disease in the CNS. This improves cure rates for limited-stage disease and prolongs survival for extensive stage disease.

Pharmacologic Therapy

Traditional chemotherapy has been the mainstay for most lung cancer patients and will be administered to the large majority of patients, despite recent advances with targeted therapy for patients with EGFR and ALK mutations. Cisplatin and carboplatin are arguably the most effective traditional chemotherapy agents regardless of histology. KEY CONCEPT *Doublet chemotherapy regimens offer superior response rates compared with single-agent chemotherapy regimens and should be used when the patient can tolerate the increased toxicity.* The effective chemotherapy agents that are added to the platinum include etoposide, paclitaxel, docetaxel, gemcitabine, vinorelbine, and pemetrexed (see Table 90–4 for regimen details).

Monoclonal antibodies targeting vascular endothelial growth factor (VEGF) signaling (bevacizumab and ramucirumab), and epidermal growth factor receptor (EGFR; cetuximab and necitumumab) have been combined with traditional chemotherapy to improve outcomes. Tyrosine kinase inhibitors (TKI) targeting EGFR such as afatinib and erlotinib can be appropriate as monotherapy (usually in those patients with an EGFR-activating mutation in exons 19 or 21). Similarly, tyrosine kinase inhibitors targeting an anaplastic leukemia kinase (ALK) gene rearrangement (gene fusions and translocations) can be treated with crizotinib or ceritinib as monotherapy. Selecting the best regimen for a specific patient is aided by patient characteristics (PS, comorbid conditions, etc), extent of tumor spread, histology, and genetics as discussed in more detail below. Preventing and managing therapy induced toxicity (see Chapter 88) is crucial to optimizing patient outcomes (eg, curing, prolonging life, or palliating symptoms). Furthermore, decisions to start chemotherapy must include the full consent and understanding of risks by the patient. Counseling on the therapeutic regimen and risk of toxicity is imperative before dosing. Lung cancer regimens and their associated toxicities are shown in Table 90–4. Refer to Chapter 88 for dosing recommendations in renal and hepatic failure.

Treatment of Small Cell Lung Cancer

SCLC typically presents as extensive disease (approximately 60%–70% of new cases) and progresses very quickly. SCLCs are very responsive to chemotherapy and radiation but have a short duration of response. Radiotherapy became the standard in 1969, when a randomized trial showed that it offered the potential for

Patient Encounter, Part 3

The patient's condition has interfered with her ability to work, but she is able to complete daily activities and has been working to this point, managing her restaurant.

What is this patients ECOG PS score?

Are there any nonpharmacologic interventions you would suggest?

Table 90–4

Chemotherapy Regimens in Lung Cancer and Associated Toxicities[13,17,19,24,33–37]

	Dose	Cycle Length (days)	Neutropenia	
			Grade III (%)	Grade IV (%)
Non–Small Cell				
Paclitaxel–carboplatin–bevacizumab	Carboplatin, dose targeted to AUC of 6 IV (day 1), paclitaxe l200 mg/m^2 IV over 3 hours (day 1), bevacizumab 15 mg/kg IV (day 1)	21		24
Cisplatin–paclitaxel	Paclitaxel 135 mg/m^2 IV over 24 hours (day 1) and cisplatin 75 mg/m^2 IV (day 2)	21	18	57
Cisplatin–docetaxel	Cisplatin 75 mg/m^2 IV (day 1) and docetaxel 75 mg/m^2 IV (day 1)	21	21	48
Cisplatin–gemcitabine	Cisplatin 100 mg/m^2 IV (day 1) and gemcitabine 1000 mg/m^2 IV (days 1, 8, and 15)	28	24	39
Cisplatin–vinorelbine–cetuximab	Cisplatin 80 mg/m^2 (day 1) and vinorelbine 25 mg/m^2 (days 1 and 8) with or without cetuximab 400 mg/m^2 initial dose; then 250 mg/m^2 weekly)	21	14	38
Cisplatin–vinorelbine	Cisplatin 80 mg/m^2 (day 1) and vinorelbine 25 mg/m^2 weekly (days 1 and 8)	21	14	38
Carboplatin–paclitaxel	Carboplatin, dose targeted to AUC of 6 IV (day 1), and paclitaxel 225 mg/m^2 IV over 3 hours (day 1)	21	20	43
Gemcitabine–paclitaxel	Paclitaxel 200 mg/m^2 IV (day 1) and gemcitabine 1000 mg/m^2 (days 1 and 8)	21	10	5
Gemcitabine–docetaxel	Gemcitabine 1100 mg/m^2 IV (days 1 and 8) and docetaxel 100 mg/m^2 IV (day 8)	21	11	11
Gemcitabine	Gemcitabine 1125 mg/m^2 (days 1 and 8)	21		19
Pemetrexed	Pemetrexed 500 mg/m^2 (day 1), vitamin B_{12} 1 mg IM 1–2 weeks before treatment initiation and every 9 weeks thereafter; folic acid 1 mg/day beginning 3 weeks before treatment initiation	21		5–6
Paclitaxel	Paclitaxel 200 mg/m^2 IV over 3 hours (day 1)	21	34	3
Docetaxel	Docetaxel 35 mg/m^2 IV over 1 hour (days 1, 8, 15)	28		5
Small Cell				
EP	Etoposide 100 mg/m^2 IV (days 1–3) and cisplatin 100 mg/m^2 IV (day 2)	28	85	18
CAV	Cyclophosphamide 800 mg/m^2 IV (day 1), doxorubicin 50 mg/m^2 (day 1), and vincristine 1.4 mg/m^2 (maximum, 2 mg) IV (day 1)	21–28	15	72
EC	Etoposide 100 mg/m^2 IV (days 1–3) and carboplatin AUC 5–6 IV (day 1)	21	10–20	5–15
IC	Irinotecan 60 mg/m^2 (days 1, 8, 15) and cisplatin 60 mg/m^2 (day 1)	28	40	25
Topotecan	Topotecan 1.5 mg/m^2 IV over 30 minutes (days 1–5)	21	18	70

	Other Significant Toxicities	Nausea/Vomiting Potential
Non–Small Cell		
Paclitaxel–carboplatin–bevacizumab	Diarrhea, fever, headache, hypertension, hemoptysis, infection, leukopenia, nausea, neuropathy, peripheral neuritis, vomiting, thrombocytopenia, thrombotic events, bleeding, proteinuria	High (day 1 only)
Cisplatin–paclitaxel	Febrile neutropenia or infection, thrombocytopenia, nausea, vomiting, diarrhea, cardiac toxicity, renal toxicity, neuropathy, weakness, hypersensitivity reactions, anemia	High (day 2 only)
Cisplatin–docetaxel	Infection, thrombocytopenia, nausea, vomiting, diarrhea, cardiac, renal, neuropathy, weakness, hypersensitivity, anemia	High (day 1 only)
Cisplatin–gemcitabine	Febrile neutropenia or infection, thrombocytopenia, nausea, vomiting, diarrhea, cardiac, renal, neuropathy, weakness, anemia	High (day 1) mild (days 8/15)
Cisplatin–vinorelbine–cetuximab	Infection, thrombocytopenia, rash, constipation, neuropathy, hepatotoxicity	High (day 1 only)
Cisplatin–vinorelbine	Neutropenia, infection, anorexia, thrombocytopenia, nausea, vomiting, dyspnea, constipation, neuropathy, anemia	High (days 1 and 8)
Carboplatin–paclitaxel	Infection, thrombocytopenia, nausea, vomiting, diarrhea, cardiac, renal, neuropathy, weakness, hypersensitivity, anemia	High (day 1 only)
Gemcitabine–paclitaxel	Alopecia, nausea and vomiting, neurotoxicity, thrombocytopenia	Moderate
Gemcitabine–docetaxel	Nausea and vomiting, diarrhea, thrombocytopenia, asthenia, neurotoxicity	Moderate
Gemcitabine	Thrombocytopenia	Mild
Pemetrexed	Anemia	Mild
Paclitaxel	Infection, nausea, vomiting, diarrhea, mucositis, arthralgia, asthenia, peripheral neuropathy, alopecia, cardiovascular	Mild (day 1 only)
Docetaxel	Fatigue, nausea, vomiting, skin toxicity, neuropathy, anemia, hypersensitivity, alopecia	Mild

(Continued)

Table 90–4

Chemotherapy Regimens in Lung Cancer and Associated Toxicities[13,17,19,24,33–37] (Continued)

Small Cell

	Other Significant Toxicities	Nausea/Vomiting Potential
EP	Infection, nausea, vomiting, thrombocytopenia, anemia	High (day 2 only)
CAV	Nausea, vomiting, thrombocytopenia, neuropathy, hepatic, renal, alopecia	High
EC	Infection, thrombocytopenia, alopecia	High (day 1 only)
IC	Fever, infection, thrombocytopenia, anemia, diarrhea, nausea and vomiting, elevated liver enzymes	High (day 1), moderate (days 8/15)
Topotecan	Neutropenic fever, neutropenic sepsis, anemia, thrombocytopenia, nausea, fatigue, vomiting, stomatitis, anorexia, diarrhea, fever	Mild (days 1–5)

AUC, area under the curve; CAV, cyclophosphamide–doxorubicin–vincristine; EC, etoposide–carboplatin; EP, etoposide–cisplatin; IC, irinotecan–cisplatin; IM, intramuscular; IV, intravenous.

See Chapter 88 for dose reductions for hepatic and renal dysfunction.

cure, whereas surgery did not.[12] In the vast majority of patients, chemotherapy with or without radiotherapy is the treatment of choice. Even after a complete response to therapy, the cancer usually recurs within 6 to 8 months, and the survival time following recurrence is typically short (~ 4 months). This yields an average survival rate of 14 to 20 months for limited disease and 8 to 13 months for extensive disease.[13] Figure 90–2 illustrates the general treatment path of SCLC.

▸ *Limited Disease*

The regimen of choice for limited-disease SCLC is etoposide–cisplatin (EP). In patients who are able to tolerate combined modality therapy, concomitant chemoradiotherapy offers the greatest survival benefit. Carboplatin may be substituted for cisplatin in patients who cannot tolerate cisplatin toxicity. Cisplatin is preferred over carboplatin because of a small study that randomized patients to cisplatin or carboplatin plus etoposide. There was a numerically higher complete response rate with cisplatin, which is believed to be requisite for cure. Consequently, the guidelines recommend that the EP regimen be used with concurrent radiotherapy.[13]

Because patients with SCLC commonly have a recurrence in the CNS, trials have been performed to evaluate the benefit of PCI. A pivotal study showed that PCI reduces the incidence of brain metastasis and increases the 3-year survival rate from 15% to 21%.[14] Patients with limited stage SCLC who achieve a complete response with treatment should be offered PCI.

▸ *Extensive Disease*

Platinum regimens, particularly EP, are the treatment of choice in extensive disease. In one Japanese study, a combination of irinotecan and cisplatin demonstrated an increased median survival time by approximately 3 months over the EP regimen. This irinotecan–cisplatin regimen also had a lower incidence of severe neutropenic side effects but exhibited higher rates of middle- to high-grade diarrhea. However, this study was repeated in the United States and did not show a similar improvement over the EP regimen.[15] Therefore, EP remains the regimen of choice for treating extensive SCLC in the United States. Because of the high sensitivity of treatment-naïve SCLC to chemotherapy, it is imperative that these patients be monitored for signs of tumor lysis syndrome and possibly treated with prophylactic therapy.

Concurrent radiotherapy is not used routinely in extensive disease; however, PCI provides significant benefit in patients responding to chemotherapy. A pivotal study demonstrated that median survival from the time of randomization increased from 5.4 to 6.7 months and 1-year survival rates increased from 13.3% to 27.1% with PCI. An additional benefit was a lower rate of brain metastases (14.6% vs 40.4%).[16]

▸ *Recurrent Disease*

The treatment of recurrent SCLC depends on the time to recurrence. If the time to recurrence is less than 6 months, second-line therapy should be considered if the patient has an acceptable PS (see Patient Care Process). The most widely accepted second-line therapies in SCLC are topotecan alone or CAV (cyclophosphamide, doxorubicin [Adriamycin], and vincristine). Relapses occurring more than 6 months after treatment warrant a repeat of the initial regimen. Patients with a poor PS (3–4) are typically managed with best supportive care, including palliative care therapies.

Treatment of Non–Small Cell Lung Cancer

The first step in treatment of NSCLC involves confirmation of the clinical stage and determination of likelihood of resection of the tumor. When the histology results are not of squamous cell histology (adenocarcinoma and large cell), tissue should be sent for genetic analysis of EGFR mutations and ALK rearrangement. Treatment options depend on the stage of disease (ie, eligibility for resection), PS, histology, and genetic findings.

▸ *Local Disease (Stages 1A, 1B, and IIA)*

Local disease encompasses stages IA through IIA and is associated with a favorable prognosis because approximately 40% to 60% of patients are expected to live more than 5 years from diagnosis. Goals of therapy are curative in local disease, and surgery is the mainstay of treatment regardless of histology or genetics. Stage IA tumors are rarely seen clinically and may be treated with surgery alone. If surgical margins are positive, radiotherapy or re-resection is recommended.[17] Stage IB, IIA, and locally advanced IIB NSCLC are treated with adjuvant chemotherapy. The rationale behind adjuvant chemotherapy is to eradicate micrometastases or other tumor cells that may have been missed during removal of the primary tumor. The recent results of five relatively large prospective trials suggest that there is benefit

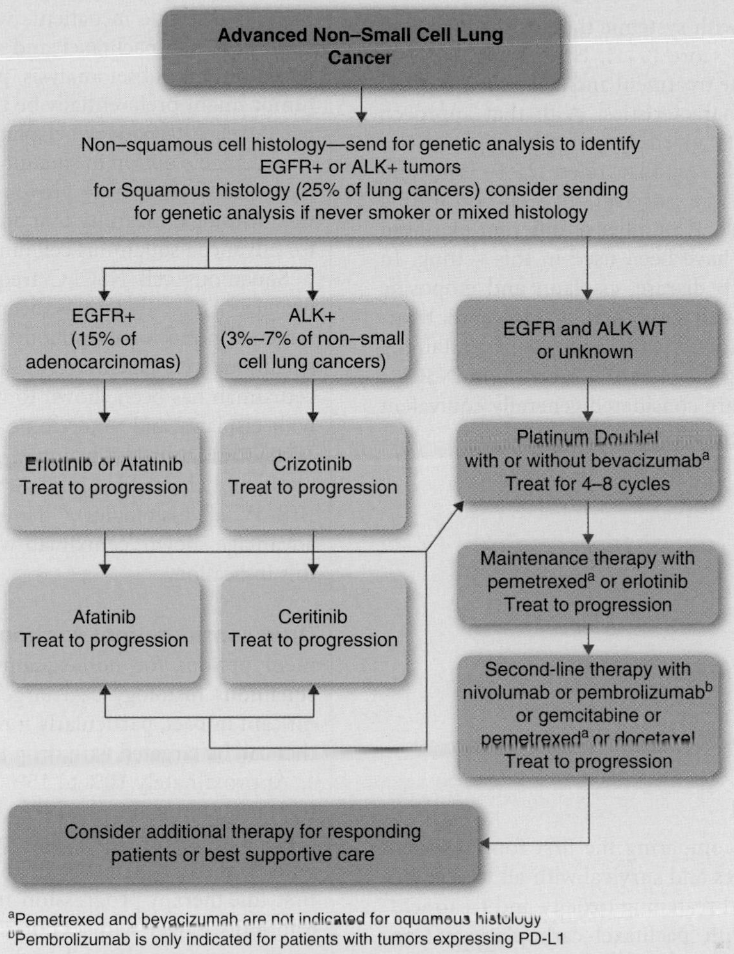

FIGURE 90–2. Advanced stage non–small cell lung cancer treatment algorithm.[13] Reproduced, with permission, from NCCN Practice Guidelines in Oncology: Non-Small Cell Lung Cancer. National Comprehensive Cancer Network; 2015; v.1.2016. www.nccn.org. Accessed November 9, 2015.

from adjuvant (postsurgical) chemotherapy leading to a survival advantage of 4% to 15%.[18,19] Consequently, adjuvant therapy has become the standard of care in resectable NSCLC and should be offered to patients after resection, particularly those with stage II or III disease.

Although the regimen of choice is unclear, studies evaluating pemetrexed in squamous cell histology demonstrate that it has minimal to no activity in this subtype. Thus, regimens containing pemetrexed should be avoided in patients with squamous cell histology. Based on prospective randomized trials, cisplatin–vinorelbine appears to be the regimen with the most evidence regardless of histology and genetics.

▶ *Locally Advanced Disease (Stages IIB and IIIA)*

Patients with locally advanced disease should also be considered for surgery, which would be followed with adjuvant treatment as outlined in local disease. However, neoadjuvant (aka. induction) chemotherapy could also be considered before surgery. The rationale behind neoadjuvant therapy is to decrease the size of the tumor so that it can be extracted more easily with clean margins, as well as to eliminate distant micrometastases before invasive local treatment. Meta-analysis of neoadjuvant trials suggests that neoadjuvant chemotherapy in all early stages improves 5-year survival by 5%.[20] However, the methods used in many of these studies did not give adjuvant chemotherapy, which could also improve survival by about the same degree. One concern of giving neoadjuvant therapy is that the toxicity of induction regimens may delay surgery, and if the tumor does not respond to the treatment, there is a risk of disease progression. Nonetheless, current data suggest that more than 90% of patients who are treated with neoadjuvant therapy maintain their scheduled surgery.[21] The utilization of neoadjuvant chemotherapy is inconsistent, but is most common in patients with locally advanced tumors (stage III).[22] Neoadjuvant chemotherapy regimens are platinum-based doublets that do not include a targeted therapy (see Table 90–4). None of the large studies prospectively controlled/individualized therapy choices based on histology or genetics, which could improve results. Three cycles of carboplatin and paclitaxel administered on a 3-week schedule is a common and supported approach. The benefit of combining neoadjuvant therapy and surgery with additional adjuvant therapy is being investigated but is of unknown value at this time. Relatively small studies have evaluated using three treatment modalities (chemotherapy, radiation, and surgery) to two treatment modalities (chemotherapy and radiation). Improvements have been shown for progression-free survival, but not overall survival. Consequently, the value of trimodal therapy is unknown and does not have a clear role.

► *Advanced or Metastatic Disease (Stages IIIB and IV)*

Advanced disease is treated with systemic therapy if the patient has an acceptable ECOG PS score (0–1). Historically, patients with NSCLC received the same treatment and had a similar prognosis regardless of tumor characteristics. With that approach platinum-containing doublets given for four to eight cycles produced the highest overall response rates (25%–35%) and survival times (30%–40% 1-year survival) in well-performing patients with advanced disease. A number of different platinum doublet treatment regimens have been used in this setting. In some patients with stage IIIB disease, cisplatin and etoposide may be given concurrently with radiotherapy. However, treating unresectable stage III patients with a platinum-containing doublet regimen and omitting the radiation is common. NSCLC chemotherapy doublets that are considered generally equivalent include:

- Paclitaxel–cisplatin
- Paclitaxel–carboplatin
- Cisplatin–gemcitabine
- Cisplatin–docetaxel
- Carboplatin–docetaxel
- Cisplatin–vinorelbine
- Gemcitabine–paclitaxel
- Gemcitabine–docetaxel
- Cisplatin–pemetrexed
- Carboplatin-nab-paclitaxel

A large randomized trial comparing the first four regimens reported similar response rates and survival with all treatments, although there were less life-threatening toxicity and treatment-related deaths associated with paclitaxel–carboplatin.[23] Consequently, some argued that paclitaxel–carboplatin was the treatment of choice.

Individualized treatment is now the standard approach. Beyond patient characteristics, tumor histology and genetic analysis (in non–squamous cell histology) for activating EGFR mutations and ALK rearrangements guide treatment selection (see Figure 90–2).

Drug Considerations for Squamous Cell NSCLC There are specific drug considerations that must be made with squamous histology. In squamous NSCLC, pemetrexed is associated with decreased efficacy. This is true for combination studies as well as monotherapy studies and the inactivity with this histology is reflected in current treatment guidelines. Furthermore, bevacizumab is associated with an increased risk of fatal hemorrhage in squamous NSCLC. In the randomized phase II study that included 13 patients with squamous cell histology, four had a life-threatening bleeds, which led to the exclusion of this population in the phase III trial. Tumor EGFR activating mutations and ALK rearrangements can identify patient most likely to respond to TKI-targeted therapy. Since the incidence of these mutations in squamous cell histology is so low, current guidelines do not recommend testing squamous cell tumors for these mutations. Although these guiding factors are well established, the best combination is still unclear. Based on subset analysis of randomized controlled trials, it appears that gemcitabine and albumin-bound nanoparticle paclitaxel (nab-paclitaxel) have greater activity in squamous histology. The recent randomized trial comparing carboplatin with nab-paclitaxel versus carboplatin with traditional paclitaxel did not find a difference in overall survival (including the squamous histology subset); however, the response rate in patients with squamous cell histology was 41% with nab-paclitaxel and 24% with traditional paclitaxel. Based on this subset analysis, patients who have a symptomatic tumor might preferentially be treated with carboplatin and nab-paclitaxel. Alternatively, cisplatin and gemcitabine appear to be an acceptable option in squamous NSCLC, although no randomized clinical trials have proven an overall survival advantage in this histology, meaning that any platinum doublet is acceptable for advanced squamous cell lung cancer.

Squamous cell NSCLC frequently overexpresses the EGFR protein. Thus, there has been interest in adding an EGFR-targeted monoclonal antibody with chemotherapy for advanced squamous cell NSCLC. The anti-EGFR monoclonal antibody cetuximab has been shown to improve survival when combined with cisplatin and vinorelbine. The FLEX trial demonstrated a 1.2-month survival advantage of cetuximab when added to cisplatin and vinorelbine in recurrent or metastatic NSCLC (stages IIIB–IV all histologies).[24] However, despite the small survival advantage shown, cetuximab was not approved by the FDA for this indication.

Drug considerations for non–squamous cell NSCLC Treatment options for non–squamous histology are broader than squamous histology and targeted therapies are making a significant impact, particularly for patients with a genetic alteration that can be targeted with drug therapy.

Approximately 10% to 15% of NSCLC patients have tumors with mutations in exon 19 and/or 21 in the EGFR gene. These mutations define a population likely to respond to treatment with EGFR TKIs (erlotinib or afatinib). In this population, first-line therapy progression-free survival is approximately 4 to 6 months longer with EGFR TKIs than platinum-doublet chemotherapy. Since afatinib and erlotinib have not been compared in a randomized trial, it is not possible to determine which one is better. However, there is evidence that afatinib works in EGFR-mutant tumors in patients who fail erlotinib or have an exon 20 T790M mutant (which predicts resistance to erlotinib). Based on these data, patients who are started on erlotinib, respond, and then progress can be treated with afatinib although going straight to chemotherapy may still be considered the standard. Since there are no data showing that patients who recur after afatinib will respond to erlotinib, patients failing afatinib first line should then go on to treatment with chemotherapy like genetic wild-type adenocarcinoma patients (see Figure 90–2).

Crizotinib is a new targeted therapy that was designed for a subset of patients with an ALK rearrangement (ALK+; ~ 5% of patients). It received accelerated approval based on a single-arm trial in the salvage setting that resulted in a 55% survival rate at 2 years.[25] Despite the lack of data in the first-line setting, the NCCN guidelines recommend that patients with a known ALK rearrangement can be treated with crizotinib in the first-line setting. Response rates are approximately 60% with a progression free survival of 8 to 10 months, and most patients have a recurrence within 12 months. Ceritinib was recently approved for patients who fail crizotinib. In this setting about half of patients respond and the duration of response is approximately 7 months. Although neither have been tested in a randomized trial as first-line therapy or against each other, based on the data and guidelines; ALK+ patients should receive first-line crizotinib, then ceritinib, and then start treatment with chemotherapy like genetic wild-type adenocarcinoma patients (see Figure 90–2).

Table 90–5

Molecularly Targeted Agents in Lung Cancer

Agent	Target	FDA-Approved in Lung Cancer	Genetic or Histologic Indication	Contraindication	Dosage	Regimen
Erlotinib	EGFR	Yes	EGFR mutations in exons 19 and 21	EGFR mutations in exon 20	150 mg orally daily	Single agent
Cetuximab	EGFR	No, used off-label	EGFR expression		400 mg/m² IV day 1, then 250 mg m² weekly thereafter	Cisplatin and vinorelbine
Afatinib	EGFR	Yes	EGFR mutations (all)		40 mg orally daily	Single agent
Bevacizumab	VEGF	Yes		Squamous cell histology	15 mg/kg IV day 1 of a 3 week cycle	Carboplatin and paclitaxel
Necitumumab	EGFR	No, investigational drug	Squamous cell histology		800 mg IV days 1 and 8 of a 3-week cycle	Gemcitabine and cisplatin
Ramucirumab	VEGFR2	Yes	Can be used in squamous cell histology		10 mg/kg IV day 1 of a 3-week cycle	Docetaxel
Crizotinib	ALK, cMET, ROS1	Yes	ALK-rearranged (translocations and fusions)		250 mg orally twice daily	Single agent
Ceritinib	ALK	Yes	ALK-rearranged (translocations and fusions) can be used in crizotinib-resistant patients		750 mg orally daily	Single agent

In summary, targeted therapy as monotherapy or in combination with chemotherapy has become a mainstay in first-line treatment of advanced NSCLC. Targeted agents utilized in NSCLC are presented in Table 90–5.

Special Populations

Patients who cannot tolerate platinum can be treated with gemcitabine–paclitaxel or gemcitabine–docetaxel. Randomized trials have produced response durations and survival times similar to the platinum-containing doublet regimens. However, these regimens are only recommended for patients who are unlikely to tolerate the toxicity of platinum regimens owing to comorbidities or other factors.[26]

Poorly performing patients, defined as those with a PS of 2 is a subject of debate. Although patients with a PS of 2 typically have inferior survival rates and higher toxicity to platinum chemotherapy than higher performing patients, low-toxicity single-agent regimens may offer a survival advantage in this subset. Use of these regimens also presents a method of providing symptomatic care for advanced stage patients. Agents such as pemetrexed, gemcitabine, and docetaxel may be used in this scenario. In patients with a PS of 3 or 4, chemotherapy typically results in high rates of toxicity and fails to convey a survival benefit. Consequently, treatment should be aimed at relief of symptoms instead of a definitive cure. Because targeted agents typically have lower rates of severe toxicity, they also have been used in appropriate subsets of patients with a poor PS (ECOG PS of 2 or 3). Unfortunately, we do not adequate clinical trial data regarding the efficacy and toxicity of targeted agents in these patients. In summary, debilitated patients should not be treated with combination chemotherapy with or without targeted agents because of historically high rates of toxicity without benefit. Single-agent therapy with less toxicity can be used to help palliate symptoms.

Duration of Therapy

Because advanced stage NSCLC is not curable, an argument can be made that the goal is to extend the number of quality days, rather than just overall survival. With this goal in mind and an assumption that quality of life is lower during chemotherapy treatment, it is important to consider the duration of therapy. Over the last decade, treatment has moved toward fewer chemotherapy cycles. Typical therapy regimens have decreased from planning eight cycles to six cycles, to four cycles, which was the standard until several years ago. It was at this time that positive data were reported from two studies using pemetrexed, erlotinib, and bevacizumab as maintenance therapy. Both key studies included patients who had a response or stable disease after four cycles of a platinum-based doublet who were then randomized to placebo or treatment.[27] The pemetrexed study reported a 3-month survival advantage with maintenance therapy. A subgroup analysis of this study demonstrated that patients with squamous histology did not benefit from therapy leaving an overall survival benefit of 5 months for the non–squamous cell group. Similarly, the erlotinib maintenance study reported a 1-month overall survival advantage, which does not appear as robust; however, the subset analysis showed benefit was much more likely in nonsmokers and those with adenocarcinoma histology and particularly in patients who had an activating mutation (exon 19 or 21). Similar to the pemetrexed study, patients whose tumor was of squamous cell histology did not appear to benefit from maintenance. In summary, the duration of therapy depends highly on histology; patients with squamous cell histology will likely be treated for four cycles, but patients with non–squamous cell histology will be treated until progression.[27]

▶ *Recurrent and Progressive Disease*

Although patients frequently experience a response to initial therapy, disease recurs in most cases. If the recurrence is

Patient Encounter, Part 4

The patient undergoes surgery for her disease, which is successful, with negative margins. After 1 year, however, the patient returns for routine follow-up and is found to have recurrent disease, with metastases present in both the brain and in the liver. Molecular diagnostics reveals an ALK rearrangement (ALK-EML4 translocation/fusion).

What is the patient's new clinical stage?

Discuss the significance of the genetic alteration identified in the tumor.

Based on the information provided, develop a care plan for this patient. Include (a) treatment goals, (b) monitoring parameters for anticipated toxicities, and (c) a follow-up plan to determine response to treatment and surveillance.

Patient Care Process

Patient Assessment:

- Determine stage and histology of cancer.
- Perform mutation analysis if clinically indicated.

Therapy Evaluation:

- Evaluate the appropriateness of a patient's regimen at every visit (every week, 3 weeks, or 4 weeks).
- Inquire about toxicity or issues.
- Include a medication reconciliation process.
- Laboratory and/or radiology evaluations can be prompted by the initial assessment or at a scheduled interval for the treatment regimen.
- Findings of tumor growth or significant toxicity should prompt a change in the therapeutic plan.

Care Plan Development:

- Grade and monitor toxicity—Grade 3 or 4 toxicity (see Chapter 88) requires a change in therapy with the next cycle of treatment. Common changes include a chemotherapy dose reduction or pharmacologic intervention to prevent or treat the toxicity.
- Manage toxicity—KEY CONCEPT *Knowing when and how to treat adverse events from chemotherapy is an important aspect of patient care. Unmanaged events may cause delays in chemotherapy administration and reduced chemotherapy doses and may contribute to treatment failure.* This includes managing neutropenic episodes (See Chapter 99) and chemotherapy-induced nausea and vomiting (see Chapter 99). The emetogenic potential of selected chemotherapy regimens are listed in Chapter 99.
- Counsel patients on appropriate use and adherence of oral medications.

Follow-Up Evaluation:

- Monitor for recurrence. Follow recommendations of the NCCN, as outlined in Outcome Evaluation.
- Smoking cessation plans. For NSCLC patients, all long-term care plans should include options and recommendations for smoking cessation (see Chapter 36).

localized, surgery options may be assessed. If the patient's PS remains acceptable (0–1), second-line systemic chemotherapy has been shown to improve survival. Although platinum doublets may be used at this point in care, a single-agent therapy with docetaxel, pemetrexed, erlotinib, or crizotinib is recommended, depending on the tumor genotype.[25,28] A recent phase III trial tested the addition of ramucirumab (a VEGFR2-targeted monoclonal antibody) to docetaxel as second-line therapy regardless of histology. The results show that ramucirumab increases overall survival and progression-free survival by approximately 1.5 months.[29] Currently ramucirumab is not approved for lung cancer, but is approved for gastric cancer and might be used off label with docetaxel.

Recurrences in poorly performing patients (3–4) usually are not treated with chemotherapy and are instead treated with supportive care. Additional recurrences (eg, third-line therapy) may be treated with single-agent therapy not previously used or best supportive care.

Progression on targeted TKIs such as erlotinib or crizotinib in appropriately (genetically) selected patients after an initial response occurs frequently. This phenomenon is a sign of acquired resistance of the tumor to the molecular effects of the agent. Order of therapy for TKIs is discussed previously in "Drug considerations for non–squamous cell NSCLC." An overwhelming amount of clinical and preclinical data suggests that patients with molecularly targetable tumors should never lose the opportunity to be treated with TKIs, and perhaps the best opportunity of maintaining quality of life and survival is to enroll in clinical trials testing these second-generation agents. Furthermore, it is important to note that patients who initially benefit from erlotinib and acquire resistance to therapy may benefit from retreatment with erlotinib after other lines of therapy.

OUTCOME EVALUATION

Evaluating outcomes is a goal-oriented process and should begin from that perspective. Patients with localized disease are treated with localized therapy with or without systemic therapy with curative intent as the goal. Monitoring for toxicity and recurrence on a regular basis is essential.

Following surgery or pharmacologic treatment, the patient should be monitored regularly to detect recurrence or progression of disease. Methods include a physical examination and chest x-ray every 3 to 4 months for 2 years. If no disease is detected during this time, follow-up frequency can be prolonged to every 6 months for 3 years and then annually. Low-dose spiral CT scanning is also recommended annually.

Smoking cessation counseling with or without pharmacologic treatment should be a priority. Although studies have shown that patients who continue to smoke through treatment in NSCLC do not perform more poorly compared with those that quit before treatment, those who respond to treatment and continue to smoke probably have an increased risk of developing secondary malignancies.[30] In contrast to NSCLC, some data suggest that SCLC patients with limited stage disease have poorer outcomes if they continue to smoke during treatment.[31]

For those with advanced disease, the goal of treatment is to prolong the duration of life, particularly the number of quality days. Ultimately, most lung cancer patients succumb to their disease. Palliative care involves management of symptoms and improvement of quality of life when curative treatment options are no longer available. Often, problematic metastases can be removed by surgery (depending on location) or can be treated with radiotherapy to reduce tumor size. In selecting options at this point in treatment, it is important to keep the goals of therapy (ie, maximizing the duration and quality of life) in mind. Low-toxicity single-agent chemotherapy, targeted therapy, and best supportive care (including fatigue and pain management) are commonly the mainstays of palliative care.

Abbreviations Introduced in This Chapter

5-FDG	5-Fluorodeoxyglucose
ALK	Anaplastic lymphoma kinase
CAV	Cyclophosphamide, doxorubicin [Adriamycin], vincristine
CT	Computed tomography
ECOG	Eastern Cooperative Oncology Group
EGF	Epidermal growth factor
EGFR	Epidermal growth factor receptor
EML4	Echinoderm microtubule-associated protein-like 4
EP	Etoposide, cisplatin
ETS	Environmental tobacco smoke
NSCLC	Non–small cell lung cancer
PCI	Prophylactic cranial irradiation
PET	Positron-emission tomography
PS	Performance status
SCLC	Small cell lung cancer
TNM	Tumor, node, and metastasis staging
VEGF	Vascular endothelial-derived growth factor
VEGFR	Vascular endothelial-derived growth factor receptor

REFERENCES

1. Siegel R, Ma J, Zou Z, Jemal A. Cancer statistics, 2014. CA Cancer J Clin. 2014 Jan-Feb;64(1):9–29.
2. Alberg AJ, Brock MV, Samet JM. Epidemiology of lung cancer: Looking to the future. J Clin Oncol. 2005 May 10;23(14): 3175–3185.
3. Westmaas JL, Brandon TH. Reducing risk in smokers. Curr Opin Pulm Med. 2004 Jul;10(4):284–288.
4. Ginsberg MS. Epidemiology of lung cancer. Semin Roentgenol. 2005 Apr;40(2):83–89.
5. Buchner FL, Bueno-de-Mesquita HB, Ros MM, et al. Variety in fruit and vegetable consumption and the risk of lung cancer in the European prospective investigation into cancer and nutrition. Cancer Epidemiol Biomarkers Prev. 2010 Sep;19(9):2278–2286.
6. Karp DD, Lee SJ, Keller SM, et al. Randomized, double-blind, placebo-controlled, phase III chemoprevention trial of selenium supplementation in patients with resected stage I non-small-cell lung cancer: ECOG 5597. J Clin Oncol. 2013 Nov 20;31(33):4179–4187.
7. Mao JT, Roth MD, Fishbein MC, et al. Lung cancer chemoprevention with celecoxib in former smokers. Cancer Prev Res (Phila). 2011 Jul;4(7):984–993.
8. Micke P, Faldum A, Metz T, et al. Staging small cell lung cancer: Veterans Administration Lung Study Group versus International Association for the Study of Lung Cancer—what limits limited disease? Lung Cancer 2002 Sep;37(3):271–276.
9. Fox W, Scadding JG. Medical Research Council comparative trial of surgery and radiotherapy for primary treatment of small-celled or oat-celled carcinoma of bronchus. Ten-year follow-up. Lancet. 1973 Jul 14;2(7820):63–65.
10. Jeremic B, Shibamoto Y, Acimovic L, Milisavljevic S. Hyperfractionated radiotherapy for clinical stage II non-small cell lung cancer. Radiother Oncol. 1999 May;51(2):141–145.
11. Spira A, Ettinger DS. Multidisciplinary Management of Lung Cancer. N Engl J Med. 2004 January 22;350(4):379–392.
12. Miller AB, Fox W, Tall R. Five-year follow-up of the Medical Research Council comparative trial of surgery and radiotherapy for the primary treatment of small-celled or oat-celled carcinoma of the bronchus. Lancet. 1969 Sep 6;2(7619):501–505.
13. NCCN Practice Guidelines in Oncology: Non-Small Cell Lung Cancer. National Comprehensive Cancer Network; 2015; v.1.2016. www.nccn.org. Accessed November 9, 2015.
14. Auperin A, Arriagada R, Pignon JP, et al. Prophylactic cranial irradiation for patients with small-cell lung cancer in complete remission. Prophylactic Cranial Irradiation Overview Collaborative Group. N Engl J Med. 1999 Aug 12;341(7):476–484.
15. Hanna N, Bunn PA, Jr., Langer C, et al. Randomized phase III trial comparing irinotecan/cisplatin with etoposide/cisplatin in patients with previously untreated extensive-stage disease small-cell lung cancer. J Clin Oncol. 2006 May 1;24(13):2038–2043.
16. Slotman B, Faivre-Finn C, Kramer G, et al. Prophylactic cranial irradiation in extensive small-cell lung cancer. N Engl J Med. 2007 Aug 16;357(7):664–672.
17. NCCN Practice Guidelines in Oncology: Non-small cell lung cancer. National Comprehensive Cancer Network; 2014 [updated 2014; cited 2014 Sept 1]; v.2.2014. www.nccn.org.
18. Arriagada R, Bergman B, Dunant A, et al. Cisplatin-based adjuvant chemotherapy in patients with completely resected non-small-cell lung cancer. N Engl J Med. 2004 Jan 22;350(4): 351–360.
19. Winton T, Livingston R, Johnson D, et al. Vinorelbine plus cisplatin vs. observation in resected non-small-cell lung cancer. N Engl J Med. 2005 Jun 23;352(25):2589–2597.
20. Preoperative chemotherapy for non-small-cell lung cancer: A systematic review and meta-analysis of individual participant data. Lancet. 2014 May 3;383(9928):1561–1571.
21. Belani CP. Adjuvant and neoadjuvant therapy in non-small cell lung cancer. Semin Oncol. 2005 Apr;32(2 Suppl 2):S9–S15.
22. De Marinis F, Gebbia V, De Petris L. Neoadjuvant chemotherapy for stage IIIA-N2 non-small cell lung cancer. Ann Oncol. 2005 May;16 Suppl 4:iv116–iv122.
23. Schiller JH, Harrington D, Belani CP, et al. Comparison of four chemotherapy regimens for advanced non-small-cell lung cancer. N Engl J Med. 2002 Jan 10;346(2):92–98.
24. Cetuximab plus chemotherapy in patients with advanced non-small-cell lung cancer (FLEX): an open-label randomised phase III trial. Pirker R, Pereira JR, Szczesna A, von Pawel J, Krzakowski M, Ramlau R, Vynnychenko I, Park K, Yu CT, Ganul V, Roh JK, Bajetta E, O'Byrne K, de Marinis F, Eberhardt W, Goddemeier T, Emig M, Gatzemeier U; FLEX Study Team. Lancet. 2009 May 2;373(9674):1525–31. doi: 10.1016/S0140-6736(09)60569-9.
25. Shaw AT, Yeap BY, Solomon BJ, et al. Effect of crizotinib on overall survival in patients with advanced non-small-cell lung cancer harbouring ALK gene rearrangement: A retrospective analysis. Lancet Oncol. 2011 Oct;12(11):1004–1012.
26. Azzoli CG, Baker S, Jr., Temin S, et al. American Society of Clinical Oncology Clinical Practice Guideline update on chemotherapy for stage IV non-small-cell lung cancer. J Clin Oncol. 2009 Dec 20;27(36):6251–6266.
27. Stinchcombe TE, Socinski MA. Maintenance therapy in advanced non-small cell lung cancer: Current status and future implications. J Thorac Oncol. 2011 Jan;6(1):174–182.
28. Pfister DG, Johnson DH, Azzoli CG, et al. American Society of Clinical Oncology treatment of unresectable non-small-cell lung

cancer guideline: Update 2003. J Clin Oncol. 2004 January 15, 2004;22(2):330–353.
29. Garon EB, Ciuleanu TE, Arrieta O, et al. Ramucirumab plus docetaxel versus placebo plus docetaxel for second-line treatment of stage IV non-small-cell lung cancer after disease progression on platinum-based therapy (REVEL): A multicentre, double-blind, randomised phase 3 trial. Lancet. 2014 Aug 23;384(9944):665–673.
30. Tsao AS, Liu D, Lee JJ, et al. Smoking affects treatment outcome in patients with advanced nonsmall cell lung cancer. Cancer. 2006 Jun 1;106(11):2428–2436.
31. Videtic GM, Stitt LW, Dar AR, et al. Continued cigarette smoking by patients receiving concurrent chemoradiotherapy for limited-stage small-cell lung cancer is associated with decreased survival. J Clin Oncol. 2003 Apr 15;21(8):1544–1549.
32. Ruckdeschel JC, Schwartz AG, Bepler G, et al. Cancer of the Lung: NSCLC and SCLC. In: Abeloff MD, Armitage JO, Niederhuber JE, Kastan MB, McKenna WG, editors. Clinical Oncology, 3rd ed. Orlando: Churchill Livingston; 2004.
33. Hanna N, Shepherd FA, Fossella FV, et al. Randomized phase III trial of pemetrexed versus docetaxel in patients with non-small-cell lung cancer previously treated with chemotherapy. J Clin Oncol. 2004 May 1;22(9):1589–1597.
34. Kosmidis P, Mylonakis N, Nicolaides C, et al. Paclitaxel plus carboplatin versus gemcitabine plus paclitaxel in advanced non-small-cell lung cancer: A phase III randomized trial. J Clin Oncol. 2002 Sep 1;20(17):3578–3585.
35. Noda K, Nishiwaki Y, Kawahara M, et al. Irinotecan plus cisplatin compared with etoposide plus cisplatin for extensive small-cell lung cancer. N Engl J Med. 2002 Jan 10;346(2):85–91.
36. Scagliotti GV, Kortsik C, Dark GG, et al. Pemetrexed combined with oxaliplatin or carboplatin as first-line treatment in advanced non-small cell lung cancer: A multicenter, randomized, phase II trial. Clin Cancer Res. 2005 Jan 15;11(2 Pt 1):690–696.
37. Shepherd FA, Dancey J, Ramlau R, et al. Prospective randomized trial of docetaxel versus best supportive care in patients with non-small-cell lung cancer previously treated with platinum-based chemotherapy. J Clin Oncol. 2000 May;18(10):2095–2103.

91 Colorectal Cancer

Emily B. Borders and Patrick J. Medina

LEARNING OBJECTIVES

Upon completion of the chapter, the reader will be able to:

1. Identify the risk factors for colorectal cancer.
2. Recognize the signs and symptoms of colorectal cancer.
3. Describe the treatment options for colorectal cancer based on patient-specific factors, such as stage of disease, age of patient, genetic mutations, and previous treatment received.
4. Outline the pharmacologic principles for agents used to treat colorectal cancer.
5. Develop a monitoring plan to assess the efficacy and toxicity of agents used in colorectal cancer.
6. Educate patients about the adverse effects of chemotherapy that require specific patient counseling.
7. Outline preventive and screening strategies for individuals at average and high risk for colorectal cancer

INTRODUCTION

Colorectal cancer is one of the four most common cancers diagnosed in the United States and includes cancers of the colon and rectum. In 2015, an estimated 139,970 new cases of colon cancer with an estimated 50,710 deaths, making colorectal cancer the second leading cause of cancer-related deaths in the United States.[1] The prognosis is primarily determined by the stage of disease with the majority of patients with early stage (I or II) disease cured. Treatment options for colorectal cancer include surgery, radiation, chemotherapy, and targeted molecular therapies.

EPIDEMIOLOGY AND ETIOLOGY

Colorectal cancer occurs more frequently in industrialized regions such as North America and Europe, while the lowest rates are seen in less-developed areas, suggesting that environmental and dietary factors influence the development of colorectal cancer. In addition to environmental factors, colorectal cancers develop more frequently in certain families, and genetic predisposition to this cancer is well known.

The incidence of colorectal cancer in men is approximately 1.5 times greater than observed in women. Overall, colon and rectal cancers make up approximately 12% of all cancer diagnoses in men and women in the United States. The median age at diagnosis is 68 years with very few cases occurring in individuals younger than 45 years of age.[2] KEY CONCEPT *Age appears to be the biggest risk factor for the development of colorectal cancer with 70% of cases diagnosed in adults older than 65 years of age.*

Although still the second leading cause of cancer death, mortality rates for colorectal cancer have declined over the past 30 years as a result of better, and increasingly used screening modalities, and more effective treatments.

RISK FACTORS

In addition to age, dietary or environmental factors, inflammatory bowel disease, and genetic susceptibility increase the risk of colorectal cancer. Table 91–1 lists well-known risk factors for developing colorectal cancer.

KEY CONCEPT *Diets high in fat and low in fiber are associated with increased colorectal cancer risk.* While data is not entirely consistent, long-term consumption of red and processed meats is associated with an increased risk of colorectal cancer. A large pooled analysis of 13 prospective cohort studies found dietary fiber intake to be inversely associated with the risk of colorectal cancer; however, upon multivariate analysis for other dietary risk factors, the benefit was no longer observed.[3] This analysis does not consider for the known benefits of a fiber-rich diet for noncancerous conditions such as diabetes and coronary artery disease.

Foods that are high in fiber include vegetables, fruit, grains, and cereals. The protective effects of fiber may be a result of reduced absorption of carcinogens in the bowel, reduced bowel transit time, or a reduction in dietary fat intake associated with high-fiber diets.[3]

Physical inactivity and elevated body mass index (BMI) are associated with up to a twofold increase in the risk of colorectal cancer. Decreased bowel transit time and exercise-induced alterations in body glucose, insulin levels, and other hormones may reduce tumor cell growth.[4,5] Type 2 diabetes mellitus, independent of body mass size and physical activity level, is also associated with an increased risk of colorectal cancer in women and supports a role for hyperinsulinemia as a possible link between obesity, sedentary lifestyle, diabetes mellitus, and colorectal cancer.[5] Additional lifestyle choices that increase the risk of colorectal cancer include alcohol consumption and smoking that may increase the risk of colorectal cancer by generating carcinogens or their direct toxic effects on bowel tissue.[4]

Table 91–1

Risk Factors for Colorectal Cancer

General	
Age is the primary risk factor	
Dietary	
High-fat, low-fiber diets	
Lifestyle	
Alcohol	
Smoking	
Obesity or physical inactivity	
Comorbid Conditions	
Inflammatory bowel disease (ulcerative colitis and Crohn disease)	
Hereditary or Genetic	
FAP and HNPCC	
Family history	

FAP, familial adenomatous polyposis; HNPCC, hereditary nonpolyposis colorectal cancer.

Inflammatory bowel diseases, such as chronic ulcerative colitis, particularly when it involves the entire large intestine, and to lesser extent Crohn disease, confer increased risk for colorectal cancer. Overall, individuals with inflammatory bowel disease account for about 1% to 2% of all new cases of colorectal cancer each year.

Finally, as many as 10% of cases are thought to be hereditary. The two most common forms of hereditary colorectal cancer are familial adenomatous polyposis (FAP) and hereditary nonpolyposis colorectal cancer (HNPCC). FAP is a rare autosomal dominant trait that is caused by mutations of the adenomatous polyposis coli (APC) gene and accounts for 1% of all colorectal cancers. The disease is manifested by hundreds to thousands of polyps arising during adolescence.[6] The risk of developing colorectal cancer for individuals with untreated FAP is virtually 100%, and patients require early screening for the disease and likely prophylactic total colectomy. HNPCC, also an autosomal dominant syndrome, accounts for up to 5% of colorectal cancer cases.[6] In contrast to FAP, juvenile polyps occur rarely, and the average age of colorectal cancer in these patients is closer to that of average risk patients, with most patients diagnosed in their 40s. Testing for HNPCC mutations is available but reserved for individuals who meet strict diagnostic criteria.

Up to 25% of patients who develop colorectal cancer have a family history of colorectal cancer unrelated to a mutation described earlier.[7] First-degree relatives of patients diagnosed with colorectal cancer have an increased risk of the disease that is at least two to four times that of persons in the general population without a family history.

Summary of Risk Factors

In summary, the true association between most dietary factors and the risk of colorectal cancer is unclear. The protective effects of fiber and a diet low in fat are not completely known at this time. Physical inactivity, alcohol use, and smoking appear to increase the risk of colorectal cancer. Clinical risk factors and genetic mutations are well-known risks for colorectal cancer.

SCREENING

KEY CONCEPT *Effective colorectal cancer screening programs incorporate annual fecal occult blood testing in combination with regular examination of the entire colon starting at age 50 years for average-risk individuals and should be recommended by all health care providers.* Appropriate screening of patients at normal and high risk for colorectal cancer leads to the detection of smaller, localized lesions and higher cure rates.[8] Screening techniques include fecal occult blood tests (FOBTs) and imaging of the colon. The use of FOBTs annually in combination with digital rectal examinations has led to diagnosis of early stages of disease and may reduce colorectal cancer mortality by up to one-third.[8] However, FOBT using a single stool sample collected during a digital rectal examination is not a recommended option for screening because this method has a decreased sensitivity for detecting advanced disease.[7] Recommendations for adequate FOBT require the patient to collect two stool samples from three consecutive specimens using at-home testing procedures.[8] Two main methods are available to detect occult blood in the feces: guaiac dye and immunochemical methods. The Hemoccult II is the most commonly used FOBT in the United States and is a guaiac-based test. Proper counseling by health care providers is required to receive accurate test results. Consumption of red meat, blood sausages, peroxidase-containing vegetables, iron products, or NSAIDS may result in false-positive results. Vitamin C and dehydrated samples may lead to false-negative results. These products should be avoided for 3 days prior to testing. Fecal immunochemical tests (FITs) (InSure and others), which use antibodies to detect hemoglobin, are also available for use. Though more expensive, an advantage of FITs is that they do not react with dietary factors or medications. Both FOBTs can be recommended in screening protocols for patients.

In addition, imaging of the colon with a sigmoidoscopy, colonoscopy, or double-contrast barium enema is required every 5 to 10 years in most individuals. Colonoscopy is the preferred procedure as it allows for greater visualization of the entire colon and simultaneous removal of lesions found during screening.[8] A sigmoidoscopy only examines the lower half of the colon, and a double-contrast barium enema requires a supplemental colonoscopy to remove any lesions found during the screening process. Several revisions to the colorectal cancer screening guidelines have been made in an attempt to increase the compliance to screening guidelines. These include the use of computed tomographic colonography (CTC) and stool DNA testing as acceptable screening methods. CTC, also known as "virtual colonoscopy," uses integrated two- and three-dimensional images

Patient Encounter, Part 1

A 66-year-old woman presents to your clinic with a chief complaint of abdominal discomfort and changes in her bowel habits with up to six loose stools per day. She also states she has felt tired and has had a reduced appetite over the past month. She has a medical history positive for hypertension, type 2 diabetes mellitus, peripheral neuropathy from her diabetes, and obesity. She states that she consumes a moderate amount of alcohol (two or three beers most days of the week after work), is a current smoker (one pack per day for 32 years), and does not follow any particular diet.

What risk factors does this patient have for colon cancer?

Does she have clinical symptoms suggestive of colon cancer?

What additional tests need to be ordered to diagnosis colon cancer?

Table 91–2

Colon Cancer Screening Guidelines

Average risk	Annual FOBT or FIT after age 50 years Stool DNA testing may be used as an alternative *and* One of the following after age 50 years: Sigmoidoscopy every 5 years Colonoscopy every 10 years Barium enema every 5 years CTC every 5 years
Family history	Screening at ages 40 years or 10 years before the youngest case in the immediate family, whichever is earlier
HNPCC	Screening at age 20–25 years or 10 years before the youngest case in the immediate family, whichever is earlier
FAP	Screening at ages 10–12 years
IBD	8 years after the onset of pancolitis; 12–15 years after onset of left-sided colitis

CTC, computed tomographic colonography; FAP, familial adenomatous polyposis; FIT, fecal immunochemical tests; FOBT, fecal occult blood tests; HNPCC, hereditary nonpolyposis colorectal cancer; IBD, inflammatory bowel disease.

to detect and characterize polyps. Although noninvasive compared with colonoscopy, adequate bowel preparation, which is often cited as the reason for noncompliance, is still required. In addition, any lesions found on examination require a follow-up colonoscopy.

Stool DNA testing detects molecular markers associated with advanced colorectal cancer. Because this test is not dependent on the detection of bleeding, which can be sporadic, it requires only a single stool collection. How often and what molecular markers to test for are undergoing further evaluation. KEY CONCEPT *Table 91–2 is a summary of the current American Cancer Society guidelines for screening and surveillance for early detection of colorectal polyps and cancer.*[8]

COLORECTAL CANCER PREVENTION

There are currently no pharmacologic agents approved for colorectal cancer prevention. Strategies under investigation to prevent colorectal cancer include pharmacologic and surgical interventions and involve either preventing the initial development of colorectal cancer (primary prevention) or preventing cancer in patients who demonstrate early signs of colorectal cancer (secondary prevention).

The most widely studied agents for the chemoprevention of colorectal cancer are agents that inhibit COX-2 (aspirin, NSAIDs, and selective COX-2 inhibitors) and calcium supplementation.[9] Individual studies have demonstrated that regular (at least two doses per week) nonsteroidal anti-inflammatory drug (NSAID) and aspirin use is associated with a 20% to 40% reduction in risk of colorectal cancer in individuals at average risk.[10,11] However, a meta-analysis of over 40 trials suggests the benefit of these agents may be limited to individuals at high risk for developing colorectal cancer.[12] Chronic use of aspirin and other NSAIDs are associated with significant potential adverse effects, including gastrointestinal (GI) and cardiovascular toxicities. These risks limit health care professionals from routine recommendations for use in patients of average risk for colorectal cancer.

The risk of colorectal cancer appears to be inversely related to calcium and folate intake. Calcium supplementation appears to be associated with a moderate reduction in risk of recurrent colorectal adenomas with prospective studies demonstrating a nonstatistical decrease in adenoma recurrence, its role as a chemoprevention agent in the average-risk patient remains under investigation.[9,12]

Additional agents, including selenium and folic acid, show promise as chemopreventive agents in colorectal cancer and preliminary, and confirmatory studies evaluating their effectiveness have been completed or are ongoing.[9] Exogenous hormone use, particularly postmenopausal hormone replacement therapy, is associated with a significant reduction in colorectal cancer risk in most studies with the greatest benefit in women who are on current hormone replacement therapy.[13] Unfortunately, the known risks of hormone replacement therapy outweigh this benefit, and routine use of hormone replacement therapy to prevent colorectal cancer is not recommended.

Surgical resection remains an option to prevent colorectal cancer in individuals at extremely high risk for its development such as patients diagnosed with FAP. Individuals with FAP who are found to have polyps on screening examinations require total abdominal colectomy. In addition, removal of noncancerous polyps detected during screening colonoscopy is considered the standard of care to prevent the progression of premalignant polyps to cancer.

PATHOPHYSIOLOGY

Anatomy and Bowel Function

The large intestine consists of the cecum; ascending, transverse, descending, and sigmoid colon; and rectum (Figure 91–1).

Four major tissue layers, from the lumen outward, form the large intestine: the mucosa, submucosa, muscularis externa, and serosa. Complete replacement of surface epithelial cells occurs every 7 to 10 days with the total number of epithelial cells remaining constant in normal colonic tissue. As patients age, abnormal cells accumulate on the surface epithelium and

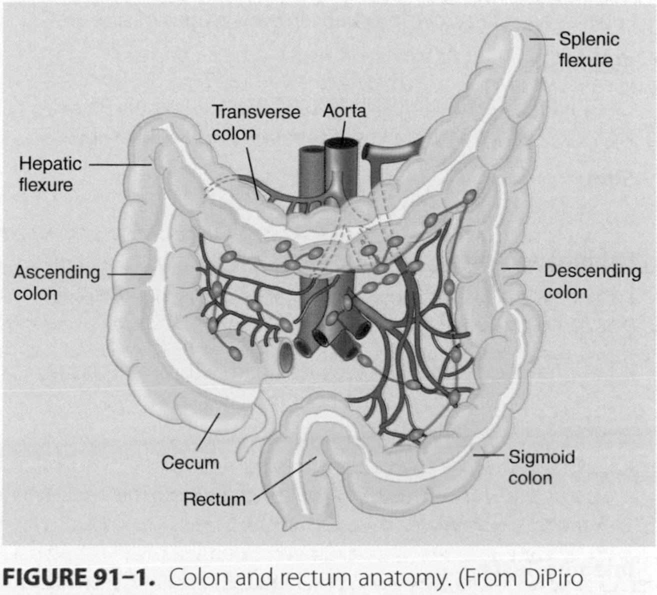

FIGURE 91–1. Colon and rectum anatomy. (From DiPiro JT, Talbert RL, Yee GC, et al, eds. Pharmacotherapy: A Pathophysiologic Approach, 9th ed. New York: McGraw-Hill, 2014; Figure. 107–2.)

protrude into the stream of fecal matter; their contact with fecal mutagens can lead to further cell mutations and eventual adenoma formation.[6]

Colorectal Tumorigenesis

The development of a colorectal neoplasm is a multistep process of several genetic and phenotypic alterations of normal bowel epithelium leading to unregulated cell growth, proliferation, and tumor development. A genetic model has been proposed for colorectal tumorigenesis that describes a process of transformation from adenoma to carcinoma. This model of tumor development reflects an accumulation of mutations within colonic epithelium that gives a selective growth advantage to the cancer cells.[6] Genetic changes include activating mutations of **oncogenes**, mutations of **tumor suppressor genes**, and defects in **DNA mismatch repair genes**.

Additional genes and protein receptors are believed important in colorectal tumorigenesis. COX-2, which is induced in colorectal cancer cells, influences apoptosis and other cellular functions in colon cells, and overexpression of the EGFR, a transmembrane glycoprotein involved in signaling pathways that affect cell growth, differentiation, proliferation, and angiogenesis, occurs in the majority of colon cancers.[14] These mechanisms are potentially important because of the availability of pharmacologic agents targeted to inhibit these processes.

More than 90% of colorectal cancers that develop are adenocarcinomas and are assigned a grade of I to III based on how similar they are compared with normal colorectal cells. Grade I tumors most closely resemble normal cellular structure, but grade III tumors have frequently lost the characteristics of mature normal cells. Grade III tumors are associated with a worse prognosis than grade I tumors.[15]

Clinical Presentation and Diagnosis of Colorectal Cancer

General

Patients are often asymptomatic in early stages of disease

Symptoms

Changes in bowel habits, abdominal pain, anorexia, nausea and vomiting, weakness (if anemia is severe), and tenesmus

Signs

Blood in stool and weight loss

Laboratory Tests

- Patients may have a low hemoglobin level from blood loss
- Positive FOBT
- Liver function tests (INR, activated partial thromboplastin time, and bilirubin) may be abnormal if disease has metastasized to the liver
- CEA level may be high; normal level is less than 2.5 ng/mL (2.5 mcg/L) in nonsmokers and less than 5 ng/mL (5 mcg/L) in smokers

Imaging Tests

Chest x-ray, CT scan, or PET scan results may be positive if cancer has spread to the lungs, liver, or peritoneal cavity

CLINICAL PRESENTATION AND DIAGNOSIS

The signs and symptoms associated with colorectal cancer can be extremely varied, subtle, and nonspecific. Most patients are asymptomatic but may develop changes in bowel or eating habits, fatigue, abdominal pain, and blood in the stool.

TREATMENT

Desired Outcomes

Patients are staged with the tumor, node, metastasis (TNM) classification system (TNM) (See Chapter 88) to determine treatment options and assess prognosis. Figure 91–2 depicts how the three categories are used in combination to determine the stage of disease. KEY CONCEPT *The stage of colorectal cancer upon diagnosis is the most important prognostic factor for survival and disease recurrence. Stages I, II, and III disease are considered potentially curable and are aggressively treated in an attempt to cure these patients. Patients who develop stage IV disease are treated to reduce symptoms, avoid disease-related complications, and prolong survival.*

General Approach to Treatment

The treatment approaches for colorectal cancer reflect two primary treatment goals: curative therapy for localized disease (stages I–III) and palliative therapy for metastatic cancer (stage IV). Surgical resection of the primary tumor is the most important part of therapy for patients in whom cure is possible.[16] Depending on the stage of disease and whether the tumor originated in the colon or rectum, further **adjuvant** chemotherapy or chemotherapy plus radiation may be needed after surgery to cure these patients. In the metastatic setting, pharmacologic intervention is the main treatment option.

Pharmacogenetic and pharmacogenomic testing has become an integral component to designing the optimal pharmacologic intervention for patients with colorectal cancer. The choice of treatment agents is largely dictated by individualized patient and tumor-specific factors. For example, data have demonstrated specific tumor characteristics that may assist clinicians in predicting who will respond to EGFR inhibitors. Early immunohistochemical staining for EGFR status is not useful in predicting response because both EGFR-positive and EGFR-negative patients respond at the same rate. However, *RAS* gene mutation status has demonstrated predictive value. Patients should be tested for both *KRAS* and *NRAS*, patients with mutated *RAS* are unlikely to benefit from cetuximab or panitumumab therapy.[15] In particular, testing for *RAS* mutational status is now part of the disease workup to define patients who may derive benefit from cetuximab or panitumumab. Characteristics of the tumor are also vital in making treatment decisions for patients with stages II and III disease. The degree of **microsatellite instability (MSI)** within a tumor tells clinicians information about both prognosis and treatment options. More detail on specific pharmacogenetic and pharmacogenomic information is provided the pertinent pharmacologic therapy sections.

Nonpharmacologic Therapy

▶ *Operable Disease (Stages I–III)*

Surgery Individuals with stages I to III colorectal cancer should undergo a complete surgical resection of the tumor mass with removal of regional lymph nodes as a curative approach for their disease.[16] Surgery for rectal cancer depends on the region of tumor involvement with attempts to retain rectal

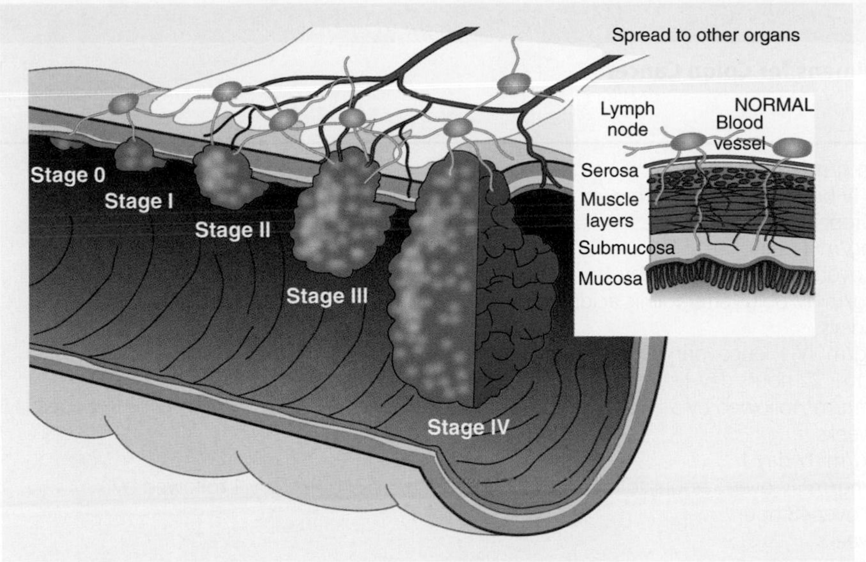

FIGURE 91–2. Stage I: cancer is confined to the lining of the colon. Stage II: cancer may penetrate the wall of the colon into the abdominal cavity but does not invade any local lymph nodes. Stage III: cancer invades one or more lymph nodes but has not spread to distant organs. Stage IV: cancer has spread to distant locations in the body, which may include the liver, lungs, or other sites. (From http://www.cancer.gov/cancertopics/pdq/treatment/colon/Patient/page2.)

function as a goal of the surgical procedure. Overall, surgery for colorectal cancer is associated with low morbidity and mortality rates. Common complications include infection, anastomotic leakage, obstruction, adhesion formation, and malabsorption syndromes.

Radiation Therapy There is currently no role for adjuvant radiation in colon cancer. However, patients who receive surgery for rectal cancer receive radiation therapy to reduce local tumor recurrence. Adjuvant radiation plus chemotherapy is considered standard treatment for patients with stage II or III rectal cancer after the surgical procedure is complete.[17] Preoperative radiation may be used to reduce the initial size of rectal cancers to make the surgical procedure easier.

► *Metastatic Disease (Stage IV)*

Surgery Unlike stages I to III disease, the benefit of surgical resection in most patients with metastatic disease is limited to symptomatic improvement. Select patients who have from one to three small nodules isolated to the liver, lungs, or abdomen may have a prolongation of survival, although cure is rare. Five-year survival for patients who undergo surgical resection of metastases isolated to the liver is approximately double that of patients who are not surgical candidates with approximately 33% of patients alive at 5 years.[18] Alternatives to surgery include destroying the tumor through freezing and thawing (cryoablation), heat (radiofrequency), or alcohol injection, although these appear to be less successful than surgical resection.[16,18] Because the majority of these patients will relapse, many practitioners offer adjuvant chemotherapy to select patients following potentially curative resection, but further studies are needed to determine an optimal treatment regimen.[18]

Radiation Symptom reduction is the primary goal of radiation for patients with advanced or metastatic colorectal cancer.

Pharmacologic Therapy

Table 91–3 lists common chemotherapy regimens used in colorectal cancer and the abbreviations used in the literature to describe them.

Patient Encounter, Part 2

PMH: Hypertension since age 40 years; obesity; the patient is 55% over her ideal body weight

FH: Father died at age 60 years after a stroke. Mother died at age 75 years with breast cancer; older sister with breast cancer; maternal aunt died at age 47 years from rectal cancer

SH: Works in a department store. Married with three grown children

Meds: Atenelol 50 mg daily; glyburide 10 mg daily; gabapentin 300 mg three times a day; aspirin 81 mg daily

ROS: (+) Abdominal cramping, loss of appetite, diarrhea, and fatigue

PE:

VS: 154/88 mm Hg, P 80, RR 17, T 37.1°C (98.8°F), Ht 168 cm (66 in), Wt 89 kg (196 lb)

Abd: Distended and tender to touch, (+) bowel sounds

Labs: Positive hemoglobin 11.8 g/dL (118 g/L or 7.32 mmol/L) decreased from 13.4 g/dL (134 g/L or 8.32 mmol/L) last year

Imaging and Diagnostic Studies

- Colonoscopy revealed multiple polyps in her transverse colon
- Biopsy revealed four polyps positive for adenocarcinoma of the colon
- Staging CT scan negative for disease outside of her colon.
- Three lymph nodes positive for disease

Because the patient has stage III colon cancer, how does this affect the goal of your treatment plan compared with stage IV disease?

What nonpharmacologic and pharmacologic options are available to this patient?

Table 91–3

Dosing Schedules of Chemotherapy Regimens for Colon Cancer[a]

Regimen	Dosing
5-FU + leucovorin (continuous infusion)	Leucovorin 200 mg/m² IV 5-FU 400 mg/m² IV bolus and then 600 mg/m² of 5-FU as a 22-hour continuous infusion on days 1 and 2; repeat every 2 weeks
FOLFIRI	Irinotecan 180 mg/m² IV day 1 Folinic acid (leucovorin) 400 mg/m² IV day 1 5-FU 400–500 mg/m² IV bolus after folinic acid; then 2400–3000 mg/m² of 5-FU IV over 46 hours Repeat every 14 days
FOLFOX4	Oxaliplatin 85 mg/m² IV + leucovorin 200 mg/m² IV followed by 5-FU 400 mg/m² IV bolus and then 5-FU 600 mg/m² IV over 22 hours day 1 Leucovorin 200 mg/m², followed by 5-FU 400 mg/m² IV bolus and then 5-FU 600 mg/m² IV over 22 hours day 2 Repeat every 2 weeks
mFOLFOX6	Oxaliplatin 85 mg/m² IV day 1 Leucovorin 400 mg/m² IV over 2 hours, followed by 5-FU 400 mg/m² IV bolus day 1 followed by 2400 mg/m² IV over 48 hours Repeat every 2 weeks
FOLFOXIRI	Irinotecan 165 mg/m² IV day 1 Oxaliplatin 85 mg/m² IV day 1 Leucovorin 200 mg/m² IV over 2 hours, followed by 5-FU 3200 mg/m² IV over 48 hours Repeat every 2 weeks
Bevacizumab + 5-FU regimen	Bevacizumab 5 mg/kg every 2 weeks + a 5-FU–containing regimen (FOLFOX, FOLFIRI, or 5-FU + leucovorin) Bevacizumab 7.5 mg/kg every 3 weeks with CapeOX
Cetuximab ± irinotecan	Cetuximab 400 mg/m² first infusion, then 250 mg/m² weekly ± irinotecan 125 mg/m² every week for 4 weeks Repeat irinotecan every 6 weeks (after a 2-week break)
Panitumumab	6 mg/kg every 2 weeks
Capecitabine	1250 mg/m² twice a day orally for 14 days Repeat every 3 weeks
CapeOX	Capecitabine 1000 mg/m² twice a day orally for 14 days Oxaliplatin 130 mg/m² IV on day 1 Repeat every 3 weeks

5-FU, 5-fluorouracil; CapeOX, capecitabine–oxaliplatin; IV, intravenous.

[a]Note that many variations exist, and current literature should be checked before administering any chemotherapy regimen.

▶ *Operable Disease (Stages I–III)*

KEY CONCEPT *Adjuvant chemotherapy is administered after tumor resection to decrease relapse rates and improve survival in patients with colon cancer by eliminating micrometastatic disease that is undetected on imaging studies. Patients diagnosed with stage I colon or rectal cancer are usually cured by surgical resection, and adjuvant chemotherapy is not indicated in these patients.[16] The role of adjuvant chemotherapy for stage II colon cancer is controversial but may benefit certain high-risk groups. Adjuvant chemotherapy is standard therapy for patients with stage III colon cancer.* Table 91–4 lists adjuvant treatment regimens based on stage and performance status (PS). Adjuvant chemotherapy for patients with stage II disease has not been shown to be superior to surgery alone with the possible exception of high-risk patients, including those with inadequate nodes sampled for staging, bowel perforation upon diagnosis, T4 lesions, and those with unfavorable histology.[15] The risks and benefits of adjuvant chemotherapy should be discussed with medically fit patients who have stage II disease with high-risk features. However, the American Society of Clinical Oncology does not recommend the routine use of adjuvant chemotherapy in the general patient population unless part of a clinical trial.[19]

There is currently insufficient data to recommend the use of tumor gene profiling to determine need for adjuvant therapy in stage II disease, but it is an area of active research.[15] An additional consideration for deciding on adjuvant therapy is the status of MSI within the tumor. MSI results from defective **DNA mismatch repair (dMMR) genes** leading to damaged DNA. Patient' with tumors that display high levels of MSI may have better prognosis than patients with microsatellite-stable

Table 91–4

Treatment Regimens for Adjuvant Colon Cancer

Stage II[a]	Stage III
High Risk	**Good Performance Status**
• Capecitabine or 5-FU plus leucovorin • FOLFOX • CapeOx • FLOX	• FOLFOX • CapeOX • FLOX • Capecitabine or 5-FU plus leucovorin
Low Risk[b]	**Poor Performance Status**
• Observation or clinical trial • Capecitabine or 5-FU plus leucovorin	• Capecitabine

5-FU, 5-fluorouracil.

[a]Individualized assessment of patient risk is necessary to determine if treatment is required. Clinical trials or observation may be an appropriate option.

[b]T3 lesions may be considered high risk by some clinicians.

(MSS) tumors. Despite being associated with a better prognosis, tumors that display high levels of MSI do not respond as well to certain chemotherapy, including 5-fluorouracil (5-FU).[20] It is recommended that stage II patients should be tested for the status of MSI if 5-FU is being considered for therapy, and an alternative therapy should be considered if high levels of MSI are displayed.[15] In general, patients with stage II colon cancer should be enrolled into clinical trials to assess the impact of new agents and prognostic models.

Adjuvant chemotherapy is standard therapy for patients with stage III colon cancer. The presence of lymph node involvement in the resected specimen places patients with stage III colon cancer at high risk for relapse; the risk of death within 5 years of surgical resection alone is as high as 70%.[16] In this population of patients, adjuvant chemotherapy significantly decreases the risk of cancer recurrence and death and is considered the standard of care.

KEY CONCEPT *5-FU, leucovorin, and oxaliplatin (FOLFOX)–based chemotherapy is the standard regimen used in adjuvant colon cancer. It is usually given for 6 months.* Refer to Tables 91–3 and 91–4 for recommended treatment regimens and schedules. 5-FU alone results in a small improvement in survival that can vary based on the method of 5-FU administration and the status of MSI.[20]

The combination of 5-FU plus leucovorin has undergone extensive study in the adjuvant setting with decreased rates of recurrence and improved survival seen in patients receiving 5-FU plus leucovorin compared with surgery alone. Though various schedules of 5-FU and leucovorin can be administered, continuous infusions may be less toxic and have improved response rates (although no survival advantage) compared with bolus regimens. Capecitabine is an oral prodrug of 5-FU that is also effective in the adjuvant setting and is being used as a replacement in certain regimens for 5-FU. Data suggest that capecitabine is at least equivalent to bolus 5-FU and leucovorin in efficacy and is better tolerated by patients in the adjuvant setting.[21] An increase in hand–foot syndrome and decreased mucositis and neutropenia are seen with capecitabine compared with bolus 5-FU.

More often, 5-FU or capecitabine is administered as part of a combination regimen with oxaliplatin and leucovorin (FOLFOX or CapeOx). FOLFOX is considered standard of care for patients with stage III disease unless their PS is so poor that clinicians do not believe the patients could tolerate intensive combination therapy. Every effort should be made to minimize adverse treatment effects and use this regimen in patients with stage III colon cancer because this is the only regimen demonstrated to improve overall survival in these patients.[16,22] Several variations on the original FOLFOX regimen have been studied with mFOLFOX6 being the most routinely used in clinical practice (Refer to Table 91–4). CapeOx resulted in improved DFS compared with bolus 5-FU–leucovorin, but no overall survival benefit in stage III patients and is considered an acceptable adjuvant regimen in this patient population.[15,23]

Targeted therapies, including cetuximab and bevacizumab, have been evaluated for their role in their adjuvant treatment of colon cancer. At this time, no targeted agents are approved for use as adjuvant therapy in stage II or III colorectal cancer patients. Additionally, irinotecan should not be used in the adjuvant setting because its addition to 5-FU–based regimens has increased toxicity without therapeutic benefit.[15]

▸ *Metastatic Disease (Stage IV)*

Traditional chemotherapy and targeted biological therapies are the mainstay of treatment for metastatic colon or rectal cancer and have improved the median survival time of these patients to more than 2 years.[16] Most often, a combination of chemotherapy agents with biological therapies is administered to these patients. Currently, metastatic colorectal cancer is incurable, and treatment goals are to reduce patients' symptoms, improve quality of life, and extend survival. Combination chemotherapy regimens have been demonstrated to result in prolongation of survival with tolerable adverse effects. Similar to the adjuvant setting, 5-FU plus leucovorin continues to be in most first-line chemotherapy regimens used for metastatic colorectal cancer. A variety of continuous intravenous (IV) infusion 5-FU and bolus regimens can be used; however, compared with IV bolus 5-FU, response rates with continuous infusion 5-FU are approximately doubled. In a large meta-analysis of patients with advanced colorectal cancer, continuous infusions of 5-FU had a significantly higher tumor response rate, a small increase in survival, and lower incidence of myelosuppression, diarrhea, and mucositis when compared with bolus regimens.[24]

Additional agents including irinotecan and oxaliplatin have been added to the 5-FU and leucovorin regimen with superior response and survival rates compared to the two drugs used alone.[25,26] A large European study compared a combined bolus and infusional 5-FU regimen plus irinotecan (FOLFIRI) with the FOLFOX regimen (using a slightly different schedule) with crossover to the opposite arm upon relapse.[27] No difference in patient survival was seen with either regimen, and toxicity was as expected. Neuropathy and neutropenia were more common with FOLFOX, while diarrhea, nausea, vomiting, dehydration, and febrile neutropenia were more common with FOLFIRI. Based on improved survival data with the FOLFOX and FOLFIRI regimens, irinotecan-based regimens should only be administered outlined as described in Table 91–3.

Capecitabine also has activity in the metastatic setting. When combined with oxaliplatin in regimens known as CapeOx or XELOX, capecitabine appears to be as safe as 5-FU–based regimens.[15] Additionally, **progression-free survival** (PFS) with capecitabine and oxaliplatin is similar to that of FOLFOX and is considered noninferior to the FOLFOX regimen as first-line therapy in advanced disease.[28] This noninferiority with capecitabine may be specific to its use with oxaliplatin because capecitabine in combination with irinotecan (CAPIRI) demonstrated decreased PFS compared with FOLFIRI and the routine substitution of 5-FU with capecitabine in irinotecan-based regimens is not recommended.[15,29]

5-FU plus leucovorin, or capecitabine alone, is appropriate first-line treatment options for individuals for whom three-drug combination regimens are believed to toxic. The site(s) of tumor involvement, history of prior chemotherapy, and patient-specific factors help define the appropriate management strategy. KEY CONCEPT *The most important factor in patient survival is not the initial regimen but whether or not patients receive all three active chemotherapy drugs (5-FU, irinotecan, and oxaliplatin) at some point in their treatment course.*[30] Some clinicians choose to use all three agents in combination in the first-line setting in a regimen termed FOLFOXIRI, although only in patients who are able to tolerate intensive therapy.

Targeted or biologic agents have been approved for use in metastatic colorectal cancer. Bevacizumab in combination with IV 5-FU–based chemotherapy (either FOLFOX or FOLFIRI) is approved by the FDA for initial treatment of patients with metastatic colorectal cancer. Results from randomized trials show increased benefit compared with chemotherapy alone.[15] The efficacy of bevacizumab in this patient population shows the relevance of angiogenesis as an important target for the treatment of metastatic colorectal cancer. The addition of bevacizumab to first-line oxaliplatin-based chemotherapy has also been demonstrated to improve PFS but did not positively impact response rates or overall survival.[31] Similar results were demonstrated with bevacizumab in combination with capecitabine and oxaliplatin.[42]

Based on these results, bevacizumab is recommended as part of 5-FU–based chemotherapy regimens used for the first-line treatment of metastatic colorectal cancer unless contraindicated. Bevacizumab is contraindicated in patients with GI perforation or fistulas involving a major organ, recent (within 28 days) major surgeries or open wounds, wound dehiscence requiring medical intervention, hypertensive crisis or uncontrolled severe hypertension, hypertensive encephalopathy—serious bleeding, a severe arterial thromboembolic event, moderate or severe proteinuria (urine protein excretion 2 g/24 hours or more), nephrotic syndrome, and reversible posterior leukoencephalopathy syndrome.

The EGFR inhibitors, cetuximab and panitumumab, demonstrate improved PFS as first-line therapy in the metastatic setting when individually combined with either the FOLFOX or FOLFIRI regimens in *KRAS* wild-type individuals.[32–35] KEY CONCEPT *Before using these agents, testing for KRAS mutation status should occur. Extensive literature exists demonstrating poor response rates of EGFR inhibitors in patients whose tumors have a mutation in codon 12 or codon 13 of the KRAS gene.*[15,36] Consequently, cetuximab or panitumumab may be used in the first-line setting in combination with traditional chemotherapy agents in *KRAS* WT patients only.[15]

Attempts to combine the vascular endothelial growth factor (VEGF) inhibitor bevacizumab with cetuximab and panitumumab as part of traditional chemotherapy regimens have resulted in inferior outcomes to regimens with bevacizumab alone.[37] Based on these results, the use of bevacizumab with either EGFR inhibitor is not recommended.[15]

KEY CONCEPT *In summary, most practitioners select first-line treatment for metastatic colorectal cancer from among these treatments: oxaliplatin plus 5-FU plus leucovorin (FOLFOX); irinotecan plus 5-FU plus leucovorin (FOLFIRI); capecitabine plus oxaliplatin (CapeOx or XELOX); oxaliplatin plus irinotecan plus 5-FU plus leucovorin (FOLFOXIRI); bevacizumab plus 5-FU– or capecitabine-based chemotherapy (FOLFIRI or FOLFOX or CapeOx or FOLFOXIRI); or cetuximab or panitumumab plus 5-FU–based chemotherapy (FOLFOX or FOLFIRI) in KRAS* WT patients.[15]

▸ *Second-Line Therapy*

KEY CONCEPT *Treatment of relapsed or refractory metastatic disease uses agents not given in the first-line setting. Patients who receive all effective chemotherapy options have improved outcomes compared with those who do not.* Because most patients will have received a combination of 5-FU or capecitabine with either irinotecan or oxaliplatin, second-line therapy with the alternate regimen should be considered.[15] For example, a patient who received FOLFOX plus bevacizumab as first-line therapy for metastatic disease should be offered FOLFIRI as part of their second-line regimen. EGFR inhibitors are an additional option for use in the second-line setting in patients with WT *KRAS* only. Patients who did not have an EGFR inhibitor in their first-line regimens are candidates for single-agent cetuximab or panitumumab or either agent in combination with 5-FU and irinotecan (FOLFIRI + EGFR inhibitor). Additionally cetuximab plus irinotecan can be used without the inclusion of 5-FU. The use of EGFR inhibitors may be beneficial as monotherapy, but response rates and PFS appear to be increased in combination with irinotecan-based chemotherapy.[38–42] The results appear to be best when irinotecan is continued because of synergy demonstrated between the two classes of agents.[15,38]

If targeted agents such as bevacizumab were not part of the initial regimen, addition to the second-line regimen should be strongly considered. The addition of bevacizumab to FOLFOX has been shown to increase overall survival.[43] Bevacizumab as monotherapy was shown to be inferior to FOLFOX4 in efficacy and should not be considered as a treatment option in the second-line setting. In patients receiving bevacizumab as part of first-line therapy, continuation of bevacizumab with second-line therapy is associated with increased survival.[44] Based on these findings, continuation of bevacizumab in combination with traditional second-line chemotherapy regimens (5-FU-irinotecan or 5-FU-oxaliplatin based) can be considered in patients treated with a first-line bevacizumab containing regimen. A second agent targeting VEGF, ziv-aflibercept, in combination with FOLFIRI can also be considered for use in the second-line setting in patients who have progressed following an oxaliplatin-based first-line regimen. A modest increase in overall and PFS was found in patients receiving FOLFIRI plus ziv-aflibercept compared to FOLFIRI alone.[45] Adverse events and warnings for use with ziv-aflibercept are similar to those with bevacizumab and described in the section of specific agents. Table 91–5 lists treatment options for first- and second-line treatment of metastatic colorectal cancer. Patients with good PS are treated more aggressively than those with poor PS because of their ability to better tolerate chemotherapy.

Table 91–5

Treatment Options for Metastatic Colon Cancer[a]

First-Line Therapy	Second-Line Therapy
Good Performance Status	**If First-Line Irinotecan**
• FOLFOX or FOLFIRI with bevacizumab	• FOLFOX with or without bevacizumab[b]
• FOLFOX or FOLFIRI with cetuximab or panitumumab[c]	• Irinotecan with or without cetuximab[c,d]
• FOLFOXIRI with or without bevacizumab	• Capecitabine or 5-FU plus leucovorin
• 5-FU + leucovorin or capecitabine with or without bevacizumab	
Poor Performance Status	**If First-Line Oxaliplatin**
• Capecitabine or 5-FU plus leucovorin with or without bevacizumab	• FOLFIRI with or without bevacizumab
	• FOLFIRI with ziv-aflibercept
	• Irinotecan with ziv-aflibercept
	• FOLFIRI or irinotecan with or without cetuximab or panitumumab[c,d]

5-FU, 5-fluorouracil.

[a]CapeOX may replace FOLFOX in selected patients.

[b]Bevacizumab may be given if not part of the first-line therapy.

[c]If KRAS wild type.

[d]Cetuximab or panitumumab may be given if not part of first-line therapy.

Patient Encounter, Part 3

Based on the information presented, create a care plan for this patient's colon cancer.

Your plan should include:

(a) The patient's drug- and nondrug-related needs and problems.

(b) The goals of therapy.

(c) A treatment plan specific to HB that includes strategies to prevent adverse effects of chemotherapy.

(d) A follow-up plan to determine whether the goals have been achieved and the adverse effects of chemotherapy have been minimized.

(e) A plan for treatment options when the initial therapy is no longer achieving the goals of therapy.

▸ *Salvage Therapy*

Third-line options for patients with metastatic colorectal cancer are limited. Panitumumab is approved for patients who have progressed after 5-FU, oxaliplatin, and irinotecan. Compared with best supportive care, it improves time to disease progression.[15] Based on improvement in PFS compared to best supportive care, the multiple tyrosine kinase inhibitor, regorafenib, was approved as a single agent for metastatic colorectal cancer in the third- or fourth-line setting.[46] Patients who fail standard treatment for metastatic colorectal cancer should be encouraged to participate in a clinical trial evaluating new treatment approaches for this incurable disease.

SPECIFIC AGENTS USED IN COLORECTAL CANCER

Table 91–6 lists all FDA-approved drugs used in colorectal cancer along with their mechanisms of action, common toxicities, and recommended dose adjustments for hepatic and renal dysfunction as well pharmacogenetic considerations.

5-Fluorouracil

5-Fluorouracil (5-FU) acts as a "false" pyrimidine inhibiting the formation of the DNA base thymidine as described in Chapter 88.[16]

5-FU is commonly used in the adjuvant and metastatic treatment of colon and rectal cancers with common regimens listed in Table 91–3. Clinical studies comparing efficacy of bolus and continuous infusion schedules generally favor continuous infusion of 5-FU. This is consistent with evidence that suggests that the duration of infusion may be an important determinant of the biologic activity of 5-FU, particularly because of its short plasma half-life, S-phase specificity, and relatively slow growth of colon tumors.[16,47]

Clinically significant differences in toxicity also differ based on the dose, route, and schedule of 5-FU administration. Leukopenia and mucositis are the primary dose-limiting toxicities of bolus 5-FU, whereas palmar-plantar erythrodysesthesia ("hand–foot syndrome") and diarrhea occur most frequently with continuous infusions of 5-FU.[16,47] Health care practitioners can offer valuable patient advice to decrease the impact of these adverse effects. Patients can be informed to suck on ice chips before and for up to 30 minutes after 5-FU boluses to decrease the incidence of mucositis. Hand–foot syndrome, characterized by painful swelling and redness of the soles of the feet and palms of the hand, can be minimized with loose-fitting clothing and keeping skin moist. Additional toxicities include moderate nausea and vomiting, skin discoloration, nail changes, photosensitivity, and neurologic toxicity.

An additional determinate of 5-FU toxicity, regardless of the method of administration, is related to its catabolism and pharmacogenomic factors. Dihydropyrimidine dehydrogenase (DPD) is the main enzyme responsible for the catabolism of 5-FU to inactive metabolites.[48] A number of polymorphisms in DPD have been identified in which patients have a complete or near-complete deficiency of this enzyme. This results in unusually severe toxicity, including death, after the administration of 5-FU. Approximately 3% of patients have a complete lack of DPD activity with other patients demonstrating a partial deficiency in enzyme activity. Although patients may be tested for level of DPD activity, it is not routinely done but may be considered in patients who develop severe toxicity after 5-FU administration. The response to 5-FU is also influenced by the status of MSI within the tumor. Tumors with high levels of MSI are generally more resistant to 5-FU despite being associated with better prognosis.

Leucovorin is commonly given with 5-FU. Leucovorin acts to increase the affinity of 5-FU to thymidine synthase, thus increasing the pharmacologic activity of 5-FU.[16] Leucovorin is most effective when administered before 5-FU and can be given by IV bolus or as a continuous infusion. Health care practitioners can also expect an increase in 5-FU toxicities (leukopenia, mucositis, and diarrhea) when leucovorin is given in combination with 5-FU.

Capecitabine

Capecitabine (Xeloda) is an oral prodrug of 5-FU that is designed to be selectively activated by tumor cells. Capecitabine undergoes a three-step conversion to 5-FU, the last step being phosphorylation by thymidine phosphorylase (TP). TP levels are reported to be higher in tumor cells than normal tissues; therefore, the systemic exposure of active drug is minimized, and tumor concentrations of the active drugs are optimized.[16,22] After the drug is converted to 5-FU, it has the same mechanism of action. The current FDA-approved indication for capecitabine is for use in metastatic and adjuvant colorectal cancer when monotherapy is desired, although it is actively being investigated as a replacement for 5-FU in most combinations of colon and rectal cancer regimens. Capecitabine has been demonstrated to be at least equivalent to bolus IV 5-FU in the metastatic and adjuvant setting with improved patient tolerability.[22,49] Hand–foot syndrome and diarrhea are common with capecitabine because its toxicities (and pharmacologic activity) appear to mimic those of continuous infusions of 5-FU. Both irinotecan and oxaliplatin have been combined with capecitabine. Capecitabine in combination with oxaliplatin appears to be as safe and effective as IV-based 5-FU in the treatment of patients with colorectal cancer.[15,47] Combinations with irinotecan have had mixed results and are not routinely recommended.[15,29]

The dose of capecitabine ranges from 1000 to 1250 mg/m^2 twice a day when used by itself; lower doses are often used when it is given in combination with irinotecan or oxaliplatin or in patients with renal insufficiency. The dose should be taken on a full stomach with breakfast and dinner. Capecitabine administered with warfarin can result in significant increases in patients' international normalized ratio (INR) and requires close monitoring.

Table 91–6

FDA-Approved Drugs Used in Colon Cancer

Generic Name (Trade Name)	Mechanism of Action	Common Toxicities	Dosing Adjustments for Renal or Hepatic Dysfunction or Pharmacogenetic Considerations
5-FU	Inhibition of the enzyme thymidylate synthase, the rate-limiting step in thymidine formation	*Dose limiting:* Myelosuppression and mucositis with bolus administration Diarrhea and hand–foot syndrome with continuous infusion *Additional toxicities:* Skin discoloration, nail changes, photosensitivity, and neurologic toxicity	Do not give if bilirubin greater than 5 mg/dL (86 μmol/L) DPD deficiency may result in increased toxicity. Testing not routine, but may be considered in those with excessive toxicity
Capecitabine (Xeloda)	Orally active prodrug of 5-FU. Once activated, the mechanism of action is the same	Similar to continuous infusion 5-FU	CrCl 30–50 mL/min (0.50–0.83 mL/s) decrease starting dose to 75% of the original dose Do not give if CrCl < 30 mL/min (0.50 mL/s)
Irinotecan (Camptosar)	Topoisomerase inhibitor that forms a complex with the covalently bound DNA topoisomerase enzyme and interferes with the DNA breakage-resealing process	*Dose limiting:* Early and late diarrhea *Additional toxicities:* Neutropenia, nausea, and vomiting	Decrease dose one level in patients with a homozygous UGT1A1*28 allele. Having this allele decreases the hepatic metabolism of irinotecan and increases the toxicity
Oxaliplatin (Eloxatin)	Similar to other platinum analogues (cisplatin) in that it binds to the N-7 position of guanine, which results in cross-linking of DNA and double-stranded DNA breaks	*Dose limiting:* Acute (within first 2 days) and persistent (> 14 days) neuropathies *Additional toxicities:* Anaphylactic-like reactions, dyspnea, nausea, vomiting	No formal dose adjustment, though use with caution in patients with mild to moderate renal dysfunction
Bevacizumab (Avastin)	Monoclonal antibody that binds to VEGF and inhibits angiogenesis	*Dose limiting:* Hypertension, bleeding episodes, thrombotic events *Additional toxicities:* Rare perforation of the bowel, proteinuria	None
Ziv-aflibercept (Zaltrap)	Recombinant fusion protein that binds to VEGF and inhibits angiogenesis	*Dose limiting:* Hypertension, bleeding episodes, thrombotic events, infection, diarrhea *Additional toxicities:* Rare perforation of the bowel, proteinuria	None
Regorafenib (Stivarga)	Multiple protein kinase inhibitor, including VEGF KIT, PDGFR, RET, FGFR, TIE2, DDR2, TrkA, Eph2A, RAF-1, BRAF, SAPK2, PTK5, and Abl	*Dose limiting:* Hypertension, hand-foot skin reaction *Additional toxicities:* GI perforation, impaired wound healing, hemorrhage, RPLS, fatigue, electrolyte imbalance, hepatotoxicity	Do not use if Child-Pugh Class C hepatic impairment; Specific recommendations exist for hepatotoxicity developing while on therapy
Cetuximab (Erbitux)	Binds to the cell surface EGFR, preventing EGF and TGF-α binding. This decreased cell proliferation of cancer cells	*Dose limiting:* Infusion-related reactions, acneiform skin rash *Additional toxicities:* Diarrhea, hypomagnesemia, hypocalcemia, interstitial lung disease	*KRAS* WT only
Panitumumab (Vectibix)	Similar to cetuximab	*Dose limiting:* Acneiform skin rash *Additional toxicities:* Infusion-related reactions, diarrhea, hypomagnesemia, hypocalcemia, interstitial lung disease	*KRAS* WT only

5-FU, 5-fluorouracil; CrCl, creatinine clearance; EGF, epidermal growth factor; EGFR, epidermal growth factor receptor; RPLS, Reversible posterior leukoencephalopathy syndrome; TGF, transforming growth factor; VEGF, vascular endothelial growth factor; WT, wild type.

The convenience of oral administration, potentially requiring fewer clinic visits, and an improvement in toxicity make capecitabine a useful alternative to IV 5-FU both by itself and incorporated into other regimens used in colorectal cancer.

Irinotecan

Irinotecan (Camptosar) is a topoisomerase-I inhibitor that forms a complex with the covalently bound DNA topoisomerase I enzyme and interferes with the DNA breakage–resealing process.[49] Binding permits uncoiling of the double-stranded DNA, but it prevents subsequent resealing of the DNA, resulting in double-stranded DNA breaks. Irinotecan is a prodrug that is converted by carboxylesterases to its active form, SN-38. Irinotecan is indicated for the first-line treatment of metastatic colorectal cancer in combination with 5-FU and leucovorin or as a single agent in patients who fail first-line therapies. Irinotecan is not recommended as part of the adjuvant treatment of colorectal cancer at this time.

The major toxicity of irinotecan is diarrhea, which can occur both early and late in therapy.[15,47] The early diarrhea is a cholinergic reaction that occurs in the first 24 hours (often during the infusion) in up to 10% of patients and responds to atropine 0.25 to 1 mg IV. The late diarrhea seen in a larger percent of patients occurs 7 to 14 days after the irinotecan infusion. Health care practitioners have to be diligent in counseling patients on this adverse reaction and counseling them on the proper use of antidiarrheals. At the first change in bowel habits, an intensive loperamide regimen should be started by patients (4 mg initially followed by 2 mg every 2 hours until diarrhea free for 12 hours). If diarrhea does not stop or if it worsens, patients should be instructed to call their health care provider immediately. Late-onset diarrhea may require hospitalization or discontinuation of therapy, and fatalities have been reported. Additional toxicities with irinotecan include leukopenia (including neutropenic fever) and moderate nausea and vomiting. Toxicities of irinotecan appear to be greater when the drug is given weekly compared with other administration schedules.

Similar to 5-FU, a pharmacogenomic abnormality is associated with irinotecan toxicity. UDP-glucuronosyltransferase (UGT1A1) is an enzyme that is responsible for the glucuronidation of SN-38 to inactive metabolites, and reduced or deficient levels of this enzyme correlate with irinotecan-induced diarrhea and neutropenia.[15,47] The FDA approved a blood test that detects variations in this gene. This test may assist health care providers in predicting which patients may develop severe toxicities from "normal" doses of irinotecan and can be ordered before patients receive irinotecan.[15] The package insert recommends dose reductions of one level in patients who are UGT1A1 homozygous variants. Irinotecan is administered as an IV bolus over 60 to 90 minutes in a variety of dosing schedules.

Oxaliplatin

Oxaliplatin (Eloxatin) is similar to other platinum analogues (cisplatin) in that it binds to the N-7 position of guanine that results in cross-linking of DNA and double-stranded DNA breaks.[47] Oxaliplatin differs from cisplatin in that the DNA damage induced by oxaliplatin may not be as easily recognized by DNA repair genes often seen in colorectal cancer. Oxaliplatin, in combination with 5-FU-based regimens, is indicated for the first- and second-line treatment of metastatic colorectal cancer as well as the adjuvant treatment of colorectal cancer.

The dose-limiting toxicity of oxaliplatin is acute and chronic neuropathy.[16] Acute neuropathies occur within 1 to 2 days of dosing, resolve within 2 weeks, and usually occur peripherally. These acute neuropathies occur in almost all patients to some degree and are exacerbated by exposure to cold temperature or cold objects. Health care providers should instruct patients to avoid cold drinks, avoid use of ice, and cover skin before exposure to cold or cold objects. In addition, carbamazepine, gabapentin, amifostine, and calcium and magnesium infusions have been used to both prevent and treat oxaliplatin-induced neuropathies, although use of these agents is not widely accepted.[16] Persistent neuropathies generally occur after eight cycles of oxaliplatin and are characterized by defects that can interfere with daily activities (eg, writing, buttoning, swallowing, and walking). Patients may receive predefined breaks from oxaliplatin to decrease the onset of these toxicities with reinitiation of therapy.[26] This strategy varies among protocols but involves administering a certain number of predefined oxaliplatin cycles and then stopping. Maintenance therapy with another agent is usually administered and then the oxaliplatin-based regimen is restarted based on the protocol. These neuropathies occur in up to half of patients receiving oxaliplatin but usually resolve with dosage reductions or after oxaliplatin is stopped.[16] A recent phase III trial in the adjuvant setting demonstrated a decrease in greater than grade 2 chronic sensory neuropathies in patients receiving IV calcium and magnesium infusions before and after oxaliplatin infusion.[47] Oxaliplatin has minimal renal, myelosuppressive effects, and nausea and vomiting when compared with other platinum drugs. Oxaliplatin is given IV in a variety of dosing schedules with a typical dose of 85 mg/m^2 IV every 2 weeks.

Bevacizumab

Bevacizumab (Avastin) is a recombinant, humanized monoclonal antibody that inhibits VEGF. VEGF is a proangiogenic growth factor found in many cancers, including colorectal, and is thought to promote blood vessel formation and metastasis of the tumor by binding to VEGF receptors on tumors. Bevacizumab inhibits circulating VEGF, preventing it from binding to receptors and decreasing the formation of new blood vessels.[15,16] Additionally, bevacizumab may allow for increased concentrations of traditional chemotherapy such as irinotecan to reach the tumor to exert its pharmacologic effect. Bevacizumab is not effective alone and must be used in combination with other agents effective in colorectal cancer. It is indicated for first-line and second-line treatment of patients with metastatic colorectal cancer in combination with IV 5-FU–based regimens. Bevacizumab is also approved for use in combination with 5-FU-irinotecan or 5-FU-oxaliplatin-based chemotherapy for treatment of patients with metastatic colorectal cancer whose disease has progressed on a first-line bevacizumab-containing regimen.

Adverse effects associated with bevacizumab include hypertension, which is common but easily managed with oral antihypertensive agents. Thrombotic events (including myocardial infarctions, pulmonary embolisms, and deep vein thrombosis) occur more frequently in the elderly patients with cardiovascular risk factors and need to be monitored routinely. Because bevacizumab interferes with normal wound healing, it should not be given shortly before or after surgical procedures.[15] Initiation within 28 days of surgery is not recommended to allow for proper wound healing and decrease the risk of bleeding. The amount of time needed after bevacizumab discontinuation to perform elective surgical procedures is less clear, but health care providers should take into consideration bevacizumab's half-life of approximately 20 days when making clinical decisions.[33] Patients should have their urine checked for protein before each dose of bevacizumab to check for potential kidney damage. Patients who have developed 2+ protein on the urinalysis require additional testing before receiving therapy. These patients will have their 24-hour urine collected and assessed for protein. Therapy is interrupted if urine protein excretion exceeds 2 g/24 hours or more and resumed when urine protein excretion decreases to less than 2 g/24 hours.

Finally, there is a risk of GI perforation that is rare but potentially fatal. Patients complaining of abdominal pain associated with vomiting or constipation should be counseled to call their physician immediately. Bevacizumab is commonly given at a dose of 5 mg/kg IV every 14 days until disease progression. Once disease progresses and salvage chemotherapy is initiated, the benefit of continuing bevacizumab is unclear.

Ziv-aflibercept

Ziv-aflibercept (Zaltrap) is a soluble recombinant fusion protein developed by fusing sections of the VEGFR-1 and VEGFR-2 immunoglobulin domains to the F_c portion of human IgG1 antibody. This results in trapping the VEGF-A, VEGF-B, and PIGF ligands before they get to the native transmembrane receptors, and therefore, inhibiting the angiogenic process.[49] It is FDA approved for the treatment of metastatic colorectal cancer in combination with FOLFIRI after progression on an oxaliplatin-based regimen. The dose is 4 mg/kg as an IV infusion over 1 hour every 2 weeks in combination with FOLFIRI.

Toxicities include severe and potentially fatal hemorrhage, GI perforation, and compromised wound healing for which the FDA has given ziv-aflibercept a black-box warning. Other adverse effects common to VEGF inhibition (thromboembolic events, hypertension, proteinuria) are seen. As a result ziv-aflibercept shares similar monitoring parameters and warnings to those mentioned in the bevacizumab section. Finally additional warnings for neutropenia, diarrhea and dehydration, and reversible posterior leukoencephalopathy syndrome (RPLS) require monitoring patients for signs and symptoms of these toxicities.

Regorafenib

Regorafenib (Stivarga) is an oral medication that inhibits multiple protein kinases. Its main mechanism of action in colorectal cancer appears to be related to inhibition of vascular endothelial receptors involved in angiogenesis. The importance of additional protein kinase inhibited by regorafenib is unknown in colorectal cancer. Regorafenib is FDA approved as a single agent for metastatic colorectal cancer in the third- or fourth-line setting.[46] The dose of regorafenib is 160 mg orally, once daily for the first 21 days of each 28-day cycle and it must be taken with a low-fat breakfast to improve absorption.

Adverse effects for regorafenib include those typical for VEGF inhibition (hemorrhage, hypertension, wound healing complications, GI perforation) mentioned with bevacizumab and ziv-aflibercept. Regorafenib has a black-box warning for hepatotoxicity that requires baseline liver function tests (ALT, AST, and bilirubin), then every 2 weeks during the first 2 months of therapy, and then monthly. In patients with elevated liver function tests holding doses, dose reductions, or permanent discontinuation of regorafenib may be necessary. Also, asthenia, fatigue, decreased appetite, hand-foot syndrome, diarrhea, mucositis, weight loss, infection, and dysphonia occurred in over 30% of patients. Refer to chapter 99 on supportive care for management. Finally, regorafenib is a substrate of CYP3A4 and patients should be screened for potential drug interactions.

Cetuximab and Panitumumab

Cetuximab (Erbitux) and panitumumab (Vectibix) are monoclonal antibodies directed against the EGFR. Cetuximab is a chimeric antibody, whereas panitumumab is a fully human monoclonal antibody. EGFR is overexpressed in colorectal cancers and leads to an increase in tumor proliferation and growth.[47] Cetuximab received FDA approval for use in EGFR-expressing metastatic colorectal cancer in irinotecan-relapsed or irinotecan-refractory patients. Cetuximab should be administered in combination with irinotecan but can be used as a single agent in patients who cannot tolerate irinotecan-based chemotherapy. Panitumumab is approved as monotherapy agent and as first-line therapy in combination with FOLFOX in metastatic colorectal cancer.

Both agents are well tolerated with infusion-related reactions being the dose-limiting toxicity of cetuximab and rash most commonly seen with panitumumab. Patients receiving cetuximab require premedication with acetaminophen and diphenhydramine and may require modifications to their administration schedule or permanent discontinuation if they develop severe allergic toxicity. A skin rash and diarrhea are also commonly seen with both agents, and health care practitioners should provide counseling to patients about these adverse effects. Treatment options include common medications used to treat acne (doxycycline), topical and systemic steroids, and general skin care. Patients may be offered these agents prophylactically, upon initiation of therapy, to decrease the potential impact the rash has on their quality of life. Development of rash may be a surrogate marker of response, and clinicians should attempt to minimize the complications of the rash before discontinuing therapy.[15] Other toxicities common to both agents include low magnesium, calcium, and potassium levels that require checking levels and replacement therapy as clinically indicated. A rare adverse effect (less than 1%), interstitial lung disease is seen with all agents that inhibit EGFR, and patients should be instructed to report any new-onset shortness of breath. Cetuximab has an initial loading dose of 400 mg/m^2 IV infusion. Weekly doses of 250 mg/m^2 are then administered starting the following week. Panitumumab is given 6 mg/kg every 2 weeks.

RECTAL CANCER

Although often treated similarly to colon cancer, there are some important differences in the treatment of rectal cancer, especially in the adjuvant setting. Rectal cancer involves tumors found in the distal 15 cm of the large bowel and, as such, is very distinct from colon cancer in that it has a propensity for both local and distant recurrence. The higher incidence of local failure and poorer overall prognosis associated with rectal cancer are attributable to limitations in surgical techniques.

Patient Encounter, Part 4

Despite completing six cycles of adjuvant chemotherapy, the patient's disease progresses, and a CT scan reveals metastases to her bone and liver. The tumor is sent for pharmacogenomic profiling and is found to be positive for the wild type *KRAS* gene (no mutation detected).

What pharmacologic treatment options are available for the treatment of her metastatic disease?

Therefore, multimodality therapies with a combination of chemotherapy, radiation, and surgery are at the forefront in the treatment of rectal cancer with the main goal of survival and quality of life by preserving the function of the anal sphincter. In addition, because treatment with surgery, radiation, or systemic chemotherapy at the time of the recurrence is often suboptimal, adjuvant therapy after tumor resection is an important aspect of treatment of the primary tumor. Similar to adjuvant therapy for colon cancer, 5-FU provides the basis for chemotherapy regimens for rectal cancer.

KEY CONCEPT *Adjuvant therapy consisting of 5-FU–based chemotherapy in combination with radiation therapy should be offered to patients with stage II or III cancer of the rectum.*[50] Radiation therapy decreases the rate of local recurrences, but 5-FU decreases the risk of distant tumor recurrence as well as acting as a radiosensitizer. Toxicities from combined modality therapy include severe hematologic toxicity, enteritis, and diarrhea. Additional trials have sought to determine optimal combinations of concurrent radiation and 5-FU. Similar to tumors in the colon, continuous infusions of 5-FU appear to be superior to bolus doses. However, leucovorin does not appear to improve efficacy of adjuvant treatment for rectal cancer. Use of oral alternatives to 5-FU that are also known to enhance radiation effects, such as capecitabine, are under investigation with preliminary data suggesting the combination of capecitabine and radiation is likely to be safe and effective. In addition, based on the efficacy in colon cancer, FOLFOX regimens have moved into clinical trials in the adjuvant setting.

Another unique aspect of rectal cancer is the use of neoadjuvant therapy. Preoperative radiation (with or without chemotherapy) is given to downstage the tumor before surgical resection to improve sphincter preservation.[50]

KEY CONCEPT *Metastatic rectal cancer is treated with similar regimens as outlined in the colon cancer section are used for palliation of symptoms.*[50]

OUTCOME EVALUATION

The goals of monitoring are to evaluate whether the patient is receiving any benefit from the management of the disease, detect recurrence, and minimize the adverse effects of treatment. During treatment for active disease, patients should undergo monitoring for measurable tumor response, progression, or new metastases; these tests may include chest CT scans or x-rays, abdominal or pelvic CT scans or x-rays, depending on the site of disease being evaluated for response; and carcinoembryonic antigen (CEA) measurements every 3 months if the CEA level is or was previously elevated.[17] A PET scan can be considered to identify localized sites of metastatic disease when a rising CEA level suggests metastatic disease but results of CT scans and other imaging studies are negative. Symptoms of recurrence such as pain, changes in bowel habits, rectal bleeding, pelvic masses, anorexia, and weight loss develop in fewer than 50% of patients. Patients who undergo curative surgical resection, with or without adjuvant therapy, require close follow-up because early detection and treatment of recurrence could still result in patient cures. In addition, early treatment for asymptomatic metastatic colorectal cancer appears superior to delayed therapy. Colorectal cancer surveillance guidelines published by the American Society of Clinical Oncology recommend against routinely monitoring liver function tests, complete blood count (CBC), FOBT, CT scans, annual chest x-rays, or pelvic imaging in asymptomatic patients.[55]

In addition, a CBC should be obtained before each course of chemotherapy administration to ensure that hematologic values are adequate. In particular, white blood cell counts and absolute neutrophil counts can be decreased in patients receiving chemotherapy such as irinotecan and 5-FU. Baseline liver function tests and an assessment of renal function should be evaluated

Patient Care Process

Patient Assessment:

- Based on a review of symptoms and presenting signs and symptoms, determine what signs and symptoms the patient is experiencing are related to their colon cancer diagnosis.
- Review the medication history (including prescription and OTC medications) to identify agents that may worsen the patient's symptoms of colon cancer. Identify agents that effect bowel function (resulting in diarrhea or constipation) or agents such as NSAIDs that may cause GI bleeding.
- Review all laboratory and imaging studies, focus on the CBC, serum creatinine, and hepatic function.
- Determine performance status of the patient (see Chapter 88).

Therapy Evaluation:

- Determine if the patient requires chemotherapy to treat the colon cancer. If you determine they need therapy, evaluate treatment options for the patient.
- Review the chemotherapy order and assess efficacy, dosages, drug-interactions, and possible adverse effects from the regimen (see Tables 91–3 and 91–5).

Care Plan Development:

- Discuss lifestyle modifications that may assist in symptom and disease management.
- Calculate the body surface area (BSA) and determine if doses are optimal and correct for this patient. Evaluate laboratory values to assist in this process.
- Review supportive care options to decrease the impact of adverse effects for this patient (see Chapters 88 and 99).
- Counsel patient on potential adverse effects of the regimen.

Follow-up Evaluation:

- Follow up when the patient is scheduled for their next round of chemotherapy. Assess the patient for adverse effects of the regimen or other supportive care measures that may need to be added (eg, pain management).
- Review medication history, physical examination, laboratory results, and other imaging and diagnostic tests to evaluate if the patient should continue on their current chemotherapy regimen.

before and periodically during therapy. Other selected laboratory tests include checking for the presence of protein in the urine in patients receiving bevacizumab and monitoring of magnesium, calcium, and potassium in patients receiving cetuximab or panitumumab.

Patients should be evaluated during every treatment visit for the presence of anticipated side effects from their treatment, and health care practitioners should anticipate these adverse reactions and aggressively treat and prevent them from occurring. These generally include loose stools or diarrhea from irinotecan, 5-FU, and capecitabine; hand-foot syndrome from 5-FU and capecitabine; nausea or vomiting from irinotecan, 5-FU, and oxaliplatin; mouth sores from 5-FU; neuropathies from oxaliplatin; bleeding and hypertension from bevacizumab; and skin rash associated with cetuximab and panitumumab.

SUMMARY

Recent advances in the treatment of cancer of the colon and rectum now offer the potential to improve patient survival, but for many patients, improved DFS and PFS represent equally important therapeutic outcomes. In the absence of the ability of a specific treatment to demonstrate improved survival, important outcome measures should include the effects of the treatment on patient symptoms, daily activities, PS, and other quality-of-life indicators. Individualized patient care to balance the risks associated with treatment and benefits of a specific treatment regimen is necessary to optimize patient outcomes.

Abbreviations Introduced in This Chapter

APC	Adenomatous polyposis coli
CapeOX	Capecitabine and oxaliplatin
CBC	Complete blood count
CEA	Carcinoembryonic antigen
COX-2	Cyclooxygenase-2
CTC	Computed tomographic colonoscopy
DFS	Disease-free survival
DPD	Dihydropyrimidine dehydrogenase
EGFR	Epidermal growth factor receptor
FAP	Familial adenomatous polyposis
FIT	Fecal immunochemical test
FOBT	Fecal occult blood test
FOLFIRI	Folinic acid, fluorouracil, and infusional irinotecan
FOLFOX	Folinic acid, fluorouracil, and oxaliplatin
GI	Gastrointestinal
HNPCC	Hereditary nonpolyposis colorectal cancer
INR	International normalized ratio
MSI	Mircrosatellite instability
NSAID	Nonsteroidal anti-inflammatory drug
PET	Positron emission tomography
PFS	Progression-free survival
TNM	Tumor, node, metastasis
TP	Thymidine phosphorylase
UGT	UDP-glucuronosyltransferase
VEGF	Vascular endothelial growth factor

REFERENCES

1. Siegel R, Ma J, Zou Z, Jemal A. Cancer statistics, 2014. CA Cancer J Clin. 2014;64:9–29.
2. Ries LAG, Eisner MP, Kosary CL, et al., eds. SEER Cancer Statistics Review, 1975–2011. Bethesda, MD: National Cancer Institute. http://seer.cancer.gov/csr/1975_2011. Accessed October 10, 2015.
3. Park Y, Hunter DJ, Spiegelman D, et al. Dietary fiber intake and risk of colorectal cancer: A pooled analysis of prospective cohort studies. JAMA. 2005;294:2849–2857.
4. Giovannucci E. Modifiable risk factors for colon cancer. Gastroenterol Clin North Am. 2002;31:925–943.
5. Giovannucci E. Metabolic syndrome, hyperinsulinemia, and colon cancer: A review. Am J Clin Nutr. 2007;86(Suppl):S836–S842.
6. Calvert PM, Frucht H. The genetics of colorectal cancer. Ann Intern Med. 2003;137:603–612.
7. NCCN Guidelines—Colorectal Cancer Screening v.1. 2014. http://www.nccn.org.
8. Levin B, Lieberman DA, McFarland B, et al. Screening and surveillance for the early detection of colorectal cancer and adenomatous polyps, 2008: A joint guideline from the American Cancer Society, the US Multi-Society Task Force on Colorectal Cancer, and the American College of Radiology. American Cancer Society guidelines for the early detection of cancer. CA Cancer J Clin. 2008;58:130–160.
9. Hawk ET, Levin B. Colorectal cancer prevention. J Clin Oncol. 2005;23:378–391.
10. Chan AT, Giovannucci EL, Meyerhardt JA, et al. Long-term use of aspirin and nonsteroidal anti-inflammatory drugs and risk of colorectal cancer. JAMA. 2005;294:914–923.
11. Chan AT, Ogino S, Fuchs CS. Aspirin and the risk of colorectal cancer in relation to the expression of COX-2. N Engl J Med. 2007;356:2131–2142.
12. Cooper K, Squires H, Carrol C. Chemoprevention of colorectal cancer: Systematic review and economic evaluation. Health Techno Assess. 2010;14:1–206.
13. Nelson HD, Humphrey LL, Nygren P, et al. Postmenopausal hormone replacement therapy: Scientific review. JAMA. 2002;288:872–881.
14. Grunwald V, Hidalgo M. Developing inhibitors of the epidermal growth factor receptor for cancer treatment. J Natl Cancer Inst. 2003;95:851–867.
15. NCCN Guidelines—Colon Cancer v.2. 2014. http://www.nccn.org.
16. Libutti SK, Saltz LB, Tepper JE. Colon cancer. In: DeVita VT, Lawrence TS, Rosenberg SA, eds. Cancer: Principles and Practice of Oncology, 9th ed. Philadelphia: Lippincott Williams & Wilkins, 2011:1084–1126.
17. Libutti SK, Tepper JE, Saltz LB. Rectal cancer. In: DeVita VT, Lawrence TS, Rosenberg SA, eds. Cancer: Principles and Practice of Oncology, 9th ed. Philadelphia: Lippincott Williams & Wilkins, 2011:1127–1141.
18. Simmonds PC, Primrose JN, Colquitt JL, et al. Surgical resection of hepatic metastases from colorectal cancer: A systematic review of published studies. Br J Cancer 2006;94:982–999.
19. Benson AB, Schrag D, Somerfield MR, et al. American Society of Clinical Oncology recommendations of adjuvant chemotherapy for stage II colon cancer. J Clin Oncol. 2004;22:3408–3419.
20. Sargent DJ, Marsoni S, Monges G, et al. Defective mismatch repair as a predictive marker for lack of efficacy of fluorouracil-based adjuvant therapy in colon cancer. J Clin Oncol. 2010;28:3219–3226.
21. Twelves C, Wong A, Nowacki MP, et al. Capecitabine as adjuvant treatment for stage III colon cancer. N Engl J Med. 2005;352:2696–2704.
22. Andre T, Boni C, Navarro M, et al. Improved overall survival with oxaliplatin, fluorouracil, and leucovorin as adjuvant treatment in stage II or III colon cancer in the MOSAIC trial. J Clin Oncol. 2009;27:3109–3116.
23. Haller DG, Tabernero J, Maroun J, et al. Capecitabine plus oxaliplatin compared with fluorouracil and folinic acid as adjuvant therapy for stage III colon cancer. J Clin Oncol. 2011;29:1465–1471.

24. Saltz LB, Cox JV, Blanke C, et al. Efficacy of intravenous continuous infusion of fluorouracil compared with bolus administration in advanced colorectal cancer. Meta-analysis Group in Cancer. J Clin Oncol. 1998;16:301–308.
25. Saltz LB, Cox JV, Blanke C, et al. Irinotecan plus fluorouracil and leucovorin for metastatic colorectal cancer. N Engl J Med. 2000; 343:905–914.
26. Goldberg RM, Sargent DJ, Morton RF, et al. A randomized controlled trial of fluorouracil plus leucovorin, irinotecan, and oxaliplatin combinations in patients with previously untreated metastatic colorectal cancer. J Clin Oncol. 2004;22:23–30.
27. Tournigand C, André T, Achille E, et al. FOLFIRI followed by FOLFOX6 or the reverse sequence in advanced colorectal cancer: A randomized GERCOR study. J Clin Oncol. 2004;22:229–237.
28. Cassidy J, Clarke S, Diaz-Rubio E, et al. Randomized phase III study of capecitabine plus oxaliplatin compared with fluorouracil/folinic acid plus oxaliplatin as first-line therapy for metastatic colorectal cancer. J Clin Oncol. 2008;26:2006–2012.
29. Fuchs CS, Marshall J, Barrueco J. Randomized, controlled trial of irinotecan plus infusional, bolus, or oral fluoropyrimidines in first-line treatment of metastatic colorectal cancer: Updated results from the BICC-C study. J Clin Oncol. 2008;26:689–690.
30. Grothey A, Sargent D, Goldberg RM, Schmoll H. Survival of patients with advanced colorectal cancer improves with the availability of fluorouracil-leucovorin, irinotecan, and oxaliplatin in the course of treatment. J Clin Oncol. 2004;22:1204–1214.
31. Saltz LB, Clarke S, Díaz-Rubio E, et al. Bevacizumab in combination with oxaliplatin-based chemotherapy as first-line therapy in metastatic colorectal cancer: A randomized phase III study. J Clin Oncol. 2008;20:2013–2019.
32. Bokemeyer C, Bondarenko I, Makhson A, et al. Fluorouracil, leucovorin, and oxaliplatin with and without cetuximab in the first-line treatment of metastatic colorectal cancer. J Clin Oncol. 2009;27:663–671.
33. Van Cutsem E, Kohne CH, Hitre E, et al. Cetuximab and chemotherapy as initial treatment for metastatic colorectal cancer. N Engl J Med. 2009;360:1408–1417.
34. Douillard JY, Siena S, Cassidy J, et al. Randomized, phase III trial of panitumumab with infusional fluorouracil, leucovorin, and oxaliplatin (FOLFOX4) versus FOLFOX4 alone as first-line treatment in patients with previously untreated metastatic colorectal cancer: The PRIME study. J Clin Oncol. 2010;28: 4697–4705.
35. Tol J, Koopman M, Cats A, et al. Chemotherapy, bevacizumab, and cetuximab in metastatic colorectal cancer. N Engl J Med. 2009;360:563–572.
36. Amado RG, Wolf M, Peters m, et al. Wild-type KRAS is required for panitumumab efficacy in patients with metastatic colotrectal cancer. J Clin Oncol. 2008;26:1626–1634.
37. Hecht JR, Mitchell E, Chidiac T, et al. A randomized phase IIIB trial of chemotherapy, bevacizumab, and panitumumab compared with chemotherapy and bevacizumab alone for metastatic colorectal cancer. J Clin Oncol. 2009;27:672–680.
38. Cunningham D, Humblet Y, Siena S, et al. Cetuximab monotherapy and cetuximab plus irinotecan in irinotecan-refractory metastatic colorectal cancer. N Engl J Med. 2004;351: 337–345.
39. Jonker DJ, O'Callaghan CJ, Karapetis CS, et al. Cetuximab for the treatment of colorectal cancer. N Engl J Med. 2007;357: 2040–2048.
40. Karapetis CS, Khambata-Ford S, Jonker DJ, et al. *KRAS* mutations and benefit from cetuximab in advanced colorectal cancer. N Engl J Med. 2008;359:1757–1765.
41. Peeters M, Price TJ, Cervantes A, et al. Randomized phase III study of panitumumab with fluorouracil, leucovorin, and irinotecan (FOLFIRI) compared with FOLFIRI alone as second-line treatment in patients with metastatic colorectal cancer. J Clin Oncol. 2010;28:4706–4713.
42. Sobrero AF, Maurel J, Febrenbacher L, et al. EPIC: Phase III trial of cetuximab plus irinotecan after fluoropyrimidine and oxaliplatin failure in patients with metastatic colorectal cancer. J Clin Oncol. 2008;26(14):2311–2319.
43. Giantonio BJ, Catalano PJ, Meropol NJ, et al. Bevacizumab in combination with oxaliplatin, fluorouracil, and leucovorin (FOLFOX4) for previously treated metastatic colorectal cancer: Results from the Eastern Cooperative Oncology Group Study E3200. J Clin Oncol. 2007;25:1539–1544.
44. Bennouna J, Sastre J, Arnold D, et al. Continuation of bevacizumab after first progression in metastatic colorectal cancer (ML18147): A randomised phase 3 trial. Lancet Oncol. 2013;14:29–37.
45. Van Cutsem E, Tabernero J, Lakomy R. Addition of aflibercept to fluorouracil, leucovorin and irinotecan improves survival in a phase III randomized trial in patients with metastatic colorectal cancer previously treated with an oxaliplatin-based regimen. J Clin Oncol. 2012;30:3499–3506.
46. Wilhelm SM, Dumas J, Adnane L, et al. Regorafenib (BAY 73-4506): A new oral multikinase inhibitor of angiogenic, stromal and oncogenic receptor tyrosine kinases with potent preclinical antitumor activity. Int J Cancer. 2011;129:245–255.
47. Wolpin BM, Mayer RJ. Systemic treatment of colorectal. Gastroenterology. 2008;134:1296–1310.
48. Mercier C, Ciccolini J. Profiling dihydropyrimidine dehydrogenase deficiency in patients with cancer undergoing 5-fluorouracil/capecitabine therapy. Clin Colorectal Cancer. 2006; 6:288–296.
49. Mitchell EP. Targeted therapy for metastatic colorectal cancer: Role of aflibercept. Clin Colorectal Cancer. 2013;12:73–85.
50. NCCN Guidelines—Rectal Cancer v.1. 2014, http://www.nccn.org.

92 Prostate Cancer

Trevor McKibbin

LEARNING OBJECTIVES

Upon completion of the chapter, the reader will be able to:

1. List the risk factors associated with the development of prostate cancer.
2. Discuss the benefits and risks associated with screening for prostate cancer.
3. Determine the prognostic- and patient-specific data needed to determine appropriate treatment options.
4. Recommend an initial treatment for prostate cancer on the basis of stage, Gleason score, prostate-specific antigen, patient age, and symptoms.
5. State adverse effects associated with androgen deprivation therapy.
6. List adverse effects associated with treatment options for castrate-resistant prostate cancer.
7. Determine an appropriate treatment for a patient with metastatic castrate-resistant prostate cancer.
8. Understand the role of immunotherapy in the treatment of metastatic castrate-resistant prostate cancer.

INTRODUCTION

Prostate cancer is the most commonly diagnosed cancer in US men and the second leading cause of cancer-related death in men.[1] The disease course varies from a slow growing, asymptomatic tumor that may not require treatment to a rapidly progressing, aggressive tumor resulting in distant metastasis, morbidity, and mortality.

EPIDEMIOLOGY AND ETIOLOGY

KEY CONCEPT *Prostate cancer is the most frequently diagnosed cancer among US men and represents the second leading cause of cancer-related deaths in all men.*[1] In the United States alone, it was predicted that more than 280,000 new cases of prostatic cancer will be diagnosed and more than 27,000 men would die from this disease in 2015.[1] Although prostate cancer incidence increased during the late 1980s and early 1990s, owing to widespread prostate-specific antigen (PSA) screening, deaths from prostate cancer have been declining since 1995.[2] In the United States, 1 in 6 men will be diagnosed with prostate cancer, with 1 in 35 eventually succumbing to the disease.

The widely accepted risk factors for prostate cancer are age, race, and family history of prostate cancer (Table 92–1). Age is the greatest predictor of risk, the disease is rare under the age of 40, but the incidence sharply increases with each subsequent decade of life.[2] In an evaluation of autopsies from men in Michigan dying of unrelated causes, prostate cancer was identified in 2%, 29%, 32%, 55%, and 64% of men in their third, fourth, fifth, sixth, and eighth decades of life, respectively.[3] Men of older age have had a greater lifetime exposure to testosterone, a known growth signal for the prostate.

Race

The incidence of clinical prostate cancer varies across geographic regions. Scandinavian countries and the United States report the highest incidence of prostate cancer, but the disease is less common in Japan and other Asian countries.[2] African American men have the highest rate of prostate cancer in the world, and prostate cancer mortality in African Americans is approximately twice that seen in the white population. Hormonal, dietary, and genetic differences, as well as differences in access to health care, may contribute to the variability in incidence and mortality in these populations.[2] Testosterone, commonly implicated in the pathogenesis of prostate cancer, is 15% higher in African American men compared with white men. Activity of 5-α-reductase, the enzyme that converts testosterone to its more active form, dihydrotestosterone (DHT), in the prostate is decreased in Japanese men compared with African Americans and whites.[2,3] In addition, genetic variations in the androgen receptor exist. Activation of the androgen receptor is inversely correlated with trinucleotide (CAG) repeat length. Shorter CAG repeat sequences have been found in African Americans. The combination of increased testosterone and increased androgen receptor activation may account for the increased risk of prostate cancer in African American men.[2]

Family History

Men with a brother or father with prostate cancer have twice the risk for prostate cancer compared to the rest of the population.[2] Genome-wide scans have identified potential prostate cancer susceptibility candidate genes, and there appears to be a familial clustering of a prostate cancer syndrome. Common exposure

Table 92–1

Risk Factors Associated with Prostate Cancer

Factor	Possible Relationship
Probable Risk Factors	
Age	More than 70% of cases are diagnosed in men older than 65 years
Race	African Americans have a higher incidence and death rate
Genetic	Familial prostate cancer inherited in an autosomal dominant manner
	Mutations in *p53*, *Rb*, E-cadherin, α-catenin, androgen receptor, *KAI1*, and microsatellite instability; loss of heterozygosity at 1, 2q, 12p, 15q, 16p, and 16q; *BRCA1* and *BRCA2* mutations
	Candidate prostate cancer gene locus identified on chromosome 1
Possible Risk Factors	
Environmental	Clinical carcinoma incidence varies worldwide
	Latent carcinoma similar between regions' nationalized men adopt intermediate incidence rates between that of the United States and their native country
Occupational	Increased risk associated with cadmium exposure
Dietary	Increased risk associated with high-meat and high-fat diets
	Decreased intake of 1,25-dihydroxyvitamin D, lycopene, and β-carotene increases risk
Hormonal	Does not occur in castrated men
	Low incidence in cirrhotic patients
	Up to 80% are hormonally dependent
	African Americans have 15% increased testosterone
	Japanese have decreased 5-α-reductase activities
	Polymorphic expression of the androgen receptor

to environmental and other risk factors may also contribute to increased risk among patients with first-degree relatives with prostate cancer.[2] Male carriers of germline mutations of *BRCA1* and *BRCA2* are known to have an increased risk for developing prostate cancer, although sequencing of these genes is not commonly performed.[4] However, as evidence has accumulated that several additional germline DNA sequence variants may be associated with prostate cancer, the possibility that genetic testing might be used to aid in prostate cancer screening, detection, diagnosis, or risk stratification has emerged. In one analysis, five such sequence variants, three single nucleotide polymorphisms (SNPs) at 8q24 and one each at 17q12 and 17q24.3, were found to have a marked association with prostate cancer, especially for men with a family history of the disease, showing a 9.46-fold increased risk (with 95% confidence interval of 3.62–24.72) for a prostate cancer diagnosis.

Diet

A number of epidemiologic studies support an association between high fat intake and risk of prostate cancer.[5] A strong correlation between national per capita fat consumption and national prostate cancer mortality has been reported, and prospective case-control studies suggest that a high-fat diet doubles the risk of prostate cancer. Dietary factors that are potentially protective for prostate cancer include retinol, carotenoids, lycopene, calcium, and vitamin D consumption.[5] Tomatoes, pink grapefruit, and watermelon are rich in lycopenes, antioxidants that help prevent damage to DNA. Studies suggest that lycopenes may help lower prostate cancer risk, but prospective clinical trials are needed. A large trial of selenium and vitamin E supplementation to prevent prostate cancer failed to show any benefit.[6]

Other Factors

Benign prostatic hyperplasia (BPH) is a common problem among elderly men, affecting more than 40% of men older than the age of 70 years. BPH results in the urinary symptoms of hesitancy and frequency. Because prostate cancer affects a similar age group and often has similar presenting symptoms, the presence of BPH often complicates the diagnosis of prostate cancer, although it does not appear to increase the risk of prostate cancer.[2,9]

Smoking has been associated with an increased risk of aggressive prostate cancer and smokers with prostate cancer have an increased mortality resulting from the disease compared with nonsmokers with prostate cancer.[2]

PATHOPHYSIOLOGY

The prostate gland is a solid, round, walnut-shaped organ positioned between the neck of the bladder and the urogenital diaphragm (Figure 92–1). Adenocarcinoma, the major pathologic cell type, accounts for more than 95% of prostate cancer cases.[7] Much rarer tumor types include small cell neuroendocrine cancers, sarcomas, and transitional cell carcinomas.

Prostate cancer can be graded systematically according to the histologic appearance of the malignant cell and then grouped into categories of well, moderately, or poorly differentiated grades.[7] Gland architecture is examined and then rated on the Gleason scale of 1 (well differentiated) to 5 (poorly differentiated). Two different specimens are examined, and the score for

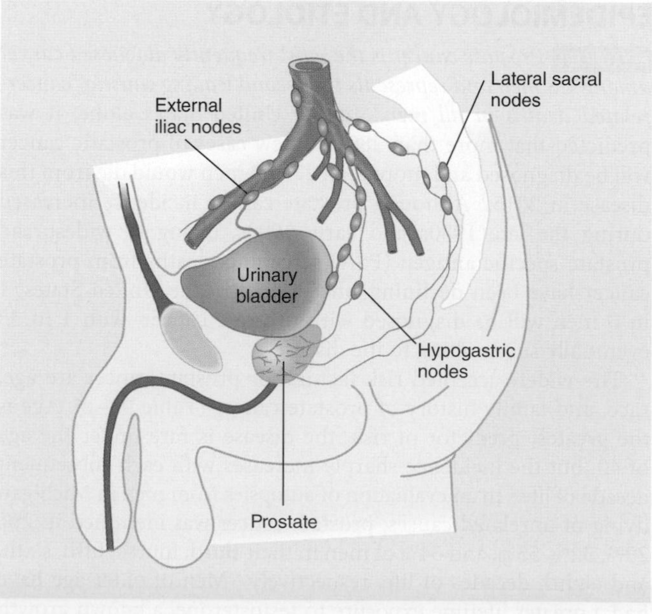

FIGURE 92–1. The prostate gland. (From DiPiro JT, Talbert RL, Yee GC, et al, eds. Pharmacotherapy: A Pathophysiologic Approach, 6th ed. New York: McGraw-Hill, 2005:1856.)

each specimen is added. Groupings for total Gleason score are 2 to 4 for well differentiated, 5 or 6 for moderately differentiated, and 7 to 10 for poorly differentiated tumors. Poorly differentiated tumors grow rapidly (poor prognosis), while well-differentiated tumors grow slowly (better prognosis).

Metastatic spread can occur by local extension, lymphatic drainage, or hematogenous dissemination.[7,8] Lymph node metastases are more common in patients with large, undifferentiated tumors that invade the seminal vesicles. The pelvic and abdominal lymph node groups are the most common sites of lymph node involvement (see Figure 92–1). Skeletal metastases from hematogenous spread are the most common sites of distant spread. Typically, the bone lesions are osteoblastic or a combination of osteoblastic and osteolytic. The most common site of bone involvement is the lumbar spine. Other sites of bone involvement include the proximal femurs, pelvis, thoracic spine, ribs, sternum, skull, and humerus. The lung, liver, brain, and adrenal glands are the most common sites of visceral involvement, although, these organs usually are not involved initially. About 25% to 35% of patients have evidence of lymphangitic or nodular pulmonary infiltrates at autopsy.

Normal growth and differentiation of the prostate depends on the presence of androgens, specifically DHT.[8,9] The testes and the adrenal glands are the major sources of circulating androgens. Hormonal regulation of androgen synthesis is mediated through a series of biochemical interactions among the hypothalamus, pituitary, adrenal glands, and testes (**Figure 92–2**).

Testosterone, the major androgenic hormone, accounts for 95% of the androgen concentration.[9] The primary source of testosterone is the testes; however, 3% to 5% of testosterone is derived from direct adrenal cortical secretion of testosterone or C19 steroids such as androstenedione. In the prostate 5-α-reductase converts testosterone to a more active form, DHT.[10]

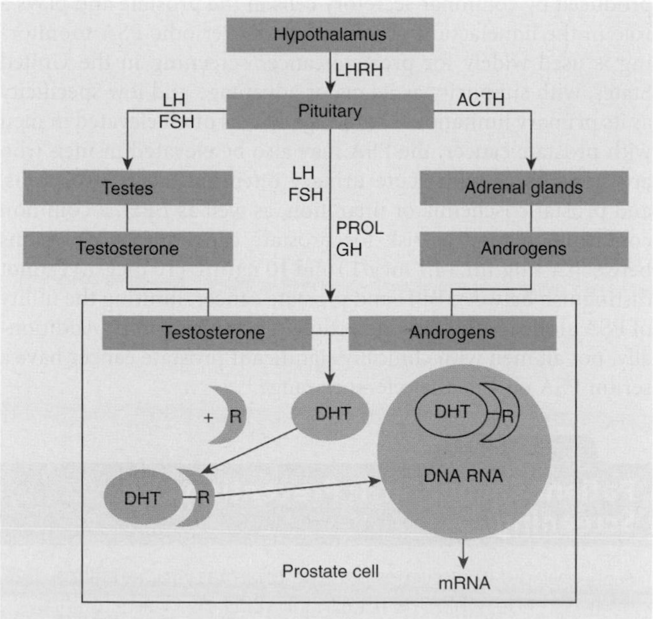

FIGURE 92–2. Hormonal regulation of the prostate gland. (ACTH, adrenocorticotropic hormone; DHT, dihydrotestosterone; FSH, follicle-stimulating hormone; GH, growth hormone; LH, luteinizing hormone; LHRH, luteinizing hormone–releasing hormone; PROL, prolactin; R, receptor.) (From DiPiro JT, Talbert RL, Yee GC, et al, eds. Pharmacotherapy: A Pathophysiologic Approach, 6th ed. New York: McGraw-Hill, 2005:1856.)

Table 92–2

Hormonal Manipulations in Prostate Cancer

Androgen Source Ablation	Antiandrogens
Orchiectomy	Flutamide
Adrenalectomy	Bicalutamide
Hypophysectomy	Nilutamide
	Enzalutamide
LHRH or LH inhibition	
Estrogens	Progesterones
LHRH agonists	5-α-Reductase inhibition
Progesterones[a]	Finasteride[b]
Cyproteroneacetate[b]	Dutasteride[b]
Gonadotropin receptor antagonists	
Degarelix	
Androgen synthesis inhibition	
Abiraterone	
Aminoglutethimide	
Ketoconazole	
Progesterones[a]	

LH, luteinizing hormone; LHRH, luteinizing hormone–releasing hormone.

[a]Minor mechanisms of action.

[b]Investigational compounds or use.

In early stage prostate cancers, aberrant tumor cell proliferation is promoted by the presence of androgens, namely testosterone and dihydrotestosterone. Blockade and reduction in the level of circulating androgens induces tumor regression in most patients. Hormonal manipulations to reduce circulating androgens can occur through several mechanisms (**Table 92–2**).[8-10] The testes, the organs primarily responsible for androgen production, can be removed surgically (orchiectomy). Hormonal pathways that modulate prostatic growth can be interrupted at several steps (see Figure 92–2). Interference with gonadotropin-releasing hormone (GnRH) or LH (by estrogens, GnRH agonists, direct GnRH antagonists, progesterones, and cyproterone acetate) can reduce testosterone secretion by the testes. Estrogen administration reduces androgens by directly inhibiting LH release, acting directly on the prostate cell, or decreasing free androgens by increasing steroid-binding globulin levels.[11]

The physiologic response to GnRH depends on both the dose and the mode of administration. Intermittent pulsed GnRH administration, which mimics the endogenous release pattern, causes sustained release of both LH and FSH, but high dose or continuous administration of GnRH inhibits gonadotropin release via receptor downregulation.[11] Structural modification of the naturally occurring GnRH and innovative delivery have produced a series of GnRH agonists that cause a similar down-regulation of pituitary receptors and a decrease in testosterone production.[12]

Androgen synthesis can also be inhibited in the testes or adrenal gland.[11] Aminoglutethimide inhibits the desmolase–enzyme complex in the adrenal gland, thereby preventing the conversion of cholesterol to pregnenolone. Pregnenolone is the precursor substrate for all adrenal-derived steroids, including androgens, glucocorticoids, and mineralocorticoids. Abiraterone is a specific and potent inhibitor of CYP17A1, decreasing the conversion of pregnenolone to dihydroepiandrosterone (DHEA), a required precursor for testosterone. Ketoconazole, an imidazole antifungal agent, causes a dose-related reversible reduction in serum cortisol and testosterone concentration through a similar mechanism. Megestrol is a synthetic derivative of progesterone that exhibits a secondary mechanism of action by inhibiting the synthesis of androgens. This inhibition appears to occur at the adrenal level, but circulating levels of testosterone also are reduced, suggesting that inhibition at the testicular level also may occur.[10,11]

Antiandrogens inhibit the formation of the DHT–receptor complex and thereby interfere with androgen-mediated action at the cellular level. Megestrol acetate, a progestational agent, also is available and has antiandrogen actions.[11] Finally, the conversion of testosterone to DHT may be inhibited by 5-α-reductase inhibitors.

In advanced stages of the disease, prostate cancer cells may be able to survive and proliferate without the signals normally provided by circulating androgens.[9,11] When this occurs, these tumors are referred to as **castrate resistant** and were formally known as hormone refractory or androgen independent. Because tumors remain amenable to secondary hormonal manipulations, and because the reintroduction of androgens can continue to promote tumor growth, the term castrate resistant more accurately reflects the clinical picture.

PREVENTION AND EARLY DETECTION

Chemoprevention

Significant decreases in the risk of prostate cancer have been demonstrated by the 5-α-reductase inhibitors finasteride and dutasteride.[13,14] Finasteride selectively inhibits the 5-α-reductase type-II isoenzyme, whereas dutasteride inhibits both type I and type II. Both finasteride and dutasteride lower the PSA by approximately 50%.[9,13] This lowering may vary across individuals or within the same individual over time. Although no prospective studies have validated a specific threshold for PSA monitoring in patients receiving a 5-α-reductase inhibitor, common clinical practice is to lower the PSA threshold by one-half, for example, a PSA of 4 ng/mL (4 mcg/L) for a man on dutasteride would be considered the same as a PSA of 8 ng/mL (8 mcg/L) for a man not on dutasteride.

The Prostate Cancer Prevention Trial compared 5 mg/day of finasteride for 7 years with placebo for the prevention of prostate cancer in men 55 years of age or older with normal digital rectal examination findings and a PSA of 3.0 ng/mL (3.0 mcg/L) or less. When compared with placebo, the prevalence of prostate cancer was reduced for those on finasteride by 24.8%. However, in those who did develop prostate cancer, there was an increase in the number of high-grade (Gleason grade, 7–10) tumors detected at biopsy in the finasteride group. Overall, finasteride did reduce the frequency of prostate cancer; however, the prostate cancers that were diagnosed in the finasteride group were more aggressive. There were no differences in overall survival. Common adverse events included decreased libido, erectile dysfunction, and gynecomastia.[13]

Dutasteride was evaluated in a different population of men.[19] The study randomized men that were 50 to 75 years of age with PSA levels of 2.5 to 10 ng/mL (2.5–10 mcg/L) and a recent negative prostate biopsy result to dutasteride 0.5 mg/day or placebo. Treatment with dutasteride resulted in a significant reduction in the risk for prostate cancer (RR reduction of 22.8%) as well as a reduction in acute urinary retention. There were no significant differences in overall survival.[15]

5-α-Reductase inhibitors decrease the period prevalence of for-cause prostate cancer by approximately 26% (RR, 0.74; 95% CI, 0.67–0.83). The absolute risk reduction is about 1.4%, although this may vary with the age of the treated population. On the basis of these outcomes, the ASCO and AUA guidelines recommend that asymptomatic men with a PSA less than or equal to 3 ng/mL (3 mcg/L) who are regularly screened with PSA may benefit from a discussion of both the benefits of 5-α-reductase inhibitors for 7 years for the prevention of prostate cancer and the potential risks (including adverse effects and the possibility of high-grade prostate cancer). Men who are taking 5-α-reductase inhibitors for benign conditions such as lower urinary tract symptoms may benefit from a similar discussion.[16]

Screening

Early detection of potentially curable prostate cancers is the goal of prostate cancer screening. For cancer screening to be beneficial, it must reliably detect cancer at an early stage, and identify those cancers that would benefit from an early intervention and decrease mortality. Whether prostate cancer screening fits these criteria has generated considerable controversy.[17,18] Digital rectal examination (DRE) has been recommended since the early 1900s for the detection of prostate cancer. The primary advantage of DRE is its specificity, reported at greater than 85%, for prostate cancer. Other advantages of DRE include low cost, safety, and ease of performance. However, DRE is relatively insensitive and is subject to interobserver variability. DRE as a single-screening method has poor compliance and had little effect on preventing metastatic prostate cancer in one large case-control study.

KEY CONCEPT *Prostate-specific antigen (PSA) is a useful marker for detecting prostate cancer at early stages, predicting outcome for localized disease, monitoring disease-free status, and monitoring response to treatment of advanced-stage disease.* PSA is a member of the human kallikrein gene family of serine proteases. PSA is produced by columnar secretory cells in the prostate and plays a role in the liquefaction of seminal fluid. Periodic PSA monitoring is used widely for prostate cancer screening in the United States, with simplicity as its major advantage and low specificity as its primary limitation.[19] Although PSA is often elevated in men with prostate cancer, the PSA may also be elevated in men who are smokers or with acute urinary retention, acute prostatitis, and prostatic ischemia or infarction, as well as BPH, a common condition in men at risk for prostate cancer. PSA elevations between 4.1 ng/mL (4.1 mcg/L) and 10 ng/mL (10 mcg/L) cannot distinguish between BPH and prostate cancer, limiting the utility of PSA alone for the early detection of prostate cancer. Additionally, not all men with clinically significant prostate cancer have a serum PSA outside the reference range.[17]

Patient Encounter 1: Prevention and Screening

A 56-year-old man comes into the pharmacy for a refill of his finasteride, which he is taking for BPH. He wants to know what he can do to reduce his risk of prostate cancer.

This patient does not have a family history of prostate cancer. He has never been screened for prostate cancer.

What do you recommend for prostate cancer screening?

What do you recommend for prostate cancer chemoprevention?

The benefit of prostate cancer screening is controversial. PSA measurements can identify small, subclinical prostate cancers, in which no intervention may be required. Detecting prostate cancer in those not needing therapy subjects some patients to unnecessary workups and psychological stress related to a cancer diagnosis.[18] Currently, the American College of Physicians recommends that rather than screening all men for prostate cancer as a matter of routine, physicians should describe the potential benefits and known risks of screening, diagnosis, and treatment; listen to the patient's concerns; and then decide on an individual's screening method.[17] The US Preventative Task Force rates PSA screening for prostate cancer a grade D, intended to "discourage the use of the service."[20]

CLINICAL PRESENTATION AND DIAGNOSIS (Table 92–3)

KEY CONCEPT *The prognosis for patients with prostate cancer depends on the histologic grade and stage of the prostate cancer*[20,2,23] Details of staging is discussed in Chapter 88. One of the most important prognostic criteria appears to be the histologic grade, assessed by Gleason score. Poorly differentiated tumors are highly associated with both regional lymph node involvement and distant metastases. Once the tumor has spread into locoregional lymph nodes, there is a significantly increased risk of recurrence of disease after curative intent therapy.[23]

TREATMENT

Desired Outcome

The desired outcome in early stage prostate cancer is to minimize morbidity and mortality from prostate cancer with consideration that some degree of morbidity may be caused by the toxicity of treatment.[23] Early stage disease may be treated with surgery, radiation, or observation. Although surgery and radiation are curative, they are associated with significant morbidity and a low rate of mortality. Because the overall goal is to minimize morbidity and mortality associated with the disease, observation is appropriate in selected individuals with a low risk of rapid disease progression. Advanced prostate cancer (metastatic spread) is not curable, and treatment of advanced disease should focus on providing symptom relief and maintaining quality of life.

Table 92–3

Diagnostic and Staging and Classification Systems Workup for Prostate Cancer

Initial tests	DRE PSA TRUS if either DRE is positive or PSA is elevated Biopsy
Staging tests	Gleason score on biopsy specimen Bone scan CBC Liver function tests Serum phosphatases (acid/alkaline) Excretory urography Chest radiography
Additional staging tests (depends on tumor classification, PSA, and Gleason score)	Skeletal films Lymph node evaluation Pelvic CT ^{111}In-labeled capromab pendetide scan Bipedal lymphangiogram Transrectal MRI

CBC, complete blood count; CT, computed tomography; DRE, digital rectal examination; MRI, magnetic resonance imaging; PSA, prostate-specific antigen; TRUS, transrectal ultrasonography.

Clinical Presentation of Prostate Cancer[21,22]

Localized Disease

Asymptomatic

Locally Invasive Disease

Ureteral dysfunction, frequency, hesitancy, and dribbling

Impotence

Advanced Disease

Back pain

Cord compression

Lower extremity edema

Pathologic fractures

Anemia

Weight loss

General Approach to Treatment

The initial treatment for prostate cancer depends on the disease stage, Gleason score, presence of symptoms, and life expectancy of the patient.[22] For asymptomatic patients, determining risk for disease progression and recurrence are critical for determining treatment options. Asymptomatic patients with a low risk of recurrence, those with a T_1 or T_{2a} tumor, with a Gleason score of 2 through 6, and a PSA of less than 10 ng/mL (10 mcg/L) may be managed by active surveillance. However, radiation or radical prostatectomy may also be offered (Table 92–4). Because patients with asymptomatic, early stage disease generally have an excellent 10-year survival rate, immediate morbidities of prostatectomy or radiation must be balanced with the lower likelihood of dying from prostate cancer. In general, more aggressive treatments of early stage prostate cancer are reserved for younger men, although patient preference is a major consideration in all treatment decisions. In a patient with a life expectancy of less than 10 years, observation or radiation therapy alone may be preferred. In those with a life expectancy of equal to or greater than 10 years, radiation (**external beam** or **brachytherapy**), or radical **prostatectomy** with a pelvic lymph node dissection may be offered; however, observation can still be used.[23]

Radical prostatectomy and radiation therapy generally are considered therapeutically equivalent for localized prostate cancer.[23] Complications from radical prostatectomy include blood loss, stricture formation, incontinence, lymphocele, fistula formation, anesthetic risk, and impotence. Nerve-sparing radical prostatectomy can be performed in many patients; 50% to 80% regain sexual potency within the first year. Acute complications from radiation therapy include cystitis, proctitis, hematuria, urinary retention, penoscrotal edema, and impotence (30% incidence).[23] Chronic complications include proctitis, diarrhea, cystitis, enteritis, impotence, urethral stricture, and incontinence. Because radiation and prostatectomy have significant and immediate morbidity compared with observation alone, some patients may elect to postpone therapy.[23]

Table 92–4

Management of Prostate Cancer with Low and Intermediate Recurrence Risk

Recurrence Risk	Expected Survival (years)	Initial Therapy
Low		
T_1-T_{2a} and Gleason 2–6 and PSA < 10 ng/mL (10 mcg/L) and < 5% tumor in specimen	< 10	Expectant management or radiation therapy
	10 or more	Expectant management or radical prostatectomy with or without pelvic lymph node dissection or radiation therapy
Intermediate		
T_{2b} or Gleason 7 or PSA 10–20 ng/mL (10–20 mcg/L)	< 10	Expectant management or radical prostatectomy with or without pelvic lymph node dissection or radiation therapy with or without 4–6 months of androgen deprivation therapy
	10 or more	Radical prostatectomy with or without pelvic lymph node dissection or radiation therapy with or without 4–6 months of androgen deprivation therapy

PSA, prostate-specific antigen.

Individuals with T_{2b} disease or a Gleason score of 7 or a PSA ranging from 10 to 20 ng/mL (10 to 20 mcg/L) are considered at intermediate risk for prostate cancer recurrence. Individuals with less than a 10-year expected survival may be offered observation, radiation therapy, or radical prostatectomy with or without a pelvic lymph node dissection, and those with a greater than or equal to 10-year life expectancy may be offered either radical prostatectomy with or without a pelvic lymph node dissection or radiation therapy (see Table 92–4).

The patients at high risk of recurrence (stages T_{2c}, a Gleason score ranging from 8 to 10, or a PSA value greater than 20 ng/mL [20 mcg/L]) should be treated with androgen deprivation therapy for 2 to 3 years combined with radiation therapy (Table 92–5).[24] Selected individuals with a low tumor volume may receive a radical prostatectomy with or without a pelvic lymph node dissection.

Patients with T_{3b} and T_4 disease have a very high risk of recurrence and are usually not candidates for radical prostatectomy because of extensive local spread of the disease.[23]

Table 92–5

Management of Prostate Cancer with High and Very High Recurrence Risk

Recurrence Risk	Initial Therapy[a]
High	
T_{2c} or T_{3a}, Gleason 8–10, PSA > 20 ng/mL (20 mcg/L)	Androgen ablation[b] (2–3 years) and radiation therapy, or radiation therapy or radical prostatectomy with or without pelvic lymph node dissection
Locally Advanced, Very High	
T_{3b-T4}	Androgen ablation[b] (2–3 years) or radiation therapy + androgen ablation (2–3 years)
Very High	
Any T, N_1	Androgen ablation[b] or radiation therapy + androgen ablation
Any T, Any N, M_1	Androgen ablation[b]

[a]Androgen ablation = serum testosterone levels less than 50 ng/dL (1.74 nmol/L).

[b]Luteinizing hormone–releasing hormone agonist (medical castrations or surgical are equivalent).

KEY CONCEPT *Androgen deprivation with a GnRH agonist should be used with radiation therapy for patients with locally advanced prostate cancer to improve outcomes over radiation therapy alone.*

KEY CONCEPT *Androgen deprivation therapy, with either orchiectomy, a GnRH agonist alone or a GnRH agonist plus an antiandrogen (combined androgen blockade), can be used to provide palliation for patients with advanced prostate cancer.* Secondary hormonal manipulations, cytotoxic chemotherapy, immunotherapy, or supportive care is used for patients who progress after initial therapy.[26]

Nonpharmacologic Therapy

▶ *Observation*

Observation or active surveillance involves monitoring the course of disease and initiating treatment if the cancer progresses or the patient becomes symptomatic. A PSA and a DRE are performed every 6 months with a repeat biopsy at any sign of disease progression. The advantages of observation are avoiding the adverse effects associated with definitive therapies such as radiation and radical prostatectomy and minimizing the risk of unnecessary therapies. The major disadvantage of observation is the risk that the cancer progresses and requires a more intensive therapy or metastasizes, making the disease incurable.

Patient Encounter 2: Initial Presentation and Treatment

A 58-year-old man presents to the clinic for follow-up of routine screening with DRE and PSA.

Physical examination is positive for a 1-cm nodule in the prostate, and his laboratory study results reveal the following: PSA, 22 ng/mL (22 mcg/L); PSA from 2 years ago was 2.4 ng/mL (2.4 mcg/L).

A prostate biopsy by TRUS reveals adenocarcinoma of the prostate with a Gleason score of 7. CT scanning and bone scan reveal disease that is metastatic to regional lymph nodes and the lumbar vertebrae.

Based on his metastatic disease, what are treatment options for this patient?

► *Orchiectomy*

Bilateral orchiectomy, or removal of the testes, rapidly reduces circulating androgens to castrate levels (ie, serum testosterone levels less than 50 ng/dL [1.74 nmol/L]).[23] However, many patients find this procedure psychologically unacceptable, and others are not surgical candidates. Orchiectomy may be preferred in the initial treatment of patients with impending spinal cord compression or ureteral obstruction.

► *Radiation*

The two commonly used methods for radiation therapy are external-beam radiotherapy and brachytherapy.[23,25] In external-beam radiotherapy, doses of 70 to 75 Gy are delivered in 35 to 41 fractions in patients with low-grade prostate cancer and 75 to 80 Gy for those with intermediate- or high-grade prostate cancer. Brachytherapy involves the permanent implantation of radioactive beads of 145 Gy 125-iodine or 124 Gy of 103-palladium and is generally reserved for individuals with low-risk cancers. Radiation therapy may be used to treat local or locally advanced prostate cancer with curative intent. In later stages of disease short courses of external beam radiation therapy can be used to palliate symptoms.[25]

► *Radical Prostatectomy*

Radical prostatectomy is performed in patients who are surgical candidates with disease that requires definitive therapy based on risk factors and patient preference; additionally, the disease must be amenable to complete surgical resection. Complications from radical prostatectomy include blood loss, stricture formation, incontinence, lymphocele, fistula formation, anesthetic risk, and impotence. Nerve-sparing radical prostatectomy can be performed in many patients; 50% to 80% regain sexual potency within the first year. Acute complications from radical prostatectomy and radiation therapy include cystitis, proctitis, hematuria, urinary retention, penoscrotal edema, and impotence (30% incidence).[23] Chronic complications include proctitis, diarrhea, cystitis, enteritis, impotence, urethral stricture, and incontinence. Because radiation and prostatectomy have significant and immediate mortality when compared with observation alone, many patients may elect to postpone therapy until symptoms develop.

Pharmacologic Therapy

► *Gonadotropin-Releasing Hormone Agonists*

GnRH agonists are a reversible method of androgen deprivation and are as effective as orchiectomy in treating prostate cancer.[23] Currently available GnRH agonists include leuprolide, leuprolide depot, leuprolide implant, triptorelin depot, triptorelin implant, and goserelin acetate implant. Leuprolide acetate is administered once daily, whereas leuprolide depot and goserelin acetate implant can be administered once monthly, once every 12 weeks, or once every 16 weeks (leuprolide depot). The leuprolide depot formulation contains leuprolide acetate in coated pellets. The dose is administered intramuscularly, and the coating dissolves at different rates to allow sustained leuprolide levels throughout the dosing interval. Goserelin acetate implant contains goserelin acetate dispersed in a plastic matrix of D,L-lactic and glycolic acid copolymer and is administered subcutaneously. Hydrolysis of the copolymer material provides continuous release of goserelin over the dosing period. Another formulation of leuprolide is a miniosmotic pump implanted intramuscularly that delivers 120 mcg of leuprolide daily for 12 months. After 12 months, the implant is removed, and a different implant can be placed. Triptorelin LA is administered as an intramuscular injection of 11.25 mg every 84 days. Triptorelin depot is administered once every 28 days as a 3.75-mg dose.

Several randomized trials have demonstrated that leuprolide, goserelin, and triptorelin are effective agents when used alone in patients with advanced prostate cancer. Response rates around 80% have been reported, with a lower incidence of adverse effects compared with estrogens. The choice between the three GnRH agonists is usually made on the basis of cost and patient and physician preference for a dosing schedule.

The most common adverse effects reported with GnRH agonist therapy include vasomotor symptoms such as hot flashes, erectile impotence, decreased libido, and injection site reactions. Long-term adverse effects include decreased bone mineral density and metabolic syndrome.[29] Disease flare-up in the first weeks of therapy can be caused by an initial induction of LH and FSH by the GnRH agonist, leading to an initial phase of increased testosterone production.[23] It manifests clinically as an exacerbation of disease-related symptoms, usually increased bone pain or urinary symptoms. This flare reaction usually resolves after 2 weeks and has a similar onset and duration pattern for the depot GnRH products. Initiating an antiandrogen before the administration of the GnRH agonist and continuing for 2 to 4 weeks is a frequently used strategy to minimize this initial tumor flare.

GnRH agonist monotherapy can be used as initial therapy of advanced prostate cancer, with response rates similar to orchiectomy.[23] They are preferred to orchiectomy for the adjuvant treatment of locally advanced prostate cancer as they are reversible. There is a lower incidence of cardiovascular-related adverse effects associated with GnRH therapy than with estrogen administration. A short course of concomitant antiandrogen therapy may need to be considered before initiating the GnRH agonist. Caution should be exercised if initiating GnRH agonist monotherapy in patients with widely metastatic disease involving the spinal cord or having the potential for ureteral obstruction because irreversible complications may occur.

Another potentially serious complication of androgen deprivation therapy is a resultant decrease in bone-mineral density, leading to an increased risk for osteoporosis, osteopenia, and an increased risk for skeletal fractures.[27] Most clinicians recommend that men starting long-term androgen deprivation therapy should have a baseline bone mineral density test and be initiated on a calcium and vitamin D supplement.

► *Gonadotropin-Releasing Hormone Antagonists*

An alternative to GnRH agonists is the GnRH antagonist, degarelix.[12] Degarelix reversibly binds to GnRH receptors on cells in the pituitary gland, reducing the production of testosterone to castrate levels. The major advantage of direct GnRH agonists is the speed at which they can achieve the drop in testosterone levels; castrate levels are achieved in 7 days or less with degarelix, compared with 28 days with leuprolide, eliminating the tumor flare seen and need for antiandrogens with GnRH agonists. Degarelix is equivalent to leuprolide in lowering testosterone levels for up to 1 year and is approved by the Food and Drug Administration for the treatment of advanced prostate cancer. Degarelix is available as 40 mg/mL and 20-mg/mL vials for subcutaneous injection, and the starting dose is 240 mg followed by 80 mg every 28 days. The starting dose should be split into two injections of 120 mg.

The most frequently reported adverse reactions are injection site reactions, including pain (28%), erythema (17%), swelling (6%), induration (4%), and nodule (3%). Most adverse effects were transient and mild to moderate, leading to discontinuation

Table 92–6

First-Generation Antiandrogens

Antiandrogen	Usual Dose	Adverse Effects
Flutamide	750 mg/day	Gynecomastia Hot flushes GI disturbances (diarrhea) Liver function test abnormalities Breast tenderness Methemoglobinemia
Bicalutamide	50 mg/day	Gynecomastia Hot flushes GI disturbances (diarrhea) Liver function test abnormalities Breast tenderness
Nilutamide	300 mg/day for first month; then 150 mg/day	Gynecomastia Hot flushes GI disturbances (nausea or constipation) Liver function test abnormalities Breast tenderness Visual disturbances (impaired dark adaptation) Alcohol intolerance Interstitial pneumonitis

GI, gastrointestinal.

in fewer than 1% of study subjects. Other adverse effects included elevations in lever function tests, which occurred in approximately 10% of study subjects. Similar to other methods of androgen deprivation therapy, osteoporosis may develop, and calcium and vitamin D supplementation should be considered. Degarelix is not approved in combination with antiandrogens.

Antiandrogens

The first generation of nonsteroidal antiandrogens include flutamide, bicalutamide, and nilutamide (Table 92–6). Monotherapy with first-generation antiandrogens is less effective than GnRH agonist therapy. Therefore, for advanced prostate cancer, all currently available antiandrogens are indicated only in combination with androgen-deprivation therapy, flutamide and bicalutamide are indicated in combination with a GnRH agonist, and nilutamide is indicated in combination with orchiectomy. Enzalutamide is a second-generation antiandrogen that is indicated in metastatic castrate-resistant prostate cancer.

The most common antiandrogen-related adverse effects are listed in Table 92–6. Diarrhea is reported more frequently with flutamide than bicalutamide.[21, 28] Few clinical trials have made direct comparisons among the first-generation antiandrogens.

Combined Androgen Blockade

Although up to 80% of patients with advanced prostate cancer respond to initial hormonal manipulation, almost all patients progress within 2 to 4 years after initiating therapy.[12, 29] Multiple mechanisms have been proposed to explain this tumor resistance. The tumor could be heterogeneously composed of cells that are hormone dependent and hormone independent, or the tumor could be stimulated by extratesticular androgens that are converted intracellularly to DHT. The rationale for combination GnRH agonists and first-generation antiandrogens is to interfere with multiple hormonal pathways to more completely eliminate androgen action. In clinical trials, combination hormonal therapy, also referred to as combined androgen blockade (CAB), has been used. The combination of GnRH agonists or orchiectomy with antiandrogens is the most extensively studied CAB approach.

Many studies comparing CAB with conventional medical or surgical castration have been performed.[29] CAB likely results in a small extension in overall survival compared to GnRH agonist alone or orchiectomy. However, adverse effects such as diarrhea, elevated liver function test results, and anemia are more common in those patients who receive CAB. Because the benefits of CAB are relatively small and the increased adverse effects are not insignificant, it is appropriate to use either GnRH agonist monotherapy or CAB as initial therapy for metastatic prostate cancer.[23] CAB may be most beneficial for improving survival in patients with minimal disease and for preventing tumor flare. All other patients may be started on GnRH monotherapy, and an antiandrogen may be added after several months if androgen ablation is incomplete, or if disease progression occurs despite a castrate level of testosterone.[32]

There is considerable debate concerning when to start hormonal-deprivation therapy in patients with advanced prostate cancer. The original recommendation to start therapy when symptoms appeared was based on trials in which no overall survival difference was demonstrated in patients who either started DES initially or crossed over to active treatment when symptoms appeared; the excess mortality rate was attributed to estrogen administration. Because GnRH agonists and antiandrogens have less cardiovascular toxicity, it is not clear whether delaying therapy is justified with these agents.[32] Thus, early intervention before symptoms appear is appropriate.

Secondary Therapies

Secondary or salvage therapies for patients who progress after their initial therapy depend on what was used for initial management. For patients initially diagnosed with localized prostate cancer, radiotherapy may be used for local disease recurrence after radical prostatectomy. Alternatively, androgen deprivation therapy can be used in patients who progress after either radiation therapy or radical prostatectomy.[32]

In patients treated initially with one hormonal modality, secondary hormonal manipulations may be attempted. This may include adding an antiandrogen for a patient who either incompletely suppresses testosterone secretion with a GnRH agonist or experiences disease progression while a castrate level of testosterone is maintained. In patients who have progression while receiving CAB, withdrawing antiandrogens, or using agents that inhibit androgen synthesis may be attempted.[32]

For patients who initially received a GnRH agonist alone, castration testosterone levels should be documented. Patients with inadequate testosterone suppression more than 20 ng/dL [0.7 nmol/L]) can be treated by adding an antiandrogen or performing an orchiectomy. If castration testosterone levels have been achieved, the patient is considered to have castrate-resistant disease, and palliative salvage therapy can be used. Supportive care, enzalutamide, abiraterone, radiaum-223, chemotherapy, immunotherapy, and local radiotherapy can be used in patients who have failed androgen deprivation.[26, 30, 31]

KEY CONCEPT *Antiandrogen withdrawal for patients having progressive disease while receiving combined hormonal blockade with a GnRH agonist plus an antiandrogen can provide additional symptomatic relief.* If the patient initially received CAB with a GnRH agonist with an antiandrogen, then anti androgen withdrawal is the first salvage manipulation.[32] Objective and subjective responses have been reported following the discontinuation of flutamide, bicalutamide, or nilutamide in patients receiving these agents as part of CAB. Patient responses to androgen withdrawal manifest as significant PSA reductions and improved clinical symptoms. Androgen withdrawal responses lasting 3 to 14 months have been reported in up to 35% of patients, and predicting response seems to be most closely related to longer antiandrogen exposure times. Incomplete cross-resistance has been noted in some patients who received bicalutamide after they had progressed while receiving flutamide, suggesting that patients who fail one antiandrogen may still respond to another agent.[32]

KEY CONCEPT *Once advanced prostate cancer progresses despite castrate levels of testosterone, it is known as castration-resistant prostate cancer.*[32] Previously, this was termed hormone refractory or androgen-independent prostate cancer. Castration resistant more accurately describes the cancer because it may continue to respond to treatments inhibiting the androgen pathways such as enzalutamide or abiraterone. Further, androgens remain a growth signal for the cancer and androgen deprivation therapy is continued throughout the treatment course of castrate-resistant prostate cancer.

Enzalutamide

Despite initial responses to androgen deprivation therapy and first-generation antiandrogens, disease resistance eventually develops. Enzalutamide is a second-generation antiandrogen that is effective in castrate-resistant prostate cancer, even when first-generation antiandrogens have failed.[3] This may be because enzalutamide prevents the androgen receptor from entering the cell nucleus, further inhibiting androgen signaling. Enzalutamide improves overall survival in castrate-resistant prostate cancer compared to placebo.[10,11] Primary adverse effects include fatigue, diarrhea, hot flashes, and musculoskeletal pain.[33] A rare incidence of seizures was also noted. Enzalutamide is effective in patients that have failed previous chemotherapy, or in patients that are chemotherapy naive.[26] Like other therapies for castrate-resistant prostate cancer, androgen deprivation therapy is continued. Enzalutamide is a strong CYP3A4 inducer and a moderate CYP2C9 and CYP2C19 inducer. Enzalutamide is known to decrease exposure and effect of multiple CYP enzyme substrates, including midazolam (CYP3A4 substrate), warfarin (CYP2C9 substrate), and omeprazole (CYP2C19 substrate).

Abiraterone

Despite androgen deprivation therapy with GnRH agonists, direct antagonists, or orchiectomy. Androgen synthesis can continue to occur in the periphery (namely the adrenal glands) or within the tumor. The family of cytochrome P450 of enzymes plays a critical role in the synthesis of androgens. CYP17A1 inhibition prevents the conversion of pregnenolone to DHEA, a requisite precursor for testosterone. Abiraterone acetate is a potent and specific inhibitor of CYP17A1 resulting in further reduction of testosterone when combined with continued androgen deprivation. Inhibition of CYP17A1 results in mineral corticoid excess, which contributes to the primary adverse effects of abiraterone. These include fluid retention, hypokalemia, and hypertension.[34] Less common significant adverse effects include hepatotoxicity. Abiraterone should be administered on an empty stomach either 2 hours after or 1 hour before a meal, as food significantly increases absorption. Abiraterone is effective in castration-resistant prostate cancer in chemotherapy naïve patients, as well as in patients with disease progression on docetaxel, not previously treated with abiraterone.[25,26,34]

Androgen synthesis inhibitors, such as aminoglutethimide 250 mg orally every 6 hours or ketoconazole 400 mg orally three times a day, can provide symptomatic relief for a short time in approximately 50% of patients with progressive disease despite previous androgen-ablation therapy.[26] Adverse effects during aminoglutethimide therapy occur in approximately 50% of patients. Central nervous system effects that include lethargy, ataxia, and dizziness are the major adverse reactions. A generalized morbilliform, pruritic rash has been reported in up to 30% of patients treated. The rash is usually self-limiting and resolves within 5 to 8 days with continued therapy. Adverse effects from ketoconazole include diarrhea, transient rises in liver and renal function tests, and hypoadrenalism. Additionally, ketoconazole is a strong inhibitor of CYP1A2 and CYP3A4. Absorption of ketoconazole requires gastric acidity; therefore, ketoconazole should not be administered with H_2-blockers, proton pump inhibitors, or antacids. Ketoconazole should be combined with replacement doses of hydrocortisone to prevent symptomatic hypoadrenalism.

Zoledronic Acid and Denosumab

Skeletal metastases from hematogenous spread are the most common sites of distant spread of prostate cancer. Typically, the bone lesions are osteoblastic or a combination of osteoblastic and osteolytic. Bisphosphonates may prevent skeletal-related events and improve bone mineral density. Zoledronic acid at a dose of 4 mg every 3 weeks reduces the incidence of skeletal-related (such as the need for palliative radiation or pathologic fracture) events by 25% compared with placebo.[35]

Denosumab, a monoclonal antibody targeted against the receptor activator of nuclear factor kappa-B (NF-*κB*), also

Patient Encounter 3: Progressive Disease

A 66-year-old man who was initially diagnosed with metastatic prostate cancer 5 years ago presents to the clinic. He was initially started on leuprolide and has progressed through treatment as described in the treatment summary below.

Treatment Summary

Date	PSA	Intervention
1/10/14	25 ng/mL (25 mcg/L)	Started leuprolide 7.5 mg IM every month
3/10/14	2 ng/mL (2 mcg/L)	Continued leuprolide
6/2/14	22 ng/mL (22 mcg/L)	Added bicalutamide 50 mg orally daily
9/2/14	5 ng/mL (5 mcg/L)	Continued leuprolide and bicalutamide
10/2/14	32 ng/mL (32 mcg/L)	Continued leuprolide; stopped bicalutamide
11/1/14	7 ng/mL (7 mcg/L)	Continued leuprolide

Today he presents to the clinic with bone pain and a serum PSA of 67 ng/mL (67 mcg/L).

Why was bicalutamide discontinued on 10/2/14?

How would you characterize the patient's disease?

What treatments are options for him?

decreases the incidence of skeletal-related events in patients with castrate-resistant prostate cancer with bone metastasis. Denosumab is a subcutaneous injection administered at a dose of 120 mg every 4 weeks. While it may cause a higher incidence of hypocalcemia compared to zoledronic acid, it also provides greater protection against skeletal-related events, such as fracture. Similar to zoledronic acid, patients should be counseled to take calcium and vitamin D supplementation.[35] Both denosumab and zoledronic acid also associated with a low but significant rate of osteonecrosis of the jaw.[36] Dental procedures should be avoided while receiving these agents and dental screening prior to initiation is recommended.[37]

KEY CONCEPT *Chemotherapy with docetaxel and prednisone improves survival in patients with castrate-resistant prostate cancer.*

Docetaxel 75 mg/m^2 every 3 weeks combined with prednisone 5 mg twice a day improves survival in hormone-refractory metastatic prostate cancer.[38] The most common adverse events reported with this regimen are nausea, alopecia, and bone marrow suppression. In addition, fluid retention and peripheral neuropathy, known effects of docetaxel, are observed. Docetaxel is hepatically eliminated; patients with hepatic impairment may not be eligible for treatment with docetaxel because of an increased risk for toxicity.[38]

The combination of estramustine (280 mg three times a day, days 1 to 5) and docetaxel 60 mg/m^2 on day 2 every 3 weeks also improves survival in hormone-refractory metastatic prostate cancer.[39] Estramustine causes a decrease in testosterone and a corresponding increase in estrogen; therefore, the adverse effects of estramustine include an increase in thromboembolic events, gynecomastia, and decreased libido (Table 92–7). Estramustine is an oral capsule and should be refrigerated. Calcium inhibits the absorption of estramustine. Although both the docetaxel–prednisone and the docetaxel–estramustine regimens are effective in hormone-refractory prostate cancer, the docetaxel/prednisone regimen reported similar efficacy without the cardiovascular adverse effects associated with estramustine.[25,26] In addition, androgen deprivation is continued when chemotherapy is initiated.

The regimen of mitoxantrone plus prednisone has been shown to be effective in reducing pain from bone metastasis and was a standard therapy before the development of docetaxel and prednisone.[26] Now, therapy with mitoxantrone is relegated to a salvage therapy after failure of other therapies.

KEY CONCEPT *Chemotherapy with cabazitaxel and prednisone improves survival in patients with castrate-resistant prostate cancer who have either progressed or are intolerant to docetaxel.*

Cabazitaxel is an antimicrotubule taxane with demonstrated activity in docetaxel-resistant cell lines and animal models of human cancer. A partial explanation is that docetaxel is a substrate for P-glycoprotein multidrug resistance transporter while cabazitaxel has low affinity. In patients previously treated with docetaxel and prednisone, treatment with cabazitaxel 25 mg/m^2 every 3 weeks with prednisone 10 mg/day significantly improved progression-free survival and overall survival compared with mitoxantrone and prednisone.[40] Neutropenia, febrile neutropenia, neuropathy, and diarrhea are the most significant toxicities. Hypersensitivity reactions may occur, and premedication with an antihistamine, a corticosteroid, and an H_2 antagonist is recommended. Cabazitaxel is extensively hepatically metabolized and should be avoided in patients with hepatic dysfunction (Table 92–8).

KEY CONCEPT *Immunotherapy with sipuleucel-T improves survival in patients with castrate-resistant prostate cancer with minimally symptomatic disease.*

Sipuleucel-T is a patient-specific anticancer vaccine.[41] Patients eligible for treatment first undergo leukapheresis to collect dendritic cells, which are sent to a central processing laboratory. These are then cultured and stimulated with a fusion protein of prostatic phosphatase and granulocyte macrophage colony-stimulating factor. The cultured cells are then returned and injected into the patient. This procedure is performed three times—at 0, 2, and 4 weeks. Treatment is well tolerated with common adverse effects of moderate and transient chills, fever, and transient influenza-like symptoms. Although disease progression was not improved by sipuleucel-T, overall survival was significantly improved from 21.7 months with placebo to 25.8 months with sipuleucel-T.[41] Because disease progression was not slowed by sipuleucel-T, it does not offer significant relief from disease-related symptoms. In symptomatic patients, or those with rapidly progressing disease an alternative treatment that delays tumor progression is more appropriate.

Radium-223

Radium-223 is an alpha particle emitting, calcium-mimetic, radiopharmaceutical that provides significant palliation to patients with castrate-resistant prostate cancer with bone metastasis.[42] Radium is taken up into the osseous metastatic loci of prostate cancer, where it emits primarily alpha irradiation. Alpha irradiation, as opposed to beta, consists of higher energy, dispersed into a smaller radius of approximately 1 cell length. Radium-223 results in lower rates of myelosuppression compared to alpha emitting radiopharmaceuticals. When given to patients with a high bone disease burden and limited visceral

Table 92–7

First-Line Chemotherapy for Metastatic Castrate-Resistant Prostate Cancer

Chemotherapy	Usual Dose	Adverse Effects	Dose Adjustments
Docetaxel	75 mg/m^2 every 3 weeks	Fluid retention, alopecia, mucositis, myelosuppression, hypersensitivity	*Hepatic* If AST/ALT is > 1.5 × the upper limit of normal and ALP is > 2.5 upper limit of normal, do not administer *Hematologic* Ensure CBC recovered
Estramustine	280 mg three times a day on days 1–5	Edema, gynecomastia, leukopenia, increased risk of thromboembolic events	*Hematologic* Ensure CBC recovered

ALP, alkaline phosphatase; ALT, alanine aminotransferase; AST, aspartate aminotransferase; CBC, complete blood count.

Table 92–8

Second-Line Therapy for Metastatic Castrate Resistant Prostate Cancer

Chemotherapy	Usual Dose	Adverse Effects	Dose Adjustments
Cabazitaxel	25 mg/m² every 3 weeks	Myelosuppression, neuropathy, diarrhea	*Hepatic* Extensively hepatically metabolized, usage should be avoided in hepatic dysfunction (ALT/AST > 1.5 × ULN or bilirubin > ULN) *Hematologic* Ensure CBC recovered
Abiraterone	1000 mg once daily	Edema, hypokalemia, hypertension, hepatotoxicity	*Hepatic* Moderate hepatic impairment (Child-Pugh class B), reduce the starting dose to 250 mg once daily; for development of hepatotoxicity during treatment, hold until recovery; retreatment may be initiated at a reduced dose
Enzalutamide	160 mg once daily	Edema, hypertension fatigue, hot flashes, seizures	Strong CYP2C8 inhibitors, avoid or reduce dose to 80 mg once daily

ALT, alanine aminotransferase; AST, aspartate aminotransferase; CBC, complete blood count.

disease, Radium-223 can significantly improve survival and improve palliation of pain. Primary adverse effects include moderate myelosuppression; exposure to radiation to caregivers is minimal. Plastic gloves are sufficient for shielding personnel from the radiation during administration to the patient.

Other radiopharmaceuticals that have been used for the treatment of bone metastases include strontium 89.[43] While palliation can be achieved, no survival benefit has been proven and a higher rate of hematologic adverse events is reported compared to Radium-223.

Patient Care Process

Patient Assessment:

- Obtain complete past medical history, family history, and social history.
- Obtain complete list of any concomitant prescription and over-the-counter medications; be sure to include herbal, vitamin, and mineral supplements.
- Verify completion of prostate cancer workup and staging.

Therapy Evaluation:

- Using information obtained, identify appropriate treatment options.

Care Plan Development:

- Discuss the benefits and risks of appropriate treatment options with the health care team and patient.
- If drug therapy is selected, review patient medical history for drug–drug and drug–herbal interactions.
- Initiate therapy.

Follow-up Evaluation:

- If patient is asymptomatic, monitor PSA and circulating androgens for castration level of testosterone. If patient is symptomatic, monitor symptoms for improvement or worsening.
- Monitor for any new symptoms and adverse events from therapy.

OUTCOME EVALUATION

Monitoring of prostate cancer depends on the stage of the cancer. When definitive, curative therapy is attempted, objective parameters to assess tumor response include assessment of the tumor size, evaluation of involved lymph nodes, and the response of tumor markers such as PSA to treatment. Following definitive therapy, the PSA level is checked every 6 months for the first 5 years and then annually.[23] Local recurrence in the absence of a rising PSA may occur, so the DRE and radiologic studies are also performed. In the metastatic setting, clinical benefit responses can be documented by evaluating performance status changes, weight changes, quality of life, and analgesic requirements, in addition to the PSA or and radiologic studies to objectively measure tumor response.

Abbreviations Introduced in This Chapter

BPH	Benign prostatic hyperplasia
CAB	Combined androgen blockade
DES	Diethylstilbestrol
DHT	Dihydrotestosterone
DRE	Digital rectal examination
FSH	Follicle-stimulating hormone
GnRH	Gonadotropin-releasing hormone
IM	Intramuscular
LH	Luteinizing hormone
LHRH	Luteinizing hormone–releasing hormone
NCI	National Cancer Institute
PSA	Prostate-specific antigen

REFERENCES

1. Siegel R, Ma J, Zou A, Jemal A. Cancer statistics, 2014. CA Cancer J Clin. 2014;64:9–29.
2. Brawley OW. Prostate cancer epidemiology in the United States. Worl J Urol. 2012;30:195–200.
3. Sakr WA, Grignon DJ, Crissman JD, et al. High grade prostatic intraepithelial neoplasia (HGPIN) and prostatic adenocarcinoma

between the ages of 20-69: An autopsy study of 249 cases. In Vivo. 1994;8:439–443.
4. Liede A, Karlan BY, Narod SA. Cancer risks for male carriers of germline mutations in BRCA1 or BRCA2: A review of the literature. J Clin Oncol. 2004;22:735–742.
5. Fleshner N, Zlotta AR. Prostate cancer prevention: Past present, and future. Cancer. 2007;110:1889–1899.
6. Lippman SM, Klein EA, Goodman PJ, et al. Effect of selenium and vitamin E on risk of prostate cancer and other cancers: The Selenium and Vitamin E Cancer Prevention Trial (SELECT). JAMA. 2009;301:39–51.
7. Iczkowski KA. Current prostate biopsy interpretation: Criteria for cancer, atypical small acinar proliferation, high-grade prostatic intraepithelial neoplasia, and use of immunostains. Arch Pathol Lab Med. 2006;130:835–843.
8. De Marzo AM, Meeker AK, Zha S, et al. Human prostate cancer precursors and pathobiology. Urology. 2003;62:55–62.
9. Nieto M, Finn S, Loda M, Hahn WC. Prostate cancer: Re-focusing on androgen receptor signaling. Int J Biochem Cell Biol. 2007; 39:1562–1568.
10. Shafi AA, Yen AE, Weigel NL. Androgen receptors in hormone-dependent and castration-resistant prostate cancer. Pharmacol Ther. 2013;140:223–238.
11. Sharifi N. Mechanisms of androgen receptor activation in castration-resistant prostate cancer. Endocrinology. 2013;154: 4010–4017.
12. Carter NJ, Keam SJ. Degarelix: A review of its use in patients with prostate cancer. Drugs. 2014;74:699–712.
13. Thompson IM, Goodman PJ, Tangen CM, et al. The influence of finasteride on the development of prostate cancer. N Engl J Med. 2003;349:215–224.
14. Musquera M, Fleshner NE, Finelli A, Zlotta AR. The REDUCE trial: Chemoprevention in prostate cancer using a dual 5alpha-reductase inhibitor, dutasteride. Expert Rev Anticancer Ther. 2008;8:1073–1079.
15. Andriole GL, Bostwick DG, Brawley OW, et al. Effect of dutasteride on the risk of prostate cancer. N Engl J Med. 2010; 362:1192–1202.
16. Kramer BS, Hagerty KL, Justman S, et al. Use of 5-alpha-reductase inhibitors for prostate cancer chemoprevention: American Society of Clinical Oncology/American Urological Association 2008 Clinical Practice Guideline. J Clin Oncol. 2009; 27:1502–1516.
17. Hayes JH, Barry J. Screening for prostate cancer with the prosate-specific antigen test: A review of current efidence. JAMA. 2014; 311:1143–1149.
18. Brawley OW. Prostate cancer screening: What we know, don't know, and believe. Ann Intern Med. 2012;157:135–136.
19. Schmid HP, Prikler L, Semjonow A. Problems with prostate-specific antigen screening: A critical review. Recent Results Cancer Res. 2003;163:226–231; discussion 64–66.
20. Screening for prostate cancer: U.S. Preventive Services Task Force recommendation statement. Ann Intern Med. 2008;149:185–191.
21. Simmons MN, Berglund RK, Jones JS. A practical guide to prostate cancer diagnosis and management. Cleve Clin J Med. 2011;78:321–331.
22. Cuzick J, Thorat MA, Andriole G, et al. Prevention and detection of early prostate cancer. Lancet Oncol. 2014;15:e484–e492.
23. Heidenreich A, Bellmunt J, Bolla M, et al. EAU guidelines on prostate cancer. Part 1: Screening, diagnosis, and treatment of clinically localised disease. Eur Urol. 2011;59:61–71.
24. Sumey C, Flaig TW. Adjuvant medical therapy for prostate cancer. Epert Opin Pharmacother. 2011;12:73–84.
25. Martin NE, D'Amico AV. Progress and controversies: Radiation therapy for prostate cancer. CA Cancer J Clin. 2014;64:389–407.
26. Basch E, Loblaw A, Oliver TK, et al. Systemic therapy in men with metastatic castration-resistant prostate cancer: American Society of Clinical Oncology and Cancer Care Ontario clinical practice guideline. J Clin Oncol. 2014;32:epub ahead of print.
27. Ahmadi H, Daneshmand S. Androgen deprivation therapy for prostate cancer: Long-term safety and patient outcomes. Patient Relat Outcome Meas. 2014;5:63–70.
28. Eisenberger MA, Blumenstein BA, Crawford ED, et al. Bilateral orchiectomy with or without flutamide for metastatic prostate cancer. N Engl J Med. 1998;339:1036–1042.
29. Weckermann D, Harzmann R. Hormone therapy in prostate cancer: GnRH antagonists versus GnRH analogues. Eur Urol. 2004;46:279–283; discussion 83–84.
30. Suzman DL, Antonarakis ES. Castration-resistant prostate cancer: Latest evidence and therapeutic implications. Ther Adv Med Oncol. 2014;6:167–179.
31. Fitzpatrick JM, Bellmunt J, Fizazi K, et al. Optimal management of metastatic castration-resistant prostate cancer: Highlights from a European expert consensus panel. Eur J Cancer. 2014; 50:1617–1627.
32. Heidenreich A, Bastian PG, Bellmunt J, et al. EAU Guidelines on prostate cancer. Part II: Treatment of advanced, relapsing and castration-resistant prostate cancer. Eur Urol. 2014;65:467–479.
33. Scher HI, Fizazi K, SAad F, et al. Increased survival with enzalutamide in prostate cancer after chemotherapy. N Engl J Med. 2012;367:1187–1197.
34. de Bono JS, Logothetis CJ, Molina A, et al. Abiraterone and increased survival in metastatic prostate cancer. N Engl J Med. 2011;364:1995–2005.
35. Saad F, Gleason DM, Murray R, et al. Long-term efficacy of zoledronic acid for the prevention of skeletal complications in patients with metastatic hormone-refractory prostate cancer. J Natl Cancer Inst. 2004;96:879–882.
36. Fizazi K, Carducci M, Smith M, et al. Denosumab versus zoledronic acid for treatment of bone metastases in men with castration–resistant prostate cancer: A randomized, double-blind study. Lancet. 2011;377:813–822.
37. Ruggiero SL, Dodson TB, Fantasia J, et al. American Association of Oral and Maxillofacial Surgeons position paper on medication-related osteonecrosis of the jaw-2014 update. J Oral and Maxillofac Surg. 2014;72:1938–1956.
38. Tannock IF, de Wit R, Berry WR, et al. Docetaxel plus prednisone or mitoxantrone plus prednisone for advanced prostate cancer. N Engl J Med. 2004;351:1502–1512.
39. Petrylak DP, Tangen CM, Hussain MH, et al. Docetaxel and estramustine compared with mitoxantrone and prednisone for advanced refractory prostate cancer. N Engl J Med. 2004; 351:1513–1520.
40. de Bono JS, Oudard S, Ozguroglu M, et al. Prednisone plus cabazitaxel or mitoxantrone for metastatic castration-resistant prostate cancer progressing after docetaxel treatment: A randomised open-label trial. Lancet. 2010;376:1147–1154.
41. Kantoff PW, Higano CS, Shore ND, et al. Sipuleucel-T immunotherapy for castration-resistant prostate cancer. N Engl J Med. 2010;363:411–422.
42. Parker C, Nilsson S, Heinrich D, et al. Alpha emitter Radium-223 and survival in metastatic prostate cancer. N Engl J Med. 2013; 369:213–223.
43. Crawford ED, Kozlowski JM, Debruyne FM, et al. The use of strontium 89 for palliation of pain from bone metastases associated with hormone-refractory prostate cancer. Urology. 1994;44:481–485.

93 Skin Cancer

Kenneth Lin and Jill Kolesar

LEARNING OBJECTIVES

Upon completion of this chapter, the reader will be able to:

1. Identify the risk factors associated with skin cancer.
2. Devise a plan of lifestyle modifications for the prevention of skin cancer.
3. Discuss the role of mutation testing in patients with newly diagnosed metastatic melanoma and the impact of the test on choosing drug therapy.
4. Explain the goals of therapy for the treatment of the different stages of nonmelanoma and melanoma skin cancer.
5. Compare and contrast the pharmacologic treatment options that are available for patients diagnosed with nonmelanoma and melanoma skin cancer.
6. Suggest management options for patients experiencing adverse effects of pharmacologic therapy.

INTRODUCTION

Skin cancer is the most prevalent of all malignancies occurring in humans, and in the United States, it accounts for more than 50% of all cancers.[1] The most common cutaneous malignancies are basal cell carcinoma (BCC), squamous cell carcinoma (SCC), and malignant melanoma (MM). BCC and SCC are categorized as nonmelanoma skin cancer (NMSC). It is estimated that more than 3.5 million cases (in more than 2 million people) of BCC and SCC and more than 100,000 cases of melanomas are diagnosed in the United States each year.[1] NMSC and MM differ with regard to prognosis, metastatic potential, mortality, curability, and treatment options.[2]

MELANOMA

EPIDEMIOLOGY AND ETIOLOGY

MM is the most common serious form of skin cancer, and the lifetime risk of developing it is 1 in 37 for men and 1 in 56 for women.[1] Approximately 73,870 new cases of melanoma are predicted to occur in 2015.[3] Melanoma represents about 2% of all skin cancers in the United States, but it accounts for 75% of all skin cancer deaths.[1] The incidence of melanoma is not evenly distributed among all populations; race, gender, and age confer different rates. The annual incidence rate per 100,000 is 1 for blacks, 4 for Hispanics, and 25 for non-Hispanic whites.[3] While women are more likely to develop melanoma than men before the age of 50, the converse occurs after the age of 50, with men having double the incident rate at age 65 and triple the rate at age 80 compared to women.[4] The change in risk may be due to the different level of sun exposure, be it occupational or recreational, through the lifetime of a particular sex. Even though incidence rates have significantly increased in the last 30 years, the rate among young age groups has leveled off; the incidence rate for men and women 50 years of age or older increased 2.6% per year from 2007 to 2011 but was relatively stable for those below age 50.

RISK FACTORS

Environmental

The risk factors for developing MM can be categorized as environmental factors and host factors. KEY CONCEPT *Exposure to ultraviolet radiation (UVR) from the sun is recognized as one of the primary triggers for skin carcinogenesis.* UV radiation (specifically UVB) is absorbed by DNA in the cells in the epidermal layer and may induce DNA damage. Gene mutations, such as UVR-induced mutation to the p53 tumor suppressor gene, may occur, resulting in dysregulation of apoptosis, expansion of mutated keratinocytes, and initiation of skin cancer.[2] Other mechanisms of UV radiation–induced DNA damage include the generation of reactive oxygen species, which create breaks in DNA, leading to genetic mutations and skin cancer.[2] It is estimated that 65% to 90% of MMs are attributable to UV exposure, particularly when a person has a history of intense and blistering sunburns in childhood. If a person experienced more than one severe sunburn in childhood, the risk of developing melanoma is increased twofold.[2] Exposure to sources of artificial UV radiation such as tanning beds has also been linked to increased risk of skin cancer.[2]

Host Factors

Host risk factors for developing MM include individuals with phenotypic characteristics of red hair, light skin, blue eyes, sun sensitivity, and freckling. Family history of MM in a first-degree relative is another risk factor for developing MM, with a twofold likelihood compared with patients with no family history.[2] In individuals without a family history of MM (sporadic

Patient Encounter, Part 1

A 55-year-old woman presents to her dermatologist with a pigmented skin lesion on her left shoulder that she noticed had enlarged and changed color recently in the past few months.

History: She has the lesion since youth, and it was measured at 3 mm. She noticed the change in color and size in the past few months.

The woman reports being a "sun worshiper" all her life; she spends her weekends outdoors or at the pool and vacations at the beach. She notes that she burns initially and then eventually tans with excessive freckling. She reports using an indoor tanning bed 3 to 5 days a week for the past 20 years. She does not use sunscreen or practice sun protection measures.

What are this patient's risk factors for developing malignant melanoma?

What primary prevention measures are recommended to prevent skin cancer?

What is the recommendation to detect melanoma early in a patient?

MM), the presence of benign melanocytic nevi (benign moles) is consistently identified as the strongest risk factor for the future development of MM. The greater the number of benign nevi a person possess, the greater the susceptibility to MM growth. A personal history of MM or NMSC also increases the risk of developing subsequent MM.[5] The dysplastic nevus syndrome is another risk factor. A person with five or more dysplastic nevi has six times the risk of developing MM than a person with no dysplastic nevi.[5] Larger nevi, as in the case of congenital melanocytic nevi (larger than 20 cm), is also associated with a greater risk of developing MM.[5]

The median age of MM diagnosis is 62 years in men and 54 years in women, and as a person ages, the risk increases further, especially in men.[6] The risk of MM is also increased in patients with immunosuppression due to cancer, AIDS, a history of chronic lymphocytic leukemia, non-Hodgkin lymphoma, and after organ transplants.[2] Rare genetic syndromes such as xeroderma pigmentosum (XP) increases the risk of developing MM and NMSC 100-fold compared with the general population.[6] MM has been reported in breast-ovarian cancer families with a 2.6-fold risk in carriers of *BRCA2* mutations.[6] An association has been found between pancreatic cancer and MM with mutation in *CDKN2A*.[6]

PRIMARY PREVENTION OF SKIN CANCER

UVR exposure from the sun is the major cause of NMSC and MM. Primary prevention strategies for skin cancer aim at educating people against excessive exposure to the sun and are spearheaded by the American Academy of Dermatology, American Cancer Society, Environmental Protection Agency, and Centers for Disease Control and Prevention. The aims of these programs are to increase public awareness about the harmful effects of sun exposure and the risk of skin cancer, change attitudes about the social norms related to sun protection and tanned skin, and decrease the incidence of skin cancer and deaths related to this malignancy. The National Council on Skin Cancer Prevention recommends a variety of simple strategies to minimize exposure to UV rays:[7]

- Seek shade when outdoors, especially between the hours of 10 AM and 4 PM when UV rays are most intense.
- Wear hats with a broad enough brim to shade the face, ears, and neck.
- Wear protective clothing (especially tightly woven apparel) that covers as much as possible the arms, legs, and torso.
- Cover skin with a sunscreen lotion with a skin protection factor (SPF) of at least 30, protecting against UV radiation (both UVA and UVB).
- Apply sunscreen 15 minutes before going outdoors and reapply sunscreens every 2 hours (especially if sweating or swimming).
- Avoid intentional tanning and tanning beds.
- Take extra caution near water, sand, and snow.

The use of chemical sunscreen is only one of many strategies, and it should not be the sole agent used for cancer prevention. Sunscreen protective agents have been proven only to reduce the risk of actinic keratosis (AK) and SCC. There is no convincing evidence that sunscreen application has protective effect against BCC or MM.[8]

SECONDARY PREVENTION OF SKIN CANCER

Secondary prevention of skin cancer involves early detection of premalignant cancers for early intervention with the hope that it will reduce mortality and increase cure. Regular screening for melanoma either by skin self-examination or total skin examination performed by health care providers consistently identify smaller and thinner lesions in high-risk patients.[9] However, recommendations for melanoma screening are conflicting because there are no randomized, controlled, prospective melanoma trials demonstrating that routine screening reduces mortality.

PATHOPHYSIOLOGY

MM is a cancer that arises from melanocytes, which are cells that synthesize melanin and contribute to hair and skin pigmentation. The overwhelming majority of MMs originate from the skin, although they may also arise less commonly from mucosal epithelial tissues such as the conjunctiva, oral cavity, esophagus, vagina, female urethra, penis, and anus. Exposure to UVR is an important factor in MM development. MM may occur in individuals with either inherent genetic susceptibility or low genetic susceptibility for melanocyte proliferation. The distinguishing characteristic is that MM may develop with less solar damage and on intermittent sun exposed body sites such as the trunk for individuals with high genetic susceptibility. Conversely, in individuals with low genetic susceptibility, melanoma occurs with chronic UV exposure on commonly exposed areas such as the face and neck.[10]

Genetic Pathway to the Development of Melanoma

Recent advances in molecular profiling and genome sequencing have enabled the identification of oncogenic mutations that drive MM progression. Much attention has been focused on the BRAF melanoma oncogene and its role in MM. BRAF is a serine/threonine protein kinase that is a member of the RAF kinase family, which is a part of the RAF/MEK/ERK serine threonine cascade (also known as ERK/MAP kinase pathway or "classical" MAPK pathway).[11] Mutations in *BRAF* activates the ERK/MAP pathway and thus trigger melanocyte proliferation and clonal expansion. BRAF mutation is found in approximately one half of all MM, and *BRAF* mutant melanomas tend to occur on intermittent sun-exposed skin areas, skin phenotypes that have poor UV protection (eg, pale skin, poor tanning response, red hair, and freckling), and younger individuals (younger than 55 years) with lower cumulative UV exposure.[12] There are more than 50 mutations in *BRAF* described, but the valine to glutamic acid (*BRAF V600E*) substitution accounts for over 75% of all *BRAF* mutations. Furthermore, this *V600E* mutation is the most common BRAF mutation in MM.[11] Potent and selective BRAF kinase inhibitors are now a mainstay for treating BRAF mutation positive metastatic MM.

CLINICAL PRESENTATION, DIAGNOSIS, AND STAGING

There are four major subtypes of cutaneous MM: superficial spreading, nodular, lentigo maligna melanoma, and acral lentiginous (Table 93–1). They each vary in clinical and growth characteristics.[13,14]

Data from Surveillance, Epidemiology, and End Results (SEER) show that 84% of diagnosed MM are locally confined, 9% are diagnosed after the cancer has spread regionally, 4% are diagnosed with distant metastasis, and the remaining 3% are not staged.[15] KEY CONCEPT *Once skin cancer is diagnosed, the cancer is staged to determine if the cancer is confined to the original tumor site or has spread to other sites, such as the lymph nodes, liver, brain, lungs, or bone. The purpose of staging is to determine prognosis, categorize patients with regard to metastatic potential and survival probability, and aid in clinical decision making.* As with most solid tumors, the tumor, node, metastasis (TNM) classification is used to stage MM.[16] Staging of solid tumors is described in Chapter 88.

KEY CONCEPT *Determination of lymph node status is important in melanoma staging because it is an independent prognostic factor, and it provides guidance for therapy decisions.* For patients with MM that are at risk of spreading to the lymph nodes, a sentinel lymph node (SLN) biopsy is performed. The SLN, the first lymph node to receive lymph draining from the tumor, is identified by injecting a radioactive material, technetium-99m-labeled radiocolloids, and vital blue dye into the skin next to the tumor and tracing the flow of lymph from the tumor site to the nearest lymph node chain. Once the SLN is located, it is removed and analyzed for the presence of MM cells. If it is positive for the presence of MM, then the whole lymph node basin in that area is dissected; this is also known as lymphadenectomy. An SLN biopsy is the initial procedure to assess the status of lymph node involvement to prevent the morbidity associated with a total lymphadenectomy.

In addition to the stage of the disease and the status of disease involvement in the lymph nodes, other prognostic factors for outcome in MM include primary tumor thickness (Figure 93–1), the presence of ulceration in the primary melanoma, mitotic activity, the presence of tumor infiltrating lymphocytes (TIL), and gender. Tumor thickness is defined as thin (less than 1 mm), intermediate (1–4 mm), and thick (more than 4 mm). The 10-year survival rate is 92% for thin tumors and 63% to 80% for intermediate tumors and decreases further to 50% in patients with thick tumors.[16] Ulceration is defined as the lack of an intact dermis overlying the primary tumor on histologic evaluation. Survival rates for patients with an ulcerated melanoma are proportionately lower than those with a nonulcerated melanoma of equivalent thickness, but the survival rate is similar for a nonulcerated melanoma of the next highest level of thickness. The male sex is associated with poor prognosis and adverse outcome in MM.[17]

Skin Examination

The *ABCDE* acronym is a helpful mnemonic for recognizing the signs and symptoms of early MM (Figure 93–2). It was devised in 1985 by clinicians working in the Melanoma Clinical Cooperative Group at New York University School of Medicine and is used to educate health care professionals who are not dermatologists in differentiating common moles from cancer.[9] It is also a useful tool to educate patients to assess pigmented lesions and screen for suspicious moles. This may help identify the MM in its early stage when it is curable. Not all MMs, including nodular melanoma, have all ABCDE characteristics, and it is not meant to provide a comprehensive list of all MM features. The characteristics for each of the letters are described in the Clinical Presentation and Diagnosis box. It should be noted that evolution of a lesion is one of the most important warning signs of danger in the assessment of moles for MM.

TREATMENT

Early diagnosis of skin cancer is the key to improved prognosis. On presentation to a clinician's office, patients may offer a history of a new growth or an area of irritation. Conversely, the skin cancer may have been present for years undetected by the patient. The definitive diagnosis of any suspected cutaneous malignancy should be confirmed by a biopsy before treatment.

The modality of treatment for skin cancer depends on the size, location, and stage of the tumor; the age of the patient; and the type of skin cancer. Treatment options for skin cancer include surgery, radiation, chemotherapy, immunotherapy, and targeted therapy.

Desired Outcome

The primary goals of therapy for MM are to completely eradicate the tumor and minimize the risk of tumor recurrence and metastasis. Secondary goals of therapy include preserving normal tissue, maintaining function, and providing optimal cosmetic outcomes. Patients with local disease MM (stages I and IIA) are curable with surgical resection of the tumor. Thus, the aim is to diagnose patients at the earliest stage to increase the probability of cure. Patients with regional disease (stages IIB, IIC, and III) have a high recurrence risk, and the goal of therapy is to prevent relapse of the disease. Disseminated, metastatic MM is not curable, and the goal of therapy is local control of the disease and palliation of symptoms.

The outcome of patients diagnosed with MM depends on the stage of the disease at diagnosis. The overall 5-year survival rate for patients with localized disease (stages I and IB) is the best at 89% to 95%.[16] For patients with stage IIA to IIIA disease, the 5-year survival rate ranges from 63% to 79%.[16] In patients with more advanced regional metastatic disease (stage IIIB to IIIC), the 5-year survival rate ranges from 24% to 59%. Patients with stage IV distant metastatic disease have the worst 5-year survival rate at only 7% to 19%.[16]

Table 93–1

Characteristics of Different Types of Skin Cancer

	Malignant Melanoma				Nonmelanoma Skin Cancer	
	Superficial Spreading	**Nodular**	**Lentigo Maligna Melanoma**	**Acral Lentiginous**	**Basal Cell Carcinoma**	**Squamous Cell Carcinoma**
Frequency	70%	10%–15%	10%	Less than 10%	75%	20%
Location	Head, neck Legs in women Trunk in men	Trunk, head, neck	Sun-exposed areas, face, head, neck	Palms of the hands, soles of feet, nailbeds	Head and neck	Face, hands, forearms
Age	Fifth decade	Seventh decade	Eighth decade	Sixth decade	Incidence increases after age 40	Incidence increases after age 40
Ethnicity	White	White	White	Most frequent type in ethnic groups of color	Similar between whites and African Americans	Most common in African Americans
Clinical features	Long horizontal growth phase (5–7 years); better prognosis	Very aggressive without identifiable horizontal growth phase; deeply invasive at the time of diagnosis; associated with poor prognosis	Long horizontal growth phase (10 years); lentigo maligna is the in situ form of lentigo maligna melanoma (only 5% transform to malignant melanoma)	Aggressive, rapid progression from horizontal to vertical growth; poorer prognosis	Rarely metastasize Circumscribed types: A: Nodular BCC, most common subtype B: Adenoid BCC C: Fibroepithelioma D: Basosquamous (metatypical) Diffuse types: plaque-like with horizontal spread and poorly defined margins A: Superficial BCC; second most common type of BCC, least aggressive B: Morpheaform, most aggressive C: Micronodular	Metastasize to lymph nodes and blood Have premalignant precursors and in situ variant; usually presents as raised pink papule or plaque, often scaly and sometimes ulcerated

Data from Refs. 14 and 15.

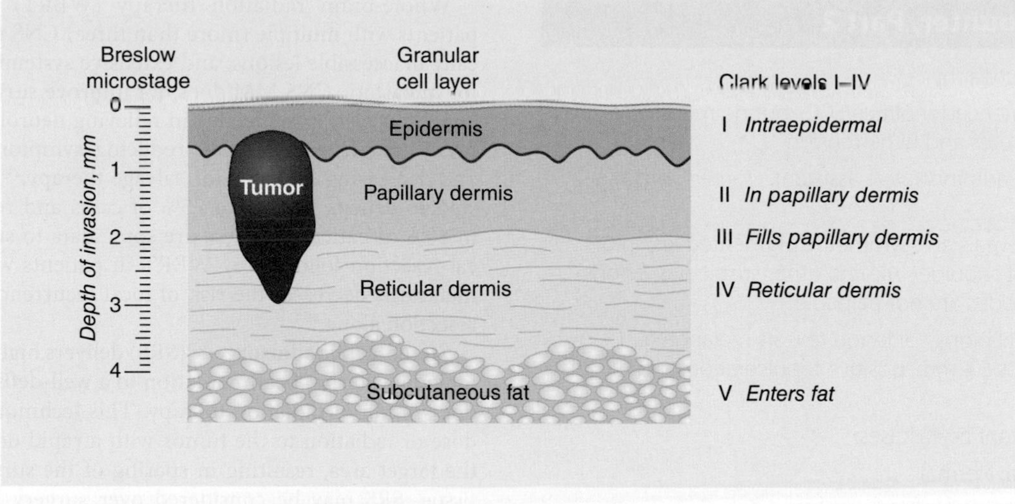

FIGURE 93–1. Skin anatomy: Breslow microstaging and Clark levels. Clark level refers to the level of penetration into the dermis. Breslow classification measures tumor thickness in millimeters from the epidermis to the deepest depth of penetration into the dermis. (From Langley RGB, Barnhill RL, Mihm Jr MC, et al. Neoplasms: Cutaneous melanoma. In: Freedberg IM, Eisen AZ, Wolff K, et al., eds. Fitzpatrick's Dermatologyin General Medicine, 6th ed. New York: McGraw-Hill; 2003:938.)

Treatment Options for Malignant Melanoma

▶ *Surgery*

KEY CONCEPT *The primary treatment modality for local/regional (stage I to III) MM is surgical excision of the tumor and a lymphadenectomy for patients with positive lymph nodes.* The goals of therapy are to optimize local control, achieve potential cure, and minimize morbidity. Achieving adequate surgical margins for the primary tumor is important in preventing local recurrence and improving overall survival. The thickness of the tumor dictates the extent of the surgical margin.[18] The most common first site of recurrence in primary melanoma after excision of the tumor is in the lymph nodes. KEY CONCEPT *For patients with metastatic MM, surgical excision is not curative. The primary goal*

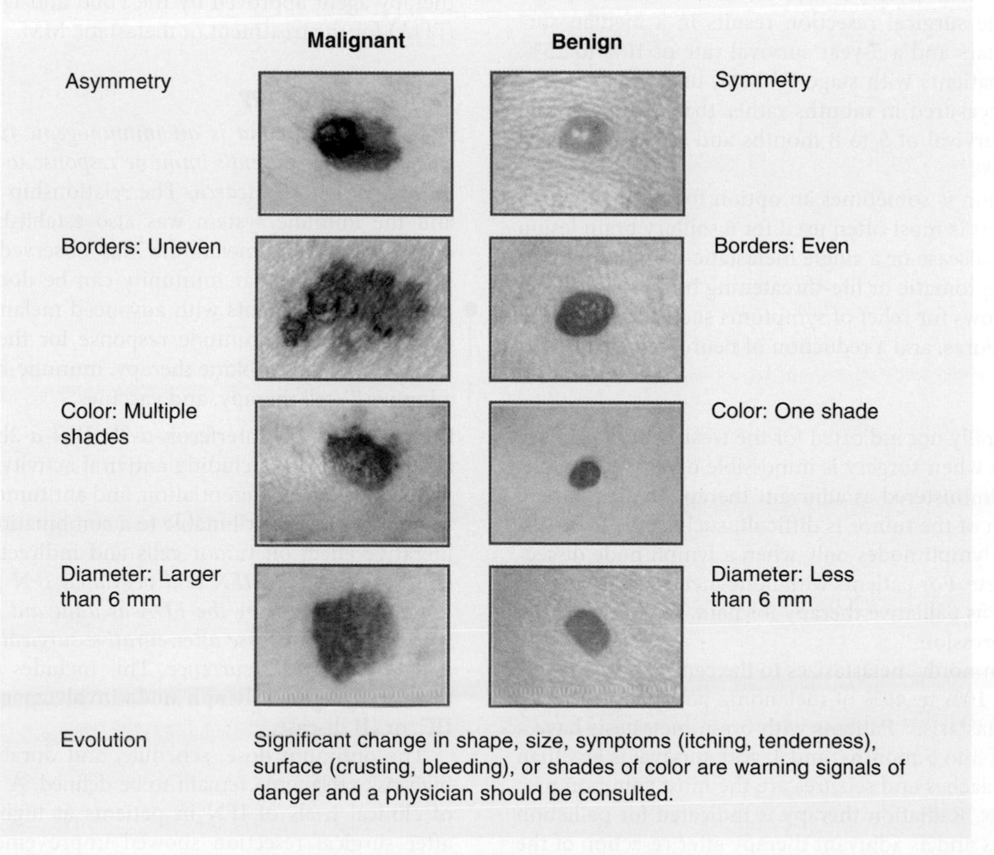

FIGURE 93–2. ABCDE features of early melanoma. (Images courtesy of the Skin Cancer Foundation, New York, www.skincancer.org.)

Patient Encounter, Part 2

PMH: Otherwise healthy

FH: Father experienced multiple SCCs but no melanoma. Mother has diabetes and hypertension

SH: Patient is an administrative assistant. Married with two children

Examination: Reveals an asymmetric pigmented lesion of 6 mm on the left shoulder with no other suspicious lesions noted. Lymph nodes are not palpable

Biopsy: Excisional biopsy of lesion reveals melanoma, Breslow thickness 5.4 mm, positive for ulceration, and mitosis 3/mm^2

CT Scan: No distant metastases

Laboratory Data: Normal

She underwent a surgical wide excision of the lesion with a 2-cm margin and sentinel lymph node biopsy. Pathology revealed negative margins and one of three nodes positive for melanoma. Her melanoma is diagnosed as stage IIIB. She underwent a lymphadenectomy of the left axilla

What is the treatment goal for this patient at this stage of her disease?

Should this patient receive adjuvant therapy?

of therapy is local control of the disease and relief of identifiable symptoms. In highly selected patients, such as those with good performance status, less aggressive tumor biology, prolonged period of disease-free interval from the time of primary tumor treatment, and limited disease that is contained within a single location, complete surgical resection results in a median survival time of 2 years and a 5-year survival rate of 10% to 25%. For most other patients with stage IV MM, unfortunately, the survival rate is measured in months rather than years, with an overall median survival of 5 to 8 months and a 5-year survival rate of less than 5%.[19]

Surgical resection is sometimes an option for patients with a brain metastases. It is most often used for a solitary brain lesion without systemic disease or a single metastatic brain lesion. For patients with symptomatic or life-threatening brain lesions, surgical resection allows for relief of symptoms such as intracranial hypertension, seizures, and a reduction of neurologic deficits.[20]

▸ Radiation

Radiation is generally not indicated for the treatment of primary melanoma except when surgery is impossible or not reasonable. It also may be administered as adjuvant therapy in areas where complete excision of the tumor is difficult, such as the face. It is indicated for the lymph nodes only when a lymph node dissection is not complete. For patients with bone metastasis, radiation may be indicated as palliative therapy for pain, fracture risks, or spinal cord compression.[21]

Melanoma commonly metastasizes to the central nervous system (CNS), with 10% to 40% of melanoma patients presenting with cerebral metastasis.[22] Patients with brain metastasis have a life expectancy of 3 to 5 months, and 1-year survival is less than 10% to 15%. Headaches and seizures are the most common presenting symptoms. Radiation therapy is indicated for palliation of CNS symptoms and as adjuvant therapy after resection of the CNS metastasis.[21]

Whole-brain radiation therapy (WBRT) is indicated for patients with multiple (more than three) CNS metastases, surgically inaccessible lesions, and extensive systemic disease. WBRT for metastatic CNS MM does not improve survival or provide a cure; however, it is effective in relieving neurologic symptoms,[22] preventing new metastasis, reducing symptomatic recurrence, and decreasing the need for salvage therapy.[21] It improves neurologic deficits in 50% to 75% of cases and relieves headaches in 80% of patients.[23] There are some data to suggest that surgical resection followed by WBRT in patients with a single CNS metastasis decreases the risk of local recurrence compared with resection alone.[21]

Stereotactic radiosurgery (SRS) delivers high doses of focused ionizing external-beam radiation to a well-defined target area in one session of radiation therapy. This technique maximizes the dose of radiation to the tumor with a rapid dose falloff outside the target area, resulting in sparing of the surrounding normal tissue. SRS may be considered over surgery for patients with fewer than three metastatic CNS lesions that are deep, nonsymptomatic, and smaller than 3 cm in size.[22]

▸ Chemotherapy

In general, cytotoxic chemotherapy is not considered a standard of care for metastatic melanoma. The major indication for systemic chemotherapy is in patients with metastatic or inoperable MM who are not candidate for immunotherapy or targeted therapy. The goal of chemotherapy is to reduce tumor size, and it is an accepted palliative therapy for stage IV melanoma. Dacarbazine, an alkylating agent, is the most active single-agent chemotherapy against MM, achieving response rates of 15% to 25% in older clinical trials.[24] More recent large-scale clinical trials have shown response rates of 5% to 12%.[25] It is the only chemotherapy agent approved by the Food and Drug Administration (FDA) for the treatment of metastatic MM.

▸ Immunotherapy

KEY CONCEPT *Melanoma is an immunogenic tumor and strategies to enhance the patient's immune response to treat the cancer are an area of active research.* The relationship between melanoma and the immune system was also established after spontaneous regression of melanoma was observed, and spontaneous serologic and cellular immunity can be documented in a high proportion of patients with advanced melanoma.[26] Strategies to enhance patients' immune response for the treatment of MM have focused on cytokine therapy, immune-modulating therapy, adoptive T-cell therapy, and vaccines.

Interferon-α-2b Interferon-α-2b (IFN-α-2b) has diverse mechanisms of action, including antiviral activity, impact on cellular metabolism and differentiation, and antitumor activity. The antitumor activity is attributable to a combination of direct antiproliferative effect on tumor cells and indirect immune-mediated effects.[27] KEY CONCEPT *IFN and pegylated IFN (peginterferon-α-2b) are both approved by the FDA as adjuvant therapy for patients who are free of disease after curative surgical resection but are at high risk of MM recurrence.* This includes patients with bulky disease or regional lymph node involvement such as stage IIB, IIC, or III disease.

The optimum dose, schedule, and duration of IFN-α-2b in high-risk melanoma remain to be defined. A recent meta-analysis of clinical trials of IFN in patients at high risk of recurrence after surgical resection showed improvements in relapse-free survival and overall survival.[28] However, IFN is associated with

Clinical Presentation of MM

Patients with skin cancer generally present with a lesion that may be located anywhere on the body. The most common sites are the head, neck, trunk, and extremities. Changes in any characteristics of a lesion are important danger warning signals. Abnormal presentations of a mole or lesion indicate the need for further assessment.

- **Asymmetry:** Half the lesion does not mirror the other half
- **Border:** Sharp, ragged, uneven, and irregular borders
- **Color:** Multiple colors of various hues of light brown, dark brown, black, red, blue, or gray
- **Diameter:** Larger than 6 mm or the size of a pencil head eraser
- **Evolving:** Significant change in shape, size, symptoms, surface, or shades of color

Other signs and symptoms to monitor for in a lesion, in addition to ABCDE, include:

- Sudden or continuous enlargement of a lesion or elevation of a lesion
- Changes in the skin surrounding the nevus
- Redness, swelling, itching, tenderness, or pain
- Ulceration: friability of the lesion with bleeding or oozing. This is a danger signal

Less Common Sites and Manifestations of MM

It is important to examine these sites for "hidden" MM:

- Nailbed
- Mucosal tissue
- Scalp
- Eye

In the nailbed, a black streak or wide variegated brown streak, elevation of nailbed, skin next to nail becomes darker, nail looks deformed or is being destroyed; size of nail streak increases over time.

Diagnostic Tests

- Dermoscopy
- Biopsy

Staging Tests (Depending on Patient's Presentation)

- Baseline chest radiography
- LDH level
- CT of chest, abdomen, pelvis
- SLN biopsy: KEY CONCEPT *The status of the SLN is one of the most powerful independent prognostic factors predicting survival. It also provides the clinician with guidance for therapy decisions and accurate staging.*
- PET
- MRI

Data from Rigel D, Russak J, Friedman R. The evolution of melanoma diagnosis: 25 years and beyond the ABCDs. CA Cancer J Clin. 2010;60(5):301–316.

substantial toxicities, and the decision for IFN therapy should be made on an individual basis after explaining to the patient the potential benefits and side effects of the therapy. The duration of high-dose IFN is for 1 year if in stage IIB to III, or peginterferon-α-2b for up to 5 years if in stage III when the decision has been made to initiate IFN; low-dose or intermediate-dose IFN is not recommended (Table 93–2).[29] Encouragement to participate in clinical trials is also reasonable for eligible patients.

HDI has substantial side effects that can be divided into acute and chronic manifestations and categorized into four major side effect groups: constitutional, neuropsychiatric, hematologic, and hepatic.[30] Patients should be educated on the side effects to expect and counseled of the interventions available to minimize the toxicities. Peginterferon-α-2b has a longer duration of action than IFN-α-2b and may be administered once a week. The side effects are similar to IFN-α-2b, although the incidence may be less. The monitoring recommendations for peginterferon-α-2b are the same as for IFN.

Interleukin 2 Interleukin-2 (IL-2) therapy is approved by the FDA for the treatment of metastatic MM. IL-2 indirectly causes tumor cell lysis by proliferating and activating cytotoxic T lymphocytes (CTLs). The overall objective response rate for patients with metastatic MM receiving high-dose IL-2 is 16%, with a complete response in 6% of patients and a partial response in 10% of patients. The median duration of response is 8.9 months for all responding patients and 5.9 months for patients with a partial response.[31] The median duration of complete response has not been reached but is at least 59 months. Disease progression is not observed in any patient responding for longer than 30 months. The data are encouraging because for the small number of patients who responded to therapy, the effect is of a long duration, and some patients may be considered to be cured of the disease. (Refer to Table 93–2 for dosing.)

High-dose IL-2 therapy is associated with significant severe toxicities and morbidity.[32] This treatment option is generally only considered in patients with good performance status who will have a better chance of tolerating and completing the therapy. With the availability of new therapies, IL-2 is no longer the primary option for patients with metastatic melanoma. Table 93–3 lists the most common side effects experienced by patients receiving IL-2 therapy and recommendations for management. All clinicians involved with the care of patients receiving IL-2 should be well educated on the monitoring and management of IL-2–specific side effects.

Immune Checkpoint Inhibitors

▸ *Ipilimumab*

T-cell activation involves two different signals: (a) the binding of the T-cell receptor to a peptide presented by the major histocompatibility complex on the antigen-presenting cell (APC) and (b) the interaction of a costimulatory receptor (CD28) on the T-cell surface with a costimulatory ligand (B7) on the APC. The costimulatory molecules enhance the immune response by promoting T-cell activation and proliferation.[33]

CTLA-4 is expressed in CD4+ and CD8+ T cells and regulatory T cells. It is a member of the immunoglobulin (Ig) super family. After T-cell activation occurs, CTLA-4 migrates to the surface of the T cell, where it has higher affinity for the B7 ligand

Table 93–2

Dosing[a] Recommendations

Interferon[a] Dosing Regimens
High dose: 20 million units/m² IV daily × 5 days per week for 4 weeks followed by 10 million units/m² SC three times per week for 48 weeks
Peginterferon: 6 mcg/kg/week SC for 8 weeks followed by 3 mcg/kg/week for up to 5 years

Interleukin-2[a] Dosing Regimen
IL-2: 600,000 International Units/kg (0.037 mg/kg) dose administered every 8 hours by an IV 15-minute infusion for a maximum of 14 doses. Following 9 days of rest, the schedule is repeated for another 14 doses, for a maximum of 28 doses

Immune Checkpoint Inhibitor[a] Dosing Regimens
Ipilimumab: 3 mg/kg IV infusion over 90 minutes every 3 weeks for four doses; permanently discontinue if treatment cannot be completed within 16 weeks
Nivolumab: 3 mg/kg IV infusion over 1 hour every 2 weeks until disease progression or unacceptable toxicity; prior to administration, evaluate liver and thyroid function and serum creatinine, and monitor periodically during treatment
Pembrolizumab: 2 mg/kg IV infusion over 30 minutes every 3 weeks; continue treatment until disease progression or unacceptable toxicity occurs

RAF-MEK-ERK (MAPK) Pathway Inhibitors[a] Dosing Regimens
Vemurafenib: 960 mg by mouth twice daily every 12 hours. Continue treatment until disease progression or unacceptable toxicity occurs
Caution should be used in patients with severe renal or hepatic impairment; no dose adjustment needed for mild to moderate renal or hepatic impairment
Dabrafenib: 150 mg by mouth every 12 hours, at least 1 hour before or at least 2 hours after a meal; continue treatment until disease progression or unacceptable toxicity occurs
Trametinib: 2 mg by mouth once daily; take at least 1 hour before or 2 hours after a meal; continue treatment until disease progression or unacceptable toxicity occurs

Chemotherapy[a] Dosing
Dacarbazine: 250 mg/m²/day IV, days 1 to 5, every 21 days

[a]The doses presented here are general. Clinicians should refer to clinical trials to determine the specific dose based on the regimen the patient is receiving.

IV, intravenous; SC, subcutaneous.

From U.S. Food and Drug Administration. Drugs@FDA FDA Approved Drug Products [Internet]. [cited 2015 Feb 22]. http://www.accessdata.fda.gov/scripts/cder/drugsatfda/.

than CD28 and preferentially binds to B7. This results in an inhibitory signal to the T cell and causes a downregulation on the immune response; in other words, CTLA-4 acts as a "brake" on the activation of the immune system.[33]

Ipilimumab is a fully human monoclonal IgG1 specific for CTLA-4. It has a high affinity for CTLA-4 and impedes binding of CTLA-4 to B7, preventing downregulation of the immune response. This results in increased proliferation of activated T cells and increases the interactions of T cells and cancer cells.[33] Ipilimumab was approved by the FDA for the treatment of unresectable or metastatic melanoma based on a phase III study demonstrating improved survival.[34] Pooled analysis of long-term survival in advanced melanoma patients found median overall survival to be 13.5 months with ipilimumab treatment-naive group compared to 10.7 months in previous treated group; 3-year survival rates were 26% and 20%, respectively.[35] Common side effects may include pruritus, rash, gastrointestinal upset, and fatigue. Because T-cell activation can lead to enterocolitis, hepatitis, dermatitis including toxic epidermal necrolysis, neuropathy, and endocrinopathy, both providers and patients are enrolled in the FDA Risk Evaluation and Mitigation Strategy (REMS) that includes a communication plan.[36] No formal studies have been done to assess cytochrome P-450 (CYP) interactions, and none are expected. Corticosteroids are the treatment of choice for ipilimumab-induced adverse events. The administration of steroids to treat the side effects did not appear to result in decreased effectiveness of ipilimumab. Interestingly, there may be a correlation between immune-related adverse events and treatment success.[37] (see Table 93–4 for adverse effects and their management).

▶ *Nivolumab*

Many tumor cells express programmed death-ligand 1 (PD-L1) that can interact with programmed death-1 (PD-1) receptor on T cells and B cells to diminish the body's immune response. Nivolumab is an IgG4 fully humanized antibody that targets PD-1 to interfere with the binding with PD-L1 and thus allow T cells to remain active to mount an immune response. The FDA-approved indication includes unresectable and metastatic MM following ipilimumab and, if BRAF V600 mutation positive, a BRAF inhibitor. Patient with confirmed, unresectable, previously treated stage III or IV melanoma without BRAF mutation in a phase III trial showed an overall rate of survival at 1 year of 72.9% in the nivolumab group compared to 42.1% in the dacarbazine group.[38] Common side effects may include rash, purities, peripheral edema, and cough while rare but serious adverse events may include ventricular arrhythmia, infection, hepatotoxicity, and neuropathy. No formal studies have been done to assess CYP interactions.[32]

▶ *Pembrolizumab*

Pembrolizumab (previously known as lambrolizumab) is an IgG4 engineered humanized antibody that is also a PD-1 inhibitor. The FDA approved indication includes unresectable

Table 93–3
IL-2 Toxicities

Toxicity (% of Patients)	Management
Cardiovascular	
Hypotension (64%), supraventricular tachycardia (17%)	Discontinue antihypertensive medications; IV fluids to maintain systolic blood pressure > 80–90 mm Hg or vasopressor support with an α-agonist such as phenylephrine as indicated; be judicious in use of IV fluids for hypotension
GI	
Vomiting and diarrhea (55%), nausea (24%), stomatitis (14%)	5-HT_3 antagonist, prochlorperazine for emesis (avoid corticosteroids), H_2-blocker for gastritis, antidiarrheal as needed (loperamide, diphenoxylate/atropine, codeine)
Neurologic	
Confusion (30%), somnolence agitation, anxiety, insomnia	Haldol for agitation, lorazepam for anxiety, zolpidem for insomnia
Pulmonary	
Dyspnea (31%), pulmonary edema, and ARDS	Advise smokers to quit 2 weeks before therapy; discontinue therapy if requiring > 4 L O_2 or 40% O_2 mask for saturation > 95% (0.95)
Hepatic	
Elevated bilirubin (51%), transaminase (39%), ALP	Consider discontinuing therapy if severe
Renal	
Oliguria (49%), elevated serum creatinine (35%), anuria (8%)	Normal saline or dopamine at renal perfusion dose of 2 mcg/kg/min for oliguria; monitor for electrolyte abnormalities and replace as indicated
Hematologic	
Thrombocytopenia (43%), anemia (29%), leukopenia (21%)	Transfuse with packed red blood cells and platelets as needed
Skin	
Rash (27%), exfoliative dermatitis (15%), pruritus	Hydroxyzine, diphenhydramine, oatmeal powder baths, Lubriderm lotion
General	
Fever and or chills (47%), malaise (34%), infection (15%)	Acetaminophen and NSAIDs around the clock for fever and chills; add meperidine if chills are severe; clindamycin or cefazolin to prevent infection
Hypothyroidism	May occur in one-third of patients; thyroid function tests

ALP, alkaline phosphatase; ARDS, adult respiratory distress syndrome; 5-HT_3, serotonin; IV, intravenous; NSAID, nonsteroidal anti-inflammatory drug.

Data from Refs. 38 and 39.

and metastatic MM following ipilimumab and, if *BRAF* V600 mutation positive, a BRAF inhibitor. A study of patients with measurable metastatic locally advanced unresectable melanoma with adequate organ function and performance score found that overall response rate from investigator-assessed immune response criteria was 37% for all examined doses; response Evaluation Criteria in Solid Tumors (RECIST) confirmed response rate was 38%.[39] Common side effects may include arthralgia and constipation/diarrhea while rare but serious adverse events may include colitis, hepatitis, pancreatitis, pneumonitis, and hypophystitis. No formal studies have been done to assess cytochrome p450 interactions interactions.[32]

RAF-MEK-ERK Pathway Targeted Therapy

▸ *Vemurafenib*

BRAF is an intermediary in signal transduction through the RAF-MEK-ERK (MAPK) pathway. Activation of *BRAF* is associated with downstream activation of ERK, elevation of cyclin D1, and an increase in cellular proliferation.[41] *BRAF* is mutated in approximately 50% of melanomas, and over 75% of these mutations are the *BRAF V600E* mutation.[11] Vemurafenib is an oral competitive small molecule serine threonine kinase inhibitor that functions by binding to the adenosine triphosphate binding domain of mutant *BRAF*.[40] KEY CONCEPT *Vemurafenib selectively targets the mutated BRAF V600E isoform and was approved by the FDA for unresectable stage IIIC or metastatic melanoma that is BRAF V600 mutation positive.* The Cobas 4800 *BRAF V600* Mutation Test is the companion FDA-approved diagnostic tool used to test for the *BRAF* V600 Mutation (see Table 93–2 for dosing).

A phase III clinical trial compared vemurafenib with dacarbazine in patients with previously untreated, unresectable stage IIIC or metastatic melanoma possessing the *BRAF V600E* mutation.[41] Data analysis at 6 months showed that overall survival was 84% and median progression-free survival (PFS) was 5.3 months for patients receiving vemurafenib compared with 64% overall survival and 1.6 months PFS for patients receiving dacarbazine. Common side effects associated with vemurafenib may include photosensitivity, rash, arthralgia, and alopecia. Rare but serious side effects may include prolonged QT interval, foot-hand syndrome, vision changes, and SCC though the latter can be excised without discontinuation of the agent.[41] Vemurafenib is metabolized by CYP3A4 and thus may interact with its inducers or inhibitors. It may increase the serum concentration of substrates of CYP1A2 and 2D6. It may decrease the serum concentration of substrates of CYP3A4.[32]

▸ *Dabrafenib*

Similar to vemurafenib, dabrafenib is also a selective inhibitor of BRAF V600E kinase. The FDA-approved indications include monotherapy for unresectable and metastatic MM with *BRAF V600E* mutation and combination therapy with trametinib for unresectable and metastatic MM with BRAF *V600E* or *V600K* mutation. Dabrafenib is unique in its activity to treat melanoma

Table 93–4

Ipilimumab Toxicities[a]

Toxicity (% of patients)	Management
Dermatologic (47%–68%)	
Maculopapular rash Pruritus Vitiligo	Do not need to stop or dose reduce ipilimumab Topical corticosteroid Urea-containing cream Antipruritic agent such as hydroxyzine For grade 3 or 4: oral corticosteroid with prednisone 1 mg/kg or dexamethasone 4 mg every 4 hours with a 4-week taper
GI (31%–46%)	
Mild diarrhea, severe diarrhea, or colitis	Loperamide, hydration, electrolyte replacement Budesonide 9 mg/day or prednisone 1 mg/kg or high-dose IV steroids: methylprednisolone 2 mg/kg once or twice daily or dexamethasone 4 mg every 4 hours; then taper over 4 weeks after symptom resolution; some patients may require 6 to 8 weeks; taper; too rapid taper may result in recrudescence or worsening of symptoms **If no response to steroids in 48 to 72 hours:** Infliximab 5 mg/kg every 2 weeks. NOTE: infliximab is contraindicated in patients with bowel perforation or sepsis Discontinue ipilimumab for severe symptoms such as colitis
Inflammatory hepatoxicity (3%–9%)	Methylprednisolone 2 mg/kg/day one to two times daily for LFT greater 8 × ULN or total bilirubin greater 5 × ULN Mycophenolate 1 g IV or 1.5 g orally two times daily if symptoms persist
Endocrine (4%–6%)	
Hypophysitis	Obtain thyroid function tests, serum cortisol levels, ACTH, testosterone, FSH, LH, prolactin Dexamethasone 4 mg every 4 hours for 7 days and taper over at least 4 weeks Hormone substitution as needed Endocrinologist consult
Neurologic (1%)	
Guillain–Barré syndrome Sensory or motor neuropathy Myasthenia gravis	If symptoms persist for more than 5 days, evaluate for neurologic disorders Corticosteroids May need to interrupt or discontinue therapy if symptoms are severe

[a]In general, for severe grade 3 or 4 ipilimumab toxicities, therapy should be discontinued permanently.

ACTH, adrenocorticotropic hormone; FSH, follicle-stimulating hormone; LH, luteinizing hormone; ULN, upper limit of normal.

Data from Kähler C, Hauschild A. Treatment and side effect management of CTLA-4 antibody therapy in metastatic melanoma. J Dtsch Dermatol Ges. 2011;9:277–285.

metastasis in the brain. A phase I trial (BREAK-I) showed patients with asymptomatic untreated brain metastasis (3 mm size or smaller) decreased brain tumor size in nine out of ten patients with *BRAF V600* mutation and previously untreated brain metastasis, with four patient achieving complete elimination. A phase II trial (BREAK–MB) showed that investigator-assessed intracranial response rate in untreated compared to previously treated but relapsed *BRAF V600E* patients were 39% and 31%, respectively.[11] Common side effects may include hypoglycemia, arthralgia, and neutropenia while rare but serious adverse events may include prolong QT interval, serious febrile reactions, uveitis, iritis, and SCC. Similar to vemurafenib, SCC can be excised without discontinuation of the agent. Dabrafenib is metabolized by CYP3A4 and 2C8 and thus may interact with its inducers or inhibitors. It may decrease the serum concentration of substrates of CYP3A4 and 2C9.[32]

Patient Encounter, Part 3

This patient presents 3 years later after treatment of her stage III melanoma with high-dose interferon. At her routine follow-up visit, a chest x-ray showed bilateral lung metastases. This patient also reports a history of increasing nonproductive cough and exertional shortness of breath in the past few weeks.

Laboratory Data: LDH two times above normal level; all other lab data are normal

CT Scan: Confirms metastasis in lung and paraaortic lymph nodes

What is the treatment of choice for this patient?

What test is used to determine if the patient should receive a BRAF inhibitor?

▶ *Trametinib*

Trametinib is a MEK 1/2 kinase inhibitor that works directly downstream of BRAF in the MAPK pathway. The FDA approved indications include monotherapy or combination therapy with dabrafenib for unresectable and metastatic MM with *BRAF V600E* or V600K mutation. Patients in a Phase III trial with metastatic melanoma with a *BRAF V600E* or V600K mutation showed a response of median PFS of 4.8 months with trametinib compared to PFS of 1.4 months with chemotherapy (dacarbazine or paclitaxel).[42] Common side effects may include dry skin and nail changes while rare but serious adverse events may include vision changes and rhabdomyolysis. No formal studies have been done to assess CYP interactions.[32]

▶ *Dabrafenib and Trametinib Combination Therapy*

Favorable synergistic effects have been found when comparing BRAF and MEK inhibitor combination to BRAF inhibitor monotherapy. A Phase III trial comparing dabrafenib and trametinib to dabrafenib alone in patients with previously untreated, unresectable stage IIIC or metastatic melanoma and either *BRAF* V600K or *V600E* mutation found an estimated median PFS of 9.3 months in the former versus 8.8 months in the latter.[43] In another phase III trial comparing dabrafenib and trametinib to vemurafenib alone in patients with metastatic melanoma and either *BRAF* V600K or *V600E* mutation found median overall survival to be 17.2 months in the vemurafenib group and was not reached for the combination group. The rate of overall survival at 12 months was 72% in the combination group compared to 65% in the vemurafenib group.[44]

Treatment options for metastatic MM include immunotherapies; ipilimumab, nivolumab, or pembrolizumab; targeted therapies; dabrafenib in combination with trametinib or vemurafenib monotherapy, or a clinical trial. Only patients determined to have mutated BRAF V600 isoform can be effectively treated with vemurafenib, dabrafenib, and/or trametinib. Even though ipilimumab and BRAF inhibitors (for *BRAF V600* mutation positive patients) are indicated before treatment with pembrolizumab or nivolumab, the latter two drugs have been shown to have higher response rate and less toxicity compared to ipilimumab and are considered part of first-line therapy. Trametinib monotherapy is only recommended for *BRAF V600* mutation positive patients who cannot tolerate BRAF inhibitor monotherapy.[29]

OUTCOME EVALUATION

After diagnosis and treatment of skin cancer, the next phase of management is appropriate follow-up with the purpose of detecting recurrent disease or new MMs.[29]

Recurrence of MM occurs after complete resection in 30% of patients diagnosed with stage I to III disease, and 80% of the patients develop recurrence within 3 years of their diagnosis of primary MM. Among patients whose melanoma recurred, the site of recurrence is local in 20% to 28% of patients; in 26% to 60%, recurrence is in regional lymph nodes; and 15 to 50% experience distant recurrence. The rate of recurrence detection by patients is reported to be 33% to 99%; thus, patients should be educated on how to perform self-examination of the skin and lymph nodes and the importance of ongoing sun protection measures.[45]

Patients who received immunotherapy for stage III or IV MM may experience fatigue and other chronic side effects. Develop a plan to order laboratory tests such as liver function tests, thyroid-stimulating hormone, and white blood cell count at baseline and on a weekly or monthly basis as indicated. Monitor and evaluate patients for side effects of IL-2, IFN, immune checkpoint inhibitors, and MAPK inhibitors and educate patients on what to expect and how the side effects will be managed. Assess patients' psychological, physical, and social functioning. Counsel patients to contact the hospital's social service department or the American Cancer Society for assistance in dealing with the disease emotionally and recommend that patients consider attending support group meetings or talking to a counselor if or before they become overwhelmed with the diagnosis.

Patient Encounter, Part 4

This patient was negative for *BRAF* mutation with analysis using the Cobas 4800 *BRAF V600* Mutation Test.

The decision was made to initiate her on ipilimumab. She is scheduled to receive 3 mg/kg every 3 weeks for a total of four cycles. At week 4, it was noted that this patient has new subcutaneous lesions and enlargement of the preexisting lesions. Furthermore, a few days after she received her second dose of ipilimumab, she experienced severe grade 3 diarrhea. She reports mild abdominal pain with no fever and no blood in her stool.

What are the most common side effects associated with ipilimumab?.

What should be done to manage the side effects of ipilimumab?

NONMELANOMA SKIN CANCER

EPIDEMIOLOGY AND ETIOLOGY

Nonmelanoma skin cancer (NMSC) accounts for more than half of all newly diagnosed cancers in the United States each year, and it was estimated that more than 3.5 million new cases of BCC and SCC (in more than 2 million people) would be diagnosed in 2011.[1] The true prevalence of NMSC may be underestimated because it is treated in outpatient settings, and no formal reporting to cancer registries is required. The incidence rate of NMSC is increasing worldwide with a yearly rise of 3% to 8% since 1960.[46] BCC is the most common form of NMSC and comprises 75% of NMSC with SCC accounting for 20%.[14] The majority of NMSCs are curable, and the mortality rate is low; cure rates approach 98%, and the overall 5-year survival rate is greater than 95%.[47] Metastasis occurs in fewer than 0.1% of BCCs compared with an average of 3.6% of SCCs. Seventy-five percent of all NMSC deaths are attributed to SCC.[47] NMSC is associated with considerable morbidity related to functional and cosmetic deformity. In addition, it is an economic burden to the health care system because costs associated with NMSC treatment are estimated at approximately $426 million per year.[14]

RISK FACTORS

The risk of developing NMSC is multifactorial (Table 93–5). The most important risk factor for NMSC is UV radiation exposure, and data from epidemiologic studies indicate that greater cumulative lifetime sun exposure is associated with a higher risk of developing SCC, but intermittent and childhood sun-exposure correlates more with BCC.[46] Most cases of BCC are sporadic; however, it occurs frequently in the rare individuals with hereditary disorders such as basal cell nevus syndrome (also known as Gorlin syndrome). It is also common in patients with genetic syndromes such as XP. The *patched* gene (*PTCH*), a tumor-suppressor gene, has been shown to be mutated in 68% of sporadic BCCs.[46] There is clear evidence linking defects of the immune system to the development of NMSC. For example, it is observed that patients receiving chronic immunosuppressant therapy for organ transplantation have a 65-fold increase in developing SCC and 10-fold increase in developing BCC.[48]

Table 93–5

Risk Factors for Developing Nonmelanoma Skin Cancer

	Basal Cell Carcinoma	Squamous Cell Carcinoma
Host Factors		
Phenotype	X	X
Fair skin		
Blonde or red hair		
Blue or green eyes		
Immunosuppression	X	X
Solid organ transplant		
HIV		
Chronic lymphocytic leukemia		
Lymphoma		
Increasing age	X	X
Environmental Factors		
UV Radiation		
Sun	X	X
Ionizing	X	X
Tanning bed		
Psoralen + UVA (PUVA)	X	X
Arsenic	X	X
Photosensitizing drugs	X	X
Human papillomavirus	X	X
Smoking		X

UVA, ultraviolet A.

Data from Refs. 46 and 48.

PATHOPHYSIOLOGY

NMSCs arise from epidermal keratinocytes and involve primarily squamous cells and basal cells of the epidermis and dermis skin layers. BCCs arise from interfollicular basal cells or keratinocytes in hair follicles or sebaceous glands.[48]

CLINICAL PRESENTATION AND PROGNOSIS

BCC is characterized as circumscribed or diffuse, and within these two groups, it is further classified according to type, degree of differentiation, and depth of invasion (see Table 93–1).[14] Nodular BCC is the most common type of BCC followed by superficial BCC. The morpheaform BCC is the most aggressive subtype.[13] BCC has indolent growth characteristics with a very low metastatic and mortality rate.[46] Paradoxically, BCCs can cause extensive local destruction and significant disfigurement. Approximately 80% of BCCs occur on the head and neck. Superficial BCC occurs predominantly on the trunk. Early-stage BCC is usually small, translucent or pearly with raised telangiectatic edges.[46] BCC may also appear as raised, yellowish-reddish lesions with a border resembling a string of pearls and telangiectasia. Dermatoscopy may distinguish between a benign and malignant lesion; however, clinical examination is usually sufficient for diagnosis of BCC. Depending on the size of the tumor, subtype, and treatment planned, a biopsy may be needed.

SCC usually presents on sun-exposed sites because of UVR damage to the skin. Unlike BCC, SCCs are preceded by premalignant lesions such as leukoplakia, actinic keratosis (AK) (a small papule that appears on areas of sun damage on the skin), or SCC in situ (Bowen disease).[46] The rate of AK progression to SCC is 1% to 10% in 10 years and may be higher if a patient has more than five AKs.[46] Patients with a Bowen lesion present with slowly enlarging erythematous scaly or crusted plaques and have a 3% to 5% risk of progressing to SCC. A typical SCC lesion has an adherent crust and ill-defined edges; the first sign of malignant SCC is induration of the lesion. The rate of metastasis for SCC is 2% to 6% and may be as high as 10% to 14% in high-risk sites such as the ear and lip and 30% in the genital area.[47] Metastasis most commonly presents 1 to 2 years after diagnosis of the primary SCC with 80% of metastasis involving the regional lymph nodes.[49]

Risk factors for NMSC are outlined in Table 93–5. If a patient possesses these factors, he or she is at high risk for disease recurrence and subsequent metastasis. Patients with NMSC have a 10-fold increased risk of developing subsequent NMSC compared with the general population.[46]

Staging for NMSC uses the TNM staging system recommended by the American Joint Committee on Cancer. It is seldom done for patients with BCC because nodal and visceral metastasis is rare for this disease.[46]

TREATMENT

KEY CONCEPT *In patients diagnosed with BCC and SCC, the primary goal of therapy is to cure the patient and to prevent recurrence.* Although NMSC has a low mortality rate, morbidity related to tissue destruction, functional impairment, and disfigurement is a significant issue. Therefore, secondary goals of therapy for NMSC are preservation of function and restoration of cosmesis. The treatment options for NMSC involve surgery, pharmacologic therapy, or a combination of both. The choice of treatment depends on factors such as tumor size, the site of the lesion, patient comorbidities, and the histologic and clinical nature of the cancer.

Nonpharmacologic Therapy

▶ *Surgery*

Surgery is the primary treatment modality for all patients diagnosed with either BCC or SCC. Full-thickness ablative procedure in the form of surgical excision of the tumor along with a margin of normal tissue surrounding the tumor is the preferred method for high-risk tumors. Obtaining negative surgical margins is critical for cure and decreasing the risk of tumor recurrence. A margin of 4 to 5 mm in well-defined BCC and SCC ensures peripheral clearance in 95% of cases. Depending on the tumor size, degree of differentiation, and invasion of surrounding structures, larger margins of resection may be necessary.[46] The two most common surgical techniques used are electrodessication and curettage (ED&C) and Mohs micrographic surgery (MMS). The indications of each of these procedures are described below.

Low-risk tumors defined as small, well-differentiated, and slow growing can be treated with superficial ablative techniques, including ED&C and cryotherapy.[46] ED&C is a simple, cost-effective technique that uses repeated cycles of using a curette to cut through malignant tissue followed by electrodesiccation, which involves the application of high voltage, low current to the skin, causing drying or desiccation of the tissue. ED&C is most appropriate for well-defined superficial lesions that are not located in areas with increased risk for metastasis. The disadvantage of this technique is that histologic confirmation of complete tumor removal is not possible.[48] This procedure is not recommended for treatment of recurrent disease, tumors of the face, and high-risk tumors.[48]

For high-risk NMSC or for tumors located in cosmetically or anatomically sensitive areas, MMS is the procedure of choice. The goal of this therapy is complete removal of the cancer with preservation of as much surrounding normal tissue as possible. MMS involves careful dissection, staining of frozen sections, and anatomic mapping of the tumor specimen. Sections are assessed immediately under the microscope by the surgeon, and the process is repeated until a tumor-free margin is attained. MMS cures 93% of primary NMSC and 90% to 94% of recurrent disease compared with 92% and 77% cure rate with standard excision for primary and recurrent disease, respectively.[49]

Cure rates for all modalities decrease with the presence of high-risk features but are still superior with MMS.[49]

Cryotherapy is a procedure used primarily for smaller, low-risk NMSCs with clearly defined margins. It involves delivering liquid nitrogen at subzero temperatures as a spray or with a supercooled metal probe to destroy the malignant tissue in a single cycle or multiple cycles.[48] This technique can achieve comparable results to conventional surgery for well differentiated, not too large, superficial tumors in older patients with BCC.[48] The procedure is contraindicated in the hair-bearing scalp, upper lip, and distal portion of lower leg because of delayed healing and high rates of recurrence.[48]

► Radiation

Radiation is not standard therapy for the treatment of skin cancer; however, there are circumstances in which radiation may be preferred. It may be offered to patients in whom surgery is not possible because the tumor is inoperable or surgery would lead to unacceptable cosmetic or functional impairment.[49] Radiation to the lip, ear, and nasal entrance for SCC may provide the best cosmetic and functional result. On the other hand, some patients may develop dyspigmentation, radiodystrophy, or telangiectasia at the site of radiation, resulting in poorer cosmetic outcomes. Radiation is contraindicated in treating BCC that recurred after radiotherapy. It should be used with caution in patients younger than 65 years because latent NMSC can develop after 15 to 20 years of radiation exposure.[46]

► Photodynamic Therapy

Photodynamic therapy (PDT) involves the topical application of a photosensitizing agent that is activated after exposure to a light source and causes tumor cell damage and death. The photosensitizer is converted to protoporphyrin IX after it is preferentially taken up by active tumor cells. Damage to cell membranes, organelles, and surrounding vasculature occurs when protoporphyrin IX is activated after exposure to a light source. Protoporphyrin IX has absorption bands at 408, 510, 543, 583, and 633 nm; therefore, blue light (corresponding to 408-nm band) and red light (corresponding to 633-nm band) are the most commonly used light source.[48] Blue light is used for superficial lesions because of its shorter wavelength and because it does not penetrate the skin as well as red light.[48]

δ-Aminolevulinic acid (ALA) and methyl aminolevulinate (MAL) are two photosensitizing agents that have FDA approval for the treatment of AK (see Table 93–6 for dosing).[29] PDT has also been shown to be effective in the treatment of SCC in situ, but it is not indicated for SCC because of its extensive invasiveness and metastatic potential.[29] In patients with superficial BCC, MAL-PDT may be considered when surgery may result in suboptimal cosmetic outcomes or complications.[29] For patients with nodular BCC, MAL-PDT may be considered but not ALA-PDT.[29,48]

Table 93–6

Topical Therapy for Nonmelanoma Skin Pre-Cancer

Methyl Aminolevulinate Hydrochloride

Actinic keratosis: apply up to 1 g (half tube) of cream topically on lesion(s) during PDT session (two sessions 1 week apart) followed by occlusive dressing for 3 hours (at least 2.5 hours and no more than 4 hours in duration) and then red light illumination for 7–10 minutes; maximum, 1 g (half tube) per treatment session.

Aminolevulinic Acid

Actinic keratosis: apply topically to target lesion(s) on face or scalp and let dry and then repeat once; 14–18 hours later, gently rinse area with water and pat dry; follow by illumination from the BLU-U(R) Blue Light Photodynamic Therapy Illuminator; may retreat a second time after 8 weeks.

Protect treated lesions from sunlight or prolonged or intense light for at least 40 hours by covering with light-opaque material; sunscreen will not protect against photosensitivity reactions caused by visible light.

Topical Fluorouracil

Actinic keratosis: cover lesions topically with 2% or 5% solution or cream twice daily for 2–6 weeks or with 0.5% microsphere formulation once daily for up to 4 weeks.

Imiquimod

Actinic keratosis: Imiquimod 5% apply topically formulation once daily five times per week for 6 weeks; apply at bedtime and leave on skin for 8 hours

The doses presented here are general. Clinicians should refer to reference materials to determine the specific dose based on the regimen the patient is receiving.

PDT, photodynamic therapy.

Reproduced, with permission, from National Comprehensive Cancer Network. Basal Cell and Squamous Cell Skin Cancer. Version 1. 2016, http://www.nccn.org.

Pharmacologic Therapy

► Fluorouracil

Nonsurgical treatment is used frequently for superficial NMSCs. Topical 5-fluorouracil has been used for the treatment of dermatologic disorders for approximately 45 years, and it has FDA approval for the treatment of AK and superficial BCC. Fluorouracil is available as solution and cream with strengths ranging from 1% to 5%. There is also a microsphere-encapsulated 0.5% cream that has reduced systemic absorption with enhanced skin retention to reduce systemic side effects. The microsphere formulation is applied only once a day, providing patient preference and convenience over the twice-daily application with the other formulations. The optimal strength of fluorouracil is still under investigation, but the FDA has approved 2% to 5% cream or solution and 0.5% microsphere formulation for AK. For superficial BCC, only the 5% strength is FDA approved for this indication. The most common side effects with topical fluorouracil are expected to occur within the initial 5 to 10 days of treatment, and it presents as erythema, irritation, burning sensation, pruritus, and pain along with hypo- or hyperpigmentation. Patients also experience inflammatory reactions that include crusting, edema, and oozing. If the reactions are severe, the fluorouracil strength or frequency of application may be reduced. To reduce inflammation, topical steroids may be used concurrent with fluorouracil application and for 1 to 2 weeks after treatment.[29] Caution should be used in administering fluorouracil to patients with dihydropyrimidine dehydrogenase deficiency, an enzyme critical in the metabolism of fluorouracil, because increased toxicity may be observed.

▸ *Imiquimod*

Imiquimod is an immune-modulating agent that works by stimulating innate and cell-mediated immune responses. It has FDA approval for the treatment of AK and for when surgical procedure is not appropriate for superficial BCC located on the trunk, neck, or extremities and when follow-up is assured. Imiquimod has been shown to have complete clearing of AK in 50% of patients and partial clearing in 75% of patients with AK compared with 5% for those treated with placebo. Cure rates for imiquimod 5% in patients with superficial BCC are greater than 90%. The response rate is much lower for nodular BCC at 75%; therefore, it should be used in these patients only if they are not able to undergo surgery, radiation, or cryotherapy and the tumor is small and in a low-risk area. Imiquimod is not recommended for the treatment of invasive SCC, but data for SCC in situ showed a 93% cure rate; thus, it may be considered for this patient population.

Imiquimod is available in 3.75% strength, which may be applied daily on larger areas of skin, the balding scalp, or the full face, and 5% strength, which may be used on areas of skin that are 25 cm^2 or smaller (see Table 93–4). Imiquimod should be applied before bedtime and left on the skin for 6 to 10 hours. The most common side effects with imiquimod involve the area of application and present as erythema, pruritus, a burning or stinging sensation, and tenderness. Less commonly, hypopigmentation, fever, diarrhea, and fatigue may also occur. Temporary discontinuation of imiquimod and application of topical steroids may be necessary to alleviate the irritation symptoms. Imiquimod may be resumed at a decreased frequency after the symptoms have resolved.[29]

▸ *Vismodegib*

Genetic alterations in hedgehog signaling pathway cause loss of function of patch homolog 1 (PTCH1), which normally acts to inhibit signaling activity of Smoothened, a transmembrane protein involved in Hedgehog signal transduction. Vismodegib is a first-in-class, oral small molecule inhibitor of the Hedgehog signaling pathway; it binds to and inhibits Smoothened (SMO). Vismodegib is approved by the FDA for the treatment of adults with metastatic BCC or locally advanced BCC that has recurred following surgery or who are not candidates for surgery or radiation.

OUTCOME EVALUATION

BCC and SCC have excellent outcomes, with cure rates approaching 98%.[47] Recurrence of NMSC is around 30% to 50% during a 5-year follow-up, and 70% to 80% of recurrence develops within the first 2 years after initial therapy.[47] Therefore, it is crucial to advise patients to schedule routine follow-up visits with their dermatologist and to educate them about the value of sun protection and total-body skin self-examination.[29]

Patients receiving topical agents such as fluorouracil or imiquimod should be educated to wash the treatment area with mild soap and water before applying the cream, use gloves to apply enough to cover the area with a 1-cm margin, and wash their hands thoroughly after each application. They should avoid sun exposure and be counseled to monitor for side effects such as pain, itching, and inflammation. They should consult their dermatologist if the side effects are intolerable.

Patient Care Process

Patient Assessment:

- Take a thorough medication history with particular attention to nonprescription or herbal medications.
- Assess sun exposure and advise patient regarding sun exposure prevention.

Therapy Evaluation:

- Determine the optimal treatment regimen for the patient incorporating diagnosis, stage, and mutation status.
- Verify regimen doses with a standardized reference and assess for dose adjustment based on height, weight, and body surface area and organ dysfunction (renal or hepatic).
- Assess appropriateness of supportive care for the regimens including need for prophylactic antiemetics.

Care Plan Development:

- Enroll patient in REMS program if they will receive ipilimumab.
- Provide patient education regarding common toxicities associated with immunotherapy such as rash, diarrhea, and hepatotoxicity.
- Provide patient education regarding common toxicities associated with targeted therapy such as hypoglycemia, arthralgia, and neutropenia.
- Advise patients receiving targeted therapies of the risk of new skin cancers.

Follow-up Evaluation:

- Schedule regular laboratory tests and skin exams to monitor for toxicities.
- Monitor patient for to therapy.

Abbreviations Introduced in This Chapter

AK	Actinic keratosis
APC	Antigen-presenting cell
BCC	Basal cell carcinoma
CNS	Central nervous system
CTL	Cytotoxic T lymphocyte
CTLA-4	Cytotoxic T-lymphocyte antigen-4
CYP	Cytochrome P-450
ED&C	Electrodessication and curettage
IFN	Interferon-α-2b
Ig	Immunoglobulin
IL-2	Interleukin 2
LFT	Liver function test

MM	Malignant melanoma
MMS	Mohs micrographic surgery
NMSC	Nonmelanoma skin cancer
PFS	Progression-free survival
REMS	Risk Evaluation and Mitigation Strategy
SCC	Squamous cell carcinoma
SEER	Surveillance, Epidemiology, and End Results
SLN	Sentinel lymph node
SPF	Skin protection factor
SRS	Stereotactic radiosurgery
TNM	Tumor, node, metastasis
UVR	Ultraviolet radiation
WBRT	Whole-brain radiation therapy
XP	Xeroderma pigmentosum

REFERENCES

1. Siegel R, Ward E, Brawley O, Jemal A. Cancer statistics, 2011: The impact of eliminating socioeconomic and racial disparities on premature cancer deaths. CA Cancer J Clin. 2011;61:212–236.
2. Narayanan D, Saladi R, Fox J. Ultraviolet radiation and skin cancer. Int J Dermatol. 2010;49(9):978–986.
3. American Cancer Society. Cancer Facts and Figures [Internet]. [cited 2015 Feb 22]. http://www.cancer.org/research/cancerfactsstatistics/cancerfactsfigures2015/index. Accessed February 22, 2015.
4. Lasithiotakisa K, Petrakisa I, Garbeb C. Cutaneous melanoma in the elderly: Epidemiology, prognosis and treatment. Melanoma Res. 2010;20:163–170.
5. Cho Y, Chiang M. Epidemiology, staging (new system), and prognosis of cutaneous melanoma. Clin Plastic Surg. 2010;37:47–53.
6. Psaty E, Scope A, Halpern A, Marghoob A. Defining the patient at high risk for melanoma. Int J Dermatol. 2010;49:362–376.
7. National Council on Skin Cancer Prevention. Skin Cancer Prevention Tips [Internet].[cited 2015 Feb 22]. http://www.skincancerprevention.org/skin-cancer/prevention-tips. Accessed February 22, 2015.
8. Gallagher R. Sunscreens in melanoma and skin cancer prevention. CMAJ. 2005;173(3):244–245.
9. Rigel D, Russak J, Friedman R. The evolution of melanoma diagnosis: 25 years and beyond the ABCDs. CA Cancer J Clin. 2010;60(5):301–316.
10. Ko J, Velez N, Tsao H. Pathways to melanoma. Semin Cutan Med Surg. 2010;29:210–217.
11. Menzies AM, Long GV, Murali R. Dabrafenib and its potential for the treatment of metastatic melanoma. Drug Des Devel Ther. 2012;6:391–405.
12. Ko J, Fisher D. A new era: Melanoma genetics and therapeutics. J Pathol. 2011;223:241–250.
13. Netscher D, Leong M, Orengo I, et al. Cutaneous malignancies: Melanoma and nonmelanoma types. Plast Reconstr Surg. 2011;127:37e.
14. Neville J, Welch E, Leff D. Management of nonmelanoma skin cancer in 2007. Nat Clin Pract Oncol. 2007;4(8):462–469.
15. National Cancer Institute. Surveillance Epidemiology and End Results (SEER) Cancer Statistics [Internet]. 2014 Apr [updated 2014 Dec 17; cited 2015 Feb 22]. http://seer.cancer.gov/csr/1975_2011/. Accessed February 22, 2015.
16. Balch C, Gershenwald J, Soong S, Thompson J, Atkins M, Byrd D, et al. Final version of 2009 AJCC melanoma staging and classification. J Clin Oncol. 2009;27:6199–6206.
17. Spatz A, Batista G, Eggermontb A. The biology behind prognostic factors of cutaneous melanoma. Curr Opin Oncol. 2010;22:163–168.
18. Ross M, Gershenwald J. Evidence-based treatment of early-stage melanoma. J Surg Oncol. 2011;104:341–353.
19. Spanknebel K, Kaufman H. Surgical treatment of stage IV melanoma. Clin Dermatol. 2004;22:240–250.
20. Tarhini A, Agarwala S. Management of brain metastases in patients with melanoma. Curr Opin Oncol. 2004;16:161–166.
21. Rao N, Yu H, Trotti III A, Sondak V. The role of radiation therapy in the management of cutaneous melanoma. Surg Oncol Clin North Am. 2011;20:115–131.
22. Bafaloukosa D, Gogas H. The treatment of brain metastases in melanoma patients. Cancer Treat Rev. 2004;30:515–520.
23. Garbe C, Peris K, Hauschild A, et al. Diagnosis and treatment of melanoma: European consensus-based interdisciplinary guideline. Eur J Cancer 2010;46:270–283.
24. Middleton M, Grob J, Aaronson N., et al. Randomized phase III study of temozolomide versus dacarbazine in the treatment of patients with advanced metastatic malignant melanoma. J Clin Oncol. 2000;18:158–166.
25. Garbe C, Eigentler T, Keilholz U, et al. Systematic review of medical treatment in melanoma: Current status and future prospects. Oncologist. 2011;16:5–24.
26. Weber J. Immunotherapy for melanoma. Curr Opin Oncol. 2011;23:163–169.
27. Jonasch E, Haluska F. Interferon in oncological practice: Review of interferon biology, clinical applications, and toxicities. Oncologist. 2001;6:34–55.
28. Mocellin S, Pasquali S, Rossi C, Nitti D. Interferon alpha adjuvant therapy in patients with high-risk melanoma: A systematic review and meta-analysis. J Natl Cancer Inst. 2010;102:493–501.
29. National Comprehensive Cancer Network. NCCN Guidelines [Internet]. [cited 2015 Feb 22]. http://www.nccn.org/professionals/physician_gls/f_guidelines.asp. Accessed February 22, 2015.
30. Hauschild A, Gogas H, Tarhini A, et al. Practical guidelines for the management of interferon-alpha-2b side effects in patients receiving adjuvant treatment for melanoma: Expert opinion. Cancer. 2008;112:982–994.
31. Atkins M, Lotze M, Dutcher J, et al. High-dose recombinant interleukin 2 therapy for patients with metastatic melanoma: Analysis of 270 patients treated between 1985 and 1993. J Clin Oncol 1999;17:2105–2116.
32. U.S. Food and Drug Administration. Drugs@FDA FDA Approved Drug Products [Internet].[cited 2015 Feb 22]. http://www.accessdata.fda.gov/scripts/cder/drugsatfda/. Accessed February 22, 2015.
33. Boasberg P, Hamid O, O'Day S. Ipilimumab: Unleashing the power of the immune system through CTLA-4 blockade. Semin Oncol. 2010;37:440–449.
34. Hodi F, O'Day S, McDermott D, et al. Improved survival with ipilimumab in patients with metastatic melanoma. N Engl J Med. 2010;363:711–723.
35. Schadendorf D, Hodi FS, Robert C, et al. Pooled Analysis of Long-Term Survival Data From Phase II and Phase III Trials of Ipilimumab in Unresectable or Metastatic Melanoma. J Clin Oncol. 2015;33(17):1889–1894.
36. U.S. Food and Drug Administration. Approved Risk Evaluation and Mitigation Strategies (REMES)[Internet]. [updated 2015 Feb 18; cited 2015 Feb 22]. http://www.fda.gov/Drugs/DrugSafety/PostmarketDrugSafetyInformationforPatientsandProviders/ucm111350.htm
37. Kähler C, Hauschild A. Treatment and side effect management of CTLA-4 antibody therapy in metastatic melanoma. J Dtsch Dermatol Ges. 2011;9:277–285.
38. Robert C, Long GV, Brady B, et al. Nivolumab in previously untreated melanoma without BRAF mutation. N Engl J Med. 2015;372(4):320–330.

39. Hamid O, Robert C, Daud A, et al. Safety and tumor responses with lambrolizumab (anti-PD-1) in melanoma. N Engl J Med. 2013;369(2):134–144.
40. Luke J, Hodi F. Vemurafenib and BRAF inhibition: A new class of treatment for metastatic melanoma. Clin Can Res. 2012;18(1):9–14.
41. Chapman P, Hauschild A, Robert C, Haanen J, Ascierto P, Larkin J, et al. Improved survival with vemurafenib in melanoma with BRAF V600E mutation. N Engl J Med 2010;364:2507–2516.
42. Flaherty KT, Robert C, Hersey P, et al. Improved survival with MEK inhibition in BRAF-mutated melanoma. N Engl J Med. 2012;367(2):107–114.
43. Long GV, Stroyakovskiy D, Gogas H, et al. Combined BRAF and MEK inhibition versus BRAF inhibition alone in melanoma. N Engl J Med. 2014;371(20):1877–1888.
44. Robert C, Karaszewska B, Schachter J, et al. Improved overall survival in melanoma with combined dabrafenib and trametinib. N Engl J Med. 2015;372(1):30–39.
45. Fields R, Coit D. Evidence-based follow-up for the patient with melanoma. Surg Oncol Clin North Am. 2011;20:181–200.
46. Madan V, Lear J, Szeimies R. Non-melanoma skin cancer. Lancet. 2010;375:673–685.
47. Kwasniak L, Garcia-Zuazaga J. Basal cell carcinoma: Evidence-based medicine and review of treatment modalities. Int J Dermatol. 2011;50:645–658.
48. LeBoeuf N, Schmults C. Update on the management of high-risk squamous cell carcinoma. Semin Cutan Med Surg. 2011;30:26–34.
49. Galiczynski E, Vidimos A. Nonsurgical treatment of non melanoma skin cancer. Dermatol Clin. 2011;29:297–309.

The author and editors wish to acknowledge and thank Dr. Trinh Pham, the primary author of this chapter in the second and third editions of this book.

94 Ovarian Cancer

Judith A. Smith

LEARNING OBJECTIVES

Upon completion of the chapter, the reader will be able to:

1. Demonstrate understanding of the etiology and risk factors associated with the development of ovarian cancer.
2. Justify the risk and benefits of the surgical and chemoprevention options available for decreasing the potential risk of developing ovarian cancer.
3. Interpret and understand the utility of the screening tests and serologic markers for diagnosing ovarian cancer.
4. Distinguish the nonspecific physical signs and symptoms of ovarian cancer.
5. Recommend the appropriate surgical and chemotherapy treatment options for newly diagnosed, persistent, and recurrent ovarian cancer patients.
6. Discuss the role of consolidation treatment for improving overall survival for ovarian cancer patients.
7. Compare and contrast chemotherapy options for women with recurrent platinum-resistant ovarian cancer.

INTRODUCTION

Ovarian cancer is relatively uncommon but is the most incurable of the gynecologic cancers. Ovarian cancer is often denoted as the "silent killer." KEY CONCEPT *The primary reason for the high mortality rate associated with ovarian cancer is the nonspecific symptoms and difficulty for early detection or screening that result in patients presenting with advanced disease.* The majority of ovarian cancers are of epithelial origin. Each time ovulation occurs, the epithelium of the ovary is broken followed by occurrence of cell repair. The incessant ovulation hypothesis proposes that the increasing number of times the ovary epithelium undergoes cell repair is associated with the increasing risk of mutations and ultimately ovarian cancer. Although the majority of patients will achieve a complete response (CR) to primary surgery and chemotherapy, disease recurs in more than 50% of patients in the first 2 years after completion of primary treatment. KEY CONCEPT *Ovarian cancers often cause metastasis via the lymphatic and blood systems to the liver, and/or lungs.* Common complications of advanced and progressive ovarian cancer include ascites and small bowel obstruction (SBO), which often are associated with the end of life.

EPIDEMIOLOGY AND ETIOLOGY

In 2015, there were an estimated 21,290 new cases of ovarian cancer diagnosed with an associated 14,180 deaths.[1] Ovarian cancer remains the number one gynecologic killer and the fifth leading cause of cancer-related death in women. Despite great efforts and extensive research, addition of new agents and routes of administration, there has been little change in the mortality rate associated with ovarian cancer over the past five decades. Again, this high mortality rate associated with ovarian cancer can be attributed to its insidious onset of nonspecific symptoms, resulting in the majority of patients not presenting until the cancer has progressed to stages III to IV disease.

As with many other disease states, a significant risk factor associated with ovarian cancer is aging. Risk of ovarian cancer increases from age 40 to 79 years, with the mean age at diagnosis being 63 years and the majority of women being diagnosed between 55 and 64 years.[2]

Ovarian cancer is a sporadic disease; fewer than 10% of ovarian cancers can be attributed to heredity. KEY CONCEPT *The majority of cases of ovarian cancer occur sporadically, thus making it difficult to screen and prevent.* Although hereditary accounts for fewer than 10% of all ovarian cancer cases, when there is a family history, it appears to be an important risk factor in the development of ovarian cancer in some patients.[3] If one family member has a diagnosis of ovarian cancer, the associated risk is about 9%, but this risk increases to greater than 50% if there are two or more first-degree relatives (ie, mother and sister) with a diagnosis of ovarian cancer or multiple cases of ovarian and breast cancer.[3] Both breast cancer activator gene 1 (*BRCA1*) and breast cancer activator gene 2 (*BRCA2*) mutations have been associated with ovarian cancer. However, *BRCA1* is more prevalent, being associated with 90% of hereditary and 10% of sporadic cases of ovarian cancer.[3] Hereditary breast and ovarian cancer (HBOC) syndrome is one of the two different forms of hereditary ovarian cancer and is associated with germline mutations in *BRCA1* and *BRCA2*.[3,4] The hereditary nonpolyposis colorectal cancer (HNPCC) or Lynch syndrome is a familial syndrome with germline mutations causing defects in enzymes involved in DNA

Patient Encounter 1, Part 1

The patient is a 66-year-old active woman, who has been in good health up until recently (about 6 weeks or so). At Thanksgiving, she mentioned to her daughter that she has had not been able to have a bowel movement in over 6 days despite use of OTC laxative medications. The following Monday she saw her gastroenterologist that completed CT scan that suggests minor colitis but no obvious reason for inability to have bowel movement. One week later, her symptoms persisted, so her physician did an exploratory laparoscopic surgery, which came back positive for an abdominal mass and thickening of the peritoneal lining and mass on right ovary extending to outside of colon wall which was removed by general surgeon and required temporary ostomy. Of note, she has been married for 41 years with only one sexual partner in her lifetime. They have three children who are all grown adults. Her first menses was when she was 11 years old and menopause was at age 54 years. She has had infrequent alcohol on social occasions only and denies any tobacco use.

Based on the results from exploratory surgery, what additional diagnostic tests would be recommended to complete her workup?

In the context of this patient, discuss why ovarian cancer is often denoted the "silent killer" and what needs to be done for earlier diagnosis of ovarian cancer.

Compare and contrast the treatment options for RH after her initial surgery.

Patient Encounter 2

A 37-year-old professional, single woman who has been in good health, presents to your clinic complaining of constipation and abdominal bloating. She explains to you that she is concerned about her cancer risk because her 64-year-old mother was recently diagnosed breast cancer and then last month, her step-sister was diagnosed with stage I ovarian cancer and underwent TAH-BSO and had genetic testing completed that revealed she was *BRCA1* positive. She is requesting to check her CA-125 level today in clinic.

Explain the association between hereditary and ovarian cancer risk.

Discuss why monitoring CA-125 is not used as a screening tool for ovarian cancer.

Describe the potential advantages and disadvantages of using oral contraceptives for prevention of ovarian cancer for this patient.

mismatch repair, which has been associated with up to 12% of hereditary ovarian cancer cases.[4]

Although it is not clearly defined, hormones and reproductive history are associated with the risk of developing ovarian cancer. Nulliparity, infertility, early menarche, or late menopause is associated with an increased risk of ovarian cancer.[5]

Ovarian cancer is associated with certain dietary and environmental factors as well. A diet that is high in galactose and animal fat and meat increases the risk of ovarian cancer, whereas a vegetable-rich diet is suggested to decrease the risk.[6,7] Although still somewhat controversial, exogenous factors such as asbestos and talcum powder use on the perineal area have also been suggested to increase the risk of ovarian cancer.[6]

Screening and Prevention

▸ *Screening*

Currently, there is no standard effective screening tool that is adequately specific or sensitive for early detection.

Pelvic examinations are effective for detecting obvious tumors present with a sensitivity of 67% for detecting all tumors; however, minimal or microscopic disease cannot be detected on physical examination.[8] Pelvic examinations are noninvasive and well accepted, but they do not usually detect ovarian cancer until it is in advanced stage. Transvaginal ultrasound (TVUS) is a component of current screening practices. Typically, it is used in combination with cancer antigen-125 (CA-125) or could be used as a single modality. TVUS releases sonic sound waves that create an image of the ovary to evaluated the size and shape and detect the presence of cystic or solid masses. Limitations of this technique are lack of specificity and an inability to detect peritoneal cancer or cancer in normal size ovaries.[2,9] Most prevention clinics use this multimodality approach to screen high-risk women and recommend yearly ultrasound in combination with CA-125 blood test every 6 months.

Serum CA-125 is the most extensively evaluated tumor marker for ovarian cancer. KEY CONCEPT *Because CA-125 is a nonspecific marker, it is not a standard recommendation for routine screening for prevention of ovarian cancer.* Unfortunately, CA-125 is nonspecific, and elevated levels can be associated with a number of other gynecologic and GI-related diseases. CA-125 levels in a woman without ovarian cancer are static or tend to decrease over time, but levels associated with malignancy continue to rise.[9,10]

▸ *Prevention*

Ovulation is considered a hostile event to the ovarian epithelium, making it more susceptible to damage and cancer. Interventions or conditions that limit the number of ovulations in a woman's reproductive history, including multiparity, have a protective effect.

Chemoprevention Investigational chemoprevention strategies used for ovarian cancer include oral contraceptives (OCs), aspirin and nonsteroidal anti-inflammatory agents, and retinoids, although none of these is currently accepted as standard treatment for the prevention of ovarian cancer. The theory that OCs reduce the number of ovulatory events is a basic explanation of its protective effect. Recent studies have suggested that progestin-induced apoptosis of the ovarian epithelium is responsible for the chemopreventive effect of OCs. The theory is that cells that have genetic damage but are not yet neoplastic have an increased chance of undergoing apoptosis.[11] OCs decrease the relative risk to less than 0.4% in women that use OCs for longer than 10 years.[12] However, the maximum protective effect of OC use in women with *BRCA* mutations has been reported to be between 3 and 5 years.[12] At the same time, OC use has been associated with an increased risk of breast cancer.[11,13] Thus, women with a family history of breast cancer would not be ideal candidates for this preventive measure.

Nonsteroidal anti-inflammatory agents, aspirin, and acetaminophen have been suggested for use in the prevention of different cancers, especially hereditary nonpolyposis colon cancer.[13] Although observational studies have linked these to a reduction of ovarian carcinoma risk, evidence is still lacking. Potential mechanisms include effects on normal ovulation shed and inhibition of ovulation.[13] Other pharmacologic interventions that have been suggested but are still being evaluated include vitamin A, lutein, and other carotenoids.[14,15] The protective effect of these agents is associated with inhibition of cell growth as well as promotion of cellular differentiation.[14]

Prophylactic Surgery Surgical strategies are also used in the prevention of ovarian cancer. The goal is to remove healthy, at-risk organs and ultimately reduce the risk of developing cancer. These surgeries include prophylactic bilateral salpingo-oophorectomy (BSO) or tubal ligation (Figure 94–1).

Prophylactic oophorectomy should be considered in any woman with a high risk of developing ovarian cancer.[16] The criteria for defining high risk includes any woman with two or more first-degree relatives with epithelial ovarian carcinoma; a family history of multiple occurrences of nonpolyposis colon cancer, endometrial cancer, and ovarian cancer; and a family history of multiple cases of breast and ovarian cancer.[17] Patients undergoing prophylactic oophorectomy need to be made aware that complete protection is not guaranteed.[17–19] Although a 67% reduction in risk has been shown, a potential 2% to 5% risk of peritoneal carcinomatosis remains.[18–20]

Tubal ligation is another procedure that has shown potential for risk reduction. However, it is not recommended as a sole procedure in prophylaxis. The protective effect may be attributable to limiting exposure of the ovary to environmental carcinogens. A case-control study conducted by Narod and colleagues[19] found that a history of tubal ligation in *BRCA*-positive women was associated with a statistically significant 63% reduction in risk.

Genetic Screening Genetic screening is another option available for high-risk patients. Patients can be screened for genes such as *BRCA1* and *BRCA2* or other genes such as those associated with HNPCC or the HBOC syndrome.[3,21] Patient and family counseling and genetic counseling should be available for the patient and family to prepare and deal with the health and psychosocial implications of the genetic test results. Before this decision, the potential preventive options should be discussed, such as prophylactic BSO and/or total hysterectomy. Cancer risk and patient's health need to be balanced, but typically surgery can be held off until after the childbearing years.[20,21]

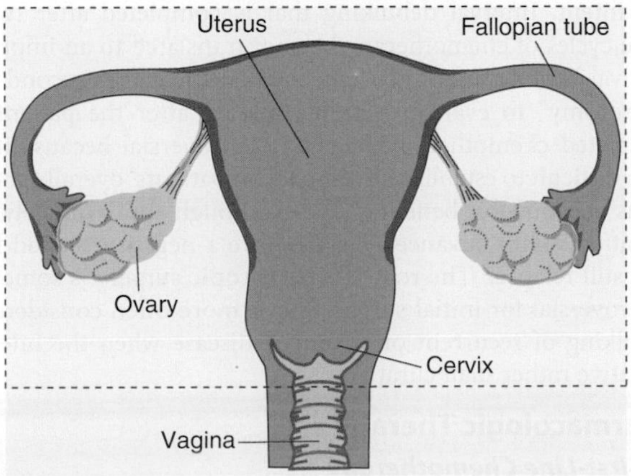

FIGURE 94–1. Diagram of female reproductive tract (uterus, fallopian tubes, ovaries, vagina). The *dashed line box* outlines what is removed during the total abdominal hysterectomy with bilateral salpingo-oophorectomy (TAH/BSO).

PATHOPHYSIOLOGY

The three current theories are the incessant ovulation hypothesis, the pituitary gonadotropin hypothesis, and the chronic inflammatory processes hypothesis.[2] The incessant ovulation hypothesis proposes that the pathogenesis of ovarian cancer is connected to continual ovulation. Ovulation is considered a "hostile" event to the ovaries, perhaps with not enough time for adequate repair. Each time ovulation occurs, the ovary epithelium is disrupted, and cell damage occurs. Thus, repeated ovulations may lead to a greater number of repairs of the ovarian epithelium and increase the possibility of aberrant repairs, mutation, and carcinogenesis.[22] The pituitary gonadotropin hypothesis associates the disease with elevations in gonadotropin and estrogen levels.[2] This leads to an increase in the number of follicles and therefore an increased risk of malignant changes. Finally, the chronic inflammatory processes may be involved with various environmental carcinogens to cause cancer.[2,13]

The three major pathologic categories of ovarian tumors include sex-cord stromal, germ cell, and epithelial. About 85% to 90% of ovarian cancers are of epithelial origin. Epithelial ovarian tumors are composed of cells that cover the surface of the ovary such as serous, mucinous, endometrioid, clear cell, and poorly differentiated adenocarcinomas. Germ cell tumors involve the precursors of ova with the most common type being dysgerminoma, which are most commonly diagnosed in women younger than the age of 40 years and generally have a better prognosis.[2] Sex-cord stromal tumors are indolent tumors that produce excess estrogen and androgens but also have a better overall prognosis.[2] Although the histologic type of the tumor is not a significant prognostic factor, it is important to know the histopathologic grade. Undifferentiated tumors are associated with a poorer prognosis than lesions that are considered to be well or moderately differentiated.

TREATMENT

Desired Outcomes

Health care providers use a multimodality approach, including surgery and chemotherapy, in initial treatment of patients with ovarian cancer with a curative intent, or restoring a normal life span. KEY CONCEPT *Although the majority of patients initially achieve a CR, disease will recur within the first 2 years in more than 50% of patients.*[2,23] CR to treatment is defined as no evidence of disease can be detected by physical examination or diagnostic tests and patient has a normalized CA-125.

The stage of disease at the time of diagnosis is the most important prognostic factor affecting overall survival in ovarian cancer patients.[24] The estimated 5-year survival rates of patients with localized, regional, distant, and unstaged ovarian cancer are 92.7%, 71.1%, 30.6%, and 26%, respectively.[24] The histology of the disease is another predominant prognostic factor influencing treatment outcomes. Clear cell and undifferentiated tumors do not respond as well to chemotherapy.[2] The extent of residual disease and tumor grade are also predictive of response to chemotherapy and overall survival.[2] There are other prognostic factors that may predict how well a patient will respond to adjuvant chemotherapy.

The treatment goals shift when a patient presents with recurrent ovarian cancer. The desired outcomes focus on relief of

Clinical Presentation and Diagnosis of Ovarian Cancer

General

Ovarian cancer typically has delay in diagnosis due to the common nonspecific signs and symptoms often initially suggesting GI-related complications. By the time symptoms become unrelenting and bothersome, patients most likely have advanced stage disease.

Symptoms

Patients may experience episodes or persistent symptoms such as abdominal pain, constipation or diarrhea, flatulence, urinary frequency, or incontinence.

Signs

The degree of abdominal swelling secondary to fluid accumulation may present like "pregnant abdomen" and irregular vaginal bleeding.

Laboratory Test

- CA-125. The normal level is less than 35 U/mL (35 kU/L). Note: This test is associated with a lack of specificity. CA-125 can be elevated in a number of other states such as different phases of the menstrual cycle, endometriosis, and nongynecologic cancers.
- NOTE: It is important to rule out other cancers associated with the abdominal cavity.
- Carcinoembryonic antigen (CEA). CEA is a marker for colon cancer. A normal value is less than 3 ng/mL (3 mcg/L).
- CA-19–9 is a marker for many GI tumors such as cholangiocarcinomas.

Chemistries with Liver Function Tests (LFTs)

- LFTs and serum creatinine might be suggestive of extent of disease. The majority of this information is needed to determine if patient is a surgical candidate. Laboratory study results should be within normal limits.

Complete Blood Count (CBC)

- Abnormalities in CBC are not associated with ovarian cancer; however, this information is needed to determine if patient is a surgical candidate. Laboratories should be within normal limits.

Other Diagnostic Tests

To characterize local disease, one or both of the following are completed:

- TVUS
- Abdominal ultrasound

To evaluate the extent of disease, only one of the following is completed:

- CT scan
- MRI
- PET scan

Chest x-ray is also often done as part of clearance for surgery.

Ovarian cancer is usually confined to the abdominal cavity, but spread can occur to the lung and liver and less commonly to the bone or brain. Disease is spread by direct extension, peritoneal seeding, lymphatic dissemination, or bloodborne metastasis. Lymphatic seeding is the most common pathway and frequently causes ascites.

symptoms such as pain or discomfort from ascites, slowing disease progression, and prevention of serious complications such as SBO. When a patient relapses, the prognostic factors are similar as after initial surgery except that the amount of time that has lapsed since the completion of chemotherapy should be considered to determine if drug resistance is emerging in the tumor. Recurrent platinum-sensitive ovarian cancer patients generally have a better prognosis than platinum-resistant patients.

Nonpharmacologic Therapy

KEY CONCEPT *Surgery is the primary treatment intervention for ovarian cancer.*[25–27] A total hysterectomy with BSO (TH-BSO) (see Figure 94–1), omentumectomy, and lymphonectomy (or lymph node dissection) is the standard initial surgical treatment of ovarian cancer.[25] The objective of the surgery is to debulk the patient to less than 1 cm of residual disease remains. Residual disease less than 1 cm correlates with better CR rates to chemotherapy and better overall survival compared with patients with bulky residual disease (larger than 1 cm).[26,27] Indeed, the size of residual tumor masses after primary surgery is found to be another important prognostic factor in patients with advanced ovarian cancer.[27]

A thorough exploratory laparotomy is essential for the accurate staging of the patient.[25–27] KEY CONCEPT *Ovarian cancer is staged surgically using the International Federation of Gynecology and Obstetrics (FIGO) staging algorithm.* For certain patients with limited stage disease, surgery may be curative.

Other surgical procedures have been evaluated to improve overall survival. Debulking surgery is intended to relieve symptoms associated with complications such as SBO and help improve the patient's quality of life but does not have a curative intent. Interval debulking that is completed after two to three cycles of chemotherapy has not translated to an improved survival benefit. Often debated, the benefit of the "second-look laparotomy" to evaluate residual disease after the patient has completed chemotherapy remains controversial because it has been difficult to establish any impact on patients' overall survival. It has questionable benefit because although approximately 40% of patients with advanced disease have a negative second look, 50% still relapse.[2] The role of laparoscopic surgery is somewhat controversial for initial surgery but is more often considered in debulking of recurrent or advanced disease when the intent is palliative rather than curative.[25]

Pharmacologic Therapy

► *First-Line Chemotherapy*

KEY CONCEPT *After initial surgery, the gold standard of care is six cycles of taxane/platinum-containing regimen for patients with advanced ovarian cancer.*[28–30] Patients with limited disease, ie, stage IA, will have observation alone after surgery

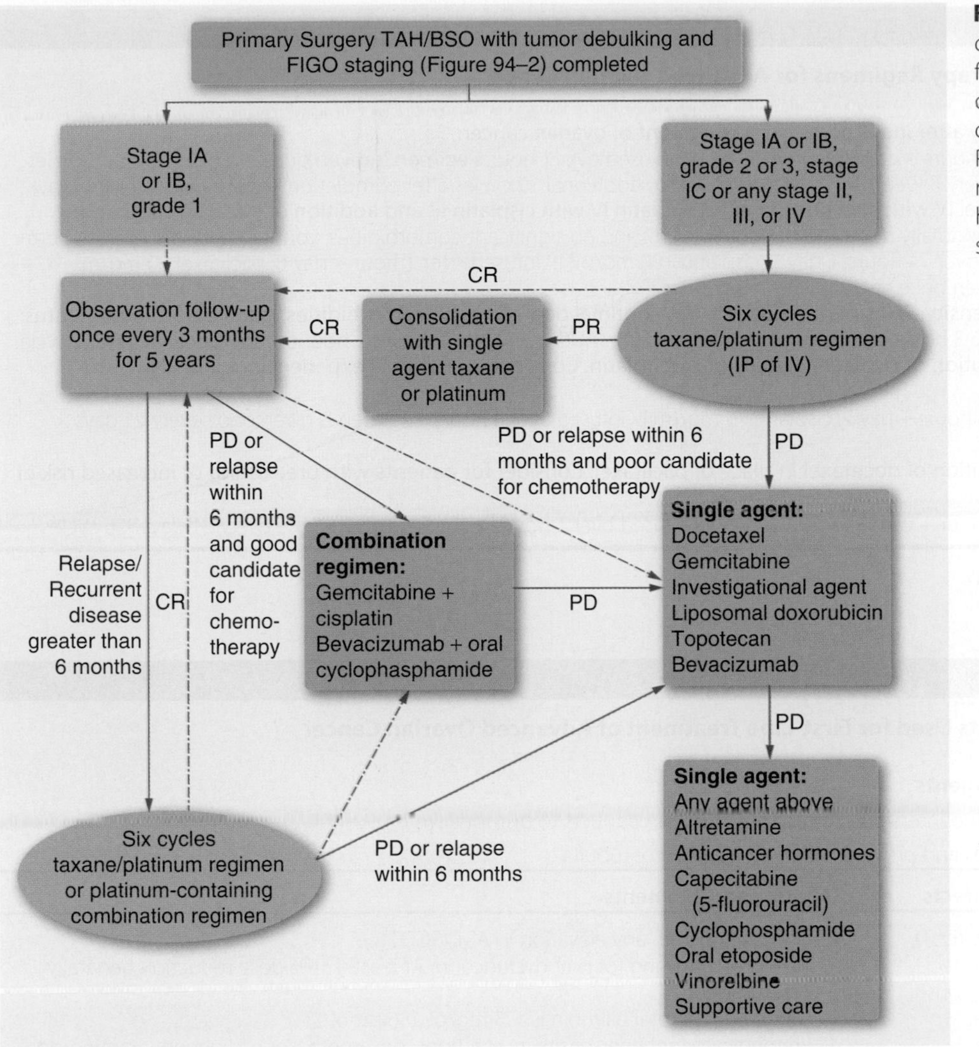

FIGURE 94–2. Summary of a chemotherapy treatment algorithm for epithelial ovarian cancer. (CR, complete response; FIGO, Federation of Gynecology and Obstetrics; PD, progressive disease; PR, partial response; TAH-BSO, total abdominal hysterectomy with bilateral salpingo-oophorectomy.)

(Figure 94–2). Most often, paclitaxel is the taxane agent used in combination with carboplatin as the preferred platinum agent.[28–30] Depending on patients' preexisting comorbidities and how well they tolerate chemotherapy regimens, substitution with docetaxel or cisplatin might be considered. The route of administration should also be discussed. Although intravenous (IV) administration is often used, intraperitoneal (IP) administration has been shown to improve overall survival and should be considered for first-line treatment; however, patient selection for IP therapy is critical[31] (Table 94–1). Close monitoring of organ function, nausea/vomiting, myelosuppression, and neuropathies is necessary for all taxane/platinum regimens (Table 94–2).

▸ *Intraperitoneal Chemotherapy*

For more than four decades, numerous investigators have evaluated the IP route for administration of chemotherapy; however, it was not until the third report of an improvement in overall survival that brought its use to the forefront in the first-line setting.[32] The principal theory supporting IP administration is to increase drug concentration in the site of disease, specifically the abdominal cavity. Patient characteristics greatly influence response and tolerability of IP chemotherapy. To be selected to receive IP chemotherapy for first-line treatment of ovarian cancer, the patient should have tumor optimally debulked and no bowel resection with primary surgery, normal renal and liver function, younger age, and no significant comorbidities.

When IP therapy is administered, the placement of an IP catheter should occur at the time of surgery unless otherwise contraindicated. During IP administration, chemotherapy is delivered to the peritoneal space in 1 L of normal saline (NS) that has been warmed followed by another liter of NS to enhance drug distribution as tolerated.[33,34] The current standard IP regimen includes the administration of paclitaxel IV on day 1 followed by cisplatin IP on day 2 and then paclitaxel IP on day 8 given on a 21-day cycle for a total of six cycles (see Table 94–2). The most common toxicities associated with IP administration include abdominal pain, myelosuppression, neurotoxicity, and catheter-related infections. The substitution of carboplatin IP in place of cisplatin remains investigational and should not be recommended outside a clinical trial protocol.

▸ *Neoadjuvant Chemotherapy*

Neoadjuvant chemotherapy is first-line treatment for patients who are poor surgical candidates or patients with bulky or significant tumor burden.[23] For patients who are poor surgical candidates because of significant comorbidities, a combination of taxane with platinum agent is administered every 21 to 28 days as tolerated with the intent to relieve symptoms and

Table 94–1

Summary of First-Line Chemotherapy Regimens for Advanced Ovarian Cancer

Gold standard first-line chemotherapy after initial surgery for treatment of ovarian cancer:
Paclitaxel 175 mg/m² IV infused over 3 hours + carboplatin AUC = 5 IV infused over 1 hour. Regimen is given once every 21 days × 6 cycles {+/− bevacizumab 7.5 mg/kg once every 3 weeks × 6 cycles followed by additional 12 cycles after completion of primary chemotherapy}
Alternative first-line regimen: Paclitaxel IV with substitution of carboplatin IV with cisplatin IP and addition of paclitaxel IP therapy:
Patient selection is critical: must have optimally debulked disease (< 1 cm) and no significant comorbidities; younger patients tolerate better
Day 1: paclitaxel 135 mg/m² IV infused over 24 hours + day 2: cisplatin 100 mg/m² IP infused over 1 hour + day 8: paclitaxel 60 mg/m² IP infused over 1 hour. Regimen is given once every 21 days × 6 cycles
Alternative first-line regimen: Dose density. Consider for patients with optimal debulking, no comorbidities, good performance status:
Paclitaxel 80 mg/m² IV infused over 1 to 3 hours once a week with carboplatin AUC = 6 IV infused over 1 hour on day 1 only of 21-day cycle.
Alternative first-line regimen: Substitution of cisplatin in place of carboplatin. Consider for patients experiencing difficulty with maintaining platelet counts:
Paclitaxel 135 mg/m² IV infused over 24 hours + day 2: cisplatin 75 mg/m² IV infused over 4 hours. Regimen is given once every 21 days × 6 cycles
Alternative first-line regimen: Substitution of docetaxel in place of paclitaxel. Consider for patients with preexisting or increased risk of neuropathies:
Docetaxel 75 mg/m² IV infused over 1 hour + carboplatin AUC = 5 IV infused over 1 hour. Regimen is given once every 21 days × 6 cycles

AUC, area under the curve; IV, intravenous.

Table 94–2

Summary of Chemotherapy Agents Used for First-Line Treatment of Advanced Ovarian Cancer

Mechanism of Action of First-Line Agents

Platinum analogues: Produce intra- and interstrand cross-links and DNA adducts to disrupt DNA replication

Taxanes agents: Stabilize microtubules and prevents depolymerization of tubulin

Agent	Common Adverse Effects	Monitoring/Comments
Paclitaxel	Peripheral neuropathy (DLT), nausea/vomiting, alopecia, hypersensitivity reactions	1. Use caution with any elevation in AST (SGOT) 2. Give proper dosing for liver dysfunction. At least a 50% dose reduction generally recommended 3. Do not give if total bilirubin is > 5 mg/dL (86 μmol/L) 4. Premedicate for hypersensitivity reactions: dexamethasone, diphenhydramine, and cimetidine
Docetaxel	Neutropenia (DLT) hyperlacrimation, fluid retention, nail disorders, myelosuppression	1. Use with caution in liver dysfunction. Patients with bilirubin greater than the ULN and/or liver transaminases > 1.5 times, the ULN should not receive docetaxel 2. Do not give if biliary tract is obstructed 3. Premedicate for hypersensitivity reactions: dexamethasone
Carboplatin	Myelosuppression (DLT), nephrotoxicity, nausea/vomiting, electrolyte wasting, diarrhea, stomatitis, hypersensitivity reactions	1. Prehydration not required 2. If using BSA dosing, then give proper dosing for renal dysfunction CrCl ≥ 60 mL/min (1.00 mL/s): no dosage adjustment needed. CrCl 41–59 mL/min (0.68–0.99 mL/s): give 250 mg/m² CrCl 16–40 mL/min (0.26–0.67 mL/s): give 200 mg/m² CrCl ≤ 15 mL/min (0.25 mL/s): do not give NOTE: Calvert formula (AUC dosing) is based on renal function, so no additional dose adjustment is needed 3. Premedicate for hypersensitivity reactions: dexamethasone, diphenhydramine, and cimetidine 4. Appropriate antiemetic regimen for prevention of acute and delayed nausea
Cisplatin	Neurotoxicity (DLT), nausea/vomiting, ototoxicity, nephrotoxicity, myelosuppression, electrolyte wasting, diarrhea	1. Prehydration and posthydration with electrolyte replacement (ie, potassium chloride 10 mEq [10 mmol] and magnesium sulfate 16 mEq [8 mmol]) required 2. Do not use if SrCr > 1.5 mg/dL (133 μmol/L) or BUN > 25 mg/dL (8.9 mmol/L) 3. Give proper dosing for renal dysfunction CrCl 46–60 mL/min (0.77–1.00 mL/s): decrease dose by 50%. CrCl 31–50 mL/min (0.51–0.83 mL/s): decrease dose by 75%. CrCl ≤ 30 mL/min (0.50 mL/s): do not use 4. Appropriate antiemetic regimen for prevention of acute and delayed nausea
Bevacizumab	Hypertension, proteinuria, infusion-related reactions, fluid retention, increase risk of thrombosis, myelosuppression	1. Monitor urine-to-creatinine baseline and every two cycles; hold therapy if ratio > 2 or measure urine protein every cycle and addition testing if positive for proteinuria 2. Use caution in patients with a history of thrombosis

AST, aspartate aminotransferase; AUC, area under the curve; BSA, body surface area; BUN, blood urea nitrogen; CrCl, creatinine clearance; DLT, dose-limiting toxicity; SrCr, serum creatinine; ULN, upper limit of normal.

slow progression of disease. In some cases, especially in elderly patients, single-agent carboplatin is used as palliative treatment instead. Chemotherapy alone has not been curative for patients with advanced ovarian cancer.[23]

In patients with bulky disease or significant tumor burden, neoadjuvant chemotherapy can be used to decrease tumor burden to increase the likelihood of optimal tumor debulking during surgery.[31] Typically, three cycles of the standard combination taxane/platinum regimen is administered once every 21 days. After surgery, patient will receive another three to six cycles depending on their response to chemotherapy.

▶ *Consolidation and Maintenance Chemotherapy*

Consolidation chemotherapy is the addition of cycles of the taxane/platinum regimen or the addition of single-agent platinum or single taxane after completion of first-line chemotherapy.[36] If the tumor has a partial response (PR) to first-line chemotherapy evident by a significant decline in CA-125 by greater than 50% presurgery level and/or tumor regression or decrease in size, then cancer is still considered taxane/platinum sensitive. Additional cycles of chemotherapy are given until CR is achieved (see Figure 94–2). In 2014, bevacizumab was finally approved to be added to the primary treatment and as consolidation treatment for ovarian cancer based on the improved overall survival observed in the ICON-7 study.[37]

Maintenance chemotherapy is similar to consolidation chemotherapy except maintenance chemotherapy is given to patients who have achieved a clinically CR.[38] Maintenance chemotherapy is used to hopefully extend progression-free and overall survival by eliminating any microscopic disease present after completion of primary chemotherapy.

For an extensive description of the common agents used in first-line, consolidation, and maintenance chemotherapy of ovarian cancer, please see Chapter 88. A brief overview of the regimens is provided in Table 94–1 and adverse effects are provided in Table 94–2.

Recurrent Chemotherapy

In the recurrent setting, platinum sensitivity of the tumor is assessed first. If recurrence occurs in less than 6 months or disease progresses while the patient is receiving a platinum-based regimen, the cancer is considered platinum resistant (see Figure 94–2). These parameters are also used to determine if tumors are taxane sensitive or resistant. However, patients resistant to paclitaxel may still respond to docetaxel.[39] If the treatment goal is palliative care, then often single therapy will be used, but curative care typically is an aggressive combination regimen (see Figure 94–2 and Table 94–3). Sometimes an investigational agent may achieve responses equivalent or surpassing standard therapy, and should be considered for most patients.

Table 94–3

Summary of Combination Chemotherapy Regimens Used for Treatment of Recurrent Ovarian Cancer

Drug(s)	Regimen Dosing	Drug Monitoring Comments[b]
Combination Regimens		
Platinum Sensitive		
Paclitaxel and carboplatin	175 mg/m² IV (3-hour infusion) AUC 5–7.5 IV every 21 days	• Monitor closely for hypersensitivity reactions
Paclitaxel and cisplatin	135 mg/m² IV (24-hour infusion) 75 mg/m² IV	• Monitor closely for hypersensitivity reactions
Docetaxel and carboplatin	75 mg/m² IV AUC 5 IV every 21 days	• Monitor closely for hypersensitivity reactions
Gemcitabine and carboplatin	800 mg/m² IV days 1 and 8 AUC 5 IV day 1 every 21 days	• Monitor platelet counts closely • Monitor closely for hypersensitivity reactions
Liposomal doxorubicin and carboplatin	30 mg/m² IV over 1–3 hour AUC 5 IV every 28 days	• Monitor closely for hypersensitivity reactions • Liposomal doxorubicin infusion start over 3 hour and decrease to 1 hour as tolerated • Counsel patient for PPE prevention
Platinum-Resistant[a]		
Gemcitabine and cisplatin	1000 mg/m² IV days 1 and 8 40 mg/m² IV days 1 and 8 every 21 days	• Monitor renal function closely • Monitor ANC closely, consider primary use of growth factor • Monitor closely for hypersensitivity reactions
Cyclophosphamide and bevacizumab	50 mg PO once daily 10 mg/kg IV once every 2 weeks every 28 days (continuous)	• Monitor for hypertension; hold therapy blood pressure greater than 140/90 mm Hg • Monitor urine-to-creatinine baseline and every two cycles; hold therapy if the ratio is greater than 2 or measure urine protein every cycle and addition testing if positive for proteinuria • Use caution in patients with history of thrombosis

[a]*Platinum resistance* = disease progression while on platinum agent or recurrence within 6 months of completion of platinum-based therapy.

[b]See Table 94–2 for specific monitoring parameters.

ANC, absolute neutrophil count; AUC, area under the curve; IV, intravenous; PO, oral; PPE, palmar-plantar erythrodysesthesia.

▸ *Platinum Sensitive*

In patients who experienced a CR to first-line chemotherapy and have had greater than a 6-month platinum-free interval, retreatment with a platinum-containing regimen is appropriate. The combination of carboplatin with gemcitabine, liposomal doxorubicin, or paclitaxel for the treatment of platinum-sensitive recurrent ovarian cancer with a curative intent is recommended.[31,40,41] (see Table 94–3). However, in patients who are unable to tolerate additional combination chemotherapy regimens, carboplatin alone or any one of the second-line agents would be appropriate[42] (see Table 94–2).

▸ *Platinum Resistant*

Recurrent or persistent ovarian cancer after platinum-based regimens has a discouraging prognosis. Second-line agents have not been successful to date, but any active agent that has not been used during initial treatment is available to use. KEY CONCEPT *Single-agent chemotherapy is standard practice for recurrent platinum-resistant ovarian cancer.* However, two combination regimens have demonstrated promising activity in the recurrent setting: (a) gemcitabine plus cisplatin because gemcitabine modulates platinum resistance allowing it to regain its cytotoxic activity, and (b) bevacizumab with metronomic oral cyclophosphamide.[43,44] Active agents include altretamine (formerly hexamethylmelamine), anastrozole, capecitabine (5-fluorouracil), cyclophosphamide, docetaxel, gemcitabine, liposomal doxorubicin, oral etoposide, vinorelbine, topotecan, bevacizumab, or investigational agents. Numerous ongoing investigational studies are evaluating the benefit of addition of bevacizumab with other cytotoxic agent to improve outcomes in the recurrent ovarian cancer setting (see Figure 94–2). KEY CONCEPT *Because the efficacy of the agents is similar, the selection of agent for treatment of recurrent platinum-resistant ovarian cancer is dependent upon residual toxicities, clinician preference, and patient convenience.* Table 94–4 gives a short summary of the adverse effects and

Table 94–4

Summary of Chemotherapy Single-Agent Regimens Used for Treatment of Progressive and Recurrent Platinum-Resistant Ovarian Cancer

Agent	Dose	Response Rate (%)	Common Adverse Effects	Monitoring/Comments
Docetaxel	75 mg/m² IV over 1 hour repeat every 21–28 days vs. 30–40 mg/m² IV over 1 hour once every week	22 NR	Neutropenia (DLT) hyperlacrimation, fluid retention, nail disorders, myelosuppression	1. Premedicate for hypersensitivity reactions with dexamethasone 2. Use with caution in liver dysfunction. Patients with bilirubin greater than the ULN and/or liver transaminases greater than 1.5 times the ULN should not receive docetaxel 3. Do not give if the biliary tract is obstructed
Gemcitabine	800 mg/m² IV infused over 30 minutes once a week on days 1, 8, and 15 followed by 1 week of rest	13.9–27	Myelosuppression (DLT), flulike symptoms, headache, somnolence, nausea/vomiting, stomatitis, diarrhea, constipation, rash	1. Use with caution in renal or liver dysfunction. No specific guidelines available
Liposomal doxorubicin	40 mg/m² IV infused over 3 hours cycle 1 and 2; then infused over 1 hr; thereafter repeat every 28 days	12.3–18	Myelosuppression, stomatitis, mucositis, alopecia, flushing, shortness of breath, hypotension, headaches, cardiotoxicity, hand–foot syndrome	1. Give proper dosing for liver dysfunction; total bilirubin 1.2–3 mg/dL (21–51 μmol/L): reduce dose by 50%; total bilirubin ≥ 3 mg/dL (51 μmol/L): reduce dose by 75% 2. Do not give if total bilirubin is > 5 mg/dL (86 μmol/L)
Topotecan	1.5 mg/m² IV infused over 30 minutes on days 1, 2, 3, 4, and 5; repeat every 21 days *OR* 4 mg/m² IV infused over 30 minutes once a week for 3 consecutive weeks followed by 1-week rest	6.5–17 31	Myelosuppression (DLT), nausea/vomiting, diarrhea, stomatitis, abdominal pain, alopecia, AST/ALT elevation	1. Give proper dosing for renal dysfunction; CrCl 40–60 mL/min (0.67–1.00 mL/s): no dosage adjustment needed; CrCl 20–39 mL/min (0.33–0.66 mL/s): reduce dose by 50% 2. Do not give if CrCl < 20 mL/min (0.33 mL/s)
Altretamine (Hexalen)	260 mg/m² PO daily for 14–21 days; repeat every 28 days	9.7	Nausea/vomiting, diarrhea, abdominal cramping, myelosuppression	1. Monitor for potential CYP450 drug interactions
Capecitabine	1800–2500 mg/m² PO as divided dose twice daily for 14 consecutive days followed by 1 week of rest	29	Myelosuppression, hand–foot syndrome, nausea/vomiting, edema, stomatitis, diarrhea, cardiotoxicity, rash	1. Monitor for PPE and recommend regular use of lotions on hands and feet 2. Use with caution in renal dysfunction; CrCl ≥ 51 mL/min (0.84 mL/s): no dose adjustment; CrCl 30–50 mL/min (0.50–0.83 mL/s): reduce dose by 25%; CrCl < 30 mL/min (0.50 mL/s): do not give 3. Use with caution in liver dysfunction; no specific guidelines available

(Continued)

Table 94–4

Summary of Chemotherapy Single-Agent Regimens Used for Treatment of Progressive and Recurrent Platinum-Resistant Ovarian Cancer (*Continued*)

Agent	Dose	Response Rate (%)	Common Adverse Effects	Monitoring/Comments
Etoposide	50 mg/m²/day PO in divided doses given daily for 3 consecutive weeks followed by 1 week of rest	18	Myelosuppression, nausea/vomiting, anorexia, alopecia, headache, fever, hypotension	1. Give proper dosing for liver dysfunction; total bilirubin 1.5–3 mg/dL (26–51 μmol/L): decrease dose by 50%; total bilirubin 3–5 mg/dL (51–86 μmol/L): decrease dose by 75% 2. Do not give if total bilirubin is > 5 mg/dL (86 μmol/L) 3. Give proper dosing for renal dysfunction; CrCl 60–45 mL/min (1.00–0.75 mL/s): reduce dose by 15%; CrCl 44–30 mL/min (0.74–0.50 mL/s): reduce dose by 20%; CrCl < 30 mL/min (0.50 mL/s): reduce dose by 25%
Letrozole	2.5 mg once daily	15	Headache, nausea, dyspepsia, skin rash	1. No protective effect on bone; recommend calcium supplementation
Tamoxifen	20 mg PO twice a day continuously until PD	10	Thrombocytopenia, anemia, thromboembolism, hot flashes, decreased libido, nausea/vomiting	1. Protective effect on bone and lipids 2. Increased risk for endometrial cancer
Vinorelbine	30 mg/m² IV infused over 15 minutes on days 1 and 8; repeat every 21 days	29	Constipation, neutropenia, anemia, thrombocytopenia, neurotoxicity	1. Consider bowel regimen to prevent constipation
Bevacizumab	15 mg/kg IV infused over 30–90 minutes every 21 days	NR	Hypertension, proteinuria, infusion-related reactions, fluid retention, increase risk of thrombosis, myelosuppression	1. Monitor urine-to-creatinine baseline and every two cycles; hold therapy if ratio > 2 or measure urine protein every cycle and addition testing if positive for proteinuria 2. Use caution in patients with a history of thrombosis

CrCl, creatinine clearance; DLT, dose-limiting toxicity; IV, intravenous; NR, not reported; PD, progressive disease; PO, oral; PPE, palmar-plantar erythrodysesthesia; ULN, upper limit of normal.

monitoring parameters for chemotherapy agents commonly used for the treatment of recurrent ovarian cancer.

OUTCOME EVALUATION

Overall survival is impacted by success of initial surgery to debulk tumor to less than 1 cm of disease and response to first-line chemotherapy. The CA-125 level should be monitored with each cycle, and at least a 50% reduction in CA-125 after four cycles of taxane/platinum chemotherapy is related to an improved prognosis. Patients who achieve CR should have follow-up examinations once every 3 months, including CA-125, physical examination, and pelvic examination, and appropriate diagnostic scans (ie, computed tomography [CT], magnetic resonance imaging [MRI], or positron emission tomography [PET] scan) should be evaluated for the detection of disease. While evaluating patient specifically assess resolution of any residual chemotherapy-related adverse effects including: neuropathies, nephrotoxicity, ototoxicity, myelosuppression, or nausea/vomiting. Younger patients with an active menstrual cycle before surgery will encounter "surgical menopause" and often experience intense hot flushes. Because there are concerns about potential of hormones in the pathogenesis of ovarian cancer, the use of hormone replacement therapy is controversial. The use of phytoestrogen supplements, such as black cohosh or soy, is also controversial. Alternative nutritional supplements with less controversy may include: omega3 (fish oil), fiber supplement, or maca root. An effective alternative has been the use of the class of serotonin reuptake inhibitors such as venlafaxine controlled-released once daily.

In the PD or recurrent setting, CA-125 levels should still be monitored with each cycle, but no change in therapy is recommended until after minimum of three cycles of chemotherapy.

Patient Encounter 1, Part 2: Completion of Primary Treatment

Your patient completed six cycles of paclitaxel 175 mg/m² IV plus carboplatin AUC 6 IV. Her CT scan findings suggest minimal residual disease and CA-125 has decreased but still above the normal range (38 U/mL [38 kU/L]) upon completion of her chemotherapy. She feels great and has no obvious symptoms of ovarian cancer at this time.

Discuss the advantages and disadvantages of treatment options for consolidation treatment with chemotherapy verses bevacizumab for this patient.

Describe the role of second-look surgery for this patient.

Patient Care Process

Patient Assessment:

- Assess patient history of nonspecific symptoms and signs to determine if patient has newly diagnosed or potential recurrence of ovarian cancer.
- Review available laboratory tests, specifically CA-125, CBC, electrolytes, LFTs and calculate estimated creatinine clearance.
- Review any recent diagnostic scans (ie, CT scan, MRI, or PET scan)
- Complete medication history (prescriptions, OTC medications and nutritional supplements) to identify any potential interactions, therapy duplication. Does patient have any new drug allergies? Any residual drug-related side effects?
- Assess patient pain to determine need for acute or chronic pain medications.

Therapy Evaluation:

- If patient is a surgery candidate, evaluate patient comorbidities and medications to determine if additional workup is necessary before tumor debulking surgery. Do any medications need to be stopped or changed before surgery (ie, aspirin, warfarin, nonsteroidal anti-inflammatory agents)?
- If patient is a chemotherapy candidate (neoadjuvant, adjuvant or recurrent) evaluate patient medications, residual toxicities, renal function and liver function to determine if any potential dose adjustments ought to be recommended for the selected chemotherapy regimen. (see Figure 94–2)
- Determine whether patient has insurance coverage for planned chemotherapy regimen and prescription coverage for supportive care medications. Assist patient in locating pharmacy to fill opioid prescription medications when needed.

Care Plan Development:

- Provide appropriate patient education on respective chemotherapy agents that will be given for treatment of ovarian cancer. What each chemotherapy agent is, route, frequency, and duration it will be administered and how it works to treat cancer.
- Explain the plan and frequency for monitoring response to treatment and treatment intent- curative verses palliative (relief of symptoms).
- What side effects to expect during chemotherapy? Precautions to take to prevent infection and how to monitor for signs and symptoms of infection; neuropathy, electrolyte wasting and bowel habits.
- Develop appropriate plan for prevention and treatment of nausea and vomiting based on emetogenic potential of regimen. Discuss nonpharmacologic interventions such as diet choices and frequency of meals. Also provide information on any drug or food interactions with chemotherapy to avoid
- Review pharmacological and non-pharmacological recommendations for blood clot prevention postsurgery.

Follow-up Evaluation:

- Patient should be evaluated 5 to 6 weeks after surgery. Evaluate wound healing, pain control/resolution, and determine if adjuvant chemotherapy required.
- Review laboratory values prior to each new cycle of chemotherapy. Recommend appropriate dose adjustments or changes for altered organ function, prolonged myelosuppression, or unacceptable toxicity.
- Assess tumor response to chemotherapy once every 3 months. Evaluate potential for recurrence or response to treatment with CT Scan/MRI once every 3 to 4 months.

In addition, appropriate diagnostic scans (ie, CT scan, MRI, or PET scan) should be evaluated once every three cycles. Patients should also have routine physical examinations with each cycle of chemotherapy to evaluate for any physical toxicity associated with chemotherapy such as neuropathies, fluid retention, palmar-plantar erythrodysesthesia, myelosuppression, or nausea/vomiting.

Unfortunately, most patients will eventually progress through all chemotherapy options, and supportive care measures should be provided to maintain patient comfort and quality of life. Common complications while developing a plan for treatment of advanced or progressive ovarian cancer include ascites, uncontrollable pain, and SBO. Precaution should be used in removal of ascites because of the potential complications associated with rapid fluid shifts. Liberal use of opioids to control pain is appropriate as ovarian cancer patients cope with PD and approaching end of life. Appropriate bowel regimens with laxatives and stool softeners should be used to prevent constipation. However, when a patient with a well-controlled bowel regimen presents with new onset of constipation, additional workup is required before altering the bowel regimen. KEY CONCEPT *In ovarian cancer patients, SBO is a common complication of progressive disease. In general, laxatives should not be used in patients with SBOs.* Before treating constipation, patients should have a physical examination and abdominal x-ray to rule out SBO. Often, palliative surgery is required to correct SBO and alleviate patient pain. Patients should not eat any solid or liquids until resolution of SBO. If inoperable SBO exists, then parenteral nutrition can be considered but weighed against ultimate treatment objectives. Overall, providing any measures needed to maintain patient comfort is the priority for patients with progressive ovarian cancer.

Abbreviations Introduced in This Chapter

AUC	Area under the curve
BRCA1	Breast cancer activator gene 1
BRCA2	Breast cancer activator gene 2
BSO	Bilateral salpingo-oophorectomy
CA-125	Cancer antigen 125
CA-19	Cancer antigen 19
CEA	Carcinoembryonic antigen
CR	Complete response
CrCl	Creatinine clearance

DLT	Dose-limiting toxicity
FIGO	International Federation of Gynecology and Obstetrics
GFR	Glomerular filtration rate
GST	Glutathione S-transferase
HBOC	Hereditary breast and ovarian cancer
HNPCC	Hereditary nonpolyposis colorectal cancer
IP	Intraperitoneal
LFT	Liver function test
NCCN	National Comprehensive Cancer Network
NS	Normal saline
OC	Oral contraceptive
PD	Progressive disease
PET	Positron emission tomography
PR	Partial response
SBO	Small bowel obstruction
SXR	Steroid xenobiotic receptor
TAH	Total abdominal hysterectomy
TVUS	Transvaginal ultrasound

REFERENCES

1. American Cancer Society, Cancer Fact & Figures 2014; Atlanta: American Cancer Society; 2014.
2. Cannistra SA. Cancer of the ovary. N Engl J Med. 2004;351: 2519–2529.
3. Lux MP, Fashing PA, Beckmann MW. Hereditary breast and ovarian cancer: review and future perspectives. J Mol Med. 2006; 84(1):16–28.
4. Lu KH, Dinh M, Kohlmann W, et al. Gynecologic cancer as a "sentinel cancer" for women with hereditary nonpolyposis colorectal cancer syndrome. Obstet Gynecol. 2005; 105:569–574.
5. Colomob N, VanGorp T, Parma G, et al. Ovarian cancer. Crit Rev Oncol Hematol. 2006;60:159–179.
6. Heintz AP, Odicino F, Maisonneuve P, et al. Carcinoma of the ovary. FIGO 26th Annual Report on the Results of Treatment in Gynecological Cancer. Int J Gynaecol Obstet. 2006; 95(Suppl):S161–S192.
7. Prentice RK, Thomson CA, Caan B, et al. Low-fat dietary pattern and cancer incidence in the Women's Health Initiative Dietary Modification randomized controlled trial. J Natl Cancer Inst. 2007;99:1534–1543.
8. Krygiou M, Tsoumpou I, Martin-Hirsch P, et al. Ovarian cancer screening. Anticancer Res. 2006;26:4793–4801.
9. Edwards BK, Brown ML, Wingo PA, et al. Annual report to the nation on the status of cancer 1975–2002, featuring population-based trends in cancer treatment. J Nat Cancer Inst. 2005;97(19):1407–1427.
10. Bast RC, Brewer M, Zou, C, et al. Prevention and early detection of ovarian cancer: mission impossible? Recent Results Cancer Res. 2007;174:91–100.
11. Whittemore AS, Balise RR, Pharoah PD, et al. Oral contraceptive use and ovarian cancer risk among carriers of BRCA1 or BRCA2 mutations. Br J Cancer. 2004;91(11):1911–1915.
12. La Vecchia C. Oral contraceptives and ovarian cancer: an update, 1998–2004. Eur J Cancer Prev. 2006;15:117–124.
13. McLaughlin JR, Risch HA, Lubinski J, et al. Reproductive risk factors for ovarian cancer in carriers of BRCA1 or BRCA2 mutations: A case control study. Lancet Oncol. 2007;8:26–34.
14. Harris RE, Beebe-Donk J, Doss H, et al. Aspirin, ibuprofen, and other non-steroidal anti-inflammatory drugs in cancer prevention: a critical review of non-selective COX-2 blockade. Oncol Rep. 2005;13:559–583.
15. Bertone ER, Hankinson SE, Newcomb PA, et al. A population-based case-control study of carotenoid and vitamin A intake and ovarian cancer. Cancer Causes Control. 2001;12:83–90.
16. Meeuwissen PAM, Seynaeve C, Brekelmans CTM, et al. Outcome of surveillance and prophylactic salpingo-oophorectomy in asymptomatic women at high risk for ovarian cancer. Gynecol Oncol. 2005;97(2):476–482.
17. Dann JL, Zorn KK. Strategies for ovarian cancer prevention. Obstet Gynecol Clin North Am. 2007;34:667–686.
18. Finch A, Beiner M, Lubinski J, et al. Salpingo-oophorectomy and the risk of ovarian, fallopian tube, and peritoneal cancers in women with a BRCA1 or BRCA2 Mutation. JAMA. 2006;296: 185–192.
19. Narod SA, Sun P, Ghadirian P, et al. Tubal ligation and risk of ovarian cancer in carriers of BRCA1 and BRCA2 mutations: a case control study. Lancet. 2001;357:1467–1470.
20. Batista LI, Lu KH, Beahm EK, et al. Coordinated prophylactic surgical management for women with hereditary breast-ovarian cancer syndrome. BMC Cancer. 2008;14(8):101–106.
21. Pavelka JC, Li AJ, Karlan BY. Hereditary ovarian cancer-assessing risk and prevention strategies. Obstet Gynecol Clin North Am. 2007;34(4):651–665.
22. Klip H, Burger CW, Kenemans P, et al. Cancer risk associated with subfertility and ovulation induction: a review. Cancer Causes Control. 2000;11:319–344.
23. Salzberg M, Thurlimann B, Bonnefois H, et al. Current concepts of treatment strategies in advanced or recurrent ovarian cancer. Oncology. 2005;68:293–298.
24. National Cancer Institute. Cancer Stat Fact Sheets. Cancer of the Ovary, 2012 http://seer.cancer.gov/statfacts/html/ovary.html.
25. Cooper A, DePriest P. Surgical management of women with ovarian cancer. Semin Oncol. 2007;34:226–233.
26. Wimberger P, Lehmann N, Kimmig R, et al. Prognostic factors for complete debulking in advanced ovarian cancer and its impact on survival. An exploratory analysis of a prospectively randomized phase III study of the Arbeitsgemeinschaft Gynaekologishce Onkologie Ovarian Cancer Study Group (AGO-OVAR). Gynecol Oncol. 2007;106:69–74.
27. Hoffman MS, Griffin D, Tebes S, et al. Sites of bowel resected to achieve optimal ovarian cancer cytoreduction: Implications regarding surgical management. Am J Obstet Gynecol. 2005;193: 582–588.
28. Ozols RF, Bundy BN, Greer BE, et al. Phase III trial of carboplatin and paclitaxel compared with cisplatin and paclitaxel in patients with optimally resected stage III ovarian cancer: a gynecologic oncology group study. J Clin Oncol. 2003;21:3194–3200.
29. Neijt JP, Engelholm SA, Tuxen MK, et al. Exploratory phase III study of paclitaxel and cisplatin versus paclitaxel and carboplatin in advanced ovarian cancer. J Clin Oncol. 2000;18: 3084–3092.
30. National Comprehensive Cancer Network (NCCN) Practice Guidelines in Oncology—Ovarian Cancer—v.1. 2012, http://www.nccn.org.
31. Armstrong DK, Bundy B, Wenzel L, et al. Intraperitoneal cisplatin and paclitaxel in ovarian cancer. N Engl J Med. 2006; 354:34–43.
32. Rao G, Crispens M, Rothenberg ML. Intraperitoneal chemotherapy for ovarian cancer: Overview and perspective. J Clin Oncol. 2007;25:2867–2872.
33. National Cancer Institute. NCI Clinical Announcement: Intraperitoneal Chemotherapy for Ovarian Cancer. January 5, 2006. http://ctep.cancer.gov/highlights/clin_annc_010506.pdf.
34. Alberts DS, Bookman MA, Chen T, et al. Proceedings of a GOG workshop on intraperitoneal therapy for ovarian cancer. Gynecol Oncol. 2006;103:783–792.
35. Katsumata N, Yasuda M, Takahashi F, Isonishi S, Jobo T, Aoki D, et al. Dose-dense paclitaxel once a week in combination with carboplatin every 3 weeks for advanced ovarian cancer: a phase 3, open-label, randomised controlled trial. Lancet. 2009; 374:1331–1338.

36. Gadducci A, Cosio S, Conte PF, et al. Consolidation and maintenance treatments for patients with advanced epithelial ovarian cancer in CR after first-line chemotherapy: a review of the literature. Crit Rev Oncol Hematol. 2005;55:153–166.
37. Perrin TJ, Swart AM, Pfisterer J et al. A phase 3 trial of bevacizumab in ovarian cancer. N Engl J Med. 2011 365;26: 2484–2496.
38. Abaid LN, Goldstein BH, Micha JP, Rettenmaier MA, Brown JV 3rd, Markman M. Improved overall survival with 12 cycles of single-agent paclitaxel maintenance therapy following a complete response to induction chemotherapy in advanced ovarian carcinoma. Oncology. 2010;78:389–393.
39. Rose PG, Blessing JA, Ball HG, et al. A phase II study of docetaxel in paclitaxel-resistant ovarian and peritoneal carcinoma: a Gynecologic Oncology Group study. Gynecol Oncol. 2003; 88:130–135.
40. Alberts DS, Liu PY, Wilczynski SP, et al. Randomized trial of pegylated liposomal doxorubicin (PLD) plus carboplatin versus carboplatin in platinum-sensitive (PS) patients with recurrent epithelial ovarian or peritoneal carcinoma after failure of initial platinum-based chemotherapy (Southwest Oncology Group Protocol S0200) Gynecol Oncol. 2008;108:90–94.
41. Pfisterer J, Plante M, Vergote I, et al. Gemcitabine plus carboplatin compared with carboplatin in patients with platinum-sensitive recurrent ovarian cancer: An intergroup trial of the AGO-OVAR, the NCIC CTG, and the EORTC GCG. J Clin Oncol. 2006;24:4699–4707.
42. Herzog TJ, Pothuri B. Ovarian cancer: a focus on management of recurrent disease. Nat Clin Pract Oncol. 2006;3:604–611.
43. Boza G, Bamias A, Koutsoukou V, et al. Biweekly gemcitabine and cisplatin in platinum-resistant/refractory, paclitaxel-pre-treated, ovarian and peritoneal carcinoma. Gynecol Oncol. 2007;104(3):580–585.
44. Garcia AA, Hirte H, Fleming G, et al. Phase II clinical trial of bevacizumab and low-dose metronomic oral cyclophosphamide in recurrent ovarian cancer: a trial of the California, Chicago, and Princess Margaret Hospital phase II consortia. J Clin Oncol. 2008;26(1):76–82.

95 Acute Leukemia

Nancy Heideman and Shirley Abraham

LEARNING OBJECTIVES

Upon completion of the chapter, the reader will be able to:

1. Describe the pathogenesis of acute leukemia.
2. Compare the classification systems for acute lymphocytic leukemia and acute myelogenous leukemia.
3. Identify the risk factors associated with a poor outcome for the acute leukemias.
4. Explain the importance of minimal residual disease and its implication on early bone marrow relapse.
5. Explain the role of induction, consolidation, and maintenance phases for acute leukemia.
6. Define the role of central nervous system preventive therapy for acute leukemia.
7. Recognize the treatment complications associated with therapy for acute leukemias.
8. Describe the late effects associated with the treatment of long-term survivors of acute leukemias.

INTRODUCTION

KEY CONCEPT *The acute leukemias are hematologic malignancies of bone marrow precursors characterized by excessive production of immature hematopoietic cells. This proliferation of "blast" cells eventually replaces normal bone marrow and leads to the failure of normal hematopoiesis and the appearance in peripheral blood as well as infiltration of other organs.* These blast cells proliferate in the marrow and inhibit normal cellular elements, resulting in anemia, neutropenia, and thrombocytopenia. Leukemia also may infiltrate other organs, including the liver, spleen, bone, skin, lymph nodes, testis and central nervous system (CNS). Virtually anywhere there is blood flow, the potential for extramedullary (outside the bone marrow) leukemia exists.

KEY CONCEPT *Acute leukemias are classified according to their cell of origin. Acute lymphocytic leukemia (ALL) arises from the lymphoid precursors. Acute nonlymphocytic leukemia (ANLL) or acute myelogenous leukemia (AML) arises from the myeloid or megakaryocytic precursors.* As a result of clinical trials defining various prognostic (risk) factors that helped guide treatment modifications, the outcomes of acute leukemias, especially ALL, has improved dramatically over the past 30 years.[1] Risk-based treatment strategies that consider multiple phenotypic and biological risk factors and attempt to match the aggressiveness of therapy with the presumed risk of relapse and death are now the standard of care. Despite the overall success in treating patients with acute leukemias, the long-term survival for patients who relapse remains dismal.

EPIDEMIOLOGY AND ETIOLOGY

Epidemiology

Leukemia is a relatively uncommon disease. The current overall age-adjusted annual incidence of acute leukemia in the United States has remained relatively stable at 10 per 100,000 in children and 1 to 2 per 100,000 in adults.[2] In 2015, it is estimated that there will be 54,270 new cases of leukemia, or 3.1% of all new cancer cases.[3]

In the pediatric population, leukemia is a common cancer, accounting for almost one-third of all childhood malignancies. ALL accounts for 75% to 80% of all cases of childhood leukemia, whereas AML accounts for no more than 20%. Males generally are affected more often than females in all but the infant age group, and its incidence is higher in whites than among other racial groups.

The incidence of AML in children is bimodal: It peaks at 2 years of age, decreases steadily thereafter to age 9 years, and then increases again at around age 16.[4] The average age of diagnosis for AML is about 65 years and is a result of an increasing incidence of AML with age.

Etiology

The causes of the acute leukemias is unknown; multiple influences related to genetics, socioeconomics, infection, environment, hematopoietic development, and chance all may play a role.[4] Table 95–1 lists the major conditions that have been associated with the acute leukemias. In most cases, however, there is no identifiable cause of the leukemia.

Although leukemia is rarely a hereditary disease, some genetic associations are evident. For example, among identical twins, the concordance for ALL in the initially unaffected twin is 20% to 25% within 1 year. Although the incidence in fraternal twins is much less, there is still a fourfold increase in the risk of leukemia in the initially unaffected twin compared with the normal population. One explanation for this association may be a shared placental circulation, which allows for transmission of disease from one twin to the other. Additionally, leukemia is known to have an increased incidence in several chromosomally abnormal populations. Patients with Down syndrome have a 20 times

Table 95–1

Clinical Conditions Associated With an Increased Frequency of Acute Leukemias

Drugs	**Chemicals**
Alkylating agents	Benzene
Epipodophyllotoxins	**Radiation**
Genetic Conditions	Ionizing radiation
Down syndrome	**Viruses**
Bloom syndrome	Epstein-Barr virus
Fanconi anemia	Human T-lymphocyte virus (HTLV-1 and HTLV-2)
Klinefelter syndrome	
Ataxia telangiectasia	**Social Habits**
Langerhans cell histiocytosis	Cigarette smoking
Shwachman syndrome	Maternal marijuana use
Severe combined immunodeficiency syndrome	Maternal ethanol use
Kostmann syndrome	
Neurofibromatosis type 1	
Familial monosomy 7	
Diamond-Blackfan anemia	

Adapted from Pieters R, Carroll WL. Biology and treatment of acute lymphoblastic leukemia. Pediatr Clin North Am. 2008;55(1):1–20.

increased risk of developing leukemia compared with the rest of the population. Patients with Klinefelter syndrome and Bloom syndrome also have an increased incidence of leukemias.[4]

Exposure to environmental agents such as agricultural chemicals, pesticides, and radiation have also been periodically associated with leukemia, but none is conclusively related to the development of leukemia. An increased frequency of ALL is associated with higher socioeconomic status. It is postulated that less social contact in early infancy and thus a late exposure to some common infectious agents may have some impact.[4]

Risk factors for the development of AML include exposure to environmental toxins, Hispanic ethnicity, and genetics.[5] Of greater concern is the increased prevalence of AML as a secondary malignancy, resulting from chemotherapy and radiation treatment for other cancers. Alkylating agents, such as ifosfamide and cyclophosphamide, and topoisomerase inhibitors, such as etoposide, are linked to an increased risk of AML and **myelodysplastic syndrome** (MDS).[5]

PATHOPHYSIOLOGY

Hematopoiesis is defined as the development and maturation of blood cells and their precursors. In utero, hematopoiesis may occur in the liver, spleen, and bone marrow; after birth, this process occurs exclusively in the bone marrow. All blood cells are generated from a common hematopoietic precursor, or stem cell. These stem cells are self-renewing and pluripotent and thus are able to commit to any one of the different lines of maturation that give rise to platelet-producing megakaryocytes, lymphoid, erythroid, and myeloid cells. The myeloid cell line produces monocytes, basophils, neutrophils, and eosinophils, whereas the lymphoid stem cell differentiates to form circulating B and T lymphocytes, natural killer (NK) cells, and dendritic cells. In contrast to the ordered development of normal cells, the development of leukemia seems to represent an arrest in differentiation at an early phase in the continuum of stem cell to mature cell.[1]

Both AML and ALL are presumed to arise from clonal expansion of these "arrested" cells. As these cells expand, they acquire one and often more chromosomal aberrations, including translocations, inversions, deletions, point mutations, and amplifications.[4] The translocation t(12;21) or *TEL–AML1* is found in approximately 25% of cases of pediatric ALL and is associated with a favorable prognosis.[6] This translocation is uncommon in adults. Another example is the t(9;22) translocation (Philadelphia chromosome, Ph^+), which results in the *BCR–ABL* fusion protein. This translocation produces a novel kinase that leads to uncontrolled proliferation, survival, and self-renewal of cells. It is uncommon in childhood ALL and commonly found in adult ALL, especially in older patients.

Patients with MDS or AML as a secondary neoplasm are often characterized by having had prior alkylator-based or etoposide-based chemotherapy. Patients who have received treatment for Hodgkin disease or solid tumors are most at risk for this problem because they often treated with these agents. Patients with MDS have an abnormal bone marrow and a variety of cytopenias involving one or more of their marrow cell lines. They are at high risk of converting to overt leukemia over time. A variety of complex cytogentic findings and monosomies of chromosome 5 or 7, and 11q23 translocations are often present in this population.[5]

Leukemia Classification

Classification methods for leukemia have evolved from simple schemes that were largely phenotypic and considered only age, gender, white blood cell (WBC) count, and blast morphology to now-complex methods that include biological features such as cell-surface receptors, DNA content (ploidy; more or less than normal chromosomal DNA content), and a variety of cytogenetic abnormalities.

For all newly diagnosed patients with leukemia, an aspirate of the liquid marrow and a bone marrow core biopsy are obtained. Analysis of the leukemic cell surface markers (immunophenotyping) establish three types of ALL, pre-B, mature B, and T-cell precursor ALL. There are eight subtypes of AML (M0 to M7) as classified by the French-American-British (FAB) scheme (Tables 95–2 and 95–3).

Immunophenotyping by **flow cytometry** has taken on an increasingly important role in the diagnosis of leukemia. Owing to the ease of application, sensitivity, and quantifiable results, flow cytometry is the preferred method for leukemic lineage as well as prognostic assignment.[7] This approach takes advantage of the development of diagnostic monoclonal antibodies (MABs) to many cell-surface antigens that are differentially expressed during hematopoietic differentiation. The antigens are referred to as antibody cluster determinants (CDs) that define cells at various stages of development and can easily separate ALL from AML and T-cell from pre–B-cell ALL.[4,7] The combined approach of flow cytometric identification and cytogenetic DNA content, much of which is also revealed by flow cytometry and fluorescent in situ hybridization (**FISH**; microscopic, fluorescence identification of chromosomal features) has facilitated diagnosis and delineation of specific subtypes of the acute leukemias. Common immunophenotypic markers seen in AML and ALL are provided in Table 95–4.

Prognostic Factors

KEY CONCEPT *The goal of treatment is to match treatment to risk and minimize overtreatment or undertreatment. Patients with leukemia are sorted into prognostic categories based on clinical and biological features that mirror their risk of relapse. Risk assessment is an important factor in the selection of treatment.* Age, WBC, leukemic cell-surface markers, DNA content, and specific

Table 95–2

Morphologic (FAB) Classification of AML

Subtype		Adults (%)	Frequency of FAB Subtype: Children Older Than 2 Years (%)	Frequency of FAB Subtype: Children Younger Than 2 Years (%)
M0	Acute myeloblastic leukemia without maturation	5	Low	Low
M1	Acute myeloblastic leukemia with minimal maturation	15	17	7
M2	Acute myeloblastic leukemia with maturation	25		27
M3	Acute promyelocytic leukemia	10		5
M4	Acute myelomonocytic leukemia	25	30	26
M5a	Acute monoblastic leukemia, poorly differentiated	5	52	26
M5b	Acute monoblastic leukemia, well differentiated	5		
M6	Acute erythroleukemia	5		2
M7	Acute megakaryoblastic leukemia	5		7

FAB, French-American-British.

cytogenetic abnormalities predict response to therapy and are used to assign risk and associated treatment.[4] On the basis of these prognostic variables, patients are assigned to standard-, high-, or very-high-risk groups that determine the aggressiveness of treatment.

Table 95–3

WHO Classification of AML and Related Neoplasms

AML with recurrent genetic abnormalities:
AML with t(8;21)(q22;q22); *RUNX1-RUNX1T1*
AML with inv(16)(p13.1q22) or t(16;16)(p13.1;q22); *CBFB-MYH11*
Acute promyelocytic leukemia (APL) with t(15;17)(q22;q12); *PML-RARA*
AML with t(9;11)(p22;q23); *MLLT3-MLL*
AML with t(6;9)(p23;q34); *DEK-NUP214*
AML with inv(3)(q21q26.2) or t(3;3)(q21;q26.2); *RPN1-EVI1*
AML (megakaryoblastic) with t(1;22)(p13;q13); *RBM15-MKL1*
Provisional entity: AML with mutated NPM1
Provisional entity: AML with mutated CEBPA

AML with myelodysplasia-related change

Therapy-related myeloid neoplasms

AML, not otherwise specified:
Undifferentiated AML (M0)
AML with minimal differentiation (M1)
AML without maturation (M2)
AML with maturation (M2)
Acute myelomonocytic leukemia (M3)
Acute monoblastic/monocytic leukemia (M4)
Acute erythroid leukemia (M5)
Pure erythroid leukemia (M6)
Erythroleukemia, erythroid/myeloid (M6)
Acute megakaryoblastic leukemia (M7)

Acute basophilic leukemia

Acute panmyelosis with myelofibrosis

Myeloid sarcoma

Myeloid proliferations related to Down syndrome:
Transient abnormal myelopoiesis
Myeloid leukemia associated with Down syndrome
Blastic plasmacytoid dendritic cell neoplasm

AML, acute myeloid leukemia.

▶ *Prognostic Factors in ALL*

In both children and adults with ALL, clinical trials have identified several risk factors that correlate with outcome (Table 95–5). Prognostic features include age, WBC count, cytogenetic abnormalities, ploidy (DNA content), leukemic cell immunophenotype, and degree of initial response to therapy, and minimal residual disease (MRD; the degree of subclinical disease remaining at various times after starting treatment)[4,7,8] When these factors are combined, they predict groups of patients with varying degrees of risk for treatment failure.

The importance of age is evident in both children and adults. Children younger than 1 year or older than 10 years of age have a poorer outcome than others. Likewise, in adults, there is a steady decline in the rate of survival with increasing age.

Similar to age, the WBC count at presentation is a reliable indicator of complete response (CR) rate and outcome. The WBC count is indicative of tumor burden, although the underlying biological mechanisms that account for the unfavorable outcomes associated with an elevated WBC count are unclear. Patients with WBC counts of less than $50 \times 10^3/\text{mm}^3$ ($50 \times 10^9/\text{L}$) are considered being at standard risk and have a better outcome than those with a higher WBC counts at presentation, which is associated with higher risk of treatment failure (see Table 95–5).

Specific chromosomal abnormalities in leukemic cells also possess prognostic significance. Blast cells with a translocation of parts of chromosome 12 and 21 (the *TEL-AML1* fusion) or trisomies of 4, 10, and 17 are considered to have favorable genetic features.[4] The presence of the Philadelphia chromosome (Ph^+), the result of a specific translocation between chromosome 9 and

Table 95–4

Common Immunophenotypes in Acute Leukemia

Leukemia	Common Immunophenotypes
AML	CD13, CD15, CD33, CD14, CD64, CD65, and C-KIT
B-cell ALL	CD19, CD20, CD10, CD22, CD79a, HLA-DR, Tdt
T-cell ALL	CD2, CD3, CD4, CD5, CD7, Tdt

ALL, acute lymphoblastic leukemia; AML, acute myeloid leukemia; CD, cluster determinants.

Adapted from Pieters R, Carroll WL. Biology and treatment of acute lymphoblastic leukemia. Pediatr Clin North Am. 2008;55(1):1–20.

Patient Encounter 1, Part 1

An 8-year-old boy presents to the pediatric emergency department with his father with a history of aches, chills, and fevers for the past 4 to 5 days. He has had several colds over the past few weeks that do not seem to be improving. He has also had diffuse body and bone pain in his legs over the past couple of weeks. Physical examination reveals pallor, cervical lymphadenopathy, and hepatosplenomegaly. Electrolytes and uric acid are within normal limits. A complete blood count (CBC) shows a normochromic, normocytic anemia with a hemoglobin of 7.0 g/dL (70 g/L, 4.34 mmol/L; reference range, 11.7 to 15.7 g/dL, 7.26 to 9.74 mmol/L), hematocrit of 21% (0.21; reference range, 35%–47% or 0.35–0.47), and WBC count of $4.1 \times 10^3/\text{mm}^3$ ($4.1 \times 10^9/\text{L}$). The differential on the WBC count reveals 65% (0.65) lymphocytes (reference range, 20%–40% or 0.2–0.4), 13% (0.13) neutrophils (reference range, 55%–62% or 0.55–0.62), and 22% (0.22) lymphoblasts (normal amount, 0%). Flow cytometry from the peripheral blood is consistent with pre–B-cell ALL.

What information is consistent with the diagnosis of ALL?

What are the prognostic factors for this patient?

What is the role of flow cytometry in identifying ALL?

22, t(9;22)(q34;q11.2), is a high-risk feature, which is present in about 3% of children but is much more common in adults with ALL. This translocation results in a novel tyrosine kinase that drives cell proliferation.[7,8]

Among children younger than 1 year of age, as many as 70% possess a poor prognostic genotype represented by the presence of the *MLL* (11q22) gene rearrangement. This finding is rare among older patients. Leukemias with the *MLL* gene rearrangement are highly resistant to the key antileukemic drugs such as glucocorticoids and L-asparaginase.[9]

The DNA content of blast cells, hyper-, hypo-, or diploid, corresponding to increased, decreased, or normal chromosome numbers, has been considered prognostic. Lower risk patients with hyperdiploidy (greater than 50 chromosomes per leukemic cell) generally include approximately 25% of children who have B-cell lineage ALL.[6] These children are between the ages of 1 and 9 years, but the higher risk patients with normal diploidy (50 chromosomes) generally are older. Hypodiploid ALL with less than 44 chromosomes occurs in 1% to 5% of pediatric patients with ALL and is an independent risk factor for poor prognosis with declining prognosis with decreased chromosome number.[10]

Patients with cell-surface markers indicating that the blasts are early in the B-cell lineage (CD markers) are considered favorable and standard risk, whereas those with mature B-cell and T-cell blasts are considered high risk. T-cell ALL is found in approximately 15% of childhood ALL. Compared with B-lineage ALL, T-cell ALL is relatively resistant to different classes of drugs, including methotrexate and cytarabine.

Patients completing induction treatment and in apparent remission still harbor malignant cells in their bone marrow even though they appear disease free by peripheral blood and bone marrow morphology. Assuming that most patients present with about a 10^{11} leukemic cell burden at diagnosis, at least 10^9 cells remain after initial treatment. These residual leukemic cells are below the limits of detection using standard morphologic examination. Measurement of this population of cells has become an increasingly significant prognostic factor and a determinant of the aggressiveness of postinduction therapy. Through flow cytometric analysis and polymerase chain reaction, it is possible to detect one leukemic cell among 10^6 normal cells, representing 1000-fold greater sensitivity than morphologic examination.[11,12]

KEY CONCEPT *Minimal residual disease (MRD) is a quantitative assessment of subclinical remnant of leukemic burden remaining at the end of the initial phase of treatment (induction) when a patient may appear to be in a complete morphologic remission. This measure has become one of the strongest predictors of outcome for patients with acute leukemia. The elimination of MRD is a principal objective of postinduction leukemia therapy.* Several studies in children, in whom ALL is common, have evaluated disease levels at the end of induction and correlated these values with event-free survival (EFS). For a patient with detectable MRD less than 0.1% at the end of induction, EFS is 88% at 3 years. Conversely, a patient with high MRD (greater than 1%) has a 3-year EFS of only 30%.[13] Assessment of MRD is also emerging as an important indicator of disease recurrence in the adult population and in patients with AML.

Table 95–5

Prognostic Factors in ALL

	Risk for Leukemic Relapse	
Factor	**Standard/Low**	**High**
Immunologic phenotype	pre–B cell	Null cell, T cell, pre–B cell, mature B cell
WBC count at diagnosis	$< 50 \times 10^3$ mm^3	$> 50 \times 10^3/\text{mm}^3$ ($50 \times 10^9/\text{L}$)
Patient age	1–10 years	< 1 year or > 10 years
Cytogenetics	Normal karyotype, t(12;21), trisomy 4,10,17	t(9;22); t(4;11); t(17;19), iAmp21, ph-like
Ploidy	Hyperdiploidy	Hypodiploidy, near haploid
CNS leukemia	Absent	Present
MRD at end of induction	< 0.01%	> 0.01%

WBC, white blood cell.

Adapted from Pieters R, Carroll WL. Biology and treatment of acute lymphoblastic leukemia. Pediatr Clin North Am. 2008;55(1):1–20.

▶ *Prognostic Factors in AML*

The major prognostic factors in newly diagnosed AML are age, subtype, chromosome status, ethnicity, and body mass index.

Older adults with AML (greater than 60 years), compared with younger patients with the same disease, have a dismal prognosis and represent a distinct population in terms of disease biology, treatment-related complications, and overall survival (OS). These older patients have a higher incidence of unfavorable chromosomal abnormalities, such as aberrations of chromosomes 5, 7, or 8, FLT_3-internal tandem duplication (ITD) and fewer abnormalities that are associated with a more favorable outcome, such as t(8;21) or inv(16) (Table 95–6).[5,13]

Recent studies suggest that ethnicity may be an important predictor of outcome in children with AML. Investigators found that African Americans treated with chemotherapy had a significantly worse outcome than whites, perhaps suggesting race-related pharmacogenetic differences. Body mass index may also affect the prognosis of children with AML. Underweight patients and

Table 95–6

Risk Category According to Cytogenetic Abnormalities Present

	Risk Category		
Disease	**Good Risk**	**Intermediate Risk**	**High Risk**
AML	t(8;21) (q22;q22); inv(16); t(15;17); t(9;11) trisomy 21	Normal karyotype; trisomy 8; 11q23; del(7q); del(9q); trisomy 22	Complex karyotype; –5; –7; del (5q); inv(3P)
Probability of relapse	25% or less	50%	70% or more
4-Year survival	70% or more	40%–50%	20% or less
ALL	Hyperdiploidy; t(12;21), trisomy 4, 10, 17		t(9;22); t(8;14); t(4;11); t(17;19), hypodiploid, near haploid
Probability of relapse	Less than 10%	Less than 20%	30-40%
4-Year survival	More than 80%	More than 60%	40-50%

ALL, acute lymphocytic leukemia; AML, acute myelogenous leukemia.

Adapted from Pieters R, Carroll WL. Biology and treatment of acute lymphoblastic leukemia. Pediatr Clin North Am. 2008;55(1):1–20.

overweight patients were less likely to survive than normal weight patients because of a greater risk of treatment-related deaths.[15] Current clinical trials in adults and pediatrics strongly suggest that patients with detectable MRD at the end of induction therapy or consolidation is strongly associated with the risk of relapse.[14]

TREATMENT

Desired Outcome

The primary objective in treating patients with acute leukemia is to achieve a continuous complete remission (CCR). Remission is defined as the absence of all clinical evidence of leukemia with the restoration of normal hematopoiesis. For both ALL and AML, remission induction is achieved with the use of myelosuppressive chemotherapy that initially induces a state of bone marrow aplasia as the leukemic cells die followed by a slow return and proliferation of normal cells. After this period, hematopoiesis is restored. Failure to achieve remission in the first 7 to 14 days of therapy is highly predictive of later disease recurrence. This again represents the growing importance of MRD in prognosis and treatment.

Nonpharmacologic Therapy

This year, roughly 1.6 million people will be diagnosed with cancer in the United States and Canada. With improvements in detection and treatment, approximately two-thirds of those diagnosed with the disease can expect to be alive in 5 years. With improving longevity, the cumulative adverse effects of both the disease and treatment are becoming an increasingly important issue. "Late-effects" data show that both adult and pediatric cancer survivors are at greater risk for developing second malignancies, cardiovascular disease, diabetes, and osteoporosis than those in the general population. With respect to the growing population of pediatric cancer survivors, data confirm that they are eight times more likely than their siblings to have a severe or life-threatening chronic health condition. For example, the survivors of pediatric ALL have an increased risk of obesity, osteopenia, and associated comorbidities. Thus, it is important to provide supportive care and intervention and counseling related to nutrition, smoking cessation, and exercise as a part of their active treatment. Health care professionals should think beyond the immediate treatment-related issues of their patients and provide appropriate, active assistance to promote healthy lifestyles and encourage patients to take active roles in pursuing general preventive health strategies.[15]

Patient Encounter 1, Part 2

The patient is admitted to the pediatric oncology service. A bone marrow biopsy and aspirate is done, which shows 85% replacement with precursor B-cell blasts. FISH analysis performed on the peripheral blood is positive for the BCR/ABL translocation (Ph$^+$) in 5.5% of the cells examined. He is started on intravenous hydration with sodium bicarbonate and allopurinol. A diagnostic lumbar puncture (LP) is performed, which is negative for CNS leukemia. During the LP, the patient receives IT cytarabine.

What is the role of CNS prophylaxis for this patient?

What is the BCR/ABL translocation?

How does the presence of this chromosomal abnormality change this patient's risk status?

Pharmacologic Therapy: ALL

The treatment for ALL consists of four main elements: remission induction (the initial tumor reduction leading to morphologic remission), CNS-directed treatment, intensive postremission consolidation regimens, followed by a prolonged maintenance phase (Table 95–7).

► *Remission Induction*

KEY CONCEPT *The initial treatment for acute leukemias is called induction. The purpose of induction is to induce a remission, a state in which there is no identifiable leukemic cells in the bone marrow or peripheral blood with light microscopy.*

KEY CONCEPT *Current induction therapy for ALL typically consists of vincristine, L-asparaginase, and a steroid (prednisone or dexamethasone). An anthracycline is added for higher risk patients.* Although induction treatment produces 95% CR in children, it declines to no more than 60% in patients older than 60 years of age.

Adults, unlike children, are universally considered to be at high risk for relapse; therefore, their induction regimens include an anthracycline (daunorubicin or doxorubicin) in addition to the standard steroid and vincristine treatment that have been the backbone of treatment for this disease for the last 40 years.[16,17]

Clinical Presentation and Diagnosis of ALL[3,6,11]

General

- Typically, patients have symptoms for 1 to 3 months before presentation. These include fatigue, fever, and pallor, but patients generally are in no obvious distress.

Symptoms

- The patient may present with weakness, malaise, bleeding, and weight loss.
- Neutropenic patients are often febrile and highly susceptible to infection.
- Anemia usually presents as pallor, tiredness, and general fatigue.
- Patients with thrombocytopenia usually present with bruising, petechiae, and ecchymosis.
- Patients often present with bone pain secondary to expansion of the marrow cavity from leukemic infiltration.
- CNS involvement is common at diagnosis.

Signs

- Temperature may be elevated secondary to an infection associated with a low WBC count.
- Petechiae and bleeding are indicative of thrombocytopenia.
- Patients may present with organ involvement, such as peripheral adenopathy, hepatomegaly, and splenomegaly.
- T-lineage ALL may present with a mediastinal mass.

Laboratory Tests

- CBC with differential is performed.
- The anemia is usually normochromic and normocytic. Approximately 50% of children present with platelet counts of less than $50 \times 10^3/mm^3$ ($50 \times 10^9/L$). The WBC count may be normal, decreased, or high. About 20% of patients have WBC counts over $100 \times 10^3/mm^3$ ($100 \times 10^9/L$), which places them at risk for leukostasis.
- Uric acid is increased in approximately 50% of patients secondary to rapid cellular turnover.
- Electrolytes: Potassium and phosphorus often are elevated. Calcium usually is low.
- Coagulation disorders: Elevated prothrombin time, partial thromboplastin time, D-dimers; hypofibrinogenemia.

Other Laboratory Tests

Flow cytometric evaluation of bone marrow and peripheral blood is performed to characterize the type of leukemia as well as to detect specific chromosomal rearrangements. The bone marrow at diagnosis usually is hypercellular, with normal hematopoiesis being replaced by leukemic blasts. At diagnosis, a LP is performed to determine if CNS leukemia is present.

Dexamethasone often replaces prednisone as the steroid of treatment because of its longer half-life and better CNS penetration.[17] Although dexamethasone possesses more favorable pharmacologic characteristics than prednisone, its use may be associated with more aseptic osteonecrosis of the femoral and humoral heads as well as an increase in life-threatening infections and septic deaths.[17]

► *CNS Prophylaxis*

KEY CONCEPT *Leukemic invasion of the CNS is considered to be an almost universal event in patients even in those whose cerebrospinal fluid (CSF) cytology shows no apparent disease. Thus, all patients with ALL and AML leukemia receive intrathecal (IT) chemotherapy. Although this is often referred to as "prophylaxis," it more realistically represents treatment.* CNS prophylaxis relies on IT chemotherapy (eg, methotrexate, cytarabine, and corticosteroids), systemic chemotherapy with dexamethasone and high-dose methotrexate, and craniospinal irradiation (XRT) in selected high-risk patients.[16] Cranial radiation use diminished substantially after the efficacy of IT treatment was evident, and the toxicities associated with radiation; learning disabilities, growth retardation, and secondary malignancies (particularly with the use of 6-mercaptopurine), were recognized. IT therapy has replaced cranial XRT as CNS prophylaxis for all except the very high-risk patients and those with T-cell ALL who are at higher risk of CNS disease.

Inexplicably, the treatment of CNS leukemia has not impacted the OS of adults as it has for childhood ALL. With IT chemotherapy alone, the incidence of CNS relapse in adults is 9% to 13% compared with less than 3% in children.[5,12]

► *Postremission Consolidation Regimens*

Consolidation After completion of induction and restoration of normal hematopoiesis, patients begin consolidation. The goal of consolidation is to administer dose-intensive chemotherapy in an effort to further reduce the burden of residual leukemic cells. It is in this and subsequent treatment phases that the remaining leukemic burden is eliminated. Several regimens use agents and schedules designed to minimize the development of drug cross-resistance. Studies have demonstrated that consolidation is an effective strategy in the prevention of relapse in children with ALL, but its benefits in adults are less clear.

In children, the intensity of the consolidation treatment is now determined not only by the child's risk classification but also by the degree of cytoreduction during induction (MRD). Patients who respond slowly to induction therapy (as determined by bone marrow examination early in induction) are at higher risk of relapse and are treated with more aggressive regimens.[18]

Delayed Intensification The Berlin-Frankfurt-Munster (BFM) Study Group introduced a treatment element called delayed intensification (or reinduction) therapy. This therapy consisted of repetition of the initial remission induction therapy administered approximately 3 months after remission. This, similar to consolidation, has been adopted as a component of treatment for children by virtually all institutions.[15]

Intensification regimens may vary in their aggressiveness and the drugs they use depending on the patient's risk group and immunophenotype. For example, the use of high-dose methotrexate (5 g/m^2) appears to improve outcome in patients with T-cell ALL. The use of intensive asparaginase treatment in T-cell ALL patients also has improved outcomes significantly.[17]

Table 95–7

Representative Chemotherapy Regimens for Adult ALL

Remission Induction		CNS Prophylaxis		Consolidation		Maintenance
Drug and Dose	**Days**	**Prophylaxis**	**Days**	**Drug and Dose**	**Days**	**Drug, Dose, and Timing**
German or Hoelzer Regimen (Adult)[a]						
PRED (po) 60 mg/m^2	1–28	Cranial irradiation		DEX (po) 10 mg/m^2	1–28	MP (po) 60 mg/m^2 daily and
VCR (IV) 1.5 mg/m^2[b]	1, 8, 15, 22	MTX (IT) 10 mg/m^2[c]	31, 38, 45, 52	VCR (IV) 1.5 mg/m^2[b]	1, 8, 15, 22	MTX (po/IV) 20 mg/m^2 weekly, weeks 10–18 and 29–130
DNR (IV) 25 mg/m^2	1, 8, 15, 22			DOX (IV) 25 mg/m^2	1, 8, 15, 22	
ASP (IV) 5000 units/m^2	1–14			CTX (IV) 650 mg/m^2[d]	29	
CTX (IV) 650 mg/m^2[d]	29, 43, 57			Ara-C (IV) 75 mg/m^2	31–34, 38–41	
Ara-C (IV) 75 mg/m^2	31–34, 38–41, 45–48, 52–55			TG (po) 60 mg/m^2	29–42	
MP (po) 60 mg/m^2	29–57					
CALGB 8811 (Adult)[e]						
Course I (4 Weeks)				**Course II: Early Intensification (4 Weeks)**		**Course V (Continues until 24 months from diagnosis)**
CTX (IV) 1200 mg/m^2	1			MTX (IT) 15 mg	1	VCR (IV) 2 mg day 1 monthly
DNR (IV) 45 mg/m^2	1, 2, 3			CTX (IV) 1000 mg/m^2	1	
VCR (IV) 2 mg	1, 8, 15, 22			MP (po) 60 mg/m^2	1–14	PRED (po) 60 mg/m^2 days 1–5 monthly
PRED (po) 60 mg/m^2	1–21			Ara-C (SC) 75 mg/m^2	1–4, 8–11	
ASP (SC) 6000 units/m^2	5, 8, 11, 15, 18, 22			VCR (IV) 2 mg	15, 22	MTX (po) 20 mg/m^2 days 1, 8, 15, 22 monthly
				ASP (SC) 6000 units/m^2	15, 18, 22, 25	MP (po) 60 mg/m^2 days 1–28 monthly
Induction chemotherapy for patients 60 years old or older, use:						
CTX (IV) 800 mg/m^2	1					
DNR (IV) 30 mg/m^2	1–3					
PRED (po) 60 mg/m^2	1–7					
Course III (12 Weeks)				**Course IV: Late Intensification (8 Weeks)**		
MTX (IT) 15 mg	1, 8, 15, 22, 29	Cranial irradiation				
MP (po) 60 mg/m^2	1–70					
MTX (po) 20 mg/m^2	36, 43, 50, 57, 64			DOX (IV) 30 mg/m^2	1, 8, 15	
				VCR (IV) 2 mg	1, 8, 15	
				DEX (po) 10 mg/m^2	1–14	
				CTX (IV) 1000 mg/m^2	29	
				TG (po) 60 mg/m^2	29–42	
				Ara-C (SC) 75 mg/m^2	29–32, 36–39	

ASP, asparaginase; C, cytarabine; CALGB, Cancer and Leukemia Group B; CTX, cyclophosphamide; DEX, dexamethasone; DNR, daunorubicin; DOX, doxorubicin; IT, intrathecal; MP, mercaptopurine; MTX, methotrexate; po, oral; PRED, prednisone; SC, subcutaneous; TG, thioguanine; VCR, vincristine.

[a]Holzer D, Thiel E, Ludwig WD, et al. Follow-up of the first two successive German multicentre trials for adult ALL (01/81 and 2/84). Leukemia. 1993;7(Suppl 2):130–134.

[b]Maximum single dose, 2 mg.

[c]Maximum single dose, 15 mg.

[d]Maximum single dose, 1000 mg.

[e]Larson RA, Dodge RK, Burns CP, et al. A five-drug remission induction regimen with intensive consolidation for adults with acute lymphocytic leukemia. Cancer and leukemia Group B study 8811. Blood. 1995;85:2025–2037.

Adapted from Leather HL, Bickert B. Acute leukemias. In: DiPiro JT, Talbert RL, Yee GC, et al., eds. Pharmacotherapy: A Pathophysiologic Approach, 6th ed. New York: McGraw-Hill, 2005:2191–2213.

► *Maintenance*

The purpose of maintenance therapy is to further eliminate leukemic cells and produce an enduring CCR. The two most important agents in maintenance chemotherapy are a combination of oral methotrexate and 6-mercaptopurine. Improved outcome is associated with increasing 6-mercaptopurine doses to the limits of individual tolerance based on absolute neutrophil count (ANC). The benefit of adding intermittent "pulses" of vincristine and a steroid (usually dexamethasone) to the antimetabolite backbone remains unclear, but it is common practice in most modern treatment regimens.[17] The goal is to induce a moderate immunosuppression and leukemic cell kill.

6-Mercaptopurine is a key agent in maintenance therapy. It has a complex metabolism and is initially cleared by thiopurine methyltransferase (TPMT). TPMT activity is variable with about 90% of patients having normal activity, about 10% having intermediate activity, and fewer than 1% having very low or no activity. These enzymatic polymorphisms are inherited in an autosomal recessive fashion and have a profound influence on 6-mercaptopurine tolerance.[20,21]

TPMT screening is recommended for children starting therapy with 6-mercaptopurine. Children who possess alleles that have diminished activity require 6-mercaptopurine dose reductions of 50% to 90% to prevent severe immunosuppression and infection. Despite these reductions, these children have equivalent OS when compared with those receiving full-dose 6-mercaptopurine. The optimal duration of maintenance therapy in both children and adults is unknown, but most regimens are given for 2 to 3 years; extension of the regimen beyond 3 years has not shown any additional benefit.

ALL in Infants and Young Children

Infants and children younger than 1 year of age account for approximately 5% of all children with ALL and have the worst outcome of any group with this disease. These patients have several poor prognostic features at diagnosis, including hyperleukocytosis, hepatomegaly, splenomegaly, and CNS leukemia.[9]

A characteristic finding in up to 70% in this group is a chromosomal translocation involving the *MLL* gene located at 11q23. There are multiple possible rearrangements of this gene with other chromosomes, and all confer a poor prognosis. In vitro, blasts of these patients showed greater drug resistance to prednisolone and L-asparaginase than those from other patients, although they are more sensitive to cytarabine.[22] Based on this information, several studies are testing the efficacy of intensified chemotherapy that includes high-dose cytarabine. Another achievement is the prevention of CNS relapse using IT cytarabine in conjunction with high-dose systemic cytarabine. This combination has eliminated the need for cranial XRT in this young population. Even with major advances in cure rates for the general pediatric ALL population, in whom survival is 80% or more, the long-term survival of infants is only about 40% (Tables 95-8).

ALL in Adolescents and Young Adults

As noted previously, age is an important prognostic factor in ALL. Adolescents and adult patients have generally been shown to have poorer survival than children. However, the group of patients between late adolescence and age 30 years (adolescents and young adults) have a substantially better outcome than older adult patients, most likely because of the use of using

Table 95–8

Representative Chemotherapy Regimens for Pediatric ALL

Induction (1 month)
IT cytarabine on day 0
Prednisone 40 mg/m²/day or dexamethasone 6 mg/m²/day po for 28 days
Vincristine 1.5 mg/m²/dose (maximum, 2 mg) IV weekly for four doses
Pegaspargase 2500 units/m²/dose IM for one dose or asparaginase 6000 units/m²/dose IM Monday, Wednesday, and Friday for six doses
IT methotrexate weekly for two to four doses
Consolidation (1 month)
Mercaptopurine 50–75 mg/m²/dose po at bedtime for 28 days
Vincristine 1.5 mg/m²/dose (maximum, 2 mg) IV on day 0
IT methotrexate weekly for one to three doses
Patients with CNS or testicular disease may receive radiation
Interim Maintenance (one or two cycles) (2 months)
Methotrexate 20 mg/m²/dose po at bedtime weekly
Mercaptopurine 75 mg/m²/dose po daily on days 0–49
Vincristine 1.5 mg/m²/dose (maximum, 2 mg) IV on days 0 and 28
Dexamethasone 6 mg/m²/day po on days 0–4 and 28–32
Delayed Intensification (one or two cycles) (2 months)
Dexamethasone 10 mg/m²/day po on days 0–6 and 14–20
Vincristine 1.5 mg/m²/dose (maximum, 2 mg) IV weekly for three doses
Pegaspargase 2500 units/m²/dose IM for one dose
Doxorubicin 25 mg/m²/dose IV on days 0, 7, and 14
Cyclophosphamide 1000 mg/m²/dose IV on day 28
Thioguanine 60 mg/m²/dose po at bedtime on days 28–41
Cytarabine 75 mg/m²/dose SC or IV on days 28–31 and 35–38
IT methotrexate on days 0 and 28
Consolidation Option (2- to 3-week intervals for six courses on weeks 5–24)
Mercaptopurine 50 mg/m²/dose po at bedtime
Prednisone 40 mg/m²/day for 7 days on weeks 8 and 17
Vincristine 1.5 mg/m²/dose (maximum, 2 mg) IV on the first day of weeks 8, 9, 17, and 18
Methotrexate 200 mg/m²/dose IV + 800 mg/m²/dose over 24 hours on day 1 of weeks 7, 10, 13, 16, 19, and 22
IT methotrexate on weeks 5, 6, 9, 12, 15, and 18
Late Intensification (weeks 25–52)
Methotrexate 20 mg/m²/dose IM weekly or 25 mg/m²/dose po every 6 hours for four doses every other week
Mercaptopurine 75 mg/m²/dose po at bedtime
Prednisone 40 mg/m²/day po for 7 days on weeks 25 and 41
Vincristine 1.4 mg/m²w/dose (maximum, 2 mg) IV on the first day of weeks 25, 26, 41, and 42
IT methotrexate on day 1 of weeks 25, 33, 41, and 49
Maintenance (12-week cycles)
Methotrexate 20 mg/m²/dose po at bedtime or IM weekly with dose escalation as tolerated
Mercaptopurine 75 mg/m²/dose po at bedtime on days 0–83
Vincristine 1.5 mg/m²/dose (maximum, 2 mg) IV on days 0, 28, and 56
Dexamethasone 6 mg/m²/day po on days 0–4, 28–32, and 56–60
IT methotrexate on day 0

IM, intramuscular; IT, intrathecal; po, oral; SC, subcutaneous.

Adapted from Leather HL, Bickert B. Acute Leukemias. In: DiPiro JT, Talbert RL, Yee GC, et al, eds. Pharmacotherapy: A Pathophysiologic Approach, 6th ed. New York: McGraw-Hill; 2005:2458–2511.

Patient Encounter 1, Part 3

This patient begins induction therapy with vincristine, prednisone, daunorubicin, and asparaginase. According to his protocol, he will begin dasatinib in the middle of his induction treatment, on day 15. He has a bone marrow on day 29 showing a morphologic remission, and his MRD on day 29 was less that 0.1%. He is now ready to begin consolidation.

What is the role of dasatinib for Ph+ ALL?

What is the significance of an MRD of 0.1%?

What is the purpose of consolidation therapy?

Patient Encounter 2

The patient is a 6-year-old boy who had completed his treatment for standard risk preB-ALL 1 year ago. For the past 3 weeks, he has been complaining of worsening headaches. A CT scan was done which was within normal limits. CBC at this visit shows WBC 6.6 K/mm^3, hemoglobin 10.1 g/dL, hematocrit 30%, platelet 75K, differential 14% neutrophils, 52% lymphocytes, 3% variant lymphocytes, 1% metamyelocyte, 30% blasts. Uric acid is 3.7 mg/dL, LDH 1947 Units/L. On examination, patient is well appearing, no significant lymphadenopathy, no hepatosplenomegaly, testicular and neurologic exam is normal.

What is the principal form of treatment failure in patients with ALL?

What are the important predictors of second remission?

pediatric ALL regimens. Retrospective studies show that survival is improved from 30% to 40% with standard adult therapy to as high as 65% with pediatric protocols.[2,23] The reasons for this are not entirely clear, and multiple factors are likely to play a role. Among the likely explanations is that pediatric protocols use more aggressive and prolonged postremission consolidation therapy before maintenance. Other proposed explanations are the potential differences in disease biology in this versus older age patients, more intense CNS prophylaxis, and the greater degree of social support and better compliance fostered in a pediatric environment. Current and planned trials are focusing on the potential of extending this treatment approach to patients age 40 years and possibly older.

ALL in Adults

The incidence of ALL in adults ages 30 to 60 years is only 2 per 100,000 persons per year compared with almost 10 per 100,000 in children. The conventional risk factors such as high WBC counts, older age, and CNS disease hold true in adults as in children. However, the significance of cytogenetic and molecular markers that are so important in children seems to be less predictive of outcome in adults. An exception is the adverse prognostic factor, the presence of the *BCR-ABL* translocation (Ph$^+$) just as in childhood ALL. This occurs in 15% to 30% of adults and is even more common in patients older than 60 years of age.[23] The use of imatinib or dasatinib, both potent inhibitors of the Ph$^+$-associated BCR-ABL tyrosine kinase, has now become a standard of practice for all patient groups with Ph$^+$ disease.[7] Results show that the combination of these agents with conventional chemotherapy improves remission rates as well as OS compared with the use of conventional chemotherapy alone.[7,8,23]

Currently, the induction and consolidation regimens in adults is similar to the regimens in pediatric patients, but the more aggressive postinduction regimens are not as well tolerated in this population, particularly in elderly patients (age greater than 60 years) and are associated with a much higher incidence of toxicity and treatment-related deaths.[7] Some investigators are studying "moderate-dose" consolidation regimens that are better tolerated, although long-term efficacy data is lacking. Even though remissions are achieved in 80% to 90% of adult patients, 5 years disease-free survivals are only in the 30% to 40% range. Among elderly patients, the outcome is even poorer with no more than 20% having long-term survival.

Relapsed ALL

Relapse is the recurrence of leukemic cells at any site after remission has been achieved. KEY CONCEPT *Bone marrow relapse is the major form of treatment failure in 15% to 20% of patients with ALL. Most relapses have the same immunophenotype and cytogenetic changes seen of the original disease.* Extramedullary sites of relapse include the CNS and the testicles.[24] Extramedullary relapse, although once common, has decreased to 5% or less because of effective prophylaxis. Site of relapse and the length of the first remission are important predictors of second remission and OS. Marrow relapses occurring less than 18 to 24 months into first remission are associated with a poor survival, but longer periods of remission (greater than 36 months) have a much higher chance of survival.[24] Treatment strategies for relapsed ALL include chemotherapy or allogeneic hematopoietic stem cell transplant (allo-HSCT). Even though patients undergoing allo-HSCT are less likely to relapse, treatment-related toxicity leads to a higher incidence of morbidity and mortality compared with chemotherapy alone.[6] Clofarabine, a next-generation deoxyadenosine analogue, has shown considerable activity in children and adults with refractory acute leukemias. Of interest, this is the only anticancer drug to receive primary indication for use in pediatrics in the past 10 years.[23]

Treatment of AML

As with ALL, the primary aim in treating patients with AML is to induce remission and thereafter prevent relapse. Treatment of AML is conventionally divided into two phases: induction and consolidation. The prognosis of children with AML has improved dramatically over the past 30 years. Rates of complete remission as high as 80% to 90% and overall survival rates of 60% now are reported. This improvement is a result of better understanding of the biology of AML and the development of molecular targets that are used in combination with conventional chemotherapy.[14]

KEY CONCEPT *The current induction therapy for AML usually consists of a combination of cytarabine, daunorubicin, and etoposide. The second phase of treatment for AML is called* ***consolidation****. The purpose of this phase is to further enhance remission with more cytoreduction.*[11]

▶ *Remission Induction*

The goal of induction chemotherapy in AML is essentially identical to that in ALL—"empty" the bone marrow of all hematopoietic precursors and allow repopulation with normal cells. The combination of an anthracycline (eg, daunorubicin, doxorubicin,

Clinical Presentation and Diagnosis of AML[3,6,11]

General

- Patients may have symptoms of AML for 1 to 3 months before presentation. These include fatigue, fever, and pallor, but patients generally are in no obvious distress.

Symptoms

- The patient may present with weakness, bone pain, malaise, bleeding, and weight loss.
- Neutropenic patients are often febrile and highly susceptible to infection.
- Anemia usually presents as pallor, tiredness, and general fatigue.
- Patients with thrombocytopenia usually present with bruising, petechiae, and ecchymosis.
- Chloromas (localized leukemic deposits named after their color) may be seen, especially in the periorbital regions and as skin infiltrates.
- Gum hypertrophy is indicative of AML M4 and AML M5 subtypes.
- Disseminated intravascular coagulation may be present in all AML subtypes, but is common in AML M3 and is associated with generalized bleeding or hemorrhage.
- Lymphadenopathy, massive hepatosplenomegaly, and bone pain are not as common in AML as in ALL.

Signs

- Temperature may be elevated secondary to an infection associated with a low WBC count.
- Petechiae and bleeding are indicative of thrombocytopenia.

Laboratory Tests

- CBC with differential is performed.
- The anemia is usually normochromic and normocytic.
- Approximately 50% of children present with platelet counts of less than $50 \times 10^3/mm^3$ ($50 \times 10^9/L$).
- The WBC count may be normal, decreased, or high. About 20% of patients have WBC counts of over $100 \times 10^3/mm^3$ ($100 \times 10^9/L$), which places them at risk for leukostasis.
- Uric acid is increased in approximately 50% of patients secondary to rapid cellular turnover.
- Electrolytes: Potassium and phosphorus are often elevated. Calcium is usually low.
- Coagulation disorders: Elevated prothrombin time, partial thromboplastin time, D-dimers; hypofibrinogenemia.

Other Diagnostic Tests

Flow cytometric evaluation of bone marrow and peripheral blood to characterize the type of leukemia, as well as to detect specific chromosomal rearrangements. The bone marrow at diagnosis usually is hypercellular, with normal hematopoiesis being replaced by leukemic blasts. The presence of greater than 20% blasts in the bone marrow is diagnostic for AML. At diagnosis, a LP is performed to determine if CNS leukemia is present. The CNS is involved at diagnosis in approximately 15% of patients.[14]

or idarubicin) and the antimetabolite cytarabine forms the backbone of AML induction therapy. The most common induction regimen (7 + 3) combines daunorubicin for 3 days with cytarabine on days 1 to 7.[13] The remission rate for this combination is approximately 80% in children and younger adults but declines to 40% to 50% in patients older than 60 years of age.[5,13] Paving the way for more innovative therapies, gemtuzumab ozogamicin, a humanized anti-CD33 antibody, has shown it improved the outcome of pediatric and younger adults patient (age less than 60 years) when added to conventional 7 + 3 chemotherapy.[26,27] Sorafenib, a tyrosine kinase inhibitor, has shown promise in adults with FLT_3 positive ITD. Bortezomib, a proteasome inhibitor, has shown to selectively reduce the leukemic stem cells that are a cause of resistance for AML.[14]

▸ *Postremission Chemotherapy*

In AML, postremission chemotherapy is often referred to as consolidation therapy. Several cycles of intensive postremission chemotherapy combining non–cross-resistant agents given every 4 to 6 weeks substantially improves DFS. Without postremission treatment, all patients would relapse within several weeks. This is analogous to the consolidation and other phases of postremission chemotherapy in ALL. The use of high-dose cytarabine in postremission therapy seems to be important for improving survival, but the most effective dose has yet to be determined.[14] Although the optimal number of courses remains to be determined, at least four are probably required.[13]

Allogeneic Hematopoietic Stem Cell Transplantation Hematopoietic stem cell transplantation (HSCT) is the most effective treatment for AML. Its promising benefit must be weighed against the potential risk of transplantation related sequelae. HSCT has become a less attractive option as the results of increasingly intensive chemotherapy and postrelapse salvage therapy have improved.[14]

The availability of HLA-matched sibling donors determines whether patients undergo HSCT as postremission treatment. To facilitate this process, it is important to obtain HLA typing on all younger patients and siblings shortly after diagnosis. Patients who do not have an HLA-matched sibling proceed to postremission therapy with chemotherapy alone.

Complications and benefits of allogeneic HSCT are described in Chapter 98. Transplant-related mortality following matched-sibling allo-HSCT is 20% to 30% in most series. Complications from transplantation increase with age; therefore, patients older than 60 years of age are uncommonly considered to receive a myeloablative allo-HSCT. Because the average age of AML patients is 65 years, most patients with this disease are not candidates for this form of therapy. For older patients up to 70 years of age, a reduced-intensity (mini or nonmyeloablative allogeneic) transplant may be an option. These transplants use less intensive preparative regimens and rely on the allogeneic graft-versus-leukemia (GVL) effect to eliminate their disease.[13]

The role of HSCT, particularly whether it should be performed during the first CR or reserved for second remission, remains the most controversial issue in pediatric AML. In certain institutions, HSCT is often reserved for patients that are considered high risk.[14] Some types of AML patients may be curable with conventional-dose chemotherapy alone.

Autologous Hematopoietic Stem Cell Transplantation Because the majority of AML patients lack a HLA-identical donor, investigators began to consider the use of the patient's own bone marrow, obtained while in CR, as a source of hematopoietic regeneration. However, relapse continues to be a problem secondary to the presence of residual disease in the graft. Despite the reduced morbidity and mortality associated with auto-HSCT, this type of transplant does not compare favorably to standard postremission chemotherapy.[13]

▸ *CNS Therapy*

The prevalence of CNS disease at diagnosis of AML is approximately 15%.[14] Features associated with the risk of CNS leukemia include hyperleukocytosis, monocytic, or myelomonocytic leukemia (FAB M4 or M5), and young age. Adequate CNS prophylaxis is an essential component of therapy. Studies have shown that patients with CNS disease at diagnosis can be cured with IT therapy alone without the use of cranial XRT. In most cases, IT cytarabine with or without methotrexate and systemic high-dose cytarabine provide effective treatment.

AML in Infants

AML in infants younger than 12 months of age shows clinical and biological characteristics different from those of older children. The disease phenotype is more commonly monoblastic or myelomonoblastic (M4, M5), and the patients usually present with hyperleukocytosis. Extramedullary involvement is common, often involving skin and other organs. As in infant ALL, there is a high incidence of translocations involving the *MLL* gene in infant AML. The number of infant AML trials reported is limited, but the EFS of this population is similar to that of older children with AML. This is in marked contrast to the outcomes for infants with ALL for whom the EFS is much lower than in older children.[28]

AML in the Elderly

AML is the most common acute leukemia in the elderly. Compared with younger patients with the same disease, older adults have a poor prognosis and represent a distinct population with regard to the biology of their disease. Older adults have a lower incidence of favorable chromosomal aberrations and a higher incidence of unfavorable aberrations.[5,13] Fms-like tyrosine kinase 3 (FLT_3) which is an AML oncogene plays an important role in AML pathogenesis and was associated with a poor outcome. FLT_3-ITD is common in adults, but is only found in 12% of the pediatric population.[14] The elderly also have a much higher incidence of comorbidities, such as type 2 diabetes, obesity, and other physiologic limitations. Thus, the poor prognosis of AML in the elderly is only partly the result of unfavorable biology.

In older adults, in contrast to children, AML is more likely to arise from a proximal bone marrow–stem cell disorder, such as MDS, or present as a secondary, prior treatment-related leukemia. These forms of AML are notoriously poorly responsive to conventional chemotherapy and thus have a lower CR rate and poorer survival.[29]

As previously noted, age is an important prognostic factor. Older adults are not as tolerant of or as responsive to remission induction and consolidation chemotherapy as younger patients. Furthermore, long-term survival for patients older than 60 years is only 5% to 15% compared with 30% DFS for younger adults.[5,13]

Relapsed AML

Even though 75% to 85% of patients with AML achieve a remission, only about 50% survive. Patients who relapse usually respond poorly to additional treatment and have a shorter duration of remission. This is probably related to drug resistance induced during induction and certain chromosomal abnormalities.

Even though there is no standard therapy for relapse, most studies have shown that high-dose cytarabine-containing regimens have considerable activity in obtaining a second remission. Cytarabine has been used in combination with mitoxantrone, etoposide, fludarabine, 2-chlorodeoxyadenosine, and (more recently) clofarabine.[5,13] The targeted immunotherapy agent gemtuzumab has induced remissions who have recurrent CD33+ AML alone or in combination with standard chemotherapy.[14]

After a patient has achieved a second remission with conven tional chemotherapy, allo-HSCT is the therapy of choice. For patients without an HLA-matched sibling, a matched unrelated donor (MUD) or cord blood transplant may be a reasonable alternative. The combination of myeloablative high-dose chemotherapy and the GVL effect is thought to offer the best chance of survival in AML.

Complications of Treatment

▸ *Tumor Lysis Syndrome*

Tumor lysis syndrome (TLS) is an oncologic emergency that is characterized by metabolic abnormalities resulting from the death of blast cells and the release of large amounts of purines, pyrimidines, and intracellular potassium and phosphorus. Uric acid, the ultimate breakdown product of purines, is poorly soluble in plasma and urine. Deposition of uric acid and calcium phosphate crystals in the renal tubules can lead to acute renal failure. Many patients with acute leukemia, especially those with a high tumor burden, are at risk for TLS during the first several days of chemotherapy. Measures to prevent TLS include aggressive hydration, alkalinization to help solubilize uric acid, and allopurinol to reduce uric acid production. Hyperhydration and alkalinization is generally an effective method of dealing with this issue. However, on some occasions, the use of rasburicase is indicated. Rasburicase is a urate oxidase that catalyzes the oxidation of uric acid to allantoin, which is much more soluble than uric acid and excreted more easily.[30,31] Given its high cost, rasburicase generally is restricted to patients with high WBC counts (greater than $50 \times 10^3/mm^3$, $50 \times 10^9/L$) and uric acid levels greater than 8 mg/dL (476 μmol/L).

▸ *Infection*

Infection is a primary cause of death in acute leukemia patients. Both the disease and aggressive chemotherapy cause severe myelosuppression, placing the patient at risk for sepsis.

The therapy for AML is extremely myelosuppressive. Children with AML have a 10% to 20% induction mortality rate secondary to infection and bleeding complications. Therefore, patients receiving induction therapy usually are hospitalized for the first 4 to 6 weeks of therapy. The induction therapy for ALL is far less myelosuppressive, and these patients recover their neutrophil counts quicker and usually do not require prolonged hospitalizations.[6]

It is important to recognize that symptoms and signs of infection may be absent in a severely immunosuppressed or neutropenic patient. Fever (greater than 38.3°C [100.9°F]) in a neutropenic patient is a medical emergency. Because the progression of infection in neutropenic patients can be rapid, empirical antibiotic therapy should be administered quickly when fever is documented. Currently, the most commonly used initial antibiotic agent is cefepime, a fourth-generation cephalosporin that has good antipseudomonal coverage as well as adequate coverage against *Streptococcus viridans* and pneumococci.[32]

Disseminated fungal infections most commonly caused by Candida and Aspergillus species can be life threatening in children with AML. From the results of clinical trials in adults, many pediatric institutions recommend antifungal prophylaxis with voriconazole, posaconazole, micafungin, or caspofungin. Fluconazole and itraconazole are not considered ideal, because they are not effective against aspergillus species and other molds.[32]

Trimethoprim–sulfamethoxazole is started in all patients with any acute leukemia for the prevention of *Pneumocystis jiroveci* pneumonia (PJP). Patients normally continue this therapy for 6 months after completion of treatment. The use of additional antibiotic prophylaxis is not encouraged because of concerns for antibiotic resistance.

Of note is that up to 10% of patients seem to exhibit excessive myelosuppression with trimethoprim–sulfa antibiotics (presumably the result of the antifolate trimethoprim in combination with other systemic cytotoxic agents). Changing to another anti-PJP agent such as dapsone or inhaled pentamidine may help to alleviate this problem.

▶ *Secondary Malignancies*

Secondary malignancies are a risk of the successful treatment of a prior cancer or the use of cytotoxic agents in a variety of autoimmune diseases. The chemotherapy agents used, especially alkylating agents and topoisomerase II inhibitors, predispose patients to secondary hematopoietic neoplasms. As the aggressiveness of treatment and the number of survivors of AML increase, the risk of secondary neoplasms also may rise. There are two different types of second malignancies: acute leukemia, which is generally myeloid in origin, or MDS. There are also reports of secondary solid tumors, especially within regions of prior radiation exposure. The latency period between the end of treatment and the development of a secondary leukemia is generally in the range of 5 to 10 years. For those patients who develop secondary solid malignancies, the latency may be as long as 10 to 20 years.

The incidence of second cancers attributed to alkylators peaks 4 to 6 years after exposure and plateaus after 10 to 15 years. Higher cumulative doses and older age at the time of treatment are risk factors for this type of cancer.

Epipodophyllotoxins (etoposide and others) can induce a second malignancy characterized by balanced chromosomal translocations and short latency periods (2–4 years). The risk of this leukemia is related to schedule (dose intensity) and the concomitant use of other agents (L-asparaginase, alkylating agents, and possibly antimetabolites). The prognosis for topoisomerase II inhibitor–related secondary leukemia is extremely poor. Only about 10% of these patients survive after salvage chemotherapy, and only 20% survive after HSCT.

Ionizing radiation therapy is also a cause of secondary malignancies. These secondary tumors generally develop within or adjacent to the previous radiation field. These cancers often have a prolonged latency, typically 15 or more years, but shorter latencies (5–14 years) are known. Higher doses of radiation and younger age are associated with an increased risk of secondary malignancy.

Unlike children, adults may have other factors that predispose them to secondary malignancies. Lifestyle choices such as tobacco use, alcohol use, and diet have been implicated in influencing the development of secondary neoplasms in the adult population.

Now that 80% or more of children survive their primary cancers, the incidence of secondary neoplasms may increase. Recognizing this potential, many treatment regimens for children are being modified appropriately to reduce exposure to alkylators, topoisomerase inhibitors, and radiation. Late effects clinics screen for secondary malignancies and other disease and treatment-related disabilities that accompany childhood cancer. Similar screening and educational opportunities are not as established in adult survivors.

▶ *Late Effects*

With increased success in pediatric clinical trials, the OS rate for pediatric cancers has increased markedly over the last 35 years. For some diseases (acute lymphoblastic leukemia, Wilms tumor, low-grade and common germ cell tumors), the OS rate is now at or above 80%. KEY CONCEPT *Despite this significant increase in survival, many patients, particularly pediatric cancer survivors, have disease-related or treatment-related disabilities. As many as 50% to 60% of these survivors are estimated to have at least one chronic or late-occurring complication of treatment.*[33] In leukemia, the intensified use of methotrexate may be responsible for some sporadic neurotoxicity seen in children and adults. Likewise, the use of pharmacologic doses of glucocorticoids has been associated with avascular necrosis of bone in older children and adults. High cumulative doses of anthracyclines can cause irreversible cardiomyopathy. Cranial XRT is now less frequently used for CNS leukemia prophylaxis but can cause neuropsychological and neuroendocrine abnormalities that may lead to obesity, short stature, or precocious puberty.[4] As newer and more intensive treatments enter clinical trials, close observation for long-term side effects will assume even greater importance.

Supportive Care

Because of the need for repeated venous access, a central venous catheter or infusion port is placed before starting treatment. These devices are useful not only for delivery of chemotherapy but also to support patients during periods of myelosuppression. Infection and bleeding complications are the primary causes of mortality in patients with leukemia.

Platelet transfusions are a common tool to prevent hemorrhage. Patients with uncomplicated thrombocytopenia can be transfused when the platelet count falls below $10 \times 10^3/mm^3$ ($10 \times 10^9/L$). Patients who are either highly febrile or actively bleeding may require transfusions at higher levels. Red blood cell transfusions generally are not necessary for a hemoglobin concentration greater than 8 g/dL (80 g/L, 4.97 mmol/L).

There is much controversy regarding the routine use of colony-stimulating factors (eg, granulocyte colony-stimulating factor [G-CSF] and granulocyte-macrophage colony-stimulating factor [GM-CSF]) in neutropenic patients. Even though several clinical trials have shown the time to ANC recovery is decreased with a colony-stimulating factor, none have demonstrated that CSFs statistically influence infection-related mortality. At present, the use of colony-stimulating factors (G-CSF most commonly) generally is limited to those chemotherapy regimens that place the patient at highest risk for prolonged neutropenia.

OUTCOME EVALUATION

Developing strategies for the treatment and monitoring of acute leukemias begins with risk stratification. Understanding the likely risk of relapse determines the aggressiveness and length

Patient Care Process

Patient Assessment:

- Based on the physical exam and review of systems does the patient have the symptoms and physical findings of acute leukemia?
- Review the medical history. Is the patient receiving any medications that would be contraindicated or cause adverse effects prior to starting induction therapy?
- Review the laboratory features especially serum electrolytes and uric acid.
- Measure serum electrolytes and uric acid every 6 to 8 hours during the first 3 to 4 days of therapy. Patient may require frequent blood and platelet transfusions.

Therapy Evaluation:

- Evaluate the response to treatment by performing a bone marrow and LP.
- Does the patient demonstrate any residual leukemia as defined by the presence of blasts in the bone marrow or CSF?
- Determine the significance of the presence MRD at the end of induction.

Care Plan Development:

- Provide patient education on the potential side effects of the drug therapy for acute leukemia.
- Address the importance of medication compliance.
- Discuss the warning signs to report immediately to the health care provider (eg, fever, bruising, or bleeding).

Follow-up Evaluation:

- Follow-up with weekly CBCs and electrolytes to assess the effectiveness of therapy for any adverse effects associated with treatment.
- Provide education regarding the long-term sequelae associated with the treatment for acute leukemia.

of therapy. Remission status and MRD after the induction phase of treatment must be closely observed. Failure to obtain morphologic bone marrow remission by day 28 is a very adverse prognostic sign and dictates further induction treatment. For those who have a morphologic remission, quantification of MRD has become an increasingly important prognostic factor. Levels of residual less than 0.01% appear to be associated with better outcomes.

A clinician is generally charged with developing a plan to educate patients and families about their drugs and doses. This is a critical responsibility; it is imperative that the patients and their families understand why they are receiving their medications and how to take them. Frank, open discussion (with the family or patient in possession of their prescriptions) go a long way toward preventing errors that occur as a result of "assuming" that they understand their medications. If modifications are necessary secondary to toxicity or inadequate response, establish a plan for treatment change. Remember that individual patients often do not fit the "average" patient profile, and dose modifications are frequently needed. The practitioner should be familiar with dosing ranges, WBC count, and other parameters that indicate appropriate treatment response. Based on response to prior phases of treatment, the clinician should recognize potential toxicities in subsequent phases of treatment with the same or different drugs at similar or different doses.

Abbreviations Introduced in This Chapter

ALL	Acute lymphocytic/lymphoblastic leukemia
allo-HSCT	Allogeneic hematopoietic stem cell transplantation
AML	Acute myelogenous leukemia
ANC	Absolute neutrophil count
ANLL	Acute nonlymphocytic leukemia
BFM	Berlin-Frankfurt-Munster
CCR	Continuous complete remission
CD	Cluster determinants
CR	Complete remission
CSF	Cerebrospinal fluid
CSF	Colony-stimulating factor
DFS	Disease-free survival
EFS	Event-free survival
FISH	Fluorescent in situ hybridization
G-CSF	Granulocyte colony-stimulating factor
GM-CSF	Granulocyte-macrophage colony-stimulating factor
GVL	Graft-versus-leukemia
HLA	Human leukocyte antigen
HSCT	Hematopoietic stem cell transplantation
ITD	Internal tandem duplication
MAB	Monoclonal antibody
MDS	Myelodysplastic syndrome
MRD	Minimal residual disease
MUD	Matched unrelated donor
OS	Overall survival
Ph^+	Philadelphia chromosome
TLS	Tumor lysis syndrome
XRT	Irradiation

REFERENCES

1. Pui CH, Relling MV, Downing JR. Acute lymphocytic leukemia. N Engl J Med. 2004;350(15):1535–1548.
2. Ribera JM, Oriol A. Acute lymphoblastic leukemia in adolescents and young adults. Hematol Oncol Clin North Am. 2009;23:1033–1042.
3. SEER Stat Fact sheet: Leukemia (2014), National Cancer Institute.
4. Campana D, Pui CH. Childhood leukemia. In: Abeloff MD, Armitage JO, Niederhuber JE, et al, eds. Clinical Oncology, 4th ed. Philadelphia: Elsevier, 2008:2139–2169.
5. Applebaum FR. Acute myeloid leukemia in adults. In: Abeloff MD, Armitage JO, Niederhuber JE, et al, eds. Clinical Oncology, 4th ed. Philadelphia: Elsevier, 2008:2215–2134.
6. Pieters R, Carroll WL. Biology and treatment of acute lymphoblastic leukemia. Pediatr Clin North Am. 2008;55(1):1–20.
7. Faderl S, O'Brien S, Pui CH, et al. Adult acute lymphoblastic leukemia: Concepts and strategies. Cancer. 2010;116:1165–1176.
8. Bassan R, Hoelzer D. Modern therapy of acute lymphoblastic leukemia. J. Clin Oncol. 2011;29:532–543.
9. Silverman LB. Acute lymphoblastic leukemia in infancy. Pediatr Blood Cancer. 2007;49:1070–1073.
10. Teachy DT, Hunger SP. Predicting relapse risk in childhood acute lymphoblastic leukaemia. Br J Haematol. 2013;162:606–620.
11. Mandrell BN, Pritchard M. Understanding the clinical implications of minimal residual disease in childhood leukemia. J Pediatr Oncol Nurs. 2006;23:38–44.

12. Margolin JE, Rabin KR, Steuber CP, et al. Acute lymphoblastic leukemia. In: Pizzo R, Poplack DG, eds. Principles and Practice of Pediatric Oncology 6th ed. Philadelphia: Lippincott Williams & Wilkins, 2011:518–565.
13. Shipley JL, Butera JN. Acute myelogenous leukemia. Exp Hematol. 2009;37:649–658.
14. Rubnitz Je, Gibson B, Smith FO. Acute myeloid leukemia. Hematol Oncol Clin North Am. 2010;24:35–63.
15. Rubnitz JE, Gibson B, Smith FO. Acute myeloid leukemia. Pediatr Clin North Am. 2008;55:21–51.
16. Hoelzer D, Gokbudet N. Acute lymphoid leukemia in adults. In: Abeloff MD, Armitage JO, Niederhuber JE, et al, eds. Clinical Oncology, 4th ed. Philadelphia: Elsevier, 2008:2191–2213.
17. Rabin KR, Poplack DG. Management strategies in acute lymphoblastic leukemia. Oncology. 2011;15:328–347.
18. Pieters R, Carroll WL. Biology and treatment of acute lymphoblastic leukemia. Hematol Oncol Clin North Am. 2010;24:1–18.
19. Pui CH, Campana D, et al. Treating childhood acute lymphoblastic leukemia without cranial irradiation. N Engl J Med. 2009;360:2730–2741.
20. Karran P, Attard N. Thiopurines in current medical practice: Molecular mechanisms and contributions to therapy related cancer. Nat Rev Cancer. 2008;8:24–36.
21. Wang L, Weinshilboum R. Thiopurine S-methyltransferase pharmacogenetics; Insights challenges and future directions. Oncogene. 2006;25:1629–1638.
22. Pui CH, Relling MV, Campana D, et al. Childhood acute lymphoblastic leukemia. Rev Clin Exp Hematol. 2002;6:161–180.
23. Larson S, Stock W. Progress in the treatment of adults with acute lymphoblastic leukemia. Curr Opin Hematol. 2008;15:400–407.
24. Ribera JM, Oriol A. Acute lymphoblastic leukemia in adolescents and young adults. Hematol Oncol Clin North Am. 2009;23:1033–1042.
25. Jeha S. Clofarabine for the treatment of acute lymphoblastic leukemia. Expert Rev Anticancer Ther. 2007;7:113–118.
26. Cooper TM, Franklin J, Gerbing RB, et al. AAML03P1, a pilot study of the safety of gemtuzumab ozogamicin in combination with chemotherapy for newly diagnosed childhood acute myeloid leukemia: A report from the Children's Oncology Group. Cancer. 2011;118(3):761–769.
27. Burnett AK, Hills RK, Milligan D, et al. Identification of patients with acute myeloblastic leukemia who benefit from the addition of gemtuzumab ozogamicin: Results of the MRC AML15 trial. J Clin Oncol. 2011;29:369–377.
28. Ishii E, Kawasaki H, Isoyama K, Eguchi-Ishimae M, Eguchi M. Recent advances in the treatment of infant acute myeloid leukemia. Leuk Lymphoma. 2003;44:741–748.
29. Foran JM, Sekeres MA. Myelodysplastic syndromes. In: Abeloff MD, Armitage JO, Niederhuber JE, et al, eds. Clinical Oncology, 4th ed. Philadelphia: Elsevier, 2008:2235–2251.
30. Coiffier B, Altman A, Pui CH, et al. Guidelines for the management of pediatric and adult tumor lysis syndrome: An evidence-based review. J Clin Oncol. 2008;26:2767–2778.
31. Davidson MB, Thakkar S, Hix JK, et al. Pathophysiology, clinical consequences, and treatment of tumor lysis syndrome. Am J Med. 2004;116:546–554.
32. Hughes WT, Armstrong D, Bodey GP, et al. 2002 guidelines for the use of antimicrobial agents in neutropenic patients with cancer. Clin Infect Dis. 2002;34:730–751.
33. Nathan PC, Wasilewski-Masker K, Janzen LA. Long-term outcomes in survivors of childhood acute lymphoblastic leukemia. Hematol Oncol Clin North Am. 2009;23:1065–1082.

96 Chronic Leukemias and Multiple Myeloma

Amy M. Pick

LEARNING OBJECTIVES

Upon completion of the chapter, the reader will be able to:

1. Explain the role of the Philadelphia chromosome in the pathophysiology of chronic myelogenous leukemia (CML).
2. Describe the natural history of CML.
3. Identify the clinical signs and symptoms and laboratory findings associated with CML.
4. Discuss treatment options for CML with special emphasis on tyrosine kinase inhibitors.
5. Describe the clinical course of chronic lymphocytic leukemia (CLL).
6. Describe patients who may be observed without treatment and those who receive aggressive treatment for CLL.
7. Discuss the various treatment options available for CLL.
8. Describe the clinical presentation of multiple myeloma.
9. Discuss the treatment options available for multiple myeloma.

INTRODUCTION

Several diseases comprise chronic leukemia. The two most common forms are chronic myelogenous leukemia (CML) and chronic lymphocytic leukemia (CLL). The slower progression of the disease contrasts it from acute leukemia, with the survival of chronic leukemia often lasting several years without treatment. This chapter covers CML and CLL. The chapter also discusses the hematologic cancer multiple myeloma.

CHRONIC MYELOGENOUS LEUKEMIA

CML is a hematologic cancer that results from an abnormal proliferation of an early myeloid **progenitor** cell. The clinical course of CML has three phases: chronic phase, accelerated phase, and **blast** crisis.[1] Criteria for these phases is largely based on the percent blasts in the peripheral blood or bone marrow. Chemotherapy can be used to control white blood cell (WBC) counts in the chronic phase, but as CML slowly progresses, the cancer becomes resistant to treatment. Blast crisis resembles acute leukemia, and immediate aggressive treatment is required.

EPIDEMIOLOGY AND ETIOLOGY

It was estimated that 6660 new cases of CML would be diagnosed in 2015, accounting for 15% of all adult leukemias.[2] The incidence of CML increases with age, the median age being 67 years.[3,4] In most newly diagnosed cases, the etiology cannot be determined, but high doses of ionizing radiation and exposure to solvents such as benzene are recognized risk factors.

PATHOPHYSIOLOGY

Cell of Origin

CML arises from a defect in an early progenitor cell. The pluripotent (noncommitted) stem cell is implicated as the origin of the disease; therefore, multiple cell lineages of hematopoiesis may be affected, including myeloid, erythroid, megakaryocyte, and (rarely) lymphoid lineages. These cells remain functional in chronic phase CML, which is why patients in this phase are at low risk for developing infections.

Ph Chromosome

KEY CONCEPT *The Philadelphia chromosome (Ph) results from a translocation between chromosomes 9 and 22, leaving a shortened chromosome 22. The Ph results in the formation of an abnormal fusion gene between the breakpoint cluster region and the Abelson proto-oncogene (BCR-ABL), which encodes an overly active tyrosine kinase. The loss of control of tyrosine kinase activity causes abnormal cellular proliferation and inhibition of apoptosis.*[1,4] Molecular tools such as quantitative and qualitative polymerase chain reaction (Q-PCR) and fluorescence in situ hybridization (FISH) are used in detection and monitoring of CML.[5]

TREATMENT

Desired Outcome

The primary goal in the treatment of CML is to eradicate the Ph positive clones. Elimination of the Ph is termed a complete cytogenetic response. International standardization of molecular

Clinical Presentation and Diagnosis of CML

Signs and Symptoms

- 30%–50% are asymptomatic at diagnosis
- Symptoms may include fatigue, fever, weight loss, and bleeding
- Organomegaly consisting of splenomegaly and hepatomegaly

Diagnostic Procedures

- Peripheral blood smear
- Bone marrow biopsy (percentage of blasts)
- Cytogenetic studies
- Molecular testing (Q-PCR and FISH to detect *BCR-ABL* transcripts)

Laboratory Findings

Peripheral blood smear

- Leukocytosis (most present with WBC count > 100 × 10^9/L [100 × 10^3/mm^3])
- Thrombocytosis (~50% of patients in chronic phase)
- Anemia
- Basophilia
- Presence of blasts

Bone marrow

- Hypercellularity with presence of blasts
- Cytogenetics including the presence of Ph

Poor Prognostic Factors

- Older age
- Splenomegaly
- High percent blasts in the blood
- High or low platelet count

response has been updated to reflect a percentage of *BCR-ABL1* compared to control gene.[3] A complete molecular response is undetectable *BCR-ABL* transcripts by the international scale. An early goal of therapy is to achieve a complete hematologic response or to normalize peripheral blood counts. A cure from CML can only come from complete eradication of the Ph clone.

General Approach to Treatment

There have been significant advances in the treatment of CML since the discovery of the Ph in 1960. The success of therapy is largely dependent on the clinical phase of the disease. Treatment decisions are based on patient's age, phase of CML, and comorbidities. Nearly all patients with CML are initially treated with a tyrosine kinase inhibitor (TKI). Depending on the clinical phase, newer TKIs or omacetaxine may be options for patients who fail to respond or do not tolerate initial TKI therapy. Hydroxyurea may be used after diagnosis to rapidly reduce high WBC counts and prevent potentially serious complications (respiratory and neurologic) associated with large numbers of circulating neutrophils. Hydroxyurea, though, does not alter the disease process. TKIs can also reduce peripheral WBC counts over several weeks; therefore, many patients are started on a TKI alone. Although allogeneic stem cell transplant is the only curative therapy for CML, transplantation is reserved for patients with TKI resistance. Figure 96–1 illustrates one approach for clinically managing newly diagnosed CML patients.

Nonpharmacologic Therapy

► *Hematopoietic Stem Cell Transplantation*

KEY CONCEPT *Allogeneic stem cell transplantation is the only curative treatment option for CML, however the TKIs have diminished the role of transplant.* Allogeneic stem cell transplant may be considered for the rare patient with BCR-ABL mutations that are resistant to or who fail TKI therapy. Transplant should also be considered for patients who present in blast crisis or who progress on a TKI in accelerated phase or blast crisis.[3] There are significant risks and long-term complications with allogeneic stem cell transplantation including early mortality and graft-versus-host disease. For patients who do not achieve a complete molecular response or have a relapse, the infusion of donor lymphocytes may place the patient back into a durable remission.[3]

Pharmacologic Therapy (Table 96–1)

The treatment of CML has dramatically changed since the introduction of TKIs. KEY CONCEPT *Nearly all patients with CML are initially treated with a TKI. These oral agents do not cure CML but are able to produce long-term disease control in the vast majority of patients.*

► *Imatinib mesylate (Gleevec)*

Imatinib mesylate (STI-571; Gleevec) is a first-generation TKI and was the first TKI to show efficacy in the treatment of CML. Imatinib inhibits phosphorylation of various proteins involved in cell proliferation. In CML, imatinib works by binding to the adenosine triphosphate–binding pocket of *BCR-ABL*.[4] The 8-year follow-up data show that the use of imatinib in chronic phase CML results in an overall survival of 85% and an estimated event-free survival of 81%.[6] As expected with more aggressive disease, lower response rates are reported in accelerated phase and blast crisis.[7] Disease progression is typically attributed to imatinib primary or secondary resistance.[8] The *ABL* mutation T315I is one mechanism of secondary resistance that results in reactivation of BCR-ABL activity. The T315I mutation renders imatinib and the second-generation TKIs ineffective; therefore, alternative therapy with agents that overcome this mutation must be selected.[3,8]

Imatinib may be used as first-line therapy in patients with CML. Standard dosing of imatinib is 400 mg/day in chronic phase CML. Studies have investigated the use of higher doses of imatinib in all phases of CML. Although these higher doses produced rapid responses compared to standard imatinib dosing, they were also associated with more serious adverse effects.[3,9]

Therapy with imatinib is generally well tolerated. Common side effects include myelosuppression (phase and dose related), rash, gastrointestinal disturbances, edema, fatigue, arthralgias, myalgias, and headaches. Congestive heart failure is a rare but serious side effect and requires careful monitoring in patients with preexisting cardiac conditions.[3,10,11] Imatinib is metabolized by CYP450 3A4, and possible drug interactions include agents that inhibit or induce 3A4, such as erythromycin, ketoconazole, and phenytoin.[3]

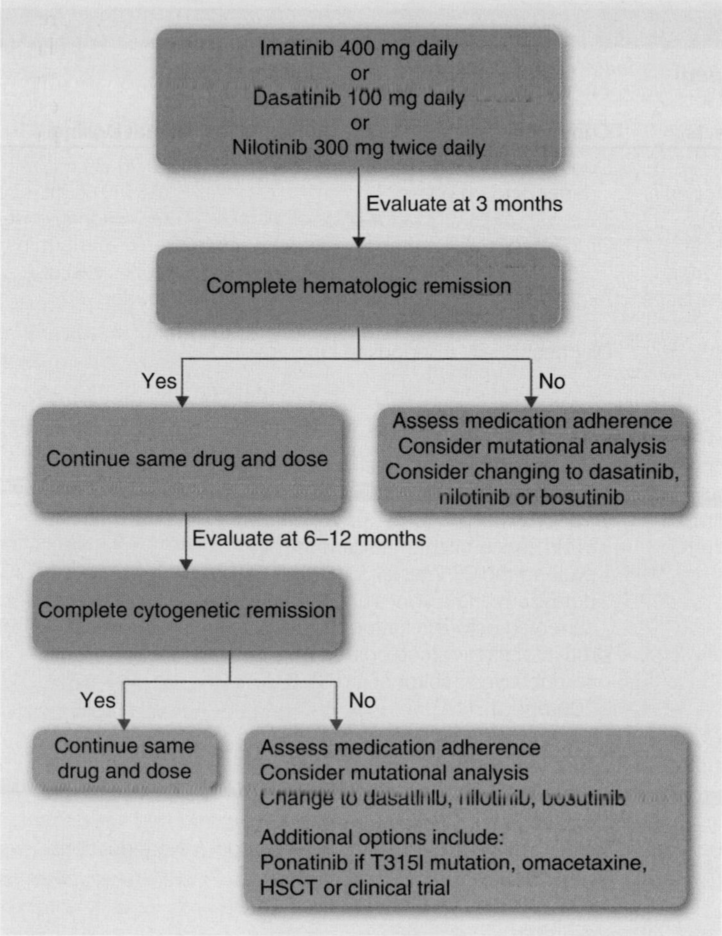

FIGURE 96–1. Algorithm for tyrosine kinase inhibitor therapy in newly diagnosed chronic myeloid leukemia (CML) patients. (HSCT, hematopoietic stem cell transplantation.)

Table 96–1

Drugs Used in CML

Drug	Adverse Effects	Comments	Renal Dosing	Hepatic Dosing
Bosutinib (Bosulif)	Diarrhea, nausea vomiting, thrombocytopenia, neutropenia, increased liver function tests, fluid retention	Dose: 500 mg po once daily Dose may be increased to 600 mg po once daily if complete hematologic response not seen at 8 weeks or complete cytogenetic response by 12 week Take with food Drug interactions: metabolized by CYP 3A4; inhibitor and substrate of P-glycoprotein	CrCl 30–50 mL/min (0.50–0.83 mL/s): 500 mg daily and may decrease to 400 mg if cannot tolerate CrCl < 30 ml/min (0.50 mL/s): 300 mg daily	Any baseline liver impairment: 200 mg daily
Dasatinib (Sprycel)	Thrombocytopenia, neutropenia, headache, rash, edema, pleural effusions	Dose: 100 mg po once daily for chronic phase CML or 140 mg po daily for accelerated phase or blast crisis Avoid concomitant medications that prolong the QT-interval; low levels of potassium and magnesium should be corrected before initiating therapy Drug interactions: metabolized by CYP 3A4 Dasatinib exhibits pH-dependent absorption; avoid medications that alter gastric pH (eg, H2 antagonists and PPIs)	No reductions	No reductions

(*Continued*)

Table 96–1

Drugs Used in CML (*Continued*)

Drug	Adverse Effects	Comments	Renal Dosing	Hepatic Dosing
Imatinib mesylate (Gleevec, STI 571)	Neutropenia, thrombocytopenia, diarrhea, rash, nausea, edema, fatigue, arthralgias, myalgias, headache, increased liver function tests, congestive heart failure (rare)	Dose range: 400–800 mg po per day depending on phase Take with meals and a full glass of water Drug interactions: metabolized by CYP 3A4; weak inhibitor of CYP 2D6 and 2C9 Avoid taking with acetaminophen to reduce hepatic toxicity Diarrhea usually responds to loperamide	CrCl 20–39 mL/min (0.33–0.66 mL/s): 50% reduction in dose CrCl < 20 mL/min (0.33 mL/s): use with caution	Mild to moderate impairment: no adjustment Severe impairment: reduce dose by 25% Discontinue imatinib if liver transaminases are > 5 × upper limit of normal or if serum bilirubin > 3 × upper limit of normal
Nilotinib (Tasigna)	Thrombocytopenia, neutropenia, elevated bilirubin, elevated serum lipase	Dose: 400 mg po twice daily Take on an empty stomach Black-box warning for QT prolongation; avoid concomitant medications that prolong the QT interval; low levels of potassium and magnesium should be corrected before initiating therapy Drug interactions: metabolized by CYP 3A4; competitive inhibitor of CYP 2C8, 2C9, 2D6, and UGT1A1 Pharmacogenomic testing of UGT1A1 polymorphisms can be used to identify patients who may have hyperbilirubinemia	No reductions	Child-Pugh class A, B, or C: 200 mg po twice daily for chronic phase CML; may increase to 300 mg if tolerating nilotinib therapy; discontinue nilotinib if experiencing grade 3 or 4 elevations in bilirubin or liver transaminases
Omacetaxine mepesuccinate (Synribo)	Myelosuppression, hyperglycemia	Dose: 1.25 mg/m^2 subcutaneous injection twice daily × 14 days, repeat every 28 days until hematologic response achieved Maintenance therapy: 1.25 mg/m^2 subcutaneous injection twice daily × 7 days every 28-day cycle Drug interactions: P-glycoprotein substrate	No reductions	No reductions
Ponatinib (Iclusig)	Arterial and venous thromboembolisms, hepatotoxicity, congestive heart failure, pancreatitis, gastrointestinal bleeding, fluid retention, myelosuppression, fatigue, headaches	Dose: 45 mg daily Black-box warnings for thromboembolism stroke, myocardial infarction, hepatotoxicity and heart failure Monitor CBC, lipase and liver function tests. Drug interactions: metabolized by CYP 3A4,2C8, 2D6 competitive inhibitor of P-glycoprotein	No reductions	Child-Pugh class A, B, or C: 30 mg daily Hold ponatinib if liver transaminases are > 3 × upper limit of normal. May resume but reduce dose when < 3 × upper limit of normal

CML, chronic myeloid leukemia; CrCl, creatinine clearance; po, oral; PPI, proton pump inhibitor.

▸ *Advanced-Generation TKIs*

There are four advanced-generation BCR-ABL TKI inhibitors. KEY CONCEPT *Dasatinib (Sprycel), nilotinib (Tasigna), bosutinib (Bosulif), and ponatinib (Iclusig) are advanced generation TKIs that may overcome imatinib resistance or intolerance.* These inhibitors are anywhere from 10 to 325 times more potent than imatinib in inhibiting BCR-ABL and are able to overcome most *BCR-ABL* mutations that lead to imatinib resistance.[12] Of the four, only ponatinib can overcome the *T315I* mutation.[13]

Dasatinib and nilotinib were initially indicated for use in CML when patients failed imatinib therapy. Their indication has now expanded to include first-line therapy based on results of trials comparing these drugs to imatinib. These study results suggest that dasatinib and nilotinib are comparable to, if not better than, imatinib in achieving faster and deeper cytogenetic and molecular responses.[6,10,14,15] These studies suggest that fewer patients may progress to accelerated or blast phase on dasatinib or nilotinib compared to imatinib. Common side effects are similar to those of imatinib.

A significant and potentially severe side effect of pleural effusions has been reported with the use of imatinib and dasatinib but not with the use of nilotinib.[6] Additional side effects include QT prolongation (dasatinib and nilotinib) and increases in indirect bilirubin (nilotinib).[3,12]

Bosutinib is used in the second-line treatment of CML when patients are resistant or intolerant to prior TKI therapy. Bosutinib overcomes most *BCR-ABL* domain mutations with the exception of the *T315I* mutation. Bosutinib is not recommended as first-line therapy since the Phase III trial comparing the efficacy of bosutinib to imatinib did not meet its primary endpoint of complete cytogenetic response at 12 months.[16] The side effects of bosutinib appear to be less severe and less common than many of the other TKIs. Gastrointestinal disturbances and rash are some of the most common nonhematologic side effects.[16]

Ponatinib is a third-generation multikinase inhibitor that overcomes the *BCR-ABL* domain mutation *T315I*. Ponatinib was initially approved for the treatment of patients in all phases that were resistant or intolerant to prior TKI therapy. In postmarketing analysis, an increase in serious arterial thrombotic events was shown in 24% of patients.[3,13] The revised label indicates the use of ponatinib in patients harboring the *T315I* mutation or have failed multiple prior TKIs. Nonhematologic side effects include rash, dry skin, and abdominal pain. Rare yet serious adverse effects include liver failure and death, which are both black-box warnings.[3,13]

► *Omacetaxine Mepesuccinate*

Omacetaxine mepesuccinate (Synribo) is a semisynthetic formulation of homoharringtonine. Omacetaxine reversibly inhibits protein synthesis thereby causing cell death.[17] Unlike TKIs, the mechanism of action affects both normal and malignant hematopoietic cells. Omacetaxine is a subcutaneous injection indicated for patients in chronic or accelerated phase CML who are resistant or intolerant to two or more TKIs.[3] It may be used in patients with the *T315I* mutation. Nonhematologic adverse reactions include gastrointestinal disturbances, fatigue and hyperglycemia. Febrile neutropenia, infections, and cerebral hemorrhage are a few of the serious adverse reactions.[17]

OUTCOME EVALUATION

Successful treatment for CML depends on the elimination of the Ph. Nearly all newly diagnosed CML patients will be placed on a TKI. First-line treatment options include imatinib, dasatinib, and nilotinib. Which agent to use depends on several factors, including mutational status, disease risk score, age, comorbid conditions, and medication safety profile. Patients should be counseled on the importance of medication adherence. Patients should understand that poorer outcomes may result if they are not adherent to daily TKI therapy. Historically, if patients fail to obtain a cytogenetic response within 6 to 12 months, a change in therapy is recommended. Research is evaluating the use of early molecular responses in the treatment management of CML. If TKI treatment failure occurs, patients should undergo *BCR-ABL* domain mutation testing. Second-line chronic phase CML therapy should be determined based on mutational analysis with second-generations TKIs (including bosutinib). These agents may also be used in patients who have accelerated phase CML. Ponatinib may be considered if the *T315I* mutational status is present with an understanding that it is associated with serious vascular effects. Omacetaxine, allogeneic stem cell transplantation and clinical trials are options for those patients that do not respond to a TKI.

Patient Encounter 1

A 48-year-old man presents to his primary care physician with complaints of worsening fatigue and left upper quadrant pain. His medical history consists of type 2 diabetes managed with metformin and gastroesophageal reflux disease treated with omeprazole. A CBC is drawn and shows the following:

Total WBC: 70×10^9/L (70×10^3/mm^3), (4% [0.04] blasts, 86% [0.86] segs, 10% [0.10] lymphs)

Hgb/Hct: 8.3 g/dL (83 g/L; 5.15 mmol/L)/25% (0.25)

Platelets: 489×10^9/L (489×10^3/mm^3)

The patient is referred to an oncologist for further workup. A bone marrow biopsy is performed and reveals hypercellular marrow with 5% (0.05) blasts. FISH analysis is positive for *Ph*.

What information is suggestive of CML?

What are the first-line treatment options for chronic phase CML patient?

Which specific treatment do you recommend for this patient and why?

Identify your treatment goals for this patient.

Assuming this patient has suboptimal response to your initial therapy, what would you recommend for second-line therapy?

What factors may contribute to this patient's having a suboptimal response?

Some patients will not respond to treatment and will progress to blast crisis where they will receive treatment for acute leukemia. Although its use is limited, allogeneic transplant offers the only cure for CML and may be useful in patients with advanced disease.

CHRONIC LYMPHOCYTIC LEUKEMIA

CLL is a cancer that results in the accumulation of functionally incompetent lymphocytes.[18] CLL is usually considered an indolent, incurable disease, and treatment should only be initiated when patients have symptoms. However, a subset of patients will have aggressive disease, and these individuals need to be treated aggressively.

EPIDEMIOLOGY AND ETIOLOGY

CLL is the most common type of leukemia diagnosed in adults, accounting for 30% of all adult leukemias. It was estimated that in 2015, 14,620 new cases would be diagnosed in the United States.[2] The median age at diagnosis is the sixth decade of life with the incidence increasing with age. The etiology of CLL is unknown, but hereditary factors may have a role, with family members of CLL patients having a twofold to sevenfold increased risk of CLL.[18]

PATHOPHYSIOLOGY

Cell of Origin

CLL is characterized by small, relatively incompetent B lymphocytes that accumulate in the blood and bone marrow over time. The lack of apoptotic mechanisms leads to the persistence and accumulation of B lymphocytes. The exact cell of origin is controversial but has been described as an antigen-activated B lymphocyte.[18] Chromosomal abnormalities have been identified in 40% to 50% cases of CLL and often correlate with progressive disease. Numerous tyrosine kinases appear to be involved in CLL, including the activation of Bruton tyrosine kinase (BTK).[19] Detection of some of these markers may predict clinical course and prognosis and may influence treatment decisions.[18,19]

Clinical Course

KEY CONCEPT *CLL can have a variable clinical course with survival ranging from months to decades. Low-risk disease is asymptomatic, and median survival times exceed 10 years. Intermediate risk is associated with lymphadenopathy and has median survival times of about 7 years.* High-risk patients with anemia have median survival times of only 3 years.[20] The typical low-risk patient is an asymptomatic elderly patient who is diagnosed on routine blood draw. The typical high-risk patient is a symptomatic middle-aged patient.

Clinical Presentation and Diagnosis of CLL

Signs and Symptoms (50% are asymptomatic at diagnosis)[16]

- Lymphadenopathy
- Organomegaly consisting of splenomegaly and hepatomegaly
- Fatigue, weight loss, night sweats, fevers
- Chronic infections caused by immature lymphocytes

Diagnostic Procedures

- Peripheral blood smear
- Bone marrow biopsy
- Cytogenetic studies
- Molecular testing

Laboratory Findings

Peripheral-blood

- Leukocytosis (WBC count > 100×10^9/L [100×10^3/mm^3])
- Lymphocytosis (absolute lymph count > 5×10^9/L [5×10^3/mm^3])
- Anemia
- Thrombocytopenia
- Hypogammaglobinemia

Bone marrow

- Must have at least 30% (0.30) lymphocytes

Molecular markers

- Cytogenetic abnormalities

Poor Prognostic Factors

- Lymphocytosis with accompanying:
  - Anemia (hemoglobin ≤ 11.0 g/dL [110 g/L; 6.83 mmol/L])
  - Thrombocytopenia (platelets < 100×10^9/L [100×10^3/mm^3])
- ZAP-70 and CD38 antigen expression
- Cytogenetics such as deletions of chromosomes 17p and 11q (deletion of 13q is favorable)

PROGNOSTIC FACTORS

Two staging systems, Rai's and Binet's, have been developed to help practitioners determine the overall prognosis of patients with CLL. They are comparable systems and are useful to broadly determine good, intermediate, and poor prognostic disease.[20] Risk stratification criteria included in these systems are lymphadenopathy, splenomegaly, hepatomegaly, and cytopenias. Increasingly, a number of biological markers of the disease such as deletions of chromosome 17p and 13q and mutational status of immunoglobulin heavy chain variable region gene (IgVH) are being used to predict the likely clinical course.[21] These biological markers are not included in the Rai's or Binet's staging systems.

TREATMENT

Desired Outcomes

The primary goals in the treatment of CLL are to provide palliation of symptoms and improve overall survival. Because the current treatments for CLL are not curative, reduction in tumor burden and improvement in disease symptoms are reasonable end points, particularly in older patients. A complete response (CR) to therapy can be defined as a resolution of lymphadenopathy and organomegaly, normalization of peripheral blood counts, and elimination of lymphoblasts in the bone marrow.

Nonpharmacologic Therapy

KEY CONCEPT *Asymptomatic early stage CLL can be observed without treatment until evidence of disease progression.* Past studies with chlorambucil suggest that chemotherapy does not improve overall survival in early stage CLL although there is question whether this remains true with the development of newer therapies. In addition, deferring therapy until a patient becomes symptomatic does not alter overall survival.[20] For this reason, the notion of "watch and wait" is considered reasonable for older patients with low risk disease. Several factors will influence this approach, including life expectancy, disease characteristics, and ability to tolerate therapy.[20,22]

▶ *Hematopoietic Stem Cell Transplantation*

The use of hematopoietic stem cell transplantation (HSCT) in CLL is limited. Allogeneic transplantation offers longer disease-free remissions than **autologous** transplantation but is associated with high treatment morbidity and mortality. Several factors must be considered before allogeneic stem cell transplantation. The lack of a donor, older age, and poor performance status make transplant an uncommon procedure in this population. Allogeneic transplantation remains an option for younger patients with aggressive disease who have failed prior therapies. Although its use is currently limited, HSCT may someday be an important component in achieving a cure for CLL.[20,22]

Pharmacologic Therapy (Table 96–2)

CLL treatment is typically initiated in the symptomatic patient. Numerous agents can be used as initial therapy in the treatment of symptomatic or advanced CLL. Many of the chemotherapy regimens have not been compared directly with one another, so

Table 96–2

Drugs Used in CLL

Drug	Adverse Effects	Comments	Renal Dosing	Hepatic Dosing
Alemtuzumab (Campath)	Infusion reactions: fever, chills, nausea, vomiting; hypotension; prolonged immunosuppression (resulting in infectious complications)	Antiviral and PCP prophylaxis should be initiated during treatment Consider antifungal prophylaxis Premedicate with acetaminophen, diphenhydramine with or without a steroid to alleviate infusion-related reactions SC dosing may lessen acute toxicity	No reductions	No reductions
Bendamustine (Treanda)	Myelosuppression, fever, nausea, vomiting, infusion reactions, tumor lysis syndrome	Consider using allopurinol for tumor lysis syndrome during first few cycles of therapy	CrCl < 40 mL/min (0.67 mL/s): do not use	Mild impairment: use with caution Moderate to severe impairment: do not use
Chlorambucil (Leukeran)	Myelosuppression; allergic reactions (skin rash); secondary malignancies	Take on an empty stomach because food decreases absorption Dose range: 4–10 mg po daily	No reductions	No reductions
Fludarabine (Fludara)	Myelosuppression; prolonged immunosuppression, resulting in secondary infectious complications; edema; neurotoxicity	Dose: 20 mg/m^2 IV daily for 5 days Often given in combination	CrCl 30–70 mL/min (0.50–1.17 mL/s): 20% reduction of dose (IV and po) CrCl < 30 mL/min (0.50 mL/s): do not use IV; reduce dose of oral by 50%	No reductions
Ibrutinib (Imbruvica)	Risk of bleeding, neutropenia, thrombocytopenia	Dose: 420 mg po once daily Avoid the use of concomitant CYP 3A4 inhibitors/inducers Drug metabolism: CYP 3A4 and 2D6	No reductions in CrCl > 25 ml/min (0.42 mL/s) Insufficient data in < 25 ml/min (0.42 mL/s)	Insufficient data exists
Idelalisib (Zydelig)	Black-box warnings: Severe hepatotoxicity, diarrhea, colitis, pneumonitis, intestinal perforation Serious allergic reactions	Dose: 150 mg po twice daily Drug metabolism: CYP 3A4; strong inhibitor of 3A4, 2C8, 2C9, 2C19	No reductions in CrCl > 15 ml/min (0.25 mL/s) Insufficient data in < 15 ml/min (0.25 mL/s)	Insufficient data exists
Obinutuzumab (Gazyva)	Infusion reactions, reactivation of hepatitis B, progressive multifocal encephalopathy, tumor lysis syndrome, neutropenia	Premedicate with acetaminophen, IV antihistamine, and an IV steroid to alleviate infusion-related reactions Consider antimicrobial, antiviral and antifungal prophylaxis Hold antihypertensives 12 hours prior, during and after due to the risk of hypotension	No reductions in CrCl > 30 ml/min (0.50 mL/s) Insufficient data in < 30 ml/min (0.50 mL/s)	No reductions
Ofatumumab (Arzerra)	Severe infusion-reactions: bronchospasm, edema, fever, chills, rigors, hypotension; prolonged myelosuppression	Premedicate with acetaminophen, IV antihistamine, and an IV steroid to alleviate infusion-related reactions Rate of infusion should be increased gradually to minimize reactions Monitor for reactivation of hepatitis B	No reductions	No reductions
Pentostatin (Nipent)	Myelosuppression; infectious complications	Fatal pulmonary toxicity when given with fludarabine	Hold dose if serum creatinine increases	No reductions
Rituximab (Rituxan)	Infusion reactions: fever, chills, rigors, hypotension	Premedicate with acetaminophen, diphenhydramine with or without a steroid to alleviate infusion related reactions Rate of infusion should be increased gradually to minimize reactions Monitor for reactivation of hepatitis B	No reductions	No reductions

CrCl, creatinine clearance; IV, intravenous; po, oral; PCP, pneumocystis pneumonia; SC, subcutaneous.

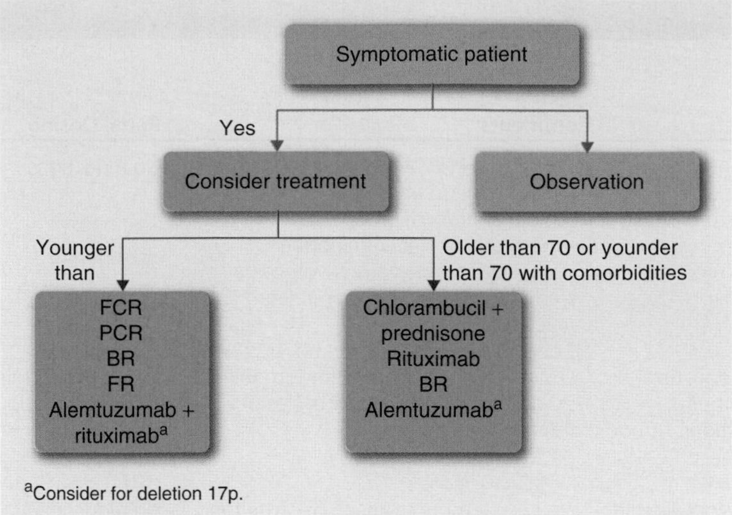

FIGURE 96–2. Algorithm for initial therapy in newly diagnosed chronic lymphocytic leukemia (CLL) patients. B, bendamustine; C, cyclophosphamide; F, fludarabine; P pentostatin; R, rituximab.

there is not one preferred regimen. Selection of the appropriate chemotherapy depends on the individual patient and practitioner's preference. Figure 96–2 illustrates one approach for initial therapy in newly diagnosed patients with CLL.

► *Cytotoxic Chemotherapy*

Historically, chlorambucil (Leukeran), an oral alkylating agent, was considered the standard treatment for CLL. Today, the treatment for CLL has changed with the development of the purine analogs. There are three purine analogs used in the treatment of CLL: fludarabine (Fludara), pentostatin (Nipent), and cladribine (Leustatin) with fludarabine being the most studied. KEY CONCEPT *Fludarabine-based chemoimmunotherapy is commonly used as first-line therapy for younger patients with CLL.* Randomized clinical trials have shown that fludarabine is superior to chlorambucil in achieving higher response rates and producing a longer duration of response.[20,22] Fludarabine is effective in previously untreated patients as well as patients who have chlorambucil-resistant disease. Although fludarabine is one of the most effective agents in the treatment of CLL, it is rarely used as a sole agent. Instead fludarabine is given in combination with other drugs to improve response rates.[19,20,22]

Fludarabine is associated with more toxicities than chlorambucil, including myelosuppression and prolonged immunosuppression.[23] Resultant infectious complications may occur during the periods of prolonged immunosuppression. Clinicians should consider antibacterial and antiviral prophylaxis for *Pneumocystis* and varicella zoster when using fludarabine-based therapy.[22] Today, chlorambucil remains a practical option for symptomatic elderly patients who require palliative therapy because of the ease of oral administration, low cost and limited side-effect profile.

Bendamustine (Treanda) is an alkylating agent used in the treatment of CLL. As first-line therapy for CLL, bendamustine was shown to have superior overall response rates, CRs, and longer progression-free survival than chlorambucil.[22] Bendamustine is usually given in combination with rituximab as first-line therapy.[19,22]

► *Monoclonal Antibodies*

KEY CONCEPT *Combination chemoimmunotherapy with anti-CD20 monoclonal antibodies are widely used in the treatment of CLL.* Rituximab (Rituxan) is a naked chimeric monoclonal antibody directed against the CD20 antigen on B-lymphocytes.[19,20] Similar to other B-cell malignancies, CLL expresses CD20 antigens. Dose escalation studies suggest that higher doses are required than those used in non-Hodgkin lymphoma.[24] The higher dose required in CLL is probably a combined effect of lower CD20 antigen expression and higher concentrations of soluble CD20 antigen than in non-Hodgkin lymphoma.[24] Rituximab is given in combination with other therapies since these combinations result in higher CRs than rituximab alone.[19] The most common side effects of rituximab include infusion reactions consisting of fever, chills, hypotension, nausea, vomiting, and headache.[18] Premedication with diphenhydramine and acetaminophen is recommended to minimize infusion reactions.

Ofatumumab (Arzerra) and obinutuzumab (Gazyva) are two newer biologics in this class. Ofatumumab is a CD20 antigen-directed monoclonal antibody that is approved in CLL patients who fail fludarabine and alemtuzumab.[25] Obinutuzumab is different than the other two having a higher binding affinity to the CD20 epitope and causing direct cell death.[25] It is approved in combination with chlorambucil for the treatment of previously untreated CLL. Premedications are similar to rituximab with the addition of a corticosteroid to reduce the incidence of infusion reactions. The rate of infusion and titration depends on patient tolerability of the medication. Table 96-2 lists some of the adverse effects seen with the anti-CD20 monoclonal antibodies.

Alemtuzumab (Campath) is a humanized monoclonal antibody directed against the CD52 antigen.[20] CD52 antigen is expressed on the majority of B and T lymphocytes. Alemtuzumab may be used as single agent or combination therapy in the treatment of CLL. Studies have shown alemtuzumab to be effective in fludarabine-resistant disease, in patients with the deletion of 17p, and as front-line therapy.[22] Infusion-related reactions can be significant and typically occur with the initial dose and lessen in severity with subsequent doses. To limit acute allergic reactions, subcutaneous administration may be given instead of IV dosing.[18,22] Premedication with oral antihistamines and acetaminophen is recommended. Alemtuzumab also suppresses the T cells, resulting in prolonged immunosuppression. Infectious complications may occur from the reactivation of cytomegalovirus and herpes virus and from infection with *Pneumocystis*. These infections have been shown to occur with both the IV and subcutaneous routes of administrations. Patients should receive trimethoprim–sulfamethoxazole and acyclovir or an equivalent antiviral to prevent these infections.[18,20]

► *Small-Molecule Inhibitors*

An understanding of the B-cell receptor signaling pathways of CLL has led to the approval of newer oral targeted therapies.[26] Ibrutinib (Imbruvica) is an inhibitor of BTK which is an essential enzyme in the B-cell receptor pathway. Ibrutinib has been shown to have an improved progression free survival, response rate and overall survival compared to ofatumumab in previously treated patients with CLL.[27] Ibrutinib has also been studied in previously untreated patients with CLL and in patients with the del 17p.[22] Idelalisib (Zydelig) targets phosphatidylinositol-3-kinase (PI3-K), an essential lipid kinase that is a regulator of the B-cell receptor pathway and involved in cellular survival and proliferation. Idelalisib has been studied as monotherapy as well as combination therapy with rituximab in patients with relapsed disease.[28] Nonhematologic side effects for both drugs may be found in Table 96-2. Black-box warnings for idelalisib include hepatotoxicity, colitis, pneumonitis, and intestinal perforation.

► *Chemoimmunotherapy*

Chemoimmunotherapy is the standard for younger patients with symptomatic CLL. The regimen is often selected based on age and cytogenetics. Combination therapy generally consists of an anti-CD20 antibody in combination with chemotherapy. The combination of fludarabine, cyclophosphamide, and rituximab improves CR rates compared with fludarabine alone (70% vs 20%, respectively) but at the expense of increased infections.[19,22] Rituximab is often added to bendamustine, lenalidomide, and alemtuzumab.[22] A recent multiple-treatment meta-analysis was not able to show a significant survival benefit of one regimen compared to another.[29]

Patient Encounter 2

A 42-year-old man presents to his health care provider for his annual well-check. Physical exam reveals cervical lymph node enlargement and splenomegaly. Blood work reports the following:

WBC: 85×10^9/L (85×10^3/mm^3)

Hgb: 10.9 g/dL (109 g/L; 6.77 mmol/L)

Platelets: 200×10^9/L (20×10^3/mm^3)

Peripheral Smear: Lymphocytosis with small, mature-appearing cells suggestive of chronic lymphocytic leukemia

Prognostic Markers: Positive for CD38 expression, negative for ZAP-70, deletion 11q

What information supports the diagnosis of CLL?

Identify your treatment goals for this patient.

What treatment approach do you recommend?

Would your treatment options change if this patient were asymptomatic? If so, what would be your new treatment?

Would your treatment options change if this patient were a symptomatic, 86-year-old man?

OUTCOME EVALUATION

Successful outcomes depend on the appropriate treatment selection for a specific patient. Risk-versus-benefit should be determined in the treatment of older CLL patients. Because CLL is incurable, watch and wait is a reasonable approach for those with indolent disease. Treatment can then begin when the patient becomes symptomatic. Aggressive chemoimmunotherapy with fludarabine is often reserved for younger patients with high-risk CLL, with the goal being prolonged disease-free survival. A desirable response to therapy includes a reduction in lymphocytes, decrease in stage of the disease, and resolution of symptoms.

MULTIPLE MYELOMA

Multiple myeloma (MM) is a malignancy of the plasma cell and is characterized by an abnormal production of a monoclonal protein in the bone marrow. Features of the disease include bone lesions, anemia, and renal insufficiency.[30] Multiple myeloma is an incurable disease; however, advancements in the treatment of myeloma have significantly extended survival.

EPIDEMIOLOGY AND ETIOLOGY

Multiple myeloma (MM) is the second most common hematologic malignancy. It is estimated that approximately 26,850 new cases of MM would be reported in 2015, accounting for 1% to 2% of all cancers.[2] The median age at diagnosis is 70 years, and fewer than 2% are diagnosed before the age of 40 years.[30,31] The incidence of myeloma is highest in African Americans, lowest in Asians, and occurs more frequently in men than women.[31] The etiology of MM remains largely unknown although a exposure to ionizing radiation and genetic factors have been implicated.[31]

PATHOPHYSIOLOGY

The pathogenesis of MM is quite complex with multiple-step models created to postulate the process. Myeloma must be distinguished from a condition called monoclonal gammopathy of unknown significance (MGUS), which is characterized by a monoclonal immunoglobulin without malignant plasma cells. Yearly, about 1% of patients with MGUS will develop MM. Chromosomal abnormalities and changes in gene expression lead to cell cycle dysregulation and appear to be involved early in the disease process.[30] The pathophysiology of MM involves complex bone marrow microenvironment, and cytokine interactions. Interleukin-6, tumor necrosis factor, vascular endothelial growth factor, and stromal-derived factor-1 support the establishment and proliferation of myeloma cells.[30,31] The understanding of these interactions has led to novel agents used in the treatment of MM.

PROGNOSTIC FACTORS

Prognostic factors for myeloma include tumor, treatment, and patient related factors. The International Staging System is used to predict outcomes after therapy. Staging is stratified based on the levels of serum β_2-microglobulinemia and serum albumin. High β_2-microglobulinemia and low albumin are poor prognostic factors and are indicative of high tumor load.[32] Although cytogenetic abnormalities are not included in the International Staging System, many abnormalities are associated with poor outcomes. The Mayo Stratification for Myeloma and Risk-Adapted

Clinical Presentation and Diagnosis of Multiple Myeloma

Signs and Symptoms

- "CRAB"
  - "C"—hyperCalcemia
  - "R"—Renal failure (serum creatinine > 2 mg/dL [177 μmol/L])
  - "A"—Anemia (fatigue)
  - "B"—Bone disease (pain, lesions, fractures)
- Weight loss
- Recurrent infections

Diagnostic Procedures

- Laboratory
  - CBC, chemistry panel, β_2 microglobulin
  - Peripheral blood smear
  - Serum protein electrophoresis and immunofixation
  - Urine protein electrophoresis and immunofixation
  - Serum free light chains
- Radiologic evaluation (MRI, bone densitometry)
- Bone marrow biopsy
  - Cytogenetic studies
  - Molecular testing

Laboratory Findings

- Peripheral blood
  - Monoclonal protein in serum (usually IgG or IgA)
  - High β_2-microglobulin
  - Low platelets and hemoglobin
  - High creatinine, urea, lactate dehydrogenase, C-reactive protein, and calcium
  - Rouleaux formation
- Urinalysis
  - Urinary free light chains (Bence-Jones Protein)
- Bone marrow
  - Plasma cells (10% or more)
  - Abnormal cytogenetics
- Radiologic findings
  - Bone lesions, fractures, osteoporosis

Poor Prognostic Factors

- High serum β_2-microglobulin and low serum albumin
- Elevated C-reactive protein
- Elevated lactate dehydrogenase
- IgA isotype
- Low platelet count
- Chromosome 13 deletions and other cytogenetic abnormalities

Patient Encounter 3

A 58-year-old woman presents to her health care provider with complaints of extreme fatigue and severe right and left hip pain. Her past medical history includes controlled hypertension. Workup reveals:

Radiology: X-ray of right and left hips: Osteolytic lesions

Labs: Hemoglobin: 7.2 g/dL (72 g/L; 4.47 mmol/L); platelets: 220×10^9/L (220×10^3/mm^3); corrected calcium: 11.8 mg/dL (2.95 mmol/L); serum creatinine: 1.8 mg/dL (159 μmol/L); serum IgG: 4200 mg/dL (42 g/L) (normal: 620–1500 mg/dL (6.2–15 g/L); serum IgM: 80 mg/dL (8 g/L) (normal: 50–200 mg/dL (0.5–2 g/L); bone marrow: 83% plasma cell infiltrates

What information is suggestive of multiple myeloma?

What treatment options are available for this patient?

Assuming this patient is a candidate for autologous stem cell transplantation, what would be an appropriate induction regimen?

Assuming this patient is a not a candidate for autologous stem cell transplantation, what would be an appropriate induction regimen?

What may be used for maintenance therapy after an autologous stem cell transplantation?

Therapy classification incorporates tumor biology to stratify patients according to their disease risk.[33] Chromosomal changes are being used to predict high-risk patients with perhaps the most important being deletions of the long arm of chromosome 13 and translocation of chromosomes 4 and 14.[30,34] Older patients, renal impairment, and other comorbidities also predict for poorer outcomes.[31]

TREATMENT

Desired Outcomes

The primary goal in the treatment of MM is to prolong progression free and overall survival while minimizing complications associated with the disease. A watch and wait approach is an option for asymptomatic patients (smoldering myeloma) who have no lytic lesions in the bone. When symptoms occur, treatment is required. The treatment of MM often includes induction, transplantation, and maintenance therapy. All patients should be evaluated early on to see if they are transplant eligible candidates. Autologous stem cell transplantation prolongs overall survival in patients who can tolerate high-dose chemotherapy. Regardless of transplant eligibility, all patients will be placed on initial induction therapy to reduce tumor burden. Maintenance therapy following transplant with immunomodulators or proteasome inhibitors is being used to prolong the duration of response. Almost all patients become refractory to initial treatment and require the use of salvage therapies. Figure 96–3

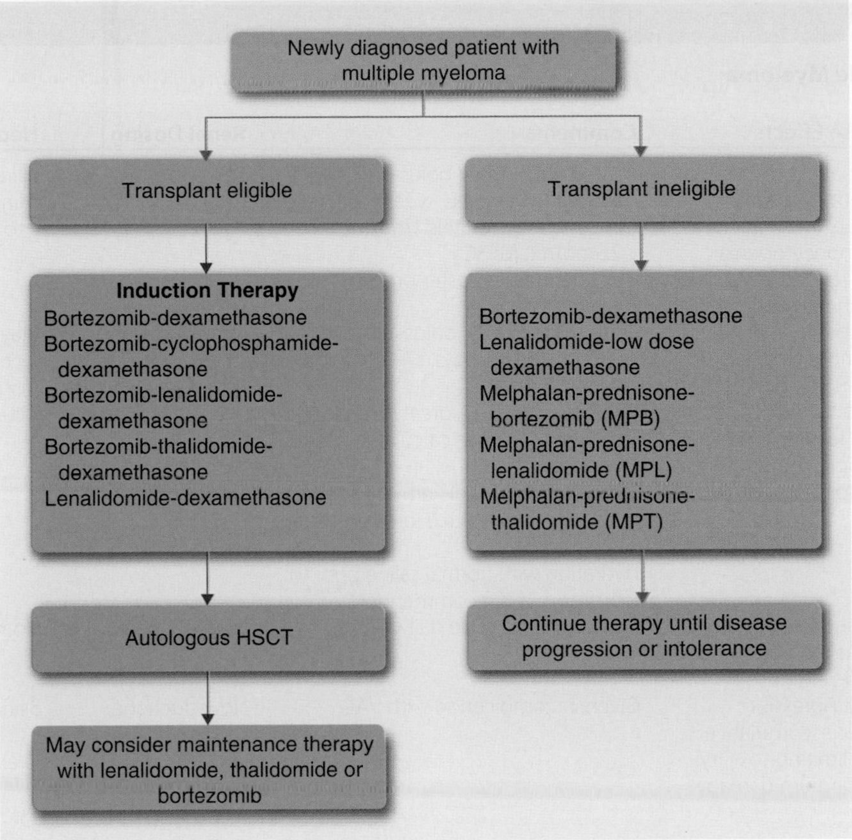

FIGURE 96–3. Possible approach for treatment in newly diagnosed patients with multiple myeloma. (HSCT, hematopoietic stem cell transplantation.)

illustrates possible treatment approaches for transplant-eligible and transplant-ineligible patients.

Nonpharmacologic Therapy

▸ *Autologous Stem Cell Transplantation*

KEY CONCEPT *Autologous stem cell transplantation results in higher response rates and extends progression-free survival compared with those who receive conventional chemotherapy.* Although these initial trials did not include the immunomodulators, stem cell transplant remains the standard of care and should be considered in all patients who can tolerate high-dose chemotherapy.[34–36] High-dose melphalan is the most common preparative regimen. Two sequential transplants (tandem transplants) improve overall survival in patients who do not have a good partial response after one transplant.[31] The use of maintenance therapy after autologous transplantation with lenalidomide or bortezomib may be used in select patients to extend progression-free survival.[34,35] Since the studies supporting the use of transplant were conducted prior to the development of many of the novel agents used in the treatment of myeloma; the future role of stem cell transplantation may evolve.

Pharmacologic Therapy (Table 96–3)

Symptomatic MM requires treatment. There are five main classes of drugs used in the treatment of multiple myeloma: alkylating agents, anthracyclines, corticosteroids, immunomodulatory agents, and proteasome inhibitors. Drugs from these classes are used in combination and are the backbone for numerous chemotherapeutic regimens.

▸ *Conventional-Dose Chemotherapy*

The use of conventional-dose chemotherapy with alkylating agents or anthracyclines has declined with the advent of immunomodulators and proteasome inhibitors. The combination of melphalan and prednisone (MP) was once the most common initial treatment combination for myeloma. Today, melphalan-based therapy may be considered as initial therapy in transplant-ineligible patients.[34] Melphalan is toxic to progenitor cells and should be avoided in transplant eligible patients.[31,34] The anthracycline doxorubicin is also incorporated into treatment regimens. Currently, the combination of doxorubicin, bortezomib, and dexamethasone may be selected for induction therapy in patients who are transplant eligible. This regimen minimizes the risk of secondary malignancies that are associated with chronic alkylating therapy.[34]

▸ *Immunomodulatory Drugs*

KEY CONCEPT *Thalidomide (Thalomid), lenalidomide (Revlimid), and pomalidomide (Pomalyst) are used in the treatment of MM. Depending on the agent, they may be used as monotherapy or combination therapy.* The precise mechanism of action is unknown, but its antimyeloma activity may be attributable to its antiangiogenic and anticytokine properties.[37] Response rates are improved when an immunomodulatory agent is added to a treatment regimen. Thalidomide and steroid combinations produce

Table 96–3

Drugs Used in Multiple Myeloma

Drug	Adverse Effects	Comments	Renal Dosing	Hepatic Dosing
Bortezomib (Velcade)	Constipation; decreased appetite; asthenia; fatigue; fever; thrombocytopenia; dose related, reversible peripheral neuropathy	Dose: 1.3 mg/m² IV bolus or SC twice weekly for 2 weeks; week 3 off; repeat Concentration for IV is 1mg/mL and 2.5mg/mL for SC Consider herpes zoster prophylaxis with daily acyclovir	No reductions	Bilirubin > 1.5 × the upper limit of normal: reduce dose to 0.7 mg/m²
Carfilzomib (Kyprolis)	Neutropenia, thrombocytopenia, cardiac toxicity including cardiac arrest, congestive heart failure, infusion-reactions, tumor lysis syndrome	Dose: 20 mg/m² IV bolus on days 1, 2, 8, 9, 16 and 16; days 17–28 off; repeat every 28 days Patients with a BSA greater than 2.2 m² should have dose calculated based on 2.2 m² Premedicate with dexamethasone 4 mg prior to reduce infusion-related reactions Hydration with normal saline prior to carfilzomib is recommended	No reductions	May need to dose reduce or hold dose depending on degree of hepatic dysfunction
Dexamethasone	Hyperglycemia, edema, adrenal cortical insufficiency	Dose given po once daily	No reductions	No reductions
Doxorubicin (Adriamycin)	Myelosuppression; alopecia; cumulative dose-limiting toxicity: myocardium damage	Given in combination with VAD	No reductions	Bilirubin 1.2–3 mg/dL (21–51 μmol/L): 50% reduction in dose Bilirubin 3.1–5 mg/dL (53–85 μmol/L): 75% reduction in dose Bilirubin > 5 mg/dL (85 μmol/L): use with caution
Lenalidomide (Revlimid)	Possible birth defects neutropenia, thrombocytopenia, DVT, PE, pruritus, fatigue	Dose: 25 mg taken with water once daily Women of childbearing age must use two forms of contraception Pregnancy test must be taken before and during use Enrollment into monitoring program required	CrCl 30–60 mL/min (0.50–1.00 mL/s): 10 mg/day CrCl < 30 mL/min (0.50 mL/s): 15 mg every 48 hours Dialysis and CrCl < 30 mL/min (0.50 mL/s): 5 mg every 24 hours given after dialysis	No reductions
Melphalan (Alkeran)	Myelosuppression, secondary malignancies, pulmonary fibrosis, sterility, alopecia	Dose given po once daily IV formulation used for stem cell transplantation	No recommendation but may consider an initial dose reduction	No reductions
Pomalidomide (Pomalyst)	Severe birth defects, DVT, neutropenia	Dose: 4 mg po daily on days 1–21; off 21–28 and repeat Drug metabolism: CYP 1A2 and 3A4	Do not use if SCr > 3 mg/dL (265 μmol/L)	Do not use if bilirubin > 2 mg/dL (34 μmol/L) and AST/ALT > 3 × the upper limit of normal
Thalidomide (Thalomid)	Severe birth defects, peripheral neuropathy, DVT, somnolence, constipation	Titrate initial doses; doses are taken nightly Women of childbearing age must use two forms of contraception Pregnancy test must be taken before and during use Enrollment into monitoring program required	No reductions	No reductions
Vincristine (Oncovin)	Dose-limiting toxicity: peripheral neuropathies; paresthesias, constipation, alopecia	Given in combination with doxorubicin and dexamethasone (VAD)	No reductions	Bilirubin > 3 mg/dL (51 μmol/L): 50% reduction in dose

DVT, deep venous thrombosis; IV, intravenous; PE, pulmonary embolism; po, oral; SC, subcutaneous; VAD, vincristine–dexamethasone.

responses in 60% to 80% of previously untreated patients.[31,34] Responses can be improved to 94% with the addition of a third agent, bortezomib, but adding a fourth agent does not further improve responses.[38,39] The addition of thalidomide to MP also improves overall response and overall survival in newly diagnosed patients.[40] This combination (MPT) can be used as initial therapy in patients who are not transplant eligible. Thalidomide is also used as maintenance therapy as an attempt to control disease posttransplant although the studies have not shown a consistent OS benefit.[41] Common side effects of thalidomide therapy include somnolence, constipation, peripheral neuropathy, and deep venous thrombosis (DVT). Standard dose warfarin or low-molecular-weight heparins are recommended to prevent DVT.[34,42] There are substantial teratogenic effects of thalidomide if it is used during pregnancy, so distribution of the drug is closely monitored through the STEPS program.

Lenalidomide is more potent and has a more favorable safety profile over thalidomide.[34] The combination of lenalidomide, bortezomib, and dexamethasone has emerged as the one of the most commonly used induction regimens in the treatment of transplant-eligible patients with myeloma. Phase III trials showed that lenalidomide in combination with dexamethasone produced higher response rates and a longer time to progression than dexamethasone alone in relapsed and refractory

Patient Care Process

CHRONIC MYELOID LEUKEMIA

Patient Assessment:

- Review laboratory values and determine the stage of CML depending on the percent blasts in the peripheral blood or bone marrow.
- Review medical history, including patient's age, comorbid conditions and current medications to avoid drug–drug interactions.

Therapy Evaluation:

- If hematologic, cytogenetic and molecular goals are not achieved, determine whether a change in medication is warranted.
- If the patient experiences intolerance to therapy including any severe adverse effects, a change in medication may be warranted.
- Determine whether one of the first-line TKIs may be more cost-effective than the other agents.

Care Plan Development:

- Discuss the importance of medication adherence and long-term outcomes.
- Address any concerns about the selected medication including cost and management of adverse effects.

Follow-up Evaluation:

- TKI therapy should be frequently monitored. Follow-up may be scheduled every 3 months to determine whether goals of therapy are being met.
- Out of office follow up (ie, phone calls) may be helpful to reinforce the importance of adherence and to identify and manage any adverse effects.

CHRONIC LYMPHOCYTIC LEUKEMIA

Patient Assessment:

- Review history of present illness, physical exams, and laboratory values to determine whether immediate treatment is necessary.

Therapy Evaluation:

- Depending on the therapy, assess efficacy, adverse effects, and patient adherence.
- If patients continue to have disease progression, another regimen may be utilized.
- Monitor WBC count and signs of infection if the patient is receiving aggressive chemoimmunotherapy.

Care Plan Development:

- Address any concerns about the selected medication including cost and management of adverse effects.
- Supportive care medication such as remedications for the prevention of infusion reactions, prophylactic trimethoprim–sulfamethoxazole and an antiviral (acyclovir, famciclovir, or valacyclovir) may be recommended for certain medications.

Follow-up Evaluation:

- Asymptomatic patients will be routinely follow-up to determine when they require treatment.
- Routine follow-ups during and postchemotherapy will be needed to assess treatment efficacy.

MULTIPLE MYELOMA

Patient Assessment:

- Review medical history, including patient's age, comorbid conditions and current medications to determine whether the patient is transplant eligible.

Therapy Evaluation:

- If patients continue to have disease progression or have relapsed disease, another regimen may be utilized.
- Monitor myeloma monoclonal protein in urine and serum, renal function, hemoglobin, and platelets.
- Assess safety of medications including the monitoring of peripheral neuropathy. Dose reduction may be necessary to prevent permanent neurologic damage.
- Supportive care including bisphosphonates, pain medications and prophylactic anticoagulation may be required depending on the medication selected.

Care Plan Development:

- Discuss the importance of medication adherence if oral therapy is chosen.

Follow-up Evaluation:

- Frequent follow-up is needed to determine efficacy or if another regimen should be used.
- Maintenance therapy posttransplantation requires additional follow-up and monitoring of adverse effects.

myeloma.[34,43] Low-dose dexamethasone with lenalidomide offers improved overall survival compared with high-dose dexamethasone.[43] The combination of melphalan, prednisone, and lenalidomide (MPL) may be used as initial therapy in transplant ineligible patients. The response rate appears to be quite high at 81% with 24% achieving a CR.[44] Lenalidomide lacks many of the common side effects seen with thalidomide. Significant adverse effects of lenalidomide include myelosuppression and DVTs. DVT prophylaxis is recommended with lenalidomide–dexamethasone combinations.[34,42] Stem cells should be collected shortly after starting lenalidomide because CD34-positive stem cell counts tend to decrease with prolonged lenalidomide exposure.[34] Maintenance lenalidomide after stem cell transplantation has been associated with an increase in progression free survival, however, with an increase in the incidence of secondary malignancies.[34]

Pomalidomide is the newest immunomodulatory agent used in the treatment of refractory or progressive MM. It was shown to increase PFS and OS when used in combination with dexamethasone in patients that were refractory to bortezomib and lenalidomide.[45] Adverse effects for pomalidomide include myelosuppression and an increase in infections.

▶ *Proteasome Inhibitors*

Bortezomib (Velcade) and carfilzomib (Kyprolis) are proteosome inhibitors approved for the treatment of MM. Proteosome inhibitors induce myeloma cell death by modulating nuclear factor kappa-B products, including inflammatory cytokines and adhesion molecules that support myeloma cell growth. These drugs also disrupt the myeloma microenvironment by inhibiting the binding of myeloma cells to the bone marrow stromal cells.[31] KEY CONCEPT *Bortezomib-based regimens are frequently used as induction therapy in transplant-eligible patients.* The response rates have been reported as high as 97% in newly diagnosed myeloma.[30] Bortezomib can also be given in combination with a corticosteroid and melphalan (MPB) in patients who are not transplant eligible. Superior response rates and survival are seen with the combination MPB compared MP.[44] Side effects of bortezomib include fatigue, nausea, peripheral neuropathy, and hematologic effects.[44] The incidence of DVT is lower than the immunomodulators; thus, bortezomib does not routinely require prophylactic anticoagulation. However, prophylactic acyclovir should be considered to reduce the risk of herpes zoster reactivations.[34] Carfilzomib is a newer second-generation proteasome inhibitor that is used in the treatment of refractory MM. Studies are also examining carfilzomib as primary therapy in combination regimens with an immunomodulator and dexamethasone.[46]

▶ *Bisphosphonates*

Bone disease is a common manifestation of MM. Bisphosphonates should be initiated in symptomatic patients with bone lesions to slow osteopenia and reduce the fracture risk associated with the disease. Pamidronate 90 mg and zolendronic acid 4 mg have equivalent efficacy in the management of osteolytic lesions.[47] The use of zolendronic acid decreases pain and bone-related complications and improves quality of life. Osteonecrosis of the jaw is a major concern with bisphosphonate therapy. Risk factors are unclear, but osteonecrosis of the jaw is more common in patients receiving IV administration of bisphosphonates and having dental procedures performed. It is recommended that patients have dental restoration work before starting bisphosphonate therapy. Several consensus guidelines have been published on the use of bisphosphonates and myeloma. Recommendations on the duration of therapy and which bisphosphonate to use have largely been left up to the practitioner.[34,48]

OUTCOME EVALUATION

Newly diagnosed, asymptomatic patients with MM may be observed without treatment. This asymptomatic period may last for months to a couple years. All patients with MM become symptomatic, and when this occurs, treatment is required. All patients should be evaluated for an autologous stem cell transplant. For patients who are eligible for transplant, induction therapy often consists of thalidomide or lenalidomide, bortezomib, and dexamethasone. Maintenance therapy with an immunomodulatory agent may be used posttransplant. There are numerous treatment options for transplant ineligible patients including MPT, MPB, or MPL. Nearly all patients progress at some point, and second-line therapy usually includes bortezomib. Monthly bisphosphonates should be given to patients who have bone lesions with the hope of reducing pain and fractures.

Abbreviations Introduced in This Chapter

CLL	Chronic lymphocytic leukemia
CML	Chronic myelogenous leukemia
CR	Complete response
DVT	Deep venous thrombosis
FISH	Fluorescence in situ hybridization
HSCT	Hematopoietic stem cell transplantation
MGUS	Monoclonal gammopathy of unknown significance
MP	Melphalan–prednisone
MPB	Melphalan–prednisone–bortezomib
MPL	Melphalan–prednisone–lenalidomide
MPT	Melphalan–prednisone–thalidomide
Ph	Philadelphia chromosome
Q-PCR	Qualitative and quantitative polymerase chain reaction
TKI	Tyrosine kinase inhibitor
WBC	White blood cell

REFERENCES

1. Pinilla-Ibarz J, Bello C. Modern approaches to treating chronic myelogenous leukemia. Curr Oncol Rep. 2008;10:365–371.
2. Siegel R, Ma J, Zou Z, Jemal A. Cancer statistics, 2014. CA Cancer J Clin. 2014;64:9–29.
3. National Comprehensive Cancer Network Clinical Practice Guidelines in Oncology [Internet]. Chronic Myelogenous Leukemia, version 3. 2014. http://www.nccn.org.
4. Kantargian HM, Cortes J, La Rosee P, Hochhaus A. Optimizing therapy for patients with chronic myelogenous leukemia in chronic phase. Cancer. 2010;116:1419–1430.
5. Aguayo A, Couban S. State-of-the-art in the management of chronic myelogenous leukemia in the era of the tyrosine kinase inhibitors: Evolutionary trends in diagnosis, monitoring and treatment. Leuk Lymphoma. 2009:50(Suppl 2):1–8.
6. Khan DL, Bixby DL. BCR-ABL inhibitors: Updates in the management of patients with chronic-phase chronic myeloid leukemia. Hematology. 2014;19(5):249–258.
7. Martin M, Dipersio JF, Uy GL. Management of the advances phases of chronic myelogenous leukemia in the era of tyrosine kinase inhibitors. Leuk Lymphoma. 2009;50(1):14–23.
8. Jabbour EJ, Cortes JE, Kantarjian HM. Resistance to tyrosine kinase inhibition therapy for chronic myelogenous leukemia:

A clinical perspective and emerging treatment options. Clinical Lymphoma Myeloma Leuk. 2013;13(5):515–529.
9. Gafter Gvili A, Leader A, Gurion R, et al. High-dose imatinib for newly diagnosed chronic phase chronic myeloid leukemia patients: Systematic review and meta-analysis. Am J Hematol. 2011;86:657–662.
10. Marin D. Initial choice of therapy among plenty for newly diagnosed chronic myeloid leukemia. Hematology. 2012; 115–121.
11. Jabbour EJ, Kanterjian J. CME information: Chronic myeloid leukemia: 2014 update on diagnosis, monitoring and management. Am J Hematol. 2014;89(5):547–556.
12. Santos FPS, Ravandi F. Advances in treatment of chronic myelogenous leukemia-new treatment options with tyrosine kinase inhibitors. Leuk Lymphoma. 2009;50(Suppl 2):16–26.
13. Ponatinib: A review of its use in adults with chronic myeloid leukaemia or Philadelphia chromosome-positive acute lymphoblastic leukaemia. Drugs. 2014;74:793–806.
14. Kantarjian H, Shah NP, Hochhaus A, et al. Dasatinib versus imatinib in newly diagnosed chronic-phase chronic myeloid leukemia. N Engl J Med. 2010;362:2260–2270.
15. Saglio G, Kim DW, Issaragrisil S, et al. Nilotinib versus imatinib for newly diagnosed chronic myeloid leukemia. N Engl J Med. 2010;362:2251–2259.
16. Cortes JE, Kim DW, Kantarjian HM, et al. Bosutinib versus imatinib in newly diagnosed chronic-phase chronic myeloid leukemia: Results from the BELA trial. J Clin Oncol. 2012;30:3486–3492.
17. Alvandi F, Kwitkowski VE, Ko CW, et al. U.S. Food and Drug Administration approval summary: Omacetaxine mepesuccinate as treatment for chronic myeloid leukemia. Oncologist. 2014;19:94–99.
18. Wierda WG, O'Brien S. Chronic lymphocytic leukemias. In: Devita VT, Hellman S, Rosenberg SA, eds. Cancer: Principles and Practice of Oncology, 9th ed. Philadelphia: Lippincott, 2011.
19. Hallek M. Signaling the end of chronic lymphocytic leukemia. Blood. 2013;122(23)3723–3734.
20. Kaufman M, Campian JL, Rai KR. Management of chronic lymphocytic leukemia: An update. Community Oncology. 2009;6(6):271–278.
21. Chiorazzi N. Implications of new prognostic markers in chronic lymphocytic leukemia. Hematology Am Soc Hematol Educ Program. 2012;2012:78–87.
22. National Comprehensive Cancer Network Clinical Practice Guidelines in Oncology. Non-Hodgkin's Lymphoma, version 3. 2014, http://www.nccn.org.
23. Wierda WG. Current and investigational therapies for patients with CLL. Hematology Am Soc Hematol Educ Program. 2006:285–294.
24. Hillmen P. Advancing therapy for chronic lymphocytic leukemia—the role of rituximab. Semin Oncol. 2004;31(Suppl 2):22–26.
25. Shah A. Obinutuzumab: A novel anti-CD20 monoclonal antibody for previously untreated chronic lymphocytic leukemia. Ann Pharmacother. 2014;48(10):1–6.
26. O'Brien S. Targeted agents in chronic lymphocytic leukemia. Clin Adv Hematol Oncol. 2014;12(1) (Suppl 3):9–11.
27. Byrd JC, Brown JR, O'Brien S, et al. Ibrutinib versus ofatumumab in previously treated chronic lymphoid leukemia. N Eng J Med 2004;371(3):213-23.
28. Furman RR, Sharman JP, Coutre SE. Idelalisib and rituximab in relapsed chronic lymphocytic leukemia. N Engl J Med. 2014;370(11):997–1007.
29. Terasawa T, Trikalinos NA, Djulbegovic B, Trikalinos TA. Comparative efficacy of first-line therapies for advanced-stage chronic lymphocytic leukemia: A multiple-treatment meta-analysis. Cancer Treat Rev. 2013;39(4):340–349.
30. Palumbo A, Anderson K. Multiple myeloma. N Engl J Med. 2011;364:1046–1060.
31. Munshi NC, Anderson KC. Plasma cell neoplasms. In: Devita VT, Hellman S, Rosenberg SA, eds. Cancer: Principles and Practice of Oncology, 9th ed. Philadelphia: Lippincott, 2011.
32. Greipp PR, San Miguel J, Durie BGM, et al. International staging system for multiple myeloma. J Clin Oncol. 2005;23: 3412–3420.
33. Mikhael JR, Dingli D, Roy V, et al. Management of newly diagnosed symptomatic multiple myeloma: Updated Mayo Stratification of Myeloma and Risk-Adapted Therapy (mSMART) consensus guidelines 2013. Mayo Clin Proc. 2013;88(4): 360–376.
34. National Comprehensive Cancer Network Clinical Practice Guidelines in Oncology [Internet]. Multiple Myeloma, version 2. 2014. http://www.nccn.org.
35. Kumar S. Treatment of newly diagnosed multiple myeloma in transplant-eligible patients. Curr Hematol Malig Rep. 2011;6: 104–112.
36. Child JA, Morgan GJ, Davies FE, et al. High-dose chemotherapy with hematopoietic stem-cell rescue for multiple myeloma. N Engl J Med. 2003;348:1875–1883.
37. Lacy MQ. New immunomodulatory drugs in myeloma. Curr Hematol Malig Rep. 2011;6:120–125.
38. Kaufman JL, Nooka A, Vrana M, et al. Bortezomib, thalidomide, and dexamethasone as induction therapy for patients symptomatic multiple myeloma: A retrospective study. Cancer. 2010;116(13):3134–3151.
39. Palumbo A, Bringhen S, Rossi D, et al. Bortezomib-melphalan-prednisone-thalidomide followed by maintenance with bortezomib-thalidomide compared with bortezomib-melphalan-prednisone for initial treatment of multiple myeloma: A randomized controlled trial. J Clin Oncol. 2010;28: 5101–5109.
40. Facon T, Mary JY, Hulin C, et al. Melphalan and prednisone plus thalidomide versus melphalan and prednisone alone or reduced-intensity autologous stem cell transplantation in elderly patients with multiple myeloma (IFM 99–06): A randomized trial. Lancet. 2007;370:1209–1218.
41. Morgan GJ, Gregory WM, Davies FE, et al. National Cancer Research Institute Haematological Oncology Clinical Studies Group. The role of maintenance thalidomide therapy in multiple myeloma: MRC Myeloma IX results and meta-analysis. Blood. 2012;119(1):7–15.
42. Palumbo A, Rajkumar SV, Dimopoulous MA, et al. Prevention of thalidomide- and lenalidomide-associated thrombosis in myeloma. Leukemia. 2008;22(2):414–423.
43. Rajkumar SV, Jacobus S, Callander NS, et al. Lenolidomide plus high-dose dexamethasone versus lenalidomide plus low-dose dexamethasone as initial therapy for newly diagnosed multiple myeloma: An open-label randomized controlled trial. Lancet Oncol. 2010;11:29–37.
44. Kyle RA, Rajkumar SV. Multiple myeloma. Blood. 2008; 111(6):2962–2972.
45. Leleu X, Attal M, Arnulf B, et al. Pomalidomide plus low-dose dexamethasone is active and well tolerated in bortezomib and lenalidomide refractory multiple myeloma: Intergroupe Francophone du Myélome 2009-02. Blood. 2013;121(11):1968–1975.
46. Rajkumar SV. Doublets, triplets or quadruplets of novel agents in newly diagnosed myeloma. Hematology Am Soc Hematol Educ Program. 2012;2012:354–361.
47. Rosen LS, Gordon D, Kaminski M, et al. Long-term efficacy and safety of zoledronic acid compared with pamidronate

disodium in the treatment of skeletal complications in patients with advanced multiple myeloma or breast carcinoma: A randomized, double-blind, multicenter, comparative trial. Cancer. 2003;98:1735–1744.

48. Lacy MQ, Dispenzieri A, Gertz MA, et al. Mayo clinic consensus statement for the use of bisphosphonates in multiple myeloma. Mayo Clin Proc. 2006;81:1047–1053.

49. Kyle Ra, Yee GC, Somerfield MR, et al. American Society of Clinical Oncology 2007 clinical practice guideline update on the role of bisphosphonates in multiple myeloma. J Clin Oncol. 2007;25:2462–2472.

97

Malignant Lymphomas

Keith A. Hecht and Susanne E. Liewer

LEARNING OBJECTIVES

Upon completion of the chapter, the reader will be able to:

1. Discuss the underlying pathophysiologic mechanisms of the lymphomas and how they relate to presenting symptoms of the disease.
2. Differentiate the pathologic findings of Hodgkin lymphoma (HL), follicular indolent non-Hodgkin lymphoma (NHL), and diffuse aggressive NHL and how this information yields a specific diagnosis.
3. Describe the general staging criteria for the lymphomas and how it relates to prognosis; evaluate the role of the prognostic systems such as the International Prognostic Score for HL, the Follicular Lymphoma International Prognostic Index, and the International Prognostic Index for diffuse, aggressive NHL.
4. Compare and contrast the treatment algorithms for early and advanced stage disease for HL.
5. Delineate the clinical course of follicular indolent and diffuse aggressive NHL and the implications for disease classification schemes and treatment goals.
6. Outline the general treatment approach to follicular indolent and diffuse aggressive NHL for localized and advanced disease.
7. Interpret the current role for monoclonal antibody therapy in NHL.
8. Assess the role of autologous hematopoietic stem cell transplantation for relapsed lymphomas.

INTRODUCTION

The malignant lymphomas are a clonal disorder of hematopoiesis with the primary malignant cells consisting of lymphocytes of B-, T-, or natural killer (NK) cell origin. Lymphoma cells predominate in the lymph nodes; however, they can infiltrate lymphoid and nonlymphoid tissues, such as the bone marrow, central nervous system (CNS), gastrointestinal (GI) tract, liver, mediastinum, skin, and spleen. An overview of the lymph node regions is depicted in Figure 97–1. KEY CONCEPT *There are two broad classifications of lymphoma, Hodgkin lymphoma (HL) and non-Hodgkin lymphoma (NHL), and both contain numerous histologic subtypes that are pathologically distinct disease entities.*

The clinical course varies widely among histologies of lymphoma. More aggressive lymphoma subtypes are highly proliferating tumor cells that require aggressive therapeutic intervention with chemotherapy, radiation therapy, or both. By contrast, certain subtypes of NHL are characterized by a disease course that flares and remits intermittently over a period of years regardless of treatment.

HODGKIN LYMPHOMA

EPIDEMIOLOGY AND ETIOLOGY

Approximately 9050 new cases of HL were estimated to be diagnosed in the United States in 2015, with 1150 deaths attributed to the disease.[1] The incidence of HL is bimodal, with its peaks occurring in the third decade of life and in patients older than 50 years of age.[2] The precise cause of HL is unknown, but certain associations have been reported and provide insight about possible etiologic factors. Epstein-Barr virus (EBV) has been associated with HL, its viral genome is detected in Reed-Sternberg (RS) cells in up to 40% of cases in developed countries. Other viruses (cytomegalovirus, human herpes viruses, HIV, and adenoviruses) have been associated with HL; however, data is conflicting.[2] Other possible risk factors identified include woodworking and a familial history of HL.

PATHOPHYSIOLOGY

Pluripotent stem cells in the bone marrow are able to differentiate to both lymphoid and myeloid progenitor cells. Lymphoid progenitor cells undergo normal gene rearrangement to yield either B-cell or T-cell lineage precursor cells. Normal maturation for naive B cells includes expression of cell surface antibody or the cells typically undergo apoptosis. These cells are differentiated from other B cells, such as memory cells, by virtue of cell surface antigen ($CD5^+$ or $CD5^-$ and $CD27^-$) and bound antibody (IgM+ and IgD+). When naive B cells recognize antigen with their cell surface antibody, they accumulate in the lymph nodes, spleen, or other lymphoid tissue. The DNA of these B cells is susceptible to three different types of genetic modification: receptor editing, somatic hypermutation, and class switching within the germinal center of the lymph node. Germinal centers are microanatomic structures located within lymph nodes that develop

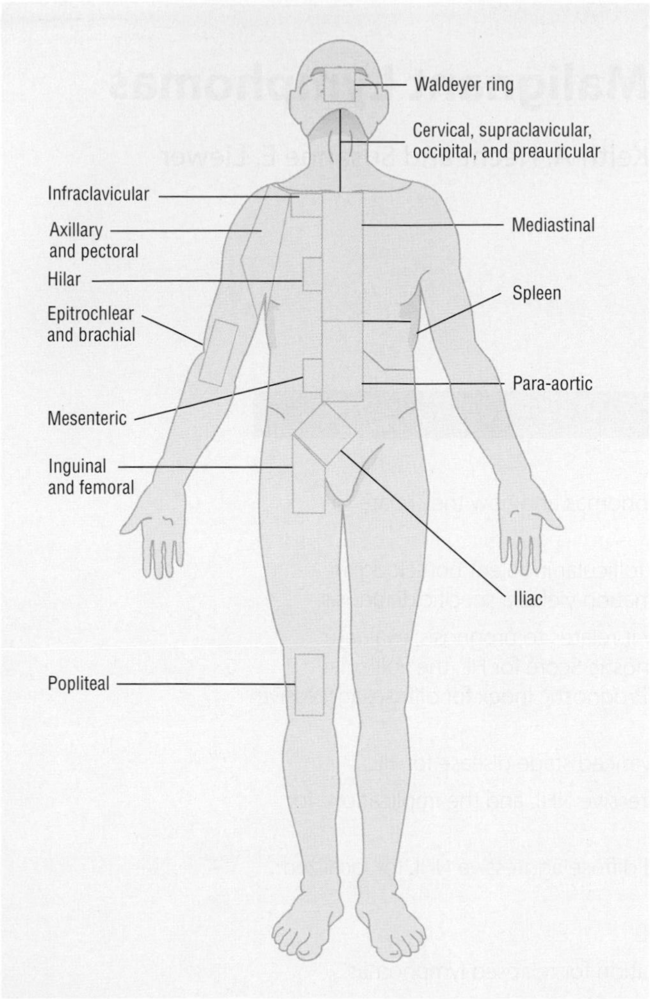

FIGURE 97–1. Representation of the anatomic regions used in the staging of Hodgkin disease. (From Rosenberg SA. Staging of Hodgkin disease. Radiology. 1966;87:146.)

with clonal B-cell expansion secondary to antigen stimulation. Under normal circumstances, these genetic changes allow for adaptation of the immune system to the repeated exposure to environmental antigens.

The pathophysiology of HL is defined by the presence of the RS cell in a grouping of lymph nodes. The RS cell is a morphologically large cell with a multinucleated structure possessing pronounced eosinophilic nucleoli, thought to be B- cell in origin.[3] In the affected lymph nodes, the RS cells are contained within an inflammatory background that is believed to be essential for their survival.

RS cells have lost the expression of most B-cell markers. Common cell-surface antigens expressed by RS cells include CD30 and CD15, but other common B-cell antigens, such as CD20 are inconsistently expressed.[4] The Janus kinase-signal transduction and transcription (JAK-STAT) signaling pathway has also been found to be active in HL. Additionally, the overexpression of nuclear factor kappa-B (NF-κB), a proliferative and antiapoptotic transcription factor nuclear factor is believed to contribute to the expansion and survival of RS cells.[5]

HL is classified into disease subtypes based on the number and morphologic appearance of RS cells and the background cellular milieu. These are listed in the World Health Organization (WHO) classification of lymphoid neoplastic diseases in Table 97–1.[6] Nodular sclerosing (70%) is the most common

Table 97–1

WHO Classification of Lymphoid Neoplasms

B-Cell Neoplasms
Precursor B-cell neoplasm
Precursor B-lymphoblastic leukemia/lymphoma
Mature (peripheral) B-cell neoplasms
B-cell chronic lymphocytic leukemia/small lymphocytic lymphoma
B-cell prolymphocytic leukemia
Lymphoplasmacytic lymphoma
Splenic marginal zone B-cell lymphoma (+/– villous lymphocytes)
Hairy cell leukemia
Plasma cell myeloma/plasmacytoma
Extranodal marginal zone B-cell lymphoma of MALT type
Nodal marginal zone B-cell lymphoma (+/– monocytoid B cells)
Follicular lymphoma
Mantle cell lymphoma
Diffuse large B-cell lymphoma
Mediastinal large B-cell lymphoma
Primary effusion lymphoma
Burkitt lymphoma/Burkitt cell leukemia
T-Cell and NK-Cell Neoplasms
Precursor T-cell neoplasm
Precursor T-lymphoblastic lymphoma/ALL
Mature (peripheral) T-cell neoplasms
T-cell prolymphocytic leukemia
T-cell granular lymphocytic leukemia
Aggressive NK cell leukemia
Adult T-cell lymphoma/leukemia (HTLV1+)
Extranodal NK/T-cell lymphoma, nasal type
Enteropathy-type T-cell lymphoma
Hepatosplenic gamma-delta T-cell lymphoma
Subcutaneous panniculitis-like T-cell lymphoma
Mycosis fungoides/Sézary syndrome
Anaplastic large-cell lymphoma, T/null cell, primary cutaneous type
Peripheral T-cell lymphoma, not otherwise characterized
Angioimmunoblastic T-cell lymphoma
Anaplastic large-cell lymphoma, T/null cell, primary systemic type
HL
Nodular lymphocyte-predominant HL
Classical HL
Nodular sclerosis HL
Lymphocyte-rich classical HL
Mixed cellularity HL
Lymphocyte depletion HL

ALL, acute myeloid leukemia; HL, Hodgkin lymphoma; MALT, mucosa-associated lymphoid tissue; NK, natural killer.

form of HL. It is more common in young adults and is marked by the presence of the RS variant cell, the lacunar cell. The second most common form of HL is the mixed-cellularity variant (20%), with others accounting for the remainder of cases.[4] Factors identified as negative disease prognostic indicators are listed in Table 97–2.

TREATMENT OF HL

Desired Outcome

Staging of HL with a standard classification is necessary to guide treatment. The extent and location of involvement, localized or disseminated extranodal disease, and B symptoms are factors in assignment of stage. The Cotswold staging system,

Table 97–2

Negative Prognostic Factors for HL

International Prognostic Score—Advanced HL	
Albumin < 4 g/dL (40 g/L)	
Hemoglobin < 10.5 g/dL (105 g/L; 6.52 mmol/L)	
Male sex	
Age > 45 years	
Stage IV disease	
WBC ≥ 15,000/mm³ (15 × 10⁹/L)	
Lymphocytopenia (count < 600/mm³ [0.6 × 10⁹/L], < 8% [0.08] of WBC count, or both)	

WBC, white blood cell.

a revision of the original Ann Arbor classification, is outlined in Table 97–3.[7]

KEY CONCEPT *The principal goal in treating HL is to cure the patient of the primary malignancy.* HL is sensitive to both radiation and chemotherapy, resulting in an 80% rate of cure with modern therapy. Treatment strategy is generally divided into approaches for early stage I/II localized disease and stage III/IV advanced disease. Patients with early stage I/II disease are further classified into favorable, unfavorable with bulky disease, and unfavorable with nonbulky disease. Regardless of stage, all patients are treated with curative intent. Other goals during treatment include:

- Complete resolution of disease symptoms
- Incorporation of supportive care measures to optimize quality of life during therapy
- Minimization of acute and long-term treatment-related toxicity

Table 97–3

Cotswold Staging Classification for Hodgkin Disease (1989 Revision of Ann Arbor Staging)[a]

Stage	Description
I	Involvement of a single lymph node region or lymphoid structure (eg, spleen, thymus, Waldeyer ring)
II	Involvement of two or more lymph node regions on the same side of the diaphragm; the number of anatomic sites is indicated by a subscript
III	Involvement of lymph node regions or structure on both sides of the diaphragm III_1: With or without involvement of splenic, hilar, celiac, or portal nodes III_2: Involvement of para-aortic, iliac, or mesenteric
IV	Involvement of extranodal site(s) beyond that designated E
Designations Applicable to All Stages	
A	No symptoms
B	Fever, night sweats, and weight loss
X	Bulky disease: greater than one-third the width of the mediastinum or > 10 cm maximal dimension of nodal mass
E	Involvement of a single extranodal site, contiguous or proximal to a known nodal site
CS	Clinical stage
PS	Pathologic stage

[a]Also used for non-Hodgkin lymphoma.

Clinical Presentation and Diagnosis of Malignant Lymphomas

General

Nonspecific; can range from an asymptomatic patient with a less aggressive lymphoma to a patient who is gravely ill with advanced disease.

KEY CONCEPT Symptoms

- *Lymphadenopathy, generally in the cervical, axillary, supraclavicular, or inguinal lymph nodes*
- *Splenomegaly*
- *Shortness of breath, dry cough, chest pressure (patients with mediastinal mass)*
- *GI complications (nausea, vomiting, early satiety, constipation, and diarrhea)*
- *Back, chest, or abdominal pain*

Signs

- Fever[a]
- Night sweats[a]
- Weight loss greater than 10% within last 6 months[a]
- Pruritus

Laboratory Tests

- LDH
- ESR
- Serum chemistries
- CBC with differential

KEY CONCEPT Other Diagnostic Tests

- *Physical examination with careful attention to lymph node inspection.*
- *Imaging—chest x-ray, chest CT, abdominal or pelvic CT; integrated PET and CT is recommended as part of the initial workup.*
- *Bone marrow biopsy.*
- *Biopsy of suspected lymph node(s)—either open lymph node biopsy (preferred) or core biopsy; fine-needle aspiration should only be performed if preferred biopsy methods are unobtainable.*
- *Hematopathology evaluation of biopsy specimen—morphologic inspection, immunohistochemistry for cell surface antigens to characterize lymphoma cells, cytogenetic analysis.*

[a]Known collectively as B symptoms.

CBC, complete blood count; CT, computed tomography; ESR, erythroid sedimentation rate; LDH, lactate dehydrogenase; PET, positron emission tomography.

Patient Encounter, Part 1: Initial Evaluation

A 52-year-old woman with a medical history of hypertension and hypothyroidism presents to the oncologist upon recommendation of her primary care provider for suspicion of new onset lymphoma. She was in her usual state of health until 2 months ago when she started experiencing fevers and night seats. Upon physical examination the oncologist notes palpable lymph nodes in the left and right inguinal areas as well as the right axilla area. The patient reports that she has reduced exercise tolerance but no other impairments of his activities of daily living. Complete blood count revealed a WBC of 16, 000/mm^3 (16 × 10^9/L), hemoglobin of 9 g/dL (90 g/L; 5.59 mmol/L) and platelets were 165,000/mm^3 (165 × 10^9/L). The chemistry panel was unremarkable.

What tests should be performed to confirm a diagnosis of lymphoma and determine its overall stage?

Based on the information provided, what is her International Prognostic Score, and how does it impact treatment selection?

Nonpharmacologic Therapy

Radiation therapy is effective in the treatment of HL and has cured patients of their disease. Historically, patients with favorable early stage I/II disease were treated with radiation alone. However, long-term toxicities associated with this practice have precluded this approach. Current treatment strategies combine radiation with chemotherapy. This has been reported to reduce the irradiated volume and dose as well as the number of cycles of chemotherapy.

Historically in the treatment of HL, the radiation fields were large and often included the lungs, liver, heart, and breast. Today, the use of involved-field radiotherapy (IFRT) limits radiation to the involved area. In addition to the smaller radiation volumes, other organs such as the breast, heart, and lungs have reduced exposure.[8]

Treatment with radiotherapy produces significant toxicity of acute and delayed onset. Acute effects of irradiation include nausea, vomiting, anorexia, xerostomia, dysgeusia, pharyngitis, dry cough, fatigue, diarrhea, and rash. These effects are typically transient, resolving shortly after completion of treatment. Delayed effects from radiotherapy are concerning in as they may be permanent and present months to years after therapy. Pneumonitis, pericarditis, hypothyroidism, infertility (with pelvic field irradiation), coronary artery disease, deformities in bone and muscle growth in children, herpes zoster reactivation, and Lhermitte sign are not uncommon. Patients cured with radiotherapy are at increased risk for new cancers of the breast, lung, and stomach, as well as melanoma and new NHL, depending on the radiation field.

Pharmacologic Therapy

▶ *Early Stage Disease*

KEY CONCEPT *Initial treatment of HL includes combination chemotherapy, these regimens are effective and have acceptable long-term toxicities.* Combined modality therapy of two to four cycles ABVD (doxorubicin, bleomycin, vinblastine, and dacarbazine) plus 20 to 30 Gy (Gray, the absorbed radiation dose) of IFRT or two cycles Stanford V chemotherapy plus 30 Gy of IRFT is the preferred treatment of patients with favorable stage I/II HL. Patients with favorable disease have: an erythrocyte sedimentation rate less than 50 mm/hour, no extralymphatic lesions, and one or two lymph nodes involved. Restaging should occur after a minimum of two cycles of chemotherapy. IFRT should be initiated within 3 weeks for patients who achieve a complete response (CR) or a partial response (PR). After completion of IFRT, no further treatment is necessary for patients with a CR, further restaging is required for patients with PR to therapy.

ABVD or Stanford V followed by IFRT is recommended for patients with unfavorable, bulky disease. Four cycles of ABVD are given before restaging. For patients with a CR, IFRT is administered alone or in combination with two more cycles of ABVD. Patients with a PR will receive two additional cycles of chemotherapy. If there is response, patients then receive IFRT followed by end of treatment assessment to determine disease response. Patients with unfavorable, nonbulky disease receive ABVD for two cycles followed by interim staging. Two to four more cycles are recommended guided by the response to chemotherapy. The use of the Stanford V regimen should be considered for patients with mediastinal disease, bulky disease, B symptoms, or unfavorable nonbulky disease.[9] A listing of chemotherapy regimens used in HL is presented in Table 97–4.

Table 97–4

Common Treatment Regimens in HL

MOPP—Every 28 Days
Mechlorethamine 6 m/m^2 IV × 1, days 1 and 8
Vincristine 1.4 mg/m^2 IV × 1, days 1 and 8
Procarbazine 100 mg/day po, days 1–14
Prednisone 40 mg/day po, days 1–14

ABVD—Every 28 Days
Doxorubicin 25 mg/m^2 IV × 1, days 1 and 15
Bleomycin 10 units IV × 1, days 1 and 15
Vinblastine 6 mg/m^2 × 1, days 1 and 15
Dacarbazine 375 mg/m^2 IV × 1, days 1 and 15

Stanford V
Doxorubicin 25 mg/m^2 IV weeks 1, 3, 5, 7, 9, and 11
Vinblastine 6 mg/m^2 IV weeks 1, 3, 5, 7, 9, and 11
Mechlorethamine 6 mg/m^2 IV weeks 1, 5, and 9
Etoposide 60 mg/m^2 IV weeks 3, 7, and 11
Vincristine 1.4 mg/m^2 IV weeks 2, 4, 6, 8, 10, and 12
Bleomycin 5 mg/m^2 IV weeks 2, 4, 6, and 8
Prednisone 40 mg po every other day for 12 weeks, start taper at week 10

BEACOPP (Escalated)—Every 21 Days
Bleomycin 10 mg/m^2 IV, day 8
Etoposide 200 mg/m^2 IV daily × days 1–3
Doxorubicin 35 mg/m^2, day 1
Cyclophosphamide 1200 mg/m^2 IV, day 1
Vincristine 1.4 mg/m^2 IV, day 8
Procarbazine 100 mg/m^2 po daily, days 1–7
Prednisone 40 mg po daily, days 1–14

BEAM (High-Dose With Autologous SCT)a
Carmustine 300 mg/m^2 IV × 1 day
Etoposide 100–200 mg/m^2 IV every 12 hours × 4 days
Cytarabine 100–200 mg/m^2 IV every 12 hours × 4 day
Melphalan 140 mg/m^2 IV × 1 day

[a]Used for both Hodgkin lymphoma and non-Hodgkin lymphoma.
IV, intravenous; po, oral; SCT, stem cell transplantation.

▸ *Advanced Disease*

Patients with advanced disease can be further classified into two groups based on IPS. (see Table 97–2) Patients with three or fewer poor prognostic factors are considered to have favorable disease while patients with four or more factors have unfavorable disease. Patients who have at least four of the criteria may warrant more aggressive treatment.

Trials have focused on the use of multiagent chemotherapy for six to eight total cycles. The combination chemotherapy regimen MOPP (mechlorethamine, vincristine, procarbazine, and prednisone) is of historical significance because it was the first chemotherapy regimen to cure HL in the 1960s. However, significant toxicity, including sterility and secondary leukemia led to the development of new regimens. ABVD was compared with MOPP or ABVD–MOPP alternating.[10] This pivotal phase III trial comparing these regimens in patients with stage III/IV HL documented a higher CR in the ABVD arms. A recent update of the data shows superior 18-year freedom from progression in the ABVD arms compared to MOPP though a survival advantage has yet to be demonstrated.[11] ABVD is now considered standard therapy for initial treatment of stage III or IV HL. Further information on ABVD may be found in Table 97–5.

Additional regimens such as Stanford V and BEACOPP were developed to improve the outcomes of patients with advanced HL. Except in patients with high risk disease (IPS greater than 3) the Stanford V regimen has demonstrated similar response rates to ABVD reported for event-free survival, overall survival, and toxicity.[12] A dose-escalated regimen of BEACOPP (with colony-stimulating factor [CSF] support) was compared with a standard-dose BEACOPP and also COPP (cyclophosphamide substituted for mechlorethamine in MOPP) alternating with ABVD. The dose-escalated BEACOPP was superior to the other arms in both freedom from treatment failure and overall survival at 10 years.[13] However, the escalated BEACOPP regimen is associated with more toxicity including infertility and more cases of secondary leukemia. Currently, neither BEACOPP regimen is widely used in the United States but is considered for advanced HL with a high number of poor prognostic factors.

Despite the high success rate in treating HL, approximately 5% to 10% of patients will be refractory to initial treatment and 10% to 30% will relapse after initial response. Patients relapsing after treatment should be offered additional therapy as durable responses have been reported. The duration of remission after chemotherapy remains a vital prognostic factor for likelihood of response to future treatment.[14] For healthy patients, the definitive therapy after relapse is high-dose chemotherapy with autologous stem cell transplantation (SCT).[15] This treatment offers a cure rate of approximately 40%.

Several studies have reported the importance of giving conventional chemotherapy before SCT. The purpose of the initial treatment after relapse is to decrease the tumor bulk before high-dose chemotherapy. The safety profile of autologous SCT continues to improve as refinements in supportive care are realized. Current estimates of mortality from autologous SCT for HL are approximately 5%. Morbidity commonly associated with preparative regimens in HL, aside from infectious and bleeding complications, includes the additive pulmonary toxicity of bleomycin coupled with carmustine, inducing potentially fatal pulmonary pneumonitis.

Patients who are not candidates for autologous SCT may receive standard salvage chemotherapy, such as etoposide, methylprednisolone, cytarabine, and cisplatin (ESHAP) or dexamethasone, cytarabine, and cisplatin (DHAP). Newer regimens such as GVD (gemcitabine, vinorelbine, and pegylated liposomal doxorubicin), IGEV (ifosfamide, gemcitabine, and vinorelbine) and GCD (gemcitabine, carboplatin, and dexamethasone) have also been effective for relapsed refractory HL. Brentuximab vedotin is a monoclonal antibody approved for the treatment of relapsed or refractory HL. It targets CD-30 and is linked to a microtubule-disrupting agent, monomethylauristatin E.[16] This agent has been effective in heavily pretreated HL patients. Clinical trials are currently ongoing to further define the role of brentuximab.

NON-HODGKIN LYMPHOMA

EPIDEMIOLOGY AND ETIOLOGY

Approximately 71850 cases of NHL were estimated to be diagnosed in the United States in 2015, with an estimated 19,790 deaths. These figures represent a stabilization in the incidence of

Table 97–5

Practical Information for ABVD and CHOP

Regimen	Drug Class	Pharmacokinetics	Unique Toxicities
ABVD			
Doxorubicin	Anthracycline	Hepatic metabolism[a]	Highly emetogenic Cardiomyopathy Maximum cummulative lifetime dose, 550 mg/m^2
Bleomycin	Antitumor antibiotic	Renal clearance[a]	Pulmonary fibrosis Maximum cummulative lifetime dose, 400 mg
Vinblastine	Vinca alkaloid	CYP 3A4/5 metabolism[a]	Neuropathy, constipation
Dacarbazine	Alkylating agent	Hepatic metabolism[a]	Myelosuppression
CHOP			
Cyclophosphamide	Alkylating agent	Prodrug; CYP3A4/5, 2D6	Highly emetogenic Hemorrhagic cystitis
Doxorubicin	Anthracycline	Hepatic metabolism	Cardiomyopathy
Vincristine	Vinca alkaloid	CYP3A4/5	Neuropathy, constipation
Prednisone	Corticosteroid	100% oral bioavailability	Hyperglycemia, osteopenia

[a]See dose adjustments (Chapter 88).

NHL since 1998 that follows a dramatic increase that had nearly doubled the number of cases in the United States since 1950.[2,17] The increase may be related to the development of aggressive NHL in patients with HIV, although the overall increase is independent of HIV disease, particularly for patients older than 65 years of age. The median age for diagnosis is 50 years, although children and young adults may also be affected. The etiology of certain aggressive NHL subtypes is related to specific endemic geographic factors. Follicular or low-grade lymphoma is more common in the United States and Europe and is relatively uncommon in the Caribbean, Far East, Middle East, or Africa. The human T-cell leukemia virus I induces T-cell lymphoma or leukemia in both Japan and the Caribbean. Human herpes virus 8, and hepatitis C have been implicated in inducing NHL. Lymphomas of the GI tract are more prevalent in patients with celiac sprue, inflammatory bowel disease, or *Helicobacter pylori* infection. The incidence of Burkitt NHL is 7 cases per 100,000 people in Africa compared with 0.1 per 100,000 in the United States. Malaria or EBV is thought to contribute to the chronic B-lymphocyte stimulation that leads to malignant transformation in Burkitt NHL. EBV has been shown to transform lymphocytes in vitro to a monoclonal malignant population, which is believed to drive the development of disease in patients who are in a chronically immunosuppressed state. Patients with congenital diseases such as Wiskott-Aldrich syndrome, common variable hypogammaglobinemia; X-linked lymphoproliferative syndrome.[18] Environmental factors have been identified as contributing to the development of NHL. Certain occupations such as wood and forestry workers, butchers, exterminators, grain millers, machinists, mechanics, painters, printers, and industrial workers have a higher prevalence of disease. Industrial chemicals such as pesticides, herbicides, organic chemicals (eg, benzene), solvents, and wood preservatives are also associated with NHL.

PATHOPHYSIOLOGY

The pathophysiology of NHL is governed by numerous environmental and genetic events culminating with a monoclonal population of malignant lymphocytes. B cells represent the cells of origin in excess of 90% of cases. Figure 97–2 outlines normal B-cell

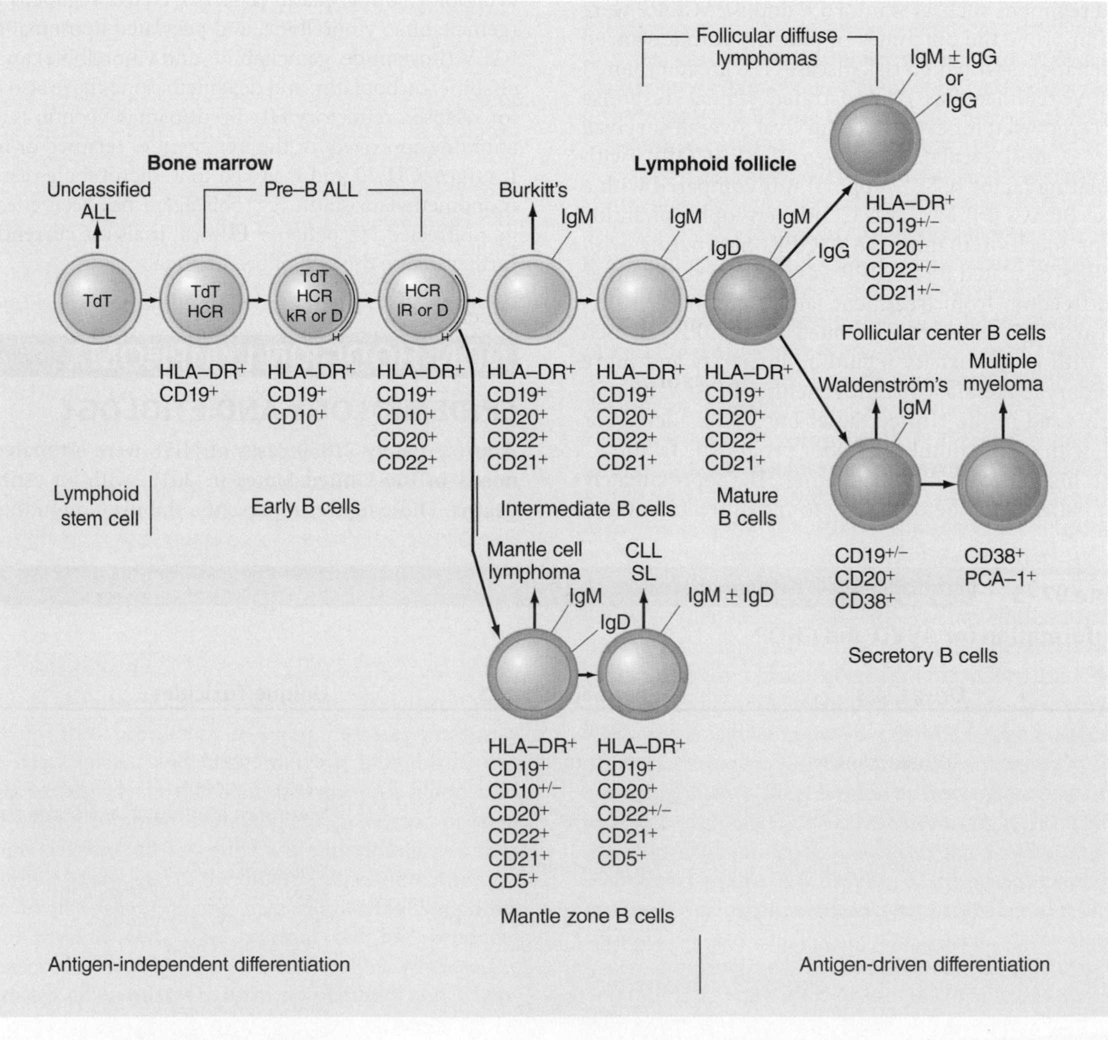

FIGURE 97–2. Pathway of normal B-cell differentiation and relationship to B-cell lymphocytes. (ALL, acute lymphoblastic leukemia; HLA, human leukocyte antigen; HCR, human chemokine receptor; Ig, immunoglobulin; TdT, terminal deoxynucleotidyl transferase.) (From Longo DL. Longo D.L. Chapter 110. Malignancies of Lymphoid Cells. In: Longo DL, Fauci AS, Kasper DL, Hauser SL, Jameson J, Loscalzo J. Longo D.L., Fauci A.S., Kasper D.L., Hauser S.L., Jameson J, Loscalzo J eds. *Harrison's Principles of Internal Medicine, 18e.* New York, NY: McGraw-Hill; 2012.)

maturation with accompanying cell-surface antigens. Evolving data are correlating chromosomal mutations with specific disease subtypes. Cytogenetic abnormalities involving translocations of antigen receptor genes are prevalent in NHL. These include T-cell receptor genes in T-cell lymphomas and immunoglobulin genes in B-cell lymphomas. The principal defect appears to be an error in the assembly of the regulatory gene segment of an antigen receptor gene, resulting in inappropriate binding to an oncogene. This results in dysregulation of cell growth and proliferation, leading to the malignant clone of lymphocytes. Oncogenes identified in different lymphomatous diseases include *c-myc, bcl-1, bcl-2, bcl-3, NF-κB,* and *bcl-6*.[19] Classic translocations for NHL include t(8;14) in Burkitt lymphoma, t(14;18) in follicular lymphomas, t(11;14) mantle cell lymphoma, and t(11;18)/t(1;14) in mucosa-associated lymphoid tissue (MALT).

KEY CONCEPT *Characterization of the morphology of the lymphocytes, the reactivity of the other cells in the lymph node, and the lymph node architecture are essential in obtaining a diagnosis and predicting disease course.* The nodal presentation of NHL is divided into two main categories: follicular, corresponding to low-grade disease, and diffuse, corresponding to aggressive disease. A follicular disease pattern in the inspected lymph node is indicative of a more indolent or low-grade progression that has survival measured in years if left untreated. In contrast, a diffuse pattern of lymph node infiltration is a marker of highly aggressive disease, resulting in death within weeks to months if untreated. Follicular NHL is the most common indolent subtype, comprising 22% of NHL. Diffuse, large B-cell lymphoma is the most common aggressive histology, comprising 31% of NHL. The cells of origin for follicular NHL tend to be more mature, nondividing lymphocytes, whereas aggressive NHL is derived from rapidly dividing lymphoid precursors. A unique feature of the biology of NHL is that follicular low-grade histologies can undergo further malignant transformation, transforming further into a diffuse, large B-cell lymphoma population. This syndrome, called Richter transformation, may occur in up to 20% of follicular low-grade lymphoma patients and involves multiple genetic events, including abnormalities of chromosomes 11 and 12 and tumor suppressor genes. Richter transformation may also occur in patients with chronic lymphocytic leukemia, which results in a transformation to diffuse lymphoma.[20]

The classification of NHL has undergone several revisions as the histology, molecular biology, and clinical course have been more precisely defined. Classification schemes such as the Working Formulation categorize disease on aggressiveness into three categories: low grade—survival estimated in years without treatment, intermediate grade—survival estimated in months without treatment, and high grade—survival measured in days to weeks for untreated disease (Table 97–6). This scheme is limited in its clinical applicability because the large number of distinct diseases that are not categorized by this classification. The WHO has updated a classification scheme published in 1994 by the International Lymphoma Study Group called the *Revised European American Classification of Lymphoid Neoplasms* (REAL) that broadly categorizes histologic subtypes into B- and T-cell subtypes. This newer classification incorporates immunologic morphologic and genetic and clinical attributes of various NHL histologies.

Prognostic factors present at diagnosis have been identified for NHL. Age, the presence of B symptoms, performance status, number of nodal and extranodal sites, lactate dehydrogenase level, bulky disease (greater than 10 cm), advanced stage, and β_2-microglobulin concentration have been shown to be important prognostic features in NHL. Table 97–7 shows the International

Table 97–6

Working Formulation for NHL

Classification	Immunophenotype
Low Grade	
Small lymphocytic	100% B cell
Follicular, small cleaved cell	100% B cell
Follicular, mixed small cleaved cell and large cell	100% B cell
Intermediate Grade	
Follicular, large cell	100% B cell
Diffuse, small cleaved cell	75% B cell, 20% T cell, 5% null cell
Diffuse, mixed small and large cell	75% B cell, 20% T cell, 5% null cell
Diffuse, large cell	70% B cell, 20% T cell, 10% null cell
Diffuse, large cell	70% B cell, 20% T cell, 10% null cell
High Grade	
Immunoblastic	50% B cell, 50% T cell
Lymphoblastic	5% B cell, 95% T cell
Diffuse, small noncleaved cell	100% B cell

[a]Lymphomas not included in the working formulation: *Mycosis fungoides*, mantle cell lymphoma, monocytoid B-cell lymphoma, mucosa-associated lymphoid tissue, anaplastic large cell lymphoma, angiocentric lymphoma, angioimmunoblastic lymphadenopathy, Castleman disease, adult T-cell leukemia/lymphoma.

Prognostic Index (IPI), a predictive model for aggressive NHL to be treated with doxorubicin-containing chemotherapy regimens.[21] This index is used as a tool to identify patients who may benefit from a more intense treatment regimen. Additionally, patients with diffuse aggressive B-cell lymphoma that is of germinal center type carry a better prognosis than other patients.[22] A model similar to the IPI, the Follicular Lymphoma International Prognostic Index (FLIPI), is used to help guide treatment decisions in follicular lymphoma.[23]

TREATMENT OF NHL

Desired Outcome

Treatment of NHL depends primarily on histologic subtype (follicular low grade versus diffuse aggressive) and staging (local stage I/II versus advanced stage III/IV) to guide treatment with observation, chemotherapy, radiation, or chemotherapy and radiation. The Cotswold modification of the Ann Arbor staging system for HL is used in NHL as well.

Treatment goals depend on the patient's specific subtype of NHL. For follicular low-grade NHL, the disease is considered to be incurable with standard therapies. Many patients with follicular lymphoma are older than 60 years of age, making allogeneic SCT impractical due to high treatment-related mortality for older patients.

KEY CONCEPT *The treatment goals for low-grade NHL include:*

- *Observation of the disease until the patient exhibits obvious progression that limits functional capacity or is life threatening*
- *Treatment that induces remission with manageable toxicity*
- *Judicious selection of treatment options to avoid long-term toxicity*
- *Prevention of infectious complications*

Table 97–7

Negative Prognostic Factors for NHL

International Prognostic Index—Diffuse, Aggressive NHL

Criteria	Risk Group	Number of criteria
Age 60 years or older		
Stage III/IV disease	Low	0–1
Extranodal disease greater than one site	Low-intermediate	2
ECOG performance status 2 or greater	High-intermediate	3
Serum LDH > 1 × normal limit	High	4–5

Follicular Lymphoma International Prognostic Index

Criteria	Risk Group	Number of criteria
Age 60 years or older		
Stage III/IV disease	Low	0–1
Hemoglobin < 12.0 g/dL (120 g/L; 7.45 mmol/L)	Intermediate	2
Serum LDH > 1 × normal limit	High	3 or more
Number of nodal sites ≥ 5[a]		

[a]The nodal map used in the Follicular Lymphoma International Prognostic Index is different than the nodal map used in conventional staging.

Table 97–8

Chemotherapy Regimens for Low-Grade, Follicular NHL

Fludarabine/Rituximab
Fludarabine 25 mg/m^2 IV days 1–5 every 28 days
Rituximab 375 mg/m^2 IV, days 1 and 5 of week 1 and 26; single dose 72 hours before fludarabine cycles 2, 4, and 6

Bendamustine/Rituximab—Every 28 Days
Bendamustine 90 mg/m^2 IV days 1 and 2
Rituximab 375 mg/m^2 IV, day 1

rCVP—Every 21 Days
Rituximab 375 mg/m^2 IV, day 1
Cyclophosphamide 750 mg/m^2 IV, day 1
Vincristine 1.4 mg/m^2 IV, day 1
Prednisone 40 mg/m^2 po daily, days 1–5

rCHOP—Every 21 Days
Rituximab 375 mg/m^2 IV, day 1
Cyclophosphamide 750 mg/m^2 IV, day 1
Doxorubicin 50 mg/m^2 IV, day 1
Vincristine 1.4 mg/m^2 IV, day 1
Prednisone 100 mg/day po, days 1–5

IV, intravenous; po, oral.

The intent of treatment for patients with aggressive histologies is cure of the malignancy. Some histologic subtypes exhibit an aggressive clinical course and are not considered to be curable. These patients are still treated with curative-intent chemotherapy or may be considered for a clinical trial.

Nonpharmacologic Therapy

For patients with low-grade follicular NHL, deferring initiation of therapy until progression of disease is a standard approach. The median survival time is 6 to 10 years. Some patients may be asymptomatic for several years after initial diagnosis, making observation a reasonable approach. Radiation therapy has a limited role in NHL relative to HL. NHL is more often a systemic disease, and radiation typically has been reserved for consolidation after chemotherapy in patients presenting with a large extranodal mass. However, IFRT without systemic therapy is a treatment option for patients with stage I/II follicular lymphoma.

For early-stage diffuse, aggressive NHL, combined-modality therapy was tested versus a longer course of chemotherapy.[24] Overall survival favored the CHOP–radiation arm for 5 years (82% vs 72%). There was a trend toward increased toxicity, particularly hematologic and cardiac toxicity, in the CHOP alone arm. The results of this trial have established combined-modality therapy as first-line treatment for early stage NHL.

Pharmacologic Therapy

► *Follicular Low-Grade NHL*

The management of low-grade lymphomas is an area of controversy, especially in patients presenting with early stage disease. Typical indications for treatment include cytopenias, recurrent infections, threatened end-organ function, disease progression over at least 6 months, or patient preference. In these patients, chemotherapy such as fludarabine or bendamustine is typically offered initially. In patients in whom a more rapid response is desired, such as patients with advanced disease, multiagent chemotherapy such as CVP (cyclophosphamide, vincristine, and prednisone) or CHOP may be used. These regimens, detailed in Table 97–8, have not been associated with an improvement in overall survival, making it impossible to select an unequivocal first-line regimen.[25–27]

Rituximab is also an integral component in drug therapy for this disease. Rituximab is a chimeric monoclonal antibody that binds specifically to CD20 expressed on B lymphocytes.[28] NHL of B-cell origin expresses CD20 in greater than 90% of cases. The initial clinical experience with rituximab involved 166 patients with CD20+ low-grade lymphoma treated with four doses of 375 mg/m^2 of rituximab weekly.[29] The overall response rate was 48%, with CR in 6% of patients. The median follow-up of 12 months demonstrated a median time to progression of 13 months. This established rituximab as a viable treatment option in patients with indolent follicular NHL, typically added to chemotherapy in most patients. Additionally, rituximab was examined as maintenance therapy administered every 8 weeks for 2 years after rituximab-containing multiagent chemotherapy. Compared with observation, rituximab increased 3-year PFS (74.9 vs 57.6 months).[30]

Other strategies for treatment of low-grade lymphomas include the combination of monoclonal antibodies directed against CD20 with a radiopharmaceutical attached and a new kinase inhibitor active against B-cells. Ibritumomab-yttrium 90 is a monoclonal antibody targeting CD20 that delivers radioactive yttrium. It is indicated for the treatment of relapsed follicular lymphoma or as consolidation after response to initial chemotherapy. Idelalisib is a small molecule that inhibits PI3Kδ kinase found in B-cells, inducing apoptosis and inhibiting chemotaxis. It was approved for follicular lymphoma based on a phase I study in patients who had failed multiple prior therapies. These heavily pretreated patients had an overall response rate of 45%.[31] High-dose chemotherapy is being evaluated for low-grade follicular NHL, but its role is currently limited to clinical trials.

▶ *Diffuse, Aggressive NHL*

KEY CONCEPT *The mainstay of therapy for diffuse, aggressive NHL has been anthracycline-based combination chemotherapy, generally consisting of four or more drugs.* Therapy options for intermediate- and high-grade NHL generally are segregated between localized (stage I/II) and advanced (stage III/IV) disease. Combined-modality therapy with an abbreviated course of CHOP and local radiation is considered a standard of care for stage I/II disease.

The standard therapy for disseminated disease since the 1970s has been CHOP. This regimen conferred a response of 50% to 60%, with long-term survival of approximately 30%. However, the 1980s were notable for the development of newer combination chemotherapy regimens that incorporated increasing numbers of agents with varying schedules. A phase III clinical trial compared CHOP to three more intensive regimens in patients with intermediate or high-grade NHL (Working Formulation Classification).[32] There were no significant differences in response rate or overall survival between the groups. Severe toxicity and death were higher in the advanced-generation treatment programs relative to CHOP. This pivotal trial has cemented CHOP as first-line chemotherapy in diffuse NHL.

Rituximab is also routinely used to treat diffuse, aggressive NHL. Another study randomized patients 60 to 80 years of age with newly diagnosed disease to either CHOP for eight cycles or CHOP plus rituximab for eight cycles.[33] Two year follow-up showed rituximab improved CR (76% vs 63%) and median event-free survival (57% vs 38%) and long-term follow-up confirmed benefit was with an increase in 10-year survival (43% vs 27.6%). Similar findings have been reported in younger patients, making CHOP plus rituximab first-line therapy for advanced-stage diffuse, aggressive NHL (Table 97–9).

▶ *Special Populations*

There are histologic subtypes of diffuse, aggressive NHL that respond less well to treatment with conventional regimens such as CHOP. Burkitt lymphoma, lymphoblastic lymphoma, mantle cell lymphoma, and primary CNS lymphoma are examples of disease that benefit from more intensive therapy. Regimens such as hyper-CVAD, which alternate cycles of hyperfractionated cyclophosphamide, doxorubicin, vincristine, and dexamethasone with high-dose cytarabine and methotrexate, may be substituted for CHOP.

Patients with CNS NHL have disease that is poorly responsive to therapy because of inadequate penetration of standard doses of chemotherapy across the blood–brain barrier. High-dose methotrexate, ranging from 2500 to 8000 mg/m^2 is a mainstay of therapy. Treatment may also include intrathecal chemotherapy. Drugs that are commonly instilled intrathecally include

Table 97–9

Treatment Regimens for Diffuse, Aggressive NHL

rCHOP—Every 21 Days[a]

EPOCH-Rituximab—Every 21 Days
Rituximab 375 mg/m^2 IV, day 1
Etoposide 50 mg/m^2/day CIVI days 1–4
Prednisone 60 mg/m^2/day po, days 1–5
Vincristine 0.4 mg/m^2/day CIVI days 1–4
Cyclophosphamide 750 mg/m^2 IV day 5
Doxorubicin 10 mg/m^2/day CIVI days 1–4

RCEOP—Every 21 Days[b]
Rituximab 375 mg/m^2 IV, day 1
Cyclophosphamide 750 mg/m^2 IV, day 1
Etoposide 50 mg/m^2 IV, day 1
Etoposide 100 mg/m^2 po days 2–3
Vincristine 1.4 mg/m^2 IV, day 1
Prednisone 100 mg/day po, days 1–5

CNOP-Rituximab—Every 21 Days[b]
Rituximab 375 mg/m^2 IV, day 1
Cyclophosphamide 750 mg/m^2 IV, day 1
Mitoxantrone 10 mg/m^2 IV, day 1
Vincristine 1.4 mg/m^2 IV, day 1
Prednisone 100 mg/day po, days 1–5

Hyper-CVAD
Part A: The following drugs given on course 1, 3, 5 and 7
Cyclophosphamide 300 mg/m^2 IV every 12 hours, days 1–3 (with Mesna)
Doxorubicin 50 mg/m^2 IV, day 1
Vincristine 1.4 mg/m^2 IV, days 1,11
Dexamethasone 40 mg/day po, days 1–4 and 11–14
Methotrexate 15 mg intrathecal, day 2
Cytarabine 30 mg intrathecal, day 2
Hydrocortisone 15 mg intrathecal, day 2

Part B: The following drugs are given on courses 2, 4, 6, and 8
Methotrexate 1000 mg/m^2 IV over 24 hours, day 1
Cytarabine 3000 mg/m^2 IV every 12 hours, days 2 and 3
Leucovorin 25 mg IV × 1; then 25 mg po every 6 hours for seven doses
Methotrexate 15 mg intrathecal, day 2

Bendamustine/Rituximab—Every 28 Days[a]

ESHAP
Etoposide 40 mg/m^2 IV per day continuous infusion, days 1–4
Cisplatin 25 mg/m^2 IV per day continuous infusion, days 1–4
Cytarabine 2000 mg/m^2 IV × 1, day 5
Methylprednisone 250 mg IV every 12 hours, days 1–4

DHAP
Dexamethasone 40 mg po or IV daily, days 1–4
Cisplatin 100 mg/m^2 IV continuous infusion, day 1
Cytarabine 2000 mg/m^2 IV every 12 hours for two doses on day 2

ICE
Etoposide 100 mg/m^2 IV daily, days 1–3
Carboplatin AUC 5 (maximum dose, 800 mg) IV, day 2
Ifosfamide 5000 mg/m^2 IV continuous infusion × 1 on day 2 (with 100% replacement with Mesna)

[a]Refer to Table 97–8 for regimen.
[b]Data is limited, use only for patients who are unable to receiving an anthracycline.
AUC, area under the curve; CIVI, continuous intravenous infusion; IV, intravenous; po, oral.

Patient Encounter, Part 2: Treatment Selection

Complete evaluation revealed stage IV Hodgkin lymphoma and therapy is scheduled to begin immediately.

What therapy (or therapies) is (are) most appropriate for this patient?

At this time is this patient an appropriate candidate for stem cell transplant?

What other information (eg, laboratory studies, diagnostic tests) is needed prior to initiating chemotherapy?

methotrexate, cytarabine (conventional formulation and liposomal products), and corticosteroids.

The recent appreciation of *H. pylori* colonization and MALT has spurred the more aggressive treatment of this organism with antibiotics. In patients with localized disease, aggressive, combination therapy for *H. pylori* has been shown to induce MALT remission. Patients with advanced disease may require combination chemotherapy, such as CHOP.

Mantle cell lymphoma, which comprises 6% of NHL cases, is defined by a chromosomal translocation of t(11;14)(q13;32). This translocation results in the overexpression of cyclin D1 coupled with NF-κB, which plays a critical role in intracellular protein regulation and protranscription factors leading to increased cell survival. Bortezomib, a proteasome inhibitor, disrupts the regulation and degradation of proteins required for cell cycle regulation. It is approved by the FDA for the treatment of patients with mantle cell lymphoma who have failed prior chemotherapy. A study conducted in 155 patients demonstrated that bortezomib resulted in 31% overall response rate with a median survival of 9.3 months.[34] Bortezomib is well tolerated, with peripheral neuropathy, thrombocytopenia, neutropenia, and nausea reported most frequently.

With more than half of patients with NHL expected to relapse, salvage therapy plays a major role in the attempt to cure recurrence. Multiple drug regimens such as ESHAP and DHAP can induce a CR, but the long-term cure rate with these regimens is less than 10%. Salvage therapy can induce remissions with subsequent relapses; however, the chance for a CR and the duration of remission is further diminished.

High-dose chemotherapy with autologous SCT has been studied as an alternative to standard dose regimens in the setting of first relapse.[35] The best-studied indication for SCT is for patients with intermediate- or high-grade disease that fails to respond to first-line therapy. A 3- to 5-year survival of greater than 40% is achieved in patients who have good performance and disease that demonstrates a significant response to one or two cycles of salvage chemotherapy. The procedure-related mortality rate has ranged from 5% to 10% in published reports. However, as with HL, with more broad application of peripheral blood stem cells and improved supportive care, the mortality rate continues to decline. The role of allogeneic SCT in this setting is limited because of donor availability, the older age of patients, and the high treatment-related morbidity and mortality. Additionally, outcomes between autologous and allogeneic transplant appear similar.

Patients with HIV-related lymphoma represent a therapeutic dilemma considering many have high-grade NHL. A common presentation is that of extranodal disease, frequently in the GI tract, CNS, or bone marrow. Therapy for this population thus far has fared poorly, with a median survival time of 6 to 12 months, which decreases to 3 months with CNS involvement.[36] The addition of rituximab to chemotherapy has failed to improve overall survival in this patient population and is associated with increased infectious complications.[37]

Patient Encounter, Part 3: Creating a Care Plan

Based on the information presented, create a care plan for this patient, including the goals of therapy, antineoplastic therapy plan, and necessary supportive care.

OUTCOME EVALUATION

Treatment response in lymphomas is measured using the response evaluation criteria in solid tumors (RECIST), a uniform criteria assessing tumor response developed by the National Cancer Institute. Lymphomas may have residual masses after completion of treatment, adding to the difficulty in establishing a definitive remission from treatment. Clinical trials with limited numbers of patients have been published suggesting the value of positron emission tomography (PET) scans to rule out whether residual tumor masses after treatment contain viable tumor.[38] Integrated PET–computed tomography (CT) scanning is recommended as part of the initial workup and to evaluate for residual disease at the end of treatment.[39]

Long-term follow-up monitors patients for continued disease remission or relapse with careful examination of the original areas of involvement and imaging studies including chest x-rays and CT scans to detect recurrence. Patients also require long-term monitoring for toxicities of their treatment.

Most patients treated for lymphoma with chemotherapy or radiation notice a regression of palpable lymphadenopathy within days. This is because of the high sensitivity of the rapidly proliferating malignant lymphocytes to chemotherapy and radiotherapy. This necessitates implementation of tumor lysis syndrome precautions with aggressive intravenous hydration and allopurinol. Rasburicase should be considered for patients with moderate to high tumor burdens. Most chemotherapy treatments for lymphoma have a significant risk of infectious complications. Combination regimens for both HL and NHL are associated with rates of severe leukopenia and/or neutropenia ranging from 20% to 100% of patients. Consideration must be given to supportive care with prophylactic antibiotics and CSFs. Most chemotherapy regimens discussed in this section are highly emetogenic. Antiemetic regimens are available to control chemotherapy-induced nausea and vomiting well for most standard-dose regimens.[40]

Advances in the treatment of lymphoma have increased the number of long-term survivors. Identification of long-term complications of lymphoma therapy is vital to patient follow-up and may influence treatment decisions in newly diagnosed patients. Outcomes associated with the treatment of HL make up the majority of data. However, advances in NHL treatment have provided more information regarding long-term toxicities. Two leading causes of death associated with lymphoma treatment are secondary malignancies and cardiovascular disease.

The use of combined modality of irradiation with doxorubicin-based therapy has been reported to increase the risk of cardiac dysfunction. Treatment-related pulmonary toxicity, hypothyroidism, and infertility have been associated with lymphoma therapy as well. Lymphoma survivors have an increased risk for developing myelodysplasia, acute myelogenous leukemia, and various solid tumors.[41]

A limitation of rituximab is severe, potentially fatal infusion-related reactions. Deaths have been reported resulting from the profound hypotension and circulatory collapse seen with the drug, particularly on the first dose. The package labeling recommends premedication with acetaminophen and diphenhydramine before each infusion. The initial infusion should be given slowly, at 50 mg/hour. The infusion rate may be increased as tolerated to a maximum of 400 mg/hour. In the absence of infusion reactions, subsequent doses may be started at a higher rate and titrated more aggressively. Reactivation of hepatitis B infections has occurred in patients treated with rituximab. Patients at high risk for hepatitis B should be screened and monitored carefully for reactivation of hepatitis. If hepatitis occurs, rituximab should be discontinued, and patients should be treated appropriately. Other associated toxicities of rituximab include fever, chills, headache, asthenia, nausea, vomiting, angioedema, bronchospasm, and skin reactions. KEY CONCEPT *Rituximab is an effective treatment option for patients with various forms of NHL in combination with chemotherapy or as a single agent as long as patients are monitored appropriately.* The radiolabeled CD-20 antibody causes more myelosuppression than rituximab alone and has a long-term risk of inducing secondary leukemias.[42]

Patient Care Process

Patient Assessment:

- Take a thorough medication history with particular attention to nonprescription or herbal medications.
- Before initiation of treatment assess patient for risk of tumor lysis syndrome.

Therapy Evaluation:

- Determine the optimal treatment regimen for the patient incorporating diagnosis, stage, and prognostic indicators.
- Verify chemotherapy regimen doses with a standardized reference and assess for dose adjustment based on height, weight, and body surface area and organ dysfunction (renal or hepatic).
- Assess appropriateness of supportive care for the chemotherapy regimens including need for prophylactic antiemetics and use of colony-stimulating factors.

Care Plan Development:

- Provide patient education regarding common toxicities associated with chemotherapy such as nausea/vomiting, mucositis, myelosuppression, and alopecia.
- For doxorubicin-containing regimens, maintain records of the cumulative doxorubicin dosage received by the patient to monitor for cardiac toxicity risk.
- For bleomycin-containing regimens, maintain records of the cumulative bleomycin dosage received by the patient to monitor for pulmonary fibrosis.
- Educate patients regarding the short- and long-term complications associated with radiation therapy.
- Provide contact numbers for patient in the event of a fever and a response plan if the patient is considered to be at risk for neutropenic fever.

Follow-Up Evaluation:

- Schedule regulatory laboratory tests including complete blood count and blood chemistries to monitor for chemotherapy toxicities.
- Monitor patient for signs and symptoms of response of tumor to chemotherapy.
- Develop a plan to monitor for long term complications of chemotherapy such as cardiotoxicity and secondary malignanacies.

Abbreviations Introduced in This Chapter

Bcl-1	Important in the regulation of mitosis
Bcl-2	A regulator of apoptosis
Bcl 3	A regulator of nuclear transcription factor
Bcl-6	Regulates cell differentiation
c-myc	Regulator of gene transcription
ABVD	Doxorubicin, bleomycin, vinblastine, and dacarbazine
CHOP	Cyclophosphamide, doxorubicin, vincristine, and prednisone
CSFs	Colony-stimulating factors
CVP	Cyclophosphamide, vincristine, and prednisone
EBV	Epstein-Barr virus
FLIPI	Follicular lymphoma international prognostic index
HL	Hodgkin lymphoma
IFRT	Involved field radiation therapy
IPI	International Prognostic Index
LDH	Lactate dehydrogenase
MALT	Mucosa-associated lymphoid tissue
MOPP	Mechlorethamine, vincristine, procarbazine, and prednisone
NHL	Non-Hodgkin lymphoma
PET	Positron emission tomography
RECIST	Response evaluation criteria in solid tumors
RS	Reed-Sternberg
SCT	Stem cell transplant

REFERENCES

1. Siegel R, Ma J, Zou Z, Jemal A. Cancer statistics, 2014. CA Cancer J Clin. 2014;64:9–29.
2. Caporaso NE, Goldin LR, Anderson WF, Landgren O. Current insight on trends, causes and mechanisms of Hodgkin's lymphoma. Cancer J, 2009;15(2):117–123.
3. Kuppers R, Hansmann ML. The Hodgkin and Reed/Sternberg cell. Int J Biochem Cell Biol. 2005;37:511–517.
4. Eberle FC, Mani H, Jaffe ES. Histopathology of Hodgkin lymphoma. Cancer J. 2009;15(2):129–137.
5. Kuppers R. Molecular biology of Hodgkin lymphoma. Hematology Am Soc Hematol Educ Program. 2009:491–496.

6. Campo E, Swerdlow SH, Harris NL, et al. The 2008 WHO classification of lymphoid neoplasms and beyond: Evolving concepts and practical applications. Blood. 2011;117(19): 5019–5032.
7. Lister TA, Crowther D, Sutcliffe SB, et al. Report of a committee convened to discuss the evaluation and staging of patients with Hodgkin's disease: Cotswold meeting. J Clin Oncol. 1989;7: 1630–1636.
8. Yahalom J. Role of radiation therapy in Hodgkin's lymphoma. Cancer J. 2009;15(2):155–160.
9. Advani RH, Hoppe RT, Baer DM, et al. Efficacy of abbreviated Stanford V chemotherapy and involved field radiotherapy in early stage Hodgkin disease: Mature results of the G4 trial. Blood. 2009;114:1670a.
10. Canellos GP, Anderson JR, Propert KJ, et al. Chemotherapy of advanced Hodgkin disease with MOPP, ABVD, or MOPP alternating with ABVD. N Engl J Med. 1992;327:1478–1484.
11. Canellos GP, Niedzwiecki D, Johnson JL. Long-term follow-up of survival in Hodgkin's lymphoma. N Engl J Med. 2009;361: 2390–2391.
12. Hoskin PJ, Lowry L, Horwich A, et al. Randomized comparison of the stanford V regimen and ABVD in the treatment of advanced Hodgkin's Lymphoma: United Kingdom National Cancer Research Institute Lymphoma Group Study ISRCTN 64141244. J Clin Oncol. 2009;27(32):5390–5396.
13. Engert A, Diehl V, Franklin J, et al. Escalated-dose BEACOPP in the treatment of patients with advance-stage Hodgkin's lymphoma: 10 years of follow-up of the GHSG HD9 study. J Clin Oncol. 2009;27:4548–4554.
14. Quddus F, Armitage JO. Salvage therapy for Hodgkin lymphoma. Cancer J. 2009;15(2):161–163.
15. Linch DC, Winfield D, Goldstone AH, et al. Dose intensification with autologous bone-marrow transplantation in relapsed and resistant Hodgkin's disease: Results of a BLNI randomised trial. Lancet. 1993;341:1051–1054.
16. Chen R, Gopal AK, Smith SE. Results of a pivotal phase 2 study of brentuximabvedotin (SGN-35) in patients with relapsed or refractory Hodgkin lymphoma. ASH Annual Meeting Abstracts. 2010;116:283.
17. Fisher SG, Fisher RI. The epidemiology of non-Hodgkin lymphoma. Oncogene. 2004;23:6524–6534.
18. Evans LS, Hancock BW. Non-Hodgkin lymphoma. Lancet. 2003; 362:139–146.
19. Kuppers R, Klein U, Hansmann ML, Rajewsky K. Cellular origin of human B-cell lymphomas. N Engl J Med. 1999;341:1520–1529.
20. Tsimberidou AM, Keating MJ. Richter syndrome: Biology, incidence and therapeutic strategies. Cancer. 2005;103:216–228.
21. The International non-Hodgkin Lymphoma Prognostic Factors Project. A predictive model for aggressive non-Hodgkin lymphoma. N Engl J Med. 1993;329:987–994.
22. van Imhoff GW, Boerma EJ, van der Holt B, et al. Prognostic impact of germinal center-associated proteins and chromosomal breakpoints in poor risk diffuse large B-cell lymphoma. J Clin Oncol. 2006;24:4135–4142.
23. Solal-Celigny P, Roy P, Colombat P, et al. Follicular lymphoma international prognostic index. Blood. 2004;104:1258–1265.
24. Miller TP, Dahlberg S, Cassady JR, et al. Chemotherapy alone compared with chemotherapy plus radiotherapy for localized intermediate-and high-grade non-Hodgkin lymphoma. N Engl J Med. 1998;339:21–26.
25. Hagenbeek A, Eghbali H, Monfardini S, et al. Phase III intergroup study of fludarabine phosphate compared with cyclophosphamide, vincristine, and prednisone chemotherapy in newly diagnosed patients with stage III and IV low-grade malignant Non-Hodgkin lymphoma. J Clin Oncol. 2006;24:1590–1596.
26. Marcus R, Imrie K, Belch A, et al. CVP chemotherapy plus rituximab compared with CVP as first-line treatment for advanced follicular lymphoma. Blood. 2005;105:1417–1423.
27. Peterson BA, Petroni GR, Frizzera G, et al. Prolonged single-agent versus combination chemotherapy in indolent follicular lymphomas: A study of the cancer and leukemia group B. J Clin Oncol. 2003;21:5–15.
28. McCune SL, Gockerman JP, Rizzieri DA. Monoclonal antibody therapy in the treatment of non-Hodgkin lymphoma. JAMA. 2001;286:1149–1152.
29. McLaughlin P, Grillo-López AJ, Link BK, et al. Rituximab chimeric anti-CD20 monoclonal antibody therapy for relapsed indolent lymphoma: Half of patients respond to a four dose treatment program. J Clin Oncol. 1998;16:2825–2833.
30. Salles G, Seymour JF, Offner F, et al. Rituximab maintenance for 2 years in patients with high tumor burden follicular lymphoma responding to rituximab plus chemotherapy (PRIMA). Lancet. 2010;377:42–51.
31. Flinn IW, Kahl BW, Leonard JP, et al. Idelalisib, a selective inhibitor of phosphatidylinositol 3-kinase-δ, as therapy for previously treated indolent non-Hodgkin lymphoma. Blood 2014;123(22): 3406–3413.
32. Fisher RI, et al. Comparison of standard regimen (CHOP) with three intensive chemotherapy regimens for advanced non-Hodgkin lymphoma. N Engl J Med. 1993;328:1002–1006.
33. Coiffer B, Thieblemont C, Van Den Neste E, et al. Long-term outcome of patients in the LNH-98.5 trial, the first randomized study comparing rituximab-CHOP to standard CHOP chemotherapy in DLBCL patients: A study by the Groupe d'Etudes des Lymphomes de l'Adulte. Blood. 2010;116:2040–2045.
34. Kane RC, Dagher R, Farrell A, et al. Bortezomib for the treatment of mantle cell lymphoma. Clin Cancer Res. 2007;13:5291–5294.
35. Thierry P, Guglielmi C, Hagenbeek A, et al. Autologous bone marrow transplant as compared with salvage chemotherapy in relapses of chemotherapy-sensitive non-Hodgkin lymphoma. N Engl J Med. 1995;333:1540–1545.
36. Stebbing J, Marvin V, Bower M. The evidence-based treatment of AIDS-related non-Hodgkin's lymphoma. Cancer Treat Rev. 2004;30:249–253.
37. Kaplan LD, Lee JY, Ambinder RF, et al. Rituximab does not improve clinical outcome in a randomized phase III trial of CHOP with or without rituximab in patients with HIV-associated non-Hodgkin lymphoma: AIDS-Malignancies Consortium Trial 010. Blood. 2005;106:1538–1543.
38. Juweid ME, Wiseman GA, Vose JA, et al. Response assessment of aggressive non-Hodgkin's lymphoma by integrated International Workshop Criteria and fluorine-18-fluorodeoxyglucose positron emission tomography. J Clin Oncol. 2005;21:4652–4661.
39. Podoloff DA, Advani RH, Allred C, et al. NCCN task force report: positron emission tomography (PET)/computed tomography (CT) scanning in cancer. J Natl Compr Canc Netw. 2007;5(Suppl 1):S1–S22.
40. Kris MG, Hesketh PJ, Somerfield MR, et al. American Society of Clinical Oncology guideline for antiemetics in oncology: Update 2006. J Clin Oncol. 2006;17:2971–2994.
41. Ng AK, LaCasce A, Travis LB. Long-term complications of lymphoma and its treatment. J Clin Oncol. 2011;29:1885–1892.
42. Armitage JO, Carbone PP, Connors JM, Levine A, Bennett JM, Kroll S. Treatment-related myelodysplasia and acute leukemia in non-Hodgkin lymphoma patients. J Clin Oncol. 2003;21: 897–906.

98 Hematopoietic Stem Cell Transplantation

Christina Carracedo and Amber P. Lawson

LEARNING OBJECTIVES

Upon completion of the chapter, the reader will be able to:

1. Explain the rationale for using hematopoietic stem cell transplant (HSCT) to treat cancer.
2. Compare the different types of HSCTs, specifically (a) the types of donors (ie, autologous and allogeneic), (b) the source of hematopoietic cells (ie, umbilical cord, peripheral blood progenitor cells, and bone marrow), and (c) the type of preparative regimen (ie, myeloablative and nonmyeloablative).
3. List the nonhematologic toxicity to high-dose chemotherapy used in myeloablative preparative regimens, specifically busulfan-induced seizures, hemorrhagic cystitis, gastrointestinal toxicities, and sinusoidal obstruction syndrome.
4. Develop a plan for monitoring and managing engraftment of hematopoiesis.
5. Explain graft-versus-host disease (GVHD).
6. Recommend a prophylactic and treatment regimen for GVHD.
7. Choose an appropriate regimen to minimize the risk of infectious complications in HSCT patients.
8. Evaluate the long-term health care of HSCT survivors.

INTRODUCTION

KEY CONCEPT *Hematopoietic stem cell transplantation (HSCT) is a procedure used mainly to treat hematologic malignancies via high-dose chemotherapy and/or a graft-versus-tumor effect.* HSCT may be either autologous; where a patient receives their own bone marrow or allogeneic; where the patient receives bone marrow from a donor. As an alternative to bone marrow, hematopoietic stem cells may be obtained from the peripheral blood progenitor cells (PBPCs) or umbilical cord blood. Bone marrow and PBPCs contain pluripotent stem cells and postthymic lymphocytes, which are responsible for long-term hematopoietic reconstitution, called engraftment and immune recovery.[1]

The rationale of an autologous transplant is to administer myeloablative preparative regimen and eradicate the patient's malignancy. Collecting the bone marrow or PBPCs prior to administering high dose chemotherapy essentially protects the collected PBPCs from the effects of chemotherapy and can restore hematopoiesis. Allogeneic transplants use donor PBPCs to rescue the patient after myeloablative chemotherapy with of an added advantage of the donor cells generating an immunologic response towards the recipient's residual tumor, called the graft-versus-tumor effect. Unfortunately, graft-versus-host disease (GVHD) where the donor cells generate an immunologic response toward the recipient's normal tissue also occurs.

The type of HSCT performed depends on a number of factors, including the type and status of disease, availability of a compatible donor, patient age, performance status, and organ function. Examples of diseases treated with HSCT are listed in Table 98–1.

EPIDEMIOLOGY AND ETIOLOGY

Worldwide, approximately 35,000 autologous HSCTs and 25,000 allogeneic HSCTs are performed per year, with approximately one-third of allogeneic HSCTs using reduced-intensity preparative regimens. In the late 1990s, the number of allogeneic HSCTs reached a plateau, most likely related to the introduction of effective oral therapies for the treatment of newly diagnosed chronic-phase chronic myelogenous leukemia (CML), a disease that was historically managed with allogeneic HSCT. Furthermore, the limited availability of suitable donors may have also contributed to the plateau effect.[2]

The use of allogeneic PBPCs is increasing; from years 2007 through 2011, almost 80% of allogeneic HSCTs performed worldwide used PBPCs as the source of hematopoietic cells rather than bone marrow in adult patients.[2]

Autologous PBPC use has increased and essentially has replaced bone marrow as a graft source in many transplant centers. From years 2007 through 2011, approximately 99% of autologous HSCTs in adults and 94% in children used PBPCs as the source of hematopoietic cells.[2]

PATHOPHYSIOLOGY

KEY CONCEPT *Autologous HSCT, or infusion of a patient's own hematopoietic cells, allows for the administration of higher doses of chemotherapy, radiation, or both to treat the malignancy or autoimmune disorder.* In this setting, the hematopoietic cells "rescue" the recipient from otherwise dose-limiting hematopoietic toxicity. Autologous HSCT is used to treat intermediate- and

Table 98–1

Diseases Commonly Treated with HSCT

	Autologous Graft	Allogeneic Graft
Cancers	Multiple myeloma Non-Hodgkin lymphoma Hodgkin disease Neuroblastoma Germ cell tumors	Acute myeloid leukemia Acute lymphoblastic leukemia Chronic myeloid leukemia Myelodysplastic syndrome Myeloproliferative disorders Non-Hodgkin lymphoma Hodgkin disease Chronic lymphocytic leukemia Multiple myeloma
Other diseases	Autoimmune diseases Amyloidosis	Aplastic anemia Paroxysmal nocturnal hemoglobinuria Fanconi anemia Thalassemia major Sickle cell anemia Severe combined immunodeficiency Inborn errors of metabolism

high-grade non-Hodgkin lymphoma (NHL), multiple myeloma (MM), autoimmune diseases, and relapsed or refractory Hodgkin disease.[1] Patients do not benefit from an immunologic graft-versus-tumor effect while undergoing an autologous transplant; instead, the administration of high-dose chemotherapy followed by an autologous stem cell transplant in chemotherapy-sensitive malignancies relies on the preparative regimen alone to eradicate the malignant disease. Autologous HSCT circumvents the need for histocompatible donors, is associated with a lower mortality rate, and is not restricted to younger patients.[2]

KEY CONCEPT *Allogeneic HSCT involves the transplantation of hematopoietic cells obtained from a different person's (donor) bone marrow, peripheral blood, or umbilical cord blood to the recipient.* Unless the donor and the recipient are identical twins (referred to as a *syngeneic HSCT*), they are dissimilar genetically.

The transplanted donor stem cells or bone marrow is immunologically active, and thus there is potential for bidirectional graft rejection. When host-versus-graft reactions occur, cytotoxic T cells and natural killer (NK) cells belonging to the host (recipient) recognize minor histocompatibility (MHC) antigens of the graft (donor hematopoietic stem cells) and lead to a rejection response. When GVHD occurs, immunologically active cells in the graft recognize host MHC antigens and elicit an immune response. When host-versus-graft effects occur in allogeneic HSCT, they are referred to as *graft failure* or *rejection,* which results in ineffective hematopoiesis (ie, adequate absolute neutrophil count [ANC] and/or platelet counts were not obtained). Allogeneic HSCT is used to treat both nonmalignant conditions and hematologic malignancies such as acute and chronic leukemias.[1]

For both allogeneic and autologous transplants, hematopoietic cells are infused after the administration of a combination of chemotherapy and/or radiation, termed the conditioning or preparative regimen. KEY CONCEPT *A myeloablative preparative regimen involves the administration of sublethal doses of chemotherapy to the recipient to eradicate residual malignant disease. The recipient will not regain his or her own hematopoiesis and will be at risk for substantial life-threatening nonhematologic toxicity.* For those undergoing an autologous HSCT, their hematopoietic cells must be harvested and stored before the myeloablative preparative regimen is administered. After the administration of the myeloablative preparative regimen, these hematopoietic cells serve as a rescue intervention to reestablish bone marrow function and avoid long-lasting, life-threatening bone marrow aplasia. In the setting of an allogeneic HSCT, the preparative regimen is designed to suppress the recipient's immunity, eradicate residual malignancy, or create space in the marrow compartment. Improved survival outcomes have been observed with both autologous and allogeneic HSCT when the hematologic malignancy is in complete remission at the time of HSCT.[2] At most HSCT centers, age younger than 65 years and normal renal, hepatic, pulmonary, and cardiac function are considered eligibility requirements for myeloablative allogeneic HSCT.

The recognition of graft-versus-tumor effect, which likely is caused by cytotoxic T lymphocytes in the donor stem cells in those undergoing a allogeneic HSCT transplant, led to investigations with nonmyeloablative transplants, in which less toxic preparative regimens are used in the hope of expanding the availability of HSCT to recipients whose medical condition or age prohibits use of myeloablative regimens.

A myeloablative or **nonmyeloablative preparative regimen** may be used for allogeneic HSCT; only myeloablative preparative regimens are used for autologous HSCT.

Histocompatibility

Histocompatibility differences between the donor and the recipient necessitate immunosuppression after an allogeneic HSCT because considerable morbidity and mortality are associated with graft failure and GVHD. Rejection is least likely to occur with a syngeneic donor. In patients without a syngeneic donor, initial HLA typing is conducted on family members because the likelihood of complete histocompatibility between unrelated individuals is remote. Siblings are the most likely individuals to be histocompatible within a family. The chance for complete histocompatibility occurring in an individual with only one sibling is 25%. Approximately 40% of patients with more than one sibling will have an HLA-identical match. Having a matched-sibling donor is no longer a requirement for allogeneic HSCT because improved immunosuppressive regimens and the National Marrow Donor Program have allowed an increase in the use of unrelated or related matched or mismatched HSCTs. The use of alternative sources of allogeneic hematopoietic cells, such as related donors mismatched at one or more HLA loci or phenotypically (ie, serologically) matched unrelated donors, has been evaluated.[5] Establishment of the National Marrow Donor Program has helped to increase the pool of potential donors for allogeneic HSCT. Through this program, an HLA-matched unrelated volunteer donor might be identified. Recipients of an unrelated graft are more likely to experience graft failure and acute GVHD relative to recipients of a matched-sibling donor. Determination of histocompatibility between potential donors and the patient is completed before allogeneic HSCT. Initially, HLA typing is performed using blood samples and compatibility for class I MHC antigens (ie, HLA-A, HLA-B, and HLA-C) is determined through serologic and DNA-based testing methods. In vitro reactivity between donor and recipient also can be assessed in mixed-lymphocyte culture, a test used to measure compatibility of the MHC class II antigens (ie, HLA-DR, HLA-DP, and HLA-DQ). Currently, most clinical and research laboratories are also performing molecular DNA typing using polymerase chain reaction (PCR) methodology to determine the HLA allele sequence.[3]

The preparative regimen or GVHD prophylaxis may be altered based on the mismatch between the donor and the recipient. The risk of graft failure decreases with better matches such that those with a class I (ie, HLA-A, HLA-B, or HLA-C) antigen mismatch have the highest risk of rejection; those with just one class I allele mismatch have a minimal risk. Graft failure does not appear to be associated with mismatch at a single class II antigen or allele. GVHD and survival have been associated with disparity for classes I and II antigens and alleles.[4]

Stem Cell Sources

KEY CONCEPT *Bone marrow, PBPCs, and umbilical cord blood can serve as the source of hematopoietic cells. The optimal cell source differs based on the donor and recipient characteristics.*

Hematopoietic stem cells are obtained from bone marrow or peripheral blood. The technique for harvesting hematopoietic cells depends on the anatomic source (ie, bone marrow or peripheral blood). A surgical procedure is necessary for obtaining bone marrow. Multiple aspirations of marrow are obtained from the anterior and posterior iliac crests until a volume with a sufficient number of hematopoietic stem cells is collected (ie, 600–1200 mL of bone marrow). The bone marrow then is processed to remove fat or marrow emboli and usually is infused intravenously into the patient similar to a blood transfusion.

The shift to the use of PBPCs over bone marrow for HSCT is primarily because of the more rapid engraftment and decreased health care resource use. For an autologous transplant, the harvest occurs before administering the preparative regimen; therefore, autologous hematopoietic cells must be cryopreserved and stored for future use.

Allogeneic cells are usually harvested just prior to the HSCT and administered to the recipient without cryopreservation; however, they are sometimes collected and cryopreserved as well. The bone marrow may need additional processing if the donor and recipient are ABO incompatible, which occurs in up to 30% of HSCTs. Red blood cells (RBCs) may need to be removed before infusion into the recipient to prevent immune-mediated hemolytic anemia and thrombotic microangiopathic syndromes.

Transplantation with PBPCs essentially has replaced bone marrow transplantation (BMT). PBPCs are obtained by administering a mobilizing agent(s) followed by apheresis, which is an outpatient procedure similar to hemodialysis. Hematopoietic growth factors (HGFs) alone or in combination with myelosuppressive chemotherapy are used for **mobilization** of autologous PBPCs with similar results.[5] HGFs are also used to mobilize donor PBPCs for allogeneic transplants, although chemotherapy is not used in this setting.

Transplant with umbilical cord blood offers an alternative stem cell source to patients requiring an allogeneic transplant who do not have an acceptable matched related or unrelated donor. When allogeneic hematopoietic cells are obtained from umbilical cord blood, the cord blood is obtained from a consenting donor in the delivery room after birth and delivery of the placenta. The cord blood is processed, a sample is sent for HLA typing, and the cord blood is frozen and stored for future use. Numerous umbilical cord blood registries exist, with the goal of providing alternative sources of allogeneic stem cells. One potential limitation to the use of umbilical cord blood transplants is the inability to use donor-lymphocyte infusions in the event of relapse. Engraftment is slower in umbilical cord blood transplants, with a potential lower risk of GVHD and similar survival rates relative to BMT.[1,6] In children receiving an umbilical cord blood graft from an unrelated donor, cell dose (eg, nucleated cells) is related to engraftment, transplant-related morbidity, and survival.[7] Although there were initial concerns regarding whether a umbilical cord blood transplant could provide enough nucleated cells to engraft adequately within an adult, there is growing experience to indicate that a umbilical cord blood transplant is feasible when at least 1×10^7 nucleated cells per kilogram of recipient body weight are administered.[11] The prospective use of dual umbilical cord units and *ex vivo* expansion of umbilical cord units to obtain adequate engraftment are methods currently under exploration.

TREATMENT

Desired Outcome

KEY CONCEPT *Engraftment is defined as the point at which a patient can maintain a sustained ANC of greater than 500 cells/mm^3 (0.5×10^9/L) and a sustained platelet count of 20,000/mm^3 (20×10^9/L) or more lasting 3 or more consecutive days without transfusions[8] and is the desired short term outcome in a transplant.* The desired long-term outcome with HSCT is to cure the patient of his or her underlying disease while minimizing the short- and long-term morbidity associated with HSCT.

Nonpharmacologic Therapy

▸ Harvesting, Preparing, and Transplanting Autologous and Allogeneic Hematopoietic Cells

Autologous Transplants The HGFs granulocyte-macrophage colony-stimulating factor (sargramostim, Leukine) and granulocyte colony-stimulating factor (filgrastim, Neupogen) are used as mobilizing agents. The use of pegylated granulocyte colony-stimulating factor (pegfilgrastim, Neulasta) for mobilization of PBPCs appears more convenient and is promising as a mobilization agent; however, further data are needed regard ing graft composition, HSCT outcomes, and donor safety in allogeneic donations before widespread use of this agent can be recommended.

The combination of chemotherapy with an HGF enhances PBPC mobilization relative to HGF alone.[1] In addition to treating the underlying malignancy, this approach lowers the risk of tumor cell contamination and the number of apheresis collections required, but there is a greater risk of neutropenia and thrombocytopenia. The HGF is initiated after completion of chemotherapy and is continued until apheresis is complete. Many centers monitor the number of cells that express the CD34 antigen (ie, CD34+ cells) to determine when to start apheresis. The CD34 antigen is expressed on almost all unipotent and multipotent colony-forming cells and on precursors of colony-forming cells but not on mature peripheral blood cells. Apheresis is continued daily until the target number of PBPCs per kilogram of the recipient's weight is obtained. For adult recipients, the number of CD34+ cells correlates with time to engraftment. Lower yield of CD34+ cells is associated with administration of stem cell toxic drugs (eg, carmustine and melphalan) and intensive prior chemotherapy or radiotherapy, which should be avoided prior to transplant if possible.

If patients are unable to obtain an adequate yield of CD34+ cells per kilogram after mobilization attempts fail, then allogeneic transplant may be considered as an alternative. Additionally, plerixafor (Mobozil) is approved by the Food and Drug Administration (FDA) for use in combination with granulocyte colony-stimulating factor to mobilize PBPCs for collection and subsequent autologous transplantation in patients with NHL and MM. Plerixafor is an inhibitor of the CXCR4 chemokine receptor that results in more circulating PBPCs in the peripheral blood because of the inability of CXCR4 to assist in anchoring hematopoietic stem cells to the bone marrow matrix. Because administration of plerixafor with granulocyte colony-stimulating factor results in increased yield of CD34+ cells per kilogram compared to granulocyte colony-stimulating factor alone, this combination serves as an alternative mobilization strategy in patients deemed to be at risk for mobilization failure with conventional methods.

Allogeneic Transplants The allogeneic donor first undergoes mobilization therapy with an HGF to increase the number of hematopoietic cells circulating in the peripheral blood. The most commonly used regimen to mobilize allogeneic donors is a 4- to 5-day course of filgrastim, 10 mcg/kg/day, administered subcutaneously followed by apheresis on the fourth or fifth days when peripheral blood levels of CD34+ cells peak. An adequate number of hematopoietic cells usually are obtained with one to two apheresis collections, with the optimal number of CD34+ collected being a minimum of 4-8 × 10^6 cells/kg of recipient body weight. Higher numbers of CD34+ cells are associated with more rapid neutrophil and platelet engraftment; patients who receive less than 2 × 10^6/kg CD34+ cells are at risk for delayed engraftment.[5] Hematopoietic stem cells obtained from the peripheral blood are processed like bone marrow–derived stem cells and may be infused immediately into the recipient or frozen for future use. Compared with bone marrow donation, allogeneic PBPC donation leads to quicker hematopoietic recovery. Neutrophil engraftment occurs 2 to 6 days earlier, and platelet engraftment occurs approximately 6 days earlier with PBPC grafts than bone marrow grafts.[9] The donor may experience musculoskeletal pain, headache, and mild increases in hepatic enzyme or lactate dehydrogenase levels related to filgrastim administration. Hypocalcemia may also occur owing to citrate accumulation, which decreases ionized calcium concentrations during apheresis.

Allogeneic PBPC grafts contain approximately 10 times more T and B cells than bone marrow grafts. Historically, there has been significant concern that the greater T- and B-cell content of PBPCs could increase the risk of acute and/or chronic GVHD. In patients with a hematologic malignancy who have an HLA-matched sibling donor, a PBPC graft is optimal relative to bone marrow graft because the PBPC graft is associated with quicker neutrophil and platelet engraftment and potentially improved disease-free survival rates.[10] Grafts from PBPCs are likely associated with a higher incidence of acute GVHD and an approximately 20% increase in the incidence of extensive-stage and overall chronic GVHD.[10] Similar trends for engraftment and GVHD have been found with unrelated donors.[11]

T-Cell Depletion Immunocompetent T lymphocytes may be depleted from the donor bone marrow *ex vivo* before infusion (referred to as T-cell–depleted hematopoietic cells) into the recipient as a means of preventing GVHD. Depletion of T lymphocytes in donor hematopoietic cells is completed *ex vivo* using physical (eg, density-gradient fractionation) and/or immunologic (eg, antithymocyte globulin [ATG] antibodies) methods. Functional recovery of T cells in the recipient is delayed, and the risk of Epstein-Barr virus–associated lymphoproliferative disorders is higher with the use of T-cell–depleted bone marrow. The use of T-cell–depleted grafts reduces the incidence of GVHD, but graft failure and relapse are more common. The use of donor lymphocyte infusion in patients who relapse after receiving a T-cell–depleted HSCT is being investigated.

Engraftment After chemotherapy and radiation, pancytopenia lasts until the infused stem cells reestablish functional hematopoiesis. The median time to engraftment is a function of several factors, including the source of stem cells such as PBPCs, which can result in earlier engraftment than bone marrow. Myeloablative preparative regimens have significant regimen-related toxicity and morbidity and thus usually are limited to healthy, younger (ie, usually less than 50 years) patients. Alternatively, nonmyeloablative transplants are being performed with the hope of curing more patients with cancer by increasing the availability of HSCT with less regimen-related toxicity and by using the graft-versus-tumor effect.[1]

A delicate balance exists between host and donor effector cells in the bone marrow environment. Residual host-versus-graft effects may lead to graft failure, which is also known as graft rejection. Graft failure is defined as the lack of functional hematopoiesis after HSCT and can occur early (ie, lack of initial hematopoietic recovery) or late (ie, in association with recurrence of the disease or reappearance of host cells after initial donor cell engraftment). Engraftment usually is evident within the first 30 days in patients undergoing an HSCT; however, rejection can occur after initial engraftment. Therapeutic options for the treatment of graft rejection are limited; a second HSCT is the most definitive therapy, although the toxicities are formidable.[12]

▸ *Graft-Versus-Tumor Effect*

A graft-versus-tumor effect caused by the donor lymphocytes occurs after transplant. This results in lower relapse rates in patients with GVHD relative to those who did not have GVHD; a higher rate of leukemia relapse after T-cell–depleted, autologous, or syngeneic HSCT; and the effectiveness of donor lymphocyte infusions in reinducing a remission in patients who relapsed after allogeneic HSCT. Rapid taper of immunosuppression in patients with residual disease may induce a graft-versus tumor effect. In donor lymphocyte infusion, lymphocytes are collected from the peripheral blood of the donor and administered to the recipient. Eradication of the recurrent malignancy is caused by either specific targeting of the tumor antigens or GVHD, which may affect cancer cells preferentially. Patients with hematologic

Patient Encounter, Part 1

A 55-year-old woman is diagnosed with acute myeloid leukemia with complex cytogenetics. The patient achieved complete remission with induction therapy and is now being evaluated for an allogeneic stem cell transplant with a peripheral blood stem cell graft from a full HLA-matched unrelated donor. She has no siblings. Her preparative regimen consists of cyclophosphamide and TBI and her GVHD prophylaxis consists of tacrolimus, methotrexate, and ATG.

What nonhematologic toxicities are associated with the preparative regimen?

What are the advantages and disadvantages of obtaining and infusing hematopoietic stem cells from a peripheral blood stem cell source as opposed to a bone marrow source?

What are the implications for this patient of an unrelated stem cell donor?

malignancies (eg, CML and acute myelogenous leukemia [AML]) and certain solid tumors (eg, renal cell carcinoma) appear to benefit from a graft-versus-tumor effect. These data gave rise to the use of nonmyeloablative preparative regimens.

Pharmacologic Therapy

▸ *Preparative Regimens for HSCT*

Examples of commonly used preparative regimens are included in Table 98–2.

Myeloablative Preparative Regimens In both autologous and allogeneic HSCT, infusion of stem cells circumvents dose-limiting myelosuppression, maximizing the potential value of the steep dose–response curve to alkylating agents and radiation, suppressing the host immune system, and creating space in the marrow compartment to facilitate engraftment. The preparative regimen is designed to eradicate immunologically active host tissues (lymphoid tissue and macrophages) and to prevent or minimize the development of host-versus-graft reactions. Most allogeneic preparative regimens for the treatment of hematologic malignancies contain cyclophosphamide, radiation, or both. The combination of cyclophosphamide and total-body irradiation (TBI) was one of the first preparative regimens developed and is still used widely today. This regimen is immunosuppressive and has inherent activity against hematologic malignancies (eg, leukemias and lymphomas). TBI has the added advantage of being devoid of active metabolites that might interfere with the activity of donor hematopoietic cells. In addition, TBI eradicates residual malignant cells at sanctuary sites such as the central nervous system. Modifications of the cyclophosphamide–TBI preparative regimen include replacing TBI with other agents (eg, busulfan) or adding other chemotherapeutic or monoclonal agents to the existing regimen in hopes of minimizing long-term toxicities. In the case of a mismatched allogeneic HSCT with a substantially increased chance of graft rejection, ATG also may be added to the preparative regimen to further immunosuppress the recipient.

The optimal myeloablative preparative regimen remains elusive. Busulfan–cyclophosphamide (BU-CY) and cyclophosphamide–TBI (CY-TBI) are prescribed in patients with AML and CML, which represent the more common indications for allogeneic HSCT. Intravenous busulfan with pharmacokinetic monitoring may improve outcomes when utilized with BU-CY compared to Cy-TBI in AML patients although preparative regimens should be tailored to the primary disease and to the degree of HLA compatibility.[17]

Nonmyeloablative Preparative Regimens KEY CONCEPT *A nonmyeloablative preparative regimen is less toxic than a myeloablative regimen in the hope of being able to offer the benefits of an allogeneic HSCT to more patients. A nonmyeloablative HSCT is based on the concept of donor immune response having a graft-versus-tumor effect.*

Because of the severe regimen-related toxicity of a myeloablative preparative regimen, the use of HSCT traditionally was limited to younger patients with minimal comorbidities. Most patients diagnosed with cancer are elderly; therefore, myeloablative HSCT could not be offered to a substantial portion of cancer patients. The concept of donor immune response having a graft-versus-tumor effect gave rise to the theory that a strongly immunosuppressive, but not myeloablative, preparative regimen (ie, a nonmyeloablative transplant may result in a state of chimerism in which the recipient and donor are coexisting). The toxicity and efficacy of nonmyeloablative transplants are being evaluated

Table 98–2

Commonly Used Preparative Regimens for HSCT[a]

Type of HSCT	Preparative Regimen	Dose and Schedule for Adults	Dose and Schedule for Pediatric Patients
Allogeneic[13]	Myeloablative CY-TBI	CY 60 mg/kg/day IV on 2 consecutive days before TBI 1000–1575 rads (10–15.75 Gy) fractionated over 1–7 days	CY 60 mg/kg/day IV on 2 consecutive days before TBI 1000–1575 rads (10–15.75 Gy) fractionated over 1–7 days
Allogeneic, autologous[14]	Myeloablative BU-CY	BU 1 mg/kg per dose po or 0.8 mg/kg per dose IV every 6 hours × 16 doses CY 60 mg/kg/day IV daily × 2 days after BU	BU 1 mg/kg per dose po or 0.8 mg/kg per dose IV every 6 hours × 16 doses CY 120–200 mg/kg IV given over 2–4 days after BU
Autologous[15]	Myeloablative BEAM (carmustine/etoposide/-cytarabine/melphalan)	Carmustine 300 mg/m² IV Etoposide 400–800 mg/m² IV given over 4 days Cytarabine 400–1600 mg/m² IV given over 4 days Melphalan 140 mg/m² IV	Carmustine 300 mg/m² IV Etoposide 400–800 mg/m² IV given over 4 days Cytarabine 400–1600 mg/m² IV given over 4 days Melphalan 140 mg/m² IV
Allogeneic[16]	Nonmyeloablative BU-FLU	Fludarabine 30 mg/m²/day IV on day –10 to day –5 followed by busulfan 1 mg/kg/dose po every 6 hours × 8 doses on days –6 and –5	Fludarabine 30 mg/m²/day IV on day –10 to day –5 followed by busulfan 1 mg/kg/dose po every 6 hours × 8 doses on days –6 and –5

[a]BEAM, carmustine, etoposide, cytarabine, and melphalan; BU-CY, busulfan and cyclophosphamide; BU-FLU, busulfan and fludarabine; CY-TBI, cyclophosphamide–total-body irradiation; IV, intravenous; po, oral; TBI, total-body irradiation.

in patients with malignant and nonmalignant conditions who are not eligible for a myeloablative HSCT.

A nonmyeloablative preparative regimen allows for development of mixed chimerism (defined as 5%–95% peripheral donor T cells) between the host and recipient to allow for a graft-versus-tumor effect as the primary form of therapy (Figure 98–1). Chimerism is assessed within peripheral blood T cells and granulocytes and bone marrow using conventional (eg, using sex chromosomes for opposite-sex donors) and molecular (eg, variable number of tandem repeats) methods for same-sex donors.

The nonmyeloablative preparative regimen does not completely eliminate host normal and malignant cells. Donor cells eradicate residual host hematopoiesis, and the graft-versus-tumor effects generally occur after the development of full donor T-cell chimerism. After engraftment, mixed chimerism should be present and is shown by the presence of both donor- and recipient-derived cells. Autologous recovery should occur promptly if the graft is rejected. The intensity of immunosuppression required for engraftment depends on the immunocompetence of the recipient and the histocompatibility and composition of the HSCT.[18] More intensive conditioning regimens that are required for engraftment in the setting of unrelated-donor- or HLA-mismatched-related HSCT have been termed reduced-intensity myeloablative transplants. After chimerism develops, donor-lymphocyte infusion can be administered safely in patients without GVHD to eradicate malignant cells.

Nonmyeloablative preparative regimens typically consist of a purine analog (eg, fludarabine) in combination with an alkylating agent or low-dose TBI. Adverse effects in the early post-transplant period are decreased because of the lower intensity preparative regimen, thus making HSCT available to patients who in the past were not healthy or young enough to receive a myeloablative preparative regimen. The risk of GVHD remains with nonmyeloablative transplant; the GVHD prophylaxis regimens are reviewed in the GVHD section below. Presently, nonmyeloablative transplant is not indicated as first-line therapy for any malignant or nonmalignant conditions, although research is ongoing. Nonmyeloablative transplantation is being evaluated for cancers sensitive to a graft-versus-tumor effect (eg, CML and AML), in older patients, or for those with comorbidities who would not be able to tolerate a myeloablative HSCT.

Toxicities and Management of Preparative Regimens Myelosuppression is a frequent dose-limiting toxicity for antineoplastics when administered in the conventional doses used to treat cancer. However, because myelosuppression is circumvented with hematopoietic rescue in the case of patients receiving HSCT, the dose-limiting toxicities of these myeloablative preparative regimens are nonhematologic and vary with the preparative regimen used. Most patients undergoing HSCT experience toxicities commonly associated with chemotherapy (eg, alopecia, mucositis, nausea and vomiting, and infertility), albeit these toxicities are magnified in the HSCT population.

Busulfan Seizures Seizures have been reported in both adult and pediatric patients receiving high-dose busulfan for HSCT preparative regimens. Anticonvulsants are used to minimize the risk of seizures. Anticonvulsants are begun shortly before busulfan, with the loading dose completed at least 6 hours before the first busulfan dose. Oral loading and maintenance regimens generally are sufficient because target phenytoin concentrations of 10 to 20 mcg/mL (10–20 mg/L; 40–79 μmol/L) can be achieved by the peak time of seizure risk. If patients are experiencing

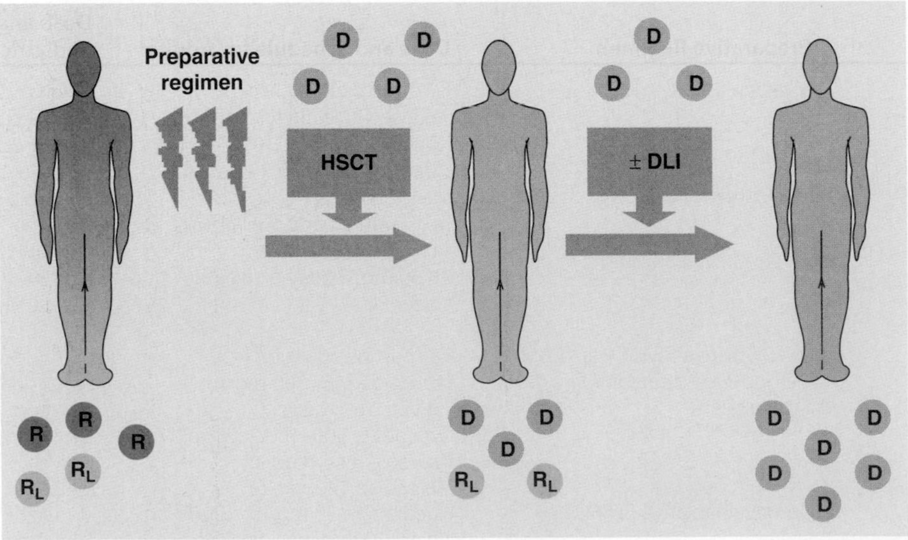

FIGURE 98–1. Schema for nonmyeloablative transplantation. Recipients (R) receive a nonmyeloablative preparative regimen and an allogeneic hematopoietic stem cell transplantation (HSCT). Initially, mixed chimerism is present with the coexistence of donor (D) cells and recipient-derived normal and leukemia or lymphoma (R_L) cells. Donor-derived T cells mediate a graft-versus-host hematopoietic effect that eradicates residual recipient-derived normal and malignant hematopoietic cells. Donor-lymphocyte infusions (DLIs) may be administered to enhance graft-versus-tumor effects.

significant vomiting or have difficulty maintaining therapeutic phenytoin concentrations, intravenous (IV) phenytoin should be substituted. Benzodiazepines such as lorazepam or clonazepam also have been used for seizure prophylaxis during high-dose busulfan therapy before HSCT. Antiseizure medications usually are discontinued 24 to 48 hours after administration of the last dose of busulfan. Seizures still can occur despite the use of prophylactic anticonvulsants and usually do not result in permanent neurologic deficits.

Adaptive Dosing of Busulfan The considerable interpatient variability in the clearance of both oral and IV busulfan along with the identified concentration–effect relationships, has led to the adaptive dosing of busulfan. Adjusting the oral busulfan dose to achieve a target concentration minimizes the toxicities of the BU-CY regimen, particularly hepatic sinusoidal obstruction syndrome (SOS; formerly referred to as veno-occlusive disease) while improving engraftment and relapse rates. Complete reviews of these relationships after oral busulfan administration are available elsewhere.[19] An IV busulfan product, Busulfex, was approved by the FDA in February 1999 in combination with cyclophosphamide as a preparative regimen before allogeneic HSCT for CML. In combination with either cyclophosphamide or fludarabine, the data available with busulfan suggests that therapeutic drug monitoring may be needed to optimize patient outcome with regards to efficacy and toxicity.[20]

Hemorrhagic Cystitis High-dose cyclophosphamide causes moderate to severe hemorrhagic cystitis; acrolein, a metabolite of cyclophosphamide, is the putative bladder toxin. Preventive measures to lower the risk of hemorrhagic cystitis include vigorous hydration, continuous bladder irrigation, or concomitant use of the uroprotectant mesna. The American Society of Clinical Oncology (ASCO) Guidelines for the Use of Chemotherapy and Radiotherapy Protectants recommends the use of Mesna (2-mercaptoethane sulfonate) plus saline diuresis or forced saline diuresis to lower the incidence of urothelial toxicity with high-dose cyclophosphamide in the setting of HSCT.[21]

Chemotherapy-Induced Gastrointestinal Effects Preparative regimens for myeloablative HSCT result in other end-organ toxicities, such as renal failure and idiopathic pneumonia syndrome. In addition, recipients of myeloablative preparative regimens are at risk for severe gastrointestinal (GI) toxicity, specifically chemotherapy-induced nausea and vomiting (CINV), diarrhea, and mucositis. CINV can be caused by administration of highly emetogenic chemotherapy over several days, TBI, and poor control of CINV before HSCT. Thus, patients who are undergoing a myeloablative HSCT should receive a prophylactic corticosteroid with a serotonin antagonist, with higher doses of serotonin antagonists potentially being needed in this patient population. In addition, these patients are at high risk for delayed CINV in the immediate posttransplant period, and these issues should be addressed accordingly as per published clinical practice guidelines.[22]

Diarrhea is also an adverse effect experienced by a majority of patients undergoing HSCT. Chemotherapy-induced diarrhea occurs because of the effects of the preparative regimen, which results in inflammation and damage to the cells lining the GI tract. Diarrhea caused by the preparative regimen is usually apparent within the first week after the initiation of chemotherapy and/or radiation. Treatment strategies for chemotherapy-induced diarrhea include the administration of antidiarrheals after excluding infectious causes of diarrhea and the prevention of dehydration.

Virtually all patients receiving a myeloablative preparative regimen experience severe mucositis owing to its effects on rapidly dividing cells of the oral epithelium and subsequent inflammation of the oropharyngeal cavity. Routine oral care protocols are indicated to reduce the severity of mucositis, which may onset within the first week of HSCT and persist for up to approximately 2 weeks. Palifermin, a keratinocytic growth factor, may be considered for patients undergoing myeloablative HSCT with TBI-based preparative regimens.[23] Patients may require parenteral opioid analgesics for pain relief owing to mucositis, and total parenteral nutrition may be necessary to prevent the development of nutritional deficiencies.

Sinusoidal Obstruction Syndrome Hepatic SOS is a life-threatening complication that may occur secondary to preparative regimens or radiation. The pathogenesis of SOS is not understood completely, but several mechanisms have been proposed. The key event appears to be endothelial damage caused by the preparative regimen. The primary site of the toxic injury is the sinusoidal endothelial cells; the endothelial damage initiates the coagulation cascade, induces thrombosis of the hepatic venules, and eventually leads to fibrous obliteration of the affected venules.[24]

The clinical manifestations of SOS are hyperbilirubinemia, jaundice, fluid retention, weight gain, and right upper quadrant abdominal pain. To make a clinical diagnosis of SOS, these features must occur in the absence of other causes of posttransplant liver failure, including GVHD, viral hepatitis, fungal abscesses, or drug reactions. Most cases of SOS occur within 3 weeks of HSCT, and the clinical diagnosis can be confirmed histologically via liver biopsy.

Patients with mild SOS have an excellent prognosis, but those with more severe disease (ie, bilirubin greater than 20 mg/dL [342 μmol/L] or weight gain greater than 15%) have a high mortality rate. Pretransplant risk factors for SOS include a mismatched or unrelated graft, increased age, prior abdominal radiation or stem cell transplant, and increased transaminases before HSCT.[24] Interpatient variability in the metabolism and clearance of the chemotherapy (ie, busulfan and cyclophosphamide) used within the preparative regimen also may be associated with a poor outcome, although the relationships vary within the various preparative regimens. The association of SOS with busulfan concentrations is discussed in the section on adaptive dosing of busulfan. Use of ursodiol, unfractionated heparin, or low-molecular-weight heparin has been associated with a lower incidence of SOS in a limited number of small, randomized studies and may be recommended for SOS prophylaxis.[24]

The mainstay of treatment for established SOS is supportive care aimed at sodium restriction, increasing intravascular volume, decreasing extracellular fluid accumulation, and minimizing factors that contribute to or exacerbate hepatotoxicity and encephalopathy. Recombinant tissue plasminogen activator administered with or without heparin has been investigated for treatment of SOS, but the life-threatening risk of bleeding precludes any potential benefit.[24] Defibrotide, an oligonucleotide with antithrombotic, anti-ischemic, and anti-inflammatory activity, is not FDA approved in the United States but has shown promising results in the treatment of SOS in clinical trials.[24]

Myelosuppression and Hematopoietic Growth Factor Use HGFs may be administered to mobilize PBPCs before an HSCT, to hasten hematopoietic recovery during the period of aplasia after an autologous HSCT, and to stimulate hematopoietic recovery when the patient fails to engraft.[25]

Autologous HSCT is associated with profound aplasia owing to the myeloablative preparative regimen. Aplasia typically lasts 7 to 14 days after an autologous PBPC transplant. During this period of aplasia, patients are at high risk for complications such as bleeding and infection. Filgrastim and sargramostim exert their effects by stimulating the proliferation of committed progenitor cells and accelerating recovery on hematopoiesis. Once engraftment occurs, HGFs may be discontinued. The anatomic source of hematopoietic cells predicts the degree of benefit, with the greatest benefit reached when bone marrow is the graft source. With autologous PBPC transplant, the effect of HGF on neutrophil recovery is variable.

The use of HGF after allogeneic HSCT—whether from bone marrow or PBPC grafts—is controversial. The amount of data with sargramostim is limited in this setting; data with filgrastim have shown more rapid neutrophil but slower platelet engraftment in those receiving grafts from bone marrow or PBPCs.[26] The effects of post-HSCT filgrastim use on acute and chronic GVHD have been conflicting, with either no effect or increases in both the incidence of acute and chronic GVHD and treatment-related mortality.[26] Thus, there is little reason to treat allogeneic BMT with filgrastim as prophylaxis after HSCT.

Clinical Presentation and Diagnosis of Sinusoidal Obstructive Syndrome

General

- Sinusoidal obstructive syndrome (SOS) usually occurs within the first 3 weeks after HSCT.
- Busulfan, cyclophosphamide, pretransplant exposure to gemtuzumab, TBI-containing preparative regimens, and pretransplant abnormalities in liver function tests may increase the risk for SOS.

Symptoms

- Patients may complain of weight gain and abdominal pain.

Signs

- Fluid retention: Weight gain caused by ascites greater than 2% compared with pretransplant weight
- Hepatomegaly: May result in right upper quadrant pain
- Hepatic: Jaundice caused by hyperbilirubinemia defined as a bilirubin greater than 2 mg/dL (34.2 μmol/L)

Laboratory Tests

- Hepatic: Elevation of bilirubin, alkaline phosphatase, and γ-glutamyltransferase (GGT)
- Hematologic: Complete blood count with differential may reveal thrombocytopenia, elevated plasminogen activator-1 levels, decreased antithrombin III, protein C, and protein S

Other Diagnostic Tests

- Reversal of blood flow in portal and hepatic veins on Doppler ultrasonography
- Liver biopsy for pathologic review

Graft Failure A delicate balance between host and donor effector cells in the bone marrow is necessary to ensure adequate engraftment because residual host-versus-graft effects may lead to graft rejection. The incidence of graft rejection is higher in patients with aplastic anemia and those undergoing HSCT with histoincompatible marrow or T-cell–depleted marrow.[1] Graft rejection is uncommon in leukemia patients receiving myeloablative preparative regimens with a histocompatible allogeneic donor.

Therapeutic options for the treatment of graft rejection or graft failure are limited. A second HSCT is the most definitive therapy, although the associated complications and toxicities may preclude its use. Graft rejection is best managed with immunosuppressants such as ATG. Primary graft failure occasionally can be treated successfully using HGFs, although patients who received purged autografts are less likely to respond.

▸ Graft-Versus-Host Disease

KEY CONCEPT *GVHD is caused by the activation of donor lymphocytes, leading to immune damage to the skin, gut, and liver in the recipient.* Immune-mediated destruction of tissues, a hallmark of GVHD, disrupts the integrity of protective mucosal barriers and thus provides an environment that favors the establishment of opportunistic infections. KEY CONCEPT *An immunosuppressive regimen is administered to prevent GVHD in recipients of an allogeneic graft; this regimen is based on the type of preparative regimen and the source of the graft.* The combination of GVHD and

Patient Encounter, Part 2

PMH: Hypertension, type 2 diabetes, hyperlipidemia, hypothyroidism, sleep apnea, and gout

FH: Father died at age of 56 years of myocardial infarction. Mother has history of hypertension. One younger sister with a history of hypertension

SH: She is a high school teacher and is married with no children. She drinks alcohol occasionally and does not smoke or use illicit drugs

Allergies: NKDA

Meds: Metformin 500 mg by mouth twice daily; lisinopril 20 mg by mouth once daily; carvedilol 12.5 mg by mouth twice daily; aspirin 81 mg by mouth once daily; atorvastatin 40 mg by mouth once nightly at bedtime; levothyroxine 75 μg by mouth once daily; allopurinol 300 mg by mouth once daily

ROS: (+) Fatigue

PE:

VS: BP 134/82, P 69, RR 18, T 37.6°C

Physical exam reveals no acute findings.

Laboratory analysis is within normal limits except for serum creatinine of 1.3 g/dL (115 μmol/L) and hemoglobin of 10.2 g/dL (102 g/L; 6.33 μmol/L).

Given this additional information, what is your assessment of the planned preparative regimen?

What infectious complications are of a concern for this patient during the early transplant period?

infectious complications are leading causes of mortality for allogeneic HSCT patients. GVHD is divided into two forms (ie, acute and chronic) based on clinical manifestations. Traditionally, the boundary between acute and chronic GVHD was set at 100 days after HSCT; however, more recent definitions hinge upon different clinical symptoms rather than the time of onset.[27,28]

Acute GVHD The degree of histocompatibility between donor and recipient is the most important factor associated with the development of acute GVHD. The pathophysiology for acute GVHD is a multistep phenomenon, including the development of an inflammatory milieu that results from host tissue damage induced by the preparative regimen; both recipient and donor antigen-presenting cells and inflammatory cytokines triggering activation of donor-derived T cells; and the activated donor T cells mediate cytotoxicity through a variety of mechanisms, which leads to tissue damage characteristic of acute GVHD.[28]

Despite prophylaxis, 20% to 80% of patients will develop acute GVHD.[29] Other factors that increase the risk of acute GVHD include increasing recipient or donor age (older than 20 years), female donor to a male recipient, and mismatches in minor histocompatibility antigens in HLA-matched transplants.[28] T-cell depletion or receipt of an umbilical cord blood graft appears to lower the risk of acute GVHD.[1]

Clinical Presentation and Staging of Acute GVHD Acute GVHD targets the skin, liver and GI tract; it must be distinguished accurately from other causes of skin, liver, or GI toxicity in HSCT patients. Other causes of toxicities affecting the skin, liver, or GI tract may include a drug reaction or an infectious process. A staging system based on clinical criteria is used to grade acute GVHD (Figure 98–2). The severity of organ involvement is scored on an ordinal scale from 0 (no symptoms) to IV (severe symptoms), and then an overall grade is established based on the number and extent of involved organs.

Immunosuppressive Prophylaxis of Acute GVHD GVHD is a leading cause of morbidity and mortality after allogeneic HSCT and thus, efforts have focused on preventing acute GVHD. The donor graft and preparative regimen influence the prophylactic regimen for acute GVHD, with two approaches having been taken by clinicians over time. One approach involves T-cell depletion, which was discussed more fully in the section on T-cell depletion earlier. The more common method is to use two-drug immunosuppressive therapy that typically consists of a calcineurin inhibitor (ie, cyclosporine or tacrolimus) with methotrexate after myeloablative HSCT. Prophylaxis of acute GVHD for nonmyeloablative preparative regimens is varied, but a calcineurin inhibitor with either methotrexate or mycophenolate mofetil is used.[16]

The calcineurin inhibitors (ie, cyclosporine and tacrolimus) should be initiated before donor cell infusion (eg, day −1) when used for GVHD prophylaxis. This schedule is recommended because of the known mechanism of action of calcineurin inhibitors, which entails blocking the proliferation of cytotoxic T cells by inhibiting production of T helper cell–derived interleukin-2 (IL-2). Administering calcineurin inhibitors before the donor cell infusion allows inhibition of IL-2 secretion to occur before a rejection response has been initiated. Studies comparing cyclosporine and tacrolimus in combination with methotrexate have shown that tacrolimus administration is associated with a lower incidence of grade II to IV acute GVHD and a similar incidence of chronic GVHD but variable effects on overall survival.[30,31]

Adaptive Dosing of the Calcineurin Inhibitors Most HSCT centers have their own standardized approach to dose adjust the calcineurin inhibitors cyclosporine and tacrolimus to target concentration ranges. Cyclosporine and tacrolimus trough concentrations are associated with acute GVHD and nephrotoxicity. Cyclosporine trough concentrations usually are maintained between 150 and 400 ng/mL (125 and 333 nmol/L) in patients undergoing allogeneic HSCT. Tacrolimus trough concentrations are targeted to a range of 10 to 20 ng/mL (10–20 mcg/L; 12.4–24.8 nmol/L).[32] Dosage adjustments to either calcineurin inhibitor also should be made for elevated serum creatinine regardless of their serum concentrations. Nephrotoxicity can occur despite low or normal concentrations of the calcineurin

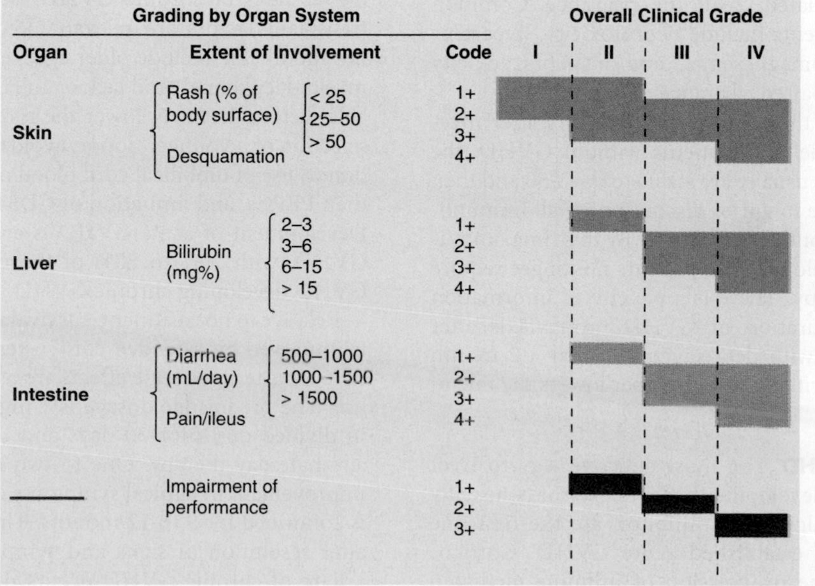

FIGURE 98–2. Staging System for graft-versus-host disease.

Clinical Presentation and Diagnosis of Acute Graft-versus-Host Disease

General

- Patients may present with any or all of the following: skin rash, GI complaints, or jaundice.
- Signs and symptoms present after engraftment when donor lymphoid elements begin to proliferate.

Symptoms

- Patients may complain of nausea, vomiting, bloody diarrhea, or itching from skin rash.

Signs

- Skin: Maculopapular skin rash on the face, truck, extremities, palms, soles, and ears which may progress to generalized total-body erythroderma, bullous formation, and skin desquamation.
- GI: Ileus, malnutrition, dehydration and electrolyte abnormalities due to nausea, vomiting, and diarrhea.
- Hepatic: Jaundice due to hyperbilirubinemia.

Laboratory Tests

- Hepatic: Elevation of bilirubin, alkaline phosphatase, and hepatic transaminases
- GI: Send stool for bacterial, viral, and parasitic cultures to rule out infectious causes

Other Diagnostic Tests

- Biopsy of affected site for pathologic review

inhibitor cyclosporine and may be a consequence of other drug- or disease-related factors known to influence the development of nephrotoxicity (eg, genetic risk factors, concurrent use of other nephrotoxic agents, and sepsis). Careful monitoring for drug interactions via CYP 3A4 and P-glycoprotein is also warranted. The calcineurin inhibitor doses are adjusted based on serum drug levels and the calculated creatinine clearance. Common adverse effects to these agents include neurotoxicity, hypertension, hyperkalemia, hypomagnesemia, and/or nephrotoxicity (which may lead to an impaired clearance of methotrexate).

Tapering schedules for the calcineurin inhibitors after myeloablative HSCT vary widely. In patients without GVHD, the calcineurin inhibitor doses usually are stable to day +50 and then are tapered slowly with the intent of discontinuing all immunosuppressive agents by 6 months after HSCT. By this time, immunologic tolerance has developed, and patients no longer require immunosuppressive therapy. There is a paucity of information regarding the optimal duration of GVHD prophylaxis after nonmyeloablative HSCT, with data suggesting that a 2-month duration of cyclosporine with a 4-month taper lowers the rate of severe acute GVHD.[33]

Treatment of Acute GVHD The most effective way to treat GVHD is to prevent its development. Corticosteroids, usually in combination with a calcineurin inhibitor, are the first-line therapy for treatment of established acute GVHD. Corticosteroids indirectly halt the progression of immune-mediated destruction of host tissues by blocking macrophage-derived IL-1 secretion. IL-1 is a primary stimulus for T helper cell–induced secretion of IL-2, which, in turn, is responsible for stimulating proliferation of cytotoxic T lymphocytes. The recommended dosage of methylprednisolone in this setting is 2 mg/kg/day; there is no advantage to higher corticosteroid doses (ie, 10 mg/kg/day).[28] A partial or complete response is seen in approximately 50% of patients treated with corticosteroids. Once a clinical improvement occurs, there is no consensus on the optimal method for tapering the corticosteroids. Patients with steroid-refractory acute GVHD have a poor prognosis, and a number of medications are being studied for salvage therapy.

Chronic GVHD Occurring in 20% to 70% of HSCT recipients surviving longer than 100 days, chronic GVHD is the most frequent and serious late complication of allogeneic HSCT.[34] Chronic GVHD is the major cause of nonrelapse mortality and morbidity. The clinical course of chronic GVHD is multifaceted, involving almost any organ in the body, and its symptoms resemble autoimmune and immunologic disorders (eg, scleroderma). Chronic GVHD symptoms usually present within 3 years of allogeneic HSCT and often are preceded by acute GVHD.[27] Traditionally, the boundary between acute and chronic GVHD was set at 100 days after HSCT; however, more recent definitions hinge on different clinical symptoms rather than the time of onset.[34] A consensus document regarding the diagnosis and scoring of chronic GVHD has been published that proposes a clinical scoring system to describe chronic GVHD as opposed to historical descriptions of chronic GVHD, which described the phenomenon as being "limited" versus "extensive" in nature.[29] The diagnosis of chronic GVHD requires distinction from acute GVHD; the presence of at least one diagnostic clinical sign of chronic GVHD or presence of at least one distinctive manifestation confirmed by pertinent biopsy or other relevant tests; and exclusion of other possible diagnoses.

Prevention and Treatment of Chronic GVHD Chronic GVHD is not a continuation of acute GVHD, and separate approaches are needed for its prevention and management. Prevention of chronic GVHD through prolonged use of immunosuppressive medications has been unsuccessful.[34] Thus, its prevention is focused on minimization of factors associated with higher rates of chronic GVHD. Several recipient, donor, and transplant factors are relevant. Recipient risk factors that are not modifiable include older age, certain diagnoses (eg, chronic myeloid leukemia), and lack of an HLA-matched donor. Modifiable factors that may lower the risk of chronic GVHD include selection of a younger donor, avoidance of a multiparous female donor, use of umbilical cord blood or bone marrow grafts rather than PBPCs, and limitation of CD34+ and T-cell dose infused.[34] Development of acute GVHD is a major predictor for chronic GVHD, with 70% to 80% of those with grade II to IV acute GVHD developing chronic GVHD.[34]

Relative to no treatment, survival in those with chronic GVHD is improved by extended corticosteroid therapy; however, multiple long-term adverse effects are associated with corticosteroid use. The prednisone dosage is 1 mg/kg/day administered orally in divided doses for 30 days and then slowly converted to an alternate day therapy. One to two months may pass before an improvement in clinical symptoms is noted, and therapy usually is continued for 9 to 12 months. Therapy can be tapered slowly after resolution of signs and symptoms of chronic GVHD. If a flare of chronic GVHD occurs during the tapering schedule or after therapy is discontinued, immunosuppressive therapy is restarted. Other potential approaches for patients who are refractory to initial therapy include etanercept (Enbrel), infliximab (Remicade), mycophenolate mofetil (Cellcept), rituximab (Rituxan), extended use of calcineurin inhibitors, or extracorporeal photochemotherapy.[34] When immunosuppressive therapy is administered for long periods, the patient must be monitored closely for chronic toxicity. Cushingoid effects, aseptic necrosis of the joints, and diabetes can develop with long-term corticosteroid use. Other severe complications include a high incidence of infection with encapsulated organisms and atypical pathogens such as *Pneumocystis jiroveci*, cytomegalovirus (CMV), and varicella zoster virus (VZV).

► *Infectious Complications*

KEY CONCEPT *Recipients of HSCT are at higher risk of bacterial, viral, and fungal infections and usually receive a prophylactic or preemptive regimen to minimize the morbidity and mortality associated with infectious complications.* After myeloablative and nonmyeloablative HSCT, opportunistic infections are a major source of morbidity and mortality. There are three periods of infectious risks, preengraftment (from 15 days prior and to 45 days after HSCT), postengraftment (engraftment to day 100 days post engraftment), and late 100 days after engraftment. From days 0 to 30 after HSCT, particularly for patients undergoing myeloablative HSCT, the primary pathogens are aerobic bacteria, *Candida* spp., and herpes simplex virus (HSV). Respiratory viruses such as respiratory syncytial virus (RSV), influenza, adenovirus, and parainfluenza virus are recognized increasingly as pathogens causing pneumonia, particularly during community outbreaks of infection with these organisms. Because of the need to administer chemotherapy, blood products, antibiotics, and other adjunctive medications, the placement of a semipermanent double- or triple-lumen central venous catheter is necessary before HSCT. However, the indwelling IV central catheters put HSCT recipients at increased risk for *Staphylococcus* infections.

The second period of infectious risk occurs after engraftment to post transplant day 100. Bacterial infections are still of concern, but pathogens such as CMV, adenovirus, and *Aspergillus* spp. are common. A common manifestation of infection is interstitial pneumonitis (IP), which can be caused by CMV, adenovirus, *Aspergillus*, and *P. jiroveci*. Suppression of the immune system from acute GVHD and corticosteroids contributes to the risk of such infections during this period. Therefore, patients undergoing nonmyeloablative transplant who are receiving corticosteroids to treat GVHD can be expected to have a similar risk for infection as those undergoing myeloablative HSCT.[35] Invasive fungal infections over the first year after HSCT occur at a similar rate in nonmyeloablative transplant compared with historical control participants receiving a myeloablative preparative regimen.[36]

During the late period (100 days after engraftment), the predominant organisms are the encapsulated bacteria (eg, *Streptococcus pneumoniae*, *Haemophilus influenzae*, and *Neisseria meningitidis*), fungi, and VZV. The encapsulated organisms commonly cause sinopulmonary infections. The risk of infection during this late period is increased in patients with chronic GVHD as a result of prolonged immunosuppression.

Prevention and Treatment of Bacterial and Fungal Infections Between the time of administration of the preparative regimen and successful engraftment, allogeneic myeloablative HSCT patients undergo a period of pancytopenia that can last from 2 to 6 weeks. The risk of infection is also reduced by aggressive use of antibacterial, antifungal, and antiviral therapy both prophylactically and for the treatment of documented infection. The antibacterial prophylactic regimens vary substantially among HSCT centers. Some HSCT centers use a prophylactic fluoroquinolone (eg, levofloxacin) on admission for HSCT and then switch to a broad-spectrum IV antibiotic (eg, cefepime) when the patient experiences his or her first neutropenic fever. Although fluoroquinolones reduce the incidence of gram-negative bacteremia, they have not been shown to affect mortality; the possibility of developing clostridium difficile-associated diarrhea exists with fluoroquinolone use and infectious causes should be ruled out if diarrhea occurs. Concerns with fluoroquinolone use in the prophylactic setting during HSCT include the emergence of resistant organisms and an increased risk for streptococcal infection. Broad-spectrum IV antibiotics should be initiated immediately at the time of the first neutropenic fever under the treatment guidelines endorsed by the Infectious Disease Society of America for management of fever of unknown origin in the neutropenic host.[37]

Prevention of HSV and VZV Patients who are HSV antibody seropositive before HSCT are at high risk for reactivation of their HSV infection. Acyclovir is highly effective in preventing HSV reactivation, and thus, prophylactic acyclovir is used commonly in HSV-seropositive patients who are undergoing an allogeneic or autologous HSCT. In the setting of HSV prophylaxis, dosing regimens for prophylactic acyclovir vary widely and most centers discontinue acyclovir at the time of hematopoietic recovery.[38] Valacyclovir (Valtrex), a prodrug of acyclovir with improved bioavailability, may allow for adequate serum concentrations to prevent HSV in patients undergoing HSCT as well.

In those with a history of VZV infection, VZV disease occurs in 30% of allogeneic HSCT recipients.[39] The appropriate duration of VZV prophylaxis is controversial. Although VZV infections are reduced by prophylactic acyclovir administered from 1 to 2 months until 1 year after HSCT, the risk of VZV persists in those on continued immunosuppression.[38]

Prevention and Preemptive Therapy of CMV Disease After allogeneic HSCT, CMV disease is common and has high morbidity and mortality rates. Allogeneic patients are at greater risk than autologous recipients primarily because the latter more efficiently reconstitute their immune system after transplantation. However, autologous HSCT recipients who are CMV seropositive before HSCT are at risk for CMV infection, and prophylaxis should be considered in a select minority of patients.[38] Infection caused by CMV is usually asymptomatic and develops when CMV replication occurs. Replication occurs primarily in body fluids such as the blood (viremia), bronchoalveolar fluid, or urine (viruria). CMV disease is symptomatic and occurs when the virus invades an organ or tissue. Pneumonia and gastritis are the most common types of CMV disease after allogeneic HSCT. The presence of a CMV infection substantially increases the risk for developing invasive CMV disease. Strategies to prevent CMV infection have resulted in dramatic reductions in the incidence of CMV disease.

Primary CMV can be prevented with CMV seromatching, which includes transplanting PBPCs or bone marrow from CMV-seronegative donors and infusing CMV-negative blood products to CMV-negative recipients. Antivirals are important in those who are CMV seropositive or have a CMV-seropositive graft, with two available approaches to minimize the morbidity associated with CMV. The first is universal prophylaxis, in which ganciclovir is begun at the time of engraftment and is continued until approximately 100 days after engraftment. The second approach is called preemptive therapy, for which ganciclovir is selectively administered based on detection of CMV reactivation.

Preemptive therapy is the most commonly used strategy for preventing CMV disease after allogeneic HSCT because ganciclovir is used only in patients at highest risk for developing CMV disease. This approach minimizes administration of ganciclovir, thus lowering the risk of ganciclovir-induced neutropenia with its subsequent increased risk of invasive bacterial and fungal infections. Preemptive strategies typically use an induction course of ganciclovir for 7 to 14 days followed by a maintenance course until 2 or 3 weeks after the last positive antigenemia result or until 100 days after HSCT.[38] Oral valganciclovir (Valcyte) is an orally bioavailable prodrug of ganciclovir that is converted to ganciclovir in vivo after intestinal absorption and has been used for preemptive therapy. Foscarnet may be given as an alternative to ganciclovir to prevent CMV disease, although its use is complicated by nephrotoxicity and electrolyte wasting.

Fungal Infections

Prevention of Fungal Infections. The widespread use of fluconazole prophylaxis since the early 1990s has led to a significant decline in the morbidity and mortality associated with invasive candidiasis in HSCT recipients. However, invasive aspergillosis (IA); zygomycetes; and fluconazole-resistant *Candida* spp., such as *Candida krusei* and *Candida glabrata*, have increased markedly in incidence.[40] Itraconazole, another azole antifungal agent, has better *in vitro* activity against fluconazole-resistant fungi (eg, *Aspergillus* and some *Candida* spp.) and is more effective than fluconazole for long-term prophylaxis of invasive fungal infections after allogeneic HSCT; however, itraconazole is used less often because of frequent GI side effects and concern for potential drug interactions.[41] Posaconazole (Noxafil) is a triazole antifungal that has been approved by the FDA for prophylaxis against IA in HSCT patients with GVHD and is now the recommended prophylactic agent for this subset of HSCT patients on immunosuppression. Posaconazole oral suspension should be given with food for adequate absorption. The posaconazole tablet can be administered without regard to food. Micafungin (Mycamine), an agent of the newer class of antifungals known as the echinocandins, has been FDA approved for prophylaxis of *Candida* infections in patients undergoing HSCT.

Risk Factors for Invasive Mold Infections. Invasive mold infections (eg, *Aspergillus* spp., *Fusarium* spp., *Zygomycetes*, and *Scedosporium* spp.) are an increasing cause of morbidity and death after allogeneic and autologous HSCT. It has been estimated that up to one-third of febrile neutropenic patients who do not respond to antibiotic therapy after 1 week are harboring a fungal infection.[37] In HSCT recipients, risk factors for invasive fungal infections include previous history of IA; recipient factors, including older age, CMV seropositivity, and type of stem cell transplant; treatment factors (eg, a fludarabine-based preparative regimen); transplant complications (eg, prolonged neutropenia, graft failure, and higher grade GVHD); and host factors (eg, diabetes, iron overload).[42] Infections with *Aspergillus* spp. remain the most common mold infections diagnosed in the HSCT population and optimal treatment must be promptly initiated if indicated.

Treatment of Invasive Aspergillosis. Early diagnosis and initiation of appropriate therapy may reduce the high mortality rate of IA. Outcomes also depend on recovery of the recipient's immune system and reduction of immunosuppression. Diagnosis is difficult with the use of computed tomography scans and cultures. Research is ongoing to evaluate the benefit of using nonculture-based methods, such as galactomannan and (1,3)-β-D-glucan antigen detection, which are components of the fungal cell wall that can be detected by commercially available assays.

Practice guidelines are available for the treatment of invasive *Aspergillus* infections in immunocompromised patients.[43] Available mold-active agents include triazole antifungals (itraconazole, voriconazole, and posaconazole), echinocandins (caspofungin, micafungin, and anidulafungin), and amphotericin B formulations.

Historically, conventional amphotericin B (c-AmB) was considered the "gold standard" antifungal therapy for any IA infection; however lipid analogs of amphotericin have shown equivalent efficacy and a reduction in side effects, albeit at a higher acquisition cost. With significant toxicity limiting the overall utility of conventional amphotericin B, voriconazole (Vfend) was compared with c-AmB for treatment of IA. For initial therapy of IA, voriconazole had higher response and survival rates than c-AmB and is now considered the primary option for patients with IA.[44]

In patients who have failed initial therapy (ie, salvage), lipid formulations of amphotericin products, itraconazole, posaconazole or an agent from the echinocandin class may be used.

The optimal duration of appropriate antifungal therapy for treating IA is individualized to the reconstitution of the patient's immune system and his or her response to antifungal treatment. Most clinicians continue aggressive antifungal therapy until the infection has stabilized radiographically and may continue with less aggressive "maintenance" therapy (eg, oral voriconazole) until immunosuppression is lessened or completed. In general, it is common to require several months of antifungal therapy to treat IA.

Pneumocystis jiroveci. After allogeneic HSCT, prophylaxis for *P. jiroveci* (formerly *P. carinii*) pneumonia (PCP) is used because *Pneumocystis* is a serious infection with a high mortality rate if left untreated. Most centers use sulfamethoxazole/trimethoprim for 6 to 12 months after HSCT;[38] aerosolized or IV pentamidine and oral dapsone are alternatives for patients who are allergic to sulfa drugs or who do not tolerate cotrimoxazole. Because PCP most often occurs after engraftment, cotrimoxazole usually is begun after neutrophil recovery because of its myelosuppressive effects. Patients receiving prophylactic cotrimoxazole should be monitored closely for rash and unexplained neutropenia or thrombocytopenia. Cotrimoxazole usually is avoided on days of methotrexate administration because the sulfonamides can displace methotrexate from plasma binding sites and decrease renal methotrexate clearance, resulting in higher methotrexate concentrations. Autologous HSCT patients do not receive posttransplant immunosuppression, and thus, their risk of developing PCP is lower.[38] PCP prophylaxis is used often after autologous HSCT in patients with a hematologic malignancy.

► *Issues of Survivorship After HSCT*

The number of long-term HSCT survivors is increasing as 5-year disease-free survival rates improve. Because nonmyeloablative preparative regimens were developed over the past decade, the late effects reported in HSCT survivors describe those resulting from myeloablative preparative regimens.[45] HSCT recipients—with either an autologous or an allogeneic graft—have a higher mortality rate than the general population.[46] KEY CONCEPT *Long-term survivors of HSCT should be monitored closely, particularly for infections and secondary malignant neoplasms.*

Survivors of HSCT are at higher risk for secondary malignant neoplasms.[45] Long-term impairment of end-organ function,

Patient Encounter, Part 3

The patient is admitted for allogeneic HSCT with a reduced-intensity preparative regimen consisting of fludarabine and busulfan. Her hospital course was complicated for neutropenic fever and gastrointestinal toxicities. Neutrophil engraftment occurred on day +12 after HSCT, and the patient was discharged from the hospital on day +14 with minimal complaints. She presents to the transplant clinic on day +22 complaining of a skin rash on her palms and trunk. She does not report diarrhea, nausea, vomiting, or any other symptoms.

What is the differential diagnosis for the patient's current condition?

How should this patient be monitored for progression of GVHD?

including the kidneys, liver, and lungs, may be caused by the preparative regimen, infectious complications, and/or post-transplant immunosuppression. Many HSCT recipients experience endocrine dysfunction, such as hypothyroidism from TBI, adrenal insufficiency from long-term corticosteroids to treat GVHD, and infertility from radiation and/or high doses of alkylating agents in myeloablative preparative regimens. Osteopenia has been found in more than half of HSCT recipients, most likely from gonadal dysfunction and/or corticosteroid administration.

Close monitoring of HSCT recipients for infections is necessary because recovery of immune function is slow, sometimes requiring more than 2 years, even in the absence of immunosuppressants.[45] Fevers should be assessed and treated rapidly to minimize the likelihood of a fatal infection. HSCT recipients—both autologous and allogeneic—lose protective antibodies to vaccine-preventable diseases; international guidelines been published regarding recommendations for reimmunization of HSCT recipients.[38]

Survivors of HSCT should be monitored routinely for signs of relapse and, if an allogeneic graft was used, chronic GVHD. They should be advised regarding revaccination and obtaining prompt medical care for fevers or signs of infection. Routine evaluations of organ function (ie, renal, hepatic, thyroid, and ovarian) and osteopenia should occur and the appropriate management strategies initiated if necessary.

OUTCOME EVALUATION

Monitor for symptoms and signs of the disease that is being treated by HSCT to assess the effectiveness of the HSCT. For example, the monitoring plan for a patient with CML would be to monitor disease response by PCR of the *BCR-ABL* transcript. The actual clinical outcome monitored, along with the frequency of monitoring, is based on the underlying disease.

Monitor for nonhematologic toxicity of the preparative regimen during its administration. Monitor these symptoms at least daily, with more frequent monitoring if the patient is experiencing these nonhematologic effects. The goal is to prevent or minimize these adverse effects. Specifically:

- *Busulfan:* Seizures, busulfan concentrations if being used with the BU-CY preparative regimen, number of vomiting episodes, and nausea by patient self-report, total bilirubin, and sudden weight changes (SOS)
- *Cyclophosphamide:* Electrocardiography during IV administration, RBCs in urine, frequency of urination, pain on urination, urinary output, number of vomiting episodes, and nausea by patient self-report, total bilirubin, and SOS
- *Etoposide:* Blood pressure, respiratory rate, serum pH, serum bicarbonate with arterial blood gases, and evaluation of anion gap if necessary

Patient Care Process

Patient Assessment:

- Assess the patient regarding the indication for HSCT, the type of preparative regimen and the type of donor.
- Review the patient's medical history and available laboratory tests. Is the preparative regimen appropriate based on this information?
- Determine the nonhematologic toxicity of the preparative regimen, the expected timing of engraftment after the graft is infused, and the need for GVHD prophylaxis.
- Conduct a medication history. Identify medications that should be continued and medications that should be stopped during the transplant period.

Therapy Evaluation:

- Determine the supportive care needs during administration of the preparative regimen, including use of indwelling central venous catheters and blood product support.
- Assess pharmacologic management of CINV, mucositis, and pain daily; adjust according to efficacy. Review new medications for drug interactions.

Care Plan Development:

- After the graft is infused, monitor the complete blood count with differential at least daily to evaluate engraftment.
- Determine the need for prophylaxis or treatment of infection during the patient's prolonged period of immunosuppression following engraftment.
- Counsel the patient regarding adherence to prophylactic antibiotic, antifungal, and antiviral regimens. Ensure that the patient is appropriately immunized after recovery from HSCT.
- Counsel the patient regarding adherence to GVHD prophylaxis and treatment. Monitor and manage for adverse drug reactions.

Follow-Up Evaluation:

- Assess the effectiveness of the HSCT for the patient's disease. Continue to monitor for nonhematologic toxicity of the preparative regimen, signs and symptoms of GVHD, and infection.
- Follow allogeneic HSCT patients closely for the first year post HSCT for long term effects of the preparative regimen and altered immunity.

- *Total-body irradiation:* Number of vomiting episodes, nausea by patient self-report, SOS, total bilirubin, and skin assessment for the presence of irritation or blister formation

Until the patient has achieved engraftment, monitor the patient for engraftment with at least daily complete blood counts with differentials; these tests may be needed more often if the patient is critically ill or had a prior low hemoglobin. Patients will require transfusion support with blood products and platelets until engraftment occurs if hemoglobin and/or platelets drop below unsafe levels.

Until engraftment has occurred, monitor the patient's temperature every 4 to 8 hours for signs of infection. Also guide monitoring signs of focal point of infection based on clinical symptoms. For example, if the patient develops shortness of breath, then imaging of the lungs should occur to assess pulmonary infection. Monitor for the toxicity of prophylaxis and/or treatment of bacterial, fungal, or viral infections.

Abbreviations Introduced in This Chapter

AML	Acute myelogenous leukemia
ANC	Absolute neutrophil count
ASCO	American Society of Clinical Oncology
ATG	Antithymocyte globulin
BMT	Bone marrow transplantation
BU-CY	Busulfan–cyclophosphamide
c-AmB	Conventional amphotericin B
CINV	Chemotherapy-induced nausea and vomiting
CML	Chronic myelogenous leukemia
CMV	Cytomegalovirus
CY-TBI	Cyclophosphamide–total-body irradiation
GVHD	Graft-versus-host disease
HGF	Hematopoietic growth factors
HLA	Human leukocyte antigen
HSCT	Hematopoietic stem cell transplant
IA	Invasive aspergillosis
IL-2	Interleukin-2
MHC	Minor histocompatibility
MM	Multiple myeloma
NHL	Non-Hodgkin lymphoma
NK	Natural killer
PBPC	Peripheral blood progenitor cells
PCP	Pneumocystis pneumonia
SOS	Sinusoidal obstruction syndrome
SCr	Serum creatinine
TBI	Total-body irradiation
VZV	Varicella zoster virus

REFERENCES

1. Copelan EA. Hematopoietic stem-cell transplantation. N Engl J Med. 2006;354:1813–1826.
2. Pasquini MC, Wang Z. Current use and ouctomes of hematopoietic stem cell transplantation: 2013 CIBMTR Summary Slides. Available at http://www.cibmtr.org.
3. Petersdorf EW, Hansen JA, Martin PJ, et al. Major-histocompatibility-complex class I alleles and antigens in hematopoietic-cell transplantation. N Engl J Med. 2001;345:1794–1800.
4. Morishima Y, Sasazuki T, Inoko H, et al. The clinical significance of human leukocyte antigen (HLA) allele compatibility in patients receiving a marrow transplant from serologically HLA-A, HLA-B, and HLA-DR matched unrelated donors. Blood. 2002;99:4200–4206.
5. Duong HK, Savani BN, Copelan E, et al. Peripheral blood progenitor cell mobilization for autologous and allogeneic hematopoietic cell transplantation: Guidelines from the American Society for Blood and Marrow Transplantation. Biol Blood Marrow Transplant. 2014;20:1262–1273.
6. Barker JN, Davies SM, DeFor T, et al. Survival after transplantation of unrelated donor umbilical cord blood is comparable to that of human leukocyte antigen-matched unrelated donor bone marrow: Results of a matched-pair analysis. Blood. 2001;97:2957–2961.
7. Rocha V, Gluckman E. Clinical use of umbilical cord blood hematopoietic stem cells. Biol Blood Marrow Transplant. 2006;12:34–41.
8. Davies SM, Kollman C, Anasetti C, et al. Engraftment and survival after unrelated-donor bone marrow transplantation: A report from the national marrow donor program. Blood. 2000;96:4096–4102.
9. Schmitz N. Peripheral blood hematopoietic cells for allogeneic transplantation. In: Blume KG, Forman SJ, Thomas ED, eds. Hematopoietic Cell Transplantation, 3rd ed. Malden, MA: Blackwell Science, 2004:588–598.
10. Stem Cell Trialists' Collaborative Group. Allogeneic peripheral blood stem-cell compared with bone marrow transplantation in the management of hematologic malignancies: An individual patient data meta-analysis of nine randomized trials. J Clin Oncol. 2005;23:5074–5087.
11. Remberger M, Ringden O, Blau IW, et al. No difference in graft-versus-host disease, relapse, and survival comparing peripheral stem cells to bone marrow using unrelated donors. Blood. 2001;98:1739–1745.
12. Wolff SN. Second hematopoietic stem cell transplantation for the treatment of graft failure, graft rejection or relapse after allogeneic transplantation. Bone Marrow Transplant. 2002;29:545–552.
13. Clift RA, Buckner CD, Thomas ED, et al. Marrow transplantation for patients in accelerated phase of chronic myeloid leukemia. Blood. 1994;84:4368–4373.
14. Woods WG, Neudorf S, Gold S, et al. Children's cancer group. A comparison of allogeneic bone marrow transplantation, autologous bone marrow transplantation, and aggressive chemotherapy in children with acute myeloid leukemia in remission. Blood. 2001;97:56–62.
15. Bierman PJ, Freedman AS. Autologous hematopoietic stem cell transplantation for non-Hodgkin lymphoma. In: Atkinson K, Champlin R, Ritz J, Fibbe WE, Ljungman P, Brenner MK, eds. Clinical Bone Marrow and Blood Stem Cell Transplantation, 3rd ed. New York: Cambridge University Press, 2004:524.
16. Baron F, Sandmaier BM. Current status of hematopoietic stem cell transplantation after nonmyeloablative conditioning. Curr Opin Hematol. 2005;12:435–443.
17. Copelan EA, Hamilton BK, Avalos B, et al. Better leukemia-free and overall survival in AML in first remission following cyclophosphamide in combination with busulfan compared with TBI. Blood. 2013;122:3863–3870.
18. Champlin R, Khouri I, Anderlini P, et al. Nonmyeloablative preparative regimens for allogeneic hematopoietic transplantation. Biology and current indications. Oncology (Williston Park). 2003;17:94–100; discussion 103–107.
19. McCune JS, Gibbs JP, Slattery JT. Plasma concentration monitoring of busulfan: Does it improve clinical outcome? Clin Pharmacokinet. 2000;39:155–165.
20. Grochow LB. Parenteral busulfan: Is therapeutic monitoring still warranted? Biol Blood Marrow Transplant. 2002;8:465–467.
21. Hensley ML, Hagerty KL, Kewalramani T, et al. American Society of Clinical Oncology 2008 clinical practice guideline update: use of chemotherapy and radiation therapy protectants. J Clin Oncol. 2008;27(1):127–145.

22. Basch E, Prestrud AA, Hesketh PJ, et al. Antiemetics: American Society of Clinical Oncology clinical practice guideline update. J Clin Oncol. 2011;29(31):4189–4198.
23. Radtke ML, Kolesar JM. Palifermin (Kepivance) for the treatment of oral mucositis in patients with hematologic malignancies requiring hematopoietic stem cell support. J Oncol Pharm Pract. 2005;11:121–125.
24. Ho VT, Revta C, Richardson PG. Hepatic veno-occlusive disease after hematopoietic stem cell transplantation: Update on defibrotide and other current investigational therapies. Bone Marrow Transplant. 2008;41:229–237.
25. Smith TJ, Khatcheressian J, Lyman GH, et al. 2006 update of recommendations for the use of white blood cell growth factors: An evidence-based clinical practice guideline. J Clin Oncol. 2006;24(19):3187–3205.
26. Ringden O, Labopin M, Gorin NC, et al. Treatment with granulocyte colony-stimulating factor after allogeneic bone marrow transplantation for acute leukemia increases the risk of graft-versus-host disease and death: A study from the Acute Leukemia Working Party of the European Group for Blood and Marrow Transplantation. J Clin Oncol. 2004;22:416–423.
27. Filipovich AH, Weisdorf D, Pavletic S, et al. National Institutes of Health consensus development project on criteria for clinical trials in chronic graft-versus-host disease: I. Diagnosis and staging working group report. Biol Blood Marrow Transplant. 2005;11:945–956.
28. Couriel D, Caldera H, Champlin R, Komanduri K. Acute graft-versus-host disease: Pathophysiology, clinical manifestations, and management. Cancer. 2004;101:1936–1946.
29. Martin PJ, Rizzo JD, Wingard JR, et al. First- and second-line systemic treatment of acute graft-versus-host disease: Recommendations of the American Society of Blood and Marrow Transplantation. Biol Blood Marrow Transplant. 2012;18:1150–1163.
30. Ratanatharathorn V, Nash RA, Przepiorka D, et al. Phase III study comparing methotrexate and tacrolimus (prograf, FK506) with methotrexate and cyclosporine for graft-versus-host disease prophylaxis after HLA-identical sibling bone marrow transplantation. Blood. 1998;92:2303–2314.
31. Nash RA, Antin JH, Karanes C, et al. Phase 3 study comparing methotrexate and tacrolimus with methotrexate and cyclosporine for prophylaxis of acute graft-versus-host disease after marrow transplantation from unrelated donors. Blood. 2000;96:2062–2068.
32. Leather HL. Drug interactions in the hematopoietic stem cell transplant (HSCT) recipient: What every transplanter needs to know. Bone Marrow Transplant. 2004;33:137–152.
33. Burroughs L, Mielcarek M, Leisenring W, et al. Extending postgrafting cyclosporine decreases the risk of severe graft-versus-host disease after nonmyeloablative hematopoietic cell transplantation. Transplantation. 2006;81:818–825.
34. Lee SJ. New approaches for preventing and treating chronic graft-versus-host disease. Blood. 2005;105:4200–4206.
35. Junghanss C, Boeckh M, Carter RA, et al. Incidence and outcome of cytomegalovirus infections following nonmyeloablative compared with myeloablative allogeneic stem cell transplantation, a matched control study. Blood. 2002;99:1978–1985.
36. Fukuda T, Boeckh M, Carter RA, et al. Risks and outcomes of invasive fungal infections in recipients of allogeneic hematopoietic stem cell transplants after nonmyeloablative conditioning. Blood. 2003;102:827–833.
37. Freifeld AG, Bow EJ, Sepkowitz KA, et al. Clinical practice guideline for the use of antimicrobial agents in neutropenic patients with cancer: 2010 update by the Infectious Diseases Society of America. Clin Infect Dis. 2011;52(4):56–93.
38. Tomblyn, M, Chiller, T, Einsele, H, et al. Guidelines for preventing infectious complications among hematopoietic cell transplantation recipients: A global perspective. Biol Blood Marrow Transplant. 2009;15:1143–1238.
39. Boeckh M, Kim HW, Flowers ME, et al. Long-term acyclovir for prevention of varicella zoster virus disease after allogeneic hematopoietic cell transplantation—a randomized double-blind placebo-controlled study. Blood. 2006;107:1800–1805.
40. Richardson M, Lass-Flörl C. Changing epidemiology of systemic fungal infections. Clin Microbiol Infect. 2008;(Suppl 4):5–24.
41. Winston DJ, Maziarz RT, Chandrasekar PH, et al. Intravenous and oral itraconazole versus intravenous and oral fluconazole for long-term antifungal prophylaxis in allogeneic hematopoietic stem-cell transplant recipients. A multicenter, randomized trial. Ann Intern Med. 2003;138:705–713.
42. Garcia-Vidal C, Upton A, Kirby KA, Marr KA. Epidemiology of invasive mold infections in allogeneic stem cell transplant recipients: Biological risk factors for infection according to time after transplantation. Clin Infect Dis. 2008;47:1041–1050.
43. Walsh TJ, Anaissie EJ, Denning DW, et al. Treatment of aspergillosis: Clinical Practice Guidelines of the Infectious Diseases Society of America. Clin Infect Dis. 2008;46(3):327–360.
44. Herbrecht R, Denning DW, Patterson TF, et al. Voriconazole versus amphotericin B for primary therapy of invasive aspergillosis. N Engl J Med. 2002;347:408–415.
45. Antin JH. Clinical practice. Long-term care after hematopoietic-cell transplantation in adults. N Engl J Med. 2002;347:36–42.
46. Bhatia S, Robison LL, Francisco L, et al. Late mortality in survivors of autologous hematopoietic-cell transplantation: Report from the Bone Marrow Transplant Survivor Study. Blood. 2005;105:4215–4222.

99 Supportive Care in Oncology

Sarah L. Scarpace

LEARNING OBJECTIVES

Upon completion of the chapter, the reader will be able to:

1. Describe the impact of various supportive care interventions on the prognosis of patients with cancer.
2. Discuss the scientific basis for providing various supportive care interventions in the oncology patient population.
3. Identify patient-related and disease-related risk factors in defining a population for whom supportive care interventions would be of benefit.
4. Recognize typical presenting signs and symptoms of common complications and emergencies that require supportive care interventions.
5. Outline appropriate prevention and management strategies for various supportive care interventions.
6. Prepare a monitoring plan to evaluate the efficacy and toxicity of pharmacotherapy interventions for supportive care problems.

INTRODUCTION

Patients with cancer are at risk for serious adverse events that result from their treatment, the cancer, or both. The management of these complications is generally referred to as supportive care (or symptom management). Examples of treatment-related complications include chemotherapy-induced nausea and vomiting (CINV), myelosuppression, febrile neutropenia (FN), hemorrhagic cystitis, mucositis, and tumor lysis syndrome (TLS). Tumor or cancer-related complications include superior vena cava (SVC) obstruction, spinal cord compression, hypercalcemia, and brain metastases. In some cases, these events can be life threatening. SVC obstruction, spinal cord compression, TLS, and hypercalcemia have traditionally been defined as oncologic emergencies. Treatment- and disease-related complications in the oncology population require rapid assessment and supportive care interventions. The onset of oncologic emergencies may herald the onset of an undiagnosed malignancy or progression or relapse of a preexisting malignancy. Optimal management of patients with various oncologic emergencies and complications requiring supportive care interventions can significantly decrease morbidity and mortality in patients with cancer. This chapter provides an overview of these issues. First, an overview of the management of common side effects of treatment is given. Later, a summary of common oncologic emergencies is presented.

CHEMOTHERAPY-INDUCED TOXICITIES: NAUSEA/VOMITING

Nausea and vomiting are among the most commonly feared toxicities by patients undergoing chemotherapy.[1] KEY CONCEPT *The optimal method of managing CINV is to provide adequate pharmacologic prophylaxis given a patient's risk level for emesis.* Insufficient control during the first cycle of chemotherapy leads to more difficulty in controlling emesis for subsequent cycles.[2]

EPIDEMIOLOGY AND ETIOLOGY

Although it is widely known that chemotherapy causes nausea and vomiting, the rate of emesis varies depending on individual patient risk factors and drug therapy regimen. Therefore, cancer treatments are stratified into varying risk levels: high, moderate, low, and minimal. Agents with a "high" emetic risk cause emesis in more than 90% of cases if not given any prophylaxis. The rates of emesis for "moderate," "low," and "minimal" are 30% to 90%, 10% to 30%, and less than 10%, respectively. Table 99–1 lists the individual agents and their risk category.[3]

PATHOPHYSIOLOGY

The pathophysiology of nausea and vomiting is described in Chapter 20. Specific to CINV, the key receptors include serotonin (5-HT_3) receptors (located in the chemoreceptor trigger zone, emetic center of the medulla, and gastrointestinal [GI] tract) and neurokinin-1 (NK1) receptors (located in the emetic center of the medulla). Serotonin plays an important role in the genesis of acute vomiting, occurring within the first 24 hours of chemotherapy, because some cancer drug therapies can stimulate a release of serotonin from enterochromaffin cells in the GI tract. Serotonin then activates the emetic response by binding to $5HT_3$ receptors in the emetic center. This short-lived release of serotonin likely explains why serotonin antagonists are more beneficial for preventing acute versus delayed vomiting.[4] Other sites that are targeted by antiemetics include dopamine, muscarinic (acetylcholine), histamine, and cannabinoid receptors.

Table 99–1

Emetogenic Potential of Chemotherapy

Risk	Agent
High emetic risk (> 90% of patients will vomit without appropriate antiemetics)	AC combination (doxorubicin or epirubicin and cyclophosphamide)
	Carmustine > 250 mg/m^2
	Cisplatin
	Cyclophosphamide > 1500 mg/m^2
	Dacarbazine
	Doxorubicin ≥ 60 mg/m^2
	Epirubicin > 90 mg/m^2
	Ifosfamide ≥ 2 g/m^2
	Mechlorethamine
	Streptozocin
Moderate emetic risk (30%–90%)	Aldesleukin > 12–15 million $units/m^2$
	Amifostine > 300 mg/m^2
	Arsenic trioxide
	Azacitidine
	Bendamustine
	Busulfan > 4 mg/m^2
	Carboplatin
	Carmustine ≤ 250 mg/m^2
	Clofarabine
	Cyclophosphamide ≤ 1500 mg/m^2
	Cytarabine > 200 mg/m^2
	Dactinomycin
	Daunorubicin
	Doxorubicin < 60 mg/m^2
	Epirubicin < 90 mg/m^2
	Etoposide (po)
	Idarubicin
	Ifosfamide < 2 g/m^2
	Irinotecan
	Imatinib (po)
	Melphalan
	Methotrexate > 250 mg/m^2
	Oxaliplatin
	Temozolamide (po)
	Vinorelbine (po)
Low emetic risk (10%–30%)	Ado-trstuzumab emtansine
	Amifostine < 300 mg/m^2
	Bexarotene
	Brentuximab
	Cabazitaxel
	Carfilzomib
	Capecitabine (po)
	Docetaxel
	Doxorubicin (liposomal)
	Eribulin
	Etoposide
	Fludarabine (po)
	5-Fluorouracil
	Gemcitabine
	Ixabepilone
	Methotrexate > 50 mg/m^2 and < 250 mg/m^2
	Mitomycin
	Mitoxantrone
	Nilotinib
	Omacetaxine
	Paclitaxel
	Pemetrexed
	Pentostatin
	Pralatrexate
	Thiotepa
	Topotecan
	Vorinostat
Minimal risk (less than 10%)	Most other agents

From Hesketh PJ. Chemotherapy-induced nausea and vomiting. N Engl J Med. 2008;358:2482–2494. Grunberg SM. Evaluation of new antiemetic agents and definition of antineoplastic agent emetogenicity state of the art. Support Care Cancer. 2010;19:S43–S47.

CLINICAL PRESENTATION AND DIAGNOSIS

CINV, although frequently discussed as one syndrome, includes two distinct clinical entities, including both nausea and vomiting. Nauseous patients may present with general GI upset and reflux and may report a sensation or desire to vomit without being able to do so.[3] In all cases, it is important that other etiologies of nausea and vomiting are ruled out before diagnosing chemotherapy as the cause.[5] Other causes of nausea and vomiting may include bowel obstruction, opioid intolerance, electrolyte imbalances, brain metastases, and vestibular dysfunction.[5]

TREATMENT

Desired Outcomes

The desired outcome is to completely prevent or minimize the severity of nausea, vomiting, and the use of breakthrough antiemetic medications. In clinical trials, a common end point is "complete response," defined as having no emesis and no breakthrough medication use within a defined period of time. If patients experience nausea or emesis, the goal is to quickly relieve the episode and prevent future nausea or vomiting, whether in the next few days or for the next cycle of chemotherapy.

General Approach to Treatment

Treatment-related factors and patient-related factors can help define a patient population at risk for developing CINV. Treatment-related factors include those chemotherapy agents with high levels of emetogenicity (see Table 99–1 for a complete listing). CINV is typically a cyclical occurrence. Although this section focuses on CINV, it can be helpful for practitioners to remember that patients undergoing concomitant radiation therapy and chemotherapy are at risk for more severe nausea and vomiting. Radiation (particularly total-body irradiation as part of a conditioning regimen for stem cell transplant) can cause a more cumulative (versus cyclical) nausea/vomiting phenomenon.

Specific patient-related factors such as female gender, age less than 50, history of motion sickness, pregnancy-induced nausea or vomiting, and poor emetic control in previous chemotherapy cycles increase the risk of emesis. Interestingly, patients

Clinical Presentation and Diagnosis of CINV

Acute Nausea/Vomiting

- Occurs within the first 24 hours after chemotherapy administration

Delayed Nausea/Vomiting

- Occurs between 24 hours and 5 days after chemotherapy administration

Anticipatory Nausea/Vomiting

- A learned, conditioned reflex response to a stimulus (sight, sound, smell) often associated with poor emetic control in a previous cycle of chemotherapy

Breakthrough Nausea/Vomiting

- Occurs despite prophylaxis with an appropriate antiemetic regimen

Differential Diagnosis

- Surgery, radiation
- Gastric outlet or bowel obstruction, constipation
- Hypercalcemia, hyperglycemia, hyponatremia, uremia
- Other drugs (opioids)

Table 99–2

Recommended Therapy by Emetic Risk

Emetic Risk Category (Incidence of Emesis without Antiemetics)	Antiemetic Regimens and Schedules
High (> 90%)	5-HT_3 serotonin receptor antagonist: day 1 Dexamethasone: days 1–4 Aprepitant: days 1–3 or fosaprepitant 150 mg IV day 1 only Or Olanzapine: Days 1–4 Palonosetron: Day 1 Dexamethasone: Day 1
Moderate (30%–90%)	5-HT_3 serotonin receptor antagonist: days 1–3 Dexamethasone: day 1 Or 5-HT_3 serotonin receptor antagonist: day 1 Dexamethasone: days 1–3
Low (10%–30%)	Dexamethasone: day 1 Or 5-HT_3 serotonin receptor antagonist: Day 1
Minimal (< 10%)	As needed

Data from Kris MG, Hesketh PJ, Somerfield MR, et al. American Society of Clinical Oncology Guidelines for Antiemesis in Oncology: Update 2006. J Clin Oncol. 2006;24:2932–2947.

with a history of alcohol abuse have a reported decreased risk of emesis.[3] It is important to design an antiemetic regimen with consideration of these patient-specific risk factors.[6] A well-designed regimen includes a prophylactic regimen and a breakthrough antiemetic drug "as needed." Although many drugs are recommended as "breakthrough" drugs, choose a drug with a different mechanism of action compared with the drugs used for prophylaxis.[5]

▶ *Nonpharmacologic Therapy*

Nonpharmacologic therapy for nausea and vomiting can be useful adjuncts to drug therapy, particularly in the setting of anticipatory nausea and vomiting. Behavior therapies such as relaxation, guided imagery, and music therapy as well as acupuncture or acupressure as useful in this setting.[5] Other general measures that can be taken include ensuring adequate sleep before treatment, eating smaller meals, and avoiding greasy foods and foods with strong odors.[5]

▶ *Pharmacologic Therapy*

Nonprescription medications such as antacids, histamine-2 receptor blockers, and proton pump inhibitors can be helpful in reducing gastroesophageal reflux associated with some cancer treatments that may trigger or exacerbate CINV.[5] Nonprescription antihistamines marketed for nausea associated with motion sickness are not usually helpful in managing CINV.

Four drug classes are highly effective in preventing CINV: corticosteroids (dexamethasone), serotonin receptor antagonists, NK1 receptor antagonists (aprepitant or fosaprepitant), and the thienobenzodiazepine, olanzapine.[7] Drugs with differing mechanisms of action are combined, depending on the emetic risk level of the chemotherapy regimen. (Table 99–2).

Intravenous (IV) antiemetics are usually administered 30 minutes before chemotherapy, and oral antiemetics are administered 60 minutes before chemotherapy. Dexamethasone is the preferred agent to prevent CINV in the delayed setting (days 2–4 after chemotherapy administration) for moderately and highly emetogenic chemotherapy and is given at dose of 4 mg orally twice daily (or 8 mg once daily) for 3 to 4 days. In some cases, the serotonin antagonists may also be continued orally for 3 to 4 days after chemotherapy or be used in place of dexamethasone. When oral aprepitant is used prechemotherapy, the aprepitant is continued as 80 mg orally once daily on days 2 and 3 of the chemotherapy cycle. No oral aprepitant is necessary when fosaprepitant is given on day 1.

Concerns of QT prolongation have resulted in the IV formulation of dolasetron to be removed from the market and dosing of ondansetron has been reduced to 16 mg IV as the 32 mg IV was reported to extend the QT interval.[8]

The other classes of antiemetics are usually prescribed "as needed" for breakthrough nausea or vomiting. The dopamine antagonists prochlorperazine and metoclopramide are usually recommended because they antagonize a different receptor than the drugs already given for prophylaxis. Other medications, including serotonin receptor antagonists, cannabinoids, dexamethasone, scopolamine, or olanzapine, may be used as alternatives to dopamine antagonists for breakthrough nausea and vomiting.[5] Breakthrough medications should have different mechanisms of action than the medications a patient is taking to prevent nausea and vomiting. For those in any risk group who experience anticipatory nausea and vomiting, the addition of lorazepam for prophylaxis and breakthrough is recommended for its antiemetic and antianxiety properties. Table 99–3 lists the doses of the antiemetic agents for prophylaxis and breakthrough use.

Table 99–3
Antiemetic Dosing

Antiemetic	Single Dose Administered Before Chemotherapy	Daily Schedule
5-HT_3 Serotonin Receptor Antagonists		
Dolasetron	po: 100 mg	100 mg po daily
Granisetron	po: 2 mg IV: 1 mg or 0.01 mg/kg Topical: 34.3-mg patch (apply 24–48 hours before chemotherapy, leave on for 7 days)	1–2 mg po daily or 1 mg two times a day
Ondansetron	po: 16–24 mg IV: 8–16 mg	8 mg po two times a day or 16 mg po daily
Palonosetron	IV: 0.25 mg	
Others		
Aprepitant	po: 125 mg	80 mg po days 2 and 3
Fosaprepitant	IV: 150 mg	No aprepitant on days 2 or 3
Dexamethasone	po: 12 mg if given with aprepitant, otherwise 20mg IV: 12mg if given with aprepitant, otherwise 20mg	8 mg po days 2–4
Olanzapine	po: 10mg	10mg po daily

Data from Kris MG, Hesketh PJ, Somerfield MR, et al. American Society of Clinical Oncology Guidelines for Antiemesis in Oncology: Update 2006. J Clin Oncol. 2006;24:2932–2947.

A prophylactic antiemetic regimen for high emetic risk levels of IV chemotherapy should be with a triple-drug combination using dexamethasone, aprepitant, and 5-HT_3 antagonist to prevent both acute and delayed emesis. Dexamethasone should be continued until day 4, and aprepitant is also administered on days 2 and 3 if the oral formulation is used. When fosaprepitant 150 mg IV is administered on day 1, no oral aprepitant is needed on days 2 and 3 of therapy. Alternatively, olanzapine in combination with palonosetron and dexamethasone can be used. A phase 3 trial of 241 patients comparing aprepitant, palonosetron, and dexamethasone to olanzapine with a palonosetron and dexamethasone for patients treated with highly emetogenic chemotherapy had similar rates of CINV control (87%–97% prevention of acute CINV, 73%–77% prevention of delayed CINV), though nausea was better controlled by the olanzapine-based regimen (69% overall vs 38% overall).[9]

For moderately emetogenic regimens, acute emesis is still of major concern, but the incidence of delayed emesis is less.

Patient Encounter 1: CINV

A 73-year-old man with non–small cell lung cancer (NSCLC) presents today for initiation of chemotherapy with cisplatin 75 mg/m^2 and paclitaxel 175 mg/m^2.

What category of emetic risk should this dose regimen fall under?

What do you recommend for preventing nausea and vomiting in this patient?

Patient Care Process: CINV

Patient Assessment:

- Evaluate patient's chemotherapy regimen and assess emetic potential.
- Using a visual analogue or numerical rating scale (0–10), have the patient rate the severity of nausea (assess nausea first; then move on to emesis).
- Daily, ask about the number of emesis episodes in the last 24 hours.
- Assess scheduled and breakthrough medication adherence.
- Assess patient for risk factors for CINV such as history of motion sickness, pregnancy-induced nausea/vomiting, anxiety, lack of sleep, etc.
- Evaluate patient's outpatient medications and determine if there are drug interactions, precautions, or other contraindications to intended antiemetic therapy.
- On subsequent cycles, evaluate continued effectiveness of initial antiemetic regimen and assess the need for breakthrough antiemetics.

Therapy Evaluation:

- Evaluate patient for complete response to therapy, especially after the first cycles—no vomiting and no nausea.
- Monitor patient diary of recording of breakthrough antiemetic use.

Care Plan Development:

- Counsel the patient on how to take the antiemetic regimen, side effects, drug interactions. Emphasize the need to take the regimen regardless of whether the patient feels nauseous or not—the goal is prevention.
- Explain which drugs are taken as prophylaxis to prevent nausea and vomiting and which are taken as needed to treat it.
- Counsel patient on nonpharmacological management of CINV—adequate sleep, small meals, stress management, etc.
- Have the patient journal when a dose is taken in relation to the chemotherapy. Encourage journaling the severity and frequency of nausea, vomiting, diet, and antiemetic adherence.

Follow-Up Evaluation:

- Ensure no episodes of nausea or vomiting at each chemotherapy visit.

Therefore, dexamethasone plus a 5-HT_3 antagonist should be given on day 1. On days 2 to 4, choose to continue either the dexamethasone or the 5-HT_3 antagonist to prevent delayed emesis. One exception is when palonosetron is given as the 5-HT_3 antagonist on day 1. Because its half-life is long, no redosing is necessary on subsequent days. Aprepitant and fosaprepitant 115 mg IV are also approved by the Food and Drug Administration (FDA) for the prevention of CINV in the moderate setting. While an NK1 receptor antagonist is not routinely used for moderately emetogenic chemotherapy, if patients have clinical risk factors or if they experienced uncontrolled emesis with previous chemotherapy cycles, the same regimen for "high-" risk levels may be used.

For low emetic risk IV chemotherapy regimens, single antiemetic prophylaxis with either dexamethasone or a dopamine antagonist is recommended. For minimal emetic risk groups, guidelines do not recommend routine prophylaxis with antiemetics; instead, patients should be provided with a drug to take as needed for nausea and vomiting. Table 99–2 summarizes regimens for antiemetic prophylaxis for the different risk levels of IV chemotherapy.

Many oral anticancer agents are now available and are typically administered daily. For highly and moderately emetogenic oral anticancer therapy, an oral 5HT_3-antagonist is administered before each dose with or without lorazepam and/or an H_2-blocker or proton pump inhibitor.[5] Low-minimal risk oral anticancer agents are given in conjunction with "as needed" antiemetics similar to the approach for IV chemotherapy.[5]

OUTCOME EVALUATION

It is often difficult to evaluate nausea and vomiting when chemotherapy is given as an outpatient. After drug administration, patients return home and may or may not report inadequate control of emesis. Subsequent chemotherapy cycles may also be poorly controlled, especially if patients do not state their experience with the previous cycle. To ameliorate this problem, patients' experiences with CINV should be assessed, particularly after the first and second cycles of chemotherapy. Patients should be asked about their previous emesis control with subsequent cycles of chemotherapy, and a prophylactic regimen may need to be adjusted. Patients should also be encouraged to self-report poor control of emesis while at home. Side effects of the antiemetic regimen should also be assessed and reported.

MUCOSITIS

Mucositis is the degradation of mucosal lining in the oral cavity and GI tract caused by damage from radiation or chemotherapy.[10] Mucositis is a common supportive care issue that deserves attention and is associated with many negative health consequences, including pain, inadequate nutritional intake, and risk for infection. Patients with mucositis often require parenteral analgesics, nutrition supplementation, and antiinfectives to treat concomitant bacterial, fungal, or viral infections. Furthermore, mucositis is associated with economic consequences, primarily increased lengths of hospital stay.[11] An understanding of the current guidelines for prevention and treatment of mucositis can help improve patient outcomes

EPIDEMIOLOGY AND ETIOLOGY

The incidence of chemotherapy or radiation-induced mucositis depends mostly on the type of chemotherapy, the type and area of radiation, and the specific cancer. Studies have reported an incidence of about 85% in head and neck cancer patients receiving chemoradiation.[10] The World Health Organization estimates that approximately 75% of patients who are treated with high-dose chemotherapy for stem cell transplantation developed oral mucositis.[10] Specific chemotherapy agents associated with moderate-severe mucositis include taxanes, anthracyclines, platinum analogues, methotrexate, and the fluoropyrimidines.

PATHOPHYSIOLOGY

The classical concept of mucositis pathophysiology asserts that direct cytotoxicity from chemotherapy or radiation to basal epithelial cells results in ulcerative lesions caused by a lack of regeneration. These lesions are further complicated by trauma or microorganism growth. However, the most recent theory of mucositis pathophysiology is more detailed and involves a multistage, dynamic process that builds upon the historical model.[11] According to this theory, there are five stages of mucositis: initiation, primary damage response, signal amplification, ulceration, and healing. It is important to note that these stages do not occur sequentially. Rather, they are dynamic and may overlap. Prevention of mucositis or treatment in early stages results in the best outcomes for patients.

CLINICAL PRESENTATION AND DIAGNOSIS

Patients with mucositis may present along a continuum of mild, painless, erythematous ulcers to those that are painful and/or bleeding that may interfere with eating and swallowing or that may require treatment with hydration, antibiotics, or even parenteral nutrition in its most severe forms.[11]

TREATMENT

Nonpharmacologic Treatment

The goal of nonpharmacologic measures to prevent mucositis is to reduce the bacterial load KEY CONCEPT *The fundamental approach to lessen the severity of mucositis begins with basic, good oral hygiene (brushing with a soft-bristled toothbrush at least twice daily, flossing, bland rinses, and saliva substitutes).*[10–12] Cryotherapy with ice chips is also helpful for almost all patients at risk for mucositis.[10] Low-level laser therapy (in centers that have the resources to offer it) is also helpful to prevent mucositis in the hematopoietic cell transplant (HCT) setting.[10]

Pharmacologic Treatment

In the setting of radiation therapy, amifostine, a free radical scavenger, at doses equal to or greater than 340 mg/m^2 intrarectal before each dose of radiation therapy for rectal cancer may be considered to prevent gastrointestinal mucositis.[10] Gelclair, Caphasol, and Biotene are gels that provide a protective barrier between damaged oral mucosa and the environment, lessening pain and irritation and are also sometimes used as part of the overall treatment of patients with mucositis.[10] Antimicrobial lozenges, sucralfate and chlorhexidine rinses, and "magic-mouthwash" compounded rinses are not generally recommended by clinical practice guidelines for mucositis prevention even though they are sometimes used in practice.[12] Ranitidine or omeprazole orally are recommended to prevent pain associated with mucositis and reflux following offending chemotherapy.[10]

Unfortunately, little evidence is available to recommend specific treatments for mucositis. Pain assessment and appropriate management are important.[10,12] Pain management may be achieved with oral morphine, topical anesthetic products, and compounded rinses that incorporate lidocaine.[10,12] In more severe cases in which infection of the oral mucosa is suspected, appropriate antibiotic therapy is necessary to prevent systemic infection.[10,12]

Clinical Presentation and Diagnosis of Mucositis

- Painful, erythematous ulcers develop on the lips, cheeks, soft palate, floor of mouth, and throughout the entire gastrointestinal (GI) tract.
- Assess mucositis using validated scales, either oral mucositis assessment scale (OMAS) or University of Nebraska oral assessment score (MUCPEAK).
- Symptoms appear within 5 to 7 days after chemotherapy and resolve in 2 to 3 weeks.
- Pain may affect ability to swallow and eat.
- The patient may have concomitant localized or systemic infection.
- Diarrhea is a symptom of mucositis in the lower GI tract can lead to electrolyte imbalances.

Palifermin is FDA approved for the prevention and treatment of mucositis in patients receiving high-dose chemotherapy as part of stem cell transplant or induction regimens for leukemia. Palifermin is administered as an IV bolus injection at a dosage of 60 mcg/kg/day for 3 consecutive days before and 3 consecutive days after myelotoxic therapy for a total of six doses. Administering palifermin within 24 hours of chemotherapy can result in an increased sensitivity of rapidly dividing epithelial cells to the cytotoxic agent. For this reason, palifermin should not be administered for 24 hours before, 24 hours after, or during the infusion of myelotoxic chemotherapy to avoid increasing the severity and the duration of oral mucositis.

OUTCOME EVALUATION

The goal of therapy is to prevent or decrease the severity and duration of mucositis. Outcomes measured in clinical trials often assess the incidence, duration, and severity of mucositis with a given intervention intended to prevent or treat mucositis. Agents that are intended to palliate the symptoms of mucositis are usually assessed by measures in pain scales and the ability to eat or drink.

HEMATOLOGIC COMPLICATIONS: FEBRILE NEUTROPENIA (FN)

INTRODUCTION

FN is a common adverse effect after administration of cytotoxic chemotherapy. The mortality rate in neutropenic patients caused by infectious complications currently remains between 5% and 10%; therefore, FN is considered a true oncologic emergency. Patients frequently require hospitalization for prompt administration of broad-spectrum antibiotics that are critical to avoid morbidity and mortality.

EPIDEMIOLOGY AND ETIOLOGY

The microorganisms responsible for infections in neutropenic patients have changed significantly in the last 50 years. From the 1960s through the mid-1980s, gram-negative organisms were the most common bacteria isolated. This pattern shifted to the gram-positive organisms in the late 1980s, which remain the most common isolates. Recent data indicate that gram-positive organisms account for 62% to 76% of all bloodstream infections.[13]

Table 99–4

Commonly Isolated Pathogens in Patients with FN

Type of Organism	Comments
Bacteria	
Gram-positive organisms	Most common isolates in FN
Coagulase-negative staphylococci (ie, *Staphylococcus epidermidis*)	Between 70% and 90% resistant to methicillin; indolent course with low mortality
Staphylococcus aureus	Some centers report greater than 50% resistance to methicillin
Enterococcus spp	Resistance to vancomycin ≥ 30%
Viridans streptococci	Increasing resistance to penicillin; result of fluoroquinolone prophylaxis; associated with mucositis
Gram-negative organisms	Infections rapidly fatal
Pseudomonas aeruginosa	High mortality rate; increasing resistance to quinolones
Escherichia coli	Increased incidence of β-lactamase–producing strains
Klebsiella spp	
Enterobacter spp	Increased incidence of β-lactamase–producing strains
Fungi	Occur primarily after prolonged neutropenia (longer than 1 week)
Yeasts	
Candida albicans	Increasing incidence (~10%); high mortality rate
Non-*albicans Candida* (*Candida krusei, Candida glabrata*)	Resistant to fluconazole; high mortality rate
Molds	Resistant to fluconazole; high mortality rate
Aspergillus spp	Pulmonary infection common
Fusarium spp	Emerging pathogen
Scedosporium spp	Emerging pathogen

FN, febrile neutropenia.

The causes of this change are attributed to the widespread use of central venous catheters and more aggressive chemotherapy regimens as well as the use of prophylactic antibiotics with relatively poor gram-positive coverage (quinolones). Commonly isolated pathogens are shown in Table 99–4. Although gram-negative infections are less common, they cause the majority of infections in sites other than the blood and are particularly virulent. It should be noted that isolates vary considerably among institutions; thus, attention to institutional isolation patterns is prudent.

Patient Encounter 2: FN

A 63-year-old woman receiving treatment for metastatic breast cancer presents today, 8 days after chemotherapy, for follow-up and laboratory check. Relevant laboratory study results include WBC count, 0.7 × 10³/mL (0.7 × 10⁹/L); HgB 9.0 g/dL (90 g/L; 5.59 mmol/L)); HCT 26.6% (0.266); PLT, 6 × 10³/mL (6 × 10⁹/L); serum chemistries within normal limits except; SCr, 1.3 mg/dL (115 μmol/L); and estimated GFR 54 mL/min/1.73m². Vitals: T 98.2°F (36.8°C); P 71 beats/min; RR 18 breaths/min; BP 116/64 mm Hg. The patient has no known drug allergies.

What risk factors for FN does this patient have?

How would you approach this patient?

Fungal infections caused by *Candida* spp. (especially *Candida albicans*) have emerged as significant pathogens, especially in patients with hematologic malignancies and those undergoing bone marrow transplantation (BMT). In addition, *Aspergillus* spp. are important pathogens in patients with prolonged and severe neutropenia.

PATHOPHYSIOLOGY

The neutrophils are the primary defense mechanism against bacterial and fungal infection. Most infections in neutropenic patients are a result of organisms contained in endogenous flora, both on the skin and within the GI tract. These organisms are provided access to the bloodstream through breakdowns in host defense barriers (**mucositis**, use of central venous catheters).

Neutropenia is defined as an absolute neutrophil count (ANC) less than 500/μL (0.50×10^9/L) cells or an ANC less than 1000/μL (1.00×10^9/L) cells with a predicted decrease to less than 500/μL (0.50×10^9/L) cells over the next 48 hours. The ANC is calculated by multiplying the total WBC by the percentage of neutrophils (segmented neutrophils plus "bands"). Fever is defined as a single oral temperature greater than or equal to 38.3°C (101°F) or a temperature greater than or equal to 38.0°C (100.4°F) for at least 1 hour. The combination of these two factors defines FN.[14] The risk of infection during the period of neutropenia depends primarily on two factors:

- The duration of the neutropenia (time period of ANC less than 500/μL [0.50×10^9/L] cells)
- The severity of the neutropenia (lowest ANC level reached [nadir])

A multitude of other risk factors for FN have been identified[15] (Table 99–5). Many of these are also risk factors for poor outcome in patients who experience FN. Cancer drug therapy regimens are also categorized as being high risk (greater than 20% incidence of FN reported in clinical trials) or intermediate risk (10%–20% risk of FN reported in clinical trials). Similar to the approach to the prevention of CINV, it is important to consider both the regimen and patient-specific risk factors when determining whether a patient should receive prophylactic therapy for FN.

Table 99–5

Risk Factors for FN

Patient Related	Therapy Related
Age 60 years or older	History of extensive chemotherapy
Poor performance status	Planned full dose intensity of chemotherapy
Bone marrow involvement by tumor	High-dose chemotherapy (ie, bone marrow transplant)
Poor nutritional status	> 20% incidence of FN reported in clinical trials with treatment regimen
Hematologic malignancy	10%–20% incidence of FN reported in clinical trials with treatment regimen plus presence of patient-specific risk factors
Elevated LDH	
Decreased hemoglobin level	
Baseline or first-cycle low neutrophil counts	
History of previous FN	
Uncontrolled or advanced stage cancer	

FN, febrile neutropenia; LDH, lactate dehydrogenase.

From Lyman GH, Lyman CH, Agboola O. Risk models for predicting chemotherapy-induced neutropenia. Oncologist. 2005;10:427–437.

Table 99–6

MASCC Risk-Index for Identifying Low-Risk Patients with FN[a]

Characteristic	Score
Burden of illness[b]	
No symptoms	5
Mild symptoms	5
Moderate symptoms	3
No hypotension	5
No COPD	4
Solid tumor or hematologic malignancy without fungal infection	4
No dehydration	3
Outpatient onset of fever	3
Age < 60 years[c]	2

[a]Note: A risk-index score of 21 or higher indicates that the patient is likely to be at low risk for complications and morbidity.

[b]Choose one symptom assessment.

[c]Does not apply to patients 16 years of age or younger.

COPD, chronic obstructive pulmonary disease; FN, febrile neutropenia; MASCC, Multinational Association for Supportive Care in Cancer.

From Klastersky J, Paesmans M, Rubenstein EB, et al. The Multinational Association for Supportive Care in Cancer risk index: A multinational scoring system for identifying low-risk febrile neutropenic patients. J Clin Oncol. 2000;18:3038–3051

It is clear that patients with FN represent a heterogenous group. Some patients are at lower risk and could potentially be treated as outpatients, thereby avoiding the risk and cost of hospitalization. The Multinational Association for Supportive Care in Cancer (MASCC) has validated a risk assessment tool that assigns a risk score to patients presenting with FN (Table 99–6).[16] Patients with a risk-index score greater than or equal to 21 are identified as low risk and are candidates for outpatient therapy (discussed under section Treatment).

PREVENTION

Three primary modalities for preventing infection in patients who are expected to become neutropenic have been utilized, the first of which is the least expensive and simplest:

- Vigilant hand hygiene
- Prophylactic antibiotics
- Colony-stimulating factors (CSFs)

The advantages and disadvantages of these strategies are discussed individually in the following sections.

Hand Hygiene

As previously discussed, most infections in neutropenic patients are a result of endogenous flora; however, prevention of further acquisition of environmental pathogens is also important. Patients who are or will become neutropenic should practice careful handwashing and avoid contact with people who neglect hand hygiene. In addition, ingestion of certain fresh fruits and vegetables as well as unprocessed dairy products should be avoided during the neutropenic period. Practitioners should also engage in vigilant hand hygiene after each patient encounter to limit the spread of infections between patients.[18]

Clinical Presentation and Diagnosis of FN[17,18]

General

- Only 50% of patients with FN have a clinically documented infection.
- Only 25% of patients with FN have a microbiologically documented infection.

Signs and Symptoms

- Fever is typically the only sign of infection, although septic patients may have chills.
- Infected catheter sites may be erythematous and tender to the touch.

Laboratory Tests

- CBC with differential
- Two blood cultures from each access site (peripheral and central), urinalysis, urine culture, chest x-ray, sputum cultures

Other Diagnostic Tests

- Detailed physical examination of the oral mucosa, sinuses, skin, catheter access sites, perineal area (no rectal examination because of the risk of bacteremia)

Prophylactic Antibiotics

Routine antibacterial prophylaxis is controversial and has been attempted primarily with sulfamethoxazole–trimethoprim (SMZ-TMP) and quinolones. SMZ-TMP offers improved prophylaxis against gram-positive organisms compared with quinolones; quinolones are more effective prophylaxis against gram-negative infections. The 2010 Infectious Diseases Society of America (IDSA) guidelines recommend fluoroquinolone prophylaxis in patients who are at high risk for "prolonged and profound" neutropenia.[14] The IDSA does not recommend routine antibiotic prophylaxis for low-risk patients because of the lack of a clear benefit on mortality rates and concerns regarding increasing antibiotic resistance. One exception is that SMZ-TMP is recommended for prophylaxis of *Pneumocystis jiroveci* (formerly *Pneumocystis carinii*) pneumonitis (PCP) in all at-risk patients (ie, hematopoietic cell transplant recipients, AIDS), regardless of the presence of neutropenia.

Two meta-analyses add fuel to the controversy of routine antibiotic prophylaxis.[19,20] Decreases in infection-related mortality and gram-negative bacteremia were demonstrated with the use of quinolones; however, overall adverse events were higher, and most of the studies were conducted in patients with hematologic malignancies (an inherently high-risk group). Although two additional randomized trials in patients with both solid tumors and hematologic malignancies demonstrated lower rates of FN, infection, and hospitalization with oral prophylactic levofloxacin compared with placebo, both the NCCN and IDSA only recommend prophylactic levofloxacin for patients with expected duration of neutropenia (defined as an ANC less than 1000/μL [1.00×10^9/L]) for more than 7 days because of the:

- Unknown long-term consequences on the development of resistant organisms
- Emergence of *Clostridium difficile* and methicillin-resistant *Staphylococcus aureus* (MRSA) from fluoroquinolone overuse
- Ability to treat lower-risk patients on an outpatient basis, reducing the need for prophylactic antibiotics.[18]

Therefore, the use of prophylactic quinolones in patients who are at high risk for infection (ie, hematologic malignancies) is reasonable; however, use should not be routine for low-risk patients. If prophylactic quinolone use is adopted, changes in local patterns of resistance should be closely monitored.

Colony-Stimulating Factors

The CSFs stimulate the maturation and differentiation of neutrophil precursors. Four agents are currently approved for use in the United States (Table 99–7). The prophylactic use of these agents decreases days of hospitalization and use of empiric antibiotics by shortening the duration of severe neutropenia (defined as ANC less than 500/μL [0.50×10^9/L]). There is little to no effect on the depth of neutrophil nadir. A recent meta-analysis found that the use of prophylactic granulocyte CSF (either filgrastim or pegfilgrastim) results in a 46% risk reduction of FN and a 48% risk reduction in infectious mortality, although absolute differences are small (3.3% vs 1.7%).[21,22] It is critical to note that patients who receive these agents may still experience FN despite the risk reduction. The primary limitation of the use of these agents is cost. CSFs are recommended beginning with the first cycle (primary prophylaxis) of chemotherapy when the risk of FN is greater than or equal to 20%, regardless if the goal of therapy is curative or palliative.[20] This is the point where the use of CSFs is cost effective when balanced against the cost of hospitalization and antimicrobials. Secondary prophylaxis refers to the subsequent prophylactic use of a CSF after a patient has had an episode of FN. This strategy should be used especially when the chemotherapy is being given in patients with the intention of cure (ie, Hodgkin lymphoma, early breast cancer). In this circumstance, administration of full doses of chemotherapy on time without delays has been shown to improve patient outcomes.

Although generally well tolerated, CSFs may cause bone pain in around 25% of patients. This may be managed with acetaminophen or nonsteroidal anti-inflammatory drugs (NSAIDs), although attention to the platelet count is warranted with the use of NSAIDs. Sargramostim in particular may result in low-grade fever and myalgias, perhaps as a result of its wider pattern of effector cell stimulation.[20]

TREATMENT

Desired Outcomes

Because rapid death may occur with certain infections in neutropenic patients, prompt and emergent treatment is indicated. The primary goal is to prevent morbidity and mortality during the neutropenic period. This is accomplished by effectively treating subclinical or established infections.

General Approach to Treatment

KEY CONCEPT *A risk assessment should be performed at presentation of FN to identify low-risk patients for potential outpatient treatment (see Table 99–6). Patients who do not meet low-risk criteria should be hospitalized for parenteral administration of broad-spectrum antibacterials.* The IDSA has published evidence-based guidelines for the management of FN (Figure 99–1).[14] The choice of initial antimicrobial agent(s) depends on the following factors:

- Presence of a central venous catheter
- Drug allergies
- Concurrent renal dysfunction or use of nephrotoxic agents

Table 99–7

Overview of CSF

Agent	Effector Cell(s)	Dosage	Common Adverse Effects	Comments[a]
Filgrastim (Neupogen GCSF, tbo-filgrastim, Granix)	Neutrophil	5 mcg/kg/day SC or IV or round to 300- *or* 480-mcg vial size	Bone pain (~25%)	Begin 1–3 days after chemotherapy
Pegfilgrastim (Neulasta)	Neutrophil	6 mg SC once	Bone pain (~25%)	Self-mediated clearance via neutrophils Once per cycle dosing Administer 1–3 days after chemotherapy
Sargramostim (Leukine GM-CSF)	Neutrophil, eosinophil, macrophage	250 mcg/m²/day SC or IV or round to 250- or 500-mcg vial size	First dose effect (hypotension, flushing) Low-grade fever Bone pain Injection site skin reaction	Indicated for use after induction chemotherapy in older patients with AML Limited experience and lack of FDA approval for prevention of FN

AML, acute myeloid leukemia; FDA, Food and Drug Administration; FN, febrile neutropenia; GC-SF, granulocyte-colony stimulating factor; GM-CSF, granulocyte-macrophage colony stimulating factor; SC, subcutaneous.

[a]No renal or hepatic dose adjustments are required for any product listed in this table.

- Use of prophylactic antibiotics
- Institutional and/or community susceptibility patterns
- Cost

KEY CONCEPT *The administration of empiric therapy should begin immediately after cultures are taken. Therapy should not be withheld until after culture results are obtained.*

As illustrated in Figure 99–1, specific criteria exist for the addition of vancomycin for coverage of resistant gram-positive organisms or agents for coverage of fungal infections. Additional agents are necessary in the setting of continued fever or declining clinical status in neutropenic patients. In general, all empiric therapy is continued until recovery of the ANC to levels above 500 cells/μL (0.500×10^9/L) in patients with negative culture results. If a specific etiology is identified, appropriate therapy should be continued until 7 days after neutropenia resolves. Specific regimens with recommended dosages are summarized in Table 99–8.

▶ *Nonpharmacologic Therapy*

Prevention of infection is key. Handwashing is critical in the prevention of disease transmission.[18,23] It is also important to ensure that patients receive annual influenza vaccines and have had a pneumonia and meningococcal vaccine, and neutropenic patients should avoid individuals with active respiratory infections.[22,23] Indwelling catheters are often sources of infection; however, the IDSA acknowledges that catheters do not always need to be removed.[14] Catheters should be removed in the following circumstances: established tunnel infection (subcutaneous tunnel or periport infection, septic emboli, hypotension associated with catheter use, or a nonpatent catheter), recurrent infection, or no response to antibiotics within 2 or 3 days.[14] Wound debridement should also be performed upon catheter removal. In the setting of peripheral blood stem cell or bone marrow transplant, the Centers for Disease Control and Prevention recommends the use of high-efficiency particulate air (HEPA) filtration systems in patient rooms, and the NCCN suggests that HEPA filters are reasonable to be considered for other patients who experience prolonged neutropenia.[18] HEPA filters are likely to be most useful in preventing mold infections. Although several small studies have attempted to evaluate the effectiveness of isolation of neutropenic patients as a mechanism for infection prevention, no clear data are available to support this practice.[18]

▶ *Pharmacologic Therapy*

There are two primary choices for the initial management of high-risk FN: monotherapy and dual therapy (see Figure 99–1) when vancomycin is not needed. Both regimens have been shown to be equivalent in randomized studies and meta-analyses. Monotherapy avoids the nephrotoxicity of the aminoglycosides and is potentially less expensive but lacks significant gram-positive coverage and may increase selection of resistant organisms. Dual therapy provides synergistic activity, decreased resistance, and dual coverage of *Pseudomonas aeruginosa* but requires therapeutic monitoring for aminoglycosides. The choice between monotherapy and dual therapy is usually provider and institution preference, although dual therapy may be preferred in an acutely symptomatic patient (eg, hypotensive).

Vancomycin adds broad-spectrum gram-positive coverage; however, the increasing emergence of vancomycin-resistant organisms (ie, *Enterococcus* spp.) prompts conservative use of this medication. Vancomycin should only be included as part of the initial therapy if the following are present:

- Severe mucositis
- Soft tissue infection

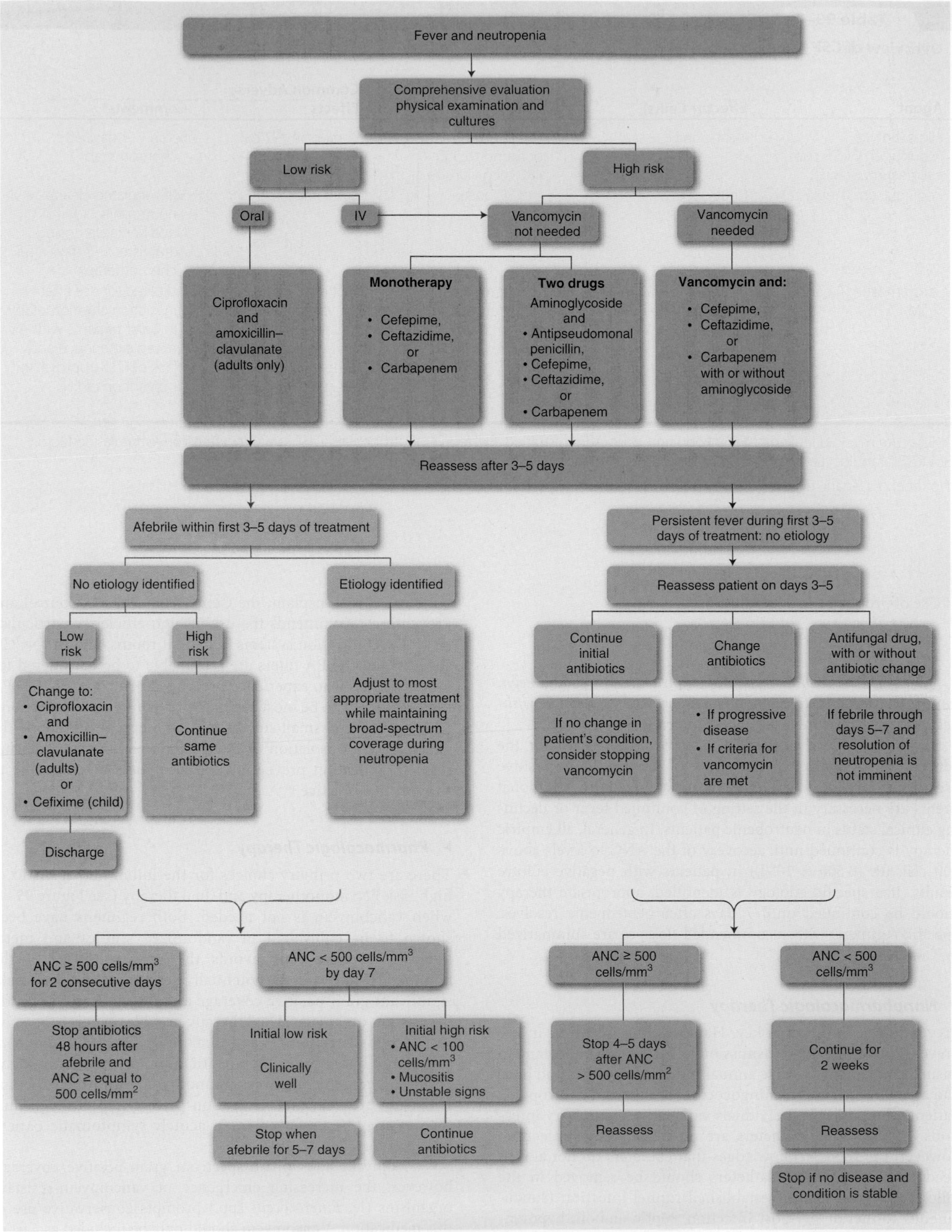

FIGURE 99–1. Management of febrile episodes in neutropenic cancer patients. (ANC, absolute neutrophil count.)

Table 99–8

Dosing Guidelines for Empiric Antimicrobial Agents in FN

Regimen Type	Agents and Dosing[a]	Comments
Antibacterial		
β-Lactam monotherapy	Cefepime 2 g IV every 8 hours Ceftazidime 2 g IV every 8 hours Imipenem 500 mg IV every 6 hours Meropenem 1 g IV every 8 hours Piperacillin–tazobactam 4.5 g IV every 6 hours	Although piperacillin–tazobactam is not recommended in the IDSA guidelines, recent data demonstrate equivalence to other monotherapy and dual therapy regimens. All these agents require renal dose adjustment, and none requires adjustment in hepatic dysfunction. All except meropenem require adjustment during dialysis.
Dual therapy with antipseudomonal β-lactam plus aminoglycoside	Cefepime, ceftazidime, imipenem, meropenem, piperacillin–tazobactam (above dosages), ticarcillin–clavulanic acid 3.1 g IV every 6 hours and gentamicin or tobramycin	Gentamicin or tobramycin 2 mg/kg loading dose followed by doses adjusted by serum concentrations; once-daily dosing of aminoglycosides may be used. Both gentamicin and tobramycin require renal dose adjustment but are dosed based on serum levels. Neither gentamicin nor tobramycin requires hepatic dose adjustment.
Empiric regimens containing vancomycin	Cefepime, ceftazidime, imipenem, meropenem (above dosages) and vancomycin 0.5–1 g every 6–12 hours with or without aminoglycoside	Vancomycin dosages may be adjusted based on serum levels and are adjusted for renal disease and dialysis. No dose adjustment is recommended for hepatic dysfunction.
Dual therapy containing fluoroquinolone	Ciprofloxacin 400 mg IV every 8 hours and piperacillin–tazobactam, ceftazidime (above dosages)	Cannot be used in patients who receive fluoroquinolone prophylaxis. Dose adjusted in renal disease and dialysis but not for hepatic dysfunction.
Low-risk po regimen	Ciprofloxacin 750 mg po every 12 hours and amoxicillin–clavulanate 500–875 mg po every 12 hours	For patients with MASCC scores ≥ 21 not receiving fluoroquinolone prophylaxis. Amoxicillin–clavulanate is adjusted in renal disease and dialysis but not hepatic dysfunction.
Antifungal		
Amphotericin B deoxycholate	0.5–1 mg/kg IV daily	Premedication with acetaminophen and diphenhydramine; 500 mL normal saline boluses before and after. No dose adjustments are recommended for renal or hepatic dysfunction or during dialysis.
Liposomal amphotericin B	3 mg/kg IV daily	Lower incidence of nephrotoxicity and infusion reactions; more expensive. No dose adjustments are recommended for renal or hepatic dysfunction or during dialysis.
Caspofungin	70 mg/kg IV loading dose on day 1 followed by 50 mg/kg IV daily	Dosage adjustment in hepatic dysfunction but not for renal disease or dialysis.
Voriconazole	6 mg/kg IV loading dose every 12 hours on day 1 followed by 4 mg/kg po or IV every 12 hours	Dosage adjustment in hepatic dysfunction; IV formulation contraindicated if creatinine clearance < 50 mL/min (0.83 mL/s); multiple drug interactions.
Posaconazole	Prophylactic: 200 mg po three times a day with food 300 mg IV twice a day on day 1, then 300 mg IV daily Salvage: 200 mg po four times a day with food; then 400 mg po two times a day when stable	Not FDA approved for primary or salvage therapy for invasive fungal infections but used clinically; no dose adjustments required for renal or hepatic dysfunction or during dialysis.

AML, acute myeloid leukemia; FDA, Food and Drug Administration; IDSA, Infectious Diseases Society of America; IV, intravenous; MDS; myelodysplastic syndrome; NCCN, National Comprehensive Cancer Network; po, oral.

[a]Dosing for adult patients; adjust doses for renal dysfunction.

- Quinolone or TMP-SMX prophylaxis
- Hypotension or septic shock
- Colonization with resistant gram-positive organisms (ie, MRSA)
- Evidence of central venous catheter infection[14]

Vancomycin may be added to the empiric regimen after 3 to 5 days in persistently febrile patients or if cultures reveal gram-positive organisms. Vancomycin should be changed if the gram-positive organism is susceptible to other antibacterials or discontinued in patients with persistent fever after 3 days with negative culture results. Linezolid, quinupristin–dalfopristin, tigecycline, and daptomycin may be used in cases of vancomycin-resistant organisms or if vancomycin is not an option because of drug allergy or intolerance.[14]

Empiric antifungal agents are typically added in persistently febrile patients after 5 to 7 days, especially if continued neutropenia is expected. Amphotericin B has historically been the drug of choice because of its broad-spectrum activity against both yeast (*Candida* spp.) and mold (*Aspergillus* spp.) infections. Because frequent toxicity (nephrotoxicity, infusion reactions) limits the use of amphotericin B, less toxic alternatives have been studied. Lipid formulations of amphotericin provide decreased toxicity, and liposomal amphotericin B (AmBisome) has been shown to be equivalent to conventional amphotericin B as empiric therapy but is significantly more expensive.;

Caspofungin is equivalent with less toxicity compared with liposomal amphotericin B in a randomized trial and is FDA approved for this indication.[14,18] Voriconazole is equivalent to liposomal amphotericin in mortality, but response was improved in those receiving liposomal amphotericin. Voriconazole does not have an indication, but it is sometimes used. Itraconazole has also been used in some institutions, but its use is complicated by poor bioavailability of oral preparations and numerous drug interactions. Posaconazole is a newer azole that is sometimes used prophylactically in neutropenic patients with acute myeloid leukemia or myelodysplastic syndrome and for patients with graft-versus-host disease while receiving intensive immunosuppressive therapy. It is not FDA approved as primary or salvage therapy for the treatment of invasive fungal infections but it is approved by the European Union for invasive aspergillosis and other fungal infections that are refractory to standard antifungal agents.

As stated earlier, low-risk patients fulfilling the MASCC criteria (see Table 99–6) may be treated empirically as an outpatient with a regimen combining amoxicillin–clavulanic acid and ciprofloxacin. Ciprofloxacin and clindamycin are reasonable alternatives for penicillin-allergic patients.

The CSF should not routinely be used for treatment of FN in conjunction with antimicrobial therapy.[14,18] However, the use of CSFs in certain high-risk patients with hypotension, documented fungal infection, pneumonia, or sepsis is reasonable. A meta-analysis demonstrated that hospitalization and neutrophil recovery are shortened and infection-related mortality is marginally improved with CSF prophylaxis in high-risk patients.[24] As with prophylactic use of these agents, cost considerations limit their use to high-risk patients.

OUTCOME EVALUATION

The success of the treatment of FN depends on the adequate recovery of the ANC and either optimal antimicrobial coverage of identified organisms or empiric coverage of unidentified organisms. Monitor the complete blood count (CBC) with differential and T_{max} (maximum temperature during previous 24 hours) daily. Assess renal and hepatic function at least twice weekly, especially in patients receiving nephrotoxic agents. Vital signs should be taken every 4 hours. Follow-up on blood and urine culture results daily because many cultures do not become positive for several days. Assess the patient daily for pain that may indicate an infectious source. Conduct daily physical examination of common sites of infection. Repeat cultures and chest x-ray in persistently febrile patients and culture developing sources of infection (ie, stool cultures for diarrhea).

Patient Care Process: FN

Patient Assessment:

- Review patient history for cytotoxic chemotherapy.
- Evaluate risk of FN with cytotoxic chemotherapy using NCCN practice guideline for myeloid growth factors.
- Obtain a complete patient history:
  a. What chemotherapy did the patient receive and when? Is the ANC on the way down (before nadir) or on the way up (after nadir)? Was the patient receiving prophylactic antibiotics, filgrastim, sargramostim, or pegfilgrastim?
  b. Did the patient have previous episodes of FN? What were the previous culture results to determine colonization status?
- Evaluate patient-specific risk factors.
- Evaluate other sources of infection, such as catheters and surgery sites.
- Assess patient for temperature, onset of fever, duration of fever.
- Ensure patient has not taken NSAIDs, acetaminophen, or other therapies which may give a false impression of a lower temperature/lack of fever.
- Assess patient for severe signs/symptoms of systemic infection such as chills, headache, disorientation, etc.
- Determine patient allergies, especially to antibiotics, antifungals, and antivirals.

Therapy Evaluation:

- Select empiric antibiotic therapy if patient meets criteria for prophylactic treatment. Do not wait for culture results. Verify patient allergies.
- Change antimicrobials once culture results are obtained, if applicable. Verify antimicrobial effectiveness against institutional nomogram.

Care Plan Development:

- Discuss with interprofessional team advantages/disadvantages of treating patient as an outpatient, if applicable.
- Counsel patients receiving cytotoxic chemotherapy or alemtuzumab to promptly report fever. Provide patients with a diet to use during the neutropenic period. Counsel patients to avoid close contact with sick friends and relatives and remind patients and caregivers of the importance of handwashing.

Follow-Up Evaluation:

- Assess the patient daily for any new signs or symptoms of infection. Evaluate the patient for adverse drug reactions, drug allergies, and interactions. Have all antibiotics been dose adjusted for renal or hepatic dysfunction?
- For patients receiving oral antibiotics either prophylactically or as treatment of FN: Counsel patients that initial or persistent fever should be promptly reported and that compliance with the regimen is critical. Patients should also have easy access to medical care and adequate caregiver support. Provide information on drug interactions and adverse effects.

CARDIOVASCULAR COMPLICATIONS: SUPERIOR VENA CAVA SYNDROME (SVCS)

INTRODUCTION

Superior vena cava syndrome (SVCS) is a relatively rare complication that, although nonmalignant, may occur in patients with cancer. SVCS is rarely immediately life threatening except in patients with airway compromise and/or laryngeal or cerebral edema. However, rapid recognition of typical presenting symptoms facilitates referral for tissue diagnosis (if unknown) and treatment.

EPIDEMIOLOGY AND ETIOLOGY

SVCS occurs in around 15,000 patients per year, 90% of which are caused by malignancy. Specific cancers most commonly associated with SVCS are listed in Table 99–9. Lung cancer is the most frequent cause, of which small cell lung cancer (SCLC) is the most frequent subtype associated with SVCS. This is thought to be because of its predilection for the central and perihilar areas of the lung. Interestingly, right-sided lung cancers are four times more likely than left-sided lesions to cause SVCS. Mediastinal masses from lymphomas are the second most common cause.

The most common nonmalignant etiology of SVCS is catheter-related thrombosis, primarily caused by the increasing use of central access devices. Other causes include benign teratoma, tuberculosis, silicosis, and sarcoidosis.

PATHOPHYSIOLOGY

The SVC is the primary drainage vein for blood return from the head, neck, and upper extremities. It is a relatively thin-walled vein that is particularly vulnerable to obstruction from adjacent tumor invasion or thrombosis. The obstruction leads to elevated venous pressure, although collateral veins partially compensate. This is one reason for the relatively slow onset of the classic symptoms of SVCS. In fact, 75% of patients have signs and symptoms for more than 1 week before seeking medical attention.[25]

Table 99–9
Tumors Most Commonly Associated with SVCS

Cause	Frequency (%)
Non–small cell lung cancer	50
Small cell lung cancer	22
Lymphoma	12
Metastatic cancer (especially breast)	9
Germ cell tumor	3
Thymoma	2
Mesothelioma	1

From Wilson LD, Detterbeck FC, Yahalom J. Superior vena cava syndrome with malignant causes. N Engl J Med. 2007;356(8):1862–1869.

Clinical Presentation and Diagnosis of SVCS[25]

General

- Presentation depends on the degree of SVCS obstruction
- Almost complete obstruction is necessary to demonstrate classic symptoms

Signs and Symptoms

- Most common: swelling of face, neck, and upper extremity edema; dyspnea; cough; dilated upper extremity veins; orthopnea
- Less common: hoarseness, dysphagia, dizziness, headache, lethargy, chest pain
- Patients with elevated ICP may have mental status changes
- Patients with airway obstruction may have shortness of breath

Diagnostic Tests

- Tissue biopsy to determine underlying malignancy (if unknown), chest x-ray, CT scan, bronchoscopy, mediastinoscopy

CLINICAL PRESENTATION AND DIAGNOSIS

TREATMENT

Desired Outcomes

KEY CONCEPT *The primary goal of treatment of SVCS is to relieve the obstruction of the SVC by treating the underlying malignancy.* In the case of SVCS caused by thrombosis, the goal is to eliminate the thrombus and prevent further clot formation. Resolution of the obstruction will rapidly relieve symptoms and restore normal SVC function. The final goal of therapy is to avoid potentially fatal complications of SVCS such as cerebral edema from rapid increases in intracranial pressure (ICP) and intracranial thrombosis or bleeding.

General Approach to Treatment

Because the majority of SVCS is not immediately life threatening, a tissue diagnosis (if malignancy is unknown) to specifically identify the cancer origin is critical because treatment approaches vary considerably according to tumor histology. Thus, therapy can typically be withheld until a definitive tissue diagnosis is established. While biopsy results are pending, supportive measures such as head elevation, diuretics, corticosteroids, and supplemental oxygen may be used.

► *Nonpharmacologic Therapy*

Radiation therapy is the treatment of choice for chemotherapy-resistant tumors such as NSCLC or in chemotherapy-refractory patients with SVCS. Between 70% and 90% of patients experience relief of symptoms. Radiation therapy may also be combined with chemotherapy for chemotherapy-sensitive tumors such as SCLC and lymphoma. In the rare emergency situations of airway obstruction or elevated ICP, empiric radiotherapy before tissue diagnosis should be used. In most patients, symptoms resolve within 1 to 3 weeks.

Patient Care Process: SVCS

Patient Assessment:

- Evaluate patient for sign/symptoms of SVCS and determine severity and duration.
- Evaluate patient for risk factors for SVCS, especially cancers known to cause SVCS and central access devices.
- Obtain head and chest CT scan to diagnose presence of obstruction.
- If possible, obtain biopsy of mass to determine cause of SVCS.
- Depending on diagnosis of cause of SVCS, evaluate appropriateness of therapy (ie, antithrombolytics if source is a thrombus vs radiation therapy and steroids if cancer is the cause).
- Determine patient's candidacy for surgery if applicable.

Therapy Evaluation:

- Verify tissue diagnosis of SVCS.
- Monitor the patient for relief of symptoms by:
  a. Daily physical assessment of signs and symptoms
  b. Daily monitoring of fluid status
    - For corticosteroid use: Monitor daily serum glucose, insomnia, fluid retention, GI upset, mental status changes, and signs and symptoms of infection.

Care Plan Development:

1. Treat underlying malignancy to relieve obstruction.
2. Consider corticosteroids.

Follow-Up Evaluation:

- Surgery provides rapid relief of symptoms within 1 to 7 days of stent placement.
- Patients who receive chemotherapy and/or radiotherapy generally experience symptom relief within 1 to 2 weeks.
- Repeat CT scans of the chest after the first cycle of chemotherapy, surgical stenting, or radiotherapy to assess tumor response.

Surgical options for the management of SVCS include stent placement and surgical bypass. SVC stenting may provide longer-term relief of symptoms than radiotherapy, so it is often used in the palliative care setting when chemotherapy has failed.[36] One disadvantage of SVC stenting is the need for anticoagulation, especially in patients at high risk for thrombosis. The role of surgical bypass is limited to patients with complete SVC obstruction or patients who are refractory to chemotherapy and radiotherapy; thus, it is rarely indicated.

▶ *Pharmacologic Therapy*

Cytotoxic chemotherapy is the treatment of choice for chemotherapy-sensitive tumors such as SCLC and lymphoma. As indicated earlier, chemotherapy may also be combined with radiotherapy, especially in patients with lymphoma who have bulky mediastinal lymphadenopathy.

Corticosteroids play a key role in the management of SVCS, particularly in cases of lymphoma, because these tumors inherently respond to corticosteroid therapy. They are also helpful in the setting of respiratory compromise. Corticosteroids benefit patients who are receiving radiation therapy by reduction of local radiation-induced inflammation and patients with increased ICP. Dexamethasone 4 mg IV or by mouth every 6 hours is a frequently used regimen. The dosage should be tapered upon completion of radiation therapy or resolution of symptoms.

The role of diuretics in the management of SVCS is controversial. Although patients may derive symptomatic relief from edema, complications such as dehydration and reduced venous blood flow may exacerbate the condition. If diuretics are used, furosemide is most frequently used with diligent monitoring of the patient's fluid status and blood pressure.

In the case of thrombosis-related SVCS, anticoagulation is controversial because there is a lack of survival benefit. However, thrombolytics (ie, alteplase) and anticoagulation with heparin and warfarin may be beneficial in patients with thrombosis caused by indwelling catheters if used within 7 days of onset of symptoms, although catheter removal may be required.[25]

OUTCOME EVALUATION

The major measure of outcome of treatment of SVCS is the relief of symptoms, regardless of the therapy used.

NEUROLOGIC COMPLICATIONS: SPINAL CORD COMPRESSION

INTRODUCTION

Although not typically life threatening, spinal cord compression is a true oncologic emergency because delays in treatment by mere hours may lead to permanent neurologic dysfunction. Practitioners must quickly recognize the signs and symptoms of this condition to facilitate rapid management strategies.

EPIDEMIOLOGY AND ETIOLOGY

Around 20,000 cancer patients experience spinal cord compression in the United States every year, most of which involves the thoracic spine (~70%). Cancers that inherently metastasize to the bone (ie, breast, prostate, and lung) are the most frequent underlying malignancies associated with this complication. Most spinal cord compression occurs in patients with a known malignancy; however, 8% to 34% of cases occur as the initial presentation of cancer, especially in patients with non-Hodgkin lymphoma, multiple myeloma, and lung cancer.[26] Recently, predictive models have been developed to predict survival from SCC from myeloma and NSCLC.[27,28]

PATHOPHYSIOLOGY

The spinal cord emerges from the brain stem at the base of the skull and terminates at the second lumbar vertebra. The thoracic spine is most vulnerable to cord compression because of natural kyphosis and because the width of the thoracic spinal canal is the smallest among the vertebrae. Most spinal cord compression is caused by adjacent vertebral metastases that compress the spinal cord or from pathologic compression fracture of the vertebra. This results in significant edema and inflammation in the affected area.

Patients with spinal cord compression are in acute, severe back and/or neck pain and may present to the emergency department

Clinical Presentation and Diagnosis of Spinal Cord Compression

General

- Once neurologic deficits appear, progression to irreversible paralysis may occur within hours to days
- Around 10% to 38% of patients present with multiple sites of spinal involvement

Signs and Symptoms

- Back pain is present in more than 90% of patients
- Initially localized and increases in intensity over several weeks
- Aggravated by movement, supine positioning, coughing, sneezing, neck flexion, straight leg raise, Valsalva maneuver, palpation of spine
- Sensory deficit
- Cervical spine compression: quadriplegia
- Thoracic spine compression: paraplegia
- Upper lumbar spine compression: bowel and bladder dysfunction (constipation and urinary retention) and abnormal extensor plantar reflexes
- Weakness

Diagnostic Tests

- MRI with gadolinium enhancement is the gold standard
- X-rays may be helpful to identify bone abnormalities

for evaluation. Diagnosis is made based on symptoms and imaging studies that show fractured vertebrae.

TREATMENT

Desired Outcomes

KEY CONCEPT *Because patients with spinal metastases are generally incurable, the primary goal of treatment of spinal cord compression is palliation. The most important prognostic factor for patients presenting with spinal cord compression is the degree of underlying neurologic dysfunction.* Only around 10% of patients who present with paralysis are able to ambulate after treatment.[26] Therefore, the goals of treatment are recovery of normal neurologic function, local tumor control, pain control, and stabilization of the spine. Therapeutic options depend primarily on the following factors:

- Underlying malignancy
- Prior therapies
- Stability of the spine at presentation
- Overall patient prognosis

▸ *Nonpharmacologic Therapy*

Radiation therapy is generally considered to be the treatment of choice for most patients. Exceptions to this include patients with prior radiation to the treatment site and patients with inherently radio-resistant tumors (ie, melanoma, renal cell carcinoma). The radiation field should include two vertebral bodies above and below the involved area.

Surgery for spinal cord compression typically involves either laminectomy for posterior lesions or decompression with fixation. Surgery is the treatment of choice for the following patients: (a) patients with unstable spine requiring stabilization, (b) immediately impending sphincter dysfunction requiring rapid spinal decompression, (c) patients who do not respond to or have received their maximum dose of radiotherapy, and (d) direct compression of the spinal cord caused by spinal bony fragments.[26] Recent evidence suggests that surgery followed by radiation therapy may be superior to radiotherapy alone in terms of increased ambulation time after treatment, maintenance of continence, and rates of nonambulatory patients becoming ambulatory.[29] Surgery is also useful for establishing a tissue diagnosis in cases of unknown malignancy. Overall, the risks and benefits of surgery must be weighed against the expected prognosis of the patient in light of the significant rehabilitation required after surgery.

▸ *Pharmacologic Therapy*

Corticosteroids play a vital role in the management of spinal cord compression. Dexamethasone is most frequently used to reduce edema, inhibit inflammation, and delay the onset of

Patient Care Process: Spinal Cord Compression

Patient Assessment:

- Take patient history of signs/symptoms of SCC.
- Obtain pain score from patient.
- Obtain imaging studies to diagnose bone fractures.
- Evaluate patient for history of radiation therapy to affected areas.

Therapy Evaluation:

- Improved symptoms of sensory loss, using physical examination every 4 hours until symptoms improve then daily
- Improved autonomic system function, including urine and bowel control, every 4 hours until symptoms improve; then daily
- Improved pain control using detailed pain assessment every 2 to 4 hours during initial titration then daily thereafter
- For corticosteroid use: serum glucose, insomnia, fluid retention, GI upset, mental status changes, signs and symptoms of infection daily

Care Plan Development:

- Treat underlying malignancy to relieve spinal cord compression
- Corticosteroids
- Pain relief

Follow-Up Evaluation:

- Evaluate patient's ability to carry out activities of daily living with minimal or no pain.
- Monitor closely for signs of compression and paralysis.

neurologic complications. Dexamethasone has been shown to improve ambulation in combination with radiation compared with radiation alone.[30] Significant controversy exists regarding the optimal dosing of dexamethasone. Oral loading doses of 10 to 100 mg followed by 4 to 24 mg orally four times daily have been used. Higher doses may be used in cases of rapidly progressing symptoms, but adverse effects, including GI bleeding and psychosis, are more severe. Steroids should be continued during radiation therapy and then tapered appropriately.

Pain management is also of critical importance in patients with spinal cord compression. Although dexamethasone will provide some benefit, opioid analgesics should also be used and titrated rapidly to achieve adequate pain control.

OUTCOME EVALUATION

Patients who receive definitive treatment with radiation and/or surgery generally derive benefit within days.

COMPLICATIONS OF BRAIN METASTASES

INTRODUCTION

Brain metastases are among the most feared complications of cancer and generally carry a poor prognosis. One serious consequence of brain metastases is elevated ICP, which can rapidly lead to fatal intracranial herniation and death. Rapid identification of the signs and symptoms of brain metastases is critical to improve long-term outcome and avoid mortality. The signs and symptoms of brain metastasis can be confused with common psychological distress or other neurologic problems (eg, headaches) that may go unrecognized. It is important that patients who are suspected to have brain metastasis are quickly referred for appropriate management.[31]

Clinical Presentation and Diagnosis of Brain Metastasis

General

- Almost all patients with brain metastases are symptomatic.
- New cerebral neurologic symptoms in a cancer patient should initiate evaluation for brain metastases.
- Other causes of brain lesions, including hemorrhage, infection, and infarct, should be ruled out.

Signs and Symptoms

- Mental status changes (most common): loss of consciousness, irritability, confusion
- Hemiparesis, aphasia, papilledema, weakness, seizure, nausea, and vomiting
- Headache: may be of gradual onset or sudden in the case of hemorrhage

Diagnostic Tests

- MRI with contrast enhancement is the gold standard.
- CT scans may be used in patients with pacemakers, but may miss small metastases.

EPIDEMIOLOGY AND ETIOLOGY

Brain metastasis is the most common neurologic complication seen in patients with cancer. Approximately 170,000 patients develop brain metastases in the United States each year.[31] Many malignancies are frequently associated with brain metastases (Table 99–10). Although melanoma is the tumor type most likely to metastasize to the brain, brain metastases caused by lung and breast cancer are seen more often because they are among the most common cancers. In addition, brain metastases may be diagnosed at the same time as the primary malignancy in around 20% of cases.[31] Around 80% of brain metastases occur in the cerebral hemispheres, 15% in the cerebellum, and 5% in the brain stem.

PATHOPHYSIOLOGY

A delicate balance of normal pressure is maintained in the brain and spinal cord by brain, blood, and cerebrospinal fluid. Because the brain is contained within a confined space (skull), any foreign mass contained within that space causes adverse sequelae. This results in either destruction or displacement of normal brain tissue with associated edema. Most brain metastases occur through hematogenous spread of the primary tumor and around 80% of patients have multiple sites of metastases within the brain.

TREATMENT

Desired Outcomes

Therapeutic modalities used for the management of brain metastases may be divided into symptomatic management and definitive management. KEY CONCEPT *The goals of treatment of brain metastases are to manage symptoms by reducing cerebral edema, treat the underlying malignancy both locally and systemically, and improve survival.*

General Approach to Treatment

Patients with brain metastases have a poor prognosis. Untreated patients generally have a median survival of 1 month. The choice of treatment depends primarily on the status of the patient's underlying malignancy and the number and sites of brain metastases. The primary definitive treatments for brain metastases are surgery and radiation therapy. Pharmacologic modalities are primarily used to control symptoms, although cytotoxic chemotherapy plays a limited role in the management.

Table 99–10

Cancers Most Frequently Associated with Brain Metastases

Type of Cancer	Frequency (%)
Lung cancer	18–64
Breast cancer	2–21
Melanoma	4–16
Colorectal cancer	2–11
Hematologic malignancies (ie, leukemia)	~10 (primarily caused by leptomeningeal spread)

From Lassman AB, DeAngelis LM. Brain metastases. Neurol Clin North Am. 2003;21:1–23.

▶ *Nonpharmacologic Therapy*

Radiation therapy is the treatment of choice for most patients with brain metastases. Most patients receive whole-brain radiation because the majority of brain metastases are multifocal. Another method known as stereotactic radiosurgery provides intense focal radiation, typically using a linear accelerator or gamma knife, in patients who cannot tolerate surgery or have lesions that are surgically inaccessible (ie, brain stem). Because brain metastases can occur in up to 50% of patients with small cell lung cancer, prophylactic cranial irradiation is recommended in patients with good performance status who at least partially respond to chemotherapy to both prevent the development of brain metastases and to prolong survival.[32] Although other cancers can metastasize to the brain, the benefits of routine prophylactic cranial irradiation have only been demonstrated in studies conducted in patients with small cell lung cancer.[32] In fact, a recent meta-analysis reported that prophylactic cranial irradiation may reduce overall survival when used in NSCLC patients even though it reduced brain metastases in these patients.[33]

Patient Care Process: Brain Metastasis

Patient Assessment:

- Determine onset and duration of signs/symptoms such as headache, nausea, visual changes, mental status changes, depression, etc.
- Evaluate the patient for drug interactions, allergies, and adverse effects with phenytoin or corticosteroid therapy.
- Obtain head CT scan to diagnose brain metastasis.

Therapy Evaluation:

- Assess the patient's symptoms for prompt referral for radiation or surgery.
- For patients receiving corticosteroids, monitor for adverse effects and drug interactions. Does the patient need GI prophylaxis for long-term treatment? Slowly taper once symptoms improve and/or radiation or surgery is completed.
- Instruct patients receiving phenytoin about symptoms of elevated serum concentrations (nystagmus, blurred vision, dizziness, drowsiness, lethargy).
- Provide patient education regarding when to take medications and the importance of compliance and to promptly report symptoms of recurrence (mental status changes, seizures).

Care Plan Development:

- Initiate treatment for underlying malignancy
- Provide symptomatic relief with mannitol and corticosteroids
- Manage seizure with phenytoin or diazepam if they develop

Follow-Up Evaluation:

- Monitor patients for improvements in presenting signs/symptoms.
- Monitor patients for response to chemotherapy.

Surgery plays a key role in the management of patients with brain metastases, particularly in patients whose systemic disease is well controlled and in patients with solitary lesions. Surgery may also benefit patients with multiple metastatic sites who have a single dominant lesion with current or impending neurologic sequelae.

In cases of elevated ICP caused by cerebral herniation, mechanical hyperventilation to decrease the arterial PCO_2 down to 25 mm Hg (3.33 kPa) acutely decreases ICP by causing cerebral vasoconstriction. Elevation of the patient's bed may also quickly reduce the ICP. It should be noted that these strategies only relieve symptoms, and definitive therapy is still required.

▶ *Pharmacologic Therapy*

Corticosteroids are a mainstay in the management of brain metastases. They reduce edema that typically surrounds sites of metastases thereby reducing ICP. A loading dose of dexamethasone 10 mg IV followed by 4 mg by mouth or IV every 6 hours is typically used. Symptom relief may occur shortly after the loading dose, although the maximum benefit may not be seen for several days (after definitive therapy).[31]

Mannitol is an agent that may be used in patients with impending cerebral herniation. Mannitol is an osmotic diuretic that shifts brain osmolarity from the brain to the blood. Doses of 100 g (1–2 g/kg) as an IV bolus should be used. Repeated doses are typically not recommended because mannitol may diffuse into brain tissue, leading to rebound increased ICP.[31]

Around 20% patients with brain metastases may present with seizures and require anticonvulsant therapy. Phenytoin is the most frequently used agent with a loading dose of 15 mg/kg followed by 300 mg by mouth daily (titrated to therapeutic levels between 10 and 20 mcg/mL [40 and 79 μmol/L]). Diazepam 5 mg IV may be used for rapid control of persistent seizures. Prophylactic anticonvulsants have frequently been used; however, a systematic review did not support their use.[32] Thus, because adverse effects and drug interactions are common, the routine use of prophylactic anticonvulsants is not recommended.

OUTCOME EVALUATION

The success of therapy is based on the ability to decrease symptoms, treat the underlying sites of disease within the brain, and prolong survival.

UROLOGIC COMPLICATIONS: HEMORRHAGIC CYSTITIS

INTRODUCTION

Hemorrhagic cystitis is defined as acute or insidious bleeding from the lining of the bladder. Although therapy with certain medications is the most common cause, it is also the most preventable. Once it occurs, hemorrhagic cystitis causes significant morbidity and mortality rates between 2% and 4%. This section focuses on preventive strategies for chemotherapeutic causes of hemorrhagic cystitis.

EPIDEMIOLOGY AND ETIOLOGY

Numerous etiologies have been linked to hemorrhagic cystitis (Table 99–11).[34] Of these, the oxazaphosphorine alkylating agents (cyclophosphamide and ifosfamide) are most

Table 99–11

Primary Causes of Hemorrhagic Cystitis

Pharmacologic	Nonpharmacologic
Cyclophosphamide	Pelvic irradiation
Chronic low doses	Viral infection
High-doses used in BMT	CMV
Ifosfamide	Papovavirus
Intravesicular thiotepa	Herpes simplex virus
Chronic oral busulfan	Adenovirus
Anabolic steroids	

BMT, bone marrow transplantation; CMV, cytomegalovirus.

From West NJ. Prevention and treatment of hemorrhagic cystitis. Pharmacotherapy. 1997;17:696–706.

frequently implicated. Hemorrhagic cystitis is the dose-limiting toxicity of ifosfamide and predisposes patients with bladder cancer. Incidence rates vary considerably but generally range between 18% and 40% with ifosfamide and 0.5% to 40% with high-dose (300 mg/m^2 or more) cyclophosphamide in the absence of prophylactic measures.[35] Chronic, low-dose oral cyclophosphamide as typically used in autoimmune disorders and chronic lymphocytic leukemia is infrequently associated with hemorrhagic cystitis.

Around 20% patients receiving pelvic irradiation may experience hemorrhagic cystitis, especially with concurrent cyclophosphamide. Viral infections commonly associated with this condition most frequently occur in bone marrow transplant recipients who may also receive cyclophosphamide.

PATHOPHYSIOLOGY

Cyclophosphamide- or ifosfamide-induced damage to the bladder wall is primarily caused by their shared metabolite known as acrolein. Acrolein causes sloughing and inflammation of the bladder lining, leading to bleeding and hemorrhage. This is most common when urine output is low because higher concentrations of acrolein come into contact with the bladder urothelium for longer periods of time.

PREVENTION

KEY CONCEPT *The use of effective prevention strategies can decrease the incidence of hemorrhagic cystitis to fewer than 5% in patients receiving cyclophosphamide or ifosfamide. Three methods are used to reduce the risk: administration of Mesna (2-mercaptoethane sulfonate), hyperhydration, and bladder irrigation with catheterization.* Mesna is the primary method used with ifosfamide; all three strategies are used with cyclophosphamide.

Mesna is a thiol compound that is rapidly oxidized in the bloodstream after administration to dimesna, which is inactive. However, after being filtered through the kidneys, dimesna is reduced back to Mesna, which binds to acrolein, leading to its inactivation and excretion. ASCO has published evidence-based guidelines for the dosing and administration of Mesna (Table 99–12).[35] The dose of oral Mesna must be double the IV dose because of its oral bioavailability between 40% and 50%. Because the half life of Mesna (~1.2 hours) is much shorter than that of ifosfamide or cyclophosphamide, prolonged administration of Mesna beyond the end of the chemotherapy infusion is critical (Figure 99–2). Patients should receive at least 2 L of IV fluids beginning 12 to 24 hours before and ending 24 to 48 hours after the last dose of chemotherapy.[34,35]

Hyperhydration with normal saline at 3 L/m^2/day with IV furosemide to maintain urine output greater than 100 mL/hour has also been used with cyclophosphamide. Continuous bladder irrigation by catheterization uses normal saline at 250 to 1000 mL/hour to flush acrolein from the bladder. Mesna is equivalent to both strategies in patients receiving high-dose cyclophosphamide and avoids the discomfort and infection risk with catheterization and the intensity of hyperhydration. Thus, Mesna is the preventive method of choice.[35]

Clinical Presentation and Diagnosis of Hemorrhagic Cystitis

General

- Presentation may be mild (microscopic hematuria) or severe (massive hemorrhage) and develops during or shortly after chemotherapy infusion

Signs and Symptoms

- Suprapubic pain and cramping, urinary urgency and frequency, dysuria and burning, hematuria
- Urinary retention leading to hydronephrosis and renal failure may occur if large blood clots obstruct the ureters or bladder outlet.

Laboratory Tests

- Urine dipsticks for blood
- Urinalysis reveals more than three RBCs per high-power field: microscopic hematuria
- CBC with differential, prothrombin time or international normalized ratio, activated partial thromboplastin time, blood urea nitrogen, creatinine

TREATMENT

Desired Outcomes

If hemorrhagic cystitis occurs, the goals of treatment are to decrease exposure to the offending etiology, establish and maintain urine outflow, avoid obstruction and renal compromise, and maintain blood and plasma volume. Restoration of normal bladder function is the ultimate goal following acute treatment.

General Approach to Treatment

The treatment of hemorrhagic cystitis first involves discontinuation of the offending agent. Agents such as anticoagulants and inhibitors of platelet function should also be discontinued. IV fluids should be aggressively administered to irrigate the bladder. Blood and platelet transfusions may be necessary to maintain normal hematologic values. Pain should be managed with opioid analgesics. Local intravesicular therapies may be necessary if hematuria does not resolve (Figure 99–3).

Table 99–12

ASCO Guidelines for the Use of Mesna with Ifosfamide and High-Dose Cyclophosphamide

Chemotherapy Schedule	Dosing Schedule for Mesna	Comments
Low-dose ifosfamide < 2 g/m²/day	Oral: 100% of total daily dose of ifosfamide given 20% IV 15 minutes before and 40% po 2 and 6 hours after start of ifosfamide	Available in 400-mg tablets Peak urinary thiol concentrations with oral Mesna is at 3 hours If patient vomits within 2 hours of administration, repeat dose po or IV
Standard-dose ifosfamide equal to 2.5 g/m²/day	Bolus: 60% of total daily dose of ifosfamide given IV in 20% increments 15 minutes before and 4 and 8 hours after start of ifosfamide Infusion: 60% of total daily dose of ifosfamide given 20% IV 15 minutes before and 40% by continuous infusion during and for 12–24 hours after end of ifosfamide	Peak urinary thiol concentrations with IV Mesna is at 1 hour Compatible with ifosfamide and cyclophosphamide by Y-site administration or when admixed in the same bag
High-dose ifosfamide > 2.5 g/m²/day	Lack of evidence for dosing, but higher doses for longer duration recommended based on longer half-life of ifosfamide at high doses	
Standard-dose cyclophosphamide	Use of Mesna is not routinely necessary	Should be combined with saline diuresis (1.5 L/m²/day of normal saline)
High-dose cyclophosphamide (BMT)	Bolus: 40% of cyclophosphamide dose given IV at hours 0, 3, 6, and 9 after cyclophosphamide Infusion: 100% of cyclophosphamide dose given by continuous infusion until 24 hours after cyclophosphamide	

ASCO, American Society of Clinical Oncology; BMT, bone marrow transplantation; IV, intravenous; Mesna, 2-mercaptoethane sulfonate; po, oral.

From Schuchter LM, Hensley ML, Meropol NJ, et al. 2002 Update of recommendations for the use of chemotherapy and radiotherapy protectants: clinical practice guidelines of the American Society of Clinical Oncology. J Clin Oncol. 2002;20:2895–2903.

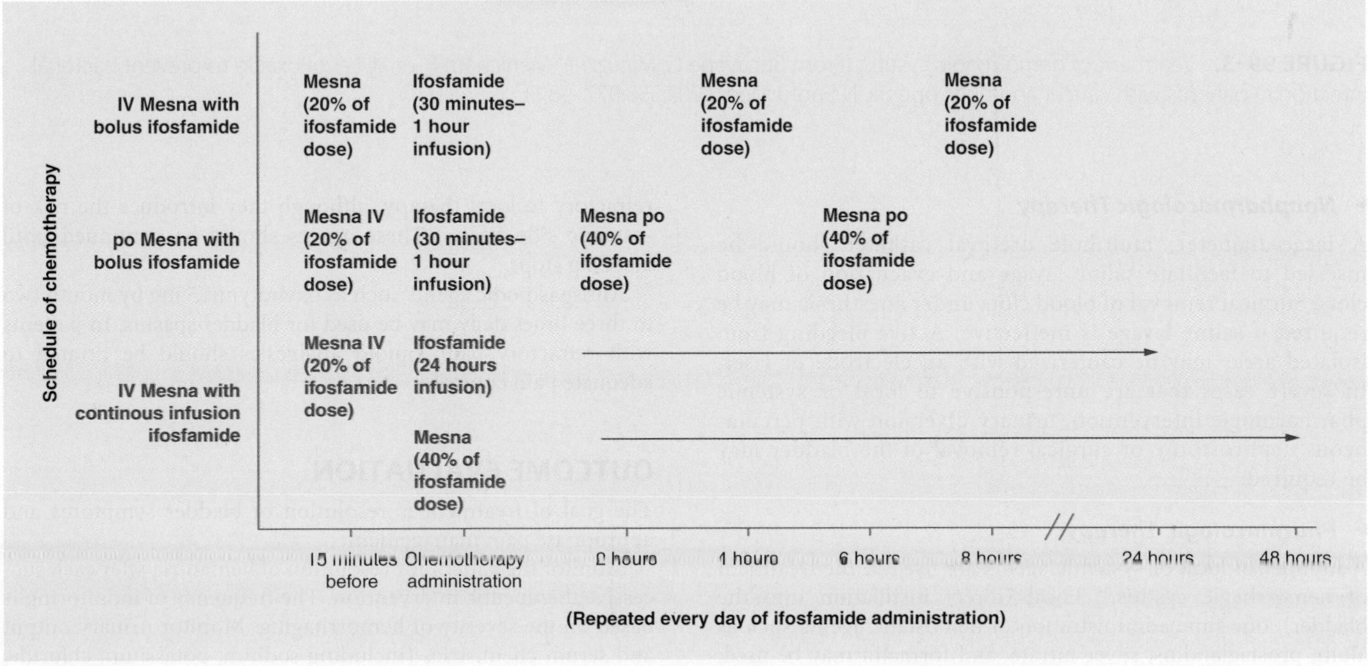

FIGURE 99–2. Examples of Mesna (2-mercaptoethane sulfonate) administration with ifosfamide. (IV, intravenous; po, oral.)

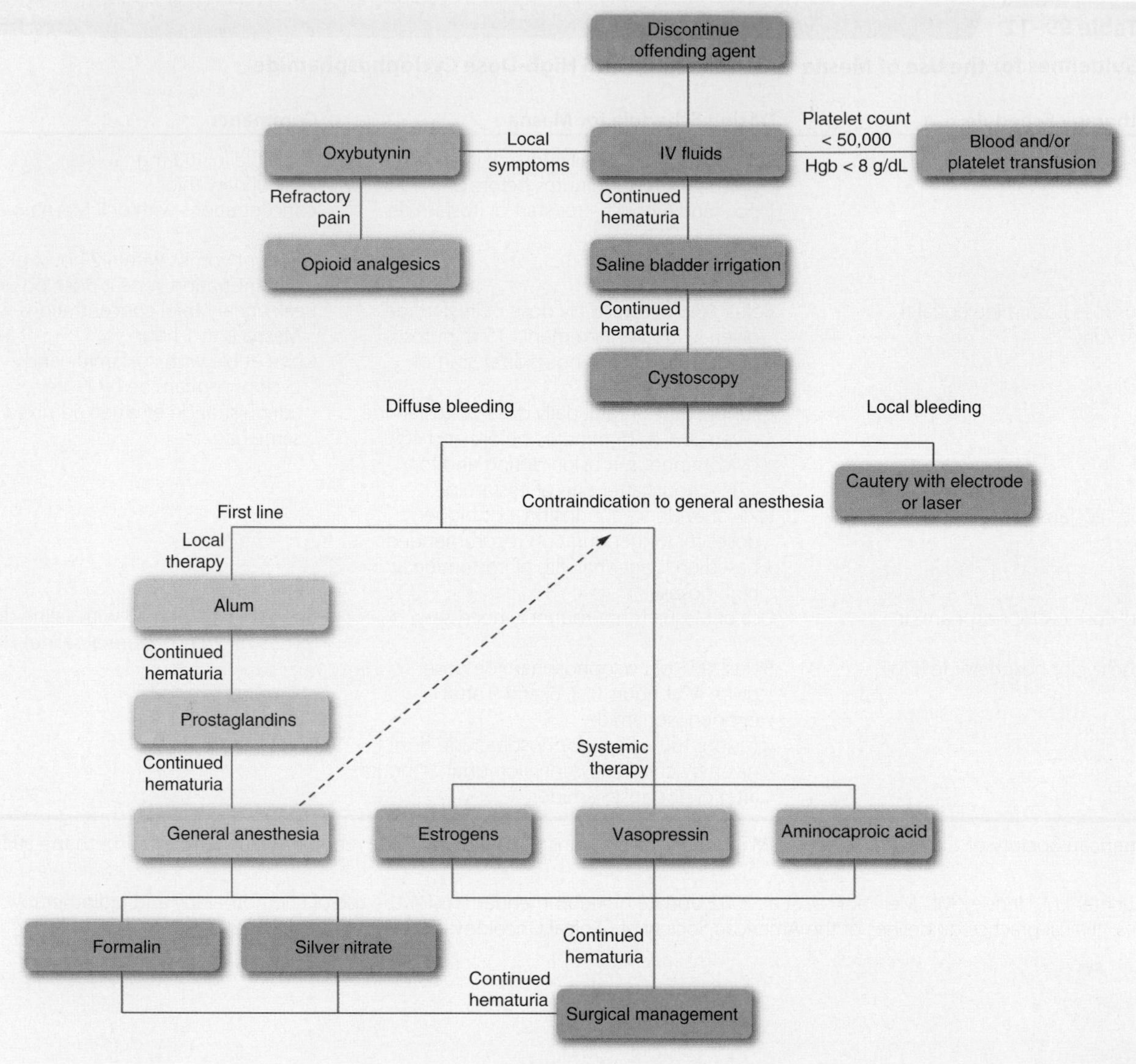

FIGURE 99–3. Treatment of hemorrhagic cystitis. (From Bucavene G, Micuzzi A, Menichetti F, et al. Levofloxacin to prevent bacterial infection in patients with cancer and neutropenia. N Engl J Med. 2005;353:977–987.)

▶ *Nonpharmacologic Therapy*

A large-diameter, multihole urethral catheter should be inserted to facilitate saline lavage and evacuation of blood clots. Surgical removal of blood clots under anesthesia may be required if saline lavage is ineffective. Active bleeding from isolated areas may be cauterized with an electrode or laser. In severe cases that are unresponsive to local or systemic pharmacologic intervention, urinary diversion with percutaneous nephrostomy or surgical removal of the bladder may be required.

▶ *Pharmacologic Therapy*

A number of local or systemic agents are used in the treatment of hemorrhagic cystitis.[34] Local (direct instillation into the bladder), one-time administration of hemostatic agents such as alum, prostaglandins, silver nitrate, and formalin may be used; however, general anesthesia is required, especially with formalin, because of pain. Systemic agents, including estrogens, vasopressin, and aminocaproic acid, may be used in patients who are refractory to local therapy, although they introduce the risk of systemic side effects. These agents should be continued until bleeding stops.

Antispasmodic agents such as oxybutynin 5 mg by mouth two to three times daily may be used for bladder spasms. In patients with refractory pain, opioid analgesics should be titrated to adequate pain control.

OUTCOME EVALUATION

The goal of treatment is resolution of bladder symptoms and appropriate pain management.

Monitor the patient for resolution of hematuria after each successive therapeutic intervention. The frequency of monitoring is based on the severity of hemorrhaging. Monitor urinary output and serum chemistries (including sodium, potassium, chloride, blood urea nitrogen, and serum creatinine) daily for renal dysfunction. Check the CBC at least daily to monitor hemoglobin and platelet count.

Patient Care Process: Hemorrhagic Cystitis

Patient Assessment:

- Assess onset and severity of symptoms of hemorrhagic cystitis such as hematuria, anuria, oliguria.
- Assess the patient receiving ifosfamide or cyclophosphamide at least daily for the development of hematuria.

Therapy Evaluation:

- Ensure administration of adequate hydration and proper doses of Mesna.

Care Plan Development:

- Initiate Mesna if indicated and assure adequate hydration.
- Counsel patient receiving oral Mesna on the importance of compliance, when to take doses, and to immediately report any episodes of vomiting for IV readministration.
- Evaluate the patient for drug interactions, allergies, and adverse effects with chemotherapy, Mesna, or systemic therapies for management.

Follow-Up Evaluation:

- Assess the quantity of urinary bleeding and promptly refer to a urologist for local or surgical management.
- Patients receiving systemic treatment should be monitored every 4 hours for resolution of hematuria. Promptly refer to urologist for refractory hematuria.

METABOLIC COMPLICATIONS: HYPERCALCEMIA OF MALIGNANCY

INTRODUCTION

Hypercalcemia is the most common metabolic abnormality experienced by patients with cancer. A small percentage of as yet undiagnosed patients present with hypercalcemia. Once hypercalcemia occurs, it is associated with a very poor prognosis because of the frequent association with advanced or metastatic disease.[36]

EPIDEMIOLOGY AND ETIOLOGY

Hypercalcemia occurs in 10% to 30% of patients with cancer during the course of their disease. The most common tumor types associated with hypercalcemia are breast cancer; squamous cell carcinomas of the head, neck, and lung; and renal cancer. Hematologic malignancies such as multiple myeloma and, rarely, lymphomas are other underlying malignancies associated with hypercalcemia.

PATHOPHYSIOLOGY

Around 99% of calcium is contained in the bones; the other 1% resides in the extracellular fluid. Of this extracellular calcium, approximately 40% is bound to albumin, and the remainder is in the ionized, physiologically active form. Normal calcium levels are maintained by three primary factors: parathyroid hormone (PTH), 1,25-dihydroxyvitamin D, and calcitonin. PTH increases renal tubular calcium resorption and promotes bone resorption. The active form of vitamin D, 1,25-dihydroxyvitamin D, regulates absorption of calcium from the GI tract. Calcitonin serves as an inhibitory factor by suppressing osteoclast activity and stimulating calcium deposition into the bones.[36]

The delicate balance maintained by these factors is altered in patients with cancer by two principal mechanisms: tumor production of humoral factors that alter calcium metabolism (humoral hypercalcemia) and by local osteolytic activity from bone metastases.[37] Humoral hypercalcemia causes around 80% of all hypercalcemia cases and is primarily mediated by systemic secretion of PTH-related protein (PTHrP). This protein mimics the action of endogenous PTH on bones. Local osteolytic activity causes 20% to 30% of hypercalcemia cases, although local osteolytic activity may also have a humoral component. Local production of various factors directly stimulates osteoclastic bone resorption, which releases growth factors and cytokines (ie, transforming growth factor-β) that are necessary for tumor growth. Thus, these metastatic tumors perpetuate their own growth through this mechanism. Calcium is also released by the osteolytic activity, resulting in hypercalcemia).[37] A third and less common mechanism is production of 1,25-dihydroxyvitamin D by tumor cells (usually lymphoma), which increases GI absorption of calcium and enhances osteoclastic bone resorption.

TREATMENT

Desired Outcomes

KEY CONCEPT *The primary goal of treatment for hypercalcemia is to control the underlying malignancy. Therapies directed at lowering the calcium level are temporary measures that are useful until anticancer therapy begins to work.* The goals of calcium-lowering therapy are to (a) lower the corrected calcium to normal levels, (b) regain fluid and electrolyte balance, (c) relieve symptoms, and (d) prevent life-threatening complications. Patients who are refractory to available therapies may have calcium-lowering therapy withheld (usually resulting in coma and death), which may be a humane approach.[36]

General Approach to Treatment

Therapeutic options for the treatment of hypercalcemia should be directed toward the level of corrected serum calcium and the presence of symptoms (Figure 99–4). Hypercalcemia may be classified as mild (corrected calcium equal to 10.5–11.9 mg/dL [2.63–2.98 mmol/L]), moderate (12–13.9 mg/dL [3.00–3.49 mmol/L]), and severe (greater than 14 mg/dL [3.50 mmol/L] or more).[36] Adequate treatment of mild or asymptomatic hypercalcemia may be achieved on an outpatient basis with nonpharmacologic measures. Moderate to severe or symptomatic hypercalcemia almost always requires pharmacologic intervention.

► *Nonpharmacologic Therapy*

Calciuric therapy in the form of hydration is a key component in the treatment of hypercalcemia, regardless of severity or presence of symptoms.[36] Mild or asymptomatic patients may be encouraged to increase their oral fluid intake (3–4 L/day). Patients with moderate to severe or symptomatic hypercalcemia should receive normal saline at 200 to 500 mL/hour according to their dehydration and cardiovascular status. Patients should

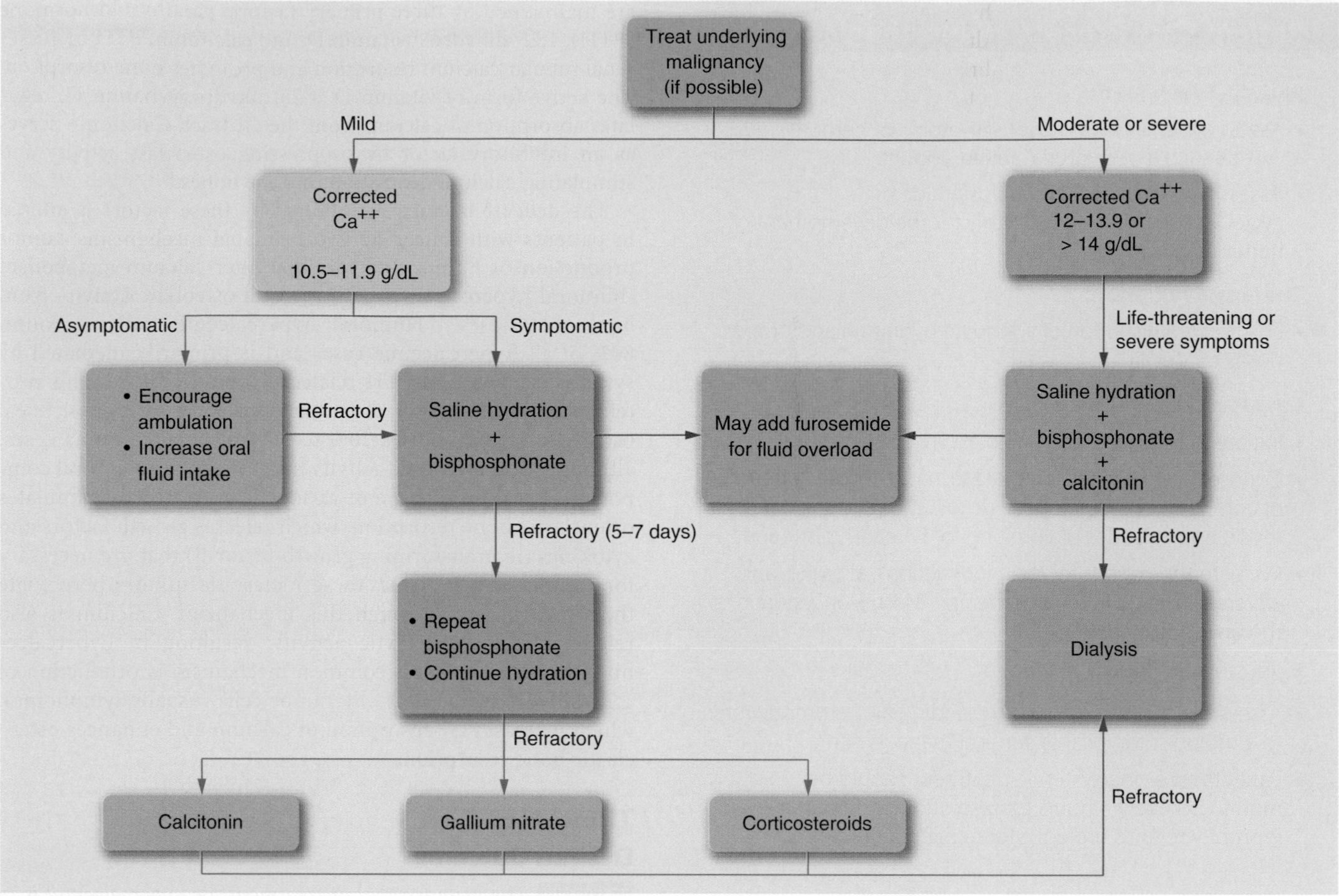

FIGURE 99–4. Treatment algorithm for the hypercalcemia of malignancy.

Clinical Presentation and Diagnosis of Hypercalcemia[36]

General

- Presence of symptoms depends not only on the calcium level but the rapidity of onset
- Normal calcium level is 8.5 to 10.5 mg/dL (2.13–2.63 mmol/L) (varies by laboratory)
- Serum calcium level *must* be corrected for albumin level using the following formula:

Corrected calcium (mg/dL) = Serum calcium + 0.8 (4 – Serum albumin) for serum calcium expressed in mg/dL and albumin in g/dL.

or

Corrected calcium (mmol/L) = Serum calcium + 0.02 (40 – serum albumin) for serum calcium expressed in mmol/L and albumin in g/L.

Signs and Symptoms

- Five primary organ systems may be affected:
- GI: anorexia, nausea, vomiting, constipation
- Musculoskeletal: weakness, bone pain, fatigue, ataxia
- CNS: confusion, headache, lethargy, seizures, coma
- Genitourinary: polydipsia, polyuria, renal failure
- Cardiac: Bradycardia, ECG abnormalities, arrhythmias

Laboratory Tests

- Elevated corrected serum calcium level (≥ 10.5 mg/dL [2.63 mmol/L]), serum albumin, low to normal serum phosphate
- Patient may have elevated blood urea nitrogen and serum creatinine
- Elevated alkaline phosphatase may indicate bone destruction
- ECG may indicate prolonged PR interval, shortened QT interval, widened T wave

Other Diagnostic Tests

- Rule out other causes of hypercalcemia, including primary hyperparathyroidism, hyperthyroidism, vitamin D intoxication, chronic renal failure be encouraged to ambulate as much as possible because immobility enhances bone resorption. Although calcium should be discontinued from parenteral feeding solutions, oral calcium supplementation minimally contributes to hypercalcemia unless it is mediated by vitamin D. In these cases, oral calcium should be discontinued. Finally, agents that may contribute to hypercalcemia (thiazide diuretics, vitamin D, lithium) or decrease renal function (NSAIDs) should be discontinued. Dialysis may be used in refractory cases or patients who cannot tolerate aggressive saline hydration.[36]

▸ *Pharmacologic Therapy*

Multiple pharmacologic interventions are available for the treatment of hypercalcemia (Table 99–13). Furosemide 20 to 40 mg/day may be added to hydration after rehydration has been achieved to avoid fluid overload and enhance renal excretion of calcium. Although effective in relieving symptoms, hydration and diuretics are temporary measures that are useful until the onset of antiresorptive therapy; thus, hydration and antiresorptive therapy should be initiated simultaneously.[36]

The antiresorptive therapy of choice for hypercalcemia of malignancy is a bisphosphonate. Because of poor oral bioavailability, only IV agents should be used. Pamidronate and zoledronic acid are most commonly used and are potent inhibitors of osteoclast activity.[35] The bisphosphonates should be administered at diagnosis of hypercalcemia because of their delayed onset of action.

Calcitonin is the drug of choice in cases of emergent hypercalcemia (patients with life-threatening electrocardiographic [ECG] changes, arrhythmias, or central nervous system [CNS] effects) because of its rapid onset of action. Calcitonin inhibits osteoclast activity and decreases renal tubular calcium resorption. Corticosteroids are useful in patients with steroid-responsive malignancies, such as lymphomas or multiple myeloma, and may delay **tachyphylaxis** to calcitonin. Gallium nitrate is another treatment option, although the 5-day

Table 99–13

Treatment Options for Hypercalcemia of Malignancy

	Agent	Dosage	Onset	Duration	Reduction in Serum Calcium Concentration	Comments
Calciuric therapy	IV normal saline	200–500 mL/hour	24–48 hours	2–3 days	0.5–2 mg/dL (0.13–0.50 mmol/L)	Avoid fluid overload, monitor electrolytes
	Furosemide	20–40 mg IV	4 hours	2–3 days		Monitor for hypokalemia, dehydration
Antiresorptive therapy	Pamidronate	60–90 mg IV over 2–24 hours[a]	24–72 hours	3–4 weeks	> 1 mg/dL (0.25 mmol/L)	Nadir not seen until after 4–7 days; may cause fever, renal dysfunction; pamidronate less expensive
	Zoledronic acid	4 mg IV over 15 minutes	24–48 hours	4+ weeks	> 1 mg/dL (0.25 mmol/L)	
	Corticosteroids	Prednisone (or equivalent) 50–100 mg/day	5–7 days	3–4 days	0.5–3 mg/dL (0.13–0.75 mmol/L)	Monitor for hyperglycemia, insomnia, immunosuppression
	Calcitonin	4–8 IU/kg SC or IM every 6–12 hours	2–4 hours	1–3 days	2–3 mg/dL (0.50–0.75 mmol/L)	Salmon-derived formulation preferred; 1-unit test dose recommended; can be given in renal failure; may cause flushing, nausea
	Gallium nitrate	100–200 mg/m² CIV daily for 5 days	24–48 hours			Do not administer if creatinine > 2.5 mg/dL (221 μmol/L); may cause renal failure
	Denosumab	120 mg SQ days 1, 8, and 15 the first month, then day 1 only	48–96 hours	4+ weeks	> 1 mg/dL (0.25 mmol/L)	Not renally cleared, may be used in patients with renal dysfunction, but reduce dose as increased risk of hypocalcemia in renally impaired

CIV, continuous intravenous infusion; IM, intramuscular; IV, intravenous; SC, subcutaneous.

[a]60 mg of pamidronate may be used in smaller patients or in patients with mild hypercalcemia or renal dysfunction. May use longer infusion time in patients with renal dysfunction.

Data from Refs. 47 and 49.

Patient Care Process: Hypercalcemia

Patient Assessment:

- Determine the disease status of the patient: Is the patient newly diagnosed or has the patient had multiple episodes of hypercalcemia and is becoming refractory to calcium-lowering therapy?
- Assess the patient's symptoms and serum calcium level to determine appropriate therapy. Is the patient taking any medications that may elevate the calcium level, inhibit its excretion, or affect renal function?
- Evaluate patient's medication history to determine if there are allergies or drug interactions that would preclude use of calcium-lowering therapies.
- Obtain renal function tests, serum calcium, albumin, electrolytes, and calculate corrected calcium level.

Therapy Evaluation:

- Initiate bisphosphonates.
- Monitor the serum calcium level, serum albumin, serum blood urea nitrogen and creatinine, and electrolytes daily during therapy.
- Assess the fluid balance by daily input and output, weights, and signs of fluid overload.
- Monitor the ECG in patients with cardiac manifestations until normalized.

Care Plan Development:

- Educate the patient regarding the importance of oral hydration and ambulation if an outpatient. Counsel to immediately report any worsening signs or symptoms.
- Develop a plan to maintain normocalcemia chronically using monthly bisphosphonates.
- Monitor patients for relief of symptoms and restoration of fluid balance.

Follow-Up Evaluation:

- Reassess patient status in terms of refractoriness to treatment to determine if treatment should be changed.
- Repeat doses of bisphosphonate after 5 to 7 days if the patient does not become normocalcemic.
- Evaluate the patient for adverse effects with calcium-lowering therapy.

Patient Encounter 3: Hypercalcemia of Malignancy

A 79-year-old man with stage IV moderately differentiated adenocarcinoma with features suggestive of a combined hepatocellular cholangiocarcinoma. The patient feels well but is fatigued and has a headache. He presents today to discuss treatment options for his disease. Relevant laboratory test results today are: calcium, 11.1 mg/dL (2.78 mmol/L) and albumin, 3.2 g/dL (32 g/L).

What is this patient's corrected calcium level?

How would you approach this patient's hypercalcemia?

administration regimen and risk of nephrotoxicity limit its use. Denosumab 120 mg subcutaneously, a RANKL inhibitor, was successful in correcting hypercalcemia in 12/15 patients with persistent hypercalcemia despite treatment with bisphosphonates and may be considered in those with bisphosphonate-resistant hypercalcemia.[37]

OUTCOME EVALUATION

The long-term success of therapy for hypercalcemia is determined primarily by the success of treatment of the underlying malignancy. The goal of treatment is to reduce serum calcium levels to normal range and to relieve patient symptoms if present.

METABOLIC COMPLICATIONS: TLS

INTRODUCTION

Although not as common as hypercalcemia, TLS may cause significant morbidity and mortality if adequate prophylaxis and treatment are not instituted. TLS is the result of rapid destruction of malignant cells with subsequent release of intracellular contents into the circulation.

EPIDEMIOLOGY AND ETIOLOGY

The overall incidence of TLS is unknown but has been linked to a number of patient- and tumor-related risk factors (Table 99–14).[38] TLS typically occurs in malignancies with high tumor burdens or high proliferative rates. Because of this, children are most

Table 99–14

Risk Factors for TLS

Disease Related
High risk
Acute lymphoblastic leukemia
High-grade non-Hodgkin lymphoma (ie, Burkitt lymphoma)
Intermediate risk
Chronic lymphocytic leukemia (especially bulky lymphadenopathy)
Acute myeloid leukemia (especially WBC count > 50,000 $10^3/\mu L$ [$50 \times 10^9/L$])
Multiple myeloma
Low risk
Low- and intermediate-grade non-Hodgkin lymphoma
Hodgkin disease
Chronic myeloid leukemia (blast crisis)
Rare
Breast cancer
Small cell lung cancer
Testicular cancer
Patient Related
Decreased urinary output, dehydration, or renal failure
Preexisting hyperuricemia
Acidic urine
WBC count > 50,000 $10^3/\mu L$ ($50 \times 10^9/L$)
LDH levels > 1500 IU/L (25.0 μkat/L)
High tumor sensitivity to treatment modalities

LDH, lactate dehydrogenase; WBC, white blood cell.

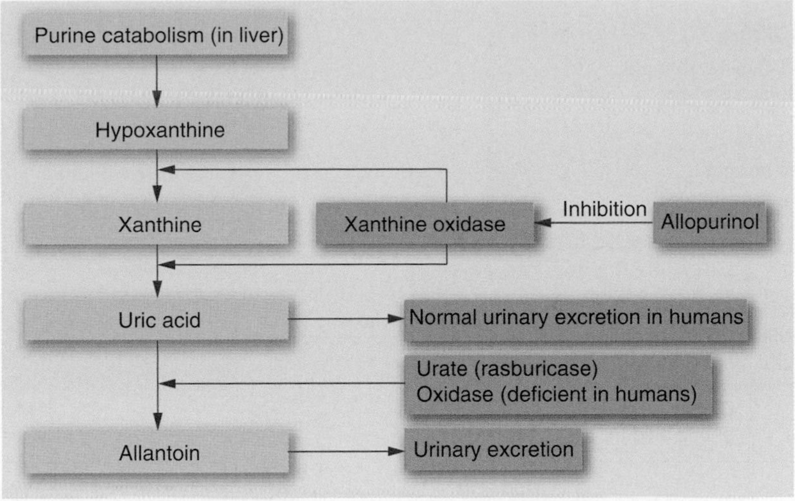

FIGURE 99–5. The role of allopurinol and rasburicase in the enzymatic degradation of purine nucleic acids.

frequently affected because they frequently have aggressive malignancies. TLS is typically induced by cancer treatment modalities, including chemotherapy, hormonal therapy, radiation, biologic therapy, or corticosteroids, although some patients may present spontaneously before treatment.[38]

PATHOPHYSIOLOGY

Patients with TLS experience a wide range of metabolic abnormalities. The massive cell lysis that occurs leads to the release of intracellular electrolytes, resulting in hyperkalemia and hyperphosphatemia. High concentrations of phosphate bind to calcium, leading to hypocalcemia and calcium phosphate precipitation in the renal tubule. Purine nucleic acids are also released, which are subsequently metabolized to uric acid through multiple enzyme-mediated steps (Figure 99–5). Uric acid is poorly soluble at urinary acidic pH, leading to crystallization in the renal tubule. The precipitation of uric acid and calcium phosphate leads to metabolic acidosis, facilitating further uric acid crystallization. Acute renal failure may be the end result.[38]

TREATMENT

Desired Outcomes

KEY CONCEPT *The primary goals of management of TLS are (a) prevention of renal failure and (b) prevention of electrolyte imbalances. Thus, the best treatment for TLS is prophylaxis to enable delivery of cytotoxic therapy for the underlying malignancy.* For patients who present with or develop TLS despite prophylaxis, treatment goals include (a) decreasing uric acid levels, (b) correcting electrolyte imbalances, and (c) preventing compromised renal function. These goals should be achieved in a cost-effective manner.

General Approach to Treatment

Prevention of TLS is generally achieved by increasing the urine output and preventing accumulation of uric acid. Prophylactic strategies should begin immediately upon presentation, preferably 48 hours prior to cytotoxic therapy. Treatment modalities primarily increase uric acid solubility, maintain electrolyte balance, and support renal output.[38]

▶ *Nonpharmacologic Therapy*

Vigorous IV hydration with dextrose 5% in water with half normal saline at 3 L/m^2/day to maintain a urine output greater than or equal to 100 mL/m^2/hour is necessary unless the patient presents with acute renal dysfunction. Alkalinization of the urine to a pH greater than or equal to 7.0 with 50 to 100 mEq/L (50–100 mmol/L) of sodium bicarbonate has been used to promote uric acid solubility for excretion. This measure is controversial because xanthine and hypoxanthine are less soluble at alkaline pH, potentially leading to crystallization, especially during and after allopurinol therapy (see Figure 99–5).[38] Medications that increase serum potassium (angiotensin-converting enzyme inhibitors, spironolactone) or block tubular resorption of uric acid (probenecid, thiazides) should be discontinued. Nephrotoxic agents such as amphotericin B or aminoglycosides should also be avoided. Hemodialysis may be required in patients who develop anuria or uncontrolled hyperkalemia, hyperphosphatemia, hypocalcemia, acidosis, or volume overload.[38]

▶ *Pharmacologic Therapy*

Pharmacologic prevention strategies for TLS are aimed at low- and high-risk patients (Figure 99–6). Allopurinol is an xanthine oxidase inhibitor that is used for prevention only because it has no effect on preexisting elevated uric acid. Rasburicase is a recombinant form of urate oxidase that is useful for both prevention and treatment, but is expensive (Table 99–15). Although the approved dose is 0.2 mg/kg/day for 5 days, recent studies using abbreviated courses (1–3 days) and/or lower doses (0.05–0.1 mg/kg/day) may be equally efficacious with significantly reduced cost.[39] Because uric acid levels generally fall within 4 hours of the first dose, one dose may be administered with frequent, serial monitoring of the uric acid level for repeat dosing if necessary (see Figure 99–6). Of note, rasburicase continues to break down uric acid in blood samples drawn from patients. This can be avoided by immediately placing the sample in an ice bath for processing to avoid falsely lowered uric acid levels.[39]

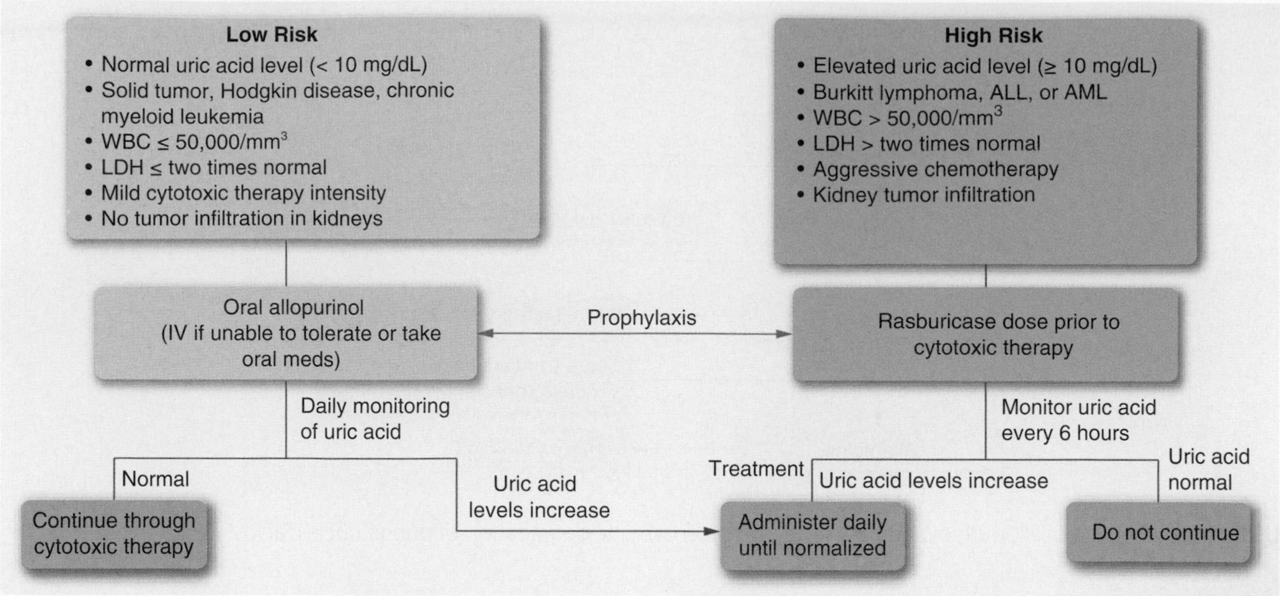

FIGURE 99–6. Prophylaxis and treatment of hyperuricemia associated with tumor lysis syndrome. (ALL, acute lymphoblastic leukemia; AML, acute myelogenous leukemia; IV, intravenous; LDH, lactate dehydrogenase; WBC, white blood cell.) (Data from Refs. 35 and 36.)

Table 99–15

Comparison of Allopurinol and Rasburicase in TLS

Drug	Dosing	AWP[a]	Comments
Oral allopurinol (Zyloprim)	Adult: 600–800 mg/day in two to three divided doses Pediatric: 10 mg/kg/day or 200–300 mg/m²/day	$0.48/day (generic)	Adjust dose for renal impairment Avoid drug interactions (mercaptopurine) Monitor for skin rash
IV allopurinol (Aloprim)	Adult: 200–400 mg/m²/day Pediatric: 200 mg/m²/day	$625–$1,250/day	As above Reserve for patients who cannot tolerate or take oral medications Maximum dose = 600 mg/day
Rasburicase (Elitek)	0.2 mg/kg/day for up to 5 days	$12,000/day	Lower doses and abbreviated schedules may be used to decrease cost (0.05–0.1 mg/kg/day) May rarely cause nausea and vomiting Contraindicated in patients with G6PD deficiency → hemolytic anemia Rare cases of hypersensitivity and antibody formation

AWP, average wholesale price; G6PD, glucose-6-phosphate dehydrogenase; po, oral.

[a]Normalized for 70-kg patient or body surface area = 1.73 m²; all costs are estimated and may vary.

From Yim BT, Sims-McCallum RP, Chong PH. Rasburicase for the treatment and prevention of hyperuricemia. Ann Pharmacother. 2003;37:1047–1054.

Clinical Presentation and Diagnosis of TLS[38]

General

- Patients present primarily with laboratory abnormalities.
- Normal uric acid is equal to 2 to 8 mg/dL (119–476 μmol/L).
- Most often occurs within 12 to 72 hours of initiation of cytotoxic therapy

Signs and Symptoms

- Most patients are asymptomatic
- Patients may develop edema, fluid overload, and oliguria, which may progress to anuria with acute renal failure
- Some patients with hyperuricemia may have nausea, vomiting, and lethargy
- Hyperkalemia: lethargy, muscle weakness, paresthesia, ECG changes, bradycardia
- Hypocalcemia: muscle cramps, tetany, irritability, paresthesias, arrhythmias

Laboratory Tests (Adults)

- Serum uric acid level greater than 8 mg/dL (476 μmol/L)
- Serum potassium greater than 6 mEq/L (6 mmol/L)
- Serum phosphorus greater than 4.5 mg/dL (1.45 mmol/L)
- Serum calcium less than 7 mg/dL (1.75 mmol/L)
- Elevated blood urea nitrogen and creatinine once renal dysfunction develops

or

- A change of greater than 25% from baseline in the above laboratory values[35]

Patient Care Process: TLS

Patient Assessment:

- Assess patient's medical history for risk factors of TLS, including cancer and chemotherapy history.
- Assess patient for signs/symptoms of TLS, including uremia, visual disturbances, muscle cramping, etc.
- Order laboratory tests: Uric acid, potassium, phosphate, calcium, electrolytes, renal function tests.

Therapy Evaluation:

- Monitor daily at-risk patients who present with normal laboratory values daily for serum uric acid, electrolytes (Na, K, Ca, Mg, Cl, PO_4), blood urea nitrogen, creatinine, and urine output.
- Monitor for signs of fluid overload during aggressive hydration.

Care Plan Development:

- Initiate allopurinol

Follow-Up Evaluation:

- Continue hydration and prophylaxis until 2 to 3 days after cytotoxic therapy.
- In patients undergoing urinary alkalinization with sodium bicarbonate, assess the urine pH every 6 hours and maintain above 7.

Electrolyte disturbances that develop in patients with TLS should be aggressively managed to avoid renal failure and cardiac sequelae. One exception pertains to the use of IV calcium for hypocalcemia. Adding calcium may cause further calcium phosphate precipitation in the presence of hyperphosphatemia and should be used cautiously.

OUTCOME EVALUATION

The most successful outcome in TLS is prevention. If the condition is not able to be prevented, the goal of therapy is to avoid renal failure and quickly return electrolytes to normal.

Abbreviations Introduced in This Chapter

ANC	Absolute neutrophil count
AWP	Average wholesale price
BMT	Bone marrow transplantation
BUN	Blood urea nitrogen
CIV	Continuous intravenous infusion
CSF	Colony-stimulating factor
G6PD	Glucose-6-phosphate dehydrogenase
ICP	Intracranial pressure
IV	Intravenous
LDH	Lactate dehydrogenase
NSAID	Nonsteroidal anti-inflammatory drug
NSCLC	Non–small cell lung cancer
PCP	*Pneumocystis jiroveci* pneumonitis (formerly *Pneumocystis carinii*)
PTHrP	Parathyroid hormone–related protein
SCLC	Small cell lung cancer
SVCS	Superior vena cava syndrome

REFERENCES

1. deBoer-Dennert M, deWit R, Schmitz PI, et al. Patient perceptions of the side effects of chemotherapy: The influence of 5HT3 antagonists. Br J Cancer. 1997;76:1055–1061.
2. Roscoe JA, Bushnnow P, Morrow GR, et al. Patient experience is a strong predictor of severe nausea after chemotherapy: A University of Rochester Community Clinical Oncology Program study of patients with breast carcinoma. Cancer. 2004;101:2701–2708.
3. Janelsins MC, tejani MA, Kamen C, et al. Current pharmacotherapy for chemotherapy-induced nausea and vomiting in cancer patients. Expert Opin Pharmacother. 2013;14(6): 757–766.
4. Geling O, Eichler HG. Should 5-hydroxytryptamine-3-receptor antagonists be administered beyond 24 hours after chemotherapy to prevent delayed emesis? Systematic re-evaluation of clinical evidence and drug cost implications. J Clin Oncol. 2005;23:1289–1294.
5. National Comprehensive Cancer Network [Internet]. Fort Washington, PA: National Comprehensive Cancer Network. Clinical practice guidelines in oncology: Antiemesis. version v.2.2014. http://www.nccn.org/professionals/physician_gls/PDF/antiemesis.pdf. Accessed Aug 31, 2014.
6. Molassioti SA, Stamataki Z, Kontopanlelis E. Development and preliminary validation of a risk prediction model for chemotherapy-related nausea and vomiting. Support Care Cancer. 2013;21(10):2759–2767.
7. Basch E, Prestrud AA, Hesketh PJ, et al. Antiemetics: ASCO clinical practice guideline update. J Clin Oncol. 2011;29 (31):4189–4198.

8. United States Food and Drug Administration. FDA Drug Safety Communication: New information regarding QT prolongation with ondansetron (Zofran) [Internet]. Rockville, MD; page last updated 2/15/2013 [cited 31 Aug 2014]. www.fda.gov/Drugs/DrugSafety/ucm310190.htm. Accessed August 31, 2014.
9. Navari RM, Gray SE, Kerr AC. Olanzapine versus aprepitant for the prevention of chemotherapy-induced nausea and vomiting: A randomized phase III trial. J Support Oncol. 2011 Sept-Oct;9(5):188–195.
10. Peterson DE, Bensadoun RJ, Roila F. Management of oral and gastrointestinal mucositis: ESMO clinical practice recommendations. Ann Oncol. 2911;22(Suppl 6):vi78–vi84.
11. Saadeh CE. Chemotherapy- and radiotherapy-induced oral mucositis: Review of preventative strategies and treatment. Pharmacotherapy. 2005;25:540–544.
12. Lalla RV, Bowen J, Barasch A, et al. MASCC/ISOO clinical practice guidelines for the management of mucositis secondary to cancer therapy. Cancer. 2014;120(10):1453–1461.
13. Wisplinghoff H, Seifert H, Wenzel RP, Edmond MB. Current trends in the epidemiology of nosocomial bloodstream infections in patients with hematological malignancies and solid neoplasms in hospitals in the United States. Clin Infect Dis. 2003;36:1103–1110.
14. Freifeld AG, Bow EJ, Sepkowitz KA, et al. Clinical practice guidelines for the use of antimicrobial agents in neutropenic patients with cancer: 2010 update by the Infectious Disease Society of America. Clin Infect Dis. 2011;52(4):e56–e93.
15. Lyman GH, Lyman CH, Agboola O. Risk models for predicting chemotherapy-induced neutropenia. Oncologist. 2005;10: 427–437.
16. Klastersky J, Paesmans M. The Multinational Association for Supportive Care in Cancer (MASCC) risk index score: 10 years of use for identifying low-risk febrile neutropenic cancer patients. Support Care Cancer. 2013;21(5):1487–1495.
17. Crawford J, Caserta C, Roila F, et al. Hematopoietic growth factors: ESMO recommendations for the applications. Ann Oncol. 2010;21(Suppl 5):v248–v251.
18. The National Comprehensive Cancer Network [Internet]. Fort Washington, PA: National Comprehensive Cancer Network. Clinical practice guidelines in oncology: Prevention and treatment of cancer-related infections. version v.2.2014, http://www.nccn.org/professionals/physician_gls/PDF/infections.pdf. Accessed Aug 31, 2014.
19. Gafter-Gvili A, Fraser A, Paul M, et al. Meta-analysis: Antibiotic prophylaxis reduces mortality in neutropenic patients. Ann Intern Med. 2005;142:979–995.
20. van de Wetering MD, de Witte MA, Kremer LCM, et al. Efficacy of oral prophylactic antibiotics in neutropenic afebrile oncology patients: A systematic review of randomized controlled trials. Eur J Cancer. 2005;41:1372–1382.
21. National Comprehensive Cancer Network [Internet]. Fort Washington, PA: National Comprehensive Cancer Network. Clinical practice guidelines in oncology: Myeloid growth factors. version, v.2.2014. http://www.nccn.org/professionals/physician_gls/PDF/myeloid_growth.pdf. Accessed Aug 31, 2014.
22. Kuderer NM, Crawford J, Dale DC, et al. Meta-analysis of prophylactic granulocyte colony-stimulating factor in cancer patients receiving chemotherapy. J Clin Oncol. 2005;23(Suppl):758S.
23. Oncology Nursing Society ONS putting evidence into practice: Prevention of infection: General. [Internet] Pittsburgh, PA: Oncology Nursing Society; [cited 31 Aug 2014]. http://www.ons.org/practice-resources/pep/prevention-infection/prevention-infection-general.
24. Clark OAC, Lyman GH, Castro AA, et al. Colony-stimulating factors for chemotherapy-induced febrile neutropenia: A meta-analysis of randomized controlled trials. J Clin Oncol. 2005;23: 4198–4214.
25. Wilson LD, Detterbeck FC, Yahalom J. Superior vena cava syndrome with malignant causes. N Engl J Med. 2007;356(8): 1862–1869.
26. Prasad D, Schiff D. Malignant spinal-cord compression. Lancet Oncol. 2005;6:15–24.
27. Douglas S, Schild SE, Rades D. A new score predicting the survival of patients with spinal cord compression from myeloma. BMC Cancer. 2012;12:425.
28. Rades D, Douglas S, Veninga T, Schild SE. A validated score for patients with metastatic spinal cord compression from non-small cell lung cancer. BMC Cancer. 2012;12:302.
29. Patchell RA, Tibbs PA, Regine WF, et al. Direct decompressive surgical resection in the treatment of spinal cord compression caused by metastatic cancer: A randomized trial. Lancet. 2005;366: 643–648.
30. Loblaw DA, Perry J, Chambers A, et al. Systematic review of the diagnosis and management of malignant extradural spinal cord compression: The Cancer Care Ontario Practice Guidelines Initiative's Neuro-Oncology Disease Site Group. J Clin Oncol. 2005;23:2028–2037.
31. Brastianos DK, Curry WT, Oh KS. Clinical discussion and review of the management of brain metastases. J Natl Compr Cancer Netw. 2013;11:1153–1164.
32. Slotman B, Faivre-Finn C, Kramer G, et al. Prophylactic cranial-irradiation in extensive small cell lung cancer. N Engl J Med. 2007;357:664–672.
33. Xie SS, Li M, Zhou CC, Song XL, Wang CH. Prophylactic cranial irradiation may impose detrimental effect on overall survival in patients with nonsmall cell lung cancer: A systematic review and meta-analysis. PLoS One. 2014;9(7):e103431.
34. West NJ. Prevention and treatment of hemorrhagic cystitis. Pharmacotherapy. 1997;17:696–706.
35. Hensley ML, Hagerty KL, Kewalramani T, et al. American Society of Clinical Oncology 2008 clinical practice guideline update: Use of chemotherapy and radiation therapy protectants. J Clin Oncol. 2009;27(1):127–145.
36. Stewart AF. Hypercalcemia associated with cancer. N Engl J Med. 2005;352:373–379.
37. Hu MI, Glezerman I, Leboulleux S, et al. Denosumab for patients with persistent or replaced hypercalcemia of malignancy despite recent bisphosphonate treatment. J Natl Cancer Inst. 2013;105(18):1417–1420.
38. Wilson FP, Berns JS. Tumor lysis syndrome: New challenges and recent advances. Adv Chronic Kidney Dis. 2014;21(1):18–26.
39. Kennedy LD, Ajiboye VO. Rasburicase for the prevention and treatment of hyperuricemia in tumor lysis syndrome. J Oncol Pharm Pract. 2010;16(3):205–213.

100 Parenteral Nutrition

Michael D. Kraft and Melissa R. Pleva

LEARNING OBJECTIVES

Upon completion of the chapter, the reader will be able to:

1. List appropriate indications for parenteral nutrition (PN) in adult patients.
2. Describe the components of PN and their role in nutrition support therapy.
3. List key elements of nutrition assessment and factors considered in assessing an adult patient's nutritional status and nutritional requirements.
4. Explain the pharmaceutical and compounding issues with PN admixtures.
5. Develop a plan to design, initiate, and adjust a PN formulation for an adult patient based on patient-specific factors.
6. Describe the etiology and risk factors for PN macronutrient-associated complications in adult patients receiving PN.
7. Describe the etiology and risk factors for refeeding syndrome.
8. Design a plan to assess the efficacy and monitor for safety, as well as fluid, electrolyte, vitamin, and trace element abnormalities in adult patients receiving PN.

INTRODUCTION

Malnutrition in hospitalized patients is associated with significant complications (eg, increased infection risk, poor wound healing, prolonged hospital stays, increased mortality), especially in surgical and critically ill patients.[1] Maintaining adequate nutritional status, especially during periods of illness and metabolic stress, is an essential part of patient care. *Nutrition support therapy* refers to the administration of nutrients via the oral, enteral, or parenteral route for therapeutic purposes.[1] KEY CONCEPT *Parenteral nutrition (PN), also called total parenteral nutrition (TPN), is the intravenous (IV) administration of fluids, macronutrients, electrolytes, vitamins, and trace elements for the purpose of weight maintenance or gain, to preserve or replete lean body mass and visceral proteins, and to support anabolism and nitrogen balance when the oral or enteral route is not feasible or adequate.* PN is a potentially lifesaving therapy in patients with intestinal failure but can be associated with significant complications.

Desired Outcomes and Goals

The goals of nutrition support therapy include:

- Correction or avoidance of nutritional deficiencies
- Weight maintenance (or weight gain in malnourished patients and growing children)
- Preservation or repletion of lean body mass and visceral proteins
- Support of anabolism and nitrogen balance and improvement of healing
- Correction or avoidance of fluid and electrolyte abnormalities
- Correction or avoidance of vitamin and trace element abnormalities
- Improving clinical outcomes

Indications for PN

PN can be a lifesaving therapy in patients with intestinal failure, but the oral or enteral route is preferred when providing nutrition support therapy. Compared with PN, enteral nutrition is associated with a lower risk of hyperglycemia and fewer infectious complications (eg, pneumonia, intra-abdominal abscess, catheter-related infections).[1–3] However, if used appropriately PN can be safe and effective and can improve nutrient delivery. Indications for PN are listed in **Table 100–1**.[1,2] PN should be reserved for patients with altered intestinal function or absorption or when the gastrointestinal (GI) tract cannot be used. The anticipated duration of adequate PN therapy should be at least 5 to 7 days because shorter durations are unlikely to have a beneficial effect on a patient's clinical and nutritional outcomes but may increase infection risk.[1,2]

PN COMPONENTS

PN should provide a *balanced* nutrition formula, including macronutrients, micronutrients, fluids, and electrolytes. Macronutrients, including amino acids, dextrose, and IV fat emulsions (IVFE), are important sources of structural and energy-yielding substrates. In a balanced PN formulation for adult patients, total daily calories are typically provided as 10% to 20% from amino

Table 100–1

Indications for Parenteral Nutrition in Adults[1,2]

- Bowel obstruction
  - Physical or mechanical (eg, tumor compressing intestinal lumen)
  - Functional (eg, ileus, colonic pseudo-obstruction)
- Major small bowel resection (eg, short-bowel syndrome)
  - Adult patients with < 100 cm of small bowel distal to the ligament of Treitz without a colon
  - Adult patients with < 50 cm of small bowel if the colon is intact
- Diffuse peritonitis
- Intestinal fistulas if EN cannot be provided above or below the fistula
- Pancreatitis—if patients have failed EN beyond the ligament of Treitz or cannot receive EN (eg, because of intestinal obstruction)
- Severe intractable vomiting
- Severe intractable diarrhea
- Preoperative nutrition support in patients with moderate to severe malnutrition who cannot tolerate EN and in whom surgery can be delayed safely for at least 7 days
- In critically ill patients without malnutrition who cannot receive oral or EN in the first 7 days of ICU admission, PN should only be initiated after the first 7 days of admission and if oral or EN is still not feasible

acids, 50% to 60% from dextrose, and 15% to 30% from IVFE. Amino acids may provide more than 20% of the total daily calories in patients with conditions that increase protein requirements (eg, severe thermal injury, healing wounds, cachexia, treatment with continuous renal replacement therapy, hypocaloric feeding). Electrolytes and micronutrients, including vitamins and trace elements, are required to support essential biochemical reactions. Patients require individual adjustments of PN components based on their nutritional status, nutritional requirements, underlying disease state(s), level of metabolic stress, clinical status, and organ functions.

Macronutrients

► *Amino Acids*

Amino acids, the building blocks of proteins, are an essential component of PN admixtures. KEY CONCEPT *Amino acids are provided to preserve or replete lean body mass and visceral proteins, to promote protein anabolism and wound healing, and as a source of energy.* Amino acids have a caloric value of 4 kcal/g (17 kJ/g).

Parenteral crystalline amino acid solutions are supplied by various manufacturers in various concentrations (eg, 7%, 8%, 8.5%, 10%, 15%, and others). Different formulations are tailored for specific age groups (eg, adults, infants) and disease states (eg, kidney or liver dysfunction). Specialized formulations for

Patient Encounter, Part 1

PG is a 59-year-old man with a history of hypertension and colon cancer, status post colon resection and colostomy, followed by chemotherapy, and subsequent colon reanastomosis. He was admitted approximately 2 weeks ago with signs and symptoms consistent with a bowel obstruction. He was taken to the OR for an exploratory laparotomy and found with multiple adhesions causing small bowel obstructions in two locations. He underwent a small bowel resection (jejunum) and extensive lysis of adhesions, and he was discharged 8 days ago. PG is readmitted with foul-smelling drainage from his surgical incision for 2 days along with nausea, decreased appetite, and decreased oral intake for the past 2 to 3 days. Since his diagnosis of colon cancer he has had weight loss, poor oral intake, and malnutrition. Most recently with his bowel obstructions and current symptoms, he reports an unintentional weight loss of about 10 lb (4.5 kg) over the past 4 to 5 weeks.

PMH: Hypertension × 10 years

Colon cancer diagnosed 2 years ago, status post colectomy, chemotherapy, and reanastomosis

Malnutrition since diagnosis of colon cancer

Past Surgical History

Colon resection with colostomy, colostomy takedown with reanastomosis 2 years ago

Exploratory laparotomy with small bowel resection and lysis of adhesions due to small bowel obstruction (greater than 100 cm of small intestine remaining, ileocecal valve intact, part of the colon remaining)

FH: Mother and father: hypertension; grandmother: chronic constipation

SH: 30 pack–year smoking history, quit 2 years ago; patient reports only occasional alcohol; no recreational drugs

Medications Prior to Admission: Hydrochlorothiazide 50 mg po daily; docusate 100 mg po twice daily

Allergies: NKDA

PE:

Ht, 178 cm (~5′10″); actual body weight, 61 kg (134 lb); ideal body weight, 73 kg (160 lb); alert and oriented × 3; mucous membranes and skin appear cool and dry; lungs clear

VS: T 37.2°C (99.0°F); HR 87 beats/min; BP 138/82 mm Hg; RR 14 breaths/min

Abd: Soft, tender around incision, faint bowel sounds, drainage of apparent enteric contents from surgical incision

Physical examination otherwise unremarkable

Diagnoses: Likely enterocutaneous fistula, probably from small bowel/jejunum (most recent surgery/small bowel resection), mild dehydration, and malnutrition

Plan: The patient was admitted to the hospital (non-ICU) for evaluation of a possible enterocutaneous fistula. The team performed a fistulogram and confirmed presence of an enterocutaneous fistula apparently originating in the proximal- to mid-jejunum. Given the patient's recent surgery, surgical intervention was deemed to not be an appropriate option at this time. A drain was placed into the fistula to control drainage and quantify output; the fistula drained approximately 600 mL in the first 24 hours. Against medical orders, the patient drank approximately 1 L of water, and the following day his fistula drained approximately 1500 mL of fluid. It is now hospital day #2

Is PN therapy indicated in this patient? Why or why not?

patients with acute kidney injury contain higher proportions of essential amino acids. Formulations for patients with hepatic encephalopathy contain higher amounts of branched-chain and lower amounts of aromatic amino acids. However, these specialized formulations have not been clearly shown to improve patient outcomes and therefore are not routinely used in clinical practice. Crystalline amino acid solutions have an acidic pH (pH ≈ 5–7) and may contain inherent electrolytes (eg, sodium, potassium, acetate, phosphate).

▶ Dextrose

KEY CONCEPT *Dextrose (D-glucose) is the major energy source, and it is vital for cellular metabolism, body protein preservation, and cellular growth.* The central nervous system, red blood cells, and the renal medulla depend primarily on dextrose as a source of energy.

Typically a 70% (70 g/100 mL) parenteral dextrose (hydrous dextrose) stock solution is used in PN compounding (a 50% stock solution is also available). Hydrous dextrose provides 3.4 kcal/g (14.2 kJ/g). A dextrose infusion rate of 2 mg/kg/min in adult patients is typically sufficient to suppress gluconeogenesis and spare body proteins from being used for energy.[4] Dextrose infusion rate in hospitalized adult patients generally should not exceed 4 to 5 mg/kg/min.[5,6] Use adjusted body weight (AdjBW) rather than actual weight in obese patients when calculating the dextrose infusion rate.

▶ Intravenous Fat Emulsions

KEY CONCEPT *Intravenous fat emulsions (IVFE) are provided to prevent or treat essential fatty acid deficiency (EFAD) and as an energy source.* IVFE particles consist of a triglyceride core surrounded by a layer of egg phospholipids (emulsifiers). These particles carry a negative charge on their surface that creates repulsive electrostatic forces between droplets and maintains the stability of the emulsion. Glycerol is added to adjust the tonicity, and water is the solvent. The negative charges on the surface of lipid particles can be disrupted by cations, especially divalent cations such as calcium, magnesium, and iron[7] and extreme pH changes, particularly acidic pH. **Creaming, coalescence,** and **oiling out** are signs of a destabilized IVFE. If there is any apparent disruption to IVFE, it should *not* be infused into a patient.

IVFEs differ in their concentration (10%, 20%, and 30%), caloric density by volume, natural source of fats/triglycerides, and ratio of phospholipids to triglycerides (PL:TG ratio). **Table 100–2** shows a comparison of standard commercially available IVFEs in the United States. Most standard IVFEs marketed in the United States contain long-chain triglycerides derived from soybean oil. Because of the addition of phospholipid emulsifiers and glycerol, the caloric density of IVFEs by weight is approximately 10 kcal/g (42 kJ/g; dietary fat is ~9 kcal/g [38 kJ/g]). Compared with the 10% IVFE, 20% and 30% IVFEs have a lower PL:TG ratio and lower phospholipid content, and this translates to better plasma clearance compared to the 10% IVFE.[8] The 30% IVFE is only approved by the Food and Drug Administration (FDA) for infusion in a total nutrient admixture (TNA) and should not be infused directly into patients nor via Y-site injection.

IVFE particles are hydrolyzed in the bloodstream by **lipoprotein lipase** to release free fatty acids and glycerol. Fatty acids are taken up into adipose tissue for storage (triglycerides), oxidized to energy in various tissues (eg, skeletal muscles), or recycled in the liver to make lipoproteins.

The essential fatty acids that cannot be produced endogenously in humans are linoleic acid (C18:2 n-6) and α-linolenic acid (C18:3 n-3) (long-chain triglycerides). Arachidonic acid (C20:4 n-6) is also essential but can be synthesized *in vivo* from linoleic acid. Adult patients should receive a minimum of 2% to 4% of total daily calories as linoleic acid and 0.25% to 0.5% of total daily calories as α-linolenic acid to prevent essential fatty acid deficiency.[6] This can be achieved by providing a minimum of ~500 mL of 20% (100 g) IVFE per week (in a single dose, or divided doses [eg, 250 mL twice a week]) for most adult patients. The typical daily dose of IVFE in adults is about 0.5 to 1 g/kg/day (or ~15%–30% of total daily calories). The maximum dose is 2.5 g/kg/day[6] or 60% of total daily calories, although doses this high are rarely used in practice and should be avoided to prevent complications.

Biochemical evidence of essential fatty acid deficiency (eg, decreased serum linoleic acid, α-linolenic acid, and arachidonic acid concentrations; elevated mead acid concentrations; elevated

Table 100–2

Comparison of Intravenous Fat Emulsions

Brand Names	Liposyn III			Intralipid			Clinolipid
Source	Soybean oil			Soybean oil			Olive and soybean oil
Concentration (%)	10	20	30	10	20	30	20
Linoleic acid (%)	54.5	54.5	54.5	44–62	44–62	44–62	13.8–22
Linolenic acid (%)	8.3	8.3	8.3	4–11	4–11	4–11	0.5–4.2
Phospholipids (egg yolk) (%)	1.2	1.2	1.8	1.2	1.2	1.2	1.2
PL:TG ratio	0.12	0.06	0.06	0.12	0.06	0.04	0.06
Caloric density[a] (kcal/mL)	1.1	2	3	1.1	2	3	2
Approximate osmolarity (mOsm/L)	284	292	293	300	350	310	260
Approximate mean pH (range)	8.3 (6.0–9.0)	8.4 (6.0–9.0)		8.0 (6.0–8.9)			(6.0–9.0)

PL, phospholipid; TG, triglyceride.

[a]1 kcal/mL is equivalent to 4.19 kJ/mL.

triene-to-tetraene ratio) can develop in well-nourished adult patients within about 2 to 4 weeks of receiving PN without IVFE, and clinical manifestations (eg, dry skin, skin desquamation, hair loss, hepatomegaly, anemia, thrombocytopenia, poor wound healing) may appear after an additional 1 to 2 weeks, although skin changes may take longer to develop.[9]

Complications and safety concerns related to the administration of IVFE include severe hypertriglyceridemia, infection, anaphylactic reactions, and infusion-related reactions. Patients with a history of hypertriglyceridemia, acute kidney injury, chronic kidney disease, hepatic dysfunction, severe metabolic stress, or pancreatitis (particularly if caused by hypertriglyceridemia) may have reduced lipid clearance and be at risk of developing hypertriglyceridemia. IVFE should be withheld in adult patients with serum triglyceride concentrations exceeding 400 mg/dL (4.52 mmol/L).

IVFEs support the growth of bacterial and fungal pathogens, but bacterial growth is slower in TNAs than in IVFE alone[10,11] due to the acidic pH of amino acid solutions and higher osmolarity of PN formulations. Because of this, the Centers for Disease Control and Prevention (CDC) recommends that TNA infusions be completed within 24 hours of initiation. Recent guidelines suggest that IVFE infusion should be completed within 12 to 24 hours if administered from the original manufacturer container, but completed within 12 hours if repackaged/transferred to another container and infused separately from a 2-in-1 PN admixture (although repackaging/transfer to another container was not recommended).[12] There is still debate about the optimal approach when infusing IVFE separately from a 2-in-1 PN admixture.

PN infusion lines must contain an appropriate filter (a 0.22-μm filter or a 1.2- μm filter). A 0.22- μm filter cannot be used on the TNA or IVFE infusion line because the average size of IVFE particles is approximately 0.4- to 0.5- μm (which cannot pass through the smaller filter intact and will clog the filter).

Patients with an allergy to eggs or specific legumes (eg, soy beans, broad beans, lentils) may develop cross-allergic reactions to IVFE. Rarely, infusion-related adverse effects may occur with rapid infusion, including fever, chills, headache, palpitations, dyspnea, chest tightness, and nausea. Extending the IVFE infusion time (eg, over 12–24 hours) can minimize infusion-related adverse events and improves IVFE clearance. Infusion rate of IVFE should not exceed 0.12 g/kg/hour.[6]

Recently the FDA approved Clinolipid for use in adult patients. Clinolipid is a mixture of refined olive and soybean oils in a 4:1 ratio. This combination reduces the amount of omega-6 fatty acids in the IVFE. This may have a positive impact on immune function and inflammation, but this is theoretical and this product has not been demonstrated to improve patient outcomes. The exact role of this IVFE product in patient care is not yet known.

▸ Fluid

KEY CONCEPT *Parenteral nutrition should not be used to treat acute fluid abnormalities. PN should be adjusted to provide maintenance fluid requirements and to minimize worsening of underlying fluid disturbances, taking into account other fluids the patient is receiving.* Daily maintenance fluid requirements for adults can be estimated with the following equation:

$$\text{Total daily fluid requirements} = 1{,}500 \text{ mL} + (20\text{mL/kg} \times [\text{Wt (kg)} - 20])^{*}$$

*For elderly patients (eg, greater than 60 years old), use 15 mL/kg for every kilogram above 20 kg.

For patients with significant fluid deficits, it is safer and more cost effective to correct fluid abnormalities using standard IV fluids (eg, 0.9% sodium chloride in water, dextrose 5% and sodium chloride 0.45% in water, lactated Ringer solution). Minimizing PN fluid volume may be indicated in patients with fluid overload, patients with oliguric or anuric acute kidney injury, or those with congestive heart failure or symptomatic pleural effusion. It is reasonable to provide total daily fluid requirements (maintenance requirements and replacement for GI or other abnormal losses) in the PN admixture in patients who require long-term PN. However, diluting a PN admixture can affect its physical and chemical properties (eg, IVFE stability, calcium–phosphate solubility/compatibility); therefore, stability and compatibility data must be confirmed before diluting a PN admixture.

Micronutrients

KEY CONCEPT *Electrolytes, vitamins, and trace elements are essential for numerous biochemical and metabolic functions and should be added to PN daily unless otherwise not indicated.*

▸ Electrolytes

KEY CONCEPT *Electrolytes are essential for many metabolic and homeostatic functions, including enzymatic and biochemical reactions, maintenance of cell membrane structure and function, neurotransmission, hormone function, muscle contraction, cardiovascular function, bone composition, and fluid homeostasis.* The causes of electrolyte abnormalities in patients receiving PN may be multifactorial, including altered absorption and distribution; excessive or inadequate intake; altered hormonal, neurologic, and homeostatic mechanisms; altered excretion and losses via the GI tract (eg, gastric, diarrhea, ostomy, enterocutaneous fistula) and kidneys; changes in fluid status and fluid shifts; and medication therapies. PN should not be used to treat acute electrolyte abnormalities but should be adjusted to meet maintenance requirements and to minimize worsening of underlying electrolyte disturbances.

Electrolytes that are included routinely in PN admixtures include sodium, potassium, phosphorus (as phosphate), calcium, magnesium, chloride, and acetate. Always assess the patient's kidney function when determining electrolyte doses in PN admixtures. Typical daily electrolyte maintenance requirements for adults with normal kidney function are listed in Table 100–3.[6,13] For additional details regarding management of fluid, electrolyte and acid–base disorders refer to Chapters 27 and 28.

▸ Calcium-Phosphate Solubility

The FDA published a safety alert in response to two deaths from microvascular pulmonary emboli associated with calcium–phosphate precipitation in PN.[14] Because calcium and phosphate can bind and precipitate in solution, caution must be exercised when mixing these two electrolytes in PN admixtures. Several factors can affect calcium–phosphate solubility, including:

- *Amino acid concentration.* Primary factor that affects pH of the PN admixture. The pH of amino acid stock solutions may vary between commercial products. In general, the higher the final amino acid concentration, the lower the pH of the final admixture. Phosphates can also bind with amino acids, leaving fewer phosphates available to bind with calcium.
- *pH.* Largely affected by the amino acid brand and concentration, to a lesser extent by the dextrose concentration; the lower the solution pH, the less chance for calcium–phosphate precipitation. Monobasic phosphates

Table 100–3

Approximate Daily Maintenance Electrolyte Requirements for Adults[6,13]

Electrolyte	Approximate Daily Maintenance Requirements[a]	Electrolyte Salts Used in PN	Maximum Concentration in PN
Sodium	1–2 mEq/kg (1–2 mmol/kg)	Chloride, acetate, phosphate	154 mEq/L (154 mmol/L, equivalent to normal saline)
Potassium	1–2 mEq/kg (1–2 mmol/kg)	Chloride, acetate, phosphate	120 mEq/L (120 mmol/L) (central PN)
Phosphorus	20–40 mmol (~10–15 mmol per 1000 kcal [2.4–3.6 mmol per 1000 kJ])	Sodium phosphate, potassium phosphate	See text section on calcium-phosphate solubility
Calcium	10–15 mEq (5–7.5 mmol)	Gluconate	
Magnesium	8–20 mEq (4–10 mmol)	Sulfate	20 mEq/L (10 mmol/L)
Chloride	[b]	Sodium, potassium	Linked to limitations of sodium and potassium. Usual ratio of chloride to acetate ~1:1–1.5:1
Acetate	[b]	Sodium, potassium	
Conversions	1 mmol potassium phosphate = 1.47 mEq potassium 1 mmol sodium phosphate = 1.33 mEq sodium 1 g of calcium gluconate = 4.65 mEq (2.32 mmol) calcium 1 g of magnesium sulfate = 8.1 mEq (4 mmol) magnesium		

[a]Electrolyte requirements are adjusted based on serum electrolyte concentrations and vary depending on kidney function, gastrointestinal losses, nutritional status, specific metabolic and endocrine functions, and medication therapy that affect electrolyte losses or retention.

[b]As needed to maintain acid–base balance; linked to amounts of sodium and potassium provided (as chloride and acetate salts).

predominate at low pH, leaving fewer free dibasic phosphates for precipitation with divalent calcium; monobasic calcium phosphate is more soluble than dibasic calcium phosphate.

- *Calcium salt.* Calcium gluconate is the preferred calcium salt in PN because it has a lower dissociation constant in solution with less free calcium available at a given time to bind phosphate.
- *Time.* The longer calcium and phosphate are in solution, the more calcium and phosphate will dissociate over time and increase the risk for calcium–phosphate precipitation.
- *Temperature.* As temperature increases, more calcium and phosphate dissociate and increase the risk of calcium-phosphate precipitation.
- *Order of mixing.* Calcium and phosphate should not be added simultaneously or consecutively when compounding PN admixtures (eg, add phosphate first, then add other PN components, and then add calcium near the end of compounding). The volume in the PN admixture at the time calcium is added (not necessarily the final volume) must be used to determine the maximum calcium that can be added.

When compounding PN admixtures, use calcium–phosphate solubility curves (based on the specific brand and final concentration of amino acids and dextrose) to determine safe and appropriate calcium and phosphate concentration limits.

▶ Acetate

Acetate is converted to bicarbonate at a 1:1 molar ratio, and this conversion appears to occur mostly outside the liver. Bicarbonate should *never* be added to or coinfused with PN admixtures. This can lead to the release of carbon dioxide and result in the formation of insoluble calcium or magnesium carbonate salts.

▶ Vitamins

Water-soluble and fat-soluble vitamins in the parenteral multivitamin products are essential cofactors for numerous biochemical reactions and metabolic processes. Parenteral multivitamins are added daily to the PN admixture. Water-soluble vitamins, with the exception of vitamin B_{12}, are generally readily excreted and not stored in the body in significant amounts. Deficiencies of water-soluble vitamins can occur rapidly in the absence of adequate vitamin supplementation in PN. Severe refractory lactic acidosis and deaths were reported in patients who received PN without added thiamine. Thiamine is an essential cofactor in carbohydrate metabolism (via the tricarboxylic acid cycle). Deficiency of thiamine pyrophosphate prevents the formation of acetyl-CoA from pyruvate, which is instead converted to lactate via anaerobic metabolism, resulting in lactic acidosis. Parenteral multivitamin products contain 150 mcg of vitamin K in accordance with FDA recommendations. A parenteral adult multivitamin formulation is available without vitamin K, but standard compounding of PN formulations should include a product that contains vitamin K unless otherwise indicated. Patients with chronic kidney disease are at risk for vitamin A accumulation and potential toxicity. Serum vitamin A concentrations should be measured in patients with chronic kidney disease when vitamin A accumulation is a concern. Not all vitamins are available individually in injectable form, so restricting vitamin A may compromise provision of other vitamins.

▶ Trace Elements

Trace elements are essential cofactors for numerous biochemical processes. Trace elements added routinely to PN include zinc, selenium, copper, manganese, and chromium (Table 100–4). Various individual and multi-ingredient parenteral trace element formulations can be added to PN admixtures. Trace element supplementation in PN should be individualized, especially for long-term PN-dependent patients, rather than using a fixed dose of multitrace element products.[15] Zinc is important for wound healing, and patients with high-output enterocutaneous fistulas, diarrhea, burns, and large open wounds may require additional zinc supplementation. Patients may lose as much as 12 to 17 mg zinc/L of GI output (eg, diarrhea, enterocutaneous

Table 100–4

Approximate Daily Maintenance Trace Element Requirements for Adults[6,a]

Zinc (Zn)	Selenium (Se)	Copper (Cu)	Manganese (Mn)	Chromium (Cr)
2.5–5 mg	20–60 mcg	0.3–0.5 mg	0.06–0.1 mg	10–15 mcg

[a]Requirements may vary based on patients' kidney function, liver function, gastrointestinal losses, nutritional status, specific metabolic and endocrine functions, serum levels, and medication therapy. Contamination of some PN ingredients with trace elements (eg, chromium, manganese) can contribute significantly to the total amount the patient receives. Monitor serum trace element levels in patients receiving long-term PN therapy.

fistula); however, 12 mg/day may be adequate to maintain positive zinc balance in these patients.[16] Patients with chronic severe diarrhea, malabsorption, high-output enterocutaneous fistula, or short-bowel syndrome may also have increased selenium losses and may require additional selenium supplementation. Chromium is a cofactor for glucose metabolism, and patients with chromium deficiency may exhibit glucose intolerance; however, chromium deficiency is a rare cause of hyperglycemia. Patients who are chronically dependent on PN may accumulate chromium[6] and manganese, resulting in high serum levels because these are known contaminants of parenteral products that are used in the making of PN, and manganese content of multitrace element products is higher than the recommended daily dose.[6,15] Patients with cholestasis (serum direct bilirubin concentrations that exceed 2 mg/dL [34.2 μmol/L]) should have manganese and possibly copper restricted to avoid accumulation and possible toxicity because both elements undergo biliary elimination. However, copper deficiency resulting in anemia, pancytopenia, and death has occurred in PN-dependent patients when copper was omitted from the PN admixture. Because copper deficiency has been reported to occur anywhere between 6 weeks and 12 months after copper elimination from PN,[17] serum copper concentrations must be regularly monitored (eg, every 6 weeks at first and then every 2–3 months thereafter) when copper is omitted from PN admixtures. Trace element status should initially be monitored periodically (eg, every 3 months) in patients at risk for trace element deficiency or accumulation. When stable, serum trace element concentrations can be monitored less frequently (eg, every 6–12 months).

PN Additives

▸ *Regular Insulin*

Regular insulin may be added to PN admixtures for glycemic control. The dose depends on the patient's clinical condition, severity of hyperglycemia, predisposing factors for hyperglycemia, renal function, and daily insulin requirements. Generally, after the patient is receiving his or her goal dextrose dose in PN, about 50% to 70% of the total insulin doses administered over the previous 24 hours as sliding scale or continuous infusion can be added to the next PN admixture. In patients with diabetes, IV insulin doses in the PN admixture to maintain euglycemia range from 0.05 to 0.2 unit of insulin per each gram of dextrose in PN (adjusted based on frequent capillary blood glucose evaluation). Caution should be used when insulin is added to PN to avoid hypoglycemia, especially when reversible causes of hyperglycemia have resolved (eg, stress, acute pancreatitis, corticosteroids therapy) or more than one form of insulin therapy is used concurrently. Adding insulin to PN (vs a continuous IV infusion) does not provide the flexibility of frequent titration.

▸ *Histamine-2 Receptor Antagonists*

Intravenous histamine-2 receptor antagonists such as ranitidine, famotidine, and cimetidine are compatible with PN admixtures and can be added when indicated.

▸ *Heparin*

Heparin (0.5–1 unit/mL of final PN volume) has been added to PN admixtures for three reasons:

- Maintain catheter patency (although this effect is debated)
- Reduce thrombophlebitis (with PPN infusion)
- Enhance lipid particle clearance as a cofactor for the lipoprotein lipase enzyme (temporary effect, and data are limited)

The benefits and necessity of adding heparin to PN are unclear, and this practice is becoming less common in adult patients. There are also concerns about the stability and compatibility of IVFE with heparin. Heparin should be omitted in patients with active bleeding, thrombocytopenia, heparin-induced thrombocytopenia (HIT), or heparin allergy.

▸ *Human Albumin*

Human albumin is a colloid used as a plasma volume expander and *not* a source of nutrition. Albumin should not be added to the PN admixture and should be administered separately from PN.

▸ *Parenteral Iron*

Chronic PN-dependent patients are at risk for iron-deficiency due to underlying clinical conditions and the lack of regular iron supplementation in PN. Parenteral iron dextran should be used with caution due to its infusion-related adverse effects. Iron dextran is compatible with 2-in-1 PN formulations, but is not commonly added to PN admixtures due to incompatibility with IVFE; Other parenteral iron formulations (eg, iron sucrose, ferric gluconate) should NOT be added to PN admixtures due to a lack of compatibility data.

NUTRITION ASSESSMENT AND NUTRIENT REQUIREMENTS

A nutrition assessment is used to determine a patient's nutritional status, identify patients with malnutrition, identify risk factors for nutrition-related problems, identify or rule out specific nutrient deficiencies, and determine nutrient requirements.[1] A complete description of nutrition assessment is beyond the scope of this chapter, and a nutrition assessment should be completed by a health care professional with appropriate training and expertise (eg, dietitian, nutrition-certified pharmacist). Briefly, key components of a nutrition assessment include[1,18]:

- Patient history
- Physical assessment, including height, weight, ideal body weight (IBW), body mass index (BMI = weight [kg]/height [m^2]), and recent weight changes (intentional or unintentional)
  - BMI is a vague indicator of total body fat mass in adults and is not an indicator of body nutrient stores. BMI categories do not account for frame size, muscle mass, bone, and water weight. Classifications of BMI:
    - Underweight, less than 18.5 kg/m^2
    - Normal, 18.5 to 24.9 kg/m^2
    - Overweight, 25 to 29.9 kg/m^2
    - Obese, more than or equal to 30 kg/m^2
- Degree of malnutrition can be classified by assessing the percentage of unintentional weight loss or percentage of usual weight. For example:
  - Severe malnutrition: greater than 5% weight loss within 1 month or greater than 10% weight loss over 6 months;
  - Moderate malnutrition: 5% to 10% weight loss over 6 months;
  - Mild malnutrition/well-nourished: less than 5% weight loss over less than or equal to 6 months
- Anthropometrics and physical examination of the musculoskeletal system (eg, biceps, triceps, quadriceps, temporalis, deltoid, and interosseus muscles) for loss of muscle mass or decreased grip strength, and examination of the skin and mucous membranes for abnormalities (eg, dry or flaky skin, bruising, edema, ascites, poorly healing wounds) and loss of subcutaneous fat
- Changes in eating habits, GI function, and associated GI symptoms
- Presence and severity of underlying and concurrent disease(s)
- Serum visceral protein concentrations (eg, albumin, prealbumin). Hypoalbuminemia at baseline or before hospitalization may indicate malnutrition, and severe hypoalbuminemia may be associated with poor outcomes. Serum albumin and prealbumin are negative acute phase proteins and therefore are not sensitive or specific indicators of nutritional status and protein stores in patients under metabolic stress or with evidence of inflammatory response (eg, postsurgery, organ failure, severe burns, trauma, sepsis). Measuring serum C-reactive protein (CRP) may help assess inflammatory response (eg, CRP greater than 2.5 mg/dL [25 mg/L]). Synthesis and distribution of albumin and prealbumin may be altered, and serum concentrations are affected by non-nutritional factors, including hydration status, kidney function, and liver function. Because prealbumin has a shorter half-life (~2 days) than albumin (~20 days), serum prealbumin concentrations may be measured usually once weekly to help evaluate the net anabolism in response to nutrition support therapy in the absence of acute stress/inflammation
- Serum concentrations of vitamins, trace elements, and iron studies as indicated

After performing a nutrition assessment, estimate the patient's daily energy and protein requirements (**Table 100–5**). Indirect calorimetry involves measuring the volumes of oxygen consumption (VO_2) and carbon dioxide production (VCO_2) to determine the resting metabolic rate (RMR) or resting energy expenditure (REE) and respiratory quotient ($RQ = VCO_2/VO_2$). The REE or RMR is the amount of calories required during 24 hours by the body in a nonactive state and is approximately 10% higher than the basal energy expenditure (BEE, metabolic activity required to maintain life) as it adjusts for the thermic effect of food and awake state. Critically ill patients may have variable energy expenditure (EE), and indirect calorimetry is a valuable tool in assessing EE in these patients. Indirect calorimetry requires specific equipment and trained personnel and therefore is not feasible in all settings.

More than 200 equations and derivations have been developed to predict EE for adults. The Harris-Benedict equations, Penn State equations (for nonobese critically ill patients receiving mechanical ventilation), and Mifflin-St. Jeor equations (for nonobese and obese noncritically ill patients) are some of the most widely used, and they take into account several variables (depending on the equation) including a patient's sex, weight, height, age, and mechanical ventilation data to determine the BEE. A "stress" or "injury" factor is sometimes applied to estimate the daily total EE (TEE), although there is debate about the appropriateness and validity of this approach. Daily energy requirements are about 100% to 130% of the RMR with adequate protein intake. Alternatively, EE can be estimated based on EE per body weight (ie, kilocalories per kilogram or in kilojoules per kilogram). However, dry weight or hospital admission weight should be used, and this estimation may not be appropriate in obese or elderly patients. There is debate over the best method to estimate energy requirements for obese patients. Indirect calorimetry would be the preferred method but may not always be available. Several equations have been developed to estimate EE in obese patients. Although there is no consensus on the weight used to estimate EE in obese patients, it is reasonable to use an AdjBW in obese patients to avoid overfeeding. AdjBW can be calculated with 25% to 50% of the difference between the actual weight and IBW added to the IBW. Using a 25% difference in calculating the AdjBW further avoids overfeeding when estimating energy requirements:

$$\text{AdjBW} = \text{IBW} + (0.25 \times [\text{Actual weight} - \text{IBW}])$$

Hypocaloric feeding is another approach for nutrient dosing in obese critically ill patients (discussed as follows).

Amino acid requirements are based on the patient's nutritional status, clinical condition(s), kidney function, and liver function. Amino acids are needed in adequate amounts to facilitate anabolism, restore lean body mass, or promote wound healing while avoiding adverse effects from excessive amino acid loading (eg, azotemia). No evidence-based data are available confirming the optimal body weight (actual, ideal, or adjusted) to use for dosing amino acids in adult patients. It is suggested to dose amino acids based on actual body weight for normal body sized or malnourished adult patients (ie, when actual weight is at or below IBW) and based on IBW or AdjBW for obese patients.

Hypocaloric nutrition support is an approach to dosing nutrition therapy for obese patients (BMI greater than or equal to 30 kg/m^2 or actual weight greater than 130% of IBW). Hypocaloric feeding involves providing high doses of protein (greater than or equal to 2–2.5 g/kg IBW/day) to support anabolism with lower amounts of total calories (average ~11–14 kcal/kg actual weight/day [~46–59 kJ/kg actual weight/day] or ~22–25 kcal/kg IBW/day [~92–105 kJ/kg IBW/day]) with primary goals to promote net protein anabolism and avoid hyperglycemia or exacerbation of metabolic stress in critically ill patients.[2,19] Other benefits could include avoiding fat weight gain

Table 100–5

Estimating Daily Nutritional Requirements in Adults[1,6,18–20]

Determining Energy Expenditure:	
Harris-Benedict equations	Men: BEE = 66.42 + 13.75 (W) + 5 (H) − 6.78 (A) Women: BEE = 655.1 + 9.65 (W) + 1.85 (H) − 4.68 (A) W = weight in kg, H = height in cm, A = age in years Energy expenditure then multiplied by a stress factor To estimate the TEE: Bed rest ≈ 1.2 × BEE Ambulatory ≈ 1.3 × BEE Anabolic ≈ 1.5 × BEE Energy requirements should also be increased ~12% with each degree of fever above 37°C (98.6°F)
Penn State equations (for critically ill nonobese adult patients receiving mechanical ventilation.)	$RMR = (0.85 \times BEE^a) + (33 \times V_E) + (175 \times T_{max}) - 6433$ $RMR = (0.96 \times BMR^b) + (31 \times V_E) + (167 \times T_{max}) - 6212$
Mifflin-St. Jeor equations (for nonobese, overweight, and obese noncritically ill adult patients)	Men BMR = (10 × Wt) + (6.25 × Ht) − (5 × Age) + 5 Women BMR = (10 × Wt) + (6.25 × Ht) − (5 × Age) − 161
Energy expenditure per body weight (ie, kcal/kg)[c]	Range of ~20–30 kcal/kg/day, possibly up to 35 kcal/kg/day Maintenance ~20–25 kcal/kg/day Repletion, postoperative wound healing, critical illness, sepsis, severe trauma, severe burns ~25–30 kcal/kg/day, possibly up to 35 kcal/kg/day
Determining Amino Acid Requirements:	
Patient Clinical Condition	**Daily Amino Acid Requirements[d] (g/kg)**
Maintenance or nonstressed	0.8–1
Repletion	1.3–2
Trauma, burns, sepsis, critical illness, wound healing	1.5–2
Hepatic failure with encephalopathy	0.8–1
Acute kidney injury, predialysis	0.8–1
Acute kidney injury receiving IHD	1.2–1.5
Chronic kidney disease receiving CAPD	1.2–1.5
Acute kidney disease receiving CRRT	1.5–2.5

BMR, basal metabolic rate; CAPD, continuous ambulatory peritoneal dialysis; CRRT, continuous renal replacement therapy; Ht, height (cm); IHD, intermittent hemodialysis; RMR, resting metabolic rate; TEE, total energy expenditure; T_{max}, maximum body temperature in degrees Celsius; V_E, minute ventilation in liters per minute; Wt, weight (kg).

[a]BEE calculated using the Harris-Benedict equation.

[b]BMR calculated using Mifflin-St. Jeor equation.

[c]One kcal/kg is equivalent to 4.184 kJ/kg.

[d]Amino acid requirements are based on actual body weight for normal body sized or malnourished adult patients and on ideal body weight (IBW) for obese patients.

or promoting fat weight loss. Most data with hypocaloric feeding are in critically ill adult patients, but this approach has been used in other patients. Hypocaloric feeding should not be used in patients with kidney or liver dysfunction. Also, the optimal safe duration of hypocaloric feeding is unknown.

Permissive underfeeding refers to providing a lower calorie nutrition support regimen to critically ill adult patients for a short period of time during the initial phase of high metabolic stress. The aims of permissive underfeeding are to avoid the burden of caloric intake on worsening metabolic stress and the negative effects of carbohydrate loading and associated hyperglycemia, increased carbon dioxide production, and fat accumulation. Typically, a permissive underfeeding PN regimen provides about 60% to 80% of daily energy requirements. Because the optimal amounts of calories for critically ill patients is not well defined, strong clinical evidence to support the use of permissive underfeeding is also lacking. Furthermore, severe underfeeding should be avoided because it can result in energy deficit to the patient with the consequences of increased infectious complications with negative outcomes.

PARENTERAL NUTRITION SAFETY

Serious and sometimes fatal adverse events have occurred with inappropriate use of PN. Shortages of key PN components have also presented challenges to meet nutritional needs of patients requiring PN therapy. The American Society for Parenteral and Enteral Nutrition (A.S.P.E.N.) has published several key PN safety documents, including comprehensive safe practice guidelines,[6] PN safety recommendations,[21] and revised guidelines that address PN ordering, order review, compounding, labeling, and dispensing.[12] A.S.P.E.N. has also provided guidance for managing shortages of PN components. These are essential resources for pharmacists and other health care professionals for the safe and efficacious use of PN therapy, and they represent the standards of practice as related to PN prescribing, compounding, stability, compatibility, labeling, administration, and quality assurance. There are several key points and recommendations in these documents to improve the safety of the PN use process, including:

- Adopting published guidelines and literature.
- Developing standardized processes for PN prescribing, order verification, compounding, labeling, dispensing, administering, and monitoring.
- Developing PN-specific policies and procedures.
- Develop education and competency assessments at least annually for all health care professionals involved in the PN use process.
- Optimizing computerized prescriber order entry (CPOE) and clinical decision support for PN orders.
- Build, test, and heed clinical decision support warnings in CPOE systems and in automated compounding devices.
- Avoiding use of handwritten PN orders and eliminate transcription of PN orders.
- Matching templates between ordering/CPOE, compounding software/automated compounding devices, and PN labels .
- PN use process and development policies, procedures, education, and competencies should include health care professionals with expertise in nutrition support, preferably from multiple disciplines.

Although application of these guidelines is voluntary, health care professionals who are involved in prescribing, compounding, dispensing, administering, and monitoring PN therapy should review and apply them to their practice.

PREPARING THE PN PRESCRIPTION: ADMINISTRATION, COMPOUNDING, AND PHARMACEUTICAL ISSUES

After performing a nutrition assessment and estimating nutritional requirements, determine the optimal route to provide nutrition support therapy (eg, oral, enteral, or parenteral). If PN is indicated, venous access for PN infusion must be obtained. Finally, formulate a PN prescription and administer PN according to safety guidelines.

Route of PN Administration: Peripheral versus Central Vein Infusion

KEY CONCEPT *PN can be administered via a smaller peripheral vein or via a larger central vein* (**Figure 100–1**). Peripheral PN (PPN) is generally is reserved for short-term administration (up to 7 days) when central venous access is not available. PN formulations are hyperosmolar, and PN infusion via a peripheral vein can cause thrombophlebitis. Factors that increase the risk of **phlebitis** include high solution osmolarity, extreme pH, rapid infusion rate, vein properties, catheter properties (eg, diameter, material), and infusion time via the same vein.[22] The osmolarity of PPN admixtures should be limited to less than or equal to 900 mOsm/L to minimize the risk of phlebitis. The approximate osmolarity of a PN admixture can be calculated from the osmolarity of the individual components:

- Amino acids ~10 mOsm/g (or 100 mOsm/L% final concentration in PN)
- Dextrose ~5 mOsm/g (or 50 mOsm/L% final concentration in PN)
- Sodium (chloride, acetate, and phosphate) = 2 mOsm/mEq (or 2 mOsm/mmol)
- Potassium (chloride, acetate, and phosphate) = 2 mOsm/mEq (or 2 mOsm/mmol)
- Calcium gluconate = 1.4 mOsm/mEq (2.8 mOsm/mmol)
- Magnesium sulfate = 1 mOsm/mEq (2 mOsm/mmol)

PPN admixtures should be coinfused with IVFE when using 2-in-1 PN because the iso-osmolarity and near-neutral pH of IVFE may decrease the risk of phlebitis (see Table 100–2). Infectious and mechanical complications may be lower with PPN compared with central venous PN administration. However, because of the risk of phlebitis, severe soft tissue damage if extravasation occurs, and osmolarity limit, PPN admixtures have

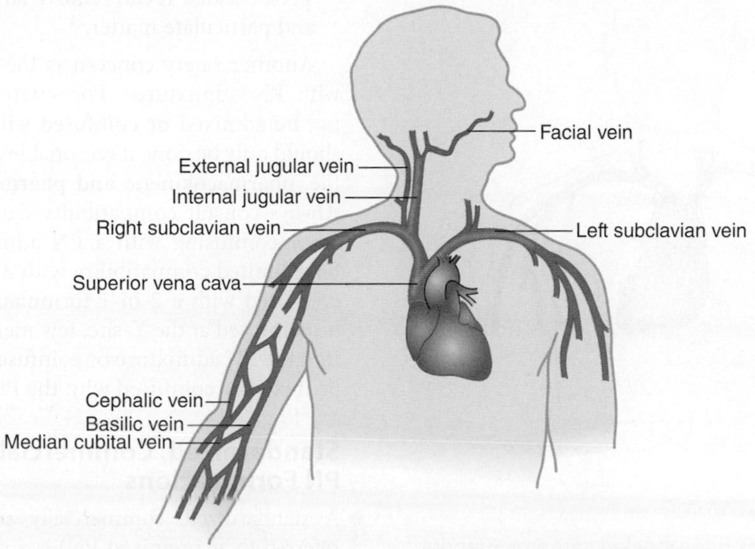

FIGURE 100–1. Selected vascular anatomy. (Reprint from Krzywda EA, Andris DA, Edmiston CE, Wallace JR. Parenteral Access Devices. In: Gottschlich MM, ed. The A.S.P.E.N. Nutrition Support Core Curriculum: A Case-Based Approach—The Adult Patient. Silver Spring, MD: American Society for Parenteral and Enteral Nutrition, 2007:300–322.)

low macronutrient concentrations and therefore usually require large fluid volumes to meet a patient's nutritional requirements. Given these limitations, every effort should be made to obtain central venous access and initiate central PN in patients who have an appropriate indication (see Table 100–1).

Central PN refers to the administration of PN via a large central vein, and the catheter tip must be positioned in the superior vena cava (**Figure 100–2**). Central PN allows the infusion of a highly concentrated, hyperosmolar nutrient admixture. The typical osmolarity of a central PN admixture is about 1500 to 2000 mOsm/L. Central veins have much higher blood flow and the PN admixture is diluted rapidly on infusion, so phlebitis is usually not a concern. Patients who require PN therapy for longer periods of time (greater than 7 days) should receive central PN. Central PN requires placement of a central venous catheter and an x-ray to confirm placement of the catheter tip. A commonly used central catheter for PN infusion is a peripherally inserted central venous catheter (PICC), which is inserted into a peripheral vein but the catheter tip is placed in the superior vena cava (**Figure 100–3**). Central venous catheter placement may be associated with complications, including **pneumothorax**, arterial injury, **air embolus**, venous thrombosis, infection, **chylothorax**, and **brachial plexus** injury.[1,22]

Types of PN Formulations: 3-in-1 versus 2-in-1

KEY CONCEPT *PN admixtures can be prepared by mixing all components into one bag, or IVFE may be infused separately (via a Y-site infusion or through a separate IV catheter or lumen). When all components are mixed together, it is referred to as a 3-in-1 admixture or TNA.*[23] *When dextrose, amino acids, and all other PN components are mixed together without IVFE, this is referred to as a 2-in-1 PN admixture.* There are various advantages and disadvantages to using either TNA or 2-in-1 PN admixtures (**Table 100–6**). With a 2-in-1 PN admixture, IVFE can be infused separately on a daily or intermittent basis. When IVFE is mixed in the PN, the TNA becomes an emulsion with respect to physical and chemical characteristics. The final concentration of IVFE in a 3-in-1 admixture should be greater than or equal to 2% (20 g/L) to prevent compromising the stability of the emulsion.[23] Electrolyte, dextrose, and amino acid concentrations may also be more limited in a 3-in-1 admixture.

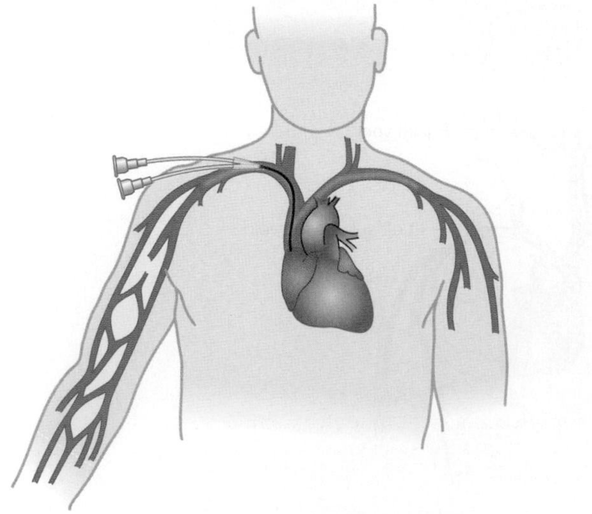

FIGURE 100–2. Percutaneous nontunneled catheter. (Reprint from Krzywda EA, Andris DA, Edmiston CE, Wallace JR. Parenteral Access Devices. In: Gottschlich MM, ed. The A.S.P.E.N. Nutrition Support Core Curriculum: A Case-Based Approach—The Adult Patient. Silver Spring, MD: American Society for Parenteral and Enteral Nutrition, 2007:300–322.)

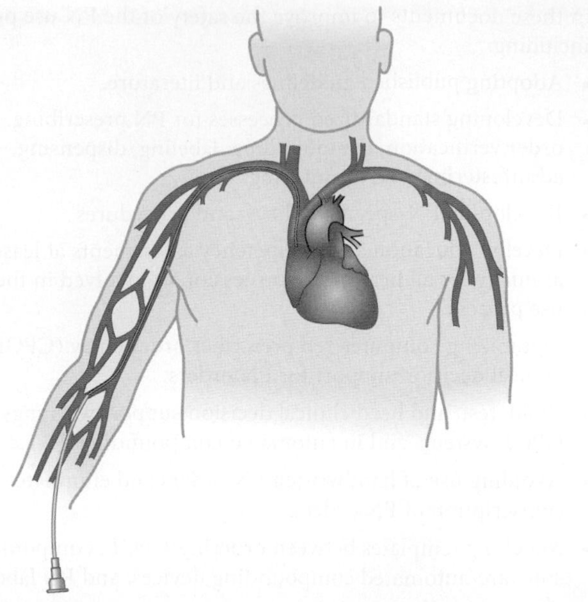

FIGURE 100–3. Peripherally inserted central venous catheter. (Reprint from Krzywda EA, Andris DA, Edmiston CE, Wallace JR. Parenteral Access Devices. In: Gottschlich MM, ed. The A.S.P.E.N. Nutrition Support Core Curriculum: A Case-Based Approach—The Adult Patient. Silver Spring, MD: American Society for Parenteral and Enteral Nutrition, 2007:300–322.)

Safety is a primary concern with PN therapy. The FDA has provided recommendations for safe infusion of PN admixtures containing calcium and phosphate:

- A 0.22- μm air-eliminating in-line filter should be used for infusion of non–IVFE-containing PN.
- A 1.2- μm in-line filter should be used for the infusion of a TNA because it can remove large and unstable fat droplets and particulate matter.[24]

Another safety concern is the coinfusion of IV medications with PN admixtures. For safety reasons, medications should not be admixed or coinfused with PN unless necessary, and it should only be done if reasonable and safe (based on toxicity profile, pharmacokinetic and pharmacodynamic considerations).[21] *Always* consult compatibility data before adding a medication to or coinfusing with a PN admixture. Many IV medications have limited compatibility with 3-in-1 formulations but may be coinfused with a 2-in-1 formulation.[25,26] Some medications can be coinfused at the Y-site, few medications can be mixed directly into the PN admixture or coinfused with IVFE, and some cannot be mixed or coinfused with the PN admixture.[25,26]

Standardized, Commercially Available (Premixed) PN Formulations

A standardized, commercially available PN formulation (also referred to as premixed PN) is a product available from a manufacturer that requires fewer compounding steps before administration.[27] These products usually contain amino acids and dextrose in a two-chamber bag, with or without electrolytes. Vitamins and trace elements must be manually added. IVFE can be added to create a TNA or infused separately. Potential advantages of premixed

Table 100–6

Potential Advantages and Disadvantages of Using 3-in-1 (TNA) or 2-in-1 PN Admixtures

	3-in-1 (TNA)	2-in-1
Advantages	Simplified regimen for patient Increased patient compliance at home Decreased labor (less nursing time) Decreased costs (fewer supplies and equipment needed) Decreased risk of contamination (caused by less manipulation and all components aseptically compounded) Inhibited bacterial growth vs separate IV lipid emulsion Minimize infusion-related reactions from IV lipid emulsions and possibly improved lipid clearance (compared to 12-hour infusion) Decreased vein irritation (with PPN)	Improved stability compared with TNA Increased number of compatible medications Decreased bacterial growth (in dextrose–amino acid component) compared with TNA Easier visual inspection Can use 0.22- μm bacterial retention filter Potential cost savings if IVFE unused (ie, not spiked or opened) and can be reused
Disadvantages	Decreased stability compared to 2-in-1 PN Cannot use 0.22- μm bacterial retention filter; must use 1.2- μm filter Increased bacterial growth compared with 2-in-1 PN Visual inspection is difficult Limited compatibility with medications	Increased labor and costs (if IV lipid emulsion infused separately) Increased vein irritation, especially if PPN is not coinfused with IV lipid emulsion

PN, parenteral nutrition; PPN, peripheral parenteral nutrition; TNA, total nutrient admixture.

PN include improvements in safety (both decreased compounding errors and microbiologic contamination) and reduced costs.[27] The safety advantages are logically related to fewer manual manipulations of the system, but clinical trial data are lacking. Cost advantages have been demonstrated in some trials, with others finding no difference or increased costs. Limitations with the use of premixed PN in the United States are related to the limited number of products available, including a lack of formulations containing IVFE (in a three-chamber bag), relatively low amino acid concentration, only 1- and 2-L volumes, limited variability in electrolyte content, and no formulations available for neonates and infants. These limitations may make premixed PN less appropriate for some patients (eg, critically ill, obese, those with organ dysfunction or who require fluid restriction).

Patient Encounter, Part 2

It is now hospital day #3. Given that PG has malnutrition, an enterocutaneous fistula originating from the jejunum with high output (greater than 500 mL/day, increased when the patient drank water), and had recent abdominal surgery, the surgery team decided to manage PG conservatively: control fistula drainage, NPO status, and begin parenteral nutrition (PN) support today. A peripherally inserted central catheter (PICC) was placed for PN therapy.

Labs: Na 134 mEq/L (134 mmol/L); K 3.3 mEq/L (3.3 mmol/L); Cl 91 mEq/L (91 mmol/L); HCO_3 26 mEq/L (26 mmol/L); BUN 12 mg/dL (4.3 mmol/L); serum creatinine 0.8 mg/dL (71 μmol/L); blood glucose 91 mg/dL (5.1 mmol/L); total Ca 8.4 mg/dL (2.10 mmol/L); ionized Ca 2.38 mEq/L (1.19 mmol/L); Mg 1.5 mg/dL (0.62 mmol/L); phosphorus 2.5 mg/dL (0.81 mmol/L); TG 129 mg/dL (1.46 mmol/L); albumin 2.9 g/dL (29 g/L); WBC count 6300/mm^3 (6.3 × 10^9/L); hemoglobin 12.4 mg/dL (124 g/L or 7.70 mmol/L); hematocrit 35.1% (0.35); platelets 204,000/mm^3 (204 × 10^9/L)

Determine appropriate nutritional goals for PG (calorie and protein requirements).

What other patient data should be collected to help formulate a PN prescription?

Formulating a PN Admixture and Regimen

After completing a full nutrition assessment; estimating the patient's daily fluid, energy, and protein requirements (see Table 100–5); and determining if PN is indicated (see Table 100–1), develop an appropriate PN prescription.

Initiating PN

Exercise caution when initiating PN to avoid hyperglycemia and fluid and electrolyte abnormalities. After the goal daily PN volume has been determined, initiate PN at a lower infusion rate (eg, ~50% of goal for anywhere from ~6 to 24 hours) on day 1 with no more than 150 to 200 g of dextrose per day (or a maximum dextrose infusion rate of ~2 mg/kg/min for the first 6–24 hours). Then increase PN to goal over the following 18 to 24 hours, provided that glycemic control is maintained and the patient does not experience significant fluid or electrolyte abnormalities. Monitor electrolytes daily and correct as needed. Advance PN more slowly and cautiously in patients with severe malnutrition and monitor for refeeding syndrome (see Complications of PN).

Cycling PN

PN should be administered over 24 hours in most hospitalized patients to minimize glucose, fluid, and electrolyte abnormalities. However, administering PN via an infusion over less than 24 hours, or *cycling PN*, may be advantageous in certain patients and situations. Cycling PN typically involves administering the same PN volume over a goal infusion time, usually over 12 to 18 hours, rather than over 24 hours. Begin with PN infusion over

Patient Encounter, Part 3

The surgical team asks for your recommendations for PN therapy for PG.

Develop a plan for a complete and balanced PN prescription (including fluid, total calories, dextrose, amino acids, IVFE, electrolytes, vitamins, trace elements, and any additives) and explain the rationale supporting your PN formulation and plan.

How should this PN admixture be initiated and titrated to goal?

Would you recommend any other treatments before initiating PN? (Hint: Is this patient at risk for refeeding syndrome?)

24 hours; then taper the PN infusion to the goal cycle over 2 to 4 days (eg, 24 hours, then 18–20 hours the next day, then 14–16 hours the next day, and then 12 hours the next day). A longer goal cycle (eg, 18 hours) may limit adverse effects related to rate of fluid and dextrose administration (hyper- and hypoglycemia). Titrate the PN infusion rate up over 1 to 2 hours to goal rate to avoid hyperglycemia and taper down over 1 to 2 hours at the end of the cycle to avoid reactive hypoglycemia. Most home infusion pumps can be programmed to cycle a given PN volume automatically over a given time. However, the pharmacist may have to develop an appropriate PN cycle if the infusion pump cannot be programmed for an automatic cycle.

Cyclic PN has the following potential advantages:

- It may improve the quality of life of patients receiving home PN by allowing the patient time off of PN to engage in normal activities of daily living.
- While data are limited, it may help prevent and alleviate PN-associated liver disease by avoiding continuous compulsive nutrient overload on the liver.[28]

Concerns with cycling PN include hyperglycemia with high infusion rates, reactive hypoglycemia when PN infusion is stopped, and fluid and electrolyte abnormalities. Random capillary blood glucose concentrations should be checked approximately 4 hours into the PN cycle (~2 hours after reaching goal rate), 15 to 60 minutes after PN stops, and intermittently during the PN cycle as needed for glycemic control. During cyclic PN infusion, the potassium infusion rate should not exceed 10 mEq/hour (10 mmol/hour) if the patient is not on a cardiac monitor. If nocturnal cyclic PN infusion interferes with patient's sleep pattern by causing overdiuresis, the PN cycle can be extended over a longer infusion time or PN can be infused during other times of the day that are most convenient to the patient.

Transition to Oral or Enteral Nutrition

The goal is to transition the patient to enteral or oral nutrition and taper off PN as soon as indicated. After initiation of enteral or oral nutrition, monitor the patient for glucose, fluid, and electrolyte abnormalities. When oral nutrition intake is inconsistent, perform calorie counts to determine the adequacy of nutrition via the oral route. When the patient is tolerating more than 50% of total estimated daily calorie and protein requirements via the oral or enteral route, decrease PN by about 50%. PN can be stopped when the patient is tolerating at least 75% of total daily calorie and protein requirements via the oral or enteral route, assuming that intestinal absorption is maintained.

Table 100–7

Complications Associated with Parenteral Nutrition

Short Term	Long Term
Hyperglycemia	Infectious complications
Hypoglycemia	Liver toxicity
Electrolyte abnormalities	Vitamin abnormalities
Refeeding syndrome	Trace element abnormalities
Acid–base disturbances	Metabolic bone disease
Hyperlipidemia	Catheter/mechanical complications
Hypercapnia	
Infectious complications	
Catheter/mechanical complications	

COMPLICATIONS OF PN

KEY CONCEPT *PN therapy is associated with significant complications, both with short- and long-term therapy (Table 100–7).* Many complications are related to overfeeding (Table 100–8).

Hyperglycemia

Hyperglycemia is one of the most common complications associated with PN therapy. The rate of dextrose oxidation may be reduced in patients with stress and hypermetabolism, patients with diabetes or acute pancreatitis, and patients receiving certain medications (eg, corticosteroids, vasopressors, octreotide, and tacrolimus).[29,30] Uncontrolled hyperglycemia can lead to fluid and electrolyte disturbances, hyperglycemic hyperosmolar nonketotic syndrome, hypertriglyceridemia, and an increased risk of infection.[31] Hyperglycemia in critically ill patients may be more a reflection of illness severity than from dextrose infusions, provided that the patient is not being overfed with dextrose.[32] Critical illness is associated with increased endogenous glucose production (caused by increased glycogenolysis and gluconeogenesis) and insulin resistance. Therefore, critically ill patients have lower tolerance for dextrose infusion compared with nonstressed patients. A portion of daily calories (~20%–30%) can be administered via IVFE to help decrease hyperglycemia, provided that the patient does not have hypertriglyceridemia. Overfeeding (with dextrose and with total calories) must always be avoided. Most recent data suggest that moderate glucose control is

Table 100–8

Consequences of Overfeeding

Source of Overfeeding	Consequences
Dextrose	Hyperglycemia, hypertriglyceridemia, hepatic steatosis, hypercapnia; hyperglycemia may cause fluid and electrolyte disturbances and increased infection risk
IV lipid emulsions	Hypertriglyceridemia, hyperlipidemia, hepatic steatosis
Amino acids	Azotemia
Total calories	Hepatic steatosis, cholestasis, hypercapnia

indicated in critically ill patients (eg, capillary glucose concentrations between ~140 and 180 mg per dL [7.8 and 10.0 mmol/L]).[33] Refer to the section on "PN Additives: Regular Insulin" regarding management of hyperglycemia with insulin.

Hypoglycemia

Hypoglycemia can occur in patients when PN is interrupted suddenly (reactive hypoglycemia), especially when patients are treated with insulin or as a result of insulin overdosing in PN.[1] It is essential to prevent hypoglycemia and, if it occurs, identify and treat it promptly. Reactive hypoglycemia typically is rare and usually can be avoided by tapering PN over 1 to 2 hours before discontinuation rather than abruptly stopping the infusion (especially if the patient is receiving insulin in PN or if the patient is not receiving oral or enteral nutrition). Reactive hypoglycemia generally occurs within 15 to 60 minutes after stopping PN (especially in neonatal patients), although it can occur later than this after discontinuing PN.[1] Capillary blood glucose concentrations should be monitored about 15 to 60 minutes after stopping PN infusion to detect any potential hypoglycemia. If PN is interrupted abruptly (eg, because of lost IV access), infusing dextrose 10% in water or dextrose 10% NaCl 0.45% in water (to avoid excessive free water) at the same rate as PN should prevent hypoglycemia. In patients with poor venous access, reduce the PN infusion rate by 50% for 1 hour before discontinuing. Another alternative to prevent reactive hypoglycemia is to provide a glucose source via the oral route (by mouth or sublingually) when feasible.

Hyperlipidemia/Hypertriglyceridemia

Patients receiving IVFE may be at risk for hyperlipidemia and hypertriglyceridemia. Hyperlipidemia in patients receiving PN may lead to a reduction in pulmonary gas diffusion and pulmonary vascular resistance.[34] Severe hypertriglyceridemia (especially serum triglyceride concentrations exceeding 1000 mg/dL or 11.30 mmol/L) can precipitate acute pancreatitis.[35] Hypertriglyceridemia may develop as a result of increased fatty acid synthesis caused by hyperglycemia, impaired IVFE clearance, in patients with history of hyperlipidemia, obesity, diabetes, alcoholism, kidney failure, liver failure, multiorgan failure, sepsis, or pancreatitis, or as a result of medications (eg, propofol, corticosteroids, cyclosporine, and sirolimus).[36,37] Hyperglycemia is probably the most common cause of hypertriglyceridemia in patients receiving PN. A higher PL:TG ratio has been proposed to cause the appearance of the abnormal lipoprotein X particles in the blood.[8,36] Lipoprotein X may compete with IVFE particles for metabolism by lipoprotein lipase. It is preferred to use IVFE with a lower PL:TG ratio, especially in patients with hypertriglyceridemia, because they have improved clearance compared with emulsions with a higher PL:TG ratio (see Table 100–2).[8,36]

Monitor serum triglyceride concentrations regularly during PN therapy (see Table 100–8). If a patient develops hypertriglyceridemia, identify and correct the underlying cause(s) if possible. Prolonging the infusion of IVFE may improve lipid clearance. If a patient is receiving propofol, IVFE should be withheld and the calories from the 10% IVFE in propofol should be taken into account (see Table 100–2). IVFE should be held when the serum is lipemic or when serum triglyceride concentrations are greater than 400 mg/dL (4.52 mmol/L). When this occurs, restart IVFE when the serum triglyceride concentration is approximately 200 to 400 mg/dL (2.26–4.52 mmol/L) (or less) and administer only two to three times per week to prevent EFAD. Avoid completely holding IVFE for more than 3 to 4 weeks due to risk of EFAD.

Hypercapnia

Hypercapnia can develop as a result of overfeeding with dextrose and/or total calories.[1,38] Excess carbon dioxide production and retention can lead to acute respiratory acidosis. Excess carbon dioxide will also stimulate an increase in respiratory rate, and this increase in respiratory workload could cause respiratory insufficiency that may require mechanical ventilation. Reducing total calorie and dextrose intake would result in resolution of hypercapnia if due to overfeeding.

Liver Complications

The incidence of liver complications associated with PN ranges from approximately 7% to 84%, and end-stage liver disease develops in as many as 15% to 40% of adult patients on long-term PN.[36] Patients may develop a mild increase in liver transaminases within 1 to 2 weeks of initiating PN, but this generally resolves as PN continues, provided overfeeding is avoided. Severe liver complications include hepatic **steatosis**, **steatohepatitis**, cholestasis, and **cholelithiasis**.[36]

Hepatic steatosis is usually a result of excessive administration of carbohydrates or fats, but deficiencies of carnitine, choline, and essential fatty acids also may contribute. Hepatic steatosis can be minimized or reversed by avoiding overfeeding, especially from dextrose and IVFE.[36] Cholestasis is a common and potentially serious complication in PN-dependent patients. Factors that predispose PN patients to cholestasis include overfeeding, bowel rest, long duration of PN, short bowel syndrome, bacterial overgrowth and translocation, and sepsis.[36] Patients may exhibit increased liver transaminases, increase alkaline phosphatase and gamma-glutamyl transferase concentrations, and mainly increased bilirubin concentrations with jaundice. The most sensitive marker of cholestasis is increased serum conjugated bilirubin concentration of greater than 2 mg/dL (34.2 μmol/L).[36] Cholestasis generally is reversible if PN is discontinued before permanent liver damage occurs. Serum liver function tests may take up to 3 months to return to normal after discontinuing PN. Steps to prevent cholestasis associated with PN include early enteral or oral feedings, using a balanced PN formulation, avoiding overfeeding, using cyclic PN infusion, and treating and avoiding sepsis.[36] Limiting soy-based IVFE infusion to one or two times weekly at a dose adequate to prevent essential fatty acid deficiency may also decrease serum bilirubin concentrations and improve cholestasis.[39] Pharmacologic treatments include ursodeoxycholic acid (ursodiol), which may improve bile flow and reduce the signs and symptoms of cholestasis. However, ursodiol is only available in an oral dosage form, and absorption may be limited in patients with intestinal resections.

Cholelithiasis can develop as a result of decreased gallbladder contractility, especially in the absence of enteral or oral intake. Lack of intestinal stimulation reduces secretion of cholecystokinin, a peptide hormone secreted in the duodenum that induces gallbladder contractility and emptying. The best prevention of cholelithiasis is early initiation of enteral or oral feeding.

Monitor liver function tests, including serum aspartate aminotransferase (AST), alanine aminotransferase (ALT), alkaline phosphatase, total bilirubin, conjugated bilirubin, unconjugated bilirubin, and γ-glutamyl transferase at the initiation of PN therapy and regularly thereafter during PN therapy. The frequency of monitoring liver function tests depends on the presence or absence of liver disease. This varies from one to two times weekly in the acute setting to once weekly, once monthly, or even one to two times per year in stable home PN patients.

Manganese Toxicity

Manganese accumulation can occur in patients with cholestasis or in patients receiving long-term PN therapy. Neurotoxicity is the most common manifestation (headache, somnolence, weakness, confusion, tremor, muscle rigidity, altered gait, and mask-like face [a Parkinson-like syndrome]), but liver toxicity also may occur.[36] Periodically monitor blood manganese concentrations in patients on long-term PN. Patients with cholestasis receiving PN may require restriction of manganese in PN to prevent accumulation and possible toxicity.

Metabolic Bone Disease

Metabolic bone disease (MBD) is a condition of bone demineralization leading to osteomalacia, osteopenia, or osteoporosis in patients receiving long-term PN. MBD may occur in as many as 40% to 100% of patients receiving long-term PN.[36] Often patients are asymptomatic, although symptoms can include bone pain, back pain, and fractures. Patients often have increased serum alkaline phosphatase concentrations, low to normal parathyroid hormone (PTH) concentrations, normal 25-hydroxyvitamin D and low 1,25 dihydroxyvitamin D concentrations, hypercalcemia or hypocalcemia, and hypercalcuria.[40] Because patients may be asymptomatic, diagnosis can be incidental. Radiographic techniques commonly used in diagnosing bone disease include quantitative computed tomography (CT) and bone mineral density.[40]

Factors that can predispose patients to developing MBD include deficiencies of phosphorus, calcium, and vitamin D; aluminum toxicity; amino acids and hyperosmolar dextrose infusions; chronic metabolic acidosis; corticosteroid therapy; and lack of mobility.[36,40] Calcium deficiency (caused by decreased intake or increased urinary excretion) is one of the major causes of MBD in patients receiving PN. Provide adequate calcium and phosphate with PN to improve bone mineralization and help to prevent MBD. Administration of amino acids and chronic metabolic acidosis also appear to play an important role. Provide adequate amounts of acetate in PN admixtures to maintain acid–base balance.

Aluminum toxicity appears to play a role in the development of MBD in patients on long-term PN, possibly by impairing calcium bone fixation, inhibiting the conversion of 25-hydroxyvitamin D to the active 1,25-dihydroxyvitamin D, and/or reducing PTH secretion.[36,40] The FDA issued a rule specifying acceptable aluminum concentrations in large-volume parenterals,[41] indicating that products contains no more than 25 mcg/L (0.93 μmol/L) of aluminum and defined a safe upper limit for parenteral aluminum intake at less than 4 to 5 mcg/kg/day. Pharmacies should use products with the lowest labeled aluminum content for the making of PN. Patients who are chronically dependent on PN should have their serum aluminum concentrations routinely monitored or whenever MBD is suspected or diagnosed.

Encourage patients on long-term PN to engage in regular low-intensity exercise. Yearly bone density measurements also should be performed on patients on long-term PN and when MBD is suspected.

Refeeding Syndrome

Refeeding syndrome describes the metabolic derangements that occur during nutritional repletion of patients who are starved, underweight, or severely malnourished.[42] Hypophosphatemia and hypokalemia (along with associated complications) are the classic signs and symptoms, but refeeding syndrome encompasses a constellation of fluid and electrolyte abnormalities affecting neurologic, cardiac, hematologic, neuromuscular, and pulmonary systems. The most severe cases of refeeding syndrome have resulted in cardiac failure, seizures, coma, and death.[42] The reintroduction of energy substrates, especially carbohydrates, increases metabolism and utilization of glucose as the predominant fuel source. This increases insulin secretion and demand for phosphorylated intermediates of glycolysis (eg, ATP and 2,3-diphosphoglycerate [2,3-DPG]), inhibits fat metabolism, and causes an intracellular shift of phosphorus, potassium, and magnesium. These changes, in combination with preexisting low total body stores of phosphorus, potassium, and magnesium and enhanced cellular uptake of phosphorus during anabolic refeeding, result in hypophosphatemia, hypokalemia, and hypomagnesemia. Vitamin deficiencies (eg, thiamine) also may exist or be precipitated during refeeding. High carbohydrate intake increases the demand for thiamine, which can precipitate thiamine deficiency and cause lactic acidosis and neurologic abnormalities,[42] as well as myocardial dysfunction and congestive heart failure. Other metabolic alterations that may occur include expansion of the extracellular water compartment and fluid intolerance.

The primary goal is preventing refeeding syndrome when initiating PN in high-risk patients (eg, prolonged lack of adequate nutritional intake, significant weight loss, or moderate to severe malnutrition). When initiating nutrition support, the rule of thumb to prevent refeeding syndrome is to "start low and go slow." Initiate PN cautiously (eg, ~25%–33% of estimated nutritional requirements on day 1) and gradually increase to goal over 3 to 5 days. Correct electrolyte abnormalities before initiating PN and provide supplemental phosphate, potassium, and magnesium in and/or outside of PN. Doses of IV phosphate up to 0.64 to 1 mmol/kg may be used to treat severe hypophosphatemia (in patients with normal kidney function), and doses can be repeated as needed until serum phosphorus concentration has normalized.[43] Provide supplemental oral or IV thiamine 100 mg/day and folic acid 1 mg/day for about 1 week in addition to the standard multivitamin in PN. Assess patients for fluid balance, signs of edema, fluid overload, and weight gain, and consider minimizing fluid and sodium intake during the first few days of PN.[42] Monitor patients closely for signs and symptoms of refeeding syndrome until they are tolerating PN at goal for a few days:

- Vital signs, mental status, and neurologic and neuromuscular function at least every 4 to 8 hours.
- Pulse oximetry and any electrocardiographic changes when indicated.
- Serum laboratory values (including sodium, potassium,, phosphorus, and magnesium) at least once a day.

Infectious Complications

Patients receiving central PN are at increased risk of developing infectious complications caused by bacterial and fungal pathogens.[1,44] Patients without malnutrition who receive early PN (eg, within 48 hours of ICU admission) may have a higher incidence of infectious complications than patients who do not receive PN or receive late PN initiation (eg, greater than 7 days after ICU admission).[2,10,45] Strict aseptic techniques must be used when placing the catheter along with continuous care of the catheter and infusion site. Catheter-related bloodstream infections are a common complication in long-term PN patients, often requiring hospital admission for parenteral antimicrobial therapy and/or removal of the catheter. Contamination of the PN admixture is

Table 100–9

Suggested Frequency of Monitoring Parameters in Hospitalized Patients Receiving PN

Parameters	Initial	Daily (Unstable)	2–3 × Weekly (Stable)	Weekly	As Indicated
BUN, creatinine	X	X	X		
Sodium, potassium, chloride, bicarbonate	X	X	X		
Glucose	X	X	X		
Calcium, phosphorus, magnesium albumin, AST, ALT, LDH, alkaline phosphatase, total bilirubin	X	X	X		
Conjugated bilirubin	X			X	X
Prealbumin[a]	X			X	X
Triglycerides	X			X	X
RBC count, hemoglobin, hematocrit, WBC count ± differential, platelets, PTT	X				X
PT or INR				X	X
Nitrogen balance					X
Zinc, selenium, chromium, copper, manganese, iron					X
TIBC, ferritin					X
Vitamin concentrations					X
Blood cultures					X
Body weight	X	X	X		

ALT, alanine aminotransferase; AST, aspartate aminotransferase; BUN, blood urea nitrogen; INR, international normalized ratio; LDH, lactate dehydrogenase; PT, prothrombin time; PTT, partial thromboplastin time; RBC, red blood cell; TIBC, total iron-binding capacity; WBC, white blood cell.

[a]Only recommended/indicated in the absence of inflammatory response.

possible but rare if protocols are followed for aseptic preparation of PN admixtures.

Mechanical Complications

Mechanical complications of PN are related to venous catheter placement and the equipment used to administer PN. A central venous catheter must be placed by a trained professional, and risks associated with placement include pneumothorax, arterial puncture, bleeding, hematoma formation, venous thrombosis, and air embolism.[1] Over time, the venous catheter may require replacement. Problems with the equipment include malfunctions of the infusion pump, IV tubing sets, and filters.

MONITORING PN THERAPY

KEY CONCEPT *When initiating PN, patients should have important baseline laboratory values checked to assess electrolyte status, organ function, and nutritional status. Thereafter, these and other nutritional parameters should be monitored routinely or as indicated (Table 100-9).* Random capillary blood glucose concentrations also should be monitored every 6 to 8 hours when initiating PN, and regular insulin should be administered to control blood glucose concentrations as needed.

SUMMARY AND CONCLUSION

PN is an effective and potentially lifesaving method of administering nutrition support to patients who cannot receive adequate oral or enteral nutrition. Administration of PN can be associated with significant adverse effects and metabolic, infectious, and mechanical complications. Optimal design, compounding, and administration of a PN regimen are essential to minimize the risk of adverse effects and complications, and patients must be monitored closely while receiving PN to optimize outcomes.

Patient Encounter, Part 4

The surgical team plans to initiate PN for PG per your recommendations. Laboratory data were listed previously.

What monitoring parameters related to PN therapy should you follow in PG after initiating PN? List monitoring parameters and frequency.

What potential complications of PN should you monitor for in PG?

What special considerations must be made when developing a plan for nutrition support therapy and a PN formulation for patients with severe malnutrition?

Abbreviations Introduced in This Chapter

AdjBW	Adjusted body weight
ALT	Alanine aminotransferase
A.S.P.E.N.	American Society for Parenteral and Enteral Nutrition
AST	Aspartate aminotransferase
ATP	Adenosine triphosphate
CT	Computed tomography
2,3-DPG	2,3-Diphosphoglycerate
FDA	Food and Drug Administration
GI	Gastrointestinal
HIT	Heparin-induced thrombocytopenia
IBW	Ideal body weight
IVFE	Intravenous fat emulsions
kcal	Kilocalorie(s)
kJ	Kilojoule(s)
LDH	Lactate dehydrogenase

MBD	Metabolic bone disease
mEq	Milliequivalents
mmol	Millimoles
mOsm	Milliosmoles
PL	Phospholipid(s)
PN	Parenteral nutrition
PPN	Peripheral parenteral nutrition
PTH	Parathyroid hormone
TG	Triglyceride
TNA	Total nutrient admixture
TPN	Total parenteral nutrition

REFERENCES

1. American Society for Parenteral and Enteral Nutrition Board of Directors and the Clinical Guidelines Task Force. Guidelines for the use of parenteral and enteral nutrition in adult and pediatric patients. JPEN J Parenter Enteral Nutr. 2002;26:1SA–138SA.
2. McClave SA, Martindale RG, Vanek VW, et al; A.S.P.E.N. Board of Directors; American College of Critical Care Medicine; Society of Critical Care Medicine. Guidelines for the Provision and Assessment of Nutrition Support Therapy in the Adult Critically Ill Patient: Society of Critical Care Medicine (SCCM) and American Society for Parenteral and Enteral Nutrition (A.S.P.E.N.). JPEN J Parenter Enteral Nutr. 2009;33:277–316.
3. Peter JV, Moran JL, Phillips-Hughes J. A metaanalysis of treatment outcomes of early enteral versus early parenteral nutrition in hospitalized patients. Crit Care Med. 2005;33:213–220.
4. Wolfe RR, Allsop JR, Burke JF. Glucose metabolism in man: Responses to intravenous glucose infusion. Metabolism. 1979;28: 210–220.
5. Rosmarin DK, Wardlaw GM, Mirtallo J. Hyperglycemia associated with high, continuous infusion rates of total parenteral nutrition dextrose. Nutr Clin Pract. 1996;11:151–156.
6. The American Society for Parenteral and Enteral Nutrition. Task Force for the Revision of Safe Practices for Parenteral Nutrition. Safe practices of parenteral nutrition. JPEN J Parenter Enteral Nutr. 2004;28(Suppl):S39–S70.
7. Driscoll DF, Bhargava HN, Li L, et al. Physicochemical stability of total nutrient admixtures. Am J Health Syst Pharm. 1995;52: 623–634.
8. Ferezou J, Bach AC. Structure and metabolic fate of triacylglycerol- and phospholipid-rich particles of commercial parenteral fat emulsions. Nutrition. 1999;15:44–50.
9. Hamilton C, Austin T, Seidner DL. Essential fatty acid deficiency in human adults during parenteral nutrition. Nutr Clin Pract. 2006;21:387–394.
10. Crocker KS, Noga R, Filibeck DJ, et al. Microbial growth comparisons of five commercial parenteral lipid emulsions. JPEN J Parenter Enteral Nutr. 1984;8:391–395.
11. D'Angio R, Quercia RA, Treiber NK, et al. The growth of microorganisms in total parenteral nutrition admixtures. JPEN J Parenter Enteral Nutr. 1987;11:394–397.
12. Boullata JI, Gilbert K, Sacks G, et. al. A.S.P.E.N. clinical guidelines: Parenteral nutrition ordering, order review, compounding, labeling, and dispensing. JPEN J Parenter Enteral Nutr 2014; 38:334–377.
13. Sheldon GF, Grzyb S. Phosphate depletion and repletion: Relation to parenteral nutrition and oxygen transport. Ann Surg. 1975; 182:683–689.
14. Food and Drug Administration. Safety alert: Hazards of precipitation associated with parenteral nutrition. Am J Hosp Pharm. 1994;51:1427–1428.
15. Btaiche IF, Carver PL, Welch KB. Dosing and monitoring of trace elements in long-term home parenteral nutrition patients. JPEN J Parenter Enteral Nutr. 2011;35(6):736–747.
16. Jeejeebhoy K. Zinc: An essential trace element for parenteral nutrition. Gastroenterology. 2009;137(5 Suppl):S7–S12.
17. Shike M. Copper in parenteral nutrition. Gastroenterology. 2009;137(5 Suppl):S13–S17.
18. Keith JN. Bedside nutrition assessment past, present, and future: A review of the Subjective Global Assessment. Nutr Clin Pract. 2008;23:410–416.
19. Dickerson RN. Specialized nutrition support in the hospitalized obese patient. Nutr Clin Pract. 2004;19:245–254.
20. Brown RO, Compher C; A.S.P.E.N. Board of Directors. A.S.P.E.N. clinical guidelines: Nutrition support in adult acute and chronic renal failure JPEN J Parenter Enteral Nutr. 2010; 34:366–377.
21. Ayers P, Adams S, Boullata J, et al; A.S.P.E.N. parenteral nutrition safety consensus recommendations. JPEN J Parenter Enteral Nutr. 2014;38:296–333.
22. Gura KM. Is there still a role for peripheral parenteral nutrition? Nutr Clin Pract. 2009;24:709–717.
23. Driscoll DF. Lipid injectable emulsions: 2006. Nutr Clin Pract. 2006;21:381–386.
24. Driscoll DF, Bacon MN, Bistrian BR. Effects of in-line filtration on lipid particle size distribution in total nutrient admixtures. JPEN J Parenter Enteral Nutr. 1996;20:296–301.
25. Trissel LA, Gilbert DL, Martinez JF, et al. Compatibility of parenteral nutrient solutions with selected drugs during simulated Y-site administration. Am J Health Syst Pharm. 1997;54:1295–1300.
26. Trissel LA, Gilbert DL, Martinez JF, et al. Compatibility of medications with three-in-one parenteral nutrition admixtures. JPEN J Parenter Enteral Nutr. 1999;23:67–74.
27. Miller SJ. Commercial premixed parenteral nutrition: Is it right for your institution? Nutr Clin Pract. 2009;24:459–469.
28. Stout SM, Cober MP. Metabolic effects of cyclic parenteral nutrition infusion in adults and children. Nutr Clin Pract. 2010;25: 277–281.
29. Watters JM, Norris SB, Kirkpatrick SM. Endogenous glucose production following injury increases with age. J Clin Endocrinol Metab. 1997;82:3005–3010.
30. Campbell IT. Limitations of nutrient intake. The effect of stressors: Trauma, sepsis and multiple organ failure. Eur J Clin Nutr. 1999; 53(Suppl 1):S143–S147.
31. Butler SO, Btaiche IF, Alaniz C. Relationship between hyperglycemia and infection in critically ill patients. Pharmacotherapy. 2005;25:963–976.
32. Atkinson M, Worthley LI. Nutrition in the critically ill patient: Part I. Essential physiology and pathophysiology. Crit Care Resusc. 2003;5:109–120.
33. The NICE-SUGAR Study Investigators. Intensive versus conventional glucose control in critically Ill patients. N Engl J Med. 2009;360:1283–1297.
34. Suchner U, Katz DP, Fürst P, et al. Effects of intravenous fat emulsions on lung function in patients with acute respiratory distress syndrome or sepsis. Crit Care Med. 2001;29:1569–1574.
35. National Cholesterol Education Program (NCEP) Expert Panel on Detection, Evaluation, and Treatment of High Blood Cholesterol in Adults (Adult Treatment Panel III). Third Report of the National Cholesterol Education Program (NCEP) Expert Panel on Detection, Evaluation, and Treatment of High Blood Cholesterol in Adults (Adult Treatment Panel III) final report. Circulation. 2002;106:3143–3421.
36. Btaiche IF, Khalidi N. Metabolic complications of parenteral nutrition in adults, part 1 and part 2. Am J Health Syst Pharm. 2004;61:1938–1949, 2050–2059.
37. Devlin JW, Lau AK, Tanios MA. Propofol-associated hypertriglyceridemia and pancreatitis in the intensive care unit: An analysis of frequency and risk factors. Pharmacotherapy. 2005;25:1348–1352.

38. McClave SA, Lowen CC, Kleber MJ, McConnell JW, Jung LY, Goldsmith LJ. Clinical use of the respirator quotient obtained from indirect calorimetry. JPEN J Parenter Enteral Nutr. 2003;27:21–26.
39. Cober MP, Teitelbaum DH. Prevention of parenteral nutrition-associated liver disease: Lipid minimization. Curr Opin Organ Transplant. 2010;15:330–333.
40. Ferrone M, Geraci M. A review of the relationship between parenteral nutrition and metabolic bone disease. Nutr Clin Pract. 2007;22:329–339.
41. Department of Health and Human Services, Food and Drug Administration. Aluminum in large and small volume parenterals used in total parenteral nutrition—FDA. Proposed rule. Fed Regist. 2000(Docket No. 90N-0056);65:4103–4111.
42. Kraft MD, Btaiche IF, Sacks GS. Review of the refeeding syndrome. Nutr Clin Pract. 2005;20:625–633.
43. Brown KA, Dickerson RN, Morgan LM, et al. A new graduated dosing regimen for phosphorus replacement in patients receiving nutrition support. JPEN J Parenter Enteral Nutr. 2006;30:209–214.
44. Beghetto MG, Victorino J, Teixeira L, de Azevedo MJ. Parenteral nutrition as a risk factor for central venous catheter-related infection. JPEN J Parenter Enteral Nutr. 2005;29:367–373.
45. Casaer MP, Mesotten D, Hermans G, et al. Early versus late parenteral nutrition in critically ill adults. N Engl J Med. 2011;365:506–517.

101 Enteral Nutrition

Sarah J. Miller

LEARNING OBJECTIVES

Upon completion of this chapter, the reader will be able to:

1. Discuss how gut structure and function impact choice of feeding route and outcome of feeding.
2. Estimate kilocalorie and protein requirements of an enteral feeding candidate and design an enteral nutrition (EN) regimen to meet these.
3. Evaluate patient-specific parameters to determine whether EN is appropriate.
4. Compare clinical efficacy, complications, and costs of EN versus parenteral nutrition (PN).
5. Formulate a monitoring plan for an EN patient.
6. Select appropriate medication administration techniques for an EN patient.

INTRODUCTION

Enteral nutrition (EN) is broadly defined as delivery of nutrients via the gastrointestinal (GI) tract. The terms *enteral nutrition* and *tube feedings* are often used synonymously. Formulas for EN usually are delivered in the form of commercially prepared liquid preparations, although some products are produced as powders for reconstitution. Nonvolitional feedings in patients who cannot meet nutritional requirements by oral intake include EN and parenteral nutrition (PN), which are collectively known as *specialized nutrition support* (SNS).

Several organizations have issued clinical guidelines on the use of EN. These include the American Society for Parenteral and Enteral Nutrition (A.S.P.E.N.), European Society for Clinical Nutrition and Metabolism (ESPEN), and a Canadian team known as Critical Care Nutrition.[1–4] A.S.P.E.N. and the Society for Critical Care Medicine (SCCM) have jointly issued guidelines for SNS in critically ill patients.[5]

GI TRACT STRUCTURE AND FUNCTION

Anatomy and Absorptive Function

With normal volitional feeding, food is ingested via the mouth. There, the process of breaking down complex foodstuffs into simpler forms that can be absorbed by the small bowel begins. Solid food is chewed in the mouth, and enzymes begin digestion. The trigger for release of many enzymes and GI hormones is the presence of food in specific regions of the GI tract. Food is swallowed and passes through the esophagus and the esophageal sphincter to the stomach, where additional digestive enzymes and acids further break it down. The stomach also serves a mixing and grinding function.

The food, now in a liquid form known as *chyme*, passes through the pyloric sphincter into the duodenum, where stomach acid is neutralized. Most absorption of digested carbohydrate and protein occurs within the jejunum. Most fat absorption occurs within the jejunum and ileum. In the small bowel, breakdown of macronutrients (ie, carbohydrate, protein, and fat) occurs both within the lumen and at the intestinal mucosal membrane surface. The absorptive units on the intestinal mucosal membrane are infoldings known as *villi*. These villi are made up of epithelial cells called *enterocytes*. Projections from these enterocytes called *microvilli* increase the surface area of the small bowel and make up the *brush-border membrane*.

Digestive substances secreted by the pancreas play a role in food breakdown. The pancreas secretes large amounts of sodium bicarbonate that neutralize stomach acid. Substances flow from the pancreas through the pancreatic duct. The pancreatic duct typically joins the hepatic duct to become the common bile duct that empties through the sphincter of Oddi into the duodenum. Bile secreted by the liver does not contain digestive enzymes, but bile salts help to emulsify fat and facilitate fat absorption. Bile flows through bile ducts into the hepatic duct and common bile duct. Bile is stored in the gallbladder until needed in the gut to aid fat digestion, at which time it empties through the cystic duct to the common bile duct to the duodenum. Pathways through which carbohydrate, protein, and fat are digested and absorbed through the small bowel are illustrated in Figure 101–1.

Remaining undigested food passes from the ileum through the ileocecal valve to the colon. A major role of the colon is fluid absorption. Some of the water and sodium absorption achieved by the colon is facilitated by short-chain fatty acids (SFCAs) formed from digestion of certain dietary fibers by colonic bacterial enzymes.

Gut Immune Function

The gut plays significant immune roles. The distal small bowel and colon host many bacteria and their endotoxins, and it is important that these organisms not gain access to the internal systems of the body. This function is known globally as the *gut barrier function*.[6] Normal flora of the gut comprises one component. The normal flora, particularly some anaerobes, helps to prevent overgrowth of potential pathogens. A second component involves

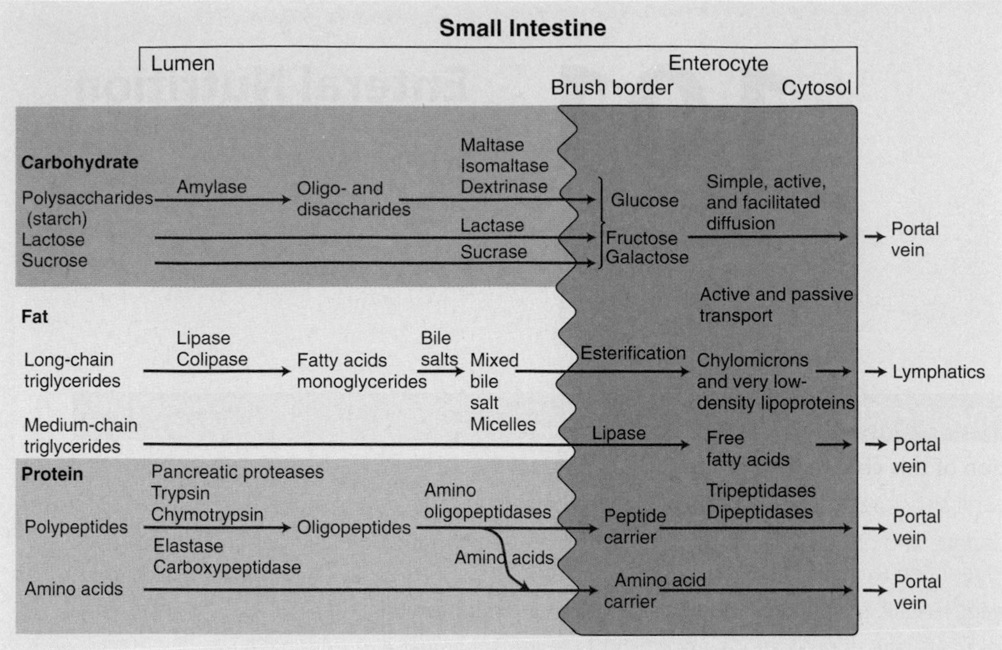

FIGURE 101–1. Schematic of carbohydrate, fat, and protein digestion. (From Kumpf VJ, Chessman KH. Enteral nutrition. In: DiPiro JT, Talbert RL, Yee GC, et al, eds. Pharmacotherapy: A Pathophysiologic Approach, 9th ed. New York: McGraw-Hill, 2014:2428.)

mechanical factors. These include a mucous layer that prevents adherence of bacteria. Peristalsis of the small bowel prevents stasis of bacteria. Gut-associated lymphoid tissue (GALT), prominent in small bowel, serves as a local immune system. Secretory immunoglobulin A produced at the mucosal surface in response to food in the gut prevents bacteria from invading the surface.

PATIENT SELECTION

In general, KEY CONCEPT *EN is the preferred route if the gut can be used safely in patients who cannot meet nutritional requirements by oral intake.* If the gut functions, EN is usually preferred over PN. The timing of SNS (either EN or PN) is controversial, but definitive guidelines for these therapies state that SNS should be started when intake has been inadequate for 7 to 14 days or if inadequate oral intake is anticipated for at least 7 to 14 days.[1] Prior nutritional status of the patient should be considered. Previously well-nourished patients can better afford not being fed for longer periods than previously poorly nourished patients. Patients in the intensive care unit (ICU) probably benefit from early EN started within 24 to 48 hours of admission to the ICU.[3,5] Ethical questions come into play when consideration is given to starting (or stopping) EN in seemingly futile situations. Methods for assessing nutritional status and designing SNS regimens are covered in Chapter 100. Generally, nonobese hospitalized patients require 20 to 35 total kcal/kg of body weight/day (84–147 kJ/kg body weight/day) and 1 to 2 g protein/kg of body weight/day. Obese patients are often fed hypocaloric, high-protein diets; guidelines state to start feedings at 1.2 g protein per kg and less than 14 kcal/kg actual body weight (59 kJ/kg actual body weight).[7]

Indications

Many potential indications for EN exist (Table 101–1). PN was used extensively in the past for many of these conditions.

Table 101–1

Potential Indications for EN

Neoplastic Disease	**GI Disease**
Chemotherapy	Inflammatory bowel disease
Radiation therapy	Short-bowel syndrome
Upper GI tumors	Esophageal motility disorder
Cancer cachexia	Pancreatitis
Organ Dysfunction	Fistulas
Liver disease/failure	Gastroesophageal reflux disease (severe)
Kidney insufficiency/failure	Esophageal or intestinal atresia
Cardiac cachexia	**Neurologic Impairment**
ARDS/ALI	Comatose state
Bronchopulmonary dysplasia	Cerebrovascular accident
Congenital heart disease	Demyelinating disease
Organ transplantation	Severe depression
Hypermetabolic States	Cerebral palsy
Closed head injury	**Other Indications**
Burns	AIDS
Trauma	Anorexia nervosa
Postoperative major surgery	Complications during pregnancy
Sepsis	Failure-to-thrive
	Geriatric patients with multiple chronic diseases
	Extreme prematurity
	Inborn errors of metabolism
	Cystic fibrosis

AIDS, acquired immune deficiency syndrome; ALI, acute lung injury; ARDS, acute respiratory distress syndrome.

From Kumpf VJ, Chessman KH. Enteral nutrition. In DiPiro JT, Talbert RL, Yee GC, et al, eds. Pharmacotherapy: A Pathophysiologic Approach, 9th ed. New York: McGraw-Hill, 2014.

Table 101–2

Contraindications and Precautions for EN

Severe hemorrhagic pancreatitis
Severe necrotizing pancreatitis
Necrotizing enterocolitis
Diffuse peritonitis
Small bowel obstruction
Paralytic ileus
Severe hemodynamic instability
Enterocutaneous fistulae
Severe diarrhea
Severe malabsorption
Severe GI hemorrhage
Intractable vomiting

Advances in EN technology now allow many patients with these conditions to receive EN. EN is administered in both institutional and home settings.

Contraindications and Precautions

EN should not be used or should be used with extreme caution in certain conditions (Table 101–2). It is possible to use EN in some patients with these conditions depending on severity of illness, location of abnormality, and experience of practitioners delivering care. Feeding in the setting of hemodynamically instability is particularly controversial; some clinicians avoid enteral feedings in this setting for fear of worsening intestinal ischemia, whereas others believe early feeding may facilitate intestinal perfusion and be beneficial.[5,8–9] Others might avoid jejunal feedings in this setting but would proceed with cautious gastric feedings.

Enteral versus Parenteral Feeding

With advent of the technique of PN by large central vein in the late 1960s, this modality quickly became popular. PN was incorporated quickly into care of patients such as critically ill patients. The relative ease of PN administration, along with the perception that critically ill patients had prolonged high-energy expenditures, led to complications of overfeeding. Dextrose overfeeding led to complications, including hyperglycemia, carbon dioxide overproduction leading to delays in weaning from mechanical ventilation, and liver abnormalities owing to hepatic steatosis.

The pendulum began to swing toward EN in the late 1980s and early 1990s as clinical studies showed better clinical outcomes with EN compared to PN. Some potential advantages of EN over PN are included here. First, EN is expected to preserve the gut barrier function better than PN. This could prevent translocation of bacteria and endotoxin from the gut lumen into the lymphatic system and systemic circulation, thus preventing infections. Some studies support that KEY CONCEPT *EN is associated with fewer infectious complications than PN.* EN is cited frequently as having a better overall safety profile than PN. Whereas PN is associated with more severe complications, such as pneumothorax and catheter sepsis, EN is associated with more nuisance complications, such as GI side effects. Another frequently cited advantage of EN over PN is that EN is less expensive. EN formulas typically are cheaper and less labor intensive to prepare than PN, although some specialty EN formulas approach the cost of PN formulas. Depending on the method of feeding tube placement, EN costs can mount if the tube must be placed by a radiologist or gastroenterologist rather than a nurse or if the tube must be replaced.

Arguments in support of EN over PN have been questioned. Part of this questioning relates to the question of whether EN is beneficial compared with PN or whether PN as commonly administered may be detrimental. Overfeeding and hyperglycemia occur easily with PN, and the potential harm of hyperglycemia, especially in critical care populations, has been demonstrated, although the exact range optimal for glycemic control in ICU patients remains controversial.[10,11] A study published in 1991 demonstrated in a mildly malnourished perioperative population that there were more infectious complications in patients randomized to receive PN compared with those randomized to receive no SNS; there was no difference in noninfectious complications between the two groups.[12] Only in severely malnourished perioperative patients were fewer noninfectious complications seen with PN; in these patients, no difference in infectious complications was seen between groups. Whether EN truly prevents infections and improves clinical outcomes or whether PN is detrimental continues to be debated and probably depends upon specific patient population. At present, EN is preferred by most experts over PN when the gut is functional. In Europe (more so than in North America), PN has been used to supplement EN during the first week of intensive care therapy when EN is not yet being tolerated at full rates.[2] This approach is currently discouraged by American and Canadian ICU guidelines.[3,5] Recent randomized controlled trials relating to this topic have yielded disparate results.[13–17]

ROUTES OF ACCESS[18]

There are several access sites for EN (Figure 101–2). Nasogastric (NG), orogastric (OG), nasoduodenal (ND), and nasojejunal (NJ) routes generally are for short-term use (less than 1 month), whereas gastrostomy, percutaneous endoscopic gastrostomy (PEG), jejunostomy, and percutaneous endoscopic jejunostomy (PEJ) tubes are preferred for longer-term treatment. Both advantages and disadvantages exist for each EN route (Table 101–3).

Gastric Feeding

Gastric feedings are used commonly. They require an intact gag reflex and normal gastric emptying for safety and success. Certain patients, such as those who have suffered head trauma, may not empty their stomachs efficiently and therefore may not be good candidates for gastric feedings. In these patients, it may be impossible to achieve a gastric tube feeding rate to provide adequate nutrients. In addition, pooling of formula in the stomach could increase risk of aspirating feeding formula into the lungs.

The NG route is used most commonly for short-term enteral access. The major advantage of this route is that the tube can be placed quickly and inexpensively by the nurse at the bedside.

Gastrostomy tubes, in which an incision is made directly through the abdominal wall, are indicated for patients who can tolerate gastric feedings but in whom long-term feedings are anticipated. The most commonly placed gastrostomy tubes are either placed by interventional radiology or are PEG tubes placed endoscopically. Gastrostomy tubes also can be placed laparoscopically or during an open procedure by a surgeon. Placement of a gastrostomy tube either endoscopically or surgically is more expensive than bedside OG or NG placement but can result in placement of a larger bore tube.

An advantage of feeding into the stomach is that feedings can be delivered either intermittently or continuously. When feeding directly into the small bowel continuous feedings must be used. Intermittent feedings into the small bowel result in GI intolerance in most patients.

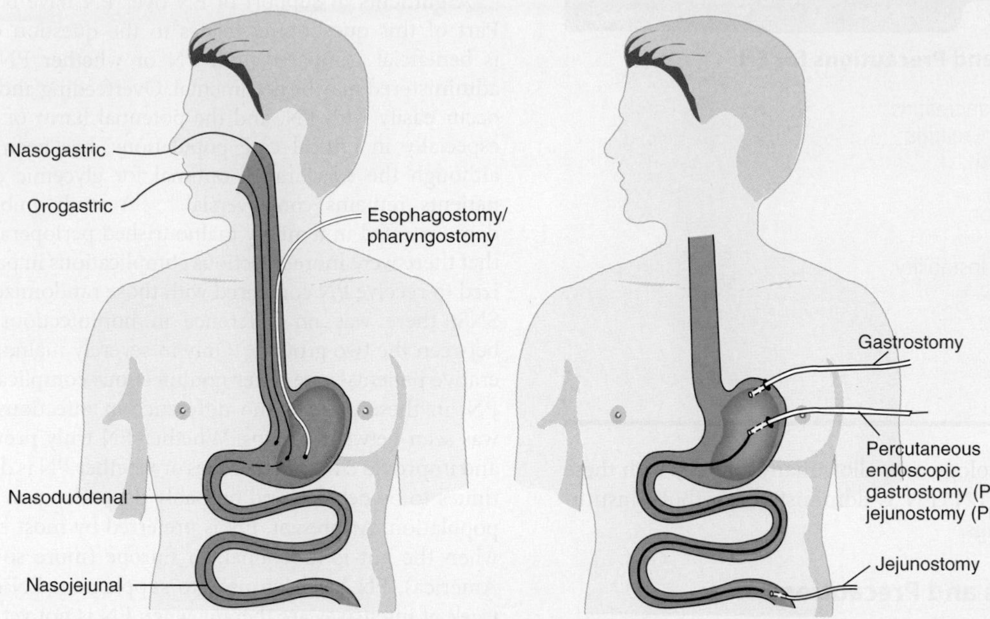

FIGURE 101–2. Access sites for tube feeding. (From Kumpf VJ, Chessman KH. Enteral nutrition. In DiPiro JT, Talbert RL, Yee GC, et al, eds. Pharmacotherapy: A Pathophysiologic Approach, 9th ed, New York: McGraw-Hill, 2014:2431.)

Table 101–3

Options and Considerations in the Selection of Enteral Access

Access	EN Duration/Patient Characteristics	Tube Placement Options	Advantages	Disadvantages
Nasogastric or orogastric	Short term Intact gag reflex Normal gastric emptying	Manually at bedside	Ease of placement Allows for all methods of administration Inexpensive Multiple commercially available tubes and sizes	Potential tube displacement Potential increased aspiration risk
Nasoduodenal or nasojejunal	Short term Impaired gastric motility or emptying High risk of GER or aspiration	Manually at bedside Fluoroscopically Endoscopically	Potential reduced aspiration risk Allows for early post injury or postoperative feeding Multiple commercially available tubes and sizes	Manual transpyloric passage requires greater skill Potential tube displacement or clogging Bolus or intermittent feeding not tolerated
Gastrostomy	Long term Normal gastric emptying	Surgically Endoscopically Radiologically Laparoscopically	Allows for all methods of administration Low-profile buttons available Large-bore tubes less likely to clog Multiple commercially available tubes and sizes	Attendant risks associated with each type of procedure Potential increased aspiration risk Risk of stoma site complications
Jejunostomy	Long term Impaired gastric motility or gastric emptying High risk of GER or aspiration	Surgically Endoscopically Radiologically Laparoscopically	Allows for early post injury or postoperative feeding Potential reduced aspiration risk Multiple commercially available tubes and sizes Low-profile buttons available	Attendant risks associated with each type of procedure Bolus or intermittent feeding not tolerated Risk of stoma site complications

EN, enteral nutrition; GER, gastroesophageal reflux.

From Kumpf VJ, Chessman KH. Enteral nutrition. In DiPiro JT, Talbert RL, Yee GC, et al, eds. Pharmacotherapy: A Pathophysiologic Approach, 9th ed. New York: McGraw-Hill, 2014.

Postpyloric Feedings

KEY CONCEPT *For patients intolerant of gastric feedings or in whom the risk of aspiration is high, feedings delivered with the tip of the tube in the jejunum are preferred.* This bypasses the problem of poor gastric emptying and adds another barrier (pyloric sphincter) through which tube feedings must traverse before aspiration into the lungs. However, **postpyloric feedings** do not preclude the possibility of aspiration. Many patients with this complication are aspirating their own nasopharyngeal secretions.

Nasoduodenal and NJ feeding tubes can be placed by trained, experienced nurses at the bedside. Although such placements typically take more time than NG or OG placements, this is still a relatively inexpensive method of placement. Bedside electromagnetic transmitter devices (eg, CORTRAK, Corpak Medsystems) may be helpful in achieving postpyloric tube placement. In some institutions, ND or NJ placements are done in radiology by a radiologist using fluoroscopy to visualize tube advancement. This procedure increases cost of EN therapy. NJ tubes generally are preferred over ND tubes; placement of the tube tip distal to the **ligament of Treitz** (located near the junction of the duodenum and the jejunum) may reduce risk of aspiration. Alternatively, during a laparotomy, the surgeon can place an ND or NJ tube.

Surgically placed jejunostomy tubes are placed through an incision in the abdominal wall, precluding the need for a tube down the nose or mouth. These tubes frequently are placed during laparotomy following abdominal trauma. Alternatively, jejunal access can be obtained by placing a jejunal extension through a PEG tube; the resulting tube is sometimes referred to as a *PEGJ tube* or *G-J tube*. Another option is to place a PEJ tube directly; this is more technically difficult than PEG placement. Tubes with both gastric and jejunal lumens are sometimes used, the gastric lumen for suctioning stomach contents and the jejunal lumen for delivery of feedings.

METHODS OF DELIVERY

Enteral feedings are delivered by several different methods. Continuous infusion must be used when duodenal or jejunal feedings are administered. For gastric feedings, bolus or intermittent feedings could be administered instead of continuous feedings. Each method has advantages and disadvantages.

In many hospitals, EN is delivered most commonly as a continuous infusion at a constant rate regulated by an infusion pump. A variation of continuous infusion is cyclic feeding, in which a constant rate is maintained over a certain number of hours daily; this method of administration is used commonly in long-term care or home settings. Sometimes EN is administered overnight.

Intermittent feedings are used commonly in long-term care or home settings. Patients frequently are started with continuous feedings; transitioned to intermittent feedings given several times a day over about 30 to 45 minutes for each feeding; and eventually changed to bolus feedings administered over less than 10 minutes per feeding. An advantage of intermittent feedings is that they may be administered by gravity flow adjusted with a roller clamp, although some institutions may use an infusion pump. Bolus feedings can be administered using a 60-mL syringe, although in some circumstances, an infusion set and pump may be used. Intermittent and bolus feedings often are given in amounts of 240 to 480 mL per feeding, corresponding to one to two cans of formula.

EN FORMULAS

One advantage of EN over PN is the availability in the United States of certain nutrients in some EN formulations (eg, glutamine, fish oils) that are not available for parenteral use. A number of EN formulas are marketed commercially. Hospitals and long-term care facilities usually limit formularies of EN formulas, stocking only a limited number of products.

Polymeric versus Oligomeric Formulas

A major criterion for categorizing EN products is whether macronutrients (particularly protein) are more intact (polymeric) or present in simpler forms (oligomeric). KEY CONCEPT *Standard EN formulas are polymeric; these are appropriate for most patients.* Oligomeric formulas should be reserved for patients with GI dysfunction.

Polymeric formulas typically contain intact proteins (most commonly casein). They have low osmolality of 300 to 500 mOsm/kg. These usually supply essential vitamins and minerals in amounts similar to the Adequate intakes (AI) or Recommended Dietary Allowances (RDA) for these nutrients when the formula is delivered in amounts adequate to meet macronutrient requirements of most patients. Many polymeric formulas are inexpensive relative to oligomeric formulas. Most modern formulas are lactose and gluten free. Products designed for use as oral supplements generally are polymeric and often have sucrose or other simple sugars added to improve taste.

Oligomeric formulas are also known as *chemically defined formulas*. These can be subcategorized based on whether the formula contains all free amino acids (elemental formulas) or peptides (peptide based) as the protein source. Some formulas contain a combination of free amino acids and small peptides. Dipeptides and tripeptides are absorbed more efficiently than free amino acids. Oligomeric formulas may be better tolerated than polymeric formulas for patients with defects in GI function and may be particularly useful with severe pancreatic dysfunction or significantly decreased GI surface area. However, adaptation of the bowel is better when intact nutrients are supplied to patients with short bowel syndrome, so those patients should be transitioned to intact nutrients as soon as possible.

Oligomeric formulas typically are more expensive than polymeric formulas and have higher osmolality. However, osmolality of these products usually does not exceed 700 mOsm/kg, a value less than that of many oral medications or a regular diet. Sometimes enteral feedings are diluted to deliver extra water required by the patient; this practice generally is discouraged because of potential risk of formula contamination. Instead, it is better to give extra water as boluses through the tube. If medications are administered through the feeding tube, generous amounts of water should be used to flush the tube before and after each medication; this practice helps provide extra fluid and prevent problems with tube occlusion.

Oligomeric formulas are less palatable than polymeric formulas and are not designed for use as oral supplements. Many oligomeric formulas provide some fat calories as medium-chain triglycerides (MCTs), a fat source that is more readily absorbed and metabolized than long-chain triglycerides (LCTs) typically found in polymeric formulas. The MCTs do not require bile salts or pancreatic enzymes for absorption. Some elemental formulas contain a low proportion of fat (less than 10% of total calories), which makes them useful in certain situations where fat needs to be restricted. The carbohydrate source in oligomeric formulas is also less complex than in polymeric formulas, consisting of oligosaccharides rather than hydrolyzed starch.

Fiber Content

Another distinguishing factor of enteral formulas is whether or not they contain fiber. Both soluble and insoluble fibers may be included. Insoluble fiber exerts an effect on gut motility by drawing water into the intestine and decreasing transit time, thus preventing constipation. Soluble fiber can help to lower blood cholesterol levels, regulate blood sugar, and prolong gastric emptying. Soluble fiber may also help control diarrhea. Cellulose gum is an example source of insoluble fiber. Oat fiber and guar gum provide primarily soluble fiber. Soy fiber provides primarily insoluble fiber but also some soluble fiber and is the most commonly used fiber source in tube feeding products. Fiber has been useful for regulating gut motility in some but not all clinical studies; it certainly can be useful in selected patients.[19] Some patients may experience GI discomfort secondary to gas production with introduction of fiber.

Fructooligosaccharides (FOS) are a form of fiber that pass through the stomach and small bowel undigested and are fermented by colonic bacteria to the SCFAs butyrate, propionate, and acetate. The SCFAs serve as a fuel source for colonocytes and also serve other important functions.[20] The FOS are thus *prebiotics* that serve as fermentable substrates for normal flora of the colon. The SCFAs are not added directly to EN products because they would be absorbed completely before reaching the colon; rather, FOS are added, allowing bacterial degradation to form SCFAs. Products containing FOS are often avoided postoperatively due to increased gas, bloating, and abdominal distention with these products.

Caloric Density

Enteral feeding formulas can be categorized based on caloric density. Standard caloric density is 1 to 1.3 kcal/mL (4.2–5.4 kJ/mL). More calorically dense formulas containing 1.5 to 2 kcal/mL (6.3–8.4 kJ/mL) are available and have a higher osmolality. Fluid-overloaded patients may benefit from more calorically dense formulas. As caloric content of a formula increases, the amount of free water decreases.

Protein Content

Protein content is an important factor in choosing an EN formula. Standard protein content in EN formulas is up to about 20% of total calories as protein. High-protein formulas containing 25% or more of total calories as protein are available for highly stressed patients with elevated protein needs. So are low-nitrogen formulas containing less than 10% of total calories as protein for use in patients requiring protein restriction. A wide range of protein is available, from about 35 to 95 g/L.

Carbohydrate Content

The most common carbohydrate source in tube feeding products is maltodextrin, a partially hydrolyzed starch that is easily digestible. Corn syrup solids are another hydrolyzed starch found in many products. Products containing simple sugars (often those intended for oral use) tend to be higher in osmolality.

Fat Content

Both MCTs and LCTs are used in tube feeding products. Corn, soy, and safflower oils are standard sources of fat, providing mainly ω-6 polyunsaturated fatty acids (PUFAs). Some newer EN products contain higher quantities of ω-3 PUFAs from sources such as fish oil (ie, docosahexanoic acid [DHA] and eicosapentaenoic acid [EPA]). Other formulas contain higher quantities of monounsaturated fatty acids (MUFAs) from canola oil and high-oleic safflower or sunflower oils. The essential fatty acid (EFA) content (mainly linoleic acid) of EN formulas is important because EFA deficiency can be induced if at least 1% to 4% of total calories are not supplied as EFAs. MCT oil does not contain EFAs.

Vitamin, Mineral, and Electrolyte Content

Most EN products contain vitamins and minerals, including major electrolytes, in amounts adequate to deliver the RDA or AI when a standard volume of formula is delivered daily. Some specialty formulas (eg, renal formulas) may have altered amounts of certain micronutrients.

Specialty Formulas

Specialty formulas designed for use in specific clinical situations generally are more expensive than standard polymeric formulas. KEY CONCEPT *Robust clinical trial data supporting use of specialty formulas in niche populations typically remain lacking in terms of improved patient outcomes.*

Stress and Trauma Formulas

Historically, formulas aimed specifically for highly stressed, critically ill patients, were enriched with branched-chain amino acids (BCAAs). The rationale was that skeletal muscle BCAAs are preferentially used for energy in critical illness. Provision of BCAAs might limit breakdown of muscle in these patients. Clinical data failed to support or refute benefit of these formulas unequivocally in terms of clinical outcomes.[3]

The newer generation of enteral feeding formulas marketed for use in these populations covers a broad spectrum of characteristics (Table 101–4). Whereas some are polymeric, others are oligomeric to address malabsorption that may accompany high stress. Some formulas marketed for use in critical illness are calorically dense (1.5–2 kcal/mL [6.3–8.4 kJ/mL]) to address fluid restrictions seen in this population, and others are less calorically dense. Most products contain generous amounts of protein to address requirements of highly stressed patients (nonprotein kilocalorie to nitrogen ratios typically between 75:1 and 125:1 [nonprotein energy to nitrogen ratio between about 300 and 500 kJ/g N]). Many products contain ingredients purported to increase immune function; the term *immunonutrition* is sometimes attached to these products.

Immune-enhancing ingredients present in some enteral feeding products include arginine, glutamine, ω-3 fatty acids, nucleic acids, and antioxidants. Few products contain all of these (see Table 101–4). Arginine is an important substrate for nitric oxide (NO) synthesis, and small amounts of NO have beneficial effects on immune function under certain conditions. Arginine has been purported to have a positive influence on lymphocyte and macrophage function. Glutamine is considered to be conditionally essential in critical illness and is a preferred fuel source for enterocytes of the small bowel. Supplementation with glutamine, either parenterally or enterally, may help maintain integrity of gut mucosa, preventing translocation of bacteria and endotoxin from the gut lumen into the lymphatic system and systemic circulation. However, a recent trial showed increased mortality with glutamine supplementation

Table 101–4

Selected Enteral Feeding Formulas Marketed for Use in High-Stress, Pulmonary Disease and Ventilator-Dependent, and Trauma Patients[a]

Product Name/Manufacturer	kcal/mL	Protein (g/L)	Enriched Ingredients[b]	Selected Specialized Indications
Impact/Nestle	1	56	Arginine, nucleotides, ω-3 fatty acids	HS, TR, PD, CI
Impact with Fiber/Nestle	1	56	Arginine, nucleotides, ω-3 fatty acids	HS, TR, PD, CI
Nutren Pulmonary/Nestle	1.5	68	56% total kcal as fat	PD, CI
Pulmocare/Abbott	1.5	62.4	55% total kcal as fat	PD
Oxepa/Abbott	1.5	62.4	55% total kcal as fat; ω-3 fatty acids	PD, CI
Isosource 1.5 Cal/Nestle	1.5	68		HS
Two Cal HN/Abbott	2	84		HS
Impact Glutamine/Nestle	1.3	78	Arginine, nucleotides, ω-3 fatty acids, glutamine	HS, TR, PD, CI
Impact Peptide 1.5/Nestle	1.5	94	Arginine, nucleotides, ω-3 fatty acids, MCT	HS, TR, PD, CI
Pivot 1.5 Cal/Abbott	1.5	93.7	Arginine, ω-3 fatty acids	HS, TR
Optimental/Abbott	1	51.5	ω-3 fatty acids	HS, TR
Vivonex Plus/Nestle	1	54	Glutamine, 100% free amino acids	TR
Vivonex RTF/Nestle	1	50	MCT, 100% free amino acids	TR
Vivonex T.E.N./Nestle	1	38	100% free amino acids	TR
Peptamen Bariatric/Nestle	1	93.2	MCT, ω-3 fatty acids	CI, PD, HS
Peptamen AF/Nestle	1.2	76	MCT, ω-3 fatty acids	HS, CI, PD
Perative/Abbott	1.3	66.7	MCT	HS
Vital AF 1.2 Cal/Abbott	1.2	75.1	MCT	HS

CI, critical illness; HS, high stress; MCT, medium-chain triglycerides; PD, pulmonary disease/ventilator dependent; TR, trauma.

[a] kcal is equivalent to 4.186 kJ.

[b]Formula considered enriched if following criteria met: arginine—greater than 10 g/1500 kcal (6,279 kJ); glutamine—greater than 10 g/1500 kcal (6279 kJ); MCT—greater than 30% of total fat; and ω-3 fatty acid—ratio of ω-6 to ω-3 less than or equal to 2:1 or greater than 1.5 g/L ω-3 fatty acids.

of patients with multiorgan failure.[21] The ω-3 fatty acids, primarily from fish oils, are included in many immunonutrition products. Metabolites of ω-6 fatty acids include mediators such as prostaglandins, leukotrienes, and thromboxanes that are primarily proinflammatory and increase coagulation. Conversely, mediators produced from ω-3 fatty acids are less proinflammatory and decrease coagulation. Limited data support nucleic acids as immunomodulators. Quantities of antioxidants (particularly vitamin C, vitamin E, and β-carotene) higher than traditionally found in standard enteral formulas are added to some immunonutrition formulas to protect body systems, including the immune system, from damage by oxygen-free radicals. KEY CONCEPT *Use of enteral immunonutrition in certain clinical settings is now widely accepted.* Commercial immunonutrition products and/or specific ingredients found in these products have generally been found to have no benefit in terms of mortality rates.[3,22,23] However, infection rates, length of stay, and length of time on a ventilator may be decreased with these products. The 2009 A.S.P.E.N./SCCM ICU Guidelines support use of these formulas in major elective surgery, trauma, burns, head and neck cancer, and mechanically ventilated patients.[5] The best timing (initiation and duration) of delivery remains to be determined. There is some concern that supplementation with arginine may be detrimental in septic patients.[3]

Pulmonary Formulas

Enteral feeding formulas designed for use in patients with chronic obstructive pulmonary disease or receiving mechanical ventilation contain higher amounts of fat (40%–55% of total kilocalories) than most formulas. The rationale for high fat content is that burning of fat for energy is associated with less carbon dioxide production compared with burning of carbohydrate. Less carbon dioxide production theoretically would be advantageous in patients with retention of this substance and might facilitate weaning from mechanical ventilation. Because part of the market targeted by the manufacturers of these products comprises mechanically ventilated patients, these products are included in Table 101–4. Carbon dioxide retention owing to carbohydrate administration was a problem previously when feeding was overzealous. However, at conservative calorie levels, standard enteral formulas usually can be given without fear of excess carbon dioxide production.

One formula, Oxepa (Nestle), has been studied specifically in critically ill patients with acute respiratory distress syndrome (ARDS), acute lung injury (ALI), and sepsis. This formula contains high quantities of the ω-3 fatty acids (EPA) and γ-linolenic acid (GLA). GLA is metabolized to a prostaglandin with vasodilatory properties. EPA is converted to prostaglandins and leukotrienes that are less proinflammatory than those derived from ω-6 fatty acids. This formula contains large quantities of antioxidants. Patients receiving this formula had improved outcomes, including fewer days of mechanical ventilation, compared with patients receiving a high-fat enteral feeding product as a control.[24] Another study using a standard enteral feeding product as a control did not show clear benefit in septic patients with ARDS or ALI.[25] However, a third study demonstrated benefit from Oxepa in patients with early sepsis even when using a standard enteral feeding control product.[26] Timing and duration of use for optimum benefit remain to be determined.

Table 101-5

Selected Enteral Feeding Formulas Marketed for Use in Diabetes and Stress-Induced Hyperglycemia[a]

Product Name/Manufacturer	kcal/mL	% kcal as Fat	% kcal as Carbohydrate	Fiber (g/L)
Glytrol/Nestle	1	42	40	15.2
Glucerna 1.0 Cal/Abbott	1	49	34.3	14.3
Glucerna 1.2 Cal/Abbott	1.2	45	35	16
Glucerna 1.5 Cal/Abbott	1.5	45	33	16

[a]One kcal is equivalent to 4.186 kJ.

Diabetic Formulas

Similar to pulmonary formulas, formulas designed for patients with diabetes or stress-induced hyperglycemia are relatively high in fat and low in carbohydrates (Table 101-5). These formulas typically contain fiber (primarily soluble) because it plays some role in glycemic control. They also may contain fructose and MUFAs. Data support improved blood sugar control with use of these formulas in patients with diabetes.[27] Whether or not a diabetic EN formula is chosen, avoidance of overfeeding and maintenance of good glycemic control with insulin or other hypoglycemic medications are important in these populations.

Renal Formulas

Products designed for use in renal failure have high caloric density (1.8–2 kcal/mL [7.5–8.4 kJ/mL]) to decrease administered fluid (Table 101-6). The products vary in amounts of nutrients of interest in renal failure patients such as protein, potassium, phosphorus, and magnesium. Products low in protein (20–35 g/L) may be appropriate in chronic renal failure patients not yet receiving dialysis. On the other hand, removal of nitrogen by dialysis, coupled with the hypercatabolic, hypermetabolic condition seen in many acute renal failure patients, makes use of higher protein formulas (80–90 g/L) appropriate in these situations. Potassium, phosphorus, and magnesium contents of EN formulas designed for use in renal failure tend to be lower than standard formulas because these renally excreted electrolytes accumulate during renal failure.

Historically, elemental formulas designed for renal failure were enriched with essential amino acids (EAAs) and contained lesser amounts of nonessential amino acids (NEAAs) than standard formulas. Theoretically, EAAs could combine with urea nitrogen in the synthesis of NEAAs, leading to a decrease in blood urea nitrogen (BUN). The only situation in which such formulas may be appropriate is in patients with chronic renal failure who are not candidates for dialysis. Even in this setting, use of these products should be limited to no more than 2 or 3 weeks.[1] These formulas have been supplanted largely by polymeric formulas with protein content similar to standard EN formulas. Many dialysis patients tolerate standard, high-protein EN formulas, although electrolytes must be monitored closely.

Hepatic Formulas

Specialized formulas for patients with hepatic insufficiency are limited in number. These are enriched with BCAAs while containing a reduced quantity of aromatic amino acids (AAAs) and methionine compared with standard formulas. These changes address high levels of AAAs and low levels of BCAAs found in the blood of patients with hepatic insufficiency. Theoretically, these products might help patients with hepatic encephalopathy (HE). Hepatic formulas have low AAA content, and this distinguishes them from the BCAA-enriched formulas historically used in patients with critical illness and stress. Improvement in mortality attributable to these products has not been consistent.[1]

The A.S.P.E.N./SCCM guidelines for the ICU recommend against the use of protein restriction to reduce risk of development of HE.[5] These guidelines recommend use of standard EN formulas for ICU patients with acute or chronic liver disease but state that the hepatic specialty formulas may be useful in improving coma grade in HE patients refractory to standard treatment with locally acting antibiotics and lactulose. An example of a specialized hepatic formula is Hepatic-Aid II (Hormel Health Labs), a product supplied as a powder for reconstitution that requires vitamin, mineral, and electrolyte supplementation. A second product is NutriHep (Nestle), supplied as a liquid formula containing the recommended amounts of key vitamins, minerals, and electrolytes.

Wound Healing Formulas

Tube feeding and oral supplement formulas designed for use in patients with wounds or decubitus ulcers typically supply high

Table 101-6

Selected Enteral Feeding Products Designed for Use in Renal Failure

Product Name/ Manufacturer	Protein/L	Characteristics
Nepro with Carb Steady/Abbott	80.6	Complete formula[a] similar to Novasource Renal for patients on dialysis
Novasource Renal/ Nestle	91.1	Complete formula similar to Nepro with Carb Steady for patients on dialysis
Suplena with Carb Steady/Abbott	44.7	Complete formula with low amounts of protein for patients not yet receiving dialysis

[a]Complete formula—contains all nutrients in amounts sufficient to meet needs of most patients in a volume equal to or less than that usually administered.

Patient Encounter, Part 1

LT is an obese 55-year-old woman with a history of diabetes mellitus and chronic obstructive pulmonary disease admitted with multiorgan failure and septic shock with a suspected pulmonary source. She meets criteria for acute respiratory distress syndrome (ARDS) and prerenal azotemia. She is placed on mechanical ventilation; started on aggressive fluid resuscitation, vasopressor therapy, and antibiotics; and systemic corticosteroid therapy. She is started on propofol for sedation while on the ventilator.

LT responds somewhat slowly to the sepsis protocol and on day 3 is still requiring both norepinephrine and vasopressin for blood pressure support. The dietitian assesses her nutritional needs. Her dry weight is 102 kg; height is 64 inches (163 cm); body mass index is 38 kg/m^2.

Is there any concern regarding starting EN at this time?

If EN is not appropriate at this time, should PN be initiated?

amounts of protein and calories. The antioxidant vitamins A, C, and E are frequently also found in high quantities as is zinc.

Modular Components

Single nutrient components are frequently administered through feeding tubes to augment the composition of the EN formula. Protein modules are probably the most commonly used. These may be supplied by the manufacturer as a powder that must be reconstituted with water or as a liquid product. Another modular component is fiber. These components are typically given as a bolus through the feeding tube rather than being added to the feeding formula.

MONITORING AND COMPLICATIONS

Although complications of EN generally are considered less serious than those of PN, some complications nevertheless can be dangerous or can lead to impaired delivery of desired nutrient load. Complications can be divided into four categories: GI, technical, infectious, and metabolic. The first three categories, along with common causes, are listed in Table 101–7. Patients on EN must be monitored for prevention of complications (Table 101–8). Monitoring of many parameters can become less frequent as patient condition stabilizes. Monitoring for efficacy of EN is also important.

GI Complications

KEY CONCEPT *GI complications are the most common complications of EN limiting the amount of feeding that patients receive.* Although diarrhea frequently is blamed on feeding formula or the method of EN administration, other possible causes usually exist (see Table 101–8). In the inpatient setting, patients receiving EN frequently are very sick. Along these lines, *Clostridium difficile* colitis must be considered as a possible cause of diarrhea, especially in patients receiving antimicrobial therapy or proton pump inhibitors.[28–30] Antibiotic therapy is a major cause of diarrhea in acutely ill patients, including those receiving EN. A medication-related cause of diarrhea is the sorbitol content of medications.[31] Large quantities of sorbitol present in oral liquid medications (often considered the dosage form of choice for administration through a feeding tube) can cause diarrhea. Unfortunately, sorbitol content of many medications is not listed on their labeling, and manufacturers frequently reformulate preparations to contain varying amounts of excipients, such as sorbitol.

Determining cause of diarrhea is important to know how to address the problem. Whereas *C. difficile* colitis should be treated

Table 101–7

Complications of Tube Feeding

Complication	Causes
GI	
Diarrhea	Drug related Antibiotic-induced bacterial overgrowth Hyperosmolar medications administered via feeding tubes Antacids containing magnesium Malabsorption Hypoalbuminemia or gut mucosal atrophy Pancreatic insufficiency Inadequate GI tract surface area Rapid GI tract transit Radiation enteritis Tube feeding related Rapid formula administration Formula hyperosmolality Low residue (fiber) content Lactose intolerance Bacterial contamination
Nausea and vomiting	Gastric dysmotility (surgery, anticholinergic drugs, diabetic gastroparesis) Rapid infusion of hyperosmolar formula
Constipation	Dehydration Drug induced (anticholinergics) Inactivity Low residue (fiber) content Obstruction or fecal impaction
Abdominal distention or cramping	Too rapid formula administration
Technical	
Occluded feeding tube lumen	Insoluble complexation of enteral formula and medication(s) Inadequate flushing of feeding tube Undissolved feeding formula
Tube displacement	Self-extubation Vomiting or coughing Inadequate fixation (jejunostomy)
Aspiration	Improper patient position Gastroparesis or atony causing regurgitation Feeding tube malpositioned Compromised lower esophageal sphincter Diminished gag reflex
Peristomal excoriation	Improper skin and tube care GI tract secretions leaking peristomally
Infectious	
Aspiration pneumonia	Same as technical—aspiration comments Prolonged use of large-bore polyvinylchloride tube

GI, gastrointestinal.

From Janson DD, Chessman KH. Enteral nutrition. In DiPiro JT, Talbert RL, Yee GC, et al, eds. Pharmacotherapy: A Pathophysiologic Approach, 5th ed. New York: McGraw-Hill, 2005.

Table 101–8

Suggested Monitoring for Patients on Enteral Nutrition

Parameter	During Initiation of EN Therapy	During Stable EN Therapy
Vital signs	Every 4–6 hours	As needed with suspected change (ie, fever)
Clinical Assessment		
Weight	Daily	Weekly
Length/height (children)	Weekly–monthly	Monthly
Head circumference (< 3 years of age)	Weekly–monthly	Monthly
Total intake/output	Daily	As needed with suspected changed in intake/output
Tube feeding intake	Daily	Daily
Enterostomy tube site assessment	Daily	Daily
GI tolerance		
Stool frequency/volume	Daily	Daily
Abdomen assessment	Daily	Daily
Nausea or vomiting	Daily	Daily
Gastric residual volumes	Every 4–8 hours (varies)	As needed when delayed gastric emptying suspected
Tube placement	Prior to starting; then ongoing	Ongoing
Laboratory		
Electrolytes, blood urea nitrogen/serum creatinine, glucose	Daily	Every 1–3 months
Calcium, magnesium, phosphorus	Three to seven times per week	Every 1–3 months
Liver function tests	Weekly	Every 1–3 months
Trace elements, vitamins	If deficiency/toxicity is suspected	If deficiency/toxicity is suspected

EN, enteral nutrition.

From Kumpf VS, Chessman KH. Enteral nutrition. In DiPiro JT, Talbert RL, Yee GC, et al, eds. Pharmacotherapy: A Pathophysiologic Approach, 9th ed. New York: McGraw-Hill, 2014.

with an appropriate antibiotic, medication-related diarrhea can be addressed by removal of the offending agent. Likewise, diarrhea secondary to malabsorption sometimes can be addressed by changing to an oligomeric EN formula. Antiperistaltic agents (eg, loperamide) may be useful in some noninfectious diarrhea.

On the other hand, constipation may occur in patients receiving EN, especially the elderly. Increased provision of fluid or fiber may be useful. Constipation may be drug related, in which case discontinuation or replacement of the offending drug may be beneficial.

Impaired gastric emptying is seen commonly in EN patients receiving gastric feedings and may be associated with nausea and vomiting. Impaired emptying may be related to disease process (eg, diabetic gastroparesis or sequelae to head injury) or to drug therapy, most notably narcotics. Gastric residual checks frequently are measured in patients receiving gastric feedings (see Table 101–8). To accomplish this, a syringe is attached to the feeding device, and as much liquid as possible is aspirated into the syringe. Debate is ongoing as to what constitutes a significant gastric aspirate, with numbers between 200 and 500 mL most commonly defended; a recent study indicated that residual checks are not necessary.[4,32–34] Approaches to the patient with delayed gastric emptying might include changing to a formula containing less fat because dietary fat is associated with slower gastric emptying. Metoclopramide often is given to patients receiving gastric feedings to facilitate gastric emptying. Erythromycin is an alternative medication that may be useful, although it is associated with drug–drug interactions. Patients with consistently high residuals are considered to be at higher risk of aspirating feedings into their lungs and should be considered for transition to postpyloric feedings. Postpyloric feedings may help relieve EN-related nausea and vomiting and are preferred for patients without an intact gag reflex. An important practice to help prevent aspiration is elevation of the head of the bed to at least 30 degrees during continuous feedings and during and for 30 to 60 minutes after intermittent and bolus feedings.

Technical Complications

Technical or mechanical complications are encountered frequently in EN patients. Tube occlusion most commonly is related to formula occlusion or medication administration through the tube. KEY CONCEPT *An important practice to help prevent medication-related occlusion is adequate water flushing of the tube before, between, and after each medication is given through the tube.* If intermittent feedings are used, water flushing after each feeding is recommended. Tube occlusion can increase cost of EN if the tube has to be removed and replaced. Clearing of occlusions using water or pancreatic enzymes plus sodium bicarbonate can be attempted, and special devices and kits (eg, DeClogger, Bionix) are available.[35]

Tube displacement is a potentially significant complication. This may be seen in an agitated patient pulling at the tube, or in some cases, the tube tip migrates spontaneously. If the tip of the tube is positioned in the tracheobronchial tree and feeding is delivered to this area, pneumonia, pneumothorax, and other problems could potentially occur. Location of the feeding tube tip should be confirmed initially by chest radiograph after placement and before use. For ongoing assessment of tube placement, auscultation and measurement of aspirate pH can be used.

Endoscopic and surgical feeding tubes can cause erosion of the exit site caused by leakage of gastric or intestinal contents onto the skin. This complication must be addressed by good wound care and repair or replacement of the access device. Similarly, NG, ND, and NJ tubes can be complicated by nasopharyngeal irritation or necrosis. This is one reason why such tubes should be considered for short-term use only.

Infectious Complications

Infectious complications of EN include aspiration pneumonia and infections related to delivery of contaminated EN formula. Although GI infections owing to industrial contamination of enteral formulas have been reported uncommonly, these formulas are more commonly seeded with organisms during the processes of transferring from can to delivery bag with ready-to-use formulas and during the process of reconstitution with powdered formulas. The so-called closed systems of delivery, wherein the formulas come from the manufacturer premixed in a delivery bag, should help decrease possibility of formula contamination. Practice recommendations from A.S.P.E.N. state that sterile water should be used for formula reconstitution, medication dilution, tube flushing, and additional water provision in acute or chronically ill patients requiring EN.[4] This recommendation can be difficult to implement, especially in home care.

Metabolic Complications

Metabolic complications of EN most commonly include disorders of fluid and electrolyte homeostasis and hyperglycemia. More severely ill patients require more frequent monitoring (see Table 101–8). Both dehydration and fluid overload can occur. Careful monitoring of fluid inputs and outputs as well as body weight is important. Dehydration may be caused by either excessive fluid losses or inadequate fluid intake. The trend in the ratio of BUN to serum creatinine can be useful in helping monitor fluid status; a ratio greater than 15:1 (60:1 for SI mmol/L:mmol/L) may be an indicator of dehydration; high ratios may also be a result of high protein provision by the feeding. Attention should be paid to free-water content of EN formulas. Free-water content varies from about 65% to 85%; percentage-free water typically drops as caloric density of the formula rises. If dehydration develops, switching to a less calorically dense formula or using larger water flushes is appropriate. Fluid overload is reflected by increases in weight, lower extremity edema, and pulmonary rales and particularly may be a problem in patients with renal or cardiac insufficiency. Use of a more calorically dense EN formula may be helpful, and diuretic therapy may be necessary. Fluid imbalances often are associated with abnormalities of sodium homeostasis that should be addressed in concert with fluid imbalance.

Hypokalemia, hypomagnesemia, and hypophosphatemia are some of the most common electrolyte abnormalities in sick, hospitalized patients. These can occur in context of the refeeding syndrome which occurs in chronically malnourished patients aggressively started on feeding. Although classically associated with PN, refeeding syndrome can also occur with aggressive EN. Careful monitoring of electrolytes, coupled with a feeding regimen increased gradually to goal rate over a period of several days, should help protect at-risk patients from this complication. Hypokalemia and hypomagnesemia also are associated with excessive losses through the GI tract or urine and are associated with various medications, including diuretics. Repletion may be accomplished enterally in nonsymptomatic patients or parenterally if the patient is symptomatic or the abnormality is severe. Enteral repletion with magnesium and phosphate can cause diarrhea. Hyperkalemia, hypermagnesemia, and hyperphosphatemia are less common and usually are associated with renal insufficiency. Hyperkalemia also is associated with medications, including potassium-sparing diuretics, angiotensin-converting enzyme inhibitors, and angiotensin receptor blockers.

Although hyperglycemia is less common with EN than PN, it can occur. Many severely ill patients (eg, septic, highly stressed) receiving EN have a metabolic milieu promoting hyperglycemia. For ICU patients with hyperglycemia receiving continuous EN, an IV insulin drip may be the most effective way to achieve good glycemic control. Scheduled intermediate or long-acting insulin plus correctional regular or rapid acting insulin is preferred after stabilization on the feeding regimen.[36,37] Administration of a higher fat, lower carbohydrate EN formula may be useful in selected patients.

Monitoring for Efficacy and Outcome Evaluation

A useful physical measurement of EN efficacy in the long-term patient is body weight. Depending on the clinical situation, the goal may be weight gain, weight maintenance, or weight loss. Whereas day-to-day fluctuations in weight generally reflect fluid changes, week-to-week variations are more useful in determining if caloric provision is appropriate.

The amount of EN actually administered is often less than the amount ordered owing to interruptions in therapy. It is imperative to monitor volume of feedings actually received and to make adjustments in rates or amounts of EN as necessary.

Biochemical markers have been used historically to help interpret EN adequacy. Use of visceral proteins such as albumin or prealbumin is limited by the effects of inflammation on serum levels of these biomarkers.[38] In the acute phase of illness characterized by a proinflammatory state, proteins known as *acute-phase reactants* are preferentially synthesized. One of these measured clinically is C-reactive protein (CRP). In some patients with significant illness, prealbumin may not rise, even though the patient is receiving appropriate EN, until CRP begins to fall. Collection of urine to measure nitrogen balance can help analyze adequacy of caloric and protein provision.

In patients with wounds (eg, decubitus ulcers), a goal of therapy is to facilitate wound healing. Monitoring status of the wound becomes part of ongoing nutritional assessment. In debilitated patients, particularly on long-term EN, measures of functional status such as grip strength and ability to perform activities of daily living become important components of nutritional assessment.

MEDICATION ADMINISTRATION IN PATIENTS RECEIVING EN

Medication Administration Through Feeding Tubes

If a patient receiving EN is alert and can swallow oral medications, then medications should be given by mouth. Many patients are not able to receive medications by this route, and the feeding tube may be considered as a delivery route. Effects of medication administration through feeding tubes on the delivery of both the drug and the EN formula nutrients have been inadequately studied.[39]

Patient Encounter, Part 2

On day 4, vasopressor requirements are minimal and enteral feeding is initiated at a low rate via nasogastric tube. Propofol is changed to dexmedetomidine on day 5. Gastric residuals range from 0 to 20 mL over the next 2 days as the tube feeding is advanced to goal rate. Blood sugar readings rise to above 200 mg/dL (11.1 mmol/L), necessitating initiation of an insulin drip on day 7; on day 9, insulin glargine subcutaneous is added as the insulin drip is titrated off.

How does propofol affect the initial EN prescription?

Design an enteral feeding regimen, including choice of formula and goal rate, appropriate for this patient at this time.

What are this patient's risk factors for hyperglycemia, and is the approach to blood sugar management rational?

KEY CONCEPT *Compatibility of medication with EN formula is of concern when administering medications through feeding tubes.* An important technical complication of EN is tube occlusion, related most commonly to medication administration. Not only must compatibility of medication and EN formula be considered, but interactions between medications and the feeding tube itself must be considered. Strict protocols for flushing the tube before, between, and after administration of medications are important.[4] The best fluid for flushing is warm water. Between 10 and 30 mL of water should be used as a flush before and after any medication administration through a feeding tube. Medications should be administered one at a time sequentially rather than being mixed together for simultaneous administration down the tube; about 5 mL of water should be used as a flush between medications. This should help prevent interactions between drugs within the tube itself that could lead to occlusion.

Different dosage forms present unique challenges for administration through feeding tubes. Certain solid dosage forms should not be crushed because crushing would alter release characteristics.[40] For example, controlled-release, extended-release, and sustained-release preparations should not be crushed, nor should sublingual dosage forms. Enteric-coated dosage forms generally are designed to protect acid-labile medications from stomach acid; when these dosage forms reach the small bowel with its higher pH, the drug is released into an environment in which it is more stable. Alternatively, enteric-coated dosage forms protect the stomach from medications that could cause irritation. Thus, crushing the enteric coating defeats the purpose of the dosage form and could lead to decreased efficacy or increased adverse events.

Medications available commercially as compressed tablets can be crushed for administration through tubes. After crushing, the fine powder should be mixed with 10 to 30 mL of fluid (usually warm water) for administration. A powdered dosage form inside a hard-gelatin capsule can be poured out and mixed with water for administration through tubes. Soft-gelatin capsules can be dissolved in warm water. Some enteric-coated and delayed-release microencapsulated products can be opened and individually coated particles administered through the tube without crushing if the tube has a large enough diameter.

If a liquid dosage form of a medication exists, it would seem rational to use this for administration through a feeding tube. This may decrease potential for tube clogging but may in some instances decrease tolerability of medication administration. Sorbitol is an excipient found in many liquid medications in amounts sufficient to cause diarrhea. If diarrhea secondary to sorbitol is suspected, contact with the manufacturer to ascertain sorbitol content may be necessary.

Another potential problem with administration of liquid medications through feeding tubes is high osmolality of some products. Dilution of hypertonic medications with 30 to 60 mL of water or administration of smaller dosages more frequently may help prevent diarrhea. Although administration of IV medications through feeding tubes may be entertained, these dosage forms frequently are hypertonic and contain problematic excipients when given via the GI tract.

It is generally not recommended to mix medications directly into EN formula because physical incompatibilities might lead to tube occlusion. Limited data currently available indicate that acidic syrups and elixirs may be most harmful, causing physical incompatibility when admixed with EN formulas. It would seem logical that medications considered absorbed better in the fasted state either should be given between feedings on an intermittent feeding schedule or feedings should be held before and after medication administration. However, not all studies have supported this notion; therefore, this issue deserves further study.[41]

Location of feeding tube tip is important when considering medication administration. This is particularly true if the medication acts locally in the GI tract. For example, sucralfate and antacids act locally in the stomach; therefore, administration through a duodenal or jejunal tube is illogical. Likewise, for medications requiring acid for best absorption, administration directly into the duodenum or jejunum may result in suboptimal absorption. Absorption of drugs when administered directly into the small bowel, especially the jejunum, is a topic where more research would be useful.

Problem Medications

▸ *Phenytoin*

Certain medications present challenges when administered through feeding tubes. The medication studied most thoroughly is phenytoin. Most studies have shown significant decreases in phenytoin absorption when administered enterally to patients receiving EN. Several mechanisms have been proposed for this interaction. Liberal dilution of phenytoin suspension before its administration down the tube may improve its delivery. Many institutions hold tube feedings for 1 or 2 hours before and after administration of phenytoin, although some EN patients subjected to this routine still require high dosages of phenytoin to achieve therapeutic serum concentrations. Holding feeding around medication administration can make meeting nutritional requirements difficult with continuous feedings, especially if phenytoin is administered several times daily. Diligent monitoring of phenytoin serum concentrations is necessary for the patient on EN receiving this medication. In some cases, use of IV phenytoin or another anticonvulsant medication may be prudent.

▸ *Warfarin*

EN formulas contain vitamin K, which can antagonize the pharmacologic activity of warfarin. Vitamin K content of EN formulas has been adjusted down over several decades, resulting in products that contain amounts of vitamin K unlikely to affect anticoagulation by warfarin significantly. However, inadequate warfarin anticoagulation in EN patients receiving formulas containing minimal vitamin K has been reported. A component of certain tube feedings, perhaps protein, may bind warfarin and result in suboptimal activity. One small study indicated a better response in terms of the international normalized ratio (INR) when feedings were held for 1 hour before and after warfarin compared with administration of the drug without

Patient Encounter, Part 3

LT is extubated on day 13. Concern regarding her swallowing strength leads to a speech pathology consult. She is switched to a standard formula tube feeding. On day 14, an order to advance oral diet as tolerated is written following the speech pathology assessment.

Was the switch to a standard tube feeding formula rational?

How should the transition from EN to oral feedings be accomplished?

Patient Care Process

Patient Assessment:

- Based on patient's disease states and severity, estimate the amount of time until adequate oral intake resumes (see Table 101–1).
- Are there any contraindications or precautions regarding use of EN (see Table 101–2)? When the GI tract is nonfunctional, either PN or no SNS is indicated.
- If inadequate intake has occurred or is anticipated for 7 to 14 days, start SNS. The threshold for starting SNS is lower for previously malnourished patients. Critically ill patients should generally be started on EN within 24 to 48 hours of ICU admission.
- Choose the appropriate type of enteral access device based upon the expected duration of use and upon whether any condition exists which precludes gastric feeding (see Table 101–3).
- Choose the method of feeding administration (eg, intermittent or continuous) based on the feeding access type (ie, gastric versus postpyloric) and other patient factors.

Therapy Evaluation:

- Adjust formula, rate of administration, and/or route of administration if intolerance develops or nutritional goals (eg, weight loss, weight maintenance, weight gain, maintenance of muscle mass, slowing of functional decline) are not met.
- Are medications being administered down the feeding tube? If so, assess the appropriateness of this route.

Care Plan Development:

- Start tube feeding at full strength and low rate and increase rate as tolerated to goal that will meet patient's nutritional requirements.
- Develop plan to include monitoring at appropriate intervals for metabolic, GI, technical, or infectious complications (see Table 101–8).
- Develop monitoring plan for adequacy of nutritional regimen. This may include serial weights, intakes and outputs, and a measure of functional status.

Follow-Up Evaluation:

If patient is to be discharged home on EN, educate patient or caregiver on enteral access device care, feeding delivery, troubleshooting, and complications to observe for (see Table 101–7).

holding feedings.[42] When tube feedings are started, changed, or discontinued, INR should be monitored closely.

▶ *Fluoroquinolones*

Absorption of antimicrobial agents such as fluoroquinolones and tetracyclines that can be bound by divalent and trivalent cations potentially could be compromised by administration with EN formulas containing these cations. Fluoroquinolones (eg, levofloxacin and ciprofloxacin) have been best studied in this regard, and results of studies are not consistent.[41] Some institutions hold tube feedings for 1 to 2 hours or more before and after enteral dosages of fluoroquinolones. Not all fluoroquinolones are affected by the interaction, suggesting that a mechanism other than chelation by divalent cations may also be significant. Because ciprofloxacin absorption has been shown to be decreased with jejunal administration, this drug probably should not be given by jejunal tube.

SUMMARY AND CONCLUSION

EN is an important method of feeding patients who cannot or should not eat enough to meet nutrient requirements for a prolonged time. When the GI tract can be used safely, EN is preferred over PN. Various types of enteral access devices are available. Whereas tubes inserted through the nose often are adequate for patients expected to receive EN for a short time, more permanent devices are preferred for longer-term patients. Choice of whether to feed into the stomach or postpylorically is patient specific. Although numerous EN formulas are available, many products are very similar, making a limited formulary feasible. Data supporting many specialized types of EN formulas are limited. Although complications of EN tend to be less serious than those of PN, adverse effects encountered can be significant, and diligent ongoing monitoring is necessary. Although medications can be administered through feeding tubes, various factors must be taken into account in each individual patient.

Abbreviations Introduced in This Chapter

AAA	Aromatic amino acid(s)
AI	Adequate intake
ALI	Acute lung injury
ARDS	Acute respiratory distress syndrome
A.S.P.E.N.	American Society for Parenteral and Enteral Nutrition
BCAA	Branched-chain amino acid(s)
BUN	Blood urea nitrogen
CRP	C-Reactive protein
DHA	Docosahexanoic acid
EAA	Essential amino acid(s)
EFA	Essential fatty acid(s)
EN	Enteral nutrition
EPA	Eicosapentaenoic acid
ESPEN	European Society for Clinical Nutrition and Metabolism
FOS	Fructooligosaccharide
GALT	Gut-associated lymphoid tissue
GI	Gastrointestinal
GLA	γ-Linolenic acid

HE	Hepatic encephalopathy
IBD	Inflammatory bowel disease
ICU	Intensive care unit
INR	International normalized ratio
LCT	Long-chain triglyceride
MCT	Medium-chain triglyceride
MUFA	Monounsaturated fatty acid
ND	Nasoduodenal
NEAA	Nonessential amino acid
NG	Nasogastric
NJ	Nasojejunal
NO	Nitric oxide
OG	Orogastric
PEG	Percutaneous endoscopic gastrostomy
PEJ	Percutaneous endoscopic jejunostomy
PN	Parenteral nutrition
PUFA	Polyunsaturated fatty acid
RDA	Recommended Dietary Allowance
SCCM	Society for Critical Care Medicine
SCFA	Short-chain fatty acid
SNS	Specialized nutrition support

REFERENCES

1. American Society for Parenteral and Enteral Nutrition Board of Directors. Guidelines for the use of parenteral and enteral nutrition in adult and pediatric patients. JPEN J Parenter Ent Nutr. 2002;26(Suppl):1SA–138SA.
2. The European Society for Clinical Nutrition and Metabolism. ESPEN Guidelines on Adult Enteral Nutrition. Clin Nutr. 2006;25:175–360.
3. Clinical Practice Guidelines. Critical Care Nutrition; [Internet]. Kingston, ON, Canada: Critical Evaluation Research Unit. 2013 [cited 2014 July 30]. http://www.criticalcarenutrition.com/index.php?option=com_content&view=category&layout=blog&id=25&Itemid=109. Accessed September 21, 2015.
4. Bankhead R, Boullata J, Brantley S, et al. Enteral nutrition practice recommendations. JPEN J Parenter Enter Nutr. 2009;33: 122–167.
5. McClave SA, Martindale RG, Vanek VW, et al. Guidelines for the provision and assessment of nutrition support therapy in the adult critically ill patient. JPEN J Parenter Ent Nutr. 2009;33: 277–316.
6. Scaldaferri F, Pizzoferrato M, Gerardi V, Lopetuso L, Gasbarrini A. The gut barrier: New acquisitions and therapeutic approaches. J Clin Gastroenterol. 2012:46(Suppl 1):S12–S17.
7. Choban P, Dickerson R, Malone A, et al. A.S.P.E.N. clinical guidelines: nutrition support of hospitalized adult patients with obesity. JPEN J Parent Ent Nutr. 2013;37:714–744.
8. Turza KC, Krenitsky J, Sawyer RG. Enteral feeding and vasoactive agents: Suggested guidelines for clinicians. Practical Gastroenterol. September 2009;11–22.
9. Wells DL. Provision of enteral nutrition during vasopressor therapy for hemodynamic instability: An evidence-based review. Nutr Clin Pract. 2012;27:521–526.
10. van den Berghe G, Wouters P, Weekers F, et al. Intensive insulin therapy in the critically ill patients. N Engl J Med. 2001;345:1359–1367.
11. The NICE-SUGAR Study Investigators. Intensive versus conventional glucose control in critically ill patients. N Engl J Med. 2009;360;1283–1297.
12. Veterans Affairs Total Parenteral Nutrition Cooperative Study Group. Perioperative total parenteral nutrition in surgical patients. N Engl J Med. 1991;325:525–532.
13. Casaer MP, Mesotten D, Hermans G, et al. Early versus late parenteral nutrition in critically ill adults. N Engl J Med. 2011;365:506–517.
14. Heidegger CP, Berger MM, Graf S, et al. Optimisation of energy provision with supplemental parenteral nutrition in critically ill patients: A randomized controlled clinical trial. Lancet. 2013:381: 385–393.
15. Doig GS, Simpson F, Sweetman EA, et al. Early parenteral nutrition in critically ill patients with short-term relative contraindications to early enteral nutrition. JAMA. 2013;309: 2130–2138.
16. Singer P, Anbar R, Cohen J, et al. The tight calorie control study (TICACOS): A prospective, randomized, controlled pilot study of nutritional support in critically ill patients. Intensive Care Med. 2011;37:601–609.
17. Casaer MP, Van den Berghe G. Nutrition in the acute phase of critical illness. New Engl J Med. 2014;370:1227–1236.
18. Blumenstein I, Shastri YM, Stein J. Gastroenteric tube feeding: Techniques, problems and solutions. World J Gastroenterol. 2014;20:8505–8524.
19. Elia M, Engfer MB, Green CJ, Silk DBA. Systematic review and meta-analysis: The clinical and physiological effects of fibre-containing enteral formulae. Aliment Pharmacol Ther. 2008;27: 120–145.
20. Robefroid M, Gibson GR, Hoyles L, et al. Prebiotic effects: Metabolic and health benefits. Br J Nutr. 2010;104(Suppl 2): S1–S63.
21. Heyland D, Muscedere J, Wischmeyer PE, et al. A randomized trial of glutamine and antioxidants in critically ill patients. N Engl J Med. 2013;368:1489–1497.
22. Braga M, Wischmeyer PE, Drover J, Heyland DK. Clinical evidence for pharmaconutriton in major elective surgery. JPEN J Parenter Enteral Nutr. 2013;37(Suppl 5):66S–72S.
23. Marik PE, Zaloga GP. Immunonutrition in critically ill patients: A systematic review and analysis of the literature. Intensive Care Med. 2008;34:1980–1990.
24. Pontes-Arruda A, Demichele S, Seth A, Singer P. The use of an inflammation-modulating diet in patients with acute lung injury or acute respiratory distress syndrome: A meta-analysis of outcome data. JPEN J Parenter Ent Nutr. 2008;32: 596–605.
25. Grau-Carmona T, Moran-Garcia V, Garcia-de-Lorenzo A, et al. Effect of an enteral diet enriched with eicosapentaenoic acid, gamma-linolenic acid and anti-oxidants on the outcome of mechanically ventilated, critically ill, septic patients. Clin Nutr. 2011;30: 578–584.
26. Pontes-Arruda A, Ferreira Martins L, Maria de Lima S, et al. Enteral nutrition with eicosapentaenoic acid, γ-linolenic acid and antioxidants in the early treatment of sepsis: Results from a multicenter, prospective, randomized, double-blinded, controlled study: The INTERSEPT Study. Crit Care. 2011;15:R144.
27. Elia M, Ceriello A, Laube H, et al. Enteral nutritional support and use of diabetes-specific formulas for patients with diabetes. Diabetes Care. 2005;28:2267–2279.
28. Howell MD, Novack V, Grgurich P, et al. Iatrogenic gastric acid suppression and the risk of nosocomial Clostridium difficile infection. Arch Intern Med. 2010;170:784–790.
29. Barletta JF, El-Ibiary SY, Davis LE, et al. Proton pump inhibitors and the risk for hospital-acquired Clostridium difficile infection. Mayo Clin Proc. 2013;88:1085–1090.
30. Stevens V, Dumyati G, Brown J, Wijngaarden E. Differential risk of Clostridium difficile infection with proton pump inhibitor use by level of antibiotic exposure. Pharmacoepidemiol Drug Saf. 2011;20:1035–1042.
31. Edes TE, Walk BE, Austin JL. Diarrhea in tube-fed patients: Feeding formula not necessarily the cause. Am J Med. 1990;88:91–93.
32. Reignier J, Mercier E, Le Gouge A, et al. Effect of not monitoring residual gastric volume on risk of ventilator-associated pneumonia in adults receiving mechanical ventilation and early

enteral feeding: A randomized controlled trial. JAMA. 2013;309: 249–256.
33. Poulard F, Dimet J, Martin-Lefevre L, et al. Impact of not measuring residual gastric volume in mechanically ventilated patients receiving early enteral feeding: A prospective before-after study. JPEN J Parenter Ent Nutr. 2010;34: 125–130.
34. DeLegge MH. Managing gastric residual volumes in the critically ill patient: An update. Curr Opin Clin Nutr Metab Care. 2011;14:193–196.
35. Lord LM. Restoring and maintaining patency of enteral feeding tubes. Nutr Clin Pract. 2003;18:422–426.
36. Cook A, Burkitt D, McDonald L, Sublett L. Evaluation of glycemic control using NPH insulin sliding scale versus insulin aspart sliding scale in continuously tube-fed patients. Nutr Clin Pract. 2009;24:718–722.
37. Dickerson RN, Wilson VC, Maish GO, et al. Transitional NPH insulin therapy for critically ill patients receiving continuous enteral nutrition and intravenous regular human insulin. JPEN J Parenter Enteral Nutr. 2013;37:506–516.
38. White JV, Guenter P, Jensen G, et al. Consensus statement: Academy of Nutrition and Dietetics and American Society for Parenteral and Enteral Nutrition: Characteristics recommended for the identification and documentation of adult malnutrition (undernutrition). JPEN J Parenter Enteral Nutr. 2012;36: 275–283.
39. Wohlt PD, Zheng L, Gunderson S, et al. Recommendations for the use of medications with continuous enteral nutrition. Am J Health-Syst Pharm. 2009;66:1458–1467.
40. Mitchell JF. Oral Dosage Forms That Should Not Be Crushed [Internet]. Horsham (PA): Institute for Safe Medication Practices; 2014. [cited 1 Aug 2014]. http://www.ismp.org/tools/donotcrush.pdf.
41. Rollins CJ. Drug-nutrient interactions. In: Mueller CM, ed. The A.S.P.E.N. Nutrition Support Core Curriculum, 2nd ed, Silver Spring, MD: A.S.P.E.N., 2012:298–312.
42. Dickerson RN, Garmon WM, Kuhl DA, et al. Vitamin K-independent warfarin resistance after concurrent administration of warfarin and continuous enteral nutrition. Pharmacotherapy. 2008;28: 308–313.

102 Overweight and Obesity

Maqual R. Graham and Daniel S. Aistrope

LEARNING OBJECTIVES

Upon completion of the chapter, the reader will be able to:

1. Explain the underlying causes of overweight and obesity.
2. Identify parameters used to diagnose obesity and other objective information that indicates the severity of disease.
3. Identify desired therapeutic goals for patients who are overweight or obese.
4. Recommend appropriate nonpharmacologic and pharmacologic therapeutic interventions for overweight or obese patients.
5. Implement a monitoring plan that will assess both the efficacy and safety of therapy initiated.
6. Educate patients about the disease state and associated risks, comprehensive lifestyle interventions, drug therapy, and surgical options necessary for effective treatment.

INTRODUCTION

Overweight and obesity are terms used to describe weight measurements greater than what is considered healthy for a given height.[1] KEY CONCEPT *Body mass index (BMI), waist circumference (WC), comorbidities, and readiness to lose weight are used in the assessment of overweight or obese patients.* The primary modality in defining overweight and obesity is the BMI, a measure of body fat based on height and weight. BMI should be used to identify adults at increased risk for cardiovascular disease (CVD) and other obesity-related disorders. Evaluation of the patient's risk status involves not only calculation of the BMI but also the measurement of WC and determination of obesity-related comorbidities and presence of CVD risk factors. KEY CONCEPT *The presence of comorbidities (CVD, type 2 diabetes mellitus, and sleep apnea) and cardiovascular risk factors (cigarette smoking, hypertension, elevated low-density lipoprotein cholesterol, low high-density lipoprotein cholesterol, impaired fasting glucose) requires identification and aggressive management for overall effective treatment of the overweight or obese patient.* Obese patients may be at very high risk for mortality if concomitant risk factors exist; therefore, high-risk patients require aggressive modification of risk factors in addition to obesity treatment.[2]

ETIOLOGY AND EPIDEMIOLOGY

Obesity is a multifactorial, complex disease that occurs because of an interaction between genotype and the environment. Although the etiology is not completely known, it involves overlapping silos of social, behavioral, and cultural influence; pathophysiology; metabolism; and genetic composition.[3] The majority of overweight or obese individuals are adults, but these diseases are also prevalent in children between 2 and 19 years of age. While the prevalence of obesity appears to be leveling off, approximately 35% of US adults 20 years of age and older are currently considered obese. The prevalence of obesity in men and women of various racial and ethnic origins differ. Thirty-six percent of non-Hispanic white adults are considered obese, where approximately 40% of Mexican Americans and 50% of non-Hispanic black Americans are obese.[4]

Thirty-two percent of children and adolescents aged 2 through 19 years are considered either overweight or obese. The prevalence of obesity among this age group remains unchanged at 17%.[5] Overweight children typically mature to overweight adults, but most obese adults were not overweight as children.[6] Overweight and obesity, when present in young adults, may be a better predictor of prevalence.[6] Adulthood overweight and obesity contribute to an increased risk of death in the presence of hypertension, dyslipidemia, diabetes mellitus, CVD, stroke, sleep apnea, gallbladder disease, osteoarthritis, and certain cancers.[2] Psychosocial functioning also may be hindered because obese patients may be at risk for discrimination if negatively stereotyped.[2] Pediatric obesity is also associated with significant health-related problems and is therefore considered a risk factor for much of the adult obesity-related morbidity and mortality.[7,8] Cardiovascular (eg, dyslipidemia and hypertension), endocrine (eg, hyperinsulinemia, impaired glucose tolerance, type 2 diabetes mellitus, and menstrual irregularities), and mental (eg, low self-esteem and depression) health problems exist for obese patients.[9]

PATHOPHYSIOLOGY

The key factor in the development of overweight and obesity is the imbalance that occurs between energy intake and energy expenditure. The extent of obesity is determined by the length of time this imbalance has been present. Energy intake is affected by environmental influences, including social, behavioral, and cultural factors, whereas genetic composition and metabolism affect energy expenditure.[10]

Energy Intake

Food intake is regulated by various receptor systems. Stimulation of the following receptors increases and decreases food intake, respectively.

▸ *Increase Food Intake*

- Serotonin 1A subtype (5-HT_{1A})
- Noradrenergic α_2
- Cannabinoid 1 (CB_1)

▸ *Decrease Food Intake*

- Serotonin 2C subtype (5-HT_{2C})
- Noradrenergic α_1 or β_2
- Histamine subtypes 1 and 3 (H_1 and H_3)
- Dopamine 1 and 2 (D1 and D2)

Identification of appetite-associated receptors is useful in the development of pharmacologic agents, however not all are targeted by currently approved anti-obesity medications. In addition to receptor-modulated food consumption, higher levels of the protein leptin are associated with decreased food intake.[11] In contrast, elevated levels of neuropeptide Y increase food intake.[11]

It is debatable whether obesity is related to total calorie intake or composition of macronutrients. Of the three macronutrients (ie, carbohydrate, protein, and fat), fat has received the most attention, given its desirable texture and its ability to augment the flavor of other foods. Food high in fat promotes weight gain, in comparison with the other macronutrients, because fat is more energy dense. When compared with carbohydrate and protein, more than twice as many calories per gram are contained in fat. In addition, fat is stored more easily by the body compared with protein and carbohydrate.[12]

Energy Expenditure

A person's metabolic rate is the primary determinant of energy expenditure. The metabolic rate is enhanced after food consumption and is directly related to the amount and type.[13] Physical inactivity may predispose an individual to overweight and obesity. In addition, endocrine-related disorders (eg, hypothyroidism and Cushing syndrome) may lower the metabolic rate, further contributing to the development of overweight and obesity.

CLINICAL PRESENTATION AND DIAGNOSIS

KEY CONCEPT *BMI, WC, comorbidities, and readiness to lose weight are used in the assessment of overweight or obese patients.* Any interaction between a patient and a health care provider presents an opportunity to evaluate the patient's height and weight; however, these parameters should be measured no less than annually. The BMI should then be calculated and classified based on current cut points for overweight and obesity. The BMI is calculated using the measured weight in kilograms divided by the height in meters squared (kg/m^2) for all adult patients regardless of gender. The greater the BMI in overweight and obese individuals, the greater the risk of CVD, type 2 diabetes mellitus and all-cause mortality.[14] The BMI distribution changes with age for children just as height and weight. Percentiles specific for age and gender are used to classify pediatric patients as overweight and obese as well as healthy and underweight. The BMI is classified according to Table 102–1. WC should also be determined no less than annually for adult patients by placing a measuring tape at the top of the right iliac crest and proceeding around the abdomen, ensuring that the tape is tight but not constricting the skin. The value is measured after normal expiration.[2] Table 102–2 defines high-risk WC.[2] Measurement of WC is not recommended for children and adolescents because reference values identifying risk are unavailable.[15] After obtaining patient appropriate parameters, further assess the adult patient for the presence of obesity-related comorbidities and cardiovascular risk factors. KEY CONCEPT *The presence of comorbidities (CVD, type 2 diabetes mellitus, and sleep apnea) and cardiovascular risk factors (cigarette smoking, hypertension, elevated low-density lipoprotein cholesterol, low high-density lipoprotein cholesterol, impaired fasting glucose) requires identification and aggressive management for overall effective treatment of the overweight or obese patient.* A patient is at very high absolute risk if diagnosed with CVD, type 2 diabetes mellitus, or sleep apnea or if three or more of the risk factors listed in Table 102–3 are present.[2] Aggressive disease management should be initiated and not limited to weight loss. If the patient is a child or adolescent and the BMI is greater than the 85th percentile, determine the patient's risk for future obesity-related problems or presence of obesity-related medical conditions such as sleep, respiratory, gastrointestinal (GI), endocrine, cardiovascular, and psychiatric disorders.[15,16]

Table 102–1

BMI Classification

Adult	
Underweight	< 18.5 kg/m^2
Normal weight	18.5–24.9 kg/m^2
Overweight	25–29.9 kg/m^2
Obesity (Class 1)	30–34.9 kg/m^2
Obesity (Class 2)	35–39.9 kg/m^2
Extreme obesity (Class 3)	≥ 40 kg/m^2
Children (Does Not Pertain to Those Less Than 2 Years of Age[a])	
Underweight	< 5th percentile
Healthy weight	5th–84th percentile
Overweight	85th–94th percentile
Obesity	≥ 95th percentile

[a]Weight for height values should be plotted and monitored over time for children younger than 2 years.

Data from Refs. 2 and 14.

Table 102–2

High-Risk Waist Circumference

Men	> 40 in (102 cm)
Women	> 35 in (89 cm)

From Department of Health and Human Services, NIH-NHLBI. Clinical guidelines on the identification, evaluation and treatment of overweight and obesity in adults. NIH publication no. 00–4084. Bethesda, MD: National Institutes of Health, 2000.

Table 102–3

Modifiable Risk Factors

- Cigarette smoking
- Hypertension
- Elevated low-density lipoprotein cholesterol
- Decreased high-density lipoprotein cholesterol
- Impaired fasting glucose

From Department of Health and Human Services, NIH-NHLBI. Clinical guidelines on the identification, evaluation and treatment of overweight and obesity in adults. NIH publication no. 00–4084. Bethesda, MD: National Institutes of Health, 2000.

TREATMENT

Desired Outcome

KEY CONCEPT *The treatment goals for overweight and obesity are to prevent additional weight gain, reduce and maintain a lower body weight, and control related risks.* A 5% to 10% weight loss as derived from the patient's current weight is the initial goal of obesity management because favorable outcomes on the negative effects of obesity have been documented.[14] A sustained loss in weight of 5% will likely reduce triglyceride and blood glucose values as well as risk for the development of type 2 diabetes mellitus.[14] Greater reductions in weight will reduce blood pressure and improve both low-density and high-density lipoprotein cholesterol. KEY CONCEPT *Weight loss is indicated for patients with a BMI of 25 to 29.9 kg/m² with one or more indicators of increased CVD risk (eg, elevated WC, prediabetes or type 2 diabetes, hypertension, dyslipidemia, current cigarette smoker) or for any patient with a BMI of 30 kg/m² or greater.* Weight loss should occur at a rate of 0.45 to 0.9 kg (1–2 lb) per week, meeting the initial weight loss goal within the first 6 months of therapy. If the patient achieves a 5% to 10% loss in weight, weight loss maintenance strategies should be considered. KEY CONCEPT *Weight maintenance occurs after successful achievement of weight loss.*

It is desirable to achieve a goal of improved long-term physical health for a child or adolescent. A BMI below the 85th percentile is warranted but is difficult to assess in frequent or short time periods. Serial weight measurements may better quantify energy balance. Goals are most likely accomplished through adaptation of lifelong healthy lifestyle habits. In doing so, weight loss or maintenance can be attained for some children. Others may need to incorporate changes that result in a negative energy balance or energy input less than energy output.[15,16]

General Approach to Treatment

KEY CONCEPT *Treatment of obesity includes comprehensive lifestyle intervention (caloric restricted diet, increased physical activity, and behavioral therapy to facilitate compliance with diet and exercise), pharmacologic treatment, surgical intervention, or a combination of modalities.* Before initiating therapy, secondary causes of obesity (eg, hypothyroidism and Cushing syndrome) must be considered. Current treatment with medications that negatively alter weight should be determined and, if present, alternative therapies should be suggested.[17,18] Table 102–4 provides a list of drugs commonly associated with weight gain. If no secondary cause exists, the presence of other cardiovascular risk factors and

Patient Encounter 1, Part 1

A 54-year-old woman presents to your weight loss clinic for an initial evaluation. She reports that her glucose was elevated upon screening while attending a community health fair. She followed up with her primary care provider who recommended weight loss as patient is unwilling to start metformin. She is not currently following any specific diet. She admits to eating foods high in sugar content, especially for breakfast. She routinely skips lunch and then snacks on potato chips, nuts, and sweetened beverages in the late afternoon. She frequently eats fast food for dinner as it is quick and requires no clean-up. Patient is recently divorced (1 year ago) and doesn't enjoy making dinner for one. This patient is not currently exercising but has adhered to a daily walking regimen in the past. The patient does not smoke or consume alcohol. Her BMI is 30.8 kg/m² and her waist circumference is 39 in (99 cm).

What classification of overweight and obesity is appropriate for this patient?

Does this patient have a high-risk waist circumference?

Does she have other risk factors that may contribute to morbidity or mortality?

What are the treatment goals for the patient?

What additional information do you need to know before creating a treatment plan for this patient?

Table 102–4

Drugs Contributing to Weight Gain

Anticonvulsants/mood stabilizers
- Carbamazepine
- Gabapentin
- Pregabalin
- Valproic acid
- Lithium

Antidepressants
- Monoamine oxidase inhibitors (phenelzine)
- Presynaptic α_2 antagonist (mirtazapine)
- Selective serotonin reuptake inhibitors (citalopram, escitalopram, fluvoxamine)
- Serotonin and norepinephrine reuptake inhibitors (duloxetine)
- Tricyclics (amitriptyline, imipramine)

Antidiabetics
- Insulin
- Meglintinides
- Sulfonylureas (glipizide, glyburide)
- Thiazolidinediones

Antipsychotics
- Atypical (clozapine, olanzapine, paliperidone, quetiapine, risperidone, ziprasidone)
- Conventional (haloperidol)

Others
- Antihistamines
- Corticosteroids
- Hormonal Contraceptives (depot injections)

Data from Refs. 17 and 18.

comorbidities must be determined to guide clinical decisions. Therapy implemented to minimize associated risk(s) may not enhance weight loss, but weight loss will positively address risk factors. Weight loss therapy should not be initiated in pregnant or lactating patients, decompensated psychiatric patients, or patients in whom reduced caloric intake can exacerbate an acute, serious illness.[2]

Four stages have been suggested for the treatment of obesity in children and adolescents. Stage 1 or Prevention Plus is the first step and includes adherence to healthy eating and activity habits. Patients should be encouraged to eat more than or equal to five servings of fruits and vegetables daily, limit consumption of sweetened drinks, decrease television or other screen time behaviors, and increase physical activity to greater than or equal to 1 hour/day. Stage 2 or Structured Weight Management incorporates Prevention Plus habits while setting specific eating and activity goals. Responsibilities include meal planning, observed physical activity or play daily for 1 hour, and documentation of energy consumption and expenditure. Comprehensive Multidisciplinary Interventions (Stage 3) is directed at increasing the intensity of healthy behaviors. To accomplish goals, the child or adolescent should work closely with the primary care provider, registered dietician, exercise specialist, and behavioral counselor. Stage 4, Tertiary Care Intervention, may be needed for severely obese adolescents. A very low-calorie diet, medication or weight control surgery may be warranted.[15]

Nonpharmacologic Therapy

Given that the imbalance between energy intake and energy expenditure is key factor for developing overweight and obesity, weight loss therapy requires the creation of an energy deficit. This may be achieved through daily caloric restriction and increased physical activity. Both therapeutic strategies are part of a comprehensive lifestyle intervention program as well as behavioral therapy to facilitate compliance diet and exercise. Comprehensive lifestyle intervention is foundational to weight loss and should be recommended for patients who have never participated in such a program. In addition, a comprehensive lifestyle intervention program is recommended for patients even when adjunctive therapy with medications or bariatric surgery have been implemented.[14]

▶ *Reduced-Calorie Diet*

Overall energy consumption and expenditure will determine the amount of weight alteration. Techniques to reduce dietary energy intake include adoption of a target energy intake less than that required for energy balance. This can usually be accomplished by reducing the energy intake by 500 kcal/day (2093 kJ/day) or greater. Recommend 1200–1500 or 1500–1800 kcals/day (5023–6279 or 6279–7534 kJ/day) for women and men, respectively. The choice of calorie-restricted diet is based on patient preference and current health status. A variety of diets, including but not limited to high protein, low carbohydrate, low fat, Mediterranean and American Heart Association (AHA) Step-1 diet, can result in weight loss if reduction in dietary intake is achieved.[14] The AHA Step-1 diet restricts daily calories to a range of 1000 to 1200 kcal (4186–5023 kJ/day) for women weighing less than 75 kg (165 lb) and 1400 to 1600 kcal (5860 6697 kJ/day) for all others. This daily limit should be considered after assessing a patient's normal daily caloric intake and ensuring that the initial caloric restriction does not exceed 500 to 1000 kcal (2093–4186 kJ/day). For example, a male patient who consumes 3000 kcal (12,557 kJ/day) should not reduce his daily caloric intake to less than 2000 kcal (8372 kJ/day) when initially implementing a dietary program. Further reduction to the target of 1600 kcal (6697 kJ/day) can be attempted when the patient has reduced calories successfully as initially recommended for a period agreeable by the practitioner and the patient.[2] Diets that are too restrictive in calorie reduction are successful initially but fail in the long term because compliance is difficult to sustain.[19] Therefore, this less aggressive approach promotes gradual weight loss and weight maintenance. Consultation with a dietician is recommended when implementing a healthy meal plan tailored to the individual's nutritional needs.

▶ *Increased Physical Activity*

Although diet and exercise contribute to weight loss, combining a reduced-calorie diet with increased physical activity results in greater weight loss compared with either therapy alone.[20] In addition, physical activity can help prevent weight regain and reduce related cardiovascular risks.[14] Slow titration of both the amount and intensity of aerobic physical activity is recommended for most patients.[2] A program that incorporates brisk walking daily is a viable option for most patients (Table 102–5). Suggest 10 minutes of physical activity 3 days/week with a target of no less than 30 minutes most days, if not every day.[2,14] Two hundred to 300 minutes per week of aerobic physical activity are recommended for weight maintenance or prevention of weight regain.[14]

▶ *Behavioral*

Nonadherence with recommended lifestyle changes may result in unsuccessful weight loss for adults.[14,20] Eliminating barriers through behavior modification is necessary to gain maximal benefit from both dietary modification and exercise. Successful behavioral therapy includes regular self-monitoring of food intake, physical activity, and weight.[14]

Targeted behaviors should be recommended to pediatric patients and their families because healthy habits help prevent excessive weight gain. These include, but are not limited to[15,16]:

- Limit the consumption of sugar-sweetened beverages.
- Limit the amount of screen time (television, computer, etc) to 2 hours or less per day.

Table 102–5

Summary of Approved Long-Term Pharmacologic Weight-Loss Agents

Drug	Class	Daily Dose (mg)
Orlistat[a]	Lipase inhibitor	360
Lorcaserin[b]	Serotonin 2C agonist	20
Phentermine-Topiramate[c]	Noradrenergic agent-antiepileptic	15/92
Naltrexone-Bupropion[d]	Opioid antagonist-antidepressant	8/90

[a]Efficacy and safety have not been determined beyond 4 years of use.

[b]Efficacy and safety have not been determined beyond 2 years of use.

[c]Efficacy and safety have not been determined beyond 1 years of use.

[d]Efficacy and safety have not been determined beyond 56 weeks of use.

Data from Refs. 23, 28, 30, and 31.

- Limit the number meals eaten at restaurants, especially those serving fast food.
- Parents should limit portion size when preparing and serving meals.

Pharmacologic Therapy

KEY CONCEPT *Pharmacotherapy in addition to comprehensive lifestyle intervention can be considered for patients with a BMI of 30 kg/m² or greater, or a BMI of 27 kg/m² or greater with other obesity-related risk factors.* Pharmacologic products promoting weight loss are classified according to their mechanisms of action, including the suppression of appetite and the suppression of fat absorption. Pharmacotherapy was indicated previously for short-term use; however, because obesity-related risks resurface with weight regain, long-term treatment may be necessary to minimize these sequelae. KEY CONCEPT *Weight will likely be regained if lifestyle changes are not continued indefinitely.* Four drugs are currently approved for long-term use in promoting weight loss and preventing weight regain.

▶ *Orlistat*

Orlistat promotes and maintains weight loss by acting locally in the GI tract. It inhibits pancreatic and gastric lipases, as well as triglyceride hydrolysis. As a result, undigested triglycerides are not absorbed, causing a caloric deficit and weight loss.[21]

Several studies have reported significant weight loss for adult patients receiving orlistat 120 mg three times a day compared with placebo.[22,23] Weight maintenance or prevention of weight regain has also been documented with continued orlistat use.[22,24]

Orlistat (120 mg three times daily) in combination with diet, exercise, and behavior modification resulted in a significant reduction in BMI and WC in adolescents. In addition, orlistat-treated subjects exhibited minimal weight increase after 1 year.[25]

The safety and efficacy of orlistat have not been determined beyond 4 years of use. Because orlistat acts locally in the GI tract, common side effects reported include oily spotting, flatus with discharge, fecal urgency, fatty or oily stools, oily evacuation, increased defecation, and fecal incontinence.[21] Other adverse events include bloating, abdominal pain, dyspepsia, nausea, vomiting, diarrhea, and headache.[26] Liver injury information is contained within orlistat's product label and includes signs, symptoms, and when to seek medical attention for severe liver disease. Signs and symptoms include itching, yellowing of the eyes or skin, dark urine, decreased appetite and light-colored stools. Orlistat should be stopped if the patient complains of these signs and symptoms. In addition, liver function tests, including aspartate transaminase (AST) and alanine aminotransferase (ALT), should be assessed.[27]

Orlistat reduces the absorption of some fat-soluble vitamins and β-carotene. Daily intake of a multivitamin containing fat-soluble vitamins, as well as β-carotene, is recommended. Patients should take the multivitamin 2 hours before or after the dose of orlistat.[21] Because the availability of vitamin K may decline in patients receiving orlistat therapy, close monitoring of coagulation status should occur with concomitant administration of warfarin.[21] Hypothyroidism has been observed in patients taking both orlistat and levothyroxine. Patients should take levothyroxine 4 hours before or after the orlistat dose and be monitored for changes in thyroid function. Administration of orlistat in conjunction with cyclosporine can result in decreased cyclosporine plasma levels. To avoid this interaction, cyclosporine should be taken 2 hours before or after the dose of orlistat. Additionally, cyclosporine levels should be monitored more frequently.[21]

Pregnant or lactating women should not take orlistat because no data exist to establish safety. Orlistat is contraindicated in patients with chronic malabsorption syndrome or cholestasis.[21]

Initiate orlistat 120 mg three times a day with a well-balanced but reduced-caloric meal containing no more than 30% of calories from fat. Orlistat may be taken during or up to 1 hour after the meal. If a meal is missed or contains little fat, the dose of orlistat may be omitted. Doses above 360 mg/day provide no greater benefit and thus are not recommended.[21]

▶ *Lorcaserin*

Lorcaserin, a 5-HT_{2C} agonist, promotes satiety and decreases food consumption; however, the exact mechanism is unknown. The safety and effectiveness of lorcaserin has been established in adults, however, no data exists for patients under the age of 18; therefore, pediatric use is not recommended.[28,29]

Common adverse reaction noted in the trials include headache, dizziness, fatigue, nausea, dry mouth, and constipation. Almost 30% of diabetic patients taking lorcaserin experienced hypoglycemia. Blood glucose should be monitored closely in patients taking an antidiabetic medication and lorcaserin.[28]

Because lorcaserin is a serotonergic drug, serotonin syndrome may occur if taken with other drugs affecting the serotonergic neurotransmitter systems including triptans, monoamine oxidase inhibitors (MAOI), selective serotonin reuptake inhibitors, serotonin-norepinephrine reuptake inhibitors, tricyclic antidepressants, bupropion, lithium, antipsychotics, St. John's wort, tryptophan, and dextromethorphan. If serotonin syndrome symptoms occur (agitation, hallucinations, tachycardia, hyperthermia, muscle rigidity, nausea/vomiting and diarrhea), discontinue lorcaserin immediately and initiate supportive care.[28]

Lorcaserin is contraindicated during pregnancy (Pregnancy Category X). Because it is unknown whether lorcaserin is excreted in human milk, the nursing mothers should avoid use while nursing or decide not to nurse.[28]

Initiate lorcaserin 10 mg twice daily in addition to a calorie-restricted diet and increased physical activity. The drug should be discontinued if the patient has not achieved a 5% weight loss by week 12 of treatment. Doses greater than 20 mg daily are not recommended and may result in the development of euphoria, altered mood, and hallucinations. Due to the potential for psychic dependence and abuse, lorcaserin is a federally controlled substance (CIV).[28]

▶ *Phentermine-topiramate*

Phentermine-topiramate is an extended-release combination product approved for weight loss. Phentermine decreases food intake by increasing norepinephrine and dopamine release in the central nervous system (CNS). Topiramate is an antiepileptic drug whose exact mechanism of action is unknown. It is thought to increase satiety and suppress appetite through multiple pathways.[30]

The safety and effectiveness of phentermine-topiramate have not been established in pediatric patients; therefore, its use is not recommended.[30]

Common adverse reactions include paresthesias, dizziness, **dysgeusia**, insomnia, constipation, and dry mouth. Phentermine-topiramate use is associated with increased heart rate. Monitor resting heart rate frequently and have patients report the presence of palpitations. Topiramate can increase a patient's risk for suicidal thoughts and behaviors. Patients should be monitored for worsening depression, thoughts of suicide, and unusual mood or behavior. Topiramate is also associated with acute myopia and secondary angle closure glaucoma. Patients should report decreased visual acuity and/or ocular pain. Phentermine-topiramate can cause mood disorders (depression and anxiety) and insomnia. Most resolve spontaneously but dose reduction or discontinuation of drug may be necessary. Cognitive impairment is also associated with use of phentermine-topiramate; patients should proceed with caution when operating hazardous machinery including driving a car until the extent of impairment is known. An increase in serum creatinine and decrease in both potassium and bicarbonate have been reported. Monitoring of serum electrolytes and creatinine are recommended at baseline and during therapy.[30]

Because topiramate is a known teratogen, use of phentermine-topiramate during pregnancy is contraindicated. All women of childbearing potential should have a documented negative pregnancy result before this drug is initiated and monthly while on therapy. Phentermine-topiramate may be excreted in human milk; nursing mothers should avoid use or discontinue nursing.[30]

Coadministration of phentermine-topiramate and MAOI could result in a hypertensive crisis. Do not initiate phentermine-topiramate within 14 days of MAOI discontinuation. Phentermine-topiramate used in patients taking an oral contraceptive may cause irregular bleeding but not an increased risk of pregnancy. Advise patients to not discontinue the oral contraceptives if spotting occurs. Alcohol can potentiate the CNS depressant effect; avoid concomitant use.[30]

Initiate phentermine-topiramate at a dose of 3.75 mg/23 mg daily for 14 days then increase to 7.5 mg/46 mg daily. Discontinue drug or increase the dose of phentermine-topiramate if a 3% weight loss is not achieved in 12 weeks. If the decision is made to increase the dose, recommend 11.25 mg/69 mg daily for 14 days then increase to 15 mg/92 mg daily. Discontinue drug if a 5% weight loss is not achieved after 12 weeks at the highest drug dose. Due to the potential for drug abuse, phentermine-topiramate is a federally controlled substance (CIV).[30]

► *Naltrexone-Bupropion*

Naltrexone-bupropion is an extended-release combination product approved for chronic weight management. The exact mechanisms by which this opioid antagonist/antidepressant combination product decreases food intake and weight are not fully known but involve two separate areas of the brain (hypothalamus and mesolimbic dopamine circuit).[31]

The safety and effectiveness of naltrexone-bupropion have not been established in patients less than 18 years; therefore, its use is not recommended.[31]

Patients taking this combination weight loss product should be monitored for emergence or worsening of suicidal thoughts and behaviors and neuropsychiatric reactions. Common adverse reactions include nausea, constipation, headache, vomiting, dizziness, and insomnia. This combination product is contraindicated in patients with elevated blood pressure, seizure disorders or in patients taking antiepileptics, in patients taking chronic opioids and in patients taking MAOI or discontinued MAOI use within 14 days. Bupropion inhibits CYP2D6 and can therefore increase the concentration of antidepressants, antipsychotics and β-blockers. When taken with a CYP2B6 inhibitor (eg, clopidogrel), the concentration of bupropion increases. Reduce maximum daily dose by half in these patients. CYP2B6 inducers may reduce bupropion efficacy.[31]

Naltrexone-bupropion is contraindicated during pregnancy as weight loss offers no benefit during pregnancy and potential for fetal harm (Pregnancy Category X). This drug is not recommended for nursing mothers.[31]

Each extended-release tablet contains 8 mg of naltrexone and 90 mg of bupropion. Patients should be advised to not cut, crush, or chew tablets. Patients should also avoid taking naltrexone-bupropion with high-fat meals to minimize the risk of enhanced bupropion absorption and subsequent seizure occurrence. To further reduce the risk of seizures, the dose must be titrated slowly. Initiate drug at one tablet every morning for 1 week, then one tablet twice daily (morning and evening) for 1 week, then two tablets in the morning and one tablet in the evening for 1 more week and then two tablets twice a day thereafter. If the patient has not lost 5% of baseline body weight following 12 weeks of maintenance therapy, naltrexone-bupropion should be discontinued.[31]

► *Phentermine*

As monotherapy, this drug is indicated for short-term use—no more than a few weeks—in addition to lifestyle modifications.[32] An average weight loss of 3.6 kg (7.9 lb) was demonstrated for patients treated with phentermine compared with placebo.[26]

Safety and efficacy have not been determined in pediatric patients less than 16 years of age.[32]

Common adverse reactions seen with phentermine use include heart palpitations, tachycardia, elevated blood pressure, stimulation, restlessness, dizziness, insomnia, **euphoria**, **dysphoria**, tremor, headache, dry mouth, constipation, and diarrhea. Phentermine should be avoided in patients with CVD, hypertension, hyperthyroidism and agitated states. Because phentermine is related to the amphetamines, the potential for abuse is high.[32]

Phentermine use should be avoided in patients concomitantly receiving or having received a MAOI within the preceding 14 days due to the potential for causing hypertensive crisis. Alcohol is not recommended for patients prescribed phentermine.[32]

The use of phentermine is contraindicated in pregnant patients as weight loss offers no benefit during pregnancy and risk of fetal harm (Pregnancy Category X). Owing to the potential for severe adverse effects in nursing infants, a decision to stop the drug or discontinue nursing must be made.[32]

Phentermine is available as an immediate- and a sustained-release product. In conjunction with a healthy lifestyle, 30 to 37.5 mg of phentermine is administered once daily, typically before breakfast or 1 to 2 hours after the morning meal. The dosage should be individualized; some patients may be managed adequately at 15 to 18.75 mg/day, but a dose of 18.75 mg twice daily may be used to minimize side effects, excluding insomnia. To lessen the risk of insomnia, dosing phentermine in the evening should be avoided.[32]

► *Diethylpropion*

This sympathomimetic amine exhibits similar pharmacologic activity as the amphetamines, resulting in CNS stimulation and appetite suppression and is indicated for short-term use in conjunction with a reduced-calorie diet and physical exercise.[33] The safety and effectiveness of diethylpropion have not been established in patients younger than 16 years; therefore, its use is not recommended.[33]

Use of diethylpropion for a period longer than 3 months is associated with an increased risk for development of pulmonary hypertension. When used as directed, reported common CNS adverse effects included overstimulation, restlessness, dizziness, insomnia, euphoria, dysphoria, tremor, headache, jitteriness, anxiety, nervousness, depression, drowsiness, malaise, **mydriasis**, and blurred vision. In addition, diethylpropion can decrease the seizure threshold. Other organ systems also can adversely be affected, resulting in tachycardia, elevated blood pressure, palpitations, dry mouth, abdominal discomfort, and constipation. Diethylpropion is contraindicated in patients with pulmonary hypertension, advanced arteriosclerosis, severe hypertension, hyperthyroidism, agitated states, or glaucoma. Because diethylpropion is related to the amphetamines, the potential for abuse is high.[33]

Use of diethylpropion should be avoided in patients receiving or having received an MAOI within the preceding 14 days to prevent hypertensive crisis. Combination with other anorectic agents should be avoided.[33]

No adequate studies have been conducted using diethylpropion in pregnant women; therefore, the drug should be used only if the benefit outweighs potential fetal risk. Use with caution in nursing mothers because the drug is excreted in breast milk.[33]

Diethylpropion is available as both an immediate- and a controlled-release product. In conjunction with a reduced-calorie diet and/or exercise, dose diethylpropion (immediate release) 25 mg three times a day before meals or 75 mg (controlled release) once a day, usually midmorning.[33]

▸ Phendimetrazine

Phendimetrazine's activity is similar to amphetamine. It suppresses appetite through stimulation of the CNS. Studies to determine efficacy were conducted over a few weeks and therefore long-term use is not indicated. Use in pregnancy has not been established; phendimetrazine should not be taken by women who are or may become pregnant. Phendimetrazine is not recommended for use in children younger than 12 years.[34]

Common adverse reactions observed in studies include heart palpitation, tachycardia, elevated blood pressure, overstimulation, restlessness, insomnia, agitation, dizziness, headache, psychotic state, blurred vision, mouth dryness, nausea, diarrhea, and constipation. Contraindications for use include advanced arteriosclerosis, symptomatic CVD, hypertension, hyperthyroidism, and glaucoma. Phendimetrazine is not recommended for patients taking other CNS stimulants including MAOI.[34]

If use is warranted, dose phendimetrazine (105 mg) in the morning, 30 to 60 minutes before the morning meal. Phendimetrazine is a federally controlled substance (CIII).[34]

▸ Surgical Intervention

KEY CONCEPT *Weight loss (bariatric) surgery is warranted when other treatment attempts have failed in severely obese patients (BMI of 40 kg/m² or greater, or 35 kg/m² or greater with obesity-related comorbidities).*[2,35] Several surgical techniques exist, however three are currently recognized as contemporary procedures: gastric bypass, which induces weight loss through both malabsorptive and restrictive mechanisms, sleeve gastrectomy and laparoscopic adjustable gastric banding (LAGB), which achieves weight loss through restriction of food intake only.[2,35]

Surgical options for obesity may produce a loss of two-thirds of excessive weight after 2 years that is sustained long term.[2] Additionally, favorable outcomes for obesity-related comorbid conditions are observed after surgery. When evaluating the various types of surgery available, long-term data suggests the average weight loss from gastric bypass after 15 years is 27%, which is significantly higher than banding (around 14%) and conventional therapy (2%).[36] Risk versus benefit must be considered as complications are inherent to any surgical procedure. The more common bariatric surgery complications are respiratory problems, wound formation, wound infections, hernia development, deep venous thrombosis, and pulmonary embolism. No differences were observed in mortality rates among various surgical procedures. Postoperative weight loss is much greater compared with pharmacologic therapies, but no comparative trials exist.[37]

Bariatric surgery is an alternative offered to adolescents because it results in substantial weight loss and medical health improvement, but also has the potential for serious complications.[38] Patients with a BMI greater than or equal to 40 kg/m² and an associated medical condition or BMI greater than or equal to 50 kg/m² at or after the age of 13 and 15 years for girls and boys, respectively; display emotional and cognitive maturity; and have implemented a behavioral-based weight-loss program are candidates for surgery.[16]

All patients undergoing bariatric surgery should be part of an comprehensive program of health education, diet, exercise, and behavioral modification before and after surgery.[2] Patients must understand and commit to a substantial change in eating patterns to maintain long-term weight reduction.[16,37]

Postoperatively, health care providers should also make considerations for medication management as these procedures may alter drug and nutrient absorption.[39]

- Medications should be transitioned to crushed or liquid formulations initially and until appropriate to restart solid dosage forms (likely variable).

Patient Encounter 1, Part 2: Medical History, Physical Exam, and Diagnostic Tests

PMH: Occasional lower back pain, occasional heartburn

FH: Father alive and 68 years of age. Mother also alive (age 65) with history of obesity

SH: (–) Tobacco, (–) alcohol

Meds: Ibuprofen 400 mg orally as needed, ranitidine 75 mg orally as needed

ROS: (+) Heartburn; (–) chest pain, nausea, vomiting, diarrhea, change in appetite, shortness of breath, or cough

PE:

VS: BP 120/84 mmHg, P 72 beats/min, RR 16 respirations/min, T 98.6° F (37.0°C), Wt 174 lb (79 kg), Ht 63 in (160 cm)

Waist Circumference: 39 in (99 cm)

CV: Normal S_1S_2; no murmurs, rubs, gallops

Abd: Obese, soft, nontender, nondistended; (+) bowel sounds

Ext: (–) Edema

Labs: All values are within normal limits except glucose (118 mg/dL [6.5 mmol/L]) and $HgbA_{1C}$ (6.0% [0.06 or 42 mmol/mol Hgb])

ECG: No evidence of past ischemia

Given this additional information, do you recommend weight loss? If so, how much weight should the patient lose and how fast?

What nonpharmacologic and pharmacologic alternatives are available for the patient?

- Certain medications should be avoided or used with caution (eg, NSAIDs, extended- or delayed-release products, oral bisphosphonates).
- Certain medications may be indicated (eg, fat soluble vitamins, iron, vitamin B_{12}).
- Alternative routes of administration may be considered.

OUTCOME EVALUATION

Successful management of overweight and obesity is determined by the ability the treatment plan has to (a) prevent weight gain, (b) reduce and maintain a lower body weight, and (c) decrease the risk of obesity-related comorbidities. Because weight is necessary to calculate the BMI, measure the patient's weight and WC. Obesity management may encompass more than weight loss or maintenance in the presence of other conditions; assess other pertinent parameters at baseline. This includes presence of hypertension, type 2 diabetes mellitus, hyperlipidemia, CVD, sleep apnea, hypothyroidism, osteoarthritis, gallbladder disease, gout, or cancer. Measure blood pressure and heart rate before implementation of any therapy, and assess basic metabolic panel, liver function tests, complete blood count, fasting lipid profile, full thyroid function tests, and other laboratory studies at baseline and as clinically indicated. Additionally, obtain an electrocardiogram if recent results are unknown.[2]

When considering various approaches to behavioral therapy for weight loss, in-person, high-intensity (defined as a minimum of 14 sessions within 6 months) behavioral therapy is the most effective. Sessions can be conducted by a pharmacist or trained interventionist for an individual or groups of patients. During each session, assess compliance with comprehensive lifestyle intervention, as well as measure weight, blood pressure, and heart rate. Measure WC intermittently. Identify presence of adverse drug reactions or drug interactions if weight loss medications have been initiated.[2,14]

Patient Encounter 2, Part 1

A 44-year-old white man presents to your CVD Risk Reduction Clinic. The patient currently denies chest pain, shortness of breath, dizziness, and lightheadedness. Upon review of previous progress notes, you discover that the patient's blood pressure has been elevated during the past three office visits. As a computer programmer, he finds himself sitting more than engaging in physical activity. He frequently eats fast food for lunch because the other guys in the office like to eat out. Evenings are spent watching TV and eating ice cream. The patient's BMI is 37.9 kg/m^2, and his waist circumference is 47 in (119 cm).

What classification of overweight and obesity is appropriate for this patient?

Does this patient have a high-risk waist circumference?

Does he have other risk factors that may contribute to morbidity or mortality?

What are the treatment goals for the patient?

What additional information do you need to know before creating a treatment plan for this patient?

Patient Encounter 2, Part 2: Medical History, Physical Exam, and Diagnostic Tests

PMH: Occasional headache

FH: Father alive and 78 years of age. Mother also alive and 77 years of age

SH: Drinks alcohol most days (socially) but denies any alcohol-related problems

Meds: None

ROS: (–) Heartburn, regurgitation; (–) chest pain, nausea, vomiting, diarrhea, change in appetite, shortness of breath, or cough

VS: BP 154/92 mmHg, P 92 beats/min, RR 15 respirations/min, T 98.7°F (37.1°C), Wt 228 lb (103.4 kg), Ht 65 in (165 cm)

Waist Circumference: 47 in (119 cm)

10-year CVD Risk: 5.3%

PE:

General: Well developed, in no acute distress

HEENT: Conjunctiva clear

CV: Regular rhythm, no S_3 or S_4 noted

Lungs: Clear to auscultation (CTA) bilaterally

Abd: Obese, soft, nontender, nondistended; (+) bowel sounds

Neuro: Normal gait, normal speech

Ext: (–) Edema

Labs: Na 142 mEq/L (142 mmol/L); K 4.6 mEq/L (4.6 mmol/L); Cl 107 mEq/L (107 mmol/L); CO_2 23 mEq/L (23 mmol/L); BUN 18 mg/dL (6.4 mmol/L); creatinine 0.9 mg/dL (80 μmol/L); glucose 72 mg/dL (4.0 mmol/L); TC 213 mg/dL (5.51 mmol/L); LDL 153 mg/dL (3.96 mmol/L); HDL 30 mg/dL (0.78 mmol/L); TG 152 mg/dL (1.72 mmol/L); AST 24 U/L (0.40 μkat/L); ALT 30 U/L (0.50 μkat/L)

Given this additional information, do you recommend weight loss? If so, how much weight should the patient lose and how fast?

What nonpharmacologic and pharmacologic options are available for the patient?

When the patient has achieved the recommended weight loss, he or she then enters the weight maintenance phase, which includes continued contact for education (no less than monthly), guidance, and risk factor assessment. Self-weighing, at least weekly, is associated with better weight maintenance over time. Counsel patient to address small weight gains before they become larger.[14]

If weight loss is not attained, further assess why the goals of therapy are unmet. Direct the interaction toward determining the motivation to lose weight, balance between caloric intake and physical activity, adherence to behavioral therapy, and determination of psychological stressors present.[2] Refer patient to a nutrition professional or for evaluation for bariatric surgery. If adjunctive pharmacotherapy has not been initiated, consider antiobesity drugs approved for long-term use.[2,14]

Patient Encounter 2, Part 3: CVD Risk Reduction 12-Week Follow-up Clinic Visit

The patient present for his 12-week follow-up visit in the CVD Risk Reduction Clinic. He states that he has been adhering to the Step-1 diet and currently jogs on a treadmill 30 minutes a day 2 days a week.

SH: Continues to drink three to four beers nightly

Meds: Lisinopril 10 mg orally every morning

ROS: (–) Heartburn, regurgitation; (–) chest pain, nausea, vomiting, diarrhea, change in appetite, shortness of breath, or cough

VS: BP 126/74 mmHg, P 84 beats/min, RR 16 breaths/min, T 98.5°F (36.9°C), Wt 221 lb (100.2 kg), Ht 65 in (165 cm)

Waist Circumference: 45 in (114)

PE:

General: Well developed, in no acute distress

HEENT: Conjunctiva clear

CV: Regular rhythm, no S_3 or S_4 noted

Lungs: CTA bilaterally

Abd: Obese, soft, nontender, nondistended; (+) bowel sounds

Neuro: Normal gait, normal speech

Ext: (–) Edema

Labs: Na 142 mEq/L (142 mmol/L); K 4.7 mEq/L (4.7 mmol/L); Cl 107 mEq/L (107 mmol/L); CO_2 23 mEq/L (23 mmol/L); BUN 18 mg/dL (6.4 mmol/L); creatinine 1.0 mg/dL (88 μmol/L); glucose 84 mg/dL (4.7 mmol/L); TC 218 mg/dL (5.64 mmol/L); LDL 155 mg/dL (4.01 mmol/L); HDL 34 mg/dL (0.88 mmol/L); TG 145 mg/dL (1.64 mmol/L); AST 20 U/L (33 μkat/L); ALT 32 U/L (0.53 μkat/L)

Calculate the patient's BMI.

What is the best weight loss option for the patient?

Patient Care Process

Patient Assessment:

- Measure weight and height.
- Calculate BMI.
- Classify BMI to identify patients at increased risk for CVD/other obesity-related conditions.
- Review medical history for secondary causes of weight gain.
- Conduct a medication history to identify drug therapy contributing to weight gain.
- Review laboratory data to identify secondary causes of weight gain, identify CVD risks and obesity-related comorbidities and to ensure safe use of medication.
- Assess current lifestyle and history of weight gain/loss over time.
- Assess need to lose weight (candidates include obese patients or overweight patients with at least one indicator of increased CVD risk:
  - Elevated WC, prediabetes or diabetes, hypertension, dyslipidemia, current cigarette smoker
- Assess readiness to make lifestyle changes.
- Determine weight loss goals.

Therapy Evaluation:

- Implement comprehensive lifestyle intervention strategies (restricted caloric-diet, increased physical activity, and behavioral therapy) with or without adjunctive therapies.
- If patient is already receiving an antiobesity medication, assess efficacy, safety, adherence, and potential drug interactions.
- Manage CVD risk factors such as hypertension, dyslipidemia, etc.

Care Plan Development:

- Implement comprehensive lifestyle intervention. If antiobesity drug is warranted, choose a medication for chronic obesity management that is deemed safe based on patient-specific parameters.
- Educate the patient regarding a comprehensive lifestyle intervention program, one that includes a balance between caloric intake and energy expenditure as well as suggest methods to modify behavior.
- Encourage self-weighing, at least weekly, for better weight loss and maintenance over time.

Follow-Up Evaluation:

- In 2 weeks, assess weight, blood pressure, heart rate, and adherence with comprehensive lifestyle intervention. Assess weight log.
- Patients should be reassessed in person no less than 14 times within a 6-month period.
- Once weight loss is achieved, continue contact with patient no less than monthly. Address small weight gains and continued adherence with comprehensive lifestyle intervention. Continually assess risk for CVD and address when necessary.

Abbreviations Introduced in This Chapter

ALT	Alanine aminotransferase
AST	Aspartate transaminase
BMI	Body mass index
CB_1	Cannabinoid receptor
CNS	Central nervous system
CVD	Cardiovascular disease
D1	Dopamine 1
D2	Dopamine 2
GI	Gastrointestinal
$5\text{-}HT_{1A}$	Serotonin 1A subtype
H_1	Histamine subtype 1
H_3	Histamine subtype 3
$5\text{-}HT_{2C}$	Serotonin 2C subtype
MAOI	Monoamine oxidase inhibitor

REFERENCES

1. CDC: Centers for Disease Control and Prevention. [Internet]. Atlanta, GA: Centers for Disease Control and Prevention. Defining Overweight and Obesity; 2010 Jun 21 [cited 2011 Oct 2]; [1 screen]. http://www.cdc.gov/nccdphp/dnpa/obesity/defining.htm
2. U.S. Department of Health and Human Services, NIH-NHLBI. Clinical guidelines on the identification, evaluation and treatment of overweight and obesity in adults. NIH publication no. 00–4084. Bethesda, MD: National Institutes of Health, 2000.
3. Lew EA, Garfinkel L. Variations in mortality by weight among 750,000 men and women. J Chronic Dis. 1979;23:563–576.
4. Flegal KM, Carroll MD, Kit BK, Ogden CL. Prevalence of obesity and trends in the distribution of body mass index among US adults, 1999-2010. JAMA. 2012;307:491–497.
5. Ogden CL, Carroll MD, Kit BK, Flegal KM. Prevalence of obesity and trends in body mass index among US children and adolescents, 1999–2010. JAMA. 2012;307:483–490.
6. Power C, Lake JK, Cole TJ. Body mass index and height from childhood to adulthood in the 1958 British born cohort. Am J Clin Nutr. 1997;66:1094–1101.
7. Freedman DS, Dietz WH, Srinivasan SR, et al. The relation of overweight to cardiovascular risk factors among children and adolescents: The Bogalusa heart study. Pediatrics. 1999;103:1175–1182.
8. Must A, Jacques PF, Dallal GE, et al. Long-term morbidity and mortality of overweight adolescents. A follow-up of the Harvard Growth Study of 1922 to 1935. N Engl J Med. 1992;327:1350–1355.
9. American Academy of Pediatrics Committee on Nutrition. Prevention of pediatric overweight and obesity. Pediatrics. 2003;112(2):424–430.
10. National Research Council. Committee on Diet and Health. Implications for reducing chronic disease risk. Washington, DC: National Academies Press, 1989.
11. Woods SC, Seeley RJ, Porte DJ, et al. Signals that regulate food intake and energy homeostasis. Science. 1998;280:1378–1383.
12. Lissner L, Levitsky DA, Strupp BJ, et al. Dietary fat and the regulation of energy intake in human subjects. Am J Clin Nutr. 1987;46:886–892.
13. Flier JS, Foster DW. Eating disorders: Obesity, anorexia nervosa, bulimia, nervosa. In: Wilson JD, Foster DW, Kronenberg HM, Larsen PR, eds. Williams' Textbook of Endocrinology, 9th ed. Philadelphia: WB Saunders, 1998:1061–1097.
14. Jenson MD, Ryan DH, Apovian CM, et al. 2013 AHA/ACC/TOS Guidelines for the management of overweight and obesity in adults: A report of the American College of Cardiology/American Heart Association Task Force on Practice Guidelines and the Obesity Society. Circulation. 2014;129:S1–S45.
15. Spear BA, Barlow SE, Ervin C, et al. Recommendations for treatment and adolescent overweight and obesity. Pediatrics. 2007;120(Suppl):S254–S288.
16. NICHQ: National Initiative for Children's Healthcare Quality. [Internet]. National Initiative for Children's Healthcare Quality. Expert committee recommendations on the assessment, prevention and treatment of child and adolescent overweight and obesity, dates unavailable [cited 2011 Oct 2]. http://www.nichq.org/documents/coan-papers-and-publications/COANImplementationGuide62607FINAL.pdf
17. Malone M. Medications associated with weight gain. Ann Pharmacother. 2005;39:2046–2055.
18. Sheehan AH. Weight gain. In: Tisdale JE, Miller DA, eds. Drug-Induced Diseases: Prevention, Detection and Management, 2nd ed. Bethesda, MD: American Society of Health-System Pharmacists; 2010.
19. Wadden TA, Foster DD, Letizia KA. One-year behavioral treatment of obesity: Comparison of moderate and severe caloric restriction and the effects of weight maintenance therapy. J Consult Clin Psychol. 1994;62:165–171.
20. Orzano AJ, Scott JG. Diagnosis and treatment of obesity in adults: an applied evidence-based review. J Am Board Fam Pract. 2004;17(5):359–369.
21. Roche Laboratories. Xenical (Orlistat) package insert. Nutley, NJ: Roche Laboratories, 2009 (January).
22. Sjöström L, Rissanen A, Andersen T, et al. Randomized placebo-controlled trial of orlistat for weight loss and prevention of weight regain in obese patients. Lancet. 1998;352:167–173.
23. Davidson MH, Hauptman J, DiGirolamo M, et al. Weight control and risk factor reduction in obese subjects treated for 2 years with orlistat: A randomized controlled trial. JAMA. 1999;281:235–242.
24. Hill JO, Hauptman J, Anderson JW, et al. Orlistat, a lipase inhibitory, for weight maintenance after conventional dieting: A 1-year study. Am J Clin Nutr. 1999;69:1108–1116.
25. Chapione JP, Hampl S, Jensen C, et al. Effect of orlistat on weight and body composition in obese adolescents: A randomized controlled trial. JAMA. 2005;293:2873–2883.
26. Li Z, Maglione M, Tu W, et al. Meta-analysis: Pharmacologic treatment of obesity. Ann Intern Med. 2005;142:532–546.
27. FDA: Food and Drug Administration. [Internet]. Silver Spring, MD: Food and Drug Administration. FDA Drug Safety Communication: Completed safety review of Xenical/Alli (orlistat) and severe liver injury; 2010 May 26 [cited 2011 Oct 2]; [1 screen]. http://www.fda.gov/Drugs/DrugSafety/PostmarketDrugSafetyInformationforPatientsandProviders/ucm213038.htm
28. Arena Pharmaceuticals. Lorcaserin (Belviq) package insert. Zofingen, Switzerland: Arena Pharmaceuticals, 2012 (August).
29. Smith SR, Weissman NJ, Anderson CM, et al. Behavioral modification and lorcaserin for overweight and obesity management (BLOOM) study group. Multi-center, placebo-controlled trial of lorcaserin for weight management. N Engl J Med. 2010;336(3):245–256.
30. Vivus, Inc. Phentermine-topiramate (Qsymia) package insert. Mountain View, CA. Vivus, Inc, 2013 (September).
31. Tekeda Pharmaceuticals America, Inc. Naltrexone-bupropion (Contrave) package insert. Deerfield, IL: Orexigen Therapeutics, 2014 (September).
32. Teva Pharmaceuticals. Adipex-P (Phentermine) package insert. Sellersville, PA: Teva Pharmaceuticals, 2012 (January).
33. Merrell Pharmaceuticals. Tenuate (Diethylpropion) package insert. Bridgewater, NJ: Merrell Pharmaceuticals, 2003 (November).

34. Valeant Pharmaceuticals North America. Bontril (Phendimetrazine) package insert. Aliso Viejo, CA; Valeant Pharmaceuticals North America. 2007 (March).
35. Snow V, Barry P, Fitterman N, et al. Pharmacologic and surgical management of obesity in primary care: A clinical practice guideline from the American College of Physicians. Ann Intern Med. 2005;142:525–531.
36. Sjöström L, Narbro K, Sjöström CD, et al. Effects of bariatric surgery on mortality in Swedish obese subjects. New Engl J Med. 357.8 (2007):741–752.
37. Maggard MA, Shugarman LR, Suttorp M, et al. Meta-analysis: Surgical treatment of obesity. Ann Intern Med. 2005;142:547–559.
38. Treadwell JR, Sun F, Schoelles K. Systematic review and meta-analysis of bariatric surgery for pediatric obesity. Ann Surg. 2008 Nov;248(5):763–776.
39. Stein J, et al. Review article: The nutritional and pharmacological consequences of obesity surgery. Aliment Pharmacol Ther. 2014; 40:582–609.

Appendix A: Conversion Factors and Anthropometrics*

CONVERSION FACTORS

SI Units

SI (*le Systéme International d'Unités*) units are used in many countries to express clinical laboratory and serum drug concentration data. Instead of using units of mass (eg, micrograms), the SI system uses moles (mol) to represent the amount of a substance. A molar solution contains 1 mole (the molecular weight of the substance in grams) of the solute in 1 L of solution. The following formula is used to convert units of mass to moles (mcg/mL to μmol/L or, by substitution of terms, mg/mL to mmol/L or ng/mL to nmol/L).

▸ *Micromoles per Liter*

$$\text{Micromoles per liter } (\mu\text{mol/L}) = \frac{\text{drug concentration (mcg/mL)} \times 1000}{\text{molecular weight of drug (g/mol)}}$$

▸ *Milliequivalents*

An equivalent weight of a substance is the weight that will combine with or replace 1 g of hydrogen; a milliequivalent is 1/1000 of an equivalent weight.

Milliequivalents per Liter

$$\text{Milliequivalents per liter (mEq/L)} = \frac{\text{weight of salt (g)} \times \text{valence of ion} \times 1000}{\text{molecular weight of salt}}$$

$$\text{Weight of salt (g)} = \frac{\text{mEq/L} \times \text{molecular weight of salt}}{\text{valence of ion} \times 1000}$$

Approximate Milliequivalents: Weight Conversions for Selected Ions

Salt	mEq/g Salt	mg Salt/mEq
Calcium carbonate ($CaCO_3$)	20.0	50.0
Calcium chloride ($CaCl_2 \cdot 2H_2O$)	13.6	73.5
Calcium gluceptate ($Ca[C_7H_{13}O_8]_2$)	4.1	245.2
Calcium gluconate ($Ca[C_6H_{11}O_7]_2 \cdot H_2O$)	4.5	224.1
Calcium lactate ($Ca[C_3H_5O_3]_2 \cdot 5H_2O$)	6.5	154.1
Magnesium gluconate ($Mg[C_6H_{11}O_7]_2 \cdot H_2O$)	4.6	216.3
Magnesium oxide (MgO)	49.6	20.2
Magnesium sulfate ($MgSO_4$)	16.6	60.2
Magnesium sulfate ($MgSO_4 \cdot 7H_2O$)	8.1	123.2
Potassium acetate ($K[C_2H_3O_2]$)	10.2	98.1
Potassium chloride (KCl)	13.4	74.6
Potassium citrate ($K_3[C_6H_5O_7] \cdot H_2O$)	9.2	108.1
Potassium iodide (KI)	6.0	166.0
Sodium acetate ($Na[C_2H_3O_2]$)	12.2	82.0
Sodium acetate ($Na[C_2H_3O_2] \cdot 3H_2O$)	7.3	136.1
Sodium bicarbonate ($NaHCO_3$)	11.9	84.0
Sodium chloride (NaCl)	17.1	58.4
Sodium citrate ($Na_3[C_6H_5O_7] \cdot 2H_2O$)	10.2	98.0
Sodium iodide (NaI)	6.7	149.9
Sodium lactate ($Na[C_3H_5O_3]$)	8.9	112.1
Zinc sulfate ($ZnSO_4 \cdot 7H_2O$)	7.0	143.8

Valences and Atomic/Molecular Weights of Selected Ions

Substance	Electrolyte	Valence	Atomic/Molecular Weight
Calcium	Ca^{2+}	2	40.1
Chloride	Cl^-	1	35.5
Magnesium	Mg^{2+}	2	24.3
Phosphate	HPO_4^{2-} (80%)	1.8	96.0[a]
(pH = 7.4)	$H_2PO_4^-$ (20%)		97.0
Potassium	K^+	1	39.1
Sodium	Na^+	1	23.0
Sulfate	SO_4^-	2	96.0[a]

[a]The atomic/molecular weight of phosphorus is only 31; that of sulfur is only 32.1.

*This appendix contains information from Appendices 1 and 2 of Smith KM, Riche DM, Henyan NN (eds.). Clinical Drug Data, 11th ed. New York: McGraw-Hill, 2010:1239–1246; With permission.

Anion Gap

The anion gap is the concentration of plasma anions not routinely measured by laboratory screening. It is useful in the evaluation of acid–base disorders. The anion gap is greater with increased plasma concentrations of endogenous species (eg, phosphate, sulfate, lactate, and ketoacids) or exogenous species (eg, salicylate, penicillin, ethylene glycol, ethanol, and methanol). The formulas for calculating the anion gap are as follows:

$$\text{Anion gap} = (Na^+ + K^+) - (Cl^- + HCO_3^-)$$

or

$$\text{Anion gap} = Na^+ - (Cl^- + HCO_3^-)$$

where the expected normal value for the first equation is 11 to 20 mmol/L and for the second equation is 7 to 16 mmol/L. Note that there is a variation in the upper and lower limits of the normal range.

Temperature

Fahrenheit to Centigrade: (°F – 32) × 5/9 = °C
Centigrade to Fahrenheit: (°C × 9/5) + 32 = °F
Centigrade to Kelvin: °C + 273 = °K

Weights and Measures

► *Metric Weight Equivalents*

1 kilogram (kg) = 1000 grams
1 gram (g) = 1000 milligrams
1 milligram (mg) = 0.001 gram
1 microgram (mcg, μg) = 0.001 milligram
1 nanogram (ng) = 0.001 microgram
1 picogram (pg) = 0.001 nanogram
1 femtogram (fg) = 0.001 picogram

► *Metric Volume Equivalents*

1 liter (L) = 1000 milliliters
1 deciliter (dL) = 100 milliliters
1 milliliter (mL) = 0.001 liter
1 microliter (μL) = 0.001 milliliter
1 nanoliter (nL) = 0.001 microliter
1 picoliter (pL) = 0.001 nanoliter
1 femtoliter (fL) = 0.001 picoliter

► *Apothecary Weight Equivalents*

1 scruple (℈) = 20 grains (gr)
60 grains (gr) = 1 dram (ʒ)
8 drams (ʒ) = 1 ounce (℥)
1 ounce (℥) = 480 grains (gr)
12 ounces (℥) = 1 pound (lb)

► *Apothecary Volume Equivalents*

60 minims (m) = 1 fluidram (fl ʒ)
8 fluidrams (fl ʒ) = 1 fluid ounce (fl ℥)
1 fluid ounce (fl ℥) = 480 minims (m)
16 fluid ounces (fl ℥) = 1 pint (pt)

► *Avoirdupois Equivalents*

1 ounce (oz) = 437.5 grains
16 ounces (oz) = 1 pound (lb)

► *Weight/Volume Equivalents*

1 mg/dL = 10 mcg/mL
1 mg/dL = 1 mg%
1 ppm = 1 mg/L

► *Conversion Equivalents*

1 gram (g) = 15.43 grains (gr)
1 grain (gr) = 64.8 milligrams (mg)
1 ounce (℥) = 31.1 grams (g)
1 ounce (oz) = 28.35 grams (g)
1 pound (lb) = 453.6 grams (g)
1 kilogram (kg) = 2.2 pounds (lb)
1 milliliter (mL) = 16.23 minims (m)
1 minim (m) = 0.06 milliliter (mL)
1 fluid ounce (fl oz) = 29.57 milliliters (mL)
1 pint (pt) = 473.2 milliliters (mL)
1 US gallon = 3.78 liters (L)
1 Canadian gallon = 4.55 liters (L)
0.1 milligram = 1/650 grain
0.12 milligram = 1/540 grain
0.15 milligram = 1/430 grain
0.2 milligram = 1/320 grain
0.3 milligram = 1/220 grain
0.4 milligram = 1/160 grain
0.5 milligram = 1/130 grain
0.6 milligram = 1/110 grain
0.8 milligram = 1/80 grain
1 milligram = 1/65 grain

► *Metric Length Conversion Equivalents*

2.54 cm = 1 inch
30.48 cm = 1 foot
1 m = 3.28 feet
1.6 km = 1 mile

ANTHROPOMETRICS

Creatinine Clearance Formulas

► *Formulas for Estimating Creatinine Clearance in Patients with Stable Renal Function*

Cockcroft-Gault Formula

Adults (age 18 years and older)[1]:

$$\text{CrCl (men)} = \frac{(140 - \text{age}) \times \text{weight}}{\text{SCr} \times 72}$$

$$\text{CrCl (women)} = 0.85 \times \text{above value}^*$$

*Some studies suggest that the predictive accuracy of this formula for women is better *without* the correction factor of 0.85.

where CrCl is creatinine clearance (in mL/min), SCr is serum creatinine (in mg/dL [or μmol/L divided by 88.4]), age is in years, and weight is in kilograms.

Traub-Johnson Formula

Children (age 1–18 years)[2]:

$$\text{CrCl} = \frac{0.48 \times \text{height} \times \text{BSA}}{\text{SCr} \times 1.73}$$

where BSA is body surface area (in m^2), CrCl is creatinine clearance (in mL/min), SCr is serum creatinine (in mg/dL [or μmol/L divided by 88.4]), and height is in centimeters.

▸ *Formula for Estimating Creatinine Clearance From a Measured Urine Collection*

$$\text{CrCl (mL/min)} = \frac{U \times V}{P \times T}$$

where U is the concentration of creatinine in a urine specimen in mg/dL, V is the volume of urine in mL, P is the concentration of creatinine in serum at the midpoint of the urine collection period in mg/dL, and T is the time of the urine collection period in minutes (eg, 6 hours = 360 minutes; 24 hours = 1440 minutes). Procedures for obtaining urine specimens should stress the importance of complete urine collection during the collection time period.

▸ *IDMS-Traceable MDRD Equation (Used for Creatinine Methods with Calibration Traceable to IDMS)*

For creatinine in mg/dL:

$$X = 175 \times \text{creatinine}^{-1.154} \times \text{age}^{-0.203} \times \text{constant}$$

For creatinine in μmol/L:

$$X = 175 \times (\text{creatinine}/88.4)^{-1.154} \times \text{age}^{-0.203} \times \text{constant}$$

where X is the glomerular filtration rate, constant for white men is 1 and for women is 0.742, and constant for African Americans is 1.212.

Ideal Body Weight

IBW is the weight expected for a non-obese person of a given height. The IBW formulas below and various life insurance tables can be used to estimate IBW. Dosing methods described in the literature may use IBW as a method in dosing obese patients.

Adults (age 18 years and older)[3]:

$$\text{IBW (men)} = 50 + (2.3 \times \text{height in inches over 5 ft})$$

$$\text{IBW (women)} = 45.5 + (2.3 \times \text{height in inches over 5 ft})$$

where IBW is in kilograms.

Children (age 1–18 years)[2] under 5-feet tall:

$$\text{IBW} = \frac{\text{height}^2 \times 1.65}{1000}$$

where IBW is in kilograms and height is in centimeters.

Children (age 1–18 years) 5 feet or taller:

$$\text{IBW (males)} = 39 + (2.27 \times \text{height in inches over 5 ft})$$

$$\text{IBW (females)} = 42.2 + (2.27 \times \text{height in inches over 5 ft})$$

where IBW is in kilograms.

REFERENCES

1. Cockcroft DW, Gault MH. Prediction of creatinine clearance from serum creatinine. Nephron. 1976;16:31–41.
2. Traub SI, Johnson CE. Comparison of methods of estimating creatinine clearance in children. Am J Hosp Pharm. 1980;37: 195–201.
3. Devine BJ. Gentamicin therapy. Drug Intell Clin Pharm. 1974; 8:650–655.

Appendix B: Common Medical Abbreviations

These are the abbreviations used commonly in medical practice both in verbal communication and in the medical record.

A&O	alert and oriented
A&O×3	awake (or alert) and oriented to person, place, and time
A&O×4	awake (or alert) and oriented to person, place, time, and situation
A&P	active and present; anterior and posterior; assessment and plans; auscultation and percussion
A&W	alive and well
A1c	hemoglobin A1c
AA	aplastic anemia; Alcoholics Anonymous
AAA	abdominal aortic aneurysm
AAO	awake, alert, and oriented
AAO×3	awake and orientated to time, place, and person
ABC	absolute band counts; absolute basophil count; apnea, bradycardia, and cytology; aspiration, biopsy, and cytology; artificial beta cells
Abd	abdomen
ABG	arterial blood gases
ABO	blood group system (A, AB, B, and O)
ABP	arterial blood pressure
ABW	actual body weight
ABx	antibiotics
AC	before meals (*ante cibos*)
ACE	angiotensin-converting enzyme
ACE-I	angiotensin-converting enzyme inhibitor
ACLS	advanced cardiac life support
ACS	acute coronary syndromes
ACTH	adrenocorticotropic hormone
AD	Alzheimer disease; right ear (*auris dextra*)
ADA	American Diabetes Association; adenosine deaminase
ADE	adverse drug effect (or event)
ADH	antidiuretic hormone
ADHD	attention-deficit hyperactivity disorder
ADL	activities of daily living
ADR	adverse drug reaction
AF	atrial fibrillation
AFB	acid-fast bacillus; aortofemoral bypass; aspirated foreign body
AFEB	afebrile
AI	aortic insufficiency
AIDS	acquired immune deficiency syndrome
AKA	above-knee amputation; alcoholic ketoacidosis; all known allergies; also known as
AKI	acute kidney injury
ALFT	abnormal liver function test
ALL	acute lymphoblastic leukemia; acute lymphocytic leukemia
ALP	alkaline phosphatase
ALS	amyotrophic lateral sclerosis
ALT	alanine transaminase (SGPT); alanine aminotransferase
AMA	against medical advice; American Medical Association; antimitochondrial antibody
AMI	acute myocardial infarction
AML	acute myelogenous leukemia
Amp	ampule
ANA	antinuclear antibody
ANC	absolute neutrophil count
ANLL	acute nonlymphocytic leukemia
AODM	adult-onset diabetes mellitus
AOM	acute otitis media
AP	anteroposterior
APAP	acetaminophen (acetyl-*p*-aminophenol)
aPTT	activated partial thromboplastin time
ARB	angiotensin receptor blocker
ARC	AIDS-related complex
ARD	acute respiratory disease; adult respiratory disease; antibiotic removal device; aphakic retinal detachment
ARDS	adult respiratory distress syndrome
ARF	acute renal failure; acute respiratory failure; acute rheumatic fever
AROM	active range of motion
AS	left ear (*auris sinistra*)
ASA	aspirin (acetylsalicylic acid)
ASCVD	arteriosclerotic cardiovascular disease
ASD	atrial septal defect
ASH	asymmetric septal hypertrophy
ASHD	arteriosclerotic heart disease
AST	aspartate transaminase (SGOT); aspartate aminotransferase
ATG	antithymocyte globulin
ATN	acute tubular necrosis
AU	each ear (*auris uterque*)
AV	arteriovenous; atrioventricular; auditory visual

AVR	aortic valve replacement
BBB	bundle branch block; blood–brain barrier
BC	blood culture
BCOP	Board Certified Oncology Pharmacist
BCP	birth control pill
BCPP	Board Certified Psychiatric Pharmacist
BCPS	Board Certified Pharmacotherapy Specialist
BE	barium enema
BG	blood glucose
bid	twice daily (*bis in die*)
BKA	below-knee amputation
BM	bone marrow; bowel movement; an isoenzyme of creatine phosphokinase
BMC	bone marrow cells
BMD	bone mineral density
BMI	body mass index
BMP	basic metabolic panel
BMR	basal metabolic rate
BMT	bone marrow transplantation
BP	blood pressure
BPD	bronchopulmonary dysplasia
BPH	benign prostatic hyperplasia
bpm	beats per minute
BR	bed rest
BS	bowel sounds; breath sounds; blood sugar
BSA	body surface area
BUN	blood urea nitrogen
Bx	biopsy
C&S	culture and sensitivity
CA	cancer; calcium
CABG	coronary artery bypass grafting
CAD	coronary artery disease
CAH	chronic active hepatitis
CAM	complementary and alternative medicine
CAPD	continuous ambulatory peritoneal dialysis
CBC	complete blood count
CBD	common bile duct
CBG	capillary blood gas; corticosteroid-binding globulin
CC	chief complaint
CCA	calcium channel antagonist
CCB	calcium channel blocker
CCE	clubbing, cyanosis, edema
CCK	cholecystokinin
CCU	coronary care unit
CF	cystic fibrosis
CFS	chronic fatigue syndrome
CFU	colony-forming unit
CHD	coronary heart disease
CHF	congestive heart failure; chronic heart failure
CHO	carbohydrate
CI	cardiac index
CIWA	Clinical Institute Withdrawal Assessment
CK	creatine kinase
CKD	chronic kidney disease
CLL	chronic lymphocytic leukemia
CM	costal margin
CMG	cystometrogram
CML	chronic myelogenous leukemia
CMV	cytomegalovirus
CN	cranial nerve
CNS	central nervous system

C/O	complains of
CO	cardiac output; carbon monoxide
COLD	chronic obstructive lung disease
COPD	chronic obstructive pulmonary disease
CP	chest pain; cerebral palsy
CPAP	continuous positive airway pressure
CPK	creatine phosphokinase (BB, MB, and MM are isoenzymes)
CPP	cerebral perfusion pressure
CPR	cardiopulmonary resuscitation
CrCl	creatinine clearance
CRF	chronic renal failure; corticotropin-releasing factor
CRH	corticotropin-releasing hormone
CRI	chronic renal insufficiency; catheter-related infection
CRNA	Certified Registered Nurse Anesthetist
CRNP	Certified Registered Nurse Practitioner
CRP	C-reactive protein
CRTT	Certified Respiratory Therapy Technician
CSF	cerebrospinal fluid; colony-stimulating factor
CT	computed tomography; chest tube
cTnI	cardiac troponin I
CTZ	chemoreceptor trigger zone
CV	cardiovascular
CVA	cerebrovascular accident
CVC	central venous catheter
CVP	central venous pressure
Cx	culture; cervix
CXR	chest x-ray
CYP	cytochrome P450
D&C	dilatation and curettage
D_5W	5% dextrose in water
DBP	diastolic blood pressure
D/C	discontinue; discharge
DCC	direct-current cardioversion
DI	diabetes insipidus
DIC	disseminated intravascular coagulation
Diff	differential
DJD	degenerative joint disease
DKA	diabetic ketoacidosis
dL	deciliter
DM	diabetes mellitus
DNA	deoxyribonucleic acid
DNR	do not resuscitate
DO	Doctor of osteopathy
DOA	dead on arrival; date of admission; duration of action
DOB	date of birth
DOE	dyspnea on exertion
DOT	directly observed therapy
DPGN	diffuse proliferative glomerulonephritis
DPI	dry powder inhaler
DRE	digital rectal examination
DRG	diagnosis-related group
DS	double strength
d/t	due to
DTP	diphtheria–tetanus–pertussis
DTR	deep tendon reflex
DVT	deep vein thrombosis
Dx	diagnosis
EBV	Epstein-Barr virus

EC	enteric coated
ECF	extracellular fluid
ECG	electrocardiogram
ECHO	echocardiogram
ECT	electroconvulsive therapy
ED	emergency department
EEG	electroencephalogram
EENT	eyes, ears, nose, throat
EF	ejection fraction
EGD	esophagogastroduodenoscopy
EIA	enzyme immunoassay
ECG	electrocardiogram
EMG	electromyogram
EMT	Emergency Medical Technician
Endo	endotracheal, endoscopy
EOMI	extraocular movements (or muscles) intact
EPO	erythropoietin
EPS	extrapyramidal symptoms
ER	emergency room
ERCP	endoscopic retrograde cholangiopancreatography
ERT	estrogen replacement therapy
ESKD	end-stage kidney disease
ESLD	end-stage liver disease
ESR	erythrocyte sedimentation rate
ESRD	end-stage renal disease
ET	endotracheal
EtOH	ethanol
FB	finger breadth; foreign body
FBS	fasting blood sugar
FDA	Food and Drug Administration
FEF	forced expiratory flow rate
FEV_1	forced expiratory volume in 1 second
FFP	fresh-frozen plasma
FH	family history
FiO_2	fraction of inspired oxygen
FOBT	fecal occult blood test
FPG	fasting plasma glucose
FPIA	fluorescence polarization immunoassay
FSH	follicle-stimulating hormone
FTA	fluorescent treponemal antibody
FT_4	free thyroxine
F/U	follow-up
FUO	fever of unknown origin
Fx	fracture
g	gram
G-CSF	granulocyte colony-stimulating factor
G6PD	glucose-6-phosphate dehydrogenase
GB	gallbladder
GBS	group B *Streptococcus*; Guillain-Barré syndrome
GC	gonococcus
GDM	gestational diabetes mellitus
GE	gastroesophageal; gastroenterology
GERD	gastroesophageal reflux disease
GFR	glomerular filtration rate
GGT	γ-glutamyl transferase
GGTP	γ-glutamyl transpeptidase
GI	gastrointestinal
GM-CSF	granulocyte-macrophage colony-stimulating factor
GN	glomerulonephritis; graduate nurse
gr	grain
GT	gastrostomy tube
gtt	drops (*guttae*)
GTT	glucose tolerance test
GU	genitourinary
GVHD	graft-versus-host disease
GVL	graft-versus-leukemia
Gyn	gynecology
H&H, H/H	hemoglobin and hematocrit
H&P	history and physical examination
HA	headache
HAART	highly active antiretroviral therapy
HAMD	Hamilton Rating Scale for Depression
HAV	hepatitis A virus
Hb, hgb	hemoglobin
HbA1c	glycosylated hemoglobin (hemoglobin A1c)
HBIG	hepatitis B immune globulin
HBP	high blood pressure
HBsAg	hepatitis B surface antigen
HBV	hepatitis B virus
HC	hydrocortisone, home care
HCG	human chorionic gonadotropin
HCO_3	bicarbonate
Hct	hematocrit
HCTZ	hydrochlorothiazide
HCV	hepatitis C virus
HD	Hodgkin's disease; hemodialysis
HDL	high-density lipoprotein
HEENT	head, eyes, ears, nose, and throat
HF	heart failure
HFA	hydrofluoroalkane
H flu	*Hemophilus influenzae*
HGH	human growth hormone
HH	hiatal hernia
Hib	*Hemophilus influenzae* type b
HIT	heparin-induced thrombocytopenia
HIV	human immunodeficiency virus
HJR	hepatojugular reflux
HLA	human leukocyte antigen; human lymphocyte antigen
HMG-CoA	hydroxy-methylglutaryl coenzyme A
H/O	history of
HOB	head of bed
HPA	hypothalamic–pituitary axis
hpf	high-power field
HPI	history of present illness
HR	heart rate
H_2RA	H_2 receptor antagonist
HRSD	Hamilton Rating Scale for Depression
HRT	hormone-replacement therapy
HS	at bedtime (*hora somni*)
HSV	herpes simplex virus
HTN	hypertension
Hx	history
I&D	incision and drainage
I&O, I/O	intake and output
IBD	inflammatory bowel disease
IBW	ideal body weight
ICD	implantable cardioverter defibrillator
ICP	intracranial pressure
ICS	intercostal space; inhaled corticosteroid
ICU	intensive care unit

ID	identification; infectious disease
IDDM	insulin-dependent diabetes mellitus
IFN	interferon
Ig	immunoglobulin
IgA	immunoglobulin A
IgD	immunoglobulin D
IHD	ischemic heart disease
IJ	internal jugular
IM	intramuscular; infectious mononucleosis
INH	isoniazid
INR	international normalized ratio
IOP	intraocular pressure
IP	intraperitoneal
IPG	impedance plethysmography
IPN	interstitial pneumonia
IRB	institutional review board
ISA	intrinsic sympathomimetic activity
ISH	isolated systolic hypertension
IT	intrathecal
ITP	idiopathic thrombocytopenic purpura
IU	international units (this can be dangerous abbreviation because it may be read as "IV" for "intravenous")
IUD	intrauterine device
IV	intravenous; Roman numeral four; symbol for class 4 controlled substances
IVC	inferior vena cava; intravenous cholangiogram
IVDA	intravenous drug abuse
IVDU	injection drug use; intravenous drug use
IVF	intravenous fluids
IVIG	intravenous immunoglobulin
IVP	intravenous pyelogram; intravenous push
JODM	juvenile-onset diabetes mellitus
JRA	juvenile rheumatoid arthritis
JVD	jugular venous distension
JVP	jugular venous pressure
K	potassium
kcal	kilocalorie
KCl	potassium chloride
KOH	potassium hydroxide
KUB	kidney, ureter, and bladder
KVO	keep vein open
L	liter
LABA	long-acting beta agonist
LAD	left anterior descending; left axis deviation
LAO	left anterior oblique
LBBB	left bundle branch block
LBP	low-back pain
LDH	lactate dehydrogenase
LDL	low-density lipoprotein
LE	lower extremity
LES	lower esophageal sphincter
LFT	liver function test
LHRH	luteinizing hormone-releasing hormone
LLE	left lower extremity
LLL	left lower lobe
LLQ	left lower quadrant (abdomen)
LMD	local medical doctor
LMP	last menstrual period
LMWH	low-molecular-weight heparin
LOS	length of stay
LP	lumbar puncture
LPN	Licensed Practical Nurse
LPT	Licensed Physical Therapist
LR	lactated Ringer's
LS	lumbosacral
LT_4	levothyroxine
LUE	left upper extremity
LUL	left upper lobe
LUQ	left upper quadrant
LUTS	lower urinary tract symptoms
LVH	left ventricular hypertrophy
MAP	mean arterial pressure
MAR	medication administration record
MB-CK	a creatine kinase isoenzyme
mcg	microgram
MCH	mean corpuscular hemoglobin
MCHC	mean corpuscular hemoglobin concentration
MCV	mean corpuscular volume
MD	Medical Doctor
MDI	metered-dose inhaler
MDRD	modification of diet in renal disease
MEFR	maximum expiratory flow rate
mEq	milliequivalent
mg	milligram
MHC	major histocompatibility complex
MI	myocardial infarction; mitral insufficiency
MIC	minimum inhibitory concentration
mL	milliliter
MM	multiple myeloma; an isoenzyme of creatine phosphokinase
MMR	measles–mumps–rubella; midline malignant reticulosis
MOM	milk of magnesia
MPV	mean platelet volume
m/r/g	murmur/rub/gallop
MRI	magnetic resonance imaging
MRSA	methicillin-resistant *Staphylococcus aureus*
MRSE	methicillin-resistant *Staphylococcus epidermitis*
MS	mental status; mitral stenosis; musculoskeletal; multiple sclerosis; morphine sulfate
MSE	mental status exam
MSW	Master of Social Work
MTD	maximum tolerated dose
MTX	methotrexate
MVA	motor vehicle accident
MVI	multivitamin
MVR	mitral valve replacement; mitral valve regurgitation
MVS	mitral valve stenosis; motor, vascular, and sensory
N&V	nausea and vomiting
NAD	no acute (or apparent) distress
N/C	noncontributory; nasal cannula
NG	nasogastric
NGT	nasogastric tube; normal glucose tolerance
NIDDM	non–insulin-dependent diabetes mellitus
NIH	National Institutes of Health
NKA	no known allergies
NKDA	no known drug allergies
NHDA	nonketotic hyperosmolar acidosis
NL	normal
NOS	not otherwise specified
NPN	nonprotein nitrogen

NPO	nothing by mouth (*nil per os*)
NS	normal saline solution (0.9% sodium chloride solution); neurosurgery
NSAID	nonsteroidal anti-inflammatory drug
NSR	normal sinus rhythm
NSS	normal saline solution
NTG	nitroglycerin
NT/ND	nontender, nondistended
NVD	nausea/vomiting/diarrhea; neck vein distension; neovascularization of the disk; neurovesicle dysfunction; nonvalvular disease
N&V	nausea and vomiting
NYHA	New York Heart Association
O&P	ova and parasites
OA	osteoarthritis
OB	obstetrics
OCD	obsessive-compulsive disorder
OD	right eye (*oculus dexter*)
OGTT	oral glucose tolerance test
OPV	oral poliovirus vaccine
OR	operating room
OR×1	oriented to time
OR×2	oriented to time and place
OR×3	oriented to time, place, and person
OS	left eye (*oculus sinister*)
OSA	obstructive sleep apnea
OT	occupational therapy
OTC	over the counter
OU	each eye (*oculus uterque*)
P	pulse; plan; percussion; pressure
P&A	percussion and auscultation
P&T	peak and trough
PA	physician assistant; posteroanterior; pulmonary artery
PAC	premature atrial contraction
$Paco_2$	arterial carbon dioxide tension
Pao_2	arterial oxygen tension
PAOP	pulmonary artery occlusion pressure
PC	after meals (*post cibum*)
PCA	patient-controlled analgesia
PCI	percutaneous coronary intervention
PCKD	polycystic kidney disease
PCN	penicillin
PCP	*Pneumocystis carinii* pneumonia (also known as *Pneumocystis jirovecii* pneumonia); pneumocystis pneumonia; primary care physician; phencyclidine
PCWP	pulmonary capillary wedge pressure
PDE	paroxysmal dyspnea on exertion
PE	physical examination; pulmonary embolism
PEEP	positive end-expiratory pressure
PEFR	peak expiratory flow rate
PEG	percutaneous endoscopic gastrostomy; polyethylene glycol
Peg-IFN	pegylated interferon
PERL	pupils equal, reactive to light
PERRLA	pupils equal, round, and reactive to light and accommodation
PERRRLA	pupils equal, round, regular, and reactive to light and accommodation
PET	positron emission tomography
PFT	pulmonary function test
pH	hydrogen ion concentration
PH	past history; personal history; pinhole; poor health; pubic hair; public health
PHx	past history
PharmD	Doctor of Pharmacy
PID	pelvic inflammatory disease
PJD	*Pneumocystis jirovecii* pneumonia (also known as *Pneumocystis carinii* pneumonia)
PKU	phenylketonuria
PMH	past medical history
PMI	past medical illness; point of maximal impulse
PMN	polymorphonuclear leukocyte
PMS	premenstrual syndrome
PND	paroxysmal nocturnal dyspnea
Po	by mouth (*per os*)
Po_2	partial pressure of oxygen
POAG	primary open-angle glaucoma
POD	postoperative day
PPBG	postprandial blood glucose
ppd	packs per day
PPI	proton pump inhibitor
PPN	peripheral parenteral nutrition
PR	per rectum
PRBC	packed red blood cell
PRERLA	pupils round, equal, reactive to light and accommodation
PRN	when necessary, as needed (*pro re nata*)
PSA	prostate-specific antigen
PSH	past surgical history
PST	paroxysmal supraventricular tachycardia
PSVT	paroxysmal supraventricular tachycardia
PT	prothrombin time; physical therapy; patient
PTA	prior to admission; percutaneous transluminal angioplasty
PTCA	percutaneous transluminal coronary angioplasty
PTE	pulmonary thromboembolism
PTH	parathyroid hormone
PTSD	posttraumatic stress disorder
PTT	partial thromboplastin time
PUD	peptic ulcer disease
PVC	premature ventricular contraction
PVD	peripheral vascular disease
PVR	peripheral vascular resistance
PVT	paroxysmal ventricular tachycardia
q	every (*quaque*)
QA	quality assurance
qday	every day (*quaque die*)
QI	quality improvement
qid	four times daily (*quater in die*)
QNS	quantity not sufficient
qod	every other day
QOL	quality of life
QS	quantity sufficient
QTc	corrected QT interval
R&M	routine and microscopic
R&R	rate and rhythm
RA	rheumatoid arthritis; right atrium
RAAS	renin–angiotensin–aldosterone system
RBC	red blood cell
RCA	right coronary artery

RCM	right costal margin
RDA	recommended daily allowance
RDS	respiratory distress syndrome
RDW	red blood cell distribution width
REM	rapid eye movement; recent event memory
RES	reticuloendothelial system
RF	rheumatoid factor; renal failure; rheumatic fever
Rh	rhesus factor in blood
RHD	rheumatic heart disease
RLE	right lower extremity
RLL	right lower lobe
RLQ	right lower quadrant
RML	right middle lobe
RN	Registered Nurse
RNA	ribonucleic acid
R/O	rule out
ROM	range of motion
ROS	review of systems
RPh	Registered Pharmacist
RR	respiratory rate; recovery room
RRR	regular rate and rhythm
RRT	Registered Respiratory Therapist
RSV	respiratory syncytial virus
RT	radiation therapy
RUE	right upper extremity
RUL	right upper lobe
RUQ	right upper quadrant
RVH	right ventricular hypertrophy
S_1	first heart sound
S_2	second heart sound
S_3	third heart sound (ventricular gallop)
S_4	fourth heart sound (atrial gallop)
SA	sinoatrial
SABA	short-acting beta agonist
SAD	seasonal affective disorder
SAH	subarachnoid hemorrhage
Sao_2	arterial oxygen percent saturation
SBE	subacute bacterial endocarditis
SBFT	small bowel follow-through
SBGM	self-blood glucose monitoring
SBO	small bowel obstruction
SBP	systolic blood pressure
SC	subcutaneous; subclavian
SCr	serum creatinine
SEM	systolic ejection murmur
SG	specific gravity
SGOT (AST)	serum glutamic oxaloacetic transaminase (aspartate transaminase)
SGPT (ALT)	serum glutamic pyruvic transaminase (alanine transaminase)
SH	social history
SIADH	syndrome of inappropriate antidiuretic hormone secretion
SIDS	sudden infant death syndrome
SJS	Stevens-Johnson syndrome
SL	sublingual
SLE	systemic lupus erythematosus
SMA-6	sequential multiple analyzer for sodium, potassium, CO_2, chloride, glucose, and BUN
SMA-7	sequential multiple analyzer for sodium, potassium, CO_2, chloride, glucose, BUN, and creatinine
SMA-12	sequential multiple analyzer for glucose, BUN, uric acid, calcium, phosphorous, total protein, albumin, cholesterol, total bilirubin, alkaline phosphatase, SGOT, and LDH
SMA-23	includes the entire SMA-12 plus sodium, potassium, CO_2, chloride, direct bilirubin, triglyceride, SGPT, indirect bilirubin, R fraction, and BUN/creatinine ratio
SMBG	self-monitoring of blood glucose
SNF	skilled nursing facility
SNS	sympathetic nervous system
SOB	shortness of breath; see order book; side of bed
S/P	status post
SPF	sun protection factor
SQ	subcutaneous
SSKI	saturated solution of potassium iodide
SSRI	selective serotonin reuptake inhibitor
STAT	immediately; at once
STEMI	ST-segment elevated myocardial infarction
STD	sexually transmitted disease
SV	stroke volume
SVC	superior vena cava
SVRI	systemic vascular resistance index
SVR	supraventricular rhythm; systemic vascular resistance
SVT	supraventricular tachycardia
SW	social worker
Sx	signs
T	temperature
T_3	triiodothyroxine
T_4	thyroxine
T&A	tonsillectomy and adenoidectomy
T&C	type and crossmatch
TB	tuberculosis
TBG	thyroid-binding globulin
TBI	total-body irradiation; traumatic brain injury
TBW	total body weight
T bili	total bilirubin
TCA	tricyclic antidepressant
TCN	tetracycline
Tdap	tetanus, diphtheria, acellular pertussis vaccine
TEE	transesophageal echocardiogram
TFT	thyroid function test
TG	triglyceride
TIA	transient ischemic attack
TIBC	total iron-binding capacity
tid	three times daily (*ter in die*)
TLC	therapeutic lifestyle changes
TMJ	Temporomandibular joint
TMP-SMX	trimethoprim–sulfamethoxazole
TNTC	too numerous to count
TOD	target organ damage
TPN	total parenteral nutrition
TPR	temperature, pulse, respiration
T PROT	total protein
TSH	thyroid-stimulating hormone
TURP	transurethral resection of the prostate
Tx	treat, treatment
UA	urinalysis, uric acid
UC	ulcerative colitis
UE	upper extremity
UFH	unfractionated heparin
UGI	upper gastrointestinal

UOQ	upper outer quadrant
UPT	urine pregnancy test
URI	upper respiratory infection
USP	United States Pharmacopeia
UTI	urinary tract infection
UV	ultraviolet
VF	ventricular fibrillation
VLDL	very low-density lipoprotein
VO	verbal order
VOD	veno-occlusive disease
V_A/Q	ventilation–perfusion
VRE	vancomycin-resistant Enterococcus
VS	vital signs
VSS	vital signs stable
VT	ventricular tachycardia
VTE	venous thromboembolism
WA	while awake
WBC	white blood cell (count)
W/C	wheelchair
WDWN	well-developed, well-nourished
WHO	World Health Organization
WNL	within normal limits
W/U	workup
yo	year old
y	year

Appendix C: Glossary

2,3-Diphosphoglycerate: A compound in red blood cells that affects oxygen binding to and release from hemoglobin.

Ablation: Destruction of part or all of an organ or structure.

Abscess: A purulent collection of fluid separated from surrounding tissue by a wall consisting of inflammatory cells and adjacent organs. It usually contains necrotic debris, bacteria, and inflammatory cells.

Absence: A primary-generalized seizure characterized by sudden and brief (i.e., several seconds in duration) loss of consciousness without muscle movements.

Acanthosis nigricans: Increased thickness and hyperpigmentation of the outer cell layers of the skin; typically observed at areas of flexure.

Acaricide: A chemical that kills mites and ticks.

Acetaldehyde: A hepatotoxic metabolic by-product of alcohol.

Acetylcholine: The neurotransmitter responsible for transmitting messages between certain nerve cells in the brain.

Achalasia: Disorder in which the esophageal sphincter is impaired, preventing normal swallowing and often causing reflux of contents and a feeling that something is caught in the throat.

Achlorhydria: Absence of free hydrochloric acid in the stomach.

Acidemia: An increase in the hydrogen ion concentration of the blood or a fall below normal in pH.

Acidosis: Any pathologic state that leads to acidemia.

Acinar cells: Exocrine glands of the pancreas that secrete digestive enzymes.

Acromegaly: A pathologic condition characterized by excessive production of growth hormone during adulthood after epiphyseal (long bone) fusions have completed.

Action potential: A rapid change in the polarity of the voltage of a cell membrane from negative to positive and back to negative; a wave of electrical discharge that travels across a cell membrane.

Acute acid-base disorder: An acid-base disturbance that has been present for minutes to hours.

Acute coronary syndrome (ACS): Ischemic chest discomfort at rest most often accompanied by ST-segment elevation, ST-segment depression, or T-wave inversion on the 12-lead electrocardiogram; caused by plaque rupture and partial or complete occlusion of the coronary artery by thrombus. Acute coronary syndromes include myocardial infarction and unstable angina.

Acute kidney injury: Characterized by a rapid decrease in kidney function and the resultant accumulation of nitrogenous waste products (e.g., creatinine and blood urea nitrogen or BUN), with or without a decrease in urine output.

Acute otitis media: Inflammation of the middle ear accompanied by fluid in the middle ear space and signs or symptoms of an acute ear infection.

Acute respiratory distress syndrome (ARDS): Occurs when fluid builds up in the alveoli of the lungs, reducing amount of oxygen delivered to other organs.

Acute tubular necrosis: Form of acute kidney injury that results from toxic or ischemic injury to the cells in the proximal tubule of the kidney.

Addiction: A primary, chronic, neurobiologic disease, with genetic, psychosocial, and environmental factors influencing its development and manifestations. It is characterized by behaviors that include one or more of the following: impaired control over substance use, compulsive use, continued use despite harm, and craving.

Adenoma: A non-malignant tumor of the epithelial tissue that is characterized by glandular structures.

Adenomatous polyposis coli (APC): A gene associated with familial adenomatous polyposis (FAP), an inherited disorder characterized by the development of myriad polyps in the colon, often occurring in adolescents and young adults ages 15 to 25.

Adjuvant chemotherapy: Treatment given after the primary surgical treatment and designed to eliminate any remaining cancer cells that are undetectable, with the goal of improving survival.

Adjuvant therapy: Treatment which follows the primary modality with the intent of reducing the risk of disease relapse and prolonging survival. The ultimate goal is to cure patients who would not otherwise be cured by the primary modality alone.

Adrenalectomy: Surgical removal of an adrenal gland.

Adrenocorticotropic hormone: A hormone secreted by the anterior pituitary that controls secretion of cortisol from the adrenal glands. Also referred to as corticotropin.

Adverse drug reaction (ADR): Any unexpected, unintended, undesired, or excessive response to a medication that requires discontinuing or changing the medication, or modifying the dose (except for minor dosage modifcations). May necessitate hospital admission and/or supportive treatment; prolong stay in a health care facility; significantly complicate diagnosis; negatively affect prognosis; or result in temporary or permanent harm, disability, or death.

Aeroallergen: An airborne substance that causes an allergic response.

Afterload: The force against which a ventricle contracts that is contributed to by the vascular resistance, especially of the arteries, and by the physical characteristics (mass and viscosity) of the blood.

Ageism: Discrimination against aged persons.

Air embolus: An obstruction in a small blood vessel caused by air that is introduced into a blood vessel and is carried through the circulation until it lodges in a smaller vessel.

Akathisia: Motor or subjective feelings of restlessness, often characterized by the urge to move limbs and inability to sit still.

Akinesia: Lack of movement.

Albuminuria: The presence of albumin (greater than 30 mg/day) in the urine, which is an early sign of chronic kidney disease (CKD).

Aldosterone: A hormone produced in and secreted by the zona glomerulosa of the adrenal cortex. Aldosterone acts on the kidneys to reabsorb sodium and excrete potassium. It is also a part of the renin-angiotensin-aldosterone system that regulates blood pressure and blood volume.

Alkalemia: A decrease in the hydrogen ion concentration of the blood or a rise above normal in pH.

Alkalosis: Any pathologic state that leads to alkalemia.

Allodynia: Pain that results from a stimulus that does not normally cause pain.

Allogeneic hematopoietic stem cell transplant: A procedure in which a person receives blood-forming stem cells (cells from which all blood cells develop) from a genetically similar, but not identical, donor.

Allogeneic transplant: Procedure by which cells from one person are transferred to another.

Allograft: Tissue or organ transplanted from a donor of the same species but different genetic makeup; recipient's immune system must be suppressed to prevent rejection of the graft.

Allograft survival: After the transplant procedure, the transplanted organ continues to have some degree of function, from excellent to poor.

Allorecognition: Recognition of the foreign antigens present on the transplant organ or the donor's antigen presenting cells.

Alopecia: Hair loss.

Alzheimer disease: Type of dementia with insidious onset and gradual progression that causes problems with memory, learning, thinking, and behavior. Symptoms eventually become severe enough to interfere with daily tasks, including self-care.

Ambulatory esophageal reflux monitoring: A telemetry capsule containing a tiny camera is swallowed, or a transnasal catheter is inserted to determine how often reflux is occurring as well as the incidence of abnormal esophageal acid exposure. The telemetry capsule provides about 48 hours of data, whereas the transnasal catheter provides about 24 hours of data.

Amenorrhea: Abnormal cessation or absence of menses.

Ampulla of Vater: Dilation of the duodenal wall at the opening of the fused pancreatic and common bile ducts.

Amylin: A 37-amino acid polypeptide hormone that is secreted from the β cells of the pancreas in response to nutrients. Mechanisms of action include slowing gastric emptying, suppressing postmeal glucagon secretion, and suppressing appetite.

Amyloid: Any of a group of chemically diverse proteins that are composed of linear non-branching aggregated fibrils.

Anaphylactic/anaphylaxis: Immediate, severe, potentially fatal hypersensitivity reaction induced by an antigen.

Anaphylactoid: An anaphylactic-like reaction, similar in signs and symptoms but not mediated by IgE. The drug causing this reaction produces direct release of inflammatory mediators by a pharmacological effect.

Anastomosis: The connection of two hollow organs to restore continuity after resection.

Anemia: Reduction in the concentration of hemoglobin that results in reduced oxygen-carrying capacity of the blood.

Anemia of chronic kidney disease: A decline in red blood cell production caused by a decrease in erythropoietin production by the progenitor cells of the kidney. As kidney function declines in chronic kidney disease, erythropoietin production also declines, resulting in decreased red blood cell production. Other contributing factors include iron deficiency and decreased red blood cell lifespan, caused by uremia.

Anergy: A reduction or lack of an immune response to a specific antigen.

Aneurysm: A blood-filled bulge which forms in the wall of a weakened blood vessel; if ruptured, may result in bleeding, shock, and/or other negative health outcome including mortality.

Angina: Discomfort in the chest or adjacent areas caused by decreased blood and oxygen supply to the myocardium (myocardial ischemia).

Angioedema: Swelling similar to urticaria (hives), but the swelling occurs beneath the skin instead of on the surface. Characterized by deep swelling around the eyes and lips and sometimes of the hands and feet. If it proceeds rapidly, it can lead to airway obstruction and suffocation, and should therefore be treated as a medical emergency.

Angiogenesis: The formation of new blood vessels. Increased blood flow to deliver nutrients is required for tumor growth.

Angiography: Examination of the blood vessels using x-rays after injection of a radiopaque substance.

Anosmia: Loss of smell.

Anterior circulation: Blood supply to the anterior section of the brain supplied by the internal carotid arteries, anterior cerebral artery, and middle cerebral artery.

Anterograde amnesia: Memory loss affecting the transfer of new information or events to long-term storage.

Antiangiogenic: Preventing or inhibiting the formation and differentiation of blood vessels.

Anticoagulant: Any substance that inhibits, suppresses, or delays the formation of blood clots. These substances occur naturally and regulate the clotting cascade. Several anticoagulants have been identified in a variety of animal tissues and have been commercially developed for medicinal use.

Antiproteinase: A substance that inhibits the enzymatic activity of a proteinase.

Anuria: Urine output of less than 50 mL over 24 hours.

Aphakic: The absence of a lens in the eye.

Aphasia: Impairment of language affecting the ability to speak and to understand speech.

Aphthous ulcer: A small superficial area of ulceration within the gastrointestinal mucosa, typically found in the oral cavity.

Apoptosis: Programmed cell death as signaled by the nuclei in normally functioning cells when age or state of cell health and condition dictates.

Arcuate scotoma: An arc-shaped area of blindness in the field of vision.

Arteriovenous malformation: A tangle of blood vessels, usually in the brain, that results in abnormal connections between arteries and veins; if ruptured, may result in hemorrhage.

Arthrocentesis: Puncture and aspiration of a joint. Certain drugs can be injected into the joint space for a local effect.

Articular: Related to a joint or joints.

Ascites: Accumulation of fluid within the peritoneal cavity.

Asterixis: A flapping tremor of the arms and hands that is seen in patients with end-stage liver disease.

Astringent: A substance that causes tissues to constrict, resulting in a drying effect of the skin.

Atelectasis: Decreased or absent air in a partial or entire lung, with resulting loss of lung volume.
Atherosclerosis: Accumulation of lipids, inflammatory cells, and cellular debris in the subendothelial space of the arterial wall.
Atherosclerotic cardiovascular disease: Disease in which plaque builds up in vessels.
Atonic seizure: A primary-generalized seizure characterized by loss of consciousness and muscle tone.
Atopy: A genetic predisposition to develop type I hypersensitivity reactions against common environmental antigens. It is seen commonly in patients with allergic rhinitis, asthma, and atopic dermatitis.
Atresia: Congenital absence of a normal opening or normally patent lumen.
Atrophic urethritis: An inflammation of the vagina (and the outer urinary tract) due to a lack of estrogen.
Attenuation: Loss of intensity or virulence.
Aura: Visual, but sometimes sensory, motor or verbal disturbance usually occurring before a migraine or seizure.
Auspitz sign: Pinpoint bleeding that occurs when a psoriatic scale or lesion is peeled off of the skin.
Autologous: A transplant using one's own stem cells.
Autologous hematopoietic stem cell transplant: A procedure in which blood-forming stem cells (cells from which all blood cells develop) are removed, stored, and later given back to the same person.
Automaticity: Ability of a cardiac fiber or tissue to spontaneously initiate depolarizations.
Avolition: Inability to initiate and persist in goal-directed activities.
Azoospermic: Having no living spermatozoa in the semen, or failure of spermatogenesis.
B2 microglobulin: A low-molecular weight protein that may be elevated in multiple myeloma.
Bacille Calmette-Guérin vaccine: A tuberculosis vaccine prepared from an attenuated strain of the closely related species *Mycobacterium bovis*, used for immunization against tuberculosis in many countries, but not in the United States.
Bacteremia: Bacteria in the bloodstream.
Bacteriuria: Presence of bacteria in urine.
Barium enema: A diagnostic test using an x-ray to view the lower gastrointestinal tract (colon and rectum) after rectal administration of barium sulfate, a chalky liquid contrast medium.
Barrett esophagus: Disorder in which the cells of the lower esophagus are damaged, most often a result of longstanding reflux.
Basal ganglia: Cluster of nerve cells deep in the brain that coordinate normal movement.
β-hydroxybutyric acid: A ketone body that is elevated in ketosis, is synthesized in the liver from acetyl-CoA, and can be used as an energy source by the brain when blood glucose is low.
Bence-Jones proteins: Light chained immunoglobulins found in the urine.
Bilateral salpingo-oophorectomy: Surgical excision (removal) of both ovaries.
Bile acids: The organic acids in bile. Bile is the yellowish-brown or green fluid secreted by the liver and discharged into the duodenum where it aids in the emulsification of fats, increases peristalsis, and retards putrefaction.
Biliary sludge: A deposit of tiny stones or crystals made up of cholesterol, calcium bilirubinate, and other calcium salts. The cholesterol and calcium bilirubinate crystals in biliary sludge can lead to gallstone formation.
Bioavailability: The amount of an agent that is absorbed orally relative to an equivalent dose administered intravenously.
Biopsy: The removal of cells or tissue for examination.
Bladder hypotonicity: Low elastic tension of the bladder.
Blast: An immature cell.
Blastospores: An asexual reproductive sphore formed by budding, often seen with yeast.
Blood urea nitrogen (BUN): A waste product in the blood produced from the breakdown of dietary proteins. The kidneys filter blood to remove urea and maintain homeostasis; a decline in kidney function results in an increase in BUN.
Body mass index (BMI): A calculation utilized to correct weight changes for height and is a direct calculation regardless of gender. It is the result of the weight in kilograms divided by the height in meters squared. If nonmetric measurements are used, it is the result of the weight in pounds multiplied by 703 and then that quantity divided by the product of height in inches squared.
Bone remodeling: The constant process of bone turnover involving bone resorption followed by bone formation.
Bouchard nodes: Hard, bony enlargement of the proximal interphalangeal (middle) joint of a finger or toe.
Brachial plexus: Collection of nerves that arises from the spine at the base of the neck from nerves that supply parts of the shoulder, arm, forearm, and hand.
Brachytherapy: A form of radiotherapy where a sealed radiation source is placed inside or next to the area requiring treatment.
Bradycardia: Slower than normal heart rate.
Bradykinesia: Slow movement.
Breakpoint: The concentration of an antimicrobial agent that can be achieved in serum after a normal or standard dose of that antimicrobial agent.
Bronchiectasis: Chronic dilation of bronchi or bronchioles as a result of inflammatory disease or obstruction associated with heavy sputum.
Bronchoalveolar lavage: Diagnostic procedure in which a scope is passed through the nose or mouth into the lungs and fluid is squirted into an area of lung then recollected for examination.
Bullectomy: Surgical removal of one or more bullae (air spaces in the lung measuring more than one centimeter in diameter in the distended state).
Bursitis: An inflammation of the bursa, the fluid-filled sac near the joint where tendons and muscles pass over bone.
Cancer survivorship: The process of living with, throughout, and beyond cancer. Begins at cancer diagnosis and includes people who are/are not receiving treatment to manage disease or to decrease the risk of recurrence.
Capillary leak: Loss of intravascular volume into the interstitial space within the body.
Carcinogenesis: The actual formation of a cancer, whereby normal cells are transformed into cancer cells.
Carcinoma: A malignant growth that arises from epithelium, found in skin or the lining of body organs. Carcinomas tend to infiltrate into adjacent tissue and spread to distant organs.
Carcinomatosis: Condition of having widespread dissemination of carcinoma (cancer) in the body.
Cardiac cachexia: Physical wasting with loss of weight and muscle mass caused by cardiac disease; a wasting syndrome that causes weakness and a loss of weight, fat, and muscle.
Cardiac index: Cardiac output normalized for body surface area (cardiac index = cardiac output/body surface area).
Cardiac output: The volume of blood ejected from the left side of the heart per unit of time [cardiac output (L/min) = stroke volume × heart rate].
Cardiac remodeling: Genome expression resulting in molecular, cellular, and interstitial changes and manifested clinically as

changes in size, shape, and function of the heart resulting from cardiac load or injury.

Carotid bruit: Abnormal sound heard when auscultating a carotid artery caused by turbulent blood flow, usually due to the presence of atherosclerotic plaques.

Carotid endarterectomy: Removal of a thrombus from the carotid artery.

Carotid intima-media thickness: A measurement of the surface between the intima and media. This is a well-validated measure of the progression of atherosclerosis. Increasing measurements over time correlate with increasing atherosclerosis, whereas a decrease in the measurement is indicative of atherosclerotic regression.

Carotids: The two main arteries in the neck.

Castrate resistant: Prostate cancers resistant to hormonal therapy.

Cataplexy: A sudden loss of muscle control with retention of clear consciousness that follows a strong emotional stimulus (e.g., elation, surprise, or anger) and is a characteristic symptom of narcolepsy.

Causalgia: Persistent burning pain, allodynia, and hyperpathia following a traumatic nerve lesion.

Cavitary lesions: A spherical, air-containing lesion found on radiograph or computed tomography. The lesion usually has a thick wall and can be found within an area of a surrounding infiltrate or mass.

CD4 and CD8: Proteins predominately found on the surface of T cells.

Central pain: Pain that results from a lesion or dysfunction in the central nervous system.

Cephalic: Of or relating to the head.

Cervicitis: Inflammation of the cervix.

Chemoprevention: The use of drugs, vitamins, or other agents to reduce the risk or delay the development or recurrence of cancer.

Chemoreceptor trigger zone (CTZ): Located in the area postrema of the fourth ventricle of the brain. It is exposed to cerebrospinal fluid and blood and is easily stimulated by circulating toxins to induce nausea and vomiting.

Chemosis: Edema of the bulbar conjunctiva.

Cheyne-Stokes respiration: Pattern of breathing with gradual increase in depth (and sometimes in rate) to a maximum, followed by a decrease resulting in apnea; the cycles ordinarily are 30 seconds to 2 minutes in duration, with 5 to 30 seconds of apnea.

Chimeric: An individual, organ, or substance composed of substances with different genetic origins.

Chloasma: Melasma characterized by irregularly shaped brown patches on the face and other areas of the skin, often seen during pregnancy or associated with the use of oral contraceptives.

Chlorpromazine equivalents: Approximate dose equivalent of a first-generation antipsychotic to 100 mg of chlorpromazine (relative potency).

Cholecystitis: Inflammation of the gallbladder.

Cholelithiasis: Formation of stones in the gallbladder (gallstones).

Cholestasis: Reduced or lack of flow of bile, or obstruction of bile flow.

Cholesteatoma: A mass of keratinized epithelial cells and cholesterol resembling a tumor that forms in the middle ear or mastoid region.

Cholinesterase inhibitor: Medication class that inhibits the acetylcholinesterase enzyme from breaking down acetylcholine, thereby increasing both the level and duration of action of the neurotransmitter acetylcholine.

Chorea: A type of dyskinesia with rhythmic dance-like movement. The increase in motor activity may be associated with fidgetiness, twitching, or flinging movements.

Chronic acid-base disorder: An acid-base disturbance that has been present for hours to days.

Chronic kidney disease (CKD): A progressive, irreversible decline in kidney function that occurs over a period of several months to years.

Chronic stable angina: Manifestation of ischemic heart disease that typically results when an atherosclerotic plaque progresses to occlude at least 70% of a major coronary artery. Patients typically present with a sensation of chest pressure or heaviness that is provoked by exertion and relieved with rest or sublingual nitroglycerin.

Chronotropic: Pertaining to the heart rate.

Chvostek sign: Noted when a tap on the patient's facial nerve adjacent to the ear produces a brief contraction of the upper lip, nose or side of the face.

Chylothorax: The presence of lymphatic fluid (chyle) in the pleural cavity.

Circadian rhythm: 24-hour cycles of behavior and physiology that are generated by endogenous biologic clocks (pacemakers).

Circulatory shock: A condition wherein the circulatory system is inadequately supplying the oxygen and vital metabolic substrates to cells throughout the body.

Cirrhosis: Hepatic fibrosis and regenerative nodules that have destroyed the architecture of the liver, scarring the liver tissues. Progressive scarring of the liver resulting in nonfunctional hepatocytes.

Clonal expansion: An immunologic response in which lymphocytes stimulated by antigen proliferate and amplify the population of relevant cells.

Closed comedo: A plugged hair follicle of sebum, keratinocytes, and bacteria that remains beneath the surface of the skin. Also referred to as a "whitehead."

Clotting cascade: A series of enzymatic reactions by clotting factors leading to the formation of a blood clot. The clotting cascade is initiated by several thrombogenic substances. Each reaction in the cascade is triggered by the preceding one and the effect is amplified by positive feedback loops.

Clotting factor: Plasma proteins found in the blood that are essential to the formation of blood clots. Clotting factors circulate in inactive forms but are activated by their predecessor in the clotting cascade or a thrombogenic substance. Each clotting factor is designated by a Roman numeral (e.g., factor VII) and by the letter "a" when activated (e.g., factor VIIa).

Clubbing: Proliferation of soft tissues, especially in the nail bed, which results in thickening and widening of finger and toe extremities.

Coalescence: Fusion of smaller lipid emulsion particles forming larger particles, resulting in destabilization of the emulsion.

Cognitive function: Executive function and mental processing such as understanding, perception, reasoning, language, and awareness. Executive function involves organization, self-regulation, attention, and problem solving.

Coitus: Sexual intercourse.

Collateral damage: The development of resistance occurring in a patient's nontargeted flora that can cause secondary infections.

Colloids: Intravenous fluids composed of water and large-molecular weight molecules used to increase volume in patients with hypovolemic shock via increased intravascular oncotic pressure.

Colonoscopy: Visual examination of the colon using a lighted, lens-equipped, flexible tube (colonoscope) inserted into the rectum.

Colony-forming units: Number of viable colonies of bacteria, yeast, or mold per unit of measurement (e.g., milliliter or gram).

Colorectal cancer: The development of malignant cells in the lining or epithelium of the first and longest portion of the large intestine.

Combined androgen blockade: The combination of both androgen receptor (AR) antagonism and inhibition or suppression of androgen production.

Comedolytic: An agent that is able to break up or destroy a comedo.

Comorbidities: Multiple disease states occurring concurrently in one patient.

Complete response: In cancer, disappearance of all targeted lesions.

Complex partial seizures: Seizures that are localized in a specific area of the brain, but there is an alteration in the patient's level of consciousness.

Complex regimen: Taking medications 3 or more times per day, or 12 or more doses per day.

Complicated acid-base disorder: The presence of two or more distinct acid-base disorders.

Concreteness: Inability to think in abstract terms. It may be a primary developmental defect or secondary to organic mental disorder or schizophrenia.

Congenital adrenal hyperplasia: A rare inherited condition resulting from a deficiency in cortisol and aldosterone synthesis with resulting excess androgen production. The clinical presentation depends on the variant of the condition but typically manifests as abnormalities in sexual development and/or adrenal insufficiency.

Conjunctival injection: Erythema of the conjunctiva.

Conjunctivitis: Inflammation of the conjunctiva.

Conjunctivitis medicamentosa: A drug-induced form of allergic conjunctivitis resulting from overuse of topical ocular vasoconstrictors.

Consolidation: Cancer treatment given after induction therapy to consolidate the gains obtained, further reduce the number of cancer cells, and enhance the likelihood of a durable complete remission.

Contiguous spread: Infection that involves bone that has come from adjacent tissues.

Continuous positive airway pressure: A technique of assisting breathing by maintaining the air pressure in the lungs and air passages constant and above atmospheric pressure throughout the breathing cycle.

Convection: The movement of dissolved solutes across a semipermeable membrane by applying a pressure gradient to the fluid transport.

Conversion (transformation): Mutated cell becomes malignant.

Cor pulmonale: Right-sided heart failure caused by lung disease.

Corneal arcus: Accumulation of lipid on the cornea.

Coronary artery bypass graft: Surgical intervention to improve coronary blood flow by removing a vein from the leg and attaching one end to the aorta and the other end to the coronary artery distal to the atherosclerotic plaque. Alternatively, an artery from the inside of the chest wall may be used to bypass the coronary occlusion.

Coronary artery disease: Narrowing of one or more of the major coronary arteries, most commonly by atherosclerotic plaques. May be referred to as coronary heart disease.

Coronary heart disease: Narrowing of one or more of the major coronary arteries, most commonly by atherosclerotic plaques. May be referred to as coronary artery disease.

Corpus luteum: The small yellow endocrine structure that develops within a ruptured ovarian follicle and secretes progesterone and estrogen.

Corticotropin-releasing hormone: A hormone released by the hypothalamus that stimulates release of adrenocorticotropic hormone by the anterior pituitary gland.

Cortisol: An adrenal gland hormone responsible for maintaining homeostasis of carbohydrate, protein, and fat metabolism.

Cosyntropin: A synthetic version of adrenocorticotropic hormone.

Counterirritant: A substance that elicits a superficial inflammatory response with the objective of reducing inflammation in deeper, adjacent structures.

C-peptide: A peptide which is made when proinsulin is split into insulin and C-peptide. They split before proinsulin is released from endocytic vesicles within the pancreas, one C-peptide for each insulin molecule. C-peptide is the abbreviation for "connecting peptide." It is used to determine if a patient has type 1 or type 2 diabetes mellitus.

Creaming: Aggregation of lipid emulsion particles that then migrate to the surface of the emulsion; can be reversed with mild agitation.

Creatinine: A waste product in the blood produced from the breakdown of protein by-products generated by muscle in the body or ingested in the diet. The kidneys filter blood to remove creatinine and maintain homeostasis; a decline in kidney function results in an increase in creatinine.

Creatinine clearance: Rate at which creatinine is filtered across the glomerulus; estimate of glomerular filtration rate.

Crepitus: A grating sound or sensation typically produced by friction between bone-on-cartilage or bone-on-bone contact.

Cretinism: Obsolete term for congenital hypothyroidism.

Cross-allergenicity: Sensitivity to one drug and then reacting to a different drug with a similar chemical structure.

Crypt abscess: Neutrophilic infiltration of the intestinal glands (crypts of Lieberkühn); a characteristic finding in patients with ulcerative colitis.

Cryptogenic (cause unknown) epilepsies: A seizure disorder that results from an underlying neurologic disorder that is often ill-defined, and other neurologic functions are often abnormal or developmentally delayed.

Crystalloids: Intravenous fluids composed of water and electrolytes (e.g., sodium, chloride, etc.) used as intravascular volume expanders for patients with hypovolemic shock.

Cutis laxis: Hypereflacidity of the skin with loss of elasticity.

Cyanosis: A dark blue or purple discoloration of the skin and mucous membranes due to deficient oxygenation of the blood.

Cyclic citrullinated peptide (CCP): A circular peptide (a ring of amino acids) containing the amino acid citrulline. Autoantibodies directed against cyclic citrullinated peptide provide the basis for a test of importance in rheumatoid arthritis.

Cyclooxygenase: An enzyme that catalyzes the conversion of arachidonic acid to prostaglandins and consists of two isoforms, generally abbreviated COX-1 and COX-2.

Cystitis: Inflammation of urinary bladder.

Cystocele: Hernial protrusion of the bladder, usually through the vaginal wall.

Cytokines: Regulatory proteins, such as interleukins and lymphokines, that are released by cells of the immune system and act as intercellular mediators in the generation of an immune response. Soluble glycoproteins released by the immune system which act through specific receptors to regulate immune responses.

Cytomegalovirus (CMV) disease: The term used when patients who are already infected with CMV present with the classically associated symptoms that resemble a viral infection and may include fever, malaise, arthralgias, and others.

Cytomegalovirus (CMV) infection: The term used when a patient has anti-CMV antibodies in the blood, when CMV antigens are detected in infected cells, or when the virus is isolated from a culture.

Decolonization: Eradication of targeted bacterial species normally found on a person's body but which have the potential to cause invasive disease.

Deep vein thrombosis: A disorder of thrombus formation causing obstruction of a deep vein in the leg, pelvis, or abdomen.

De-escalation: Decreasing antimicrobial regimen spectrum of activity to provide coverage against specific antimicrobial-sensitive pathogens recovered from culture.

Delayed peak response: The peak effects of a dose of medication take longer than expected to manifest.

Delirium: Transient brain syndrome presenting as disordered attention, cognition, psychomotor behavior, and perception.

Delirium tremens (DTs): Symptom of alcohol withdrawal characterized by hallucinations, delirium, severe agitation, fever, elevations of blood pressure and heart rate, and possible cardiac arrhythmias.

Denervation: Loss of nerve supply.

Dennie-Morgan line: A line or fold below the lower eyelids;

Dermatophyte: Any microscopic fungus that grows on the skin, scalp, and nails. May cause infections.

Desensitization: A process in which a drug to which a patient is allergic is administered in small, incremental doses to induce a state of temporary tolerance.

Desquamation: Peeling or shedding of the epidermis (superficial layer of the skin) in scales or flakes.

Detumescence: The return of the penis to a flaccid state.

Diabetes insipidus: Polyuria due to the failure of renal tubules to reabsorb water in response to antidiuretic hormone.

Diabetic ketoacidosis: A reversible but life-threatening short-term complication primarily seen in patients with type 1 diabetes caused by the relative or absolute lack of insulin that results in marked ketosis and acidosis.

Dialysate: The physiologic solution used during dialysis to remove excess fluids and waste products from the blood.

Dialysis: The process of removing fluid and waste products from the blood across a semi-permeable membrane to maintain fluid, electrolyte, and acid-base balance in patients with kidney failure.

Diaphoresis: Sweating or profuse perspiration, generally as a symptom of a disease or an adverse drug effect.

Diarthrodial joint: A freely moveable joint (e.g., knee, shoulder). Contrast with amphiarthrodial joint (a slightly movable joint; e.g., vertebral joint) and synarthrodial joint (an unmovable joint; e.g., fibrous joint).

Diastolic dysfunction: Abnormal filling of the ventricles during diastole.

Diffusion: The movement of a solute across the dialyzer membrane from an area of higher concentration (usually the blood) to a lower concentration (usually the dialysate).

Dilated cardiomyopathy: Ability of the heart to pump blood is decreased because the left ventricle is enlarged and weakened.

Diphasic dyskinesia: The motor fluctuations occur while the plasma levodopa concentrations are rising and when they are falling. In each dosing interval, the patient may experience improvement, dyskinesia and improvement (IDI) or dyskinesia, improvement, dyskinesia (DID).

Direct current cardioversion: The process of administering a synchronized electrical shock to the chest, the purpose of which is to simultaneously depolarize all of the myocardial cells, resulting in restoration of normal sinus rhythm.

Disease-free survival: Length of time after treatment duringwhich no disease is found.

Disease progression: In cancer, at least a 20% increase in the sum of the longest diameter of target lesions from baseline, including new lesions discovered during treatment.

Disseminated erythrosquamous papules: Widespread or whole body red, scaly psoriatic lesions.

Disseminated intravascular coagulopathy: Abnormal overactivity of proteins in the blood that form blood clots; over time, clotting proteins are reduced which then increases risk for serious bleeding.

DNA mismatch repair (*dMMR*) genes: Genes that control an intrinsic intracellular mechanism which corrects nucleotide insertion errors made during DNA replication, by excising the mismatched base pairs that escaped correction by the proofreading activities of DNA polymerases and replacing the mismatched bases with the correct ones.

Door-to-needle time: Time from arrival in hospital to administration of treatment in appropriate patients.

Downregulation: The process of reducing or suppressing a response to a stimulus.

Drusen: Tiny yellow or white deposits of extracellular material in the eye.

D-test: Double disk diffusion microbiological testing which indicates the presence or absence of macrolide-induced resistance to clindamycin.

Ductus arteriosus: Shunt connecting the pulmonary artery to the aortic arch that allows most of the blood from the right ventricle to bypass fetal lungs.

Duodenal enterocyte: Cells lining the duodenum, which is the first of three parts of the small intestine.

Dysarthria: Speech disorder due to weakness or incoordination of speech muscles; speech is slow, weak, and imprecise.

Dysesthesia: An unpleasant abnormal sensation.

Dysgeusia: Taste disturbance or dysfunction of the sense of taste.

Dyskinesia: Abnormal involuntary movements, which include dystonia, chorea, and akathisia.

Dyslipidemia: Elevation of the total cholesterol, low-density lipoprotein cholesterol, or triglyceride concentrations, or a decrease in high-density lipoprotein cholesterol concentration in the blood.

Dysmenorrhea: Crampy pelvic pain occurring with or just prior to menses. "Primary" dysmenorrhea implies pain in the setting of normal pelvic anatomy, while "secondary" dysmenorrhea is secondary to underlying pelvic pathology.

Dyspareunia: Painful sexual intercourse due to medical or psychological causes.

Dysphagia: Difficulty in swallowing.

Dysphonia: Impairment of the voice or difficulty speaking.

Dysphoria: An unhappy or depressed feeling.
Dyspnea: Shortness of breath or difficulty breathing.
Dystonia: A type of dyskinesia. The movement is slow and twisting. It may be associated with painful muscle contractions or spasms.
Dysuria: Difficulty or pain in urination.
Ebstein anomaly: Congenital heart defect in which the opening of the tricuspid valve is displaced toward the apex of the right ventricle of the heart.
Eburnation: A condition in which bone or cartilage becomes hardened and denser.
Ecchymosis: Passage of blood from ruptured blood vessels into subcutaneous tissue causing purple discoloration of the skin.
Echocardiogram: An ultrasound test with high-frequency sound waves to produce a graphic image of the interior heart to evaluate the heart's structures and movement.
Ectopic pregnancy: Presence of a fertilized ovum outside of the uterine cavity.
Effector cells: Cells that become active in response to initiation of the immune response.
Ejection fraction: The fraction of the volume present at the end of diastole that is pushed into the aorta during systole.
Electrocardiogram: A noninvasive recording of the electrical activity of the heart.
Electroconvulsive therapy: Administration of electric current to the brain through electrodes placed on the head to induce seizure activity in the brain; used in the treatment of certain mental disorders.
Electroencephalograph: A diagnostic test where electrodes are placed on the scalp and electrical activity in the brain is measured and recorded.
Electroencephalography: The recording of brain waves via electrodes placed on the scalp or cortex.
Embolism: The sudden blockage of a vessel caused by a blood clot or foreign material which has been brought to the site by the flow of blood.
Embolization: The process by which a blood clot or foreign material dislodges from its site of origin, flows in the blood, and blocks a distant vessel.
Emesis: Vomiting; a reflexive rapid and forceful oral expulsion of upper gastrointestinal contents due to powerful and sustained contractions in the abdominal and thoracic musculature.
Endometritis: Inflammation of the endometrium.
Endoscopic evaluation: Visual inspection of the inside of hollow organs with an endoscope; used mainly for diagnostic purposes; refers to procedures such as gastroscopy, duodenoscopy, colonoscopy, and sigmoidoscopy.
Endoscopy: A diagnostic tool used to examine the inside of the body using a lighted, flexible instrument called an endoscope.
Endothelial cell: A single layer of cells surrounding the lumen of arteries.
End-stage liver disease: Liver failure that is usually accompanied by complications such as ascites or hepatic encephalopathy.
Enteral nutrition: Delivery of nutrients via the gastrointestinal tract, either by mouth or by feeding tube.
Enthesitis: Inflammation of the sites where tendons, ligaments, or fascia attach to bone.
Enuresis: Incontinence at night.
Epilepsy: A neurological disorder characterized by recurring motor, sensory, or psychic malfunction with or without loss of consciousness or convulsive seizures.
Epistaxis: Nasal hemorrhage with blood drainage through the nostrils; a nosebleed.
Erectile dysfunction: Condition defined as the inability to achieve or maintain an erection sufficient for sexual intercourse.
Erythema multiforme: A rash characterized by papular (small raised bump) or vesicular lesions (blisters), and reddening or discoloration of the skin often in concentric zones about the lesion.
Erythematous: Flushing of the skin caused by dilation of capillaries. Erythema is often a sign of inflammation and infection.
Erythrocyte sedimentation rate: Non-specific test to indirectly measure degree of inflammation in the body due to conditions such as infections, cancers, or autoimmune diseases.
Erythrodermic psoriasis: Generalized erythema covering nearly the entire body surface area. Fever and malaise are common but, while quite rare, can be severe and even fatal; it is usually associated with a worsening of other forms of psoriasis.
Erythropoiesis stimulating agents: Agents developed by recombinant DNA technology that have the same biological activity as endogenous erythropoietin to stimulate erythropoiesis (red blood cell production) in the bone marrow. The currently available agents in the United States are epoetinalfa and darbepoetinalfa.
Erythropoietin: A hormone primarily produced by the progenitor cells of the kidney that stimulates red blood cell production in the bone marrow. Lack of this hormone leads to anemia.
Esophageal varices: Dilated blood vessels in the esophagus.
Essential fatty acid deficiency: Deficiency of linoleic acid, linolenic acid, and/or arachidonic acid, characterized by hair loss, thinning of skin, and skin desquamation. Long-chain fatty acids include trienes (containing 3 double-bonds [e.g., 5,8, 11-eicosatrienoic acid {or Mead acid}, trienoic acids]) and tetraenes (containing 4 double-bonds [e.g., arachidonic acid]). Biochemical evidence of essential fatty acid deficiency includes a triene:tetraene greater than 0.2 and low linoleic or arachidonic acid plasma concentrations.
Euphoria: A feeling of happiness and excitement.
Euthymia: Normal mood.
Euthyroid: State of normal thyroid function or hormone activity.
Euvolemia: The state of proper fluid balance.
Exanthem: Eruption of the skin.
Exfoliative dermatitis: Severe inflammation of the entire skin surface due to a reaction to certain drugs.
Exophthalmos: Abnormal protrusion of the eyeball, seen in Graves disease.
Exploratory laparotomy: Surgical incision into the abdominal cavity, performed to examine the abdominal organs and cavity in search of an abnormality and diagnosis.
External beam: An external source of radiation is pointed at a particular part of the body.
Extraction ratio: Fraction of the drug entering the liver in the blood which is irreversibly removed.
Extrapyramidal symptoms (EPS): Adverse drug effects of medications such as phenothiazines. EPS include dystonia (involuntary muscle contractions), tardive dyskinesia (repetitive, involuntary movements), and akathisia (motor restlessness or anxiety).
Extravasation: Movement of fluid from inside a blood vessel into the surrounding tissues.
Facultative anaerobe: An organism that makes adenosine triphosphate by aerobic respiration if oxygen is present, but switches to fermentation under anaerobic conditions.
Felty syndrome: An extra-articular manifestation of rheumatoid arthritis associated with splenomegaly and neutropenia.

Ferritin: A protein in the body that binds to iron; most of the iron stored in the body is bound to ferritin.

Festination: Walking with short, rapid, shuffling steps.

Fibrin: An insoluble protein that is one of the principal ingredients of a blood clot. Fibrin strands bind to one another to form a fibrin mesh. The fibrin mesh often traps platelets and other blood cells.

Fibrinolysis: A normal ongoing process that dissolves fibrin and results in the removal of small blood clots; hydrolysis of fibrin.

Fibrinolytic: Possessing the property of preventing blood clot formation.

Fibroadenoma: A benign neoplasm that commonly occurs in breast tissue and is derived from glandular epithelium.

FISH: A laboratory technique used to look at genes or chromosomes in cells and tissues. Pieces of DNA that contain a fluorescent dye are made in the laboratory and added to cells or tissues on a glass slide. When these pieces of DNA bind to specific genes or areas of chromosomes on the slide, they light up when viewed under a microscope with a special light. Also called fluorescence in situ hybridization.

Fistula: Abnormal connection between two internal organs (e.g., arteriovenous fistula is a connection between an artery and a vein), or between an internal organ and the exterior or skin (e.g., enterocutaneous fistula is a connection between the intestine and the skin).

Fistulogram: X-ray photograph (or radiograph) taken after injection of a contrast material or radiopaque material (material that will not allow passage of x-rays and will be visible in an x-ray photograph [or radiograph]).

Flexural psoriasis: Characterized by lesions found in skin folds. These lesions tend to be erythematous plaques and are often found in the axillary, genital, perineal, intergluteal, and inframammary regions. While shiny, smooth, and deep red in color, there may be skin fissures and the absence of the silvery scales.

Flight of ideas: A nearly continuous flow of rapid speech and thought that jumps from topic to topic, usually loosely connected.

Floppy iris or small pupil syndrome: The iris of the eye becomes flaccid and cannot become dilated.

Flow cytometry: A method of measuring the number of cells in a sample, the percentage of live cells in a sample, and certain characteristics of cells, such as size, shape, and the presence of tumor markers on the cell surface. The cells are stained with a light-sensitive dye, placed in a fluid, and passed in a stream before a laser or other type of light. The measurements are based on how the light-sensitive dye reacts to the light.

Foam cell: Lipid-laden white blood cell.

Forced expiratory volume in 1 second: The volume of air that a patient can forcibly exhale in the first second of forced exhalation after taking a maximal breath.

Forced vital capacity: The maximum volume of air that can be forcibly exhaled after taking a maximal breath.

Fragility fracture: A fracture resulting from a fall from standing height or less amount of trauma.

Frailty: Excess demand imposed upon reduced capacity; a common biological syndrome in the elderly.

Frank-Starling mechanism: Increase in stroke volume in response to an increase in volume of blood filling the heart (i.e., end-diastolic volume) when all other factors remain constant.

Freelite™ assay: A highly sensitive assay that determines the ratio of serum free light chain kappa to lambda.

Freezing: A sudden but temporary inability to move.

Fremitus: A palpable vibration, as felt by the hand placed on the chest during coughing or speaking.

Friction: Risk factor for pressure ulcers that is created when a patient is dragged across a surface, which can lead to superficial skin damage.

Fructooligosaccharides: Polymers of fructose that reach the colon undigested and are broken down to short chain fatty acids by bacterial enzymes.

Functional gastrointestinal disorder: A term used to describe symptoms occurring in the gastrointestinal tract in the absence of a demonstrated pathologic condition; the clinical product of psychosocial factors and altered intestinal physiology involving the brain–gut interrelationship.

Gadolinium: An intravenous contrast agent used with magnetic resonance imaging.

Gallstone (cholelithiasis): A solid formation in the gallbladder or bile duct composed of cholesterol and bile salts.

γ-Aminobutyric acid: An inhibitory neurotransmitter.

Gamma knife: A treatment using gamma rays, a type of high-energy radiation that can be tightly focused on small tumors or other lesions in the head or neck, so very little normal tissue receives radiation.

Gastrectomy: Surgical excision of part or all of the stomach.

Gastric bypass: A surgical procedure for weight loss that elicits its effectiveness through malabsorption and gastric volume limitation. The procedure involves full partitioning of the proximal gastric segment into a jejunal loop.

Gastritis: Chronic or acute inflammation of the lining of the stomach.

Gastroparesis: A form of autonomic neuropathy involving nerves of the stomach. It may include nausea, vomiting, feeling full, bloating, and lack of appetite. It may cause wide fluctuations in blood sugars due to insulin action and nutrient delivery not occurring at the same time.

Gastroschisis: Congenital abdominal wall defect in which the intestines, and sometimes other organs, develop outside the fetal abdomen through an opening in the abdominal wall.

Gastrostomy: Operative placement of a new opening into the stomach, usually associated with feeding tube placement.

Geniculate nucleus: The portion of the brain that processes visual information from the optic nerve and relays it to the cerebral cortex.

Genotype: The genetic constitution of an individual. May be used to examine the genetic structure of HIV to identify genetic mutations known to cause resistance to certain drugs.

Geriatric syndrome: Age specific presentations or differential diagnoses, including visual and hearing impairment, malnutrition and weight loss, urinary incontinence, gait impairment and falls, osteoporosis, dementia, delirium, sleep problems, and pressure ulcers; commonly seen conditions in elderly patients.

Gestational diabetes mellitus: Diabetes that occurs during pregnancy which may or may not end at delivery.

Gigantism: A condition of abnormal size or overgrowth of the entire body or of any of its parts.

Glomerular filtration rate: The volume of plasma that is filtered by the glomerulus per unit time, usually expressed as mL/min or mL/min/1.73 m^2 (and in some areas, in SI units of mL/s or mL/s/m^2), which adjusts the value for body surface area. This is the primary index used to describe overall renal function.

Glomerulonephritis: Glomerular lesions that are characterized by inflammation of the capillary loops of the glomerulus.

These lesions are generally caused by immunologic, vascular, or other idiopathic diseases. Leads to high blood pressure and possible loss of kidney function.

Glucagon: Hormone involved in carbohydrate metabolism that is produced by the pancreas and released when glucose levels in the blood are low. When blood glucose levels decrease, the liver converts stored glycogen into glucose, which is released into the bloodstream. The action of glucagon is the opposite of insulin.

Gluconeogenesis: Formation of glucose from precursors other than carbohydrates especially by the liver and kidney using amino acids from proteins, glycerol from fats, or lactate produced by muscle during anaerobic glycolysis.

Glutamate: An excitatory amino acid found in the central nervous system.

Glycogenolysis: The process by which glycogen is broken down to glucose in body tissues.

Goiter: An enlargement of the thyroid gland, causing a swelling in the front part of the neck.

Gonioscopy: Examination of the anterior chamber angle. A gonioprism or Goldman lens is used to perform gonioscopic evaluation.

Graft-versus-host disease: Disease caused when cells from a donated stem cell graft attack the normal tissue of the transplant patient. Symptoms include jaundice, skin rash or blisters, a dry mouth, or dry eyes. Also called GVHD.

Graft-versus-tumor: An immune response to a person's tumor cells by immune cells present in a donor's transplanted tissue, such as bone marrow or peripheral blood.

Grandiosity: Exaggerated sense of self-importance, ideas, plans, or abilities.

Granuloma: Unique inflammatory response composed of macrophages, giant cells, and other cells of the immune response to wall off infectious pathogens perceived as foreign but cannot be eliminated.

Gross hematuria: Visible blood in the urine.

Gummatous tumor: A soft, gummy tumor which occurs in the later stages of syphilis.

Gut-associated lymphoid tissue: Lymphoid tissue, including Peyer patches, found in the gut that are important for providing localized immunity to pathogens.

Guttate psoriasis: Psoriasis characterized a heavy or light sprinkling of teardrop-like, salmon-pink papules covered with a fine scale. These lesions are found primarily on the trunk and proximal extremities.

Haptenation: The process where a drug, usually of low molecular weight, is bound to a carrier protein or cell and becomes immunogenic.

Hashimoto disease: Condition in which the immune system attacks the thyroid gland; may result in hypothyroidism. Symptoms may include fatigue, weight gain, pale or puffy face, feeling cold, joint and muscle pain, constipation, dry and thinning hair, heavy menstrual flow or irregular periods, depression, a slowed heart rate, and problems getting pregnant and maintaining pregnancy. Occurs more commonly in women than in men.

Health literacy: Degree to which individuals have the capacity to obtain, process, and understand basic health information and services needed to make appropriate health decisions.

Heberden nodes: Hard, bony enlargement of the distal interphalangeal (terminal) joint of a finger or toe.

Hemarthrosis: Blood in the joint space.

Hematemesis: Vomiting of blood.

Hematochezia: Passage of stool that is bright red or maroon, usually because of bleeding from the lower gastrointestinal tract.

Hematogenous: Spread through the blood.

Hematoma: A localized swelling in an organ or soft tissue that is filled with clotted or partially clotted blood resulting from a break in a blood vessel wall.

Hematuria: Presence of blood or red blood cells in urine.

Hemiparesis: Weakness on one side of the body.

Hemisensory deficit: Loss of sensation on one side of the body.

Hemithorax: A single side of the trunk between the neck and the abdomen in which the heart and lungs are situated.

Hemoptysis: The expectoration of blood or blood-tinged sputum from the larynx, trachea, bronchi, or lungs.

Hemorrhagic conversion: Conversion of an ischemic stroke into a hemorrhagic stroke.

Hemostasis: Cessation of bleeding through natural (clot formation or construction of blood vessels), artificial (compression or ligation), or surgical means.

Heparin-induced thrombocytopenia: A clinical syndrome of IgG antibody production against the heparin-platelet factor 4 complex occurring in approximately 1% to 5% of patients exposed to either heparin or low-molecular weight heparin. Results in excess production of thrombin, platelet aggregation, and thrombocytopenia (due to platelet clumping), often leading to venous and arterial thrombosis, amputation of extremities, and death.

Hepatic encephalopathy: Confusion and disorientation experienced by patients with advanced liver disease due to accumulation of ammonia in the bloodstream.

Hepatic steatosis: Accumulation of fat in the liver.

Hepatocellular carcinoma: Cancer of the liver.

Hepatojugular reflex: Distention of the jugular vein induced by pressure over the liver; it suggests insufficiency of the right heart.

Hepatorenal syndrome: Acute kidney injury resulting from decreased perfusion in cirrhosis.

Hepatotoxicity: Toxicity to the liver causing damage to liver cells.

Herniation: Protrusion of the brain through the cranial wall.

Heterotopic: Placing a transplanted organ into an abnormal anatomic location.

Heterozygous: Having different alleles at a gene locus.

Hirsutism: Excess body hair, especially in females, appearing on the lower abdomen, around the nipples, around the chin and upper lip, between the breasts, and on the lower back.

Histocompatibility: Compatibility between the tissues of different individuals, so that one accepts a graft from the other without having an immune reaction.

Homeostenosis: Impaired capability to withstand stressors and decreased ability to maintain physiological and psychosocial homeostasis; a state commonly found in the elderly.

Homozygous: Having identical alleles at a gene locus.

Hormone receptor-positive: Tumors that appear to grow in the presence of estrogens; likewise, antiestrogen therapy or estrogen deprivation strategies lead to tumor regression.

Hospice: The provision of palliative care during the last six months of life as defined by federal guidelines.

Hot flashes: A feeling of warmth that is commonly accompanied by skin flushing and mild to severe perspiration.

Human leukocyte antigens (HLA): Groups of genes found on the major histocompatibility complex that contain cell-surface antigen presenting proteins. The body uses HLA to distinguish between self cells and non-self cells.

Humoral: Pertaining to or derived from a body fluid. The humoral part of the immune system includes antibodies and immunoglobulins in blood serum.

Hydramnios: Increased amniotic fluid.

Hyperalgesia: An exaggerated intensity of pain sensation.

Hypercalcemia: Excessive amount of calcium in the blood.

Hypercalciuria: Excessive amount of calcium in the urine.

Hypercapnia: Abnormally high concentration of carbon dioxide in the blood.

Hypercoagulable state: A disorder or state of excessive or frequent thrombus formation; also known as thrombophilia.

Hyperemesis gravidarum: A rare disorder of severe and persistent nausea and vomiting during pregnancy that can result in dehydration, malnutrition, weight loss, and hospitalization.

Hyperglycemic hyperosmolar nonketotic syndrome: Severe increase in serum glucose concentration without the production of ketones, leading to an increase in serum osmolality and symptoms such as increased thirst, increased urination, weakness, fatigue, confusion, and in severe cases, convulsions and/or coma.

Hyperopia: Farsightnedness.

Hyperosmolar hyperglycemic state: Blood glucose levels greater than 600 mg/dL (33.3 mmol/L) without significant ketones where extreme dehydration, insulin deficiency, hyperosmolarity, and electrolyte deficiency are common.

Hyperpigmentation: A common darkening of the skin that occurs when an excess of melanin forms deposits in the skin.

Hyperprolactinemia: A medical condition of elevated serum prolactin characterized by prolactin serum concentrations greater than 20 ng/mL (20 mcg/L; 870 pmol/L) in men or 25 ng/mL (25 mcg/L; 1087 pmol/L) in women.

Hyperthyroidism: State caused by excess production of thyroid hormone.

Hypertrichosis: Excessive growth of hair.

Hypocretin: A wake-promoting hypothalamic neuropeptide, a deficiency of which is involved in the pathophysiology of narcolepsy.

Hypogammaglobinemia: Reduced levels of antibodies.

Hypogonadism: A medical condition resulting from or characterized by abnormally decreased functional activity of the gonads, with retardation of growth and sexual development. Associated with testosterone deficiency resulting from either testicular or pituitary/hypothalamic diseases. Presenting symptoms differ according to the timing of disease onset in relation to puberty.

Hypomania: Abnormal mood elevation that does not meet the criteria for mania.

Hypomimia: Lack of facial expression. Often termed masked face.

Hypophonia: Decreased voice volume.

Hypopituitarism: A clinical disorder characterized by complete or partial deficiency in pituitary hormone production.

Hypothalamic-pituitary-adrenal axis: A neuroendocrine feedback loop that controls response to stress.

Hypothyroidism: State caused by inadequate production of thyroid hormone.

Hypovolemic shock: Circulatory shock caused by severe loss of blood volume and/or body water.

Hypoxemia: Deficiency of oxygen in the blood.

Hypoxia: Deficiency of oxygen in body tissues.

Hysterectomy: An operation to remove a woman's uterus.

Idiopathic (genetic) epilepsies: Epilepsy syndromes thought to be due to genetic alterations. Neurologic functions are completely normal apart from the occurrence of seizures.

Immunogenicity: Ability of a substance to provoke an immune response.

Immunoglobulin G index: The ratio of immunoglobulin G to protein in the serum or cerebrospinal fluid.

Immunophenotyping: A process used to identify cells, based on the types of antigens or markers on the surface of the cell. This process is used to diagnose specific types of leukemia and lymphoma by comparing the cancer cells to normal cells of the immune system.

Immunotherapy: A type of biological therapy that uses substances to stimulate or suppress the immune system to help the body fight cancer, infection, and other diseases.

Impedance pH monitoring: Detects gastroesophageal reflux based on changes in resistance to electrical current flow between two electrodes when a liquid and/or gas bolus moves between them. It can detect both acid and nonacid reflux.

Implantable cardioverter defibrillator: A device implanted into the heart transvenously with a generator implanted subcutaneously in the pectoral area that provides internal electrical cardioversion of ventricular tachycardia or defibrillation of ventricular fibrillation.

Incretrin effect: A greater insulin stimulatory effect after an oral glucose load than that caused by an intravenous glucose infusion. The majority of the effect is thought to be due to glucose-dependent insulinotropic peptide (GIP) and glucagon like peptide-1 (GLP-1). Patients with type 2 diabetes have a significant reduction of the incretin effect, implying that these patients either have decreased concentration of the incretin hormones, or a resistance to their effects. GLP-1 concentrations are reduced in patients with type 2 diabetes in response to a meal, while GIP concentrations are either normal or increased, suggesting a resistance to the actions of GIP, thus making GLP-1 a more logical target for therapeutic intervention.

Induction: The first treatment given for a disease. It is often part of a standard set of treatments, such as surgery followed by chemotherapy and radiation.

Infantile spasms (West syndrome): A seizure syndrome in infants younger than 1 year of age. It is characterized by a specific EEG pattern and spasms or jitters.

Initiation: In cancer, occurs when a carcinogenic substance encounters a normal cell to produce genetic damage, and results in a mutated cell.

Inotropic: Relating to or influencing the force of muscular contractions.

Insulin resistance: A decreased response to insulin found before or early in the diagnosis of type 2 diabetes mellitus.

Insulin-like growth factor-I (IGF-I): An anabolic peptide that acts as a direct stimulator of cell proliferation and growth in all body cells.

Integrase: Enzyme produced by HIV that enables its genetic material to be integrated into the DNA of the infected host cell.

International normalized ratio (INR): The ratio of the patient's clotting time to the clinical laboratory's mean reference value; normalized by raising it to the international sensitivity index (ISI) power to account for differences in thromboplastin reagents. Therefore, INR = (Patient's prothrombin time/laboratory's mean normal prothrombin time)^{ISI}

Intima: The inner layer of the wall of an artery or vein.

Intraarticular: Administered to or occurring in the space within joints.

Intraperitoneal: Within the peritoneal cavity.

Intrathecal: Within the meninges of the spinal cord.

Intravesicular: Administration directly into the bladder through the urethra.

Intussusception: The enfolding of one segment of the intestine within another.

Iontophoresis: Introduction of a medication into tissue through use of an electric current.

Ipsilateral: Occurring on the same side.

Ischemic heart disease: Imbalance between myocardial oxygen supply and oxygen demand.

Ischemic penumbra: Ischemic, but still viable cerebral tissue. Typically a rim of mild to moderately ischemic tissue in between normally perfused tissue and the area of evolving infarction; may remain viable for several hours.

Jejunal enterocyte: Cells lining the jejunum, which is a section of the small intestine connecting the duodenum to the ileum.

Jejunostomy: Operative placement of a new opening into the jejunum, usually associated with feeding tube placement.

Juvenile myoclonic epilepsy: An epilepsy syndrome that typically occurs during teenage years and consists of generalized tonic-seizures and myoclonic jerks. Absence seizures may also occur with this syndrome.

Kegel exercises: Specific exercises that strengthen the pelvic floor muscles and help to prevent and treat stress incontinence.

Keratinization: The sloughing of epithelial cells in the hair follicle.

Keratinocytes: The predominant cell type in the outermost layer of the skin.

Keratitis: Infection of the cornea.

Keratoconjunctivitis sicca: An eye disease caused by eye dryness, which results from either decreased tear production or increased tear film evaporation. Also known as dry eye syndrome.

Ketosis: An abnormal increase of ketone bodies present in conditions of reduced or disturbed carbohydrate metabolism.

Korotkoff sounds: The noise heard over an artery by auscultation when pressure over the artery is reduced below the systolic arterial pressure.

Kyphosis: Abnormal curvature of the spine resulting in protrusion of the upper back; hunchback.

Lactose intolerance: Inability to digest milk and some dairy products, resulting in bloating, cramping, and diarrhea; caused by enzymatic lactase deficiency.

Lag-ophthalmos: Poor closure of the upper eyelid.

Lamina cribrosa: A series of perforated sheets of connective tissue that the optic nerve passes through as it exits the eye.

Laminectomy: A surgical procedure to remove the back of one or more vertebrae, usually to give access to the spinal cord or to relieve pressure on nerves.

Laparoscopic adjustable gastric banding: A surgical procedure for weight loss that elicits its effectiveness through gastric volume limitation. The procedure involves inserting a silicone band lined with an inflatable donut-shaped balloon around the neck of the stomach to be filled with isotonic liquid thereby limiting food intake.

Laparoscopy: Abdominal exploration or surgery employing a type of endoscope called laparoscope.

Laparotomy: Surgical opening of the abdominal cavity

Latent autoimmune diabetes in adults (LADA): A slow, progressive form of type 1 diabetes mellitus for which a patient does not require insulin for a number of years. In its early stages, LADA typically presents as type 2 diabetes mellitus and is often misdiagnosed as such. However, LADA more closely resembles type 1 diabetes mellitus and shares common physiological characteristics of type 1 diabetes mellitus for metabolic dysfunction, genetics, and autoimmune features. LADA does not affect children and is classified distinctly as being separate from juvenile diabetes.

Left shift: Refers to an increase in the number of immature neutrophils (also referred to as bands). A left shift usually indicates infection or inflammation. The term originated in the days in which lab reports were written by hand and the bands were written on the left-hand side of the lab report. Also known as bandemia.

Lennox-Gastaut syndrome: An epilepsy syndrome that often appears early in life that consists of a distinct EEG pattern, mild to severe developmental delay, and multiple seizure types.

Leukocytoclastic vasculitis: Acute cutaneous vasculitis characterized by purpura (especially of the legs) and histologically by exudation of neutrophils and sometimes fibrin around dermal venules, with extravasation of red blood cells.

Leukopenia: A condition in which the number of circulating white blood cells are abnormally low due to decreased production of new cells, possibly in conjunction with medication toxicities.

Lewy bodies: Abnormal masses inside nerve cells. Their structure and composition vary depending on location.

Lhermitte sign: Tingling or shock-like sensation passing down the arms or trunk when the neck is flexed.

Libido: Conscious or unconscious sexual desire.

Ligament of Treitz: Landmark in the proximal portion of the jejunum beyond which it is preferred that postpyloric feedings be delivered for minimization of aspiration.

Linea nigra: Dark vertical line that appears on the abdomen during pregnancy.

Linear accelerator: An accelerator in which particles travel in straight lines, not in closed orbits.

Lipophilic: Having affinity for fatty substances.

Lipoprotein lipase: Enzyme located in the capillary endothelium involved in the breakdown of intravenous lipid emulsion particles.

Livedo reticularis: Purple mottling of the skin.

Liver biopsy: A procedure whereby tissue is removed from the liver and used to determine the severity of liver damage.

Locus ceruleus: Nucleus of norepinephrine containing neurons located in the brainstem that are responsible for physiological response to stress and panic.

Lower esophageal sphincter: A manometrically defined zone of the distal esophagus with an elevated basal resting pressure that prevents the reflux of gastric material from the stomach. It relaxes on swallowing to permit the free passage of food into the stomach.

Luteolysis: Death of the corpus luteum.

Lymphadenectomy: A surgical procedure in which the lymph nodes are removed and a sample of tissue is checked under a microscope for signs of cancer.

Lymphangitis: Inflammation of lymphatic channels.

Lymphatic: The network of vessels carrying tissue fluids.

Lymphoproliferative: Of or related to the growth of lymphoid tissue.

Maceration: The softening or breaking down of a solid by leaving it immersed in a liquid.

Macrophages: Large scavenger cells.

Macrovascular: Complications contributed to by diabetes that include myocardial infarctions, strokes, or peripheral vascular disease.

Macula: The central portion of the retina.

Maculopapular: A rash that contains both macules and papules. A macule is a flat discolored area of the skin, and a papule is a small raised bump. A maculopapular rash is usually a large area that is red and has small, confluent bumps.

Magnetic resonance imaging: A test that uses strong magnet fields to create a high resolution image of body parts.

Major malformation: A defect that has either cosmetic or functional significance to the child.

Manometry: Measurement of pressures and muscle contractions in the esophagus. It helps to localize the lower esophageal sphincter for ambulatory pH monitoring, evaluates peristaltic function in patients considering surgery, and identifies possible motor disorders.

Macrocytosis: Enlargement of red blood cells with near-constant hemoglobin concentration.

Mastalgia: Tenderness of the breast.

Matrix metalloproteinase: Any of a group of enzymes, normally located in the extracellular space of tissue, that function to break down proteins (e.g., collagen) and require zinc or calcium atoms as cofactors for enzymatic activity. Responsible for the degradation of connective tissue.

Meatal stenosis: Narrowing in the opening of the urethra.

Meconium: First intestinal discharge ("stool") of a newborn infant, usually green in color and consisting of epithelial cells, mucus, and bile.

Melasma: Dark skin discoloration. Patchy skin pigmentation, often seen during pregnancy.

Melena: Abnormally dark black, tarry feces containing blood (usually from gastrointestinal bleeding).

Menarche: The first menstrual cycle.

Meninges: Covering of the brain consisting of three layers.

Menopause: Permanent cessation of menses following the loss of ovarian follicular activity.

Menorrhagia: Menstrual blood loss of greater than 80 mL per cycle; a more practical definition is heavy menstrual flow associated with problems of containment of flow, unpredictably heavy flow days, or other associated symptoms.

Mesial temporal lobe epilepsy: A common epilepsy syndrome manifested by seizures arising from the mesial temporal lobe of the brain, and is often associated with an anatomical change, described as hippocampal sclerosis.

Mesocortical pathway: A neural pathway that connects the ventral tegmentum to the cortex, particularly the frontal lobes. It is one of the major dopamine pathways in the brain.

Mesothelioma: A benign or malignant tumor affecting the lining of the chest or abdomen. Commonly caused by exposure to asbestos fibers.

Metabolic acidosis: A condition in the blood and tissues that is a consequence of an accumulation of lactic acid resulting from tissue hypoxia and anaerobic metabolism. It may also be caused by a decrease in the concentration of alkaline compounds (typically bicarbonate).

Metabolic alkalosis: Alkalosis that is caused by an increase in the concentration of alkaline compounds (typically bicarbonate).

Metabolic syndrome: Constellation of cardiovascular risk factors related to hypertension, abdominal obesity, dyslipidemia, and insulin resistance diagnosed by the presence of at least three of the following criteria: increased waist circumference, elevated triglyceride concentrations, decreased high-density lipoprotein (HDL) cholesterol or active treatment to raise HDL cholesterol, elevated blood pressure, or active treatment with antihypertensive therapy, or elevated fasting glucose or active treatment for diabetes.

Metastasis: Cancer that has spread from the original site of the tumor.

Micelles: Microscopic particles of digested fat and cholesterol.

Microalbuminuria: Urinary excretion of small but abnormal amounts of albumin. Confirmed spot urine albumin to creatinine ratio of 30 to 300 mg/g (3.4 to 34 mg/mmol creatinine) is consistent with microalbuminuria. Considered an early sign of chronic kidney disease.

Microcytosis: A condition in which the erythrocytes are smaller than normal.

Micrognatia: Abnormal smallness of the jaws.

Micrographia: Small handwriting, often seen in patients with Parkinson disease.

Micrometastases: Deposits of tumor cells in distant organs that cannot be detected by any imaging techniques available.

Microsatellite instability (MSI): The condition of genetic hypermutability that results from impaired DNA mismatch repair (MMR). The presence of MSI represents phenotypic evidence that MMR is not functioning normally.

Microvascular pulmonary emboli: An obstruction in the small blood vessels in the lung caused by material (e.g., blood clot, fat, air, foreign body) that is carried through the circulation until it lodges in another small vessel.

Microvascular: Complications contributed to by diabetes that include retinopathy, neuropathy, nephropathy.

Micturition: Urination.

Minimum inhibitory concentration: The lowest concentration of an antimicrobial agent that inhibits visible bacterial growth after approximately 24-hour incubation.

Minor malformation: A defect that has neither cosmetic nor functional significance to the child.

Miosis: Pupil constriction.

Mixed acid-base disorder: See Complicated disorder.

Mixed mood episodes: Symptoms of mania and depression occurring simultaneously or in close juxtaposition.

Mobilization: Process of encouraging stem cells to emerge from the bone marrow into the peripheral blood where they can be harvested.

Mobitz type I: A type of second degree AV nodal block.

Mobitz type II: A type of second degree AV nodal block.

Möbius syndrome: Rare congenital neurological disorder characterized by facial paralysis and affects eye movement.

Monocytes: A variety of white blood cells.

Monoparesis: Slight or incomplete paralysis affecting a single extremity or part of one.

Monosodium urate: A crystallized form of uric acid that can deposit in joints leading to an inflammatory reaction and the signs and symptoms of gout.

Morphology: The science of the form and structure of organisms (plants, animals, and other forms of life).

Motor tics: An involuntary brief spasmodic muscular movement or contraction, usually of the face or extremities.

Mucositis: Inflammation of mucous membranes, typically within the oral and esophageal mucosa. Usually associated with certain chemotherapy agents and radiation therapy involving mucosal area.

Mucous colitis: A condition of the mucous membrane of the colon characterized by pain, constipation, or diarrhea (sometimes alternating), and passage of mucus or mucous shreds.

Multiparity: Condition of having given birth to multiple children.

Muscularis mucosa: The thin layer of smooth muscle found in most parts of the gastrointestinal tract.

Mydriasis: Pupil dilation.

Myelin: A protein and phospholipid sheath that surrounds the axons of certain neurons. Myelinated nerves conduct impulses more rapidly than non-myelinated nerves.

Myeloablative preparative regimen: A regimen consisting of a single agent or combination of agents expected to destroy the hematopoietic cells in the bone marrow and resulting in profound pancytopenia within one to three weeks from the time of administration. The resulting pancytopenia is long-lasting, usually irreversible, and in most instances fatal, unless hematopoiesis is restored by infusion of hematopoietic stem cells.

Myelodysplastic syndrome: One of a group of disorders characterized by abnormal development of one or more of the cell lines that are normally found in the bone marrow.

Myeloproliferative disorder: A group of diseases of the bone marrow in which excess cells, usually lymphocytes, are produced.

Myelosuppression: Reduction in white blood cells, red blood cells, and platelets.

Myocardial infarction: The formation of an infarct, an area of tissue death, due to a local lack of oxygen. Myocardial cell death secondary to prolonged ischemia.

Myocarditis: Inflammation of the heart muscle.

Myoclonic: A primary-generalized seizure characterized by a single and very brief (< 1 sec) jerk of the body, head, or arms.

Myoglobinuria: The presence of myoglobin in urine.

Myonecrosis: Necrotic damage to muscle tissue.

Myopathy: Any disease of the muscle causing weakness, pain, and tenderness.

Myringotomy: A surgical incision in the tympanic membrane to relieve pressure and drain fluid from the middle ear.

Myxedema: Hypothyroidism characterized by a relatively hard edema of subcutaneous tissue, with increased content of proteoglycans in the fluid; characterized by somnolence, slow mentation, dryness and loss of hair, increased fluid in body cavities such as the pericardial sac, subnormal temperature, hoarseness, muscle weakness, and slow return of a muscle to the neutral position after a tendon jerk.

Nail psoriasis: Nail psoriasis can be characterized by pitting, oncholysis, hyperkeratosis, and an oil-drop sign.

Nasal scotoma: An area of blindness in the nasal portion of peripheral vision.

Nascent: Immature.

Nasolacrimal occlusion: The closing of the tear duct to decrease systemic absorption of a drug.

Nausea: The subjective feeling of a need to vomit.

Necrosectomy: Surgical excision of necrotic tissue; debridement.

Necrotizing enterocolitis: Medical condition seen in premature infants, where portions of the bowel undergo necrosis.

Negative feedback: A self-regulating process that responds to influences of an original signal resulting in stabilization or reductions in the effect of fluctuations.

Nelson syndrome: A condition characterized by the aggressive growth of a pituitary tumor and hyperpigmentation of the skin.

Neoadjuvant therapy: Therapeutic strategy that precedes primary treatment modality (usually surgery). The goals are to "down-stage" tumors so that the surgical field is smaller or to transform a patient from a nonsurgical candidate to one that is surgical. Neoadjuvant therapy may improve overall survival. Strategies usually involve the use of systemic therapy with or without radiation.

Neovascular maculopathy: Proliferation of blood vessels in the macula.

Nephrolithiasis: A condition marked by the presence of renal calculi (stones) in the kidney or urinary system.

Nephron: The working unit of the kidney that filters blood to remove fluid, toxins, and drugs. Each kidney contains approximately 1 million nephrons.

Nephrostomy: Surgery to make an opening from the outside of the body to the renal pelvis (part of the kidney that collects urine). This may be done to drain urine from a blocked kidney or blocked ureter into a bag outside the body. It may also be done to look at the kidney using an endoscope (thin, lighted tube attached to a camera), to place anticancer drugs directly into the kidney, or to remove kidney stones.

Neuritic plaques: Extracellular deposits of beta amyloid in the gray matter of the brain.

Neuritis: Inflammation of a nerve.

Neurofibrillary tangles: Aggregates of hyperphosphorylated tau protein; commonly known as a primary marker of Alzheimer disease.

Neuropathic pain: Pain resulting from a lesion or dysfunction of the nervous system.

Neuropathy: An abnormal and usually degenerative state of the nervous system or nerves. Damage to the small and large nerves due to glycation end products, lack of blood and nutrients to the nerves, or chemical imbalances.

Neurotransmitters: Chemicals in the brain that allow the passage of a message between neurons or nerve cells.

Neutralizing antibodies: Antibodies that develop in response to a therapeutic agent that decrease the efficacy of the agent.

Nidus: A site of origin in which bacteria have multiplied or may multiply; a focus of infection.

Nitric oxide: An endogenous vasodilator.

NMDA antagonist: Class of medications that work to antagonize the N-methyl-D-aspartate receptor.

Nociception: Encoding and processing of noxious stimuli to the nervous system.

Nociceptors: Receptors for pain caused by injury from physical stimuli (mechanical, electrical, or thermal) or chemical stimuli (toxins); located in the skin, muscles, or in the walls of the viscera.

Nocturia: Excessive urination at night.

Nocturnal polysomnography: Electrophysiologic assessment of human sleep minimally composed of electroencephalogram, electrooculogram, and electromyogram that allows determination of sleep stage, breathing events, and muscle movements.

Nodules: An abnormal small swelling or aggregation of cells in the body. When seen with rheumatoid arthritis, nodules are subcutaneous knobs over bony prominences or extensor surfaces.

Nonmyeloablative preparative regimen: A nonmyeloablative regimen is one that will cause minimal cytopenia (but significant lymphopenia) by itself and does not require stem cell support.

Nonpolyposis: Absence of polyps.

Nonprotein kilocalorie to nitrogen ratio: Numerical value derived from dividing kilocalories from carbohydrate plus fat by the number of grams of nitrogen in the diet.

Non-REM sleep: A state of usually dreamless sleep that occurs regularly during a normal period of sleep with intervening periods of REM sleep and that consists of four distinct substages and low levels of autonomic physiological activity.

Non-ST-segment elevation myocardial infarction: A type of myocardial infarction that is limited to the sub-endocardial myocardium and is smaller and less extensive than an ST-segment elevation myocardial infarction.

Normal flora: Normal colonizing bacteria of a human host.

Nuchal rigidity: Neck stiffness.

Nuclear factor kappa-light-chain-enhancer of activated B cells (Nf-kappa-B): A protein complex that controls transcription of DNA, cytokine production, and cell survival.

Nulliparity: Condition of not having given birth to a child.

Nystagmus: Rapid, involuntary movements of the eyes.

Off time: The time when a Parkinson disease patient has poor control of his or her symptoms.

Off-label use: Use of a medication outside the scope of its approved, labeled use.

Oiling out: Continued coalescence of lipid emulsion particles, resulting in irreversible separation of the emulsion (also called "breaking" or "cracking" of the emulsion).

Oligoanovulation: The condition of having few to no ovulatory menstrual cycles.

Oligoclonal immunoglobulin G bands: Small discrete bands in the gamma globulin region of fluid electrophoresis.

Oligohydramnios: Decreased amniotic fluid.

Oligomenorrhea: Abnormally light or infrequent menstruation.

Oliguria: Reduced urine output; usually defined as less than 400 mL in 24 hours or less than 0.5 mL/kg/hour.

Omentumectomy: Excision of the double fold of the peritoneum attached to the stomach and connecting it with abdominal viscera (omentum).

On time: The time when the Parkinson disease patient has good control of his or her symptoms.

Oncogenes: Genes, when activated, that cause transformation of normal cells into cancer cells by promoting uncontrolled cell growth and multiplication leading to tumor formation.

Open comedo: A plugged hair follicle of sebum, keratinocytes, and bacteria that protrudes from the surface of the skin and appears black or brown in color. Also referred to as a "blackhead."

Opsonization: The process by which an antigen is altered so as to become more readily and more efficiently engulfed by phagocytes.

Optic neuritis: Usually monocular central visual acuity loss and ocular/periorbital pain caused by demyelination of the optic nerve.

Oral glucose tolerance test: Used to measure the body's response to glucose; may be used to screen for type 2 diabetes and gestational diabetes.

Oral rehydration solution (ORS): A liquid preparation, commercially prepared or made at home using common ingredients according to a formula developed by the World Health Organization, designed to replace fluid loss in persons with diarrhea.

Organification: Binding of iodine to tyrosine residues of thyroglobulin.

Orthopnea: Difficulty in breathing that occurs when lying down and is relieved upon changing to an upright position.

Orthostasis: Characterized by a drop in blood pressure when standing up from sitting or lying down, often causing light-headedness and dizziness.

Orthotopic transplantation: Placing a transplanted organ into the normal anatomic location.

Osmolality: A measure of the number of osmotically active particles per unit solution, independent of the weight or nature of the particle.

Osmolar gap: The difference between the measured serum osmolality and the calculated serum osmolality.

Osteoblast: Cells that secrete the matrix for bone formation.

Osteoclasts: Cells involved in bone resorption.

Osteomalacia: Softening of the bones.

Osteonecrosis: Death of bone tissue.

Osteopenia: Reduced bone density or mass.

Osteophytes: Bony outgrowths (also called bone spurs) into the joint space.

Osteoporosis: Disease of the bones characterized by a loss of bone tissue, resulting in brittle, weak bones that are susceptible to fracture (porous bones).

Ostomy: Surgical operation by which part of the abdominal wall is opened and part of the intestine is connected to the opening for intestinal draining (e.g., colostomy, ileostomy).

Otalgia: Ear pain or earache.

Otitis media with effusion: Fluid in the middle ear space with no signs or symptoms of an acute infection.

Ovulation: Periodic ripening and rupture of mature follicle and the discharge of ovum from the cortex of the ovary.

Pacemaker: A mass of fibers that possess actual or potential automaticity which initiates and determines the rate of spontaneous depolarizations.

Palliative care: The active, total care of patients whose disease is not responsive to curative treatment.

Palliative chemotherapy: Treatment given to control the symptoms of an incurable cancer.

Pancolitis: Inflammation that involves the majority of the colon in patients with inflammatory bowel disease; often used interchangeably with extensive disease.

Pancreatic pseudocysts: A cyst-like space not lined by epithelium and contained within the pancreas.

Pancreatitis: Inflammation of the pancreas.

Panhypopituitarism: A clinical disorder characterized by complete deficiency in pituitary hormone production.

Pannus: Inflamed synovial tissue that invades and destroys articular structures.

Papilledema: Swelling around the optic disk, the area where the optic nerve (the nerve that carries messages from the eye to the brain) enters the eyeball.

Paracentesis: Removal of ascitic fluid from the peritoneal space.

Paracentral scotoma: Blind spots near the center of the visual field.

Parasomnia: Undesirable physical or behavioral phenomena that occur predominantly during sleep. The most common parasomnias include sleepwalking, sleeptalking, bruxism, enuresis, and REM sleep behavior disorder.

Parenchyma: Specific cells or tissue of an organ.

Parenteral nutrition: Delivery of nutrients via the intravenous route.

Paresthesia: An abnormal touch sensation, such as burning or prickling, that occurs without an outside stimulus.

Paroxysmal: Intermittent occurrence, initiating suddenly and spontaneously, lasting minutes to hours, and terminating suddenly and spontaneously.

Partial response: In cancer, at least a 30% decrease in the sum of the longest diameter of target lesions from baseline.

Partial seizures: Seizures that begin in a localized area of the brain.

Peak expiratory flow: The maximum flow rate of air leaving the lungs upon forced exhalation. Individualized best measurements are established for each patient using a handheld peak flow meter.

Pelvic inflammatory disease: Inflammation of the endometrium, uterine tubes, and pelvic peritoneum; often due to a sexually transmitted infection.

Percutaneous coronary intervention: A minimally invasive procedure whereby access to the coronary arteries is obtained through either the femoral or radial artery up the aorta to the coronary ostia. Contrast media is used to visualize the coronary artery stenosis using a coronary angiogram. A guidewire is used to cross the stenosis and a small balloon is inflated to break up atherosclerotic plaque and restore coronary artery blood flow. A stent is often deployed at the site to prevent acute closure and restenosis of the coronary artery. Newer stents are coated with antiproliferative drugs, such as paclitaxel, sirolimus, zotarolimus, or everolimus, which further reduce the risk of restenosis of the coronary artery.

Percutaneous endoscopic gastrostomy: Gastric feeding tube placed via endoscopic technique.

Percutaneous endoscopic jejunostomy: Jejunal feeding tube placed via endoscopic technique.

Perihilar: Around the root or hilum of the lung.

Perimenopause: Also known as the climacteric, is the period of time prior to menopause when hormonal and biological changes and physical symptoms begin to occur and usually lasts for one year after the last menstrual period. The perimenopausal period may last for an average of three to five years.

Perimetry: Measurement of the field of vision.

Peripheral artery disease: Atherosclerosis of the peripheral arteries.

Peripheral resistance: The sum of resistance to blood flow by systemic blood vessels.

Peritonitis: An acute inflammatory reaction of the peritoneal lining to microorganisms or chemical irritation.

Petechiae: Tiny localized hemorrhages from the small blood vessels just beneath the surface of the skin.

Phagocytosis: The process of engulfing and ingesting an antigen by phagocytes.

Pharmacogenomics: The study of inherited genetic variations that dictate different drug responses. Pharmacogenomics explores the ways such variations can be used to predict responses to investigational products and plays an increasingly important role in drug discovery.

Phenotype: The visible or observable properties of an organism that are produced by the interaction of the genotype and the environment. May be used to evaluate the growth of HIV compared to "wild type" virus in the presence of drug to directly measure the amount of drug necessary to suppress viral replication in vitro.

Pheochromocytoma: A tumor arising from chromaffin cells, most commonly found in the adrenal medulla. The tumor causes the adrenal medulla to hypersecrete epinephrine and norepinephrine resulting in hypertension and other signs and symptoms of excessive sympathetic nervous system activity. The tumor is usually benign but may occasionally be cancerous.

Phlebitis: Inflammation of a blood vessel (e.g., vein).

Photochemotherapy: The use of psoralens in addition to ultraviolet rays for patients with a significant amount of body surface area affected (greater than 10%).

Photodynamic therapy: Treatment with drugs that become active when exposed to light.

Photophobia: Intolerance to bright light.

Phototherapy: The use of ultraviolet rays for patients with a significant amount of body surface area affected (greater than 10%).

Physical dependence: A state of adaptation that is manifested by a drug-class specific withdrawal syndrome that can be produced by abrupt cessation, rapid dose reduction, decreasing blood level of the drug, and/or administration of an antagonist.

Pilosebaceous unit: A hair follicle and the surrounding sebaceous glands.

Plaque psoriasis: Plaque psoriasis is the most common form of psoriasis and manifests as well-defined, sharply demarcated, erythematous plaques typically covered with silvery scales. These plaques are irregular, round to oval in shape, and are almost always found on the scalp, trunk, buttocks, and limbs.

Plasma cell: Antibody producing cells.

Plasmapheresis: A process of separating cells out from the plasma. This process is used to remove the monoclonal antibodies from the blood.

Pleocytosis: An increased white blood cell count in a bodily fluid, such as cerebrospinal fluid.

Pleuritis: Inflammation of the lining (pleura) around the lungs.

Pneumatic otoscopy: A diagnostic technique involving visualization of the tympanic membrane for transparency, position, and color, and its response to positive and negative air pressure to assess mobility.

Pneumothorax: The presence of air in the pleural cavity, often causing part of the lung to collapse.

Podagra: Gout involving the first metatarsophalangeal joint (great toe).

Polycythemia: An abnormal increase in the number of erythrocytes in the blood.

Polydipsia: Excessive thirst.

Polymerase chain reaction: A laboratory method used to make many copies of a specific DNA sequence.

Polyphagia: Eating excessively large amounts of food at a meal.

Polypharmacy: Taking multiple medications concurrently.

Polyps: Any growth or mass protruding from a mucous membrane.

Polyuria: Excessive excretion of urine resulting in profuse micturition.

Portal hypertension: Increased pressure in blood vessels leading to the liver; usually a result of cirrhosis.

Posterior circulation: Blood supply to the posterior section of the brain through the vertebral, basilar, and posterior cerebral arteries (i.e., brainstem, cerebellum, occipital lobe).

Postpyloric feeding: Delivery of nutrients via a tube placed with its tip past the pyloric sphincter separating the stomach from the duodenum.

Prader-Willi syndrome: A genetic disorder characterized by short stature, mental retardation, low muscle tone, abnormally small hands and feet, hypogonadism, and excessive eating leading to extreme obesity.

Prediabetes: An asymptomatic but abnormal state that precedes the development of clinically evident diabetes.

Preload: The stretched condition of the heart muscle at the end of diastole just before contraction; volume in the left ventricle at the end of diastole estimated by the pulmonary artery occlusion pressure (also known as the pulmonary artery wedge pressure or pulmonary capillary wedge pressure).

Priapism: A prolonged, painful erection lasting more than 4 hours. Considered a medical emergency.

Primary amenorrhea: Absence of menses by age 15 in the presence of normal secondary sexual development or within 5 years of thelarche (if occurs before age 10).

Primary generalized seizures: A seizure where the entire cerebral cortex is involved from the onset of the seizure.

Primary prevention: A program of activities directed at improving general well-being while also involving specific protection for selected diseases.
Prinzmetal angina: Vasospasm or contraction of the coronary arteries in the absence of significant atherosclerosis. Also referred to as variant angina.
Probiotics: Dietary supplements containing potentially beneficial bacteria that promote health by stimulating optimal mucosal immune responses.
Proctitis: Inflammation confined to the rectum in patients with inflammatory bowel disease.
Proctosigmoiditis: Inflammation involving the sigmoid colon and rectum in patients with inflammatory bowel disease.
Progenitor: A primitive cell.
Prognostic factors: Biologic or clinical indicators associated with survival independent of therapy (e.g., over-expression of HER2 is associated with increased risk of relapse and shorter survival).
Progression: In cancer, cell proliferation takes over and the tumor spreads or develops metastases.
Prolapse: A condition whereby organs fall down or slip out of place.
Promotion: Reversible process in cancer; the environment is altered by carcinogens or other factors to favor the growth of the mutated cell over the normal cell.
Proptosis: Forward displacement of the eyeball.
Prostaglandin: Any of a large group of biologically active, carbon-20, unsaturated fatty acids that are produced by the metabolism of arachidonic acid through the cyclooxygenase pathway.
Prostatectomy: An operation to remove the prostate gland and tissues surrounding it.
Prostatic hyperplasia: Enlargement of the prostate.
Protease: Enzyme that cleaves newly synthesized polyproteins into functional units of an infectious HIV virion.
Protectant: An agent that forms an occlusive barrier between the skin and surrounding moisture.
Proteinase: Any of numerous enzymes that catalyze the breakdown of proteins (also called protease).
Proteinuria: The presence of measurable amounts of protein in the urine, which is often indicative of glomerular or tubular damage in the kidney.
Proteoglycan: Any one of a class of glycoproteins of high molecular weight that are found in the extracellular matrix of connective tissue. They are made up mostly of carbohydrate consisting of various polysaccharide side chains linked to a protein and resemble polysaccharides rather than proteins with regard to their properties.
Proteolysis: Degradation of proteins in damaged tissue.
Proteosome: An enzyme complex that degrades intracellular proteins.
Prothrombin: A clotting factor that is converted to thrombin; also known as Factor II.
Prothrombin time: A measure of coagulation representing the amount of time required to form a blood clot after the addition of thromboplastin to the blood sample; also known as Quick test.
Prothrombotic state: A state of high coagulation of the blood.
Protooncogenes: Normal genes that are present in all normal cells and regulate cell function and replication, and through some genetic alteration caused by carcinogens, change into oncogenes.
Pruritis: Localized or generalized itching due to irritation of sensory nerve endings.
Pseudoaddiction: A term used to describe patient behaviors (e.g., "drug-seeking," "clock watching", or illicit drug use) that may occur when pain is undertreated. Pseudoaddiction can be distinguished from true addiction in that the behaviors resolve when pain is effectively treated.
Pseudohyphae: Chains of easily disrupted fungal cells; not a true hypha.
Pseudophakic: Refers to presence of a lens after cataract extraction.
Pseudopolyp: An area of hypertrophied gastrointestinal mucosa that resembles a polyp and contains non-malignant cells.
Psoralens: Compounds that act as photosensitizing compounds.
Psoriatic arthritis: Inflammatory arthropathy associated with psoriasis. This condition is characterized by stiffness, pain, swelling, and tenderness around the joints and ligaments.
Pulmonary artery catheter: An invasive device used to measure hemodynamic parameters directly, including cardiac output and pulmonary artery occlusion pressure; calculated parameters include stroke volume and systemic vascular resistance.
Pulmonary artery occlusion pressure: A hemodynamic measurement obtained via a catheter placed into the pulmonary artery used to evaluate patient volume status within the left ventricle.
Pulmonary embolism: A disorder of thrombus formation causing obstruction of a pulmonary artery or one of its branches and resulting in pulmonary infarction.
Pulsus paradoxus: A large fall in systolic blood pressure and pulse volume during inspiration or an abnormal variation in pulse volume during respiration in which the pulse becomes weaker with inspiration and stronger with expiration.
Punding: Stereotyped behavior with repetitive movement or actions. An adverse reaction to dopaminergic therapy.
Purkinje fibers: Specialized myocardial fibers that conduct impulses from the atrioventricular node to the ventricles.
Purpura: A small hemorrhage of the skin, mucous membrane, or serosal surface.
Purulent: Containing, consisting of, or being pus.
Pustular psoriasis: Collection of neutrophils is great enough to be seen clinically. May be generalized or localized. Often characterized by widespread sterile pustules and erythema.
Pyelonephritis: Inflammation of a kidney.
Pyuria: Presence of pus in urine when voided.
Quality indicators: A list of indicators used by long-term care facility administrators and government overseers to identify potential problems in patient care.
Quality of life: Perceived physical and mental health over time.
Radiofrequency catheter ablation: Procedure by which radiofrequency energy is delivered through a catheter positioned at the atrioventricular node for the purpose of destroying one pathway of a reentrant circuit.
Raphe nuclei: Bed of serotonin containing neurons that extend to the hypothalamus, septum, hippocampus, and cingulate gyrus.
Receptor editing: A process that occurs during the maturation of B cells, which are part of the adaptive immune system. This process forms part of central tolerance to attempt to change the specificity of the antigen receptor of self reactive immature B-cells, in order to rescue them from programmed cell death, called apoptosis.
Recombinant activated factor VII: A clotting factor manufactured via recombinant technology used off-label (not Food and Drug Administration approved) to foster clotting in

hemorrhagic shock patients with massive hemorrhage refractory to conventional therapies such as fresh frozen plasma.

Rectal prolapse: Externally visible sinking of the rectum through the anal sphincter.

Recurrence: A relapse that occurs after a clear-cut recovery.

Reentry: Circular movement of electrical impulses, a mechanism of many arrhythmias.

Refractory period: The period of time after an impulse is initiated and conducted during which cells cannot be depolarized again.

Regurgitation: A passive process without involvement of the abdominal wall and the diaphragm wherein gastric or esophageal contents move into the mouth.

Relapse: The return of symptoms, satisfying the full syndrome criteria, after a patient has responded, but prior to recovery.

REM sleep: A state of sleep that recurs cyclically several times during a normal period of sleep and is characterized by increased neuronal activity of the forebrain and midbrain, depressed muscle tone, and especially dreaming, rapid eye movements, and vascular congestion of the sex organs.

Remission: Patient has no or minimal symptoms of disease. In the case of cancer, in partial remission, some but not all signs and symptoms of cancer have disappeared. In complete remission, all signs and symptoms of cancer have disappeared, although cancer still may be in the body.

Renal osteodystrophy: Altered bone turnover that results from sustained metabolic conditions that occur in chronic kidney disease, including secondary hyperparathyroidism, hyperphosphatemia, hypocalcemia, and vitamin D deficiency. The disease can be characterized by high bone turnover, low bone turnover, or adynamic disease, or may be a mixed disorder.

Renin-angiotensin-aldosterone system: The hormonal system controlled mainly by the kidneys and adrenal glands that regulates blood pressure, blood volume, and electrolyte balance.

Resorption: The process of bone breakdown by osteoclasts.

Respiratory acidosis: Acidosis that is caused by an accumulation of carbon dioxide.

Respiratory Disturbance Index: A summary measure that quantifies the number of apneas, hypopneas, and respiratory effort-related arousals per hour of sleep.

Response: Refers to a pre-defined reduction of symptoms from baseline that generally result in significant functional improvement.

Response inhibition: Ability to stay on task or the ability to think before acting.

Restenosis: Renarrowing of the coronary artery after a percutaneous intervention.

Restriction fragment length polymorphism: Variation in the length of a restriction fragment produced by a specific restriction enzyme acting on DNA from different individuals that usually results from a genetic mutation and that may be used as a genetic marker.

Retching: A process that follows nausea and consists of diaphragm, abdominal wall, and chest wall contractions and spasmodic breathing against a closed glottis.

Reticulocytes: Immature blood cells that mature into erythrocytes.

Retinopathy: Occurs when the microvasculature nerve layer that provides blood and nutrients to the retina is damaged, and can cause blindness.

Retrograde ejaculation: Semen flows to the bladder instead of the urethra.

Reverse transcriptase: Enzyme that generates complementary DNA from an RNA template used in the replication of HIV.

Rhabdomyolysis: Destruction of skeletal muscle.

Rheumatoid factors: Antibodies reactive with the Fc region of IgG.

Rhinosinusitis: Inflammation of the mucous membranes in the nose and sinuses.

Rhonchi: Abnormal, rumbling sounds heard on auscultation of an obstructed airway. They are more prominent during expiration and may clear somewhat on coughing.

Rouleaux formation: The stacking or aggregation of red blood cells on a peripheral smear when diluted.

Rubefacient: A substance that produces redness of the skin.

Salicylism: A toxic syndrome caused by excessive doses of acetylsalicylic acid (aspirin), salicylic acid, or any other salicylate product. Signs and symptoms may include severe headache, nausea, vomiting, tinnitus (ringing in the ears), confusion, increased pulse, and increased respiratory rate.

Scleritis: Inflammation of the outer layer of the eyeball (sclera).

Scotoma: A spot in the visual field in which vision is absent or deficient.

Secondarily generalized seizure: A partial seizure (simple or complex) that spreads to the entire brain.

Secondary amenorrhea: Absence of menses for 3 cycles or 6 months in a previously menstruating woman.

Secondary hyperparathyroidism: Increased secretion of parathyroid hormone from the parathyroid glands caused by hyperphosphatemia, hypocalcemia, and vitamin D deficiency that result from decreased kidney function. Secondary hyperparathyroidism can lead to bone disease (renal osteodystrophy).

Secondary prevention: Interruption of any disease process before the emergence of recognized signs or diagnostic findings of the disorder.

Seizure: A sudden electrical disturbance of the cerebral cortex, when a population of neurons fires rapidly and repetitively for seconds to minutes and electrical discharges are excessively rapid, rhythmic, and synchronous.

Sentinel lymph node: The first lymph node to which cancer is likely to spread from the primary tumor.

Septic emboli: A detached, traveling intravascular mass of infected tissue.

Seropositive: Showing a positive reaction to a test on blood serum for a disease.

Serum sickness: A group of symptoms caused by a delayed immune response to certain medications. Arthralgias, fever, malaise, and urticaria may develop usually 7 to 14 days after exposure to the causative antigen.

Shear stress: Risk factor for pressure ulcers that is generated when the head of a patient's bed is elevated and can cause deeper blood vessels to crimp, leading to ischemia.

Sialorrhea: Drooling.

Sick sinus syndrome: Idiopathic sinus node dysfunction leading to symptomatic sinus bradycardia.

Sigmoidoscopy: Visual inspection of the sigmoid colon and rectum with a flexible tube called a sigmoidoscope.

Simple acid-base disorder: The presence of a single acid-base disorder, with or without compensation.

Simple partial seizures: Seizures in which the patient has a sensation or uncontrolled muscle movement of a portion of their body without an alteration in consciousness.

Sleep apnea: The temporary stoppage of breathing during sleep; can be caused by narrowing of the airways resulting from swelling of soft tissue.

Sleep latency: The amount of time it takes to fall asleep.

Sleeve gastrectomy: A surgical treatment for weight loss that involves constructing a small pouch in the stomach that empties through a narrow opening into the distal stomach and duodenum.

Slit-lamp biomicroscope: An instrument that allows for the microscopic examination of the cornea, anterior chamber lens and posterior chamber.

Somatic hypermutation: A cellular mechanism by which the immune system adapts to the new foreign elements that confront it (e.g., microbes), as seen during class switching.

Source control: Removal of the primary cause of an infection such as contaminated prosthetic materials (e.g., catheters), necrotic tissue, or drainage of an abscess. Antimicrobials are unlikely to be effective if the process or source that led to the infection is not controlled.

Spastic colon: A synonym for irritable bowel syndrome.

Spasticity: A motor disorder characterized by an increase in muscle tone with exaggerated tendon jerks, resulting from hyperexcitability of the stretch reflex.

Spectrum of activity: A qualitative term that describes the number of different bacterial species that are susceptible to an antimicrobial regimen. Generally, broad spectrum activity refers to regimens that possess activity against many bacterial species, whereas narrow-spectrum therapy refers to activity against a few bacterial species.

Sphincter of Oddi: Structure through which the common bile duct empties bile and pancreatic secretions into the duodenum.

Spirometry: Measurement by means of a spirometer of the air entering and leaving the lungs.

Sprain: An overstretching of supporting ligaments that results in a partial or complete tear of the ligament.

Stable disease: In cancer, neither sufficient shrinkage to qualify for partial response nor sufficient increase to qualify for progressive disease.

Stage: Estimate of tumor burden, which is not only of prognostic importance, but also has important implications regarding appropriate treatment options.

Status epilepticus: Continuous seizure activity lasting more than 5 minutes or two or more seizures without complete recovery of consciousness.

Steatohepatitis: A severe form of liver disease caused by fat deposition in the liver, characterized by hepatic inflammation that may rapidly progress to liver fibrosis and cirrhosis.

Steatorrhea: Excessive loss of fat in stool.

Steatosis: Infiltration of liver cells with fat.

Stenosis: Blockage of an artery.

Stenting: Placement of a stent to allow blood flow through an artery.

Stereotactic radiosurgery: A type of external radiation therapy that uses special equipment to position the patient and precisely give a single large dose of radiation to a tumor.

Stevens-Johnson syndrome: A severe expression of erythema multiforme (also known as erythema multiforme major). It typically involves the skin and the mucous membranes, with the potential for severe morbidity and even death.

Stimulant: Any amphetamine or amphetamine-like substance (methylphenidate) that causes an increase in dopaminergic and norepinephrine activity in the brain resulting in lessening of hyperactivity, impulsiveness, and/or inattentiveness.

Stomatitis: Inflammation of mucous membranes in the mouth.

Strain: Damage to the muscle fibers or tendon without tearing of the ligament.

Stricture: An abnormal narrowing of a body passage, especially a tube or a canal.

Stroke volume: The amount of blood ejected from the heart during systole.

ST-segment elevation myocardial infarction: A type of myocardial infarction that typically results in an injury that transects the thickness of the myocardial wall.

Subchondral: Situated beneath and supporting cartilage.

Substantia nigra: The area in the brainstem with highly pigmented cells that make dopamine.

Subtrochanteric: Below the trochanter (the bony protrusion at the end of the femur where the hip and thigh muscles attach).

Surgical site infection: Infections occurring at or near the surgical incision within 30 days of the operation; up to 1 year if a prosthesis is implanted.

Suspending agent: An additive used in the compounding of oral liquid medications to suspend drug particles throughout a liquid; enables resuspension of particles by agitation (eg, shaking well).

Symptomatic epilepsies: A seizure disorder with an identifiable cause for the seizures, such as trauma or hypoxia.

Synechia: Adhesions or the abnormal attachment of the iris to another structure. Peripheral anterior synechia refers to occurrence of synechia with the trabecular meshwork.

Synergism: Interaction between two or more factors or substances that produces an effect greater than the sum of their individual effects.

Synovitis: Inflammation of the synovial membrane, often in combination with pain and swelling of the affected joint.

Synovium: The membrane lining the internal surfaces of joints.

Systolic dysfunction: An abnormal contraction of the ventricles during systole.

T2 weighted magnetic resonance imaging: A setting of the magnetic resonance imaging machine that shows water as a bright signal.

Tachycardia: An abnormally rapid heart rate.

Tachyphylaxis: A rapidly decreasing response to a drug following its initial administration.

Tachypnea: Faster than normal respiratory rate.

Tachysystole: More than five contractions in 10 minutes, averaged over a 30-minute window.

Tangentiality: Abandoning one's ideational objective in pursuit of thoughts peripheral to the original goal. Used to describe a thought and speech pattern wherein the individual never gets to the point or answers the question.

Tardive dyskinesia: A chronic disorder of the nervous system characterized by involuntary jerky or writhing movements of the face, tongue, jaws, trunk, and limbs, usually developing as a late occurring side effect of prolonged treatment with antipsychotic drugs.

Targeted therapy: A type of treatment that uses drugs or other substances to identify and attack specific types of cancer cells with less harm to normal cells.

Tendinosis: Tendon degeneration without accompanying inflammation.

Tendonitis: Inflammation of the tendon.

Tenesmus: Difficulty with bowel evacuation despite the urgency to defecate.

Teratogenic: Causing malformations in a fetus.

Terminal secretions: The noise produced by the oscillatory movements of secretions in the upper airways in association with the inspiratory and expiratory phases of respiration. It is also known as "death rattle."

Thelarche: Onset of breast development.

Third spacing: Fluid accumulation in the interstitial space disproportionate to the intracellular and extracellular fluid spaces.

Thoracentesis: Removal of fluid that is present in the pleural space. Common procedure to determine what caused the fluid accumulation.

Thought-blocking: Speech is halted, often in mid-sentence, and then picked up later, usually at another point in the thought process.

Thrombin: An enzyme formed from prothrombin which converts fibrinogen to fibrin. It is the principal driving force in the clotting cascade.

Thrombocytopenia: A condition whereby the number of circulating platelets are abnormally low due to decreased production of new cells, possibly secondary to medication toxicities.

Thrombocytosis: Increased number of platelets in the blood.

Thrombogenesis: The process of forming a blood clot.

Thrombolysis: The process of enzymatically dissolving or breaking apart a blood clot.

Thrombolytic: An enzyme that dissolves or breaks apart blood clots.

Thrombophlebitis: Inflammation of a blood vessel (e.g., vein) associated with the stimulations of clotting and formation of a thrombus (or blood clot).

Thromboplastin: A substance that triggers the coagulation cascade. Tissue factor is a naturally occurring thromboplastin and is used in the prothrombin time test.

Thrombosis: A condition in which blood changes from a liquid to a solid state and produces a blood clot.

Thrombotic thrombocytopenic purpura: Condition characterized by formation of small clots within the circulation resulting in the consumption of platelets and a low platelet count.

Thrombus: Blood clot attached to the vessel wall and consisting of platelets, fibrin, and clotting factors. A thrombus may partially or completely occlude the lumen of a blood vessel compromising blood flow and oxygen delivery to distal tissue.

Thyroglobulin: A thyroid hormone-containing protein, usually stored in the colloid within the thyroid follicles.

Thyroid peroxidase: Enzyme that catalyzes the organification and coupling steps of thyroid hormone synthesis.

Thyroiditis: Inflammation of the thyroid gland.

Thyrotoxicosis: State caused by excess amount of thyroid hormone.

Tocolytic: Medication used to suppress premature labor.

Tolerance: A state of adaptation in which exposure to a drug induces changes that result in a diminution of one or more of the drug's effects over time.

Tonic-clonic seizure: A primary-generalized seizure characterized by a sudden loss of consciousness accompanied by tonic extension and rhythmic clonic contractions of all major muscle groups.

Tonometry: Method by which the cornea is indented or flattened by an instrument. The pressure required to achieve corneal indentation or flattening is a measure of intraocular pressure.

Tophi: Collections of monosodium urate crystals that develop in tissues and generally appear as firm nodules under the skin.

Topoisomerase-I: Enzymes that cut one of the two strands of double-stranded DNA, relax the strand, and reanneal the strand.

Torsade de pointes: Very rapid ventricular tachycardia characterized by a gradually changing QRS complex in the ECG; may change into ventricular fibrillation.

Toxic epidermal necrolysis: A life-threatening skin disorder characterized by blistering and peeling of the top layer of skin.

Toxoid: Bacterial toxin which has been inactivated.

Trained interventionist: Includes mostly health professionals such as registered dieticians, psychologists, exercise specialists, health counselors, and professionals in training who adhere to weight management protocols.

Transesophageal echocardiogram: Procedure used to generate an image of the heart via sound waves, via a probe introduced into the esophagus (rather than the traditional transthoracic view) in order to obtain a better image of the left atrium.

Transferrin saturation: The ratio of serum iron and total iron-binding capacity, multiplied by 100.

Transformation (conversion): Mutated cell becomes malignant.

Transient ischemic attack (TIA): A transient episode of neurological dysfunction caused by focal brain, spinal cord, or retinal ischemia without acute infarction. TIAs have a rapid onset and short duration, typically lasting less than 1 hour and often less than 30 minutes. The symptoms vary depending on the area of the brain affected; however, no deficit remains after the attack.

Translocation: Movement of bacteria and endotoxin from the intestinal lumen through the gut mucosa and into the lymphatic and systemic circulation.

Transmural: Existing or occurring across the entire wall of an organ or blood vessel.

Transsphenoidal pituitary microsurgery: Surgery through the nasal cavity to access the pituitary gland through the sphenoid bone.

Traveler's diarrhea: An acute infectious diarrhea that afflicts travelers during or immediately upon return from visits to other countries.

Trigeminal neuralgia: A disorder of the fifth cranial (trigeminal) nerve characterized by excruciating paroxysms of pain in the face.

Troponins T or I: Proteins found predominately in the myocardium. Troponin I and T are released into the blood from the myocytes at the time of myocardial cell necrosis secondary to infarction. These biochemical markers become elevated and are used in the diagnosis of myocardial infarction.

Trousseau sign: Noted when a blood pressure cuff is applied to a patient's upper arm and inflated.

Trypsin: A proteolytic enzyme formed in the small intestine from trypsinogen by the action of enteropeptidase, which once activated hydrolyzes peptides, amides, and esters.

Tuberoeruptive xanthomas: Small yellow-red raised papules usually presenting on the elbows, knees, back, and buttocks.

Tubulointerstitial: Involving the tubules or interstitial tissue of the kidneys.

Tumor lysis syndrome: A syndrome resulting from cytotoxic therapy, occurring generally in aggressive, rapidly proliferating lymphoproliferative disorders. It is characterized by combinations of hyperuricemia, lactic acidosis, hyperkalemia, hyperphosphatemia, and hypocalcemia.

Tumor suppressor genes: A gene that suppresses growth of cancer cells.

Tympanocentesis: Puncture of the tympanic membrane with a needle to aspirate middle ear fluid.

Tympanostomy tube: Small plastic or metal tube inserted in the eardrum to keep the middle ear aerated and improve hearing in patients with chronic middle ear effusion.

Uhthoff phenomenon: Acute worsening of multiple sclerosis symptoms on exposure to heat because high body temperatures may exceed the capacitance of the demyelinated nerve and conduction may fail.

Ultrafiltration: The movement of plasma water across a semipermeable membrane.

Uncomplicated acid-base disorder: See simple disorder.

Unstable angina: Pathogenically similar to non-ST segment myocardial infarction but without muscle damage, therefore, troponins are not elevated.

Uremia: A condition that results from accumulation of metabolic waste products and endogenous toxins in the body resulting from impaired kidney function. Symptoms of uremia include nausea, vomiting, weakness, loss of appetite, and mental confusion.

Urethral structure: Narrowing of the urethra.

Uricosuric: Pertaining to, characterized by, or promoting renal excretion of uric acid.

Urosepsis: Sepsis resulting from a urinary source.

Urticaria: Itchy, raised, swollen areas on the skin. Also known as hives.

Uveitis: An inflammation of the uvea. Uveal structures include the iris, the ciliary body, and the choroid.

Vagal maneuvers: Stimulate the activity of the parasympathetic nervous system, which inhibits atrioventricular nodal conduction. Examples of vagal maneuvers include cough, carotid sinus massage, and Valsalva.

Vagotomy: A surgical procedure that blocks vagal (cholinergic) stimulation to the stomach.

Valsalva maneuver: Vagal maneuver; patient bears down against a closed glottis, as if they were having a bowel movement.

Variceal bleeding: Varices are weak collateral blood vessels that are friable and rupture easily; often observed in the esophagus or stomach.

Vasculitis: Inflammation of the walls of blood vessels.

Vasomotor symptoms: Menopausal symptoms that include both hot flashes and night sweats.

Vasopressors: Medications that cause constriction of blood vessels, increase in vascular resistance, and increase in blood pressure.

Vasospasm: Narrowing (constriction) of a blood vessel causing a reduction in blood flow.

Ventilation/perfusion ratio (V_A/Q): A comparison of the proportion of lung tissue being ventilated by inhaled air to the rate of oxygenation of pulmonary blood.

Ventricular depolarization: Change in the membrane potential of a ventricular myocyte, resulting in loss of polarization. Under normal conditions, depolarization of ventricular myocytes is followed by ventricular contraction.

Vertigo: Sensation of spinning or feeling out of balance.

Vesicants: Chemotherapy drugs that cause significant tissue damage if extravasation occurs.

Virilization: Production or acquisition of virilism, which is masculine characteristics.

Volvulus: Twisting of the intestine causing obstruction and possible necrosis.

Vomiting: A reflexive rapid and forceful oral expulsion of upper gastrointestinal contents due to powerful and sustained contractions in the abdominal and thoracic musculature.

Waist circumference: A practical tool to measure the abdominal fat in patients with a BMI of less than 35.

Wernicke syndrome: Neurologic condition caused by thiamine deficiency and characterized by classic triad of symptoms (mental confusion, ataxia, and ophthalmoplegia).

Wheeze: A high-pitched whistling sound caused by air moving through narrowed airways. Wheezes are usually heard at the end of expiration but may be heard during inspiration and expiration in acute severe asthma.

White coat hypertension: A persistently elevated average office blood pressure of greater than 140/90 mm Hg and an average awake ambulatory reading of less than 135/85 mm Hg.

Wild-type virus: Refers to natural form of HIV virus without any genetic mutations.

Wilson disease: A disorder of copper metabolism, characterized by cirrhosis of the liver and neurological manifestations.

Xanthomas: Firm raised nodules composed of lipid-containing histocytes.

Xerostomia: Unusual dryness of the mouth.

ZAP-70 expression: An intracellular tyrosine kinase found in CLL B-cells.

Zymogen: An inactive protein precursor of an enzyme that is converted into an active form.

Appendix D: Prescription Writing Principles

Kim Hawkins, Jill Isaacs, Emily Knezevich, and Jon Knezevich

According to the International Monetary Systems (IMS) Health Report, 4 billion prescriptions were written and dispensed in the United States in 2011. This reflects a need for prescribers and dispensers to fully understand prescriptive privileges and rational prescribing.[1] The following outlines principles of pharmacotherapy, including general considerations of prescribing, rational prescribing of medications, types of prescription orders, safe prescribing practices including the importance of handwriting, adverse event reporting, and medication education.

It is essential that the prescriber and dispenser familiarize themselves with the professional guidelines, state laws, and federal laws. In addition, they must also understand the components of rational prescribing. Table D–1 below provides key elements a prescriber should understand as well as useful resources.

TYPES OF PRESCRIPTION ORDERS

Prescription orders can be provided in a variety of ways by authorized prescribers. Outpatient prescriptions may be written, verbally authorized by phone, faxed, or provided via electronic means. All outpatient prescriptions are subject to federal regulations and contain the same basic components. Laws and regulations for outpatient prescription requirements can vary from state to state, so prescribers should be knowledgeable of all applicable laws. The basic components of a prescription are listed below as well as numbered in Figure D–1.[2]

1. Prescriber information: name, address, and phone number
2. Prescriber's signature and prescriptive authority number or Drug Enforcement Administration (DEA) number (if applicable)
3. Patient information: full name and address, and weight and age if appropriate
4. Date the prescription was written
5. Superscription (Rx symbol), meaning "you take" or "recipe"
6. Inscription: medication being prescribed (name of medication, strength, and dose)
7. Signa, sig, or signature: directions to the patient (eg, take one tablet daily)
8. Subscription: dispensing instructions to the pharmacist (number, quantity, or volume to dispense)
9. Number of refills allowed
10. Generic substitution requirement: "DAW (dispense as written)" or "no substitution" if brand name medication only is desired

Further regulations are in place for prescriptions written for controlled substances. In addition to the aforementioned elements, prescriptions for controlled substances must also include the patient's full name and address as well as the full name, address, and DEA number of the prescriber. Stricter regulations exist for Schedule II controlled substances compared with Schedule III-V. Schedule II prescriptions must be written and can only be provided orally in an emergency situation. Refills are prohibited with Schedule II prescriptions.[3] Schedule II and IV prescriptions may be refilled up to five times within 6 months of when the prescription was issued.

Chart orders, orders written for hospital inpatients, are not considered prescriptions and are not subject to the same requirements. Typically chart orders include:

- Patient identifiers including name and account number
- Physician name
- Medication name, dose, route, and frequency of administration
- Date and time of order
- Physician signature
- If the order was given verbally, the person reducing the order to writing must sign the order and the ordering physician countersign

Electronic prescribing has become common practice because of government incentives aimed at moving health records to electronic databases.[4] Principles discussed previously in regard to requirements of a prescription hold true for electronic orders; however, additional considerations must be taken to ensure safe prescribing habits occur. A brief list of potential barriers and benefits is summarized in Table D–2.

Electronic prescribing is no longer a projection of the future but instead is becoming the norm. With appropriate use of this technology, patients are provided ultimately with safer and more efficient care.

Omission of any of the earlier discussed elements on a prescription order can be considered erroneous and poses a danger to patient care. Responsibility lies with the prescriber as well as the pharmacist dispensing the medication to ensure the prescriptions are not only accurate but also appropriate for the given patient.

SAFE PRESCRIBING PRACTICES

Safe prescribing should be a priority of all health care providers. To avoid inappropriate use of medications in patients, prescribers

Table D–1

Pharmacotherapy Principles

Pharmacotherapy Principle	Description	Online Resources
Prescriptive privileges	Dictated by federal and state law	
	Scope of practice and formularies vary by profession. Physicians, nurse practitioners, physician assistants, and dentists all have varying scopes of practice, which may include formularies or supervising prescribers. Each provider must become familiar with his or her profession's scope of practice.	
	Pharmacology courses in program of study and Continuing Education required	
	Prescribing legend drugs requires board examination and National Provider Identifier (NPI)	https://nppes.cms.hhs.gov/NPPES/Welcome.do
	Prescribing controlled substances requires DEA registration number	http://www.dea.gov/index.shtml
Rational prescribing	Ensure necessity of medication	
	Obtain pertinent history • Health history: comorbidities or contraindications (ie, pregnancy, hepatic failure, or renal failure) • Medication history: prior and current prescription, OTC, or herbal use; drug allergies or sensitivities; compliance issues • Family and social history	
	Select correct medication • It is important to know the following components of each medication when prescribing or dispensing: • Pharmacokinetics • Pharmacodynamics • Drug interactions • Drug-disease interactions • Interdisciplinary collaboration when necessary	http://www.jointcommission.org/

DEA, Drug Enforcement Administration; OTC, over the counter.

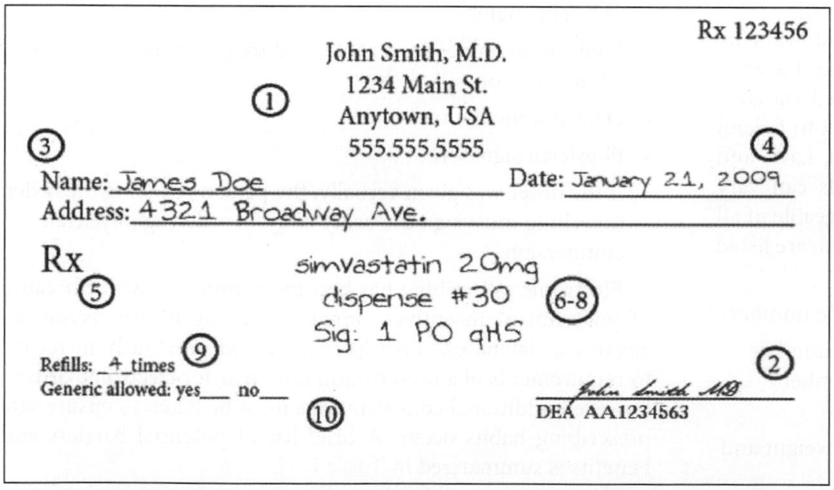

FIGURE D–1. Example of a prescription.

Table D–2

Electronic Prescribing[4–6]

Benefits	Barriers
Reduce medication errors	Cost of software programs
Reduce adverse drug events	Lack of financial benefit seen immediately
Improves efficiency	Lack of software standardization
Improved recognition of drug–drug and drug–disease interactions	Indirect costs: training personnel, reduced patient visits during training period
Improved recognition of medication allergy cross-sensitivity	
Enhanced prescriber knowledge of patient adherence	Clinician resistance: worry of worsening relationship with patient, negative impact on workflow, and fears of restrictions on prescribing habits
Enhanced prescriber knowledge of insurance coverage for medications	

Table D–3

Sound-Alike/Look-alike Medications[7,a]

Medication Name	Misinterpreted Medication Name
acetoHEXAMIDE	acetaZOLAMIDE
chlordiazePOXIDE	chlorproMAZINE
CISplatin	CARBOplatin
ePHEDrine	EPINEPHrine
hydrALAZINE	hydrOXYzine
LORazepam	ALPRAZolam
NIFEdipine	niCARdipine
RABEprazole	ARIPiprazole
risperiDONE	rOPINIRole
sulfADIAZINE	sulfaSALAzine
valACYclovir	valGANciclovir
Zantac	Xanax

[a]For additional information, please see http://www.ismp.org/tools/confuseddrugnames.pdf.

should take careful consideration in writing clear and descriptive prescriptions. This ensures appropriate communication among all interdisciplinary health care providers.

A thorough understanding of the medication prescribed, including its expected risks and benefits, should be realized by the prescriber ensuring appropriate drug selection. Providers should be aware of common errors related to prescription writing. These errors include: sound-alike/look-alike medications and inappropriate use of shorthand language and abbreviations. The Joint Commission, as well as the Institute for Safe Medication Practices (ISMP), has collected common examples of these errors seen during the ordering process. Common examples are described in Tables D–3 and D–4.

Other abbreviations are commonly used medical abbreviations used in prescription writing can be found in Appendix B: Common Medical Abbreviations.

Adverse Event Reporting

Adverse events may occur related to inappropriate prescribing, dispensing, or administrating medications. Inappropriate prescribing may be avoided by ensuring care is taken to determine

Table D–4

Error-Prone Abbreviations[8,a]

Abbreviation	Anticipated Meaning	Misinterpretation	Correction
μg	Microgram	Mistaken as "mg"	Use "mcg"
IJ	Injection	Mistaken as "IV" or "intrajugular"	Use "injection"
qd or QD	Every day	Mistaken as qid, especially if the period after the "q" or the tail of the "q" is misunderstood as an "i"	Use "daily"
U	Units	May appear as a μ or 0	Use "units"
IU	International Units	IV (intravenous)	Use "units"
bid, tid, qid	Twice daily, three times daily, four times daily	Depending on handwriting, may be misinterpreted a number of ways.	Write out the words "twice daily", etc
biw, tiw, qiw	Twice weekly, three times weekly, four times weekly	Two times per day, three times per day, four times per day	Write out the words "twice weekly", etc
Dose Designation	**Anticipated Meaning**	**Misinterpretation**	**Correction**
Trailing zero after decimal point (eg, 4.0 mg)	4 mg	Mistaken as 40 mg if the decimal point is not seen	Do not use trailing zeros for doses expressed in whole numbers
No leading zero before a decimal point (eg, .8 mg)	0.8 mg	Mistaken as 8 mg if the decimal point is NOT seen	Use zero before a decimal point when the dose is less than a whole unit
Large doses without properly placed commas(eg, 100,000 units;1,000,000 units)	100,000 units 1,000,000 units	100,000 has been mistaken as 10,000 or 1,000,000; 1,000,000 has been mistaken as 100,000	Use commas for dosing units at or above 1000 or use words such as 100 "thousand" or 1 "million" to improve readability
Drug Name Abbreviation	**Anticipated Meaning**	**Misinterpretation**	**Correction**
AZT	Zidovudine (Retrovir)	Mistaken as azathioprine or aztreonam	Use complete drug name
MS, MSO_4	Morphine sulfate	Mistaken as magnesium sulfate	Use complete drug name
PCA	Procainamide	Mistaken as patient-controlled analgesia	Use complete drug name
T3	Tylenol with codeine No. 3	Mistaken as liothyronine	Use complete drug name
Stemmed Drug Names	**Anticipated Meaning**	**Misinterpretation**	**Correction**
"Nitro" drip	Nitroglycerin infusion	Mistaken as sodium nitroprusside infusion	Use complete drug name
"IV Vanc"	Intravenous vancomycin	Mistaken as Invanz	Use complete drug name
Symbol	**Anticipated Meaning**	**Misinterpretation**	**Correction**
× 3d	For 3 days	Mistaken as three doses	Use "for 3 days"
&	And	Mistaken as "2"	Use "and"
°	Hour	Mistaken as a zero (eg, q2° seen as q 20)	Use "hr," "h," or "hour"

[a]For additional information, please see ISMP/Joint Commission List of Error-Prone Abbreviations.

all pertinent patient related issues are discussed during the encounter. Additionally, appropriate interdisciplinary care where multiple health care providers are evaluating the patient's problem and its treatment may help avoid adverse events from occurring. Inappropriate dispensing and administration may be avoided through use of clear order entry that undergoes multiple checks by a variety of providers before it reaches the patient. Movement to electronic prescribing has helped eliminate many issues with misinterpreting hand written orders, however, should they still be encountered, providers should take care to very legibly write prescriptions. If any questions remain upon receipt of a questionable order should be verified with the writing provider by the dispensing pharmacist. If adverse events related to medication use are determined, the health care provider who discovers the event is responsible for reporting it. The Food and Drug Administration's reporting system for such adverse events is MedWatch http://www.fda.gov/Safety/MedWatch/default.htm.[9] This online database archives medication-related adverse events, and providers are able to report errors seen in clinical practice.

Medication Education

After a prescription has been written, counseling patients on newly prescribed therapies is an essential responsibility of the prescriber and pharmacist. The patient should be made aware of the rationale for drug use, the dose, route, and frequency at which they should administer the medication and expectations of the prescribed drug. Expectations should include risks and benefits to avoid patient confusion about side effects or efficacy measures. Thorough discussion of medication therapy selected with the patient may identify contraindications previously unknown or a patient history of failure or success with the selected agent in the past.

CONCLUSION

Multiple principles must be exercised for appropriate drug delivery from the bedside to the patient. As a health care provider, understanding these processes helps to ensure safe medication prescribing.

REFERENCES

1. Sullivan D. Prescription writing and electronic prescribing. In: Sullivan D, ed. Guide to Clinical Documentation. Philadelphia, PA: FA Davis; 2012:207–217.
2. Enz SL, Ockerman AV. The prescription. In: Allen LV, ed. Remington: The Science and Practice of Pharmacy, 22nd ed. Philadelphia, PA: Lippincott Williams & Wilkins; 2013:1955–1970.
3. Section IX–Valid Prescription Requirements [Internet]. Office of Diversion Control. [cited 2014 Aug 28]. http://www.deadiversion.usdoj.gov/pubs/manuals/pharm2/pharm_content.htm
4. Cusack CM. Electronic health records and electronic prescribing: Promise and pitfalls. Obstet Gynecol Clin North Am. 2008;35:63–79.
5. Lapane KL, Rosen RK, Dubé C. Perceptions of e-prescribing efficiencies and inefficiencies in ambulatory care. Int J Med Inform. 2011;80:39–46.
6. Ammenwerth E, Schnell-Inderst P, Machan C, Siebert U. The effect of electronic prescribing on medication errors and adverse drug events: a systematic review. J Am Med Inform Assoc. 2008;15:585–600.
7. ISMP's List of Confused Drug Names [Internet]. Horsham (PA): Institute of Safe Medication Practices:c2014 [updated 2014; cited 2014 Aug 28]. http://ismp.org/tools/confuseddrugnames.pdf.
8. ISMP's List of Error-Prone Abbreviations, Symbols, and Dose Designations [Internet]. Horsham (PA): Institute of Safe Medication Practices:c2013 [updated 2013; cited 2014 Aug 28]. http://ismp.org/tools/errorproneabbreviations.pdf.
9. MedWatch: The FDA Safety Information and Adverse Event Reporting Program [Internet]. Bethesda (MD): The U.S. Food and Drug Administration. C2011 [updated 2014; cited 2014 Aug 28]. http://www.fda.gov/Safety/MedWatch/default.htm.

INDEX

Page numbers followed by *f*, *t*, and *a*, indicate figures, tables, and algorithms, respectively.

C

H

I

U